DISEASES/CONDITIONS AND ICD-9-CM CODES *(Continued)*

Intracerebral hemorrhage 431
Iron deficiency anemia 280.0-280.9
Irritable bowel syndrome 564.1
Jellyfish sting 989.5
Juvenile rheumatoid arthritis 714.3**
Keloids 701.4
Laryngitis 464.00
Lead poisoning 984*
Legionnaires' disease 482.84
Leishmaniasis 085*
Leprosy 030*
Lichen planus 697.0
Low back pain 724.2
Lyme disease 088.81
Lymphogranuloma venereum 099.1
Malabsorption 579*
Malaria 084.6
Measles (rubeola) 055.9
Meconium aspiration 770.1
Melanoma, malignant 172*
Ménière's disease 386.0**
Meningitis 320-322
Menopausal. 627.2
Migraine headache 346**
Mitral valve prolapse 424.0
Monilial vulvovaginitis 121.1
Multiple myeloma 203.0**
Multiple sclerosis 340
Mumps 072.9
Myasthenia gravis 358.0**
Mycoplasmal pneumonias 483.0
Mycosis fungoides 202.1**
Nausea and vomiting 787.01
Neoplasm of the vulva 239.5
Neutropenia 288.0
Nevi 216*
Newborn physiologic jaundice 774.6
Nongonococcal urethritis 099.4**
Non-Hodgkin's lymphomas 202.8**
Non-autoimmune hemolytic anemia 283.1**
Normal delivery 650
Obesity 278.0**
Obsessive-compulsive disorders 300.3
Onychomycosis 110.1
Optic neuritis 377.3**
Osteoarthritis 715**
Osteomyelitis 730**
Osteoporosis 733.00
Otitis externa 380.10
Paget's disease of bone 731.0
Panic disorder 300.01
Pap smear V72.3
Parkinsonism 332.0
Paronychia 681.0**
Partial epilepsy 345.4**
Patent ductus arteriosus 747.0
Pediculosis 132*
Pelvic inflammatory disease 614*
Peptic ulcer disease 533*
Pericarditis 432.9
Peripheral arterial disease 443.9
Peripheral neuropathies 356*
Pernicious anemia 281.0
Personality disorder 301**
Pheochromocytoma 227.0
Phobia 300.2**
Pigmentary disorders—vitiligo 709.01
Pinworms 127.4
Pityriasis rosea 696.3
Placenta previa 641**
Plague 020*
Platelet-mediated bleeding disorders 287.1
Pleural effusion 511.9
Polycythemia vera 238.4
Polymyalgia rheumatica 725
Porphyria 277.1
Postpartum hemorrhage 666.1**
Post-traumatic stress disorder 309.81
Pregnancy V22.2
Pregnancy-induced hypertension 642**
Premature beats 427.6**
Premenstrual tension syndrome (PMS) 625.4
Prescribed oral contraceptive. V25.01
Pressure ulcers 707.0
Preterm labor 644.2**
Primary glomerular disease 581-583
Primary lung abscess 513.0
Primary lung cancer 162.9
Prostate cancer 185
Prostatitis 601*
Pruritus 698.9
Pruritus ani 698.0
Pruritus vulvae 698.1
Psittacosis (ornithosis) 073*
Psoriasis 696.1
Pulmonary embolism 415.1
Pyelonephritis 590**
Q fever 083.0
Rabies 071
Rat-bite fever 026*
Relapsing fever 087*
Renal calculi 592
Reye syndrome 331.81
Rheumatic fever 390
Rheumatoid arthritis 714.0
Rib fracture 807.0**
Rocky Mountain spotted fever 082.0
Rosacea 695.3
Roseola 057.8
Rubella 056*
Salmonellosis 003.0
Sarcoidosis 135
Scabies 133.0
Schizophrenia 295**
Seborrheic dermatitis 690.1**
Septicemia 038*
Sézary's syndrome 202.2**
Shoulder dislocation 831.0**
Sickle cell anemia 282.6**
Silicosis 502
Sinusitis, chronic 473*
Skull fracture 800, 801, 803
Sleep apnea 780.57
Sleep disorders 780.50
Snakebite 989.5
Stasis ulcers 454.0
Status epilepticus 345.3
Stomach cancer 151*
Streptococcal pharyngitis 034.0
Stroke 436
Strongyloides infection 127.2
Subdural or subarachnoid hemorrhage 852**
Sunburn 692.71
Syphilis 090-097
Tachycardias 785.0
Tapeworm infections 123*
Telogen effluvium 704.02
Temporomandibular joint syndrome 524.6**
Tendonitis 726.90
Tetanus 037
Thalassemia 282.4**
Therapeutic use of blood components V59.0**
Thrombotic thrombocytopenic purpura 446.6
Thyroid cancer 193
Thyroiditis 245*
Tinea capitis 110.0
Tinnitus 388.3**
Toe fracture 826.0
Toxic shock syndrome 040.82
Toxoplasmosis 130*
Transient cerebral ischemia 435*
Trauma to the genitourinary tract 958,959
Trichinellosis 124
Trichomonal vaginitis 131.01
Trigeminal neuralgia 350.1
Tuberculosis, pulmonary 011**
Tularemia 021*
Typhoid fever 002.0
Typhus fevers 080, 081
Ulcerative colitis 556*
Urethral stricture 598*
Urinary incontinence 788.30
Urticaria 708*
Uterine inertia 661.0**
Uterine leiomyoma 218*
Varicella 052*
Venous thrombosis 453.8
Viral pneumonia 480.9
Viral respiratory infections 465.9
Vitamin deficiency 264-269
Vitamin K deficiency 269.0
Warts (verrucae) 078.10
Wegener's granulomatosis 446.4
Whooping cough (pertussis) 033*
Wrist fracture 814.0**

*4th digit needed
**5th (or 4th and 5th) digit needed

CONN'S
Current Therapy 2005

More Volumes in the Current Therapy Series

Upcoming

Current Therapy in Plastic Surgery
McCARTHY, GALIANO, AND BOUTROS, 2006

Published

Current Therapy in Colon and Rectal Surgery, 2nd Edition
FAZIO, CHURCH, AND DELANEY, 2005

Current Surgical Therapy, 8th Edition
CAMERON, 2004

Current Therapy in Thoracic and Cardiovascular Surgery
YANG AND CAMERON, 2004

Current Therapy in Allergy, Immunology and Rheumatology, 6th Edition
LICHTENSTEIN, BUSSE, AND GEHA, 2003

Gellis and Kagan's Current Pediatric Therapy, 17th Edition
BURG, INGELFINGER, POLIN, AND GERSHON, 2002

Current Therapy in Neurologic Disease, 6th Edition
JOHNSON, GRIFFIN, AND McARTHUR, 2002

Current Therapy of Infectious Disease, 2nd Edition
SCHLOSSBERG, 2001

Current Therapy in Vascular Surgery, 4th Edition
ERNST AND STANLEY, 2001

Current Ocular Therapy, 5th Edition
FRAUNFELDER AND ROY, 2000

Current Therapy in Obstetrics and Gynecology, 5th Edition
QUILLIGAN AND ZUSPAN, 2000

CONN'S Current Therapy 2005

Robert E. Rakel, MD
Professor, Department of Family and
Community Medicine
Baylor College of Medicine
Houston, Texas

Edward T. Bope, MD
Family Practice Residency Director
Riverside Family Practice Residency Program
Clinical Professor
Department of Family Medicine
The Ohio State University
Columbus, Ohio

LATEST APPROVED METHODS
OF TREATMENT FOR
THE PRACTICING PHYSICIAN

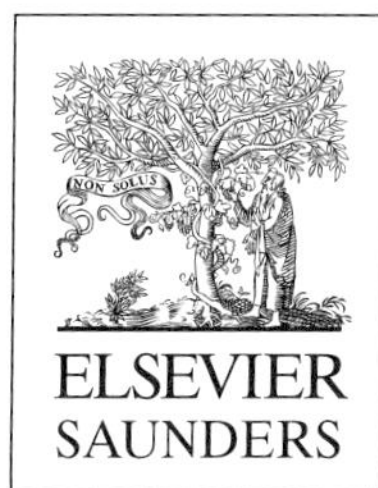

ELSEVIER
SAUNDERS

ELSEVIER
SAUNDERS

170 S. Independence Mall W 300 E
Philadelphia, Pennsylvania 19106

CONN'S CURRENT THERAPY 2005 ISBN 0-7216-3864-3

Notice

Medicine is an ever-changing field. Standard safety precautions must be followed, but as new research and clinical experience broaden our knowledge, changes in treatment and drug therapy may become necessary or appropriate. Readers are advised to check the most current product information provided by the manufacturer of each drug to be administered to verify the recommended dose, the method and duration of administration, and contraindications. It is the responsibility of the treating physician, relying on experience and knowledge of the patient, to determine dosages and the best treatment for each individual patient. Neither the Publisher nor the author assumes any liability for any injury and/or damage to persons or property arising from this publication.

The Publisher

Library of Congress Cataloging-in-Publication Data

Current therapy; latest approved methods of treatment for the practicing physician.
Editors: H. F. Conn and others
v. 28 cm. annual
ISBN 0-7216-3864-3
1. Therapeutics. 2. Therapeutics, Surgical. 3. Medicine—Practice.
I. Conn, Howard Franklin, 1908–1982 ed.

RM101.C87 616.058 49–8328 rev*

Associate Editor: Elyse O'Grady
Publishing Services Manager: Frank Polizzano
Senior Project Managers: Natalie Ware and Jeff Gunning
Design Coordinator: Gene Harris

Printed in the United States of America.

Last digit is the print number: 9 8 7 6 5 4 3 2 1

Contributors

Ali F. AbuRahma, MD
Professor of Surgery; Chief, Vascular Surgery; Medical Director, Vascular Laboratory; and Co-Medical Director, Vascular Center of Excellence, Department of Surgery, Robert C. Byrd Health Sciences Center of West Virginia University, Charleston, West Virginia
VENOUS THROMBOSIS

G. David Adamson, MD
Fertility Physicians of Northern California, Palo Alto, California
ENDOMETRIOSIS

Sharareh Ahmadi, MB
Specialist Registrar, Department of Dermatology, Mater Misericordiae Hospital, Dublin, Ireland
DISEASES OF THE MOUTH

Olufemi O. Akinjanju, MD
Professor and Chairman, Sickle Cell Foundation Nigeria, Victoria Island, Lagos, Nigeria
SICKLE CELL SYNDROME

Muhammad G. Alam, MD, MPH
Assistant Professor of Internal Medicine, University of Arkansas for Medical Sciences; Staff Physician, Medical Service, Central Arkansas Veterans Healthcare System, Little Rock, Arkansas
ACUTE RENAL FAILURE

Ezra A. Amsterdam, MD
Professor, Department of Internal Medicine,University of California, Davis, School of Medicine, Davis; Associate Chief, Division of Cardiovascular Medicine, Davis Medical Center, Sacramento, California
PREMATURE BEATS

Colonel Ian B. Anderson, CD, MDCM
Assistant Clinical Professor of Surgery, University of Calgary Faculty of Medicine; Advisor of Surgery and Wound Ballistics, Canadian Forces Medical Services; Attending Trauma and General Surgeon, Foothills Medical Centre, Calgary, Alberta, Canada
DISTURBANCES CAUSED BY COLD

Gunnar B. J. Andersson, MD, PhD
Professor and Chairman, Department of Orthopedic Surgery, Rush University Medical Center, Chicago, Illinois
LOW BACK PAIN

Raymond F. Anton, MD
Distinguished University Professor of Psychiatry, Medical University of South Carolina College of Medicine, Charleston, South Carolina
ALCOHOL USE DISORDERS

Ronald I. Apfelbaum, MD
Professor, Department of Neurosurgery, University of Utah Health Science Center, Salt Lake City, Utah
TRIGEMINAL NEURALGIA

David C. Aron, MD, MS
Professor of Medicine and Epidemiology and Biostatistics, Case Western Reserve University School of Medicine; Director, Center for Quality Improvement Research, Louis Stokes Cleveland Department of Veterans Affairs Medical Center, Cleveland, Ohio
ADRENAL INSUFFICIENCY

Louis J. Aronne, MD
Clinical Professor of Medicine, Weill-Cornell Medical College; Director, Comprehensive Weight Control Program, New York, New York
OBESITY

Bertha S. Ayi, MD
Postdoctoral Fellow, Department of Internal Medicine, University of Nebraska Medical Center, Omaha, Nebraska
BLASTOMYCOSIS

Lionel C. Bailly, MD
Senior Lecturer, Department of Psychiatry and Behavioural Sciences, University College of London Medical School, London, United Kingdom
CHRONIC FATIGUE SYNDROME

David A. Baker, MD
Professor, Department of Obstetrics, Gynecology, and Reproductive Medicine, State University of New York at Stony Brook Health Sciences Center School of Medicine, Stony Brook, New York
VULVOVAGINITIS

Kelty R. Baker, MD
Assistant Professor, Hematology-Oncology Section, Baylor College of Medicine, Houston, Texas
THROMBOTIC THROMBOCYTOPENIC PURPURA

Ashok Balasubramanyam, MD
Associate Professor of Medicine, Division of Diabetes, Endocrinology, and Metabolism, Baylor College of Medicine; Chief, Endocrine Services, Ben Taub General Hospital, Houston, Texas
CUSHING'S SYNDROME

Henry H. Balfour, Jr., MD
Professor, Department of Laboratory Medicine and Pathology and Department of Pediatrics, University of Minnesota Medical School, Minneapolis, Minnesota
VARICELLA (CHICKENPOX)

Robert A. Balk, MD
J. Baily Carter Professor of Medicine, Rush Medical College of Rush University; Director, Division of Pulmonary and Critical Care Medicine, Rush University Medical Center, Chicago, Illinois
BACTEREMIA AND SEPSIS

Roberta A. Ballard, MD
Professor of Pediatrics and Obstetrics/Gynecology, University of Pennsylvania School of Medicine; Attending Physician, Division of Neonatology, Children's Hospital of Philadelphia, Philadelphia, Pennsylvania
RESUSCITATION OF THE NEWBORN

Pradip K. Bardhan, MD
International Centre for Diarrhoeal Disease Research, Dhaka, Bangladesh
ACUTE INFECTIOUS DIARRHEA

Raymond Bégin, MD
Professor of Medicine, Pulmonology Division, Université de Sherbrooke Faculty of Medicine, Sherbrooke, Quebec, Canada
ASBESTOS AND SILICA-RELATED DISEASES

Wilma F. Bergfeld, MD
Head of Clinical Research, Department of Dermatology, Cleveland Clinic Foundation, Cleveland, Ohio
SKIN DISEASES OF PREGNANCY

Mitchell Bernstein, MD
Assistant Professor of Clinical Surgery, Columbia University College of Physicians and Surgeons; Attending Physician, Division of Colon and Rectal Surgery, St. Luke's/Roosevelt Hospital Center, New York, New York
HEMORRHOIDS, ANAL FISSURE, ANORECTAL ABSCESS, AND FISTULA

Satish Bhagwanjee, MBChB
Professor and Head, Department of Anesthesiology, University of the Witwatersrand, Johannesburg, South Africa
TETANUS

Zulfiqar A. Bhutta, MB, PhD
Husein Lalji Dewraj Professor of Pediatrics, Aga Khan University and Medical Center, Karachi, Pakistan
TYPHOID FEVER

Emil Bisaccia, MD
Professor of Clinical Dermatology, Columbia University College of Physicians and Surgeons, New York, New York
DISEASES OF THE HAIR

Jacob D. Bitran, MD
Director, Department of Hematology/Oncology, Luther General Hospital Cancer Care Center, Park Ridge, Illinois
PRIMARY LUNG CANCER

Brian Boehlecke, MD, MSPH
Professor, Department of Medicine, University of North Carolina at Chapel Hill School of Medicine, Chapel Hill, North Carolina
OBSTRUCTIVE SLEEP APNEA

Julie A. Boom, MD
Assistant Professor of Pediatrics, Baylor College of Medicine; Director, Immunization Project, Texas Children's Hospital, Houston, Texas
OFFICE-BASED IMMUNIZATION PRACTICES

Valia Boosalis, MD
Assistant Professor, Department of Medicine, Boston University School of Medicine; Staff Hematologist Oncologist, Jamaica Plain Boston Veterans Medical Center, Boston, Massachusetts
THALASSEMIA

William Z. Borer, MD
Professor, Department of Pathology, Jefferson Medical College of Thomas Jefferson University, Philadelphia, Pennsylvania
REFERENCE INTERVALS FOR THE INTERPRETATION OF LABORATORY TESTS

Kraig S. Bower, MD
Assistant Professor of Surgery, Uniformed Services University of the Health Sciences, Bethesda, Maryland; Director, Center for Refractive Surgery, Walter Reed Army Medical Center, Washington, DC
VISION CORRECTION PROCEDURES

Steven B. Brandes, MD
Assistant Professor, Division of Urologic Surgery, Washington University School of Medicine; Chief of Urology, St. Louis Veterans Affairs Medical Center, St. Louis, Missouri
TRAUMA TO THE GENITOURINARY TRACT

Denise Bratcher, DO
Associate Professor, Department of Pediatrics, University of Missouri–Kansas City School of Medicine; Staff Physician, Division of Infectious Diseases, Children's Mercy Hospital, Kansas City, Missouri
WHOOPING COUGH (PERTUSSIS)

Renier Brentjens, MD, PhD
Clinical Assistant, Department of Medicine, Leukemia Service, Memorial Sloan-Kettering Cancer Center, New York, New York
CHRONIC LEUKEMIAS

Sylvia L. Brice, MD
Associate Professor, Department of Dermatology, University of Colorado Health Sciences Center, Denver, Colorado
HUMAN HERPESVIRUSES

Gerald Brock, MD
Associate Professor, Division of Urology, University of Western Ontario Faculty of Medicine and Dentistry, London, Ontario, Canada
ERECTILE DYSFUNCTION

Adam M. Brodsky, MD
Fellow in Cardiology, Northwestern University Feinberg School of Medicine, Chicago, Illinois
ATRIAL FIBRILLATION

Charles K. Brown, MD
Professor, Department of Emergency Medicine, Brody School of Medicine at East Carolina University, Greenville, North Carolina
MARINE TRAUMA, ENVENOMATIONS, AND INTOXICATIONS

Forrest C. Brown, MD
Clinical Professor, Department of Dermatology, University of Texas Southwestern Medical Center at Dallas Southwestern Medical School; Chief, Division of Dermatology, Medical City Hospital, Dallas, Texas
PREMALIGNANT LESIONS

Barbara J. Browne, MD
Medical Director of Stroke Rehabilitation, Magee Rehabilitation Hospital, Philadelphia, Pennsylvania
REHABILITATION OF THE STROKE PATIENT

Carlo Brugnara, MD
Professor of Pathology, Harvard Medical School; Director, Hematology Laboratory, Department of Laboratory Medicine, Children's Hospital Boston, Boston, Massachusetts
NONIMMUNE HEMOLYTIC ANEMIA

Ruth Dowling Bruun, MD
Adjunct Associate Professor, Department of Psychiatry, New York University Medical Center; Executive and Medical Director, Family Counseling Service, New York, New York
GILLES DE LA TOURETTE SYNDROME

Kristina A. Bryant, MD
Assistant Professor, Department of Pediatrics, University of Louisville School of Medicine, Louisville, Kentucky
CAT-SCRATCH DISEASE

Bruce A. Buckingham, MD
Associate Professor of Pediatrics, Division of Pediatric Endocrinology and Diabetes, Stanford University School of Medicine, Stanford, California
DIABETES MELLITUS IN CHILDREN AND ADOLESCENTS

Robert Buckmire, MD
Assistant Professor, Department of Otolaryngology, University of Pittsburgh School of Medicine, Pittsburgh, Pennsylvania
HOARSENESS AND LARYNGITIS

Lucinda S. Buescher, MD
Associate Professor, Division of Dermatology, Southern Illinois University School of Medicine, Springfield, Illinois
SPIDER BITES AND SCORPION STINGS

James J. Burke II, MD
Assistant Professor, Department of Obstetrics and Gynecology, Mercer University School of Medicine, Macon; Attending Physician, Memorial Health University Medical Center, Savannah, Georgia
ENDOMETRIAL CANCER

Michael J. Burke, MD, PhD
Director of Medical Student Education; Director of Inpatient Services; Director of Electroconvulsive Therapy (ECT) Services, Department of Psychiatry and Behavioral Sciences, University of Kansas School of Medicine–Wichita, Wichita, Kansas
MOOD DISORDERS

John A. Burns, MD
Clinical Professor, Department of Ophthalmology, Ohio State University College of Medicine and Public Health, Columbus, Ohio
CONJUNCTIVITIS

John B. Buse, MD, PhD
Associate Professor of Medicine, University of North Carolina at Chapel Hill School of Medicine; Chief, Division of General Medicine and Clinical Epidemiology; Director, Diabetes Care Center, Chapel Hill, North Carolina
DIABETES MELLITUS IN ADULTS

Thomas M. Bush, MD
Clinical Associate Professor, Stanford University School of Medicine, Stanford; Chief of Rheumatology, Santa Clara Valley Medical Center, San Jose, California
CUTANEOUS VASCULITIS

John E. Buster, MD
Professor, Division of Reproductive Endocrinology and Infertility, Department of Obstetrics and Gynecology, Baylor College of Medicine, Houston, Texas
ECTOPIC PREGNANCY

Alexander Bystritsky, MD, PhD
Professor, Department of Psychiatry and Biobehavioral Sciences, David Geffen School of Medicine at UCLA; Director, Anxiety Disorders Program, Neuropsychiatric Institute and Hospital, Los Angeles, California
PANIC DISORDER

Eve Callahan, RD
Research Dietitian, Vanderbilt Center for Human Nutrition, Vanderbilt University Medical Center, Nashville, Tennessee
TOTAL PARENTERAL NUTRITION IN THE ADULT PATIENT

George P. Canellos, MD
William Rosenberg Professor of Medicine, Harvard Medical School; Senior Physician, Dana-Farber Cancer Institute, Boston, Massachusetts
HODGKIN'S DISEASE: CHEMOTHERAPY

Thomas R. Caraccio, PharmD
Associate Professor of Emergency Medicine, State University of New York at Stony Brook Health Sciences Center School of Medicine, Stony Brook; Assistant Professor of Pharmacology and Toxicology, New York College of Osteopathic Medicine, Old Westbury, New York
MEDICAL TOXICOLOGY: INGESTIONS, INHALATIONS, AND DERMAL AND OCULAR ABSORPTIONS

Richard W. Carlson, MD, PhD
Professor, Department of Medicine, Mayo Clinic College of Medicine, Rochester, Minnesota; Professor, Department of Clinical Medicine, University of Arizona College of Medicine, Tucson; Chairman, Department of Internal Medicine, Maricopa Medical Center, Phoenix, Arizona
SNAKEBITE

F. Xavier Castellanos, MD
Brooke and Daniel Neidich Professor of Child and Adolescent Psychiatry; Director, Institute for Pediatric Neuroscience; Director of Research, New York University Child Study Center, New York, New York
ATTENTION DEFICIT HYPERACTIVITY DISORDER (ADHD)

Kristin Casper, PharmD
Assistant Professor of Clinical Pharmacy, Division of Pharmacy Practice and Administration, Ohio State University College of Pharmacy, Columbus, Ohio
NEW DRUGS IN 2003 AND AGENTS PENDING FDA APPROVAL

Miriam M. Chan, RPH, PharmD
Clinical Assistant Professor of Pharmacy, Ohio State University College of Pharmacy, Columbus; Adjunct Assistant Professor of Pharmacy, Ohio Northern University, Ada; Director of Pharmacy Education, Riverside Family Practice Residency Program, Riverside Methodist Hospital, Columbus, Ohio
SOME POPULAR HERBS AND NUTRITIONAL SUPPLEMENTS; NEW DRUGS IN 2003 AND AGENTS PENDING FDA APPROVAL

Peter T. Chang, MD
Instructor of Ophthalmology, Cullen Eye Institute, Baylor College of Medicine, Houston, Texas
GLAUCOMA

Sam S. Chang, MD
Assistant Professor, Department of Urologic Surgery, Vanderbilt University Medical Center, Nashville, Tennessee
MALIGNANT TUMORS OF THE UROGENITAL TRACT

Subhash Chaudhary, MD
Professor of Pediatrics, Southern Illinois University School of Medicine, Springfield, Illinois
MUMPS

Rahul K. Chhablani, MD
Resident, Department of Medicine, Hospital of the University of Pennsylvania, Philadelphia, Pennsylvania
INFLAMMATORY BOWEL DISEASE

Daniel I. Choo, MD
Associate Professor, Department of Otolaryngology, University of Cincinnati College of Medicine; Director, Center for Hearing Deafness Research, and Head, Auditory Genetics Laboratory, Cincinnati Children's Hospital Medical Center, Cincinnati, Ohio
OTITIS MEDIA

James Christensen, MD
Professor Emeritus, Department of Internal Medicine, University of Iowa Carver College of Medicine; University of Iowa Hospitals and Clinics, Iowa City, Iowa
IRRITABLE BOWEL SYNDROME

Bart L. Clarke, MD
Assistant Professor of Medicine, Mayo Clinic College of Medicine; Consultant, Division of Endocrinology, Diabetes, Metabolism, Nutrition and Internal Medicine, Mayo Clinic, Rochester, Minnesota
PAGET'S DISEASE OF BONE

Daniel J. Clauw, MD
Professor of Medicine, Division of Rheumatology, University of Michigan Medical School; Director, Chronic Pain and Fatigue Research Center; Director, Center for the Advancement of Clinical Research, Ann Arbor, Michigan
BURSITIS, TENDINITIS, MYOFASCIAL PAIN, AND FIBROMYALGIA

Bruce A. Cohen, MD
Professor, Davee Department of Neurology, Northwestern University Feinberg School of Medicine, Chicago, Illinois
VIRAL MENINGITIS AND ENCEPHALITIS

Gary Robert Cohen, MD, MBA
Medical Director, Saint Luke's Perinatal Center, Kansas City, Missouri
HEMOLYTIC DISEASE OF THE FETUS AND NEWBORN

Jeffrey A. Cohen, MD
Director, Experimental Therapeutics, Mellen Center for Multiple Sclerosis Treatment and Research, Cleveland Clinic Foundation, Cleveland, Ohio
MULTIPLE SCLEROSIS

Denis Colin, MD, PhD
Medical Director, Le Mans Rehabilitation Hospital, Saint Saturnin, France
PRESSURE ULCERS

Robert R. Conley, MD
Professor of Psychiatry, University of Maryland School of Medicine; Chief, Inpatient Research Program, Maryland Psychiatric Research Center, Baltimore, Maryland
SCHIZOPHRENIA

Alex R. Constantinescu, MD
Medical Director, Pediatric Nephrology, Joe DiMaggio Children's Hospital, Hollywood, Florida
PARENTERAL FLUID THERAPY FOR INFANTS AND CHILDREN

Michael S. Cookson, MD
Associate Professor, Department of Urologic Surgery, Vanderbilt University Medical Center, Nashville, Tennessee
MALIGNANT TUMORS OF THE UROGENITAL TRACT

Leslie T. Cooper, MD
Assistant Professor of Medicine, Mayo Clinic College of Medicine; Consultant, Division of Cardiovascular Diseases and Internal Medicine, Mayo Clinic, Rochester, Minnesota
PERIPHERAL ARTERIAL DISEASE

Larry J. Copeland, MD
Professor and Chair, Department of Obstetrics and Gynecology, Ohio State University College of Medicine and Public Health, Columbus, Ohio
CANCER OF THE CERVIX

Jody Corey-Bloom, MD, PhD
Professor, Department of Neurosciences, University of California, San Diego, School of Medicine, La Jolla, California
ALZHEIMER'S DISEASE

Christina R. Covelli, MD
Resident, Department of Internal Medicine, University of Alabama School of Medicine at Birmingham, Birmingham, Alabama
CONSTIPATION

John F. Coyle II, MD
Clinical Professor, Department of Medicine, University of Oklahoma College of Medicine, Tulsa, Tulsa, Oklahoma
DISTURBANCES CAUSED BY HEAT

Donita R. Croft, MD, MS
Clinical Instructor, Pulmonary and Critical Care Section, University of Wisconsin Hospital and Clinics, Madison, Wisconsin
HISTOPLASMOSIS

Burke A. Cunha, MD
Professor of Medicine, State University of New York at Stony Brook Health Sciences Center School of Medicine, Stony Brook; Chief, Infectious Disease Division, Winthrop-University Hospital, Mineola, New York
BACTERIAL PNEUMONIAS; LEGIONELLOSIS (LEGIONNAIRES' DISEASE)

John J. Cush, MD
Clinical Professor of Internal Medicine, University of Texas Southwestern Medical Center at Dallas Southwestern Medical School; Chief, Rheumatology and Clinical Immunology, Presbyterian Hospital of Dallas, Dallas, Texas
RHEUMATOID ARTHRITIS

F. William Danby, MD
Lecturer, Department of Medicine (Dermatology), Dartmouth Medical School, Lebanon, New Hampshire
PRURITUS ANI AND VULVAE

Shannon Daniell, PharmD
Pharmacy Resident, Vanderbilt Center for Human Nutrition, Vanderbilt University Medical Center, Nashville, Tennessee
TOTAL PARENTERAL NUTRITION IN THE ADULT PATIENT

Kenneth R. Dardick, MD
Clinical Assistant Professor, University of Connecticut School of Medicine, Farmington; Attending Physician, Windham Community Memorial Hospital, Storrs, Connecticut
TRAVEL MEDICINE

Robert L. Deresiewicz, MD
Assistant Professor of Medicine, Harvard Medical School; Associate Physician, Channing Laboratory and the Infectious Disease Division, Brigham and Women's Hospital, Boston, Massachusetts
TOXIC SHOCK SYNDROME

Julie Deschênes, MD
Assistant Professor of Medicine, Pulmonology Division, Université de Sherbrooke Faculty of Medicine, Sherbrooke, Quebec, Canada
ASBESTOS AND SILICA-RELATED DISEASES

Marjolein de Wit, MD
Assistant Professor of Medicine, Virginia Commonwealth University School of Medicine; Division of Pulmonary and Critical Care Medicine, Department of Medicine, Virginia Commonwealth University Medical Center, Medical College of Virginia Hospitals, Richmond, Virginia
ACUTE RESPIRATORY FAILURE

Ananias C. Diokno, MD
Chief, Department of Urology, William Beaumont Hospital, Royal Oak, Michigan
BENIGN PROSTATIC HYPERPLASIA

Robert Dluhy, MD
Professor of Medicine, Harvard Medical School; Senior Physician, Division of Endocrinology, Diabetes, and Hypertension, Brigham and Women's Hospital, Boston, Massachusetts
HYPERPROLACTINEMIA

Peter Doelken, MD
Assistant Professor, Department of Pulmonology, Medical University of South Carolina College of Medicine, Charleston, South Carolina
PLEURAL EFFUSION AND EMPYEMA THORACIS

Alan B. Douglass, MD
Assistant Director, Family Practice Residency Program, Middlesex Hospital, Middletown, Connecticut
PAIN

Mark Dykewicz, MD
Professor of Medicine, Division of Allergy and Immunology, Saint Louis University School of Medicine, St. Louis, Missouri
NONALLERGIC RHINITIS

Marcia Edmonds, MD, MSc
Clinical Assistant Professor, University of Alberta Faculty of Medicine and Dentistry; Emergency Physician, Royal Alexandra Hospital and University of Alberta Hospital, Edmonton, Alberta, Canada
ACUTE BRONCHITIS

George E. Ehrlich, MD
Adjunct Professor, Department of Medicine, University of Pennsylvania School of Medicine, Philadelphia, Pennsylvania; Adjunct Professor of Clinical Medicine, New York University School of Medicine, New York, New York
OSTEOARTHRITIS

M. Patrice Eiff, MD
Associate Professor, Department of Family Medicine, Oregon Health Sciences University School of Medicine, Portland, Oregon
CONTRACEPTION

Nayef El-Daher, MD, PhD
Clinical Associate Professor of Medicine, University of Rochester School of Medicine; Head, Infectious Diseases Unit, Department of Medicine, Park Ridge Hospital, Unity Health System, Rochester, New York
PYELONEPHRITIS

Jack S. Elder, MD
Carter Kissell Professor of Urology and Professor of Pediatrics, Case Western Reserve University School of Medicine; Director of Pediatric Urology, Rainbow Babies and Children's Hospital, Cleveland, Ohio
BACTERIAL INFECTIONS OF THE URINARY TRACT IN GIRLS

Peter J. Embi, MD, MS
Associate Professor of Medicine, Division of General and Internal Medicine and Division of Immunology, University of Cincinnati College of Medicine, Cincinnati, Ohio
POLYMYALGIA RHEUMATICA AND GIANT CELL ARTERITIS

Per-Olof Eriksson, DDS, PhD
Professor, Department of Odontology, Clinical Oral Physiology, Faculty of Medicine Umeå University, Umeå; Center for Musculoskeletal Research, Gävle University, Gävle and Umeå, Sweden
MUSCULOSKELETAL DISORDERS IN THE JAW–FACE AND NECK

Gulchin A. Ergun, MD
Clinical Chief, Digestive Diseases Section, Baylor College of Medicine, Houston, Texas
DYSPHAGIA AND ESOPHAGEAL OBSTRUCTION

Geoffrey Eubank, MD
Clinical Instructor, Ohio State University College of Medicine and Public Health; Director, Neurology Education, Riverside Methodist Hospital; President, Neurological Associates, Inc., Columbus, Ohio
INTRACEREBRAL HEMORRHAGE

Janine Evans, MD
Associate Professor of Medicine, Section of Rheumatology, Department of Internal Medicine, Yale University School of Medicine, New Haven, Connecticut
LYME DISEASE

Shereen Ezzat, MD
Professor, Department of Medicine, University of Toronto Faculty of Medicine; Head, Endocrine Oncology Site Group, Mount Sinai Hospital, Toronto, Ontario, Canada
ACROMEGALY

Ronald J. Falk, MD
D. J. Thurston Professor of Medicine and Chief, Division of Nephrology and Hypertension, University of North Carolina at Chapel Hill School of Medicine, Chapel Hill, North Carolina
PRIMARY GLOMERULAR DISEASES

Adel G. Fam, MD
Professor of Medicine, University of Toronto Faculty of Medicine; Division of Rheumatology, Sunnybrook and Women's College Health Sciences Center, Toronto, Ontario, Canada
GOUT AND HYPERURICEMIA

Lameh Fananapazir, MD
Cardiovascular Branch, National Heart, Lung, and Blood Institute, National Institutes of Health, Bethesda, Maryland
HYPERTROPHIC CARDIOMYOPATHY

R. Wesley Farr, MD, MPH
Senior Medical Officer, *USS Harry S. Truman*, Norfolk, Virginia
RELAPSING FEVER

Vahab Fatourechi, MD
Professor of Medicine, Mayo Clinic College of Medicine; Consultant, Division of Endocrinology, Diabetes, Metabolism, Nutrition and Internal Medicine, Mayo Clinic, Rochester, Minnesota
HYPERTHYROIDISM

Lee D. Faucher, MD
Assistant Professor, Department of Surgery, University of Iowa Carver College of Medicine, Iowa City, Iowa
BURNS

Jerome M. Feldman, MD
Professor Emeritus, Departments of Medicine and Endocrinology, Duke University School of Medicine, Durham, North Carolina
PHEOCHROMOCYTOMA

Caraciolo J. Fernandes, MD
Assistant Professor of Pediatrics, Baylor College of Medicine; Attending Neonatologist, Department of Pediatrics, Texas Children's Hospital, Houston, Texas
CARE OF THE HIGH-RISK NEONATE

Kenneth H. Fife, MD, PhD
Professor of Medicine, Microbiology and Immunology and Pathology, Indiana University School of Medicine, Indianapolis, Indiana
CONDYLOMA ACUMINATA (GENITAL WARTS)

Jordan N. Fink, MD
Professor of Pediatrics (Allergy & Immunology) and Medicine, Medical College of Wisconsin, Milwaukee, Wisconsin
HYPERSENSITIVITY PNEUMONITIS

Dan Fintel, MD
Associate Professor of Medicine, Director, Coronary Care Unit, Northwestern University Feinberg School of Medicine, Chicago, Illinois
ATRIAL FIBRILLATION

John M. Fisk, MD
Transfusion Medicine Fellow, Yale University School of Medicine; Department of Laboratory Medicine, Blood Bank, Yale-New Haven Hospital, New Haven, Connecticut
THERAPEUTIC USE OF BLOOD COMPONENTS

Richard E. Fitzpatrick, MD
Associate Clinical Professor, Department of Dermatology, University of California, San Diego, School of Medicine, La Jolla; Dermatology Associates of San Diego County, Inc., Encinitas, California
KELOIDS

David Fivenson, MD
Medical Dermatologist, Private Practice, Ann Arbor, Michigan
VENOUS ULCERS

Matthew I. Fogg, MD
Fellow, Department of Allergy and Immunology, University of Pennsylvania School of Medicine, Philadelphia, Pennsylvania
ASTHMA IN CHILDREN

Mary E. Fontana, MD
Associate Professor of Internal Medicine, Division of Cardiovascular Medicine, Ohio State University College of Medicine and Public Health, Columbus, Ohio
MITRAL VALVE PROLAPSE

Nathan B. Fountain, MD
Associate Professor and Director, Comprehensive Epilepsy Program, Department of Neurology, University of Virginia School of Medicine, Charlottesville, Virginia
SEIZURES AND EPILEPSY IN ADOLESCENTS AND ADULTS

Lawrence S. Friedman, MD
Professor of Medicine, Harvard Medical School; Assistant Chief of Medicine, Massachusetts General Hospital, Boston; Chair, Department of Medicine, Newton-Wellesley Hospital, Newton, Massachusetts
ACUTE AND CHRONIC VIRAL HEPATITIS

Peter O. Fritsch, MD
Professor and Chairman, Department of Dermatology and Venereology, Medical University of Innsbruck, Innsbruck, Austria
ERYTHEMA MULTIFORME GROUP

George J. Fuchs, MD
Professor of Pediatrics and Chief of Pediatric Gastroenterology and Nutrition, University of Arkansas for Medical Sciences; Director of Gastroenterology, Arkansas Children's Hospital, Little Rock, Arkansas
CHOLERA

Niall T. M. Galloway, MD
Associate Professor of Urology, Emory University School of Medicine; Director, Emory Continence Center, Atlanta, Georgia
URINARY INCONTINENCE

Donald G. Gallup, MD
Professor and Chairperson, Department of Obstetrics and Gynecology, Mercer University School of Medicine, Macon; Attending Physician, Memorial Health University Medical Center, Savannah, Georgia
ENDOMETRIAL CANCER

Laura M. Gandrud, MD
Pediatric Endocrinology Fellow, Division of Pediatric Endocrinology and Diabetes, Stanford University School of Medicine, Stanford, California
DIABETES MELLITUS IN CHILDREN AND ADOLESCENTS

Jean-Pierre Gangneux, MD, PhD
Rennes Teaching Hospital and Faculté de Médecine de Rennes, Laboratoire de Parasitologie-Mycologie, Rennes, France
LEISHMANIASIS

Mark S. Gans, MD
Department of Ophthalmology, McGill University Faculty of Medicine, Montreal, Quebec, Canada
OPTIC NEURITIS

Bruce J. Gantz, MD
Professor of Otolaryngology, University of Iowa Carver College of Medicine; Head, Department of Otolaryngology—Head and Neck Surgery, University of Iowa Hospitals and Clinics, Iowa City, Iowa
ACUTE FACIAL PARALYSIS (BELL'S PALSY)

Dan Gehlbach, MD
Medical Director, Reproductive Medicine and Infertility, Shawnee Mission Medical Center, Shawnee Mission, Kansas
AMENORRHEA

Todd W. B. Gehr, MD
Professor of Medicine, Division of Nephrology, Virginia Commonwealth University School of Medicine, Richmond, Virginia
CHRONIC KIDNEY DISEASE

George J. Gianakopoulos, MD
Clinical Assistant Professor of Medicine, Ohio State University College of Medicine and Public Health; Private Practice, Infectious Diseases, Riverside Methodist Hospital, Columbus, Ohio
FOOD-BORNE ILLNESS

Gwendolyn L. Gilbert, MD
Clinical Professor, Departments of Medicine and Infectious Diseases, University of Sydney; Director, Centre for Infectious Diseases and Microbiology, Institute of Clinical Pathology and Medical Research, Westmead Hospital, Sydney, New South Wales, Australia
RAT-BITE FEVER

Curtis L. Gingrich, MD
Clinical Assistant Professor, Department of Family Medicine, Ohio State University College of Medicine and Public Health; Associate Program Director, Family Practice Residency Program, Riverside Methodist Hospital, Columbus, Ohio
BACTERIAL INFECTIONS OF THE URINARY TRACT IN WOMEN

Ondria C. Gleason, MD
Associate Professor, Department of Psychiatry, University of Oklahoma College of Medicine, Tulsa, Tulsa, Oklahoma
DELIRIUM

Matthew Bidwell Goetz, MD
Professor of Medicine, David Geffen School of Medicine at UCLA; Chief, Division of Infectious Diseases, Veterans Affairs Greater Los Angeles Healthcare System, Los Angeles, California
VIRAL AND MYCOPLASMAL PNEUMONIA

Michael R. Gold, MD, PhD
Professor of Medicine and Chief, Division of Cardiology, Medical University of South Carolina College of Medicine, Charleston, South Carolina
HEART BLOCK

Leonard H. Goldberg, MD
Staff Member, Department of Dermatology, Methodist Hospital, Houston, Texas
CANCER OF THE SKIN

Myla D. Goldman, MD
Postdoctoral Fellow, Mellen Center for Multiple Sclerosis Treatment and Research, Cleveland Clinic Foundation, Cleveland, Ohio
MULTIPLE SCLEROSIS

Philip H. Gordon, MD
Professor of Surgery and Oncology, McGill University Faculty of Medicine; Director of Colorectal Surgery, Sir Mortimer B. Davis Jewish General Hospital, Montreal, Quebec, Canada
NEOPLASMS OF THE COLON AND RECTUM

J. Andrew Grant, MD
Professor, Department of Internal Medicine, University of Texas Medical Branch at Galveston, Galveston, Texas
ASTHMA IN ADOLESCENTS AND ADULTS

H. L. Greenberg, MD
Chief Resident, Division of Dermatology, Scott & White Clinic, Texas A & M University System Health Science Center, Temple, Texas
PARASITIC DISEASES OF THE SKIN

Stephen B. Greenberg, MD
Herman Brown Teaching Professor, Baylor College of Medicine; Chief of Medicine, Ben Taub General Hospital, Houston, Texas
INFLUENZA

Joseph Greensher, MD
Professor of Pediatrics, State University of New York at Stony Brook Health Sciences Center School of Medicine, Stony Brook; Medical Director and Associate Chair, Department of Pediatrics, Long Island Regional Poison and Drug Information Center, Winthrop-University Hospital, Mineola, New York
MEDICAL TOXICOLOGY: INGESTIONS, INHALATIONS, AND DERMAL AND OCULAR ABSORPTIONS

Philip E. Greenspan, MD
Fellow, Division of Pulmonary, Critical Care, and Sleep Medicine, Mount Sinai School of Medicine of New York University, New York, New York
SARCOIDOSIS

Ronald L. Gross, MD
Professor of Ophthalmology, Baylor College of Medicine; Clifton R. McMichael Chair of Ophthalmology, Cullen Eye Institute, Houston, Texas
GLAUCOMA

John R. Guyton, MD
Associate Professor of Medicine, Duke University Medical Center, Durham, North Carolina
HYPERLIPOPROTEINEMIAS

Chul S. Ha, MD
Professor and Center Medical Director, Department of Radiation Oncology, M. D. Anderson Cancer Center, Houston, Texas
HODGKIN'S DISEASE: RADIATION THERAPY

Timothy C. Hain, MD
Professor of Neurology, Otolaryngology, and Physical Therapy, Northwestern Memorial Hospital, Chicago, Illinois
EPISODIC VERTIGO

Anna Q. Hare, BS
Clinical Associate Professor of Dermatology, Northwest Cutaneous Research Specialists, Portland, Oregon
FUNGAL INFECTIONS OF THE SKIN

Joanie Hare-Morris, MD
Maternal Fetal Medicine Specialist, Houston Perinatal Associates, Houston, Texas
HYPERTENSIVE DISORDERS OF PREGNANCY

Julie C. Harper, MD
Assistant Professor, Department of Dermatology, University of Alabama School of Medicine at Birmingham, Birmingham, Alabama
ACNE VULGARIS AND ROSACEA

Jeffrey P. Harris, MD, PhD
Professor and Chief, Division of Otolaryngology—Head and Neck Surgery, University of California, San Diego, School of Medicine, La Jolla, California
MÉNIÈRE'S DISEASE

Jay Heidecker, MD
Fellow, Department of Pulmonology, Medical University of South Carolina College of Medicine, Charleston, South Carolina
PLEURAL EFFUSION AND EMPYEMA THORACIS

Shannon Heitritter, MD
Fellow in Endocrinology, Division of Endocrinology, Diabetes, and Hypertension, Brigham and Women's Hospital, Boston, Massachusetts
HYPERPROLACTINEMIA

Chaim Hershko, MD
Professor of Medicine, Department of Hematology, Shaare Zedek Medical Center and Hebrew University Hadassah Medical School, Jerusalem, Israel
HEMOCHROMATOSIS

Irl B. Hirsch, MD
Medical Director, Diabetes Care Center, University of Washington Medical Center, Seattle, Washington
HYPEROSMOLAR HYPERGLYCEMIC SYNDROME AND DIABETIC KETOACIDOSIS

Paul Hirsch, MD, JD
Clinical Professor of Medicine (Dermatology), Keck School of Medicine of USC, Los Angeles, California
MELANOCYTIC NEVI (MOLES)

Gary S. Hoffman, MD, MS
Chairman, Department of Rheumatic and Immunologic Diseases, Center for Vasculitis Care and Research, Cleveland Clinic Foundation, Cleveland, Ohio
POLYMYALGIA RHEUMATICA AND GIANT CELL ARTERITIS

Fiona Horwood, BMedSci
Specialist Registrar in Respiratory and General Medicine, Nottingham City Hospital NHS Trust, Nottingham, United Kingdom
PSITTACOSIS (ORNITHOSIS)

John W. House, MD
Clinical Professor, Department of Otolaryngology—Head and Neck Surgery, Keck School of Medicine of USC; Private Practice, House Ear Clinic, Los Angeles, California
TINNITUS

Tamara Salam Housman, MD
Resident, Department of Dermatology, Wake Forest University Health Sciences Center, Winston-Salem, North Carolina
WARTS (VERRUCAE)

Shirley H. Huang, MD
Instructor, Department of Pediatrics, University of Pennsylvania School of Medicine; Fellow, Division of Gastroenterology and Nutrition, Children's Hospital of Philadelphia, Philadelphia, Pennsylvania
NORMAL INFANT FEEDING

Richard H. Hunt, MD
Professor of Medicine and Gastroenterology, McMaster University Medical Centre, Hamilton, Ontario, Canada
GASTROESOPHAGEAL REFLUX DISEASE

Raymond J. Hutchinson, MS, MD
Professor of Pediatrics, University of Michigan Medical School; Division of Pediatric Hematology/Oncology, University of Michigan Comprehensive Cancer Center, Ann Arbor, Michigan
ACUTE LEUKEMIA IN CHILDHOOD

Phuong N. Huynh, MD, MPH
Senior Resident, Department of Urology, William Beaumont Hospital, Royal Oak, Michigan
BENIGN PROSTATIC HYPERPLASIA

Mark D. Iannettoni, MD
Johanne L. Ehrenhaft Professor of Surgery and Chair, Department of Cardiothoracic Surgery, University of Iowa Carver College of Medicine, Iowa City, Iowa
ATELECTASIS

Michael C. Iannuzzi, MD
Chairman, Division of Pulmonary, Critical Care, and Sleep Medicine, Mount Sinai School of Medicine of New York University, New York, New York
SARCOIDOSIS

Jeffrey A. Jackson, MD
Associate Professor of Internal Medicine, Texas A & M University Health Science Center; Staff Endocrinologist, Scott & White Clinic, Temple, Texas
HYPERPARATHYROIDISM AND HYPOPARATHYROIDISM

Heidi T. Jacobe, MD
Assistant Professor and Director of Phototherapy Clinic, Department of Dermatology, University of Texas Southwestern Medical Center at Dallas Southwestern Medical School, Dallas, Texas
SUNBURN

Preeti Jaggi, MD
Fellow, Department of Infectious Diseases, Children's Memorial Hospital, Chicago, Illinois
STREPTOCOCCAL PHARYNGITIS

James J. James, MD, DrPH, MHA
Director, Center for Disaster Preparedness and Emergency Response, American Medical Association, Chicago, Illinois
TOXIC CHEMICAL AGENTS REFERENCE CHART: SYMPTOMS AND TREATMENT; BIOLOGIC AGENTS REFERENCE CHART: SYMPTOMS, TESTS, TREATMENT

Gordon Jensen, MD, PhD
Professor of Medicine, Vanderbilt University School of Medicine; Director, Vanderbilt Center for Human Nutrition, Nashville, Tennessee
TOTAL PARENTERAL NUTRITION IN THE ADULT PATIENT

Hal B. Jenson, MD
Professor and Chair, Department of Pediatrics, and Director, Center for Pediatric Research, Eastern Virginia Medical School; Senior Vice President for Academic Affairs, Children's Hospital of the King's Daughters, Norfolk, Virginia
INFECTIOUS MONONUCLEOSIS

Andrew B. Joel, MD
Fellow, Department of Urology, Georgetown University Hospital, Washington, DC
URINARY STONE DISEASE

Gerald H. Jordan, MD
Professor of Urology, Eastern Virginia Medical School; Devine Center for Genitourinary Reconstruction, Norfolk, Virginia
URETHRAL STRICTURE

Matthew H. Kanzler, MD
Clinical Professor, Stanford University School of Medicine, Stanford; Chief of Dermatology, Santa Clara Valley Medical Center, San Jose, California
CUTANEOUS VASCULITIS

Karl H. Karlson, Jr., MD
Associate Professor, Department of Pediatrics, Wake Forest University School of Medicine, Winston-Salem, North Carolina
CYSTIC FIBROSIS

Karthikeshwar Kasirajan, MD
Assistant Professor, Department of Surgery, Emory University School of Medicine, Atlanta, Georgia
ACQUIRED DISEASES OF THE AORTA

James W. Kazura, MD
Professor of International Health and Director, Center for Global Health and Diseases, Case Western Reserve University, Cleveland, Ohio
MALARIA

Dennis Kellar, MD
Fellow, Pulmonary and Critical Care Medicine, Rush Medical College of Rush University, Chicago, Illinois
BACTEREMIA AND SEPSIS

Deanna L. Kelly, PharmD
Assistant Professor of Psychiatry, University of Maryland School of Medicine; Maryland Psychiatric Research Center, Baltimore
SCHIZOPHRENIA

J. William Kelly, MD
Associate Director, Department of Internal Medicine, Greenville Memorial Hospital, Greenville, South Carolina
BACTERIAL MENINGITIS

Anita S. Kestin, MD
Clinical Assistant Professor, Department of Medicine, Brown University School of Medicine; Physician, Internal Medicine, Division of Hematology and Oncology, Rhode Island Hospital, Providence, Rhode Island
PLATELET MEDIATED BLEEDING DISORDERS

Azim J. Khan, MD
Assistant Professor of Clinical Dermatology, State University of New York at Stony Brook Health Sciences Center School of Medicine, Stony Brook, New York
DISEASES OF THE HAIR

John Khazin, DO
Chief Resident, Department of Internal Medicine, Maricopa Medical Center, Phoenix, Arizona
SNAKEBITE

Robert C. Kimbrough III, MD
Professor and Clerkship Director, Division of Infectious Diseases, Department of Internal Medicine, Texas Tech University Health Sciences Center, Lubbock, Texas
Q FEVER

Charles P. Kimmelman, MD, MBA
Associate Clinical Professor of Otorhinolaryngology, Weill-Cornell Medical College; Attending Surgeon, Department of Otolaryngology—Head and Neck Surgery, Lenox Hill Hospital and Manhattan Eye, Ear and Throat Hospital, New York, New York
OTITIS EXTERNA

Charles E. King, MD
Digestive Disorders Associates of Annapolis and Glen Burnie, Annapolis, Maryland
MALABSORPTION

Major (res) Andrew W. Kirkpatrick, CD, MD
Clinical Assistant Professor, Departments of Critical Care Medicine and Surgery, University of Calgary Faculty of Medicine; Staff Trauma, General Surgeon, and Multi-Disciplinary Intensivist, Foothills Medical Centre, Calgary, Alberta, Canada
DISTURBANCES CAUSED BY COLD

Katalin I. Koranyi, MD
Professor of Clinical Pediatrics, Section of Infectious Diseases, Department of Pediatrics, Ohio State University College of Medicine and Public Health; Children's Hospital, Columbus, Ohio
RUBELLA AND CONGENITAL RUBELLA SYNDROME

David S. Kotlyar, BS
Research Associate, Department of Medicine, Gastroenterology Division, University of Pennsylvania Health Systems, Philadelphia, Pennsylvania
CIRRHOSIS

Ertug Kovanci, MD
Fellow, Division of Reproductive Endocrinology and Infertility, Department of Obstetrics and Gynecology, Baylor College of Medicine, Houston, Texas
ECTOPIC PREGNANCY

Peter R. Kowey, MD
Professor, Department of Medicine, Jefferson Medical College at Thomas Jefferson University, Philadelphia; Chief, Division of Cardiovascular Diseases, Lankenau Hospital, Wynnewood, Pennsylvania
TACHYCARDIAS

Keith Krasinski, MD
Professor, Department of Pediatrics and Environmental Medicine, New York University School of Medicine, New York, New York
MEASLES (RUBEOLA)

John N. Krieger, MD
Professor, Department of Urology, University of Washington School of Medicine, Seattle, Washington
BACTERIAL INFECTIONS OF THE URINARY TRACT IN MALES

Abhijit V. Kshirsagar, MD, MPH
Assistant Professor of Medicine, Division of Nephrology and Hypertension, University of North Carolina at Chapel Hill School of Medicine, Chapel Hill, North Carolina
PRIMARY GLOMERULAR DISEASES

Timothy M. Kuzel, MD
Associate Professor, Department of Medicine, Division of Hematology/Oncology, Northwestern University Feinberg School of Medicine; Robert H. Lurie Comprehensive Cancer Center, Chicago, Illinois
CUTANEOUS T-CELL LYMPHOMAS (MYCOSIS FUNGOIDES AND SÉZARY SYNDROME)

Robert A. Kyle, MD
Professor of Medicine and of Laboratory Medicine, Mayo Clinic College of Medicine; Consultant, Division of Hematology and Internal Medicine, Mayo Clinic, Rochester, Minnesota
MULTIPLE MYELOMA

Christopher J. Lahart, MD
Assistant Professor, Department of Medicine, Baylor College of Medicine, Houston, Texas
TUBERCULOSIS AND OTHER MYCOBACTERIAL DISEASES

Richard A. Larson, MD
Professor of Medicine, Section of Hematology/Oncology, University of Chicago Pritzker School of Medicine, Chicago, Illinois
ACUTE LEUKEMIA IN ADULTS

Paul A. Leach, MRCS
Specialist Registrar, Department of Neurosurgery, Hope Hospital, Manchester, United Kingdom
ACUTE HEAD INJURIES IN ADULTS

Mark G. Lebwohl, MD
Chairman, Department of Dermatology, Mount Sinai School of Medicine of New York University, New York, New York
PAPULOSQUAMOUS ERUPTIONS

Sandra Lee, MD
Fellow, Dermatology Associates of San Diego County, Inc., Encinitas, California
KELOIDS

Clifford L. S. Leen, MD, MBChB
Consultant Physician and Part-time Senior Lecturer, Regional Infectious Diseases Unit, Western General Hospital, Edinburgh, United Kingdom
SALMONELLOSIS

Jose F. Leis, MD, PhD
Associate Professor of Medicine, Center for Hematologic Malignancies, Oregon Health and Science University School of Medicine, Portland, Oregon
POLYCYTHEMIA VERA

Anthony Lembo, MD
Instructor of Medicine, Division of Gastroenterology, Harvard Medical School; Director of Gastrointestinal Motility, Beth Israel Deaconess Medical Center, Boston, Massachusetts
GASEOUSNESS AND INDIGESTION

Matthew E. Levison, MD
Professor of Medicine and Public Health, Drexel University College of Medicine, Philadelphia, Pennsylvania
INFECTIVE ENDOCARDITIS

Robert Libke, MD
Chief of Infectious Diseases and Clinical Professor of Medicine, University of California, San Francisco, Fresno, School of Medicine, Fresno, California
COCCIDIOIDOMYCOSIS

Gary R. Lichtenstein, MD
Professor of Medicine, University of Pennsylvania School of Medicine; Director, Center for Inflammatory Bowel Diseases, Division of Gastroenterology, Hospital of the University of Pennsylvania, Philadelphia, Pennsylvania
INFLAMMATORY BOWEL DISEASE

Marcia Torres Lima, MD
Visiting Scientist, Division of Allergy and Clinical Immunology, Department of Internal Medicine, University of Texas–Houston Medical School, Houston, Texas
ANAPHYLAXIS AND SERUM SICKNESS

D. Scott Lind, MD
Professor, Department of Surgery, University of Florida College of Medicine; Chief, Surgical Services, North Florida–South Georgia Veterans Affairs Health System, Gainesville, Florida
DISEASES OF THE BREAST

Frank W. Ling, MD
Professor and Immediate Past Chairman, Division of Gynecologic Specialties, Department of Obstetrics and Gynecology, University of Tennessee Health Science Center, Memphis, Tennessee
UTERINE LEIOMYOMA

Michael Littner, MD
Professor of Medicine, David Geffen School of Medicine at UCLA, Los Angeles; Staff Physician, Department of Medicine, Pulmonary, Critical Care, and Sleep Medicine, Veterans Affairs Greater Los Angeles Healthcare System, Sepulveda, California
MANAGEMENT OF CHRONIC OBSTRUCTIVE PULMONARY DISEASE

Warren Lo, MD
Associate Professor, Departments of Pediatrics and Neurology, Ohio State University College of Medicine and Public Health, Columbus Ohio
ACUTE HEAD INJURIES IN CHILDREN

Gerald L. Logue, MD
Professor of Medicine, State University of New York at Buffalo School of Medicine and Biological Sciences; Hematology Division Head, Erie County Medical Center, Buffalo, New York
ADVERSE REACTIONS TO BLOOD TRANSFUSIONS

James M. Lyznicki, MS, MPH
Senior Scientist, Center for Disaster Preparedness and Emergency Response, American Medical Association, Chicago, Illinois
TOXIC CHEMICAL AGENTS REFERENCE CHART: SYMPTOMS AND TREATMENT; BIOLOGIC AGENTS REFERENCE CHART: SYMPTOMS, TESTS, TREATMENT

John Macfarlane, DM
Consultant in Respiratory Medicine, Nottingham City Hospital NHS Trust, Nottingham, United Kingdom
PSITTACOSIS (ORNITHOSIS)

Kenneth Madden, MD, PhD
Clinical Associate Professor of Neurology, University of Wisconsin Medical School, Madison; Neurologist, Cerebrovascular Disease Subspecialist, Marshfield Clinic, Marshfield, Wisconsin
ISCHEMIC CEREBROVASCULAR DISEASE

James W. Maher, MD
Professor, Department of Surgery, University of Iowa Carver College of Medicine; Director, Division of Gastrointestinal Surgery, University of Iowa Hospitals and Clinics, Iowa City, Iowa
CHOLELITHIASIS AND CHOLECYSTITIS

Tariq Mahmood, MD
Clinical Associate Professor, Department of Medicine, UMDNJ–New Jersey Medical School, Newark, New Jersey
URTICARIA AND ANGIOEDEMA

Anthony J. Mancini, MD
Associate Professor of Pediatrics and Dermatology, Northwestern University Feinberg School of Medicine; Attending Physician, Division of Dermatology, Children's Memorial Hospital, Chicago, Illinois
ATOPIC DERMATITIS

Scott C. Manning, MD
Professor, Department of Otolaryngology, University of Washington School of Medicine; Children's Hospital and Regional Medical Center, Seattle Washington
SINUSITIS

Lynette J. Margesson, MD
Assistant Professor, Departments of Medicine (Dermatology) and Obstetrics and Gynaecology, Dartmouth Medical School, Lebanon, New Hampshire
PRURITUS ANI AND VULVAE

Barry J. Marshall, MD
Clinical Professor of Microbiology, University of Western Australia, Nedlands, Western Australia, Australia
GASTRITIS AND PEPTIC ULCER DISEASE

Gailen D. Marshall, Jr., MD, PhD
Professor of Medicine and Pediatrics and Vice Chair, Department of Medicine; Director, Division of Clinical Immunology and Allergy, University of Mississippi School of Medicine, Jackson, Mississippi
ANAPHYLAXIS AND SERUM SICKNESS

Michael McGuigan, MD
Medical Director, Long Island Regional Poison and Drug Information Center, Winthrop-University Hospital, Mineola, New York
MEDICAL TOXICOLOGY: INGESTIONS, INHALATIONS, AND DERMAL AND OCULAR ABSORPTIONS

Christopher R. McHenry, MD
Professor of Surgery, Case Western Reserve University School of Medicine; Vice Chairman, Department of Surgery; Director, Division of General Surgery, MetroHealth Medical Center, Cleveland, Ohio
NECROTIZING SOFT-TISSUE INFECTIONS; THYROID CANCER

Donald McNeil, MD
Associate Professor of Clinical Medicine, Department of Immunology, Ohio State University College of Medicine and Public Health, Columbus, Ohio
ALLERGIC REACTIONS TO DRUGS

Stephanie J. Mengden Koon, MD
Resident in Dermatology, Mayo Graduate School and Mayo Clinic College of Medicine, Rochester, Minnesota
CONTACT DERMATITIS

Jeffrey D. Merrill, MD
Assistant Professor of Pediatrics, University of Pennsylvania School of Medicine; Medical Director, Neonatology Intensive Care Unit, Hospital of the University of Pennsylvania, Philadelphia, Pennsylvania
RESUSCITATION OF THE NEWBORN

Ted A. Meyer, MD, PhD
Fellow, Department of Otolaryngology—Head and Neck Surgery, University of Iowa Carver College of Medicine; University of Iowa Hospitals and Clinics, Iowa City, Iowa
ACUTE FACIAL PARALYSIS (BELL'S PALSY)

James S. Milledge, MD
Physician Emeritus, Northwick Park Hospital, Watford Road, Harrow, England, United Kingdom
HIGH-ALTITUDE SICKNESS

Deborah M. Miller, MB, ChB
Volunteer Clinical Faculty, Department of Pediatrics, University of California, San Francisco, School of Medicine, San Francisco, California
DYSFUNCTIONAL UTERINE BLEEDING

Ronald D. Miller, MD
Director, Medical Specialists for Women, Tustin, California
DYSFUNCTIONAL UTERINE BLEEDING

William F. Miser, MD, MA
Associate Professor, Department of Family Medicine, Ohio State University College of Medicine and Public Health, Columbus, Ohio
NAUSEA AND VOMITING

James E. Mitchell, MD
The NRI/Lee A Christoferson Professor and Chester Fritz Distinguished Professor, University of North Dakota School of Medicine and Health Sciences; Chairman, Department of Neurosciences, and President, Neuropsychiatric Research Institute, Fargo, North Dakota
BULIMIA NERVOSA

Joel L. Moake, MD
Professor, Hematology/Oncology Section, Baylor College of Medicine; Associate Director, Biomedical Engineering Laboratory, Rice University, Houston, Texas
THROMBOTIC THROMBOCYTOPENIC PURPURA

Howard C. Mofenson, MD
Professor of Pediatrics and Emergency Medicine, State University of New York at Stony Brook Health Sciences Center School of Medicine, Stony Brook; Professor of Pharmacology and Toxicology, New York College of Osteopathic Medicine, Old Westbury, New York
MEDICAL TOXICOLOGY: INGESTIONS, INHALATIONS, AND DERMAL AND OCULAR ABSORPTIONS

Saidi A. Mohiddin, MB, ChB
Cardiovascular Branch, National Heart, Lung, and Blood Institute, National Institutes of Health, Bethesda, Maryland
HYPERTROPHIC CARDIOMYOPATHY

Anuroop Mongia, MD
Division of Allergy and Immunology, UMDNJ–New Jersey Medical School, Newark, New Jersey
URTICARIA AND ANGIOEDEMA

Nancy A. Morin, MD
Assistant Professor of Surgery, McGill University Faculty of Medicine; Colorectal Surgeon, Sir Mortimer B. Davis Jewish General Hospital, Montreal, Quebec, Canada
NEOPLASMS OF THE COLON AND RECTUM

Patrick J. Mulrow, MD
Professor Emeritus, Department of Medicine, Medical College of Ohio, Toledo, Ohio
HYPERTENSION

Diya F. Mutasim, MD
Professor and Chairman, Department of Dermatology, University of Cincinnati College of Medicine, Cincinnati, Ohio
BULLOUS DISEASES

Tricia Cook Myers, PhD
Clinical Assistant Professor, Department of Neurosciences, University of North Dakota School of Medicine and Health Sciences, Fargo, North Dakota
BULIMIA NERVOSA

Ashwatha Narayana, MD
Assistant Attending Physician, Department of Radiation Oncology, Memorial Sloan-Kettering Cancer Center, New York, New York
BRAIN TUMORS

William H. Nealon, MD
Professor of Surgery and Director, Pancreatico-Biliary and Hepatic Surgery Service, University of Texas Medical Branch, Galveston, Texas
CHRONIC PANCREATITIS

Susan Nedorost, MD
Assistant Professor of Dermatology, Case Western Reserve University School of Medicine; University of Cleveland Hospitals, Cleveland Ohio
PRURITUS

Peter E. Newburger, MD
Professor and Vice Chair of Pediatrics, University of Massachusetts Medical School, Worcester, Massachusetts
NEUTROPENIA

J. Curtis Nickel, MD
Professor, Department of Urology, Queen's University Faculty of Health Sciences; Kingston General Hospital, Kingston, Ontario, Canada
EPIDIDYMITIS

Nigel O'Farrell, MD
Consultant Physician, Ealing Hospital, London, England
DONOVANOSIS; LYMPHOGRANULOMA VENEREUM

Jacqueline G. O'Leary, MD
Research Fellow, Department of Medicine, Harvard Medical School; Clinical and Research Fellow, Gastrointestinal Unit, Massachusetts General Hospital, Boston, Massachusetts
ACUTE AND CHRONIC VIRAL HEPATITIS

Joyce Olutade, MD, MBBS
Assistant Professor, Department of Family Medicine, University of Mississippi Medical Center, Jackson, Mississippi
DYSMENORRHEA

Debora Ortega-Carr, MD
Associate Professor, Division of Rheumatology, Allergy, and Immunology, Ohio State University College of Medicine and Public Health; Midwest Allergy and Asthma Associates, Columbus, Ohio
ALLERGIC REACTIONS TO INSECT STINGS

Charles H. Packman, MD
Clinical Professor of Medicine, University of North Carolina at Chapel Hill School of Medicine, Chapel Hill; Chief, Section of Hematology and Oncology, Carolinas Medical Center, Charlotte, North Carolina
AUTOIMMUNE HEMOLYTIC ANEMIA

Heather Paladine, MD
Assistant Professor, Department of Family Medicine, Oregon Health and Science University School of Medicine, Portland, Oregon
CONTRACEPTION

Robert M. Pascuzzi, MD
Professor and Interim Chair, Department of Neurology, Indiana University School of Medicine, Indianapolis, Indiana
MYASTHENIA GRAVIS AND RELATED DISORDERS

Sheral S. Patel, MD
Assistant Professor, Department of Pediatrics, Case Western Reserve University School of Medicine, Cleveland, Ohio
MALARIA

Sonal M. Patel, MD
Fellow, Division of Gastroenterology, Beth Israel Deaconess Medical Center, Boston, Massachusetts
GASEOUSNESS AND INDIGESTION

Susan P. Perrine, MD
Associate Professor, Department of Medicine, Pediatrics, Pharmacology, and Experimental Therapeutics, and Director, Hemoglobinopathy-Thalassemia Research Unit, Boston University School of Medicine, Boston, Massachusetts
THALASSEMIA

Robert W. Peters, MD
Professor of Medicine, University of Maryland School of Medicine; Chief, Cardiology Section, Baltimore Veterans Affairs Medical Center, Baltimore, Maryland
HEART BLOCK

George A. Petroianu, MD, PhD
Professor and Chairman, Department of Pharmacology and Therapeutics, UAE University, Al Ain, United Arab Emirates; apl. Professor, Pharmacology and Toxicology, University of Heidelberg at Mannheim, Mannheim, Germany
HICCUPS

David H. Pfizenmaier II, MD, DPM
Vascular Medicine Fellow, Mayo Graduate School, Mayo Clinic College of Medicine; Attending Physician, Mayo Clinic, Rochester, Minnesota
PERIPHERAL ARTERIAL DISEASE

Melissa Peck Piliang, MD
Resident, Department of Dermatology, Cleveland Clinic Foundation, Cleveland, Ohio
SKIN DISEASES OF PREGNANCY

Neville Pimstone, MD, PhD
Professor of Medicine, University of California, Davis, Medical Center, Sacramento, California
THE PORPHYRIAS

E. Geoffrey Playford, MB, BS
Senior Lecturer, Department of Medicine, University of Queensland; Infectious Diseases Physician, Infection Management Services, Princess Alexandra Hospital, Brisbane, Queensland, Australia
PLAGUE

Martin Poleski, MD
Clinical Professor of Medicine, Duke University Medical Center, Durham, North Carolina
DIVERTICULA OF THE ALIMENTARY TRACT

Charles A. Polnitsky, MD
Adjunct Professor, Quinnipiac University, Hamden; Medical Director, Regional Sleep Laboratory, Waterbury, Connecticut
COUGH

John Pomann, MD, MS
Resident Physician, Department of Dermatology, Henry Ford Hospital, Detroit, Michigan
VENOUS ULCERS

Michel A. Pontari, MD
Associate Professor, Department of Urology, Temple University School of Medicine, Philadelphia, Pennsylvania
PROSTATITIS

Uday Popat, MD
Assistant Professor of Medicine, Center of Cell and Gene Therapy, Baylor College of Medicine, Houston, Texas
NON-HODGKIN'S LYMPHOMA

Frank C. Powell, MD
Lecturer, Department of Dermatology, University College, Dublin, Ireland
DISEASES OF THE MOUTH

Scott W. Pyne, MD
Assistant Professor, Department of Family Medicine, Uniformed Services University of the Health Sciences, Bethesda; Director, Sports Medicine, Naval Medical Clinic, United States Naval Academy, Annapolis, Maryland
COMMON SPORTS INJURIES

Christiane Querfeld, MD
Fellow, Department of Dermatology, Northwestern University Feinberg School of Medicine, Chicago, Illinois
CUTANEOUS T-CELL LYMPHOMAS (MYCOSIS FUNGOIDES AND SÉZARY SYNDROME)

G. Andres Quiceno, MD
Assistant Medical Director, Arthritis Consultation Center, Presbyterian Hospital of Dallas, Dallas, Texas
RHEUMATOID ARTHRITIS

S. Vincent Rajkumar, MD
Associate Professor of Medicine, Mayo Clinic College of Medicine; Consultant, Division of Hematology and Internal Medicine, Mayo Clinic, Rochester, Minnesota
MULTIPLE MYELOMA

Srikanth Ramachandruni, MD
Clinical Assistant Professor, Department of Medicine, University of Florida College of Medicine, Gainesville, Florida
MANAGEMENT OF ANGINA PECTORIS

Susan M. Ramin, MD
Professor of Obstetrics, Gynecology, and Reproductive Sciences, Director, Division of Maternal-Fetal Medicine, University of Texas–Houston Medical School, Houston, Texas
ANTENATAL CARE

Annemarei Ranta, MD
Epilepsy and EEG Fellow, Department of Neurology, University of Virginia School of Medicine, Charlottesville, Virginia
SEIZURES AND EPILEPSY IN ADOLESCENTS AND ADULTS

David W. Rattner, MD
Professor of Surgery, Harvard Medical School; Chief, Division of General and Gastrointestinal Surgery, Massachusetts General Hospital, Boston, Massachusetts
ACUTE PANCREATITIS

A. Andrew Ray, MSc, MD
Resident, Division of Urology, University of Western Ontario Faculty of Medicine and Dentistry, London, Ontario, Canada
ERECTILE DYSFUNCTION

K. Rajender Reddy, MD
Professor of Medicine and Surgery, University of Pennsylvania School of Medicine; Director of Hepatology, Medical Director of Liver Transplantation, Department of Medicine, Gastroenterology Division, University of Pennsylvania Health Systems, Philadelphia, Pennsylvania
CIRRHOSIS

Gary C. Reid, MD
Clinical Associate Professor, Division of Gynecologic Oncology, Ohio State University College of Medicine and Public Health; Associate Director, Gynecologic Oncology, Riverside Methodist Hospital, Columbus, Ohio
NEOPLASMS OF THE VULVA

Andreas Otto Reiff, MD
Associate Professor of Pediatrics, Keck School of Medicine of USC; Attending Rheumatologist, Division of Rheumatology, Children's Hospital Los Angeles, Los Angeles, California
JUVENILE ARTHRITIS

Martin Reite, MD
Professor of Psychiatry, Director of Insomnia and Sleep Disorders Clinic, University of Colorado Health Sciences Center, Denver, Colorado
TREATMENT OF INSOMNIA

David C. Rhew, MD
Associate Clinical Professor, Department of Medicine, David Geffen School of Medicine at UCLA; Staff Physician, Division of Infectious Diseases, Veterans Affairs Greater Los Angeles Healthcare System, Los Angeles, California
VIRAL AND MYCOPLASMAL PNEUMONIA

Lawrence Rice, MD
Professor of Medicine and Program Director, Hematology, Department of Medicine, Baylor College of Medicine, Houston, Texas
NON-HODGKIN'S LYMPHOMA

Phoebe Rich, MD
Clinical Associate Professor of Dermatology, Northwest Cutaneous Research Specialists, Portland, Oregon
FUNGAL INFECTIONS OF THE SKIN

Bertrand Richert, MD, PhD
Associate Clinical Professor, Dermatology Department, University of Liège, Belgium
DISEASES OF THE NAILS

Alan G. Robinson, MD
Executive Associate Dean and Associate Vice Chancellor, Medical Sciences, David Geffen School of Medicine at UCLA, Los Angeles, California
DIABETES INSIPIDUS

Gail Rock, MD, PhD
Chief, Division of Hematology and Transfusion Medicine, Department of Pathology and Laboratory Medicine, Ottawa Hospital, Ottawa, Ontario, Canada
DISSEMINATED INTRAVASCULAR COAGULATION

Cameron K. Rokhsar, MD
Fellow, Dermatology Associates of San Diego County, Inc., Encinitas, California
KELOIDS

Matthew A. Romano, MD
Fellow, Section of Thoracic Surgery, University of Michigan School of Medicine, Ann Arbor, Michigan
ATELECTASIS

Ellen S. Rome, MD, MPH
Head, Section of Adolescent Medicine, Children's Hospital at the Cleveland Clinic, Cleveland, Ohio
CHANCROID

Clifford J. Rosen, MD
Director, Maine Center for Osteoporosis Research and Education, St. Joseph Hospital, Bangor, Maine
OSTEOPOROSIS

Steven T. Rosen, MD
Geneviève Teuton Professor, Department of Medicine, Division of Hematology/Oncology, Northwestern University Feinberg School of Medicine; Director, Robert H. Lurie Comprehensive Cancer Center, Chicago, Illinois
CUTANEOUS T-CELL LYMPHOMAS (MYCOSIS FUNGOIDES AND SÉZARY SYNDROME)

Jean-François Rossignol, MD, PhD
Director and Chief Science Officer, Romark Institute for Medical Research, Tampa, Florida
GIARDIASIS

Mark E. Rupp, MD
Associate Professor of Medicine, Department of Internal Medicine, University of Nebraska Medical Center, Omaha, Nebraska
BLASTOMYCOSIS

Scott A. Rutherford, AFRCS
Specialist Registrar, Department of Neurosurgery, Hope Hospital, Manchester, United Kingdom
ACUTE HEAD INJURIES IN ADULTS

Christopher W. Ryan, MD
Clinical Associate Professor of Family Medicine, State University of New York Upstate Medical University, Clinical Campus at Binghamton, Binghamton; Wilson Family Practice Residency, Johnson City, New York
HEADACHE

George R. Saade, MD
Professor, Department of Obstetrics and Gynecology, Division of Maternal Fetal Medicine, University of Texas Medical Branch at Galveston, Galveston, Texas
POSTPARTUM CARE

Carlos Salama, MD
Assistant Professor of Medicine, Mount Sinai School of Medicine of New York University; Division of Infectious Diseases, Elmhurst Hospital Center, New York, New York
MANAGEMENT OF THE HIV-INFECTED PATIENT

Susan Samson, MD, PhD
Fellow, Department of Medicine, Division of Diabetes, Endocrinology, and Metabolism, Baylor College of Medicine, Houston, Texas
CUSHING'S SYNDROME

Isaac Samuel, MD
Assistant Professor, Department of Surgery, University of Iowa Carver College of Medicine, Iowa City, Iowa
CHOLELITHIASIS AND CHOLECYSTITIS

Mark A. Sanchez, MD
Resident, Department of Internal Medicine, University of Texas Medical Branch at Galveston, Galveston, Texas
ASTHMA IN ADOLESCENTS AND ADULTS

Juan C. Sarria, MD
Assistant Professor, Division of Infectious Diseases, Department of Internal Medicine, Texas Tech University Health Sciences Center School of Medicine, Lubbock, Texas
Q FEVER

Dwight Scarborough, MD
Adjunct Assistant Professor of Dermatology, Columbia University College of Physicians and Surgeons, New York, New York
DISEASES OF THE HAIR

Anouk Scheres, PhD
Associate Research Scientist, Institute for Pediatric Neuroscience, New York University Child Study Center, New York, New York
ATTENTION DEFICIT HYPERACTIVITY DISORDER (ADHD)

Nicola E. Schiebel, MD
Assistant Professor of Emergency Medicine, Mayo Clinic College of Medicine; Consultant, Department of Emergency Medicine, Mayo Clinic, Rochester, Minnesota
CARDIAC ARREST: SUDDEN CARDIAC DEATH

Isaac Schiff, MD
Joe Vincent Meigs Professor of Gynecology, Harvard Medical School; Chief, Vincent Memorial Obstetrics and Gynecology Service, Massachusetts General Hospital, Boston, Massachusetts
MENOPAUSE

Steven M. Schlossberg, MD
Professor of Urology, Eastern Virginia Medical School; Devine Center for Genitourinary Reconstruction, Norfolk, Virginia
URETHRAL STRICTURE

George P. Schmid, MD, MSc
Medical Officer, Department of HIV/AIDS, World Health Organization, Geneva, Switzerland
GONORRHEA

Robert A. Schwartz, MD, MPH
Professor and Head, Department of Dermatology, and Professor of Medicine, Pathology, Pediatrics, Preventive Medicine, and Community Health, UMDNJ–New Jersey Medical School, Newark, New Jersey
PIGMENTARY DISORDERS

Hilliard Seigler, MD
Professor of Surgery and Immunology, Duke University Medical Center, Durham, North Carolina
MALIGNANT MELANOMA

Alberto Selman, MD
Assistant Professor of Obstetrics/Gynecology, Universidad de Chile; Director, Division of Gynecologic Oncology, Clinical Hospital, Santiago, Chile
CANCER OF THE CERVIX

Edward J. Septimus, MD
Clinical Professor, Department of Medicine, University of Texas–Houston Medical School; Associate Clinical Professor, Department of Medicine, Baylor College of Medicine; Medical Director, Infectious Diseases and Occupational Health, Memorial Hermann Healthcare System, Houston, Texas
OSTEOMYELITIS

Curtis N. Sessler, MD
Professor of Medicine, Division of Pulmonary and Critical Care Medicine, Department of Medicine, Virginia Commonwealth University Medical Center, Medical College of Virginia Hospitals, Richmond, Virginia
ACUTE RESPIRATORY FAILURE

Daniel J. Sexton, MD
Professor, Division of Infectious Diseases, Department of Medicine, Duke University Medical Center, Durham, North Carolina
RICKETTSIAL AND EHRLICHIAL INFECTIONS

Ralph Shabetai, MD
Professor of Medicine, University of California, San Diego, School of Medicine, La Jolla, California
ACUTE PERICARDITIS

Mehnaz A. Shafi, MD
Associate Professor of Medicine, Gastroenterology Section, Baylor College of Medicine, Houston, Texas
DYSPHAGIA AND ESOPHAGEAL OBSTRUCTION

Mrunal Shah, MD
Clinical Assistant Professor of Family Medicine, Ohio State University College of Medicine and Public Health; Assistant Program Director, Riverside Family Practice Residency Program, Columbus, Ohio
SYPHILIS

Sudhir V. Shah, MD
Professor of Internal Medicine, University of Arkansas for Medical Sciences; Chief of Renal Medicine, Medicine Service, Central Arkansas Veterans Healthcare System, Little Rock, Arkansas
ACUTE RENAL FAILURE

Harry Sharata, MD, PhD
Associate Professor, Department of Dermatology, University of Wisconsin Medical School; Chief of Dermatology, Veterans Affairs Hospital, Madison, Wisconsin
PARASITIC DISEASES OF THE SKIN

Mary Jo Shaver-Lewis, MD
Assistant Professor of Internal Medicine, University of Arkansas for Medical Sciences; Staff Physician, Medicine Service, Central Arkansas Veterans Healthcare System, Little Rock, Arkansas
ACUTE RENAL FAILURE

David S. Sheps, MD, MSPH
Professor, Department of Medicine, University of Florida College of Medicine, Gainesville, Florida
MANAGEMENT OF ANGINA PECTORIS

Jan L. Shifren, MD
Assistant Professor of Obstetrics, Gynecology, and Reproductive Biology, Harvard Medical School; Director, Menopause Program, Vincent Memorial Obstetrics and Gynecology Service, Massachusetts General Hospital, Boston, Massachusetts
MENOPAUSE

Lydia A. Shrier, MD, MPH
Assistant Professor of Pediatrics, Harvard Medical School; Assistant in Medicine, Children's Hospital Boston, Boston, Massachusetts
PELVIC INFLAMMATORY DISEASE

Stanford T. Shulman, MD
Professor of Pediatrics, Northwestern University Feinberg School of Medicine; Chief, Division of Infectious Diseases, Children's Memorial Hospital, Chicago, Illinois
STREPTOCOCCAL PHARYNGITIS

Emmanuel Siaw, MD, PhD
Assistant Professor of Pediatrics, University of Arkansas for Medical Sciences; Staff Gastroenterologist, Arkansas Children's Hospital, Little Rock, Arkansas
CHOLERA

Dee E. Silver, MD
Head, Section of Neurology, Scripps Memorial Hospital, La Jolla; Medical Director, Parkinson's Disease Association, San Diego, California
PARKINSONISM

Marc A. Silver, MD
Clinical Professor of Medicine, University of Illinois Medical Center, Chicago; Adjunct Professor, Department of Biomedical Engineering, Illinois Institute of Technology, Chicago; Chairman, Department of Medicine, and Director, Heart Failure Institute, Advocate Christ Medical Center, Oak Lawn, Illinois
HEART FAILURE

Peter A. Singer, MD
Professor of Clinical Medicine, Department of Medicine, Keck School of Medicine of USC, Los Angeles, California
HYPOTHYROIDISM

Edwin A. Smith, MD
Professor, Department of Medicine, Medical University of South Carolina College of Medicine, Charleston, South Carolina
CONNECTIVE TISSUE DISORDERS

Robert B. Smith III, MD
John E. Skandalakis Emeritus Professor, Department of Surgery, Emory University School of Medicine, Atlanta, Georgia
ACQUIRED DISEASES OF THE AORTA

Edward L. Snyder, MD
Professor of Laboratory Medicine, Yale University School of Medicine; Director, Transfusion, Apheresis, and Cell Therapy Services, Yale–New Haven Hospital, New Haven, Connecticut
THERAPEUTIC USE OF BLOOD COMPONENTS

Jonathan M. Spergel, MD, PhD
Assistant Professor of Pediatrics, University of Pennsylvania School of Medicine; Children's Hospital of Philadelphia, Philadelphia, Pennsylvania
ASTHMA IN CHILDREN

Virginia A. Stallings, MD
Professor, Department of Pediatrics, University of Pennsylvania School of Medicine; Director, Nutrition Center, and Deputy Director, Joseph Stokes, Jr., Research Institute, Children's Hospital of Philadelphia; Philadelphia, Pennsylvania
NORMAL INFANT FEEDING

Sharon L. Stein, MD
Clinical Fellow, Department of Surgery, Massachusetts General Hospital, Boston, Massachusetts
ACUTE PANCREATITIS

Dana Kazlow Stern, MD
Fellow, Department of Dermatology, Mount Sinai School of Medicine of New York University, New York, New York
PAPULOSQUAMOUS ERUPTIONS

Catherine Stevens-Simon, MD
Associate Professor of Pediatrics, Division of Adolescent Medicine, University of Colorado Health Science Center and Children's Hospital, Denver, Colorado
CHLAMYDIA TRACHOMATIS

Greg V. Stiegmann, MD
Professor and Head, Gastrointestinal, Tumor, and Endocrine Surgery, Department of Surgery, University of Colorado Health Sciences Center and Denver Veterans Affairs Hospitals, Denver, Colorado
BLEEDING ESOPHAGEAL VARICES

Mathias L. Stoenescu, MD
Fellow, Department of Electrophysiology, Lankenau Hospital, Wynnewood, Pennsylvania
TACHYCARDIAS

Marshall L. Stoller, MD
Professor, Department of Urology, University of California, San Francisco, School of Medicine, San Francisco, California
URINARY STONE DISEASE

Patrick A. Stone, MD
Chief Surgical Resident, Department of Surgery, Robert C. Byrd Health Sciences Center of West Virginia University, Charleston, West Virginia
VENOUS THROMBOSIS

Benjamin H. Sun, DVM, MPVM
State Public Health Veterinarian, California Department of Health Services, Sacramento, California
RABIES

Morton N. Swartz, MD
Professor, Department of Medicine, Harvard Medical School; Physician and Chief, Jackson Firm of the Medical Service, Massachusetts General Hospital, Boston, Massachusetts
ANTHRAX

Sinésio Talhari, MD, PhD
Chief, Department of Dermatology, Fundação de Medicina Tropical do Amazonas, Manaus, Brazil
LEPROSY (HANSEN'S DISEASE)

Charu Taneja, MD
Department of Surgery, Boston University Medical Center, Boston, Massachusetts; Roger Williams Medical Center, Providence, Rhode Island
GASTRIC CANCER

Herbert B. Tanowitz, MD
Professor, Departments of Pathology and Medicine, Albert Einstein College of Medicine of Yeshiva University, Bronx, New York
AMEBIASIS

Victor F. Tapson, MD
Associate Professor of Medicine, Division of Pulmonary and Critical Care, Duke University Medical Center, Durham, North Carolina
PULMONARY EMBOLISM

James Temprano, MD, MHA
Fellow, Division of Allergy and Immunology, Saint Louis University School of Medicine, St. Louis, Missouri
NONALLERGIC RHINITIS

Susan Thys-Jacobs, MD
Assistant Professor, Department of Medicine, Columbia University College of Physicians and Surgeons, New York, New York
PREMENSTRUAL SYNDROME

Joyce A. Tinsley, MD
Associate Professor of Psychiatry, Director of Psychiatric Residency Training, and Director of Addiction Psychiatry Training, University of Connecticut School of Medicine, Farmington, Connecticut
DRUG ABUSE

Glenn Tisman, MD
Whittier Cancer Research Institute, Whittier, California
PERNICIOUS ANEMIA AND OTHER MEGALOBLASTIC ANEMIAS

Anthony Toft, MD
Consultant Physician, Outpatient Department 2, Endocrine Clinic, Royal Infirmary, Edinburgh, Scotland
THYROIDITIS

John F. Toney, MD
Associate Professor of Medicine, Division of Infectious and Tropical Diseases, University of South Florida College of Medicine, Tampa, Florida
NONGONOCOCCAL URETHRITIS

Edwin Trevathan, MD, MPH
Professor of Neurology and Pediatrics and Director, Pediatric Epilepsy Center, Washington University School of Medicine, St. Louis, Missouri
EPILEPSY IN INFANTS AND CHILDREN

Dace L. Trence, MD
Director, Diabetes Care Center, University of Washington Medical Center, Seattle, Washington
HYPEROSMOLAR HYPERGLYCEMIC SYNDROME AND DIABETIC KETOACIDOSIS

Jaya R. Trivedi, MD
Assistant Professor, Department of Neurology, University of Texas Southwestern Medical Center at Dallas Southwestern Medical School, Dallas, Texas
PERIPHERAL NEUROPATHIES

Chang-Yong Tsao, MD
Professor, Departments of Pediatrics and Neurology, Ohio State University College of Medicine and Public Health, Columbus Ohio
ACUTE HEAD INJURIES IN CHILDREN

Douglas Tyler, MD
Associate Professor of Surgery, Duke University School of Medicine; Chief, Surgical Oncology, Duke University Medical Center; Chief, Surgical Services, Durham Veterans Affairs Medical Center, Durham, North Carolina
MALIGNANT MELANOMA

Jay Umbreit, MTS, MD, PhD
Professor, Department of Hematology/Oncology, Winship Cancer Institute, Emory University School of Medicine, Atlanta, Georgia
IRON DEFICIENCY

G. Nicholas Verne, MD
Assistant Professor of Medicine, University of Florida College of Medicine, Gainesville, Florida
CONSTIPATION

Alex C. Vidaeff, MD, MPH
Associate Professor of Obstetrics, Gynecology, and Reproductive Sciences, Division of Maternal-Fetal Medicine, University of Texas–Houston Medical School, Houston, Texas
ANTENATAL CARE

Ana M. Vidal, MD
Fellow, Department of Obstetrics and Gynecology, Division of Maternal Fetal Medicine, University of Texas Medical Branch at Galveston, Galveston, Texas
POSTPARTUM CARE

Philip D. Walson, MD
Professor of Pediatrics and Pharmacology, University of Cincinnati College of Medicine; Head and Director, Clinical Pharmacology Division, Clinical Trials Office, Cincinnati Children's Hospital Medical Center, Cincinnati, Ohio
FEVER

Julian Wan, MD
Department of Urology, University of Michigan Medical School, Ann Arbor, Michigan
CHILDHOOD ENURESIS

Harold J. Wanebo, MD
Professor of Surgery, Boston University Medical Center, Boston, Massachusetts; Chief of Surgical Oncology, Roger Williams Medical Center, Providence, Rhode Island
GASTRIC CANCER

Thomas T. Ward, MD
Associate Professor of Medicine, Oregon Health and Science University School of Medicine; Chief, Infectious Diseases, Portland Veterans Affairs Medical Center, Portland, Oregon
TOXOPLASMOSIS

Indira Warrier, MD
Professor of Pediatrics, Wayne State University School of Medicine; Co-Director, Hemophilia Treatment Center, Department of Hematology and Oncology, Children's Hospital of Michigan, Detroit, Michigan
HEMOPHILIA AND RELATED CONDITIONS

Peter C. Weber, MD
Professor and Program Director; Director of Implantable Hearing Devices, Head and Neck Institute, Cleveland Clinic, Cleveland, Ohio
ACUTE FACIAL PARALYSIS (BELL'S PALSY)

Michael Wein, MD
President, Florida Allergy, Asthma, and Immunology Society; Chief of Allergy, Indian River Memorial Hospital, Vero Beach, Florida
ALLERGIC RHINITIS

Myron H. Weinberger, MD
Professor, Department of Medicine, Indiana University Medical Center, Indianapolis, Indiana
PRIMARY ALDOSTERONISM

Mark Weiss, MD
Associate Attending Physician, Department of Medicine, Leukemia Service, Memorial Sloan-Kettering Cancer Center, New York, New York
CHRONIC LEUKEMIAS

Dov Weissberg, MD
Department of Thoracic Surgery, Tel Aviv University Sackler School of Medicine, Tel Aviv; E. Wolfson Medical Center, Holon, Israel
PRIMARY LUNG ABSCESS

Robert C. Welliver, Sr., MD
Professor of Pediatrics, Co-Director, Infectious Diseases, University Pediatric Associates, Inc.; Co-Director, Division of Infectious Diseases, Women and Children's Hospital of Buffalo, Buffalo, New York
VIRAL UPPER RESPIRATORY TRACT INFECTIONS

Dylan R. Wells, MD
Instructor, Division of Gynecologic Specialties, Department of Obstetrics and Gynecology, University of Tennessee Health Science Center, Memphis, Tennessee
UTERINE LEIOMYOMA

Sterling G. West, MD
Professor, Division of Rheumatology, Department of Medicine, University of Colorado School of Medicine, Denver, Colorado
ANKYLOSING SPONDYLITIS

A. Clinton White, Jr., MD
Professor, Infectious Disease Section, Department of Medicine, Baylor College of Medicine; Chief, Infectious Diseases, Ben Taub General Hospital, Houston, Texas
INTESTINAL PARASITES

David R. White, MD
Pediatric Otolaryngology Fellow, Department of Otolaryngology, Cincinnati Children's Hospital Medical Center, Cincinnati, Ohio
OTITIS MEDIA

Roger D. White, MD
Professor of Anesthesiology, Mayo Clinic College of Medicine; Consultant, Department of Anesthesiology, Mayo Clinic, Rochester, Minnesota
CARDIAC ARREST: SUDDEN CARDIAC DEATH

Richard J. Whitley, MD
Professor of Pediatrics, Microbiology, Medicine, and Neurosurgery, Departments of Pediatrics, Microbiology, and Medicine, University of Alabama School of Medicine at Birmingham, Birmingham, Alabama
SMALLPOX: A TWENTY-FIRST CENTURY VIEW

Michael G. Wilkerson, MD
Clinical Assistant Professor of Dermatology, University of Oklahoma College of Medicine, Tulsa, Tulsa, Oklahoma
BACTERIAL DISEASES OF THE SKIN

Kira Williams, MD
Chief Resident in Psychiatry, Anxiety Disorders Clinic, Department of Psychiatry and Biobehavioral Sciences; Neuropsychiatric Institute and Hospital, David Geffen School of Medicine at UCLA, Los Angeles, California
PANIC DISORDER

Phillip M. Williford, MD
Associate Professor, Department of Dermatology, Wake Forest University Health Sciences, Winston-Salem, North Carolina
WARTS (VERRUCAE)

Murray Wittner, MD, PhD
Professor, Department of Pathology, Albert Einstein College of Medicine of Yeshiva University, Bronx, New York
AMEBIASIS

Gil I. Wolfe, MD
Associate Professor, Department of Neurology, University of Texas Southwestern Medical Center at Dallas Southwestern Medical School, Dallas, Texas
PERIPHERAL NEUROPATHIES

R. Scott Wright, MD
Associate Professor of Medicine, Mayo Clinic College of Medicine; Consultant, Division of Cardiovascular Diseases and Internal Medicine, Mayo Clinic, Rochester, Minnesota
TREATMENT OF ACUTE MYOCARDIAL INFARCTION

Lawrence R. Wu, MD
Associate Clinical Professor, Department of Community and Family Medicine, Duke University Medical Center, Durham, North Carolina
ANXIETY DISORDERS

Dario Yacovino, MD
Department of Otolaryngology, Northwestern Memorial Hospital, Chicago, Illinois
EPISODIC VERTIGO

Linda Yancey, MD
Postdoctoral Fellow, Infectious Disease Section, Department of Medicine, Baylor College of Medicine, Houston, Texas
INTESTINAL PARASITES

James A. Yiannias, MD
Associate Professor of Dermatology, Mayo Clinic College of Medicine, Rochester, Minnesota; Consultant, Department of Dermatology, Mayo Clinic, Scottsdale, Arizona
CONTACT DERMATITIS

Edward J. Young, MD
Professor of Medicine, Baylor College of Medicine; Staff Physician, Michael E. DeBakey Veterans Affairs Medical Center, Houston, Texas
BRUCELLOSIS

Neal S. Young, MD
Chief, Hematology Branch, National Heart, Lung, and Blood Institute, National Institutes of Health, Bethesda, Maryland
APLASTIC ANEMIA

Thomas W. Young, MD
Assistant Professor, Department of Pediatrics, Division of Cardiology, Medical College of Georgia School of Medicine, Augusta, Georgia
CONGENITAL HEART DISEASE

Yuhong Yuan, MD, PhD
Research Associate, Division of Gastroenterology, McMaster University Medical Centre, Hamilton, Ontario, Canada
GASTROESOPHAGEAL REFLUX DISEASE

Hamayun Zafar, PT, PhD
Assistant Professor, Department of Odontology, Clinical Oral Physiology, Umeå University Faculty of Medicine, Umeå; Center for Musculoskeletal Research, Gävle University, Gävle and Umeå, Sweden
MUSCULOSKELETAL DISORDERS IN THE JAW–FACE AND NECK

Jami Star Zeltzer, MD
University of Massachusetts Medical School, Worcester, Massachusetts
VAGINAL BLEEDING IN LATE PREGNANCY

Donald Zimmerman, MD
Professor of Pediatrics, Northwestern University Feinberg School of Medicine; Head, Division of Endocrinology, Children's Memorial Hospital, Chicago, Illinois
DISEASES OF THE PITUITARY GLAND

Preface

This is the 57th edition of *Conn's Current Therapy*. The goal remains unchanged since Howard Conn published the first edition in 1949: to provide the practicing physician and other health professionals with a concise reference to the most recent advances in therapy. Specific information on the treatment of conditions the practicing physician commonly encounters in a clinical setting is presented by international authorities in the field who see these problems frequently and often have conducted research leading to changes in therapy.

Every year we turn to new authorities who provide their method for treating problems frequently encountered in practice, and some less common problems that can be serious if not managed properly. Many of these authorities reside outside the United States. This year 33 authors are from other countries such as Sweden (Temporomandibular Disorders), Belgium (Diseases of the Nails), Nigeria (Sickle Cell Disease), Brazil (Leprosy), Pakistan (Typhoid Fever), South Africa (Tetanus), Bangladesh (Acute Infectious Diarrhea), Australia (Gastric and Peptic Ulcer Disease), Israel (Hemochromatosis), France (Pressure Ulcers), and Austria (Erythema Multiforme). There are also many authors from Canada and the United Kingdom.

In response to the potential for worldwide bioterrorism, we have updated the Reference Tables on "Biologic Agents" and "Toxic Chemical Agents." The table on "Popular Herbs and Nutritional Supplements" and the table on "New Drugs in 2004 and Agents Pending FDA Approval" have also been updated.

Our greatest challenge each year is to meet the tight deadlines required in an annual publication to ensure that the information is current. This year 92% of the authors are new, and the other 8% have thoroughly updated their material. Because each new authority presents his or her preferred method for managing the problem, the reader is encouraged to compare this with the methods presented in previous editions that may provide alternatives for consideration. The drugs recommended are the most effective according to their experience, even though some have not yet been FDA approved for that indication.

A new crisp and clean format has been used in this edition, making the text even more easy to read. We hope that you agree and that this book continues to assist you in providing high-quality medical care.

Our special thanks to Norma Kessler, our editorial assistant, who organizes the manuscripts and galley proofs and ensures that all deadlines are met.

Robert E. Rakel, MD

Edward T. Bope, MD

Contents

SECTION 3
Diseases of the Head and Neck

SECTION 4
The Respiratory System

SECTION 5
The Cardiovascular System

SECTION 6
The Blood and Spleen

SECTION 7
The Digestive System

SECTION 8
Metabolic Diseases

SECTION 9 The Endocrine System

SECTION 10 The Urogenital Tract

SECTION 11
The Sexually Transmitted Diseases

SECTION 12
Diseases of Allergy

SECTION 13
Diseases of the Skin

SECTION 14 The Nervous System

SECTION 15 The Locomotor System

SECTION **16**

Obstetrics and Gynecology

SECTION **17**

Psychiatric Disorders

SECTION **18**

Physical and Chemical Injuries

SECTION 19
Appendices and Index

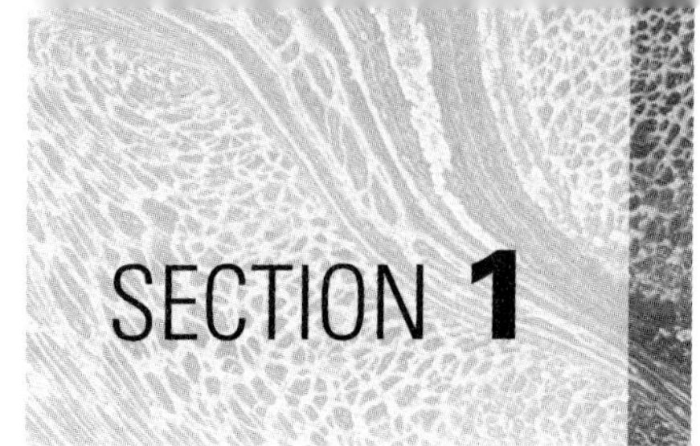

Symptomatic Care Pending Diagnosis

PAIN

METHOD OF

Alan B. Douglass, MD

Pain is an almost ubiquitous human condition, and a common reason for seeking medical care. Ninety percent of patients with advanced cancer, 45% to 80% of nursing home patients, and 25% to 50% of community adults report daily pain. Pain is a major cause of lost productivity, with United States (U.S.) annual costs of more than 60 billion dollars in lost work alone. Improving pain assessment and management is currently a U.S. national priority.

The literature clearly documents that 90% of pain can be adequately controlled using standard techniques such as the World Health Organization (WHO) pain ladder and the Agency for Healthcare Policy and Research (AHCPR) (now known as the Agency for Healthcare Research and Quality [AHRQ]) guidelines. However, undertreatment is rife. More than one half of patients, even those at the end of life, do not receive adequate analgesia.

Pain is defined by the International Association for the Study of Pain as "an unpleasant sensory and emotional experience associated with actual or potential tissue damage, or described in terms of such damage." Pain is a complex and subjective sensory, emotional, and cognitive phenomenon. The degree of pain experienced by a patient does not always correlate well with identifiable tissue injury, making assessment challenging.

Acute pain often follows an injury, but may also arise de novo as the result of structural degeneration, infection, or metabolic changes. Acute pain tends to abate as tissues heal, and generally responds well to analgesics and other therapies. Chronic pain persists over time and is generally defined as lasting longer than 3 to 6 months, or 1 month longer than the usual time required for an injury to heal. The management of chronic pain is often complex.

Pain is generally divided into two broad categories: nociceptive and neuropathic. Nociceptive pain is pain induced when nociceptive receptors are stimulated by a tissue injury process. Nociceptive pain is further divided into visceral and somatic pain. Visceral pain originates in internal organs. It is often poorly localized and described as cramping, squeezing, or colicky in nature if originating from a hollow viscus, or aching and dull if originating from a solid organ. Somatic pain is more easily localized, and usually described as achy, throbbing, or dull.

Neuropathic pain is pain induced by pathophysiologic changes to the central and peripheral nervous system. Neuropathic pain is typically described as a sharp, tingling, burning, or electric sensation and it often radiates. Pain of neuropathic origin may be associated with dysesthesias (unpleasant abnormal sensations), hyperalgesia (mildly painful stimuli perceived as very painful), or allodynia (nonpainful stimuli perceived as painful). Neuropathic pain usually requires a multimodal approach to therapy and tends to be more refractory to treatment.

Patient Assessment

Pain is a subjective, complex, multidimensional experience that is perceived only by the patient. Patient response to pain involves physical, psychological, and cognitive facets. Pain assessment is always challenging for clinicians because there is no single objective measurement available. Consequently, the patient's assessment of the severity and quality of their pain should be considered the best available assessment tool.

Pain reporting by patients can be subject to exaggeration, minimization, and misinterpretation. Many factors can influence the pain perception of others. Generally speaking, family members tend to overestimate, while health care professionals tend to underestimate. Reduced cognitive ability, reduced level of consciousness, and stoicism can result in underreporting. Cultural, ethnic, and gender factors on the part of both patients and caregivers can all affect pain interpretation and communication.

Effective pain management begins with comprehensive patient assessment. A number of validated pain assessment tools of varying length and complexity are available. Simple examples include the numerical rating scale (1 to 10) and visual analogue scale. Special instruments, such as the faces scale, are available for rating discomfort in young children, the cognitively impaired, and when language barriers are present. Frequent re-evaluation is an essential part of effective pain management.

Pharmacologic Management

Medication is the mainstay of pain management. The pharmacologic management of pain has long been based on the WHO analgesic ladder, where the selection of agent is dependent on the severity and type of pain experienced. Patients with mild pain are treated with Step 1 nonopioid agents such as acetaminophen or nonsteroidal anti-inflammatory drugs (NSAIDs), with or without the addition of adjuvant medications. Pain that is moderate in intensity is treated with Step 2 weak opioids in addition to Step 1 medications. Severe pain is treated with Step 3 strong opioids, such as morphine, in addition to adjuvants and appropriate adjuvants. Some authors recommend a fourth step in the ladder, representing interventional pain-management techniques. It is important to note that if pain is initially severe, the treating physician does not have to proceed up the ladder sequentially, but may begin with either Step 2 or Step 3.

ACETAMINOPHEN

Full-dose acetaminophen (Tylenol) is an effective, well-tolerated analgesic in a variety of pain scenarios. Although 4 g/day is listed as the maximal safe dosage, many experts advocate maximum dosages of 2 to 3 g/day. Furthermore, in alcoholism, fasting states, hepatic disease, the presence of certain medications (especially anticonvulsants), or in the frail elderly, liver toxicity can occur at recommended doses. Toxicity increases when acetaminophen is taken in conjunction with a NSAID. Particular care should be taken when patients are taking combination analgesics containing acetaminophen that daily dose limits are not inadvertently exceeded.

NSAIDs

There is strong evidence for the efficacy of NSAIDs in acute and chronic pain. The efficacy of all NSAIDs appears roughly equivalent, but patient response to any particular agent is highly idiosyncratic. Non-acetylated salicylates (choline magnesium trisalicylate [Trilisate], salsalate [Disalcid]) and cyclooxygenase (COX)-2–specific inhibitors are effective and may have fewer gastrointestinal side effects than traditional NSAIDs. Salicylates have the additional advantage of low cost. If traditional NSAIDs are chosen, gastric cytoprotection should be considered based on the patient's risk profile. Clinicians should also be aware of potential nephrotoxicity in the elderly and in patients with renal disease. NSAIDs should be particularly considered when inflammation is believed to be playing a substantial role in the production of the pain process.

OPIOIDs

Opioids are an effective option in the management of moderate to severe pain. They are often the drug of choice in acute and chronic cancer pain. Opioids have recently become more accepted in the long-term management of severe chronic noncancer pain, although concerns have been raised about the safety and efficacy of prolonged, high-dose opioid therapy.

Traditionally, it was believed that opioids had the advantage over other agents of the absence of a ceiling effect. Recent research suggests a ceiling may exist, but it is variable, and often determined by side effects such as myoclonus. Doses can be escalated by 50% to 100% in a 24-hour period for severe, uncontrolled pain. Increases of less than 25% are usually ineffective in this situation. However, smaller increases may be effective for moderate pain.

Immediate-release opioids commonly prescribed orally in the ambulatory setting include codeine, hydrocodone, and oxycodone (Roxicodone). Codeine tends to be very constipating and should be used with care in the elderly. Propoxyphene (Darvon) has limited analgesic effect and active metabolites accumulate over time. Its use should be limited to the short-term. Partial agonists such as butorphanol (Stadol) are strongly discouraged as first-line agents. They should not be given to patients taking pure opioid agonists because they may precipitate withdrawal.

Morphine, the prototypical opioid, is available in a variety of dosage forms and is widely used. Fentanyl (Duragesic) and hydromorphone (Dilaudid) are also commonly used. Hydromorphone is particularly useful because of its high potency and safety in patients with renal failure, but is available only in short-acting preparations. Methadone (Dolophine) is increasingly being used in the management of chronic pain because of its low cost and beneficial side-effect profile. However, because of its peculiar pharmacokinetics that can lead to drug accumulation and toxicity, it should be prescribed only after careful consideration and only by physicians experienced in its use. Meperidine (Demerol) is not recommended because of accumulation of active metabolites that can trigger neurotoxicity and seizures.

In patients with chronic pain the use of sustained-release morphine and oxycodone should be considered. Once at steady state, sustained-release opioids are more convenient and prevent the "peaks and valleys" associated with short-acting agents. However, many patients, particularly those with cancer pain, will require an additional short-acting agent to manage breakthrough pain.

The diversity of opioid receptors allows the transition from one opioid agonist to another when one agent ceases to be effective or side effects limit dose escalation. Opioid rotation must be done with care. Doses of different agents are not equivalent, so a conversion table (Table 1) should be used to calculate the equianalgesic doses. Alternatively, the dose of the original agent can be converted to oral morphine equivalents (Table 2) and then converted to the correct dosage of the new agent. To account for the phenomenon of incomplete cross-tolerance, the equianalgesic dose of the new agent should be decreased by 25% to 50%.

Opioids can be delivered by a variety of routes, including orally, rectally, intravenously, and subcutaneously. The intramuscular route is not recommended because of the pain associated with injections and wide fluctuations in blood levels. Fentanyl (Duragesic) is highly lipophilic and can be delivered transdermally through a 72-hour patch. Butorphanol (Stadol NS), a mixed agonist–antagonist, can be delivered intranasally. Interventional delivery of a variety of agents through the intrathecal or epidural route is also possible. Patient-controlled analgesia through the intravenous or epidural route can be very effective. When changing from one route to another doses must be recalculated, even if the same agent is used (see Table 1).

TABLE 1 Single-Dose Opioid Equianalgesic Doses in Milligrams

Drug	Oral Dose	Parenteral Dose
Morphine	15	5
Meperidine (Demerol)	150	50
Hydromorphone (Dilaudid)	3.75	0.75
Oxycodone (Roxicodone)	10	NA
Hydrocodone	15	NA
Codeine	90	NA

TABLE 2 Oral Morphine Equivalents (OME)

Drug	OME
Morphine	1
Codeine 30 mg	1-2
Hydrocodone 5 mg	2
Oxycodone 5 mg	5
Hydromorphone 4 mg	15

The most common side effect of opioid therapy is constipation, which, once established, can be severe and difficult to treat. All patients started on an opioid should receive a prophylactic bowel regime with a stimulant laxative. Use of a stool softener alone is rarely effective. Nausea and vomiting are common, but usually transient. Sedation and impaired psychomotor function occur in a dose-dependent fashion and are most common when initiating therapy. Symptoms typically dissipate over time, and patients on long-term opioid therapy are often capable of carrying out their usual daily activities, including working and driving.

There is current debate over the long-term use of opioids in the management of chronic noncancer pain. Clearly, some patients can benefit from this approach. Recent research on prolonged, high-dose opioid therapy has raised concerns of opioid-induced abnormal pain sensitivity, hormonal changes, including changes in libido and fertility, and immune suppression. Daily doses of more than 180 mg of daily morphine equivalent have not been validated as effective in clinical trials, and may present an increased risk of toxicity. The decision on an appropriate dose in a given patient should be individualized, with a focus on efficacy, avoiding potential toxicities, and functional improvement.

Both physicians and patients are often leery of the use of opioids because of fears of addiction and abuse. The nature of addiction and its risk in the use of opioids for pain management is frequently misunderstood, and confusion over definitions worsens the problem. The result often is undertreatment of pain.

Addiction is a primary, chronic, neurobiologic disease with genetic, psychosocial, and environmental risk factors. It is characterized by behaviors such as impaired control over drug use, cravings and excessive or compulsive drug use, and persistent use despite adverse consequences. Addiction occurs very infrequently in patients receiving opioid analgesia, and the risk is generally overrated. *Psuedoaddiction* is the manifestation of opioid-seeking behaviors that superficially appear similar to addiction, but in reality are driven by undertreatment of pain. Unlike addiction, symptoms of pseudoaddiction disappear when pain is effectively treated.

There are two terms that describe the physiologic adaptation to chronic opioid therapy. Both are universal and predictable. *Dependence* is adaptation to a medication that results in a class-specific withdrawal syndrome if that medication is abruptly discontinued. This abstinence syndrome should not be confused with addiction. *Tolerance* is the development of diminution of drug effect over time, resulting in the need for increasing dosages to achieve the same analgesic effect. Tolerance occurs most commonly early in the course of opioid therapy. In cancer patients, an increasing need for opioid therapy usually reflects progressive disease rather than tolerance.

ADJUVANT ANALGESICS

Anticonvulsants are effective treatments for all types of neuropathic pain. In some patients, responses can be complete and dramatic. They are often used in combination with analgesics. All require gradual dose titration to maximize response while minimizing side effects. Gabapentin (Neurontin)[1] is commonly prescribed and has few drug interactions, although sedation and ataxia can be problematic at higher doses. Topiramate (Topamax)[1], because of its several mechanisms of action, may be more effective than existing anticonvulsants, but is not as well studied. Older anticonvulsants, such as carbamazepine (Tegretol), are as effective as and less expensive than newer agents, but are associated with more side effects and adverse reactions.

Tricyclic antidepressants can be effective adjuvants in the management of headache and neuropathic pain, although it is unusual for responses to be complete. Amitriptyline (Elavil)[1] has been most extensively studied. However, secondary amines such as nortriptyline (Pamelor)[1] and desipramine (Norpramin)[1] are also effective and have less anticholinergic side effects. Small doses (10 to 25 mg at bedtime) can be effective in some patients, but the response is generally dose-dependent and greatest in the 100 to 150 mg/day range. Dose-limiting side effects include dry mouth, sedation, weight gain, constipation, and urinary retention. Serious side effects, including cardiac rhythm disturbances, have been reported, so patients should be evaluated for cardiac abnormalities prior to initiating therapy.

Serotonin reuptake inhibitors have not been demonstrated to have an independent analgesic effect beyond their antidepressant action, although research is ongoing. Venlafaxine (Effexor)[1], an atypical antidepressant, is effective in reducing pain, but has not yet been studied in nondepressed patients.

[1]Not FDA approved for this indication.

Corticosteroids are highly useful agents in the management of a variety of painful cancer syndromes, including bone, visceral, and neuropathic pain, as well as headaches caused by increased intracranial pressure and soft-tissue infiltration by tumor. In addition to their analgesic actions, they have a number of beneficial secondary effects, such as antiemetic activity, improved mood, energy, and sense of well-being, and appetite stimulation. Choice of agent is empiric. There is no therapeutic dose ceiling, but toxicities are related to dose and duration of therapy. To minimize problems, including hyperglycemia, immunosuppression, myopathy, osteoporosis, and gastrointestinal toxicity, short-term use at the lowest effective dose is recommended.

Topical anesthetics such as transdermal lidocaine (Lidoderm) have been shown to be effective in neuropathic pain with minimal side effects.

Muscle relaxants can sometimes be helpful in acute musculoskeletal pain. Side effects, such as sedation and the potential for abuse of some agents limit their use. They have a limited role in long-term pain management.

In addition to their role in the management of hypercalcemia, bisphosphonates can substantially reduce cancer-related bone pain caused by osteolytic metastases either alone or in combination with radiation therapy. Pamidronate (Aredia)[1] and zoledronic acid (Zometa)[1] are available only in intravenous form.

Nonpharmacologic Management

Although pharmacologic therapies are clearly a mainstay of pain management, optimal care often also involves the use of nonpharmacologic strategies that complement and supplement medications.

PHYSICAL MODALITIES

There is substantial high-quality evidence that a variety of physical modalities can be effective in the management of both acute and chronic pain. Physical rehabilitation, such as stretching, exercise, and ergonomic attention, is of benefit in many pain situations, and can prevent maladaptive deconditioning. Thermotherapy and neurostimulatory approaches can have independent analgesic effects. In certain musculoskeletal problems massage, mobilization, and manipulation can be helpful.

PSYCHOLOGICAL METHODS

In appropriate clinical settings, individual counseling, group therapy, relaxation training, biofeedback, and support groups can all be useful adjuncts. Treatment of coincident depression and anxiety has

[1]Not FDA approved for this indication.

clearly been shown to improve pain control, quality of life, and functionality.

ALTERNATIVE MODALITIES

Americans are turning to alternative therapies in ever-increasing numbers. Studies of the treatment efficacy of a variety of alternative modalities are ongoing, but strong evidence currently exists to support only a limited number of therapies. Physicians should discuss alternative therapies openly with patients, and be knowledgeable about evidence of efficacy, side effects, and the potential for interactions with other conventional therapies.

INTERVENTIONAL APPROACHES

Interventional pain specialists offer a variety of diagnostic and therapeutic techniques that can be helpful in the care of some patients. These include diagnostic facet and nerve blocks, therapeutic rhizotomies and nerve ablations, and selective joint and epidural injections. Referral to an interventionalist is appropriate if a structural defect is likely and a potentially beneficial procedure is available. Good communication between treating physicians is critical for overall treatment success.

NAUSEA AND VOMITING

METHOD OF
William F. Miser, MD, MA

Nausea and vomiting are common, anxiety-provoking symptoms that often prompt patients to seek medical attention. The causes are myriad and range from benign, self-limiting conditions to chronic, potentially life-threatening disorders. The challenge for clinicians is to determine, in a cost-effective and orderly manner, the most likely causes and to decide whether or not further intervention is required. However, current evidence suggests there is a lack of consistency in the management of these symptoms in clinical practice.

Definitions

The sensation of *nausea* is purely subjective, the degree of which can only be judged by the individual. It is a vague, unpleasant feeling described as being "sick to the stomach" or "queasy," and is often associated with a flushed feeling, fatigue, and an urge to vomit. *Vomiting* (emesis) is a physical event that results in a quick and forceful expulsion of the stomach's contents in a retrograde fashion up to and out of the mouth. This emptying can either be voluntary or involuntary. *Retching* is repetitive, spasmodic contractions of the diaphragm and abdominal wall muscles that may or may not result in the evacuation of gastric contents. In contrast, *regurgitation* is a passive, retrograde flow of gastric and esophageal contents into the mouth, with a water that has a brash or acidic taste, most often the results of gastroesophageal reflux. Some individuals may experience *rumination,* which, likewise, is an effortless regurgitation of recently ingested food into the mouth, followed by either a spitting out or a rechewing and reswallowing. Although nausea and vomiting may be associated symptoms, *dyspepsia* is marked by chronic or recurrent epigastric discomfort with early satiety. Most instances of nausea and vomiting are acute with rapid resolution. *Chronic nausea and vomiting*, defined as the persistence of these symptoms for more than 1 month, present a diagnostic challenge to clinicians.

Differential Diagnosis

The causes for nausea and vomiting are numerous (Table 1). The key organs involved are the brain (chemoreceptor trigger zone, cerebral cortex, vestibular apparatus, and vomiting center), and the gastrointestinal tract. Neurotransmitter receptors that mediate nausea include dopamine, serotonin, acetylcholine, and histamine.

A common cause of nausea is an adverse reaction to a recently prescribed medication. Patients will often complain about their new medicine making them "sick." Almost any medication can cause nausea, but nonsteroidal anti-inflammatory drugs (NSAIDs), opioids, aspirin, and alcohol are probably the best known causes because of concomitant local gastric irritation. The most "notorious" drugs that cause nausea and vomiting are chemotherapeutic agents, particularly cisplatin (Platinol-AQ), cyclophosphamide (Cytoxan), dacarbazine (DTIC-Dome), and nitrogen mustard. Postchemotherapy nausea and vomiting (PCNV) can be acute (within 24 hours of administration), delayed (beyond 1 day of administration), or anticipatory; the latter is most common if the nausea and vomiting were not well controlled during previous courses of therapy.

Nausea and vomiting caused by viral infections (e.g., Norwalk virus, reoviruses, and adenoviruses) are of an acute onset, usually occurring in the autumn and winter. Bacterial infections (e.g., *Staphylococcus aureus, Salmonella sp., Bacillus aureus,* and *Clostridium perfringens*) are associated with contaminated water or food, and accompanied by abdominal cramping, fever, and profuse diarrhea.

TABLE 1 Differential Diagnosis of Nausea and Vomiting

Medications

Analgesics—acetaminophen, aspirin, nonsteroidal anti-inflammatory drugs (NSAIDs), rheumatologic and antigout drugs, opioids (codeine, morphine, oxycodone [Roxicodone])
Anesthetic agents—halothane, fentanyl (Sublimaze)
Antiasthmatics—theophylline
Anticonvulsants—phenobarbital, phenytoin (Dilantin)
Antidepressants—selective serotonin reuptake inhibitors (SSRIs)
Antimicrobials—acyclovir (Zovirax), erythromycin, itraconazole (Sporanox), metronidazole (Flagyl), sulfonamides, tetracycline
Antiparkinsonian drugs—levodopa (Dopar), carbidopa (Lodosyn)
Cancer chemotherapy—cisplatin (Platinol-AQ), cyclophosphamide (Cytoxan), dacarbazine (DTIC-Dome), nitrogen mustard
Cardiovascular agents—antiarrhythmics, antihypertensives, β-blockers, calcium channel antagonists, digoxin, diuretics
Corticosteroids—prednisone
Diabetic drugs—sulfonylureas, metformin (Glucophage)
Ergot alkaloids—dihydroergotamine (Migranal), ergotamine (Ergomar), methysergide (Sansert)[1]
Gastrointestinal agents—azathioprine (Imuran), sulfasalazine (Azulfidine)
Hormonal agents—estrogen, progesterone, oral contraceptives
Iron replacement—ferrous sulfate
Substance abuse—alcohol, nicotine

Infectious Causes

Gastroenteritis—viral, bacterial, parasitic
Other—otitis media, systemic sepsis

Gastrointestinal Disorders

Functional disorders—chronic intestinal pseudo-obstruction, gastroparesis, irritable bowel syndrome, nonulcer dyspepsia
Mechanical obstruction—gastric outlet obstruction, small-bowel obstruction
Organic gastrointestinal disorders
  Appendicitis
  Hepatobiliary disease—biliary colic, cholecystitis, hepatitis, neoplasia
  Inflammatory bowel disease—Crohn's disease
  Mesenteric ischemia
  Peptic diseases—esophagitis, gastritis, *Helicobacter pylori*, nonulcer dyspepsia, peptic ulcer disease
  Pancreatic disease—pancreatitis, pancreatic adenocarcinoma
  Paralytic ileus
  Peritoneal irritation—peritonitis, metastases
  Postoperative gastric surgery
  Retroperitoneal fibrosis

Central Nervous System (CNS) Disorders

Increased intracranial pressure—abscess, hemorrhage, hydrocephalus, infarction, malignancy, meningitis, pseudotumor cerebri
Demyelinating disorders
Labyrinthine disorders—labyrinthitis, Meniere's disease, motion sickness
Migraine headaches
Parkinsonian disorders
Seizures—complex partial

Psychological/Psychiatric disorders

Anxiety
Depression
Eating disorders—anorexia nervosa, bulimia nervosa
Pain
Psychogenic vomiting

Medical Conditions

Cardiac—acute myocardial infarction, congestive heart failure
Genitourinary—acute nephritis, nephrolithiasis, ovarian torsion, pyelonephritis, testicular torsion
Endocrinologic and metabolic conditions—acute intermittent porphyria, Addison's disease, diabetic ketoacidosis, hypercalcemia, hyperparathyroidism, hyperthyroidism, hypoparathyroidism, uremia
Pregnancy—hyperemesis gravidarum, morning sickness

Postoperative Nausea and Vomiting

Radiation Therapy

Idiopathic Conditions

Cyclic vomiting syndrome
Gastric dysrhythmias

[1]Not FDA approved for this indication.

Other infectious agents, such as cytomegalovirus and herpes simplex virus, can cause nausea and vomiting in those who are immunocompromised.

Small-bowel obstruction can also be acute and is associated with intermittent abdominal pain. Mesenteric ischemia can result in unexplained nausea. Gastroparesis, which is frequently seen in those with uncontrolled diabetes mellitus, scleroderma, amyloidosis, and systemic lupus erythematosus, causes nausea because of an inability to clear secretions and retained food. Lesions within the central nervous system, especially those involving the brainstem where the structures mediating vomiting (vomiting center) are located, can be a cause of nongastrointestinal vomiting. Psychogenic vomiting is usually associated with a previous history of psychiatric illness or social stressors and is often suspected when an individual maintains adequate nutrition despite a reported prolonged course of vomiting.

Pregnancy is another common cause of nausea and vomiting, particularly in the first trimester. Typically, younger, primigravida women are the most prone to "morning sickness," which often resolves by the end of the first trimester. Hyperemesis gravidarum, marked by intractable vomiting, weight loss, and ketosis, occurs in up to 5% of pregnancies. Postoperative nausea and vomiting (PONV) complicates up to half of all surgeries and is associated with several risk factors, including type of inhalation anesthetic used (particularly nitrous oxide), female gender, and younger patients. Concomitant use of opiate medication postoperatively can worsen this condition.

A rare condition causing nausea and vomiting is cyclic vomiting, also known as "abdominal migraine" or "abdominal epilepsy." Individuals with this condition typically have discrete, acute episodes of vomiting lasting up to 20 hours, with frequent attacks during the year. This condition usually starts early in life and is more common in girls. Associated conditions include migraine headaches and motion sickness.

Clinical Approach to Patients with Nausea and Vomiting

Because the differential diagnosis for the causes of nausea and vomiting is so great, the clinician must arrive at the diagnosis in an orderly and careful fashion. Several questions that need to be addressed as one evaluates the patient include: Is this an emergency situation (e.g., mechanical obstruction, perforation, peritonitis) that requires immediate attention? Does the patient need to be hospitalized to correct electrolyte abnormalities or dehydration or to treat intractable, incapacitating symptoms? Are there any clues clinically that would suggest a self-limited condition (e.g., viral gastroenteritis)? Was a medication recently started that could be the source of symptoms, and if so, can it be safely discontinued? Is there a need to empirically prescribe an antiemetic? A comprehensive history and physical examination will often answer these questions, and help pinpoint the cause of the nausea and vomiting.

INITIAL HISTORY

The first step in making a proper diagnosis is to obtain a clear description of the patient's symptoms. The clinician should obtain a history of the duration, frequency, and severity of the nausea and vomiting, and the nature of any other associated symptoms. An acute onset of symptoms suggests conditions such as viral gastroenteritis, pancreatitis, biliary tract disease, or an adverse reaction to a medication. The nausea and vomiting caused by acute viral gastroenteritis are often accompanied by low-grade fever, malaise, headache, and diarrhea. Typically, the symptoms are self-limited and will resolve within 5 days. A more insidious onset of nausea and vomiting is seen in conditions such as gastroparesis, gastroesophageal reflux disease (GERD), metabolic disorders, and pregnancy.

The timing and characteristics of the vomiting can also provide clues as to the potential diagnosis. Early morning vomiting, especially before breakfast, can be seen with pregnancy, alcohol ingestion, uremia, and increased intracranial pressure. Projectile vomiting characterizes this latter condition. If fever accompanies the vomiting, one must consider acute gastroenteritis, appendicitis, hepatitis, or cholecystitis. Vomiting consisting of partially digested food or chyme caused by mechanical outlet obstruction or gastroparesis is usually delayed 1 hour or longer after eating, while the vomiting caused by psychiatric conditions such as bulimia or anorexia usually occurs during or right after eating. Bilious vomiting suggests small-bowel obstruction, while hematemesis (coffee-ground or black emesis) can be a result of peptic ulcer disease or esophageal varices. Sometimes the pressure generated by vomiting can be so great that it results in linear tears of the esophageal mucosa in the region of the gastroesophageal junction (Mallory-Weiss syndrome) or, rarely, rupture of the esophagus (Boerhaave's syndrome); these conditions will also result in hematemesis.

While taking the patient's history, the clinician should also ask about other associated symptoms. If abdominal pain is present, a precise description of the location may help to isolate the more serious causes. An organic cause, such as from an obstruction, usually causes abdominal pain, which precedes the vomiting. Significant weight loss may be associated with malignancy or chronic peptic ulcer disease with gastric outlet obstruction. A history of recent travel or similar symptoms found in family or friends points toward an infectious cause. Vertigo suggests Meniere's disease, benign positional labyrinthitis, or motion sickness. A headache with fever, stiff neck, or focal neurologic symptoms indicates a central nervous system disorder.

PHYSICAL EXAMINATION

After obtaining a detailed history, the clinician next must search for physical examination clues that indicate consequences or complications from the vomiting, and for signs that help to identify the potential cause of the symptoms. Dry mucus membranes with normal vital signs are a result of mild dehydration. In contrast, orthostatic changes in the vital signs, with a postural lowering of the blood pressure with increased heart rate, suggest significant dehydration. Other physical examination clues can include jaundice, lymphadenopathy, abdominal masses, and occult blood in the stool.

A careful abdominal examination can detect distension or hernias. Specific areas of abdominal tenderness provide clues as to potential causes. Midepigastric pain is seen with peptic ulcer disease, right upper quadrant pain occurs with hepatobiliary disease, and right lower quadrant tenderness suggests the possibility of appendicitis. Auscultation of the abdomen may detect the increased bowel sounds seen with obstruction, or absent bowel sounds that occur with an ileus. Examining the fingernails and teeth may disclose findings suggestive of self-induced vomiting. A thorough neurologic examination should also be done, including an examination of the cranial nerves, looking for nystagmus, a funduscopic examination to rule out increased intracranial pressure, and observation of the patient's gait to evaluate cerebellar function.

LABORATORY AND OTHER DIAGNOSTIC EVALUATIONS

Findings from the history and physical examination will help guide what further laboratory and diagnostic studies are required. Basic laboratory studies, if done, should include a complete blood count, looking for anemia or an elevated white blood count suggesting infection, and electrolytes, which may detect hypokalemia, hyponatremia, metabolic alkalosis, or uremia. A pregnancy test should be done in women of childbearing age who are still menstruating. Further laboratory tests might include screening for hyperthyroidism and drug toxicity (e.g., salicylates, digoxin, and theophylline).

The clinical picture should direct other diagnostic testing. If the symptoms suggest a mechanical obstruction, radiographic studies, such as upright and supine abdominal radiographs, should be obtained. However, the results of these films may be nonspecific or normal with intermittent small-bowel obstruction. Esophagogastroduodenoscopy (EGD) can detect abnormalities in the esophageal, gastric, or duodenal mucosa suggestive of esophagitis or peptic ulcer disease. Further gastrointestinal studies, such as an upper gastrointestinal barium study, small bowel follow-through, and enteroclysis, may sometimes be needed to detect underlying disorders such as gastroparesis or small-bowel obstruction. Other diagnostic studies that might help in making the diagnosis include an abdominal ultrasound of the right upper quadrant or an abdominal CT scan. Tests of gastric motility function include gastric emptying scintigraphy, antroduodenal manometry, and electrogastrography.

If a gastrointestinal disorder is not found, the clinician should consider systemic illness, central nervous system disorders, or psychological conditions. The clinician should obtain a head imaging study in those cases in which the nausea and vomiting are severe, unexplained, and chronic. Magnetic resonance imaging (MRI) of the brain is superior to computed tomographic (CT) scanning to detect lesions in the posterior fossa. In those patients with chronic, unexplained nausea and vomiting, a psychological evaluation should be performed. Rarely, some causes of nausea and vomiting remain undiagnosed despite this thorough evaluation, in which case, consultation with a gastroenterologist is warranted.

Management of Nausea and Vomiting

Goals in managing nausea and vomiting include (a) identifying and correcting any fluid, electrolyte, acid-base, and/or nutritional deficiencies that are a result of the nausea and vomiting; (b) identifying and eliminating, if possible, the underlying cause of the symptoms; and (c) suppressing or eliminating the symptoms if the underlying cause cannot be quickly identified. If oral rehydration is not possible, the individual may need intravenous hydration with normal saline solution and appropriate potassium replacement.

Initially in acute nausea and vomiting, the best treatment is often nutritional discretion. When nauseated, individuals should slowly drink small amounts of clear, cool liquids that contain some caloric content, preferably 30 to 60 minutes before and after meals. If vomiting occurs, solid foods should be avoided. To avoid dehydration, salty rehydration solutions such as Gatorade or bullion are good choices, while sweetened and acidic juices (e.g., orange or grapefruit juices) should be avoided. The goal is to consume 1 to 2 L of fluid during the day in multiple, small (1-4 ounces) amounts.

If liquids are well tolerated, individuals may cautiously advance their diet to include a variety of easily digested foods such as crackers, dry toast, broth-based soups with rice or noodles, and hard candy. The goal is to ingest approximately 1500 calories daily. Creamy, milk-based liquids should be avoided at this time. Once this is tolerated, individuals may try other mild-flavored, low-fat foods such as plain pasta, baked potatoes, chicken, fish, vegetables, and fruit. They should eat the food slowly and stop once satisfied. Also, they should rest, either sitting or laying down slightly propped up, after eating, because activity may increase the nausea and lead to vomiting.

Typically, if the nausea is mild, dietary changes may be all that is needed because the symptoms are usu-ally short-lived and resolve spontaneously. However, if symptoms persist despite dietary changes, or if the nausea and vomiting are severe, the individual may require treatment empirically with an antiemetic while the cause of the symptoms is sought.

There are a wide variety of antiemetic agents available (Table 2). Many of these drugs act primarily within the central nervous system (CNS) to suppress the nausea and prevent vomiting. This mechanism of action also explains the potential CNS side effects that can occur with these medicines. As such, one must weigh the potential benefit of relieving the symptoms against the potential risk of developing other intolerant symptoms.

Except in the cases of PCNV and PONV, there are relatively few randomized trials that provide insight into which are the antiemetics of choice. One of the most widely used drugs for moderate to severe nausea and vomiting is prochlorperazine (Compazine). It is available in oral, rectal, and parenteral forms. However, side effects are common and include sedation, extrapyramidal symptoms, including dystonic and tardive dyskinesias. Metoclopramide (Reglan), provides both antiemetic and prokinetic activities and is useful in GERD and gastroparesis. However, it, too, has associated significant side effects which include fatigue and extrapyramidal symptoms such as oculogyric crisis, opisthotonos, akathisia, dyskinesia, and dystonia.

Normally, antiemetics should be avoided in the nausea and vomiting of pregnancy, especially during the first trimester. Pyridoxine (vitamin B_6)[1] has been used with some success. In severe cases of hyperemesis gravidarum marked by weight loss, ketosis, and dehydration, the patient should be hospitalized and

[1]Not FDA approved for this indication.

TABLE 2 Commonly Used Medications for Nausea and Vomiting

Class/Medication	Usual Dosage	Route(s)	Adverse Effects
Anticholinergic			
Scopolamine (Transderm Scop)	1 patch every 3 days	Transdermal	Dry mouth, drowsiness, impaired eye accommodation; rare: disorientation, memory disturbance, dizziness, hallucinations
Antihistamines			
Diphendydramine (Benadryl)	25–50 mg q 4-6 h	IM, IV, PO	Sedation, dry mouth, constipation, confusion, blurred vision, urinary retention
Hydroxyzine (Atarax, Vistaril)	25–100 mg q 6 h	IM, PO[1]	
Meclizine (Antivert)	25–50 mg q 6 h	PO	
Promethazine (Phenergan)	12.5–25 mg q 4-6 h	IM, IV, PO, PR	
Benzamides			
Metoclopramide (Reglan)	5–15 mg q 6 h	IM, IV, PO	Sedation, restlessness, diarrhea, agitation, central nervous depression, extrapyramidal effects, hypotension, neuroleptic syndrome, supraventricular tachycardia
Trimethobenzamide (Tigan)	250 mg q 6–8 h	IM, PO, PR	
Benzodiazepines			
Lorazepam (Ativan)[1]	0.5–2.5 mg q 8–12 h	IM, IV, PO	Sedation, amnesia, respiratory depression, ataxia, blurred vision, hallucinations, emotional reactions
Butyrophenones			
Droperidol (Inapsine)	0.625–1.25 mg q 3–4 h[3]	IM, IV	Sedation, hypotension, tachycardia, extrapyramidal effects, dizziness, blood pressure increase, hallucinations, chills, QT prolongation, torsades de pointes
Haloperidol (Haldol)[1]	0.5-5 mg q 8 h	IM, IV, PO	
Cannabinoids			
Dronabinol (Marinol)	2.5–5 mg q 8 h	PO	Drowsiness, euphoria, vision difficulties, somnolence, vasodilation, abnormal thinking, dysphoria, diarrhea, flushing, tremor, myalgias
Corticosteroids			
Dexamethasone (Decadron)[1]	4 mg q 6 h	IM, IV, PO	Gastrointestinal upset, anxiety, insomnia, hyperglycemia, facial flushing, euphoria, perineal itching
Phenothiazines			
Chlorpromazine (Thorazine)	10–25 mg q 4–6 h	IM, PO, PR	Sedation, lethargy, skin irritation, cardiovascular effects, extrapyramidal effects, cholestatic jaundice, hyperprolactinemia, neuroleptic malignant syndrome, blood abnormalities
Prochlorperazine (Compazine)	5–10 (25 PR) mg q 6 h	IM, IV, PO, PR	
Thiethylperazine (Torecan)	10–20 mg q 6 h[3]	IM, IV, PO	
5-HT$_3$ Serotonin Antagonists			
Ondansetron (Zofran)	8 mg q 8 h	IV, PO	Headache, constipation, fever, asthenia, arrhythmias, diarrhea, dizziness, ataxia, tremor, somnolence, thirst, nervousness, elevated hepatic transaminases
Granisetron (Kytril)	2 mg per 24 h	IV, PO	
Dolasetron (Anzemet)	100 mg per 24 h	IV, PO	

Abbreviations: IM = intramuscular; IV = intravenous; PO = orally; PR = per rectum; q = every; h = hours
[1]Not FDA approved for this indication.
[3]Exceeds dosage recommended by manufacturer.

given intravenous fluids. In severe cases, meclizine (Antivert)[1] or promethazine (Phenergan)[1] may be used.

The 5-HT$_3$ serotonin antagonists ondansetron (Zofran), granisetron (Kytril), and dolasetron (Anzemet) have both central and peripheral activities, and are usually very well tolerated with few adverse effects. These drugs, along with corticosteroids, are highly effective in PCNV. At equivalent doses, each of these drugs has equivalent safety and efficacy and can be interchanged based on availability, cost and convenience. Single doses are effective, and their oral forms are equally effective and are as safe as their intravenous forms.

Nonpharmacologic options for nausea and vomiting exist. Studies of accupressure, using the P6 (Neiguan) point, located 5 cm proximal to the palmar aspect of the wrist between the flexor carpii radialis and the palmaris longus tendons, show favorable results. In addition, some studies suggest that ginger (*Zingiber officinale Roscoe*)[1] may help.

[1]Not FDA approved for this indication.

GASEOUSNESS AND INDIGESTION

METHOD OF

Sonal M. Patel, MD, and Anthony Lembo, MD

Gaseousness

Excessive "gas" can cause significant discomfort and embarrassment. The symptoms of gaseousness can refer to excessive belching (or eructation), flatus, or even abdominal bloating. These symptoms are especially prominent in patients with irritable bowel syndrome (IBS). In most cases, gaseousness is not caused by an increased volume of gas within the gastrointestinal tract. Recent studies in patients with IBS demonstrate that it is not increased gas production but rather the altered transit of gas or the location of trapping of gas within the gastrointestinal (GI) tract that creates symptoms of gaseousness. Most patients who complain of excessive gas actually have symptoms that fall within range of normal and can be reassured. However, the patient's perception that his or her symptoms are abnormal can make successful treatment of gaseousness difficult.

EXCESSIVE BELCHING (ERUCTATION)

Symptoms and Physiology

Occasional belching is a normal physiologic process, which allows for swallowed air to be removed from the stomach. The normal frequency of belching has not been well documented but patients who complain of it usually have repetitive and uncontrollable episodes of belching.

Involuntary belching usually occurs after meals and is the release of swallowed air after gastric distension. The most common cause of excessive, repetitive belching is excessive air swallowing (aerophagia). Swallowing food, or even saliva, can result in some air entering the upper gastrointestinal tract. Air can also be swallowed by itself consciously and unconsciously. Factors that can result in increased aerophagia include stress, gastroesophageal reflux, increased salivary production from excessive sucking on hard candy or chewing gum, and cigarette smoking. Rarely, other upper gastrointestinal diseases such as peptic ulcer disease (PUD), gastroesophageal reflux disease (GERD), and cholecystitis can present with excessive belching.

Patient Treatment

Although belching is usually the result of excessive air swallowing, a complete history and physical examination are important to exclude the rare causes of upper gastrointestinal disorders that may produce these symptoms (e.g., GERD, PUD, or cholecystitis). If other associated gastrointestinal symptoms are present, appropriate diagnostic tests should follow. In most patients, no other diagnostic testing is necessary. Rather, the patient should be reassured that the symptom is not associated with an organic disorder. In this group of patients, treatment is focused on techniques that reduce air swallowing. Dietary modifications, such as avoiding sucking on hard candies or chewing gum, eating slowly with small swallows, and avoiding carbonated beverages, can be suggested, although they have not been sufficiently tested and are usually disappointing in practice. Another technique is to hold an object (such as a pencil) between one's teeth. Simethicone (Mylicon) and activated charcoal preparations (Charcoal Plus) are ineffective. Stress management may be helpful in those patients whose excessive air swallowing seems exacerbated by underlying stress. Other forms of psychotherapy (e.g., cognitive behavioral therapy) should be considered in patients who remain symptomatic.

EXCESSIVE FLATUS

Symptoms and Physiology

The range of normal volume and frequency of flatus varies widely. Adults pass flatus on average 10 to 14 times per day for a total volume of 400 to 2500 mL per day. Because flatus volume is difficult to measure, clinicians rely on the frequency of flatulence to estimate volume. To do this, patients record the number of flatulence "episodes" per day over the course of one week (normal is less than 22 per day). Most individuals can evacuate relatively large volumes of gas without any difficulty. Recent evidence demonstrates that when gas is infused into the proximal small bowel there exists a minority of patients who are "gas retainers." These patients develop symptoms such as bloating, pressure, or cramping in response to gas in their small bowel. Furthermore, the location of gas retention may be important. Specifically, gas trapped in the jejunum seems to create a worsening of symptoms in "gas retainers." Although helpful in understanding the physiology, impaired transit alone does not explain gas related symptoms. Visceral hypersensitivity, as seen in IBS, may also help explain why some patients perceive that they have excessive flatus.

Rectal gas comes from either swallowed air or from bacterial fermentation. Malabsorption of carbohydrates, which can occur in patients with celiac sprue, pancreatic insufficiency, and short-bowel syndrome, can result in increased flatus production. Lactose and fructose are simple sugars commonly found in many foods that are commonly malabsorbed. Likewise, many common starches found in various fruits, vegetables, and flours are not fully absorbed by healthy patients.

Patient Management

The first step is to determine if excessive flatulence is present by having the patient record the frequency of rectal gas passage for 2 weeks. Patients who pass flatus more than 22 times per day without signs of malabsorption should undergo dietary modification. Specifically, patients should be advised to restrict lactose- and fructose-containing foods. It is virtually impossible to restrict all carbohydrates, but certain carbohydrates that may be malabsorbed include fructose (soft drinks), lactose (dairy), trehalose (mushrooms), raffinose and stachyose (legumes), and resistant starches (fruits, flours, vegetables). A patient diary of foods associated with concomitant symptoms may be instrumental in determining any salient offending carbohydrates. Hydrogen breath testing can be helpful in the diagnosis of lactose and fructose intolerances. Patients not responding to dietary modifications should be advised to reduce behaviors associated with excessive air swallowing, including stress, smoking, chewing gum, or sucking on candy. α-D-Galactosidase enzyme (Beano), which facilitates oligosaccharide digestion and is available over the counter, can be a helpful treatment. Pharmacologic treatments for noxious flatus odor are zinc acetate[1], bismuth subsalicylate (Pepto-Bismol)[1], and carbohydrate laxatives[1]. The charcoal cushion, which decreases flatus odor immediately after passage, is another treatment option for noxious flatus.

Indigestion (Dyspepsia)

DEFINITION AND EPIDEMIOLOGY

Indigestion, or dyspepsia, is defined as a persistent or recurrent pain or discomfort centered in the upper abdomen. Other associated characteristics include postprandial fullness, upper abdominal bloating, early satiety, anorexia, nausea, and vomiting. Its prevalence in the United States is estimated to be as high as 40%. Dyspepsia is responsible for substantial health care costs and considerable time loss from work. Dyspepsia has a number of possible etiologies. Symptoms and causes can overlap, which can make the initial diagnosis difficult. The most common cause of dyspepsia encountered in primary care practice is functional dyspepsia; however, more serious conditions should always be considered in the initial evaluation.

DIFFERENTIAL DIAGNOSIS

PUD accounts for 15% to 25% of patients with dyspepsia; 30% to 60% of these patients will be positive for *Helicobacter pylori* if tested. Nonsteroidal anti-inflammatory drug (NSAID) use accounts for the majority of the remaining patients.

[1]Not FDA approved for this indication.

GERD is defined as epigastric burning that radiates substernally. Heartburn and regurgitation are the most common symptoms. The symptom of substernal radiation is somewhat specific for GERD; however, many patients with GERD may not have the classic radiation, but solely complain of epigastric pain or discomfort.

Functional or nonulcer dyspepsia (NUD) accounts for up to 60% of patients who present with dyspepsia. This syndrome is a diagnosis of exclusion when other organic etiologies have been excluded. Although up to 40% of patients with IBS can also have dyspeptic symptoms, isolated functional dyspepsia appears to be a separate syndrome. Various theories or factors that have not been conclusively implicated include, *H. pylori* infection, visceral hypersensitivity, and abnormal motility.

Biliary or pancreatic disease can be mistaken for dyspepsia, but a proper history and physical examination should point to these disease processes with further diagnostic tests such as blood work and imaging.

Although gastric and esophageal malignancies are rare (<2%) in patients presenting with dyspepsia, the risk increases with age.

PATIENT MANAGEMENT

Patients who present with dyspepsia who are older than age 45 years should undergo an upper endoscopy to rule out serious processes such as malignancy. Also, any patient who has any alarming features, such as unexplained weight loss, anemia, GI bleeding (hematemesis or melena), or significant examination (tenderness, lymphadenopathy or jaundice), should also undergo an upper endoscopy.

For patients who are younger than age 45 years and without alarming symptoms, empiric testing for *H. pylori* infection either by serology or breath test is a reasonable first step. However, this strategy may not suit all patients or physicians. Alternatively, upper endoscopy with biopsies for *H. pylori* may provide the patient added reassurance if the study is negative. If the patient is positive for *H. pylori* infection, the patient should be treated with eradication therapy.

Treatment of functional dyspepsia can be challenging. Important aspects of the therapy include explanation and reassurance. Acid suppression with either an H_2 blocker or proton pump inhibitor should be the first-line of therapy. If these do not provide any relief, a promotility agent such as metoclopramide (Reglan)[1] or erythromycin (E-Mycin)[1] can be considered. Tricyclic antidepressants such as amitriptyline (Elavil)[1] have also been used with some anecdotal success. Other behavioral therapies, such as biofeedback or hypnosis, have not been studied, but may be reserved for severely refractory patients.

[1]Not FDA approved for this indication.

HICCUPS

METHOD OF

Georg A. Petroianu, MD, PhD

Hiccup (hiccough or Latin *singultus*) is caused by an involuntary, usually repetitive and rhythmical, spasmodic contraction of the diaphragm (or hemidiaphragm) and accessory inspiratory muscles followed shortly (within 35 milliseconds) by the sudden closure of the glottis. The forcefully inspired air meeting a closed glottis causes the typical hiccup sound. The term describing hiccups in most languages contains the sounds /h/ and /k/, the word being an onomatopoeic reflection of the sound produced during the event. Occasional hiccups are generally perceived as being "funny"; however, hiccupping of extended duration can be incapacitating. Although its most common direct consequence is esophagitis as a consequence of concomitant relaxation of the lower esophageal sphincter favoring reflux, extended hiccupping can also lead to wound dehiscence, depression, weight loss, malnutrition, insomnia, and exhaustion. Cases of hiccupping over many years are regularly reported: the record in hiccupping is apparently held by an American who hiccupped for 68 years (more than 430 million hiccups). A case of familial intractable hiccup, in which several members of a patient's family suffered from the same affliction, has also been documented. Also documented is the similarity to yawning with respect to contagiousness: hiccupping can spread to others in the same room, as was described to have happened at the Charité Hospital in Berlin in 1897. The hiccup frequency distribution is apparently bimodal, with the frequency either under 7 per minute or above 60 per minute.

Classifications

Most classifications use (different) purely arbitrary time limits to categorize hiccupping. Generally, hiccups lasting less than 1 day are considered transient (acute), those lasting less than 1 week are labeled persistent, and hiccupping for more than 1 week is described as chronic. A simplified categorization draws the line at 48 hours: any hiccupping episode lasting longer is described as chronic. The practical value of these classifications is questionable; by the time the practitioner sees the patient, almost invariably the case involves persistent or chronic hiccup forms requiring drug therapy. The exceptions (in terms of time span between appearance and presentation) are hiccup forms presenting immediately postoperatively or in critical care units. Brief episodes of hiccupping, as experienced by the vast majority of people at some point in time, are certainly physiologic. The point of transition to a pathologic form is not well defined. The "rule of thumb" of hiccup therapy, however, is that the longer the duration of the hiccupping, the less amenable it will be to nonpharmacologic interventions.

Etiologic classifications are also fraught with problems. Hiccup is not a disease, but a symptom. Literally there is no known disease that has not been associated with hiccups. The medical literature is rich in case reports demonstrating the most unusual links, ranging from ants in the external auditory canal to sarcoidosis, and from multiple sclerosis to subphrenic abscess. In practice, while the categories psychogenic, organic, and idiopathic are most commonly used, the situation most commonly encountered is that of hiccup of unknown (idiopathic) origin. In this context, "idiopathic" describes one's inability to demonstrate, rather than the absence of, an organic origin.

Epidemiology

During intrauterine life, hiccups are universally present, their incidence peaking in the third trimester. They can also be seen regularly in the newborn, the frequency of occurrence decreasing slowly over the first year of life. In adults, occasional transient hiccup is also so frequent that it can be viewed as physiologic. Persistent and chronic idiopathic singultus, the pathologic forms, are rare, their prevalence being estimated at 1:100,000 persons. Males are almost exclusively affected (the male:female patient ratio is approximately 80:1), suggesting a hormone (estrogen) protective effect. The incidence increases with age. The psychogenic form, although less frequent overall by one order of magnitude, is believed to be more prevalent in females, with an even distribution among all age groups; however, data to support this view are almost nonexistent.

Pathophysiology

The universality of hiccups during fetal life begs the question of purposefulness. Already in 1887, it was suggested that hiccups might represent a necessary and vital primitive reflex that would permit intrauterine training of the diaphragm without aspiration of amniotic fluid. During intra- and postpartum maturation, higher centers would then suppress this primitive reflex. Immaturity or damage to the central nervous system would favor the persistence or reappearance of the reflex. The putative reflex arch includes autonomic afferent fibers (the majority vagal fibers) from the digestive tract to a putative medullary hiccup center and motor efferent fibers through the phrenic nerve (diaphragm) and other branches of the vagus nerve to the intrinsic muscles of the larynx adducting the vocal cords. In an analogy with the vomiting center, the assumed role of the medullary hiccup center is to coordinate and fine-tune the sequence of events required for hiccupping; it is therefore a "pattern generator." Needless to say, the concept described, although useful for the purpose of designing a quasi-rational treatment protocol for hiccup, is anything but proven or generally accepted.

Another school of thought, questioning the assumption that hiccupping is a reflex phenomenon, suggests, instead, a similarity with cardiac arrhythmias, making hiccups a consequence of arrhythmias of the breathing center. Still other researchers work on the assumption that hiccup is a myoclonic event, or that it represents brainstem seizures. These views are not necessarily mutually exclusive, because hiccup is not primarily a disease but a symptom, possibly representing different pathophysiologies. Whatever view one might prefer, we must not forget that all these are mere working hypotheses, not (or only minimally) backed by solid evidence.

Evaluation of the Hiccup Patient

Hiccup is a symptom associated with a multitude of pathologies. The practitioner must take the hiccupping patient seriously and for the purpose of finding and treating hidden pathology, persistent and chronic hiccups should be investigated. No consensus exists, however, concerning the extent of such investigations. Even the most enthusiastic users of modern imaging technologies will, in most cases, end up with a working diagnosis of chronic idiopathic singultus. Nonetheless, a detailed history, a thorough physical examination, and basic laboratory and diagnostic procedures are essential.

HISTORY

Ask about previous episodes, as well as precipitating and alleviating factors. The patient who describes vomiting as a "cure" for previous hiccup episodes gives a telltale sign that acidity is an etiologic factor, and omeprazole (Prilosec)[1] is a drug to consider. If the patient indicates that hyperventilation is a "sure bet" to worsen his or her hiccups, then you can assume that drugs lowering the excitability of the nervous system are likely to help. Elucidating present drug consumption (medical and recreational) is essential: benzodiazepines, barbiturates, alcohol, and steroids are well-known hiccup inducers.

PHYSICAL EXAMINATION

Foreign bodies in the external auditory canal can induce hiccups, so look in the ears. Examine the neck, chest, and abdomen looking for possible sources of irritation (infection, neoplastic processes, or both) to the vagus and phrenic nerves and the diaphragm. Perform a neurologic examination, keeping in mind the association of hiccup with multiple sclerosis and intracranial processes.

LABORATORY AND DIAGNOSTIC PROCEDURES

An upright chest x-ray, together with a complete blood count (CBC) with differential, will help exclude neoplastic or infectious disease. An electrocardiogram (ECG) will help to exclude pericarditis and malfunctioning pacemakers, while electrolytes and urea determinations will exclude known metabolic causes (hyponatremia and uremia).

To what extent magnetic resonance imaging (MRI), ultrasound scanning, or endoscopic examinations are necessary is a judgment call, and no generalizations are possible; certainly they might occasionally be indicated.

Nonpharmacologic Interventions

A multitude of nonpharmacologic interventions to terminate hiccup belong to the public domain hiccup "mythology" or have been described in the medical literature as case reports. Although usually effective in terminating bouts of acute hiccup, they are mostly ineffective in cases of hiccupping that has been present for an extended period. Some of them, if practiced too enthusiastically, can be dangerous to the patient, and their necessity may be difficult to explain convincingly to jurors, should a court case develop (e.g., rectal massage).

VALSALVA MANEUVER

Named after Italian anatomist Antonio Maria Valsalva (1666-1723), the maneuver—expiratory effort against a closed glottis—is used not only to terminate paroxysmal supraventricular tachycardia, but also to terminate bouts of singultus.

ASCHNER'S OCULOCARDIAC REFLEX

Compression of the eyeball is answered with a decrease in pulse rate. The same maneuver can also terminate hiccup attacks.

Osler's maneuver (traction on the tongue), carotid massage, irritation of the external ear channel, application of bitter substances to the back of the tongue (Angostura therapy), drinking ice water, scaring the patient, and rectal massage are additional well-known possible cures for hiccup. The common denominator of these maneuvers (also used to terminate paroxysmal supraventricular tachycardia) is their ability to directly or indirectly increase efferent vagal activity; the increased parasympathetic tone has a limiting effect on hiccupping. Interestingly, estrogens are also considered to be parasympathomimetic, which offers a plausible explanation of why the singultus prevalence in females is much lower than in males.

Another very attractive (but possibly expensive) nonpharmacologic avenue in treating acute (transient) hiccup is that of promising financial rewards if

[1]Not FDA approved for this indication.

the patient manages to produce a hiccup on demand. Of course, focusing the patient's attention on the hiccup decreases the likelihood of the event, as we know from other autonomically controlled body functions, where the rule applies that "the more we want to, the less we can."

Pharmacologic Interventions

Probably only a few drugs in the *Physician's Desk Reference* have not been tried in the therapy of singultus, and anyone who looks hard enough at the literature will be able to find somewhere anecdotal support for the use of almost any drug. However, prospective controlled studies to support the use of a particular therapy are very few and rare. Before adhering too enthusiastically to the use of a particular drug, one must not forget the well-publicized success of an intravenous therapy for singultus in the 1960s: the only problem with the therapy was the fact that the patient stopped hiccupping before the drug could be injected.

Conceptually, all drugs with the potential of success in the therapy of chronic hiccups work either by decreasing the input from the gastrointestinal tract to a (putative) hiccup center, or by decreasing the excitability of the nervous system and therefore the output from the (putative) hiccup center.

SEDATIVE-HYPNOTICS

Both benzodiazepine and barbiturate γ-aminobutyric acid receptor type A ($GABA_A$) agonists have been tried for the treatment of hiccups. The consensus is that these substances not only are ineffective, but can actually worsen the clinical picture, producing a situation similar to the paradoxical excitation seen with the use of sedatives and explained by inhibitory effects on inhibitory centers.

ANTIEMETICS

Following up on the analogy between the vomiting center and hiccup center as pattern generators, "setron" class antiemetics (5-HT_3 receptor antagonists) have been tried, with no success. Anecdotal evidence hints at possible worsening of the hiccup under the influence of ondansetron (Zofran)[1].

ANALEPTICS

The use of analeptics derives from the concept that hiccup is a suppressed primitive reflex. Analeptics potentiate the central suppression. Although success has been reported with methylphenidate (Ritalin)[1], caffeine[1] produced failure.

[1]Not FDA approved for this indication.

ANTICONVULSANTS

Anticonvulsants (Phenytoin [Dilantin][1], carbamazepine [Tegretol][1], valproate [Depakene][1], and gabapentin [Neurontin][1]) have been used to try to suppress hiccups. Considering the multitude of pharmacodynamic effects of anticonvulsants, it is not surprising that some success was achieved.

ANTIPSYCHOTICS

Historically, chlorpromazine (Thorazine) has been the most widely used drug for the treatment of hiccup, and it is the only drug approved by the FDA for the disorder. Aliphatic phenothiazines, like chlorpromazine, have strong sedative, hypotensive, and anticholinergic properties, and mild to moderate extrapyramidal effects. For hiccup control, results are mixed at best, and in view of the side effects, routine use is not warranted. Haloperidol (Haldol)[1], a butyrophenone derivative, has also been used for hiccup control; again, results are mixed at best, and the possibility of developing tardive dyskinesia weighs heavily against the routine use of this drug.

ANTIDEPRESSANTS

The tertiary amine tricyclic antidepressant amitriptyline (Elavil) is one of the oldest players in the therapy of hiccup; its use was being suggested in the mid-1960s. As with anticonvulsants, considering the multitude of pharmacodynamic effects of tricyclic antidepressants, it is not surprising that some success was achieved with these drugs. Their effectiveness is not related to their ability to inhibit monoamine uptake, but probably to their sodium channel blocking properties.

CALCIUM CHANNEL BLOCKERS

Nifedipine (Procardia[1]) is the dihydropyridine derivative most commonly used for hiccup control. Nimodipine (Nimotop[1]) has also been tried for the same purpose. Interestingly, anecdotal reports about the use of calcium for the same purpose also exist.

SODIUM CHANNEL BLOCKERS

The local anesthetic, class Ib antidysrhythmic lidocaine (Xylocaine) and its oral analogue mexiletine (Mexitil) have been used for hiccup control, with mixed results.

$GABA_B$ AGONISTS

Among the substances acting on the nervous system, baclofen (Lioresal) has by far the best credentials in the treatment of chronic hiccup. It is one

[1]Not FDA approved for this indication.

of the very few substances proven in clinical studies (albeit with small patient numbers) to be efficacious. This γ-aminobutyric acid receptor type B ($GABA_B$) agonist, which is normally used to lower an increased muscle tone (spasticity), has also been shown to suppress hiccups in an animal (cat) hiccup model. $GABA_B$ agonists, by reducing transmitter release, are generally able to depress complex reflexes.

ANTACIDS

Lowering the acidity of the stomach using H_2-receptor blockers ("-tidine" class drugs) or proton pump inhibitors ("-prazole" class drugs) conceptually decreases the input from the gastrointestinal tract to the hiccup center. In a limited number of trials, omeprazole (Prilosec) was shown to be effective in hiccup treatment.

GASTROKINETIC DRUGS

One of the few reliable methods to induce a physiologic hiccup in people is rapidly drinking an ice-cold can of beer on a hot summer day. Although it is highly debatable whether it has to be beer, stomach distension by carbon dioxide induces hiccups. Conversely, reducing stomach distension by using a gastrokinetic drug is helpful in alleviating hiccups. The strongest evidence available for the usefulness of a gastrokinetic drug was for cisapride (Propulsid); however, this selective serotonin 5-HT_4-receptor agonist was withdrawn from the market because of its propensity to prolong the QT-interval and induce torsades de pointes. The available alternatives include the related benzamide metoclopramide (Reglan[1]), a mixed dopamine receptor antagonist, 5-HT_4-receptor agonist and cholinesterase inhibitor, with a long tradition in the treatment of hiccups, going back to the late 1960s, and the new 5-HT_4-partial agonist tegaserod (Zelnorm[1]). Interestingly enough, recent research revealed that the breathing center in the brainstem is under serotoninergic control through a certain subtype of 5-HT_4 receptor, opening the possibility that 5-HT_4 agonists might also influence hiccupping by activating the rhythm-generating respiratory neurons.

Physical Interventions

PHRENIC NERVECTOMY

Irreversible surgical destruction of the phrenic nerve cannot be recommended. Even if hiccup relief is achieved after unilateral local anesthetic blockade of the phrenic nerve without serious compromise in respiratory function, the long-term effects of phrenic nerve destruction are unpredictable. Possible effects include both hiccup reappearance—even after bilateral phrenic nerve transection—and deterioration in respiratory function. More recently, diaphragmatic (phrenic) pacing has been described; however, experience is very limited.

HYPERCAPNIA

Rebreathing into a paper bag is a well-known and reliable remedy for hyperventilation tetany. The increase in blood carbon dioxide (CO_2) levels (hypercapnia) thus induced leads to mild acidosis and to a liberation of calcium ions from the protein binding. The increase in free calcium decreases neuronal excitability, thus terminating not only the tetany, but possibly also hiccupping. A more high-tech version of this is the induction of normoxic hypercapnia in ventilated patients.

POSITIVE END EXPIRATORY PRESSURE

Also practicable only in intubated patients is the application of high positive end expiratory pressure (PEEP), a high-tech version of the Valsalva maneuver.

NASOGASTRIC TUBE

Gastric decompression through a nasogastric (NG) tube can terminate hiccups.

Treatment

The treatment algorithm described is based on the assumption that correctable organic causes have been excluded or treated.

PATIENT PRESENTING WITH NEWLY DEVELOPED SINGULTUS

These patients are treatment naïve, and a therapeutic attempt with metoclopramide (Reglan) 10 mg three times a day (tid) PO is warranted. If the results are not satisfactory, omeprazole (Prilosec) 20 mg PO daily can be added. If results are still not satisfactory, follow the routine for long-established singultus.

PATIENT PRESENTING WITH LONG-ESTABLISHED SINGULTUS

Start therapy with omeprazole (Prilosec)[1] 20 mg PO daily. If after 7 to 14 days no satisfactory change has occurred, introduce baclofen (Lioresal)[1]. With baclofen, a "start low, go very slow" approach is indicated to avoid excessive drowsiness, weakness, and fatigue. The maximum daily dose is 45 mg. Quite often these hiccup patients are already on a proton pump inhibitor (PPI) when presenting. In these cases, immediate introduction of baclofen and continuation of the PPI are recommended. In this author's experience, the time of response to the combination

[1]Not FDA approved for this indication.

[1]Not FDA approved for this indication.

therapy omeprazole and baclofen is unpredictable; however, all changes that were observed happened within the first 6 months, and the majority, within the first 6 weeks. If the desired result is achieved, continue therapy for another 6 months, after which a very cautious weaning from baclofen should be attempted. The NNT (number needed to treat) with the described combination is estimated to be less than two. In cases where the combination therapy omeprazole and baclofen is not (or not entirely) satisfactory, the addition of gabapentin (Neurontin)[1] "on the top" can be attempted. As with baclofen, a "start low, go slow" approach is indicated with gabapentin, the maximum dose of 400 mg tid used in such cases being reached after 3 weeks. In the past, the drug combination used for chronic idiopathic singultus also included cisapride; however, cisapride has been taken off the market. Although there is a reluctance to use metoclopramide routinely, if required (if it is believed that gastroparesis is possibly contributory), metoclopramide (Reglan)[1] 10 mg tid PO can be added. Tegaserod (Zelnorm)[1] is an attractive alternative because it lacks any dopaminergic effects; however, the experience with this drug for the treatment of hiccups is extremely limited.

In addition to any pharmacologic therapy, the practitioner must convey to the patient the belief that the practitioner understands and appreciates the seriousness of the condition. Compliance with the treatment is required from the patient, who must understand that success can take time. Lifestyle and habit changes are also required. The hiccup patient must limit the size of meals and avoid carbonated beverages and "gas-forming" foods.

The approach presented here represents this author's experience in the treatment of chronic singultus. The views expressed are neither guidelines nor regulations. With the exception of chlorpromazine (Thorazine), all drug use mentioned is "off label."

[1]Not FDA approved for this indication.

ACUTE INFECTIOUS DIARRHEA

METHOD OF

Pradip K. Bardhan, MD

Acute diarrhea is defined as the passage of three or more abnormally loose or watery stools per 24 hours, with or without other gastrointestinal symptoms such as vomiting or abdominal cramps. However, recent changes in consistency and character of stools are more important rather than the number of stools. Frequent passage of formed stools, defecation immediately after taking food because of the initiation of gastrocolic reflex, and passage of pasty stools in a breast-fed infant do not constitute diarrhea. The worldwide annual mortality from diarrhea is currently estimated to be between 2 and 3 million, which is a significant decrease from about 5 million in the early 1990s. Widespread use of oral rehydration therapy is likely to be the cause for this decrease in diarrheal mortality. In the poorer developing countries, diarrheal diseases are very common and are a leading cause of death because the dehydration, if not treated with appropriate rehydration, may quickly lead to death. In contrast, diarrhea in the developed industrialized countries affects people once or twice per year and is usually a mild disease. However, certain situations, such as a high purging rate, presence of signs of invasive disease, or electrolyte imbalance resulting from persistent diarrheal fluid loss, denote a more severe form of the disease, which if untreated, may lead to death.

A multitude of microbial infectious agents may cause diarrhea, but it may also occur as a consequence of noninfectious causes, such as use of laxatives, lactose intolerance, irritable bowel syndrome, inflammatory bowel diseases, and malabsorption.

Clinical Evaluation

The goal of clinical evaluation of patients with acute diarrhea is to determine the type of diarrhea, the likely cause of the diarrhea, the severity of the illness, and the treatment strategy. Information regarding the age of the patient (different pathogens are more commonly isolated from certain age groups); duration of symptoms (because chronic symptoms suggest more chronic conditions, which may require a different work-up strategy); type of diarrhea (presence of blood in the stool points toward invasive diarrhea); other signs and symptoms of invasive diarrhea (e.g., fever, marked abdominal cramps, tenesmus); history of recent intake of unsafe and possibly contaminated foods, beverages, or water; history of recent travel, especially to developing countries; signs and symptoms of dehydration (to decide urgency and method of rehydration therapy); history of antibiotic use (certain pathogens are more commonly associated with diarrhea after use of antibiotics); and evidence of any systemic illness should be sought from all patients presenting with diarrhea. Most mild cases of acute watery diarrhea can be managed without specific laboratory tests. Laboratory investigations may be useful in the evaluation of certain patients to determine the presence of blood or pus cells in the stool, and also to evaluate cases suspected of having infection, with *Shigella, Salmonella, Campylobacter,*

Vibrio, Clostridium difficile, Entamoeba histolytica, or *Giardia lamblia* bacteria, or rotavirus. However, it should be noted that a diarrheal pathogen is only rarely isolated from patients in the United States. Initially, a broad differential diagnosis is considered, because diarrhea may be the initial presentation of noninfectious and potentially life-threatening diseases, including inflammatory bowel diseases, mesenteric vascular disease, intestinal obstruction, and gastrointestinal hemorrhage. Inquiries should be made regarding use of medications that may cause diarrhea, such as angiotensin-converting enzyme (ACE) inhibitors, metformin (Glucophage), proton pump inhibitors (PPI), and magnesium-containing antacids. Whatever the cause, the crucial management of fluids and electrolytes should continue during clinical evaluation and laboratory investigations searching for etiology.

Clinical Syndromes

According to the clinical presentation of the patient, the diarrheal syndrome is divided into acute diarrhea, persistent diarrhea, and invasive diarrhea. Acute diarrhea is defined when the duration of diarrhea is less than 14 days, and persistent diarrhea is when the duration of diarrhea persists for more than 14 days. When patients with either acute or persistent diarrhea present with blood with or without mucus, the disease is called invasive diarrhea, inflammatory diarrhea, or dysentery. Classification into these syndromes helps to identify the pathophysiologic mechanisms, the probable infectious agents causing the illness, the clinical and laboratory investigations that may help to further characterize the illness, and the treatment needed.

ACUTE WATERY DIARRHEA

This is the predominant diarrheal syndrome characterized by the sudden onset of loose or watery stools. This may be accompanied by nausea, vomiting, anorexia, and abdominal cramps. A low-grade fever is also commonly observed, although fever higher than 102°F (38.9°C) suggests an invasive illness. The stools generally are watery and voluminous but without blood or mucus. A fecal leukocyte test, if performed, is negative for pus cells.

Diarrhea in Infants

Acute watery diarrhea is common in infants during the first 18 months of life, and continues to cause a large proportion of pediatric hospital admissions in the United States. The diarrhea is often preceded by vomiting, and the infant may be irritable, lethargic, and reluctant to feed. Dehydration caused by excessive loss of fluids in diarrhea stool without adequate replacement is the most important complication. Loss of large volumes of stool, as well as oliguria, may remain unrecognized because of the use of disposable diapers. In the developed countries, rotavirus is the most common cause of the infantile diarrhea syndrome, where it usually occurs during a winter season. In developing countries, rotavirus and enterotoxigenic *Escherichia coli* are the major causes. Whatever be the particular pathogen, the vital part of the management strategy is the administration of rehydration solutions to correct dehydration and maintain hydration until resolution of the diarrhea. Antibiotics and antidiarrheal drugs (e.g., diphenoxylate with atropine [Lomotil] or loperamide [Imodium]) should not be used in the common infantile diarrhea.

Traveler's Diarrhea

Traveler's diarrhea is a syndrome that is acquired when a person travels from industrialized countries to the tropical developing countries. This definition also includes illnesses occurring during the first 7 to 10 days after travelers return to their homes. Up to 50% of travelers develop one or more episodes of diarrhea or loose stools during travel to developing countries, although the majority of them are mild to moderate in nature. Bacterial pathogens are responsible for at least 80% of traveler's diarrhea. The most common agent causing this syndrome is enterotoxigenic *E. coli*, but other bacteria and, rarely, viruses and parasites can also cause these symptoms.

The watery diarrhea is usually accompanied by abdominal cramps and may also be accompanied by nausea, vomiting, anorexia, fever, fecal urgency, and the inability to carry out planned activities. Symptoms of traveler's diarrhea usually resolve within 3 to 5 days and are self-limited in otherwise healthy people. Treatment includes maintenance of fluids with oral rehydration solution and, in severe cases, use of an antibiotic such as ciprofloxacin (Cipro) or norfloxacin (Noroxin)[1]. The antibiotic may be given for 1 to 3 days. Loperamide (Imodium)* may be combined with the antibiotic. Combination therapy represents the treatment of choice for afebrile, nondysenteric traveler's diarrhea. Bismuth subsalicylate (Pepto-Bismol) may be used to provide some symptomatic relief for mild cases.

Preventive measures consist of traveler's education (behavioral modification) and chemoprophylaxis. Travelers should be instructed to avoid potentially contaminated food and water, and should follow rules to ensure that food and water are hygienic (e.g., "cook it, peel it, or forget it"). Chemoprophylactic measures are generally not recommended, and are considered

[1]Not FDA approved for this indication.

*Not FDA approved for use with antibiotic.

only for those travelers who have an underlying medical illness. Prophylaxis may be used for short-term travel in patients with hypochlorhydria (e.g., patients using PPIs), inflammatory bowel diseases, or HIV infection, or in persons who are otherwise immunosuppressed. Doxycycline (Vibramycin)[1] (100 mg/day with food) reduces the risk of traveler's diarrhea significantly. Frequently, doxycycline is used to prevent malaria and if given for this purpose, will also prevent most episodes of traveler's diarrhea. Prophylactic norfloxacin[1] (100 mg) or ciprofloxacin[1] (250 mg) daily will prevent nearly all episodes of diarrhea. Bismuth subsalicylate[1] is moderately effective in the prevention of traveler's diarrhea, with protection rates of approximately 65%, and the dosage recommended for prophylaxis is two tablets orally with meals and at bedtime. The prophylactic agent should be started on the day of travel and continued daily until 2 days after leaving the countries at risk.

INVASIVE DIARRHEA (DYSENTERY)

Invasive diarrheas are caused by infection as a consequence of pathogens that are capable of mucosal invasion in the distal small intestine and colon. This causes local and systemic inflammatory responses, with mucosal ulceration and hemorrhage, clinically manifested as dysentery. The patient tends to have the feeling of fecal urgency, but the volume is very small because the urgency is secondary to proctitis. Frequently, only small amounts of mucus or pus are passed. Because of the inflammation, patients with invasive diarrhea generally suffer from abdominal cramps which can be quite severe, which is often accompanied by fever and tenesmus. Some patients may complain of nausea and vomiting in the early stage of the disease. A fecal microscopic examination will reveal many polymorphonuclear leukocytes. In the case of shigellosis or salmonellosis, the illness may start as typical watery diarrhea progressing to bloody diarrhea. The most common causes for dysentery are *Shigella, Campylobacter,* and *Salmonella.* Amebic colitis may cause bloody stools, and stool microscopic examination is needed to identify the hematophagous trophozoites of amebiasis. Some invasive pathogens, such as *Salmonella* spp., *Shigella* spp., and *Entamoeba histolytica,* may invade the bloodstream or may be carried by the lymphatic system to distant organs, (e.g., liver, spleen, joints, and central nervous system).

Antimicrobial therapy is indicated for patients with shigellosis, although they are of questionable benefit in infections with *Campylobacter* and *Salmonella.* Treatment options have changed markedly over the years as a result of an increasing drug resistance of *Shigella* organisms. *Shigella* are now commonly resistant to ampicillin and cotrimoxazole (Bactrim)[1], and the newer quinolones have become the drugs of choice for most patients. In developing countries, knowledge of the antibiotic sensitivities of local or endemic strains should guide immediate therapy. When possible, culture and sensitivity tests should be carried out.

[1]Not FDA approved for this indication.

Specific Pathogens

There are numerous causes of acute infectious diarrhea. Viral, bacterial, and protozoal agents differ according to the setting in which diarrhea occurs, and the presence of specific pathogens is suspected based on epidemiologic setting and clinical presentation.

VIRUSES

Rotavirus

Rotaviruses (groups A and C) are the most common causes of pediatric diarrhea in developed countries. The illness causes watery diarrhea, which is often preceded by vomiting. Rotavirus should be suspected in infants and young children, especially during the winter season, although rotavirus infection occurs throughout the year in tropical countries. According to surveillance reports, nearly every infant is infected with rotavirus before the infant is 2 years old, and in 15% to 20% of infants, the diarrhea is severe enough to seek care from a health care provider. The mode of transmission is probably from person to person through airborne droplets. Rotavirus infection causes structural damage in the small intestinal mucosa, and recent evidence suggests that one of the nonstructural viral proteins (NSP4) may act as an enterotoxin. Case series of infants brought to medical attention describe 3 to 5 days of watery diarrhea and 2 to 3 days of vomiting. Mild fever is common. The infection is self-limiting, but the illness can continue for several days, and total fluid losses during the illness can be life-threatening unless treated promptly and properly. Maintenance of fluids and electrolytes using oral rehydration solution is the treatment of choice, but some children may require intravenous fluids because of a high purging rate or frequent episodes of vomiting. Antibiotics are not indicated. Antiemetics and antidiarrheal agents are not recommended for young children. Although rotavirus infection may occur in some children more than once, the first attack is usually the most severe and subsequent infections are generally mild or asymptomatic. Rapid antigen testing by stool enzyme-link immunosorbent assays and latex agglutination assays are available to confirm the diagnosis.

A live, oral vaccine tetravalent vaccine (RotaShield) for rotavirus was introduced to prevent this common infection. Unfortunately, intussusception, a serious adverse event, occurred in a very small proportion of vaccinated infants and the vaccine was subsequently withdrawn. The other vaccines, based on human and bovine strains, are still under development.

Group B rotaviruses may be responsible for 5% to 10% of sporadic diarrheal episodes in adults. Rarely, rotaviruses can cause mild diarrhea in family members handling diapers of sick infants. Rotavirus infection can cause persistent diarrhea in immunocompromised patients, and in such patients, passive oral immunoglobulins[1] have proved useful by reducing the duration of diarrhea and viral shedding.

Adenovirus

Certain enteric adenoviruses, mainly subgroup F, serotypes 40 and 41, may be the second most common cause of viral diarrhea in infants in both industrialized and developing countries. They are transmitted by the fecal–oral route. These viruses cause diarrhea throughout the year, affecting mostly children younger than age 4 years. They also frequently cause diarrhea in immunocompromised patients. Reinfections and asymptomatic infections are common. Antigen testing by stool enzyme-link immunosorbent assays is available for diagnosis.

Norwalk-Like Virus

Norwalk-like virus may cause acute watery diarrhea in any age group. They are accountable for up to 5% of childhood diarrhea in the developing countries. They can be transmitted through water, food, or person-to-person contact. Generally, the illnesses occur in outbreaks and can affect people in camps and dormitories, who experience acute vomiting and diarrhea. There may be associated fever, headache, and abdominal cramps. The illness is usually short-lived Commercial diagnostic tests are not yet available.

Other Viruses

Other viruses like caliciviruses, astroviruses, and coronaviruses can also cause acute watery diarrhea that is frequently associated with vomiting. There may also be a mild fever and abdominal cramps. There are no commercial diagnostic tests.

BACTERIA

Vibrio cholerae

Cholera is caused by *Vibrio cholerae* serotype 01 or 0139. Cholera has major public health importance because of it can cause severe watery diarrhea leading rapidly to severe dehydration, and can spread through contaminated food and water. Death as a consequence of severe dehydration can occur within a few hours of onset of symptoms, even in previously healthy individuals. Travelers suspected of having cholera should have a stool culture performed using specific media for this organism, and positive cases should be reported to the authorities. In endemic countries, the numbers of cases are too great to culture all cases; consequently, specimens from a sample of cases should be tested to confirm the type of organism and the antibiotic sensitivity patterns. Cases occurring in an area not previously infected should be confirmed and reported to the authorities.

Symptoms include severe watery diarrhea, and often the stool is so watery it loses its fecal character and resembles "rice water." Serious cases usually also have repeated copious vomiting, and with increasing dehydration they develop classic signs of acute dehydration proceeding to shock, coma, and death unless treated rapidly. The cholera patients lose large amounts of bicarbonate in their stool, and then they develop severe metabolic acidosis. The patients may suffer from painful muscle cramps, and sometimes signs of tetany, including carpopedal spasm, are present.

The symptoms of cholera result from the enterotoxin produced by *V. cholerae* that stimulates adenylate cyclase, resulting in increased levels of intracellular cyclic AMP, chloride secretion, and tremendous outpouring of fluids and electrolytes into the gut lumen. There is essentially no inflammation in the gut and the intestinal mucosal cells remain healthy, but the cholera toxin maximally stimulates their cyclic AMP system. GM_1 ganglioside present on the surface of the mucosal cells acts as the receptor for the toxin.

V. cholerae that are not serotype 01 or 0139, as well as other *Vibrio* species, may also cause diarrhea (as well as systemic infections) in individual patients, but do not cause epidemic cholera.

The treatment of cholera includes rapid rehydration, correction of acidosis. Antibiotics are used to shorten the illness and decrease stool outputs. In severely dehydrated cholera patients, the dehydration has occurred in a short time, and most of the fluid deficit is from the circulatory volume. In these situations intravenous fluids need to be given rapidly (in less than 4 hours) to completely restore circulatory volumes, the amount calculated to be approximately 10% of the body weight. Slow or insufficient rehydration may lead to acute renal failure or other complications of shock. The most appropriate intravenous rehydration fluid is either Ringer's lactate solution or other polyelectrolyte solution (e.g., Dhaka solution[2]) that includes a base to correct the acidosis, as well as potassium to correct the potassium deficit.

Oral rehydration can be started as soon as the patient is able to drink, even while the intravenous fluids are being given. The best oral rehydration solution (ORS) for cholera and other severely purging patients is one prepared with rice powder. Rice ORS is prepared commercially (CeraLyte)[2], or it can be prepared with homemade ingredients. The electrolytes should be those conforming to the recently

[1]Not FDA approved for this indication.

[2]Not available in the United States.

recommended standard oral rehydration solution of the World Health Organization, which contains 75 mEq of sodium, 20 mEq of potassium, and 10 mEq of citrate.

Doxycycline (Vibramycin) (300 mg as a single dose) and tetracycline (500 mg four times daily [qid]) are the antibiotics of choice for adults, and trimethoprim-sulfamethoxazole (Bactrim)[1] is preferred for children. Other antibiotics can be used for resistant strains.

Enterotoxigenic *Escherichia coli*

Enterotoxigenic *E. coli* (ETEC) pathogens are among the most common causes of infantile and childhood diarrhea in the world, and also are the leading causes of traveler's diarrhea. However, they are relatively uncommon in the industrialized countries, and their occurrences can be usually related to food- or water-borne outbreaks. This group of *E. coli* causes illness through the production of a heat-labile enterotoxin (LT), or a heat-stable enterotoxin (ST), or both. Either of these toxins leads to secretion of fluids from the small intestines. The LT acts like the cholera toxin, whereas the ST stimulates small intestinal secretion of water and electrolytes through the guanylate cyclase–cyclic guanosine monophosphate (GMP) system. Frequently, the ETEC also express specific colonization factor pili that allow them to colonize the small intestine. Transmission occurs through the ingestion of contaminated food and drinks, with peaks during the warm, wet seasons.

In general, the illness is less severe than cholera, but individual patients may have an illness that is indistinguishable from cholera. The cardinal symptoms are watery diarrhea and vomiting. Fever (usually mild) and abdominal cramps are also frequently present. Most ETEC diarrhea episodes are self-limiting, and the diarrhea resolves within 4 to 5 days, although few cases may persist for 2 weeks or more.

Treatment is aimed at correction of dehydration along the same guidelines as for other watery diarrheas. Antibiotics are not recommended for most cases in endemic settings. However, appropriate antibiotics may be used in patients suffering from moderate to severe traveler's diarrhea caused by these organisms. Antibiotic regimens found useful include doxycycline (Vibramycin)[1], trimethoprim-sulfamethoxazole (Bactrim), and various quinolones, including ciprofloxacin (Cipro).

Enteropathogenic *Escherichia coli*

Enteropathogenic *E. coli* (EPEC) remains an important cause of watery diarrhea in infants and young children in many developing countries, although it has become uncommon in the developed industrialized countries since the 1960s. EPEC is able to induce a characteristic attaching and effacing lesion in the small intestinal mucosa. It has a short incubation period and causes a self-limited water diarrhea. Vomiting, abdominal pain, and fever may be associated with the diarrhea. The treatment is focused at maintenance of hydration.

Enterohemorrhagic *Escherichia coli*

The prototype of enterohemorrhagic *E. coli* (EHEC) is the *E. coli* O157:H7, which is commonly associated with hemolytic uremic syndrome (HUS) in North America. EHEC produces the phage-encoded cytotoxin Shiga-like toxins I and II. The principal mode of transmission is through undercooked or contaminated ground beef, although transmission can also be by ingestion of processed meat, unpasteurized milk, raw fruits and vegetables, and swimming in contaminated waters. The onset of illness with EHEC infection is acute watery diarrhea with vomiting and crampy abdominal pain. The diarrhea becomes bloody, usually within 3 to 4 days, in approximately 85% to 90% of cases. However, fever is often absent or low grade, which is unlike other bloody diarrheas. During outbreaks of EHEC, up to 10% of patients may develop HUS, and 1% will die. Besides HUS, other complications, such as rectal prolapse, intussusception, appendicitis, and pseudomembranous colitis, may also be noted. Routine stool culture cannot detect *E. coli* O157:H7; suspicious colonies are screened with a commercially available antisera. Treatment is symptomatic, and antibiotics are not indicated, because there is evidence that patients receiving them may have worse outcomes than untreated patients.

Other Diarrheogenic Forms of *Escherichia coli*

Other forms of *E. coli* that may cause diarrheal illness include enteroaggregative *E. coli* (EAggEC), diffusely adhering *E. coli* (DAEC), and enteroinvasive *E. coli* (EIEC). The EAggEC has a typical pattern of adherence to the intestinal mucosa. It is associated with persistent diarrhea in the pediatric population in the developing countries, and sporadic diarrhea in the developed countries. The diarrhea caused by EHEC is typically watery and sometimes mixed with mucus; vomiting may be absent or mild. The acute diarrhea is self-limiting, and treatment is aimed at correction of dehydration. Antibiotics and nutritional therapy may be required in the more persistent cases. The diarrhea caused by DAEC is very similar to that caused by ETEC. The watery diarrhea is self-limiting, and vomiting or abdominal pain is uncommon. The diagnosis is usually made by DNA probing. Treatment of diarrhea caused by DAEC is similar to the guidelines followed in ETEC diarrhea. The EIEC are very similar to *Shigellae* in terms of the biochemical properties, virulence characteristics, and clinical presentation. In developed countries, it causes uncommon food-borne outbreaks, although in

[1]Not FDA approved for this indication.

certain developing countries, it may be associated with up to 5% of diarrheal episodes. The management of patients with EIEC infection is also similar to the guidelines followed to manage patients with shigellosis.

Shigella spp.

Among the organisms causing invasive diarrhea or bloody diarrhea, *Shigellae* are the most common, although they may also cause a watery diarrhea syndrome. The genus is divided into four species and multiple serotypes. *Shigella flexneri* is more common in the developing countries, whereas *Shigella sonnei* is the most common species in industrialized countries. *Shigella dysenteriae* serotype O1 is noted in the developed countries almost exclusively in travelers, but in developing countries it may cause epidemics of dysentery. These epidemics are major public health emergencies because of the severity of the disease, the rapidity of the spread of the disease, and the resistance to the usual antibiotics often seen among the epidemic strains. *Shigella boydii* is generally less common, but the disease is similar to that caused by *S. flexneri*.

Shigellae are highly contagious because of low infectious inoculum, transmission is fecal–oral, and humans are the only natural hosts. After an incubation of 1 to 4 days, the disease starts with an acute onset of fever, malaise, headache, occasional vomiting, and watery diarrhea, progressing to bloody diarrhea within hours to days. Most episodes of shigellosis in an otherwise healthy host usually resolve within 1 week. In some patients, there occasionally may be some unusual extraintestinal manifestations, including seizure, arthritis, HUS, and thrombotic thrombocytopenic purpura.

Diagnosis is confirmed by stool culture. Because of the fastidious nature of *Shigellae*, they are best isolated from fresh stool samples processed promptly. Patients presenting with acute invasive diarrhea should be assumed to have shigellosis and should be treated accordingly, based on the local antibiotic sensitivity patterns. Unfortunately, resistance to formerly effective antibiotics are being increasingly noted among *Shigella* isolates. Ampicillin or trimethoprim-sulfamethoxazole is effective in sensitive strains, but other antibiotics, such as one of the new quinolones[1] or pivmecillinam[2] are necessary to treat resistant strains. Nalidixic acid (NegGram)[1] is still useful against many strains, but *S. dysenteriae* is now frequently resistant to this drug as well.

Campylobacter jejuni

Campylobacter jejuni is the most commonly isolated bacterial pathogen isolated in the United States from patients with diarrhea. In the developing countries, *Campylobacter* bacteria can be isolated from up to 15% of healthy people. The organism is usually transmitted from poultry, although transmission can occur through unpasteurized milk and contaminated water. It can cause either watery diarrhea or dysentery. The illness starts with an abrupt onset of watery diarrhea, which may progress to bloody diarrhea. There are usually some abdominal cramps, which in some patients may mimic appendicitis. The organism can be isolated from stool. Use of antibiotics is controversial, especially if the start of treatment is delayed. Erythromycin[1] is generally used if the treatment can begin within the first few days of the onset. Occasionally, *Campylobacter* infection can lead to systemic illness with bacteremia, which is a definite indication for using antibiotics according to the local sensitivity patterns.

Rarely, infection with *Campylobacter* has been associated with the subsequent development of Guillain-Barré syndrome. It is possible that an autoimmune process is initiated by certain strains expressing gangliosides through the process of molecular mimicry.

Salmonella spp.

Typhoid fever caused by *Salmonella entericus* serovars *typhi* and *paratyphi* continues to be a global health problem, although in the developed countries considerable success has been noted in controlling this disease through better sanitation, water supply, and food handling. This systemic illness is characterized by fever and gastrointestinal symptoms, but may be complicated with altered mentation, perforation, and ileus. The symptoms in uncomplicated typhoid fever usually resolve by the fourth week without antimicrobial treatment, although relapse may occur in some patients. Diagnosis is made by isolation of *Salmonella typhi* or *Salmonella paratyphi* from blood, stool, urine, bone marrow, or rose spots. Chloramphenicol (Chloromycetin) is the drug of choice, but with the emergence of multi-drug resistant strains of *S. typhi*, treatment with a fluoroquinolone[1] or a third-generation cephalosporin (e.g., ceftriaxone [Rocephin][1]) may be necessary.

In contrast to typhoid, nontyphoidal *Salmonella* infections are apparently rising in the developed countries. *Salmonella* species are frequently associated with foodborne outbreaks and *Salmonella enteritidis* is the most common cause of food-borne outbreaks in the United States. The infection leads to acute diarrhea that is generally watery but may progress to dysentery. Fever, headache, abdominal pain, and vomiting may be present. The illness may continue for up to 1 week. Treatment is with appropriate rehydration; except in complicated cases, antibiotics are generally not needed. Rarely, septicemia, meningitis, and osteomyelitis may occur.

---

[1]Not FDA approved for this indication.
[2]Not available in the United States.

[1]Not FDA approved for this indication.

Clostridium difficile

Clostridium difficile is an anaerobic organism that can produce an enterotoxin leading to an illness ranging from mild diarrhea to a severe and often fatal pseudomembranous colitis. It most commonly occurs after the use of an antibiotic that modifies the intestinal flora and selects for this organism. This can become a severe infection, especially in the elderly and otherwise compromised hosts. Culturing the organism or detecting the toxin from stool specimens by enzyme-linked immunosorbent assay or by tissue culture assay is employed in detecting this infection. In the majority of cases the disease is self-limited and responds to withdrawal of the offending antibiotic. Recommended treatment for severe disease is with metronidazole (Flagyl)[1], or vancomycin (Vancocin), which is generally used for patients whose treatment with metronidazole has failed. Relapse may happen in approximately 40% of patients despite treatment.

PARASITES

Giardia lamblia

This is the most common cause of parasitic diarrhea in the developed countries, whereas in the developing countries, it is a relatively minor cause of diarrhea. Transmission occurs from person to person through the fecal–oral route. Occasionally, outbreaks may occur through drinking of contaminated water or in a daycare setting. Diagnosis is made through microscopic examination of duodenal aspirates or stool samples revealing trophozoites or cysts of *G. lamblia*. The treatment of choice is metronidazole.[1]

Entamoeba histolytica

This is an infrequent cause of diarrhea in the developing countries. In the developed world, persons at risk for contracting infection with *E. histolytica* include travelers returning from foreign countries, persons having anal intercourse, and institutionalized persons. Transmission is mostly by the fecal–oral route. The clinical presentation ranges from asymptomatic infection to amebic colitis with accompanying bloody diarrhea, fever, abdominal pain, and tenesmus. The disease may have a more chronic course than the bacterial invasive diarrheas, and may need to be distinguished from inflammatory bowel diseases, because inappropriate treatment with antimotility agents and steroids will worsen the condition. Occasionally, complications such as toxic megacolon and perforation may occur, particularly when amebic colitis is noted in young children and elderly patients. Diagnosis is made by demonstration of cysts or trophozoites in fresh stool samples, or colonic mucosal biopsy samples. Metronidazole[1] remains the drug of choice.

[1]Not FDA approved for this indication.

Other Parasites

Cryptosporidium parvum is an important cause of diarrhea in immunocompromised hosts and is also implicated as a cause of childhood diarrhea in the developing countries. Diagnosis is confirmed by antigen enzyme immunoassay. Treatment is mostly supportive. *Cyclospora*, formerly known as blue-green algae, can cause diarrhea in travelers and in immunocompromised hosts. The illness is self-limiting and is associated with nonbloody, watery diarrhea, which may be preceded by flulike symptoms. Treatment may be necessary in patients having relapse or who are immunocompromised, and trimethoprim-sulfamethoxazole (Bactrim)[1] is the drug of choice. Other protozoa (*Blastocystis hominis, Balantidium coli*) and helminths (*Strongyloides stercoralis, Trichuris trichuria*) are also associated with diarrhea in the developing countries.

LABORATORY FINDINGS

Mild episodes of diarrhea are usually self-limited and do not require laboratory evaluation.

Fecal Microscopy

This relatively simple test provides information about the presence of fecal leukocytes and erythrocytes. The presence of fecal leukocytes implies colonic and rectal inflammation, pointing toward invasive diarrhea. Fecal microscopic examination is also the most practical way to look for intestinal parasites and helminths. The indications for suspecting presence of parasites include persistent diarrhea, diarrhea in homosexual men, AIDS-associated diarrhea, and regular exposure to daycare centers.

Stool Cultures

Stool cultures should be performed when the isolation of a pathogen will make a meaningful and practical contribution toward case management. Stool cultures are indicated in patients who present with invasive diarrhea, persistent diarrhea, severe dehydration, high fever (temperature of 102°F [38.9°C]), and during outbreaks.

Special Tests

Enzyme-linked immunosorbent assays are available for the detection of several viruses causing diarrhea including rotaviruses. They may be done when there is confusion about clinical diagnosis and laboratory confirmation is needed, or when a deviation from the usual clinical course is present or suspected. Enzyme-linked immunosorbent assays for *C. difficile* toxin should be performed on all cases with suspicion

[1]Not FDA approved for this indication.

TABLE 1 Clinical Assessment of Dehydration

	Diagnosis		
Assessment	**No Dehydration**	**Some Dehydration**	**Severe Dehydration**
Diagnostic criteria	No significant signs/symptoms	At least two signs/symptoms, including one key (*) sign present	Criteria for "some dehydration" plus one of these key (*) signs/symptoms present
Signs/symptoms			
Condition	Normal	Irritable/less active*	Lethargic/comatose*
Eyes	Normal	Sunken	
Mucosa	Normal	Dry	
Thirst	Normal	Thirsty*	Unable to drink*†
Skin turgor	Normal	Reduced*	
Radial pulse	Normal		Uncountable/absent*
Body-weight loss	0%-4%	5%-9%	≥10%

†The patients are unable to swallow; not a refusal to drink.

of infection with *E. coli* O157:H7, including hamburger-associated diarrhea. Examinations of samples from the proximal small intestinal contents obtained by the string test (Entero-Test) may be done when the presence of *G. lamblia* or *Strongyloides stercoralis* is suspected.

Flexible Sigmoidoscopy and Colonoscopy

Endoscopic examinations are usually not required for the work-up of patients with acute diarrhea. Endoscopic examinations with histologic examinations of mucosal biopsies may be needed in certain patients, (e.g., homosexual men, patients with AIDS, patients developing diarrhea after antibiotic therapy, or patients with persistent diarrhea, or in situations where chronic inflammatory bowel diseases need to be ruled out).

Management

Patients presenting with acute diarrhea should be assessed quickly to decide the nature and pattern of diarrhea, the degree of dehydration (Table 1), and the presence of any other associated symptoms, particularly in children, so that appropriate treatment can be started without any delay. Although most patients with acute infectious diarrhea can be treated in an outpatient clinic or at home, some patients will still need hospitalization, mainly for intravenous rehydration. Presence of severe dehydration, shock, toxic state, neurologic change, suspected surgical problem, severe vomiting, immunodeficiency, and malnutrition will generally require hospitalization.

The most essential part in the effective clinical management of acute diarrhea is the management of dehydration. Diarrheal patients lose a substantial amount of fluid in stool that is isotonic, containing large amounts of electrolytes. In patients with severe purging, losses of sodium, potassium, and bicarbonate are significant; they need to be replenished by a rehydration solution that has an electrolyte content similar to the diarrheal fluid that is lost.

REHYDRATION

The management of dehydration has three components: prevention of dehydration; prompt rehydration therapy by oral or intravenous rehydration fluids in the presence of dehydration; and maintaining hydration during the course of the illness. Dehydration may be absent in many diarrheal patients at the early stage of the disease, and although they may not require the standard ORS, they should be encouraged to drink larger amounts of appropriate fluids at home, in addition to their normal daily requirements. Oral rehydration therapy (ORT), if initiated early at home to prevent dehydration, will substantially decrease the number of visits to treatment facilities. In dehydrated patients, the degree of dehydration should be quickly assessed, and the mode of rehydration decided. Most patients (>90%) will improve with the standard oral solutions containing the proper mixture of salts and carbohydrates (Table 2). Several studies have found that complex carbohydrates (e.g., rice starch) are more effective in severely purging patients. Although almost any fluid can be used with mild cases, the fluid loss from significant purging should be replaced with oral rehydration solution (e.g., CeraLyte[1], Pedialyte, Infalyte) that contains the proper concentrations of electrolytes and carbohydrates. Soft drinks, sports drinks, and many other commonly used fluids are inappropriate for replacing significant fluid loss from diarrhea, because they do not have the proper composition of salts, may have excess sugars, or may be hypertonic. ORS should be offered in adequate

[1]Not FDA approved for this indication.

TABLE 2 The Composition of the New Oral Rehydration Solution Recommended by the World Health Organization

Glucose	75 mmol/L
Sodium	75 mmol/L
Potassium	20 mmol/L
Chloride	65 mmol/L
Citrate	10 mmol/L

TABLE 3 Recommended Antibiotics for Use in Patients With Common Diarrheal Pathogens

Syndrome	Antimicrobial Agent	Adults	Children
Acute watery diarrhea with no complications		No antibiotic recommended	No antibiotic recommended
Cholera	Doxycycline (Vibramycin), single dose	300 mg	Not recommended
	Tetracycline qid for 3 days	500 mg per dose	12.5 mg/kg per dose
	Ciprofloxacin (Cipro)[1] bid for 3 days	500 mg per dose	Not recommended
	Trimethoprim-sulfamethoxazole (Bactrim)[1] bid for 3 days	TMP 160 mg and SMX 800 mg	TMP 5 mg/kg and SMX 25 mg/kg
Traveler's diarrhea	Ciprofloxacin bid for up to 3 days	500 mg	Not recommended
	Trimethoprim-sulfamethoxazole bid for 3 days	TMP 160 mg and SMX 800 mg	TMP 5 mg/kg and SMX 25 mg/kg
Shigellosis	Ciprofloxacin bid for 5 days	500 mg	Not recommended
	Trimethoprim-sulfamethoxazole bid for 5 days	TMP 160 mg and SMX 800 mg	TMP 5 mg/kg and SMX 25 mg/kg
	Nalidixic acid (NegGram)[1] qid for 5 days	1 g	15 mg/kg
		400 mg	125 mg/kg
	Pivmecillinam[2] qid for 5 days		
Giardiasis	Metronidazole (Flagyl)[1] tid for 5 days	250 mg	5 mg/kg
Cyclospora	Trimethoprim-sulfamethoxazole[1] bid for 3 days	TMP 160 mg and SMX 800 mg	TMP 5 mg/kg and SMX 25 mg/kg
Rotavirus		No antibiotic recommended	No antibiotic recommended

Abbreviations: bid = twice daily; qid = four times a day; SMX = sulfamethoxazole; tid = three times a day; TMP = trimethoprim.
[1]Not FDA approved for this indication.
[2]Not available in the United States.

amounts to replace the fluid loss. It is assumed that a mildly dehydrated patient loses approximately 5% of body weight, and this volume should be offered to correct the loss. Additional solution should then be given to make up for continuing losses until the illness subsides. If vomiting is a problem, the fluids can still be generally given in smaller amounts, but more frequently. Additional water and other fluids should be given in addition to the oral rehydration solution to make up for normal physiologic fluid replacement. In some patients who present with dehydration, the patient may be unable to drink (painful oral lesion, lethargy, severe or persistent vomiting) or ORT may be contraindicated (paralytic ileus). In such cases, intravenous rehydration therapy is necessary until the dehydration is corrected and the patient is able to drink. Then ORS can be started.

More aggressive rehydration with intravenous fluids is needed in patients presenting with severe dehydration. The preferable intravenous solution is either Ringer's lactate solution (sodium 130 mEq/L, potassium 4 mEq/L, chloride 109 mEq/L, and lactate 28 mEq/L) or the Dhaka solution[1] (sodium 133 mEq/L, potassium 13 mEq/L, chloride 98 mEq/L, and lactate 48 mEq/L) where available. Normal saline (0.9% sodium chloride) can be used in an emergency if the above solutions are not available; however, in such cases, ORS should be started as soon as the patient is able to drink, because the potassium and bicarbonate lost in the stool are not replaced by infusing normal saline. Patients with severe dehydration can be assumed to have lost approximately 10% of their body weight, a loss which needs to be corrected. Patients with shock need very rapid administration of fluids—within 1 to 4 hours.

[1]Not FDA approved for this indication.

A slower rehydration should be done in infants and malnourished children. Administration of oral rehydration solution can begin as soon as the patient is able to drink to make up for ongoing stool losses.

The maintenance phase is for the replacement of ongoing losses of water and electrolytes as long as the diarrhea continues. The goal is to prevent dehydration. ORS is adequate for the maintenance of hydration in most of the patients.

SYMPTOMATIC MANAGEMENT

For symptomatic relief bismuth subsalicylate (Pepto-Bismol) and loperamide (Imodium) are often used, especially in traveler's diarrhea. However, they neither correct the fluid loss nor restore the electrolyte balance. Bismuth subsalicylate is given in a dose of 2 tablets (or 1 tablespoon) every 6 to 8 hours until symptoms subside. Patients should be warned that their stool will blacken and to avoid overdosing with salicylate. The dose of loperamide is a 4-mg initial dose, followed by 2 mg every 6 hours until the diarrhea stops. Loperamide should not be given to children or to patients with dysentery.

ANTIMICROBIAL AGENTS

Because most cases of acute diarrhea are self-limiting, antimicrobial agents generally are not required, except in a few conditions. These include cholera, shigellosis, severe traveler's diarrhea, *C. difficile* enterocolitis, amebiasis, giardiasis, and *Cyclospora* infection. Specific antiviral agents may be necessary in immunosuppressed patients depending on specific infections. Table 3 summarizes the most common antimicrobial agents.

CONSTIPATION

METHOD OF

Christina R. Covelli, MD, and

G. Nicholas Verne, MD

Constipation is among the most common gastrointestinal symptoms in the general population. The prevalence of constipation in Western countries ranges from 2% to 27%. Self-reported constipation is more prevalent in women, nonwhites, and those older than age 65 years. It accounts for 2.5 million physician visits annually in the United States, 20,000 hospitalizations each year, and 3 million prescriptions for laxatives each year. Risk factors for constipation include physical inactivity, limited education, history of sexual abuse, low income, and symptoms of depression.

Defining constipation appears to be a simple task, but the term often means a different complex of symptoms to patients and physicians. From a medical perspective, constipation is the inability to evacuate stool completely and spontaneously more than three times per week. Most patients define it as passage of hard stools, a sense of incomplete bowel evacuation, a sense of excessive straining, and excessive time spent in unsuccessful defecation, although the frequency of defecation is within the normal range. For clinical purposes, the physician should use a combination of objective and subjective criteria when addressing these complaints.

Etiology and Pathophysiology

Constipation is believed to be disordered movement through the colon and anorectum. Causes are multifactorial and can result from neurologic or systemic disorders, or as a side effect of numerous drugs. Constipation is classified into three broad categories: normal-transit constipation, slow-transit constipation, and disorders of rectal evacuation. In normal-transit constipation ("functional constipation"), patients believe they are constipated, yet stool frequency and colonic transit are normal. These patients respond to dietary fiber supplementation, risk factor modification, or the addition of an osmotic laxative. Slow-transit constipation ("colonic inertia") occurs as a primary motor disorder that involves less-than-normal movement of contents from the proximal to distal colon and rectum. Defecatory disorders include pelvic floor dyssynergia and structural abnormalities such as rectal intussusception and rectocele.

Evaluation

The initial work-up should consist of a thorough history and physical examination with a digital rectal examination. An important part of the history includes defining the nature and duration of the symptoms. A recent change in bowel habits makes an identifiable cause more likely and requires investigation, whereas long-standing complaints suggest a functional origin. Any patient with occult gastrointestinal bleeding or anemia, particularly those older than age 35 years, or those with recent and persistent changes in bowel habits, should have their colon examined with a flexible sigmoidoscopy, barium enema, or colonoscopy to determine the cause. Potentially constipating medications should be considered with the prospect of changing to other medications without risk factors (Table 1). Signs of systemic disease, such as diabetes and hypothyroidism, should be appraised and the patient's other medical problems should be weighed as potential secondary causes of constipation (Table 2). Studies of colonic motility and rectosphincteric function should be reserved for patients with severe symptoms who fail conservative management and who have had structural abnormalities ruled out with a colonoscopic or barium enema examination.

Treatment of Chronic Constipation

GENERAL MEASURES

Initial management involves patient education, which should include reassurance and an explanation of normal bowel habits. Medications known to cause constipation should be minimized, and metabolic abnormalities (e.g., hypothyroidism) should be corrected. Regular exercise, increases in fiber and fluid

TABLE 1 Medications Commonly Associated with Constipation

Anticholinergics
Antihistamines
Tricyclic antidepressants
Antipsychotics
Neuroleptic agents
Antiparkinsonian drugs
Antihypertensives:
Clonidine (Catapres)
Calcium channel blockers
Cation-containing agents:
Iron supplements
Calcium (antacids [Tums], supplements)
Aluminum (antacids, sucralfate [Carafate])
Bismuth
Diuretics
Opiates:
Morphine
Diphenoxylate with codeine (Lomotil)
Codeine
Nonsteroidal anti-inflammatory agents
Resins
Cholestyramine (Questran)
Sympathomimetics
Serotonin type 3 antagonists
Ondansetron (Zofran)
Granisetron (Kytril)

TABLE 2 Constipation Associated with Systemic Disease

Endocrine and Metabolic Disorders
Diabetes mellitus
Hypothyroidism
Hypercalcemia
Chronic renal insufficiency
Central Nervous System Disorders
Dementia
Parkinson's disease
Multiple sclerosis
Spinal cord lesions
Cerebrovascular accidents
Neuromuscular Diseases
Progressive systemic sclerosis
Muscular dystrophy
Hirschsprung's disease
Chagas' disease *(Trypanosoma cruzi)*
Autonomic neuropathy
Others
Amyloidosis
Dermatomyositis
Depression

intake (1500 mL/day), and reduction in the use of laxatives and cathartics are also beneficial. Because colonic motor activity is more active after waking and after a meal, patients should be encouraged to attempt defecation after meals when there is increased colonic motility, especially each day 30 minutes after breakfast. Patients should not strain for more than 5 minutes, pushing at a level of 5 to 7, assuming a maximum straining effort of 10. In general, a trial of a high-fiber diet, fiber supplementation, regular exercise, and an increase in fluid intake will be successful in most patients and is the most natural approach.

FIBER

Increased dietary fiber is the cornerstone of treating constipation. Fiber serves to increase stool bulk and water content. The goal is to increase dietary fiber to 20 to 30 g daily, which can be achieved through diet and with the aid of fiber supplements such as psyllium (Metamucil) or methylcellulose (Citrucel). Initially, patients are encouraged to increase their intake of fruits, vegetables, and high-fiber breakfast cereals or raw bran. Cereals such as Fiber One and All Bran contain more than 10 g of fiber. Patients with poor dietary habits can sprinkle 1 to 2 tablespoons of bran powder over foods, or can mix it with fluids twice daily, providing an inexpensive means of consuming 10 to 20 g of fiber daily.

Although there is a wide variety of pharmaceutical fiber supplements, they are more expensive than bran powder. Preparations include psyllium (Metamucil) and methylcellulose (Citrucel), both providing natural fibers derived from vegetable matter. They exert their laxative effect by increasing stool bulk and absorbing water to decrease colonic transit time. It is recommended that these agents be adequately diluted with water and be consumed before meals and at bedtime for maximal effect. Polycarbophil (FiberCon) is another fiber supplement; it is a synthetic fiber that may be less gas producing than natural fibers.

Patient compliance with the use of fiber supplements is poor because of their side effects, which include bloating, flatulence, and distension. Patients should be warned that increasing fiber intake can cause these symptoms, but that they will subside after several days of therapy. To improve compliance, instruct patients to slowly increase fiber intake to 20 to 25 g per day over a period of 1 to 2 weeks.

PHARMACOLOGIC THERAPY

Table 3 summarizes the pharmacologic management of constipation.

Osmotic laxatives, such as milk of magnesia, sorbitol, lactulose (Chronulac), or polyethylene glycol (MiraLax), can be used in patients with continued symptoms despite the general measures outlined above. A small daily dose of an osmotic laxative can be effectively used to soften stool with minimal adverse effects. Osmotic laxatives are safe to use long-term and do not promote dependency. There are two different categories of osmotic laxatives: poorly absorbed sugars such as lactulose or sorbitol, and saline laxatives such as magnesium salts. They function by increasing osmotic retention of fluid in the lumen of the intestine. They are titrated to a dose that results in semisolid to soft stools and can take several days to work. Care must be taken in patients with renal insufficiency and cardiac dysfunction when using osmotic laxatives because they may cause volume overload and electrolyte abnormalities from absorption of sodium, magnesium, and phosphorus. Lactulose and sorbitol may cause significant bloating, flatulence, and abdominal discomfort because of bacterial metabolism of unabsorbed carbohydrates. Polyethylene glycol causes less bloating and flatulence because it is a large polymer that is not degraded by bacteria; it is commonly used to purge the colon prior to colonoscopy. It has been very successful in treating patients with chronic constipation, and is well tolerated. Polyethylene glycol is available by prescription only and is comparable in price to lactulose, both of which are less expensive than sorbitol.

Emollient laxatives consist of docusate sodium (Colace) or mineral oil. Docusates soften feces by reducing surface tension, thus allowing fecal mass to be penetrated by intestinal fluids. Mineral oil is an effective emollient in enemas to soften fecal impactions, but it should be avoided in the elderly, the neurologically impaired, and in those with impaired swallowing, because of its aspiration risk and resultant lipoid pneumonitis.

Stimulant laxatives should be used in patients with severe constipation who do not respond to fiber

TABLE 3 Pharmacologic Management of Constipation.

Medication	Maximal Recommended Doses
Bulk Laxatives	
Psyllium (Metamucil)	Titrate up to 20 g/day[3]
Methylcellulose (Citrucel)	Titrate up to 20 g/day[3]
Polycarbophil (FiberCon)	Titrate up to 20 g/day[3]
Osmotic Laxatives	
Unabsorbed Sugars	
Lactulose (Cephulac, Chronulac)	15-30 mL once or twice daily
Sorbitol 70% (Cytosol)	15-30 mL once or twice daily
Polyethylene glycol (MiraLax)	17-36 g once or twice daily
Polyethylene glycol and electrolytes (GoLYTELY, NuLYTELY)[1]	17-36 g once or twice daily
Salts	
Magnesium hydroxide (Milk of Magnesia)	15-30 mL once or twice daily
Magnesium Citrate (Evac-Q-Mag)	150-300 mL as needed
Sodium phosphate (Fleet Enemas, Fleet Phospho-Soda)	10-25 mL with 12 oz (360 mL) of water as needed
Stimulant Laxatives	
Bisacodyl (Dulcolax)	5-10 mg suppository every night
Senna (Ex-Lax, Senokot)	70-100 g daily[3]
Cascara sagrada (Colamin)	2-5 mL daily
Aloe (casanthranol)[1]*	30-60 mg daily
Castor oil (Purge, Emulsoil)	15-30 mL daily
Stool Softeners	
Mineral Oil	5-15 mL orally at night for children, 15-45 mL for adults
Docusate sodium (Colace)	100 mg twice daily
Rectal enema or suppository	
Glycerin bisacodyl suppository	10 mg daily
Tap-water enema	500 mL daily
Phosphate enema (Fleet Enema)	120 mL daily
Mineral oil retention enema (Fleet Mineral Oil Enema)	100 mL daily
Prokinetic agent	
5-HT_4-receptor agonist Tegaserod (Zelnorm)[1]	6 mg twice daily

[1]Not FDA approved for this indication.
[3]Exceeds dosage recommended by the manufacturer.
*Available as a dietary supplement.

or osmotic laxatives. Common preparations of stimulant laxatives include senna (Ex-Lax), cascara sagrada, castor oil, and bisacodyl (Dulcolax). They increase intestinal motility and stimulate fluid secretion in the bowel lumen. They result in a bowel movement within 6 to 12 hours of oral ingestion or 15 to 60 minutes after rectal administration. It was believed that stimulant laxatives cause "cathartic colon," also described as loss of haustration and dilation of the colon, with long-time use, but there is no supporting evidence for this theory. Chronic use of anthraquinones (senna, cascara sagrada, aloe), which are widely used and may be abused, can cause melanosis coli, a brown-black pigmentation of the colonic mucosa. It has no clinical consequence and will regress if the patient stops taking stimulant laxatives. Often patients will have abused stimulant laxatives for many years before being seen for their constipation, and it can be difficult to change their habits because fiber and other conservative means do not produce the rapid results to which the patients have become accustomed.

Self-administration of *enemas* is an alternative means for patients who do not respond to oral laxatives for acute constipation. There are tap-water enemas, sodium phosphate enemas (Fleet enema), saline enemas, and oil-retention enemas. Tap-water and Fleet enemas are easy to administer and are relatively safe. Oil-retention enemas are useful for hard and impacted stool. Caution should be observed because some enema solutions can irritate the mucosa of the colon, including tap-water enemas. Fluid and electrolyte abnormalities can be seen with the administration of enemas. Volume overload and dilutional hyponatremia may occur in the elderly, children, and patients with megacolon after the administration of a tap-water enema. Sodium phosphate enemas may induce hyperphosphatemia and hypocalcemia in patients with renal insufficiency as a consequence of the absorption of large amounts of phosphate in the Fleet enema preparations.

Tegaserod (Zelnorm) is a colonic *prokinetic agent* that was recently approved for use in women with constipation predominant irritable bowel syndrome. It is a serotonin (5-HT_4) receptor agonist that accelerates transit through the small bowel and colon. In constipated patients, it improves stool consistency, frequency, and abdominal pain.

Treatment of Fecal Impaction

Patients with stool impaction and patients with hard stools that are difficult to expel require either twice-daily enemas for 3 days or digital disimpaction. Occasionally, sedation or anesthesia is required for manual disimpaction. Some patients may benefit from mineral oil enemas (Fleet Mineral Oil) to soften hard-stool impactions, which will ease rectal evacuation with manual disimpaction. An effective alternative approach is to drink 4 to 8 L of polyethylene glycol (GoLYTELY) to clean out the colon, specifically the hard stool that cannot be reached manually. Once the colon has been evacuated, these patients will require long-term therapy directed at maintaining regular, soft bowel movements. This can be accomplished by using a bowel regimen of laxatives and suppositories. Sorbitol and polyethylene glycol can be used initially to produce a bowel movement once a day to every other day. A stimulant laxative, such as bisacodyl or glycerin suppository, can be used to prevent recurrence of impaction if there is no bowel movement after 2 days. Once the patient is having regular bowel movements, laxative use can be weaned. After establishing a bowel regimen, it is important to assess for an underlying colonic or motility disorder.

Biofeedback

Neuromuscular conditioning using biofeedback techniques can be beneficial in the treatment of constipation caused by defecatory disorders, particularly by pelvic floor dyssynergia. Patients are taught, through trial and error with visual and auditory feedback, to relax the pelvic floor muscles and the external anal sphincter during straining with defecation. Biofeedback appears to be effective in up to 67% of patients with pelvic outlet dysfunction, as demonstrated in a recent systemic review of biofeedback studies, although data from controlled studies are lacking. Biofeedback also has overall excellent long-term results.

Surgical Approaches

Select patients with colonic inertia or intractable slow-transit constipation who fail an aggressive trial of medical therapy and do not have a defecatory disorder may require surgical intervention with total colonic resection and ileorectostomy. A recent review of 32 studies demonstrated that 39% to 100% of patients were satisfied after colectomy. The most common reported complications were small-bowel obstruction, diarrhea, and incontinence. It is recommended that motility studies of the upper gastrointestinal tract be performed prior to colectomy to rule out a generalized motility disorder. Patients should also undergo psychiatric evaluation prior to considering surgery, because coexisting psychiatric disorders have a less-favorable outcome after colectomy. Some anatomic problems, such as rectal prolapse and vaginal rectocele, may benefit from surgical resection.

FEVER

METHOD OF

Philip D. Walson, MD

Fever is the single most common symptom treated by primary care physicians. In the majority of visits, patients receive medications. Numerous studies have increased our knowledge about the pathophysiology of fever, as well as of the risks and benefits of treating it. Unfortunately, as many as 91% of parents and caregivers, as well as many health providers, harbor misconceptions about the dangers of, and the need to treat, fever. The unrealistic concerns of parents was termed "fever phobia" by Barton Schmitt in 1980. This "phobia" can result in many unnecessary diagnostic and therapeutic interventions.

Fever is a common manifestation of many medical conditions, both trivial and serious. Only in very rare situations, and only when extremely high (i.e., above 106°F [41.1°C]), can elevated body temperature cause harm, and it may even be protective. Treatment of fever can cause delay in seeking needed, disease-specific treatment or prolong recovery from disease. However, fever treatment can also have benefits, providing patients comfort, improving oral intake, and allowing for sleep, as well as discouraging unnecessary diagnostic evaluation or dangerous therapeutic interventions.

Pathophysiology of Fever

Both the decision whether to treat fever or not and the choice of methods used to lower body temperature require an appreciation of the pathophysiology of fever. There are multiple causes of elevated body temperature. Infectious causes of fever are the most common and are the only causes associated with an altered "setpoint" of the central "thermostat," located in the preoptic anterior hypothalamic region. It is important clinically to distinguish these infectious causes of fever from hyperthermia. Hyperthermia results from excessive heat production, altered heat dissipation, or pharmacologic or physiologic alterations in homeostatic temperature regulatory mechanisms. A risk:benefit analysis of lowering temperature depends on the underlying cause(s) of temperature elevation. True hyperthermia should be treated only by external cooling, whether it was caused by, for example, chemicals (e.g., salicylates, nitrophenol, anticholinergics, stimulants, anesthetics), dehydration, elevated environmental temperature or wrapping, excessive exercise, head trauma, or neurosurgery. Other noninfectious causes of fever, such as malignancy, hyperthyroidism, autoimmune diseases, and so forth, should receive disease-specific treatment.

This discussion deals with the symptomatic treatment of infection-associated fever caused by increases in inflammatory mediators (i.e., cytokines such as interleukin-1, interleukin-8, and tumor necrosis factor) that are released from cells, especially white blood cells, in response to infection. These mediators act on the central "thermostat" to reset the body temperature by causing production of prostaglandin E_2. There are many patient-specific factors that alter the response to these mediators. For example, patients who are very young or very old, malnourished, treated with certain drugs (i.e., steroids or nonsteroidal anti-inflammatory drugs [NSAIDs]), or have renal diseases can all have altered fever responses.

Definition of Fever

The definition of fever is arbitrary, in part because temperature variability, both between and within individuals, is rather large. "Normal," baseline temperatures differ between individuals. They also vary during the day by almost 3.6°F (2°C) (from 96.8°F [36°C] to 100°F [37.8°C]) in the same individual, with the highest temperatures at night. Some temperature variabilities are the results of differences in measurement techniques, patient age, environmental temperature, dress, body composition, exercise, and metabolic state. In older children and adults, an oral temperature above 99.5°F (37.5°C), a rectal temperature above 100.4°F (38°C), or an axillary temperature above 99°F (37.2°C) is generally accepted to constitute a fever.

Tympanic membrane temperature measurements are capable of predicting core, or rectal temperatures, but not all studies have validated the accuracy of tympanic measurements, especially in inexperienced hands. Accurate measurement of body temperature is not trivial, especially in ill or uncooperative patients. The site of measurement, the equipment used, the ambient temperature, the skill of the observer, and the cooperation of the subject all can have major effects on the accuracy of temperature measurements. For example, consumption of liquids, location and duration of the thermometer in the mouth, and mouth breathing all alter oral temperature measurements, especially if electronic temperature devices are used without disabling their automatic timing devices. Electronic temperature probes that are ingested orally and transmit core temperatures to a radio receiver device have even been used experimentally to obtain accurate measurements. Fortunately, there is seldom any need to obtain very accurate temperatures in the vast majority of clinical situations.

Risks and Benefits of Fever

Fever is associated with some harmful clinical effects such as fetal damage from fever in pregnancy, increased metabolic needs in malnutrition, and increased cardiac demand with borderline cardiac function. However, most of the misconceptions concerning fever are the result of other, weak, noncausal associations. There is a sound evolutionary theory that fever is beneficial, and despite some contrary opinions, there are also some data to support this theory. Fever has been shown in animal studies to enhance the immune response to many infectious agents and to some malignancies. Use of antipyretic drugs to lower fever increases both morbidity and mortality in infected laboratory animals, and prolongs varicella infection in humans. Much of the fear of fever is the result of concern that high fever can cause "brain damage." There are simply no data to support these fears, which appear to be perpetuated by the common association between fever and conditions such as brain trauma, central nervous system (CNS) infections, neurosurgery, hyperthermia, and febrile convulsions. Febrile convulsions are a special cause of fear. Yet in previously normal children, almost all simple febrile convulsions are associated with neither recurrence of seizures (febrile or otherwise) nor with any "brain damage." Most, if not *all*, children who are found to have "brain damage" after a high fever, with or without convulsions, were either suffering from a disease known to cause damage (e.g., meningitis) or had abnormal brain development prior to the onset of fever and convulsions. It is the presence of abnormal development preceding the seizure, not the recurrence of high fever or the clinical characteristics of the febrile seizures themselves, that is most predictive of seizure recurrence or "brain damage." There is also no evidence that parents can prevent recurrent febrile convulsions with the use of antipyretic drugs. Prescribing or using such therapy can lead to failure, frustration, and parental guilt.

Clinical Aspects of Treatment Decisions

In addition to the risks of symptomatic therapies (see later), the major risk of fever treatment involves delays in diagnosis and initiation of specific treatment. The physician must always first attempt to diagnose the cause of the fever and determine what benefit, if any, would come from specific or nonspecific therapy.

Treatment of hyperthermia requires cooling and specific therapy as mentioned previously. Fevers from drugs or toxins require specific toxicologic management. Malignancies and autoimmune diseases need specific drug therapy. Symptomatic therapy can also be used but can be dangerous. For example, shock can occur in Hodgkin's lymphoma patients given antipyretics. In infectious causes of fever, treatment decisions involve the type and seriousness of the infection, and which, if any, specific and nonspecific therapy is needed. The assessment of the febrile patient is a critically important, complicated, clinical process that is often transparent to the patient or parent. The need for therapy depends on a clinical assessment of how ill the patient is, rather than how high the temperature is. This is especially true in patients who have any decreased ability to generate a febrile response or to tolerate delay in specific treatment (e.g., elderly, malnourished, immunocompromised, newborn, or renal patients). In all patients, the decision to treat and what to use are based on the patient's history, physical findings, and, occasionally, on laboratory test results.

There is a general misconception that trivial causes of fever respond more readily to antipyretic medication than do serious infections. In fact, there is no difference in the response of fever to symptomatic therapy between children with serious as opposed to trivial illnesses. Whether symptomatic therapy is given or not, the physician must continually assess the patient's overall clinical condition and not just whether the temperature decreases.

Nonpharmacologic Therapy

A number of nondrug therapies are available. If used, they should make the patient more comfortable rather than just lower the reading on a thermometer. Overwrapped patients should have extra clothing removed. Activities that raise the body temperature, such as shivering, crying, and excessive motor activity should be minimized. Excessive environmental temperature (i.e., above 77°F [25°C]) should be avoided, but the child should not become chilled enough to shiver. Extra fluids should be encouraged to prevent dehydration. Sponge bathing is controversial. If attempted, only comfortable temperature water should be used and only small portions of the body exposed to the water. The sponging should be stopped if the child becomes too upset or inconsolable, and the child should be held and comforted by a competent adult at all times. Ice water and alcohol bathing must *not* be used. Alcohol is absorbed through the skin and lungs and can cause a chemical pneumonitis or ketosis; both ice water and alcohol can cause shivering, discomfort, and increased motor activity.

Antipyretics/analgesics are commonly used for the symptomatic treatment of fever. Their major advantage is their ability to control pain. They may make patients more comfortable even when the fever is not controlled. Studies in adults demonstrate that there is only a modest correlation between improvement in subjective feelings of wellness and temperature decrease. Parents and patients should be encouraged to think of these drugs as pain killers rather than as fever reducers. The goal of therapy with antipyretic/analgesics is to make patients more comfortable. If this were understood, caretakers would be less likely to treat thermometer readings and less likely to awaken quietly sleeping patients in order to dose them again or to continue to dose comfortable, awake patients with minimally elevated temperatures.

There are two general classes of antipyretics/analgesics: acetaminophen (Tylenol) and nonsteroidal anti-inflammatory drugs (NSAIDs) (e.g., salicylates, ibuprofen [Advil], and the newer relatively selective cyclooxygenase^{-2} [COX^{-2}] inhibitors).

The choice of drug is based on a number of things, including the clinical situation, cost, availability, dosage forms, patient age, drug allergies, and other patient characteristics that influence the relative safety of the individual agents.

There are a number of prescription and over-the-counter NSAIDs that are effective antipyretics/analgesics; some have specific benefits such as parenteral dosage forms (e.g., ketorolac [Toradol]) or prolonged durations of action (e.g., naproxen [Naprosyn]). Although the drugs are useful in selected clinical situations, the relative safety and efficacy of these alternatives have not yet been sufficiently studied to recommend them for routine symptomatic fever therapy. This includes the many parenteral antipyretics that are marketed in other countries (e.g., antipyrine, propacetamol), but are not available in the United States.

Pharmacotherapeutic Agents

ACETAMINOPHEN

Acetaminophen (Tylenol) can be very inexpensive and is available in a wide variety of brands and dosage forms. Although it does have the ability to inhibit certain peripheral prostaglandin synthetic enzymes, it is not generally classified as an NSAID. It has been available chemically for more than a century and used clinically for almost 60 years. It is rapidly and well absorbed orally and rectally. Parenteral dosage forms are available in some European, but not North American, countries. It is a very effective antipyretic and analgesic, but its anti-inflammatory activity is weak. There is a 1- to 3-hour delay between the attainment of maximal plasma concentrations and therapeutic effects. Clearance is largely by hepatic metabolism to inactive and nontoxic metabolites. However, in overdose, its usual metabolic pathways can be saturated and a toxic quinone produced. This metabolite can be detoxified by endogenous glutathione. However, when production of the toxic metabolite exceeds glutathione stores, such as in overdosed malnourished patients or patients whose hepatic metabolizing enzymes are induced (by cigarettes, anticonvulsants, etc.), these detoxification mechanisms can be overwhelmed, leading to hepatic or even renal toxicity. Except for rare, poorly substantiated reports of hepatotoxicity in alcoholic patients who took therapeutic doses chronically, the drug appears to be very safe in patients taking usual therapeutic doses. Even in overdose, if diagnosed and treated (especially if within 12 to 24 hours), the use of acetylcysteine (Mucomyst) (as a glutathione substitute) is remarkably effective in preventing serious morbidity or mortality. However, if the diagnosis of overdose is delayed, especially in patients taking enzyme-inducing drugs, in pregnant women, and in malnourished patients, serious or even fatal hepatic or renal toxicity can occur. Yet despite its potential to produce toxicity in overdose, acetaminophen is by far the safest analgesic/antipyretic drug to use therapeutically, especially in patients with gastrointestinal (GI) ulcers, bleeding problems, allergies, asthma, or renal diseases, and in pregnant or elderly patients. Therapeutic acetaminophen use can be problematic only in patients at risk for chronic, accidental, or intentional overdose or who are pregnant. Dosing is generally 10 to 15 mg per kg every 4 to 6 hours for 3 to 4 days. There is good theoretical and clinical evidence that at least 15 mg per kg, and probably

20 to 30 mg per kg[3], can be given safely, especially as a "loading dose," and be effective for up to 8 hours (therefore not changing the total daily mg per kg exposure). Doses in adults are from 325 to 650 mg every 3 to 4 hours. There are multiple dosage forms available, including drops, elixirs, syrups, tablets, capsules, caplets, chewable tablets, and suppositories, and even prolonged-release preparations that allow for less frequent dosing. It is not known whether double-dosing of a rapid-release preparation would be more effective or less safe than use of these less frequent, higher dose, prolonged-release products.

IBUPROFEN

Ibuprofen (Advil) is a classic NSAID that works as a reversible inhibitor of prostaglandin synthesis. Of note, it is available as a racemic mixture of two optical (R and S) isomers, which differ in pharmacokinetics, as well as in therapeutic and toxic effects. The R isomer is converted enzymatically in the body to the more active and less toxic S isomer. It is unclear whether the use of pure S isomer would improve the therapeutic ratio, and this could increase costs significantly. Although used for decades as an anti-inflammatory and analgesic, ibuprofen has more recently been widely used as an antipyretic. It is rapidly absorbed, but the percentage absorbed can differ between preparations and can be decreased by food. Ibuprofen at the doses used for antipyresis produces a more rapid temperature fall and longer duration of action (usually 5 to 6 and up to 8 hours) than acetaminophen after the first dose, especially in children with higher (i.e., above 102.5°F [39.2°C]) temperatures. This advantage may not be maintained with repeated dosing.

The toxicity of ibuprofen is similar to that of all NSAIDs. GI upset is much more common than with acetaminophen but is usually minor, especially in children. Serious GI, renal, pulmonary, allergic, and bone marrow toxicity occurs rarely. Patients with hypovolemia or renal disease can develop renal failure after taking ibuprofen. Asthmatic patients can develop bronchospasm. If taken by a pregnant woman in the third trimester, fetal toxicity can occur (e.g., closure of the ductus arteriosus, delayed labor, decreased fetal urine output, oligohydramnios, bleeding, etc.). Sudden, previously silent, life-threatening GI hemorrhage (especially in the elderly), GI ulcers, hepatic damage, platelet dysfunction, hypertension, rashes, worsening of psoriasis, bone marrow suppression, headaches, confusion, and even aseptic meningitis all can occur. Toxicity after single therapeutic doses is much more common than with acetaminophen, but less common than with other NSAIDs, including salicylates or naproxen. The risk of Reye's syndrome is unknown. The major advantage of ibuprofen, in addition to its longer duration of action and excellent efficacy, is its safety in overdose. Although ibuprofen can produce life-threatening toxicity in certain susceptible populations (e.g., ulcer or renal patients, pregnant women, or asthmatics), it appears to be extremely safe when taken in overdose by most of the general population. Except for mild acidosis and some CNS changes, there are few reports of serious, nonidiosyncratic, acute, or long-term toxicity after even massive overdoses.

Ibuprofen is available both by prescription and over the counter in a number of liquid and solid dosage forms from a number of manufacturers at a variety of prices. Over-the-counter dosing recommendations result in about 5 to 10 mg per kg per dose, which is given every 6 to 8 hours. Higher temperatures may respond better to the higher dosages, but after the first dose, repeat doses as little as 2.5 mg per kg[*] may be equally effective. The adult over-the-counter dose is 200 to 400 mg given every 4 to 6 hours.

SALICYLATES

Aspirin—acetylated salicylic acid—is the classic NSAID. Although still important analgesic and antiplatelet drugs, the salicylates are seldom used as only antipyretics because of safety concerns. Use is especially rare in children. Fear of drug-induced Reye's syndrome has stopped salicylate use in all but very rare childhood diseases (e.g., for Kawasaki disease, arthritis, or inflammatory bowel diseases), or as components of various preparations (e.g., topical methylsalicylate and bismuth subsalicylate preparations).

All salicylates are rapidly and well absorbed, and both metabolized and excreted renally as both metabolites and unchanged drugs. The metabolism and distribution of salicylates are saturable, as well as time, dose, duration, and pH-dependent processes. This is part of the reason that toxicity is so problematic. The onset of different effects are variable. Noncompetitive antiplatelet effects occur very rapidly; platelet prostaglandin synthetase is irreversibly acetylated when aspirin is rapidly deacetylated (half-life about 15 minutes). This results in inhibition of platelet function that persists for the life of the affected platelet, because platelets cannot resynthesize the prostaglandin synthetase. The antipyretic and additional antiplatelet effects of salicylates are reversible, last only about 3 to 4 hours, and are slower in onset.

Aspirin and other salicylates are very inexpensive and effective antipyretics, analgesics, and anti-inflammatory drugs. They are probably the standard in terms of efficacy against which other drugs (at least in adults) should be compared. Toxicity, rather than cost or efficacy, limits their more widespread use. Adverse effects from salicylates are common and can be serious after both therapeutic use and with accidental and intentional overdose. They produce the same GI, hepatic, renal, allergic, platelet, fetal,

[3]Exceeds dosage recommended by the manufacturer.

*Less than dosage recommended by the manufacturer.

and pulmonary toxicity as ibuprofen. Asthmatic patients with nasal polyps are especially prone to aspirin induced bronchospasm. Unique to aspirin as an NSAID is its ability to produce irreversible (in addition to reversible) platelet dysfunction. This has been used to prevent conditions associated with platelet adhesion such as myocardial dysfunction and intracardiac valve replacement. Salicylate toxicity from therapeutic, accidental, or suicidal overdose is common and often life-threatening. Because there are safer, inexpensive, equally effective drugs available, the use of salicylates for symptomatic antipyresis cannot be recommended, especially in children.

COMBINATIONS

Use of combinations of two antipyretics for fever, although a common clinical practice, is mentioned only to seriously question this approach. The combination of aspirin and acetaminophen was historically shown to be more effective at lowering temperature than either drug alone. Similar data are not available for acetaminophen plus ibuprofen. However, more than one half of pediatricians use this approach, many of whom cite as the source of this unproven practice recommendations from the American Academy of Pediatrics that simply do not exist. There is no reason to believe that it is necessary to lower temperature more than can be done with adequate doses of a single drug. Combinations have not been proven to produce quicker or longer-lasting responses, and studies show that lowering of temperature does not correlate well with comfort provided. It is also not known whether the current practice of alternating usual therapeutic doses of acetaminophen with ibuprofen is either more effective or as safe as the use of a single drug alone at usual, or at increased, doses. Combining drugs is more expensive, adds toxicity, could delay proper diagnosis or therapy, and contributes to the impression that lowering temperature, rather than controlling symptoms, is the primary goal of therapy. This practice perpetuates unnecessary "fever phobia."

Proper treatment of fever can be inexpensive and effective, and can relieve discomfort and anxiety. However, much needs to be done to educate patients, parents, and health providers about rational fever evaluation and treatment.

Acknowledgment

This work was supported by a cooperative agreement from the Agency for Healthcare Research and Quality for the UNC Center for Education and Research on Therapeutics (award number U18 HS 10397).

COUGH

Charles A. Polnitsky, MD

Cough is a source of concern to patients, contacts, and health care providers. It ranges from a barely audible, self-limited minor irritation to a persistent problem that results in major disruption of daily activities and restful sleep. Cough is the third most common reason for an office visit, resulting in approximately 30 million patient contacts annually. Because there are numerous and diverse etiologies for cough—and because studies indicate that up to 50% of chronic cases may be multifactorial—it is essential to work through a list of possible causes and avoid the temptation to prescribe a nonspecific remedy.

Pathophysiology

The stimulation of airway receptors by irritants, foreign bodies, and mucus triggers cough. It is the result of a reflex arc that begins in the pharynx, larynx and bronchial airways. Signals carried mainly through the vagus nerve arrive in the medullary cough center where the response is generated. A deep inspiration is followed by forceful contraction of the diaphragm and accessory muscles. It has been recently questioned whether glottic closure is essential for maximal effectiveness, but when vocal cord apposition is possible, it contributes to expiratory pressure that may reach 300 mm Hg. Peak expiratory flow can be as high as 500 mph. The rapid expulsion of air carries along mucus, purulent secretions, aspirated liquids and food matter, and any other foreign bodies that might have found their way into the respiratory tract. Extrapolation from animal studies has provided much of the data, and full understanding of the cough reflex in humans is yet to be gained. The production of a cough can also be volitional.

For cough to be maximally effective, the reflex arc must not be impeded (as in depressed mental status or mucosal sensory fatigue associated with immobility) and respiratory muscle strength must be preserved. It is also important to have a potential vital capacity that is not reduced by restrictive lung or chest wall conditions, loss of pulmonary elastic recoil (emphysema), or limited expiratory airflow (bronchospasm, mucus plugging). Also, mucus viscosity and adhesiveness must not be excessive.

Complications

Persistent cough can induce respiratory mucosal irritation, producing a self-propagating situation in which bronchial receptors continue to signal even after the original illness or condition has passed. The consequences of severe or chronic cough are multiple, and adversely impact upon many major organ systems (Table 1).

Acute Cough

Acute, self-limited cough is usually associated with a symptom complex that is easily identified, such as typical viral upper respiratory tract infection (RTI), acute bacterial sinusitis, pertussis, acute exacerbation of chronic bronchitis (AECB), and pneumonia. The cough of viral RTI may persist for 6 weeks or longer. It can be alleviated by an ipratropium bromide metered-dose inhaler (Atrovent MDI)[1], 2 to 4 puffs qid (4 times per day), or by inhaled albuterol MDI (Proventil)[1], 2 inhalations qid. More severe symptoms can be suppressed by an inhaled corticosteroid (triamcinolone [Azmacort MDI][1] 2 to 4 inhalations qid; budesonide [Pulmicort DPI][1] 2 to 4 inhalations daily). Cough suppression by dextromethorphan (Benylin), codeine, and more potent narcotics is widely believed to be effective, although controlled trials are few and have failed to provide positive evidence. There is considerable variability in patients' expectations and practitioners' responses to complaints suggesting infection of the sinuses. The misdiagnosis of nasal and sinus congestion caused by a viral respiratory tract infection results in the frequent but inappropriate prescription of antibiotics. A placebo-controlled, double-blind trial of antibiotic treatment in 252 adults showed no therapeutic advantage, and those receiving placebo had significantly fewer adverse effects. In most cases, the condition resolves in 5 to 10 days. Sinus infection syndromes that fail to improve—or worsen—during this interval are likely to be bacterial (*Streptococcus pneumoniae*, *Haemophilus influenzae*, and *Moraxella catarrhalis*) in origin and should be treated with an antibiotic (amoxicillin clavulanate [Augmentin] 875 mg bid [twice a day]), usually in a regimen including saline irrigation and topical or systemic decongestants. Antibiotic treatment of early pertussis is important. Timely diagnosis is often made in children, but in adults, the acute infectious phase has usually passed before the entity is considered. Treatment specifics of AECB and pneumonia are beyond the scope of this article. Several other diagnostic entities require special mention.

[1]Not FDA approved for this indication.

TABLE 1 Complications of Cough

General
Ruptured conjunctival and nasal veins
Displacement of IV and gastrostomy tubes
Sleep deprivation
Social alienation
Neurologic
Headache
Vertebral artery dissection
Air embolism
Cardiovascular
Hypotension; syncope
Bradycardia; ventricular ectopy
Pulmonary
Pneumothorax
Laryngeal trauma
Bronchial rupture
Rib fracture
Asthma exacerbation
Gastrointestinal
Gastroesophageal reflux; emesis
Splenic rupture
Inguinal herniation
Urinary
Incontinence
Bladder inversion

ACUTE BRONCHITIS

Acute bronchitis, an acute respiratory illness with cough (either productive or nonproductive) occurring in an otherwise healthy adult in whom pneumonia has been excluded, occurs approximately 12 million times annually in the United States. The prodrome can include myalgias and malaise. Low-grade fever (<38°C [100.5°F]) is common; purulent sputum has been reported in up to 48% of typical cohorts. The cough usually persists for 1 to 3 weeks although it can be present for as long as 6 weeks. Viruses, particularly influenza, parainfluenza, adenovirus, rhinovirus, coronavirus, and, in the elderly, respiratory syncytial virus (RSV) are nearly always the cause. Other occasional organisms include *Mycoplasma, Chlamydia,* and *Bordetella*. Significantly, the bacterial pathogens that most commonly cause pneumonia (*S. pneumoniae*, *H. influenzae*, and *M. catarrhalis*) are rarely, if ever found. Despite this microbiologic profile, studies show that 70% to 90% of these cases are inappropriately treated with antibiotics, a practice that is considered to be the most significant factor in the development of resistant bacteria. Inhaled albuterol (Proventil)[1] palliates the cough.

FOREIGN BODY ASPIRATION

Individuals of all ages and clinical conditions are at risk of aspiration. Children are notorious for choking on small objects, parts of toys, and food such as candy. Bronchoscopists are frequently called upon to remove dental amalgam, broken teeth, ballpoint pen parts, and tongue studs from the airways of adolescents and adults. The elderly are at additional risk of food and pill aspiration because of depressed cough

[1]Not FDA approved for this indication.

and gag reflexes, as well as altered mental status secondary to illness and medication effects. In most cases, the history clearly indicates that a foreign body has been inhaled, but this is not always the case. The physical examination may reveal a localized wheeze. The chest radiograph will show the object if it is not radiolucent; it may reveal atelectasis if there is a completely obstructed airway; or it can be normal. If discovered early, most objects can be removed endoscopically. Once local inflammation and edema have surrounded a foreign body, surgical resection may be the only option.

Definition of Chronic Cough

The American College of Chest Physicians considers a cough to be chronic if it persists for >8 weeks, occurs in an otherwise healthy nonsmoker who has not had an irritant exposure, is not taking an angiotensin-converting enzyme (ACE) inhibitor, and who has a normal chest film. Studies show that in nearly 100% of such cases, an etiology can be found. Most significantly, abolition of cough has been accomplished in 84% to 98% of individuals in various reported studies.

Diagnostic Approach

A comprehensive history and physical examination are the most important bases for evaluation. Smokers should have a chest film. If the patient is taking an ACE inhibitor, this medication should be discontinued; an angiotensin-receptor blocking agent can be substituted. It is best to avoid adding a β-blocker, because it may complicate the picture by inducing bronchospasm. If the cough does not disappear, all remaining individuals should have a chest film done. If it is negative (or shows known stable abnormalities), attention is focused on the three most common causes of chronic cough: postnasal drip (PND), asthma, and gastroesophageal reflux (GER). In one survey of 30 patients, this triad accounted for 48%, 20%, and 17% of cases, respectively, accounting for 85% of the total. Other groups have reported these three entities to cause 72% to 100% of cough complaints. Figure 1 is a simplified algorithm for treating chronic cough.

POSTNASAL DRIP SYNDROME

Excess mucus production by the nasal mucosa and sinuses can be caused by nonspecific stimuli, IgE-mediated allergy, or chronic bacterial infection. Vasomotor rhinitis (VMR, also known as perennial rhinitis) is a nonspecific, nonallergic, noninfectious condition that affects 5% to 10% of the population. Symptoms include nasal congestion, rhinorrhea, an irritated or tickling feeling in the throat, a need to clear the throat, sneezing, and cough. There is individual variation in specific complaints, but no seasonal association. Precipitating factors include odors, exposure to various irritants, variations in humidity and temperature, certain foods, and alcohol.

Clear or opalescent mucus adherent to the posterior pharyngeal may be seen, but its absence does not rule out the diagnosis. By default, the condition has historically been treated with topical steroids and/or oral antihistamines and decongestants, with inconsistent results. More recently, the topical nasal

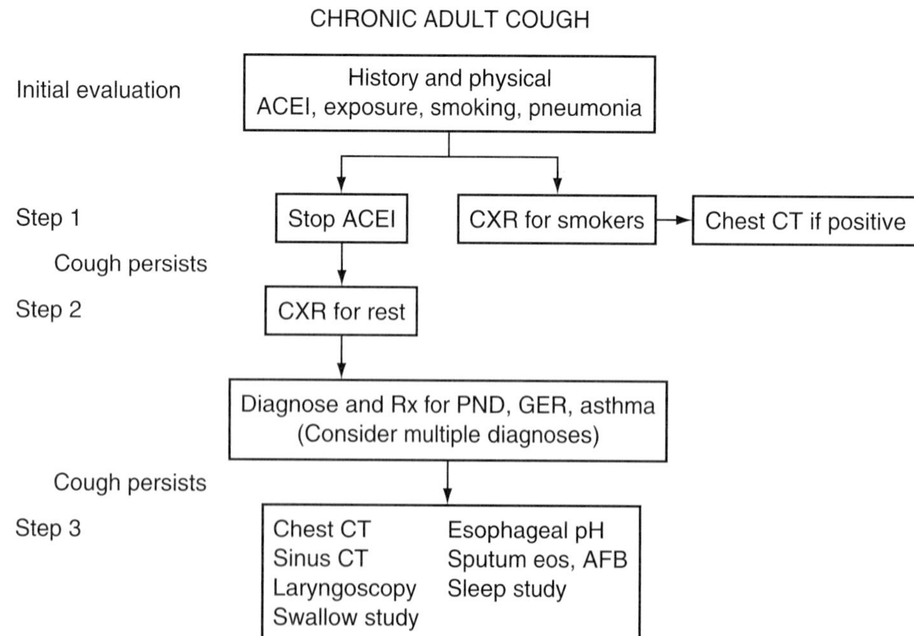

FIGURE 1 Simplified algorithm for the evaluation of chronic cough in an adult. ACEI = angiotensin-converting enzyme inhibitor; AFB = acid fast bacillus; CT = computed tomography; CXR = chest x-ray; GER = gastroesophageal reflux; PND = postnasal drip.

antihistamine azelastine (Astelin) was shown to be of benefit in randomized, placebo-controlled trials. Topical saline sprays (AYR, Simply Saline)[1] have also been employed with some success and have the additional advantages of being drug-free and relatively inexpensive. Avoidance of known stimuli should also be recommended.

Seasonal rhinitis ("hay fever") and perennial allergic rhinitis are IgE mediated and show inflammatory changes in histology. Prevalence is increasing worldwide, along with asthma. Allergen exposure results in congestion, rhinorrhea, conjunctivitis, lethargy, headache, and poor concentration ability. The nasal mucosa is classically pale and boggy; polyps may be present; secretions are watery and increased. Diagnosis is usually made by examination in the context of an atopic history. In some cases, allergen skin or radioallergosorbent assay test (RAST) testing is confirmatory and helps to identify substances that should be avoided. Treatment options are many and include ophthalmic and nasal topical chromoids (Crolom ophthalmic; NasalCrom nasal spray) and ketotifen (Zaditor ophthalmic); topical nasal steroids (budesonide [Rhinocort], flunisolide [Nasalide]); and systemic antihistamines. The older, sedating antihistamine diphenhydramine (Benadryl) is more potent, but its use is limited in many individuals because of side effects. Second-generation antihistamines such as loratadine (Claritin OTC) and fexofenadine (Allegra), with or without pseudoephedrine, are most commonly used. The combination with decongestant adds convenience, but some people experience discomforting tremors, palpitations, or anxiety from sympathomimetics. Adding small doses of as-needed daytime over-the-counter pseudoephedrine can solve this problem. Other pharmacologic treatments include leukotriene receptor antagonists such as montelukast (Singulair). Avoidance of allergens is an important component of treatment, but is often difficult to achieve. A recent study indicated that the use of dust mite barrier bed coverings as a single measure reduced household levels of mite antigen, but did not result in amelioration of rhinitis symptoms. When a combined routine of environmental control and medical treatment has failed, desensitization should be considered. As a final resort, therapy with injectable monoclonal anti-IgE antibody omalizumab (Xolair)[1] can be considered. The full side-effect profile may not be known for this new modality, and the cost can be prohibitive ($10,000 or more per year).

CHRONIC SINUSITIS

When symptoms of sinus pain, purulent discharge, and congestion persist beyond 12 weeks, the condition is classified as chronic rhinosinusitis. In this case, microbial flora may include mixed aerobic and anaerobic bacteria as well as fungi. Most patients with this diagnosis require consultation with an otolaryngologist. Antibiotic therapy for 6 weeks or longer may be necessary, and may require combinations to cover staphylococcus, anaerobes, and pseudomonas. If the condition fails to improve or becomes recurrent, a coronal sinus computed tomography (CT) to evaluate the ostiomeatal complexes and rule out neoplasm is usually performed. Endoscopic examination and surgery are frequently necessary.

ASTHMA

Cough frequently accompanies asthma, especially if it is suboptimally controlled. Current standards for diagnosis and treatment of asthma in children and adults are found in the National Asthma Education and Prevention Program (NAEPP) reports from the National Heart, Lung, and Blood Institute (http://www.nhlbi.nih.gov). The difficulty lies in the fact that for many individuals, especially children, cough is the *only* manifestation of asthma. Peak flow and spirometric values may be normal. Testing before and after bronchodilator administration should be routine; if significant bronchodilation occurs, it indicates an underlying relative bronchospasm. When these conventional tests are normal, abnormal bronchial hyperreactivity can be demonstrated by provocation spirometry, usually employing methacholine. The test is safe and may be essential to confirm the suspicion of cough variant asthma. Treatment is the same as for conventional wheezing asthma. Because the condition typically is present on a daily basis, it meets NAEPP criteria for daily maintenance therapy with an anti-inflammatory agent (inhaled corticosteroids such as low-dose budesonide [Pulmicort] 200 μg) with a long-acting β-agonist (formoterol [Foradil] or salmeterol [Serevent]) if needed for additional control. Combination products are available, but their use trades slight convenience for reduced dosage flexibility. All asthmatics should also have a short-acting beta agonist (albuterol) inhaler for rescue treatment. Under no circumstances should a long-acting beta agonist be employed as monotherapy. Published reports have indicated that although they may provide excellent symptomatic relief from the bronchospastic component of asthma, they have no anti-inflammatory effect. Asthmatics employing them as a single maintenance agent have experienced a small but significant increase in severe and fatal attacks. For severe, oral steroid-dependent asthma, monoclonal anti-IgE antibody (Xolair) improves control and reduces or eliminates chronic systemic steroid needs.

Finally, the "one airway" hypothesis should be mentioned. Uncontrolled allergic rhinitis may seriously compromise the control of asthma. In cases where both conditions contribute to cough, failure to treat upper airway atopy may result in failure to eliminate cough.

[1]Not FDA approved for this indication.

GASTROESOPHAGEAL REFLUX

Gastric acid reflux into the esophagus, frequently accompanied by microaspiration during sleep, is responsible for 21% to 41% of cough complaints. When symptomatic, diagnosis is fairly straightforward once angina and other possible chest pain etiologies are ruled out. GER, however, is clinically silent in 50% to 75% of coughers. Esophageal pH monitoring has classically been advocated as a necessary diagnostic step before treatment is begun. The test is not widely available, is cumbersome to perform, and is costly. In one series, an empiric trial of antireflux therapy with omeprazole 40 mg (Prilosec) or a similar proton pump inhibitor (PPI), occasionally supplemented by a promotility agent (metoclopramide) along with behavior modification (weight reduction, high-protein antireflux diet, and elevation of the head of the bed), successfully diagnosed and treated the condition in 79%. Six to 8 weeks of treatment were needed. Other investigators indicate that up to 3 months of treatment, frequently with higher doses, were required for remission of cough. Considering the excellent results from appropriate empiric treatment regimens, many practitioners now reserve pH testing for nonresponders. Histamine-2 antagonists such as ranitidine (Zantac) are not recommended for initial acid suppressive therapy; they are significantly less potent than the PPIs and have not yielded comparable results in clinical trials. A small series of eight patients were reported to be refractory to intensive therapy that resulted in documented elimination of esophageal acid. They were improved by antireflux surgery. It should be noted that there is a continuing debate over medical versus surgical treatment of chronic GER in general.

OTHER CAUSES

The remaining group of patients whose cough is not caused by what has been called the "pathologic triad" have a wide variety of diagnoses (Table 2), several of which require specific mention. Eosinophilic bronchitis, characterized by persistent cough, sputum eosinophilia, normal spirometry, and absence of reactivity on methacholine challenge, was found in 13% of one reported series and 10% of another. Diagnosis was confirmed by cell count on induced sputum. Improvement began within 3 weeks of treatment with inhaled budesonide (Pulmicort)[1] 400 μg bid. The chronic bronchitis of smokers and some workers with industrial exposure is characterized by daily sputum production. Many individuals become unaware of the cough and deny or minimize it even when queried; observation during the interview or information from a household member may indicate its presence. Elimination of the irritant may lead to resolution, although many smokers with chronic asthmatic bronchitis continue to be symptomatic even after smoking cessation. For both current and former smokers, provision of a β_2-agonist inhaler (albuterol)[1] may improve sputum clearance and alleviate some of the cough. It will not change the progression of any underlying chronic obstructive pulmonary disease (COPD). Obstructive sleep apnea (OSA) has been linked to cough through several mechanisms. Forceful inspiratory effort during apnea fosters GER, which in turn stimulates cough or exacerbates asthma. The inspiratory gasp that terminates an apnea also results in aspiration of pharyngeal secretions and refluxed gastric material. Infection with the *Mycobacterium avium* and *Mycobacterium intracellulare* complex (MAC) can cause chronic cough in several non-HIV populations. Persons of both genders with COPD, healed cavitary tuberculosis, bronchiectasis, and other scarring lung diseases become infected with atypical mycobacteria and present with persistent cough, weight loss, dyspnea, hemoptysis, and infiltrates or nodules on chest radiography. Nonsmoking women older than age 50 years, without a history of lung disease, are also predisposed. Diagnosis requires that other causes be ruled out, after which multiple sputum cultures growing MAC must be obtained. Bronchoscopic washings and biopsy are needed when expectorated sputum is not adequate. Treatment with macrolides and antituberculous drugs until sputum clears may take 1 year or more. In some refractory cases, surgical resection is needed. In appropriate circumstances, other diagnostic modalities are indicated.

TABLE 2 Differential Diagnosis of Cough

"Pathologic Triad"
Postnasal drip syndrome
Gastroesophageal reflux
Asthma
Upper Airway
Chronic sinusitis
Vocal cord lesions
Irritation through auricular branch of vagus
Chronic aspiration
Obstructive sleep apnea
Lower Airway
Chronic obstructive pulmonary disease
Chronic bronchitis
Smoking; environmental exposure
Eosinophilic bronchitis
Bronchiectasis
Foreign body aspiration
Bronchiectasis
Tuberculosis and atypical mycobacteria
Sarcoidosis
Interstitial lung diseases
Pediatric Specific
Congenital heart disease
Tracheoesophageal fistula
Bronchial cysts

[1]Not FDA approved for this indication.

These include chest CT and fiberoptic examination of vocal cords and swallowing function. A few points about ACE inhibitors deserve mention, although it is assumed that a diagnosis of chronicity will not be made until the drug has been withdrawn and the cough persists. The onset of cough may be within a week of institution or may occur 6 months or more after the drug was begun. Sputum production is rare. Pulmonary function tests are normal in the absence of other lung conditions. Cough resolves within several days of drug discontinuation or substitution with another drug of the same class. Angiotensin-receptor blockers have not been shown to be protussive.

Chronic Cough in Children

The "pathologic triad" (PND, asthma, and GER) tops the list of causes in children as well as adults. Children are also prone to developing postinfectious coughs that may persist for months following viral infections and pertussis. Cardiac and pulmonary congenital abnormalities usually present in infancy, although a delayed onset of cystic fibrosis is not unusual. Active and passive inhalation of tobacco smoke and recreational drugs should be considered under many circumstances. Foreign bodies in the tracheobronchial tree or ear are more common in infants and children. Habit or psychogenic cough may begin with an illness and become persistent. In patients of all ages, this diagnosis remains one of exclusion.

Nonspecific Treatment

There is little objective evidence that medications other than morphine effectively suppress chronic cough. In general, treatment of the underlying cause improves or eliminates the problem. Some patients with a bronchiectatic form of chronic bronchitis benefit from monthly 5-day courses of rotating antibiotics, aimed at reducing the bacterial burden of their colonized airways. Choices include doxycycline (Vibramycin) 100 mg, cefuroxime (Ceftin) 250 mg, levofloxacin 250 mg (Levaquin), and clarithromycin (Biaxin) 250 mg bid. Those with extremely viscid sputum sometimes benefit from the regular use of oral guaifenesin in adequate doses (Humibid LA, 1200 mg po [by mouth] every 12 hours). Inhaled ipratropium (Atrovent)[1] and albuterol (Proventil)[1], either alone or in combination (Combivent MDI[1]; DuoNeb nebulizer solution[1]) are frequently effective. Although the indications for the use of inhaled steroids in COPD patients without demonstrable response to bronchodilators remains the subject of fierce international debate, many clinicians and researchers have observed the amelioration of symptoms and reduction of exacerbations with their use. Finally, some investigators report improved sputum clearance in bronchiectasis and COPD patients employing a handheld mucus clearance device (Flutter).

[1]Not FDA approved for this indication.

TREATMENT OF INSOMNIA

METHOD OF
Martin Reite, MD

Three things should be remembered when considering treatment of an insomnia complaint. First, insomnia is more often a symptom, than a specific disorder. Second, it is important to perform a systematic differential diagnosis, keeping in mind the possibility that there will very likely be more than one cause of an insomnia complaint. Finally, the cause of the complaint can usually be determined, and most patients complaining of insomnia can be helped. Also, insomnia must not be trivialized.

Insomnia is among the most frequent complaints in the population; untreated insomnia is associated with increases in new-onset anxiety and depression, increased daytime sleepiness, and increased health-related concerns.

Insomnia can include difficulty in getting to sleep (sleep-onset insomnia), difficulty staying asleep (sleep-maintenance insomnia), or early morning awakening (terminal insomnia). Because such subtypes are not stable over time, this method of subtyping may have little clinical usefulness. As a rule, insomnia complaints are more frequent in women, elderly persons, and patients of lower socioeconomic status.

Screening for Sleep Complaints

Three routine questions, illustrated in Table 1, will detect most significant sleep problems. A positive answer to any of these questions merits consideration of a more detailed sleep history to determine whether in fact a sleep disorder is likely present. Table 2 outlines the items to be covered in a sleep history.

Sources of diagnostic information should include the bed partner whenever possible because many sleep-related symptoms are apparent only to the bed partner. A several-week daily sleep diary can also be useful at this stage of the evaluation because it can

TABLE 1 Detection of Specific Sleep Disorders

Are you content with your sleep? (identifies most insomnia complaints)
Are you excessively sleepy during the day? (identifies most disorders of excessive sleepiness)
Does your bed partner complain about your sleep? (identifies most parasomnia disorders)

provide a detailed daily description of sleep/wake activity patterns.

Transient and Short-Term Insomnia

Transient (1 to several days) and short-term (up to 3 weeks) insomnias are typically stress related, and respond well to pharmacologic (short-term hypnotic) intervention. They should be considered for active treatment, because untreated short-term insomnia can lead to a state of "conditioned arousal" resulting in a chronic insomnia.

Differential Diagnosis of the Chronic Insomnia Complaint

The differential diagnosis of a chronic insomnia complaint can represent a more challenging task and requires a thorough differential diagnostic evaluation, which includes systematically considering the conditions or combinations of conditions that are most likely to result in insomnia complaints. General practice parameters for the evaluation of chronic insomnia complaints can be found at: http://www.aasmnet.org/PDF/ChronicParameter.pdf (available as of March 29, 2004). Table 3 lists the common causes of insomnia (not necessarily listed in order of frequency). Each is briefly discussed below.

MEDICAL CONDITIONS AND TREATMENT

Medical conditions, and in susceptible patients, many pharmacologic treatments of medical conditions, can result in insomnia complaints. The endocrinopathies are notorious for being associated with sleep-related complaints, as are conditions associated with chronic pain, breathing difficulties, cardiac arrhythmias, arthritis, renal failure, and central nervous system (CNS) disorders. Table 4 lists the more commonly used medications that can result in insomnia complaints.

The treatment of insomnia associated with medical conditions is first to isolate and appropriately treat the medical condition and the symptoms (e.g., pain) causing the insomnia. If the insomnia complaint persists, evaluate the possibility of an additional cause for the sleep complaint. Supplementary use of a short half-life hypnotic agent (e.g., zolpidem [Ambien], 5-10 mg at bedtime) may be helpful. Insomnia complaints associated with fibromyalgia and chronic fatigue syndrome are frequently resistant to treatment, although small doses of amitriptyline (Elavil)[1] (10-50 mg at bedtime) or cyclobenzaprine (Flexeril)[1] (10 mg three times a day) have been reported to be helpful; occasionally, zolpidem (5-10 mg) will help with the associated insomnia complaints.

Dementing illnesses are often associated with severe insomnia complaints that are quite disruptive to patients and families and often are the factors precipitating institutional care. Sleep is often disturbed in such disorders on the basis of disease-associated CNS lesions, and different specific pathophysiologies (not yet well understood) may respond to different treatments. Until such specific treatments can be based on specific pathophysiology, we should adhere to optimal environmental circadian principles (quiet, dark nocturnal environment; bright, socially stimulating daytime environment). Appropriate use of hypnotics may be helpful, although responses may be variable.

TABLE 2 Sleep History Questionnaire

When did the symptoms start, and what was going on at the time?
What has been the symptom pattern across time?
Are symptoms stress or situationally related?
What is your typical daily schedule, hour by hour?
What medications and treatments have been and are currently being used to date?
Is there a presence of familial sleep-related symptoms?

TABLE 3 Common Causes of Insomnia

Medical conditions and/or pharmacologic treatment of medical conditions
Psychiatric disorders (especially depression, anxiety, and post-traumatic stress disorder [PTSD])
Substance abuse disorders
Circadian rhythm disorders presenting as insomnia
Periodic limb movements in sleep (PLMS)
Central sleep apnea
The primary insomnia, conditioned insomnia, and sleep-state misperception group

[1]Not FDA approved for this indication.

TABLE 4 Medications Often Associated with Insomnia

Anticholinergics
Antidepressants
Antihypertensives
Antineoplastic agents
Bronchodilators
CNS stimulants
Corticosteroids
Decongestants
Diuretics
Histamine-2 (H_2) blockers
Smoking cessation aids

TABLE 5 Effect of Antidepressants on Sleep Scale*

		Effects on EEG Sleep			
Drug	**Trade Name**	**Continuity**	**SWS**	**REM**	**Sedation Effects**
TCAs					
Amitriptyline	Elavil	I (3)	I (1)	D (3)	4
Doxepin	Sinequan	I (3)	I (2)	D (2)	4
Imipramine	Tofranil	I (0-1)	I (1)	D (2)	2
Nortriptyline	Pamelor	I (1)	I (1)	D (2)	2
Desipramine	Norpramin	(0)	I (1)	D (2)	1
Clomipramine	Anafranil	I (0-1)	I (1)	D (4)	0
MAOIs					
Phenelzine	Nardil	D (1)	(0)	D (4)	0
Tranylcypromine	Parnate	D (2)	(0)	D (4)	0
SSRIs					
Fluoxetine	Prozac	D (1)	D (0-1)	D (0-1)	0
Paroxetine	Paxil	D (1)	D (0-1)	D (2)	0
Sertraline	Zoloft	(0)	(0)	D (2)	0
Citalopram	Celexa	D (1)	(0)	D (1)	ND
Fluvoxamine	Luvox	D (1)	(0)	D (1)	ND
Escitalopram	Lexapro	(0)	(0)	D (2)	0
Other					
Bupropion	Wellbutrin	D (0-1)	(0)	I (1)	0
Venlafaxine	Effexor	D (1)	D (1)	D (3)	2
Trazodone	Desyrel	I (3)	I (0-1)	D (1)	4
Mirtazapine	Remeron	I (3)	I (2)	(0)	3
Nefazodone	Serzone	I (1)	(0)	I (1)	1

Abbreviations: EEG = electroencephalogram; MAOIs = monoamine oxidase inhibitors; REM = rapid eye movement; SSRIs = selective serotonin reuptake inhibitors; SWS = slow-wave sleep; TCAs = tricyclic antidepressants.
*Scale 0-4: 0 = no significant effect; I = increase and D = decrease.

PSYCHIATRIC DISORDERS

Psychiatric disorders, especially those associated with anxiety or depression, frequently include insomnia (delayed sleep onset, frequent awakening, or early morning awakening) as an associated symptom. Effective treatment of the psychiatric condition will often relieve the insomnia complaint, although a supplemental hypnotic might be indicated early in treatment. Different antidepressant agents have quite different effects on sleep as illustrated in Table 5, and the initial choice of an antidepressant might profitably take such effects into account.

If, for a patient already complaining of insomnia, an antidepressant with a known high incidence of insomnia side effects is chosen, it may be useful to augment it with a hypnotic agent early in the course of treatment.

SUBSTANCE USE SLEEP DISORDERS

Alcohol abuse remains a significant problem in the etiology of sleep complaints, as do stimulants and other drugs of abuse. Treatment includes withdrawal of the offending substance, with long-term abstinence as the goal. Treatment of substance abuse-related insomnia should emphasize behavioral treatment strategies to the fullest extent possible, because psychoactive agents have already proved to be a problem.

CIRCADIAN RHYTHM DISORDERS

Disturbances in the regulation of the circadian system frequently present as sleep-related complaints, although the source of the problem lies in the circadian system rather than sleep pathology. Sleep per se may be adequate, but it occurs at the wrong time. Delayed sleep-phase syndrome (DSPS) is the most common, and is likely a genetically based disorder with frequent onset in adolescence or early adulthood. These individuals cannot get to sleep (because of phase delay in the body temperature rhythm) until 3 to 4 a.m., and if allowed to sleep, 8 to 9 hours may do well. If they have to arise at 7 a.m. for school or work, they will be sleep deprived and complain of insomnia.

Early morning bright-light exposure, with restriction of light exposure in the evening, has been found to be effective for phase-advancing the circadian system in DSPS. Evening bright-light treatment is effective in treating advanced sleep-phase syndrome. Low-dose (1-3 mg) melatonin[1]* at bedtime may help regulate circadian rhythms in some individuals.

Jet lag and shift-work–related sleep problems also fall in the category of circadian rhythm problems.

[1]Not FDA approved for this indication.
*Available as a dietary supplement.

TABLE 6 Beginning Dose Schedules for PMLS and RLS

Drug	Dose (mg)	Administration
Dopa Agonists		
Carbidopa/Levodopa (Sinemet)[1]	25/100-50/200	Bedtime/ symptom onset
Controlled-release Carbidopa/Levodopa (Sinemet CR)[1]	25/100-50/200	Bedtime/ symptom onset
Bromocriptine (Parlodel)[1]	2.5–5	Bedtime
Baclofen (Lioresal)[1]	20–40	Bedtime
Pergolide (Permax)[1]	0.05	Bedtime/ symptom onset
Pramipexole (Mirapex)[1]	0.125	Bedtime
Ropinirole (Requip)[1]	0.25	Bedtime
Other Agents		
Oxycodone (Roxicodone)[1]	5–15	Bedtime
Codeine[1]	10–60	Bedtime
Triazolam (Halcion)[1]	0.125–0.25	Bedtime
Temazepam (Restoril)[1]	15–30	Bedtime
Clonazepam (Klonopin)[1]	0.5–1.5	Bedtime
Gabapentin (Neurontin)[1]	100–300	Bedtime

[1]Not FDA approved for this indication.

A detailed discussion of these problem areas is beyond the scope of this article, but recently emerging data suggest that properly timed bright-light exposure, supplemented with melatonin[1*] administration and appropriate hypnotic use, can significantly reduce associated symptoms.

PERIODIC LIMB MOVEMENTS OF SLEEP AND RESTLESS LEGS SYNDROME

Both restless legs syndrome (RLS) and periodic limb movements of sleep (PLMS) are associated with a variety of medical conditions, including iron deficiency, but they may occur in otherwise healthy individuals (especially the elderly). A polysomnogram (PSG) is usually required for accurate diagnosis of a PLMS disorder, quantifying both the number of events and their association with awakenings or arousals. Table 6 lists the drugs currently used in the treatment of PLMS and RLS.

CENTRAL SLEEP APNEA

Central sleep apnea with frequent arousals is a relatively rare cause of chronic insomnia except at higher altitudes, and may require a PSG for accurate diagnosis. Both oxygen and continuous positive airway pressure (CPAP) can be used in the treatment of central apnea in patients with medical disorders. The efficacy of pharmacologic agents in the treatment of central sleep apnea has yet to be clearly established in well-controlled studies. Acetazolamide (Diamox)[1] (250 mg twice a day) may be effective for the prevention of high altitude-induced central apnea.

[1]Not FDA approved for this indication.
*Available as a dietary supplement.

THE PRIMARY INSOMNIA, CONDITIONED INSOMNIA, AND SLEEP-STATE MISPERCEPTION SYNDROME GROUP

Although there are several more rare causes of a chronic insomnia complaint, most often it is generally safe to assume that once the aforementioned specific causes have been systematically excluded or appropriately treated (and the insomnia complaints remain), we are in all probability left with either a primary insomnia disorder (DSM-IV 307.42), a conditioned insomnia, or a sleep-state misperception syndrome (SSMS), or some combination thereof.

A treatment approach that combines both behavioral and pharmacologic approaches is generally recommended. Such a combined treatment approach offers the advantage of a pharmacologic agent that can produce rapid relief of the sleep complaint, along with behavioral strategies, which take longer to become effective but provide long-term strategies that are under a patient's control. Active and continued involvement of the patient is important for any chronic insomnia treatment.

Sleep Laboratory Studies

All night PSG, which monitors multiple physiologic variables during sleep, are rarely needed in the evaluation of insomnia complaints, except for symptoms associated with PLMS or for a sleep-related breathing disorder, where a PSG is usually required for accurate diagnosis. A recent review of the use of PSG in the insomnia complaints can be found at: http://www.aasmnet.org/PDF/260616.pdf (available as of March 29, 2004).

The 24-hour recording of activity (Actigraphy) can also be useful in the diagnosis of circadian rhythm-based sleep complaints (e.g., see: http://www.aasmnet.org/PDF/ 260315.pdf [available as of March 29, 2004]).

Treatment

After completing the evaluation of a chronic insomnia complaint and arriving at a diagnostic formulation, a treatment plan should be developed addressing all likely contributing causes. The treatment plan will likely include both behavioral and pharmacologic components, and should be discussed in detail with the patient. Patients might be encouraged to visit the web pages of the American Sleep Disorders Association (www.asda.org) and the National Sleep Foundation (www.nsf.org) to learn more about factors influencing sleep. Patient education facilitates effective treatment.

[1]Not FDA approved for this indication.

TABLE 7 Good Sleep Hygiene

Establish a regular sleep schedule that does not vary by more than 1 hour.
Maintain a state of good aerobic fitness with regular exercise (but not within 3 hours of sleep onset).
Do not use caffeine or alcohol to excess.
Ensure a quiet, dark, cool bedroom.
Provide a time to wind down in the evening before sleeping.
Consider a high-tryptophan snack (milk, cookies, banana) before bed.
Use the bedroom for sleep and sex but not for reviewing or thinking about the affairs of the day.
Minimize exposure to late evening bright light to avoid phase-delaying the circadian system.

BEHAVIORAL TREATMENTS

Behavioral treatment strategies are aimed at (a) breaking bad sleep habits and replacing them with sleep-promoting habits; (b) directly decreasing physiologic arousal levels using cognitively based or learned strategies; and (c) providing the patient with several types of cognitive strategies to deal with sleep difficulties, thus promoting a sense of competence and diminishing anxiety about sleep. First and foremost among the behavioral strategies is good sleep hygiene—the behaviors and habits that foster good sleep. Table 7 highlights the principles of good sleep hygiene. It is helpful to prepare a handout for patients summarizing good sleep hygiene practices that they can take with them. Table 8 lists additional behavioral strategies.

PHARMACOLOGIC TREATMENTS

Benzodiazepine (BZ) compounds and newer nonbenzodiazepine agents active at the level of the benzodiazepine receptor are the most commonly used hypnotic agents today. Older hypnotic agents (chloral hydrate, paraldehyde [Paral], barbiturates) may have limited usefulness for very short-term use in specific patients, but they cannot be recommended for the treatment of chronic insomnia.

BZ agents activate all BZ receptors (hypnotic, anxiolytic, muscle relaxant, anticonvulsant), and different agents demonstrate relatively little receptor specificity.

TABLE 8 Other Behavioral Strategies for the Treatment of Insomnia

1. Biofeedback (EMG and EEG): teaches subjects to decrease autonomic arousal
2. Progressive relaxation: training in systematic total body relaxation
3. Sleep restriction: good for subjects spending excessive time in bed with poorly consolidated sleep
4. Yoga, transcendental mediation (TM): self-control strategies
5. Cognitive behavioral therapy (several types): improved self-confidence and self-control

The benzodiazepine compounds differ substantially in terms of half-life and are illustrated in Table 9. The clinician can choose the agent with a half-life most appropriate for the clinical situation.

Long half-life BZ agents may be associated with residual daytime sedation and impairments in psychomotor performance. All BZ agents interfere with memory consolidation, the more potent agents (e.g., triazolam [Halcion]) most prominently. All BZ agents are prone to the development of tolerance, dependence, and rebound insomnia in response to rapid withdrawal. BZ agents also tend to decrease stages 3 to 4 sleep, and increase fast activity in the waking and sleeping electroencephalogram (EEG). These results may continue after drug discontinuation. Clearly useful for the treatment of insomnia associated with anxiety, the use of long-term BZ treatment of primary insomnia is problematic, especially in light of the research and development of new, apparently safe and effective nonbenzodiazepine agents designed to be selectively more active on the hypnotic receptor.

Newer non-BZ agents selectively active at the $omega_1$ (primarily hypnotic) BZ receptor include the imidazopyridine zolpidem (Ambien), and the cyclopyralone zaleplon (Sonata) that are effective and relatively safe hypnotics that do not alter sleep architecture, and do not appear to induce significant tolerance, dependence, or withdrawal. Both agents have a rapid onset of action, but differ in half-life and duration of action. Zolpidem (5-10 mg) can be taken if the patient has 6 to 7 hours to sleep. Zaleplon can be taken if the patient has 4 hours available for sleep.

Antidepressant agents, especially sedative tricyclics, are frequently used at low doses to manage chronic insomnia despite the relative lack of well-controlled double-blind studies demonstrating efficacy. These agents are clearly indicated in insomnia that accompanies depressive disorders, where their effectiveness is clear. These agents are normally taken about one hour before bedtime so their sedative effects have time to emerge. This effectively teaches the patient to take a pill to sleep, which is counterproductive for treating insomnia. The new non-BZ hypnotics with their rapid onset of action can be placed at the bedside and are taken if the patient has not fallen asleep within 30 minutes.

Several agents more directly involved in modulating γ-aminobutyric acid (GABA) activity, such as tiagabine (Gabitril)[1] and sodium oxybate (Xyrem)[1], have been used in limited studies to promote slow-wave sleep, but there is insufficient published data to make specific recommendations as to their potential usefulness in insomnia at this time.

LONG-TERM USE OF HYPNOTIC AGENTS

Current thinking suggests we might best conceptualize primary insomnia as a chronic disorder that

[1]Not FDA approved for this indication.

TABLE 9 Benzodiazepines

Name		Dose (mg)			
Generic	Trade Name	Adult	Elderly	Onset	Half-Life (Hours)
Triazolam	Halcion	0.125-0.25	0.125-0.25	Rapid	1.5-5.5
Estazolam	ProSom	1-2	0.5-1	Rapid	20-30
Temazepam	Restoril	15-30	7.5-15	Intermediate	8-20
Quazepam	Doral	7.5-15	7.5	Intermediate	15-120
Flurazepam	Dalmane	15-30	7.5	Intermediate	36-250

will likely require long-term treatment. Considering the known adverse effects of chronic sleep loss, in the context of the present availability of relatively safe and effective hypnotic agents, there would appear to be no reason to withhold or severely limit pharmacologic treatment in those responsible patients for whom a comprehensive and thorough diagnostic evaluation has established the presence of a primary insomnia disorder. It should go without saying, however, that behavioral treatment also should be actively implemented in those patients who are being considered for long-term pharmacologic management.

PRURITUS

METHOD OF

Susan Nedorost, MD

Pruritus (itch) is the most troublesome symptom of many diseases. Pruritus may also be useful as a diagnostic clue. The best treatment for pruritus is to thoroughly investigate and treat the underlying cause. Antihistamines are useful for the itch of urticaria (hives) and their sedative effect is helpful to allow sleep in a variety of pruritic conditions. Systemic and topical corticosteroids suppress itch from most causes of pruritus, but they have significant side effects when used chronically and should not be prescribed without a diagnostic investigation and should not be refilled without a confirmed diagnosis. Table 1 shows the history that should be obtained from all patients with itch.

Diagnosis of Pruritic Rash

Table 2 divides these diagnoses in a somewhat artificial fashion between those that are generalized and those more localized, and those typically diagnosed when present for less than 2 weeks and those usually diagnosed when present for longer than 2 weeks. The rapidity of diagnosis is a function of both the tempo of development of the rash and the difficulty of making the diagnosis. The first step in examining the skin is to look for lesions that have not been scratched and have not been treated with a topical medication. If a skin biopsy is required for diagnoses, these "primary" skin lesions are desirable for histologic examination as well.

All dermatologic diagnoses begin with close observation of morphology and distribution.

Papulosquamous lesions are usually mildly to moderately pruritic and may be distinguished by character of the scale and by distribution. Pityriasis rosea begins with one larger plaque, and then multiple smaller lesions develop oriented along skin cleavage lines. Pityriasis rosea scale is fine; the rash affects the torso and proximal extremities. Psoriasis often occurs with a family history. Psoriasis "Koebnerizes" such that rash occurs in scratches and appears linear; scale is coarse; rash especially affects extensor surfaces. Lichen planus is purple in color with very fine scale; it heals with brown postinflammatory color. The volar wrists and oral mucosa are areas of predilection. Lichen planus also "Koebnerizes."

Urticaria is intensely itchy and may affect any area of skin or mucous membrane. Causes include medications, occult infection (e.g., sinusitis, dental abscess, tinea pedis), foods, and autoimmune ("idiopathic") diseases. Insect bites may appear as nonevanescent "papular urticaria." Insect bites are diagnosed by pattern: chiggers bite in areas of snug clothing; mosquitoes bite exposed skin; fleas bite below the knee; Cheyletiella mites bite where pets have contact with skin.

Vesicular rashes are intensely pruritic. Vesicles caused by varicella are associated with fever and usually with cough in adults. Because of vaccine availability, this is seen rarely now; however, coxsackievirus infections may have a similar appearance. Other pruritic vesicular rashes are miliaria, which consists of tiny vesicles in follicular distribution with a history of exposure to heat and often occlusion of the affected area, and dermatitis herpetiformis, which consists of

TABLE 1 History Required to Evaluate Pruritus

History of present condition: initial appearance and exact location first noticed on skin; duration of individual lesions and of the entire episode
Prior medical problems and review of systems: may be directly relevant to etiology and may contraindicate some systemic treatments of itch
Medication (prescription and over-the-counter): same relevance as prior medical history and, additionally, some bullous and lichenoid primary diagnoses may be drugs-induced
Environment: includes conditions of recent temperature and ambient humidity, occupations and hobbies, pets, prior topical treatments and personal care products applied to skin

fragile tiny blisters outnumbered by excoriations. Dermatitis herpetiformis is caused by hypersensitivity to gluten and sometimes associated with celiac sprue.

Folliculitis is mildly to moderately pruritic and appears as pustules. This may be a result of *Candida* and is often intertriginous and often in diabetics following a history of heat exposure. Staphylococcal folliculitis is more common in patients with a history of atopy; pseudomonas folliculitis follows exposure to a hot tub or other standing water.

Bullae are also intensely itchy. Acute presentation may be caused by plant dermatitis (e.g., poison ivy) with some of the bullae in linear streaks. Chronic bullae over urticarial bases suggest bullous pemphigoid, which is usually seen in people over 50 years of age.

Dermatitis is very itchy and features a variable proportion of vesicles, oozing excoriations, and scale. Atopic dermatitis is often seen with a family history of eczema, asthma, and/or allergic rhinitis. This form of eczema begins before adolescence with accentuation in flexural areas. It is worsened by extremes of humidity, staphylococcal infection, and scratching. Irritant contact dermatitis develops and resolves rapidly after exposure to the offending substance (e.g., detergent, solvent, fiberglass). Allergic contact dermatitis develops days after exposure and may last for weeks. Common causes are fragrance, metals, preservatives, rubber, clothing dyes and finishes, and adhesives. Allergic contact dermatitis should always be considered in a diagnostic work-up of occupational skin disease, or in adult-onset eczema. Refer for diagnosis to a dermatologist skilled in patch testing. Scabies is a dermatitis caused by mite infestation and favors flexural areas but spares the face. Xerosis is a wintertime itch in low humidity climates, especially affecting the lower legs and the back.

Polymorphic eruptions suggest medications as a cause. Morbilliform drug eruptions typically have mixed features of urticaria and dermatitis. Pustular drug eruptions may feature both pustules and urticaria, often with fever and leukocytosis. Bullous drug eruptions may produce a burn-like condition and require urgent dermatologic referral, especially if mucous membranes are involved. Drug hypersensitivity syndrome (as seen with anticonvulsants) may cause facial edema, lymphadenopathy, and organ dysfunction.

Photodermatoses are distributed on the face, dorsal forearms and hands, and lateral neck. These may be allergic reactions to the sun itself (polymorphous light eruption or chronic actinic dermatitis), or photoaggravated allergic contact dermatitis such as that to sunscreen, or provocation of connective-tissue diseases such as dermatomyositis or lupus. Dermatologic referral is indicated for skin biopsy and/or photo patch testing.

Generalized itch without rash, or with only secondary skin findings related to chronic scratching, should prompt a work-up for systemic causes of itch as outlined in Table 3.

Treatment of Itch

Lotions containing menthol or camphor cause a cooling sensation when applied to the skin that counteracts itching. Chilling these preparations may further enhance this effect. Heat exacerbates itch, so use of central air conditioning, exercising in front of a fan, and reducing the number of bed covers during sleep may be helpful. Dry skin also itches more, so in low humidity conditions, minimal cleansers should be used and liquid cleansers containing emollients or synthetic detergent bars are preferred. Emollients should be applied to damp skin immediately after bathing. Ointments are strongly preferred to lotions

TABLE 2 Pruritic Rashes

Generalized, Diagnosed within 2 Weeks of Onset	Generalized, Diagnosed More than 2 Weeks After Onset	Localized, Diagnosed within 2 Weeks of Onset	Localized, Diagnosed More than 2 Weeks After Onset
Drug eruption	Bullous pemphigoid	Folliculitis (yeast, bacteria)	Allergic contact dermatitis other than plant*
Pityriasis rosea	Dermatitis herpetiformis	Irritant contact dermatitis	Atopic dermatitis*
Viral exanthem	Scabies	Insect bites	Lichen planus*
Urticaria	Xerosis	Miliaria rubra	Psoriasis*
		Plant dermatitis*	Photodermatoses

*May also be generalized.

TABLE 3 Causes of Generalized Itch without Rash or with Only "Secondary" Features Such as Prurigo Nodularis or Lichen Simplex Chronicus (Bumps or Thickening from Chronic Scratching)

Medications	Opioids, ketoconazole (Nizoral), and cocaine are examples
Hematopoietic malignancy may first present as itch without rash; solid tumors with hypercalcemia may also cause itch	Examination should include palpation of lymph nodes, complete blood count, metabolic profile, and chest radiograph
Renal disease and cholestatic liver disease are often associated with itch; thyroid disease is also common	Thyroid function tests should be performed, especially in patients with weight or hair changes, or with temperature intolerance
HIV infection may present with pruritus	
Subtle physical urticarias such as those caused by cold or pressure may appear as invisible rash	Stroking the skin and observing for a wheal will detect dermatographism
Central nervous system disease	Stroke, brain tumor or abscess, multiple sclerosis
Psychogenic	Delusions of parasitosis

because they are more occlusive, less likely to sting upon application to broken skin, and contain fewer preservatives that may cause secondary sensitization (allergic contact dermatitis). However, patients may not accept ointments because they do not vanish into the skin upon application and may leave oil spots on clothing. Creams may be used as an alternative.

Antihistamines are effective for the itch of urticaria, but higher-than-usual dosages may be required. A nonsedating antihistamine should be used in the morning and a sedating antihistamine at night. Sedating antihistamines may also aid sleep in other pruritic conditions, but should not be used round-the-clock because they may impair reflexes while driving and interfere with learning. Topical antihistamines are not recommended because of the risk of sensitization.

Systemic corticosteroids are effective for most pruritus caused by rash, although they may worsen some conditions such as scabies and psoriasis. They have significant side effects and should be used as monotherapy only for self-limited conditions such as severe plant dermatitis. For chronic severe dermatoses such as the bullous disorders, immunosuppressives such as mycophenolate mofetil (CellCept[1]) are used as steroid-sparing agents.

Topical corticosteroids are helpful for dermatitis and lichenoid disorders, but should be used only intermittently to avoid tachyphylaxis and long-term side effects such as cutaneous atrophy. Extra caution must be used when corticosteroids are applied to the face because they may cause acne rosacea, telangiectasias, cataracts, and glaucoma. As with vehicles for emollients, ointments are the most effective form, followed by creams. Lotions should be reserved for hairy areas or special situations, such as around ostomy sites where other vehicles interfere with adhesion. Topical tacrolimus (Protopic) and pimecrolimus (Elidel) are as effective as moderate-potency corticosteroids for atopic dermatitis and do not have as many long-term side effects. However, they may sting upon application, can cause cutaneous dissemination of herpesvirus, and should not be used on sun-exposed skin.

Treatment of secondary infection helps to alleviate itch. Atopic dermatitis is particularly prone to exacerbation by staphylococcal infection. Systemic cephalosporins or azithromycin (Z-pack) are effective in most communities, but the prescriber must be knowledgeable about local resistance patterns.

Phototherapy is useful for the papulosquamous disorders and some cases of itch caused by systemic disease. Natural sunlight or narrow-band ultraviolet B wavelengths are effective; PUVA (psoralen plus ultraviolet A[*]) is effective but has more side effects, such as nausea from the psoralen and an increased risk of cutaneous malignancy.

Some systemic causes of itch appear to be mediated by the central nervous system as evidenced by response to the opiate antagonist naltrexone (ReVia[1]), which is effective in itch caused by primary biliary cirrhosis. Chronic itch is a miserable condition that interferes with sleep and concentration and can strain family relationships. Stress worsens itch, and referral for psychotherapy may be indicated for patients with chronic symptoms.

[1]Not FDA approved for this indication.

[*]Not FDA approved for itch.

[1]Not FDA approved for this indication.

TINNITUS

METHOD OF

John W. House, MD

When discussing tinnitus it is important to understand that it is a symptom and not a disease. Many patients are under the misimpression that they have a "disease" and are concerned about the future of their ailment. In fact, 80% of patients with hearing loss have associated tinnitus. In this country, there are about 20 to 30 million people who experience tinnitus. Most of these patients are not particularly concerned about their tinnitus. They have learned to live with it and are not aware of it much of the time. In my experience, only approximately 5% of patients are disturbed by it and require some form of therapy. When dealing with patients who have tinnitus it is important to evaluate them to determine the etiology of the symptom.

Tinnitus is defined as one or more sounds perceived by the patient in the absence of an external source of the sound. It may be perceived in one ear, both ears, or in the head. Tinnitus usually is benign, but may represent a serious underlying pathology. The tinnitus may be constant, intermittent, steady state, or pulsatile. The frequency of the tinnitus is variable from one patient to another and may vary within the same patient. At times, it may be barely perceptible or may be described as quite loud. It is interesting to note that when we perform tinnitus-matching tests the average relative loudness, regardless of the patient's perception of the tinnitus, is only 5 decibels above their hearing threshold. The two types of tinnitus are *objective* and *subjective*.

Objective Tinnitus

This type of tinnitus can be heard by an observer and is uncommon. Objective tinnitus may be of vascular or muscular origin. Vascular tinnitus may arise from either venous, arterial causes, or vascular tumors, such as glomus tympanicums or glomus jugulare tumors. The arterial causes include conditions that cause turbulent flow, such as arterial sclerosis associated with aging, aberrant carotid artery, arterial–venous fistula or an arterial–venous malformation. It may also be associated with conditions that cause an increase in blood flow around the ears, such as anemia, hyperthyroidism, or Paget's disease. The venous causes include a large or exposed jugular bulb on one side and benign intracranial hypertension. The venous type of tinnitus is easily differentiated from the arterial type. Typically, the sound will stop or be reduced when light pressure is applied over the internal jugular vein on the involved side. In addition, the patient may report that the sound is reduced when they turn their head toward the involved ear and increased when they turn their head away from it. Evaluation includes radiographic and ultrasound studies, as indicated. High-resolution computed tomography (CT) scanning with contrast and bone program is helpful in identifying erosive lesions or tumors. Magnetic resonance angiography (MRA) and magnetic resonance venography (MRV) are helpful in defining vascular lesions or aberrant vessels. Standard angiography is being performed less often because of the effectiveness of MRA, MRV, and ultrasound studies. This type of tinnitus responds well to treatment aimed at the vascular lesion or correction of the anemia or hyperthyroidism.

The three causes of muscular tinnitus are myoclonic activity of the stapedial muscle, of the tensor tympani muscle, and of the palatal muscle. These types of tinnitus are characterized by brief periods of clicking, popping, or banging sounds in the ear. Palatal myoclonus can be differentiated from the other causes by observing rhythmic contractions of the soft palate that are synchronized with the patient's sounds. While observing the palate, it is important not to have the patient open the mouth widely, because this usually stops the myoclonus. It may be possible to observe movement of the tympanic membrane either with the microscope or the tympanometer. Treatment is often successful and is aimed at the offending muscle. By cutting the tendon to the stapedial or tensor tympani muscle, the symptoms are relieved. If the cause is the palatal muscle, treatment is more difficult and palliative. Placing the patient on muscle relaxants or performing a myringotomy with tubes may help. Botulinum toxin (Botox)[1] injections into the levator palatini muscle help to relieve the sound in some patients.

Subjective Tinnitus

The vast majority of tinnitus is subjective in which only the patient is able to hear the sound. It is usually associated with some type of hearing loss. In my experience, approximately 90% of tinnitus patients have a sensorineural hearing loss, approximately 5% have a conductive loss, and approximately 5% have normal hearing.

Because tinnitus is a symptom, the underlying cause must be determined by a history, physical examination, audiogram, and any additional tests that are indicated. The physical examination includes otoscopy, and, at times, auscultation and palpation around the ear and neck. The remainder of the head and neck examination is performed. Tuning fork tests (Rinne and Weber) are routinely performed to determine if the hearing loss is conductive or sensorineural. The possible causes of a conductive hearing loss with tinnitus are cerumen impaction, otitis externa, otitis media (acute and chronic), chronic otitis media with effusion (serous otitis), and otosclerosis.

[1]Not FDA approved for this indication.

Some of the causes of sensorineural hearing loss associated with tinnitus include presbycusis (age-related hearing loss), noise-induced hearing loss, ototoxic medications, sudden hearing loss as a result of either vascular or viral causes, Meniere's disease, and cerebellopontine angle tumors (acoustic neuromas or meningiomas). The latter are usually associated with unilateral symptoms (hearing loss with or without tinnitus). Patients having unilateral complaints must have a neurotologic evaluation that would include an MRI with gadolinium to rule out a tumor. Blood tests may be indicated if there is a fluctuating or rapidly progressive hearing loss associated with the tinnitus. This would include a complete blood cell count (CBC) with sedimentation rate, a fluorescent treponemal antibody (FTA), and possibly an antinuclear antibody (ANA) test. These tests are performed to rule out syphilitic or autoimmune hearing loss.

Treatment

Because tinnitus is a symptom and not a disease, there is no one treatment that is effective for all. Victor Goodhill, MD, in 1950, put it very well: "Any management which is based upon a single panacea for the treatment of a symptom and not a disease will result in failure." The important steps in the management of the patient with tinnitus are the evaluation, the examination, and the explanation. The explanation is very helpful when it is accompanied by reassurance that the tinnitus does not represent serious pathology and that the patient is not going deaf. Approximately 95% of the patients seen in my office who have tinnitus are not particularly bothered by it; on the other hand, 5% of my patients are driven to distraction by their tinnitus.

If the tinnitus is associated with a hearing loss, amplification with a hearing aid will usually help. The normal environmental sounds mask out the tinnitus and at the same time improve the patient's hearing. At night, a noise generator, fan, air conditioner, or a radio tuned to an FM station can help to mask the tinnitus. Tinnitus maskers are wearable devices that generate sound to help mask the tinnitus. These have limited success in helping reduce aggravation of the tinnitus. For those patients with tinnitus and a hearing loss who find that a masker or hearing aid alone are not helpful, a tinnitus instrument (combined hearing aid and masker) may help to both mask the tinnitus and provide amplification. A new promising tinnitus treatment is auditory habituation as proposed and developed by Pawel Jastreboff, PhD. This therapy involves retraining the auditory system to ignore the tinnitus sounds. Therapeutic noise devices are used that emit stable, broadband noise that is softer than the patient's tinnitus. The theory is not to cover up the tinnitus but to help the patient learn to ignore it. This training takes time (as long as 1 year), and requires the therapist to spend a great deal of time counseling the patient.

I have found that for approximately 80% of a selected group of patients, biofeedback training helps to reduce the tinnitus by teaching the patient relaxation techniques. Muscle tension and stress worsen the perceived tinnitus. The biofeedback consists of monitoring muscle tension and skin temperature. When the patients are able to learn to relax the muscles and increase circulation in the skin that their tinnitus was reduced. In addition, the patients recognized the relationship between their stress level and the perceived loudness of the tinnitus.

Over the years many medications have been tried for the treatment of tinnitus. There is not a single medication that works uniformly in reducing tinnitus. Both my group and Robert Dobie, MD, have found that antidepressants are effective in some patients. Most of our severe tinnitus sufferers have sleep problems, are anxious, and are depressed. Small doses of either amitriptyline (Elavil)[1] or nortriptyline (Pamelor)[1] given at bedtime seems to help the patient get through the night and reduces the aggravation of the tinnitus during the day.

[1]Not FDA approved for this indication.

TABLE 1 Medications Proposed to Help Tinnitus*

Anesthetics
Lidocaine[1] (IV—temporary relief in about 80%)
Procaine (Novocain)[1]
Tocainide (Tonocard)[1] (oral lidocaine analog)
Flecainide (Tambocor)[1]
Mexiletine (Mexitil)[1] (oral lidocaine analog)
Antianxiety
Alprazolam (Xanax)[1]
Diazepam (Valium)[1]
Clonazepam (Klonopin)[1]
Anticonvulsants
Carbamazepine (Tegretol)[1]
Phenytoin (Dilantin)[1]
Primidone (Mysoline)[1]
Gabapentin (Neurontin)[1]
Antidepressants
Amitriptyline (Elavil)[1]
Nortriptyline (Pamelor)[1]
Diuretics (in Meniere's Disease)
Triamterene/HCTZ (Dyazide)[1]
Vitamins and Herbs
Niacin
Misoprostol (Cytotec)[1] (synthetic prostaglandin)
Magnesium
Vitamin B_{12}
Ginkgo biloba

[1]Not FDA approved for this indication.
*Results are inconsistent.

Other medications that might be helpful include antianxiety agents such as alprazolam (Xanax)[1], clonazepam (Klonopin)[1], and diazepam (Valium)[1]. Recently, Abe Schulman, MD, reported some success in relieving severe tinnitus by combining clonazepam and gabapentin (Neurontin)[1]. Because of the potential for abuse and dependence, I rarely prescribe this category of medication.

Table 1 lists additional medications that have been mentioned as possibly helping tinnitus. My group recently completed a double-blinded study using a combination of ginkgo biloba[1], magnesium[1], and vitamin B_{12}[1]. We found that the active treatment group did no better than the placebo group.

In conclusion, there is no sure cure for tinnitus. Many patients have tinnitus, but most learn to ignore it. Most patients find that after an evaluation and explanation with reassurance, they can live with it and learn to ignore it. There is no magical cure, but many avenues of treatment are available to help a patient cope with and overcome the problem of tinnitus.

[1]Not FDA approved for this indication.

LOW BACK PAIN

METHOD OF

Gunnar B.J. Andersson, MD, PhD

Back pain is so common that more than 85% of the population in the industrial world will experience it at some time during their lives. Although there are minor differences between countries in the prevalence and incidence of back pain, there are remarkable similarities. In the United States, approximately 15% of all adults will have a back episode in a given year and in about one-third of these, the pain is severe and chronic. Back pain is the most frequent cause of activity limitation in people younger than age 45 years, the second most common reason for patient visits, the fifth ranking reason for hospitalization, and the third most common reason for surgical procedures. Approximately 2% of the U.S. workforce report compensation back injuries each year. Over the past few decades, there has been a large increase in the number of surgical procedures for back-related conditions.

Back pain remains, however, a generally benign condition. Some 60% of patients recover in 1 week, and approximately 90% recover in 6 weeks. After 12 weeks, additional recovery is typically slow. Advanced age, pain radiating into the leg, and psychosocial and occupational factors have all been identified as increasing the risk for chronicity. Recurrence is common, almost part of the natural history. Again, prognosis is typically excellent. Prevention strategies that include education, lifestyle changes, and ergonomic and protective equipment have not proven significantly effective.

Causes of Back Pain

Most patients with back pain will never know the precise origin of their pain. Indeed, excluding degenerative changes, 85% of patients are given a symptom diagnosis only. Many textbooks classify back patients into more or less well-defined categories as illustrated in Table 1. Although this is certainly helpful, it is often more useful to classify a patient according to the patient's presenting symptoms. By this method you can early on focus on those patients who require particular attention. Whenever a patient is evaluated for back pain, the history and physical examination

TABLE 1 Causes of Low Back Pain

Developmental
Scoliosis
Spondylolisthesis
Infectious
Discitis
Vertebral osteomyelitis
Inflammatory
Seronegative spondyloarthropathies
Polymyalgia rheumatica
Traumatic
Fractures
Metabolic
Osteoporosis
Osteomalacia
Hyperparathyroidism
Neoplastic
Primary
Metastatic
Degenerative
Herniated disc
Degenerative disc disease
Facet arthropathy
Spinal stenosis
Spondylolisthesis
Referred
Vasculogenic
Aortic aneurysm, ischemia
Viscerogenic
Gastrointestinal, genitourinary, pancreas
Hip osteoarthritis
Unknown
Musculoligamentous overuse
Psychosocial factors

TABLE 2 The "Red Flags" of Low Back Pain

Possible Condition	History	Physical
Fracture	Major trauma	
	Minor Trauma (older patient)	
Tumor	Age <15 or >50 years	
	Known cancer	
	Unexplained weight loss	
	Night pain	
Infection	Recent fever or chills	Fever
	Recent bacterial infection (UTI)	
	Intravenous drug use	
	Immune suppression	
	Unrelenting pain	
Cauda equina syndrome	Saddle numbness	Weak anal sphincter
	Urinary retention, incontinence	Perianal sensory loss
	Severe (progressive) lupus erythematosus	Flaccid motor weakness
	Neurologic deficit	Hyporeflexia

should always consider the so-called "red flags" (Table 2). Patients can usually easily be divided into six categories:

- Back pain only
- Back pain and leg pain, or leg pain mainly
- Back pain, leg pain, and inability to void
- Back and/or leg symptoms with walking
- Severe unremitting back pain (with or without leg pain)
- Back pain in the morning that improves through the day

Back pain only is the most frequent presentation. Patients often associate the onset with a lift, a movement, or other physical activity, but frequently the pain developed for no obvious reason. The pain pattern is usually mechanical—increasing with activity, decreasing with rest. The source of the pain may be the muscles, ligaments, facet joints, discs, or bone. Generally, the possibility of muscle and ligament being the source is higher in the young, while disc problems are more frequent in the 35- to 55-year-old age group, and bone-related pain is more common in the elderly, >55 years old, (osteoporosis). When leg pain is present, the probability of a nerve root involvement increases, particularly when the pain is radicular. One cause of radicular pain is a disc herniation, which usually results in pain radiating below the knee. Narrowing of the spinal canal (central stenosis), or more often nerve root foramina (foraminal stenosis), can also cause radiculopathy. Inability to void or loss of bowel and bladder control suggests a cauda equina syndrome, which constitutes an emergency. Back and leg symptoms, which occur when walking, suggest the possibility of spinal stenosis, particularly in the elderly population. Stenosis patients often describe how their pain decreases when they bend forwards (for example to push the grocery cart), or sit down, which enlarges the spinal canal and neuroforamina. Severe, unremitting pain is one of the "red flags" (see Table 2). These patients have the greatest chance of having a life-threatening or disabling problem (tumor, infection, or fracture). Some patients, for secondary gain reasons, will tell you their pain is "present all the time." On further discussion this can often be resolved. Morning pain and stiffness that improves over the day suggests inflammatory disease of which ankylosing spondylitis is the most common.

It is important to appreciate that degenerative changes do not equal pain, and are the result of normal aging. Discs degenerate early, and by age 40 years, nuclear fissures and annular cracks are the rule, not the exception. Disc degeneration is almost a prerequisite for a disc herniation, and occurs most often at the L4 and L5 discs, and only rarely, and late in life at discs L1 and L2. The degenerative disc process shifts the loads in the facet joints causing osteoarthritis. The combination of disc degeneration and facet osteoarthritis, in turn, causes spinal stenosis, because the discs often bulge and lose height and the facet joints enlarge in response to the osteoarthritis.

History and physical examination are sufficient to exclude red flags and to provide treatment. In the absence of "red flags," radiographs are not particularly helpful. Thus it is rare that a need for radiographs exists in the first 4 to 6 weeks (at the end of which time 90% of patients have recovered). In patients with severe symptoms, particularly of a radicular nature, a magnetic resonance imaging (MRI) examination may also be helpful; but again, only when symptom resolution over 4 to 6 weeks does not occur. Most positive findings on imaging are incidental, and of limited value to treatment.

Treatment

Because back pain has such a favorable natural history, treatment can often be simplified to pain medication, education, and activity alteration. Patients who present without "red flags" should be advised that "there is no evidence of a severe underlying problem," and that "a rapid recovery can be expected." Many patients are concerned when experiencing back pain because they may have friends, relatives, or coworkers who have developed chronic or recurrent back problems. They need to know that this is the exception, not the rule. Patients with leg pain (particularly when radicular) have a slower recovery, and a greater chance of future need for a specific treatment. Yet, the prognosis is excellent in these patients as well.

Pain relief is the primary concern, and usually the reason for the physician visit. Activity alteration, analgesics and/or nonsteroidal anti-inflammatory drugs (NSAIDs), and various physical methods are available for symptomatic relief. Bedrest, long a cornerstone of back care, is almost never indicated, and if it is, then only for 1 to 2 days. Prolonged bedrest actually leads to deconditioning and is worse than a gradual return to normal activities, which is the advice of choice. Temporary activity limitations, including avoiding heavy lifts, bending and twisting of the back, and prolonged sitting are indicated in patients with acute pain.

Analgesics, preferably acetaminophen (Tylenol), and NSAIDs are reasonably safe drugs, helpful in accomplishing pain relief. NSAIDs have higher complication risks, but are sometimes more effective. Muscle relaxants offer no particular advantages over NSAIDs, and may cause drowsiness. A combination of NSAIDs and muscle relaxants may produce added beneficial effect. Opioids are rarely indicated, but are occasionally necessary to manage patients with very severe acute symptoms. They should be used sparingly and for short periods only. Steroids are not recommended for the treatment of acute lower back pain. In patients with radiculopathy, oral steroids[1], epidural injections, or root blocks with steroids[1] may be used in an attempt to avoid surgery. Antidepressants[1] may be useful in patients with chronic back pain, but are not helpful in the acute stages of pain.

Physical agents and modalities are often used, including ice, heat, diathermy, and ultrasound. They have no documented effect on back pain, as such, but carry little risk of complications. Self-application of cold or heat often results in short-term symptomatic relief. Physiologically it makes more sense to use cold in the acute stages of back pain, and heat in the later stages. Ultrasound and diathermy should not be used on pregnant women because of theoretical risks to the fetus. Transcutaneous electrical nerve stimulation (TENS) has no role in the treatment of acute back pain. Acupuncture is also not recommended as a first-line treatment.

Corsets, braces, and back belts are widely used, but there is no evidence of effectiveness in acute back pain. In patients with chronic and recurrent problems, there is conflicting evidence, as is also the case with the preventive use of back belts in industry. Continuous use of corsets can result in weakening of the trunk muscles and should be avoided. Traction has no documented effect on either back pain or sciatica.

Aerobic exercise programs (walking, biking, and swimming) should be started early in patients with acute back pain (after 1-2 weeks), and continue indefinitely in patients with recurrent or chronic problems. Trunk muscle exercises and stretching are not particularly helpful during the first 2 weeks of acute pain, but can subsequently be initiated. It is often beneficial to have a physical therapist's advice on the proper exercise routines. There is no specific advantage to one of the many alternative philosophies used by therapists; the response is not universal. Although exercise programs cannot prevent recurrences, it appears that maintaining good physical fitness allows for a more rapid recovery. Furthermore, exercise improves mood, increases pain tolerance, and prevents deconditioning.

Spinal manipulation (chiropractic, osteopathic, or other) can reduce pain and perhaps even speed recovery if applied during the first month of pain. Manipulations should not be used in patients with neurologic deficits, and should not be continued if a few attempts are unsuccessful. The use of spinal manipulation in chronic back pain is controversial because studies remain inconclusive. Manipulation has no preventive value.

Surgery is indicated primarily in patients with herniated discs, spinal stenosis, and spondylolisthesis. Even in those conditions, nonoperative treatment is often successful and surgery should not be performed without appropriate attempts at such treatment. The cauda equina syndrome remains the exception and should be addressed surgically.

Back pain is a benign condition with excellent prognosis. In the majority of patients, no specific work-up is required and treatment is directed at reducing pain. Activity should be resumed early to avoid deconditioning.

[1]Not FDA approved for this indication.

SECTION 2

The Infectious Diseases

MANAGEMENT OF THE HIV-INFECTED PATIENT

METHOD OF
Carlos Salama, MD

In 1981, a cluster of cases of *Pneumocystis carinii* pneumonia (PCP) and Kaposi's sarcoma (KS) in previously healthy young gay men led to the recognition of a newly described entity known as AIDS. Three years later, the retrovirus HIV was recognized as the cause of this syndrome. HIV primarily infects and destroys CD4 cells, leading to a progressive destruction of the immune system. The clinical manifestations of this syndrome are variable; but eventually most patients have a depletion in their CD4 count to below 200 cells/μL, placing them at considerable risk for opportunistic infections. In the 22 years since the initial description of this syndrome, millions have died. However, there have been great advances in our understanding of HIV, its pathogenesis, genetics, and immunology. These have led to enormous strides in the treatment of HIV infection and the opportunistic infections associated with it. Most of these advances have come from and benefited patients in the developed world. Unfortunately, more than 95% of people who have HIV and AIDS live in developing nations, primarily in sub-Saharan Africa, where access to antiretroviral therapy remains exceedingly limited and AIDS kills thousands of people every day.

Transmission

Transmission of HIV occurs through contact with blood or genital secretions. This primarily occurs via sexual intercourse, intravenous drug use, transfusion of blood products, and mother-to-infant vertical transmission.

Sexual transmission remains the most common route of infection worldwide. Although rates of infection in the developed world are highest among gay men, the epidemic in the developing world is driven by heterosexual transmission. Sexual transmission occurs when infected body fluids come into contact with mucous membranes during anal, vaginal, or oral intercourse. Rates of transmission are highest among receptive partners, especially via receptive anal intercourse. High viral burden in the source patient, lack of circumcision, and the presence of sexually transmitted diseases, especially ulcerative ones such as herpes, syphilis, and chancroid, all significantly increase rates of transmission. Abstinence and consistent use of condoms are the best known ways to reduce sexual transmission.

Vertical transmission may occur in utero, peripartum, or through breast-feeding. Among untreated HIV-infected mothers, the vertical transmission rate is ~30%, and is most influenced by the viral burden of the mother. Peripartum transmission accounts for the majority of cases; it occurs as the infant passes through the birth canal and comes into contact with infected blood. Antiretroviral therapy dramatically reduces the HIV vertical transmission rate by reducing the maternal viral burden.

Transmission among injection drug users results from needle sharing between HIV-positive and -negative individuals. Needle-exchange programs and education of drug users to prevent the sharing of needles have been effective ways to curtail transmission. Other forms of drug use (e.g., crack-cocaine), although not directly associated with HIV transmission, may serve to increase risky sexual behavior and lead to increased transmission rates.

Epidemiology

Now in the third decade of the AIDS pandemic, worldwide cases of HIV/AIDS continue to climb at alarming rates, with 5 million new cases estimated in 2002 (14,000 new cases per day). As of December 2002, there were 42 million known HIV-infected persons worldwide; 29.4 million of these (70%) were in sub-Saharan Africa. Half of all infected adults are women, while children (<15 years old) account for 8% of the total (3.2 million). Since the start of the pandemic, it is estimated that 26 million individuals have died of AIDS-related diseases, including 3.1 million in 2002. An estimated 10,000 individuals continue to die every day. Thirteen million children have lost one or more of their parents to AIDS, a figure expected to rise to 25 million by 2010.

In many developing nations, unsafe sexual practices continue to fuel the epidemic. The lack of effective health care and public health infrastructure, an often-absent political will, and a largely uneducated population combine to make it difficult to slow transmission rates. In sub-Saharan Africa where death rates due to AIDS have been so high for so long, particularly in the economically productive age group (15–44 years), local economies have been devastated by the depletion of the work force.

The most explosive growth of HIV infection rates is now occurring in India and the former Soviet republics of Eastern Europe. In the latter, HIV prevalence has tripled in three years from 400,000 cases in 1999 to 1.2 million cases in 2002, with the majority of infections seen in intravenous drug users. There is fear that an ongoing outbreak of sexually transmitted diseases in the general population will converge with the HIV epidemic in intravenous drug users and cause a catastrophic spike in new infections.

In the industrialized world, HIV prevalence has increased slightly, as a result of patients living longer with effective therapy. As of 2001, there were 816,149 individuals living with HIV in the United States; 467,910 had died since the beginning of the epidemic. The new infection rate in the United States has remained steady at ~40,000 cases per year, with African Americans and Latinos disproportionately affected. For example, although African Americans currently represent only 12% of the U.S. population, they account for more than 40% of currently infected Americans and 50% of all new HIV infections. After years of decline in the incidence of infections seen in men who have sex with men (MSM), the past few years have seen a reversal in this trend, most prominently in African American and Latino men. In a study of HIV prevalence in multiple U.S. cities, 32% of young (ages 23–29 years) African American MSM were HIV infected. Although only 17.5% of all HIV-positive adults in the United States are women, 80% of all female AIDS cases in 2000 were African American and Latino women.

Natural History

Untreated, the vast majority of individuals infected with HIV progress to AIDS. Clinical progression depends on the infecting virus (tropism), host immunity (cytotoxic T-lymphocyte activity), and host genetic factors (CCR5); the combination of these factors influence the host's ability to control viral replication, as demonstrated in the baseline viral load. The Multicenter AIDS Cohort Study followed the clinical progression of 1604 HIV-infected gay men over a prolonged period. Higher baseline viral loads resulted in more rapid progression to AIDS and the appearance of AIDS-defining illnesses. Infection with T-cell tropic (syncytia-inducing) virus leads to a faster progression to AIDS than infection with macrophage tropic virus. Individuals lacking both genes for the CCR5 receptor are immune from infection with macrophage tropic virus (the overwhelming virus involved in sexual transmission), while those lacking one gene have a slower progression rate to AIDS. Although progression is related to viral burden, the risk for opportunistic infection is most closely dependent on the CD4 count (Table 1).

The advent of highly active antiretroviral therapy (HAART) has completely altered disease progression in HIV patients. Those who can remain adherent with their antiretroviral therapy can sustain durable virus suppression and arrest the progression of disease indefinitely. Even modest reductions of viral burden can result in significant CD4 increases and enormous clinical benefit for the patient. However, regimens that do not completely suppress viral burden are likely to eventually fail, lead to antiretroviral resistance, and limit future treatment options.

Life Cycle and Kinetics of HIV Infection

HIV binds, fuses with, and enters the host cell through a complex interaction between its transmembrane proteins (gp 120 and gp 41), the chemokine coreceptors (CCR5 or CXCR4), and the host cell

TABLE 1 Correlation of $CD4^+$ Count and HIV Complications

$CD4^+$ Count	Infectious Complications	Noninfectious Complications
>500/mm³	Acute retroviral syndrome Candidal vaginitis	Persistent, generalized lymphadenopathy Guillain-Barré syndrome Myopathy Aseptic meningitis
200–500/mm³	Pneumococcal and other bacterial pneumonia Pulmonary tuberculosis Herpes zoster Thrush (oropharyngeal candidiasis) Kaposi's sarcoma Oral hairy leukoplakia	Cervical carcinoma (and CSIL) B-cell lymphoma Anemia Mononeuritis multiplex Idiopathic thrombocytopenic purpura Hodgkin's disease
<200/mm³	*Pneumocystis carinii* pneumonia Disseminated histoplasmosis Coccidioidomycosis Miliary/extrapulmonary TB Progressive multifocal leukoencephalopathy	Wasting Peripheral neuropathy HIV-associated dementia Cardiomyopathy Vacuolar myelopathy Progressive polyradiculopathy Non-Hodgkin's lymphoma
<100/mm³	Disseminated herpes simplex Toxoplasmosis Cryptococcosis Microsporidiosis *Candida* esophagitis	
<50/mm³	Disseminated CMV Disseminated *Mycobacterium ovium complex*	CNS lymphoma

Abbreviations: CMV = cytomegalovirus; CNS = central nervous system; CSIL = cervical squamous intraepithelial lesion; TB = tuberculosis.
Adapted from Hanson DL, Chu SY, Ferizo KM, Ward JW: Distribution of $CD4^+$ T lymphocytes at diagnosis of acquired immunodeficiency syndrome-defining and other human immunodeficiency virus-related illnesses. The Adult and Adolescent Spectrum of HIV Disease Project Group. Arch Intern Med 155:1537–1542, 1995, Copyright 1995, American Medical Association.

CD4 receptor. Once inside the CD4 cell, viral RNA is converted to DNA by reverse transcriptase. Proviral DNA enters the nucleus and gets integrated into the host chromosomal DNA via the integrase enzyme. Once integrated, proviral DNA may remain latent or undergo transcription into newly formed viral RNA particles. During the latter, virus that is produced is immature and must be cleaved by HIV protease in order to allow for maturation of virus into infective virions.

CD4 cells in which proviral DNA remains inactive are called latent (nonreplicating) CD4 cells. Because viral replication is not active in these cells, therapy aimed at points in the life cycle of HIV cannot reach these viral particles. Thus, these cells serve to sequester HIV and re-ignite viral replication in patients who have stopped therapy after long periods of viral suppression.

The viral kinetics seen in patients with HIV infection differs according to disease stage (primary, latent asymptomatic, advanced). *Primary infection* is heralded by an acute burst of viremia with viral loads often in the millions of copies/mL. As the host develops an HIV-specific immune response, signs and symptoms of acute HIV infection appear, resulting in the partial containment of HIV and the eventual development (within 6 months) of a viral setpoint. The *asymptomatic period* is a steady-state period between the host immunity and viral replication. During this period, the host immunity attempts to keep up with the immense viral turnover and cell destruction occurring primarily in lymphatic tissues. Eventually, as lymphoid architecture is damaged through continued viral turnover, the steady state is lost. No longer able to contain replication, the viral burden rises above the previously established setpoint, CD4 count drops, and the patient progresses to *advanced AIDS*. HAART rapidly extinguishes viral replication in the active pool. However, latently infected CD4 cells may re-ignite replication within days of drug discontinuation.

Acute HIV Syndrome

Primary HIV infection is an acute, transient, nonspecific mononucleosis-like illness occurring in 40% to 90% of infected individuals. It is associated with extremely high rates of viral replication, often over 1 million copies/mL, resulting in the development of a potent HIV-specific immune response. The nonspecific nature of acute retroviral infection and private nature of high-risk activity make diagnosis difficult, as some clinicians may feel uncomfortable discussing drug use or sexual orientation and practices with their patients. Without obtaining such information, HIV testing may not be considered.

The clinical features occur 2 to 6 weeks after exposure and usually last for 2 to 10 days. The most common findings include fever, fatigue, lymphadenopathy, sore throat, rash, and, less commonly, mucosal ulcerations. The latter two findings are helpful in the diagnoses, since diffuse rash and oral lesions can help differentiate acute HIV from infectious mononucleosis. Therefore, any adult with a febrile exanthem and a history of a new sexual partner or high-risk sexual behavior should be tested for HIV. Diagnosis is made with a positive HIV-1 RNA polymerase chain reaction (PCR) and a negative or indeterminate HIV antibody test. HIV antibody tests become positive approximately 20 to 60 days after acute infection. Chronic antiretroviral therapy of all patients with acute HIV remains controversial, because viral setpoints are not established until ~6 months after infection. Treating all patients with acute HIV will undoubtedly result in unnecessary therapy for some individuals, many of whom may develop antiretroviral resistance along the way. However, early therapy may alter disease progression by preserving HIV-specific immunity and possibly lowering viral setpoints. As a result, all patients with acute retroviral syndrome should be referred for clinical trials.

Mathematical models have shown that a significant proportion of new infections result from exposure to recently infected individuals. Identification and testing of patients with primary HIV infection can result in lower infection rates through appropriate counseling to alter high-risk behavior.

HIV Testing

Patients infected with HIV usually remain asymptomatic for many years before developing AIDS. Identification of asymptomatic patients is critical to decreasing new infections by counseling patients to notify partners, use condoms, stop drug use, and prevent high-risk sexual activity. Early diagnosis also saves lives, as many patients are still not diagnosed until they present with an AIDS-defining illness. The CDC now recommends HIV screening of all persons in high-prevalence medical settings. Specific conditions that should prompt physicians to offer HIV testing are listed in Table 2.

TABLE 2 Situations in Which HIV Testing Should Be Offered*

Perform HIV testing on all persons who request testing and all pregnant women
Certain Infections
Severe herpetic lesions
Shingles
Community-acquired pneumonia
Recurrent bacterial infection
Infection with unusual organisms
Atypical features of common infections
Other STDs
Oropharyngeal candidiasis
Recurrent vulvovaginal candidiasis
Tuberculosis
Symptoms
Weight loss
Chronic diarrhea
Laboratory Tests
For: ITP, TTP, anemia, leukopenia
Unexplained renal insufficiency
Dermatologic Conditions
Severe psoriasis
Seborrheic dermatitis
Extensive HPV infection
Molluscum contagiosum
Oral leukoplakia
Neurologic Conditions
Neuropathies
Dementia
Guillain-Barré syndrome
Aseptic meningitis
Malignancies
Non-Hodgkin's lymphoma
Hodgkin's disease
Cervical carcinoma
Anal carcinoma

Abbreviations: HPV = human papillomavirus; ITP = idiopathic thrombocytopenic purpura; STDs = sexually transmitted diseases; TTP = thrombotic thrombocytopenic purpura.

*This list is in addition to persons who report known HIV risk factors and those who have an infection or condition listed in Table 1.

Management of Patients Infected with HIV

Management of HIV patients is sufficiently complicated to warrant that all HIV-infected patients be cared for by clinicians with expertise in the field. This goal is easily attainable in large cities where HIV infection is common and experienced HIV practitioners abound. In areas of lower HIV prevalence, this may be more difficult. Nevertheless, an attempt should be made to match up HIV patients with experienced HIV caregivers.

INITIAL EVALUATION

A thorough history and review of systems should focus on common presentations seen in patients with symptomatic HIV disease, including fever, weight loss, respiratory symptoms, diarrhea, odynophagia, visual problems, and skin lesions. The history should be guided by the CD4 count when known. Other important questions should focus around sexual orientation and activity, history of sexually transmitted diseases, history of drug use, mental illness, partner HIV status, partner notification, and condom use. Patients who are not newly diagnosed should be questioned about their past antiretroviral (ARV) use, since the success of future regimens will depend heavily on past ARV.

Examination should be thorough and guided by the CD4 count (for possible opportunistic infections). Women should have pelvic examinations with Papanicolaou (Pap) smears to evaluate for cervical dysplasia, and gay men should be evaluated for anal lesions. All patients with advanced AIDS should have dilated funduscopic examinations performed by an ophthalmologist.

All patients should have basic blood work (CBC, chemistries, liver function tests, lipids), counts, and viral load. The CD4 count instructs the clinician about the patient's current immune status, whereas the HIV-1 RNA PCR (viral load) may be a predictor of future CD4 decline. Other important blood tests include syphilis, toxoplasmosis, cytomegalovirus, and hepatitis B and hepatitis C serologies. MSM and patients with underlying liver disease also should be tested for hepatitis A serology. All patients must have a purified protein derivative (PPD) test, pneumococcal polysaccharide vaccine (Pneumovax 23), and a yearly influenza vaccination. Patients with negative hepatitis A and B serologies should be vaccinated, and those with a positive rapid plasma reagin (RPR) or PPD test should be treated with appropriate antibiotics. A baseline chest x-ray (CXR) is helpful given the high rates of respiratory infections in patients with AIDS, and is mandatory in patients with a positive PPD (yearly).

Prophylactic antibiotics save lives in patients with AIDS. Patients with CD4 counts below 200 cells/μL should be offered trimethoprim-sulfamethoxazole (Bactrim) to prevent reactivation disease with *Pneumocystis carinii* pneumoniae (PCP). Patients with AIDS have a significantly higher incidence of allergy to sulfa drugs. When sulfa allergy is present, prophylaxis with dapsone[1] (cross-allergy common) or atovaquone (Mepron) is recommended. Dapsone is preferable due to significantly lower cost, but G6PD deficiency should be ruled out first. In patients with positive serology for toxoplasmosis, prophylaxis is recommended when the CD4 count falls below 100 cells/μL. This is also achieved with Bactrim, or with the addition of weekly pyrimethamine (Daraprim) in sulfa allergic patients. Prophylaxis for mycobacterium avium complex (MAC) is recommended for patients with CD4 counts below 50 cells/μL, although it is not clear that MAC prophylaxis affects survival in the post-HAART era. In patients with CD4 counts below 100 cells/μL, where antiretroviral therapy is unlikely to succeed (resistance, nonadherence), prophylaxis against Cryptococcus should be considered with fluconazole (Diflucan), given the high morbidity and mortality rates associated with this pathogen.

[1]Not FDA approved for this indication.

THE ANTIRETROVIRALS

There are four classes of antiretroviral medications: nucleoside/nucleotide reverse transcriptase inhibitors, non-nucleoside reverse transcriptase inhibitors, protease inhibitors, and the newly released fusion inhibitor (enfuvirtide [Fuzeon]). All act against enzymes or proteins in the life cycle of HIV. Dosing and adverse events related with each are included in Table 3 (NRTI), Table 4 (NNRTI), and Table 5 (PI). For enfuvirtide (Fuzeon, T-20), the dose is 90 mg subcutaneously twice daily, and side effects include local injection site reactions, increased rate of bacterial pneumonia, and hypersensitivity reaction. Some complications of ARV therapy are potentially fatal. Abacavir (Ziagen) therapy can cause a hypersensitivity reaction in approximately 4% of individuals; re-exposure can result in a more fulminant allergic reaction and death. Nevirapine (Viramune) and efavirenz (Sustiva) therapy may rarely result in a potentially fatal Stevens-Johnson

TABLE 3 Nucleoside Reverse Transcriptase Inhibitors[a]

NRTI[b]	Dose	Selected Side Effects
Zidovudine (AZT, Retrovir, Combivir, Trizivir)	300 mg q12h Combivir or Trizivir, 1 tablet q12h[c]	GI upset, headache, anemia,[d] myopathy
Lamivudine (3TC, Epivir, Combivir, Trizivir)	150 mg q12h or 300 mg qd Combivir or Trizivir, 1 tablet q12h[c]	Minimal
Stavudine (d4T, Zerit)	40 mg q12h (if >60 kg), 30 mg q12h (if <60 kg)	Neuropathy, pancreatitis, lipodystrophy
Didanosine (ddI, Videx, Videx EC)[e]	200 mg q12h or 400 mg/d (if >60 kg); 125 mg q12h or 250 mg/d (if <60 kg)	Neuropathy, GI upset,[e] pancreatitis
Abacavir (ABC, Ziagen, Trizivir)	300 mg q12h or 600 mg/d, or Trizivir, 1 tablet q12h[c]	Hypersensitivity reaction[f]
Dideoxycytidine (ddC, zalcitabine [Hivid])[g]	0.75 mg tid	Peripheral neuropathy (17%–30%), pancreatitis stematitis
Tenofovir (viread)	300 mg PO qd	Rare cases of renal failure
Emtricitabine (Emtriva)	200 mg/d	Minimal

[a]Lactic acidosis is a rare complication of the NRII class, much more commonly associated with stavudine, didanosine, and dideoxycytidine.
[b]Renal adjustments are available for all NRTIs except abacavir.
[c]Combivir is one tablet that contains 300 mg of zidovudine and 150 mg of lamivudine. Trizivir is Combivir with the addition of abacavir, 300 mg.
[d]Can treat AZT-associated anemia with erythropoietin; check the hematocrit 2 to 4 weeks after starting treatment and then every 3 months.
[e]Should be taken on an empty stomach. Doses are for tablets (chewed or dissolved), not powder. Videx EC is preferable because of improved tolerability.
[f]The hypersensitivity reaction is characterized by abdominal pain, nausea, vomiting, fever, rash, and malaise. Do not rechallenge; the drug can be fatal if the patient discontinues and then restarts abacavir therapy. Most reactions occur within 6 weeks. Patients must be extensively educated about this side effect.
[g]ddC should be avoided because of its side effect profile and decreased efficacy.

TABLE 4 Nonnucleoside Reverse Transcriptase Inhibitors

NNRTI	Dose	Selected Side Effects
Efavirenz (Sustiva)	600 mg qhs	CNS effects*, rash
Nevirapine (Viramune)	200 mg/d × 14d, then 200 mg bid	Rash, hepatitis† or 40 mg qd§
Delavirdine (Rescriptor)‡	400 mg q8h	Rash, headache

*CNS effects occur in 25% to 40% and consist of a feeling of dizziness, disconnected feeling, and strange dreams, all of which usually decrease within 2 weeks. It is recommended that efavirenz be given at bedtime; the drug is contraindicated in pregnancy.

†The rash and hepatitis are more common in women. The hepatitis occurs within the first 4 weeks and can be fatal. Stevens-Johnson reaction is reported. Check liver function 2 to 4 weeks after starting therapy.

‡This regimen is used much less commonly because of dosing every 8 hours and rash.

§400 mg/d of viramune has higher rates of hepatitis.

syndrome. Nevirapine use has also been associated with rare events of acute fulminant liver failure, particularly in women with CD4 counts >250 cells/μL. The nucleoside analogues, particularly stavudine (Zerit), didanosine (Videx), and zalcitabine (Hivid) may cause life-threatening lactic acidosis.

DEFINING UNDETECTABLE VIRAL LOAD

An undetectable viral load <50 copies/mL is the virologic goal of antiretroviral therapy and the major outcomes measurement of most clinical trials assessing HIV therapy success. Before initiating antiretroviral therapy, all patients should have their pretherapy baseline viral load checked (range: 400-750,000 copies/mL). Approximately 4 weeks after therapy initiation, the first post-therapy viral load is performed to assess for treatment response. Rarely will the viral load be undetectable (<400 copies/mL) at this point; however, a significant (≥1 log) decrease is expected, otherwise nonresponse to therapy should be considered (due to either nonadherence or preexistent resistance). Close monitoring of the viral load should continue, and by 6 months, the viral load should be undetectable in the vast majority of cases. Once the viral load is consistently below 400 copies/mL, an ultra-sensitive viral load may be performed (range: 50-75,000 copies/mL). In the stable patient on therapy, the viral load and CD4 count are measured every 3 months. If virus becomes again detectable, it should be promptly reconfirmed and followed up with a resistance test.

WHEN TO START THERAPY

The decision regarding when to initiate antiretroviral therapy in the asymptomatic HIV patient is one of the hardest for the HIV clinician, since ARV exposure can result in resistance in a large number of patients. Whether to initiate therapy depends most heavily on three factors: the current immune status of the patient, the likely rate of progression to AIDS if untreated, and the patient's motivation to remain adherent with medication.

All patients with symptomatic AIDS and all asymptomatic patients with CD4 counts below 200 cells/μL

TABLE 5 Protease Inhibitors

Protease Inhibitors	Dose	Selected Side Effects
Nelfinavir (Viracept)[a]	1250 mg q12h or 750 mg q8h	Diarrhea, GI upset
Indinavir (Crixivan)[b]	800 mg q12h (with ritonavir, 100 or 200 mg q12h) or 800 mg q8h	GI upset, increased bilirubin, nephrolithiasis (take with 48 oz of water daily)
Saquinavir SGC (Fortovase)[c]	400 mg q12h (with ritonavir, 400 mg q12h) or 1200 mg q8h	GI upset
Saquinavir HGC (Invirase)	400 mg q12h (with ritonavir, 400 mg PO q12h) or 1000–2000 mg q12h–qd (with ritonavir 100–200 mg q12h–qd)	GI upset
Amprenavir (Agenerase)[d]	1200 mg q12h or 600–1200 mg q12h–qd (with ritonavir, 100–200 mg q12h–qd)	Rash, GI intolerance
Lopinavir/ritonavir (Kaletra)[e]	400/100 mg q 12h	GI upset, diarrhea
Ritonavir (Norvir)[f]	600 mg q12h (not recommended)	GI upset
Atazanavir (Reyataz)	400 mg/d or 300 mg/d (with ritonavir 100 mg/d)	Indirect hyperbilirubinemia
Fos-Amprenavir (Lexiva)	1400 mg q12h or 700 mg q12h (with ritonavir 100 mg q12h) or 1400 mg qd (with ritonavir 200 mg qd)	Rash, GI intolerance

[a]Must be taken with food.

[b]An indinavir/ritonavir combination is preferred because of an improved dosing schedule and pharmacokinetic profile. Indinavir (Crixivan) given alone must be taken on an empty stomach and separated from didanosine (ddI).

[c]Saquinavir/ritonavir is preferred because of a smaller pill burden and an improved pharmacokinetic profile.

[d]Amprenavir alone is 8 pills every 12 hours. Co-administration with ritonavir can decrease the pill burden.

[e]Increase the dose to 533/133 mg every 12 hours when co-administered with efavirenz and nevirapine.

[f]Ritonavir is poorly tolerated at full dose and is primarily used to enhance serum levels of other protease inhibitors through cytochrome P-450 blockade.

should be offered antiretroviral therapy; treatment of this group has been shown to improve survival and quality of life. No such benefits have been shown among patients with CD4 counts above 350 cells/μL, and therapy may be safely deferred under most circumstances. Use caution with patients in this subgroup who have very high viral loads, because CD4 depletion may occur rapidly; consequently, high-viral-load (>100,000 copies/mL) patients, regardless of CD4 counts, should be strongly considered for antiretroviral treatment. A debate remains regarding the need for immediate treatment of patients with CD4 counts between 200 and 350 cells/μL, although most clinicians favor treatment in this situation, particularly in high-viral-load patients. When therapy is deferred, close monitoring and trending of CD4 and viral load are imperative.

Adherence

Strict adherence to antiretroviral therapy is among the most important factors determining the durability of a specific regimen. Although even modest reduction in virus load has been associated with outstanding improvement in many outcomes measurements, all regimens that fail to suppress virus maximally will eventually fail, lead to resistance, and possibly limit future therapeutic options. Data from centers utilizing directly observed therapy (DOT) have taught us that when taken every day, approved therapeutic regimens work well; Fischl and colleagues documented a 100% rate of undetectable viral load (<400 copies/μL) at 48 weeks among incarcerated patients on DOT. Although the potency of a regimen when taken 100% adherently may not dramatically differ between one regimen and another, in somewhat less adherent patients, some regimens may be more forgiving than others. This is particularly the case with regimens that contain medications with improved genetic barriers to resistance, such as boosted protease inhibitors.

Adherence is impossible to predict for patients initiating therapy. Although patients with mental illness or a history of dependence on alcohol or drugs can be predicted to have higher rates of nonadherence, a large number of these individuals are successfully adherent with their medications. The inverse may be true of patients in groups (i.e., professionals) historically believed to have higher rates of good adherence. Clinicians should not make assumptions about patients based on their socioeconomic status, lifestyle choices, or history of mental disease. In addition, some patients learn from their first or second treatment failure while others become more adherent when they become ill; it is crucial for clinicians caring for HIV-infected individuals to never give up on patients as a result of past nonadherence problems.

Many strategies may be employed to improve adherence, including:

- Educating patients about the connection between strict ARV adherence and resistance emergence.
- Using a team approach that uses the clinician, nurse, social worker, adherence counselor, and pharmacist to reinforce the importance of taking medications on schedule.
- Treating substance abuse and mental illness.
- Ensuring that the patient has the necessary social support.
- Choosing regimens that are easy to take, dosed no more than twice per day, and have little or no dietary requirements.
- Ensuring, once therapy is initiated, that patients visit weekly with either the clinician or a member of the adherence team for the first 2 to 4 weeks. This can help deal with problems as they arise, such as adverse events, incompletely filled prescriptions, and missed doses. These quick and easy visits will help patients gain confidence, answer their questions, and improve patient–clinician relationships.

First Regimen

Once the decision has been made to treat, there are many first line regimens that have been shown to be effective. In order to make the best choice for the initial regimen, the clinician should inquire about the patient's lifestyle, eating habits, work situation and hours, available social support, and family history of heart disease and diabetes. A resistance test may be performed, particularly in areas with high rates of antiretroviral resistance. Most antiretroviral regimens are made up of three medications, the backbone of which contains two nucleoside reverse transcriptase inhibitors: lamivudine (epivir) or emtricibatine (emtriva) and either zidovudine (retrovir), stavudine (zerit), tenofovir (viread), abacavir (ziagen), or didanosine (videx). The third drug in the cocktail may be another nucleoside analogue, a non-nucleoside reverse transcriptase inhibitor (NNRTI), or a protease inhibitor (PI)—unboosted or boosted with ritonavir (norvir).

NNRTI- and boosted PI-based regimens are the best studied, most efficacious and durable regimens, and are the recommended first choices when initiating antiretroviral therapy in naïve patients. The advantages of using NNRTI-based regimens (efavirenz or nevirapine) include low pill burden, no dietary restrictions, lack of gastrointestinal side effects, and outstanding outcomes data. Their major disadvantage rests with the poor genetic barrier to resistance. A patient who misses a few doses in the first month of therapy may rapidly develop NNRTI resistance (i.e., K103N) leading to loss of efficacy for the entire NNRTI class (cross-resistance). Protease inhibitor regimens have the advantage of being more resilient to resistance development. However, PI pill burdens remain relatively high, most continue to have dietary restrictions, they contribute to higher rates of lipid abnormalities and insulin resistance, and they are associated with high rates of gastrointestinal disturbances.

The triple-nucleoside Trizivir (fixed-dose zidovudine/lamivudine/abacavir) has the advantage of being extremely easy to take (one pill twice daily, no dietary restrictions), but has recently been shown to be less durable than NNRTI-based regimens, and is therefore only recommended when PI- or NNRTI-based regimens cannot be used. If trizivir is to be used alone, it should be used only in patients with baseline viral loads below 100,000 copies/mL and without pre-existing resistance mutations. Recent data have shown that triple nucleoside regimens that do not contain a thymidine analogue have unacceptable rates of virologic failure and should never be used. The quadruple nucleoside regimen of trizivir and tenofovir (viread) has gained popularity, but little data is available regarding its long-term efficacy. The use of first line regimens that contain three drug classes (NRTI, NNRTI, and PI) have the disadvantage of potentially leading to a widely resistant virus if virologic failure occurs.

See Table 6 for the most recent Department of Health and Human Services (DHHS) antiretroviral therapy guidelines.

Resistance and Resistance Testing

Resistance to antiretroviral therapy has become common. A recent study showed that a majority of patients who have taken antiretrovirals have resistance to at least one medication.

The reverse transcriptase gene (RT) naturally makes numerous errors during viral transcription, resulting in the development of mutant strains of HIV. In the absence of drug pressure (ARV), these strains are unable to effectively compete with wild-type virus. In the presence of ARV, mutant HIV strains survive if they have an improved ability to replicate in the presence of the antiretroviral therapy

TABLE 6 Antiretroviral Regimens Recommended for Treatment of HIV-1 Infection in Antiretroviral Naïve Patients[a]

NNRTI-Based Regimens[b]		**Pills Per Day**
Preferred Regimens	**Efavirenz + lamivudine + (zidovudine or tenofovir DF or stavudine[c]); do not use for pregnant women or women with pregnancy potential**	3–5
	Efavirenz + emtricitabine + (zidovudine or tenofovir DF or stavudine[c]); do not use for pregnant women or women with pregnancy potential[d]	3–4
Alternative Regimens	Efavirenz + (lamivudine or emtricitabine) + didanosine; do not use for pregnant women or women with pregnancy potential[d]	3
	Nevirapine + (lamivudine or emtricitabine) + (zidovudine or stavudine[c] or didanosine)	4–5
PI-Based Regimens[b]		**Pills Per Day**
Preferred Regimens	**Lopinavir/ritonavir (co-formulated as Kaletra) + lamivudine + (zidovudine or stavudine)**	**8–10**
Alternative Regimens	Amprenavir/ritonavir[e] + (lamivudine or emtricitabine[1]) + (zidovudine or stavudine)	12–14
	Atazanavir + (lamivudine or emtricitabine) + (zidovudine or stavudine[c])	4–5
	Indinavir + (lamivudine or emtricitabine[1]) + (zidovudine or stavudine[c])	8–10
	Indinavir/ritonavir[e] + (lamivudine or emtricitabine) + (zidovudine or stavudine[c])	8–11
	Lopinavir/ritonavir (co-formulated as Kaletra) + emtricitabine + (zidovudine or stavudine[c])	8–9
	Nelfinavir[f] + (lamivudine or emtricitabine[1]) + (zidovudine or stavudine[c])	6–14
	Saquinavir (SGC or HGC)/ritonavir[e] (lamivudine or emtricitabine) + (zidovudine or stavudine)	14–16
Triple NRTI Regimen[b]—Only when an NNRTI- or PI-based regimen cannot or should not be used as first line therapy		**Pills Per Day**
Only as an alternative to NNRTI- or PI-based regimen	Abacavir + lamivudine + zidovudine (or stavudine[c])	2–6

Abbreviations: SGC = soft gel capsule; HGC = hard gel capsule.

[a]This table is a guide to treatment regimens for patients who have no previous experience with HIV therapy. Regimens should be individualized based on the advantages and disadvantages of each combination such as pill burden, dosing frequency, toxicities, and drug-drug interactions; and patient variables, such as pregnancy, co-morbid conditions, and level of plasma HIV-RNA. Preferred regimens are in bold type; regimens are designated as preferred for use in treatment-naïve patients when clinical trial data suggests optimal and durable efficacy with acceptable tolerability and ease of use. Alternative regimens are those where clinical trial data show efficacy, but it is considered alternative due to disadvantages compared to the preferred agent, in terms of antiviral activity, demonstrated durable effect, tolerability or ease of use. In some cases, based on individual patient characteristics, a regimen listed as an alternative regimen may actually be the preferred regimen for a selected patient. Clinicians initiating antiretroviral regimens in the HIV-1-infected pregnant patient should refer to *"Recommendations for Use of Antiretroviral Drugs in Pregnant HIV-1-Infected Women for Maternal Health and Interventions to Reduce Perinatal HIV-1 Transmission in the United States"* at http://www.aidsinfo.nih.gov/guidelines/.

[b]The generic and brand names for all the drugs listed are: abacavir (ziagen), amprenavir (Agenerase), atazanavir (Reyataz), didanosine (Videx), efavirenz (Sustiva), emtricitabine (Emtriva), indinavir (Crixivan), lamivudine (Epivir), lopinavir/ritonavir (Kaletra), nelfinavir (Viracept), nevirapine (Viramune), saquinavir HGC (Invirase), saquinavir SGC (Fortovase), stavudine (Zerit), tenofovir (Viread), zidovudine (Retrovir).

[c]Higher incidence of lipoatrophy, hyperlipidemia, and mitochondrial toxicities reported with stavudine than with other NRTIs.

[d]Women with childbearing potential implies women who want to conceive or those who are not using effective contraception.

[e]Low-dose (100–400 mg) ritonavir.

[f]Nelfinavir available in 250 mg or 625 mg tablet.

being used (natural selection of resistant mutants). Once this occurs, these mutants go on to infect latent CD4 cells and long-lived cells (monocytes) and are archived. Every time the antiretroviral is reintroduced, the archived strain reemerges.

Maximal viral suppression (<50 copies/mL) is critical to the prevention of resistance emergence, by virtually halting replication of virus in the active pool. Absence of viral turnover leads to inactivity of RT. When RT is inactive, it makes fewer errors in transcription and resistance is less likely to emerge.

Resistance testing should be performed to assess baseline resistance in every patient naïve to antiretroviral therapy, including those with acute and chronic infection. Among therapy-experienced patients, resistance testing should be performed in patients who are failing an antiretroviral regimen while they are still on the failing regimen (drug pressure).

There are two types of resistance tests: genotypic testing (GT) and phenotypic testing (PT). In GT, the reverse transcriptase and protease genes are sequenced and compared with those of wild-type virus; differences are reported as codon mutations, which the clinician must interpret to choose the best possible regimen. For proper interpretation clinicians must have sufficient knowledge of specific mutations and corresponding resistance associated with them. Given the complexity of this technology, all results of genotypic resistance tests should be interpreted with the aid of an expert in HIV resistance. PT is a direct measurement of the ability of virus to grow in the presence of specific medications. A minimum viral load of 500-1000 copies/mL is usually necessary to perform both tests.

Resistance Pathways

The choice of nucleoside backbone is important with regard to the pathway to nucleoside resistance. The first nucleoside mutation to occur when lamivudine (Epivir) is part of a regimen is M184V. Although this mutation causes high-level resistance to lamivudine, it also has many significant advantages associated with it:

- It slows the accumulation of thymidine analogue mutations.
- It prevents the development of pan-nucleoside resistance mutations (Q151M, 69 sss).
- It resensitizes the virus to zidovudine (Retrovir).
- It causes hypersusceptibility of the virus to tenofovir.
- It significantly reduces viral fitness.

Thymidine analogues (zidovudine [Retrovir] or stavudine [Zerit]) have been a core component of the nucleoside backbone since the introduction of HAART. However, the toxicity of thymidine analogues and desire by clinicians to use once-daily therapy has led to the development of thymidine analogue-sparing regimens. Such regimens usually combine a two-drug nucleoside backbone (lamivudine [Epivir] with tenofovir [Viread], abacavir [Ziagen], or didanosine [Videx]) with an NNRTI to create a low pill burden once-daily regimen. Although these regimens are highly potent and offer some clear advantages, failures of thymidine analogue-sparing regimens often occur with the rapid development of multiple mutations: M184V (lamivudine) with either K65R (tenofovir) or L74V (abacavir), and K103N (when NNRTI is used). Virologic failure occurring with a conventional backbone of a thymidine analogue and lamivudine usually occurs with the development of the M184V mutation, followed by the slow accumulation of thymidine analogue mutations (TAMs). Even when tenofovir and abacavir are included in the thymidine analogue-containing regimens, K65R and L74V rarely occur. Although the presence of multiple TAMs very significantly affects resistance to the entire nucleoside class, their slow accumulation gives the patient and clinician time to adjust therapy.

Intensification, Change in Therapy, Salvage

Changes to antiretroviral regimens may be made due to adverse events, to decrease pill burden, for simplification (q12h to qd, remove dietary restrictions), or as a result of virologic failure. When there is resistance, one or more drugs in the regimen may be changed, depending on the results of resistance test. Any time such a change is made, the underlying reason for virologic failure must be identified and addressed. In salvage situations, the clinician must do his or her best to construct a regimen that the patient will tolerate, be able to adhere to, and be efficacious. Many, but not all, patients who end up with a salvage regimen, do so because of past nonadherence, making this task ever more difficult. Virologic outcomes in salvage situations are better when new drug classes are available, thus making early judicious use of ARV important. The use of resistance testing and a close review of past ARV are critical to choosing a successful regimen. If possible, enrolling the patient in an adherence or partial DOT program may be helpful.

Among patients with adherence difficulties, dual-boosted PI regimens (i.e., lopinavir/ritonavir [Kaletra] plus saquinavir [Invirase] or amprenavir [Agenerase]) may be particularly valuable, as they are relatively resilient to resistance development, are extremely potent, and may be effective without a nucleoside backbone.

Postexposure Prophylaxis (PEP)

Health care workers and victims of sexual assault exposed to blood or genital secretions of individuals who are HIV-infected can decrease the risk of becoming infected by taking postexposure antiretroviral prophylaxis. The risk of seroconversion after percutaneous exposure to HIV-positive blood is 1:324. The three most important factors contributing to this risk include inoculum size (device size, visible blood, hollow bore needle), source viral burden, and host immunity.

A CDC run, retrospective case control study using national surveillance data from the United States, the

United Kingdom, France, and Italy from 1988 through 1994 demonstrated an estimated 81% decrease in transmission with the use of zidovudine (Retrovir) alone. For sexual assaults, the risk of transmission is probably lower, and may depend on the type of intercourse (anal vs. vaginal), the degree of brutality, and the number of assailants involved. Current guidelines of PEP recommend using a full-scale antiretroviral regimen (i.e., zidovudine, lamivudine, tenofovir) for a full month to decrease the risk of transmission for both health care workers and victims of sexual assaults. Therapy must be initiated as soon as possible after exposure, since HIV has been found to drain into regional lymph nodes within 48 hours of vaginal intercourse. When in doubt, therapy should be started and then be reevaluated. Avoid potentially life-threatening medications, such as abacavir and nevirapine, given the low risk of transmission even in untreated individuals. Every health care facility should have a systematic approach for identification and prophylaxis of health care workers in the timeliest manner possible.

Therapy of the Pregnant Patient

An attempt should be made to test all pregnant women for HIV; if positive, these women should be offered antiretroviral therapy to reduce the possibility of vertical transmission. Treatment should be initiated at week 14 (to avoid first trimester ARV exposure), include zidovudine when possible, and continue through the baby's birth, as per the landmark ACTG 076 trial. The goal of therapy is to achieve an undetectable viral load, thereby dramatically reducing the risk of vertical transmission. After birth, zidovudine therapy is continued in the newborn for 6 weeks and mothers are instructed not to nurse, thus avoiding further postpartum exposure. In developed countries, antiretroviral therapy invariably means three or more active agents chosen with the aid of a genotypic resistance test. In developing countries, prophylaxis of vertical transmission may consist of one dose of nevirapine (Viramune) immediately prior to birth. Although not as effective, it is a cost-effective means of preventing most cases of HIV vertical transmission. Those already on antiretrovirals when they become pregnant should remain on therapy. Medications may be adjusted according to risk for teratogenicity, particularly when efavirenz (Sustiva) is part of the regimen. Patients with persistently elevated viral loads (>1000 copies/mL) at time of delivery may benefit from elective cesarean section. Once the baby is born, the mother's own need for antiretroviral medication may be reassessed.

Complications of Antiretroviral (ARV) Therapy

IMMUNE RECONSTITUTION SYNDROME (IRS)

HIV potently stimulates immune cells to release cytokines; cytokines work to further activate T-lymphocytes, including CD4 cells, to combat HIV. Thus, uncontrolled viral replication is a state of constant cytokine secretion and leads to CD4 cells being drawn to and sequestered within lymphatic tissues. Effective antiretroviral therapy shuts down viral replication, thereby greatly diminishing immune cell activation and cytokine release; this makes it possible for memory CD4 cells previously trapped within lymphatics to redistribute into the peripheral circulation. This abrupt, rapid, and abundant transfer of memory CD4 cells allows for a restoration of pathogen-specific immune reactivity, and may result in a paradoxical immune-mediated inflammatory reaction against previously diagnosed or latent opportunistic infectious agents.

The clinical manifestations of IRS are inflammatory in nature. Cases have been described with a multitude of opportunistic pathogens, most commonly MAC and TB. Patients present with fever and localized immune-mediated disease shortly after commencing antiretroviral therapy. The immune-mediated illness varies according to infection type: patients with MAC and TB may develop localized necrotic lymphadenopathy or pulmonary infiltrates; those with a history of cytomegalovirus (CMV) retinitis may develop an immune mediated vitritis; patients with cryptococcal disease may get worsening meningitis and/or raised intracranial pressure. The diagnosis is made clinically, although cultures in cases of mycobacterial IRS are often positive and granuloma formation may be seen on biopsy. Treatment of the offending pathogen results in improvement of most cases, and anti-inflammatory agents may be used as adjuncts; continuation of antiretroviral therapy is recommended.

PERIPHERAL NEUROPATHY

Peripheral neuropathy in patients with HIV may result from antiretrovirals (stavudine [Zerit], didanosine [Videx], dideoxycytidine [Hivid]) or from HIV itself. The pain associated with neuropathy may be severe enough to limit function. Treatment is aimed at symptomatic pain relief with gabapentin (Neurontin)[1] or tricyclic antidepressants (Elavil)[1]. When pain is caused by ARV, replacement of the offending agent is also an option. Even after withdrawal of the offending antiretroviral, it may take weeks or months for the pain to completely resolve.

LACTIC ACIDOSIS

Lactic acidosis is a rare, life-threatening complication of therapy with nucleoside reverse transcriptase inhibitors, usually occurring at least 6 months after their initiation, and more commonly found in females and obese individuals. The nucleosides that most commonly cause this adverse event are the so-called

[1]Not FDA approved for this indication.

d-drugs: stavudine (d4T/Zerit), didanosine (ddI/Videx) and dideoxycytidine (ddC/HIVID). The syndrome occurs when nucleoside analogues damage the mitochondria of cells, resulting in the accumulation of lactate. The most common symptoms are malaise, fatigue, nausea, vomiting, anorexia, abdominal pain, and eventual tachypnea (as the patient attempts to breathe off acid). Treatment involves withdrawal of antiretrovirals and supportive care. When lactic acidosis results from stavudine, didanosine, or dideoxycytidine, re-introduction of alternate nucleoside analogues known to have significantly lower risks for lactic acidosis (zidovudine [Retrovir], tenofovir [Viread], abacavir [Ziagen], lamivudine [Epivir]) may be carefully considered on a case-by-case basis.

METABOLIC COMPLICATIONS

The metabolic complications of antiretroviral therapy include: lipid abnormalities, insulin resistance/ diabetes mellitus, and lipodystrophy. Lipid elevations and insulin resistance may increase the risk of heart disease in these patients.

Lipid abnormalities may occur from exposure to nucleoside analogues, PIs, and NNRTIs. The most significant lipid increases occur with protease inhibitors boosted with ritonavir (Norvir) , particularly lopinavir/ritonavir (Kaletra); the only protease inhibitor to not cause lipid increases is atazanavir (Reyataz). Among the nucleosides and NNRTIs, increases in lipid levels are more common with stavudine (Zerit) and efavirenz (Sustiva). Treatment is with diet, exercise, and lipid-lowering agents. Discontinuation of the offending agent may occasionally be necessary, particularly when triglyceride levels increase to the thousands, risking pancreatitis.

Insulin resistance and diabetes mellitus are most closely associated with PI use. Treatment includes diet/weight loss, exercise, and when necessary, hypoglycemic agents, as in HIV-negative individuals. Those predisposed to diabetes through family history or from being overweight should be counseled about the risks of insulin resistance even before antiretrovirals are initiated.

Lipodystrophy is the redistribution of fat from the periphery (peripheral lipoatrophy) to the trunk (central fat accumulation). Peripheral lipoatrophy is the loss of subcutaneous fat from the face, arms, legs, and buttocks, resulting in a sunken facial appearance (especially cheeks) and bulging veins in the extremities. This syndrome has a very negative impact on the body image of patients with AIDS and frequently leads to patients wanting to discontinue therapy. The cause is unknown, but antiretroviral therapy is widely believed to be responsible. Although stavudine (Zerit) is most closely associated with this syndrome, regimens lacking stavudine are known to cause it as well. Patients starting ARV regimens with low nadir CD4 counts may be at the greatest risk of developing lipoatrophy. Treatments that have been attempted to restore subcutaneous fat have included growth hormone, anabolic steroids, metformin (Glucophage)[1], and thiazolidinediones, without significant success. ARV withdrawal or replacement has been generally unsuccessful as well. Some patients have sought localized injections to the cheek area to fill in areas of subcutaneous fat loss. Central fat accumulation may occur with or without peripheral lipoatrophy. Patients accumulate fat in the abdomen, neck, breasts, dorsocervical area (buffalo hump), and viscera. Some patients may also develop multiple lipomas. The exact cause is unknown. Besides liposuction of specific areas (high recurrence), there is no effective therapy.

DRUG INTERACTIONS

Drug interactions are common with antiretroviral agents, making pharmacists an integral part of the HIV management team. A few of the more important interactions are discussed here. Ritonavir (Norvir) strongly interacts with the cytochrome P-450 system, thereby affecting the levels of many medications, including statins, oral contraceptives, other PIs, and methadone. Some effects are desirable (PI boosting), while others are not (methadone withdrawal, inactivity of oral contraceptives). NNRTIs can also significantly decrease methadone levels, precipitating withdrawal. Rifampin is a potent inducer of cytochrome P-450; when co-administered with protease inhibitors, PI levels may be significantly decreased, leading to treatment failure. Tenofovir (Viread) is known to dramatically decrease levels of atazanavir (Reyataz), while raising levels of didanosine (Videx). Co-administration of these agents without proper adjustments in doses (didanosine) or appropriate boosting (atazanavir) could lead to severe toxicities or early drug failure. Atazanavir levels are also lowered by efavirenz (Sustiva), so ritonavir boosting is recommended.

Infectious Syndromes and Malignancies in Patients with HIV/AIDS

THE AIDS PATIENT WITH PNEUMONIA

Community-acquired pneumonia (CAP) is very common among HIV-infected individuals. Etiologies of CAP that are strongly associated with HIV infection include Pneumococcal pneumonia, *Pneumocystis carinii* pneumonia, tuberculosis, *Cryptococcus neoformans, Histoplasma capsulatum, Rhodococcus equi, Penicillium marneffei* (southeast Asia), and *Pseudomonas aeruginosa*. The presenting history and nature of infiltrates (focal or disseminated) on a chest film can be extremely useful in differentiating between etiologic agents. The clinician should elicit the following: abrupt or insidious presentation, presence of

[1]Not FDA approved for this indication.

pyogenic features, current and nadir CD4 counts, place or country of origin, exposure to tuberculosis, history of smoking, and use of prophylactic antibiotics (i.e., Bactrim). For many of these etiologies, the pneumonia may be part of a disseminated illness. In many underdeveloped countries, TB is the single biggest killer of patients with AIDS. As such, patients originating from high-risk areas, those potentially exposed, and anyone else with the remote possibility of having active pulmonary tuberculosis should be placed into respiratory isolation.

Patients presenting with abrupt symptoms of fever, cough, purulent sputum, relative leucocytosis and focal infiltrates usually have bacterial pneumonia. Pneumococcal pneumonia and bacteremia are remarkably common among patients with HIV/AIDS; this results from a variety of immunologic defects, most notably altered antibody production against pneumococcal capsular polysaccharides. The diagnosis may be confirmed by sputum gram stain, sputum culture, or blood culture. Although penicillin is still effective in a majority of cases, the increasing incidence of resistance to penicillin has made empiric therapy with ceftriaxone (Rocephin), expanded spectrum fluoroquinolones, or vancomycin (Vancocin) the recommended standard of care. If cultures are available and penicillin susceptibility is confirmed, completion of therapy with penicillin is advisable. All patients with pneumococcal pneumonia, particularly when accompanied by bacteremia, should be evaluated for the possibility of HIV infection. All HIV patients should be vaccinated with the pneumococcal vaccine (Pneumovax). Other pyogenic bacteria with higher infection rates in AIDS patients include Haemophilus influenza and *Pseudomonas aeruginosa*. The latter often presents with cavitary disease and bacteremia, and carries a high mortality rate.

The differential diagnosis for AIDS patients with diffuse bilateral pneumonia is extensive, including *Pneumocystis carinii* pneumonia (PCP), tuberculosis, pulmonary cryptococcosis, endemic mycosis (Histoplasma, coccidioidomycosis), and diffuse bacterial (pneumococcal) pneumonia. Kaposi's sarcoma may cause diffuse pulmonary involvement, but patients seldom have symptoms of infection, such as fever. PCP continues to be a common AIDS-defining illness with a high mortality rate. The risk for PCP occurs when the CD4 count falls below 200 cells/μL. Patients with PCP often have an insidious presentation, with fever, progressive dyspnea, and nonproductive cough for weeks; pneumothorax may occasionally occur. The dyspnea is initially exertional, but progresses to dyspnea at rest; patients with normal oxygen saturation should be ambulated to evaluate for exertional desaturation. Hypoxemia and elevated LDH are common, resulting from diffuse lung inflammation. The chest radiograph classically reveals diffuse bilateral infiltrates, although a clear CXR may also be seen. The diagnosis of PCP is made with a Giemsa-stained evaluation of pulmonary secretions, either as a result of induced sputum (yield depends on institution) or via bronchoalveolar lavage (>95% sensitivity). In CXR-negative cases, a positive gallium scan is suggestive. When PCP is suspected, empiric therapy with trimethoprim-sulfamethoxazole (Bactrim) should not be delayed until the diagnosis is confirmed. Total duration of therapy is 21 days. In cases of moderate-to-severe hypoxia (Po_2 <70 mm Hg or A-a gradient >35 mm Hg), the use of corticosteroids can blunt the overwhelming inflammatory response seen in the lungs as a result of antibiotic therapy, thereby improving survival. Even in cases where the patient appears well, the presence of significant hypoxemia can result in acute respiratory distress syndrome (ARDS) once PCP therapy is initiated. The use of PCP prophylaxis is highly efficacious for primary and secondary prophylaxis. All patients with CD4 counts <200 cells/μL, CD4% <14, or a history of oral candidiasis should be given prophylaxis. Table 7 lists therapeutic and prophylactic regimens used for PCP.

CENTRAL NERVOUS SYSTEM INFECTIONS IN PATIENTS WITH AIDS

Patients with AIDS may develop a variety of CNS infections, including meningitis, encephalitis (HIV, CMV), and focal brain lesions (FBLs). CNS complications of AIDS are often devastating, can result in prolonged hospitalizations, and use an abundance of resources.

Meningitis in AIDS patients is caused by a variety of agents, most commonly *Cryptococcus neoformans*, *Streptococcus pneumoniae*, *Mycobacterium tuberculosis*, and *Treponema pallidum* (syphilis). HIV itself may cause aseptic meningitis during primary infection. *Cryptococcus neoformans* is a ubiquitous fungus that causes meningitis, pneumonitis, or a disseminated febrile illness in patients with CD4 counts below 100 cells/μL. Patients with cryptococcal meningitis typically have an indolent presentation with fever and headaches, but often may develop acute or sub-acute mental status changes. Neck stiffness and photophobia are uncommon features. Occasionally, focal neurologic findings may be present, usually because of elevated intracranial pressure, vasculitis, or cryptococcoma formation. The cerebrospinal fluid (CSF) findings usually reveal a lymphocytic pleocytosis, high protein, and low or normal glucose. The diagnosis may be made in a variety of ways: a newly positive serum cryptococcal antigen in a patient with a clinical picture consistent with meningitis, a positive CSF India ink or cryptococcal antigen, and growth of *Cryptococcus neoformans* in CSF culture. Virtually all AIDS patients with cryptococcal disease have a positive serum cryptococcal antigen. Poor prognostic features include low or no CSF cellular response, increased CSF opening pressure, abnormal mental status at presentation, extremely elevated cryptococcal antigen, and positive blood culture for yeast. Patients with

TABLE 7 Treatment of *Pneumocystis carinii* Pneumonia

Regimens[a]	Side Effects
Acute Infection	
Primary	
Trimethoprim-sulfamethoxazole (Bactrim, Septra), 15 mg/kg IV or PO trimethoprim and 75 mg/kg/d of sulfamethoxazole divided q6–8h × 21 d[b]	Neutropenia, rash, GI upset, increased creatinine and potassium
Alternatives	
Atovaquone (Mepron), 750 mg PO bid	GI upset, rash
Clindamycin (Cleocin), 600 mg IV q8h or 300–450 mg PO q6h + primaquine, 30 mg base PO qd × 21 d[c]	GI upset, neutropenia, diarrhea, *Clostridium difficile*
Pentamidine (Pentam), 4 mg/kg IV qd × 21 d[d]	Pancreatitis, hypoglycemia or hyperglycemia, rash, neutropenia, decreased blood pressure, conduction abnormalities
Trimethoprim (Proloprim), 15 mg/kg PO divided q6, + dapsone, 100 mg PO qd × 21 d[c]	Rash, pruritis, N/V, hemolytic anemia (dapsone)
Trimetrexate (NeuTrexin), 45 mg/m² IV qd, and folinic acid (leucovorin), 20 mg/m² PO/IV q6h, ± dapsone, 100 mg PO qd	Neutropenia, rash, fever
Prophylaxis[e]	
Primary	
Trimethoprim-sulfamethoxazole (Bactrim, Septra), 1 DS or 1 SS tablet PO qd[f]	Rash, pruritus, hepatitis, neutropenia, hyperkalemia
Alternatives	
Dapsone, 100 mg PO qd	Rash, neutropenia, hemolytic anemia
Dapsone, 50 mg PO qd, pyrimethamine (Daraprim), 50 mg PO qwk, and + leucovorin, 25 mg PO qwk; or dapsone, 200 mg PO qwk, pyrimethamine, 75 mg PO qwk, and leucovorin, 25 mg PO qwk[g]	Rash, N/V, hemolytic anemia, megaloblastic anemia, neutropenia
Atovaquone (Mepron), 750 mg PO bid (liquid) or 1500 mg PO qd	GI upset, rash
Aerosolized pentamidine (NebuPent), 300 mg aerosolized via Respirgard II Nebulizer[h]	Cough (can give inhaled β-agonist)
Trimethoprim/sulfamethoxazole, 1 DS 3 × weekly	Neutropenia, rash, GI upset, increased creatinine and potassium

Abbreviations: DS = double strength; GI = gastrointestinal; HAART = highly active antiretroviral therapy; N/V = nausea/vomiting; PCP = *Pneumocystis carinii* pneumonia; SS = single strength.

[a]Check arterial blood gases before starting therapy. When Pao_2 is less than 70 or the alveolar-arterial gradient is greater than 35, use prednisone, 40 mg orally twice daily for 7 days, then 20 mg twice daily for 7 days, and then 10 mg twice daily for 7 days regardless of the regimen (administer 30 minutes before the first dose of antibiotic).

[b]This regimen has the most experience in the treatment of PCP and should be used if possible.

[c]Consider using these regimens for patients with mild to moderate PCP who are allergic to sulfonamides. These regimens are equally efficacious.

[d]This regimen can be used for patients who are allergic to sulfonamides and have moderate to severe disease.

[e]Secondary prophylaxis required after treatment. Primary and secondary PCP prophylaxis can be stopped after the patient has started HAART and is controlling viral replication with a $CD4^+$ count greater than 200 for 3 to 6 months.

[f]Most efficacious PCP prophylaxis regimen.

[g]Only trimethoprim-sulfamethoxazole at a dose of 1 DS daily and dapsone/pyrimethamine/leucovorin protect against toxoplasmosis.

[h]*Pneumocystis* infection in the apices and in extrapulmonary sites can develop in patients receiving this regimen, and it is less effective when the $CD4^+$ count is less than 50.

elevated intracranial pressure may suffer visual or hearing impairments, if they survive the infection. This makes the measurement of intracranial pressure an important component of performing the lumbar puncture, because patients with elevated pressures should be singled out for repeated taps to decrease symptoms and prevent complications. The gold standard treatment of cryptococcal meningitis is amphotericin B (Fungizone), followed by oral fluconazole (Diflucan) once clinical improvement has occurred. The duration of amphotericin B therapy is controversial; the potential for renal complications must be weighed against the need for longer courses of therapy. At least 2 weeks is advisable. High-dose fluconazole (400 mg/day) should be continued for 12 weeks, followed by maintenance therapy until there has been sufficient immune reconstitution.

HIV encephalopathy is one of the most common neurological complications of AIDS. It is usually seen in patients with low CD4 counts, follows a chronic course, and leads to a global cognitive and motor decline. Diffuse cerebral atrophy with bilateral, nonenhancing white matter hypodensities (leukoencephalopathy) are usually seen on brain MRI. Lumbar puncture may be performed to exclude the possibility of progressive multifocal leukoencephalopathy (PML) or CMV encephalitis. Some improvement may be seen with HAART.

FBLs are common in patients with AIDS. The differential diagnosis includes acute toxoplasmosis, primary CNS lymphoma (PCNSL), PML, brain abscess, tuberculoma, and cryptococcoma, as well as malignancies and infections not related to HIV, such as brain metastases, primary brain tumors, and neurocysticercosis. Toxoplasmosis and PCNSL are the most common FBLs seen with AIDS, mostly occurring in patients with very advanced immunosuppression. Patients may present with a host of clinical findings, including altered mentation, seizures, focal neurologic findings, and headaches. Contrast imaging studies of the brain usually reveal one or more ring-enhancing lesions. Toxoplasmosis is much more common than PCNSL, and screening all patients with *Toxoplasma gondii* antibody titer is standard. The diagnosis of toxoplasmosis is virtually always presumptive, and relies primarily on its response to initial antiparasitic therapy with oral sulfadiazine, pyrimethamine (Daraprim), and folinic acid (Leucovorin). In patients allergic to sulfa drugs, clindamycin (Cleocin) may be substituted. Systemic therapy with corticosteroids should be avoided unless there is imminent brain herniation, as PCNSL is steroid-sensitive and dual-therapy with antiparasitics and steroids could cloud the diagnosis. A repeat imaging study is usually performed after a 2-week interval if the patient's clinical status is stable. If there is improvement, the diagnosis of toxoplasmosis is confirmed and long-term therapy is continued. If there is no improvement, further work-ups are recommended, including: CSF for EBV PCR, cytology, flow cytometry, SPECT thallium scanning, and/or brain biopsy to primarily exclude the diagnosis of lymphoma. While toxoplasmosis is treatable in most cases, primary CNS non-Hodgkin's lymphoma has a high mortality rate, with death usually occurring within 1 year of diagnosis. Radiation therapy is often used as a palliative measure.

PML is a progressive, demyelinating illness caused by the JC virus in patients with very advanced AIDS. Patients present with focal neurologic abnormalities, gait disturbances, and worsening cognitive dysfunction. Diagnosis is made by contrast CT or MRI of the brain, usually revealing focal, nonenhancing white matter demyelinating lesions. The presence of a positive JC virus PCR in the CSF confirms the diagnosis. Although there is no specific therapy for this illness, some patients may improve with aggressive antiretroviral therapy.

TUBERCULOSIS IN PATIENTS WITH HIV

HIV patients infected with tuberculosis develop active disease at dramatically higher rates than their HIV-negative counterparts. Disease may result from recent infection or reactivation. Reactivation is more common with lower CD4 counts, but may occur at any CD4 level. In the absence of HAART, it is likely that a majority of HIV patients infected with TB will eventually reactivate their disease; the risk for active disease is extreme (up to 40%) during the first two years after infection, and approximately 5% to 10% per year for the remainder of the patient's life. Although the use of HAART has clearly changed disease progression of TB, yearly PPD testing is still recommended and all HIV patients with a positive PPD (>5 mm) or a known TB exposure should receive chemoprophylaxis for 9 months. When active tuberculosis does occur, it tends to have a more aggressive course, with higher rates of dissemination and death. Pulmonary involvement is most common; lymphangitis, meningitis, and disseminated disease also occur with increased frequency. Given the high rates of TB in the developing world, immigrants from high-risk nations with AIDS and a respiratory illness should be isolated until a diagnosis of TB is excluded. See the article on tuberculosis for a more in-depth review.

MUCOCUTANEOUS CANDIDIASIS IN PATIENTS WITH AIDS

Candida albicans infection is common in patients with AIDS, primarily causing oral, vaginal, and esophageal disease. Oral candidiasis is rarely seen in normal hosts receiving antibiotics or corticosteroids (including inhalers). Patients without an acceptable reason for oral candida and women with recurrent vaginal candidiasis should be tested for HIV. Diagnosis is made by visualization of candida and may be confirmed with a potassium hydroxide (KOH) preparation. Oral and vaginal candidiasis should be treated with topical agents when possible. Keeping in mind that resistance to therapy may occur with recurrent therapy, the goal should be the improvement of the host immunity with antiretroviral therapy. Among topical agents, clotrimazole (Gyne-Lotrimin) is more reliable than nystatin. Among oral medications, fluconazole (Diflucan) is the treatment of choice, but recurrent use may lead to resistance. Some fluconazole-resistant cases may still respond to itraconazole (Sporanox) or voriconazole (Vfend).

Patients with esophageal candidiasis usually present with odynophagia and retrosternal pain. On examination, oral candida is often present and should prompt the clinician to empirically treat. Treatment is primarily with fluconazole, but again, ARV is critical for increasing CD4 counts, improving underlying immunity, and avoiding long-term use of fluconazole. If complete azole resistance does occur, intravenous amphotericin B (Fungizone), caspofungin (Cansidas)[1], or voriconazole (Vfend) must be used. When there is no response to antifungal therapy, other etiologies must be considered. The differential diagnosis of esophagitis in the AIDS patient includes CMV, herpes simplex virus (HSV), and idiopathic aphthous ulcers. Diagnosis is by endoscopy with biopsy. Treatment is aimed at the specific virus identified, or tapering doses of steroids for idiopathic ulcers.

[1]Not FDA approved for this indication.

DISSEMINATED MAC

In the pre-HAART era, disseminated *Mycobacterium avium-intracellulare* complex (MAC) infection was extremely common among patients with CD4 counts <50 cells/μL. However, the incidence of this disease has declined dramatically with widespread ARV use. Patients typically present with high fever, weight loss, night sweats, and anorexia. Examination and laboratory findings may include lymphadenopathy, hepatosplenomegaly, elevated alkaline phosphatase, and bone marrow suppression. Diagnosis is confirmed with mycobacterial blood culture, and treatment is with ethambutol (Myambutol) and a macrolide (clarithromycin [Biaxin] or azithromycin [Zithromax]); rifabutin (Mycobutin) and fluoroquinolones are effective substitutes. Although patients with disseminated MAC may have significant morbidity and are frequently hospitalized, the direct mortality is low. MAC prophylaxis is recommended for patients with CD4 counts of less than 50 cells/μL, but in patients willing and able to take ARV, prophylaxis may not be necessary.

CYTOMEGALOVIRUS DISEASE IN AIDS PATIENTS

Cytomegalovirus is a ubiquitous virus that is usually sexually transmitted and commonly found in patients with HIV. Latent CMV disease can reactivate when CD4 counts drop below 50 cells/μL, primarily resulting in retinitis, esophagitis, and colitis (less commonly adrenal or CNS disease). CMV colitis presents with abdominal pain, fever, and diarrhea (sometimes bloody), while esophagitis typically causes odynophagia and retrosternal pain. Both are diagnosed with endoscopy, which shows ulceration of the mucosa. Biopsy of these lesions reveals cytomegalic inclusion bodies. Treatment is with oral valganciclovir (Valcyte). Intravenous therapy is reserved for patients unable to tolerate oral therapy or with absorption problems. The major complication of valganciclovir is bone marrow suppression, particularly when combined with other bone marrow suppressing medications such as trimethoprim-sulfamethoxazole (Bactrim) and zidovudine (Retrovir).

The retina is the most common site of end-organ involvement in patients with AIDS, accounting for the vast majority of invasive CMV disease. However, the incidence of CMV retinitis has dropped dramatically with the advent of HAART. Nevertheless, all patients with advanced AIDS should be screened for CMV retinitis by an ophthalmologist. Patients with retinitis may be asymptomatic (picked up on screening), have floaters, or have decreased visual acuity (involvement of macula). The diagnosis is clinical: funduscopic examination reveals retinal inflammation ("pizza pie" appearance). Patients with untreated CMV retinitis eventually progress to complete visual loss of the affected eye. HAART may slow or stop disease progression even in the absence of specific CMV therapy. Specific therapy of CMV retinitis may include implanted, intravenous, or oral antiviral therapy. The treatment of choice today is oral valganciclovir (Valcyte). When implants are used, the use of concomitant oral therapy is necessary to protect the other eye. Therapy is guided by weekly eye examinations performed by an ophthalmologist.

MALIGNANCIES IN PATIENTS WITH AIDS

Kaposi's sarcoma (KS) is the most common malignancy affecting patients with AIDS, although the incidence has significantly declined with the widespread use of HAART. Originally an endemic malignancy of southern Africa and the Mediterranean area, the sudden appearance of KS among young, previously healthy gay men led to the original descriptions of AIDS in the United States. KS is caused by infection with human herpes virus 8 and is almost exclusively seen in gay men. Disease may be cutaneous, mucosal (oral), or disseminate widely to viscera, most notably the gastrointestinal tract and lungs. Cutaneous disease is most commonly seen in the lower extremities and face, but may occur anywhere in the body; drainage to regional lymph nodes with significant lymphedema may occur. The diagnosis is made by visualization of typical raised purple nodular lesions, but should be confirmed by biopsy to differentiate it from Bartonella infection. Indications for therapy of cutaneous KS lesions include pain, regional lymph node involvement, and for cosmetic reasons. Most lesions do not require therapy. Gastrointestinal KS is infrequently symptomatic, but lung involvement usually is, presenting with dyspnea, nonproductive cough, and diffuse bilateral infiltrates (often nodular); fever is less common. Gallium scan is typically negative and diagnosis is made with bronchoscopy. Treatment of KS usually involves irradiation of cutaneous lesions or systemic chemotherapy for visceral disease. Antiretroviral therapy is effective in improving host immunity against KS, delaying disease progression, and occasionally leading to disease regression.

Other malignancies have been described with increased frequency in AIDS patients, including Hodgkin's and non-Hodgkin's lymphoma (NHL), and human papillomavirus (HPV)-related anal and cervical squamous cell carcinoma. The lymphomas are discussed in detail elsewhere. HPV-related malignancies are more common and have faster rates of progression from dysplasia to cancer in patients with AIDS. A routine gynecologic evaluation and Pap smear should be performed every 6 to 12 months to evaluate for cervical dysplasia. If dysplasia is identified, the patient should undergo colposcopy and appropriate therapy. Anal carcinomas are more difficult to diagnose early, as there is no current standard for performing anal Pap smears and long-term data regarding their outcomes are not available. Anal inspection and digital examination of the anal verge should be performed yearly on patients with a history of receptive anal intercourse. When lesions are found, referral for anoscopy should be made.

HEPATITIS C VIRUS

Hepatitis C virus (HCV) is both common and more aggressive in patients with AIDS, with a more rapid progression to end-organ damage. With the success of HAART, cirrhosis related to hepatitis C is now one of the leading causes of death in patients with HIV. Hepatitis C infection may be acquired through sharing of intravenous needles, blood transfusion, sexual intercourse (uncommon), and vertically from mother to infant. Eighty percent of patients infected with hepatitis C become chronically infected, of which ~20% develop cirrhosis or hepatocellular carcinoma. Chronically infected patients are asymptomatic for years until end-organ damage develops.

All HIV patients should be screened with a hepatitis C antibody. If positive, HCV RNA confirms chronic infection. Testing for HCV subtype may also be helpful, as it may have implications on response to therapy; most U.S. subtypes are 1a and 1b, whereas Europeans are more commonly infected with subtypes 2 and 3. The decision of whom to treat, however, depends on the likelihood of disease progression, which can only be determined with liver biopsy. When a liver biopsy reveals mild disease, therapy may be deferred and a repeat biopsy should be performed in 3 to 5 years. When significant liver disease is found, therapy with interferon injections (peginterferon alpha-2a [Pegasys]) and ribavirin (Rebetol) oral therapy should be considered. Potential side effects resulting from the above therapy include bone marrow suppression, hemolytic anemia, flu-like symptoms, depression, weight loss, and insomnia. Patients with a history of depression should be pretreated with antidepressants. The overall response rate for pegylated interferon and ribavirin in non-HIV patients is ~55%, but depends on viral subtypes. Subtypes 1a and 1b have a response rate of ~45%, while subtypes 2 and 3 respond at ~80%. Similar outcomes data are not yet available for co-infected patients. All patients with confirmed HCV chronic infection should completely avoid alcohol and be vaccinated against hepatitis A and B, if they are not immune. Patients with recent (<1 year) hepatitis C infection have much better response rates (>90%), regardless of viral subtype, so therapy should not be delayed.

SYPHILIS

Syphilis has a more rapid progression in patients with HIV infection. Progression from primary to secondary and tertiary syphilis may occur within a few months of acute infection. Given the high-risk sexual activity associated with both syphilis and HIV infection, syphilis is more common among HIV patients and leads to increased HIV transmission rates. As a result, all patients with HIV infection are screened yearly for infection with syphilis. Treatment according to stage is generally similar to HIV-uninfected patients, but lumbar puncture should be more aggressively pursued in HIV-infected patients with latent syphilis.

AMEBIASIS

METHOD OF

Herbert B. Tanowitz, MD, and

Murray Wittner MD, PhD

Amebiasis usually refers to an infection caused by the protozoan parasite *Entamoeba histolytica*. This parasite is an important cause of morbidity and mortality in the tropical and subtropical worlds. Although it is found worldwide, it is most prevalent where there is poor sanitation such as that which occurs in the underdeveloped areas. It is estimated that the annual number of cases of intestinal amebiasis (amebic colitis) and amebic liver abscess is 40 to 50 million, with a mortality of approximately 100,000 worldwide. In the developed areas of the world, invasive amebiasis (intestinal and liver) is observed in certain high-risk groups such as returning travelers and immigrants from endemic areas, patients in mental institutions, migrant workers, and individuals who engage in oral-anal sex. The infection is acquired from the ingestion of water or food that has been contaminated with the tetranucleate cyst of *E. histolytica*. Person-to-person transmission can occur via the fecal-oral route, which perpetuates the life cycle. There is a noninvasive species, *Entamoeba dispar*, that is morphologically indistinguishable from the pathogenic *E. histolytica*.

Intestinal Amebiasis

There are several clinical classifications of amebiasis based on pathogenesis and for purposes of therapy. The vast majority of individuals infected with *E. dispar* complex are asymptomatic, and some patients carrying *E. histolytica* are also asymptomatic. Intestinal amebiasis is a term that encompasses the entire spectrum of clinical intestinal disease. Thus, individuals may have mild diarrhea with cramping abdominal pain to severe colitis manifested by fever, abdominal tenderness, fulminate bloody diarrhea, necrotizing colitis, toxic megacolon, and intestinal perforation. The symptoms are usually more severe in children, the aged, pregnant women, and the immunocompromised. Intestinal amebiasis must be distinguished from other etiologies such as inflammatory bowel disease and bacterial causes of dysentery.

The diagnosis and treatment of intestinal amebiasis must be based on tests that distinguish *E. histolytica* from *E. dispar*. The examination of three stools is recommended. It is important that the individual has not ingested laxatives, bismuth-containing compounds, or antacids in the recent past. In addition, hypertonic or barium enemas may interfere with the diagnosis by stool examination. As noted, light microscopy cannot distinguish *E. histolytica* from *E. dispar* except when ingested erythrocytes are observed within trophozoites. This is an almost pathognomonic finding for *E. histolytica*. Other tests that may aide in the diagnosis include a stool antigen assay such as the one distributed by TechLab. Serology and stool polymerase chain reaction tests can be helpful in making a diagnosis.

Amebic Liver Abscess

The most serious complication of amebiasis is amebic liver abscess. It is more common in men and rare in children. The majority of patients with amebic liver abscess present with signs and symptoms that evolve over 2 to 4 weeks. These include fever, chills, right upper quadrant abdominal pain, and right-sided pleuritic chest pain. Up to 40% of patients with amebic liver abscess have other gastrointestinal symptoms. The complications of an amebic liver abscess include rupture into the peritoneal or pleural cavity or pericardium. The diagnosis is established by the demonstration of a space-occupying lesion of the liver by ultrasonography, computed tomography (CT) scan, or magnetic resonance imaging (MRI). Amebic serology is positive in virtually all patients but may be negative during the first week of illness.

Therapy of Amebiasis

In the treatment of intestinal amebiasis the aim is to eradicate cysts and lumen-dwelling trophozoites with lumen-active agents and to treat invasive intestinal disease with tissue-active agents. The drug of choice for asymptomatic cyst passers is iodoquinol (Yodoxin) or paromomycin (Humatin). Iodoquinol can cause gastrointestinal side effects and interfere with thyroid function because of its high iodine content. Prolonged use and high doses have rarely led to neurotoxicity. Paromomycin is a nonabsorbable aminoglycoside that has minor gastrointestinal side effects and is safe in pregnancy. Metronidazole (Flagyl) should not be used to treat cyst passers.

Metronidazole (Flagyl) is the drug of choice for intestinal diseases ranging from mild intestinal disease to frank amebic colitis. Although most experts recommend a 7- to 10-day course of therapy, there are data that indicate a single dose of 2.4 g may be efficacious for intestinal amebiasis. Although metronidazole has not been demonstrated to be teratogenic in humans, it is generally withheld during pregnancy unless the patient has severe colitis. The common side effects of metronidazole are nausea, a metallic taste in the mouth, headache, abdominal pain, and dark-colored urine. Neurological side effects include paresthesias, insomnia, and ataxia. Outside the United States and Canada, tinidazole (Fasigyn)[2] is the drug of choice for invasive amebiasis (Table 1).

[2]Not available in the United States.

TABLE 1 Drug Treatment of Amebiasis

Drug	Adult Dose	Pediatric Dose
Asymptomatic Intestinal Colonization		
Drug of Choice		
Iodoquinol (Yodoxin)	650 mg tid × 20 d	30-40 mg/kg/d (max 2 g) in 3 doses × 20 d
or		
Paromomycin (Humatin) in 3 doses × 7 d	25-35 mg/kg/d	Same as the adult dose
Alternatives		
Diloxanide furoate (Furamide) 500 mg tid ×10 d	20 mg/kg/d in 3 doses × 10 d	
Nitazoxanide (Alinia)	None	500 mg tid × 3 d <12 y
Mild-to-Moderate Intestinal Disease		
Drug of Choice		
Metronidazole (Flagyl)	500-750 mg tid × 7-10 d	30-50 mg/kg/d in 3 doses × 7-10 d
or		
Tinidazole (Fasigyn)	2 gm/d in 3 divided doses	50 mg/kg (max 2 g) qd × 3 d
Alternative		
Nitazoxanide (Alinia)	None	500 mg tid × 3 d <12 y
Severe Intestinal Disease and Amebic Liver Abscess		
Drug of Choice		
Metronidazole (Flagyl)	500-750 mg tid × 7-10 d	30-50 mg/kg/d in 3 doses × 7-10 d
or		
Tinidazole (Fasigyn)	800 mg tid × 5 d	60 mg/kg (max 2 g) qd × 5 d

Notes: A luminal agent used in the treatment of asymptomatic cyst passers should be used following treatment of invasive intestinal disease and amebic liver abscess.
Diloxanide furoate is available from Panorama Compounding Pharmacy, Van Nuys, CA, 1-800-247-9767.

It is believed to have fewer side effects. A luminal agent used in the treatment of asymptomatic cyst passers should be used following treatment of invasive intestinal disease and amebic liver abscess even if not observed on stool examination. Follow-up stool examination should be performed 3 to 4 weeks following the completion of therapy. Nitazoxanide (Alinia)[1] can be used for the treatment of mild-to-moderate intestinal amebiasis in children who are 1 to 11 years of age. Side effects include abdominal pain and headaches.

The medical therapy of amebic liver abscess consists of either metronidazole or tinidazole (see Table 1). As an alternative to the 7- to 10-day course for metronidazole or the 5-day course for tinidazole, some have suggested a single dose of 2.5 g[3] of metronidazole orally or a single dose of 2 g[3] of tinidazole. Metronidazole can be used intravenously in those individuals who cannot tolerate the oral route. Amebic liver abscess can usually be managed by medical therapy without percutaneous drainage. However, drainage of the abscess may be considered for individuals with a high risk of rupture (diameter >5-10 cm) or a left-lobe lesion. Patients treated by percutaneous drainage should still receive the full course of treatment. Bacterial infection of amebic abscesses is uncommon, but when suspected or diagnosed appropriate antibiotics should be added. The serology may not fall for at least 2 to 3 years following successful therapy of amebic liver abscess.

[1]Not FDA approved for this indication.
[3]Exceeds dosage recommended by the manufacturer.

GIARDIASIS

METHOD OF

Jean-François Rossignol, MD, PhD

Giardiasis is the most common human intestinal protozoan infection, and is widely recognized as a common cause of persistent diarrhea and enteritis. In the United States, it is the most frequently reported intestinal protozoan, and it is responsible for 4600 hospitalizations every year. That equals two hospitalized patients per 100,000 persons, a figure almost identical to shigellosis. *Giardia intestinalis* (syn. *duodenalis* or *lamblia*) is the organism responsible. This flagellate was first discovered by van Leeuwenhoek in 1681, who found it in his own stools; but was first recognizably described by Lambl in 1859, who gave it the name *intestinalis*. In 1915, because he was not sure about the availability of the name *intestinalis*, Stiles proposed naming it *Giardia lamblia* in honor of Professor Giard of Paris and Dr. F. Lambl of Prague.

Like most other species of this genus, *G. intestinalis* has both trophic and cystic stages. Transmission of *G. intestinalis* is usually by viable cysts that are swallowed with water, but in some circumstances it is by intimate contact, much like the intestinal nematode pinworms. It is commonly contracted in day care settings, in recreational water (swimming pools, water parks, lakes, rivers, and streams), by ingestion of contaminated food, and by contact with animals; and it is recognized as the leading cause of post-travel diarrhea. In the United States the true incidence of giardiasis ranges from 46 to 926 cases per 100,000 population. *G. intestinalis* is typically more prevalent in children than it is in adults. In northern Peru for instance, the incidence of symptomatic giardiasis in nearly 5000 screened inhabitants was 37% in children ages 1 to 11 years, but only 2.1% in people older than 12 years of age.

The pathogenicity of *G. intestinalis* was intensely debated during the first half of the 20th century largely because the parasite could coexist with its human host without producing symptomatic disease. The presence of *G. intestinalis* in the glandular crypts of the duodenal-jejunal mucosa ordinarily causes no apparent irritation. The parasite does not invade the tissue, but feeds on the mucous secretions, and in many cases is strictly commensal in its relationship to the host. Occasionally, the gallbladder and, more specifically, the ampulla of Vater, can become parasitized, resulting in cholangiopathy. Such cases are more frequent in diabetic and immunocompromised patients, such as those with AIDS. Generally, in young children and immunologically naive adults, particularly travelers, giardiasis can produce serious diarrheal disease with intestinal malabsorption, marked weight loss, and, in infants and young children, impairment of growth and development. Most typically, the disease begins with an acute phase lasting 3 or 4 days that looks like a traveler's diarrhea. Light acute infections can sometimes be self-limiting by spontaneous elimination of the parasite, but most often, a subacute or chronic infection develops with persistent and recurrent symptoms, such as foul-smelling greasy stools, foul-smelling gas, distention, anorexia, weight loss, and marked fatigue. Approximately 15% of infected adults and up to 50% of infected young children (0 to 3 years of age) will become asymptomatic cyst passers, though the duration of this asymptomatic phase is unknown. Nevertheless, the clinical diversity of giardiasis suggests that there may be relatively virulent and avirulent biotypes, and recent studies indicate that there is a marked phenotypic and genotypic heterogeneity in isolates of *G. intestinalis*.

Because of the variability of symptoms, giardiasis should be considered when diagnosing most cases of diarrhea, but particularly when symptoms last more than 5 to 7 days. Diagnosis is based on microscopic examination of a stool specimen. Diarrheic stools will usually reveal numerous active trophozoites, and semiformed or formed stools will contain cysts of this organism. In the case of light infection where few cysts are present, the Faust zinc sulfate centrifugal concentration is the best technique, but a Ritchie ether centrifugal sedimentation method is also acceptable. These will greatly enhance the sensitivity of the stool examination. Widely used to confirm microscopy and approved in the United States, Merifluor *Cryptosporidium/Giardia* (Meridian Bioscience, Inc., Cincinnati, OH) is a direct immunofluorescent detection procedure using monoclonal antibodies to detect both *G. intestinalis* and *Cryptosporidium parvum* antigens present in a stool specimen. There are also a number of enzyme-linked immunoassays available in the United States for fresh or fresh-frozen unfixed fecal specimens. It is usual for infections to have alternating periods of high, low, and no excretion of cysts. This pattern of excretion, coupled with the potential for technician error, inevitably results in a high number of false-negative examinations. Consequently, several techniques should be used to diagnose *G. intestinalis*, and they should be carried out on serial stool specimens (at least three) collected at least 24 hours apart. When the organism cannot be found in the stool but there is strong historical and clinical evidence of giardiasis, duodenal fluid can be obtained using the duodenal string test (Entero-Test from HDC Corporation, Milpitas, CA), or by endoscopy, in which case a small bowel biopsy can be performed at the same time. In view of difficulties that can be involved in obtaining a clear diagnosis of giardiasis, empirical treatment may be appropriate in some cases, particularly where exposure risks and symptoms (e.g., persistent diarrhea) are suggestive.

Treatment

There is only one drug, nitazoxanide (Alinia), specifically approved by the U.S. Food and Drug Administration for treating giardiasis. Nitazoxanide is available as 500 mg tablets and as a 100 mg/5 mL pediatric suspension. Other drugs available in the United States that can be used for treating giardiasis include metronidazole (Flagyl)[1] in 250 mg and 500 mg tablets, paromomycin (Humatin)[1] in 250 mg capsules, and albendazole (Albenza)[1] in 200 mg tablets.

Nitazoxanide is a broad-spectrum antiparasitic drug effective against a wide range of protozoa and helminths. In the United States, it is the first approved treatment for infection caused by *Cryptosporidium parvum* in immunocompetent patients. It is also highly effective against *G. intestinalis* with a dose of 500 mg twice a day for 3 consecutive days for people who are ages 12 years and older, a 200 mg/10 mL suspension twice a day for 3 consecutive days for children ages 4 to 11 years, and a 100 mg/5 mL suspension for children who are 1 to 3 years old. Nitazoxanide is effective against the biliary stages of *C. parvum* and *G. intestinalis* mainly observed in AIDS or severely immunosuppressed individuals. It is also active against metronidazole-resistant isolates of *G. intestinalis*. Nitazoxanide was studied in 245 adults, adolescents, and children with symptomatic giardiasis using metronidazole and placebo as controls. It was found to be as effective as metronidazole, with cure rates ranging from 85% to 95%. Parasitological examinations used both microscopic and immunofluorescent techniques. In controlled and uncontrolled clinical studies carried out in a total of 1280 HIV-negative patients receiving the 3-day dose, the most frequent adverse events reported regardless of causality were abdominal pain (7.8%), diarrhea (2.1%), vomiting (1.1%), and headache (1.1%). These were typically mild and transient in nature. In placebo-controlled studies, the rates of occurrence of these events did not differ significantly from those of placebo, and none of the 1280 patients discontinued therapy because of adverse events. Nitazoxanide has not been found to be mutagenic or teratogenic in laboratory animals.

Metronidazole (Flagyl)[1] and its related derivatives tinidazole, secnidazole[2], and ornidazole[2] are nitroimidazole compounds, which are highly effective against *G. intestinalis*. In the United States, only metronidazole is available, but it is not approved for this indication. It is listed on the World Health Organization's essential drug list for the treatment of giardiasis and amebiasis. The adult dose is 250 mg 3 times a day for 5 to 7 consecutive days. Cure rates are high, almost constantly above 85%. At this dose level, and with divided doses every 6 hours, tolerance is good, with only mild and transient clinical side effects. These drugs may cause symptoms of epigastric or abdominal pain and diarrhea. Metallic taste and dark urine have also been reported. Alcohol is contraindicated during treatment with metronidazole because it interacts with aldehyde dehydrogenase and could cause severe vomiting, flushing, headache, and gastrointestinal pain. Nitroimidazoles are highly

[1]Not FDA approved for this indication.

[1]Not FDA approved for this indication.

[2]Not available in the United States.

mutagenic and carcinogenic in laboratory animals. They are probably safe in adults, though high doses in children should be avoided in the presence of alternative treatment.

Albendazole (Albenza)[1], a benzimidazole carbamate anthelminthic that is highly effective against a broad range of intestinal nematodes, was first reported to be effective against giardiasis in 1986. Although not approved for this indication in the United States, several trials carried out in Asia and South America reported that a dose of 400 mg/day for 5 to 7 consecutive days was 90% effective in treating giardiasis, while a 3-day treatment at the same dose level was not effective. The combination albendazole-metronidazole is now proposed in Europe for the treatment of patients with giardiasis who fail to respond to metronidazole. Paromomycin (Humatin),[1] a poorly absorbed aminoglycoside antibiotic, has shown some variable results in the treatment of giardiasis and is not approved in the United States for this indication. However, it is the only drug that is used to treat giardiasis in pregnancy. Practically not absorbed from the gastrointestinal tract, it is probably quite safe in this specific indication. The recommended dose is 500 mg 3 times a day for 7 consecutive days.

Two older drugs have been removed from the market. Quinacrine, an acridine derivative first described in 1934 for its antimalarial properties, has been used at a dose of 100 mg 3 times a day for 5 to 7 consecutive days. While effective in treating giardiasis, the toxicity profile of the drug was poor. Dizziness, headache, and vomiting were frequent, and occasionally it caused toxic psychosis, blood dyscrasia, urticaria, severe exfoliative dermatitis, yellow staining of skin and sclera, blue and black nail pigmentation, and adverse ocular effects (e.g., abnormalities in visual acuity, visual field, retinal macular areas, or other visual symptoms similar to those seen with another antimalarial, chloroquine). It is no longer available in the United States, except in a few compounding pharmacies. Furazolidone (Furoxone) is a nitrofuran derivative that was approved for use in the treatment of giardiasis in the United States as tablets and pediatric suspensions. It is highly mutagenic and carcinogenic in laboratory animals, and is no longer available.

Giardiasis is the most prevalent intestinal parasitic infection in the United States. Sometimes difficult to diagnose, repeated fecal examinations are needed to identify the parasite. In persistent diarrhea with clinical symptoms suggesting giardiasis, and in the presence of a strong history, presumptive treatment may be considered. There is no need to treat asymptomatic carriers, except young children, particularly those in day care centers, and food handlers, because they are both potential sources of infection to others.

[1]Not FDA approved for this indication.

Although *G. intestinalis* is not as opportunistic as *C. parvum* in AIDS, it could become a serious problem in this population because of the dissemination of the parasite in the biliary tree. Nitazoxanide, the only approved drug for this indication, is the drug of choice, and metronidazole is the alternate second-line treatment.

BACTEREMIA AND SEPSIS

METHOD OF

Dennis Kellar, MD, and Robert A. Balk, MD

Sepsis has been defined as the systemic inflammatory response to an infection. The true incidence of sepsis is unknown, in part because of the lack of a uniformly accepted definition. The Centers for Disease Control and Prevention (CDC) had previously reported a dramatic 139% increase in the septicemia discharge diagnosis over a decade of monitoring. Using discharge coding data from seven states, it has been recently suggested that there are more than 750,000 episodes of severe sepsis each year in the United States. Severe sepsis accounts for 1 of every 10 intensive care unit (ICU) admissions and represents 2% to 3% of all hospital admissions. Furthermore, the U.S. incidence of sepsis is projected to rise at a rate of 1.5% per year. Factors responsible for this increase include the continued growth in the number of elderly patients, an increased number of immunocompromised patients, the increased use of invasive procedures and devices to care for patients, the growing problem with resistant microorganisms, and a greater awareness and recognition of this disorder.

Sepsis is now reported to be the tenth most common cause of death in the United States and is one of the two most common causes of death in the noncoronary ICU. Using the extrapolated annual incidence of 750,000 episodes of sepsis in the United States and a relatively conservative mortality estimate of 28%, there would be an annual mortality of greater than 220,000. This surprisingly high mortality rate has been projected despite our enhanced understanding of the pathophysiologic alterations that occur in sepsis, our technologic improvements in monitoring and support of the critically ill patient, and our use of more potent antibiotic therapy. There have also been multiple attempts to improve the outcome of the septic patient using innovative therapeutic strategies that are designed to target selected aspects of the pathophysiologic response to the causative microorganism(s).

A recent epidemiologic review of sepsis in the United States reported that sepsis is more common in males and in the non-white population. Over the past 22 years gram-positive organisms have become the predominant cause of sepsis, but there has also been a dramatic increase in the number of episodes of fungal sepsis. Over this observation period, the incidence and number of sepsis-related deaths have increased, while the actual sepsis mortality rate has improved.

Definitions of SIRS and SEPSIS

The approach to management of patients with severe sepsis and septic shock begins with prompt recognition of the septic process (Table 1). As mentioned, in the past there has been difficulty in identifying septic patients, in part related to the lack of a uniformly accepted definition. In 1991, the American College of Chest Physicians and the Society of Critical Care Medicine convened a consensus conference that was charged with developing a set of definitions that would assist the medical community in communication about sepsis and would provide for the early recognition of the septic patient. The definition would incorporate predominantly readily available clinical criteria that would facilitate patient identification and enrollment in investigational trials of innovative therapeutic agents. The consensus conference recognized that there were patients with presumed sepsis based on their clinical presentation who lacked a positive culture or other evidence of a documented infection. These individuals were classified as having the systemic inflammatory response syndrome or SIRS. SIRS can result from a diverse group of insults, such as trauma, burns, or pancreatitis. Sepsis was defined as the SIRS response to a documented infection.

TABLE 1 Diagnostic Criteria For Sepsis

Infection (documented or suspected) and some of the following:
General Variables
Fever (core temperature >38.3°C [101°F])
Hypothermia (core temperature <36°C [96.8°F])
Heart rate >90 min^{-1} or >2 SD above the normal value for age
Tachypnea
Altered mental status
Significant edema or positive fluid balance (>20 mL/kg over 24 h)
Hyperglycemia (plasma glucose >120 mg/dL, or 7.7 mmol/L) in the absence of diabetes
Inflammatory Variables
Leukocytosis (WBC count >12000 μL^{-1})
Leukopenia (WBC count <4000 μL^{-1})
Normal WBC count with >10% immature forms (bands)
Plasma C-reactive protein >2 SD above the normal value
Plasma procalcitonin >2 SD above the normal value
Hemodynamic Variables
Arterial hypotension (SBP <90 mm Hg, MAP <70, or an SBP decrease >40 mm Hg in adults or <2 SD below normal for age)
Svo_2 >70%
Cardiac index >3.5 L/min–1M^2
Organ Dysfunction Variables
Arterial hypoxemia (Pao_2/Fio_2 <3000)
Acute oliguria (Urine output <0.5 mL/kg/hr or 45 mmol/L for at least 2 hours.)
Creatinine increase >0.5 mg/dL
Coagulation abnormalities (INR >1.5 or aPTT >60 secs)
Ileus (absent bowel sounds)
Thrombocytopenia (platelet count <100,000 μL^{-1})
Hyperbilirubinemia (plasma total bilirubin >4 mg/dL or 70 mmol/L)
Tissue Perfusion Variables
Hyperlactatemia (>1 mmol/L)
Decreased capillary refill or mottling

From Levy et al: 2001 SCCM/ESICM/ACCP/ATS/SIS International sepsis definitions conference, *Crit Care Med* 2003;31:1250-1256.

SIRS was defined as a widespread systemic inflammatory response to a variety of insults, including, but not limited to, infection. SIRS was operationally defined by the presence of two or more of the following:

- temperature >38°C (100.4°F) or <36°C (96.8°F),
- heart rate >90 beats per minute,
- respiratory rate >20 breaths per minute or $PaCO_2$<32 mm Hg,
- white blood cell count >12,000 cells/mm^3, or <4000 cells/mm^3 or >10% immature band forms.

Sepsis is the systemic inflammatory response to a documented infection. The diagnosis of sepsis requires the presence of at least two of the these SIRS criteria, plus an infection. Signs of infection include an inflammatory response to the presence of microorganisms or the invasion of normally sterile host tissue by those organisms. There is a continuum of injury severity in SIRS and sepsis. Severe SIRS and severe sepsis are defined by the presence of organ dysfunction or hypoperfusion as a result of the inflammatory response. Hypoperfusion and perfusion abnormalities may include, but are not limited to, lactic acidosis, oliguria, or an acute alteration in mental status. Sepsis-induced hypotension occurs when systolic blood pressure falls to <90 mm Hg or there is a reduction of ≥40 mm Hg from baseline systolic pressure in the absence of other causes for hypotension.

Septic shock is a subset of severe sepsis with hypotension despite adequate fluid resuscitation, along with the presence of perfusion abnormalities. Patients receiving inotropic or vasopressor agents may no longer be hypotensive by the time they manifest hypoperfusion abnormalities or organ dysfunction, yet they would still be considered to have septic shock. When there is multiple dysfunction of organ systems present, it is termed multiple organ dysfunction syndrome, or MODS. The definition of MODS is the alteration of organ function such that normal homeostasis cannot be maintained without intervention. Unfortunately, there are no uniformly agreed-upon

TABLE 2 PIRO Staging of Sepsis

Predisposition
Premorbid conditions that influence likelihood of infection, sepsis, morbidity, survival (i.e., age, sex, hormonal state, genetic polymorphisms for TNF, IL-10, IL-6, IL-1ra, TLR)
Insult/Infection
Insult or organism associated with the sepsis response (i.e., type of organism, sensitivity pattern, community or nosocomial acquisition)
Response
Clinical manifestations of the SIRS response (Procalcitonin, IL-6, HLA-DR, TNF, PAF, C-RP, etc.)
Organ Dysfunction
Type and number of dysfunctional organs (reversible vs. irreversible dysfunction)
Severity of dysfunction (judged by scoring systems, i.e., MODS, LODS, SOFA, etc.)

From Levy et al: 2001 SCCM/ESICM/ACCP/ATS/SIS International sepsis definitions conference, *Crit Care Med* 2003;31:1250-1256.

definitions to define the dysfunction or failure of specific organ systems. However, most would agree that the need for organ support or replacement therapy does signify the presence of specific organ failure.

Validation of these consensus conference definitions came from a prospective evaluation of University of Iowa patients who met the SIRS criteria, sepsis, severe sepsis, and septic shock definitions. They demonstrated an increase in mortality as patients moved down this continuum of injury severity.

In 2001, the International Sepsis Definitions Conference convened to revisit the ACCP-SCCM Consensus Conference Sepsis Definitions. Representatives from the Society of Critical Care Medicine, American College of Chest Physicians, European Society of Intensive Care Medicine, American Thoracic Society, and the Surgical Infection Society re-affirmed the basic validity of the 1991 definitions. To enhance the clinician's ability to recognize severe sepsis and to possibly enhance the specificity of the clinical diagnosis of sepsis, the conference provided a listing of common signs and symptoms of sepsis that are included in Table 1. In addition, the International Sepsis Definitions Conference developed a classification scheme for sepsis modeled after the TNM system used in cancer staging (Table 2). It is hoped that the PIRO classification system would aid in stratifying septic patients on the basis of the predisposing condition(s), the nature of the insult, the nature and magnitude of the host's response, and the degree of concomitant organ dysfunction. The potential utility of the proposed staging systems is the ability to discriminate the morbidity associated with the infection from the morbidity arising from the response to the infection.

Pathogenesis of Sepsis

The septic response begins as a normal physiologic response to an infection that attempts to wall off and eliminate the offending microbiologic organism(s). The pathologic process we clinically recognize as sepsis is the result of an excessive and uncontrolled physiologic response that may culminate in endothelial cell injury, MODS, or death. The normal response to infection involves a process that serves to localize and contain an invading organism usually resulting in the initiation of repair of injured host tissue. When this inflammatory response to infection becomes generalized and extends to healthy host tissue this becomes SIRS. With the onset of SIRS, normal host tissue, whether infected or not, becomes damaged. This results in the release of proinflammatory and anti-inflammatory molecules and mediators that are capable of producing injury or altering the host's immune response. These contrasting elements help facilitate host tissue repair in healing. However, when there is an imbalance in the complex and intricate septic cascade, either a SIRS or a compensatory anti-inflammatory response syndrome (CARS) can predominate. If the SIRS response predominates there is a predisposition for an exaggerated proinflammatory response that can culminate in the production of MODS. In contrast, when the anti-inflammatory CARS response predominates, there is a state of immune suppression that can result in secondary or nosocomial infections. These additional inflammatory insults may supply additional "hits" to the immune system and have been termed the "multiple hits hypothesis" for the production of multiple organ dysfunction or failure. The sepsis cascade has been categorized into five stages by Bone and colleagues, which are listed in Table 3.

Host factors responsible for important first-line of defense against the infectious insult include epithelial barriers, mucociliary flow, pH of body fluids, urine volume, and secretory immunoglobulins. Overall immune function of the host is also a key consideration. Chronic diseases such as diabetes mellitus, HIV infection, and chronic alcoholism commonly predispose the host to an infectious insult. The adaptive and innate immunity of the host also provide key defenses against infectious insults. The adaptive arm of host immunity is composed of specialized B cells and T cells. Receptors unique to each of these cell lines result in a proliferation of immune response when stimulated. The innate arm of the immune response uses receptors that recognize highly conserved antigenic regions in large groups of microorganisms. A group of cell surface receptors that have become of particular interest are the toll-like receptors (TLR). For example, activation of TLR-4 by circulating endotoxin from the gram-negative bacterial cell wall induces the transcription of a number of inflammatory

TABLE 3 The Five Stages of Sepsis

The infectious insult
Preliminary systemic response
Overwhelming systemic response
The compensatory anti-inflammatory reaction
Immunomodulatory failure

and immune response genes. Gram-negative organisms contain a component of endotoxin within the cell wall that is responsible for many of the manifestations of sepsis. Gram-positive organisms produce exotoxins that may function as superantigens. The result is a massive activation of T cells, with an overproduction of cytokines and an out-of-control immune response.

Mediators of the host inflammatory response are initially found in high concentrations locally, at the nidus of infection. In severe infections proinflammatory cytokines will produce systemic symptoms. This usually becomes the telltale sign that the infection is unable to be contained locally. Some of the more common primary pro- and anti-inflammatory molecules and mediators are listed in Table 4. Included in the list of proinflammatory cytokines are tumor necrosis factor (TNF)-α, interleukin (IL)-1, IL-6, and interferon-γ.

An overwhelming systemic inflammatory response results when the host is unable to contain the proinflammatory response locally. The massive, uncontrolled production of proinflammatory molecules and cytokines produce SIRS. Endothelial dysfunction typically ensues from the inflammatory response coupled with the activation of the coagulation syndrome. The result is microvascular thrombi and upregulation of endothelial adhesion molecules, causing microvascular permeability, vasodilatation organ dysfunction, and shock.

The overwhelming response is then followed by CARS, which down-regulates the proinflammatory cascade. The balance that ensues during the mixed antagonistic response syndrome (MARS) will determine the clinical manifestations and outcome of the response to the infection. The principle mediators of the CARS response include IL-4, IL-10, and transforming growth factor (TGF)-β. In some cases the compensatory reaction can lead to excessive production of counterregulatory cytokines, leading to immune suppression. This can be recognized by a decreased production of IL-6 and TNF-α by monocytes. The final result may be immunomodulatory failure, progression of infection, or superinfection along with coagulation activation, abnormalities of fibrinolysis leading to MODS and death.

TABLE 4 Potential Molecules Involved in the Pathogenesis of Sepsis and SIRS

Proinflammatory Molecules and Cells
Polymorphonuclear leukocytes (PMNLs)
Tissue macrophages and monocytes
Platelets
Arachidonic acid metabolites
Prostaglandins, prostacyclin, thromboxane
Leukotriene
Cytokines (interleukins 1, 2, 6, 8, 15, TNF, G-CSF)
Soluble adhesion molecules
Platelet activating factor (PAF)
Complement and activation of the complement cascade
Various kinins (i.e., Bradykinin)
Endorphins
Histamine and serotonin
Proteolytic enzymes
Elastase and lysosomal enzymes
Protein kinase, tyrosine kinase
Toxic oxygen metabolites
Superoxide, hydroxyl radical, hydrogen peroxide, peroxynitrite, etc.
Endotoxin and other bacterial and microbial toxins
Activation of the coagulation cascade
Neopterin
Plasminogen activator inhibitor-1 (PAI-1)
CD-14
Toll-like receptors 2 and 4
NfκB
Vasoactive neuropeptides
Monocyte chemoattractant protein (MCP)-1 and 2
Potential Anti-Inflammatory Molecules
Interleukin-1 receptor antagonist (Il-irs)
Type II interleukin-1 receptor
IL-4
IL-10
IL-13
Transforming growth factor β (TGF-β)
IκB
Glucocorticoid receptors
Epinephrine
Soluble TNF receptor (BTNFr)
Leukotriene B_4 receptor antagonist
Soluble CD-14
Lipopolysaccharide (LPS) binding protein

Management of Severe Sepsis and Septic Shock

Management of sepsis and septic shock begins with prompt recognition of the process (Table 5). Along with recognition and determination of a probable site of infection the initial management begins with an assessment of the physiologic derangements. In critically ill patients the general management involves source control, restoration, and maintenance of normal hemodynamic function, adequate oxygenation, ventilation, tissue oxygen delivery, and prevention of complications. Recently, the assessment of adrenal function and detection of occult adrenal insufficiency in vasopressor-dependent patients with septic shock have been important for defining a potential role for physiologic adrenal replacement therapy. It is also important to evaluate for the presence of complications of critical illness and to administer preventive strategies where appropriate.

SOURCE CONTROL

Prompt, effective management of the source of the infection is the cornerstone of sepsis management. Early initiation of appropriate, effective, antimicrobial therapy is essential for a favorable outcome in the septic patient. Necessary specimens should be sent for culture and sensitivity testing as early as possible, because this information will guide subsequent antimicrobial therapy and allow for good antimicrobial stewardship. The initial antimicrobial therapy is empiric and should be directed toward the organisms that are likely to be causing the infection that has

TABLE 5 Basic Management Principles for Severe Sepsis and Septic Shock

Identify the Cause and Source of Infection
Obtain suitable material for needed cultures, gram stains, and diagnostic studies.
Initiate Appropriate Antibiotic Therapy
Initial therapy will be empiric, but tailored therapy may be started when more data is available. Survival is improved when the initial antibiotic therapy is effective against the isolated organism(s).
Surgical Drainage where Appropriate
Restore and maintain hemodynamic function
Early goal-directed therapeutic approach
Fluids are the initial choice for volume resuscitation and may include:
Crystalloids
Colloids
Volume expanders
Blood products
If hypotension and poor perfusion persist than **vasoactive agents** should be used as necessary to ensure adequate hemodynamic function
Hemodynamic monitoring is frequently required to ensure the adequacy and effectiveness of therapy
Physiologic dose corticosteroid replacement therapy may be beneficial for vasopressor-dependent patients with "inadequate cortisol response"
Support Oxygenation and Ventilation
Supplemental oxygen as needed to ensure that the patient has adequate arterial oxygen saturation
Ensure "adequate" tissue oxygen delivery
Ventilator support as necessary
Use lung protective ventilator support strategy
Antithrombotic, Profibrinolytic, Anti-Inflammatory Therapy
Drotrecogin alfa (activated); use as per package insert recommendations
Metabolic Support
Early nutritional support
Enteral route is preferred to maintain intestinal mucosal barrier function
Control hyperglycemia to decrease infectious complications
Prevent Complications of Critical Illness
DVT/PE prophylaxis
Stress-related gastrointestinal bleeding
Prevent organ system dysfunction
Prevent nosocomial and secondary infections
Critical illness polyneuropathy
Anemia of critical illness

Adapted from Balk RA: Optimum treatment of patients with severe sepsis and septic shock: evidence in support of the recommendations, *Dis Mon* 2004;50:168-213.

given rise to the septic response. A review of nosocomial infections suggests that the urinary tract, respiratory system, and bloodstream are the three most common sources of hospital-acquired infections. Clinical trials of new agents for the treatment of sepsis have observed that the respiratory tract and the abdomen are the most common sources of infection. After identification of the likely site and cause of the infection, the initial antibiotic selection should be made taking into account the antibiogram of the institution or specific unit where the infection was acquired. When the results of the various cultures and their sensitivity patterns, are available, the antimicrobial therapy should then be appropriately tailored. It has been well documented that the use of early effective antimicrobial therapy will decrease mortality, particularly in patients with gram-negative bacteremia, elderly patients with *Streptococcus pneumoniae* infection, and critically ill patients with bloodstream infections or hospital-acquired pneumonia. The use of early effective antibiotic therapy in critically ill patients has been associated with significant reductions in infection-related and all-cause mortality rates. This benefit was present despite the addition of effective antibiotics after the culture and sensitivity data was available. This observation underscores the importance of initiating the correct initial empiric therapy. Correct antibiotic decisions become even more important in this era of increasing antibiotic resistance. It is important to know the ecology of organisms in your institution along with the antibiogram for the institution. Several recently published reviews assist with the initial empiric antibiotic selection.

HEMODYNAMIC MANAGEMENT

Sepsis is characterized by vasodilatory or distributive shock, and there is an increase in vascular capacitance along with the decrease in the systemic vascular resistance. Septic patients are typically intravascularly volume depleted related to the presence of increased permeability as a result of endothelial cell injury along with an increase in fluid loss coupled with a decrease in fluid replacement. Early recognition of significant hemodynamic derangements and restoration of normal organ perfusion are vital in preventing organ dysfunction and failure. The goal of hemodynamic resuscitation should be to either raise the mean arterial pressure above 60-65 mm Hg or achieve a systolic blood pressure of ≥90 mm Hg. The resuscitative efforts and the adequacy of tissue perfusion can be assessed at the bedside by monitoring heart rate, blood pressure, orthostatic blood pressure changes, mental status, hourly urine output, and skin perfusion. The initial hemodynamic resuscitation should take the form of fluid volume replacement. The fluid resuscitation can be accomplished with a variety of fluids, including crystalloid, colloid, blood, synthetic starches, and hypertonic saline. Most clinicians accomplish the fluid resuscitation with intravenous infusion of either crystalloid or colloid. Bolus infusions are typically administered using the clinical response or measurements of central venous pressure or pulmonary capillary wedge pressure as a guide. In many instances, adequate volume resuscitation may be sufficient to restore normal perfusion pressure. The choice of crystalloids versus colloids for fluid resuscitation has been the subject of numerous studies and reviews. Currently there is no clear benefit of one fluid over the other. Crystalloids tend to be cheaper and more readily available, but a larger volume is required. Generally, it may take significant liters of fluid to adequately resuscitate patients with severe septic shock. Colloids are typically more expensive and may be associated with coagulation abnormalities, but smaller volumes are needed.

Invasive vascular monitoring may be used to aid in the determination of adequate hemodynamic resuscitation. If a central venous catheter is present, the central venous pressure can be measured to assess the adequacy of the intravascular volume status. In selected patients with hemodynamic insufficiency, the insertion of pulmonary artery catheters to measure the left- (and right-) sided filling pressures and the various hemodynamic parameters may be beneficial. A sphygmomanometer may not be reliable for blood pressure measurement in hypotensive septic patients. Insertion of an arterial line may be required, especially if the patient does not respond to volume resuscitation and requires the addition of vasopressor therapy for hemodynamic resuscitation.

VASOPRESSOR MANAGEMENT

If adequate fluid resuscitation is not sufficient to restore adequate hemodynamic function, then vasopressor or inotropic therapy will be necessary. There is a wide variety of vasoactive medications that are useful in the hemodynamic resuscitation of septic shock. Table 6 lists some of the more commonly used agents. Despite a wide range of possible agents, dopamine (Intropin) and norepinephrine (Levophed) are typically used in most clinical units. Some centers prefer to use phenylephrine (Neo-Synephrine) in patients with tachycardia or a history of arrhythmias because this pure alpha agent will cause less tachycardia and arrhythmias.

Unfortunately, there is a lack of large, prospective, randomized, protocol-controlled clinical trials that have compared dopamine with norepinephrine for the management of patients with septic shock. Therefore, until such data are available to guide the decision process, there is no clear benefit of one vasopressor strategy over the other. Therefore, either agent is acceptable in the management of hypotensive patients. Dopamine has been the preferred agent in many units, in part related to its ease of use, the concept that it improves splanchnic and renal perfusion, and its safety record. Recent clinical trial results have revealed that there is no specific beneficial effect of so-called renal dose dopamine in preventing the development of renal failure or in decreasing the need for renal replacement therapy. In addition, the use of dopamine has been associated with an increased incidence of arrhythmias and a decrease in the gastric intramucosal pH (an indicator of splanchnic oxygen delivery and utilization). Norepinephrine is a potent vasoconstrictor that also has some increase in inotropic and chronotropic effect on the heart. There is no decrease in renal or splanchnic perfusion as was once thought and, in fact, there is an increase in the perfusion of these vascular beds as a result of the increased cardiac output and vasoconstriction. A large observational study of French septic shock patients who required high doses of vasopressor therapy demonstrated a significant improvement in

TABLE 6 Vasoactive Agents Commonly Used in the Management of Severe Sepsis

Drug	Receptor Activity	Dose	Effect	Notes
Norepinephrine (Levophed)	α_1: 3+, α_2: 2+, β_1: 2+	0.03–1.5 µg/kg/min	Vasoconstriction	Little change in heart rate or CI May decrease lactate
Epinephrine	α_1: 3+, α_2: 3+, β_1: 3+, β_2: 2+	0.1–0.5 µg/kg/min	Increase stroke volume and CI	Unpredictable dose-response Decrease splanchnic blood flow Increase oxygen consumption and delivery
Dopamine (Intropin)	α_1: 3+, α_2: 3+, β_1: 3+, β_2: 2+	<5 µg/kg/min	Vasodilation	Dopaminergic effects predominate Dilation of renal, mesenteric, and coronary arteries Increased glomerular filtration rate (GFR) Sodium excretion
Dopamine	α_1: 3+, α_2: 3+, β_1: 3+, β_2: 2+	5–10 µg/kg/min	↑ Inotropy and chronotropy	β-adrenergic effects predominate Increased CI primarily due to increased stroke volume
Dopamine	α_1: 3+, α_2: 3+, β_1: 3+, b_2: 2+	>10 µg/kg/min	Vasoconstriction	α-adrenergic effects predominate
Dobutamine (Dobutrex)	α_1: 1+, α_2: 1+, β_1: 3+, β_2: 2+	2–20 µg/kg/min	↑ Inotropy and chronotropy	25%–50% increase in CI Decreases PAOP
Phenylephrine (Neo-Synephrine)	α_1: 3+	0.5–8 µg/kg/min	Vasoconstriction	Increase MAP without change in heart rate CI may decrease
Vasopressin (Pitressin)	V_1	0.04 units/min	Vasoconstriction	"Hormone replacement therapy." May potentiate the vasoconstrictor effect of endogenous catecholamines or act directly on a V_1 receptor

Modified from Steel A, Blbari D: Choice of catecholamine: does it matter? *Curr Opin Crit Care* 2000;6:847-853.

survival with the use of norepinephrine as compared with high doses of dopamine with or without the addition of epinephrine.

Recently there has been renewed interest in the use of vasopressin (Pitressin)[1] in patients with vasodilatory shock. The initial release of stored vasopressin from the posterior pituitary during hypotension depletes the body's store of the hormone. As the shock state persists, there is a state of vasopressin deficiency, which some view as a hormone deficiency state that is amenable to replacement therapy. Some centers are now infusing vasopressin as a hormone replacement therapy in a constant, nonescalating dose to augment dopamine or norepinephrine's pressor effects. The importance of early goal-oriented hemodynamic resuscitation was emphasized in a recent trial comparing this technique with more traditional resuscitation efforts. The early goal-oriented protocol was associated with significant improvement in ICU and hospital survival and significantly less death from sudden hemodynamic collapse.

Some patients with severe sepsis and septic shock have a reversible biventricular myocardial dysfunction, which has been attributed to circulating TNF-α, IL-1, or nitric oxide that are elaborated as part of the SIRS response. Ventricular dilatation and a reduced ejection fraction comprise this myocardial depression. Inotropic agents such as dobutamine (Dobutrex) or epinephrine can improve the myocardial contractility and hemodynamic function in these patients. By increasing stroke volume and heart rate, dobutamine increases the cardiac index. While epinephrine can also increase the cardiac index, its use should be limited in the septic patient because it can impair splanchnic blood flow and increase systemic and regional lactate concentrations.

SUPPORT OXYGENATION AND VENTILATION

Abnormalities of the respiratory system are some of the most common signs of organ system involvement in sepsis. Septic patients should be assessed for adequacy of oxygenation, oxygen delivery, ventilation, and the ability to protect the airway. Septic patients commonly have abnormalities of oxygenation and increased work of breathing. Patients who are hypoxemic should be given supplemental oxygen with a goal of achieving arterial oxygen saturation ≥90%.

Another decision to make in caring for the septic patient is the need and timing for endotracheal intubation and ventilatory support. Acute lung injury and ARDS are relatively common manifestations of pulmonary dysfunction in the patient with severe sepsis and septic shock. Up to 35% of septic patients may manifest ARDS. The goal of mechanical ventilation is to maintain the Pa_{O_2} in the 55 to 70 mm Hg range while keeping the FI_{O_2} below 60% (0.6). The traditional approach to mechanically ventilating patients with acute lung injury (ALI) and ARDS has been to employ

[1]Not FDA approved for this indication.

tidal volumes in the 10 to 15 mL/kg range. The Acute Respiratory Distress Syndrome Network (ARDSNet) trial of low tidal volume ventilation of 6 mL/kg ideal body weight, coupled with maintaining an end-inspiratory plateau pressure ≤30 cm H_2O, and a nomogram for positive end-expiratory pressure (PEEP) titration based on FI_{O_2} and oxygenation goals demonstrated an overall decrease in hospital mortality along with an increase in ventilator-free and organ failure-free days.

The risk of infection and ventilator-associated complications increases with the duration of ventilatory support. Patients should be removed from the ventilator as soon as they no longer need mechanical ventilatory support. The use of weaning protocols implemented by trained ICU support staff have been shown to speed the weaning process and improve the overall process of extubating the critically ill patient. It is also important to use sedation and analgesia appropriately in this critically ill population. Excessive sedation and analgesia have been linked to prolonged stays on mechanical ventilatory support and increased complications.

In a large, multicenter controlled trial conducted in critically ill patients without ischemic cardiac disease or acute blood loss, the restrictive practice of packed red blood cell transfusions in the management of anemia and low hemoglobin levels (Hb levels between 7.0 and 9.0 g/dL) was shown to provide adequate oxygen delivery to the tissues and in a subgroup of younger patients and less ill patients was found to be associated with a lower mortality rate compared with a more liberal transfusion policy with Hb levels maintained in the 10.0 to 12.0 g/dL range. The use of weekly recombinant erythropoietin has also been shown to reduce the need for transfusions in critically ill patients. Aggressive use of packed red blood cell transfusions in an effort to achieve supernormal oxygen delivery states should be discouraged.

SUPPORTIVE CARE FOR THE CRITICALLY ILL PATIENT

Patients with severe sepsis and septic shock are critically ill and susceptible to the multiple complications common in the critically ill population. These complications include deep vein thrombosis and pulmonary emboli, stress-related gastrointestinal bleeding, nosocomial infections, MODS, and critical illness polyneuropathy/myopathy. Patients in the ICU with sepsis or septic shock should receive prophylaxis for deep vein thrombosis with unfractionated or low-molecular-weight heparin or pneumatic compression devices if they have a coagulopathy or increased risk of bleeding. Prophylaxis for stress-related gastrointestinal bleeding may be accomplished with H_2-receptor blockers, proton pump inhibitors[1], sucralfate (Carafate)[1], or early enteral feeding.

Nutritional support of the patient with severe sepsis is important from multiple standpoints. Proper

[1]Not FDA approved for this indication.

nutrition is important to maintain the necessary immune function during the catabolic septic metabolic process. Enteral administration of nutrition may prevent stress-related gastrointestinal bleeding and may prevent the translocation of bowel organisms or endotoxin by maintaining the integrity of the gastrointestinal tract's mucosal barrier function. Nutritional requirements during severe sepsis and septic shock have been addressed by numerous organizations and medical societies. Adequate nutrition is responsible for improved wound healing, decreasing susceptibility of critically ill patients to infection and optimizing immune function. The following nutritional guidelines have been recommended for patients with sepsis:

- daily caloric intake, 25 to 30 kcal/kg/usual body weight per day
- protein, 1.3 to 2.0 g/kg per day
- glucose, 30% to 70% of total nonprotein calories to maintain serum glucose <225 mg/dL
- lipids, 15% to 30% of total nonprotein calories
- Omega-6 polyunsaturated fatty acids should be reduced in septic patients, maintaining that level which avoids deficiency of essential fatty acids (7% of total calories, generally 1 g/kg per day).

Metabolic management also includes correction of electrolyte abnormalities as well as tight control of blood sugar, which may require constant insulin infusion. In a report of postsurgical predominantly ventilated patients, tight glucose control aimed at keeping the blood sugar between 90 and 110 mg/dL was associated with a significant improvement in ICU and hospital survival. There were four times more deaths from multiple organ failure secondary to a proven septic focus in the group that did not receive the tight glucose control.

Innovative Therapies in Severe Sepsis and Septic Shock

Severe sepsis and septic shock have continued to be associated with a significant mortality rate despite the improvements in our understanding of the septic process, the use of powerful antibiotic agents, and the provision of basic sepsis management. Technologic advances have also brought forward antibodies, receptor blockers, and other innovative agents designed to interrupt or block aspects of the septic cascade. The majority of innovative experimental strategies were directed at various components of the proinflammatory response evident during the initial phases of SIRS and sepsis. Lack of success with the majority of these trials has led to a shift in the target for interruption toward a later stage aspect of the septic cascade. A number of these recent strategies have taken aim at the coagulation system in an effort to inhibit the generation of thrombin and fibrin, which may be instrumental in the disorder of the microcirculation that may be at least partially responsible for the organ system dysfunction and MODS seen in severe sepsis and SIRS.

CORTICOSTEROID THERAPY

Experimental studies in animal models of sepsis and septic shock have demonstrated improved survival with the pretreatment or early treatment with high doses of corticosteroids. The use of high doses of corticosteroids in humans with severe sepsis and septic shock has not been associated with significant improvements in survival except in one study. As a result of multiple trials of high-dose steroids in patients with severe sepsis showing no benefit and potential harm this practice has been abandoned. Recently, the observation that basal cortisol levels and the cortisol response to the administration of adrenocorticotropic hormone (corticotropin; ACTH) could predict survival in patients with severe sepsis and septic shock has drawn attention back to the use of steroid therapy. A French study of patients with septic shock demonstrated that a basal cortisol level of ≤34 μg/dL along with the ability to increase the cortisol level by ≥9 μg/dL was associated with a 74% survival rate. In comparison, patients who had a basal cortisol level of >34 μg/dL and were unable to increase their cortisol level by ≥9 μg/dL had an 18% survival rate. The investigators proposed that some patients with septic shock have a state of relative adrenal insufficiency or problems with their glucocorticoid receptors that can be improved with the use of more physiologic corticosteroid replacement therapy. A recent multicenter, prospective, randomized, controlled trial of 300 patients with vasopressor-dependent septic shock who were all receiving mechanical ventilatory support and were resuscitated according to a defined protocol demonstrated improved survival rates in those patients who failed to increase their basal cortisol level by >9 μg/dL and were given physiologic corticosteroid replacement therapy. For this trial the physiologic corticosteroid replacement therapy consisted of 50 mg of hydrocortisone (Solu-Cortef)[1] intravenously administered every 6 hours for 7 days combined with once daily fludrocortisone (Florinef)[1] given enterally at 50 μg per day. The authors of this trial concluded that physiologic corticosteroid therapy is beneficial and should be administered to vasopressor-dependent patients in septic shock who manifest relative adrenal insufficiency as defined by the failure to increase the cortisol level by more than 9 μg/dL after ACTH stimulation.

HIGH-VOLUME CONTINUOUS VENOVENOUS HEMOFILTRATION THERAPY

The use of high-volume, continuous hemofiltration (either continuous arteriovenous or venovenous) has been reported to benefit the hemodynamic course and outcome in patients with intractable circulatory failure resulting from septic shock. The use of this form of management is expensive, requires defined expertise, and may be associated with metabolic and coagulation abnormalities. Further studies are needed to

[1]Not FDA approved for this indication.

determine if this mode of therapy improves outcome in septic patients. Its use should probably be limited to patients with renal indications for hemofiltration.

ANTITHROMBOTIC THERAPY

Newer therapies have been directed toward inhibitors of the coagulation system as a potential therapeutic strategy for patients with severe sepsis and septic shock. Earlier therapies targeting the proinflammatory stage have shown little benefit in reducing mortality. Among the therapies that have been used are antithrombin, tissue factor pathway inhibitor (TFPI), and activated protein C replacement therapy.

Antithrombin III (AT) is an endogenous serine protease that has antithrombotic and anti-inflammatory properties. In an early trial in a small number of patients the administration of AT[1] to patients with septic shock and disseminated intravascular coagulation demonstrated a trend toward improved survival. Subsequently a large multicenter, prospective, randomized, double-blind, placebo-controlled trial was conducted which unfortunately showed no difference in mortality compared to placebo at 30, 60, and 90 days.

Tissue factor pathway inhibitor (TFPI) inhibits Factor VIIa within the Factor VIIa/tissue factor complex, after first binding and inactivating Factor Xa. Recently, a Phase 3 multicenter, prospective, randomized, double-blind, placebo-controlled trial has been completed and reportedly failed to demonstrate a significant benefit in the primary endpoint, which was 28-day all-cause mortality.

As with antithrombin, the Protein C system is one of the endogenous antithrombotic agents. Drotrecogin alfa (activated) (Xigris) is recombinant human activated protein C. A recent Phase 3 trial was stopped after the second interim analysis demonstrated a significant survival benefit associated with the use of activated protein C versus placebo in 1690 patients with severe sepsis and septic shock. Treatment with a 96-hour infusion of drotrecogin alfa (activated) produced a 6.1% absolute risk reduction and a 19.4% relative risk reduction in the 28-day all-cause mortality in patients with severe sepsis (P = .005). The use of drotrecogin alfa (activated) was accompanied by a significant reduction in D-dimer and IL-6 levels, supporting a beneficial effect on coagulation and inflammation, respectively. There was also restoration of the normal fibrinolytic pathway with the use of activated protein C. The drotrecogin alfa (activated)-treated population did experience more serious bleeding complications (3.5%) compared with the placebo group (2.0%), and this difference trended toward significance. These results suggest that for every 66 patients treated with drotrecogin alfa (activated), one additional serious bleeding event would occur. The number needed to treat to save an additional life was 16. A recent pharmacoeconomic analysis concluded that this agent is beneficial in patients with severe sepsis and septic shock who had a high risk of mortality and were young or had a high likelihood of surviving were it not for the complicating septic process.

The Food and Drug Administration (FDA) and 19 other regulatory bodies in other countries (including the European Union) have approved the use of drotrecogin alfa (activated) for the treatment of severe sepsis in adult patients with a high risk of mortality. The FDA gives the example of using the Acute Physiology and Chronic Health Evaluation (APACHE) II to estimate the risk of death (APACHE II score ≥25) and other means such as the number of dysfunctional organs to determine the target population of patients. Currently, the safety and efficacy of drotrecogin alfa (activated) in pediatric patients has not been determined. Contraindications for the use of drotrecogin alfa (activated) include patients with known sensitivity to drotrecogin alfa (activated) and those patients with a high risk of death from or significant morbidity associated with bleeding. This group would include patients with active internal bleeding, recent (within 3 months) hemorrhagic stroke, recent (within 2 months) intracranial or intraspinal surgery or severe head trauma, trauma with increased risk of life-threatening bleeding, the presence of an epidural catheter, an intracranial neoplasm, or mass lesion or evidence of cerebral herniation.

[1]Not FDA approved for this indication.

Prognosis

Despite the tremendous advances in our appreciation of the pathophysiologic processes that comprise the septic response coupled with improved antibiotics and technologic support of the critically ill, the mortality rate for patients with severe sepsis and septic shock remains high. Clinical trials have reported placebo-group mortality rates attributable to severe sepsis and septic shock of 20% to 50%, with mortality rates up to 80% to 85% with septic shock and multiple organ failure. This high rate of morbidity and mortality demands an aggressive approach for early diagnosis and treatment in an attempt to improve the outcome of these critically ill patients. A number of factors have been found to impact survival including, age, comorbid condition, site and type of infection, severity of illness, the number, and specific organ system failures. In addition, a patient's genetic makeup or gender may have a dramatic impact on whether or not they develop sepsis, as well as the severity, clinical manifestations, and outcome of the sepsis. It has also been demonstrated that survivors of sepsis have increased 6- and 12-month mortality rates compared with matched non-septic critically ill patients. There is also a reduced quality of life and more health-related issues in those patients who have survived an episode of sepsis. These observations underscore the importance of early aggressive management of the septic patient and suggest that our future focus should also be directed toward prevention of sepsis.

BRUCELLOSIS

METHOD OF

Edward J. Young, MD

Brucellosis is a disease of animals (zoonosis) that under certain conditions is transmittable to humans. Although brucellosis exists worldwide, it is especially prevalent in the Mediterranean basin, the Arabian Peninsula, the Indian subcontinent, in parts of Mexico, and in Central and South America. Programs to control brucellosis in cattle have dramatically reduced the incidence of human infection in the United States.

Brucellosis is transmitted to humans by direct contact with infected animals, their secretions, and their carcasses. Other modes of transmission include inhalation of contaminated aerosols and ingestion of unpasteurized milk and other dairy products, such as cheese. Whereas brucellosis was once principally an occupational disease of those in the livestock industry—farmers, ranchers, veterinarians, and abattoir workers—the epidemiology of the disease in the United States has changed in recent years. Currently, the majority of cases occur in persons of Hispanic descent, with ingestion of unpasteurized goat's milk cheese as the vehicle of transmission. The disease has long been recognized to be a risk for laboratory personnel, and biohazard level 3 precautions are recommended when handling clinical specimens.

On the basis of genetic identity, *Brucella* is considered a monospecific genus; however, for epidemiological purposes, the pathogenic species are classified according to their preferred natural hosts, namely, *Brucella abortus* (cattle), *Brucella melitensis* (goats and sheep), *Brucella suis* (swine), and *Brucella canis* (dogs). Recently discovered isolates of brucellae from marine mammals are still being characterized, including their potential to cause human infection.

Brucellosis is a systemic disease that can involve any organ or tissue of the body. Symptoms are largely nonspecific and usually begin within 2 to 3 weeks after inoculation or ingestion. In about one half of cases the onset of illness is insidious, developing slowly over weeks to months after exposure. The disease is characterized by a plethora of somatic complaints, such as fatigue, malaise, body aches, and depression. In contrast, there is a paucity of abnormal physical findings, most notably fever, sweats, lymphadenopathy, and hepatosplenomegaly. Fever often waxes and wanes over time, giving rise to the term *undulant fever*. When symptoms related to a single organ predominate, the disease is termed focal or localized. Osteoarticular localization is the most frequent complication. The diagnosis of brucellosis is made with certainty when brucellae are isolated from blood, bone marrow, or other tissues. In the absence of bacteriologic confirmation, a presumptive diagnosis can be made on the basis of high or rising levels of specific antibodies in the serum, cerebrospinal fluid, or other body fluids. Although no single titer is always diagnostic, most patients will have titers >1:160 in the serum. A variety of serologic tests have been employed, including agglutination, Coombs' test, and enzyme-linked immunoabsorbent assay (ELISA).

Treatment

Antimicrobial therapy relieves symptoms, shortens the duration of illness, and decreases the incidence of complications of brucellosis. A variety of drugs are active against *Brucella* in vitro; however, the results of routine susceptibility tests do not always predict clinical efficacy. Moreover, the intracellular localization of brucellae appears to offer some protection for the organism against certain classes of drugs. Consequently, despite showing activity in vitro, β-lactam antibiotics (e.g., penicillins, cephalosporins, macrolides, and quinolones) are generally ineffective. The tetracyclines are the most effective class of antibiotics for the treatment of human brucellosis with most strains inhibited by 0.1 μg/mL or less. Because tetracyclines are bacteriostatic they are usually used in combination with other drugs, such as an aminoglycoside, rifampin (Rifadin), or trimethoprim-sulfamethoxazole (Bactrim). Although resistance to antibiotics is not a major problem, treatment failure or relapse is common unless antimicrobial therapy is continued for prolonged periods of time.

The combination of a tetracycline and an aminoglycoside is the most effective therapy for human brucellosis. The traditional regimen is tetracycline HCl (500 mg four times daily orally), administered for 6 weeks, in combination with streptomycin (1 g per day intramuscularly), administered for 2 to 3 weeks. Currently, a doxycycline (Vibramycin) oral dose of 100 mg twice a day for 6 weeks has largely replaced tetracycline HCl because of its longer half-life and fewer adverse side effects. Moreover, gentamicin (Garamycin)[1] administered as a single intramuscular dose of 5 mg/kg/d for 2 weeks is now used in place of streptomycin.

Rifampin (Rifadin)[1] has good activity against *Brucella* (MIC_{90} 1 μg/Ml), penetrates cell membranes, and, in combination with a tetracycline, provides a fully oral regimen. The combination of doxycycline (100 mg twice daily by mouth) and rifampin (15 mg/kg/d orally) with each drug administered for 45 days is an acceptable regimen; however, when compared to the regimen of doxycycline plus an aminoglycoside, the failure/relapse rate is higher. Some clinicians treat with doxycycline for 6 weeks in combination with gentamicin for the first 2 weeks followed by rifampin for the remaining 4 weeks; however, this approach has never been subjected to a formal study.

Cotrimoxazole (Bactrim, Septra)[1] in a fixed combination of 80 mg of trimethoprim and 400 mg

[1]Not FDA approved for this indication.

of sulfamethoxazole is also active against *Brucella*. The usual dose is four tablets (or two tablets of the double-strength dose) daily for 45 days[3]; however, some authorities have reported unacceptably high rates of relapse with this drug.

Fluoroquinolones have shown poor results when used as monotherapy for human brucellosis. Their role in combination therapy with other drugs remains to be fully elucidated.

Special Situations

CHILDHOOD BRUCELLOSIS

Tetracyclines are contraindicated for children 8 years of age or younger because of the potential for irreversible staining of teeth. Doxycycline (Vibramycin) appears to bind less well to enamel than other tetracyclines, but this does not entirely obviate the concern. Nevertheless, some clinicians have treated children with doxycycline plus streptomycin or gentamicin with satisfactory results. An alternative approach is to use co-trimoxazole (Bactrim) in combination with rifampin (Rifadin) for 6 weeks, but experience with this regimen is limited.

PREGNANCY

Brucellosis during pregnancy can result in spontaneous abortion, but prompt antimicrobial therapy can be lifesaving to the fetus. The same problems with the choice of antibiotics in childhood also apply to pregnancy. Nevertheless, doxycycline (Vibramycin) plus an aminoglycoside has been used successfully despite the lack of approval for these drugs in pregnancy. Co-trimoxazole (Bactrim) has also been used in this setting and in combination with rifampin (Rifadin) appears to be a safer alternative.

OSTEOARTICULAR BRUCELLOSIS

Complications involving bones and joints occur in up to 60% of patients in some series. Rarely does this present special treatment problems except in cases of spondylitis and osteomyelitis, for which therapy for 8 weeks may be required. Surgical intervention is rarely necessary except to drain septic joints and large paraspinal abscesses. The indications for drainage of spinal abscess include neurological dysfunction, persistent fever and pain after prolonged antimicrobial therapy, and spinal instability. Only a few cases of *Brucella* infection of bone prostheses have been reported. Approximately 50% of these cases required removal of the prosthesis, and the remainder were cured with prolonged antibiotic therapy.

[3]Exceeds dosage recommended by the manufacturer.

NEUROBRUCELLOSIS

A variety of neurological syndromes have been reported in patients with brucellosis, of which acute or chronic meningitis is the most frequent. Although central nervous system (CNS) involvement occurs in fewer than 5% of cases, it poses special problems owing to the need to achieve bactericidal concentrations of drugs in the cerebrospinal fluid (CSF). Most drugs commonly used to treat brucellosis do not cross the blood-brain barrier well. Most authorities recommend doxycycline, streptomycin, and rifampin (Rifadin)[1] for CNS infection. Co-trimoxazole (Bactrim)[1] has also been used, but it should not be monotherapy. There is no unanimity of opinion on the length of treatment; however, continuation for 6 to 8 months is often recommended depending on the clinical response. Although the value of adding corticosteroids has not been proven, some authorities advise their use in complicated cases.

ENDOCARDITIS

Another complication of brucellosis requiring bactericidal concentrations of antibiotics is endocarditis. Although rare, endocarditis is reportedly the most frequent cause of fatal brucellosis. Some patients have been treated successfully with antibiotics alone, but the majority require valve replacement surgery as well. Triple therapy using doxycycline, an aminoglycoside, and rifampin (Rifadin)[1] or co-trimoxazole (Bactrim)[1] is generally recommended with treatment continued for periods ranging from 6 weeks to 9 months. Prosthetic valve endocarditis invariably requires replacement of the infected valve.

FOCAL INFECTION

In addition to the complications listed above, deep tissue abscess caused by either acute brucellosis or reactivation of previous disease, such as hepatosplenic suppuration, may require surgical drainage in addition to antimicrobial chemotherapy.

RELAPSE

Most patients are cured by a complete course of antibiotic therapy as long as treatment is continued for at least 6 weeks. In some cases, relapse of symptoms occurs following the completion of therapy, usually within the first 6 months. Because relapse is rarely caused by the emergence of antibiotic-resistant strains, most patients are cured by repeating therapy with the same drugs. Some patients will experience a delayed convalescence and voice subjective complaints of ill health in spite of declining titers of antibodies and the absence of objective signs of infection. Such patients can be a challenge to manage.

[1]Not FDA approved for this indication.

The presence of localized disease must always be ruled out. When this is done, there is little evidence to support additional courses of antibiotics.

PROPHYLAXIS

Persons in high-risk occupations are advised to use precautions when handling potentially infected animals or their carcasses. Dairy products made from unpasteurized milk should be avoided, especially those originating in *Brucella*-endemic areas. Attenuated live *Brucella* vaccines are available for immunizing livestock, but vaccination of humans is not recommended. Accidental self-inoculation with veterinary vaccines (*B. abortus* strain 19 and *B. melitensis* strain Rev-1) can cause human infection; however, *B. abortus* strain RB-51 appears to be less pathogenic for humans. There are no data to support using antibiotic prophylaxis in persons exposed to brucellosis in the laboratory or elsewhere. Each case must be considered individually, and if antibiotic treatment is deemed necessary, a full 6-week course using two drugs is probably indicated.

VARICELLA (CHICKENPOX)

METHOD OF

Henry H. Balfour, Jr., MD

Chickenpox is both preventable and treatable. Like measles, mumps, and rubella, chickenpox is preventable by immunization with a live, attenuated vaccine. Unlike measles, mumps, and rubella, it can be successfully treated with specific antiviral therapy. Chickenpox is a mild disease for most children, but it can be serious and sometimes fatal for adults and immunocompromised patients of any age.

Etiology and Epidemiology

Chickenpox (also called varicella) usually results from primary infection with varicella-zoster virus, a human herpesvirus. Shingles (also called herpes zoster) occurs when varicella-zoster virus, which has remained clinically latent in dorsal root ganglia after causing chickenpox, reactivates and travels down afferent sensory nerves to produce a painful dermatomal rash. Varicella-zoster virus is spread most readily by droplets aerosolized when an infected person talks, coughs or sneezes. This virus also may be contracted by direct contact with the skin lesions of a patient who has either chickenpox or shingles. Persons with chickenpox are most likely to transmit the virus during the tail end of their incubation period and for the first 2 days of the rash. Chickenpox is quite contagious: when introduced into a household, 86% of susceptible children will contract it. In temperate climates, chickenpox is a seasonal illness that most commonly affects young children during the months of October through May. Children are infected less frequently in the tropics, leaving them susceptible to adult-onset chickenpox. Varicella-zoster virus is heat-labile, which may explain its apparent reduced infectivity among children in rural tropical settings. The incubation period of chickenpox is 14 days with a range of 10 to 21 days. Second cases are well documented but are uncommon. There were 4,000,000 cases of chickenpox annually in the United States until a live, attenuated vaccine was approved in 1995. Since then, the yearly incidence has steadily fallen.

Clinical Course

OTHERWISE HEALTHY CHILDREN

Children have a mild or unapparent prodrome of low grade fever, malaise, and respiratory symptoms. A day or two later, a pruritic rash develops in the scalp and on the face. The rash quickly spreads to the trunk and then to the extremities. Skin lesions are usually most numerous on the trunk. The rash evolves rapidly from maculopapules to superficial vesicles and then more slowly to pustules which finally crust. I have actually seen papules turn into vesicles during the course of a physical examination. Vesicles form on mucosal surfaces as well as the skin but these rapidly rupture to become shallow ulcers. Lesions are frequently at different stages of development in the same area. New skin lesions continue to form for a median of 3 days after the onset of rash. The appearance of new lesions for more than 7 days suggests that the patient has an underlying immunocompromised condition. Children who are not treated with antiviral therapy average 350 to 400 skin lesions. Oral acyclovir (Zovirax) therapy results in 50 to 100 fewer lesions. A reduction in the total number of lesions is first appreciated on the fourth day after the onset of rash. The lesions usually crust within a week. When the crusts are shed, a small pit sometimes surrounded by hypopigmentation may remain. In controlled clinical treatment trials, children who received placebo averaged 33 of these residual lesions when examined 28 days after onset of illness as compared with 13 lesions among their acyclovir-treated counterparts. The vast majority of the residual lesions heal in several months without leaving a scar.

ADOLESCENTS AND ADULTS

The prodrome in adults and adolescents is more pronounced than it is in children. The evolution and distribution of the rash is similar to that of younger patients, except that the lesions are more numerous and may be more pruritic. Patients are often systemically ill.

PREGNANT WOMEN AND NEWBORN INFANTS

Pregnant women with chickenpox are prone to develop viral pneumonia. If chickenpox occurs during the first 20 weeks of pregnancy, there is a 1% to 2% risk of fetal damage resulting in ocular and central nervous system abnormalities, cicatricial skin lesions, and limb hypoplasia. If a mother develops chickenpox within 7 days before or after delivery, her infant may develop neonatal chickenpox. This disease resembles bacterial sepsis and can be fatal. Until the age of 28 days, neonates who contract chickenpox from any source are at some risk for a severe illness. In contrast, infants whose mothers have shingles during pregnancy rarely if ever sustain a clinically significant varicella-zoster virus infection.

IMMUNOCOMPROMISED HOSTS

Chickenpox in an immunocompromised patient is serious. Among 127 children with cancer not given prophylaxis or antiviral therapy, 28% developed chickenpox pneumonia and the overall mortality rate was 7%. Immunocompromised hosts have a prolonged course and may continue to form new skin lesions for several weeks unless treated with antiviral drugs. Rather than following its usual evolution, the rash often stalls at the vesicular or even papulovesicular stage. Vesicles may become bullous or hemorrhagic. The virus may substantially damage visceral organs, especially the lungs, liver, gastrointestinal tract, bone marrow, or central nervous system. Signs and symptoms of visceral involvement mean that the illness is potentially life-threatening.

Complications

In immunocompetent children, the most common complication is bacterial infection of skin lesions, which may progress to cellulitis or even necrotizing fasciitis. If patients become septic, suppurative arthritis, osteomyelitis, or bacterial pneumonia may result. Rare complications due to the virus itself include arthritis, carditis, cerebellar ataxia, encephalitis, glomerulonephritis, hepatitis, orchitis, pneumonia, thrombocytopenia, uveitis, and vasculitis.

In the immunocompromised host, the virus has a predilection for the lungs, liver, gastrointestinal tract, central nervous system, and bone marrow. Any evidence of visceral involvement (such as dyspnea or abdominal pain) should prompt admission to the hospital for antiviral therapy as described below.

Diagnosis

Chickenpox is almost always a clinical diagnosis. Most patients give a history of exposure to chickenpox 2 weeks before they present with characteristic skin lesions concentrated on the face and trunk. In atypical cases, the diagnosis may be confirmed by submitting lesion aspirates or swabs to a diagnostic virology laboratory for culture or antigen detection. Conditions most often confused with chickenpox are skin infections due to herpes simplex virus, streptococci, or staphylococci. If the central nervous system is involved and the diagnosis is uncertain, cerebrospinal fluid should be submitted for detection of varicella-zoster virus by a sensitive and specific diagnostic technique such as polymerase chain reaction.

Prevention

A live, attenuated vaccine (Varivax) is approved in the United States for prevention of chickenpox and should be part of routine childhood immunizations (Table 1). Chickenpox vaccine had a protective efficacy of 95% over a 7-year follow-up period in children who participated in a placebo-controlled research study. If vaccinees develop chickenpox after exposure to wild virus, their illness is usually mild. The United States has opted for a strategy of universal chickenpox immunization, whereas some other countries offer vaccine only to persons at high risk of exposure (as listed in Table 1). There are advantages and disadvantages to both approaches. Success of the universal immunization plan depends upon achieving herd immunity. If the velocity of transmission is slowed but not stopped, the result could be an increase in the age at which susceptible individuals contract chickenpox. Adults are sicker than children and are at greater risk for complications. Therefore, it is important that every effort be made to maximize acceptance and uptake of chickenpox vaccine in the United States.

Although chickenpox vaccine is approved only for otherwise healthy persons, certain immunocompromised patients may be safely and effectively immunized. They include children with acute leukemia in remission, transplant candidates, and HIV-infected individuals with CD4 cell counts >200/µL or CD4 percentages of at least 25%. Before immunizing such patients, it would be prudent to consult an infectious disease specialist.

Chickenpox vaccine can also provide post-exposure protection if given within 4 days of the exposure. If more than 4 days have elapsed and prophylaxis is deemed necessary, the best approach is to prescribe

TABLE 1 Prevention of Chickenpox

Prophylaxis	Clinical Category	Dosage	Comments
Pre-exposure			
Chickenpox vaccine (Varivax)	Healthy child 1-12 years old	1 dose (0.5 mL SC)*	Give after age 15 mo if possible
	Healthy susceptible person ≥13 years old†	2 doses, 4-8 weeks apart	It may be cost-effective to screen patients for antibody and only immunize the seronegatives, because ~80% of persons in this age group are seropositive
Post-exposure			
Varicella-zoster immune globulin (VZIG) MUST BE GIVEN WITHIN 96 HR OF EXPOSURE	Premature newborn	1 vial (1.25 mL) IM	Gestational age <28 wk: all hospital exposures; gestational age >28 wk: hospital exposures if mother is seronegative
	Term newborn	1 vial IM	If exposed in hospital when <28 days old
	Pregnant woman	5 vials IM	Or one large vial (6.25 mL)
	Infant with maternal chickenpox	1 vial IM	If mother develops chickenpox 7 days before or after delivery
	Immunocompromised host	1 vial/10 kg of body weight IM	
Acyclovir (Zovirax)[1]	Susceptible household member	20 mg/kg (maximum 800 mg) 4 times daily for 7 days	Best results when initiated 7-9 days post-exposure
	Pregnant woman Immunocompromised host	800 mg orally 5 times daily for 7-10 days	An option when the exposure is not recognized until the 5th day

[1]Not FDA approved for this indication.
*Based on recent data, 2 doses given at least 3 months apart may be more efficacious.
†Susceptible persons to target for immunization include women of childbearing age (unless pregnant), workers in environments where transmission is likely (healthcare, day care, elementary and middle school), and residents in households with children who haven't had chickenpox.

oral acyclovir. Postexposure prophylaxis using varicella-zoster immune globulin (VZIG) or acyclovir (Zovirax)[1] is appropriate in certain settings as outlined in Table 1. VZIG is expensive and pain at injection site is a frequent complaint. Because VZIG is passive prophylaxis, it must be repeated after each exposure until the patient develops chickenpox or persistent antibodies to varicella-zoster virus indicating that a subclinical infection has stimulated active immunity.

Treatment

ANTIVIRAL THERAPY

Acyclovir (Zovirax) is the mainstay of specific treatment (Table 2). Both valacyclovir (Valtrex)[1] and famciclovir (Famvir)[1] should be at least as effective as acyclovir, but they have not yet been studied appropriately in patients with chickenpox. Acyclovir shortens the clinical course by 25% to 30% in otherwise healthy persons. Many children and their parents find this desirable. My rationale for treating all children over the age of 24 months is that it is impossible to predict exactly which child is destined to have a severe case of chickenpox. Since oral acyclovir therapy is safe, the risk-to-benefit ratio favors treatment. Therapy is especially worthwhile in adolescents, adults, and children who represent secondary cases in their household, because patients in these categories tend to be sicker. Acyclovir is most effective when started within 24 hours of onset of rash, but recent data have shown a benefit if it is initiated on the second and perhaps even third day of the rash.

Immunocompromised patients with chickenpox should always be given antiviral therapy. The standard of care is acyclovir administered intravenously at a dose of 10 mg/kg every 8 hours (Table 2). There are data to support switching from intravenous to oral acyclovir once the patient has ceased forming new lesions and has no evidence of visceral disease. Antiviral therapy should be initiated as soon as possible, because it may not prevent spread to visceral organs if given more than 2 days after onset of rash. However, immunocompromised patients who present late in their clinical course should still be treated with intravenous acyclovir unless they have stopped forming new skin lesions and have no evidence of visceral disease.

Which immunocompromised patients are at risk for visceral chickenpox? Solid organ and bone marrow transplant recipients, patients receiving cytotoxic drugs or chronic corticosteroid therapy for malignancies or autoimmune diseases, and persons with AIDS who have <200 CD4 cells are at high risk. Patients who take aspirin regularly or use intermittent corticosteroids, as well as those with chronic cutaneous, cardiac, or pulmonary disease are at some risk.

[1]Not FDA approved for this indication.

TABLE 2 Antiviral Therapy for Chickenpox

Clinical Category	Treatment of Choice	Alternative Treatment	Comments
Otherwise healthy child	Oral acyclovir (Zovirax), 20 mg/kg (maximum 800 mg) 4 times daily for 5 days	None	Treatment most effective when initiated within 24 hr of onset of rash; secondary household cases tend to be sicker than index case
Otherwise healthy adolescent or adult	Oral acyclovir, 800 mg 4 times daily for 5 days	Valacyclovir (Valtrex),[1] 1000 mg 3 times daily for 5 days Famciclovir (Famvir),[1] 500 mg 3 times daily for 5 days	Both valacyclovir and famciclovir should be at least as effective as acyclovir but controlled trials have not been reported and these drugs are not approved for treatment of chickenpox
Pregnant woman	Oral acyclovir, 800 mg 4 times daily for 5 days	Intravenous acyclovir, 10 mg/kg every 8 hr for 7 days if there is evidence of visceral chickenpox	Acyclovir is not approved for use in pregnancy (Pregnancy Category B)
Neonatal chickenpox	Intravenous acyclovir,[1] 10 mg/kg every 8 hr for 7 days	None	
Immunocompromised host	Intravenous acyclovir,[1] 10 mg/kg every 8 hr for 10 days	Switch to oral acyclovir, 800 mg 5 times a day to complete 10-day course	The switch from intravenous to oral acyclovir should not be made until the patient is afebrile, has ceased forming new lesions, and has no evidence of visceral chickenpox

[1]Not approved for this indication.

Many clinicians elect to treat mildly immunocompromised patients with oral rather than intravenous acyclovir. If oral acyclovir is prescribed, these patients should be followed closely and admitted to the hospital for intravenous acyclovir if evidence of visceral disease develops.

SYMPTOMATIC RELIEF

Pruritus is the chief complaint, especially in adolescents and adults. Patients should avoid sunlight, especially in the summer, because it aggravates the rash, intensifying itching. Pruritus may be relieved with cold compresses applied periodically to the itchiest spots. Colloidal oatmeal baths (Aveeno) and oral diphenhydramine hydrochloride (Benadryl) may also be helpful. If fever is a problem, acetaminophen (Tylenol) is preferred. Aspirin should not be given to patients younger than age 18 years because its use in children with acute viral illnesses has been associated with Reye syndrome.

CHOLERA

METHOD OF

Emmanuel Siaw, MD, PhD, and

George J. Fuchs, MD

Cholera, caused by *Vibrio cholerae*, is the prototypical noninflammatory secretory diarrheal disease and most extreme watery diarrhea known to man. The seventh pandemic of cholera that began in Indonesia in 1961 remains with us in the twenty-first century. As a result, cholera continues to kill millions of people worldwide each year because of severe dehydration. With the ability of *V. cholerae* to mutate into new strains and develop antimicrobial resistance, as well as increased regional and global travel, cholera promises to be of major, ongoing relevance to both developing and developed countries for years to come.

Organism and Pathophysiology

V. cholerae organisms are gram-negative curved rods subdivided into serogroups based on their cell wall O antigens. Members of the O1 group are responsible for clinical and epidemic disease, whereas non-O1 organisms cause sporadic disease or are nonpathogenic. *V. cholerae* O1 is further categorized into two biotypes, classical and El Tor, each of which has three serotypes (Ogawa, Inaba, and Hikojima) based on antigenic differences. *V. cholerae* O1 was the only known cause of epidemic cholera until 1992 when a new strain of non-O1 was isolated from India and neighboring countries during a large cholera outbreak. This new organism, subsequently named *V. cholerae*

O139 Bengal, was found to have clinical and epidemiologic characteristics similar to *V. cholerae* O1. The pathogenicity of cholera related to both *V. cholerae* O1 and O139 depends on its colonization in the small bowel and production of cholera toxin (CT). *V. cholerae* organisms are quickly killed by gastric acid, but ingestion of a large number of them or disruption of the gastric barrier rapidly precipitates disease. Once in the small intestine, the bacteria secrete the enzyme mucinase, which dissolves the protective glycoprotein coating over the intestinal epithelia and enables the organisms to adhere to the intestinal wall. From this position the organism multiplies and secretes CT comprised of an A (enzymatic) subunit and five B (binding) subunits. CT binds to a G_{M1} ganglioside epithelial cell membrane receptor. This stimulates adenylate cyclase, which results in increased intracellular amounts of cyclic AMP that activate electrolyte secretory pathways. The dual effect of CT-enhanced chloride secretion in crypt cells combined with CT inhibition of sodium absorption in villous cells manifests as a massive outpouring of watery stool without the signs of inflammation.

Epidemiology

More countries than ever are affected by cholera, which largely reflects extension of the seventh pandemic to the countries of the former Soviet Union and South America where cholera had not been reported for decades. Although cholera remains a disease primarily of underdeveloped countries, the emergence of *V. cholerae* O139 Bengal as a second etiologic agent of cholera in South Asia in early 1992 and the subsequent, nearly global spread of the disease has ensured scientific and public interest among developed countries as well. It was initially thought that the rapid emergence and predominance of *V. cholerae* O139 might herald the start of the eighth pandemic of cholera. However, the prevalence of *V. cholerae* O139 subsequently decreased dramatically, and *V. cholerae* O1 remains the dominant cholera strain in most areas of the world where cholera is endemic. Cholera also remains endemic in the gulf states of the United States, although very few cases are reported each year. In South Asia, cholera exhibits a bimodal seasonal pattern in which epidemics occur immediately before or early in the monsoon season and again as the monsoon season is ending. In between, the disease is endemic at low rates during which the organism seems to enigmatically disappear from the aquatic environment in which it normally thrives. *V. cholerae* has a unique ability to assume a noncultural but viable form in response to changes in the salinity and temperature of its environment. When ambient conditions are favorable as a result of climactic changes, the organisms blossom and become pathogenic once again. Marine shellfish and plankton are the main reservoirs of *V. cholerae*, with cholera spread via the fecal–oral route with man as the other natural reservoir. Poor sanitation and hygiene, therefore, are the primary risk factors; risk of infection decreases markedly with basic attention to the quality of ingested food and water. In cholera-endemic areas, infection rates are highest in children 2 to 4 years old, because older children and adults more often have vibriocidal antibodies from previous infections. However, in nonendemic, newly infected regions, adults and children are affected equally. In infants, inadequate breastfeeding practices further increase disease rates because of increased exposure and the lack of benefit of protective breast milk antibodies. Persons with hypochlorhydria resulting from malnutrition, medication (e.g., antacids, H_2 receptor antagonists, proton pump inhibitors), or gastric surgery are also at increased risk. *Helicobacter pylori*, a cause of atrophic gastritis and hypochlorhydria, is highly prevalent in the developing countries, and *H. pylori* infection may undermine the gastric barrier to *V. cholerae*. Although overall risk of cholera does not appear to be significantly increased among *H. pylori*-seropositive adults, risk of life-threatening cholera is significantly elevated (relative risk: 1.61), but only in persons lacking pre-existing natural vibriocidal antibodies.

Clinical Picture

Clinical disease has its onset after an incubation period of 18 hours to 5 days. The presentation of archetypal cholera occurs in approximately 10% of cholera cases, while the remaining 90% are comparatively mild and indistinguishable from other forms of acute watery diarrheal diseases. In severe disease, patients present with extreme watery diarrhea of short duration and characteristically have prominent abdominal cramping and vomiting, metabolic acidosis, hurried respiration, cold and clammy skin, poor skin turgor, and wrinkling of the skin, especially of the hands and feet (*washerwoman*). As the illness progresses, signs of advanced intravascular fluid depletion and collapse predominate, including depressed mentation and obtundation, hypovolemic shock, and renal failure. As impressive as the disease itself, so too is the recovery, which is usually rapid with proper treatment. If treatment is inadequate, however, mortality rates are high (approaching 50% in severe disease), and death can occur within hours from the onset of symptoms.

The diagnosis of cholera is generally made on a clinical basis without the need of laboratory tests, particularly where the disease is endemic, in part because treatment of watery diarrhea is the same regardless of etiology. Stool darkfield examination or culture is reserved for a definitive case diagnosis or for characterizing outbreaks and tracking the spread of endemic and epidemic disease. Different monoclonal, antibody-based, rapid immunodiagnostic kits for *V. cholerae* O1 and O139 have been developed in recent years, some of which compare favorably in sensitivity and specificity with conventional culture methods with the advantage of yielding results within minutes.

TABLE 1 Composition of Cholera Stool and Rehydration Solutions Used to Treat Cholera

	Concentration (mmol/L)			
	Na^+	K^+	Cl^-	HCO_3^-
Cholera Stool				
Adults	130	20	100	45
Children	100	30	90	30
ORS				
WHO (current)	75	20	65	30*
WHO (previous)	90	20	80	30*
Rice	90/75†	20	65	30*
Intravenous				
Lactated Ringer's	131	4	109	28
Dhaka solution	133	13	98	48
Normal saline‡	154	0	154	0

*Trisodium citrate (10 mmol/L) is now commonly used.
†Higher/lower osmolarity solution.
‡Only used if other, more appropriate solutions are not available.

Treatment

Management of the cholera patient is one of the most straightforward yet gratifying of any illness. It is not uncommon for a patient arriving with severe diarrhea and dehydration in a comatose condition to be discharged from the hospital/clinic and walking unassisted within 12 to 18 hours. Most cases can be treated adequately with oral rehydration solution (ORS) alone, but those with severe dehydration usually require initial rehydration with an intravenous isotonic solution such as lactated Ringer's that contains sodium, potassium, and a base in concentrations similar to that excreted in cholera stool. Initial replacement therapy can be achieved within approximately 3 hours in adults, and 4 hours and 6 hours in children and young infants, respectively. If they are malnourished, however, rehydration time is extended. Timely and appropriate intervention is crucial. The primary objective is rapid replacement of fluid and electrolyte deficits and, once achieved, maintenance of fluid balance through the replacement of ongoing stool losses with oral or, in the case of severe illness, parenteral solutions. It is important that children continue to be fed during diarrhea, and breast-feeding of infants should not be discontinued.

The development of oral rehydration solution (ORS) was a dramatic breakthrough in the treatment of cholera, reducing cholera mortality from more than 50% to less than 1%. As a general guideline, 5 to 10 mL/kg of ORS should be administered to children after each ongoing diarrheal bowel movement. The World Health Organization (WHO) and UNICEF historically recommended an ORS with 90 mmol sodium, 20 mmol potassium, 80 to 100 mmol chloride, 30 mmol bicarbonate, and 111 mmol of glucose per liter of water. This was designed to approximate stool losses (Table 1). More recently, the recommended solution for watery diarrhea has changed to an ORS that contains less sodium (75 mmol/L), although its use in cholera is controversial because the hyposmolar ORS results in more hyponatremia and little benefit in terms of reduced stool output compared to the higher sodium solution. The substitution of glucose with rice cereal provides more sodium-cotransporting substrate to intestinal epithelia without increasing osmolarity. Such rice-based ORS has been shown to be superior in the treatment of cholera, but not in noncholera, acute watery diarrhea.

Severely malnourished children (weight for age <60%, weight for length <70%, or any malnutrition with nutritional edema) have excess total body sodium despite a characteristic paradoxical hyponatremia, marked depletion of total body potassium, and impaired cardiac output. Because of the unique metabolic disturbances of severe malnutrition, a modified oral rehydration solution for malnourished children (termed ReSoMal) with reduced sodium (45 mmol/L) and increased potassium (40 mmol/L) and glucose (125 mmol/L) concentrations was proposed as having advantages in minimizing fluid overload and consequences of potassium deficiency, both of which are

TABLE 2 Antimicrobial Therapy for Cholera*

Antibiotic	Administration	Dose	
		CHILDREN	ADULTS
Doxycycline	Single dose		300 mg
Tetracycline	Four times per day for 3 d	12.5 mg/kg	500 mg
Erythromycin†1	Four times per day for 3 d	12.5 mg/kg	500 mg
Furazolidone (Furoxone)†	Four times per day for 3 d	1.25 mg/kg	100 mg
TMP-SMX (Bactrim)1	Twice per day for 3 d	TMP 5mg/kg, SMX 25 mg/kg	TMP 160 mg, SMX 800 mg
Ciprofloxacin (Cipro)1	Single dose		1 g
Azithromycin (Zithromax)1	Single dose	20 mg/kg, max 1 g	1 g

Abbreviation: TMP-SMX = trimethoprim-sulfamethoxazole.
1Not FDA approved for this indication.
*Specific therapy dependent on local *V. cholerae* resistance patterns.
†Indicated in pregnant women.

life-threatening in these children. However, the use of ReSoMal, while significantly improving potassium status, unexpectedly resulted in hyponatremia including symptomatic hyponatremia with seizure indicating that further modification will be needed. To avert fluid overload, it is crucial to extend the rehydration time using an appropriate solution for up to 10 hours, introduce oral rehydration therapy (ORT) early, and avoid intravenous infusion where possible. However, severely malnourished children with cholera who have severe dehydration should be hydrated as follows:

- The first hour administer 20 mL/kg of intravenous lactated Ringer's solution or a similar fluid with 5% dextrose and 20 mmol potassium per liter.
- The second hour administer 10 mL/kg of the same solution together with ORS of 10 mL/kg/h.
- At the end of the second hour, the IV can be discontinued and the ORS continued with 10 mL/kg/h for the next 2 hours.
- At the end of the 2 hours, reduce the ORS to 5 mL/kg/h for the next 10 hours or until diarrhea is resolved.

For infants older than 2 months, the selected intravenous fluid should be diluted by 50% (1/2 strength) and have a concentration of 5% dextrose and 20 mmol potassium per liter.

As an adjuvant to fluid replacement, antimicrobial agents significantly reduce stool volume, shorten the duration of diarrhea (often to within 48 hours), and markedly reduce vibrio excretion, which has implications for nosocomial or secondary spread of the disease (Table 2). Although a variety of antibiotics are efficacious, *V. cholerae* are resistant to inexpensive and commonly available antimicrobials such as tetracycline/doxycycline (Vibramycin), furazolidone (Furoxone), and trimethoprim-sulfamethoxazole (Bactrim)[1], and there have been rare reports of resistance to erythromycin[1] and ciprofloxacin (Cipro)[1]. Treatment options, therefore, are heavily dependent on local *V. cholerae* resistance patterns, especially because resistance is not stable and can fluctuate with periods of sensitivity. Presently, tetracycline, or its congener doxycycline, is the first-line agent in adults in most regions. Tetracycline/doxycycline can also be used in children because the short courses required to treat cholera are unlikely to discolor teeth, although erythromycin or furazolidone are often preferred for children younger than 8 years old and for pregnant women. Single-dose azithromycin (Zithromax)[1] or ciprofloxacin[1] therapy are also effective, but cost, availability, and concern about the emergence of resistant organisms with use of these broader-spectrum agents are barriers to their widespread use. To date, there are no antisecretory agents available that have a combined satisfactory efficacy and safety profile to enable them to be recommended.

[1]Not FDA approved for this indication.

Prevention

To prevent illness and epidemic spread, consumption of clean water and knowledge and practice of good hygiene behaviors are essential. Abstention from raw or undercooked seafood and insisting on cooked foods heated to the point of steaming are also advised for travelers. Such practices assume even greater importance for individuals taking gastric acid suppression medication. Development of an effective vaccine to prevent cholera continues to be an elusive goal, although several candidate vaccines are on the horizon that result in higher levels of protective efficacy compared to earlier oral and parenteral vaccines.

FOOD-BORNE ILLNESS

METHOD OF

George J. Gianakopoulos, MD

Food-borne illness remains an important and continually changing health problem in all countries of the world. In the United States over the last 20 years, several "new kids on the block" have emerged to take our attention, including *Escherichia coli* 0157:H7, *Campylobacter jejuni, Listeria monocytogenes, Cyclospora*, and *Cryptosporidium*. The CDC recently reported that they estimate food-borne diseases will cause 76 million illnesses with 5000 associated deaths in the next year in the United States alone. There is a palpable paranoia in the United States when it comes to the perceived lack of safety in our food supply. This is because food-borne diseases are common and the notion that our food supply comes from places with less rigid sanitary standards than that of the United States. Technology and food science practices of the 21st century have not eradicated or reduced food-borne diseases because of the mass production and processing of meats, fruits and vegetables as well as the loss of smaller farmers and producers. Other contributing factors may include migrating and moving populations, more restaurants and "fast foods," and less emphasis on traditional home lifestyle and family meals.

Table 1 lists food-borne illnesses and their characteristics. The CDC web site at www.CDC.gov has an exhaustive list of articles on the subject and detailed chapters are available in the infectious disease textbooks in any medical library. The office physician will come into contact mostly with viral, bacterial and protozoal causes of food-borne illnesses. Included in this chapter's tables are toxin-associated syndromes from mushrooms and seafood.

TABLE 1 Food-Borne Illnesses

Etiologic Agent	Estimated U.S. Food-Borne Cases/Year*	Incubation	Signs and Symptoms	Associated Foods	Treatment
Viral Agents					
Calicivirus (Norwalk-like agents)	~9,200,000	24–48 h	Nausea, vomiting, watery diarrhea; may be fever	Fecally contaminated foods, ready-to-eat foods touched by infected food workers, shellfish	Fluids, antimotility agents
Rotavirus, astrovirus	~39,000 each	1–3 d	Vomiting, watery diarrhea, low-grade fever	Same	Same
Hepatitis A	~4200	30 d (range, 15–50 d)	Dark urine, jaundice, flulike symptoms, diarrhea	Same	Same
Bacterial Agents					
Campylobacter jejuni	~2,000,000	2–5 d	Diarrhea, cramps, fever, vomiting; may be bloody diarrhea Sequela: Guillain-Barré syndrome	Raw and undercooked poultry, unpasteurized milk, contaminated water	Fluids; antibiotics (ciprofloxacin [Cipro]), 500 mg PO bid × 3 d, or azithromycin 500 mg PO qd × 3 d
Salmonella (nontyphoidal)	~1,300,000	1–3 d	Diarrhea, fever, abdominal cramps, vomiting; occasional bloody diarrhea Sequela: septicemia	Raw or undercooked poultry, contaminated eggs (*Salmonella enteritidis*), unpasteurized milk or juice, contaminated raw fruits or vegetables	Fluids; antibiotics *not* indicated unless extraintestinal spread (or immunocompromised host at risk for extraintestinal spread); for invasive/extraintestinal disease, ciprofloxacin, 500 mg PO bid × 5–7 d
Clostridium perfringens	~250,000	8–16 h	Watery diarrhea, nausea, abdominal cramps; fever rare	Meats, poultry, gravy; often precooked	Fluids, supportive care
Staphylococcal food poisoning	~190,000	1–6 h	Sudden onset of severe nausea and vomiting; may be diarrhea	Unrefrigerated or improperly refrigerated meat, potato and egg salad, cream pastries	Fluids, supportive care
Escherichia coli 0157:H7 and STEC	~94,000	1–8 d	Diarrhea, often bloody; abdominal pain and vomiting; little or no fever Sequela: hemolytic-uremic syndrome	Undercooked beef (esp. hamburger), unpasteurized milk and juice, raw fruits and vegetables (sprouts)	Fluids, supportive care; *antibiotics contraindicated*
Shigella	~90,000	24–48 h	Abdominal cramps, fever, diarrhea; stool may contain blood and mucus	Fecally contaminated food or water, ready-to-eat foods touched by infected food workers	Fluids, supportive care. Treat with ciprofloxacin, 500 mg PO bid × 3 d, or TMP/SMZ (Bactrim), DS PO bid × 3 d
Yersinia enterocolitica	~87,000	24–48 h	Diarrhea and vomiting, fever, abdominal pain; may cause pseudoappendicitis syndrome	Undercooked pork, unpasteurized milk	Fluids, supportive care; antibiotics if suggestion of invasive disease (ciprofloxacin, 500 mg PO bid × 3 d, TMP/SMZ, DS PO bid × 3 d, or ceftriaxone [Rocephin], 2.0 g IV qd)
Food-borne streptococcus	~51,000	24–48 h	Pharyngitis	Contamination of foods by infected food workers	Pen V PO × 10 d, or azithromycin, 500 mg PO qd × 5 d
Bacillus cereus	~27,000	Emetic toxin: 1–6 h	Sudden onset of nausea and vomiting; diarrhea may be present	Improperly refrigerated/ rewarmed cooked and fried rice	Fluids, supportive care

		Diarrheal toxin: 10–16 h	Abdominal cramps, watery diarrhea, nausea	Meats, stews, gravies; often precooked	
E. coli, enterotoxigenic	~24,000	1–3 d	Watery diarrhea, abdominal cramps, some vomiting	Water or food contaminated with human feces	Fluids; antibiotics in severe cases (ciprofloxacin, 500 mg PO bid × 3 d; TMP/SMZ)
Vibrio cholerae (nonepidemic/non-01/0139), *Vibrio parahaemolyticus*	~5200	6–72 h	Watery diarrhea; occasionally bloody diarrhea	Raw or undercooked shellfish, seafood	Fluids; doxycycline, 100 mg pO bid × 3 d in severe cases
Vibrio vulnificus		1–4 d	Sepsis in patients with liver disease or those who are immunocompromised; possible diarrhea	Same	Minocycline (Minocin), 100 mg PO q12 h, and cefotaxime (Claforan), 2.0 g IV q8h
Listeria	~2500	GI: 9–48 h; invasive disease: 2–6 wk	Fever, muscle aches, and nausea or diarrhea. Pregnant women may have mild flulike illness, with infection leading to premature delivery or still birth. Elderly or immuno-compromised patients may have bacteremia or meningitis	Fresh soft cheese, unpasteurized milk, ready-to-eat deli meats, hot dogs	Fluids for gastroenteritis; for invasive disease, ampicillin, 2 g IV q4–6h, or TMP/SMZ
Botulism	~60	12–72 h	Blurred vision, dysphagia, descending muscle weakness; may be vomiting, diarrhea	Home-canned foods with low acid content; foods where anaerobic growth possible	Supportive care. Botulinum antitoxin helpful if given early in course of illness. Call (404) 639-2206 or (404) 639-3753 workdays or (404) 639-2888 nights and weekends
Parasitic Agents					
Giardia lamblia	~200,000	1–4 wk	Acute or chronic diarrhea, flatulence, bloating	Untreated surface water, contamination of foods by water or infected food worker	Metronidazole (Flagyl), 250 mg PO tid × 5 d
Toxoplasma gondii	~110,000	6–10 d	Generally asymptomatic; cervical lymphadenopathy and/or flulike illness may develop in 20% Immunocompromised patients: CNS disease Pregnant women: fetal CNS infection	Undercooked meats, including pork, lamb, venison; contact with cat fecal material	Asymptomatic infections: no treatment Pregnant women (first 18 weeks' gestation): spiramycin,† 3 g qd, obtained from FDA, (301) 827-2335 Immunocompromised hosts: pyrimethamine (Daraprim) plus sulfadiazine, folinic acid
Cryptosporidium parvum	~30,000	2–28 d	Cramping, abdominal pain, watery diarrhea; fever and vomiting may be present and may be relapsing	Contaminated water, vegetables, fruits, unpasteurized milk	Supportive care
Cyclospora cayetanensis	~15,000	1–11 d	Fatigue, protracted diarrhea; often relapsing	Imported berries, contaminated water, lettuce	TMP/SMZ, DS PO bid × 7 d

Continued

TABLE 1 Food-Borne Illnesses—cont'd

Etiologic Agent	Estimated U.S. Food-Borne Cases/Year*	Incubation	Signs and Symptoms	Associated Foods	Treatment
Natural Toxins					
Ciguatera fish poisoning		GI: 2–12 h	Abdominal pain, nausea, vomiting, diarrhea; in severe cases, may be hypotension and bradycardia	Large predacious tropical reef fish: barracuda, grouper, red snapper, amberjack	Supportive care, atropine and blood pressure support; IV mannitol (20% solution, 1 g/kg piggybacked over 30 min) reported to be lifesaving in severe cases
		Neurologic: 12 h–5 d	Paresthesias, pain and weakness in legs, temperature reversal		In chronic cases, amitriptyline[1] (Elavil) may be beneficial
Scombroid (histamine toxicity)		1 min–3 h	Flushing, rash; burning sensation of skin mouth	Improperly refrigerated "scombroid" fish, including tuna, mahi-mahi	
Paralytic shellfish poisoning		30 min–3 h	Paresthesias, ataxia, dysphagia, mental status changes, hypotension; respiratory paralysis in severe cases	Scallops, mussels, clams, cockles harvested from beds exposed to blooms of the dinoflagellate *Alexandrium*; occurs primarily in Alaska, Pacific Northwest, California, and Maine	Supportive care

[1]Not FDA approved for this indication.
*Estimates of disease incidence (rounded to two significant figures) from Mead PS, Slutsker L, Dietz V, et al: Food-related illness and death in the United States. *Emerg Infect Dis* 5:607-625, 1999.
†Investigational drug in the United States.
Abbreviations: CNS = central nervous system; DS = double-strength tablet; FDA = Food and Drug Administration; STEC = Shiga toxin–producing *E. coli*; TMP/SMZ = trimethoprim/sulfamethoxazole. Adapted from Diagnosis and management of foodborne illnesses: A primer for physicians. MMWR Morb Mortal Wkly Rep 50 (RR02):1-69, 2001.

Food-borne diseases cause the most morbidity–mortality in the very young and the very old. This reflects the immaturity of the infant's immune system and the waning immunity seen with aging that predisposes to other diseases. Also of note is the role of normal intestinal microflora and microenvironment or lack thereof in the susceptible host. The stomach's low pH is classically one of the "lines of first defense" of the alimentary canal and when altered by age, disease or antacids, may predispose to symptomatic infection with various organisms. This concept has been well documented with salmonellosis and it is even postulated that alteration of normal gut flora with antibiotics disrupts colonization resistance and creates an environment suitable for allowing symptomatic salmonellosis.

Salmonella will be handled extensively in a separate chapter. It, along with *Campylobacter*, is one of the most common bacterial causes of acute infectious colitis. Foods most commonly associated with salmonellosis include poultry and dairy products but also sources of *Salmonella* include reptiles and exotic pets, such as iguanas. Tens of thousands of these kinds of animals are being imported each year. There are many well-documented outbreaks of nontyphoidal *Salmonella* associated with pets. Classic typhoid fever is rare in the United States but can be seen in expatriates, travelers and migrant workers. *Salmonella* has a "tropism" for vascular endothelium and can cause mycotic aneurysm formation, particularly in patients with pre-existing atherosclerosis. Positive blood cultures for *Salmonella* should always be treated with at least two weeks of a susceptibility directed antimicrobial, typically ciprofloxacin (Cipro). Careful follow-up of patients with documented positive blood cultures for *Salmonella* species is prudent. If persistently positive blood cultures are noted, a search for an endovascular sanctuary site such as a pre-existing aneurysm should be undertaken.

Campylobacter is probably underappreciated by many primary care physicians as one of the most common causes of symptomatic and prolonged diarrhea syndromes. In adolescents and young adults, it is the most common cause of bacterial infectious colitis. This is essentially a zoonotic infection that can also contaminate food and water in a classic fecal–oral model. There also is an association between Guillain-Barré syndrome and *Campylobacter* infection. A high percentage of individuals who have Guillain-Barré syndrome have either serologic or historical evidence of a recent *Campylobacter* infection. *Campylobacter* are commonly found as commensals in the gut flora of cows, sheep, fowl, as well as dogs and cats. A higher percentage of poultry probably are contaminated with *Campylobacter* than compared with *Salmonella*.

Diagnosis

When first evaluating a patient with possible food-borne disease, historical factors will help narrow the differential diagnosis. The most common bacterial causes, *Campylobacter*, *Salmonella*, *E. coli*, and *Shigella* do have a summer/fall seasonality and are most commonly seen among children. There is a second peak in the incidence of disease seen in young adults, particularly with *Campylobacter* associated illnesses. *Staphylococcus aureus* toxin-mediated food poisoning syndromes occur typically in the summer months. Water conditions supportive for *Vibrio* infections are seen at the end of the summer. As far as chemical food poisoning syndromes are concerned, ciguatera is most commonly a spring-summer disease; paralytic seafood poisoning is often associated with summer-fall red tide and mushroom hunters are out in the warm months. The office clinician has little means at his or her disposal, other than the history and stool studies upon which to make a diagnosis. Health departments utilize powerful molecular typing methods allowing the tracking of food-associated illnesses and it is not unusual to see sporadic emergence of illnesses from a single source of contaminated food, that is, single individuals can become ill even when multiple individuals have eaten from the same source.

The presence of the following should prompt stool cultures, ova, and parasitic screenings:

1. crampy abdominal pain with tenesmus and fever,
2. bloody diarrhea,
3. prolonged diarrhea greater than seven days,
4. neurologic symptoms such as paresthesia, weakness or cranial nerve palsies,
5. the above symptoms in an immunocompromised patient,
6. pertinent travel history.

Blood cultures can be valuable and the physician should have a low threshold to order when any of the above symptoms are present in the immunocompromised host or when the degree of toxicity so dictates. Typhoid fever is associated with greater than 95% positive blood culture rate. It is not unusual to see positive blood cultures in older patients with *Campylobacter* colitis.

Evaluation of patients in whom food-borne illness is suspected must include a differential diagnosis of noninfectious, non–food-borne illnesses, such as inflammatory bowel disease, irritable bowel syndrome, malignancies and importantly a history of previous antibiotic administration since the diagnosis of *Clostridium difficile* colitis is so common. The use of antibiotics in the patient with *C. difficile* may precede the diarrheal illness and the seeking of medical attention by many weeks. The presentation of *C. difficile* can be subtle particularly in nursing home patients and a high index of suspicion is required. Occasionally in the elderly debilitated patient, the presentation of antibiotic associated colitis is characterized by paralytic ileus, toxic megacolon or perforation but minimal or no diarrhea. Any suspicion of this condition warrants a baseline complete blood cell count (CBC), electrolytes, renal function testing and close follow-up. *C. difficile* is just one consequence of the overuse of our once-thought-invincible arsenal of antibiotics. Sadly, vancomycin-resistant enterococci, methicillin-resistant staphylococci and penicillin-resistant pneumococci are terms that have entered the day-to-day conversations in virtually all hospitals and nursing homes across the country. Strategy for long-term control of these problems must first and foremost begin by emphasizing judicious antibiotic prescription and not by assuming the major pharmaceutical companies will be able to solve the problem with new antibiotics.

Other important historical issues to help define the pathogen in food-associated illnesses include the specific symptoms themselves. As outlined below and as seen in Table 1, vomiting, nausea, abdominal pain, diarrhea, bloody diarrhea, neurologic symptoms, and systemic inflammatory response syndrome caused by bacteremia may help define the etiology in addition to laboratory testing. Recent travel suggests an enterotoxigenic *E. coli* (traveler's diarrhea), amebiasis, or giardiasis. Ingestion of seafood with neurologic symptoms and/or rapid onset symptoms suggests natural toxin ingestion associated with various shellfish and seafood (see Table 1). *Vibrio vulnificus* infection in patients with underlying liver disease is usually not subtle and is also associated with raw shellfish and undercooked seafood. *Campylobacter* and *Salmonella* exposures may be suspected with exposure to poultry, eggs and not uncommonly seen in epidemic settings in extended care facilities and subacute nursing facilities. Livestock handlers and participants in state fair livestock exhibitions have been infected with *E. coli* 0157:H7 outbreaks. Deli meats, soft cheeses and unpasteurized dairy products can transmit *L. monocytogenes*. *Listeria* can cause severe sepsis syndromes and meningitis in pregnant women, as well as groups more classically at risk such as the elderly and immunocompromised.

When a practitioner makes the diagnosis of a diarrhea-associated syndrome based upon a positive stool culture, the lab usually notifies the local health department. This may happen as a routine from the laboratory testing facility. If the lab is not automatically reporting the positive culture, then a call to the local or State Health Department is appropriate. Local and State Health officials will then report to the CDC who compile the data nationally. Patients recovering from a food-borne illness should be educated regarding hand washing and may be allowed back to work or school once the symptoms have abated and/or stool surveillance cultures are negative. There may be local health regulations with more specific requirements.

Treatment

Once the diagnosis is made, specific treatment regimens are outlined in Table 1. However, in the office setting, a clear diagnosis is initially often not apparent. A simple approach in this initial setting is to categorize patients into groups that cause (a) short incubation nausea and vomiting, (b) "classic" gastroenteritis with diarrhea, (c) gastroenteritis with a neurologic syndrome, (d) and the patient systemically ill with infectious colitis.

SHORT INCUBATION VOMITING SYNDROME/"CLASSIC" GASTROENTERITIS WITH DIARRHEA

Most food-borne illnesses in this category are self-limited and antibiotic administration is not indicated. Supportive care is the mainstay of treatment in most viral and toxin mediated food-borne illness syndromes. Enteral or parenteral rehydration with a solution that contains both sugar and salt in physiologic proportions is the key component of treatment. The World Health Organization suggests an enteral rehydration solution containing 3.5 g NaCl, 1.5 KCl, 2.5 g $NaCHO_3$ and 20 g glucose/L boiled water. In the United States, "clear liquids" or Pedialyte are reasonable alternatives. Care must be taken when giving parenteral hypotonic fluid resuscitation in the dehydrated patient to avoid rapid shifts in serum sodium. Bismuth subsalicylate (Pepto-Bismol) is a time-honored over-the-counter medicine that is very useful in treating symptoms of viral gastroenteritis. Diarrhea symptoms can be ameliorated with over-the-counter medications such as loperamide (Imodium); see package insert for instructions. For intractable nausea and vomiting promethazine (Phenergan) or prochlorperazine (Compazine) can be taken by mouth or per rectum.

The self-limited nature of many causes of infectious colitis and food-borne diseases in the healthy host is testament to the robust nature of the immune system. The overprescription of antibiotics and possibly the heavy use of antibiotics in food animals contributes to the continued escalation of resistance to common antibiotics and there is no end in sight. *Salmonella* testing routinely shows multiresistance patterns and some strains were even resistant to previously thought first-line drugs such as ciprofloxacin and trimethoprim-sulfamethoxazole (Bactrim). *Salmonella* DT104 is one of the most notorious of these resistant strains with very high mortality rates associated with its infections in the United Kingdom. The CDC surveys resistance patterns and *Shigella* also routinely exhibits a multiresistant pattern to commonly prescribed antimicrobials, including tetracycline, ampicillin, and in up to 10% of the strains, trimethoprim-sulfamethoxazole. *Shigella* isolates from foreign countries sometimes can show the most extensive resistance patterns and sensitivity testing should direct care in these situations.

GASTROENTERITIS WITH A NEUROLOGIC SYNDROME

One of the most feared toxin-associated illnesses remains botulinum toxin poisoning. Fatalities are still seen with botulism as well as with some mushroom ingestion syndromes. *Clostridium botulinum* toxin ingestion produces descending paralysis characterized initially by diplopia, dysphasia, and sometimes neurologic respiratory failure. Botulinal spore germination in improperly preserved foods remains the most common vehicle for disease. Treatment includes supportive care and antitoxin administration. The antitoxin is available through the CDC at 404-329-2888.

Ciguatera fish poisoning is caused when a toxin produced by tiny dinoflagellates is concentrated as it moves up the food chain in larger tropical reef fish such as barracuda and grouper. The larger fish are then eaten and a disease occurs characterized by gastroenteritis as well as paresthesia and weakness. When symptoms are severe, hospitalization with mannitol administration may be indicated (see Table 1). Similar toxin-associated syndromes have been described and include paralytic shellfish poisoning (clams and mussels), neurotoxic shellfish poisoning, amnesic shellfish poisoning, and histamine toxicity seen with improper storage of fish after being caught.

Table 2 lists food-borne illnesses associated with mushroom consumption. These also produce gastroenteritis with associated neurologic symptoms. In these scenarios, treatment includes gastric lavage with activated charcoal administration to aid removal of toxin and cathartics (e.g., magnesium citrate) to speed gut transit time. Ingestion of *Amanita phalloides* ("death-cap" mushrooms) can result in death and intensive support including hemodialysis and liver transplantation has been described. *A. phalloides* is endemic along the West Coast and Mid-Atlantic Coast.

THE SYSTEMICALLY ILL PATIENT WITH INFECTIOUS COLITIS

Antimicrobial chemotherapy is indicated for systemic syndromes, even before a specific diagnosis can be made. The initial antibiotic prescription should be directed against the most common pathogens and the quinolone class of antimicrobials is often first prescribed. However, depending on the severity of the illness and risk factors of the host, a broader spectrum "cocktail" may be appropriate. The risk of death from bacterial disease is highest with infections from *E. coli* 0157:H7, *Listeria* (in immunocompromised hosts), and *V. vulnificus* (in hosts with chronic liver disease). Antiperistaltics are probably contraindicated in patients acutely ill with high fever, bloody diarrhea, fecal leukocytes, or evidence of a systemic inflammatory response syndrome. Nontyphoidal, nonsystemic salmonellosis syndromes classically are not treated with antimicrobials. Antibiotic intervention in *E. coli* 0157:H7 infection is yet unsettled. It is thought they have minimal use in these cases and generally these are followed carefully for the development of hemolytic uremic syndrome. These cases can be severe with extended intensive care unit stays and hemodialysis.

Organisms and Foods

The two classic preformed toxin mediated food poisoning syndromes are associated with outbreaks of *S. aureus* and of *Bacillus cereus* food poisoning. The mechanisms are slightly different. Staphylococcal food poisonings are associated with contamination of food during preparation by a food handler. The food handler presumably contaminates the food from a cutaneous source such as an infected boil, the organism then replicates under suboptimal storage conditions and the toxin is produced. Individuals become ill almost immediately after ingesting the preformed enterotoxin. Symptom onset is within 6 hours and includes nausea, vomiting, and occasional diarrhea. In contrast, *B. cereus* short incubation food poisoning syndromes are often associated with foods contaminated by the organism such as fried rice that has been cooked and then held for extended periods. Illnesses from both organisms are of short duration and spontaneously abate within 12 to 18 hours.

TABLE 2 Mushroom Syndromes

Syndrome (Toxin)	Incubation	Symptoms	Mushrooms
Anticholinergic syndrome (muscarine)	30 min–2 h	Sweating, salivation, lacrimation, bradycardia, hypotension	*Inocybe* species
Delirium (ibotenic acid, muscimol isoxazole)	20–90 min	Dizziness, ataxia, incoordination, hyperactivity	*Clitocybe* species *Amanita* species
Hallucination (psilocin, psilocybin)	30–60 min	Mood elevation, hallucination	*Psilocybe* species *Panaeolus* species
Disulfiram-like (coprine)	30 min after alcohol	Headache, nausea, vomiting	*Coprinus* species
Hepatic failure (gyromitrin)	2–12 h	Nausea, vomiting, hemolysis, hepatic failure, seizures	*Gyromitra* species
Hepatorenal (amatoxins and phallotoxins)	6–24 h	Abdominal pain, vomiting, diarrhea, renal and hepatic failure	*Amanita phalloides*
Nephritis (orellanine)	3–5 d	Thirst, nausea, headache, abdominal pain, renal failure	*Corinarius* species

Clostridium perfringens outbreaks and long incubation *B. cereus* food poisoning are associated with in vivo toxin production from the consumed organism. Because the toxin is not preformed in these syndromes, abdominal cramping and diarrhea predominate the clinical picture as opposed to vomiting. Both of these organisms have been isolated from raw meat, poultry and fish and so it is not uncommon to see outbreaks when large quantities of food are prepared in institutional settings, including nursing facilities. *B. cereus* has also been isolated from dried foods including beans, cereals, spices, and mixes.

E. coli 0157:H7 outbreaks have classically been associated with undercooked ground beef, raw milk, and foods that are associated with meat production. However, increasingly outbreaks have been seen with many other food groups. Often fertilizer or manure is contaminated with *E. coli* 0157:H7, which then contaminates food or water and in this way foods not associated with cattle production have been implicated in outbreaks. Raw eggs have been implicated and considered a major source of salmonellosis in the United States as well as unpasteurized orange juice products, milk, and other fresh produce. *Shigella* outbreaks are less common but associated with preprepared potato and egg salads, as well as fresh produce, including salad bars at restaurants. *Campylobacter* infections most often follow ingestion of undercooked poultry but are also considered a zoonotic infection associated with many domesticated animals.

Yersiniosis, although rare, can be seen with contaminated tofu, raw pork, and contaminated dairy products. Traveler's diarrhea from enterotoxigenic *E. coli* is a notorious condition with well-known risk factors. "If it is not cooked or you cannot peel it, do not eat it!" Well-documented outbreaks in foreign countries make salads less glamorous while dining at the seaside resort.

Botulism outbreaks continue and are associated with home canning of various foods. Honey can be the source of *C. botulinum* in cases of infant infections and this natural food should be avoided in very small children. Other distasteful documented scenarios include Norwalk virus and Snow Mountain agent associated with shellfish and salad foods that have been contaminated by a fecal–oral mechanism possibly by a food handler. Norwalk-like agents are thought responsible for recent cruise ship outbreaks and a food handler or passenger source is thought responsible as opposed to contaminated food. Investigations of viral gastroenteritis outbreaks have implicated the fisherman who harvested the foods while ill from the same virus, which caused the outbreak. They contaminated the water where they were working because of lack of toilet facilities on the boat. There have been well-publicized *Cyclospora* outbreaks following imported raspberry consumption. They were imported from a Central American farm and the contamination occurred when sewage contaminated runoff went into the fields where the raspberries were grown.

Prevention

Proper processing and preparation most directly impacts the incidence of food-borne disease. Usually as consumers, we cannot control whether a food product is contaminated. Therefore most of the effort to prevent disease for an individual will revolve around food choices, preparation, storage, as well as careful attention to the food preparation area. If a meat product is contaminated with a pathogen such as *E. coli* 0157:H7, proper food handling and preparation can mitigate the risk of becoming ill after consumption. The same can be said for cooked vegetables. However, contaminated fruits that are not cooked essentially cannot be sterilized regardless of how much they are washed or rinsed; if contaminated, they will still transmit the organism. Food-borne disease from the common bacterial pathogens is usually transmitted as a result of contaminated food of animal origin as opposed to contamination from a food handler or a person harvesting seafood, that is, an outbreak of salmonellosis or *Campylobacter* is likely related to food contaminated with its own indigenous flora during processing. This could not be said of staphylococcal food poisoning, viral gastroenteritis outbreaks, hepatitis A, or *Shigella* infections which are often a result of contamination by the food handler.

Our role as primary care givers includes diagnosis; treatment and education particularly to the high-risk hosts discussed above. A laundry list of foods to be avoided given to the HIV patient, the elderly, the pregnant, and those with severe chronic medical conditions may cause undue paranoia, but a few guidelines such as careful food preparation, avoiding unpasteurized dairy products and raw shellfish is prudent and practical. Also, the clinician can play a role in detection of outbreaks and assist in reporting institutional illness that may reflect breakdown in the efforts to avoid food-borne disease.

NECROTIZING SOFT-TISSUE INFECTIONS

METHOD OF

Christopher R. McHenry, MD

Soft-tissue infections may involve one or more layers of the skin, the superficial fascia, the subcutaneous tissue, the deep fascia, and the muscle. Non-necrotizing or superficial soft-tissue infections primarily involve the epidermis or dermis of the skin and usually respond to antibiotic treatment alone. In contrast, necrotizing soft-tissue infections usually involve the superficial fascia and the subcutaneous tissue but can also affect the deep fascia, muscle, and skin. They are a spectrum of rare diseases characterized by progressive soft-tissue necrosis, systemic toxicity, and high morbidity and mortality. Necrotizing soft-tissue infections most commonly involve the lower extremity. They also frequently involve the groin, perineum, and abdomen. They may rarely involve the head or neck, usually as a consequence of soft-tissue trauma or dental infection.

One of the earliest descriptions of necrotizing soft-tissue infection appeared in 1871 when Joseph Jones, MD, a surgeon in the confederate army, used the term *hospital gangrene* to describe a serious soft-tissue infection that afflicted more than 2600 Civil War soldiers and was associated with a 46% mortality rate. In 1883, Fournier described a gangrenous infection involving the scrotum, now referred to as Fournier's gangrene. In 1924, Melaney published a classic description of necrotizing fasciitis, identifying the pathogenic role of streptococcal bacteria and introducing the term hemolytic streptococcal gangrene. Two years later, Brewer and Melaney described a progressive, polymicrobic, synergistic gangrene that occurred following appendectomy. In 1952, Wilson introduced the term *necrotizing fasciitis* to describe the characteristic pathologic feature of fascial necrosis.

Necrotizing soft-tissue infections most often occur in patients who have associated conditions that compromise their ability to contain infection and predispose them to tissue necrosis, such as diabetes mellitus, immunosuppression, chronic debilitating diseases, advanced age, malnutrition, and obesity. Necrotizing soft-tissue infection may be classified as primary or secondary. Primary, or idiopathic, infections, which account for 10% to 15% of all necrotizing soft-tissue infections, are defined as infections that occur in the absence of a known portal of entry for bacteria. It is thought that such infections result from hematogenous bacterial spread or from bacterial invasion through small, unrecognized breaks in the epidermis. Secondary necrotizing soft-tissue infections are much more common, accounting for 85% to 90% of these types of infections. They result from some factor predisposing to bacterial inoculation such as human, insect, or animal bites; blunt or penetrating soft-tissue trauma; burns; contaminated operations, particularly those involving the colon; intravenous drug abuse; and occult infections such as diverticulitis. Secondary necrotizing soft-tissue infections are further classified as postoperative, post-traumatic, or a consequence of an inadequately treated cutaneous infection (most commonly perirectal abscess or folliculitis, but also a Bartholin cyst abscess, ischemic leg ulcer, or a decubitus ulcer).

Necrotizing soft-tissue infection is characterized as cellulitis, necrotizing fasciitis, or myonecrosis, which is determined by whether the deepest layer involved with necrosis is subcutaneous tissue, fascia, or underlying muscle. The necrotizing soft-tissue infection that affects the superficial fascia and the subcutaneous tissue is categorized as necrotizing cellulitis, and it can be further divided into clostridial or nonclostridial types. Clostridial cellulitis is most commonly caused by *Clostridium perfringens*, whereas nonclostridial cellulitis is usually a mixed infection caused by the combination of anaerobes and gram-negative aerobes.

Necrotizing fasciitis involves the deep fascia, and it is subdivided into monomicrobic (25%) and polymicrobic infections (75%). Polymicrobic infections are caused by the synergistic activity of facultative aerobes (most commonly *Escherichia coli* and streptococcal species), in combination with anaerobes (most commonly *Bacteroides* species). Monomicrobic infections are principally caused by *Streptococcus pyogenes* and, less commonly, by *C. perfringens*, *Staphylococcus aureus*, *Pseudomonas aeruginosa*, and *Vibrio vulnificus*. Exposure to seawater or ingestion of raw seafood is a prerequisite for fulminant infections caused by *Vibrio* organisms.

Monomicrobic necrotizing fasciitis tends to be a more fulminant infection, characterized by acute onset and rapid progression. The more fulminant course is related to production of bacterial exotoxins, which are powerful proteolytic enzymes that are responsible for tissue destruction and systemic manifestations. Pyrogenic exotoxins A and B are important in the pathogenicity of infections caused by *S. pyogenes*. Alpha toxin, a lecithinase enzyme produced by *C. perfringens*, is responsible for intravascular hemolysis and acute renal failure. The collagenase enzyme, elaborated by *P. aeruginosa*, is responsible for local tissue damage and necrosis.

A necrotizing soft-tissue infection is classified as myonecrosis when the principal layer of involvement is the muscle. Myonecrosis may be further subdivided into clostridial or nonclostridial types. Myonecrosis caused by *C. perfringens*, known as gas gangrene, accounts for 70% of clostridial myonecrosis. *Clostridium septicum* is the principal cause for metastatic gas gangrene, which usually occurs in patients with underlying carcinoma of the colon.

Nonclostridial myonecrosis is a synergistic infection caused by the combination of facultative aerobes and anaerobes.

The diagnosis of necrotizing soft-tissue infection is primarily clinical and is made on the basis of a history and a physical examination. The clinical course may be acute and fulminant or subtle and slowly progressive. Patients may complain of severe pain that is often out of proportion to local physical findings. Characteristic physical features include edema and tenderness that extend beyond the limits of cutaneous erythema. Lymphangitis or lymphadenitis, features associated with simple non-necrotizing cellulitis, are characteristically absent. Crepitance is present in 10% to 15% of patients. Blebs, bullae, and cutaneous anesthesia appear with progression of necrotizing soft-tissue infections. Cellulitis that is refractory to antibiotic therapy suggests the possibility of a necrotizing soft-tissue infection. As the infection progresses, the patient may experience disseminated intravascular coagulation, acute renal failure secondary to shock or rhabdomyolysis, cardiovascular collapse, or other manifestations of systemic toxicity.

Imaging studies are of value for patients in whom the diagnosis is not clear from physical examination. A plain x-ray can demonstrate soft-tissue gas. However, this is an unusual finding and standard radiographs are seldom diagnostic. Magnetic resonance imaging (MRI) may be performed to evaluate patients with pain in the absence of characteristic physical findings. The findings on MRI that are suggestive of necrotizing soft-tissue infection include:

- Soft-tissue gas
- Inflammatory changes or edema of the deep soft tissues
- High signal intensity on T2-weighted images and contrast enhancement after gadolinium administration
- Low signal intensity on T1-weighted images with the absence of gadolinium enhancement, which is indicative of necrosis. Because MRI is a very sensitive test, necrotizing fasciitis can be excluded when no deep fascial involvement is revealed on MRI. The specificity of MRI, however, is not as high as the sensitivity, so false-positive imaging can be problematic.

There are certain diagnostic barriers that may delay recognition and treatment of necrotizing soft-tissue infection. Early on the skin appears normal, masking the underlying necrosis. Up to 20% of necrotizing soft-tissue infections can be idiopathic without a predisposing factor or a known portal of entry for bacterial inoculation. Only 30% of necrotizing soft-tissue infections have soft-tissue gas, either palpable or present on a radiographic study. Finally, the clinical presentation for necrotizing soft-tissue infection can be extremely variable.

Other modalities used to establish a diagnosis of necrotizing soft-tissue infection include fine-needle aspiration biopsy and incisional biopsy, which can both be performed at the patient's bedside. A fine-needle aspiration biopsy specimen is submitted for cytologic analysis, and an incisional biopsy is submitted for frozen section examination. Both specimens are also sent for culture and antimicrobial sensitivity testing. The delineation of necrosis in either specimen is indicative of a necrotizing soft-tissue infection. A normal serum creatinine phosphokinase level excludes the presence of muscle necrosis. Persistent postoperative creatinine phosphokinase elevation and myoglobinuria are indicative of residual dead muscle.

For patients who have one or more obvious clinical signs of necrotizing soft-tissue infection, operative exploration should be performed immediately to confirm the diagnosis and complete the necessary débridement. In the absence of obvious clinical signs of necrotizing soft-tissue infection, MRI is recommended for patients with a white blood cell count of >15,000, pain that is out of proportion to physical findings, the presence of bullae, blebs, or cellulitis that is refractory to antibiotic therapy. When MRI demonstrates soft-tissue gas, operative exploration is performed. When edema, inflammation, or gadolinium enhancement of the deep soft tissue is demonstrated on MRI, a biopsy and frozen tissue section examination are obtained. Operative exploration and débridement are performed when necrosis is demonstrated on frozen section examination. In the absence of signs suggestive of a necrotizing soft-tissue infection or when biopsy is negative, patients are treated with antibiotics. Patients who fail to respond to antibiotic treatment undergo full thickness tissue biopsy, and tissue is sent for frozen section examination and culture. When the frozen section examination is positive for necrosis, débridement is performed. When the frozen section examination is negative, a reassessment of antibiotic treatment is completed.

The single most important factor in treatment of necrotizing soft-tissue infection is early and complete débridement. The time that elapses before the initial operative débridement is the most important factor influencing patient mortality. All patients are treated with intravenous antibiotics. Because most necrotizing soft-tissue infections are polymicrobic, the initial antibiotic regimen should be effective against a diverse group of pathogens. Piperacillin-tazobactam (Zosyn) and clindamycin (Cleocin) in combination is one such regimen. Antimicrobial therapy is then modified based on culture and antibiotic susceptibility results.

Before initiation of general anesthesia, patients are resuscitated with intravenous fluids. Patients with traumatic wounds should receive tetanus toxoid or human tetanus immunoglobulin, depending on their immunization status. Intravenous calcium may be necessary to correct hypocalcemia, which can result from calcium precipitation related to extensive fat necrosis. Packed red blood cell transfusion may be required to correct anemia related to intravascular hemolysis in patients with clostridial infections.

Routine reexploration should be performed within 24 hours, either at the bedside or in the operating room, to ensure that all necrotic tissue has been eradicated. Repeated débridements are the performed until the infection is controlled. Following the operation, open wounds are managed with wet-to-dry dressing changes using normal saline solution, topical antiseptic, or antimicrobial agents.

Amputation may be necessary as a life-saving measure in patients with persistent infection despite repeated débridement. This is especially true for clostridial myonecrosis that is causing severe systemic toxicity and for patients where circumferential necrotizing fasciitis results in a nonfunctioning extremity. In patients with necrotizing fasciitis involving the perineum, a diverting colostomy may be necessary to prevent tissue contamination and to control wound sepsis. Early enteral nutrition and prompt recognition of nosocomial infection reduce the subsequent development of organ system failure.

To date, no prospective randomized study has evaluated the role of hyperbaric oxygen in patients with necrotizing soft-tissue infection. Although its therapeutic role is controversial, the use of hyperbaric oxygen should not delay operative débridement, nor should it substitute for complete débridement of all nonviable tissue.

Once wound sepsis is controlled, soft-tissue coverage is imperative. Soft-tissue coverage is usually accomplished by split-thickness skin grafting. However, it may require more complex reconstructive procedures. Soft-tissue coverage is necessary to preserve limb function and to protect exposed tendons, nerve, and bones.

In summary, necrotizing soft-tissue infection is a rare group of deep soft-tissue infections characterized by progressive necrosis and systemic toxicity. It is associated with a mortality of approximately 30%. The single most important factor in improving outcome is early recognition and complete débridement.

TOXIC SHOCK SYNDROME

METHOD OF

Robert L. Deresiewicz, MD

Staphylococcal toxic shock syndrome (TSS) is an acute, severe, febrile illness characterized by fever, hypotension, rash, multiorgan dysfunction, and convalescent-stage desquamation. It results from intoxication by any of several related *Staphylococcus aureus* exotoxins, most commonly TSS toxin type-1 (TSST-1). A related and clinically indistinguishable illness, toxic shock-like syndrome (TSLS) may follow infection by toxigenic strains of *Streptococcus pyogenes*.

TSS was first described in a pediatric population but became widely known in 1980 following a large outbreak among young, menstruating women, the overwhelming majority of whom were tampon users. Menstrual cases presently account for about half of TSS cases reported in the United States. The remainder are attributable to staphylococcal colonization or infection of diverse body sites, and occur in patients of either gender and any age. With prompt recognition and proper management the outcome is usually good; the principal challenge, as with many rare and severe diseases, is to recognize the illness and promptly intervene.

Etiology and Pathogenesis

Virtually all menstrual TSS cases and about 60% of nonmenstrual cases are caused by TSST-1. Most of the remainder are caused by staphylococcal enterotoxin B (SEB), and a small fraction by enterotoxin C. Coagulase-negative staphylococci do not produce TSS toxins and, therefore, cannot cause TSS. The TSS toxins are encoded by variable genetic elements, meaning that the genetic capability to produce one or more of the toxins is present in only a subset of strains. Approximately 10% to 20% of human *S. aureus* isolates produce TSST-1 and 7% to 14% produce SEB.

Necessary steps in the pathogenesis of TSS are colonization of a nonimmune host by a toxigenic strain, toxin production, toxin absorption, and intoxication. Approximately 4% to 10% of people harbor toxigenic staphylococci at any site at any given time, including approximately 1% to 4% of postmenarcheal women who carry TSST-1–producing staphylococci in the vagina. Most people acquire protective levels of antibodies to TSST-1 and SEB during youth and adolescence, presumably consequent to benign staphylococcal colonization or trivial infection. By adulthood, more than 90% of people are immune to each toxin.

Toxigenic staphylococci that have the genetic capability to produce a TSS toxin actually do so only at limited times. The risk of TSS associated with the use of tampons or certain surgical dressings likely results from changes that these products cause to the local microenvironment, and the stimulus to toxin production resulting therefrom. For example, tampon use introduces oxygen into the normally anaerobic vagina; oxygen is required for TSST-1 synthesis, at least in vitro. Once produced, TSST-1 is rapidly transported across the vaginal mucosa.

The TSS toxins are superantigens—V_β-restricted T-cell mitogens—whose toxicity to humans is thought to derive from their ability to stimulate certain immune cells and thereby provoke exuberant, dysregulated cytokine release. How cytokine release culminates in the various manifestations of TSS remains uncertain. An important sequelae, however, is the development of capillary leak syndrome, which may be principally responsible for the hypotension and end-organ damage that occurs in TSS.

Epidemiology

TSS is principally a disease of the first three decades of life. As noted, cases may be classified as menstrual or nonmenstrual. Menstrual cases peak in incidence between the third and fifth days of menses. The vast majority are in tampon users. Nonmenstrual cases include those related to colonization or infection of the female genitourinary tract (e.g., puerperal cases and cases associated with barrier contraceptive use, septic abortion, and nonobstetric gynecologic surgery); those associated with skin or soft-tissue infections (including both primary staphylococcal infections such as folliculitis, cellulitis, and furunculosis, and secondary infections such as of burns, bites, varicella lesions, or surgical wounds); and those related to infections of the respiratory tract (e.g., staphylococcal pharyngitis, tracheitis, sinusitis, or pneumonia) the musculoskeletal system (e.g., osteomyelitis, septic arthritis), or, rarely, the bloodstream. In postoperative cases, the illness may manifest within hours of the surgical procedure or may be delayed for days or weeks.

The number of TSS cases reported annually to the Centers for Disease Control and Prevention (CDC) has dropped considerably since the early 1980s. The drop is partly attributable to the development of safer tampons and tampon usage practices, but likely also reflects substantial under-reporting. The true frequency of menstrual TSS is probably at least 1 per 100,000 women per year, and is likely higher among women in their teens and early twenties. According to a recent study, the incidence of postoperative (nonmenstrual) TSS is 3 cases per 100,000 women.

Mortality also appears to have diminished over time. For the 10 years ended in 1996, the minimum case fatality rate for definite or probable menstrual cases reported to the CDC was 1.8%; for nonmenstrual cases the minimum rate was 5.5%.

Clinical Manifestations

Mild prodromal, flu-like symptoms occur in a minority of patients. The acute illness begins precipitously, with high fever, chills, headache, severe myalgias, muscle tenderness, abdominal pain, nausea, vomiting, and profuse watery diarrhea. Oral, conjunctival, and vaginal mucosal irritation also typically occurs. Orthostasis or hypotension and the characteristic macular erythroderma develop during the next 2 days. The erythroderma is usually generalized, often intense, and blanches with pressure. However, it may be locally distributed, mild, or fleeting; and it may be subtle, particularly in the presence of severe hypotension. On admission patients appear toxic, with hypotension, tachycardia, and oliguria. Examination may reveal conjunctival suffusion; tender, beefy-red oral or vaginal mucosa; and a strawberry tongue. Peripheral cyanosis and edema are common as is diffuse abdominal tenderness. Rales may be present. The liver, spleen, and lymph nodes are usually unremarkable. Encephalopathy as evidenced by confusion, disorientation, agitation, or somnolence is also common, but the neurologic examination is typically nonfocal. The site of staphylococcal toxin production may be purulent or erythematous, or it may appear entirely benign. Laboratory studies reflect multiorgan dysfunction. Frequent findings include leukocytosis, thrombocytopenia, coagulopathy, azotemia, transaminitis, hypoalbuminemia, hypocalcemia, hypophosphatemia, and pyuria. Disseminated intravascular coagulation is not a common feature of TSS.

Like many other toxin-mediated diseases, TSS follows a fairly predictable course. The early manifestations of fever, erythroderma, gastrointestinal distress, and blood chemistry abnormalities resolve within the first few days of illness. In severe cases, hypotension may persist and may be complicated by myocardial dysfunction, pulmonary edema, rhabdomyolysis, hepatic damage, renal failure, or peripheral gangrene.

Desquamation is a late event in TSS. Superficial flaking of the skin on the trunk and extremities begins about a week into the illness. The characteristic full-thickness desquamation of the palms, soles, and digits follows in the second week and may continue for up to 1 month. Late sequelae of TSS include postfebrile telogen effluvium (reversible loss of the hair and nails), prolonged weakness or fatigue, memory loss, emotional changes, and impaired ability to concentrate. Fatalities typically occur within the first few days of illness, most commonly from refractory shock, respiratory failure, or cardiac arrhythmia.

Although not included in the case definition of TSS, mild systemic intoxications by the TSS toxins probably occur. Such cases lack two or more criteria for TSS but have certain clinical or epidemiologic features suggestive of the diagnosis (e.g., erythroderma, severe gastrointestinal disturbance, and/or convalescent desquamation). The occurrence of such an illness during menses in a young tampon user should prompt a search for evidence of TSST-1 involvement, particularly if the illness is recurrent. Compatible findings include the isolation of TSST-1–producing *S. aureus* from the vagina, and the demonstration of a nonprotective titer of serum anti-TSST-1 antibodies. Although such findings do not prove that an illness was TSST-1–related (certainly most perimenstrual flu-like illness is not attributable to TSST-1), they should, nevertheless, prompt discontinuation of tampon use until seroconversion has been documented. An attempt to eradicate vaginal staphylococcal carriage in such circumstances is also reasonable.

Diagnosis

The diagnosis of TSS is made exclusively on clinical grounds (Table 1). A host of possibilities other than TSS should be considered in the patient acutely ill with fever, rash, and hypotension. These include severe group A streptococcal infections (scarlet fever, necrotizing fasciitis, streptococcal TSLS), Kawasaki syndrome (particularly in children younger than 4 years of age), staphylococcal scalded skin syndrome, Rocky Mountain spotted fever, leptospirosis, meningococcemia, exanthematous viral syndromes, and severe allergic drug reactions.

In menstrual TSS cases, particularly when a purulent vaginal discharge is present, the diagnosis may be readily apparent. The challenge is to recognize subtle cases including nonmenstrual cases and cases in which the rash is evanescent. A careful history with attention to past health, possible infectious exposures, travel, vocation, avocation, vaccination status, menstrual status, and medication usage often considerably narrows the diagnostic possibilities. Backdrops particularly suggestive of TSS include the menstruating or postpartum female, the female who uses barrier contraceptive methods, the postoperative patient, the patient with varicella-zoster infection, and the patient with chemical or thermal burns.

Laboratory evaluation should include a complete blood count and differential, serum electrolytes, calcium, phosphate, albumin levels, liver and renal function tests, creatine phosphokinase level, coagulation studies, and urinalysis. A chest radiograph and an electrocardiogram should also be obtained. In females, vaginal culture should be performed. Blood, urine, and respiratory tract cultures should also be obtained, as should cultures of all wounds, regardless of how benign they might appear. The laboratory should be instructed to speciate any staphylococci isolated from mucosal sites. *S. aureus* isolates (mucosal or otherwise) should be referred for TSST-1 testing, if possible.

Acute and convalescent sera should be tested for antibody to TSST-1, particularly in suspected menstrual cases. The absence initially of a protective titer to TSST-1 supports the clinical diagnosis of TSS, and seroconversion, if it occurs, confirms it. The majority of patients, however, do not seroconvert following TSS; such patients, particularly those whose illness occurred in the perimenstrual period, are at risk for recurrent disease.

Treatment

With prompt treatment, the serious consequences of TSS (organ failure, limb loss, death) can often be avoided. Treatment involves four components:

1. Decontamination of the site of toxin production
2. Administration of antistaphylococcal antibiotics
3. Fluid resuscitation
4. General supportive care

The nidus of toxin production should be carefully sought. If present, vaginal tampons or other types of

TABLE 1 Staphylococcal Toxic Shock Syndrome: Case Definition

Criteria	Definition
1. Fever	Temperature ≥102°F (38.9°C)
2. Rash	Diffuse macular erythroderma *(sunburn* rash)
3. Hypotension	Systolic blood pressure ≤90 mm Hg (adults) or <5th percentile for age (children younger than 16 years of age) Orthostatic hypotension (orthostatic drop in diastolic blood pressure ≥15 mm Hg, orthostatic dizziness, or orthostatic syncope)
4. Organ involvement (at least 3 of the defined organ systems)	**GI** (vomiting or diarrhea at onset of illness) **Muscular** (severe myalgias or serum creatine phosphokinase level at least twice the upper limit of normal) **Mucous membranes** (vaginal, oropharyngeal, or conjunctival hyperemia) **Renal** (blood urea nitrogen or creatinine at least twice the upper limit of normal, or pyuria [≥5 leukocytes per high-power field] in the absence of urinary tract infection) **Hepatic** (total serum bilirubin or transaminase level [alanine aminotransferase or aspartate aminotransferase] at least twice the upper limit of normal) **Hematologic** (thrombocytopenia [platelets ≤100,000 per μL]) **CNS** (disorientation or alteration in consciousness in the absence of focal neurologic signs at a time when fever and hypotension are absent)
5. Desquamation	1 to 2 weeks after onset of illness (typically of palms and soles)
6. Evidence against alternative diagnosis	If obtained, negative cultures of blood, throat, or cerebrospinal fluid*; absence of a rise in antibody titers to the agents of Rocky Mountain spotted fever, leptospirosis, or rubeola

Abbreviations: CNS = central nervous system; GI = gastrointestinal.
*Blood cultures may be positive for *Staphylococcus aureus*.
Adapted from Reingold AL, Hargrett NY, Shands KN, et al: Toxic shock syndrome surveillance in the United States, 1980 to 1981. *Ann Intern Med*, 96 (Part 2):875-880, 1982.

foreign bodies should be removed. Purulent foci should be drained and débrided and cutaneous lesions copiously irrigated. Thorough lavage lowers the burden of organisms and potentially slows toxin accretion. For TSS occurring in the postoperative period, the surgical wound *must* be explored, even if it appears uninfected.

Antibiotic administration offers a second opportunity to interrupt intoxication. While β-lactamase–resistant semisynthetic penicillins or first-generation cephalosporins have historically been given for TSS, growing evidence suggests that clindamycin (Cleocin) is superior. Under conditions of saturating (stationary phase) growth, staphylococci produce only low levels of penicillin-binding proteins. Penicillin-binding proteins are the molecular targets of β-lactam antibiotics. β lactams are, therefore, relatively ineffective against such cells. On the other hand, TSST-1 is essentially only produced under those saturating conditions. Organisms producing TSST-1 are likely to be relatively resistant to β lactams. In addition, β-lactam levels fluctuate widely during dosing, and may fall below the minimum inhibitory concentration for *S. aureus* toward the end of each dosing interval. Subinhibitory concentrations of β lactams may actually enhance TSST-1 production.

Clindamycin, on the other hand, is a protein synthesis inhibitor; its antistaphylococcal activity is independent of growth phase. Moreover, clindamycin potentially suppresses TSST-1 production in vitro, even at concentrations insufficient to inhibit staphylococcal growth. The great majority of *S. aureus* strains causing TSS, particularly menstrual TSS, remain susceptible to clindamycin (and to methicillin). I suggest clindamycin 900 mg intravenously every 8 hours for suspected cases of TSS. In the critically ill patient in whom clindamycin- or methicillin-resistant infection may be a concern, it is reasonable to co-administer vancomycin (Vancocin) 1 g intravenously every 12 hours until microbiologic data are available. If the diagnosis of TSS is initially uncertain, broader empiric coverage is prudent. Antibiotics should be administered for at least 10 days but can be given orally once the patient has stabilized.

Aggressive fluid resuscitation should be initiated to reverse hypotension and forestall end-organ damage. Adult patients may require up to 10 liters of crystalloid for the first 24 hours to maintain adequate cardiac filling. The principal mechanism of hypotension in TSS is capillary leak syndrome. Fluid therapy is, therefore, typically complicated by massive weight gain and peripheral edema. Pressors and central hemodynamic monitoring may be useful in cases of refractory hypotension, particularly if oxygenation is impaired.

In addition to the specific interventions outlined above, intensive care should be provided. Metabolic abnormalities should be corrected, and potential complications should be diligently sought. A final therapeutic option, especially for refractory cases or cases associated with an undrainable purulent focus, is pooled human immunoglobulin.[1] All commercial preparations contain anti-TSST-1 at concentrations sufficient to generate protective titers after a single intravenous dose of 400 mg/kg. Evidence supporting this therapy in humans is strictly anecdotal, but the approach makes sense on theoretical grounds.

---

[1]Not FDA approved for this indication.

INFLUENZA

METHOD OF

Stephen B. Greenberg, MD

Influenza is an acute respiratory illness occurring in yearly outbreaks and epidemics throughout the world. Epidemics typically occur in the winter season and are associated with increased morbidity and mortality. People are infected by aerosol or close contact. After an incubation period of 1 to 3 days, upper and lower respiratory tract signs and symptoms develop. These include sore throat and cough as well as systemic complaints of fever, headache, and myalgias. Although school-aged children have the highest attack rates, mortality is highest in people older than age 65 years.

Influenzavirus is an RNA virus from the orthomyxovirus family. Influenza types A and B are responsible for epidemic and pandemic disease. Influenza C is an uncommon cause of respiratory illness. The two surface glycoproteins, hemagglutinin (HA) and neuraminidase (NA), are important in the pathogenesis of this infection. Changes or mutations in one or both of these proteins are the major reasons for the repeated epidemics of influenza. Minor changes in HA or NA, or "antigenic drift," occur in both influenza A and B viruses. A major change in HA or "antigenic shift" is associated with a worldwide epidemic or pandemic. These pandemic strains are thought to occur when exchange (reassortment) of genes between human and avian influenza A viruses occurs during a dual infection and results in a new strain that can replicate in people who are susceptible.

Excess mortality from epidemic influenza has ranged between 10,000 and 40,000 deaths annually in the United States. Far greater numbers of deaths have been documented in those worldwide outbreaks that were recorded in 1918 (H1N1), 1957 (H2N2), 1968 (H3N2), and 1977 (H1N1). In 1918, it is estimated that more than 500,000 deaths occurred in the U.S. secondary to pandemic influenza.

Influenza is monitored each year by the Centers for Disease Control and Prevention (CDC) and the

World Health Organization. Information can be found through the CDC at (888)232-3228 or at its web site: http://www.cdc.gov/ncidod/diseases/flu/weekly.htm. An epidemic of influenza is heralded by an increase in school absenteeism and visits to health care facilities. Increases are also recorded in industrial absenteeism, hospitalization for pneumonia and influenza, and total deaths.

Clinical Manifestations

Influenza-associated illness usually begins with the abrupt onset of fever, headache, myalgias, sore throat, and cough. Other presentations can include a "common cold" syndrome or systemic signs and symptoms without much respiratory tract involvement. Other signs and symptoms can include hoarseness and tracheal pain. Typically, the acute illness lasts 3 to 5 days with cough and malaise persisting for several weeks.

There are few physical findings in influenza. Hyperemia in the oropharynx is common. Mild cervical lymphadenopathy is seen most frequently in children. The chest examination is usually normal in uncomplicated influenza, even though ventilatory defects have been described in patients undergoing pulmonary function testing.

Common complications of influenza include otitis media, sinusitis, bronchitis, and pneumonia. The major serious complication of influenza is pneumonia that occurs in patients with underlying cardiovascular or pulmonary problems, patients with diabetes mellitus, renal diseases or immunosuppression, patients in nursing homes or chronic care facilities, and in individuals older than age 65 years. Three patterns of pneumonia have been reported: (a) primary viral; (b) secondary bacterial; or (c) mixed viral and bacterial. In primary influenza pneumonia, symptoms persist in a patient with acute influenza and include fever, tachypnea, and dyspnea. Primary viral pneumonia is the most severe but least common pneumonia complication of influenza. Because the influenza virus affects the integrity of the tracheobronchial epithelium, there is a predisposition for bacterial superinfections of the lungs. Although the most frequently detected bacterial cause is *Streptococcus pneumoniae, Staphylococcus aureus* is second in frequency (approximately 20% of cases). With secondary bacterial pneumonia, there is an exacerbation of fever and respiratory symptoms after an initial improvement in what appears to be acute influenza. Many patients have features of both viral and bacterial pneumonia. One can recover both influenza virus and bacterial pathogens from the sputum of such patients.

Other complications of influenza include myositis, rhabdomyolysis, Reye syndrome, central nervous system involvement, myocarditis, and exacerbations of asthma and chronic obstructive pulmonary disease. Acute myositis presents with tenderness of the affected muscles with marked elevation of serum creatine phosphokinase levels. Myoglobinuria and acute renal failure have been reported in such cases. Reye syndrome is reported in children with influenza B, and less frequently with influenza A. It presents with nausea and vomiting followed by change in mental status. Hepatomegaly and elevated blood ammonia levels are noted. An association with the use of aspirin has been noted in Reye syndrome cases. Central nervous system diseases associated with influenza also include encephalitis, transverse myelitis, and Guillain-Barré syndrome (GBS). Cases of toxic shock syndrome have also been reported in association with *S. aureus* infection and acute influenza.

Diagnosis

Other respiratory viruses and infectious agents can give a clinical syndrome similar to influenza virus. Where influenza virus is known to be circulating in a community, influenza illness is likely to be caused by influenza virus in approximately 60% to 70% of cases. To make a specific diagnosis, one of several virus specific assays would be necessary.

Laboratory diagnosis requires detection of virus or viral antigen from throat swabs, nasal washes, or sputum. Virus isolation using embryonated eggs or cell culture monolayers is the gold standard for detecting influenza virus. After a respiratory sample is obtained, it should be placed in viral transport medium and taken immediately to the laboratory. Influenza viruses are usually isolated within 3 to 7 days of tissue culture inoculation.

Rapid viral diagnostic tests are becoming available in many laboratories. Some tests will distinguish between type A and B viruses and others do not. Immunofluorescence tests require expensive equipment, technical expertise, and take longer than enzyme immunoassays to perform. Enzyme immunoassay techniques can provide results within 30 minutes of collection and can be performed in physician offices. Although the specificity of these rapid tests is high, the sensitivity has ranged between 60% and 90%, with better results being observed in specimens from children.

Nucleic acid detection methods such as reverse-transcriptase polymerase chain reaction (RT-PCR) assays are sensitive and specific but not available except in research laboratories. The use of RT-PCR may allow for the detection of influenza infection more quickly and aid in the use of specific antiviral treatment.

Influenza can be diagnosed retrospectively using serologic methods. Paired sera collected 2 to 4 weeks apart can demonstrate a more than fourfold antibody rise demonstrating that an acute illness has occurred. Serologic methods include hemagglutination-inhibition, complement fixation, and enzyme immunoabsorbent assay.

Prevention and Treatment

VACCINE

The primary method of preventing influenza and its severe complications is influenza vaccination. The target groups recommended for annual vaccination include (a) people older than 65 years of age, (b) people of any age with certain chronic medical conditions, and (c) people who live with or care for people at high risk. Vaccination has led to fewer influenza-related respiratory illnesses and physician visits, hospitalizations, and deaths among high-risk individuals, otitis media among children, and lower work absenteeism among adults. Although the optimal time to receive influenza vaccine is during October and November, vaccination efforts in October should be for high-risk people and health care workers. Depending on supply of vaccine, other groups should receive vaccine in November. For as long as vaccine supplies are available, all targeted groups should receive vaccine into December and later. Influenza vaccination of healthy children ages 6 to 23 months is supported by the Advisory Committee on Immunization Practices.

Special populations should receive consideration for influenza vaccination. Because of the documented influenza-associated excess deaths among pregnant women, women who will be beyond the first trimester of pregnancy during the influenza season should be vaccinated. Regardless of the stage of pregnancy, pregnant women with medical conditions that increase the risk for complications from influenza should be vaccinated before the influenza season. There is limited information on the frequency and severity of influenza illness as well as the benefits of influenza vaccination among people with HIV infection. However, vaccine should be offered to HIV-infected people, including HIV-infected pregnant women. Breast-feeding mothers can receive influenza vaccine. Persons at high risk for complications of influenza should consider influenza vaccine if they were not vaccinated in the preceding fall or winter and plan to travel to the tropics, or with an organized tourist group at any time of year, or plan to travel to the Southern Hemisphere during April through September. People providing essential community services should also consider vaccination. Students or people in closed institutional settings should be encouraged to be vaccinated.

Certain individuals should not be vaccinated. Those known to have anaphylactic hypersensitivity to eggs or to other components of the vaccine should not receive the influenza vaccine. Those with an acute febrile illness should not be vaccinated until symptoms have lessened.

Dosage recommendations depend on the age of the person. Children younger than 9 years of age who are previously unvaccinated should receive two doses more than 1 month apart. All other individuals should receive one dose. Only FDA-approved influenza vaccine should be used in children ages 6 months to 3 years. The intramuscular route is recommended. Adults and older children should be vaccinated in the deltoid muscle; infants and young children should be vaccinated in the anterolateral area of the thigh.

TABLE 1 Influenza Vaccine Dose by Age Group*

Age Group	Dose†	Number of Doses‡
6–35 months	0.25 mL	1 or 2
3–8 years	0.50 mL	1 or 2
≥9 years	0.50 mL	1

*Check with each manufacturer for FDA approval by age.
†Intramuscular administration in deltoid muscle for adults and older children and anterolateral thigh for infants and young children.
‡Two doses given 1 month apart for children younger than 9 years of age who are receiving influenza vaccine for the first time.

The inactivated influenza virus vaccine is composed of virus antigens from three influenza virus strains: A/H1N1, A/H3N2, and B. Based on worldwide surveillance of new strains, the virus strains for vaccine development are selected to be those most likely to circulate in the upcoming season. Each vaccine strain is grown in embryonated chicken eggs, inactivated with a chemical agent, and partially purified. Vaccines are made from whole virus, disrupted virus particles (subvirion), or purified surface HA or NA antigens. Whole virus vaccine is not available in the United States. Split-virus vaccines contain subvirion or purified surface antigens. The vaccine contains 15 μg of HA antigen from each of the candidate strains in a 0.50 mL dose. Table 1 contains the recommended doses of vaccine to be used for different age groups.

People receiving vaccine should be told that the vaccine contains noninfectious killed viruses and cannot cause influenza and that incubating or coincidental respiratory illness unrelated to influenza vaccination can occur around the time of vaccination. The most frequent side effect is soreness at the vaccination site lasting less than 2 days. Systemic reactions including fever, malaise, and myalgia can begin 6 to 12 hours after vaccination, especially in individuals who have no prior exposure to the influenza virus antigens in the vaccine. Immediate reactions such as hives, angioedema, or anaphylaxis are rare. Recent studies have suggested no substantial increase in GBS associated with influenza vaccination. Most authorities believe the potential benefit of influenza vaccination, significantly outweighs the possible but low risks for vaccine associated GBS. Although there are no studies evaluating the simultaneous administration of influenza vaccine and other childhood vaccines, it is recommended that children at high risk for influenza-related complications receive influenza vaccine when receiving other routine vaccinations.

Live, attenuated intranasal influenza vaccine (LAIV) is approved for use in healthy children and adults from 5 through 49 years of age. The currently approved LAIV is FluMist. Because the safety of LAIVs has not been evaluated in other groups, it should not be used by individuals at risk for influenza or its complications. LAIV is administered intranasally by sprayer, is more expensive than inactivated influenza vaccine, and contains the same annual recommended antigens as the inactivated trivalent influenza vaccine. The potential advantages of LAIVs include broad mucosal and systemic immune responses, ease, and acceptability of administration.

Antivirals

Four licensed influenza antiviral agents are an adjunct to influenza vaccine for controlling and preventing influenza and are not substitutes for vaccination. The four drugs have different pharmacokinetics, side effects, routes of administration, approved age groups, dosages, and costs. When administered within 2 days of illness onset, both amantadine (Symmetrel) and rimantadine (Flumadine) reduce the duration of influenza A illness, and zanamivir (Relenza) and oseltamivir (Tamiflu) reduce the duration of influenza A and B illness by 1 day. No studies have demonstrated the effectiveness of any of these four antiviral agents in preventing serious complications of influenza. There are only limited data on the effectiveness of these four antiviral agents for treatment of influenza among persons at high risk for serious complications of influenza. Few studies have been published on the efficacy of influenza antivirals in pediatric patients.

Amantadine (Symmetrel) and rimantadine (Flumadine) are M2 inhibitors that block proton ion channels in the virus membrane and prevent uncoating of virus and initiation of viral replication. Zanamivir (Relenza) and oseltamivir (Tamiflu) are neuraminidase inhibitors that block the activity of the viral NA or sialidase. Neuraminidase removes sialic acid residues from the surface of the infected cell and also helps virus pass through the overlying mucus layer to the respiratory epithelium.

Amantadine and rimantadine are approved for the chemoprophylaxis of influenza A but not B infections. Both drugs are effective in preventing illness from influenza A infections in approximately 70% to 90% of individuals. Amantadine and rimantadine do not inhibit the antibody response to vaccines. Only oseltamivir, among the neuraminidase inhibitors, has been approved for prophylaxis. However, oseltamivir and zanamivir have been shown to prevent influenza illness when given to people as chemoprophylaxis after a household member was diagnosed with influenza. No studies have demonstrated the effectiveness of these four antiviral agents in preventing influenza in severely immunocompromised persons. When any of these drugs are taken as chemoprophylaxis, it must be taken each day for the duration of influenza activity or at least during the period of peak activity in the community.

Chemoprophylaxis should be considered (a) for people at high risk who are vaccinated after influenza activity has begun, (b) for people who provide care to those at high risk, (c) for people who are expected to have an inadequate antibody response to influenza vaccine, and (d) for people who should not be vaccinated. Use of these drugs for treatment and prophylaxis of influenza is important in institutional outbreak control. Table 2 lists the FDA's approved indications for each drug and recommended drug doses by age group.

All four drugs are administered orally. Amantadine and rimantadine are available in tablet or syrup form. Oseltamivir is available in capsule or oral suspension. Zanamivir is available as a drug powder given by oral inhalation using a plastic device. Amantadine is excreted unchanged in the urine (90%) and thus dosages need to be reduced with renal insufficiency. Rimantadine is metabolized by the liver (approximately 75%) and therefore should be used with caution in patients with liver disease. Most of the orally inhaled zanamivir is deposited in the oropharynx with less than 20% being systemically absorbed. Approximately 80% of oseltamivir is absorbed systemically.

Amantadine and rimantadine can cause central nervous system (CNS) and gastrointestinal side effects.

TABLE 2 Approved Indications for Influenza Antiviral Medications

		Age Group (y)				
Indication	**Antiviral Agent**	**1-6**	**7-9**	**10-12**	**13-64**	**≥65**
Treatment						
	Amantadine (Symmetrel)	5 mg/kg/d*	5 mg/kg/d*	100 mg bid	100 mg bid	≤100 mg/d
	Rimantadine (Flumadine)	Not approved	Not approved	Not approved	100 mg bid	100 mg bid
	Zanamivir (Relenza)	Not approved	Not approved	10 mg bid	10 mg bid	10 mg bid
	Oseltamivir (Tamiflu)	Varies by weight	Varies by weight	Varies by weight	75 mg bid	75 mg bid
Prophylaxis						
	Amantadine	5 mg/kg/d*	5 mg/kg/d*	100 mg bid	100 mg bid	≤100 mg/d
	Rimantadine	5 mg/kg/d*	5 mg/kg/d*	100 mg bid	100 mg bid	100 mg/d
	Zanamivir	Not approved	Not approved	Not approved	Not approved	Not approved
	Oseltamivir	Not approved	Not approved	Not approved	75 mg/d	75 mg/d

*Up to 150 mg per day.

The CNS side effects include nervousness, anxiety, insomnia, difficulty concentrating, and lightheadedness and are more frequent with amantadine than with rimantadine. Gastrointestinal side effects are usually nausea and anorexia and occur in 1% to 3% of people taking either drug. Lowering the dosage of amantadine in those with renal insufficiency, seizure disorders, or certain psychiatric disorders can reduce the incidence and severity of side effects.

Zanamivir is currently not recommended for treating patients with chronic airway disease because of the potential for decline in respiratory function. Oseltamivir was associated with nausea (10%) and vomiting (9%), although only a small number of patients discontinued the drug because of these side effects. Oseltamivir is recommended to be taken with food to decrease these side effects.

No studies have been completed on the safety or efficacy of these antiviral drugs in pregnant women. There is limited information on drug-drug interactions with these drugs. Amantadine should be given cautiously to patients receiving drugs that also affect the CNS. No published data are available that address the safety and efficacy of combination therapy with any of these antiviral drugs.

Drug-resistant viruses have been reported in patients given either amantadine or rimantadine for therapy. Resistant strains have been recovered from patients within 2 to 3 days of starting therapy. The frequency of transmission of resistant viruses is unknown but already reported. In vitro resistance to zanamivir and oseltamivir has been demonstrated, and clinical isolates with demonstrated resistance have appeared but are infrequent. Surveillance for neuraminidase inhibitor-resistant influenza virus is ongoing.

OTHER MEASURES

Symptom management of influenza should include oral hydration, acetaminophen for fever and headache, nasal decongestant, and cough suppressant. Antibiotics should be given only for secondary bacterial infections.

LEISHMANIASIS

METHOD OF

Jean-Pierre Gangneux, MD, PhD

Leishmania parasites are kinetoplastid protozoa members of the family Trypanosomatidae. They are transmitted by phlebotomine sandflies and are responsible for a broad spectrum of human diseases: localized and disseminated cutaneous leishmaniasis (LCL and DCL), mucocutaneous leishmaniasis (MCL), and visceral leishmaniasis (VL). Variability of the disease outcome results from a complex host-parasite relationship. The host's genetic background and immunologic status and the parasite's intrinsic pathogenicity represent three main components that determine the clinical expression but also the therapeutic response.

Out of 350 million people at risk in 88 endemic countries, there is an estimated prevalence of 12 million cases with an incidence of 1.5 million cases annually of dermal and mucosal infections and 0.5 million cases annually of visceral infections. Difficulties remain for the control and treatment of leishmaniasis and new strategies are needed. Evaluation of optimal chemotherapeutic protocols or identification of new vaccine candidates is of prime interest but we should also take into account the host diversity, the parasite polymorphism, and the vector and reservoir controls.

Life Cycle and Pathophysiology

Leishmania are dimorphic parasites. The flagellated promastigotes multiply in the female sandfly's intestinal tract and are transmitted during bloodsucking. More than 20 species of the *Leishmania* genus are transmitted to humans by sandfly vectors, members of the *Phlebotomus* genus (in the Old World) and of the *Lutzomyia* genus (in the New World). In the mammalian host, promastigotes are engulfed by phagocytic cells, and proliferate as nonflagellated obligate intracellular amastigotes. Experimental and clinical data suggest that an efficient host immune response involves a CD4+ T helper 1 cell-mediated response, leading to macrophage activation and elimination of intracellular amastigotes through nitrogen oxidation products. It has been shown that the course of *Leishmania* infection is under genetic control, in particular with the NRAMP1, TNF-α, TNF-β, and MHC genes implicated.

Besides, the clinical expression of *Leishmania* infection also depends on the causing species and on the strain's intrinsic virulence. Anthropophilic species belong to both *Leishmania* and *Viannia* subgenus. It is convenient to classify species upon their geographical distribution and their tropism (dermal, mucosal, or visceral) (Table 1). However, this schematic view does not reflect the role of host factors on the outcome as mentioned previously, and for example, visceralizing diseases have been observed with typical dermotropic species such as *L. major* or *L. amazonensis* in immunosuppressed patients. Because microscopic examination does not allow for the differentiation between *Leishmania* species, identification of isolates mainly relies on the reference method of isoenzymatic characterization. More recently, molecular tools proved to be relevant in distinguishing closely related strains in epidemiologic studies.

TABLE 1 Geographic Distributions, Vectors, and Clinical Forms of Major Anthropophilic Species of the *Leishmania* Genus

	Old World Leishmaniasis	New World Leishmaniasis
Vectors	*Phlebotomus* genus	*Lutzomyia* genus
Parasites	***Leishmania* sub-genus** —*L. donovani:* VL, rarely LCL, PKDL and oronasal leishmaniasis —*L. infantum:* VL, rarely LCL and oronasal leishmaniasis —*L. major, L. tropica, L. killicki, L. arabica:* LCL —*L. aethiopica:* LCL, DCL	***Leishmania* sub-genus** —*L. chagasi:* VL, rarely LCL —*L. venezuelensis:* LCL —*L. mexicana, L. amazonensis:* LCL, DCL ***Viannia* sub-genus** —*L. braziliensis:* LCL, MCL —*L. braziliensis panamensis, L. guyanensis:* LCL, rarely MCL —*L. peruviana, L. naiffi, L. lainsoni, L. shawi, L. colombiensis:* LCL

DCL = diffuse cutaneous leishmaniasis; LCL = localized cutaneous leishmaniasis; MCL = mucocutaneous leishmaniasis; PKDL = post-Kala Azar dermal leishmaniasis; VL = visceral leishmaniasis.

Clinical Manifestations and Diagnosis

VISCERAL LEISHMANIASIS

This life-threatening form corresponds to the generalized involvement of the reticuloendothelial system. After an incubation period of 2 to 12 months, VL presents itself with chronic fever (Kala Azar = "black fever" in Hindi), hepatosplenomegaly, and weight loss. Biologic signs are pancytopenia and hypergammaglobulinemia. If untreated, the infection evolves to a fatal form with cachexia and secondary complications, such as bacterial and viral infections, epistaxis, gingival bleeding, or petechiae. Nodules and hypo- or hyperpigmented macules named post-kala-azar dermal leishmaniasis (PKDL) may occur after treatment in the Indian and African forms of VL. India, Bangladesh, Nepal, and Sudan in the Old World (*L. donovani* and *L. infantum*) and Brazil (*L. chagasi*) in the New World are the major epidemic and endemic foci of VL. In the Mediterranean basin, VL resulting from *L. infantum* occurs sporadically in children and immunosuppressed patients (HIV infected patients, and patients undergoing organ transplantation). Atypical presentation of VL, gastrointestinal involvement, and concurrent opportunistic infection are usual in immunosuppressed patients. The diagnosis is based mainly on the demonstration of the parasite in blood buffy coat or bone marrow, lymph nodes, spleen, or liver aspirates. Two complementary methods are used: a Giemsa colored smear showing intracellular amastigotes or a promastigote growth in an axenic culture medium (Novy-Mac Neal-Nicolle, or various liquid media such as Schneider's *Drosophila* medium or RPMI medium supplemented with fetal calf serum). A positive culture allows a species identification by enzymatic characterization. Reference laboratories also use polymerase chain reaction for the diagnosis and a molecular identification. In case of negative parasitologic diagnosis, serology may contribute to help the decision to treat. Detection of anti-*Leishmania* antibodies is mainly performed using direct/indirect agglutination or indirect immunofluorescence assays, and detection of specific antibodies against recombinant K39 antigen are mainly performed using strip-test or ELISA assays.

CUTANEOUS AND MUCOCUTANEOUS LEISHMANIASIS

LCL is the most common clinical expression of *Leishmania* infection. The lesion generally heals spontaneously within 1 month to 3 years. Except the nations of the Pacific region, including Australia and New Zealand, CL is found in all tropical and subtropical regions of the World. The situation in Southwest/ Central Asia (Afganistan, Pakistan, Iraq) appears to be particularly severe. The incubation period varies from 1 week to several months after the infected insect bite. The localized lesions progressively evolve from erythematous papules to nodules and noduloulcerative lesions. Less typical lesions may include verrucous, eczematous, psoriasiform, varicelliform, keloidal, erysipeloid, and sporotrichoid morphologies. Inflammatory satellite papules and regional lymphadenopathy may be present during New World CL. Four major complicated cutaneous forms are described, depending on the causative species:

- *Leishmaniasis recidivans* (LR) is an oligoparasitic and recurrent localized form resembling lupus vulgaris. It corresponds to the development of new lesions within the scar of a healed acute lesion. *L. tropica* is the most causative species.
- DCL is an anergic polyparasitic form of CL resembling lepromatous leprosy. *L. aethiopica* in the Old World and *L. mexicana* and *L. amazonensis* in the New World are the principal causative species.
- PKDL manifests itself by skin lesions after resolution of VL or during relapses. This form is frequently disfiguring mainly caused by *L. donovani* in India and East Africa.

- MCL, also known as Espundia, is a rare but severe event after *L. braziliensis* (more rarely *L. panamensis* and *L. guyanensis*) infection. It corresponds to oronasal mucosa tropism of the parasite after hematogenous or lymphatic dissemination from the skin, abutting on chronic disease with a risk of facial mutilation. Without treatment, no spontaneous healing is observed and relapses are observed even under treatment.

The diagnosis is based on the demonstration of the parasite in Giemsa-stained tissue smears or biopsies or on the identification of promastigotes in culture, thus allowing a species identification. PCR may improve the sensibility of the diagnosis.

Chemotherapeutic Treatments

PENTAVALENT ANTIMONY DERIVATIVES (SB^V)

Organic pentavalent antimonials have been the first-line therapy for VL since their introduction in 1937. Sodium stibogluconate (Pentostam-100 mg SB^v/mL)[1] and meglumine antimonate (Glucantime-85 mg SB^v/mL)[1] are administered intravenously or intramuscularly, in doses of 20 mg SB^v/kg per day for 28 d for the treatment of VL. However, response rates have been decreasing, particularly in India, but also in the Mediterranean basin and to a small extent in East Africa. In HIV–co-infected patients, relapses after initial treatment are almost ineluctable. These trends incite to lengthen duration of therapy or to increase doses, with a higher risk of reversible side effects (nausea, vomiting, myalgias, arthralgias, raised hepatic transaminase levels, subclinical pancreatitis, and minor electrocardiographic changes) and of severe cardiotoxicity (concave ST segment, prolongation of the QT, arrhythmia, and sudden death). Old World CL with multiple lesions at risk of disfiguring scars and New World CL at risk of mucosal metastasis should be treated with parenteral SB^v in doses of 20 mg SB^v/kg per day for 20 days. Localized CL is easy to treat with well-tolerated intralesional injections of 0.2 to 1 mL SB^v per lesion per week for 4 or 5 weeks, particularly during *L. tropica* infections.

[1]Not FDA approved for this indication.

AMPHOTERICIN B (AMB) AND LIPID FORMULATIONS OF AMB

During the past decade, deoxycholate AmB (Fungizone) has been considered to be an efficient alternative in the treatment of Old and New World VL (0.5 mg/kg daily for 28 days or 1 mg/kg daily for 20 days). In a recent Indian study, 1 mg AmB/kg daily for 20 days appeared far superior to sodium antimony gluconate (SAG, registered in India) as a first-line drug against VL. However, its use is limited because of infusion-related reactions and nephrotoxicity. Liposomal AmB (AmBisome) in a simplified therapeutic protocol (Table 2) proved effective and much better tolerated than the deoxycholate formulation. Although it is costly, liposomal AmB is now a first-line treatment recommended for children as well as for adults and is a candidate of special interest for secondary prophylaxis in immunosuppressed patients because of its tolerance and long tissue half-life (3 to 4 mg/kg/d on days 0, 1, 2, 3, 4, and 10; total dose: 18 to 24 mg/kg). Shorter high-dose regimens with liposomal AmB were recently assessed and proved effective and more affordable (e.g., 10 mg/kg daily for 2 days for Mediterranean VL in children). AmB lipid Complex (Abelcet), another lipid formulation of AmB, has been less evaluated but also proved effective. During CL and MCL, deoxycholate Amb is considered by some authors as a valuable alternative in case of resistance to first-line therapy with antimonials. Available data are insufficient to draw conclusions on lipid formulations of AmB for CL and MCL treatment.

MILTEFOSINE[1]

Since 1997, only hexadecylphosphocholine (miltefosine, Miltex) has emerged as a new anti-*Leishmania* drug. Miltefosine, originally developed as an oral antineoplastic agent, is the first orally administered treatment that proved effective for VL

[1]Not FDA approved for this indication.

TABLE 2 Recommendations on Drug Regimens to be Used in the Treatment of Mediterranean Zoonotic Visceral Leishmaniasis (WHO Conference, Roma, Italy, 1995)

Drug	Posology
Pentavalent derivative antimony (SB^v) • meglumine antimonate = Glucantime* • sodium stibogluconate = Pentostam*	20 mg SB^V/kg/d during 20–28 d
Pentavalent derivative antimony + Allopurinol**	20 mg sbV/kg/d + 15 mg/kg/d during 20–28 d
Liposomal amphotericin B = AmBisome	3 mg/kg/d on d 0, 1, 2, 3, 4 and 10 (total dose:18 mg/kg)
Aminosidine = paromomycin (Humatin)[1]	12–16 mg/kg/d during 14–63 d

[1]Not FDA approved for this indication.
*Investigational drug in the United States.

including those with antimony-resistant infections. The treatment is 100 mg per day for 28 days in adults and children >10 years old, 50 mg per day for 28 days in children 6 to 9 years old, and 2.5 mg/kg/d for 28 days in children 3 to 5 years old. Even shorter courses of treatment (100 mg per day for 3 weeks) allowed high-level efficacy in preliminary series of patients. Since 2002, miltefosine (Impavido) is registered in India and in the European Community for the treatment of Kala Azar. Unfortunately, this promising treatment for the twenty-first century did not prevent relapses in the first few HIV–co-infected patients treated with it. This phospholipid derivative also proved effective for the treatment of New World CL at the dose of 2.25 to 2.5 mg/kg per day for 3 to 4 weeks. Little is known on the interest of a topical formulation of miltefosine.

PENTAMIDINE ISETHIONATE

Discovered in 1939, pentamidine isethionate (Pentacarinat) has been used for a long time as an alternative of choice for patients intolerant to or presenting with a refractory VL to antimonials. High cure rates were reported using a classical regimen (15 parenteral injections of 4 mg/kg on alternate day), but its efficacy has diminished over the years, particularly in India. This declining activity with an estimated cure rate lower than 70%, together with the drug toxicity (from reversible hypoglycemia to definitive insulin-dependent diabetes mellitus and cardiac toxicity), have led to its decreased use. Treatment regimens based on 3 to 4 intramuscular injections of 3 to 4 mg/kg on alternate days allow a cure rate of more than 80% either during Old World or New World CL. Similar cure rates are obtained only after at least eight injections during the treatment of MCL, DCL, or LR.

AMINOSIDINE

Aminosidine sulfate[†] is an aminoglycoside antibiotic, with an identical chemical structure to paromomycin (Humatin)[1] and erythromycin (Monomycin). In VL, several studies reported a favorable outcome after administration of aminosidine alone or combined with pentavalent derivatives of antimony in African and Indian Kala Azar. It is considered as a valuable alternative drug in case of unresponsiveness to antimonials or can be used in combination with antimonials to reduce the duration of therapy (see Table 2). However, the parenteral formulation is not currently produced. Limited documented cases and experimental data are not in favor of using aminosidine for the treatment of Mediterranean *L. infantum* VL. Against *Leishmania major*, it has good in vitro activity and clinical trials have been performed with various formulations containing 15% aminosidine for the topical treatment of Old World and New World CL. Results are ranging from more than 85% cure rate to same rate as obtained with placebo, depending on the design of the study, the causing species, and the ointment formulation (methyl benzethonium chloride, urea or urea + 0.5% gentamicin).

[†]Available as an orphan drug only.

[1]Not FDA approved for this indication.

OTHER MEDICATIONS

Allopurinol (Zyloprim)[1], metronidazole (Flagyl)[1], ergosterol biosynthesis inhibitors (ketoconazole [Nizoral][1], itraconazole [Sporanox][1], fluconazole [Diflucan][1], terbinafine [Lamisil][1]), or dapsone[1] have been used either for the treatment of VL or CL in monotherapy or combined with antimonials. However, only limited data are available with these drugs that proved inconsistently effective, mainly depending on the causal species. Recent studies suggest that fluconazole could be a treatment of prime interest for LCL resulting from *L. major*. Clinical trials are in prospect with the primaquine analogue WR6026 (Sitamaquine). This compound previously developed in the field of malaria and pneumocystosis showed antileishmanial activity and has the advantage of being taken orally.

Strategies for Optimal Treatment and Control of Leishmaniasis

The declining activity and the toxicity of traditional leishmanicidal drugs, and the high rates of relapses in immunosuppressed patients stress the need for alternative compounds screening and for the optimization of therapeutic protocols.

- Drug adaptation to the presumed causative species of the parasite and drug monitoring resistance are relevant strategies because it's now admitted that the therapeutic response varies with the *Leishmania* species.
- A powerful drug delivery system can optimize tolerance and action of traditional drugs. For example, liposomes loaded with amphotericin B proved particularly effective in targeting the infected macrophages, permitting drug delivery into the parasitophorous vacuole.
- Multitherapy is an interesting approach to increase efficacy and tolerance, and to avoid the emergence of drug resistance. Principal protocols used in patients with refractory VL included antimonials combined with aminosidine, allopurinol, or immunotherapy. Other drug combinations were also experimentally evaluated.
- In immunosuppressed patients, mainly HIV-coinfected patients, a partial or complete restoration of immune functions remains the only warrant against relapses. Secondary prophylaxis proved inconsistently effective and no consensus has still been adopted.

[1]Not FDA approved for this indication.

Although "historical" immunization with parasites from active human lesions to produce self-cure CL and induce lifelong protection against reinfection have been reported, the development of a *Leishmania* vaccine will not be an easy task. First-generation vaccines with killed *Leishmania* showed no evidence of significant protection against VL during the past 50 years. More recently, native and recombinant antigens were screened and tested for second-generation vaccines. Their interest will depend on their potentiality to protect against all clinical forms of leishmaniasis, independently to the causative species.

Before disposing of an effective vaccine, the vector and reservoir controls remain of prime interest. To decrease the risk of being bitten, long pants and long-sleeved shirts should be worn; insect repellents containing diethyltoluamide (DEET) on uncovered skin and fine-mesh insecticide-impregnated bed-nets should be used. Besides, a better knowledge on the ecology of reservoir host species and of phlebotomine sandflies can direct towards new strategies of control of leishmaniasis.

LEPROSY (HANSEN'S DISEASE)

METHOD OF

Sinésio Talhari, MD, PhD

Leprosy is an infectious disease caused by *Mycobacterium leprae* and transmitted from man to man through prolonged and close contact with patients presenting the multibacillary (MB) types of the disease. Heavily infected MB patients have abundant organisms in the nasal mucosa. Transmission is believed to occur principally through the nasal mucosa (aerosol) and skin-to-skin transmission. The median incubation time is 2 to 5 years, but it may be as long as 20 years.

There are rare cases of leprosy that are probably transmitted through contact with infected nine-banded armadillos in the United States. Up to now the nine-banded armadillo and some African monkeys are among the few animals naturally infected with *M. leprae*.

More than 95% of adults are resistant to the infection. Leprosy is a curable disease, but it still represents a serious public health problem in many tropical countries including India, Brazil, Nepal, Mozambique, and Tanzania. In 2002, there were 18 endemic countries. Leprosy cannot be considered a tropical disease because it was previously endemic in some European countries. It is mostly related to poverty and a deficient health infrastructure.

According to the World Health Organization (WHO), the disease is defined as endemic in countries with a prevalence rate of 1 or more patients per 10,000 people. Until the 1980s, there were more than 5 million registered patients with leprosy around the world.

After successful implementation of multidrug therapy (MDT), a highly effective treatment regimen introduced by WHO in 1981, the World Health Assembly declared, in 1991, that the endemic countries would achieve the elimination target of leprosy (less than 1 patient per 10,000 people) by the year 2000. After a huge effort by these nations, coordinated by WHO, the target was reached. Leprosy was eliminated as a global health problem, but the major endemic countries did not reach the elimination goal. In 2003 there were 523,605 leprosy patients registered in the world, and the global prevalence was 0.84.

It was believed that after the elimination of leprosy the transmission would be very low and the disease would disappear naturally. Unfortunately, this has not been observed in most of the countries that reached the elimination goal years ago. A total of 612,110 new patients were diagnosed in 2002, and this is very close to the incidence rate (new patients/10,000/per year) observed since the introduction of MDT. There is no adequate explanation for this fact.

Classification of Leprosy and Diagnosis

In most patients, leprosy initiates as macular and hypochromic lesions. This initial type of leprosy is indeterminate (I) leprosy (Figure 1). The baciloscopy (skin smear and Ziehl-Nielsen staining) is negative and the histopathology of these lesions shows a nonspecific

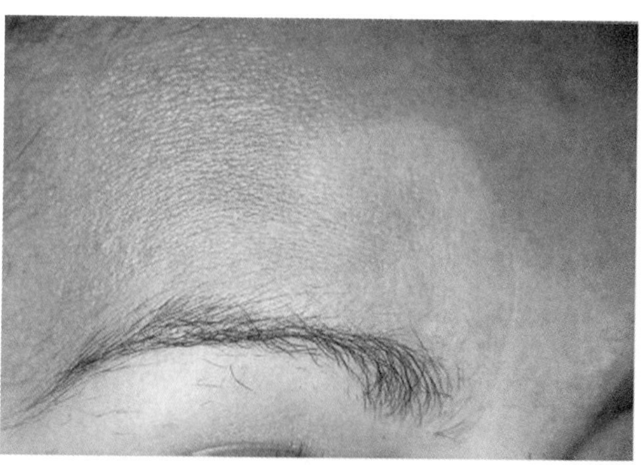

FIGURE 1 Indeterminate leprosy.

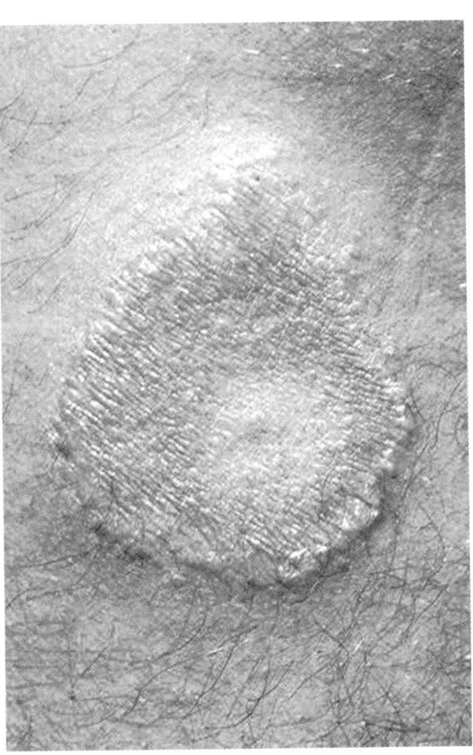

FIGURE 2 Tuberculoid leprosy.

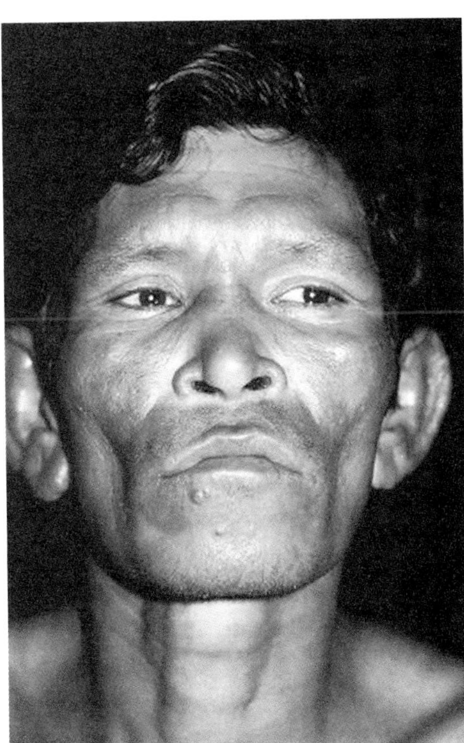

FIGURE 3 Lepromatous leprosy.

lympho-histiocytic infiltration around small nerves and annexes. Scarce or no *M. leprae* are observed through special stainings for acid-fast bacilli (Wade or Fite-Faraco method).

A very important clinical characteristic of leprosy lesions is the impairing of sensation (anesthesia). In the hypochromic lesions the patient cannot differentiate between cold and hot water (thermal sensation). Usually two test tubes are used for this purpose.

The number of lesions depends on the genetically determined cellular immunity of the patient. Without treatment the patients with few lesions (usually five or less) evolve into polar tuberculoid (TT) leprosy (Figure 2). The skin smear of this form of leprosy is negative, and the histopathology shows a granulomatous infiltrate that typically is located around the nerves and annexes. Very rarely, bacilli are observed.

In TT leprosy, sensation is absent in most of the lesions. Besides thermal sensation, the patient cannot feel pain when a needle is slightly pressed on the suspected area or touch when a piece of cotton or paper is passed over the lesion. It is very important to remember that the innervation of the face is from multiple sources so it is not often anesthetic.

There are patients with countless numbers of hypochromic lesions. Without treatment these patients evolve to a nonresistant form of the disease called polar lepromatous (LL) leprosy. A diffuse infiltration of the hypochromic lesions and the apparently normal skin slowly involves the whole body. The infiltrated face and ears get the typical aspect known as leonine facies (Figure 3); the hands and feet become edematous, cyanotic, and in some patients an ictiosis-like aspect appears on the legs. Gradually, papules and nodules appear over the infiltrated areas, and after years without treatment the patient becomes completely disfigured by the disease. A skin smear of LL leprosy is positive with a very large number of bacilli and microcolonies called globi. The histopathology shows a high number of foamy macrophages in the dermis in which numbers of bacilli are incorporated. Some patients may develop LL leprosy without noticing the hypochromic lesions.

A large number of patients do not fit in the TT and LL polar types of leprosy. These patients belong to a group designated borderline (B) leprosy. There are borderline types of patients near the polar TT called borderline tuberculoid (BT) leprosy (Figure 4). Another group close to the LL form is borderline lepromatous (BL), and another group is known as borderline-borderline (BB). BB and BL leprosy reveal a positive skin smear, and BT usually has a negative skin smear. The histopathology shows a great variation of infiltrate.

The so-called Ridley-Jopling classification of leprosy consists of the polar forms and the borderline groups TT, BT, BB, BL, and LL. This is a very useful classification for research purposes, but not feasible at the peripheral level and in most health centers.

With the exception of the indeterminate type, all types of leprosy may develop peripheral nerve involvement (enlarged and/or painful). The most frequent nerves affected by *M. leprae* are the ulnar, median,

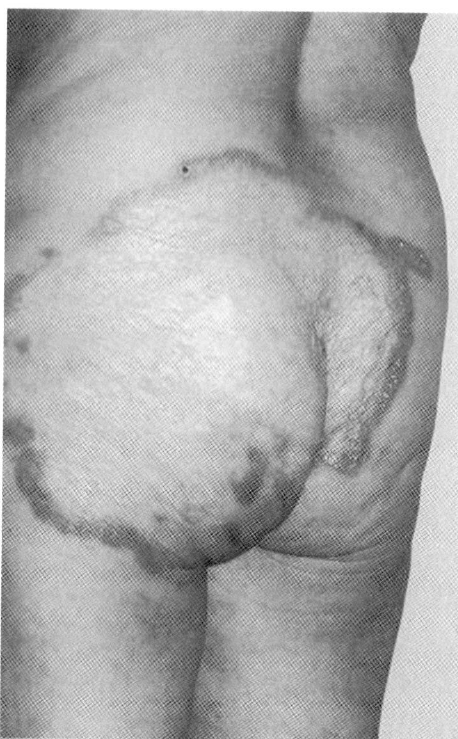

FIGURE 4 Borderline tuberculoid leprosy.

radial, cutaneous branch of the radial, common peroneal, posterior tibial, anterior tibial, great auricular nerve, and supraorbital.

For treatment, WHO recommends classifying the patients as having either paucibacillary (PB) or multibacillary (MB) leprosy. PB leprosy is designated for patients with a negative skin smear, and it comprises indeterminate, TT, and most BT leprosies. MB patients have a positive skin smear and include BB, BL, LL, and a few BT leprosies.

In rural or difficult-to-reach areas WHO suggests using the operational classification, which is determined by the number of lesions. With operational classification, PB patients have five lesions or less, and MB patients have more than five skin lesions. The WHO definition of a case of leprosy, which is very important for operational classification, is, "A case of leprosy is defined as a person having one or more of the following features, and who has yet to complete a full course of treatment:

- Hypopigmented or reddish skin lesion (s) with definite loss of sensation;
- Involvement of the peripheral nerves, as demonstrated by definite thickening with loss of sensation;
- Skin smear positive for acid-fast bacilli."

Treatment

The current treatment recommended by WHO and accepted by all endemic countries is MDT.

PAUCIBACILLARY LEPROSY

The recommended treatment for adults with PB leprosy is a combination of:

- Rifampin (Rifadin):[1] 600 mg once a month, supervised
- Dapsone: 100 mg daily, self-administered

PB patients should complete 6 monthly doses of this treatment within a 9-month period. The efficacy of the MDT for PB leprosy is approximately 99%.

Single Skin Lesion

The recommended treatment for adults (it is not recommended for children) with this kind of single-lesion PB leprosy, without trunk nerve involvement, is a supervised single-dose treatment with the following drugs:

- Rifampin (Rifadin) 600 mg
- Ofloxacin (Floxin)[1] 400 mg
- Minocycline (Minocin)[1] 100 mg

This treatment regimen is strongly supported by WHO but not well accepted by many specialists in leprosy, who prefer to give the standard PB treatment. It is estimated that the efficacy of this regimen is more than 99%.

MULTIBACILLARY LEPROSY

The recommended treatment for adults with MB leprosy is:

- Rifampin 600 mg once a month, supervised
- Clofazimine (Lamprene) 300 mg once a month, supervised, and 50 mg daily, self-administered
- Dapsone 100 mg daily, self-administered

MB patients should complete 12 monthly doses within an 18-month period. The efficacy of the MDT for MB leprosy is approximately 99%.

ALTERNATIVE REGIMENS

Ofloxacin (Floxin), 400 mg daily, or minocycline (Minocin), 100 mg daily, are recommended as substitutes for patients who do not accept clofazimine (Lamprene) (although there is no proven resistance to clofazimine). For these patients, WHO suggests a therapeutic regimen with a combination of 600 mg rifampin, 400 mg ofloxacin, and 100 mg minocycline, given once a month for 24 months.

In place of rifampin (because of adverse effects or resistance), it is possible to use ofloxacin, 400 mg daily; minocycline, 100 mg daily; and 50 mg daily of clofazimine for the first 6 months. This should be followed by daily administration of clofazimine, 50 mg; ofloxacin, 400 mg; or minocycline, 100 mg for an additional 18 months.

[1]Not FDA approved for this indication.

If dapsone cannot be included in the standard MDT because of side effects or resistance, it may be replaced by 50 mg of clofazimine for PB patients. In MB patients, dapsone should be stopped and treatment continued only with rifampin 600 mg once a month and clofazimine 50 mg daily for 12 months.

Standard MDT is also used for children, with adjusted doses. Dapsone is given at 1 mg/kg/day, rifampin at 10 mg/kg/day, and clofazimine at 1 mg/kg/day. Minocycline and fluoroquinolones should be avoided in children and pregnant women.

There is no reported resistance to the combined drugs. Relapses with MDT are less than 1%.

TREATMENT OF PATIENTS WITH LEPROSY AND HIV

Patients with leprosy and HIV are treated with the same regimens. Up to now there has been no contraindication for the association of MDT with the current antiretroviral treatment.

PATIENTS WITH LEPROSY AND TUBERCULOSIS

If the patient has tuberculosis and leprosy simultaneously, the treatment with the monthly supervised doses is not necessary in the first 3 months. After this time the standard MDT should be given.

DURATION OF THE MULTIDRUG THERAPY TREATMENT

Until 1994 it was recommended that MDT be given until skin smears become negative. Based on the knowledge acquired since the introduction of MDT, the WHO Study Group on Chemotherapy of Leprosy recommended treating MB patients with standard MDT for 24 months. After a new evaluation of the MDT regimen in 1998, WHO recommended the standard MDT for 12 months.

There is a new WHO recommendation for treating MB leprosy with 6 months of MDT. This proposal is not well accepted by most of the specialists in leprosy and endemic countries such as Brazil. Additional research is necessary before the implementation of this recommendation.

In the United States, the U.S. National Hansen's Disease Programs (NHDP) recommend 12 months for PB treatment (with rifampin and dapsone given daily), and 24 months of MDT for MB patients. Rifampin is given daily, and monthly supervised doses of clofazimine are recommended to be given for 12 months.

Side Effects Of Multidrug Therapy

MDT is relatively safe. For more than 20 years it has been a worldwide recommended treatment for leprosy, and very few side effects have been reported. In a study conducted in India with 45,439 patients under MDT, the most important adverse effects were 15 cases with hepatitis (2 patients died), 3 cases with kidney failure, and 4 cases with severe allergic reactions.

Thrombocytopenia, dapsone syndrome, hemolytic anemia, flu-like syndrome, gastric intolerance, and respiratory failure are also among the very important adverse side effects observed. The flu-like syndrome is related to the monthly doses of rifampin and sometimes may be severe. In severe cases the drug should be stopped. Marrow suppression, interstitial nephritis, and drug interactions are the most frequently observed side effects related to rifampin.

The most important side effects related to clofazimine are skin pigmentation and xerosis.

Methemoglobinemia, anemia, hemolysis (glucose-6-phosphate dehydrogenase [G6PD] deficiency), and agranulocytosis are among other adverse effects related to dapsone.

Standard MDT may be used during pregnancy and lactation.

TREATMENT OF REACTIONS

Before, during, and after treatment, approximately 30% to 50% of all leprosy patients can develop leprosy reactions. Reactions are immunologically mediated episodes of acute or subacute inflammation. The two types of reactions are type 1 (reversal reaction) and type 2.

The type 1 reaction (TH1) is the result of spontaneous enhancement of cellular immunity and delayed hypersensitivity to *M. leprae* antigens. This reaction occurs in the borderline group. The pre-existing cutaneous lesions become more erythematous, infiltrated, swollen, and may ulcerate (Figure 5). New lesions may occur during these episodes. The peripheral nerves may also be involved during the reaction, becoming thickened and painful. The patients with plaque lesions over the peripheral trunk nerves are more susceptible to developing severe neuritis (see Figure 5). Without prompt treatment, subsequent paralysis and deformity may occur. Severe type 1 reaction is a matter of urgency, and the patient must receive prompt treatment.

Type 2 reaction (TH2) occurs in LL and some BL (they also develop type 1) patients. This reaction is related to antigen–antibody complexes. TH2 is dependent on tumor necrosis factor-alfa (TNF-alfa), and is characterized by erythematous, nodular lesions. The most frequent clinical picture is known as erythema nodosum leprosum (ENL). Fever, malaise, iridocyclitis, orchitis, arthritis, myositis, some degree of sensory and motor neuropathy and ulcerated cutaneous lesions are quite frequent in severe type 2 reaction.

Treatment of Type 1 Reaction

Prednisone (or other corticosteroids) is indicated for patients with widespread lesions and/or nerve involvement. The recommended dosage is 1 to 2 mg/kg/day

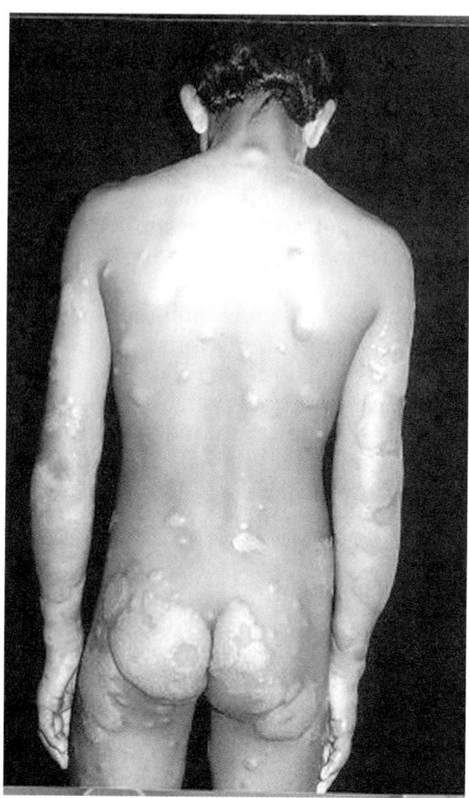

FIGURE 5 Borderline leprosy type 1 reaction.

Prevention and Control Measures

Although a specific vaccine is not yet available, the Bacille Calmette-Guérin (BCG) vaccine gives protection against multibacillary leprosy. The protection varies from 30% to 70% according to the studies conducted in India, Malawi, Venezuela, Brazil, and other countries. In Brazil, BCG is recommended by the Ministry of Health for all the leprosy contacts.

Chemoprophylaxis for leprosy is not advisable according to studies using one or a combination of such drugs, because they failed to demonstrate any protective effect.

At present, the only practical method of prevention is early detection, prompt treatment with MDT, and dermatoneurologic examination of contacts.

until the reaction is controlled. After that, the corticosteroid is slowly tapered off and stopped after 2 to 4 months up to 6 months. All the adverse effects of corticosteroids should be considered but this is the best drug to control the type 1 reaction.

Cyclosporine (Neoral)[1] and azathioprine (Imuran)[1] are alternative drugs for patients who cannot receive corticosteroids.

Treatment of Type 2 Reaction

Thalidomide (Thalomid) is the drug of choice for type 2 reaction. Depending on the severity of the reaction, a total dosage of 100 to 300 mg/day is indicated. The drug is slowly tapered off and stopped after 1 to 4 months. Unfortunately, because of its teratogenic effect, this drug should *never* be used for women of childbearing age. Another important adverse effect of thalidomide is peripheral neuropathy. For patients who cannot take thalidomide, the second choice is prednisone at the same dosage and tapered off as recommended for type 1 reaction.

Corticosteroids are not the best choice for type 2 reaction because frequently patients find it very difficult to stop the drug.

Alternative drugs to treat erythema nodosum leprosum (ENL)/type 2 reaction are clofazimine, cyclosporine[1], azathioprine (Imuran) [1], and pentoxifylline (Trental)[1].

[1]Not FDA approved for this indication.

MALARIA

METHOD OF

Sheral S. Patel, MD, and James W. Kazura, MD

Human malaria is caused by one of four intraerythrocytic protozoan species of the genus *Plasmodium*, namely *Plasmodium falciparum, Plasmodium vivax, Plasmodium ovale,* or *Plasmodium malariae.* The infection is transmitted through the bite of the female anopheline mosquito. While malaria is endemic throughout tropical areas of the world, its incidence is increasing in travelers returning from these regions to nonendemic countries. Early diagnosis and treatment are necessary to prevent complications, particularly from *P. falciparum* in nonimmune individuals. Appropriate chemoprophylaxis and personal protective measures play important roles in preventing malaria infection and disease.

Description of Organism

LIFE CYCLE

Human infection begins when an infected female anopheline mosquito injects sporozoites into the vertebrate host during the process of blood feeding. The sporozoites then travel from the site of inoculation in skin capillaries to the liver via the bloodstream. In the liver, they pass through endothelial cells and ultimately invade hepatocytes where they mature to tissue schizonts. In some species (*P. vivax* and *P. ovale*), hepatic schizonts may become dormant and are called hypnozoites. Hepatic schizonts amplify the infection during a period of 8 to 25 days and produce 10,000 to 30,000 merozoites, which are released into the bloodstream. Each merozoite can invade an erythrocyte, begin asexual replication, and release 24 to 32 new merozoites in 48 to 72 hours to invade additional erythrocytes. While hepatic schizonts are found with all four malaria species, hypnozoites are present only in the relapsing malarias, *P. vivax* and *P. ovale.* Hypnozoites can remain dormant in the liver for 6 to 11 months and cause no symptoms during this time. Symptomatic parasitemia occurs when a proportion of hypnozoites mature and release merozoites that can then lead to blood-stage infection. Intraerythrocytic malaria parasites develop into gametocytes, the sexual forms necessary to complete the life cycle in the anopheline vector. When gametocytes are taken up by a female anopheline mosquito during blood feeding, the male and female gametocytes mature to gametes and fuse to produce zygotes. The diploid zygote matures to an ookinete, which undergoes a meiotic reduction division that produces haploid sporozoites. The sporozoites migrate to the salivary gland of the mosquito and subsequently reinfect humans.

RECURRENT AND PERSISTENT MALARIA INFECTIONS

Recurrent malaria infections develop in several ways. First, relapses from the activation of dormant hypnozoites in the liver occur with *P. vivax* and *P. ovale.* Second, recrudescence of blood-stage infection may result from incomplete treatment or partially effective host immune responses to pre-existing infection. As is the case for relapse, recrudescence is caused by the same parasite clones that produced the initial infection. Recrudescence may occur with any species but is most common with *P. falciparum* because of drug resistance. Finally, reinfection or simultaneous infection with multiple parasite strains or species can occur in areas of intense transmission. Persistent infections are frequently associated with *P. malariae,* which can remain in the bloodstream at undetectable levels for 20 to 30 years.

TRANSMISSION

Natural mosquito-borne transmission of malaria requires contact between human hosts with infectious gametocytes in their blood and anopheline mosquitoes that are competent to allow further development of the parasite. Less common modes of transmission include transfusion of infected blood or blood products and sharing contaminated syringes or needles. Infection of newborns at or near the time of birth (congenital malaria) occurs occasionally when mothers are infected. In endemic areas, congenital malaria may be difficult to distinguish from natural mosquito-borne transmission when the diagnosis is made 2 to 3 weeks after birth.

Epidemiology

Malaria is endemic throughout tropical areas where nearly one half of the world's population lives. There are at least 300 to 500 million malaria cases per year, resulting in 1.5 to 2.7 million deaths each year. Most deaths attributable to malaria occur in infants and children less than 5 years of age. *P. falciparum* and *P. malariae* have a worldwide distribution. *P. vivax* is prevalent on the Indian subcontinent, Central and South America, Southeast Asia, and Oceania but rare in sub-Saharan Africa. *P. ovale* is most common in western Africa but is found in other areas of the world.

The risk of malaria infection for travelers is highest in sub-Saharan Africa, Papua New Guinea, the Solomon Islands, and Vanuatu. Intermediate risk of infection is present in Haiti and the Indian subcontinent. Travelers to most areas of Southeast Asia and South America have a low but still significant risk of malaria infection. Transmission is also possible in temperate areas, such as the United States, where *Anopheles* species mosquitoes are present. Outbreaks have been documented in people working or residing near international airports, presumably from mosquitoes inadvertently transported by airplanes flying from tropical climates. Most of the approximately 1200 cases of malaria reported in the United States each year are acquired abroad.

Chloroquine-resistant *P. falciparum* has spread through most parts of the world, particularly sub-Saharan Africa, Southeast Asia, and South America. *P. falciparum* is also becoming resistant to other antimalarial drugs, such as pyrimethamine-sulfadoxine (Fansidar), mefloquine (Lariam), and halofantrine (Halfan). Partial *P. falciparum* resistance to quinine or quinidine has been described in Southeast Asia. Chloroquine-resistant *P. vivax* has been described in Southeast Asia, India, the South Pacific, South and Central America, and Somalia.

Clinical Manifestations

POPULATIONS AT RISK

The clinical consequences of *Plasmodium* infection can vary widely from asymptomatic parasitemia to severe disease and death. Nonimmune individuals, including tourists and children 6 months to 9 years of age living in endemic areas, are at the greatest risk for complications and death, especially from *P. falciparum.* Pregnant women also have an increased risk of complications particularly during their first pregnancy. Persons who live their entire lives in endemic areas are regularly reinfected and become semi-immune. They rarely develop serious complications after childhood.

MAJOR CLINICAL FINDINGS

The classic presentation is the malarial paroxysm, which is associated with red blood cell lysis and the release of merozoites at the end of a period of intraerythrocytic asexual reproduction. This includes high fever with chills, rigors, sweats, and headache. If appropriate therapy is not administered, paroxysms can recur in a cyclic pattern—every 48 hours with *P. vivax* and *P. ovale*, and every 72 hours with *P. malariae*. Despite a regular 48-hour asexual erythrocytic cycle of replication, fever and chills typically occur without any periodicity in *P. falciparum* infections because erythrocyte lysis is not synchronized.

Other clinical manifestations of uncomplicated malaria include nausea, vomiting, diarrhea, cough, arthralgia, as well as abdominal and back pain. Pallor, jaundice, and hepatosplenomegaly may be found on physical examination. Anemia and thrombocytopenia can also occur.

Congenital malaria secondary to perinatal transmission is usually caused by *P. vivax* and *P. falciparum*. Clinical manifestations are similar to neonatal sepsis and include fever, poor appetite, irritability, and lethargy.

COMPLICATIONS OF *PLASMODIUM FALCIPARUM*

P. falciparum infection has the greatest risk of complications and death for several reasons. It can invade erythrocytes of all ages and produce overwhelming parasitemias. In addition, *P. falciparum*-infected erythrocytes adhere to endothelial cells in vivo and cause microvascular pathology not observed with *P. vivax, P. ovale,* or *P. malariae*. Finally, *P. falciparum* is often resistant to antimalarials.

Infection with *P. falciparum* most commonly manifests as a febrile, nonspecific, influenza-like illness without localizing signs (i.e., uncomplicated malaria described above). More severe disease presents as one or more of the following syndromes (Table 1):

- Cerebral malaria—This is defined as an acute major neurologic event (i.e., rapid onset of seizures, obtundation, coma) in a subject with *P. falciparum* infection with the major alternative etiology being bacterial meningitis. Cerebral malaria has a high mortality rate, killing 15% to 30% of the affected children in endemic areas and a greater proportion of nonimmune adults such as travelers. Despite the high mortality rate, well-documented neurologic sequelae are observed in fewer than 10% of the survivors. It is known, however, that subtle cognitive and motor deficits persist in a large proportion of children.
- Severe anemia—In nonimmune individuals, severe anemia (hemoglobin <5-7 g/100 mL) can develop rapidly (in days) as a result of overwhelming parasitemia (>10^6 parasitized red blood cells [RBC]/µL or >20% circulating RBCs) and hemolysis. In semi-immune individuals, severe anemia develops more slowly, often as a result of persistent or recurrent infection.
- Metabolic complications—Hypoglycemia and acidosis are frequent complications of *P. falciparum* infections and depress central nervous system function. Hypoglycemia can be associated with quinine treatment.
- Renal failure—Malaria-associated renal failure is caused by acute tubular necrosis and is typically oliguric and often reversible. Renal failure is rare in children younger than 8 years of age and more frequent in nonimmune persons treated with quinine or quinidine (blackwater fever).
- Pulmonary edema—Noncardiogenic pulmonary edema typically occurs late in the course of severe malaria, especially in individuals who already have other complications such as cerebral malaria or renal failure. It is rare in children.
- Diarrhea—A common presentation of *P. falciparum* infection in children living in endemic areas is diarrhea. It is associated with cytoadherence of parasitized red blood cells to endothelial cells in the microvasculature of the gastrointestinal tract.
- Vascular collapse and shock—This can be associated with hypothermia and adrenal insufficiency.

TABLE 1 Complications of *Plasmodium* Infection

Complications of *P. falciparum*
Cerebral malaria: seizures, obtundation, coma
Severe anemia
Metabolic: hypoglycemia, acidosis
Renal failure
Pulmonary edema
Diarrhea
Shock
Complications of *P. vivax* and *P. ovale*
Anemia
Splenic rupture
Complications of *P. malariae*
Immune complex glomerulonephritis

COMPLICATIONS OF *PLASMODIUM VIVAX* AND *PLASMODIUM OVALE*

Unlike *P. falciparum* infection, peripheral sequestration in deep vascular beds or the placenta does not occur with *P. vivax, P. ovale,* or *P. malariae*. Thus, microvascular changes in the major organs are not observed, and all stages of the parasite circulate in the peripheral blood. Anemia can result from acute parasitemia. Hypersplenism and splenic rupture are important late complications of *P. vivax* infection (see Table 1). Because of latent hepatic stages, relapse can occur from both *P. vivax* and *P. ovale* for as long as 3 to 5 years after the primary infection.

COMPLICATIONS OF *PLASMODIUM MALARIAE*

P. malariae typically results in low parasitemia and mild symptoms such as weakness, low-grade fever, and fatigue. Chronic asymptomatic parasitemia can last for several years. Infection with *P. malariae* can cause a nephritic syndrome from immune complex deposition in the kidneys (see Table 1).

Pathogenesis

PLASMODIUM FALCIPARUM

The pathogenic factors for *P. falciparum* are many:

- Microvascular sequestration—During the maturation of *P. falciparum* parasites to trophozoite- and schizont-stage parasites, malaria-infected host RBCs develop knobs on their surface by which they mediate adherence to the microvascular endothelium. Because of cytoadherence, only young ring stages of *P. falciparum* are detected in the peripheral bloodstream. The parasitized erythrocytes remain sequestered in the peripheral microvasculature until red blood cell lysis, when newly released merozoites infect additional erythrocytes.
- Cerebral malaria—Because cerebral malaria is a clinical diagnosis, it can have multiple etiologies including hypoglycemia, hypoxia, lactic acidosis, and microvascular sequestration.
- Renal failure—Although hemolysis associated with severe malaria can cause renal failure, there may be other contributing factors including hypotension, microvascular obstruction of the cortex by parasitized erythrocytes, and free malaria pigment or heme. In addition, a number of reports have linked quinine or quinidine treatment to renal failure, suggesting that antimalarials that rapidly lyse large numbers of infected red blood cells may precipitate renal failure in patients with hyperparasitemia.
- Anemia—At least three mechanisms are thought to be involved in the pathogenesis of anemia due to malaria. These include red blood cell lysis with release of mature intraerythrocytic parasites, cytokine suppression of erythropoiesis, and splenic destruction of erythrocytes.
- Metabolic complications—Decreased oral intake, depletion of liver glycogen, parasite consumption of glucose, insulin release from the pancreas by quinine or quinidine, and inhibition of gluconeogenesis may all contribute to malaria-associated hypoglycemia. Because these metabolic complications are generally associated with high parasitemia, they are important problems with *P. falciparum* but not with *P. vivax, P. ovale*, and *P. malariae* infections.
- Pulmonary edema—The pulmonary pathology observed in patients with *P. falciparum* infection is due to a capillary leak syndrome rather than congestive heart failure. Sequestration in the lungs is uncommon.
- Diarrhea—The pathogenesis of watery diarrhea observed in children with *P. falciparum* infection is unknown; but may result from cytoadherent-infected red blood cells in the microvasculature of the small and large intestine in these children. Cytokines could also contribute to a secretory diarrhea.

PLASMODIUM VIVAX

The most important factors in the pathogenesis of *P. vivax* infection are its invasion of reticulocytes, which limits the parasite invasion to young red blood cells and results in lower levels of parasitemia compared with *P. falciparum,* and the fact that cytoadherence does not occur. People lacking expression of the Duffy blood group antigen, including many black people in Africa, are protected from infection with *P. vivax* because *P. vivax* parasites use this antigen as a receptor for invasion of erythrocytes.

PLASMODIUM MALARIAE

The most striking syndrome *P. malariae* infection produces are immune complexes containing parasite antigen (*P. malariae*), host antibody (against *P. malariae*), and complement.

Diagnosis

HISTORY

Fever in travelers returning from endemic countries should alert the physician to the possibility of malaria regardless of associated symptoms. Typical paroxysms of fever and chills may not occur. Other symptoms such as malaise, fatigue, diarrhea, headache, myalgias, or sore throat may lead to incorrect alternative diagnoses. Semi-immune individuals may have a greater frequency of asymptomatic infection but may present with fever and persistent malaise.

MICROSCOPY

The gold standard for clinical malaria diagnosis is microscopic examination of a Giemsa-stained thin and thick blood smear. The thin smear aids in species identification and determination of the degree of parasitemia, while the thick smear allows for concentration of the blood to find parasites present in low numbers. If the initial blood smears are negative for plasmodia and malaria infection remains in the differential diagnosis, blood smears should be repeated every 12 to 24 hours during a 72-hour period. The presence of malaria on a blood smear from semi-immune individuals may not be conclusive of malaria because other infections can be superimposed on low-grade parasitemia. False-positive results can occur when inexperienced microscopists misidentify platelets or stain debris for parasites. Low parasitemia can give a false-negative result.

OTHER DIAGNOSTIC METHODS

There are several alternative methods now available for the diagnosis of malaria infection with equal or greater sensitivity than microscopy. These include (a) fluorescence microscopy that identifies parasites stained by acridine orange, (b) an enzyme-linked immunosorbent assay for a histidine-rich *P. falciparum* antigen, (c) an immunoassay for *Plasmodium* species-specific lactate dehydrogenase isoenzymes, (d) DNA probes for parasite-specific sequences, and (e) polymerase chain reaction amplification of parasite-specific DNA or RNA sequences. Commercially available kits, which can be performed within 10 minutes, are available for the enzyme-linked immunosorbent assay of histidine-rich protein 2 or parasite lactate dehydrogenase. The latter tests have the greatest diagnostic specificity in the nonimmune individual (e.g., a returning traveler) rather than in residents of endemic areas, because the latter are likely to harbor asymptomatic infection.

Treatment

CONSIDERATIONS FOR TREATMENT

Effective therapy for individuals with malaria includes appropriate antimalarial chemotherapy as well as supportive care. This should be considered as an emergency because *P. falciparum* malaria can progress rapidly and be lethal. Factors influencing the choice of antimalaria agents include the immune status of the host, the infecting species, drug resistance, and disease severity. Nonimmune hosts are at increased risk of severe complications and death, particularly from *P. falciparum*. Semi-immune hosts are at lower risk of serious complication and death. Asymptomatic infections routinely occur in these individuals. Resistance to antimalarials for *P. falciparum* and *P. vivax* are well-known and depend on the geographic location where the infection was acquired.

RESISTANCE

Chloroquine-resistant *P. falciparum* has spread throughout most of the world including South America, Southeast Asia, and sub-Saharan Africa. In many areas, *P. falciparum* is resistant to other drugs such as pyrimethamine-sulfadoxine (Fansidar), mefloquine (Lariam), and halofantrine (Halfan); and is partially resistant to quinine and quinidine in addition to chloroquine. More recently, chloroquine-resistant *P. vivax* has been reported in Southeast Asia and South America. Primaquine-resistant *P. vivax* strains have been reported in Southeast Asia, India, the South Pacific, South and Central America, and Somalia. Some strains will respond to higher doses and longer courses of primaquine treatment.

TREATMENT OF CHLOROQUINE-SUSCEPTIBLE *PLASMODIUM FALCIPARUM, PLASMODIUM VIVAX, PLASMODIUM OVALE,* AND *PLASMODIUM MALARIAE*

Chloroquine is the drug of choice for infections due to chloroquine-susceptible malaria (Table 2). It has excellent oral absorption and can be given by nasogastric tube to obtunded or comatose patients. If patients are unable to take oral chloroquine, parenteral treatment with quinidine or quinine is recommended. Intramuscular dosing is generally not advised because of secondary concerns for inadvertent intravenous administration and cardiac arrhythmias. Chloroquine is as efficacious as quinine[2] or quinidine for the treatment of cerebral malaria caused by a chloroquine-susceptible *P. falciparum* parasite.

TREATMENT OF CHLOROQUINE-RESISTANT *PLASMODIUM FALCIPARUM*

Chloroquine-resistant *P. falciparum* infections usually respond to therapy with mefloquine (Lariam), halofantrine (Halfan), quinine[2], quinidine, artemisinin[2], or pyrimethamine-sulfadoxine (Fansidar) (see Table 2). In general, treatment should not be given with the same drug that was used for chemoprophylaxis. In addition, because parasite resistance to mefloquine and halofantrine can be linked, halofantrine should not be used for treating malaria in individuals who were taking mefloquine prophylaxis. Individuals treated with pyrimethamine-sulfadoxine should be watched carefully because resistance of *P. falciparum* to this drug is common in areas of chloroquine resistance, particularly sub-Saharan Africa. Quinidine is preferred for parenteral therapy in the United States because it is more active than quinine, its serum and plasma levels can be followed, and parenteral quinine is no longer available in the United States. Artemisinin derivatives may clear parasitemia and coma more rapidly than quinine or quinidine and should be considered for use when the level of parasitemia is extraordinarily high. Additional drugs, such as mefloquine, doxycycline[1], tetracycline[1], or

[1]Not FDA approved for this indication.

[2]Not available in the United States.

TABLE 2 Treatment

Infection	Generic Name	Trade Name	Adult Dosage	Pediatric Dosage	Comments
Chloroquine-resistant *P. falciparum*					
Oral					
Drugs of choice	Quinine sulfate plus		650 mg q8h × 3–7 d	25 mg/kg/d in 3 doses × 3–7 d	In Southeast Asia, continue treatment for 7 days because of increased relative resistance to quinine.
	Doxycycline[1]	Vibramycin, Vibra-Tabs, Doryx, Periostat and others	100 mg bid × 7 d	2 mg/kg/d × 7 d	Adverse effects: gastrointestinal upset, vaginal candidiasis, photosensitivity, allergic reactions, blood dyscrasias, azotemia in renal diseases, hepatitis. Contraindicated in pregnancy and in children <8 yrs.
	or plus Tetracycline[1]	Achromycin, Sumycin, Panmycin, and others	250 mg qid × 7 d	6.25 mg/kg qid × 7 d	Adverse effects: gastrointestinal upset, vaginal candidiasis, photosensitivity, allergic reactions, blood dyscrasias, azotemia in renal diseases, hepatitis. Contraindicated in pregnancy and in children <8 yrs.
	or plus Pyrimethamine-sulfadoxine	Fansidar	3 tablets at once on last day of quinine	<1 yr: 1/4 tablet; 1–3 yrs: 1/2 tablet; 4–8 yrs: 1 tablet; 9–14 yrs: 2 tablets	Fansidar tablet contains 25 mg pyrimethamine and 500 mg sulfadoxine. Resistance reported from Southeast Asia, the Amazon basin, sub-Saharan Africa, Bangladesh, and Oceania.
	or plus Clindamycin[1]	Cleocin and others	900 mg tid × 5 d	20–40 mg/kg/d in 3 doses × 5 d	For use in pregnancy.
OR	Atovaquone/ proguanil	Malarone	2 adult tablets (500 mg atovaquone /200 mg proguanil bid × 3d daily[3]	11–20 kg: 1 adult tablets/d × 3d; 21–30 kg: 2 adult tablets/d × 3 d; 31–40 kg: 3 adult tablets/d × 3 d; >40 kg: 2 adult tablets bid × 3 d[3]	Take with food or milk. Adult tablets contain 250 mg atovaquone/ 100 mg proguanil (Malarone). Pediatric tablets contain 62.5 mg atovaquone/ 25 mg proguanil (Malarone Pediatric). Adverse effects: nausea, vomiting, abdominal pain, diarrhea, increased transaminase levels, seizures. Approved for once a day dosing but can be divided in two to reduce nausea and vomiting.
Alternatives:	Mefloquine	Lariam, Mephaquin	750 mg followed by 500 mg 12 h later	<45 kg: 15 mg/kg followed by 10 mg/kg 8–12 h later	In the U.S., 250 mg tablet of mefloquine contains 228 mg mefloquine base. Outside the U.S., each 275 mg tablet contains 250 mg base. Adverse effects: dizziness, diarrhea, nausea, vivid dreams, nightmares, irritability, mood alterations, headache, insomnia, anxiety, seizures, and psychosis. Contraindicated for treatment in pregnancy. Do not give with quinine, quinidine, or halofantrine. In areas of reported resistance (such as Thailand-Myanmar and Cambodia borders and the Amazon basin), 25 mg/kg should be used[3].
	Halofantrine	Halfan	500 mg q6h × 3 doses; repeat in 1 wk[1]	<40 kg: 8 mg/kg q6h × 3 doses; repeat in 1 wk[1]	Available in the U.S. only from the manufacturer. May be effective in multiple drug-resistant *P. falciparum* malaria. A single repeat 250 mg dose can be used to treat recurrent mild-to-moderate infections in adults. Do not take 1 h before or 2 h after meals because food increases absorption. Contraindicated in patients with cardiac conduction abnormalities, pregnancy, or use with other drugs that can affect the QT interval such as quinine, quinidine, and mefloquine.

Continued

TABLE 2 Treatment—cont'd

Infection	Generic Name	Trade Name	Adult Dosage	Pediatric Dosage	Comments
OR	Artesunate[2] plus	-	4 mg/kg/d × 3 d		Available in the U.S. only from the manufacturer as an orphan drug from the WHO.
	Mefloquine	Lariam, Mephaquin	750 mg followed by 500 mg 12 h later	15 mg/kg followed 8–12 h later by 10 mg/kg	In the U.S., 250 mg tablet of mefloquine contains 228 mg mefloquine base. Outside the U.S., each 275 mg tablet contains 250 mg base. Adverse effects: dizziness, diarrhea, nausea, vivid dreams, nightmares, irritability, mood alterations, headache, insomnia, anxiety, seizures, and psychosis. Contraindicated for treatment in pregnancy. Do not give with quinine, quinidine, or halofantrine. In areas of reported resistance (such as Thailand-Myanmar and Cambodia borders and the Amazon basin). 25 mg/kg should be used.[3]
Choloriquine-resistant P. vivax					
Oral					
Drugs of choice	Quinine sulfate plus	-	650 mg q8h × 3-7 d	25 mg/kg/d in 3 doses × 3-7 d	In Southeast increased relative resistance to quinine, thus treatment should be continued for 7 days.
	Doxycycline	Vibramycin, Vibra-Tabs, Doryx, Periostat and others	100 mg bid × 7 d	2 mg/kg/d × 7 d	Adverse effects: gastrointestinal upset, vaginal candidiasis, photosensitivity, allergic reactions, blood dyscrasias, azotemia in renal diseases, hepatitis. Contraindicated in pregnancy and in children <8 yrs.
OR	Mefloquine	Lariam, Mephaquin	750 mg followed by 500 mg 12 h later	15 mg/kg followed 8–12 h later by 10 mg/kg	In the U.S., 250 mg tablet of mefloquine contains 228 mg mefloquine base. Outside the U.S., each 275 mg tablet contains 250 mg base. Adverse effects: dizziness, diarrhea, nausea, vivid dreams, nightmares, irritability, mood alterations, headache, insomnia, anxiety, seizures, and psychosis. Contraindicated for treatment in pregnancy. Do not give with quinine, quinidine, or halofantrine. In areas of reported resistance (such as Thailand-Myanmar and Cambodia borders and the Amazon basin), 25 mg/kg should used.[3]
Alternatives	Halofantrine	Halfan	500 mg q6h × 3 doses; repeat in 1 wk	<40 kg: 8 mg/kg q6h × 3 doses; repeat in 1 wk	Available in the U.S. only from the manufacturer. May be effective in multiple drug-resistant *P. falciparum* malaria. A single repeat 250 mg dose can be used to treat recurrent mild-to-moderate infections in adults. Do not take 1 h before or 2 h after meals because food increases absorption. Contraindicated in patients with cardiac conduction abnormalities, pregnancy, or use with other drugs that can affect the QT interval such as quinine, quinidine, and mefloquine.
	Chloroquine phosphate	Aralen	25 mg base/kg in 3 doses over 48 h		If chloroquine phosphate is not available, hydroxychloroquine sulfate is effective, (400 mg of hydroxychloroquine sulfate is equivalent to 500 mg of chloroquine sulfate). Adverse effects: pruritis in black-skinned patients, nausea, headache, skin eruptions, reversible corneal opacity, nail and mucous membrane discoloration, nerve deafness, photophobia, myopathy, retinopathy (with daily use), blood dyscrasias, psychosis, seizures, alopecia. In pregnancy, chloroquine prophylaxis has been used extensively and safely.

plus	Primaquine phosphate[1]	-	2.5 mg base/kg in 3 doses over 48 h		Take with food. Can cause methemoglobinemia and hemolytic anemia, especially in patients with glucose-6-phosphate dehydrogenase (G6PD) deficiency. Screen for G6PD deficiency before treatment. Contraindicated in pregnancy.
All *Plasmodium* except Chloroquine-resistant *P. falcinarum* and Chloroquine-resistant *P. vivax*					
ORAL					
Drug of choice	Chloroquine phosphate	Aralen	1 gram (600 mg base), then 500 mg (300 mg base) 6 hrs later, then 500 mg (300 mg base) at 24 and 48 h	10 mg base/kg (max. 600 mg base), then 5 mg base/kg 6 h later, then 5 mg base/kg at 24 and 48 h	If chloroquine phosphate is not available hydroxychloroquine sulfate is effective, (400 mg of hydroxychloroquine sulfate is equivalent to 500 mg of chloroquine sulfate). Adverse effects: pruritis in black-skinned patients, nausea, headache, skin eruptions, reversible corneal opacity, nail and mucous membrane discoloration, nerve deafness, photophobia, myopathy, retinopathy (with daily use), blood dyscrasias, psychosis, seizures, alopecia. In pregnancy, chloroquine prophylaxis has been used extensively and safely.
All *Plasmodium*					
PARENTERAL					
Drug of choice	Quinidine gluconate	-	10 mg/kg loading dose (max. 600 mg) in normal saline slowly for 1 to 2 h followed by continuous infusion of 0.02 mg/kg/min until oral therapy can be started or parasitemia is <1%	Same as adult dose	Continuous EKG, blood pressure, and glucose monitoring are recommended especially in pregnant women and children. The loading dose should be decreased or omitted in patients who have received quinine or mefloquine. For problems with quinidine availability, call the manufacturer (Eli Lilly, 800-821-0538) or the CDC Malaria Hotline (770-488-7788). If >48 h of parenteral therapy is required, the quinine or qunidine dose should be decreased by 1/3 to 1/2.
OR	Quinine dihydrochloride (IV)[2]	-	20 mg/kg loading dose IV in 5% dextrose over 4 h followed by 10 mg/kg over 2-4 h q8h (max. 1800 mg/d) until oral therapy can be started or parasitemia is <1%	Same as adult dose	Not available in the U.S. Continuous ECG, blood pressure, and glucose monitoring are recommended especially in pregnant women and children. The loading dose should be decreased or omitted in patients who have received quinine or mefloquine. If >48 h of parenteral therapy is required, the quinine or quinidine dose should be decreased by 1/3 to 1/2.
OR	Quinine dihydrochloride (IM)[2]	-	10 mg/kg q8h (max. 1800 mg/day)	Same as adult dose	Use only if unable to give oral or intravenous treatment.
Alternative:	Artemether[2]	-	3.2 mg/kg IM, then 1.6 mg/kg daily × 5–7 d	Same as adult dose	Available in the U.S. only from the manufacturer.
Prevention of relapses: *P. vivax* and *P. ovale* only					
Drug of choice	Primaquine phosphate	-	26.3 mg (15 mg base)/d × 14 d or 79 mg (45 mg/base)/wk × 8 wk[3]	0.3 mg base/kg/d × 14 d	Take with food. Can cause hemolytic anemia, especially in patients with glucose-6-phosphate dehydrogenase deficiency, methemoglobinemia. Screen for G-6-PD deficiency before treatment. Contraindicated in pregnancy. Relapses have been reported with this regimen and should be treated with a second 14-day course of 30 mg base/day. In Southeast Asia and Somalla, the higher dose (30 mg base/day)[3] should be used initially.

[1]Not FDA approved for this indication.
[2]Not available in the United States.
[3]Exceeds dosage recommended by the manufacturer.

pyrimethamine-sulfadoxine, are often given after the initial treatment with artemisinin derivatives to prevent recrudescence 3 to 4 weeks later.

TREATMENT OF CHLOROQUINE-RESISTANT *PLASMODIUM VIVAX*

Infections due to chloroquine-resistant *P. vivax* respond to oral treatment with mefloquine, halofantrine, atovaquone plus proguanil (Malarone), or quinine sulfate plus either pyrimethamine-sulfadoxine or doxycycline[1] (see Table 2).

ERADICATION OF *PLASMODIUM VIVAX* OR *PLASMODIUM OVALE* HYPNOZOITES

In order to prevent relapse, primaquine is used to eradicate the hypnozoites in individuals with *P. vivax* or *P. ovale* infection. Individuals receiving primaquine should have a normal glucose-6-phopshate dehydrogenase (G6PD) level because of the risk of methemoglobinemia and hemolysis in G6PD-deficient individuals.

SUPPORTIVE CARE

Components of severe malaria include parasitemia levels noted in greater than 1% to 5% of red blood cells, signs of central nervous system or end-organ involvement, shock, acidosis, and/or hypoglycemia. Admission to the intensive care unit is usually required for patients with severe malaria to help manage hypoglycemia, acidosis, seizures, pulmonary edema, renal failure, and other complications. Exchange transfusions are useful adjuncts to therapy particularly when parasitemias exceed 5% or are rising rapidly. Sequential blood smears are useful in monitoring response to therapy. Nonimmune individuals, particularly those who have returned from malaria endemic areas to nonendemic areas, should be hospitalized until a response to treatment has been observed and time has elapsed to be certain that complications from severe disease are unlikely. If reliable follow-up is possible, individuals with partial immunity and uncomplicated *P. falciparum* infection and some nonimmune individuals with *P. vivax, P. ovale,* or *P. malariae* infection may be treated as outpatients.

Prevention

CHEMOPROPHYLAXIS

Antimalarials should be used to prevent infection in nonimmune individuals (including children) who are traveling to malaria-endemic areas. Factors influencing the choice of chemoprophylaxis include transmission intensity, resistance patterns in the endemic country, pregnancy, underlying medical conditions, and allergies (Table 3). Dosages for children should be based on body weight. Current information regarding country-specific risks, antimalarial resistance, and recommendations for travelers is available through the Centers for Disease Control (see Resources). In general, travelers should start chemoprophylaxis 1 to 2 weeks (chloroquine or mefloquine [Lariam]) or 1 to 2 days (doxycycline or atovaquone/proguanil [Malarone]) before travel to obtain effective serum concentrations. Chemoprophylaxis should be continued while in malaria-endemic areas and for 4 weeks (chloroquine, doxycycline, or mefloquine) or 7 days (atovaquone/proguanil) after leaving such areas. With the exception of pregnant women, routine chemoprophylaxis is not recommended for residents of malaria endemic areas because of the emergence of parasite resistance and prevention of the development of partial immunity in the host.

[1]Not FDA approved for this indication.

CHEMOPROPHYLAXIS OF CHLOROQUINE-SUSCEPTIBLE *PLASMODIUM FALCIPARUM, PLASMODIUM VIVAX, PLASMODIUM OVALE,* AND *PLASMODIUM. MALARIAE*

The chemoprophylactic drug of choice for the prevention of chloroquine-susceptible plasmodia infections is chloroquine (see Table 3). Transient side effects such as headache, dizziness, and blurred vision can occur. Many side effects can be reduced by taking half the dose twice a week rather than the full dose once a week. Overdose can lead to arrhythmias. Atovaquone/proguanil (Malarone), doxycycline, or mefloquine (Lariam) can be used for travelers unable to take chloroquine.

CHEMOPROPHYLAXIS OF CHLOROQUINE-RESISTANT *PLASMODIUM FALCIPARUM*

Three options exist for malaria chemoprophylaxis for travelers to areas endemic for chloroquine-resistant *P. falciparum*. These include atovaquone/proguanil (Malarone), doxycycline, and mefloquine (Lariam) (see Table 3). Doxycycline may produce a photosensitive drug eruption and increase the risk of monilial vaginitis. Because of the risk of dental staining, doxycycline should be avoided in children younger than 8 years of age and pregnant women. Mefloquine can cause headache, nausea, dizziness, and vivid dreams and is contraindicated in persons with active depression or a history of psychosis or convulsions. Mefloquine is not recommended in individuals with cardiac conduction abnormalities. In areas where mefloquine-resistant strains of *P. falciparum* have been reported (Thailand-Myanmar and Thailand-Cambodia borders), doxycycline or atovaquone/proguanil can be used. In rare instances, primaquine[1] can be used for malaria chemoprophylaxis for travelers unable to tolerate other chemoprophylactic regimens.

[1]Not FDA approved for this indication.

TABLE 3 Prevention of Malaria (*Plasmodium falciparum, P. vivax, P. ovale,* and *P. malariae*)

Infection	Drug: Generic Name	Drug: Trade Name	Adult Dosage	Pediatric Dosage	Comments
Chloroquine-Sensitive Areas					
Drug of choice	Chloroquine phosphate	Aralen	300 mg base (500 mg salt), once/wk; beginning 1-2 wk before exposure and continuing until 4 wk after exposure	5 mg/kg base (8.3 mg/kg salt) once/wk, up to adult dose of 300 mg base; beginning 1-2 wk before exposure and continuing until 4 wk after exposure	Adverse effects: pruritus in black-skinned patients, nausea, headache, skin eruptions, reversible corneal opacity, nail and mucous membrane discoloration, nerve deafness, photophobia, myopathy, retinopathy (with daily use), blood dyscrasias, psychosis, seizures, alopecia. In pregnancy, chloroquine prophylaxis has been used extensively and safely.
OR	Hydroxychloroquine sulfate	Plaquenil	310 mg base (400 mg salt), once/wk; beginning 1-2 wk before exposure and continuing until 4 wk after exposure	5 mg/kg base (6.5 mg/kg salt) once/wk, up to 400 mg (310 mg base); beginning 1-2 wk before exposure and continuing until 4 wk after exposure	If chloroquine phosphate is not available, hydroxychloroquine sulfate is effective (400 mg of hydroxychloroquine sulfate is equivalent to 500 mg of chloroquine sulfate).
Chloroquine-Resistant Areas					
Drug of choice	Mefloquine	Lariam, Mephaquin	250 mg salt (228 mg base) once/wk; beginning 1-2 wk before exposure and continuing until 4 wk after exposure	<15 kg: 5 mg/kg salt (4.6 mg/kg base); 15-19 kg: {1/4} tablet; 20-30 kg: 1/2 tablet; 31-45 kg: {3/4} tablet; >45 kg: 1 tablet; beginning 1-2 wk before exposure and continuing until 4 wk after exposure.	In the U.S., the 250 mg tablet of mefloquine contains 228 mg mefloquine base. Outside the U.S., each 275 mg tablet contains 250 mg base. Adverse effects: dizziness, diarrhea, nausea, vivid dreams, nightmares, irritability, mood alterations, headache, insomnia, anxiety, seizures, and psychosis. Contraindicated in persons with active depression, a recent history of depression, generalized anxiety disorder, psychosis, schizophrenia, other major psychiatric disorders, or seizures. Not recommended for persons with cardiac conduction abnormalities. Use with caution in travelers involved in tasks requiring fine motor coordination and spatial discrimination. For areas where *P. vivax* and *P. ovale* are found, some experts recommend primaquine phosphate 26.3 mg (max: 15 mg base)/d or, for children, 0.3 mg base/kg/d during the last 2 wk of prophylaxis. Others prefer to avoid the risk of toxicity and rely on surveillance to detect cases.
OR	Doxycycline	Vibramycin, Vibra-Tabs, Doryx, Periostat, and others	100 mg/d; beginning 1-2 d before exposure and continuing until 4 wk after exposure	≥8 yrs: 2 mg/kg/d, up to 100 mg/d; beginning 1-2 d before exposure and continuing until 4 wk after exposure	Strict compliance with daily dosing required. Take with food. Adverse effects include gastrointestinal upset, vaginal candidiasis, photosensitivity, allergic reactions, blood dyscrasias, azotemia in renal diseases, hepatitis. Contraindicated in children <8 yrs and pregnant women. For areas where *P. vivax* and *P. ovale* are found, some experts recommend primaquine phosphate 26.3 mg (15 mg base)/d or, for children, 0.3 mg base/kg/d (max: 15 mg base)/d during the last 2 wk of prophylaxis.

Continued

TABLE 3 Prevention of Malaria (Plasmodium falciparum, P. vivax, P. ovale, and P. malariae)—cont'd

Infection	Drug: Generic Name	Drug: Trade Name	Adult Dosage	Pediatric Dosage	Comments
					Others prefer to avoid the risk of toxicity and rely on surveillance to detect cases.
OR	Atovaquone/ proguanil	Malarone	250 mg atovaquone/100 mg proguanil (1 adult tablet)/d; beginning 1-2 d before exposure and continuing until 7 d after exposure	11-20 kg: 62.5 mg atovaquone/25 mg proguanil (1 pediatric tablet); 21-30 kg: 125 mg/ 50 mg (2 pediatric tablets); 31-40 kg: 187.5 mg/75 mg (3 pediatric tablets); >40 kg: 250 mg/ 100 mg (4 pediatric tablets); beginning 1-2 d before exposure and continuing 7 d after exposure	Take with food or milk. Adult tablets contain 250 mg atovaquone/100 mg proguanil (Malarone). Pediatric tablets contain 62.5 mg atovaquone/25 mg proguanil (Malarone Pediatric). Adverse effects: nausea, vomiting, abdominal pain, diarrhea, increased transaminase levels, seizures. Approved for 1 dose/d but dose can be divided in two to reduce nausea and vomiting. Contraindicated in persons with severe renal impairment (creatine clearance <30 mL/min). Not recommended for children <11 kg, pregnant women, and women breast-feeding infants. For areas where *P. vivax* and *P. ovale* are found, some experts recommend primaquine phosphate 26.3 mg (max: 15 mg base)/d or, for children, 0.3 mg base/kg/d max: 15 mg base/d during the last 2 wk of prophylaxis. Others prefer to avoid the risk of toxicity and rely on surveillance to detect cases. Adverse effects: nausea, vomiting, abdominal pain, diarrhea, increased transaminase levels, seizures.
Alternatives	Primaquine phosphate	-	30 mg base (52.6 mg salt)/d; beginning 1 d before departure and continued until 7 d after exposure	0.5 mg/kg base (1 mg/kg salt)/d; beginning 1 d before departure and continued until 7 d after exposure	Take with food. Can cause methemoglobinemia and hemolytic anemia, especially in patients with glucose-6-phosphate dehydrogenase (G6PD) deficiency. Screen for G6PD deficiency before treatment. Contraindicated in pregnancy.
	Chloroquine phosphate	Aralen	500 mg (300 mg base) once/wk; beginning 1-2 wk before exposure and continuing until 4 wk after exposure	5 mg/kg base once/wk, up to adult dose of 300 mg base; beginning 1-2 wk before exposure and continuing unitl 4 wk after exposure	Adverse effects: pruritus in black-skinned patients, nausea, headache, skin eruptions, reversible corneal opacity, nail and mucous membrane discoloration, nerve deafness, photophobia, myopathy, retinopathy (with daily use), blood dyscrasias, psychosis, seizures, alopecia. In pregnancy, chloroquine prophylaxis has been used extensively and safely.
	plus Proguanil[2]	Paludrine	200 mg once/d; beginning 1-2 d before exposure and continuing until 4 wk after exposure	<2 yrs: 50 mg once/d; 2-6 yrs: 100 mg once/d; 7-10 yrs: 150 mg once/d; >10 yrs: 200 mg once/d; beginning 1-2 wk before exposure and continuing until 4 wk after exposure	Not available alone in the U.S. but is widely available in Canada and Europe and is recommended mainly for use in sub-Saharan Africa. Adverse effects include anorexia, nausea, mouth ulcers. Has been used in pregnancy without evidence of toxicity.

Presumptive Treatment					
	Atovaquone/proguanil	Malarone	2 adult tablets bid × 3d[3] or 4 adult tablets once/d × 3 d	11-20 kg: 1 adult tablet/d × 3d; 21-30 kg: 2 adult tablet/d × 3 d; 31-40 kg: 3 adult tablet/d × 3 d; >40 kg: 2 adult tablets bid × 3d or 4 adult tablets once/d × 3 d	Not recommended for self-treatment in persons on atovaquone/proguanil prophylaxis. Take with food or milk. Adult tablets contain 250 mg atovaquone/100 mg proguanil (Malarone). Pediatric tablets contain 62.5 mg atovaquone/25 mg proguanil (Malarone Pediatric). Adverse effects: nausea, vomiting, abdominal pain, diarrhea, increased transaminase levels, seizures. Approved for once/d dosing but dose usually divided in two to reduce nausea and vomiting. Contraindicated in persons with severe renal impairment (creatine clearance <30 mL/min). Not recommended for children <11 kg, pregnant women, and women breast-feeding infants.
OR	Pyrimethamine-sulfadoxine	Fansidar	Carry a single dose (3 tablets) for self-treatment of febrile illness when medical care is not immediately available	<1 yr: 1/4 tablet; 1-3 yrs: 1/2 tablet; 4-8 yrs: 1 tablet; 9-14 yrs: 2 tablets	Fansidar tablet contains 25 mg pyrimethamine and 500 mg sulfadoxine. Resistance reported from Southeast Asia, the Amazon basin, sub-Saharan Africa, Bangladesh, and Oceania.

[2]Not available in the United States
[3]Exceeds dosage recommended by the manufacturer.

A normal G6PD level must be documented when using primaquine because it can cause methemoglobinemia and hemolysis in G6PD-deficient individuals.

PREVENTION OF INFECTION DUE TO CHLOROQUINE-RESISTANT *PLASMODIUM VIVAX*

Because the prevalence of chloroquine-resistant *P. vivax* is unknown, chloroquine is still recommended for chemoprophylaxis against *P. vivax.*

PREVENTION OF RELAPSES OF *PLASMODIUM VIVAX* AND *PLASMODIUM OVALE*

Because *P. vivax* and *P. ovale* produce hypnozoites that remain dormant for several years, terminal prophylaxis with primaquine is recommended in some situations (see Table 3). This is generally reserved for individuals with prolonged exposure in malaria-endemic areas such as missionaries, Peace Corps volunteers, and military personnel. If chloroquine, doxycycline, or mefloquine was used for primary prophylaxis, primaquine can be given during the last 2 weeks of postexposure prophylaxis. If atovaquone/proguanil (Malarone) is used, primaquine can be given during the final 7 days of atovaquone/proguanil prophylaxis and then for an additional 7 days or for a total of 14 days after atovaquone/proguanil is stopped. Individuals should have a normal G6PD level documented prior to giving primaquine.

CHEMOPROPHYLAXIS DURING PREGNANCY

Pregnant women are at increased risk for severe malaria. Malaria can increase the risk for complications during pregnancy including prematurity and miscarriage. Women who are pregnant or likely to become pregnant should be advised to avoid travel to areas with malaria transmission if possible. Chloroquine prophylaxis can be used for pregnant women traveling to areas where chloroquine-susceptible *P. falciparum* is present. The drug has been used extensively for chemoprophylaxis in pregnant women without any known harmful effects to the fetus or mother. In areas with chloroquine-resistant *P. falciparum,* mefloquine (Lariam) can be used. Mefloquine at prophylactic doses appears to be safe in the second and third trimester, and limited data suggest that it is also safe during the first trimester. Atovaquone/proguanil (Malarone) is not currently recommended for malaria chemoprophylaxis in pregnant women. Doxycycline and tetracycline are contraindicated because of the risk of dental staining and inhibition of bone growth in the fetus. Primaquine should not be used as the infant may be G6PD deficient and develop a hemolytic anemia in utero.

CHEMOPROPHYLAXIS WHILE BREAST-FEEDING

Most antimalarial drugs are not excreted in breast milk in sufficient amounts to protect the infant from malaria. Therefore, both the mother and child should receive malaria chemoprophylaxis. Breast-feeding infants of mothers who are taking primaquine should be tested for G6PD levels because the amount of primaquine that enters breast milk is unknown.

PRESUMPTIVE SELF-TREATMENT

Long-term travelers taking effective prophylaxis and working in very remote areas may decide to take along a dose of antimalarials for self-treatment (see Table 3). Prompt self-treatment should be started if the individual has fever, chills, and influenza-like illnesses if medical care is not available within 24 hours. Travelers must be instructed that this is only a temporary measure and prompt medical evaluation is necessary.

PERSONAL PROTECTIVE MEASURES

In addition to chemoprophylaxis, personal protective measures are recommended for all travelers to malaria-endemic areas. This includes using insecticide-impregnated (permethrin or deltamethrin) bed nets, staying in well-screened areas, wearing protective clothing, particularly at dusk, and using insect repellant containing diethyltoluamide (DEET).

Resources

Detailed and updated recommendations regarding malaria prevention are available on the Centers for Disease Control (CDC) Web site *http://www.cdc.gov/travel.* Recommendations are also available 24 hours a day from the CDC voice information service (1-877-394-8747) or the fax information service (1-888-232-3299). Assistance with the diagnosis and treatment of malaria is available to health-care professionals through the CDC Malaria Hotline at 770-488-7788 from 8:00 AM to 4:30 PM Eastern Standard Time. After business hours or on holidays, call the CDC Emergency Operation Center at 770-488-7100 and ask the operator to page the person on call for the Malaria Epidemiology Branch. The World Health Organization has information available from its publication, *International Travel and Health,* at *http://www.who.int/ith/index.html.*

BACTERIAL MENINGITIS

METHOD OF

J. William Kelly, MD

Acute bacterial meningitis is a medical emergency requiring rapid decisive action to prevent death or permanent neurologic sequelae. Since the introduction of antibiotics, the mortality rate has remained between 5% and 40%; of the survivors 10% to 30% suffer significant residual neurologic deficits. The prognosis is affected by the timeliness of therapy; therefore presumptive diagnosis and empiric therapy are necessary. This article focuses on these aspects of initial management.

Diagnosis

Acute bacterial meningitis must be considered in the differential diagnosis of any patient presenting with fever, headache, and signs of meningeal irritation. The presentation may be quite subtle, particularly in the very young and very old, and in patients who have received antibiotics; therefore, particular care is required to avoid overlooking patients whose only symptoms are changes in mental status. Once suspicion has been raised, the diagnosis of bacterial meningitis rests on the cerebrospinal fluid (CSF) examination. There has been considerable debate during the last few years regarding the need for obtaining a computed tomographic (CT) scan of the head of all patients before performing a lumbar puncture. Two recent studies indicated that lumbar puncture may be safely performed on patients who have normal mental status, no focal neurologic signs, and no papilledema. The physician's clinical impression in the studies was predictive of the CT findings. If there are signs or symptoms suggestive of an intracranial mass, blood cultures should be obtained and empiric antibiotics administered while one awaits the results of a CT scan. The classic CSF findings in bacterial meningitis include a cell count of more than 1000 white blood cells (WBCs) per mm^3, with a predominance of neutrophils, and a protein concentration of more than 150 mg/dL. These values are not absolute, and any single parameter may be normal in 10% to 30% of patients with proven bacterial meningitis.

The most valuable study is a careful examination of a Gram-stained sediment of centrifuged CSF. In patients who have not received antibiotics, the CSF Gram stain is positive in 80% to 90% of culture-confirmed cases. In patients who have been previously treated, the Gram stain is positive in 60% to 70% of cases. The protein, glucose, and cell counts are usually not significantly altered by one or two doses of antibiotics. In patients who have negative CSF Gram stains, especially those whose stains may have been rendered negative by prior antibiotics, latex agglutination methods to detect bacterial antigens may also be used, rather than depending on the Gram stain alone. Clinical judgment is required, and no single test should be the basis for withholding antibiotics.

Antibiotic Selection

The timeliness of therapy is a prime predictor of outcome in bacterial meningitis. The presence of hypotension, altered mental status, or seizures at the time of the initial antibiotic administration has been shown to be predictive of a poor outcome (death or neurologic sequelae). In one study, 15% of patients developed these symptoms while awaiting antibiotics and these patients had a significantly worse outcome. Because prompt administration of antibiotics is critical, the choice of antibiotics usually must be made before the results of CSF cultures are known. If organisms are seen on the Gram stain, therapy may be directed by the morphology. (Table 1 lists

TABLE 1 Cerebrospinal Fluid Gram Stain Morphology and Antibiotic Recommendations

Morphology	Common Pathogens	Treatment of Choice	Alternative Therapy
Gram-positive cocci in short chains and pairs	*Streptococcus pneumoniae* (group B streptococcus)	Ceftriaxone (Rocephin)* plus vancomycin (Vancocin)	Chloramphenicol (Chloromycetin)
Gram-positive cocci in clusters	*Staphylococcus aureus*	Vancomycin	Nafcillin (Unipen)
Gram-positive bacilli	*Listeria monocytogenes*	Ampicillin plus aminoglycoside†	Trimethoprim-sulfamethoxazole (Bactrim)
Gram-negative cocci	*Neisseria meningitidis*	Ceftriaxone*	Penicillin G or chloramphenicol
Gram-negative coccobacilli	*Haemophilus influenzae*	Ceftriaxone*	Ampicillin plus chloramphenicol
Gram-negative bacilli	*Escherichia coli, Klebsiella*, and *Pseudomonas aeruginosa*	Ceftazidime (Fortaz)	‡

*Cefotaxime (Claforan) may be substituted for ceftriaxone.
†Gentamicin (Garamycin), tobramycin (Nebcin), and amikacin (Amikin) may all be used based on local susceptibilities.
‡No alternative therapy has been clinically proven reliable. Infectious disease consultation is recommended in these difficult cases.

TABLE 2 Antibiotic Recommendations by Age Groups

Age Group	Common Pathogens	Empiric Drug of Choice
Neonate (<1 mo)	Group B streptococcus, *Escherichia coli*, and *Listeria monocytogenes*	Ampicillin plus aminoglycoside*
Infants (1-3 mo)	*Haemophilus influenzae, Neisseria meningitidis, Streptococcus pneumoniae,* Group B streptococci, and *L. monocytogenes*	Ampicillin plus ceftriaxone (Rocephin)†
Young children (3 mo-7 y)	*H. influenzae, S. pneumoniae,* and *N. meningitidis*	Ceftriaxone† plus vancomycin (Vancocin)
Older children and adults (7-50 y)	*S. pneumoniae* and *N. meningitidis*	Ceftriaxone† plus vancomycin
Older adults (>50 y)	*S. pneumoniae, N. meningitidis, and L. monocytogenes*	Ceftriaxone† plus ampicillin

*Gentamicin (Garamycin), tobramycin (Nebcin), and amikacin (Amikin) may all be used based on local susceptibilities.
†Cefotaxime (Claforan) may be substituted for ceftriaxone.

likely CSF pathogens and treatments of choice based on the CSF Gram stain morphology.) When the Gram stain fails to show any organisms, antibiotics must be chosen empirically on the basis of the patient's age (Table 2) and other epidemiologic clues (Table 3). Once culture results are known, these empiric choices can be modified according to the culture and sensitivity data.

It is important that the antibiotics used are rapidly bactericidal and have adequate penetration into the CSF. It is also important that antibiotics be given in maximal doses (Table 4), because the bactericidal activity of antibiotics in the CSF is dose dependent, and CSF penetration under the best of conditions is only a fraction of the serum level. Finally, care should be taken not to use combinations of bacteriostatic and bactericidal drugs to avoid antagonizing the bactericidal activity of the therapy.

Special Considerations

During the past 15 years there has been a steady increase in the percentage of strains of *Streptococcus pneumoniae* that are resistant to penicillin and cephalosporins. At present, approximately 40% of pneumococci demonstrate relative resistance, while 10% to 15% have high-level resistance to penicillin and frequently have resistance to third-generation cephalosporins such as ceftriaxone (Rocephin) and cefotaxime (Claforan). For this reason, vancomycin (Vancocin) is generally recommended for empiric therapy for meningitis because *S. pneumoniae* is the most common cause of bacterial meningitis. Vancomycin penetration into the CSF may be variable, therefore, consideration should be given for repeat lumbar puncture and CSF culture at 48 hours, particularly if the patient is not responding appropriately to antibiotic therapy.

Meningitis caused by resistant gram-negative bacilli such as *Pseudomonas aeruginosa* should be treated with a cephalosporin with antipseudomonal activity such as ceftazidime (Fortaz) or cefepime (Maxipime). Carbapenems, such as imipenem (Primaxin) or meropenem (Merrem), have been used in patients with meningitis caused by cephalosporin-resistant, gram-negative bacilli. Meropenem appears to have less tendency to cause seizures and may be a better choice in meningitis because 30% of patients with meningitis may present with seizures.

Patients with ventriculoatrial and ventriculoperitoneal shunt-associated meningitis usually require removal of the shunt as well as antibiotics to clear the infection. Certain patients with low-virulence

TABLE 3 Antibiotic Recommendations for Special Hosts

Condition	Common Pathogens	Antibiotic Recommendation
Impaired cellular immunity	*Listeria monocytogenes* and *Streptococcus pneumoniae*	Ampicillin plus ceftriaxone (Rocephin)*
Closed head trauma	*S. pneumoniae*	Ceftriaxone* plus vancomycin (Vancocin)
Asplenia	*S. pneumoniae* and *Neisseria meningitidis*	Ceftriaxone* plus vancomycin
Terminal complement deficiency	*N. meningitidis*	Ceftriaxone*
Neurosurgical procedures/CSF shunts	*Staphylococcus aureus, Staphylococcus epidermidis,* and Gram-negative bacilli	Vancomycin plus ceftriaxone*
Patients >65 years old	*S. pneumoniae* and *L. monocytogenes*	Ceftriaxone* plus ampicillin
Recurrent meningitis	*S. pneumoniae*	Ceftriaxone* plus vancomycin
Alcoholic patients	*S. pneumoniae* and Gram-negative bacilli	Ceftriaxone* plus vancomycin

*Cefotaxime (Claforan) may be substituted for ceftriaxone.

TABLE 4 Antibiotic Doses in Bacterial Meningitis

Antibiotic	Daily Adult Dose	Daily Pediatric Dose	Dose Interval
Amikacin (Amikin)	15 mg/kg	20 mg/kg	8 h
Ampicillin (Polycillin)	12 g	200 mg/kg	4 h
Cefotaxime (Claforan)	12 g	200 mg/kg	4 h
Ceftazidime (Fortaz)	6 g	150 mg/kg	8 h
Ceftriaxone (Rocephin)	4 g	100 mg/kg*	12 h
Chloramphenicol (Chloromycetin)	4 g	75 mg/kg†	6 h
Gentamicin (Garamycin)	5 mg/kg	7.5 mg/kg	8 h
Nafcillin (Unipen)	12 g	200 mg/kg	4 h
Penicillin G	24 million units	250,000 U/kg	4 h
Tobramycin (Nebcin)	5 mg/kg	6 mg/kg	8 h
Trimethoprim-sulfamethoxazole (Bactrim)	10 mg/kg‡	10 mg/kg	8 h
Vancomycin (Vancocin)	2 g§	40-60 mg/kg	12 h

*Ceftriaxone is not recommended for neonates because it may displace bilirubin from albumin-binding sites.
†Ideally, serum levels should be monitored in pediatrics.
‡Dosing based on trimethoprim component.
§Vancomycin levels may be useful to assure adequate dosing to penetrate CSF.

organisms, such as coagulase-negative staphylococci, and with exquisitely sensitive organisms can be treated with antibiotics alone. Infectious disease consultation should be obtained to assist in these decisions.

Because of the extreme sensitivity of *Neisseria meningitidis* to antibiotics, uncomplicated meningococcal meningitis may be treated with as little as 7 days of antibiotics. Pneumococcal meningitis is generally treated with a 2-week course of antibiotics. Gram-negative meningitis usually requires 3 weeks of therapy. All patients with meningitis should be monitored carefully and treatment extended in those who are slow to respond.

Repeated lumbar punctures are not necessary in patients with bacterial meningitis who respond well to therapy. Follow-up cultures to assess sterilization of the CSF may be indicated in patients who are infected with more resistant organisms, such as penicillin-resistant pneumococci or resistant gram-negative bacilli, in patients who have an inadequate clinical response, or in patients who deteriorate on therapy.

Adjunctive Therapy

Great attention has been given to the use of corticosteroids in bacterial meningitis. Corticosteroids have been shown to reduce the incidence of death and permanent neurologic sequelae in children with bacterial meningitis. The effect was most pronounced in children with meningitis caused by *Haemophilus influenzae* and *S. pneumoniae*. Present recommendations are for dexamethasone (Decadron)[1] 0.15 mg/kg/dose, or 10 mg for adults, every 6 hours for the first 4 days of treatment. Steroids should be given just before or at the time of the first dose of antibiotics.

Use of corticosteroids in adults has been more controversial. A recent study in adults found that corticosteroids significantly reduced the risk for unfavorable outcomes, particularly in patients with pneumococcal meningitis. There has been concern that dexamethasone may decrease the penetration of antibiotics, especially vancomycin, into the CSF. One study in children did not show this to be the case. Dexamethasone is probably indicated in adults with pneumococcal meningitis, if given prior to the first dose of antibiotics. For the first 4 days of therapy, 10 mg every 6 hours should be given. If the meningitis is found not to be pneumococcal, the dexamethasone should be discontinued. In patients with meningitis caused by *S. pneumoniae* that is highly resistant to penicillin and cephalosporins, vancomycin should not be used as a single agent if corticosteroids are given. The addition of rifampin (Rifadin)[1] is often recommended in these situations.

Prevention

Prophylactic antibiotics are employed in documented cases of meningitis caused by *N. meningitidis* and *H. influenzae* to eliminate nasopharyngeal carriage of the organisms among contacts and prevent spread of invasive disease. In cases of meningococcal meningitis, prophylaxis is indicated only for household or intimate contacts of the index case. Chemoprophylaxis is not necessary for casual contacts or medical personnel unless there is direct exposure to respiratory secretions. The recommended agent is rifampin (Rifadin) at a dose of 10 mg/kg (or 600 mg in adults) twice a day for 2 days. Ciprofloxacin (Cipro)[1] 500 mg as a single dose is also effective and is often used in adult contacts.

Chemoprophylaxis for *H. influenzae* meningitis is recommended for all household contacts of an index case if one of the contacts is an unvaccinated child younger than 4 years old. It is also necessary for the

[1]Not FDA approved for this indication.

[1]Not FDA approved for this indication.

index case to receive prophylaxis, because *Haemophilus* organisms are not reliably eradicated from the nasopharynx by intravenous antibiotics. The preferred regimen for prophylaxis against *H. influenzae* is rifampin,[1] 20 mg/kg (or 600 mg in adults) once a day for 4 days.

The widespread use of the vaccine against *H. influenzae* in children resulted in a 94% reduction in *H. influenzae* meningitis between 1987 and 1995. The pneumococcal polysaccharide vaccine (Pneumovax 23) is recommended for patients >65 years old and chronically ill patients and has been shown to be effective in preventing invasive pneumococcal disease. Clear proof of its effectiveness in preventing pneumococcal meningitis is still lacking. Interest in the meningococcal polysaccharide vaccine (Menomune-A/C/Y/W-135) has increased following several apparent clusters of meningococcal meningitis among college students. Recommendations regarding the widespread use of the vaccine for college students have been mixed; however, in view of the excellent safety record of the vaccine, its use may be warranted especially for freshmen living in college dormitories.

[1]Not FDA approved for this indication.

INFECTIOUS MONONUCLEOSIS

METHOD OF

Hal B. Jenson, MD

Infectious mononucleosis connotes a self-limited clinical syndrome usually caused by Epstein-Barr virus (EBV) with prominent manifestations of fever, fatigue and malaise, tender lymphadenopathy, and sore throat. It was originally described as glandular fever in the late nineteenth century and is still known by this name in Europe. Easy transmissibility and the characteristic mononuclear response with atypical-appearing lymphocytes led to the term infectious mononucleosis.

Etiology

EBV was discovered in 1964 in cells of Burkitt lymphoma, and identified in 1968 by serologic studies as the principal cause of infectious mononucleosis. EBV is an enveloped, double-stranded DNA virus of the *Herpesviridae* family with a genome of approximately 172,000 base pairs encoding about 100 gene products. Approximately 10% of cases of infectious mononucleosis are caused by other agents, principally cytomegalovirus (CMV) and *Toxoplasma gondii*, and occasionally attributed to adenovirus, hepatitis A, hepatitis B, human immunodeficiency virus, and rubella virus.

Epidemiology

EBV infection is present in 95% or more of adults worldwide. In developing countries and in socioeconomically disadvantaged populations of developed countries, primary infection usually occurs during infancy and early childhood, with 95% to 100% of children being seropositive by 2 to 4 years of age. Infection in young children is generally asymptomatic or only mildly and nonspecifically symptomatic. Among affluent populations in developed countries, early childhood infection is still most frequent but approximately 33% to 50% of infections occur during adolescence and early adulthood. Primary EBV infection in adolescents and young adults is manifest in approximately 59% of cases by fever, pharyngitis, and generalized lymphadenopathy, which is the characteristic triad of infectious mononucleosis. Thus, the clinical disease of EBV-associated infectious mononucleosis is most commonly observed among 15- to 25-year-old individuals in higher socioeconomic groups in industrialized countries, despite the higher incidence of EBV infection among young children.

EBV shows no sex predilection and no seasonal variation. The peak age-specific incidence for cases outside of childhood is approximately 18 years for men and 16 years for women. No substantive evidence for adverse outcome of in utero or congenital infection has been found. Outbreaks are uncommon, although college and military populations experience high incidence rates.

Pathophysiology

EBV is usually transmitted person-to-person via salivary secretions from infected individuals. The efficiency of transmission is low and appears to require close contact such as sexual contact or kissing, hence the moniker *kissing disease*. Environmental sources and fomites do not seem to be important. Post-transfusion infectious mononucleosis is most commonly attributable to CMV.

EBV infection begins with local viral replication in the epithelium of the oropharynx, resulting in hypertrophy and inflammation of pharyngeal lymphoid tissue. Viral infection spreads to B lymphocytes and is quickly followed by an intense CD8 T lymphocyte immune response. The circulating atypical lymphocytes that are characteristic of infectious mononucleosis are CD8 T lymphocytes that exhibit both suppressor and cytotoxic functions. A relative as well as absolute increase in CD8 lymphocytes results in a lymphocytosis with transient reversal of the normal 2:1, CD4:CD8 T-lymphocyte ratio. The entire lymphoreticular system becomes involved. Lymph nodes throughout the body show moderate enlargement and increased numbers of active lymphoid follicles. Hepatocytes may demonstrate minimal swelling associated with lymphocytic and monocytic portal infiltration. The spleen is enlarged with hyperplasia of the red pulp, and the bone marrow is usually normocellular to mildly hypercellular. Many of the clinical manifestations of infectious mononucleosis may result, at least in part, from the host immune response.

After primary infection, EBV establishes lifelong infection of the host that is latently maintained by multiple episomal copies in the nuclei of resting B lymphocytes. In contrast, epithelial mucosal cells are lytically infected and release infectious viral particles. EBV can be cultured from the oropharynx of 75% to 100% of persons during the acute phase of infectious mononucleosis and is subsequently shed sporadically for life in salivary secretions. Approximately 10% to 25% of asymptomatic seropositive healthy adults are shedding virus in oral secretions at any given time. The prevalence of oral shedding is as high as 50% in the presence of immunosuppression such as with organ transplant or cancer chemotherapy, and is as high as 80% to 90% among persons infected with acquired immunodeficiency syndrome.

EBV was the first virus to be identified as a human tumor virus, and has been closely associated, although not necessarily causally, with Burkitt lymphoma in Africa, nasopharyngeal carcinoma, some types of Hodgkin's disease, B cell lymphoproliferations and leiomyosarcomas in cancer patients, solid organ and bone marrow transplant recipients, and persons with immunodeficiency disorders including X-linked lymphoproliferative syndrome and the acquired immunodeficiency syndrome. The precise etiologic role of EBV in the development of these tumors remains to be defined, however.

Clinical Manifestations

The incubation period of EBV-associated infectious mononucleosis is approximately 30 to 60 days. The cardinal symptoms of infectious mononucleosis in adolescents and adults include fever, easy fatigability and malaise, cervical or generalized tender lymphadenopathy, and sore throat, with the additional signs of splenomegaly and hepatomegaly. Minor symptoms often include headache and myalgias. The onset of symptoms may be abrupt or gradual with symptoms that progressively develop slowly over several days and persist for a variable period. Primary EBV infection in young children is usually asymptomatic. There is gradual spontaneous resolution and a total duration of usually 1 to 4 weeks, although lymphadenopathy and fatigue may persist for up to 6 weeks.

Lymphadenopathy is bilateral and usually diffuse, and is most prominent in the anterior and posterior cervical, submandibular, and occipital lymph nodes, and less frequently involves the axillary and inguinal lymph nodes. The nodes are freely mobile and mildly but not exquisitely tender. Tonsillar enlargement with pharyngeal erythema, which may be exudative, are usually present. A few petechiae at the junction of the hard and soft palate are occasionally evident. Splenomegaly is present in up to 59% of patients by physical examination and up to 100% of patients by ultrasonography. Hepatomegaly is present in up to 10% of patients.

Hepatomegaly and hepatic tenderness occur in 10% to 15% of cases, with mild jaundice in approximately 5% of cases. Lymphocytic infiltration of the liver and proliferation of Kupffer cells results in mild intrahepatic cholestasis but with maintenance of the lobular architecture, and without necrosis. Mild, transient elevations in hepatic transaminases occur in 50% to 80% of cases during the second to fourth weeks of illness with levels that are usually up to four times normal.

Various rashes have been described in approximately 5% of cases. An unusual but nonspecific maculopapular, erythematous rash following administration of ampicillin consistently occurs in adolescents and adults with infectious mononucleosis.

Autoimmune hemolytic anemia occurs in approximately 3% of cases, with onset during the first 2 weeks of illness and lasting for less than 4 weeks. Mild thrombocytopenia and neutropenia are common. Severe neutropenia to less than 1000 neutrophils/mm^3 and typically lasting a few days to 1 to 2 weeks occurs in approximately 3% of cases.

Severe neurologic manifestations, primarily meningoencephalitis, occur in up to 5% of cases. Most neurologic symptoms resolve without sequelae in 1 week to 3 months. Guillain-Barré syndrome, facial nerve palsy, optic neuritis, and transverse myelitis may occur.

Visual hallucinations and acute psychotic reactions are reported occasionally, and auditory and gustatory hallucinations are reported rarely. An "Alice-in-Wonderland" syndrome of metamorphopsia, which is the distortion of perception of sizes, shapes, and spatial relationships of objects, has been described, especially in children.

EBV infection in immunosuppressed persons, such as solid organ and bone marrow transplant recipients or those with AIDS, may result in progressive lymphoproliferation and extranodal lymphoma. The incidence of malignant lymphoproliferations in transplant recipients is approximately 1% in adults and 4% in children, presumably reflecting an increased incidence of primary infection in seronegative children.

Unregulated EBV replication in persons with AIDS may lead to lymphocytic interstitial pneumonitis and oral hairy leukoplakia. Lymphoid interstitial pneumonitis has been described primarily in children with AIDS, and has decreased in incidence with highly active antiretroviral therapy. The causal role for EBV is not firmly established, but it is plausible and supported by studies confirming the presence of EBV and a characteristic peribronchial infiltration of cytotoxic T lymphocytes directed against alveolar epithelial cells. Corticosteroid therapy is beneficial in both clinical and radiographic improvement. Oral hairy leukoplakia occurs almost exclusively in adults with AIDS. The lesions appear as white, raised lesions from 5 to 30 mm with a corrugated, rough surface along the lateral margins of the tongue. EBV is found by in situ hybridization in the upper layers of the epithelium.

The X-linked lymphoproliferative (XLP) syndrome, also known as Duncan syndrome, is a rare X-linked disorder that has been reported in 272 males in 80 kindreds. The defective gene product is known as SAP for SLAM-associated protein. SLAM (signaling lymphocyte activate molecule) is upregulated on both T and B cells with infection. SAP inhibits the upregulation of SLAM, preventing uncontrolled lymphoproliferation of EBV infection in immunocompetent hosts. Males with XLP syndrome are healthy until they acquire EBV infection. About 66% of affected males develop fulminating and fatal infectious mononucleosis with primary EBV infections. The survivors typically develop either hypogammaglobulinemia or B cell lymphoma, or both, with a mortality rate approaching 85% by 10 years of age.

Diagnosis

A clinical diagnosis of infectious mononucleosis is based on the pattern of typical clinical symptoms in the presence of absolute lymphocytosis, which usually peaks during the first and second weeks of illness, with more than 5% atypical lymphocytes—the hallmark laboratory finding of infectious mononucleosis. The diagnosis is confirmed by a positive heterophile antibody test or by definitive EBV-specific serologic tests (Figure 1). Approximately 80% of children at 4 years of age or older and 90% of adolescents and older patients with primary EBV infection have heterophile antibodies; children younger than 4 years of age and adults older than 40 years of age have lower heterophile antibody responses that may not be detectable. Heterophile-negative infectious mononucleosis in adults implies an illness that is not caused by EBV.

The heterophile antibodies in human serum are associated with acute infectious mononucleosis—also known as Bunnell-Davidsohn antibodies, agglutinate sheep and horse erythrocytes, among others—and are adsorbed by beef red blood cells but not guinea pig kidney cells. These immunoglobulin (Ig) M antibodies have no affinity against any EBV antigens. This antibody response usually peaks in the second and third weeks of illness, and can be detected for up to 6 to 9 months after resolution of symptoms, especially in adults. Approximately 20% of patients have a positive heterophile test for 18 months or longer. The most widely used method for detection of heterophile antibodies is the qualitative, rapid slide test.

EBV-specific serologic testing is usually used for definitive diagnosis, and is indicated if the heterophile antibody test is negative or if a positive heterophile antibody test is associated with clinical or laboratory findings uncharacteristic of infectious mononucleosis. Several distinct EBV-associated antigen systems have been characterized (Table 1 and see Figure 1). The viral capsid antigen (VCA), early antigen (EA),

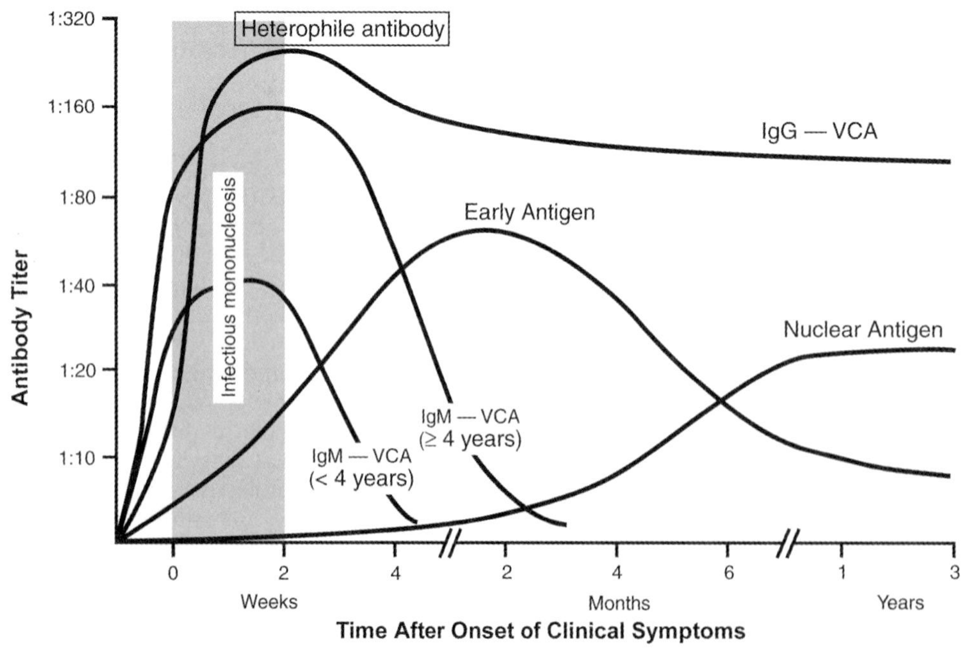

FIGURE 1 Schematic of the development of antibodies to various Epstein-Barr virus antigens in patients with infectious mononucleosis. The titers are geometric mean values expressed as reciprocals of the serum dilution. The immunoglobulin (Ig) M response to viral capsid antigen (VCA) is less in children younger than 4 years of age. IgG = immunoglobulin G. Reprinted with permission from Jenson HB, Ench Y: Epstein-Barr virus. In Rose NR, Hamilton RG, Detrick B (eds): Manual of Clinical Laboratory Immunology, 6th ed. Washington, DC, American Society for Microbiology, 2002.

TABLE 1 Correlation of Clinical Status and Serologic Responses to EBV Infection*

Clinical Status	Heterophile Antibodies (Qualitative Test)	Serologic Response EBV-Specific Antibody				
		IgM-VCA	IgG-VCA	EA-D	EA-R	EBNA
Negative reaction	–	<1:8†	<1:10†	<1:10†	<1:10†	<1:2.5†
Susceptible	–	–	–	–	–‡	–
Acute primary infection: infectious mononucleosis	+	1:32 to 1:256	1:160 to 1:640	1:40 to 1:160	–‡	– to 1:2.5
Recent primary infection: infectious mononucleosis	+/–	– to 1:32	1:320 to 1:1,280	1:40 to 1:160	–‡	1:5 to 1:10
Remote infection	–	–	1:40 to 1:160	–§	– to 1:40	1:10 to 1:40
Reactivation: immunosuppressed or immunocompromised	–	–	1:320 to 1:1,280	–§	1:80 to 1:320	– to 1:160
Burkitt lymphoma	–	–	1:320 to 1:1,280	–§	1:80 to 1:320	1:10 to 1:80
Nasopharyngeal carcinoma	–	–	1:320 to 1:1,280	1:40 to 1:160	–¶	1:20 to 1:160

*The data were obtained from numerous studies. Individual responses outside the characteristic range may occur.
†Or the lowest test dilution.
‡In young children and adults with asymptomatic seroconversion, the antiearly antigen response may be mainly to the EA-R component.
§A minority of individuals will have the antiearly antigen response mainly to the EA-D component.
¶A minority of individuals will have the antiearly antigen response mainly to the EA-R component.
Abbreviations: – = negative; + = positive; EA-D = diffuse staining component of EA; EA-R = cytoplasmic restricted component of early antigen; EBNA = EBV-determined nuclear antigens; EBV = Epstein-Barr virus; IgM = immunoglobulin M; IgG = immunoglobulin G; VCA = viral capsid antigen.
Table data from Jenson HB, Ench Y: Epstein-Barr virus. In Rose NR, Hamilton RG, Detrick B (eds): Manual of Clinical Laboratory Immunology, 6th ed. Washington, DC, American Society for Microbiology, 2002.

and EBV nuclear antigen (EBNA) systems are the most useful for diagnosis. The acute phase of infectious mononucleosis is characterized by rapid IgM and IgG antibody responses to VCA in all cases. The IgM response to VCA is transient, whereas the IgG response to VCA usually peaks during the acute illness, declines slightly over the next few weeks to months, and then remains at a relatively stable level for life. An IgG response to the EA complex is seen in most cases. EA antibodies are usually present for several months but may persist at low titers for several years following resolution of the acute infection, and therefore cannot be used to confirm acute infection. EBNA antibodies emerge after 2 to 4 months following the onset of illness and persist for life. The presence of EBNA antibodies indicates remote EBV infection.

The detection of IgM antibody to VCA is the most valuable and specific serologic test for the diagnosis of acute EBV infection, and is sufficient to confirm an acute EBV infection. The IgM-VCA antibody response is detectable for up to 4 months after clinical onset of the infectious mononucleosis, and in a few cases even longer. More than 80% of patients with infectious mononucleosis develop a transient antibody response to the EA-D (EA-diffuse) component. In some adults and especially in young children, however, this response may be directed mainly against the EA-R (EA-restricted) component.

Latent or quiescent EBV infection is characterized concomitant presence of moderate but stable titers of IgG antibodies to VCA and EBNA, and the absence of IgM antibody to VCA. Antibodies to EA are usually absent, but may be intermittently present at low titers, predominantly to the EA-R component, in up to 10% of healthy persons following EBV infection.

High titers of IgG antibody to VCA and EA are considered to indicate enhanced EBV activity or reactivation. Characteristic antibody profiles have been noted in persons with Burkitt lymphoma, nasopharyngeal carcinoma, and immunosuppression or immunodeficient states (see Table 1).

Assessment of plasma viral load by real time polymerase chain reaction (PCR) quantitative assay for detection of EBV DNA is of value for assessment of life-threatening infections such as post-transplant lymphoproliferative disorder. EBV can be cultured in peripheral blood lymphocytes, cultured alone, or co-cultivated with human umbilical cord lymphocytes, using the transformation assay, which requires 6 to 8 weeks and does not discern the quantitative level of EBV replication. In situ hybridization for EBERs (EBV-encoded RNAs), which are expressed in excess of 10^6 copies per cell in latently infected lymphocytes, is a very sensitive method for EBV detection in tissue samples.

Treatment

There is no effective specific treatment for EBV-associated infectious mononucleosis. Randomized clinical trials of acyclovir treatment of infectious mononucleosis show no clinical benefit. There is significant reduction in the rate of oropharyngeal EBV shedding during 10 days of therapy, but no difference in oropharyngeal shedding at 3 weeks. Persons with fulminating disease and immunocompromised persons may benefit from acyclovir therapy.

Rest and symptomatic therapy are the mainstays of management. Acetaminophen or ibuprofen should be used for fever. Intravenous hydration may be necessary, especially in young children if tonsillar hypertrophy interferes with swallowing. Subcapsular splenic hemorrhage and spontaneous rupture of the spleen are celebrated but rare complications of infectious mononucleosis, occurring in less than 0.5% of cases in adults. The highest incidence is during the second and third week of illness, and is rarely fatal. Because blunt abdominal trauma may predispose to splenic rupture, it is customary and prudent to advise exclusion from contact sports and strenuous physical activities for the first 2 to 3 weeks of illness, or if splenomegaly is present on physical examination at least until the splenomegaly is resolved. Although approximately 50% of patients with splenic rupture have a history of abdominal trauma, such recommendations have not been documented to reduce the incidence of splenic rupture.

Transient psychologic distress, somatization, and functional disability are common during acute infection, and depressive symptoms appear to occur more frequently with infectious mononucleosis than with other viral illnesses.

The benefit of corticosteroids for complications of infectious mononucleosis is advocated based on anecdotal experience but has not been critically evaluated and remains controversial. Corticosteroids are unnecessary in mild, uncomplicated cases and should not be routinely administered to all persons with infectious mononucleosis. Indications include incipient upper airway obstruction, autoimmune hemolytic anemia or neutropenia, thrombocytopenia with hemorrhage, and meningoencephalitis and other neurologic complications. Tonsillar hypertrophy and progressive airway obstruction with respiratory symptoms occurs in less than 5% of all cases, but are the most common indications for hospitalization for infectious mononucleosis. Younger children appear to be at greater risk. Intravenous dexamethasone (Decadron) (0.25 mg/kg every 6 hours), methylprednisolone (Solu-Medrol)[1] (1 mg/kg every 6 hours), and oral prednisone (40 mg daily) given for 1 to 3 days have all been used with equivalent results of dramatic subjective improvement within 24 hours and objective improvement within 72 hours. Corticosteroid therapy may hasten resolution of complications in some but not all cases of infectious mononucleosis. Reluctance to use corticosteroids is based on the unknown long-term effects of administering an immunomodulator for a virus that establishes intracellular latency and is associated with several malignancies, especially since the normal immune response is usually quite effective in facilitating recovery. Intravenous immunoglobulin[1] may be as good or better than corticosteroids for treatment of thrombocytopenia or hemolytic anemia associated with infectious mononucleosis.

[1]Not FDA approved for this indication.

Unusually severe immune responses during infectious mononucleosis may occur with exaggerated symptoms of persistent or intermittent fever, generalized lymphadenopathy, and hepatosplenomegaly with extremely high antibody titers and high viral burdens. Most cases of fatal infectious mononucleosis are the consequence of an apparently uncontrolled lymphoproliferative response to primary EBV infection and demonstrate hemophagocytic lymphohistiocytosis. EBV is considered to be the principal cause of severe cases of virus-associated hemophagocytic syndrome, a nonmalignant generalized histiocytic proliferation with marked hemophagocytic lymphohistiocytosis. Treatment with etoposide (VePesid)[1], which reduces both monocyte and macrophage activity, and corticosteroids may be an effective therapy.

Polyclonal post-transplant lymphoproliferative disease is best managed by reducing the immunosuppression to a minimal level, combined with acyclovir (Zovirax)[1]. Monoclonal post-transplant lymphoproliferative disease has been treated with rituximab (Rituxan)[1]. The future treatments of choice for both of these diseases are adoptive transfer of EBV-specific immunity by infusion of unmodified lymphocytes from human leukocyte antigen (HLA)-matched healthy EBV-seropositive donors, or in vitro expansion of HLA-matched reactivated EBV-specific cytotoxic T lymphocytes. Use of adoptive therapy requires strategy planning to generate cell lines prospectively from individuals at risk of severe EBV infection, such as before organ transplantation or from HLA-matched seropositive donors.

Prognosis

The clinical course of infectious mononucleosis in healthy persons is usually 1 to 4 weeks, with maximal fever, lymphadenopathy, and sore throat occurring during the first 2 weeks of illness and then gradually resolving. The disease is much milder during the third week. The constitutional symptoms of malaise and fatigue may resolve more slowly, with convalescence over several weeks to even months in otherwise unremarkable cases. Unusual persistence of fatigue for months to a few years following infection with EBV or influenza virus infection is well-recognized.

[1]Not FDA approved for this indication.

Both biologic and psychologic determinants are important in the clinical expression of infectious mononucleosis in adolescents and adults. Several studies of convalescence after acute systemic infection support the view that symptomatic recovery critically depends on the emotional state and attitude of the patient. An individual with a propensity for depression is more likely to respond to acute infection with depression-like symptoms than a person who does not have such a vulnerability. There is no evidence for a causative role for EBV in the pathogenesis of chronic fatigue syndrome.

Prevention

EBV is ubiquitous. Because intimate contact is necessary for transmission, isolation of patients with infectious mononucleosis is unnecessary. Individuals with infectious mononucleosis should not donate blood during acute illnesses for a minimum of 6 months. There is no vaccine against EBV, although numerous approaches are under investigation.

CHRONIC FATIGUE SYNDROME

METHOD OF

Lionel C. Bailly, MD

Severe fatigue goes far beyond the normal physiological experience of tiredness and can be distressing and debilitating. It usually poses a significant challenge to the medical profession. To be able to provide the best-adapted treatment or health care management of debilitating fatigue, using the best evidence available, health professionals should pay particular attention to a positive diagnosis of the condition that generates fatigue in their patients. In addition to the many organic and psychiatric disorders that cause fatigue, a specific condition has been described. This is chronic fatigue syndrome (CFS), and it remains highly contentious because the etiology and pathogenesis of CFS are not clearly elucidated, and uncertainty continues to surround these issues.

Why a Controversy?

Patients with CFS suffer from symptoms that some medical experts believe are not signs of a recognized illness. They may find it hard to justify their suffering as legitimate in the eyes of a public that values the opinions of medical experts. From the health professional's point of view, because CFS symptoms do not conform to the codified rational explanation of diseases, the syndrome falls into a mysterious or unsubstantiated disease category. Sufferers are reclassified as "difficult, illness-focused, demanding, medializing," and then passed to the medical domain of imagined illnesses. The patients may then become frustrated and begin to question the professional's expertise. Some patients are concerned that their illness is not taken seriously, that some general practitioners show indifference, or that they do not always understand the illness and its possible severity.

Controversy

- Doctors are frustrated to have no explanation for CFS sufferers' symptoms.
- Patients are upset to be treated like simulators.

Terminology

Several names have been suggested for this syndrome but none is fully satisfactory. *Chronic fatigue syndrome* (CFS) is the most commonly accepted term by professionals, but fatigue, although invariably present, may not be the major symptom. In the United Kingdom (UK), the term *myalgic encephalomyelitis* has been suggested, but myalgic is inappropriate for those patients with little muscle pain, and encephalomyelitis describes an inflammation of the brain and spinal cord for which there is no evidence. The term *immune dysfunction* is also unsatisfactory, because the relevance of observed abnormalities and an immune cause for the disease are not established.

- Of all the terms suggested, chronic fatigue syndrome (CFS) is the most commonly accepted by professionals.

Etiology

The etiology and pathogenesis of CFS are not clearly elucidated, and uncertainty continues to surround these issues. Although CFS has certain characteristic features, the condition may be heterogeneous both in causative factors and in its clinical nature. The heterogeneity could represent the range of a single condition, or could mean that several distinct diseases are being bracketed together because of the similarity of their clinical appearance.

Research has demonstrated immune, endocrine, musculoskeletal, and neurologic abnormalities, but to what extent these abnormalities are part of the primary disease process or secondary consequences remains the subject of debate.

Etiology

- The etiology and pathogenesis of CFS are not clearly elucidated.
- Immune, endocrine, musculoskeletal, and neurologic abnormalities could be causes or consequences of the disease.

Diagnostic Process

No laboratory test has yet been found that has the sensitivity and specificity to constitute a diagnostic test for CFS. Until such a test is found, the diagnosis of CFS will be based on clinical findings. Because fatigue can be caused by many conditions other than CFS, it is of utmost importance to safely establish a diagnosis for CFS; otherwise, the risk is either to apply the wrong treatment programs to CFS patients or to miss applying appropriate treatments for other fatigue-inducing illnesses. Diagnosis is based on the recognition of the typical symptom pattern together with exclusion of alternative conditions. When a clinically evaluated, unexplained chronic fatigue case fails to meet the criteria for CFS, the diagnostic category idiopathic chronic fatigue is used.

Positive Diagnosis

The diagnosis is based on the recognition of typical symptoms of CFS and the exclusion of other conditions, which would better explain the presence of disabling fatigue.

RECOGNITION OF TYPICAL SYMPTOMS OF CHRONIC FATIGUE SYNDROME*

1. Persistent or relapsing chronic fatigue:

- Clinically evaluated
- Unexplained
- Not the result of ongoing exertion
- Not substantially alleviated by rest
- Substantial reduction in previous levels of occupational, educational, social, or personal activities

2. The concurrent occurrence of four or more of the following symptoms, which must not have predated the fatigue:

- Self-reported impairment in short-term memory
- Self-reported impairment in concentration
- Sore throat
- Tender cervical or axillary lymph nodes
- Muscle pain
- Multijoint pain without joint swelling or redness
- Headaches of a new type, pattern, or severity
- Unrefreshing sleep
- Postexertional malaise lasting more than 24 hours

3. Duration:

- Six or more consecutive months

EXCLUSION OF ALTERNATIVE CONDITIONS

Any of the following active medical conditions may explain the presence of chronic fatigue:

- Addison's disease
- Anemia (hematological conditions and other causes)
- Chronic infections (e.g., Lyme disease, hepatitis C, tuberculosis, parasitic disease)
- Celiac disease
- Hypopituitarism
- Iatrogenic conditions (side effects of beta blockers, interferon, etc.)
- Immunodeficiency
- Malignancy
- Multiple sclerosis
- Myasthenia gravis
- Obesity (severe as defined by a body mass index ≥45)
- Primary sleep disorder (e.g., sleep apnea, narcolepsy, restless leg syndrome)
- Rheumatic diseases (e.g., Sjögren's disease)
- Thyroid disease

Any of the following previously diagnosed medical conditions, if not resolved beyond reasonable clinical doubt and exhibit continued activity, may explain the chronic fatigue illness:

- Treated malignancy
- Hepatitis B or C
- Mononucleosis
- Parasitic infection

Any past or present diagnosis of the following psychiatric conditions may explain the chronic fatigue illness:

- Alcohol or other substance abuse within 2 years prior to the onset of the chronic fatigue
- Anorexia nervosa or bulimia nervosa
- Bipolar affective disorders
- Conversion disorder
- Delusional disorders of any subtype
- Dementia of any subtype
- Hypochondriasis
- Major depressive disorder
- Neurasthenia
- Pain disorder
- Schizophrenia of any subtype
- Somatization disorder

Chronic Fatigue and Psychiatric Disorders

A variety of psychiatric conditions can generate fatigue.

*Adapted from Fukuda, et al (1994) *Ann Intern Med*, 121:953-959.

Fatigue in Psychiatric Conditions

- Is genuinely experienced
- Is not intentionally produced or feigned
- Is beyond the patient's control
- Causes impairment that is real

Because fatigue is a well-documented symptom of many psychiatric conditions, it is important to differentiate between CFS and these conditions. General practitioners may need the opinion of a psychiatrist or clinical psychologist to rule out some unusual psychiatric disorders. Patients are often reluctant to consider the possibility of a psychiatric condition, or to accept a referral to a psychiatrist or clinical psychologist for diagnostic purposes. It is important, however, that such a diagnostic is carried out, first to ensure that the sufferers receive the most appropriate treatment, and second to ensure that research into CFS is not compromised by the inclusion of non-CFS sufferers.

The psychiatric disorder most difficult to distinguish from CFS is neurasthenia. Neurasthenia is defined in the International Classification of Diseases 10 (ICD-10) as a neurotic disorder whose main feature is a complaint of increased fatigue after mental effort, often associated with some decrease in occupational performance or coping efficiency in daily tasks. The mental fatigability is typically described as an unpleasant intrusion of distracting associations or recollections, difficulty in concentrating, and generally inefficient thinking. In a recent epidemiologic study, 1.5% of a large sample of the Australian general population met the ICD-10 neurasthenia criteria in the past year.

ICD-10 Diagnostic Guidelines for Neurasthenia:

- Persistent and distressing complaints of increased fatigue after mental effort, or persistent and distressing complaints of bodily weakness and exhaustion after minimal effort, or persistent and distressing complaints of bodily weakness and exhaustion after minimal effort

- At least two of the following:

  Feeling of muscular aches and pains
  Dizziness
  Tension headaches
  Sleep disturbance
  Inability to relax
  Irritability
  Dyspepsia

- Any autonomic or depressive symptoms present that are not sufficiently persistent and severe to fulfill the criteria for any of the more specific disorders in this classification

No research has been carried out into the treatment of neurasthenia, but anecdotal evidence suggests that pharmacologic agents are not very helpful, and that psychodynamic psychotherapy and cognitive behavioral therapy produce the best results.

Another psychiatric condition that leads to increased fatigability and diminished activity is depression, and it is important to rule this out. This often presents a chicken-and-egg conundrum, as CFS sufferers can become depressed *because* of their illness. Typically when fatigue is the consequence of depression, depressive symptoms are present before the fatigue becomes the main complaint. Antidepressant medication is also likely to lead to major and fast improvement in cases of fatigue secondary to depression, while CFS sufferers who become depressed do not see any major improvement in their fatigue with the antidepressant treatment.

Individuals with somatization disorder usually describe their complaints in colorful, exaggerated terms, but are unable to provide specific factual information. They often seek treatment from several physicians concurrently, which may lead to complicated and sometimes hazardous combinations of treatments. They commonly display prominent anxiety symptoms and depressive moods, and may also show impulsive and antisocial behavior, make suicide threats and attempts, and experience marital discord. The history of their physical complaints begins before the age of 30 years.

The essential feature of conversion disorder is the presence of symptoms or deficits affecting voluntary motor or sensory functions, which are not explained by a neurologic or other general medical condition. Psychological factors are judged to be associated with the symptom or deficit, a judgment based on the observation that the initiation or exacerbation of the symptom or deficit is preceded by conflicts or other stressors.

Subjects with pain disorder experience pain of sufficient severity to cause significant distress or impairment in social, occupational or other important areas of functioning. Psychological factors are judged to play a significant role in the onset, severity, exacerbation, or maintenance of the pain. The pain is not better accounted for by mood, psychotic, or anxiety disorders and does not meet the criteria for dyspareunia.

Hypochondriasis is the preoccupation with fears of having, or the idea that one has, a serious disease. This fear is based on the person's misinterpretation of bodily symptoms. The preoccupation persists despite appropriate medical evaluation and reassurance. The preoccupation causes clinically significant distress or impairment in social, occupational, or other important areas of functioning.

Prognosis of Chronic Fatigue Syndrome

Severity of illness is a major factor of chronicity. The more severely affected patients tend to be ill longer. Individuals for whom the onset of the illness is acute appear to have a better prognosis than those for whom the onset is gradual. Epidemic or *clustered* disease seems to have a better prognosis than sporadic disease. In children, as among adults, the prognosis appears worse for more severe cases. Overall, the duration of the disease appears to be shorter in younger people than in adults, and a high proportion of children appear to recover.

Management of Chronic Fatigue Syndrome

NONPHARMACOLOGIC MANAGEMENT

As CFS is a chronic illness of unknown etiology, the aim of the professional is to develop a supportive relationship and provide information and education to assist the patients and their families, and to guide them toward self-management with support. Management plans and therapeutic approaches require continual assessment, supervision, and reevaluation. The frequency of the evaluation is based on the severity of the illness, on the plan agreed to jointly between clinician and patient, and, in the case of children, the child and parents.

Patients with CFS and their families need clear clinical communication on options, progress, and prognosis. Information on the nature of the condition and self-management seems to facilitate adjustment to the illness and a better outcome. Such education is particularly important for anticipating and managing fluctuations or more substantial remissions and relapses.

A key component in the successful management of a long-term illness is to involve patients as partners in care, whatever their age. Taking a patient's views into consideration leads to higher satisfaction, better compliance with treatment, and greater continuity of care. A partnership approach to management acknowledges that the patient must continue to cope with the illness throughout its duration, rather than just during intermittent clinical interventions.

It appears that CFS may be ameliorated by graded exercise, psychotherapy/cognitive behavioral therapy, and pacing. These therapies may improve the patients' levels of functioning, but there is no evidence that CFS can be cured. Overall, the evidence available is patchy and there is a clear need for a good randomized, controlled study of therapeutic intervention for CFS.

Nonpharmacologic Management

- Professional:

  Support, information, and education
  Patient self-management with support

- Patient:

  Graded exercise
  Pacing
  Psychotherapy/cognitive behavioral therapy

Graded exercise is a form of structured activity management that aims for gradual but progressive increases in aerobic activities such as walking or swimming. It is possible that inactivity is a factor that maintains the illness through physical deconditioning and its physiological consequences. Graded and supervised increases in exercise can help reverse the impact of inactivity. In addition, the gradual exposure of the patient to an activity that has been avoided may help restore the patient's self-esteem and confidence. Several randomized, controlled trials found varying degrees of improvement in fatigue and disability with differing graded exercise regimens compared with no treatment and two control treatments.

Randomized, controlled trials evaluating cognitive behavioral therapy found a positive overall effect for the intervention, with the majority of those who had the therapy demonstrating varying degrees of improvement in both function and fatigue. Qualitative studies of psychodynamic psychotherapy suggest that it may be helpful if applied appropriately by a clinician with experience of CFS, but that a too-rigid approach may jeopardize the possibility of success.

Pacing is an energy management strategy that involves living within the physical and mental limitations imposed by the illness. Patients are encouraged to achieve an appropriate balance between rest and activity by avoiding performing activities to a degree that exacerbates symptoms, or interspersing activity with periods of rest. The aim is to prevent patients from entering a vicious cycle of overactivity and setbacks, while assisting them to set realistic goals for increasing activity when appropriate.

One limitation of all trials of treatment effectiveness is that none of them have been able to include either children or people who were unable to attend outpatient clinics.

PHARMACOLOGIC THERAPY

Large, randomized, controlled trials of the pharmacologic treatment of CFS have failed to prove that any one particular agent is beneficial to sufferers. Until the etiology and pathogenesis are found it is unlikely that any definitive treatment will be identified. Pharmacologic management of CFS primarily involves the treatment of associated symptoms. In addition to their unpleasantness, some symptoms may exacerbate the impact of the illness and impede recovery and/or adaptation. Mood, sleep disturbances, and pain are the main symptoms that require treatment.

Mood Disturbances

Up to 50% of patients suffering from CFS experience major depression in the months and years after the onset of illness, and antidepressant agents are indicated. Selective serotonin reuptake inhibitors (SSRIs) are the most commonly prescribed antidepressants, but the evidence of efficiency from randomized, controlled trials is not encouraging.

Sleep Disturbances

Because of the chronicity of the symptoms, the prescription of hypnotic agents is not encouraged. Many professionals have tried low doses of sedative tricyclic antidepressants at bedtime (for example, amitriptyline [Elavil][1] at doses of 10-25 mg). Despite the absence of scientific evaluation of this treatment, anecdotal evidence is encouraging. It is important to remember that such low doses of tricyclic antidepressants have no therapeutic effect on symptoms of depression.

Pain

Patients experiencing headaches, myalgia, or arthralgia usually benefit from the simple prescription of nonsteroidal anti-inflammatory drugs (NSAIDs) such as ibuprofen or naproxen. More powerful NSAIDs are sometimes prescribed.

Pharmacologic Therapy

- No particular pharmacologic agent has yet been proven able to cure CFS.
- Pharmacologic management involves treatment of associated symptoms such as:

  Mood disturbances
  Sleep disturbances
  Pain

Severe fatigue is a common complaint at general practitioners' offices, although in many cases organic and psychiatric disorders may be the causes. However, besides these known disorders, a specific condition called chronic fatigue syndrome (CFS) has been described. CFS remains highly contentious because its etiology and pathogenesis have not been elucidated. No laboratory test has yet been found that has the sensitivity and specificity to constitute a diagnostic test for CFS, and, until such a test is found, the diagnosis of CFS will be based on clinical findings. Clinically, the diagnosis is based on the recognition of a clinically evaluated, unexplained, persistent or relapsing fatigue that is not the result of ongoing exertion, is not substantially alleviated by rest, and is not caused by another condition. Before confirming the diagnosis of something as contentious as CFS, it is important to rule out any active medical conditions, previously diagnosed medical conditions whose resolution has not been documented, and psychiatric disorders that may explain the chronic fatigue. As CFS is a chronic illness of unknown etiology, the aim of the professional should be to develop a supportive relationship that helps the patient toward self-management with support, and to provide information and education to assist the patients' families and caregivers. Management plans and therapeutic approaches require continual assessment, supervision, and reevaluation. A key component to successful management of long-term illnesses is to involve patients as partners in care, whatever their ages. There is no cure for CFS, but graded exercise, psychotherapy/ cognitive behavioral therapy, and pacing seem to be beneficial in modifying the illness. Large, randomized, controlled trials of pharmacologic treatment of CFS have failed to prove that one particular agent is beneficial to CFS sufferers, and pharmacologic management of CFS primarily involves the treatment of associated symptoms. Mood, sleep disturbances, and pain are the main symptoms that require treatment.

[1]Not FDA approved for this indication.

MUMPS

METHOD OF

Subhash Chaudhary, MD

Mumps (epidemic parotitis) is an acute, communicable disease caused by the RNA virus *Rubulavirus* in the *Paramyxoviridae* family. In the United States, as a result of administering the recommended two doses of the measles-mumps-rubella (MMR) vaccine to a high percentage of the population, there were only 266 reported cases for 2001 (an all-time low). This far exceeds the Healthy People 2001 objective of fewer than 500 cases per year.

In the prevaccine era, mumps was mainly a disease of young children with peaks between January and May and periodic outbreaks in young adults in the military. Since 1981, a majority of the cases have been in children 10 years of age or older with little seasonal variation. Now most cases of parotitis in immunized persons are not because of mumps. The virus is spread by respiratory droplets with an incubation period of 16 to 18 days. The prodromal phase of 1 to 2 days (which exhibits fever, headache, anorexia, and vomiting) is followed by painful enlargement in one (25%) or both parotid glands. The swelling of the glands reaches a peak in about 3 days and is associated with severe pain. Other salivary glands may be involved with (10%) or without (rare) involvement of the parotids. In approximately 33% of cases, swelling of the gland may not be clinically apparent. The fever and swelling resolve in 7 to 10 days. The patient is contagious 1 to 2 days before to 5 days after the onset of parotid swelling. In most infected children, systemic symptoms are mild but a variety of complications are known to occur.

Complications

In children, meningitis and mild meningoencephalitis are the most frequent complications. Typically meningitis develops 5 days after the onset of illness, but occasionally it can precede parotitis. Pleocytosis in cerebrospinal fluid may be seen in greater than 50% of cases, but signs and symptoms occur in fewer than 10% of children. Prognosis in central nervous system (CNS) disease is good. Rarely ataxia, facial palsy, hearing loss, Guillain-Barré syndrome, and transverse myelitis may be seen. Epididymo-orchitis and oophoritis almost never occur in prepubertal children. Approximately 33% of postpubertal males develop orchitis with the highest rates at 15 to 29 years of age. It manifests as painful swelling of one or both testes, chills, and recurrence of fever during the first 8 days of illness. The involved testicle may atrophy, but sterility occurs only in some patients with bilateral involvement. Oophoritis occurs in about 7% of postpubertal female patients. Pancreatitis is seen but severe involvement is rare. There are many cases of temporal association of diabetes mellitus although a causal relationship has not been confirmed. Increased fetal mortality has been reported with mumps during the first trimester, but there is no evidence of increased risk of fetal malformations. Other rare complications include thyroiditis, arthritis, mastitis, glomerulonephritis, myocarditis, endocardial fibroelastosis, and thrombocytopenia.

Diagnosis

During an outbreak diagnosis is straightforward. Because mumps is uncommon now, parotitis of unknown etiology lasting more than 2 days should be investigated to rule out mumps. Mumps and other viruses causing parotitis can be grown from saliva, throat swabs, or mouth washings using primary monkey kidney tissue culture. Diagnosis can also be confirmed by a greater than fourfold increase in antibody titer between acute and convalescent serum specimens by any standard serologic assay. Determination of the presence of mumps-specific immunoglobulin M (IgM) antibody by enzyme immunoassay is more helpful.

Purulent parotitis can be differentiated from mumps by expression of pus from Stensen's duct in addition to exquisite tenderness and leukocytosis with neutrophilic predominance. Lymphadenitis should be differentiated from parotitis. Cervical lymph nodes are below the ramus of the mandible, and enlarged preparotid nodes, which are associated with conjunctivitis, are anterior to the parotid.

Management

Supportive therapy is indicated because the illness is self-limited and no specific antiviral therapy is available. Adequate hydration and nutrition should be maintained. Acidic foods (orange juice) may cause discomfort and vomiting, and should be avoided. Acetaminophen and nonsteroidal anti-inflammatory drugs (NSAIDs) may be given for headache and discomfort. Narcotic analgesics like codeine, scrotal support, and ice may help patients with orchitis. There is no role for steroids in the management of mumps.

Prevention

Live-virus vaccine administered by subcutaneous injection as a monovalent vaccine (Mumpsvax) or, preferably, combined MMR should be given routinely at 12 to 15 months, with a second dose at 4 to 6 years of age. A single dose of the vaccine induces protective and long-lasting antibody in more than 95% of susceptible individuals. It is particularly important to vaccinate children approaching puberty, adolescents, and adults born after 1957 who have not had the mumps illness or mumps vaccine. Vaccine given after exposure does not prevent infection but will hinder subsequent exposures. Adverse events are rare, and there is no evidence that there is an increase in adverse events following reimmunization. The mumps vaccine can be given to children with minor illnesses with or without fever. Persons with a history of anaphylactic or other immediate reaction to egg ingestion, neomycin, or gelatin may be at increased risk of immediate-type hypersensitivity reaction after immunizations. The mumps vaccine should be given at least 2 weeks before or at least 3 months after administration of immune globulin. The vaccine is contraindicated in pregnant women, immunodeficient individuals, patients on immunosuppressive therapy, and those who have had an immediate hypersensitivity reaction to a previous dose of vaccine. MMR vaccine can be given to HIV-infected children unless they are severely immunosuppressed.

Infection Control

Droplet precautions, in addition to standard precautions, should be followed for 9 days after the onset of parotid swelling. During school outbreaks, students who continue to be exempted from mumps immunization should be excluded until at least 26 days after the onset of parotitis in the last person with mumps.

PLAGUE

METHOD OF

E. Geoffrey Playford, MB, BS

Epidemiology

Plague is a zoonotic disease caused by the gram-negative bacillus *Yersinia pestis* whose usual life cycle involves rodents as its principal host and fleas as its primary vector. Certain species of rodents are responsible for the stable maintenance of enzootic foci of infection, whereas other mammals, such as domestic rats and mice, squirrels, and prairie dogs, contribute to spreading or epizootic infection. Following ingestion, plague bacilli multiply within the flea midgut and eventually cause obstruction. The cycle is then completed with the regurgitation of subsequent blood meals, together with plague bacilli, into new mammalian hosts.

Humans are occasionally infected as incidental hosts via bites from infected fleas. Fleas from some mammals, such as squirrels, are more likely to transmit plague than others, such as domestic cats and dogs. Less commonly, human acquisition follows direct contact with infected mammals, particularly cats, or the inhalation of infected material. Human-to-human transmission may result from contact with a case of pneumonic plague.

Enzootic plague exists in semi-arid areas of all continents except Australia and Antarctica. Most human cases have been reported from Africa, Vietnam, Peru, Myanmar, and China. Within the United States, a large enzootic focus exists in the southwestern and Pacific coastal regions; around 10 cases are reported annually, principally from New Mexico, Arizona, Colorado, Utah, and California. Infection usually occurs during summer months when interaction between humans, rodents, and their fleas is most likely.

Several aspects of plague are of major contemporary concern—the increasing encroachment of humans into rural enzootic regions, the increasing importance of domestic cats as sources for human infection, and the potential use of plague as a biological warfare or bioterrorism agent.

Clinical Features

Plague presents as one of three primary forms—bubonic, septicemic, or pneumonic. Bubonic plague accounts for more than 75% of U.S. plague cases. Two to 6 days following a flea bite, it manifests with an abrupt onset of prominent systemic complaints (fever, headaches, and chills), followed by swollen tender regional lymphadenopathy (buboes), often with a marked overlying inflammation. Gastrointestinal symptoms (nausea, vomiting, and diarrhea) are often also prominent. Although commonest in inguinal and femoral nodes, buboes may form in other anatomical sites depending upon the flea bite location. Skin lesions at the site of flea bites occur infrequently. A fulminant and progressive clinical course with prostration, lethargy, delirium, high-grade fevers, and hemodynamic instability typically follows. Although such clinical features are generally distinctive, bubonic plague may be confused with other causes of regional lymphadenitis, including pyogenic infections (*Streptococcus pyogenes* and *Staphylococcus aureus*), cat-scratch disease, tularemia, and rat-bite fever. Bacteremia and secondary septicemic plague occur relatively commonly and, untreated, the mortality of bubonic plague exceeds 40%. However, with appropriate treatment, mortality averages 14%, with most deaths associated with delayed presentation or recognition.

Primary septicemic plague involves plague bacteremia, with rapidly progressive shock and disseminated intravascular coagulopathy, but without palpable lymphadenopathy. It is clinically indistinguishable from other causes of gram-negative septicemia. Overall, septicemic plague accounts for 10% of U.S. plague cases and has a mortality rate of 30% to 50%. Pneumonic plague presents as a rapidly overwhelming pneumonia. It has a very high mortality rate and may result in human-to-human transmission. Primary pneumonic plague is rare (2% of U.S. cases) and is typically acquired from infected cats, whereas secondary pneumonic plague complicates up to 10% of bubonic or septicemic plague cases.

Diagnosis

The diagnosis of bubonic plague should be considered in any patient exposed to fleas, rodents, or other animals in the southwestern United States (or other areas of plague endemicity) presenting with tender regional lymphadenitis, fever, and prostration. Although clinical features are less specific with other forms of plague, it should be considered in anyone with an appropriate exposure history. As soon as plague is clinically suspected, appropriate diagnostic specimens should be collected, specific antibiotic therapy commenced, and public health authorities notified. As all forms of plague may progress rapidly to death, antibiotic therapy should not be delayed, although several sets of blood cultures should be obtained first. Wherever possible, buboes should be aspirated—saline may need to be injected and re-aspirated into the node, as liquified material may not be present. Other specimens, such as sputum, skin biopsies, and cerebrospinal fluid (CSF), should be collected where clinically appropriate. Personal protective equipment including gloves, mask, eyewear, and gown should be used for these procedures. A rapid presumptive diagnosis may be obtained from stained smears of blood, bubo aspirate, or other specimens, as distinctive plague bacilli are often present in large numbers. Some laboratories also perform a direct immunofluorescence stain (DFA) on bubo aspirates.

All specimens should also be cultured using appropriate bacteriologic media to provide a definitive diagnosis. It is vital that clinicians directly contact laboratories and communicate clinical suspicions of plague to facilitate the timely and appropriate testing of specimens and the implementation of laboratory biohazard precautions. Although not rapid, serology is useful in situations where clinical specimens are either unavailable or nondiagnostic. Although elevated antibody titers on a single sample provides presumptive evidence of infection, a fourfold rise in antibody titers on paired serum specimens collected during acute and convalescent phases is diagnostic.

Treatment

Antibiotics with demonstrated clinical efficacy for plague include streptomycin, gentamicin (Garamycin)[1], doxycycline (Vibramycin), and chloramphenicol (Chloromycetin)[1]. Streptomycin (15 mg/kg, up to 2 g, every 12 hours intramuscularly) is the traditional antibiotic of choice and usually leads to defervescence within 3 days, although a full 10-day course is required to minimize the risk of relapse. Gentamicin (5 mg/kg/day or in 3 divided doses intravenously) appears to be a satisfactory alternative to streptomycin. Both agents require parenteral administration, may cause nephrotoxicity and ototoxicity, and may precipitate endotoxemic shock from rapid bacteriolysis when initially administered. Doxycycline (2.2 mg/kg for children ≥8 years of age, up to 100 mg, every 12 hours intravenously or orally) is an alternative for uncomplicated bubonic plague following defervescence from streptomycin therapy. It is, however, contraindicated in pregnant females and children younger than 8 years of age. No role for combination antibiotic therapy has been demonstrated in bubonic plague. Chloramphenicol (25 mg/kg every 6 hours intravenously) is recommended for plague meningitis when there is high CSF penetration. Fluoroquinolones appear highly active in animal models, although human data are lacking. Beta-lactam agents, including penicillins and cephalosporins, and macrolides are ineffective. Antibiotic-resistant strains are very rare and do not appear to be increasing in frequency.

Most patients require fluid resuscitation, if not more intensive hemodynamic support, particularly during the initial few days of therapy. Buboes usually recede with antibiotic therapy, although surgical drainage is occasionally required.

An effective insecticide should be applied to all patients and their clothing. Patients with bubonic plague should be managed with contact precautions for any secretions or drainages for at least 48 hours after instituting antibiotic therapy. The possibility of pneumonic plague should be considered in all patients; those with a cough, chest radiograph changes, septicemic plague, or in whom a high clinical index of suspicion exists should be strictly placed in respiratory isolation.

[1]Not FDA approved for this indication.

Prevention

Plague may be acquired in any recreational, occupational, or domestic situation where exposure to infected rodents and their fleas occurs; its prevention therefore relies on rodent and flea control within domestic environments, personal protective measures and insecticides to prevent flea bites, and avoidance of sick or dead animals. Where close exposure to a person or an animal with pneumonic plague or direct handling of infected material has occurred, postexposure prophylaxis is appropriate. Recommended prophylactic regimens include doxycycline (2.2 mg/kg for children ≥8 years, up to 100 mg, every 12 hours) or ciprofloxacin[1] (20 mg/kg, up to 500 mg, every 12 hours). A formalin-killed vaccine, used previously in laboratory workers and others at greatest risk, is no longer available.

Public Health Implications

All suspected plague cases should be reported to local public health authorities as a matter of urgency, as they may herald a larger epidemic. Primary pneumonic plague, in particular, is rare and a single case should prompt strong consideration of bioterrorism or a biological warfare exposure. All U.S. cases are investigated by the Centers for Disease Control and Prevention. Although urban plague is potentially controllable through a coordinated public health program, rural plague ultimately defies effective control given its widespread distribution through wild rodent reservoirs.

[1]Not FDA approved for this indication.

ANTHRAX

METHOD OF
Morton N. Swartz, MD

Anthrax is primarily a zoonotic illness caused by *Bacillus anthracis*, but humans may acquire the disease following various forms of contact with the microorganism. *B. anthracis* is an aerobic, nonmotile, nonhemolytic, gram-positive, spore-forming bacillus species. Its pathogenic potential stems from an antiphagocytic capsule and two toxins that are responsible for most of the clinical manifestations of anthrax. Edema toxin, an adenylate cyclase, is responsible for localized edema, and for impairment of neutrophil function. The lethal toxin, a metalloprotease, causes the release of tumor necrosis factor (alpha) and interleukin-1 (beta) by macrophages, thought to account for sudden death in anthrax.

Epidemiology

B. anthracis is distributed widely about the world in soil as highly resistant spores. Herbivores acquire anthrax infection by grazing on contaminated soil or ingesting contaminated feed. In ordinary circumstances humans acquire the infection following exposure to anthrax-infected animals or from contact with contaminated animal products (wool, hides, goat hair), particularly in plants sorting wool from Africa and Asia. The commonest form is cutaneous anthrax, of which approximately 2000 cases are reported worldwide annually. Epizootics have occurred among herbivores; and in Zimbabwe between 1979 and 1985 an epidemic of human anthrax, almost all cutaneous, was directly related to such an epizootic in cattle. In the United States from 1944 to 1994 there were 224 cases of cutaneous anthrax. During the 20 years before 2001 the incidence declined to less than one case per year.

A second, highly fatal form of anthrax, inhalation anthrax, follows deposition of aerosolized spores in alveolar spaces. Cases of woolsorter's disease have occurred in workers in enclosed factory spaces where processing wool generated numerous aerosolized anthrax spores. From 1976 until 2001 there were no cases of inhalation anthrax in the United States. However, the possibility that inhalation anthrax might be employed as a biological weapon was brought to public attention in 1979 when 66 people in Sverdlovsk, U.S.S.R., died from inhalation anthrax as a result of the accidental release of weaponed anthrax spores from a military research facility. A third form of anthrax, gastrointestinal anthrax, is rare, with no cases reported in the United States. It is caused by ingestion of poorly cooked infected meat.

Bioterrorism-related anthrax suddenly burst on the scene in the United States in the autumn of 2001 when *B. anthracis* spores were sent through the mail in five letters addressed to media outlets (in Florida and New York City) and to a U.S. senator (in Washington, D.C.). Twenty-two individuals developed anthrax (half, cutaneous; half, inhalation), with five fatalities among those with inhalation anthrax. In addition to office workers, the largest group of individuals infected were postal service employees, particularly those who worked in mail-sorting centers. From prior animal inhalation data, the human median lethal dose (LD_{50}) had been estimated to be 2500 to 55,000 inhaled *B. anthracis* spores. Recent primate data suggest that an infecting dose may be only one to three spores. This may explain the two cases of fatal inhalation anthrax (in Connecticut and New York City) where the individuals had no exposure to the previously noted sites, raising the possibility that some of the mail addressed to them had gotten lightly cross-contaminated by spores released from other letters by automated mail sorting machines.

Whichever form of anthrax develops in an infected body, a prerequisite is that spores germinate into vegetative forms following ingestion by macrophages. Following inhalation, the spores are deposited in alveolar spaces and then carried by lymphatics to mediastinal lymph nodes where germination ensues up to 60 days later. In cutaneous anthrax, infection is initiated upon introduction of the spores through a break in the skin; in gastrointestinal anthrax, it is initiated through the mucosa.

Clinical Manifestations

INHALATION ANTHRAX

Inhalation anthrax consists of hemorrhagic thoracic lymphadenitis and mediastinitis; typical bronchopneumonia is absent. However, in most fatal cases of inhalation anthrax in Sverdlovsk, a focal, necrotizing, pulmonary lesion was observed, suggestive of the focal Ghon lesion of primary tuberculosis. Inhalation anthrax is typically a biphasic illness, following an occupational/environmental exposure: a 2- to 5-day prodromal, viral-like syndrome followed by worsening symptoms and development of marked dyspnea, cyanosis, respiratory failure, and hypotension. Initial symptoms consist of fever, chills, sweats, malaise and fatigue, nonproductive cough, mild shortness of breath, chest discomfort or pleuritic pain, nausea, vomiting, diarrhea, abdominal pain, headache, myalgia, and sore throat. Although distinguishing early inhalation anthrax from influenza-like illness may be difficult, the presence of nasal congestion might suggest a viral respiratory infection, whereas a persistent tachycardia (heart rate >100/min.) might suggest a bacterial process such as inhalation anthrax.

If untreated, the second phase of illness is rapidly progressive during the course of 24 to 48 hours resulting in hypothermia, shock, and death. In some patients, markedly enlarged intrathoracic lymph nodes, mediastinal widening, and subcutaneous edema may produce extrinsic obstruction of the trachea and stridor. In the recent bioterrorism-associated outbreak, with the availability of antimicrobial therapy and intensive care, mortality was 45%.

Blood cultures usually show growth in 6 to 24 hours, but prior administration of antimicrobials (even 1 or 2 doses) may prevent isolation. The intensity of bacteremia in the late stage of inhalation anthrax may be so great that bacilli are visible on Gram or Wright-Giemsa stains of peripheral blood. Anthrax meningitis can follow bacteremia and is characterized by nuchal rigidity, altered sensorium, and a polymorphonuclear pleocytosis, often with hemorrhagic cerebrospinal fluid (CSF) containing gram-positive bacilli. Although it is rare, patients treated with antibiotics have survived.

Initial laboratory results include a peripheral white blood count that is normal or elevated, but often with a neutrophilia and shift to the left. Chest radiographs show mediastinal widening, pleural effusions, and pulmonary infiltrates (likely secondary to the effusions and representing atelectasis) in the majority of cases. Computerized tomography (CT) of the chest is more sensitive in delineating mediastinal widening and pleural effusions.

CUTANEOUS ANTHRAX

Cutaneous anthrax accounts for more than 95% of naturally occurring human anthrax and for half the cases in the 2001 bioterrorism outbreak. The initial lesion, occurring 1 to 8 days after exposure to the spore, is a painless or pruritic papule, usually on the upper extremities, face, and neck. Small vesicles appear about the papule and may become confluent, forming a bulla that discharges clear or serosanguineous fluid and ulcerates. There is low-grade fever or none at all. Gram stain of the fluid shows gram-positive bacilli and relatively few neutrophils. A painless black eschar develops with extensive surrounding gelatinous edema. Regional lymphadenopathy is often present. Lymphangitis can occur from the initial process or because of secondary infection. Bacteremia is rare, but without antimicrobial therapy, mortality can reach 20%. The edema may become massive, particularly with lesions on the face or neck, and suggest cellulitis.

GASTROINTESTINAL ANTHRAX

Gastrointestinal anthrax still occurs in less-developed countries. Symptoms develop 2 to 5 days after ingestion of spores or of vegetative bacilli in undercooked meat. Symptoms consist of nausea, vomiting, fever, and abdominal pain; manifestations progress rapidly to bloody diarrhea, findings of an acute abdomen, or features of sepsis. Intestinal lesions occur in the terminal ileum or caecum and are ulcerative in nature, associated with hemorrhagic, mesenteric lymphadenitis. Marked ascites may be present. Hematemesis may occur associated with gastric ulceration. An oropharyngeal form of the disease produces oral or esophageal ulcers with fever, sore throat, dysphagia, and, occasionally, respiratory distress caused by local lymphadenitis and edema. Untreated gastrointestinal anthrax has a mortality rate of more than 50%.

Differential Diagnosis

In the past an important factor in considering the diagnosis of anthrax was exposure and environmental history (farm animals, animal products from abroad). Because of 2001's anthrax outbreak, attention has focused on the possible connection of any patient with clinical findings suggestive of anthrax to airborne spread of anthrax spores via bioterrorism.

Inhalation anthrax is suggested by prominent influenza-like symptoms in a patient with a widened mediastinum. The latter might also suggest lymphoma, tularemia, histoplasmosis, or other causes of mediastinal lymphadenopathy. Dissection of the aorta lacks fever, has a different quality of chest pain, and doesn't suggest lymphadenopathy radiologically. Fever, dyspnea, and pulmonary infiltrates might initially suggest the diagnosis of pneumonia.

Differential diagnosis of cutaneous anthrax includes:

- Ecthyma (usually lacking edema)
- Staphylococcal furuncle (painful)
- Ecthyma gangrenosum (usually in patients with neutropenia and *Pseudomonas aeruginosa* bacteremia)
- Brown recluse spider bite (in rural areas; painful during incipient necrosis)
- Orf (exposure to sheep; scab but no large eschar or gelatinous edema)
- Cellulitis (gelatinous edema of anthrax on face or neck in adults or on extremities in infants may suggest cellulitis)
- Other infection-associated eschars at the sites of tick and mite bites (tularemia, rickettsial spotted fevers, scrub typhus)

Laboratory Diagnosis

In inhalation anthrax, sputum Gram stain and culture usually do not reveal the organism. The finding of gram-positive bacilli on a stained smear of CSF of a patient with meningitis, particularly if hemorrhagic, is suggestive of anthrax. Blood cultures are usually positive within 24 hours, showing relatively large gram-positive rods. *B. anthracis* must be distinguished from other *Bacillus* species (*B. subtilis*, *B. cereus*) that are likely contaminants. Colonial morphology, lack of motility, and biochemical tests provide a provisional identification, which should be confirmed (by gamma phage lysis or direct fluorescence-antibody staining of cell-wall polysaccharide or of capsular antigen) at a level-B laboratory of the Laboratory Response Network (LRN). The predictive value of nasal swab testing for anthrax spores is undetermined, and is not recommended to rule out aerosol exposure or infection.

In suspected cutaneous anthrax, a direct Gram-stained smear of vesicular fluid, or fluid from beneath the eschar, may show the organism, and *B. anthracis* may grow on culture. If negative, a skin biopsy should be performed for immunohistochemical staining and PCR testing for *B. anthracis*, but only after administering the first dose of an antimicrobial (ciprofloxacin or doxycycline).

Serologic testing for immunoglobulin (Ig) G, anti-PA (protective antigen) antibody is not helpful in the diagnosis of an active case but might be of epidemiologic value.

Antimicrobial Therapy

For many decades penicillin was the drug of choice, and almost all naturally occurring strains are susceptible. With the 2001 anthrax outbreak, because of concern that strains used in terrorist attacks could well have been deliberately modified to be resistant to commonly used penicillins and tetracyclines, recommendations were made for initial therapy for suspected inhalation anthrax with two antimicrobials intravenously (Table 1). Ciprofloxacin (Cipro), doxycycline (Vibramycin), and penicillin have been approved by the FDA for this indication, for the former two on the basis of efficacy in a monkey model. In vitro studies indicate susceptibility of *B. anthracis* strains to many antimicrobials including other fluoroquinolones[1], various tetracyclines, clindamycin (Cleocin)[1], imipenem (Primaxin)[1], rifampin (Rifadin)[1], chloramphenicol (Chloromycetin)[1], aminoglycosides, cefazolin (Ancef)[1], vancomycin (Vancocin)[1], macrolides[1], and linezolid (Zylox)[1]. They are resistant to cefuroxime (Ceftin) and extended-spectrum cephalosporins and trimethoprim-sulfamethoxazole (Bactrim). Although the anthrax attack strain proved susceptible to most antimicrobials (including penicillin), penicillin was not recommended for therapy of inhalational anthrax because of evidence of an inducible β lactamase that might become problematic with prolonged treatment.

[1]Not FDA approved for this indication.

TABLE 1 Recommendations for Antimicrobial Therapy Where Risk of Bioterrorism Exists

	Inhalational (Also Gastrointestinal) Anthrax		
Age Group	**Initial Treatment (Intravenous)**	**Follow-up Treatment (Oral)**	**Duration**
Adults	Ciprofloxacin (Cipro), 400 mg every 12h, *or* doxycycline (Vibramycin), 100 mg every 12 h, and 1 or 2 additional antimicrobials*	Switch to oral therapy (1 or 2 drugs) based on clinical course: Ciprofloxacin, 500 mg PO every 12 h, *or* doxycycline, 100 mg PO every 12 h	Continue for 60 days total
Children	Ciprofloxacin, 10-15 mg/kg every 12 h (not to exceed 1 g/d), *or* doxycycline† as follows: • >8y and >45 kg, 100 mg every 12 h • >8y and ≤45 kg, 2.2 mg/kg every 12 h • 8y, 2.2 mg/kg every 12 h *plus* 1 or 2 additional antimicrobials	Switch to oral route (1 or 2 drugs) based on clinical course as follows: Ciprofloxacin, 10-15 mg/kg PO every 12 h (not to exceed 1g/day), *or* doxycycline† as follows: • >8y and >45kg, 100 mg PO every 12 h • >8y and ≤45 kg, 2.2 mg/kg PO every 12 h • 8y, 2.2 mg/kg PO every 12 h	Continue for 60 days total
	Cutaneous Anthrax		
	Initial Treatment (Oral)		
Adults	Ciprofloxacin 500 mg every 12 h *or* doxycycline 100 mg every 12 h		60 days‡§
Children	Ciprofloxacin 10-15 mg/kg every 12 h (not to exceed 1 g/day) *or* doxycycline† as follows: • >8y and >45 kg: 100 mg every 12 h • >8y and ≤45 kg: 2.2 mg/kg every 12 h • ≤8y: 2.2 mg/kg every 12 h		60 days‡§

*Includes rifampin (Rifadin),[1] vancomycin (Vancocin),[1] penicillin, ampicillin,[1] imipenem (Primaxin),[1] clindamycin (Cleocin),[1] chloramphenicol (Chloromycetin),[1] and clarithromycin (Biaxin).[1]

†Use of tetracyclines warranted in children because of seriousness of the infection.

‡Previously treatment recommended for cutaneous anthrax was for 7-10 days, but increased to 60 days in setting of bioterrorism risks because of likelihood of aerosol exposure.

§Amoxicillin 500 mg orally every 8 h for adults or 80 mg/kg/day, divided every 8 h, for children is an option for completion of treatment after clinical improvement.

Modified from Morb Mortal Wkly Rep (MMWR), 50:917-918, 2001.

TABLE 2 Recommendations for Antimicrobial Postexposure Prophylaxis*

Age Group	Initial Treatment	Optimal Treatment (if Strain Proven Susceptible)
Adults	Ciprofloxacin (Cipro), 500 mg orally every 12 h, *or* doxycycline (Vibramycin), 100 mg orally every 12 h	Amoxicillin,[1] 500 mg orally every 8 h, *or* doxycycline, 100 mg orally every 12 h
Children	Ciprofloxacin, 10-15 mg/kg orally every 12 h (not to exceed 1 g/day)	Amoxicillin,[1] 500 mg orally every 8 h in children >20 kg; 80 mg/kg orally divided into 3 doses (every 8 h) in children <20 kg (maximum 500 mg/dose)

*Given for at least 60 days.
[1]Not FDA approved for this indication.
Note: Prophylaxis recommendations may change with time and based on antimicrobial susceptibility results during a biologic attack. Before instituting prophylaxis, physicians should consult with an infectious disease specialist and with public health authorities. Check for updates and revisions of recommendations at http://www.bt.cdc.gov/Health Professionals/index.asp. This information is adapted from CDC and Working Group on Civilian Biodefense recommendations.

Treatment for at least 60 days is indicated because of the possibility of delayed spore germination. The choice of clindamycin as the second drug to be used with ciprofloxacin or doxycycline might have the theoretical advantage of reducing toxin production. Treatment of anthrax meningitis should include ciprofloxacin plus one or more drugs with the capacity to enter the CSF in effective concentrations (penicillin, chloramphenicol, rifampin).

Thoracentesis is indicated for sizable pleural effusions.

Corticosteroids may be considered for adjunctive therapy for patients with marked edema of the face and neck and for meningitis (initially, as for bacterial meningitis of other etiologies).

For cutaneous anthrax, oral fluoroquinolones or doxycycline are the drugs of choice; amoxicillin is an alternative during pregnancy, lactation, or for treating children (see Table 1). Previously, treatment for cutaneous anthrax was administered for 7 to 10 days. However, after the bioterrorism attack in 2001, treatment was recommended for 60 days because of the possibility of concomitant inhalational exposure.

Postexposure (Bioterrorism Risk) Prophylaxis

Only when public health authorities have ascertained there is risk of exposure of the population to release of *B. anthracis* spores as a biological weapon is postexposure prophylaxis indicated for defined high-risk groups (determined by site, timing, and conditions of exposure). Because a strain of *B. anthracis* has been produced abroad that is resistant to many antibiotics (penicillin, chloramphenicol, macrolides, doxycycline, and rifampin), a fluoroquinolone is the recommended drug of choice administered for 60 days (Table 2). Careful monitoring for adverse drug reactions is necessary because of the prolonged duration of administration. Postexposure prophylaxis has been provided in primates by combining immunization with antimicrobials. If the vaccine was available for use in humans in a program of combined prophylaxis, administration at 0, 2, and 4 weeks might reduce the duration of postexposure antimicrobial prophylaxis to 30 to 45 days.

Vaccination

Anthrax vaccine absorbed (AVA), consisting of a cell-free filtrate of an attenuated, nonencapsulated strain of *B. anthracis,* is licensed for use in the U.S. military. The vaccine is administered at 0, 2, and 4 weeks and again at 6, 12, and 18 months. Annual boosters are necessary. It provides complete protection against aerosol exposure in monkeys at 8 weeks, and 88% protection at 100 weeks. In a human trial, a similar vaccine was protective against cutaneous anthrax. Systemic reactions (mainly headache, myalgia, and fever) occurred in approximately 1% of vaccine recipients in the military.

PSITTACOSIS (ORNITHOSIS)

METHOD OF

Fiona Horwood, BMedSci, and

John Macfarlane, DM

Psittacosis is an uncommon cause of community-acquired pneumonia. The causative organism, *Chlamydia psittaci* is a gram-negative, obligate, intracellular coccus. It derives its name from the Greek for parrot (psittacosis), after a human outbreak in Paris in the 1890s from infected imported parrots. Ornithosis is perhaps a more accurate term, as *C. psittaci* infection is associated with most bird species. There are no accurate figures for the incidence of psittacosis because it is difficult to diagnose and is, therefore, underreported. However, 813 cases were reported to the Communicable Disease Centre of England and Wales from 1988 to 1998, and the incidence is increasing.

Epidemiology

C. psittaci is hosted by many avian species. Most cases of psittacosis are sporadic with no seasonal variation. Human infection is acquired by inhalation of aerosol from dried feces or respiratory secretions of infected birds. This may occur even after exposure to infected birds so brief that some patients may not even recall the event.

Infected mammals may also transmit *C. psittaci* to humans by exposure to birth fluids and placentae of infected sheep, goats, or cattle. Human-to-human transmission has never been reported, so an infected person does not require specific isolation.

Pathogenesis

C. psittaci enters the body via the respiratory tract and travels via the blood to the reticuloendothelial cells of the liver and spleen where it replicates. Large numbers of the organism then cause secondary bacteriemia and invade the lungs and other organs hematogenously. Occasionally, immediate infection of the respiratory epithelial cells may occur causing pneumonia without the bacteremic stage.

Clinical Features

Psittacosis tends to occur in adults of working age. The incubation period is 5 to 14 days. The spectrum of illness varies from subclinical to severe pneumonia with systemic illness and organ failure. If treated with appropriate antibiotics, the mortality rate is less than 1%; before the antibiotic era it was 15% to 20% of cases.

Psittacosis characteristically presents with a sudden onset of fevers, chills, headache, malaise, and myalgia. Respiratory symptoms are a nonproductive cough, dyspnea, chest tightness, pleuritic chest pain, and hemoptysis. These may be accompanied by sore throat, nausea, vomiting, and abdominal pain. The presence of splenomegaly and a pale macular rash (Horder spots) in a case of community-acquired pneumonia suggests the possibility of *C. psittaci* infection.

There have been case reports of extrapulmonary complications of psittacosis affecting all organ systems of the body. Amongst the most common are epistaxis, hepatitis, endocarditis, acute renal failure, arthritis, and encephalitis.

Auscultation findings of the chest often underestimate the extent of lung involvement. Chest radiograph features are variable but characteristically show patchy infiltrates in the lower lobes radiating from the hila. Bilateral shadowing is present in approximately 12% of cases, small pleural effusions may also be seen and often the changes are slow to clear.

Diagnosis

The laboratory confirmation of *C. psittaci* infection may be achieved in one of the following ways:

- Complement fixation tests—Complement fixation identifies the chlamydia family but is not species specific. Two serum samples are required, one during the acute phase and a second in the convalescent phase, two weeks after the fever abates. Both samples should be analyzed simultaneously and in the same laboratory. A fourfold change in antibody level (rise or fall) is diagnostic, but a single reciprocal titer of 32 is very suggestive when accompanied by a compatible clinical syndrome.
- Microimmunofluorescence (MIF)—This tool is species specific and so may be used once chlamydia infection has been identified by complement fixation. It detects *C. psittaci* immunoglobulin (Ig) M and IgG to identify recent or current infection.
- Culture

C. psittaci may be cultured from sputum on specific cell lines. This is technically difficult and potentially hazardous to the laboratory personnel and is rarely used in clinical practice.

Enzyme-linked immunoabsorbent assay (ELISA), polymerase chain reaction (PCR), and direct immunofluorescence techniques have been developed but tend to be used in research only.

Treatment

The antibiotic group of choice for the treatment of psittacosis is the tetracyclines, either tetracycline

(Sumycin) or doxycycline (Vibramycin). Most patients respond to oral therapy, but in severe cases intravenous doxycycline is necessary. Symptoms often subside within 2 to 3 days, but because the infection is prone to relapse, treatment should be continued for 3 weeks.

For those who cannot take tetracycline, for example, pregnant women and young children, erythromycin (E-Mycin)[1] is the drug of choice. Chloramphenicol (Chloromycetin) and high-dose penicillin have been effective in some cases.

Prevention

Since psittacosis is primarily contracted from birds, prevention is aimed at controlling disease in susceptible species. This is achieved by quarantining imported birds and treating suspected infections in all birds early with tetracycline-impregnated feed.

[1]Not FDA approved for this indication.

Q FEVER

METHOD OF

Juan C. Sarria, MD, and

Robert C. Kimbrough III, MD

Q fever is a worldwide zoonosis caused by the intracellular pathogen *Coxiella burnetii*. This agent is highly infectious and rather resistant in harsh environmental conditions. In fact, a single organism is enough to cause an infection. Because of these attributes, it is considered a potential biological warfare threat. A wide variety of wild and domestic animals can be infected; however, sheep, goats, cattle, and cats are the primary reservoirs of *C. burnetii*. These animals, when infected, shed organisms in urine, feces, milk, and birth products. Humans acquire infection through inhalation of contaminated aerosols from infected animal products. This usually occurs when the animal gives birth, because organisms are concentrated in high numbers in the products of conception. Uncommon modes of transmission include ingestion of contaminated milk and tick bites. In the United States, most cases result from occupational exposure involving veterinarians, farmers, dairy workers, or meat handlers.

Clinical Features

The clinical spectrum of Q fever is wide and nonspecific. Acute infections may be asymptomatic or manifest as a self-limited febrile illness that resolves without any treatment. Thrombocytopenia and a slight elevation (2-3 times normal) of the hepatic transaminases are common laboratory findings. Other acute manifestations of Q fever include pneumonia, hepatitis, and meningoencephalitis. A less common but more serious form of the disease is chronic Q fever, characterized by infection that persists for more than 6 months. The predominant clinical syndrome of chronic Q fever is culture-negative endocarditis. Fever of unknown origin, endovascular infections, uterine infections, and osteomyelitis are also well-documented chronic manifestations of *C. burnetii* infection. Individuals at high risk of developing chronic Q fever are those with pre-existing valvular heart disease, aneurysms or vascular grafts, and to a lesser extent, immunocompromised hosts and pregnant women.

Diagnosis

Diagnosis of Q fever remains based on serology in the appropriate epidemiologic and clinical settings. Most laboratories use the indirect immunofluorescence assay (IFA). *C. burnetii* exists in two antigenic phases, called phase I and phase II. This antigenic difference is important in diagnosis. During acute infection, the antibody response is directed primarily against phase II antigen, whereas in chronic infections the predominant response is directed against phase I. *C. burnetii* may also be identified in infected tissues by using immunohistochemical staining. Because of the fastidious nature and special growth requirements of the organism, routine culture is not feasible. Moreover, because of the risk of human contamination, isolation must be performed in biosafety level 3 laboratories. The use of polymerase chain reaction (PCR) for detecting *C. burnetii* has been problematic because of frequent DNA contamination.

Treatment

The optimal treatment of Q fever is still debated. Doxycycline (Vibramycin) is considered the drug of choice because of its excellent in vitro activity and clinical effectiveness. Other active agents include quinolones[1], trimethoprim-sulfamethoxazole (Bactrim)[1], and macrolides[1] (Table 1). Antibiotic courses of 14 to 21 days have been used to treat patients with acute Q fever with good clinical outcomes. A consensus is emerging that combination

[1]Not FDA approved for this indication.

TABLE 1 Treatment of Q Fever

Drug Name	Oral Adult Dosage	Comment
Doxycycline (Vibramycin)	100 mg twice a day	First-line therapy
Quinolone (various)[1]	Varies with drug	Good in vitro activity; consider in meningitis
Trimethoprim-sulfamethoxazole (Bactrim or Septra)[1]	1 double-strength tablet twice a day	Alternative in children and pregnancy
Macrolide (various)[1]	Varies with drug	Susceptibility is variable; clinical failures have occurred; alternative in children and pregnancy
Rifampin (Rifadin)[1]	300 mg twice a day	Use only as part of combination regimens
Hydroxychloroquine (Plaquenil)[1]	200 mg daily	Enhances intracellular bactericidal effect of doxycycline

[1]Not FDA approved for this indication.

antibiotic therapy is necessary to treat chronic Q fever, however, comparative data are lacking. Regimens commonly used include doxycycline plus ciprofloxacin (Cipro)[1], doxycycline plus rifampin (Rifadin)[1], doxycycline plus hydroxychloroquine (Plaquenil)[1], and ciprofloxacin plus rifampin. The optimal duration of therapy in chronic Q fever is unknown, but prolonged courses of 1 to 4 years have been proposed to prevent relapses. Some authorities have recommended life-long treatment in chronic Q fever endocarditis. Antibody titers can be used to monitor response and decide when to discontinue treatment. Surgery to remove infected tissues, such as heart valves or bone sequestra, or foreign material is required in many of these infections. In the case of Q fever in pregnant women, antibiotic treatment should be continued until delivery to avoid fetal death.

Prevention

Preventive efforts should be directed primarily toward high risk groups. Counseling persons with pre-existing cardiovascular disease or immunosuppression about hazardous exposures is imperative. In the occupational setting, inhalation of aerosolized body fluids and products of conception from animals should be minimized. In hospitalized patients, isolation is not necessary since transmission has not been documented during clinical care of infected patients. A vaccine (Q-Vax)[2] has been developed but is not commercially available in the United States. To enhance surveillance efforts, health care providers should report cases of Q fever to state health departments.

[1]Not FDA approved for this indication.
[2]Not available in the United States.

RABIES

METHOD OF
Benjamin H. Sun, DVM, MPVM

Rabies is a preventable viral infection that is most often transmitted through a bite from an infected mammal. Once introduced, the rabies virus migrates to the central nervous system (CNS) and causes a fatal encephalomyelitis. While dogs are the primary rabies reservoir in many regions of the world, several wild mammals (e.g., bats, raccoons, skunks, and foxes) are the most important reservoirs in the United States. Although human rabies is very rare in the United States, potential exposures to humans should promptly be assessed and managed. Because there is no effective treatment for the disease, essential prevention strategies include controlling rabies in animals, preventing exposures, and applying appropriate rabies postexposure prophylaxis (PEP) measures.

Etiology

Rabies virus belongs to the genus *Lyssavirus* in the family Rhabdoviridae, RNA viruses that have a distinctive bullet shape. Other viruses in the genus include Lagos bat virus, Mokola virus, Duvenhage virus, European bat viruses 1 and 2, and Australian bat virus.

Transmission

Animal bites are the most frequent route of rabies transmission. Rabies is transmitted only when the virus is introduced into a bite wound, nonintact skin, or onto a mucous membrane. Infectious material from a rabid animal includes saliva, neurologic tissue, and cerebrospinal fluid. Contact with the fur, urine, blood, or feces from a rabid animal does not constitute an exposure to rabies. Contact with dried saliva does not constitute a rabies exposure because the rabies virus is inactivated by desiccation or exposure to ultraviolet light. The likelihood of developing rabies varies with the nature and degree of exposure. If no exposure has occurred, rabies PEP is unnecessary.

Pathogenesis

Although the incubation period for rabies averages from 1 to 3 months, it can be highly variable and in rare instances, may be greater than 1 year. Rabies is a neurotropic virus that, following primary introduction, will directly or indirectly enter into peripheral nerves. This stage may last from a few days to months and is the time that the host immune defenses play a key role. Following peripheral nerve uptake, the virus is transported to the CNS via retrograde axoplasmic flow. Rapid replication and dissemination of the virus in the CNS occurs during the final stages of the disease; the virus spreads centrifugally via peripheral nerves to various tissues, including the salivary glands. Intracytoplasmic inclusions in the CNS, known as Negri bodies, are formed and are a classic histological feature, although this may be an inconsistent finding.

Clinical Features

Rabies is an acute, severe, and rapidly progressive encephalomyelitis that is incurable and should be considered in the differential diagnosis of such cases in animals and humans, regardless of whether there is a history of an animal bite or other exposure. Initial prodromal symptoms include nonspecific flu-like signs such as malaise, fever, or headache, lasting for days. Some patients have reported discomfort or paresthesia at the exposure site. Signs will progress rapidly within days to symptoms of anxiety, confusion, agitation, and cerebral dysfunction; which further progresses to delirium, hallucination, insomnia, and abnormal behavior. Autonomic dysfunction signs are also common (e.g., body temperature fluctuations, lacrimation, hypersalivation, and cardiac arrhythmias). The disease is almost always fatal once symptoms appear, and case management is palliative. An aggressive, experimental therapy approach for patients has been published for cases in the early disease stages that includes a combination of rabies vaccine, rabies immunoglobulin, monoclonal antibodies[1], ribavirin (Rebetol)[1], interferon[1], and ketamine (Ketalar)[1]. The clinical course of rabies from onset to death typically ranges between several days up to several weeks with supportive care.

Epidemiology

HUMAN RABIES

An estimated 50,000 people die of rabies annually worldwide. The majority of cases occur in Asia, Africa, Eastern Europe, and Latin America where rabies is endemic in dogs. In the United States, an average of 1 to 4 cases are reported annually with only 38 cases reported during the period between 1990 and 2003. Of these 38 cases, 29 were caused by virus variants associated with insectivorous bats indigenous to the United States. Only 3 of these 29 case-patients reported a definitive bat bite in the history and an approximate 12 others reported some sort of bat contact. Seven of the 38 cases were imported cases associated with canine rabies virus variants not present in the United States.

ANIMAL RABIES

Approximately 7000 to 9000 rabid animals are reported annually in the United States from all states except Hawaii. Wild animals account for more than 90% of the rabid animals reported in the United States with the most common species being raccoons, followed by skunks, insectivorous bats, and foxes. These species, except for bats, represent the terrestrial rabies reservoirs in the United States, which are found in distinct geographic regions. Rabies in domestic animals represents spillover from the wildlife reservoirs, with cats followed by dogs and cattle being the most frequently reported domestic rabid animals. Rabies in dogs has dramatically declined in the United States since the 1940s, when mass rabies vaccination programs were instituted.

Diagnosis

The direct fluorescent antibody (DFA) test performed on specific fresh brain areas is the most frequently used test to diagnose rabies. This test typically takes less than one day to perform in animals, and medical decisions regarding PEP of exposed persons can usually await the test results if the animal is tested in a timely fashion. There is no available test to determine if a patient has been exposed to rabies or to definitively rule out if a person or animal has rabies antemortem. Tests using serology, reverse transcriptase polymerase chain reaction, DFA, and virus culture are available typically at the state health department to aid in the antemortem diagnosis in humans. Specimens include serum, spinal fluid, nuchal skin biopsies, brain biopsies, and saliva.

Assessment of Potential Rabies Exposures

When seeing a patient with an animal bite, the most difficult decision the health care provider is confronted with is determining whether or not a possible rabies exposure has occurred. This risk assessment is based upon several factors surrounding the exposure situation, which include:

- The animal species involved
- The type of exposure (e.g., bite vs. nonbite)

[1]Not FDA approved for this indication.

- The local animal rabies epidemiology
- The circumstances of the exposure (e.g., provoked or unprovoked bite)
- The health status, vaccination history, and disposition of the exposing animal

The Advisory Committee on Immunization Practices (ACIP) has published detailed recommendations on human rabies prevention, which are widely available. Local public health officials should be consulted for assistance in evaluating unusual exposures and to obtain information on the local animal rabies epidemiology.

If a person is bitten by a healthy dog, cat, or ferret, the animal should be held for a 10-day observation period following the bite regardless of the animal's vaccination status, and rabies PEP usually should not be administered. If the animal develops clinical signs consistent with rabies during this period, the animal should be euthanized and tested for rabies; PEP should be administered to the bite victim immediately if it tests positive. No PEP is necessary if the dog, cat, or ferret is healthy at the end of the 10-day period. Wild animal bites represent the highest risk of rabies transmission, and there are no established observation periods for these species. If available, the wild animal should be euthanized and tested and PEP administered accordingly.

Special consideration should be given to exposure situations involving bats. Bites from bats may be very small and not result in a visible wound. If the bat is not available for testing, or if the test result is positive, PEP is appropriate for persons with a bite, scratch, or mucous membrane exposure, and for encounters where a definitive exposure cannot be excluded (e.g., waking up with a bat in the same room, or a bat found in the same room with a child or a mentally disabled or intoxicated person).

Rabies in small rodents and lagomorphs (e.g., rabbits and hares) is extremely rare, and most exposures to these species do not represent a significant exposure to rabies unless the animal appears to be ill or if there are unusual circumstances surrounding the exposure, in which case the animal should be tested.

Postexposure Management

Administration of rabies PEP following a potential exposure is a medical urgency, not a medical emergency. Rabies PEP is highly effective if administered in a timely manner. It includes thorough wound treatment, modern cell-culture rabies vaccinations, and the administration of human rabies immunoglobulin (RIG) for previously nonimmunized persons. Several factors that determine the risk of rabies and the incubation period include the dose of virus inoculated, the rabies virus variant, the anatomic location of the exposure, the nature of the exposure, whether timely and appropriate PEP was administered, and whether prompt and thorough wound cleansing took place. Immediate wound treatment has been shown to markedly reduce the likelihood of rabies and consists of thorough washing of all bite wounds and scratches with soap, water, and a virucidal agent such as povidone-iodine irrigation. The need for a tetanus-diphtheria (Td) booster should also be assessed.

Following wound treatment, rabies PEP consists of both passive and active immunizations. The three equally safe and efficacious rabies vaccines currently licensed in the United States are human diploid cell vaccine (HDCV-Imovax Rabies), purified chick embryo cell (PCEC-RabAvert), and rabies vaccine adsorbed (RVA). Two RIGs are currently licensed in the United States, Imogam Rabies-HT and BayRab. The administration schedules and dosages for these products are all the same. Vaccination schedules, routes, and doses are listed in Table 1 and are categorized by the prior vaccination status of the patient. RIG is only administered once to previously unvaccinated persons at the beginning of the five-dose rabies

TABLE 1 Rabies Postexposure Prophylaxis

Vaccination Status	Rabies Biologic*	Schedule	Dose‡	Route
Not previously vaccinated	RIG	Day 0†	20 IU/kg body weight	Infiltrate full dose, if anatomically feasible, in and around the wound; give remainder IM at site distant from the vaccine.
	Vaccine	Days 0‡, 3, 7, 14, and 28	1 mL	HDCV, RVA, or PCEC given IM in deltoid area or anterolateral thigh in infants; avoid gluteal administration.
Previously vaccinated§	RIG	Do not administer		
	Vaccine	Days 0† and 3	1 mL	HDCV, RVA, or PCEC given IM in deltoid area or anterolateral thigh in infants; avoid gluteal administration.

Abbreviations: HDCV, human diploid cell vaccine; IM, intramuscular; PCEC, purified chick embryo cell; RIG, rabies immunoglobulin; RVA, rabies vaccine adsorbed.

*Thorough wound cleansing should always be performed.

†Day 0 is the day of first vaccine administration. RIG may be administered through day 7.

‡Doses are for all ages and sizes, including children.

§This includes any person with a history of completed preexposure vaccination with HDCV, RVA, or PCEC; prior postexposure vaccination with HDCV, RVA, or PCEC; or prior rabies vaccination with a different rabies vaccine and documented antibody response.

vaccination schedule to provide immediate antibodies until an active immune response develops following the multiple rabies vaccinations. RIG may be administered through the seventh day following the first rabies vaccination. It is important to note that for persons previously vaccinated for rabies (e.g., received preexposure prophylaxis or completed PEP series), RIG should not be administered and only two booster vaccinations should be given, one on day 0 and the other on day 3. Serologic testing is not needed to document seroconversion unless the patient is immunocompromised.

Preexposure Management

Preexposure rabies vaccination is indicated for people who, because of their occupation, activities, or travel destinations, are at a high risk for potential rabies exposure. Occupations with a higher rabies exposure risk include, but are not limited to, veterinarians and staff, animal and wildlife handlers, and laboratory workers who handle rabies virus. Globally, dogs are the primary reservoir in many regions of the world. International travelers should consider preexposure rabies vaccination if they are likely to come into contact with animals in regions where canine rabies is enzootic and timely access to medical care and rabies biologics may be limited. Travelers should inquire about the rabies status of areas that they are visiting and also consult the Centers for Disease Control and Prevention Yellow Book that discusses regions reporting rabies.

Preexposure prophylaxis does not eliminate the need for postexposure prophylaxis; it simplifies the PEP therapy by eliminating the need for RIG and three doses of rabies vaccine (see Table 1). This may be important for persons traveling to areas with limited rabies biologics or for persons at high risk for adverse reactions. In addition, preexposure prophylaxis may provide protection where PEP is delayed or for persons with unapparent rabies exposures. Previously rabies-immunized persons must receive a rabies vaccine booster, on day 0 and day 3, following every potential rabies exposure. Serologic testing by the rapid fluorescent focus inhibition test (RFFIT) is recommended periodically (every 6 months for laboratory workers and every 2 years for persons at frequent risk) to measure the viral neutralizing antibody levels for previously immunized persons; a single rabies booster is recommended for persons with inadequate titers.

Adverse Reactions and Precautions

Approximately 30% to 74% of rabies vaccine recipients have reported mild, local reactions consisting of pain, erythema, and swelling at the injection site; systemic reactions of headache, nausea, abdominal pain, muscle aches, and dizziness have been reported among 5% to 40% of vaccine recipients. Severe reactions are extremely rare, and three cases of a transient Guillain-Barré syndrome have been reported. Local pain or a low-grade fever has been reported following receipt of RIG administration. Because of the incurable and fatal nature of the disease, rabies PEP should not be interrupted or discontinued in pregnancy cases or when there are local or mild systemic reactions. Such reactions are typically managed successfully with anti-inflammatory and antipyretic agents. Management of serious reactions should be reported to local health officials, and they should be consulted about the situation.

Immunosuppressive conditions or agents may interfere with the development of active immunity following rabies vaccination. Immunosuppressive agents should be postponed if possible during PEP, and a follow-up titer should be collected 2 to 4 weeks following PEP completion to be evaluated for an adequate immune response.

Infection Control

Standard infection control precautions are adequate to prevent rabies exposure to health care workers. Human-to-human rabies transmission is a concern, although no cases have been reported among health care workers exposed to a patient with rabies. A systematic and careful risk assessment should occur following the identification of a positive or probable case of rabies. This evaluation should be based upon contact with the patient's secretions and will limit unnecessary PEP.

Rabies Management Review

- Timely wound management and rabies postexposure prophylaxis are effective in preventing rabies.
- All mammal exposures should be evaluated as soon as possible to determine if a possible rabies exposure occurred, and special attention should be paid to bat interactions.
- Rabies should be considered in the differential diagnosis of patients presenting with an acute, rapidly progressing encephalomyelitis without an apparent cause and regardless of a history of animal contact.
- Rabies preexposure prophylaxis for higher risk individuals will simplify postexposure prophylaxis and may offer some additional protection for travelers or unapparent exposures.
- In the United States, 76% of human rabies cases reported during the period 1990–2003 were associated with insectivorous bat rabies virus variants; only 10% of the patients reported a bat bite.

RAT-BITE FEVER

METHOD OF

Gwendolyn L. Gilbert, MD

Rat-bite fever is an uncommon zoonosis caused by one of two unusual bacteria, *Streptobacillus moniliformis* or *Spirillum minus*, either of which may be carried asymptomatically in the oropharynges or conjunctivae of rodents. A bite or scratch from a rat or mouse is the usual cause of sporadic human disease; for example in children living in rat-infested dwellings or laboratory workers handling infected rodents. Less commonly, it follows the bite of a dog or other animal that feeds on or has contact with rodents. Both organisms apparently have worldwide distribution, but the prevalence of carriage in rodents varies widely. Most recognized cases of rat-bite fever in the United States are caused by *S. moniliformis*, whereas *S. minus* has been more widely recognized in Europe and Asia. The incidence of rat-bite fever is unknown, and many cases are probably missed because the disease responds rapidly to empirical antibiotic therapy and the organisms are difficult to culture.

Rat-Bite Fever Caused by *Streptobacillus Moniliformis*—Streptobacillary Fever

CLINICAL FEATURES

The typical clinical presentation of rat-bite fever caused by *S. moniliformis* is an abrupt onset of an influenza-like illness with fever, chills, headache, and myalgia 3 to 21 days after a bite. The bite wound is usually unremarkable and heals readily, although there may be associated lymphadenopathy. The illness is characterized by rash, arthralgia, arthritis (in approximately 50% of cases), splenomegaly, and, uncommonly, cough or sore throat. The rash is typically erythematous and maculopapular, involves the palms and soles, and begins several days into the illness as fever is starting to wane. It lasts for up to a week and may desquamate. Less commonly the rash is petechial or pustular. Arthritis may be migratory and transient or persistent; it can mimic rheumatoid arthritis or present as an inflammatory, sterile joint effusion or septic arthritis of one or more large joints. *S. moniliformis* can cause inflammation or abscess formation in almost any organ, including subcutaneous tissue, female genital tract, prostate, brain, and pericardium. It is a rare cause of endocarditis, meningitis, and chorioamnionitis. Recovery is the rule, but, if not treated the illness runs a relapsing course and can be fatal, usually as a result of endocarditis.

S. moniliformis can also cause an epidemic illness, known as Haverhill fever, which is not associated with rodent bites or direct animal contact, but with ingestion of contaminated milk or water. The organism is sometimes excreted in the urine of rodents, which is assumed to be the source of contamination.

BACTERIOLOGY AND DIAGNOSIS

The diagnosis of rat-bite fever may be suspected because of a history of bite injury. However, this often is not elicited until isolation of an unusual, fastidious gram-negative bacillus prompts specific questioning. *S. moniliformis* can be isolated from blood, although it is inhibited to varying degrees by sodium polyanethol sulfonate (SPS), an additive in most commercial blood culture media. Pediatric and anaerobic blood culture media generally have low concentrations of SPS and so are more likely to support the growth of *S. moniliformis*. The organism may also be identified by Gram stain and culture of fluid from a joint, pustular skin lesion, or abscess. Apart from culture, the results of laboratory investigations are usually unhelpful.

S. moniliformis is the only species in its genus. It is a highly pleomorphic, nonhemolytic, nonmotile gram-negative bacillus. It is facultatively anaerobic and produces classical puffball colonies at the base of broth cultures after 3 to 5 days of incubation. Direct smears of pus and young cultures usually show relatively uniform coccobacilli or short rods (0.5-1 μm in diameter) with occasional long, curved or looping filaments, which may show bulbous, yeast-like swellings, giving a string-of-beads appearance—hence *moniliformis*. Older cultures show degenerative changes with fragmentation, granule formation, and irregular staining. Cell-wall-deficient L forms develop readily in culture (and probably in vivo also).

Subculture on chocolate or supplemented blood agar shows small round translucent colonies after 2 to 3 days of incubation. In older cultures, smaller rough transitional colonies appear and, later, the typical fried egg (mycoplasma-like) colonies of L forms. The organism is biochemically quite inactive, and special media are required to demonstrate sugar fermentation reactions. It has a distinct fatty acid profile on gas chromatography and can also be identified by polymerase chain reaction (PCR) of the 16S rRNA gene, using universal bacterial primers and amplicon sequencing or species-specific PCR, if available.

TREATMENT

S. moniliformis is susceptible to β-lactam antibiotics, tetracycline, aminoglycosides[1], erythromycin (E-Mycin)[1], and clindamycin (Cleocin)[1]. Intravenous benzylpenicillin (Penicillin G)[1] (1.2 g every 6 hours for 7 days for adults; 30 mg/kg every 6 hours for children)

[1]Not FDA approved for this indication.

followed by oral amoxicillin[1] for 1 week is appropriate therapy for uncomplicated infection. Endocarditis should be treated with a higher dose (1.8-2.4 g every 4 hours) for 4 to 6 weeks. Patients with a history of penicillin allergy can be treated with a cephalosporin[1] (if minor allergy only) or tetracycline. Penicillin treatment occasionally fails, possibly because of development of L forms in vivo; if so, tetracycline should be added.

Rat-Bite Fever Caused by *Spirillum Minus*—Spirillary Fever

CLINICAL FEATURES

Spirillary rat-bite fever was first recognized in Japan where it is also known as sodoku (rat poison). The clinical features overlap with those of streptobacillary fever, with some differences. Spirillary fever also usually follows a bite, which initially heals promptly. After a longer incubation period (1-5 weeks), a purplish induration develops at the wound site, usually without suppuration, but sometimes followed by ulceration and eschar formation. This is associated with high fever, a dark purplish, maculopapular or urticarial rash, leukocytosis, and sometimes vomiting and diarrhea. Local and systemic symptoms remit spontaneously after several days but recur intermittently with asymptomatic intervals. Without treatment, recurrences may continue for months and cause chronic anemia and weight loss. In contrast to streptobacillary fever, arthritis is uncommon.

BACTERIOLOGY AND DIAGNOSIS

S. minus is an unusual, tiny (0.2 μm diameter), spiral bacillus. It has bipolar flagella and is actively motile and so can be seen by darkfield or phase contrast microscopy in blood or a wound aspirate. In tissue sections it is visualized using Giemsa or Wright stains. *S. minus* can be amplified from clinical specimens by intraperitoneal inoculation of mice and regular examination of tail vein blood for motile spiral organisms. Limited in vitro broth culture has been reported, but not long-term culture on solid media. Little is known about the taxonomy of *S. minus* or its relationship to other spiral bacteria; even its Gram stain reaction is uncertain. Approximately 50% of patients with spirillary rat-bite fever have false-positive nontreponemal serologic tests for syphilis (e.g., rapid plasma reagin test).

TREATMENT

Penicillin is the drug of choice for spirillary fever, in similar doses to those used for streptobacillary fever. The organism is also susceptible to tetracycline, chloramphenicol (Chloromycetin)[1], and streptomycin[1], but there is little data relating to clinical effectiveness.

[1]Not FDA approved for this indication.

RELAPSING FEVER

METHOD OF

R. Wesley Farr, MD, MPH

Relapsing fevers are arthropod-borne spirochetal infections characterized by recurrent febrile episodes followed by asymptomatic periods. The tick-borne variety is seen worldwide including the western United States. The louse-borne variety is seen in the developing world, but not in the United States unless imported.

Etiology, Epidemiology, and Pathophysiology

Various rodent ticks and the human body louse are the vectors by which humans acquire the spirochetal bacteria that causes relapsing fever. These microbes are members of the *Borrelia* spirochete genus and are 8 to 30 μm long with a helix of 3 to 10 loose spirals. They cannot be cultivated in standard media but, unlike other spirochetes causing human disease, they can be readily detected with Giemsa and Wright stains.

Louse-borne disease is caused by *Borrelia recurrentis* and is endemic in the highlands of Africa, in South America, and in the Far East. It is not observed endemically in the United States. This form of relapsing fever usually occurs in the setting of overcrowding where dissemination of body lice results in epidemics. Untreated, the mortality rate may reach 40%, partly because of related host factors such as malnutrition and concurrent illnesses.

More than a dozen species of *Borrelia* produce the tick-borne variety of relapsing fever. The vectors are soft ticks of the genus *Ornithodoros*. The natural reservoirs are rodents and other small mammals residing in warm areas throughout the world at elevations of 1500 to 9600 feet. The ticks usually feed at night, have a painless bite, and feed for 5 to 20 minutes; hence, exposures to the vector may go unnoticed. Most cases in North America have occurred in the western forests; the number of reported cases there is growing because of increased intrusion of humans into the vectors' environments. From 1977 to 2000, 450 cases occurred in 11 western states with more than one half reported in 11 counties. Sixty-two visitors lodging in cabins at Grand Canyon National Park in Arizona, in 1979, constituted the largest outbreak of the disease in the Western Hemisphere. The second largest outbreak of 17 cases occurred there in 1990. The characteristic pattern of fevers interspersed with asymptomatic periods is related to the human immune response to the spirochete's ability to reconfigure its outer membrane antigens. A single borrelial spirochete may produce up to 40 different variants or serotype progeny by this multiphasic antigen variation during the same infection. A different gene, activated to evade the host's serospecific antibody encodes each surface antigen. Thus, after the first serotype wanes and the fever subsides because of an effective antibody response by the host, another antigen is expressed by a new bacterial variant. Several days later, as this new serotype multiplies, another febrile episode ensues necessitating a new specific antibody response to clear the new variant. This cycle of genetic recombination and antigen expression followed by specific antibody response is repeated, and is responsible for the periodicity distinctive in this disease.

Symptoms, Signs, and Diagnosis

Tick-borne and louse-borne relapsing fevers have similar manifestations that develop after approximately a 1-week incubation period. Symptoms begin suddenly with high fever, rigors, myalgia, arthralgia, weakness, and a severe headache. Nausea, abdominal pain, diarrhea, vomiting, or nonproductive cough is sometimes reported. During the febrile episodes, patients are acutely ill with lethargy, tachycardia, tachypnea, and occasionally confusion. Nonspecific maculopapular rashes may be seen; petechial rashes are less common. Hepatosplenomegaly is frequent in louse-borne disease, but is unusual in the tick-borne variety. Lymphadenopathy, which usually affects the cervical chains is not dramatic. Jaundice or mucosal bleeding is an infrequent sign of louse-borne relapsing fever and portends a worse prognosis. Myocarditis is a rare phenomenon. Central nervous system (CNS) involvement, manifesting as meningitis or cranial nerve deficits, is occasionally seen, particularly in louse-borne disease. Laboratory parameters are nonspecific. Hemograms are usually normal, although thrombocytopenia has been reported. Liver enzymes may be elevated, especially in severe cases of louse-borne relapsing fever. Positive serologic tests for Lyme disease and syphilis occur in less than 5% of patients.

The most useful laboratory study is a thick or thin smear of peripheral blood with a Wright or Giemsa stain. Organisms may be detected only during febrile episodes. Repeated examinations may be necessary to demonstrate spirochetes. Darkfield and fluorescence microscopy may increase the sensitivity but require more laboratory expertise. Serologic tests are not widely available except in reference laboratories, and they often lack specificity.

The acute clinical syndrome lasts 1 to 6 days and then terminates as abruptly as it begins. Hypotension and shock have been observed in the primary episode. Subsequent relapses, occurring 7 to 10 days later, are usually less severe. In tick-borne disease, relapses may recur for several weeks; fewer relapses occur in louse-borne disease. The early stages of relapsing fever may simulate other disorders, so geographic and epidemiologic factors are important in the diagnosis. Tick-borne disease may be confused with Colorado tick fever or Rocky Mountain spotted fever. Early louse-borne relapsing fever may resemble malaria, dengue fever, typhoid fever, or leptospirosis.

Treatment

Tetracycline or doxycycline (Vibramycin) is the drug of choice and is usually given orally. Erythromycin (E-Mycin)[1] is used in pregnant women and children. A single 500-mg dose of tetracycline or erythromycin is satisfactory for most episodes of louse-borne disease. A 500-mg oral dose of tetracycline or erythromycin four times daily for 7 to 10 days is given for the tick-borne variety because it has a higher rate of treatment failure and relapse. Penicillin[1] or ceftriaxone (Rocephin)[1] is recommended if CNS involvement is present. Chloramphenicol (Chloromycetin)[1] is another effective alternative therapy (Table 1).

Hospitalization may be necessary for very ill patients. Observation for 12 hours as a precaution in anticipation of a Jarisch-Herxheimer reaction (JHR) is also recommended. Frequently seen within 3 hours after treatment with recommended antibiotics and other antibiotics such as ciprofloxacin (Cipro)[1], the JHR elicits fever, increased rigors, and hypotension persisting for up to 24 hours. Management of JHR consists of supportive care. The JHR is associated with the systemic appearance of cytokines, such as tumor necrosis factor (TNF-alpha), interleukin-6, and interleukin-8. Corticosteroids, acetaminophen, pentoxifylline (Trental),[1] and recombinant human interleukin-10* fail to prevent or modify the JHR. Uncomplicated, adequately treated relapsing fever has a mortality rate of less than 5%.

Prevention

Minimizing overcrowding and maintaining good hygiene best prevent louse-borne relapsing fever.

[1]Not FDA approved for this indication.
*Investigational drug in the United States.

TABLE 1 Preferred Therapy for Relapsing Fever

	Drug	Adult Dosage	Duration
Louse-borne relapsing fever	Tetracycline*	500 mg PO	1 dose
	Doxycycline*	100 mg q12h PO	2 doses
Tick-borne relapsing fever	Doxycycline[1]	100 mg q12h PO or IV	7-14 d
	Erythromycin[1]	500 mg q6h PO or IV	7-14 d
Alternative drugs	Chloramphenicol (Chloromycetin)[1]	500 mg q6h PO or IV	
	Penicillin V[1]	500 mg q6h PO	
	Penicillin G[1,†]	5 million units q6h IV	
	Ceftriaxone (Rocephin)[1,†]	2 g/d IV	

[1]Not FDA approved for this indication.
*Substitute erythromycin, 500 mg PO, for pregnant women. In children younger than 8 years old, give 40 mg/kg/day in divided doses q6-8h.
†Use in patients with central nervous system manifestations.

Malathion-type insecticides may be necessary to successfully delouse crowded housing facilities. Rodent-proofing of lodging facilities and the use of insect repellents may reduce the risk of tick-borne disease if vector habitats cannot be avoided. Cases should also be reported to state and local health departments.

LYME DISEASE

METHOD OF

Janine Evans, MD

Epidemiology

Lyme disease (LD), a systemic illness caused by the spirochete *Borrelia burgdorferi*, is the most common tick-borne disease in the United States. More than 128,000 cases have been reported to health authorities in the United States since 1982, when a systematic national surveillance was initiated. It is likely that the true number of cases of Lyme disease is significantly greater because many do not satisfy the Centers for Disease Control and Prevention (CDC) case definition, and Lyme disease is often underreported. Although cases of LD have been reported from 48 states in the United States, the disease occurs in distinct and geographically limited areas. More than 90% of reported cases come from eight states located in the Northeast, the upper Midwest, and the Pacific Coast.

Lyme disease occurs worldwide. However, most cases occur in temperate regions and coincide with the distribution of the principal vector, ticks of the *Ixodes ricinus* complex, which are *Ixodes scapularis* in the eastern and upper midwestern United States, *Ixodes pacificus* in California, *Ixodes ricinus* in Europe, and *Ixodes persulcatus* in Eastern Europe and Asia.

I. scapularis has a three-stage, 2-year life cycle. Transovarial passage of *B. burgdorferi* occurs at a low rate. Ticks become infected with spirochetes by feeding upon a spirochetemic animal, typically small mammals, during larval and nymphal stages. In highly endemic areas, 20% to more than 60% of *I. scapularis* carry *B. burgdorferi*. Man is only an incidental host of the tick; contact is typically made in areas of underbrush or high grasses, but may occur in well-mowed lawns in endemic areas. Lyme disease occurs predominantly during May through July when nymphal *I. scapularis* feed. Animal models show that transmission is unlikely to occur before a minimum of 36 hours of tick attachment and feeding.

B. burgdorferi is a genetically and phenotypically divergent species. To date, 11 different genospecies have been identified, and only three have been associated with human disease. The three genospecies pathologic to humans are:

- Species I, *Borrelia burgdorferi sensu stricto*, which includes all strains studied thus far from the United States and some European and Asian strains.
- Species II, *Borrelia garinii*
- Species III, *Borrelia afzelii*, which is found in Europe and Asia. *B. afzelii* seems primarily associated with a chronic skin lesion, *acrodermatitis chronica atrophicans*, which is rare in the United States.

Clinical Manifestations

Lyme disease primarily affects the skin, heart, joints, and nervous system. Clinical features of Lyme disease are typically divided into three general stages—early localized, early disseminated, and late persistent infection. These stages may overlap, and most patients do not exhibit all of them. Seroconversion can occur in asymptomatic individuals, but is rare with strict surveillance. The illness usually begins with a skin lesion, erythema migrans (EM), and associated symptoms (early localized), which are sometimes followed weeks to months later by neurologic or cardiac abnormalities (early disseminated) and weeks to years by arthritis. Chronic neurologic and skin involvement also may occur years after onset (late persistent).

Early Localized Disease

Erythema migrans, the hallmark of early localized disease, appears as an expanding erythematous papule or macule, sometimes with central clearing, at the site of a deer tick bite. EM lesions have been reported in 60% to 90% of individuals with well-documented LD. Typically the lesion is flat, warm, and not painful. Sometimes it may become indurated, warm, and pruritic. The outer borders are red, generally well demarcated, and without scaling. Variations such as multiple rings may occur. Central clearing is associated with lesions that have been present for longer duration. With time the lesion expands centrifugally, presumably related to the outward migration of the organisms. With time EM lesions may become quite large (greater than 5 cm). Lesions are often located in intertriginous areas such as the groin, buttocks, axilla, popliteal fossa, as well as the waist and thigh, and in areas where clothing ends. EM lesions occur approximately 1 to 36 days (median 7-10 days) after a deer tick bite. Only 14% to 32% of patients with EM recall a tick bite. If untreated, the rash disappears without scarring several days to weeks after onset; in treated patients resolution typically occurs faster. Most patients (up to 80%) have associated systemic complaints including fatigue, myalgias, arthralgias, headache, fever, chills, and stiff neck. In early localized disease these symptoms tend to be mild. The most common objective physical findings associated with this stage are fever and lymphadenopathy. Occasionally, LD can produce a febrile, flu-like syndrome (exhibiting myalgias, arthralgias, headache, stiff neck, and/or fatigue) without an associated EM rash.

EM-like skin rashes have been reported from many southern U.S. states. Infected individuals develop an expanding circular skin lesion at the site of a tick bite. Associated symptoms include generalized fatigue, headache, stiff neck, and fever. The illness, referred to as *southern tick-associated rash illness* (STARI), is caused by an as-yet-uncharacterized spirochete. The Lone Star tick (*Amblyomma americanum*) appears to be the important vector in the transmission of LD-like infections, because it accounts for 95% of the human tick bites in some regions with reported cases. It is uncertain if *B. burgdorferi* infection is the responsible agent because it has rarely been isolated from local reservoir animals, patients typically do not have serologic evidence of exposure, and cultures of biopsy specimens failed to grow the organism. It is possible these rashes are secondary to a different, related spirochetal infection.

Early Disseminated Disease

In some patients the spirochetes disseminate hematogenously to multiple sites causing characteristic clinical features. Secondary annular lesions, sites of metastatic foci of *Borrelia* in the skin, develop within days of onset of EM in about one half of U.S. patients. They are similar in appearance to EM, but are generally smaller, migrate less, and lack indurated centers.

Cardiac involvement occurs in up to 10% of untreated patients. Transient and varying degrees of atrioventricular block several weeks to months after a tick bite are the most common manifestations. Other features are pericarditis, myocarditis, ventricular tachycardia, and, rarely, a dilated cardiomyopathy; valvular disease is not seen. Carditis is typically mild and self-limited, although patients may present quite dramatically in complete heart block, and some require the insertion of a temporary pacemaker. In most cases, carditis resolves completely, even without treatment with antibiotics. Treatment of carditis is indicated to prevent the development of late manifestations of the disease.

In addition to musculoskeletal flu-like symptoms, mild hepatitis, splenomegaly, sore throat, nonproductive cough, testicular swelling, conjunctivitis, and regional and generalized lymphadenopathy may sometimes occur during early stages.

Early neurologic involvement occurs in 15% to 20% of untreated patients and appears within 2 to 8 weeks after the onset of disease. Manifestations include cranial nerve palsies, meningitis, or meningoencephalitis, chorea, and peripheral neuritis or radiculoneuritis, in various combinations. Unilateral or bilateral seventh nerve palsies are the most common neurologic abnormalities. Presenting symptoms depend upon the area of the nervous system involved. Patients with meningitis present with fever, headache, and a stiff neck; those with Bannwarth syndrome (primarily in Europe) develop severe and migrating radicular pain lasting weeks to several months; and those with encephalitis have concentration deficits, emotional lability, and fatigue. Analysis of cerebrospinal fluid (CSF) from patients with early central nervous system (CNS) symptoms typically reveals a lymphocytic pleocytosis. Specific antibodies against *B. burgdorferi* may also be present and concentrated in the CSF relative to the serum concentration; they are useful to confirm disease. In general, neurologic abnormalities last for months but usually resolve completely.

In Europe, patients occasionally develop a solitary cutaneous lesion called *Borrelia* lymphocytoma with follicles resembling those seen in lymph nodes. It has been reported to occur in less than 10% of individuals in most series. Lymphocytomas appear most often as a red or violaceous solitary lesion on the ear or nipple; sometimes more widespread lesions may be seen. Patients usually have associated regional lymphadenopathy, but generalized symptoms are typically absent. Lesions promptly resolve with antibiotic therapy; if untreated they may last months and even years.

Late Disease

Late manifestations of Lyme disease typically occur months to years after the initial infection (mean of 6 months). In the United States, arthritis is the dominant feature of late Lyme disease, reported in approximately 60% of untreated individuals. The initial pattern of involvement may be migratory arthralgias (early) followed later by intermittent attacks of arthritis. Large joints, particularly the knee, are most commonly involved. Swelling is often prominent, with large effusions and Baker's cysts. However, small joints may be affected, and a few patients have had symmetrical polyarthritis. Attacks of arthritis, which generally last from weeks to months, typically recur for several years and decrease in frequency over time. Systemic symptoms such as fever do not accompany bouts of arthritis in most cases.

Synovial fluid specimens usually demonstrate white blood cell counts that vary from 500 to 110,000 cells/mm^3, with an average of 25,000 cells/mm^3, predominantly polymorphonuclear leukocytes. Joint fluid protein ranges from 3 to 8 g/dL.

A small subgroup of Lyme arthritis patients develop a prolonged, potentially erosive arthritis unresponsive to antibiotics. These patients often have major histocompatibility class II gene products, human leukocyte antigen (HLA)-DR4, accompanied by strong serum immunoglobulin (Ig) G responses to *Borrelia* outer surface proteins A or B (OspA or OspB). Repeated courses of treatment with antibiotics have not improved clinical outcomes.

A chronic neurologic syndrome may occur months to years after disease onset and involve the central or peripheral nervous systems. Typically, the neurologic features consist of a radiculoneuropathy, encephalopathy, or, rarely, encephalomyelitis. Peripheral nervous system involvement is characterized by paresthesias and electrophysiologic evidence of axonal polyneuropathy. Lyme encephalopathy, a rare neuropsychiatric disorder, predominantly affects memory and concentration. Cognitive dysfunction, headache, affective changes, seizures, ataxia, and chronic fatigue have all been reported. Because these complaints are often nonspecific and may be associated with post-Lyme syndromes, it is important to look for and document evidence of ongoing *B. burgdorferi* infection. Lymphocytic pleocytosis is uncommon in late neurologic disease, but increased intrathecal, *B. burgdorferi*-specific antibodies and/or elevated CSF protein may well be present. Polymerase chain reaction assays have been applied to CSF specimens but are not very sensitive. Single-photon emission computed tomography (SPECT) may detect reduced cerebral perfusion, especially in frontal subcortical and cortical regions, but are nonspecific and abnormalities should not be used as the sole criterion for diagnosis. Careful evaluation with neuropsychological testing can help to distinguish cognitive abnormalities in Lyme disease from those associated with chronic fatigue states and depression.

Other late findings (years) associated with this infection include a chronic skin lesion, acrodermatitis chronica atrophicans (ACA), well known in Europe but rare in the United States. ACA lesions appear as violaceous infiltrated plaques or nodules, especially on extensor surfaces, that eventually become atrophic. One third of patients experience an associated polyneuropathy, usually sensory. *B. burgdorferi* has been isolated from ACA skin biopsy specimens.

Ocular lesions in Lyme disease are rare, but have involved every portion of the eye and vary depending on the stage of disease. The most common opthalmic presentations in early disease include conjunctivitis, photophobia, and neuroophthalmologic manifestations caused by cranial nerve palsies. The most severe ocular manifestations occur in late stages and include episcleritis, symblepharon, keratitis, iritis, choroiditis, panuveitis, and retinal vasculitis.

Children

Children have the highest incidence of Lyme disease, likely because of a greater risk of exposure. The clinical spectrum is similar to that of adults. Most children present for medical attention with EM lesions. Younger children typically have EM lesions on either the head or neck, while in older children the extremities are the most common site. Children appear to recover more completely from active infection with *B. burgdorferi*. Most studies have indicated that long-term outcomes in children are excellent.

Pregnancy

Intrauterine transmission of *B. burgdorferi* is uncommon, usually occurring in cases of obvious disseminated infection during pregnancy. No uniform pattern of congenital anomaly has been reported. Prenatal exposure to Lyme disease has not been found to be associated with an increased risk of adverse pregnancy outcome.

Diagnosis

The diagnosis of Lyme disease relies upon the presence of characteristic clinical features and supporting serologic test results. Although spirochetes have been isolated from a variety of patient specimens, culture or direct visualization of *B. burgdorferi* is difficult and frequently yields negative results. In response to the need of a uniform definition, the CDC, in association with state health departments, developed a national surveillance case definition for Lyme disease. The criteria were intended to be used for epidemiologic surveillance and for comparing treatment results in different trials. Because the criteria are biased toward certainty in the diagnosis of Lyme disease, strict application in clinical practice may result in underdiagnosis and unnecessary delay in treatment. Serologic confirmation is the most practical and widely used laboratory aid currently available. Laboratory testing is best used to confirm a diagnosis of Lyme disease. Valid interpretation of test results depends upon sound clinical evidence that Lyme disease is present. Disease predictive value calculations demonstrate that when tests are ordered without regard for clinical features (i.e., used as a screening test), the positive predictive value was only 7%, even with ideal testing conditions. The positive predictive value rises to more than 96% when patients with a good clinical history for Lyme disease are tested.

IgM antibodies generally develop within 2 to 4 weeks after the onset of infection, peak after 6 to 8 weeks of illness, and decline to the normal range after 4 to 6 months of illness, in most patients. Antibodies of the IgG class are usually measured within 6 to 8 weeks after the onset of disease and peak after 4 to 6 months. In some patients, IgG levels remain elevated indefinitely.

An immunologic response can be detected within weeks of the onset of the disease using either an indirect immunofluorescence assay (IFA) or an enzyme-linked immunosorbent assay (ELISA). ELISA tests are preferred because they are more sensitive and reproducible. Most ELISA assays use extracts of sonicated whole *B. burgdorferi* as antigen. Purified *B. burgdorferi* proteins have also been used as substrates. Currently available commercial tests vary in sensitivity and specificity, consequently, identical serum samples sent simultaneously to different laboratories may yield different results. In the best of circumstances false-positive and false-negative results occur.

Immunoblotting is advocated as a method of distinguishing true-positive ELISA results. Antibodies directed against specific *Borrelia* proteins are identified. Because many proteins on *B. burgdorferi* are shared with other organisms, false-positive results may also occur with immunoblots. Criteria for the interpretation of immunoblot results have been established.

When serologic testing is indicated, authorities recommend testing initially with a sensitive first test, either an ELISA or an indirect fluorescent antibody (IFA) test, followed by testing with the more specific Western immunoblot (WB) test to corroborate equivocal or positive results obtained with the first test. Although antibiotic treatment in early localized disease may blunt or abrogate the antibody response, patients with early disseminated or late-stage disease usually have strong serologic reactivity.

B. burgdorferi can be cultured from 80% or more of biopsy specimens taken from early EM lesions. However, the diagnostic usefulness of this procedure is limited because of the need for a special bacteriologic medium (modified Barbour-Stoenner-Kelly medium) and protracted observation of cultures.

Polymerase chain reaction (PCR) is used to amplify genomic DNA *of B. burgdorferi*. Sensitive and specific PCR assays have been developed. Recent application of a PCR method on skin biopsy specimens resulted in an 80% positive rate from patients with EM lesions and a 92% positive rate from ACA patients. PCR of synovial fluid specimens have proven valuable in studying patients with Lyme arthritis. PCR techniques are also applied to blood, urine, and CSF specimens but, to date, the results are disappointing. The major problem in using the PCR technique is the issue of false-positive results. Proper handling of specimens is required to avoid contamination. Interpretation of PCR results is only reliable when performed in laboratories where appropriate precautions are taken.

Treatment

The goals of antibiotic therapy in Lyme disease are to eradicate the causative organism and reduce the risk of developing serious late manifestations of infection. Lyme disease is most responsive to treatment with antibiotics early in the course of infection. Current treatment recommendations are based on the results of published scientific studies and on clinical experience. The appropriate endpoint in antibiotic treatment is not always clear because of the persistence of certain symptoms and the difficulty of proving when the organism has been fully eradicated. Better understanding of the etiology of persistent symptoms following treatment will likely result in improved therapies. Additional courses of antibiotics do not benefit patients with persistent symptoms, in most cases. The treatment regimens outlined here represent guidelines.

Treatment of early stages of Lyme disease with oral antibiotics is adequate in the majority of patients. In patients with acute disseminated Lyme disease but without meningitis, oral doxycycline (Vibramycin)[1] appears to be equally as effective as parenteral ceftriaxone (Rocephin)[1] in preventing the late manifestations of disease. Initial studies of treatment for early Lyme disease reported therapy with phenoxymethyl penicillin (Penicillin VK)[1], erythromycin[1], and tetracycline[1] (250 mg four times a day for 1-20 days), shortened the duration of symptoms of early Lyme disease. Phenoxymethyl penicillin and tetracycline were superior to erythromycin[1] in preventing serious late manifestations of disease. Subsequent clinical trials have proven amoxicillin and

[1]Not FDA approved for this indication.

doxycycline to be equally efficacious. Concomitant use of probenecid[1] has not been definitively shown to improve clinical outcome and is associated with a higher incidence of side effects. Doxycycline is effective in treating the agent of human granulocytic ehrlichiosis (HGE), an organism also transmitted by *Ixodes scapularis* ticks; amoxicillin is not. Cefuroxime axetil (Ceftin), an oral, second-generation cephalosporin, is effective in treating early Lyme disease; azithromycin (Zithromax), an azalide analogue of erythromycin, is somewhat less effective. The prognosis for patients treated during the early stages of Lyme disease is excellent. Jarisch-Herxheimer–like reactions, which present with increased discomfort in skin lesions and temperature elevation occurring within hours after the start of antibiotic treatment, have been encountered in 14% of patients treated during early Lyme disease. They typically occur within 2 to 4 hours of starting therapy, are more common in disseminated disease, and are presumably caused by rapid killing of a large number of spirochetes.

Minor symptoms, including arthralgia, fatigue, headaches, and transient facial palsy, are common following treatment and generally resolve in 6 months. The etiology of these symptoms is unclear; it may be the result of retained antigen rather than persistence of live spirochetes. Persistent symptoms are more common in adults, patients with disseminated or late stages of disease, and individuals that have had long delays before receiving antibiotic therapy.

The optimal treatment of Lyme carditis is unknown, and, to date, no studies have been performed focusing specifically on treatment of carditis. Several oral and intravenous antibiotic regimens have been successful. Thirty-day courses of oral antibiotics—amoxicillin[1] (500 mg orally 3 to 4 times a day) or doxycycline (Vibramycin)[1] (100 mg twice a day)—are likely sufficient to treat milder forms of cardiac involvement such as first-degree heart block with PR intervals on EKG less than 0.3 sec. Hospitalization with cardiac monitoring is indicated for patients with first-degree heart block with longer PR intervals, higher-degree heart block, or evidence of global ventricular impairment. Intravenous antibiotics such as penicillin (Penicillin G)[1] or ceftriaxone (Rocephin)[1] are recommended for such patients. Insertion of a temporary pacemaker should be considered in patients with severe and symptomatic heart block, although permanent pacing is rarely indicated. The use of adjuvant corticosteroids or salicylates should be reserved for patients with prolonged dense heart block to speed recovery and reduce the risk of permanent conduction system defects.

Intravenous antibiotics are recommended for all cases of neuroborreliosis except isolated seventh nerve palsy. Patients presenting with a Bell-like palsy who have features that suggest possible CNS involvement, such as high fever, headache, or stiff neck, should undergo a lumbar puncture looking for evidence of more extensive disease. The most experience in the treatment of CNS Lyme disease has been with aqueous penicillin (Penicillin G)[1] and third-generation cephalosporins. Although optimal duration of therapy is unknown, it is recommended that patients be treated for 2 to 4 weeks. The risk of relapse of Lyme encephalopathy is reduced when intravenous antibiotics are extended to 4 weeks.

Lyme arthritis has been successfully treated with both oral and parenteral antibiotics, but failures have occurred with both regimens. Unless CNS involvement is present, first-line treatment with 1 or 2 months of doxycycline (Vibramycin)[1] (100 mg twice a day) or amoxicillin[1] (500 mg 3 times a day) is recommended. Complete resolution of arthritis may be delayed as long as 3 months or more following completion of treatment with antibiotics. In patients who do not respond to one or more courses of antibiotics, immunomodulatory therapy or arthroscopic synovectomy is recommended. Persistent Lyme arthritis eventually resolves after several years regardless of the regimen chosen.

Prevention

Recommended personal protective measures against tick bites include avoiding areas highly infested with deer ticks; wearing light-colored clothing, long-sleeve shirts, and long pants; tucking pant legs into socks; using a tick repellent on clothing and exposed skin; and performing regular body checks for ticks. These strategies require significant self-motivation.

The risk of infection from a deer tick bite in a Lyme disease endemic area is low. In mice, infected ticks have been attached for more than 36 hours before significant risk of developing Lyme disease occurred. In a controlled, double-blind study in patients with tick bites, no patient asymptomatically seroconverted, no treated patient developed EM, and the 2 of 182 untreated patients who did develop EM were successfully treated with oral antibiotics. These results support marking and watching a tick bite, and should EM develop, treating it early when antibiotics are most effective.

A single 200-mg dose of doxycycline (Vibramycin)[1], if given within 72 hours after an *I. scapularis* tick bite was shown to reduce the development of Lyme disease. Treatment with the antibiotic produced more frequent adverse effects when compared with placebo. It is reasonable to consider prophylaxis in individuals in highly endemic areas who have bites associated with partially or fully engorged ticks.

The results of two large clinical trials reported that vaccination using recombinant OspA preparations was

[1]Not FDA approved for this indication.

[1]Not FDA approved for this indication.

TABLE 1 Treatment Guidelines

Antibiotic Regimen	Comments
Erythema Migrans	
Amoxicillin1, 500 mg tid for 14-21 d	Pediatric dose, 50 mg/kg/day divided into 3 doses
Doxycycline (Vibramycin)[1], 100 mg bid for 14-21 d	Effective against human granulocytic ehrlichiosis; not recommended for children younger than 9 years of age or for pregnant or lactating women
Cefuroxime axetil (Ceftin)[1], 500 mg bid for 21 d	
Tetracycline[1], 500 mg qid for 14-21 d	Not recommended for children younger than 9 years of age or for pregnant or lactating women
Azithromycin (Zithromax)[1], 500 mg/d for 7-10 d	Less effective than other regimens
Early Disseminated Disease (without neurologic, cardiac, or joint involvement)	
Initial treatment is the same as for erythema migrans except duration of treatment may be extended to 21-28 d.	
Neuroborreliosis and Isolated Seventh Nerve Palsy	
Initial treatment is the same as for erythema migrans except duration of treatment is 21-28 d. The need for cerebral spinal fluid examination remains controversial.	
All Other Neurologic Manifestations (including meningitis, radiculoneuritis, peripheral neuropathy, encephalomyelitis, chronic encephalopathy)	
Ceftriaxone (Rocephin)[1], 2 g/d for 14-30 d	30-day regimen associated with fewer relapses in patients with chronic encephalopathy
Penicillin G[1], 20 million units/d for 14-28 d	Pediatric dose, 200,000-400,000 U/kg/d given in divided doses every 4 h
Cefotaxime sodium (Claforan)[1], 2 g every 8 h for 14-28 d	Pediatric dose, 90-180 mg/kg/d
Doxycycline[1], 100 mg bid (oral or IV) for 14-28 d	No published experience in the United States
Carditis	
Doxycycline[1], 100 mg orally bid for 21 d	For first-degree heart block; PR interval <0.3 sec
Amoxicillin[1], 500 mg tid for 21 d	For first-degree heart block; PR interval <0.3 sec
Ceftriaxone[1], 2 g/d for 14-30 d	Optimal duration of therapy unknown
Penicillin G[1], 20 million units daily for 14-30 d	Optimal duration of therapy unknown; given in divided doses every 4 h
Arthritis	
Amoxicillin[1], 500 mg qid for 30-60 d	Oral regimens limited to patients without evidence of neurologic involvement; may extend oral treatment for 60 d if no response to 30 d course
Doxycycline, 100[1] mg bid for 30-60 d	
Cefuroxime axetil, 500 mg bid for 30-60 d	For patients with doxycycline and penicillin allergies
Ceftriaxone[1], 2 g/d for 14-30 d	
Lyme Disease in Pregnancy	
Amoxicillin[1], 500 mg 500 mg tid for 21 d	For early localized disease only
Penicillin G[1], 20 million units daily for 14-28 d	Given in divided doses every 4 h
Ceftriaxone[1], 2 g/d for 14-28 d	
Asymptomatic Tick Bite	
No treatment or single dose of 200 mg doxycycline[1]	For pregnant women, consider 10 d course of amoxicillin[1]

Abbreviations: bid, twice per day; IV, intravenous; PR, pulse rate; qid, four times per day; tid, three times per day.
[1]Not FDA approved for this indication.

safe and efficacious. LYMErix[2] (SmithKline Beecham, Philadelphia, PA), a recombinant OspA vaccine, was approved by the Food and Drug Administration (FDA) for the prevention of Lyme disease in 1999 for use in individuals older than age 16 years. Recommendations for the use of the Lyme disease vaccine were made by the CDC and the Committee on Infectious Disease. The production and sales of LYMErix were halted in early 2002 by the sponsor, GlaxoSmithKline, reportedly because of poor sales.

Lyme disease is the most common tick-borne disease in the United States. The overall trend has been an average annual increase in cases since surveillance was initiated by the CDC in 1982. Most individuals with Lyme disease are diagnosed early with erythema migrans and respond well to short courses of oral antibiotics. In patients who present with later stages of illness, the diagnosis is based upon sound clinical evidence of disease and supported by serologic testing. The stage and organ system involved guide the selection of an antibiotic regimen. Successful eradication of the infecting organism, *B. burgdorferi*, appears to occur in the majority of patients with Lyme disease using these treatment guidelines (Table 1). Patients with persistent symptoms following antibiotic therapy, particularly those with previous evidence of disseminated disease, pose a difficult management problem. Most persistent symptoms are likely caused by retained antigens and are not the results of persistent infection or noninfectious sequelae such as fibromyalgia. In the former patients, resolution of symptoms occurs during the course of weeks to months and does not require prolonged courses of antibiotics; in the latter, treatment is related to the associated syndrome. Rarely, persistent or recurrent symptoms are caused by continued or recurrent infection and require additional courses of antibiotics. Such patients require careful diagnostic evaluation to determine the need for additional treatment.

RUBELLA AND CONGENITAL RUBELLA SYNDROME

METHOD OF

Katalin I. Koranyi, MD

Epidemiology

Rubella is a self-limited viral illness caused by an RNA virus from the Togaviridae family. Postnatal rubella is usually a mild disease characterized by a maculopapular rash and lymphadenopathy. The disease is often asymptomatic and complications are infrequent. The primary concern with this disease is congenital rubella syndrome resulting from infection of the fetus in utero. The most commonly associated anomalies with congenital rubella syndrome include eye, cardiac, auditory, and neurologic complications. Congenital rubella syndrome was first described in 1941. During the worldwide rubella pandemic from 1962 to 1964, the United States reported 12.5 million cases of postnatally acquired rubella, 11,000 fetal deaths, and 20,000 infants born with congenital rubella syndrome. The estimated cost to the U.S. economy was approximately $2 billion. Since the 1969 introduction of the rubella vaccine, the incidence of rubella and congenital rubella syndrome has declined by 99% in the United States. Many of the cases that have occurred developed in unimmunized young adults in colleges and occupational settings. Also, unimmunized, susceptible persons, particularly women of childbearing age coming into the United States from developing countries, accounted for most of the congenital rubella syndrome cases reported in the country. Before the use of rubella vaccine, rubella epidemics occurred in 6- to 9-year cycles, which is still the epidemiologic phenomenon occurring in countries that do not have the vaccine (primarily developing countries). According to the World Health Organization (WHO), worldwide eradication of rubella is feasible with worldwide vaccine coverage. Unfortunately, only approximately 36% of all countries currently have rubella immunization programs. The incubation period is usually 16 to 18 days. Postnatal rubella is usually spread by direct or droplet contact from nasopharyngeal secretions. The virus is communicable a few days before through 5 to 7 days after the onset of the rash.

Clinical Features

POSTNATALLY ACQUIRED RUBELLA

After an incubation period of 14 to 21 days (usually 16-18 days), the first manifestation that appears in children is usually a rash. Adolescents and adults may have nonspecific prodrome symptoms 1 to 5 days before the onset of the rash, consisting of fever, sore throat, and arthralgia. From 25% to 50% of individuals infected with rubella virus are asymptomatic. Therefore, a lack of history of past rubella is unreliable. The rash is a fine, pink maculopapular eruption that begins behind the ears and on the face and then spreads downward. In contrast to measles, the rash does not coalesce and it seldom involves the palms and the soles. The rash usually fades in 1 to 3 days and is not followed by desquamation. Occasionally, a palatal enanthem is seen in the oropharyngeal examination. Lymphadenopathy, particularly postauricular but also suboccipital and cervical, is found. Fever, if present, is usually low grade. Arthralgia or arthritis is occasionally seen in adolescents and adults. The evanescent nature of the rash and the lack of specific signs and symptoms make clinical diagnosis of postnatally acquired rubella difficult, and it usually needs to be confirmed by laboratory tests. Immunity is usually lifelong, but reinfection has been documented on rare occasions.

CONGENITAL RUBELLA

The greatest risk for congenital infection is during the first trimester. Between 40% and 90% of conception products obtained from women with clinical rubella during the first trimester were found to be infected. Fetal infections may lead to miscarriages, stillbirths, and infants born with congenital rubella syndrome. Maternal infection after 16 weeks of gestation rarely causes congenital abnormalities. The newborn with congenital rubella syndrome may be asymptomatic at birth and have defects manifested later in life, or the symptoms may be manifested at birth. The clinical manifestations are variable; one identical twin may be infected and the other spared. Maternal infection may lead to maternal viremia, placental infection, and then fetal viremia, but there may be no transplacental infection. The disease is more severe with multisystem involvement if infection occurs during the first 8 weeks of gestation. Fetal infection is chronic, and the virus persists throughout fetal life and after birth. Some infants with congenital rubella continue to shed virus in nasal pharyngeal secretions and urine for 1 year or more. The classic triad of congenital rubella syndrome characterized by cataracts, deafness, and congenital heart disease was described in 1941. During the pandemic of 1960-1962 the spectrum of rubella embryopathy was expanded to include most organ systems. The most common manifestations are ophthalmologic (cataracts, congenital glaucoma, retinitis), cardiac (patent ductus arteriosus, peripheral pulmonary artery stenosis), auditory (sensory neurodeafness), and neurologic (meningoencephalitis, microcephaly, mental retardation). Physical examination of infants with congenital rubella at birth often shows hepatosplenomegaly, jaundice, and purpuric skin lesions ("blueberry muffin" appearance). Growth retardation, radiolucent bone disease, and thrombocytopenia also may be apparent. The early clinical manifestations of congenital rubella are transient and often resolve in a few weeks; however, progressive or permanent manifestations of congenital rubella can occur in any organ. Deafness is usually bilateral and may be progressive. Clinical manifestations of congenital rubella may not be apparent at birth, particularly when infection occurs later during pregnancy (i.e., after 16 weeks), with manifestations occurring later on in life. The late onset manifestations may not be apparent until 2 years of age or older. These findings include hypogammaglobulinemia, endocrine manifestations (diabetes, thyroiditis, hypothyroidism, growth hormone deficiency), pneumonitis, and progressive panencephalitis. The purpuric rash seen at birth usually disappears in a few weeks, but a chronic rash may be present later. Permanent neurologic defects including microcephaly, behavioral problems, developmental delay, and chronic encephalitis may not be present at birth but appear later in life. The degree of mental retardation varies from mild to moderate. Progressive panencephalitis is a rare complication that usually becomes apparent in the second decade of life.

Diagnosis

The clinical diagnosis of rubella is difficult because of overlap with other viral infections, including parvovirus B19 in the spring and enteroviral exanthems in the summertime. An accurate diagnosis is important particularly during pregnancy or during an outbreak. Serologic tests for rubella-specific immunoglobulin (Ig) M and IgG antibodies usually result in an accurate diagnosis if the rubella infection is recent, past, or does not exist. A fourfold or greater rise of rubella-specific IgG antibodies in paired sera, or the presence of rubella-specific IgM antibodies in a single sample indicate recent infection. Rubella-specific IgM antibodies in the fetus usually become detectable after 22 weeks of gestation. If maternal rubella infection is proven, chorionic villus, amniotic fluid culture, or polymerase chain reaction amplification for rubella virus should be performed on the fetus by an experienced perinatologist. After birth, if the infant is suspected to have congenital rubella, cultures of the pharyngeal secretions, urine, and cerebrospinal fluid (CSF) need to be done. The persistent nature of congenital rubella infection allows these cultures to remain positive for weeks to months. Rubella-specific IgM antibody present in a newborn is highly suggestive of congenital infection. However, false-positive and false-negative results with IgM antibodies can occur. Maternal rubella-specific IgG antibody usually disappears from the infant's serum after 6 months of age. Therefore, persistence of rubella-specific IgG antibody in the infant beyond 6 months of age or an increase in titer is also suggestive of congenital infection.

Treatment and Management

For postnatal rubella, only symptomatic treatment is indicated. Symptoms usually resolve in a few days. Rubella-specific IgG antibodies should be determined during the first prenatal visit and nonimmune women should receive rubella vaccine soon after delivery. If serologic tests in a pregnant woman indicate rubella infection in the first trimester, expert advice needs to be sought. Some perinatologists will recommend further testing of the fetus to determine if fetal infection has occurred. Other experts might advise termination of the pregnancy. The main control measure to prevent rubella is active immunization with rubella vaccine.

Vaccine

In the United States, immunization of all infants with rubella vaccine, which is usually a combination of measles, mumps, and rubella (MMR), is recommended at 12 months of age. Selective vaccination of prepubertal women or women of reproductive age is also recommended. In some countries only selective rubella vaccination is practiced. The rubella vaccine is a live, attenuated virus vaccine of the RA27/3 strain grown in human diploid cell cultures. A single dose at 12 months of age or older induces protective antibody that prevents rubella in 95% of the recipients. The current recommendation of 2 doses for the MMR vaccine improves its efficacy for those individuals with primary vaccine failures. Rubella vaccine is contraindicated during pregnancy or for women who are considering pregnancy within 3 months of vaccine administration. None of the 226 seronegative women who were inadvertently vaccinated with rubella vaccine during the first trimester of pregnancy delivered a baby with congenital defects; 2% of the infants, however, had serologically confirmed rubella infection. The MMR vaccine is generally well tolerated in children. Rash occurs in about 5% of immunized persons, fever may be seen in 5% to 15% from 5 to 12 days after immunization. Mild lymphadenopathy and arthralgia of the small peripheral joints may also occur. Thrombocytopenia following immunization with MMR is very rare. In addition to pregnancy, contraindications to rubella vaccination include immunosuppressive states, except HIV-infected children with relatively normal immune function. Passive immunization with immunoglobulin for postexposure prophylaxis is generally not recommended. It should be considered only for the susceptible pregnant woman if termination of the pregnancy cannot be considered. Health care workers, childcare workers, and college students should be screened for rubella immunity, and those susceptible should be vaccinated to prevent possible infection and congenital rubella. All instances of suspected or proven congenital rubella infection should be investigated and reported to the local or state health department or to the Centers for Disease Control and Prevention. Isolation of persons with postnatal rubella is indicated for 7 days after the onset of rash. Some level of contact isolation is indicated for newborns suspected to have congenital rubella. Infants with congenital rubella are considered infectious until 1 year of age, or until multiple urine and nasopharyngeal cultures for rubella virus are negative.

MEASLES (RUBEOLA)

METHOD OF

Keith Krasinski, MD

Measles virus is a linear, single-stranded, negative-sense, 15.9-kilodalton, enveloped, human RNA *Morbillivirus* of the *Paramyxoviridae* family. A single serotype is recognized with a great deal of homogeneity among isolates of a given outbreak; however, genetic sequencing studies indicate relatively stable differences among strains in the viral nucleoprotein and hemagglutinin genes.

Epidemiology

Although measles is vaccine preventable, it and its complications continue to be important causes of morbidity and mortality worldwide, with an estimated 40 million cases resulting in more than 770,000 deaths, principally affecting children in the developing world. Case fatality rates are increased in children younger than 5 years of age and among the immunocompromised. Infected individuals shed measles virus in respiratory secretions for approximately 2 days before the development of respiratory symptoms and 3 to 4 days before the development of rash; they continue to shed virus for approximately 4 days after the development of rash. The virus is spread by direct or indirect contact with virus-containing droplets, typically in crowded situations such as classrooms, daycare centers, and residential care settings. Less commonly, measles virus is spread by the airborne route, with documented transmission in domed stadiums and in physicians' offices resulting from virus exposure hours after the index case has left. Measles is among the most contagious of diseases with more than 90% of closely exposed and 25% of community-exposed susceptibles developing infection. Measles occurs worldwide. In the prevaccine era in developed countries (and still among unimmunized populations), measles was epidemic, with biennial cycles occurring in winter and spring in temperate climates; it tended to be a disease of infancy and childhood. The availability and use of a single-dose measles vaccine strategy has been associated with a 100-fold reduction in the incidence of measles and a change in the epidemiology to unimmunized preschool children and young adults. Improved efforts at immunization and use of a two-dose strategy has resulted in further reductions of measles. Passive maternal-to-infant transfer of immunoglobulins generally results in immunity in the first 4 to 5 months of life or longer; however, susceptible mothers deliver susceptible infants. One consequence of immunization is lower concentrations of measles-specific immunoglobulins, compared with concentrations that result from natural infection. Thus, less antibody is passed transplacentally, resulting in an earlier age of susceptibility of infants because of earlier waning of passive immunity. Although primary vaccine failure occurs in up to 5% of individuals immunized at or after 12 months of age and waning immunity contributes to the susceptible population, the overwhelming cause of continued transmission of measles is failure to immunize.

Pathogenesis

Measles virus attaches to the respiratory epithelium via its hemagglutinin. The virus replicates at the site of infection and in macrophages and regional lymph nodes, resulting in a primary viremia with extensive systemic spread to many organs and tissues. Subsequently, a secondary viremia develops coincident with clinical symptomatology. The human host responds with the development of a mononuclear cell response, the generation of specific T cell-mediated cytotoxic responses, and the production of specific immunoglobulin (Ig) M and IgG antibodies. Measles causes well-recognized suppression of cell-mediated immunity that may contribute to its complications. Immunologic abnormalities include depressed lymphoproliferative responses to mitogens, decreased natural killer cell activity, and altered production of cytokines, all at a time of intense immune activation. Measles binds to the CD46 receptor of monocyte/macrophages, interacting with the complement system at the binding site of C3b, causing cell aggregation and apoptosis.

Pathologically, multinucleated giant cells develop in pharyngeal and bronchial mucosa as well as in the reticuloendothelial system, where they are known as Warthin-Finkeldey cells. The lungs develop peribronchiolar inflammation. The cutaneous and mucosal rashes also demonstrate focal syncytial epithelial giant cells with intranuclear aggregates of virus particles. When acute encephalomyelitis occurs, lymphocytic cellular infiltrates with perivascular hemorrhages occur and may be followed by demyelination.

Clinical Findings

The incubation period to clinical illness generally ranges from 8 to 12 days, but may be as short as 7 days or as long as 18 days. It first manifests as fever, malaise, and mild respiratory involvement; which is followed, in approximately 24 hours, by progressive cough, coryza, and conjunctivitis accompanied by photophobia and occasionally by nausea and rising fever. Koplik spots develop 3 to 4 days after respiratory symptoms and are characterized as fine, irregular, bright red spots with a bluish-white center on buccal mucous membranes. During the next 1 to 2 days, Koplik spots increase in number, coalesce, and then begin to slough. Concurrent with their regression, an erythematous macular rash appears at the hairline and in the next 3 days spreads cephalocaudal on the entire body, finally affecting the palms and soles. The rash may become hemorrhagic. It begins to fade by the third day in the order in which it appeared, leaving a brownish discoloration and then a fine desquamation at the sites of greatest involvement. In the absence of complications, fever also regresses. Vomiting and diarrhea may also occur and tend to be severe in malnourished children. Measles is usually accompanied by postauricular, cervical, and occipital lymphadenopathy and in more severe cases by generalized lymphadenopathy including splenomegaly. Some manifestations of bronchitis, bronchiolitis, or pneumonia are typically present and may be severe, particularly in immunodeficient patients who may exhibit disease without the typical enanthem or exanthem. Severe laryngotracheobronchitis may also occur and sometimes requires intubation. Modified measles may occur following exposure in individuals with passively acquired humoral immunity, such as those who have used exogenous immunoglobulins and occasionally in infants with maternal antibody. Following an incubation period that can be prolonged to as much as 14 to 20 days, disease tends to be milder and of shorter duration. A syndrome of atypical measles occurs following measles exposure in individuals immunized with inactivated measles virus vaccine, which was used between 1963 and 1967. The inactivated vaccine failed to induce immunity to the fusion protein of the virus, and immunized persons are incapable of preventing the cell-to-cell spread of virus. Atypical measles manifests as fever; pneumonia, which may be associated with consolidation or pleural effusion; and unusual rashes. Urticaria; maculopapular, petechial, or purpuric rashes; and occasionally vesicles, with a tendency to centrifugal distribution, have all been described. There may be associated edema, pain, and hyperesthesias of the extremities. Confirmation of the clinical diagnosis of measles is usually established with the detection of IgG antibodies in samples collected 2 to 4 weeks after acute illness. Enzyme immunoassays are the most convenient and frequently used tests, although hemagglutination inhibition and neutralization assays are still performed. IgM antibodies may be detected as early as 72 hours after onset of rash; however, measles IgM assays may be less sensitive and less specific than IgG assays. Reassessment for IgM antibodies frequently establishes the diagnosis when tests conducted in the first 72 hours are negative. Measles virus is recoverable in culture from respiratory secretions, urine, and blood, and a sensitive reverse transcriptase-nested polymerase chain reaction test can be used for diagnosis. Except in the presence of immunodeficiency or central nervous system disease, nucleic acid testing is rarely necessary for clinical purposes.

Complications

Otitis media is a common concomitant of measles. Viral pneumonia and supervening bacterial pneumonia with expected pathogens of children occur commonly and may be life-threatening. The well-known exacerbation of tuberculosis following measles and reactivation of herpes simplex virus may also occur. Although electrocardiographic changes are also common, myocarditis is rare. Acute encephalomyelitis, apparently mediated by autoimmune mechanisms, is characterized by fever, headache, vomiting, changes in mental status, personality changes, seizures, and coma and occurs in approximately 0.1% of measles cases between 2 to 6 days after the onset of rash. The course is variable and carries a 15% mortality rate with 33% of survivors exhibiting evidence of brain damage. Cerebellar ataxia, retrobulbar neuritis, and hemiplegia may also occur. Subacute sclerosing panen-cephalitis (SSPE) is a rare (1 per 100,000 cases) complication of measles, with a long incubation period averaging 10.4 years. SSPE begins insidiously, first with subtle and then progressive mental deterioration, followed by motor dysfunction, seizures, coma, and death, all occurring in succession during a period of approximately 2 years. SSPE appears to result from persistence of measles virus that escapes immune surveillance because of defects in expression of viral matrix and/or hemagglutinin or fusion genes. Immunosuppressed patients exhibit another central nervous system (CNS) syndrome characterized by generalized seizures and altered consciousness occurring weeks to 7 months after measles and progressing to death within 3 months in 85% of those affected. In this syndrome intact measles virus can be demonstrated. Neutropenia and thrombocytopenia occur with measles. Keratoconjunctivitis is common, and corneal ulcerations may occur that can be aggravated by vitamin A deficiency and may result in blindness. Appendicitis, often with rupture, also occurs. Infection during pregnancy is associated with excess fetal loss and prematurity; however, no congenital malformations have been identified. Putative associations of measles with Crohn's disease, Paget's disease of bone, autoimmune hepatitis, multiple sclerosis, and otosclerosis are unsupported.

Treatment

Symptomatic therapy is indicated. Antipyretics are used for the management of high fever. Appropriate antibiotics are used for the management of bacterial complications, but are not used routinely for the purpose of prophylaxis during acute measles because of problems with emergence of resistance. Because severe measles is associated with a low serum concentration of vitamin A and outcome is improved with the administration of vitamin A[1], consideration should be given to the use of vitamin A in children 6 months to 2 years of age who have severe measles or its complications as well as in children older than 6 months who have immunodeficiency, ophthalmologic evidence of vitamin A deficiency, impaired intestinal absorption, or malnutrition, or who have immigrated from areas with high mortality. A single oral dose of 200,000 IU (100,000 IU for those younger than 1 year of age) is used with possible side effects of vomiting and headache. For those with night blindness, Bitot's spots, or xerophthalmia the dose should be repeated in 24 hours and again in 4 weeks. Ribavirin (Virazole)[1] has activity in vitro against the virus and has been used in severe respiratory illness, CNS disease, and immunodeficiency.

[1]Not FDA approved for this indication.

Prevention

Measles vaccine is safe and effective in preventing measles and its complications, with 95% of vaccines demonstrating serologic evidence of immunity. Susceptible individuals are those born after 1956 who have no documentation of measles vaccination or serologic evidence of immunity; they should be immunized using a two-dose regimen. Generally, the first dose is given at or after 12 months and the second at 5 years of age before school entry. If the second dose is not given at 5 years, it should be given as soon after as practical. Measles-rubella (MMR) vaccine is the preferred product, given in a dose of 0.5 mL subcutaneously. A monovalent product (Attenuvax) is also available and deserves consideration for immunization of children 6 to 12 months of age during an outbreak situation. Children vaccinated in this manner should be revaccinated with a two-dose MMR or measles-rubella (MR) regimen as above. Adverse consequences of immunization include fever (5%-15%), transient rashes (5%), and transient thrombocytopenia (1/25,000-1/2,000,000). Children predisposed to seizures or with seizure disorders should be immunized despite the possibility of a slight increase in risk of a seizure. Measles vaccination is generally contraindicated in individuals who are significantly immunocompromised; however, asymptomatic and mildly symptomatic individuals infected with the human immunodeficiency virus without severe depression of CD4 count should be immunized, and the two-dose regimen should be accelerated to induce immunity before the progression of the underlying immunodeficiency. Individuals on high dose steroids, but who are not otherwise immunologically compromised, should be immunized after a minimum of 1 month after interruption or discontinuation of steroid use. Measles vaccine may suppress delayed-type hypersensitivity, but it does not aggravate tuberculosis; therefore, tuberculin testing is not a precondition for immunization. To avoid false-negative, purified protein derivative (PPD) responses, tuberculin testing is not performed in the 6 weeks following vaccination. Hypersensitivity to measles vaccine is rare. Children with egg allergies may be immunized safely. Children with a history of anaphylaxis to eggs have also been immunized safely. When anaphylaxis can be anticipated, prudence dictates vaccination in a setting in which it can be managed adequately. Anaphylaxis to measles vaccine or to neomycin is a contraindication. Minor illnesses with or without fever are not contraindications to vaccination. Because exogenous antibody may interfere with the vaccine take, an immunization delay following the administration of antibodies—3 months for low-dose immunoglobulin-containing products and up to 11 months for very high doses—is recommended. Vaccine administered within 72 hours after exposure may prevent measles. IG (Immune Globulin), 0.25 mL/kg within 6 days after exposure, may also prevent measles. The immunoglobulin dose is increased to 0.5 mL/kg in immunodeficient individuals, who should receive prophylaxis despite prior active immunization. The maximum dose is 15 mL. Unimmunized, exposed individuals who are given immunoglobulin should be actively immunized beginning at 5-, 6-, or 12-month intervals depending on the dose of immunoglobulin. In hospital settings, exposed, susceptible individuals should be managed with infection control precautions from the fifth through the twenty-first day after contacts, or if they develop disease, through the fifth day of rash. All suspected cases of measles should be reported promptly to the public health authorities before the diagnosis is established.

TETANUS

METHOD OF

Satish Bhagwanjee, MBChB

Tetanus was first described in ancient Egypt more than 3000 years ago. Despite the availability of active and passive immunization, tetanus is estimated to cause up to one million fatalities annually. The majority of these deaths occur in developing countries in Africa and Asia where the disease is endemic. These deaths in these countries are primarily because of ineffective vaccination programs as well as the lack of clinical facilities to offer mechanical ventilation and invasive monitoring. As many as 40% of these fatalities occur following neonatal and maternal tetanus as a result of unhygienic delivery practices. In developed countries, fatalities from tetanus are less common and tend to occur in the older patient.

In the severe form of the disease, prehospital deaths occur from airway obstruction and respiratory failure. Sympathetic overactivity (SOA) is a major cause of mortality in the early hospital phase. Late in the disease, death results from complications associated with prolonged intensive care.

Prevention

In developed countries where effective immunization programs and adequate standards of living are evident, the incidence of the disease has fallen dramatically. In developing countries, neither of these is satisfied. Overcoming the lack of effective immunization programs, installing basic health care provisions, and attempting to achieve minimum basic standards of living are priorities of the World Health Organization (WHO) in its efforts to eradicate this disease. Active immunization involves administration of tetanus toxoid (as diphtheria, tetanus toxoids, and acellular pertussis [DtaP]) at least four times to children, with booster doses (as tetanus-diphtheria [Td]) every 5 to 10 years to ensure ongoing immunity. Reactions to immunization are rare, but commonly include fever and local tenderness when they do occur. Guillain-Barré syndrome is a rare complication. Passive immunization with tetanus immunoglobulin (BayTet) is indicated particularly for the immunocompromised and those at extremes of age. The risk of neonatal tetanus can be minimized by immunization of mothers during pregnancy. In addition, education regarding safe care of the mother and child during childbirth is essential to change hazardous practices in unsophisticated communities.

Pathogenesis

The causative organism is *Clostridium tetani*, an anaerobic spore-forming, gram-positive bacillus that is extremely stable even in harsh environmental conditions. The organism is widely distributed in the environment and gains access to the host via breaches in the skin. Disease is produced by the toxin that enters peripheral nerves at the site of injury and migrates to the central nervous system (CNS) via retrograde axonal transport. The toxin prevents release of the inhibitory neurotransmitters γ-aminobutyric acid (GABA) and glycine. The motor neurons are, therefore, uninhibited and produce the severe spasms typical of tetanus following minimal stimulation. The effect of the toxin is seen primarily at the level of the spinal cord, brainstem, and peripheral nerves. Recent data suggest that cortical disinhibition may also occur, which may explain the neurological deficit observed in neonates.

Clinical Features

Several mechanisms of entry have been described including minor trauma, nonsterile injections, compound fractures, and postpartum infections. The incubation period varies from hours to months, depending on the site of entry and the quantity of toxin released. Several classification systems have been described. For the purpose of this discussion a simple, clinically relevant approach is appropriate (Table 1). Prognosis is related to whether the disease is localized or generalized, and to the extent of organ system involvement.

TABLE 1 Classification of Tetanus

Localized	Disease limited to site of injury
Generalized	Wide distribution of spasms
Cephalic	Variant of localized, involving cranial nerves
Neonatal	Generalized disease in the neonate

TABLE 2 Complications of Tetanus

Early (First Few Days)	Intermediate (Few Days to 2 Weeks)	Late (Beyond 2 Weeks)
Airway loss/hypoxemia Respiratory failure Severe spasms/fractures	SOA Respiratory failure and barotrauma Renal failure Gastrointestinal failure	Nosocomial sepsis Nutritional disturbances Cardiomyopathy Thromboembolism

Abbreviation: SOA = sympathetic overactivity.

Lack of immunization and extremes of age are associated with a poor prognosis.

In the localized form, pain and spasm occur close to (and is limited to) the site of injury. This is usually self-limiting. Generalized tetanus is characterized by generalized spasms and severe pain, trismus, risus sardonicus, and opisthotonus. The major complications associated with the severe form of the disease are listed in Table 2. Spasms may be triggered by minimal stimulation, produce excruciating pain, and, in the most severe form, produce fractures. Effective ventilation is not possible during severe spasms and may, therefore, result in respiratory failure. Laryngeal spasm causes loss of the airway and hypoxemia. SOA is a common later complication characterized by wide swings in pulse and blood pressure. Sudden cardiac arrest, dysrhythmias, intracranial hemorrhage, and gastrointestinal dysfunction are complications associated with SOA. Renal failure occurs following hypovolemia and severe vasoconstriction. Barotrauma is a common iatrogenic complication of mechanical ventilation when spasms are poorly controlled. Cardiomyopathy occurs late and is a consequence of excessive catecholamine stimulation. Cephalic tetanus is characterized by cranial nerve involvement and early loss of the airway. Neonatal tetanus is usually generalized and commonly results from contamination of the umbilical stump. Severe spasms and SOA are common and are rapidly fatal if untreated. The diagnosis is made on the clinical presentation and by excluding other diagnoses. In developed countries where the disease is uncommon, the diagnosis may be easily missed. The characteristic severe spasms without loss of consciousness are pathognomonic of the disease. There are no specific confirmatory laboratory tests. The differential diagnoses include strychnine poisoning, dystonic reactions, and meningitis. In neonates, hypoglycemia, seizures, and hypocalcemia should also be considered. The complications related to prolonged intensive care management of these patients include nosocomial sepsis, thromboembolic disease, and nutritional disturbances.

Management

GENERAL PRINCIPLES

While the site of initial injury is often not identifiable when the patient presents with spasms, when a site is evident, effective local débridement is the mainstay of initial management. Penicillin is the classic antibiotic prescribed for eradication of the organism. The disadvantage with this drug is that it is structurally similar to GABA and it may act as a competitive antagonist, thereby enhancing CNS excitability. Metronidazole (Flagyl) is a safe alternative. Lastly, the occurrence of spasms implies inadequate immunization. Consequently, active immunization with tetanus toxoid (Td) and passive immunization with tetanus immunoglobulin (BayTet) are mandatory.

LOCALIZED TETANUS

The mild form of the disease lends itself to conservative management in a ward environment. The patient should be nursed in a quiet area with adequate sedation using a benzodiazepine such as diazepam (Valium). Stimulation should be kept to a minimum to minimize the risk of provoking further spasms. Clinical assessment to ensure nonprogression is the only indication for stimulation. The natural history is for resolution of symptoms within 7 to 14 days.

CEPHALIC TETANUS

These patients are at high risk for major complications, including loss of the airway and inadequate ventilation, and should be given the same treatment as generalized tetanus patients.

GENERALIZED AND NEONATAL TETANUS

The mortality rate in these patients is high, therefore, care should be provided in an intensive/critical care unit. Transfer should occur as soon as the diagnosis is made.

Airway Management

The airway should be secured as soon as generalized spasms are noted. This is ideally performed in an operating room environment, although that is not always feasible. A skilled anesthesiologist should perform intubation using an induction dose of a benzodiazepine such as midazolam (Versed). Alternatively, thiopental (Pentothal)[1] or propofol (Diprivan)[1] may be used. The muscle relaxant of choice is succinylcholine (Anectine), which will allow for rapid airway control. It is common for tracheotomy to be performed at this

[1]Not FDA approved for this indication.

time, although there is insufficient data to support this practice. The intervention must be based on the standard practice at the institution.

Management of Sympathetic Overactivity (SOA)

A plethora of drugs and techniques are used to control this devastating complication. The perfect approach has not been described; treatment must be individualized. The principles of management are:

- Ensure adequacy of the preload
- Prevent wide swings in pulse and blood pressure
- Minimize catecholamine secretion

The first step in effective management is to ensure adequacy of the preload with appropriate volume replacement guided by central venous pressure measurements and measures of perfusion. This ensures hemodynamic control and prevents complications such as renal failure. The steps described below are important to prevent delayed cardiac sequelae. Adequate sedation using the benzodiazepines is essential to minimize sensory stimulation (auditory, visual, tactile). Benzodiazepines also augment GABA activity in the CNS, as do midazolam (Versed)[1] and diazepam (Valium)[1]. Major tranquilizers such as chlorpromazine (Thorazine) are sometimes used as adjuncts for sedation. High-dose morphine[1] produces sedation and cardiovascular stability. The effect is thought to be based on replacing depleted endogenous opioids and histamine release. Beta-blockade with drugs such as propranolol (Inderal)[1] is advocated as a means of controlling sympathetic discharge. Rebound bradycardia and hypotension limit the usefulness of this approach, because sympathetic discharge is generally transient. The short-acting beta-blocker, esmolol (Brevibloc)[1], has the advantage of a short half-life but is generally unavailable in resource-constrained countries. Alpha-blockade has not been shown to be beneficial. Atropine[1] is used to block cholinergic excess associated with autonomic disturbance. The effect is peripheral and central, blocking both nicotinic and muscarinic receptors. This approach reduces sweating and secretions. Neuraxial blockade using intrathecal baclofen (Lioresal intrathecal)[1] has been used in a small series of patients. Serious adverse effects described with this approach include coma and respiratory depression. Epidural blockade using bupivacaine (Marcaine)[1] with and without opiates is employed successfully. The advantages of this approach are a reduction in the need for ventilation and improvement in renal

[1]Not FDA approved for this indication.

function, but a possible, serious complication, epidural abscess, limits the use of the technique to patients with refractory SOA. Magnesium sulfate[1] is used to treat both spasm and SOA with good effect. The benefit is based on a reduction in catecholamine release, peripheral vasodilatation, and reduced myocardial responsiveness to circulating catecholamines. It must, however, be used in conjunction with parenteral sedation such as a benzodiazepine. Given that most patients are treated in circumstances with seriously constrained resources, a rational sequential approach to treat SOA is as follows:

- Adequate sedation with a benzodiazepine
- Addition of a parenteral opiate
- Addition of parenteral magnesium sulphate
- Epidural bupivacaine plus opiate

Ventilation

The major respiratory complications are barotrauma and nosocomial pneumonia. A lung-protective ventilatory strategy (limiting plateau pressure to 30 cmH_2O, and limiting tidal volume to 6-8 mL/kg) and appropriate use of positive-end expiratory pressure (PEEP) are essential to prevent these complications. In addition, effective sedation and control of spasms are essential. The long-term use of muscle relaxants should be discouraged to prevent the development of the polyneuropathy of critical illness.

General Intensive Care Management

Nasogastric feeding should be commenced as soon as possible to ensure adequate nutritional status and to minimize the occurrence of nosocomial sepsis. These patients are often in the intensive care unit (ICU) for several weeks and are prone to develop ICU-related complications. Nosocomial sepsis is a serious threat to life as there are often multiple episodes with associated hemodynamic consequences. Thromboembolic events are late complications that require attention to prophylaxis against deep vein thrombosis.

Although a preventable disease, tetanus is still an important cause of morbidity and mortality, particularly in developing countries. The importance of effective immunization programs and education in prevention cannot be overemphasized. Insights into the pathogenesis of the disease have allowed clinicians to offer effective therapy for patients afflicted with it. The choice of therapy is, however, often dependent on existing resources. A systematic approach to total patient care results in improved outcomes even in resource-constrained environments.

[1]Not FDA approved for this indication.

WHOOPING COUGH (PERTUSSIS)

METHOD OF

Denise Bratcher, DO

Pertussis, or whooping cough, is a highly contagious, acute respiratory tract infection caused by *Bordetella pertussis*. It is a prolonged cough illness that lasts at least 2 weeks and is characterized by paroxysms of coughing, inspiratory "whoops," and post-tussive vomiting. In the prevaccine era, pertussis was a common cause of morbidity and mortality among children, with an average of 175,000 cases reported per year in the United States. Following the introduction of pertussis vaccines in the 1940s, the incidence of pertussis fell to a historic low of 1010 cases in 1976. Since the 1980s, reported pertussis incidence has increased with peaks occurring every 3 to 4 years. Despite effective vaccines, pertussis continues to occur in the United States among all age groups.

Microbiology and Pathophysiology

B. pertussis is a small, gram-negative, aerobic, pleomorphic coccobacillus that grows optimally at 95°F to 98.6°F (35°C to 37°C). The organism is fastidious and requires media containing protective substances such as charcoal, blood, or starch. *B. pertussis* produces multiple virulence factors, which serve as antigens and are responsible for its pathogenesis. These include pertussis toxin, adenylate cyclase toxin, tracheal cytotoxin, fimbriae, filamentous hemagglutinin, agglutinogens, and pertactin. The organism attaches to ciliated respiratory epithelium, evades host defenses, produces toxins that paralyze the respiratory cilia, and causes inflammation of the respiratory tract.

Epidemiology

B. pertussis is exclusively a human pathogen and is the sole cause of epidemic pertussis. Transmission occurs person-to-person via aerosolized droplets from patients with disease or by contact with their secretions. Most cases occur in summer and early fall. Pertussis is highly contagious, infecting 80% to 90% of susceptible contacts. Individuals with pertussis are most contagious during the catarrhal period and the first 2 weeks after onset of the cough.

As a result of waning immunity following natural disease or vaccine, the prevalence of pertussis in adolescents and adults is increasing. The peak incidence of reported cases typically occurs among 1 to 5 year olds, many of whom are inadequately immunized. An increase in reported cases among those 10 years of age and older has been noted since 1993. This increase may be, in part, because of a greater awareness of pertussis and the potential for disease in older children and adults, as well as improved diagnostic techniques. Despite continued high levels of vaccination coverage, the number of reported pertussis cases in the United States has increased steadily since the 1980s.

Immunity

Immunity to pertussis, whether following natural infection or vaccination, is not persistent. As a result, adolescents and adults in the United States are inadequately protected against *B. pertussis* and may be important sources of pertussis for infants and young children.

Clinical Symptoms

The incubation period of pertussis is usually 7 to 10 days, but ranges between 4 days to 3 weeks. Classic pertussis is a prolonged illness that presents in three stages—catarrhal, paroxysmal, and convalescent—with each lasting approximately 2 weeks. The stages may be shorter in immunized children, and symptoms may vary in young infants. Pertussis is more severe when it occurs during the first 6 months of life.

The first stage, the catarrhal stage, is the most contagious and presents with nonspecific symptoms similar to the common cold, including rhinorrhea, sneezing, possibly a low-grade fever, and an occasional cough that gradually becomes more severe. Young infants may have minimal symptoms in this stage.

As symptoms progress, bursts of numerous, rapid coughs mark the paroxysmal stage. A long, inspiratory effort accompanied by the characteristic high-pitched whoop follows the cough. Post-tussive emesis is common, and exhaustion following a coughing episode is typical. Paroxysms are more frequent at night, occurring with minimal provocation such as during feedings, while laughing, or with change of position during sleep. Between coughing attacks, patients usually appear completely normal. Young infants frequently present with apnea, choking, gasping, or color changes ranging from a reddened face to cyanosis; cough and whoop are frequently absent. Infants may appear very ill and distressed during the paroxysmal stage and require close observation and supportive care. Older children and adults can have atypical manifestations, with prolonged cough with paroxysms but no whoop, or without paroxysms. The paroxysmal stage usually lasts 1 to 6 weeks. Cultures obtained in the early paroxysmal stage are frequently positive.

The cough gradually disappears over 2 to 3 weeks during the convalescent period. The cough may initially become louder with a detectable whoop among young infants as they grow and gain strength during convalescence. Milder paroxysms may recur with subsequent respiratory infections for many months following a pertussis infection.

Complications

Complications occur most commonly among young infants with pertussis. Infants and children with underlying conditions, such as cardiopulmonary disease, neuromuscular disease, prematurity, or immune deficiency, are also at higher risk for severe disease. The most common complication is secondary bacterial pneumonia. Otitis media also occurs as a secondary bacterial complication. Hypoxia or effects of pertussis toxin may contribute to neurologic complications including seizures and encephalopathy. Other problems related to the forceful coughing include subconjunctival hemorrhages, upper body petechiae, subdural hematomas, umbilical and inguinal hernias, rectal prolapse, subcutaneous emphysema, rib fractures, and pneumothorax. In the 4-year period between 1997 and 2000, the case-fatality rate caused by pertussis in the United States was 0.2%, with 90% of deaths occurring in children younger than 6 months of age.

Diagnosis

A clinical diagnosis is typically made based on the history and characteristic cough, although patients are often examined several times before the correct diagnosis is considered. Supportive laboratory features include an absolute lymphocytosis (>10,000 lymphocytes/mm^3), which is characteristic of pertussis in the late catarrhal and paroxysmal stages but less common among adults and immunized children. Absolute lymphocyte counts of >20,000 lymphocytes/mm^3 are common. Chest radiographs may be normal but often show peribronchial consolidation, interstitial edema, or variable atelectasis. The presence of fever and consolidation in a child with pertussis suggests a secondary bacterial infection.

Isolation of *B. pertussis* from a culture of nasal secretions remains the gold standard for laboratory diagnosis, particularly as it provides isolates for genotypic analysis and antimicrobial susceptibility testing. A nasopharyngeal specimen is obtained by inserting a small, flexible Dacron or calcium alginate swab through the nose into the posterior nasopharynx where it is held for a few seconds of cough. Nasal aspirates may enhance recovery of *B. pertussis* and are preferred if polymerase chain reaction (PCR) is being performed in conjunction with culture. The specimen is transferred to *Bordetella*-specific transport media and subsequently plated on fresh Bordet-Gengou media, Regan-Lowe charcoal agar, or Stainer-Scholte agar. Cultures are incubated at 95°F to 98.6°F (35°C to 37°C) in a humid environment and examined daily for at least 7 days. Continued observation for up to 12 days may enhance recovery. Cultures are usually positive if obtained in the catarrhal or early paroxysmal stage of disease in unimmunized children. Success in isolating *B. pertussis* diminishes if patients have received pertussis vaccine or recent antimicrobials with pertussis activity or if specimens are obtained beyond the first 3 weeks of symptoms.

PCR has consistently shown greater sensitivity than culture or direct fluorescent antibody (DFA) and more rapid detection than culture. PCR is more sensitive among persons with mild or atypical symptoms and those who have received prior antimicrobial therapy. Currently, no standardized, universally accepted PCR technique exists, and potential variability among adolescent and adult patients requires further study. The Centers for Disease Control and Prevention recommend using PCR as a presumptive assay in conjunction with culture.

DFA testing has a low sensitivity and variable specificity, requiring experienced laboratory personnel for consistent results. DFA testing should only be performed as an adjunct to culture or PCR.

Serologic testing methods are difficult to interpret as a lack of association between antibody levels and immunity to pertussis exists. These methods are not standardized, are not widely available, and are usually not helpful during acute illness.

Treatment

Medical management of pertussis is primarily supportive. Infants and children with severe paroxysms associated with cyanosis or apnea require hospitalization and frequently require intubation, mechanical ventilation, and intensive care. Infants younger than 3 months of age are admitted routinely for observation of their paroxysmal episodes, their need for supportive interventions, and their ability to feed appropriately. Continuous monitoring of heart rate, respiratory rate, and oxygen saturation is indicated. Once assured that no supportive intervention is required during paroxysms, that nutrition is adequate, and that their symptoms are improving or not progressing, infants can be managed at home. Infants between 3 and 6 months of age are frequently hospitalized unless their witnessed paroxysms are not severe.

Supportive care includes minimizing stimuli and supplemental oxygen, if needed and only during paroxysmal episodes. Airway suctioning should be accomplished with caution as it may precipitate a paroxysm. Intravenous fluids and nutritional support are indicated if the child is unable to take adequate nutrition. Data from well-controlled, prospective clinical trials are not available to determine the role of corticosteroids or bronchodilators, such as albuterol (Proventil)[1]. Aerosol treatments may also trigger paroxysms. Therefore, their use is not indicated. Cough suppressants are of no benefit. Pertussis immunoglobulin has shown promise in reducing coughing episodes and is currently undergoing clinical trials.

---

[1]Not FDA approved for this indication.

When pertussis is suspected or confirmed, antimicrobial therapy is always warranted, even in those who have coughed for weeks. Antimicrobial agents given during the catarrhal stage may ameliorate the disease, especially among young infants. Once cough is established, antimicrobial therapy may have no discernible effect on the course of illness, but it can eradicate the organism from secretions and decrease communicability.

Erythromycin estolate (Ilosone) (40-50 mg/kg/d, orally, in 4 divided doses; maximum 2 g/d) for 14 days is the drug of choice. Although more expensive, clarithromycin (Biaxin)[1] (15 mg/kg/d, orally, in 2 divided doses; maximum 500 mg every 12h) for 7 days and azithromycin (Zithromax)[1] (10-12 mg/kg/d, orally, in a single daily dose; maximum 500 mg/d) for 5 days have similar efficacy and are better tolerated. Resistance to erythromycin and other macrolides has been reported rarely. Trimethoprim-sulfamethoxazole (Bactrim)[1] (8 mg/kg/d trimethoprim, orally, in 2 divided doses) is an alternative therapy with modest activity.

To limit secondary transmission of pertussis, household and daycare contacts of a pertussis patient should receive a 14-day course of erythromycin regardless of their immunization status or age. Treatment regimens listed above are appropriate for chemoprophylaxis.

An association between orally administered erythromycin and infantile hypertrophic pyloric stenosis was reported in infants younger than 2 weeks of age. The American Academy of Pediatrics continues to recommend the use of erythromycin for prophylaxis and treatment of pertussis, because the disease in neonates can be life-threatening and alternative therapies are not well studied. Parents of newborn infants should be informed about the potential risks if erythromycin is prescribed.

Prevention and Control

Universal immunization with pertussis vaccine provides 80% to 90% protection against the disease and is recommended for children younger than 7 years of age. Acellular pertussis vaccines in combination with diphtheria and tetanus toxoids (DTaP) are preferred for routine childhood immunization in the United States due to their lower rates of reactogenicity. Five doses of DTaP are routinely recommended for children at ages 2, 4, 6, and between 12 and 18 months, followed by a booster at 4 to 6 years of age. Four DTaP vaccines are currently licensed in the United States; completion of the primary series with the same DTaP product is recommended, when feasible. Clinical trials are ongoing to determine the safety and efficacy of acellular pertussis vaccines in adolescents and adults with a goal of reducing the reservoir of pertussis.

Following a pertussis exposure, all close contacts younger than 7 years of age who have received fewer than four doses of pertussis vaccine should complete the primary series with minimal intervals between injections. If the third DTaP dose was administered more than 6 months before exposure, a fourth dose should be given. If the primary series is completed but the fourth dose was given more than 3 years prior to exposure, a booster dose of DTaP is indicated.

Using standard and droplet precautions, patients with pertussis are isolated for 5 days after initiation of appropriate antimicrobial therapy, including daycare and school exclusion. If antimicrobial therapy is not given, precautions should continue until 3 weeks after the onset of paroxysms.

[1]Not FDA approved for this indication.

OFFICE-BASED IMMUNIZATION PRACTICES

METHOD OF

Julie A. Boom, MD

The rates of most vaccine-preventable diseases in the United States are at record low levels. In 2002, there were no cases of paralytic polio, only 22 cases of tetanus, and 36 cases of measles. However, pertussis incidence has been on a gradual rise since the 1980s. In 2001, 6,051 pertussis cases were reported. In 2002, this number rose to 7,845. Of the 10,650 children ages 3 months to 14 years who were diagnosed with pertussis between 1990 and 1996, 54% were not appropriately immunized against diphtheria, tetanus toxoids, and pertussis (DTP vaccine). This recent increase in pertussis disease rates is of great concern as disease levels are often a late indicator of the soundness of the immunization system. In 2002, the National Immunization Survey conducted by the Centers for Disease Control and Prevention found that nationally, only 74.8% of children between the ages of 19 months and 35 months have been vaccinated with four doses of diphtheria, tetanus, acellular pertussis vaccine (DTaP); three doses of polio vaccine; one dose of measles-containing vaccine; three of *Haemophilus influenzae* type b vaccine; and three doses of hepatitis B vaccine.

The reasons for low immunization coverage levels are multifactorial and include:

- Fragmentation of medical records
- Missed opportunities for vaccination
- Lack of reminder and recall systems
- Lack of provider education
- Growing complacency regarding the need for immunization

Therefore, improving immunization coverage levels for all children is important for providers caring for children. Importantly, before the administration of each dose of every vaccine, all providers must provide to the parent, legal guardian, or adult vaccine recipient a copy of the relevant Vaccine Information Statement (VIS) provided by the Centers for Disease Control and Prevention (CDC). Copies of the VIS are available on the CDC's web site at http://www.cdc.gov/nip/publications/VIS. The VIS is available in multiple languages at http://www.immunize.org. The health care provider should record in the medical record the edition date of the materials given.

Diphtheria, Tetanus, and Acellular Pertussis Vaccine

Since the early 1990s, new outbreaks of diphtheria have occurred in the newly independent states of the former Soviet Union because of low immunization coverage levels. Diphtheria is a toxin-mediated disease caused by *Corynebacterium diphtheriae*. The aerobic, nonspore-forming, gram-positive bacillus, *C. diphtheriae*, produces toxin when the bacillus is infected by a bacteriophage that carries the genetic information for the toxin. Susceptible persons who live in crowded conditions may acquire the disease through colonization of the nasopharynx. The bacillus toxin causes local tissue destruction and membrane formation. The toxin then may be hematologically spread and result in severe complications—myocarditis, neuritis, otitis media, and respiratory insufficiency—which are caused by membrane formation and airway obstruction. The case fatality rate is 5% to 10%, with rates up to 20% in children younger than age 5 years and adults older than age 40 years. Case fatality rates in epidemics may range from 3% to 23%.

Tetanus is a toxin-mediated disease caused by *Clostridium tetani*. This gram-positive, anaerobic bacillus can produce spores. The organism is sensitive to heat and oxygen, whereas the spores are very heat resistant and antiseptic resistant. Susceptible persons may acquire the disease through an open contaminated wound. If an anaerobic environment exists, such as in a deep puncture wound, *C. tetani* spores may germinate and produce toxins. Tetanus toxin, tetanospasmin, binds gangliosides at the myoneural junction, thereby blocking inhibitory impulses to motor neurons. Symptom onset is gradual and usually follows a descending pattern, including trismus (lockjaw), neck stiffness, difficulty swallowing, muscle rigidity, and spasms. Complications include laryngospasm, spinal and long-bone fractures, autonomic nervous system hyperactivity, and nosocomial infections resulting from prolonged hospitalization. This disease is fatal in 11% of reported cases, and most fatal in persons older than 60 years of age.

Pertussis, or whooping cough, is caused by the bacterium *Bordetella pertussis*. *B. pertussis* is an aerobic, gram-negative bacillus, which produces many biologically harmful products, including pertussis toxin, filamentous hemagglutinin, agglutinogens, adenylate cyclase, pertactin, and tracheal toxin. The disease is characterized by three classic stages. The *catarrhal stage* is characterized by mild upper respiratory symptoms. After 1 to 2 weeks, the *paroxysmal stage* begins. This stage is characterized by episodes of continuous, rapid coughs followed by a long inspiratory effort, which produces the high-pitched whoop. These attacks may be accompanied by cyanosis, vomiting, and exhaustion. The paroxysmal stage is followed by the *convalescent stage* during which time symptoms improve over weeks to months. Complications are worst in young infants and include secondary bacterial pneumonia, seizures, and encephalopathy. Apnea is common in infants younger than 6 months of age. The case fatality rate is 0.2%, with most deaths occurring in infants younger than 6 months of age.

Since 1996, the DTaP vaccine has been recommended for all doses of the primary pediatric series. The whole-cell vaccine (DTP) is no longer recommended for use in the United States, because studies show that the acellular pertussis vaccine is significantly more effective with fewer mild and serious adverse events. The primary series of DTaP consists of four doses of vaccine beginning at 6 weeks to 2 months of age. The first three doses are given at 4- to 8-week intervals, with the fourth dose given at 15 to 18 months of age (Figure 1). The fourth dose may be given earlier if the following three criteria are met:

1. The child is at least 12 months of age.
2. At least 6 months have elapsed since the third dose.
3. The child is unlikely to return for vaccination at 15 to 18 months of age.

A fifth dose is recommended after 4 years of age but before school entry. The fifth dose is not necessary if the fourth dose was given on or after the fourth birthday. DTaP is not recommended for children older than 7 years of age because vaccine reactions are thought to be greater in older age groups. DTaP may cause local reactions including pain, redness, or swelling, especially after the fourth or fifth dose. Approximately 1% to 4% of children may experience swelling of an entire arm or thigh following the fourth or fifth dose of DTaP. The pathogenesis of this swelling is unknown and the swelling resolves without sequelae. Moderate to severe illness is a precaution

RECOMMENDED CHILDHOOD IMMUNIZATION SCHEDULE
UNITED STATES, JANUARY–JUNE 2004

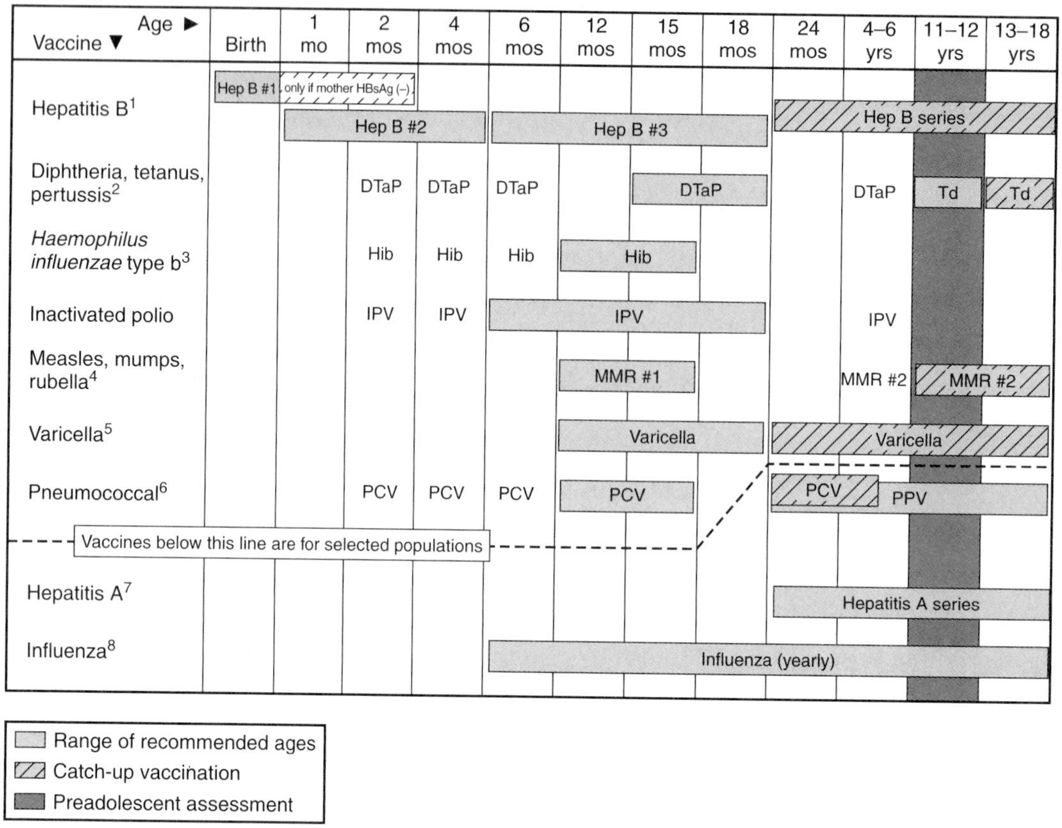

Vaccine ▼ / Age ►	Birth	1 mo	2 mos	4 mos	6 mos	12 mos	15 mos	18 mos	24 mos	4–6 yrs	11–12 yrs	13–18 yrs
Hepatitis B[1]	Hep B #1	only if mother HBsAg (–)	Hep B #2			Hep B #3					Hep B series	
Diphtheria, tetanus, pertussis[2]			DTaP	DTaP	DTaP		DTaP			DTaP	Td	Td
Haemophilus influenzae type b[3]			Hib	Hib	Hib	Hib						
Inactivated polio			IPV	IPV		IPV				IPV		
Measles, mumps, rubella[4]						MMR #1				MMR #2	MMR #2	
Varicella[5]							Varicella				Varicella	
Pneumococcal[6]			PCV	PCV	PCV	PCV			PCV	PPV		
Vaccines below this line are for selected populations												
Hepatitis A[7]											Hepatitis A series	
Influenza[8]									Influenza (yearly)			

Range of recommended ages
Catch-up vaccination
Preadolescent assessment

This schedule indicates the recommended ages for routine administration of currently licensed childhood vaccines, as of December 1, 2003, for children through age 18 years. Any dose not given at the recommended age should be given at any subsequent visit when indicated and feasible. The shaded hash marked areas indicate age groups that warrant special effort to administer those vaccines not previously given. Additional vaccines may be licensed and recommended during the year. Licensed combination vaccines may be used whenever any components of the combination are indicated and the vaccine's other components are not contraindicated. Providers should consult the manufacturers' package inserts for detailed recommendations. Clinically significant adverse events that follow immunization should be reported to the Vaccine Adverse Event Reporting System (VAERS). Guidance about how to obtain and complete a VAERS form can be found on the Internet: http://www.vaers.org/ or by calling 1-800-822-7967.

1. Hepatitis B (HepB) vaccine. All infants should receive the first dose of hepatitis B vaccine soon after birth and before hospital discharge; the first dose may also be given by age 2 months if the infant's mother is hepatitis B surface antigen (HBsAg) negative. Only monovalent HepB can be used for the birth dose. Monovalent or combination vaccine containing HepB may be used to complete the series. Four doses of vaccine may be administered when a birth dose is given. The second dose should be given at least 4 weeks after the dose, except for combination vaccines which cannot be administered before age 6 weeks. The third dose should be given at least 16 weeks after the first dose and at least 8 weeks after the second dose. The last dose in the vaccination series (third or fourth dose) should not be administered before age 24 weeks.

Infants born to HBsAg-positive mothers should receive HepB and 0.5 mL of Hepatitis B Immune Globulin (HBIG) within 12 hours of birth at separate sites. The second dose is recommended at age 1 to 2 months. The last dose in the immunization series should not be administered before age 24 weeks. These infants should be tested for HBsAg and antibody to HBsAg (anti-HBs) at age 9 to 15 months.

Infants born to mothers whose HBsAg status is unknown should receive the first dose of the HepB series within 12 hours of birth. Material blood should be drawn as soon as possible to determine the mother's HBsAg status: if the HBsAg test is positive, the infant should receive HBIG as soon as possible (no later than age 1 week). The second dose is recommended at age 1 to 2 months. The last dose in the immunization series should not be administered before age 24 weeks.

2. Diphtheria and tetanus toxoids and acellular pertussis (DTaP) vaccine. The fourth dose of DTaP may be administered as early as age 12 months, provided 6 months have elapsed since the third dose and the child is unlikely to return at age 15 to 18 months. The final dose in the series should be given at age ≥4 years. Tetanus and diphtheria toxoids (Td) is recommended at age 11 to 12 years if at least 5 years have elapsed since the last dose of tetanus and diphtheria toxoid-containing vaccine. Subsequent routine Td boosters are recommended every 10 years.

3. *Haemophilus influenzae* type b (Hib) conjugate vaccine. Three Hib conjugate vaccines are licensed for infant use. If PRP-OMP (PedvaxHIB or ComVax [Merck]) is administered at ages 2 and 4 months, a dose at age 6 months is not required. DTaP/Hib combination products should not be used for primary immunization in infants at ages 2, 4 or 6 months but can be used as boosters following any Hib vaccine. The final dose in the series should be given at age ≥12 months.

4. Measles, mumps, and rubella vaccine (MMR). The second dose of MMR is recommended routinely at age 4 to 6 years but may be administered during any visit, provided at least 4 weeks have elapsed since the first dose and both doses are administered beginning at or after age 12 months. Those who have not previously received the second dose should complete the schedule by the 11- to 12-year-old visit.

5. Varicella vaccine. Varicella vaccine is recommended at any visit at or after age 12 months for susceptible children (i.e., those who lack a reliable history of chickenpox). Susceptible persons age ≥13 years should receive 2 doses, given at least 4 weeks apart.

6. Pneumococcal vaccine. The heptavalent pneumococcal conjugate vaccine (PCV) is recommended for all children age 2 to 23 months. It is also recommended for certain children age 24 to 59 months. The final dose in the series should be given at age ≥12 months. Pneumococcal polysaccharide vaccine (PPV) is recommended in addition to PCV for certain high-risk groups. See *MMWR* 2000;49(RR-9):1-38.

7. Hepatitis A vaccine. Hepatitis A vaccine is recommended for children and adolescents in selected states and regions and for certain high-risk groups: consult your local public health authority. Children and adolescents in these states, regions, and high-risk groups who have not been immunized against hepatitis A can begin the hepatitis A immunization series during any visit. The 2 doses in the series should be administered at least 6 months apart. See *MMWR* 1999;48(RR-12):1-37.

8. Influenza vaccine. Influenza vaccine is recommended annually for children age ≥6 months with certain risk factors (including but not limited to children with asthma, cardiac disease, sickle cell disease, human immunodeficiency virus infection, and diabetes; and household members of persons in high-risk groups [see *MMWR* 2003;52(RR-8):1-36]) and can be administered to all others wishing to obtain immunity. In addition, healthy children age 6 to 23 months are encouraged to receive influenza vaccine if feasible, because children in this age group are at substantially increased risk of influenza-related hospitalizations. For healthy persons age 5 to 49 years, the intranasally administered live-attenuated influenza vaccine (LAIV) is an acceptable alternative to the intramuscular trivalent inactivated influenza vaccine (TIV). See *MMWR* 2003;52(RR-13);1-8. Children receiving TIV should be administered a dosage appropriate for their age (0.25 mL if age 6 to 35 months or 0.5 mL if age ≥3 years). Children age ≤8 years who are receiving influenza vaccine for the first time should receive 2 doses (separated by at least 4 weeks for TIV and at least weeks for LAIV).

For additional information about vaccines, including precautions and contraindications for immunization and vaccine shortages, please visit the National Immunization Program Web site at www.cdc.gov/nip/ or call the National Immunization Information Hotline at 800-232-2522 (English) or 800-232-0233 (Spanish).

Approved by the Advisory Committtee on Immunization Practices (www.cdc.gov/nip/acip), the American Academy of Pediatrics (www.aap.org), and the American Academy of Family Physicians (www.aafp.org).

FIGURE 1 Recommended childhood and adolescent immunization schedule, United States, 2004.

to vaccination. Precautions to future doses of pertussis vaccine include:

- Temperature more than 40.5°C (104.9°F) that occurs within 48 hours of vaccination with no other identifiable cause
- Collapse or shock-like state (also known as a hypotonic-hyporesponsive episode) within 48 hours of vaccination
- Persistent, inconsolable crying lasting more than 3 hours within 48 hours of vaccination
- Seizures with or without fever occurring within 3 days of vaccination

Contraindications to further vaccinations with DTaP include severe allergic reaction (anaphylaxis) and encephalopathy with no other identifiable causes occurring within 7 days of vaccination.

Polio Vaccine

Polio virus is an enterovirus that is spread via the fecal–oral and respiratory routes. It enters the mouth and multiplies in the pharynx and gastrointestinal tract. The virus then spreads through the local lymphoid tissue to the bloodstream and may spread to the central nervous system (CNS). In less than 1% of cases, the virus then replicates and destroys neurons in the anterior horn and brainstem resulting in flaccid paralysis. Ninety-five percent of persons with polio infection may actually be asymptomatic. Approximately 4% to 8% of persons have a minor, nonspecific illness characterized by upper respiratory symptoms, gastrointestinal symptoms, or an influenza-like illness. Nonparalytic aseptic meningitis occurs in 1% to 2% of infections. The death-to-case rate is 2% to 5% for persons with paralytic polio; the rates are higher in adults and those with bulbar involvement. Since July 1999, inactivated polio vaccine (IPV) has been exclusively recommended by the Advisory Committee on Immunization Practices (ACIP). Oral polio vaccine (OPV) is no longer routinely available in the United States as its use was associated with 8 to 10 cases of vaccine-associated paralytic polio (VAPP) each year in the United States. The primary series of IPV consists of three doses beginning at 6 to 8 weeks of age. The second dose is usually given at 4 months, and the third dose between 6 and 18 months of age (see Figure 1). A fourth dose is recommended on or after the fourth birthday before school entry. A fourth dose is not necessary if the third dose was given on or after the fourth birthday. A minimum interval of 4 weeks should separate all doses of the series. Minor local reactions including pain or redness may occur. Allergic reactions may occur in persons sensitive to streptomycin, polymyxin B, and neomycin because IPV may contain trace amounts of these antibiotics.

Haemophilus influenzae Type b Vaccines

H. influenzae type b (Hib) is a gram-negative coccobacillus that has six capsular subtypes (a through f). It enters the nasopharynx where it may colonize. In younger persons, the organism (especially types b and f) may then cause invasive disease. Hib disease peak attack times in unvaccinated children are at 6 and 18 months of age; the disease is uncommon after 5 years of age. The most common types of invasive disease include meningitis, epiglottitis, septic arthritis, cellulitis, pneumonia, osteomyelitis, purulent pericarditis, endocarditis, and neonatal sepsis.

Since 1990, three polysaccharide-protein conjugate vaccines have been licensed for use in infants. All infants should receive a primary series of conjugate Hib vaccine (see Figure 1); the number of doses depends on the type of vaccine used and the age that the Hib series is initiated (Table 1). Regardless of the type of Hib protein conjugate vaccine used, a booster dose is recommended at 12 to 15 months. The minimum interval between doses is 4 weeks, with the optimal interval being 8 weeks. Children who initiate the Hib series after 7 months of age may not require the full series. Only one dose is needed between 15 and 59 months of age (see Table 1). Hib vaccine should not be given before 6 weeks of age because early doses

TABLE 1 Detailed Vaccination Schedule for *Haemophilus influenzae* Type b Conjugate Vaccines

Vaccine	Age at 1st Dose (Months)	Primary Series	Booster
HbOC (Hibtiter)/PRP-T (ActHIB)	2-6	3 doses, 2 months apart	12-15 months*
	7-11	2 doses, 2 months apart	12-15 months*
	12-14	1 dose	2 months later
	15-59	1 dose	—
PRP-OMP (PedvaxHIB)	2-6	2 doses, 2 months apart	12-15 months*
	7-11	2 doses, 2 months apart	12-15 months*
	12-14	1 dose	2 months later
	15-59	1 dose	—
PRP-D (Connaught)*	15-59	1 dose	—

*At least 2 months after previous dose.

Abbreviations: HbOC = hepatitis B oligosaccharide-CRM197 vaccine; PRP-D = polyribosylribitol phosphate-diphtheria toxoid conjugate vaccine; PRP-OMP = polyribosybribitol phosphate polysaccharide-Neisseria meningitidis outer membrane protein complex; PRP-T = polysaccharide tetanus conjugate vaccine.

may induce immunologic tolerance to additional doses of Hib vaccine.

Adverse events are uncommon after Hib vaccination; 5% to 30% of vaccine recipients report swelling, redness, or pain. Fever and irritability are infrequent. Precautions include moderate-to-severe illness. Contraindications include anaphylaxis to a prior dose and age younger than 6 weeks because of the risk of immunologic tolerance.

Measles Vaccine

In the United States between 1989 and 1991, a dramatic resurgence of measles recurred because of low immunization coverage levels of preschool age children in urban areas. The measles virus is a paramyxovirus that results in an acute viral systemic infection. The virus enters the nasopharynx and subsequently causes a primary viremia and infection of the reticuloendothelial system. The incubation period ranges from 7 to 18 days. The prodrome of measles classically includes a stepwise increase in fever (≥38.3°C [100.9°F]), followed by cough, coryza, conjunctivitis, and Koplik spots on the mucous membranes. The classic measles rash begins at the hairline and proceeds with a downward, distal spread. Complications include diarrhea, otitis media, laryngotracheobronchitis, pneumonia, encephalitis, and death. Death is usually secondary to neurologic and respiratory complications.

Currently, the first dose of a measles-containing vaccine (MMR) should be given on or after the first birthday (see Figure 1). Ninety-five percent of children respond to the first dose. A second dose is recommended at ages 4 to 6 years to produce immunity in children who failed to respond to the first dose (primary vaccine failure). The second dose may be given a minimum of 4 weeks after the first dose, as long as the first dose was given on or after 1 year of age. Adverse reactions may include fever (≥39.4°C [102.9°F] or higher) or rash 6 to 12 days after vaccination. Rarely, thrombocytopenia, lymphadenopathy, or allergic reactions may occur. Contraindications to MMR include:

- Allergy to gelatin or neomycin
- Severe allergic reaction after a prior dose
- Pregnancy
- Immunosuppression
- Moderate to severe illness
- Persons receiving large daily doses of steroids (>2 mg/kg per day or >20 mg per day) for 14 days or more
- HIV infection with severe immunosuppression
- Recipients of antibody-containing blood products

Egg allergy is not a contraindication to MMR vaccination, and skin testing to eggs is not indicated. If a tuberculin skin test (TST) is needed at the time of MMR vaccination, it should be placed simultaneously or separated by more than 4 weeks to eliminate any theoretical concern of the suppression of the TST reactivity after vaccination. If a child is due for both MMR and varicella vaccines, they either should be given simultaneously or separated by more than 28 days.

Varicella Vaccine

Varicella zoster is a herpesvirus that results in the disease commonly known as chicken pox. The virus enters through the respiratory tract and conjunctiva followed by a primary and secondary viremia. Clinical features begin after an incubation period ranging from 10 to 21 days. A mild prodrome of fever and malaise is followed by a generalized, pruritic rash. Classically, the rash follows a centripetal distribution with skin lesions in multiple stages of development (papules, vesicles, and crusts). Complications of varicella include secondary bacterial infection of skin lesions, arthritis, hepatitis, thrombocytopenia, pneumonia, and CNS involvement (ranging from aseptic meningitis to encephalitis). Death occurs in approximately 1 per 60,000 cases. Complications are highest in persons older than 15 years and younger than 1 year of age.

The varicella zoster vaccine is a live attenuated viral vaccine. Routine vaccination is recommended at 12 to 18 months of age (see Figure 1). The vaccine is highly recommended by the thirteenth birthday, because severe complications from varicella disease are more frequent after this age. Children older than age 13 years, who have not been immunized or had natural disease, should receive two doses of varicella vaccine separated by 4 to 8 weeks, as seroconversion rates in children older than 13 years of age after a single dose are lower than those in younger children. Contraindications and precautions are similar to those for MMR vaccine and include severe allergy to a prior dose, allergy to neomycin or gelatin, immunosuppression, pregnancy, moderate-to-severe illness, or receipt of an antibody-containing blood product. Salicylates should be avoided for 6 weeks after the varicella vaccine because of an association between aspirin use and Reye syndrome after chickenpox. If a child is due for both MMR and varicella vaccines, they either should be given simultaneously or separated by 28 days or more.

Hepatitis A Vaccine

Hepatitis A is a picornavirus that is spread by the fecal–oral route. A long incubation period of 15 to 50 days may be followed by the abrupt onset of fever, malaise, anorexia, nausea, and jaundice. Children younger than 6 years of age are symptomatic in 30% of cases, compared with older children and adults who are symptomatic in more than 70% of cases. Fulminant hepatitis A is rare, but may occur in those with underlying liver disease. Hepatitis A vaccine is an inactivated whole virus vaccine. Currently, it is not licensed for children younger than 2 years of age. Routine hepatitis A vaccination is recommended for children older than 2 years of age who live in states, counties, or communities where the annual hepatitis A disease rate between 1987 and 1997 was greater than 20 per 100,000 persons (twice the national average).

Health care providers should contact their local health department to determine if hepatitis A vaccine is recommended in their area. Children ages 2 to 18 years should receive an initial dose followed by a booster dose 6 to 12 months later (see Figure 1). Adverse reactions are mild and may include pain, erythema, or swelling at the injection site. Low-grade fever, fatigue, and malaise are even less common. Contraindications and precautions include severe allergic reaction after a previous dose, allergy to alum, or, in the case of the Havrix vaccine, allergy to 2-phenoxyethanol.

Hepatitis B Vaccine

Hepatitis B virus (HBV) is a hepadnavirus. This virus is transmitted by parenteral or mucosal exposure from infected bodily fluids. After a prolonged incubation period ranging from 6 weeks to 6 months, the typical illness is characterized by a 3- to 10-day prodromal phase (i.e., malaise, anorexia, nausea, and abdominal pains) followed by a 1- to 3-week icteric period and a convalescent period in which malaise and fatigue may persist for weeks to months. Young children may be asymptomatic. Complications may include chronic HBV infection, which may result in chronic liver disease. Fulminant hepatitis may occur in 1% to 2% of persons.

Hepatitis B vaccination is recommended for all infants before hospital discharge. The primary dose may be given at 2 months of age if the infant's mother is hepatitis B surface antigen (HBsAg)-negative. The second dose is recommended 1 to 4 months after the first dose with a 1-month minimum interval between doses 1 and 2. The third dose is recommended at age 6 to 18 months with a 2-month minimum interval between the second and third doses (see Figure 1). The minimum interval between doses 1 and 3 is 4 months. The third dose should not be given to infants before they are 6 months of age. Children not vaccinated during infancy should be vaccinated at 11 to 12 years of age.

Adult hepatitis B vaccine candidates are many and include:

- Alaskan natives
- Blood product recipients
- Health care workers
- Heterosexuals with multiple partners; prostitutes
- Household members who live with HBV carriers
- Immigrants from HBV endemic areas
- Institutionalized individuals
- Intravenous drug users
- Men who have sex with men
- Pacific Islanders
- Persons on hemodialysis
- Persons with other sexually transmitted diseases
- Prison inmates

Contraindications to hepatitis B vaccine include serious allergic reaction to a previous dose or vaccine component or moderate to severe illness. Adverse events after vaccination include pain at the injection site and fever. Of note, no causal links between demyelinating disease, rheumatologic illnesses, or autoimmune diseases and hepatitis B vaccination have been found.

Influenza Vaccine

Influenza is an RNA virus with three antigenic strains—A, B, and C. Influenza type A affects all age groups and results in moderate-to-severe illness. Influenza type B primarily affects children and causes milder disease than type A. Influenza type C is rarely associated with human illness.

Influenza type A has subtypes that are determined by the surface antigens hemagglutinin (H1, H2, and H3) and neuraminidase (N1 and N2). The hemagglutinin and neuraminidase antigens periodically change. When major changes occur in one or both surface antigens (antigenic shift), worldwide pandemics may result from the large number of individuals with no prior immunologic experience to the new antigens. When minor changes occur in the surface antigens (antigenic drift), persons who are incompletely protected may transmit or develop disease. Antigenic drift occurs annually, however, antigenic shift occurs at intervals of 10 years or more.

Influenza virus is spread by respiratory transmission. The virus attaches and penetrates respiratory epithelial cells. After an incubation period of 1 to 5 days (average 2 days), infected persons may develop the abrupt onset of fever, sore throat, myalgia, and nonproductive cough. Symptoms usually last from 2 to 3 days and rarely longer than 5 days. Attack rates are highest among school-age children. Complications of influenza include secondary bacterial pneumonia, myocarditis, worsening of chronic bronchitis, myositis, Reye syndrome, and possibly death.

Currently, two types of influenza vaccine are available for use, an inactivated trivalent intramuscular influenza vaccine (TIV); and the live, attenuated, intranasal, trivalent, cold-adapted, vaccine (LAIV). Optimally, the vaccine is administered annually between early October and mid-November. Inactivated vaccine (TIV) is recommended for at-risk individuals including:

- All children ages 6 to 23 months
- Close contacts of children ages 0 to 6 months
- Health care workers
- Household contacts of persons at increased risk
- Persons ages 6 months to 18 years receiving chronic aspirin therapy
- Persons older than 50 years of age

TABLE 2 Inactivated Influenza Vaccine Dosage, by Age Group—United States

Age Group	Dosage	Number of Doses	Route
6-35 months	0.25 mL	1* or 2	IM
3-8 years	0.50 mL	1* or 2	IM
>9 years	0.50 mL	1	IM

*Only one dose is needed if the child received influenza vaccine during a previous influenza season.

- Persons older than 6 months of age with chronic illness (i.e., chronic pulmonary disease such as asthma, emphysema, bronchopulmonary dysplasia, or chronic bronchitis; cardiovascular disease such as congenital heart disease or congestive heart failure; metabolic disease including diabetes mellitus, renal dysfunction, hemoglobinopathies, and immunosuppression)
- Residents of long-term care facilities
- Women who are pregnant

Because the composition of the influenza vaccine changes yearly and immunity declines 1 year following immunization, yearly revaccination is recommended. Table 2 gives information regarding influenza dosages.

LAIV may be used as an alternative to TIV for vaccinating healthy persons ages 5 to 49 years (Table 3). LAIV should not be used in children younger than age 5 years; adults older than age 50 years; persons with asthma, reactive airways disease, chronic disease (defined previously); children or adolescents receiving aspirin or salicylates; persons with a history of Guillain-Barré syndrome, pregnant women; or persons with history of hypersensitivity or anaphylaxis to eggs or any components of LAIV.

Following influenza vaccination, local reactions such as soreness, erythema, and induration may occur. The vaccine only contains inactivated products and cannot cause influenza disease. Fever, malaise, and myalgias occur in less than 1% of vaccine recipients. Allergic reactions are rare; however, egg allergy and thimerosal sensitivity are contraindications to immunization.

Pneumococcal Vaccines

Streptococcus pneumoniae is a gram-positive organism that may result in serious invasive diseases such as pneumonia, bacteremia, and meningitis. Although many different serotypes exist, ten of the most common serotypes produce approximately 62% of the invasive diseases. Pneumococci are commonly found in the respiratory tract. Asymptomatic carriage rates vary depending on age, environment, and presence of upper respiratory tract infections. The highest rates of invasive disease are found in children younger than 2 years of age, persons with functional or anatomic asplenia such as in sickle cell disease, and

TABLE 3 Live Attenuated Influenza Vaccine (LAIV) Compared With Inactivated Influenza Vaccine

Characteristic	LAIV	Inactivated Trivalent Influenza Vaccine (TIV)
Route of administration	Intranasal spray	Intramuscular injection
Type of vaccine	Live virus	Killed virus
Number of included virus strains	3 (2 influenza A, 1 influenza B)	Same as LAIV
Vaccine virus strains updated	Annually	Same as LAIV
Frequency of administration	Annually	Same as LAIV
Can be administered to children and adults at high risk* for complications resulting from influenza infection	No	Yes
Can be administered to family members or close contacts of immunosuppressed persons	Inactivated influenza vaccine preferred	Yes†
Can be administered to family members or close contacts of persons at high risk but who are immunocompetent	Yes	Yes
Can be simultaneously administered with other vaccines	Yes‡	Yes§
If not simultaneously administered, can be administered within 4 weeks of another live vaccine	Prudent to space 4 wk apart	Yes
If not simultaneously administered, can be administered within 4 weeks of an inactivated vaccine	Yes	Yes

*Populations at high risk from complications of influenza infection include persons ages ≥65 years; residents of nursing homes and other facilities that house persons with chronic medical conditions; adults and children with chronic disorders of the pulmonary or cardiovascular systems; adults and children with chronic metabolic diseases (including diabetes mellitus), renal dysfunction, hemoglobinopathies, or immunosuppression; children and adolescents receiving long-term aspirin therapy (at risk for developing Reye syndrome after wild-type influenza infection); and women who will be in the second or third trimester of pregnancy during influenza season.

†Immunosuppressed persons include, but are not limited to, persons with human immunodeficiency virus, malignancy, or those receiving immunosuppressive therapies.

‡No data are available regarding effect on safety or efficacy.

§Inactivated influenza vaccine coadministration with pnuemococcal polysaccharide vaccine has been evaluated systematically only among adults.

Source: http://www.cdc.gov/mmwr/PDF/rr/rr5213.pdf

persons with HIV. Children of certain ethnic groups (Alaskan native, Native American, and African American) and children in daycare are also at increased risk.

Two pneumococcal vaccines are available in the United States, the 23-valent polysaccharide vaccine and the 7-valent polysaccharide conjugate vaccine. The 23-valent polysaccharide vaccine, which may be given to individuals older than 2 years of age, protects against 60% to 70% of invasive forms of pneumococcal disease. The 23-valent vaccine is recommended for all adults older than 65 years and persons older than 2 years who are immunocompromised or who have chronic diseases such as heart disease, lung disease, diabetes, liver disease, or cerebrospinal fluid leaks. The most common adverse events are local reactions occurring in 30% to 50% of recipients. Fever and myalgias occur in fewer than 1% of recipients. Severe systemic adverse events are rare.

A series of four 7-valent polysaccharide conjugate vaccines are recommended for infants. This vaccine has been shown to reduce invasive pneumococcal disease by 89%. Primary series doses are given at 2, 4, and 6 months of age (see Figure 1). Children who begin vaccination who are older than 7 months of age require fewer doses (Table 4). After vaccination, local reactions occur in 10% to 20% of recipients with fever and myalgias occurring in 15% to 24% of recipients. For both types of pneumococcal vaccines, serious allergic reaction to a prior dose is a contraindication. Moderate-to-severe illness is a temporary contraindication to immunization.

Reporting Adverse Events

Health care providers are encouraged to report any clinically significant adverse event following the administration of any vaccine licensed in the United States to the Vaccine Adverse Events Reporting System (VAERS). VAERS is a national vaccine safety surveillance program that is sponsored by the CDC and the Food and Drug Administration. A copy of the Reportable Events Table can be found at http://www.vaers.org/pubs.htm. Providers may obtain a VAERS report form by calling 1-800-822-7967 or by visiting http://www.vaers.org.

TABLE 4 Recommended Schedule of Doses for PCV7, Including Primary Series and Catch-up Immunizations, in Previously Unvaccinated Children*

Age at First Dose	Primary Series	Booster Dose†
2-6 mo	3 doses, 6-8 wk apart	1 dose at 12-15 mo of age
7-11 mo	2 doses, 6-8 wk apart	1 dose at 12-15 mo of age
12-23 mo	2 doses, 6-8 wk apart	
≥24 mo	1 dose	

*Recommendations for high-risk groups are given in Table 3.
†Booster doses should be given at least 6 to 8 weeks after the final dose of the primary series.
Abbreviation: PCV7 = pneumococcal 7-valent conjugate vaccine.

TRAVEL MEDICINE

METHOD OF

Kenneth R. Dardick, MD

All our patients travel. It is estimated that 40 million Americans will travel abroad each year; 8 to 10 million Americans and more than 1 million Canadians will visit underdeveloped or tropical areas. Many more will stay within the United States or visit nearby destinations such as Mexico, Canada, or Europe. Physicians must be prepared to identify travel-related issues when they arise. Some patients will ask, "What shots do I need?" which is not the best starting point. Other patients are simply in the office for a cold or sprained ankle. Only by taking a complete history will the physician discover that the patient is about to take a long trip. Maybe the patient with diarrhea has just returned from a stay in the tropics. The practice of travel medicine comprises pretravel counseling, risk assessment for travelers with unique needs, and the care of travelers who return home with symptoms of illness or injury.

Physicians with expertise in travel medicine may be found among members of the American Society of Tropical Medicine and Hygiene's (ASTMH) clinical interest group, the American Committee on Clinical Tropical Medicine and Traveler's Health (ACCTMTH), or the International Society of Travel Medicine (ISTM). The ACCTMTH offers an examination leading to a Certificate in Clinical Tropical Medicine and Traveler's Health under the auspices of the American Society of Tropical Medicine and Hygiene. The ISTM offers a Certificate of Knowledge Examination leading to a Certificate in Travel Health.

Sources of Information

There are more than 200 countries and international entities worldwide. Each has its own unique set of factors including geography, climate, regulations, illnesses, and social customs, which may impact the traveler. The physician providing medical care to the traveler cannot possibly keep all this in memory. Outbreaks occur and are reported on an almost daily basis. Books and guides, even those published monthly or yearly cannot keep track of all this. It is essential to have access to an online source or sources of reliable information. Some are free, others require a paid subscription (Table 1).

Pretravel Counseling

Health issues while traveling are common. Overall, 20% of travelers may become ill, but as many as 39% in one recent study had at least one medical or health problem, and 9% consulted a health professional while abroad. More than 50% of travelers to the tropics become ill, but only 0.2% to 0.5% require hospitalization. Frequency of illness is not related to the duration of the trip.

Depending on the trip and the individual's itinerary and medical history, it may require as much as 6 months to 1 year or as little as 1 to 2 days to prepare the traveler. A formal consultation is an excellent way to begin. Plan to spend about 30 to 45 minutes with the traveler. Many patients do not object to this, but one study found that 60% to 80% of patients in Great Britain would pay nothing for travel health advice. Health insurance may not cover expenses for medical consultations, immunizations, or prescriptions related to travel.

Avoid the temptation to give advice over the telephone. You will probably not have enough time to get into all the issues in the depth required. Remember, it is not good enough to simply state whether "shots are needed"; that is only a small part of the process. Avoid the temptation to schedule patients just for a shot; invariably there will be questions about other travel health concerns, and either your nurse, assistant, or you will then be in the delicate position of telling the patient there isn't time to discuss these other important issues right then and there. It is much better to schedule the visit as a formal *travel consult* right up front.

TABLE 1 Sources of Travel Health Information

CDC Traveler's Health: www.cdc.gov/travel
CDC biweekly updates on quarantinable diseases ("blue sheet"): www.cdc.gov/travel/blusheet.htm
CDC automated fax information line: 888-232-3299 (document #000005—document directory)
CDC telephone information: Division of Global Migration and Quarantine, 404-498-1600; Division of Vector-Borne Diseases, 970-221-6400; Division of Parasitic Diseases, 770-488-7775
World Health Organization: www.who.int/ith
American Society of Tropical Medicine and Hygiene: www.astmh.org
International Society of Travel Medicine: www.istm.org
ProMED (listserv of emerging diseases): www.promedmail.org
CIA World Factbook: www.cia.gov/cia/publications/factbook/index.html
GIDEON (Global Infectious Disease Epidemiology Network) $: www.gideononline.com
Travax (Shoreland) $: www.shoreland.com
TravelCare (International SOS) $: www.travelcare.com

Abbreviation: $ = paid subscription.

Even so, much of the advice physicians give to prospective travelers will be ignored. We must pay special attention to giving health advice in ways it will be understood and acted upon. A recent study of Dutch travelers to malarious areas found that only 16% followed advice to avoid mosquito bites during the trip. Those who failed to follow doctors' advice tended to be younger, more experienced, and going on adventure trips.

Pretravel advice includes:

- General issues for any traveler
- Environmental health, vector-borne illnesses
- Immunizations, both recommended and required
- Personal issues for individual circumstances

General Issues

ACCIDENTS

Accidents are common both at home and on the road. In a 1987 study of 90 deaths among Swiss travelers, most were related to accidents, drowning, or the act of travel. Accidents are the most common cause of death for Peace Corps workers. Morbidity and mortality rates from accidents are worse than those in the United States for comparable accidents (roughly twice the accident mortality—80% of deaths occur out of hospital). Prevention can be difficult for many reasons:

- Seat belts are not always available.
- Others may do the driving.
- Alcohol use is common.
- A sense of adventure and invulnerability often prevails.
- Driving on the "other side" of the road creates confusion.

INSURANCE AND MEDICAL ASSISTANCE

Insurance is not the same as medical assistance. Insurance pays for medical bills and hospital expenses after the fact, while medical assistance helps obtain care and coordinates services such as finding a doctor, paying up-front fees, communicating with the traveler's own physician at home, and arranging the return home. Many insurance companies provide medical assistance coverage (see the United States Department of State web site for a comprehensive listing of these companies at www.travel.state.gov/medical.html). These policies are often coupled with other coverages sold by travel agents.

Note that Medicare is not valid outside the United States. Supplemental travel policies are essential for medical coverage of Medicare beneficiaries while traveling. Commercial health insurance coverage outside the United States may have other limitations such as the need for prior authorization for diagnosis and treatment as well as issues of out-of-network coverage. In any case the traveler will have to pay for any services first and then attempt to be reimbursed by his or her medical policy. Supplemental health insurance policies can cover these and other gaps.

TRAVEL KIT

Prepare a list of generic drug names, doses, and indications for your patient in case a replacement prescription is needed. Medications should be carried with the traveler, not checked through with luggage. All medications should be carried in original pharmacy bottles (not loose in a ziplock plastic bag, very suspicious). Those traveling with needles and syringes should have a letter on the medical practice letterhead indicating the need for the injectable drugs (e.g., diabetes). Travelers should take an extra pair of glasses, contact lenses, and a copy of their vision prescription. Those with a cardiac condition should carry a copy of a recent electrocardiogram (ECG) and, if relevant, pacemaker information. Other items are related to the duration of travel and availability of common supplies at the destination (e.g., bandages, antibacterial ointment, antidiarrheal medication, antibiotics for presumptive treatment of skin or respiratory infections).

JET LAG

Jet lag is caused by an imbalance between the traveler's diurnal rhythm and the real time at the destination. It is not a problem with north-south travel, only east-west travel across more than 5 time zones. The biological clock prefers a longer day, so westward travel is usually handled better. Common symptoms of jet lag are fatigue, malaise, headache, anorexia, and difficulty concentrating. Jet lag is compounded by the fatigue that all travelers experience and by dehydration. There is no easy way to avoid jet lag; most travelers do not have the luxury of breaking up their trip with intermediate stops to allow the biological clock to adjust. The use of short-acting hypnotic drugs is controversial; amnesia has been reported with triazolam (Halcion), especially when mixed with alcohol. Melatonin[1,*] may be effective in reducing symptoms of jet lag, but may take 2 to 3 days of daily administration to reach full effect. Typical doses for eastward travel are 3 to 5 mg daily at destination bedtime on the day of travel, and then nightly for 3 to 5 nights. When traveling westward omit the dose on the day of travel, but continue melatonin 3 to 5 mg nightly for 3 to 5 nights after arrival.

DEEP VENOUS THROMBOSIS

There is good evidence that jet travelers on long-haul flights (>8 hours duration) are at increased risk of developing deep venous thrombosis (DVT), which may be symptomless. This can be prevented by wearing moderate compression (20-30 mm Hg) elastic stockings. High-risk travelers (prior history of DVT, pregnant women, hypercoagulable states) should be advised to wear elastic stockings, drink ample fluids, and walk up and down the aisles every 30 to 60 minutes, if possible.

MOTION SICKNESS

All forms of travel may induce the familiar symptoms of motion sickness (nausea, diaphoresis, anorexia, lethargy, vomiting). These symptoms are triggered by an imbalance among visual, rotatory, and kinesthetic cues in the inner ear (labyrinth) and brain. All travelers are susceptible to motion sickness in certain circumstances, but some are clearly more susceptible than others. Those at greatest risk are children 5 to 12 years of age and women. Travel in small aircraft, small boats, and cars may pose the greatest risks. Motion sickness is often aggravated by up and down movements of the head and neck. A number of strategies are known to help reduce the symptoms of motion sickness (Table 2).

There are many effective medications but no one solution is best for all travelers. Children do best with common antihistamines such as dimenhydrinate (Dramamine), diphenhydramine (Benadryl), or promethazine (Phenergan). Drowsiness is the most common side effect for all of these drugs. A little-known fact is that dimenhydrinate is actually the theophylline salt of diphenhydramine, a pharmacological attempt to make it less sedating. The antihistamines are highly effective if taken before the onset of symptoms.

Adults can use the same antihistamines as children, as well as meclizine (Bonine or Antivert, ages 12 and older). The most effective single medication for prevention of motion sickness is scopolamine. The transdermal patch (Transderm Scop), introduced in 1981, was the first transdermal medication,. A single patch provides 72 hours of prevention and is applied at least 6 to 8 hours before travel. For longer trips,

TABLE 2 Strategies for Minimizing Motion Sickness Symptoms

Sit in the front seat of a car (note that this is not acceptable for children who must sit in car seats in the back for safety reasons).
Avoid strong odors, perfumes, colognes, or smoke; maintain adequate ventilation.
Sit over the wings in a plane or amidships in a boat (the most stable areas).
Eat and drink lightly, if at all.
Do not read or play video games; look at the distant horizon.
On a boat stay on deck, watch the horizon, do not lie down; the ideal position is in a deck chair with a cushion around the neck for stability.
Children may benefit from a cushion to raise them up to look out the window.

[1]Not FDA approved for this indication.
*Available as a dietary supplement.

additional patches should be applied every 72 hours. Scopolamine cannot be used by those younger than 12 years of age or by those with glaucoma, urinary retention, or pyloric obstruction. Elderly patients may develop hallucinations. More than 60% of patients using scopolamine develop dry mouth. Other side effects may include blurred vision and bradycardia. Sedation is seen much less commonly with scopolamine than with antihistamines.

Nonpharmacologic measures to prevent motion sickness, such as ginger[1,*] and acupuncture (at the P6/Neiguan acupuncture point), may reduce symptoms but have not been shown to prevent motion sickness. Wristband acupressure has not been shown to be effective.

HIGH ALTITUDE (ALSO SEE HIGH ALTITUDE SICKNESS CHAPTER)

High altitude is not just a problem for mountain climbers. Many who travel to hike or sightsee are susceptible to the clinical syndromes of altitude illness. There are no reliable screening tests for altitude illness, but those who have had problems in the past are more likely to have problems in the future. Anyone traveling to destinations above 1219 m (4000 ft) may be at risk for acute mountain sickness (AMS), but the risk is greatest with abrupt ascent above 2743 m (9000 ft).

Symptoms are variable and include headache, fatigue, anorexia, nausea, and vomiting. AMS can be prevented with acetazolamide (adult dose 125 mg twice a day, starting 2 days before ascent and continuing for 2-3 days after reaching maximal altitude). Ginkgo biloba[4,*] (various preparations; 100 mg twice a day, starting 5 days prior to ascent and continuing for 2-3 days after reaching maximal altitude) may also be effective for prevention.

High-altitude cerebral edema (HACE) is more severe than AMS, comprising symptoms of severe lethargy, confusion, and ataxia. AMS may progress to HACE.

High-altitude pulmonary edema (HAPE) is manifest by dyspnea on exertion, progressing to dyspnea at rest. HAPE and HACE may occur alone or in tandem. Rapid descent is critical in managing both HAPE and HACE. Medications including dexamethasone (Decadron) and nifedipine (Adalat)[1] are effective treatments for HAPE and HACE. A pressurization (Gamov) bag can simulate a descent of 1500 to 1800 m (5000-6000 ft), which can be lifesaving if actual emergency descent cannot be achieved.

SEXUALLY TRANSMITTED DISEASES

The relationship between sexually transmitted diseases (STDs) and travel is not a new one. Columbus was said to have brought syphilis home to the Old World from the New World. United States military personnel brought home penicillin-resistant gonorrhea (PPNG) from Southeast Asia. Travelers on jet aircraft from Africa to Europe and the Americas spread HIV rapidly. Condoms and abstinence (not necessarily in that order) are the most effective means of prevention. In a study of Dutch expatriates in HIV-endemic areas, 41% of the men and 31% of the women had sex with casual or steady local partners, and 23% had unprotected sex with local partners. It is important to remind travelers of their responsibility to practice safe sex to protect themselves from acquiring or spreading venereal diseases worldwide.

[1]Not FDA approved for this indication.

[4]Not yet approved for use in the United States.

*Available as a dietary supplement.

Environmental Health (Enteric, Vector-Borne)

Travel exposes the individual to a variety of infectious diseases. Some are related to poor sanitation or hygiene; others are acquired by exposure to vectors. Many of these diseases are not vaccine preventable. The traveler must be educated about other preventive measures to avoid disease; these include behavioral measures as well as preventive or presumptive treatment medication in some cases.

TRAVELER'S DIARRHEA

Traveler's diarrhea (TD) is one of the major illnesses causing significant morbidity in travelers. Most illness is caused by enterotoxigenic *Escherichia coli*; some is caused by other enteric bacteria. There is no generally agreed-upon definition of TD, but most people "know it when it happens," an abrupt onset of an increase in watery stools with or without fever, cramps, and usually lasting 3 to 5 days. More than 90% of cases last less than 1 week, but nearly 1% may last 3 months or longer. TD is rarely life threatening, but in an area where cholera is present, a TD syndrome may be the early clinical presentation of cholera. Fluid replacement is an important part of the early management of all cases of TD. Prevention of traveler's diarrhea and other enteric infections is based on a number of well-established principles (Table 3).

Self-treatment of mild traveler's diarrhea can promptly relieve symptoms of most cases. Up to 80% of patients will be cured with as little as a single dose of antibiotics. If there is no fever, the person can take both an antibiotic and loperamide (Imodium AD) (see list below). If there is fever, the person should take only the antibiotic. In most parts of the world a fluoroquinolone is an excellent choice, but in Southeast Asia, because of an increasing prevalence of quinolone-resistant *Campylobacter* infection, azithromycin (Zithromax)[1] is a better choice.

[1]Not FDA approved for this indication.

TABLE 3 "Boil It, Peel It, Cook It, or Forget It!"—Advice for the Prevention of Traveler's Diarrhea

Cooked food that has been held at room temperature for several hours constitutes one of the greatest risks of food-borne illness. Make sure your food has been thoroughly cooked and is still hot when served.
Avoid any uncooked food, apart from fruits and vegetables that can be peeled or shelled. Avoid fruits with damaged skin.
Ice cream from unreliable sources is frequently contaminated and can cause illness. If in doubt, avoid it.
In some countries, certain species of fish and shellfish may contain poisonous biotoxins even when they are well cooked. Local people can advise you about this.
Unpasteurized milk should be boiled before consumption.
When the safety of drinking water is doubtful, have it boiled or disinfect it with reliable, slow-release, disinfectant tablets. These are generally available in pharmacies. Iodine tablets may be effective for purification, but it is affected by the temperature and clarity of the water and may impart an objectionable taste. Or, drink bottled water.
Filters may be used to purify water in some settings (hiking), but be aware that small filter pore size (0.1-0.3 micron) can remove bacteria and protozoa, but not viruses. Filters with a small pore size are readily clogged and less effective for large volumes of water; they are not effective in water with heavy sediment. Neither the FDA nor the CDC certifies filters, but the following are useful sources of information:
www.cdc.gov/ncidod/dpd/parasites/cryptosporidiosis/factsht_crypto_prevent_water.htm
www.NSF.org/certified/dwtu (click on "cyst reduction")
Avoid ice unless you are sure that it is made from safe water.
Beverages such as hot tea or coffee, wine, beer, and carbonated soft drinks or fruit juices that are either bottled or otherwise packaged are usually safe to drink.

Adapted from WHO and CDC publications.

The dosages for self-treatment of TD are:

1. Antibiotic

- Ciprofloxacin (Cipro) 500 mg, 2 tablets initially, then 1 tablet twice a day.
- Doxycycline monohydrate (Vibramycin)[1] 100 mg, 1 tablet twice a day.
- Azithromycin (Zithromax) 250 mg, one tablet daily.
- Take the antibiotic until symptoms are gone (as little as a single dose of antibiotics may be curative). Do not exceed 3 days of treatment. There is no clear preference among these antibiotics except that azithromycin may be favored in areas of Southeast Asia where there is increasing resistance to fluoroquinolones and an increase in prevalence of *Campylobacter* infection. Azithromycin may also be preferred for children and women who might be pregnant.

2. Loperamide

- Take 4 mg (2 capsules or 4 teaspoons) initially, followed by 2 mg (1 capsule or 2 teaspoons) after each loose stool, up to a maximum of 16 mg (8 capsules or 16 teaspoons) per day.
- Do not take loperamide in the presence of fever or bloody dysentery syndrome.

[1]Not FDA approved for this indication.

MALARIA

Malaria is one of the most significant health risks to travelers, not because of the large number of cases or morbidity, but because it can be fatal and should be largely preventable. From 1985 to 2001, the Centers for Disease Control and Prevention (CDC) reported an average of about 600 cases of malaria per year in the United States civilians, with 4 fatalities per year. Approximately 94% of the U.S. malaria cases were caused by *Plasmodium falciparum*, and 71% were contracted in sub-Saharan Africa. Transmission is predominantly by the bite of an infected anopheline mosquito (usually in the dusk-to-dawn hours), but malaria can also be transmitted by blood transfusion. It is estimated that worldwide there are 300 to 500 million cases annually with up to 1 million deaths. The risk of acquiring malaria while traveling is specific to location and itinerary. For example, two visitors to the same location will have very different risks if one hikes and sleeps out doors at night while the other remains predominantly in an air-conditioned environment, uses adequate repellents, and wears long sleeves and trousers.

Education of the traveler is paramount. The use of personal protective measures—applying insect repellents on the skin (diethyltoluamide [DEET]) and clothing (permethrin), sleeping under bed nets (even more effective if treated with permethrin), remaining in screened areas, and wearing long sleeves and pants—greatly reduces the likelihood of being bitten by mosquitoes. Recent publications have emphasized the safety and effectiveness of DEET repellents.

Malaria, dengue, leishmaniasis, filariasis, and other vector-borne infections are best prevented by avoiding insect bites. Protective measures to avoid mosquito exposure are advised by the CDC in addition to taking prophylactic antimalarial medication (Table 4).

TABLE 4 Personal Protective Measures to Avoid Insect Bites

Sleep inside screened areas
Wear clothing that covers arms and legs
Avoid outdoor activities in the evening when mosquitoes are most active. (Note that day-biting mosquitoes may transmit dengue, yellow fever, filaria, and Japanese encephalitis. Sandflies, which transmit leishmaniasis; deerflies, which transmit onchocerciasis; and tsetse flies, which transmit African trypanosomiasis may also bite during the day.)
Apply repellent as follows:
- DEET (diethyltoluamide) is now available in low-concentration slow-release formulations that keep the DEET on the skin surface and prevent absorption. Ultrathon, Sawyer controlled release, and Sawyer Family are products that contain DEET in nonabsorbable formulations.
- Permethrin (Permanone) is a synthetic derivative of chrysanthemum. It is applied to clothing; one soaking application may last up to 4-8 wks or longer, even with laundering.
- Use a pyrethrum-containing insect spray in living and sleeping areas at night.

TABLE 5 Malaria Preventive Medication According to Travel Destination

Region of Travel	Preferred Medication for Malaria Prevention
Areas of the world with chloroquine-sensitive malaria (Central America west of the Panama Canal, the Middle East, and Egypt)	Chloroquine
Mefloquine-resistance areas of Southeast Asia (Thailand-Myanmar and Thailand-Cambodian borders, eastern Myanmar)	Atovaquone/proguanil (Malarone) or doxycycline
All other areas	Atovaquone/proguanil, mefloquine (Lariam), or doxycycline

MEDICATION

Travelers to areas at high risk for malaria transmission must be counseled about proper preventive medication. The decision about which medication is best for each individual traveler depends on factors such as the local pattern of malaria transmission, season of the year, activities of the traveler, presence of drug resistance (Table 5), availability of competent local medical care, and contraindications to a particular drug. A 2002 CDC summary of malaria in travelers documented that fewer than 20% of those infected with malaria had taken proper medication. Travelers returning home to visit friends or relatives have a high risk of developing malaria.

Various medications are available for the prevention of malaria among travelers. An understanding of the factors listed above is critical in being able to properly prescribe the optimal medication for each traveler (Table 6).

DENGUE

Dengue is a flavivirus infection found in most tropical countries and many tropical urban centers; more than 2.5 billion people live in areas at risk for dengue infection. Dengue is transmitted by the bite of an infected day-biting *Aedes aegypti* mosquito, the same mosquito vector as yellow fever. There are four serotypes of dengue (DEN1-4) and no cross-immunity among them. In fact, it is the subsequent infection with different serotypes that may increase the risk of developing dengue hemorrhagic fever (DHF). There are an estimated 50 to 100 million cases per year with 200 to 500,000 cases of DHF, which has a case-to-fatality ratio (CFR) of 5%. Repellents are an effective preventive measure (see Table 4). Dengue infection produces an acute febrile illness with a typical incubation period of 4 to 7 days (range: 3-14 days). High fever is accompanied by headache, myalgias, and arthralgias ("breakbone fever"); a rash may appear 3 to 5 days after the onset of fever.

LEISHMANIASIS

Leishmaniasis is a protozoan infection transmitted by the bite of an infected phlebotomine sandfly. These flies are quite small and easily pass through typical mosquito netting. They cannot bite through most clothing. Preventive measures include using repellents and wearing trousers and long-sleeved shirts. All nonhealing papular–ulcerative lesions in travelers who have visited endemic countries should be considered suspicious for diagnosis of leishmaniasis. Leishmaniasis can also present as a systemic syndrome of splenomegaly, anemia, fever, and weight loss. Contact the CDC Division of Parasitic Diseases (770-488-7775) for assistance in the diagnosis and treatment of suspected cases of leishmaniasis.

SCHISTOSOMIASIS

Schistosomiasis is a potentially serious systemic infection. It is acquired by swimming in fresh water inhabited by certain species of snails carrying the infective cercariae. These cercariae penetrate the skin and subsequently invade various body organs including the lungs, spinal cord, portal veins, and the urinary bladder. Although there is some evidence that application of DEET repellent on the skin may prevent infection, the most important advice for travelers is to be aware of the presence of this infection in certain freshwater areas (not saltwater) and to avoid swimming or wading in these locations.

Immunizations

Although the first question asked is often, "I'm taking a trip, what shots do I need?" it must be understood that advice for travelers may or may not include immunizations. There are only limited situations in which vaccination is required for entry to a country. Yellow fever vaccine (YF-VAX) may be a legal requirement for some travelers; some visitors to Saudi Arabia on Haj (pilgrimage) may be required to have proof of meningococcal vaccination.

All other vaccine advice should be based on factors such as these:

- Prevalence of a vaccine-preventable disease
- Itinerary and risk behaviors that increase the traveler's risk of acquiring a particular disease
- Effectiveness and side effects of the vaccine
- Personal medical history of the traveler, which may increase susceptibility to a particular disease or increase risk from the vaccine (immune status, pregnancy, age)

It is important to obtain accurate, up-to-date information for the traveler. Because books become quickly

TABLE 6 Drugs Used in Malaria Prophylaxis

Drug	Usage	Adult Dose	Pediatric Dose	Adverse Reactions	Contraindications
Chloroquine phospate (Aralen)	In areas with chloroquine-sensitive *P. falciparum*	300 mg base (500 mg salt) orally 1/wk	5 mg/kg base (8.3 mg/kg salt), orally 1/wk, up to max adult dose of 300 mg base	Mild nausea, blurred vision, headache, psoriasis flare-ups; itching in dark-skinned persons; very rarely agranulocytosis, photosensitivity, neuropsychiatric effects.	Patients hypersensitive to 4-aminoquinolone derivatives; patients with retinal or field changes attributable to drug therapy; patients with psoriasis; use with caution in patients with liver disease, and/or alcoholism.
Atovaquone/ proguanil (Malarone)	In areas with chloroquine-resistant *P. falciparum*	Each tablet contains atovaquone 250 mg/ proguanil 100 mg; adults, adolescents, and children ≥3 years of age weighing >40 kg: 1 tablet orally 1/d	Each pediatric tablet contains atovaquone 62.5 mg/proguanil 25 mg; children ≥3 y and 31-40 kg: 3 oral tablets 1/d; ≥3 y and 21-30 kg: 2 oral tablets 1/d; ≥3 y and 11-20 kg: 1 tablet orally 1/d; children <3y or <11 kg: safety and efficacy not established	Abdominal pain, nausea/vomiting, headache, diarrhea, asthenia, anorexia, dizziness, pruritus.	Any known hypersensitivity to proguanil or atovaquone.
Mefloquine HCl (Lariam)	In areas with chloroquine-resistant *P. falciparum*	228 mg base (250 mg salt) orally, 1/wk	<15 kg, 4.6 mg/kg base (5 mg/kg salt), orally 1/wk; 15-19 kg: 1/4 tab/wk; 20-30 kg: 1/2 tab/wk; 31-45 kg: 3/4 tab/wk; >45 kg: 1 tab/wk	Adverse reactions include nausea/vomiting, diarrhea, dizziness, difficulty sleeping, and bad dreams.	Patients who are hypersensitive to related compounds, such as quinine; patients with active depression or with history of seizures or severe psychiatric disorders; use with caution in patients with cardiac conduction abnormalities. Do not combine with halofantrine (Halfan).
Doxycycline monohydrate (Adoxa) or hyclate (Vibramycin) (monohydrate may be better tolerated)	In areas with chloroquine-resistant *P. falciparum*	100 mg orally 1/d	>8 years of age: 2 mg/kg orally 1/d, up to adult dose of 100 mg	Photosensitivity reactions to doxycycline after sunlight (ultraviolet). Discontinue at first sign of erythema; skin reactions can increase when used with sulfonamide, sulfonylureas, or thiazide diuretics; gastrointestinal upset	Patients hypersensitive to any of the tetracyclines; some commercially available preparations contain sulfites that can result in increased asthmatic attacks in such persons, as well as anaphylaxis
Hydroxychloro-quine sulfate (Plaquenil)	Alternative to chloroquine	310 mg base (400 mg salt) orally 1/wk	5 mg/kg base (6.5 mg/kg salt), orally 1/wk, up to max adult dose of 310 mg base	Same as chloroquine	Same as chloroquine

Adapted with permission from Dardick K: Educating travelers about malaria: Dealing with resistance and patient noncompliance. *Cleve Clin J Med* 69(6):469, 2002.

out of date, the Internet and a subscription service (see Table 1) remain the most reliable sources of such information for proper health advice, including immunizations, for the traveler.

Routine immunizations such as tetanus, diphtheria, pertussis (in children), *Haemophilus* influenza, measles-mumps-rubella (MMR), polio, varicella, hepatitis B, and influenza should all be maintained according to the usual schedules. The risk of acquiring these diseases is generally no greater while traveling than while at home, but infants who are not protected against measles may be exposed to a greater risk of measles in many parts of the world where infant vaccination is less complete than in the United States. Travelers have been known to import measles back to the United States. There have been outbreaks of diphtheria (Eastern Europe) and influenza (late summer on cruises), and the prevalence of hepatitis B in East Asia is far greater than in North America or Europe.

Other immunization considerations more directly associated with travel (Table 7) are:

- Conditions of poor hygiene and sanitation increase the risk of hepatitis A and typhoid.
- Hepatitis A is perhaps the most common vaccine-preventable disease among travelers with considerable morbidity and some mortality in those older than 40 years of age.
- Typhoid fever is most commonly acquired on the Indian subcontinent, often by those returning to their native land to visit family.
- Japanese encephalitis is a risk for travelers who will be spending extended time in certain rural areas of Asia where exposure to mosquitoes is considerable, especially in areas devoted to rice farming and pig farming.
- Meningococcal disease is found in the sub-Saharan belt of Africa; vaccination may be appropriate for those spending extended periods in crowded cities during epidemic periods.
- Rabies vaccine should be strongly advised for those who will spend extended periods of time in developing countries or rural areas other than North America, Europe, Australia, Japan, and other islands designated as "rabies-free." Pre-exposure vaccination precludes the need for postexposure human rabies immunoglobulin (BayRab), which may be difficult to obtain or of questionable safety. It also reduces the number of postexposure shots from 5 to 2.
- Vaccines against diseases such as cholera, anthrax, and plague are of limited effectiveness and rarely advised for travelers except for unique circumstances such as field biologists or laboratory workers.
- Tick-borne encephalitis vaccine is not available in the United States. It may be obtained in Canada or in Europe for a traveler who will be exposed in areas of Eastern or Central Europe while hiking or camping.

The CDC offers the following vaccine information:

- Except for oral typhoid vaccine (Vivotif Berna), it is unnecessary to restart an interrupted series of vaccine or toxoid, or to add extra doses. Simply pick up with the next dose in the series.
- It is okay to give any combination of vaccines on the same day including all live virus vaccines and yellow fever vaccine (YF-VAX).
- Live virus vaccines not given concurrently should be given more than 28 days apart. If live virus vaccines are given less than 28 days apart, the second vaccine should be readministered after 4 to 6 weeks.
- Immunoglobulin is now given infrequently. If it is administered it may interfere with the immune response to certain vaccines. Refer to Table 1-1 in *CDC Health Information for International Travel 2003–2004* for detailed information on the use of immunoglobulin.
- Immunosuppressed travelers should not receive live virus vaccines (yellow fever, measles, mumps, rubella, varicella), including patients with AIDS, leukemia, lymphoma, generalized malignancy or those taking systemic steroids, alkylating drugs, antimetabolites and radiation therapy.
- The following patients are *not* considered immunosuppressed and may receive live virus vaccines:

Patients taking low-dose steroids (<20 mg prednisone per day)
Patients on short-term (<2 weeks) steroid therapy
Patients receiving steroid injections in joints, tendons, or bursae
Patients who have asymptomatic HIV infection with established laboratory verification of adequate immune system function (CD4 >200)

Yellow fever is a flavivirus transmitted by the bite of the *Aedes aegypti* mosquito. It exists in both South America (approximately 10% of the cases) and sub-Saharan Africa (approximately 90% of the cases). The World Health Organization (WHO) reports that in 2003 there were 200,000 cases with 30,000 deaths. Lately there may be an increased risk of yellow fever infection to the 3 million who visit endemic areas annually because the infection is spreading and is under-reported. It has been estimated that an unvaccinated traveler spending 2 weeks in a yellow fever zone in Africa has a 1 in 267 chance of contracting the illness and 1 in 1333 risk of death. Rates in South America are one tenth the rates in Africa.

The yellow fever vaccine (YF-VAX) is an attenuated strain (17D), which has been in widespread use for more than 60 years. More than 400 million doses have been given with an excellent safety record. A single dose yields protective antibodies in more than 99% of recipients in 1 month; the immunity may last for decades, but repeat vaccination is required every 10 years. Mild adverse effects may be seen in up to

TABLE 7 Travel Immunization Doses

Vaccine Name	Dosage	Comments
	Inactivated or Recombinant Antigens	
Hepatitis A vaccine—Havrix	Age 2-18 y, 720 EL.U., 0.5 mL, 2 doses at 0, 6-12 mo; age ≥19 y, 1440 EL.U., 1.0 mL, 2 doses at 0, 6-12 mo	2 doses provide life-long immunity; Havrix or Vaqta may be substituted for the 2 nd dose of the other. Giving the 2nd dose at a longer interval does not interfere with immune response; it may give an even better result.
Hepatitis A vaccine—Vaqta	Age 2-18 y, 25 U, 0.5 mL, 2 doses at 0, 6-18 mo; age ≥19 y, 50 U, 1.0 mL, 2 doses at 0, 6-12 mo	
Hepatitis B vaccine—Engerix-B	Age 0-19 y, 10 µg, 3 doses at 0, 1, 6 mo, or 4 doses at 0, 1, 2, 12 mo; age ≥20 y, 20 µg, 3 doses at 0, 1, 6 mo, or 4 doses at 0, 1, 2, 12 mo	May also be given in a non-FDA-approved schedule of 0, 7, 14 d with a booster 6 mo later. No need to restart a series that has been interrupted. Engerix-B and Recombivax-HB may be used interchangeably in the 3-dose schedule only.
Hepatitis B vaccine—Recombivax-HB	Age 0-19 y, 5 µg, 3 doses at 0, 1, 6 mo; age 11-15 y 10 µg; 2 doses at 0, 4-6 mo; age ≥20 y, 10 µg; 3 doses at 0, 1, 6 mo	
Hepatitis A/hepatitis B—Twinrix (combined vaccine)	Age ≥18 y, 720 EL.U./20 µg, 1.0 mL, 3 doses at 0, 1, 6 mo	
Meningococcal polysaccharide vaccine—Menomune (quadrivalent A,C,Y,W-135)	Age ≥2 y, but may be given for short-term protection against group A to infants >3mo, 1 dose, 0.5 mL	Revaccination of a single 0.5 mL dose administered subcutaneously may be indicated for individuals at high risk of infection, particularly children who were first vaccinated when they were less than 4 y of age; such children should be considered for revaccination after 2 or 3 y if they remain at high risk. Although the need for revaccination in older children and adults has not been determined, antibody levels decline rapidly over 2-3 y, and if indications still exist for immunization, revaccination may be considered within 3-5 y.
Typhoid vaccine, injectable—Typhim Vi	Age ≥2 y, 0.5 mL	Booster dose every 2 y.
Japanese encephalitis virus vaccine—JE Vax	Age 1-2 y, 0.5 mL; ≥3 y 1.0 mL, 3 doses on d 0, 7, 30	Adverse reactions to JE vaccine manifesting as generalized urticaria or angioedema may occur within minutes following vaccination. Most reactions occur in 48 h, but can be as late as 17 d after vaccination. Vaccinated persons should be observed for 30 min after vaccination and warned about the possibility of delayed generalized urticaria, often in a generalized distribution or angioedema of the extremities, face, and oropharynx, especially of the lips. They should be advised to remain in areas where they have ready access to medical care and should not embark on international travel within 10 d after receiving a dose of JE vaccine. Booster dose: 1 dose at 24 mo, but the full duration of protection is not known.
Rabies vaccine—Imovax (human diploid cell vaccine); HDCV; RVA (rabies vaccine adsorbed); RabAvert (purified chick embryo cell vaccine [PCEC])	All ages, 1.0 mL, 3 doses at 0, 7, and 21 or 28 d	The full course should be given with the same product. Travelers who are immunosuppressed should avoid travel to areas at risk for rabies and postpone vaccination. If this cannot be avoided, antibody titers should be checked after vaccination. Booster doses are not advised for travelers other than those with frequent exposure to rabies (spelunkers, veterinarians, rabies diagnostic laboratory workers, animal control workers in rabies-epizootic areas).
	Live-Attenuated Vaccines	
Typhoid vaccine, oral (attenuated bacteria)—Vivotif	Age ≥6 y, 1 capsule, 4 doses on d 0, 2, 4, 6	Booster dose, same as the initial 4-capsule dose after 5 years. Do not take with antibiotics which kill the attenuated bacterium.
Yellow Fever (attenuated virus vaccine)—YF-VAX	Age ≥9 mo, 0.5 mL	Booster dose every 10 years. Yellow fever vaccination may be required for international travel. Some countries in Africa require evidence of vaccination from all entering travelers and some countries may waive the requirements for travelers staying less than 2 wks that are coming from areas where there is no current evidence of significant risk for contracting yellow fever. Some countries require an individual, even if only in transit, to have a valid International Certificate of Vaccination if the individual has been in countries either known or thought to harbor yellow fever virus. The certificate becomes valid 10 d after vaccination with YF-VAX.

From CDC and package inserts.

25% of recipients (fever, myalgias), with 1% of recipients curtailing daily activities. Immediate hypersensitivity reactions are seen in less than 1 per 100,000; these are mostly because of egg protein allergies. Disseminated systemic reactions (viscerotropic) have been seen lately with seven cases (six deaths) reported from 1996 to 2000. It is estimated that there is a viscerotropic reaction risk of 1/400,000 to 1/500,000 vaccine recipients older than 60 years of age. The vaccine is contraindicated during pregnancy and in infants younger than 6 months of age, but there is limited data on its use during lactation. It is not recommended for infants 6 to 8 months of age except during outbreaks. Those who are immunosuppressed should not receive yellow fever vaccine.

Simultaneous administration of yellow fever vaccine with all others is acceptable, except data are not available on interactions of the yellow fever vaccine with the rabies vaccine and the Japanese encephalitis vaccine. If other live virus vaccines cannot be given at the same time as the yellow fever vaccine, they should be given more than 4 weeks later.

HEPATITIS A (SEE ACUTE AND CHRONIC VIRAL HEPATITIS CHAPTER)

Hepatitis A is an enteric viral infection that is a risk to travelers visiting tropical or poorly developed areas. Infections are usually asymptomatic (>70%) in those younger than 6 years of age, and the CFR is low (<0.3%). Those older than 50 years of age have both greater morbidity and mortality (CFR 1.8%). Completion of the two-dose series of hepatitis A immunization appears to provide life-long protection. The vaccine (Havrix, Vaqta is a recombinant DNA vaccine and should be offered to all travelers to tropical or underdeveloped areas outside of the United States, Canada, Western Europe, Australia, New Zealand, and Japan.

HEPATITIS B (SEE ACUTE AND CHRONIC VIRAL HEPATITIS CHAPTER)

Hepatitis B is a blood-borne viral infection that poses a risk to travelers who have blood and body-fluid exposure in areas of the world with rates of hepatitis B infection in excess of 2%. These areas comprise much of the world except North America, northern and western Europe, Australia, New Zealand, and southeast South America. The usual dosing schedule is 3 doses given in a 6 to 12 month period, but there is a non-FDA–approved accelerated schedule. Adolescents, 11 to 15 years old, may receive a two-dose schedule. A combination hepatitis A–hepatitis B vaccine (Twinrix) is also available. This vaccine is contraindicated for those allergic to yeast, but may be given during pregnancy or lactation.

INFLUENZA (SEE INFLUENZA CHAPTER)

Influenza is a common viral respiratory infection worldwide. Outbreaks may occur among travelers out of the usual seasonal pattern. There have been well-documented outbreaks among passengers on cruise ships during the summer months. North American travelers may be at risk of influenza infection while traveling to the southern hemisphere from April to September. Influenza vaccine is recommended for all travelers during the influenza season (including the North American summer for travel to the southern hemisphere).

MENINGOCOCCAL DISEASE

Neisseria meningitidis is an encapsulated gram-negative bacterium that can produce both meningitis and disseminated sepsis (meningococcemia). Travelers to Saudi Arabia on Haj (pilgrimage) may be required to show proof of this vaccination. Areas of sub-Saharan Africa in the so-called meningitis belt have both endemic and epidemic meningococcal disease. Travelers to these countries with extended itineraries may be at increased risk and should consider vaccination with the polysaccharide capsular meningococcal vaccine (Menomune-A/C/Y/W-135).

RABIES (SEE RABIES CHAPTER)

Perhaps the most important things to remember about rabies are these:

- Rabies infection is invariably fatal.
- There is no treatment for rabies infection, only prevention; there is a limited time window of opportunity for vaccination after suspected exposure.
- Pre-exposure immunization and postexposure immunization (and rabies immunoglobulin, if needed), when followed properly, protect against rabies infection.
- After suspected rabies exposure, those who have been properly prepared with pre-exposure immunization do not require rabies immunoglobulin (RIG) (BayRab) and only require two doses of rabies vaccine instead of the usual five doses.

TYPHOID (SEE TYPHOID FEVER CHAPTER)

Typhoid is a member of the salmonella family that produces both intestinal and enteric fever syndromes. There are an estimated 2.6 cases per million U.S. citizens or residents traveling abroad. Two vaccines are available, oral (Vivotif Berna) and injectable (Typhim Vi). Both have equivalent efficacy, about 70% protection; and the side effects of the two vaccines are comparable. The advantage of the injectable vaccine is that it is given in the office with no concerns about compliance or interference from antibiotics. These are both possible problems with the oral vaccine, which must be taken as four doses during a 7-day period—noncompliance is common. Also, the injectable vaccine can be given to children who cannot swallow the oral capsule; it cannot be crushed or broken because that would destroy the enteric coating, which is important for its dissolution. The oral vaccine provides protection for 5 years as opposed to only 2 years for the injectable vaccine. Pregnant women should not receive the oral vaccine; it is a live, attenuated bacterial vaccine.

Individual Health Considerations

HEALTH CARE WORKERS

Health care workers at risk of blood and body-fluid exposure should receive hepatitis B vaccinations and consider carrying a 1- to 2-week course of highly active retroviral therapy (HAART) with them in case they cannot receive prompt care after exposure.

HIV-INFECTED AND IMMUNOSUPPRESSED TRAVELERS

Travel to tropical and developing destinations may pose an increased risk of infectious diseases especially to those with CD4 counts less than 200. The CDC advises these travelers to pay particular attention to:

- Knowledge of the diseases present in the destination country
- Sources of medical care and need for supplemental insurance
- Adequate supply of medications which may not be available in the travel destination
- Chemoprophylaxis for traveler's diarrhea, a fluoroquinolone for nonpregnant persons, azithromycin for pregnant women and children
- Safe sex practices
- Risk from live virus vaccines (measles, varicella, yellow fever) balanced against the risk of the disease

PREGNANCY

According to the American College of Obstetrics and Gynecology the safest time to travel during pregnancy is during weeks 18 to 24. Travel no more than 300 miles from home during the third trimester. Be sure that health insurance covers pregnancy-related health problems while traveling as well as delivery, complications, and newborn care. The CDC advises that the greatest risks for the pregnant traveler are motor vehicle accidents (be sure to wear seat belts), hepatitis E (follow food and water precautions) and scuba diving (risk of decompression). It is safe for pregnant women to travel up to 36 weeks of gestation. International travel may be allowed until the week 32 of gestation, depending on each airline's individual policy. Those with placental abnormalities, severe anemia, sickle disease or trait, or those with a history of DVT probably should not fly. Getting up to walk frequently and wearing 20- to 30-mm compression stockings will help to prevent thrombosis.

Malaria is a more severe infection in pregnancy. Travel to a malarial zone should be deferred until after pregnancy if possible. If travel cannot be avoided, then the usual principles of mosquito avoidance and chemoprophylaxis should be followed. There is no evidence of any risk to the pregnant woman or developing fetus from recommended use of DEET or permethrin. Antimalarial chemoprevention with standard doses of chloroquine and mefloquine (Lariam) are not believed to be a significant risk to the mother or developing fetus or child. It is malaria that kills, not the preventive measures.

BREAST FEEDING

Breast feeding should be encouraged for infants who are traveling. Breast milk is a safe and convenient source of food. Women who are breast feeding should obtain any necessary immunization, as there is no evidence of any risk from immunization in this setting. Although some immunity may be passed to the unimmunized infant, it cannot be relied upon for protection of the child. The infant should receive any necessary immunizations, but some (meningococcal, yellow fever, typhoid) cannot be administered; therefore, risk of infection in the young infant must be considered. Traveler's diarrhea can pose a particular risk if the mother becomes dehydrated. Breast feeding should be continued, oral rehydration solution administered, and antibiotics considered for treatment. Bismuth must be avoided. The use of iodine for water treatment is acceptable but must be limited in time to avoid thyroid toxicity.

POST-TRAVEL

All who travel must be educated about which signs or symptoms following travel require evaluation. This is particularly important for those who have visited malarial zones. The majority of life-threatening malaria cases manifest themselves within 1 month of the traveler's return home, but some cases of *P. falciparum* malaria may take longer to develop.

Other parasitic diseases, including tapeworms and helminths, may not be apparent for months or years after the return home. Cutaneous leishmaniasis typically develops 2 to 6 months after the return home. Some infections, such as tuberculosis or strongyloidiasis, may only be apparent years later when the patient's immune system is impaired by malignancy, immunosuppressant drugs, or age. Symptoms of cough and fever, which would ordinarily be considered a routine respiratory infection, may take on new significance if the traveler has visited an area of the world experiencing an outbreak of a "new" infection such as severe acute respiratory syndrome (SARS). Physicians must always include a travel history in the evaluation of unusual symptoms.

There is no indication for routine laboratory testing for returned travelers. Those who have lived abroad for an extended period of time (missionaries, Peace

Corps and other humanitarian volunteers, expatriates) may benefit from tuberculin testing, a complete blood count (CBC) (to check for eosinophilia, a sign of intestinal helminth infection), and stool testing for parasites (three samples taken during a few days). Those who have lived in areas endemic for relapsing (vivax or ovale) malaria should be considered for terminal prophylaxis with primaquine.

TOXOPLASMOSIS

METHOD OF

Thomas T. Ward, MD

Toxoplasmosis is the disease caused by infection with the obligate intracellular protozoan *Toxoplasma gondii*. Toxoplasmosis is a worldwide zoonosis and causes infection in both birds and mammals. Cats, the definitive hosts for *T. gondii*, are the animals in which the parasite maintains an enteroepithelial sexual cycle. Human beings and domestic animals are secondary hosts and are important in maintaining an extraintestinal asexual cycle of transmission. Although most human infection is asymptomatic, self-limited clinical disease can infrequently occur after primary infection in immunocompetent persons. Because of the persistence of dormant cyst forms, all infection becomes chronic and latent. Primary infection during pregnancy can result in transplacental transmission of infection to the fetus; resultant congenital toxoplasmosis has varied clinical manifestations. Reactivation of dormant cysts is an important cause of infection in immunocompromised patients with defective T-cell-mediated immunity, including those patients with advanced HIV infection, hematologic malignancies, and bone marrow and solid-organ transplants.

T. gondii exists in three forms: the oocyst, the tissue cyst, and the tachyzoite. Oocysts are formed only in infected felines; these cats excrete large numbers of cysts for approximately 2 weeks after infection. Oocysts may remain viable in the soil for months and are an important environmental reservoir for infection of incidental hosts. Tachyzoites occur with acute infection in incidental hosts; their presence is required for the histologic confirmation of active disease. Tissue cysts occur after replication of tachyzoites and likely persist for the life of the incidental host. Dormant cysts are most commonly located in skeletal and smooth muscle, heart, brain, and eye. The presence of tissue cysts in histologic sections is indicative of past infection, but by itself it does not signify active infection.

The human incidence of seropositivity for *T. gondii* antibody varies greatly throughout the world. Within the United States, seropositivity increases with age, and the overall seroprevalence is approximately 15%. Within Western Europe, seroprevalence ranges between 50% and 70%. Human transmission occurs by oral exposure to oocysts that have contaminated water sources, vegetables, or other food products or, even more commonly, by ingesting poorly cooked or raw meat that contains tissue cysts. As many as 25% of lamb or pork samples have been shown to contain tissue cysts.

After human ingestion of either oocysts or tissue cysts, specialized forms of *T. gondii* emerge that penetrate the intestinal mucosa, establish intracellular infection within white blood cells, and enter the blood and lymphatic circulations to result in widespread dissemination throughout the body. Intact cell-mediated immunity leads to clearance of intracellular tachyzoites and the formation of dormant tissue cysts. Impaired cell-mediated immunity leads to either uncontrolled, primary infection (as in the fetus) or reactivation of infection later in life (as in AIDS and other immunosuppressed conditions).

Diagnosis

The diagnosis of *T. gondii* infection can be established by serologic tests, amplification of specific nucleic acid sequences, or histologic demonstration of the parasite or its antigens. Rarely employed reference or research methods for diagnosis include isolation of the organism, specific immunoglobulin (Ig) G avidity tests, various antigen detection tests, and lymphocyte transformation tests.

IgG antibodies appear in immunocompetent individuals within 2 to 3 weeks after infection. A negative IgG test essentially excludes previous or past infection with *T. gondii*. IgG antibody may persist in high titers for years after infection; therefore, a single positive IgG titer does not differentiate whether infection is recently acquired, chronic and latent, or chronic and reactivated. Sequential IgG antibody tests that increase by more than two tube dilutions are consistent with recent infection. Specific IgM and IgA antibody tests are usually positive during the first 6 months after acquisition of infection, and negative tests have a high predictive value for excluding recent infection. A positive IgM test can indicate recent onset of infection; however both false-positive results and persistently positive IgM antibody test results in chronically infected individuals can occur. When therapeutic decisions will be based on the interpretation of a positive IgM antibody test, confirmatory testing by a reference laboratory should be performed if feasible. Serologic tests can be more difficult to interpret in immunocompromised patients.

Polymerase chain reaction (PCR) for detection of specific *T. gondii* nucleic acid sequences has been successfully employed using vitreous and aqueous humor, bronchoalveolar lavage fluid, peripheral blood buffy coat preparations, cerebrospinal fluid, and amniotic fluid after 18 weeks of gestation. False-positive brain tissue PCR tests may occur in patients with HIV infection and suspected toxoplasmic encephalitis.

Specific histopathologic findings on resected lymph nodes can be strongly suggestive of the diagnosis of toxoplasmosis in immunocompetent patients. Demonstration of tachyzoites in tissue is invariably diagnostic of active infection. Although the presence of a single cyst does not differentiate between active and chronic or latent infection, multiple cysts present on cytopathologic examination suggest the presence of active disease. Staining for specific antigens (e.g., immunoperoxidase techniques) is highly specific for active infection when positive, and it is much more sensitive than hematoxylin and eosin or Wright-Giemsa staining alone. Tests employing direct fluorescent antibody tests can be nonspecific and are best avoided.

Clinical Manifestations

Most patients with acute *T. gondii* infection do not have symptomatic disease. Clinical manifestations of acute infection occasionally occur in immunocompetent adults, as does reactivation of infection within the retina of the eye. Infection during pregnancy results in congenital toxoplasmosis at an incidence of approximately 1 in 8000 live births in the United States; the frequency in which *T. gondii* causes spontaneous abortion is unknown. Reactivation infection from dormant cysts is the cause of toxoplasmic infections in patients with AIDS, patients with bone marrow or solid-organ transplantations, and other immunosuppressed hosts. The clinical syndromes in each of the foregoing settings are sufficiently distinct to warrant separate comment.

ACUTE INFECTION IN IMMUNOCOMPETENT PATIENTS

Approximately 15% of immunocompetent patients who become infected have either regional lymphadenopathy or a mononucleosis-like syndrome characterized by generalized adenopathy and constitutional symptoms. Toxoplasmic lymphadenopathy is largely a self-limited disease in immunocompetent patients, and it rarely requires therapy. Epstein-Barr virus and cytomegalovirus infections are much more common causes of the mononucleosis syndrome. Other causes of lymphadenopathy that need to be considered include cat-scratch disease, lymphoma or metastatic malignancy, sarcoidosis, tuberculosis, and the deep mycoses. Serologic testing and lymph node biopsy are most beneficial in establishing a diagnosis. Infections acquired by blood transfusion or through a laboratory accident may be severe and should be treated.

OCULAR TOXOPLASMOSIS IN IMMUNOCOMPETENT PATIENTS

Approximately 33% of all cases of chorioretinitis within the Unites States are caused by *T. gondii*. Most cases are believed to result from unrecognized congenital infection that reactivates, most commonly during the second and third decades of life. Retinal clinical findings are highly suggestive of *T. gondii* infection when evaluated by ophthalmologists experienced in managing this infection. Serologic testing is usually positive for prior exposure to toxoplasmosis, but in difficult cases, PCR testing may be performed on samples of aqueous or vitreous humor to confirm the diagnosis. Control of the host inflammatory response by the concomitant use of corticosteroids may be required in some patients receiving therapy for toxoplasmosis. Relapse of infection requiring repeated treatment is not uncommon.

CONGENITAL TOXOPLASMOSIS

Congenital toxoplasmosis results from transplacental spread of *T. gondii* infection that is asymptomatically acquired either during pregnancy or shortly before the onset of gestation. The risk of fetal infection varies with the stage of trimester; it is highest during the second and third trimesters. Approximately 60% of maternal infections acquired during the third trimester will result in fetal infection. Fetal infection occurring during the first trimester is believed to result frequently in spontaneous abortion. Clinical manifestations of congenital toxoplasmosis are varied. There may be no sequelae, or clinical disease may become manifest at birth or at various times after birth. Children may be born with the nonspecific manifestations of the TORCH (toxoplasmosis, other infections, rubella, cytomegalovirus, and herpes simplex) syndrome, including chorioretinitis, hydrocephalus, intracranial calcifications, hepatosplenomegaly, rash, anemia, and/or jaundice. Other infectious causes such as herpes simplex, cytomegalovirus, rubella, and syphilis should be considered and excluded. In those infants born with subclinical congenital infection, studies suggest that most will eventually demonstrate evidence of clinical disease even though they appear normal at birth. Years or decades later, previously subclinically infected children may develop chorioretinitis, seizure disorders, or psychomotor and mental retardation. Early recognition and treatment of congenital infection reduce the likelihood of subsequent sequelae; therefore, congenital *T. gondii* infection should always be treated regardless of whether there are symptoms at birth. Treatment of acute maternal infection diagnosed during pregnancy reduces the risk of fetal infection by approximately 60%.

Because congenital toxoplasmosis occurs almost exclusively in women infected during pregnancy, it is important that such infection be recognized and treated aggressively. In some countries where there is a higher seroprevalence of *T. gondii* infection (e.g., France), routine screening for acquisition of infection during pregnancy is performed. Routine pregnancy screening is not currently advocated in the United States. Women who have IgG antibody but who lack specific IgM antibody are believed to have evidence of past, chronic infection and are not at risk of transmitting congenital infection. A positive IgM test requires further confirmatory testing through a reference laboratory to determine whether infection has been recently acquired. Confirmation of acutely acquired maternal infection during pregnancy mandates testing during and after pregnancy to determine whether fetal or congenital infection has occurred. PCR testing of amniotic fluid at 18 weeks of gestation and beyond is approximately 60% sensitive and 100% specific in diagnosing fetal infection. Diagnosis of congenital toxoplasmosis at birth is usually confirmed by the presence of specific IgA (or IgM) in fetal serum, with careful attention to exclusion of maternal contamination of fetal blood. In children with suspected congenital toxoplasmosis, it is important to perform ophthalmologic evaluation and neuroimaging studies and to examine the cerebrospinal fluid for pleocytosis or elevated protein concentrations.

TOXOPLASMOSIS IN AIDS AND IMMUNOCOMPROMISED PATIENTS

In immunocompromised patients, toxoplasmosis almost always occurs as reactivation infection. One exception is infection after heart transplantation, in which primary infection can occur when a seronegative host receives a donor heart from a seropositive donor. The central nervous system is the most commonly affected site, resulting in necrotizing focal or multifocal encephalitis and, less frequently, focal spinal cord involvement. Other forms of infection include chorioretinitis, myocarditis, and pneumonia. Active toxoplasmosis in immunodeficient patients can cause significant morbidity and mortality and always requires therapy. The duration of therapy is largely dependent on the degree of chronic immunosuppression, and, on occasion, lifelong maintenance therapy is indicated.

In natural history studies of HIV infection performed before effective antiretroviral therapy, it was observed that approximately one third of toxoplasmosis seropositive patients with AIDS developed toxoplasmic encephalitis before death. Daily receipt of one tablet of double-strength trimethoprim (160 mg)-sulfamethoxazole (800 mg) (Bactrim DS) largely eliminates the risk of disease. Most episodes of toxoplasmic encephalitis complicating AIDS occur in patients with CD4 counts of less than 100 cell/mm^3, and infection is uncommon if the CD4 count exceeds 200 cell/mm^3. Patients with toxoplasmic encephalitis most commonly present with focal neurologic abnormalities of subacute (weeks) onset, often with fevers, headache, or subtle mental status or memory changes. Motor palsies are the most common focal abnormalities, although cranial nerve abnormalities, visual field defects, and seizure disorders can be the major presenting symptoms. Neuroradiologic imaging is best performed using magnetic resonance imaging, with the most common finding being multiple, ring-enhancing cerebral lesions. Involvement of the basal ganglion area is common. Computed tomography is, in general, less sensitive in defining disease and its extent. Single lesions on magnetic resonance imaging are unusual in toxoplasmic encephalitis and suggest possible central nervous system lymphoma. Multifocal leukoencephalopathy resulting from JC virus can also cause neuroradiologic findings that resemble toxoplasmosis. PCR can be performed on cerebrospinal fluid for Epstein-Barr virus, JC virus, and toxoplasmosis.

A definitive diagnosis of toxoplasmic encephalitis is made by brain biopsy and by the histologic demonstration of tachyzoites. However, to avoid the morbidity associated with brain biopsy, in patients with HIV infection who are toxoplasmosis seropositive and who have consistent neuroradiologic findings, it is now standard practice to treat these patients for toxoplasmosis empirically and to observe the clinical response. Although neuroradiologic resolution is delayed, most patients with toxoplasmic encephalitis demonstrate clinical improvement within 7 days of initiating therapy. Failure to respond clinically to empirical therapy, seronegativity to *T. gondii* antibody, and the presence of a single lesion on magnetic resonance imaging all are findings that suggest the possibility of an alternative diagnosis and warrant consideration of performing a brain biopsy.

Tissue biopsies with histologic examination are usually necessary for diagnosing toxoplasmosis at other sites in immunocompromised patients. PCR testing on bronchoalveolar lavage fluid can be positive in cases of pneumonitis. Endomyocardial biopsy should be performed if toxoplasmosis is a consideration in the seronegative heart recipient of a seropositive donor.

Therapy

Treatment of toxoplasmosis is summarized in Table 1. Most infections in immunologically normal adults are self-limited and do not require therapy. In ocular, central nervous system, and congenital toxoplasmosis, first-line therapy is the combination of pyrimethamine (Daraprim), and sulfadiazine, with folinic acid (leucovorin, not folic acid). Treatment duration is based on time of clinical resolution, but it is usually approximately 6 weeks in ocular and central nervous system infections and 12 months in congenital infection. In patients with AIDS who have persistently low CD4 counts (less than 200 cells/mm^3),

TABLE 1 Therapy of Toxoplasmic Infection

	Adult Doses	Pediatric Doses
Immunologically Normal		
Acute lymphadenopathy	No treatment	No treatment
Acute chorioretinitis	Pyrimethamine (Daraprim) 100 mg PO bid on day 1, then 25 mg PO qd + Sulfadiazine 1 g PO qid + Folinic acid (leucovorin) 5 mg PO qd	
Pregnancy	Spiramycin[2] 1.0 g PO q8h (see text)	
Congenital toxoplasmosis		Pyrimethamine 2 mg/k for 2 d, then 1 mg/kg PO qd + Sulfadiazine 50 mg/kg PO bid + Folinic acid 10 mg 3 × wk PO
AIDS and Immunologically Impaired		
Encephalitis and other tissue sites of infection	Pyrimethamine 200 mg PO × one dose, then 75 mg PO qd + Sulfadiazine 1 g PO qid + Folinic acid 5-10 mg PO qd	

[2]Not available in the United States except from the FDA.

and in other patients with continued profound immunosuppression, long-term maintenance therapy with pyrimethamine-sulfadiazine-folinic acid should be continued at the same doses used for primary therapy. Spiramycin[1,2] (3 g per day) is the drug of choice for pregnant women with acquired primary *T. gondii* infection. Spiramycin should be continued until term if there is no evidence of fetal infection. Spiramycin does not cross the placenta and will not treat infection in the fetus. If fetal infection is demonstrated to be present by amniotic fluid PCR, pyrimethamine-sulfadiazine-folinic acid should be administered during the second and third trimesters. Pyrimethamine is potentially teratogenic and should not be administered during the first 16 weeks of pregnancy.

Allergic reactions to sulfonamides are common in patients with HIV infection. Alternative drugs to sulfadiazine that may be employed in combination therapy include clindamycin (Cleocin)[1] 600 to 1200 mg every 6 hours intravenously or orally; clarithromycin (Biaxin)[1] 1 g every 12 hours orally; atovaquone (Mepron)[1] 750 mg every 6 hours orally; azithromycin (Zithromax)[1] 1200 to 1500 mg per day orally; and dapsone[1] 100 mg per day orally. Alternatively, increasing experience suggests that trimethoprim-sulfamethoxazole (Bactrim, Septra)[1] 5 mg/kg trimethoprim component every 6 hours orally or intravenously (20 mg/kg per day total) is equally effective as the pyrimethamine-containing combination regimens in those patients who are not allergic to sulfa agents.

[1]Not FDA approved for this indication.

[2]Not available in the United States except from the FDA (call 301-827-2335).

Corticosteroids can be administered to patients with ocular toxoplasmosis in whom a brisk inflammatory response is believed to be contributing to ocular pathology. Similarly, in toxoplasmic encephalitis with cerebral edema or significant mass effect, short-duration corticosteroids may be concomitantly employed with antitoxoplasmic antimicrobial therapy.

Prevention

Prevention of *T. gondii* infection is of major importance in pregnant women and immunodeficient patients who have not been previously exposed. Risk of primary infection can be reduced by not eating undercooked meat and by taking proper precautions when disposing of or cleaning cat litter material. Cysts in meat are killed at 60°C (140°F) or higher. Hands should be thoroughly washed after soil contamination, and all fruits and vegetables should be washed before they are eaten.

Primary prophylaxis should be administered in patients with AIDS who have CD4 counts of less than 100 cells/mm^3 and who are seropositive for toxoplasmosis antibody. Trimethoprim (160 mg)-sulfamethoxazole (800 mg)[1] as one double-strength tablet daily is highly effective for prevention of toxoplasmosis infection. Alternative prophylactic regimens include either (a) pyrimethamine 50 to 75 mg orally per week plus dapsone[1] 50 mg per day or 200 mg per week; or (b) pyrimethamine-sulfadoxine (Fansidar)[1] at three tablets every 2 weeks. Dapsone alone is not effective at preventing toxoplasmosis.

[1]Not FDA approved for this indication.

CAT-SCRATCH DISEASE

METHOD OF

Kristina A. Bryant, MD

Cat-scratch disease (CSD) is a zoonosis caused by infection with *Bartonella henselae*, a small, pleomorphic, gram-negative bacillus. An estimated 22,000 cases occur annually in the United States, with the highest age-specific incidence in children less than 10 years of age. CSD has a seasonal predilection, with the majority of cases diagnosed in the fall and winter. Seroprevalence studies suggest that infection is most common in warm, humid regions. Most cases of CSD are sporadic, although clusters of cases within families have been reported. Infection appears to confer lifelong immunity, as reports of reinfection are rare.

Cats are the primary animal reservoir for *B. henselae* and contact with cats, especially kittens, is the most important risk factor for infection. Bacteremia is common among kittens. Infection typically occurs after a cat bite or scratch, although occasionally an individual with confirmed CSD denies cat contact. The cat flea (*Ctenocephalides felis*) is involved in transmission between felines, but the role of fleas in transmission to humans remains uncertain. Rarely, dogs have been implicated in *B. henselae* transmission. Although *B. henselae* has been identified in ticks, the role of ticks in transmission of infection to humans is unknown. Human-to-human transmission does not occur.

Clinical Features

CSD commonly presents as regional lymphadenopathy after a cat bite or scratch. Three to 10 days following bacterial inoculation, reddish-brown papules appear at the site of the bites or in the line of the scratch. One to 2 weeks later, adenopathy occurs in the nodes that drain the affected area. Axillary nodes are most commonly involved, followed by nodes that drain the neck and jaw (cervical and submandibular). Affected lymph nodes are variably tender and remain enlarged for 2 to 3 months. Constitutional symptoms, including low-grade fever and malaise, accompany lymphadenopathy in less than 50% of patients. CSD may mimic acute bacterial lymphadenitis that is caused by *Staphylococcus aureus* or group A streptococcus, glandular tularemia, and tuberculous or nontuberculous mycobacteria.

Parinaud's oculoglandular syndrome (preauricular adenopathy and conjunctivitis) is the most common form of atypical CSD and results from inoculation of the organism directly into the eye. Less common manifestations of *B. henselae* infection include encephalopathy with or without status epilepticus, aseptic meningitis, stellate neuroretinitis, pneumonia, and hepatosplenic granulomas. Osteomyelitis may occur as a result of hematogenous spread or direct extension from an involved lymph node. Vertebral infection is more common than long bone disease. Terminal ileitis and mesenteric adenitis mimicking Crohn's disease have been described in individuals with high immunoglobulin (Ig) M titers to *B. henselae*. Recent attention has focused on CSD as a cause of fever of unknown origin, accounting for up to 5% of cases in some series. Seroprevalence studies suggest that infection may be asymptomatic.

Severe, disseminated disease may occur in immunocompromised individuals, especially those with HIV infection. *B. henselae* and a related species, *Bartonella quintana*, are the cause of bacillary angiomatosis, a rare vasoproliferative disorder characterized by vascular tumors of the skin and subcutaneous tissue. Reticuloendothelial lesions in the visceral organs are seen with bacillary peliosis. *Bartonella* infections may also cause persistent or relapsing fever with bacteremia in immunocompromised hosts.

Diagnosis

Although *B. henselae* may be cultured on chocolate or blood-enriched agar plates, this organism is fastidious and requires incubation periods of up to 6 weeks. Culture is rarely helpful in the diagnosis of typical CSD. Histologic demonstration of microabscesses and granulomas with central necrosis in lymph node tissue suggests the diagnosis of CSD. Gram-negative organisms may be visualized by Warthin-Starry silver staining, although this stain is not specific for *B. henselae*. Detection of DNA sequences by polymerase chain reaction (PCR) testing is sensitive and specific, although testing is expensive and not widely available. Visualization of multiple, round hypodense lesions in the liver and spleen by computerized tomography (CT) should prompt further testing for CSD.

Serology is the mainstay of diagnosis for CSD. Indirect immunofluorescence antibody (IFA) testing for antibodies to *B. henselae* is available through the Centers for Disease Control and some commercial laboratories; results from commercial laboratories are not universally reliable. A single titer greater than or equal to 1:64, or a fourfold rise between acute and convalescent titers, is diagnostic. Enzyme immunoassays for *B. henselae* antibody detection have also been developed. Antibody titers peak 6 to 8 weeks after the onset of illness and decline thereafter. The cat-scratch skin test is no longer available or recommended for diagnosis.

Treatment

Case reports and retrospective analyses of patients treated for CSD suggest that gentamicin

(Garamycin)[1], azithromycin (Zithromax)[1], rifampin (Rifadin, Rimactane)[1], trimethoprim-sulfamethoxazole (Bactrim, Septra)[1], and ciprofloxacin (Cipro)[1] are clinically efficacious. Only azithromycin has been studied in a prospective, randomized trial. Twenty-nine patients with lymphadenopathy and serologic evidence of *B. henselae* infection were randomized to receive oral azithromycin or placebo for 5 days. Patients who received azithromycin experienced a greater decrease in lymph node volume during the first 30 days of therapy, although long-term results were similar in both groups.

Treatment of typical CSD is supportive. Regional lymphadenitis typically resolves without antimicrobial therapy, although occasionally nodes will suppurate and require surgical drainage. The optimal antimicrobial regimen and duration of therapy for atypical CSD in immunocompetent hosts have not been defined, although some experts advocate treatment with gentamicin, rifampin, or azithromycin. Anecdotal reports suggest a role for corticosteroids in selected clinical scenarios, including eye disease and severe systemic disease unresponsive to antibiotic therapy.

Prevention

Prevention of CSD requires education of cat owners, elimination of fleas from household pets, and avoidance of traumatic injury from cats. Cats harboring *B. henselae* rarely appear ill. Vaccines to prevent feline infection are not commercially available. In general, the diagnosis of CSD does not require removal of the family pet, even if the kitten or cat is the suspected source of infection. Immunocompromised individuals should be counseled about the risks of *B. henselae* transmission from cats, especially those younger than 1 year of age.

[1]Not FDA approved for this indication.

SALMONELLOSIS

METHOD OF

Clifford L. S. Leen, MBChB, MD

Until recently all *Salmonella* species were given names based on the Kaufmann-White typing system, with the species defined by the O antigens (the polysaccharide component of their lipopolysaccharide [LPS]) and the H antigens (flagella). The genus has now been reorganized into two species, *Salmonella bongori* and *Salmonella enterica*. *S. enterica* is subdivided into additional subgroups. All *Salmonella* that are isolated from humans and other warm-blooded animals, including *Salmonella typhi*, are included in the *S. enterica* subgroup 1. The other subgroups are made up of *Salmonella* serotypes that are usually isolated from cold-blooded hosts or the environment. However, because no general agreement has been reached on a new naming convention, and because most clinicians are familiar with the old serologically defined names, the old nomenclature will be used in this article. *Salmonella typhimurium* and *Salmonella enteritidis* are the most common species causing human disease.

Epidemiology

The number of cases of nontyphoid *Salmonella* infections has increased during the past few years, with a threefold increase in the United States. This may be an underestimate, because most cases of gastroenteritis are managed without diagnostic stool cultures, and there is under-reporting of diagnosed cases.

Almost all *Salmonella* infections are acquired orally, although infection transmitted via contaminated blood products has been reported.

Host Factors

The infective dose of nontyphi *Salmonella* is very low, approximately 10^5 organisms. Conditions that lead to low gastric acid, such as pernicious anemia; or the use of antacids, H-2 blockers, or proton pump inhibitors predispose individuals to salmonellosis. Other risk factors include extremes of age, recent use of antibiotics, increased gastric transit (as in gastroenterostomy), diabetes, malignancy, rheumatological disorders, sickle-cell disease, HIV, and iatrogenic immunodeficiency.

Clinical Features

The four clinical syndromes arising from infection with nontyphoid *Salmonella* are gastroenteritis, bacteriemia, enteric fever, and asymptomatic fecal excretion. Enteric fever is not discussed in this article.

Gastroenteritis

This is the most common manifestation of *Salmonella* infection and occurs after an incubation period of 12 to 96 hours. Gastroenteritis caused by *Salmonella* cannot be reliably distinguished from that caused by other pathogens. The illness is usually self-limiting and consists of nausea, vomiting, crampy abdominal pain, and watery diarrhea.

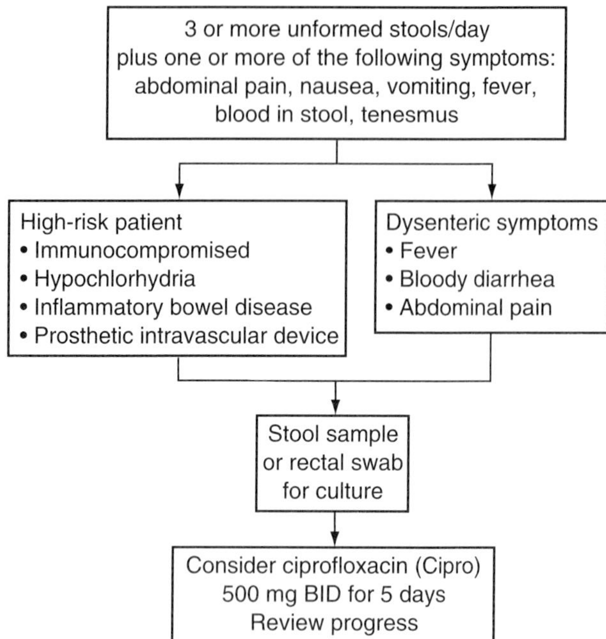

FIGURE 1 Algorithm for empiric therapy of gastroenteritis.

Other symptoms include fever, urgency of defecation, and tenesmus. The stools may be frankly bloody, reflecting significant mucosal inflammation. The illness usually resolves within 4 to 6 days but may last up to 14 days. Fever may be present in 50% of patients and persist for 1 to 2 days. Approximately 5% of patients with gastroenteritis have positive blood cultures.

TREATMENT OF ACUTE NONTYPHOID *SALMONELLA* GASTROENTERITIS

Salmonella are facultative, intracellular pathogens, and although they are susceptible to most antibiotics that are active against gram-negative organisms, only the antibiotics that are highly active intracellularly, such as the quinolones, tend to be useful in the treatment of salmonellosis. There is an increasing prevalence of antibiotic-resistant *Salmonella* throughout the world; these include resistance to ampicillin, trimethoprim-sulfamethoxazole. Furthermore, 6% of all *Salmonella* cases in England proved to be quinolone resistant in 1995. A study of stored *Salmonella* isolates shows that resistance to nalidixic acid is a predictor for poor clinical response to other quinolones. An outbreak of salmonellosis caused by multidrug and quinolone-resistant *Salmonella* linked to a swine herd lends supporting evidence of a link between antimicrobial resistance in human isolates with agricultural use of antibiotics. The emergence of *Salmonella* resistant to third-generation cephalosporins and other extended-spectrum beta-lactamases (ESBLs) is of major concern. In a case report, all but one of the resistances to 13 antibiotics were carried on a conjugative plasmid, and the clinical isolate from the child was indistinguishable from one that was isolated from the family's cattle. Resistance to third-generation cephalosporins is a growing concern for children for whom the cephalosporin antibiotics are the current drugs of choice for the treatment of invasive salmonellosis.

The quinolone group of antimicrobial agents are active against *Salmonellae* because they have:

- High bactericidal activity against *Salmonella*, including multiresistant strains
- Rapid oral absorption resulting in wide tissue distribution with high concentrations in bile, the gallbladder wall, and feces
- Excellent intracellular penetration and concentration in neutrophils and macrophages
- Cephalosporins have high serum levels and long serum half-lives but have poor intracellular penetration. However, they are particularly helpful for treating systemic infections in children where the therapeutic choices are very limited.

Because the illness is self-limiting, treatment is generally based on symptom relief and replacement of fluid and electrolyte losses. Antipyretics and antiemetics are usually effective, but antimotility agents are usually contraindicated particularly when dysenteric symptoms are present. Antisecretory agents are not helpful because they have insignificant effects on stool water losses.

Studies indicate that oral treatment with ciprofloxacin (Cipro)[1] (500 mg twice daily for 5 days) or norfloxacin (Noroxin) (400 mg twice daily for 5 days) can shorten both the duration of fever and diarrhea and lessen the severity of the diarrhea; the benefit is greatest for those with severe illness. These studies were conducted within the first 3 days of onset of symptoms and may not be applicable if treatment with quinolone is started late, particularly when microbiological isolation is delayed. The effect of quinolones on fecal clearance of *Salmonella* is unclear but they do not appear to prolong carriage. As a result, antibiotic therapy is not routinely recommended for the empiric treatment of mild-to-moderate, presumed or proven *Salmonella* gastroenteritis in healthy persons.

Empiric antibiotics are indicated for those who are severely ill and for high-risk patients who are prone to systemic invasive disease or severe local disease. However, management is complicated, as those with bloody diarrhea may have infection with other pathogens including shigella or enterohemorrhagic *Escherichia coli* (EHEC), and antibiotic treatment of EHEC may increase the risk of hemolytic uremic syndrome. An algorithm for the possible use of empiric antibiotics is shown in Figure 1. Additional patients who could be considered at risk of severe complications include patients with underlying atherosclerotic lesions and infants younger than 3 months of age.

---

[1]Not FDA approved for this indication.

Antibiotics are also useful when rapid interruption of fecal shedding is required to reduce transmission of *Salmonella* infection in institutions.

Follow-up fecal cultures are not routinely indicated, but meticulous personal hygiene is important to prevent spread of infection. Good hand hygiene and the firming up of stools are important criteria for return to work. Local health departments should be consulted about food handlers and health care workers with *Salmonella* as each department may have different criteria for return to work.

Bacteriemia

Most nontyphoid *Salmonella* serotypes can cause a primary bacteriemia and extraintestinal infections in the absence of diarrhea. Most invasive serotypes carry virulence plasmids. Extraintestinal infections are found in 10% to 20% of bacteriemia cases. While *Salmonella choleraesuis* can cause invasive infection in previously healthy persons, bacteriemia can occur in persons with underlying immune defects. Host factors that are associated with invasive infections include defects in T cell immunity. These include, HIV, systemic lupus erythematosus (SLE), lymphomas, and immunosuppression with steroids or for transplantation; conditions associated with iron overload, congenital defects in interferon (IFN)-γ, and interleukin (IL)-12 signaling. Metastatic infections include meningitis, osteomyelitis, septic arthritis, and, less frequently, aortitis, endocarditis, pyelonephritis, and pneumonia. Infection in other rare sites like the prostate and thyroid have also been reported.

A mycotic aneurysm results from *Salmonella* infection of an artery previously affected by arteriosclerosis. Diagnosis of endovascular infection is very difficult, but must be suspected in any person with bacteriemia without an obvious source. Classical features such as fever, pain, and tender palpable mass are uncommon. If suspected, the diagnosis should be further explored using computerized tomography (CT), magnetic resonance imaging (MRI), or white cell or gallium scanning.

Salmonella meningitis is a rare cause of bacterial meningitis, and usually occurs in children younger than 1 year of age. It carries a high mortality rate and high rates of complications including seizures and hydrocephalus. In young children with sickle cell disease, *Salmonella* osteomyelitis affects the long bones; but in adults with this condition, it tends to involve the vertebrae. Monoarticular infection caused by *Salmonella* tends to involve the knee or hip joints, which is usually a result of adjoining osteomyelitis. Approximately 5% of nontyphoid *Salmonella* cases involves the urinary tract, and this is more common in patients who have abnormal renal tracts, particularly those with obstructive uropathy.

Salmonellosis in AIDS can be an invasive disease presenting as bacteriemia. The risk of nontyphoid bacteriemia increases as the CD4 cell count decreases, and AIDS patients have a 100-fold increased risk compared with HIV patients without AIDS. Metastatic complications occur at the same frequency as other immunocompromised patients but may also involve very unusual sites such as muscles. Recurrent bacteriemia is described and before highly active antiretroviral therapy (HAART) it often required lifelong antibiotic therapy.

TREATMENT OF INVASIVE SALMONELLOSIS

Treatment of *Salmonella* bacteriemia is usually with a single antibacterial agent, either a third-generation cephalosporin or a quinolone. In view of the changing resistance pattern in human *Salmonella* isolates, life-threatening infections should probably be treated with a combination of a quinolone and a third-generation cephalosporin until the susceptibility to antimicrobial agents is confirmed. If there is no suspicion of endovascular focus, *Salmonella* bacteriemia can usually be successfully treated with a 14-day course of antibiotics.

Any suspicion of an endovascular infection warrants further investigation. If endocarditis or infectious arteritis is confirmed, surgery should be considered. However, for the hemodynamically stable patient, medical treatment alone may be considered for both native and prosthetic endocarditis in view of some case reports of successful prolonged medical treatment without surgery.

For endovascular infection, surgical intervention is recommended for patients who are able to have surgery. Antibiotic therapy should be continued for a minimum of 6 weeks after surgery, although many clinicians may elect to continue the antibiotics for a few months. In cases where the focus of infection cannot be removed surgically, lifelong suppressive treatment is recommended, as there is a high risk of recurrence once the antibiotic is stopped. There is no consensus on whether the choice of antibiotics should be a third-generation cephalosporin or a quinolone. Some clinicians favor cephalosporins because high serum levels of cephalosporins relative to minimum bactericidal concentrations may lead to adequate antibiotic penetration and, therefore, kill the *Salmonella* in the vegetation or devitalized tissue. Other clinicians favor quinolones because of their intracellular activity against *Salmonella*. Unfortunately, it is unlikely that any clinical trial will be undertaken to resolve this issue. Certainly the long-term use of an oral quinolone after an initial period of treatment with an intravenous cephalosporin (ceftriaxone [Rocephin] 2 to 3 g twice daily) would be a good compromise.

Focal infections such as arthritis and abscesses should be drained or surgically treated whenever possible. Antibiotic treatment should be carried out for a minimum of 4 to 6 weeks.

The use of ceftriaxone or ciprofloxacin leads to adequate therapeutic concentration in the cerebrospinal fluid (CSF) even when the blood-brain barrier is intact. A minimum of 4 to 6 weeks treatment with either agent is recommended for the treatment of *Salmonella* meningitis, brain abscess, or subdural empyema.

AIDS patients with invasive disease will benefit from long-term quinolone treatment until their immune systems can be reconstituted with the use of HAART. Because zidovudine (Retrovir) has been shown to have in vitro activity against gram-negative organisms, including *Salmonella*, it is possible that its inclusion in the HAART regimen may have additional benefits to its anti-HIV activity.

Asymptomatic Fecal Excretion

Following acute gastroenteritis, most patients will excrete *Salmonella* in their stools for a mean duration of 4 weeks for adults and 7 weeks for young children. However, up to 1% of patients may continue to excrete nontyphoid *Salmonella* for 1 year after acute infection. Patients older than 50 years of age with biliary tract disease are predisposed to long-term carriage. Management of chronic carriage of greater than a 1-year duration is extrapolated from experience with *S. typhi*. Quinolones are useful in eradicating chronic carriage, but the optimal duration and dose have not been established. Regimens that have been tried include ciprofloxacin (Cipro)[1] (500 mg twice a day for up to 28 days) and ofloxacin (Floxin)[1] (400 mg once daily for 7 days). Failure and relapse following treatment are not uncommon. Cholecystectomy may be considered particularly when antibiotics have failed to eradicate carriage and when gallbladder pathology is present.

During an outbreak of infection in an institution, antibiotics may be used to reduce fecal shedding in order to limit transmission and the need for prolonged isolation.

Special Consideration for Children and Pregnant Women

The finding of cartilage dysplasia in animal studies of quinolones has given rise to concerns regarding their use in children and pregnant women. However, there is now increasing evidence that they may be safely administered to children with severe, pathogen-resistant infections. For example, quinolones are now routinely given to children in areas of the world where multidrug-resistant *S. typhi* is common. Alternative agents include azithromycin (Zithromax)[1] and aztreonam (Azactam)[1], although experience with their use is limited. Where resistance is limited, third-generation cephalosporins are used rather than quinolone.

[1]Not FDA approved for this indication.

Antibiotic treatment is not usually indicated in young, healthy individuals with mild-to-moderate gastroenteritis caused by *Salmonella*. In the immunocompromised individual, *Salmonella* can cause severe, invasive disease in the form of bacteriemia and focal disease. This needs careful clinical evaluation to identify the focus of infection. Management includes prolonged antibiotic use and surgical intervention for endovascular infections if possible. Resistance to current antimicrobial agents is increasing worldwide and knowledge of antimicrobial susceptibility is essential for optimal management of invasive salmonellosis.

TYPHOID FEVER

METHOD OF

Zulfiqar A. Bhutta, MB, PhD

Despite vast advances in public health and hygiene in much of the developed world, typhoid fever remains endemic in many developing countries. Probably because of the ease of modern travel, cases are also reported in most developed countries.

Etiology

Typhoid fever is caused by *Salmonella typhi*, a gram-negative bacterium. A very similar but often less severe disease is caused by *Salmonella* serotype *paratyphi* A. The ratio of disease caused by *S. typhi* to that caused by *S. paratyphi* is approximately 10:1, although the proportion of *S. paratyphi* infections is increasing in some parts of the world. Although *S. typhi* shares many genes with *Escherichia coli* and at least 90% with *Salmonella typhimurium*, there are several unique gene clusters known as pathogenicity islands and others that have been acquired during evolution. One of the specific genes is for the polysaccharide capsule Vi. This is present in approximately 90% of all freshly isolated *S. typhi* and has a protective effect against the bactericidal action of the serum of infected patients.

Epidemiology

Although accurate community-based figures are unavailable, it is estimated that more than 16 million cases occur annually, with more than 0.6 million deaths. The vast majority of cases occur in Asia. Given the paucity of microbiological facilities in developing countries, these figures may largely represent the clinical syndrome. Regional incidence rates vary from 100 to 1000 cases per 100,000 population, and there may be differences in the spectrum of the disorder. Recent population-based studies from south Asia also indicate that, contrary to previous views, the disease may largely affect children younger than 5 years of age. In contrast, data from sub-Saharan Africa and HIV-endemic areas indicate that nontyphoidal *Salmonella* bacteremia far outstrips typhoid fever as a cause of community-acquired bacteremia.

In recent years typhoid fever has been notable for the emergence of drug resistance. Following sporadic outbreaks of chloramphenicol-resistant typhoid, many strains of *S. typhi* have developed plasmid-mediated, multidrug resistance (MDR) to all of the three primary antimicrobials (ampicillin [Chloromycetin], chloramphenicol, and trimethoprim-sulfamethoxazole [Septra]). More troubling, chromosomally acquired quinolone resistance in *S. typhi* has been recently described in various parts of Asia and may be a consequence of widespread and indiscriminate use of these agents.

Pathogenesis

The disease occurs by the ingestion of the organism, and a variety of sources of fecal contamination have been reported including street vendor foods and contamination of water reservoirs. A larger infecting dose leads to a shorter incubation period and more severe infection. The organism crosses the intestinal mucosal barrier after attachment to the microvilli by an intricate mechanism involving membrane ruffling, actin rearrangement, and internalization in an intracellular vacuole. Once inside the intestinal cells, *S. typhi* find their way into the circulation and reside within the macrophages of the reticuloendothelial system. The clinical syndrome is produced by a release of proinflammatory cytokines (interleukin [IL]-6, IL-1β, and tumor necrosis factor [TNF]-α) from the infected cells. Some 1% to 5% of patients with acute typhoid infection may become chronic carriers of the infection in the gallbladder, depending on age, sex, and treatment regimen.

Clinical Features

Typhoid fever usually presents with high grade fever and a wide variety of associated symptoms such as abdominal pain, hepatosplenomegaly, diarrhea, and constipation. In the absence of localizing signs, the early stage of the disease may be difficult to differentiate from other endemic diseases including malaria and dengue fever. The classic stepladder rise of fever is relatively rare, but the presentation of typhoid fever may be tampered with by coexisting morbidities and early administration of antibiotics. In malaria-endemic areas and in parts of the world where schistosomiasis is common, the presentation of typhoid may also be atypical.

Although data from South America and parts of Africa suggest that typhoid may present as a mild illness in young children, this may vary in different parts of the world. There is emerging evidence from south Asia that the presentation of typhoid may be more dramatic in children younger than 5 years of age, with comparatively higher rates of complications and hospitalization. Diarrhea, toxicity, and complications such as disseminated intravascular complications are also more common in infancy, with higher case fatality rates. However, some of the other features of typhoid fever seen in adults, such as relative bradycardia, are rare, and rose spots may only be visible at an early stage of the illness in fair-skinned children.

It is also recognized that MDR typhoid is a more severe clinical illness with higher rates of toxicity, complications, and case fatality rates. This may be related to the increased virulence of MDR *S. typhi* as well as a higher number of circulating bacteria. These findings may have implications for treatment algorithms, especially in endemic areas with high rates of MDR typhoid.

Diagnosis

The mainstay of the diagnosis of typhoid fever is a positive culture from the blood or another anatomic site. However, the sensitivity of blood cultures in diagnosing typhoid fever in many parts of the developing world is limited because widespread use of antibiotics may render bacteriologic confirmation difficult. Although bone marrow cultures may increase the likelihood of bacteriologic confirmation of typhoid, these are difficult to obtain and relatively invasive.

The serological diagnosis of typhoid is also fraught with problems because a single Widal test may be positive in only 50% of cases in endemic areas, and serial tests may be required in cases presenting in the first week of illness. Newer serological tests such as a dot-enzyme-linked immunoabsorbent assay (ELISA) (Typhidot) and the TUBEX tests are promising, but require further evaluation in large scale studies in community settings. In much of the developing world, the mainstay of diagnosis of typhoid remains clinical, and several diagnostic algorithms have been evaluated in endemic areas.

Therapy

An early diagnosis of typhoid fever and institution of appropriate treatment are essential. The vast majority of typhoid patients can be managed at home with oral antibiotics and close medical follow-up for complications or failure to respond to therapy. However, patients with persistent vomiting, severe diarrhea, and abdominal distension may require hospitalization and parenteral antibiotic therapy. The general principles of management of typhoid include:

- Adequate rest, hydration, and attention to correction of fluid–electrolyte imbalance
- Antipyretic therapy (acetaminophen, 120-750 mg orally every 4-6 hours[3]) as required
- Soft, easily digestible diet unless the patient has abdominal distension or ileus
- Antibiotic therapy (the right choice, dosage, and duration)
- Antibiotics are critical to curing typhoid with minimal complications. Traditional therapy with either chloramphenicol (Chloromycetin) or amoxicillin[1] is associated with relapse rates of 5% to 15% and 4% to 8%, respectively; whereas the newer quinolones and third-generation cephalosporins are associated with higher cure rates.

[3]Exceeds dosage recommended by the manufacturer.
[1]Not FDA approved for this indication.

Some authorities have recommended treatment with second-line agents in all cases of typhoid. Others have questioned this on the basis of adequate response to therapy among sensitive cases with first-line agents. Blanket administration of second-line agents such as fluoroquinolones and third-generation cephalosporins in all cases of suspected typhoid is expensive and may lead to the rapid development of further resistance. Table 1 gives the recommended therapy for typhoid fever based on a recent consensus document by the World Health Organization (2003).

Preventive Strategies for Typhoid

Of the major risk factors for outbreaks of typhoid, contamination of water supplies with sewage is the most important. During outbreaks, therefore, a combination of central chlorination and domestic water purification are important. In endemic situations consumption of street vendor foods, especially ice cream and cut-up fruit, has been recognized as an important risk factor. The human-to-human spread by chronic carriers is also important, and attempts

TABLE 1 Treatment of Typhoid Fever Based on Diagnosis, Treatment, and Prevention

Uncomplicated Typhoid Fever						
	Optimal Therapy			**Alternative Effective Drugs**		
Susceptibility	**Antibiotic**	**Daily Dose (mg/kg)**	**Days**	**Antibiotic**	**Daily Dose (mg/kg)**	**Days**
Fully sensitive	Fluoroquinolone; e.g., ofloxacin (Floxin)[1] or ciprofloxacin (Cipro)	15	5-7*	Chloramphenicol (Chloromycetin) Amoxicillin[1] TMP-SMX (Bactrim)[1]	50-75[3] 75-100[1] 8/40	14-21 14 14
Multidrug resistance	Fluoroquinolone or cefixime (Suprax)[1]	15 15-20[3]	5-7 7-14	Azithromycin (Zithromax)[1] Cefixime	8-10[3] 15-20[3]	7 7-14
Quinolone resistance†	Azithromycin (Rocephin)[1] or ceftriaxone (Rocephin)[1]	8-10[3] 75[3]	7 10-14	Cefixime[1]	20[3]	7-14
Severe Typhoid Fever						
	Optimal Parenteral Drug			**Alternative Effective Parenteral Drug**		
Susceptibility	**Antibiotic**	**Daily Dose (mg/kg)**	**Days**	**Antibiotic**	**Daily Dose (mg/kg)**	**Days**
Fully sensitive	Fluoroquinolone; e.g., ofloxacin[1]	15	10-14	Chloramphenicol Ampicillin[1] TMP-SMX	100[3] 100[3] 8/40	14-21 14 14
Multidrug-resistant	Fluoroquinolone	15	10-14	Ceftriaxone[1] or cefotaxime (Claforan)[1]	60[3] 80[3]	10-14
Quinolone-resistant	Ceftriaxone[1] or cefotaxime[1]	60[3] 80[3]	10-14	Fluoroquinolone	20[3]	14

Abbreviation: TMX-SMX = trimethoprim-sulfamethoxazole.
[1]Not FDA approved for this indication.
[3]Exceeds dosage recommended by the manufacturer.
*Three-day courses are also effective and are particularly so in epidemic containment.
†The optimum treatment for quinolone-resistant typhoid fever has not been determined. Azithromycin, the third-generation cephalosporins, or a 10-14 day course of high-dose fluoroquinolones, is effective.
Source: World Health Organization (WHO)/Vaccines and Biologicals/03.07

should be made to target food handlers and high-risk groups for *S. typhi* carriage screening.

The classic heat-inactivated whole cell vaccine is associated with an unacceptably high rate of side effects. Two newer vaccines that offer protection from school-age children and older people are the Vi polysaccharide vaccine (Typhim Vi) and the orally administrable, attenuated Ty21a vaccine (Vivotif Berna). Both offer a protective efficacy of 70% to 80% for at least 3 to 5 years. In younger children the experimental Vi conjugate vaccine has been shown to have a protective efficacy exceeding 90% and may offer protection in parts of the world where a large proportion of preschool children are at risk for the disease.

RICKETTSIAL AND EHRLICHIAL INFECTIONS

METHOD OF

Daniel J. Sexton, MD

Rocky Mountain Spotted Fever

Rocky Mountain spotted fever (RMSF) is caused by an obligate intracellular bacterium called *Rickettsia rickettsii*. RMSF occurs in western Canada, much of the United States, Mexico, Central America, Brazil, and Columbia. This disease occurs predominately between April and September but in southern areas of the United States or in Mexico or Central America, illness may occur during autumn and occasionally even in mid-winter.

In the eastern United States RMSF is transmitted by *Dermacentor variabilis* (the American dog tick), and in the western United States by *Dermacentor andersoni* (the wood tick) is the principal vector. RMSF may occur after contact with ticks in rural, suburban, and even highly urbanized areas such as New York City. Rarely, transmission may occur from crushing or removing infected ticks from humans or animals. Infection can be experimentally induced with aerosols of infected tick tissues or by mucosal contact. Most tick bites are painless and frequently tick bites are unnoticed or undetected. Thus many patients with RMSF have no knowledge of a tick bite before the onset of their illness.

After inoculation, *R. rickettsii* proliferates intracellularly and then subsequently spreads throughout the body via the bloodstream or lymphatics. *R. rickettsii* has a tropism for endothelial cells that ultimately results in widespread rickettsia-induced vasculitis that may in turn lead to innumerable minute foci of hemorrhage, increased vascular permeability, edema, and the activation of the humoral inflammatory and coagulation mechanisms. Vascular thrombosis and hemorrhage may occur in severe cases, resulting in widespread organ dysfunction often with hypovolemia and shock.

Host factors associated with increased severity of fatal outcome of RMSF include increasing age, male gender, and the presence of glucose-6-phosphate dehydrogenase deficiency. Black race and alcohol use have also been associated with a more severe disease and a higher fatality rate, but it is difficult to exclude the role of delay in seeking or receiving antimicrobial therapy in these patients. Delay in effective therapy has been associated with a significantly worse outcome—particularly if a delay in therapy exceeds 6 days.

The incubation period for RMSF ranges from 2 to 14 days. In the early phases of illness, symptoms are nonspecific. Most adult patients initially complain of headache, myalgias, malaise, and anorexia. Children may have prominent abdominal pain in the early phase of illness. Prominent gastrointestinal symptoms in children and adults with RMSF may lead to erroneous diagnoses such as acute appendicitis, cholecystitis, and even bowel obstruction.

Most patients with RMSF develop a rash between the third and fifth days of illness. However, rash is often absent when patients first contact a physician. In one study, 14% of patients had a rash on the first day of illness and less than one half of all patients developed a rash during the first 3 days of illness. In a small percentage of patients, rash is delayed in onset for more than 5 days, and it may be atypical (e.g., confined to only one body region). Rash never occurs in up to 10% of patients. These cases of "spotless RMSF" may be severe and then fatal.

Most adult patients with RMSF complain of intense headache. Cough, abdominal pain, bleeding, edema (especially in children), confusion, and focal neurologic findings (including seizures) may occur in severe cases. Gangrene of the ears, digits, and scrotum may also develop in severe cases.

Most patients with RMSF have normal white counts at presentation, but the white count in individual patients may be low, normal or elevated; thus it is not diagnostically useful. As illness progresses, most patients develop thrombocytopenia that may be severe. Low platelet counts may be accompanied by reduced fibrinogen concentrations and elevated fibrin split products. However, true disseminated intravascular coagulation is rare. Other laboratory abnormalities in severe cases include hyponatremia and elevated levels of aminotransferases (transaminases), bilirubin, and creatinine. Jaundice and renal failure may occasionally be severe and confuse the clinical presentation.

Misdiagnosis is common. In early phases, RMSF may be mistaken for undifferentiated viral illnesses. If oral antibiotics or other drugs are administered empirically during this phase of illness, subsequent skin rash may be incorrectly diagnosed as a drug eruption. RMSF has been confused with measles, meningococcemia, infectious mononucleosis, hepatitis, leptospirosis, streptococcal infections, and viral meningitis. In addition, the clinical features of RMSF overlap with those of monocytic and granulocytic ehrlichiosis.

There is no completely reliable diagnostic test for RMSF in the early phase of illness when therapy should begin. Thus it is imperative that therapy be based on individual clinical features and the epidemiologic setting. Any patient with suggestive symptoms in an endemic area who presents with a compatible illness in the spring or early summer warrants empirical therapy.

Diagnosis can be confirmed by biopsy of a skin lesion and use of direct immunofluorescent or immunoenzymatic staining methods. The sensitivity of detecting *R. rickettsii* in skin biopsy by direct immunofluorescent staining is approximately 70% with a specificity of 100%. However, sensitivity rapidly declines after antirickettsial therapy is begun. Moreover, such testing is available only in specialized medical centers. *Rickettsia* can be recovered from blood inoculated into tissue cultures or laboratory animals, but these techniques are available only in a small number of research facilities.

The mainstay of diagnosis of RMSF remains serologic testing. Indirect fluorescent antibody (IFA) testing is available through all state health departments and through several large reference laboratories. The minimum diagnostic titer in most laboratories is 1:64. Antibodies typically appear 10 to 12 days after the onset of illness but the optimal time to obtain a convalescent antibody titer is 14 to 21 days after the onset of symptoms.

The preferred treatment for RMSF is doxycycline (Vibramycin), 100 mg intravenously or orally every 12 hours for adults and children who weigh more than 45 kg. The dose for children older than 8 years of age who weigh less than 45 kg and for children less than 8 years of age is 3 mg/kg body weight in two divided doses (maximum dose 200 mg per day). Adjunctive measures such as oxygen therapy, mechanical ventilation, and hemodialysis are useful in severe cases. Although there are no published studies on the optimal duration of therapy for RMSF, doxycycline therapy is usually continued for 5 to 10 days or until the patient has been afebrile for at least 48 hours. Doxycycline is also the treatment of choice for children with RMSF as the risk of dental staining is minimal when short doses of therapy are given. Doxycycline should not be used in pregnant women (who should be treated with chloramphenicol [Chloromycetin] 500 mg intravenously every 6 hours).

Prevention of RMSF is difficult because of the ubiquity of ticks. However, persons exposed to tick-infested habitats should periodically inspect their body and clothes for ticks and remove any crawling or attached ticks. Fingers should be shielded with a cloth, tissue or paper towels, or gloves during tick removal when possible.

Ehrlichiosis

Ehrlichia are obligate intracellular bacteria that grow within membrane-bound vacuoles in human and animal leukocytes. Ehrlichia replicate within phagosomes in the host cell to produce intracellular colonies called morula. These morula are visible by light microscopy and can be stained with gram, Giemsa, Wright, or silver stains. *Ehrlichia* belonged to the family *Rickettsiaceae*. The *Ehrlichia* genus is complex and includes both human and animal pathogens. There are four genogroups of *Ehrlichia* that cause human disease: *Ehrlichia chaffeensis* (the agent of human monocytic ehrlichiosis), *Ehrlichia ewingii*, the *Anaplasma phagocytophila* genogroup (which includes the human granulocytic *Ehrlichia* agent [HGE]), and the *Ehrlichia sennetsu* genogroup.

As yet there is no clear understanding of the mechanism by which *Ehrlichia* produces human disease. Current knowledge about the pathogenic lesions of human monocytic ehrlichiosis is based on a small number of autopsies and bone marrow or liver biopsies. Humans infected with *Ehrlichia* do not show cell or tissue necrosis, abscess formation, or a severe inflammatory response. *Ehrlichia* do not produce vasculitis, thrombosis, or acute or chronic endothelial injury as seen in rickettsial infections. The major cellular target of *E. chaffeensis* is the mononuclear cell and macrophages; the major targets of the HGE agent are granulocytes. Patients with HGE infection may develop secondary opportunistic infections such as cryptococcal pneumonia or invasive aspergillus pneumonia.

Cases of HME have been recognized in the southeastern, south-central, and mid-Atlantic regions of the United States. Since *E. chaffeensis* was first isolated from a soldier at Fort Chaffee, Arkansas, in 1990, a few cases of HME have been recognized in New England and the Pacific Northwest, and isolated cases have recently been reported in Europe, Africa, and Mexico. In some locations, HME is more common than RMSF.

HGE was first described in 1994; since then, cases have been described in Wisconsin, Minnesota, New England, California, Florida, North Carolina, and Western Europe. *E. ewingii* infection was first described in 1999 in patients from Missouri and Oklahoma.

The principal vector of *E. chaffeensis* is the Lone Star tick (*Amblyomma americanum*). HGE is primarily transmitted by *Ixodes scapularis* (the tick that also is the vector of Lyme disease and babesiosis).

Ixodes pacificus, the black-legged tick, is the primary infector of HGE in the western United States. White tail deer are the principal animal reservoirs for *E. chaffeensis* infection; deer and the white-footed mouse are the principal animal hosts for HGE.

Most ehrlichial diseases have an incubation period of 7 to 14 days but shorter incubation periods occasionally occur. Most patients are febrile but self-limiting mild or unapparent infections probably occur. Nonspecific symptoms such as malaise, myalgias, headaches, and chills are present in most cases. Nausea, vomiting, joint pain, and cough may occur in some patients. Rash is uncommon in ehrlichiosis but a faint rash may occur in a small number of patients. When rash is striking, co-infection with another rickettsial or other tick-borne pathogens should be suspected. Neurologic symptoms may occur in patients with ehrlichiosis and include mental status changes, stiff neck, and focal neurologic findings.

The most common laboratory abnormality in patients with HME is leukopenia. Thrombocytopenia and elevated plasma levels of aminotransferases (transaminases), lactate dehydrogenase, and alkaline phosphatase are commonly present. Anemia and an elevated plasma creatinine concentration may also occur. Leukopenia in patients with HGE can be caused by lymphopenia or neutropenia. Lymphopenia tends to occur in early stages of infection followed by lymphocytosis with atypical lymphocytes in the later phases of illness. The initial neutrophil count in patients with HGE is inversely related to the duration of symptoms before treatment is given.

Thrombocytopenia is present in many patients with HGE and HME and is a useful diagnostic clue. Patients with both HME and HGE may develop pleocytosis, and cerebral spinal fluid abnormalities may mimic the changes of viral or aseptic meningitis.

Rarely subacute or chronic infection with *E. chaffeensis* may occur. Such patients may present subacutely with unexplained fever that may last for up to 6 to 8 weeks in untreated cases.

Complications of severe ehrlichiosis include seizures, comas, renal and respiratory failure, and congestive heart failure. Patients with ehrlichiosis who are co-infected with HIV may have an unusually severe course that ends fatally, and patients with HGE may develop fungal superinfections late in the course of illness.

Differential diagnosis of ehrlichiosis is similar to that of RMSF. Both diseases may mimic an array of common viral illnesses such as mononucleosis as well as thrombotic thrombocytopenia purpura, hematologic malignancy, cholangitis, and even community-acquired pneumonia. Diagnosis of ehrlichiosis is based primarily on serologic testing as culture of *Ehrlichia* is extremely difficult even in research laboratories. There are four primary methods to diagnose both HME and HGE: (a) examination of the peripheral blood or buffy coat for the presence of characteristic morulae in lymphocytes or granulocytes; (b) indirect fluorescent antibody testing; (c) polymerase chain reaction testing of bone marrow, spinal fluid, or tissue samples; and (d) the synthesis of the history, clinical and laboratory, and epidemiologic features of an individual case.

All patients who present with a nonspecific febrile illness in the spring or summer months and have a recent history of tick bite or tick exposure should be evaluated for the possibility of ehrlichiosis. Although only a minority of patients with HME have morulae detectable in smears of their blood, a blood film should be examined in all patients with suspected infection. Morulae are more frequently seen in patients with HGE. In some studies more than two thirds of such patients have detectable morulae after careful microscopic examination. Serologic testing for ehrlichiosis is available in most state health departments. The minimum diagnostic IFA titer in most laboratories is 1:64; a fourfold-antibody rise is considered confirmatory of recent infection.

Although there are no controlled trials that examined the efficacy of antimicrobial therapy for ehrlichiosis, tetracycline and chloramphenicol (Chloromycetin) both appear to be effective agents in treatment. Of these, doxycycline (Vibramycin) is preferred. Most patients treated with doxycycline defervesce within 48 hours of initiation of therapy. Doxycycline can be administered either orally or intravenously at a dose of 200 mg per day in two divided doses in adults and children older than 8 years of age. The dose of doxycycline for children older than 8 years of age who weigh less than 45 kg and for children less than 8 years of age is 3 mg/kg body weight in two divided doses (maximum dose 200 mg per day). Therapy should be continued for at least 7 days or from 3 to 5 days after defervescence has occurred. Although all tetracyclines can cause dental staining in children, the risk of such staining after the use of doxycycline is minimal if a short course of therapy is administered. Because chloramphenicol (Chloromycetin) is not readily available in many parts of the United States and because of its risk of hematologic toxicity, doxycycline should be administered to all patients with noted or suspected infection except for women who are pregnant. Patients who are intolerant or allergic to tetracyclines and pregnant women can be treated with rifampin (Rifadin)[1] for 7 to 10 days, but the efficacy of such therapy is currently based on only anecdotal information. The possibility of perinatal transmission in HGE should be considered when HGE occurs in women near delivery.

[1]Not FDA approved for this indication.

SMALLPOX: A TWENTY-FIRST CENTURY VIEW

METHOD OF

Richard J. Whitley, MD

The events of September 11, 2001, along with the subsequent identification of anthrax in the United States Postal System, have generated a new sense of awareness for the potential of biological terrorism, if not warfare. Among the agents identified as "Class A Bioterrorist Threats" by the U.S. Centers for Disease Control and Prevention (CDC), smallpox is one of the most dangerous. The ease of transmission of smallpox, the lack of immunity in the population at large to this agent, and the rapidity of its spread, if released, all have generated significant concern for its deployment. A vaccine directed against smallpox* is available, but it is also associated with significant adverse events, some of which are life-threatening. No antiviral drug has proven efficacious for therapy of human disease, although one licensed drug, cidofovir (Vistide)[1], does have in vitro activity. Heightened awareness should lead to the development of a vaccine without significant adverse events as well as safe and efficacious antiviral drugs. The availability of a vaccine and antiviral drugs that are safe would significantly remove any major threat of smallpox deployment by terrorists.

History

Smallpox is one of the oldest recorded infections of mankind. Likely, this agent, also known as variola, evolved by adaptation to humans from a rodent cowpox-like virus through an intermediate host, such as cattle. The earliest descriptions of smallpox date back to 10,000 BC in Asia and India. The infection's subsequent spread can be traced eastward to Pacific Rim countries and westward to Europe and North Africa. By the seventeenth century, smallpox was introduced into North America from Europe. At its peak, namely when the World Health Organization (WHO) decided to initiate an eradication program, 10 to 15 million cases occurred annually, with an attendant fatality rate estimated to be 20% to 40%.

The WHO program against smallpox became one of the first effective preventive measures for an infectious disease, namely immunization. Interestingly, as early as 1000 AD, dried smallpox scab material was used in China for intranasal inhalation in order to develop protective immunity. In India, the same material was used to generate pustules to cause variolation, resulting in disease protection. Importantly, and surprisingly, the mortality following vaccination by such procedures, even if the material contained live virus, was approximately 2% rather than the customary 30%. Prevention by vaccination, however, was not introduced as a standard procedure until the late eighteenth century when Edward Jenner recognized that milkmaids who acquired cowpox were resistant to smallpox. By the middle-to-late nineteenth century, the use of vaccinia for the prevention of smallpox was routine. By the 1950s most industrialized countries had eliminated endemic smallpox by the use of vaccine prepared on the skin of either cattle or sheep and suspended in bactericidal concentrations of glycerol.

As early as 1958, the possibility of global eradication was suggested. Eradication was accomplished in a few developing countries by 1965, and in 1967 WHO launched its *Intensified Eradication Program*. Using the unique epidemiologic intervention principle of Foege and colleagues known as ring vaccination, cases gradually decreased in West Africa. The success of ring vaccination can be attributed to several factors, including:

- An intense sociologic desire to rid itself of this scourge
- A very long incubation period (12 days) during which a vaccine can induce immune responses
- The lack of an animal reservoir
- Henderson and colleagues facilitated the WHO program leading to global eradication with the last case occurring in Somalia in October of 1977. Routine smallpox vaccination of civilians was discontinued in the United States in 1972.

With the worldwide eradication of smallpox, the WHO launched an effort to destroy the remaining stocks of virus known to exist at the CDC in the United States and in Koltsovo, Russia, at the State Center of Virology and Biotechnology (VECTOR). As the issues concerning smallpox destruction were publicly debated, societies of the western world developed an increasing concern that stocks of smallpox existed in the hands of individuals for its clandestine use in an offensive biowarfare program, particularly in individuals and countries such as Iraq, Korea, Iran, and Libya. Polar positions existed in the United States regarding the destruction of the smallpox samples. Ultimately, following an Institute of Medicine Advisory Committee, a recommendation to maintain the stocks for purposes of antiviral and vaccine development was put forward by then President Clinton and supported by the Department of Defense and the United States Congress. This recommendation receives continued support from the Department of Health and Human Services and the Department of Defense.

Initially, scientists believed that the possibility of the reappearance of smallpox was miniscule; however,

[1]Not FDA approved for this indication.

*Licensed for restricted use and available only from the CDC.

the safety of the population at large changed dramatically after the events of September 11, 2001, with the complete destruction of the World Trade Centers in New York City and the other tragic events of that day. Further, the subsequent deaths related to anthrax in postal workers and community members heightened awareness of the possibility that disease-causing microbes for bioterrorism could be deployed, particularly in developed societies. Because of waning immunity to smallpox, it is one of the most likely for consideration as a microbe of bioterrorism.

Bioterrorist Use

Likely, smallpox was first deployed as a biological weapon during the French and Indian Wars (1754-1767) by British forces in North America. Apparently, blankets contaminated with smallpox virus (obtained from infected patients) were distributed to American Indians. The resulting epidemics led to a mortality of greater than 50% in the effected tribes.

More recently, the potential spread of smallpox, if used as a biological weapon, was illustrated by two European smallpox outbreaks in the 1970s. These outbreaks were not thought to be intentional. The first occurred in Meschede, Germany, in 1970 when aerosol deployment led to a widespread outbreak, even when low doses of smallpox were released.

The second outbreak occurred in Yugoslavia in 1972. In spite of routine immunization, a single case led to a logarithmic increase in the number of person-to-person transmissions. From these two European events, it is anticipated that exposure of a limited number of individuals would result in an expansion factor of ten- to twentyfold. Inactivation of aerosol virus takes place during a period of approximately 48 hours.

Epidemiology

At the beginning of the twentieth century, smallpox existed worldwide; however, its distribution was not uniform—areas of endemicity existed. Two principle forms of the disease exist, variola major and, the much milder form, variola minor (or alastrim). In 1970, 1300 new cases of variola major occurred in 1000 villages in Southwest India and in 1973, an additional 10,000 new cases occurred in India.

Smallpox is a viral disease that is unique to humans; no known animal reservoirs exist. To sustain itself, the virus must be transmitted from person to person. It is caused by variola virus, a large DNA virus that belongs to the *Orthopoxvirus* family. The mechanism of spread is by droplet, aerosol, or direct person-to-person contact. Typically, an infected individual will cough or sneeze, which transmits the virus to the oral mucosa of a susceptible host. Direct contact is also a route of transmission, including contact with contaminated clothing or bed linens. The incubation period is, on average, 12 to 14 days with a range of 7 to 17 days. The disease is characterized by seasonal distribution with spread occurring during the late winter and early spring, a time when chickenpox is prevalent in most communities. However, it can be transmitted in any climate and in any part of the world. As would be expected, transmission within families is increased by overcrowding during rainy periods. On the other hand, transmission between communities increases during dry periods because of the greater mobility of individuals. The transmission of smallpox among populations is slower than those of chickenpox or measles. As noted, spread is primarily to family members and friends who are in close contact, but not among classroom contacts. The reason for this latter observation is that transmission did not occur until the onset of rash. Because disease onset was abrupt with fever and malaise, confinement occurred early in the course of illness.

After the early descriptions of smallpox, the distinction between variola major and variola minor was defined on epidemiologic grounds. In Asia, for example, variola major was associated with a mortality of 30% or higher. In contrast, in South America and sub-Saharan Africa, a similar clinical entity resulted in a mortality of 1% or lower, and was designated variola minor. Importantly, through the end of the nineteenth century, variola major predominated throughout the world. However, at the turn of the century, variola minor was detected at the very southern extremes of Africa and, subsequently, Florida. The distinction between these two strains relates to genetic and growth characteristics of the causative viruses in vitro.

Smallpox was typically a disease of children; nearly 33% of cases occurred in children younger than 5 years of age, and nearly 75% in individuals younger than 14 years of age. However, in rural communities where vaccination and natural infection were less common, disease incidence paralleled the age distribution. Both sexes are equally affected. The incidence of smallpox was higher in lower socioeconomic groups, presumably secondary to overcrowding.

Patients suffering from smallpox are most infectious during the early stages of illness, namely the first 7 to 10 days after the onset of lesions but not before. Transmission occurs most frequently 4 to 6 days after the onset of cutaneous lesions. At that time, the skin lesions are in a papulovesicular stage. However, as scabs form, infectivity wanes rapidly. Patients are considered infectious until all the crusts have separated.

Clinical Manifestations

Issues relevant to clinical variola are summarized in Table 1. Infection is initiated by viral replication on the respiratory mucosa. Primary viremia leads to seeding of the reticuloendothelial system. Secondary viremia results in clinical disease associated with fever, malaise, and myalgia. Virus localizes in small

TABLE 1 Smallpox

Clinical	Flu-like symptoms with 2 to 4 day prodrome of fever and myalgia Rash prominent on face and extremities including palms and soles Pustular lesions become scabs over one to two weeks Rash onset is synchronous
Mode of transmission	Person-to-person
Incubation period	1 day to 8 weeks (average 5 days)
Communicability	Contagious at onset of rash and remains infectious until scabs separate (about 3 weeks)
Infection control practices	Contact and airborne precautions N95 respirator Private room or cohort Discharge when noninfectious
Prevention	Live-virus intradermal vaccine that does not confer lifelong immunity Contact CDC Previously vaccinated person should be considered susceptible
Supply assessment	Number of airborne precautions rooms available Number of N95 respirators available Vaccine availability
Postexposure Prophylaxis	Smallpox vaccine within 3 days of exposure If greater than 3 days, vaccine and vaccinia immunoglobulin (VIG) Instruct exposed individuals to monitor self for flu-like symptoms or rash for 7 to 17 days
Treatment	There is no licensed antiviral for smallpox (cidofovir [Vistide][1] is experimental) Supportive care

[1]Not FDA approved for this indication.
Source: Whitley RJ, Smallpox: A potential agent of bioterrorism, *Antiviral Res* 57:7-12, 2003.

blood vessels of the dermis. The incubation period for smallpox is characteristically 12 days. The first clinical sign of infection is a prodromal illness that lasts 2 to 4 days, characterized by malaise, headache, high fever, vomiting, and delirium. Likely, prodrome coincides with the phase of secondary viremia. As prodrome progresses to the third or fourth day, buccal and pharyngeal lesions begin to appear. Rash begins on the face, spreads to the forearms and hands, and then to the lower limbs and trunk. Lesions are always more numerous on the face than other areas of the body. Lesions begin as macules and quickly evolve to papules and, subsequently, to vesicles by about the fifth day of illness. Pustules appear about the eighth day of illness. The pustules are usually round and tense and deeply embedded in the dermis. Pustules are followed by scabs and, ultimately, scars.

Hemorrhagic smallpox does occur; it is the most serious form of disease and is usually fatal. As would be anticipated, hemorrhages into the skin or mucous membranes characterize this clinical presentation. Secondary bacterial infection is not common. Death usually occurs during the second week and is attributed to immune complex mediated shock.

The illness associated with variola minor is less severe with few constitutional symptoms and a less pronounced rash.

The disease most commonly confused with smallpox is chickenpox. During the first 2 to 3 days of rash, it may be difficult to distinguish these two entities. Chickenpox is characterized by the development of a rash that involves lesions in all stages of development—maculopapules, vesicles, pustules, and scabs. Nevertheless, smallpox lesions do not demonstrate all stages of evolution simultaneously. The lesions of chickenpox tend to involve the extremities to a greater extent than the trunk.

Diagnosis

The identification of a single suspected case of smallpox should be treated as an international health emergency and brought immediately to the attention of national officials through local and state health departments. As discussed above, the clinical findings resemble those encountered with chickenpox. Laboratory confirmation of the diagnosis in a smallpox outbreak is important. Specimens should only be collected by someone who has been recently vaccinated. Vesicular/pustular fluid should be harvested and transmitted immediately to state or local health department laboratories for confirmation. Laboratory examination requires high containment (BL-4) facilities and should only be undertaken by experienced personnel. Typical approaches to the identification of the agent include electronmicroscopy, polymerase chain reaction, and isolation in cell culture. Differentiation from chickenpox can be accomplished by staining of scraped skin lesions with monoclonal antibodies directed against varicella zoster virus. A potentially confusing diagnosis, and one that occurs with global travel, is that of monkeypox, which would be identified in typical diagnostic assays. From 1970 to 1986, there were 400 cases of monkeypox worldwide with recent outbreaks in sub-Saharan Africa. This disease closely resembles chickenpox but has a 5% to 10% mortality. Monkeypox is indistinguishable from smallpox with the exception of the enlargement of cervical and inguinal lymph nodes. Also, monkeypox resolves more promptly.

Vaccination

In the United States, vaccination against smallpox was discontinued in 1972. Thus, a significant portion of the American population is susceptible to smallpox. Persistence of detectable antibodies as detected by enzyme-linked immunoabsorbent assay (ELISA), particularly for older individuals, is approximately 5 to 10 years. However, persistence of neutralizing antibody has been documented in a few individuals for longer than 10 years after vaccination. Regardless, the following can be concluded. First, immunity is not lifelong. Second, some persistence of immunity has been documented in a limited number of individuals. In studies performed in Scandinavia, individuals exposed to smallpox but immunized as children had a lower mortality upon exposure to variola major than those not vaccinated. The implications of these findings are unclear.

Vaccination consists of the administration of vaccinia virus grown on scarified scabs of calves. Vaccine production for smallpox is, likely, the crudest of all vaccines available. After purification, virus is freeze-dried in rubber-stopped vials that contain enough vaccine for at least 50 doses. Vaccine is administered with a bifurcated needle. Vaccine should be stored at –20°C (–4°F). Currently, there are approximately 90 to 100 million doses of vaccine* available for administration in the United States.

Vaccination is not without complications. First, and most importantly, no immunocompromised host should be vaccinated, as illustrated by an immunocompromised military recruit who was inadvertently vaccinated. Second, the rate of postvaccine encephalitis is approximately 2.3 to 2.9 cases per one million vaccinations with an associated 25% mortality. In addition, vaccinia gangrenosum occurs in approximately 2.6 cases per one million vaccinations and is associated with a high mortality. Generalized vaccinia is usually not fatal but occurs in as many as 290 individuals per one million vaccinations. Vaccine complications are summarized in Table 2.

*Available only from the CDC.

Postexposure Prophylaxis and Treatment

Postexposure vaccine prophylaxis is the ideal method for disease prevention. However, given the vaccines currently available, it is not without both contraindications (immunocompromised hosts) and complications (encephalitis, etc.). However, adequate protective immune responses appear induced in the normal host within four days. For individuals in whom the vaccine is contraindicated, there is a limited supply of vaccinia immunoglobulin (VIG)* that is available through the CDC.

At the present time, no antiviral drug has been shown to be effective in the prevention or treatment of smallpox. However, cidofovir (Vistide)[1], a licensed phosphonate analog, has in vitro activity against monkeypox, vaccinia, and variola, and is active against other pox viruses as well. While this drug is active in vitro, cidofovir does have significant nephrotoxicity. In addition, lipid products of cidofovir that are orally bioavailable are being investigated. Cidofovir administration should be by physicians experienced with its use. In the opinion of this author, cidofovir is a logical current choice of treatment. With the availability of vaccinia immunoglobulin, smallpox would at least be ameliorated if an outbreak occurred.

*Investigative drug in the United States.
[1]Not FDA approved for this indication.

TABLE 2 Complications of Smallpox Vaccination in the United States for 1968

		Number of Cases						
Vaccination Status	Estimated No. of Vaccinations	Postvaccinial Encephalitis*	Progressive Vaccinia*	Eczema Vaccinia*	Generalized Vaccinia	Accidental Infection	Other	Total
Primary vaccination†	5,594,000	16 (4)	5 (2)	58	131	142	66	418
Revaccination	8,574,000	0	6 (2)	8	10	7	9	40
Contacts	. . .‡	0	0	60 (1)	2	44	8	114
Total	14,168,000	16 (4)	11 (4)	126 (1)	143	193	83	572

*Data in parentheses indicate number of deaths attributable to vaccination.
†Data include 31 patients with unknown vaccination status.
‡Ellipses indicate contacts were not vaccinated.
Source: Henderson, DA, Inglesby, TV, Gartlett, JG, Ascher, MS, Eitzen, E, Jahrling, PB, Hauer, J, Layton, M, McDade, J, Osterholm, MT, O'Toole, T, Parker, G, Perl, T, Russell, PK, Tonat, K, and the Working Group on Civilian Biodefense 1999. Smallpox as a biological weapon, *JAMA* 281:2127-2137.

Development of New Vaccines

The original smallpox eradication campaigns used vaccines that were derived from many vaccinia virus strains, including the New York calf lymph virus, a New York City chorioallantoic membrane strain; EM-63 (USSR); and Temple of Heaven (China). By the late 1960s, more than 70 manufacturers used 15 principal strains of vaccinia virus for the development of vaccines. The Lister, or Elestree, strain, derived from sheep in the United Kingdom, became the most prevalently used throughout the world. Historically, most of these vaccines were produced in live animals. More recently, the use of primary cell substrates, particularly embryonated chicken egg-produced smallpox vaccine, avoids some of the potential problems associated with vaccine production in animals. These problems include harvesting, contamination, adventitious agents, allogenicity, and accompanying animal proteins. In addition, the Food and Drug Administration (FDA) has licensed live-virus vaccines that are produced in diploid cell substrates (e.g., MRC-5, WI-38). The MRC-5 cell line was used for the preparation of a vaccine evaluated in a phase I clinical trial. Likely, the FDA will consider acceptable the production of live smallpox vaccines produced in these diploid cell substrates.

Alternatively, the continuous Vero cell line has been used to prepare inactivated virus vaccines, particularly the inactivated polio vaccine. While the FDA has not yet licensed this substrate for live virus production, international experience suggests that it may be a suitable substrate for a smallpox vaccine. The selection of cell substrates of vaccine production in Vero cells has recently been addressed in an FDA letter (http://www.fda.gov/cber/letters.htm).

Strains selected for vaccine production warrant note. The LC16m8, an attenuated vaccinia virus strain, was developed in Japan for primary vaccination in 1975. It was derived by passing the Lister strain 36 times through primary rabbit kidney cells at low temperature. Initial studies indicated lower reactive genicity with acceptable immunogenicity. Of note, there was lower neurovirulence in a monkey assay. The most highly attenuated vaccinia strain is the Ankara. It has been passaged more than 570 times in chicken embryo fibroblasts. This virus is host restricted, being unable to replicate in human and other mammalian cells. Thus, for all intents and purposes it behaves like an inactivated virus, making it acceptable in high-risk individuals. It has been safely used in more than 100,000 persons in Turkey and Germany; however, its effectiveness in the prevention of smallpox is unknown.

Each of these constructs, as well as genetically engineered viruses, are being considered for use in humans. Of note, the recent availability of vaccinia pools at the Adventis Laboratory in Swiftwater, Pennsylvania, removes some of the intense pressure for the immediate development of new constructs.

Management of a Smallpox Outbreak

As soon as a diagnosis of smallpox is entertained, suspected infected individuals should be isolated and all household contacts vaccinated, if vaccine is available. Because of the potential of aerosol transmission, if feasible, patients should be managed in the home environment to prevent person-to-person spread. Vaccination administered within the first few days after exposure (up to 4 days) may prevent or significantly ameliorate subsequent illness. Currently, the more effective method of vaccine deployment to prevent the appearance of new cases, namely ring vaccination versus universal, is under discussion.

Because of aerosol transmission, smallpox transmission within the hospital environment has been recognized as a problem for some time. As a consequence, many health care providers have established two facilities for the delivery of health-related services during epidemics of smallpox with standby hospitals that deal only with patients having smallpox.

The potential use of smallpox has ominous implications, particularly given its rapidity of spread among susceptible individuals. As we have learned from the deployment of anthrax in North America during the fall of 2001 and early 2002, aerosol release of a potentially life-threatening agent is both feasible and devastating. Recognizing that improved vaccines take time to develop and there currently is no antiviral therapy for smallpox, research efforts to develop treatments and improve vaccines should be and is a high priority to the United Stated research establishment. As reported in *Emerging Infectious Diseases* in July, 2002, all of the vaccines and treatments discussed in this article are actively being investigated by a team of researchers from the CDC.

SECTION 3

Diseases of the Head and Neck

VISION CORRECTION PROCEDURES

METHOD OF

Kraig S. Bower, MD

Refractive errors are the most frequent eye problems in the United States. Nearly one half of the U.S. population requires vision correction of some kind at a cost of more than $15 billion annually. Since the Food and Drug Administration (FDA) approved the first excimer laser for refractive surgery in 1995, laser eye surgery has been performed on more than 6 million people worldwide. Almost 2 million more are expected to undergo treatment in the coming year. This article describes the different refractive problems and various surgeries used to treat them.

Corneal Anatomy

The cornea is 550 ± 50 μm thick and has five distinct layers. The outermost layer is stratified squamous epithelium, approximately five cell layers thick, coated by a thin tear film. It provides a smooth optical surface and barrier against infection. Beneath the epithelium, Bowman's membrane serves as a barrier and for structural purposes. The stroma, which accounts for 90% of the corneal thickness, is made up of uniform and regularly spaced collagen fibrils. The endothelium and its basement membrane (Descemet's membrane) form the innermost layers. Endothelial cells remove fluid from the cornea via an active sodium-potassium–adenosine-triphosphatase (ATPase) pump. Corneal dehydration, lack of vascularity, and regular collagen arrangement provide corneal transparency.

Optics, Refraction, and Vision

Refraction refers to the way the eye focuses light, the source of vision. Three elements determine the eye's ability to focus—the shape of the cornea, the power of the lens, and the length of the eyeball. The cornea is responsible for two thirds of the total focusing power. The lens, which lies behind the pupil, accounts for one third and can change its shape to adjust focusing power.

In an eye with normal vision, the power of the cornea and lens perfectly matches the length of the eye. Light rays from a distant object are focused precisely on a light-sensitive membrane called the retina, and a clear image is perceived. Objects viewed up close require additional focusing power by the lens in a process known as accommodation.

Refractive Error

Refractive errors occur when light entering the eye does not focus on the retina. They are normal differences in visual ability rather than true diseases. The three basic types of refractive errors are myopia, hyperopia, and astigmatism.

In myopia, the cornea and lens are too powerful for the length of the globe. Distant objects cannot be seen clearly because light rays are focused in front of the retina. However, because the myopic eye has a focal point close to the eye, near objects can be seen clearly without corrective lenses—hence the term *nearsighted*.

In hyperopia, the cornea and lens are too weak or the eyeball is too short. Light rays reach the retina before they are focused to a single point, resulting in a blurry image. Accommodation may bring a distant object into focus but may be inadequate for near vision—hence the term *farsighted*.

Astigmatism often occurs with either myopia or hyperopia. It is an irregular curvature of the cornea in which the refractive power of the eye varies in different meridians. Light rays cannot be brought to a single point and objects are blurry at any distance.

Another refractive problem, presbyopia, occurs as the aging lens loses its ability to accommodate. This change occurs in everybody, usually around age 45 years, resulting in eyestrain with prolonged nearwork. Myopes frequently notice that it is easier to remove their glasses to read. Hyperopes who rely on accommodation have increasing difficulty focusing. Once presbyopia develops, additional focusing power is necessary in the form of reading glasses or bifocals.

Corrective lenses alter the path of light rays entering the eye. Myopia is treated with concave lenses with minus (divergent) power. Hyperopia requires convex lenses with plus (convergent) power. Astigmatism is corrected with cylindrical lenses. Glasses have been used for centuries and are simple, relatively inexpensive, and safe. Contact lenses are an option for those who find glasses unacceptable. Problems with contacts, such as intolerance, infection, inconvenience, and cost, limit their use in some people.

Refractive Surgery

Refractive surgery is a modern alternative to glasses or contact lenses. Procedures are generally permanent and irreversible. They are performed in otherwise healthy eyes and do not treat reduced vision from cataract, glaucoma, macular degeneration, and other disorders that may require other medical or surgical treatments. Myopia, hyperopia, and astigmatism are the refractive problems most commonly treated with surgery. Table 1 lists the indications and contraindications for refractive surgery.

TABLE 1 Eligibility Criteria for Refractive Surgery

Indications
Age 18 years or older
Myopia ≤14.00 D
Astigmatism ≤4.00 D
Hyperopia ≤+6.00 D
Stable refraction at least 1 year*
Reasonable expectations
Medical Contraindications
Uncontrolled vascular disease
Autoimmune disease
Immune suppressed/immune compromised
Pregnant or nursing
Keloid formation†
Diabetes†
Isotretinoin (Accutane), sumatriptan (Imitrex), or amiodarone
Ocular Contraindications
Keratoconus
Herpetic keratitis
Progressive myopia
Cataract
Corneal disease‡
Glaucoma‡
Amblyopia‡

*No more than a 0.5 D change in the 12 months preceding surgery.
†Relative contraindications. Well-controlled diabetes mellitus is not an absolute contraindication to surgery, but fluctuating refractions caused by uncontrolled blood sugar levels, diabetic cataract, or diabetic retinopathy may recommend against refractive surgery.
‡Other eye problems including previous infections, scarring, surgery, trauma, glaucoma, dry eye, or blepharitis must be carefully evaluated to determine whether they pose an increased risk or will significantly alter the results of refractive surgery.
Abbreviation: D = diopter.

All patients require a complete eye examination by a provider experienced in refractive surgery. Evaluation includes refraction, slit-lamp examination, intraocular pressure testing, and a dilated examination to rule out cataracts or retinal abnormality. Computerized videokeratography and wavefront aberrometry, measurements of corneal curvature, shape and thickness, and the pupil size are also needed for a successful visual outcome. Patients must review information about the surgery and discuss risks, benefits, alternatives, expected outcomes, and potential complications with their surgeon before deciding to have surgery. Based on the patient's expectations and examination findings, the surgeon and patient must select the correct surgical procedure to maximize results while minimizing risks.

Excimer Laser Procedures

Lasers have been used in medicine and surgery for decades. One of the most important advances in refractive surgery is the excimer laser. In 1995, the FDA approved the first excimer laser to treat mild and moderate myopia. Since then, additional lasers have been approved for an expanded therapeutic range (Table 2).

The excimer laser combines argon (Ar) and fluoride (F) gases to generate a beam of ultraviolet light with a 193-nm wavelength. This has sufficient energy to break molecular bonds within corneal collagen in a process called ablative photodecomposition, or *photoablation*. The laser removes microscopic amounts of corneal tissue with little risk of thermal damage to surrounding tissues. A computer programmed with the patient's prescription controls the laser beam to reshape the cornea with great precision. In myopia, the laser flattens the central cornea to decrease its focusing power. In hyperopia, the laser indirectly steepens the central cornea by flattening the periphery. Astigmatism is treated with an elliptical or cylindrical beam to flatten the steepest corneal meridian.

PHOTOREFRACTIVE KERATECTOMY (PRK)

Excimer laser PRK is approved for myopia and hyperopia (see Table 2). The desired correction is

TABLE 2 FDA-Approved Lasers for Refractive Surgery in the United States

Company and Model	Procedure	Indication	Range (D = Diopters)
Alcon - LADARVision	LASIK*	Myopia	Less than –9.0 D with or without astigmatism from –0.5 to –3.0 D
Alcon (Autonomous) - LADARVision	LASIK	Hyperopia	Less than +6.0 D with or without astigmatism less than –6.0 D
Alcon (Autonomous) - LADARVision	PRK†	Myopia	From –1.0 to –10.0 D with or without astigmatism less than –4.00 D
Alcon (Autonomous) - LADARVision	PRK	Hyperopia	Less than +6.0 D with or without astigmatism less than –6.0 D
Alcon (Autonomous) - LADARVision	WFG‡ LASIK	Myopia	Up to –7.0 D with or without astigmatism less than 0.5 D
Bausch & Lomb Surgical - Technolas 217A	LASIK	Myopia	Less than –11.0 D with or without astigmatism less than –3.0 D
Bausch & Lomb Surgical - Technolas 217A	LASIK	Hyperopia	Between +1.0 and +4.0 D with or without astigmatism up to 2.0 D
Bausch & Lomb Surgical - Technolas 217A	PRK	Myopia	From –1.0 to –10.0 D with or without astigmatism less than –4.5 D
LaserSight - LaserScan LSX	LASIK	Myopia	From –0.5 to –6.0 D with or without astigmatism up to 4.5 D
LaserSight - LaserScan LSX	PRK	Myopia	From –1.0 to –6.0 D with or without astigmatism less than 1.0 D
Nidek - EC5000	LASIK	Myopia	From –1.0 to –14.0 D with or without astigmatism less than 4.0 D
Nidek - EC5000	PRK	Myopia	From –1.0 to –10.0 D with or without astigmatism from –0.5 D to –4.0 D
Refractec - ViewPoint CK System	CK§	Hyperopia	From +0.75 to +3.25 D with or without astigmatism up to 0.75 D
Summit - Apex Plus	LASIK	Myopia	Less than –14.0 D with or without astigmatism from 0.5 to 5.00 D
Summit - Apex Plus	PRK	Myopia	From –1.0 to –7.0 D with or without astigmatism from –1.0 to –4.0 D
Summit - Apex Plus	PRK	Hyperopia	From +1.5 to +4.0 D with or without astigmatism less than –1.0 D
Sunrise - Hyperion	LTK¶	Hyperopia	From + 0.75 to +2.5 D with or without astigmatism less than 0.75 D
VISX - Star S2 & S3	LASIK	Myopia	Less than –14.0 D with or without astigmatism between –0.5 and –5.0 D
VISX - Star S2 & S3	LASIK	Hyperopia	Between +0.5 and +5.0 D with or without astigmatism up to –3.0 D
VISX - Star S2 & S3	LASIK	Mixed astigmatism	Up to 6.0 D; cylinder > than sphere and of opposite sign
VISX - Star S2 & S3	PRK	Myopia	From 0 to –12.0 D with or without astigmatism from 0 to –4.0 D
VISX - Star S2 & S3	PRK	Hyperopia	From +0.5 to +6.0 D with or without astigmatism +0.5 to +4.0 D
VISX - S4 & WaveScan	WFG LASIK	Myopia	Up to –6.0 D with or without astigmatism up to –3.0 D

*Laser in situ keratomileusis.
†Photorefractive keratectomy.
‡Wavefront guided.
§Conductive keratoplasty.
¶Laser thermal keratoplasty.
Abbreviations: CK = conductive keratoplasty; LASIK= laser-assisted in-situ keratomileusis; PRK = photorefractive keratectomy; WFG = wavefront-guided (surgery).

programmed into the laser's computer, and the patient is given topical anesthetic drops (0.5% proparacaine [Alcaine]). The eyelids are swabbed with 1% povidone iodine solution and draped with adhesive plastic drapes. A speculum gently retracts the eyelids. The corneal epithelium is removed using a soft-bristled rotary brush, the laser, or an instrument that resembles a spatula. The patient views a fixation target while the surgeon aligns the laser and delivers the laser treatment. Immediately after treatment the cornea is irrigated with chilled saline and a contact lens is placed to protect the cornea. After surgery, the patient uses topical nonsteroidal anti-inflammatory drugs (NSAIDs) for 48 hours, antibiotic drops for 1 week, steroid drops for 1 month, and oral analgesics as needed.

For the first few days, patients experience blurred vision and moderate discomfort as the corneal surface heals. The contact lens is removed after the epithelium has healed, usually in 3 to 5 days. Mild blurriness is common for several weeks as the cornea heals. Once the healing process is complete, 96% of treated eyes are 20/40 or better—sufficient to drive legally without corrective lenses. Two thirds have unaided vision of 20/20 or better. Potential problems include over- or undercorrection, astigmatism, scarring, glare, and corneal haze (Table 3). The latter is more common after treating higher degrees of myopia.

LASER-ASSISTED IN-SITU KERATOMILEUSIS (LASIK)

LASIK is an effective treatment for myopia and hyperopia (see Table 2). After topical anesthesia and lid preparation similar to PRK, the surgeon uses an instrument called a microkeratome to create a hinged corneal flap 8.5 to 9.5 mm in diameter with a thickness of 130 to 180 µm (160 µm average). The flap is folded back to expose the underlying tissue to the laser. After ablation the surgeon returns the flap to its original position and irrigates under the flap with saline solution. The flap seals without the need for sutures. Topical antibiotic, NSAID, and steroid drops are applied, and the eyelid speculum and drapes are carefully removed. The flap is inspected by slit-lamp examination to confirm good position and stability before the patient leaves the office.

Visual results are comparable with PRK. Advantages of LASIK include quicker postoperative visual recovery with less discomfort and lower risk of corneal haze. A disadvantage is the potential for corneal flap complications (see Table 3). Although such complications

TABLE 3 Complications of Refractive Surgery

Excimer Laser Procedures	Nonexcimer Corneal Procedures	Intraocular Procedures
Possible with All	**Laser Thermal Keratoplasty**	**Phakic Intraocular Lenses**
Overcorrection	Overcorrection/undercorrection	Angle supported
Undercorrection	Astigmatism	Endophthalmitis
Astigmatism	Regression	Uveitis
Central island	Infection	Glaucoma
Decentration	Corneal scarring	Cystoid macular edema
Regression	Corneal edema	Decentration
Infection	**Conductive Keratoplasty**	Pupillary changes
Dry eye	Overcorrection/undercorrection	Corneal decompensation
Glare/halos	Astigmatism	Iris supported
More Likely with PRK	Regression	Endophthalmitis
Delayed epithelial healing	Infection	Uveitis
Corneal haze	Corneal abrasion	Dislocation
Scarring	Corneal scarring	Iris atrophy
Recurrent erosion	Corneal edema	Corneal decompensation
Steroid–induced glaucoma	**Intacs**	Cystoid macular edema
More Likely with LASIK	Intolerance/foreign-body sensation	Glare and edge effects
Intraoperative flap complications	Infection	Posterior chamber
Ocular penetration	Overcorrection/undercorrection	Endophthalmitis
Recurrent erosion	Astigmatism	Pupillary block
Traumatic flap dislocation	Glare/halos	Anterior subcapsular cataract
Epithelial ingrowth	Abnormal wound healing	Pigment dispersion
Interface debris	**Radial Keratotomy**	Iris atrophy
Flap striae	Wound leak, ocular penetration	Open-angle glaucoma
Diffuse lamellar keratitis	Infection	Edge effect and glare
More Likely with LASEK	Overcorrection/undercorrection	**Clear Lens Extraction**
Same as PRK	Astigmatism	Endophthalmitis
Sloughed flap	Glare and starburst effects	Glaucoma
	Fluctuating vision	Corneal decompensation
	Ocular rupture with blunt trauma	Retinal detachment
	Progressive hyperopia	

may result in the loss of vision, they are, fortunately, rare (<0.1% of surgeries).

LASER EPITHELIAL KERATOMILEUSIS (LASEK)

LASEK is a modification of the PRK technique that may address the shortcomings of LASIK and PRK. In LASEK, a 20% alcohol solution is applied for 25 to 35 seconds to separate the epithelium from Bowman's membrane. The loosened epithelium is retained as an intact flap that is returned to position after the laser ablation is complete. The early postoperative course is similar to PRK. LASEK may result in less corneal haze than PRK, and offers an alternative for patients with high myopia who are unable or unwilling to undergo LASIK. This typically includes patients with thin corneas and patients at increased risk of flap trauma, such as athletes in contact sports and military personnel.

WAVEFRONT-GUIDED SURGERY

Since the 1800s, doctors have described optical imperfections (aberrations) in terms of myopia, hyperopia, and astigmatism, and have used simple letter charts to measure and express vision (e.g., 20/20, 20/40, etc.). Using modern diagnostic tools that allow analysis of the visual system in more detail, we now know that simple refractive errors are not the only optical aberrations. Higher-order aberrations may be associated with night vision difficulties or reduced contrast sensitivity despite eye chart vision of 20/20 or better.

An exciting advance in ophthalmology is wavefront technology. Astronomers use wavefront technology to identify atmospheric distortions (aberrations) of incoming light and to correct these aberrations to produce clear images of distant stars and other celestial bodies beyond earth's atmosphere. In the same way, a wavefront capture device, called an aberrometer, analyzes light rays reflected from the retina to identify all aberrations, lower *and* higher order, of the eye. These aberrations are then displayed as a three-dimensional wavefront map.

Wavefront-guided (WFG) surgery makes it possible to address higher-order aberrations while treating lower-order refractive errors with the excimer laser. In clinical trials for myopia without astigmatism, WFG LASIK reduced higher-order aberrations, improved contrast sensitivity, and resulted in a quality of vision superior to conventional LASIK. Two wavefront-guided laser systems have FDA approval for LASIK (see Table 2) and others are currently under investigation. Additional clinical trials will determine the effectiveness of WFG PRK, WFG treatment for hyperopia, and customized treatment of eyes with special visual disorders.

Intraocular Procedures

Excimer laser procedures have limits in treating high myopia and high hyperopia, which require removal of significantly more corneal tissue to achieve the desired treatment effect. Although the FDA approved a therapeutic range of –14.00 to +6.00 D (diopters), in most cases the realistic limits of laser keratectomy are –10.00 D of myopia to +5.00 D of hyperopia. One must look beyond the cornea to treat refractive errors outside of this range.

CLEAR LENS EXTRACTION

The success of modern cataract surgery has resulted in interest in lens extraction as a means of treating refractive error. Predictability and stability of results are the chief advantages. There is a significant risk of retinal detachment after intraocular surgery in the highly myopic eye, and this procedure is not generally recommended. Results of clear lens extraction for high hyperopia have been promising, with significant improvement in unaided vision and few complications. Current formulas for calculating intraocular lens (IOL) power allow most patients to achieve a postoperative refraction within 1.00 D of the refractive goal. A drawback to refractive clear lens extraction in younger patients is the loss of accommodation that comes with removal of the crystalline lens.

PHAKIC INTRAOCULAR LENS

Phakic IOLs are implanted in the eye without removing the patient's natural lens. They may prove to be a powerful surgical option for individuals with refractive errors not amenable to laser treatment. Unlike clear lens extraction, the patient keeps the natural lens allowing accommodation.

There are three lens types based on their location in the eye—angle supported (in front of the iris), iris supported, and posterior chamber. Most phakic IOLs provide good short-term results, but long-term safety data are lacking. All are intraocular procedures with a higher risk profile than the excimer laser. Most significant is the risk of postoperative endophthalmitis. Additional complications are listed in Table 3.

Surgery for Hyperopia

The excimer laser is approved for hyperopia up to +6.00 D with up to 4.00 D of astigmatism (see Table 2). The technique is the same as for myopic PRK and LASIK, but a larger ablation is required and, therefore, a larger epithelial defect or flap, respectively, is possible. Surgery is safe and effective, although results are generally not as good as those seen with myopic treatments. Higher levels of hyperopia are better addressed with clear lens extraction.

Thermal keratoplasty offers an alternative to the excimer laser for hyperopia. A series of thermal spots tightens the peripheral cornea, which, in turn, leads to central corneal steepening. Treatment occurs outside of the visual axis with risk of no flap complications or compromise of the structural integrity of the cornea. The FDA has approved two systems for the treatment of low-to-moderate hyperopia (see Table 2).

LASER THERMAL KERATOPLASTY (LTK)

The Hyperion LTK system uses a holmium:YAG (yttrium-aluminum-garnet) laser as a heat source to treat low hyperopia without astigmatism. After topical anesthetic drops, an eyelid speculum is placed and the cornea carefully dried. The patient is positioned at the laser console and instructed to view a fixation light during the treatment, which takes less than 5 seconds. Following surgery, the patient is treated with topical NSAID for 48 hours, topical antibiotic drops for a week, and oral analgesics as needed. The most common complication is hyperopic regression. This can be retreated with LTK, CK, or the excimer laser.

CONDUCTIVE KERATOPLASTY (CK)

CK uses a radiofrequency probe that is inserted into the peripheral corneal stroma. Resistance to current along the probe results in localized heat and collagen shrinkage. The Refractec ViewPoint CK System is approved for the treatment of mild-to-moderate hyperopia. The eye is anesthetized with 0.5% proparacaine (Alcaine) drops, and the cornea is marked for the treatment. The treatment pattern, determined by the patient's preoperative refraction, takes 8 to 32 spots. Additional spots can be placed to steepen the flattest meridian in astigmatic eyes. The treatment takes about 5 minutes to perform. Postoperative topical antibiotics, topical NSAIDs, and oral analgesics are given. Results are promising, with 51% of eyes demonstrating uncorrected visual acuity (UCVA) 20/20 or better and 91% 20/40 or better at 12 months postoperatively. Importantly, there is less hyperopic regression than with LTK.

Surgery for Presbyopia

" . . . in this world nothing can be said to be certain, except death and taxes."

Benjamin Franklin (Letter to Jean-Baptiste Leroy, November 13, 1789)

Franklin, the inventor of bifocal glasses, no doubt suffered from another certainty in this world, presbyopia. Dependence on reading glasses remains a potential source of dissatisfaction in older patients following otherwise successful refractive surgery. A *cure* for presbyopia is a highly sought-after goal.

One approach is monovision, which intentionally creates mild myopia in one eye to achieve reading vision. This was traditionally done with contact lenses and can be the target correction with the laser as well, but not all patients tolerate monovision.

Another approach is to increase accommodation through surgery to the sclera. Scleral expansion surgeries are under continued investigation, but at the present time do not offer a safe, reproducible, effective, and stable alternative.

Multifocal lenses mimic accommodation by allowing for both distance and near vision at the same time. They tend to compromise the quality of both, and continue to have limited acceptance. Accommodating IOLs are designed to increase their optical power by shifting position as the patient attempts to accommodate. They have a promising future, but are not presently approved or readily available in the United States.

Other Procedures

INTRASTROMAL CORNEAL RINGS (INTACS)

Intacs are clear plastic rings threaded into the outer part of the cornea to alter its shape. Potential advantages include avoidance of the visual axis and reversibility by removing the rings. FDA clinical trials demonstrated efficacy equal to PRK and LASIK after 12 months; however, long-term results and safety are unknown. Intacs have not gained widespread acceptance by patients or surgeons as an alternative to excimer laser surgery. Currently, Intacs are primarily being used for the "off-label" treatment of keratoconus.

INCISIONAL SURGERY

Radial keratotomy (RK) uses radial or spoke-like corneal incisions to alter corneal curvature. Although more than 1 million Americans have had this procedure since the late 1970s, RK has significant limitations (see Table 3) and has been abandoned since the advent of the excimer laser. Astigmatic keratotomy (AK) and limbal relaxing incisions (LRI) use transverse or arcuate incisions in the peripheral cornea to flatten the steep corneal meridian. Indications

TABLE 4 Evaluating the Results of Refractive Surgery

Term	Definition/Measurement
Predictability	Ability to achieve target of emmetropia (±0.50 or 1.00 D)
Efficacy	Percentage that meet UCVA goal (≥20/20, 20/25 or 20/40)
Stability	Long-term maintenance of the surgical effect over time
Safety	Preservation of preoperative BSCVA Side effects and complications
Patient satisfaction	Patient expectations and how well the outcome matches those expectations

Abbreviations: BSCVA = best spectacle-corrected visual acuity; UCVA = uncorrected visual acuity.

include isolated astigmatism, often in association with cataract surgery or following corneal surgery.

The excimer laser has revolutionized ophthalmology and is the procedure of choice for most patients desiring refractive surgery. Current and emerging procedures must be evaluated in terms of predictability, efficacy, stability, and safety (Table 4) before they find their place in the refractive surgery armamentarium.

CONJUNCTIVITIS

METHOD OF

John A. Burns, MD

Conjunctivitis is inflammation of the conjunctiva from multiple causes including allergic, atopic, bacterial, viral, fungal, and secondary agents.

Anatomy

Conjunctiva is a transparent mucous membrane covering the posterior surface of the eyelids (palpebral conjunctiva) and the sclera (bulbar conjunctiva) up to the limbus of the cornea. It is composed of superficial epithelium, basement epithelial cells, superficial stroma, and a deep fibrous layer. Blood vessels course through the stromal layer. Goblet cells are also present and produce the mucous component of the tear film. Two different types of accessory lacrimal glands are also located within the stroma of the conjunctiva and produce part of the aqueous tear film.

Red Eye

Conjunctivitis is one of a number of pathologic conditions that will produce a red eye. It is imperative, when establishing a diagnosis of conjunctivitis, that the other pathologic alternatives are ruled out. In general, conjunctivitis will not produce significant change in vision, is not associated with pain, is associated with a diffuse injection of both the bulbar and palpebral conjunctiva, is frequently more intensive in the cul-de-sac, and is not associated with abnormal pupillary movements. The type of discharge will vary greatly, depending upon the etiology of the conjunctivitis. Prior to establishing the diagnosis of conjunctivitis, one should rule out the other potential causes of a red eye (Table 1).

History

The signs and symptoms identified via history will vary greatly, depending upon the etiology of the conjunctivitis being diagnosed. Such history, however, should include the age and sex of the patient, a history of present illnesses, an ocular history, medical history, and social history. The history for conjunctivitis should elicit the signs and symptoms associated with the specific disease being studiod including:

- If the patient has itching, discharge, irritation, pain, photophobia, or blurred vision.
- The duration of symptoms.
- Whether the condition started unilaterally or bilaterally and whether it has remained so.
- Character of any discharge present.
- Whether the patient has been exposed to other individuals with infectious diseases and/or conjunctivitis.
- Whether there is a history of trauma, which could be mechanical, chemical, toxic agents, or unusual light exposure (i.e., ultraviolet light, welding torches, flash burns, or high altitude travel).
- Whether the patient is a contact lens wearer and, if so, the type of lens (rigid versus soft).
- A careful history of past allergies and present exposure to topical and systemic medications as well as personal care products.

Physical Examination

A physical examination should include recording the visual acuity in each eye separately, optimally with glasses correction. An external examination should also be carried out using bright illumination and, if available, a slit lamp. The external examination should include an evaluation of the skin to confirm that it is either normal or has been changed by the disease process, evaluation of regional lymphadenopathy with specific attention being paid to the preauricular area. Evaluation of the eyelids should be specific including discoloration, malposition, and swelling. The lid margins should be evaluated for inflammation, ulceration, nodules, vesicles, or keratinization. The lashes should be inspected to rule out nits, lice, and/or crust. The tarsal plates and conjunctiva should be inspected for the presence of papilla (small elevations of the palpebral conjunctiva that contain the central tufts of blood vessels), follicles (tiny, glistening, translucent elevations on the palpebral conjunctival surface), cicatricial changes causing shortening of the cul-de-sac. Membranes and pseudomembranes may also be present, as well as hemorrhages and/or foreign material. The bulbar conjunctiva should specifically be inspected for ciliary flush, chemosis (blister-like edema of the conjunctiva), ulceration,

TABLE 1 Potential Causes of Red Eye

	Visual Acuity	Pain	Site of Injection	Discharge	Pupillary Status
Conjunctivitis	Usually associated with no or minimal reduction	None or subtle foreign body sensation	Diffuse injection of the bulbar and palpebral conjunctiva	Variable, watery, mucoid, mucopurulent	Normal
Scleritis	Unaffected or minimal decrease	Mild	Segmental	Watery	Usually unaffected
Iritis	Mild-to-moderate reduction in vision	Moderate to severe, associated with photophobia	Ciliary flush	Watery	Mild-to-moderate myosis
Keratitis	Mild-to-severe reduction in vision	May be associated with photophobia	Segmental ciliary flush	Watery and/or mucoid	Normal
Glaucoma	Mild-to-marked reduction in vision	Moderate-to-severe pain, usually located in eyebrow; may be associated with nausea and vomiting	Ciliary, but also diffuse on the bulbar conjunctiva	Watery	Mild dilation to fixed and dilated pupil

phlyctenules (wedge-shaped nodular lesions usually located at the corneal edge and associated with increased segmental injection). The cornea should be inspected for epithelial erosions, abrasions, dendritic lesions, filaments, and true ulceration. To facilitate evaluation of the bulbar and palpebral conjunctiva and cornea, fluorescein should be placed on the surface of the eye. The status of the pupil should be carefully noted.

Bacterial Conjunctivitis

In the adult, the most common causes of bacterial conjunctivitis are *Streptococcus pneumoniae, Staphylococcus aureus*, and *Haemophilus influenzae*. Common characteristics of each include unilateral development, although bilateral spread is possible; an onset over 1 to 2 days; mucopurulent discharge; and a diffuse injection with the greatest injection frequently in the cul-de-sac.

Most forms will respond rapidly to empirical treatment with topical antibiotics. Common preparations used are bacitracin-polymyxin-B (Polysporin) and/or erythromycin drops or ointment. Cultures are usually not indicated because most patients respond rapidly to appropriate topical therapy. Most authorities prefer to reserve topical immunoglycosides and fluoroquinolones for nonresponsive cases.

Ophthalmia neonatorum, or conjunctivitis in the newborn, is an acute form of conjunctivitis usually caused by *Neisseria gonorrhoeae* or *Neisseria meningitidis*. This form of conjunctivitis can occur as rapidly as 12 hours after birth and may rapidly lead to conjunctival and/or corneal scarring. Because of the potential severe complications associated with ophthalmia neonatorum, all children in the United States are prophylactically treated to prevent occurrence of this infection. For many years, standard treatment was a drop of topical 1% silver nitrate placed in each eye, however, this is no longer available. Children should now be treated with an application of 3.5 g neomycin ointment (Neosporin) and/or tobramycin 0.3%[1,2]. If ophthalmia neonatorum is suspected, immediate conjunctival scraping and culture should be carried out and topical, as well as systemic, therapy is indicated. Infants should be treated with ceftriaxone, (Rocephin)[1] 25 to 50 mg/kg IV or IM single dose, not to exceed 125 mg. Children weighing less than 45 kg should be treated with ceftriaxone[1], 125 mg IM as a single dose. Referral to an ophthalmologist is recommended.

Viral Conjunctivitis

Most viral conjunctivitis is caused by adenovirus serotypes 8, 11, and 19. Serotypes 3, 4, and 7 are sometimes responsible for pharyngoconjunctival fever. Viral conjunctivitis is usually acute in onset, associated with follicles, begins unilaterally, and is frequently associated with unilateral preauricular adenopathy. At least 50% of cases will become bilateral. Discharge is usually watery, and the patient may have associated mild photophobia and/or foreign body sensation.

Adenoviral keratoconjunctivitis and conjunctivitis are highly contagious, so the patient must be carefully warned to avoid contact with partners and siblings during the first 4 to 7 days. Children should be kept home from school until minimally symptomatic.

Specific treatment is not available. Symptomatic treatment can be used including cold compresses and artificial tears to provide symptomatic relief. Topical antihistamines may be useful if patients have significant itching. The use of topical steroids is generally discouraged because some authorities are suspicious that its use can lead to chronicity of the infection. Conversely, if conjunctival scarring or membrane

[1]Not FDA approved for this indication.

[2]Not available in the United States.

formation is noted, then steroids are indicated to decrease this cicatricial reaction.

Herpes simplex virus may produce keratoconjunctivitis with associated vesicles of the periocular skin or lid margin. The conjunctivitis is usually follicular and may be associated with palpable preauricular nodes. Herpes simplex conjunctivitis should be aggressively treated to prevent corneal infections and/or complications. Topical trifluridine (Viroptic) 1%, 8 times a day; vidarabine (Vira-A) 3% ointment, 5 times a day; and oral acyclovir (Zovirax)[1] 5 times daily should be continued until the conjunctivitis resolves. Oral valacyclovir (Valtrex) and famciclovir (Famvir)[1] are alternative oral treatments. Topical steroids should not be used because of the increased probability of corneal infection or worsening if infection is already present.

Chlamydial Conjunctivitis

Neonates, children, and adults all are susceptible to this form of conjunctivitis. In the infant, eyelid edema, bulbar conjunctival injection, and a purulent discharge are characteristic. It usually occurs 5 to 19 days following birth. Fifty percent of infants who have conjunctivitis have multiple sites of infection including the nasopharynx, genital tract, and/or lungs; this requires systemic therapy. In the adult, the presentation is usually bilateral conjunctival injection and a follicular reaction on the tarsal plate as well as on the bulbar conjunctiva. All age groups should be treated with oral medications. Children who weigh less than 45 kg should be treated with erythromycin suspension, 30 to 50 mg/kg per day orally in four divided doses for 2 weeks. Children who weigh more than 45 kg and adults should be treated with azithromycin (Zithromax)[1], 1 g orally in a single dose. It is imperative that sexual partners be evaluated to prevent reinfection.

Molluscum contagiosum is caused by pox virus. Infections frequently occur on the eyelids and appear as smooth umbilicated, dome-shaped skin nodules. If a lesion is adjacent to the eye, viral particles will contaminate the tears resulting in palpebral and conjunctival injection. The associated conjunctivitis cannot be successfully treated with topical medications. Each individual cutaneous lesion must be eradicated by curettage, cryotherapy, or excision. Conjunctivitis will then spontaneously regress.

Seasonal Allergic Conjunctivitis

Seasonal allergic conjunctivitis is caused by environmental allergens. As the name implies, it occurs at specific times of the year and is associated with moderate conjunctival injection, a watery discharge, and itching (its hallmark symptom). It is always bilateral. Cases may be mild, moderate, or severe. If mild, observation, artificial tears, cold compresses, and avoiding increased histamine release caused by eyelid rubbing are appropriate treatments. For more severe cases, topical vasoconstrictors, antihistamines, mast cell stabilizers, and nonsteroidal anti-inflammatory topical agents are used. Only in the most severe cases, which are nonresponsive to the aforementioned treatments, should topical steroids be used; but *only* after a dilated fundus examination—to evaluate the patient's lens and optic nerve—and a glaucoma test are performed. Desensitization by an allergist is frequently not indicated unless the patient has significant systemic symptoms in addition to those associated with this seasonal allergic conjunctivitis.

Giant Follicular Conjunctivitis

Giant follicular conjunctivitis is directly associated with the wear of contact lenses, most frequently the soft type. It becomes more common with long-term wear. The conjunctivitis is limited to the conjunctiva overlying the upper lid tarsal plate and the tissue just above it. Very large follicles, clearly visible to the naked eye, occur across the tarsal plate. The greatest incidence is usually seen at the upper edge. The cause is felt to be an autoimmune reaction to the proteins precipitated in the lens and/or an abrasive effect on the contact lens from the underside of the lid, and/or an allergic reaction to the chemicals used to clean the contact lenses. The condition does not respond to medical therapy without discontinuation of the contact lenses. It usually responds to discontinuation of the lenses, mast cell stabilizing agents, and, frequently, refitting with a different composition lens. The diagnosis is derived from information that the patient is a contact lens wearer and examination of the lid, which is everted to observe the changes on the tarsal plate.

Medicine-Induced Conjunctivitis

Numerous ophthalmic medications have the potential to cause allergic conjunctivitis as well as the preservatives used to make the multidose containers safe for long-term use. The most common medications causing allergic conjunctivitis are neomycin, topical sulfonamides, and all topical glaucoma medications. The risk of allergic response is obviously increased with long-term use associated with chronic ocular conditions. The condition may be unilateral or bilateral, but will be present only in the eye or eyes where medication is instilled. Varying degrees of conjunctival injection, tarsoconjunctival follicles, and itching may be present. The condition does become progressively worse if the causative medication is not discontinued. The hallmark of the condition is an associated contact dermatitis of the eyelids associated with erythema and a dry, thick eyelid skin.

[1]Not FDA approved for this indication.

Treatment should begin with discontinuation of the offending medication and, if the symptoms are acute, topical ophthalmic steroids as well as topical steroid creams applied to the lid surface, both of which should be of short duration. If there is recurrence after an alternate medication is prescribed, it is usually an indication that the preservative is the offending agent.

There are numerous other causes of conjunctivitis that cannot be covered in this article, but if it is suspected, require additional literature review. They include conjunctivitis secondary to floppy lid syndrome, ocular cicatricial pemphigoid, vernal trachoma, Stevens-Johnson syndrome, and *Acanthamoeba* keratoconjunctivitis.

Consultation

Most forms of conjunctivitis are correctly diagnosed and respond to appropriate medical therapy. However, there are exceptions. If a patient is experiencing visual loss, moderate or severe pain, significant recurrent episodes, or lack of appropriate response to therapy, then immediate consultation with an ophthalmologist is indicated.

Definitions

Ciliary flush: Marked injection at the junction of the cornea at the limbus (the junction of the cornea and sclera) with little or no injection in the cul-de-sac or palpebral conjunctiva.

Glaucoma: Glaucoma associated with a red eye; usually indicates a sudden marked elevation of pressure and a palpable change in firmness of the globe should be identifiable by digital compression of the globe.

Photophobia: Pain caused by direct light stimulation of the eye.

Segmental injection: Injection usually limited to a single quadrant of the bulbar conjunctiva.

OPTIC NEURITIS

METHOD OF

Mark S. Gans, MD

Optic neuritis refers to inflammation of the optic nerve. It is the most frequent acute optic neuropathy involving patients from the age of approximately 20 to 50 years old. Although an underlying source of this inflammation may be present in some individuals, the most common etiology of this diagnosis is idiopathic or demyelinating disease.

Clinical Features of Demyelinating Optic Neuritis

Patients usually present with monocular visual loss and a distinct periorbital pain, which is precipitated by eye movement. The visual dysfunction can progress over the course of 1 to 10 days and invariably involves central vision as well as the peripheral visual field. The extent of visual acuity loss ranges from no light perception to 20/25. In addition, approximately 33% of patients note *positive* visual phenomena such as intermittent patterns of lights.

The diagnosis of optic neuritis is based on the above symptoms and the presence of signs of optic nerve dysfunction in the involved eye. These signs include:

- A relative afferent pupillary defect, which may be quantified with neutral density filters
- A subjective loss of light brightness or perception of red desaturation
- A diminution of color vision, which may be measured with Ishihara color plates or more precisely with Hardy-Rand-Rittler pseudochromatic plates
- A visual field defect

The visual field defects vary significantly from patient to patient with respect to both the extent and pattern of loss. The pattern of the initial visual field defect may be central, cecocentral, altitudinal, arcuate, and, rarely, hemianopic.

Funduscopy performed upon the acute optic neuritis patient reveals a normal optic nerve 66% of the time. Optic neuritis in the presence of a normal-appearing optic nerve is termed retrobulbar optic neuritis. In the remainder of the patients the optic nerve will appear edematous, and this entity is termed papillitis. Although the extent of the edema ranges from mild to massive swelling of the optic nerve it does not relate to the level of visual loss.

As with other optic neuropathies, repeat funduscopy 4 to 6 weeks following the onset of visual loss will reveal pallor of the involved optic nerve regardless of its presenting appearance.

Clinical Course

Regardless of the presenting visual acuity loss, patients usually notice some improvement in their vision approximately 2 to 3 weeks from the onset of optic neuritis. Although the bulk of visual recovery occurs within the first 1 to 2 months, the final status of the patient's visual function may take up to 1 year to stabilize. Less than 10% of patients remain with a visual acuity of less than 20/40. In contrast to the bulk of optic neuritis patients, individuals whose initial visual acuity was light perception or no light perception recover to 20/40 or better less than 66% of the time. There does not appear to be any other factors that affect the final visual outcome of these patients.

Despite this excellent visual acuity prognosis, patients may notice the relatively poor quality of the involved eye's visual function as compared with the uninvolved eye. The vision may appear to be less distinct, colors less rich, and lights not as bright. In addition, during exercise or other activities that raise body temperature, patients may recognize a transient drop in the visual function of the involved eye. This is termed the Uhthoff syndrome.

The Optic Neuritis Treatment Trial (ONTT)

The Optic Neuritis Treatment Trial (ONTT) was a multicenter, controlled study of 455 patients with typical acute unilateral optic neuritis funded by the National Institute of Health (NIH) to determine the role of corticosteroids in the treatment of this disorder. From the evidence in this study it is clear that the use of oral prednisone alone will result in an increased rate of recurrent optic neuritis over the next 5 years. Although treatment with intravenous methylprednisolone (250 mg every 6 hours for 3 days) followed by oral prednisone (1 mg/kg/day for 11 days) was demonstrated to hasten the recovery of visual function in the short term, it did not have an effect on the ultimate level of visual recovery in patients treated in this manner.

In addition to directing us in the therapy of these patients, the ONTT revealed valuable information regarding the correlation between brain magnetic resonance imaging (MRI) and the prognosis for developing multiple sclerosis in these patients. It was demonstrated that patients with normal MRIs, one or two typical lesions on MRI, or more than two typical lesions on MRI had a 16%, 37%, or 51%, respectively, cumulative risk of developing multiple sclerosis over 5 years. At 10 years of follow-up the ONTT group determined that a single MRI demyelinating lesion on presentation put the optic neuritis patient at a 56% risk of developing multiple sclerosis. Treatment with corticosteroids did not alter this prognosis.

Controlled High-Risk Avonex Multiple Sclerosis Study (CHAMPS)

Following the ONTT, treatment modalities other than corticosteroids were studied to determine their effect on the prognosis with respect to multiple sclerosis in these patients. One of the earlier studies was termed the CHAMPS study. This study was designed to determine whether interferon β-1a (Avonex) therapy would help patients with a first acute demyelinating event and MRI signal abnormalities typically associated with multiple sclerosis. The study randomized 383 patients into Avonex-treated and placebo-treated groups. At 18 months, treatment with Avonex was associated with a significant reduction of new demyelinating MRI lesions, and at 3 years a 44% drop in the cumulative risk of developing clinically definite multiple sclerosis was demonstrated in this group. Since this study, other similar therapeutic compounds have been introduced to this population with similar results.

GLAUCOMA

METHOD OF

Ronald L. Gross, MD, and Peter T. Chang, MD

Glaucoma is a leading cause of irreversible blindness in the United States and the world. In the United States alone, an estimated 120,000 people are blind from glaucoma. It is the leading cause of irreversible blindness among African Americans, and it numbers among the two most common causes overall. More than 2.2 million Americans age 40 years and older, or approximately 2% of the population, have glaucoma; it is estimated that an equal number remain undiagnosed.

Glaucoma refers to a group of conditions characterized by typical loss of visual field because of optic nerve degeneration and damage. Elevated intraocular pressure is the most important risk factor. The progressive damage to the optic nerve can be slowed or halted by an adequate reduction in intraocular pressure. In most cases, the elevated pressure is caused by reduced outflow of aqueous humor. Aqueous humor is produced by the ciliary body in the posterior chamber and normally passes through the pupil into the anterior chamber of the eye, exiting through the trabecular meshwork and Schlemm canal into the episcleral venous circulation. An obstruction to outflow increases aqueous humor volume, raising the intraocular pressure, damaging retinal ganglion cells and their axons in the optic nerve. This results in the typical findings of an increased size of the optic cup, often with a localized area of thinning of the neural rim tissue. Visual field testing evaluates the function of the optic nerve and exhibits characteristic abnormalities in glaucoma. Although intraocular pressure plays an important role in glaucoma, the site of damage is the optic nerve. Its appearance and function are the key factors in the diagnosis and the treatment of glaucoma. Other local or systemic factors that affect the optic nerve, such as vasospasm and systemic hypotension, may exacerbate the condition.

Increasing age is also a major risk factor for glaucoma, which affects 8% of the population older than age 70 years, and nearly 15% of the population older than age 80 years. Glaucoma is 5 to 15 times more likely to occur in African Americans than in whites; glaucoma also has an earlier onset and more aggressive course in African Americans. Immediate family members of affected patients have a 10- to 15-fold higher risk of developing glaucoma than the general population. Patients with myopia, diabetes, and systemic hypertension are also more likely to be affected.

Glaucoma Suspects

Patients with elevated intraocular pressure without the characteristic optic nerve appearance or visual field abnormality are glaucoma suspects with ocular hypertension. Only 10% to 20% of these patients will eventually develop glaucoma, but they are at increased risk compared with the general population. Older individuals, those with large optic cups, vasospastic conditions, and thin corneas also appear to be at greater risk. A recent clinical trial showed that a 20% reduction in the intraocular pressure decreases the cumulative probability of developing glaucoma from 9.5% to 4.4% at 60 months into the study.

Primary Open-Angle Glaucoma

The most common form of glaucoma, affecting nearly 66% of patients, is primary open-angle glaucoma (POAG). The disease is bilateral but may be asymmetrical. It is caused by increased resistance to aqueous humor outflow through the trabecular meshwork that results in a mild-to-moderate elevation of intraocular pressure. It is a chronic disease, and because intraocular pressures are not markedly elevated, it is often asymptomatic. There is no pain or redness in the eye. The visual field loss tends to be peripheral and slowly progressive, so the patient may have no visual complaint until the disease process is very advanced. When the central vision is affected, the disease is far more progressed and more difficult to control.

POAG is insidious; therefore, early diagnosis and treatment are crucial in preventing visual loss. Patients older than 35 years should be evaluated with a complete eye examination every 2 to 3 years. Older adults, African Americans, individuals with a family history of glaucoma, and persons with other ocular or systemic problems (e.g., ocular trauma, myopia, diabetes, systemic hypertension) are at an increased risk and should be evaluated more frequently.

Glaucoma screening consists of four components:

1. Medical and family history
2. Vision testing
3. Examination of the optic nerve
4. Measurement of intraocular pressure

Medical history that increases the likelihood of glaucoma includes the presence of diabetes, systemic hypertension, and vasospastic diseases such as migraines or Raynaud's phenomenon. Systemic hypotension, migraines, and cardiac arrhythmias are associated with increased risk of progressive glaucoma damage. As stated earlier, family history is relevant. Confrontation visual field testing is a poor predictor of glaucoma. By the time an abnormality is typically detected, the disease is far advanced. Formal visual field testing is much more sensitive, but is often cumbersome for screening.

Examination of the optic nerve is greatly enhanced by pupillary dilatation. The optic nerve is composed of retinal ganglion cell axons. The surface of a normal optic nerve is normally flat or slightly elevated with a small, central, pale, and depressed physiologic cup. This cup is surrounded by neural rim tissue that is normally orange-red. The appearance of the normal optic nerve and its cup varies among individuals. It is important to document the appearance of the optic nerve so that any change can be recognized. Early glaucomatous damage to the nerve fibers often occurs at the inferior and superior poles of the optic disk and results in a vertical elongation of the optic cup, with narrowing of the neural rim and pallor of the optic nerve. Glaucoma should be suspected:

- If the optic cup represents greater than one third of the surface of the disk, extends to the rim of the disk, or is larger vertically than horizontally.
- If there is asymmetry between the optic disks of the patient's eyes.
- If a flame-shaped hemorrhage is present in the nerve fiber layer near the border of the optic disk.
- If there is a definite change in the appearance of the optic disk from that of a previous evaluation.

Intraocular pressure measurement is also important in the evaluation of glaucoma. Applanation tonometry (AT) is the best way to measure intraocular pressure. This method requires topical anesthesia but is painless and accurate. A pressure above 21 mm Hg is suggestive of glaucoma and warrants further evaluation. Intraocular pressure normally fluctuates in everyone, but to a greater degree in patients with glaucoma. Therefore, patients with glaucomatous damage may not have elevated pressures at a given time of measurement. Conversely, patients with elevated intraocular pressures do not necessarily have glaucomatous damage. Therefore intraocular pressure measurement alone is neither sensitive nor specific for glaucoma.

TREATMENT

The only proven treatment of glaucoma is reducing intraocular pressure. Medical therapy is often instituted initially, using the minimal concentration, frequency, and number of medications to control the disease while minimizing side effects. These topically administered drugs may, however, cause systemic effects.

Medications

β-Blockers

β-Blockers decrease intraocular pressure by reducing the production of aqueous humor. The potential side effects of ocular drops are the same as for the systemic use of these agents and include exacerbation of reactive airway disease, bradycardia, systemic hypotension, decreased libido, and altered mentation. Patients who are already taking oral β-blockers may experience additive side effects while having less benefit from intraocular pressure lowering. These agents are contraindicated in patients with heart block or heart failure, asthma, or obstructive lung disease.

Sympathomimetic Agents

Sympathomimetic drugs, such as epinephrine (Epifrin) and dipivefrin (Propine), increase aqueous humor outflow. Their potential side effects include systemic hypertension, headache, cardiac palpitation, and arrhythmias. Alpha-adrenergic agonists, such as apraclonidine (Iopidine) and brimonidine (Alphagan), also decrease aqueous humor production. Systemic effects may include dry mouth and somnolence. The most common problem, however, is development of a local allergic response.

Parasympathomimetic Agents

Miotics such as pilocarpine (Pilocar) improve aqueous humor outflow through the trabecular meshwork. These agents often have ocular side effects caused by ciliary body spasm and pupillary miosis. Systemic cholinergic effects are rare. Cholinesterase inhibitors, such as echothiophate (Phospholine Iodide), are topical agents but can inhibit systemic cholinesterase. Patients taking these drugs should not receive agents such as succinylcholine (Anectine) during general anesthesia.

Carbonic Anhydrase Inhibitors

Carbonic anhydrase inhibitors reduce intraocular pressure by decreasing aqueous humor production. For long-term use, the topically applied form is preferred because of improved safety profile. Topical agents include dorzolamide (Trusopt) and brinzolamide (Azopt). The long-term use of oral carbonic anhydrase inhibitors is controversial, as they can cause urinary frequency, anorexia, nausea, depression, malaise, peripheral neuropathy, kidney stones, and, rarely, blood dyscrasias. Oral acetazolamide (Diamox) and methazolamide (Neptazane) may lower serum potassium concentration and should be used with caution in patients taking non–potassium-sparing diuretics or digoxin. Carbonic anhydrase inhibitors are sulfonamides and are consequently contraindicated in patients allergic or sensitive to these medications.

Prostaglandin Analogues

The newest class of antiglaucoma agents that increase aqueous humor outflow, prostaglandins, appear to have few, if any, systemic effects and have become the mainstay of glaucoma treatment. This class includes latanoprost (Xalatan), travoprost (Travatan), bimatoprost (Lumigan), and unoprostone (Rescula). They require only once daily dosing, except for unoprostone (twice daily). Iris hyperpigmentation caused by an increase in the production of melanin occurs in some patients and is irreversible. Eyelash changes (increased thickness, length, and number) are common. Darkening of periocular skin may also occur but appears to be reversible. These agents should be used with caution in patients predisposed to ocular inflammation.

Topical Application and Treatment Duration

To reduce the systemic absorption of ophthalmic drops, nasolacrimal duct compression or simple eyelid closure should be performed for 3 to 5 minutes after instillation of each drop.

Treatment is gradually advanced until intraocular pressure has been substantially reduced in comparison with the level at which damage occurred. Approximately 50% of patients require more than one medication to achieve this target pressure range. The patient is then followed closely with evaluation of the intraocular pressure, optic nerve, and visual field to be sure that no further damage occurs. Patients should understand that the medications only treat not cure glaucoma. The decision as to the most appropriate therapy for each patient is individualized based on severity of disease, medical status, and the patient's needs. Compliance with therapy remains a concern. Cessation of treatment leads to an immediate increase in the intraocular pressure to the previous untreated level.

Other Modalities

If medical therapy is unsuccessful in adequately lowering intraocular pressure, surgical methods are considered. Laser trabeculoplasty can be used to treat the trabecular meshwork to increase aqueous humor outflow. Initial treatment is successful in approximately 80% of patients with POAG, with 50% of the 80% showing a treatment effect for up to 5 years. Other conventional surgical procedures, such as trabeculectomy and aqueous shunt, are designed to provide alternative aqueous humor outflow; ciliodestructive procedures reduce production of aqueous humor.

Primary Angle-Closure Glaucoma

Primary angle-closure glaucoma (PACG) is a true ocular emergency. In contrast to POAG, the onset is acute with severe symptoms. Patients at risk are those with narrow iridocorneal angles, almost always in an eye that is hyperopic, resulting in close apposition of the lens-iris diaphragm and the cornea. When an attack occurs, flow of the aqueous humor through the pupil is completely stopped. Aqueous humor continues to be secreted by the ciliary body, creating an escalating pressure gradient between the posterior and anterior chambers of the eye. This forces the peripheral iris anteriorly, blocking the trabecular meshwork and preventing outflow. Within a very short time, the intraocular pressure can rise to a dangerously high level.

The acute attack may be precipitated by physical or emotional stress or by dilatation of the pupil in response to dim lighting or the use of eye drops. The predisposition to angle closure is uncommon (1% of the population), and the majority of patients at risk never have an attack. Physicians should not hesitate to dilate a pupil to facilitate an examination of the posterior segment of the eye. Antihistamines and other medications with autonomic effects may dilate the pupil slightly, which could precipitate an attack in a predisposed patient. When such agents are used in their recommended dosage, however, this effect is rare.

Unlike patients with POAG, a patient with PACG exhibits severe symptoms, including ocular pain and redness, blurred vision, rainbow-colored halos around lights, headaches, and, frequently, nausea and vomiting. Usually only one eye is affected. On examination, the eye is red, the pupil is mid-dilated, the cornea is cloudy, and the eye is quite firm on tactile tension.

TREATMENT

If an acute attack of PACG is suspected, the patient should be immediately referred to an ophthalmologist; in the meantime or if an immediate referral is not possible, treatment should be instituted. It should include a topical β-blocker, 1 drop every 30 minutes; pilocarpine (Pilocar) 2%, 1 drop every 15 minutes for 1 hour; and also acetazolamide (Diamox) tablets (250 mg × 2), if not contraindicated. Osmotic diuretics, such as glycerin orally or mannitol (Osmitrol) intravenously, 1 to 1.5 g/kg, can be given if necessary.

Medical therapy is usually effective in lowering intraocular pressure and breaking the attack. Laser peripheral iridotomy may be performed to make an opening in the iris, which allows the flow of aqueous humor and prevents future attacks. Sequelae of the attack may lead to a chronic glaucoma and require long-term treatment. The contralateral eye should be evaluated for the risk of acute attack and receive prophylactic iridotomy, if indicated.

Primary Developmental Glaucoma

Primary developmental glaucoma is a rare condition in which glaucoma is caused by an abnormal development of the anterior segment, including the outflow channels. In 75% of the affected patients, the condition is bilateral. Patients with developmental glaucoma usually present within the first year of life, initially with excessive tearing. In addition, the infant with developmental glaucoma may have enlarged eyes as a result of the increased intraocular pressure in eyes that are immature and relatively elastic. Photophobia, or light sensitivity, is a common symptom, as is frequent blinking or blepharospasm. The treatment of developmental glaucoma is primarily surgical. Developmental glaucoma must also be considered among the differential diagnosis of a cloudy cornea at birth.

Secondary Glaucoma

One of the most common forms of secondary glaucoma, that is the group of glaucomas in which a specific etiology can be identified, is steroid-induced glaucoma. It occurs when corticosteroid eye drops or, less commonly, systemic or inhaled corticosteroids are used, usually for several weeks. In 15% of normal patients and 95% of patients with POAG, intraocular pressure may increase by 15 mm Hg after treatment with long-term topical corticosteroids. Once this effect is identified, discontinuation of the steroid with treatment of the intraocular pressure will usually alleviate the problem. However, it may take weeks to months for the normalization of intraocular pressure. Any concentration or type of corticosteroid may cause the pressure rise. Other ocular complications can result from steroid use, including cataract formation and exacerbation of herpetic infections. Therefore, great care should be exercised when prescribing these drops.

Secondary glaucoma may also be caused by ocular trauma, retinal vascular occlusion, ocular inflammation, intraocular tumor, diabetes, cardiovascular disease, and advanced cases of cataract. Any patient suspected of having a secondary glaucoma should be referred to an ophthalmologist for a prompt evaluation.

OTITIS EXTERNA

METHOD OF

Charles P. Kimmelman, MD, MBA

Otitis externa, or external otitis, is an inflammatory condition of the external auditory canal (EAC) and is among the most common of human afflictions. The EAC is a cul-de-sac ending medially at the tympanic membrane, creating a warm, moist tubular volume conducive to the growth of microbes. Continuous exfoliation of skin provides a nourishing matrix for sustaining these organisms. Under the proper conditions, they proliferate and lead to the most common form of otitis externa.

Because this is such a frequent ailment, clinicians have a tendency to assume that all external ear inflammations are the same. Nothing could be further from the truth, and, in fact, some external canal processes can be life-threatening. It behooves the astute clinician to understand the various causes and treatments of external otitis and to recognize when referral to an otologist is necessary.

Anatomy and Physiology of the External Ear

The EAC functions as a resonator to amplify incoming sound and to protect the deeper and fragile structures of the middle ear. It is anatomically divided into a lateral cartilaginous and a medial bony region. The skin of the cartilaginous canal is thicker and replete with adnexa (hair follicles, sebaceous glands, and apocrine sweat glands). The continuous exfoliation of stratified squamous epithelium would lead to obstruction of the canal from the first month of life were it not for the lateral migration of canal skin from medial to lateral, automatically *cleaning* the canal. Cerumen, or ear wax, is produced by the admixture of skin, sebum, and apocrine secretion and is of variable consistency, which is determined by heredity, hormonal milieu, moisture, and drugs. Because of the self-cleansing capability of the ear canal, instrumentation by the patient is rarely necessary; hence, cotton applicators should not be used because they traumatize the delicate skin. Furthermore, excessive removal of wax is unwarranted. Ear wax is not dirt; on the contrary, it is beneficial and protects and defends the fragile skin from drying, infection, and trauma.

The medial bony canal possesses extremely thin skin without adnexa. The canal is usually coiled, so that its entire circumference is often not visible. At the end of the canal is the tympanic membrane, whose lateral surface squamous epithelium is contiguous with that of the canal. Inflammation of the canal skin thus readily extends onto the lateral surface of the drum head.

The EAC is extremely well innervated by branches of the cervical plexus, vagus nerve, facial nerve, mandibular division of the trigeminal nerve, and glossopharyngeal nerve. Thus, even mild stimulation of the skin of the bony canal is painful. Manipulation of the canal can stimulate a vagal reflex leading to cough and, rarely, bradycardia with syncope (Arnold's reflex). Acoustic tumors within the internal auditory canal may compress sensory fibers running with the facial nerve, leading to anesthesia of a small portion of the EAC (Hitselberger's sign). EAC inflammation can also disturb auditory function. It is obvious that ear canal disorders, from cerumen impaction to neoplasms, readily gain the attention of the sufferer.

Pathology of the External Auditory Canal

External otitis is, by definition, an inflammation of the skin of the external auditory canal. It usually begins in the cartilaginous region and initially involves the hair follicles and sebaceous glands (pilosebaceous unit). The resulting cellulitis may spread rapidly to adjacent areas, with edema, fluid transudation, and squamous desquamation leading to canal obstruction. Bacterial or fungal organisms thrive in this environment and add to the obstruction and inflammation. If unchecked, the inflammation may progress to abscess formation, chondronecrosis, cellulitis of the surrounding skin, and even osteomyelitis of the temporal bone in special instances.

Neoplasms of the skin of the canal (squamous cell carcinoma and, occasionally, basal cell carcinoma), its glandular tissue (adenoid cystic carcinoma), the bone (osteoma, exostosis) all can simulate or secondarily cause external otitis. Contact dermatitis from toiletries and otic drops, skin disorders (eczema, psoriasis), hypertrichosis of the canal, and trauma from misguided attempts at cleaning are common causes of canal inflammation.

Etiology of External Otitis

INFECTION

Under certain conditions, such as excessive moisture, excessive removal of cerumen, canal trauma from scratching or instrumentation, the defense of the canal is reduced to the point that the resident flora invades the pilosebaceous unit. The most common organisms, in order of frequency, are *Pseudomonas aeruginosa*, *Staphylococcus epidermidis*, and *Staphylococcus aureus*. Fungi, such as *Aspergillus* and *Candida* species, usually accompany the bacteria and may dominate at the start of the infection, or assume it once bacteria are eliminated.

More rarely, viruses (herpes zoster oticus, herpes simplex) infect the ear canal and may be misinterpreted as bacterial processes. In their early stages the viruses cause canal pain, swelling, and erythema. The characteristic bullae develop after several days. Mycobacteria can also cause inflammation of the external canal and temporal bone.

Immunodeficiencies may allow *garden variety* external otitis to assume the monumental proportions of so-called *malignant external otitis*, more appropriately termed *necrotizing external otitis*. Inability to control the infection permits the invasion of EAC organisms into soft tissues, characteristically resulting in granulation tissue on the floor at the bony cartilaginous junction. CT scans demonstrate the extent of involvement from soft tissue thickening of the external canal, middle ear, and mastoid system to bone destruction of the external canal extending deeper into the temporal bone and skull base. There may be abscess formation. Both gallium and bone scans will reveal the extent of destructive inflammation, but the gallium scan is more useful for monitoring response to treatment. The predominant organism is *Pseudomonas*, which, if unchecked, invades bone and spreads along vascular and fascial planes leading to osteomyelitis of the skull base. Inflammation of the cranial nerve foramina results in facial paralysis, hoarseness, trapezius weakness, and throat pain. Extension through the fissures of the cartilaginous canal (fissures of Santorini) can lead to facial and temporomandibular joint involvement. Without treatment, the process inexorably extends intracranially causing death. Most patients are elderly diabetics, but HIV patients and children with debilitation (e.g., dehydration) or congenital immunodeficiencies may also develop this severe form of external otitis.

TRAUMA

Direct injury from foreign bodies leads to abrasion or laceration of the delicate skin. A foreign body or accumulated blood impairs the canal's self-cleaning mechanism and fosters bacterial growth. During the cold winter months insects seek warmth in the external canal. Attempts by the patient and physicians to remove the unwanted visitor can injure the canal. Head and facial trauma may lacerate the skin of the canal or fracture the bony canal. Thermal burns and radiation injury will create a canal that is less resistant to minor trauma, leading to frequent infections that can occasionally progress to bone exposure and sequestration.

IMMUNE MEDIATED

Contact dermatitis usually is caused by lotions, cosmetics, or ototopical drugs placed in the external canals. Paradoxically, in certain patients the very drops used to treat the ear canal can intensify the inflammation and induce a chronic inflammatory state. Neomycin, often used to treat bacterial external otitis, can evoke a severe inflammatory response in sensitive individuals, causing extreme swelling, bulla formation, and otorrhea. The rash may extend onto the face and/or neck. Immediate cessation of ear drops, delicate canal débridement, and application of corticosteroid creams are used in these cases.

Eczema of the canal is common, especially during childhood. Autoimmune disorders such as pemphigus and systemic lupus may cause inflammation of the canal skin.

NEOPLASMS

Squamous cell carcinoma may simulate an inflammatory process in its early stages. Children may develop rhabdomyosarcoma and Langerhans cell histiocytosis of the canal region. There may be swelling, otorrhea, bleeding, and surrounding erythema. It is typical for these rare lesions to be treated as infections for weeks and occasionally months before a definitive diagnosis is made.

Treatment of External Otitis

The treatment of external otitis obviously depends on the etiology. In *all* cases the first therapeutic effort should be débridement of the canal to remove obstructing crusts and desquamations. In some limited cases this alone is all the treatment that is needed. Most cases are infectious, and, therefore, topical antimicrobials are commonly used. If canal swelling is severe, the insertion of an expansile "wick" (gauze, compressed sponge) is useful to stent the canal and deliver ototopicals by capillary action. Addition of an anti-inflammatory agent, such as hydrocortisone or dexamethasone, will speed resolution and lessen the duration of discomfort. Keeping the ear dry is a must, as a wet canal fosters microbial growth and reduces protective responses. If pain is severe, systemic analgesics such as ibuprofen or codeine should be given to the patient.

The otic preparations discussed in the following sections are my preferences.

ACIDIFYING AGENTS

The normal pH of skin is acidic and restoration of the pH can help the defenses of the external canal. In cases of mild external otitis or hypersensitivity, an anhydrous acetic acid preparation with hydrocortisone (VoSol HC) is applied as 3 to 4 drops four times per day. It is also useful for otomycotic infections.

TOPICAL ANTIBIOTICS

Fluoroquinolones are the preferred choice, including ciprofloxacin and hydrocortisone (Cipro HC), three drops twice daily for 7 days; ciprofloxacin and dexamethasone (Ciprodex), three drops twice daily for 7 days; and ofloxacin (Floxin), five drops twice daily. The old standard neomycin, polymyxin, hydrocortisone (Cortisporin Otic) drop is used less frequently because of contact dermatitis to neomycin, but it is still effective. Ophthalmic topical antibiotics, such as gentamicin (Garamycin)[1] and tobramycin (Tobrex)[1], may also be useful but should be avoided when the tympanic membrane is perforated or contains a tympanostomy tube.

Otomycosis of the ear canal can be treated with acidifying agents, such as acetic acid (VoSol), drying agents (gentian violet, Cresylate), and antifungal antibiotics (clotrimazole [Lotrimin AF] solution, ketoconazole [Nizoral][1] cream, amphotericin[1] [Fungizone]). As with all cases of external otitis, frequent (even daily) débridement of the external canal is mandatory to remove infectious material and allow access of the drops to the surface of the canal skin.

SYSTEMIC ANTIBIOTICS

In cases of severe inflammation or when there is inflammatory extension to the pinna, middle ear, or face, a systemic antibiotic should be given. Because of the prevalence of *Pseudomonas*, ciprofloxacin (Cipro), 500 mg twice daily, or Levofloxacin (Levaquin), 500 mg daily, for 7 to 10 days is prescribed.

Malignant (necrotizing) external otitis is managed with topical and systemic treatment. Ciprofloxacin is given as a first-line agent both by drop and orally after granulation tissue débridement-biopsy and culture and sensitivity specimens are taken. In cases of abscess or cranial nerve dysfunction, intravenous therapy should be initiated with an aminoglycoside (tobramycin [Nebcin]) along with an antipseudomonal penicillin (piperacillin/tazobactam [Zosyn]). Third-generation cephalosporins (ceftazidime [Fortaz], cefepime [Maxipime]) and aztreonam (Azactam) have also been used alone or in combination with aminoglycosides.

Herpes zoster oticus requires topical cleaning, antibiotic treatment of secondary bacterial infection of ruptured vesicles, and systemic antiviral therapy with famciclovir (Famvir). If facial nerve palsy is present, systemic corticosteroids are given.

SURGICAL PROCEDURES

Abscess formation within the canal, caused by furuncles or carbuncles, may require incision and drainage to evacuate purulent sebaceous debris if spontaneous drainage or resolution does not occur with topical or oral antistaphylococcal medication. Biopsy of suspicious lesions and obstructing granulation tissue should be performed under the operating microscope. Abscesses of the subperichondrial space of the pinna must be incised and drained to prevent cartilage injury and resultant deformity of the pinna.

[1]Not FDA approved for this indication.

OTITIS MEDIA

METHOD OF

David R. White, MD, and Daniel I. Choo, MD

Otitis media is a general term meaning inflammation of the middle ear. Otitis media is divided into three groups

1. Acute otitis media
2. Chronic otitis media with effusion
3. Chronic suppurative otitis media

Acute otitis media refers to acute infection of the middle ear, lasting up to 3 weeks. Chronic otitis media with effusion is defined as otitis media with effusion present for 3 months or longer. Chronic suppurative otitis media is defined as infection of the middle ear with purulent otorrhea lasting 3 months or longer.

Acute Otitis Media

Acute otitis media (AOM) is the most common diagnosis made in the United States in the pediatric population. Incidence peaks between 6 and 12 months of age, gradually tapering off until 7 years of age, after which AOM is uncommon. Risk factors include recent upper respiratory infection, attendance in daycare centers, formula feeding (breast feeding has a protective effect), and exposure to tobacco smoke.

AOM can be accompanied by earache, irritability, and fever. Earache has a high specificity in children older than 2 years of age, but can be difficult to assess in younger children. Pneumatic otoscopy classically reveals an injected, bulging, immobile tympanic membrane with pus in the middle ear space. Tympanometry is usually unnecessary, but reveals a *flat* or type B tympanogram.

Streptococcus pneumoniae, *Hemophilus influenzae*, and *Moraxella catarrhalis* are responsible for the great majority of AOM. These pathogens colonize the nasopharynx and enter the middle ear via the eustachian tube. In the United States, significant rates of penicillin resistance exist for each pathogen, with *S. pneumoniae* rates ranging from 10% to 40%, *H. influenzae* 20% to 40%, and *M. catarrhalis* approaching 100%.

Approximately 80% of AOM episodes resolve spontaneously without antibiotic treatment. First-line treatment of AOM with amoxicillin (Amoxil), 40 to 80 mg/kg per day for 10 days, is successful in approximately 92% of all cases. Second-line therapy consists of treatment with amoxicillin/clavulanate (Augmentin) or second-generation cephalosporins. Daily ceftriaxone, given intramuscularly for 3 days, is an appropriate third-line treatment. Failure to respond to multiple courses of treatment is an indication for tympanocentesis, which is both therapeutic and provides culture and sensitivity information.

Surgical placement of tympanostomy tubes is recommended when medical therapy fails, when complications of AOM develop, and when recurrent acute otitis media (RAOM) is present. RAOM is defined as 3 to 4 separate episodes of AOM with complete resolution between episodes in a 6-month interval or 4 to 5 such episodes within 1 year. Tympanostomy tubes decrease the total amount of time with active AOM. They also allow treatment of AOM episodes with topical antibiotic drops that achieve extremely high concentrations of antibiotics in the middle ear and reduce the need for systemic antibiotics. Antibiotic prophylaxis with amoxicillin or trimethoprim-sulfamethoxazole (Bactrim) is effective in reducing the number of AOM episodes. This practice, however, promotes antibiotic resistance and should be reserved for poor surgical candidates.

The primary argument for antibiotic treatment of AOM is avoidance of complications such as acute mastoiditis, facial nerve palsy, chronic tympanic membrane perforation, labyrinthitis, meningitis, sigmoid sinus thrombosis, and intracranial abscesses. Otolaryngology consultation should be obtained when these complications are suspected.

Chronic Otitis Media with Effusion

Chronic otitis media with effusion (COME) is the most common cause of conductive hearing loss in children. Middle ear effusions (MEE) are present in up to 50% of children 1 month after resolution of AOM. After 3 months, 90% of these effusions spontaneously clear. MEE lasting longer than 3 months is unlikely to resolve spontaneously, and may result in reversible conductive hearing loss for prolonged periods of time. Down syndrome, craniofacial abnormalities, prematurity, allergy, Eskimo/Native American race, tobacco smoke exposure, and enrollment in daycare centers have been implicated as risk factors for COME.

Eustachian tube dysfunction is considered the primary cause of COME. Poor middle ear ventilation and clearance may result from the immature tubal cartilage, poor tensor veli palatini function, or short tubal length seen in early childhood. As children age, COME incidence decreases with 90% resolution by 7 years of age. Several studies indicate, however, that speech and language, cognitive, and behavioral development are adversely affected because of the conductive hearing loss that accompanies COME during childhood.

A history of AOM may be the only indication that COME is present, because hearing loss can be difficult for parents to identify in young children and because COME is often asymptomatic. Physical diagnosis and tympanometry are the primary methods of identifying COME. Pneumatic otoscopy reveals an immobile tympanic membrane with fluid in the middle ear space. Bubbles, air-fluid levels, or dullness of the tympanic membrane may also be present. Tympanometry typically reveals a type B or *flat* tympanogram.

Antibiotic treatment results in only a 15% increase in resolution of COME. For MEE lasting more than 3 months, primary treatment is surgical placement of tympanostomy tubes allowing removal of the effusion, ventilation of the middle ear, and resolution of associated conductive hearing loss. Two thirds of COME cases resolve after only one set of tympanostomy tubes, which typically last 9 to 12 months. When a second set of tympanostomy tubes is required, simultaneous adenoidectomy has been demonstrated to further lower the rate of COME resolution. Presence of a unilateral effusion in an adult should raise suspicion for a nasopharyngeal mass, requiring an otolaryngology consultation for nasopharyngoscopy.

Chronic Suppurative Otitis Media

Chronic suppurative otitis media (CSOM) represents an indolent infectious process of the middle ear. A tympanic membrane perforation or an indwelling tympanostomy tube accompanies CSOM. Upon presentation, most cases of CSOM have already failed to respond to first- and second-line antimicrobial therapies. Risk factors include autoimmune disorders, previous tympanostomy tube placement, and history of acute otitis media.

Diagnosis is based on history of 3 months of purulent otorrhea, presence of tympanic membrane perforation or tympanostomy tube, and absence of other pathology such as cholesteatoma. Tympanometry is unnecessary. Computed tomography may be useful in ruling out cholesteatoma and determining the extent of mastoid involvement.

Initial therapy includes careful aural cleaning (suctioning of the debris and drainage from the external auditory canal) and use of topical quinolones. Because *Pseudomonas aeruginosa* and *Staphylococcus aureus* are common pathogens in CSOM, culture and sensitivity of otorrhea may be necessary to identify resistance patterns and guide antibiotic treatment. Initial treatment with quinolone antimicrobials is appropriate given this microbial profile and the sensitivities of these bacteria. Fungal superinfection (typically *Candida*) may also be present. Mycobacterial infection should also be considered in high-risk populations. Intravenous antibiotic therapy may be required for treatment of resistant organisms.

Failure of CSOM to respond to antibiotic therapy warrants surgical intervention. CSOM with indwelling tympanostomy tubes can be associated with biofilms on the tubes, allowing colonization of the tube with a reservoir of bacteria unreachable by antibiotics.

Removing the tubes or replacing them with ionized, coated fluoroplastic tubes, which allow less biofilm accumulation, can be effective in stopping the purulent otorrhea. CSOM may also result from sequestered granulation tissue or unrecognized cholesteatoma in the mastoid cavity. Tympanomastoidectomy can be diagnostic and therapeutic in these cases.

AOM is a common diagnosis that typically responds to short-term antimicrobial therapy, but the clinician must be aware of the potential for development of complications. COME and CSOM patients that fail in initial antimicrobial treatment should be considered candidates for otolaryngology referral.

EPISODIC VERTIGO

METHOD OF

Timothy C. Hain, MD, and Dario Yacovino, MD

Illusory rotation (vertigo) is nearly always caused by vestibular system dysfunction. Management of vertigo is easiest when an accurate localization, mechanism, and etiologic diagnosis are available; and specific treatment is sometimes available for conditions in which an etiology can be established. Unfortunately, however, we are unable to establish an etiologic diagnosis in the majority of patients with vertigo and even establishing the site of lesion is often impossible. In cases where a specific treatment is not available, symptomatic relief may be provided by antiemetics and drugs that depress peripheral vestibular function. Unfortunately, these medications are problematic as specific agents do not exist that will selectively ablate vestibular function—all vestibular suppressant medications have side effects that limit their use. Furthermore, reduction of vertigo is accomplished by reducing vestibular function on *both* the normal and abnormal sides. Thus, vestibular suppressants can induce ataxia.

The inability of available medications to effectively suppress vertigo without unacceptable side effects has lead clinicians to attempt other modes of treatment. Recently, greater emphasis has been placed upon vestibular rehabilitation therapy in which recovery is promoted by exercises aimed at facilitating central adaptive mechanisms.

This article concentrates on common conditions that account for most referrals to a dizziness clinic. The objective is to define the role of medication or vestibular exercises in these disorders.

Pathophysiology

The peripheral vestibular apparatus, which consists of the semicircular canals and otolith organs, senses angular and linear acceleration. Angular acceleration is caused by rotation of the head and is registered by the canals. Linear acceleration, which is caused by translation of the head as well as changes in the orientation of the head to gravity, is registered by the otoliths. Accordingly, illusions of rotation, translation, or tilt and symptoms initiated or aggravated by head movement are the hallmarks of vestibular system disease.

Symptoms of semicircular canal disturbance include a sensation of rotation as if the body might be spinning, cartwheeling, or tumbling. Symptoms of otolith disturbance include sensations of tilt, levitation, or impulsion. If an otolithic disturbance is severe enough, the patient falls to the ground (e.g., the *otolithic crisis of Tumarkin* experienced by patients with Ménière's disease). Symptoms of autonomic overactivity such as sweating, pallor, nausea, and vomiting nearly always accompany vertigo of labyrinthine origin.

Central vestibular lesions, which also can cause vertigo, usually involve structures where afferent activities from both labyrinths have been combined. The resulting pattern of imbalance in vestibular activity may more closely resemble naturally induced sensations of rotation and usually is associated with milder symptoms than peripheral vestibular imbalance.

Acute Peripheral Vestibular Imbalance

Vestibular neuritis and labyrinthitis are examples of acute peripheral vestibular disorders. These conditions generally result in distress caused by sensation of movement, nausea, and malaise for only 2 to 3 days. Even patients with vestibular nerve section are usually up and about by 1 week. Accordingly, even untreated, most patients with symptoms caused by a transient and incomplete paresis of vestibular function on one side will be ready to go back to their regular activities after several weeks. There are, however, exceptions to this general rule such as patients in occupations where good balance is essential.

In treatment, the dilemma of the physician is that while patients seek to be treated with a medication that will completely suppress their vertigo and somatic responses to vestibular imbalance, such treatment can harm the patient by denying the nervous system the ability to compensate for a vestibular lesion. If the vestibular imbalance is covered up by a vestibular suppressant medication, little repair activity may be initiated. Even bedrest may be poorly conceived.

TABLE 1 Drugs Used for Nausea

Drug	Dose	Comment
Prochlorperazine (Compazine)	10 IM or PO q4-6h or 25 mg rectally q 12 h	May produce extrapyramidal reaction
Promethazine (Phenergan)	25 mg PO q4-6h or 25 mg rectally q6h	Sedating
Odansetron (Zofran)	4 mg PO q8 or 8 mg PO q8	Not sedating; available in an orally disintegrating form

Animal studies have clearly shown that after experimental vestibular lesions immobilization delays recovery.

The strategy, therefore, is to use as few medications as possible and to encourage head movement and early ambulation. Antiemetics such as promethazine (Phenergan) may be essential—these may be prescribed as suppositories. Brief usage of meclizine (Antivert) and/or a low dose of a benzodiazepine can also help. Tables 1 and 2 list commonly available drugs and dosages.

In the acute phase, generally the first few days, patients should be warned that sudden head movements and changing the position of the head relative to the gravitational axis may cause increased vertigo. However, once the patient is able to sit up and walk, he or she should be encouraged to attempt as much normal activity as is possible without triggering emesis. Medications, particularly sedatives, should be stopped as soon as possible as they may retard eventual compensation. Most patients spontaneously recover, without the need for a formal vestibular rehabilitation program, perhaps because their vestibular impairment is transient rather than permanent.

Patients who don't recover may have a severe and fixed vestibular loss. Patients who have sustained a unilateral, complete vestibular loss whether caused by head trauma, surgery, or a viral neuritis, are faced with the prospect of going through life with half of their vestibular system ablated. Surprisingly enough, these patients usually do well, testifying to the amazingly effective compensatory machinery that can be brought to bear by the central nervous system (CNS). Recovery that does not occur in a timely fashion can signify a failure of central vestibular compensation such as in cerebellar disorders, a disease process that is fluctuating such as Ménière's disease, or substitution of another process such as a phobia.

Even such patients should largely recover after 2 months, except for those with vertigo elicited by rapid head movement. They can benefit from the addition of a physical therapy program incorporating the gait training and visual-vestibular exercises outlined in Table 3. This is to ensure that they get adequate sensory input regarding their impaired vestibular system and develop appropriate strategies to deal with sensitivity to head motion and disequilibrium.

Benign Paroxysmal Positional Vertigo

Benign paroxysmal positional vertigo (BPPV) is the single most common cause of vertigo. The diagnosis is easily made through a history of vertigo elicited by changes of head position with respect to gravity combined with a typical nystagmus pattern (an upbeating-torsional nystagmus) that appears on positional testing. The cause is currently thought to be loose debris in the labyrinthine system, and which settles to the bottom of the ear causing nystagmus for certain head positions. These patients are sometimes troubled by mild gait ataxia, but they are always most concerned by the inability to control vertigo that arises when they roll over in bed at night, or when they get up in the morning.

Drugs are not very useful in BPPV because although the vertigo is severe, it lasts only seconds. Nevertheless, meclizine in a dose of 12.5 to 25 mg taken at the hour of sleep may improve rest by preventing awakening by vertigo that occurs as the patient rolls over.

There are presently two very effective approaches to treatment—exercise and surgery. Numerous studies over the last decade have documented that more than 90% of patients benefit from exercises for BPPV (Table 3). If the diseased side is known, perhaps from positional testing, and the patient has a classic nystagmus (upbeating-torsional vector) the Epley maneuver is very effective, usually curing the patient of their symptoms on the first application in the

TABLE 2 Drugs Used to Decrease Vertigo

Drug	Dose	Comment
Diazepam (Valium)[1]	5-10 mg (1 dose) given acutely; 2 mg bid	Sedating; respiratory depressant
Dimenhydrinate (Dramamine)	50 mg q4-6h	Sedating
Meclizine (Antivert)	25 mg q4-6h[3]	Sedating
Scopolamine (Transderm Scōp)	Patch q3d	Anticholinergic side effects

[1]Not FDA approved for this indication.
[3]Exceeds dosage recommended by the manufacturer.

TABLE 3 Vestibular Exercises

Gait Training Exercises

Begin with feet a comfortable distance apart; progress to tandem position, eyes-closed tandem, and head-up tandem.
Repeat while standing on a slab of foam rubber about 4 inches off the floor.
Walk across the room with eyes open and then repeat with eyes closed.
Walk heel-toe across the room with eyes open and then repeat with eyes closed.

Visual-Vestibular Exercises

View a small target (about 2 in. by 2 in.) containing written material (for example, a match cover). Fix the target to the wall or other solid object—do *not* use a hand held object. While trying to keep the words on the target in clear focus, move your head (approximately ±45 degrees) from side to side, then move head and then up and down (about ± 30 degrees) at progressively higher speeds in both directions. The speed of the head movement should be increased until the words on the target can no longer be read.
Repeat above with a large-patterned target.
Hold a small target or a patterned piece of cardboard at arm's length. While trying to keep the pattern or target in focus, move the head and target horizontally in opposite directions about 20 degrees to either side.
Perform any game involving simultaneous movement of the head and use of vision.

Exercises for Benign Paroxysmal Positional Vertigo (BPPV) (Brandt-Daroff Maneuver)

Position yourself sitting up in bed with the legs on the floor (see Figure 1). Close your eyes and suddenly tilt yourself to one side so that one side of your body is against the bed. Turn the head slightly upward and wait for the vertigo to subside. Sit back up and wait for 30 seconds before tilting to the opposite side. If vertigo is also present in this position, wait until it subsides and then sit up again. Perform this exercise five times in the morning and five times at night until you have 2 days with no vertigo.

office (Figure 1). A home variant of the Epley maneuver can be used effectively for persons with persistent symptoms.

If the *bad ear* side is unknown, the Brandt-Daroff exercises can be used (Figure 2). These consist of the process of repeatedly bringing on their symptoms for 2 weeks or until they can no longer bring on their symptoms. Compliance may be a problem with these exercises, however.

These exercise approaches are successful presumably either because the debris is dissolved or moved to an insensitive portion of the labyrinth, because the patient learns to tolerate the symptoms, or because the disease process remits spontaneously. If the exercises provoke nausea, patients can be premeditated with antiemetics such as promethazine (Phenergan), meclizine (Antivert), or ondansetron (Zofran). If patients do not benefit from the exercises, the diagnosis should be reconsidered as central positional nystagmus can be mistaken for BPPV.

A second treatment approach is to surgically plug the posterior semicircular canal. In our view, this procedure should be considered only in patients who have been symptomatic for more than 6 months or have an intractable recurrent pattern. Also they should be patients in whom the side of lesion is certain and who have not benefited from the exercises. In this refractory group, the surgery eliminates symptoms in approximately 90% of cases.

Ménière's Disease

A diagnosis of Ménière's disease should be considered in patients who combine intermittent vertigo with a static or intermittent hearing deficit, aural fullness, and an episodic multifrequency "roaring" tinnitus. Ménière's disease is probable when spontaneous nystagmus is observed on at least one occasion, fluctuations in hearing can be documented on audiometry, and studies necessary to exclude structural lesions of the labyrinth have been performed. Ménière's disease can be difficult to distinguish from migraine-associated vertigo. Migraine should be seriously considered as an alternative diagnosis when hearing fluctuates in both ears together as well as in situations where there are no hearing symptoms (so-called vestibular Ménière).

Two levels of therapy can be considered. For patients who have infrequent episodes, vestibular suppressants, possibly combined with an antiemetic, are used for the acute attack, and no medications are used in the interim. Oral meclizine and a small dose of a benzodiazepine such as lorazepam (Ativan)[1] or clonazepam (Klonopin)[1] are the most useful agents for mild attacks. In the emergency room where patients with severe attacks present, prochlorperazine (Compazine) (which can be given intramuscularly) and diazepam (Valium)[1] are the most useful agents. Dehydrated patients can be rehydrated and sent home on antiemetics. Vestibular exercises are not used acutely, as adaptations made during the transient vestibular imbalance are inappropriate when the patient has recovered.

Over the long term, salt restriction and use of a mild sodium-wasting diuretic such as a hydrochlorothiazide/triamterene (Dyazide)[1] combination may reduce the frequency of attacks and should be tried. Some patients will respond to verapamil (Calan SR)[1] (120 mg sustained release), administered in a way similar to that used for migraine prophylaxis. There are a very large number of unproven and controversial treatments for Ménière's disease, and the physician who treats these patients should be prepared to discuss lipoflavenoids (a vitamin preparation), betahistine[1,2] (a medication sometimes considered a placebo), endolymphatic shunt surgery, as well as devices that claim effects through pressurization of the middle ear (Meniett device).

For patients who have hearing loss confined to one ear and who are troubled by frequent attacks of vertigo, a chemical labyrinthectomy using gentamicin

[1]Not FDA approved for this indication.
[2]Not available in the United States.

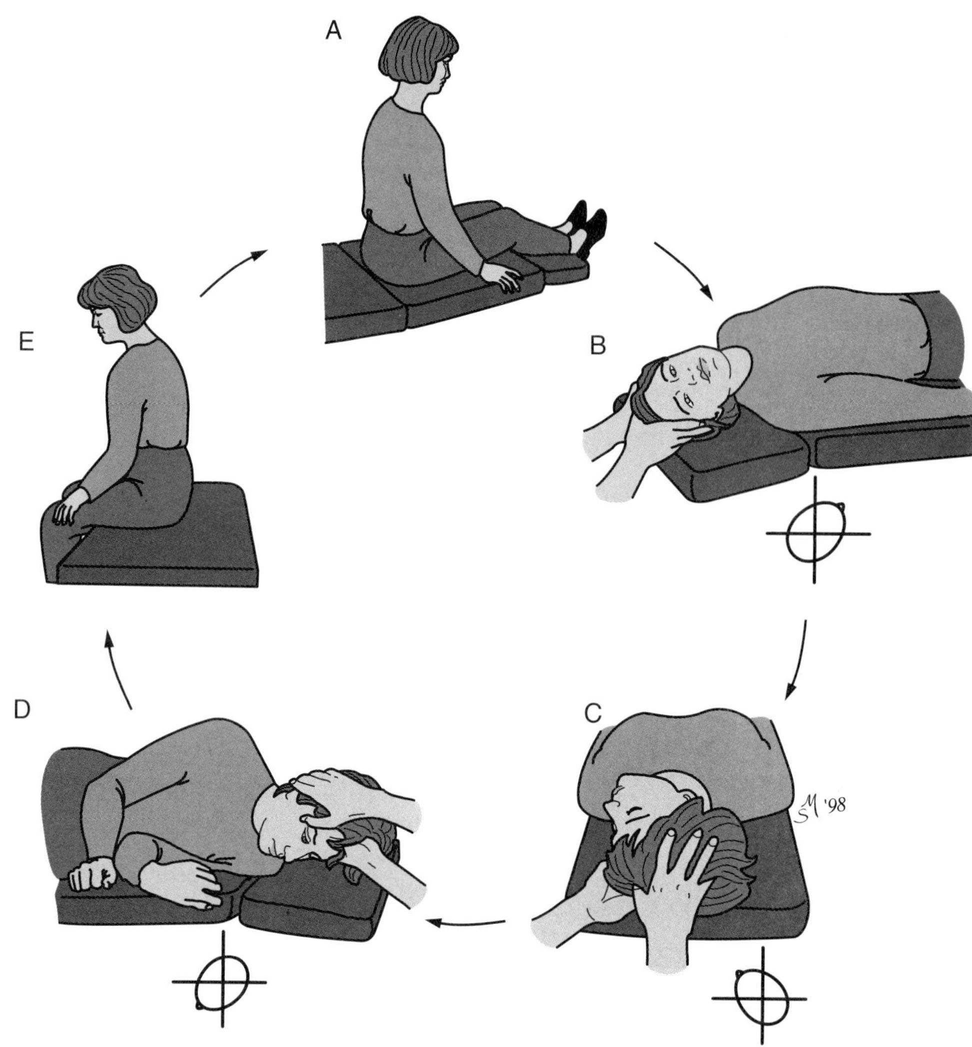

FIGURE 1 Epley maneuver as office treatment of BPPV. The patient is initially brought from sitting (A) down into the head-hanging position (B) on the symptomatic side. After 30 seconds the head is turned to the opposite side (C). After another 30 seconds, the body is rolled onto the uninvolved side (D). The head is carried with it so that the nose is pointed 45 degrees downward with respect to horizontal. After another 30 seconds the patient is moved to a sitting up position (E) with the head tucked 30 degrees.

(Garamycin) can be considered. This procedure must be considered with caution as approximately 50% of patients with Ménière's disease will eventually develop disease on both sides—in such cases, unilateral vestibular ablation will be ineffective. Nevertheless, given the ineffectiveness of drug therapy, it may be the only practical form of relief to offer.

Ototoxicity

Ototoxic antibiotics can cause oscillopsia, ataxia, and vertigo. Usually the diagnosis can be made by obtaining a history—a patient becomes infected and is placed on ototoxic antibiotics for several weeks. After recovering from infection, the patient attempts to get up out of bed and discovers symptoms of ataxia. On examination, the patient can read the vision chart when the head is still, but drops four or more lines of acuity when the head is gently oscillated.

The treatment strategy for these patients is purely a physical therapy approach with several available avenues of adaptation to the illness's deficits. First, there is considerable plasticity of the vestibulo-ocular reflex, and by having the patient perform maneuvers that exaggerate the mismatch between head movements and compensatory eye responses, that is, activities that elicit oscillopsia, improvement in their symptoms may result. From Table 3, the visual-vestibular exercises would be used in this situation.

Cognitive strategies provide a second avenue of help. Patients can *spot*, that is, fixate a reference target before making a head movement, and use their intact visual pursuit mechanism to provide visual stability. Before walking across a room in the dark, patients do better if they can form a mental map of the room before turning out the lights.

A final strategy is to improve nonvestibular methods of obtaining orientation information and to develop better motor programs for dealing with instability. Improving vision through proper glasses or cataract removal if indicated, and use of appropriate shoes (no high heels) can be very useful. The gait training exercises outlined in Table 3 may be used. Of course, medications are ototoxic or which suppress the vestibular system (such as those of

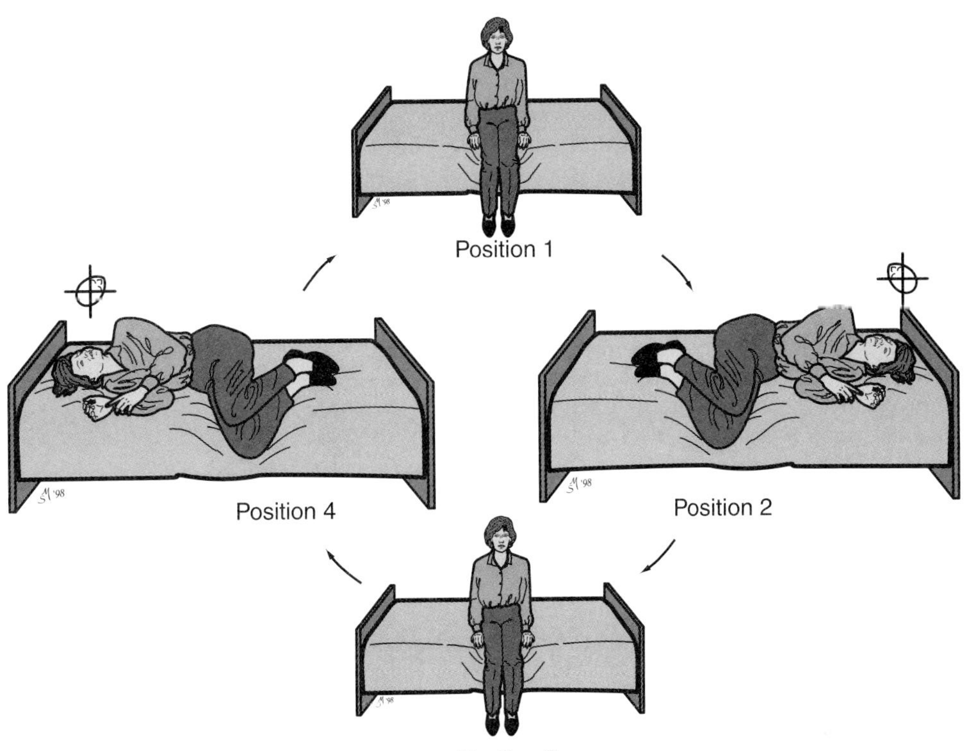

FIGURE 2 Brandt-Daroff positioning exercises for treatment of benign paroxysmal positional vertigo. See Table 3 for details.

Table 2) and their pharmacologic relatives should be avoided.

Central Vertigo

The majority of patients with central vertigo have migraine-associated vertigo, and most of these are women of childbearing age. They can be treated with the usual prophylactic medications. Because of its favorable side effect profile, verapamil (Calan)[1], starting with a dose of 120 mg sustained release, is generally the most helpful agent, followed by propranolol (Inderal) and amitriptyline (Elavil). Both verapamil and amitriptyline[1] have pharmacologic effects outside of migraine prophylaxis that are often useful in managing other types of vertigo.

An unusual but interesting central vertigo syndrome is mal de debarquement—a prolonged land-sickness that typically occurs after getting off of a 7-day cruise. The main symptom is a constant rocking sensation. Mal de debarquement typically responds very well to a low dose of clonazepam (Klonopin)[1] (0.5 mg twice daily).

The next most common group are older persons with small infarcts in the cerebellum, pons, and lateral medulla. The vestibular nucleus is a large target for vascular lesions. These patients can present with vertigo without other localizing symptoms. Furthermore, while patients with peripheral vestibular asymmetry typically recover within months, patients with central vertigo may continue to be distressed by ataxia, nausea, and illusions of motion for years. Presumably the persistence of their symptoms reflects a lesion in the central mechanisms that usually compensate for vestibular lesions. After addressing the underlying cause, symptomatic treatment may include vestibular suppressants such as meclizine (Antivert) or scopolamine (Transderm-Scōp), or clonazepam[1] in a dose of 0.5 mg twice daily. These agents are generally much less effective than in peripheral disorders, but lacking a method of predicting which agent will be useful, brief trials are in order. Gabapentin (Neurontin)[1] in a dose of 300 to 600 mg per day in divided doses is often useful in persons with nystagmus. Gait training and visual-vestibular exercises such as those outlined in Table 3 should be attempted.

Vertigo of Unknown Origin

A common group of patients are those who experience vertigo but in whom there is no clue as to the origin. Some of these patients have psychogenic causes of vertigo, and the others simply have disorders for which our diagnostic technology is not adequate. There are probably a large number of the latter, because, although there are three semicircular canals and two otolith organs on each side of the head, we have specific tests only for the lateral semicircular

[1]Not FDA approved for this indication.

[1]Not FDA approved for this indication.

canals—we have no practical clinical method for assessing function of the vertical canals or of the otolith organs.

The approach to these patients is to manage them symptomatically and follow them at 3- to 6-month intervals. Patients may benefit from vestibular suppressants and vestibular physical therapy.

One should see these patients when they are acutely dizzy, hoping to be able to establish on which side the lesion is located through observation of a nystagmus or hearing loss. Often a trial of salt restriction and diuretics is useful because it is generally impossible to exclude the possibility of Ménière's disease. In patients with frequent headaches, an attempt at migraine prophylaxis is worthwhile.

Controversial Vestibular Disorders

Cervical vertigo is a condition that is generally agreed to exist but the diagnosis is made by exclusion—which means that it is essentially a variant of vertigo of unknown origin. Cervical vertigo is diagnosed most often in patients with whiplash injuries. Treatment includes physical therapy and measures intended to reduce neck pain and spasm.

Microvascular compression syndrome, also called disabling positional vertigo and vestibular paroxysmia, is attributed to compression of the eighth nerve by blood vessels within the cerebellopontine angle. As such blood vessels occur commonly in asymptomatic persons, imaging procedures cannot establish the diagnosis. Response of vertigo to oxcarbazepine (Trileptal)[1] is suggestive of this syndrome.

Psychogenic vertigo certainly exists, but clinicians often have difficulty in assessing its significance. Anxiety and vertigo are so often intertwined and it is frequently difficult to separate cause from effect. Persons who are unsteady are often (justifiably) afraid of heights or open spaces without an available support. Individuals with anxiety may also present with lightheadedness or simply be overly sensitive to bodily symptoms that most people ignore. Effective management of vertigo requires a willingness of the clinician to consider and treat anxiety, panic, or depression along with nystagmus and ataxia.

[1]Not FDA approved for this indication.

MÉNIÈRE'S DISEASE

METHOD OF
Jeffrey P. Harris, MD, PhD*

Ménière's disease is a chronic illness that affects approximately 97,000 Americans annually, with symptoms that wax and wane throughout their lifetimes. Patients often experience a period of intense symptoms followed by years of remission, with relapse in later stages of the disease. Since it was first described by Prosper Ménière in 1861, this illness has defied scientific investigation into its etiology and cure.

This disorder is often described as severe episodic vertigo, fluctuating hearing loss, roaring tinnitus, and a feeling of aural pressure. The characteristics are so unique that just the description of the attack by the patient can lead to a correct diagnosis of the condition. Selective tests can be performed to rule out other conditions in the short list of differential diagnoses. Unfortunately, the common perception by patients, primary care physicians, and often by general otolaryngologists is that there is no effective treatment for this disorder. The patient usually has no choice but to find a way to deal with the attacks until the disease burns itself out, which then coincides with the development of severe hearing and vestibular loss.

I have evaluated a group of patients with Ménière's disease and performed quality of life evaluations, both between attacks and within days of an acute spell. The results were eye opening. These patients, most of whom were middle-aged, were found to be severely impaired by their illness—their self-rated Quality of Well-being (QWB) was worse than adults with life-threatening illnesses (i.e., AIDS, cancer, renal, and pulmonary diseases). On days with acute symptoms, Ménière's patients were much more severely affected, scoring worse than noninstitutionalized Alzheimer's patients and elderly patients with severe obstructive pulmonary disease. Additionally, these patients were clinically depressed on the Center for Epidemiologic Studies (CES) depression scale and were also one standard deviation below the mean for the general population on the Medical outcomes study SF-12 (short form), a widely used general health measure. Taken together, these findings underscore the importance of attempting to aggressively treat these patients rather than letting the disease run its course.

Histopathology

Ménière's disease is characterized by the presence of endolymphatic hydrops seen on temporal bone

**Financial disclosure*: The author holds the patent for the Otoblot test and has a financial interest in OTO Immune Diagnostics, Inc.

studies. During the early phases of the illness there are normal numbers of hair cells and neurons in the organ of Corti. But with repeated attacks of an admixture of endolymph and perilymph caused by ruptures of Reissner's membrane, there is increasing damage to both of these structures, as well as derangements within the membranous labyrinth caused by the presence of swollen endolymphatic membranes. One such alteration is the contact of the saccular membrane with the undersurface of the stapes footplate. This is thought to lead to a positive Hennebert's sign (dizziness or nystagmus induced by pneumo-otoscopy) in approximately 30% of patients. Occasionally one will see bone or detritus blocking the outflow channels of the endolymphatic compartment or its duct, which may be interfering with the longitudinal flow of the inner ear fluid.

Epidemiology

SEX DISTRIBUTION

There is a slight increased female preponderance among Ménière's patients, although there are some exceptions, such as in Sweden where the incidence is 57% males to 43% females. In Japan in the 1970s, there was an equal male-to-female incidence, but that has changed over the last 30 years to a female predominance. The reasons for this are unknown.

AGE

The patients who develop this condition are often in the prime of their working lives. The average age of onset has been reported to range between 38 and 50 years of age. The disease is rare in children.

BILATERALITY

This is a very important statistic because the illness can lead to severe hearing loss in the affected ear and can influence the treatment decision-making process, especially if destructive procedures are being considered. The incidence of bilaterality has been reported to range from as low as 2% to as high as 47%. Most practitioners inform patients that the incidence is approximately 20% to 30%, with an increased incidence the longer they are followed. However, this depends upon the criteria being used that determine when the second ear is affected. For instance, a second ear may show a hearing loss but no symptoms of dizziness; to some physicians, this would be considered bilateral disease. In one temporal bone cadaver study, the histopathologic evidence of endolymphatic hydrops seen in the second ear of Ménière's patients was reported to be approximately 30%.

HEREDITARY FACTORS

There are some families that have a strong history of Ménière's disease. This has been reported in approximately 5% to 14% of Ménière's patients. It is not known whether common structural or biochemical factors present in the temporal bones of these family members might be responsible for their development of the illness, but given the rapid identification of mutations that lead to derangements of gene products in the ear, it is reasonable to expect that soon one will be identified that has relevance to inner ear fluid homeostasis.

NATURAL HISTORY

The presenting symptoms of Ménière's disease are variable. Approximately 40% of the cases present with a sudden hearing loss, and approximately 50% report acute vertigo as their initial symptom. The incidence of these two symptoms occurring simultaneously ranges from 7% to 44%. When hearing loss is the presenting symptom, most of these patients begin to exhibit vertigo within 2 years. However, when vertigo is the initial symptom, fewer of these cases develop into Ménière's disease.

The audiograms of patients with Ménière's disease have a typical appearance. They often start with a low frequency hearing loss averaging 35 dB, with fluctuations back to near normal range. As the illness progresses, one begins to see associated high frequency losses that result in a tent-like or peaked audiogram centered on 2000 Hz. Further along in the illness, the peak diminishes to a flat audiogram with further losses in the high frequencies and an associated loss in word identification scores.

Over time, the hearing and vestibular losses plateau and the attacks abate. In this stage, hearing is reduced to the 50 to 60 dB range and the word identification scores are 50% to 60%. While these patients find the hearing loss disabling, hearing aids are usually not helpful because of distortion and poor word discrimination. At this point there is still caloric function but it too is reduced on average by 50%. It is rare that the caloric function is not maintained to some degree, but if it is 100% lost, one should investigate for other retrocochlear pathology such as an acoustic neuroma, or possibly even autoimmune inner ear disease.

Patients sometimes have a recrudescence of their illness later after a period of relative calm. This may result in a frightening disorder characterized by a sudden drop attack known as the otolithic crisis of Tumarkin. During these spells the patient is thrown to the ground without losing consciousness or having a change in hearing. If this occurs, the illness has moved to a dangerous phase because these sudden drop attacks can cause serious injury. The patient should be treated aggressively at this point.

Evaluation (Table 1)

When patients present with the classic symptoms of complex episodic vertigo, fluctuating hearing loss, roaring tinnitus, and aural pressure, a thorough

TABLE 1 Classification of Ménière's Disease

Typical Ménière's Disease (Classic)

Episodic vertigo, fluctuating sensorineural hearing loss, roaring tinnitus, and aural pressure

Atypical Ménière's Disease

Cochlear Ménière's: Characteristic auditory symptoms without the vertiginous episodes
Vestibular Ménière's disease variant: Characteristic vestibular symptoms without signs of hearing loss
Otolithic crisis of Tumarkin: Sudden fleeting drop attacks without loss of consciousness often seen in late stage
Lermoyez syndrome: Hearing improvement with attacks of vertigo rather than the reverse

otoneurologic examination is required. Otoscopy and tuning fork examinations are unremarkable in most patients until hearing loss is manifested. Patients may also report distortion and intolerance to loud sounds. Occasionally patients will complain of a fleeting dull ache in their mastoid tip region. Patients will not usually exhibit spontaneous nystagmus unless they are in the throes of an acute attack during the visit. In such a situation, patients will have an irritative nystagmus within the early moments of the attack, evolving into a paralytic nystagmus as the attack progresses.

It is mandatory that patients undergo a complete audiogram that includes word identification scores. Patients may also have an electronystagmogram (ENG), with results that can range from normal to reduced vestibular responses on the ipsilateral ear. Quite often even the most symptomatic patients may have normal ENGs, but this should not reduce the need to treat them or consider them to be minimally affected. Electrocochleography (ECoG) can be performed either with a noninvasive canal wick electrode or with a transtympanic electrode. The latter gives more accurate results but may cause some injury to the tympanic membrane and, very rarely, to the inner ear. The value of the ECoG is controversial because if patients are asymptomatic, it may be normal. So its value for confirming the diagnosis is only when it is positive, not negative.

All patients with unexplained asymmetrical hearing loss should have magnetic resonance imaging (MRI) with gadolinium or a fast spin-echo sequence to rule out a retrocochlear process such as an acoustic neuroma (vestibular schwannoma) or other cerebellopontine angle (CPA) mass. Acoustic neuromas can sometimes present identically as a new case of Ménière's disease. To rule out syphilis and autoimmunity, the following laboratory tests should be ordered:

- Fluorescent treponemal antibody absorption (FTA-ABS)
- Antinuclear antibody (ANA)
- Erythrocyte sedimentation rate (ESR)
- Rheumatoid factor (RF)
- C-reactive protein (CRP)
- C1q immune complex detection
- Otoblot test (anti-68 kD antibody)

TABLE 2 Treatment of Ménière's Disease

Medical

Low-salt diet (<1200 mg NaCl daily)
Diuretics (hydrochlorothiazide, 25 mg/KCl bid)
Vestibular sedatives (diazepam [Valium][1], promethazine [Phenergan][1], meclizine [Antivert][1], prochlorperazine [Compazine])
Steroids for autoimmune variant (60 mg prednisone[1], tapered over 3 to 4 weeks)
Intratympanic gentamicin (Garamycin)[1] (low-dose titration method)

Surgical

Pressure equalizing tube with or without Meniett device
Endolymphatic sac shunt or decompression
Vestibular nerve section (good hearing)
Labyrinthectomy (poor hearing)

[1]Not FDA approved for this indication.
Abbreviations: bid = twice daily; KCl = potassium chloride; NaCl = sodium chloride.

The Otoblot test is especially important in cases of bilateral Ménière's disease.

Treatment (Table 2)

MEDICAL THERAPY

The first step in managing a patient with Ménière's disease is to explain their illness to them. The patients need to be engaged in their therapy to understand how they can take control of this condition. This often includes a change in lifestyle, reduction of stress, increased exercise, and a reduced intake of salt and processed foods.

The patient should be given vestibular sedatives (diazepam [Valium][1], promethazine [Phenergan][1], meclizine [Antivert][1], prochlorperazine [Compazine][1]) to reduce the symptoms of an acute attack of vertigo. They should also be given a diuretic along with a 1200-mg NaCl diet. My diuretic of choice is hydrochlorothiazide (HCTZ)[1], 25 mg, twice daily, with a potassium supplement (also twice daily). If they are sulfa allergic, I prescribe bumetanide (Bumex)[1], 1 mg, twice daily. I do not believe that the combination of triamterine and HCTZ (Dyazide) is as effective as HCTZ alone. If patients have strong allergic histories, I will refer them for allergy testing and desensitization.

Additionally, if their evaluation shows any form of autoimmunity or a positive Otoblot, high-dose prednisone[1] (60 mg) is administered for a 3- to 4-week taper. If a response is seen, they are be referred to rheumatology for better-tolerated immunosuppressive agents such as methotrexate (Rheumatrex)[1], etanercept (Enbrel)[1], or infliximab (Remicade)[1]. Repeated bursts of prednisone are given for relapses. Under this type of management, up to 80% of patients will improve and can be managed medically.

[1]Not FDA approved for this indication.

Recently, there has also been a trend toward intratympanic injections of methylprednisolone (Solu-Medrol)[1] to control patients with steroid responsive Ménière's disease.

ENDOLYMPHATIC SAC SURGERY

Patients who fail medical management may then be considered for surgical therapy. This option has a wide range of differing opinions by specialists dealing with this disorder. Many otologists recommend endolymphatic sac shunt surgery or endolymphatic sac decompression as the next step. This outpatient procedure involves a mastoidectomy to expose the endolymphatic sac; the site is then opened and a silastic drain is placed into the mastoid, or, alternatively, the sac is left decompressed. This procedure has few risks to hearing or to other structures and usually has a 65% to 80% improvement in vertigo. This has not been shown to statistically improve hearing or stop tinnitus, though both sometimes improve. Because this procedure is not destructive and carries little risk to hearing, patients and practitioners alike often choose this option. In controlled studies, this procedure was found to be no more effective than sham surgery performed on the ears under general anesthesia. However, both groups of patients statistically improved over their baseline status, so the value of this surgery is controversial.

INTRATYMPANIC GENTAMICIN

Vestibular ablation through chemical means has recently had a resurgence in popularity. Once used only systemically for bilateral cases, it has now become a well-accepted and effective method to stop vestibular attacks in Ménière's disease. Low doses of gentamicin (Garamycin)[1] are injected into the middle ear, with gradual vestibular ablation occurring. The goal is not to destroy the vestibular end organ completely, but to titrate the dose until symptoms occur, and then watch for possible recurrence. By this low-dose titration method, the risk to hearing is reduced to approximately 6% and the overall effective vertigo control is 92%. Repeated doses can be administered as needed for new symptoms.

The only drawback to this method is the temporary instability patients develop as a consequence of vestibular injury incurred by the gentamicin. Patients often experience disequilibrium for a variable period following the treatment. There have also been reports of incidences of severe hearing loss associated with intratympanic (IT) gentamicin, but usually with higher cumulative doses. Round window microcatheters have also been developed for this treatment, but they require a surgical procedure. This method has not been found to be more effective than direct injections into the middle ear or through a pressure equalizing tube.

[1]Not FDA approved for this indication.

VESTIBULAR NERVE SECTIONING

Sectioning of the vestibular nerve was once a popular procedure, but it has been employed less over the last decade. In this surgery, the posterior fossa or the middle fossa approach exposes the vestibular nerve for its selective sectioning, sparing both the cochlear nerve and the facial nerve. This procedure has been recommended when symptoms are severe and hearing is still quite serviceable. It involves a craniotomy and thus has the inherent risks of meningitis, cerebrospinal fluid (CSF) leak, and neurologic injury.

The goal is to spare hearing and obtain complete deafferentation of the vestibular end organs. This procedure has a 90% chance to relieve vertigo spells, but there is a period of adaptation involved, as there is with chemical ablation. In these cases, the disease will progress with unremitting hearing deterioration, aural fullness, and tinnitus; this procedure does little to change inner ear pathophysiology. Some patients also report persistent disequilibrium even after a successful vestibular nerve section, but it is markedly improved over what it was preoperatively.

LABYRINTHECTOMY

When hearing is reduced by the illness to unserviceable levels (defined as at least 50 dB speech reception threshold (SRT) and a less than 50% word identification score), a labyrinthectomy can be recommended. This procedure is the gold standard of procedures in Ménière's disease with which other methods must be compared. In this operation, the five vestibular end organs are systematically removed under direct microscopic control in an approach usually through the mastoid. By removing these end organs the inner ear can no longer generate vestibular attacks; but the residual hearing is destroyed as a consequence of the procedure. Patients will be unsteady for several weeks following the surgery and must undergo central adaptation for the loss of vestibular function through vestibular exercises or physical therapy. This procedure is effective in approximately 95% of cases. One must be certain there is adequate vestibular function on the contralateral side before the vestibular tissue is removed, otherwise the patient may end up with a form of Dandy-Walker syndrome where disabling oscillopsia and ataxia are experienced.

LOW PRESSURE, MIDDLE EAR PRESSURE (THE MENIETT DEVICE)

It has been found that low-pressure pulses delivered through a pressure equalizing tube in the tympanic membrane can be transmitted into the inner ear, reducing inner ear pressure and presumably reducing endolymphatic hydrops. In recent clinical trials, there has been a reduction in vestibular attacks after a period ranging from 6 weeks to 4 months.

Patients still experience occasional attacks, but they are fewer than before treatment. No change occurs in their hearing, tinnitus, or activities of daily living. The device carries the high price of approximately $3500, which is variably covered by insurance. It is being marketed as an intermediate step in the management of this illness—when medical management fails and before surgery is recommended. It should be noted that some patients who receive a pressure equalizing tube into their tympanic membrane report that this alone is effective in controlling Ménière's disease. The device is relatively new and only time will tell if it is effective.

SINUSITIS

METHOD OF

Scott C. Manning, MD

Background and Diagnosis

Rhinosinusitis is the most commonly reported chronic condition of adults on health surveys, affecting up to 14% of the U.S. population. On validated general health outcome measures, a history of sinusitis is associated with significant increases in scores for body pain, impaired social functioning, and general health problems. As with respiratory tract disease in general, health statistics show an increasing prevalence of sinusitis as an ambulatory clinic primary diagnosis over the past 2 decades. Rhinosinusitis now accounts for approximately 12% of all antibiotic prescriptions in the United States, and it represents the fifth most common diagnosis for which antibiotics are prescribed.

Despite its prevalence, no specific symptom or sign defines sinusitis. For adults, the most common symptoms include congestion, facial pressure, nasal discharge, dental pain, cough, loss of smell, and headache. Headache as the principal symptom actually correlates with a greater likelihood of normal sinus imaging findings. For children, the most common symptoms include congestion, nighttime cough, fatigue, and irritability. Persistent of symptoms beyond the usual 7- to 10-day course of a viral upper respiratory infection most commonly defines clinical rhinosinusitis.

Imaging studies are helpful to confirm (or rule out) sinusitis, but they must be interpreted in light of clinical signs and symptoms. Air-fluid levels, frontal or sphenoid disease, and complete sinus opacification correlate more strongly with clinical symptoms. The finding of clear sinuses on imaging correlates with the absence of symptoms (except headache). Computed tomography (CT) demonstrates sinus anatomy in more detail than plain radiographs, but findings of mucosal thickening on CT in general do not correlate well with clinical signs and symptoms, especially in children. In fact, up to 70% of young children undergoing CT for non–sinus-related diagnoses in the winter have findings of sinus mucosal thickening.

Children and adults are estimated to average eight and four viral upper respiratory tract infections, respectively, per year, and approximately 2% of these episodes are believed to progress to bacterial infections of the sinus cavities. The second most common predisposing condition is allergic rhinitis, present in at least 60% of patients with chronic or recurrent rhinosinusitis. Gastroesophageal reflux, cigarette smoking, other environmental pollutants, and immunodeficiency are also potential predisposing conditions. Healthy sinuses are a consequence of adequate local and systemic immune defenses, mucociliary function, and sinus drainage and ventilation.

Acute Sinusitis

Acute sinusitis is usually defined as upper respiratory signs and symptoms persisting beyond the usual course of a viral illness, but for less than 3 weeks. In placebo-controlled studies, the rate of spontaneous resolution of symptoms is at least 40%. The most commonly cultured organisms in radiographically documented acute sinusitis cases are *Streptococcus pneumoniae* and nontypeable *Haemophilus influenzae.* While unusual in adults, *Moraxella catarrhalis* is cultured from approximately 20% of pediatric cases. *Staphylococcus aureus* can be cultured from approximately 30% of healthy noses, but it is unusual in specimens obtained from maxillary sinus taps in acute sinusitis. The usual recommendation for initial antibiotic therapy for uncomplicated pediatric acute sinusitis is still amoxicillin (Amoxil), although at higher doses (80 mg/kg/day for pediatric patients), in order to overcome the intermediate penicillin resistance of *S. pneumoniae.* The fact that studies usually fail to show improved outcomes for acute pediatric sinusitis with other drugs despite a growing incidence of β-lactamase resistance with *M. catarrhalis* and *H. influenzae* may in part be because of the lower virulence and higher spontaneous resolution rates of those organisms versus *S. pneumoniae*. Backup drugs for amoxicillin failure for acute sinusitis include amoxicillin/clavulanate, cefuroxime, cefdinir, and macrolides. The usual recommended treatment time course is 10 days.

Chronic Sinusitis

Chronic sinusitis is classically defined as persistence of symptoms beyond 3 months, but a far more common history is that of symptoms that improve with therapy and then recur. In contrast to acute sinusitis, nontypeable *H. influenzae* is more commonly cultured in maxillary tap studies along with *S. aureus*, gram-negative bacteria, and anaerobes. Chronic infections are also much more likely to be polymicrobial. Although maxillary sinus puncture and culture remain the gold standard for antimicrobial selection, it is not commonly performed in routine clinical settings. However, culture of purulent secretions from the middle meatus or nasal vestibule under direct visualization with an endoscope or otoscope correlates well with maxillary tap results and should be performed routinely to identify the organism(s) and sensitivity profile(s). For empiric therapy of adult chronic sinusitis, after considering prevailing resistance patterns, drug concentrations in sinus fluid and other pharmacodynamic and pharmacokinetic properties, a recent practice management consortium has recommended fluoroquinolones, amoxicillin/clavulanate, high-dose amoxicillin, or cefdinir as initial therapy. Patients with chronic sinusitis are commonly treated for 2 to 3 weeks (poor concentration levels in sinus fluid) to achieve bacterial eradication and recovery of mucosal defense.

Although study data are limited, topical antibiotic therapy holds promise as a way to potentially overcome microbial resistance with high antibiotic concentration. One empiric regimen is mupirocin[1] ointment or cream (Bactroban) (5 g in 45 mL nasal saline), at a dose of two squirts in each nostril twice a day. Some clinicians recommend gentamicin (Garamycin)[1] (1 g in 1 L of saline) nasal irrigation if the patient is demonstrated to have a gram-negative infection. A few commercial enterprises have begun supplying compounded antibiotic powder or solution (based upon culture and sensitivity results) delivered nasally via a nebulizer.

Care must be used in targeting appropriate antimicrobial therapy to identified organisms for limited defined periods. Antibiotic overuse and *shotgunning* multiple antibiotics without culture guidance have been shown to alter normal flora competitive inhibition and to increase the potential for resistant polymicrobial infection.

Perhaps the most significant new insights into chronic sinusitis involve the concept of the upper and lower airways as a unified system with eosinophilic inflammation in the background of a large percentage of cases of respiratory tract illness. Chronic or recurrent sinusitis is strongly associated with allergic rhinitis and bronchial hyperreactivity. Strategies designed to help reduce nasal inflammation can improve mucociliary function and improve sinus ventilation and are often necessary to break a cycle of recurrent disease. Daily nasal saline lavages can help to remove allergens and bacteria. Topical cromolyn sodium (Intal)[1] can help by stabilizing mast cells but works best when started before a known allergy season. Topical nasal steroids are the most potent treatment for nasal congestion and have been shown to potentiate the treatment benefit of antibiotics in placebo-controlled trials of adult chronic sinusitis. Azelastine hydrochloride (Astelin)[1] is approved by the Food and Drug Administration (FDA) for age 12 years and older as an antihistamine nasal spray; it is particularly beneficial for symptoms of eustachian tube dysfunction. Leukotriene inhibitors (montelukast [Singulair]) recently received FDA approval for seasonal rhinitis, and study data show particular benefit when these medications are combined with oral antihistamines. Immunotherapy is generally considered for documented allergens when patients desire greater symptom relief after trying pharmacologic therapy.

[1]Not FDA approved for this indication.

Fungal disease has received significant attention recently as a possible cause of chronic sinusitis in immunocompetent patients. This conclusion is based upon the culture of fungal organisms from nasal secretions of affected patients. All normal control patients also grew fungi from nasal secretions using careful culturing techniques, which is not surprising given the ubiquitous nature of fungal spores. True allergic fungal sinusitis is characterized by nasal polyps, atopic history, and allergic mucin within sinus cavities (eosinophils, scattered fungal elements, and Charcot-Leyden crystals). Treatment usually consists of surgery, topical and systemic steroids, and immunotherapy.

Adjunctive Therapy

Common oral decongestants include phenylpropanolamine[2] and pseudoephedrine. They have not been shown to change the course of clinical respiratory tract disease, and they must be used with caution in patients younger than 3 years and older than 65 years of age, and those with a history of thyroid disease, hypertension, or depression (interaction with monoamine oxidase inhibitors). Similarly, the topical alpha agonists, such as oxymetazoline (Afrin), have not been shown to shorten the course of sinusitis, and they can lead to symptomatic rebound congestion within 1 week of use.

Guaifenesin (Robitussin) is the most commonly used mucolytic, and it is often found in combination with decongestants. High doses (up to 2400 mg per day in adults) are required for a mucous thinning effect, but side effects such as abdominal pain and nausea are common at those doses.

Daily use of nasal saline has been shown to be better than no therapy in prospective controlled studies for relief of nasal symptoms. Among nutritional therapies, vitamin C[1] and echinacea[1] have mild antihistamine effects at high doses, but, along

[1]Not FDA approved for this indication.
[2]Not available in the United States.

TABLE 1 Treatment Options for Chronic Rhinosinusitis

REDUCE VIRAL EXPOSURE
Handwashing, alcohol hand lotions
Smaller daycare
ENVIRONMENTAL IRRITANTS
Daily use of nasal saline lavages
Cessation (or avoidance) of smoking (cigarette smoke)
Avoidance of paint, perfume, chlorine (patients with chemical sensitivities)
ALLERGY MANAGEMENT
Environmental measures for dust mite and mold
Oral antihistamines
Nasal antihistamines
Leukotriene receptor antagonists (montelukast [Singulair])
Nasal steroids
Systemic steroid burst
Allergy immunotherapy
GASTROESOPHAGEAL REFLUX MANAGEMENT
H_2 blockers
Proton pump inhibitors
ANTIBIOTIC THERAPY
Topical antibiotic sprays
High-dose amoxicillin (Amoxil)
Fluoroquinolones
Amoxicillin/clavulanate (Augmentin)
Cefdinir (Omnicef)
SURGERY
Adenoidectomy (usually young children)
Inferior turbinate reduction (chronic congestion)
Endoscopic ethmoidectomy, middle meatus antrostomies

with zinc[1] and goldenseal[1], they have not been shown to prevent or to speed resolution of sinusitis.

Sinusitis is a potential endpoint of many etiologic pathways. The problem of chronic sinusitis is rarely solved simply by trying to match an antibiotic to the suspected bacterial culprit. Strategies to reduce underlying mucosal inflammation to help restore sinus ventilation and local mucociliary defense are necessary to break a cycle of recurrent infection. Referral to an otolaryngologist should be considered for refractory symptoms, persistent polyposis, disease in an immunocompromised patient, or concern for developing orbital or intracranial infection. In general, surgery is reserved for the small percentage of patients with image-documented, persistent symptomatic disease after completing an appropriate hierarchy of medical options (Table 1).

[1]Not FDA approved for this indication.

NONALLERGIC RHINITIS

METHOD OF

James Temprano, MD, MHA, and
Mark Dykewicz, MD

Rhinitis is an inflammation of the membranes that line the nose. Symptoms include rhinorrhea, sneezing, nasal congestion, itching of the nose, postnasal drainage, and conjunctivitis. Rhinitis can be categorized as allergic, nonallergic, or both (Table 1). Allergic rhinitis is characterized by immunoglobulin (Ig) E and allergen reactions in the nose, however, the nonallergic forms of rhinitis do not result from these events. Nonallergic rhinitis encompasses several different pathologic forms of rhinitis and includes:

- Nonallergic rhinitis with eosinophilia
- Vasomotor rhinitis
- Infectious rhinitis
- Occupational rhinitis
- Hormonal rhinitis
- Drug-induced rhinitis
- Atrophic rhinitis
- Gustatory or food-related rhinitis
- Mechanical or anatomic rhinitis

Nonallergic rhinitis has been estimated to comprise approximately 30% to 50% of patients presenting with rhinitis symptoms. Nonallergic rhinitis more commonly affects females, patients during adult life, and those with perennial symptoms. Additionally, patients with nonallergic rhinitis are less likely to have nasal or ocular pruritus than those with allergic rhinitis.

Pathophysiology and Classification

VASOMOTOR RHINITIS

Vasomotor rhinitis (VMR) is a noneosinophilic nonallergic rhinitis that is characterized by chronic nasal symptoms that are not immunologic or infectious in etiology. It is the most common form of nonallergic rhinitis, comprising 61% in one study. VMR is a diagnosis of exclusion, so other causes of rhinitis (allergy, infection, anatomic abnormalities, and nonallergic rhinitis with eosinophilia syndrome [NARES]) must be ruled out. Although the etiology of VMR is not known, biopsies of nasal mucosa reveal findings similar to normal individuals; namely, a noninflammatory cellular infiltration. However, mast cell activation through a nonimmunologic pathway may contribute to the symptoms found in VMR.

TABLE 1 Nonallergic and Allergic Rhinitis

	Nonallergic Rhinitis	Allergic Rhinitis
Historical features:		
Age of onset	>20-30 y	<20-30 y
Timing	Usually perennial but may vary with weather changes	Seasonal or perennial
Exacerbating factors	Temperature, humidity, irritants (perfumes, scents, tobacco smoke)	Allergen exposure
Prominent associated symptoms or diseases	Postnasal drainage Congestion Anosmia (NARES)	Pruritus Sneezing Postnasal drainage Congestion Ocular symptoms Asthma
Physical examination	Variable, but nasal mucosa is often erythematous	Variable, but often pale nasal mucosa and turbinates boggy
Nasal cytology	Nasal eosinophils positive in NARES Nasal eosinophils negative in VMR	Nasal eosinophils positive
Skin tests	Negative (may be positive without correlating history of symptoms upon acute allergen exposure)	Positive
Serum total IgE	Normal	Elevated
Response to oral antihistamines	Usually not beneficial	Usually beneficial

Abbreviations: Ig = immunoglobulin; NARES = nonallergic rhinitis with eosinophilia syndrome; VMR = vasomotor rhinitis.

Patients typically present in adult life with a variety of symptoms. Patients are less commonly affected by pruritus, conjunctival symptoms, and sneezing. Their symptoms are more likely to be perennial and precipitated by environmental factors such as tobacco smoke, odors, perfumes, weather changes, and cold air. Additionally, patients may have sinusitis complaints such as headache and postnasal drip. Although allergy skin testing is usually negative, patients may have concurrent allergic rhinitis with positive skin tests.

NONALLERGIC RHINITIS WITH EOSINOPHILIA SYNDROME

Nonallergic rhinitis with eosinophilia syndrome consists of marked nasal eosinophilia (>25%) on nasal smear and perennial symptoms, but lacks a clinically significant positive skin test and/or specific IgE antibodies in the serum. NARES represents 15% to 33% of adults with nonallergic rhinitis. Although the pathophysiology is not completely understood, the presence of eosinophilia may lead to nasal mucosa dysfunction secondary to the release of eosinophilic substances such as major basic protein and eosinophilic cationic protein. The subsequent damage to the nasal mucosa from these proteins may prolong mucociliary clearance and lead to an increased risk of infection. Severe forms of NARES have been associated with asthma, sinusitis, and aspirin sensitivity. The presence of nasal eosinophilia in nonallergic rhinitis usually correlates with a good response to treatment with intranasal glucocorticoids. Blood eosinophilia nonallergic rhinitis syndrome (BENARS) is an associated disorder that has elevated levels of blood eosinophils in conjunction with the features characteristic of NARES. The frequency of this disorder has been purported to be 4% in those with nonallergic rhinitis.

BASOPHILIC/METACHROMATIC NASAL DISEASE

Similar to NARES, nasal mastocytosis—basophilic/metachromatic nasal disease—requires a histologic diagnosis. Although the etiology is unknown, the syndrome is characterized by mast cell infiltration (>2000/mm^3) without nasal eosinophilia. Patients are more likely to present with rhinorrhea and nasal congestion without an associated pruritus or sneezing.

INFECTIOUS RHINITIS

Infectious rhinitis can be subdivided into acute and chronic forms. Acute infectious rhinitis is of recent onset and is usually secondary to infection by one of many different viruses. Most commonly, human rhinovirus is the etiologic agent. It can also be caused by bacterial or fungal organisms, or become complicated by a bacterial infection with subsequent sinus involvement. Chronic forms also exist, most commonly associated with bacterial sinusitis, and are characterized by mucopurulent nasal discharge, inflammation of the nose and paranasal sinuses with facial pain and pressure, postnasal drainage with cough, and olfactory disturbances. The bacterial organisms that are most commonly involved in chronic rhinosinusitis are *Streptococcus pneumoniae*, *Staphylococcus aureus*, *Haemophilus influenzae*, and *Moraxella catarrhalis*.

OCCUPATIONAL RHINITIS

Occupational rhinitis is sneezing, nasal discharge, and nasal obstruction that are found in association with the workplace. Causes of occupational rhinitis can be of allergic or nonallergic origin. Common triggers include detergents, formalin, chlorine, and ammonia. Common workplace aeroallergens include psyllium (ingredient in bulk laxatives), guar gum (used as a food thickening agent, fixator of dyes to fabrics, rubber cable insulator), latex, western red cedar, trimellitic anhydride (industrial chemical used as a plasticizer), and diisocyanates (foundry workers, foam makers, and spray painters) to name a few. Symptoms usually resolve upon removal from the workplace, but patients may have an isolated late reaction that does not become apparent until leaving the workplace. Additionally, it may take several days for symptoms to resolve in patients who have chronic exposure. Occupational rhinitis may coexist with occupational asthma.

ENDOCRINE OR HORMONAL RHINITIS

Pregnancy, hypothyroidism, and acromegaly can be causes of nonallergic rhinitis. The exact mechanism and causal effect in which pregnancy contributes to rhinitis symptoms are not known but are likely multifactorial. Possible mechanisms that may increase nasal congestion and obstruction during pregnancy are an increase in the circulating plasma volume and progesterone-induced smooth muscle relaxation. Additionally, increased nasal mucous gland hyperactivity occurs, which leads to increased rhinorrhea. Acromegaly causes turbinate hypertrophy, and hypothyroidism can lead to myxedematous deposits in the turbinates leading to rhinitis.

DRUG-INDUCED RHINITIS

Several medications can be a cause of nonallergic rhinitis, including antihypertensives (angiotensin-converting enzyme inhibitors, reserpine, guanethidine, phentolamine, methyldopa, hydralazine, clonidine, α_1-adrenergic antagonists, β blockers), chlorpromazine, aspirin, NSAIDs, and oral contraceptives. Rhinitis medicamentosa results from the overuse of topical nasal decongestants or vasoconstrictor nasal medications such as oxymetazoline or phenylephrine. This form of rhinitis can also be the result of cocaine abuse, which is characterized by nasal congestion. Physical examination demonstrates a reddened, congested nasal mucosa that may have areas of punctate bleeding. The rebound swelling present in this disorder is caused by interstitial edema rather than vasodilation.

ATROPHIC RHINITIS

This disorder is most commonly seen in undeveloped countries where hygiene is poor, but it is also seen as a rare complication of radical nasal tissue removal to relieve an obstruction. Symptoms most notably consist of nasal congestion, severe crusting, a foul odor in the nose, and *Klebsiella pneumoniae ozaenae* colonization. The nasal cavities also become enlarged, and squamous metaplasia of the nasal epithelium is seen on microscopic examination.

GUSTATORY OR FOOD-RELATED RHINITIS

There are multiple mechanisms that can account for rhinitis that occurs after the ingestion of foods or alcohol. Food allergy is an unusual cause of rhinitis without an associated gastrointestinal, dermatologic, or systemic reaction. The oral allergy syndrome is characterized by oral allergic reactions to foods that have cross-reacting allergenic determinants to tree pollens to which the patient is sensitive. Rhinorrhea after the ingestion of spicy foods likely occurs as a consequence of the capsaicin content in these foods that stimulates sensory nerve fibers. Other etiologies include vagally mediated mechanisms and nasal vasodilation.

MECHANICAL OR ANATOMIC RHINITIS

There are several conditions that can produce symptoms consistent with rhinitis. Some of the more common causes include nasal septal deviation, tumors, enlarged nasal turbinates, dysfunctional nasal valve, and, especially in children, adenoidal hypertrophy. It is important to exclude these causes during the workup of nonallergic rhinitis as these conditions account for approximately 5% to 10% of chronic nasal disorders. Nasal septal deviation, when moderate to severe, can be complicated by sinusitis, snoring, sleep apnea, and fatigue.

A rare cause of rhinorrhea is a cerebrospinal (CSF) fluid leak. This usually occurs within 48 hours of trauma or as a complication of surgery; delayed onset can be seen however. A CSF leak can be distinguished from rhinorrhea by testing for the presence of glucose in the nasal secretions. CSF contains glucose, while nasal mucous does not.

Granulomatous and vasculitic diseases may also be causes of rhinitis symptoms. Etiologies include Churg-Strauss vasculitis, systemic lupus erythematosus, relapsing polychondritis, Sjögren's syndrome, sarcoidosis, and Wegener's granulomatosis.

NASAL POLYPS

Nasal polyps may present with nasal obstruction, rhinorrhea, anosmia, and snoring. Nasal polyps are pale, gelatinous outgrowths of the nasal mucosa that are often associated with aspirin sensitivity, intrinsic asthma, and chronic sinusitis. They are also seen in cystic fibrosis (especially when found in children), ciliary dyskinesis, or Kartagener's syndrome (bronchiectasis, chronic sinusitis, and nasal polyps), Young's syndrome (sinopulmonary disease, azoospermia, and nasal polyps), and Churg-Strauss syndrome. Although nasal polyps may occur in patients with allergic rhinitis, allergy as the underlying etiology of nasal polyps has not been established.

Diagnosis

The first step in diagnosis should be a careful history with attention to seasonal variation, coexisting symptoms or illnesses, exacerbating factors, responses to medications, and possible environmental exposures. Concomitant symptoms that should be inquired about include the presence of conjunctivitis, pruritus, asthma, postnasal drip, sneezing, and congestion.

Although physical examination is not diagnostic of allergic or nonallergic rhinitis, an inspection of the nose should be made to exclude mechanical or anatomic factors as causes of the patient's symptoms. Particular attention should be made to detect the presence of septal deviation or perforations, nasal polyps, enlarged nasal turbinates, and tumors.

Testing for specific IgE antibodies is an integral part of the evaluation of rhinitis. This can be performed through skin testing or in vitro tests. It is important to note that the presence of a positive test is not sufficient to make a diagnosis of allergic rhinitis and does not rule out the possibility of a coexisting nonallergic etiology. A diagnosis of allergic rhinitis should be made by correlating a positive test with a history of symptoms upon exposure to a corresponding allergen. However, a negative test will give firm support to a diagnosis of a nonallergic cause of the patient's symptoms. Another adjunct in the evaluation of rhinitis is the use of rhinopharyngoscopy or CT scanning. This can be used to further define any possible anatomic factors that may be causing or contributing to the patient's symptoms.

Management

The first step in the management of rhinitis of any cause is to control environmental factors that may be contributing to the patient's symptoms. The patient and clinician should identify any possible inciting factors (irritants, medications, occupational exposures) and institute proper avoidance measures. Although nonallergic rhinitis is usually more difficult to treat than allergic rhinitis, there are also several forms of pharmacologic therapy available. The patient's underlying form of rhinitis should be considered in order to tailor specific treatment.

The mainstays of treatment of nonallergic rhinitis are topical glucocorticoids and topical antihistamines. Intranasal glucocorticoids are used as a first-line therapy in the treatment of nonallergic rhinitis. The intranasal glucocorticoid preparations have not been shown to cause significant systemic side effects in adults. Patients should be taught proper technique and avoid spraying directly on the nasal septum as irritation and bleeding may occur. Additionally, the clinician should periodically examine the nasal septum for mucosal erosions that may precede the development of septal perforations.

Azelastine (Astelin) nasal spray is a topical antihistamine that is used for both allergic and nonallergic rhinitis. Azelastine nasal spray has been shown to improve all symptoms of VMR (congestion, rhinorrhea, postnasal drainage, and sneezing). Oral antihistamines are not indicated for treatment of nonallergic rhinitis. Patients should be counseled on possible side effects such as bitter taste and sedation (secondary to significant systemic absorption).

Symptom-directed therapies are also beneficial in the treatment of nonallergic rhinitis. Decongestants are of benefit in patients with mostly obstructive symptoms, however, they are not effective in the treatment of pruritus, rhinorrhea, or sneezing. Side effects include insomnia, nervousness, loss of appetite, and urinary retention in males. These agents should also be used cautiously in patients who have hypertension, hyperthyroidism, angina, or arrhythmias.

Intranasal anticholinergics (e.g., ipratropium bromide [Atrovent]) are effective in patients that complain chiefly of rhinorrhea. These agents do not have a significant effect on other symptoms of rhinitis. Side effects are usually minimal, but may include nasal dryness or epistaxis. Systemic anticholinergic effects have not been associated with its use.

Intranasal saline can be an important adjunct to therapy. Frequent irrigation of the nose with saline can relieve symptoms of nasal congestion, sneezing, and postnasal drip. It may be of additional benefit when used in conjunction with other therapies.

Surgical management may also be considered in select populations. These are generally patients who are refractory to medical therapy or who have an anatomic or mechanical etiology for their rhinitis symptoms. Turbinectomy or parasympathectomy may be options.

Special Considerations

Certain causes of rhinitis deserve special attention with regard to treatment. Hormonal rhinitis associated with pregnancy is often initially treated with nasal saline and avoidance measures secondary to concerns for safety. However, intranasal steroids are often required for symptom relief. Decongestants should be avoided in the first trimester of pregnancy, because there is a risk of gastroschisis in the newborn.

The treatment of rhinitis medicamentosa requires discontinuation of the topical decongestant and treatment of the patient's underlying rhinitis. Initially, a topical corticosteroid should be used, but a short course of oral steroids may be required to allow discontinuation of the nasal decongestant.

HOARSENESS AND LARYNGITIS

METHOD OF

Robert Buckmire, MD

Hoarseness is a nonspecific complaint that connotes a subjective change in voice production. As a presenting complaint, hoarseness often means something different to patients than it does to the clinician. Further questioning is required to appropriately determine the patient's specific voice-related complaints. Common specific complaints include complete intermittent voice loss (aphonia), loss of vocal range, vocal fatigue, and generalized change in voice quality (dysphonia). If the patient is a singer, a more complete delineation of voice symptoms and complaints is warranted. The voice complaints of singers often involve loss of singing endurance, pitch control, and a reduction of vocal range. These discrete deficits may not be as readily apparent in the speaking voice.

Laryngitis is another nonspecific complaint that connotes a generalized, persistent change in voice quality. When used in a medical setting, laryngitis suggests an inflammatory process of the vocal folds commonly caused by infection or vocal trauma (coughing, screaming).

Hoarseness is a common early symptom of laryngeal cancer. Therefore, any persistent voice change lasting longer than 2 weeks in duration requires detailed evaluation to ascertain the etiology. This article focuses on the most common causes of persistent voice changes and their treatments.

Muscle Tension Dysphonia

Muscle tension dysphonia (MTD) is a common voice disorder characterized by inappropriate or excessive use of the intralaryngeal and extralaryngeal musculature during speech. Patients with this disorder typically present with hoarseness and vocal fatigue as primary complaints. Other associated symptoms may include loss of vocal range and frequent sore throats exacerbated by voice use. The cause of this disorder is unknown, but it is often associated with periods of vocal overuse, misuse, or immediately following viral upper respiratory symptoms. The condition specifically involves a maladaptive compensatory behavior, overusing the extralaryngeal muscles (such as the strap muscles), as well as the intralaryngeal muscles, resulting in the common symptom profile. Muscle tension dysphonia is most often successfully treated with behavioral voice therapy. The therapeutic regimen is designed to produce a more efficient and appropriate technique for voice production. The prognosis for improvement of dysphonia from MTD with voice therapy is excellent. A typical course of therapy requires only 8 to 12 sessions.

Neurologic Voice Disorders

There are a variety of neurologic disorders that affect voice quality and voice production. Parkinson's disease, essential tremor, and spasmodic dysphonia are all fairly common neurogenic causes of dysphonia. *Parkinson's disease* causes a classic constellation of communication difficulties consisting of soft voice and rapid and slurred speech. One of the major communication disorder components of Parkinson's disease appears to involve an inability of patients to monitor their own vocal volume. The Lee Silverman Voice Training Program (LSVT) was specifically developed to address improving the communication disorder associated with Parkinson's disease and has been shown to be highly efficacious. LSVT is administered by a speech pathologist and requires a specialized form of speech therapy four times per week for 1 month (approximately 16 to 20 sessions). The improvement gained from the LSVT program is best maintained when the patient continues the home exercises on a long-term basis.

Essential tremor resulting in hoarseness can occur, specifically in the larynx or, more diffusely, throughout the upper aerodigestive tract and head and neck region. This causes a periodic alteration (tremor) to the voice production that is often mistakenly associated with an aging voice. When this tremor is quite severe, it can significantly disrupt normal communication ability. It is primarily treated with pharmacologic agents for the essential tremor. Adjunctive treatment with voice therapy techniques and intralaryngeal botulinum toxin (Botox) injection are helpful in selected patients with this disorder.

Spasmodic dysphonia is a focal dystonia of the laryngeal musculature, with an unknown etiology. The voice symptoms of this disorder are characterized by severe disruption of the normal fluency of voice production and voice breaks. Patients typically feel as if they cannot "get their voice out" and have a strained/strangled voice quality and sensation. This disorder is treated successfully with intralaryngeal botulinum toxin injections and occasionally with voice therapy after the injections.

Voice Disorders Associated with Aging

Voice disorders related to the aging process have recently gained greater visibility because a growing portion of the aging population remains highly active. These voice problems are typically related to a loss of muscle bulk or atrophy of the vocal fold musculature, resulting in a weak voice, decreased vocal range, and vocal fatigue. After exclusion of focal neurologic or specific anatomic voice pathology, the treatment for this condition is voice therapy. In general, eight to ten sessions of voice therapy are highly successful (>85%). Some patients who have a voice disorder associated with severe symptoms caused by the aging process and have significant vocal demands require vocal fold augmentation by such means as medialization thyroplasty or injection laryngoplasty. When necessary, these surgical techniques are usually successful in improving the specific voice complaints of elderly voice users.

Vocal Fold Lesions

Vocal fold polyps, nodules, and cysts are common benign lesions of the true vocal folds that cause dysphonia. They can reliably be distinguished from one another only by a thorough laryngoscopic examination including videostrobolaryngoscopy.

VOCAL NODULES

Vocal nodules (often referred to in the singing community as nodes) are localized, benign, superficial growths on the medial surface of the true vocal cords that are commonly believed to be the result of a pattern of vocal misuse and abuse. Nodules are bilateral in nature and are classically located at the junction of the anterior third and the middle third of the vocal fold. They are most often seen in women 20 to 50 years of age, but are also commonly seen in children (boys more often than girls) who are prone to excessive loud talking or screaming.

Treatment

Treatment for nodules always involves a course of behavioral voice therapy. Patient compliance is paramount because the therapy is designed to correct the etiologic vocal behaviors. Surgical intervention is inappropriate as a first-line therapy. It may be considered, however, in the rare case in which the patient strictly complies with the prescribed course of therapy but is still left with an unacceptable vocal impairment. (If performed, surgery must be limited to the most superficial layers of the vocal fold, preserving the uninvolved surrounding lamina propria.)

VOCAL FOLD POLYPS

Vocal fold polyps are generally unilateral and have a broad spectrum of appearances from pedunculated to sessile. They too are believed to result from vocal abuse, however, they can arise from a single episode of abusive behavior or hemorrhage. Polyps typically involve the free (medial) edge of the vocal fold mucosa. Their mass contributes to altered vocal fold vibration and interferes with glottic closure, both of which cause the resultant symptom of dysphonia.

Treatment

Most experts believe that these lesions are most directly related to vocal use, vocal technique, and their resultant phonotrauma. Treatment is aimed at correcting the underlying causative factors, largely through voice therapy and vocal education. Following voice therapy, if significant dysphonia persists, surgery is indicated. The recommended technique is a minimally invasive, microlaryngoscopic procedure, preserving the uninvolved epithelial cover and surrounding submucosal tissue. When voice therapy and surgery are used appropriately and combined with a compliant patient, the voice outcome is usually excellent.

VOCAL FOLD CYSTS

Vocal fold cysts are focal abnormalities of the superficial lamina propria and are predominantly unilateral. Intracordal mucous retention cysts are believed to arise after blockage of a glandular duct. Another type of cyst found in the vocal folds, epidermoid cysts, is similar to those found in the skin and tends to be smaller in size. Both varieties appear as well-circumscribed spherical masses beneath intact, normal-appearing epithelial lining.

Treatment

Treatment of these lesions consists of a surgical microlarynologic approach with creation of a flap of the overlying epithelium that will be entirely preserved and returned after removal of the lesion. This approach allows for the expedient return of proper glottic closure and vocal fold vibration previously interrupted by this intracordal mass lesion. Pre- and postoperative voice therapy is a key component to successful treatment.

RECURRENT RESPIRATORY PAPILLOMA

Recurrent respiratory papilloma (RRP) is a benign neoplastic lesion most commonly affecting the glottis and resulting in dysphonia and occasionally airway embarrassment. This papillomatous alteration of the squamous epithelium affects both children and adults and is caused by the human papilloma virus. Lesions may be self-limited or progressive, and, depending upon the site of involvement as well as the size of the patient's airway, symptoms may range from mild dysphonia to frank stridor and airway obstruction. Malignant transformation to squamous cell carcinoma is exceedingly rare, but has been documented. The course of disease typically involves recurrence and unpredictable remissions. Death from this disease is usually associated with complications of repeated surgical therapy or respiratory failure caused by distal spread of extralaryngeal disease. Aggressive cases in children may require extremely frequent surgical treatments (1 to 2 per month) and/or tracheotomy to preserve the airway.

Treatment

Surgical excision of RRP lesions is the mainstay of therapy with either CO_2 laser or cold steel excision.

Adjuvant medical therapy is also available. The most common of these medications is interferon alfa-2b (Intron A). Typical doses include 5 million U/m^2 of body surface in a subcutaneous injection daily to initiate therapy, and then 3 million U/m^2 3 days a week over 6 months. This treatment regimen has been shown to effectively slow RRP growth, but it is not curative. Cidofovir (Vistide)[1], a nucleoside analogue, antiviral agent, has been administered by injection and has shown some significant success in topical treatment of recurrent papillomatous lesions. Several different concentrations of the medication have been used clinically in both adults and children. Long-term recurrence rates and frequency as well as local tissue side effects, such as postinjection scar formation, remain to be fully quantified.

VOCAL FOLD GRANULOMA

Vocal fold granuloma is characterized by a mass lesion of the glottis located posteriorly near the vocal process of the arytenoids. Granulomata may take on a myriad of appearances from irregular to smooth and pedunculated to broad based. They are multifactorial in origin; common correlates include intubation trauma, laryngopharyngeal reflux disease, and vocally abusive behaviors.

Treatment

Treatment of granulomata is similarly multifactorial. Surgical removal of these lesions without further therapy leads to frequent recurrences. Multifaceted treatments, including behavioral modification and gastric acid-lowering medications (proton pump inhibitors), are now the mainstays of therapy. Omeprazole (Prilosec)[1], 20 to 40 mg twice daily, is a typical starting dose. Adjunctive intralaryngeal botulinum toxin injections have also been used successfully in selected recalcitrant cases. Medical therapy for gastroesophageal reflux disease (GERD) in conjunction with behavioral voice therapy to eliminate vocally traumatic behaviors has, for the most part, supplanted surgical excision for these lesions and should always be employed prior to surgical intervention.

LEUKOPLAKIA AND ERYTHROPLAKIA

Leukoplakia and erythroplakia refer to discrete areas of abnormal epithelium within the larynx. The normal vocal fold epithelium is a nonkeratinized stratified squamous cell lining. Alterations in this covering epithelium often appear as discolored (whitish or erythematous) plaques. The altered stiffness and thickness of these areas cause dysphonia that is often the only associated symptom. These changes are often associated with a history of tobacco use.

Treatment

Because of the risk of premalignant change or frank malignancy, these lesions must be biopsied and submitted for histologic evaluation. Complete excision by delicate phonomicrosurgical techniques is ideal for the evaluation of surgical margins and to achieve an optimal postoperative voice result. In the case of a circumscribed, superficially invasive carcinoma, this may serve as both a diagnostic and therapeutic modality.

VOCAL FOLD PARALYSIS (VOCAL FOLD IMMOBILITY)

Normal vocal fold motion involves wide abduction (away from the midline) during inspiration as well as coordinated glottic closure during phonation and swallowing. When a unilateral vocal fold is found to be immobile, the glottis is generally incompetent in adduction resulting in some level of dysphonia. Associated vocal fatigue and potential aspiration during swallowing may also be present. In cases of bilateral immobility, the vocal folds are generally found in the paramedian position allowing for good voice but poor air exchange, and, therefore, patients suffer from airway compromise. When either condition is diagnosed, a search for the cause should be instituted. History of systemic disease and past surgical interventions should be elicited. Imaging of the course of neural supply to the larynx, including chest radiograph and computed tomography (CT) or magnetic resonance imaging (MRI) from the skull base through the mediastinum, are necessary to rule out occult neoplastic lesions. Common etiologies of vocal fold immobility include paralysis secondary to vagal or recurrent laryngeal nerve injury from thyroid, carotid, or chest surgery. It must be borne in mind, however, that vocal folds may also be immobile secondary to cricoarytenoid joint dysfunction with an entirely intact nerve supply. A laryngeal electromyogram (EMG) performed within 6 months after the onset of this diagnosis is helpful in establishing the status of the neural innervation as well as providing important prognostic information in a timely manner.

Treatment

Treatment for unilateral vocal fold immobility is dependent upon the resultant deficits and physiologic impact. Dysphonia in the absence of aspiration may be amenable to both voice therapy and surgical intervention. The therapeutic decision-making is generally based upon the patient's desire for an improved voice and the glottic configuration on laryngoscopic examination. Small glottic chinks associated with an immobile vocal fold in the paramedian position may be well treated with voice therapy alone. Significant dysphonia secondary to a larger glottic gap may be treated with injection laryngoplasty techniques (fat, gelfoam, or collagen) or medialization laryngoplasty.

[1]Not FDA approved for this indication.

Larger levels of glottic incompetence are more likely to require medialization thyroplasty (laryngeal framework surgery) designed to statically position the immobile vocal fold in a phonatory posture. Patients may also benefit from an additional arytenoid adduction procedure to better close the posterior glottic chink. Aspiration is an indication for surgical intervention whether temporary or permanent in scope. This decision must be based upon the mechanism of injury and the likelihood of recovery. Procedures to improve closure are employed early in the course of the disease to avoid the potentially devastating complications of aspiration pneumonia.

Laryngopharyngeal Reflux Disease

Reflux laryngitis is caused by the effects of gastric secretions on the mucosal lining of the larynx. The classically described changes include interarytenoid edema and erythema, as well as posterior laryngeal pachydermia (heaped up thickened tissue). In severe cases, posterior glottic ulceration and granulation tissue are seen. These changes may be associated with symptoms of heartburn or dyspepsia, but absence of symptoms in no way excludes the clinical diagnosis. Commonly associated pharyngeal symptoms include excessive thick pharyngeal mucus, throat clearing, globus sensation, and dysphonia. Dysphonia is a result of altered glottic closure and inflammation from the posterior glottic changes. Objective confirmation of pathologic reflux disease may be established by means of a multiple channel, ambulatory pH probe.

TREATMENT

Ideal treatment of reflux laryngitis is multifactorial. Lifestyle changes such as elevation of the head of bed, avoiding meals several hours prior to recumbency, and weight reduction programs are important in the management of this condition. Diet should include avoidance of acidic foods and foods that promote reflux (tomato-based foods, caffeine, alcohol, etc.). Adjuvant medical therapy involves lowering the amount of gastric acid production. Antacids, H_2 blockers, and proton pump inhibitors are effective medications, although cases of medication resistance are occasionally seen. Surgical intervention addressing the lower esophageal sphincter is also available for particularly refractory cases. With significant glottic changes, aggressive medical therapy might begin with omeprazole (Prilosec)[1], 20 mg orally twice daily, in conjunction with the previously mentioned lifestyle and dietary modifications.

Acute Laryngitis

The term *laryngitis* refers to a nonspecific inflammatory condition affecting the larynx and resulting in dysphonia or hoarseness. The causes of this condition are numerous and include all forms of infection or trauma including viral and bacterial pathogens, intubation trauma, blunt neck trauma, vocal trauma, and laryngopharyngeal reflux disease, to name a few. In general, an acute voice change persisting for more than 2 weeks duration is an indication for a laryngeal examination.

TREATMENT

The therapeutic modality chosen is entirely dependent upon the suspected cause of the laryngitis. By far the most common transient cause of this complaint is an inflammation associated with an upper respiratory viral infection. Treatment for this condition should be expectant with attention to good hydration and reduced voice use (not voice rest). Bacterial and fungal laryngotracheitis are diagnosed by laryngeal visualization in association with appropriate symptoms. Bacterial infection is suspected with prolonged symptoms of dysphonia, productive cough, and fever and is generally well treated by full course therapy with a broad spectrum oral antibiotic that covers oropharyngeal flora. Treatment of fungal laryngitis typically requires a systemic antifungal such as fluconazole (Diflucan), 200 mg orally the first day followed by 100 mg daily for the rest of the prescribed course. These infections are uncommon unless concurrent steroid use or some form of immunosuppression is present. Topical antifungal preparations (Nystatin oral suspension [Nilstat]) may be sufficient for the treatment of mild cases.

[1]Not FDA approved for this indication.

STREPTOCOCCAL PHARYNGITIS

METHOD OF

Preeti Jaggi, MD, and Stanford T. Shulman, MD

Acute pharyngitis, inflammation of the posterior pharynx, is usually caused by viral pathogens. However, it is important to consider that beta-hemolytic streptococci cause acute bacterial pharyngitis in both children and adults. Group A [β-hemolytic] streptococci (GAS) account for approximately 15% to 30% of acute pharyngitis in children and 5% to 10% in adults. Children 5 to 11 years of age have the highest incidence of GAS pharyngitis, although it occurs in other age groups as well. The major justification for accurate diagnosis and treatment of GAS pharyngitis is the prevention of acute rheumatic fever (ARF) and rheumatic heart disease (RHD). In temperate climates, GAS pharyngitis is more common during the winter and early spring months. The incubation period for streptococcal pharyngitis is short (2 to 5 days). Transmission occurs with close contact via inhalation of organisms in large droplets or by direct contact with respiratory secretions.

Distinguishing Viral from Group A Streptococci Pharyngitis

One of the most crucial decisions to make in evaluating a patient with pharyngitis is whether to perform a bacterial culture (or rapid antigen test) of the throat for GAS. The clinician must keep in mind two important principles. First, accurate detection and treatment of GAS pharyngitis are needed to prevent ARF and other complications. Second, the practice of unnecessarily performing pharyngeal bacterial cultures in patients who present with typical viral pharyngitis symptoms will result in the misdiagnosis of GAS pharyngitis in asymptomatic chronic GAS carriers who have an intercurrent viral illness. Treatment of the GAS carrier state with antimicrobials is unlikely to terminate carriage, results in patient apprehension, and contributes to the increasing problem of antibiotic resistance.

Pharyngitis that is accompanied by rhinitis, stridor, hoarseness, conjunctivitis, cough, and/or diarrhea is highly likely to have a viral etiology; it is generally unnecessary to obtain a bacterial throat culture when these symptoms are present. Symptoms such as an abrupt onset of fever, throat pain, headache, abdominal pain and dysphagia, and signs such as exudative pharyngitis, palatal petechiae, uvulitis, and tender anterior cervical nodes are suggestive of GAS pharyngitis. In addition, the absence of rhinitis, hoarseness, conjunctivitis, and cough are more suggestive of GAS pharyngitis. Patients who have symptoms persisting longer than 4 to 5 days at the time of presentation are unlikely to have GAS pharyngitis, as it is a self-limited illness that usually lasts 3 to 5 days.

If it is determined that the constellation of signs and symptoms suggests GAS pharyngitis, patients should be tested for GAS using a throat swab of the posterior pharynx. Relying on clinical impression alone to decide if treatment is warranted results in the gross over-diagnosis of GAS pharyngitis and is strongly discouraged. Children younger than 3 years of age uncommonly develop GAS pharyngitis and almost never develop acute rheumatic fever. A positive throat culture from a patient with exudative pharyngitis in this age group is much more likely to be viral than streptococcal in origin.

Throat Cultures

Throat culture has long served as the gold standard for diagnosis of GAS pharyngitis. One of the most important factors resulting in a false-negative throat culture is inadequate specimen acquisition. It is optimal to rub both tonsils and the posterior pharyngeal wall with a cotton or synthetic fiber-tipped swab. Specimens should be inoculated promptly or placed in transport media, then inoculated onto 5% sheep blood agar and incubated in an aerobic chamber with 5% to 10% CO_2 at 37°C for at least 24 hours. If there are no β-hemolytic bacteria growing after 24 hours, the plate should be reincubated for another 24 hours.

By microscopy, GAS appear as gram-positive cocci in pairs and chains. On blood agar, they form gray-white colonies with a zone of β hemolysis (a clear rim that surrounds the colonies). Normal oral flora may be a hemolytic (with a green rim that surrounds the colonies) or γ-hemolytic (with no zone of hemolysis). Other β-hemolytic streptococci include groups B (*Streptococcus agalactiae*), C, G, and F.

Because the throat culture results in delayed diagnosis, rapid antigen detection systems for identification of GAS have been developed to allow prompt diagnosis of GAS pharyngitis. Standard rapid antigen tests generally have a very high specificity rate (95% to 98%), but their sensitivity rate varies from 70% to 90%. Sensitivity rate varies with inoculum quantity and technical expertise in processing and interpreting the sample. A presumptive diagnosis of GAS pharyngitis can, therefore, be made with a positive standard rapid antigen test for GAS (and confirmatory testing is not needed), but many experts believe a negative test should be confirmed by a throat culture. Standard rapid antigen detection tests use enzyme-linked immunoabsorbent assays (ELISA); another category of a highly sensitive rapid antigen detection system has been developed using optical immunoassay (OIA) technology. Rapid antigen tests using OIA have been shown in some studies, but not others, to be as sensitive as a throat culture performed in the office setting; some experts recommend that a backup throat culture is not needed if a high-sensitivity rapid antigen test is negative. This, however, remains controversial; therefore, if physicians wish to rely upon a high-sensitivity rapid antigen test alone, they may consider confirming the reliability of the assay in comparative studies with throat cultures among their own patients before implementing this test without backup cultures in daily practice.

Serologic testing for acute GAS pharyngitis is not generally useful, as antistreptococcal antibodies rise only weeks after infection. Antibodies against streptolysin O, deoxyribonuclease B (DNAse B), hyaluronidase, and streptokinase are sometimes used to confirm a recent (but not current) GAS infection. Assessing these antistreptococcal antibodies is most useful for those in whom the likelihood of culturing GAS is poor but confirmation of a recent GAS illness is needed, such as in ARF or poststreptococcal glomerulonephritis.

Initial Therapy (Table 1)

Accurate diagnosis and treatment of acute GAS pharyngitis reduce suppurative complications (such as retropharyngeal or peritonsillar abscesses) and transmission of GAS, and, to a limited degree, shortens the duration of pharyngeal symptoms. In addition, it reduces the risk of acute rheumatic fever. Therapy has not been shown to reduce the risk of acute poststreptococcal glomerulonephritis. Prevention of acute rheumatic fever is most effective if therapy is initiated within 9 days of onset of symptoms. Although GAS pharyngitis is self-limited, appropriate treatment leads to resolution of symptoms approximately 1 day earlier than without antibiotic therapy.

GAS remain universally sensitive to penicillin, and this drug remains the first-line therapy for GAS pharyngitis (as recommended by the American Academy of Pediatrics, the American Heart Association, and the Infectious Disease Society of America) because of its narrow spectrum, low cost, and proven efficacy. A clinical isolate of GAS that is resistant to penicillin or a cephalosporin *in vitro* has never been documented. Parenteral therapy can be given if needed to ensure compliance, and a single intramuscular dose of benzathine penicillin G (Bicillin L-A) is bactericidal for up to 28 days. However, parenteral penicillin is a painful injection and is associated with more serious allergic reactions than is oral therapy. Therefore, many prefer to use oral penicillin V, which must be continued for 10 days to ensure eradication of GAS. Decreasing the frequency of penicillin to once daily is inadequate to eradicate GAS, although twice-daily regimens of 500 mg in adults and 250 mg per dose in children achieve similar cure rates for GAS pharyngitis as thrice-daily dosing.

An alternative medication used primarily because of its increased palatability and higher compliance is amoxicillin (Amoxil). Previously published and ongoing studies show that once-daily amoxicillin at 50 mg/kg (up to 750 mg once daily) in children and adults has bacteriologic cure rates equal to those

TABLE 1 Treatment Regimens for Group A Streptococci (GAS) Pharyngitis

	Medication	Pediatric Dosage	Adult Dosage	Duration
First-line therapy	Penicillin VK (Veetids)	If ≤27 kg, 400,000 U (250 mg) bid or tid If >27 kg, 800,000 U (500 mg) bid or tid	500 mg bid or tid	10 d
	Intramuscular penicillin G benzathine (Bicillin L-A)	≤27 kg, 600,000 U >27 kg, 1.2 million U single dose *or* 900,000 U benzathine penicillin G + 300,000 U procaine penicillin	1.2 million units single dose	1 d
	Amoxicillin (Amoxil)	50 mg/kg divided bid *or* once daily regimen of 50 mg/kg qd (maximum 750 mg)	500 mg bid *or* once daily regimen of 750 mg qd	10 d
Drugs for penicillin-allergic patients *and* short-course regimens	Erythromycin estolate (Ilosone)	20-40 mg/kg divided bid or qid	500 mg bid	10 d
	Erythromycin ethylsuccinate (EES)	40 mg/kg/day divided bid or qid (maximum 1 g/day)	500 mg bid	10 d
	Clarithromycin (Biaxin)	7.5 mg/kg/dose bid	250 mg bid	10 d
	Cephalexin (Keflex)	25-50 mg/kg/day divided bid	500 mg bid	10 d
	Clindamycin (Cleocin)	10-20 mg/kg/day divided tid	150 mg tid	10 d
	Cefpodoxime (Vantin)	10 mg/kg/day up to 200 mg/day divided bid	200 mg/day divided bid	5 d
	Cefdinir (Omnicef)	14 mg/kg/day divided bid (not to exceed adult dosage)	600 mg qd or divided bid	5 d
	Azithromycin (Zithromax)	12 mg/kg/day qd × 5 d (not to exceed adult dose)	500 mg qd × 1 day, then 250 mg qd × 4 d	5 d

achieved with thrice-daily penicillin dosing. Although once-daily amoxicillin treatment for GAS pharyngitis is not currently approved by the FDA, it appears to be an excellent alternative to penicillin.

For individuals who are allergic to penicillin, the drug of choice is erythromycin; other macrolide antibiotics, such as clarithromycin (Biaxin) and azithromycin (Zithromax) are acceptable (though more costly) alternatives. Azithromycin is often chosen because it has once-daily dosing and the treatment course is only 5 days, though it provides 10 days of antimicrobial activity. Treatment with azithromycin, 10 mg/kg for 3 days, for acute GAS pharyngitis is associated with inadequate bacterial eradication and is not currently advised. Areas of the world with heavy macrolide use have shown a direct relationship between overall macrolide usage and GAS macrolide resistance. In 2000-2001, a high rate of macrolide-resistant GAS (up to 48%) was described in Pittsburgh, Pennsylvania, raising concerns about the increasing U.S. macrolide-resistance rates. However, our ongoing nationwide surveillance has not confirmed this high rate of resistance in other parts of the country. Our studies indicate that the U.S. macrolide-resistance rate is approximately 4%. First-generation cephalosporins may be used for those who are allergic to penicillin if there is no history of immediate severe hypersensitivity to the penicillins, but these agents have broader antimicrobial activity than is necessary and are more expensive. Clindamycin (Cleocin) may be used if other antibiotics are not an option. Tetracyclines and sulfonamides should *not* be used for treating GAS pharyngitis because they are ineffective in eradicating the organism.

Post-Therapy Issues

Streptococcal pharyngitis patients are considered noncontagious 24 hours after initiation of treatment. In the United States, it is unnecessary to re-culture the posterior pharynx routinely following GAS pharyngitis, as the incidence of acute rheumatic fever remains low in almost all areas. In select circumstances, such as an outbreak of rheumatic fever in a community, a past history of ARF or RHD, or a household contact with a history of ARF, it may be prudent to re-culture a patient with GAS pharyngitis following therapy. Asymptomatic contacts of patients with streptococcal pharyngitis should not be cultured unless there are extenuating circumstances.

Clinical treatment failure of GAS pharyngitis is rare. If a patient returns for evaluation with recurrent symptoms of GAS pharyngitis within a few weeks of treatment, the possibilities to consider are a chronic pharyngeal carrier state with intercurrent viral pharyngitis, noncompliance with medication, or a new infection with a different strain of GAS. Recurrent pharyngitis caused by the same GAS strain is thought to be uncommon.

Treatment of Group A Streptococci Pharyngitis Chronic Carriers

A chronic GAS carrier is one who harbors the organism over a period of months with no symptoms or sequelae and who does not mount a rise in antistreptococcal antibodies. As many as 25% of school-age children can be carriers, especially in the springtime. The mechanisms by which GAS maintains a carrier state are not well understood, but it is clear that simply adhering to the pharyngeal epithelium is not sufficient to initiate disease. Eradication of GAS carriage may be indicated if there is an outbreak of ARF, poststreptococcal glomerulonephritis, or invasive GAS disease. Benzathine penicillin combined with rifampin (Rifadin), 10 mg/kg twice daily for 4 days of treatment, can be used. Oral clindamycin[1], given as 20 mg/kg per day in three divided doses for 10 days, has been the most effective regimen for eradicating the carrier state.

Recurrent Pharyngitis

The Infectious Disease Society of America currently recommends that continuous antimicrobial prophylaxis *not* be prescribed for recurrent pharyngitis except to prevent the recurrence of rheumatic fever in patients who have experienced a previous episode of ARF or who have rheumatic heart disease. Tonsillectomy may decrease the number of recurrences of symptomatic pharyngitis in some patients with severe, prolonged, recurrent pharyngitis, but only for a limited time, and generally is *not* recommended except in rare circumstances.

Non-Group A Streptococcal Pharyngitis

Groups C and G streptococci have been associated with acute self-limited pharyngitis (especially in teens and young adults) and rarely even acute poststreptococcal nephritis, but they do not cause rheumatic fever. Treatment of these organisms with antimicrobials has not been proven beneficial, and they generally do not require treatment. Many laboratories do not identify these organisms on throat culture.

[1]Not FDA approved for this indication.

SECTION 4

The Respiratory System

ACUTE RESPIRATORY FAILURE

METHOD OF

Marjolein de Wit, MD, and Curtis N. Sessler, MD

Respiration, the process of breathing, consists of the movement of gases into and out of alveoli coupled with gas exchange of O_2 and CO_2 molecules across the alveolar–capillary membrane. Acute respiratory failure (ARF) ensues when one or more of these processes falters, typically resulting in hypoxemia and/or hypercapnia. Such derangements can develop gradually, in which case compensatory responses and adaptation are more likely to occur, thus blunting the clinical impact. This distinction between ARF and chronic respiratory failure or insufficiency is somewhat arbitrary since there may be a continuum from chronic to acute respiratory failure.

Arterial Blood Gas Analysis

The measurement of arterial oxygen partial pressure ($Pa{O_2}$) and arterial partial pressure of carbon dioxide ($Pa{CO_2}$), as well as the hydrogen ion concentration (pH), using arterial blood gas (ABG) analysis is central to the diagnosis and management of ARF. The normal range of $Pa{O_2}$ varies with age, owing to structural changes in the lungs with advancing age, and can be calculated from the regression equation

$$Pa{O_2} = 100.1 - 0.323 \times (\text{age in years})$$

when breathing ambient air at sea level. Generally, an acute decrease in $Pa{O_2}$ to less than 55 mm Hg is considered to be consistent with hypoxemic respiratory failure. However, since $Pa{O_2}$ is highly dependent upon the percentage (or fraction, $F{I}{O_2}$) of the inhaled oxygen, expression of oxygenation as the ratio of $Pa{O_2}$ to $F{I}{O_2}$ (P/F ratio) is widely used. The P/F ratio should be greater than 500 mm Hg with normal gas exchange. A P/F ratio less than 200 mm Hg, along with additional clinical and radiographic features, is consistent with the diagnosis of acute respiratory distress syndrome (ARDS). The normal $Pa{CO_2}$ is 40 ± 5 mm Hg, and elevations above the normal range denote hypercapnia.

Evaluation of $Paco_2$ in the context of the pH is crucial, because $Paco_2$ may become elevated purely as a compensatory mechanism for metabolic alkalosis. Further, gradual onset of hypercapnia from inadequate ventilation would trigger compensatory processes to blunt the systemic acidosis, whereas acute hypercapnia is typically accompanied by incomplete compensation and a more acidemic state.

Clinical Manifestations

Clinical manifestations of ARF reflect the underlying causative conditions (for example, pneumonia, ARDS, chronic obstructive pulmonary disease (COPD), asthma, drug overdose, neuromuscular disease) that produce ARF, the signs and symptoms of respiratory distress, and findings related to hypoxemia and hypercapnia. Hypoxemia is often accompanied by tachypnea, tachycardia, hypertension, cardiac arrhythmias, tremor, and alterations in mentation such as anxiety, delirium, and agitation. Progressive bradycardia culminating in asystole can be seen with severe or protracted hypoxemia. Signs and symptoms of hypercapnia include tachypnea or bradypnea, tachycardia, hypertension, cardiac arrhythmias, conjunctival injection, papilledema, asterixis, and progressive obtundation.

Causative and Predisposing Clinical Conditions

A wide variety of clinical conditions can play a role in the development of ARF (Table 1). Hypoxemic respiratory failure is primarily the result of ventilation–perfusion mismatching and venous admixture or shunting, most often resulting from disorders of the lung parenchyma, airways, or vasculature. Hypercapnic respiratory failure develops because of alveolar hypoventilation, increased dead space ventilation, and/or increased CO_2 production.

Management

Care of the patient who has impending or established ARF includes initial evaluation and stabilization, evaluation and management of the underlying conditions, support of oxygenation and ventilation, and prevention and management of complications.

INITIAL EVALUATION AND STABILIZATION

Basic life-support measures include management of the airway and breathing. Life-threatening respiratory distress requires immediate attention, often including endotracheal (ET) intubation followed by mechanical ventilation (MV). Initial evaluation also includes a clinical estimation of the work of breathing and distress, measurement of oxygenation using pulse oximetry or ABG analysis, and measurement of acid–base status. The need for endotracheal intubation, ventilatory support, and/or supplemental oxygen is assessed. Once emergent issues are addressed, a more deliberate evaluation includes a careful history to identify causative conditions. Physical examination may reveal evidence of respiratory distress and findings caused by contributing conditions. Management steps for causative conditions such as

TABLE 1 Clinical Conditions Associated With Acute Respiratory Failure

Hypoxemic Failure

Diseases of the Conducting Airways

Chronic bronchitis
Asthma
Bronchiolitis
Upper airway obstruction

Diseases of the Gas Exchange Units

Emphysema
Infectious pneumonia
Pneumonitis
Acute lung injury/acute respiratory distress syndrome (ARDS)
Pulmonary edema
Alveolar hemorrhage
Pulmonary embolism
Interstitial lung disease
Neoplasm
Lung contusion
Atelectasis

Hypercapnic Failure

Diseases of Central Respiratory Control

Illicit drugs (e.g., narcotics and sedatives)
Medications (e.g., anesthetics, sedatives)
Meningoencephalitis
Central alveolar hypoventilation
Trauma
Cerebrovascular accident
Severe alkalosis
Myxedema

Diseases of the Spinal Cord, Nerves, and Muscles

Spinal cord trauma
Myasthenia gravis
Guillain-Barré syndrome
Multiple sclerosis
Medications (certain antibiotics, neuromuscular blocking agents)
Severe electrolyte abnormalities (e.g., hypophosphatemia, hypokalemia, hypomagnesemia)

Diseases Affecting Primarily the Chest Wall and Thoracic Cage

Trauma (e.g., flail chest)
Kyphoscoliosis
Ankylosing spondylitis
Scleroderma
Pleural disease (massive effusion, pneumothorax)

Diseases that Increase Physiologic Dead Space

Chronic obstructive pulmonary disease
Severe asthma

administration of inhaled bronchodilators for bronchospasm, management of upper airway obstruction, and needle decompression and/or tube thoracostomy drainage of the pneumothorax may be necessary.

SUPPORT OF OXYGENATION

In many ARF cases hypoxemia is present and administration of supplemental oxygen (administered via nasal cannula, face tent or shield, or face mask) is indicated. The effective percentage of oxygen in the inhaled gases depends upon the oxygen flow rate, whether or not re-breathing of exhaled gases occurs, and the patient's minute ventilation. Nasal cannula can deliver up to about 40% oxygen. Standard face masks can deliver up to 40% to 50% oxygen, and Venturi masks permit more precise titration of FIO_2. Non-rebreather masks provide up to 60% oxygen, with higher levels attained when combined with high-flow nasal cannula. The most effective means of providing supplemental oxygen is by positive pressure ventilation.

SUPPORT OF VENTILATION

Ventilatory insufficiency requires institution of measures to improve the mechanics or drive to breathe, along with mechanical ventilatory support. Although MV is typically delivered through an artificial airway (ET or tracheostomy tube), which serves as a conduit for gas delivery by positive pressure ventilation, MV can also be provided through a tightly fitting nasal or full face (oronasal) mask known as noninvasive positive-pressure ventilation (NPPV). In some cases of ARF, the presence of apnea, overt respiratory distress, or cardiopulmonary arrest mandates emergent endotracheal intubation. Endotracheal intubation is usually required for patients who have altered mental status, upper airway obstruction, inability to protect their airway, copious or tenacious respiratory secretions, and refractory hypoxemia. In other situations, particularly hypercapnic respiratory failure superimposed upon COPD, NPPV should be considered because it has been associated with better outcomes, including lower infection rates and lower mortality.

Noninvasive Positive Pressure Ventilation

The difference between conventional MV and NPPV is the interface; NPPV uses an oronasal mask or nasal mask. The oronasal mask may be more effective for patients who are mouth breathers, and is often preferred during the early phase of treatment. Careful attention must be given to avoid air leaks, eye irritation, and nasal bridge abrasions, and to identify poor tolerance. Respiratory therapists and nurses experience a higher workload during the first 6 to 8 hours of NPPV, but over time the additional workload is minimal at most. Close patient monitoring in addition to careful mask fitting and fine ventilator adjustments are necessary to prevent NPPV failure. The most frequently applied ventilatory mode combines pressure support (PS) and positive end-expiratory pressure (PEEP), but all conventional modes can be used with NPPV. NPPV may be delivered using an ICU ventilator or ventilators with more limited modes.

NPPV has been most thoroughly studied in three areas:

1. Prevention of ET intubation
2. Aid to weaning and extubation
3. Prevention of reintubation

Patients with chronic lung disease who experience hypercapnic respiratory failure are the most likely to benefit from NPPV. It should be considered a first-line treatment for patients with COPD exacerbations and is effective at decreasing the need for endotracheal intubation, duration of MV, and mortality. Patients with cardiogenic pulmonary edema may benefit from NPPV by decreasing both the work of breathing and left ventricular afterload. However, patients with ischemic heart disease may have a higher risk of acute myocardial infarction, indicating the need for close monitoring. NPPV has been effectively used as an aid to extubation in patients with COPD, as well as other forms of ARF. In this setting the ET tube is removed before conventional weaning criteria are satisfied, and patients are immediately placed on NPPV. The amount and time of NPPV support are gradually diminished over time. The third area has focused on prevention of reintubation, with less compelling evidence. In particular, NPPV should not be used in most non-COPD patients with ARF since one large study showed an increased mortality in those who received NPPV compared with conventional mechanical ventilation. We recommend prompt reintubation in this setting.

Mechanical Ventilation

Mechanical ventilation through an ET or tracheostomy tube allows delivery of breaths with high levels of positive pressure, as well as direct access to the lower airways compared with NPPV. Although oxygenation and ventilation are physiologically closely related, from a clinical standpoint they may be thought of separately (Figure 1). Effective oxygenation depends upon the FIO_2 and on alveolar recruitment and retention, which are achieved through inspiratory delivery of a positive pressure breath and PEEP that prevents subsequent alveolar collapse. Increasing PEEP is particularly effective for improving oxygenation in conditions with diffuse lung disease such as ARDS.

Ventilation is dependent upon respiratory rate and tidal volume (V_T). The operator generally has three options for breath delivery rate—assist control (AC) mode, synchronized intermittent mandatory ventilation (SIMV) mode, and spontaneous mode. In the AC and SIMV modes, a minimum number of mandatory breaths is specified, which are either ventilator-initiated or patient-initiated. Modern ventilators are

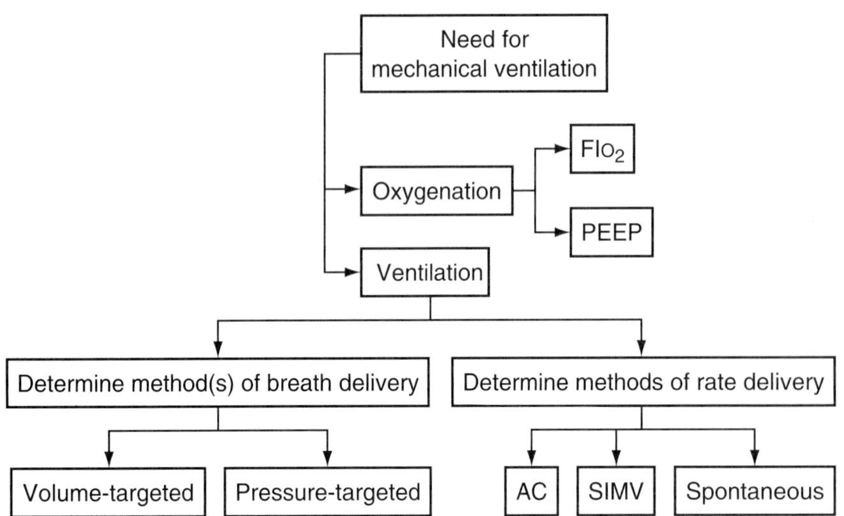

FIGURE 1 The principle components of mechanical ventilation are displayed. Primary parameters that influence oxygenation include adjustment of FIO_2 and PEEP. Modern ventilators allow selection of a method of rate delivery (mode of ventilation), as well as the method of breath delivery (e.g., pressure-targeted or volume-targeted). AC = assist control; FIO_2 = fraction of inspired gas that is oxygen; PEEP = positive end-expiratory pressure; SIMV = synchronized intermittent mandatory ventilation.

able to synchronize mandatory breaths with patient inspiratory effort in both the SIMV and AC modes, producing a patient-triggered breath. In AC, patients who breathe above the preset rate are given an assisted breath that has features similar to ventilator-initiated mandatory breaths. Thus, the tachypneic patient risks hyperventilation with the AC mode. In the SIMV mode, breaths in excess of the preset number of breaths do not trigger an assisted breath, but result in spontaneous breaths that should be supported with pressure support (PS). The spontaneous mode requires the patient to initiate all breaths, thus it is not suitable for patients who are apneic or hypoventilating.

In addition to selecting the rate mode, the clinician must set breaths to be volume-targeted or pressure-targeted, as airway pressure and V_T are interdependent. In volume-targeted ventilation, the V_T is preset and the airway pressure is variable, whereas in pressure-targeted ventilation, the preset inspiratory airway pressure results in a variable V_T. Traditionally, with volume-targeted ventilation, one must specify a flow rate (the velocity at which the V_T is delivered); however, newer ventilators are able to administer variable flow rates to adjust to patient demands. Pressure-targeted mandatory breaths apply a predetermined pressure for a preset time, with longer times resulting in larger V_T. The inspiratory time may also be set using the ratio of inspiratory time to expiratory time (I:E ratio). Spontaneous pressure-targeted breaths apply predetermined pressure for the duration of the patient's inspiratory cycle resulting in variable times. The spontaneous breaths in SIMV should be augmented with PS (usually 7 cm H_2O) to overcome the resistance of the tube and ventilatory circuit.

Spontaneous mode breaths can be pressure-targeted (typically 5 to 30 cm H_2O); this is called pressure support ventilation (PSV) in traditional terminology. In newer ventilators, support of spontaneous breaths with a volume-targeted delivery is possible, but not yet widely used. Older terminology implied that AC and SIMV were applied in a volume-targeted mode. The older term, pressure control ventilation (PCV), refers to pressure-targeted AC ventilation. In an international survey, the most common modes of ventilation were volume-targeted AC (60%), followed by volume-targeted SIMV + PS (10%-20%), PCV (10%-20%), and PSV (10%).

Positive end-expiratory pressure is often applied during passive exhalation. The majority of patients benefit from low-level PEEP (5 cm H_2O). Patients with significant airflow obstruction may experience worsening of air trapping with PEEP, whereas patients with ARDS benefit from high levels. Continuous positive airway pressure (CPAP), as the name implies, has the same pressure applied throughout the entire respiratory cycle. High pressures of CPAP (i.e., >10 cm H_2O) may cause discomfort as it forces patients to exhale against an elevated pressure.

Monitoring

Airway pressure, volumes, and other parameters are monitored during ventilation. Elevation in peak inspiratory pressure (PIP) can be detected, as can disconnection or apnea. Because

$$\text{PIP} = \text{flow} \times \text{resistance} + \text{plateau pressure (Pplat)}$$

$$\text{where Pplat} = V_T/\text{compliance (C)} + \text{PEEP}$$

the etiology of elevated PIP may be caused by increased airway resistance or elevated Pplat. Rarely, a high flow rate alone is responsible for high PIP, as this is an operator-set parameter. Increased airway resistance may be caused by biting on the ET tube, a small-diameter ET tube, secretions, or bronchospasm. Elevated Pplat may be caused by underlying lung disease (ARDS, pulmonary edema, pneumonia), pleural disease (pneumothorax), chest wall disease (obesity, kyphoscoliosis), abdominal disease (abdominal distention, obesity, or recumbent position), or lung overinflation (auto-PEEP, excessive V_T). Evaluation using physical examination, chest radiograph review, and overview of airflow graphics helps to uncover the underlying etiology.

Mechanical Ventilation During Status Asthmaticus

Mechanical ventilation in the setting of severe airflow obstruction deserves particular comment, because prolonged exhalation and the propensity for dynamic hyperinflation mandate the use of specific ventilatory strategies. Ventilatory support with large V_T and/or short exhalation time causes incomplete exhalation with each cycle, increased intrathoracic pressure (so-called auto-PEEP or intrinsic-PEEP), and increased intrathoracic volume (dynamic hyperinflation). The combination of airflow obstruction and anxiety resulting in tachypnea is prone to aggravate a cycle of respiratory distress that may culminate in severe air-trapping, resulting in hypotension from reduced cardiac output and gas exchange compromise (Figure 2). The patient who has evidence of hemodynamic compromise from air-trapping should be briefly disconnected from MV; thereby allowing passive exhalation to occur, which provides rapid, temporary relief from dynamic hyperinflation.

Controlling the respiratory rate, by administering sedative medications and by reducing the preset rate, is crucial because expiratory time is inversely related to respiratory rate. The AC mode is generally avoided because each inspiratory effort will produce an assisted breath, potentially worsening the hyperinflation. Additional measures include delivery of smaller V_T and increasing the inspiratory flow rate (thereby shortening inspiratory time and lengthening expiratory time). These measures may result in alveolar hypoventilation and CO_2 retention; however, this *permissive* hypercapnia may be blunted through reduced dead space ventilation as hyperinflation is relieved. Permissive hypercapnia should be avoided in patients with increased intracranial pressure or significant myocardial dysfunction. Some experts recommend giving sodium bicarbonate to buffer the respiratory acidosis if pH is less than 7.1 to 7.25.

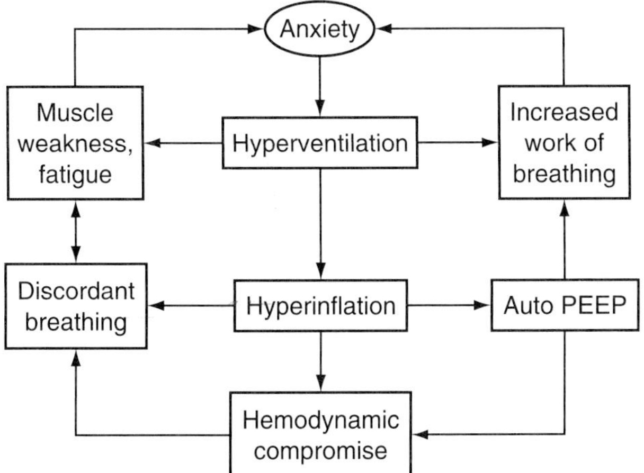

FIGURE 2 The cycle of anxiety, hyperinflation, increased work of breathing, muscle fatigue, and hemodynamic compromise seen in ventilated patients with airflow obstruction.

Mechanical Ventilation During ARDS

A strategy of lung-protective ventilation is now widely accepted as the preferred approach to MV for ARDS. This approach is based upon evidence from human clinical trials and animal experiments, which shows that MV can promote lung injury from excessive stretch and overdistention of alveoli at peak inspiration, as well as from the repetitive recruitment and collapse of alveoli. Further, computerized tomography (CT) studies of ARDS patients demonstrate reduced amounts of functional lung tissue, suggesting small V_T may be more appropriate. Most importantly, a large, NIH-sponsored, multicenter, randomized clinical trial of patients with ARDS showed improved survival for patients ventilated with smaller (6 mL/kg predicted body weight [PBW]) versus larger (12 mL/kg PBW) V_T. Guidelines for lung protective ventilation, which emphasize smaller V_T, limited Pplat, and relatively high levels of PEEP are presented in Table 2. Increasing the mean airway pressure in general, and PEEP in particular, will often improve oxygenation in ARDS through alveolar recruitment and retention. Application of excessive PEEP, however, can impair oxygen delivery by reducing cardiac output. In addition to raising the PEEP level, mean airway pressure can be elevated by

TABLE 2 Mechanical Ventilation of Patients Who Have Acute Respiratory Distress Syndrome (ARDS)*

Set initial mode: assist-control, volume-targeted.
Set initial tidal volume (V_T): 8 mL/kg predicted body weight (PBW).†
Set initial mandatory respiratory rate to maintain baseline minute ventilation.
Make V_T adjustments.
Reduce V_T to 7 mL/kg after 1-2 hours, then to 6 mL/kg 1-2 hours later.
Check inspiratory plateau pressure (Pplat) every 4 hours and after ventilator changes.
If Pplat >30 cm H_2O, decrease V_T by 1 mL/kg.
If Pplat <25 cm H_2O and V_T <6 mL/kg, increase V_T by 1 mL/kg until Pplat >25 cm H_2O or VT = 6 mL/kg.
If breath stacking or severe dyspnea, increase V_T to 7-8 mL/kg if Pplat <30 cm H_2O
Use FiO_2–PEEP combination to achieve oxygenation goal:

FiO_2	0.3	0.4	0.4	0.5	0.5	0.6	0.7	0.7	0.7	0.8	0.9	0.9	0.9	1
PEEP	5	5	8	8	10	10	10	12	14	14	14	16	18	20-24

Adjust respiratory rate (maximum = 35 breaths/min) to achieve pH = 7.3-7.45

*Modified from http://www.ardsnet.org/6mL.html.
†Predicted body weight formulas:
Male = 50 + 2.3 (height[inches] – 60).
Female = 45.5 + 2.3 (height[inches] – 60).

increasing Pplat, by increasing inspiratory time or I:E ratio, and by increasing the respiratory rate.

There are ancillary ventilatory strategies for use in the hypoxemic patient with ARDS, including recruitment maneuvers, prone positioning, high-frequency oscillatory ventilation (HFOV), and inhaled nitric oxide (NO). These techniques all improve oxygenation; however, none have improved survival or significantly reduce duration of MV. Recruitment maneuvers (40 cm H_2O positive airway pressure applied for 40 sec, for example) open collapsed alveoli and transiently improve oxygenation, particularly after endotracheal suctioning or disconnection with loss of PEEP. Prone positioning allows more uniform alveolar ventilation in ARDS, improves oxygenation, and may be particularly effective with severe ARDS, but is cumbersome to perform. HFOV may be the ultimate example of lung-protective ventilation since very small V_T (100-150 mL) are delivered rapidly (180-300 breaths/min), with high PEEP and acceptable Pplat. HFOV requires a specialized ventilator and experienced personnel, however, and has not been compared directly with lung-protective strategies. Inhaled NO improves ventilation–perfusion matching, thus improving oxygenation; but it is expensive, the effects are temporary, and outcomes are not improved.

Discontinuation of Mechanical Ventilation

Assessment of readiness for discontinuation of MV and extubation should be undertaken daily, once the cause of respiratory failure is treated. Three methods for discontinuation of MV have been widely used:

1. PS weaning (the amount of PS is decreased over time)
2. SIMV weaning (the mandatory rate is decreased over time)
3. T-piece weaning (the duration of unsupported breathing is increased over time)

Research has demonstrated that SIMV is the least effective method and therefore should not be used as a weaning mode. Studies have found conflicting results when comparing T-piece and PS weaning. These strategies all gradually decrease the amount of support needed (thus the term *weaning*). However, most patients can tolerate a daily abrupt withdrawal of support that can indicate their readiness for independent breathing and extubation—the spontaneous breathing trial (SBT).

Clinicians should screen patients daily for the elements listed in section A of Table 3—satisfying these parameters indicates the SBT should be safe. Excessive sedation is an important cause of delayed extubation, and strategies such as algorithms to reduce the use of continuous infusion sedatives and/or daily interruption of all sedative medications are used to shorten duration of MV. Some experts also recommend doing a rapid shallow breathing index (RSBI). Although earlier research showed an RSBI of greater than 105 to be an accurate predictor of successful extubation, recent research suggests that this approach can actually delay weaning unnecessarily. For patients (i.e., women, people who are a small size, and those with pre-existing lung disease) with smaller V_T, we prefer using a higher threshold, such as an RSBI of greater than 125, or omission of RSBI testing altogether.

Patients who pass all elements of the daily screen undergo an SBT (see Table 3, section B). The patient receives minimal support (CPAP 5 cm H_2O or PS

TABLE 3 Discontinuation of Mechanical Ventilation and Endotracheal Tube Removal

The Patient Who Successfully Meets Criteria A, B, and C Has a Low Likelihood of Extubation Failure

A. Screening Evaluation

The patient should meet all of the following criteria:

- Ability to handle secretions (i.e., suctioning not more frequently than every 2 hours)
- Absence of upper airway obstruction
- Adequate neurologic status (not excessively sedated)
- Ability to initiate an inspiratory effort
- pH ≥7.25
- Adequate oxygenation (P/F ratio >150-200)
- PEEP ≤5-8 cm H_2O
- Hemodynamic stability (i.e., absence of cardiac ischemia and no more than minimal vasopressor use [for example, no more than dopamine 5 mcg/kg/min])

Another but optional consideration is the patient's rapid shallow breathing index (RSBI)* (see text for discussion).

B. Spontaneous Breathing Trial (SBT)

The patient who passes the screening tests (part A) proceeds to spontaneous breathing at low-level ventilatory support (CPAP = 5 cm H_2O, PSV = 5-7 cm H_2O + PEEP 5 cm H_2O, or automatic tube compensation), with baseline FIO_2 and PEEP = 5 cm H_2O for 30 to 120 min duration. If any of the following criteria are met, the SBT is aborted and the patient is placed back on adequate ventilator support to achieve comfortable breathing and satisfactory gas exchange.

Clinical criteria for failing an SBT include any of the following:

- Respiratory rate >35 breaths per minute for 5 minutes
- Heart rate >140 beats per minute or >20% change in either direction from baseline
- Systolic BP <90 or >180 mm Hg or >20% change in either direction from baseline
- Reduced oxygen saturation to <90%
- Increased anxiety or diaphoresis

C. Upper Airway Patency

Demonstration of adequate airflow around the ET tube should be done in patients who have upper airway obstruction. Some clinicians perform this step in all patients before extubation. In one technique, the patient is placed on assist control ventilation with 10-12 mL/kg V_T breaths, and the exhaled V_T (average of 4 to 6 breaths) is measured before and after cuff deflation. A "leak" volume (V_T with cuff inflated – V_T with cuff deflated) >130 mL is associated with a low likelihood of postextubation stridor.

*RSBI is calculated as f/V_T, where f = respiratory rate and V_T = the average V_T (in liters) after 2 min of spontaneous breathing with no, or minimal, pressure support.

Abbreviations: CPAP = continuous positive-airway pressure; PEEP = positive end-expiratory pressure; PSV = pressure support ventilation.

TABLE 4 Common Factors Contributing to Failure to Discontinuation of Mechanical Ventilation

Hemodynamic instability
Ischemic heart disease
Infection
Impaired mental status
Malnutrition
Overfeeding
Neuromuscular disorders
Psychological factors
Airflow obstruction
Increased endotracheal tube resistance
Excessive respiratory secretions
Respiratory depressant medications
Metabolic alkalosis
Electrolyte imbalance

5-7 cm H_2O + PEEP 5 cm H_2O) to overcome the resistance of the ET tube. Studies evaluating SBT have excluded tracheostomized patients. With newer ventilators, an automatic tube compensation (ATC) setting in the spontaneous mode can be used. The type (ET or tracheostomy) and diameter of the tube are programmed into the ventilator, and the amount of pressure necessary to overcome the resistance of the tube (usually 2-5 cm H_2O) is applied to patient-triggered breaths. ATC has not been adequately studied for SBT. Criteria for failure of SBT are listed in Table 3. Patients who fail an SBT should be placed back on a nonfatiguing mode of MV. Clinicians should evaluate potential causes of failure to pass SBT (Table 4). A patient who passes a 2-hour SBT should have the ET tube removed if there is no concern for upper airway obstruction (see Table 3, section C). Extension of SBT beyond 2 hours may produce respiratory muscle fatigue and is thus avoided.

COMPLICATIONS OF MECHANICAL VENTILATION

Common complications of mechanical ventilation and endotracheal intubation are displayed in Table 5. It is noteworthy that air leaks typically develop from rupture of alveoli that abut relatively fixed structures like the bronchi and vessels, and air tracks medially along these structures often resulting in pneumomediastinum and/or subcutaneous emphysema before pneumothorax occurs. Tension pneumothorax is an important complication for which prevention, timely evaluation, and management are crucial. Ventilator-associated lung injury (VALI), a state of heightened lung inflammation and injury, is caused by alveolar overdistention and cyclic alveolar wall stretch through collapse and recruitment. There is increasing evidence that this pulmonary inflammation can be the engine for systemic inflammatory and organ dysfunction. Ventilator-associated pneumonia is common, is associated with increased mortality, and the risk can be reduced using multidisciplinary programs that promote backrest elevation, avoidance of nasal tubes, and other measures.

TABLE 5 Complications of Mechanical Ventilation

Oxygen toxicity
Pulmonary barotrauma (air leak)
Pneumothorax
Pneumomediastinum/pneumopericardium/subcutaneous emphysema
Subdiaphragmatic air collections (retroperitoneal, within bowel wall, scrotal)
Pulmonary air cysts or cavities (can be with tension)
Pulmonary interstitial emphysema
Systemic air embolism
Alveolar overdistention
Hemodynamic compromise (hypotension) from increased intrathoracic pressure
Ventilator-associated lung injury (VALI)
Multiple organ dysfunction
Tracheomalacia
Vocal cord damage and dysfunction
Lip, oral cavity, nasal, pharyngeal damage
Unplanned extubation
Endotracheal tube malposition
Bronchial intubation
Esophageal intubation
Ventilator-associated pneumonia
Gastrointestinal bleeding from stress ulceration/gastritis

Acute respiratory failure, consisting of hypoxemia and/or hypercapnia, represents a serious, often life-threatening condition that can be effectively managed through stabilization of the airway and breathing, management of the underlying conditions, provision of effective oxygenation and ventilation, and careful avoidance of complications. Advances in the mechanical ventilatory management, including use of noninvasive techniques, lung-protective strategies for ARDS, and timely discontinuation of MV are leading to better outcomes.

ATELECTASIS

METHOD OF

Matthew A. Romano, MD, and

Mark D. Iannettoni, MD

Definition and Diagnosis

Atelectasis is the collapse of previously inflated lung parenchyma and the consequent collapse of alveoli. Conceptually, it is seen as diminished gas within the lung associated with reduced lung volume. The term *lung collapse* is often used synonymously with atelectasis, especially with complete atelectasis. Atelectasis is the most common pulmonary complication. In the surgical patient, it is most often associated with a recent surgical procedure that results in a pain-induced decreased respiratory excursion or with direct lung injury. As with any variety of pulmonary dysfunction; dyspnea, tachypnea, and tachycardia may be prominent clinical features of alveolar collapse, especially in the acute setting. The response appears to be mediated in part by vagal stretch receptors in the lung. This mechanism may be responsible for the nonproductive cough associated with atelectasis. Fever is almost always present. When the collapsed lung tissue reinflates, the fever promptly resolves. If large portions of lung are atelectatic, clinical examination may reveal dullness to percussion, decreased breath sounds, and elevation of the diaphragm. Changes seen with chest radiographs are areas of volume loss, which may be manifested by elevation of the diaphragm. The key approach to atelectasis should be early prevention.

Classification and Etiology

By convention, the classification of atelectasis is centered on the alterations of the mechanisms that maintain lung expansion. Commonly, atelectasis has been classified into four types:

1. Obstructive
2. Compressive
3. Cicatrization
4. Adhesive

Obstructive atelectasis occurs from bronchial obstruction, thereby blocking the communication between the alveoli and the trachea. Because collapse results from resorption of gas from the alveoli, this type of atelectasis is also referred to as resorption atelectasis. *Compressive* atelectasis, also known as relaxation or passive atelectasis, can be seen with space-occupying lesions. The lung has a natural tendency to collapse and does so when removed from the chest. While the lungs are in the thoracic cavity, this tendency is opposed by the chest wall. When the thorax contains a space-occupying process, the lung retracts and its volume decreases. *Cicatrization* atelectasis occurs because of scarring of the pulmonary parenchyma. Maintaining lung volume depends on a balance between the applied force and opposing elastic forces. If the lung is stiffer than normal (i.e., compliance is decreased), lung volume is decreased. Finally, *adhesive* atelectasis is seen when there is a lack or interference with surfactant. In this situation, there is an alteration of the alveolar surface tension and subsequent collapse. The etiologies that lead to each type of atelectasis are numerous (Table 1).

TABLE 1 Etiology of Atelectasis

Etiology of Atelectasis
Obstructive Atelectasis
Foreign bodies
Bronchial neoplasms
Infection
Airway edema
Excessive mucus
Impaired mucociliary clearance
Compressive Atelectasis
Pneumothorax
Hemothorax
Hydrothorax
Excessive elevation of diaphragm
Cicatrization Atelectasis
Abscess
Inflammatory or fibrotic process
Previous infection with scar formation
Adhesive Atelectasis
Acute respiratory distress syndrome (ARDS)
Surfactant denaturation

Pathophysiology

Atelectasis develops at different rates. This may, in part, be related to the presence of collateral ventilation. Collateral ventilation is age dependent. In adults, especially those with chronic obstructive pulmonary disease, collateral channels are often well developed. This is not the case in young children. Additionally, the location of the obstruction affects collateral pathways. If the obstruction is at the level of a lobar bronchus, the development of atelectasis is readily explained by the absence of a parenchymal bridge from the involved lobe to a contiguous lobe. However, if the obstruction is in a segmental or subsegmental bronchus, intralobe collateral pathways may prevent the development of atelectasis. The percent of inspired gas also affects the rate at which atelectasis develops. Atmospheric air contains approximately 21% oxygen, and the remainder is mainly nitrogen. Because oxygen is absorbed much more rapidly than nitrogen, when a lobe is filled with a very high concentration of oxygen at the moment of occlusion (a situation that might occur during general anesthesia), collapse occurs much more rapidly. Ultimately, the sequela of each type of atelectasis may follow the same course. The loss of volume with continued perfusion of the collapsed segment results in a ventilation perfusion mismatch and subsequent shunt formation. The extent of alveolar collapse and right-to-left shunt is reflected in arterial blood gas pressures. Hypoxemia of variable severity is typical and is initially accompanied by mild hypocapnia. As the atelectasis becomes more severe, hypercapnia and impending respiratory failure supervene.

Treatment of Atelectasis and Risk Factors

The primary method of treating atelectasis is prevention of the factors that place a patient at risk for developing collapse. The management should be aggressive with frequent clinical assessment. It is essential to identify and alleviate the underlying disease process. Aggressive pulmonary toilet and maintenance of airway patency are essential in the management. Pain associated with chest wall injury or surgical procedures in the torso often results in shallow breathing and is the major cause of atelectasis in the postoperative patient. Intraoperative infiltration of the incision with local anesthetic or use of continuous epidural anesthesia relieves pain and permits increased ventilatory effort without discomfort. Tracheal suction, deep breathing maneuvers, and airway humidification are also indicated for prevention and treatment of postoperative atelectasis. Incentive spirometry is useful to prevent small airway collapse. Early and frequent ambulation of hospitalized patients also facilitates airway expansion. Bronchoscopy is an effective means of removing debris from larger airways, especially if a lobe or entire lung is collapsed. Additionally, bronchoscopy permits the collection of sputum for bacterial culture. Bronchodilators may be a beneficial therapy if a component of reactive airway disease is present. Aerosolized or systemic steroids may be administered in refractory cases. In severe cases, mechanical assistance may be necessary with intermittent positive-pressure breathing (IPPB). However, with close observation and preemptive measures to maintain airway expansion, atelectasis may be avoided, therefore minimizing the need for intervention.

MANAGEMENT OF CHRONIC OBSTRUCTIVE PULMONARY DISEASE

METHOD OF
Michael Littner, MD

Chronic obstructive pulmonary disease (COPD) is defined, in part, by the American Thoracic Society (ATS) and the European Respiratory Society (ERS) as a preventable and treatable disease state characterized by airflow limitation that is not fully reversible. Cigarette smoking is overwhelmingly the most common cause of COPD. COPD is increasing in prevalence and is the fourth leading cause of mortality in the United States.

Classification, Diagnosis, and Severity

Obstructive pulmonary function is when the forced expiratory volume (FEV) in one second divided by the slow, or forced, vital capacity (SVC, or FVC) (FEV1/SVC or FEV1/FVC) times 100 is less than 70%. The Global Initiative for Obstructive Lung Disease (GOLD) and ATS-ERS also require an FEV_1 that is less than 80% predicted to confirm a diagnosis of COPD. COPD by GOLD and ATS-ERS criteria occurs in approximately 15% of long-time smokers. All values for diagnostic purposes are postbronchodilator.

The clinical–pathologic condition most associated with COPD is one or a combination of chronic bronchitis and emphysema. Chronic bronchitis (chronic cough and sputum) occurs in approximately 30% of long-time smokers. The prevalence of emphysema (pathologically enlarged airspaces) is not fully defined.

Symptoms also include dyspnea, exacerbations, and fatigue.

Current guidelines require confirming spirometry (i.e., FEV_1 and FVC) to make a diagnosis of COPD.

Several FEV_1 severity classifications of COPD have been proposed including those of GOLD (Table 1), which is similar to those of ATS-ERS. Once diagnosed and classified, initiation and escalation of therapy are based primarily on symptoms such as dyspnea and exacerbations.

Etiology and Pathophysiology

In the United States, it is estimated that 85% of COPD is from cigarette smoking. Chronic exposure to noxious occupational and environmental fumes

TABLE 1 Staging of COPD Severity

COPD Stage	Spirometry and Symptoms
0: At risk	Normal spirometry ($FEV_1/FVC \geq 70\%$, $FEV_1 \geq 80\%$ predicted) Cough, sputum production
I: Mild	$FEV_1/FVC < 70\%$, $FEV_1 \geq 80\%$ predicted No requirement for cough, sputum production
II: Moderate*	$FEV_1/FVC < 70\%$, $FEV_1 \geq 50\%$ and $< 80\%$ predicted No requirement for cough, sputum production
III: Severe	$FEV_1/FVC < 70\%$, $FEV_1 \geq 30\%$ and $< 50\%$ predicted No requirement for cough, sputum production
IV: Very severe	$FEV_1/FVC < 70\%$, $FEV_1 \leq 30\%$ or $FEV_1 < 50\%$ predicted, with chronic respiratory failure ($Pa_{O_2} < 60$ mm Hg, $Pa_{CO_2} > 50$ mm Hg breathing room air at sea level)

*Stages II and higher confirm a diagnosis of chronic obstructive pulmonary disease (COPD) (i.e., obstruction that is not fully reversible) according to the Global Initiative for Obstructive Lung Disease (GOLD) and the American Thoracic Society-European Respiratory Society (ATS-ERS).

Abbreviations: FEV_1 = forced expiratory volume in 1 sec; FVC = forced vital capacity; Pa_{O_2} = partial pressure arterial oxygen; Pa_{CO_2} = partial pressure of arterial carbon dioxide.

Source: Table modeled after GOLD.

and gases may contribute to the remaining 15%. The pathologic result may include squamous metaplasia of the respiratory epithelium, ciliary loss and dysfunction, inflammation and fibrosis of airways, mucous gland hyperplasia and hypersecretion, increased airway smooth muscle, loss of alveolar attachments, and reflex bronchoconstriction from vagally mediated release of acetylcholine.

The pathologic changes are thought to result from an inflammatory cascade that begins with oxidant stress and other pulmonary irritants leading to attraction and stimulation of neutrophils and lymphocytes. This results in mediators including interleukin-8 (IL-8), cytotoxic lymphocytes (CD8+ cells), and release of various proteases. Fortunately, most (85%) individuals at risk have anti-inflammatory defenses such as antioxidants and antiproteases that prevent the development of significant COPD.

The pathologic changes lead to reduction in airflow from increased airway resistance and decreased elastic recoil of the lungs (emphysema).

Evaluation of the Stable Patient

A complete history and physical examination should be performed. Although physical examination is useful in characterizing COPD (e.g., use of accessory respiratory muscles), the most important information generally comes from the history. Determine the patient's smoking history and symptoms of COPD, distinguish COPD from asthma and other lung diseases, and determine whether there are coexistent conditions such as coronary artery disease. Determine when the patient first noted symptoms, if these are stable or changing, if there are any unusual symptoms such as hemoptysis, and what are the number and severity of exacerbations.

Spirometry before and after inhalation of a bronchodilator should always be performed. The postbronchodilator value should be used for diagnosis and severity of obstruction and *not* to determine if the patient is likely to respond to maintenance bronchodilator therapy.

Often, there is confusion about whether a patient has asthma or COPD. The presence or absence of reversibility to bronchodilators should not be the deciding factor in most cases. Asthma is often distinguished from COPD by the company it keeps such as peripheral blood and sputum eosinophilia, early age of onset before substantial smoking history, elevated serum IGE levels, the presence of other allergic signs and symptoms such as hay fever and allergic rhinitis, and the absence of a significant (>10 pack-years) smoking history. If there is strong evidence of both asthma and COPD, the diagnosis of both should be made and managed accordingly.

Apart from asthma, the differential diagnosis includes bronchiectasis, bronchiolitis, upper airway obstruction (e.g., from a tumor), postviral airway inflammation, eosinophilic bronchitis, and congestive heart failure.

Laboratory studies should include, in addition to spirometry, a chest radiograph, oximetry at rest and during exercise for possible hypoxemia, and a complete blood count (CBC) for polycythemia. Serum α_1-antitrypsin levels are recommended for COPD patients who are younger than 45 years of age with a strong family history of COPD. Arterial blood gases are generally obtained only in borderline cases of hypoxemia (arterial oxygen saturation = 92% by pulse oximetry) and to determine the presence of hypercapnia. Patients with very low FEV_1 levels (<30% predicted) are particularly at risk of having hypercapnia. More specialized testing such as computed tomography (CT) should be reserved for patients with difficult-to-diagnose disease (e.g., possible interstitial lung disease) or to diagnose and quantify emphysema if this is required for management (e.g., lung volume reduction surgery).

Treatment of the Stable Patient

SMOKING CESSATION

The most important treatment is initiation and maintenance of smoking cessation. Smoking cessation is the only intervention that reduces the rate of decline of pulmonary function. All patients who smoke should be counseled to stop smoking at every visit.

A five-step, brief intervention process, known as the "5 As" is:

- **Ask:** Systematically identify tobacco users.
- **Advise:** Strongly urge all tobacco users to quit.
- **Assess:** Determine willingness to make a quit attempt.

- **Assist:** Help the patient by providing information, giving referrals to smoking cessation programs, and recommending use of approved pharmacotherapy.
- **Arrange:** Schedule follow-up contact, either in person or by telephone.

More intensive smoking cessation programs include group sessions and adjunctive support with FDA-approved pharmacotherapy including nicotine replacement therapy and/or bupropion (Zyban). One-year quit rates with intensive programs are, at best, approximately 30%.

PHARMACOLOGIC THERAPY

Pharmacologic treatment is primarily directed at relaxing airway smooth muscle with bronchodilators. Attempts to reduce inflammation have not been obviously successful, but inhaled corticosteroids and phosphodiesterase inhibition (e.g., theophylline) may have a limited anti-inflammatory effect.

Short-Acting Inhaled Bronchodilators

Short-acting anticholinergic (ipratropium [Atrovent]) has a duration of about 3 to 6 hours with a slow (15-30 minute) onset of action. A maximum benefit is achieved with 144 μg by metered-dose-inhaler (MDI) or 500 μg from a nebulizer. However, with the MDI this is eight inhalations, which is generally impractical. There is no benefit of using a nebulizer versus using an MDI if both are used correctly.

In patients with mild symptoms, 36 μg (2 inhalations) four times a day is a standard FDA-approved dose. In patients with moderate-to-severe symptoms, 72 μg (4 inhalations) four times a day[3] can be considered. Higher doses can be used, but combination therapy is preferred.

Short-acting β-agonists (e.g., albuterol [Proventil], pirbuterol [Maxair], metaproterenol [Alupent]) have a rapid onset (up to 2 min) and a duration of approximately 3 to 6 hours. A maximum benefit is achieved at generally four times the typical dose of two inhalations. However, such higher doses may have obvious side effects, such as tremor and tachycardia, and are not recommended routinely. Dosing should generally be as needed and not for scheduled maintenance because studies show no difference in outcome. In patients whose as-needed dose amounts to routine scheduled maintenance, a combination with ipratropium may be used for convenience.

Long-Acting Inhaled Bronchodilators

Currently, the only long-acting inhaled bronchodilators available in the United States are salmeterol (Serevent) and formoterol (Foradil) (β_2-adrenergic agents) and tiotropium (Spiriva) (inhaled anticolinergic). Salmeterol has a delayed onset of action (up to an hour) and a 12-hour duration of action. Formoterol has a rapid onset of action (up to 2 min) and a 12-hour duration of action. Both are used twice daily, ideally 12 hours apart. The dose is fixed at 50 μg each use for salmeterol, and 12 μg each use for formoterol. Regular use of higher doses is potentially dangerous because of β-adrenergic side effects and because both drugs are generally less effective on outcomes, such as health status, when higher-than-approved doses are administered.

Side Effects of Ipratropium and Tiotropium

The main side effect of ipratropium is dry mouth, which is mild and almost always tolerable. There are rare reports of systemic anticholinergic effects such as urinary retention and supraventricular tachycardia. Tiotropium (Spiriva) has a delayed onset of action (up to one hour) and 24 hours or more duration of action. The dose is 18 μg once daily. Its use with ipratropium is not approved.

Side Effects of β-Agonists

Tremor, tachycardia, nervousness, headaches, and other troublesome side effects are common but tolerable with β-agonists. In addition, electrolyte disturbances such as hypokalemia can result. Overuse of long-acting β_2-agonists has been associated with death. A recent study in asthma patients suggests an increased mortality from respiratory events in African Americans who used salmeterol. The relevance to COPD is unknown.

Oral Bronchodilators

Theophylline (Slo-Phyllin) can be effective, but side effects of nausea, vomiting, and cardiac and central nervous system stimulation limit its use. There are a number of drug interactions with antibiotics and other medications that may lead to changes in levels of theophylline or the interacting medication. Many side effects can be reduced or avoided by using low doses that produce serum levels of less than 12 μg/mL. Only sustained release formulations (once or twice daily) are recommended and generally only in combination with other bronchodilators.

Oral β-agonists are not generally recommended for treatment of COPD.

Corticosteroids

Oral corticosteroids are not recommended for treatment of stable COPD patients because of the high incidence of side effects and an 80% to 90% lack of efficacy.

Inhaled corticosteroids do not reduce the rate of decline of pulmonary function and should not be used for this purpose. The use of inhaled corticosteroids is controversial and none used alone has an FDA indication for COPD. Evidence to date suggests

[3]Exceeds dosage recommended by the manufacturer.

that inhaled corticosteroids, when used alone, produce a slight overall increase in FEV_1, improve dyspnea and health status, and reduce COPD exacerbations in patients with frequent exacerbations. The effect is most consistently demonstrated in patients with chronic cough and sputum production. The increase in FEV_1 is far inferior to that of bronchodilators. Inhaled corticosteroids, used alone, are not generally superior to bronchodilators in reducing exacerbations and improving dyspnea and health status.

Oral corticosteroids are associated with the usual side effects including systemic hypertension, glucose intolerance, osteoporosis, weight gain, mood changes, and cataracts. Inhaled corticosteroids are associated with dysphonia and oral candidiasis, and skin bruising in older patients. In addition, a decrease in bone density has been reported and there may be an association with glaucoma and cataracts.

Inhalers

There are currently two types, MDIs and dry powder.

Combination Therapy

The most consistent effect is improvement in FEV_1. In addition, less consistent effects have been noted on exacerbations, dyspnea, and health status. The combination of albuterol and ipratropium (Combivent) is superior to either alone. The combination of a long-acting β_2-agonist and a long- or short-acting anticholinergic is superior to the long-acting β_2-agonist used alone. When a long-acting β_2-agonist is used, a short-acting β_2-agonist should also be used for rescue. A combination of a long-acting β_2-agonist and oral theophylline is superior to a long-acting β_2-agonist used alone. A combination of a short-acting β_2-agonist, short-acting anticholinergic, and theophylline is superior to the short-acting anticholinergic or a combination of oral theophylline and a short-acting β_2-agonist. A combination of an inhaled steroid and a long-acting β_2-agonist is superior to either alone in maintaining baseline pulmonary function in patients with chronic bronchitis.

Step Therapy

Because no pharmacologic therapy has disease modifying effects, all treatment is directed toward reducing dyspnea, improving ability to perform activities, improving health status, and preventing exacerbations. This leads to the concept of step therapy in which treatment begins with one agent and then other agents are added to titrate to symptomatic relief with the least side effects. There are a number of possible approaches, but what is presented here is a modification of the methods adopted by the Department of Veterans Affairs/Department of Defense VA/DoD (Table 2).

Other Therapies

Infusion therapy with α_1-antitrypsin (Prolastin) for patients with moderate-to-severe emphysema and severe deficiency should be considered. Mucolytics[1] continue to be under investigation and are not recommended for treatment of stable COPD at this time. Antibiotics are not recommended for treatment of stable COPD. The use of leukotriene modifiers such as montelukast (Singulair),[1] zafirlukast (Accolate),[1] or zileuton (Zyflo)[1] is *strongly discouraged* for treatment of COPD in the absence of a clear-cut diagnosis of asthma or other FDA-approved indication.

Vaccinations

Vaccination against influenza can reduce serious illness and death in COPD by approximately 50% and is recommended for all COPD patients unless otherwise contraindicated. Vaccination against pneumococcal disease reduces bacteremia in vaccinated patients with pneumonia and is recommended for patients with COPD.

Long-Term Oxygen Therapy

To qualify for long-term oxygen therapy (LTOT), patients must have an arterial oxygen saturation that is less than or equal to 88% or partial pressure arterial oxygen (PaO_2) that is less than or equal to 55 mm Hg at rest, or a saturation of 89% (PaO_2 of 56-59 mm Hg) with evidence of complications of hypoxemia such as polycythemia or cor pulmonale. Oxygen therapy to continuously increase PaO_2 to greater than or equal to 60 mm Hg (arterial oxygen saturation ≥90%) reduces mortality in these COPD patients. In patients without hypoxemia at rest, exercise may produce hypoxemia and increasing dyspnea. Oxygen during exercise often reduces dyspnea in such patients. Patients who are hypoxemic only during sleep have an increase in mortality, and nocturnal oxygen may be used. However, there have been no definitive studies to document benefit.

NONPHARMACOLOGIC INTERVENTIONS

Pulmonary Rehabilitation

Pulmonary rehabilitation is an intensive multidisciplinary program of exercise training, education, psychosocial/behavioral intervention, and nutritional therapy. Although each component adds to the program's effectiveness, most outcomes depend heavily on cardiovascular conditioning, which should be maintained. Benefits include improvements in dyspnea, exercise ability, health status, and health care use.

Lung Volume Reduction Surgery

Lung volume reduction surgery removes predominantly emphysematous portions of the lungs. When effective, patients have an increase in FEV_1 and

[1]Not FDA approved for this indication.

TABLE 2 Step Pharmacotherapy of COPD

Step	Symptoms and FEV_1	Therapy
1	Asymptomatic *and* FEV_1 >50% of predicted*	No bronchodilator medication indicated.
2a	Symptoms less than daily *and* FEV_1 ≥50% of predicted*	**Inhaled short-acting β_2-agonist**[†] (2 puffs prn up to 12 puffs/d).
2b	Asymptomatic *and* FEV_1 <50% of predicted*	**Inhaled short-acting anticholinergic** (Atrovent) (2 puffs qid). Consider using combination of inhaler containing a short-acting β_2-agonist and an anticholinergic (Combivent) (2 puffs qid). Consider use of an inhaled long-acting anticholinergic, tiotropium (Spiriva) (18 µg inhaled qd) as an alternative to an inhaled short-acting anticholinergic (Atrovent) or combination inhaler (Combivent). Consider using an inhaled long-acting β_2-agonist bid as an alternative to inhaled anticholinergic or combination inhaler.
2c	Symptoms appear less than daily *and* FEV_1 <50% of predicted *or* daily symptoms*	**Inhaled short-acting anticholinergic** (Atrovent) (2 puffs qid) **Short-acting β_2-agonist** (2 puffs prn up to 12 puffs/d) Consider use of combination inhaler containing a short-acting β_2-agonist and an anticholinergic (Combivent) (2 puffs qid and prn up to 12 puffs/d). Consider use of an inhaled long-acting anticholinergic, tiotropium (Spiriva) (18 µg inhaled qd) as an alternative to an inhaled short-acting anticholinergic (Atrovent) or combination inhaler (Combivent). Consider use of an inhaled long-acting β_2-agonist bid as an alternative to an inhaled anticholinergic or combination inhaler.
3	Symptoms not controlled*	**Increase dose of an inhaled short-acting anticholinergic** (Atrovent) (3-6 puffs qid) and **continue inhaled short-acting β_2 agonist** (2-4 puffs prn up to 12 puffs/d). Consider use of a long-acting inhaled anticholinergic, tiotropium (Spiriva) (18 µg inhaled qd) as an alternative to an inhaled short-acting anticholinergic. Consider use of an inhaled long-acting β_2-agonist bid with inhaled short-acting β_2 agonist prn for rescue as an alternative to frequent use of inhaled short-acting β_2-agonist.
4	Symptoms not controlled*	If not already implemented, consider adding **long-acting inhaled β_2-agonist** with inhaled short-acting β_2 agonist prn for rescue and/or inhaled long-acting anticholinergic, tiotropium (Spiriva) (18 µg inhaled qd).
5	Symptoms not controlled*	Consider adding **theophylline trial** (slow-release theophylline [Theo-24] adjusted to level of 5-2 µg/mL).
6	Symptoms not controlled*	Consider adding **corticosteroids** (high-dose inhaled steroids).[‡] Consider specialist consultation.
7	Symptoms not controlled*	**Refer to specialist promptly**.

[1]Not FDA approved for this indication.

*Symptoms include dyspnea, exacerbations, and inability to maintain lifestyle at optimal levels, including recreational activities. Use the lowest level of therapy that satisfactorily relieves symptoms and maximizes activity level. Assure compliance and proper use of medications before escalating therapy. Symptoms of dyspnea, general well-being, and improved exercise tolerance should be monitored. If asymptomatic patients with FEV_1 <50% show no improvement, discontinue therapy.

[†]Bolded recommendations are preferred; short-acting inhaled β_2-agonist should be used as needed for rescue at each step, if appropriate.

[‡]Addition of high-dose inhaled steroids (equivalent to 880 µg/d by MDI, or 1000 µg/d of the dry powder of fluticasone [Flovent], or 1200 µg/d of triamcinolone [Azmacort][1]) may improve dyspnea and health status and reduce exacerbations. Substantial improvement in pulmonary function is limited to a minority of patients (perhaps 10%). When combined with salmeterol, the FDA has approved 250 µg/50 µg (fluticasone/salmeterol [Advair]) twice daily for chronic obstructive pulmonary disease (COPD) to improve pulmonary function.

Abbreviations: FEV_1 = forced expiratory volume in 1 sec; prn = as needed; qid = 4 times daily.

Source: Modified from Department of Veterans Affairs/Department of Defense (VA/DoD) guidelines.

improvements in exercise capacity, health status, and dyspnea. The National Emphysema Therapy Trial (NETT) provided criteria to select those who are likely to benefit (in order of degree of benefit). These are patients with predominant upper-lobe emphysema and low workload capacity, predominant upper-lobe emphysema and high workload capacity, and nonupper lobe predominant emphysema with low workload capacity. The Centers for Medicare & Medicaid Services (CMS) has announced its intention to provide coverage for patients who meet these and other criteria.

Lung Transplantation

Lung transplantation (usually single lung) results in improved pulmonary function, exercise capacity, and health status in patients with very severe COPD. The 5-year survival rate is approximately 40%. Some suggested criteria are FEV_1 less than or equal to 25% predicted (without reversibility), and/or resting room air with partial pressure of arterial carbon dioxide ($PaCO_2$) greater than 55 mm Hg, and/or elevated $PaCO_2$ with progressive deterioration requiring long-term oxygen therapy. Elevated pulmonary artery pressure with progressive deterioration is also a potential indication.

Therapies on the Near Horizon

Oral phosphodiesterase 4 (PDE4) inhibitors* are being developed and are similar to theophylline

*Investigational drug in the United States.

without many of the side effects, particularly those of the cardiac and CNS.

Management of Exacerbations

Evaluation

All definitions of exacerbations include worsening of symptoms from baseline variability. These symptoms include dyspnea and increased sputum production, with purulent sputum being the most indicative of an infectious, often bacterial, etiology. Bacterial pathogens include *Haemophilus influenzae*, *Streptococcus pneumoniae*, and *Moraxella catarrhalis*. Exacerbations of COPD can be classified as mild, moderate, or severe. Exacerbations if treated with bronchodilators alone are considered mild, if treated with antibiotics and/or oral corticosteroids are moderate to severe, and if hospitalized are severe. Referral to an urgent care or emergency department should be considered if the patient has dyspnea at rest, rapid respiratory rate, tachycardia of more than 110, and use of accessory muscles of respiration.

Hospitalization should be considered if a patient is in impending or actual acute or acute-on-chronic respiratory failure despite optimal therapy. This decision is tempered by factors such as home support and ability of the patient to implement self-treatment.

THERAPY

Management includes pharmacotherapy, supportive treatment for hypoxemia and dehydration, and, in very severe cases, mechanical ventilatory support.

Bronchodilator therapy is with ipratropium (Atrovent) and albuterol (Proventil) in escalating doses to stabilize the patient. Oral or intravenous corticosteroids are often necessary and are effective compared with placebo. No benefit has been demonstrated beyond a 2-week course. Theophylline is generally not recommended because the efficacy is marginal and there may be significant side effects. Antibiotics are indicated if the patient's sputum is yellow or green. Which antibiotic to use depends on severity of the exacerbation, response of the patient to previous therapy, and local sensitivities of likely organisms.

Mechanical Ventilatory Support for Acute Respiratory Failure

Mechanical ventilation should be considered when, despite optimal medical therapy and oxygen administration, the patient remains in severe respiratory distress with unresponsive dyspnea, has a respiratory rate of greater than or equal to 25, is in impending or actual acute hypercapnic respiratory failure ($Paco_2$ $\geq$45 mm Hg), or presents with a significant increase in $Paco_2$ over baseline.

Noninvasive Ventilation

Noninvasive (without endotracheal intubation) positive-pressure ventilation (NPPV) is preferred and should be offered to cooperative and alert patients who are able to tolerate the necessary nasal or facial mask. Patients with cardiovascular instability, copious or viscous secretions, recent facial or gastroesophageal surgery, craniofacial trauma, high aspiration risk, and extreme obesity are not candidates. Patients who are not candidates should be considered for immediate intubation to provide access for mechanical ventilation. The benefits of NPPV are the avoidance of the complications of intubation and possibly a reduction in mortality. It is important that NPPV not delay intubation in appropriate patients.

Invasive Ventilation

Intubation should be considered in patients in whom NPPV is not indicated or who fail to resolve or stabilize arterial blood gases or hydrogen ion concentration (pH). Patients with life-threatening hypoxemia despite administration of supplemental oxygen, rapid respiratory rate (>35 breaths per minute), and conditions that are unlikely to resolve in the near or immediate future, such as sepsis and pneumonia, should be intubated immediately.

Advance directives, a living will or equivalent, should be discussed with patients regarding their wishes with respect to end-of-life care.

CYSTIC FIBROSIS

METHOD OF

Karl H. Karlson, Jr., MD

Cystic fibrosis (CF) is an autosomal recessive disease that affects approximately 1 in 2500 live births in the United States; 1 in 20 Caucasians is a carrier for the gene, whereas it is less common in African Americans. The most common genetic defect is the Delta F-508 allele, although hundreds of alleles associated with CF are known. They control various stages of development of the CF transmembrane conductance regulator (CFTR) protein, which acts as a chloride channel. This chloride channel dysfunction leads to thickened, tenacious mucus resulting in the pulmonary and gastrointestinal manifestations of the disease that are the primary problems in CF. A quantitative pilocarpine iontophoresis (sweat test) analysis of quantitative

TABLE 1 Intravenous Antibiotics for Acute Exacerbations

Amikacin (Amikin) 15-30 mg/kg/day divided q8h
Gentamicin (Garamycin) 2.5-3.3 mg/kg/dose q8h
Tobramycin (Nebcin, Tobrex) 2.5-3.3 mg/kg/dose q6-8h
Ceftazidime (Fortaz) 50-75 mg/kg/dose q8h
Aztreonam (Azactam) 50 mg/kg/dose q6-8h
Imipenem and Cilastatin 60-100 mg/kg/day divided q6h
Meropenem (Merrem) 50-70 mg/kg/day divided q8h
Piperacillin and Tazobactum (Zosyn) 300-400 mg/kg/day divided q4-6h
Ticarcillin (Ticar) 200-400 mg/kg/day divided q4-6h
Ticarcillin-Clavulanate (Timentin) 200-400 mg/kg/day divided q4-6h
Ciprofloxacin (Cipro) 20-30 mg/kg/day divided q12h

sweat chloride concentrations has long been the diagnostic test of choice.

A sweat chloride of 60 mEq or greater is consistent with the diagnosis of CF. Recently, gene probe analysis has been available for the most common alleles. The diagnosis of CF depends on the combination of the characteristic clinical presentation of CF and the confirmation of the diagnosis by either a sweat test or a gene probe. Because CF is an autosomal recessive disease, patients who have it, as well as their families, should receive genetic counseling about the one-in-four chance that subsequent children will have the disease. Also, siblings of the affected patient should be evaluated for CF. Cystic Fibrosis Centers provide diagnostic and therapeutic services for CF patients, who usually visit the Centers at 3-month intervals.

The respiratory tract manifestations of CF include chronic cough, recurrent bronchitis or pneumonia, chronic sinusitis, nasal polyposis, and hemoptysis. The most common organisms associated with the chronic infection of CF are *Pseudomonas aeruginosa* and *Staphylococcus aureus*. Antibiotic therapy aimed specifically at the offending organism is the mainstay of the pulmonary therapy in CF (Table 1). Pulmonary exacerbations are characterized by increased cough and sputum production, decreased exercise tolerance and activity, decreased appetite, weight loss, low-grade fever, and general malaise. In patients who have milder pulmonary exacerbations, oral antibiotics may be useful. For more serious exacerbations, intravenous antibiotics are used. The use of tobramycin solution for inhalation (TOBI) at a dose of 300 mg twice a day, given in cycles of 28 days on/28 days off, is effective long-term therapy. Azithromycin (Zithromax)[1] has recently been found to have both antimicrobial and anti-inflammatory effects in the CF lung. Although more study is needed to evaluate the efficacy of this drug in CF patients, it is being used in some patients for long-term therapy. However, because it can mask the effects of mycobacterial infections, it is important that tuberculosis be ruled out before the institution of long-term azithromycin therapy. Early intervention with aggressive antibiotic therapy is now used to decrease the likelihood of the early airway infection in CF proceeding to chronic suppurative lung disease.

[1]Not FDA approved for this indication.

Bronchoscopy with bronchoalveolar lavage for culture is used in some infants with CF to identify the organisms in the lower respiratory tract. If *Pseudomonas aeruginosa* is identified in the lower airway, then antibiotics are used to eradicate the infection even in children who are relatively asymptomatic.

In addition to antibiotics, several other treatments are used to control the pulmonary manifestations of CF. Ibuprofen[1] at high doses (20-30 mg/kg per dose twice daily)[3] with close monitoring of blood levels is used to decrease inflammation. Prednisone given orally every other day, however, is associated with side effects that outweigh the benefits.

There are several methods of chest physical therapy, which are used to clear mucus from the airways. The most conventional, hand-chest physical therapy, has been used longest.

High frequency oscillation of the chest enhances mucus clearance. Either external compression of the chest wall using a vest that is pneumatically inflated or oscillating positive expiratory pressure (PEP) devices through which the patient exhales, such as the Flutter and the Acapella, can be used. There are other PEP breathing exercises that can enhance mucus clearance. Many studies document that mucus clearance improves pulmonary function in CF, but there are insufficient data comparing various methods to show that one is superior to another.

Aerosolized bronchodilator therapy with albuterol (Proventil) is often used as an adjunct to other pulmonary therapies in CF before chest physical therapy. Some CF patients, however, have a paradoxical increase in airway resistance after aerosolized β-agonist therapy and thus need to be monitored carefully. Inhaled dornase alfa (Pulmozyme) (DNase) at a dose of 2.5 mg once daily by aerosol is associated with long-term improvement of pulmonary function in CF patients. Although inflammation is a major problem in the CF lung, the role of inhaled steroids is not yet known.

Abdominal pain, poorly formed stools, excessive flatus, poor weight gain, and abdominal protuberance are gastrointestinal manifestations of CF. Treatment of the gastrointestinal manifestations of CF includes pancreatic enzyme supplementation (Viokase), vitamin supplementation, and adequate caloric intake. Satisfactory weight gain is the goal of adequate nutritional therapy. Supplemental enzymes, also aimed at achieving satisfactory weight gain, are given orally and titrated against the patient's clinical symptoms. The maximum dose for enzyme supplementation is limited to 2500 lipase units per kilogram per dose to avoid colonic strictures. Supplemental vitamins are specifically designed to replace the fat-soluble vitamins that are poorly absorbed. Oral nutritional

[1]Not FDA approved for this indication.
[3]Exceeds dosage recommended by the manufacturer.

supplementation is used to reach the goal of one and a half to two times the standard caloric intake. In the more malnourished patients, nocturnal feedings given via a feeding gastrostomy are indicated. Because patients with CF lose excessive amounts of salt in their sweat, salt supplementation is also necessary in their diets.

Pulmonary complications of CF include pneumothorax and hemoptysis. Chest tube drainage is the initial therapy of pneumothorax. Chemical pleurodesis, physical abrasion of the pleura, or pleurectomy can decrease the likelihood of a recurrent pneumothorax; however, lung transplantation after pleural ablation can be complicated. Therefore, pleural ablation is generally reserved for selected cases that have not responded to more conservative therapy. Hemoptysis is a complication often associated with infection, and patients with hemoptysis are treated vigorously with antibiotics to control the infection. In patients who have a relatively small amount of hemoptysis, chest physical therapy is withheld until the hemoptysis resolves. In patients who experience massive hemoptysis, embolization of the involved bronchial artery may be indicated. Bronchoscopy prior to embolization can sometimes be helpful in localizing the area of bleeding.

Gastrointestinal complications include distal intestinal obstruction syndrome (DIOS), or meconium ileus equivalent, and cirrhosis. Typically, DIOS presents as an acute abdomen, and abdominal films reveal a pattern consistent with obstruction of the distal small intestine. An enema with contrast solutions such as Gastrografin can be both diagnostic and therapeutic. Adequate IV fluid therapy needs to be provided to these patients. GoLYTELY given either orally or by a nasogastric tube, up to 1000 cc per hour over several hours, also can be used but is contraindicated in complete bowel obstruction. The liver involvement initially involves fatty infiltration of the liver that then can progress to cirrhosis. Liver enzymes are often mildly elevated in CF.

Ursodeoxycholic acid (Actigall, Urso),[1] 15 to 20 mg/kg per day,[3] is used to slow the progression of liver disease and improve liver function studies. Esophageal varices from portal hypertension associated with cirrhosis can present with acute bleeding. Standard treatment includes endoscopic band ligation or sclerotherapy to control the bleeding. Occasionally patients with portal hypertension need to have shunt procedures. Gastroesophageal reflux is common in patients who have CF. Therapy with proton pump inhibitors can be helpful in controlling the symptoms. In addition, the decrease in the gastric acidity can increase the effectiveness of enzyme therapy.

Insulin-dependent diabetes is a complication of the pancreatic involvement. Treatment involves titration of the insulin doses using blood glucose levels.

Lung transplantation is indicated in patients with advanced lung disease. Patients with a forced expiratory volume at one second (FEV_1) between 30% and 35% predicted are candidates for evaluation at a transplant center. Liver transplantation is beneficial in selected patients with advanced liver involvement.

[1]Not FDA approved for this indication.
[3]Exceeds dosage recommended by the manufacturer.

OBSTRUCTIVE SLEEP APNEA

METHOD OF

Brian Boehlecke, MD, MSPH

Obstructive sleep apnea syndrome (OSAS) comprises a constellation of symptoms and physiologic changes associated with recurrent episodes of apnea and/or hypopnea during sleep. Bed partners report observing loud snoring, gasping or choking, and pauses in breathing followed by "snorting" and/or body jerking. The patient usually has excessive daytime somnolence (EDS) and may complain of non-refreshing sleep, morning headaches, decreased ability to concentrate, poor memory, irritability or frank mood disturbance, and/or impotence. Evidence is accumulating that OSAS is associated with increased risk for hypertension, cardiovascular disease and stroke, and insulin resistance. Patients with OSAS report reduced quality of life on standardized questionnaires and have an increased risk of motor vehicle accidents. These consequences are felt to be related to the sleep disturbance (recurrent micro-arousals, and reduced deep and rapid eye movement sleep) and the oxyhemoglobin desaturation associated with the apneas and hypopneas. The most commonly used measure of severity is the number of apneas plus hypopneas per hour of sleep (the apnea-hypopnea index [AHI]) during an overnight sleep study (polysomnogram [PSG]). Also clinically important is the severity of oxyhemoglobin desaturations indicated by the lowest arterial oxyhemoglobin saturation (S_PO_2) and the percent of time that it is below 90% saturation. The objective of treatment is to ameliorate current symptoms and physiologic abnormalities with the goal of reducing the risks of future morbidity and mortality.

Basis for Treatment

Recurrent sleep-related upper airway narrowing or complete closure causes the hypopneas and apneas characteristic of OSAS. Both anatomic abnormalities (e.g., large tongue and/or tonsils, redundant pharyngeal tissue, submucosal fat deposition, and/or retrognathia) and inadequate upper airway muscle tone during inspiration (increased collapsibility) can compromise upper airway patency. Maintaining adequate airway patency ameliorates obstructive apneas and hypopneas and reduces or eliminates the associated arousals and oxyhemoglobin desaturations. Reducing the AHI to near normal levels and maintaining oxyhemoglobin saturation at 90% or greater for most of the night has been shown to reduce daytime somnolence and improve self-rated quality of life in patients with OSAS. Although less consistently demonstrated, improvements in cognition and mood have also been found. Likewise, reduction in nocturnal and daytime blood pressure, especially in those classified as hypertensive, often occurs within a relatively short time after starting effective treatment. From these findings it is postulated but not yet proven that risk for cardiovascular disorders will also be decreased.

Whom to Treat

The severity of sleep disordered breathing (SDB) has been graded using the AHI as mild (5-15), moderate (>15-30), or severe (>30). Although those with higher grades of SDB tend to have more severe symptoms, an individual patient's symptoms are often not consistent with the grade of SDB demonstrated on his or her PSG. This may be caused by perceptual differences, individual variability in susceptibility to the effects of sleep disturbance and hypoxemia, and/or contributions by factors other than the events tallied in the AHI. The latter might include arousals associated with increased respiratory effort without airflow reduction (upper airway resistance syndrome [UARS]) or poor quality of sleep from pain or psychological distress. Likewise, although it is logical to assume that those with the most severe SDB are at greatest risk for long term adverse consequences and mortality, this has yet to be definitively demonstrated. Therefore, decisions on whom to treat and the optimal modality must still rely on clinical judgment applied to an individual patient's overall circumstances. Guidelines for determining initial management based on the AHI and the presence or absence of symptoms and co-morbid conditions potentially caused or aggravated by sleep disordered breathing are given in the Treatment Guidelines section of this article. Because nasal continuous positive airway pressure (CPAP) is the most efficacious therapy for OSAS, has few serious side effects, and is easily discontinued if the patient cannot tolerate it or does not improve, it is shown as the initial specific therapy of choice for OSAS. Basic measures to reduce sleep disturbance and sleep disordered breathing are always indicated and may suffice in some instances. Alternate therapies may be indicated if CPAP is not tolerated or is not fully effective.

Treatment Guidelines

Management is initially based on the AHI:

- *AHI less than 5*: No specific treatment for OSAS (SDB unlikely to account for symptoms or significantly increase risk for cardiovascular disease or insulin resistance). Recommend basic measures (good sleep hygiene, weight loss if indicated, avoidance of respiratory depressants and alcohol, oxygen if clinically significant hypoxia not caused by OSAS is present). Evaluate for UARS if symptoms and risk factors consistent with this diagnosis are present.
- *AHI > 5 to 15*: If symptoms (e.g., EDS, morning headaches) or co-morbid condition(s) (e.g., hypertension, insulin resistance, depression), possibly caused or aggravated by sleep disordered breathing, are present, start nasal CPAP after adequate titration. If no improvement in symptoms or objective improvement in co-morbid conditions occurs in 2 months, evaluate for causes of treatment failure and consider reverting to basic measures. If no symptoms or co-morbid conditions are present at baseline, recommend basic measures.
- *AHI equal 15 to 30*: Start nasal CPAP after adequate titration. If no subjective improvement (e.g., improved alertness or mood even if not recognized as a problem before treatment) or objective improvement in co-morbid conditions (e.g., reduction in need for antihypertensive medication or improved insulin sensitivity) occurs in 2 months, evaluate for causes of treatment failure. Consider reverting to basic measures.
- *AHI greater than 30*: Start nasal CPAP after adequate titration. If no subjective or objective improvement occurs in 2 months, evaluate for causes of treatment failure. Consider reverting to basic measures if no symptoms are present. However if co-morbid conditions are present and/or there is a strong family history of early cardiovascular disease and the patient is tolerating therapy, consider continuing CPAP for 6 months and re-evaluate.

Optimal CPAP pressure for a patient is best identified by an in-laboratory titration attended by a qualified sleep technologist. Because a patient's initial experience with CPAP is a major determinant of long-term use, the technician should be attentive to correcting any difficulty the patient experiences during titration and should provide encouragement and support to facilitate adaptation. Ideally one would like to identify a pressure that abolishes all sleep-related disordered breathing events and prevents significant oxyhemoglobin desaturations. However, the pressure needed to achieve this endpoint may not be tolerable for the patient. If prescribed at this pressure, CPAP may be rejected outright, underused, or discontinued. The optimal pressure for effective treatment is often a compromise between the lowest level that produces nearly complete reversal of the sleep disordered breathing events and the highest one likely to be accepted and adhered to by the patient. Selection of this level requires clinical judgment and consideration for readjustment based on patient response during the first few weeks of treatment. An attempt should be made to identify a pressure that reduces the AHI to less than 15 and abolishes oxyhemoglobin desaturations that are below 88%. In some cases supplemental oxygen will be needed to maintain adequate saturation at a tolerable CPAP pressure.

Problems that may compromise patient acceptance or adherence to treatment should be addressed promptly. Discomfort from the interface or air leaks because of poor mask fit are common initial problems amenable to adjustments or changes in equipment. If mouth opening cannot be prevented by use of a chin strap, a full face mask is indicated. If the patient has a sense of claustrophobia or cannot tolerate a nasal mask for other reasons, nasal pillows or a nasal cannula type of interface should be tried. Humidification reduces nasal drying and congestion; some patients, especially those with pre-existing nasal problems, may require a heated humidifier. Persistent rhinitis may respond to nasal steroids. Oral nonsedating antihistamine therapy may be added if allergic rhinitis is present. Significant rhinorrhea may respond to ipratropium (Atrovent) nasal spray. If anatomic nasal obstruction is present (e.g., deviated nasal septum or marked turbinate enlargement), referral for evaluation for surgery or radiofrequency ablation by an otorhinolaryngologist is indicated.

If the patient cannot tolerate the pressure required to achieve an acceptable AHI, use of machines that reduce the pressure during part of the exhalation (*flexible* CPAP) or have separately adjustable pressures during inhalation and exhalation (*bilevel* positive airway pressure) may improve tolerance. Autotitrating CPAP machines, which continuously adjust the pressure based on automated detection of apneas and flow limitation, may be efficacious when significant changes in optimal pressure occur with position changes or varying nasal obstruction throughout the night. Some patients find these machines easier to tolerate than conventional CPAP if the average pressure used is significantly lower than that required for adequate therapy for the most severe airway compromise during sleep. However, improvement in compliance or overall therapeutic outcomes has not been clearly demonstrated and some patients have their sleep disturbed when changes in pressure are initiated by the machine.

It is important to see the patient for a follow-up visit early in the course of CPAP treatment to address any problems. In some cases, temporary use of a benzodiazepine medication or a short-acting hypnotic may ease acclimatizations to CPAP.

Basic measures including weight loss, if indicated, should be recommended for all patients with OSAS. In some cases relatively modest weight loss will significantly improve sleep quality and reduce the CPAP pressure required. Sedatives and alcohol should be avoided. Good sleep hygiene with relatively constant bedtime and rise times and adequate time in bed is important. If airway obstruction is significantly worse in the supine position, efforts to maintain sleep in the lateral position are useful. A foam wedge or body pillow behind the back is most effective. Elevation of the head of the bed is also helpful and can ameliorate symptoms of gastroesophageal reflux commonly present in patients with OSAS.

Other Therapies

Oral devices to hold the tongue forward or reposition the mandible to increase airway size have been used with variable success. They are more easily tolerated than CPAP by some patients. However, they are less efficacious than CPAP for reducing the AHI and maintaining oxyhemoglobin saturation. They should generally be considered only for patients with mild-to-(at most) moderate OSAS who are intolerant of CPAP. Patients must have adequate dentition to use mandibular repositioning devices.

Several surgical procedures to reduce upper airway narrowing have been developed. Uvulopalatopharyngoplasty (UPPP) removes the uvula and redundant pharyngeal tissue. It appears to be most effective in milder cases of OSAS and results in a *cure* in 50% or less of cases. Use of CPAP after UPPP may be complicated by increased mouth leaks due to lack of a seal of the soft palate against the back of the tongue.

Genioglossus/hyoid advancement has produced significant reduction in the AHI, but the success rate has been similar to UPPP. Maxillomandibular advancement can increase upper airway dimensions and improve OSAS, especially in patients with significant retrognathia. However, this is extensive surgery and may require adjustment of dental occlusion. Laser-assisted uvulopalatoplasty is not recommended. In general, surgical procedures should be considered as second-line therapy for those who do not respond to basic measures and cannot tolerate CPAP.

Residual Sleepiness on Continuous Positive Airway Pressure

Excessive daytime sleepiness despite a patient's report of compliance with CPAP requires careful evaluation to determine appropriate management. Documentation of CPAP use with a recording CPAP device or, at minimum, a patient log should be created. Equipment should be checked for function and correct pressure setting. The patient should be carefully questioned regarding possible mask leaks or mouth opening (often suggested by morning dry mouth and nose), which cause inadequate pressure maintenance. Adequate sleep hygiene with sufficient time in bed should be evaluated by a patient log maintained for 2 weeks. Other factors that may contribute to inadequate or non-refreshing sleep should be considered. These include chronic pain, psychological conditions (e.g., anxiety or mood disorders), medications, need for frequent nocturnal urination, or periodic limb movements of sleep (PLMS). If no clear cause is identified, a repeat PSG on CPAP is indicated to evaluate adequacy of the prescribed pressure and to look for other causes of sleep disturbance such as PLMS. Persistent spontaneous arousals on CPAP at the prescribed pressure may be indicative of UARS, and attempts to eliminate them with increased pressure may be warranted. The PSG may be followed by a Multiple Sleep Latency Test (MSLT) to objectively evaluate daytime sleepiness and look for multiple episodes of sleep onset REM suggestive of narcolepsy. Lack of short sleep latency may indicate misperception of fatigue as sleepiness by the patient.

Lengthening of the sleep period by 30 minutes to 1 hour may be helpful. If excessive sleepiness is documented despite adequate sleep with no recognized disruptions, treatment with a stimulant may be indicated. Modafinil (Provigil), 100 to 400 mg in the morning, may increase daytime alertness without causing overstimulation or sleep disturbance. Scheduled naps up to 30 minutes long often improve alertness without residual grogginess interfering with rapid resumption of activities or interfering with sleep onset at the usual bedtime.

PRIMARY LUNG CANCER

METHOD OF
Jacob D. Bitran, MD

Epidemiology

Lung cancer is a health care problem of global proportions. Trillions of dollars are spent globally in providing care to victims of lung cancer and in lost wages that would be better spent on preventive medicine, prenatal care, and nourishing the world's youth.

Lung cancer is lethal. Within the United States, we are witnessing an epidemic of lung cancer. In 2004, it was estimated that lung cancer will be diagnosed in 170,400 individuals (90,200 men and 80,200 women) and 154,900 will die of it. Among U.S. women, lung cancer is the leading cause of cancer-related deaths and was projected to account for an estimated 65,700 deaths in 2004. Although the incidence of lung cancer has decreased in U.S. men, it is increasing at an alarming rate among U.S. women, with 80,200 cases in 2004 versus 73,000 in 1995. The increased incidence in women is clearly related to the fact that more women are smoking. In addition, given the popularity of smoking among teenage girls, it is likely that the epidemic of lung cancer will continue into the twenty-first century. Lung cancer is preventable in the majority of instances, and preventive efforts need to be redoubled to curb the rising tide of smoking among women and teenage girls.

Cigarette smoking accounts for 85% of all lung cancer; the remaining 15% is thought to be linked to either environmental exposure or genetic factors. Environmental exposure to arsenic, asbestos, bis(chloromethyl)ether, chromium, nickel, radon, and vinyl chloride and passive exposure to smoke (secondhand smoke) have been implicated in the increased risk for lung cancer. Most recently, an increased risk for primary lung cancer has been described in patients treated with external beam radiation therapy for Hodgkin's disease and breast cancer. Genetic factors that may contribute to an increased risk of lung cancer include genotypes inducing the synthesis of high levels of 4-debrisoquin hydroxylase and relative deficiency of the MU phenotype of glutathione transferase. Adults who survive childhood retinoblastoma have a 15-fold increased incidence of small cell lung cancer (SCLC) when compared with the general population. It is believed that the polycyclic aromatic hydrocarbons and N-nitrosamines in cigarette smoke lead to DNA damage by methylation. In turn, the DNA methylation leads to altered gene expression and contributes to the neoplastic process.

Symptoms and Signs

The symptoms and signs of lung cancer can vary from complete absence of any symptoms or signs (an incidental lesion found on a chest radiograph that has been obtained for another reason) to the presence of a new or changed cough, dyspnea, hemoptysis, chest pain, shoulder pain, superior vena cava syndrome, Horner's syndrome, Pancoast's syndrome, supraclavicular or cervical lymphadenopathy, unresolving pneumonia or pneumonitis, bone pain, headache, paresis or paralysis, confusion, ataxia, or abdominal pain. Systemic symptoms can include fatigue, weight loss, or cachexia. Paraneoplastic syndromes that are often associated with primary lung cancer include ectopic adrenocorticotropic hormone (ACTH) syndrome,

Eaton-Lambert syndrome, dermatomyositis, and acanthosis nigricans.

Histologic Classification

It is likely that all lung cancers arise from a common pluripotent cell. Furthermore, it is likely that the phenotypic (histologic) appearance is a function of the altered gene expression associated with a variety of genetic mutations. The pathologic appearance of a primary lung cancer is of particular importance both for diagnostic purposes and in developing the therapeutic approach. Lung cancer is basically composed of four different subtypes: SCLC and squamous cell carcinoma, adenocarcinoma, and large cell lung cancer, all of which are referred to as non-small cell lung cancer (NSCLC). Most pathologists use the World Health Organization classification of lung cancer (Table 1). Many lung cancers, if examined closely, have mixed histologic features.

SCLC accounts for 25% of the lung cancer diagnosed in the United States. The presence of neurosecretory granules on electron microscopy and overexpression of the neural cell adhesion molecule (NCAM) is characteristic of SCLC. Most often, SCLC is manifested as a central (hilar) lesion. Adenocarcinoma accounts for 40% of all the lung cancer diagnosed in the United States, and it is the most frequent lung cancer in women. It is associated with cigarette smoking and pulmonary injury and can arise in a central or peripheral location. Squamous cell lung cancer accounts for 25% of all lung cancers and has been declining in the past 2 decades. It stains positively for keratin and is most often manifested as a central lesion. Large cell lung cancer accounts for about 3% of all lung cancers and has an anaplastic appearance. It is thought to represent a continuum of neuroendocrine tumors that include carcinoid and SCLC. Yet despite this view, large cell cancers are treated clinically as NSCLC. The use of immunohistochemical stains (carcinoembryonic antigen, cytokeratin-7, and TTF-1) permits accurate differentiation of poorly differentiated adenocarcinoma or anaplastic squamous cell lung cancer from large cell lung cancer. Bronchoalveolar carcinoma of the lung is classified as a subtype of adenocarcinoma. The neoplastic cells in bronchoalveolar carcinoma are type II pneumocytes. Patients with bronchoalveolar carcinoma usually have alveolar infiltrates or lobar consolidation that is often initially diagnosed as pneumonia. Unresolved pneumonia infiltrates in an adult may be a manifestation of bronchoalveolar carcinoma.

TABLE 1 World Health Organization Histologic Classification of Epithelial Bronchogenic Carcinoma

I. Malignant
  A. Squamous cell (epidermal) and spindle cell carcinoma
  B. Small cell
    1. Oat cell carcinoma (lymphocytic-like)
    2. Intermediate cell type
    3. Combined oat cell carcinoma (mixed histologic types, small with squamous cell carcinoma or adenocarcinoma)
  C. Adenocarcinoma
    1. Acinar
    2. Papillary
    3. Bronchoalveolar
    4. Mucinous secreting
  D. Large cell
    1. Giant cell
    2. Clear cell
  E. Adenosquamous carcinoma
    1. Carcinoid
    2. Bronchial gland carcinoma
    3. Adenoid cystic
    4. Mucoepidermoid
  F. Others

Adapted from World Health Organization: Histological Typing of Lung Tumors, 2nd ed. Geneva, WHO, 1981.

Biology of Primary Lung Cancer

Lung cancers arise from mutations in the bronchial epithelium over the course of a person's life. Lung cancer represents the culmination of 10 to 20 such mutational events. In the past decade, scientists have begun to define these events and construct a hypothesis of how lung cancer develops. It appears that one of the earliest events that leads to bronchial epithelial hyperplasia is allelic loss on the short arm of chromosome 3 (3p), where at least three tumor suppressor genes are present. Allelic loss of 3p, coupled with allelic loss on the short arm of chromosome 9 (9p), leads to dysplasia. Mutational events that convert epithelial dysplasia into carcinoma in situ include mutation of the gene for p53 (chromosome 17) and mutational activation of the K-ras oncogene (chromosome 12). At this point, further mutational events and the loss of antecedent cytogenetic events will determine the progression of carcinoma in situ and the ultimate phenotypic appearance (histologic type) of the lung cancer. Deletion of 3p, coupled with myc oncogene (N-, c-, and L-myc, chromosome 8q24) activation, mutation of the gene encoding retinoblastoma (chromosome 13), and loss of K-ras activation, will lead to the SCLC phenotype. In contrast, persistence of K-ras activation, allelic loss of chromosome 1, and overexpression of c-erb-2 and/or bcl-2 will lead to the NSCLC phenotype.

Growth factors that serve as paracrine (autocrine) promoters of cellular growth include gastrin-releasing peptide (SCLC), epidermal growth factor (SCLC and NSCLC), insulin-like growth factor type I (SCLC and NSCLC), transforming growth factor-β1 (NSCLC), bombesin, and cholecystokinin (SCLC).

Screening for Lung Cancer

Screening for lung cancer has been an area of investigation for almost 2 decades. Based on the findings of the Mayo Lung Project, screening of smokers by chest radiography and sputum cytology is not recommended. More recently, the Early Lung Cancer Action Project has published the results of low-dose computed tomography (CT) in patients at high risk for lung cancer. These results show that low-dose CT of the chest is superior to chest radiography at baseline. The results of this study have led to controlled clinical trials to evaluate whether low-dose spiral CT can decrease mortality from lung cancer in high-risk populations.

Diagnostic Methods and Staging of Lung Cancer

Patients with lung cancer usually have an abnormal chest radiograph. Stage 0 lung cancer (carcinoma in situ) is exceedingly rare and represents an incidental finding in a patient undergoing bronchoscopy for another indication. If a suspicious lesion is found on chest radiography, obtaining old chest radiographs for comparative purposes is essential. If a lesion has been stable on the chest radiograph for 2 years, further workup is not necessary. New lesions need to be investigated, however. A thorough history and physical examination are keys to the investigation of a pulmonary nodule or hilar mass (Figure 1). Particular attention should be paid to the lymph node examination (cervical and supraclavicular), the lung examination (localized rales or rhonchi, absent breath sounds), the abdomen (organomegaly), and the neurologic examination. The presence of lymphadenopathy or organomegaly will provide staging information and locate a potential area for biopsy to determine the histologic diagnosis. In the event that the findings on physical examination are entirely normal, CT of the chest to the level of the adrenals should be performed while the physician attempts to arrive at a histologic diagnosis. CT confirms the presence and extent of the pulmonary mass, evaluates the mediastinum for the presence or absence of any lymphadenopathy, and confirms or excludes the presence of other pulmonary nodules. Positron emission tomography (PET) with 2-fluorodeoxyglucose (2-FDG) is necessary for evaluating solitary pulmonary nodules and for staging of the lung cancer. PET scanning of the hilum and mediastinum is more sensitive than CT. The sensitivity and specificity of PET scans of the hilum and mediastinum are 85% and 89%, respectively. The absence of any uptake of 2-FDG on a PET scan excludes a malignant neoplastic process with a 99% level of confidence.

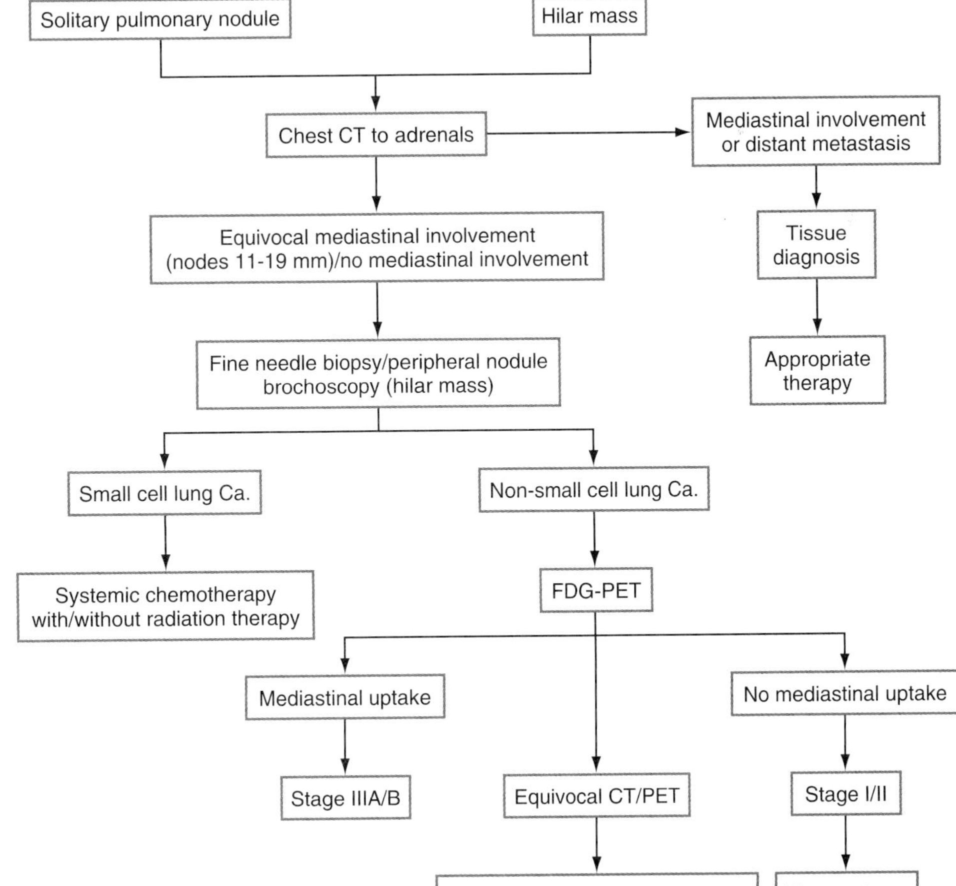

FIGURE 1 Clinical/pathological staging of lung cancer. CT, computed tomography; FDG, flourodeoxyglucose; PET. positron emission tomography.

After a histologic diagnosis of lung cancer has been established, further workup is based on the symptoms and signs. Complaints of back pain should prompt a technetium Tc 99m bone scan. A complaint of headache should prompt CT scanning or magnetic resonance imaging (MRI) of the brain. At the completion of clinical staging, patients are placed into a clinical stage as described in Table 2. Patients with clinical stage I and II NSCLC require further pathologic staging; patients with clinical stage IIIA, IIIB, and IV NSCLC will not require further pathologic staging, and treatment decisions can be based on the clinical stage. Patients with SCLC of any stage (with the exception of stage I) are treated with chemotherapy.

PATHOLOGIC STAGING

Fiberoptic bronchoscopy is a very accurate and safe technique for rendering a diagnosis of lung cancer in patients with central (hilar) lesions. The bronchoscope can directly visualize the tracheobronchial tree, and hilar masses can be sampled by directed biopsy and/or brush biopsy. Location of the mass relative to the carina is noted, and the carina can be inspected and sampled. Clinical staging of the mediastinum is provided by CT scanning of the chest. The presence of enlarged mediastinal lymph nodes (2 cm or larger) is considered pathologic, and histologic confirmation is not always necessary. Mediastinal lymph nodes that are 1 cm or smaller are considered normal, and mediastinoscopy is a low-yield procedure. Mediastinal nodes that are 1.1 to 1.9 cm are considered intermediate in size and represent a "gray area." Such nodes may be reactive or harbor metastases. PET scanning of the mediastinum in patients with nodes of normal or intermediate size can determine the presence or absence of metastases.

At present, patients with clinical stage I or II lung cancer and mediastinal nodes of indeterminate size and/or equivocal PET scans of the mediastinum require mediastinoscopy (for right-sided lesions) or mediastinotomy (for the left hilar regions) for pathologic confirmation. Mediastinoscopy is a surgical procedure performed under general anesthesia in which a hollow, rigid instrument is introduced through a small incision in the suprasternal notch and advanced along the pretracheal plane to the level of the carina. Enlarged lymph nodes can be visualized and sampled for biopsy. On the right side, the upper margin of the hilum may be reached, whereas the aortic arch precludes access to the left hilum. Contraindications to mediastinoscopy include superior vena caval obstruction, mediastinal surgery, and previous radiotherapy. A limited parasternal mediastinoscopy can be performed for pathologic or diagnostic staging of left hilar or aortopulmonary window lesions. Figure 1 summarizes the clinical and pathologic staging of lung cancer.

Once pathologic staging has been completed and patients have been segregated into clinical/pathologic stages I to IV, the physician is ready to make treatment decisions regarding which patients are surgical candidates and which are better suited for alternative therapies.

TABLE 2 International Staging System for Lung Cancer

Primary Tumor (T)	
T0	No evidence of primary tumor
TX	Cancer cell in bronchopulmonary secretions; no tumor seen on chest radiography or bronchoscopy
Tis	Carcinoma in situ
T1	Tumor ≤3 cm in greatest dimension, surrounded by lung tissue; no bronchoscopic evidence of tumor proximal to the lobar bronchus
T2	Tumor >3 cm in greatest diameter or tumor of any size that involves the visceral pleura or is associated with atelectasis extending to the hilum (but not involving the entire lung); must be ≥2 cm from the carina
T3	Tumor involves the chest wall, diaphragm, mediastinal pleura, or pericardium or is <2 cm from the carina (but does not involve it)
T4	Tumor involves the carina or trachea or invades the mediastinum, heart, great vessels, esophagus, or vertebrae; or malignant pleural effusion is present
Nodal Involvement (N)	
N0	No demonstrable lymph node involvement
N1	Ipsilateral peribronchial or hilar nodes involved
N2	Metastases to the ipsilateral mediastinal nodes or subcarinal nodes
N3	Metastases to the contralateral hilar, mediastinal, or scalene or supraclavicular nodes
Distant Metastasis (M)	
M0	No (known) distant metastasis
M1	Distant metastasis present—specify site(s)
Stage 0	Tis
Stage IA	T1, N0, M0
Stage IB	T2, N0, M0
Stage IIA	T1, N1, M0
Stage IIB	T2, N1, M0
Stage IIIA	T3,N0 or N1, M0; or T1-3, N2, M0
Stage IIIB	Any T, N3, M0; or T4, any N, M0
Stage IV	Any T, any N, M1

Adapted from Mountain CF: Revisions in the international staging system for lung cancer. Chest 111:1710-1717, 1997.

Preoperative Assessment

It is obvious that in planning treatment, one needs to consider the overall health of the patient, the patient's age, and other co-morbid conditions that preclude lung resection. In patients who are identified as potential surgical candidates, preoperative assessment of pulmonary function and estimation of postoperative pulmonary function are necessary. All surgical candidates should have initial pulmonary function tests. Patients who have a preoperative forced expiratory volume in 1 second (FEV_1) of greater than 1.2 L and a diffusing capacity for carbon monoxide (DLCO) of greater than 80% and do not have hypercapnia or cor pulmonale are clearly surgical candidates, independent of the extent of lung resection (lobectomy versus pneumonectomy). Patients who have an FEV_1 of 0.5 L or less are inoperable, and no further assessment is required. Those with an FEV_1 of 0.8 to 1.2 L or a DLCO of less than 60% are considered borderline operative candidates in whom thoracotomy is deemed high risk. Such patients should undergo quantitative ventilation/perfusion lung scans to estimate postoperative pulmonary function. In general, patients who are estimated to have a postoperative FEV_1 of less than 0.5 L are not operative candidates.

Non-Small Cell Lung Cancer

TREATMENT OF STAGES IA, IB, IIA, AND IIB

Patients with stage I or II NSCLC account for only 20% to 25% of all patients with newly diagnosed NSCLC. The preferred treatment of such patients who are medically fit is surgical resection. The preferred surgical resection is lobectomy and a sampling of the mediastinal lymph nodes. Segmental pulmonary resection is an appropriate alternative if patients do not have the pulmonary reserve to undergo lobectomy; however, several series have reported a higher local recurrence rate after segmental resection. Pneumonectomy does not confer any advantage over lobectomy and is indicated only if lobectomy results in incomplete resection. The operative mortality (which includes the 30-day postoperative period) associated with pneumonectomy, lobectomy, and segmental resection is 6.2%, 2.9%, and 1%, respectively. Causes of death include pneumonia, respiratory failure, myocardial infarction, pulmonary embolism, bronchopleural fistula, and empyema. Video-assisted thoracoscopic lobectomy is undergoing evaluation, but at present, its role in the treatment of stages IA, IB, IIA, and IIB NSCLC is unclear.

Surgical resection in patients with stages IA, IB, IIA, and IIB NSCLC leads to an excellent disease-free survival rate of 60% to 80% for stage I NSCLC and 35% to 50% for stage II. Patients with stage I or II squamous cell carcinoma have better disease-free survival than do those with stage I or II adenocarcinoma. Additional prognostic factors that may predict recurrence and survival are the presence of K-ras mutations at codon 12 (adenocarcinoma, a factor indicating a poor prognosis) and overexpression of bcl-2 (positive prognostic factor). Patients with stage I or II NSCLC who either are medically unfit or, for whatever reason, are not surgical candidates should be treated with radiotherapy, at least 60 Gy in 30 fractions (2-Gy fractions). The disease-free survival rate for patients with stage I or II NSCLC treated with radiotherapy is 17% to 32% at 5 years.

Although several studies have adjuvant chemotherapy or postoperative radiotherapy in patients with stage I or II NSCLC, none of the published studies have yielded a survival benefit. However, a recent CALGB trial employing carboplatin and paclitaxel as adjuvant therapy has shown a survival benefit. This study requires publication and confirmation before adjuvant chemotherapy becomes the standard of care. Patients who have been successfully treated for stage I or II NSCLC have a 2% to 3% risk per year of a second primary lung cancer developing. In 10 years, the risk is 20% to 30%. Currently, ongoing studies are investigating neoadjuvant (preoperative) chemotherapy in stage I and II NSCLC. Because such patients represent a high-risk group, they should be monitored at a minimum of every 3 to 4 months for the first 24 months and then every 6 months thereafter.

TREATMENT OF STAGES IIIA AND IIIB

Stage III:T3, N0-1, M0

Patients with stage IIIA NSCLC represent a subset of differing cohorts: T3, N0, M0; T3, N1, M0; T1-3, N2, M0; and T1-3, N3, M0. Accordingly, a uniform treatment approach to all patients with stage IIIA cannot be recommended. Rather, the treatment approach will vary with the subset of patients. For patients with NSCLC who have tumor directly extending into the chest wall (T3, N0-1, M0), it is generally agreed that surgical resection of the primary lung cancer and the involved chest wall is indicated. The 5-year survival rate of such patients is approximately 50%. To date, adjuvant postoperative radiotherapy to the chest wall or the resected tumor bed has had no role in management. For patients with Pancoast's tumor (superior sulcus tumors) (T3, N0-1, M0), treatment consists of preoperative radiotherapy of 30 to 45 Gy, followed if possible by lung resection along with resection of usually the first two ribs. The 5-year survival rate of patients with Pancoast's tumor is 35% to 45%. Whereas some reports advocate the use of radiotherapy and chemotherapy in the treatment of Pancoast's tumor, no randomized trials have compared the potential additive effect of chemotherapy, and its use cannot be recommended at this time.

Stage IIIA (T1-3, N2, M0) and Stage IIIB

Patients with mediastinal nodal (N2) involvement are detected in two ways. The most common is detection of mediastinal nodal involvement by chest radiography, chest CT, or mediastinoscopy. Such patients are not candidates for surgery; they have inoperable lung cancer and should be treated as described in the following paragraphs. The other smaller group of N2 patients are those who have clinical-pathologic stage I or II NSCLC at the time of lung resection and are found on mediastinal nodal sampling to have involved mediastinal lymph nodes. The 5-year survival rate of this subset of patients is poor, 9% to 12%. No compelling data indicate that this subset of patients have had their natural history altered with the use of postoperative adjuvant chemotherapy, radiotherapy, or both. The recommendation for such patients is close follow-up, and treatment decisions can be made at the time of relapse.

As already stated, the vast majority of stage IIIA patients, T1-3, N2, M0, and stage IIIB patients are detected at the time of clinical staging. Patients with stage IIIA and IIIB NSCLC are best treated with either initial cisplatin-based chemotherapy followed by radiation therapy or concurrent chemotherapy and radiotherapy. Numerous prospective randomized trials and meta-analyses have demonstrated improved median survival when chemotherapy is added to radiation therapy. A recent prospective randomized study from Japan addressed the issue of whether chemotherapy should be used sequentially or concurrently with radiation therapy. The study showed that concurrent chemotherapy plus radiotherapy leads to improved median survival and 5-year relapse-free survival.

Patients with unresectable stage IIIA or IIIB NSCLC who have good overall physical status should be encouraged to participate in the current generation of clinical trials, which are designed to determine the optimal initial chemotherapy and optimal radiotherapy regimens. For patients who choose not to enroll in such studies, initial chemotherapy with a cisplatin- or carboplatin-based regimen followed by radiotherapy represents standard care. Patients who are debilitated from stage IIIA/IIIB NSCLC are best treated with palliative radiotherapy alone.

The concept of neoadjuvant chemotherapy (preoperative) is not new, and a number of feasibility studies have addressed this concept in stage IIIA patients with NSCLC. In most of these feasibility studies, surgical resection has been attempted after neoadjuvant chemotherapy. In 1994, two small prospective randomized studies showed a survival benefit with the use of neoadjuvant chemotherapy followed by surgical resection in a selected group of patients with stage IIIA NSCLC. Subsequently, two larger multi-institutional trials have confirmed the benefit of neoadjuvant chemotherapy followed by surgical resection versus surgery alone. Patients who received neoadjuvant chemotherapy had a median survival in the range of 26 to 64 months, and the 3- to 5-year survival rate was 25% to 30%. These results were better than those of the surgery control arm. Patients treated with surgery alone had a median survival of 8 to 12 months and a 3-year survival rate of 0% to 5%. However, this approach carries with it significant morbidity and a treatment-related mortality of 10% to 15%. Furthermore, it is unknown whether this treatment approach is better or worse than the sequence of chemotherapy followed by radiotherapy in patients with stage IIIA NSCLC. A large multi-institutional phase III trial is currently addressing this question. At present, the standard approach in patients with stage IIIA/IIIB NSCLC is initial chemotherapy followed by radiotherapy.

TREATMENT OF STAGE IV

After sequential staging, about 40% to 50% of patients with NSCLC will be found to have stage IV disease. For such patients, no curative therapy is available, and the goal should be palliation and improved quality of life. Seven randomized clinical trials have attempted to answer the question of whether multiagent chemotherapy is better than the best supportive care in NSCLC. These seven trials used a variety of chemotherapy regimens. During the past 8 years, three meta-analyses of these randomized trials have been performed, and the following conclusions have been reached:

1. Patients without debility from NSCLC (good performance status) have a 35% and 27% reduction in mortality from NSCLC at 3 and 6 months, respectively, which is statistically significant; however, the reduction in risk diminishes with time.
2. Median survival increases from 3.9 to 6.7 months, a net gain of 12 weeks.

Because none of the studies performed a quality-of-life analysis, conclusions cannot be drawn. However, a trial carried out by the National Cancer Institute of Canada and reported by Rapp and colleagues analyzed the cost of care and concluded that the best supportive care was more expensive than one of the chemotherapy arms (CAP: cyclophosphamide [Cytoxan],[1] doxorubicin [Adriamycin],[1] and cisplatin [Platinol-AQ][1]). Patients in the supportive care group required more radiotherapy and days in the hospital than did patients receiving CAP. The net savings with CAP chemotherapy was $6172 per year of life gained when compared with best supportive care. These data suggest that patients receiving chemotherapy experience palliation of symptoms and spend less time in the hospital. Thus, in patients who have a good performance status, the current recommendation is that they receive chemotherapy, preferably on an ambulatory basis. Such patients should be encouraged to enroll in clinical trials so that we can advance the state of the art. If patients decide to not enroll in such studies, medical oncologists can choose a variety of drugs in an attempt to provide palliation. During the past few years, many new chemotherapeutic agents have been developed and released. Many of these new drugs are active in NSCLC (>15% response rate) and include paclitaxel (Taxol), docetaxel (Taxotere), gemcitabine (Gemzar), irinotecan (CPT-11 [Camptosar]),[1] and topotecan (Hycamtin).[1] The current generation of clinical trials is exploring the use of small molecules that interfere with epidermal growth factor receptor (EGFR) signal/transduction. IRESSA, an EGFR antagonist, interferes with the tyrosine kinase activated by EGFR. In phase II studies, it has provided clinical benefit, and the Food and Drug Administration approved it recently. It is expected that better treatments will be forthcoming for stage IV NSCLC.

---

[1]Not FDA approved for this indication.

Small Cell Lung Cancer

SCLC represents 20% to 25% of all lung cancers in the United States; the incidence of SCLC in 2002 was estimated to be between 33,000 and 42,000 men and women. SCLC is a distinct clinical-pathologic entity and is almost always associated with cigarette smoking. It has a characteristic histologic appearance consisting of the presence of neuroendocrine granules (electron dense) on electron microscopy and a distinctive cytogenetic alteration, deletion of the short arm of chromosome 3 (3p14-21), which in turn leads to overexpression of the c-myc oncogene. SCLC is associated with peptide secretion, such as gastrin-releasing peptide (bombesin), and it stains positively for neuron-specific enolase and chromogranin A. SCLS is characterized clinically by rapid tumor growth and progression. It is responsive to both chemotherapy and radiotherapy, and a large percentage of patients attain a complete response, which represents complete disappearance of all clinical disease. Other clinical features include ectopic production of hormones, such as antidiuretic hormone and corticotropin (ACTH). As stated previously, patients with SCLC may be characterized as having limited disease (encompassed within a single radiation therapy stage I, II, IIIA, IIIB) or extensive disease (stage IV).

Staging in SCLC consists of a thorough history and physical examination, chest radiography, CT of the chest to the level of the adrenals, bone marrow aspiration and biopsy (to detect occult bone marrow involvement), MRI or CT of the brain, and bone scanning. PET scans are sensitive in detecting occult metastases in patients with SCLC and thus complement the aforementioned staging procedures.

TREATMENT

Treatment of patients with SCLC is determined by whether they have limited or extensive disease. Patients with extensive disease represent about 67% of all those with SCLC, and treatment of such patients is chemotherapy with the intent of providing palliation. The chemotherapy regimens in clinical use include cisplatin (Platinol-AQ)[1] plus etoposide (VePesid)(PE), carboplatin[1] plus etoposide, and more recently, cisplatin[1] plus irinotecan.[1] A recent multicenter Japanese trial compared cisplatin plus weekly irinotecan with PE.

The cisplatin plus irinotecan combination led to superior median survival when compared with PE, 12.8 versus 9.4 months. Moreover, the 2-year survival rate for the cisplatin plus irinotecan combination was 19.5%, as opposed to 5.2% for the PE group. Clearly, patients with extensive SCLC and a good performance status should receive cisplatin plus irinotecan. For elderly patients or those debilitated by SCLC (poor performance status), a British trial conducted by the Medical Research Council Lung Cancer Working Party showed that oral etoposide resulted in greater toxic effects and an inferior survival than cyclophosphamide, Adriamycin (doxorubicin), and vincristine (CAV) did. Thus, even in the elderly or patients with poor performance status, multidrug chemotherapy remains the treatment of choice. The dismal survival of patients with SCLC underscores the importance of finding new and active agents. In the past 5 years, investigators have initiated phase II studies in previously untreated patients with extensive SCLC with the aim of identifying new agents. The design of these studies has been to use the single agent for three or four courses and obviously to continue its use if patients have a complete or partial response; however, if patients have either stable or progressive disease during the time that the phase II agent is administered, they rapidly cross over to a conventional chemotherapy program such as PE or CAV. It is clear from analyses of such trials that the use of a phase II agent in previously untreated patients with extensive SCLC does not jeopardize their ability to respond to a more conventional program, nor does it decrease their median survival. As a result of such studies, newer active chemotherapeutic agents for SCLC include paclitaxel (Taxol),[1] docetaxel (Taxotere),[1] topotecan (Hycamtin), JM-216[†] (an oral carboplatin analogue), and gemcitabine (Gemzar).[1]

Patients with SCLC who are found to have limited disease (approximately one third of patients with SCLC) are treated with concurrent chemotherapy and radiotherapy. In the past 9 years, a number of important trials have established the beneficial role of administering concurrent radiotherapy and chemotherapy in patients with limited SCLC. On the basis of a meta-analysis of 13 randomized trials that included over 2100 patients, the use of radiotherapy decreased mortality from SCLC by 14% and increased survival at 3 years by 5.4%. A randomized trial conducted in Canada addressed the issue of the timing of thoracic irradiation in limited SCLC and concluded that patients who received chemotherapy and radiotherapy beginning on the first day of treatment had better survival than when the thoracic radiotherapy was delayed. On the basis of the aforementioned meta-analysis and the Canadian trial, the current recommendation is to begin cisplatin (Platinol-AQ)[1] and etoposide (PE) (VePesid) with concurrent thoracic irradiation (through a portal that includes the chest primary, the mediastinum, and both supraclavicular fossae up to a total dose of 55 Gy). The PE regimen is given every 3 to 4 weeks for a total of six courses. Continuation of PE beyond six courses does not lead to a survival benefit as demonstrated by several randomized trials. Prophylactic cranial irradiation (PCI), 25 Gy in 10 fractions, is administered to these patients because the brain represents a pharmacologic

[1]Not FDA approved for this indication.

[1]Not FDA approved for this indication.
[†]Investigational drug in the United States.

sanctuary and numerous randomized studies have shown that PCI decreases the frequency and morbidity of central nervous system relapse. Concurrent radiotherapy and PE lead to a 70% to 90% complete response rate (complete clinical disappearance of all disease). The median survival for all patients with limited SCLC who are undergoing such treatment is 17 to 20 months; 2- and 4-year disease-free survival rates are 40% and 15% to 30%, respectively. This approach is not without toxic effects, including myelosuppression, esophagitis, and pulmonary fibrosis, which is usually radiographically apparent but generally asymptomatic. The use of PCI can lead to cognitive defects and a slight decrease in IQ. The 5-year disease-free survival rate for patients with limited SCLC is 12% ± 2%. A stepwise decrease in the disease-free survival rate is observed between years 2 and 5 as a result of the development of a second non-small cell primary lung cancer. Late relapse (>3 years) of SCLC is distinctly unusual. Patients with limited SCLC who do relapse usually do so within the first 24 to 36 months. Such patients may be candidates for phase II clinical trials or CAV if they have previously received PE. Survival after relapse is generally limited, 4 to 6 months.

THE ROLE OF SURGERY

Ever since publication of the British Medical Research Council randomized trial in which surgical resection was compared with radiotherapy for SCLC, surgery has been abandoned as a mode of treatment for most patients with SCLC. To date, no study has demonstrated that the use of surgery in addition to chemoradiotherapy in patients with limited SCLC has conferred a survival advantage. The only subset of patients with SCLC who should be approached surgically are patients with small peripheral lesions (solitary pulmonary nodule). Such patients should undergo pulmonary resection even if preoperative biopsy shows SCLC. After resection, patients should receive postoperative adjuvant chemotherapy with either cisplatin (Platinol-AQ)[1] and etoposide (PE) (VePesid) or cyclophosphamide (Cytoxan),[1] doxorubicin (Adriamycin), and vincristine (Oncovin)[1] (CAV). The 5-year survival rate in this small subset of patients with SCLC is 50% to 60%.

Future Directions

The advances made in the past decade in the treatment of lung cancer have been small but incremental. The most fundamental advances have been in understanding the molecular events that lead to the malignant lung cancer phenotype. With a better understanding of the stepwise intracellular molecular events that result in a malignant phenotype, there is no doubt that novel compounds and treatments will be developed to delay and reverse the progression to malignant transformation. Clinical trials have brought about small, but significant incremental survival in stage IIIA and IIIB NSCLC. Clinical trials require the support of the entire medical community, including physicians, nurses, patients, insurers, and managed health care organizations. The sad comment is that only 1.4% of Americans in whom lung cancer is diagnosed participate in a clinical trial. Finally, identification of new drugs and novel antineoplastic compounds can only happen by supporting and enrolling patients in phase I and phase II studies. Progress in the treatment of lung cancer cannot occur without clinical research.

[1]Not FDA approved for this indication.

COCCIDIOIDOMYCOSIS

METHOD OF
Robert Libke, MD

Coccidioidomycosis is an illness caused by the fungus *Coccidioides immitis*. This fungus grows in soil in conditions found in the arid and semiarid regions of the southwestern United States and in a few places in Central and South America. Under proper conditions the fungus produces an abundance of arthroconidia, which are very light and easily carried in the air. Infection occurs when arthroconidia are inhaled and converted in the host to spherules, which reproduce by endosporulation. The primary infection is, therefore, almost always in the lung. In the great majority of cases the infection is quickly contained by host defenses and remains confined to a limited area of the lung. In a few cases the organism is more aggressive and rapidly produces a diffuse pneumonia with an adult respiratory distress syndrome (ARDS)-like picture that may be fatal. In other cases the pulmonary legions heal but the organism is spread to other organs in the body through the blood or lymphatic channels. When this happens, the disease is considered to be disseminated and takes on a different character.

The pathology of infection with *C. immitis* is dimorphic. The initial reaction of the body to the arthroconidia and to the endospores is an acute inflammatory reaction similar to that seen in acute bacterial infections. Reaction to the mature coccidioidal spherules is a granulomatous one similar to that seen in tuberculosis. Clinically, coccidioidomycosis reflects both of those processes; it can have features of both acute and chronic infection.

Clinical Manifestations

The primary infection in the lung is asymptomatic in the majority of instances. When symptomatic, it resembles many other acute lower respiratory tract infections. In some cases, however, clues are present that raise the suspicion of coccidioidomycosis. These include a radiological finding of hilar adenopathy on the side of the airspace consolidation, significant eosinophilia in the differential leukocyte count, certain dermatoses (erythema nodosum, erythema multiform, or a morbilliform maculopapular eruption), and a failure to show a clinical response to conventional antibiotic therapy. Recovery from the primary pulmonary infection may be complete or may leave chronic residuals of either a cavity or a granuloma. Some cavities heal spontaneously within 2 years of the primary infection. Others are complicated by secondary infection, recurrent hemoptysis, or, rarely, rupture into the pleural space. Occasionally these complications are severe enough to warrant lobectomy, but this is the exception rather than the rule (except in cavity rupture). Unlike tuberculosis, the chronic cavitary residuals of primary pulmonary coccidioidomycosis rarely progress. When they do, the progressive fibrocavitary disease may be indistinguishable from tuberculosis in radiographs.

The residual granuloma is significant because of the difficulty of distinguishing it from a carcinoma of the lung when it is first discovered on a routine chest radiograph. If the patient is younger than 40 years of age or the lesion is calcified (coccidioidal granuloma calcify in less than 20% of cases), the lesion can be considered benign and possibly followed with serial chest radiographs. Occasionally organisms recovered from the lesion by computerized tomography (CT)-guided fine-needle aspiration allow the pathologist to make the diagnosis without tissue biopsy. Otherwise, enough tissue must be obtained by transbronchial, thoracoscopic, or open biopsy to allow the pathologist to make a diagnosis.

Dissemination is considered to occur when clinically apparent lesions are found outside the thoracic cavity. The most common sites of dissemination are the skin, lymph nodes, skeleton, synovia, and central nervous system (CNS). Almost any organ, however, can be involved. Dissemination may be focal, multifocal, or diffuse. The two most serious forms are diffuse dissemination and focal dissemination to the CNS. Before the advent of effective therapy, those two forms were almost always fatal. Even now, with effective antifungal agents, these two conditions carry a significant mortality. Dissemination usually occurs with the primary infection and only rarely as a late complication of a chronic pulmonary lesion. Cumulative clinical experience since the first description of coccidioidomycosis now allows the clinician to predict with some accuracy the likelihood of dissemination. Coccidioidomycosis is unique among infectious illnesses in that humans have a genetically determined resistance to dissemination of the organism. This resistance is found most commonly in whites and least frequently in Filipinos. In between, in descending order of frequency of inherited resistance, are Asians, Native Americans, Hispanics, and African Americans. Infection in infancy and infection in the second or third trimester of pregnancy carry a high risk of dissemination, as does infection in persons with immunocompromised status. Clinical clues to the development of dissemination are (one or more of) a rapid rise in complement-fixing antibodies to a titer of 1:32 or greater, a prolonged febrile primary illness (greater than 4 weeks), and the development of mediastinal adenopathy on the chest radiograph. The risk of dissemination is so high in the latter two circumstances that treatment is advisable before clinically overt evidence of dissemination occurs. The same can be said for infection in infants and in immunocompromised patients. Otherwise, the risk of dissemination is a matter of clinical judgment in weighing the number of unfavorable factors such as race, pregnancy, co-morbid illnesses, and complement-fixation titers.

Diagnosis

The diagnosis of coccidioidomycosis is established by finding the distinctive organism microscopically, by culture of tissue or body fluids, or by serology. Skin test results were used in the past but reagents are no longer available. Serologic reactions are the tests most frequently used for the diagnosis of coccidioidal infection. The best are both specific and sensitive. Some of the serologic tests are designed to detect immunoglobulin (Ig) M antibodies (the earliest and most evanescent); others detect IgG antibodies (which persist much longer and are quantitatively related to the severity of the infection), and others detect both. The most reliable techniques for detecting IgM antibodies are the tube precipitin test, the immunodiffusion technique, and an enzyme immunoassay. The most reliable tests for IgG antibodies are the complement fixation test and an immunodiffusion test. The magnitude of the complement fixation titer or IgG quantitative immunodiffusion has the great advantage of being related to the severity of infection and, therefore, is useful in following the progression or resolution of the disease. In patients with extra pulmonary spread, biopsy of lesions or aspiration of fluid from abscesses or joints not only establishes the diagnosis of coccidioidomycosis but also confirms the presence of dissemination in some cases.

Cerebrospinal fluid (CSF) examinations are needed to evaluate for coccidioidal meningitis. Differential and total cell counts and glucose and protein measurements, along with CSF complement fixation titers, should be done. Fungal cultures of CSF are rarely positive in patients with proven meningitis and should not be relied upon for diagnosis.

Treatment

PRIMARY PULMONARY DISEASE

Treatment is not usually necessary for patients with uncomplicated primary infection. However, patients who:

- Have prolonged signs and symptoms
- Have diabetes
- Are in the third trimester of pregnancy
- Are of Filipino ancestry
- Are immunocompromised

should receive treatment for primary coccidioidomycosis with an azole. If the infection appears to be unusually severe and is progressing to an ARDS-like picture, however, it is prudent to undertake immediate diagnostic tests and initiate treatment with intravenous amphotericin B (Fungizone) or, if pre-existing renal disease is present, a lipid complex form of amphotericin (Abelcet). After control of toxicity and disease progression is arrested, change to an oral form of therapy is possible (Table 1).

DISSEMINATED DISEASE

Disseminated disease is always an indication for treatment. There are several classes of antifungal agents now available, including amphotericin B, lipid complex forms of amphotericin, azoles, and echinocandins. The azoles have the advantage of being sufficiently absorbed from the gastrointestinal tract to achieve serum concentrations that are effective. Fluconazole (Diflucan)[1] is not dependent on gastric acidity for absorption and has the additional theoretical advantage of readily passing the blood-brain barrier to achieve good concentration in the CSF. Itraconazole (Sporanox)[1] and fluconazole appear to be equally effective for nonmeningeal disseminated disease.

[1]Not FDA approved for this indication.

TABLE 1 Antifungal Agents

Drug	Dose (mg/d)	Route
Ketoconazole (Nizoral)	200-400	PO
Fluconazole (Diflucan)[1]	200-2000[3]	PO/IV
Itraconazole (Sporanox)[1]	200-800[3]	PO/IV
Amphotericin B (Fungizone)	0.3-1.5 mg/kg	IV
Lipid complex amphotericins (AmBisome, Abelcet, Amphotec)	3-6 mg/kg	IV

[1]Not FDA approved for this indication.
[3]Exceeds dosage recommended by the manufacturer.

Treatment with fluconazole (Diflucan) should start with 400 mg per day and be gradually increased to a tolerable dose up to a maximum of 800 mg per day.[3] Patients with meningitis may be treated with doses up to 2000 mg per day.[3] Itraconazole (Sporanox) is usually given at 400 mg per day but may be increased to 800 mg per day.[3] Because the half-lives of both of those drugs are very long, they can be administered in one dose or divided into a twice daily dosage schedule. The length of treatment is entirely dependent on the clinical course and should probably be continued for several months following complete clinical resolution. Relapse following cessation of therapy is common, and some patients may require lifelong treatment. When given for threatened rather than clinically evident dissemination, the course of treatment can often be shortened. Fluconazole[1] is preferred in the treatment of coccidioidal meningitis in doses of 600 to 2000 mg per day.[3] Control of disease with improvement in CSF parameters has occurred in the majority of patients, but relapse has been frequent when therapy has been stopped. When treating patients who have coccidioidal meningitis with fluconazole, it is prudent to continue the treatment indefinitely, possibly lifelong.

When dissemination is diffuse and rapid or an ARDS-like pulmonary picture develops, mortality is high regardless of the type of therapy used. Initial control of severe dissemination with intravenous amphotericin B is recommended because it may have more rapid onset of action than agents. Amphotericin B is given intravenously in a concentration of 0.1 mg/mL during a period of 1 to 2 hours daily. It is customary to start with a small dose of 10 mg and increase it by 20-mg increments up to a daily dose of 50 mg. The dosage can be escalated more rapidly when the patient is desperately ill or when the clinical course is deteriorating rapidly. Toxic side effects are almost universal and should be anticipated by giving premeditation of acetaminophen, 650 mg, and diphenhydramine (Benadryl), 50 mg, to lessen the rigors that frequently accompany the intravenous infusion. When this combination fails to control rigors, 25 mg of meperidine (Demerol)[1] given as a slow intravenous bolus is often successful. Nausea and vomiting can frequently be ameliorated with antiemetics such as prochlorperazine (Compazine) or trimethobenzamide (Tigan). Renal tubular acidosis with hypokalemia, hypomagnesemia, mild metabolic acidosis, and azotemia are also predictable results of continued amphotericin treatment. The metabolic acidosis is rarely significant enough to require attention, but the serum potassium, magnesium, and creatinine levels must be monitored frequently until the response to treatment appears to be stable. Potassium can be replaced orally but sometimes requires very

[1]Not FDA approved for this indication.
[3]Exceeds dosage recommended by the manufacturer.

large doses. Magnesium replacement may also be required and usually can be done orally. Daily amphotericin should be discontinued when the serum creatinine exceeds 3.0 and can be restarted and given less frequently when the creatinine drops below 2.5. After an accumulated dose of 0.5 gram of amphotericin has been given and disease control is apparent, administration can often be reduced to three times a week instead of daily. This makes outpatient administration quite practical for most patients. The clinical course and response to treatment should determine the total dosage of amphotericin. For disseminated disease, anywhere from 1 to 4 or more grams may be required.

Newer lipid complex forms of amphotericin (Abelcet, Amphotec, and AmBisome) have reduced side effects compared with the older colloidal dispersion form of amphotericin B (Fungizone). These forms of amphotericin may be considered if patients have severe immediate reactions such as hypotension, bronchospasm, and persistent uncontrollable rigors to the standard form of amphotericin. In addition, patients with pre-existing renal dysfunction may be candidates for treatment with these newer agents since they are less nephrotoxic. Doses of 3 to 6 mg/kg of the liposomal formulations are given IV for 1 to 2 hours daily. The possibility of reduced side effects must be balanced with the dramatic increase in cost of the lipid forms.

When patients fail to respond to azole therapy for meningitis, intrathecal (cisternal or intraventricular)* amphotericin B[1] may be necessary. Cisternal injection is the preferred route of administration whenever possible. The starting dose is 0.05 mg, and this is increased daily by 0.1 mg to a maximum of 0.5 mg per day for an indefinite period of time as determined by the lumbar fluid parameters as well as the clinical response. It is desirable to continue intrathecal therapy until the lumbar fluid returns to normal and then for an additional 3 to 6 months. After achieving a stable dose, the frequency of administration can be reduced to three times a week and after lumbar fluid parameters have returned to normal, to once or twice a week.

The newer azoles (voriconazole [Vfend][1] and posaconazole[†]) and the echinocandin (caspofungin [Cancidas][1]) have promising in vitro and animal data regarding *C. immitis*, but experience in treatment of human infections is limited.

[1]Not FDA approved for this indication.
*Not FDA approved for this route of administration.
[†]Investigational drug in the United States.

HISTOPLASMOSIS

METHOD OF
Donita R. Croft, MD, MS

Epidemiology and Pathogenesis

Histoplasmosis is caused by the dimorphic fungus *Histoplasma capsulatum*, which lives as a mold in soil. It grows especially well in moist soil that is rich with the droppings of birds or bats. The majority of histoplasmosis cases occur sporadically, although clusters of illness have been associated with high-dose exposures such as during construction when contaminated soil is disturbed or during public gatherings near bird nests or bat roosts. Histoplasmosis is the most common endemic respiratory mycotic infection in the United States, where it is most prevalent in the Ohio and Mississippi River Valleys. The incubation period is 3 to 17 days.

Human infections result from the inhalation of airborne mold spores into the lungs where the fungus converts to its pathogenic yeast form. Macrophages ingest the organisms and disseminate them to regional lymph nodes and hematogenously. Cellular immunity develops in immunocompetent hosts approximately 10 to 14 days after exposure, and the infection is controlled in most cases. Airborne person-to-person transmission does not occur.

Clinical Manifestations

The severity of illness depends on exposure dose and host immune status. The majority of infections are asymptomatic or result in mild, self-limited illnesses; although acute, even life-threatening pulmonary infections can occur especially after heavy fungal exposure. Chronic indolent pulmonary infections or inflammatory sequelae can develop. Pulmonary histoplasmosis can progress to disseminated disease particularly in persons who are immunosuppressed and do not mount an appropriate cell-mediated response. At high risk for disseminated histoplasmosis are people with AIDS or other immunosuppressive illnesses, people at the extremes of age, and people being treated with immunosuppressive medications.

Fever, chills, myalgias, fatigue, chest pain, and cough with radiographic evidence of pulmonary infiltrates and hilar adenopathy are common features of symptomatic acute histoplasmosis. Persons with heavy exposure histories may present with diffuse pulmonary infiltrates and progress to respiratory failure. Pericarditis, arthritis, and erythema nodosum are systemic inflammatory reactions complicating approximately 5% to 10% of acute histoplasmosis cases.

Chronic pulmonary histoplasmosis affects persons with underlying pulmonary disease. Fevers, sweats, fatigue, chest pain, dyspnea, and a productive cough with radiographic findings of fibrotic apical infiltrates with cavitation are typical features.

The long-term complications broncholithiasis, granulomatous mediastinitis, and fibrosing mediastinitis occur rarely after histoplasmosis. Broncholithiasis occurs when calcified lymph nodes erode into adjacent bronchi. This manifests by the expectoration of small stones or gritty material and can be complicated by massive hemoptysis and bronchopleural fistulas. Mediastinal granulomas, which are enlarging caseous mediastinal lymph nodes, can compress nearby compliant structures (pulmonary vessels, esophagus, and the airway) and result in dyspnea, dysphagia, chest pain, and cough. Fibrosing mediastinitis is caused by an excessive fibrotic reaction leading to progressive entrapment and distortion of the great vessels, heart, esophagus, and airway. It is progressive and has a high mortality rate.

The presenting signs and symptoms of disseminated histoplasmosis, which depend on the severity of the host's immunodeficiency, range from fevers, night sweats, weight loss, rash, anemia, and dyspnea, to shock, coagulopathy, and respiratory, renal, or hepatic failure. The reticuloendothelial system, skin, gastrointestinal tract, and central nervous system (CNS) are frequently affected during disseminated histoplasmosis. The chronicity of disseminated histoplasmosis varies from weeks (acute infections) to months (subacute infections) to years of intermittent signs and symptoms (chronic infections).

Diagnostic Evaluation

The diagnosis of histoplasmosis can be difficult and requires a high index of suspicion. The growth of the *H. capsulatum* from tissue or body fluid culture is the diagnostic gold standard; however, other proven diagnostic methods include tests for antibodies or antigens and fungal stains of tissue or body fluids. All of these methods have strengths and limitations and must be interpreted in the context of the patient's illness. Skin test reactivity to *H. capsulatum* antigens is useful for epidemiologic studies but is not helpful in individual patient evaluations.

Fungal cultures are positive primarily in patients with disseminated disease or chronic pulmonary histoplasmosis and tend to be negative in patients with acute pulmonary histoplasmosis. The clinical usefulness of culture during severe infections is limited because the growth of *H. capsulatum* requires up to 4 weeks in culture medium.

Antibodies are detected in the serum of 90% of persons with histoplasmosis. Although serologic tests are frequently used to diagnose acute histoplasmosis, persons with mild illness might not seroconvert. The clinical usefulness of this test is also limited because it takes 2 to 6 weeks for antibodies to be produced. Immunosuppressed patients could have impaired antibody production leading to false-negative results.

Antigen detection provides rapid results and is more sensitive when testing bronchoalveolar lavage fluid or urine rather than other body fluids. Because of the high fungal burden, it is most useful in patients with disseminated histoplasmosis in immunosuppressed hosts or acute pulmonary histoplasmosis after heavy fungal exposure. Antigen testing is helpful in monitoring treatment and diagnosing relapses. During chronic pulmonary histoplasmosis, antigen detection is generally unhelpful because of the fungal burden.

Fungal stains of tissue or body fluids may be useful especially during infections with a high fungal burden. The sensitivity of fungal stains is less than 50% for all types of histoplasmosis.

Radiographic findings in patients with a compatible illness are the most useful means of diagnosing granulomatous or fibrosing mediastinitis. Positive serologic tests can support these diagnoses and antigens are rarely detected.

Treatment

Because the majority of patients with histoplasmosis have mild self-limited illnesses, most require no therapy. However, patients with severe or prolonged signs and symptoms or immunosuppressed patients with disseminated disease generally do require treatment. Treatment options for histoplasmosis include amphotericin B (Fungizone), amphotericin B lipid formulations (Amphotec), and the azole antifungal agents itraconazole (Sporanox), fluconazole (Diflucan)[1], and ketoconazole (Nizoral). The dosages and representative, potential adverse effects of these medications are included in Table 1.

Amphotericin B is very effective for the treatment of histoplasmosis, but its toxicities and intravenous administration limit its use to severe infections. Potential adverse effects are infusion-related reactions and chronic toxicities especially nephrotoxicity. Infusion-related reactions may be decreased by premedications including acetaminophen (Tylenol), 650 to 1000 mg orally, diphenhydramine (Benadryl), 25 mg orally or IV, nonsteroidal anti-inflammatory agents (NSAIDs), and meperidine (Demerol), 25 to 50 mg IM or IV. Volume expansion with 500 to 1000 mL of intravenous saline may decrease the risk of nephrotoxicity. The amphotericin B lipid formulations may also decrease the risk of nephrotoxicity but are considerably more expensive.

Azoles are preferred for the treatment of mild cases of histoplasmosis because of their more favorable adverse effects profiles and their ease of administration. Itraconazole (Sporanox) is generally the recommended

[1]Not FDA approved for this indication.

TABLE 1 Antifungal Options for Histoplasmosis Treatment with Dosages and Representative, Potential Adverse Effects

Antifungal Agent	Recommended Dosage	Potential Adverse Effects
Amphotericin B (Fungizone)	0.7-1 mg/kg IV once daily	Infusion-related reactions: fevers, chills, headaches, rigors, hypotension, nausea, vomiting, phlebitis Chronic toxicities: hypokalemia, hypomagnesemia, renal tubular acidosis, anemia, renal insufficiency and failure
Amphotericin B lipid formulations (Amphotec)	3 mg/kg IV once daily	Similar to Amphotericin B
Itraconazole (Sporanox)	Loading dose: 200 mg PO 3 times daily for 3 days Maintenance dose: 200 mg PO once to twice daily	Headache, nausea, edema, rash, congestive heart failure, hepatotoxicity Absorption affected by gastric acidity, avoid medications that decrease gastric acidity Pharmacokinetic reactions with other medication metabolized by cytochrome P450 system
Fluconazole (Diflucan)	Immunocompetent host: 400 mg PO once daily Immunosuppressed host: 800 mg PO once daily	Headache, nausea, abdominal discomfort, edema, hepatoxicity Pharmacokinetic reactions with other medication metabolized by cytochrome P450 system
Ketoconazole (Nizoral)	200 mg, 400 mg, or 800 mg PO once daily (toxicity more common with 800 mg dose)	Nausea, vomiting, abdominal pain, hepatotoxicity, leukopenia, thrombocytopenia Pharmacokinetic reactions with other medication metabolized by cytochrome P450 system

azole because it is highly effective and well tolerated. Absorption of itraconazole is enhanced by increased gastric acidity, and it is best absorbed with food and an acidic beverage such as cola or cranberry juice. The liquid suspension of the medication has greater bioavailability than the capsules. An intravenous preparation is available for use when the medication cannot be taken orally. Fluconazole (Diflucan)[1] is less active against *H. capsulatum* than itraconazole, but it has fewer adverse effects and penetrates the meninges. It is typically used only for patients who cannot use itraconazole or have meningitis. Ketoconazole (Nizoral) is also less effective and less well-tolerated than itraconazole, but it has the advantage of being less expensive.

The treatment of histoplasmosis varies by the clinical syndrome. Antifungal therapy is not necessary for most cases of acute pulmonary histoplasmosis, although it is recommended for prolonged or severe cases. Specific indications for treatment are symptoms that have not improved during the first month of the infection, fever for greater than 3 weeks, or hypoxemia associated with radiographic evidence of diffuse pulmonary disease. Treatment with itraconazole (Sporanox) is recommended for 8 to 12 weeks. Patients ill enough to require hospitalization may receive initial therapy with several days of amphotericin B with transition to complete the 8- to 12-week therapy with itraconazole. These severely ill patients should also be treated initially with prednisone, 60 mg orally daily for 1 to 2 weeks, to reduce the inflammatory response, but this should be used concurrently with antifungal therapy. Histoplasmosis pericarditis may be treated with 2 to 12 weeks of NSAIDs without antifungal therapy, or prednisone may be used concurrently with antifungal therapy. Pericardial drainage is necessary with pericardial tamponade. Rheumatologic syndromes complicating acute histoplasmosis are not an indication for treatment with antifungal therapy and may be treated with 2 to 12 weeks of NSAIDs.

Antifungal therapy is recommended for all cases of chronic pulmonary histoplasmosis because of the progressive pulmonary disease risk. The recommended therapy is itraconazole for 12 to 24 months. Ketoconazole is also effective but fluconazole[1] is less effective. For severely debilitated patients, treatment may be initiated with amphotericin B then transitioned to complete azole therapy. Treated patients must be evaluated carefully for relapse.

Treatment is also indicated for all cases of progressive disseminated histoplasmosis. Most immunocompetent patients or immunosuppressed patients without AIDS can be effectively treated with itraconazole for 6 to 18 months. Severely ill patients may have initial amphotericin B therapy with transition to itraconazole after the patient becomes afebrile. Ketoconazole is used when itraconazole use is not possible, as it is quite effective but not as well tolerated. Fluconazole[1] use is discouraged because of possible fungal resistance. Treated patients must be carefully evaluated for relapses. Patients with immunosuppression from AIDS have a high rate of relapse and must be treated with lifelong maintenance therapy. In the context of AIDS, induction treatment is itraconazole, 200 mg orally three times daily for 3 days, then 200 mg two times daily for

[1]Not FDA approved for this indication.

[1]Not FDA approved for this indication.

12 weeks; then maintenance therapy at 200 mg once to twice daily for life. Amphotericin B can be used initially for patients ill enough to require hospitalization with transition to azole therapy when stable. Higher relapse rates occur with fluconazole than with itraconazole, but it may be used when itraconazole is not tolerated. Antigen detection in serum or urine should be checked every 3 to 6 months during maintenance therapy to evaluate for relapses. As prophylaxis, patients with CD4 counts less than 150 μL should receive itraconazole orally at a dose of 200 mg daily.

Treatment of patients with localized manifestations of histoplasmosis can be particularly challenging. Because of its high mortality rate, CNS histoplasmosis should be treated aggressively. Amphotericin B treatment up to a total dose of 35 mg/kg for 3 to 4 months is recommended. Fluconazole[1] may be used for another 9 to12 months to reduce relapse risk.

Granulomatous mediastinitis accompanied by severe obstruction should be treated initially with amphotericin B. Itraconazole may be used to complete therapy and for patients with milder illness persistent for more than 1 month. Treatment for 6 to 12 months is recommended. Surgical resection should be considered only for those with major obstruction who do not respond to antifungal therapy.

The optimal treatment for fibrosing mediastinitis is unknown, although given its grave consequences it is reasonable to treat with a 12-week trial of itraconazole. With significant improvement, the trial should be extended to 12 months of therapy. Intravascular stents have been helpful for major vascular obstruction; however, surgical interventions are problematic and should be last resort considerations.

[1]Not FDA approved for this indication.

BLASTOMYCOSIS

METHOD OF

Bertha S. Ayi, MD, and Mark E. Rupp, MD

Epidemiology, Clinical Manifestations, and Diagnosis

Blastomycosis is a pyogranulomatous disease caused by *Blastomyces dermatitidis*, a thermally dimorphic fungus that grows as a budding yeast in human tissues. It occurs naturally in soil from warm, moist, wooded areas that are rich in organic content. In North America, this endemic mycosis is found in the Ohio and Mississippi River basins and in the Canadian provinces surrounding the St. Lawrence River and the Great Lakes. *B. dermatitidis* is geographically widely distributed, and blastomycosis has been described in Poland, Saudi Arabia, Israel, Lebanon, and India. However, the epidemiology of blastomycosis remains incompletely defined because of difficulty in isolating the organism from soil and the lack of sensitive serologic and dermatologic tests. In contrast to previous reports suggesting a high incidence in healthy middle-aged men with outdoor occupations, analysis of more recent data does not suggest any predilection for a particular age, gender, race, or time of year.

The major route of inoculation appears to be inhalation. Outbreaks of blastomycosis have been linked to activities in which soil is disturbed, presumably resulting in aerosolization of conidia. Rare cases of perinatal or sexual transmission have been reported. Primary cutaneous disease has been described following bite wounds or other means of direct inoculation. The incubation period is estimated to range from 30 to 45 days. The primary pneumonia is asymptomatic in about one half of infected patients. Symptomatic patients experience a pulmonary disease that may mimic bacterial pneumonia with the acute onset of cough, fever, chills, fleeting chest pain, myalgia, and arthralgia. As the disease progresses, the initial dry cough often becomes productive of purulent sputum. Radiographic studies may demonstrate a localized or diffuse infiltrate. Pleural effusions rarely develop. Immunocompromised patients are more likely to present with progressive diffuse infiltrates or miliary lung disease. Chronic pneumonia is a common presentation, occurring in approximately 90% of symptomatic cases. Patients often have a low-grade fever, weight loss, productive cough, hemoptysis, and pleuritic chest pain; which may mimic carcinoma, tuberculosis, or any of the endemic mycoses such as histoplasmosis. Radiographic imaging reveals alveolar infiltrates, mass lesions, fibronodular infiltrates, or cavitation. Acute respiratory distress syndrome (ARDS) may occur and is associated with a high mortality rate.

Hematogenous spread may result in disseminated disease and can stem from either symptomatic or asymptomatic primary pneumonia. Extrapulmonary disease may involve a multitude of body sites including the skin, bones and joints, genitourinary tract, central nervous system (CNS), lymphatic tissue, or larynx. Adrenal insufficiency, caused by destruction of the adrenals, has been observed. After the pulmonary tract, the skin is the next most frequent site of involvement, thus the organism is aptly named *dermatitidis*. Cutaneous disease takes the appearance of verrucous papules, plaques, ulcers, or nodules and must be differentiated from squamous cell carcinoma, atypical mycobacterial infection, pyoderma gangrenosum, or giant keratoacanthoma. Pustules resembling disseminated pyogenic bacterial infection have occasionally been noted. In otherwise healthy persons, CNS involvement is uncommon (<5%). In immunocompromised patients blastomycosis is often complicated by CNS disease, which may present as a localized mass or meningitis. Approximately 40% of AIDS patients with blastomycosis have CNS involvement. Disease in immunosuppressed hosts tends to be more fulminant and more commonly results in dissemination or relapse. A mortality rate of 30% to 40% is noted. Aggressive treatment as well as chronic suppressive therapy in survivors are necessary.

The diagnosis of blastomycosis is usually established by examining clinical specimens or histological sections under a wet mount with 10% potassium hydroxide. The round, single, broad-based budding yeasts, with a double refractile wall, are often readily identified and distinguished from other fungal pathogens. Large volume specimens, such as urine, pleural fluid, or cerebrospinal fluid (CSF), may be centrifuged prior to examination. Calcofluor white stain may be used to enhance visualization. Tissues may be stained with periodic acid-Schiff or Gomori methenamine silver (GMS) for better visualization. Unlike *Candida* or *Aspergillus*, colonization with *B. dermatitidis* does not occur and visualization or recovery of the fungus is proof of infection.

The diagnostic gold standard is isolation of the organism from cultures of clinical specimens. *B. dermatitidis* is not particularly difficult to recover on standard mycologic media within a 2- to 4-week incubation period. In addition, DNA probes are currently available to speed the identification of *B. dermatitidis*. Serologic tests for *B. dermatitidis* are available and include complement fixation, immunodiffusion, and enzyme-linked immunosorbent assays. However, these studies are neither sensitive nor specific and serologic tests should not be used to make a diagnosis, rule out disease, or follow therapy. Blastomycin skin testing is no better than serologic studies and should not be used as a diagnostic tool.

Treatment

Spontaneous resolution of chronic or disseminated blastomycosis is rare, and untreated disease is associated with mortality rates of 60% to 80%. Controversy continues on whether all cases of acute pulmonary blastomycosis require treatment. Available agents include amphotericin B, itraconazole, ketoconazole, and fluconazole. There is limited data available regarding the efficacy of the newer triazole agents or echinocandins. With therapy, mortality is reduced to less than 10%.

PNEUMONIA

Ketoconazole (Nizoral) was the first azole agent to be used as an alternative to amphotericin B for the treatment of blastomycosis. At a dose of 400 to 800 mg per day, ketoconazole achieves cure rates of 70% to 85%. However, the higher dose level is poorly tolerated. In addition, relapses occur in 10% to 14% of cases, necessitating a 1- to 2-year follow-up period. Itraconazole (Sporanox) has proven efficacy, is better tolerated than ketoconazole, and is the agent of choice for patients with mild-to-moderate disease. Itraconazole, at a dose of 200 to 400 mg per day, is recommended for 6 months. Use of the oral suspension results in greater bioavailability. Although there have been no randomized, prospective, comparative trials to assess which is most efficacious, based on outcomes in noncomparative trials, itraconazole is the preferred oral agent. Fluconazole (Diflucan)[1] appears to be less efficacious than itraconazole and ketoconazole. To achieve a cure rate of 85% or higher, doses of 400 to 800 mg[3] are required for approximately 9 months. Because of its enhanced penetration, some clinicians use fluconazole in the treatment of CNS disease. However, clinical experience is limited. Amphotericin B (Fungizone) was the first drug shown to be clinically effective against *B. dermatitidis*, and it remains the drug of choice for patients with severe or progressive disease and for immunocompromised patients. Amphotericin B should be administered at a dose of 0.7 to 1 mg/kg per day for a total of 2 to 2.5 grams. In patients who achieve clinical stability after the delivery of approximately 500 mg of amphotericin B (Amphotec), many clinicians opt to switch to the better-tolerated alternative of oral itraconazole at 200 to 400 mg per day. Although lipid formulations of amphotericin B have not been fully assessed for use in blastomycosis, they may be used in patients who cannot tolerate amphotericin deoxycholate because of renal toxicity or infusion-related events.

CENTRAL NERVOUS SYSTEM DISEASE

Because of limited blood-brain barrier penetration, ketoconazole or itraconazole cannot be recommended for the treatment of CNS disease. Amphotericin B, at a total dose of 2 to 2.5 grams, is the preferred regimen.

EXTRAPULMONARY DISEASE

All extrapulmonary diseases require therapy. Depending on the severity of symptoms, as well as the immune status of the patient, therapy may be initiated with either amphotericin B or itraconazole.

[1]Not FDA approved for this indication.

[3]Exceeds dosage recommended by the manufacturer.

For life-threatening disease, a total of 2 to 2.5 g of amphotericin B is generally recommended. Patients with mild-to-moderate disease may be treated with itraconazole at 200 to 400 mg per day. Standard therapy for bone involvement is associated with a high relapse rates. Therefore, 1 year of treatment is suggested. Immunocompromised patients with disseminated disease may require chronic suppressive therapy with itraconazole. Ketoconazole should not be used as chronic suppressive therapy because of the high relapse rate and greater toxicity. Because of the teratogenicity and embryotoxicity of the azole drugs, amphoterin B is the treatment of choice for pregnant women. The recommended dose is 0.7 mg/kg per day up to a total administered dose of 1.5 to 2.5 g. Blastomycosis in children may be more difficult to treat, and amphotericin B is preferred at a total administered dose less than or equal to 30 mg/kg. Itraconazole at 5 to 7 mg/kg per day is an alternative.

RECENTLY DEVELOPED ANTIFUNGAL AGENTS

Newer azoles such as voriconazole (Vfend)[1] and posaconazole* are active against *B. dermatitidis* in tests conducted in vitro and in animal models. However, there are limited data in humans and clear recommendations cannot be offered. Likewise, there are minimal data regarding the activity of echinocandins versus *B. dermatitidis*.

[1]Not FDA approved for this indication.

*Investigational drug in the United States.

PLEURAL EFFUSION AND EMPYEMA THORACIS

METHOD OF

Jay Heidecker, MD, and Peter Doelken, MD

Pathogenesis

The pleural space is approximately 10 to 20 μm in width and separates the parietal and visceral pleura. Under normal conditions, approximately 7 mL of pleural fluid are formed per day. Pleural effusions accumulate because of pathologic states that result in dysequilibrium between pleural fluid formation and removal. Pleural effusion may be caused by disease within the pleura itself; these effusions are usually exudative. Alternatively, pleural effusion can be caused by systemic or local hydrostatic or oncotic imbalances resulting in a transudate. Some of the mechanisms of pleural fluid accumulation are:

- Increased hydrostatic pressure in the microvasculature (e.g., congestive heart failure)
- Decreased oncotic pressure in the microvasculature (e.g., hypoalbuminemia)
- Decreased hydrostatic pressure in the pleural space (e.g., lobar or lung atelectasis or trapped lung)
- Increased permeability of the microvasculature causing leakage of fluid and protein (e.g., parapneumonic effusion)
- Obstructed or disrupted thoracic duct causing a chylothorax
- Fluid movement from extrapleural spaces to the pleural space (e.g., hepatic hydrothorax, urinothorax, duropleural fistula)
- Iatrogenic complications (e.g., extravascular migration of a central venous catheter)
- Trauma resulting in a hemothorax

Diagnosis

Pleural effusions can be symptomatic by compromising ventilatory function resulting in dyspnea. Pleuritis may accompany pleural effusion because of an inflammatory process of the pleura. Pleural effusions can be detected on physical examination. The physical examination may reveal decreased or absent breath sounds, dullness to percussion, and an absence of egophony. On chest radiography, small pleural effusions may blunt the costophrenic angle or cause an absence of lung markings behind the ipsilateral diaphragm. Larger pleural effusions obscure the entire hemidiaphragm on the affected side, may track up along the chest wall, and may show a meniscus. Pleural effusions may result in a veil-like radiopacity, much like a breast shadow in semierect or supine radiographs. Ultrasonography is routinely used when evaluating pleural effusions because it reliably detects even minute amounts of pleural fluid and can easily distinguish fluid from lung consolidation and soft tissue. Safe access sites can be determined for thoracentesis in free-flowing and loculated effusions. There are three dynamic signs that indicate pleural fluid is accessible to thoracentesis. The first is movement of structures such as the flapping of collapsed lung within the fluid during respiration. The second is a swirling motion that indicates there is particulate matter within the pleural effusion. The third is a dynamic change in the shape of the pleural space during respiration. Sonographically complex effusions have (one or more of) debris, fibrin fronds, and fully developed septations. On chest radiograph, they will appear to be non–free-flowing on lateral decubitus films

Ultrasound is performed at the bedside immediately preceding the procedure to avoid positional fluid shifts between the time of sonography and the procedure. Sonographically guided thoracentesis and catheter insertion has an excellent safety record with complication rates of less than 3%. This is likely because it avoids lung and other major organ punctures. If ultrasonography is not available, a lateral decubitus film can help distinguish between a free-flowing pleural effusion and an alveolar filling process. Layering 1 cm of pleural fluid on a lateral decubitus film can indicate a pleural effusion that can be safely drained by thoracentesis. Computed tomography (CT) scanning should be used when evaluating loculated pleural effusions.

Thoracentesis

There are different indications for diagnostic and therapeutic thoracentesis as well as chest tubes. A diagnostic thoracentesis should be performed on all undiagnosed unilateral pleural effusions, on bilateral pleural effusions felt not to be from congestive heart failure, and in febrile patients with pleural effusions. Therapeutic thoracentesis should be performed on patients with significant dyspnea that is felt secondary to the pleural effusion. It should also be performed on patients with large parapneumonic effusions. Relative contraindications to thoracentesis and chest of tube placement are uncorrected thrombocytopenia of less than 50, uremia with creatinine greater than 6 mg/dL, and coagulopathy with an international normalized ratio (INR) greater than 1.6. Routine measurement of prothrombin time (PT), partial thromboplastin time (PTT), and INR and platelet counts are not necessary if there is no history to suggest an underlying bleeding disorder. Thoracentesis on ventilated patients can be safely performed with ultrasound guidance. If coagulopathy or thrombocytopenia is found, preprocedural fresh-frozen plasma (FFP) or platelets, respectively, must be given or the procedure should be aborted. Chest tubes should be placed in patients with empyema, complicated parapneumonic effusion, hemothorax, tension pneumothorax, and for pleurodesis and certain symptomatic pleural effusions such as malignant pleural effusions. Large-bore chest tubes are often placed instead of small-bore chest tubes. The indications for placement of a large-bore chest tube include traumatic hemothorax and pneumothorax in mechanically ventilated patients. Chest tubes should not be placed into patients with effusions from congestive heart failure, nephrotic syndrome, cirrhosis, and chylothorax.

TABLE 1 Complications of Thoracentesis

Major	Minor
Pneumothorax	Pain at puncture site
Arterial laceration	Seroma at puncture site
Hemothorax	Hematoma at puncture site
Re-expansion pulmonary edema	Cough
Hypotension	Vasovagal reaction

Ultrasonography is used for pleural effusions. The effusion is localized by ultrasound, and the rib below the proposed thoracentesis site is palpated. The superior portion of the rib is anesthetized with lidocaine (Xylocaine). The needle is advanced over the rib in a direction perpendicular to the chest wall until pleural fluid is withdrawn. Thereby, the intercostal neurovascular bundle under the rib above is avoided. The needle is withdrawn slightly and a bolus of lidocaine is given to anesthetize the parietal pleura. The pleural effusion is sampled for at least 20 cc for a diagnostic thoracentesis, or a thoracentesis catheter is inserted for large-volume thoracentesis or to obtain pleural pressure measurements. Complications of thoracentesis are listed in Table 1. Large-volume thoracentesis can be performed with the assistance of pleural manometry. If manometry is not available, no more than 1 to 1.5 L of pleural fluid should be drained. If more fluid is drained, the risk of development of clinically significant re-expansion pulmonary edema may be increased, especially in long-standing effusions. If the patient develops chest pain during the procedure, further fluid should not be withdrawn. The effusion may be drained in a stepwise fashion with repeat thoracentesis. Conversely, a pigtail small-bore chest tube can be placed for stepwise drainage. Postprocedural radiographs are obtained for mechanically ventilated patients and patients with marginal respiratory status. Otherwise, postprocedural radiographs are not necessary unless the procedure is complicated or the patient develops chest pain or dyspnea following the thoracentesis. For patients with sonographically complex pleural effusions, small-bore chest tubes are used to facilitate drainage.

Pleural Fluid Analysis

Every unilateral undiagnosed pleural effusion should be sampled. Bilateral effusions felt to be secondary to congestive heart failure can be managed with appropriate heart failure treatment in the absence of fever or disparate-sized pleural effusions as long as decrease of the effusion occurs with therapy. All pleural fluid sampled should be sent for hydrogen ion concentration (pH), protein, lactic dehydrogenase (LDH), glucose, and cell count; and a sample should be saved. Concomitant serum protein and LDH should also be drawn. Effusions are classified as exudative if the pleural fluid/serum protein

TABLE 2 Pleural Effusions Classified as Transudates or Exudates

Transudates	Exudates	Rare Exudates
Congestive heart failure	Parapneumonic effusion	Hepatic and abdominal abscesses
Constrictive pericarditis	Empyema	Asbestos effusion
Cirrhosis	Malignant effusion	Radiation pleuritis
Peritoneal dialysis	Tuberculosis	Meigs syndrome
Atelectasis	Fungal infection	Lymphangiomyomatosis
Nephrotic syndrome	Collagen vascular pleurisy	Yellow nail syndrome
Urinothorax	Pulmonary embolism	Mesothelioma
Nontraumatic duropleural	Pancreatitis	Postendoscopic sclerotherapy
Fistula	Uremic effusion	Esophageal perforation
Trapped lung	Trapped lung	Sarcoid
	Postcardiac injury syndrome	Amiodarone (Cordarone)
	Chylothorax	Dantrolene (Dantrium)
	Pseudochylothorax	Methysergide (Sansert)
		Paclitaxel (Taxol)

ratio is less than 0.5, or the pleural fluid/LDH ratio is greater than 0.6, or the pleural fluid LDH is greater than 66% of the upper limits of normal. Otherwise, the pleural effusion is a transudate. Notable transudates and exudates are listed in Table 2. Other laboratory tests should be ordered based upon the clinical situation. Specific disease processes and the diagnostic test on pleural fluid analysis are listed in Table 3. The pleural fluid cell count can also be of diagnostic use. Specifically, a high lymphocyte or eosinophil cell count narrow the differential diagnosis to a limited number of disease processes. These conditions are listed in Table 4.

Management of the pleural effusion is dependent upon its etiology. Transudative effusions and many exudative effusions respond to treatment of the underlying disorder. Notably, ascitic effusions and chylothorax should not be drained by chest tube as the resulting loss of protein and chylomicrons, respectively, can adversely affect the nutritional status of the patient. Trapped lung can only be definitively treated by thoracotomy and stripping of the visceral peel that limits the lung's expansion. For many pleural effusions, complete evacuation of the pleural space followed by treatment of the underlying disorder is sufficient to prevent reaccumulation of the effusion.

For malignant and lymphomatous effusions, patients often have shortened expected survival and significant dyspnea from their effusion. For these patients, complete drainage followed by pleurodesis can significantly improve quality of life. To perform pleurodesis, a fibrosing agent like talc or doxycycline (Vibramycin)[1] is placed into the pleural space. The chest tube should be clamped while the talc or doxycycline is left in the pleural space for 2 hours. It should

[1]Not FDA approved for this indication.

TABLE 3 Specific Diagnoses Obtained by Pleural Fluid Analysis

Effusion Type	Diagnostic Test
Peritoneal dialysis	Protein <1, glucose >300; pleural fluid/serum glucose >1
Urinothorax	Pleural fluid/serum creatinine ratio >1
Malignant	Cytology
Lymphoma	Flow cytometry
Tuberculous	AFB (low sensitivity, increased by culture of fluid and pleura); excellent specificity with ADA levels and PCR
Fungal	Culture of fluid or tissue
Esophageal perforation	pH <6 and increased amylase
Mesothelioma	Increased hyaluronic acid, typical cytology, ultrasound-guided pleural biopsy, thoracoscopy if necessary
Rheumatoid	Glucose <30, pH = 7, LDH >1000, positive RF in pleural fluid
Lupus pleuritis	ANA >1:160 or lupus erythematosus cells in pleural fluid
Pancreatitis	Pleural fluid/serum amylase ratio >1.0
Trapped lung	Negative pleural pressure or high elastance of pleural space by manometry
Chylothorax	Elevated triglycerides or chylomicrons; lymphoma most common cause
Cholesterol effusion	Cholesterol >200, pleural fluid/serum cholesterol >1, cholesterol crystals; TB most common cause

Abbreviations: ADA = adenosine deaminase; AFB = acid-fast bacillus; ANA = antinuclear antibody; PCR = polymerase chain reaction; pH = hydrogen ion concentration; RF = rheumatoid factor; TB = tuberculosis.

TABLE 4 Effusions Suggested by Cell Count

Effusions with Greater than 80% Lymphocytes	Effusions with Greater than 10% Eosinophils
Tuberculous pleurisy	Hemothorax
Lymphoma	Pulmonary infarction
Sarcoid	Pneumothorax
Chronic rheumatoid pleurisy	Previous thoracentesis
Chylothorax	Parasitic disease
Yellow nail syndrome	Fungal infection
	Drugs
	Asbestos pleurisy

then be drained from the chest tube. Complications include chest pain, re-expansion pulmonary edema, and, rarely, ARDS. Infection in the pleural space is an absolute contraindication to pleurodesis. Some of these patients have lung entrapment associated with malignancy and will have an unsuccessful pleurodesis. Trapped lung occurs when the inflammatory process causing the pleural effusion causes a peel over the visceral pleura, preventing the lung from expanding fully. This creates a negative pressure gradient, which causes a persistent fluid filled pleural space. In trapped lung found by manometry or video-assisted thoracic surgery (VATS), pleurodesis should not be performed because complete apposition of the pleural surfaces will not occur and pleurodesis will fail. However, for patients with malignant effusions, VATS and thoracoscopy have shown increased morbidity and length of hospital stay.

An alternative to pleurodesis is a tunneled catheter that is placed into the pleural space (sterile conditions must be maintained). The patient can periodically drain the effusion at home using this type of system. For persistent, symptomatic, large effusions, this technique has several advantages over repeat thoracentesis, including decreased pain, decreased hospitalizations, and increased patient autonomy. Up to 40% of patients may experience spontaneous pleurodesis after several weeks of drainage.

Parapneumonic Effusion and Empyema Thoracis

Forty percent of bacterial pneumonias are associated with a pleural effusion. The pneumonic process causes infiltration of inflammatory mediators that increase the permeability of the pleural capillaries. Protein and fluid then migrate into the pleural space. At this point, the fluid is characterized by moderate neutrophil counts, protein, normal glucose, and pH greater than 7.3. These parapneumonic effusions are classified as simple or uncomplicated, and they usually resolve with appropriate antibiotic therapy. Simple effusions can progress when there is bacterial invasion into the pleural space. This causes increased neutrophil recruitment and migration of clotting factors into the space. The fluid becomes gelatinous, the pH and glucose drop, the LDH rises, and fibrous adhesions develop. At this stage drainage is often unsuccessful. The final stage occurs when fibroblasts migrate into the pleural space and lay down collagen.

As mentioned, all pleural fluid sampled should be sent for LDH, glucose, protein, cell count, and pH. When there is suspicion of parapneumonic effusion, Gram stain and culture should also be sent. Numerous studies have verified that the pH is most predictive of a complicated pleural space requiring drainage. To obtain a valid pH, it is important to immediately place the pleural fluid sample on ice and deliver it to the arterial blood gas (ABG) analyzer within 30 minutes. Parapneumonic effusions are classified as simple when LDH is less than 1000, glucose is normal, and pH is less than 7.2. They are classified as complicated when LDH is greater than 1000, glucose is low, pH is less than 7.2, or the effusion is loculated. Empyema is defined by presence of pus, positive gram stain, or culture. Complicated parapneumonic effusions and empyemas should be drained with a chest tube.

Optimal management of complicated parapneumonic effusions and empyema is controversial. However, if a patient with a chest tube has persistent fever or decreased drainage of the tube with persistence of the effusion, additional measures must be taken. Proper chest tube placement should be assured with posteroanterior (PA) and lateral chest radiograph (CXR) or CT scan. If the tube is properly positioned but there is inadequate drainage, there are three main options: intrapleural fibrinolytic therapy, VATS, and thoracotomy.

Both urokinase (Abbokinase)[1] and streptokinase (Streptase)[1] appear to be efficacious at drainage in selected patients. Streptokinase is associated with the risk of development of antibodies as it is a bacterial protein and should only be given during one hospitalization. Fibrinolytics, if used, are instilled up to four times per day. Recent studies show decreased hospital stay and cost with use of early VATS procedure. Experience shows that a patient with inadequate drainage from a chest tube should be given a trial of fibrinolytics; however, if adequate drainage is not quickly achieved, VATS should be performed. Thoracotomy is reserved for those patients for whom VATS cannot achieve complete drainage or lung expansion.

[1]Not FDA approved for this indication.

PRIMARY LUNG ABSCESS

METHOD OF

Dov Weissberg, MD

Lung abscess is a localized collection of pus and necrotic debris contained in a cavity formed by the disintegration of the surrounding lung parenchyma. A very large lung abscess involving at least one entire lobe is often referred to as pulmonary gangrene as it is the same pathologic process; the definition depends on the extent of the abscess. Lung abscess can be either acute (duration of less than 6 weeks) or chronic. The most common cause of primary lung abscess is aspiration of oropharyngeal contents, which is often related to impaired consciousness accompanied by a suppressed cough reflex. Other conditions associated with aspiration include anesthesia, neurologic disorders, alcoholism, drug and narcotic abuse, periodontal disease, dysphagia, and nasogastric tube interference with cardiac sphincter.

Etiology

The majority of patients with lung abscess are infected with multiple anaerobic bacteria. The most commonly isolated organisms are *Prevotella, Fusobacterium nucleatum, Peptostreptococcus,* and *Bacteroides fragilis*. These are often mixed with aerobes: *Pseudomonas aeruginosa, Staphylococcus aureus*, streptococci, *Klebsiella pneumoniae,* and *Haemophilus influenzae*.

Symptoms and Signs

Patients with lung abscess usually present with cough, fever, dyspnea, and occasionally chest pain of pleural origin. Malaise, weight loss, and anemia are common. Cough with expectoration of foul-smelling sputum suggests anaerobic infection.

Radiologic Diagnosis

The typical radiographic appearance of lung abscess is a cavity with air-fluid level. This picture must be differentiated from several other pulmonary pathologic processes. A cavitating neoplasm (particularly squamous cell carcinoma) can be confused with a lung abscess, however, it is recognizable by an irregular thick-walled cavity that does not respond to antibiotic therapy. Other processes mimicking lung abscess include loculated interlobar empyema, infected cysts and bullae, and other thoracic infections, such as tuberculosis and fungal infections. Bacteriologic studies are important, but reliable results can be difficult to obtain. Expectorated sputum cannot be used for culture, because of contamination by organisms frequently present in the oral cavity and the upper airways. However, good anaerobic and aerobic cultures can be obtained from empyema liquid (often accompanying lung abscess), bronchoalveolar lavage, and brushings from the involved segment or lobe.

Management

Antibiotics and drainage are the standard treatment of primary lung abscess (Figure 1). For most patients, penicillin up to 20 million units per day intravenously (IV) is sufficient. It should be used in combination with metronidazole (Flagyl), 2 g per day IV, in four divided doses. Once the febrile reaction subsides, this can be changed to an oral regimen. However, some patients present with organisms that produce β lactamases and are resistant to penicillin G. For these patients, and for those who are allergic to penicillin, amoxicillin/clavulanate (Augmentin) or clindamycin (Cleocin) is indicated. Clindamycin should be administered intravenously, 600 mg every 6 hours until improvement, then 300 mg orally every 6 hours. Depending on the offending organism, an aminoglycoside, a cephalosporin (Ceclor) or, in extremely difficult, toxic cases, imipenem/cilastatin (Primaxin) may be appropriate.

Chest physiotherapy consisting of coughing, chest percussion, and postural drainage are important and should be used in parallel with antibiotics. Bronchoscopy may be necessary to remove viscous secretions and establish bronchial drainage.

Abscess that does not respond to treatment with antibiotics and physical therapy should be drained. This is best done by percutaneous insertion of a drainage catheter into the abscess cavity. Although it is difficult to provide a rigid time limit, the waiting period for the resolution of abscess before initiating drainage should not exceed 1 month. In the presence of sepsis, with the patient's condition deteriorating, the postponement should not be that long, and the abscess should be drained without delay under antibiotic coverage. The drainage is effective in more than 90% of patients and is best done under imaging control (ultrasound or computed tomography [CT]). The procedure should be performed under general endobronchial anesthesia, with the tube placed in the bronchus contralateral to the abscess. Complications (contamination of pleura with pus, bleeding, pneumothorax) are rare.

In the past, lobectomy used to be the standard therapy for those patients who did not respond to antibiotics and physiotherapy, however, at present this is rarely indicated as percutaneous tube drainage is nearly always possible. Today, the indications for lobectomy should be restricted to cases with massive necrosis involving at least one entire lobe, and to patients with a major, life-threatening hemorrhage.

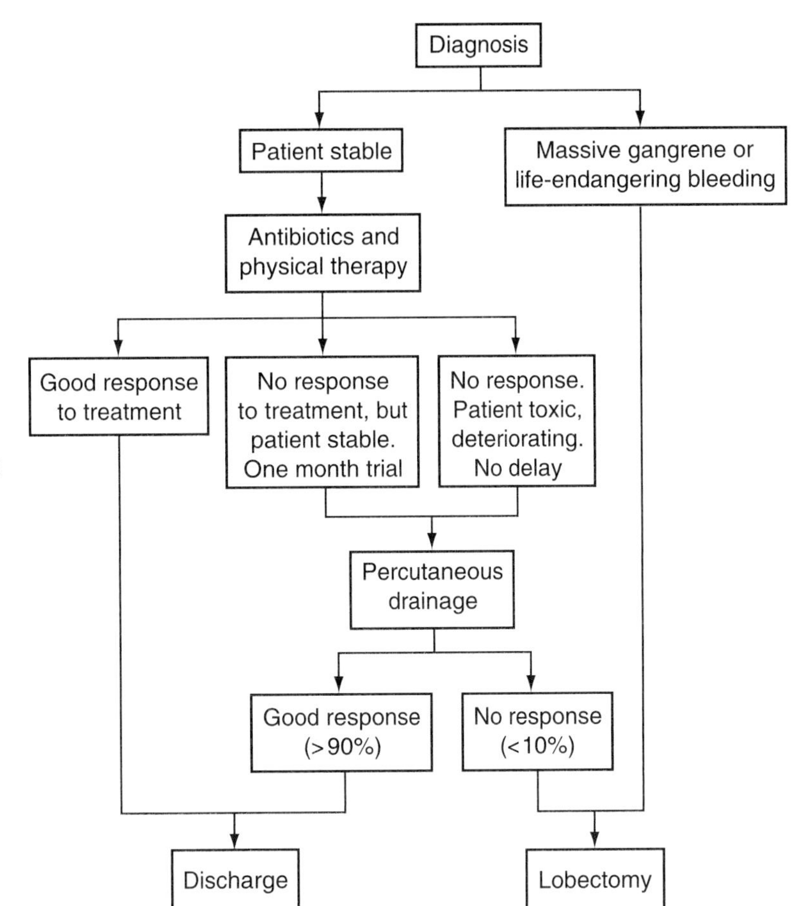

FIGURE 1 Algorithm of management of primary lung abscess.

ACUTE BRONCHITIS

METHOD OF

Marcia Edmonds, MD, MSc

Acute bronchitis, one of the most common respiratory infections diagnosed by family physicians, is frequently seen in the family physician's office and in hospital emergency rooms. Each year in the United States, acute bronchitis accounts for more than 300 million dollars in costs for physician visits and prescriptions, and is a common reason for lost time from work. Despite this, controversy still exists as to which clinical features suggest the diagnosis of acute bronchitis, and there are no confirmatory laboratory investigations. The majority of cases of acute bronchitis in healthy individuals are caused by viral etiologies, and current guidelines recommend withholding antibiotics in patients with this diagnosis, but recent studies suggest that physicians still prescribe antibiotics for acute bronchitis 42% to 79% of the time.

Acute bronchitis can be defined as acute inflammation of the bronchial tree, which presents clinically as a cough, with or without sputum production, with evidence of concurrent upper airway infection. Following a viral infection, the cough may be prolonged, with 45% of patients still coughing after 2 weeks, and 25% after 3 weeks. Acute bronchitis should be differentiated from chronic bronchitis, which is characterized by ongoing excessive secretion of bronchial mucus, manifested by a productive cough for 3 months or more in at least 2 consecutive years in the absence of other diseases to account for the symptoms. Cigarette smoking is by far the most important cause of chronic bronchitis. Patients with an exacerbation of chronic bronchitis present with increased sputum purulence, volume, and/or increased dyspnea as compared with their baseline status. A bacterial etiology is far more likely in chronic bronchitis than acute bronchitis.

The diagnosis of acute bronchitis is made on history and physical examination since no diagnostic test is currently available to make a definitive diagnosis. The incidence of acute bronchitis is likely overestimated, as other conditions may mimic the symptoms of acute bronchitis, particularly the cough (Table 1). A chest radiograph may be done in select cases to look for evidence of pneumonia or foreign body aspiration.

TABLE 1 Differential Diagnoses of Acute Bronchitis

Pneumonia
Acute exacerbation of chronic bronchitis
Pertussis
Postnasal drip
Asthma
Foreign body aspiration
Pulmonary edema
Sinusitis

Indications for a chest radiograph in patients presenting with a clinical syndrome compatible with acute bronchitis include abnormal vital signs, (pulse >100, respiratory rate >24, or temperature >38°C [100.4°F]), or focal findings on chest examination. Advanced age may be another reason to request a chest radiograph. Patients with a presentation compatible with influenza including fever, without suspicion of complications, do not require a chest radiograph. Although pulmonary function testing may be abnormal in patients with acute bronchitis, it is not routinely recommended. Pulmonary function tests may be helpful if asthma is suspected based on the clinical presentation, and a trial of asthma therapies may be worthwhile in these patients.

The usual cause of acute bronchitis is predominantly viral. More than 180 viruses have been implicated in acute bronchitis, with the most common ones including rhinoviruses, adenoviruses, influenza, respiratory syncytial virus, and coronaviruses. Rapid tests are available for influenza, and cultures may also be performed, although the sensitivity of the tests is similar to the sensitivity of a clinical diagnosis during a known epidemic. Testing for influenza may be most useful to document the presence of influenza in a community at the start of a season, or when the diagnosis is in question.

Although both *Mycoplasma pneumoniae* and *Chlamydia pneumoniae* have been implicated as possible bacterial agents in acute bronchitis, both agents tend to cause self-limited disease. As well, clear diagnosis of these two conditions is problematic, both clinically and in the laboratory, and the role of antibiotics in their treatment is unclear. Sputum cultures and serologic testing for these agents are generally unhelpful as they do not enhance the clinical diagnosis or change management. Sputum cultures for other bacterial agents are also not useful in most cases, as acute bronchitis is not usually caused by bacteria, and the cultures will usually grow oropharyngeal flora. Cultures may be useful in patients with airway violations such as tracheostomy or endotracheal intubation, or in those with an exacerbation of chronic bronchitis, where a bacterial etiology is more likely.

If *Bordetella pertussis* is suspected, specific testing for it is important. A prominent barking cough that is severe, persistent, and often associated with vomiting is characteristic of pertussis, particularly in an unimmunized patient. Although immunization is highly effective in preventing severe disease, a less severe infection can occur in subjects who are adequately vaccinated, but these patients can still transmit the disease. Nasopharyngeal cultures specific for pertussis should be performed when this is suspected.

Treatment of acute bronchitis is primarily symptomatic. Although there is ongoing controversy, most trials do not show a convincing benefit of antibiotic therapy in acute bronchitis, and meta-analyses suggest that any benefit of antibiotics may be offset by their side effects. Although outcomes such as time to return to work or normal activities have not been extensively investigated, and the power to detect uncommon complications is limited, consensus statements agree that antibiotics are not indicated in acute bronchitis. As well, the unnecessary use of antibiotics may contribute to antibiotic resistance. Although the overall use of antibiotics for acute bronchitis has declined somewhat in recent years, the use of broad-spectrum antibiotics has become more common. In the majority of cases, antibiotic therapy is still not indicated. Patients with pertussis should be treated with an antibiotic (erythromycin base [E-Mycin], 500 mg orally four times per day for 10 days, or azithromycin [Zithromax][1], 500 mg orally on day 1 and then 250 mg orally daily for 4 days) to decrease illness severity and duration, and prevent spread. Routine use of antibiotics directed at *M. pneumoniae* or *C. pneumoniae* is not recommended, as treatable infections are infrequent, difficult to diagnose, and usually self-limited.

Providing written information to patients and families about the self-limited nature of acute bronchitis may help to decrease antibiotic use without increasing physician visits. Explaining the expected duration of the illness (anticipate 2 to 3 weeks of coughing with eventual complete resolution) and the lack of any proven benefit of antibiotics with their potential for harm may increase patient satisfaction with symptomatic treatments.

In patients with known or suspected influenza, antiviral medications may be of help if started early in the course of the illness. Their efficacy is limited and the appropriate clinical niche for these drugs is a source of ongoing controversy. Oseltamivir (Tamiflu), 75 mg orally twice daily, or zanamivir (Relenza), 10 mg inhaled twice daily, are moderately effective in reducing illness severity and duration (by approximately 1 day), particularly if started during the first day of illness. They are not beneficial if started more than 48 hours into the illness. Amantadine (Symmetrel) or rimantadine (Flumadine) are active against influenza A, although their clinical use is limited by side effects and minimal efficacy. These agents may have a role in prophylaxis during influenza outbreaks.

Some studies suggest a modest benefit of bronchodilators (such as albuterol [Ventolin][1], 180 μg

[1]Not FDA approved for this indication.

inhaled every 4 hours as needed) on the cough of acute bronchitis, although a meta-analysis did not confirm this benefit. A trial of these medications may still be worthwhile in select patients with ongoing symptoms. There is no evidence for the use of anticholinergics or long-acting β-agonists in acute bronchitis. Corticosteroids (inhaled or oral) have not been adequately studied and are not recommended. Antitussive medications may help with symptom relief, although they will not shorten the course of illness and are of limited efficacy.

Patients presenting with an episode of acute bronchitis may be receptive to interventions to decrease their risk of recurrent episodes. It is an excellent opportunity to discuss smoking cessation in patients who are currently smoking. It also provides the opportunity to discuss the need for pneumococcal vaccinations, where indicated, and yearly influenza vaccinations.

Acute bronchitis is generally a self-limited illness that is diagnosed clinically in most cases and does not require antibiotic therapy. Treatment remains primarily symptomatic.

BACTERIAL PNEUMONIAS

METHOD OF

Burke A. Cunha, MD

Community-Acquired Pneumonias

Eighty-five percent of community-acquired pneumonias (CAPs) are caused by *Streptococcus pneumoniae*, *Haemophilus influenzae*, or *Moraxella catarrhalis*. The clinical manifestations overlap considerably and cannot be distinguished readily on clinical grounds. For this reason, antibiotics for typical bacterial CAPs should cover all three of these key pathogens. It is equally important to recognize that other pathogens are uncommon and should be covered only under certain circumstances. *Staphylococcus aureus* CAP, for example, occurs only in the postviral influenza setting. *Klebsiella pneumoniae* CAP occurs almost exclusively in chronic alcoholics, and *Pseudomonas aeruginosa* causes CAP only in patients with bronchiectasis or cystic fibrosis but not in normal hosts. Therefore, *S. aureus, K. pneumoniae*, and *P. aeruginosa* coverage need not be included in empiric therapy regimens of CAPs. Typical bacterial CAPs have clinical findings confined to the lungs.

Community-Acquired Atypical Pneumonias

Atypical CAPs are distinguished from the typical CAPs by their extrapulmonary manifestations. The atypical pneumonias may be classified as zoonotic (e.g., psittacosis, tularemia, Q fever) or nonzoonotic (e.g., legionnaires' disease, *Mycoplasma pneumoniae* pneumonia, *Chlamydia pneumoniae* pneumonia). Epidemiologic contact histories regarding animal or bird contact quickly rule in or rule out the zoonotic atypical pathogens.

M. pneumoniae and *C. pneumoniae* pneumonia occur in young adults or in adults who have had recent contact with infected young adults and are usually mild in normal adults. In contrast, legionnaires' disease may be severe. Clinical diagnostic approaches should distinguish *Legionella* from typical CAPs, because β lactams used to treat typical CAPs are ineffective against *Legionella*. Legionnaires' disease may be treated with macrolides, doxycycline, or quinolones.

Diagnostic Approach

No single clinical or laboratory feature is diagnostic of any atypical CAP, but the pattern of organ involvement is characteristic. No patient has all the extrapulmonary findings associated with a particular atypical organism, but most patients have enough clinical and laboratory manifestations to permit an accurate presumptive clinical diagnosis.

SEVERE COMMUNITY-ACQUIRED PNEUMONIA

Patients with severe CAP do not require a different therapeutic approach than patients with mild-to-moderate CAP. Severe CAP is caused by the same pathogens that cause mild-to-moderate CAP. Because the organisms causing severe CAP are the same as those causing mild-to-moderate CAP, antimicrobial therapy is the same for both CAP groups regardless of severity.

The severity of CAP depends on the degree of the patient's immunocompromise status as well as cardiopulmonary function. Patients with significant cardiopulmonary disease are likely to have a severe CAP because they have little cardiopulmonary reserve. Predictably, CAP will be serious regardless of the infecting pathogen. Even mild CAP caused by a low-virulence pathogen (e.g., *M. catarrhalis*) can present as severe CAP in a patient with borderline pulmonary function. Superimposed on pre-existing pulmonary disease, CAP caused by any pathogen will be severe. CAP is also severe in patients with clinically significant coronary artery disease, valvular heart disease, or congestive heart failure.

Immunocompromised patients, especially those with impaired humoral immunity/B-lymphocyte function, are prone to severe CAP. Fulminant pneumococcal pneumonia with bacteremia/shock is well known in asplenics. The usual treatment for overwhelming pneumococcal sepsis is penicillin given at the same dose and dosing interval as for patients with an intact immune system and mild-to-moderate disease. The antibiotic approach is the same for mild-to-moderate and severe CAP because antibiotic therapy is directed against the pathogen and is not affected by co-morbidities or host factors.

Prognostic/severity indices have been developed for patients with CAP. Importantly, the severity indices have no bearing on the selection of initial empirical therapy for the treatment of CAP because antibiotic therapy is independent of disease severity. Additional antibiotic should not be given for severity or co-morbid factors (Table 1).

COMMUNITY-ACQUIRED PNEUMONIA IN COMPROMISED HOSTS

Compromised hosts with CAP are most often infected with the usual bacterial pathogens. Viral pneumonias are common in transplant and HIV-infected patients, but the clinical radiologic presentation is distinct from bacterial CAP. Viral pneumonia or *Pneumocystis carinii* pneumonia (PCP) are rarely focal, segmental, or lobar on chest radiograph, and a segmental/lobar infiltrate should be assumed to be bacterial until proven otherwise.

If therapy with a respiratory quinolone (e.g., levofloxacin [Levaquin], gatifloxacin [Tequin], or moxifloxacin [Avelox]) does not result in clinical improvement in 72 hours in a compromised host with CAP, the patient should have diagnostic bronchoscopy (Table 2).

TABLE 1 Severe Community-Acquired Pneumonia (CAP) With Shock

- CAP does not present with shock in normal hosts.
- If CAP presents with shock, look for "mimics of pneumonia" with pulmonary infiltrates, fever, leukocytosis, and hypotension, (e.g., acute myocardial infarction [MI], acute pulmonary embolism [PE]).
- If CAP presents with shock but no evidence of acute MI, acute PE, etc., then consider an exacerbation of pre-existing advanced cardiopulmonary disease (e.g., coronary insufficiency, hypoxemia in emphysema) as the cause of shock.
- If CAP presents with shock without a cardiopulmonary explanation, look for impaired or absent splenic function.
- Disorders associated with impaired splenic function are:

Amyloidosis	Rheumatoid arthritis
Celiac disease	Sézary syndrome
Chronic active hepatitis	Sickle cell trait/disease
Chronic alcoholism	Splenectomy
Congenital asplenia	Splenic infarcts
Fanconi syndrome	Splenic malignancies
Hyposplenism of old age	Steroid therapy
IgA deficiency	Systemic lupus
Intestinal lymphangiectasia	Systemic lupus erythematosus
Intravenous gamma globulin therapy	Systemic mastocytosis
Myeloproliferative disorders	Systemic necrotizing vasculitis
Non-Hodgkin lymphoma	Thyroiditis
Regional enteritis	Ulcerative colitis
Waldenström macroglobulinemia	

- Howell-Jolly bodies in the peripheral smear are indicative of splenic dysfunction.
- If CAP presents with shock but no evidence of cardiopulmonary/splenic dysfunction, rule out GI bleed, acute pancreatitis, and volume depletion as a cause.

TABLE 2 Therapeutic Approach to Community-Acquired Pneumonia (CAP)

- CAP is caused by single, not multiple, pathogens.
- Antibiotic coverage should be directed against both typical and atypical causes of CAP.
- Antibiotic coverage should be directed against these pathogens only in specific circumstances:
  - *Klebsiella pneumoniae* (only in chronic alcoholics)
  - *Staphylococcus aureus* (only in postviral influenza pneumonia)
  - *Pseudomonas aeruginosa* (only in cystic fibrosis/bronchiectasis)
- Most compromised hosts (especially organ transplant recipients, febrile leukopenics, and patients with HIV infection) with CAP usually have the same bacterial pathogens as do normal hosts and should be treated the same as normal hosts.
- CAP therapies that have a high degree of antipneumococcal activity and low resistance potential are used:
  - β-Lactams
  - Respiratory quinolones
  - Doxycycline
  - Telithromycin (Ketek)
- Appropriate monotherapy is used for severe CAP. Do not add additional antibiotics if the patient is critically ill. Severity is a function of underlying cardiopulmonary disease/impaired splenic function. Antibiotics do not correct co-morbidities.

THERAPEUTIC CONSIDERATIONS

Intravenous-to-Oral Switch Therapy

Critically ill patients with CAP are treated intravenously until clinically improved. In the treatment of typical bacterial CAP, 2 days of intravenous (IV) therapy followed by 12 days of oral therapy is therapeutically equivalent to a full 14-day course of intravenous antibiotics. The majority of hospitalized patients can take oral antibiotics after 48 to 72 hours. Switching patients to an appropriate oral antibiotic after 48 to 72 hours has several clinical advantages—the length of stay is decreased, the costs of therapy are lower, and the incidence of IV-line infection is reduced.

When selecting an antibiotic for an IV-to-oral switch, the same considerations used to select an antibiotic for oral therapy alone apply. Oral antibiotics should have

TABLE 3 Empiric Monotherapy for Community-Acquired Pneumonia (CAP)

Typical Coverage	Atypical Coverage	Typical and Atypical Coverage
Mild-to-Moderate CAP (PO Therapy)		
Amoxicillin (high dose)/clavulanate (Augmentin)	Respiratory quinolone*	Respiratory quinolone*
Doxycycline (Vibramycin)	Doxycycline	Doxycycline
Telithromycin (Ketek)	Azithromycin (Zithromax)	Telithromycin
	Telithromycin	
Severe CAP (Initial IV Therapy)		
Ceftriaxone (Rocephin)	Doxycycline	Doxycycline
Cefepime (Maxipime)	Respiratory quinolone*	Respiratory quinolone*
Respiratory quinolone		
IV/PO Switch Therapy for CAP		
Amoxicillin (high dose)/ clavulanate	Respiratory quinolone*	Respiratory quinolone*
Doxycycline	Doxycycline	Doxycycline
Telithromycin	Azithromycin	Telithromycin
	Telithromycin	

*Respiratory quinolones: levofloxacin (Levoquin), gatifloxacin (Tequin), and moxifloxacin (Avelox).

the same therapeutic spectrum as their IV counterparts, and bioavailability should be 90%, which would achieve the same serum and tissue levels as their IV counterparts. With the exception of those who cannot take oral medications, all patients with CAP should be switched to an appropriate oral antibiotic after 48 to 72 hours after clinical improvement. As with oral antibiotics, the total duration of therapy for typical CAPs is 14 days (Tables 3 and 4).

TABLE 4 Therapeutic Approach to Nosocomial Pneumonias

- Direct coverage against *Pseudomonas aeruginosa*, which also covers most other nosocomial pathogens:
  - *Pseudomonas aeruginosa*
  - *Klebsiella pneumoniae*
  - *Serratia marcescens*
  - *Escherichia coli*
- Do not cover/treat colonizers in respiratory secretions:
  - *Enterobacter* spp.
  - *Citrobacter* spp.
  - *Enterococcus* spp.
  - *Flavobacterium meningosepticum*
  - *Pseudomonas cepacia*
  - *Xanthomonas maltophilia*
  - *Staphylococcus aureus*
- Use monotherapy for nosocomial pneumonia, not double-drug therapy. Monotherapy is equivalent to combination therapy.
- Avoid covering/treating noninfectious conditions that mimic nosocomial pneumonia. Many patients are needlessly treated for unexplained or undiagnosed pulmonary infiltrates, fever, or leukocytosis because of positive respiratory secretion cultures (colonizers).
- Give a full 14-day course and then discontinue antibiotics. Do not continue antibiotic therapy for persistent low-grade fever/pulmonary infiltrates (suggests a noninfectious disease etiology). Obtain an infectious disease consultation/perform a definitive diagnostic procedure.

Oral Antibiotic Treatment of Community-Acquired Pneumonia

Patients admitted to the hospital with mild-to-moderate CAPs may be treated entirely with oral antibiotics. The choice of an oral antibiotic depends on the therapeutic spectrum, tissue penetration, resistance potential, safety profile, and cost. The ideal antibiotic for oral therapy has the same spectrum of activity as its IV counterpart. Antibiotics with high bioavailability (e.g., 90% absorption) are equivalent to their intravenous counterparts attaining the same blood and tissue levels. Patients with moderate CAP who are able to take oral medications and do not require hospitalization may be treated entirely with oral antibiotics. The duration of oral antibiotic therapy to treat CAP is the same as that with intravenous preparations, that is, usually 14 days for typical pathogens and 2 to 4 weeks for legionnaires' disease. Treatment may be shortened in healthy, immunocompetent hosts and extended in patients with impaired host defenses.

Nosocomial Pneumonias

Nosocomial pneumonias may be acquired via inhalation or hematogenous dissemination to the lungs from a distant source. The former type usually demonstrates a segmental or lobar distribution on the chest film. In contrast, hematogenously acquired nosocomial pneumonia presents with bilateral, symmetrical, interstitial alveolar infiltrates resembling left ventricular failure, adult respiratory distress syndrome, or massive bilateral aspiration. The diagnosis of nosocomial pneumonia is difficult because there are many conditions with similar presentations. Many patients in the critical care unit or other hospital settings who have pulmonary infiltrates and fever, with or without leukocytosis, are treated empirically for hospital-acquired pneumonia but do not have a nosocomial pneumonia. The recovery of respiratory pathogens from respiratory secretions in an intubated patient with fever, leukocytosis, and pulmonary infiltrates is insufficient for the diagnosis.

There are many disorders that present with findings that mimic hospital-acquired pneumonia (e.g., pulmonary embolism and collagen vascular diseases such as systemic lupus erythematosus). Clinicians should try to rule out conditions that mimic nosocomial pneumonia and initiate appropriate therapy.

NOSOCOMIAL ASPIRATION PNEUMONIA

Community-acquired aspiration pneumonia is caused by aspirated oral anaerobic flora. If aspiration occurs after 7 days of hospitalization, the patient has hospital-acquired aspiration pneumonia. After a week or more of hospitalization, the predominant oropharyngeal flora are replaced by the aerobic gram-negative bacilli acquired from the hospital environment. Anaerobes are not important in nosocomial pneumonia.

Nosocomial pulmonary pathogens include *P. aeruginosa*, *Serratia marcescens*, and *K. pneumoniae*. Antibiotic therapy of nosocomial aspiration pneumonia should be directed against the usual hospital-acquired respiratory pathogens. Nosocomial aspiration pneumonia is treated as hospital-acquired pneumonia; there is no need to add antianaerobic coverage.

THERAPEUTIC CONSIDERATIONS

Monotherapy Versus Combination Therapy

Antimicrobial therapy should be directed primarily against *P. aeruginosa*, because such coverage will cover the other nosocomial pathogens, including *S. marcescens* and *K. pneumoniae*. Several therapeutic empiric approaches are used for the treatment of nosocomial pneumonias. Traditionally, two antibiotics with antipseudomonal activity are given in a full 14-day course of therapy regardless of whether *P. aeruginosa* is shown to be the pathogen. Alternately, two antipseudomonal antibiotics are given for the first 72 hours while waiting for blood cultures to show whether *P. aeruginosa* is the pathogen. If *P. aeruginosa* is not cultured, then one of the antipseudomonal antibiotics is discontinued and the 14-day course of therapy is completed with the other antipseudomonal antibiotic.

The preferred initial approach is to use a single antipseudomonal agent with a high degree of activity against *P. aeruginosa* and with a low resistance potential. If *P. aeruginosa* is cultured from the blood, then a second antipseudomonal antibiotic is added. This is the most cost-effective and logical approach because it minimizes needless double-drug therapy. Monotherapy with an anti-*P. aeruginosa* antibiotic with a high degree of anti-*P. aeruginosa* activity and minimal resistance potential is the preferred therapeutic approach.

Antibiotic Resistance

The use of combination therapy does not eliminate resistance problems; for example, the addition of any antipseudomonal antibiotic to ceftazidime (Fortaz) does not prevent the ceftazidime-resistant *P. aeruginosa*. Preferentially selecting antibiotics with a low resistance potential is the best strategy to prevent the emergence of antibiotic resistance in the critical care unit.

Optimal Therapeutic Approach

Therapy of nosocomial pneumonia is ordinarily continued for 14 days, but a longer course may be necessary in patients with impaired cardiopulmonary function. Patients with persistent or increasing pulmonary infiltrates should not be treated for longer than 14 days. Treating persistent leukocytosis, low-grade fever, and unresolved pulmonary infiltrates beyond 14 days should be discouraged. If pulmonary infiltrates are still present in normal hosts after 2 weeks of effective antipseudomonal therapy, the process is most likely noninfectious and not remediable to further antibiotic therapy. Such patients should undergo diagnostic bronchoscopy/lung biopsy for a definitive diagnosis.

VIRAL UPPER RESPIRATORY TRACT INFECTIONS

METHOD OF
Robert C. Welliver, Sr., MD

Epidemiology

Viral infections of the upper respiratory tract (commonly known as colds) represent one of the most common reasons for requests for medical attention. Colds also result in considerable absenteeism from school and work. Infants and young children suffer 6.7 to 8.3 colds annually, whereas adults generally sustain 4 colds per year. Rhinoviruses are the most commonly recognized cause of colds, whereas respiratory syncytial virus (RSV), parainfluenza viruses, coronaviruses, influenza virus types A and B, adenovirus, enteroviruses, and the recently-discovered human metapneumovirus are all important etiologic agents. Transmission occurs by large droplet spread or by direct contact with secretions in the case of rhinovirus infections and RSV, but small droplets (i.e., in coughs) may transmit influenza and coronavirus infections. Infection with some of these agents induces persistent serotype-specific immunity, but there are more than 100 potentially pathogenic serotypes of rhinoviruses, and more than 70 unique serotypes of enteroviruses and adenoviruses. Other cold viruses are capable of causing reinfection almost annually despite the presence of pre-existing neutralizing antibody.

Clinical Manifestations

Symptoms of colds include nasal discharge and obstruction, sneezing, sore throat, muscle or joint aches, and cough. Fever is often present, especially in children, but is usually not striking. The rhinorrhea may be watery initially, but then attains a white color and contains leukocytes (predominantly neutrophils). The presence of a green tint to the nasal discharge occurs commonly in children and is of no significance, but may suggest a sinus infection when it occurs in an adult. Pharyngitis is usually not severe, but exudates may be present on tonsils, and the anterior cervical lymph nodes may be enlarged and mildly painful. More severe adenitis suggests the presence of bacterial infection. Colds caused by influenza viruses are often characterized by more intense myalgia and headache, and easy fatigability is frequently present. Perhaps, surprisingly, a 1-year survey in our emergency department indicated that fevers greater than 39°C (102.2°F) are unusual with influenza virus infection in adolescents and adults. Laryngitis may be more frequent with colds caused by parainfluenza viruses. Conjunctivitis is particularly common with adenovirus colds, and rashes are most frequently associated with enterovirus infections. However, colds caused by other viruses are essentially indistinguishable clinically. Symptoms resolve spontaneously in 5 to 7 days in adults, although they may persist for 10 to 14 days in infants and preschool children. More prolonged persistence of symptoms suggests the presence of sinusitis.

Management

Rest and maintenance of adequate fluid intake in order to avoid dehydration are the mainstays of therapy for colds. Because colds are almost always self-limited, one should resist the temptation to overmedicate with so-called *cold remedies* that contain numerous (largely ineffective) compounds aimed at treating all the possible symptoms of colds. A high rate of occurrence of the placebo effect complicates the evaluation of any modality in the treatment of colds.

Nasal obstruction may be caused by blockage of the nostril by thick mucus, in which case warm humidified air or saline nose drops (Ocean Spray) may be effective in liquefying the secretion. Swelling of the nasal mucous membranes may also cause nasal obstruction. In this case topical administration of decongestants such as 0.25% phenylephrine nose drops (Neo-Synephrine) (2 drops in each nostril in older children, 4 drops in each nostril for adults, up to four times a day) or 0.05% oxymetazoline nasal sprays (Afrin) (twice a day), may provide temporary relief. These medications should not be administered to infants and young children, as they may cause supraventricular tachycardia. These compounds should not be administered to patients also taking monoamine oxidase inhibitors. In any case, administration of these medications for more than 4 to 5 days should be avoided. Prolonged use results in a rebound vasodilatation and, therefore, nasal obstruction as a result of the medication itself. Oral formulations of decongestants are available, but are no more effective than topical preparations and cause more side effects.

Antihistamines are frequently included in cold remedies in the hope that drying of secretions will occur. The theoretical basis for this is unsound, as histamine has not been demonstrated to cause any of the symptoms of colds. The results of controlled studies do not show any beneficial effects of antihistamines in colds.

Sore throat with colds is usually not severe, and may be relieved somewhat by saline gargles ($\frac{1}{2}$ teaspoon of salt in 4 ounces of warm water). Effective analgesia can be obtained with either acetaminophen (Tylenol) (10 to 15 mg/kg in children up to 650 mg, and 650 mg in adults, given every 4 to 6 hours) or ibuprofen (Motrin) (10 mg/kg in children up to 200 or 400 mg given every 6 to 8 hours, and 400 to 600 mg in adults given every 6 hours). The effect of ibuprofen is apparently longer lasting in children than that of acetaminophen, and both agents have similar safety profiles. Compounds containing salicylates (i.e., aspirin) should be avoided because of the association of the use of these agents with the occurrence of Reye syndrome.

Constitutional symptoms such as fever, malaise, and headache may be managed with the doses of acetaminophen and ibuprofen listed above.

Cough is usually not prominent with colds, although it may occasionally prevent sleep. Cough suppressants such as dextromethorphan (Robitussin Cough) and codeine may be effective in these circumstances. The dose for children older than 5 years is 1 mg/kg up to 60 mg, and for adults the dose is 15 to 60 mg; both child and adult doses are given every 6 hours if necessary. These compounds induce side effects such as drowsiness and bronchoconstriction, and may also be ineffective in children younger than 5 years of age. Therefore they should not be prescribed for these younger children. These compounds also should not be administered to patients taking monoamine oxidase inhibitors.

Specific antiviral therapy is presently available only for influenza virus infections, but the efficacy of amantadine (Symmetrel), rimantadine (Flumadine), oseltamivir (Tamiflu), and zanamivir (Relenza) is so limited that the general use of these drugs in the treatment of influenza virus infections cannot be supported.

Prevention

In many cases, the viruses causing colds are acquired by direct contact with the secretions on the hands of infected persons. Inoculation of the eye or nasal mucous membranes (but probably not the oropharynx) then transmits the infection to the recipient. Therefore handwashing, avoiding contact of the ocular and nasal mucosa with the hands, and, of course, avoiding exposure to infected persons will reduce the frequency of colds.

Various compounds have been advocated to reduce the rate of acquiring colds. These include zinc lozenges (Halls Zinc Defense)*, vitamin C, Echinacea*, and others. Controlled clinical trials do not support the use of these compounds for cold prevention, nor do they indicate that interferon gamma[1], pleconaril[†], or blockers of the epithelial cell receptor for rhinovirus prevent colds. In contrast, the prompt administration of oseltamivir (Tamiflu)[1] (2 mg/kg every 12 hours orally)[3] or zanamivir (Relenza)[1] (10 mg inhaled every 12 hours) to household contacts of influenza virus-infected subjects prevents the development of infection caused by this virus. An efficient strategy for the use of this compound has not been developed.

[1]Not FDA approved for this indication.

[3]Exceeds dosage recommended by the manufacturer.

*Available as a dietary supplement; not yet approved in the United States.

[†]Investigational drug in the United States.

VIRAL AND MYCOPLASMAL PNEUMONIA

METHOD OF

David C. Rhew, MD, and

Matthew Bidwell Goetz, MD

The term *atypical pneumonia* originated in the mid-1940s to represent pneumonias in which the causative agent could not be identified using routine Gram stain or culture of respiratory specimens. Mycoplasmal and viral infections represent common causes of atypical pneumonia and account for approximately 2% to 7% of pneumonias requiring hospitalization. Other atypical pathogens include *Legionella*, *Chlamydia*, fungal, mycobacterial, and others. This article describes in greater detail the diagnostic and management principles for treating patients with pneumonias caused by *Mycoplasma pneumoniae* and respiratory viruses, including influenzas A and B, respiratory syncytial virus (RSV), parainfluenza viruses, adenovirus, hantavirus, and severe acute respiratory syndrome (SARS)-associated coronavirus.

Mycoplasma Pneumoniae

Although *Streptococcus pneumoniae* is the most common pathogen isolated from patients with community-acquired pneumonia, a study by Marston and colleagues has demonstrated that *M. pneumoniae* is seen in 32.5% of adult patients admitted to the hospital with community-acquired pneumonia (CAP), with *S. pneumoniae* in 12.6% of cases. Other studies indicate that the incidence of *M. pneumoniae* ranges from 2% to 30% and that *M. pneumoniae* is usually the second or third most common pathogen in adult CAP. Overall estimates are that *M. pneumonia* accounts for 8% to 11% of cases of CAP in persons treated as outpatients and 1% to 8% of cases of CAP among patients who are hospitalized.

M. pneumoniae infection is common in children and young adults and often does not require hospitalization in these patients. Severe disease may occur in older adults as a result of reinfection with *M. pneumoniae* and/or coinfection with other bacteria or viruses. *M. pneumoniae* also causes outbreaks in closed settings (e.g., summer camps and college dormitories) and can cause community-wide epidemics.

The clinical manifestations of *M. pneumoniae* infection consist of pharyngitis and bronchitis, which can progress to pneumonia in 5% to 10% of cases. Infection may be accompanied by a persistent cough, likely related to cilial dysfunction. The cough may be so persistent as to keep the patient up at night and be so severe as to cause chest pain due to muscle strain. Other symptoms associated with *M. pneumoniae* include fever, malaise, and headache. Physical examination of the lung is generally negative, but may occasionally demonstrate wheezing. Nonpulmonary findings associated with *M. pneumoniae* infection include bullous myringitis, rashes (erythema multiforme, Stevens-Johnson syndrome), Raynaud phenomenon, and cardiac, neurologic, rheumatologic, and renal abnormalities.

A variety of tests may be applied to diagnose *M. pneumoniae* infection. Cold agglutinin titers of greater than 1:32 are highly suggestive of mycoplasmal infection, but are not diagnostic. Other conditions, in particular viral infections and lymphoma, may also cause elevations in cold agglutinin titers. Complement-fixing antibodies are specific, but not sensitive for diagnosing mycoplasmal infection, especially early in the disease course. Mycoplasmal culture on special media is difficult to perform and requires 1 to 2 weeks for final results. Rapid tests for diagnosing *M. pneumoniae*, such as polymerase chain reaction (PCR) and enzyme-linked immunoassay (ELISA) tests, are not well established.

Ideally, the treatment of infections should be pathogen-directed. However, no component of the history or physical examination has sufficient sensitivity or specificity to rule out or rule in the diagnosis of *M. pneumoniae* infection. Furthermore, there are no currently available tests to reliably make the diagnosis of *M. pneumoniae* in a rapid manner. For these reasons, the initial treatment of patients with community-acquired pneumonia is usually empiric, and most authorities recommend an initial regimen that includes an agent that has activity against atypical bacterial pathogens including *M. pneumoniae*. These agents are doxycycline (Vibramycin), macrolide (erythromycin, clarithromycin [Biaxin], azithromycin [Zithromax], or dirithromycin [Dynabac]), or a respiratory fluoroquinolone (e.g., levofloxacin [Levaquin], gatifloxacin [Tequin], moxifloxacin [Avelox]) (Table 1). Several large retrospective analyses have demonstrated that patients hospitalized with CAP who are treated with an initial regimen that has activity against atypical pathogens have lower severity-adjusted, 30-day mortality rates than those not receiving regimens with atypical activity.

Influenza Viruses

There are three influenza viruses, A, B, and C. Influenza A, and less commonly B, can cause epidemics with significant mortality in persons aged 65 or older and other high-risk patients. Influenza A can also trigger pandemics that can cause significant mortality in young persons. Influenza C causes cold-like, but not influenza-like, symptoms. Influenza C also occurs year-round, unlike influenza A and B, which occur in a seasonal pattern.

While rates of influenza infection are highest in children, mortality and serious morbidity are highest in persons who are 65 years of age and older and in those with high-risk conditions (Table 2).

A population study of influenza-related deaths in the United States demonstrated that the percentage of deaths due to influenza has significantly increased from 1976 to 1999, presumably due to the aging population. Furthermore, in this study 90% of all influenza-associated respiratory and circulatory deaths occurred in persons 65 years of age and older.

During outbreaks, influenza may cause up to 10% of cases of pneumonia among hospitalized patients. Influenza-associated pneumonia may occur in two forms. The first is a severe primary viral form characterized by diffuse interstitial infiltrates and

TABLE 1 Antibiotics for Community-Acquired Pneumonia with Atypical Activity

Antibiotic	Dose (Adult)
Doxycycline	100 mg PO or IV every 12 h
Erythromycin	Mild-to-moderate infection: 250 to 500 mg (base, estolate, stearate) or 400-800 mg (ethylsuccinate) PO every 6 h Severe infection: 1-4 g/d IV in divided doses every 6 h
Clarithromycin (Biaxin)	250 to 500 mg PO every 12 h
Azithromycin (Zithromax)	Mild: 500 mg PO on day 1, followed by 250 mg PO on days 2-5; Moderate-severe: 500 mg IV daily for at least 2d, followed by 500 mg PO once a day
Levofloxacin (Levaquin)	500 mg PO or IV every 24 h or 750 mg PO or IV every 24 h (may allow for shorter duration of therapy)
Gatifloxacin (Tequin)	400 mg PO or IV every 24 h
Moxifloxacin (Avelox)	400 mg PO every 24 h

TABLE 2 High-Risks for Complications Caused by Influenza

Age 65 or older
Resident of nursing home or long-term care facility
Chronic cardiopulmonary disease (including asthma)
Chronic metabolic disease (diabetes mellitus)
Renal dysfunction
Hemoglobinopathies
Immunosuppression (e.g., infected with HIV or receiving immunosuppressive medications)
Children and adolescents receiving long-term aspirin therapy (and at risk for Reyes syndrome after influenza infection)
Women who will be in their second or third trimester of pregnancy during the influenza season

Adapted from: Prevention and control of influenza: Recommendations of the Advisory Committee on Immunization Practices (ACIP). MMWR 52(RR-8):1-36, April 25, 2003.

hypoxia. The second is a bacterial pneumonia superimposed or subsequent to an influenza infection. While rates of bacterial coinfection with *Staphylococcus aureus* are higher in influenza-associated pneumonia than in routine CAP (i.e., 19% in conjunction with influenza versus 6% without influenza), coinfection with *S. aureus* is still less frequent than coinfection with *S. pneumoniae* (48%).

The presumptive diagnosis of influenza is based on clinical grounds. Influenza occurs in the United States between the months of October and mid-May, with peak activity in December and January. Clinical clues to the diagnosis of influenza include the presence of fever, cough, myalgias, and weakness. However, cough and fever are the two most predictive symptoms. A retrospective pooled analysis of signs and symptoms of patients enrolled in eight phase 2 and phase 3 trials of zanamivir (Relenza) demonstrated that the presence of fever and cough is associated with a sensitivity of 64%, specificity of 67%, positive predictive value (PPV) of 79%, and negative predictive value (NPV) of 49% for diagnosing influenza infection when influenza is endemic. The addition of other symptoms does not increase the PPV for diagnosing influenza.

The diagnosis of influenza can be confirmed by sending a nasopharyngeal swab specimen for viral culture, rapid antigen assay direct immunofluorescence stain, or PCR. For epidemiological purposes, influenza acute and convalescent serologic studies may be useful. The timeliness and rapid availability of the antigen detection assays make them clinically useful.

Anti-influenza agents include amantadine (Symmetrel), rimantadine (Flumadine), and the neuraminidase inhibitors (zanamivir [Relenza] or oseltamivir [Tamiflu]) (Table 3). In otherwise healthy adults, administration of amantadine or rimantadine within 48 hours of symptom onset results in a decrease in uncomplicated influenza illness. Similarly, a meta-analysis of randomized controlled trials has demonstrated that neuraminidase inhibitors (zanamivir or oseltamivir) when administered within 48 hours of symptom onset reduce the median duration of symptoms by up to 1 day and reduce the odds for complications requiring antibiotics by 29% to 43% in children and healthy adults. All anti-influenza agents lose effectiveness if treatment is delayed for more than 48 hours after symptom onset. On the basis of these data, anti-influenza agents have been recommended for the following types of patients with influenza-like symptoms, many of whom are at high-risk for complications due to influenza:

- Immunosuppressed patients (vaccinated or unvaccinated)
- Elderly nursing home patients (vaccinated or unvaccinated)
- Other high-risk patients (e.g., chronic cardiopulmonary disease, diabetes mellitus, chronic renal or liver disease, the elderly) who are unvaccinated
- Unvaccinated patients with suspected influenza-associated pneumonia
- Unvaccinated household contacts of immunosuppressed patients
- High-risk patients who have received an influenza vaccine that does not match with the circulating virus strain

There have been no studies that directly compare the effectiveness of anti-influenza agents. Important considerations are that rimantadine has significantly less central nervous system (CNS) toxicity than amantadine in elderly nursing home residents (1.9% versus 18.6% [$P < 0.01$] in a retrospective analysis), and that amantadine and rimantadine are active only against influenza A, and not B, while the neuraminidase inhibitors are active against both types of influenza. However, this advantage is small unless influenza B is known to be the predominant influenza strain in the community. On average, influenza A is responsible for more than 80% of all influenza-related deaths annually. Furthermore, amantadine and rimantadine are less expensive than the neuraminidase inhibitors.

Presently, two influenza vaccines are approved for use in the United States. The first vaccine is a trivalent inactivated vaccine (Fluzone), which is administered intramuscularly. The second is a trivalent live-attenuated, cold-adapted vaccine (FluMist), which is administered intranasally. A meta-analysis of cohort studies shows that the inactivated influenza vaccine reduces risk of mortality by 32%, risk of hospitalization by 50%, and risk of pneumonia by 47% in elderly persons. A randomized, double-blind, controlled trial shows that inactivated influenza vaccine when administered to healthy working adults results in 25% fewer respiratory illnesses, 43% fewer days of sick leave, and 44% fewer visits to the physician's office for respiratory complaints as compared with those receiving placebo. Furthermore, randomized clinical trials show that administering the inactivated influenza vaccine to health care workers in nursing homes reduces the mortality of the nursing home residents. The Advisory Committee on Immunization

TABLE 3 Anti-Influenza Agents

Agent	Treatment Dose (Adult)	Prophylactic Dose (Adult)
Amantadine (Symmetrel)	200 mg/qd PO (persons age ≥65: 100 mg/qd PO)	200 mg/qd PO (persons age ≥ 65: 100 mg/qd PO)
Rimantadine (Flumadine)	100 mg PO bid (persons with hepatic failure, renal failure [CrCl <10 mL/min], or who are elderly nursing home patients: 100 mg/qd PO)	100 mg PO bid (persons with hepatic failure, renal failure [CrCl <10 mL/min], or who are elderly nursing home patients: 100 mg/qd PO)
Zanamivir (Relenza)	2 inhalations (5 mg per inhalation) bid 12 h apart for 5 d	No Food and Drug Administration (FDA) indication
Oseltamivir (Tamiflu)	75 mg bid for 5 d	75 mg/qd for at least 7 d

Practices recommends annual vaccination with the inactivated influenza vaccine for high-risk patients (see Table 2), persons 50 to 64 years of age (as these patients have an elevated prevalence of chronic medical conditions), and persons who live with or care for elderly or debilitated persons (e.g., health care workers). The live-attenuated, cold-adapted vaccine is indicated for use only in healthy persons ages 5 to 49. Randomized controlled trials show that the live-attenuated, cold-adapted vaccine is protective in healthy young children as well as in healthy adults.

Respiratory Syncytial Virus

Like influenza virus, respiratory syncytial virus (RSV) infection occurs primarily in the winter months (December 8 to March 31) and is associated with significant morbidity and mortality. In a U.S. national surveillance study of the years 1976 to 1999, RSV was the most common viral cause of death in children ages 5 and younger, especially in those less than 1 year of age. Rates of death due to RSV were even higher in persons 65 years of age and older (6.6 deaths per 100,000 persons in persons 65 and older versus 5.4 deaths per 100,000 in children younger than 1 year). In patients with chronic lung disease, RSV accounts for 33% of acute respiratory hospitalizations in children and 9% of hospitalizations in adults. RSV is also responsible for 9% of deaths in those who are 65 years of age or older with chronic lung disease. A retrospective cohort study of nursing home residents shows that RSV results in 15 hospitalizations and 17 deaths per 1,000 persons.

RSV typically causes bronchiolitis, but it also causes 50% of pneumonias in infants and 4.4% of pneumonias in adults. RSV is second only to influenza as the most common viral cause of CAP in adults. Serious RSV-associated pneumonia occurs in premature infants (birth at gestational age younger than 36 weeks) and children with chronic lung disease (e.g., bronchopulmonary dysplasia, cystic fibrosis). RSV also causes serious pneumonia in the elderly and immunosuppressed patients and is a major cause of morbidity and mortality in patients receiving allogeneic bone marrow transplants.

The seasonal prevalence of RSV overlaps that of influenza. However, RSV is usually associated with a less abrupt onset of illness, more prolonged upper respiratory tract signs and symptoms, and a high incidence of wheezing (seen in 50% to 5% of patients with RSV pneumonia). The diagnosis of RSV can be made by detecting RSV antigens using either immunofluorescence or enzyme immunoassay, or through viral culture. Sterile specimens may be obtained from a nasal washing. The enzyme immunoassay has a rapid turn-around time (15 to 30 minutes) and is commonly used.

A systematic review of randomized clinical trials demonstrates that the majority of studies involving ribavirin (Virazole), corticosteroids, and bronchodilators for patients with RSV infection do not conclusively show improvement in outcomes with these agents. Two (40%) of 5 randomized clinical trials show benefit with ribavirin, while 3 (60%) show no benefit. The American Academy of Pediatrics recommends that early use of ribavirin should be reserved for treatment in high-risk infants and immunocompromised patients. Three (19%) of 16 randomized clinical trials show benefit with corticosteroids, while 13 (81%) show no benefit. Twelve (48%) of 25 randomized clinical trials show improvement with bronchodilators in RSV infection, while 13 (52%) show no benefit. Some experts recommend that if bronchodilators are to be used and no benefit is seen after 1 to 2 treatments, then bronchodilators should be discontinued. On the other hand, 8 (80%) of 10 randomized clinical trials show that inhaled racemic epinephrine improves outcomes for patients with RSV infection.

Treatment of RSV pneumonia with immunoglobulin and RSV antibody remains unestablished. However, use of these agents as prophylaxis for RSV in patients at greatest risk for severe RSV disease has been previously studied. A meta-analysis of randomized clinical trials shows that prophylaxis with RSV-immunoglobulin (RespiGam) or monoclonal antibody (Xolair) decreases the incidence of RSV hospitalizations and admissions to the intensive care unit, but does not prevent mechanical ventilation or improve mortality for children with prematurity, bronchopulmonary dysplasia, or congenital heart disease.

Parainfluenza Viruses

Parainfluenza viruses, especially serotypes 1, 2, and 3, rank second only to RSV as the most common cause of viral lower respiratory tract infections in young children. Parainfluenza virus serotypes 1 and 2 are associated with croup, while serotype 3 is associated with pneumonia and bronchiolitis. It has been estimated that parainfluenza infection in children results in 250,000 visits to the emergency department and 70,000 hospitalizations annually. Parainfluenza also causes serious infection in the elderly and in immunosuppressed adults.

In the immunocompromised host, certain clinical features may help distinguish infection due to parainfluenza or RSV from other opportunistic pathogens. These features include the presence of upper respiratory tract signs, sinusitis, and wheezing. Parainfluenza viruses may be detected using viral cell culture, antigen detection using immunofluorescence or ELISA, amplification of RNA using PCR, or serology.

Treatment of parainfluenza is primarily supportive. Uncontrolled studies do not show a benefit to administering ribavirin (Virazole) to bone marrow transplant patients with parainfluenza virus pneumonia.

Adenovirus

Adenovirus causes upper and lower respiratory tract infections, gastrointestinal illness, conjunctivitis, cystitis, and rash. Infection with adenovirus is common in children, immunosuppressed patients, and young adult military recruits. Morbidity and mortality are particularly high in lung transplant patients. Adenovirus serotypes 4 and 7 are associated with outbreaks of pneumonia in young military recruits, and deaths have been reported in this group of young, previously healthy persons.

Adenovirus may be detected using viral cell culture, antigen detection using immunofluorescence or ELISA, amplification of RNA using PCR, or serology. Serotyping may be performed using hemagglutination-inhibition or neutralization with type-specific antisera. Since there is no specific antiviral treatment for adenovirus, treatment for adenovirus infections is generally supportive. Vaccines for adenovirus serotypes 4 and 7 used to be provided to military recruits to prevent adenovirus respiratory illness. However, in 1996 the manufacturer ceased production of the vaccine.

Hantavirus

Hantavirus pulmonary syndrome (HPS) is caused by a virus of the genus *Bunyaviridae* called the Sin Nombre virus (SNV) and is associated with a case fatality rate as high as 76%. SNV is transmitted by the urine, feces, and saliva of rodents. While originally localized to the southwestern United States, SNV has also been identified in humans and rodents in all regions of the United States as well as in Canada, Central America, South America, and Europe. HPS infection initially presents as a brief prodromal influenza-like illness that rapidly progresses to increased permeability (noncardiac) pulmonary edema and low-cardiac output shock. The most common prodromal symptoms and signs are listed in Table 4.

TABLE 4 Symptoms and Signs of Hantavirus Pulmonary Syndrome

Symptoms	Frequency (%)
Fever	100
Myalgia	100
Headache	71
Cough	71
Nausea or vomiting	71
Signs	
Tachypnea (RR ≧ 20)	100
Tachycardia (HR ≧ 100)	94
Temperature ≧ 38.1°C (100.6°F)	75

Adapted from: Duchin JS, Koster FT, Peters CJ, et al: Hantavirus pulmonary syndrome: a clinical description of 17 patients with a newly recognized disease. The Hantavirus Study Group. N Engl J Med, 1994; 330(14):949-955.

Significant hematologic laboratory findings include thrombocytopenia, leukocytosis with a left shift and presence of immunoblasts, and elevated hematocrit. A retrospective study of 17 patients with HPS by Duchin and colleagues has shown that elevations in hematocrit, lactate dehydrogenase, partial thromboplastin time (PTT), or white blood cell count suggest the diagnosis of SNV pneumonia in at-risk patients and that the presence of increasing numbers of these factors correlates with disease severity.

In the presence of a clinical picture consistent with HPS, a definitive diagnosis of HPS may be confirmed with positive serology, antigen detection using immunohistochemistry, or amplification of RNA using PCR for SNV. Treatment of HPS is primarily supportive and often consists of volume resuscitation with crystalloids or colloids, administration of inotropic agents such as dobutamine (Dobutrex) or dopamine (Intropin), mechanical ventilation, and possibly extracorporeal membrane oxygenation (ECMO). While a case report has shown that ribavirin may help in the treatment of HPS, an open label study has shown that ribavirin (Virazole)[1] does not appear to improve survival in patients with HPS. Randomized controlled trial data are needed to establish whether ribavirin offers any benefit to patients with HPS.

Severe Acute Respiratory Syndrome

Severe acute respiratory syndrome (SARS) is caused by a highly virulent strain of coronavirus and is associated with significant morbidity and

[1]Not FDA approved for this indication.

mortality in immunocompetent persons. The case definition as defined by the Centers for Disease Control and Prevention (CDC) consists of epidemiologic evidence of exposure to SARS along with clinical symptoms of moderate to severe respiratory illness (see *http://www.cdc.gov/ncidod/sars/casedefinition.htm*). Epidemiological evidence consists of travel or residence within 10 days in a region in which community transmission of SARS has been reported or exposure to a person who has or is suspected to have SARS. A current listing of regions where community transmission of SARS has been reported is available on the CDC (*http://www.cdc.gov/ncidod/sars/index.htm*) and World Health Organization (*http://www.who.int/csr/sars/en/*) Web sites. Patients with moderate-to-severe SARS demonstrate a temperature greater than 100.4°F (38°C) and one or more findings of respiratory illness (e.g., cough, shortness of breath, difficulty breathing, or hypoxia). Severe disease is defined by the presence of either pneumonia on chest radiograph or respiratory distress syndrome. Laboratory evidence can either confirm or refute a diagnosis of SARS in patients who fulfill epidemiologic and clinical criteria for SARS. Presence of antibody to SARS-associated coronavirus in the serum, detection of SARS-associated coronavirus RNA via PCR, or isolation of the SARS virus confirms a SARS diagnosis. Absence of antibody to SARS-associated coronavirus for more than 28 days after symptom onset excludes the diagnosis of SARS.

The CDC currently recommends that patients with SARS should receive empiric coverage for community-acquired pneumonia pathogens. Furthermore, until further data are available regarding the transmissibility of SARS, strict respiratory and contact precautions, including eye protection, should be instituted. The benefits of antivirals, ribavirin (Virazole)[1], and corticosteroids have not yet been well established.

Other Viral Pneumonias

Pneumonias caused by viruses such as cytomegalovirus (CMV), varicella zoster virus, and others may occur in patients who are immunocompromised. These include patients with AIDS, bone marrow transplantation, and those receiving cytotoxic chemotherapy or immunosuppressive drugs. The diagnosis of CMV pneumonia often requires the presence of intranuclear inclusion bodies on the histopathology of a bronchial specimen. Other viral pneumonias may be diagnosed with viral cultures or by identifying the virus through direct (e.g., PCR) or indirect (e.g., serology) diagnostic techniques. When appropriate, antiviral treatment is directed at the specific virus.

[1]Not FDA approved for this indication.

LEGIONELLOSIS (LEGIONNAIRES' DISEASE)

METHOD OF

Burke A. Cunha, MD

Legionnaires' disease presents as a community-acquired pneumonia (CAP) and rarely as episodic outbreaks of nosocomial pneumonias. Legionnaires' disease is a nonzoonotic, atypical pneumonia. Atypical pneumonias are systemic infectious diseases with characteristic extrapulmonary findings. Typical CAP pathogens (e.g., *Streptococcus pneumoniae*, *Haemophilus influenzae*, and *Moraxella catarrhalis*) have findings that are confined to the lungs. What distinguishes atypical pathogens (e.g., *Legionella*, *Mycoplasma pneumoniae*, *Chlamydia pneumoniae*, tularemia, psittacosis, and Q fever) from their typical counterparts is the presence or absence of extrapulmonary features, which is the best way clinically to distinguish typical from atypical CAPs.

Diagnostic Considerations

ZOONOTIC ATYPICAL COMMUNITY-ACQUIRED PNEUMONIA

Clinicians confronted with CAP should determine if extrapulmonary findings are present. If the patient has CAP plus extrapulmonary findings, then the patient has an atypical pneumonia. After it has been determined that the patient has an atypical pneumonia, the clinician's next task it to differentiate zoonotic atypical pneumonias (Q fever, psittacosis, and tularemia) from the nonzoonotic atypical pneumonias (Legionnaires' disease, *M. pneumoniae*, *C. pneumoniae*). The appropriate epidemiologic contact questions for each zoonotic atypical pathogen will rule in or exclude from diagnostic consideration the zoonotic atypical CAPs. If there has been no recent intimate contact with well or sick psittacine birds or parrots, then the psittacosis is effectively eliminated from further diagnostic consideration. If the patient has been bitten by a deer fly, or has recently been skinning or handling the meat of freshly killed rabbits or deer, then tularemia is a possible diagnostic consideration especially in the presence of a bluish ulcer on the extremity at the point of contact. If the patient lacks the appropriate contact history for tularemia, then tularemia may be eliminated from the list of diagnostic possibilities. Close contact with a parturient cat or sheep is the appropriate history for epidemiological acquisition of Q fever pneumonia. If there has been no such contact, the

TABLE 1 Extrapulmonary Manifestations of Legionnaires' Disease

Common	Uncommon
Neurologic	
Confusion Headache	Insomnia Disorientation Lethargy
Cardiac	
Relative bradycardia	Endocarditis
Gastrointestinal	
Loose stools/diarrhea	Nausea Vomiting Abdominal pain
Renal	
Hematuria	Renal failure

Table reproduced with permission from Cunha BA: Clinical features of legionnaires' disease. Semin Respir Infect 13:116-127, 1998.

likelihood of Q fever is very low. Because all of the zoonotic atypical pneumonias require the appropriate vector for transmission, a negative contact history with the vectors mentioned above effectively eliminates these pathogens from further diagnostic consideration.

NONZOONOTIC ATYPICAL CAPS

Using this approach, the clinician has limited diagnostic possibilities to nonzoonotic atypical CAPs. Because each atypical pathogen has its own characteristic pattern of organ involvement, it is possible to make a presumptive clinical diagnosis. Using this approach, legionnaires' disease may be readily differentiated from *M. pneumoniae* and *C. pneumoniae* (Table 1). The extrapulmonary involvement with legionnaires' disease typically involves the central nervous system (CNS), heart, gastrointestinal (GI) tract, liver, and kidneys. CNS manifestations include mental confusion, headache, change in mental status, lethargy, or stupor. Cardiac involvement is manifested by relative bradycardia. Hepatic involvement is limited to chemical hepatitis, manifested as mild elevations of the serum transaminases. GI involvement typically takes the form of loose stools or diarrhea. Some patients develop abdominal pain, which may be so severe as to mimic a surgical abdomen. Abdominal pain may be generalized or localized. Renal involvement is characterized by microscopic hematuria. Other nonspecific laboratory findings that suggest legionnaires' disease include early/transient mild hypophosphatemia. Hyponatremia is common in legionnaires' disease, but is the least specific abnormality.

THE CLINICAL APPROACH WITH LEGIONNAIRES' DISEASE

While all patients with legionnaires' disease do not have all of these findings, each patient has sufficient extrapulmonary findings to provide a syndromic clinical presumptive diagnosis. Importantly, diagnostic findings do not have equal diagnostic significance. Mental status changes, particularly encephalopathy, are important in patients with CAP; they suggest legionnaires' disease because CNS involvement with other atypical pathogens is rare. Encephalopathy and relative bradycardia in patients not taking β-blockers and in a patient with CAP suggest the possibility of legionnaires' disease if psittacosis and Q fever have been eliminated epidemiologically. Abdominal pain mimicking a surgical abdomen is not a feature of any other CAP and immediately suggests the possibility of legionnaires' disease. None of these findings taken alone are specific, but the pattern of extrapulmonary findings comprise a syndrome complex. It is the association of multiple characteristic nonspecific extrapulmonary findings that gives diagnostic specificity to the diagnostic approach. Taking into account the diagnostic weights of the various symptoms, signs, and laboratory abnormalities of legionnaires' disease, a weighted diagnostic point system has been developed. This point system takes into account the variability of clinical presentations permitting an accurate diagnosis (Table 2). The findings on a chest radiograph of legionnaires' disease are nonspecific.

It is not difficult to differentiate legionnaires' disease from *M. pneumoniae* pneumonia because of the characteristic patterns of extrapulmonary organ involvement. *M. pneumoniae* pneumonia does not present with headache or encephalopathy except in rare cases of mycoplasmal meningoencephalitis. Relative bradycardia occurs regularly in legionnaires' disease and is not a feature of *M. pneumonia* pneumonia. Although both *Legionella* and *M. pneumonia* often present with loose stools or diarrhea, only legionnaires' disease is associated with sharp abdominal pain. Hepatic and renal involvement are not features of *M. pneumoniae* CAP.

Antimicrobial *Legionella* Therapy

MACROLIDES

Erythromycin and tetracycline[1] were the initial agents used to treat legionnaires' disease. Trimethoprim-sulfamethoxazole (TMP-SMX) (Bactrim)[1] was effective against some *Legionella* species such as *L. micdadei*. Rifampin (Rifadin)[1] also had a high degree of anti-*Legionella* activity in vivo.

Because erythromycin is only modestly active against *Legionella* in vitro, rifampin is commonly added to erythromycin to treat severe cases of legionnaires' disease. Treatment of legionnaires' disease is generally successful but numerous treatment failures have been reported with erythromycin. Erythromycin is associated with exacerbating liver dysfunction or

[1]Not FDA approved for this indication.

TABLE 2 Community-Acquired Pneumonia

	Qualifying Conditions	Point Score*
Clinical Findings†		
Headache	Acute onset	+1
Mental confusion/encephalopathic	Acute onset	+5
Ear pain	Acute onset	−3
Sore throat	Acute onset	−3
Hoarseness	Acute onset	−3
Hemoptysis	Mild-to-moderate	−1
Chest pain	Pleuritic	−2
Loose stools/diarrhea	Not due to erythromycin/diarrheal causing drugs	−3
Abdominal pain	With or without diarrhea	+5
Relative bradycardia	Adults, temperature ≥ 38.9°C (102°F) if no β-blockers, pacemaker, or arrhythmias	+5
Lack of response to β-lactam therapy	After 72 hours	+5
Laboratory Findings†		
↓ Na	Otherwise unexplained	+1
↓ PO_4	Excluding other causes of hypophosphatemia	+5
↑ SGOT/SGPT	Otherwise unexplained	+4
↑Total bilirubin	Otherwise unexplained	+2
↑CPK/aldolase	Otherwise unexplained	+4
↑CRP (>30)	Otherwise unexplained	+4
↑ Cold agglutinin titer ≥1:64	Otherwise unexplained	+4
↑ Creatinine	Otherwise unexplained	+1
Microscopic hematuria	Otherwise unexplained	+2

*Diagnostic Point System: Legionellosis highly probable = ≥10; legionellosis probable = 5-10; legionellosis unlikely = ≤5.
†Acute and associated with the community-acquired pneumonia.
Abbreviations: CKP = creatine phosphokinase; CRP = C-reactive protein; SGOT = serum glutamic-oxaloacetic transaminase; SGPT = serum glutamic-pyruvic transaminase.
Table reproduced with permission from Cunha BA: Clinical features of legionnaires' disease. Semin Respir Infect 13:116-127, 1998.

may worsen or cause diarrhea in the patient with legionnaires' disease. Phlebitis is a common problem with intravenous erythromycin. Erythromycin also may cause cardiac abnormalities, (e.g., ↑QTc interval [torsades de pointes]) and has high potential for drug interactions with other medications.

Newer macrolides (e.g., clarithromycin [Biaxin] [1], azithromycin [Zithromax][1]) have a high degree of anti-*Legionella* activity. Similarly, ketolides (e.g., telithromycin [Ketek]*) also have anti-*Legionella* activity. Of the tetracyclines and macrolides available, doxycycline (Vibramycin)[1] and azithromycin are the two most frequently used antimicrobials in the treatment of legionnaires' disease.

DOXCYCLINE

If doxycycline (Vibramycin)[1] is used, the clinician should remember that it has a very long half-life, $t_{1/2}$ 22 hours, and it is highly lipid soluble. These pharmacokinetic characteristics make it mandatory that doxycycline be administered with a loading dose regimen. The usual dose of doxycycline, 100 mg (IV/PO) every 12 hours, is not adequate for patients that are moderately ill with legionnaires' disease. If one uses doxycycline in this fashion, it will be 4 to 5 days before steady state kinetics is achieved and a therapeutic response is manifest. Some physicians reporting disappointing therapeutic response to doxycycline have used doxycycline in the usual manner without a loading dose regimen. It is not that doxycycline has not been effective after 4 to 5 days, it is that the patient has not received adequate therapy. With a loading regimen of 200 mg (IV/PO) every 12 hours[3], a therapeutic response will be noted within 72 hours in the patient with legionnaires' disease. After the loading regimen, the patient is switched to oral doxycycline; a dose of 100 mg (PO) every 12 hours is sufficient to complete the course of therapy. If doxycycline is used, always use the loading regimen described to treat legionnaires' disease, which results in very rapid and high serum and lung levels. It is not necessary to add rifampin to doxycycline.

QUINOLONES

Fluoroquinolones are highly active against all strains of *Legionella*. Ciprofloxacin (Cipro) [1] has anti-*Legionella* activity and is used successfully to treat legionnaires' disease. The newer respiratory quinolones, such as levofloxacin (Levaquin), gatifloxacin (Tequin), and moxifloxacin (Avelox) [1], also

[1]Not FDA approved for this indication.
*Investigational drug in the United States.

[1]Not FDA approved for this indication.
[3]Exceeds dosage recommended by the manufacturer.

have a high intrinsic activity against *Legionella*. Because of the high anti-*Legionella* activity of the respiratory fluoroquinolones, the addition of rifampin is not necessary. In normal and compromised hosts with legionnaires' disease, for both moderately and severely ill patients, a respiratory quinolone offers optimal anti-*Legionella* activity.

In compromised hosts with legionnaires' disease, the same therapy is used as for normal hosts. Legionnaires' disease in HIV patients also is optimally treated with a respiratory quinolone; alternately, doxycycline or a macrolide may be used if the patient is intolerant of quinolones. In organ transplants, optimal therapy is a respiratory quinolone plus azithromycin (Zithromax)[1]. There is synergy between respiratory quinolones and azithromycin that provides the highest degree of anti-*Legionella* activity needed in the transplant patient. Oral therapy can be completed with either one of these antibiotics.

DURATION OF THERAPY

The duration of therapy (IV/PO) for *Legionella* is 2 to 4 weeks. Two weeks of therapy may be associated with relapse.

[1]Not FDA approved for this indication.

PULMONARY EMBOLISM

METHOD OF

Victor F. Tapson, MD

Venous thromboembolism (VTE) represents the spectrum of deep venous thrombosis (DVT) and the potentially fatal entity of pulmonary embolism (PE) with the latter responsible for as many as 60,000 to 200,000 deaths in the United States every year. Most commonly, PE results from DVT that develops in the legs, but upper extremity thrombosis is common, particularly in patients with central venous catheters, and these clots may embolize also. The risk of PE is higher in patients with proximal DVT than in patients with only calf-vein thrombosis. The diagnosis should be suspected in patients presenting with dyspnea, chest pain (particularly, but not only, pleuritic), hemoptysis, and syncope; other nonspecific symptoms and signs may be present as well, and the diagnosis may be particularly elusive in patients with underlying cardiopulmonary disease. Leg pain, tenderness, swelling, and Homans' sign may suggest the diagnosis of DVT (with or without PE) but these findings are neither sensitive nor specific. The presence of risk factors for DVT, and thus PE, such as prior VTE, cancer, older age, obesity, surgery, trauma, and acute medical illness should raise the suspicion for DVT and PE if a consistent clinical scenario is present. Such risk factors should also prompt the use of prophylactic measures. Hospitalized patients are frequently at risk because such individuals have underlying disease that may increase the risk for VTE, and because they are immobilized to varying degrees, rendering them susceptible.

The Diagnostic Approach to Acute Pulmonary Embolism

The chest radiograph and electrocardiogram (ECG) may offer clues to alternative diagnoses, but they are nonspecific for PE. For suspected PE, ventilation-perfusion scanning followed by pulmonary arteriography has been the gold-standard approach for decades. Spiral (helical) computed tomography (CT) scanning is used increasingly, and in many hospitals is the procedure of choice for suspected PE. When PE is suspected, leg studies may be useful if a scan cannot be easily obtained or interpreted. There should be a low threshold for proceeding with a diagnostic evaluation when PE is suspected. In severely ill patients who may be candidates for aggressive treatment, such as thrombolytic therapy or open embolectomy, bedside echocardiographic evaluation for massive central emboli and evaluation of right ventricular function may hasten therapeutic interventions. For the diagnosis of suspected DVT, ultrasound is the appropriate initial test with magnetic resonance imaging (MRI), or a venography is sometimes necessary. D-dimer testing is most useful when there is a relatively low suspicion for DVT or PE. The enzyme-linked immunoabsorbent assay (ELISA)-based assays are the most sensitive. A negative test in the latter setting may eliminate the need for further evaluation. If clinical suspicion is higher, objective radiographic imaging is crucial.

Initial Therapy for Acute Pulmonary Embolism

When there is a high clinical suspicion for acute DVT or PE, initiation of therapy should be considered even before confirmation of the diagnosis, as long as the risk of anticoagulation appears to be minimal. Confirmatory diagnostic testing should be arranged as soon as possible if anticoagulation is to be continued. The issue of bedrest is frequently raised in patients with acute DVT and/or PE. At present, there is no convincing data suggesting that bedrest is necessary, although in patients with extensive, symptomatic DVT, bedrest is advisable until the initial inflammation and swelling begin to subside.

Options for initial treatment include anticoagulation with heparin or low-molecular weight heparin (LMWH), thrombolytic therapy, and inferior vena cava filter (IVCF) placement. The approaches to anticoagulation for DVT and for PE are essentially the same. Massive PE may occasionally be treated with surgical embolectomy. Each therapeutic approach has specific indications as well as advantages and disadvantages.

UNFRACTIONATED HEPARIN

By accelerating the action of antithrombin III, heparin and LMWH exert a prompt antithrombotic effect that prevents thrombus extension. They do not directly dissolve the thrombus, but allow the fibrinolytic system to proceed unopposed and more readily reduce the size of the thromboembolic burden. While thrombus growth can be prevented, early recurrence may sometimes develop even when anticoagulation is therapeutic. Specific settings may require alternative therapies as when direct thrombin inhibitors are used for heparin-induced thrombocytopenia with or without proven thrombosis.

When continuous intravenous unfractionated heparin (UFH) is initiated, the activated partial thromboplastin time (aPTT) must be followed at 6-hour intervals until it is consistently in the therapeutic range of 1.5 to 2.0 times the control value. This range corresponds to a heparin level of 0.2 to 0.4 μ/mL as measured by protamine sulfate titration. Because achieving a therapeutic aPTT within 24 hours after PE reduces the recurrence rate, it is clear that the traditional heparin regimen, consisting of a 5000 unit bolus at 1000 units/hour, is often inadequate. Heparin should be administered in one of several ways. An intravenous bolus of 5000 units followed by a maintenance dose of 30,000 to 40,000 units per 24 hours by continuous infusion is one approach. The lower dose is administered if the patient is considered at high risk for bleeding. This aggressive approach decreases the risk of subtherapeutic anticoagulation. An alternative regimen, consisting of a bolus of 80 U/kg followed by 18 U/kg per hour is recommended by the American College of Chest Physicians in their 2001 Consensus Conference on Antithrombotic Therapy. Subsequent adjusting of heparin should also be weight-based.

Warfarin (Coumadin) is generally initiated the same day as parenteral anticoagulation unless the risk of bleeding suggests that the longer acting oral anticoagulant should be temporarily withheld. It is possible that early initiation of warfarin, *without* heparin or LMWH may intensify hypercoagulability and increase the clot burden caused by the short half-life of anticoagulation factors that are inhibited by warfarin. Factor VII is the primary clotting factor affecting the prothrombin time; it has a half-life of approximately 6 hours. Definitive anticoagulation requires the depletion of factor II (thrombin), which takes approximately 5 days. Thus, at least 5 days of intravenous heparin or subcutaneous LMWH is recommended. Heparin is maintained at a therapeutic level until two consecutive therapeutic international normalized ratio (INR) values of 2.0 to 3.0 have been documented at least 24 hours apart. The first several doses of warfarin should be 5 or 10 mg, depending on the size of the patient, and it is generally administered in the evening. Subsequent dosing is based upon the INR value.

LOW-MOLECULAR-WEIGHT HEPARIN

The LMWH preparations have tremendous advantages compared with unfractionated heparin and have had a substantial impact upon the treatment of thromboembolic disease. Among the differences between these two substances is the greater bioavailability of the LMWHs and more predictable dosing. They can be subcutaneously administered once or twice per day even at therapeutic doses and do not require monitoring in most settings. Intravenous LMWH is never required for therapy of DVT or PE. Subcutaneous LMWH is replacing standard heparin in many settings. Numerous clinical trials strongly suggest the efficacy and safety of LMWH for treatment of established acute DVT and PE. These trials, which used recurrent symptomatic VTE and bleeding as outcome measures, indicate that LMWH preparations are at least as effective and as safe as unfractionated heparin. At least one meta-analysis suggests that LMWH preparations result in less bleeding and lower mortality than unfractionated heparin for the treatment of acute VTE. The lower mortality is not entirely explained by a reduction in fatal PE. Presently, the two LMWH preparations that are FDA-approved for treatment of DVT with or without PE are enoxaparin (Lovenox) and tinzaparin (Innohep). A comparison of LMWH with standard, unfractionated heparin is provided in Table 1.

Unlike unfractionated heparin, LMWHs do not require monitoring in most settings. This is supported by extensive experience from large clinical trials. However, monitoring appears appropriate in a few clinical settings such as in morbidly obese patients (>150 kg [331 lb]), very small patients (<40 kg [88 lb]), pregnant patients, and those with renal insufficiency. Because these drugs are renally metabolized, monitoring is particularly important when the creatinine clearance is less than 30 mL/minute. A patient might be expected to require a dose of two thirds of the usual dose when the creatinine clearance is less than 30 mL/minute. With more severe renal insufficiency, standard heparin

TABLE 1 Comparison of LMWH with Unfractionated Heparin

Characteristic	UFH*	LMWH
Mean molecular weight	12,000-15,000	4,000-6,000
Protein binding	Substantial	Minimal
Bioavailability	Substantial	Much lower/less predictable
Heparin-induced thrombocytopenia	Incidence 3%-4%	Much less common†
Anti-Xa activity	Substantial	Substantial
Anti-IIa activity	Substantial	Minimal
Monitoring	aPTT every 6 h	None in most settings†
Outpatient therapy	Difficult	Simplified

*LMWH should not be used for treatment of established heparin-induced thrombocytopenia (HIT).

†In certain circumstances, the anti-Xa level is appropriate to monitor. This should be considered when weight ≥150 kg or ≤40 kg, creatinine clearance <30 mL/min, and in pregnant patients.

Abbreviations: aPTT = activated partial thromboplastin time; LMWH = low-molecular-weight heparin; UFH = unfractionated heparin.

TABLE 2 Initiation of LMWH for Therapy of Acute Deep Venous Thrombosis and Pulmonary Embolism

- Begin LMWH by subcutaneous administration.*
- Determine whether monitoring is needed (extremes of weight, renal insufficiency, pregnancy).
- Administer warfarin from day 1; initial dose 5-10 mg, adjusted according to INR.
- Check platelet count between days 3 and 5.
- Stop LMWH after ≥5 days of combined therapy and when INR is ≥2.0 for 2 consecutive days.
- Anticoagulate with warfarin for ≥3 months (goal, INR = 2.0-3.0).

*Enoxaparin (Lovenox) and tinzaparin (Innohep) are the two LMWHs that are FDA-approved for treatment of VTE. While LMWH preparations are sometimes used for patients presenting with PE in the United States, and while clinical trials support this use, the FDA approval reads "established DVT with or without PE."

Abbreviations: INR = international normalized ratio; LMWH = low-molecular-weight heparin.

should be considered. The LMWHs have a more profound effect with regard to inhibiting clotting factor Xa relative to thrombin, and when patients on these drugs are monitored, it is the anti-Xa level (sometimes referred to as an LMWH level) that should be checked and not the aPTT. The steps for anticoagulating with LMWH are outlined in Table 2.

OTHER AGENTS FOR INITIAL THERAPY

A very-low-molecular-weight (pentasaccharide) heparin (fondaparinux [Arixtra][1]) has proven effective for the treatment of both DVT and PE in two separate large, randomized trials. Like the LMWHs, fondaparinux is administered subcutaneously. It is a pure factor Xa inhibitor. However, at present this agent does not have the FDA-approved indication for treatment of acute DVT or PE. Another agent, an oral direct thrombin inhibitor called ximelagatran (Exanta)*, has proven effective for the treatment of acute DVT and PE, both for long-term management instead of warfarin, and as initial therapy. It has not yet been evaluated for FDA approval in the United States.

OUTPATIENT THERAPY OF ACUTE DEEP VENOUS THROMBOSIS AND PULMONARY EMBOLISM

Patients with acute DVT can be treated as outpatients if they meet certain criteria. While outpatient treatment of PE has been studied and is feasible, it is not commonly practiced in the United States. A Canadian clinical trial evaluated patients with proven PE for possible outpatient treatment. Criteria for admission included hemodynamic instability, hypoxemia requiring oxygen therapy, admission for another medical reason, severe pain requiring parenteral analgesia, or high risk of major bleeding. Certainly, in the setting of either DVT or PE when inpatient therapy is initiated, therapy may be completed in the outpatient setting in appropriate, stable individuals. It is clear that at least 30% to 40% of patients with acute, proximal DVT, have *silent* PE. Many patients treated for DVT also have asymptomatic PE, unknown to the treating clinician. The criteria for outpatient therapy for acute DVT are given in Table 3.

PREGNANCY AND ACUTE VTE: LOW-MOLECULAR-WEIGHT HEPARIN

Increasing experience suggests that LMWHs are safe and effective for VTE in pregnancy. The advantages of

[1]Not FDA approved for this indication.

*Investigational drug in the United States.

TABLE 3 Criteria for Outpatient Therapy of Acute DVT/PE*

- DVT/PE that is stable and not massive/extensive
- Low risk of bleeding
- Education complete/compliance with injections
- Follow-up assured
- Other medical problems stable
- Reimbursement available

*Patients with symptomatic PE are generally treated as inpatients. However, the use of low-molecular-weight heparin (LMWH) as a bridge can facilitate earlier hospital discharge. The two LMWH preparations approved for treatment of acute venous thromboembolism (VTE) are approved for acute DVT with or without PE. Thus, although data supports the use of LMWH preparations for acute PE, treatment of acute PE may be considered off-label in the United States.

Abbreviations: DVT = deep venous thrombosis; PE = pulmonary embolism.

these preparations compared with UFH include the same advantages evident in the nonpregnant population. These include a longer plasma half-life coupled with substantially increased bioavailability and, thus, a more predictable dose response. Once- or twice-daily subcutaneous administration facilitates treatment. While anti-factor Xa monitoring is not generally required with LMWH use, it is appropriate in pregnancy, particularly in view of the usual progressive weight gain. Evidence indicates that LMWHs do not cross the placenta.

Long-Term Therapy for Pulmonary Embolism

The duration of therapy is the same for acute DVT and for PE. Anticoagulant therapy should be stopped when the benefit no longer clearly outweighs the risk. This assessment needs to be individualized. Patients with VTE provoked by a transient risk factor have a lower (approximately 33%) risk of recurrence than those with an unprovoked VTE or a persistent risk factor. Three months of anticoagulation is adequate treatment for VTE provoked by a transient risk factor; the subsequent risk of recurrence is approximately 3% per patient-year. Three months of anticoagulation is inadequate for an unprovoked (idiopathic) episode of VTE; the subsequent early risk of recurrence varies from 5% to 25% per patient-year. Idiopathic VTE can be somewhat difficult to define in some settings. Clearly, VTE in the complete absence of any temporary or permanent risk factor would be classified as idiopathic. Prolonged travel appears to be a risk factor for acute VTE. However, it would be unusual for an otherwise healthy young patient without VTE risk factors to develop PE, for example, after a 6-hour car ride. Such a patient might be considered for more prolonged treatment. Idiopathic VTE should be treated for at least 6 months to 1 year, with the shorter duration reserved for patients considered at higher risk of bleeding. If patients are not candidates for long-term anticoagulant therapy, it is reasonable to stop therapy for an unprovoked VTE after 6 months and to use aggressive prophylaxis at times of superimposed high risk.

INTENSITY OF WARFARIN THERAPY

While lower INR values (range of 1.5 to 2.0) have proven superior to placebo for long-term therapy, normal-intensity warfarin with a target INR of 2.5 (range of 2.0 to 3.0) is shown to result in less recurrences than low-intensity warfarin. Thus, current evidence suggests that normal-intensity warfarin is appropriate for long-term anticoagulation. It is reasonable to stop therapy for an unprovoked VTE after 6 months and to use aggressive prophylaxis at times of superimposed high risk.

Other Forms of Therapy

INFERIOR VENA CAVA FILTER PLACEMENT

Placement of an IVCF is the standard of care when a patient fails therapeutic anticoagulation or develops significant bleeding while being anticoagulated for acute VTE. If a patient is felt to have suffered a recurrent event, it is important to be certain that the anticoagulation was truly in the therapeutic range before proceeding with a filter. Temporary filters are now available that can be removed within two weeks if a bleeding complication has resolved and a patient can safely be anticoagulated. Lifetime anticoagulation, when deemed safe, is appropriate when a filter must remain in place.

THROMBOLYTIC THERAPY

Based upon the potential for serious bleeding complications, thrombolytic therapy must be used cautiously. These agents activate plasminogen to form plasmin, which then results in fibrinolysis as well as fibrinogenolysis. Because anticoagulants do not actively lyse emboli, thrombolytic agents are considered in certain settings to hasten the reduction in thromboembolic burden. Clinical studies have culminated in the approval of streptokinase (Streptase), urokinase (Abbokinase), and recombinant tissue-type plasminogen activator (tPA) (Activase) for the treatment of massive PE. The specific regimens are shown in Table 4.

For several decades, the clearly accepted scenario in which thrombolytic therapy was recommended was for patients with hemodynamic instability (hypotension). Those with severely compromised oxygenation have also been considered. Although thrombolytic therapy may result in rapid improvement of right ventricular function in patients with acute PE, it remains controversial as to whether or not patients with echocardiographic right ventricular dysfunction but without hypotension should receive this form of treatment. Several large studies suggest that such patients should be considered. There are no clear data proving that one thrombolytic agent is superior to the others, but in massive PE more rapidly infused regimens may be favored.

Coagulation assays are unnecessary during thrombolysis because the approved regimens are

TABLE 4 Thrombolytic Therapy for Acute Pulmonary Embolism: Approved Regimens

- Streptokinase (Streptase): 250,000 U IV (loading dose over 30 min); then 100,000 U/h for 24h*
- Urokinase (Abbokinase): 2000 U/lb IV (loading dose over 10 min); then 2,000 U/lb/h for 12 to 24 h
- Tissue-type plasminogen activator (Activase): 100 mg IV for 2 h

*Streptokinase administered over 24 to 72 h at this loading dose and rate has also been approved for use in patients with extensive deep venous thrombosis (DVT).

administered as fixed doses. Heparin is generally withheld until the thrombolytic infusion is completed. The aPTT is then determined and heparin is initiated without a loading dose if this value is less than twice the upper limit of normal. If the aPTT exceeds this value, the test is repeated every 4 hours until it is safe to proceed with heparin. While a number of investigators have employed standard or low-dose intrapulmonary arterial thrombolytic infusions in order to deliver a high concentration of drug in close proximity to the clot, intravenous therapy appears adequate in most cases. Thrombolytic therapy for DVT is more controversial. Local thrombolytic therapy can be considered in patients with proximal occlusive DVT associated with significant swelling and symptoms when there are no contraindications. Many vascular radiology or vascular medicine departments have established protocols for this form of therapy.

Hemorrhage is the primary adverse effect associated with thrombolytic therapy. If possible, invasive procedures should be minimized. The most devastating complication associated with thrombolytics is the development of intracranial hemorrhage, which occurs in less than 1% of patients. Retroperitoneal hemorrhage may result from a vascular puncture above the inguinal ligament and may be life-threatening. Thrombolytic therapy is contraindicated in the presence of any previous intracranial surgery or pathology, in patients having surgery in the previous 10 to 14 days, and in patients with active bleeding or recent significant bleeding.

HEMODYNAMIC MANAGEMENT OF MASSIVE PULMONARY EMBOLISM

Massive PE should always be suspected in the setting of the sudden onset of hypotension or extreme hypoxemia. The presence of electromechanical dissociation or sudden cardiac arrest should always make massive embolism a consideration. Once PE associated with hypotension and/or severe hypoxemia is suspected, supportive treatment is immediately initiated. Intravenous saline should be infused rapidly but cautiously because right ventricular function is often markedly compromised. Dopamine (Intropin) and norepinephrine (Levophed) (one or the other) are the favored choices of vasoactive therapy in massive PE and should be administered if the blood pressure is not rapidly restored. Dobutamine (Dobutrex) may offer inotropy, but hypotension is one of the potential risks. Oxygen therapy is administered, and thrombolytic therapy is considered as described above. Intubation and institution of mechanical ventilation are instituted as needed to support respiratory failure.

PULMONARY EMBOLECTOMY

A candidate for acute embolectomy should meet the following criteria:

- Massive PE (detected by ventilation-perfusion scan, angiography, or CT scan)
- Hemodynamic instability (shock) despite anticoagulation/resuscitative efforts
- Failure of thrombolytic therapy or a contraindication to its use

Operative mortality in the era of rapidly available cardiopulmonary bypass ranged from 10% to 75% in an uncontrolled, retrospective case series. Embolectomy should only be undertaken when a patient meets all three criteria and an experienced surgical team is immediately available. Catheter-directed embolectomy (fragmentation, suction, low-dose thrombolytic therapy) is sometimes performed at experienced centers.

The treatment of acute venous thromboembolism should be aggressive, with caution regarding the potential for bleeding. Therapy for PE unequivocally reduces mortality.

SARCOIDOSIS

METHOD OF

Philip E. Greenspan, MD, and

Michael C. Iannuzzi, MD

Sarcoidosis, a multisystem disorder of unknown etiology, occurs in a genetically susceptible host following exposure to an as-yet unidentified environmental agent. The diagnosis of sarcoidosis is best established in the presence of compatible clinical-radiologic findings by histologically demonstrating noncaseating epithelioid granulomas in multiple organs. Because the symptoms of sarcoidosis vary widely, delay in diagnosis is usual. Sarcoidosis frequently mimics more common organ-specific diseases, resulting in patient evaluation by multiple subspecialists who fail to consider a unifying systemic diagnosis such as sarcoidosis.

Based on more than a century of clinical experience, symptomatic organ dysfunction secondary to granuloma accumulation is managed by immunosuppression. Recently, however, specific anticytokine therapy has become possible. This article reviews the indications for treatment, as well as some of the major

TABLE 1 Indications for Treatment by Site of Involvement

Neurologic: Brain, spinal cord
Ophthalmologic: Posterior uveitis, unresolving anterior uveitis
Cardiac: Arrhythmias, heart block, cardiomyopathy
Pulmonary: Progressive decrement of pulmonary function (regardless of chest radiograph staging)
Spleen: Symptomatic splenomegaly leading to pressure symptoms or cytopenia
Liver: Cholestatic jaundice not relieved by ursodiol (Actigall)
Endocrine: Hypercalcemia/hypercalciuria
Dermatologic: Disfiguring skin lesions not responsive to topical therapy

agents currently used. In addition, treatment algorithms for specific sites affected by sarcoidosis are reviewed.

Indications for Treatment

The decision to treat sarcoidosis (Table 1) is complicated by the fact that spontaneous remission frequently occurs. Approximately two thirds of patients remit spontaneously, while only 10% to 30% progress to chronic disease. Thus, for the vast majority of patients, treatment with potent immunosuppressives could lead to greater harm than good. For asymptomatic patients, 85% of spontaneous remissions occur within the first 2 to 3 years. Failure to remit within that time portends a chronic or progressive disease course. Newly diagnosed patients should be followed every 3 months during the first 2 years to determine whether active or progressive disease is present. Even for the subgroup of patients who fail to remit, immunosuppression is indicated only for sarcoidosis that impairs organ function or results in uncontrollable symptoms.

As most patients with sarcoidosis have pulmonary findings, a descriptive system for chest radiography has been established:

- Stage 0—normal image
- Sage I—bilateral hilar lymphadenopathy
- Stage II—bilateral hilar lymphadenopathy with parenchymal changes
- Stage III—parenchymal infiltrates without bilateral hilar lymphadenopathy
- Stage IV—advanced fibrosis

While this staging system is useful for descriptive purposes, the scoring of chest radiography in sarcoidosis is of little prognostic value unless end-stage fibrotic changes are present (stage IV). Furthermore, evaluation by chest computed tomography (CT) has demonstrated that often hilar adenopathy is present in patients with a stage III radiograph and parenchymal changes present in patients with a stage II radiograph. In general, treatment decisions are not based on chest radiograph staging. Because of the risks inherent in placing a patient on an immunosuppressive regimen, indication for treatment remains progressive clinical dysfunction in any organ system.

Corticosteroids

Corticosteroids act broadly to inhibit multiple proinflammatory cytokines. As steroids are the most effective means of diminishing granulomas, they remain the first-line agent for the treatment of sarcoidosis. While steroids undoubtedly improve the manifestations of sarcoidosis, because of the large percentage of patients who spontaneously remit without any therapy, it remains unclear whether steroids actually change the natural history of the disease. For example, a recent meta-analysis found that following treatment with oral corticosteroids, chest radiograph findings may improve in radiographic stage II and stage III disease, but it is not clear whether this improvement is maintained beyond the first 2 years, during which patients would manifest a high spontaneous rate of remission with or without treatment.

While no randomized, controlled trials have demonstrated a long-term benefit for steroid use, there clearly remains a role for these agents in this disease. A British Thoracic Society study looked at patients with persistent abnormal chest radiographs in the absence of pulmonary symptoms. It determined that those randomized to 18 months of steroids had improved diffusing capacity and dyspnea scores up to 5 years after stopping therapy. This study has been criticized because asymptomatic patients were excluded from the trial—the asymptomatic are the very people in whom the benefits of steroids remain most in question.

Despite the absence of an optimum of evidence-based literature, steroids remain a cornerstone of therapy of the symptomatic patient. Progressive organ dysfunction secondary to granuloma formation (particularly in key areas such as neurologic, ophthalmologic, cardiac, pulmonary, or endocrinologic systems) merits aggressive, yet judicious, treatment with systemic corticosteroids.

The optimal dosing and duration of steroids have not been determined by randomized, controlled trials. While steroids are helpful in minimizing the damage done by sarcoidosis, their well-known side effects dictate that they be used only at the minimal dose necessary to benefit the patient. Once the need for steroids has been established, one approach is to start prednisone at 40 mg per day for about 2 to 3 weeks and then taper by 5 mg every 2 to 3 weeks, until a dose of 15 to 25 mg is reached. Patients should then be maintained at this dose for about 3 to 6 months before further tapering the medication. This affords one the opportunity to assess disease activity and progression. Higher doses (e.g., 1 mg/kg per day) of corticosteroids should be reserved for life-threatening or cardiac sarcoidosis. Patients should be followed closely for *objective* improvements in their sarcoidosis (e.g., pulmonary function tests [PFTs] for pulmonary disease, neurologic examinations, and/or magnetic resonance imaging [MRI] with gadolinium for central nervous system [CNS] manifestations). Benefit from steroid use should be expected within 3 months after starting therapy. Those who do not demonstrate clear improvement within 3 months are either inadequately dosed, and may have already had significant fibrosis and organ destruction, or are noncompliant with their medications. To assess noncompliance, long-lasting intramuscular (IM) steroids in the form of triamcinolone (Kenalog) can be given. If the questionably compliant patient remains symptomatic after IM steroid use, one can be confident of a steroid failure and should consider using other agents. If patients experience a worsening of their sarcoidosis during the taper period, reinstitute prednisone at 40 mg per day and follow the above tapering schedule. Some patients will relapse as the steroids are tapered. These patients may require a prolonged or even indefinite course of therapy. For nonresponders and for those who develop unacceptable or debilitating side effects from the steroids, adding steroid sparing agents should be considered.

Methotrexate (Rheumatrex)

Methotrexate[1] is a folic acid analogue that inhibits dihydrofolate reductase and transmethylation reactions. Its net effect is to inhibit purine metabolism and polyamine synthesis. One should begin with 10 to 12.5 mg per week with frequent monitoring for mucositis, nausea, and hematologic, liver, and pulmonary toxicity. If tolerated, the dose can be increased up to 15 mg per week. Folic acid (1 mg per day) should be given to minimize toxicity. Patients taking methotrexate should not expect any additional objective improvement in their sarcoidosis for at least 3 to 6 months. Of note, liver function tests (LFTs) are not predictive of biopsy-proven hepatotoxicity. Cirrhosis can develop in patients taking methotrexate, even in the absence of abnormal liver function tests. Methotrexate is also highly teratogenic, so birth control may need to be discussed.

Because of its potentially debilitating side effects, such as nausea, vomiting, diarrhea, and mucositis, along with its more insidious pulmonary, bone marrow, and hepatic toxicity; methotrexate necessitates the monitoring of complete blood counts, plus renal and liver function profiles (even with the limited sensitivity of LFT's). Given the complexity of its use, methotrexate should be used only for either organ-threatening disease that does not respond to other agents, or for unacceptable steroid side effects. For patients placed on methotrexate, a lack of response after 6 to 9 months indicates that the drug should be discontinued.

[1]Not FDA approved for this indication.

Azathioprine (Imuran)

Azathioprine[1] is a purine analog that is converted to 6-mercaptopurine. It is an RNA/DNA inhibitory agent that decreases T- and B-cell proliferation and cytotoxic T-cell function. As with methotrexate, patients should not expect any improvement in their disease for 3 to 6 months.

Like other immunomodulatory agents, azathioprine necessitates close monitoring for toxicity. Side effects include nausea, abdominal pain, and severe pancytopenias (especially in patients with an undiagnosed methyltransferase deficiency). The elimination of azathioprine is markedly influenced by polymorphisms in the enzymes responsible for their metabolism. Patients who are deficient in thiopurine methyltransferase (TPMT) are at an increased risk for toxicity because of the accumulation of toxic metabolites. Before initiation of therapy, in order to decrease the risk of severe and possibly preventable adverse effects, and to identify patients who might benefit from higher doses of azathioprine, TPMT genotyping (now commercially available) should be considered. Measuring the TPMT activity at baseline is not a substitute for monitoring white blood cell counts throughout therapy, because drug therapy and other conditions may still cause myelosuppression in these patients. After initiating azathioprine at 50 mg orally per day, a complete blood count should be performed within 2 weeks to rule out acute bone marrow toxicity. While monitoring the complete blood cell count, the dose of the medication can be increased to a maximum of 200 mg, generally by increasing the dose by 50 mg every 2 weeks. After the target dose is reached, blood counts should be monitored every 4 to 6 weeks. Azathioprine is associated with an increased risk of hepatitis, lymphoma, and cervical carcinoma. Patients should have their liver function carefully followed, and females should receive regular gynecologic examinations. As with methotrexate, azathioprine should be reserved only for progressive organ dysfunction not well controlled with safer agents.

Cyclophosphamide (Cytoxan)

Cyclophosphamide[1] is a nitrogen mustard alkylating agent that has broad immunosuppressive abilities. A small study of patients with intractable neurosarcoidosis demonstrated some response to this agent. It is dosed orally at 50 to 150 mg per day, or via pulse dosing at 500 to 2000 mg intravenously (IV) every 2 weeks.

[1]Not FDA approved for this indication.

Cyclophosphamide's toxicities include alopecia, gastrointestinal (GI) disturbances, pancytopenias, transitional cell carcinoma of the bladder, and hemorrhagic cystitis (which has an incidence of 5% to 10% of patients per year taking cyclophosphamide). GI tolerance of the medication can be increased by adding IV dexamethasone (Decadron)[1] and granisetron (Kytril), while the increased ingestion of water (8 to 10 glasses per day) can help prevent hemorrhagic cystitis because of enhanced clearance. Should hemorrhagic cystitis develop despite the added water intake, the medication must be discontinued. Finally, the use of cyclophosphamide is also associated with secondary malignancies, such as lymphomas and leukemias. As with the noncorticosteroid agents previously mentioned, cyclophosphamide should be restricted only to patients with organ-threatening disease (particularly neurosarcoidosis), which is demonstrably refractory to other immunomodulatory agents.

Antimalarials

The mechanism by which antimalarial drugs such as chloroquine (Aralen)[1] and hydroxychloroquine (Plaquenil)[1] ameliorate sarcoidosis remains unclear, but they likely act by inhibiting antigen presentation and granuloma formation. These agents inhibit tumor necrosis factor (TNF)-α and interleukin (IL)-6. Hydroxychloroquine, while less potent than chloroquine, is more frequently prescribed because of its markedly decreased incidence of ocular toxicity.

Hydroxychloroquine can be used as primary therapy for cutaneous sarcoidosis, mild hypercalciuria, or hypercalcemia. In addition, hydroxychloroquine is useful as a steroid-sparing adjunct.

Hydroxychloroquine is well tolerated by most patients (less than 10% of patients report having to discontinue the medication because of adverse effects). The starting dose is usually 200 mg orally twice a day. Once the disease process is in remission, the dose can be maintained at 200 mg per day. One must allow a 6-month trial to determine whether the medication is efficacious. Side effects include nausea and vomiting, skin rashes, and insomnia. The most worrisome side effect is ocular toxicity (less so with hydroxychloroquine than with chloroquine). Patients should undergo a baseline ophthalmologic examination before starting the medicine and should thereafter be seen by an ophthalmologist every 6 months to rule out drug-induced ocular toxicity. LFTs should also be routinely monitored every 3 months. Antimalarials are contraindicated in pregnancy.

[1]Not FDA approved for this indication.

Nonsteroidal Anti-Inflammatory Agents

Nonsteroidal anti-inflammatory drugs (NSAIDs) are useful for the 25% to 40% of patients with musculoskeletal complaints such as myalgias and arthralgias. In particular, NSAIDs are helpful in the setting of pain from erythema nodosum/Löfgren's syndrome. This class of drugs has no role as a steroid-sparing agent in other more insidious forms of the disease.

Novel Agents

As our knowledge of the basic science of sarcoidosis grows, other immunomodulatory agents are being studied in small groups of patients. One example is infliximab (Remicade)[1], a chimeric monoclonal antibody to TNF-α. Thalidomide (Thalomid)[1], a decades-old agent with well-known side effects, has also been shown to block TNF-α production. Use of these drugs to inhibit cytokines (such as TNF-α), while based on sound principles of basic science, requires further study pending their use as standard agents in the treatment of sarcoidosis.

Organ Transplantation

Of the few patients who die as a direct result of their sarcoidosis (direct mortality from sarcoidosis is 1% to 5%), 75% do so secondary to advanced lung disease. For patients with end-stage sarcoidosis, hypoxemia necessitates an aggressive workup and treatment for pulmonary hypertension. In addition, consideration should be made for the early referral to a lung transplant center (the wait for a lung can be up to 1.5 years). No formal guidelines currently exist for lung transplantation in sarcoidosis. Despite the fact that the disease may recur in the transplanted lung, several small series suggest that patients may do relatively well post-transplant (with a 2-year survival of approximately 70%). Transplantation should also remain an option for sarcoid involvement of other organs (e.g., heart, liver, kidneys). For sarcoidosis patients, post-transplant immunosuppression has the added benefit of reducing the incidence and intensity of postoperative disease remission.

Treatment of Specific Sites (Table 2)

PULMONARY

More than 90% of sarcoidosis patients manifest lung involvement. Patients often present after having been incorrectly diagnosed and treated for more common syndromes (e.g., obstructive lung disease). Most symptomatic patients present with dyspnea or

[1]Not FDA approved for this indication.

TABLE 2 Therapy for Sarcoidosis

First Line

Corticosteroids
- Uncomplicated superficial (e.g., conjunctivitis, dermatologic): Topical.
- Parenchymal: Initially 40 mg PO qd prednisone for 6 weeks followed by a 3-6 months of gradual tapering (triamcinolone [Kenalog] IM for poorly compliant).
- CNS/cardiac: 1 mg/kg/qd prednisone.

Second Line (for Steroid Resistance/Failure)

Methotrexate (Rheumatrex)[1]
- Initially 10-12.5 mg PO/wk; may titrate to 15 mg PO/wk.

Azathioprine (Imuran)[1]
- Initially 50 mg PO qd to maximum 200 mg PO qd.

Cyclophosphamide (Cytoxan)[1] (reserve for CNS sarcoidosis refractory to other agents)
- For PO, start 50 mg qd to maximum 150 mg qd.
- For IV pulse dosing, begin 500 mg IV every 2 weeks to maximum 2000 mg every 2 weeks.

Hydroxychloroquine (Plaquenil)[1]
- 200 mg PO bid.

[1]Not FDA approved for this indication.
Abbreviations: bid = twice daily; IM = intramuscularly; IV = intravenously; PO = by mouth; qd = once daily.

dry cough. Chest radiographs, while part of the standard of care for sarcoidosis management, must be placed in context. The linear staging system previously described (stages 0-IV) does not correlate with a worsening in prognosis. CT scans are generally overused and are not helpful in the routine management of sarcoidosis. CT does have a role in the diagnosis of secondary complications such as bronchiectasis, aspergillosis, or interstitial fibrosis. Gallium scans can be useful diagnostic adjuncts; the classic "panda" (parotid/lacrimals) and "lambda" (bilateral hilar lymphadenopathy) signs are pathognomonic for sarcoidosis. Gallium scans are most useful in helping to identify affected sites for biopsy.

Upon diagnosis and follow-up, all patients should undergo pulmonary physiology testing to assess impairment. A restrictive pattern with decreased vital and diffusing capacities is usual. Patients may present with obstructive defects as well. Patients should be followed every 3 months during this crucial period with serial PFTs and chest radiography. Asymptomatic patients without a decrement in pulmonary function should not be treated, even if chest films demonstrate up to stage III abnormalities. Given the risks of therapy, only the symptomatic patient with objective or symptomatic deterioration in his or her pulmonary function merits treatment.

Patients should be started on 40 mg per day of prednisone. To help clarify steroid responsiveness in poorly compliant patients, IM triamcinolone (Kenalog) may be considered. For responders who remit upon initiation of a taper, a prolonged course at a higher dose might be necessary. For those who demonstrate an inability to be weaned off corticosteroids, other agents such as hydroxychloroquine (Plaquenil)[1], may be used in an attempt to decrease steroid dependence. Inhaled corticosteroids have not demonstrated a consistent benefit in pulmonary sarcoidosis, although they may decrease the symptom of cough. For complete steroid nonresponders, consider other agents, such as azathioprine (Imuran)[1] or methotrexate (Rheumatrex)[1].

CARDIAC

While autopsy studies of patients with sarcoidosis in the United States show a 10% to 20% involvement of granulomas in the heart, only 5% of all patients with sarcoidosis present with cardiac symptoms. Unfortunately, the most common presentation is sudden cardiac death. Diagnostic modalities include thallium-201 scanning, cardiac MRIs with gadolinium, and positron emission tomography (PET) scanning. These examinations (although generally of low sensitivity), when positive, can be useful in the demonstration of defects that correspond to granulomatous involvement, or fibrous scarring. Invasive endomyocardial biopsies, while helpful when positive, are generally not performed because of the low yield and the high risk of this procedure. The low sensitivity of these objective diagnostic modalities, coupled with the life-threatening nature of cardiac involvement, necessitates a low threshold for the administration of steroid therapy upon the clinical suspicion of cardiac sarcoidosis. Patients should be treated for a prolonged period of time after the resolution of arrhythmias. Those who manifest complete heart blocks or ventricular arrhythmias should be considered for pacemakers/defibrillators.

NEUROSARCOIDOSIS

Neurosarcoidosis affects 5% to 10% of patients, with more than half of these individuals having CNS involvement. Early and more responsive lesions include cranial nerve defects, particularly facial palsies, as well as hypothalamic and pituitary processes. Later and less responsive lesions include space-occupying masses, peripheral neuropathies, and neuromuscular disease. Often, histologic confirmation of granulomatous disease is difficult to obtain. Cerebrospinal fluid (CSF) findings are nonspecific and include lymphocytosis (80% of patients), increased angiotensin converting enzyme (ACE) (50% of patients), and increased CD4/CD8 ratio. The utility of lumbar puncture is useful only in excluding infectious causes of CNS disease. Gadolinium-enhanced MRI appears to be more sensitive than CSF analysis in detecting neurologic involvement. Patients with neurosarcoidosis merit high-dose steroids (prednisone 1 mg/kg per day). Combination therapy with hydroxychloroquine (Plaquenil)[1] at the time of the initiating steroid

[1]Not FDA approved for this indication.

therapy should be considered given some evidence that hydroxychloroquine is effective in neurosarcoidosis, and that neurosarcoidosis patients tend to have a more chronic course. Patients not responding to steroids/hydroxychloroquine can be given cyclophosphamide (Cytoxan)[1]. Radiation therapy should be used for unremitting, focal space-occupying lesions that do not respond to medical therapy.

OPHTHALMOLOGIC SARCOIDOSIS

Ocular manifestations occur in 11% to 83% of patients with sarcoidosis. After the lung, it is the second most common site of disease. Anterior uveitis is more common than posterior uveitis and chronic anterior uveitis, which tends to occur without symptoms, is more common than acute anterior uveitis. Thus slit-lamp examination should be routine. Topical steroids can be used to treat anterior uveitis, but systemic steroids and occasionally methotrexate (Rheumatrex)[1] are required for posterior uveitis.

CUTANEOUS SARCOIDOSIS

Involvement of the skin occurs in 25% of sarcoidosis patients. Screening for sarcoidosis is indicated in any patient with granulomas on skin biopsy. Many skin lesions can be associated with sarcoidosis (e.g., macules, plaques, subcutaneous nodules, and scars). Lesions are typically located on the head, neck, extremities, periorbital areas, and lips, but are rare in the buccal mucosa.

Two important lesions associated with sarcoidosis are erythema nodosum and lupus pernio. Erythema nodosum (which is commonly located on the anterior tibial areas), although nonspecific, is a hallmark of acute sarcoidosis. It is a favorable prognostic indicator, with a greater than 80% overall disease remission rate within 2 years. Erythema nodosum should not be biopsied for the purpose of diagnosis. Only septal panniculitis will be found. Lupus pernio, which is sarcoid-specific, is characterized by indurated plaques on the nose, cheeks, lips, and ears. It is associated with bone cysts, pulmonary fibrosis, and, unfortunately, portends a prolonged and progressive course.

Dermatologic involvement is typically asymptomatic, and the major indication for treating cutaneous sarcoidosis is disfigurement. Cutaneous disease not responding to topical steroids can be treated by systemic corticosteroids, hydroxychloroquine (Plaquenil)[1], and even methotrexate (Rheumatrex)[1] for severe and unremitting cases. Trials are currently ongoing for the use of thalidomide (Thalomid)[1] and infliximab (Remicade)[1] for cutaneous sarcoidosis.

[1]Not FDA approved for this indication.

HEPATIC AND SPLENIC SARCOIDOSIS

Granulomas are found in 50% to 80% of liver biopsy specimens, and liver function profiles are often elevated (particularly alkaline phosphatase). Treatment is rarely indicated as hepatic granulomas rarely cause liver dysfunction. For the relief of cholestatic symptoms, or for persistently and markedly elevated alkaline phosphatase, a trial of ursodiol (Actigall)[1] can be considered. This is given at 15 to 20 mg/kg in two to four divided doses[3].

Splenic involvement is seen in 10% to 50% of patients with sarcoidosis. Splenomegaly is typically clinically silent, but some patients can present with abdominal pressure symptoms, as well as cytopenias. Corticosteroids are usually effective in diminishing splenomegaly, while splenectomy is reserved for steroid refractory hypersplenism, which engenders cytopenias, splenic rupture, and infarction.

DISORDERS OF CALCIUM HOMEOSTASIS

Hypercalcemia occurs in 2% to 10% of patients with sarcoidosis. Because hypercalciuria is more common than hypercalcemia, a 24-hour urine collection for calcium should be obtained routinely. This endocrinologic abnormality is secondary to the increased production of 1,25 dihydroxycholecalciferol (1,25-[OH]2-D3 [calcitriol]) by granulomas. Unchecked hypercalcemia and hypercalciuria can cause nephrocalcinosis, renal calculi, and even renal failure. Calcium dysregulation is an indication for systemic corticosteroid use. Low-dose prednisone and hydroxychloroquine (Plaquenil)[1], taken together, are effective.

Sarcoidologists are currently focusing on the identification of antigen(s) that initiate the cytokine cascade leading to granuloma formation. In addition, researchers are hoping to develop less toxic and more directed immunomodulatory agents. Until such investigations unlock further secrets of this fascinating disease, the care of the patient with sarcoidosis remains an art form. Clinicians, in partnership with sarcoidosis patients, must constantly balance the risk-to-benefit ratios of watchful waiting versus aggressive therapy. While the best treatment for most asymptomatic patients with sarcoidosis is no treatment, those manifesting progressive and debilitating disease of key organ systems require immunosuppression with systemic corticosteroids, other immunomodulatory agents, or transplants.

[1]Not FDA approved for this indication.

[3]Exceeds dosage recommended by the manufacturer.

ASBESTOS AND SILICA-RELATED DISEASES

METHOD OF
Raymond Bégin, MD, and Julie Deschênes, MD

Asbestos Exposure

Asbestos refers to fibrous, hydrous silicate minerals that are almost indestructible and heat resistant. There are six types, chrysotile and the five amphiboles (crocidolite, amosite, anthophyllite, tremolite, and actinolite), which are more rigid than chrysotile and not cylindrical. All six types can produce all asbestos-related diseases.

Chrysotile represents 95% of the world production of asbestos and is used in asbestos cement products for:

- The building construction industry (molded sheet, flat sheet, pipes, shingles, clapboard)
- Asbestos paper for insulation and filtering products
- Friction materials for brake linings and clutch facings
- Gaskets
- Tiles
- Textile products (whisk, yarn, tape, felt)
- Spray products for decorative and acoustic purposes
- Fireproofing in heating systems

The major end users of the past have been in the building construction, shipbuilding, automobile, and railroad equipment industries. The mill tailings of the mining process are used in road construction and for the extraction of magnesium.

Asbestos fibers in lung samples document past exposure to asbestos. At least two asbestos bodies (AB) seen in fibrotic lungs establish asbestosis, but fibrosis from chrysotile exposure alone occurs without AB. On lung lavage sample, more than one AB per mL corresponds to a nontrivial exposure. On lung tissue sample, more than one AB per visual field is significant.

Asbestos fiber induces fibrosis and cancers. Fibrosis formation starts with inflammation that then evolves into a fibrosing and damaging repair process leaving permanent scars. The cancer starts with damaging of the DNA of the target cells, which form increasingly altered tissue, and then become a clinically detected cancer.

Silica Exposure

In developed countries, the incidence of silicosis is 10 cases per 1 million males. It is caused by inhalation and retention of free silica generating a pathologic tissue reaction. There are three forms of free silica, crystalline, amorphous, and cryptocrystalline. The crystalline forms, quartz, tridymite, and cristobalite, are responsible for the pathogeneses of silicosis. Occupational exposure to silica particles is associated with:

- Mining, quarrying, and tunneling
- Stonecutting, engraving, and polishing
- Glass manufacturing
- Use of silica-containing abrasives (scouring powders, polishers, toothpastes, sandpaper) and fillers
- Foundry work
- Manufacturing of ceramics and refractories
- Sandblasting
- Grinding pottery
- Vitreous enameling

Also, quartz is in resonators, transducers, laser technology, watches, and color television circuits.

Silica is initially ingested by alveolar macrophages, which are activated to release inflammatory mediators (cytokines, acid arachidonic [AA] metabolites) that have chemotactic activity for inflammatory cells in the alveolar wall and epithelial surface. Hypertrophy, hyperplasia, and activation of type II pneumocytes produce surfactant-related substances found in the silicotic nodules. Following these events, the lung initiates an alveolitis, which if sustained can evolve into a silicotic nodule. The inflammatory phase is followed by a reparative phase, which may result in the development of fibrosis.

Diseases associated with asbestosis exposure are asbestosis, benign asbestos pleurisy, pleural plaques, pachypleuritis, rounded atelectasis, bronchogenic carcinoma, and malignant mesothelioma.

Asbestos-Related Diseases

ASBESTOSIS

Asbestosis is an interstitial fibrosis of the lung parenchyma. The severity and the extension of the fibrotic process can be graded in four and three grades, respectively. The symptoms and signs are those of other interstitial lung fibrosis. Crepitations are the most important physical findings (absent in 10% to 15% of patients). Standard films may be normal in 10% of patients. Asbestosis is manifested by diffuse reticulolinear infiltrates at lung bases, often accompanied by pleural manifestations. The changes seen on high-resolution computed tomography (HRCT) are:

- Thickenings of the interlobar and interlobular septa in the periphery of the lung
- Parenchymal bands extending from the pleural surface in the parenchyma

- Honeycombing
- Small cystic zones of lung destruction with thick wall, mostly located in posterior and nondependent areas of the lung
- Curvilinear lines in nondependent areas, parallel to the pleural surface but located at 1 cm from the latter
- Ground glass or haze-like, nondependent subpleural densities, reflecting possibly alveolitis

Bronchoalveolar lavage eliminates other diseases and documents past asbestos exposure. Several asbestos workers develop a macrophagic and neutrophilic fibrosing alveolitis before radiographic asbestosis. The lung functions are restrictive.

The most sensitive and specific method of diagnosis is histopathology, coupled with mineralogic assessment. Otherwise, the diagnosis is based on clinical findings. An abnormal chest radiograph or computed tomography (CT) scan suggestive of a diffuse interstitial lung disease with a significant history of asbestos exposure establishes clinical asbestosis.

The evolution of asbestosis has improved with early recognition; only 20% to 40% of patients will develop a severe form of the disease.

BENIGN PLEURISY

Benign pleurisy is an inflammatory, exudative, and transient inflammation of the pleura. It is defined by four criteria: asbestos exposure; radiographic or thoracocentesis confirmation of effusion; absence of other causes of effusion; and absence of tumor in follow-up of at least 3 years. The diagnosis is one of exception. It can be asymptomatic in 66% of cases and recurrent in some 28% of cases. Some have shortness of breath or chest pain, with or without fever. The pleural fluid is usually an exudate with or without blood staining. Physical findings are those of pleural effusion. The lung function restriction is proportional to the severity of the disease. The latency period is usually less than 20 years, and it is often the first manifestation of asbestos-related diseases. The outcome is either toward a regression with minimal or no pleural scar, one or many recurrences of the effusion, and, in a few cases, an evolution to diffuse pachypleuritis and/or rounded atelectasis. It is not a precursor of mesothelioma.

PLEURAL PLAQUES

Pleural plaques are avascular hyaline masses formed by collagen fibers. They are asymptomatic and are the most frequent manifestation of asbestos exposure. The development and progression of pleural plaques appear to be in direct relation with amphibole. Latency time for the production of plaques is in the range of 3 to 57 years.

On chest radiograph, asbestos-related pleural plaques are usually seen on both hemithorax, although to variable extent. Plaques are thin, linear with sharp margins, and appear as discrete opacities arising from the parietal pleura, with irregular, geographic contours. They may be located at costal margins, in the parasternal and paravertebral diaphragm, in pericardium, and mediastinum. The CT scan can recognize plaques much earlier and at a less well-defined stage than a chest radiograph.

Pleural plaques in asbestos workers are markers of exposure. They can enlarge very slowly and/or calcify and become confluent. Multiples pleural plaques can produce a restrictive syndrome.

PACHYPLEURITIS

Pachypleuritis is a disease of the visceral pleura, often associated with lung fibrosis. Dyspnea and dry cough are the main symptoms. There is a history of past benign pleuritis in more than 30% of cases. Pachypleuritis can progress in the interlobar and interlobular fissures and produce a retracted mass, a pseudotumor, or a round atelectasis. It can cause significant restriction.

On plain chest radiograph, there is a diffuse pleural thickening extending on more than 25% of the pleural surface with usually blunting of the costodiaphragmatic angle. On CT there is a pleural thickening (5 cm in width, 8 cm in length, 3 mm in thickness). Pachypleuritis affects mainly visceral pleura in posterolateral areas of the lower zones.

ROUNDED ATELECTASIS (PSEUDOTUMOR, FOLD LUNG, BLESOVSKY SYNDROME)

The rounded atelectasis is a retracted mass mimicking a carcinoma or a confluence of pneumoconiosis on the plain chest radiograph. It rarely can progress to respiratory failure and death. Chest pain in the area may be present.

The CT scan shows a round lesion of 2 to 7 cm diameter, pleural-based location, curvilinear shadows extending toward hilum (comet's tail sign), intrapulmonary location, pleural thickening adjacent to lesion, thickening of interlobar fissure (separated from diaphragm by lung tissue), and low progression.

LUNG CARCINOMA

In workers exposed to asbestosis fibers, there is a fivefold increase in lung cancer. There is an important synergy between cigarette smoking and asbestos exposure when evaluating the risk of developing lung cancer. Cancer resulting from asbestos usually has a latency period of 20 years. The greater the dose or the longer the exposure, the shorter the latency period, and the greater the risk of developing lung cancer. The clinical presentation and pathology of the asbestos-related cancers are not distinct from those associated with cigarette smoking. Fiber counts in lung tissues help to establish causality.

MALIGNANT MESOTHELIOMA

There is a clear association between asbestos and mesothelioma, but no association with cigarette smoking. Malignant mesothelioma may be of peritoneal origin in less than 25% of cases. Tumor develops by direct extension, invading the adjacent structures. Death is usually caused by restriction of these vital structures.

Mesothelioma has a histochemical profile distinct from that of adenocarcinoma. It has three histologic presentations: epithelial (50%), sarcomatoid (16%), and mixed (34%). Mesothelioma has a latency period of 20 to 50 years. The chief complaint is usually chest pain, occasionally pleuritic, requiring progressively higher doses of analgesics. Cough, dyspnea, weight loss, fever, and fatigue are often present in the late phase. There is restriction of lung functions. Most people die within 24 months of diagnosis.

The radiologic findings are multiple circumscribed thickening of pleura with irregular nodulated surfaces, multiple pleural nodules or masses or plaque-like opacities, and pleural effusion. Positron emission tomography (PET) is used to exclude nonmalignant disease and to stage the extension. Biopsy with closed pleural biopsy or video-assisted thoracic surgery (VATS) is needed for diagnosis.

The tumor is neither chemico-sensitive nor radiosensitive. Radiotherapy may be used for pain palliation or prophylaxis following thoracic procedure. Extrapleural pneumonectomy (EPP), which consists of surgical removal of ipsilateral pleura, lung, hemidiaphragm, and pericardium with diaphragm and pericardium reconstruction, could benefit patients with limited disease (stage I or, rarely, stage II) of the epithelial form. Pleurectomy with decortication could be used, but with less success in removing all of the tumor. Pleurodesis is used for palliation. Single-modality therapy does not change the median survival, but multimodality treatment, which is EPP followed by sequential chemotherapy (intrapleural or systemic) and radiation, has led to prolonged survival. Hyperthermia with intrapleural chemotherapy could potentiate the action of the agent on the tumor. Immunotherapy (with interleukin [IL]-2[1] and various interferons) and gene therapy, alone or as adjuvant, show encouraging response rates, but it has various adverse effects. In the future, antiproliferative, immune, and photodynamic therapies, as well as angiogenesis inhibitors and vaccines, appear promising.

Silica-Related Diseases

CHRONIC SILICOSIS (SIMPLE)

Chronic silicosis is the most common presentation. This is seen in workers with 15 to 20 years of low-intensity exposure to silica. The chest radiograph is characterized by less than 10-mm round, nonconfluent opacities seen predominantly in the upper lung fields or more diffusely. Usually, simple silicosis is symptomless, and the pulmonary function tests are normal. The disease will progress to confluent silicosis in 20% to 30% of patients. The intensity and duration of exposure appear to influence the outcome.

CONFLUENT SILICOSIS (COMPLICATED SILICOSIS OR PROGRESSIVE MASSIVE FIBROSIS)

In confluent silicosis, there are coalescence of adjacent silicotic nodules and fibrosis to form large masses of disease, surrounded by adjacent paracicatricial emphysema. Progression is the rule. The patient often has exercise dyspnea and nonproductive cough. On chest radiograph, the opacities become confluent, forming nodular opacities of more than 10 mm, with reduced amounts of nodules and rarefaction of the vascular markings around these large opacities. Progressive massive fibrosis (PMF) is often associated with lung distortion and shift of the mediastinum and the trachea to the affected side. The lung functions show a mixed pattern of restrictive and obstructive changes. The course may be complicated by avascular necrosis, cavitation, tuberculosis, pneumothorax, hypoxia, and pulmonary hypertension.

ACUTE SILICOPROTEINOSIS

Acute silicoproteinosis, an uncommon form of silicosis, is a rapidly progressive disease developing after massive silica exposure of short duration. This occurs in unprotected or confined sandblasting work, silica flour work, or ceramic work. Patients present with severe dyspnea, generalized weakness, weight loss, and fever. On the radiograph, profuse ground glass-like round opacities, poorly demarcated silicotic nodules or loose granulomas, and interstitial fibrosing pneumonitis are seen. Liver and kidneys may be involved. Acute respiratory failure develops with a severe decrease in diffusing capacity for carbon monoxide, hypoxemia, and restriction. Rapid progression to respiratory failure and death is the rule.

ACCELERATED SILICOSIS

Accelerated silicosis has an intermediate rate of progression between that of simple silicosis and that of acute silicoproteinosis. It usually appears after 5 to 10 years of high-intensity silica exposure. The patient presents with dyspnea and cough. The initial chest radiograph show dense nodular infiltrates with some confluence. Lung functions are restrictive. Death occurs within 10 years.

In acute or accelerated silicosis, the use of high-dose prednisolone (Prelone)[1] (1 mg/kg per day) tapered gradually over 12 months may result in shorter

[1]Not FDA approved for this indication.

reduction of the alveolitis and provide some clinical improvement. Such treatment may accelerate infections such as tuberculosis. Alternatively, one may consider massive whole lung lavage under general anesthesia to improve gas exchange and remove alveolar materials. Both treatments' efficacies have not been proven.

END-STAGE SILICOSIS

Patients with end-stage silicosis have advanced lung infiltrations, confluence, airway distortion, emphysematous changes, and severe deterioration of lung functions with dyspnea, hypoxemia, and cor pulmonale.

SILICOSIS AND AUTOIMMUNE DISEASES

Up to 25% of patients exposed to silica have a positive rheumatoid factor. A definitely increased incidence of scleroderma has been reported in persons with more than 3 years of exposure (even in those without silicosis), with high intensity of exposure being a contributor. Rheumatoid nodules have been seen pathologically in up to 2% of silicosis. Silicosis is also associated with systemic rheumatoid arthritis, dermatopolymyositis, systemic lupus erythematosus, and immunoglobulins.

COMPLICATIONS

Patients with silicosis are at greater risks for tuberculosis (which remains the most prevalent complication) and atypical mycobacteria. Silicosis, but not silica exposure alone, is likely associated with an increased incidence of lung cancer.

Fungal colonization of a cavity may cause recurrent hemoptysis. Acute or chronic bronchitis and segmental atelectasis might result from distortion or compression of the airways by adjacent nodes (middle lobe collapse). Enlarged silicotic lymph nodes may cause irreversible paralysis of the left recurrent laryngeal nerve and dysphagia associated with oesophageale compression. Acute glomerulonephritis has been associated with acute silicosis.

Treatment

No treatment affects silicosis and asbestosis; treatment is given for the complications. This is why prevention remains the cornerstone of eliminating the pneumoconiosis maladies associated with these materials.

Prevention

Prevention is done through legislative regulation of hygiene at work places; education of workers on the risks of their jobs; and control of the silica dust and asbestosis fiber levels by ventilation and exhaust systems, process enclosures, and personal protection with appropriate respirators. The current U.S. standard for asbestos fiber is 0.1 fiber per cc of air, and for silica it is 0.05 mg/m^3 of air.

HYPERSENSITIVITY PNEUMONITIS

METHOD OF
Jordan N. Fink, MD

Hypersensitivity pneumonitis (HP), or extrinsic allergic alveolitis, is an immunologic inflammatory lung disease that is caused by the interaction of environmental foreign organic substances, which are immunogenic, with the pulmonary parenchyma and the immune system. It differs from asthma in its symptom presentation, physical and radiographic findings, nonimmunoglobulin (Ig) E immunologic pathogenesis, and disease progression.

Etiology

A number of organic antigens of approximately 5 µm or smaller, which are derived from bacteria, fungi, protozoans, or plant or animal proteins as well as some reactive chemicals, cause HP. Examples of these include thermophilic species found in moldy hay, compost, or humidifiers, fungi from moldy wood dusts, amoebae-contaminating ventilation systems, and avian or laboratory animal proteins. Bacterial contamination of metalworking fluids is linked with HP in machinists.

Chemicals such as isocyanates (used in the plastics and paint industries as catalysts) and epoxy resins are another group of possible causative agents of HP. Medications such as amiodarone (Cordarone), gold (Solganal), and β blockers have also been reported.

Clinical Presentation

The clinical features of HP are divided into acute and chronic forms. The type of organic dust inhaled is less important than the nature, intensity, and frequency of inhalation or the immune response of the host. Sensitization of susceptible individuals occurs after repeated exposure to offending agents. After a variable latency period, the symptoms occur acutely or insidiously after further exposure. This repeated exposure to antigens, which is usually intermittent, is essential to induce HP.

In the acute form, flu-like symptoms with fever, chills, headache, malaise, cough, and dyspnea may occur approximately 4 to 6 hours after inhalation of the offending agent. These symptoms may persist for up to 24 hours, and spontaneous recovery follows. In some acute reactions symptoms may persist for 5 to 7 days, resolving slowly. Physical examination during an episode may reveal an acutely ill patient with dyspnea. Bibasilar end-inspiratory rales are prominent and may persist for weeks after the cessation of exposure. Wheezing is not prominent. Pulmonary function abnormalities include a restrictive pattern, decreased diffusing capacity, and decreased oxygen saturation.

Chest radiographs may reveal diffuse, bilateral, patchy parenchymal densities. A ground-glass appearance of the parenchyma is also seen. Lesions are present most frequently in the lower lobes. These abnormalities resolve with therapy, but will recur with additional exposures. Thus, the patient may appear to have multiple episodes of pneumonia. Laboratory studies may show a leukocytosis, left shift, and mild eosinophilia. Precipitating antibodies of the IgG type against the offending agent and rheumatoid factor reflecting a nonspecific inflammatory response may be demonstrated. Lung biopsy specimens demonstrate lymphocytic infiltration of the alveolar walls with plasma cells and macrophages occluding the alveolar spaces and intraalveolar foamy macrophages and granulomas. Lavage of the bronchoalveolar spaces demonstrates a lymphocytosis usually with marked increase in T cells bearing the CD8 marker indicative of suppressor cells. As the disease progresses, the alveolar spaces become obliterated and interstitial infiltration with fibroblasts occurs.

The chronic form of HP may appear with progressive dyspnea, cough, weakness, cyanosis on exertion, and occasional weight loss. Physical examination may reveal fine bibasilar rales and clubbing of the fingers. Pulmonary function tests may show restrictive or obstructive defects and decreased diffusing capacity. Chest radiographs may demonstrate reticulonodular infiltrates, and, in advanced disease, fibrosis with honeycombing may be present. Laboratory findings may be similar to those of the acute disease. Lung biopsy demonstrates interstitial fibrosis of varying degrees, lymphocytic alveolitis, and alveolar septal wall thickening.

Diagnosis

The differential diagnosis of HP includes infectious diseases as well as other interstitial pulmonary disorders. Chronic aspergillosis, sarcoidosis, chronic granulomatous infections, chronic bronchitis, drug reactions, collagen vascular diseases, and inorganic respiratory dust syndromes including berylliosis, silicosis, and asbestosis should be considered, as should idiopathic pulmonary fibrosis. These diseases may progress with time and may appear with constitutional symptoms or may result in pulmonary fibrosis as well.

The diagnosis of HP is made by consideration of the symptom complex; physical examination; and radiographic, laboratory, and pulmonary function findings; together with a carefully obtained environmental, occupational, and medication exposure history. Bronchoalveolar lavage may be helpful, although berylliosis and tuberculosis also have lymphocytosis with increased CD8 T cells. Lung biopsy may be necessary in some cases to solidify the diagnosis. In some cases, a purposeful and controlled challenge with the suspected offending agent may be performed.

Treatment

Avoidance or removal from exposure to the offending agent is of extreme importance. Patients with the acute form of HP spontaneously improve after avoidance measures are instituted. Avoidance techniques may include the installation of air filtration systems, the wearing of protective masks, or a change of occupation or hobby. Treatment with corticosteroids can dramatically improve acute HP. Daily steroid therapy is recommended with gradual tapering once pulmonary functions have stabilized and strict avoidance of the offending agent has been accomplished. The usual therapy is prednisone, 40 to 60 mg per day until there is objective evidence of improvement, then gradual tapering over several months with pulmonary function and chest radiograph follow-up. The effect of treatment with long-term corticosteroids, if avoidance of exposure is not accomplished, has not been established. Inhaled steroids and cromolyn sodium (Intal) have been tried but are usually of little benefit.

Prognosis

Factors important in the prognosis of HP are related to the reversibility of the disease, the degree of permanent respiratory impairment, avoidance, and the patient's age. More than four episodes of recurrent acute symptoms of low-grade exposure may result in progressive pulmonary disease and irreversible fibrosis. Digital clubbing when associated with fibrosis may be a poor prognostic sign. Chest radiographic progression and persistent diffusion capacity reduction may also be related to a poor clinical outcome.

TUBERCULOSIS AND OTHER MYCOBACTERIAL DISEASES

METHOD OF

Christopher J. Lahart, MD

Tuberculosis (TB) is a curable and preventable disease. TB is the cause of more deaths each year worldwide than any other infectious disease. Although apparently contradictory, both of these statements about TB are accurate and, unfortunately, will remain accurate for years to come. The World Health Organization (WHO) has estimated that during 2001 there were 8.5 million new cases of tuberculosis with 1.9 million deaths. The vast majority of these cases and deaths occur in the developing world. In the United States, the Centers for Disease Control and Prevention (CDC) reported a total of 15,075 cases in 2002 and 749 deaths in 2001. Within the United States tuberculosis cases are not evenly distributed, with a concentration in urban and medically underserved areas. The top five states in numbers of TB cases (California, Texas, New York, Florida, and Illinois) account for more than 52% of the national cases, while the five states with the lowest occurrence have less than 1%. There are fewer than 50 cases in each of 14 states. In 2002, for the first time since nation-of-birth data were collected, more than 50% of the TB cases in the United States were in persons born outside of the country. This highlights the worldwide issues of resource distribution and the ability of infectious diseases to transcend national borders. In recognition of this, the CDC has increased efforts of collaboration with international organizations to improve TB control in countries heavily impacted by the disease.

Case identification and treatment are important aspects of tuberculosis control efforts. Another is identification of individuals with latent tuberculosis infection who are at high risk of progressing to active disease. With an estimated 25% of the human population infected by *Mycobacterium tuberculosis*, this is an enormous task. It is even more important in areas with a low prevalence of active TB, such as the United States, where a high percentage of the annual cases arise from these latently infected people. It is estimated that 10% of the U.S. population has latent TB infection, providing a reservoir of more than 25 million individuals from which active cases may arise. Primary care physicians are on the front line of this challenge and must learn to assess a patient's risk and then test for latent tuberculosis infection when warranted.

An additional challenge to TB control in the United States is presented by the increasing infrequency of the disease itself. Fewer cases mean fewer physicians familiar with the disease's presentation, complications, and treatment. Despite a decreasing chance of encountering TB, practitioners must remind themselves to *think TB* when confronted with patients who have symptoms and signs suggestive of TB.

Pathogenesis of Tuberculosis

The human disease termed *tuberculosis* is caused by the organism *M. tuberculosis*. Archeological findings have determined the presence of this disease since before recorded history, and it is more prevalent now than ever before. Transmission of *M. tuberculosis* is from person-to-person with no intermediate host or environmental reservoir. A person with respiratory tract tuberculosis expels airborne particles that contain *M. tuberculosis*. This occurs during coughing and sneezing, but also during normal speech and respiration. The particles of greatest importance are generally only 1 to 5 μm in size and can remain suspended in air for a considerable period of time. Another individual inhales them along with ambient air. Organism-containing particles of appropriate size make their way to the pulmonary alveoli where the organisms are promptly ingested by alveolar macrophages. *M. tuberculosis* can survive and multiply within macrophages, are released with cell death, and spread to regional lymph nodes and hematogenously to other well-perfused organ systems. The resulting immune response from this initial infection induces cell-mediated immunity as well as granuloma formation. Delayed-type hypersensitivity reaction is developed to certain tuberculin antigens and forms the basis of tuberculin skin testing. Latent tuberculosis infection (LTBI) is thus established; this condition is present in 25 million persons in the United States and 1.5 billion persons worldwide.

The immune response generated by this initial infection is able to perpetuate this latency as a lifelong condition in 90% of those infected. Only 10% will progress from latent infection to active disease. Half of this progression (5% of the infected total) will occur within the first 2 years following infection. The remaining half will occur during the remaining lifetime, often associated with the development of other medical complications such as diabetes, malignancy, renal failure, or immunosuppressive diseases or therapy. The proportions progressing to active disease and the time course of progression are dramatically altered by HIV infection. This interaction between TB and HIV is a critical driving force of the TB epidemic in the developing world, but also of major importance in the United States. This is elaborated upon in a separate section of this article, highlighting the recommendations for HIV testing and special considerations for both TB and HIV therapy.

Diagnosis of Latent Tuberculosis Infection

TUBERCULIN SKIN TESTING

Although 25 million persons in the United States have latent tuberculosis infection, mass screening is not recommended. Rather, practitioners must assess the risk of an individual to progress to active disease if they were latently infected and then test for latent infection in those at high risk. The diagnosis of LTBI is based upon purified protein derivative (PPD) tuberculin skin testing to elicit the delayed-type hypersensitivity reaction. This reaction is usually present within 2 to 12 weeks following infection. Tuberculin is injected intradermally on the volar aspect of either forearm and the intensity of the reaction is assessed within 48 to 72 hours by measuring the amount of induration around the injection site. Prior vaccination with bacilli Calmette-Guérin (BCG) is not a contraindication to tuberculin skin testing, and a significant reaction should not be ascribed to such vaccination. Persons receive this vaccination because they reside in a country with a high burden of TB, and the significant tuberculin reaction is more likely a reaction to LTBI than to BCG.

Because of the sensitivity and specificity of the tuberculin skin test, as well as the prevalence of LTBI in different groups, the interpretation of the skin test reaction incorporates three different cutpoints for significance of reaction (Table 1). For those at highest risk of developing active TB and those with immunosuppressive conditions that may impair their response, 5 mm of induration indicates a significant reaction. Persons with an increased likelihood of recent infection or other social or clinical conditions associated with higher risk of progression exhibit a significant reaction at the 10-mm level. For those with no perceived risk factors or who are entering into a longitudinal screening program such as for employment, 15 mm is a significant reaction size. Results of tuberculin skin testing should be recorded in millimeters of induration and not as *positive* or *negative*. Depending upon certain life events, what was once considered to be an insignificant reaction could very well be considered significant with the development of a new clinical diagnosis (e.g., HIV infection).

If sequential tuberculin skin testing is anticipated, such as annual screening in the health care industry, special consideration must be given to the boosting phenomenon. In some individuals the cellular immune response to tuberculin may be lost over a period of years. The initial application of tuberculin may not elicit a significant response, but the second application may. If this second tuberculin exposure is part of the annual re-examination, it may be misinterpreted to signify recent tuberculosis infection during the past year of employment. Repercussions of such a misinterpretation include investigations of lapses in TB control within the facility and placement of the individual in a high-risk category for progression because of recent infection. However, the infection may have been remote, the risk of progression low, and there may have been no TB transmission in the facility. To prevent this mishap, a two-stage approach to the initial tuberculin screening needs to be used. A second tuberculin test should be done shortly following the initial one to assess the presence or absence of boosting.

TABLE 1 Targeted Skin Testing to Identify Persons With Latent Tuberculosis Infection Who Would Benefit From Treatment: Criteria for PPD Positivity for Specific Disease Risk Factors

Positive Result	Risk for Disease After Infection*
5 mm	HIV Infection
5 mm	Fibrotic changes on chest radiograph consistent with old healed TB
5 mm	Recent contact with infectious TB case
5 mm	Organ transplantation or other immunosuppression†
10 mm	Medical conditions Diabetes mellitus End-stage renal disease Silicosis Immunosuppressive therapy Hematologic or reticuloendothelial diseases Cancers of the head, neck, and lung Intestinal bypass or gastrectomy Chronic malabsorption Body weight 10% or more below ideal
10 mm	History of inadequately treated TB in the past
10 mm	TB infection within 2 y (skin test increase by 10 or more mm)
10 mm	Illicit injection of drugs or cocaine use
10 mm	Children <4 y old, children and adolescents exposed to high-risk adults
10 mm	Foreign individuals from high prevalence countries who have resided in the United States <5 y.
10 mm	Prolonged travel/residence in a high-prevalence region
10 mm	Residents or employees of high risk group settings‡
10 mm	Health care workers serving high risk persons
10 mm	Mycobacteriology laboratory personnel
15 mm	No risk factors§

*Includes individuals with a high likelihood of recent infection and thus more at risk for disease.
†Fifteen mg of prednisone or more per day for 1 month or more.
‡Prisons, jails, shelters, health care facilities, nursing homes; low-risk individuals being tested for the first time for longitudinal screening programs are not included.
§Includes those being tested for the first time as part of a longitudinal screening program.
Abbreviations: PPD = purified protein derivative; TB = tuberculosis.

CHEST RADIOGRAPHS

Once the diagnosis of LTBI has been considered, care must be taken to not miss a diagnosis of active disease. A missed diagnosis can have serious consequences, because the treatment regimens for LTBI are inadequate for active disease and would foster drug resistance. All persons diagnosed with LTBI in whom treatment is being considered should have a chest radiograph performed. A single posterior-anterior exposure is appropriate for persons older than 5 years of age. For children younger than 5, the only manifestation of active TB may be small pleural effusions or adenopathy, so a lateral projection of the chest should also be obtained. Pregnant women with LTBI or with recent contact with active TB cases are at risk for progression to active disease and congenital TB in the infant. Chest radiography should be performed with the use of proper shielding in the radiology suite.

SPUTUM EXAMINATION

In a person with LTBI and a chest radiograph that is clear of changes for tuberculosis, no sputum examination for mycobacterial smear or culture is necessary. However, a special consideration is the HIV-infected person with or without respiratory symptoms. If symptoms are present, sputum specimens from 3 consecutive days should be submitted, unless the respiratory symptoms are explained by an alternate diagnosis and resolve with treatment. If no symptoms are present but the HIV infection is advanced, as indicated by an AIDS diagnosis, sputum should be examined if recent contact with a TB case is suspected.

Persons with chest radiographs that are suggestive of prior or healed TB infection, but with no history of prior TB treatment, should have sputum samples sent for examination on 3 consecutive days. Initiation of treatment for LTBI can await the results of these examinations, or treatment for active TB disease can be initiated and subsequently tapered to treatment of LTBI once results are final and negative.

Treatment of Latent Tuberculosis Infection

Because the decision to test for LTBI should be based upon the identification of those at high risk of progression to active disease, the decision to test is also a decision to treat those in whom LTBI is diagnosed. The primary contraindication to the treatment of LTBI with a recommended single-drug regimen is the inability to rule out active TB disease. If active TB remains a clinical consideration, multidrug therapy should be initiated and maintained until active disease is no longer a consideration. Other contraindications to treatment are the presence of active hepatitis or end-stage liver disease.

PRETREATMENT EVALUATION

The major pretreatment evaluation is to eliminate active disease from consideration. The evaluation in preparation of LTBI treatment is an assessment of the risk of hepatic disease. Persons with a history or physical examination indicative of liver disease or regular excessive use of alcohol should have baseline liver function tests (LFTs). The presence of risk factors for hepatitis B or C infection or diagnosed HIV infection should also prompt baseline LFTs. Pregnant women and those in the immediate postpartum period should also undergo such testing. Routine baseline testing is not indicated. If rifampin is to be used, a baseline complete blood count (CBC) should be obtained.

TREATMENT REGIMENS

A common misunderstanding is that isoniazid (INH) therapy for LTBI is not recommended for persons older than 35 years of age. Current recommendations do not include consideration of age. Individuals at high risk, regardless of age, should receive treatment of LTBI because the risk of active TB is higher than the risk of treatment-related complications. Practitioners must assess individual patients for their risk of a treatment-related complication.

There are four recommended regimens for treatment of LTBI. Medications used to treat LTBI are the same as those used to treat active TB (Table 2). The preferred regimen consists of isoniazid given daily for 9 months (which can be self-administered by the patient), or, alternately, the drug may be taken on a twice-weekly dosing schedule given as part of a directly observed protocol. It should be emphasized that because of the concern for the development of drug resistance, any intermittent therapy, whether for latent or active TB, should only be prescribed as part of a directly observed therapy. A second, but less preferred regimen, is isoniazid given for 6 months. This also can be given daily or twice weekly, but should be reserved for those unable to complete a full 9-month course. It is also not preferred for those with HIV infection or fibrotic lesions on chest radiograph. The 6-month regimen results in slightly higher rates of active disease despite treatment of LTBI.

A third regimen, better studied in the HIV-infected population, consists of rifampin (Rifadin) plus pyrazinamide administered for 2 months. This also can be prescribed as daily therapy or twice weekly. Caution must be taken with this regimen because of its higher rate of hepatotoxicity, especially in the non–HIV-infected patient. This regimen can be considered for patients who are close contacts with a person who has isoniazid-resistant TB. Patients should be evaluated every 2 weeks while on this regimen to minimize the chance of continued treatment administration during development of hepatitis. Although well studied in the HIV-infected, the use of rifampin can complicate treatment of HIV infection because of the significant drug–drug interactions between rifampin and many HIV medications. The fourth regimen consists of rifampin alone, administered for 4 months as daily therapy.

TABLE 2 First-Line Antituberculosis Drugs

		Dose: mg/kg (Maximum)*					
		Daily		2 Times/wk†		3 Times/wk†	
Drug	**Form**	**Adults**	**Children**	**Adults**	**Children**	**Adults**	**Children**
Isoniazid	100-300-mg tablets Intramuscular Syrup, 50 mg/5 mL	5 (300 mg)	10–20	15 (900 mg)	20–40	15 (900 mg)	20–40
Rifampin (Rifadin)	150-300 mg capsules Intravenous 10 mg/kg	10 (600 mg)§	10–20§	10 (600 mg)§	10–20§	10 (600 mg)§	10–20§
Rifabutin (Mycobutin)[1]	150-mg capsules Intravenous‡	5 (300 mg)§	10–20§	5 (300 mg)§	10–20§	5 (300 mg)§	Unknown
Pyrazinamide	500-mg tablets.	15–30 (2 g)	15–20	50–70 (4 g)	50–70	50–70 (4 g)	50–70
Rifamate	Fixed-combination capsules containing 150 mg isoniazid, 300 mg rifampin	2 capsules					
Rifater	Fixed-combination capsules containing 50 mg isoniazid, 120 mg rifampin, 300 mg pyrazinamide	<45 kg; 4 tablets 45–54 kg: 5 tablets >54 kg: 6 tablets					
Ethambutol (Myambutol)	100-400-mg tablets	15–25	15–25 (1 g)	50	50 (4 g)	25–30	25–30
Streptomycin	Intramuscular Intravenous	15 (1 g) Age >60 y	20–40 (1 g) 10 (750 mg)	25–30 (1.5 g)	25–30 (1.5 g)	25–30 (1.5 g)	25–30 (1.5 g)

*Maximal doses for children are the same as those for adults.
†Directly observed therapy should be used with intermittent dosing.
‡Not available in the United States.
§Complex drug interactions occur with many medications, including those used for HIV infection; refer to the text.
[1]Not FDA approved for this indication.

MONITORING DURING TREATMENT OF LATENT TUBERCULOSIS INFECTION

After the initial clinical evaluation and the initiation of treatment for LTBI, patients should receive monthly follow-up evaluations if they are receiving isoniazid or rifampin alone. If they are receiving rifampin and pyrazinamide, they should be evaluated at weeks 2, 4, 6, and 8. The evaluation should include examination for symptoms and signs of hepatitis. Routine laboratory monitoring is not recommended. Only patients with abnormal baseline LFTs or who are at risk for hepatic disease should be retested routinely during therapy. Follow-up chest radiographs are not indicated.

Diagnosis of Active Tuberculosis Disease

Control of tuberculosis depends upon the prompt recognition of active TB disease and the initiation of effective therapy. Because TB is generally a slowly progressive disease of a rather indolent nature, it is uncommon for the individual suspected of TB to require hospitalization. The patient suspected of infectious TB should preferably be evaluated as an outpatient, remaining in the environment in which they have resided instead of bringing them into a new environment with potential new contacts, many of whom may be immunosuppressed. Should a TB suspect need hospitalization because of the severity of illness, co-morbidities, or to facilitate evaluation, he or she should be placed in strict respiratory isolation until 3 sputum specimens are smear negative for acid-fast bacilli. Unfortunately, studies show significant delays in the diagnosis of active TB in hospitalized patients with up to 50% of the cases not suspected at the time of admission. Consideration of TB must remain prominent in clinicians' minds.

CLINICAL FEATURES

Active TB typically presents as a chronic illness with progression of symptoms occurring over a period of weeks to months. Symptoms often include chronic cough, fever, night sweats, and weight loss. Some patients may minimize these symptoms, but will present themselves within days of the development of hemoptysis. Approximately 80% of TB cases have pulmonary involvement, with 72% having pulmonary alone and 8% having both pulmonary and extrapulmonary. Twenty percent have only extrapulmonary disease, which is characterized by constitutional symptoms plus symptoms referable to the organ system involved. Many of the so-called *extrapulmonary* cases actually involve intrathoracic sites that are separate from the pulmonary parenchyma, such as mediastinal lymph nodes and pleural disease. Other sites include bones and joints, the genitourinary system, the central nervous system (CNS), the meninges, and peritoneal TB. Granulomas may be seen in the liver or spleen.

RADIOGRAPHS

The typical chest radiograph of active TB shows unilateral or bilateral upper lobe involvement with fibronodular disease and/or cavitation. Such findings should always raise suspicion of TB. Although this is the typical appearance of adult reactivation disease from the latent state, TB disease caused by progression of initial infection may be seen in children or the immunosuppressed, especially advanced HIV infection. This picture includes middle and lower lobe infiltrates, pleural effusions, and hilar adenopathy.

SPUTUM EXAMINATION

In pulmonary TB, sputum specimens have positive acid-fast bacilli (AFB) smears in 45% of the cases and culture positive for *M. tuberculosis* in 70% of the cases. When pulmonary TB is considered, sputum should be submitted for examination. Because of specimen quality issues and test sensitivity, a sputum specimen from each of 3 consecutive days is recommended. The initial culture positive specimen should have drug susceptibility testing performed as a routine procedure. Most mycobacteriology laboratories will do this without a specific request, but the practitioner must confirm this. Up to 17% of TB cases in the United States are based upon clinical and radiographic suspicions when sputum specimens remain smear and culture negative. In these instances, appropriate diagnostic studies should be performed to evaluate other possible diagnoses; however, if TB remains the leading diagnostic concern, therapy should be initiated. Clinical and radiographic responses to TB treatment at 2 months should be assessed to provide further support for the TB diagnosis.

Treatment of Active Tuberculosis

Current regimens for treatment of active TB have a 97% success rate in the initial treatment and less than a 5% relapse rate. The success of these regimens depends upon the use of appropriate multidrug therapy to eliminate the emergence of drug-resistant organisms, the extended duration of therapy to reach the slowly replicating mycobacteria and to prevent later relapse, and maximum adherence to the regimen dosing and duration. Adherence is best addressed through the use of directly observed therapy. Directly observed therapy uses the resources of the local public health authority to deliver therapy to the patient with the public health worker observing the patient taking the medication. In addition to verifying treatment administration, the worker also inquires about potential side effects and serves as a resource for the patient, further enhancing adherence.

PRETREATMENT EVALUATION

Much like treatment of LTBI, active TB patients must be assessed for the presence or potential for hepatic disease. Baseline LFTs should be obtained along with a CBC with a platelet count. Most patients also receive ethambutol (Myambutol) as part of their initial regimen, so testing of visual acuity and color vision should be performed and recorded.

TREATMENT REGIMENS

There are four recommended regimens for treating active TB. Three of the regimens use typical four-drug therapy, including isoniazid, rifampin, pyrazinamide, and ethambutol. The fourth regimen is for patients who are unable to take pyrazinamide (severe liver disease, gout, and pregnancy) and includes the remaining three drugs. Each regimen has a 2-month initial phase followed by a 4- or 7-month continuation phase. Six months is the minimal acceptable duration of treatment for any case of culture-positive TB. The differences between the regimens are how intermittent some of the dosing frequencies are and how soon in the course of treatment the intermittent administration begins. For all treatment, directly observed therapy is recommended, but for any intermittent therapy it is absolutely necessary.

Regimen 1 is the daily administration of all four drugs for the initial 2 months of treatment. In regimen 2 the same medications are administered daily for the first 2 weeks, followed by twice-weekly dosing for 6 weeks. Regimen 3 consists of the same four drugs administered three times weekly for 8 weeks. Regimen 4 is isoniazid, rifampin, and ethambutol administered daily for 8 weeks. A special exception are patients with advanced HIV infection. These patients should never receive medications less than three times per week because of the higher rate of relapse seen in that setting. The usual prescription for these patients is daily therapy for 2 weeks followed by thrice-weekly dosing to completion.

After the initial 2-month phase there is a second decision point. By this time drug susceptibility results should be known and if the organism is pansensitive, both pyrazinamide and ethambutol should be discontinued. Pyrazinamide is used to hasten early sterilization, and the early phase is completed. Ethambutol is used to protect the other medications in the setting of possible drug resistance and can actually be discontinued as soon as susceptibility results demonstrate no resistance. Most patients will continue therapy for 4 additional months (regimens 1, 2, and 3). Those who should continue for 7 months include persons with cavitary disease whose sputum culture obtained at the 2-month interval remains positive and those who did not receive pyrazinamide (regimen 4). For all four regimens, the continuation phase can consist of isoniazid and rifampin given daily, twice weekly, or thrice weekly; the exceptions are regimen 3, which continues on the thrice-weekly schedule, and the patient with advanced HIV infection who should not receive twice-weekly dosing.

Rifapentine (Priftin) is a recently approved antituberculosis medication that allows for once-weekly dosing in the continuation phase of therapy. Rifapentine (10 mg/kg, 600 mg maximum) can be given with isoniazid (900 mg) once per week for the final 4 months in persons known to be HIV-negative, persons with noncavitary pulmonary disease, and persons who have negative sputum cultures after the initial 2 months. This can only be done via directly observed therapy.

MONITORING THERAPY

Therapy is often initiated before culture results are finalized. Drug susceptibility results will further lag the culture results. A sputum specimen for AFB smear and culture should be submitted at monthly intervals until two consecutive cultures are negative. If a culture obtained after 3 months of treatment is reported as positive, drug susceptibility testing should be repeated on that isolate to assess acquired drug resistance. If AFB cultures have been negative throughout the evaluation, a repeat chest radiograph at 2 months should be done to check for response to therapy. No other chest radiographs are needed during the course of therapy. A chest radiograph at the time of completion of therapy should be done to serve as the new baseline study with which future radiographs will be compared.

PARADOXICAL REACTIONS

Although more typically seen in the current era with HIV co-infection, paradoxical reactions have been described with antituberculosis therapy before the HIV epidemic. A paradoxical reaction appears to indicate a worsening of disease or failure of treatment when in actuality it is occurring during adequate therapy. Symptoms occur weeks into therapy and may include a return of cough or fever, enlarging lymph nodes, a chest radiograph with worsening of prior infiltrates or development of new infiltrates, effusions, or adenopathy. In the HIV-infected TB case, paradoxical reactions are related to the initiation of effective anti-HIV therapy. This may occur in the early, mid, or late stages of TB treatment, but are more common as the HIV therapy initiation is closer to the initiation of TB therapy. In the more advanced HIV-infected, care must be taken not to assume these symptoms are related to TB. They may also signify an immune reconstitution reaction to other disseminated infections such as histoplasmosis, cryptococcus, or *Mycobacterium avium* complex. These events should prompt a review of all data, including laboratory results of cultures and sensitivities, and assessment of adherence to therapy. In patients with no prior HIV testing, it should be recommended again at this time. Records of adherence from public health administered directly observed therapy are invaluable to evaluate the possibility of treatment failure. If all other etiologies are ruled out, consideration may be given to administration of steroids to moderate the reaction.

Tuberculosis and HIV Co-Infection

HIV infection alters the natural history and presentation of tuberculosis. In the non–HIV-infected person there is a 10% lifetime risk of developing TB after infection. If a person with LTBI becomes infected with HIV, the risk for active TB approaches 7% per year. A person without HIV who is newly infected by TB has a 5% risk of developing TB in the next 1 to 2 years. Depending upon the degree of immunosuppression, an HIV-infected person has up to a 40% risk of developing active TB within the first year after infection. Additionally, HIV-related TB is more likely to present as primary infection with noncavitating pulmonary infiltrates in the middle and lower lobes, pleural effusions, and hilar adenopathy. Because of this dramatic alteration of ability to control TB infection, many active cases of TB are in persons with HIV infection. Thus, all patients with active TB should be tested for HIV infection. In many U.S. urban areas, the HIV rate in TB cases may be 20%. Also, to properly interpret a tuberculin skin test a person's risk for HIV needs to be assessed. As noted in Table 1, a 5-mm reaction is significant if HIV infection is known, but is not significant for the majority of those tested.

Performing HIV testing in TB cases can help make an earlier diagnosis of HIV infection, preventing an opportunistic infection in the future. Should a person with TB be diagnosed with HIV, a question about the timing of therapy for HIV arises. The therapies for HIV and TB have multiple drug–drug interactions. If a person with HIV/TB does not have an imminent need for HIV therapy, it is likely best to complete treatment of TB prior to starting HIV therapy. If it is determined that HIV therapy is necessary before the completion of TB therapy, treatment should be done in consultation with a healthcare provider experienced in such dual therapy. The primary concern in dual therapy is the interaction of rifampin with HIV medications in the protease inhibitor and non-nucleoside reverse transcriptase inhibitor classes. Rifampin induces the hepatic cytochrome P450 metabolic pathway, which results in accelerated metabolism and reduced drug levels of these HIV medications. Such lowered drug levels can result in treatment failure because of HIV drug resistance. In general, rifabutin (Mycobutin) can be substituted for rifampin without altering the antituberculosis efficacy, but it greatly reduces the degree of enzyme induction. Much is still to be learned about these drug interactions; the practitioner supervising the treatment of either TB or

HIV, or both, needs to consult the most recent guidelines available through the CDC or the AIDS Treatment Information Service of the National Institutes of Health (NIH) at www.AIDSinfo.nih.gov.

Disease Caused by Nontuberculous Mycobacteria

Once considered the realm of pulmonary consultants, nontuberculous mycobacteria (NTM) are becoming more important causes of pulmonary disease, especially as TB becomes less common, the general population ages, and the prevalence of chronic obstructive pulmonary disease (COPD) increases. Many of the NTM are ubiquitous in the environment and can colonize airways, may cause transient infection, or even contaminate clinical specimens. A decision to make a diagnosis of disease caused by NTM involves an analysis of symptoms, radiographic findings, and culture data (Table 3).

CLINICAL AND RADIOGRAPHIC FEATURES

Much like TB, disease caused by NTM is characterized by a slow progression over time and is symptomatic with chronic cough, fever, night sweats, and weight loss. Hemoptysis may also occur. Radiographic findings are also similar to TB with the most common finding being upper lobe pulmonary disease that is fibrotic and/or cavitary. There is often evidence of underlying pulmonary disease such as COPD, healed TB, silicosis, or even malignancy. Tuberculin skin tests may exhibit some cross-reactivity to NTM, but the recommended cut-points (see Table 1) take this into consideration. A significant reaction to tuberculin skin testing should be interpreted to indicate LTBI, even in the setting of confirmed NTM. Upon presentation there is usually no way to distinguish NTM from TB. In the interest of the patient and public health, anti-TB therapy is often to be initiated before receiving the laboratory report of the final culture results. Respiratory isolation should be maintained in institutional settings until TB is ruled out.

TABLE 3 Criteria for Diagnosing Pulmonary Disease Caused by Nontuberculous Mycobacteria* in HIV-Positive and HIV-Negative Individuals

Symptoms	Cough, fatigue, sputum, weight loss, hemoptysis not solely explained by an underlying condition.
and Radiographic abnormalities	Cavities, infiltrates, nodules. High-resolution computed tomography, and multifocal bronchiectasis and/or multiple tiny nodules. Radiographic findings not explained by another condition.
and Sputum/bronchial washings grow NTM	3 sputum/bronchial washing specimens are available from previous 12 mo *and* 3 cultures are positive but AFB smears are negative or 2 cultures are positive and 1 AFB smear is positive *or* 1 bronchial washing is available *and* culture is positive with a 2+, 3+, or 4+ AFB smear *or* 2+, 3+, or 4+ growth on solid media.
or Lung biopsy	Culture positive for NTM *or* Lung biopsy shows granulomas and/or positive AFB *and* 1 or more sputum/bronchial washing are culture-positive for NTM.

*These criteria apply best to disease caused by *Mycobacterium avium* complex, *Mycobacterium* kansasii, and *Mycobacterium abscessus*.

Abbreviations: AFB = acid-fast bacillus; NTM = nontuberculous mycobacteria.

TREATMENT REGIMENS

Like the treatment of active TB, treatment of NTM requires prolonged multidrug therapy. Because of the lack of person-to-person transmission and thus any public health concerns, there is no option for directly observed therapy via local public health authorities. Often, TB is suspected and such therapy will be initiated and this can be done through directly observed therapy. Once NTM is diagnosed, directly observed therapy will no longer be provided. The two most common disease-causing NTM are *M. avium* complex (MAC) and *Mycobacterium kansasii*. Both can be successfully controlled initially by any of the four–drug anti-TB regimens, but therapy can be tailored to the causative organism once it is identified. MAC therapy uses a macrolide antibiotic, either clarithromycin (Biaxin) (500 mg twice daily) or azithromycin (Zithromax) (250 mg once daily), plus ethambutol (Myambutol)[1] (25 mg/kg once daily) plus either rifampin (Rifadin)[1] (600 mg once daily) or rifabutin (300 mg once daily). In HIV-infected patients with disseminated MAC, effective therapy has been only a macrolide plus ethambutol, which allows for the more important anti-HIV therapy to continue without the drug interactions of the rifamycins. *M. kansasii* is treated with antituberculous doses of isoniazid[1] plus rifampin[1] plus ethambutol[1].

Duration of therapy is generally recommended to be 12 months of therapy after culture conversion, which often occurs around month 6. Thus, 18 months of therapy is usually taken as a full course. With the amount of underlying lung disease present in many patients, therapy is often extended because of persistent positive cultures. In patients with advanced HIV infection, therapy was formerly considered lifelong. The increasing efficacy of anti-HIV therapy has allowed recovery of some immune function and these relatively low-grade pathogens are often contained by the reconstituted immunity. Still, therapy is continued as long as cultures are positive; discontinuation is considered after at least 12 months of therapy, with negative cultures, and upon recovery of the CD4+ lymphocyte count.

[1]Not FDA approved for this indication.

SECTION **5**

The Cardiovascular System

ACQUIRED DISEASES OF THE AORTA

METHOD OF

Karthikeshwar Kasirajan, MD, and Robert B. Smith III, MD

Acquired diseases of the aorta range from occlusive disease to aneurysmal degeneration. The majority of these are secondary to atherosclerosis and have the same risk factors. Less common disorders that occur more commonly in the thoracic aorta (dissection, penetrating ulcers, intramural hematoma) are being recognized with increasing frequency, especially due to better imaging modalities. New imaging techniques such as computed tomography (CT), magnetic resonance angiogram (MRA), transesophageal echocardiography (TEE), and intravascular ultrasound (IVUS) have improved the detection of diseases of the aorta. These techniques not only provide a better visualization of the aorta but also a better understanding of the pathogenesis of aortic diseases, which have led to new strategies for decision-making and patient management.

Aneurysms of the Aorta

THORACIC AND THORACOABDOMINAL AORTIC ANEURYSM

The incidence of thoracic aortic aneurysms is reported to be 10.4% per 100,000 person-years. However, the prevalence of thoracic and thoracoabdominal aortic aneurysms in the United States is difficult to determine precisely, because of under-reporting of these aneurysms in mortality statistics. In a study from Malmö, Sweden, which has a stable urban population and an autopsy rate of 83%, the overall incidence of thoracic aortic aneurysms between 1958 and 1985 was 489 per 100,000 autopsies in men and 437 per 100,000 autopsies in women. The prevalence of asymptomatic thoracic aneurysms was about 400 per 100,000 autopsies in 65-year-olds and about 670 per 100,000 autopsies in 80-year-olds. Thoracoabdominal aneurysms made up 5% of all asymptomatic thoracic aneurysms.

Fatalities following rupture of thoracic aneurysms have been reported to be as high as 74% to 94%. Aneurysms limited to the descending thoracic aorta comprise a subgroup of this, with an incidence of 2.21 per 100,000 patient-years, and a reported fatality rate from rupture of 40%.

Indications for Surgery

Ascending Aorta

Degenerative aneurysms that are confined to the ascending aorta are treated by graft replacement of the involved segment when the diameter of the aorta exceeds 5.0 to 5.5 cm or if symptoms are present.

Aortic Arch

The aortic arch is anatomically defined as the segment of the thoracic aorta that extends from the proximal origin of the innominate artery to the distal origin of the left subclavian artery. Because of the risk of neurologic injury, elective surgery is generally advised only for aneurysms that are more than 5.5 to 6.0 cm in diameter. Patients with symptoms attributable to the aneurysm and those with documented progressive enlargement should undergo surgical treatment. Aneurysms of the aortic arch are often associated with aneurysms of the ascending or descending aorta, and these associated dilatations may be the principal indication for surgery.

Descending Thoracic Aorta

For patients with degenerative or chronic aneurysm, elective resection is advisable if the aneurysm exceeds 5 to 6 cm in diameter or if symptoms are present.

Thoracoabdominal Aneurysms

Elective surgery is indicated in symptomatic patients and patients whose aneurysm or chronic dissection exceeds 5 to 6 cm in diameter.

Preoperative Evaluation

Myocardial infarction, respiratory failure, renal failure, and stroke are the principal causes of death and morbidity after operations on the thoracic aorta. Because of the high prevalence of coronary atherosclerotic heart disease in older persons, assessment of cardiac function is essential in patients in whom elective operation is contemplated, particularly those older than age 50 years and those with a history of myocardial infarction. Patients with symptoms or electrocardiographic changes indicative of myocardial ischemia or infarction should undergo stress testing and coronary arteriography when indicated. Patients with valvular heart disease are evaluated with echocardiography and cardiac catheterization. Clinically significant coronary artery disease should be treated with angioplasty or bypass grafting, and valvular heart disease should be treated with valve replacement or repair before or, in some cases, during the procedure on the thoracic aorta.

History of smoking and the presence of chronic pulmonary disease are important predictors of respiratory failure. Pulmonary function tests should be performed, when possible, in patients with these risk factors. Spirometric tests and arterial blood gas analysis should be performed in patients with chronic pulmonary disease. If reversible restrictive disease or excessive sputum production is present, antibiotics and bronchodilators should be administered. Cessation of smoking is highly recommended.

The presence of preoperative renal dysfunction is the most important predictor of acute renal failure. Adequate preoperative hydration and avoidance of hypotension, low cardiac output, and hypovolemia in the perioperative period are important mechanisms for reducing the incidence of this complication. To minimize the risk of stroke or reversible ischemic neurologic deficits, duplex imaging of the carotid arteries and angiography of the brachiocephalic and intracranial arteries, when indicated, should be performed preoperatively in patients with a history of stroke, transient ischemic attacks, or other risk factors for cerebrovascular disease. Patients with greater than 80% stenosis of one or both common or internal carotid arteries should be considered for carotid endarterectomy before elective operations on the thoracic aorta.

Preoperative Aortic Imaging

Computed Tomography

This is the most commonly used noninvasive technique for the diagnosis of thoracic aortic disease. It provides information about the size, location, extent of the disease, and, for endograft patients, the status of the proximal and distal landing vessels. It is also valuable for follow-up information. Additionally, approximately 25% of patients have aneurysms in more than one area of the aorta; hence, both the thoracic and the abdominal aorta should be examined. The main disadvantage of the technique is that it requires the use of a radiopaque contrast agent, and this may be contraindicated in patients with allergies to contrast agents or with renal insufficiency.

Magnetic Resonance Imaging

Magnetic resonance imaging (MRI) is emerging as the premier imaging method for the diagnosis of diseases of the thoracic aorta. Standard techniques do not require the use of contrast medium. In certain applications, a single study can provide information similar to that obtained from a combination of echocardiography, CT, and angiography. The current disadvantages include greater cost, inaccessibility to patients who are connected to ventilators and monitoring devices, and limited availability.

Transesophageal Echocardiography

Transesophageal echocardiography with color Doppler imaging is being used with increasing frequency for the diagnosis of thoracic aortic disease and for the care of patients who undergo surgery of the thoracic aorta. It is distinctly superior to transthoracic echocardiography for these purposes.

During operations on the thoracic aorta, transesophageal echocardiography is invaluable for assessing the presence of atherosclerosis in the thoracic aorta; it establishes the competency of the aortic valve before cardiopulmonary bypass and the adequacy of reparative procedures on the valve. It also provides information about ventricular performance and the function of the mitral and tricuspid valves.

Aortography

Aortography is usually required for most patients undergoing elective operations on the thoracic aorta. It provides information about the location of the aneurysm, length of the aneurysm, access vessels for endograft insertion, and the relation of the aneurysm to the major branches of the aorta in the chest and upper abdomen. It can also detect the presence of aortic regurgitation. Selective injections of the coronary, brachiocephalic, visceral, and renal arteries provide important information that permits more accurate assessment of operative risk and may demonstrate the need for modifications in operative technique. The major disadvantages of aortography are the risk of allergic reactions to contrast medium and the risk of renal failure in patients with impaired renal function.

Treatment and Results

The most commonly performed procedure for the ascending aorta is replacement of the ascending aorta and the aortic valve with a composite graft containing a Dacron graft and mechanical valve prosthesis. The coronary arteries are implanted in the Dacron graft. Alternative treatments include the use of aortic allografts and procedures that remove the diseased aorta but preserve the aortic valve. Although not widely practiced clinically, the concept of wrapping the aorta may be a reasonable alternative to replacement in older, higher risk patients with limited life expectancy undergoing operations for other cardiac pathologies. In a comparative series, the early and late results among 390 patients undergoing separate valve graft repair (255 patients) or composite root replacement (135) were compared. The type of operation was not predictive of either early or late mortality on multivariate analysis. Data from these studies indicate that an average of 5% of patients develop recurrent aortic root aneurysms 6 to 9 years after supracoronary graft replacement.

Operations on the aortic arch usually require the use of hypothermic cardiopulmonary bypass and a period of circulatory arrest. With current techniques, a period of circulatory arrest of up to 30 to 40 minutes at a body temperature of 15°C to 18°C (27°F to 32°F) is well tolerated by the majority of patients. Focal or diffuse neurologic deficits are the major complications associated with resection of aneurysms of the aortic arch and occur in 3% to 18% of patients. Permanent neurologic injury occurs less frequently.

Descending thoracic aortic aneurysms have traditionally been repaired by open surgical graft replacement. Morbidity and mortality associated with this procedure continue to be significant despite considerable improvements in management strategies. In a recent report involving 224 patients, the 30-day mortality rate was 14.3%. The major cause of death was cardiac problems (50%). In addition to the cardiac mortality, two other dreaded complications, renal failure and paraplegia, have been reported to be as high as 26% and 18%, respectively. Endovascular stent grafting of the descending thoracic aorta is receiving increasing attention, as it is a promising, less-invasive alternative to open surgical repair. Given a choice, most patients would opt for a simpler, less invasive, less painful procedure, but most vascular surgeons prefer a curative procedure as opposed to palliation, since endovascular stent-grafting does not provide definitive freedom from rupture. However, in an older, sicker population, lack of certainty about a long-term cure after endovascular stent-graft repair seems less relevant (Figure 1). Thus, the decision to recommend one type of thoracic aortic aneurysm treatment over another is quite subjective, varies among institutions, and is governed by anatomic factors, co-morbid conditions, the technical skills of the operator, and the availability and accessibility of the resources. In properly selected patients, endovascular repair appears to be comparable with the conventional open repair.

Thoracoabdominal aneurysms involving the visceral vessels are not amenable to endograft repair with the currently generation of devices. Aneurysm replacement with reimplantation of the visceral vessels is the current standard of care. With current techniques, elective resection of thoracoabdominal aortic aneurysms can be accomplished with an operative mortality of 7% to 12%.

Aortic Dissection

Aortic dissection is defined as a disruption of the aortic wall, forming an intimal flap and therefore separating a true from a false lumen (Figure 2). Aortic dissection is differentiated into type A and type B according to the Stanford classification. In type A the ascending and descending aorta are involved, while in type B only the descending aorta is involved. In type A dissection the patient is monitored for emergency signs including pericardial effusion, pleural effusion, periaortic fluid extravasation, and compression of the left atrium. A mortality of more than 50% results when these signs are present, so surgical treatment has to start without delay. Surgery in aortic dissection type B is restricted to patients with signs of aortic expansion, persistence or recurrence of chest pain, and emergency signs.

Imaging is the same as for thoracic aneurysms. Currently, the preferred imaging modality is MRA (Figure 3). Use of an MRA fulfills all diagnostic requirements; tears are detected and side branch involvement, even of coronary arteries, can be evaluated.

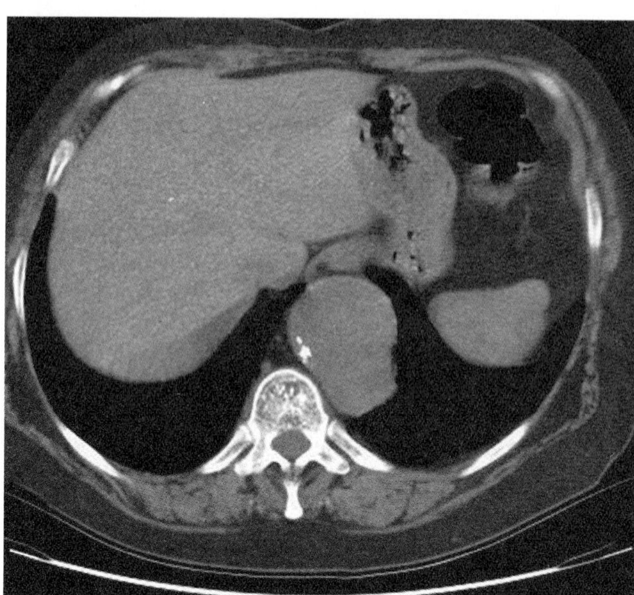
A

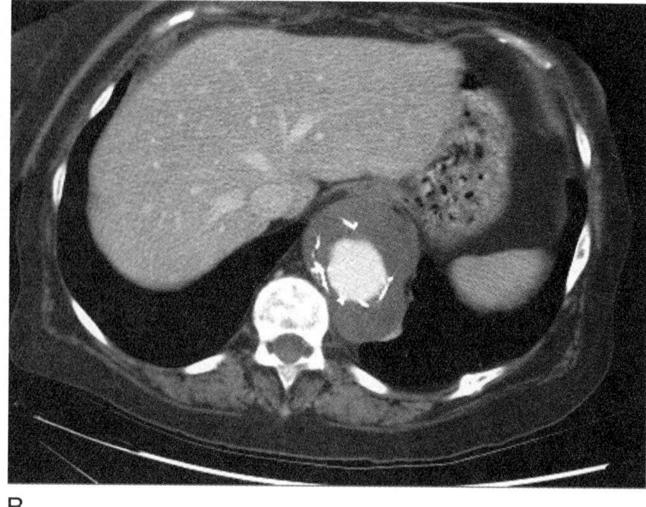
B

FIGURE 1 A. Preoperative computed tomogram in a high-risk patient with a symptomatic thoracic aneurysm. B. Endograft exclusion of the thoracic aneurysm.

TREATMENT

Surgery is indicated in type A dissection because it has a high mortality rate, which can be reduced but not completely eliminated by operation. The perioperative surgical mortality continues to be as high as 20% to 35%. Treatment includes replacement of the ascending aorta with or without aortic valve prosthesis. Surgery in acute type B dissection has a mortality of more than 30%. The major morbidity is the high rate (up to 30%) of paraplegia, which can be observed after this procedure, despite the availability of more sophisticated techniques for spinal cord protection. Open surgical graft replacement of the entry flap is rapidly being replaced with endovascular stent graft placement for sealing the entry tear. Endovascular

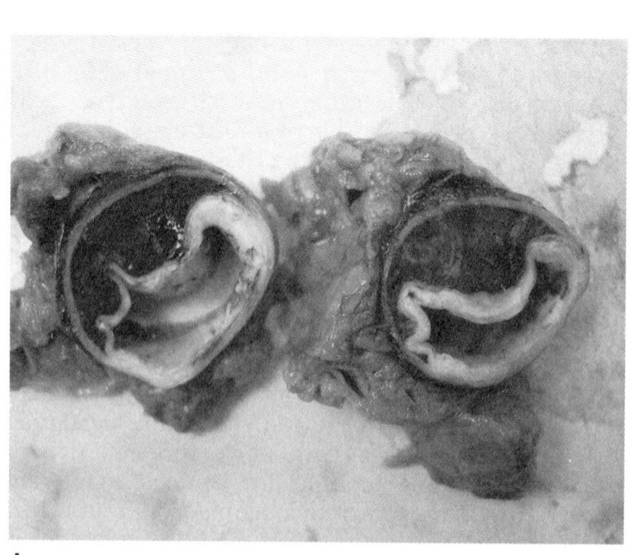
A

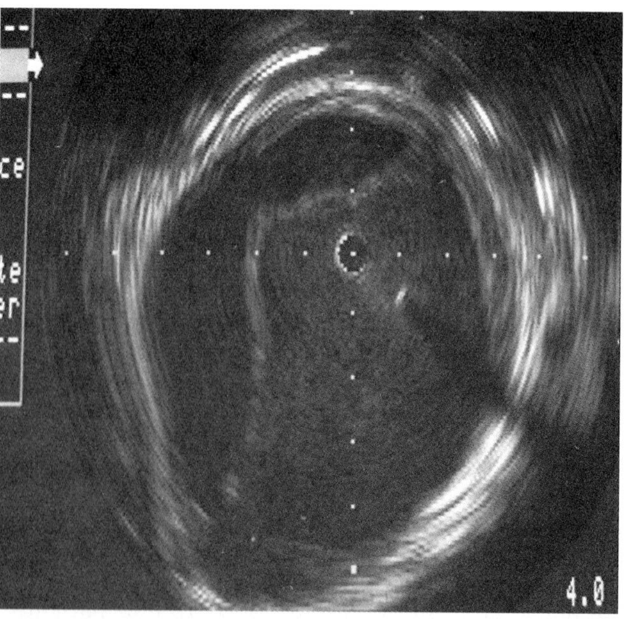

B

FIGURE 2 A. Cross-section of the aorta in a deceased patient with aortic dissection. B. Intravascular ultrasound demonstrates a true and false lumen in the same patient with dissection.

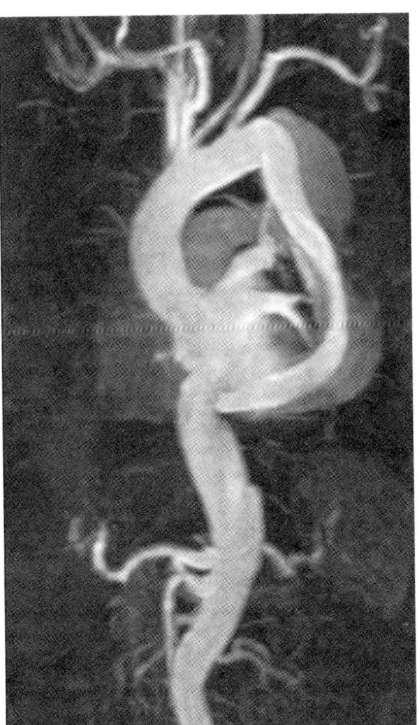

FIGURE 3 Magnetic resonance angiogram (MRA) in a patient with a type B dissection.

stent-grafting poses both advantages and limitations. For example, the avoidance of thoracotomy potentially reduces the incidence of pulmonary complications, and patients with severe pulmonary compromise may not tolerate the single-lung ventilation that is needed for the ideal exposure of the descending thoracic aorta for open repair. In addition, avoiding the cross-clamping of the aorta may reduce complications such as paraplegia, renal failure, myocardial infarction, heart failure, and downstream embolization. Spinal cord ischemia with resultant paraplegia is of significant concern to all surgeons treating descending thoracic aortic aneurysms, and the endovascular stent-graft has the potential to reduce this complication in patients who are at high risk for spinal cord ischemia.

Penetrating Thoracic Ulcers and Intramural Hematoma

When patients with a diagnosis of penetrating thoracic ulcers have been followed conservatively, the majority have progressive aortic enlargement, with formation of saccular or fusiform pseudoaneurysms and intraluminal thrombus. Dissection, embolization, and rupture can also occur. In a series of 13 patients with intramural hematomas who were not treated surgically, the 30-day mortality rate was 46%. The highest mortality rate (71%) occurred among patients in whom the hematoma originated in the ascending aorta and aortic arch. Patients with severe atherosclerosis (plaques greater than 4 mm in depth) of the ascending aorta and arch have a high prevalence of atheromatous emboli in the cerebral circulation. These emboli are probably a major cause of cerebral infarction. Patients with severe ascending aortic atherosclerosis are at risk for embolization and stroke after manipulation of the ascending aorta during coronary-artery bypass grafting and other cardiac surgical procedures. When severe atheromatous disease is present in the distal aortic arch and the descending thoracic aorta, embolization to the visceral, renal, and peripheral arteries can occur.

Patients with symptomatic penetrating ulcers or intramural hematomas need to be repaired with open surgical graft replacement or endograft coverage if in a favorable location (Figure 4).

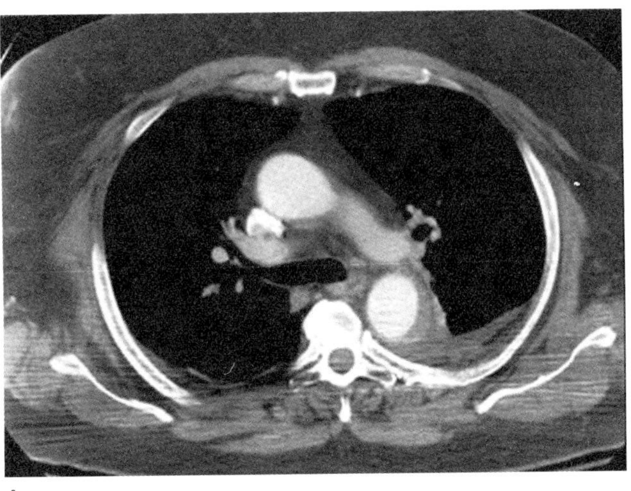

A

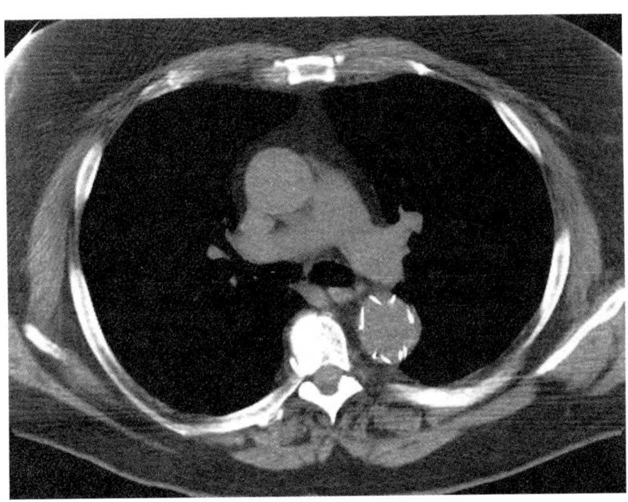

B

FIGURE 4 A. Penetrating ulcer with an expanding intramural hematoma. B. Disappearance of the intramural hematoma following endograft placement at 1-month follow-up visit.

Abdominal Aortic Aneurysms

Abdominal aortic aneurysm (AAA) remains the 13th leading cause of death for males in the United States. The prevalence of abdominal aortic aneurysms among men is about three times greater than in women, and women younger than 55 years of age rarely have such aneurysms. Aneurysms greater than 4 cm are found in about 1% of men 55 to 64 years of age, and the prevalence increases by 2% to 4% per decade thereafter. Atherosclerosis is considered to be the main etiology for abdominal aortic aneurysms, as studies show a positive relation between aneurysms and other cardiovascular diseases and related markers. Smoking is the strongest independent risk factor. Compared with persons who have never smoked, the incidence of aneurysm is increased by a factor of six among those who have smoked for more than 40 years and by a factor of seven among those who have smoked more than 20 cigarettes per day. The risk of rupture of a 5- to 6-cm aneurysm is approximately 20% within 5 years.

Currently, it is recommended that treatment be considered when aneurysms reach a diameter of 5 cm or when aneurysms of any size are symptomatic. The presence of acute abdominal, back or, flank pain in a patient with a known aneurysm is an indication for emergency surgery, as this may indicate an impending rupture (Figure 5). Screening intervals of 12 months are recommended for aneurysms with diameters of 3 to 4.4 cm, and 6-month intervals for aneurysms greater than 4.5 cm.

IMAGING AND TREATMENT

Preoperative risk factor evaluation for AAA is similar to patients with thoracic aortic aneurysm. CT scan is reliable in estimating the size of the aneurysm and gives details for evaluation for endograft placement. Routine preoperative angiograms are not required unless the aneurysm is juxtarenal or suprarenal, in order to evaluate the status of the visceral vessels in relation to the aneurysm. Treatment is either by open surgical graft placement or by endograft exclusion. Conventional open repair of aneurysms by replacement with a graft is a major surgical procedure. However, the expectation that endovascular repair poses less operative risk than conventional repair remains unproven in patients with minimal systemic risk factors. However, patients' preferences for treatment, including the potential timing of any corrective procedure, should be considered. Endografts have the advantages of earlier returns to work and shorter hospital stays. Endovascular repair is becoming the clear choice for repair in higher risk patients with abdominal aortic aneurysms who have suitable anatomic criteria. Yet open aneurysm repair remains the gold standard for the healthy or younger patient in whom durability is a concern, given that studies have only begun to examine the long-term results of endovascular repair. The future holds promise because such endovascular treatment offers the economic advantages of short hospital stays or even treatment as an outpatient, as well as elimination of the need for postoperative intensive care. Of more importance is the potential for improved patient care. If endovascular grafting proves effective and durable, selective screening of the elderly to identify the most suitable candidates for such therapy, even those with abdominal aortic aneurysms of less than 4 cm in diameter, may substantially reduce the mortality rate from this disease.

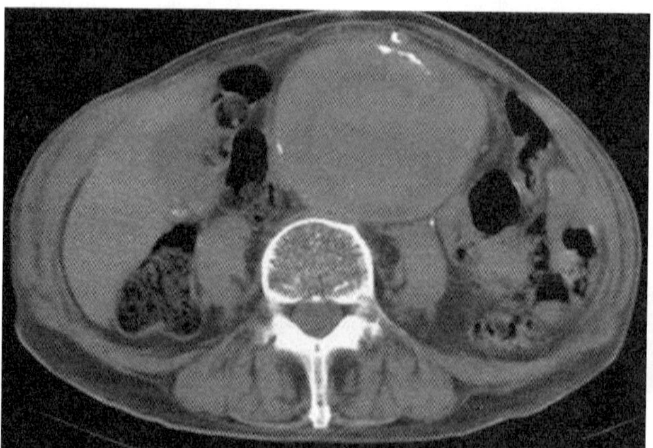

FIGURE 5 Symptomatic infrarenal abdominal aortic aneurysm.

Aortoiliac Occlusive Disease

Occlusive disease of the aorta is rarely seen in the suprarenal aortic segments; occlusion or stenosis is more common at the location of the aortic bifurcation. Such patients often have claudication symptoms but rarely does proximal aortic occlusive disease result in tissue gangrene, unless accompanied by distal embolization or infrainguinal occlusive disease. Most patients have significant atherosclerotic risk factors, especially a history of smoking.

DIAGNOSIS

Symptoms of buttock claudication with diminished femoral pulses on clinical examination are highly indicative of aortoiliac occlusive disease. The next study is usually a noninvasive measurement of ankle-brachial index and a pulse volume recording (PVR). A diminished thigh pressure and waveform suggest proximal occlusive disease. An angiogram is then obtained depending on the need for intervention, which is based on the severity of symptoms. Occasionally, for patients with absent femoral pulses, a transbrachial aortogram may be required for access (Figure 6). Patients with elevated creatinine levels or who are allergic to contrast agents can be evaluated with an MRA. If open surgical intervention is contemplated, cardiac stress testing is mandatory and a coronary angiogram is obtained if indicated.

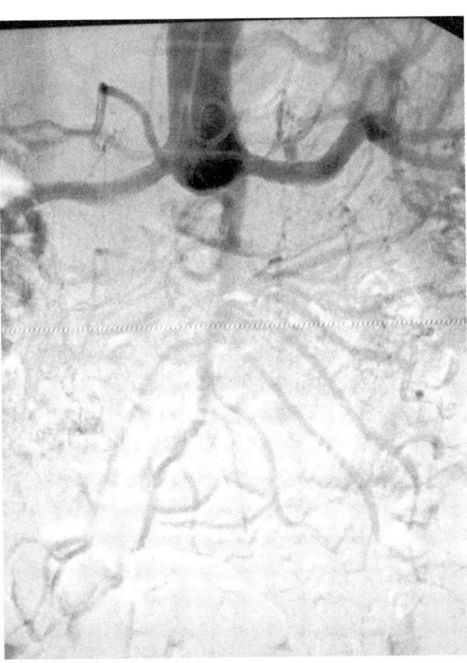

FIGURE 6 Transbrachial abdominal aortogram in a patient with total aortic occlusion.

As atherosclerosis is a global process, the presence of peripheral vaso-occlusive disease is often an indicator of significant coronary artery disease. Identification and correction of coronary artery disease takes a high priority in these patients to minimize perioperative complications and improve long-term survival. Patients with a history of smoking are also evaluated with pulmonary function tests. Smoking cessation and risk factor optimization are beneficial for decreasing procedural complications and improving long-term survival.

TREATMENT

Revascularization for aorto-occlusive disease has traditionally been achieved in good-risk patients by aortobifemoral bypass grafting (ABF), or in higher risk patients by femorofemoral (FF) or axillobifemoral (AxBF) bypass grafting. Although these procedures are very effective (5-year patencies of 70% to 80%) and low risk (30-day mortalities of 1% or less for ABF; 2% to 5% for FF, AxBF), they are not performed without significant morbidity or hospital stays. Hence, less invasive techniques such as balloon angioplasty and stenting have received increasing attention. In the presence of iliac occlusive disease, angioplasty and stents are the preferred option to treat stenosis, and open surgery is reserved for patients with an occlusive disease pattern. Angioplasty for short segment stenosis in the aortoiliac location has patency rates comparable with open surgery (5-year patency of more than 80%), with less morbidity and mortality.

MANAGEMENT OF ANGINA PECTORIS

METHOD OF

Srikanth Ramachandruni, MD, and
David S. Sheps, MD, MSPH

Classical angina is pain or discomfort usually caused by coronary ischemia. It typically occurs in patients with coronary artery disease (CAD) involving one or more epicardial arteries. Classical angina occurs with exertion or emotional distress and is relieved by rest or nitroglycerin. Atypical angina has other features.

Diagnosis

Careful characterization of a patient's chest pain should be part of the detailed history and physical examination with which a physician establishes the probable presence of significant CAD as defined by a 70% or greater diameter stenosis of one or more major epicardial artery segments, or a 50% or greater diameter stenosis of the left main coronary artery. The physician should determine whether the patient's chest pain is *squeezing, dull aching, crushing, pressure-like, burning,* or *heavy*. Some patients report their physical symptoms as just *discomfort* and *tightness*. The pain of myocardial ischemia may radiate to the neck, throat, lower jaw, teeth, upper extremity, or shoulder. Noncoronary explanations of the chest pain must be ruled out. Pain made worse by movement and respirations may be musculoskeletal in origin. Pain increasing with deep inspiration is pleural based and usually worsens with lying down. Constant pain over several days and related to swallowing suggests gastrointestinal causes. Other causes of chest pain of great concern are aortic dissection, a hemodynamically significant pulmonary embolus, a ruptured abdominal aortic aneurysm, or critical aortic stenosis (particularly if the patient has a history of exertional dyspnea).

Pain that is typically aggravated by exertion and other activities such as cold, emotional stress, and sexual intercourse usually indicates ischemic origin. The onset of ischemic pain is most often gradual with an increasing intensity over time. The pain from myocardial ischemia generally lasts for a few minutes; more prolonged pain may be a sign of myocardial infarction (MI). A wide extension of chest pain radiation increases the probability that it is caused by MI.

The type and extent of chest pain evaluation the physician chooses to perform should be guided by his or her knowledge of the patient's risk factors and consequent disease likelihood. Table 1 identifies key precipitating conditions for angina. Table 2 lists the

TABLE 1 Conditions Known to Precipitate Angina

1. Hyperthermia
2. Hyperthyroidism
3. Uncontrolled tachyarrhythmia
4. Cocaine abuse
5. Anemia
6. Pulmonary conditions
7. Increased blood viscosity (leukemias, polycythemias, thrombocytosis, and hypergammaglobulinemia)

risk factors predictive of angina; of the factors shown, diabetes increases risk the most.

The physical examination may also aid risk stratification by determining the presence or absence of signs and symptoms that could alter the probability of severe CAD. Complete cardiac examination, including auscultation and palpation, should be performed in both the sitting and supine positions to establish the presence of a pericardial rub or signs of acute aortic insufficiency or aortic stenosis. Evidence of atherosclerosis/vascular disease (such as abnormal fundi, carotid bruit, and/or absence of pedal pulses) combined with male gender and previous MI nearly double the risk for severe CAD. In addition to peripheral vascular disease, signs and symptoms related to congestive heart failure (CHF), which reflect poor left ventricular (LV) function, convey an adverse prognosis. (It need also be recognized that patients with decreased LV function may not have any signs or symptoms of CHF.) Presence of an S_4 is also indicative of increased diastolic resistance from long-standing hypertension. A mitral regurgitation (MR) murmur may be indicative of papillary muscle rupture from MI. A marked difference in blood pressure between the two arms suggests the presence of aortic dissection.

Electrocardiography (ECG) and chest radiograph are initial diagnostic tests that can provide valuable information. ECG changes such as ST segment elevation, ST segment depression, new Q waves, and T-wave abnormalities suggest the likelihood of ischemia. Q waves in multiple leads indicate poor LV function and adverse prognosis. Likewise, the presence of the following suggest a poor prognosis:

- ST–T-wave abnormalities in V1-V3
- Left bundle branch block
- Bifascicular block
- Second and third degree atrioventricular (AV) blocks
- Presence of LV hypertrophy
- Atrial fibrillation
- Ventricular tachyarrhythmia

TABLE 2 Predictors of Coronary Artery Disease

1. Smoking ≥½ pack of cigarettes per day within 5 years, or at least 25 pack-years
2. Q wave or ST–T-wave changes
3. Hyperlipidemia (cholesterol level >200 mg/dL)
4. Diabetes (glucose >140)
5. Family history of coronary artery disease
6. Hypertension
7. Obesity

Chest radiograph can exclude pneumothorax and pneumomediastinum. Fasting glucose, fasting lipid panel, and hemoglobin are other tests recommended for inclusion in the diagnostic workup. Stress testing is also an important part of the diagnostic workup.

The stratification of disease likelihood is important in assessing stress test results (Table 3). For example, in patients with an otherwise low probability of CAD (5%), the positive predictive value of an abnormal test result is only 21%; whereas, in patients with a high probability of CAD (90%), a positive test result raises the probability of disease to 98% and a negative test result lowers probability to 83%. Stress testing is most useful in patients with an intermediate pretest likelihood of disease. The flow chart in Figure 1 describes the risk stratification of patients with symptoms of angina.

Echocardiography to assess LV function is strongly indicated in patients with a prior MI, pathological Q waves, systolic murmur suggesting MR, or symptoms or signs suggestive of heart failure. A rest ejection fraction (EF) of less than 35% is associated with an annual mortality rate greater than 3% per year. Electron-beam computed tomography (EBCT) yields a calcium score that in a few studies appears to correlate well with atherosclerosis documented by coronary angiography. However, the role of EBCT needs to be further clarified in terms of risk stratifying patients and is not currently recommended as a screening test by the American Heart Association/American College of Cardiology (AHA/ACC) guidelines.

Treatment

Treatment involves modification of major cardiovascular risk factors, pharmacological therapy, and coronary revascularization.

TABLE 3 Probabilities* of Coronary Artery Disease (CAD) Based on Age, Gender, and Symptomatic Presentation

	Nonanginal Chest Pain		Atypical Chest Pain		Typical Chest Pain	
Age	**Men**	**Women**	**Men**	**Women**	**Men**	**Women**
30-39	4%	2%	34%	12%	76%	26%
40-49	13%	3%	51%	22%	87%	55%
50-59	20%	7%	65%	31%	93%	73%
60-69	27%	14%	72%	51%	94%	86%

*Based on percent of significant CAD (>70% narrowing of dominant coronary artery) found with cardiac catheterization.

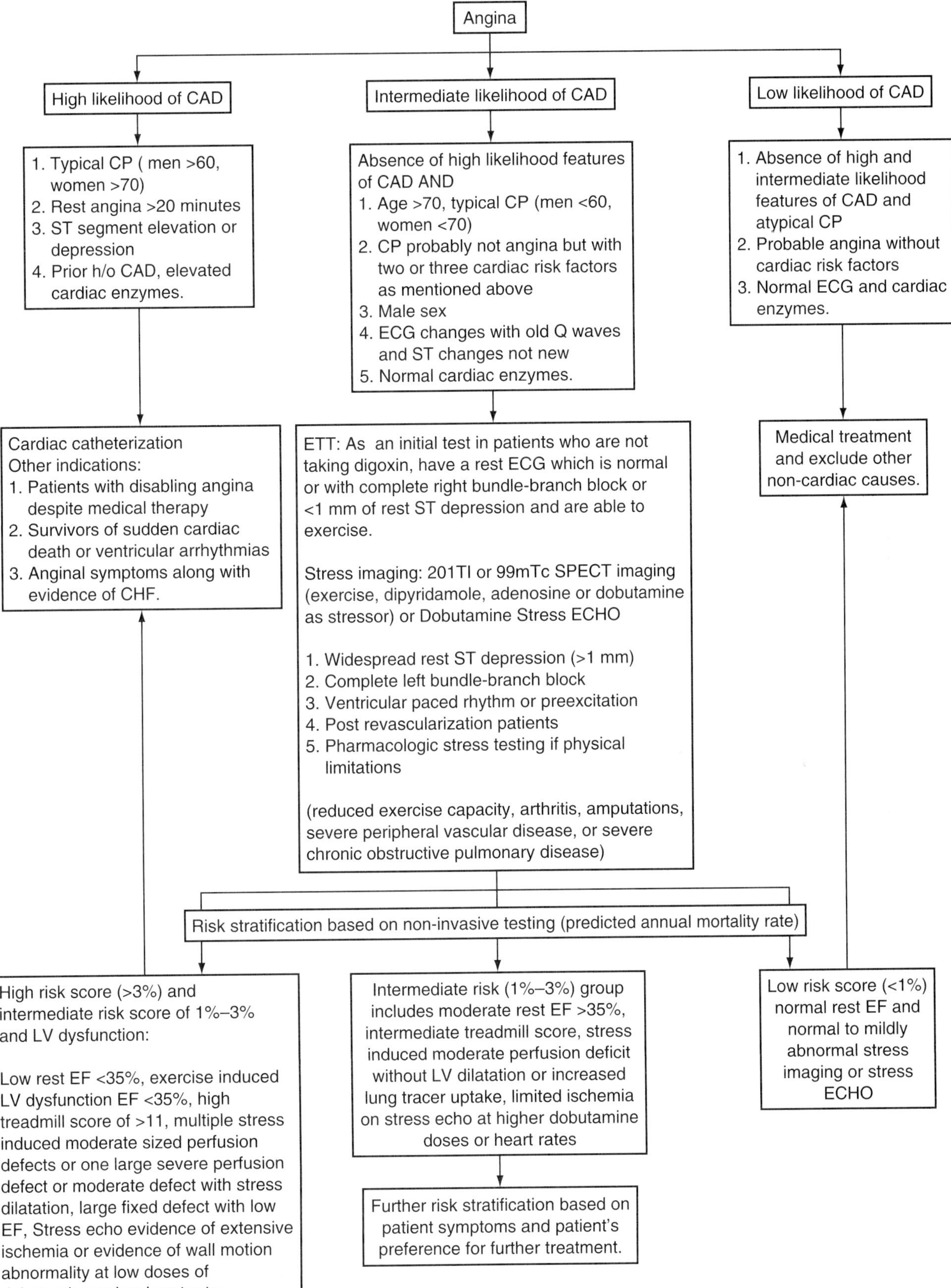

FIGURE 1 Angina algorithm.

MODIFICATION OF CARDIOVASCULAR RISK FACTORS

Hypertension

There is a continuous, graded relationship between blood pressure and the risk of CAD. Guidelines for classifying hypertension from the seventh report of the Joint National Committee on Prevention, Detection, Evaluation, and Treatment of High Blood Pressure (JNC VII) appear in Table 4. Lifestyle modifications are indicated for all patients with blood pressure above 140/90 mm Hg or—in patients with diabetes or chronic kidney disease—above 130/80 mm Hg. Patients with Stage 1 hypertension can be treated with lifestyle modifications alone for up to 1 year, if they have no other risk factors, or for up to 6 months, if they have other risk factors. Treating hypertension has been linked to left ventricular hypertrophy (LVH) regression in several studies. In the Framingham Heart Study, LVH regression was associated with low cardiovascular mortality. Low salt intake, weight loss in obese individuals, moderation in alcohol intake, and a regular exercise regimen will lower blood pressure in the long term.

Diabetes

Cardiovascular disease is the most prevalent and detrimental complication of diabetes mellitus. In diabetics, microalbuminuria is a major predictor of cardiovascular events, most likely as a marker of generalized endothelial dysfunction in diabetes. The beneficial roles of angiotensin-converting enzyme inhibitors and angiotensin II blockers in patients with microalbuminuria are well established.

Lipid Abnormalities

Total cholesterol level has a continuous and graded relationship to the development of CAD events, beginning at levels of less than 180 mg/dL. Epidemiologic studies indicate a 2% to 3% increase in risk for coronary events per 1% increase in LDL-cholesterol level.

TABLE 4 Classification of Hypertension*

Category	Systolic Blood Pressure (mm Hg)	Diastolic Blood Pressure (mm Hg)	Treatment
Normal	<120	<80	None necessary
Prehypertension	120-139	80-89	None necessary
Stage 1 hypertension	140-159	80-99	Thiazides, CEI, ARB, BB, CCB
Stage 2 hypertension	≥160	≥100	Two-drug combination

*Based on guidelines contained in the seventh Report of the Joint National Committee on Prevention, Detection, Evaluation, and Treatment of High Blood Pressure.

Abbreviations: ARB = angiotensin receptor blocker; BB = β blocker; CCB = calcium channel blocker; CEI = converting enzyme inhibitor.

Measurements of LDL and HDL cholesterol are warranted in all patients with coronary disease. The publication of the Scandinavian Simvastatin Survival Study (4S), the Cholesterol And Recurrent Events (CARE) trial, and the Long-term Intervention with Pravastatin in Ischemic Disease (LIPID) trial supported the proposition that, in patients with established CAD and elevated LDL, statins reduced total and cardiac mortality and markedly reduced cardiovascular events. The Veteran's Administration HDL Intervention Trial (VA-HIT) showed the cardiovascular benefit of raising HDL-C. Lowering LDL to less than 100 *may* be beneficial in patients with CAD. Further studies are needed in this area, however.

Exercise

Several research studies have confirmed the benefits of a moderate amount of exercise for enhancing cardiovascular health. A lifelong appropriate physical activity regimen should include 30 to 60 minutes at least 5 days per week.

In addition to the above risk modification treatments, smoking cessation has an additive effect in improving cardiovascular mortality and morbidity.

PHARMACOLOGIC THERAPY

Antiplatelet Agents

The use of antithrombotic medication, especially aspirin (80 to 325 mg daily), is now well established. Aspirin decreased cardiovascular mortality by 30% to 40% in the Physicians' Health Study and the Swedish Angina Pectoris Aspirin Trial (SAPAT). The recent Clopidogrel in Unstable Angina and Recurrent Events (CURE) trial showed that the addition of 75 mg of clopidogrel (Plavix) resulted in a 16% reduction in cardiovascular events above that obtained with aspirin. Dipyridamole (Persantine) can enhance exercise-induced myocardial ischemia, and thus should be avoided. Ticlopidine (Ticlid) has not been shown to decrease adverse cardiovascular events.

Antianginal Medications

β Blockers or nitrates should be used for the initial treatment of stable angina. A calcium channel blocker should be considered if there are contraindications or adverse reactions to either β blockers of nitrates or if symptoms are not well controlled with a combination of these agents.

β Blockers

Cardioselective β blockers (atenolol [Tenormin] and metoprolol [Lopressor] are the most commonly used) offer the advantage of not interfering with bronchodilatation or peripheral vasodilatation. The dosage of β blockers is usually titrated to reduce heart rate at rest to 55 to 60 beats per minute. In one study, atenolol effectively suppressed angina and also reduced both resting and exercise-stressed heart

TABLE 5 Commonly Used β Blockers

Drug Name	Class	Dosage
Atenolol (Tenormin)	Cardioselective	25 mg to 100 mg qd
Metoprolol (Lopressor)	Cardioselective	25 mg bid to 100 mg bid
Carvedilol (Coreg)	Cardioselective	25 mg bid to 50 mg bid
Nadolol (Corgard)	Nonselective	25 mg qd to 240 mg qd
Propranolol (Inderal)	Nonselective	40 mg bid to 120 mg bid
Pindolol (Visken)[1]	Intrinsic sympathomimetic	5 mg bid to 30 mg bid

[1]Not FDA approved for this indication.

rates for 24 hours after ingestion when given in a 100-mg or 200-mg dose once daily. In the Carvedilol-Angina Study, 122 patients were randomized to receive carvedilol (Coreg) or placebo. Carvedilol* at doses of either 25 mg or 50 mg twice daily was found to be effective and safe in treating patients with chronic stable angina. In patients with pure vasospastic (Prinzmetal) angina without fixed, obstructive lesions, β blockers are ineffective and may increase the tendency to induce coronary vasospasm from unopposed α-receptor activity; thus, they should not be used, and calcium channel blockers are preferred. Commonly used β blocker preparations are listed in Table 5.

Calcium Channel Antagonists

Both of the two main categories of calcium channel blockers—the dihydropyridines (nifedipine [Adalat], amlodipine [Norvasc], nicardipine [Cardene], nitrendipine*, and others) and the nondihydropyridines (including verapamil [Verelan] and diltiazem [Cardizem])—cause coronary vasodilatation and reduce blood pressure. The dihydropyridines exert a greater effect than nondihydropyridines on vasodilatation, have a smaller inhibitory effect on both the sinus and AV nodes, and have a smaller negative inotropic effect. Addition of calcium channel blockade to β blockade reduces symptomatic and asymptomatic ischemic events in patients with chronic stable angina even further.

In patients with vasospastic (Prinzmetal) angina, calcium antagonists significantly reduce the incidence of angina. Long-acting nifedipine, diltiazem, and verapamil all appear to completely abolish the recurrence of angina in approximately 70% of patients; in another 20% of patients, the frequency of angina is reduced substantially. Amlodipine is also effective in vasospastic angina.

Nitroglycerin and Nitrates

Long-acting nitrate preparations such as isosorbide dinitrate (Isordil), mononitrates, transdermal nitroglycerin patches, and nitroglycerin ointment are used to prevent recurrence of angina. Nitrates are especially useful in patients with CHF, particularly at night in those with significant orthopnea or paroxysmal nocturnal dyspnea. In addition, patients with exertional dyspnea may benefit if nitrates are taken before exertion. Tolerance has been a major problem with the use of nitrates as chronic antianginal therapy. All long-acting nitrates, including isosorbide dinitrates and mononitrates, appear to be equally effective when a sufficient nitrate-free interval is provided. Sublingual nitroglycerin is the agent of choice in acute anginal episodes, with the usual dose being 0.3 mg to 0.4 mg repeated every 5 minutes for a total of three doses. A physician should be contacted if angina persists after rest and three sublingual nitroglycerin tablets. Isosorbide dinitrate is usually prescribed 10 mg to 40 mg three times a day (8 AM, 1 PM, and 6 PM) with a 14-hour drug-free interval. Isosorbide mononitrate is usually started at 30 mg a day and titrated up to 120 mg a day. Transdermal nitroglycerin (0.2 mg to 0.8 mg per hour) is applied 12 hours a day, preferably from 8 AM to 8 PM. Nocturnal anginal symptoms respond to nighttime application. Commonly used nitrate preparations are listed in Table 6.

Angiotensin-Converting Enzyme Inhibitors

Angiotensin-converting enzyme (ACE) inhibitors should be used as a routine secondary prevention for patients with known CAD, particularly in diabetics without severe renal disease. The Heart Outcomes Prevention Evaluation (HOPE) trial has now

*Investigational drug in the United States.

TABLE 6 Common Nitrate Preparations

Drug Name	Route of Administration	Dosage	Onset of Action	Duration of Action
Nitroglycerin	Sublingual tablet	0.15-0.9 mg	2-5 min	15-30 min
	Sublingual spray (Nitrolingual)	0.4 mg	2-5 min	15-30 min
	Transdermal patch	0.2-0.8 mg q12h	30 min	8-14 h
	Intravenous	5-200 μg/min	2-5 min	During infusion; tolerance develops after 7-8 h
Isosorbide dinitrate (Isordil)	Oral	5-80 mg bid to tid	30 min	8 h
	Slow release	40-80 mg/qd		
Isosorbide mononitrate (Imdur)	Oral	20-40 mg bid	30 min	12-24 h
	Extended release	60-240 mg/d		

confirmed that Ramipril (Altace), 10 mg per day, significantly reduces the rates of death, MI, and stroke in a broad range (diabetes, hypertension, vascular disease, CAD) of high-risk patients not known to have a low ejection fraction or heart failure.

CORONARY REVASCULARIZATION

Patients with persistent symptoms despite adequate medical therapy and patients with high-risk coronary anatomy (based on lesion location and severity, number of diseased vessels, and presence of LV dysfunction) should be considered for revascularization (see Figure 1). The Bypass Angioplasty Revascularization Investigation (BARI), which compared percutaneous transluminal coronary angioplasty (PTCA) with coronary artery bypass grafting (CABG), showed that the benefit of CABG over PTCA is more pronounced in treated diabetics. Other techniques available in patients with refractory angina even after revascularization, or in patients not amenable to complete revascularization, are spinal cord stimulation and enhanced external counter pulsation.

Unstable Angina

Three main presentations of unstable angina (UA), as previously described, are angina at rest, new onset angina, and increasing angina. The process central to the initiation of an acute coronary syndrome is disruption of an atheromatous plaque. Fissuring or rupture of these plaques—with consequent exposure of core constituents such as lipid, smooth muscle, and foam cells—leads to the local generation of thrombin and deposition of fibrin. This in turn promotes platelet aggregation and adhesion and the formation of intracoronary thrombus. UA and non-ST segment elevation myocardial infarction (NSTEMI) are generally associated with white, platelet-rich, and only partially occlusive thrombus, in contrast to fibrin-rich reddish thrombus in ST segment elevation MI (STEMI). Microthrombi can detach and embolize downstream, causing myocardial ischemia and infarction.

TREATMENT

On the basis of clinical characteristics and laboratory markers on admission, patients can generally be categorized as low risk, intermediate risk, or high risk. Patients at low or intermediate risk (i.e., those without pain at the time of evaluation, those who have an unchanged or normal electrocardiogram, and those whose condition is hemodynamically stable) should be treated with aspirin and assessed further. Serial ECGs should be obtained once a day or with any change in symptoms. Continuous ECG monitoring, three sets of serum troponins, and creatine kinase myocardial band (CK-MB) should be drawn every 8 hours. Low-risk patients with a negative stress test can be managed as outpatients. ECG changes during chest pain suggest the probability of CAD. High-risk patients urgently require simultaneous evaluation and treatment (Table 7).

Medical therapy should be adjusted rapidly to relieve manifestations of ischemia and should include antiplatelet therapy (aspirin or clopidogrel [Plavix], if aspirin is contraindicated), antithrombotic therapy (unfractionated heparin or low-molecular-weight heparin), β blockers, nitrates, and possibly calcium channel blockers. Early administration of glycoprotein (GP) IIb/IIIa inhibitors may be particularly important, especially in high-risk patients with positive troponin tests or those in whom implantation of coronary stents is anticipated. The use of calcium channel blockers, especially the nondihydropyridines, should be reserved for patients in whom β blockers are contraindicated or those with refractory symptoms despite aggressive treatment with aspirin, nitrates, and β blockers. A meta-analysis of the Efficacy Safety Subcutaneous Enoxaparin in Non–Q-wave Coronary Events (ESSENCE) and the Thrombolysis in Myocardial Infarction (TIMI) 11B trials, which compared enoxaparin (Lovenox) with unfractionated heparin, demonstrated that enoxaparin improved outcomes, reducing death and ischemic events by 20%. These findings, coupled with the simplicity of subcutaneous administration and elimination of the need for anticoagulation monitoring, make enoxaparin an excellent candidate to replace unfractionated heparin as the antithrombin for the acute phase management of high-risk UA/non–Q-wave MI. Lepirudin (Refludan)[1] rather than heparin can be used in patients with a history of heparin-associated thrombocytopenia.

A 2002 meta-analysis of randomized trials concluded that intravenous GP IIb/IIIa inhibitors were of

[1]Not FDA approved for this indication.

TABLE 7 Indicators of High Risk in Patients with Coronary Artery Disease Assessed for Unstable Angina

1. Recurrent angina/ischemia at rest or with low-level activities despite intensive anti-ischemic therapy
2. Elevated TnT or TnI
3. New or presumably new ST segment depression
4. Recurrent angina/ischemia with CHF symptoms, an S_3 gallop, pulmonary edema, worsening rales, or new or worsening MR
5. High-risk findings on noninvasive stress testing
6. Depressed LV systolic function (e.g., EF <0.40 on noninvasive study)
7. Hemodynamic instability
8. Sustained ventricular tachycardia
9. PCI within 6 months
10. Prior CABG

Abbreviations: CABG = coronary artery bypass graft; CHF = congestive heart failure; EF = ejection fraction; LV = left ventricular; PCI = percutaneous coronary intervention; MR = mitral regurgitation; TnI = troponin I; TnT = troponin T.

TABLE 8 Computation of Thrombolysis in Myocardial Infarction (TIMI) Risk Score

Assign 1 point for each of the following:

1. Age ≥65 years
2. Presence of at least 3 risk factors for coronary artery disease
3. Prior coronary stenosis of ≥50%
4. Presence of ST segment deviation on admission ECG
5. At least 2 anginal episodes in prior 24 hours
6. Elevated serum cardiac biomarkers
7. Use of aspirin in previous 7 days

Rates of composite end points (all-cause mortality, MI, severe recurrent ischemia) at the end of 14 days, based on number of risk factors present in patients presenting with acute coronary syndrome in TIMI IIB and Efficacy Safety Subcutaneous Enoxaparin in Non–Q-wave Coronary Events (ESSENCE). Score of 0-1 = 4.7%; 2 = 8.3%; 3 = 13.2%; 4 = 19.9%; 5 = 26.2%; 6-7 = 40.9%.

substantial benefit in patients with a non-ST–segment elevation acute coronary syndrome (ACS) undergoing percutaneous coronary intervention (PCI), and also is recommended in almost all patients with NSTEMI and many with UA.

The TIMI risk score (Table 8), developed by using data from the TIMI 11B and ESSENCE trials, stratifies patients with UA or an NSTEMI into high, intermediate, and low-risk groups. A higher TIMI risk score correlated significantly with increased numbers of events (all-cause mortality, new or recurrent MI, or severe recurrent ischemia requiring revascularization) at 14 days. A score of 0/1 versus 7 corresponds to a 4.7% versus 40% event rate. The most recent major trials (Fast Revascularization During Instability in Coronary Disease [FRISC] II trial, Randomized Intervention Trial of Unstable Angina [RITA] 3 trial, Medicine versus Angiography in Thrombolytic Exclusion [MATE] trial, and TACTICS-TIMI 18) show a consistent benefit from an early invasive strategy, reducing death or MI in moderate- and high-risk groups and recurrent and refractory angina in all patients. Conversely, the TIMI IIIB and Veterans Affairs Non–Q-Wave Myocardial Infarction Strategies In-Hospital [VANQWISH] trials showed no significant benefit of early invasive strategy. Two other situations that warrant an early invasive approach because of high risk for subsequent ischemic events are new angina following an acute MI—either NSTEMI or STEMI and angina after PCI (now mostly involving stenting) or CABG. Prior to discharge, patients who have been medically treated should undergo non-invasive assessment for residual inducible ischemia.

Variant Angina or Prinzmetal Angina

Variant angina is chest pain occurring at rest associated with ST segment elevation, and coronary artery spasm is its underlying pathophysiological mechanism. Risk factors include cigarette smoking, cocaine, insulin resistance, and hyperinsulinemia. Patients tend to be young and lack classic cardiac risk factors. The chest pain is often severe and may be accompanied by dizziness and syncope. Arrhythmias are also common during variant angina.

Exercise testing has limited diagnostic value. Catheterization findings commonly reveal significant proximal coronary obstruction of at least one major coronary artery or normal coronaries. Spasm occurs usually within 1 cm of fixed obstruction. The remainder of this patient population will have normal coronaries. Ergonovine can cause focal spasm in Prinzmetal angina as opposed to diffuse reduction in coronary caliber in others; the test is only performed in patients with normal coronaries.

Nitrates and calcium channel blockers are mainstays of treatment, often in high dosages. Prazosin (Minipress), a selective α-receptor blocker, is also used to control the symptoms. β blockers are contraindicated, as they can cause unopposed α-receptor mediated vasospasm.

CARDIAC ARREST: SUDDEN CARDIAC DEATH

METHOD OF

Nicola E. Schiebel, MD, and

Roger D. White, MD

Sudden cardiac death (SCD) is the term used to denote unexpected cardiovascular collapse culminating in cardiorespiratory arrest. According to the American Heart Association (AHA), SCD claims approximately 250,000 lives each year. Although it may follow the onset of ischemic signs and/or symptoms, it may occur without preceding warning signs of impending collapse and without a prior history of ischemic cardiac disease. The majority of these events occur outside the hospital and, therefore, are out-of-hospital cardiac arrests. Whereas there are many possible causes of out-of-hospital cardiac arrest, coronary artery disease, often without acute myocardial infarction, is the most frequent cause.

At onset, ventricular tachyarrhythmias are the presenting electrical derangement in more than 80% of these episodes, most commonly monomorphic ventricular tachycardia (VT) that then degenerates into ventricular fibrillation (VF) (Figure 1). Without defibrillation, VF will progress to asystole, and as a result VF is the initial rhythm identified in only approximately 40% to 50% of out-of-hospital cardiac arrests in most emergency medical services

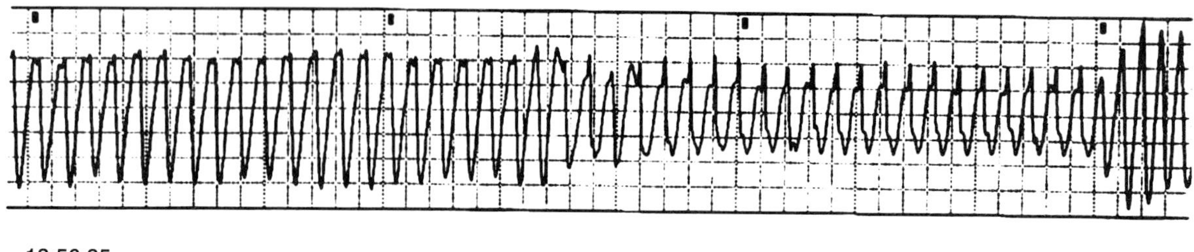

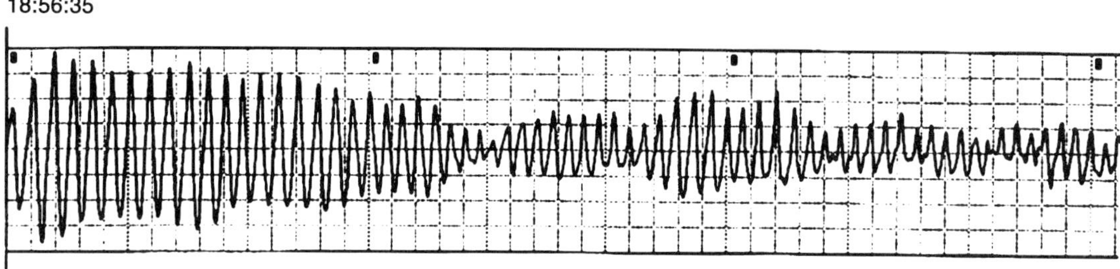

FIGURE 1 Degeneration of fast monomorphic ventricular tachycardia into ventricular fibrillation in out-of-hospital cardiac arrest.

(EMS) systems. Bradyarrhythmias initiate cardiac arrest in 18% of patients. The most frequent presenting SCD arrhythmia, VF, is, fortunately, also the most treatable; therefore, an aggressive effort is warranted in treating patients experiencing SCD. In well-organized EMS systems, 40% or more of patients in out-of-hospital cardiac arrest with VF as the presenting rhythm can be resuscitated and discharged without neurologic impairment. The likelihood of survival is directly dependent on rapid and sequential implementation of the AHA chain of survival; its critical links are rapid EMS access by calling for help (911 telephone call), prompt bystander cardiopulmonary resuscitation (CPR), early defibrillation, and follow-up advanced cardiac life support (ACLS) care.

Early defibrillation has emerged as the most critical lifesaving intervention that has the potential for substantially increasing survival from SCD caused by VF. A major national initiative is needed to implement this intervention on a widespread scale to improve survival from cardiac arrest. The thrust of this presentation is to describe an approach to cardiac arrest that will maximize the likelihood of survival by emphasis on the strategic employment of early defibrillation. However, because the benefit of rapid defibrillation frequently depends on the integration of the other components of the chain of survival, these components need to be understood as well.

The victim who is most likely to survive cardiac arrest is one whose arrest is witnessed and caused by VF, for whom EMS is called immediately (early access), who receives prompt CPR by bystanders (early CPR), who is defibrillated within 6 to 8 minutes of collapse (early defibrillation), and, finally, who receives follow-up stabilizing ACLS treatment (early advanced care) as needed. The last might include administration of antiarrhythmic drugs, endotracheal intubation, or other definitive interventions. Each of these components is discussed in this article; the information will help physicians and emergency personnel to develop an action plan that will enable as many patients as possible to be among those most likely to survive a cardiac arrest.

Early Access

As soon as a victim is observed to be unresponsive, the EMS system should be called, ideally by the universal emergency number 911. If this number is not yet established in one's community, then all citizens should have posted by their telephones the number to call to access the EMS system.

Early Cardiopulmonary Resuscitation

Preservation of cerebral and myocardial viability during the arrested state is totally dependent on delivery of oxygenated blood to the brain and heart by ventilation and external chest compressions. It is a regrettable experience for an arrested patient to have spontaneous circulation restored by defibrillation only to die or vegetate from irreversible ischemic brain injury. Whereas it is acknowledged that CPR is largely a *holding* function, awaiting more definitive interventions, it can be a major determinant of whether a patient awakens without neurologic deficit after cardiac arrest. High-quality CPR also exerts beneficial effects on myocardial perfusion during the arrested state and can directly influence resuscitation success. Three minutes of CPR prior to defibrillation enhances survival to hospital discharge when delay of defibrillation exceeds 5 minutes in out-of-hospital cardiac arrest.

It behooves all physicians to avail themselves of the opportunity to learn this skill and to periodically (every 1 to 2 years) be updated in the performance of CPR.

New CPR techniques are being investigated clinically. They include interposed abdominal compression CPR, active compression–decompression CPR, circumferential thoracic compression (vest CPR), and mechanical piston devices. These CPR adjuncts require additional personnel, training, or equipment with maximum benefits reported when commenced early in cardiac arrest. Although limited data suggest some benefit for in-hospital settings where this specialized care can occur early, no adjunct has been shown to be consistently superior to standard (AHA) manual CPR for prehospital basic life support (BLS).

Early Defibrillation

The termination of ventricular fibrillation by externally applied electricity was a major breakthrough in cardiac resuscitation. First described in 1956, it proved to be a remarkably effective treatment for an otherwise universally fatal arrhythmia. Since then, the most significant advance in improving the chances for survival from VF cardiac arrest is the implementation of early defibrillation programs in out-of-hospital settings. Automated external defibrillators (AEDs) make possible the delivery of defibrillatory shocks rapidly, effectively, and safely. AEDs are attached to the chest wall by means of cables connected to adhesive conductive electrode pads that are used to both monitor the rhythm and deliver shocks. A microprocessor-based algorithm program automatically analyzes the rhythm. If a treatable rhythm (VF or pulseless VT with a rate beyond the cutoff) is detected, the AED capacitor is automatically charged, and the operator is requested visually (screen display) and audibly (voice synthesizer) to deliver a shock. After the shock, most devices are programmed to reanalyze the rhythm to determine whether a shockable rhythm is still present. If so, the cycle is repeated, and again a third time if needed. Thus, a total of three shocks can be delivered rapidly and without interruption if needed. After a third shock, or after any shock that terminates VF, the device calls for a pulse check. If none is present, CPR is performed for 1 minute, then the analyze-shock cycle can be repeated. The algorithms that analyze the rhythm have high degrees of both specificity and sensitivity, both in the range of 97% to 100%. AEDs are lightweight and easy to operate. New versions require minimal maintenance. AEDs are available with event documentation systems such as event cards that store times and electrocardiographic data for a subsequent printout and review (Figure 2).

Improved survival from VF cardiac arrest depends on early defibrillation. All areas for care of patients should be equipped with AEDs, including physicians' offices. In out-of-hospital settings, AEDs are carried

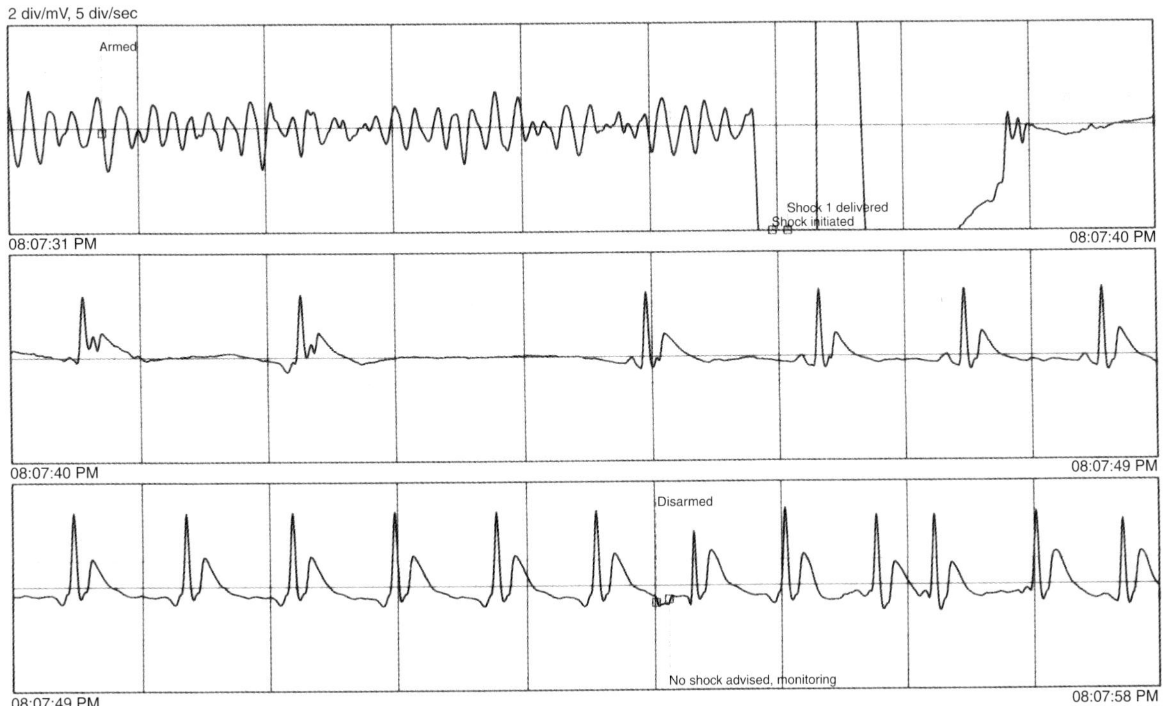

FIGURE 2 Termination of ventricular fibrillation with one 150-joule biphasic truncated exponential waveform shock in out-of-hospital cardiac arrest. An organized rhythm with sustained pulses followed the single shock. Data were obtained from the data card inside the automated external defibrillator, which was operated by a police officer.

in BLS ambulances and by many first-responder EMS personnel, such as firefighters and police officers. It is evident that physicians seeing patients in their offices or in outpatient clinics would be well advised to consider placement of AEDs in those settings and to have office or clinic staff, as well as themselves, trained in their proper operation and maintenance. There is a form of VT that can lead to cardiac arrest that necessitates an awareness of modes of presentation, etiology, and intervention. This is torsades de pointes, a form of polymorphic ventricular tachycardia (PVT) caused by prolonged repolarization, manifest electrocardiographically as QT-interval prolongation. It is characterized by typical *twisting of the points* QRS complexes on the electrocardiogram. The patient may have paroxysms of this tachycardia, between which the QT-interval prolongation is evident. When the disorder is suspected, a search should be made for a cause (Table 1 and Figure 3). Sustained episodes of torsades de pointes can cause cardiac arrest and should be treated with defibrillation using the same doses of energy as specified for VF and pulseless VT. Magnesium sulfate[1] (1 to 2 g intravenously) can be injected to control the episodes of torsades de pointes, or, if it is available, overdrive atrial or ventricular pacing can suppress the tachycardia. PVT can occur without QT prolongation (e.g., after acute myocardial infarction), in which case standard antiarrhythmic therapy with lidocaine, amiodarone, procainamide, or sotalol is used. It is essential in this scenario to aggressively treat the ischemia as well as any electrolyte abnormalities. The primary care physician must, therefore, be alert not only to the electrocardiographic appearance of PVT but also to the etiologic mechanisms that define the PVT as torsades de pointes and thus lead to treatment variations.

[1]Not FDA approved for this indication.

TABLE 1 Causes of Torsades de Pointes

Congenital Prolonged QT Syndromes
Romano-Ward
Jervell and Lange-Nielsen
Acquired Prolonged ET Interval
Drug induced
Quinidine
Procainamide (Pronestyl)
Disopyramide (Norpace)
Sotalol (Betapace)
Bepridil (Vascor)
Amiodarone (Cordarone)
Phenothiazines
Thioridazine (Mellaril)
Chlorpromazine (Thorazine)
Tricyclic antidepressants
Amitriptyline
Imipramine
Cisapride (Propulsid)
Lithium
Terfenadine (Seldane) and astemizole (Hismanal) in combination with ketoconazole (Nizoral), itraconazole (Sporanox), erythromycin, or hepatic disease
Electrolyte derangements
Hypokalemia
Hypomagnesemia
Hypocalcemia
Neurologic
Subarachnoid hemorrhage
Cerebrovascular accident
Bradycardia of any cause
Sinus or junctional
Atrioventricular block
Any combination of the above (e.g., subarachnoid hemorrhage with bradycardia and hypokalemia)

Early Advanced Cardiac Life Support Care

In many patients experiencing VF cardiac arrest, prompt defibrillation is all that is required to restore a spontaneous circulation. After this, supplemental oxygen and an intravenous line can be initiated with fluid and medications administered as needed. In some patients, more definitive and aggressive interventions will be required, such as airway control, ventilation, and vasopressor support for circulation. Whereas endotracheal intubation is the intervention of choice for airway protection and for both oxygenation and ventilation, persons who are not trained in this skill should not attempt it. Instead, a mask with a one-way valve can be used to ventilate the patient with a mouth-to-mask technique. Bag-valve mask devices can deliver higher flow oxygen, but are technically difficult for one person to use without proper training and practice. Another airway option is a multilumen airway such as the esophageal-tracheal tube (Combitube). This device can be inserted by trained persons to protect the airway if endotracheal intubation cannot be accomplished. The laryngeal mask airway (LMA) is another adjunctive device composed of a tube with a cuffed mask-like projection at the distal end. Although it does not ensure absolute protection from aspiration, regurgitation is less likely with the LMA than with a bag-valve mask device, and it provides equivalent ventilation with the endotracheal tube. All of these airway skills are incorporated in the AHA ACLS training program. Primary care physicians are strongly encouraged to avail themselves of this training opportunity to become thoroughly acquainted with all of these ACLS procedures and devices.

Drug Therapy

On close review of the literature to date, there is little evidence that the administration of any drug during cardiac arrest improves survival to hospital discharge. As a result, the International Guidelines for 2000 stress that during cardiac arrest "drug administration must be secondary to other interventions." Once CPR, defibrillation, and proper airway

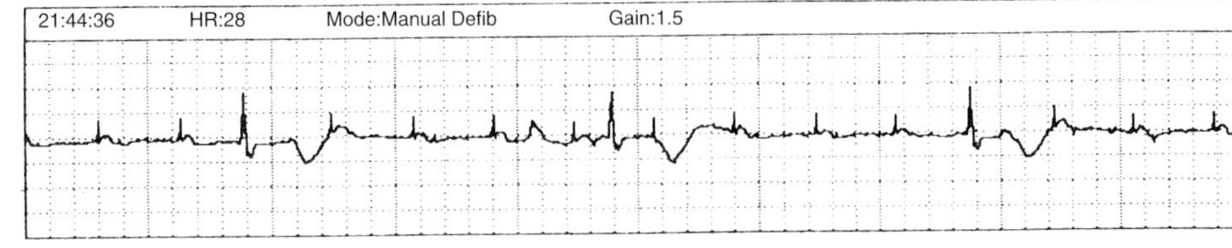

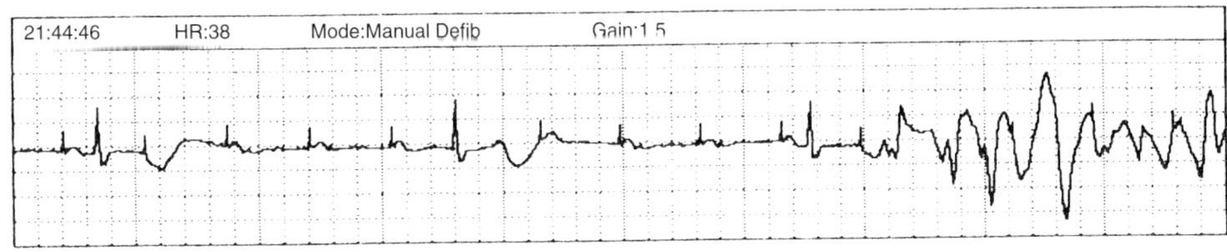

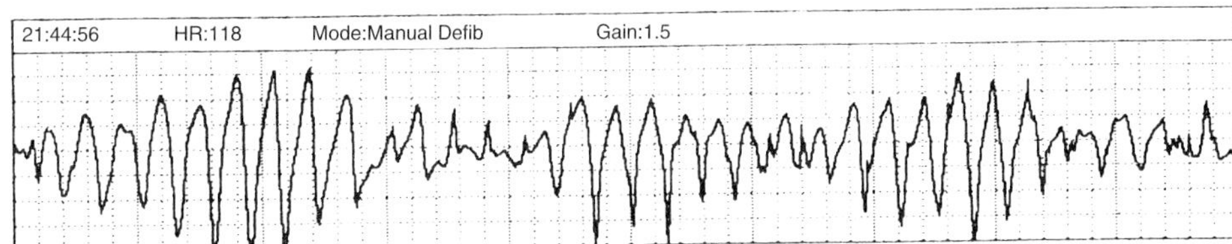

FIGURE 3 Onset of torsades de pointes ventricular tachycardia in the presence of bradycardia caused by dual-chamber pacemaker malfunction. Only the atrial pacing lead is functional, causing loss of a ventricular-paced rhythm and a very slow ventricular escape rhythm.

management are established, certain drugs are considered by standard practice to be potentially useful. These drugs include epinephrine, vasopressin, amiodarone, and lidocaine.

EPINEPHRINE

Historically, epinephrine has been used in resuscitation of all cardiac arrest rhythms. Although considerable animal data exist supporting its use, no randomized, prospective, placebo-controlled trials have ever been done in humans to determine its efficacy. Given the widespread acceptance of epinephrine as a *standard of care* in refractory VF, asystole, and PEA, it is doubtful that better quality evidence of its efficacy will be available in the near future.

Despite the paucity of evidence supporting the use of epinephrine in cardiac arrest, considerable research has been done comparing high-dose epinephrine (0.07 to 0.20 mg/kg)[3] with standard-dose epinephrine (1 mg every 3 to 5 minutes). The findings on multiple randomized trials are consistently the same. High-dose protocols result in higher rates of return of spontaneous circulation (ROSC) during initial resuscitation. However, no differences can be found when survival to hospital discharge and final neurologic outcome are compared. The higher doses have not clearly been shown to be harmful, but would likely confer added costs to health care systems by increasing hospitalization in hopeless situations. The use of high-dose epinephrine is, therefore, strongly discouraged, and when administered should be given in the standard dose.

VASOPRESSIN

Vasopressin (Pitressin)[1] (40 U IV, single dose only) was introduced in the 2000 guidelines as an acceptable alternative to epinephrine in refractory VF and pulseless VT. It is a naturally occurring hormone that in high doses acts as a potent nonadrenergic vasoconstrictor. The theoretical advantage to vasopressin is that it lacks some of the potentially detrimental β-adrenergic effects of epinephrine in the postresuscitation setting. Unfortunately, vasopressin has not been shown in human trials to increase survival to discharge.

AMIODARONE AND LIDOCAINE

The use of lidocaine (Xylocaine)[1] (1 mg/kg boluses up to 3 mg/kg) for refractory VF and pulseless VT is largely based on historical use of the drug to prevent VF in acute MI. Only one retrospective prehospital trial provides some supporting evidence for its use in VF and pulseless VT, demonstrating an improved survival to hospital admission rate. Another retrospective study suggests that lidocaine has a detrimental effect on ROSC. More recently, the prophylactic use of lidocaine in acute MI has been shown to be associated with increased morbidity and to cause more serious

[3]Exceeds dosage recommended by the manufacturer.

[1]Not FDA approved for this indication.

arrhythmias than it prevents. Additionally, it has been established in experimental models that lidocaine increases energy requirements for defibrillation. More studies need to be done to determine the role of lidocaine in cardiac arrest, and it should be recognized that current practice has no sound evidence base.

Amiodarone (Cordarone) (150 to 300 mg IV) modestly increases survival to hospital admission in out-of-hospital VF cardiac arrest that is refractory to initial defibrillation. However, it has not been shown to increase survival rate to hospital discharge.

Other Forms of Cardiac Arrest (Pulseless Electrical Activity and Asystole)

As discussed, VF is the most common and treatable presenting rhythm in SCD and cardiac arrest. However, other presentations include bradyarrhythmias with pulselessness (pulseless electrical activity) and asystole. These, of course, are not treatable with defibrillation. In pulseless electrical activity, which by definition is some form of electrical activity on the electrocardiogram without palpable pulses, a concerted effort must be made to identify a potentially correctable cause, such as:

- Hypovolemia (e.g., exsanguination from concealed or evident hemorrhage)
- Tension pneumothorax after trauma or attempted subclavian venous puncture
- Acute pulmonary thromboembolism
- Cardiac tamponade from trauma or secondary to ventricular rupture with acute myocardial infarction

Survival after left ventricular rupture and tamponade is dependent on suspicion, diagnosis, and immediate intervention.

Asystole is most commonly an irreversible derangement secondary to long-standing hypoxia. However, even here a rapid search should be initiated for a treatable cause. For example, successful resuscitation has been described after prolonged asystolic cardiac arrest associated with hyperkalemia. External pacing can be tried, but it has not been shown to alter outcome from this form of arrest.

Termination of Resuscitation

Physicians involved in resuscitation invariably will be called upon to make the difficult decision of when to stop resuscitative efforts. Multiple factors come into play, with the ultimate decision involving a complex interaction of patient and physician variables. The most important single factor associated with poor outcomes is prolonged time of resuscitation. As time spent increases, the chance of neurologically intact survival diminishes. A simple clinical decision aid has been derived and recently validated for in-hospital arrests. It involves assessing three simple parameters—whether the arrest was witnessed *or* the initial cardiac rhythm was either VF or VT *or* patients regained a pulse during the first 10 minutes of chest compressions. If none of these three variables was present the aid predicts no chance of discharge. Ideally, prospective testing in another hospital setting would further ensure its validity, but it does provide clinicians with some parameters to help them make complex decisions on individual cases.

SCD and cardiac arrest are most commonly the consequence of coronary artery disease. VF is the most frequent presenting rhythm, and VF is often correctable with rapid interventions centered on early defibrillation. AEDs provide a means for rapid delivery of defibrillatory shocks to persons in VF cardiac arrest and constitute the single most important means for improving survival from VF arrests. All areas of care for patients, including physicians' offices and outpatient clinics, should be equipped with AEDs. In pulseless electrical activity or asystolic arrest, a rapid assessment should be made to determine whether a potentially correctable cause of arrest is present.

ATRIAL FIBRILLATION

METHOD OF

Adam M. Brodsky, MD, and Dan Fintel, MD

Atrial fibrillation is the most common sustained arrhythmia, affecting 0.4% of the general population. The prevalence of atrial fibrillation increases with age, such that 2% to 5% of those older than 60 years, of age and more than 6% of those older than 80 years of age are afflicted. This rhythm disturbance carries with it a relative risk of death of 1.5 in males and 1.9 in females, largely because of increased cardiovascular and stroke-related mortality. The average incidence of stroke in all patients with nonrheumatic atrial fibrillation is approximately 5% per year, and is two to seven times that of those without atrial fibrillation.

Atrial fibrillation is characterized by uncoordinated depolarization of the atria leading to an irregular ventricular rate. P waves are absent on the electrocardiogram and coarse or fine atrial fibrillatory waves may be seen. Often the irregular ventricular rate is rapid, with rates higher than 120 beats per minute. Atrial fibrillation may be characterized by its temporal pattern as paroxysmal, persistent, or permanent. Paroxysmal atrial fibrillation spontaneously terminates and is often recurrent. Persistent atrial fibrillation is not self-terminating, although it may be terminated by pharmacologic or electrical cardioversion. Permanent atrial fibrillation is chronic and occurs when the decision has been made not to attempt cardioversion. Atrial fibrillation may also be characterized by its etiology, as primary or secondary. Secondary atrial fibrillation may be caused by a wide variety of medical and surgical insults including myocardial infarction, cardiac surgery, rheumatic heart disease, hyperthyroidism, pulmonary embolism, pneumonia, myocarditis, pericarditis, alcohol intoxication, and electrocution. Primary atrial fibrillation that occurs in the absence of any cardiovascular or stroke-related risk factors in patients younger than 60 years of age is referred to as lone atrial fibrillation. Atrial fibrillation may be considered acute if it has occurred within 48 hours.

The exact mechanism and pathophysiology underlying atrial fibrillation remain unclear. The electrophysiologic prerequisite for atrial fibrillation seems to be a combination of enhanced automaticity and reentry. In many cases, initiation of the arrhythmia is thought to be caused by rapid bursts of electrical activity emanating from atrial tissue extending into the pulmonary veins. The multiple wavelet hypothesis is felt to be responsible for rhythm maintenance. This hypothesis describes multiple depolarization wavefronts of varying wavelengths propagating at varying speeds throughout the atria. Electrophysiologic remodeling is also known to occur, such that there is a decreased chance for successful cardioversion if the fibrillation has been long-standing.

Clinical Features

There are three hemodynamic consequences of atrial fibrillation. First, the loss of the atrial component of ventricular filling during late diastole may significantly reduce the cardiac output. This effect is more pronounced in patients with diastolic dysfunction or restrictive cardiomyopathy. Second, the irregular ventricular rate may independently reduce cardiac output. Third, the often rapid ventricular rate allows less time for diastolic filling, thereby reducing the stroke volume. Additionally, a persistently elevated ventricular rate may cause a reversible, tachycardia-induced cardiomyopathy, with a significantly reduced ejection fraction and frank signs of heart failure.

Clinically, atrial fibrillation manifests with a variety of symptoms including palpitations, chest discomfort, syncope, dizziness, fatigue, dyspnea, and exercise intolerance. Physical examination usually reveals an irregularly irregular pulse and irregular venous pulsations. Appropriate tests in a patient with suspected atrial fibrillation include an electrocardiogram, which will document the absence of P waves and an irregular ventricular rhythm. Because atrial fibrillation may be paroxysmal, ambulatory monitoring with either a halter monitor or loop recorder may be necessary to establish a diagnosis. A chest radiograph and echocardiogram are useful to exclude associated cardiac and pulmonary abnormalities. Other tests that may be indicated include exercise stress testing to assess the ventricular rate during and after exercise, transesophageal echocardiography to rule out atrial thrombi prior to cardioversion, and invasive electrophysiologic testing if catheter-based ablation is considered.

Management

Successful treatment of atrial fibrillation must combine management of the arrhythmia itself and any associated symptoms as well as minimization of the risk of stroke, the most feared complication of atrial fibrillation. Management issues include control of the ventricular rate during atrial fibrillation, cardioversion from atrial fibrillation to sinus rhythm, and long-term maintenance of sinus rhythm. The first decision to be made, and one which will often be revisited, is whether or not to proceed to cardioversion at all or to simply achieve rate control without attempted cardioversion. For patients with atrial fibrillation who are hemodynamically unstable, cardioversion is often an immediate necessity. For patients who have failed multiple attempts at maintenance of sinus rhythm following cardioversion, simple rate control may be the best option. A long-held suspicion was that the risk of stroke could be significantly reduced if sinus rhythm could be restored. This suspicion led to the belief that cardioversion and maintenance of sinus rhythm were of paramount importance. However, recent studies such as the Atrial Fibrillation Follow-up Investigation of Rhythm Management (AFFIRM) and Rate Control versus Electrical Cardioversion for Persistent Atrial Fibrillation (RACE) trials demonstrated no reductions in either mortality or stroke rates between those patients managed with simple rate control and anticoagulation, compared with those in whom a strategy of cardioversion with rhythm maintenance using antiarrhythmic drugs was employed. This new knowledge has led to the current feeling that a strategy of simple rate control may be acceptable in certain patients, especially if they have no symptoms related to their arrhythmia.

CARDIOVERSION

Cardioversion may be accomplished electrically or pharmacologically. Electrical cardioversion consists of a single discharge of electricity. The discharge must be synchronized with the electrocardiogram so as not to fall during the T-wave, possibly inducing ventricular fibrillation. Electrical cardioversion must be distinguished from defibrillation, which is not synchronized. Recent data suggest that a biphasic energy

TABLE 1 Drugs Used for Pharmacologic Cardioversion of Atrial Fibrillation

Drug	Dosage	Comments
Amiodarone (Cordarone)[1]	5 mg/kg IV bolus, then 0.25-1.0 mg/min infusion	IV form may cause hypotension. May use PO but cardioversion may not occur for days to weeks.
Dofetilide (Tikosyn)	0.5 mg PO bid (for normal creatinine)	May be used in patients with heart disease. Must be dosed according to renal function.
Flecainide (Tambocor)	300 mg PO single dose	Must be avoided in patients with underlying heart disease. May regularize AF leading to 1:1 conduction; therefore must use with nodal blockers.
Ibutilide (Corvert)	1 mg IV over 10 min, may repeat once if unsuccessful	Risk of torsade de pointes in up to 8% of patients.
Procainamide (Pronestyl)[1]	10-15 mg/kg IV bolus followed by 1-4 mg/min infusion	May cause hypotension. Long-term use is associated with drug-induced lupus in 30% of patients.
Propafenone (Rythmol)[1]	450-600 mg PO single dose	Should be avoided in patients with underlying heart disease. May regularize AF leading to 1:1 conduction, therefore must use with nodal blockers.
Quinidine sulfate	200 mg PO followed by 400 mg PO 1-2 h later	May cause ventricular arrhythmias. May increase ventricular response rate due to vagolytic effects.

[1]Not FDA approved for this indication.
Abbreviation: AF = atrial fibrillation.

discharge is more often successful and requires less energy than a simple monophasic discharge. In patients with pacemakers or internal cardioverter-defibrillators (ICDs), there is a small risk of damage to the generator or, if the electricity is conducted through the pacemaker or ICD leads, myocardial damage at the lead tips. Therefore, the paddles should be placed as far away as is practical from the generator. The pacer or ICD should also be interrogated before and after the cardioversion. In general, cardioversion is a very safe procedure. Possible risks include arrhythmia, minor skin irritation, postcardioversion bradycardia (especially if the ventricular rate is slow during atrial fibrillation). To reduce the threat of arrhythmia, potassium levels should be normal and digoxin toxicity must be carefully avoided. The risk of embolism during cardioversion in unanticoagulated patients is 1% to 7%; however, this risk may be reduced by proper anticoagulation verified by weekly blood tests for 4 weeks prior to and 4 weeks after cardioversion.

There are several drugs available for pharmacological cardioversion (Table 1), however, these drugs are at best only 30% to 70% effective. If one agent has failed, another one may be tried. Pharmacological cardioversion carries the same risk of embolic stroke as does electrical cardioversion, therefore, proper anticoagulation is important. In addition to their use as primary agents for cardioversion, these drugs may also be used to enhance the success rate of electrical cardioversion. Digoxin (Lanoxin), calcium channel blockers, and β blockers are not effective for cardioversion.

MAINTENANCE OF SINUS RHYTHM

Once successful cardioversion has been achieved, several oral drugs are available to help maintain sinus rhythm (Table 2). Many of the drugs listed in Table 2 have side effects, and most must be initiated in a monitored setting because of their proarrhythmic potential. It is important to note that recurrences are common despite long-term pharmacotherapy. Nevertheless, if recurrences are symptomatic and bothersome to the patient, then antiarrhythmic drug therapy may be useful even if only to lower the frequency and/or duration of such recurrences. The question of when it is safe to discontinue an antiarrhythmic agent in a patient in whom sinus rhythm has been maintained is a difficult one because of the high rate of recurrences in general. Some patients have successfully discontinued antiarrhythmic therapy after 6 months to 1 year of documented sinus rhythm, however, the risk of recurrence is ever-present. The most important risk factor for the recurrence of atrial fibrillation is left atrial size. A history of prior recurrences, duration of atrial fibrillation, and age are other risk factors that should be considered.

Nonpharmacological modalities to maintain sinus rhythm include the surgical maze procedure, during which a series of lesions are made in the atria and around the pulmonary veins to create electrically isolated islands of atrial tissue that are incapable of sustaining the arrhythmia. This is often performed in conjunction with left atrial appendage exclusion or excision, thus reducing the risk of embolism. The maze procedure is very effective at preventing atrial fibrillation, however, it is most often limited to patients undergoing open heart surgery for other reasons such as valve replacement or coronary artery bypass grafting. Atrial dual-site or site-specific pacing, although less effective overall, may be an attractive option in certain cases, and atrial antitachycardia pacing strategies have also been employed successfully in some patients. Catheter-based techniques include pulmonary vein isolation, during which a series of lesions are made using radiofrequency ablation to electrically isolate the pulmonary veins, thereby blocking the initiation of the arrhythmia in many cases. Pulmonary vein stenosis is one risk of this procedure.

TABLE 2 Drugs Used for Maintenance of Sinus Rhythm

Drug	Dosage	Comments
Amiodarone (Cordarone)[1]	200 mg PO QD after loading	Long-term use associated with pulmonary fibrosis, corneal deposits, thyroid abnormalities. Has β-blocking effects. May be used in patients with underlying heart disease.
Disopyramide (Norpace)[1]	100-150 mg PO qid or 200-300 mg controlled-release PO bid	Avoid in patients with systolic heart failure due to negative inotropic effects. Anticholinergic side effects are common.
Dofetilide (Tikosyn)	0.5 mg PO bid for normal creatinine	Must be initiated in a monitored setting due to proarrhythmic potential. May be used in patients with heart disease. Dose according to renal function.
Flecainide (Tambocor)	50-100 mg PO bid	Should be avoided in patients with underlying heart disease. May regularize AF leading to 1:1 conduction, therefore must use with nodal blockers.
Propafenone (Rythmol)[1]	150-300 mg PO tid	Should be avoided in patients with underlying heart disease. May cause a metallic taste. May regularize AF leading to 1:1 conduction, therefore must use with nodal blockers.
Quinidine	Sulfate: 200-400 mg PO qid Gluconate: 324-648 mg PO tid	May increase ventricular response rate during atrial fibrillation due to vagolytic effect. Has GI side effects. Must be initiated in a monitored setting due to proarrhythmic potential.
Sotalol (Betapace)	120-160 mg PO bid	Has β-blocking properties. Must be initiated in a monitored setting because of proarrhythmic potential.

[1]Not FDA approved for this indication.
Abbreviations: AF = atrial fibrillation; GI = gastrointestinal.

RATE CONTROL

Atrial fibrillation recurs in up to 50% of patients 1 year after successful cardioversion. While further attempts at cardioversion may be tried, a significant proportion of these patients will eventually progress to permanent atrial fibrillation. These patients, as well as those who have chosen not to pursue cardioversion, must be maintained on therapy to control the ventricular response rate. Therapy should be adjusted to achieve a rate of 60 to 80 beats per minute at rest and 90 to 115 beats per minute during exercise. The most common agents used are β blockers and calcium channel blockers. An advantage of β blockers is their benefit to patients with ischemic heart disease and reduced ventricular function. At higher doses, however, β blockers may aggravate bronchospastic disease. The most common calcium channel blockers used are diltiazem (Cardizem) or verapamil (Calan, Isoptin, Verelan). Digoxin has also been used for rate control; however, because its primary method of action is through an enhanced vagal effect on the atrioventricular (AV) node, any increase in sympathetic tone will quickly overwhelm its rate control ability. Digoxin is, therefore, less useful in young or active patients and should be reserved for older, less active patients, especially those with concomitant systolic heart failure. Some of the antiarrhythmic agents, such as amiodarone (Cordarone)[1] and sotalol (Betapace), will also act to lower the ventricular rate during relapses of atrial fibrillation. In rare cases when pharmacologic rate control is not possible or has failed, AV node ablation with pacemaker implantation should be considered.

[1]Not FDA approved for this indication.

PREVENTION OF THROMBOEMBOLISM

Prevention of thromboembolism is of paramount importance in patients with atrial fibrillation. The primary risk factors for stroke in patients with atrial fibrillation are hypertension, ejection fraction of less than 35%, and history of heart failure. Other risk factors include prior history of stroke, age older than 65, coronary artery disease, and diabetes. The risk of stroke varies, from less than 1% per year in patients with lone atrial fibrillation (patients younger than 60 years of age with no risk factors for stroke), to greater than 8% per year in those older than 75 years of age with one or more risk factors for stroke. Therapeutic options to reduce the risk of stroke include aspirin or warfarin (Coumadin). A general strategy for antithrombotic therapy in patients with atrial fibrillation is presented in Table 3. Because many thrombi in atrial fibrillation originate in the left atrial appendage, left atrial exclusion or excision is an option that may be performed at the time of open heart surgery to reduce the risk of stroke. This is often performed as part of the maze procedure, as described above. Newer, catheter-based techniques for left atrial appendage exclusion are currently under investigation.

Most patients who are older than age 65 and have one or more other risk factors should be offered warfarin therapy. Those at lower risk may be offered aspirin therapy. There is some disagreement as to what constitutes appropriate therapy for patients in the intermediate risk group (younger patients with only one risk factor or patients older than age 65 with no risk factors); however, many clinicians recommend anticoagulation with warfarin (Coumadin) as the most prudent option for this group. Because warfarin

TABLE 3 Anticoagulation in Patients with Atrial Fibrillation

Risk Factors*	Antithrombotic Therapy	Target INR
Age <65, no risk factors	Aspirin 325 mg/d	N/A
Age <65, one or more risk factors	Warfarin (Coumadin)	2.5 (range 2-3)
Age 65-75, no risk factors	Aspirin 325 mg/d or warfarin	2.5 (range 2-3)
Age 65-75, one or more risk factors	Warfarin	2.5 (range 2-3)
Age >75	Warfarin	2.0 (range 1.8-2.5)
Rheumatic heart disease, prosthetic heart valve, or thrombus visible on echocardiogram	Warfarin	3.0 (range 2.5-3.5)

*Risk factors include heart failure, ejection fraction <35%, hypertension, diabetes, coronary artery disease, and prior history of stroke.
Abbreviations: INR = international normalized ratio.

therapy requires monthly blood tests at a minimum, has attendant bleeding risks, and interacts with many foods and drugs, quality of life issues must be carefully addressed and patient preferences taken into account. Ximelagatran (Exanta)*[,4], an oral direct thrombin inhibitor that does not require dose adjustments or blood tests and has few drug interactions, is currently under investigation and appears to be a promising new alternative to warfarin. If approved by the FDA, this drug will remove many of the negative lifestyle factors associated with long-term warfarin use. For those patients with atrial fibrillation as well as coronary artery disease, 81 mg of aspirin may be taken in addition to warfarin, although this may increase the bleeding risk slightly. The combination of warfarin, aspirin, and clopidogrel (Plavix) is becoming a more common necessity despite the increased bleeding risks, as coronary stenting has become more common and as the recommended duration of therapy with clopidogrel has increased to up to 3 to 6 months for patients receiving drug-eluting stents or brachytherapy.

The few weeks surrounding cardioversion are a particularly high-risk period for thromboembolism. Left atrial stunning is known to be present after cardioversion such that atrial contractile function may not fully return for several weeks. For this reason, one should assure full anticoagulation for at least 4 weeks prior to and 4 weeks after cardioversion. Transesophageal echocardiography (TEE) may be performed before cardioversion to rule out the presence of thrombus in the atria and specifically in the left atrial appendage. If no thrombus is found and spontaneous echo contrast (indicating stasis within the atrium) is not seen, then cardioversion may proceed even without prior anticoagulation. However, TEE does not obviate the need for anticoagulation during and after cardioversion.

After successful cardioversion patients are often eager to know when it is safe to discontinue anticoagulation. Until recently conventional wisdom held that if sinus rhythm was successfully maintained for 6 months to 1 year, documented by either serial electrocardiograms or ambulatory monitoring, one could contemplate discontinuing warfarin therapy. However, the recent AFFIRM trial compared the strategy of rhythm control (maintenance of sinus rhythm with antiarrhythmic drug therapy) versus rate control plus anticoagulation and found no difference in mortality between the two groups. In fact, there was a trend toward higher mortality in the rhythm control group. Both groups suffered ischemic strokes at a similar rate, and 33% of the strokes in the rhythm control group occurred in patients who either had subtherapeutic INRs or in whom warfarin had been discontinued. While not conclusive, this trial suggests that it may never be safe to discontinue warfarin therapy. It is unclear whether the stroke rate in the rhythm control group was primarily caused by undetected recurrences of atrial fibrillation. If so, then more effective treatments to prevent atrial fibrillation may reduce the stroke rate, making the discontinuation of anticoagulation more acceptable. Alternatively, atrial fibrillation may be a marker for a systemically increased stroke risk. Supporting this theory is the observation that up to 25% of strokes in patients with atrial fibrillation are caused by cerebrovascular disease or embolism emanating from the aortic arch. Thus one must give careful consideration before discontinuing warfarin, even after successful cardioversion.

*Investigational drug in the United States.

[4]Not yet approved for use in the United States.

PREMATURE BEATS

METHOD OF

Ezra A. Amsterdam, MD

Premature cardiac beats are the most frequent disturbances of cardiac rhythm and one of the most frequent causes of an irregular pulse. They originate from all areas of the heart; in descending order of frequency, they occur in the ventricles, atria, and atrioventricular (AV) junctional tissue. Although premature beats are a frequent manifestation of cardiac disease, they also occur in the absence of structural abnormalities of the heart and can be provoked by numerous cardiac and extracardiac factors.

However, the prevalence and complexity of premature beats increase in the presence of heart disease, particularly in association with acute cardiac and noncardiac provoking factors. Although premature beats are frequently an incidental finding in both patients with cardiac disease and healthy persons, they commonly produce symptoms and can occasionally impair hemodynamic function. Moreover, they may also be harbingers of sustained tachyarrhythmias. Their prognostic importance varies from nil to ominous and depends on the setting—the presence or absence of cardiac disease—in which they occur. Symptomatic premature beats may be distressing to the patient, whereas asymptomatic premature beats may indicate increased prognostic risk to the physician if they are associated with structural heart disease. The essence of management of these rhythm disturbances is recognition that the patient, rather than the arrhythmia, is the primary consideration. Thus, depending on the circumstances of the individual patient, premature beats may require: (a) no specific treatment, (b) correction or elimination of cardiac or extracardiac provoking factors, or (c) pharmacologic or other therapy.

A premature beat is defined by its occurrence earlier in the cardiac cycle than the anticipated normal sinus beat, and it is further described by its origin from the atrium (atrial premature beat [APB]), AV junction (junctional premature beat [JPB]), or ventricle (ventricular premature beat or contraction [PVC]). Various terms, in addition to premature beats, have been applied to these ectopic forms, the most common of which are premature ventricular beat, premature ventricular depolarization, extrasystole, and ventricular ectopic depolarization. These alternative terms have also been applied to APBs and JPBs. Because an ectopic depolarization may be early (premature) or late (in which case it is an escape beat), and the prefix extra provides no information on timing, it is more precise to use the term premature to indicate an abnormally early beat.

Documentation of premature beats requires electrocardiographic (ECG) demonstration to determine their timing and morphology accurately. Morphology reflects their site of origin (atrium, junction, ventricle). By common consensus, three or more consecutive premature beats define tachycardia. For example, three consecutive PVCs comprise ventricular tachycardia. Two consecutive premature beats are referred to as coupled premature beats or a couplet (coupled PVCs). Single premature beats that occur after every other normal sinus beat are described as occurring in bigeminy; trigeminy and quadrigeminy indicate occurrence after every third and fourth normal beat, respectively. The focus in this chapter is on nonrepetitive premature beats.

Mechanisms

Premature beats are caused by the same mechanisms that are primarily responsible for most cardiac arrhythmias: (a) disorders of impulse conduction, represented by reentry; and (b) disorders of impulse generation, comprising abnormal automaticity and triggered activity.

REENTRY

This mechanism is generally considered to account for the majority of cardiac arrhythmias. It is considered an abnormality of impulse conduction and involves reexcitation of an area of myocardium by an impulse that returns to the latter focus after traversing a circuitous route. It requires unidirectional block and may include a region of inexcitable tissue, such as a myocardial scar. Reentry accounts for what has been classically termed the circus movement that underlies many arrhythmias. If the circus movement results in endless loop impulse conduction, a sustained arrhythmia will result. Isolated premature beats occur when the impulse following the reentry pathway dissipates after a single cycle. Reentry is associated with structural, functional, or metabolic abnormalities of the myocardium (e.g., ischemia, fibrosis, drug toxicity).

ABNORMAL AUTOMATICITY

This mechanism refers to (a) the occurrence of spontaneous depolarization in cardiac tissue, such as atrial and ventricular muscle that normally lacks intrinsic automaticity; and (b) increased automaticity in the His-Purkinje system, which is automatic under physiologic conditions. Conditions that can cause an abnormal increase in automaticity include ischemia, metabolic abnormalities, and drug toxicity (e.g., digitalis, catecholamine, methylxanthines).

TRIGGERED ACTIVITY

This mechanism is defined as the generation of action potentials resulting from afterdepolarizations. Triggered activity differs from automaticity in that it is dependent on the previous action potential rather than representing a spontaneous depolarization. Afterdepolarizations may occur during repolarization (early afterdepolarizations) or after repolarization (delayed afterdepolarizations). Afterdepolarizations may be subthreshold and not result in a premature beat. When individual triggered action potentials reach the threshold for depolarization of the cell, premature beats appear, whereas repetitive triggered activity results in a sustained arrhythmia. Triggered activity can be caused by ischemia, digitalis, and catecholamines.

General Concepts

PVCs are detected during evaluation prompted by symptoms or as incidental findings on physical examination or ECG. Appropriate management is predicated on a thorough evaluation that includes a complete history, physical examination, and relevant laboratory studies, including a standard 12-lead ECG, and, in selected patients, special techniques such as ambulatory ECG monitoring and cardiac stress testing. These methods will provide evidence not only of the presence or absence of premature beats, but also of cardiac and noncardiac conditions that may be causative factors for ectopic beats.

HISTORY

Symptoms

Symptoms are frequently suggested by complaints of palpitations, variably described by patients as an irregularity, skipped beats, or pounding. Occasionally, symptoms of dizziness, presyncope, or syncope may be related to PVCs, although they are more likely to indicate sustained tachycardia or bradyarrhythmia.

Palpitation is defined as an unpleasant perception of the heartbeat as rapid or forceful. A "skipped beat" suggests an awareness of the compensatory pause frequently associated with premature beats, and a forceful sensation is commonly related to the increased contractility and augmented ejection of the post-extrasystolic beat.

There is a frequent discrepancy between palpitations and documented arrhythmia. Thus, in many patients with and without cardiac disease, palpitations do not correlate with premature beats, but rather, they represent an unpleasant awareness of the heartbeat unassociated with any abnormality of cardiac rhythm. In these cases, the symptom is commonly attributable to anxiety. Moreover, most patients with premature beats, even in relatively high frequency, are not aware of the irregular cardiac activity. By contrast, many more patients with sustained arrhythmias are aware of the abnormality. In this regard, one study that evaluated patients with palpitations reported that the symptom had a cardiac origin in less than one half of the group. The next largest category was psychiatric conditions, most of which were related to panic disorder.

Arrhythmogenic Factors

Important potential causes of premature beats revealed by the clinical evaluation include structural heart disease (ischemic, valvular, hypertensive, primary myocardial, right ventricular dysplasia, mitral valve prolapse), noncardiac disease (pulmonary disease, hyperthyroidism, electrolyte abnormalities), drugs (digitalis, diuretics, psychotropics, sympathomimetics), and habits (caffeine, nicotine, alcohol, cocaine, amphetamines). Optimizing therapy and/or eliminating provoking factors may be sufficient to alleviate premature beats.

PHYSICAL EXAMINATION

The physical examination provides direct evidence of premature beats by detection of an irregular pulse, and therefore in selected patients it is important in indicating the need for further, objective evaluation by ECG and other methods. However, its utility resides in positive findings, because the brevity of the examination renders it insensitive to recognition of even relatively frequent premature beats. Isolated premature beats are distinguished by interruption of a regular rhythm by intermittent, singly occurring premature beats. However, the physical examination is limited beyond this point. It cannot provide the site of origin of the abnormal beat, because all types, by definition, occur early, and each may or may not be associated with a compensatory pause. The latter characteristic is worth emphasizing; it is a common misconception that a compensatory pause is diagnostic of PVCs. Moreover, frequent premature beats of any site of origin may result in an irregularly irregular rhythm indistinguishable from atrial fibrillation, atrial flutter with variable conduction, and multifocal atrial tachycardia. PVCs may be useful in the clinical diagnosis of hypertrophic obstructive cardiomyopathy. In this disease, the pulse of the post-PVC sinus beat, assessed by physical examination, is smaller than the pulse associated with sinus rhythm, whereas in physiologically normal persons and those with systolic murmurs not related to hypertrophic obstructive cardiomyopathy, the post PVC pulse is greater than that in sinus rhythm. This phenomenon is the result of the increased obstruction to left ventricular outflow caused by the augmented contractility of the post-PVC beat (a result of the force-frequency relation of cardiac muscle). The physical examination can reveal the characteristic click murmur of mitral valve prolapse, a condition commonly associated with premature beats.

ELECTROCARDIOGRAM AND AMBULATORY MONITORING

The definitive diagnosis of premature beats requires ECG documentation. The 12-lead ECG is a simple, relatively inexpensive office method by which abnormal beats may be detected. If the rhythm is regular and symptoms are intermittent, ambulatory monitoring is the most accurate means of detecting and quantifying abnormal cardiac rhythm and its relation to symptoms and daily activity. However, this is an expensive method and should be reserved for selected patients with significant symptoms or evidence of cardiac disease. In this regard, it has been found that the diagnostic yield and cost-effectiveness of transtelephonic event monitors are superior to those of 48-hour continuous ambulatory monitoring in the assessment of patients with palpitations. An event recorder provides direct correlation of symptoms and cardiac rhythm in that, rather than yielding a continuous record, it is an ambulatory monitor that is activated by the patient when symptoms occur. The resting ECG can also provide important evidence of cardiac abnormalities that are potential causes of premature beats. Thus, pathologic Q waves indicate prior myocardial infarction or cardiomyopathy.

Enlargement of ventricles or atria can be detected, and ST-T abnormalities may indicate ischemia or fibrosis. Conduction abnormalities such as left bundle branch block are also suggestive of structural heart disease. It is essential to search for ECG patterns associated with arrhythmias (e.g., long QT syndrome, Brugada's syndrome, right ventricular dysplasia, Wolf-Parkinson-White syndrome).

EXERCISE TESTING

This type of testing is useful in selected patients. It is indicated in those with symptoms related to exertion, in whom it provides objective evidence of exercise capacity; occurrence of symptoms; response of heart rate, rhythm, and blood pressure; and evidence of myocardial ischemia. It thereby can confirm or exclude, in a controlled setting, the presence or absence of cardiac rhythm abnormalities during exertional stress and their potential causes. Exercise testing is also useful in patients whose symptoms do not occur during exertion, to evaluate their threshold for arrhythmias and to detect evidence of cardiac disease. Premature beats in most patients, with or without cardiac disease, decrease during exercise and reappear as the heart rate declines after exercise. Exercise-induced reduction in premature beats, therefore, is not evidence of the absence of cardiac disease. However, an increase in the frequency of premature beats during exercise is associated with an increased probability of underlying cardiac disease.

ECHOCARDIOGRAPHY

This method provides noninvasive evaluation of cardiac systolic and diastolic function, chamber dimensions, wall thickness, and valve structure and function. Intracardiac thrombi and pericardial disease are also detectable by echocardiography. Abnormalities of all these aspects of cardiac structure and function may be relevant to the origin of premature beats. In addition, the single most important factor relative to the prognostic significance of PVCs is left ventricular systolic function. Therefore, this single test provides extensive information on cardiac status in a patient with premature beats. In selected patients, stress echocardiography provides a noninvasive approach to the detection of inducible myocardial ischemia and thereby evidence of coronary artery disease.

SUMMARY OF THE GENERAL APPROACH TO THE PATIENT

Evaluation should be thorough, to confirm or exclude the presence of premature beats in patients with compatible symptoms. The correlation between symptoms and objective evidence of premature beats is frequently weak. Patients with persistent symptoms and no evidence of premature beats on screening studies require further testing by methods such as an event recorder or ambulatory ECG monitoring. Exercise testing and echocardiography provide important information of value in selected patients. The former method is useful in patients with exercise-related symptoms suggestive of premature beats, and the latter provides noninvasive cardiac evaluation for detection of the cause of premature beats and the prognostic significance of PVCs. Elimination of provoking factors is essential and may obviate the need for further therapy in many patients.

Atrial Premature Beats

CLINICAL FEATURES

APBs can be detected by prolonged ECG monitoring in approximately 10% of persons without evidence of cardiac disease. However, the prevalence of APBs rises to 80% or more in patients with disease involving the atria, such as dilation or fibrosis. The mechanism is usually automatic foci or reentry foci in the atrium, which are promoted by structural disease, but automatic foci may result from excessive adrenergic activity. Provoking factors include most of the causes enumerated earlier and, in addition, noncardiac conditions such as infection, fever, and emotional stress, which involve sympathetic stimulation. APBs may cause symptoms, but the patient is usually not aware of them unless they are of high frequency.

ELECTROCARDIOGRAM

APBs are recognized on the ECG by the premature appearance and altered morphology of the P wave compared with the sinus P wave. Depending on the site of origin in the atrium and the ECG lead, alterations may include increased or decreased amplitude, widening, notching, or superimposition on the preceding T wave. APBs may be associated with (a) a compensatory pause before the next sinus P wave, (b) a pause that is greater than compensatory, or (c) no pause. These outcomes depend on the timing of the APB and on whether it penetrates and resets the sinus node. Very early APBs may be nonconducted (blocked) and hidden in the T wave. This can result in significant bradycardia if the APBs are bigeminal. Failure to recognize this abnormality may result in inappropriate therapy, such as a pacemaker, when the proper approach is an antiarrhythmic agent to abolish the APBs and to restore sinus rhythm. APBs may also result in aberrant conduction in the His-Purkinje system, owing to impulse conduction before these fibers are fully recovered from the preceding impulse. This yields a widened QRS complex that suggests a ventricular premature beat if the premature P wave is not identified.

MANAGEMENT

The clinical approach to most patients with APBs consists primarily of identifying and eliminating provoking factors and optimizing treatment of underlying cardiac disease, if present. Specific antiarrhythmic therapy is usually not required unless the APBs precipitate tachycardias, in which case digitalis, a β blocker, or a calcium channel blocker that inhibits AV node conduction can be used.

Junctional Premature Beats

CLINICAL FEATURES

JPBs are less frequent than the other two forms of premature beats. They result from abnormal automaticity or reentry mechanisms and are induced by the previously noted provoking factors, most prominent among which are digitalis toxicity, myocardial infarction, and myocarditis. They may also occur in the absence of cardiac disease.

ELECTROCARDIOGRAM

Because the AV junction is located between the atria and ventricles, a JPB depolarizes in both anterograde (to the ventricles) and retrograde (to the atria) directions and can therefore produce both a P wave and a QRS complex. Their sequence on the ECG depends on both the site of origin of JPB in the junctional tissue and the conductivity of the pathways. If the retrograde impulse reaches the atria before the anterograde impulse reaches the ventricles, the result will be a premature, inverted P wave followed by a premature QRS complex; if the atria and ventricles are simultaneously depolarized, the P waves will be lost in the premature QRS complex; and if the ventricles are depolarized initially, a premature QRS complex will precede the premature, inverted P wave. Aberrant conduction within the ventricles may produce a wide QRS that is indistinguishable from a ventricular premature beat.

MANAGEMENT

Isolated JPBs are managed by correction of the underlying process. Specific antiarrhythmic therapy is usually not warranted unless sustained tachycardia occurs.

Ventricular Premature Beats

CLINICAL FEATURES

PVCs are the most frequent form of premature beat. They are associated with increased prognostic risk in patients with left ventricular dysfunction and are therefore a continuing therapeutic challenge. Drug therapy to suppress PVCs to prevent serious ventricular arrhythmias has been unsuccessful and is associated with increased mortality related to proarrhythmia. PVCs encompass the entire spectrum of provoking factors, but significant impairment of left ventricular function is the most important and most difficult to treat. PVCs originate at any site in the His-Purkinje (ventricular) conducting system and depolarize the right and left ventricles consecutively (rather than nearly simultaneously as occurs normally) by abnormal routes, thus accounting for the altered QRS complex in the ECG.

ELECTROCARDIOGRAM

A PVC is characterized on the ECG by a premature, bizarre, wide (0.12 seconds or longer) QRS complex. The ST segment and T wave are usually directed opposite to the dominant deflection of the QRS, representing a secondary repolarization abnormality. (In the simplest terms, abnormal depolarization results in abnormal repolarization.) A retrograde P wave may be seen but is commonly obscured in the wide QRS complex. Retrograde activation of the atria may also be precluded by their prior depolarization by the normal sinus beat before the arrival of the retrograde impulse. A PVC usually results in a compensatory pause before the next sinus beat, but depending on the timing of the PVC and conduction velocity of the impulses, there may be no pause.

A wide QRS complex may represent a beat of supraventricular origin when aberrant conduction is present. This phenomenon occurs when a premature beat arises from a supraventricular focus before the nodal and infranodal conducting pathways (AV node, junctional tissues, and bundle branches) are completely repolarized. This abnormal conduction is reflected by aberration-distortion and widening of the QRS complex, which can be difficult to distinguish from PVCs. This is an important distinction because of the different clinical implications of supraventricular premature beats and PVCs. Morphologic criteria have been developed to aid in discrimination of aberrantly conducted beats and PVCs. Although these criteria are helpful, they are not definitive.

Descriptors favoring aberration include antecedent P wave, right bundle branch block pattern, triphasic QRS configuration in V_1 (rsRN), and initial QRS identical to the normally conducted beats. Descriptors favoring ventricular origin include fusion beats, capture beats, QRS complex of 140 milliseconds or longer, left axis deviation, AV dissociation, and certain configurational characteristics of the QRS (V_1: monophasic or biphasic or R>R′; V_6: QS or rS; concordance: similar QRS polarity in V_1 to V_6).

MANAGEMENT

In patients with and without cardiac disease, symptoms from isolated PVCs are unusual, even when the abnormal beats are frequent. The therapeutic dilemma posed by PVCs is primarily related to their importance as a risk factor for sudden death in patients with left ventricular dysfunction, a finding indicating they may be triggers for initiating lethal ventricular tachyarrhythmias. Alternatively, PVCs may be markers of electrical instability and high risk without having an initiating role. In studies of survivors of myocardial infarction, it has been established that the presence of high-grade PVCs (more than 10 per hour) increases the risk of death. Thus, the long-term mortality rate in patients with the combination of left ventricular ejection fraction of less than 40% and greater than 10 PVCs per hour was 1.5 to 2.1 times higher than the mortality rate in patients with the same ejection fraction and fewer than 10 PVCs per hour. However, as previously indicated, drug therapy to reduce mortality by eliminating or decreasing the frequency of high-grade PVCs in patients with left ventricular dysfunction, with the goal of preventing lethal arrhythmias, not only has failed to achieve this end but also has been associated with an increase in mortality.

The deleterious outcomes of drug therapy were obtained in the Cardiac Arrhythmia Suppression Trial, and they resulted in a general policy of refraining from the use of antiarrhythmic therapy in patients with asymptomatic PVCs. Amiodarone (Cordarone) has the best record of efficacy and safety for drug therapy of high-grade PVCs but it is recommended only in high-risk patients. Noninvasive techniques such as the signal-averaged ECG have been useful in identifying those patients within this population who are at the highest risk. The approach to high-grade PVCs in patients with left ventricular dysfunction comprises vigorous management of the underlying disease with the appropriate cardioprotective agents (aspirin, β-adrenergic blockade, and lipid-lowering therapy for coronary artery disease; angiotensin-converting enzyme inhibitors, a diuretic, and digitalis for left ventricular dysfunction), optimization of anti-ischemic therapy, and correction of metabolic abnormalities.

In patients with acute coronary events (myocardial infarction, unstable angina), asymptomatic PVCs may presage the development of sustained ventricular arrhythmias. Therefore, in selected patients in this setting, it is reasonable to use antiarrhythmic drug therapy (e.g., β blockade, amiodarone). However, the first approach is elimination of provoking factors (ischemia, pain, cardiac failure, metabolic abnormalities). Patients with PVCs that impair hemodynamic function require therapy.

In patients without evidence of structural heart disease, it is clear the PVCs impose no increase in prognostic risk. Distressing palpitations should be managed by correction of provoking factors and reassurance to the patient. This approach should result in the need for drug therapy in a very small minority of this group who have intolerable palpitations associated with anxiety. The most appropriate drug is a β blocker because of its efficacy and safety. This approach is particularly useful in patients in whom PVCs are related to adrenergic stimulation associated with exercise or emotional stress.

In summary, specific drug therapy for asymptomatic, isolated PVCs is not currently indicated in patients with or without cardiac disease. In the former, drug therapy has not been beneficial and has been associated with increased mortality. In patients without cardiac disease, PVCs are not a risk factor for more serious arrhythmias, and drug therapy should be avoided in all but exceptional cases.

HEART BLOCK

METHOD OF

Robert W. Peters, MD, and
Michael R. Gold, MD, PhD

The term heart block encompasses a wide variety of disorders of diverse etiologies. Until the early 1960s heart block was largely an electrocardiographic curiosity that was devoid of any true therapeutic implications. The development and refinement of permanent pacing techniques have had a major impact upon the natural history of heart block. Although medications may occasionally be helpful in individuals with mild symptoms, in most cases, advanced heart block requires permanent pacing, or, depending on the presence, type, and severity of underlying heart disease, an implantable cardioverter defibrillator (ICD) with bradycardia pacing capabilities. In this article, we briefly review some aspects of the basic anatomy and physiology as well as the histopathology and pathophysiology of the conduction system. The bulk of our discussion, however, focuses on the clinical aspects, including etiology, diagnosis, and treatment of individuals with conduction system disease.

Functional Anatomy of the Specialized Conduction System

The atrioventricular (AV) node is a small ovoid structure embedded in the interatrial septum. It consists of a combination of small, star-like P cells (thought to be the site of impulse initiation), Purkinje cells, muscle cells, and atrial transitional cells imbedded in a loose framework of collagen. The embryologic development of the AV node is separate from the His-Purkinje system, and it has been suggested that this phylogenetic separation may be a protective adaptation in that it blocks conduction and allows the AV node to prevent very rapid atrial rates (as might occur in atrial flutter or fibrillation) from being conducted to the ventricles. The AV node has extensive autonomic innervation (both sympathetic and parasympathetic) and an abundant blood supply, mostly from the large AV nodal artery that emanates from the right coronary artery 90% of the time.

The AV node terminates in a poorly defined group of Purkinje fibers that converge into a distinct band (the common bundle of His) and descend through the membranous septum before dividing into the bundle branches near the crest of the muscular septum. These Purkinje fibers are separated by a collagenous framework embedded with P cells (especially in the proximal aspect). The His bundle has relatively sparse autonomic innervation, but it does have an abundant blood supply, usually from branches of both the AV nodal artery and the left anterior descending coronary artery.

The right bundle branch originates from the His bundle, usually as a slender bundle of Purkinje fibers that descends to the base of the anterior papillary muscle where it trifurcates. In contrast, the left bundle branch spreads out, sometimes in a fan-like fashion, over the left ventricle. In at least some individuals, the left bundle branch divides into two distinct fascicles—a broad anterior superior fascicle that courses along the left ventricular outflow tract, and a shorter group of fibers (the posterior inferior fascicle) that extends along the posterior septum toward the posterior papillary muscle. In others there is also a separate septal fascicle that activates the septum directly. As with the His bundle, there is sparse autonomic innervation of the bundle branches but abundant blood supply from branches of both the left and right coronary arteries. There is considerable interindividual variation in the anatomy and also in the blood supply of the bundle branches, which is reinforced by multiple anastomoses.

Histopathology of the Specialized Conduction System

Because the AV node and His bundle evolve embryologically as separate entities, congenital AV block is most likely related to failure of fusion of the embryonic primordia. Acquired AV node disease may be caused by a variety of etiologies. Because of the abundant blood supply and extensive fiber network entering the AV node from the atria, acquired complete AV nodal block is relatively uncommon. Even in the setting of acute myocardial infarction, necrosis of the AV node is rare and most cases of complete AV block resolve spontaneously. Because the His bundle and bundle branches also possess a very ample blood supply, frank necrosis of these areas is similarly uncommon. Most frequently, postmortem examinations of the conduction system in patients with advanced heart block have revealed nonspecific degenerative changes and fibrosis.

The standard 12-lead electrocardiogram tends to be a relatively poor indicator of the site of heart block. Disease within the conduction system is often diffuse, and individuals who clinically appear to have heart block at the level of the AV node often have extensive disease within the His-Purkinje system as well. Similarly, patients who present with block of a single bundle branch (e.g., right bundle-branch block [RBBB]) often have severe involvement of the other bundle branch.

Physiology of the Specialized Conduction System

The AV node is strategically located between the heart's major receiving and pumping chambers, the atria and the ventricles. The cells in the AV node involved in impulse transmission differ from those of the His-Purkinje system in that they are characterized by the calcium-dependent slow response, decreasing conduction velocity, and prolonging refractoriness. These characteristics help to explain some of the major properties of the AV node that are relevant clinically. These include serving as an area of conduction delay, assuring appropriate timing, and allowing the atria to fully *prime* the ventricles, acting as a filter to prevent dangerously rapid rates from being transmitted to the ventricles, and functioning as a subsidiary pacemaker in the event of sinus node dysfunction.

As described above, the His bundle consists of a group of parallel Purkinje fibers that conduct impulses rapidly to the ventricles. The collagenous septae that compartmentalize the His bundle provide the substrate for longitudinal dissociation of the fascicles. Thus, bundle-branch block or even isolated fascicular can be produced by lesions within the common bundle, proximal to its division into the various fascicles.

Purkinje cells have been demonstrated to have a progressive increase in refractory periods as they extend distally, to a point approximately 2 mm from their termination in the ventricular muscle, after which they progressively decrease. This *gate* serves to prevent propagation of premature impulses traveling in either direction. The bundle-branch/fascicle system provides for synchronous and coordinated contraction of the ventricles that maximizes cardiac output. It follows then that intraventricular conduction defects may deleteriously affect cardiac performance, especially in individuals with preexisting left ventricular dysfunction. This observation has led to a variety of newer pacing techniques aimed at *resynchronizing* ventricular contraction, most recently using biventricular pacing.

Electrocardiographic Aspects of Heart Block (Table 1)

Heart block has been conventionally divided into first, second, and third-degree AV blocks. In first-degree AV block, the pulmonary regurgitation (PR) interval is prolonged but the delay can be at the level of the AV node, the His-Purkinje system, or both. Second-degree AV block has traditionally been divided into:

- Type I block, defined as having a gradual PR interval prolongation followed by a nonconducted sinus P wave

TABLE 1 Electrocardiographic Manifestations of AV Block

Type of Block	Electrocardiogram	Location of Block
First-degree	PR prolongation	AVN = HPS
Second-degree		
Type I	PR prolongs progressively before nonconducted P wave	AV node (narrow QRS) AVN = HPS (wide QRS)
Type II	Sudden nonconducted P wave without PR prolongation	Always HPS
2:1 AV block	Nonconducted P wave every other beat	AVN = HPS
Higher degrees of AV block	Multiple consecutive nonconducted P waves	AVN (narrow QRS) HPS (wide QRS)
Third-degree AV block	All P waves nonconducted	
Narrow QRS		AVN>HPS
Wide QRS		HPS>AVN

Abbreviations: AV = atrioventricular; AVN = atrioventricular node; HPS = His-Purkinje system; PR = PR interval; QRS = electrocardiographic wave.

- Type II block, defined as having no progressive PR prolongation

Type I block usually occurs at the level of the AV node, especially when the electrocardiographic wave (QRS) complex is narrow, whereas type II block occurs almost exclusively within the His-Purkinje system or, occasionally, within the common bundle itself. On occasion, differentiating between type I and type II second-degree AV blocks can be difficult, and this differentiation has been the source of some controversy. High-degree AV block is characterized by two or more (consecutive) nonconducted sinus P waves, culminating in complete (third-degree) AV block where none of the P waves are conducted to the ventricles.

Clinical Aspects of Atrioventricular Block (Table 2)

ATRIOVENTRICULAR NODAL BLOCK

There are many disease processes capable of producing high-grade AV block at the level of the AV node. In general, prognosis seems most closely related to the specific etiology and to the presence and severity of organic heart disease. Chronic high-grade block at the AV node is usually associated with a low incidence of syncope and sudden cardiac death, so a trial of medical therapy (generally oral theophylline[1], 200 to 300 mg every 12 hours) may be warranted in individuals with relatively mild symptoms. (Oral ephedrine[1] and sublingual isoproterenol [Isuprel] have also been tried in the past but were largely abandoned because of poor patient tolerance.) Patients who are more symptomatic (e.g., recurrent syncope, severe exercise intolerance associated with a slow ventricular rate) usually require permanent pacing. The need for permanent pacing in AV block is addressed in detail in a 2002 update of the joint guidelines from the American College of Cardiology (ACC), the American Heart Association (AHA), and the North American Society for Pacing and Electrophysiology (NASPE); therefore, the issue is addressed only briefly in this article.

A few clinical situations are worthy of specific comment. Although there have been no controlled clinical trials, complete AV block caused by radiofrequency catheter ablation is generally associated with an absent or unreliable escape rhythm, and permanent pacing seems mandatory. Although it had been thought for years that congenital AV block was associated with a low incidence of symptoms or sudden cardiac death, recent studies suggest that most individuals will eventually require pacemakers, and permanent pacemaker implantation, even in childhood, is becoming more common. Lastly, AV block in the setting of progressive neuromuscular diseases (such as myotonic muscular dystrophy or Kearns-Sayre syndrome) is considered potentially malignant, regardless of the site of block, because of the diffuse nature and unpredictable progression of conduction

TABLE 2 Etiology of Chronic Conduction System Disease

Ischemic (acute myocardial infarction, acute ischemia, reperfusion, coronary artery spasm)
Congenital (endocardial cushion defect)
Valvular (calcific aortic stenosis)
Traumatic (traumatic injury, following open heart surgery, radiofrequency, alcohol, or surgical ablation)
Benign tumors (fibroma, etc.)
Malignant tumors (leiomyosarcoma, etc.)
Benign infiltrative (amyloid, sarcoid, hemochromatosis, carcinoid)
Malignant infiltrative (leukemia, lymphoma, myeloma)
Connective tissue disorders (rheumatoid arthritis, systemic lupus erythematosus, scleroderma)
Infectious (diphtheria, viral myocarditis, bacterial endocarditis, Lyme disease, Chagas' disease, luetic)
Degenerative (Lev's disease, Lenègre's disease)
Neuromuscular (Friedreich's ataxia, Kearns-Sayre syndrome, myotonic dystrophy, Erb's dystrophy)
Metabolic (myxedema, thyrotoxicosis, Paget's disease)

[1]Not FDA approved for this indication.

TABLE 3 Class I Indications for Permanent Pacing in Chronic Heart Block

Acquired AV Block

High-grade or complete AV block at any anatomic location associated with any of the following:

1. Symptomatic bradycardia (including heart failure)
2. Arrhythmias and other conditions requiring drugs that result in symptomatic bradycardia
3. Documented asystole ≥3 seconds
4. Escape rate <40 beats/min in awake, symptom-free patients
5. Following catheter ablation of the AV junction
6. Postoperative AV block not expected to resolve after cardiac surgery
7. Neuromuscular diseases with AV block, with or without symptoms, because of the possibility of unpredictable progression

Chronic Bifascicular or Trifascicular Block and the Following:

1. Intermittent second- or third-degree AV block
2. Alternating bundle-branch block

Congenital Heart Disease

1. Advanced second- or third-degree AV block with symptomatic bradycardia, congestive heart failure, or low cardiac output
2. Postoperative second- or third-degree AV block that is not expected to resolve or persists ≥7 days after cardiac surgery
3. Third-degree AV block with a wide QRS complex escape rhythm, complex ventricular ectopy, or ventricular dysfunction
4. Sustained pause-dependent ventricular tachycardia, with or without prolonged QT, in which the efficacy of pacing is thoroughly documented

Abbreviations: QRS = electrocardiographic wave; QT = electrocardiographic interval from the beginning of QRS complex to end of the T wave.

system disease. Permanent pacing is generally recommended in this situation.

INFRANODAL BLOCK

Although less common than AV nodal block, there are also a large number of diseases that may be associated with chronic infranodal block. Histologic examination of the conduction system in most of these cases generally reveals nonspecific sclerodegenerative changes. Because the escape rhythm in patients with high-grade infranodal block tends to be slow and unreliable, permanent pacing is usually recommended for these individuals.

A summary of the class I indications for permanent pacing in chronic AV block (conditions for which there is evidence and/or general agreement that a procedure is beneficial, useful, and effective) is provided in Table 3.

BUNDLE-BRANCH BLOCK

Bundle-branch block is a relatively common electrocardiographic abnormality with a differential diagnosis similar to that for AV block. Patients with bundle-branch block are at increased risk of progression to high-grade AV block and sudden cardiac death (Framingham). However, the risk of these complications is low, considering the size of the population at risk, and does not warrant routine prophylactic permanent pacemaker insertion. Examination of the data from a number of large prospective epidemiologic studies suggests that prognosis is most closely related to the presence and severity of underlying cardiovascular disease.

In the late 1970s, several large prospective studies used intracardiac recordings in an attempt to identify patients with bundle-branch block who were at especially high risk of complications. In general, the populations examined in these studies were referral-based (not randomly selected) and potentially biased toward patients with symptoms (e.g., syncope, seizures) suggestive of intermittent high-degree block. Although there is no universal agreement, an infranodal conduction time interval of more than 100 msec is generally considered a class IIa indication for permanent pacing (conditions for which there is conflicting evidence and/or a divergence of opinion, but the weight of evidence is in favor of usefulness/efficacy of a procedure), especially in symptomatic individuals. Unfortunately, this finding is relatively nonspecific and insensitive. In the setting of significant organic heart disease, the patient with recurrent syncope should undergo complete electrophysiologic evaluation to exclude other arrhythmic causes such as sinus node disease or ventricular tachycardia.

ADDITIONAL TECHNIQUES INCLUDING STRESSING THE CONDUCTION SYSTEM

Despite the above observations, there remain a number of patients with conduction system disease and recurrent syncope of unknown causes. Performing 24-hour ambulatory electrocardiographic recordings (Holter monitor) may be helpful, especially in individuals with frequent symptoms. Also, 30-day event recorders and loop recorders are now routinely employed; and recently the implantable loop recorder, with a battery lasting up to 2 years, has been demonstrated to be especially effective in identifying individuals with recurrent syncope caused by intermittent high-degree AV block.

There are now a variety of means of stressing the conduction system to help identify individuals who are likely to require permanent pacing. Exercise-induced AV block (which is almost always infranodal) is specific but extremely insensitive. Atrial pacing-induced infranodal block (with intact AV nodal conduction) improves the diagnostic yield but remains relatively insensitive. Various pharmacologic agents have also been suggested, including intravenous procainamide (Pronestyl)[1], disopyramide (Norpace)[1], ajmaline[2], and flecainide (Tambocor)[1]. They appear to improve sensitivity, but the specificity remains untested.

---

[1]Not FDA approved for this indication.

[2]Not available in the United States.

In summary, in patients with documented symptomatic irreversible second- or third-degree AV block, with or without coexisting bundle-branch block, permanent pacing is indicated. In addition, there are various subgroups (e.g., degenerative neuromuscular diseases, congenital AV block, etc.) in which permanent pacing in asymptomatic individuals should be strongly considered. Patients with clinical evidence of conduction system disease and recurrent symptoms, but in whom a high-degree block has not been documented, should undergo ambulatory electrocardiographic recordings. Individuals with negative studies should have complete electrophysiologic evaluations, with provocative maneuvers if necessary. Finally, if the cause of symptoms has still not been elucidated, an implantable loop recorder should be considered.

Acute Myocardial Infarction and Acute Ischemic Syndromes

The significance of heart block in the setting of acute myocardial infarction and in acute ischemic syndromes is largely dependent upon the site of the infarct (and/or ischemia) and the clinical status of the patient. As discussed in the section on functional anatomy, inferior wall myocardial infarction is generally caused by involvement of the right coronary artery, usually the major (but not the only) blood supply of the AV node. AV block in this setting, even when complete, is often well tolerated because of the presence of a relatively rapid, reliable escape rhythm. Because the blood supply of the AV node is so abundant, AV block is usually caused by hypervagotonia or by edema and/or ischemia rather than frank necrosis, and tends to be transient. Accordingly, treatment is usually directed at symptomatic relief. The truly asymptomatic patient should be observed carefully but warrants no specific therapy. In the patient demonstrating signs or symptoms of hypoperfusion, intravenous atropine (0.5 to 1.0 mg), low-dose isoproterenol (1 to 4 mg/min), or oral theophylline[1] (200 to 300 mg every 12 hours) may be helpful, with temporary pacing as an alternative if pharmacotherapy is ineffective or associated with unacceptable side effects. In the vast majority of instances, conduction abnormalities resolve spontaneously and permanent pacing is unnecessary.

In acute anterior myocardial infarction, heart block is usually associated with occlusive disease in the proximal portion of the left anterior descending coronary artery. Unlike inferior wall myocardial infarction, heart block in this setting is caused by disease in the His-Purkinje system. The resulting idioventricular escape rhythm is slow and unreliable, so even a single nonconducted sinus P wave mandates emergency temporary pacing. Complete heart block is usually caused by extensive necrosis of the His-Purkinje system. Because the infarct is frequently very large, mortality, even with temporary pacing, is extremely high because of severe left ventricular dysfunction. Similarly, because the blood supply of the bundle branches is so abundant, bundle-branch block in anterior wall infarction is also associated with very large infarcts and the mortality is correspondingly high. The class I indications for temporary and permanent pacing in patients with conduction system disease associated with acute myocardial infarction are listed in Table 4.

TABLE 4 Class I Indications for Pacing with Heart Block and Acute Myocardial Infarction

Temporary Pacing

1. Symptomatic bradycardia (including type I second-degree AV block)
2. Bilateral bundle-branch block/alternating bundle-branch block or RBBB with alternating LAFB and LPFB
3. Bifascicular block of new or indeterminate age and first-degree AV block
4. Type II second-degree AV block

Permanent Pacing

1. Persistent second-degree AV block within the His-Purkinje system with bilateral bundle branch block
2. Third-degree AV block within the His-Purkinje system
3. Transient second- or third-degree AV block within the His-Purkinje system with coexisting bundle-branch block
4. Persistent symptomatic second- or third-degree block at any location

Abbreviations: LAFB = left anterior fascicular block; LPFB = left posterior fascicular block; RBBB = right bundle-branch block.

Regardless of the site of infarction, patients with high-degree AV block have an increased mortality. The use of thrombolytic agents and, more recently, acute angioplasty have had a major impact upon mortality in acute myocardial infarction, but so far have not been shown to diminish mortality in patients with complete AV block.

Heart block is a relatively common condition of diverse etiologies displaying various clinical manifestations. Some knowledge of the functional anatomy, histopathology, and physiology of the specialized conduction system may provide considerable insight for the clinician dealing with patients with conduction system disease. The development of permanent pacing techniques has made definitive therapy available. Based upon accumulated information, a combined task force from the ACC/AHA/NASPE has recently provided up-to-date and relatively detailed indications for pacemaker implantation. These recommendations are not intended as rigid rules to be blindly implemented but are meant to assist the clinician as general guidelines, and to be interpreted in light of a particular clinical setting. The recommendations will doubtless continue to evolve along with the evolution of pacing techniques and as our understanding of the conduction system continues to grow.

[1]Not FDA approved for this indication.

TACHYCARDIAS

METHOD OF
Mathias L. Stoenescu, MD, and
Peter R. Kowey, MD

The category of *tachycardias* encompasses a heterogeneous group of heart rhythms, which have in common a rate exceeding 100 beats per minute (bpm). Another group of rhythms displaying rates higher than expected, but generally less than 100 bpm, are called *accelerated rhythms* (e.g., accelerated idioventricular rhythm, accelerated junctional rhythm, etc.). Some in this latter group may represent escape rhythms manifesting a faster rate than the typical escape rate emanating from that particular focus. The interest in tachycardias has increased proportionally to the advances in understanding their mechanisms and devising more effective treatments. New antiarrhythmic drugs, ablation techniques, and antiarrhythmic devices have started to play major roles in our therapeutic approach. In this context, knowing the mechanism has become vital.

The mechanism underlying a majority of tachycardias is *reentry*. Two pathways—one with a fast conduction speed and longer refractoriness, the other with slower conduction but a shorter refractory period—constitute a potential reentry circuit. An impulse that encounters a unidirectional block in the fast pathway during its longer refractory period will instead take the route of the slow-conducting pathway. Because of its shorter refractory period, this pathway has already recovered and hence will conduct the impulse. Arriving at the lower junction of the two pathways, the impulse, which has traveled relatively slowly through the slow pathway, will find the fast pathway recovered and will return to its origin via this pathway, thus establishing a reentry circuit. If this cycle repeats itself, a reentrant tachycardia has been established (Figure 1).

Increased automaticity represents another mechanism generating tachycardias. Myocytes displaying spontaneous pacemaker activity override the natural pacemaker cells of the heart by reaching the threshold for activation faster than normal pacemaker cells (steeper phase 4 slope).

Triggered activity is the third mechanism that results in tachycardias and is related to increased automaticity. The difference is that cells do not exhibit increased automaticity spontaneously, but as a result of preceding stimuli, like pacing. This mechanism depends on previous depolarizations to generate delayed afterdepolarizations. These are potentials, which occur after repolarization (phase 4) has taken place. They fluctuate in amplitude and may reach the depolarization threshold, producing a sustained arrhythmia.

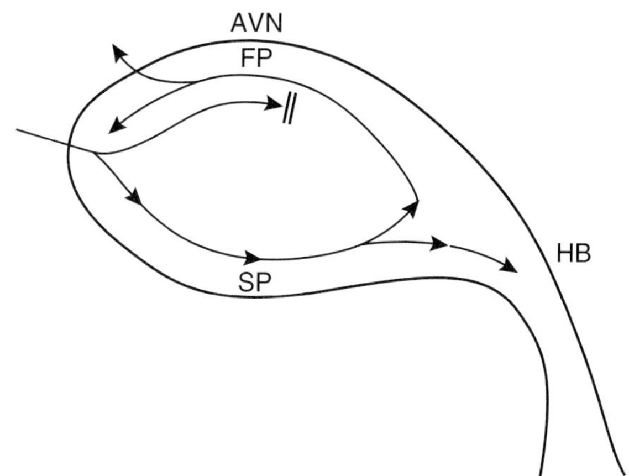

FIGURE 1 In typical atrioventricular nodal reentry tachycardias (AVNRT), the impulse encounters unidirectional block in the fast pathway and takes the route of the slow pathway instead. It returns via the now recovered FP to complete the reentry circuit within the AVN. AVN = atrioventricular node; FP = fast pathway; HB = His bundle; SP = slow pathway.

Several classifications have been proposed, each based on different aspects of the tachycardias. Considering the site of origin, two major categories emerge:

1. *SVT (supraventricular tachycardias)* from the sinus node, the atria, and the atrioventricular (AV) junction
2. *VT (ventricular tachycardias)* from all sites below the AV junction

A second classification applicable to SVTs considers the relation between P waves and R waves on the electrocardiogram (ECG) during the tachycardia. If the RP interval is longer than the PR interval, the tachycardia falls into the category of *long RP*; whereas an RP interval shorter than the PR interval represents a *short RP* category (Table 1). A third classification takes the morphology of the electrocardiographic QRS complex during tachycardia into account—*narrow QRS* (less than 100 ms) versus *wide QRS* (greater than 100 ms). A majority of SVTs, but not all, exhibit a narrow QRS; and a majority of VTs exhibit a wide QRS with a few notable exceptions. ECG criteria that are useful in discriminating

TABLE 1 Classification of Supraventricular Tachycardias Based on P-Wave to R-Wave Relationship

Long RP (RP > PR)	Short RP (RP < PR)	Others
SANRT	—	Atrial flutter
AT	—	Atrial fibrillation
PJRT	NPJT	
AVNRT (atypical)	AVNRT (typical)	

Abbreviations: AT = atrial tachycardia; AVNRT = atrioventricular nodal reentry tachycardias; NPJT = nonparoxysmal junctional tachycardia; PJRT = permanent junctional reciprocating tachycardia; SANRT = sinoatrial node reentry tachycardia.

TABLE 2 ECG Criteria in Favor of Ventricle Tachycardias

AV dissociation
Capture beats
Fusion beats
RS nadir interval >100 ms
QRS >140 ms
Right axis deviation (–90 degrees to +180 degrees)
Left axis shift during tachycardia (compared with SR)

Abbreviations: AV = atrioventricular; QRS = electrocardiographic wave; SR = sinus rhythm.

between SVT with aberrant conduction displaying wide QRS morphology and VT are listed in Table 2.

A fourth classification pertinent to SVTs looks at the dependency of a tachycardia on the AV node. This has obvious therapeutic implications. An AV node, independent tachycardia for instance cannot be terminated by AV nodal blocking drugs, although ventricular rate control may be achieved by slowing AV conduction.

History

The clinical diagnosis is greatly aided by a detailed history. Palpitations and their description (i.e., rapid versus slow, regular versus irregular), syncope, presyncope, lightheadedness, angina, and dyspnea should be inquired about. The duration and frequency of these symptoms and the circumstances leading to their onset and termination are all significant. For example, abrupt onset or offset suggests a reentrant mechanism. A careful drug history must include all prescription drugs in addition to all over-the-counter (OTC) substances. The use of alcohol, tobacco, recreational drugs, and caffeine should not be ignored. A search for symptoms associated with conditions causing dysrhythmias should be conducted, particularly electrolyte abnormalities, thyroid dysfunction, coronary artery disease (CAD), congestive heart failure (CHF), and pulmonary disease. The family history is helpful when dealing with syncope, idiopathic dilated cardiomyopathy, hypertrophic cardiomyopathy, long QT syndromes, and preexcitation syndromes.

Physical Examination

Determining the heart rate and ascertaining whether the pulse is regular or irregular are helpful, and educating patients and relatives in taking the pulse is worth the time investment. Blood pressure (BP) change related to the tachycardia should be the first physical sign examined as it guides the whole approach to the tachycardia. For example, a tachycardia causing hypotension is by definition unstable and requires prompt treatment (usually cardioversion), whereas the absence of any significant BP drop generally allows for more time to evaluate and treat a dysrhythmia. The jugular venous pulse may reveal cannon waves as a manifestation of the right atrium contracting when the tricuspid valve is closed, as is the case with AV dissociation. Auscultatory findings, albeit rather nonspecific, may provide clues to associated conditions like valvular heart disease, congenital anomalies, and others.

Finally, the response to maneuvers like Valsalva or carotid sinus massage (CSM) may help in diagnosing and also in terminating certain tachycardias. In atrial flutter, for example, CSM by slowing conduction in the AV node will demonstrate the presence of flutter waves, previously hidden in the QRS complexes. Atrioventricular nodal reentry tachycardias (AVNRTs) and atrioventricular reentry tachycardias (AVRTs), on the other hand, may terminate abruptly, as CSM slows conduction in the AV node, which represents one limb of their reentry circuit.

Electrocardiography

One cannot overstate the importance of obtaining a 12-lead ECG during the tachycardia, if the circumstances allow it. Rhythm strips are helpful and often represent the only documentation of the arrhythmia in question, but their diagnostic yield is overshadowed by the 12-lead ECG. This has the ability to provide more accurate information regarding P wave and QRS axis and morphology. Two newer technologies—the first allowing both patient-triggered as well as continuous monitoring over longer periods of time, and the second represented by implantable loop recorders—have emerged to complement Holter monitoring for outpatient use. They constitute invaluable tools in the often frustrating attempt to document a specific tachycardia.

Sinus Tachycardia

Sinus tachycardia can be physiologic, in response to exercise or certain states (anxiety, fever, hypovolemia, etc.), or nonphysiologic. Physiologic sinus tachycardia arises in the sinus node and, because it is not reentrant, has a gradual onset and termination.

INAPPROPRIATE SINUS TACHYCARDIA

Inappropriate sinus tachycardia is a chronic condition manifested as a resting heart rate of more than 100 bpm without an obvious cause. There is a variant showing an inappropriate increase in the sinus rate in response to exercise, with heart rates disproportionate to the level of exercise. The morphology of the P waves is identical to that of normal sinus rhythm given their common origin in the sinus node. If the patient is symptomatic, both variants respond well to β blockers and only in the rare case of drug treatment failures is a catheter-based intervention necessary for modification or ablation of the sinus node.

SINOATRIAL NODE REENTRY TACHYCARDIA

Sinoatrial node reentry tachycardia (SANRT) has a sudden onset and termination, which often represents the only clue to its diagnosis. Because it originates in the sinus node or its close proximity, it has virtually identical morphology to the normal sinus rhythm. It is a long RP type of SVT with a P wave in front of each QRS complex and constant PR intervals. CSM can terminate it. Both β blockers and calcium channel blockers (CCBs), like diltiazem (Cardizem) or verapamil (Calan), can prevent or decrease the frequency of paroxysms and, administered intravenously, can terminate this tachycardia. Refractory cases are amenable to ablation.

ATRIAL TACHYCARDIA

Two mechanisms underlie the atrial tachycardia (AT) form of SVT. A spatially restricted circuit called micro-reentry causes *the paroxysmal type of atrial tachycardia*, which can be induced and terminated by pacing. The other is the truly *focal* or *automatic atrial tachycardia* caused by increased automaticity within a given atrial focus. Both account for approximately 4% of SVTs. The rate of AT is usually 120 to 250 bpm and is subject to autonomic nervous influences. The RP interval is long, and the P wave morphology and axis depend on their site of origin in the right or left atrium; they are usually different from the P waves in normal sinus rhythm. Occasionally, the tachycardia stems from an area close to the sinus node making the P wave morphology indistinguishable from that of sinus rhythm. Vagal maneuvers commonly fail to terminate this AV–node-independent tachycardia; but by inducing transient AV block, they expose the P waves and thus help in the diagnosis. When AT presents in conjunction with AV block, digitalis toxicity should be suspected.

Acutely administered intravenous CCBs, such as diltiazem (5 to 20 mg bolus) or verapamil (5 mg bolus repeated to a maximum of 20 mg), are effective in terminating AT. β–blockers given intravenously are somewhat less effective, and adenosine (Adenocard) is rarely effective. The CCBs and the β blockers have the advantage of decreasing the ventricular rate even if they fail to terminate the tachycardia. Prophylactic treatment to prevent recurrences is based on oral preparations of the same CCBs or β blockers, and sometimes combinations of both classes prove useful. Amiodarone (Cordarone) should be reserved for only the most refractory cases and when other less toxic alternatives are contraindicated. Class I C drugs like flecainide (Tambocor) and propafenone (Rythmol) have also been successfully employed to maintain sinus rhythm, but structural heart disease prohibits their use.

MULTIFOCAL ATRIAL TACHYCARDIA

Multifocal atrial tachycardia (MAT) is a separate entity from the ATs described above. The mechanism seems to be abnormal automaticity. The diagnosis rests on the electrocardiographic criteria of identifying at least three different P wave morphologies and a ventricular rate exceeding 100 bpm. Both atrial and ventricular rates are irregular and the PR interval varies in length. It is often associated with pulmonary disease (usually chronic obstructive pulmonary disease [COPD]), but can also be encountered in a variety of acute illnesses. It can be associated with use of theophylline and digoxin. It is sometimes mistaken for atrial fibrillation, which is unfortunate, especially when attempts are made to control the rate with digoxin, which, as mentioned, may be a causative factor. Treatment is based on addressing the primary cause or stopping the offending drug. Rate control can usually be successfully achieved with CCBs and β blockers; the latter, however, have to be used with caution in patients with pulmonary diseases.

ATRIOVENTRICULAR NODAL REENTRY TACHYCARDIA

AVNRT is a narrow-complex SVT caused by a reentrant circuit within the AV node. Two pathways—one with a short refractory period, but slow conduction, and one with rapid conduction and longer refractoriness—form the two limbs of the circuit. In sinus rhythm the impulse travels down the fast pathway to depolarize the ventricles, but cannot conduct retrogradely up the slow pathway, as this is now refractory. A premature atrial depolarization may, however, find the fast pathway refractory and instead take the route of the slow pathway to depolarize the ventricles. The longer conduction time will allow the fast pathway to recover, and the impulse can now travel back up the fast pathway to establish a reentrant circuit (see Figure 1). AVNRT is the most common type of SVT (60%). The atria and ventricles are depolarized almost simultaneously, hence the P waves fall within the QRS or shortly thereafter (less than 70 ms) making this a very short RP tachycardia. Rates of 150 to 250 bpm are usual.

A variant, called *atypical AVNRT*, occurs when the direction of reentry is reversed causing inverted P waves in the inferior leads II, III, and AVF and a long RP interval. It represents less than 10% of AVNRTs.

Both variants start and end abruptly and may terminate in response to vagal maneuvers, which delay conduction in the slow pathway, thus interrupting the reentrant circuit. Drugs that block conduction in the AV node—adenosine (Adenocard), verapamil (Isoptin), diltiazem (Cardizem), and β blockers like metoprolol (Lopressor)[1]—given intravenously are effective in terminating AVNRT, and the latter three in oral formulations prevent recurrences. CCBs should be avoided in wide-complex tachycardias, because they may induce dangerous hypotension in VT or AF with Wolff-Parkinson-White (WPW) syndrome. The frequency and severity of symptoms

[1]Not FDA approved for this indication.

(palpitations felt often in the neck, dyspnea, lightheadedness, and syncope) should guide referral for catheter ablation procedures, which are safe and effective.

BYPASS TRACT MEDIATED TACHYCARDIAS

Accessory pathways (APs), or bypass tracts, are strands of myocardial tissue with conduction properties that can be similar to the His Purkinje system. They frequently form an invisible connection between atria and ventricles bypassing the AV node. When impulses travel fast down the AP, they depolarize the ventricles somewhat prematurely and fuse with the impulses traveling slower through the AV node. This is called preexcitation, and the resulting QRS complexes exhibit a delta wave (a slurring of the initial part of the complex), which becomes wide. The PR interval is short. Patients who have APs, which conduct antegradely, have the *WPW syndrome,* with SVTs escaping the protective blocking properties of the AV node and conducting rapidly to the ventricles. Atrial fibrillation in this setting can result in ventricular rates exceeding 250 bpm, which can cause sudden death by degenerating into ventricular fibrillation. The possibility of WPW should be raised by the combination of an irregular wide-complex tachycardia in a young patient, especially when the ventricular rate is very rapid.

When APs conduct only retrogradely, as is more commonly the case, they are called *concealed pathways,* because the ECG does not provide any hints of their presence. Because there is no preexcitation, there is no delta wave. Tachycardias can take the route of the AV node down (descending limb) and complete the reentry circuit retrogradely via the AP (ascending limb), as is the case with *orthodromic atrioventricular reentry tachycardia (O-AVRT)* (Figure 2). This is a short RP and AV–node-dependent tachycardia and it represents the second most frequent reentrant SVT. The risk of sudden death is minimized in patients with only concealed bypass tracts by the inability to conduct antegradely at rapid rates, but some APs may also have the ability to conduct antegradely as well as retrogradely. A rare variant of O-AVRT is *permanent junctional reciprocating tachycardia (PJRT),* which is caused by an AP with slow retrograde conduction leading to an incessant tachycardia with a long RP interval, especially in children and young adults. If unrecognized, it can cause tachycardia-induced cardiomyopathies.

When the direction of the impulse is reversed in the reentry circuit and travels down the fast AP and retrogradely through the AV node, a less common atrioventricular reentry tachycardia (AVRT) ensues, called *antidromic AVRT* or *ART*. In contrast to O-AVRT there is preexcitation with wide QRS complexes.

Asymptomatic patients generally do not require treatment. In symptomatic patients catheter mapping and ablation are safe and more effective than

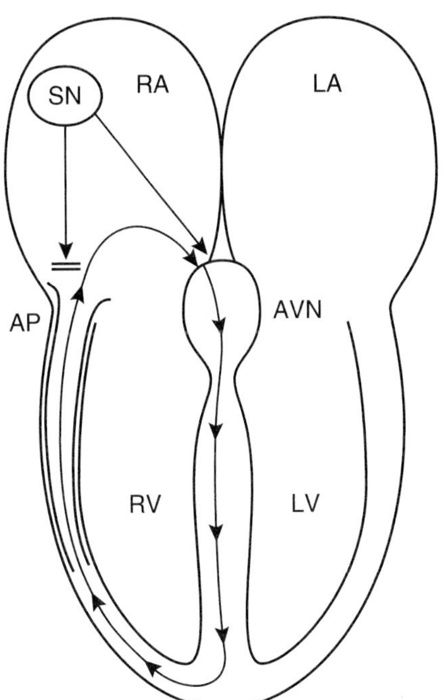

FIGURE 2 Reentry circuit taken by orthodromic atrioventricular reentry tachycardias (AVRT). Antegrade unidirectional block channels the impulse down the AVN; this then returns up via the accessory pathway to complete the reentry circuit. AP = accessory pathway; AVN = atrioventricular node; LA = left atrium; LV = left ventricle; RA = right atrium; RV = right ventricle; SN = sinoatrial node.

drug treatment, providing a definitive cure. The drug treatment of AVRT is aimed at slowing AV conduction, thus breaking or preventing reentrant circuits. Both β blockers and CCBs can be used, provided there is no preexcitation. In the latter case they represent a hazard, because by slowing conduction antegradely in the AV node they may accelerate conduction via the AP. Here, drugs that slow conduction in the AP, such as IV procainamide (class IA), may terminate the tachycardia and the class IC flecainide (Tambocor) and propafenone (Rythmol) can prevent recurrences. DC cardioversion may be necessary if the tachycardia is unstable as may be the case with rapidly conducted atrial fibrillation caused by preexcitation.

NONPAROXYSMAL JUNCTIONAL TACHYCARDIA

Nonparoxysmal junctional tachycardia (NPJT) is an uncommon form of SVT that is caused by increased AV node automaticity. It is associated with valve surgery, digitalis toxicity, myocardial infarction, and myocarditis. It is a narrow-complex tachycardia with rates between 70 and 130 bpm. The P waves are inverted in the inferior leads and usually follow the QRS complexes (short RP), but occasionally they can precede them (long RP). Treatment is only necessary in symptomatic cases.

ATRIAL FLUTTER

The mechanism of atrial flutter is reentry, which can follow a path through the isthmus—a narrow band of tissue located between the tricuspid annulus and the os of the inferior vena cava in the right atrium. When viewed from the tip of the heart, *isthmus-dependent flutter* proceeds in a counterclockwise direction (*typical flutter*) (Figure 3). It can also follow the opposite direction, resulting in *clockwise isthmus-dependent flutter*. Some authors call this *atypical flutter*. We would like to reserve the term *atypical flutter* for *nonisthmus-dependent flutter*, which often centers around the pulmonary veins in the left atrium or around scars; the atrial rates for nonisthmus-dependent flutter range from 300 to 450 bpm and are higher than in isthmus-dependent flutter (220 to 300 bpm).

Counterclockwise flutter is characterized by a saw-toothed pattern of flutter waves on the ECG. They are upright in V1 and negative in II, III, and AVF. Clockwise flutter has negative flutter waves in V1 and positive waves in II, III, and AVF. Atrial flutter is usually associated with some degree of AV block. In the case of 2:1 conduction, the flutter waves may be buried in the QRS complex; CSM, by increasing the AV block, may unmask the flutter waves. Adenosine may achieve the same effect, but because flutter is independent of the AV node it will not terminate it. A narrow-complex tachycardia with a rate close to 150 bpm should raise the suspicion of atrial flutter with 2:1 conduction. AV conduction can be irregular and flutter may be confused with atrial fibrillation.

Like atrial fibrillation, flutter increases the risk of embolic events and requires anticoagulation for prevention. When the onset is longer than 48 hours prior, DC cardioversion can only be safely performed after 3 weeks of full anticoagulation with warfarin (Coumadin) and should be followed by another 4 weeks of anticoagulation until mechanical systole as well as electrical systole are restored. Transesophageal echocardiography (TEE)-guided cardioversion followed by 4 weeks of warfarin is also acceptable. Isthmus-dependent flutter is amenable to catheter ablation. Alternatively, rate control with drugs that block AV nodal conduction in conjunction with anticoagulation offers a long-term treatment option. Ibutilide (Corvert) has been successful in chemically cardioverting atrial flutter, but it has to be used carefully, as it prolongs the QT interval; the risk of thromboembolism is present with chemical cardioversion as well as electrical. Drugs used in maintaining sinus rhythm include the class IC drugs flecainide and propafenone in the absence of structural heart disease and the class III representatives amiodarone (Cordarone), sotalol (Betapace), and dofetilide (Tikosyn), which all prolong the QT interval.

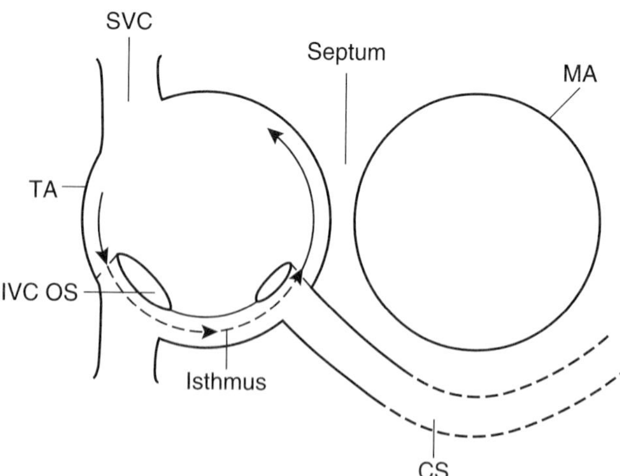

FIGURE 3 View of the heart from the apex in LAO view. The arrow represents the counterclockwise direction of the typical atrial flutter circuit. CS = coronary sinus; IVC = inferior vena cava; MA = mitral annulus; SVC = superior vena cava; TA = tricuspid annulus.

ATRIAL FIBRILLATION

Atrial fibrillation is discussed in a separate article, titled *Atrial Fibrillation*.

VENTRICULAR TACHYCARDIA

Ventricular tachycardia (VT) is a run of three or more consecutive ventricular complexes. If the run lasts longer than 30 seconds and causes hemodynamic compromise, it is called *sustained*; a shorter run is considered *nonsustained (NSVT)*. If all the complexes have the same morphology, the VT is *monomorphic*. Changing of QRS morphologies during the tachycardia is characteristic of *polymorphic VT*. Polymorphic VT in the setting of a baseline prolonged QT interval in sinus rhythm is called *torsade de pointes*, suggesting a rotation of the axis of the QRS complexes around the isoelectric baseline.

VT is usually a wide-complex tachycardia, which raises the question of differentiation from SVT with aberrant conduction or preexcitation. Clinically, a history of ischemic heart disease in a patient with a wide-complex tachycardia makes the diagnosis of VT likely. Termination of a wide-complex tachycardia with vagal maneuvers favors SVT with aberrancy. Multiple electrocardiographic criteria are suggested as a means to differentiate VT from SVT with aberrancy. Some of the more reliable criteria in favor of VT are summarized in Table 2. *AV dissociation*, especially when the ventricular rate is faster than the atrial rate, is diagnostic of VT. *Capture beats*, which are supraventricular in origin and have a narrow QRS, are conducted through the AV node and depolarize the ventricles somewhat prematurely within the VT cycle; and they are also diagnostic of VT. *Fusion beats* are QRS complexes generated by two different sources, of which at least one is ventricular in origin; their morphology is a combination of that of the two sites. If RS complexes are present in any precordial lead during the tachycardia, measuring the interval from the beginning of the R wave to the nadir of the S wave is suggestive of VT, if the interval is greater than 100 ms. Other ECG clues suggestive of VT are far leftward shifts in axis during the tachycardia, extreme right axis deviation, QRS concordance in the precordial leads (all QRS complexes negative or positive) and absence of RS complexes in V1-V6.

The clinical management of VT focuses on two aspects—treatment of the acute episode and long-term management. The latter emphasizes risk-stratification for sudden cardiac death (SCD), risk modification, and tachycardia prevention.

ACUTE MANAGEMENT

This depends on the degree of hemodynamic compromise, which is largely a function of the rate and the left ventricle (LV) function. Slower rates may be tolerated relatively well without significant hypotension. Intravenous amiodarone (150 mg bolus, followed by infusion of 1 mg/min for 6 hours, then 0.5 mg/min) has recently superseded lidocaine as first line for treatment of VT. Procainamide represents an alternative. Both can cause hypotension so close BP monitoring is required. Unstable VT causing hypotension requires DC cardioversion.

CHRONIC MANAGEMENT

VT in the setting of structural heart disease represents a significant risk of sudden death. A majority of patients with VT have a history of prior MI and ischemic heart disease. Reentrant VT circuits tend to form around scar tissue. A second large group is patients with nonischemic cardiomyopathies followed by other less frequent etiologies. Several tools are available in assisting in risk stratification. The ejection fraction is one of the easiest to obtain and, if decreased, represents a strong predictor of poor prognosis in both ischemic and nonischemic groups. Sustained VT in both groups requires implantation of an internal cardioverter-defibrillator (ICD) for sudden death prevention, whereas asymptomatic NSVT in patients with ischemic heart disease and decreased EF (less than 40%) requires an invasive electrophysiologic study (EPS). If monomorphic VT is inducible, an implantable cardioverter-defibrillator (ICD) implantation is recommended. It is less clear what course of action to take in patients with normal systolic LV function. No doubt they have a lower risk. In those with ischemia, EPS may further define their risk. In the case of nonischemic cardiomyopathies and NSVT, EPS seems to be a poor predictor of risk. If systolic LV function is poor and there is a history of syncope, ICD implantation may be required. The drug prophylaxis of VT in patients with structural heart disease is limited to the Class III drugs amiodarone, sotalol, and dofetilide[1]. If tolerated, β blockers may also be indicated.

[1]Not FDA approved for this indication.

Other Types of Ventricular Tachycardias

RIGHT VENTRICULAR OUTFLOW TACHYCARDIA

Right ventricular outflow tachycardia (RVOT) originates from a focus of triggered activity around the right ventricular outflow tract and, therefore, has a left bundle-branch block (LBBB) morphology with an inferior axis. It is most common in young patients and can be triggered by exercise. It responds to IV adenosine and verapamil (Calan), and can be prevented by treatment with β blockers and CCBs. It is also amenable to catheter ablation.

IDIOPATHIC LEFT VENTRICLE-VENTRICULAR TACHYCARDIA

Idiopathic left ventricle-ventricular tachycardia (LV-VT) is also most common in young adults. It has a right bundle-branch block (RBBB) and left anterior fascicular block (LAFB) morphology. It can also be exercise induced and responds to CCBs or can be ablated.

ARRHYTHMOGENIC RIGHT VENTRICULAR DYSPLASIA

Arrhythmogenic right ventricular dysplasia (ARVD) is a familial form of infiltrative cardiomyopathy affecting the right ventricle (RV) and is best diagnosed by its characteristic appearance on MRI showing fatty infiltration. It is associated with monomorphic VT, and affected patients are at risk of sudden death. Prophylactic ICD implantation is recommended, but catheter ablation can be used in an adjunctive role.

Infiltrative cardiomyopathies like sarcoidosis, hypertrophic cardiomyopathies, and the newly described Brugada syndrome can all predispose to sudden cardiac death, and ICD implantation is recommended for patients at risk.

POLYMORPHIC VENTRICULAR TACHYCARDIA AND VENTRICULAR FIBRILLATION

Polymorphic VT can occur in acute ischemic states without baseline QT interval prolongation and can rapidly degenerate into ventricular fibrillation VF. Alternatively polymorphic VT can be associated with acquired long QT syndromes caused by electrolyte disturbances (hypokalemia, hypomagnesemia), drugs (class I A and II antiarrhythmics, phenothiazines, tricyclics, and antibiotics like erythromycin, fluoroquinolones, and others), or congenital long QT syndromes. A family history of sudden death and symptoms of syncope and near syncope can alert the physician to the presence of the latter. ICD is the preferred form of therapy for patients at risk.

Ventricular fibrillation is a rapid and disorganized form of ventricular arrhythmia, usually ischemic in origin. It is invariably unstable, and prompt electrical defibrillation is imperative. It is well documented that the earlier electrical defibrillation takes place, the more likely it is to succeed and the better the prognosis. This fact has led to efforts to educate the public in cardiopulmonary resuscitation (CPR) and to introduce automatic external defibrillators in strategic locations in the community.

CONGENITAL HEART DISEASE

METHOD OF

Thomas W. Young, MD

Approximately 0.8% of newborn babies have congenital heart disease (CHD), not including bicuspid aortic valve and patent ductus arteriosus in premature infants. CHD may range in severity from asymptomatic to immediately life-threatening. During the past 50 years there have been remarkable advances in the medical and surgical management of CHD, with close to 90% of patients now surviving into adulthood. There have been considerable advances in diagnostic modalities as well. Chest radiography (CXR), electrocardiography (ECG), and cardiac catheterization were once the major modalities. Echocardiography has become the diagnostic study of choice in most forms of CHD, and fetal echocardiography can often diagnose CHD before birth. Magnetic resonance imaging (MRI) is used with increasing frequency. Diagnostic cardiac catheterization is used less frequently, although catheter-based interventional procedures are becoming much more common. In the future, in utero intervention may prevent the development of some serious CHD. An in-depth discussion of the myriad forms of CHD is beyond the scope of this article. Several representative disorders are briefly detailed.

Acyanotic Congenital Heart Disease

CHD can be classified as acyanotic or cyanotic. Acyanotic heart disease consists of left-to-right shunt lesions, obstructive lesions, and regurgitant lesions. In left-to-right shunt lesions, blood from the left side of the heart prematurely reenters the pulmonary circulation in a process dependent on both the systemic and pulmonary vascular resistances (SVR and PVR, respectively). A volume (and possibly pressure) load is placed on the heart, and pulmonary congestion can occur. Symptoms develop after the normal fall in PVR that occurs during early infancy. Congestive heart failure (CHF) may develop early in infancy, manifesting as feeding difficulty, poor weight gain, tachypnea, and frequent respiratory infections. Symptoms may develop later in life, with dyspnea and decreasing exercise tolerance as frequent complaints. The presence of a heart murmur often results in the diagnosis of CHD in an asymptomatic patient. Medical therapy for congestive heart failure consists of digoxin and diuretics, with intravenous inotropes and mechanical ventilation reserved for seriously ill patients. Afterload reduction, often with angiotensin-converting enzyme (ACE) inhibitors, may be used to decrease SVR and lessen the left-to-right shunt. Eventually, more definitive therapy may be required. Over time, a large left-to-right shunt can result in irreversible and progressive changes in the pulmonary vasculature, causing pulmonary vascular obstructive disease (PVOD). As PVR increases, CHF resolves and the shunt may reverse to right-to-left, causing progressive cyanosis.

Obstructive and regurgitant lesions are also frequently diagnosed because of a murmur on examination. Obstructive CHD results in a pressure load on the heart. Regurgitant lesions place a volume load on the heart. In both, the heart undergoes progressive hypertrophy to adapt to the increased demands.

Left-to-Right Shunt Lesions

VENTRICULAR SEPTAL DEFECTS

In a ventricular septal defect (VSD), a communication exists between the right and left ventricles (RV and LV, respectively). This is the most common form of CHD. Frequently isolated, VSDs are also often associated with other forms of CHD. Perimembranous VSDs are the most common type. Along with muscular VSDs, perimembranous VSDs frequently become smaller with time, often closing on their own during childhood. Inlet defects are less common and are often associated with abnormal atrioventricular valves. Outlet VSDs (also called supracristal or conoseptal defects), uncommon in the western world, comprise approximately 33% of VSDs seen in the Far East.

A holosystolic murmur is heard. A diastolic rumble at the apex suggests a large left-to-right shunt. ECG may suggest left atrial and left ventricular enlargement, and CXR can reveal cardiomegaly and increased pulmonary vascular markings.

Defect size is the principle determinant of clinical course. Most VSDs present at birth either close spontaneously or become too small to warrant surgical closure. Small defects are hemodynamically insignificant, with very little chance of developing into CHF or PVOD. There is a risk of endocarditis, and subacute bacterial endocarditis prophylaxis (SBEP) is necessary. Larger defects often result in CHF. Symptomatic perimembranous or muscular VSDs in infancy may become smaller with time, allowing for the withdrawal of therapy. Over time, PVOD will develop in larger defects. Progressive aortic insufficiency (AI) can occur in outlet, and, less frequently, perimembranous VSDs. Both right and left ventricular outflow obstruction can also arise.

Surgical closure is the definitive treatment. Heart failure not responsive to medical management may prompt surgical repair in infancy. More commonly, larger defects are closed in early childhood to lessen the volume load on the heart and to prevent PVOD. The risk of AI in outlet defects often prompts earlier repair. Significant elevation of PVR not adequately responsive to pulmonary vasodilators is a contraindication to closure. Catheter-based closure of some VSDs is now possible.

ATRIAL SEPTAL DEFECTS

In an atrial septal defect (ASD), a left-to-right shunt exists at the atrial level. The most common type is the secundum ASD, located at the level of the fossa ovalis. Primum ASDs are often associated with abnormal atrioventricular valves. Sinus venosus defects may be associated with partial anomalous pulmonary venous return. Truly rare is the unroofed coronary sinus form of ASD.

Patients are usually asymptomatic in childhood. Small secundum defects frequently close in childhood. A fixed, split second heart sound with a systolic ejection murmur is the classic examination finding. CXR and ECG often suggest right atrial (RA) and RV enlargement.

Larger defects often manifest in early adulthood with decreasing exercise tolerance. In older patients, atrial arrhythmias and worsening CHF become more significant. Transient reversal of the shunt can result in paradoxical emboli to the brain. PVOD can also develop and is more common in females.

Surgical correction can be performed in hemodynamically significant defects with minimal morbidity and mortality. ASD repair in childhood or early adulthood normalizes life expectancy. Repair in older patients is still justified, although atrial arrhythmias may persist. PVOD is a contraindication to repair. Catheter-based device closure of amenable secundum ASDs is becoming a standard of care. SBEP is not needed in simple ASDs.

ATRIOVENTRICULAR CANAL DEFECTS

Atrioventricular canal defects (AVC) result from abnormal development of the endocardial cushion and are often called endocardial cushion defects. In a complete AVC, a large primum ASD and inlet VSD are found. A single, large atrioventricular valve is present. In partial AVC, the VSD is absent or small and the atrioventricular valve is divided into two functional, albeit abnormal, valves. Approximately 50% of Down syndrome patients have congenital heart disease, with complete AVC and VSD being the most common forms.

Complete AVC defects usually present in early infancy with significant heart failure caused by the large shunt and significant atrioventricular valve regurgitation. PVOD can develop in early childhood if surgical correction is delayed. Physical examination reveals a regurgitant systolic murmur. The electrocardiographic wave (QRS) axis on ECG is *superior*, between –40 degrees and –150 degrees. Cardiomegaly is common on CXR. Partial defects may not be clinically evident in childhood, instead presenting with exercise intolerance, atrial arrhythmia, or paradoxical emboli in adulthood. PVOD can also develop.

Complete surgical repair is the definitive therapy and consists of patch closure of the septal defects and construction of two separate atrioventricular valves. This is usually performed in infancy to treat heart failure and to prevent PVOD. Heart block may occur spontaneously or as a complication of surgery. Atrioventricular valve regurgitation and stenosis and atrial arrhythmias are potential long-term complications.

PATENT DUCTUS ARTERIOSUS

A patent ductus arteriosus (PDA) is the abnormal persistence of the normal fetal ductus, which connects the proximal left pulmonary artery to the proximal descending aorta, just distal to the origin of the left subclavian artery. It is more common in premature infants.

The classic physical examination finding is a continuous machinery-like murmur in the left infraclavicular area and bounding pulses. ECG and CXR may reveal left atrial (LA) and LV volume overload.

Moderate-to-large defects result in CHF and can eventually cause PVOD. Small defects are hemodynamically insignificant but pose a risk for endocarditis. *Silent* PDAs, which are not clinically evident, are diagnosed when echocardiography or cardiac catheterization is performed for another reason.

Definitive therapy involves closure. Premature infants often respond to indomethacin (Indocin)[1]. Full-term infants and older patients do not. Surgical closure via a left thoracotomy is accomplished with minimal morbidity and mortality. Even small defects are fixed to prevent subacute bacterial endocarditis (SBE). Catheter-based closure with various devices has become commonplace. Larger defects and symptomatic defects in small infants may still require surgery. The silent PDA does not require SBEP and should not be closed.

Obstructive Lesions

PULMONARY STENOSIS

In pulmonary stenosis (PS), there is obstruction to right ventricular outflow. Valvular PS is the most common form. Dysplastic, thickened leaflets can be

[1]Not FDA approved for this indication.

seen in Noonan's syndrome. Supravalvular PS can be seen in William's and rubella syndromes. Subvalvular PS, often caused by acquired hypertrophy of RV muscle bundles, usually exists in the presence of a VSD.

In valvular PS, a systolic ejection click is appreciated. A systolic ejection murmur radiating to the lung fields and varying with respiration is the hallmark finding. ECG and CXR may reveal right ventricular hypertrophy (RVH).

Mild PS is well tolerated, with no need for activity restriction or therapy other than SBEP. Mild PS occasionally becomes more severe with time. Moderate and severe PS often progress and may cause exercise intolerance and right-sided heart failure. Severe PS can present in the newborn as cyanosis caused by a right-to-left patent foramen ovale (PFO) shunt and poor pulmonary perfusion.

Balloon valvuloplasty in the cardiac catheterization laboratory is now the standard of care for significant valvular PS. Excellent results are expected, and redevelopment of significant stenosis is unlikely. Dysplastic valves are less amenable to balloon dilation. Surgery is sometimes required.

AORTIC STENOSIS

Congenital aortic stenosis (AS) is usually valvular. Subaortic stenosis is often associated with a VSD or other CHD. Supravalvular stenosis may be seen in William's syndrome.

The vast majority of patients with congenital valvular AS have a bicuspid aortic valve (BAV), a finding in 1% to 2% of the general population. Neonates born with critical AS, often associated with other left side of the heart obstructive lesions, present acutely with congestive heart failure and poor systemic perfusion. Clinical progression may coincide with the closure of the ductus arteriosus, and reopening the ductus with an infusion of prostaglandin E (PGE) may allow stabilization before surgical correction.

The majority of patients born with a BAV have no AS and go undiagnosed until AS or aortic insufficiency (AI) develops in adulthood. A systolic ejection click may be the only physical examination finding. Patients with mild-to-moderate AS are usually asymptomatic. A systolic ejection murmur radiating to the carotid arteries is heard. Progression of mild-to-moderate AS may occur in childhood but is more common later in life as the valve calcifies. AI may be more hemodynamically significant than AS. Valve calcification is worsened by hyperlipidemia. The hallmark symptoms of AS are angina, syncope, and CHF. Their presence suggests severe disease with a poor long-term prognosis. The risk of sudden death is significant, and exercise should be limited in moderate-to-severe AS. SBEP is required, even in BAV patients without AS or AI.

The definitive therapy for significant AS is surgery. Balloon angioplasty in the catheterization laboratory may be useful in young patients without significant calcification. Balloon dilation and surgical valvuloplasty and commissurotomy may be complicated by worsening AI. Replacement of the aortic valve may be necessary. Bioprosthetic valves have relatively short lifetimes, necessitating reoperation. Mechanical valves require chronic anticoagulation. In children, somatic growth may limit the life span of either option. The Ross procedure, in which the patient's native pulmonary valve is used to replace the diseased aortic valve and a homograft is used to replace the pulmonary valve, may be an attractive option. Early diagnosis of BAV allows for prevention of SBE, promotion of a healthy lifestyle, and control of hyperlipidemia, hopefully delaying or preventing the onset of significant obstruction.

COARCTATION OF THE AORTA

Coarctation of the aorta (COA) describes an obstruction to blood flow within the aortic lumen. It is more common in males and in females with Turner's syndrome. COA almost always exists at the level of the ligamentum arteriosus' insertion into the proximal descending aorta, just distal to the origin of the left subclavian artery. A bicuspid aortic valve is present in the majority of patients. Coexisting CHD is common.

Blood supply to the descending aorta may be dependent on the PDA in the neonate with critical COA. With closure of the ductus, CHF and decreased systemic perfusion develops. A murmur and differential pulses may not be evident because of depressed cardiac output. Initial medical management consists of PGE to open the PDA, inotropes, and mechanical ventilation. Surgical repair is performed once the patient is stabilized.

More commonly, patients are relatively asymptomatic as children. Leg pain and weakness may be reported. Often, a COA is discovered during a workup for hypertension (HTN) or a murmur. In COA, arm blood pressures are higher than leg pressures. Pulses in the legs are weak and delayed. A systolic ejection murmur, sometimes localized to the left infrascapular area, is often heard. LVH may be present on ECG. The workup of systemic hypertension should always include arm and leg blood pressures to screen for a COA.

With time, extensive collateral vessels may develop linking the proximal to the distal aorta. Long-term complications of untreated COA include intracranial hemorrhage caused by rupture of berry aneurysms, LV failure, endocarditis, aortic aneurysm rupture and dissection, and the sequelae of BAV and chronic systemic HTN. Systemic HTN may persist in corrected patients.

Primary therapy consists of surgical repair. The use of balloon angioplasty with or without stent placement is controversial in native coarctation, but is an excellent option in surgically repaired patients with recoarctation.

Interrupted aortic arch (IAA) is a severe form of COA, where a segment of the aorta is absent or atretic and the distal aorta is fed exclusively by a PDA. A VSD is usually present. Closure of the PDA results in shock. DiGeorge syndrome is a common association. PGE infusion is used to maintain the PDA until surgical repair can be performed.

Regurgitant Lesions

Lengthy discussion of mitral and aortic insufficiency is beyond the scope of this article. AI frequently complicates BAV, and both mitral and aortic insufficiency can result from acute rheumatic fever. Afterload reduction with ACE inhibitors are frequently used to improve forward flow. Valve repair or replacement is sometimes required.

Cyanotic Congenital Heart Disease

Cyanosis in the newborn is a frequent concern and can be caused by lung disease, central nervous system (CNS) depression and cardiac pathology. A "hyperoxitest" is useful. Providing 100% oxygen is unlikely to improve PO_2 significantly in cyanotic CHD, while dramatic improvement may be seen with lung and CNS disease. If cyanotic congenital heart disease is suspected, PGE is started while awaiting consultant evaluation. The cyanosis is caused by unoxygenated blood bypassing the pulmonary circulation and entering into the systemic circulation.

TETRALOGY OF FALLOT

Tetralogy of Fallot (TOF) is the most common form of cyanotic CHD. It is caused by an anterior malalignment of the infundibular septum. This produces the *tetralogy*—a large VSD, subvalvular PS, an aortic overriding of the septum, and RV hypertrophy. A right aortic arch is frequently present. Additional RV outflow obstruction may exist at the pulmonary valve and pulmonary artery levels, and coronary artery anomalies are not uncommon. DiGeorge syndrome is common. Cyanosis occurs because of right-to-left VSD shunting. Some newborns have minimal obstruction and no cyanosis (acyanotic, or *pink* TOF), although progressive cyanosis develops with time. Hypercyanotic spells secondary to an acute worsening of pulmonary blood flow obstruction or a decrease in SVR produce marked cyanosis and may be life-threatening. Patients may learn to squat or bend their knees in an attempt to increase SVR and pulmonary blood flow. If untreated, most patients with TOF die prior to adolescence.

Varying levels of cyanosis are found on examination. The second heart sound is single, and a long, harsh systolic ejection murmur is heard. ECG reveals RVH. The CXR may show RVH with a hypoplastic main pulmonary artery (MPA) segment (boot-shaped heart) and decreased pulmonary blood flow.

Surgical repair consists of closing the VSD and relieving RV outflow obstruction. This is often performed electively between 3 to 6 months of age, although neonatal repair is advocated by some. Complicating factors may necessitate palliation with a modified Blalock-Taussig shunt (BTS), which is a synthetic tube that connects the innominate or subclavian artery to the pulmonary arteries, to allow adequate pulmonary blood flow prior to definitive repair.

Successful repair carries an excellent prognosis. RBBB is common on ECG. Problems with atrial and ventricular arrhythmias as well as pulmonary and aortic insufficiency may complicate long-term care. There is an increased risk of sudden death in patients after TOF repair.

In TOF with pulmonary atresia, pulmonary blood flow is dependent either on a PDA supplying the pulmonary arteries or aorta to pulmonary collateral vessels. Surgical repair can be challenging. In TOF with absent valve, marked in utero pulmonary insufficiency results in massively dilated pulmonary arteries. This can cause life-threatening airway compromise.

TRANSPOSITION OF THE GREAT ARTERIES

In dextrotransposition of the great arteries (D-TGA), the aorta arises from the RV and the pulmonary artery arises from the LV (ventriculoarterial discordance). Oxygenated blood returning via the pulmonary veins is ejected back to the lungs, and unoxygenated blood returning via the systemic veins is ejected to the body. Some mixing occurs at the atrial level (PFO or ASD) and at the PDA. Many patients also have a VSD, and coronary abnormalities can rarely affect surgical options. D-TGA is more common in males and in infants of diabetic mothers. It is the most common form of cyanotic CHD presenting in the newborn.

Patients are cyanotic. The second heart sound is single. Often no murmur is heard. The classic CXR pattern is described as an "egg on a string" caused by a narrowed mediastinum. If left untreated, the vast majority will die within the first year of life.

Initial therapy includes supplemental oxygen and PGE to maintain ductal patency. In a balloon atrial septostomy, a balloon tipped catheter is inserted into the femoral or umbilical vein and advanced across the PFO into the left atrium. The balloon is inflated and rapidly pulled back into the right atrium, ripping the foramen open. This can vastly improve mixing at the atrial level, allowing discontinuation of PGE while awaiting definitive surgery.

Until about two decades ago, a Mustard or Senning procedure was used to baffle systemic venous blood across the mitral valve and pulmonary venous blood across the tricuspid valve. This results in unoxygenated blood circulating to the lungs and oxygenated blood circulating to the body. This approach carries relatively low short-term mortality as problems frequently arise with age. RV failure and severe tricuspid insufficiency can occur. Baffle obstruction and atrial arrhythmias are also very common, and sudden death is a significant risk.

The arterial switch operation is now the procedure of choice. The great arteries are transected and reconnected with the proximal end of the opposite great artery. The coronaries are also moved. Thus, the LV pumps to the aorta, and the RV pumps to the pulmonary artery. Problems related to coronary obstruction and pulmonary artery stenosis can occasionally complicate this procedure, but it is generally well tolerated. SBEP is lifelong in D-TGA.

In congenitally corrected transposition of the great arteries (L-TGA), there is ventriculoarterial discordance. However, the LV is connected to the right atrium, the RV is connected to the left atrium (ventricular inversion), and oxygenation is normal. Associated forms of CHD are common. With age, failure of the systemic RV and arrhythmias may necessitate complicated surgery and/or electrophysiology procedures.

TOTAL ANOMALOUS PULMONARY VENOUS RETURN

In total anomalous pulmonary venous return (TAPVR), the pulmonary veins drain into the right side of the heart instead of into the left atrium. There is complete mixing of pulmonary and systemic venous return. An ASD or PFO is necessary. Cyanosis is present. The pulmonary veins can drain (often via complicated routes) into the SVC, coronary sinus, or directly into the right atrium. In infradiaphragmatic TAPVR, the pulmonary vein confluence courses inferiorly across the diaphragm, eventually draining into the inferior vena cava (IVC). Obstruction in the common pulmonary vein can occur in any type of TAPVR, but is most common in the infradiaphragmatic type.

If no obstruction is present, patients present with cyanosis and CHF. As PVR falls, CHF worsens as cyanosis improves. The right side of the heart is dilated. The diagnosis may be missed in the newborn period. Obstructed TAPVR produces a very ill newborn with marked cyanosis. Little or no cardiomegaly and significant pulmonary edema are present on CXR.

Surgery involves anastomosing the pulmonary veins with the left atrium and ligating any additional drainage routes. Results are excellent in unobstructed TAPVR, but mortality is high in obstructed disease. Rarely, pulmonary venous obstruction can occur at the anastomosis. This is very challenging to treat.

In partial anomalous pulmonary venous return (PAPVR), some, but not all, of the pulmonary veins drain into the RA. These patients are not cyanotic. They instead present with ASD physiology. Surgical repair is indicated if the left-to-right shunt is significant. If only one pulmonary vein drains anomalously, surgery usually is not needed.

TRUNCUS ARTERIOSUS

In truncus arteriosus (TA), a single great artery arises from the heart and gives rise to the coronary arteries, aorta, and pulmonary arteries. It is more common in infants of diabetic mothers and in DiGeorge syndrome. A VSD is always present, and there may be associated interruption of the aorta. A right-sided aortic arch is common. The single semilunar valve (the truncal valve) is frequently abnormal, and significant insufficiency and stenosis can occur.

Patients have cyanosis (often mild because of a large amount of pulmonary blood flow) and will develop CHF as the PVR falls. Significant truncal valve insufficiency produces severe CHF early in the newborn period. Bounding pulses are common. A systolic ejection click, single second heart sound, and loud harsh systolic murmur are the common cardiac findings. Cardiomegaly with increased pulmonary vascular markings is seen on CXR.

The vast majority will not survive past their first birthday if surgery is not performed. The VSD is closed, the pulmonary arteries are removed from the truncal artery, and a homograft is used to connect the RV to the pulmonary arteries. The need for intervention on a regurgitant truncal valve increases mortality. With age, patients with repaired TA will need RV-to-pulmonary artery homograft revisions, and truncal insufficiency may worsen. SBEP is required.

SINGLE VENTRICLE

The term *single ventricle* can be used to describe a heterogeneous assortment of lesions where there is functionally only one ventricle. Two examples are tricuspid atresia and hypoplastic left heart syndrome (HLHS). Other examples include double-inlet left ventricle and unbalanced AVC defects.

In tricuspid atresia, the RV is hypoplastic and pulmonary blood flow is often dependent on a PDA. Babies are cyanotic at birth and closure of the ductus is catastrophic. PGE is started while awaiting a modified Blalock-Taussig shunt to provide a stable source of pulmonary blood flow.

In HLHS, there is hypoplasia or atresia of the mitral and aortic valves. The LV is hypoplastic. Frequently, the ascending aorta and arch are small as well. Patients are cyanotic at birth, although this may be subtle. Systemic perfusion is dependent on the PDA. Constriction of the ductus compromises systemic and coronary perfusion. As the PVR falls, blood preferentially circulates to the lungs rather than the body and shock worsens. PGE is started while awaiting the Norwood stage I procedure, which produces an adequately sized "aorta" attached to the RV utilizing the proximal main pulmonary artery and a modified BTS to provide pulmonary perfusion. Surgical mortality rates range from 20% to 40%.

Further staged surgical intervention is identical in tricuspid atresia and HLHS and is guided by the concept that systemic venous blood will flow to the lungs if PVR is low. In a bidirectional Glenn or hemi-Fontan procedure, the SVC is attached to the pulmonary artery. Later, the Fontan procedure is completed as IVC flow is directed into the pulmonary artery.

Systemic venous return now flows directly to the lungs, and cyanosis is abolished. The single functional ventricle (the LV in tricuspid atresia and the RV in HLHS) now solely supplies the systemic circulation. Although surgical mortality in the staged Fontan is low, many patients die between procedures or are deemed poor surgical candidates.

A well-functioning Fontan physiology requires a low PVR. Anything that impedes flow will result in elevation of the central venous pressure (CVP) and compromise of cardiac output. Pulmonary artery stenosis, distal pulmonary vascular disease, pulmonary venous obstruction, atrioventricular valve insufficiency, and an elevated ventricular end diastolic pressure are all poorly tolerated, as are positive pressure ventilation and airway diseases.

Numerous long-term complications accompany the Fontan procedure. Atrial arrhythmia, clot formation, protein losing enteropathy, and recurrent effusions are common as patients age. Progressive ventricular failure, especially with a systemic right RV, can also occur. There has been an evolution in surgical technique, and long-term outcomes are improving. Chronic anticoagulation and afterload reduction are frequently prescribed. Interventional catheterization, electrophysiology procedures, and repeat surgery may be needed. Heart transplant or Fontan revision is occasionally required in poorly functioning Fontan procedure patients.

EBSTEIN'S ANOMALY

Ebstein's anomaly is defined by abnormal downward displacement of tricuspid valve (TV) leaflets, resulting in an atrialized segment of RV and tricuspid insufficiency. An ASD or PFO is usually present. Maternal lithium use may increase the risk. Severe disease can cause fetal demise. Newborns may be cyanotic because of right-to-left atrial shunting and decreased pulmonary blood flow. Older patients present with exercise intolerance, cyanosis, a murmur, or arrhythmia. There is an increased risk of sudden death because of atrial and ventricular arrhythmia. The majority of untreated patients will not survive past early adulthood without intervention, although very mild disease may allow a normal life expectancy.

Physical examination often reveals a quadruple rhythm consisting of split first and second heart sounds along with an S3 and an S4 and the regurgitant murmur of tricuspid insufficiency. Cyanosis may be present. ECG may show RA enlargement, RBBB, and first-degree heart block. The pre-excitation pattern of Wolff-Parkinson-White syndrome is common. CXR reveals cardiomegaly.

Cyanotic neonates often become fully saturated as the newborn PVR falls. The need for surgery in the newborn period carries a very poor prognosis. Progressive cyanosis, RV and LV failure, and arrhythmia (both reentrant SVT and atrial fibrillation and flutter) may prompt surgical intervention later in life. Repair of the valve is preferred, although valve replacement may be needed.

Other Issues

DIGEORGE SYNDROME

CHD is associated with numerous genetic syndromes. DiGeorge syndrome deserves special attention. DiGeorge syndrome is most often caused by a submicroscopic chromosomal deletion at 22q11. The term "CATCH-22" has been used to describe associated findings, representing:

- **C**ardiac defects
- **A**bnormal facies
- **T**hymic hypoplasia
- **C**left palate
- **H**ypocalcemia

There is a wide variation in expression. TA, TOF, and interrupted aortic arch are frequently associated with 22q11 microdeletion, which can be diagnosed with fluorescent in situ hybridization (FISH). Recognition is important for several reasons. Hypocalcemia and immune compromise caused by parathyroid and thymic hypoplasia, respectively, can greatly affect pre- and postoperative care. Developmental delay and psychiatric problems are common, and early intervention can be instituted. Genetic counseling with regard to future pregnancies is another important issue.

CHRONIC CYANOSIS

Patients with chronic cyanosis are frequently encountered in a pediatric cardiology practice. Most of these are young infants and children awaiting surgical repair with the goal of normal oxygenation. These children tolerate mild-to-moderate cyanosis well. However, older children and adults with chronic cyanosis are still encountered. Some have complex unrepaired or palliated cyanotic CHD. Others have left-to-right shunt lesions complicated by PVOD and Eisenmenger's syndrome. Care of these patients is challenging.

Chronic cyanosis produces a secondary erythrocytosis mediated by erythropoietin. In the past, frequent phlebotomy was common to prevent symptoms of polycythemia-related hyperviscosity, including headaches, myalgias, fatigue, and, rarely, stroke. A threshold hematocrit of 65% to 70% was often used. Currently, phlebotomy is used infrequently. Iron deficiency and dehydration are recognized as significant contributors to morbidity, and phlebotomy may significantly worsen symptoms. Dehydration should be treated. Iron deficiency warrants a course of iron therapy. Low-dose iron (ferrous sulfate 325 mg per day orally for adults) can be given until the hematocrit is noted to rise. Treatment of dehydration and iron deficiency may significantly improve symptoms.

Continued symptoms rather than a specific hematocrit should prompt phlebotomy. A slow exchange of 250 to 500 mL of the patient's blood for isotonic saline is usually well tolerated and may temporarily improve symptoms.

These patients have a bleeding disorder not completely explained by their baseline thrombocytopenia, and mucocutaneous hemorrhage is common. Medications that increase bleeding tendency (including nonsteroidal anti-inflammatory drugs [NSAIDs]) are avoided if possible. A phlebotomy exchange may be indicated before surgery to improve hemostasis.

Gallstones are frequent because of increased bilirubin metabolism. Likewise, hyperuricemia is common secondary to increased uric acid production and decreased renal clearance. Uric acid nephropathy is rare, and asymptomatic hyperuricemia is not treated. Episodes of gout may prompt therapy with allopurinol (Zyloprim).

Proteinuria secondary to renal glomerular changes can be seen. Bony changes are also frequently encountered.

PREGNANCY

Pregnancy is usually well tolerated in patients with well-repaired CHD. Unrepaired CHD may be more problematic. Pregnancy is characterized by a high cardiac output and stroke volume and a low SVR. Left-to-right shunt and regurgitant lesions tend to handle pregnancy well. Severe valve stenosis and COA, hypertrophic cardiomyopathy, and Marfan's syndrome patients with dilated ascending aortas do not. Cyanotic CHD and Eisenmenger's syndrome tolerate pregnancy poorly, as the drop in SVR may be accompanied by a significant worsening in cyanosis.

Warfarin (Coumadin) is teratogenic in the first trimester, and heparin should be used in patients requiring anticoagulation. Many centers restart Coumadin after the first trimester, discontinuing it and restarting heparin shortly before delivery. In all pregnant patients with CHD, care to prevent deep venous thrombosis is essential because of the hypercoagulable state of pregnancy and the potential for right-to-left shunting of emboli.

A partnered approach between the cardiologist and the high-risk obstetrician is needed. A fetal ultrasound is performed because of the increased risk of CHD in offspring of mothers with CHD. Vaginal delivery is usually well tolerated. Many physicians provide SBEP despite the American Heart Association's guidelines stating that it is not needed in an uncomplicated vaginal delivery.

HYPERTROPHIC CARDIOMYOPATHY

METHOD OF
Lameh Fananapazir, MD, and
Saidi A. Mohiddin, MB, ChB

Hypertrophic cardiomyopathy (HCM), a myocardial disease with a prevalence of approximately 1 case per 500 of the population, is characterized by left ventricular (LV) hypertrophy. It may, however, masquerade as other diseases, and mild and asymptomatic cases are often undetected. Significant advances have been made in elucidating the genetic causes of HCM, in explaining the clinical correlates of specific molecular defects, in improving risk stratification through identification of mechanisms of syncope and cardiac arrest, and in devising new strategies to improve symptoms and prognosis.

Genetics and Molecular Causes of Hypertrophic Cardiomyopathy

Most cases of HCM are inherited (familial HCM [FHC]) as an autosomal dominant disease. Hence, half of the parents, siblings, and children are at risk of inheriting the disease mutation. However, fewer than half actually develop HCM, as the disease penetrance (number of subjects with HCM ÷ number of subjects with disease mutation × 100) is often less than 100%. Indeed, HCM may skip one or more generations in some families. Truly sporadic HCM, proven by the demonstration of the absence of an identified disease mutation in both parents, is uncommon and is likely to present below the age of puberty. Most of the molecular defects that have been identified to date are missense mutations (single base-pair substitution) changing the identity of an evolutionarily conserved amino acid in one of several genes that encode contractile proteins of the sarcomere (Table 1). However, the sarcomeric protein, myosin-binding protein C, is prone to deletion mutations that also cause HCM. Occasionally, HCM is associated with double homozygous or double heterozygous disease-causing mutations. Known genetic defects probably account for approximately 50% of cases of HCM, and few of these have been adequately characterized clinically. Mutations in different protein domains are likely to have distinct effects on the function of the actomyosin molecular motor. Hence, several gene-specific clinical correlates of the molecular defects have been described. For example, some cardiac actin mutations are associated with apical HCM; and several mutations, such as the missense mutation of β-myosin amino acid residue 403 that results in the substitution of arginine with

TABLE 1 Genetic Heterogeneity in Hypertrophic Cardiomyopathy (HCM)

Gene/Disease	Number of Mutations	Features
Sarcomeric HCM		
β-myosin heavy chain	>100	Most common cause of HCM, variable disease penetrance and phenotype
Cardiac myosin binding protein C	>50	Second most common cause of HCM
α-tropomyosin	>6	Mild LVH and high risk of sudden death in some pedigrees
Cardiac troponin T	>20	Mild LVH and high risk of sudden death in some pedigrees
Cardiac troponin I	>10	
α cardiac actin	>6	
Essential light chain of myosin	3	Midcavity HCM
Regulatory light chain of myosin	>10	Midcavity HCM
Titin	1	
Nonsarcomeric		
PRKAG2, subunit of AMPK	>5	Glycogen granules, AV bypass tracts, WPW, and sinus node disease
Sorcin	1	Asymmetric LVH and hypertension
Cardiac ryanodine		
Myosin VI (unconventional myosin)	1	Sensorineural deafness
Muscle LIM protein gene	3	Variable phenotype
Component of Multisystem Syndrome		
McLeod syndrome (XK)	>15	Neuroacanthocytosis
Friedreich ataxia (FRDA)	>15	Expanded trinucleotide repeat and missense mutations
Leopard syndrome (PTPN11)	2	Biventricular outflow obstruction
Mitochondrial DNA deletions (e.g., MELAS, MERFF, Kearns-Sayre)		LVH, LV systolic dysfunction, AV node disease
Alpha-B crystallin myopathy (CRYAB)	1	Skeletal myopathy, lens opacities

Abbreviations: AMPK = adenosine monophosphate-activated protein kinase; AV = atrioventricular; LVH = left ventricle hypertrophy; MELAS = myopathy, encephalopathy, lactic acidosis, and stroke-like episodes syndrome; MERFF = myoclonic epilepsy and ragged red fiber disease; PRKAG2 = protein kinase AMP-activated gamma 2; WPW = Wolff-Parkinson-White syndrome.

glutamine (Arg403Glut), are associated with severe LV hypertrophy and a high incidence of sudden death. Other cardiac actin mutations, such as the β-myosin mutation Leucine908Valine, are associated with mild LV hypertrophy and a relatively benign prognosis. Sinisterly, some genetic defects, such as the Alanine95Valine α-tropomyosin mutation, are associated with mild LV hypertrophy but a poor outcome. Recently, several nonsarcomeric genes have been shown to cause HCM associated with distinct phenotypes, and patterns of LV hypertrophy similar to those of HCM are a feature of several multisystem diseases.

MODIFIERS OF PHENOTYPE EXPRESSION

A notable feature of HCM is its marked phenotypic heterogeneity. Disease penetrance, severity, and distribution of cardiac hypertrophy; presence or absence of ventricular obstruction; LV systolic and diastolic dysfunction; myocardial perfusion abnormalities; arrhythmia; and risk of sudden death vary considerably even in affected members of the same family. This phenotypic heterogeneity is attributed to variable expressions of genes that are activated secondarily and that modulate the severity of the hypertrophic response. It is thought likely that hormones and growth factors, which act through endocrine, paracrine, or autocrine mechanisms, contribute to the hypertrophy and hyperplasia of myocytes, other cell types (smooth-muscle cells, endothelial cells, and fibroblasts), and interstitial fibrosis. Several of these, including the components of the renin–angiotensin system, endothelin, and insulin growth factor are currently under investigation as their inhibition may reduce LV hypertrophy and cardiac fibrosis, and improve long-term outcome.

Clinical Presentations and Investigations

Although HCM is occasionally detected in utero or in infancy, the disease usually develops during the period of rapid body growth in puberty. Significant increases in LV wall thickness after the age of 18 years are unusual. Occasionally, HCM is diagnosed for the first time in those over 65 years of age, although in most cases it is thought that the LV hypertrophy has been present for decades. Severe LV hypertrophy may be asymptomatic in some patients, but complaints of chest discomfort, dyspnea, palpitations, fatigue, presyncope, and syncope are common. Symptoms are frequently induced by postural changes or by exertion, dehydration, arrhythmia, and vasodilating drugs. Clinical examination may also be normal, and must not be solely relied upon when screening at-risk family members. Patients with obstructive HCM may have a bifid arterial pulse and there is often a prominent LV apical impulse. Auscultation may reveal an added third or fourth heart sound, and in patients with obstruction, a harsh systolic murmur at mid-sternum radiates to the axilla, increases in intensity on assuming an upright posture and becomes fainter with squatting. Additionally, there may be signs of secondary right heart failure. The 12-lead electrocardiogram is highly variable and may be normal. The most common finding, however, is voltage criteria for LV hypertrophy with "strain" pattern. Electrocardiographic changes frequently precede echocardiographically detectable LV hypertrophy. Two-dimensional echocardiography is the primary method for diagnosing HCM and the usual diagnostic criteria require the demonstration of LV wall thickness of greater than 13 mm (usually asymmetric hypertrophy of the septum) in the absence of another cause for cardiac hypertrophy. In athletes, who may have physiologic LV hypertrophy, wall thickness should exceed 15 mm. Echocardiography also establishes the severity and distribution of left and right ventricular hypertrophy; establishes the presence or absence of LV obstruction and its site and severity (LV outflow tract or intra-LV cavity), and the presence or absence of mitral valve regurgitation and aberrant papillary muscles; and provides estimates of LV systolic function, pulmonary arterial pressure, and the severity of left atrial enlargement. Magnetic resonance imaging provides a more accurate definition of regional cardiac wall thickness and LV mass and systolic function. Several distinct morphologic types of HCM are recognized. *Asymmetric septal hypertrophy* (ASH) is the most common variety and primarily affects the intraventricular septum. ASH associated with LV outflow obstruction is traditionally termed *idiopathic hypertrophic subaortic stenosis* (IHSS). In *reversed ASH*, the posterior LV wall is of greater thickness than the septum. In contrast, the septal, posterior, and free walls of the LV have a similar degree of hypertrophy in *concentric HCM*. *Apical HCM* or *Japanese HCM* affects predominantly the LV apex and is associated with giant T wave inversions. In *midcavity obstructive HCM*, an uncommon variety, LV hypertrophy at the level of the papillary muscles causes these to become apposed in systole, and a pressure gradient develops between the basal LV cavity and an aneurysmal apical segment. HCM that presents in the elderly is often characterized by mitral annular calcification and marked narrowing of the LV outflow tract caused by anterior migration of the mitral valve annulus. Genetic testing may identify the responsible disease mutation, which may help determine the description of the mutation-specific natural history in the affected pedigree, determine the disease penetrance, and obtain a preclinical diagnosis. With adequate precautions, treadmill exercise testing is safe and objectively establishes exercise tolerance. Exercise-induced arrhythmia and a hypotensive blood pressure response may identify patients at increased risk for sudden death (Table 2). Myocardial perfusion defects detected by exercise thallium scintigraphy and arrhythmias detected by ambulatory electrocardiographic or Holter monitoring also assist risk stratification. Exercise radionuclide angiography estimates LV ejection fraction and often demonstrates indices of abnormal LV diastolic dysfunction (prolongation of isovolumic relaxation, reduced rate and extent of rapid filling, and increased contribution of atrial systole to LV end diastolic volume). Cardiac catheterization is valuable at providing estimates of cardiac output, ventricular filling pressures, and LV pressure gradients under basal conditions and following provocation. These hemodynamic indices are valuable for guiding symptomatic therapy and for assessing the efficacy of therapeutic interventions. Coronary artery angiography excludes congenital and acquired coronary disease and assesses the suitability of septal arteries for alcohol septal ablation (see Management section). Electrophysiologic studies often provide evidence of sinus node, atrioventricular node, and His-Purkinje disease, and also help identify patients prone to atrial and ventricular arrhythmias and sudden death.

TABLE 2 Clinical Indicators of Increased Risk of Sudden Death in Hypertrophic Cardiomyopathy (HCM)

Young age (<20 years)
Cardiac arrest
Presyncope and syncope, particularly if not associated with LV outflow obstruction
Myocardial ischemia, particularly in the young and if associated with exercise-induced presyncope, syncope, or hypotension
Genetic mutation associated with a poor prognosis
Family history of multiple sudden deaths in close relatives
Disease progression to LV wall thinning and impaired LV systolic function
Induction of sustained ventricular arrhythmia at electrophysiologic study
Spontaneous sustained ventricular tachycardia
Nonsustained ventricular tachycardia during ambulatory Holter monitoring, if associated with symptoms of impaired consciousness
Markedly enlarged left atrium and atrial fibrillation
Severe cardiac hypertrophy (LV wall thickness >30 mm)
LV outflow obstruction/midcavity obstructive HCM

Abbreviation: LV = left ventricle.

Pathophysiology

The genetically induced myocardial hypertrophy in HCM is frequently severe, the magnitude of which may predict adverse outcome. It is often associated with dynamic LV outflow obstruction, LV diastolic dysfunction, myocardial perfusion abnormalities, disabling symptoms, heart failure, arrhythmia, and an increased risk of sudden death.

OBSTRUCTIVE HYPERTROPHIC CARDIOMYOPATHY

In approximately 33% of HCM patients, hypertrophy generates high blood velocities in the LV outflow tract, which is narrowed by septal hypertrophy. This increased flow velocity creates a negative pressure that pulls the mitral valve toward the septum; this is systolic anterior motion (SAM) of the mitral valve—the most important determinant of the severity of LV outflow obstruction. SAM is often associated with mitral regurgitation. An intraventricular pressure gradient in patients with pure midcavity obstructive HCM results from systolic apposition of hypertrophied papillary muscles and does not result from SAM. Patients with the uncommon midcavity variant commonly also have SAM and LV outflow tract obstruction. Patients with midcavity obstructive HCM may present with sustained monomorphic ventricular tachycardia (VT) arising from an apical LV aneurysm. LV pressure gradients may be present under basal conditions, or may only become apparent after maneuvers that decrease preload or afterload, or increase myocardial contractility—for example, following sudden adoption of an erect posture, during Valsalva maneuver, after premature ventricular complexes, with catecholaminergic stimulation (isoproterenol or dobutamine infusion), and with digoxin therapy. LV outflow obstruction is the most common cause of presyncope and syncope and is an important determinant of clinical outcome in HCM.

MYOCARDIAL ISCHEMIA

Anginal chest pain is common in HCM, and exercise thallium scintigraphy demonstrates reversible myocardial perfusion abnormalities in approximately 66% of adult HCM patients. Chest pain may be accompanied by myocardial damage. In children, myocardial ischemia may not be associated with chest pain, but with exercise-induced symptoms of impaired consciousness and cardiac arrest. The etiology of myocardial ischemia may be related to:

- Blood supply/demand mismatch
- Disease of intramural arteries and small myocardial vessels
- Mitochondrial dysfunction
- Compression of intramyocardial vessels caused by high LV pressures.

Myocardial bridging and systolic compression of a coronary artery are believed to be related to the severity of LV hypertrophy and are not of hemodynamic or prognostic significance.

LV SYSTOLIC DYSFUNCTION

HCM patients characteristically have high LV ejection fractions, and the enhanced LV systolic function is probably, in part, caused by lower systolic wall stresses secondary to increased wall thickness, smaller end-diastolic volumes, and mitral regurgitation. Additionally, in vitro research indicates that several HCM mutations may enhance the velocity of cycling of the actomyosin molecular motor, and it has been suggested that there is an increase in myocyte contractility. The disease progresses to LV wall thinning and impaired LV systolic function in a minority of patients. Although these patients may present with overt heart failure, most have mild-to-moderate symptoms of heart failure but nevertheless are at high risk for sudden death (see Table 2).

LV DIASTOLIC DYSFUNCTION

LV diastolic dysfunction is common in HCM and an important cause of symptoms that result from the elevated ventricular filling pressures and a reduced capacity to increase stroke volume. LV diastolic dysfunction commonly causes overt pulmonary edema despite high LV ejection fractions. Several mechanisms that may explain LV diastolic dysfunction are:

- Hyperplasia and hypertrophy of cardiac cells, and myofiber disarray
- Interstitial fibrillar collagen, an elastic element of considerable stiffness
- Myocardial ischemia
- Increased intracellular Ca^{2+} and an increased responsiveness of the myofilament to Ca^{2+}

LV stiffness results in elevated right and left atrial pressures and progressive atrial enlargement that predispose to atrial arrhythmias, which in turn are poorly tolerated in the presence of LV diastolic dysfunction.

ARRHYTHMIA

Both supraventricular and ventricular arrhythmias are common in HCM. The myocardial substrate may be myofiber disarray, interstitial fibrosis and gross scarring, myocardial ischemia/infarction, and accessory atrioventricular bypass tracts. Arrhythmias may have serious hemodynamic consequences caused by induction of acute myocardial ischemia, loss of atrial transport mechanism, aggravation of LV obstruction, and/or abbreviation of diastolic filling time. Wolff-Parkinson-White (WPW) syndrome occurs in less than 5% of HCM cases, and some cases have been associated with mutations affecting the function of adenosine monophosphate (AMP) kinase, a protein involved in the homeostatic control of myocellular adenosine triphosphate (ATP) concentrations (see Table 1). Sinus node disease is present in approximately 66% of HCM patients and may present as sinus bradycardia or inappropriate sinus tachycardia (sinus node reentry). Other supraventricular tachycardias include paroxysmal atrioventricular tachycardia caused by an accessory atrioventricular pathway, atrial flutter, and atrial fibrillation. The incidence of atrial fibrillation increases with age and with progressive left atrial enlargement, and it complicates the disease in approximately 10% of all HCM patients. His-Purkinje conduction abnormalities occur in approximately 33% of HCM patients, and occasionally hemodynamic collapse is caused by onset of complete heart block. Nonsustained VT is present in approximately 33% of the patients after several days of ambulatory electrocardiographic monitoring, and tends to be pleomorphic and of brief duration. Sustained monomorphic and polymorphic VTs are uncommon and often precipitate cardiac arrest. Sustained monomorphic VT may indicate old myocardial infarction, or midcavity obstructive HCM associated with an apical LV aneurysm.

SUDDEN DEATH

HCM is the most common cause of sudden death in otherwise healthy young individuals such as athletes. The cumulative annual incidence of sudden death in HCM patients is 1% to 2%. Several indicators of increased risk for sudden death have been identified, but generally have low positive predictive values (see Table 2). Mechanisms of cardiac arrest that have been identified are:

- Arrhythmogenic LV substrate
- Heart block
- Supraventricular tachycardia
- Myocardial ischemia
- LV outflow obstruction

Some athletes are at increased risk for sudden death and competitive sports are discouraged. However, as it is unclear that this advice is heeded or indeed prevents sudden death, investigations should be directed at identifying treatable abnormalities.

MISCELLANEOUS FEATURES

Mitral valve prolapse is common in HCM, and may be associated with significant mitral regurgitation. Some of the sarcomeric genes are also expressed in skeletal muscle, and may cause a mild, nonprogressive skeletal myopathy. β-myosin mutations are associated with hypertrophied skeletal myofibers, a predominance of type I or slow fibers, and loss of mitochondria from the centers of many slow fibers (appearances likened to those of central core disease, a mitochondrial myopathy). Mutations of the myosin light chains and α-tropomyosin are associated with a ragged, red-fiber pattern (also seen in mitochondrial myopathies). Despite involvement of skeletal muscle, there is no clinical skeletal myopathy associated with the sarcomeric mutations, and the histological abnormalities may be compatible with a high level of athletic achievement. This may be caused by the property of skeletal muscle to regenerate from the transformation of satellite cells, in contrast to cardiac muscle, which has little or no capacity to regenerate in response to injury. HCM associated with several novel nonsarcomeric genes is often associated with specific cardiac phenotypes (see Table 1).

Management

Asymptomatic adult patients may not require specific therapy unless features indicating increased risk for sudden death are present (Figure 1; see Table 2). There is no uniform consensus on the management of children with HCM. However, a more aggressive approach to investigating and treating identified cardiac abnormalities may be justified because of difficulties in eliciting symptoms in severely affected children, rapid disease progression with body growth, and a sudden death rate higher than in adults (2% to 6% per year) with sudden death often presenting despite the absence of symptoms.

OUTFLOW TRACT AND MIDCAVITY LEFT VENTRICLE OBSTRUCTION

Symptomatic patients with LV obstruction are initially treated with a β blocker, such as atenolol (Tenormin[1], 100 mg per day); a calcium antagonist, such as verapamil[1] (Calan, 180 to 240 mg per day); and/or disopyramide (Norpace[1], 200 to 400 mg daily), an antiarrhythmic drug with negative inotropic properties (see Figure 1). However, β blockers may cause bradycardia, particularly, in patients with sinus node disease or conduction abnormality. Because of its vasodilatory properties, verapamil is contraindicated in patients with severe LV outflow obstruction, low filling pressures, and hypotension. Disopyramide is often not tolerated in those over 65 because of anticholinergic side effects. Both verapamil and disopyramide may aggravate congestive heart failure, and should be avoided in patients with pulmonary hypertension. LV myotomy and myectomy have been standard therapies in patients with drug-refractory symptoms. The operative mortality (2% to 5%) and the success of the procedure depend on the skill and experience of the surgeon. Complications include heart block, ventricular septal defect, late aortic regurgitation, LV dysfunction, and 1% to 2% cumulative annual mortality. Alternative, nonsurgical, therapies for the relief of drug-refractory symptoms associated with LV outflow obstruction include dual chamber pacemaker (DDD) therapy and percutaneous transluminal alcohol septal ablation (PTSA). The relief of LV obstruction in DDD pacemaker therapy relies on the altered pattern of ventricular contraction that results from pacing at the apex of the right ventricle. The resultant *paradoxic motion* of the septum moves it away from the mitral valve apparatus to lessen the severity of SAM and the outflow obstruction. Procedural risks associated with DDD therapy are relatively minimal, but some researchers have expressed concerns about its efficacy. At PTSA, the septal myocardium adjacent to the increased outflow tract blood velocities responsible for SAM is identified. The septal artery that perfuses

[1]Not FDA approved for this indication.

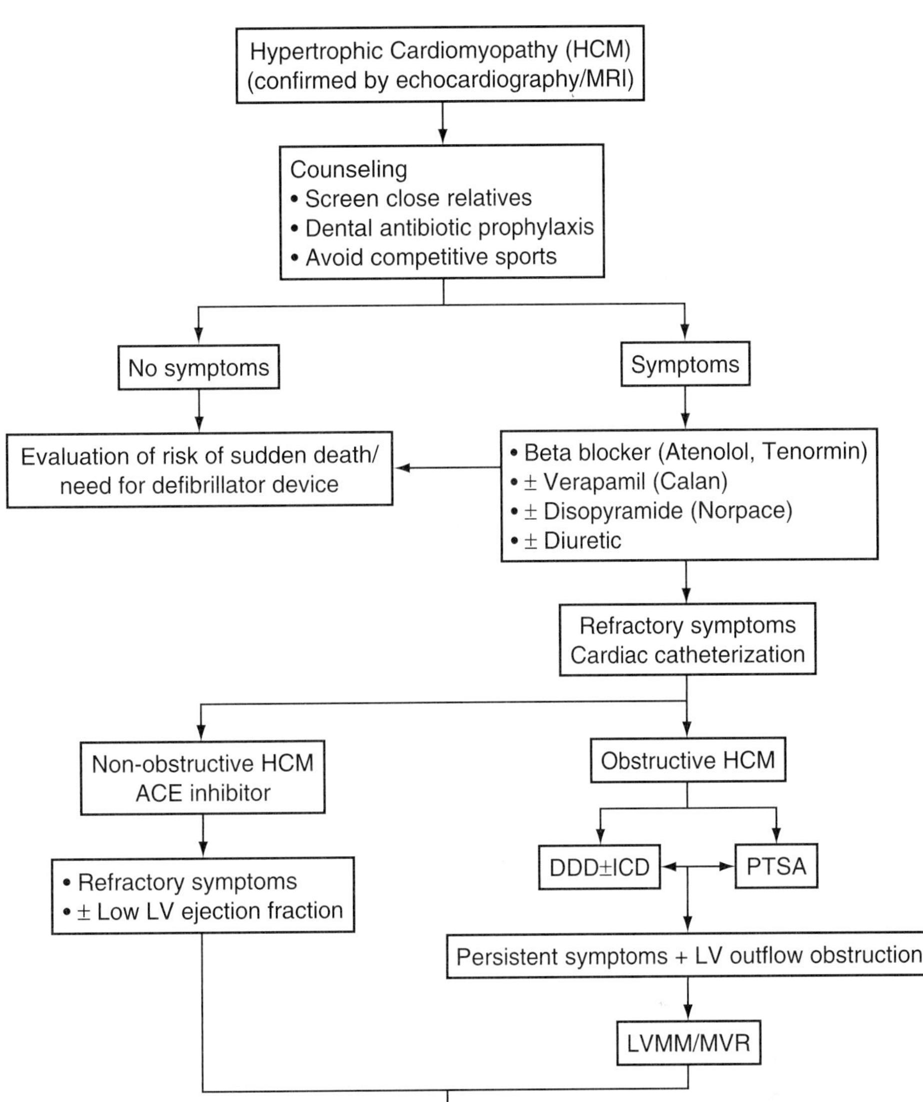

FIGURE 1 Management of hypertrophic cardiomyopathy.

this region is catheterized, isolated, and alcohol infused to ablate and thin the dependent myocardium, widening the outflow tract and reducing the outflow velocities and the resultant SAM. Complications of PTSA include heart block and extensive myocardial infarcts, and there are concerns about the arrhythmogenic potential of the resulting scar. The choice between these three effective therapies for drug refractory symptoms of obstructive HCM has depended on the expertise and experience of referral centers and on patient choices. Currently, none of them is the treatment of choice by consensus.

LV DIASTOLIC DYSFUNCTION

Treatment of associated LV outflow obstruction and myocardial ischemia (e.g., with verapamil) may improve LV diastolic dysfunction. Congestive heart failure should be treated with judicious doses of diuretics. Angiotensin converting enzyme (ACE) inhibitors may help symptoms and prevent heart failure in the absence of LV outflow obstruction, particularly, if there is LV dysfunction. Patients with severe LV diastolic dysfunction and heart failure should be referred for cardiac transplantation.

ARRHYTHMIA

Verapamil[1] and/or β blockers are prescribed to control ventricular rates in patients with atrial fibrillation. The role of catheter-based or surgical treatments for atrial fibrillation are not established in HCM. Disopyramide (Norpace)[1] or sotalol[1] (Sotacor[2] or Betapace) in those under 30 years of age and amiodarone (Cordarone)[1] in low doses in those over 65 years of age may be valuable in maintaining

[1]Not FDA approved for this indication.

[2]Not available in the United States.

sinus rhythm. All patients with paroxysmal or chronic atrial fibrillation require anticoagulation because of a high risk of thromboembolic disease. Catheter ablation of the atrioventricular node combined with implantation of a rate-responsive, dual switch-mode pacemaker/defibrillator is an attractive alternative therapy in symptomatic patients who have chronic or paroxysmal atrial fibrillation but do not tolerate drugs with negative inotropic effects. Nonsustained VT has been considered an important predictor of sudden death, but it is relatively common and its prognostic importance in asymptomatic patients has been questioned. Defibrillators may improve prognosis in high-risk patients but they are not without complication in HCM, most commonly painful inappropriate shocks. The provision of DDD pacemaker capability in current defibrillator devices allows management of bradyarrhythmias, LV outflow obstruction, the termination of atrial fibrillation, and protection against sudden death.

GENETIC COUNSELING, PREGNANCY, WORK-RELATED ISSUES, AND PSYCHOLOGICAL SUPPORT

Patients should be counseled about the mode of inheritance of HCM, including the fact that as penetrance may be limited, not every child who inherits the disease-causing gene develops HCM. Reassurance is necessary that most affected individuals lead full and relatively normal lives. The pros and cons of genetic testing should be discussed, including the fact that many genetic causes of HCM are unknown and the natural history is variable and has been described for only a few mutations. However, determination that the disease mutation has not been inherited in a child eliminates the need for regular screening evaluations that are normally performed until the age of 18 to 20 years. Also, the genetic diagnosis of HCM at a presymptomatic stage allows a child to be advised against pursuing careers that are incompatible with the diagnosis of HCM, such as athletics and aviation. Pregnancy is usually well tolerated in patients with obstructive HCM, probably because the obstruction lessens as a result of the volume expansion of pregnancy. If possible, verapamil, β blockers, and other drugs should be withdrawn at least during the first trimester to avoid their potential teratogenic effects. Prolonged labor should be avoided. Finally, it is important to consider the psychological burden of the diagnosis of an inherited disease that may be lethal, may be transmitted to one's children before the development of the disease, and for which there is no cure at present.

HEART FAILURE

METHOD OF

Marc A. Silver, MD

Heart failure is an epidemic in the United States. Every day, clinicians face the task of caring for more patients with heart failure in all its forms. Heart failure is the primary reason for hospitalization of Americans older than 65 years, and although 6 million Americans are estimated to have symptomatic heart failure, that number is expected to double over the next 7 years. Many millions more have asymptomatic left ventricular dysfunction or existing medical conditions that make it quite likely that heart failure will develop and they will die.

It is truly in the hands of primary care physicians, who care for most heart failure patients, as well as those with common precursors of heart failure, to better understand heart failure and its natural history and thereby make an impact on this challenging epidemic. Therefore, with this concept in mind, I will discuss heart failure from the perspective of understanding its natural history or stages, as well as a chronic disease process amenable to strategic planning.

Definitions

All clinicians define heart failure differently. Some choose to think about heart failure only when the patient has advanced disease characterized by significant volume overload and exercise limitation. Others consider heart failure to be present only when the left ventricle is dilated. Though broad by intent, heart failure is usually defined as a complex clinical syndrome that affects cardiac function (its ability to fill and/or eject blood) and is often preceded by and certainly accompanied by systemic neurohormonal abnormalities that participate in and perpetuate the dysfunction of the heart, as well as other target organs, including the vasculature and muscles.

Although a wide range of signs and symptoms may accompany the heart failure syndrome of whatever cause, once symptomatic, patients usually have evidence of dyspnea, fatigue, and sodium and water retention manifested as congestion in the lungs, legs, and gut.

It is useful, however, to think about heart failure not only as a symptomatic disease but also as a disease whose development begins decades before the patient crosses the threshold of clinical symptoms.

Classification and Stages of Heart Failure

Although many clinicians bristle at the concept of prescribed sets of recommendations or guidelines to be applied to a diverse disease process such as heart

TABLE 1 Stages of Heart Failure

Stage A

Patients who are at increased risk for heart failure because of associated medical conditions (e.g., hypertension, coronary artery disease, or diabetes mellitus)
Heart structure and function: Not yet affected
Potential therapies: Treatment of hypertension, smoking cessation, and weight loss; ACE inhibitors in appropriate patients

Stage B

Patients who have abnormal heart structure and/or function but who have not manifested signs or symptoms
Heart structure and function: Abnormal
Potential therapies: Same, plus ACE inhibitors and β blockers in all appropriate patients

Stage C

Patients with symptomatic heart failure. These patients indeed have advanced heart failure. Note that signs and symptoms develop as late phenomena after significant perturbation of many homeostatic mechanisms and the consumption of large cardiac reserves
Heart structure and function: Abnormal
Potential therapies: Same, plus ACE inhibitors, β blockers, and digoxin and diuretics in most patients; also, coronary revascularization and repair of mitral regurgitation in select patients

Stage D

Patients with extremely advanced heart failure
Heart structure and function: Extremely abnormal
Potential therapies: Same, consideration of advanced therapies including investigational therapies, as well as end-of-life counseling and hospice

Abbreviation: ACE = angiotensin-converting enzyme.

TABLE 2 New York Heart Associated Functional Classification of Heart Failure

I. Symptoms occur only at a level that would cause normal individuals to become symptomatic
II. Symptoms occur with ordinary exertion or moderate levels of activity
III. Symptoms occur with less than ordinary degrees of activity
IV. Symptoms occur even at rest

This classification scheme is generally applied to patients once they are or have been symptomatic with heart failure (stages C and D). Note that in general, the classification implies the patient's worst level of functioning related to a heart failure symptom (e.g., fatigue, dyspnea, exercise intolerance).

failure, these guidelines are frequently a place where available evidence is evaluated in a critical way and balanced with consensus to provide the readers with a distillation of what might work for them when they are caring for a patient with a disease process.

Recently, one of the well-accepted standard guidelines for heart failure has been revised. Within the 2001 Revision of the American College of Cardiology/American Heart Association Guidelines for the Evaluation and Management of Chronic Heart Failure for the Adult (executive summary and full text available at http://www.acc.org/clinical/guidelines/failure/hf_index.htm), aside from detailed information on the testing and therapies currently supported by evidence, appears a new classification for heart failure (Table 1). The classification most clinicians are familiar with is that of the New York Heart Association (NYHA) (Table 2). The NYHA classification is generally applied to patients who at some point become symptomatic. Although they may revert to a symptom-free status (NYHA functional class I), it is still implied that the patient has overt heart failure. Even though the NYHA classification is of great value and carries prognostic value, it also tends to allow us to think of a patient with mild or moderate symptoms (i.e., NYHA functional class II to III) as having a mild or moderate disease, but indeed, patients in this category have a markedly shortened life span and by definition have less than optimal functional status.

The new classification, on the other hand (see Table 1), identifies four stages of heart failure based on the spectrum of common clinical syndromes from which they have evolved. By so doing, it is hoped that the clinician will recognize the patient's increased risk for the clinical syndrome and then act aggressively to reduce the risk and/or intervene earlier just as one would with a patient at risk for cancer.

The classification addresses four stages. Unlike the NYHA classification, in which a patient may easily pass back and forth through several functional classes over a period of days to weeks, as the patient passes through each stage of the new classification, there is no longer any hope of reverting to an earlier stage, which should act as an impetus to capture the patient at the earliest stage and prevent progression to the next stage by the use of proper diagnostics and therapeutics.

Stage A refers to patients who by virtue of having other common clinical conditions are at increased risk of heart failure ultimately developing. These conditions include hypertension, diabetes mellitus, and coronary artery disease. Similarly, patients with a family history of heart failure would have an increased risk. Clearly, the heart failure syndrome will not develop in all these patients, but acknowledging their "at-risk" status gives the clinician and the patient fair warning of the potential risk of development of heart failure and may serve as an early warning detection system for the insidious progression to more advanced heart failure. Progression to the next stage is preventable, and disease progression is usually measured in years or decades.

Stage B refers to patients in whom structural and even functional abnormalities in heart function have already developed, but because of enormous cardiac reserve, the signs or symptoms that usually bring these patients to medical attention have not developed. This stage has also been referred to as "asymptomatic left ventricular dysfunction." Progression to the next stage may be slowed and again may be measured in years.

Stage C represents most of what we call heart failure today, specifically, a patient who has structural and functional disease but who has now progressed and used up enough cardiac reserve to actually have signs and symptoms of the disease. By looking at heart failure in this perspective, it becomes clear that any symptomatic heart failure indeed represents a serious condition that the clinician must diagnose and treat accordingly. In this stage of the disease, clinicians can intervene to improve symptoms and quality of life, as well as improve, but not completely abolish the increased mortality. Progression to the next stage is quite variable but is usually measured in months to years.

Stage D represents very advanced disease in which even standard measures cannot overcome the severity of the disease and advanced measures need to be undertaken. During this stage, despite best efforts, patients usually have increased use of resources, decreased quality of life, and progressive limitation. Although many advanced resources are being applied during this stage, including heart transplantation and ventricular restraint and assist devices, generally, these patients ultimately die of either progressive heart failure or sudden cardiac death.

Steps for Appropriate Heart Failure Management

Physicians often take a reflex approach to initiating drug therapy in a patient with symptomatic heart failure. For example, a patient who is volume overloaded might be treated with diuretics as monotherapy while overlooking the need to not only treat the current symptoms but also plan a strategy to limit progression of disease. Therefore, a useful approach in planning patient care involves two broad steps. The first is assessment of the information needed to create a management plan, and the second is an understanding of the therapeutic targets in heart failure treatment.

An assessment of what is known or yet needed to be known to best make the diagnosis and treat a patient with heart failure is a very useful step. This assessment generally involves an understanding of the etiology of the heart failure, the current stage or functional class, and so forth. However, even after a detailed history and physical examination and collection of some diagnostic data, a gap can remain in the information needed to complete the therapeutic plan. Generally, the clinician can group the areas that need to be completed into three main categories: diagnostics, therapeutics, and prognostics. In fact, it is useful to consider these three areas each time a patient is seen in the office or hospital. Even though one often initiates treatment without complete information in each of these areas, not asking what other information is needed often leads to an incomplete understanding of the disease syndrome, as well as suboptimal therapy.

Diagnostics refers to any additional information that allows a better understanding of the etiology, status, degree of limitation, and signs and symptoms of a patient. For example, an echocardiogram allows assessment of the nature and degree of left ventricular function and may lead to consideration of myocardial ischemia (wall motion abnormalities) or valvular disease (valvular regurgitation or stenosis) as a therapeutic target. Often, in this category are tests that might reveal an easily addressable cause of the heart failure and even a form of heart failure that is potentially reversible (such as hyperthyroidism).

Therapeutics refers to the design of the treatment strategy based on what is currently known about the patient and that patient's disease. It is also useful to write down a therapeutic plan, including the one or two next steps one might take for the patient should the signs or symptoms not abate with the current regimen. For example, one might begin with using angiotensin-converting enzyme (ACE) inhibitors but indicate that if the patient is found to have underlying coronary artery disease, the addition of long-acting nitrates will be considered.

Prognostics refers to focusing in on what is known about the patient's heart failure in terms of predicting what might be the path of progression in the near future. Though imperfect, many pieces of information are closely linked to survival and disease progression, including functional status, exercise tolerance, and left ventricular ejection fraction. In considering any additional prognostics, the clinician should always ask what might be done differently given the result. Over the years we have become more willing to intervene earlier with therapeutics, which can alter progression of the disease, and we are therefore less dependent on a bad set of prognostic markers to make these decisions. Nevertheless, awareness of a low peak oxygen consumption, a low right ventricular ejection fraction, or a markedly elevated neurohormonal marker often serves to alert the physician and the patient and family to review the current therapeutic plan and broaden considerations to include the next level of care and treatment, which might consist of investigational therapies and evaluation for heart transplantation. The role of measurement of B-type natriuretic peptide in this regard is of some interest and may prove to be a prognostic marker against which we target our therapies.

TREATMENT TARGETS

In designing the drug treatment plan, we take into consideration the following treatment targets for patients with heart failure: improved survival, improved symptoms, slowing and/or reversal of disease progression, improved functional status and quality of life, avoidance of troublesome adverse events, and decreased use of resources, including hospitalization. With the recognition that not all these targets are concordant or attainable, the drug regimen reflects these targets and our understanding of the ability of drugs to address them.

In general, patients with symptomatic heart failure are managed with a core group of four drug classes,

TABLE 3 Common Heart Failure Drugs and Their Therapeutic Targets

Drug	Dose	Comment
Loop diuretics (expressed as furosemide [Lasix] equivalent units)	40-100 mg once or twice daily	Many factors affect the doses required, such as patient compliance with dietary restrictions, fluid intake, and associated titration of other medication, including ACE inhibitors and β blockers
ACE inhibitors (expressed as enalapril [Vasotec] equivalent units)	10-20 mg twice daily	Higher doses seem to have an impact on hospitalization rates. Be aware of adverse events that will limit use, including hyperkalemia. To allow adequate titration of β blockers, reduced doses may be used
β Blockers (expressed as carvedilol [Coreg] equivalent units)	25-50 mg twice daily	Dependent on body size. Although data suggest clinical improvement and decreased mortality with smaller doses, the target remains full dose
Digoxin	0.125-0.25 mg daily	Adjustment needed for renal function. Routine measurement of serum levels is not required unless done to confirm toxicity

including diuretics, an ACE inhibitor, a β blocker, and usually digoxin. The former and the latter are generally applied to relieve symptoms or to improve functional status or exercise tolerance, whereas the middle two are also administered with the specific intention of altering disease progression, reversing the structural and/or functional abnormalities of the heart and other target organs, and improving medium- and long-term survival.

Increasing evidence supports the initiation of ACE inhibitors and β blockers jointly when caring for a symptomatic patient. Diuretics often need to be adjusted up or down, depending on a patient's level of compensation, as well as where they are in terms of other (β blocker) titration. Target doses for most of the commonly used drugs come from clinical trials suggesting their benefit (ACE inhibitors) or from tradition, as well as from attempts to balance drug efficacy with drug safety (digoxin and diuretics). Target doses are listed in Table 3. Excellent details and practical considerations of implementing and titrating heart failure drugs can be found in recent guidelines (http://www.acc.org/clinical/guidelines/failure/hf_index.htm).

NONPHARMACOLOGIC MEASURES

An enormous armamentarium outside routine drug therapy is available to clinicians caring for patients with heart failure. In general, most nonpharmacologic measures should be used in a simultaneous fashion with the initiation and titration of drug therapy. Although most of these therapies either have not or will not undergo rigorous clinical investigation, they nonetheless remain therapeutic cornerstones of complete heart failure care. Often, dramatic functional improvement can be observed with more careful attention to nonpharmacologic therapies. Of particular interest is an understanding that sleep-disordered breathing (including obstructive and central forms of sleep apnea) may be present in nearly 40% of heart failure patients. Increasing evidence suggests that therapy that includes continuous positive airway pressure may alter symptoms, disease progression, and even survival (Table 4). As far as dietary advice, generally admonitions for avoidance of excessive sodium intake and fluid are given along with specific information on lowering dietary saturated fat. However, emerging information is that the patient with heart failure suffers a significant energy imbalance and may well benefit from nutritional assessment, including measurement of nitrogen balance.

Use of Disease Management and Other Resources

Perhaps one of the greatest tools at hand for clinicians caring for patients with heart failure, as well as for their families, is provision of a thorough understanding of the heart failure syndrome and how self-empowered actions might have a significant impact on how they feel, what they can do, and how long they might live. Studies have repeatedly demonstrated the benefits of a structured disease management program in reducing symptoms, improving functional status, and in particular, reducing heart failure hospitalizations. Frequently, the clinician can best serve the patient by fostering and supporting a heart failure disease management program. Though not present in all communities yet, the resources required (a physician and/or a nurse champion) are often available everywhere. Abundant educational, patient-oriented books and materials are available to support these programs.

TABLE 4 Nonpharmacologic Therapies for Patients with Heart Failure

Therapy
Definitely Helps Reduce Symptoms or Improve Functional Status
Salt restriction (target, 2.3 g of salt/d)
Exercise
Stress reduction
Screening for depression
Smoking cessation
Weight loss
Treatment of documented sleep-disordered breathing
May Be of Use in Selected Patients
Fluid restriction
Avoidance of alcohol

Disease management programs are often part of a larger specialized heart failure center. Within these structures abide advanced strategies, including investigational therapies. It is incumbent on the clinician to be aware of these local and regional resources and refer patients when appropriate. Even with advanced disease, these centers can often offer improved outcomes and strategies not available to all clinicians.

Another area within the disease management spectrum that can be used is the home care programs that exist in most communities. These services frequently provide a link between intensive hospital-based care and infrequent, less intensive office-based care. In addition, for many patients with advanced disease, home care meets the constraints of patients and families.

For patients with advanced disease, physicians often begin discussions surrounding end-of-life issues too late. Generally, patients who have advanced disease requiring frequent hospitalization and treatment are aware of their likelihood of death and, in fact, value regaining some of the mastery and control of their lives through discussion of end-of-life planning and preferences. For some, hospice care will be the choice made, whereas for others, referral to specialized centers and participation in emerging therapies through clinical trials might be the correct choice. Understanding comes only with an open and frank discussion with each patient and family.

Emerging and Emerged New Therapeutic Areas

Because of the intense interest in heart failure, a variety of additional therapies have recently undergone or are currently undergoing clinical investigation that the clinician should be aware of. These therapies include new application of biventricular pacemakers, aggressive mitral valve repair for patients with ongoing mitral valve regurgitation, and the use of left ventricular assist devices as bridges to heart recovery, as well as destination or permanent therapies. Moreover, several new cardiac restraint devices are being applied with some success. Within years, genomic therapies will broaden, as will areas of vascular and myogenic regeneration. Again, although most clinicians will not be aware of all these newly emerging therapies, what they can offer their patients are interest and referrals to specialized centers where suitable therapies can be sought.

MITRAL VALVE PROLAPSE

METHOD OF
Mary E. Fontana, MD

In mitral valve prolapse (MVP), the primary defect is one of collagen dissolution accompanied by elastin fragmentation, mucopolysaccharide infiltration, and myxomatous degeneration. The extent of involvement ranges from one scallop of the posterior leaflet to both leaflets and chordae. Annular enlargement and calcification can further impair leaflet function. The degree of valve dysfunction influences the clinical presentation. The anatomic description of the enlarged, redundant, floppy myxomatous mitral valve leaflets with the elongated chordae that characterize the severe end of the mitral valve prolapse spectrum was first expressed in the 1940s.

Physical Examination

The auscultatory correlates of the anatomic spectrum of MVP were defined in the 1960s and 1970s. The milder forms are identified by one or more nonejection systolic clicks, with or without the mid-late systolic murmur, which is best heard at the apex. The postural auscultatory pattern differentiates MVP from other causes of clicks and late systolic murmurs. The systolic clicks move toward and often into the first heart sound; the murmur is longer and often louder, or it initially appears with the assumption of upright posture, particularly if a markedly increased heart rate occurs. A honking or whooping sound may be heard within this murmur, particularly in the upright position. Prompt squatting returns the auscultatory pattern to what it was in the supine position. Any maneuver, such as Valsalva's strain, anxiety, or exercise, that reduces ventricular volume exaggerates the prolapse and the clinical findings. Maneuvers that increase volume, such as Valsalva's release, handgrip, β blocker therapy, and pregnancy, have the opposite effect. The presence of the click or late systolic murmur with typical postural variation indicates the diagnosis of MVP. After pansystolic regurgitation occurs (usually a floppy, redundant valve with or without chordal rupture), creating a pansystolic murmur, the postural auscultatory changes may be lost. In a patient with an apical, high-pitched pansystolic murmur with or without an S_3 gallop, diastolic filling rumble, or apical thrill, echocardiography is required to establish MVP as the cause of the mitral regurgitation.

There is a frequent association of MVP with heritable connective tissue disorders, such as Marfan syndrome and Ehlers-Danlos syndrome. Lens displacement (which often requires slit-lamp examination), arachnodactyly, marked joint laxity, very long limbs compared with trunk length, and cigarette paper scars suggest these diagnoses. Low body weight and skeletal abnormalities, such as pectus carinatum or excavatum, straight back or scoliosis, and an arm span greater than height are commonly seen in patients with MVP, with or without a genetically transmitted connective tissue disease.

Mitral Valve Prolapse Syndrome

Mitral valve prolapse is estimated to affect 3% to 4% of the population, making it the most common congenital heart abnormality. Most patients are asymptomatic, and because only patients with symptoms seek medical attention, the incidence seems higher. Chest pain and palpitations are the most common presenting symptoms, with dyspnea, anxiety, fatigue, lightheadedness, syncope, and focal neurologic signs also occurring. These symptoms in conjunction with the auscultatory diagnosis of MVP constitute the mitral valve prolapse syndrome. Autonomic dysfunction is thought to play a major role in producing symptoms.

The chest pain is usually not typical of angina pectoris. It may be sharp, dull, or pressing, and it may last seconds or hours. There is usually no specific relationship to exertion, and exacerbations may occur over days, weeks, or months, with long remissions in between. Palpitations most often correlate with sinus tachycardia. Often there is no correlation with specific arrhythmias seen on ambulatory monitoring. Atrial or ventricular premature beats, supraventricular and ventricular tachycardias, ventricular fibrillation, and all degrees of AV block have been documented in symptomatic patients with MVP.

Dyspnea and fatigue in mild MVP disease have no hemodynamic correlates. These symptoms in a patient with left ventricular enlargement and severe mitral regurgitation, with or without atrial arrhythmias, are caused by elevated left atrial pressure, with or without left ventricular dysfunction, and low forward cardiac output.

Anxiety is very common in patients with MVP who present to physicians. This anxiety can be related to a hyperadrenergic state, concern over symptoms, or specific neuroendocrine abnormalities (e.g., hyperthyroidism); and it is often contributed to by physicians who label patients with heart disease without proper knowledge or explanations of the problem to the patient.

Postural lightheadedness and syncope may be associated with documented orthostatic hypotension. It is important to document pulse rates and blood pressures in the supine and upright positions in patients with these symptoms. Focal neurologic signs do occur in MVP. Possible mechanisms include emboli from surface erosions on a myxomatous valve or from the atriovalvular junction, endocardial friction lesions, and coexisting mitral annular calcifications. Abnormal platelet function has also been found in some patients. Vasospasm should be considered, because other vasospastic disorders (e.g., migraine) are associated with MVP. In older patients with floppy valves, large atria, and atrial arrhythmias, the incidence is higher, and the source is more convincingly embolic. Older patients may have coexisting cerebrovascular disease.

Diagnostic Testing

After MVP is suspected on clinical examination, Doppler echocardiography should be done to define the anatomic characteristics of the valve, chamber size, left ventricular function, severity of mitral regurgitation, and associated lesions, which may include atrial septal defect or hypertrophic cardiomyopathy. In patients with severe mitral regurgitation in whom surgical intervention is contemplated, and in patients with focal neurologic signs, transesophageal echocardiography should be done to define mitral valve anatomy and possible embolic sources.

Some patients with typical clicks or murmurs have negative echocardiograms. Echocardiography is routinely done in the supine position, and all scallops of the leaflets may not be visualized. Rarely, a patient has classic MVP by echocardiography and a negative clinical examination. The ventricular volume and inotropic state of the patient with milder forms of MVP are influenced by the physical and emotional states at the time of examination, and it is complicated by the wide use of β-blocking agents for chest pain and palpitations. Serial examinations may be required under different conditions and without β blocker therapy to be sure of the clinical diagnosis. The finding of mild MVP by echocardiography with the symptom complex but no auscultatory findings does not establish the diagnosis. Physicians must not use MVP as a convenient explanation of symptoms that are common in the general population.

An electrocardiogram should be obtained. Although normal in most patients, ST-T wave changes may be seen, especially in the inferior leads, which may suggest coronary disease in patients with chest pain. The ST-T wave changes often normalize with exercise and may be caused by autonomic dysfunction. The finding of a short PR interval or delta waves of the Wolff-Parkinson-White syndrome suggests supraventricular tachycardia as the cause of palpitations. A long QT interval is highly significant in a patient with neurologic signs or syncope. Patients with lightheadedness, syncope, and palpitations should undergo ambulatory monitoring. A 24-hour Holter monitor is effective for frequent symptoms, but event monitoring for 1 month is invaluable for sporadic symptoms. Treadmill exercise testing should also be performed to look for exercise-induced arrhythmias. Patients with chest pain suggesting angina and those older than 40 years of age should have a stress myocardial perfusion imaging examination. Cardiac catheterization studies are indicated for those with protracted symptoms unresponsive to simple therapeutic measures and for evaluating associated conditions, such as atrial septal defect, coronary disease, pulmonary hypertension, and left ventricular diastolic and systolic dysfunction. Tilt testing should be done for patients with severe orthostatic symptoms, with isoproterenol provocation, if initial studies are negative. Electrophysiologic testing is performed for patients with recurrent, unexplained syncope or symptomatic complex ventricular ectopy; sudden-death survivors; and those with Wolff-Parkinson-White syndrome.

Management

For most patients with MVP, drug therapy is not required. If none of the markers of a high-risk profile are present, the patients should be reassured of the benign nature of MVP. They should be encouraged to live normal, active lives. A regular mild or moderate aerobic exercise program is encouraged. The training effect of exercise appears to benefit the MVP symptom complex. The explanation of MVP and the benign prognosis are often therapeutic.

Identification of the high-risk patient is important. Patients at higher risk for progression and complications are those with mitral systolic murmur; thick, redundant, floppy, mitral valve leaflets; left ventricular enlargement; a recognized, heritable disorder of connective tissue, such as Marfan or Ehlers-Danlos syndromes; or long QT syndrome. Complications of progression to severe mitral regurgitation (e.g., myxomatous degeneration, annular dilatation, chordal elongation, rupture), infective endocarditis, uncontrolled atrial or ventricular arrhythmias, and sudden death occur more often and at a younger age in these patients. The clinician must categorize patients for proper treatment. Most of the discussion that follows refers to the milder end of the anatomic spectrum of MVP (i.e., the click-late murmur group), which occurs predominantly in adult females younger than 40 years of age.

In patient populations with endocarditis, MVP is the most frequent associated diagnosis. A patient with MVP who has a murmur of mitral regurgitation must receive antibiotic prophylaxis for dental and surgical procedures. Thick, redundant leaflets further increase endocarditis risk. Current endocarditis recommendations do not include patients with isolated systolic clicks. Problems with excluding this group include the dynamic nature of the findings in MVP, because a murmur may be heard under certain conditions and not others, and mitral regurgitation may be found by color-flow Doppler in some patients in whom it cannot be heard. Therefore, unless the patient clearly does not have a murmur on multiple consecutive examinations under different conditions and does not have thickened leaflets or mitral regurgitation by echocardiography, prophylaxis should be given according to the current American Heart Association recommendations—2 g of amoxicillin (Amoxil) orally 1 hour before a procedure or, if the patient has a penicillin allergy, 600 mg of clindamycin (Cleocin) are given.

Patients with MVP with palpitations associated with excessive tachycardia and milder tachyarrhythmias should be treated with reassurance and the elimination of catecholamine-stimulating compounds, such as caffeine, alcohol, and other drugs containing catecholamine derivatives. If the symptoms of palpitations, dyspnea, anxiety, or fatigue are not improved by avoiding these agents, β-blocking agents provide the greatest symptomatic relief. This is consistent with the hyperadrenergic state found in many of these symptomatic individuals. Marked tachycardia (>20 beats per minute increase) on standing is improved with low-dose β blockade, such as 25 to 50 mg of metoprolol succinate (Toprol-XL) daily, or metoprolol tartrate (Lopressor) at a dose of 25 to 50 mg twice daily. Any of the β-blocking agents can be used, with the choice governed by side effects, need for β_1 specificity, and pharmacokinetics. Therapy should be started with minimum doses and titrated. Patients with atrial flutter or atrial fibrillation unresponsive to β blockade can be given a class IC agent such as propafenone (Rythmol), 150 mg three times daily, or a class III agent such as sotalol (Betapace), 80 to 160 mg twice daily, to maintain sinus rhythm. Amiodarone (Cordarone) can be used in refractory cases, or ablation or maze procedure can be considered. Patients with Wolff-Parkinson-White syndrome require electrophysiologic testing and catheter ablation. Frequent ventricular ectopic beats and nonsustained ventricular tachycardia require treatment if symptomatic for patient and physician comfort, because prognosis does not appear to be worsened by their presence.

The chest pain has no unifying pathophysiologic explanation. Some possible causes for myocardial ischemia are:

- Excessive stretching or tension of chordae tendineae
- Reduced subendocardial blood flow caused by shortened diastole with tachycardia
- Coronary artery vasoregulatory abnormalities
- Microembolism

Potentially vasoconstricting compounds, such as cigarettes, should be eliminated. Therapy with β-blocking drugs is most beneficial. Calcium channel blockers and nitrates may be useful in infrequent cases of typical angina pectoris with normal coronary arteries. Anti-inflammatory agents can be tried for neuromusculoskeletal components. Therapeutic benefit may result from a normal coronary arteriogram performed in refractory cases.

Orthostatic symptoms are treated by increasing fluid intake, increasing salt intake, and avoiding diuretics and dehydration. In more severe cases of orthostatic hypotension or syncope, salt-retaining steroids, such as fludrocortisone (Florinef) (0.1 mg orally one to three times daily), and support stockings may be of benefit. For patients not responding to simple measures, tilt testing can identify significant autonomic abnormalities and guide therapy. A hypervagal state is the most common finding in MVP patients. Therapy with β-blocking agents, selective serotonin uptake inhibitors, such as sertraline hydrochloride (Zoloft)[1], 50 to 150 mg daily, or an $alpha_1$ agonist midodrine (ProAmatine)[1], 5 to 10 mg three times daily, may be beneficial. Sudden death is rare in MVP. In survivors and in patients with symptomatic complex arrhythmias, electrophysiologic testing is done to guide antiarrhythmic therapy.

A documented focal neurologic event dictates the use of aspirin (81 to 325 mg) daily, even if the embolic source cannot be identified. A transthoracic echo with saline contrast injection or transesophageal echo should be done to exclude other causes such a patent foramen ovale or atrial septal defect (ASD). Prophylactic antiplatelet drugs are not indicated. Anticoagulation with warfarin (Coumadin) is indicated if the patient has recurrent episodes, cardiac enlargement (particularly left atrial enlargement), atrial fibrillation, severe mitral regurgitation, or congestive heart failure. Patients experiencing focal neurologic signs should avoid vasoconstrictors and agents that enhance coagulability, such as cigarettes and oral contraceptives.

The pattern of inheritance of MVP is autosomal dominant. This should be explained to the patient. This is particularly important in those identified as having a heritable connective tissue disorder. In these cases, the family should be screened to identify high-risk members. Pregnancy is well tolerated in women with MVP. The increased blood volume in pregnancy may actually improve symptoms. A patient with a connective issue disorder with an aortic root of greater than 4 cm has an increased risk of aortic complications during pregnancy.

Competitive sports should be restricted for those with MVP who have moderate left ventricular enlargement, any degree of left ventricular dysfunction, uncontrolled supraventricular or ventricular tachyarrhythmias, a long QT interval, unexplained syncope, prior sudden death, or an enlarged aortic root.

The largest group of patients requiring mitral valve regurgitation surgery are those with:

- A floppy myxomatous mitral valve with severe regurgitation
- Disruption caused by ruptured chordae resulting in a flail leaflet
- Previously mild MVP with valve disruption as a result of bacterial endocarditis

Valvular disruption with acute, severe mitral regurgitation is symptomatic from high left atrial pressure, which results in pulmonary congestion. The surgical decision is easy in those cases. Progressive regurgitation with MVP may not be symptomatic until significant left ventricular dysfunction occurs, when surgery is a higher risk and the results are poorer. Surgery in the absence of symptoms is indicated when:

- Serial echocardiograms demonstrate enlargement of the left ventricle to twice normal.
- There is an end-systolic left ventricle (LV) dimension of more than 45 mm.
- There is a fall in LV ejection fraction to low-normal.

Posterior leaflet prolapse is most common, especially the middle scallop, which makes repair the preferred operation. Resection of the middle scallop with placement of an annuloplasty ring results in a competent valve in most cases with an operative mortality of 1% to 2% and a good long-term durability. Anterior leaflet prolapse and chordal repair or transposition can also be addressed. Valve replacement increases mortality 2 to 3 times. Refractory arrhythmias are not an indication for mitral valve repair or replacement.

Women with mild MVP predominate in the under 40 age group. Patients older than 60 years of age with significant mitral valve regurgitation that requires intervention are predominantly men. Floppy, redundant, myxomatous mitral valves with regurgitation in younger patients, particularly in those with heritable connective tissue disorders, indicate progression at a faster rate. Until more information is known, asymptomatic patients with milder forms of MVP should be seen every 2 to 3 years, with echocardiography performed approximately every 5 years to help define the natural history of the disease. Asymptomatic patients with evidence of myxomatous degeneration on echocardiogram and with a murmur of mitral regurgitation should be evaluated annually, even if there are no symptoms. Patients who have symptoms with mild MVP with a click and late systolic murmur or with more severe mitral regurgitation are seen every 6 months or more often if symptoms change.

INFECTIVE ENDOCARDITIS

METHOD OF

Matthew E. Levison, MD

Definition

A vegetation, or a lesion resulting from the deposition of platelets and fibrin on the endothelial surface of the heart, is the hallmark of endocarditis. Infection is the most common cause, and the usual pathogen is one of a variety of bacterial species, in

[1]Not FDA approved for this indication.

which case microscopic bacterial colonies are buried beneath the surface of fibrin, in the absence of an inflammatory reaction. Other types of microorganisms such as fungi may also be involved, so the more general term infective rather than bacterial endocarditis is preferred. Usually, the heart valve is the site of the vegetation, but in certain instances, vegetations may occur on other parts of the endocardium. Involvement of extracardiac sites, which can produce an illness clinically similar to endocarditis, is properly termed endarteritis.

Host

In population-based studies, the age- and sex-adjusted incidence of endocarditis is about 5 per 100,000 person-years. The incidence rate in the Philadelphia region is approximately 12 per 100,000 person-years, with the excess incidence attributed almost entirely to the increased frequency of intravenous drug use in this region, where endocarditis in intravenous drug users represents 46% of all cases. Other significant risk factors are (a) advancing age (in part because of the increased prevalence of predisposing cardiac lesions, e.g., degenerative cardiac lesions and prosthetic cardiac valves, and circumstances that may lead to bacteremia, e.g., invasive urologic procedures, anorectal and colonic disease, and use of intravascular catheters in the elderly) and (b) male gender (in part because of the increased prevalence of certain cardiac lesions in males, such as bicuspid aortic valves). The incidence rate ratio for those 65 years or older is almost 9 times that of those younger than 65 years, and the rate for males is 2.5 times that for females.

Pathogenesis of Bacterial Endocarditis

The following sequence of events is thought to result in endocarditis: the normal endothelium is nonthrombogenic, but when damaged, the endothelium is a potent inducer of blood coagulation. The turbulent blood flow produced by certain types of congenital or acquired heart disease, especially flow from a high- to a low-pressure chamber or across a narrowed orifice, traumatizes the downstream endothelium. Such blood flow creates a predisposition for the deposition of platelets and fibrin on the surface of the endothelium, the so-called nonbacterial thrombotic endocarditis lesion (NBTE). Episodes of bacteremia with microbial species capable of survival in the bloodstream, adherence to the NBTE, and proliferation at this site can then result in infective endocarditis.

RISK FACTORS FOR BACTEREMIA

Trauma to mucosal surfaces populated with a dense endogenous flora (including the gingival crevice, oropharynx, terminal ileum, colon, distal part of the urethra, and vagina) releases many different microbial species into the bloodstream. The intensity of the resulting bacteremia is directly related to the magnitude of the trauma, the density of the microbial flora, and the presence of inflammation or infection at the site of skin or mucosal injury. For example, spontaneous and procedure-induced bacteremia occurs more frequently in the presence of periodontal and periapical infection and is a likely consequence of the hyperemia and more abundant microflora in infected tissues surrounding the teeth. Optimal oral hygiene fostered by regular personal and professional care is therefore important in patients who are at risk for endocarditis.

The specific microbial species entering the circulation depend on the unique endogenous microflora colonizing the particular traumatized site. However, only a few bacterial species that gain access to the bloodstream in this manner—specifically, viridans streptococci, staphylococci, and enterococci—are commonly capable of causing endocarditis. Viridans streptococci and enterococci account for about 65% of cases of bacterial endocarditis.

Bacteremia caused by viridans and other oral streptococci occurs in 18% to 85% of dental extractions and periodontal procedures. Bacteremia caused by oral streptococci also follows esophageal dilation and sclerotherapy for esophageal varices. Enterococcal bacteremia occurs somewhat less frequently and follows genitourinary and gastrointestinal invasive procedures such as prostatic surgery, endoscopic retrograde cholangiopancreatography for biliary obstruction, biliary tract surgery, surgery on the lower intestinal mucosa, and urethral dilation.

A history of such procedures within the preceding 2 months has been found in 25% of patients with viridans streptococcal endocarditis and in 40% of those with enterococcal endocarditis. However, these procedures (particularly dental procedures) are common in the general population, which makes assessment of the risk of the procedure for the development of endocarditis difficult; the mere temporal association of a particularly common procedure, such as a dental procedure, with a rare disease such as endocarditis does not necessarily infer causation. Minor mucosal trauma as routine as bowel movements, brushing teeth, chewing hard candy, or other everyday experiences causes an asymptomatic bacteremia characterized by small numbers (usually <10 colony-forming units [CFU]/mL of blood) and very short duration (15 to 30 minutes). Although transient bacteremia is a common, everyday event and each event may be associated with only a very small risk for endocarditis, the cumulative risk of these transient episodes of low-grade bacteremia may be sufficient to account in large part for the 75% of patients with viridans streptococcal endocarditis or the 60% of patients with enterococcal endocarditis who fail to recall a medical or dental procedure that preceded the onset of their endocarditis. Indeed, transient bacteremia from everyday events may additionally be responsible for some cases of endocarditis in patients who give a history of a preceding procedure. One recent study of patients with endocarditis that used age- and sex-matched, population-based controls and sought to quantify the risk attributable to various procedures failed to demonstrate a relationship between recent dental procedures and endocarditis from oral organisms.

CARDIAC RISK FACTORS

Predisposing cardiac lesions are found in about three fourths of patients with infective endocarditis. Patients without a predisposing cardiac risk factor more likely have nosocomial endocarditis, have endocarditis caused by more virulent organisms such as *Staphylococcus aureus*, or are intravenous drug users.

The degree of risk for endocarditis in these cardiac lesions has commonly been inferred from the relative frequencies at which particular cardiac lesions occur in patients with endocarditis. However, inferring risk from these distributions can be problematic. Mitral valve prolapse (MVP) is now among the more frequent cardiac lesions found in patients with endocarditis. Various degenerative valvular lesions, cyanotic congenital heart disease, bicuspid aortic valves, rheumatic valvular heart disease, prosthetic cardiac valves, and previous endocarditis are other conditions that have been identified as cardiac risk factors for endocarditis (Table 1). However, because the relative frequency of various lesions in case series of endocarditis also reflects the prevalence of the particular cardiac abnormality in the general population, the lesions found more frequently in the population at large are also most likely to be common in case series of patients with endocarditis. The high prevalence of MVP in the general population, estimated to be between 2% and 21%, will lead to a greater representation in series of patients with endocarditis than will a rarer, but more risky cardiac abnormality such as valvular rheumatic heart disease.

TABLE 1 Cardiac Conditions Associated with Endocarditis

High Risk	Moderate Risk	Low Risk
Prosthetic valve	Valvular RHD	Nonvalvular RHD
Previous endocarditis	Other CHD	Secundum ASD
Cyanotic CHD	Marfan's syndrome	Surgery >6 mo ago, no residua of ASD, VSD, PDA
Surgical conduits or systemic/pulmonary shunts	Hypertrophic cardiomyopathy	
	MVP with regurgitation	Kawasaki disease
		Pacemakers, CABG
	MVP/thick leaflets	MVP/no regurgitation

Abbreviations: ASD = atrial septal defect; CABG = coronary artery bypass graft; CHD = congenital heart disease; MVP = mitral valve prolapse; PDA = patent ductus arteriosus; RHD = rheumatic heart disease; VSD = ventricular septal defect.

The true degree of the risk for endocarditis of a cardiac lesion can be determined only by measuring the incidence rate of endocarditis in those who have a particular cardiac abnormality. The highest incidence rates (300 to 740/100,000 patient-years) occur in persons with previous native valve endocarditis and prosthetic cardiac valves. For prosthetic valve endocarditis (PVE), the risk is greatest during the first few postoperative months as a result of intraoperative and perioperative contamination, and it probably does not vary by site of placement or type of prosthetic valve material. The incidence rate is approximately 400/100,000 patient-years for those with valvular rheumatic heart disease; 100 to 200/100,000 patient-years for individuals with uncorrected congenital lesions, especially those associated with cyanosis, including single-ventricle states, transposition of the great arteries, patent ductus arteriosus, ventricular septal defects, tetralogy of Fallot, and tricuspid or pulmonary stenosis or atresia; and 50/100,000 patient-years (only about tenfold higher than that of the general population) for patients who have MVP with murmur. Other lesions associated with endocarditis include Marfan's syndrome and hypertrophic cardiomyopathy.

Cardiac lesions that pose no greater risk than that of the general population include secundum atrial septal defects, atherosclerosis, previous coronary artery bypass graft surgery, MVP without murmur, previous rheumatic heart disease without valvular dysfunction, cardiac pacemakers and implanted defibrillators, and syphilitic aortitis.

Clinical Features

Symptoms usually begin within 2 weeks of the inciting bacteremia. In the preantibiotic era, when endocarditis was uniformly fatal, a short duration of illness of less than 6 weeks before death was typical for acute endocarditis; in contrast, subacute and chronic endocarditis had a more indolent course, with death occurring in 6 weeks to 2 years. Such a distinction based on chronicity has continued to prove useful in the antibiotic era. Chronicity is now used in reference to the duration of illness before diagnosis. Acute endocarditis is usually caused by *Staphylococcus aureus*, especially when accompanied by marked signs of general infection and suppurative embolic phenomena, and it has a rapidly fatal course if treatment is delayed. Acute infection may develop on a previously normal valve. Therefore, a diagnosis of acute endocarditis can serve as an effective guide to empirical antibiotic therapy, even before the results of blood culture are available. In contrast, subacute endocarditis, commonly caused by streptococci and enterococci, often develops on previously damaged endocardium, has less dramatic clinical manifestations of general infection, and is characterized by nonsuppurative peripheral vascular phenomena.

Clinical manifestations result from (a) the valvular infection itself, (b) embolization of fragments of the vegetation, (c) suppurative complications that result from hematogenous spread of infection, or (d) an immunologic response to the infection in the form of immune complex vasculitis. Systemic manifestations of endocarditis most commonly include fever and other symptoms that may accompany fever, such as drenching night sweats, arthralgia, myalgia, pain in the low back region and thighs, and weight loss. Fever is usually low grade, with temperature peaks rarely exceeding 39.4°C (103°F), but may be high and spiking in acute endocarditis. Fever may be absent in a few patients, such as those who are very elderly or severely debilitated, have significant renal or heart failure, or are taking antipyretics or antibiotics.

Cardiac manifestations include murmurs, valve ring abscess, myocardial infarction, myocardial abscess, and diffuse myocarditis. Murmurs of valvular insufficiency can be due to destruction or distortion of the valve and its supporting structures or, more rarely, valvular stenosis as a result of large vegetations. Murmurs are likely to be absent in tricuspid endocarditis or may be absent when a patient is first seen with acute endocarditis. PVE may result in regurgitant systolic or diastolic murmurs as a result of dehiscence of the valve at the annulus, the usual site in PVE, or muffling of the usual crisp prosthetic valve clicks. Valve ring abscesses may result from local extension of the infection from the valve ring of the noncoronary cusp of the aortic valve. A valve ring abscess can lead to (a) persistent fever despite appropriate antimicrobial therapy, (b) heart block as a result of the destruction of conduction pathways in the area of the atrioventricular node and bundle of His in the upper interventricular septum, (c) pericarditis or hemopericardium as a result of burrowing abscesses into the pericardium, or (d) shunts between cardiac chambers or between the heart and aorta as a consequence of burrowing abscesses into other cardiac chambers or the aorta. Myocardial infarction can result from coronary artery embolization, and myocardial abscess can occur as a consequence of bacteremia. Diffuse myocarditis is possibly due to immune complex vasculitis.

Congestive heart failure, the most common complication of endocarditis, develops in about 60% of patients as a consequence of valvular or myocardial involvement, or it may precede the onset of endocarditis and be caused by the underlying cardiac lesion. Congestive heart failure may develop dramatically in patients with acute *S. aureus* endocarditis with the sudden onset of an aortic diastolic murmur or rupture of the mitral valve chordae. It occurs more frequently with left-sided than right-sided endocarditis and more often with aortic involvement than mitral involvement.

Extracardiac manifestations include (a) embolic events that result in infarction of numerous organs, such as the lung in right-sided endocarditis or the brain, spleen, or kidneys in left-sided endocarditis; (b) suppurative complications, such as abscesses, septic infarcts, and mycotic aneurysms; and (c) immunologic reactions to the valvular infection, including glomerulonephritis, sterile meningitis or polyarthritis, and a variety of vascular phenomena such as mucocutaneous petechiae, splinter hemorrhages, Roth's spots, and Osler's nodes. The development of clinically apparent splenomegaly and many of the various nonsuppurative peripheral vascular phenomena is related to the duration of illness before diagnosis. The frequency of these clinical manifestations (<50%) is currently less than in the past because of an earlier diagnosis and a consequent shorter duration of illness before initiation of antimicrobial therapy.

Systemic embolization, often a devastating complication when the cerebral circulation is involved, occurs in about 20% to 40% of patients with left-sided endocarditis. Embolization is more frequent with *S. aureus* and fungal endocarditis, vegetations of the anterior leaflet of the mitral valve, and vegetations larger than 1 cm in diameter. Frank cerebral abscess is rare but occurs in 1% to 5% of patients with *S. aureus* endocarditis. Septic pulmonary emboli that appear as multiple round infiltrates commonly occur in patients with tricuspid valve *S. aureus* endocarditis and may cavitate or be complicated by empyema. The frequency of embolization decreases dramatically during the first 2 weeks of antimicrobial therapy as the vegetation heals.

Mycotic aneurysms are an unusual but important complication of endocarditis. Mycotic aneurysms are commonly asymptomatic but can become clinically evident in 3% to 5% of patients, even months or years after completion of successful therapy. These aneurysms characteristically develop at arterial bifurcations, such as in the middle cerebral, splenic, superior mesenteric, pulmonary, coronary, and extremity arteries, the abdominal aorta, and the sinus of Valsalva. In a patient with endocarditis, unremitting headache, visual disturbance, cranial nerve palsy, meningeal signs, or a focal neurologic deficit is suggestive of impending rupture of a cerebral mycotic aneurysm. Signs of blood loss at any site in a patient with endocarditis should suggest rupture of a mycotic aneurysm.

NOSOCOMIAL ENDOCARDITIS

Nosocomial endocarditis, defined as endocarditis following a hospital-based procedure performed within 4 weeks before the onset of symptoms, accounts for 10% to 30% of cases of endocarditis. The clinical features of nosocomial endocarditis are similar to those of community-acquired endocarditis. The source of the bacteremia can be identified in more than 90% of cases of nosocomial endocarditis. The most important bacteremia-inducing event during hospitalization that results in endocarditis is the use of an intravascular device, which is present in up to 50% of cases. *S. aureus* bacteremia is much more frequently complicated by endocarditis (10% to 30% of the time) than nosocomial enterococcal bacteremia is (<1%).

A major predisposing cardiac lesion for nosocomial endocarditis is a prosthetic cardiac valve. Although blood cultures are usually positive, the diagnosis of endocarditis is frequently delayed because of failure to recognize the presence of endocardial infection, which frequently is evident only on transesophageal echocardiography (TEE).

Echocardiography

Echocardiography has become second only to culture of blood in the investigation of patients who are clinically suspected of having endocarditis. Echocardiography can visualize valvular vegetations, satellite vegetations, flail valves, ruptured chordae, perivalvular abscesses, fistulas, valvular perforations, and mycotic aneurysms. Echocardiography is also relied on to identify predisposing cardiac lesions and the causes and severity of congestive heart failure by assessment of ventricular size, wall motion, and dynamic function. Two-dimensional transthoracic echocardiography (TTE) and TEE, the two types of echocardiography currently in use, are safe and may be performed at the bedside. TTE is rapid, noninvasive, and relatively inexpensive. TEE is invasive, requires sedation, and is slightly more expensive. TTE can give more general information regarding cardiac structure and function that cannot be obtained with TEE; however, TEE is frequently helpful in situations where TTE is not, such as in the presence of obesity, emphysema, and prosthetic cardiac valves, which may obscure the TTE image. Hemodynamic complications such as central or perivalvular regurgitant flow in the presence of a prosthetic valve can easily be detected and semiquantitated by the addition of color-flow Doppler. The sensitivity of TEE is greater (90% to 100%) than that of TTE (<80%), and vegetations as small as 1 mm can be detected. TEE also has a specificity (i.e., true-negative rate), positive predictive accuracy (the probability of endocarditis when the echocardiogram is positive), and a negative predicative accuracy (the probability of no endocarditis when the echocardiogram is negative) of 95% to 100%. However, the frequency of a falsely positive finding of vegetations, such as nonspecific valvular thickening or rupture of a valve leaflet or the mitral valve chordae, which can simulate a vegetation in patients likely to be studied by echocardiography, though very low, may be greater than the frequency of endocarditis in low-risk populations. Therefore, echocardiography should be performed only for the diagnosis of endocarditis in patients in whom such a diagnosis is likely on clinical grounds. The use of TEE as the initial diagnostic test is recommended in patients with at least "possible endocarditis" according to clinical criteria (see Duke criteria, Table 2), in patients with suspected complicated infective endocarditis (e.g., valve ring abscess), and in those with suspected PVE.

TABLE 2 Modified (Duke) Criteria for the Diagnosis of Infective Endocarditis

1. Definite diagnosis of infective endocarditis
   A. Pathologic criteria
      a. Microorganisms demonstrated by culture or histologic examination of vegetations, vegetations that have embolized, or an intracardiac abscess specimen, or
      b. Pathologic lesions: vegetations, or intracardiac abscess confirmed by histologic examination showing active endocarditis
   B. Clinical criteria
      a. 2 major criteria *or*
      b. 1 major/3 minor *or*
      c. 5 minor
2. Possible diagnosis
   a. 1 major and 1 minor criterion *or*
   b. 3 minor
3. No endocarditis
   a. Firm alternative diagnosis
   b. Clinical resolution after ≤4 d of antimicrobial therapy, or
   c. No pathologic evidence of infective endocarditis at surgery or autopsy with ≤4 d of antimicrobial therapy

or

   d. Does not meet criteria for possible infective endocarditis, as above

Major Criteria

1. Blood Culture
   a. 2 separate blood cultures positive for
      i. Viridans streptococci, *Streptococcus bovis*, HACEK, *Staphylococcus aureus*, or
      ii. Community-acquired enterococci in the absence of a primary focus
   b. Microorganisms consistent with endocarditis isolated from
      i. at least 2 blood cultures drawn >12 h apart, or
      ii. all of 3 blood cultures or a majority of 4 or more separate blood cultures with 1st and last ≥1 h apart
   c. Single positive blood culture for *Coxiella brunetti* or antiphase 1 IgG antibody titer>1:800
2. Endocardial involvement
   a. Echocardiography: oscillating intracardiac mass on a valve or supporting structure, in the path of a regurgitant jet stream, or on implanted material in the absence of an alternative anatomic explanation, valve ring abscess, or new partial dehiscence of a prosthetic valve
   b. New regurgitant murmur (increasing or changing pre-existing murmur not sufficient)

Minor Criteria

1. Predisposing heart condition or intravenous drug use
2. Fever, temperature >38°C (100.4°F)
3. Major arterial emboli, septic pulmonary infarcts, mycotic aneurysm, intracranial hemorrhage, conjunctival hemorrhage, and Janeway's lesions
4. Immunologic phenomena: glomerulonephritis, Roth's spot, Osler's node, and rheumatoid factor
5. Positive blood culture, but does not meet major criterion, (excludes single positive culture for coagulase-negative staphylococcus and organisms that do not cause endocarditis) or serologic evidence of active infection by organism consistent with infective endocarditis

Modified from Li JS, Sexton DJ, Mick N, et al: Proposed modification to the Duke criteria for the diagnosis of infective endocarditis. Clin Infect Dis 30:633–638, 2000.

Sequential echocardiography during the course of antimicrobial therapy is used to assess healing of vegetations, detect the development or progression of complications, and guide decisions regarding the necessity and timing of surgery. The finding of early closure of the mitral valve as a consequence of elevated left ventricular end-diastolic pressure in association with acute aortic valve endocarditis has been used to predict the need for surgery, and detection of a vegetation, especially a large one (i.e., >10 mm in largest dimension), has been found to signify a poorer outcome, such as a greater likelihood of embolization, congestive heart failure, the need for surgery, and death. However, for assessment of the need for surgical intervention, echocardiographic results must be viewed in light of the specific clinical situation, especially the patient's hemodynamic status, previous embolic events, and the type of pathogen involved, such as antibiotic-resistant gram-negative bacilli or fungi.

OTHER INVESTIGATIVE PROCEDURES

Cardiac catheterization can provide important information and should not be avoided when indicated in selected patients with endocarditis for fear of dislodging emboli. Coronary angiography is used to assess the presence of significant coronary artery disease before elective placement of prosthetic cardiac valves in patients who are older than age 40 years and have additional atherogenic risk factors. Contrast-enhanced computed tomography (CT) or magnetic resonance imaging (MRI) can best evaluate abscesses or infarcts of the intra-abdominal organs (spleen or liver). Contrast-enhanced CT or MRI of the head may provide evidence of a bleeding mycotic aneurysm. Magnetic resonance angiography for the detection of intracranial aneurysms is promising, but four-vessel cerebral angiography is the standard for detection of aneurysms smaller than 5 mm.

Electrocardiographic Manifestations

A baseline electrocardiogram (ECG) should be obtained to assess the presence of conduction abnormalities, which develop in about 10% to 20% of patients with endocarditis as a consequence of burrowing valve ring abscesses. Prolongation of the PR interval may be the initial indication of the sudden development of more severe conduction abnormalities, such as complete heart block. Other abnormalities that can be detected by ECG include myocardial infarction and pericarditis.

Hematologic Manifestations

Progressive anemia of chronic disease with normochromic, normocytic indices routinely develops in patients with subacute endocarditis, and normal platelet, white blood cell, and differential counts. In acute endocarditis caused by *S. aureus*, anemia may be initially absent, although the white blood cell count is usually elevated with a shift to the left and the platelet count is often low. PVE with an unstable prosthesis may cause acute hemolysis. The erythrocyte sedimentation rate is routinely elevated in endocarditis, except in those with hypofibrinogenemia secondary to disseminated intravascular coagulation or congestive heart failure.

Renal Manifestations

Proteinuria and microscopic hematuria are common findings that occur in up to 50% of patients. Renal emboli or focal glomerulonephritis can cause microscopic hematuria, but gross hematuria usually indicates renal infarction. Renal failure that develops in a patient with endocarditis is usually due to diffuse immune complex glomerulonephritis.

Other Laboratory Manifestations

Serologic evidence of circulating immune complexes, as detected by Raji cell radioimmunoassay, may be found in patients with endocarditis, the frequency of which is related to the duration of illness. Occasional false-positive nontreponemal serologic tests for syphilis occur. Cerebrospinal fluid may show polymorphonuclear leukocytes and a moderately elevated protein concentration in up to 15% of patients, but a normal glucose value. Frank bacterial meningitis, though unusual, occurs in *S. aureus* endocarditis.

Diagnosis

Definitive diagnosis of infective endocarditis depends on microbiologic or pathologic proof of infection by histology or culture of vegetations obtained at the time of surgery or autopsy or by histology or culture of vegetations obtained at the time of surgical removal of an arterial embolus. In lieu of surgery or autopsy, a definitive diagnosis can be established by demonstration of (a) a characteristic vegetation, valve ring abscess, or new prosthetic valve dehiscence with echocardiography and (b) intravascular infection with multiple separate blood cultures obtained over a period of time that are positive for a microorganism consistent with endocarditis. However, blood culture or echocardiography is usually performed only after the diagnosis is suspected on the basis of the history and physical findings. Because the clinical manifestations are numerous and no single clinical finding is pathognomonic of endocarditis, a constellation of signs and symptoms, in addition to the presence of certain risk factors, has been suggested as a set of diagnostic criteria for general clinical use. Risk factors include the presence of a prosthetic cardiac valve or other predisposing cardiac conditions and intravenous drug use. The diagnosis can be ranked in order of the probability that endocarditis is present by distinguishing between major and minor criteria, which allows for weighting of clinical, microbiologic, and echocardiographic findings, as has been done by the Duke endocarditis group (see Table 2).

MICROBIOLOGIC INVESTIGATION

Isolation of a pathogen from several blood cultures obtained over an extended period is important both to confirm the diagnosis of endocarditis and to enable determination of the optimal antibiotic regimen. Bacteremia in endocarditis is characterized by a constant number of organisms per milliliter of blood (usually 20 to 200 CFU/mL), unrelated to the height of the patient's temperature or the site of blood sampling (e.g., arterial versus venous blood), except for a slight fall in numbers across the hepatic or splenic circulation. Less than 5% of patients with endocarditis have sterile blood cultures if adequate culture methods are used. The proper method of obtaining blood for culture includes (a) disinfection of the skin with 70% isopropyl alcohol and then 2% iodine or iodophor solution, with the disinfectant allowed to remain on the skin for at least one minute, and (b) withdrawal of 10 mL to 20 mL of blood per blood culture in an adult through the least contaminated site, preferably an antecubital vein rather than, for example, the femoral vein. Three blood cultures should be obtained in this manner at least one hour apart to demonstrate that the bacteremia is continuous. The clinical microbiology laboratory should be advised of the suspected diagnosis of endocarditis because some organisms require special media or more prolonged incubation (up to 3 weeks) for detection. In the absence of previous antibiotic therapy, the first three blood cultures are expected to be positive in over 95% of patients. Previous antibiotic therapy and infection with fastidious bacteria (such as *Abiotrophia* species, the HACEK [*Haemophilus spp., Actinobacillus actinomycetemcomitans, Cardiobacterium hominis, Eikenella corrodens*, and *Kingella kingae*] group of organisms, *Neisseria, Brucella, Legionella*, and fungi, *Bartonella, Tropheryma, Chlamydia, Coxiella*, and *Rickettsia*) and fungi can result in negative cultures. Gram stain of the blood cultures may identify some pathogens that may not otherwise be apparent. Abiotrophia species require subculture on pyridoxal- or L-cysteine–enriched agar or on plates streaked with *S. aureus*. Serology may be required for *Bartonella, Brucella, Chlamydia, Mycoplasma, Legionella*, and *Coxiella* (although antibodies for *Bartonella* and *Chlamydia* are often cross-reactive); polymerase chain reaction on cardiac valvular tissue for *Bartonella, Tropheryma*, and *Coxiella*; special stains or fluorescent antibody staining on tissue for *Bartonella, Tropheryma, Legionella, Coxiella, Chlamydia*, and fungi; and special media or the lysis centrifugation system for *Bartonella, Legionella, Brucella*, and fungi. Fungal endocarditis, which is likely to have negative blood cultures, tends to be complicated by large vegetations and embolization, in which case the organisms can be identified by Gram stain and culture of the surgically removed emboli.

In acute endocarditis, for which empirical antibiotic therapy should be initiated as soon as possible, two to three blood samples should be drawn 1 hour apart for culture before initiation of empirical therapy. In the face of a preceding course of antibiotic therapy, further antibiotic treatment should be withheld and blood cultures repeated until positive if clinical conditions permit. The longer the duration since the last dose of antibiotic or the shorter the preceding course of the antibiotic, the more likely that the blood culture will be positive. Bacteriuria with either enterococci or *S. aureus* occurs in endocarditis caused by the respective organism.

A variety of in vitro tests must be performed on the pathogen isolated from blood to assess its susceptibility to potential bactericidal drugs (Table 3). Enterococci are routinely tested for β-lactamase production (which predicts resistance to penicillin and ampicillin) and for high-level gentamicin and streptomycin resistance (which predicts lack of synergy with a combination of the respective aminoglycoside and a cell wall-active drug such as vancomycin, penicillin, or ampicillin), in addition to susceptibility to penicillin and vancomycin. Synergism between cell-wall–active antibiotics and aminoglycosides has been demonstrated for other microorganisms, including viridans streptococci, staphylococci, *Pseudomonas aeruginosa*, and aerobic enteric gram-negative bacilli, and its presence can be assessed by a special in vitro test, the so-called time-kill assay.

For nonstandard regimens or unusual pathogens, peak serum bactericidal activity may be assayed against the patient's pathogen early in the course of therapy, and if inadequate, the dose of antibiotic is increased (though not at the cost of toxicity) and the serum retested. Measurement of vancomycin or aminoglycoside serum levels is helpful to ensure adequate but nontoxic antibiotic levels.

Organisms should be retained in the laboratory for susceptibility testing of additional antibiotics if the need arises, and organisms obtained at surgery or relapse should be retested for antimicrobial susceptibility.

DIAGNOSTIC STRATEGIES IN SPECIAL SITUATIONS

Intravenous Drug Users

Because outpatient follow-up in this population is rarely possible, admission of febrile intravenous drug users without a clinically apparent source for their fever is indicated for at least one week until the results of blood culture are available. Blood cultures will usually become positive within 1 week if fungi, fastidious gram-negative bacilli or streptococci, or anaerobes are involved or the patient has recently taken antibiotics. After obtaining blood for culture, empirical antimicrobial therapy should be initiated. Once the blood cultures are found to be positive, evidence of endocarditis should be sought initially by

TABLE 3 In Vitro Assays

Organism	Test	Result
Viridans streptococci	Broth dilution test	Penicillin MIC
Enterococci	Broth dilution test	Penicillin MIC Vancomycin (Vancocin) MIC
	Growth in	High-level resistance*
	500 μg/mL of gentamicin	Gentamicin (Garamycin)
	1000 μg/mL of streptomycin	Streptomycin
	Nitrocefin degradation	β-Lactamase production
Staphylococcus aureus, coagulase-negative staphylococci	Nitrocefin degradation	β-Lactamase production
	Oxacillin/methicillin sensitivity	MRSA/MRSE
	Broth dilution test	Vancomycin MIC Rifampin (Rimactane) MIC TMP/SMX (Bactrim) MIC
Other pathogens	Broth dilution tests	Antibiotic MIC/MBC† Time-kill studies†
All pathogens	Serum antibiotic concentrations	Peak and trough vancomycin‡ and aminoglycoside§ concentrations

*The choice of an aminoglycoside should be based on in vitro high-level aminoglycoside susceptibility testing. If the strain is susceptible to high levels of gentamicin, gentamicin is preferred because determination of gentamicin serum levels is more generally available.
†May be useful for nonstandard antimicrobial regimens or unusual pathogens.
‡Vancomycin peak serum levels obtained 1 hour after completion of a 1- to 2-hour infusion should be in the range of 30 to 45 μg/mL. Vancomycin trough levels obtained just before the next dose should be 10 to 15 μg/mL.
§Gentamicin peak serum levels obtained 1 hour after the start of a 20- to 30-minute IV infusion or IM injection of 1 mg/kg should be about 3 μg/mL, and the trough level should be less than 1 μg/mL. The streptomycin peak serum level 1 hour after IM administration of 15 mg/kg is about 15 to 20 μg/mL, and the trough should be about 5 μg/mL.
Abbreviations: MBC = minimal bactericidal concentration; MIC = minimal inhibitory concentration; MRSA = methicillin-resistant *S. aureus*; MRSE = methicillin-resistant coagulase-negative staphylococci; TMP/SMX = trimethoprim-sulfamethoxazole.
From Levison ME: In vitro assays. In Kaye D (ed): Infective Endocarditis, 2nd ed. New York, Raven, 1992, pp 151–167.

TTE and, if negative, by TEE. Even if the patient has another potential source for the bacteremia and no echocardiographic or clinical evidence of endocarditis, but the organism isolated is likely to be a cause of endocarditis, such as *S. aureus*, the diagnosis of endocarditis should nevertheless be suspected. If no apparent source for the bacteremia can be found, the patient should still be considered to possibly have endocarditis even if echocardiographic and clinical evidence is lacking. In patients with negative echocardiographic results, if the clinical course dictates and another diagnosis is still not apparent, TEE should be repeated in about 1 week. If blood cultures remain negative after 1 week of incubation, the patient may be discharged from the hospital without echocardiography, unless clinical evidence of left-sided or right-sided endocarditis is detected, in which case the diagnosis of endocarditis should nevertheless be suspected.

Nosocomial Native Valve Endocarditis

In patients with bacteremia related to intravascular devices, such as an arteriovenous graft for hemodialysis, indwelling central intravenous catheter, cardiac assist balloon pump, or pacemaker wire, removal of the intravascular device is usually required, especially with *S. aureus* or fungi or if a tunnel or exit site infection is present. In patients with *S. aureus* bacteremia, echocardiography should be performed to detect vegetations and to assess for complications of valve infection because of the high frequency of endocarditis in these patients. Catheter-associated, coagulase-negative staphylococcal nosocomial bacteremia, which rarely eventuates in native valve endocarditis, should not be investigated with echocardiography after the initiation of antibiotic therapy unless the patient has a prosthetic cardiac valve. Indeed, catheter removal may not be necessary to cure coagulase-negative, staphylococcal catheter-associated bacteremia. The necessity of echocardiography to detect occult native valve endocarditis after catheter removal and initiation of antibiotic therapy for nosocomial fungemia or enterococcal bacteremia is unresolved.

Prosthetic Valve Endocarditis

The diagnosis of PVE is usually suspected because of fever and confirmed by the presence of multiple blood cultures positive for the same microorganism. In a recent study, 43% of patients with a prosthetic valve in whom fever and bacteremia developed had PVE, or it developed later. Any organism in blood cultures in these patients must be taken seriously as a potential cause of endocarditis, including streptococci, enterococci, staphylococci, enteric gram-negative bacilli, atypical mycobacteria, and fungi, regardless of whether a portal of entry can be identified (such as an intravascular device, undrained abscess, wound infection, or genitourologic or gastrointestinal disease or procedure). In those with clinical evidence suggestive of PVE, empirical antibiotic therapy can be initiated after three to four sets of blood cultures are obtained. After antimicrobial therapy is started, blood cultures should be repeated to assess for clearance of bacteremia. The source of the bacteremia should be sought and eliminated (e.g., drainage of abscesses or removal of intravascular devices). Echocardiographic evidence of endocarditis, such as valvular vegetations, new prosthetic valve dysfunction, and perivalvular infection, should be sought by TEE. New conduction abnormalities, which can occur as a result of perivalvular extension of infection, should be sought by ECG. Serial ECG and echocardiograms should be obtained if initially unrevealing. An annular location and perivalvular extension of the infection are likely when the aortic valve is involved and when infection develops within the first 12 months after surgery.

Antibiotic Therapy

PRINCIPLES

Effective antimicrobial therapy for endocarditis optimally requires identification of the specific pathogen and assessment of its susceptibility to various antimicrobial agents. Therefore, every effort must be made to isolate the pathogen before initiation of antimicrobial therapy, if clinically feasible. In patients who are in immediate danger of death, empirical antibiotic therapy should be started as soon as possible after obtaining blood cultures. Empirical therapy should be targeted at the most likely pathogens in that particular clinical setting. Specific antimicrobial therapy that is anticipated to be the most effective and least toxic, inconvenient, and costly is instituted once the results of antimicrobial susceptibility testing of the isolated pathogen become available. Minimal requirements for an effective antimicrobial regimen include the following:

Bactericidal Activity

Bacteriostatic agents are not able to clear pathogens from infected tissues unaided by host defenses, such as polymorphonuclear leukocytes, antibody, and complement. Because host defenses are not thought to operate within vegetations (except in tricuspid valve vegetations, where polymorphonuclear leukocytes may aid the effect of an antimicrobial agent), clearance of bacteria from these vegetations requires a bactericidal antibiotic. In fact, complete eradication of pathogens from the vegetation is thought to be essential to cure endocarditis. If any bacteria remain after completion of antibiotic therapy, the residual organisms will multiply and cause a relapse. If the pathogen cannot be eliminated completely by antimicrobial therapy, the infected vegetation may need to be excised surgically to effect a cure. For microorganisms without predictable susceptibility, the bactericidal activity of an antimicrobial agent for the particular patient's pathogen must be assessed by determination of the minimal inhibitory (MIC) and minimal bactericidal (MBC) concentrations of the antimicrobial agents in vitro (see Table 3).

High Concentrations of the Antimicrobial Agent in the Vegetation

Optimally, the antimicrobial agent should have a minimal "inoculum effect"; specifically, it should exhibit the least reduction in potency when tested against microbial inocula, such as the microbial densities of 10^8 to 10^{10} CFU/g that exist in vegetations, which are higher than the standard inocula of 10^5 to 10^6 CFU/mL used to perform the MIC and MBC tests. If the inoculum effect is considerable, such as a rise in MIC and MBC at high inocula, as is usually seen with β-lactam antibiotics, the doses of the antimicrobial agent must be adjusted to compensate for the reduction in potency that would be anticipated in vivo in the vegetation. Doses of the antimicrobial agent must also be large enough to achieve concentrations of the antimicrobial agent in blood to facilitate passive diffusion of the agent into the depths of the vegetation where the microcolonies of the pathogen are located. Dosing that is sufficiently large to attain bactericidal activity against the patient's pathogen in a greater than 1:8 dilution of the patient's serum at the peak time after administration of the antimicrobial agent has traditionally guided therapy (although more recent data suggest that dilutions >1:64 have more predictive accuracy for bacteriologic cure). Serum bactericidal activity can be quantitated by the in vitro serum bactericidal test. However, the methodology of the test in general has not been well standardized, and scant clinical data are available to validate this recommendation. Despite high concentrations in blood, some antimicrobial agents fail to penetrate vegetations deeply enough (e.g., amphotericin B), or they penetrate vegetations unevenly (e.g., teicoplanin). Although amphotericin B is a fungicidal agent, cure of fungal endocarditis usually requires valve surgery.

Prolonged Duration of Antimicrobial Therapy

More than 90% of the microbial population in the vegetation are nongrowing and metabolically inactive once the infection has become well established. Nongrowing organisms are more likely to be found in the central portions of the microcolonies in the deeper regions of the vegetation. Because bactericidal drugs such as the β-lactam are active only against growing microorganisms, each dose is able to effect a reduction in microbial count in only that minor portion (less than 10%) of the population that happens to be growing at the time of drug administration. The duration of drug therapy must therefore be prolonged to result in complete clearance of the pathogen from the vegetation.

The duration of therapy varies with the specific pathogen, the site of the infection, and the type of antibiotic. For example, bacterial clearance is more rapid for viridans streptococci than for staphylococci, in tricuspid than in aortic vegetations, with antistaphylococcal β-lactams than with vancomycin, and with combinations of a cell wall-active agent plus an aminoglycoside than with a single drug. More rapid clearance in these special circumstances may permit a shorter course of therapy to achieve cure.

The duration of antimicrobial therapy after valve replacement depends to some extent on evidence of active infection at the time of surgery. In patients with positive intraoperative cultures or Gram stain, a full course of postoperative therapy is reasonable; otherwise, an additional 2 weeks plus the time remaining on the regimen is routinely recommended for that type of endocarditis.

Dosing Should Be Frequent Enough to Prevent Regrowth of Microorganisms Between Doses

The organisms that remain after brief in vitro exposure to an aminoglycoside or a β-lactam antibiotic frequently exhibit a postexposure delay in further growth in vitro, the so-called postantibiotic effect. Unfortunately, no such effect occurs with enterococci or *P. aeruginosa* in the rat model of endocarditis despite a postantibiotic effect in vitro. Thus, even though a bactericidal effect can be achieved in the vegetation in the early portions of a dosing interval when levels of the drug are high, if antibiotic levels are not maintained in the vegetation at least above the MIC during the rest of the dosing interval, regrowth of residual organisms may occur and efficacy may be compromised.

Standardized regimens have been recommended for the most common pathogens on native and prosthetic valves-viridans streptococci, enterococci, staphylococci, and HACEK organisms (Table 4). Staphylococci that are sensitive to methicillin or oxacillin can be treated with an antistaphylococcal β-lactam such as nafcillin or cefazolin, or vancomycin; a β-lactam is always preferable over vancomycin because of the relatively slow bactericidal action of vancomycin. Ceftriaxone has relatively poor

TABLE 4 Standard Antibiotic Therapy for Infective Endocarditis Caused by Common Pathogens (Doses are for Adults with Normal Renal Function)

A. Penicillin-susceptible viridans streptococci and *Streptococcus bovis* (MIC equal to or less than 0.12 μg/mL)
  1. Aqueous penicillin G, 18 million U daily IV continuously or in 4 or 6 equally divided doses, or ceftriaxone (Rocephin), 2 g IV or IM q24h, or vancomycin (Vancocin), 15 mg/kg IV q12h for 4 wk (Vancomycin is recommended only for patients unable to tolerate penicillin or ceftriaxone (e.g., for patients with immediate-type allergic reactions to penicillin; i.e., urticaria, angioedema, or anaphylaxis). The dosage of vancomycin is adjusted to obtain a peak level in serum 1 h after completion of a 1 h IV infusion of 30-45 μg/mL and a trough concentration of 10-15 μg/mL. These regimens are preferred in patients more than 65 y old and those with 8th cranial nerve or renal impairment
  2. Aqueous penicillin, 18 million U daily IV continuously or in 4 or 6 equally divided doses, or ceftriaxone, 2 g IV or IM q24h, plus gentamicin, 3 mg/kg IV* or IM q24h (administered at the time of ceftriaxone) for 2 wk. (The 2-week regimen is appropriate for uncomplicated cases of endocarditis in patients at low risk for adverse events from aminoglycosides. For prosthetic valve endocarditis: aqueous penicillin G, 24 MU daily IV continuously or in 4 or 6 equally divided doses or ceftriaxone, 2 g IV or IM q24h for 6 wk with or without gentamicin, 3 mg/mg IV or IM once daily for the first 2 weeks, or vancomycin alone, 15 mg/kg IV q12h for 6 wk. Gentamicin should not be given to patients with creatinine clearance <30 mL/min.

B. Relatively penicillin-resistant viridans streptococci, and *S. bovis* (MIC >0.12 – less than or equal to 0.5 μg/mL)
  1. Aqueous penicillin, 24 MU daily IV either continuously or in 4 or 6 equally divided doses, or ceftriaxone, 2 g IV or IM q24h for 4 wk, plus gentamicin, 3 mg/kg IV or IM q 24h for the first 2 wk.
  2. Vancomycin, 15 mg/kg IV q12h (Vancomycin is recommended only for patients unable to tolerate penicillin or ceftriaxone (e.g., patients with immediate-type allergic reactions to penicillin; i.e., urticaria, angioedema, or anaphylaxis). Vancomycin use may enhance the nephrotoxicity of gentamicin. When vancomycin is chosen, the addition of gentamicin is not recommended. For prosthetic valve endocarditis: aqueous penicillin G, 24 MU daily IV continuously or in 4 or 6 equally divided doses or ceftriaxone, 2 g IV or IM q24h with gentamicin, 2 mg/kg IV or IM once daily for 6 weeks, or vancomycin alone, 15/mg/kg IV q12h for 6 wk.

C. Penicillin-resistant viridans streptococci and *S. bovis* (MIC >0.5 μg/mL), enterococci susceptible to penicillin, vancomycin and aminoglycoside, and *Abiotrophia*[†] (nutritionally variant streptococci)
  1. Aqueous penicillin, 24 MU daily IV either continuously or in 4 or 6 equally divided doses or ampicillin, 2 g IV q4h plus gentamicin, 1 mg/kg IV or IM q8h (or streptomycin, 7.5 mg/kg IM q12h[‡]) for 4-6 wk (The 4-week regimen is recommended for patients with symptoms of illness less than 3 months in duration, and the 6-week regimen is recommended for patients with symptoms more than 3 months in duration).
  2. Vancomycin, 15 mg/kg IV q12h, plus gentamicin, 1 mg/kg IV or IM q8h (or streptomycin, 7.5 mg/kg IM q12h[‡]) for 6 wk (For patients with immediate-type allergic reactions to penicillin, i.e., urticaria, angioedema, or anaphylaxis). For prosthetic valve endocarditis due to steptococci with MIC >0.5 μg/mL: aqueous penicillin G, 24 MU daily IV continuously or in 4 or 6 equally divided doses or ceftriaxone, 2 g IV or IM q24h with gentamicin, 3 mg/kg IV or IM once daily for 6 weeks, or vancomycin alone, 15/mg/kg IV q12h for 6 weeks. For prosthetic valve endocarditis caused by enterococci susceptible to penicillin, aminoglycoside and vancomycin and *Abiotrophia* species: aqueous penicillin G, 24 MU daily IV continuously or in 4 or 6 equally divided doses or ampicillin, 2 g IV or IM q4h, or vancomycin, 15/mg/kg IV q12h, each with gentamicin, 3 mg/kg IV or IM daily in 3 equally divided doses for at least 6 weeks.[§]

TABLE 4 Standard Antibiotic Therapy for Infective Endocarditis Caused by Common Pathogens (Doses are for Adults with Normal Renal Function)—cont'd

D. Methicillin/gentamicin-susceptible staphylococci—uncomplicated right-sided disease, native valve only
Nafcillin (Unipen), 2 g q4h IV, with gentamicin, 1 mg/kg q8h IV/IM for 2 wk (Vancomycin is less rapidly bactericidal than antistaphylococcal β-lactam antibiotics, as reflected by slower clearance of staphylococci from vegetations and blood. Consequently, vancomycin is not effective in the short-course [2-wk] regimen and should not be used in other antistaphylococcal regimens unless the organism is methicillin resistant or the patient has an immediate-type penicillin allergy that precludes use of β-lactam antibiotic.)

E. Methicillin-susceptible staphylococci—native valve complicated right-sided or left-sided Nafcillin, 2 g q4h or cefazolin (Ancef), 2 g q8h IV, for 4-6 wk, or vancomycin, 15 mg/kg q12h IV for 6 wk, with or without gentamicin, 1 mg/kg q8h IV/IM for the first 3-5d only. (The additional benefit of an aminoglycoside has not been clearly established. Use gentamicin only if the isolate is gentamicin susceptible. Cefazolin [Kefzol] or vancomycin should be used in penicillin-allergic patients. Cefazolin should be avoided in those with immediate-type penicillin hypersensitivity.)

F. Methicillin-resistant staphylococci—native valve
Vancomycin, 15 mg/kg q12h for 6 wk

G. Methicillin-resistant staphylococci—prosthetic valve
Vancomycin, 15 mg/kg q12h, plus rifampin (Rifadin)[1] 300 mg q8h for 6 wk or longer, plus gentamicin, 1 mg/kg q8h IV/IM for the first 2 wk (Rifampin should be added in cases of rifampin-susceptible, staphylococcal PVE; combination therapy is essential to prevent the emergence of rifampin resistance. If the isolate is gentamicin resistant, use another aminoglycoside to which the isolate is sensitive. If resistant to all aminoglycosides, substitute a fluoroquinolone to which the isolate is sensitive.)

H. Methicillin-susceptible staphylococci—prosthetic valve
Nafcillin or oxacillin, 2 g q4h IV plus rifampin[1], 300 mg for q8h for 6 wk or longer, plus gentamicin, 1 mg/kg q8h IV/IM for the first 2 wk (Rifampin should be added in cases of rifampin-susceptible, staphylococcal PVE; combination therapy is essential to prevent the emergence of rifampin resistance. If gentamicin resistant, an alternative third agent should be added after in vitro susceptibility testing results are known. Cefazolin or vancomycin should be used in penicillin-allergic patients. Cefazolin should be avoided in those with immediate-type penicillin hypersensitivity.)

I. HACEK organisms
Ceftriaxone[1], 2 g IV q24h for 4 wk or ciprofloxacin 750 mg po or 400 mg IV q12h for 4 weeks in patients unable to tolerate cephalosporin therapy.

[1]Not FDA approved for this indication.
*Exceeds dosage recommended by the manufacturer.
†Because of technical difficulties in susceptibility testing of *Abiotrophia* species, many experts recommend treating infection by these strains with the standard regimen recommended for enterococci. Six weeks of therapy is recommended for patients with enterococcal endocarditis who have had more than 3 months of symptoms before therapy. Six to 8 weeks of therapy is recommended for prosthetic valve endocarditis. Cephalosporins are not acceptable alternatives for treatment of enterococcal endocarditis.
‡The choice of aminoglycoside for treatment of enterococcal endocarditis is based upon in vitro susceptibility to high levels of gentamicin and streptomycin. If the strain is susceptible to both aminoglycosides, gentamicin is preferred because of the availability of assays for the determination of gentamicin serum concentrations in most laboratories, unlike that of streptomycin.
§If gentamicin is administered in three equally divided doses per day, adjust dose to achieve peak and trough serum levels of ~3 μg/mL and <1 μg/mL, respectively. The dose of streptomycin administered q12h is adjusted to achieve peak and trough serum levels of ~20 μg/mL and <5 μg/mL, respectively.
Abbreviations: PVE = prosthetic valve endocarditis; VRE = vancomycin-resistant enterococci.
Adapted from Wilson WR, Karchmer AW, Dajani AS, et al: Antibiotic treatment of adults with infective endocarditis due to streptococci, enterococci, staphylococci and HACEK microorganisms. JAMA 274:1706, 1995.

antistaphylococcal activity and should not be used for this indication despite the ease of its once-daily regimen. Methicillin (or oxacillin)-resistant *S. aureus* (MRSA) is cross-resistant to all β-lactams; in addition, these strains are frequently resistant to other classes of antibiotics, except usually vancomycin. In the event that vancomycin is not tolerated, many MRSA are sensitive to trimethoprim-sulfamethoxazole, which has been shown to be effective in one series of cases. Strains should be tested for susceptibility to rifampin or gentamicin if the use of these drugs is planned. Linezolid, daptomycin, and quinupristin- dalfopristin (Synercid) are active against MRSA, but linezolid has limited bactericidal activity and Synercid is not bactericidal against strains that have constitutive MLSb-type resistance (clindamycin- and erythromycin-resistant phenotype), a frequent finding in MRSA. MLSb resistance is due to methylation of the ribosomal target that results in decreased affinity of this target that is common to antibiotics of these classes.

Ticarcillin, aztreonam, antistaphylococcal penicillins such as nafcillin and methicillin, the cephalosporins, and the carbapenems have no or limited activity against enterococci. Linezolid and Synercid have only inhibitory activity against enterococci, and the activity of Synercid is limited to *Enterococcus faecium*. Enterococci should be routinely tested for high-level resistance to gentamicin and streptomycin because they frequently exhibit this type of resistance to one or both aminoglycosides. Only the aminoglycoside to which the enterococcal strain is sensitive should be chosen for combination with a cell wall-active antimicrobial agent (penicillin, ampicillin, or vancomycin). β-Lactam–gentamicin combinations are preferable to vancomycin-gentamicin because of the increased risk of nephrotoxicity with the vancomycin-gentamicin combination. No reliable bactericidal regimen is available to treat infective endocarditis caused by enterococcal strains that are resistant to high levels of both aminoglycosides in vitro and thus lack penicillin-aminoglycoside synergy. Endocarditis from these strains can be treated with penicillin or vancomycin alone for 8 to 12 weeks, but the relapse rate is high. If the enterococcus is β-lactamase positive (detected by a nitrocefin strip because MIC testing of β-lactamase-positive strains may fail to disclose this type of penicillin resistance), ampicillin-sulbactam or vancomycin can be used alone for 8 to 12 weeks because most of these strains are also highly aminoglycoside resistant. If the enterococcus has a penicillin MIC greater than 16 μg/mL, vancomycin can be used in combination with an aminoglycoside if the strain is highly aminoglycoside susceptible. If the enterococcus is vancomycin resistant (MIC >4 μg/mL), infectious disease consultation should be sought because these strains are usually multidrug resistant.

In vitro susceptibility testing should be performed on gram-negative bacilli, anaerobes, and diphtheroids and the patient treated with the regimen that demonstrates the best bactericidal activity. Therapy for endocarditis attributable to these organisms should be developed in consultation with an infectious disease specialist. Bactericidal activity against anaerobic gram-negative bacilli can frequently be achieved with metronidazole, aerobic enteric gram-negative bacilli or *P. aeruginosa* is often cleared with a cell wall-active agent-aminoglycoside combination or ciprofloxacin, and bactericidal activity against diphtheroids can frequently be attained with a vancomycin-aminoglycoside combination. *Bartonella* endocarditis has been treated with doxycycline and aminoglycoside plus valve replacement, and doxycycline[1] plus hydroxychloroquine and valve replacement have been successful in treating *Coxiella* endocarditis (although reinfection of the prosthetic valve is common). Blood culture-negative endocarditis is generally treated empirically with vancomycin, ceftriaxone, and gentamicin.

Surgical Therapy

Replacement of an infected valve with a prosthesis is indicated in the following situations:

1. Increasing or refractory congestive heart failure secondary to valvular dysfunction. The prognosis of patients with congestive heart failure and infective endocarditis is grave. In patients who are hemodynamically unstable, emergency cardiac valve replacement should not be delayed to allow further antibiotic therapy. Delayed surgery in conjunction with worsening of congestive heart failure increases operative mortality from 6% to 8% in patients with mild or no congestive heart failure to 17% to 33% in those with severe congestive heart failure. The incidence of reinfection of a newly placed cardiac valvular prosthesis is estimated to be 2% to 3%, far less than the mortality associated with uncontrolled congestive heart failure. Although the frequency of operative mortality and PVE is higher when a prosthetic valve is implanted in the presence of active infection, the overall outcome is better if the valve replacement is prompt, before the development of severe congestive heart failure or spread of the infection into perivalvular tissue. If the patient is hemodynamically stable, valve replacement is best delayed until a course of antimicrobial therapy is completed, or at least until after 7 days of antibiotic therapy has been given.
2. Multiple clinically significant emboli despite antibiotic therapy for 2 weeks. However, the first or second embolic episode may so impair the patient that prosthetic valve replacement at that point may be futile. The use of a variety of factors, such as the large size or continued enlargement of vegetations with medical therapy, location on the anterior leaflet of the mitral valve, and fungi or *S. aureus* as the pathogen, to predict significant embolization as an indication for valve replacement remains unresolved.
3. Endocarditis caused by certain pathogens that rarely respond to medical therapy alone, such as fungi, enterococci for which no synergistic bactericidal combination is available (e.g., high-level ampicillin/aminoglycoside/vancomycin-resistant enterococci or β-lactamase-producing/high-level aminoglycoside-resistant *Enterococcus faecalis*), and β-lactam- or fluoroquinolone-resistant gram-negative bacilli.
4. Uncontrolled bacteremia despite optimal antibiotic therapy. However, it should be remembered that the average duration of S. aureus bacteremia in patients receiving vancomycin therapy is 8 days, with bacteremia persisting for several weeks in some patients before its ultimate resolution.
5. Indications for surgical treatment of a valve ring abscess, which may heal with antimicrobial therapy alone, include further extension of infection into the myocardium, the development of prosthetic valve dehiscence, heart block, congestive heart failure, or persistence of bacteremia despite medical therapy. Patients with valve ring abscess should be monitored for the development of conduction abnormalities, which may require placement of a transvenous pacemaker because of the risk of a high-grade heart block.
6. The surgical indications for PVE are the same as those outlined for native valve endocarditis. Some patients without evidence of infection at the annulus may be treated medically. To avoid the complications of prosthetic valve replacement (e.g., PVE, bleeding, thromboembolic events, and valve deterioration), new surgical options that have been proposed as an alternative to a prosthetic valve include valve débridement, valvuloplasty, and repair or replacement of the perivalvular structure with a pulmonary root autograft. Prosthetic valve replacement in an intravenous drug user is problematic because the prosthetic valve places the patient at continued

[1]Not FDA approved for this indication.

risk for PVE. Alternatively, tricuspid valve resection without prosthetic replacement can be tolerated hemodynamically for extended periods in many of these patients.

Intrathoracic, intra-abdominal, or peripheral mycotic aneurysms usually require surgical excision, whereas cerebral aneurysms may heal with medical therapy alone. Cerebral aneurysms should be monitored closely with serial angiograms and generally require surgery if accessible and enlarging or bleeding. Myocardial revascularization should be performed at the time of elective valve surgery if significant coronary artery disease is present. However, patients who require emergency placement of a prosthetic valve for hemodynamic decompensation secondary to acute endocarditis cannot usually tolerate the dye load necessary for coronary angiography and the additional bypass surgery.

Anticoagulant Therapy

Although anticoagulant therapy may impede further enlargement of a vegetation, it is relatively contraindicated in endocarditis because of the increased risk of intracranial hemorrhage from either occult mycotic aneurysms, cerebral emboli, or cerebral immune vasculitis. Anticoagulation may be used for an over-riding indication that is separate from endocarditis, but for deep vein thrombophlebitis of the lower extremities, an inferior vena cava filter would be preferable to anticoagulation. Anticoagulation may be continued with caution during treatment of PVE; however, anticoagulation is particularly problematic when *S. aureus* is the pathogen because of the increased risk of cerebral embolism with this organism, in addition to being problematic in patients with endocarditis who undergo prosthetic valve replacement within 1 month after a neurologic event. In these latter patients, use of a bioprosthesis that will not require anticoagulation is preferable to a mechanical prosthesis.

Shorter Inpatient Therapy

The use of shorter courses of antibiotic therapy and oral regimens and the administration of parenteral antibiotic therapy at home have been investigated in selected patients as a means of shortening the duration of hospitalization. The usual candidate for outpatient therapy is a patient with endocarditis due to a highly penicillin-sensitive viridans streptococcus, when the duration of illness is less than 3 months, and when there is low risk for serious complication, such as CHF or emboli. Such patients can be treated with 4 weeks of a β-lactam alone or 2 weeks of a β-lactam plus an aminoglycoside (see Table 4). Close monitoring on a regular basis is required to assess response to therapy and possible development of adverse drug effects. Easy access to medical care in the event of complication and a support system at home are essential. Having a focal infection that would require more than 2 weeks of antimicrobial therapy, PVE, or significant renal or eighth nerve impairment would preclude the use of short-course β-lactam–aminoglycoside combination therapy. Absorption of orally administered agents may be unreliable, so the oral route is not generally recommended. Before considering outpatient therapy, most patients should first be evaluated and stabilized in the hospital; only rarely can some patients be managed entirely as outpatients. The standard regimens used to treat penicillin-sensitive streptococci require either continuous infusion of penicillin or frequent intravenous administration. A single daily dose of ceftriaxone is an attractive alternative to penicillin. Because of its long half-life and good potency against these streptococci, serum levels of ceftriaxone remain well above the MIC and MBC for over 24 hours.

Response to Therapy

Once receiving appropriate antimicrobial therapy, most patients will note a sense of well-being, lessened fatigue, and improved appetite, and their temperature will usually fall to normal levels within 2 to 5 days. The erythrocyte sedimentation rate, anemia, and renal function may take weeks to months to improve. Circulating immune complexes and related serologic findings, including hypocomplementemia, mixed cryoglobulinemia, and rheumatoid factor, also tend to resolve gradually with effective antibiotic therapy. A variety of tests are performed to monitor both the antimicrobial effects (see Table 3) and the potential toxicities of the drugs used to treat the infection. Blood cultures for streptococci and enterococci should become sterile after 1 to 2 days of appropriate therapy and cultures for *S. aureus*, after 3 to 5 days; however, with vancomycin therapy, blood cultures for *S. aureus* may take 10 to 14 days to become sterile. Blood cultures are performed daily until sterile. If no organism is isolated from blood but the patient has a good clinical response to an empirical antimicrobial regimen, the empirical therapy should be continued. If no organism is isolated and no clinical response to empirical therapy is seen after 1 to 2 weeks, endocarditis due to a fastidious pathogen, or a diagnosis other than infective endocarditis should be considered, such as antiphospholipid antibody syndrome, which requires anticoagulants rather than antibiotic therapy.

If the pathogen is initially isolated from blood and appropriate antimicrobial therapy is started but fever persists or recurs, blood cultures should be repeated to assess for persistent or relapsing infection, among other possibilities (Table 5), most commonly pulmonary or systemic embolization. Blood cultures are repeated 2 and 4 weeks after therapy has been completed because relapse is most common within

TABLE 5 Reasons for Inadequate Clinical Response

Inadequate therapy: wrong drug, wrong dose
Infarcts secondary to emboli
Metastatic abscesses of the spleen, kidney, brain etc., which may require surgical drainage
Suppurative thrombophlebitis at the site of an IV catheter, with or without superinfecting endocarditis
Other superinfections, e.g., *Clostridium difficile* colitis, urinary tract infection
Febrile reaction to the antimicrobial agent or another drug
Another unrelated febrile illness

1 month. The relapse rate is less than 1% to 2% for native valve endocarditis caused by viridans streptococci, 8% to 12% for enterococci, and higher for *S. aureus* and other pathogens or PVE.

Outcomes

Factors that affect mortality include the infecting organism (the mortality of endocarditis from fungi, *P. aeruginosa*, and aerobic enteric gram-negative bacilli > staphylococci > enterococci > streptococci), the site of infection (aortic > mitral and left-sided > tricuspid infection), PVE versus native valve endocarditis (early onset PVE > late-onset PVE > native valve endocarditis), age (higher in the elderly and very young), gender (men > women), and the presence of certain complications such as heart or renal failure, rupture of a mycotic aneurysm, cardiac arrhythmias and conduction abnormalities, perivalvular extension, cerebral emboli, and perhaps, severe immunosuppression from HIV infection. Heart failure remains the leading cause of death. However, with increasing use of prosthetic valve replacement for heart failure, the leading cause of death may shift to neurologic complications from embolic episodes or mycotic aneurysms or to uncontrolled infection with antibiotic-resistant microorganisms. After cure of one episode of endocarditis, patients still have a greatly increased risk of reinfection.

Prevention

The effect of endocarditis prophylaxis with antimicrobial agents has been estimated to be modest, with less than 10% of all cases being preventable by prophylaxis. For example, only about half of cases have recognizable predisposing cardiac lesions, most cases do not follow an invasive procedure, and only about two thirds of cases are due to microorganisms (viridans streptococci and enterococci) against which prophylactic regimens are directed. However, in patients who are known to have a risky cardiac lesion and are about to undergo a procedure that is likely to induce bacteremia with organisms having predictable susceptibility to antibiotics with minimal inconvenience, toxicity, and cost, the American Heart Association has made the recommendations shown in Table 6. Additional preventive measures are to minimize invasive procedures; avoid unnecessary use of intravascular catheters, a major predisposing event for nosocomial endocarditis; aggressively treat focal infections; and maintain good dental hygiene in patients at increased risk for endocarditis.

TABLE 6 Chemoprophylaxis of Endocarditis

Chemoprophylaxis Recommended for High- and Medium-Risk Patients
Dental procedures
Dental and periodontal procedures known to induce mucosal bleeding
Dental implant placement and reimplantation of avulsed teeth
Endodontic instrumentation or surgery only beyond the apex
Subgingival placement of antibiotic fibers or strips
Initial placement of orthodontic bands but not brackets
Intraligamentary local anesthetic injections
Respiratory tract
Tonsillectomy and adenoidectomy
Bronchoscopy with a rigid bronchoscope
Surgery on the respiratory mucosa
Genitourinary tract
Prostate surgery
Cystoscopy or urethral dilation
Chemoprophylaxis Recommended for High-Risk, Optional for Medium-Risk Patients
Esophageal dilation or sclerotherapy for esophageal varices
Biliary tract surgery
Endoscopic retrograde cholangiography with biliary obstruction
Surgery on the intestinal mucosa
Chemoprophylaxis Optional for High-Risk Patients
Bronchoscopy with a flexible bronchoscope, with or without biopsy
Transesophageal echocardiography
Endoscopy with or without gastrointestinal biopsy
Vaginal hysterectomy
Vaginal delivery

TABLE 6 Chemoprophylaxis of Endocarditis—cont'd

Prophylactic Regimens	
*Dental, Oral, Respiratory Tract, and Esophageal Procedures in Patients at High and Moderate Risk**	
STANDARD REGIMEN	
Amoxicillin (Amoxil)†	2.0 g orally 1 h before the procedure
AMOXICILLIN/PENICILLIN-ALLERGIC PATIENTS	
Clindamycin (Cleocin)†	600 mg orally 1 h before the procedure
or	
Cephalexin (Keflex)† or cefadroxil (Duricef)†‡	2.0 g orally 1 h before the procedure
or	
Azithromycin (Zithromax)† or clarithromycin (Biaxin)†	500 mg orally 1 h before the procedure
PATIENTS UNABLE TO TAKE ORAL MEDICATIONS	
Ampicillin†	IV or IM administration of ampicillin, 2 g within 30 min before the procedure
AMPICILLIN/PENCILLIN-ALLERGIC PATIENTS UNABLE TO TAKE ORAL MEDICATIONS	
Clindamycin†	IV administration of clindamycin, 600 mg within 30 min before the procedure
or	
Cefazolin (Kefzol)‡	IV administration of cefazolin, 1.0 g within 30 min before the procedure
Genitourinary/Gastrointestinal (Excluding Esophageal) Procedures in Patients at High Risk§	
STANDARD REGIMEN	
Ampicillin,† amoxicillin,† plus gentamicin (Garamycin)	IV or IM administration of ampicillin, 2 g, plus gentamicin, 1.5 mg/kg (not to exceed 120 mg) within 30 min of starting the procedure; 6 h later, ampicillin, 1.0 g IV/IM, or amoxicillin, 1 g orally
AMPICILLIN†/AMOXICILLIN/PENICILLIN-ALLERGIC PATIENTS	
Vancomycin (Vancocin) plus gentamicin	IV administration of vancomycin 1.0 g over 1-2 h, plus gentamicin, 1.5 mg/kg IV/IM (not to exceed 120 mg); complete infusion or injection within 30 min of starting the procedure
Genitourinary/Gastrointestinal (Excluding Esophageal) Procedures in Patients at Moderate Risk	
STANDARD REGIMEN	
Ampicillin† or amoxicillin†	IV or IM administration of ampicillin, 2 g within 30 min of starting the procedure, or amoxicillin, 2 g orally 1 hr before the procedure
AMPICILLIN/AMOXICILLIN/PENICILLIN-ALLERGIC PATIENTS	
Vancomycin	IV administration of vancomycin, 1.0 g over 1-2 h; complete infusion within 30 min of starting the procedure

*Doses in the table are for adults.
†Not FDA approved for this indication.
‡Cephalosporins should not be used in individuals with immediate-type hypersensitivity reactions to penicillin (urticaria, angioedema, or anaphylaxis).
§No second dose of vancomycin or gentamicin is recommended.
Adapted from Dajani AS, Taubert KA, Wilson W, et al: Prevention of bacterial endocarditis. Recommendations of the American Heart Association. JAMA 277:1794, 1997.

HYPERTENSION

METHOD OF

Patrick J. Mulrow, MD

Hypertension, or elevated blood pressure, is a worldwide epidemic. In Western Europe and North America, the prevalence for this condition is more than 20% of the adult population, and it increases with age. In the United States, more than 50% of the population 65 years of age or older has hypertension, and this approaches 90% for those older than 80 years of age. Thus, approximately 50 million people in the United States and approximately 1 billion people worldwide have hypertension. Hypertension is the most common diagnosis for patient office visits in the United States.

The relationship between blood pressure and cardiovascular disease is continuous and independent of other risk factors. The higher the blood pressure, the greater the risk of stroke, heart attacks, heart failure, and kidney failure. An increase of 20 mm Hg systolic blood pressure or 10 mm Hg diastolic blood pressure doubles the risk of cardiovascular disease from the blood pressure range of 115/75 to 185/115 mm Hg.

The health benefits of lowering blood pressure have been demonstrated time and time again. In clinical trials, antihypertensive treatment has reduced stroke incidence by approximately 40%, heart attacks by approximately 25%, and heart failure by more than 50%. Despite the demonstration of health benefits, in study after study the control of hypertension to goal levels of less than 140/90 mm Hg is only approximately 30% in the United States and much less in many countries around the world. This failure to adequately treat hypertension persists despite the availability of multiple drugs and lifestyle modifications known to be effective in preventing and treating hypertension.

This failure to apply the fruits of clinical science to clinical practice is because of many factors, but it is clear that physicians are part of the problem. Physicians frequently do not follow up and aggressively treat hypertension. In clinical trials—notably the Antihypertensive and Lipid Lowering Treatment to Prevent Heart Attack Trial (ALLHAT study)—approximately 66% of hypertension patients can be treated to reach goal blood pressure levels. The success of clinical trials in achieving a higher patient success rate is because of the health care team approach to the management and follow-up of the hypertensive patient.

Classifications of Blood Pressures

The definition of hypertension has changed over the years. A blood pressure of greater than 160/95 mm Hg was often used as the cut-off point, but it is clear from numerous epidemiologic studies that there is a continuous cardiovascular disease risk in blood pressure from 120 mm Hg systolic on up. The consensus is that 140/90 mm Hg in the general population is a cut-off point and a treatment goal. However, in certain conditions, such as diabetes mellitus or underlying renal disease, 130/80 mm Hg or lower is the goal.

Table 1 summarizes the recommendations from the Seventh Report of the Joint National Committee on Prevention, Detection, Evaluation, and Treatment of High Blood Pressure (JNC 7). A new category, called *prehypertensive*, has been added because patients with prehypertension are at twice the risk of developing hypertension compared with those with lower levels. For this extremely large population of potential hypertensive patients, prevention of hypertension by lifestyle modification is strongly recommended. It should be remembered that even a controlled hypertensive patient has more cardiovascular events than someone who has never had hypertension. Therefore, it is best to prevent the development of hypertension.

Measurement of Blood Pressure

Blood pressure is an extremely variable hemodynamic measurement. Its measurement is the basis for diagnosing and classifying hypertensive patients. We can measure many blood elements very accurately, but frequently the results are of no consequence or are unimportant. Blood pressure measurement is often poorly measured in the doctor's office or clinic. There are two important components to measuring blood pressure, the preparation of the patient and the actual measurement. Here are some suggestions:

- Patients should be seated quietly for 5 minutes with feet on the floor and the arm supported at the level of the heart. The blood pressure in both arms should be measured at the first visit. Standing blood pressure is indicated sometimes, especially in those patients over 65 years of age and those prone to postural hypotension, such as diabetics.

TABLE 1 Classification and Management of Blood Pressure for Adults

				Initial Drug Therapy	
BP Classification	**Systolic BP (mm Hg)**	**Diastolic BP (mm Hg)**	**Lifestyle Modification**	**Without Compelling Indications**	**With Compelling Indications***
Normal	<120	<80	Encourage		
Prehypertension	120-139	80-89	Yes	No antihypertensive drug indicated	Drug(s) for compelling indications
Stage 1 hypertension	140-159	90-99	Yes	Thiazide-type diuretics for most May consider ACEI, ARB, BB, CCB, or combination	Drug(s) for the compelling indications Other antihypertensive-drugs (diuretics, ACEI, ARB, BB, CCB) as needed
Stage 2 hypertension	>160	>100	Yes	Two-drug combination for most (usually thiazide-type diuretic and ACEI, ARB, BB, or CCB)	

*Compelling indications are diabetes mellitus, heart failure, coronary artery disease, and chronic kidney disease.

Abbreviations: ACEI = angiotensin-converting enzyme inhibitor; ARB = angiotensin-receptor blocker; BB = β blocker; BP = blood pressure; CCB = calcium channel blocker.

Modified from: U.S. Department of Health and Human Services, National Heart Institutes of Health, National Heart, Lung, and Blood Institute: JNC 7 Express, The Seventh Report of the Joint National Committee on Prevention, Detection, Evaluation, and Treatment of High Blood Pressure (Publication No. 03-5233). May 2003, p 3.

- Patients should refrain from smoking or ingesting caffeine for at least 30 minutes before the measurement.
- An appropriate size arm cuff should be used. The cuff bladder should encircle at least 80% of the arm.
- A properly calibrated instrument should be used, and the instrument should be validated at regular intervals.
- An average of two or more readings should be taken at each sitting.
- If the auscultatory method is used, systolic blood pressure is the point at which the first of two or more successive sounds are heard. Diastolic pressure is the point before the disappearance of sounds.
- The physician should inform the patient of the blood pressure level.

AMBULATORY AND SELF-MEASUREMENT OF BLOOD PRESSURE

A number of publications have reported the usefulness of ambulatory blood pressure monitoring (ABPM) in certain conditions. The measurement is somewhat complex and should be done in the office of the specialist. ABPM is warranted for patients who need evaluation for white-coat hypertension and resistant hypertension, and in patients with unusual reactions to blood pressure medications. The ambulatory blood pressure values are lower than clinical readings. A blood pressure measured by ABPM that is more than 135/85 mm Hg is defined as hypertension. There should be a nocturnal dip in blood pressure.

Self-measurement of blood pressure is more practical and useful in monitoring the response to antihypertensive medication and in evaluating white-coat hypertension. I have many of my patients measure their blood pressure at least weekly at home, record the results, and bring the record to the office for evaluation. Oscillometric blood pressure measurement instruments are becoming more reliable and easy to use. The patient needs to be instructed in the office on how to measure the blood pressure at home.

Types of Blood Pressure: Systolic or Diastolic

Traditionally, hypertension has been classified based on the diastolic blood pressure. Numerous reports, especially from the Framingham study, have emphasized that *systolic* hypertension is a greater risk for causing cardiovascular disease than *diastolic* hypertension. A combination of a high systolic and low diastolic blood pressure (widened pulse pressure) is a major predictor of cardiovascular disease. The widened pulse pressure reflects atheromatous thickening and stiffening of the major capacitance vessels. With aging, systolic blood pressure tends to increase even in the normotensive patient, while diastolic tends to fall. Most elderly (65 years of age or older) hypertensive patients have primarily systolic hypertension with only minor elevations of diastolic blood pressure. It is imperative, therefore, to control systolic hypertension to below goal levels of 140. A blood pressure of 150/80 mm Hg is too high in a 65-year-old patient.

Evaluation of the Hypertensive Patient

To make the diagnosis of hypertension, an accurate blood pressure measurement should be made on at least two separate occasions, one or more weeks apart. Obviously, if the blood pressure is very high under nonstress conditions, a diagnosis can be made on one visit and treatment started.

DIAGNOSTIC EVALUATION

There are two components to the diagnostic workup:

1. Evaluation of the patient for the presence of cardiovascular risk factors (Table 2) and organ damage
2. Evaluation for secondary causes of hypertension

A thorough medical history, physical examination, and routine laboratory studies should be performed. Before starting treatment, I usually include a urinalysis, serum electrolytes including calcium, creatinine, blood glucose, hematocrit, a fasting lipid profile, and an electrocardiogram.

Secondary causes of hypertension also should be evaluated. How extensive the evaluation should be is a subject of debate. Unless there is some obvious reason to suspect a secondary cause or the patient has resistant hypertension, or there is sudden onset of type 2 hypertension in the young (under 30) or in the patient over 55 years of age, I do not routinely do special diagnostic tests. Recently, the evidence is becoming compelling that approximately 7% to 8% of the hypertensive population has primary aldosteronism. Blood tests for measuring the serum aldosterone to renin ratio are being recommended by many experts. A ratio greater than 25 should be pursued with more extensive testing. I have been doing these ratios recently, but my practice is more a tertiary rather than a primary practice, where many patients have stage 1 hypertension. Secondary causes of hypertension should be pursued when the above criteria are noted, as listed in Table 3.

TABLE 2 Major Cardiovascular Risk Factors

Obesity (body mass index >30 kg/m^2)
Dyslipidemia
Cigarette smoking
Diabetes mellitus
Family history of premature cardiovascular disease (CVD)
Age (men >55 years, women >65 years)
Microalbuminuria
Decreased renal function
Left ventricular hypertrophy (LVH)

TABLE 3 Causes of Secondary Hypertension

Coarctation of the aorta
Cushing's syndrome
Drug induced (e.g., nonsteroidal anti-inflammatory drugs, estrogen, sympathomimetics, certain herbal medications)
Hyperparathyroidism
Hyperthyroidism
Pheochromocytoma
Primary aldosteronism
Renal disease
Renovascular disease
Sleep apnea

Treatment of the Hypertensive Patient

The goal of therapy is to reduce cardiovascular complications. In the usual hypertensive patient, the blood pressure goal is less than 140/90 mm Hg. However, in patients with diabetes or renal disease and hypertension, the blood pressure goal is less than 130/80 mm Hg.

LIFESTYLE MODIFICATION

Lifestyle modification such as weight reduction, low-sodium diet, reduced alcohol intake, cessation of smoking, and increased physical activity should be an adjunct to all drug therapy. In the hypertensive patient, lifestyle modifications can reduce blood pressure, enhance the blood pressure lowering effects of antihypertensive drugs, and decrease cardiovascular risk. As little as 10 to 20 pounds weight loss can significantly reduce blood pressure. A low-sodium diet of less than 100 meq per day can be quite effective. Reduction in excess alcohol intake can also lower the blood pressure. Physical activity, such as brisk walking for 30 minutes daily, can reduce blood pressure. Certain diets (Dietary Approaches to Stop Hypertension [DASH]) that are high in fruits, vegetables, and low-fat dairy products may be as effective as monotherapy in lowering the blood pressure. Smoking cessation may not lower the blood pressure, but it does decrease the cardiovascular complications.

Although lifestyle modification can be extremely effective, every physician knows how difficult it is for some patients to adhere to these lifestyle changes. I give patients in stage 1 hypertension (140-159/90-99 mm Hg), without diabetes or other cardiovascular risk factors or end-organ damage, a 4-month trial of lifestyle changes. If goal blood pressure is not achieved, I start pharmacologic therapy.

WHITE-COAT HYPERTENSION

Some patients have a blood pressure that is high in the office, but normal when measured at home or at work. However, to be certain of the diagnosis of this benign condition, the blood pressure should be monitored frequently over several months. Patients with true white-coat hypertension show little if any evidence of end-organ damage from the blood pressure. If the diagnosis is not certain, drugs that diminish sympathetic activity such as β blockers or α-adrenergic drugs may be effective. Ambulatory blood pressure measurement can be helpful in making the diagnosis, because these patients on 24-hour monitoring show normal blood pressures. In my opinion, one should err on the side of treating the patient if there is doubt about the diagnosis.

DRUG TREATMENT OF HYPERTENSION

The efficacy of various antihypertensive agents in lowering blood pressure is about the same when the proper dose is used. A single drug usually reduces blood pressure 8 to 12 mm Hg compared with placebo.

Clinical outcome trials demonstrate the ability of angiotensin-converting enzyme (ACE) inhibitors, angiotensin receptor blockers (ARB), β blockers, calcium channel blockers, and thiazide diuretics to reduce the complications of hypertension.

Classes of Antihypertensive Drugs (Table 4)

Thiazide Diuretics

Thiazide diuretics have been shown in many studies to be useful in lowering blood pressure and preventing cardiovascular complications. In low doses they have few complications, hypokalemia being the most serious. In my opinion, it is the first-line drug in most hypertensive patients; if two or more drugs are needed, a thiazide diuretic is usually one of the drugs. Loop diuretics are good diuretics, but poor antihypertensive agents unless renal failure is present. In patients with chronic renal disease, loop diuretics can be used instead of thiazide diuretics, because thiazides are ineffective in producing a diuresis. Volume retention plays an important role in the development of hypertension in the patient with chronic renal failure. All thiazide diuretics appear to be equally effective. Potassium-sparing compounds such as triamterene (Dyrenium), amiloride (Midamor), and spironolactone (Aldactone) are sometimes added alone or in a combination pill to lessen the potassium-losing effect of diuretics, especially when large doses are used. I usually start with 12.5 mg of hydrochlorothiazide. To avoid cutting the 25 mg pill in half, 15 mg of chlorthalidone can be used.

TABLE 4 Classes of Antihypertensive Drugs

Diuretics
β Blockers
Calcium channel blockers (CCBs)
Angiotensin-converting enzyme (ACE) inhibitors
Angiotensin receptor blocker (ARB)
α-Adrenergic blocking drugs
Central α-adrenergic agonists
Direct vasodilators
Combination products

Adverse Effects. Hypokalemia is a common problem when large doses of thiazide diuretics are used. The mechanism is diuresis → volume depletion → increased renin → increased aldosterone → increased kidney loss of potassium. With low doses, especially in the elderly and diabetics with low renin levels, hypokalemia is not as common. When needed, I usually recommend a combination pill, triamterene plus hydrochlorothiazide (Dyazide) or amiloride plus hydrochlorothiazide (Moduretic) to prevent the hypokalemia. If several drugs are needed, ACE inhibitors or angiotensin-receptor blockers (ARBs) can block the renin-angiotensin system and lessen K loss. K supplements, 10 to 20 mEq per day, may be useful in some patients, but serum levels of K should be monitored to prevent serious hyperkalemia when multiple K-sparing drugs are used.

Hyponatremia is seen in the elderly, especially women. Some patients are exquisitely sensitive to very low doses of thiazides, and the hyponatremia can cause serious neurologic problems. Mild hyponatremia with a serum concentration of sodium of more than 130 mEq/L usually is of no consequence. Hyperuricemia can occur and lead to gout, especially in males. This complication may cause the discontinuation of diuretics; but if a diuretic is needed, allopurinol (Zyloprim) can be added to the regimen to reduce uric acid production.

β Blockers

β Blockers are not usually a first-line drug except in young people under 30 years of age with a hyperdynamic circulation or in hyperthyroidism. β Blockers are included in the treatment of patients with ischemic heart disease, postmyocardial infarction, and patients with certain arrhythmias. I do not use them unless there is some cardiovascular reason for adding it to the blood pressure regimen. Labetalol (Trandate), a combination of α and β drugs, may be used. Labetalol combines an α-adrenergic receptor blockade and a β blocker. It lowers blood pressure faster than other β blockers. Carvedilol (Coreg) is another α blocker and nonselective β blocker that lowers blood pressure by a peripheral vasodilatation while maintaining cardiac output. It is promoted as especially effective in treating patients with hypertension and congestive heart failure. These patients are usually on multiple drugs, including a diuretic and an ACE inhibitor.

Adverse Events. The major adverse events are bronchospasm, fatigue, and Raynaud's phenomenon. There is some concern that long-term treatment of patients with β blockers may cause a higher incidence of type 2 diabetes.

Calcium Channel Antagonist

Calcium channel blockers (CCBs) have been shown to be very effective in treating hypertension in patients, especially in patients older than 65 years of age and African Americans. They cause vasodilatation, which decreases peripheral resistance. Short-acting CCBs such as nifedipine (Procardia) should not be used to treat hypertensive patients. There is concern that the reflex tachycardia may lead to cardiovascular events. However, the long-acting dihydropyridines, such as amlodipine (Norvasc), and nondihydropyridines, such as verapamil (Calan), and diltiazem (Cardizem), are effective. There is debate over the use of CCBs in diabetic patients with proteinuria, because the CCBs may increase protein excretion. I do not use them except as a third add on in patients with proteinuria. Usually I give an ACE inhibitor or an ARB plus a thiazide diuretic, and if the blood pressure is not controlled, I add a CCB or a β blocker.

Verapamil, diltiazem, and amlodipine cause little or no reflex increase in heart rate. However, verapamil and diltiazem can actually slow the heart rate and have an adverse effect on atrioventricular (AV) conduction. They should be used with caution in patients taking a β blocker. Amlodipine causes significant peripheral edema, especially in high doses, but combining it with an ACE inhibitor reduces the edema.

I prefer CCBs such as amlodipine as a second drug, usually added to a diuretic in elderly patients and in African Americans. However, if significant proteinuria is present, an ACE inhibitor or ARB should be used instead.

Angiotensin-Converting Inhibitors

ACE inhibitors were originally introduced as antihypertensive drugs, but are now considered to have significant effects in preventing cardiovascular events in patients with underlying cardiovascular disease. They are now recommended as an adjunct therapy for patients with left ventricular dysfunction, recent myocardial infarction, or stroke; and to preserve renal function in diabetic patients. They also appear to increase sensitivity to insulin and reduce the development of diabetes mellitus. The ACE inhibitors are less effective in lowering blood pressure in African American patients. However, there is a broad range of response with many African Americans showing good hypotensive effects. Furthermore, ACE inhibitors confer renal protection in African Americans.

Adverse Events. A common adverse effect of an ACE inhibitor is a dry cough. Approximately 10% of the patients note a dry cough, and in a few patients it is especially annoying at night, requiring the drug to be discontinued. Cough is a side effect for all ACE inhibitors and is not related to dose.

Angioedema is an uncommon but serious side effect. Patients with bilateral renal vascular disease may develop acute renal failure from ACE inhibitors. Also, hyperkalemia may occur, especially in the patient taking K supplements or K-sparing diuretics, or who has poor renal function. I measure serum K and creatinine levels about 1 week after starting an ACE inhibitor. I measure creatinine and electrolytes periodically thereafter. ACE inhibitors are contraindicated in pregnancy.

There are numerous ACE inhibitor preparations on the market. I believe they are all equally effective when given in the proper dose. I prefer the ones that are long acting and need only once-a-day medication. This applies to most of the ACE inhibitors. In patients with diabetes, renal disease, and proteinuria, I recommend increasing the dose to the maximum dose to reduce proteinuria and protect the kidneys.

Angiotensin Receptor Blocker

By blocking the binding of angiotensin II to its receptor (AT_1), ARBs can lower blood pressure. They have few side effects. In contrast to ACE inhibitors, ARBs do not cause a cough. The ARBs have been shown to have renal protection in patients with diabetes mellitus type 2. Compared with the β blocker atenolol (Tenormin), the ARB losartan (Cozaar) is more effective in reducing left ventricular hypertrophy (LVH) and the incidence of stroke in patients with hypertension and LVH. However, this protective effect is not seen in African Americans. Like ACE inhibitors, the beneficial cardiovascular effects of ARBs appear to be beyond just lowering blood pressure. Usually ARBs are given with a diuretic.

As with ACE inhibitors, all ARBs seem to be equally effective when the proper dose is used. Perhaps the only unique feature of one of the ARBs is the mild uricosuric effect of losartan.

α-Adrenergic Blocking Drugs

α-Adrenergic blocking drugs were once considered to be heart friendly because of their favorable effects on blood lipids and glucose metabolism. However, in the ALLHAT study, the doxazosin (Cardura) arm was discontinued because of the twofold increase in the risk of heart failure when compared with diuretics. Therefore, α-adrenergic drugs are not recommended as first-line drugs. In patients who do not have the risk for heart failure, they may be beneficial as an add-on drug or be useful for symptomatic relief of prostatism in men. However, they may cause significant hypotension. I rarely use these drugs.

Central α-Adrenergic Agonists

Central α-adrenergic agonist drugs are not recommended as first-line drugs. They are not used as much today because of their side effects of sedation, dry mouth, and depression. Clonidine (Catapres) is used more frequently because it can be applied to the skin as a patch, but there is some concern about reflex tachycardia and rebound hypertension when it is discontinued. Occasionally I will use guanfacine (Tenex) at bedtime because it is a longer acting drug. It would be a fourth-line add-on in patients with resistant hypertension. In other words, I do not recommend these drugs as routine medications, but do add them as a third- or fourth-line add-on in certain patients.

Peripheral Adrenergic Neuron Antagonists

Reserpine in low doses is the only drug in this category that is still in use. Low doses are effective as antihypertensive drugs with few significant side effects. The reported side effects of depression and sedation were overemphasized by physicians because too large a dose was used. Reserpine is cheap and often combined with a diuretic. However, no outcome studies have been performed with reserpine. Nevertheless, this is a commonly prescribed drug in many developing countries because it is inexpensive.

Direct Vasodilators

Direct vasodilators such as hydralazine (Apresoline) cause reflex tachycardia, and when used should be given with a β blocker to prevent the tachycardia. Hydralazine has to be given 3 or 4 times each day and is rarely used today. Minoxidil (Loniten), a potent drug, is reserved for severe resistant hypertension. It can cause significant fluid retention and its chronic use can cause disfiguring hirsutism.

Combination Products (Table 5)

More than 50% of hypertensive patients need two or more antihypertensive drugs to attain goal blood pressures. In diabetics with a lower goal, three or more drugs may be needed. Also, patients with stage 2 hypertension (blood pressure greater than 160/100 mm Hg) usually require two drugs as initial therapy. Combination products may improve compliance. Also, combining antihypertensive drugs with different mechanisms of action may allow smaller doses of each drug to be used and thus lessen dose-dependent side effects. Although there are no prospective drug studies comparing the efficacy of combination therapy with monotherapy, in most monotherapy trials the majority of the subjects are taking one or more drugs in addition to the study drug. Diuretics plus ACE inhibitors or ARBs are frequent combinations. The combination of an ACE with a CCB lessens the edema seen with the large doses of dihydropyridine CCBs. Of course, for many years potassium-sparing drugs have been combined with thiazide diuretics.

Compliance

Good blood pressure control requires patient and physician compliance. The physicians must educate

TABLE 5 Combination Drugs

Diuretics and potassium-sparing drugs such as hydrochlorothiazide plus triamterene (Maxzide) or amiloride (Moduretic) or spironolactone (Aldactazide)
Various ACE inhibitors plus thiazide
Various ARBs plus thiazide
Various β blockers plus thiazide
Centrally acting drugs such as reserpine or clonidine or methyldopa plus thiazide diuretics
Calcium channel blockers plus ACE inhibitors in various combinations

Abbreviations: ACE = angiotensin-converting enzyme; ARB = angiotensin-receptor blocker.

the patients, prescribe appropriate medication, and follow the patient carefully. Hypertensive patients usually have several cardiovascular risk factors that need to be assessed and treated. All members of the health care team—physician, nurse, and other health professionals—must work together to improve lifestyle and detect and control blood pressure. We have the knowledge and the modalities to control hypertension if we apply what we know to our clinical practice.

First Choice of Drug

The recent JNC7 guidelines in hypertension recommend low-dose diuretics as the first step in treatment for most hypertensive patients, including those at risk such as elderly hypertensives and hypertensives with cardiovascular risk factors. Diuretics are also recommended as the second drug choice when the initial drug does not lower the blood pressure to goal levels. Because most patients require two or more drugs, a diuretic is usually a component of the regimen. These recommendations are based on a number of long-term clinical studies that demonstrate the beneficial effects of diuretics in preventing cardiovascular complications in hypertensive patients. However, despite the evidence the use of diuretics declined in the United States until the recent ALLHAT study gave a major boost to diuretics. In this study, thiazide was compared with a CCB, an ACE inhibitor, and an α-adrenergic blocker. The latter drug was discontinued early in the study because of poor outcome compared with a diuretic. The major finding of this study is that the diuretic is as good as, if not better than, other drugs in lowering blood pressure and preventing cardiovascular complications. Thiazide diuretics are cheap and, in low doses, relatively free of side effects. A thiazide diuretic is my first-line drug for treating hypertension. I usually start with 12.5 mg of hydrochlorothiazide and occasionally the longer acting one, chlorthalidone. I emphasize thiazide diuretics because nonthiazide diuretics have not been shown to be effective antihypertensive agents.

HYPERTENSION AND CO-MORBID CONDITIONS

Patients with hypertension tend to have multiple metabolic abnormalities such as diabetes mellitus, obesity, dyslipidemia and insulin resistance, as well as underlying vascular disease. Therefore, in addition to antihypertensive medication, these patients receive several other medications and diets to decrease the cardiovascular complications.

Diabetes

Two or more drugs are usually needed to meet the target goal of less than 130/80 mm Hg in diabetic patients. ACE inhibitors and ARBs, in addition to lowering blood pressure, also slow the progression of diabetic nephropathy. Diuretics are usually required as a second-line drug to reduce the blood pressure to goal levels. There is some concern that CCBs may increase proteinuria. Nevertheless, all these drugs—thiazide diuretics, ARBs, ACE inhibitors, and CCBs—have been shown in clinical trials to reduce cardiovascular disease and stroke in diabetic subjects. Although ACE inhibitors and ARBs may have beneficial vascular effects, it is important to control the blood pressure to goal levels. This may mean the use of two or more medications. I usually recommend starting with an ACE inhibitor and then adding a small dose of a thiazide diuretic, if necessary. If a third drug is needed, I usually add either the CCB amlodipine (Norvasc) or the β blocker atenolol (Tenormin), depending upon the cardiovascular situation.

Ischemic Heart Disease

In patients with hypertension and ischemic heart disease, the first-line drug therapy is usually a β blocker. CCBs are a reasonable alternative drug. For patients with a myocardial infarction and hypertension, a β blocker and an ACE inhibitor should be started and other drugs then added to control the blood pressure to goal levels.

Heart Failure

In patients with hypertension and heart failure, loop diuretics along with ACE inhibitors and β blockers are recommended. ARBs may be substituted for ACE inhibitors, and small doses of the aldosterone antagonist spironolactone (Aldactone) should be added. Close monitoring of the serum K levels is required.

Chronic Renal Disease

Hypertensive male patients with creatinine greater than 1.5 mg/dL and hypertensive female patients with creatinine greater than 1.3 mg/dL will progress to chronic renal failure unless treated aggressively. Treatment with ARBs and ACE inhibitors show favorable responses in both diabetic and nondiabetic kidney disease. The blood pressure goal is less than 130/80. When renal failure is more advanced (creatinine 2.5 to 3), loop diuretics such as furosemide (Lasix) may be needed for diuresis. The renin angiotensin system inhibitors may cause a limited rise in serum creatinine, but blood pressure drugs should be maintained unless there is a doubling of the creatinine or significant hyperkalemia.

RESISTANT HYPERTENSION

Resistant hypertension is defined as the failure to reach goal blood pressure on three blood pressure medications. Adding an adequate diuretic dose to the drug regimen usually controls resistant hypertension. In addition, the physician should obtain a history for the possibility of certain drugs and over-the-counter

TABLE 6 Causes of Resistant Hypertension

Volume overload
Failure to take drugs
Inadequate drug doses
Drug-induced hypertension (nonsteroidal anti-inflammatory drugs, sympathomimetics, estrogens, oral contraceptives, adrenal glucocorticoids, amphetamines, cyclosporine, erythropoietin, over-the-counter drugs such as ephedra)
Excess adrenal glucocorticoid production
Excess adrenal glucocorticoid administration
Excess alcohol intake
Poor blood pressure measurement, especially in obese subjects
Secondary causes of hypertension

medications that may contribute to hypertension, as well as excessive alcohol intake. Table 6 indicates some of the causes of resistant hypertension.

TREATMENT OF ACUTE MYOCARDIAL INFARCTION

METHOD OF

R. Scott Wright, MD

Approximately 2 million individuals annually suffer an acute myocardial infarction (AMI) in the United States and 30% to 50% die before reaching a hospital. Approximately 50% of patients with AMI have ST segment elevation (STE) on their electrocardiogram (ECG). This article focuses on the treatment of patients presenting with ST segment elevation acute myocardial infarction (STEMI). Patients with non-ST elevation MI (Non-STEMI) and with unstable angina are addressed on pages 334-335 (Angina Pectoris).

Pathophysiology

Coronary artery disease (CAD) is responsible for almost all STEMI. Rupture of an atherosclerotic plaque results in thrombotic occlusion of the coronary vessel, producing the acute infarct. Certain features predispose the plaque to "vulnerability" or rupture including a thin fibrous cap, lack of calcification, local inflammation, negative arterial remodeling, and exposure to increased sheer stress. Following plaque rupture, coronary blood flow is reduced or arrested and myocardial necrosis occurs producing chest pain (angina pectoris) and ST segment elevation on the ECG. The diagnosis of STEMI is confirmed by the typical electrocardiographic changes and by the appropriate rise and fall of plasma cardiac biomarkers.

Clinical Presentation

Chest pain is the most common symptom of AMI. It is described as an intense sensation, much like a pressure or weight on the chest. It is described as substernal in location. The chest pain can radiate into the left arm or shoulder region, or to the left jaw or neck. Diaphoresis, dyspnea, nausea, and vomiting are often accompanying symptoms with STEMI.

Atypical symptoms also occur including abdominal pain, back pain, unexplained syncope, confusion, and unexplained dyspnea. Those over 65 years of age and women are more likely to present with atypical symptoms. Other conditions can mimic AMI including acute cholecystitis, peptic ulcer disease, esophagitis, aortic dissection, acute pericarditis, acute pulmonary embolism, and musculoskeletal chest pain. Table 1 outlines the features of each of these conditions.

Given the significant risk of mortality during the initial hours of STEMI, a high index of suspicion should be maintained in any adult with unexplained chest pain, abdominal pain, nausea, diaphoresis, or syncope who presents to the emergency room.

Evaluation of Suspected Acute Myocardial Infarction

A comprehensive approach is necessary in the evaluation of the patient with suspected STEMI. The patient with chest pain or suspected STEMI should be evaluated in the emergency room or transported to the nearest emergency room via emergency medical services. The initial evaluation should include a focused physical examination, an ECG, establishment of an intravenous line, analysis for plasma biomarkers of myocardial necrosis, and a chest radiograph.

Electrocardiographic Findings

An ECG should be obtained in every patient with suspected STEMI, ideally, within 10 minutes of emergency room arrival. Most hospitals use the standard 12-lead ECG, although recent work has suggested that a 15-lead ECG, which incorporates the posterior leads V_7-V_8-V_9, is a better diagnostic tool. The posterior leads should be considered when the presenting ECG has inferior (leads II, III, aVF [augmented voltage unipolar left foot lead]) ST segment elevation or significant precordial (V_1-V_2-V_3) ST segment depression accompanied by an R/S ratio greater than 0.8. The diagnosis of acute posterior STE AMI is established by either the demonstration of ST segment elevation in the posterior precordial leads (V_7-V_8-V_9)

TABLE 1 Differential Diagnosis of Chest Pain

Condition	Symptoms	Location of Symptoms	Physical Examination Findings	ECG Findings
Acute MI	Chest pressure or tightness	Midprecordium; radiation into neck, jaw, shoulder, or arm	Diaphoresis; S_4 gallop; elevated JVP (with heart failure); rales in lung fields	ST segment elevation in ≧ 2 contiguous leads; or new LBBB; or ST depression in $V_1 + V_2$ with R/S ratio >0.8
Acute pericarditis	Chest pain that worsens with inspiration or position changes; mild dyspnea	Precordial region	Loud rub diaphoresis	Diffuse ST segment elevation; PR depression
Aortic dissection	Chest pain of a tearing nature	Precordium but radiates into the back	Differential pulses (upper extremity > lower extremity); Aortic regurgitation murmur	ST depression and T wave inversion; ST elevation in the inferior leads (if RCA involved)
Pulmonary embolism	Pleuritic chest pain; Dyspnea	Chest region	Diaphoresis; tachycardia; dyspnea	Sinus tachycardia; new RBBB; S1Q3 pattern; normal ECG
Cholecystitis	Upper abdominal pain plus chest pain	RUQ of abdomen	Tenderness in the RUQ	Normal or nonspecific ST; T changes; ST elevation in inferior leads
Esophagitis	Burning chest pain	Mid or upper precordial region	Normal examination	Normal or nonspecific ST; T changes
Peptic ulcer disease	Abdominal or chest pain	Upper abdomen or lower precordial region	Mild tenderness in upper abdomen	Nonspecific or normal ECG
Chest wall pain	Chest pain that tears or is positional; can be continuous for hours	Lateral chest or precordium	Palpable discomfort or no abnormalities	Normal ECG

Abbreviations: ECG = electrocardiogram; JVP = jugular venous pulse; LBBB = left bundle-branch block; MI = myocardial infarction; PR = PR interval; RBBB = right bundle-branch block; RCA = right coronary artery; RUQ = right upper quadrant.

or by the presence of more than 2 mm ST depression accompanied by an R/S ratio greater than 0.8 in leads V_1-V_2-V_3.

The diagnosis of right ventricular AMI is facilitated by finding ST elevation (greater than 1 mm) on the right-sided precordial leads V_3R and V_4R. I recommend that the right-sided precordial leads be obtained whenever acute right ventricular infarction is suspected (such as in nearly all patients with inferior wall STEMI).

Patients presenting with a new left bundle-branch block (LBBB) and the clinical symptoms typical of STEMI should be considered to have the clinical equivalent of STEMI. Several studies have demonstrated that patients with a new LBBB-associated AMI have high mortality risks compared with other patients suffering AMI. Acute reperfusion therapy should be considered in patients presenting with a new LBBB associated AMI.

One may also see ST segment depression on the ECG of a patient suffering STEMI. The presence of concurrent ST segment depression is a high-risk marker and often reflects an underlying substrate for more extensive coronary artery disease. These electrocardiographic changes should not be ignored, or simply referred to as reciprocal changes accompanying the STEMI pattern, given their prognostic and diagnostic utility.

The rapid diagnosis of STEMI facilitates the triage of those patients to acute reperfusion therapy who will benefit from it the most. Previous work has demonstrated that the presence of STEMI is most commonly associated with complete coronary artery occlusion, and that prompt use of acute reperfusion therapy is associated with significant reductions in short- and long-term mortality risks.

Biomarkers

Plasma biomarkers including creatine kinase (CK), the MB isoform of creatine kinase (CK-MB), myoglobin, and the cardiac troponins (cTnT, and/or cTnI) are all very helpful in the diagnosis of AMI. The gold standard of diagnosis is now an elevation of a cardiac troponin (cTnT or cTnI). Newer biomarkers including plasma myoglobin and the cardiac CK-MB isoforms and more established biomarkers such as CK and CK-MB are also helpful at identifying the myocardial necrosis that accompanies STEMI.

The most recent AHA/ACC/ESC* guidelines for diagnosis of AMI prespecifies the presence of a rapid rise and fall of a cardiac troponin in the setting of typical clinical symptoms. The cardiac troponins are

*American Heart Association/American College of Cardiology/European Society of Cardiology.

the most specific biomarkers for acute myocyte necrosis, because the assays used measure the cardiac-specific isoforms. The cardiac troponins appear in plasma 4 to 6 hours after the onset of necrosis. Myoglobin appears earlier but is less specific. The troponins may remain elevated for several days, while CK-MB tends to normalize after 36 to 48 hours.

It is ideal to draw a cardiac biomarker profile in patients within 20 minutes of arrival at the hospital with chest pain, and then perform serial sampling every 6 to 8 hours until it is clear that elevation of the cardiac troponin has occurred. Our practice is to sample for cTnT and, once elevated, to confirm the acute nature of the risk by sampling for CK-MB if the clinical nature is not clear cut. The need for sampling for CK-MB in patients with new onset STEMI appears nonexistent. It is important to frequently sample after any degree of cTn biomarker elevation to document the peak and decline of the biomarker profile. If there is recurrent chest pain during the hospitalization, it is prudent to resample for troponin as well CK and CK-MB to look for evidence of reinfarction. The diagnosis of reinfarction may not always be reliably made with the troponin biomarkers because of the persistence of the initial elevation.

Additional biomarkers have emerged that offer prognostic data in patients with STEMI. Patients with elevations of C-reactive protein (CRP) and B-type natriuretic peptide (BNP) have increased short- and long-term risks for mortality and reinfarction. The use of these biomarkers is discussed later in this article.

TABLE 2 Strategies in the Initial Management of Suspected Acute Myocardial Infarction (MI)

Time Frame	Goal to Achieve in the Management of Suspected Acute MI in the Emergency Department
10 min	Obtain 12-lead ECG. Administer supplemental oxygen (2-4 L by nasal cannula) Administer aspirin (four 81 mg tablets chewed) Obtain focused history and physical examination
20 min	Review 12-lead ECG (call for cardiology consultation if unclear) Review chest radiograph Obtain blood chemistries (CBC, lipids, and cardiac biomarkers) Administer heparin Administer β blockers Consider IV nitroglycerin
30 min	Initiate reperfusion strategy Administer narcotic analgesia Transfer to coronary care unit (CCU)

Abbreviations: CBC = complete blood count; ECG = electrocardiogram.

Treatment of Acute Myocardial Infarction

INITIAL TREATMENT OF SUSPECTED ACUTE MYOCARDIAL INFARCTION

The initial evaluation and management of a patient with suspected STEMI should be standardized in every hospital. Myocardial necrosis and salvage are time dependent. Delays in the accurate diagnosis and initiation of treatment of AMI can result in greater myocardial necrosis and elevated mortality rates. Table 2 suggests goals that should be achieved in every patient within 30 minutes of hospital arrival.

Aspirin

Aspirin should be administered to all patients with AMI unless contraindicated by a known allergy. The patient should chew 325 mg of aspirin immediately. Chewed aspirin is absorbed from the buccal mucosa and inhibits platelet aggregation within minutes. Aspirin reduced 35-day AMI mortality by 23% in the Second International Study of Infarct Survival (ISIS)-2 study. Aspirin should be continued indefinitely. For the rare patient with aspirin intolerance or allergy, one can consider substitution with clopidogrel (Plavix), 75 mg per day. Clopidogrel inhibits platelet aggregation via a cAMP-dependent pathway, and is currently being tested in combination with intravenous fibrinolytic therapy in patients with STE AMI. Clopidogrel is routinely administered following percutaneous coronary intervention (PCI) in patients with STEMI. We generally continue it for a minimum of 3 months following PCI and often continue it for up to 1 year in high-risk patients.

Oxygen

Oxygen should be administered by nasal cannula to any patient presenting with suspected AMI. Administration of supplemental oxygen improves arterial oxygen saturation and increases oxygen delivery to the ischemic myocardium. No randomized trials have tested its efficacy. Oxygen therapy need not be continued beyond the initial few hours of hospitalization unless clinically indicated.

Analgesia

Intravenous morphine can be administered in small doses (1 to 5 mg IV administered 1 mg per minute) to alleviate or reduce the discomfort associated with the AMI as well as to reduce myocardial oxygen demand. Morphine sulfate also reduces the acute anxiety response frequently observed with AMI. Use of intravenous morphine sulfate can reduce cardiac preload, especially in patients who are volume dependent, and it can result in hypotension. For this reason, it should be used with caution in suspected acute right ventricle (RV) infarct patients. If hypotension develops, the patient should receive intravenous saline to restore cardiac preload.

REPERFUSION THERAPY

Acute reperfusion therapy (Table 3) should be initiated in all patients with suspected AMI who

TABLE 3 STEMI Fibrinolytic Therapy

Indications	Relative Contraindications
1. Typical chest pain >30 min but <12h	1. H/O stroke
and	2. Active bleeding
	3. BP >180 systolic
2. ST ↑ in >2 contiguous leads	4. Major surgery/trauma in last 3-6 months
a. ≥1 mm in limb leads	
b. ≥2 mm in chest leads	5. Recent noncompressible vascular puncture
or	6. Possible intracranial event/ unclear mental status
ST ↓ in only V_1 and V_2 >2 mm	
or	7. Pregnancy
New LBBB	

t-PA (alteplase [Activase])-15 mg bolus then 0.75 mg/kg for 30 min (not >50 mg) then 0.5 mg/kg over 60 min (not >35 mg). Total dose ≤ 100 mg.
SK (streptokinase [Streptase]) - IV SK 1.5 million units infused over 60 min.
Reteplase (Retavase) - 2 IV bolus doses of 10 U given 30 min apart.
TNK-tPA (tenecteplase [TNKase]) – Weight adjusted: <60 kg: 30 mg; 60-70 kg: 35 mg; 70-80 kg: 40 mg; 80-90 kg: 45 mg, >90 kg: 50 mg (not to exceed 50 mg) given as a single IV bolus.
Abbreviations: H/O = history of; LBBB = left bundle-branch block; ST = ST segment; STEMI = ST elevation myocardial infarction.

present within 6 to 12 hours of symptom onset and meet any of the following ECG criteria:

- ST segment elevation greater than 1 mm in two contiguous limb leads or greater than 2 mm in two contiguous precordial ECG leads
- New left bundle-branch block (LBBB)
- ST segment depression of greater than 2 mm in leads V_1 + V_2 with R/S ratio greater than 0.8 (acute posterior MI), or ST segment elevation greater than 2 mm in the posterior leads V_7, V_8, or V_9
- ST segment elevation of greater than 1 mm in lead V_1 + V_3R or V_4R (acute RV infarction)

Intravenous fibrinolytic therapy should not be administered in patients with ST segment depression MI as the available data suggests no benefit and potential harm. Acute posterior MI is an exception.

Fibrinolytic Therapy

Table 3 lists the currently available intravenous fibrinolytic agents for treatment of AMI. Recombinant tissue-type plasminogen activator (t-PA) (alteplase [Activase]), reteplase (Retavase), and tenecteplase (TNKase) are fibrin-specific agents; while streptokinase (Streptase) is a nonspecific agent. The fibrin-specific agents have been demonstrated to establish reperfusion more quickly and effectively than streptokinase, although all are effective in AMI at limiting infarct size and reducing short- and long-term mortality. The GUSTO-1 (Global Utilization of Streptokinase and Tissue Plasminogen Activator for Occluded Coronary Arteries) trial demonstrated that recombinant t-PA was associated with reduced 30-day mortality compared with intravenous streptokinase. The GUSTO-1 trial demonstrated that the enhanced fibrinolytic efficacy of alteplase compared with streptokinase came at a greater risk of intracranial hemorrhage, especially in those older than the age of 70 years.

One of the oldest available intravenous fibrinolytic agents is streptokinase (Streptase). Intravenous streptokinase should be administered as 1.5 million units over 30 to 60 minutes. Intravenous fluids can be administered if hypotension develops during the infusion of streptokinase. It is best not to administer streptokinase more than once to any individual patient out of concern of the development of circulating antibodies, which reduce efficacy. The use of streptokinase in the United States has diminished greatly over the past few years.

Intravenous t-PA (alteplase [Activase]) is a widely used intravenous fibrinolytic agent. It is administered in a weight-adjusted dose (see Table 3), given as a 15 mg bolus, followed by a 0.75 mg/kg dose infused over 30 minutes (not to exceed 50 mg), which is then followed by a 0.50 mg/kg dose infused over 60 minutes (not to exceed 35 mg). The total infusion time for intravenous t-PA should be 90 minutes, and the total dose should not exceed 100 mg.

Reteplase (r-PA [Retavase]) is a fibrin-specific agent modified from wild-type alteplase. The GUSTO-3 trial compared intravenous t-PA with reteplase and demonstrated no significant differences between reteplase and t-PA with regard to reduction in rates of mortality and risk of hemorrhage. Most clinicians accept the agents as clinically equivalent. Intravenous reteplase is given as two 10-unit boluses administered 30 minutes apart. Intravenous reteplase does not require weight based dosing, which some feel simplifies its usage compared with t-PA and tenecteplase.

Tenecteplase (TNKase) is the most recent FDA-approved intravenous fibrinolytic agent. Tenecteplase is derived from t-PA with specific amino acid substitutions that prolong its plasma half-life and allow it to be administered as a single bolus over a few seconds. It has been extensively tested in comparison with t-PA. The Assessment of the Safety and Efficacy of a New Thrombolytic (ASSENT) 2 trial demonstrated equivalency with t-PA with regard to improved survival at 30 days and 1 year in patients with STEMI. Additionally, there were fewer major bleeding episodes reported in the tenecteplase group as well as a reduced need for blood transfusions.

Finally, there are additional intravenous fibrinolytic agents being tested in phase 2 and 3 clinical trials including staphylokinase* (SAK STAR), a highly fibrin-specific, 136 amino acid protein secreted by some strains of *Staphylococcus aureus*. It remains unclear when any of the newer agents might be brought to market.

Selection of a Fibrinolytic Agent

The use of a bolus fibrinolytic agent (tenecteplase or reteplase) is often easier than one requiring a

*Investigational drug in the United States.

prolonged infusion (streptokinase or t-PA), and evidence suggests that use of a bolus fibrinolytic is accompanied by a reduced risk for dosing errors, infusion errors, and complications from such errors. Data has demonstrated an association between increased short-term mortality risks and dosing and/or infusion errors during initial treatment of STEMI. More importantly, it is crucial for every hospital system to have in place a well-designed, well-organized approach to initiation of acute reperfusion therapy in STEMI, so that errors from delay of initiation of reperfusion therapy, errors from dosing and infusion rate administration, and errors from failure to use proper adjunctive anticoagulation and antiplatelet therapies are minimized.

The fibrin-specific agents should be administered concurrently with IV unfractionated heparin (UFH) to reduce the risk of late reocclusion of the infarct-related artery following fibrinolysis. A common mistake encountered in clinical practice is the failure of treating centers to administer IV UFH in a timely manner with the intravenous fibrinolytic agent. I recommend that IV UFH be administered as a bolus immediately before use of the fibrinolytic agent to ensure it is not forgotten during the acute treatment of STEMI. Some even advocate use of intravenous UFH following streptokinase to simplify hospital protocols and maintain consistency for the nursing staff, but in general IV UFH is not needed in combination with streptokinase unless there is a concurrent clinical need for heparin anticoagulation such as anterior MI with LV thrombus or atrial fibrillation.

Intravenous fibrinolytic therapy should be administered as early as possible in STEMI. The agents should be maintained in the emergency department, and door-to-needle times should be kept as low as possible, ideally no longer than 30 minutes. Each emergency department must have a well thought out and planned strategy for triage and treatment of patients with STEMI. The decision to administer fibrinolytic therapy should be made by the evaluating physician in the great majority of cases. There is typically no need for a cardiac consultation unless the treating physician is concerned because the patient has a relative contraindication.

Contraindications to intravenous fibrinolytic therapy must be considered before initiation of therapy. Absolute contraindications include:

- History of intracranial hemorrhage
- Uncontrolled hypertension, defined as systolic blood pressure (SBP) greater than 180 mm Hg or diastolic blood pressure (DBP) greater than 100 mm Hg
- Recent surgery (1 month or less)
- Recent vascular puncture in a noncompressible region (less than 2 weeks)
- Unclear mental status
- Active gastrointestinal (GI) bleeding
- Aortic dissection
- Acute pericarditis
- Prolonged (greater than 10 minutes) cardiopulmonary resuscitation.

Relative contraindications to intravenous fibrinolytic therapy include:

- Prior stroke (nonhemorrhagic)
- Major surgery (3 months or less)
- Pregnancy
- Bleeding diathesis
- Active peptic ulcer disease

Minor hemorrhage, menstruation, and diabetic retinopathy are not contraindications to fibrinolytic therapy.

Primary Percutaneous Coronary Revascularization

Primary percutaneous coronary revascularization (PCR) is an effective treatment strategy in STEMI. It should be initiated within 75 to 90 minutes of hospital arrival. Primary PCR, when performed at a center with significant expertise and experience, is more effective at establishing coronary reperfusion than intravenous fibrinolytic therapy, and it is associated with a reduced risk of stroke and intracranial hemorrhage. A recent meta-analysis suggested that primary PCR is superior to fibrinolysis with regard to reductions in early mortality, repeat MI, and stroke. There are very few contraindications to the use of primary PCR. The only absolute contraindication to primary PCR is when concurrent heparin therapy cannot be given.

The limitation to primary PCR is that most hospitals in the United States are not equipped to perform it 24 hours per day, and many centers lack the necessary expertise. It is very appropriate to use intravenous fibrinolytic therapy when primary PCR is unavailable, or when the angioplasty operator cannot achieve the thrombolysis in myocardial infarction (TIMI-3)-3 flow rates that are observed with lytic therapy. The decision of using fibrinolysis versus primary PCR should be based on what is most readily available for the patient. For patients who present more than 45 minutes away from a center with available primary PCR, it is best to administer intravenous fibrinolytic therapy rather than delaying reperfusion therapy with a center-to-center transfer. Myocardial salvage and mortality reduction are time-dependent processes. Indeed, recent data demonstrates that patients who receive intravenous fibrinolytic therapy within 60 minutes of symptom onset have very low in-hospital mortality and salvage large amounts of myocardium.

Transfer for Primary Percutaneous Coronary Revascularization or Start Fibrinolytic Therapy?

A current debate among cardiologists is whether to treat STEMI patients presenting at hospitals without catheterization laboratory facilities with an intravenous fibrinolytic agent or start adjunctive anticoagulation and antiplatelet therapies and transfer to a center equipped for primary PCI. Data from the DANish Trial in Acute Myocardial Infarction (DANAMI)-2 suggests lower 30-day and 1-year mortalities in patients who were randomized to a transfer strategy rather than receiving intravenous fibrinolysis. Equally provocative was data from the Comparison of Angioplasty and Prehospital Thrombolysis in Acute Myocardial Infarction (CAPTIM) group in France where early use of intravenous fibrinolytic therapy for STEMI was associated with slightly lower 30-day mortality risks than the patients who were randomized to a strategy of transfer for primary PCI. There is no international consensus on this issue yet. It is our practice to continue to recommend use of intravenous fibrinolytic therapy for patients who present more than 30 minutes away from a PCI center unless they are presenting late in the course of STEMI (more than 6 hours from symptom onset).

A subset of STEMI patients present in cardiogenic shock at the time of initial presentation with their STEMI. Data from the SHould we emergently revascularize Occluded Coronaries for Cardiogenic ShocK (SHOCK) trial suggests that an aggressive treatment approach in younger shock patients, including early use of primary PCI, improves survival at 30 days. A decision about initial reperfusion therapy in patients with STEMI presenting in shock should be discussed with a consulting cardiologist. However, in general, the earlier one can initiate reperfusion therapy in these patients the greater the likelihood of reperfusion and salvage of ischemic and infarcting myocardium.

As in all clinical decisions, one must individualize decisions regarding therapies by taking into account the individual issues unique to each patient encounter.

Rescue or Early Nonrescue Primary Percutaneous Coronary Revascularization

The use of rescue PCI remains an important clinical tool for patients with ongoing ischemia following intravenous fibrinolytic therapy. Criteria for consideration of use of rescue PCI include failure of ST segment elevation to resolve more than 70% within 90 minutes of initiation of fibrinolytic therapy, patients with ongoing chest pain or ischemia, and patients with evidence of reinfarction (re-ST elevation or reelevation of cardiac biomarkers). There are several ongoing or recently completed clinical trials examining the role of rescue PCI following intravenous fibrinolytic therapy, and it is expected that data from these studies will enhance understanding in the future regarding the optimal use of rescue PCI.

There is no consensus regarding the early (less than 24 hours) elective use of PCI following intravenous fibrinolytic therapy, especially in patients in whom successful reperfusion has occurred. Some centers practice it routinely and others use an ischemia-driven approach. There are randomized clinical trials examining the benefit of elective PCI following successful fibrinolysis that will provide better insight into this issue in the near term.

ANTITHROMBOTIC THERAPIES

Unfractionated Heparin

Intravenous unfractionated heparin[1] (UFH) should be used at the onset of hospital presentation for STEMI and just preceding administration of intravenous fibrinolytic therapy. Failure to use UFH at the time of initiation of fibrinolytic therapy is a common mistake encountered in clinical practice today. Some centers have wrongly believed that the newer fibrin-specific fibrinolytic agents do not require concomitant use of UFH. Use of a fibrin-specific fibrinolytic agent (t-PA, reteplase, tenecteplase) requires concurrent use of UFH. Heparin is administered intravenously as a 60 units/kg bolus (not to exceed 4000 units) and as an infusion of 12 units/kg per hour (not to exceed 1000 units per hour). The heparin dose should be adjusted to keep the activated partial thromboplastin time (APTT) between 50 and 70 seconds. It is important to avoid wide swings in the APTT values, especially to values greater than 80 seconds. Over-anticoagulation at 12 hours following initiation of intravenous fibrinolysis has been associated with significantly higher risks of short-term mortality. I recommend frequent sampling of the APTT during the initial 48 hours of treatment of STEMI, when UFH is typically administered. At a minimum, the APTT should be evaluated 4 to 6 hours following heparin bolus and then checked every 6 to 8 hours thereafter.

Most clinicians now continue UFH for 48 to 72 hours following use of intravenous fibrinolytic therapy, but there is little outcome data to drive this decision. It is very reasonable to continue heparin for 5 to 7 days in patients with large anterior infarctions and in patients with atrial fibrillation. Warfarin (Coumadin) can be used when there is a need for chronic anticoagulation (atrial fibrillation, left ventricular EF less than 30%) with a target international normalized ratio (INR) of prothrombin time range of 2.0 to 3.0. Some patients will present with an AMI who are on chronic warfarin therapy. These patients should receive intravenous UFH in a manner similar to those not on warfarin but with the understanding that their short-term bleeding risks are increased.

Low-Molecular-Weight Heparins

Some centers are using low-molecular-weight heparins (LMWH) (enoxaparin [Lovenox][1] or dalteparin [Fragmin][1]) in place of intravenous UFH. Low-molecular-weight agents have not been adequately tested in combination with intravenous fibrinolytic agents or with primary PCR, and cannot be recommended for widespread use. There are several ongoing clinical trials testing the initial use of a LMWH with use of fibrinolytic therapy. Certainly, the low-molecular-weight agents can be substituted for UFH

[1]Not FDA approved for this indication.

on day 2 and beyond for those who require extended heparin therapy.

Hirudin and Bivalirudin

Direct thrombin inhibitors like hirudin[1] and bivalirudin[2] continue to occupy an evolving role in the treatment of patients with AMI. Both have been demonstrated to be more efficacious than intravenous UFH, especially in patients receiving fibrinolytic therapy with streptokinase. Despite the proven efficacy, their use is not widespread in the management of AMI.

Glycoprotein IIb/IIIa Antagonists

There is a growing use of the potent platelet glycoprotein IIb/IIIa[1] receptor antagonists in AMI. Most of the data demonstrating efficacy has occurred in patients with non-ST elevation MI. These agents are now being tested in STEMI.

Use with Fibrinolytic Therapy

Recently, the combination of a glycoprotein IIb/IIIa receptor antagonist with an intravenous fibrinolytic agent has been tested to see if the combination would enhance *fibrinoplatelet lysis*. The data have suggested mixed results. As a consequence, the use of such combination therapy is not clinically used widespread nor is it recommended in the near-term. Ongoing studies to optimally define how the combination of a fibrinolytic agent and a glycoprotein IIb/IIIa antagonist might be used will provide further insight. This strategy of combined therapy should not be routinely used until the final results of these trials are reported.

Use with Primary Percutaneous Coronary Revascularization

This strategy of facilitated PCI, using a glycoprotein IIb/IIIa antagonist with PCI has been tested and remains under investigation. There is clear data that use of an intravenous glycoprotein IIb/IIIa antagonist during PCI in the catheterization laboratory reduces complication and mortality risks. Some are now testing the *upstream* use of these agents in emergency department (ED) settings before transfer of patients to the catheterization laboratory for primary PCI.

[1]Not FDA approved for this indication.

[2]Not available in the United States.

Use Following Failed Fibrinolysis

The use of an intravenous glycoprotein IIb/IIIa antagonist in patients with failed fibrinolytic therapy is an area of emerging interest. Post-hoc data from clinical trial registries suggest that use of a glycoprotein IIb/IIIa antagonist in this setting is accompanied by increased risk of bleeding at the time of and following rescue PCI. Despite these risks, there are occasions when it may be appropriate to use a glycoprotein IIb/IIIa antagonist along with intravenous UFH in a patient with re-STEMI or failed fibrinolysis as a temporizing strategy to bridge to rescue PCI.

ADJUNCT MEDICAL THERAPY (Table 4)

Aspirin

Aspirin and/or clopidogrel (Plavix) should be continued in all patients with STEMI (without allergies to these agents) at time of hospital discharge. Many patients will be on both agents for a period of 3 to 12 months. It is my practice to reduce the aspirin dose to 81 mg when the patient is concurrently taking clopidogrel. It is expected that aspirin will be continued indefinitely in most patients who have suffered STEMI. Most patients with STEMI will not need clopidogrel therapy for longer than 1 year following hospital discharge.

β Blockers

β blockers are an important adjunct therapy in AMI as they reduce heart rate, lower blood pressure, reduce cardiac contractility, and reduce myocardial oxygen demand. They also reduce myocardial infarct size, alleviate the pain of AMI, reduce the likelihood of developing complications of AMI, and also reduce mortality from AMI. β Blockers remain underused in clinical practice despite the data demonstrating efficacy from their use in AMI; they should be given to all patients with AMI unless there is a strong contraindication to treatment.

TABLE 4 STEMI Adjunctive Therapy

	Hypotension <80 SYS	Heart Block >1°AV	Bleeding	Severe COPD	Severe Asthma	Renal Failure	History of CHF
β-Blocker	No	No	Yes	Yes	No	Yes	Yes
NTG IV[1]	No	Yes	Yes	Yes	Yes	Yes	Yes
Heparin[1]	Yes	Yes	*	Yes	Yes	Yes	Yes
ASA chew	Yes	Yes	Yes	Yes	Yes	Yes	Yes
Statin	Yes	Yes	Yes	Yes	Yes	Yes	Yes
Ace inhibitor or ARB[1]	No	Yes	Yes	Yes	Yes	Yes*	Yes

*Use if benefits outweigh risks.
[1]Not FDA approved for this indication.
Abbreviations: STEMI = ST elevation myocardial infarction; SYS = systolic; AV = atrioventricular; COPD = chronic obstructive pulmonary disease; CHF = congestive heart failure; NTG = nitroglycerin; ASA = aspirin; ARB = angiotensin receptor blocker.

Contraindications to treatment with a β-blocker include:

- Asthma
- Known allergy
- Presence of high-grade atrioventricular (AV) block at time of presentation
- Cardiogenic shock, hypotension, or severe pulmonary edema
- Heart rate less than 60 at time of evaluation

The presence of mild-to-moderate heart failure, known obstructive airway disease (in the absence of asthma), known peripheral vascular disease, diabetes mellitus, and a history of cardiomyopathy are not contraindications to treatment with β blockers.

β-Blockade can be administered intravenously in the emergency room and then as an oral preparation 6 to 8 hours later. Intravenous agents include metoprolol (Lopressor) (5 to 15 mg IV), atenolol (Tenormin) (5 to 10 mg), and esmolol (Brevibloc)[1] (500 µg/kg bolus, 50 to 100 µg/kg per minute infusion). Esmolol has the shortest half-life and is usually very well tolerated. It is the agent of choice when faced with the marginal patient who appears borderline at best with regard to tolerating the β blocker.

When initiating oral β blocker therapy, it is best to start at the lower end of the dosing range and titrate upward during the hospital stay. It should be noted that the elderly are more sensitive to medications, and it is best to advance medications more slowly in them. We believe it is important to continue the β blocker at hospital discharge given the strong data from randomized trials and large observational databases that consistently demonstrate efficacy in patients post-MI who were discharged on β blockers.

Angiotensin-Converting Enzyme Inhibitors/Angiotensin Receptor Blockers

Angiotensin-converting enzyme (ACE) inhibitors reduce blood pressure and cardiac afterload, resulting in a reduction in myocardial oxygen demand and an improvement in ventriculoarterial coupling. ACE inhibitors favorably alter remodeling following AMI. Multiple randomized trials have demonstrated that these agents reduce short-term mortality in all patients with AMI, and long-term mortality in patients with reduced left ventricular function (LV EF less than 0.40). It is important to start ACE inhibitors during the first day of hospitalization for the AMI, as much of the reduction in mortality occurs in the initial 24 hours. ACE inhibitors should be continued in all patients for 6 weeks, and permanently in those patients with reduced left ventricular function (EF less than 0.40), anterior MI, or transient CHF during hospitalization. Some experts now advocate use of ACE inhibitors in all patients post-MI given the recent data with regard to secondary prevention.

[1]Not FDA approved for this indication.

It is best to start with the lowest dose of the ACE inhibitor and titrate up slowly as the blood pressure allows. It is wise to use a short-acting agent initially, and then switch to a one-per-day agent once it is established that the patient tolerates ACE inhibition. One must use caution with initiating ACE inhibition in patients with moderate renal insufficiency (glomerular filtration rate [GFR] less than 50 cc/min), diabetes mellitus, or pre-existing hyperkalemia because these agents may exacerbate hyperkalemia or worsen renal insufficiency. ACE inhibitors are contraindicated in patients with known renal artery stenosis or a known history of anaphylaxis to the agents.

Angiotensin receptor blockers (ARBs) have emerged as potent agents that reduce afterload similarly to ACE inhibitors. The recent Valsartan in Acute Myocardial Infarction Trial (VALIANT) has shed considerable insight regarding the use of ARBs in the AMI setting. In VALIANT, patients with post-MI CHF or decreased LV systolic function were randomized to captopril[1], valsartan[1], or to a combination of captopril and valsartan. The VALIANT data demonstrate that use of an ARB is comparable (non-inferior) with that of an ACE inhibitor with regard to short- and long-term mortality risk reduction and prevention of recurrent CHF. No benefit from a combination of ACE and ARB therapy is noted in the trial results. The VALIANT data suggest that use of an ARB (valsartan) is comparable with use of an ACE inhibitor (captopril) with regard to mortality and morbidity risk reduction and with a slight benefit with regard to medication-associated side effects.

Lipid-Lowering Treatment

Hyperlipidemia is an established risk factor for CAD. Most patients with AMI have an elevated LDL cholesterol (greater than 100 mg/dL). There are three randomized trials that demonstrate a robust secondary prevention benefit for treatment with statin agents in patients with hyperlipidemia and CAD, including two (Cholesterol and Recurrent Events Study [CARE] and Lipid) that used post-STEMI patients. Both trials show that initiation of statin therapy within 3 months of hospital discharge is associated with improved long-term survival.

Two clinical trials (Plasminogen-activator Angioplasty Compatibility Trial [PACT] and Prevention of Reinfarction with Cerivastatin Study [PRINCESS]) examine whether initiation of therapy during the hospitalization for STEMI compared with initiation following a trial of nonpharmacologic therapy is superior, but neither has published their results. Most clinicians have extrapolated data from the Myocardial Ischemia Reduction with Aggressive Cholesterol Lowering (MIRACL) trial (STEMI and non-STEMI) that demonstrates that initiation of statin therapy (atorvastatin [Lipitor]) within 96 hours of hospitalization for AMI results in improved

[1]Not FDA approved for this indication.

clinical outcomes by 16 weeks following hospital discharge. It is now our clinical practice to initiate statin therapy in all patients with STEMI by time of hospital discharge unless their LDL cholesterol is low at time of assessment.

It is prudent to check the patient's lipid profile during the initial 24 hours of hospitalization. The inflammatory response of the AMI reduces total and LDL cholesterol values by up to 20% within 48 hours after symptom onset. The current National Cholesterol Education Panel (NCEP) Guidelines suggest a target LDL cholesterol of less than 100 mg/dL in all patients with known CAD. It is appropriate to counsel and educate the patient and spouse about the need for a strict low-fat, low-cholesterol diet during the hospitalization and to make plans to recheck the lipid profile 6 to 12 weeks following discharge. The clinician may need to up-titrate the statin dose if the LDL remains elevated at that time (LDL greater than 100 mg/dL). Most recently, clinical evidence has emerged regarding treatment of a low HDL cholesterol (less than 40 mg/dL) in patients with CAD. One should not overlook a low HDL cholesterol at time of hospitalization. The first line of treatment in most patients should be a statin agent, a low saturated fat died, and a prescription for a vigorous exercise program. If the HDL remains low at follow-up, one might consider the addition of niacin or a fibrate to the treatment regimen.

Nitrates

Nitroglycerin dilates the coronary arteries, improves coronary and collateral blood flow to the ischemic region of the myocardium, reduces cardiac preload (which results in reduced myocardial oxygen demand), and controls hypertension associated with the acute anxiety response during AMI. Nitroglycerin also reduces ischemic mitral regurgitation and is effective treatment for symptomatic CHF. Nitroglycerin has been demonstrated to reduce infarct size in experimental models of AMI. Despite these beneficial actions, GISSI-3 (Gruppo Italiano per lo Studio della Sopravvivenza nell'Infarto miocardico) and ISIS-4 failed to demonstrate any reduction in mortality from the use of nitroglycerin in AMI.

It is reasonable to initiate therapy with intravenous nitroglycerin[1] during the initial management phase of AMI if the symptoms of chest pain do not improve after treatment with aspirin, β blockers, and antithrombotic therapies. Caution must be exercised in patients who are volume-depleted and in the elderly. Many patients experience significant relief of anginal symptoms once the nitroglycerin is started. The nitroglycerin dose can be reduced or discontinued if necessary to allow upward titration of the doses of β blockers and ACE inhibitors following initial stabilization.

[1]Not FDA approved for this indication.

Calcium Blockers

Calcium channel blockers (CCBs) have been widely tested in AMI. There is no long-term benefit from use of these agents in acute ST elevation MI. Both diltiazem (Cardizem)[1] and verapamil (Calan)[1] have shown a short-term benefit in non-Q wave MI, but long-term follow-up studies are not supportive of their use. The dihydropyridine class of calcium antagonists should not be used in the absence of concurrent β-blockade in AMI because of their propensity for reflex tachycardia and some evidence that they may increase mortality in AMI. The new generation dihydropyridines, such as amlodipine (Norvasc)[1] and felodipine (Plendil)[1], have not been studied in AMI.

Agents to Limit Infarct Size

There have been several trials examining new strategies to limit infarct size in patients with AMI. A variety of mechanisms have been tested, or are undergoing clinical evaluation. Strategies include:

- Inhibition of the Na/H exchange pump
- Adenosine infusions
- Adenosine-like agonist infusions
- Leukocyte arresting agents
- Use of glucose/potassium/insulin infusions
- Novel strategies to cool the patient prior to use of reperfusion therapy

Most of the data remains preliminary and further work is necessary. Nevertheless, this area of therapeutic intervention remains an exciting venue for additional clinical testing.

Diet

Dietary instruction should be provided to all patients convalescing from AMI. Recently, research findings have emerged that highlight the important contribution of dietary management. First and foremost, patients who are obese should be instructed on caloric restriction as part of a comprehensive management program for obesity management. Those with glucose intolerance should be admonished to lose weight, exercise vigorously, restrict calories, consider substituting complex fiber and more protein for simple carbohydrates, and be instructed to return for early reassessment of glycemic control. A recent large randomized trial of AMI success documented a striking benefit from adherence to a Mediterranean-type diet—independent of cholesterol levels. While the mechanisms of benefit remain unclear, one should consider incorporating these observations into the dietary instruction that is routinely provided to patients while convalescing in the hospital.

Obesity Management

Obesity is a newly recognized risk factor for the development of CAD and AMI, and is an emerging

[1]Not FDA approved for this indication.

epidemic in western society. It is a complex, yet common problem and needs to be addressed prior to hospital discharge following STEMI. A multifactorial approach is warranted including caloric restriction, vigorous exercise, treatment of accompanying medical conditions (diabetes, obstructive sleep apnea) and scheduled follow-up to enhance patient motivation for lifestyle change.

Diabetes Management

Diabetes as a co-morbid condition during time of STEMI increases the short- and long-term risks for death and CHF. Recent work has emerged demonstrating that tighter glycemic control during hospitalization for STEMI may reduce short-term mortality risks. The data suggest that use of insulin protocols during the initial 48 to 72 hours of hospitalization for STEMI results in tighter glycemic control. There are ongoing trials examining whether use of a glucose, insulin, and potassium (GIK) strategy in STEMI improves survival. Long-term management of diabetes following STEMI is less well defined, but in general tighter glycemic control often results in reduced complication risks. Diabetic patients suffering STEMI should be counseled on the optimal management strategies for diabetes and encouraged to exercise vigorously to reduce long-term mortality and complication risks.

Smoking Cessation

Cigarette smoking remains a prevalent risk factor among patients with AMI. It is crucial to address tobacco use while the patient is hospitalized. We recommend that a coordinated effort aimed at promoting smoking cessation be initiated in the hospital and continued into the outpatient arena. There is little data regarding initiation of nicotine replacement therapy (NRT) in the immediate post-MI population. If possible, NRT should be delayed until the patient is dismissed to home, but certainly NRT is preferable to resumption of cigarette smoking.

TARGETED SECONDARY PREVENTION

It is important to initiate appropriate secondary prevention measures in the post-MI patient. It is crucial to target intervention for patients with dyslipidemia, hypertension, diabetes mellitus, and obesity. It is important to encourage patients to stop cigarette smoking. Finally, particular attention must be given to management of psychosocial stress and depression, conditions often overlooked but very prevalent in the post-MI population. The period of hospitalization for AMI allows for a unique opportunity to fully evaluate the patient's risk profile and is often a very opportune time to encourage the patient to contemplate the need for action on risk factor modification.

It is reasonable to allow patients with uncomplicated MI to resume driving an automobile in 1 to 2 weeks and return to work in 2 to 4 weeks. Patients with a complicated STEMI may need to complete 4 to 6 weeks of cardiac rehabilitation before resuming full activities.

Some patients, especially those who are obese and often younger, have concurrent obstructive apnea that will manifest itself during hospitalization for STEMI. It is crucial to address this issue and refer the patient for sleep testing in a timely manner.

Sildenafil (Viagra) and Other Agents Used in the Treatment of Erectile Dysfunction

Many patients with CAD and STEMI suffer from erectile dysfunction. Patients who are immediately post-MI should be cautioned about the use of sildenafil or any other agent in this class of compounds. Patients should be warned about all of the potential side effects including the theoretical possibility of developing angina while using the agent. Patients must be cautioned about the absolute contraindication of taking sildenafil or any agent within this class within 24 hours of nitrate use (oral, topical, sublingual). Following an appropriate convalescence from the STEMI, it is expected that most patients could safely resume use of these agents. Individual circumstances may need to be tailored by the treating physician.

RISK STRATIFICATION

It is important to risk stratify patients with AMI prior to hospital discharge. The GUSTO-1 trial suggested that advanced age, anterior MI location, lower systolic blood pressure at hospital admission, higher Killip Class at hospital admission, and elevated heart rate predicted 90% of the prognostic data regarding 30-day survival. All of these factors are identified on the initial history and physical examination and carry no additional cost to the patient. There are additional ways to risk stratify before hospital discharge with regard to intermediate and long-term survival. Some advocate using risk scoring systems such as the TIMI score, the Primary Angioplasty in Myocardial Infarction trial (PAMI) score, the Mayo score, and others. Some suggest using simple clinical markers as defined in the GUSTO-1 criteria.

High-risk clinical features following STEMI include:

- Presence of CHF or left ventricular systolic dysfunction
- Advanced age
- Renal failure with an estimated GFR less than 50 cc/min
- Presence of mitral regurgitation
- Concurrent ST depression on the presenting ECG and/or the presence of multivessel CAD at time of coronary arteriography
- Diabetes (recognized, unrecognized, or glucose more than 200 mg/dL) at time of presentation with STEMI

- Significant co-morbidities including history of stroke, severe peripheral vascular disease, and severe COPD
- Unrecognized severe diastolic heart failure

All of these co-morbidities must be taken into account when making management decisions in patients with STEMI.

There are biochemical markers that also help stratify patients with STEMI. Elevations of plasma CRP and BNP are associated with increased risks for reinfarction and death, respectively, in patients with STEMI. An elevation of BNP also often helps identify patients with subclinical CHF or systolic left ventricular dysfunction in the setting of STEMI.

It is my practice with regard to risk stratification to routinely measure plasma glucose, plasma creatinine for the estimation of GFR, lipids, and CRP and BNP at the time of hospitalization for STEMI; and to assess cardiac function as outlined in the next section.

Assessment of Left Ventricular Function

Left ventricular function remains one of the best predictors of long-term survival in CAD. It is important to assess LV function following AMI, but there are no data to provide guidance about the proper timing of such assessment. It is clear that left ventricular function may improve in the days to weeks following the AMI, particularly in patients who have received reperfusion therapy. Those patients with a borderline reduction in LV function ($0.40 < EF < 0.55$) should have reassessment at some point in follow-up to determine if there is compelling evidence to continue ACE inhibitors, which may favorably alter remodeling and prevent the onset of CHF symptoms. Early assessment of severe left ventricular dysfunction allows the clinician to more aggressively treat the patient with newer pharmacologic therapies or with surgical revascularization. There are a variety of techniques available to assess LV function including echocardiography, left ventriculography, radionuclide angiography, and cardiac MRI. Some of these techniques can perform both systolic and diastolic function assessments, some can directly quantify infarct size, and some can concurrently assess valvular function. Of all of these, echocardiography remains the most widely available and least invasive technique.

Stress Testing, Holter Monitoring, and Signal-Averaged Electrocardiogram

Treadmill stress testing is an excellent risk stratification tool for patients with AMI. It can identify patients with inducible ischemia following intravenous fibrinolytic therapy who may need catheterization. Treadmill stress testing can also identify patients with exercise-induced arrhythmias. Treadmill testing can be performed at 3 to 4 days following onset of the MI, or be delayed for up to 1 week.

The widespread use of Holter monitoring and signal averaged ECG analysis cannot be recommended in patients who have received intravenous fibrinolytic therapy or primary PCR. These tests may have a role in identifying patients at high risk of arrhythmias who did not receive primary reperfusion therapy, or when reperfusion therapy failed, or was administered late. It is also important to look for ventricular arrhythmias in patients with LV dysfunction.

Angiography

Coronary angiography is frequently performed following AMI. It is indicated in patients with spontaneous or inducible ischemia, recurrent chest pain, and in patients for whom revascularization strategies are being considered for a variety of reasons. There is little data to support the practice of routine angiography following successful fibrinolytic therapy in the absence of ischemia. It is reasonable to perform angiography in patients with heart failure if there is an intention to consider immediate or delayed surgical revascularization for treatment of left ventricular dysfunction. Figure 1 outlines our strategy with regard to decision-making for catheterization.

REVASCULARIZATION STRATEGIES

Percutaneous Coronary Revascularization

Percutaneous coronary revascularization is frequently performed in the post-MI population in the United States. The presence of inducible or spontaneous ischemia is an indication for consideration of early revascularization. To date, there are little data supporting revascularization in the absence of inducible ischemia (see earlier section on use of rescue PCI). However, there are ongoing randomized trials that will evaluate the role of the *open-artery* concept, and the need for revascularization in patients several days post-MI who do not have inducible ischemia.

Coronary Artery Bypass Grafting

The use of coronary artery bypass grafting (CABG) in the AMI and post-MI settings has declined as the use of primary PCR has increased. It is reasonable to consider CABG for patients with inducible or spontaneous ischemia who have multivessel CAD. It is also reasonable to plan for elective CABG for patients with ischemic left ventricular dysfunction and multivessel CAD. The mortality rates associated with CABG are reduced if the acute infarct is allowed several weeks to heal.

Intra-aortic Balloon Counterpulsation

Intra-aortic balloon counterpulsation (IABP) therapy reduces cardiac afterload and improves coronary artery perfusion and systolic blood pressure. The IABP catheter is advanced into the central aorta and

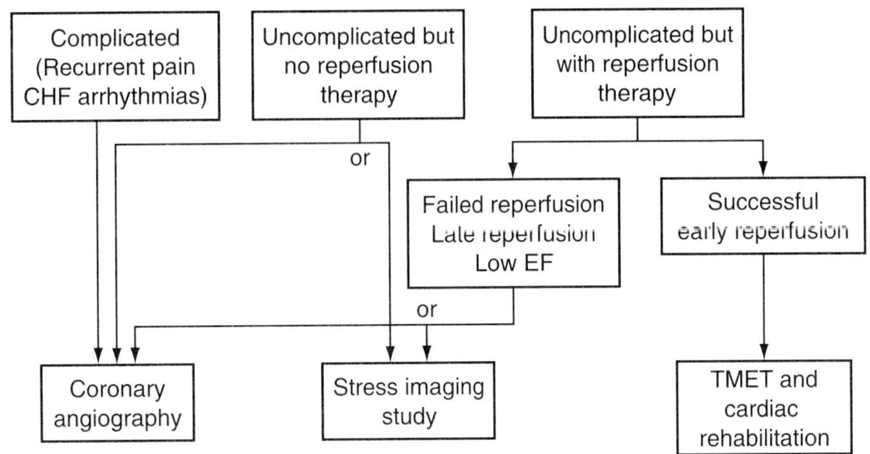

FIGURE 1 Flow chart of reperfusion treatment decisions for acute ST elevation myocardial infarction.

is actively inflated during diastole and rapidly deflated during systole. This action reduces systemic vascular resistance, augments the systolic blood pressure, and improves coronary artery perfusion. The use of IABP in AMI should be reserved for patients with cardiogenic shock, severe heart failure with borderline hemodynamic stability, acute ventricular septal defect or papillary muscle rupture, and as a bridge to high-risk percutaneous revascularization, surgical revascularization, or heart transplantation. The use of IABP is contraindicated in patients with aortic regurgitation or aortic dissection, and it should be used with extreme caution in patients with significant peripheral vascular disease.

Special Situations

CARDIOGENIC SHOCK

Cardiogenic shock is a consequence of inadequate perfusion pressure to the vital organs from ventricular dysfunction. Typically, there is systemic hypotension (SBP less than 80 mm Hg) with a reduced cardiac index (less than 2.2 L/min) in the setting of adequate cardiac preload (pulmonary capillary wedge pressure [PCWP] greater than 16 mm Hg). Shock requires pressor support with agents like dopamine, dobutamine, phenylephrine, and norepinephrine to the blood pressure plus IABP. It is associated with an increased in-hospital mortality risk. Recently, the SHOCK trial demonstrated that a strategy of early angiography and revascularization was associated with a lower 6-month mortality when compared with a less aggressive approach that included early use of IABP and delayed revascularization after initial medical stabilization. The patient with cardiogenic shock should undergo early angiography and percutaneous and/or surgical revascularization in an attempt to reduce the risk of mortality. Despite the use of aggressive revascularization techniques, more than 50% of patients with shock will die during the hospitalization period. It is best to transfer patients with cardiogenic shock to centers with available catheterization laboratories and expertise in managing the situation.

RIGHT VENTRICULAR INFARCTION

Right ventricular infarction (RVI) occurs in up to 40% of patients with acute inferior MI. The mechanism is typically occlusion of the proximal right coronary artery, but not in every situation. Patients may present with unexplained hypotension or with nitrate-induced hypotension, but in the majority the only sign of an RVI is an elevated jugular venous pressure (JVP) without any evidence of hemodynamic compromise. Typical findings on physical examination include elevated JVP, a positive Kussmaul sign, and the presence of right-sided gallops. Additionally, conduction disturbances are common. The diagnosis is established by the presence of a greater than 1 mm ST segment elevation in leads V_1, V_3R, or V_4R; or by demonstration of RV dysfunction by echocardiography.

The treatment of RV infarction is supportive. These patients often require intravenous fluid resuscitation, especially if there has been aggressive diuresis in the emergency room at the time of presentation. The use of inotropic support, often with intravenous dobutamine, is frequently necessary. A pulmonary artery catheter to guide resuscitation is frequently indicated. There can be associated bradycardia or heart block with acute RV infarcts, and the use of temporary atrial and ventricular pacing is sometimes warranted. Recent work suggests that early revascularization with PCR is beneficial in this population.

It is crucial to avoid volume depletion by using intravenous fluid resuscitation, and restricting use of diuretics. You may need to use intravenous inotropes to support the blood pressure and temporary A-V sequential transvenous pacing to treat high-grade AV block.

COMPLICATIONS OF ACUTE MYOCARDIAL INFARCTION

There are a variety of complications that can arise as a consequence of AMI including mechanical complications, electrical complications, and ischemic complications. The nature, diagnosis, and treatment strategies for a variety of AMI complications are presented in Table 5.

TABLE 5 Complications of Acute Myocardial Infarction (MI)

Complications of Acute MI	Clinical Findings	ECG Findings	Treatment
Mechanical			
Ventricular septal defect (VSD)	New systolic murmur that radiates across precordium; may be able to remain supine; elevated JVP; increased RV impulse	Typical septal Q waves; Can see: -Marked ST segment elevation -Bradyarrhythmias -Heart block -Tachyarrhythmias	IABP; Percutaneous closure or urgent surgical repair; Observation
Papillary muscle rupture	New systolic murmur (may be unimpressive in intensity); unable to be supine, often sitting upright; can present as flash pulmonary edema	Resolving ST segment elevation; No need for development of Q waves	IABP; Emergent mitral valve replacement or repair surgery
Ischemic mitral regurgitation	New or more intense holosystolic murmur; may develop CHF symptoms	Resolving ST elevation; pathologic Q waves often	ACE inhibitors or ARBs; diuretics; possible surgical revascularization ± MV repair
Free wall rupture	Recurrent CP; possible unexplained vomiting, pleuritic CP, restlessness and/or agitation, and bradycardia	Re-ST ↑ or failure of ST segments to return to baseline	Emergent surgical repair
Hyperdynamic LVOT obstruction	Unexplained hypotension; unresponsive to IV pressors; possible systolic murmur	ST ↑ or resolution of ST ↑	TEE-confirmed diagnosis; IV fluids to expand volume; IV β blockers; IV phenylephrine to support BP; D/C diuretics, nitrates.
Ischemic			
Postinfarction angina	Recurrent chest pain—hours to days after resolution of initial symptoms	ST depression or re-ST elevation that is transient; T wave inversion	Stabilization with medical therapy; Angiography and revascularization
Infarct extension	Recurrent chest pain with reelevation of biomarkers	ST re-elevation; development of Q waves	Urgent angiography and revascularization
Infarct expansion	Heart failure; Arrhythmia	Q-waves; echo-demonstrated LV aneurysm	ACE inhibitors; ARBs; nitrates; surgical resection
Acute pericarditis	New onset of pleuritic or positional chest pain associated with a new rub	dDiffuse or regional ST elevation with PR depression	Aspirin or indomethacin 25-50 mg tid; No steroids
Electrical			
Ventricular premature contraction (VPC)	Palpitations possible; often asymptomatic	Unifocal or multifocal VPCs	β blockers; K^+, Mg^{2+} within normal limits
Ventricular tachycardia	Palpitations; hemodynamic collapse; syncope; sudden cardiac death	Sustained monomorphic VT	β blockers, nitrates for ischemia; possible revascularization; possible EPS ± amiodarone or PCD
Torsades de pointes	Loss of consciousness; sudden cardiac death	Polymorphic VT	Hypokalemia and hypomagnesemia treatment; bradycardia avoidance; possible temporary pacing; possible antiarrhythmic treatment with IV phenytoin
Ventricular fibrillation	Unexpected, associated with sudden hemodynamic collapse	VF	DC cardioversion; CPR; IV lidocaine; IV bretylium; IV amiodarone; IV magnesium; if occurring beyond first 24h, EPS ± antiarrhythmic ± PCD
Atrial fibrillation	Often marked by onset of palpitations, dyspnea, and angina; poor prognostic sign when occurring with acute MI	Atrial fibrillation ± rapid ventricular response	IV heparin; IV β blockers or oral β blocker for rate control; DC cardioversion; Sotalol or amiodarone antiarrhythmic therapy

TABLE 5 Complications of Acute Myocardial Infarction (MI)—cont'd

Complications of Acute MI	Clinical Findings	ECG Findings	Treatment
2° AV block Mobitz I	Often asymptomatic, can be accompanied by LOC	Mobitz I more frequent with inferior MI	Observation; ↓ or discontinue β blocker
2° AV block Mobitz II	Often asymptomatic; can be accompanied by LOC	Mobitz II more frequent with inferior MI	With: Inferior MI, possible temp PM before proceeding with permanent PM Anterior MI, permanent pacing
3° AV block	Near syncope or syncope	A-V dissociation	Permanent pacing

Abbreviations: ACE = angiotensin-converting enzyme; ARB = angiotensin receptor blockers; AV = atrioventricular; CHF = congestive heart failure; CP = chest pain; DC = dual chamber; EPS = exophthalmos-producing substance; IAPB = intra-aortic balloon counterpulsation; JVP = jugular venous pulse; LOC = loss of consciousness; LVOT = left ventricular outflow tract; MV = mitral valve; PCD = programmable cardioverter-defibrillator; PM = pacemaker; TEE = transesophageal echocardiography; RV = right ventricle; VF = ventricular fibrillation; VT = ventricular tachycardia.

ACUTE PERICARDITIS

METHOD OF

Ralph Shabetai, MD

A common cause of acute pericarditis is viral infection. In many cases, even exhaustive investigation fails to disclose the cause, and clinicians generally do not include viral studies in their evaluation; therefore, for practical purposes, viral and idiopathic pericarditis are considered as the same, so treatment is also the same. Acute pericarditis may conveniently be categorized as simple and complicated (Table 1). Antiviral therapy has yet to find a place in the treatment of acute pericarditis, therefore treatment of simple pericarditis comprises anti-inflammatory and analgesic agents. Treatment of complicated pericarditis requires, in addition, recognition and management of the etiology and treatment of complications such as persistent pericardial effusion, cardiac tamponade, and tuberculosis or purulent infection.

TABLE 1 Features Suggesting that Acute Pericarditis Requires Hospital Admission for Investigation of Etiology and to Provide Optimal Treatment Safely

Persisting large pericardial effusion
Cardiac tamponade; elevated jugular pressure
Suspected purulent pericardial effusion
Tuberculous pericarditis, known or suspected
Failure to respond promptly to anti-inflammatory treatment
Large pericardial effusion in end-stage renal disease or dialyzed patients
Traumatic pericardial effusion

Simple Pericarditis

Frequently, this is a benign condition that often affects the relatively young and responds quickly to simple treatment. Hospital admission is unnecessary provided the patient can be observed closely as an outpatient for the ensuing several days and at decreasing intervals thereafter. Furthermore, detailed evaluation to determine etiology or to exclude other conditions, such as ischemic heart disease, is not justified. Nonsteroidal agents should be employed. Steroid treatment is not only unnecessary, but invites complications. The choice of agent can be left to the practitioner and often is influenced by the patient's prior experience with this class of drug. While newer nonsteroidal agents are often recommended by *experts*, evidence that they are more effective than aspirin is lacking. Very few patients need to be treated with an expensive cyclooxygenase (COX)-2 drug.

Aspirin[1] should be started at high dose, for example, one gram three of four times daily for 1 week to 10 days. Ibuprofen (Motrin)[1] starting with 800 to 1200 mg thrice daily, or indomethacin (Indocin)[1] starting with 50 mg daily taken three times daily is an acceptable alternative. Whichever drug is selected, resolution of chest pain, ST elevation, and PR depression and fever should be anticipated within 48 hours or less. After 2 weeks, the dose can be halved and then tapered over the ensuing 2 to 4 weeks and then stopped. If the patient relates gastric intolerance to these drugs or a history of gastrointestinal problems, prophylaxis with a mucosal protective agent such as omeprazole (Prilosec), 20 mg, or misoprostol (Cytotec), 100 to 200 μg four times daily, with food, is prescribed.

Complex and High-Risk Acute Pericarditis

Most cases that fall into this category (see Table 1) should be admitted to the hospital for close

[1]Not FDA approved for this indication.

observation, including, where indicated, hemodynamic monitoring. Many, perhaps the majority, will not have idiopathic or viral pericarditis; therefore, a thorough search for the etiology is required. Patients who fail to respond to anti-inflammatory immunosuppressive treatment after 24 hours should be treated for complicated acute pericarditis.

RECURRENT PERICARDITIS

In 20% to 30% of cases, acute pericarditis recurs. The recurrences may be single or multiple, may occur soon after the initial episode or after months or years. It is considered to be an autoimmune phenomenon. Pain is often severe and tries the patience of patient and practitioner alike. The patient should be informed that the illness is not another infection, and that long-term sequelae are rare and recurrences eventually cease. As with the initial episode, every effort should be made to avoid treatment with prednisone[1], but resorting to steroidal treatment cannot always be avoided. When prednisone must be given, the starting dose, which is 1 to 2 mg/kg per day, is maintained for about 3 weeks, after which it is tapered by 5 mg every 3 days. If another recurrence is diagnosed, the patient is returned to the lowest dose that suppresses pericardial pain, and maintained there for 3 weeks, after which tapering is attempted again. Patients who require long or repeated courses of high-dose prednisone should have bone density levels monitored. A nonsteroidal anti-inflammatory agent (NSAID) should be given as well. Some reports claim that colchicine[1] (1 mg daily) facilitates avoidance of, and weaning from, prednisone. After multiple recurrences over a period of years, some patients report recurrence of pain, but all objective evidence of pericarditis is absent. Although the explanation is not clear, these patients should be treated for pain, often with help from a pain clinic.

PURULENT PERICARDITIS

Patients with purulent pericarditis are very sick, often with multisystem disease, and frequently are already in an intensive care unit before the diagnosis is suspected. The correct diagnosis is often missed, or made too late. A high index of suspicion is the key to improving this situation. Mortality is alarmingly high, even in the antibiotic era. Any reasonable suspicion of purulent pericarditis mandates exploration of the pericardium via pericardiocentesis or surgical operation. When the diagnosis is confirmed, an infectious disease specialist and a cardiac surgeon must immediately be brought into the treating team. When thick pus is found, and especially if adhesions and organization of the effusion are present, surgical drainage is usually optimal. Cardiologists should defer to the infectious disease specialist for identification and classification of the infecting organism, and direction of the antibiotic regimen, be it supplementary to surgical treatment or the primary modality. The sooner in the course that treatment is begun and the more thorough its supervision, the less likely is the infection to progress to constrictive pericarditis.

TUBERCULOUS PERICARDITIS

Clues to the correct diagnosis include immunosuppressed patients, especially those with AIDS, immigrants from countries where the prevalence of tuberculosis is high, patients who fail to respond to NSAID therapy, patients who have had contact with known cases, and those who have had a recent conversion to a positive tuberculin test. Pericardial effusion is present in the majority. The effusion may be large and can cause cardiac tamponade. Treatment of large or persistent pericardial effusion and cardiac tamponade is reviewed later in this article. Samples should be taken for microscopic examination, culture, and, where suspicion is high, polymerase chain reaction (PCR). In view of the emergence of resistant strains of *Mycobacterium tuberculosis*, and the possibility of infection by mimics such as the bacillus of avian tuberculosis, in these cases too, a cardiologist and an infectious disease specialist should ideally participate in management.

A recommended regimen for adults comprises isoniazid (300 mg daily), rifampin (Rifadin) (600 mg daily), pyrazinamide (15 to 30 mg/kg daily to a total of 2 g per day), and either ethambutol (Myambutol) (15 to 25 mg/kg daily), or streptomycin (20 to 40 mg/kg up to 1 g daily). After 8 weeks, treatment is only with isoniazid and rifampin daily or twice weekly. If the twice-weekly regimen is selected, drug administration should be monitored. Empirical treatment for suspected tubercular pericarditis is seldom warranted, but may be appropriate in immunosuppressed patients. The acute phase frequently leads to effusive-constrictive pericarditis and subsequent constrictive pericarditis. Prednisone is thought to lessen the chance of this complication.

Pericardial Effusion

Any pericarditis can cause pericardial effusion, and any effusion may cause cardiac tamponade. The volume of effusion varies from small to massive. Not all effusions need specific treatment. Examples are small effusion during acute viral pericarditis and small effusion during acute myocardial infarction.

Management of a large chronic pericardial effusion, *not compromising hemodynamics,* and for which the cause cannot be elucidated, is tailored to the patient's circumstances and the physician's preferences. Treatment can be expectant, but it is critically important that the primary care physician following the case be skilled in detecting the early signs of tamponade. In practice, this generally means that the patient is referred to a cardiologist. The patient

[1]Not FDA approved for this indication.

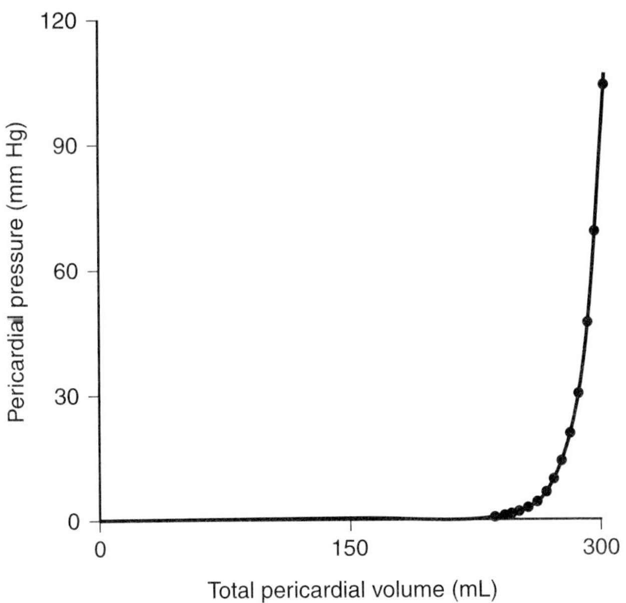

FIGURE 1 Pericardial pressure-volume curve of a normal canine pericardium. The volume does not begin at zero because the volume of the heart has been added. The curve was constructed by infusing fluid into the pericardium. Its J shape shows that the pericardium is compliant when slightly stretched, but rapidly loses compliance and resists with increasing pressure any attempt to increase its volume. Removing a small volume of fluid produces dramatic relief.

must be highly reliable, faithfully keep medical appointments, and not travel frequently or for long periods to places where state of the art cardiology is not readily accessible; otherwise, pericardiectomy is the safest option. The patient is followed for increase in jugular pressure and other signs of tamponade, which, when found and are at least of moderate severity, call for removal of pericardial fluid. Should the effusion recur after one or two extensive draining procedures, pericardiectomy is a reasonable option.

Cardiac Tamponade

Normal pericardial pressure is zero or a few mm Hg lower. Cardiac tamponade is the result of pericardial effusion that has created a significant increase in pericardial pressure, thereby impairing diastolic filling. The increase in pericardial pressure ranges from 3 to 10 to as much as 40 or more mm Hg. Diastolic function is impaired in direct proportion to the severity of this abnormal constraint on chamber filling and compliance. Pericardial pressure of about 7 mm Hg denotes mild tamponade. Often pericardiocentesis is not indicated for mild tamponade, but the patient should be observed and, in cases of borderline severity, monitored until it is clear that the situation is stable. Many such cases respond to NSAID.

Severe tamponade, pericardial pressure of 15 to 40 mm Hg, may be acute, in which case the effusion is *small,* because the normal pericardium is extremely stiff and quickly limits the volume of effusion and fiercely resists distension in the face of a rapid effusion of fluid or blood. For the same reason, aspiration of a small amount of fluid dramatically improves the patient (Figure 1). When tamponade is not acute, the elevation of pericardial pressure can be just as high as it is in acute tamponade, but the effusion varies enormously in size, depending on the rate at which the effusion accumulated. The reason is that when the effusion accumulates over weeks or months, the pericardium remodels and becomes more compliant (Figure 2). As with acute tamponade, it is the earlier aliquots of pericardial fluid aspirated that cause pericardial pressure to drop substantially,

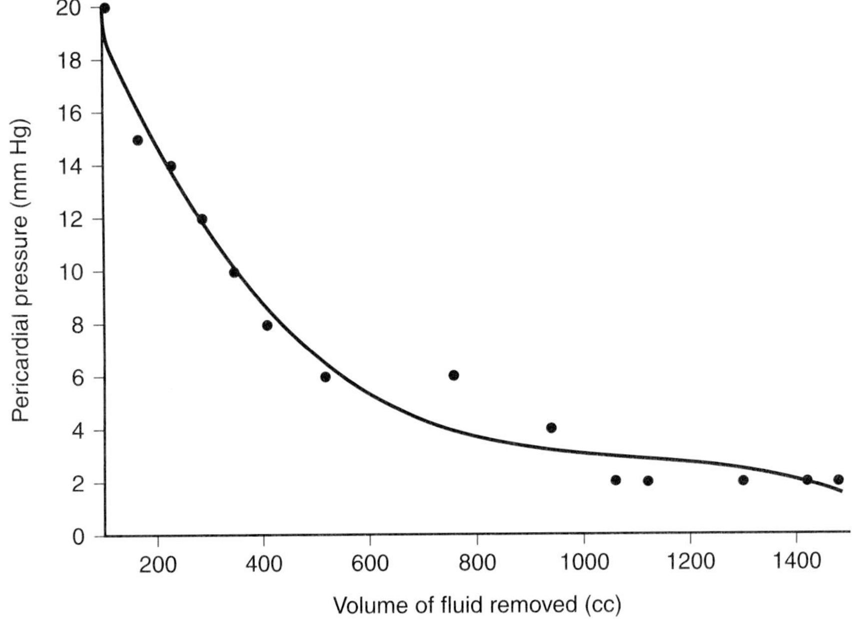

FIGURE 2 Pericardial pressure curve constructed from data obtained during pericardiocentesis of subacute cardiac tamponade. The direction of the curve is opposite from that of the normal curve, as shown in Figure 1, because fluid is being infused in the former, but aspirated in the latter. Note that the pericardial pressure is severely elevated, but that the volume of the effusion is much greater than could be infused into a normal pericardium. Removal of several hundred mL lowered pericardial pressure to 6 mm Hg. The residual effusion did not impair diastolic function.

TABLE 2 Tamponade in Renal Disease Compared with Typical Tamponade

Variable	Classic Tamponade	Tamponade in Renal Disease
Jugular pressure	Elevated	May be low (low pressure tamponade)
Pulsus paradoxus	Usually present	Often absent
Diastolic pressures equalized	RA = pericardial = wedge	RA = pericardial; wedge considerably higher
Reason for atypical findings	Usually absent except in localized tamponade postcardiac surgery	BP+, LVH, CAD, dialysis shunt

Abbreviations: BP+ = hypertension; CAD = coronary arterial disease; LVH = left ventricular hypertrophy; RA = right atrial pressure; Wedge = pulmonary wedge pressure.

but the volume removed is much more than in acute tamponade.

Circulation cannot be maintained when pericardial pressure significantly exceeds cardiac diastolic pressures. The patient with severe tamponade (pericardial pressure 18 or more mm Hg) has severe diastolic dysfunction with dyspnea, anxiety, hypotension, tachycardia, and a profound drop of blood pressure with each inspiration (severe pulsus paradoxus). Inspection of the neck veins shows the central venous press identical to pericardial pressure and thus provides direct evidence of the severity of tamponade. When pericardial pressure is lowered to a nearly normal value, the symptoms and signs quickly and dramatically disappear. Pericardiocentesis for severe acute tamponade is urgent and lifesaving but hazardous, and therefore must be undertaken only by a physician experienced in treating this syndrome. The alternative is surgical drainage. Less severe and less acute tamponade, in which the findings are often less dramatic, is treated by elective pericardiocentesis. Again, only those skilled and experienced with the technique should perform the procedure unsupervised.

UREMIC AND DIALYSIS-RELATED PERICARDIAL EFFUSION AND TAMPONADE

Pre-existing heart disease and hypertension and the volume status greatly modify the findings (Table 2). Uncomplicated effusion often responds well to increased dialysis intensity. Large, nonresponsive effusion may require pericardiocentesis or subxiphoid pericardiotomy.

Patients receiving dialysis may be either hypovolemic or hypervolemic. Hypovolemia is responsible for the paradox of low-pressure tamponade in which central venous pressure is normal or only modestly elevated, because central pressure was very low before tamponade supervened and thus pericardial pressure need not be very high before it compresses the heart. These patients respond to fluid infusion and subsequent pericardiocentesis. Unlike patients with classic tamponade, increased dialysis intensity *worsens* the tamponade. The correct therapeutic choice depends on accurate evaluation of the clinical and echocardiographic findings, and often is beyond the scope of even highly competent primary care physicians.

Constrictive Pericarditis

With constrictive pericarditis, cardiac volume is restrained and diastolic function is impeded by a pericardium that is rigid, often abnormally thick and sometimes calcified (Figure 3). As with tamponade, central venous pressure is elevated in proportion to the severity of compression. Euvolemic patients with a venous pressure less than 10 mm Hg do not need specific treatment, but should be followed for increasing pericardial constriction. Patients with venous pressure around 10 cm H_2O who develop edema require salt restriction and occasional low-dose diuretics. Those with higher venous pressure and more impressive edema are best treated by pericardiectomy. Venous pressure of 15 or more cm H_2O is often associated with anasarca and demands radical pericardiectomy. It is a mistake to treat them with escalating doses of diuretic. The need for high-dose diuretic is an indication for pericardiectomy. The operative mortality in good hands has dropped to 5%.

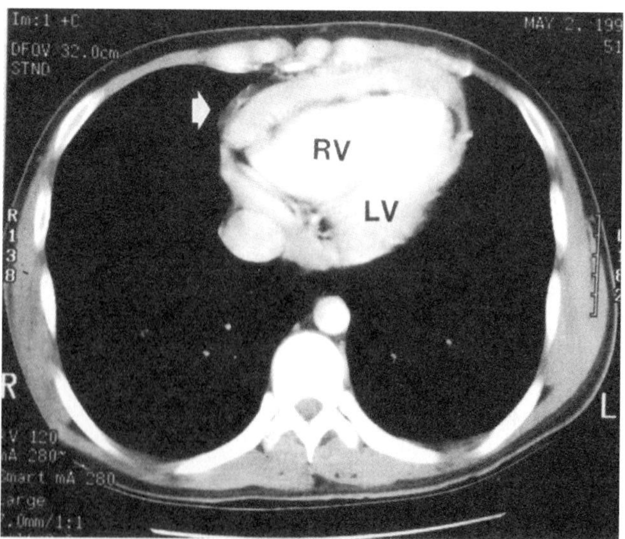

FIGURE 3 Severe constrictive pericarditis. The computer-assisted tomogram shows an extremely thick pericardium caused by mesothelioma. The jugular pressure was 25 mm Hg. As in tamponade, the abnormal external restraint greatly impairs diastolic function. There is no fluid to aspirate; therefore, pericardiectomy is the only effective remedy.

It is critically important to distinguish anasarca caused by cirrhosis, or other noncardiovascular causes, from constrictive pericarditis, but all too often this distinction is not made. The clue lies in the jugular pressure. In anasarca secondary to constrictive pericarditis, pulsation of the internal jugular veins is visible to the ear lobes when the patient is sitting straight up. In patients in whom it is difficult to determine the jugular pressure at the bedside, an echocardiogram quickly shows a dilated inferior vena cava when the jugular pressure is greatly elevated. In patients with anasarca not caused by cardiac or pericardial disease, jugular pressure is normal, or nearly normal, and the size of the inferior vena cava is normal.

Patients with late-stage constrictive pericarditis with anasarca, cachexia, and atrial fibrillation are at high operative risk, and even when the operation is successfully accomplished, the outcome often is disappointing. Consideration should be given to managing them with salt restriction and larger diuretic doses, and by controlling the heart rate. Aspiration of pleural effusion or ascites may be a useful adjunct. The primary care physician is often ideally suited for managing these patients.

Ionizing radiation is a cause of severe constrictive pericarditis, but it also injures the myocardium; therefore, the outcome of pericardiectomy becomes less satisfactory than for pericardiectomy in general. Physicians referring these patients for treatment should be aware of this unfortunate fact and should conduct frank discussions with the cardiac surgeon and family.

Neoplastic Pericardial Disease

Malignancy may cause either pericardial effusion with or without tamponade, constrictive pericarditis, or even both (effusive-constrictive pericarditis). Technical details are not relevant to this article. Pericardiocentesis may be required for patient comfort. The drainage catheter should be left in place until its yield is 50 mL per day to prevent recurrence. This step may also obviate the need to inject a sclerosing agent into the pericardium. In patients expected to survive several months or longer, surgical or balloon pericardiotomy is often performed when pericardial effusions recurs.

The topic of how to manage neoplastic pericardial disease is of paramount importance to family physicians. For far advanced cases with poor prognosis, it is sometimes legitimate to withhold all procedures. Left to the cardiologist, emergency room physician, or the cardiac surgeon, inappropriately radical treatment may be advised, even carried out, before the primary care physician has been consulted. In patients with advanced neoplastic pericardial disease, the oncologist, but more especially the physician who best knows the patient and the family, should retain firm control to the end.

PERIPHERAL ARTERIAL DISEASE

METHOD OF

David H. Pfizenmaier II, MD, DPM, and

Leslie T. Cooper, MD

Peripheral arterial disease (PAD) traditionally refers to disorders of the extracranial, noncardiac arteries. Most commonly, PAD is attributed to a systemic atherosclerotic process that leads to increased cardiovascular and cerebrovascular events. PAD is present in approximately 10 million people in the United States, and more than one half are undiagnosed. People with PAD have a 10-year mortality that is six times higher than in people without PAD. With the increasingly aging population, the recognition and control of PAD becomes paramount to the primary care provider.

This article reviews relevant aspects of risk factors, diagnosis, and presentations of atherosclerotic and nonatherosclerotic PAD. A concise review of the vascular physical examination is provided to emphasize the importance of PAD detection.

Risk Factors for Peripheral Arterial Disease

Risk factors for the development of PAD are the same as those associated with the development of coronary artery disease. Cigarette smoking entails the highest relative risk (2.5 to 10.0), followed by diabetes (3.0 to 4.0), homocysteine (1.7 to 2.6), age in 10-year increments (1.6 to 2.4), hypertension (1.5 to 2.5), and cholesterol elevation (1.1).

Recognition and modification of risk factors are key elements to decreasing mortality and increasing cardiovascular event-free survival in PAD.

Vascular Physical Examination

Screening for and evaluation of vascular disease begins with a thorough clinical assessment of the peripheral circulation. A satisfactory pulse examination includes palpation of the carotid, brachial, radial, ulnar, femoral, popliteal, dorsalis pedis, and posterior tibial arteries. Using the pads of the fingers, palpation of the arterial pulse strength is typically graded using a five-point scale (Table 1). Zero of 4 means the pulse is absent, while 4 of 4 signifies a normal pulse.

Temporal artery tenderness and thickening may signify temporal arteritis, especially in a patient reporting jaw claudication. It is best palpated by gently pressing the second and third fingers anterior and

TABLE 1 Pulse Strength Assessment

Clinical Finding	Grade
Aneurysm (bounding)	5
Normal (easily palpable)	4
Mildly decreased	3
Moderately decreased	2
Severely decreased (faint)	1
Absent	0

slightly superior to the ear. During the examination, the physician should:

- Examine the neck for jugular venous distention and carotid pulsation.
- Avoid compression of the carotid sinus, as bradycardia and syncope may result.
- Auscultate the carotid arteries for bruits, which may signify internal carotid artery (ICA) stenosis, external carotid stenosis, or an unusually tortuous vessel. Perform subsequent ultrasonography to further evaluate for stenosis, especially if the bruit is new.
- Perform bilateral blood pressure measurements as part of the upper extremity vascular examination. Proximal arterial stenosis should be suspected if a difference of more than 10 mm Hg exists.
- Perform the Allen's test, after palpation of ulnar and radial pulses, to exclude distal ulnar or palmar arch occlusion.
- Inspect the hands for edema, rubor, pallor, telangiectasias, and ulceration.
- Palpate the abdomen for aortic size. If width exceeds 3 cm, consider further evaluation with ultrasonography or computed tomography (CT) to evaluate for an abdominal aortic aneurysm (AAA). Bruits of the abdomen suggest arterial stenosis or arteriovenous fistula. Celiac or superior mesenteric artery bruits are best heard at the midline above the umbilicus, and may decrease with inspiration in cases of median arcuate ligament syndrome.
- Auscultate the lateral abdomen for renal artery bruits and the lower quadrants proximal to the inguinal ligaments for iliac artery bruits.

As with the upper extremities, the lower extremities should be carefully inspected for edema, rubor, pallor, and ulceration. A femoral artery bruit suggests atherosclerotic arterial occlusive disease and, therefore, an increased risk of cardiovascular death. Palpation of the popliteal artery and pulse is performed with the fingertips of both hands placed into the lateral third of the popliteal fossa with the knees bent and relaxed. If the estimated width of the popliteal artery exceeds 1 cm, an aneurysm should be excluded by ultrasonography. If a popliteal aneurysm is confirmed, then the patient should also be screened for an AAA, because approximately 33% of patients with a popliteal aneurysm also have AAA. The dorsalis pedis and posterior tibial pulses should be palpated and, if decreased, the legs should be elevated for up to 1 minute to evaluate for elevational pallor. This finding suggests advanced lower-extremity PAD.

Lower-Extremity Peripheral Arterial Disease

Intermittent claudication (IC) is the most common symptomatic presentation of lower-extremity PAD. Symptoms of IC include muscle aching, burning, or cramping that is consistently exacerbated by activity and relieved by several minutes of rest. The location of symptoms can suggest the level of arterial occlusion (Table 2).

Claudication may be caused by nonatherosclerotic conditions such as arterial dissection, popliteal entrapment syndrome, Takayasu arteritis, fibromuscular dysplasia, atheroembolism, and medial cystic disease. IC must also be differentiated from pseudoclaudication, which results from spinal stenosis. Usually IC develops within a predictable distance and improves with standing at rest, whereas pseudoclaudication occurs at variable distances and improves with sitting or bending forward at the hips.

An easy-to-perform, sensitive (95%), and specific (100%) test for lower-extremity PAD is the ankle-brachial index (ABI). With the patient supine, systolic blood pressure measurements of the brachial, dorsalis pedis, and posterior tibial arteries are performed bilaterally. The ABI is calculated for each leg by dividing the higher of the two ankle systolic pressures by the higher brachial systolic pressure. Signs, symptoms, and survival tend to correlate with the degree of arterial occlusive disease and the resultant ABI (Table 3).

A diagnosis of PAD can be made if the ABI is less than 0.95 or if ischemic limb symptoms are present. Patients with PAD have twice the risk of coronary artery disease than those with a normal ABI, as well as increased risk of myocardial infarction, stroke, and death. ABI values greater than 1.3 may be because of noncompressible vessels, as would be seen in calcified diabetic arteries. The gold standard for the anatomic localization of PAD is conventional iodinated contrast angiography. Magnetic resonance angiography (MRA) may be an acceptable alternative, especially in patients with impaired renal function or contrast dye allergy. CT angiography may also evolve into an acceptable alternative.

TABLE 2 Symptomatic Distribution by Location of Peripheral Arterial Disease (PAD)

Area of Claudication	Probable Level of Arterial Occlusion
Buttock, thigh, calf	Aortoiliac
Buttock	Internal iliac
Thigh	External iliac
Calf	Superficial femoral
Arch of the foot	Infrapopliteal vessels

TABLE 3 Implications of Ankle-Brachial Index Stratification

Resting ABI	Degree of PAD	5-Year Survival	Sign or Symptom
>1.3	Indeterminate	Unknown	Variable
0.95-1.3	Normal		None
0.71-0.94	Mild	91%	Asymptomatic or claudication
0.5-0.7	Moderate	71%	Nonpalpable pulses and claudication
<0.5	Severe	63%	Ischemic rest pain, nonhealing ulcer

Abbreviations: ABI = Ankle-Brachial Index; PAD = peripheral arterial disease.

Treatment of lower-extremity PAD begins with aggressive risk factor modification and promotion of foot care. Smoking cessation decreases the risks of surgical bypass and amputation. Guidelines for optimal treatment of diabetes, hypertension, and hyperlipidemia should be followed. A proven effective therapy for IC is a structured walking program of at least 30 minutes per day.

Pharmacotherapy for symptomatic PAD is generally limited and displays variable effectiveness. Antiplatelet therapy is recommended, though placebo-controlled studies are lacking. Pentoxifylline (Trental), 400 mg orally three times daily, has been studied in several randomized claudication trials and was associated with a modest improvement in walking distance during 2 to 26 weeks of use. Cilostazol (Pletal), 100 mg orally twice daily, is a phosphodiesterase III inhibitor for claudication that also has been associated with improvement in walking distance. Cilostazol is contraindicated for patients with heart failure of any severity. It is metabolized by hepatic cytochrome P450 3A4 and 2C19, and, therefore, dose reductions of cilostazol may be required with coadministration of drugs that inhibit these enzymes, such as omeprazole (Prilosec), clarithromycin (Biaxin), erythromycin (EES), itraconazole (Sporanox), fluoxetine (Prozac), sertraline (Zoloft), and diltiazem (Cardizem).

Revascularization with surgical bypass and/or angioplasty is usually reserved for patients who fail medical management or who progress to critical limb ischemia (CLI). CLI is defined as rest pain or ulceration caused by PAD. The pain in CLI is worse with elevation and improved with dependency. Persistent dependency of the lower extremity leads to the typical appearance of rubor and edema.

Acute Peripheral Arterial Occlusion

The clinical hallmarks of acute peripheral arterial occlusion include the six *P*s: pallor, polar (cold), pulselessness, pain, paresthesia, and paralysis. Embolization, thrombosis in situ, and dissection are usually the intravascular mechanisms of occlusion. Extra-arterial causes of occlusion involve extrinsic compression from compartment syndrome, phlegmasia (from extensive deep venous thrombosis [DVT]), or hematoma. The onset of neurologic and muscular symptoms signifies impending limb loss and warrants urgent consultation with a vascular surgeon. Surgical embolectomy and intra-arterial thrombolysis are the most common treatments for acute intravascular peripheral arterial occlusion.

Extracranial Atheroembolic Disease

Blue toe syndrome and livedo reticularis are sequelae of atheromatous embolization to the lower extremities. Risk factors for atheroemboli include trauma from an invasive vascular procedure or catheterization, proximal aneurysmal disease, and severe PAD. The use of anticoagulants and/or thrombolytics may also predispose to an atheroembolic shower, and, therefore, use of these agents as a therapy for atheroemboli is often debated. Complications include severe pain, ulceration, gangrene, limb loss, and renal failure. Treatment is usually supportive with limb protection and warmth, pain control, and optimal wound care. Anecdotally, hydroxymethylglutaryl coenzyme A (HMG-CoA) reductase inhibitors (statins) and antiplatelet agents may be implemented to attempt to reduce recurrence. Patients experiencing recurrent emboli from diffuse atheromatous aortic lesions or ulcers may require aortic surgery.

Nonatherosclerotic Peripheral Arterial Disease

Although most cases of PAD are atherosclerotic, nonatherosclerotic causes of arterial occlusive disease exist and should be considered in the differential diagnosis.

Thromboangiitis obliterans (Buerger's disease) is a segmental inflammatory disease that involves occlusion of the small- and medium-sized arteries and superficial veins of the upper and lower extremities, resulting in digital ischemia and superficial thrombophlebitis. Raynaud's phenomenon may also be seen in approximately 40% of patients. This disease usually affects patients before the age of 50 years and is always associated with tobacco exposure. Suspect Buerger's disease in a case of a smoker with digital ischemia and isolated infrapopliteal and/or forearm arterial occlusive disease. Tobacco cessation is the foundation of treatment.

Fibromuscular dysplasia (FMD) is a noninflammatory cause of arterial occlusion. It is seen more often in women and usually involves the renal arteries, though other peripheral arteries can be involved. Medial FMD produces the classic *string of beads* appearance angiographically, which is diagnostic. Suspect FMD in a case of a 20- to 40-year-old female with rapidly progressive hypertension and a renal artery bruit. Treatment usually involves percutaneous angioplasty or surgical revascularization.

Takayasu arteritis (TA) is an inflammatory vasculitis that usually involves the aorta and its large branches. It can cause aneurysmal and occlusive disease, most commonly in women before the age of 40 years. Suspect TA in a case of a young woman with a vague history of fatigue, arthralgias, and low-grade fever who develops arm claudication and has asymmetric upper extremity blood pressures and pulses. The diagnosis is made via angiography or post-operative pathology analysis. Treatment for active disease begins with high-dose steroids and often includes agents such as methotrexate (Rheumatrex)[1], azathioprine (Imuran)[1], cyclophosphamide (Cytoxan)[1], or mycophenolate mofetil (CellCept)[1].

Giant cell arteritis (GCA) is an inflammatory vasculitis of large- and medium-sized vessels. It usually occurs in women after the age of 50 years and is associated with polymyalgia rheumatica in approximately 33% to 50% of patients. Unlike TA, GCA is associated with high erythrocyte sedimentation rates (>100 mm per hour). Suspect GCA in a case of a middle-aged patient with myalgias and temporal headaches who relates abrupt visual loss and/or jaw claudication. Diagnosis is confirmed with temporal artery biopsy, but a negative result does not exclude GCA. Contrast angiography shows long, tapered narrowing of involved vessels. Treatment is with high-dose steroids, which may be started before a biopsy is obtained.

Popliteal entrapment syndrome (PES) may result from compression of the popliteal artery by aberrant gastrocnemius or popliteus muscles. Anatomic PES leads to occlusive or aneurysmal disease of the popliteal artery and may present with claudication. Suspect PES in a 15- to 50-year-old male having few atherosclerotic risk factors who displays diminished pedal pulses with dorsiflexion and plantarflexion of the ankle. Diagnosis can be obtained by using magnetic resonance imaging/magnetic resonance angiography (MRI/MRA) to define the muscular/arterial relationships, and by using contrast angiography with dorsiflexion and plantarflexion views to determine the extent of dynamic and fixed stenosis. Treatment usually involves vascular repair with musculotendinous resection.

Aneurysmal Arterial Disease

The most common aneurysmal disease of the arteries involves the aorta, which is covered in the article, *Acquired Diseases of the Aorta.* Risk factors for aneurysmal disease in peripheral arteries are similar to those of the aorta—increasing age, hypertension, tobacco smoking, family history of aneurysms, and underlying connective tissue diseases such as Marfan's and Ehlers-Danlos syndromes. Once aneurysms become symptomatic, the risk of rupture increases substantially. While surgical repair remains the standard of care, the use of percutaneous stent grafts is gaining in clinical application and acceptance.

Extracranial Cerebrovascular Disease

Atherosclerosis of the carotid arteries leads to stenosis and increases the risk of stroke via embolization of thrombotic material to the intracranial circulation. In fact, the risk of ischemic stroke is strongly associated with the degree of internal carotid artery (ICA) stenosis. Other risk factors for ischemic stroke include hypertension, male gender, increasing age, tobacco smoking, and diabetes.

ICA stenosis should be suspected in patients with systemic PAD or known risk factors, especially if a bruit is present on examination. The diagnosis is established using duplex ultrasonography to provide anatomic and hemodynamic assessments of severity. MRA or contrast angiography may be necessary in cases where duplex imaging is suboptimal or for surgical planning.

Treatment recommendations for carotid atherosclerosis have been developed based on data collected from several large, prospective, randomized trials (North American Symptomatic Carotid Endarterectomy Trial [NASCET], European Carotid Surgery Trial [ECST], Veterans Affairs Cooperative Study, asymptomatic carotid atherosclerosis study [ACAS]) and upon consensus statements from the American Heart Association. For patients with symptomatic disease (TIA or stroke), carotid endarterectomy (CEA) should be considered in those with 70% to 99% stenosis. In selected cases, CEA may benefit symptomatic patients with 30% to 69% stenosis. For asymptomatic carotid disease, CEA recommendations vary based on expected level of surgical risk and anticipated life expectancy. In patients with a surgical risk less than 3% and a life expectancy of at least 5 years, CEA should be considered in those with 60% stenosis. CEA is considered acceptable in patients with greater than 75% stenosis that have a surgical risk of 3% to 5% and a contralateral stenosis of 75% to 100%.

While surgical CEA is considered to be the standard of care, percutaneous carotid angioplasty and stenting have been gaining acceptance as viable alternatives, though prospective studies are pending.

Arterial Skin Ulceration

Advanced PAD can lead to reduced perfusion of the skin and subsequent ulceration. Ischemic wounds typically involve the distal extremities. Arterial ulcers

[1]Not FDA approved for this indication.

often lack granulation tissue and display either a dry, yellow base or a dark eschar over the wound surface. Unless neuropathy is present, these wounds are often quite painful. Symptomatically, ischemic ulcers usually display pain that tends to improve with dependency and worsen with elevation.

Cutaneous vasculitis or small-vessel occlusive disease can also lead to ulceration. These wounds usually appear *punched-out* with a sharply demarcated edge and have a fibrotic yellow base or eschar. These ulcers tend to be extremely painful—regardless of dependency, elevation, or pressure.

Treatment of ischemic ulcers involves optimal hygiene and protection. An abundance of wound care products exists, each with variable indications and effectiveness. The key to healing ischemic ulcers is to improve tissue perfusion. Ulcers secondary to large- and medium-sized vessel PAD may improve after surgery or angioplasty. This approach, however, is not an option for ulcers secondary to small vessel disease. Enhancing circulating blood flow in the extremities with the use of an intermittent pneumatic compression pump can be an effective therapeutic option for improving pain and wound healing in patients with nonsurgical PAD.

VENOUS THROMBOSIS

METHOD OF

Ali F. AbuRahma, MD, and Patrick A. Stone, MD

Deep venous thrombosis (DVT) was recognized by Rudolph Virchow in 1846 to be associated with embolic sequelae in the lungs. Prior to the twentieth century, venous ligation was the predominate therapy for DVT. It wasn't until 1937 that heparin was introduced into practice, and the diagnosis and treatment of DVT have continued to progress. Despite the increased awareness of this disease and improvement in prophylaxis, approximately 80 cases per 100,000 people are diagnosed annually in the United States. Approximately 600,000 patients are hospitalized yearly with a diagnosis of DVT and/or pulmonary emboli (PE). Thrombosis of the deep venous system results in fatal PE in 200,000 patients each year, and is the leading cause of preventable in-hospital mortality. Of those patients who do not succumb to PE, continued morbidity from chronic venous insufficiency occurs in up to 66%, with at least a 5% ulceration rate during an 8-year follow-up. Health care costs have been estimated to be more than two billion dollars each year in acute treatment alone.

Pathophysiology and Risk Factors

Virchow formulated the triad of venous stasis, endothelial injury, and hypercoagulable state. Usually two of the three inciting events are needed for venous thrombosis to occur. Evidence is accumulating that an inflammatory response is related to thrombosis by initiation or amplification. Once thrombosis occurs within a deep vein, the vein will either recanalize or scar, or the thrombus will dislodge and embolize. The most common site of DVT is in the soleal veins within the calf or behind the valve pockets. Determining those at highest risk is important in the decision to use DVT prophylaxis.

Recognized risk factors for the development of thrombus in the deep venous system have been thoroughly evaluated by epidemiologic findings. As previously published in the Handbook of Venous Disorders by Gloviczki et al, and modified by the American Venous Forum, the highest risk factors are age, surgery, trauma, malignancy, previous DVT, immobilization, primary hypercoagulable states, oral contraceptives, hormone therapy, and pregnancy. Multiple risk factors appear to have an exponential rather than additive risk of developing thrombosis.

AGE

DVT occurs in both the young and the elderly. The risk with age appears to increase nearly two times for each 10 years of increasing age. The influence of age on the incidence of venous thrombosis is likely to be multifactorial. The number of risk factors increases with age; three or more risk factors are generally present in a few percent of hospitalized patients younger than 40 years, but in more than 30% of patients ages 40 years and older. Venous thrombosis is generally rare in children younger than 10 years of age, and almost always is associated with recognized thrombotic risk factors. Multiple risk factors are often required to precipitate DVT in children including spinal cord injuries, prolonged orthopedic immobilization, and hypercoagulable states.

SURGERY

The increased risk of DVT with surgery is dependent on the length and type of surgery (i.e., general surgery, neurosurgery, orthopedic surgery, gynecological surgery, etc.) and the duration of postoperative immobilization. The overall incidence of DVT is approximately 20% in patients undergoing general surgical procedures, 25% for elective neurosurgical procedures, and 50% to 60% among those undergoing orthopedic procedures, such as hip fractures and hip and knee replacements. Accordingly, patients can be classified as being at low, moderate, or high risk for thromboembolic complications as seen in Table 1.

TABLE 1 Risk of Postoperative Deep Venous Thrombosis

Category	Characteristics
Low	Age <40 years, no other risk factors, uncomplicated abdominal/thoracic surgery Age >40 years, no other risk factors, minor elective abdominal/thoracic surgery <30 min
Moderate	Age >40 years, abdominal/thoracic surgery >30 min
High	History of recent thromboembolism Abdominal or pelvic procedure for malignancy Major lower extremity orthopedic procedure

From Hull RD, Raskob GE, Hirsh J: Prophylaxis of venous thromboembolism. Chest 89(5) Suppl:374S-383S, 1986.

Approximately 50% of postoperative lower extremity DVT cases develop at the time of surgery, with the remaining one half occurring primarily in the next several days; however, the risk of thromboembolic events does not end at hospital discharge, and may be delayed up to 6 weeks after surgery. Surgery is generally accompanied by a transient hypercoagulable state secondary to the release of tissue factor, and increased plasminogen activator inhibitor levels, which are also associated with a decrease in fibrinolytic activity on the first postoperative day.

MALIGNANCY

DVT may be a herald for undetected malignancy and found in up to 25% of those with idiopathic DVT. Approximately 15% of malignancies are complicated by venous thromboembolism. Carcinoma of the lung is more prevalent and considered to be the most common malignancy associated with venous thromboembolism, accounting for 25% of cases. An association between mucin-secreting gastrointestinal malignancy and thrombosis has also long been recognized. Another wide variety of malignancies has been associated with DVT, including genitourinary malignancies. Thrombotic events during malignancy are likely to involve multiple factors, including the release of substances that activate coagulation. Tissue factor and cancer procoagulant, cysteine protease activator of factor X, are the primary tumor cell procoagulants; associated macrophages may also produce procoagulants as well as inflammatory cytokines. Approximately 90% of patients with malignancies have abnormal coagulation studies, including elevation of coagulation factors (e.g., fibrinogen or fibrin degradation products and thrombocytosis). In addition, the level of coagulation prohibitors antithrombin, protein C, and protein S may also be reduced in malignancy. Chemotherapeutic agents used for treatment of some malignancies may also be associated with an increasing incidence of DVT.

TRAUMA

Trauma patients have a significantly increased risk for DVT, especially those with increased age, blood transfusions, fracture of the femur or tibia, and spinal cord injury. The prevalence of DVT among autopsied trauma patients has been reported to be 60% to 65%, compared with a 58% incidence in injured patients in a modern series using venography. Lower DVT rates of 4% to 20% have been noted in studies using duplex ultrasonography, although many of these patients were receiving prophylaxis. Several risk factors may be responsible for a high incidence of DVT in trauma patients, including immobilization by skeletal fixation, paralysis, venous stasis in critically ill patients, mechanical injury, and central venous cannulation. Trauma patients may also be associated with hypercoagulable states following depletion of coagulation inhibitors and components of the fibrinolytic system.

IMMOBILIZATION

The longer the immobilization, the higher the risk of thrombosis. Advancing age and inactivity of the calf muscle pump exacerbates stasis in the soleal veins and behind the valve cusps. Both preoperative and postoperative immobilization is associated with an increasing incidence of DVT. DVT among stroke patients is significantly more common in paralyzed limbs than in nonparalyzed limbs. Immobilization has been extended to include prolonged travel, the *economy class syndrome*, which arises after sitting in a cramped position during extended aircraft flights. Further evidence includes PE as the second leading cause of death in those traveling.

HISTORY OF VENOUS THROMBOEMBOLISM

Approximately 25% of patients presenting with an acute DVT have a previous history of venous thrombosis. Several population-based studies have demonstrated that recurrent thromboembolic events occur once in every 10 to 50 patients with a previous episode of thromboembolism, depending on age and sex. Primary hypercoagulable states appear to have a significant role in many recurrences.

PRIMARY HYPERCOAGULABLE STATES

Deficiencies of antithrombin III, protein C, and protein S can cause hypocoagulable states. Also, resistance to activated protein C (factor V Leiden is considered to be the most common cause of hypercoagulable states. Overall, 40% to 50% of patients with lower extremity DVT can be characterized as thrombophilic on this basis, and a family history is associated with a relative risk of 2.9 for venous thromboembolism. Primary deficiencies of protein C, protein S, and antithrombin are present in approximately 0.5% of healthy subjects. Approximately 25% of individuals with factor V Leiden mutation sustain a thrombosis by the age of 50 years, and the prevalence of activated protein C resistance among DVT patients has varied from 10% to 65%.

ORAL CONTRACEPTIVES AND HORMONE THERAPY

The use of oral contraceptives has been established as an independent risk factor for DVT. Most reports indicate an odds ratio of 3 to 11.0 for idiopathic thrombosis with an unweighted summary relative risk among 18 controlled studies of 2.9. The increased risk of thromboembolic events appears to decrease soon after these contraceptives are discontinued. It has been estimated that the use of third generation oral contraceptives may act synergistically with factor V Leiden mutation, increasing the thromboembolic risk 30- to 50-fold. Hormonal therapy also increases the risk of venous thromboembolic events when used for lactation suppression, treatment for carcinoma of the prostate, or postmenopausal replacement therapy.

CENTRAL VENOUS CATHETERS

The increasing use of central venous catheters for hemodynamic monitoring, infusion catheters, and pacemakers has been associated with increasing incidences of thromboembolic events. This is particularly noticeable in upper extremity venous thrombosis, where as many as 60% of thrombi are related to central venous cannulation.

Diagnosis

Clinical evaluation is notoriously inaccurate in the diagnosis of DVT. Pain with plantar extension has been traditionally taught as a classic finding of DVT, as described by Homan, but also has minimal usefulness. Approximately 50% of patients with DVT are asymptomatic. Findings suggestive of thrombus in the deep veins include more than 3 cm calf or thigh swelling, tenderness along the distribution of the deep veins, unilateral pitting edema, erythema, and dilated nonvaricose veins in the symptomatic extremity only. Massive thrombosis of the deep and superficial system can result in phlegmasia alba dolens (pale or white leg) and phlegmasia cerulean dolens (blue leg) with the later a high risk of limb loss if not addressed promptly.

Wells and colleagues have demonstrated that categorizing the patient's pretest probability of DVT into low, moderate, or high probability improves diagnostic accuracy. They demonstrated that combining the use of a model of clinical probability of DVT with venous duplex ultrasound examination decreased the number of false-positive and false-negative diagnoses; they used ascending venography as the definitive diagnostic test. As indicated in Table 2, patients with a high clinical suspicion of DVT have an 85% chance of having venography-proven DVT. Wells et al. also suggested that patients with low pretest probability and a negative noninvasive test result, do not require treatment or additional testing, and those with high pretest probability and positive noninvasive test results should be treated.

TABLE 2 Clinical Signs, Symptoms, and Risk Factors of Deep Vein Thrombosis (DVT)*

Major
Acute cancer
Paralysis/paresis
Recent cast immobilization of lower extremities
Bedridden for 3 days
Major operation within 4 weeks
Tenderness in distribution of the deep venous system
Swelling of thigh or calf (>3 cm)
Family history of DVT (≥ first-degree relatives)
Minor
History of recent trauma to symptomatic leg
Unilateral pitting edema (symptomatic leg)
Dilated (nonvaricose) superficial veins, symptomatic leg only
Hospitalization within the prior 6 months
Erythema
Clinical probability
High
≥3 major points and no alternative diagnosis
≥2 major point and >2 minor points and no alternative diagnosis
Low
1 major point and ≥2 minor points and an alternative diagnosis
1 major point and ≥1 minor point and no alternative diagnosis
0 major points and ≥3 minor points and an alternative diagnosis
0 major points and ≥2 minor points and no alternative diagnosis
Moderate
All other combinations

*Used to develop a clinical model for predicting the pretest probability of DVT.

Overall, the ultimate test to diagnose DVT should be accurate, inexpensive, and noninvasive. Blood tests have been performed for the past two decades with attempts to find a reliable marker to identify those with DVT. D-Dimer has been extensively evaluated and found to have an extremely high negative predictive value. Most recently, Wells and colleagues reported that D-dimer had a negative predictive value of nearly 100% of those with low risk as determined by clinical predictors. Except in this small group of patients, an objective test is needed to assess these patients.

Venous duplex imaging has become the study of choice for evaluation of DVT. Duplex findings suggestive of acute DVT include enlargement of the vein, noncompressible vein, absence of spontaneous phasic signal, and the presence of echogenic thrombus in the lumen. The sensitivity and specificity are near 100% in detecting thrombus from the groin to the popliteal vein; however, the veins above the inguinal ligament and calf veins are more difficult to visualize. Despite the mentioned drawbacks, duplex is extremely safe, painless, and easy to repeat. Magnetic resonance venography (MRV) has been used increasingly in the evaluation of suspected DVT. Some authors recommend MRV as the study of choice for suspected iliac vein or inferior vena caval thrombosis. Gadolinium, as a contrast agent, extravasates into the area of inflammation with acute thrombi. The limitations of its use are the cost and contraindications in patients with metallic implants and those with claustrophobia.

Venography has been used as the gold standard for evaluation of extremity DVT. However, it has many disadvantages, including contrast induced phlebitis and high cost; therefore, its use has become extremely selective. In recent years, duplex technology has become increasingly considered the gold standard for the diagnosis of DVT.

DIAGNOSTIC STRATEGIES FOR PATIENTS WITH DVT

Patients with clinical suspicion of DVT should initially be examined using venous duplex imaging. If the test is positive, the patient should be treated for DVT. If the test is negative, the patient should then be classified according to the level of clinical suspicion for DVT, as previously indicated in Table 2. A low clinical suspicion of DVT accompanied by a negative duplex image can effectively exclude DVT, and no further evaluation is necessary. For patients with moderate clinical suspicion, a negative duplex test should be followed by another test in a few days or a D-dimer test. A negative D-dimer test would most probably exclude the presence of DVT. However, a positive D-dimer test following a normal venous duplex image requires further evaluation with ascending venography or MRV. Patients with a high clinical suspicion of DVT, despite a negative venous duplex image, should undergo an additional investigation using ascending venography, MRV, or a second venous duplex image. For those patients with inconclusive venous duplex imaging, which is infrequent, the following can be pursued:

- For patients with a low clinical suspicion, a second duplex image in a few days is appropriate.
- For those with a moderate or high clinical suspicion, the D-dimer test, MRV, or ascending venography can be used.
- If the D-dimer test is negative and the patient's clinical status remains stable or improved, the patient can be observed.
- If the clinical suspicion of DVT increases with time or if the D-dimer test is positive, ascending venography or MRV is indicated.

Treatment

Once the diagnosis of DVT has been made, the treatment and treatment duration are determined based on the site of thrombosis. Isolated calf vein thrombosis has been an area of controversy for some time. However, increasing evidence supports the use of anticoagulation therapy secondary to the risk of propagation up to 30%, and an increase in recurrence as well as post-thrombotic syndrome in those without anticoagulation. Femoral-popliteal DVT carries a more complicated natural history with up to 40% of patients having asymptomatic PE by routine ventilation/perfusion scans. These patients are generally treated with routine anticoagulation. Anticoagulation does not lyse the thrombus, but allows for physiologic fibrinolysis of the affected vein. Iliofemoral DVT, which has the most serious manifestation of this DVT, is also associated with severe post-thrombotic sequelae. Eliminating the thrombus by either thrombectomy or thrombolysis improves both the short- and long-term venous function and overall morbidity. Vena cava filters may be placed in those patients with a free-floating thrombus or nonocclusive thrombus in their vena cava before thrombolysis. Anticoagulation is the mainstay of treatment in the United States unless contraindications are present. Heparin, low-molecular-weight heparin (LMWH), and warfarin (Coumadin) compounds are used in the treatment of DVT.

Heparin is an unfractionated product that binds to antithrombin III and augments the inhibition of Xa and thrombin. The anticoagulation effect varies widely in those treated and, therefore, requires measurement of response to treatment by a partial thromboplastin time (PTT) level, with titration based on laboratory results. An elevation in the PTT to a level of 1.5 to 2 times that of the control value is needed for treatment. There is a proven decrease in recurrent thrombosis, if a therapeutic level is achieved within the first 24 hours of diagnosis, by as high as six times that of patients taking longer to achieve therapeutic levels.

More recently, LMWH has grown very popular for prophylaxis and treatment, with a longer half-life, 90% bioavailability, and a more predictable anticoagulation response than unfractionated heparin. This class of anticoagulation can be administered once or twice daily, without the need for routine laboratory monitoring. In a meta-analysis comparison between LMWH and unfractionated heparin, patients with LMWH had a decrease in major bleeding. With these findings, the use of this class of drugs has allowed for safe outpatient treatment of DVT and for use as a bridge to therapeutic oral anticoagulation in those patients who are in the hospital with no other reason for continued hospitalization. Heparin is generally given for 5 days while oral anticoagulation is initiated.

Warfarin (Coumadin) therapy is inexpensive and used for long-term treatment after the patient is discharged. The drug is started after therapeutic effect with heparin or LMWH, secondary to the paradoxical effect on the coagulation cascade, until therapeutic levels are obtained, which are verified with a prothrombin time (PT) and international normalization ratio (INR). The mechanism of action of warfarin is inhibition of the vitamin K-dependent carboxylation of the clotting factors II, VII, IX, and X. The time to peak effect is up to 72 hours after administration and close evaluation of the PT is needed. A troublesome consequence of this drug is its high level of interaction with other medications; therefore, close evaluations must be made of all new and old medications. The recommended goal of therapy is to achieve an INR of 2.0 to 3.0. Warfarin compounds cross the placenta and are contraindicated during pregnancy, secondary to teratogenic effects. Both unfractionated heparin and LMWH can be used in this population.

The recommended length of treatment depends on the etiology and presence of recurrence. The length of treatment for a first episode of DVT is 3 to 6 months, and those with recurrence require lifelong anticoagulation, particularly those with cancer or hypercoagulable states. Ultrasound follow-up in patients with DVT revealed a statistically significant increase in recurrence in those with residual thrombus. The ongoing incidence of recurrent DVT is 5% to 6% per year. A recent multicenter study, the Prevention of Recurrent Venous Thromboembolism (PREVENT) trial, showed a reduction of recurrent DVT or PE by 64% in those with low-dose warfarin therapy, compared with those taking placebo. An INR goal of 1.5 to 2.0 was achieved in the studied patients, with an average follow-up of 2 years.

The major adverse effect of all anticoagulation therapy is bleeding. Other complications of heparin therapy include osteoporosis and thrombocytopenia. Patients with bleeding while on heparin require cessation of anticoagulation, use of fresh frozen plasma, and the use of protamine. A dreaded possible complication of heparin-induced thrombocytopenia (HIT) is venous as well as arterial thrombosis resulting in limb loss or death. This complication is secondary to immunoglobulin (Ig) G antibodies binding to the platelet membrane, with a stimulating effect on platelets. HIT occurs in up to approximately 2% of patients receiving heparin, and typically develops 2 to 10 days after therapy is initiated. A drop of more than 50% of the platelet count should raise a high level of suspicion for this complication. In these patients, direct thrombin inhibitors (lepirudin [Refludan]) are used, and warfarin therapy is instituted after several days of treatment. With warfarin therapy, skin necrosis can develop, usually within 10 days of therapy and most often in women in areas of abundant subcutaneous tissue. Patients with congenital deficiencies of protein C and malignancies are especially prone to warfarin-induced skin necrosis. Prompt cessation of warfarin therapy and initiation of alternative anticoagulate are required.

Prevention of DVT

Prophylaxis in high-risk patients has been used to decrease the incidence of DVT. The importance of prevention is paramount; as seen in orthopedic patients in the National Confidential E[I]nquiry into Perioperative Deaths (NCEPOD) study, which indicated PE as the cause of death in 35% of patients at autopsy following hip replacement. Graduated compression stockings and intermittent leg compression devices have shown to decrease the incidence of DVT in moderate-risk surgical patients. Their use is routine in surgical and trauma patients, with good reason, because approximately 50% of DVT occurs intraoperatively. With the ease of administration of LMWH products, and with no need for frequent laboratory work to assess the level of anticoagulation, anticoagulation therapy has become increasingly popular as a means of prophylaxis. Randomized control trials have shown LMWH to have an equal or greater effectiveness and similar or less bleeding complications than traditional unfractionated heparin. Even subtherapeutic doses of oral anticoagulation have shown a decreased incidence of thrombosis in patients with indwelling catheters.

SPECIFIC DVT PROPHYLAXIS RECOMMENDATION

Low-Risk Patients

These patients do not usually need specific prophylactic measures, except for ambulation.

Moderate-Risk Patients

General Surgical, Thoracic, or Gynecologic Procedures

The use of subcutaneous low-dose unfractionated heparin (5000 units every 8 to 12 hours) or subcutaneous LMWH is recommended in this group of patients. Intermittent pneumatic compression (IPC) devices can also be effective. Neurosurgical patients should receive IPC, however, a low-dose heparin is also an acceptable alternative.

High-Risk Patients

Patients with elective hip replacement can be treated with LMWH or warfarin adjusted to maintain an INR of 2 to 3. Other effective approaches include adjusted-dose subcutaneous unfractionated heparin and IPC. For patients with elective knee replacement, the prophylaxis of choice is LMWH once or twice daily postoperatively. For patients with hip fractures, either warfarin with an INR of 2 to 3 or a fixed dose of subcutaneous LMWH started preoperatively is effective. The combined use of IPC with LMWH or warfarin may prove of additional benefit in certain patients with hip fractures.

Multiple Trauma

LMWH is the prophylaxis of choice. IPC has been recommended, when feasible, because it eliminates any risk for bleeding. Other alternatives include low-dose unfractionated heparin or warfarin. Insertion of an IVC filter has been recommended for very high-risk patients when anticoagulation may be contraindicated.

Acute Spinal Cord Injury Associated with Paralysis

LMWH is the most effective prophylaxis in these patients.

Other Medical Conditions

These medical patients should be classified as low, moderate, or high risk for venous thromboembolic events, and depending on their medical condition and risk, they can be treated based on the previous outlines as suggested.

Pregnancy

Subcutaneous, low-dose heparin is the prophylaxis of choice for pregnant patients who are at high risks for DVT and PE. For those undergoing an emergency caesarean section, prophylaxis with low-dose unfractionated heparin is recommended.

Superficial Thrombophlebitis

Some consider thrombosis of the superficial veins a benign process. The most common etiologies include direct injury, stasis within varicose veins, and in association with malignancy. The incidence of DVT has been reported to be 11% in these patients. This diagnosis is easier to make in the superficial system than in the deep system. A painful cord is often palpated with erythema along the course of the underlying vein. Duplex is accurate and critical in assessing the extension of the thrombus. Anti-inflammatory agents are the mainstay of treatment and compression, bed rest and warm compresses are also part of first-line therapy. If extension occurs to the saphenofemoral junction, then ligation or anticoagulation with warfarin can be performed with the known concomitant presence of DVT in 40% of patients. The prognosis depends on etiology, deep venous involvement, and thrombus load. Follow-up duplex is recommended, and if the process persists, a hypercoagulable state workup and malignancy search should be sought.

Axillary-Subclavian Vein Thrombosis

Thrombosis of the axillary or subclavian vein (ASVT) accounts for 1% to 2% of all DVT. ASVT can be either primary (effort vein thrombosis) or secondary. Primary ASVT is more commonly reported in young men 40 years of age or less, but may occur at any age or in any sex. Secondary ASVT may be related to:

- Iatrogenic (secondary to insertion of Hickman catheters, pacemakers, central venous pressure lines, or other vascular catheterizations)
- Malignancy (both from direct obstruction by tumor or it metastatic nodes or secondary to hypercoagulability states associated with certain tumors)
- Direct trauma
- Heart disease (stasis) and nephrotic syndrome
- Infections

In a review of reported phlebograms in patients with permanent pacemaker electrodes, evidence of venous thrombosis was observed in 31%. Total occlusion was present in 15%, but arm or facial edema was reported in only 5%.

EFFORT SUBCLAVIAN VEIN THROMBOSIS

The most frequently reported examples of subclavian venous thrombosis are those related to effort or positioning of the arm and external compression of the vein in the costoclavicular space.

Paget, in 1875, and von Schroetter, in 1884, described cases of upper arm swelling attributable to thrombosis of the main veins of the upper extremity. Hughes, in his excellent collective review of 320 reported cases, coined the term *Paget-Schroetter syndrome*. The thrombosis may occur in the axillary or subclavian vein and may be related to injury or effort but may also be spontaneous. This syndrome is therefore best described as a primary ASVT.

The pathophysiology of effort vein thrombosis has been postulated to be multifactorial. First, external compression of the axillary-subclavian vein contributes to stasis of blood flow. Factors causing external compression include anomalous subclavius or anterior scalene muscle, congenital fibromuscular bands or narrowing of the costoclavicular space from depression of the shoulder. Second, the stress of exercise may temporarily cause hypercoagulability. Third, repetitive shoulder-arm motion may cause microscopic intimal tears in the vessel wall. These three factors satisfy Virchow's classic triad for thrombosis—stasis, hypercoagulability, and intimal damage. The most important factor in explaining the high thrombosis rate in the axillary-subclavian vein compared with other major veins, seems to be its relatively fixed position in the thoracic outlet, exposing it to repeated trauma during arm movement.

The commonly observed activities are those associated with hyperabduction and external rotation of the arm or with activities in which the shoulders are held in the backward and downward positions. Hyperabduction actions described include throwing a baseball or football, playing tennis, painting ceilings, chopping wood, rowing a boat, and washing walls. Depression of the shoulder, as occurs with carrying heavy objects or in a figure-eight splint, has preceded thrombosis. It has also been observed following positioning of the arms during sleep or under anesthesia in which the arm is positioned in hyperabduction or the shoulders are depressed. Direct compression of the axillary vein by hanging on a ladder rung or falling asleep with an arm over the back of a chair has been described. However, there are some cases described in which no inciting effort or position is remembered. Roos emphasized the central role of the first rib as the major limiting structure in the thoracic outlet.

Effort vein thrombosis presents clinically, predominately in middle-aged men, with abrupt swelling of the involved upper extremity. The involved extremity is most often the person's dominate arm. Recent trauma or unusual exertion can be documented in the majority of cases. Venous hypertension of the upper extremity after the onset of subclavian vein thrombosis causes long-term disability consisting of arm pain and swelling exacerbated by exercise. These symptoms persist for a long time in a large percentage of patients and appear uninfluenced by standard anticoagulant therapy. Venous duplex imaging has been recently used in the diagnosis of this entity with excellent accuracy. Venography can be used to confirm the diagnosis.

Several investigators have employed oral anticoagulation as the sole therapy for patients with subclavian vein thrombosis, with a reported clinical success rate of 4% to 100% (mean 49%). With early conservative therapy of effort vein thrombosis, complete resolution of symptoms occurs in 15% to 30% of patients. Adams and DeWeese reported residual symptoms in up to 70% of conservatively treated patients, including swelling, pain, disability, and even a rare case of venous gangrene. PE has also been observed in 12% to 36% of patients with ASVT.

The use of lytic therapy may ultimately improve the efficacy of oral anticoagulation therapy and may partially explain the improved results of more current oral anticoagulation series compared with historical studies. Although thrombolytic therapy is costly, its use is justified when one considers the potential loss of productivity in relatively young males with effort ASVT who are treated with anticoagulation therapy.

Symptoms associated with effort subclavian vein thrombosis are sufficiently dramatic that most patients present promptly for treatment. Lytic therapy can reduce the size or completely lyse the clots, and it is most effective for fresh clots (5 to 7 days old). However, the results of lytic therapy in clot resolution of ASVT have been somewhat mixed. Some authorities have reported good results, with clot resolution ranging from 57% to 100%, while others have had limited success. In our series, initial thrombolysis was achieved in the majority (93%) of patients. When using adjunctive therapy, 13 (87%) patients who had initial lytic therapy experienced complete resolution of their symptoms and patent veins. However, more objective data regarding subclavian vein lumen patency following lytic therapy and anticoagulation are needed, including a comprehensive follow-up with duplex scanning of the subclavian vein, before any recommendation regarding surgery versus lytic therapy can be made.

Although initial lytic therapy has been gaining wider acceptance, proponents of early surgical thrombectomy and initial surgical repair remain. At the other end of the spectrum, some authorities have suggested treating the thrombotic process alone, without addressing the underlying anatomical abnormality. However, Machleder refutes this approach, arguing that if the underlying anatomical abnormality is not corrected, the recurrence rate and/or residual symptoms will be rather high.

First rib resection may seem the logical treatment for effort vein thrombosis, because the major cause of this disorder seems to be a fixed position of the axillary-subclavian vein in the thoracic outlet. However, no anatomical abnormality is apparent in some cases. For this reason, we believe that first rib resection should be reserved for patients in whom an anatomical abnormality can be identified or if reocclusion of the vein occurs after treatment. In our series, 7 of 23 patients had supplementary first rib or cervical rib resection in the present series, and all symptoms were resolved.

The timing of first rib resection following initial successful lytic therapy is controversial. Some authorities advocate first rib resection shortly after the vein has been opened and a few days of heparin therapy have been administered. The rationale for this is to decompress the vein before it reoccludes. The second option, which was chosen in our series, is to maintain warfarin therapy for 2 to 3 months and then perform a first rib resection for persistent and significant symptoms. At this time, there is insufficient data for favoring one option over the other.

It is generally felt that the clinical outcome is very good following effort subclavian vein thrombosis treatment that includes at least catheter-directed lytic and oral anticoagulation therapy. Balloon angioplasty appears to be ineffective regardless of etiology. Stent placement may enhance the results of angioplasty in selected patients without effort vein thrombosis, and surgery may improve symptom resolution in effort vein thrombosis patients with external compression or intrinsic venous abnormalities.

Deep Venous Thrombosis in Pregnancy

The incidence of antepartum DVT is estimated to occur in 0.5% or less of deliveries. Postpartum DVT is 3 to 5 times more common than antepartum. One out of 2000 pregnancies is complicated by a PE. Twenty percent of untreated DVT may be complicated by a PE, which carries a 15% mortality rate. In contrast, if treated, the incidence of PE is less than 5% with less than a 1% mortality rate.

Pregnancy is considered to be an acquired hypercoagulable state, or a low grade of chronic disseminated intravascular coagulation (DIC) within the placenta. There are increases of several clotting factors (factors I, V, VII, VIII, IX, X, and XII), which are associated with decreased fibrinolytic activities and increased fibrinolytic inhibitors. Decreases in antithrombin III and proteins C and S have been observed.

A clinical diagnosis is generally invalid in 50% of cases, and the diagnosis is primarily made using a color duplex ultrasound.

TREATMENT

The choice of therapy has been widely debated. Warfarin passes through the placenta to the fetus and may cause fetal complications and/or death. Heparin, in contrast, does not cross the placenta, but its long-term use may be impractical and may increase the risk of complications.

Conventional Therapy (for Proximal Iliofemoral Popliteal DVT)

Full-dose IV heparin is administered for several days followed by subcutaneous heparin every 12 hours until delivery. Then subcutaneous heparin or warfarin is used for 6 weeks postpartum.

Distal below-knee isolated DVT can be treated using compression stockings and heat with follow-up duplex ultrasounds.

Peripartum Management of DVT

Several options can be considered for peripartum management:

- Continue heparin treatment as antepartum for high-risk patients.
- Decrease heparin dose to 5000 units subcutaneous every 12 hours (PTT of 1.5) for recent thromboembolic disease.
- Discontinue IV heparin 4 to 6 hours before delivery and insertion of IVC filter.
- Resume heparin 6 hours after delivery and continue for 6 to 8 weeks.
- Warfarin therapy is acceptable in nonlactating mothers.

Alternative Therapies of DVT in Pregnancy

Alternative therapies during pregnancy include low-dose heparin and IVC filter, iliofemoral venous thrombectomy, and LMWH. In a recent Medline review of LMWH, it was concluded that they are generally safe and effective, however, the benefits remain inconclusive.

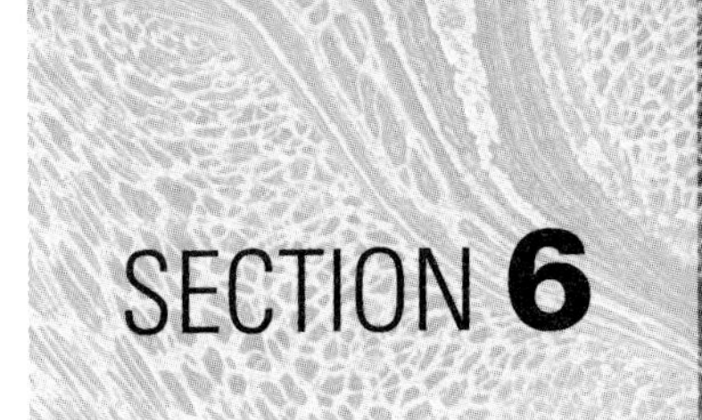

The Blood and Spleen

APLASTIC ANEMIA

METHOD OF

Neal S. Young, MD

Aplastic anemia is pancytopenia with bone marrow hypocellularity. The disease, first described by Ehrlich over a century ago, appears infrequently but is not rare. Formal epidemiologic studies in Europe found an incidence (annual new cases) of about 2 per million; the rate is two- to threefold higher in Asia.

Aplastic anemia can be constitutional or acquired. Inherited marrow failure usually manifests in the first decade or two of life but can appear later; therefore, these pediatric syndromes enter into the differential diagnosis of pancytopenia in the adult. Fanconi anemia is often, but not always, associated with short stature and specific physical anomalies of the skeletal and urogenital systems. The diagnosis rests on the characteristic susceptibility of chromosomes to chemicals like mitomycin C and diepoxybutane, detected by cytogenetic analysis of blood cells. At least eight separate genes have been identified as altered in different Fanconi subtypes. Physical anomalies in dyskeratosis congenita include abnormal nails and skin as well as mucous membrane findings. The responsible genes encode for members of the telomerase complex, which also may be mutated in patients with apparently acquired aplastic anemia; short telomeres are a characteristic finding and contribute to the diminished stem cell pool.

Acquired aplastic anemia occurs predominantly in young adults (15 to 25 years old) and also among older persons over the age of 60 years. Aplastic anemia has many clinical associations. Direct toxicity to marrow clearly occurs in three circumstances—following acute irradiation, after treatment with myelosuppressive drugs (especially alkylators and nitrosoureas), and with benzene exposure. High doses of these agents are required to produce irreversible marrow failure; for example, the dose of radiation predicted to result in death from hematologic causes in 50% of an exposed population is probably in excess of 2.5 Gy. Except in cancer patients undergoing chemotherapy, direct toxicity is an infrequent etiology of acquired aplastic anemia. Pesticides, insecticides, and many drugs have also been associated with bone marrow failure, but here the relationship is idiosyncratic, meaning that despite their wide use, they only occasionally are linked to disease in an individual. In formal epidemiologic studies, nonsteroidal anti-inflammatory drugs, anticonvulsants, and sulfa drugs have been most strongly incriminated. Historically, chloramphenicol appeared to initiate an epidemic of aplastic anemia on its introduction in the 1950s, but this drug is now infrequent in medical practice in the United States and Europe. Although a suggestive history of drug or chemical exposure may be obtained from a patient, establishing an etiologic relationship by laboratory studies in an individual case is difficult. Aplastic anemia also occurs in the setting of viral infections. In the hepatitis/aplasia syndrome, severe bone marrow failure follows an uncomplicated episode of hepatitis, which is seronegative for the known hepatitis viruses. Rarely, aplastic anemia is a sequela of infectious mononucleosis, and Epstein-Barr virus can be demonstrated in the marrow in these cases. Cytopenias in patients with AIDS are usually accompanied by a cellular, dysplastic bone marrow. Rarely, aplastic anemia occurs in relation to pregnancy and may be resolved or improved by its termination. Aplastic anemia is associated with the collagen vascular disease eosinophilic fasciitis. Transfusion-associated graft-versus-host disease that develops after infusion of blood products containing viable lymphocytes into an immunocompromised host, produces fatal marrow aplasia. However, despite the large numbers of clinical associations, in most series, the majority of cases of plastic anemia are labeled idiopathic.

Aplastic anemia is closely linked to several clonal hematologic diseases. Paroxysmal nocturnal hemoglobinuria (PNH) is strongly associated with aplastic anemia. In a high proportion of patients, especially young persons, PNH evolves to aplasia; and, conversely, a significant proportion of aplastic anemia patients develop a positive acidified serum lysis (Ham) test months to years after successful immunosuppressive therapy, sometimes with clinical hemolysis. PNH is now known to be secondary to a defect in the *PIG-A* gene, the protein product of which participates in the synthesis of the glycosylphosphatidylinositol (GPI) anchor, which links a large family of proteins to the cell membrane. Absence of certain cell-surface proteins leads to increased complement sensitivity of red cells, but the relationship of GPI-linked proteins to hematopoietic failure is unknown. Detection of absent GPI-linked proteins by flow cytometry is more sensitive than the Ham test for the diagnosis of PNH, and use of this test has shown that a very large proportion of aplastic anemia patients have an expanded clone of PNH cells at the time they first present with pancytopenia. Acquired aplastic anemia—especially when blood count suppression is incomplete or the marrow is only moderately hypocellular—must also be distinguished from myelodysplasia (hypocellular in about 20% of cases), aleukemic leukemia (especially in the very young and the very old), and myelofibrosis. Some patients with aplastic anemia appear to evolve to a myelodysplastic marrow appearance, accompanied by stereotypical cytogenetic aneuploidy (monosomy 7 or trisomy 8).

Aplastic anemia is characterized by a severe defect of hematopoietic progenitors and probably also stem cells. Marrow stroma and hematopoietic growth factor production are usually normal, consistent with the success of marrow transplantation and the relative ineffectiveness of growth factor administration in this disease. Hematopoietic cell destruction in most cases of aplastic anemia is probably immunologic, mediated by activated cytotoxic lymphocytes overexpressing type 1 cytokines, especially gamma-interferon, which in turn induce apoptosis in their marrow targets; a variety of chemical, viral, and even endogenous *self* antigens might incite such an abnormal immune system response in some individuals. The high rate of clinical responses to and sometimes dependence on immunosuppressive therapy is consistent with an immune hypothesis.

Diagnosis and Laboratory Features

Prompt diagnosis is important in order to avoid unnecessary complications and to provide the appropriate definitive therapy. In a classic case, there is abrupt onset of bleeding symptoms; blood counts show severe thrombocytopenia, neutropenia, and anemia, and the marrow is empty.

Typically blood counts are uniformly low; lymphocytes are usually better preserved than neutrophils but are commonly also reduced in number. The absolute or corrected reticulocyte count is very low. Red cells on the blood smear appear normal, but macrocytosis is the rule on automated cell analysis. The differential diagnosis is more difficult in moderate aplastic anemia, in which blood counts and marrow cellularity are better preserved; these cases can be hard to distinguish from hypocellular myelodysplasia. Atypically, aplastic anemia may present with only two or even a single affected hematopoietic lineage and so resemble pure red cell aplasia, amegakaryocytic thrombocytopenia, or a chronic neutropenia. Fever, night sweats, weight loss, and other constitutional symptoms are unusual in aplastic anemia, and the presence of lymphadenopathy or hepatosplenomegaly should suggest alternative diagnoses. Patients with Fanconi anemia may have short stature, café au lait spots, and abnormal formation of the hand; dyskeratosis congenita can be diagnosed from the peculiar nail changes and leukoplakia.

The diagnosis of aplastic anemia rests on the bone marrow examination. At least a 1-cm biopsy specimen should be obtained from the iliac crest, and the sternum should be aspirated if no spicules are obtained from the hip site. In general, the bone marrow is aspirable but watery. The biopsy specimen may appear white rather than red. On microscopic examination, hematopoietic precursor cells of all types are markedly reduced or absent, and the aspirate smear shows only residual lymphocytes, plasma cells, and fibroblastoid stromal cells. There may be a few small *hot spots* of erythropoietic activity. The biopsy specimen is largely replaced by fat. Megakaryocytes are absent. A careful search should be made for blast cells, adjacent to the spicule, or infiltrating carcinoma, at the edge of the smear. Mild abnormalities of erythroid differentiation, called *megaloblastoid* changes, occur commonly, but marked dysmyelopoiesis or aberrant megakaryocytes point to myelodysplasia.

Some other laboratory tests are important. In a young patient or an older individual with an unusual family history or physical findings, Fanconi anemia should be excluded by chromosomal analysis of a peripheral blood specimen. Bone marrow cytogenetics are usually normal in aplasia but abnormal in myelodysplasia. Magnetic resonance imaging of marrow has also been proposed to help in this differential diagnosis. Flow cytometry has replaced the Ham test to diagnose PNH. Elevated serum transaminases suggest a recent bout of hepatitis, and such a finding should be followed by specific serologic assays.

Tissue typing to determine HLA antigens should be performed as early as possible in patients who may require a stem cell transplantation; this information is also useful for the selection of platelet donors.

Clinical Features

Most patients seek medical help because of minor bleeding into the skin and from the gums or nose; symptoms related to anemia such as dizziness, fatigue, shortness of breath, and a pounding sensation in the ears are common. The first physical examination in acquired aplastic anemia is often remarkably normal, with the exception of pallor, petechiae, and ecchymoses. Aplastic anemia may be fulminant with death in a matter of days as a result of intracranial bleeding or overwhelming infection, but more often the course is insidious. Symptoms and medical complications arise from the alterations in blood components. Thrombocytopenic bleeding rarely is massive or life-threatening in the absence of concomitant infection; fatal intracranial bleeding is now very unusual with the effective employment of platelet transfusions. Infection is uncommon at presentation but becomes problematic as the disease progresses and is the major cause of morbidity and mortality in aplastic anemia. Neutropenia predisposes to bacterial infections, most commonly with organisms that originate in the patient's gut or enter via intravenous catheters. Many, perhaps most, febrile or septic episodes do not yield culture evidence of a specific organism. Local infections of skin, sinuses, and the perianal areas occur. As neutropenia persists, fatal fungal disease may develop, especially aspergillosis of the lungs and sinuses. Death usually results from invasive fungal disease or overwhelming bacterial sepsis.

The prognosis in aplastic anemia depends on the blood counts. Severe disease has been defined as the presence of two of the following three criteria:

1. Absolute neutrophil count (ANC) below 500 per mm^3
2. Platelets below 20,000 per mm^3
3. Corrected reticulocyte count of less than 1% (corresponding to an absolute reticulocyte count in automated blood counters of less than 40,000 to 60,000 mm^3)

Extreme neutropenia (ANC less than 200/mm^3) carries an especially high mortality.

Treatment

Aplastic anemia is a hematologic emergency. The patient requires the most fastidious attention to the bleeding and infectious complications of the disease, and the correct, definitive therapy should be instituted quickly. Moderate aplastic anemia can be observed, but there is no place for watchful waiting or trials of low-dose corticosteroids or novel growth factors in severe aplastic anemia.

Supportive therapy consists of appropriate transfusions and aggressive treatment of infections. The patient should be warned to avoid aspirin and other nonsteroidal anti-inflammatory drugs (NSAIDs) that inhibit platelet function. Menses should be suppressed. Dental attention to gingivitis can alleviate much gum oozing. Active bleeding responds to platelet transfusions, and one or two transfusions weekly can alleviate symptoms. All transfused products should be depleted of donor leukocytes, and family donors should never be employed for a patient who may need to undergo marrow transplantation. Massive hemorrhage is unusual and requires much more frequent transfusion for control. The effectiveness of platelet transfusion is most easily assessed by a 1-hour post-transfusion blood count. A minority of patients become refractory to random donor platelet transfusions; refractoriness does not correlate with the number of units received. Some refractory patients will show adequate increments using histocompatible donors. Inhibitors of fibrinolysis may be useful in controlling mucosal bleeding in some cases despite their ineffectiveness in controlled trials. Whether platelet transfusions in chronic thrombocytopenia are better administered prophylactically or solely on demand for symptoms remains unsettled. Mucosal hemorrhage increases at platelet counts below 5000 per mm^3, and 10,000 per mm^3 is therefore a reasonable trigger value for preventive platelet infusions.

Red cell transfusions are given to maintain the hemoglobin at a level compatible with full activity, at least 7 g/dL in general and 9 g/dL in older persons with cardiopulmonary impairment. Transfusional hemosiderosis in chronic aplastic anemia should be treated with iron chelation therapy. In patients with a prognosis of survival for years, subcutaneous deferoxamine (Desferal) infusions can be begun after transfusion of about 50 units of erythrocytes.

Fever, local areas of inflammation, and symptoms suggestive of sepsis in a severely neutropenic patient require careful clinical assessment. Treatment of infection, either documented or suspected, consists of broad-spectrum parenteral antibiotics administered for at least a week. The specific combination of antibiotics is less important than their prompt application. Persistent fever is addressed by modification of the regimen, as for example the addition of vancomycin for a suspected catheter infection or empiric institution of antifungal antibiotics. The threshold for treatment should be low, because neglect or delay in starting antibiotics is likely be fatal in a granulocytopenic individual.

HEMATOPOIETIC STEM CELL TRANSPLANTATION

Transplantation is curative therapy for aplastic anemia and should be the first consideration in every suitable candidate. The preferred donor is a histocompatible sibling, who unfortunately is available only in a minority of cases. Bone marrow and also cytokine-mobilized peripheral blood can be employed as a source of hematopoietic stem cells. In minimally transfused young patients, transplantation has a high success rate (probably more than 80% have long-term survival). Among all young recipients, 5-year survival is 65% to 70%. The outcome of transplantation is affected by the recipient's age, prior transfusion history, and clinical condition. Age correlates with the major complication of graft-versus-host disease. Although older aplastic patients have been successfully transplanted, morbidity and mortality are increased in adults, especially those older than 40 years of age. Transfusions lead to allosensitization and an increased risk of graft rejection. However, especially when leucocyte-depleted blood products are used, limited numbers of blood transfusions do not appear to adversely affect outcome. A patient who is infected, is refractory to platelet transfusions, or has active liver disease has a poor prognosis with transplant. Transplantation from alternative donors, sometimes mismatched family members but more often histocompatible nonfamily members, has been successful, particularly in very young patients. The current approximately 50% risk of transplant-related mortality for matched unrelated procedure may be improved by more precise, fine genetic matching of donor and recipient.

IMMUNOSUPPRESSION

Immunosuppression is effective in the majority of patients with aplastic anemia and is the first therapy in older patients and those without a sibling marrow donor. Horse antithymocyte globulin (ATG or Atgam) and rabbit antithymocyte globulin (Thymoglobulin)[1] are both commercially available in the United States. Response rates to ATG vary depending on patient selection, but hematologic remission rates are about 50%. ATG is administered intravenously; a recommended schedule is 40 mg/kg per day for 4 days for Atgam and at 3.5 mg/kg per day for 5 days for Thymoglobulin. Methylprednisolone (Solu-Medrol) at about 1 mg/kg per day is also given to alleviate symptoms of serum sickness, but should be rapidly tapered beginning about 2 weeks after the first dose of ATG. Extremely high doses of corticosteroids are no more effective than ATG and have more associated complications, especially aseptic necrosis in major joints.

[1]Not FDA approved for this indication.

Cyclosporine (Sandimmune)[1] is also effective in aplastic anemia. Cyclosporine can salvage approximately 50% of patients who have failed ATG therapy. When cyclosporine is added to ATG as first therapy, hematologic remission rates increase to 65% to 75%, and both children and absolutely neutropenic patients respond to combined immunosuppression. We administer cyclosporine orally at a dose of 12 mg/kg per day in adults and 15 mg/kg per day in children, with dose adjustments to blood drug levels or creatinine, for 3 to 6 months. Prophylaxis for *Pneumocystis pneumoniae* infection during cyclosporine therapy is advisable.

Patients who experience relapse usually respond to a second course of immunosuppression. Occasionally, adequate blood counts depend on continued cyclosporine treatment. Some patients who have responded to immunosuppression therapy will later develop clonal hematologic abnormalities, most frequently clinical evidence of PNH as a result of clonal expansion but also marrow failure as a result of the appearance of myelodysplasia and even acute leukemia. Although immunosuppression cannot be considered curative therapy for most patients, it should be noted that long-term survival in patients receiving transplants and those treated by immunosuppression is equivalent.

ATG and cyclosporine are standard regimens for aplastic anemia. Other immunosuppressive modalities have been successfully employed. High-dose cyclophosphamide (Cytoxan)[1] can induce hematologic remissions, but in our experience it is associated with unacceptable early toxicity caused by prolonged neutropenia, invasive fungal infections, and death. An anti-interleukin-2 receptor monoclonal antibody (daclizumab [Zenapax][1] from Protein Design Laboratories)[1] is effective in some moderate aplastic anemia cases. Other agents are in development; for example, a monoclonal antibody to the C5a complement component (Eculizumab[1] from Alexion) may correct hemolysis in PNH.

HEMATOPOIETIC GROWTH FACTORS

Growth factors can be used as an adjunct to definitive treatment by marrow transplantation or immunosuppression. Both granulocyte colony-stimulating factor (G-CSF) (filgrastim [Neupogen])[1] and granulocyte-macrophage colony-stimulating factor (GM-CSF) (sargramostim [Leukine])[1] may occasionally increase neutrophil numbers and even marrow cellularity. Addition of G-CSF or GM-CSF to antibiotics is reasonable in an infected neutropenic patient. Severely neutropenic patients are less likely to respond than those with moderately depressed

[1]Not FDA approved for this indication.

granulocyte numbers; and neither platelets nor reticulocytes are affected. Interleukin-1* and interleukin-3* have not been active in aplastic anemia.

ANDROGENS

Male hormones have not proven to be generally effective in randomized trials. Nevertheless, occasional patients appear to improve or demonstrate dependence on androgen therapy. A trial of androgens is appropriate only in patients with moderate disease or in severely affected patients who have failed immunosuppression. We prefer nandrolone decanoate (Deca-Durabolin),[1] a formulation with little hepatotoxicity, administered intramuscularly at a dose of 5 mg per week[3] for 3 months (prolonged pressure at the injection site will prevent local hemorrhage).

*Investigational drug in the United States.
[1]Not FDA approved for this indication.
[3]Exceeds dosage recommended by the manufacturer.

IRON DEFICIENCY

METHOD OF
Jay Umbreit, MTS, MD, PhD

Iron deficiency is the most common nutritional deficiency. In children of both sexes ages 1 to 2 years, the prevalence is 7%. For females 16 to 19 years of age, it is as high as 19%. Iron deficiency increases in minority populations and is as high as 22% in Hispanic women. Iron deficiency in its most severe form results in iron deficiency anemia. In infants and preschool children, iron deficiency anemia results in decreased motor activity, social inattention, and decreased social interaction. These defects persist if the deficiency is not corrected. Among pregnant women, iron deficiency anemia during the first two trimesters results in increased incidence of preterm labor and low birth weight. The prevalence of anemia in low-income pregnant females in the first, second, and third trimesters is 9%, 14%, and 37%, respectively. Evidence is considered strong that iron deficiency anemia results in decreased work productivity, increased child mortality, increased maternal mortality, and slowed child development. The effects of mild-to-moderate anemia are less well established as is the effect on susceptibility to infectious disease.

There is data that indicate neuropsychological effects of iron deficiency occur without overt anemia and may respond to iron therapy. Nonanemia iron deficiency probably does reduce work capacity. This suggests that iron deficiency anemia is only part of the overall syndrome of iron deficiency.

Diet predicts iron status into infancy and early childhood. Between 20% and 40% of infants fed nonfortified formula or cow's milk, and 15% to 20% of breast-fed infants are at risk. After the age of 24 months, the risk of iron deficiency decreases with the decreased dependence on milk. In older children the risk for deficiency is related to limited access to food because of family income, low-iron diets, or medical conditions such as bleeding or inflammatory disease. During adolescence (12 to 18 years of age), iron requirements increase because of growth. Among females menstrual blood loss becomes important, and heavy loss (greater than 80 mL per month) is a significant risk factor. Other risk factors for this population include the use of an intrauterine device, high parity, and low iron intake. Data from the Health and Nutrition Examination Survey (HANES) III indicated that 11% of nonpregnant women ages 16 to 49 have iron deficiency and 3% to 5% iron deficiency anemia. Among pregnant women the expansion of the blood volume, growth of the fetus, and other maternal tissues increase the demand for iron threefold. In the absence of iron supplements, many pregnant women are unable to maintain iron stores, although prevalence data across the entire population are not available. While some iron is returned by contraction of the blood volume after delivery, the iron in the fetal and supportive tissues is lost.

Worldwide the problem of anemia is magnified. In children younger than 5 years, it may reach 49% and probably 25% of adult females.

Dietary iron is present in two forms, as inorganic iron and heme-iron. In meat, 50% of the iron is heme, and 15% to 35% of this is bioavailable. While most iron in the diet is inorganic iron, its absorption ranges from 2% to 20%, so that most dietary iron is from heme. In developed countries perhaps 66% of the iron is derived from heme. Men absorb and excrete approximately 1 mg of iron daily. Women during their childbearing years need to absorb approximately 2 mg per day because of menstrual bleeding and childbirth losses. Nonheme (inorganic) iron absorption is facilitated by meat and ascorbic acid, but inhibited by phytates, some dietary fibers and lignins, phenolic polymers, and calcium. Gastric acid is required to maintain the common ferric form of inorganic iron soluble, and achlorhydria may be a significant cause of iron deficiency in the elderly. Perhaps 30% of the elderly have achlorhydria. Gastric atrophy and *Helicobacter pylori* gastric infestation may result in altered pH and iron deficiency. Pharmacologic iron is ferrous iron that is soluble at a neutral pH, and its absorption is unaffected by low gastric acidity. Unusual dietary habits resulting in ingestion of chelators such as starch or clay are still seen in clinical practice.

The most common etiology of iron deficiency is bleeding, and a bleeding source should be investigated in all cases of iron deficiency. One mL of blood contains 0.5 mg of iron. Occult bleeding may be caused by gastrointestinal (GI) loss, but the usual stool test requires a 20-mL-per-day loss for detection. Bleeding into the hip joint space or intra-abdominally may be initially undetected. Menstrual loss may not be reported as bleeding. Rarely, hemosiderinuria may cause iron deficiency. Pregnancy by itself can result in iron deficiency. During a full-term pregnancy the fetus takes up approximately 400 mg of iron, and the placenta and uterus take up approximately 150 mg. Additionally, 300 to 400 mg is needed to increase the red cell mass. Iron lost in milk during lactation is approximately 30 mg per month. During the first 6 months of life, approximately 50 g of new hemoglobin is made. A growing child obtains enough iron for this hemoglobin synthesis by absorbing approximately 0.5 mg of iron per day in excess of daily loss. By adulthood a 70-kg man ultimately achieves iron stores of about 4000 mg. Women achieve a lower level (about 3000 mg) due to continued losses in menstrual bleeding and childbirth. The majority (66%) of this iron is stored as hemoglobin, but about 1000 mg (25%) is stored as ferritin or hemosiderin.

Iron is transported in the plasma bound to transferrin. This protein binds a specific receptor on the cell surface, the transferrin receptor (TfR), with high affinity, and the complex is internalized via a clathrin-coated pit. A small amount of TfR is found in a soluble form in the plasma (serum transferring receptor [sTfR]). The body is able to detect iron deficiency and compensate to a limited extent by increased intestinal absorption. But the mechanism by which the cell detects the body stores of iron is not known. Hepcidin may be the communicator between iron stores and the intestinal absorption mechanism. The pathophysiology of iron deficiency is largely unknown. In iron deficiency there is an increase in red-cell-free porphyrin. Ribonucleotide reductase (RR) is a nonheme-iron protein commonly stated to be the most sensitive enzyme to iron deficiency, and lack of iron is reported to stop DNA synthesis. Other essential heme proteins might be involved, in particular those of the respiratory chain in the genesis of loss of energy and central nervous system (CNS) function. Severely anemic rats with a 50% decrease in hemoglobin have an almost 50% reduction in myoglobin and cytochrome c, a decrease in iron-sulfur content, pyruvate dehydrogenase, and other tricarboxylic acid (TCA) cycle enzymes. Perinatal iron deficiency in rats decreases cytochrome c oxidase activity in the neonatal brain. In contrast, in milder anemias, which would be more physiologic with hemoglobins in a 6- to 12-g/dL range, there is increased platelet count and increased serum transaminase consistent with cell damage, but no decrease in the activities of TCA enzymes or cytochrome oxidase activity, suggesting this is not an important mechanism. On the other hand, abnormalities in lipid composition are observed, consistent with effects on the lipid desaturase activities.

A variety of genes are increased in iron deficiency based on limited DNA microarray data, including Rb; p21; cdk2; cyclins A, D3, and E1; myc; iNOS; and FasL, none of which are known to be involved in iron metabolism, but may help account for the symptoms and signs. Many of the proteins involved in iron homeostasis may be regulated at the translational (rather than transcriptional) level, and would not be detected on gene expression analysis. The messenger RNAs (mRNAs) of ferritin, transferrin receptor, aminolevulinic acid synthetase, ferroprotein, m-aconitase, and divalent metal transporter-1 (DMT-1) are regulated by an iron responsive element (IRE) on the mRNA.

Individuals with iron deficiency may experience no symptoms. Findings common to all anemias may be present, or those rather specific to iron's effects on rapidly turning over epithelial cells; glossitis gastric atrophy, stomatitis, ice eating (pagophagia), and leg cramping. The esophageal web syndrome (Plummer-Vinson syndrome) is still reported, and at least some cases appear to respond to iron therapy. Koilonychia, or spoon nails, are more commonly caused by fungal infection or hereditary variation.

Definitive diagnosis requires laboratory tests. A bone marrow smear with no stainable iron is definitive. A low serum iron level, elevated total iron-binding capacity (transferrin), and a low serum ferritin concentration are considered diagnostic for iron deficiency. Serum iron binding capacity should be less than 10%. In advanced iron deficiency the ferritin levels are 0.6 to 12 ng/mL, serum iron is 7 to 60 µg/dL, and total iron-binding capacity (TIBC) is increased to 450 to 500 µg/dL with absent stores in the marrow. However, serum iron is subject to diurnal variations, with higher concentrations late in the day, and may be increased after meat ingestion. Oral contraceptives increase serum transferrin and result in low transferrin saturation. The serum ferritin reflects body stores and is not affected by recent iron ingestion. When present as a microcytic anemia, the anemia of chronic disease may be mistaken for iron deficiency. This anemia classically has low serum iron, low iron binding capacity, elevated ferritin, and saturation of iron-binding capacity more than 10%.

Perhaps a better estimate of body stores is obtained by the ratio of sTfR to serum ferritin (R/F ratio). Studies of the R/F ratio show age dependence; and in males there is a gaussian distribution, but in females a bimodal distribution. Ferritin is an *acute phase reactant* and in the presence of infection or inflammation the ferritin may be high and the serum iron and transferrin low. The R/F ratio is also affected by inflammation. In the elderly, the R/F ratio may be more sensitive than the classic blood tests, and may be more sensitive in distinguishing iron deficiency anemia from anemia of chronic disease. A major problem is the lack of standardization of the sTfR assay.

In individuals treated with recombinant erythropoietin the increased production of red blood cells (RBCs) exhausted iron stores rapidly, resulting in serum iron being reduced and transferrin becoming desaturated. A functional deficiency resulting from decreased body stores without anemia is suggested by rapid development of the phenotype of iron deficiency upon erythropoietin therapy. In healthy individuals iron stores determine the response to erythropoietin, and baseline ferritin values less than 1000 μg/L have been associated with *functional* iron deficiency. But ferritin concentrations are not correlated to body stores in the setting of hyperthyroidism, malignancy, inflammation, hepatocellular disease malignancies, alcohol, and oral contraception use. The percentage of hypochromic RBC and reticulocyte hypochromic cells may be useful in the identification of functional iron deficiency, and in predicting response to erythropoietin and IV iron treatments. The percentage is not useful in the settings of thalassemia or chemotherapy-treated patients.

Oral iron is the preferred treatment for nutritional iron deficiency. Ferrous iron salts are preferred because of their increased solubility and availability at the pH of the duodenum and jejunum. Standard therapy for iron deficiency anemia in adults is oral administration of a 300-mg tablet of ferrous sulfate (60 mg of elemental iron) three or four times daily. Absorption is enhanced by administration of the iron on an empty stomach. The major side effects of oral iron therapy are epigastric distress, heartburn, nausea, vomiting, and diarrhea. Administering the tablets with meals, decreasing the dose of iron, or gradual escalation of the dose can reduce these symptoms. Other preparations containing less iron, such as ferrous gluconate tablets (320 mg with 36 mg of elemental iron) or the oral administration of carbonyl iron (Ircon) may reduce intolerance. Pediatric liquid preparations of iron (Fer-In-Sol) can be used with the dose modified to avoid side effects. The response of the anemia to iron deficiency should be determined. Reticulocytosis may be observed as early as 4 days after treatment and will reach a maximum at 7 to 10 days. Ferritin responds within a few days. An increase in the hematocrit and hemoglobin is delayed. Therapy needs to continue for 2 to 3 months after correction of the anemia to restore the body's store of iron.

Noncompliance is the most common cause of failure to respond. Inability to absorb enteric-coated iron tablets or malabsorption of iron caused by high transit times may occasionally cause treatment failure. True malabsorption of ferrous sulfate is extremely rare, but may be diagnosed by administering an oral dose of liquid ferrous sulfate (50 to 60 mg of iron) in a fasted state and obtaining a serum iron level before administration and 1 and 2 hours later. An increase in the serum iron concentration of 100 μg/100 mL should be attained. Iron for intramuscular or intravenous administration was available in the form of iron dextran (INFeD, Watson Pharm, Inc.), but had a high toxicity rate, and is now rarely indicated. In contrast, iron sucrose appears safer. The iron is delivered to endogenous iron-binding proteins with a half-life of 90 minutes, and it becomes rapidly available for erythropoiesis. Some formulations can cause anaphylactoid reactions. Some parenteral preparations, such as ferric gluconate and ferric citrate, deliver iron to many proteins rather than specifically iron-binding proteins and are deposited in the parenchyma of the liver resulting in necrosis. Oral iron products have been largely abandoned in patients with end-stage renal disease, most of whom are being treated with erythropoietin. Parenteral iron can be administered by slow intravenous injection, intravenous drip infusion, or injection into the dialyzer. The most frequently adverse effects reported during treatment in hemodialysis patients are hypotension, cramps, and nausea. Some dialysis centers have tried oral heme-iron. Some authorities are recommending the combination of erythropoietin (Epogen)[1] and intravenous iron (iron sucrose [Venofor],[1] 200 mg IV, and recombinant human erythropoietin [rhEPO], 300 U/kg twice a week) for rapid reversal of anemia in pregnant patients.

[1]Not FDA approved for this indication.

AUTOIMMUNE HEMOLYTIC ANEMIA

METHOD OF

Charles H. Packman, MD

The autoimmune hemolytic anemias (AIHAs) are characterized by shortened red blood cell (RBC) survival mediated by autoantibodies. The entities that constitute AIHA are classified primarily by the temperature at which the autoantibodies bind most efficiently to the patient's RBCs. In adults, most cases (80% to 90%) are mediated by antibodies that react optimally with RBCs at 37°C (98.6°F) (warm-reactive autoantibodies). Patients with cryopathic hemolytic syndromes exhibit autoantibodies that bind more avidly to RBCs at temperatures below 37°C (98.6°F) (cold-reactive autoantibodies). The warm- and cold-antibody distinctions are further classified by the presence or absence of underlying disease. When no recognizable underlying disease is evident, the AIHA is designated *primary* or *idiopathic*. The term *secondary* is used when the AIHA is a manifestation or complication of an underlying disorder. Primary (idiopathic) AIHA and secondary AIHA occur with approximately equal frequency. Finally, certain drugs may also cause immune destruction of RBCs by three different mechanisms. Some drugs induce formation of true autoantibodies directed against RBC antigens. In the hapten-drug adsorption mechanism, antibodies seemingly are directed only against the drug, which binds tightly to the RBC membrane. In some, if not all, cases mediated by the ternary (immune) complex mechanism, antibodies may recognize both a drug

TABLE 1 Diseases Characterized by Immune-Mediated Red Blood Cell Destruction

I. Autoimmune hemolytic anemia due to warm-reactive autoantibodies
   A. Primary (idiopathic)
   B. Secondary
      1. Lymphoproliferative disorders
      2. Connective tissue disorders (especially systemic lupus erythematosus)
      3. Nonlymphoid neoplasms (e.g., ovarian tumors)
      4. Chronic inflammatory diseases (e.g., ulcerative colitis)

II. Autoimmune hemolytic anemia due to cold-reactive autoantibodies (cryopathic hemolytic syndromes)
   A. Primary (idiopathic) cold agglutinin disease
   B. Secondary cold agglutinin disease
      1. Lymphoproliferative disorders
      2. Infections (*Mycoplasma pneumoniae* infection, infectious mononucleosis)
   C. Paroxysmal cold hemoglobulinuria (primary or associated with syphilis)
   D. Donath-Landsteiner hemolytic anemia (associated with viral syndromes)

III. Drug-induced immune hemolytic anemia
   A. Hapten—drug adsorption
   B. Ternary (immune) complex
   C. True autoantibody induction

or its metabolite and an epitope of a specific RBC antigen. The classification of the immune hemolytic anemias is shown in Table 1.

Clinical Features and Diagnosis

The annual incidence of AIHA is approximately 1 or 2 cases per 100,000 population. It occurs in people of all ages, with a peak incidence in the seventh decade. No racial predisposition is known, and familial occurrence is rare.

In warm-antibody AIHA, the presenting complaints are usually referable to the anemia itself. The onset of symptoms is typically insidious over months, but occasional patients may experience sudden symptoms of severe anemia and jaundice over a few days. In secondary cases, the symptoms and signs of the underlying disease may overshadow the hemolytic anemia. The physical examination is often normal. Modest splenomegaly may be noted in patients with relatively severe hemolytic anemia. Patients with acute hemolysis may exhibit fever, pallor, hyperpnea, angina, tachycardia, hepatosplenomegaly, heart failure, and jaundice. In secondary cases, other physical findings may be contributed by the associated disorder.

Patients with cold agglutinin disease usually exhibit chronic hemolytic anemia with or without jaundice, but some patients experience episodic, acute hemolysis with hemoglobinuria induced by chilling. Acrocyanosis is sometimes seen, owing to sludging of RBCs in the cutaneous circulation. Hemolysis in patients with *Mycoplasma pneumoniae* infections is acute at onset, often appearing as the patient is recovering from pneumonia, and lasting 1 to 3 weeks. Hemolytic anemia in infectious mononucleosis can occur at any time within the first 3 weeks of illness. Splenomegaly, which is most characteristic of lymphoma and infectious mononucleosis, may also occur in idiopathic cold agglutinin disease.

Paroxysmal cold hemoglobinuria (PCH) is a chronic illness characterized by periodic episodes of massive hemolysis after cold exposure. It occurs in an idiopathic form and in patients with congenital or tertiary syphilis. Donath-Landsteiner hemolytic anemia is a related disorder that occurs more commonly in children or young adults; it manifests as an acute, self-limited hemolytic anemia usually after a viral syndrome. In both diseases, paroxysms are characterized by prominent constitutional symptoms, including aching pains in the back or legs, abdominal cramps, headaches, and chills and fever occurring a few minutes to several hours after cold exposure. The urine typically contains hemoglobin. The constitutional symptoms and hemoglobinuria generally last a few hours.

Drug-induced immune hemolytic anemias are usually slow in onset. However, those caused by the ternary (immune) complex mechanism are characterized by a rapid onset after only a few days of drug exposure, or after a single dose in patients who have taken the drug previously. Some common drugs implicated in immune RBC injury are shown in Table 2.

Laboratory Features

GENERAL

In both warm-antibody and cold-antibody AIHA, the anemia can be mild or severe, with hemoglobin levels occasionally as low as 3 to 4 g/dL. Patients with

TABLE 2 Drug-Induced Immune Hematologic Anemia

Mechanism	Examples of Causative Drugs*
Hapten-drug adsorption	Penicillins Cephalosporins Tolbutamide
Ternary (immune complex)	Quinine Quinidine Cephalosporins Chlorpropamide
True autoantibody induction	Methyldopa Levodopa Cephalosporins Procainamide
Uncertain	Acetaminophen Thiazides Ibuprofen Erythromycin Omeprazole

*Listed are examples of commonly used drugs that are well documented to cause immune hemolysis. The list is incomplete; many other drugs have been implicated. In general, in patients with immune hemolytic anemia, any recently ingested drug should be considered etiologically suspect until proved otherwise.

drug-induced immune hemolysis mediated by the hapten-drug adsorption mechanism or by true autoantibodies usually exhibit mildly depressed hemoglobin levels, whereas those with hemolysis mediated by the tertiary (immune) complex mechanism may have severe, life-threatening anemia. Polychromasia on the blood smear indicates reticulocytosis, reflecting an increased rate of RBC production. Spherocytes are usually seen as well. Most patients exhibit mild leukocytosis and neutrophilia; occasionally, leucopenia and neutropenia are noted. Platelet counts are usually normal. Although not usually indicated, marrow examination may reveal an underlying lymphoproliferative disorder.

The reticulocyte count is usually elevated, but transient reticulocytopenia may be seen early in approximately 30% of patients with AIHA for unknown reasons. Usually, reticulocytes appear in the circulation of such patients in a few days. Reticulocytopenia may also be seen in patients with compromised marrow function related to infection, toxic chemicals, or nutritional deficiency. These patients must be monitored carefully and transfused promptly, because life-threatening anemia may develop quickly in patients with hemolysis and decreased RBC production.

Total bilirubin is often mildly increased, up to 5 mg/dL, and is chiefly unconjugated (indirect). Bile is not detected in the urine unless serum conjugated (direct) bilirubin is increased. Serum haptoglobin levels are typically low, and lactate dehydrogenase levels are usually elevated. In warm-antibody AIHA and in cold agglutinin disease, hemoglobinuria is encountered only in those uncommon patients who develop hyperacute hemolysis. In patients with PCH or Donath-Landsteiner hemolytic anemia, hemoglobinuria is characteristic, starting shortly after chilling. Hemoglobinuria may be a prominent feature of drug-induced hemolysis because of the ternary (immune) complex mechanism and may cause renal failure.

SEROLOGIC FEATURES

The diagnosis of AIHA depends on the demonstration of an immune response directed against autologous RBCs. The evidence for this usually comes in the form of a direct antiglobulin reaction (Coombs test) or demonstration of direct agglutinins or hemolysins in the patient's serum.

Warm-Antibody and the Direct Antiglobulin Test

Most patients with warm-antibody AIHA exhibit neither direct agglutinins nor hemolysins. Rather, their RBCs are coated with nonagglutinating antibodies, almost always of the immunoglobulin (Ig) G class, and/or complement components. Antibodies and complement components on patient RBCs are detected by antiglobulin serum (Coombs reagent), which cross-links the RBCs to produce visible agglutination. This procedure is called the direct antiglobulin (Coombs) test. The *broad-spectrum* antiglobulin (Coombs) reagent detects both immunoglobulin and complement components (principally C3). More specific reagents that detect *only* IgG or complement may be used to refine the pattern of RBC coating. Three *major* patterns of direct antiglobulin reaction have been noted in warm-antibody AIHA—RBCs coated with IgG alone, RBCs coated with IgG plus complement components, and RBCs coated with complement components alone.

In patients with warm-antibody AIHA, the autoantibody exists in a reversible, dynamic equilibrium between RBCs and plasma. If sufficient *free* autoantibody is present in the plasma or serum of the patients, it may be detected by the indirect antiglobulin test. In general, the presence of plasma autoantibody may be viewed as *overflow* or excess above that bound to RBCs. Thus, patients with a positive indirect antiglobulin test caused by a warm-reactive autoantibody must also have a positive direct antiglobulin test. A patient who exhibits a positive *indirect* antiglobulin reaction but a negative *direct* antiglobulin reaction probably does not have an autoimmune process but rather an alloantibody stimulated by prior transfusion or pregnancy.

Cryopathic Hemolytic Syndromes: Direct Agglutinins and Hemolysins

Direct agglutinins, as the name implies, directly agglutinate normal or autologous human RBCs. These antibodies, largely of the IgM class, are present in patients with cold agglutinin disease. Cold agglutinins cause RBCs to agglutinate maximally at 0°C to 5°C (32°F to 41°F). In patients with chronic cold agglutinin disease, the serum cold agglutinin titers are commonly 1:10,000 or higher and may reach 1:1,000,000 or more. The direct antiglobulin test is positive only with anticomplement reagents. This is because the cold agglutinin autoantibody molecules readily dissociate from the RBCs during the washing steps of the antiglobulin test procedure and are not detected. In contrast, complement components are covalently bound to target RBCs and cannot be washed off.

In PCH and Donath-Landsteiner hemolytic anemia, the patient's serum contains hemolysins, antibodies that lyse RBCs in the presence of complement. The direct antiglobulin reaction may be positive during or briefly after an acute attack, because of the coating of surviving RBCs with complement. The antibody is a nonagglutinating IgG that binds only in the cold. It is detected by the biphasic Donath-Landsteiner test, in which the patient's fresh serum is incubated with RBCs initially at 4°C (39°F) and then warmed to 37°C (98.6°F). Intense hemolysis follows.

Drug-Induced Immune Hemolytic Anemia

The serologic findings in drug-induced immune hemolytic anemia vary according to the mechanism.

When hemolysis is mediated through the hapten-drug adsorption mechanism, the direct antiglobulin test is positive for IgG alone. The indirect antiglobulin test may be positive, but only when the test RBCs have been previously coated with the drug.

In hemolysis mediated by the ternary (immune) complex mechanism, the direct antiglobulin test is positive only for complement components. The drug does not bind in measurable quantity to the RBC membrane, but if the drug is included in a mixture of reagent RBCs, patient serum as a source of antibody, and fresh blood-group-specific serum as a source of complement, the cells become coated with complement components, which can then be detected by an antiglobulin reagent. The term *ternary complex* is derived from the observation that in certain of these cases, a trimolecular complex of antibody, drug, or metabolite and a specific RBC membrane antigen must be present for complement deposition and hemolysis to occur, indicating that the RBC membrane antigen is necessary and that the RBC itself is not just an innocent bystander.

In patients with drug-induced immune hemolysis mediated by autoantibody induction, the direct antiglobulin reaction is generally positive for IgG alone. The direct antiglobulin test may be positive in as many as 25% to 30% of patients receiving methyldopa (Aldomet), formerly the most common drug to induce autoantibodies, but less than 1% of these patients actually have hemolysis. The indirect antiglobulin reaction is almost always positive in those who do have hemolysis.

Treatment

WARM-ANTIBODY AUTOIMMUNE HEMOLYTIC ANEMIA

Transfusion

The clinical consequences of anemia are related to both the severity of the anemia and the rapidity with which it develops. Most patients with AIHA are in little danger of circulatory failure, because the anemia usually develops over a sufficient time to allow cardiovascular compensation to occur. It is not usually necessary to transfuse these patients. The best guide to the need of blood transfusion is the patient's clinical condition rather than a predetermined hematocrit or hemoglobin level. In patients with significant co-morbid disease such as coronary artery disease with angina, or in patients who suddenly develop severe anemia and exhibit signs and symptoms of circulatory failure, transfusion is often required and may prove lifesaving. As noted previously, transfusion should be considered early in a patient with AIHA and reticulocytopenia, because the anemia may become severe quite rapidly.

Transfusion of RBCs in AIHA presents two problems, the issue of cross-matching and the likelihood of rapid hemolysis of transfused cells. It is usually impossible to find a truly serocompatible donor blood. The autoantibody in the patient's serum usually reacts with all potential donor RBCs except in those unusual cases in which the autoantibody exhibits specificity for a defined blood group antigen and binds only to cells exhibiting that antigen. Without such specificity, candidate units of blood should be chosen on the basis of least incompatibility with the patient's serum in cross-match testing. Furthermore, before such an incompatible unit is transfused, it is also essential to assay the patient's serum for an alloantibody that would cause a severe hemolytic transfusion reaction directed toward the donor RBCs. Alloantibodies are more likely found in patients with a history of pregnancy or prior transfusion. Once selected, packed RBCs should be infused slowly while the patient is monitored for evidence of a hemolytic transfusion reaction. The transfused cells are often destroyed as rapidly as the patient's own cells. Nonetheless, the temporarily increased hemoglobin level may maintain the patient's oxygen-carrying capacity during the time required for more definitive therapy to become effective.

Corticosteroids

Corticosteroids cause cessation or slowing of hemolysis in about two thirds of patients. Approximately 20% of patients with warm-antibody AIHA achieve a complete remission with corticosteroids. Approximately 10% show minimal or no response. Treatment is initiated with oral prednisone, 1 to 2 mg/kg daily. Critically ill patients with severe hemolysis should receive intravenous methylprednisolone, 2 to 4 mg/kg in divided doses for the first 24 to 48 hours. High dose of prednisone may be required for 10 to 14 days. When the hemoglobin level begins to increase, the prednisone dose may be decreased in fairly large steps to approximately 30 mg per day. With continued response, the prednisone dose is further deceased by 5 mg per day each week, to a dose of 15 to 20 mg daily. This dose should be continued for 8 to 12 weeks after the acute hemolytic episode has subsided. The patient may then be weaned from the drug during 4 to 8 weeks. If continued corticosteroid therapy is needed, treatment on an alternate-day schedule may be helpful, for example, 20 to 40 mg of prednisone every other day. Alternate-day therapy causes fewer corticosteroid side effects but should be attempted only after the patient maintains a stable hemoglobin level with daily prednisone in a dose range of 15 to 20 mg per day. Many patients achieve complete remission of hemolysis, but relapses often occur after discontinuation of corticosteroids. Patients should be followed up for several years after treatment. If relapse occurs, the patient may require further corticosteroid therapy and eventually splenectomy, or immunosuppression.

Splenectomy

Approximately 30% of patients with warm-antibody AIHA require prednisone in doses greater than 15 mg daily to maintain an acceptable hemoglobin concentration. Such patients are candidates for splenectomy. It is usually reasonable to continue corticosteroids for 4 to 8 weeks and wait for a response. If the patient's clinical condition deteriorates, the anemia is extremely severe, or there is no response to prednisone, splenectomy should be done sooner. Approximately 66% of splenectomized patients have a partial or complete remission, but relapses are disappointingly common. After splenectomy, some patients may require further prednisone therapy to maintain an acceptable hemoglobin level, albeit at lower dosage than required before splenectomy.

After splenectomy, there is a slightly increased risk of sepsis caused by encapsulated organisms, more likely in children than in adults. Vaccines against pneumococcus, meningococcus, and *Haemophilus influenzae* are generally given 2 weeks before surgery. Prophylactic penicillin (250 to 500 mg daily) is also of value in children.

Cytotoxic Immunosuppressive Drugs

Cytotoxic immunosuppressive therapy is not universally accepted, but responses to immunosuppressive drugs have been observed in some patients who do not respond to corticosteroids. It is important to note that most patients with warm-antibody AIHA respond to corticosteroids and/or splenectomy. Cytotoxic immunosuppressive therapy is usually considered only for those patients who have no response to corticosteroids and splenectomy, or for those patients who are poor surgical risks. The most commonly used drugs are cyclophosphamide (Cytoxan),[1] 1.5 to 2 mg/kg, or azathioprine (Imuran),[1] 1.5 to 2 mg/kg given daily. If the patient tolerates the drug, treatment may be continued for up to 6 months in hopes of a response. When response occurs, the drug dose may be slowly decreased during 2 to 3 months. If there is no response, the alternative drug may be similarly tried. Cyclophosphamide and azathioprine cause marrow suppression, so the patient's blood counts must be monitored closely during therapy. Both agents increase the risk of subsequent severe hemorrhagic cystitis. Women of childbearing age should avoid pregnancy while taking cytotoxic immunosuppressive agents.

The anti-B-lymphocyte monoclonal antibody rituximab (Rituxan),* 375 mg/m^2 intravenously, weekly for 4 to 8 weeks, has been used with success in patients refractory to other therapies according to several case reports and small series of patients.

Other Therapies

Plasma exchange (plasmapheresis) has been used in warm-antibody AIHA. Improvement has been noted in a few cases, but its use remains controversial. The literature contains anecdotal reports of short-term successful treatment with high-dose intravenous gamma globulin, as well as reports of treatment failures. Danazol (Danocrine),* a nonvirilizing androgen, is also reported as useful in uncontrolled studies and in case reports. These therapies may be tried in cases unresponsive to other therapies.

Cryopathic Hemolytic Syndromes

Keeping the patient warm, particularly the extremities, provides symptomatic relief. This may be the only measure required in patients with mild chronic hemolysis, who generally have a benign course and survive for many years. When a cold agglutinin is associated with a lymphoproliferative disorder, treatment of the underlying neoplasm often corrects the hemolysis. Successful therapy with cyclophosphamide* or chlorambucil (Leukeran) has been reported in a few instances. Rituximab (Rituxan),* has been used successfully in one large series and in multiple case reports. Splenectomy and corticosteroids are generally disappointing, although exceptions have been reported. RBC transfusions, as in warm-antibody AIHA, are generally reserved for patients who have severe anemia and are in danger of cardiorespiratory complications. The use of washed RBCs may avoid replenishing depleted complement components, which could reactivate the hemolytic process. Plasma exchange (with replacement by albumin-containing saline) has been tried in refractory cases. The procedure may temporarily slow the rate of hemolysis but does not provide long-term benefit. The postinfectious forms of cold agglutinin disease are usually self-limited, with recovery expected in a few weeks.

Acute attacks in both chronic and transient forms of PCH may be prevented by avoidance of cold. Corticosteroids and splenectomy have not been useful. PCH associated with syphilis often responds to effective treatment of the syphilis. Patients with chronic idiopathic PCH may survive for many years in spite of occasional paroxysms of hemolysis. Donath-Landsteiner hemolytic anemia is usually self-limited.

DRUG-INDUCED IMMUNE HEMOLYTIC ANEMIA

Discontinuation of the offending drug is usually all that is required. This measure is particularly important and potentially lifesaving in patients with severe hemolysis mediated by the ternary (immune) complex mechanism. In such patients, hemoglobinuria may lead to renal failure requiring a period of dialysis. Corticosteroids are generally unnecessary and of questionable efficacy. Transfusions should be reserved for the unusual circumstance of severe, life-threatening anemia. Cross-matching may present a problem, as with warm-antibody AIHA, in patients with a strongly positive indirect antiglobulin test.

[1]Not FDA approved for this indication.

*Investigational drug in the United States.

*Investigational drug in the United States.

Patients with hemolytic anemia caused by the hapten-drug adsorption mechanism should have a compatible cross-match, because the serum antibody reacts only with drug-coated cells. In hemolysis caused by ternary complex or hapten-drug adsorption mechanisms, the direct antiglobulin test becomes negative once the drug is cleared from circulation, usually a few days after it is discontinued. Hemolysis induced by methyldopa ceases promptly after the drug is discontinued. However, the autoantibodies may remain in the circulation for weeks or months, as evidenced by a persistently positive direct antiglobulin test.

NONIMMUNE HEMOLYTIC ANEMIA

METHOD OF

Carlo Brugnara, MD

Several congenital and acquired diseases lead to premature destruction of the erythrocyte in the absence of antibody-mediated hemolysis. I address here congenital anemias characterized by abnormal red cell morphology or abnormal metabolism and acquired nonimmune hemolytic anemias.

Congenital Nonimmune Hemolytic Anemias

HEMOLYTIC ANEMIAS CAUSED BY RED CELL MEMBRANE ABNORMALITIES

The functional integrity and proper survival of the human erythrocyte are critically dependent on several integral membrane proteins and their interaction with the underlying cytoskeleton. Genetic alterations in these critical components result in chronic hemolytic anemia, reduced red cell survival, and characteristic morphologic abnormalities of the erythrocyte.

Hereditary Spherocytosis and Elliptocytosis

Clinical Manifestations

Hereditary spherocytosis (HS) arises as a chronic hemolytic anemia, with jaundice and splenomegaly. Severity of this disease varies from mild to severe. Thirty percent of the cases are mild, with Hb levels higher than 11 g/dL, reticulocyte counts below 6%, and bilirubin levels around 1 to 2 mg/dL. In neonates with HS, early neonatal icterus is common; Hb values are usually normal at birth but decrease sharply in the first 3 weeks of life, frequently to levels that require blood transfusion. The erythropoietic response to hemolysis is delayed in neonatal HS; reticulocytosis appropriate for the level of anemia appears only several months after birth. Bilirubin gallstones are a frequent and sometimes early complication. Severe anemia caused by acute red cell aplasia (parvovirus B19 infection) is another potential complication.

Hereditary elliptocytosis (HE) is characterized by chronic hemolysis and elliptic erythrocytes. In some cases elliptocytes coexist with spherocytes or poikilocytes. A subtype of HE is hereditary pyropoikilocytosis, with extreme poikilocytosis and bizarre-shaped erythrocytes. Most cases of HE are clinically mild and asymptomatic.

Molecular and Cellular Bases of the Disease

Mutations affecting ankyrin, band 3 anion exchanger, β- or α-spectrin, and protein 4.1 or 4.2 have been shown to produce HS or HE. One person in every 5000 in Europe or North America is born with HS. However, a large number of mild cases are undiagnosed and the incidence could be as high as 1 in 2000. The incidence of HS is lower in blacks. Seventy-five percent of the HS-HE cases display an autosomal dominant pattern of transmission (one parent carries the abnormality). In the remaining cases of HS, both parents are clinically and hematologically normal. Most of these cases are autosomal recessive, although de novo mutations resulting in dominant HS have been demonstrated. Coinheritance of HS and Gilbert's syndrome results in higher levels of bilirubin and greater risk for developing gallstones.

Laboratory Diagnosis

HS and HE are chronic hemolytic anemias with abnormal erythrocyte morphology (presence of hyperchromic spherocytes, uniformly dark and round cells, and/or microspherocytes for HS; presence of elliptocytes in HE). High mean corpuscular hemoglobin concentration (MCHC) indicates the presence of spherocytes and low mean cell volume (MCV) in conjunction with high MCHC that of microspherocytes, the latter being a good indicator of disease severity. Osmotic fragility (un-incubated) is characteristically increased in HS; in borderline cases overnight incubation (incubated osmotic fragility) can demonstrate increased fragility. Marked reticulocytosis or the presence of a significant number of fetal erythrocytes, which are more osmotically resistant than adult erythrocytes, may mask the increased fragility of HS erythrocytes. Additional biochemical markers of hemolysis are decreased haptoglobin and increased serum lactate dehydrogenase (LDH) and bilirubin levels.

All cases of hereditary pyropoikilocytosis and many of HE exhibit abnormal erythrocyte thermal sensitivity, with increased fragmentation at temperatures of 44°C to 46°C.

Treatment

Because shortened red cell survival and anemia are due to the splenic sequestration of spherocytes, splenectomy is the preferred therapy for severe HS. To prevent postsplenectomy infections, vaccination against pneumococcus, *Haemophilus influenzae*, and meningococcus should be performed before surgery, with boosters every 5 years. Oral penicillin[1] should be administered for at least 1 year after surgery and in very young children continued up to 5 to 6 years of age. The surgical risk associated with splenectomy, the risk of postsplenectomy sepsis, and the higher incidence of myocardial infarction in splenectomized patients after age 40 should be carefully considered in patients with mild to moderate anemia. For young patients and adults with gallstones and mild HS, the best therapeutic strategy involves combination of prophylactic splenectomy and satellite cholecystectomy. Isolated cholecystectomy should be performed laparoscopically.

Subtotal splenectomy has emerged as a treatment option for young children with HS. This procedure removes approximately 90% of the enlarged spleen, leaving a remnant that is approximately one quarter of a normal spleen. Subtotal splenectomy leads to a therapeutic decrease of hemolytic rate in most cases while at the same time maintaining adequate phagocytic function. Although there is some regrowth of the remaining spleen, this does not diminish the beneficial effects of subtotal splenectomy.

Hereditary Stomatocytosis and Xerocytosis

Hereditary stomatocytosis and xerocytosis are rare genetic disorders of still unidentified membrane proteins, mostly dominantly inherited. The severity of hemolysis can range from mild to severe. There have been reports of several cases of strikingly severe thrombotic complications following splenectomy in patients with hereditary stomatocytosis. Iron overload is a common complication of hereditary stomatocytosis.

HEMOLYTIC ANEMIAS CAUSED BY RED CELL METABOLISM ABNORMALITIES

The two genetic defects in red cell metabolisms associated with significant hemolysis affect either glucose-6-phosphate dehydrogenase (G6PD) or pyruvate kinase (PK). The production of reduced nicotinamide adenine dinucleotide phosphate (NADPH) by the pentose phosphate pathway plays a central role in providing this essential coenzyme to reductive processes and to protect against oxidant damage. G6PD catalyzes the first step of this pathway. NADPH is the essential hydrogen donor that supports the regeneration of reduced glutathione (GSH) from oxidized glutathione and the activity of catalase, which degrades H_2O_2.

PK catalyzes an essential step in ATP synthesis. PK defects result in (1) ATP deficiency with early demise of reticulocyte and erythrocytes and (2) marked increases in glycolytic intermediates above the defect, resulting in a marked elevation in 2,3-diphosphoglycerate that favors the compensation of the anemia.

Glucose-6-Phosphate Dehydrogenase Deficiency

Clinical Manifestations

At steady state, in the absence of offending agents, no hematologic or serum biochemical abnormalities are present. A typical presentation is that of a hemolytic crisis, with anemia, jaundice, and dark urines, precipitated by a variety of offending agents, including antimalarial drugs (primaquine, pamaquine[2]), sulfonamides and sulfones, nitrofurans, and antihelmintics. Hemolysis usually resolves in a few days, with return to baseline Hb levels in a few weeks. An acute hemolytic attack after ingestion of fava beans (favism) is typical in children, with severe symptomatic anemia, fever, abdominal pain, nausea, and more rarely vomiting.

Severe neonatal jaundice is a frequent neonatal complication of G6PD deficiency. A small fraction of patients present with chronic hemolytic anemia, with reticulocytosis and normal red cell indices.

Molecular and Cellular Bases of the Disease

The gene of G6PD resides toward the end of the long arm of chromosome X. Approximately 500 mutations have been described that result in qualitative or quantitative changes in G6PD. High-incidence areas for G6PD deficiency are Africa, the Mediterranean countries, the Middle East, and Southeast Asia. Although this X-linked disease mostly affects males, the incidence of G6PD deficiency is sufficiently high to produce cases of symptomatic females. G6PD deficiency cells are unable to regenerate large quantities of GSH and thus compensate the increased generation of oxidized glutathione by an oxidizing agent. When GSH is depleted, SH residues of Hb are oxidized and denatured Hb precipitates on the inner side of the membrane.

Laboratory Diagnosis

Moderate to severe anemia characterizes hemolytic attacks; staining with methyl violet reveals the presence of Heinz bodies (precipitates of denatured Hb, more prominent within the first 24 hours of an acute episode). Haptoglobin levels are extremely low, free Hb may be present in serum, unconjugated bilirubin

[1]Not FDA approved for this indication.

[2]Not available in the United States.

is elevated, and urines are dark because of the presence of hemoglobinuria. The direct antiglobulin test is negative, ruling out autoimmune hemolysis.

Several semiquantitative screening tests are available for the initial identification of a deficiency in G6PD. Samples with less than 30% of the normal activity should be considered deficient. Specific quantitative determination of G6PD activity is available in several reference or specialized laboratories. However, false-negative results may be obtained in the presence of reticulocytes or leukocytes (increased G6PD activity) and immediately after acute hemolysis because the destruction of older cells leaves behind a relatively "young" population with higher G6PD activity. After a severe hemolytic episode, it may be necessary to wait 2 to 3 weeks before performing G6PD activity studies.

Treatment

Transfusion should be considered if the anemia is severe and the hemolysis is persistent (continuous hemoglobinuria). Acute renal failure may complicate a severe hemolytic episode. Drugs and/or food known to generate oxidative insults should be avoided.

Pyruvate Kinase Deficiency

PK deficiency affects mostly people of northern European and Mediterranean ancestry. Transmission is autosomal dominant. Anemia is seen only in the presence of homozygous defects. The clinical severity of the chronic hemolysis varies, with exacerbations of hemolysis during pregnancy or infections; aplastic crises related to parvovirus infections are a potential complication.

Acquired Nonimmune Hemolytic Anemias

PAROXYSMAL NOCTURNAL HEMOGLOBINURIA

Clinical Manifestations

Paroxysmal nocturnal hemoglobinuria (PNH) is a rare acquired disease that usually arises as hemolytic anemia in a previously healthy subject, in many cases associated with the report of dark urine (sign of hemoglobinuria and intravascular hemolysis). Anemia is characterized by paroxysmal hemolytic crises and in less than half of the cases is accompanied by the classical nocturnal hemoglobinuria. Deep vein thrombosis can be the initial presentation and less frequently cytopenia and bone marrow failure, from mild degrees all the way to severe aplastic anemia. In "florid PNH," hemolysis and thrombotic complications are prominent; in "aplastic anemia with a PNH clone" the picture is that of severe aplastic anemia with the incidental finding of a PNH clone. PNH is a chronic disorder, with a median survival time of 8 to 10 years.

Molecular and Cellular Bases of the Disease

PNH erythrocytes lack membrane proteins, which use a glycosyl phosphatidylinositol (GPI) anchor embedded into the membrane to attach to the cell membrane. Acquired mutations in the PIG-A gene (phosphatidyl inositol glycan complementation group A), a critical component in the biosynthetic process of GPI anchors, have been demonstrated in most patients with PNH. The PIG-A gene is located on the short arm of the X chromosome, and a single (one-hit) mutation can induce the PNH phenotype. Thus, PNH is a clonal disorder. However, because PNH clones and PIG-A mutations can be seen in hematologically normal subjects, it is possible that additional factors determine the expansion of these clones in PNH. The absence of proteins that limit complement activation and insertion in red cells (CD55, CD59, C8-binding protein) explains the chronic intravascular hemolysis of PNH and its exacerbation with concomitant viral or bacterial infections. The pathophysiology of thrombotic complications of PNH is not clear: the hypercoagulable state of PNH seems to be due to platelet hyperactivity (platelets also arise from the PNH clone) rather than activation of the coagulation factors cascade because it is not prevented by warfarin (Coumadin) or heparin prophylaxis. The aplastic anemia associated with PNH is most likely due to autoimmunity because it responds to immunosuppressive therapy in the majority of cases.

Laboratory Diagnosis

The classical tests based on the hemolysis of PNH erythrocytes in the presence of acidified serum or low ionic strength (Ham test, sugar-water test, sucrose hemolysis) have been replaced by specific flow cytometric determination of CD59/55 on red cells. On the basis of the expansion of the PNH clone, the proportion of cells defective in CD59/55 and the extent of CD59/55 depletion vary among subjects and in the same subject over time. The severity of the disease is usually related to the proportion of CD59/55-deficient cells.

Treatment

Allogeneic bone marrow transplantation (BMT) should be considered in young patients, especially if an HLA-identical sibling is available. A less aggressive treatment course, which is the only option for patients who are not candidates for BMT, is based on immunosuppressive therapy with antilymphocyte globulin (ALG) or antithymocyte globulin (ATG)[1] and cyclosporine (Neoral)[1]. Supportive treatment with chronic red blood cell transfusion is another therapeutic option for PNH patients. If PNH arises as "aplastic anemia with a PNH clone," the therapy

[1]Not FDA approved for this indication.

should be similar to that of other aplastic anemias and is detailed elsewhere.

TRAUMATIC (ANGIOPATHIC) HEMOLYTIC ANEMIAS

Clinical Manifestations

Erythrocytes undergo mechanical damage when exposed to disturbances of the blood flow, which generate high shear stress. Traumatic hemolysis can be seen in 5% to 15% of heart valve surgical replacements, more commonly with mechanical (carbon alloy) valves. Rarely, traumatic hemolysis may be seen in congenital heart defects, such as patent ductus arteriosus or ventricular septal defects. These clinical situations are defined as macroangiopathic hemolytic anemias to distinguish them from traumatic anemias associated with disseminated intravascular coagulation and thrombotic thrombocytopenic purpura-hemolytic-uremic syndromes (microangiopathic anemias). In microangiopathic anemias, intravascular activation of the coagulation cascade in small vessels leads to formation of fibrin aggregates that disrupt blood flow and cause traumatic hemolysis. Acute, self-limited traumatic hemolysis can be seen after strenuous physical exercise or activities that impose local damage on circulating blood cells (long-distance running, drumming, karate).

Laboratory Diagnosis

The hallmark of traumatic hemolysis is the presence on the peripheral smear of schistocytes (fragmented red cells) and sometimes "helmet," "burr," or "triangle" cells. Haptoglobin is decreased and indirect bilirubin and serum LDH are increased. Additional laboratory abnormalities may be present depending on the underlying disease.

Treatment

Severe anemia may require transfusion. Anemia usually resolves with the resolution of the underlying disease.

PERNICIOUS ANEMIA AND OTHER MEGALOBLASTIC ANEMIAS

METHOD OF
Glenn Tisman, MD

The clinical portrait of vitamin B_{12} and folate deficiencies has changed during the last three decades. In the past the clinician was on the lookout for overt megaloblastic anemia before thinking of folate or B_{12} deficiency. Neurologic compromise associated with B_{12} deficiency was a secondary concern. Today, because of the advent of newer, sensitive laboratory testing and awareness of damage from metabolic perturbations caused by early folate and B_{12} deficiencies, other disorders strongly associated with deficiency of these vitamins have taken center stage. These include birth defects, diffuse atherosclerosis, coronary artery disease, venous and arterial thrombosis, increased risk of breast and colon cancer, and subtle-to-marked neuropsychiatric compromise.

Before deficiency of these vitamins causes clinically detectable hematologic change, patients present with measurable perturbations in cell metabolism resulting in elevated concentrations of blood homocysteine and methylmalonic acid. Half or more of the general population older than 69 years have laboratory abnormalities of hidden or overt B_{12} or folate deficiency.

As vitamin deficiency progresses, blood cell nuclear maturation is impaired and red cells become large and oval in shape (macroovalocytosis). White blood cell precursors enlarge, producing giant metamyelocytes and bands. Mature granulocytes display hypersegmented nuclei. If anemia is present, the clinical picture is one of megaloblastic anemia. An early clinical sign of B_{12} deficiency includes subtle loss of vibratory sensation of the index toes to the 265 vibrations per second (vps) tuning fork. Both B_{12} and folate deficiencies may present with atrophy of the tongue mucosa and angular stomatitis.

Causes of folate and B_{12} deficiencies are so diverse that deficiency of these vitamins should be pursued in any elderly patient, in patients with hyperhomocysteinemia, unexplained neuropsychiatric dysfunction, or, in those with anemia, leukopenia, thrombocytopenia, or stomatitis.

This article discusses the diagnosis, clinical spectrum, and treatment of B_{12} and folate deficiencies.

Laboratory Evaluation of Suspected Folate or B_{12} Deficiency

Evaluation begins with the suspicion of deficiency followed by a review of a stained blood smear. Morphologic changes of folate and B_{12} deficiencies are identical. Although many disorders may cause red blood cell (RBC) macrocytosis (Table 1), only megaloblastic anemia presents with macroovalocytic RBCs. Macroovalocytosis may be accompanied by teardrop-shaped RBCs, and the mean corpuscular volume (MCV) is usually greater than 95 fL. Although macrocytosis is a hallmark of folate and B_{12} deficiency, these deficiencies only account for 10% of macrocytosis cases. Many B_{12}- and folate-deficient patients display a normal MCV.

B_{12} deficiency may cause very large ovalocytes (MCV greater than 120 fL), yet it presents with normal-sized red cells in 33% of patients. Consider that iron deficiency decreases the MCV. Thus iron deficiency coupled with folate or B_{12} deficiency will present a dimorphic picture of the peripheral blood. In such cases, both large and small ovalocytic RBCs are present and the MCV may be normal.

Measurement of Serum Vitamin and Metabolite Levels

B_{12}

Normal total serum B_{12} levels range between 200 to 900 pg/mL. However, marked clinical B_{12} deficiency has been reported with serum levels well within the lower normal range of 200 to 375 pg/mL.

FOLATE

The World Health Organization (WHO) defines the lower limit of normal for serum folate as 13.6 nmol/L (6 ng/mL). Levels below 6 ng/mL induce a rapid and steep rise in serum homocysteine. The National Health and Nutrition Evaluation Surveys II (NHANES II) study defined the lower limit as 6.8 nmol/L or 3 ng/mL.

The lower limit of normal for RBC folate is 317 nmol/L or 160 ng/mL. Erythrocyte folate is an indirect measure of folate stores for the past 60 to 90 days. It is helpful in determining true folate deficiency in patients given a large dietary or medicinal source of folate before blood for the assay is collected. Under such circumstances, serum levels are normal while RBC folate remains low.

TABLE 1 Causes of Macrocytosis Without Ovalocytosis

Reticulocytosis
Drug effects (alcohol)
Liver disease
Hypothyroidism
Myeloproliferative diseases
Myelodysplastic syndromes
Aplastic anemia
Chronic lung disease
Cold agglutinin disease

THE METABOLITES: BLOOD HOMOCYSTEINE AND METHYLMALONIC ACID

Elevations of both homocysteine and methylmalonic acid are sensitive metabolic markers of B_{12} deficiency and occur in more than 90% of cases, while elevated homocysteine alone accompanies folate deficiency. Normal serum total homocysteine levels vary between 5.1 to 13.9 μmol/L. Normal blood methylmalonic acid ranges between 73 and 376 nmol/L.

These metabolites are useful in determining early vitamin deficiency where anemia and clinical signs are absent, and may indicate insufficiency with otherwise normal serum vitamin levels. Homocysteine is elevated in 20% of patients with normal serum B_{12} and folate. Unfortunately, renal failure may cause elevation of both metabolites, while hypothyroidism, diabetes mellitus, rheumatoid arthritis, and certain drugs (anticonvulsants, methotrexate [Rheumatrex], and cycloserine [Seromycin]) may cause elevation of homocysteine.

HOLOTRANSCOBALAMIN: EARLY MARKER OF B_{12} MALABSORPTION

B_{12} is transported in the serum bound to two major proteins, transcobalamin and haptocorrin. Holotranscobalamin is composed of B_{12} attached to transcobalamin and represents biologically active serum B_{12} delivered to all DNA-synthesizing cells. Normal holotranscobalamin levels are greater than 70 pg/mL. In early B_{12} malabsorption, levels range from 40 to 70 pg/mL. Normally holotranscobalamin represents only 20% of total serum B_{12}.

B_{12} bound to haptocorrin as holohaptocorrin represents the 80% of metabolically inert B_{12}. When B_{12} absorption from the gastrointestinal (GI) tract decreases, holotranscobalamin, with a metabolic half-life of only 6 minutes, rapidly falls below normal even while total serum B_{12} remains within normal limits for months. This defines B_{12} malabsorption in the presence of normal serum B_{12} levels. Tests to measure serum holotranscobalamin are now commercially available.

SERUM ANTIBODIES AND ATROPHIC GASTRITIS

If advanced chronic atrophic gastritis of pernicious anemia (PA) is present (see section titled Causes of Deficiency–B_{12}), then 90% of patients with PA will have antibody to intrinsic factor (IF) in either gastric juice or serum.

SCHILLING TEST

While the Schilling test does not diagnose B_{12} deficiency, it can be used to determine the mechanism

TABLE 2 Schilling Test Results

Condition	Oral ^{57}Co-Cbl	Oral ^{57}Co-Cbl + IF	Oral ^{57}Co-Cbl after 7-10 Days of Tetracycline	Oral ^{57}Co-Cbl + Pancreatic Extract	Oral ^{57}Co-Cbl Food Absorption
Normal	N				
Lack of IF	Low	N			
Bacterial overgrowth	Low	Low	N		
Pancreatic insufficiency	Low	Low	Low	N	
Defective ilial enterocyte transport	Low	Low	Low	Low	
Inadequate dissociation of food-bound B_{12}	N				Low
Folate deficiency	Low until folate Rx	Low until folate Rx	Low	Low	
B_{12} deficiency	Low	Possibly low until 2 mo of B_{12} Rx			

Abbreviations: ^{57}Co-Cbl = radioactively labeled cyanocobalamin; IF = intrinsic factor; Low = low Schilling test result; N = normal Schilling test result.

responsible for B_{12} malabsorption (Table 2). The test measures B_{12} absorption by the amount of orally administered ^{57}Co-labeled-B_{12} excreted in a 24-hour urine collection after injecting 1000 μg of cobalamin at baseline to bind to all blood and tissue B_{12} binding sites (normal is 8% or greater secretion).

BLOOD, BONE MARROW, AND OTHER CELLS

Blood and bone marrow changes of folate and B_{12} deficiencies are identical and morphologically indistinguishable. As vitamin depletion progresses from metabolic abnormality to overt anemia, routine blood counts may reveal depression of any or all formed elements. The appearance of a single six-lobe neutrophil or more than 5% of neutrophils with five lobes is very suggestive of folate or B_{12} deficiency (in the absence of other factors associated with hypersegmentation, such as iron deficiency, hereditary hypersegmentation, uremia, glucocorticoid ingestion, and treatment with antimetabolites).

The reticulocyte count is normal or low, and in severe cases serum lactate dehydrogenase (LDH) and total bilirubin rise and haptoglobin falls.

Bone marrow is generally hyperplastic. Nucleated RBC morphology consists of finely stippled, sieve-like open nuclear chromatin, appearing as the surface of sliced salami.

White blood cell precursor changes include enlarged (called *giant*) metamyelocytes and large band forms with hypersegmentation of neutrophils (neutrophil lobe average or Arneth count greater than 3.5 lobes/cell). The megakaryocyte is large, as is its product the platelet.

Megaloblastosis may be seen in cells lining the GI tract (buccal mucosa, tongue, enterocytes), bronchial epithelium, and cells of the uterine cervix. These changes may lead to vitamin-reversible dysplasia and possibly contribute to irreversible malignancy of the breast and colon.

Clinical Spectrum of Megaloblastic Anemias and B_{12} and Folic Acid Deficiencies

The late Dr. Victor Herbert, a brilliant pioneer researcher of folate and B_{12} metabolism, observed that deficiency of these vitamins progresses through four stages of negative vitamin balance. One may trace these orderly stages of vitamin insufficiency in most but not all patients. Occasionally tissue deficiency may be present in the absence of serum deficiency. In stages I and II, the plasma pool and then the cell stores become vitamin depleted. In stage III depletion, the metabolic markers, blood homocysteine (for folate and B_{12} depletion), and methylmalonic acid (for B_{12} depletion) are elevated. Stage IV depletion is marked by clinical signs and symptoms associated with severe anemia and possibly neurologic and psychiatric symptoms.

The degree of folate or B_{12} insufficiency combined with a patient's basic genetic repertoire determines the clinical presentation. Because the U.S. government added folic acid to grains and flour, and television advertisements and health food stores began pushing the sales of vitamin supplements, the frequency of folate deficiency has declined. Patient demographics such as age, diet, ingested medications, gestational status, alcohol ingestion, and the presence of hereditary enzyme defects (i.e., thermolabile tetrahydrofolate reductase and hereditary deficiency of folate conjugase) determine the clinical picture.

CLINICAL PRESENTATION

Folate Deficiency

A new concept in folate metabolism suggests that folate deficiency may be compartmentalized. For instance, there is evidence that bronchial mucosal cells, cells of the uterine cervix, and some esophageal mucosal cells may become deficient in folate before there are signs of anemia or depletion of folate from blood cells. Additionally, there may be folate deficiency of both red and granulocyte precursors without deficiency within lymphocytes. This compartmentalization may allow the toxic effects of hyperhomocysteinemia, dysplasia, and premalignant changes to progress in the absence of the usual signs of megaloblastic anemia.

Deficiency of folic acid at the time of conception is associated with neural tube defects of the offspring. High concentrations of homocysteine caused by folate or B_{12} deficiency have been associated with increased habitual spontaneous abortion and serious complications of pregnancy, including hypertension, preeclampsia, and placental abruption. Homocysteine is a vascular and neurotoxin and is strongly associated with atherosclerosis, coronary artery disease, and stroke.

Marked folate deficiency presents with megaloblastic anemia, leukopenia, and thrombocytopenia. Hyperhomocysteinemia may synergize with other causes of thrombophilia (factor V Leiden, estrogen and progesterone ingestion) thus increasing the incidence of thrombosis. There is an association between folate deficiency and increased incidence of cancer of the breast, ovary, and colon.

Neurologic symptoms including impaired cognitive function, depression, and recent memory loss are associated with elevated homocysteine and folate deficiency. Other unusual neurologic symptoms have been observed, including peripheral neuropathy similar to that reported for B_{12} deficiency.

Recent studies have noted the acute onset of folate deficiency in some critically ill patients manifest by thrombocytopenia and variable leukopenia in the absence of macrocytosis. Serum folate and red cell folate may be normal, but the deficiency is expressed within the rapidly proliferating bone marrow compartment requiring more folate than can be supplied.

B_{12} Deficiency

The earliest stages of B_{12} depletion, stages I and II, are manifest by the progressive decrease of serum holotranscobalamin. Neurologic compromise ranging from loss of recent memory to overt subacute combined degeneration of the spinal cord (ataxic gait, peripheral neuropathy, loss of vibratory sensation, and loss of proprioception) may occur at this stage. An early objective clinical sign is loss of vibratory sensation to the 256 vps tuning fork at the index toe. Such damage may occur while the total serum B_{12} level remains well within the normal range. If neurologic damage is detected within 6 months of the first symptoms, it will totally reverse with parenteral B_{12} therapy. Symptoms present for more than 6 months may only partially resolve.

Stage III depletion is associated with hypersegmented granulocytes and elevation of both homocysteine and methylmalonic acid. Stage IV deficiency is associated with macroovalocytic anemia, and progressive neurologic damage may be present.

TABLE 3 Causes of Folate Deficiency

Dietary Insufficiency
Tea and toast eaters, indigent populations, nursing home population, chronic alcoholics alcohol = empty calories
Destruction of Folate
Ingestion of large amounts of vitamin C in the presence of iron supplements destroys folate, heating finely minced foods
Abnormal Small-Bowel Absorption
Regional enteritis, intestinal lymphoma, surgical intestinal resection, blind loops (i.e., proximal duodenal segment of a Billroth II resection), amyloidosis, sarcoidosis, Whipple disease, scleroderma, gluten-induced enteropathy, B_{12} deficiency causing megaloblastic mucosa with decreased absorptive capacity
Genetic defect of the folate polyglutamate conjugase enzyme causes decreased absorption
Increased Need for Folate
Critically ill patients, pregnancy, psoriasis, chronic hemolysis (thalassemia)
Drugs and Chemicals
Birth control pills, alcohol, metformin, phenytoin (Dilantin), phenobarbital (Luminal), sulfonamides and methotrexate (Rheumatrex), triamterene; trimethoprim, pentamidine, Azulfidine

CAUSES OF DEFICIENCY

Folate

Usual causes of folate deficiency are given in Table 3. Dietary insufficiency is the most common cause of folate deficiency. Folic acid is absorbed in the proximal half of the small intestine. A typical deficient patient is an elderly person whose diet is inadequate in fresh fruits and vegetables, or who cooks foods diluted in copious amounts of water, or who cooks finely minced foods that are exposed to excessive heat (Mexican diet).

Increased use of folate can occur in critically ill intensive care unit (ICU) patients, during pregnancy, in patients with psoriasis or exfoliative dermatitis, in patients with leukemia, and in persons with chronic hemolysis (thalassemic syndromes).

B_{12}

The most frequent causes of vitamin B_{12} deficiency are given in Table 4. The leading cause is related to chronic atrophic gastritis of the body of the stomach resulting in either inability to liberate B_{12} from food or to ilial malabsorption.

Pernicious Anemia

There are two types of chronic atrophic gastritis. Type A, or autoimmune gastritis, involves the body of the stomach while sparing the gastrin-producing

TABLE 4 Causes of B_{12} Deficiency

Cultural/Religious Causes

Strict vegetarianism; Hinduism, Seventh-Day Adventism

Failure of B_{12} Absorption (Small Bowel)

Ilial surgery/resection, Crohn disease, hereditary anomaly of IF-B_{12} receptors as occurs in Imerslund-Grasbeck syndrome, pernicious anemia, gluten-induced enteropathy, tropical sprue

Failure of B_{12} Liberation from Food and Absorption

Chronic atrophic gastritis of the body of the stomach with varying degrees of hypochlorhydria, pepsin deficiency, and loss of intrinsic factor (pernicious anemia), gastrectomy (partial or total)

Competition in Utilization

Diphyllobothrium latum parasitic infestation, blind loop syndrome with bacterial overgrowth in stomach and small bowel; rapidly growing malignant cells

External-Beam Radiation

Pelvic or abdominal irradiation (for rectal, cervical, endometrial, and prostate cancer)

Drugs

Metformin (Glucophage), birth control pills, cancer chemotherapy, nitrous oxide anesthesia (for as little as 65 minutes), hypochlorhydria as a result of over-the-counter H_2, and proton pump inhibitor ingestion

antrum. Type B, or nonimmune gastritis, involves the antrum as well as the body. Type B is associated with *Helicobacter pylori* infection, low serum gastrin concentrations, hypochlorhydria, and decreased B_{12} absorption caused by impaired HCl-mediated release of dietary protein–bound B_{12} from food.

The advanced stage of type A body gastritis is associated with pernicious anemia (PA), a genetically predetermined, autosomal recessive, chronic, atrophic gastritis involving the body of the stomach. It results in decreased excretion of pepsin, hydrochloric acid, parietal cell intrinsic factor, and autoantibodies to IF. The end results are anemia and malabsorption of B_{12} at the terminal ileum. In type A atrophic body gastritis results in elevation of gastrin and a decrease of serum pepsinogen I.

PA occurs primarily in whites, and is more likely to occur in persons of Scandinavian and Northern European descent. Recent evidence suggests that PA also occurs in Asian, Latin American, and African American persons, although with much lower frequency. It is more frequent in women and usually occurs in women older than 40 years of age, although black women have an earlier age of onset. *H. pylori*–associated gastritis is most common in the elderly and in immigrant populations.

Intrinsic factor secreted by the parietal cell must first bind B_{12} before the vitamin can be absorbed by specific receptors of the terminal ileum. The atrophic gastritis causing PA slowly progresses over 20 to 30 years. Initial gastric damage is manifest by hypochlorhydria and inability to cleave B_{12} from food protein. As the relentless parietal cell atrophy continues, IF autoantibody and loss of IF secretion intensify the malabsorption of not only food-bound B_{12} but crystalline B_{12} as well.

There is a four- to sixfold increased risk of gastric malignancy in patients with PA (adenocarcinoma) and in those with *H. pylori* infection (adenocarcinoma and mucosa-associated lymphoid tissue lymphoma [MALToma]). Approximately 20% of relatives of PA patients develop pernicious anemia.

Many studies have demonstrated decreased B_{12} absorption caused by chronic atrophic gastritis of the body of the stomach and hypochlorhydria in as many as 20% to 49% of those older than age 64. However, advanced atrophic body gastritis leading to lack of IF or PA occurs in only 2% of those older than age 60 years. Thus there is a spectrum of gastric atrophy caused by various degrees of atrophic body gastritis, initially associated with decreased acid secretion (types A and B), and ultimately culminating in PA with failure to produce intrinsic factor (late stage type A). Patients with gastritis may be without peptic symptoms. It is not unusual for these patients to present with severe neurologic damage caused by subtle B_{12} deficiency in the absence of anemia. These patients have abnormally low serum holotranscobalamin levels.

PA may be associated with other autoimmune endocrinopathies and with antireceptor autoimmune diseases such as Hashimoto thyroiditis, type I diabetes mellitus, hypoadrenalism, primary hypoparathyroidism, vitiligo, Graves disease, myasthenia gravis, and the Lambert-Eaton syndrome.

Other Causes of B_{12} Deficiency

When *Diphyllobothrium latum* (i.e., fish tapeworm) is entrenched in the small intestine, it competes with the host for ingested B_{12}. The organism is most often found contaminating fish in Canada, Alaska, and the Baltic Sea. Traditional preparation of gefilte fish where the chef tastes the ground fish mixture before cooking may initiate infection in the chef.

Blind loop syndrome involves bacterial colonization of intestines that are deformed either because of strictures, surgical blind loops, or anastomoses. Folate deficiency may cause malabsorption of B_{12}.

Nitrous oxide anesthesia for as short as 65 minutes irreversibly inactivates cobalamin-dependent methionine synthase, thus causing acute megaloblastic hematopoiesis. This may aggravate marginal B_{12}/folate status by precipitating neurologic symptoms, or it may synergize with known inhibitors of folate metabolism (i.e., methotrexate given as chemotherapy or used in rheumatoid arthritis). Nitrous oxide has been abused as a recreational drug. Its effects are rapidly circumvented by folinic acid (leucovorin) administration.

Treatment of Megaloblastic Anemias

Anemia caused by folate or B_{12} deficiency responds to folic acid administration. This may be dangerous for patients deficient in B_{12}, however, because anemia caused by B_{12} deficiency responds to large dose of folic acid but associated neurologic damage continues to progress. Thus exact diagnosis before therapy is highly recommended. If the patient is acutely ill, a blood draw for vitamin and metabolite levels should be done, and bone marrow should be taken if possible. Blood may be administered slowly with use of diuretics or opposite arm phlebotomy to avoid congestive heart failure. Patients found to be deficient in both vitamins should simultaneously receive both.

VITAMIN REPLACEMENT AND SUPPLEMENT THERAPY

B_{12} Replacement

Initial treatment of pernicious anemia and other causes of cobalamin malabsorption require intensive parenteral therapy to restore stores to normal levels. Available preparations include cyanocobalamin and hydroxocobalamin. I treat with cyanocobalamin 1000 μg subcutaneously, intravenously, or intramuscularly daily for 7 days followed by weekly administration for an additional month and monthly thereafter. After 2 months patients with pernicious anemia, small-bowel disease, blind loop syndrome, or gastrectomy may continue parenteral therapy or convert to oral crystalline B_{12} administration with 1000 μg orally every day for life. Vegans need only 25 to 100 μg of B_{12} orally every day for life.

After initiation of treatment, serum B_{12} levels and hematologic response should be monitored closely. Serum iron usually falls within 24 hours, reticulocyte count increases by 72 hours and peaks in 7 to 10 days. Although bone marrow morphology reverts to normal within 24 to 48 hours, neutrophil hypersegmentation may linger for 2 weeks. Hemoglobin, neutrophil, and platelet counts will increase after 1 week. Failure to return to normal hematologic parameters suggests complicating factors such as folate or iron deficiency, chronic renal failure, chronic inflammation, or myelodysplastic syndrome.

Clinical symptoms rapidly improve. Occasionally, diffuse bone pain may be precipitated 24 to 72 hours following the first B_{12} injection as a result of bone marrow expansion. Serum potassium may precipitously drop, necessitating potassium replacement. Iron deficiency, if present or precipitated by therapy, must be treated to ensure a complete hematologic response. Psychiatric symptoms rapidly regress while neurologic damage, if present for less than 6 months, completely reverses, but if present longer improvement may only be slight.

Folate Supplementation During Conception and Pregnancy

The estimated mean dietary folate intake of women is approximately 200 μg per day, which is approximately equivalent to the recommended dietary allowance (RDA) for the nonpregnant state (180 μg per day). Approximately 90% of women consume less than 400 μg folate per day (the recommended dietary allowance for pregnancy is 600 μg per day). It is estimated that a supplemental dose of folate of 200 μg per day would reduce the risk of neural tube defects (NTDs) by 42%. To prevent the first occurrence of an NTD, women are recommended to consume an extra 400 μg per day in addition to usual folate intake from before conception (last menstrual period plus or minus 28 days). Approximately 50% of all pregnancies are unplanned. Thus governmental supplementation of flour and grain with folate, which increases consumption by approximately 200 μg per day, should substantially decrease birth defects for those unplanned pregnancies. A supplement of 400 μg of folic acid periconceptionally and during pregnancy and lactation is adequate to decrease the frequency of NTDs by half and will maintain adequate folate stores during the increased folate use of pregnancy and lactation.

Folate Replacement Therapy

Folate deficiency is treated with oral folic acid. Nonprescription preparations available in health food stores include 800-μg tablets. Prescription preparations include 1- and 5- mg tablets. In the absence of severe malabsorption, patients will respond to oral 100- to 200-μg doses. In the presence of severe malabsorption, daily doses as high as 2 to 5 mg may be necessary for maximum response. The time line for hematologic response is identical to that noted for B_{12} deficiency. If the cause of folate deficiency can be corrected, then after folate stores are restored (usually after 4 months of therapy), supplementation may be discontinued.

THALASSEMIA

METHOD OF

Susan P. Perrine, MD, and Valia Boosalis, MD

Pathophysiology: Basic Mechanisms of Hemoglobin Synthesis

The sequential expression of the globin genes results in production of specific types of hemoglobins at different stages of development. At 12 weeks of gestation, a transition from embryonic to fetal hemoglobin ($\alpha_2\gamma_2$) occurs; and at 28 weeks of gestation, increasing amounts of β-globin and of adult hemoglobin (Hb A, $\alpha_2\beta_2$) are produced. For intact hemoglobin tetramers to form, α-like globin proteins must equal β-like globin proteins. Thalassemia syndromes result from deficiencies in either α-globin (α-thalassemia) or β-like globin (β-thalassemia) chains. The diseases become apparent when the affected globin is required during development. During gestation, α-thalassemia is symptomatic, because α-globin is required for fetal hemoglobin (Hb F, $\alpha_2\gamma_2$). Because β-globin is not required in large amounts before birth, β-thalassemia is asymptomatic until 6 months after birth. Mutations that cause prolonged production of fetal γ-globin chains may manifest later, at 2 to 4 years of age.

The major pathologic process of thalassemia is caused by the imbalance of α and non-α chain accumulation. The unaffected chains, produced in normal amounts, precipitate during erythropoiesis. In β-thalassemia, the precipitated α-globin chains are particularly toxic, damaging cell membranes and causing rapid cell death (apoptosis). Red blood cell life span is further shortened by removal of abnormal cells in the reticuloendothelial system. In response to the hypoxia, erythropoietin levels increase, causing erythroid hyperplasia. Hypersplenism causes more severe anemia. An increase in plasma volume, from marrow and splenic expansion, also lowers hemoglobin levels.

In β-thalassemic fetuses, the unbalanced fetal (γ)-globin chains form tetramers (γ_4, hemoglobin Bart's); excess β-globin (β_4, hemoglobin H) accumulates after birth. Hemoglobin Bart's and hemoglobin H result in milder ineffective erythropoiesis but have abnormal oxygen binding. If all four α-globin genes are deleted, only hemoglobin Bart's is formed, with a massively left-shifted oxygen dissociation curve that provides almost no oxygen delivery to tissues and results in a lethal intrauterine condition, hydrops fetalis. Decreased production of α-globin from three or four abnormal α-globin genes results in a moderate hemolytic anemia, hemoglobin H disease. Deletion of only one (α-thalassemia-2) or two (α-thalassemia-1) loci is asymptomatic.

Thalassemia syndromes are graded according to severity of the anemia. *Thalassemia major*, in which severe anemia manifests during infancy, is caused by inheritance of two severely impaired β-globin alleles. This homozygous or doubly heterozygous state may have a milder manifestation when there is a higher-than-usual increase in fetal chain production or when the co-inheritance of β-thalassemia decreases the net imbalance of the synthesis of α-globin to β-globin. *Thalassemia trait* (thalassemia minor), which is caused by the inheritance of a single defective allele, is characterized by mild hypochromic, microcytic anemia. *Thalassemia intermedia* manifests as moderate anemia with total hemoglobin levels of 6.0 to 10.0 g/dL. These patients require occasional transfusions with concomitant infections, but do not require chronic transfusions.

Diagnosis

The diagnosis of severe thalassemia is usually straightforward in ethnic groups at risk (Mediterranean, African, Asian, Middle Eastern, East Indian). Thalassemia major and intermedia are marked by severe microcytic anemia; hyperbilirubinemia, elevated lactate dehydrogenase levels, and splenomegaly appear in the first few years of life (β-thalassemia). Hydrops fetalis (α-thalassemia with classic four-gene deletion) manifests as polyhydramnios and fetal distress during the second trimester. Thalassemia trait is characterized by mild anemia (hematocrit greater than 30), low mean corpuscular volume (less than 75 fL), and erythrocytosis (red blood cell [RBC] count of greater than 5×10^6 per mm^3). Quantitative hemoglobin electrophoresis demonstrates elevated hemoglobins A_2 and F. Hemoglobin A is absent in β°-thalassemia and decreased in β+-thalassemia. α-Thalassemia is best diagnosed by the presence of hemoglobin Bart's in cord blood. Hemoglobin H is unstable, and electrophoresis of fresh specimens is required for its detection. In most, but not all, β-thalassemia heterozygotes, hemoglobin A_2 levels are elevated. Basophilic stippling, target cells, fragmented cells (schistocytes), and nucleated RBCs are typical of the severe thalassemias. The reticulocyte count may be relatively low because of ineffective erythropoiesis, and MCV may become high from rapid emergence of erythroid precursors. Prenatal diagnosis of thalassemia is performed by direct polymerase chain reaction (PCR) analysis of fetal DNA obtained by amniocentesis or chorionic villus sampling. This procedure is being explored for use in preimplantation diagnosis and in vitro fertilization procedures.

Transfusion Therapy

In β-thalassemia major, RBC transfusion is the mainstay of supportive therapy. Transfusions should maintain a hemoglobin level ideally above 10.5 to 11 g/dL (range: 10.5 to 13 g/dL) to suppress endogenous erythropoiesis, with the least amount of transfused blood required. Regular transfusions are begun for a persistent decline in hemoglobin below 7 g/dL in children with two β-thalassemic mutations. A complete genotype of the patient's RBCs should be performed before transfusions are begun to facilitate identification of involved antigens in the event of isoimmunization. Ideally, transfusions of 15 mL/kg of packed RBCs (in children) should be given at 3- to 4-week intervals using fresh compatible blood from a limited donor pool, and filtered to remove white blood cells and viruses inhabiting these cells. Cytomegalovirus (CMV)-negative preparations should be used for transplantation candidates. Administering acetaminophen (Tylenol) and diphenhydramine (Benadryl) before transfusions prevents febrile reactions. Transfusion records should be meticulously maintained to assess mean pre- and post-transfusion hemoglobin levels and annual blood consumption. An increase in transfusion requirements suggests hypersplenism, isoimmunization, or an accessory spleen.

Transfusions can transmit blood-borne infections, including hepatitis viruses, HIV, and CMV. In regions where hepatitis C is endemic, 90% of patients on chronic transfusions may develop hepatitis C within 5 years; chronic infection eventually advances to cirrhosis in 85%. Patients should be vaccinated against hepatitis A and B and monitored for elevated transaminase levels and for hepatitis C antibodies, with referral to consultants for management if found. Combined therapy with interferon alfa-2a (Roferon-A) and ribavirin (Rebetol) can produce sustained responses in hepatitis C; transfusion requirements often increase during treatment. HIV testing should be performed annually.

Partial exchange transfusion by erythrocytapheresis (PET-E), in which older red blood cells are exchanged for fresh-packed red cells by pheresis, reduces iron accumulation significantly compared to simple transfusion with deferoxamine chelation. PET-E exposes patients to more units of packed RBCs and minor side effects related to citrate, but reduces transfusional iron burden, which is the long-term cause of early mortality.

Splenectomy

Massive splenomegaly is avoidable by transfusion, but splenic sequestration of donor cells can cause excessive transfusion requirements. Splenectomy should be performed if a 40% or greater increase in the transfusion requirement occurs during a 1-year period, or if a transfusion of more than 200 mL/kg per year of packed RBCs is required without isoimmunization, or if the patient develops thrombocytopenia. Splenectomy increases the risk of overwhelming sepsis with encapsulated organisms and *Yersinia*, especially in young children, so ideally should be deferred until 4 to 5 years of age. Polyvalent pneumococcal vaccine should be given at least 1 month before splenectomy. Prophylactic oral penicillin VK should be used in children younger than 10 years and for invasive (dental) procedures. Immediate medical attention should be sought and broad-spectrum antibiotics given emergently for significant fever (greater than 38.3°C [101°F]), as asplenic patients are at risk for a fulminant course and death within hours.

Complications of Transfusion Therapy

Approximately 1 mg of iron per mL of packed RBCs is administered in packed RBC transfusions, with no mechanism for elimination. Iron deposition from transfusional hemosiderosis causes dysfunction in the heart, liver, and endocrine organs. Glucose intolerance with insulin-dependent diabetes mellitus, primary hypothyroidism, hypoparathyroidism, delayed puberty, amenorrhea, and other endocrinopathies are not uncommon; digoxin refractoriness and arrhythmias result from cardiac iron deposition and hypocalcemia secondary to hypoparathyroidism. Growth retardation may respond to growth hormone before 13 years of age. Hepatic hemosiderosis and hepatitis C lead to fibrosis and cirrhosis. Cardiac dysfunction (detectable first by magnetic resonance T2* measurement of less than 20 milliseconds and reduced ejection fractions) typically presents with fatigue, arrhythmias, or pericarditis, advancing to congestive heart failure. Cardiac disease remains the major cause of death in transfused patients (60%), with infections (13%) and liver disease, including cancer, (6%) following. Osteopenia may be severe and cause fractures, especially in thalassemia intermedia. Patients should be maintained on elemental calcium (1500 mg per day) and vitamin D (400 IU per day) in adults. Osteoporosis may require bisphosphonates, such as pamidronate (Aredia)[1] or alendronate (Fosamax), and monitoring with calcium, phosphate, 1,25-hydroxyvitamin D levels, 24-hour urinary calcium and hydroxyproline, and bone mineral density (dual-energy x-ray absorptiometry scan [DEXA]) measurements annually.

Monitoring and Treatment of Iron Overload (Table 1)

The parenteral iron chelator deferoxamine mesylate (Desferal) is the only first-line chelator approved in the United States and Europe for more than 30 years. Deferoxamine can maintain negative iron balance relative to the transfusion burden, when administered five to seven times per week as a continuous subcutaneous or intravenous infusion or as twice-daily bolus subcutaneous (not intramuscular) injections of the same total dose. Urinary iron excretion is used to adjust the dosage to maintain negative iron balance. When begun within 2 years of beginning transfusions and faithfully administered, deferoxamine prolongs survival. If a significant iron burden is present before chelation therapy is begun, progressive cardiac dysfunction may not be completely prevented or reversed.

Iron overload should be documented by a challenge test or begun after 12 to 18 months of regular transfusions, as children require iron for growth, and chelation is detrimental for patients who are not overloaded with iron. To begin chelation, iron in a 24-hour urine after injection of 500 mg of deferoxamine should exceed 1 mg, or the serum ferritin level should exceed 1000 ng/mL. Small infusion pumps are used to administer doses of 25 to 40 mg/kg per day over 12 hours subcutaneously. Irritation from hypertonicity and

[1]Not FDA approved for this indication.

TABLE 1 Recommended Monitoring of Thalassemia Patients

Monitoring of Patients Undergoing Regular Transfusions
Red blood cell phenotype (before transfusions)
History, monthly physical examination
Pre- and post-transfusion CBC and record of amounts of each transfusion
Indirect antibody screen twice annually or with a positive Coombs test result on cross-match
Liver function studies (ALT, AST, bilirubin, GGT, LDH, alkaline phosphatase, albumin, total protein, and ferritin every 3 months)
Hepatitis A and B panels (before vaccine)
Hepatitis C antibody (mRNA by PCR if antibody-positive) and HIV test annually
INR and PTT annually
Liver biopsy, after 5 years of transfusions, or in hepatomegaly cases, to assess iron content and fibrosis
T2* MRI of hepatic and cardiac iron burden
Cardiac Monitoring After 5 Years of Transfusions
Echocardiogram, ECG annually
T2* MRI to evaluate cardiac iron and ventricular function
24-hour Holter or event monitor (for patients >12 years) annually
Cardiology consultation, stress test (for patients >18 years)
Endocrine and Osteoporosis Monitoring
TSH, free T_4 parathormone, calcium, inorganic phosphorus, growth hormone levels annually
Glucose tolerance test, Cortrosyn stimulation test annually
Gonadotropins and estradiol or testosterone after 12 years of age annually
Bone mineral density test or DEXA, bone age annually
24-hour urine calcium, creatinine, hydroxyproline annually
Serum calcium, phosphorus, alkaline phosphatase, 1,25-hydroxyvitamin D level twice annually
Monitoring of Effects of Deferoxamine Therapy
Ophthalmologic and hearing evaluation annually
Sitting and standing height, weight every 4-6 months until 18 years of age
Zinc, copper, selenium, vitamin C, and vitamin E levels every 4-6 months
Urinary iron excretion annually or biannually and dose adjustment

Abbreviations: ALT = alanine aminotransferase; AST = aspartate aminotransferase; CBC = complete blood cell count; DEXA = dual-energy x-ray absorptiometry (scan); ECG = electrocardiogram; GGT = g-glutamyltransferase; INR = international normalized ratio; LDH = lactate dehydrogenase; MRI = magnetic resonance imaging; PCR = polymerase chain reaction; PTT = partial thromboplastin time; TSH = thyroid-stimulating hormone.

local reactions can be prevented by increasing the diluent to produce a 10% solution, adding hydrocortisone (2 mg/mL), or with topical diphenhydramine. A topical anesthetic cream should be applied 30 to 60 minutes before insertion of the needle. Intravenous administration through an indwelling port device is often more tolerable, because such devices can be accessed once weekly without repeated needle sticks. Intravenous chelation is more effective than subcutaneous chelation, so fewer treatment days may suffice. Arrhythmias and congestive heart failure have been temporarily reversed with high-dose deferoxamine (15 mg/kg per hour maximum for 24 hours per day, 7 days per week). Anaphylactic reactions can be treated with desensitization; idiosyncratic acute respiratory distress syndromes are rare but life-threatening, necessitating rapid recognition and intensive care. Excessive doses can cause optic and acoustic neuritis, so ophthalmologic and hearing evaluations should be performed annually. Iron overload causes depletion of vitamin C, which inhibits iron release from reticuloendothelial cells. Sudden availability of vitamin C can cause a massive release of iron and serious cardiotoxicity. Vitamin C (50 mg per day in children and 100 mg per day in adults) should be given only after the first cycle of deferoxamine. Despite available deferoxamine therapy, 50% to 60% of transfused thalassemia patients die of cardiac disease before age 35 years.

New oral and long-acting iron chelators (still in clinical trials in the United States) offer major advantages and less onerous therapy. The oral chelator deferiprone[1] (L1) crosses cell membranes more readily than does deferoxamine, and, in a recent British study, prevented the onset or progression of myocardial dysfunction more effectively. Combined use of deferoxamine (2 days per week) with daily deferiprone (75 mg/kg) produces higher iron excretion than deferoxamine alone. An international trial demonstrated that deferiprone does not promote hepatic fibrosis, which had been raised previously in a trial that was confounded by hepatitis C. A new oral chelator, ICL670*, requires administration once daily and has shown efficacy similar to deferoxamine in ongoing clinical studies. The experimental chelator 40SD02*, containing deferoxamine chemically attached to a modified starch polymer, has favorable pharmacokinetics with once weekly intravenous administration.

Serial ferritin levels should be followed every 3 months, but *do not correlate directly with cardiac iron*. Liver biopsy is used to assess hepatic iron content and fibrosis, but also does not correlate with *cardiac* iron burden. Noninvasive technology is available in a few medical centers, including a superconducting quantum interference device (SQUID) and T2*, a magnetic resonance method that assesses myocardial iron and ventricular function in the same study and can detect myocardial iron before ventricular dysfunction occurs, which facilitates earlier treatment. T2* can detect hepatic iron burden, albeit with more variability when fibrosis is present.

Thalassemia Intermedia

Patients with β-thalassemia who do not develop debilitating anemia should not be committed to a lifelong transfusion regimen. When the hemoglobin levels remain above 8 g/dL, patients generally can lead a normal life. Most specialists avoid regular transfusions

[1]Not FDA approved for this indication.
*Investigational drug in the United States.

at hemoglobin levels higher than 7 g/dL, particularly in regions where the blood supply predictably results in hepatitis C transmission, although intermittent transfusions are often necessary for more severe anemia with infections. Patients should be monitored closely for signs of marrow expansion, facial deformity, splenomegaly, or growth retardation. Facial deformity can be severe, and is an indication for regular transfusions. Hypertransfusion can often be avoided by splenectomy. Anemia in thalassemia intermedia patients, particularly those with high baseline Hb F levels, often responds to experimental therapies that stimulate fetal globin production.

The hyperplastic marrow in thalassemia intermedia stimulates intestinal iron absorption and iron overload, which eventually results in the same endocrine deficiencies that occur in thalassemia major, and requires chelation therapy. The same clinical manifestations, including splenomegaly, gallstones, osteopenia, and iron overload develop more slowly in thalassemia intermedia, but cardiomyopathy does not typically develop in untransfused patients. Avoidance of iron-rich meats and regular consumption of tea can reduce iron absorption. Folic acid and antioxidant supplements should be given. Spinal cord compression syndromes from thoracic or vertebral paraspinal bone marrow masses should be suspected with acute or increasing weakness, numbness, and diminished reflexes in the lower extremities—this is a medical emergency. Diagnosis is made by magnetic resonance imaging (MRI) or computed tomography (CT); radiation therapy and steroids should be instituted emergently.

α-Thalassemia

The homozygous form of α-thalassemia is usually lethal in utero. However, prenatal diagnosis and milder variants have enabled affected fetuses to be supported to term with intrauterine transfusions, followed by postnatal transfusions. For milder hemoglobin H disease, only folic acid, antioxidants, and monitoring for severe anemia during infections or with increasing splenomegaly are necessary. Because hemoglobin H is sensitive to oxidant stress, drugs such as sulfonamides should be avoided, particularly with coexistent glucose-6-phosphate dehydrogenase (G6PD) deficiency. Iron status should be monitored.

Transplantation

Allogeneic bone marrow or stem cell transplantation is curative by replacing the patient's hematopoietic stem cells with normal stem cells that contain two normal genes or one normal and one thalassemic globin gene. Transplantation from a human leukocyte antigen (HLA)–identical related donor in patients younger than 8 years of age, without hepatic fibrosis, and with a good iron chelation history (risk class 1), has an excellent prognosis. Still, the overall mortality rate of transplantation in experienced centers is 15%. Significant morbidity may result from graft-versus-host disease (GVHD). Unrelated donors and cord blood as sources of donor cells have increased risks of GVHD and graft rejection, but provide broader availability. Relapses (graft rejection) occur in 8% of patients receiving related donor transplants. Many patients do well clinically even with mixed chimeric states. The serious risks of this curative treatment modality must be weighed against the lifelong burden of hypertransfusion and chelation. This balance may be shifted with the new oral iron chelators.

Stimulation of Fetal Globin Gene Synthesis and Erythropoiesis

A large body of evidence shows that expression of endogenous fetal globin to approximately 70% of α-globin chain synthesis ameliorates anemia in β-thalassemia enough to eliminate transfusion requirements. Chemotherapeutic agents (5-azacytidine[1] or decitabine[1], hydroxyurea[1]), short chain fatty acid derivatives (SCFADs), and human recombinant (rhu) erythropoietin (EPO) are being evaluated in phase II trials, with best responses observed in patients with baseline endogenous (untransfused) Hb F levels of greater than 50%. Combinations of these agents will likely be required to completely eliminate transfusion requirements in severe β-thalassemia patients. SCFADs, which are not mutagenic or cytotoxic, are preferable over chemotherapy for lifelong treatment. Sodium phenylbutyrate (Buphenyl)[1] and arginine butyrate[1], which require large numbers of tablets or IV infusion, respectively, have increased total hemoglobin by 1 to 4 g/dL above baseline in untransfused patients with active erythropoiesis. Patients with β+ thalassemia with baseline erythropoietin levels less than 40 mU/mL have responded best to combined therapy with butyrate and EPO. The long-acting EPO preparation, darbepoetin (Aranesp)[1], may also increase hemoglobin in some. These therapies require supplementation with oral iron to be effective, even in the presence of elevated ferritin levels, as stored iron may not be available for erythropoiesis, and several months of treatment are often required for responses to EPO. New oral short chain fatty acid derivatives, which are currently being evaluated, appear more tolerable and promising.

Gene Transfer

Gene therapy for β-thalassemia requires both a transfer of the fetal (γ) or a normal β-globin gene into repopulating hematopoietic stem cells and a

[1]Not FDA approved for this indication.

high-level expression of transferred genes solely in erythrocytes throughout life, a formidable challenge. Major DNA regulatory elements must also be introduced, and transferred genes must be integrated at sites that allow high-level expression. Problems that must be surmounted include:

- Need and production of safe, effective vectors for long-term treatment
- Prevention of silencing of transduced genes
- Difficulty in transducing rare pluripotent repopulating stem cells
- Selective expansion of transduced stem cells
- Selection of ablative chemotherapy prior to infusion of transfected cells (to create space in the marrow for expansion of transduced stem cells)

Clinical trials of gene therapy with limited endpoints are projected to begin in years 2006 to 2007.

SICKLE CELL SYNDROME

METHOD OF

Olufemi O. Akinyanju, MD

Although it is now clear that modern treatment can enhance the quality of life and increase the life span of persons with sickle cell disorder (SCD), knowledge of the pathophysiology of the disorder is incomplete. SCD is an inherited hemoglobin disorder arising from the possession of variant sickle (S) hemoglobin, alone or in combination with another variant hemoglobin (Hb). It is the most common inherited disorder in the world by virtue of the survival advantage it has conferred over the centuries on heterozygous carriers of the S gene in areas where falciparum malaria is or was endemic. The sickle cell syndrome describes the characteristic clinical manifestations in patients with SCD.

Sickle cell disorder includes the homozygotes with sickle cell anemia (Hb SS), the double heterozygotes with sickle cell hemoglobin C (Hb SC), sickle thalassemia (Hb Sb^+-thalassemia and Hb $S\beta^o$-thalassemia), and other very rare combinations with Hb S. The vast majority of patients with SCD are homozygotes (Hb SS), whereas only a relatively few are double heterozygotes. Although patients with SCD are found on many continents, more than 80% of Hb SS newborns are born in Africa. While black Africans, African Americans, and West Indians are predominantly affected, SCD is also present in some other racial groups. These include Arabs in parts of Saudi Arabia, Indians, Northern Greeks, and Portuguese.

Apart from Hb S, more than 600 other variant hemoglobins have been described in humans. Further discussion of them is beyond the scope of this article, except to state that a few of them are rather commonly found in combination with Hb S in the same individual. The most common of these, which is only found in persons of West African descent, is Hb C. Others are Hb E (which is found in indigents of Southeast Asia), Hb D, and Hb G. Among West African indigents or descendants, patients who are doubly heterozygous with Hb SC, or even homozygous with Hb CC, may be encountered.

Sickle Cell Trait

The single heterozygotes with sickle cell trait (Hb AS or Hb AC) are healthy carriers with a normal hematologic profile and a normal life expectancy. They ordinarily do not have symptoms related to SCD except for a rare hematuria caused by papillary necrosis in persons with sickle cell trait (Hb AS).

Pathogenic Mechanisms

Two basic pathogenic mechanisms are widely believed to be responsible for the clinical manifestations of the sickle cell syndrome (Figure 1). The first is that deoxygenation of the erythrocyte induces polymerization of the Hb S, rendering the cell elongated and rigid. The rigid sickled erythrocyte is unable to deform sufficiently to traverse small blood vessels in the microcirculation and consequently breaks down, thereby shortening the red cell life span from an average of 120 days to an average of 10 days. The resulting chronic hemolysis is not compensated in patients with Hb SS and Hb $S\beta^o$-thalassemia, but may be compensated in patients with Hb SC in whom anemia may therefore be absent or mild (Table 1). The compensatory effort of the bone marrow leads to expansion of the marrow-containing bones and to excess production

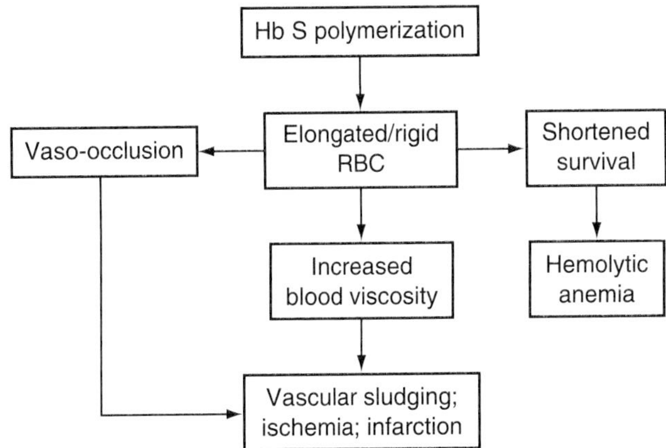

FIGURE 1 Sickle cell syndrome pathogenic mechanisms.

TABLE 1 Hemoglobin Genotypes and Usual Concentrations

Hb Genotype	Usual Range of Hb (g/dL)
AA	12-16
AS	12-16
AC	12-16
SC	9-14
Sβ⁺ thal	8-13
SS	6-10
Sβ⁰ thal	6-10

Abbreviation: Hb = hemoglobin.

of reticulocytes and variable numbers of nucleated red blood cells. Platelets are moderately-to-markedly increased, whereas leukocytes may be mildly elevated. The leukocyte count is, however, liable to error because nucleated red cells are often enumerated along with it to give a falsely high value. For this reason, the clinician should insist on a corrected white blood cell (WBC) count before making a decision based on it.

According to the second pathogenic theory, the rigid sickled cells are prone to circulatory logjams, which cause occlusion (*not thrombosis*) of small blood vessels. This vasoocclusion leads to sluggish blood flow, which, in turn, leads to more deoxygenation and more sickling and sluggish flow in a vicious circle leading eventually to ischemia and infarction in distal organs. This process is thought to cause the pain in the bones and abdomen and to cause painless infarction and necrosis in various organs. Further elucidation of the pathophysiology of several morbid events is clearly required. Some mysteries and inconsistencies requiring answers are:

- Cerebral thrombosis (*not sickle cell vasoocclusion*) with consequent neurologic deficit (e.g., stroke) is more common in children than in adolescents and adults with sickle cell anemia.
- Patients with severe lobar pneumonia tend to be spared from bone pains at a time when oxygenation of erythrocytes should be suboptimal.
- Tonsillitis, a relatively minor infection with little, if any, influence on deoxygenation, is a recognized trigger of bone pain crisis.
- The most severe and prolonged pain crisis can occur unexpectedly in a clinically stable patient.
- Severe pain lasting for several days has been known to involve the nipples of both breasts and subside without leaving any visible sign of ischemia of the tissue in a patient with Hb SC.
- Patients with Hb CC disorder, whose red cells do not sickle, are known to have typical bone pain crisis on rare occasions.
- The ingestion of certain foods or drugs triggers pain crises in some individuals.

Severity of Symptoms

There is great disparity and unpredictability in the severity and frequency of symptoms in the sickle cell syndrome. This is only partially explained by the influence of known genetic or environmental attributes because it can sometimes be seen between affected siblings sharing the same environment. Persons with Hb SS and Hb Sβ°-thalassemia generally have the most severe illness, whereas persons with Hb CC have few, if any, symptoms throughout life. Persons with Hb SC and Hb Sβ⁺-thalassemia fall somewhere between these two extremes in clinical severity. The two best-known ameliorating genetic factors are a high percentage of fetal hemoglobin (Hb F) or coexisting α-thalassemia, although the influence of the latter is still controversial. Nevertheless, the unpredictability of the clinical course of SCD makes pronouncements on the severity of the syndrome in any particular individual a risky pastime.

Concept of the Steady State and Sickle Cell Crisis

Individuals with SCD are said to be in a steady state when they are feeling and looking well and have maintained a state of well-being without acute symptoms over the preceding 2 weeks. Affected persons are in steady state most of the time, during which they tend to maintain stable hematologic levels.

A sickle cell crisis is an acute noninfectious ailment that is peculiar to, and solely attributable to, SCD. Thus infection per se is not a sickle cell crisis, although it may provoke one or arise as a sequel to one. The frequency of crises varies from person to person and from time to time in the same person. Sickle cell crises can be classified into vasoocclusive or anemic, but both types may afflict a patient simultaneously. Crisis often arises without apparent cause, but some conditions are recognized as triggers of crises (Table 2).

VASOOCCLUSIVE CRISES

These crises are the most common and certainly the most dramatic sickle cell crises (Table 3). The bones are most frequently involved, and they become mildly to excruciatingly painful and may also become swollen or tender, or both. The pain is self-limiting and lasts for an average of 4 days when moderately severe. In tropical Africa, these crises occur more frequently during the rainy season whereas in temperate or cold countries, they are more frequent during the winter.

TABLE 2 Factors That May Trigger Sickle Cell Crisis

Rapid exposure to colder weather or environment
Drenching by rain
Excessive physical exertion (e.g., competitive sports)
Late pregnancy, childbirth, and puerperium
Infection: malarial, bacterial, viral, or mycoplasma
Dehydration (e.g., after alcoholic binge, water deprivation, fever, excessive heat, sweating)
Idiosyncratic reaction (? allergic) to foods, drugs, or chemicals
Emotional or mental stress

TABLE 3 Classification of Vasoocclusive Crises

Painful	Painless
Bones	Hematuria
Abdomen	Stroke
Acute chest syndrome	Acute visual impairment (retinopathy)
Acute hepatopathy	
Priapism	

ANEMIA CRISIS

This term describes a life-threatening situation in which anemia increases so rapidly that it induces dyspnea at rest or on slight exertion, or causes heart failure. The Hb level is usually below 5.0 g/dL, and the etiology is multifactorial (Table 4).

General Treatment Strategies

GOAL

The goal of treatment is to ensure that the affected individual leads a happy and fulfilled life, free from the characteristic pains, debilitating complications, and untimely death. The objectives may be itemized as follows:

- To maintain a steady state of health
- To prevent complications
- To treat complications promptly and effectively
- To promote a healthy lifestyle
- To promote a positive self-image in the affected person

HOLISTIC TREATMENT

The strategy is to deliver holistic treatment, which takes care of the overall needs of the patient and not only the immediate clinical ones. The advantages are that the patient is more involved in his or her own management, understands its purpose and options and, therefore, complies better. The patient is also better able to cope with the medical and social consequences of the disorder or of its treatment and is more confident and eventually requires less therapeutic intervention.

TABLE 4 Classification of Crises of Anemia

Cause	Etiology
Hyperhemolysis	Infection (e.g., malaria, G6PD deficiency)
Acute red cell sequestration	Splenic, hepatic, mesenteric, or pulmonary
Chronic hypersplenism	Splenomegaly
Red cell hypoplasia	Renal failure, folate deficiency, infection
Aplastic	Epidemic parvovirus B19 infection

Abbreviation: G6PD = glucose-6-phosphate dehydrogenase.

Measures aimed at achieving the objectives include the following:

- Appropriate and continuing education of health care professionals
- Information, education, and communication activities appropriately targeted to relevant segments of the community, including resource allocators
- Delivery of genetic counseling and relevant health and nutritional education to patient and significant relatives
- Encouragement of membership in patient support and patient advocacy groups
- Infection prophylaxis
- Avoidance of crisis-provoking conditions
- Daily folic acid and multivitamin supplementation
- Access to prompt consultation for symptoms
- Pharmacologic amelioration of disease severity if necessary
- Sex education
- Supervised pregnancy and childbirth
- Regular health surveillance checks
- Family planning and family life education
- Establishment of a sickle cell center in areas of high prevalence to coordinate and monitor the delivery of clinical and other services

Establishment of an Accurate Diagnosis

This step may appear superfluous, but it is occasionally omitted for a variety of reasons. Patients may wrongly believe they have SCD because of misunderstanding or misinformation. A poorly endowed laboratory may wrongly diagnose a case of Hb SC as Hb SS; or Hb AD as Hb AS; or Hb Sβ^+-thalassemia as Hb AS. Another fairly common error is that a laboratory may understandably diagnose Hb SS as Hb AS shortly after the patient has received a blood transfusion. The physician should interpret the result in its true context.

Genetic Counseling

SCD should be sensitively managed within the community. Otherwise, affected individuals and persons with the sickle cell trait may feel stigmatized and be tempted to conceal, deny, or falsify their status. This can be counterproductive to efforts aimed at managing and controlling the disorder in the community. The importance of genetic counseling in preventing these undesirable outcomes is well established. The role of the counselor is to ensure that the clients (patient, family, or carrier) are provided with all the information necessary to assist them in reaching their own decision on any course of action. Their decision must be respected and supported by the counselor, and confidentiality maintained. Failure to do so may alienate the client. Effective counseling is thus informative, confidential, nondirective, and supportive. It requires skills that are best acquired through appropriate training and experience. Physicians who see many patients with SCD should endeavor to acquire the necessary skills, or employ the services of trained counselors, or both.

Growth and Development

Growth, puberty, and sexual development are delayed, especially in persons with Hb SS and Hb Sβ°-thalassemia. They tend to be small for their age between childhood and adolescence, after which their growth accelerates and they usually attain normal stature by young adulthood. A few of them also have a delay in overcoming nocturnal *enuresis,* which may continue until puberty or adolescence. Reassurance that dryness will be achieved sooner or later allays much anxiety. Meanwhile, limiting fluid intake a couple of hours before bedtime and emptying the bladder just before retiring can reduce its frequency. In contrast, patients with milder phenotypes such as Hb SC tend to have a normal rate of growth, sexual development, and physique.

Complications and Their Management

SPLENIC DISEASE

From the earliest age, the spleen is overburdened with products of broken-down erythrocytes, thus impairing its bacteria-filtering role. Furthermore, repeated infarction leads to early splenic necrosis and shrinkage, compromising its protective role especially against pneumococcal and other encapsulated bacteria. This so-called *autosplenectomy* occurs less commonly in patients with Hb SC and Hb Sβ⁺-thalassemia and is unknown in those with Hb CC disorder. Thus, spleens are usually not palpable in patients with Hb SS but are palpably enlarged in some patients with Hb Sβ⁺-thalassemia or Hb SC and in virtually all Hb CC patients.

The spleen may suddenly enlarge and trap a significant proportion of the circulating blood cells, thus creating a sudden severe anemia. This phenomenon, known as *acute splenic sequestration* (ASS), is common in young children and, although self-limiting, tends to be recurrent and may be fatal. Immediate blood transfusion saves lives. Parents should therefore be taught to palpate the spleen, recognize ASS, and seek urgent blood transfusion. Splenectomy should be performed after no more than two episodes.

Chronic splenomegaly is rare in Hb SS patients but it occasionally occurs. The spleen can become uncomfortably large and also retain a larger proportion of circulating blood cells, leading to chronic severe anemia and stunting. This *chronic hypersplenism* is cured by elective splenectomy, which should be preceded by pneumococcal vaccination and followed by lifelong prophylactic penicillin.

LIVER DISEASE

Like the spleen, the liver macrophages are overloaded with iron and cellular debris from excessive hemolysis. Unlike the spleen, however, the liver is spared the indignity of shrinkage in size because of its double blood supply and its remarkable powers of regeneration. It usually becomes enlarged as the child grows older. The insult to the liver occasionally results in pain, tenderness, and intrahepatic obstructive jaundice. The absence of preicteric anorexia and of very highly raised serum transaminase levels helps to distinguish this *sickle hepatopathy* from infective hepatitis. *Acute sequestration of blood cells* occasionally occurs in the liver, leading to sudden enlargement and tenderness of the organ and severe anemia. Transfusion of 1 to 2 units of blood rapidly reverses the symptoms and signs.

GALLBLADDER DISEASE

Bilirubin gallstones are found in up to 30% of patients with Hb SS. They are best demonstrated by ultrasonography, but calcified stones are visible on plain radiographs. They are usually asymptomatic and do not require treatment. Rarely, they may cause pain, infection, or extrahepatic obstructive jaundice. When possible, complications should be treated conservatively, but cholecystectomy may occasionally be necessary.

UROGENITAL DISEASE

From an early age, patients manifest *hyposthenuria,* which describes a reduced capacity of the renal tubules to concentrate urine and thus conserve body fluids. This makes patients susceptible to dehydration at times when they feel least inclined to drink, such as during a severe pain crisis or when abstinence is enforced, as before general anesthesia. At such times, attention should be paid to hydrating patients intravenously.

Hematuria resulting from papillary necrosis may occur and can be diagnosed on a plain radiograph. The bleeding is usually from the left kidney and is commonly mild and self-limiting. Hematuria can be alarming and the physician should assure the patient and family that it is self-limiting and has a good prognosis. Admission to the hospital, high fluid intake (4 to 5 liters per day with furosemide [Lasix], 40 mg twice daily), and alkalinization of the urine with sodium bicarbonate are the cornerstone of treatment. The increased urinary volume helps to prevent blood clots in the urinary tract. When blood is profuse, replacement blood transfusion is needed. We have never needed to perform nephrectomy, which is a last resort for catastrophic prolonged blood loss.

It is negligent to assume that all hematuria is caused by papillary necrosis. A thorough investigation to exclude other causes should always be carried out.

Albuminuria unrelated to infection is fairly common in adults. It should not be mistaken for preeclampsia in pregnant women, but it may herald *nephrosis* in some patients.

Chronic renal failure may be seen in some adolescent or adult patients and should be suspected when there is systemic hypertension (otherwise rare in SCD) or persistent severe anemia.

Priapism, or unwanted erection of the penis, is common in SCD. Minor priapism is defined as unwanted erection lasting more than 30 minutes but less than 3 hours. Minor priapism is often recurrent daily or weekly, usually at night or at the time of arising in the morning, and it is termed stuttering priapism. It may begin in boys as young as 5 years of age, and it usually subsides spontaneously or after urine is passed or after light exercise or a cold shower. A trial of oral hydralazine (Apresoline)[1], 25 mg, or nifedipine (Procardia)[1], 10 mg, or an antiandrogen (e.g., stilbestrol[1]), 5 mg daily for 3 to 10 days or etilefrine (adrenergic agonist) 50 to 100 mg daily may be successful in preventing further episodes of stuttering priapism. A longer course of an antiandrogen drug for up to 6 months may be necessary to prevent recurrences but should rarely be used. We can surmise from the multiple claims that an effective treatment of choice is not yet discovered. Exchange blood transfusion (EBT) may also be useful in terminating stuttering priapism that is unresponsive to conservative treatment.

Sustained or major priapism (lasting more than 3 hours) is rare, occurring in less than 2% of males. It is very painful, and the corpora cavernosa are engorged with stagnant sickle erythrocytes. The pathophysiology of priapism is not known and the engorgement may well be a consequence and not the cause of it. The treatment of major priapism is unsatisfactory. Reassurance and pain relief are important, using analgesics of commensurate potency. The patient should be well-hydrated intravenously. Oxygen inhalations should be given, and the effect of slowly administered intravenous hydralazine[1], 10 mg every 3 hours for 3 doses, should be tried while monitoring for hypotension. EBT should be performed early in the course of major priapism to give it the best chance of success. If the condition persists, the corpora cavernosa should be aspirated through a wide-bore needle. Thereafter, the Winter procedure—shunting between the corpora spongiosum and the corpora cavernosum—should be performed under local anesthesia, preferably by a urologist.

Prevention of Sickle Cell Crisis

Simple, attentive, holistic care without hydroxyurea or pneumococcal vaccination can drastically reduce the morbidity and mortality rates in the Hb SS population. We have shown this in a tightly run Sickle Cell Club and Clinic in Lagos, whose membership consequently did not meet the three-crises-per-year criterion for inclusion in a clinical trial.

Elimination of a nidus of infection can also reduce the frequency of crisis. In our experience, an increased frequency of pain crisis in patients with recurrent tonsillitis was significantly reversed after *tonsillectomy.*

When confronted with a patient experiencing intolerable severe frequent crisis, our policy is to exhaust all strategies of reversing the trend. When it is impossible to identify and eliminate or avoid the provoking factors, the patient is offered treatment with *hydroxyurea* (Hydrea), after due explanation. For monitoring purposes, the levels of total Hb, Hb F, mean corpuscular volume (MCV), and WBCs are determined initially and every 3 months thereafter while patients remain on the drug. We find an average dose of 1500 mg daily effective in a small group of our patients. Regarding efficacy, hydroxyurea has, on the whole, reduced the frequency of crisis, improved the sense of well-being, and engendered greater confidence in the pursuit of daily activities. A recent review has suggested that patients on hydroxyurea live longer than those who are not. For this reason, some sickle cell doctors have advocated its use in all persons with sickle cell anemia. Perhaps irrationally, I have not yet adopted this all-for-it approach. Time will tell.

Infection in Sickle Cell Disorder

There is increased susceptibility to infection caused by *Streptococcus pneumoniae* (pneumonia, septicemia, and meningitis) and to salmonella osteomyelitis. The susceptibility to pneumococcal infection is attributed to splenic dysfunction; occurrence is greatest in very young children with Hb SS, and markedly diminishing in older patients. The salmonellae are opportunistic bacteria that colonize bone in which defenses against bacteria have been compromised by ischemia and necrosis. Staphylococcal infection (*Staphylococcus aureus* and *Staphylococcus albus*) is also clinically important at any age. Other important pathogens in children in Africa include *Klebsiella* species, *Escherichia coli*, and *Pseudomonas* species. In countries in which it is endemic, malaria is a cause of severe anemia and death, especially in childhood and, to a lesser extent, in pregnancy.

Fever should always be regarded as indicative of infection. In bacterial infection, the WBC count usually shows neutrophilia with a shift to the left. Delay in making the diagnosis can be fatal, and the three greatest dangers are:

1. Regarding fever as an innocuous feature of sickle cell crisis.
2. Empirically treating a febrile patient for malaria and delaying consideration of the likelihood of bacterial infection. By the time the doctor discovers that the child is not responding to antimalarials, it may be too late.

[1]Not FDA approved for this indication.

3. Regarding a high corrected WBC count as being a normal feature in SCD rather than of infection.

In chronic osteomyelitis, the erythrocyte sedimentation rate tends to be raised and can be used to monitor progress. Early osteomyelitis can only be suspected and not conclusively diagnosed clinically or radiologically. Waiting for proof involves waiting for chronicity, by which time treatment is no longer an easy matter. Therefore, any persistently tender bone swelling after pain crisis should be regarded with suspicion and treated as acute osteomyelitis for 1 to 2 weeks in the first instance.

INFECTION PROPHYLAXIS

Malaria

In residents of countries in sub-Saharan Africa, malaria is best prevented throughout life by chemoprophylaxis and by adopting *mosquito bite avoidance measures* such as:

- Sleeping at night under mosquito nets impregnated with permethrin
- Wearing long-sleeved shirts and trousers in the evenings
- Eliminating nearby stagnant pools of water
- Applying topical mosquito-repellent skin lotions and sprays containing chemicals such as diethyltoluamide (DEET)

Chemoprophylaxis can be accomplished by daily oral proguanil hydrochloride (Paludrine)[1], 50 mg for children up to 5 years of age, 100 mg for older residents, and 200 mg for older visitors to the region. The long-term safety record of proguanil is excellent. The addition of chloroquine tablets (Aralen), 300 mg (base) once a week, is also advocated for nonimmune persons and visitors. Our practice is to use proguanil for prophylaxis and to reserve chloroquine for treatment.

When proguanil is not affordable, which is often in many developing countries, pyrimethamine (Daraprim) taken once a week has remained an effective alternative. The dose is 12.5 mg[3] for children up to 10 years of age and 25 mg weekly for older persons. Mefloquine (Lariam), 250 mg (125 mg for children 5 to 12 years of age) given once a week, is effective and safe over periods up to 1 year. Its long-term safety is not yet established.

Chemoprophylaxis should be started 1 week before traveling to an endemic area and continued for 1 month after leaving the area.

Pneumococcal Infections

Penicillin

Oral penicillin V, 125 mg twice daily (bid), is commenced at the age of 2 months. After the third birthday, it is increased to 250 mg bid. Erythromycin[1] at the same dose is given to patients who are allergic to or cannot tolerate penicillin. Penicillin prophylaxis has been shown to reduce the frequency of pneumococcal infection and save lives. Resistance to penicillin has not been a significant problem.

When to stop giving prophylactic penicillin has remained controversial over several years. Although a recent study suggests that it is safe to stop after the age of 5 years, previous reports of three teenage children dying from pneumococcal infection soon after they were taken off penicillin prophylaxis informs the reluctance of some sickle cell specialists to stop penicillin at any age. My own practice is to discontinue penicillin prophylaxis after the age of 10 years because, thereafter, compliance becomes a problem; moreover, the risk of pneumococcal infection is much reduced. If they develop fever after being taken off penicillin, I order blood tests for malaria or other infection but immediately start using amoxicillin (Amoxil)[1] or ceftriaxone (Rocephin)[1] and will subsequently add an antistaphylococcal agent such as dicloxacillin[1] or flucloxacillin[2] if necessary.

Children 5 to 10 years of age who have never used prophylactic penicillin are given the option of not starting but of reporting all fevers promptly to us or, if this is impossible, starting a course of amoxicillin.

Pneumococcal Vaccination

Pneumococcal vaccination (Pneumovax 23) has an additional role in the prevention of these infections. The traditional 23-valent polysaccharide vaccine (PPV) is not effective in children younger than the age of 2 years and is hence recommended from the age of 2 years and repeated 3 years later. A booster dose every 5 years may be adequate, provided there were no adverse reactions to the previous dose. The dose is 0.5 mL given into the deltoid or in older children into the thigh muscle. The vaccination is not a foolproof guarantee against pneumococcal infections.

A new 7-valent pneumococcal conjugate vaccine (PCV) has the advantage of being effective in children younger than 2 years. Three doses of 0.5 mL separated by intervals of 1 month can be given between the ages of 2 and 6 months. At the age of 2 years, PPV should still be given to those children who received PCV. A disadvantage of the conjugated vaccine is its enormous cost, which makes it inaccessible to the vast majority of my patients and to other eligible children in the developing countries.

Haemophilus influenzae Infections

The same bacterial defense defect that encourages pneumococcal infection also encourages infection caused by *Haemophilus influenzae* bacteria. The infections include pneumonia, septicemia, and meningitis. The difference is that although *H. influenzae* infection

[1]Not FDA approved for this indication.
[3]Exceeds dosage recommended by the manufacturer.

[1]Not FDA approved for this indication.
[2]Not available in the United States.

is four times more likely to occur in children with SS than in those without SCD, the risk is still much less than that of acquiring pneumococcal infection. Furthermore, it is not as fulminant or lethal as pneumococcal infection. Penicillin does not prevent the infection but for good measure, many doctors now protect infant sicklers with *H. influenzae* type b (Hib) conjugate vaccine given from the age of 6 months. The benefit from so doing has not yet been clearly demonstrated in a clinical trial.

TREATMENT OF INFECTIONS

Infections should be treated promptly with recognition that certain infections are particularly prevalent and fulminant in very young children with SCD. Malaria is obviously important in residents of countries in which it is endemic and in recent visitors to those countries. The collection of blood and other relevant specimens for full blood count, Gram staining, microscopy, and bacteriologic cultures should be completed within 60 to 90 minutes of presentation to allow for speedy commencement of treatment. *Malaria,* if diagnosed, should be treated in the standard manner.

Choice of antibiotics before bacteriologic confirmation should follow standard practice with the following exceptions. Any case of *meningitis* or suspicion of one should be treated as *pneumococcal* until proven otherwise. The same should be done for *lobar pneumonia and bacteremia* except that the spectrum should be extended to include the likelihood of staphylococcal infection if there is no clinical improvement within 36 to 48 hours of commencement. Intravenous infusion of aqueous penicillin G is still the most effective antibiotic for community-acquired lobar pneumonia in Nigeria, but this might vary in other places depending on prevailing resistance patterns. Erythromycin for 1 to 2 weeks in standard dosages for children and adults is effective in patients with *atypical pneumonia.*

All patients with *osteomyelitis* should be treated for salmonella and staphylococcal infection before evidence of causative bacteria is available. Acute osteomyelitis, defined as a case having a duration of less than 4 weeks, is curable within 4 weeks. Treatment should commence with intravenous antibiotics and may continue with oral drugs after subsidence of systemic symptoms. Chronic osteomyelitis requires prolonged treatment for 2 to 3 months with oral antibiotics and, often, surgical drainage, débridement, and sequestrectomy. Our standard antibiotics for chronic osteomyelitis have been chloramphenicol and cloxacillin or flucloxacillin[2], each given 500 mg every 6 hours. We have not had any adverse effects using chloramphenicol over the years, and its low cost and excellent absorption are assets. An alternative choice is ciprofloxacin (Cipro), 500 mg to 750 mg every 12 hours, for osteomyelitis. Septic arthritis should be treated with aspiration and the same antibiotics that are used for osteomyelitis unless culture yield dictates otherwise.

[2]Not available in the United States.

Bone Disease

Bone pain with inflammatory swelling and tenderness is the most common manifestation of sickle cell crisis. The distal bones, such as those of the hands and feet, are usually affected in infancy and early childhood up to the age of about 4 years. The resulting painful *dactylitis* and swelling of the soft tissues of the dorsa of the hands and feet constitute the *hand-foot syndrome,* which is the earliest manifestation of SCD in many patients. Other involved sites include the bones of more proximal sites in the arms and legs. The central bones of the vertebrae, ribs, and skull tend to be more involved in adolescents and adults. It is remarkable that bone pain is frequently bilateral, multisited, and symmetrical, especially in young children. Infarction of the bone marrow can, although rarely, lead to embolization of the marrow, which, if in the lungs, can cause serious problems. Full anticoagulant doses of heparin should then be administered.

When the mandible is affected, the consequent periosteal swelling may temporarily compress the mental nerves running through its foramina, causing numbness or a tingling sensation in the skin in their area of distribution, which is just beneath the lower lip. This is sometimes referred to as the *numb jaw syndrome.* The symptoms usually improve as the nerves recover from the inflammatory compression. Patients should be reassured about this common outcome. Vitamin B complex is prescribed, more for its placebo effect than for any proven efficacy.

Avascular necrosis of the head of the femur, on one or both sides, is a common disability starting in adolescence. The femoral head and nearby bones of the ischium are involved, showing variable areas of translucency and increased density on radiography. This may lead to pain, which is aggravated by walking, limping gait, and flattening of the head of the femur, with consequent shortening of the leg, secondary osteomyelitis, or subluxation of the hip joint. Avascular necrosis also affects vertebral bones and may cause mild-to-moderate kyphoscoliosis. Rarely, it affects the humeral heads and may result in severe pain and disability in the shoulder joints.

All infarcted bones lend themselves to colonization by opportunistic bacteria such as the salmonellae. Hence the high incidence, especially in early childhood, of multiple-sited salmonella osteomyelitis. Other organisms, especially the staphylococci, may also be involved.

Abdominal Pain Crisis

This describes acute, self-limiting abdominal pain that is not attributable to another disease process.

It is more common in children but care must be taken to exclude acute surgical abdomen by standard diagnostic methods. In most cases, the pain is mild to moderate and the signs are nondescript. In a severe case, the mesenteric vessels are widely occluded by sickled erythrocytes and the patient usually experiences severe generalized abdominal pain, fever, and tenderness, sometimes with rebound and some distension. The bowel sounds may become quiet and infrequent with ileus and distension and the anemia may increase. The liver may become enlarged and tender without or with jaundice of varied intensity. This clinical picture is known as the girdle syndrome. It is usually associated with staphylococcal or other bacteremia and is more common in adolescents and adults, in whom it is often fatal if not effectively treated. Vital signs should be frequently monitored and fluid balance maintained with intravenous infusion. Blood and stool cultures should be taken in an attempt to identify associated bacterial infection. Intravenous broad-spectrum antibiotics, such as a combination of cefuroxime (Zinacef), 1.5 g, gentamicin (Garamycin), 80 mg, and metronidazole (Flagyl), 500 mg, should be given every 8 hours. Analgesics and EBT are also given.

TREATMENT OF PAIN CRISES

The following methods are recommended:

- Reassurance and empathy to allay anxiety and establish rapport. Very severe pain is often accompanied by an unspoken but palpable fear of death, which should be dispelled.
- A quick history and examination to exclude any conditions that might require immediate attention or contraindicate the administration of opioid analgesics or nonsteroidal anti-inflammatory drugs (NSAIDs).
- Rapid relief of pain with analgesics of commensurate potency. This will gain the confidence of patient and relatives and facilitate thorough history taking and physical examination. With severe pain, it is best to start with an opioid drug such as parenteral morphine, 10 mg. Alternative drugs include diamorphine[2], 10 mg, and pentazocine (Talwin), 30 to 60 mg, or tramadol (Ultram), 50 to 100 mg. Adjuvant parenteral promethazine (Phenergan) is often useful to prevent vomiting and induce welcome sleep in a patient that may have been awake all night in pain.
- Oral or, where necessary, intravenous hydration, 70 to 100 mL/kg per day, with 4.3 dextrose in 0.18 normal saline or normal saline alternating with 5% dextrose in water.
- Follow-up analgesia, given with the same or other classes of analgesics before the anticipated duration of the analgesia elapses. This is done to forestall a return to the initial intensity of pain. Thus, a parenteral NSAID such as diclofenac (Voltaren), 75 mg, may be given before the duration of action of morphine is over.
- Treatment of any associated condition such as infection.
- Listening to and involving the patient in the plan and expected effect of treatment

Many studies show that fears of respiratory depression and of iatrogenic opiate addiction are mostly unfounded. Opioid drug should not be withheld unnecessarily and can be repeated every 3 hours in cases of severe pain. The physician should become familiar with the pharmacologic attributes and use of one or two analgesics in each potency class. Oral opioids or tramadol (Ultram) can be used for maintenance after the initial 2 to 4 parenteral doses. Intravenous patient-controlled analgesia using morphine or diamorphine[2] is an efficient and well-documented option (Table 5).

[2]Not available in the United States.

TABLE 5 Analgesia for Acute, Painful Crises

		Dose			
				CHILD	T
Indication	Drug	Adult	<1Y	1-5Y	6-12Y
Mild pain	Paracetamol[2]	1 g/4h	60 mg/4h	120 mg/4h	250 mg/4h
	Aspirin	600 mg/4h			
	Co-Proxamol[2]	1-2 tablet/4h			
	Naproxen	1-2 tablet/4h			
	Ibuprofen	1200-2400 mg/d		20 mg/kg/d	
Moderate pain	Dihydrocodeine[2]	60 mg/24h		1 mg/kg/6h	
	Oxycodone	40 mg/4h			
Severe pain	Pethidine[2]	1.5 mg/kg/h		0.5-1.5 mg/kg/h IV or IM	
	Morphine	0.15 mg/kg/4h		0.1 mg/kg/4h	

[2]Not available in the United States.
From World Health Organization: Guidelines for the management of sickle cell disease. WHO/HDP/SCD/GL/91.2. Geneva, WHO, 1991.

Acute Chest Syndrome

The deliberately vague term, acute chest syndrome (ACS), is used to describe any acute symptoms related to the chest. These symptoms usually include pain, tachypnea, dyspnea, and cough with or without fever. The pain may be continuous or pleuritic. Physical signs of ACS may include tenderness of some thoracic bones and abnormal breath and adventitial sounds. Pulmonary opacities may be visible on chest radiograph. The pathology can be one or more of the following:

- Thoracic bone pain crisis
- Pulmonary infarction
- Pulmonary infection
- Sequestration of erythrocytes

Conventional wisdom is that ACS is more likely to be caused by infection in children and by infarction in adults. ACS should be treated with antibiotics (as is done for pneumonia), bed rest, analgesics, and, if there is dyspnea at rest or hypoxemia, with oxygen inhalation and EBT.

Leg Ulceration

The prevalence of leg ulceration is less than 10% in West Africa but apparently much higher in the Caribbean and the United States. It is virtually unknown in patients younger than 12 years of age. Ulceration is situated around the medial or lateral malleolus of one or both ankles and arises spontaneously, although a history of preceding trauma may be obtained. It cannot be accurately attributed to the sickling phenomenon, because it is a recognized complication in all chronic, hereditary hemolytic anemias. Topical and systemic antibiotics have a limited role and should only be used when there is obvious localized infection. Healing is very slow but can be accelerated by keeping the wound surface fresh and clean, bed rest, daily dressings, or autologous skin grafting. The bane of leg ulcers is the high rate of recurrence, but permanent healing tends to occur in patients 30 years of age or older. My clinical impression, in agreement with some isolated reports, is that the use of oral hydroxyurea (Hydrea)[1] accelerates healing and may reduce recurrence. Enthusiasm for a clinical trial has been dampened by recent reports that hydroxyurea itself can induce skin ulceration.

Eye Disease

Visual loss, dimness, or blurring may be sudden and is usually caused by bleeding into the vitreous from a new growth of blood vessels, a condition termed proliferative sickle retinopathy (PSR). More than 90% of those affected have Hb SC and in many individuals, it is the first indication that they may have SCD. Altered vision is an alarming symptom for which much reassurance is required to decrease the patient's anxiety. It is important to refer the patient to an ophthalmologist with experience of the natural history of PSR. Meanwhile, bed rest with a pad over the affected eye will limit eye movements and promote cessation of the bleeding in the first few days.

Stroke

Stroke is predominantly the result of cerebral thrombosis and affects primarily children, with the median age at first occurrence being about 7 years. Mono- or hemiplegia, seizures, and intellectual disablement may result. There is a high recurrence rate of approximately 70% within 3 years of the first stroke. The goal of treatment is, therefore, to limit the damage and prevent a recurrence. The risk of developing a stroke can be predicted in 2-year-old children by routine Doppler transcranial ultrasonography, and the initial stroke can be prevented in a significant proportion of patients who are at risk by suppressive red cell hypertransfusion.

The treatment of choice for strokes is immediate EBT. This should help to limit the damage and assist recovery of function. Maintenance red cell transfusion with Hb A blood given often enough to keep the level of Hb S in circulation below 20% is effective in reducing the risk of a recurrence. The transfusions should be maintained for 3 years initially, after which, the patient should be reviewed with computed tomographic (CT) brain scans.

Intracranial hemorrhage is said to be more common in adolescents and adults with SCD, but in my practice, there is no evidence that it is more frequent than in the general population.

Treatment of Anemia Crisis

Bed rest, reassurance, and oxygen inhalation should be provided to patients in an anemia crisis. Blood should be drawn for grouping and cross-matching in readiness for transfusion and for hematologic assessment, including reticulocyte count. A clinical examination is carried out to help determine the etiology and any concurrent ailment. Once the crisis is averted, more blood and other specimens are collected, if necessary, for other investigations. Treatment is also given for any co-morbid condition. If the reticulocyte count equals 1% or less, aplastic crisis (red cell aplasia only) should be considered. The physician should be alert to signs of an epidemic of aplastic crisis among nearby affected individuals. If possible, serum should be obtained and stored in a frozen state until parvovirus B19 antibody testing can be performed.

[1]Not FDA approved for this indication.

Perioperative Care

For minor-to-moderate surgery, blood transfusion is often unnecessary, but blood should be grouped and cross-matched and held in reserve. Intravenous hydration should be given during preanesthetic starvation and oxygen during and after surgery. For elective major surgery, the Hb level should be increased gradually over a 1-month period by simple red cell transfusion to 10 to 12 g/dL. EBT is ideal for emergency surgery, to raise the Hb level while maintaining the blood volume.

Contraception

Contraception by any effective method is safer than the risks associated with pregnancy. Counseling is necessary to prevent unsafe sex with its twin disadvantages of unwanted pregnancy and sexually transmitted disease. Regular use of condoms is recommended, but in a stable monogamous relationship, the methods of choice are the low-estrogen or the progesterone-only pill. Contrary to some expressed reservations, they do not increase the risk of thrombosis in SCD. The parenteral progesterone products such as medroxyprogesterone acetate (Depo-Provera), 150 mg given every 3 months by deep intramuscular injection, or levonorgestrel (Norplant), 228 mg implanted subcutaneously every 5 years, are useful in couples who do not desire further children. These methods also have the advantage of preventing menstrual blood loss. Tubal ligation for women and ligation of the vas deferens for men is recommended when permanent contraception is appropriate.

Pregnancy

All pregnancies are at high risk and should be closely supervised by a joint hematologic and obstetric team. Patients should be counseled about limiting their exposure to the risks of childbirth; no more than two births are recommended. Folic acid, 5 mg daily, and in malaria-endemic areas, proguanil[2], 200 mg daily, are recommended throughout pregnancy. Routine iron supplementation is not necessary unless iron deficiency (rare) is demonstrated. We avoid routine blood transfusion because no advantage in outcome has been established for this practice. Red cell transfusion is, however, advised whenever the Hb level drops below 6 g/dL.

Labor, Childbirth, and the Puerperium

This is a high-risk period during which women are prone to sickle cell crises, bacterial infection, and pulmonary embolism. Adequate hydration is advised during labor and, for any perinatal sickle crisis, EBT and antibiotics (e.g., ceftriaxone [Rocephin], 2 g daily) should be given. Although not yet subjected to controlled trial, the use of prophylactic subcutaneous heparin, 5000 units every 12 hours from 36 weeks' gestation to 6 weeks' postpartum, appears to reduce the risk of death from embolism.

Infants of mothers with SCD are usually small, and most patients go into labor before the due date and have spontaneous vaginal deliveries. Assisted deliveries or cesarean sections are only performed for obstetric complications. There is no contraindication to epidural anesthesia, but general anesthesia for operative delivery should be preceded, when possible, by EBT. Even after a normal delivery, patients should remain in the hospital for 1 week of observation to ensure adequate rest and optimal hydration. Breast-feeding is advised in most patients, because it is best for the infant.

[2]Not available in the United States.

Blood Transfusion

Our patients understand and accept that we do not want to transfuse them unless it is truly necessary. A patient who is feeling tired from increased anemia is confined to bed for a few days for rest and observation and quite often spontaneously recovers. We withhold blood transfusion unless doing so would be life-threatening. One key principle is to base the need for transfusion on the patients' clinical conditions and not on their Hb levels. The indications for blood or red cell transfusion are shown in Table 6.

Simple whole blood or red cell transfusion or EBT may be given. Using red cells helps to limit unwanted expansion of the patient's blood volume, which can also be achieved by the concurrent administration of oral or intravenous furosemide (Lasix), 40 to 80 mg. EBT is given when it is advantageous to rapidly reduce the concentration of sickle cells in circulation.

EBT is performed by transfusing 1 unit (500 mL) of blood and immediately withdrawing 1 unit (500 mL) of blood from the patient. This is repeated two or three times.

TABLE 6 Blood (Red Cell) Transfusion: Indications

Replacement
Anemia crisis, Hb usually <5.0 g/dL
Anemic heart failure (with diuretic rescue)
Normal pregnancy, Hb <6.0 g/dL
Exchange
Acute CVA
Acute chest syndrome
Refractory priapism
Complicated late pregnancy, predelivery
Preoperative
Chronic hypertransfusion
Prevention of CVA recurrence

Abbreviations: CVA = cerebrovascular accident; Hb = hemoglobin.

Bone Marrow (Stem Cell) Transplantation

Bone marrow transplantation (BMT) or, more accurately, stem cell transplantation can cure the patient by changing the Hb phenotype to that of the donor. Consequently, the recipient no longer manifests the features of Hb SS. It is, however, not a generic cure or replacement, and the recipient continues to transmit only Hb S genes to his or her offspring. The procedure is very expensive and is safest and most successful when the patient is younger than 16 years of age and has a human leukocyte antigen (HLA)–compatible sibling donor.

A recent summary of the results of BMT in 48 Hb SS patients showed that 42 (88%) were surviving free from Hb SS after 2 years and that 2 (4%) had died in the process. Several patients, including some of those now enjoying disease-free survival, had initial graft failure or graft-versus-host disease. Some neurologic complications occurred among the earliest patients grafted.

The current indication for performing BMT if all other conditions have been met is that the patients have severe disease (e.g., after a stroke or repeated ACS). The truth is that many patients and their parents would prefer to receive treatment before rather than after developing a debilitating life-threatening complication. I suspect that the agreement to limit the procedure to persons with manifestly severe SCD is largely informed by economic considerations. The transplantation of umbilical cord blood–derived stem cells is practiced in some centers and avoids the need to have a matched sibling donor. It is a growing science with the promise of making phenotypic cure more widely available.

NEUTROPENIA

METHOD OF

Peter E. Newburger, MD

Neutropenia is defined as a below-normal number of peripheral blood neutrophils, as determined by calculation of the absolute neutrophil count (ANC). The ANC equals the total white blood cell count multiplied by the proportion of neutrophils (including both segmented and band forms) on the differential count. The clinical significance of neutropenia depends upon the level of depression of the ANC, as indicated in Table 1. Severe neutropenia, with ANC less than 200, is also termed *agranulocytosis,* even though eosinophils and basophils (which are also granulocytes) may remain normal in number.

Fever in the setting of ANC less than 500 is a medical emergency that compels immediate evaluation and antibiotic treatment.

Clinical Presentation

Neutropenia causes no clinical symptoms or signs per se, so the clinical presentation derives only from secondary infections. Some patients are asymptomatic, but most eventually present with fever, with or without localizing signs of infection. Stomatitis, often with thrush, also occurs commonly; periodic stomatitis occurring every 21 days is a hallmark of cyclic neutropenia. Predictable, but often asymptomatic, neutropenia follows 7 to 14 days after administration of myelosuppressive cancer chemotherapy.

Neutropenic patients can develop infection in virtually any organ system. The most common forms are cellulitis; pneumonia and lung abscess; enteritis, which can progress rapidly to peritonitis; perirectal abscess; lymphadenitis; and sepsis, which is particularly likely in patients with indwelling central venous catheters or mucositis. With agranulocytosis, clinical signs may be limited to fever and limited local inflammation; pus is formed slowly or not at all. Common pathogens include *Staphylococcus aureus* and enteric gram-negative bacilli, including *Escherichia coli,* and *Pseudomonas* species. Fungi and unusual, opportunistic, or multiple antibiotic-resistant bacteria generally cause infection only after prolonged neutropenia and broad-spectrum antibiotic therapy, but need to be considered even at initial presentation.

Evaluation

Table 2 presents a differential diagnosis of neutropenia, which can serve as a guide for diagnostic evaluation. In an acutely ill patient, the initial evaluation for infection needs to be completed rapidly (within hours at the most) and should include assessment of potential sites and causes of infection, but with minimal or no manipulation of the rectum or genitourinary tract. Unlike anemia (and, to some extent, thrombocytopenia), in which peripheral blood tests and bone marrow examination generally indicate whether the low numbers of the particular blood element derives from destruction or hypoproduction, neutropenia can only rarely be classified by its kinetics. Rather, the diagnostic approach generally requires a step-by-step evaluation of a differential diagnosis based on the history, severity, and duration of neutropenia, leukocyte and bone marrow morphology, associated hematological or congenital abnormalities, and tests for specific disorders.

Acquired neutropenia often accompanies viral infection and requires only monitoring of blood counts until recovery. However, depletion of bone marrow reserves can also reduce the ANC in bacterial sepsis in

TABLE 1 Clinical Significance of Absolute Neutrophil Counts

ANC (Neutrophils/mm³)	Clinical Significance	Treatment
>1500	Normal	None
1000-1500	Not clinically significant	None
500-1000	Very slight predisposition to infection	Outpatient antibiotic treatment for febrile illness
200-500	Significant predisposition to infection	G-CSF if symptomatic; inpatient IV antibiotics for febrile illness
<200 (agranulocytosis)	Very high risk of infection, decreased local signs of inflammation	G-CSF if responsive; aggressive IV antibiotics for febrile illness

Abbreviation: G-CSF = granulocyte colony-stimulating factor.

the newborn or in overwhelming bacteremia, as with meningococcus. Drug-induced neutropenia can be associated with a large number of agents including, but by no means limited to, antibiotics, anticonvulsants, anti-inflammatories, antithyroid drugs, diuretics, and phenothiazines. Antineutrophil antibodies may be detected by flow cytometry or agglutination assays, but false negative and borderline positive results may obscure the diagnosis of immune neutropenia. Careful review of the peripheral blood smear may reveal blasts or nucleated erythrocytes indicative of bone marrow involvement by malignancy or may demonstrate abnormal neutrophil morphology associated with a congenital form of neutropenia.

Bone marrow examination (including cytogenetics) is indicated in cases of severe neutropenia or when other bone marrow lineages are abnormal. In some of the less severe forms of congenital neutropenia, such as familial benign neutropenia, adequate bone marrow reserves of mature neutrophils can be demonstrated by steroid stimulation of their release into the peripheral blood, which is evaluated by white blood cell and differential counts just before and 6 hours after prednisone, 1 to 2 mg/kg orally (or methylprednisolone intravenously). Serial blood counts, taken twice weekly over 6 to 9 weeks, are necessary to make the diagnosis of cyclic neutropenia and to document the period of the cycles and the depths of the nadirs. Several of the syndromes listed in Table 2 include unique phenotypic features that aid in the diagnosis; most pediatric hematology texts and the Online Mendelian Inheritance in Man Web site (http://www.ncbi.nlm.nih.gov/Omim/) provide detailed descriptions. Evaluation of the immunoglobulins and cellular immunity not only contributes to the diagnosis of neutropenia associated with immunologic abnormalities, but may also indicate a need for more aggressive management if other arms of the host's defense are impaired. In newborns or infants with hypoglycemia or neurologic abnormalities, blood and urine testing may reveal a metabolic disorder such as glycogen storage disease type 1b, Barth syndrome, hyperglycinemia, tyrosinemia, or an organic acidemia. Excessive neutrophil margination in benign *pseudoneutropenia* may be demonstrated by epinephrine administration.

TABLE 2 Differential Diagnosis of Neutropenia

Acquired

- Viral bone marrow suppression
- Overwhelming bacterial sepsis
- Drug-induced
- Impaired production (chemotherapy, phenothiazines, other drugs)
- Antibody-mediated (aminopyrine, other drugs)
- Immune-mediated (alloimmune and autoimmune)
- Bone marrow aplasia, dysplasia, or replacement
- Hypersplenism
- Nutritional (folate, vitamin B_{12})

Congenital

- Congenital neutropenia
- Severe congenital neutropenia (Kostmann disease)
- Cyclic neutropenia
- Myelokathexis
- Familial benign neutropenia
- Syndromes including neutropenia
  - Cartilage-hair hypoplasia
  - Chédiak-Higashi syndrome
  - Dyskeratosis congenita
  - Fanconi anemia
  - Reticular dysgenesis
  - Shwachman-Diamond syndrome
- Neutropenia associated with immunologic abnormalities (e.g., X-linked hyper-IgM)
- Neutropenia associated with metabolic disorders (e.g., glycogen storage disease type 1b, organic acidurias)
- Pseudoneutropenia

Abbreviation: Ig = immunoglobulin.

Treatment

SUPPORTIVE CARE

Fever or other signs of infection require immediate, aggressive antibiotic therapy in the neutropenic patient with ANC less than 500. Antibiotics tailored to the susceptibility of identified organisms provide ideal treatment for infections with positive cultures. However, the initial treatment of most febrile illnesses and the entire therapy of many with negative cultures will rely on an empiric choice of antibiotics. Empirical therapy may consist of a single, broad-spectrum antibiotic (such as a third generation cephalosporin) or a combination of broad-spectrum antibiotics such as an aminoglycoside (e.g., gentamicin [Garamycin][1], tobramycin [Nebcin][1]) and either a third generation cephalosporin (e.g., ceftazidime [Fortaz][1]) or a semisynthetic penicillin with antipseudomonas activity (e.g., piperacillin [Pipracil][1], ticarcillin [Ticar][1]). Patients with indwelling central venous catheters may require substitution of an agent with better gram-positive coverage (e.g., nafcillin [Nafcil][1] or vancomycin [Vancocin][1]) for the aminoglycoside. Each institution needs to base its empirical antibiotic selection upon the identity and antibiotic susceptibilities of microorganisms in the community or hospital (depending upon the likely site of acquisition of infection), with the final choices made in consultation with the local microbiology or infectious disease division. Fever persisting for more than 5 days generally indicates the need for modification of antibiotic coverage, generally including addition of empirical antifungal therapy such as amphotericin B (Fungizone)[1] or a triazole agent.

For hospitalized patients, handwashing needs to be strictly enforced. More aggressive *reverse precautions* do little to prevent the majority of infections, which derive from the patient's own skin, mucosa, and gastrointestinal (GI) flora. Careful oral, perianal, and skin hygiene may help reduce the prevalence of infection in patients with acute or chronic neutropenia.

Prophylactic antibiotics are useful in severe chronic neutropenia, particularly for the prevention of staphylococcus colonization and infection. Cephalosporins[1] or trimethoprim-sulfamethoxazole (Bactrim)[1] are appropriate for this indication. The latter, a widely used combination, provides broad-spectrum coverage with very little toxicity, but may itself cause neutropenia.

SPECIFIC THERAPY

For patients with autoimmune neutropenia, high-dose IV gamma globulin (Gamimune N)[1], 2 g/kg, as a single dose or divided into daily doses over 3 to 4 days, may provide a transient elevation of ANC. Patients with systemic rheumatologic disorders, including Felty syndrome, may benefit from therapy with glucocorticosteroids (e.g., prednisone), but there is rarely any indication for their use in other forms of neutropenia. Administration of steroids to a patient with neutropenia may do more harm than good, particularly if there is little or no response. Steroids add immunosuppression to an already compromised host defense system and predispose the patient to fungal infection. However, brief use is safe as a diagnostic test for mobilization of bone marrow neutrophils.

Granulocyte colony-stimulating factor (G-CSF), marketed as filgrastim (Neupogen), is the most important, highly specific drug for the treatment of neutropenia. FDA-approved indications for G-CSF include neutropenia associated with cancer chemotherapy and severe congenital neutropenia. Treatment with G-CSF can correct the ANC to the normal range in most patients with severe congenital neutropenia, cyclic neutropenia, or autoimmune neutropenia. Successful correction of the peripheral blood count also prevents stomatitis and other infection-related symptoms and risks. At the initiation of therapy, or if the ANC rises far above normal, expansion of myelopoiesis may cause bone pain or splenomegaly. The major long-term risk in patients with severe congenital neutropenia (but not in other forms of neutropenia) is a conversion to myelodysplasia or leukemia. Most reported cases of myelodysplasia or secondary myeloid leukemia in severe congenital neutropenia patients, both treated and untreated, have been associated with an acquired deletion or abnormality of chromosome 7. Therefore, bone marrow cytogenetics need to be examined before initiation of G-CSF and yearly during its chronic administration. Because the risk is still uncertain, the drug should be used only for patients who are repeatedly symptomatic or have had a life-threatening infection. Sensitivity to G-CSF varies considerably in severe congenital neutropenia, so dosage needs to be titrated for each patient, usually within a range of 1 to 20 μg/kg per day, administered subcutaneously.

The use of G-CSF for acquired neutropenia is more controversial. Although it has been demonstrated to hasten recovery in drug-induced neutropenia, discontinuation of the myelosuppressive drug is usually sufficient. An empiric trial of G-CSF in other acquired forms of chronic neutropenia may be warranted for symptomatic patients. Most patients with autoimmune neutropenia respond to rather low doses of G-CSF and may experience severe bone pain at the standard 5 to 10 μg/kg per day dosage used for postchemotherapy myelosuppression.

Granulocyte transfusion, although rarely indicated, provides additional therapeutic support for newborns with sepsis and bone marrow neutrophil depletion, as well as for some older patients with prolonged agranulocytosis and life-threatening bacterial or fungal infections that persist after adequate trials of appropriate antibiotic therapy.

[1]Not FDA approved for this indication.

HEMOLYTIC DISEASE OF THE FETUS AND NEWBORN

METHOD OF

Gary Robert Cohen, MD, MBA

The term hemolytic disease of the fetus and newborn (HDN) refers to a group of conditions that are manifested during the in utero and newborn period by varying degrees of anemia. The first case of HDN was reported in the early 1600s by a French midwife who delivered a set of severely affected twins. In spite of this it took three centuries before there was even a partial understanding of the physiologic mechanism involved in this disease. The first real breakthrough did not occur until 1940, when Landsteiner and Weiner found that when rabbits were immunized with red blood cells from a *Macaca mulatta,* an antibody was produced that agglutinated red blood cells. The agglutination occurred not only in the monkey but also in the majority of human blood samples tested. The *Macaca mulatta* is commonly known as the rhesus monkey and thus the term *Rh factor* was used to designate this characteristic. With the discovery of the Rh factor, the mechanism by which an Rh-negative mother can produce antibodies that cross the placenta and cause hemolytic anemia in an Rh-positive fetus was finally explained.

Immunologic Mechanism for HDN

If the maternal immunologic system recognizes a foreign red cell antigen from a fetomaternal hemorrhage or heterologous transfusion, a sequence of events is initiated that causes the formation of antibodies to that antigen. The initial maternal exposure to a foreign red cell antigen causes a maternal B lymphocyte reaction. The B lymphocytes produce an immunoglobulin (Ig) M that does not cross the placenta and does not affect the fetus. A re-exposure to this antigen activates the immunologic memory of the mother, which causes the maternal plasma cells to produce IgG antibodies against the foreign antigen. Because IgG has a relatively small size when compared to the IgM, the IgG antibody readily crosses the placenta binding to the corresponding antigen on the membrane of the red blood cell. The antibody-antigen reaction causes a lysis and destruction of the red blood cell. As more and more cells are destroyed the fetal hemopoietic system is overburdened and the fetus becomes anemic. If the anemia continues to worsen, the fetus can become hydropic and die.

As progress in blood typing and banking techniques improved, further analysis revealed that the red blood cells contain some of the most complex and polymorphic antigens found in the body. Each of these red cell antigens has the potential to initiate an immunologic reaction that causes the formation of antibodies that may cause varying degrees of HDN. With the introduction of Rh-immunoglobulin prophylaxis, the relative frequency and importance of antibodies to non-Rh antigens has increased. Table 1 illustrates a list of the clinically significant antibodies detected in descending order of their frequency and their potential to cause hemolytic disease. The full list of potential antibodies is extensive but most of them are extremely rare and have no clinical significance.

Inheritance of Blood Group Antigens

The genetic locus of the Rh antigen has been localized on the short arm of chromosome 1. The exact number of loci is unknown but the three main loci responsible for the expression of the Rh factor are designated by CDE/-ce. A *d* has not been identified. The failure as yet to identify a small *d* explains the difference between phenotypic and genotypic identification of the antigen. Because of the unidentified *d*, the zygosity of an Rh-positive individual can be identified only by knowing the zygosity of its offspring or by knowing the other antigens in the sequence and then statistically extrapolating the probability of the D antigen sequence from population studies. The presence of the Rh antigen has been detected as early as 38 days postconception (7 weeks' gestation).

Rh-Positive, D^u-Positive, Weak or Partial D

Rh-positive (D pos) individuals can be either heterozygous or homozygous for the D antigen. Fifty-five percent of Rh-positive individuals are heterozygous for D. The most frequent phenotypic D antigen is expressed as CeDeDe or Cde. The D can also have a variable phenotypic expression. The variable

TABLE 1 Most Frequently Detected Antibodies and Their Potential to Cause Hemolytic Disease of the Fetus

Antibody (In Decreasing Order of Frequency)	Potential to Cause Severe HDN
D	Common—Mild to severe
K (Kell)	Common—Moderate to severe
E	Common—Mild to severe
Fy^a(Duffy)	Very rare—Mild to severe
Jk^a (Kidd)	Very rare—Mild to severe
c	Common—Mild to severe
C	Uncommon—Mild to severe
e	Uncommon—Mild to moderate

Abbreviation: HDN = hemolytic disease of the fetus and newborn.

expression of the D antigen was called a D^u variant. This variant was a frequent cause of mistyping between Rh-negative and Rh-positive samples. A new classification of the D^u variant now consists of two separate D variants. The first is a *weak* D, which has a reduced quantity of D antigens. The second is a *partial* D. The partial D is a qualitative difference in the structure of the epitomes of the antigen and not quantitative as in the weak D. The partial D mother has a higher risk of sensitization than the weak D variant. A mother with a weak or partial D variant can theoretically produce anti-D antibodies if exposed to the blood of a D-positive fetus. An Rh-negative (D-negative or dd) mother can also theoretically be sensitized by a weak or partial D fetus.

Rh-Negative

Rh-negative individuals lack the D antigen. There is a marked ethnic distribution of the Rh-negative phenotype. The largest single percentage of Rh-negative individuals is found in the Basque population—approximately 35% of this population is Rh-negative. The lowest percent of Rh-negative individuals is found in Asians with only 1% of the population being negative. The frequency of Rh-negative individuals in non-Basque whites approaches 15%. An Rh-negative genotype is also relatively rare in the African American population with only 8% possessing that trait. It should be noted that blacks have the highest incidence of weak and partial D variants.

Pathogenesis of Isoimmunization

Pathogenesis of maternal blood group isoimmunization can occur through heterologous blood transfusions, transplacental hemorrhage, and, theoretically, through a mechanism known as the grandmother theory. Rh sensitization from a heterologous transfusion is a rare occurrence with today's blood banking techniques. It can occasionally occur when there is incomplete antigen expression. Most often this type of mistyping causes sensitization to atypical antibodies. Sensitization from incomplete antigen expression usually produces antibodies of the IgM class, which are not clinically significant.

The most frequent cause of sensitization is through a fetomaternal hemorrhage. Transplacental hemorrhages have been detected in up to 6% of all pregnancies in the first trimester. The frequency increases to 15% in the second trimester and 40% in the third trimester. Although, transplacental fetomaternal hemorrhages are not an uncommon event, the volume is usually less than 0.1 mL of fetal blood. In approximately 1% of all deliveries the volume of the transplacental hemorrhage exceeds 5 mL. Occasionally a positive antibody screen is found without any evidence of a previous pregnancy or heterologous transfusion. To explain this finding, a mechanism has been theorized that has become known as the Grandmother Theory. If a heterozygous Rh-positive mother has a fetus that is Rh-negative, the fetus could theoretically become sensitized to its mother's Rh-positive blood.

The risk of sensitization has decreased since the introduction of Rh-immunoglobulin (RhIG). Prior to the introduction of RhIG, the risk of sensitization during the first pregnancy was estimated to be between 8% and 16%. The difference between transplacental hemorrhage rates and sensitization rates is because the average transplacental fetal blood hemorrhage is so small (<0.1 mL) that the individual may not have a demonstrable immune response as expressed by a positive antibody titer. The individuals exposed were still sensitized but required a second antigen exposure to occur before an immune response could be detected by a positive titer. There is a small measure of natural protection from sensitization if the fetus is ABO incompatible with the mother. The ABO incompatibility causes destruction of the Rh-positive cells by the anti-A or anti-B in the mother's serum before they can elicit an immune response and sensitization. Gender may play a role in both frequency and degree of sensitization. The risk of sensitization has been observed to be higher in women who carry male fetuses. In addition, male fetuses are affected more severely and at an earlier gestational age than female fetuses. The mechanism involved may be related to the presence of the H-Y antigen. This presence of a male antigen may induce a heightened T cell reaction in the female immune system.

Antibody Titers

A maternal blood type and antibody screen are routinely drawn at the first prenatal visit. If an antibody is detected, the next step is to determine the titer of the antibody by performing an indirect antiglobulin test (indirect Coombs). If the antibody that is identified is anti-D, a specimen of maternal serum is incubated with Rh-positive red blood cells. The mixture is washed, and antihuman IgG is added to agglutinate the mixture. Serial dilutions are then performed to quantitate the level of antibody present. In HDN it is important that the antihuman globulin test be performed rather than the albumin or saline test because of its increased sensitivity. It is also important that the same laboratory and technique be employed to ensure consistency of results.

The use of antibody titers as a means to detect anemia is limited depending on the clinical situation. Many centers establish a *critical* titer that serves as the breakpoint at which further evaluation is necessary. This value usually ranges between 1:8 and 1:16. Values below the critical value are not associated with intrauterine fetal death but nonetheless still can be associated with varying degrees of anemia. The absolute value is less important than the trend or pattern of titers. Unfortunately, primary fetal surveillance with titers below the established critical titer is only suited for a newly discovered anti-D antibody or when there has been no history of a previously affected infant. There is very poor correlation between an antibody titer and severity of disease if the antibody present is anything other than anti-D. For example, Kell or *c* antibodies can cause significant anemia in the fetus even when the titers are below the established critical titer.

Atypical Antibodies

The relative frequency of atypical antibodies has increased as compared to anti-D sensitization as a direct result of widespread RhIG use. Included in this is a relative increase in patients who are sensitized with anti-C, anti-c, anti-E, and anti-e antibodies. One of the more serious antibodies to be sensitized against is the Kell antibody. Kell sensitization can cause severe early onset anemia and hydrops even when the antibody titer is at a low level. The fetuses that are affected by anti-Kell antibodies may have anemia secondary not only to hemolysis but also through erythropoietic suppression. This would explain why those fetuses have lower reticulocyte counts and bilirubin levels than those found affected by anti-D sensitization. The prevalence of the Kell antigen is low, with 91% of the population being Kell-negative. The risk to the fetus is also modified by the fact that the gene can be inherited as a homozygous and heterozygous complement. The Duffy antigen system consists of two antigen groups. These groups are designated as Fy^a and Fy^b. Anti-Fy^a can cause mild-to-severe hemolytic disease while anti-Fy^b has not been shown to cause any problems in the fetus. The Kidd blood group system also consists of two components, Jk^a and Jk^b. Anti-Jk^a can cause moderate-to-severe hemolytic disease, and anti-Jk^b causes mild anemia that usually does not require treatment. Antibodies to the Lewis blood system have not been shown to cause hemolytic disease of the fetus. A rule of thumb about the significance of atypical antibodies can be found in the saying "*Kell kills, Duffy dies, and Lewis lives.*"

Rh Immunoglobulin

The widespread administration of anti-D immune globulin (RhIG) was introduced in the 1970s. Almost immediately after its introduction, the incidence of Rh sensitization fell significantly. The prophylactic prevention of sensitization by RhIG occurs because the RhIG blocks the D antigen through competitive inhibition. The standard dose of 300 μg is sufficient to block 30 mL of fetal blood or 15 mL of fetal red blood cells. A single standard dose will prevent 90% of susceptible mothers from being sensitized. To further prevent antenatal sensitization from occurring because of a potential second- or third-trimester transplacental hemorrhage, an additional dose at 28 weeks is recommended. The administration of a dose at 28 weeks in combination with a dose postpartum can reduce maternal sensitization to less than 0.1%.

The recommended time frame for administration of anti-D immune globulin after delivery or potential fetomaternal hemorrhage is 72 hours. This includes first-trimester spontaneous or induced abortions. The protective prophylactic efficacy of RhIG is variable in terms of time of administration and delivery. If delivery is delayed past 12 weeks from the 28-week dose, RhIG should be readministered. Partial protection has been demonstrated if RhIG is given up to 13 days postpartum. The American Association of Blood Banks recommends that all Rh-negative mothers who deliver Rh-positive infants be tested for excessive fetomaternal hemorrhage (>30 mL fetal blood) so that an adequate dose of RhIG can be given. The American College of Obstetricians and Gynecologists does not go as far but does recommend that those women at risk for excessive fetomaternal hemorrhages undergo testing to determine the volume of fetal blood in the maternal circulation. At-risk women are those who may have had abdominal trauma, abruptio placentae, placenta previa, or intrauterine manipulation such as the manual removal of the placenta. The standard dose of 300 μg of RhIG is given as an intramuscular injection. If multiple doses of immune RhIG need to be given, there is an intravenous formulation available. If RhIG is given postpartum, administration of rubella vaccine (Meruvax II) to rubella nonimmune mothers should be delayed because of the possible diminishment of the vaccine's efficacy in relation to the immune response to the RhIG.

From a consumer standpoint there have been a number of questions and concerns regarding the use and safety of RhIG. RhIG is obtained by cold alcohol fractionation of plasma collected from donors who have high antibody titers of anti-D antibody. Infectious morbidity is a frequent consumer concern when any blood product is used. During the preparation of RhIG, a microfiltration process is used to remove contaminants and viruses such as parvovirus B19, HIV, and hepatitis. Consumers are also concerned about the possible effect of a mercury-based preservative, thimerosal, and its potential to cause autism. Thimerosal is no longer used in the manufacture of RhIG.

Maternal Surveillance

If the mother is found to be Rh-positive at her first prenatal visit, a follow-up antibody screen is recommended at 28 weeks. If the mother is Rh-negative and her antibody screen is negative, a repeat screen is recommended at 28 weeks to detect potential sensitization before the administration of RhIG. If a mother is Rh-negative and is sensitized to either

D or an atypical antibody, the approach in terms of surveillance and treatment depends on a number of factors such as previous history, paternal antigen status, titer levels, and offending antigen.

If a mother is detected with an anti-D antibody and she has had no prior history of a pregnancy affected by HDN, the risk to the fetus depends on paternal Rh status and the level of antibody titer. Figure 1 illustrates the diagnostic pathway for this clinical situation. Paternal D status and zygosity should be documented. If the paternal D status is negative, further surveillance other than a repeat antibody screen at 28 weeks is not necessary. If the father is heterozygous, the fetus has only a 50% chance of inheriting the D antigen, and an amniocentesis is performed to determine fetal blood type by polymerase chain reaction (PCR). If the fetus is Rh-positive and the maternal titer remains below the critical titer, monthly titers are recommended until 24 weeks, at which time titers are repeated every 2 weeks. If the titers rise above the established critical level, increased fetal surveillance by either invasive or noninvasive means is indicated.

If a mother has had a previously affected infant or has an atypical antibody that causes HDN, a different pathway is necessary (Figure 2). Antibody titers are not a reliable indicator of fetal status. Determination of paternal antigen status after a potential offending antibody is found is the first step in the diagnostic pathway. If there is an antigen to match the maternal antibody, determination of fetal zygosity is recommended. This is accomplished through amniocentesis and PCR analysis of amniocytes in the amniotic fluid specimen. If the fetus is positive for the antigen, further invasive or noninvasive fetal surveillance is indicated.

Fetal Surveillance

Fetal surveillance would be ideal if it could determine which fetuses were at risk to develop HDN before becoming severely affected. In 1961, Liley proposed that the optical density of amniotic fluid at 450 nm could be used to determine which fetuses were at risk for fetal death. Serial amniocenteses are performed to measure the ΔOD450 value of amniotic fluid and plotted against the gestational age. The Liley curve is separated into three zones and extends from 27 weeks until term. Because the Liley curve was developed with 27 weeks as the starting point, its usefulness is limited for fetal surveillance before this gestational age. To address this issue, Queenan revised the ΔOD450 Gestational Age curve to extend from 14 weeks until term. He further modified the three original zones into four. The lowest zone is the Rh-negative, or *unaffected zone*. Approximately 50% of the unaffected fetuses will be in this zone as well as some mildly anemic Rh-positive fetuses. If an amniocentesis reveals a ΔOD450 value in this zone, an additional tap will be necessary within a 3- to 4-week time frame for confirmation. If the initial ΔOD450 value is in the next zone, which is designated as the *indeterminate zone*, serial amniocenteses are recommended every 2 to 4 weeks to follow their trend. The zone above the indeterminate zone is the Rh-positive, or *affected zone*. Serial titers need to be repeated every 1 to 2 weeks so that a trend in

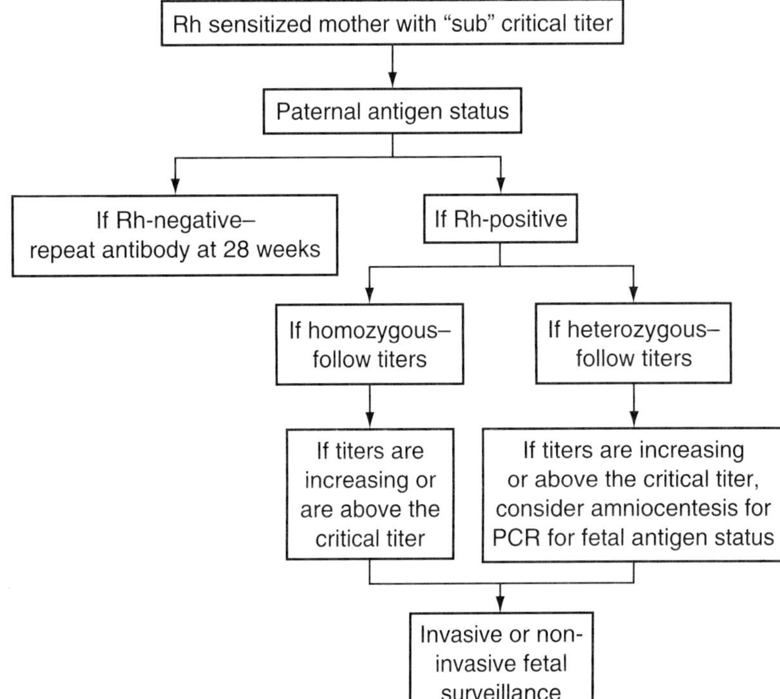

FIGURE 1 Rh sensitized mother with no prior history of an affected infant.

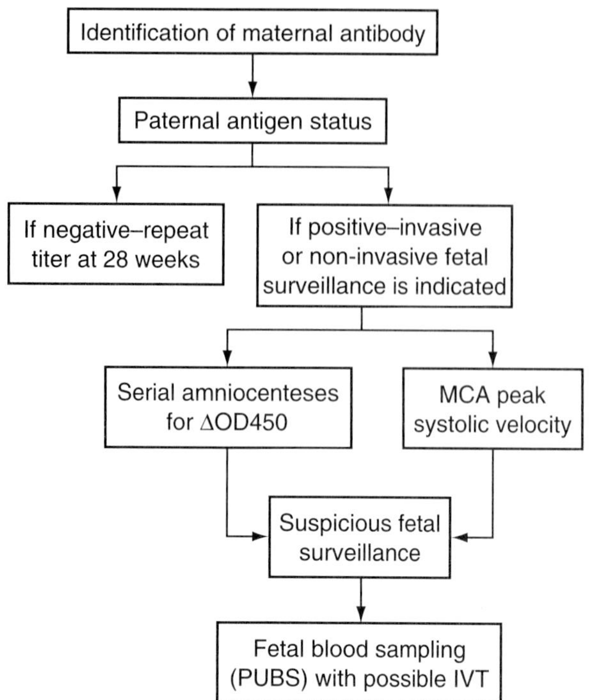

FIGURE 2 Sensitized mother with previously affected infant or atypical antibody.

values can be plotted. The trend or slope of the values is as important clinically as where the absolute measurements fall. If any of the values extend into the upper zone, which indicates potential intrauterine death, intervention is required.

Noninvasive, ultrasound-based surveillance of the fetus has also been used to predict which fetuses are at risk for developing hydrops. Serial ultrasounds of fetuses at risk for hydrops have shown that the first sign of fetal decompensation is the appearance of a small pericardial effusion or dilated right atrium. A noninvasive test that can detect fetal anemia before fetal decompensation is found in the measurement of the peak systolic velocity of the middle cerebral artery (MCA). The peak velocity of the MCA is measured with the pulse wave Doppler. The MCA closest to the transducer is visualized with color flow Doppler, and the velocity is measured while keeping the angle between the flow and beam to a minimum. The velocity is plotted against the gestational age in the same way as with ΔOD450 values. The curve used is divided into different zones of none-to-mild-to-severe anemia. The thresholds of the different zones are set by the multiples of median (MOM) of the peak systolic velocity of the MCA. At 1.35 MOM, 100% of all severely anemic fetuses are detected with only an 18% false-positive rate. After 35 weeks, the accuracy of Doppler assessment decreases because of a high false-positive return. The frequency of measurement depends on the zone in which the initial measurement is made and the subsequent slope of two weekly measurements. If any of the measurements are found to be in the upper zone and then reconfirmed on a repeat measurement, fetal blood sampling is recommended.

Intervention for either signs of fetal decompensation or abnormal fetal surveillance is now based on direct access to the fetal circulation. Percutaneous umbilical blood (PUBS) sampling can give a direct measurement of fetal hematocrit and hemoglobin. Under direct ultrasound visualization, blood can be obtained from the placental cord insertion, free loop of cord, or even the fetal portal vein. If the fetus is found to be anemic, a transfusion can be performed. This procedure is commonly known as an intrauterine transfusion, or IVT. There are a number of techniques and protocols used for direct fetal sampling and transfusions. The principle involved is to transfuse packed red blood cells with a hematocrit of greater than 75 until adequate fetal hematocrit levels are achieved. The gestational age at which direct fetal access and transfusions can be performed is determined by fetal size. A severely affected fetus may need intervention prior to 20 weeks and the earliest an IVT can be safely performed is sometime around 18 weeks. The frequency of transfusions depends on gestational age, fetal surveillance, and fetal hematocrit. After a transfusion, fetal hematocrit falls at a rate of 1% per day. The survival rate for a nonhydropic fetus after an intrauterine transfusion is greater than 90%. If hydrops is present, the survival rate is reduced to approximately 80%.

If a mother is severely sensitized with markedly elevated titers or had a prior pregnancy that was lost at a stage before an ability to intervene, intravenous immune globulin (Gamimune N)[1] has been used to delay the onset of fetal decompensation. It should be noted that intravenous immune globulin does not replace the need for fetal therapy, but rather only delays it until a gestational age is reached that therapeutic intervention is possible.

The diagnosis and treatment of hemolytic disease of the fetus and newborn has shown a number of advancements in the last decade. Fetal surveillance has been refined through the use of Doppler flow studies to evaluate fetal anemia. Intervention and survival have been impacted by the ability to directly transfuse the fetus while it is still in utero. The challenge of the future is to eliminate the condition completely, either through prevention of a mother developing antibodies or through prevention of the fetus being adversely affected by them.

[1]Not FDA approved for this indication.

HEMOPHILIA AND RELATED CONDITIONS

METHOD OF

Indira Warrier, MD

Hemophilia A (factor VIII deficiency) and hemophilia B (factor IX deficiency) are X-linked hereditary bleeding disorders affecting males almost exclusively. By contrast, von Willebrand disease (vWD) is an autosomal dominant disorder affecting males and females equally. Hemophilia A and B are characterized by joint and muscle bleeding, whereas mucocutaneous bleeding is the hallmark of vWD. Although hemophilia A and B have similar clinical manifestations and are indistinguishable clinically, factors VIII and IX activity assays can differentiate them easily. In hemophilia A, only factor VIII procoagulant activity is deficient, whereas other components of the factor VIII system (von Willebrand factor [vWf] antigen and activity) are normal. In vWD, as a result of deficiency or abnormality of vWf necessary for stability of circulating factor VIII, factor VIII activity is reduced.

Hemophilia A and hemophilia B can be classified according to clinical severity, which correlates well with measured factor assay values. Assay values of less than 0.01 unit/mL (1%) are associated with severe disease manifestations, including spontaneous bleeding into joints and soft tissues. Individuals with factor assay values of 1% to 5% are considered to have moderately severe disease, whereas individuals with values greater than 5% are known to have clinically mild disease.

The estimated incidence of hemophilia in the United States is 1 in 10,000 individuals or 1 in 5000 males. Hemophilia A/B ratio is 4:1. More than 66% of affected individuals with hemophilia A have severe disease, whereas severe disease is seen in only 32% of individuals with hemophilia B. Factors VIII and IX genes are located on the long arm of the X chromosome. Factor VIII protein is substantially larger than factor IX protein (approximately 340,000 daltons compared with 60,000 daltons), and this has significant implications in gene therapy or gene transplantation in hemophilia A. The genes encoding factor VIII and factor IX have been shown to be susceptible to new mutational events. New mutations account for 25% to 30% of newly diagnosed cases of hemophilia.

First described by von Willebrand in 1926, vWD is the most common hereditary bleeding disorder, affecting 1% of the population. It occurs when there is a quantitative or qualitative defect of vWf. The gene for vWf is located on chromosome 12. The vWf, which is a complex multimeric glycoprotein consisting of 226,000 daltons, is essential for platelet adhesion at vascular injury sites as well as platelet-to-platelet interaction (by cross-linking of glycoprotein 1 and receptors on platelets). The vWf protects factor VIII from proteolysis in the circulating plasma.

von Willebrand disease, which is genetically and phenotypically heterogeneous, has been categorized into three major types. Type 1 vWD (classic) is the most common form and is characterized by decreased levels of normal functioning vWf. The type 2 variants (2A, B, M, and N) are caused by qualitative abnormalities of vWf. Type 3 (severe) vWD is characterized by absent or nearly absent vWf. This rare form of the disease results from the inheritance of two genes for vWD and is associated with joint bleeding in addition to severe mucous membrane bleeding. In type 1 vWD, clinical bleeding manifestation varies considerably. Most affected individuals have only mild-to-moderate bleeding tendency. It is not uncommon to obtain a negative bleeding history in some affected individuals. Laboratory studies show that all three components of factor VIII/vWf complex are proportionally decreased in the plasma.

Among type 2 qualitative variants, type 2A is the most commonly observed variant. Type 2B is the next most common. For treatment purposes, it is essential to distinguish 2A from 2B. Both types have decreased high-molecular-weight multimers in plasma. In addition, in type 2A intermediate-molecular-weight multimers are also absent. Type 2B defect is characterized by increased binding of vWf to platelets. As a result, thrombocytopenia is a variable feature of type 2B vWf and occurs with release of vWf (e.g., caused by stress, inflammation, pregnancy, administration of desmopressin [deamino (8-D-arginine) vasopressin (DDAVP)]).

Inherited bleeding disorders secondary to clotting factor deficiencies other than factor VIII and IX do exist, but they are far less common than hemophilia and vWD. Factor XII deficiency (Hageman factor deficiency), although manifested with a prolonged activated partial thromboplastin time (PTT), is usually not associated with a bleeding tendency. Congenital deficiencies of fibrinogen; prothrombin; and factors V, VII, X, and XIII do cause bleeding. Some patients with factor XI deficiency also have bleeding problems. Most of these coagulation disorders are inherited in an autosomal recessive fashion.

Three inherited protein deficiencies that are not commonly detected by routine coagulation screening tests are factor XIII deficiency, α_2-antiplasmin deficiency, and plasminogen activator inhibitor (PAI) deficiency. Factor XIII deficiency is characterized by delayed bleeding after initial hemostasis (umbilical stump bleeding). The α_2-antiplasmin and other fibrinolytic system disorders must be kept in mind when evaluating an individual with a significant bleeding history and normal screening tests. Disorders of primary hemostasis (platelet number and function) can also cause significant bleeding and are discussed elsewhere.

Hemostatic Abnormalities

REPLACEMENT THERAPY

Treatment of acute hemorrhage in individuals with coagulation disorders requires prompt intravenous replacement of the deficient clotting factor. In the 1990s highly purified, virally attenuated, plasma-derived clotting factor concentrates and recombinant factor preparations became the products of choice for replacement therapy in severe hemophilia A and B. Desmopressin (DDAVP), a synthetic analog of vasopressin, has been recommended for treatment of minor bleeding episodes in mild hemophilia A and type 1 vWD.

FRESH-FROZEN PLASMA

Fresh-frozen plasma (FFP) is still the first-line treatment in several situations with relatively rare hereditary deficiencies of coagulation factors II, V, VII, XI, and XIII. Hemostasis generally can be achieved with FFP of 10 to 15 mL/kg body weight. Most clotting proteins have their hemostatic activity defined as unit of clotting activity present in milliliters of fresh plasma. An average unit of FFP of 230 mL contains approximately 200 units of activity for each of the clotting factors. Donor-retested single donor plasma and solvent detergent-treated plasma became available in the late 1990s for treating some of these rare coagulation factor deficiencies.

CRYOPRECIPITATE

Each bag of cryoprecipitate prepared from a single unit of plasma contains approximately 50% of factor VIII, vWf, and fibrinogen present in 1 unit of plasma initially. With the availability of virally attenuated factor VIII products containing vWf, cryoprecipitate is not considered as the treatment of choice for vWD. Cryoprecipitates are still used for bleeding associated with hypofibrinogenemia or afibrinogenemia, however. One of the major disadvantages of cryoprecipitate is that the plasma product is not subject to any viral attenuation process.

Factor VIII Concentrates

Plasma-derived and recombinant factor VIII concentrates produced by several different manufacturers in the United States and Europe are widely used for the treatment of hemophilia A.

PLASMA-DERIVED FACTOR VIII PRODUCTS

Currently available plasma-derived factor VIII concentrates are considered safe from HIV and similar retroviral contamination, but are not absolutely free of hepatitis C virus transmission risk. Available products can be classified into three groups:

1. Intermediate-purity products
2. High-purity products
3. Ultra-high-purity products

The intermediate-purity products undergo viral inactivation; however, there is a small percentage of other plasma proteins in the final product. Factor VIII coagulation activity per milligram of total protein may be 6 to 10 units. High-purity factor VIII concentrates have five times (50 units) more of factor VIII per milligram of protein than intermediate-purity products. These products are safe from HIV but are not absolutely safe from hepatitis C. Ultra-high-purity products include the monoclonal antibody–purified, plasma-derived factor VIII concentrates and recombinant factor VIII concentrates. These products contain 3000 units of factor VIII per milligram of protein (60 times more than high purity). Plasma-derived monoclonal preparations are virally safe.

RECOMBINANT FACTOR VIII PRODUCTS

Five recombinant factor VIII preparations currently available in the United States are produced in well-established mammalian cell lines (Chinese hamster ovary cells and baby hamster kidney cells) that are transfected with gene encoding for human factor VIII. Two currently licensed recombinant factor VIII preparations contain human albumin as a stabilizer. Both preparations have been well studied, and they appear to be effective and safe. One recombinant factor VIII preparation, from which the B domain of the gene has been removed before transfection of the hamster cell lines, has undergone clinical studies and is licensed. Some of the second- and third-generation recombinant factor VIII products without any human albumin/protein have undergone clinical studies and are now licensed in the United States. These products do not require human serum albumin for stabilization in the final lyophilized product and provide a higher level of confidence against future microbiologic contamination. Most pediatric hematologists prefer to use recombinant factor VIII products for their young patients.

Factor IX Products

Similar to factor VIII products, factor IX products available for hemophilia B are of two types, plasma derived and recombinant.

PLASMA-DERIVED FACTOR IX PRODUCTS

There are two types of plasma-derived factor IX concentrates, prothrombin complex concentrates, which contain all of the vitamin K-dependent clotting factors (factor II, VII, IX, and X), and coagulation factor IX concentrates, which are highly purified factor IX. Both currently available plasma-derived, high-purity products are subjected to viral depletion processes and have not been implicated in transmission of HIV and hepatitis virus.

Prothrombin complex concentrates (PCCs) contain all vitamin K-dependent factors, some in activated forms. These products produce thrombotic complications, such as disseminated intravascular coagulation, deep venous thrombosis, and pulmonary embolism, when given in high doses repeatedly. Because of their thrombogenic nature, these products are not used widely for hemophilia B patients undergoing surgery or for those with major hemorrhages requiring several repeated doses. However, PCCs have been used widely to treat bleeding episodes in persons with hemophilia A and B who have developed inhibitor antibodies to factor VIII or factor IX (see following sections on inhibitors).

Highly purified factor IX products with little or no other vitamin K-dependent coagulation factors have no thrombogenic potential even when used in high doses. Monoclonal immunoaffinity purified factor IX product has been studied more rigorously for viral safety with respect to hepatitis C or similar viruses.

RECOMBINANT FACTOR IX PRODUCT

Recombinant factor IX product has no human serum albumin in the final product. Although recombinant factor IX recovery may be slightly different from monoclonal factor IX because of a slightly different volume distribution, the in vivo half-life of recombinant factor IX is identical to that of plasma-derived monoclonal factor IX.

ANTIFIBRINOLYTIC THERAPY

Antifibrinolytic therapy is a useful adjuvant treatment in patients with hemorrhagic disorders. Antifibrinolytic agents epsilon-aminocaproic acid (EACA)[1] and tranexamic acid (Cyklokapron)[1] stabilize a clot by inhibiting the normal process of clot lysis by the fibrinolytic system. Their primary use in hemophilia has been in the management of oral mucosal bleeding. Antifibrinolytic therapy is usually begun in conjunction with factor replacement therapy and continued for 5 to 7 days or until the mucosal laceration is healed completely. Because there is a theoretical risk of enhanced thrombogenicity with concurrent use of PCCs and antifibrinolytic agents, patients can either use a high-purity factor IX product or use tranexamic acid as a mouthwash rather than systemically. EACA, 75 mg/kg every 6 hours (maximum 5 g per dose) orally, or tranexamic acid, 25 mg/kg every 8 hours (maximum 1.5 g) orally, is given.

Other Agents

DESMOPRESSIN

DDAVP, a synthetic analogue of the antidiuretic hormone 9-arginine vasopressin, stimulates a transient threefold-to-fourfold increase in factor VIII levels and is the treatment of choice for persons with classic type 1 vWD. It also provides an effective alternative therapy for less severe hemorrhage in most patients with mild-to-moderate hemophilia A. DDAVP can be administered intravenously at a dose of 0.3 to 0.4 μg/kg in 30 to 50 mL of normal saline for 15 to 20 minutes. When given intravenously, peak effect is observed in 30 to 60 minutes.

A concentrated intranasal form of DDAVP is available that has similar efficacy to intravenous preparation. The recommended dose for the intranasal form (Stimate) is 150 μg (1 metered dose or puff) for individuals weighing less than 50 kg (110 lb) and 300 μg (2 puffs) for individuals weighing 50 kg or more. The major side effect of DDAVP is asymptomatic facial flushing. Hyponatremic seizures have been reported in young children (<2 years old) and the elderly (>60 years old) with repeated doses of DDAVP or nonrestricted fluid intake. Fluid restriction and close monitoring of urine output are advisable after DDAVP administration.

Although the mechanism of action of DDAVP is not understood completely, it is thought to act by causing an immediate release of factor VIII or vWf from storage sites. The drug may have other mechanisms of action as well. It has been shown to enhance platelet adhesion and spreading at injury sites, thus promoting hemostasis in persons with platelet function disorders, as well as to decrease blood loss in hemostatically normal individuals undergoing surgical procedures.

For persons with type 3 vWD (severe vWD) and for those with types 1 and 2 who have an inadequate response to DDAVP, most coagulation specialists recommend the use of one of the intermediate-purity factor VIII concentrates containing high-molecular-weight vWf. Most prefer these products to cryoprecipitates because of the theoretical viral safety conferred by the viral attenuation process they undergo in preparation. Hemostatic efficacy of those products has been shown to be excellent when individuals with type 3 vWD were treated for life-threatening bleeding.

Treatment of Hemophilia A and B

Treatment guidelines for factor replacement therapy for bleeding episodes in hemophilia A and B are given in Table 1. The most common indications for treatment are acute joint hemorrhage (hemarthrosis) and bleeding into a muscle mass. Treatment consists of factor replacement, rest, elevation of the affected limb, application of ice, and compression.

Factor replacement is achieved by intravenous infusion of reconstituted lyophilized concentrates. The label on each bottle of concentrate indicates the amount of factor VIII or factor IX it contains. Factor VIII, 1 unit per kg body weight, raises the recipient's factor VIII level by 0.02 unit per mL (2%). A patient with severe hemophilia with less than 0.01 unit per mL

[1]Not FDA approved for this indication.

TABLE 1 Factor Replacement Therapy Guidelines for Severe and Moderately Severe Hemophilia A and B

Type of Bleeding	Hemophilia A (Factor VIII)	Hemophilia B (Factor IX)	Frequency of Dose	Comments
Minor				
Early joint, early soft tissue, muscle, oral mucosa	20 U/kg	30-40 U/kg	q24h as needed	Low end of dose if plasma-derived factor IX is used. Antifibrinolytic therapy essential for mucosal bleeding (use discouraged with PCC).
Major*				
Late joint and muscle	40 U/kg	60-80 U/kg	q12-24h	May need several doses. Calf and forearm bleeds are limb-threatening. Retroperitoneal/iliopsoas bleeding associated with severe blood loss.
Gastrointestinal	40 U/kg	60-80 U/kg	q12-24h	Evaluation is necessary to find the lesion including endoscopy.
Genitourinary (traumatic)	40 U/kg	60-80 U/kg	q12-24h	Spontaneous bleeding episodes do not require factor replacement. Increase hydration.
Major trauma or surgery	40-50 U/kg	80-100 U/kg	q12-24h or continuous infusion†	Duration of treatment varies depending on surgical situation and extent of trauma; inhibitor status must be assessed before surgery.
Life-threatening*				
CNS (head, neck) and major abdominal trauma	50 U/kg	100 U/kg	q8-12h or continuous infusion†	Duration of treatment and intensity vary; treat until imaging studies show complete resolution. For CNS bleed, follow with minimum of 6 mo of prophylaxis.

*Major and life-threatening hemorrhages should be treated in a comprehensive treatment center. If the patient is seen first in another hospital, initial treatment should be given, then transfer to a hemophilia treatment center should occur after first contacting the center.
†For hemophilia B, use high-purity factor IX products only for continuous infusion.
Abbreviations: CNS = central nervous system, PCC = prothrombin complex concentrate.

can expect to have a level of 0.40 unit per mL (40%) immediately after infusion of 20 units per kg body weight of factor VIII. The biologic half-life of factor VIII is approximately 12 hours. Factor IX has a large volume of distribution; 1 unit per kg body weight of factor IX raises plasma levels of factor IX by 0.01 unit per mL (1%). Pharmacokinetic studies show some variation in the factor IX recovery when recombinant factor IX concentrate is used (0.6% to 1.2%). Factor IX has a biologic half-life of approximately 24 hours.

The treatment regimen and factor replacement in hemophilia are based on volume of distribution of infused factor, the factor survival, and required hemostatic factor level. The type and extent of bleeding determine the dose and frequency of dosing and the duration of treatment. The guidelines for factor replacement therapy for treatment of hemorrhages in severe and moderately severe hemophilia A and hemophilia B (as shown in Table 1) are based on the aforementioned principles of therapy.

Complications of Treatment

RISK OF VIRAL TRANSMISSION

With the availability of recombinant factor concentrates, viral transmission is not considered a major risk. When using plasma-derived concentrates, however, one must be aware of the potential complications of their use. Despite greatly improved donor screening methods and viral reduction methods, there remains a slight risk of hepatitis virus transmission with the use of FFP, cryoprecipitate, and other blood components. Estimated frequency of hepatitis C virus-contaminated units is 1 in 103,000. Although rare, transmissions of hepatitis C virus, hepatitis A virus, and human parvovirus B19 have been reported with some of the existing plasma-derived factor VIII products. All patients with a diagnosis of a coagulation disorder should be immunized against hepatitis B and hepatitis A because safe and effective vaccines are available for prevention of these viral infections.

INHIBITOR DEVELOPMENT

A serious and potentially life-threatening complication of hemophilia is the development of neutralizing antibodies to factor VIII or IX, which makes replacement therapy ineffective. These antibodies, referred to as *inhibitors*, occur almost always after the patient has had some exposure to factor replacement. The inhibitors can be detected by routine screening or by testing for inhibitor at the time the

TABLE 2 Guidelines for Treatment of Bleeding in Hemophiliacs with High Titer Antibodies

Type of Bleeding	Factor VIII Inhibitor	Factor IX Inhibitor	Repeat Dosing	Comments
Minor				
Early joint, early soft tissue, muscle, oral mucosa	PCC or APCC, 50-100 U/kg	PCC or APCC, 75-100 U/kg	q24h as needed	For oral mucosal bleeding use antifibrinolytic therapy with caution; allow 3-4 h between PCC and antifibrinolytic agent.
Major*				
Late joint and muscle, gastrointestinal, genitourinary, major trauma, and surgery	Hyate C[†], 100 U/kg, or		q8h for several days	Monitor platelet count and factor VIII response.
	APCC, 75-100 U/kg, or	APCC, 75-100 U/kg, or	q12-24h	Do not exceed 4-6 doses.
	rFVIIa, 90 μg/kg	rFVIIa, 90 μg/kg	q2h until bleeding stops, then taper	Monitor PT and platelet count. Limb-threatening compartment syndrome with calf and forearm bleeds. Significant blood loss with iliopsoas and thigh bleed.
Life-threatening*				
CNS (head, neck) and major abdominal trauma	rFVIIa, 90 μg/kg or	rFVIIa 90 μg/kg, or	q2h for 48-72 h, then taper over 5-7 d if bleeding is controlled	Monitor PT and platelet count. Duration of treatment as per imaging studies.
	Hyate C, 100 U/kg, or		q12-24h	
	APCC, 75-100 U/kg	APCC, 75-100 U/kg	q12-24h	

*Major and life-threatening hemorrhages should be treated in a comprehensive treatment center. The patient must be transferred to a treatment center after initial treatment if seen at another hospital.

[†]Porcine factor VIII.

Abbreviations: APCC = activated prothrombin complex concentrate; CNS = central nervous system; PCC = prothrombin complex concentrate; PT = prothrombin time; rFVIIa = recombinant activated factor VII.

patient shows a poor clinical response to usual factor replacement therapy. Some patients develop antibodies in low titer and can be treated with higher amounts of factor products, whereas most have high titer antibodies. Patients with high-titer antibodies have a brisk anamnestic response to factor replacement therapy and cannot be treated with their usual factor replacement. Inhibitors develop in 15% to 30% of patients with hemophilia A and 1% to 3% of patients with hemophilia B. Most of these inhibitors occur in childhood.

Treatment of bleeding episodes in inhibitor patients can be challenging. Currently available treatment modalities for factor VIII inhibitors include the use of bypassing agents (PCC, activated PCC), porcine factor VIII, and recombinant factor VIIa, in addition to temporary removal of antibody by plasmapheresis (used only in life-threatening or limb-threatening situations). In hemophilia B with inhibitors, treatment of bleeding episodes consists of the use of bypassing agents and recombinant factor VIIa. An unusual complication of concurrent anaphylaxis to factor IX along with inhibitor development has been described in hemophilia B inhibitor patients. In these patients, recombinant factor VIIa is the drug of choice for treatment of bleeding episodes. Eradication of the inhibitors by *immune tolerance induction* has been attempted in hemophilia A and B with varying success. A variety of regimens have been tried, some requiring regular daily doses of factor with or without immune modulatory drugs (cyclophosphamide [Cytoxan][1], steroids, immune globulin intravenous). The overall success rate reported by various regimens in hemophilia A inhibitor patients has been 60% to 80%. This process is often time-consuming, requiring central venous lines in young children with associated complications (infections and, rarely, thrombosis). In hemophilia B, experience with immune tolerance therapy is limited, and the overall success rate is not good. Nephrotic syndrome has been reported as a unique complication of immune tolerance induction in hemophilia B inhibitor patients who also have had anaphylaxis to factor IX products. Guidelines for treatment of bleeding episodes in inhibitor patients are presented in Table 2.

THROMBOGENICITY

Thrombogenicity is a potential complication of PCCs resulting from their contamination with trace amounts of active proteases (factor Xa or VIIa) in addition to zymogen overload (factors II, VII, and IX, which the hemophilic patient already has in adequate amounts). Disseminated intravascular

[1]Not FDA approved for this indication.

coagulation and thromboembolic complications have been reported when large doses of PCCs have been used repeatedly more often than every 6 hours. The hemophilic patients at greatest risk for this complication are those undergoing orthopedic procedures with prolonged immobilization, those with major crush injuries, and those with large intramuscular bleeds. Neonates and patients with significant hepatocellular disease are also at risk. Low antithrombin III and decreased clearance of intermediates predispose these patients to PCC-induced thrombogenicity.

ACUTE MYOCARDIAL INFARCTION

More than 30 hemophiliacs with inhibitors have been reported to have had acute myocardial infarction while receiving large repeated doses of PCCs for treatment of bleeding. Myocardial transmural hemorrhage was the most consistent finding at autopsy. The exact pathophysiology of this complication is not clear. This complication is not associated with the use of purified factor IX concentrates.

COMPLICATION OF DDAVP TREATMENT

As mentioned earlier, the most commonly observed side effect of DDAVP treatment is facial flushing. Occasionally, headache has been associated with DDAVP administration. Hyponatremic seizures are rare and occur in children (<2 years old) and the elderly (>60 years old) with repeated doses of DDAVP or unrestricted fluid intake. Thrombosis is rarely reported as a complication of DDAVP treatment.

ALLERGIC REACTION

Allergic reactions to plasma, cryoprecipitate, and plasma-derived concentrates include urticaria, rashes, headache, emesis, angioedema, and collapse. These allergic reactions are observed to occur less often with purer factor concentrates. Hemophilia B inhibitor patients are reported to have immunoglobulin (Ig) E–mediated allergic reactions more often than hemophilia A patients. Genetic and immunologic factors may be involved in inducing this complication.

Treatment of von Willebrand Disease

Treatment of various types of vWD is discussed in an earlier section, Desmopressin, except for the dosing recommendation for plasma-derived vWf-containing factor VIII products. Current dosing regimen is based on the amount of ristocetin cofactor units contained in the concentrates. For most of the minor bleeding episodes in type 2 and 3 vWD patients the dose of concentrate recommended is 40 IU/kg. For treatment of major and life-threatening hemorrhages, the recommended dose is 80 IU/kg. Treatment of serious bleeding requires several doses of factor concentrates.

PROPHYLAXIS

Recurrent joint bleeding leading to the development of target joints, chronic synovitis, and chronic arthropathy is the hallmark of hemophilia. With the advent of newer and safer concentrates, prophylaxis against this complication has been attempted in the United States. *Primary prophylaxis* involves the institution of bleeding prevention starting at an early age, before a target joint has developed, whereas *secondary prophylaxis* is usually started at a later age to prevent further progression of joint damage in a target joint. An orthopedic outcome study in the United States revealed that secondary prophylaxis improved clinical orthopedic outcome, but did not prevent eventual radiographic progression of hemophilic arthropathy. Recommendation for either primary or secondary prophylaxis must be made after careful consideration of patient and family and only after consulting professionals at the regional comprehensive treatment center.

Preventative Care and Comprehensive Care

Genetic counseling is an integral part of comprehensive care of hemophilia. Women who are potential carriers must be advised against having their male infants circumcised until the diagnosis of hemophilia is excluded by laboratory testing. In male infants of potential carriers, blood must be obtained for factor assays from the umbilical cord. When a cord blood sample is not available, blood must be obtained from a peripheral vein, not from femoral or jugular veins.

Diagnosis of hemophilia should not prevent the child from receiving routine childhood immunizations, including hepatitis B vaccine. Hepatitis A vaccine is also recommended for children with hemophilia. All injectable vaccines should be given subcutaneously rather than by deep intramuscular injections to avoid intramuscular bleeding requiring factor replacement therapy.

Prophylactic dental care and teaching proper brushing and flossing methods are usually included when children are seen in the comprehensive hemophilia treatment center annually. Comprehensive hemophilia treatment centers are special treatment centers established to provide multidisciplinary care of hemophilia including psychosocial, orthopedic, nutritional support, dental support, physical therapy, and genetic counseling. These treatment centers also provide ongoing education to hemophilia patients regarding management of their bleeding disorder and updates regarding any new developments in the field of hemophilia.

PLATELET MEDIATED BLEEDING DISORDERS

METHOD OF

Anita S. Kestin, MD

Virtually every physician can expect to encounter patients with quantitative or qualitative platelet disorders. This article outlines the key disorders that compromise platelet number and function and delineates the conditions requiring urgent action or particular vigilance.

Biologic

In the hemostatic system as a whole, platelets are the first responders once bleeding has occurred (Figure 1). Platelets are formed in the bone marrow. Megakaryocytes, which are derived from a pluripotent stem cell, give rise to platelets by cytoplasmic shedding. Under usual conditions, platelets survive in the circulation for 8 to 10 days. Thrombopoietin, a cytokine produced in the liver, influences the differentiation and maturation of the megakaryocyte and influences the total platelet count.

Thrombocytopenia is generally thought to occur when the platelet count falls below 150,000 (normal platelet count is 150,000 to 400,000).

Table 1 describes the typical presenting symptoms of platelet disorders.

The relationship between thrombocytopenia and bleeding risk is given here as a general guideline; a hematologist should be consulted in the management of these problems. Bleeding risk in the thrombocytopenic patient is not determined solely by the platelet count. Medications (e.g., aspirin, nonsteroidal anti-inflammatory drugs [NSAIDs]) and intercurrent illnesses (e.g., uremia, coagulopathy, cancer, liver disease) can also influence the bleeding tendency in thrombocytopenic individuals. Excessive surgical bleeding often occurs in patients with platelet counts less than 50,000, but attainment of a higher platelet count may be necessary in certain surgical settings. Spontaneous bleeding is a serious risk when the platelet count falls below 10,000, but maintenance of a higher platelet count may be advisable, particularly if other hemostatic compromises exist or if platelets for transfusion are not available in a timely manner.

CLASSIFICATION OF PLATELET DISORDERS

Diseases that can impair competency are listed in Tables 2, 3, and 4. It is important to note that certain conditions may be associated with both qualitative and quantitative disorders. Similarly, a given individual may demonstrate abnormalities both in platelet function and platelet quantity.

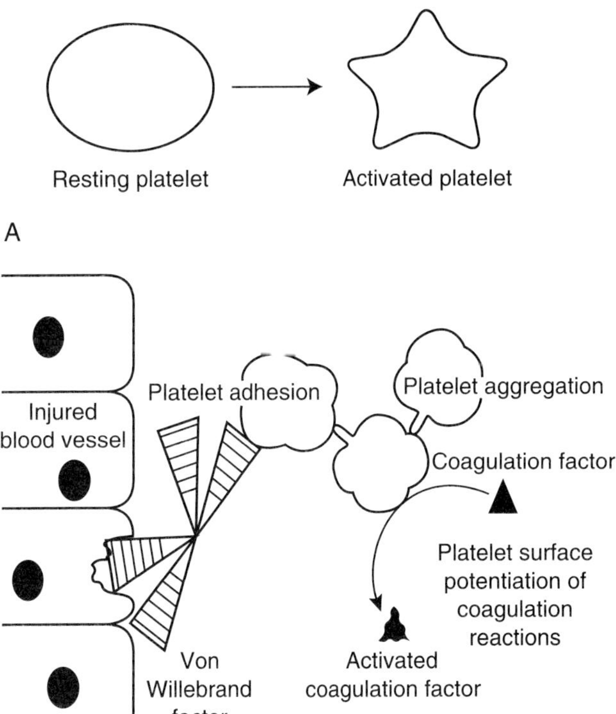

FIGURE 1 A, Platelets circulate in a resting state but become activated upon exposure to thrombin. B, Activated platelets are then able to adhere to von Willebrand factor and thereby to damaged blood vessels, to aggregate with other platelets, and to offer their surface as a nidus for potentiation of coagulation reactions.

Thrombocytopenia

APPROACH TO THE PATIENT WITH THROMBOCYTOPENIA

When a patient presents with symptoms suspect for thrombocytopenia:

1. Exclude spurious thrombocytopenia (a benign finding) or lab error. The platelet count should be repeated and the smear should be examined to see

TABLE 1 Platelet Disorders: Common Presentations

1. Asymptomatic thrombocytopenia; low platelet count on CBC
2. Excessive bleeding during surgery
3. Mucocutaneous bleeding:
   - Epistaxis
   - Menorrhagia
   - Petechiae
   - Bleeding from gums
   - Ecchymoses
4. Laboratory evidence of abnormal platelet function

Abbreviation: CBC = complete blood count.

TABLE 2 Classification of Thrombocytopenic Disorders

Increased Destruction	Immune	Immune thrombocytopenia (ITP)
		Neonatal alloimmune thrombocytopenia (NAIT)
		Sepsis/infection
		Medications
		Post-transfusion purpura (PTP)
		Second-degree maternal ITP
		Second-degree maternal lupus
		HIV-related
		Heparin-induced thrombocytopenia (HIT)
		Second-degree lymphoproliferative disorder
	Nonimmune	Hemolytic uremic syndrome (HUS)
		Thrombotic thrombocytopenia purpura (TTP)
		Preeclampsia
		Sepsis/infection
		Disseminated intravascular coagulation (DIC)
		Bypass surgery-pump
		Burns
		Medications
		von Willebrand disease (vWD) type IIb
Decreased Production	Malignant bone marrow disorders	Leukemia
		Multiple myeloma (MM)
		Myelofibrosis (MF)
		Carcinoma in marrow
		Aplastic anemia (AA)
		Paroxysmal nocturnal hemoglobinuria (PNH)
		Lymphoproliferative disorder
	Nutritional	Vitamin B_{12} or folate deficiency
	Toxic	Radiation
		Chemotherapy
		Medications
		Ethanol
	Infections	Cytomegalovirus (CMV)
		HIV
	Congenital (genetic)	Wiskott-Aldrich
		Thrombocytopenia-absent radius (TAR)
		May-Hegglin
		Numerous genetic syndromes
Sequestration		Splenic pooling

whether the platelet count is accurate. Platelet agglutination in ethylenediaminetetraacetic acid (EDTA) is a relatively common cause of a low platelet count; examination of the smear will reveal clumps of platelets rather than an even distribution of isolated platelets.

2. Assess the urgency of the clinical situation. Situations requiring urgent evaluation or action are listed in Table 5. These situations should be managed by a physician familiar with the clinical problem, generally a hematologist.
3. Determine the results of prior blood counts; the smear should be reviewed (Table 6).
4. Obtain a complete history and review the medical record.
5. Perform a complete physical exam.
6. Review the patient's medication list to identify (and eliminate if possible) medications that can cause thrombocytopenia and medications that can impair hemostasis.
7. Rule out bone marrow disorders; the likelihood of this possibility is increased if neutropenia,

TABLE 3 Platelet Function Defects

Acquired Defects	Congenital Defects
1. Uremia	1. Bernard-Soulier syndrome
2. Liver disease	2. Glanzmann thrombasthenia
3. Medications (especially antiplatelet agents)	3. von Willebrand disease, platelet type
4. Dysproteinemias (Waldenström syndrome, myeloma)	4. α-Granule deficiency (gray platelet syndrome)
5. Myeloproliferative syndromes (especially essential thrombasthenia)	5. Dense granule deficiency
6. Coronary bypass/hypothermia	
7. ITP with antibodies directed against a functional site	
8. Myelodysplastic syndromes, acute leukemia	

TABLE 4 Causes of Thrombocytosis*

Platelet Function Normal
Iron deficiency
Connective tissue syndromes
Acute inflammation
Postsplenectomy
Acute hemorrhage
Malignancy
Platelet Function May Be Abnormal
Myeloproliferative disorders (MPD) (e.g., essential thrombocytosis, chronic myelogenous leukemia, polycythemia vera, agnogenic myeloid metaplasia/myelofibrosis)

*This table delineates the differential diagnosis of disorders which can cause thrombocytosis. As indicated in the text, when thrombocytosis is secondary to another disease process, platelet function will usually be normal. In contrast, primary thrombocytosis can be associated with platelet dysfunction.

anemia, or immature cells (e.g., blasts, myelocytes) are also present.

8. Bear in mind that if urgent correction of the platelet count appears necessary, there are two situations in which platelet transfusion is considered to be contraindicated—thrombotic thrombocytopenic purpura/hemolytic uremic syndrome (TTP/HUS) and heparin-induced thrombocytopenia (HIT). Both of these are discussed later in this article.
9. Obtain hematologic evaluation, especially if the cause of the thrombocytopenia is not apparent or the physician is not experienced in the management of these disorders.

SPECIAL CLINICAL SCENARIOS

There are several clinical situations involving thrombocytopenia that require special consideration.

Intensive Care Setting

Thrombocytopenia that first presents in the patient in an intensive care unit (ICU) is often caused by more than one process. Infections, medications, transfusion, transplantation, disseminated intravascular coagulation (DIC), and intercurrent illness can contribute to thrombocytopenia.

TABLE 5 Situations Requiring Urgent Evaluation or Action

Active bleeding
Severe thrombocytopenia
Steeply falling platelet count
Neurologic symptoms
Recent or impending surgery
Concomitant or recent heparin use
Pregnancy
Neonates, children
Possible TTP/HUS
Concomitant coagulopathy
Presence of immature cells or plasma cells on smear

Abbreviations: HUS = hemolytic uremic syndrome; TTP = thrombotic thrombocytopenic purpura.

TABLE 6 Morphologic Findings on Peripheral Smear in Key Disorders*

Disorder	Morphology
DIC	Schistocytes
Acute leukemia	Blasts
TTP/HUS	Schistocytes
Liver disease	Targets cells
Vitamin B_{12} or folate deficiency	Hypersegmented polymorphonuclear leukocytes
MM	Rouleaux
ITP	Large platelets
Myelofibrosis, cancer in marrow	Tear drops, nucleated red cells
Uremia	Burr cells
Chronic lymphocytic leukemia	Smudge cells, monomorphic mature lymphocytes
Chronic myelogenous leukemia	Immature white cells, eosinophilia, basophilia, tear drops, nucleated red cells
Infection	Toxic granulations, Döhle bodies, vacuoles

*Examination of the smear is an important component of the workup.
Abbreviations: DIC = disseminated intravascular coagulation; HUS = hemolytic uremic syndrome; ITP = idiopathic thrombocytopenic purpura; MM = multiple myeloma; TTP = thrombotic thrombocytopenic purpura.

Heparin Therapy

Thrombocytopenia that develops in a patient on heparin therapy should always prompt an evaluation for possible HIT. In contrast to most cases of drug-induced thrombocytopenia, in which the clinician needs to be concerned about bleeding, patients with HIT are at increased risk of thrombosis either in the venous or the arterial circulation. Thrombotic events can represent a serious threat to life or limb; patients suspected of having HIT should be evaluated and managed by a physician familiar with the syndrome. Heparin should be discontinued if patients are thought to have HIT and an alternative anticoagulant (but not low molecular weight heparin or warfarin), such as a thrombin inhibitor (lepirudin [Refludan], argatroban or bivalirudin [Angiomax][1]), should be administered. Platelet transfusion should be avoided. Although testing may prove helpful, HIT remains a clinical diagnosis.

Bypass Surgery

Patients who undergo coronary artery bypass surgery typically develop a reduction in platelet count on the order of 50%.

Malignancy

Patients with cancer are often thrombocytopenic (Table 7). Platelet support of the patient undergoing active therapy is an important clinical task.

[1]Not FDA approved for this indication.

TABLE 7 Causes of Thrombocytopenia in Pregnant Women*

Disorder	Clinical Features
Gestational thrombocytopenia	Mild, asymptomatic, self-limited; tends to present in the third trimester Fetus is not thrombocytopenic Nature of relationship to ITP is unclear
ITP	More severe; onset earlier in pregnancy Fetus is at risk for thrombocytopenia Antecedent history of thrombocytopenia may be found
Preeclampsia	Edema, proteinuria, hypertension Typical onset late in pregnancy Common syndrome Can progress to eclampsia (seizures) Symptoms abate after delivery
HELLP syndrome	Hemolysis (schistocytes), elevated liver enzymes Onset late in pregnancy Symptoms abate after delivery
TTP-HUS	Renal failure, fever, mental status changes Hemolysis (schistocytes) Variable onset during pregnancy/ postpartum Symptoms generally do not abate after delivery

*The differential diagnosis of thrombocytopenia in pregnancy includes these important entities as well as many of the items listed in Table 2.

Abbreviations: HELLP = hemolysis, elevated liver enzymes, low platelets; HUS = hemolytic uremic syndrome; ITP = idiopathic thrombocytopenic purpura; TTP = thrombotic thrombocytopenic purpura.

Neonates and Children

The following describes conditions that are diagnosed or identified principally in neonates/children.

Conditions Found in Neonates

Antibody-mediated thrombocytopenia can develop in pregnant women who lack a key common platelet antigen (e.g., HPA-1a) when they are exposed to fetal blood containing this antigen. This disorder, neonatal alloimmune thrombocytopenia (NAIT), reflects discordance between mother and father as regards a common platelet antigen. Maternal antibodies react with the platelets in the neonatal circulation causing severe neonatal thrombocytopenia and thus placing the fetus at risk for bleeding. If transfusion of platelets is required, platelets should be obtained from the mother or from another individual who lacks the critical antigen. This disorder generally will recur in a subsequent pregnancy, the assistance of an individual familiar with management of NAIT should be sought in all future pregnancies.

The fetus is also at risk of developing thrombocytopenia if the mother has an autoimmune disorder such as idiopathic thrombocytopenic purpura (ITP) or systemic lupus erythematosus. In contrast, maternal gestational thrombocytopenia does not confer a risk of fetal thrombocytopenia.

Necrotizing enterocolitis, most common in premature neonates, can lead to enhanced platelet destruction.

Maternal preeclampsia can result in transient fetal thrombocytopenia.

Conditions Found in Children

ITP is relatively common in children and differs in several key respects from ITP in adults. ITP in children is usually detected when an otherwise well child presents with signs of mucocutaneous bleeding or ecchymosis. Examination of the smear is of critical importance. Large platelet forms may be present, but the cells seen on the smear should be otherwise unremarkable. Bone marrow examination is mandatory if any signs of a bone marrow disorder are present (see Table 6). It is, in fact, incumbent upon the clinician caring for a child with presumed ITP to ensure that thrombocytopenia is not caused by a bone marrow disorder. ITP in children is usually transient and generally abates even if treatment is not given. Solicitation of assistance from an individual familiar with childhood ITP is essential. Cornerstones of management include avoidance of medications that can impair platelet function and temporary abstention from activities that can increase the risk of bleeding. Decisions regarding the appropriate indications for active treatment in ITP are complex, and evidence is less than ideal. Guidelines published by the American Society of Hematology can serve as a basis for treatment decisions. Pharmacologic treatment of ITP typically involves corticosteroids, intravenous gammaglobulin (IGIV [Gamimune N]), splenectomy, anti-Rh_o immune globulin (Rh_oGAM)[1], platelet transfusion and, in rare cases, immunosuppressive agents. A minority of children with ITP develop chronic ITP.

The cardinal features of HUS include renal dysfunction, microangiopathic anemia, and thrombocytopenia. HUS shares a number of features with TTP (Table 9). In children with HUS, renal dysfunction is a prominent feature, and a history of preceding gastroenteritis (caused by certain strains of *Escherichia coli* or *Shigella*) is often elicited. Peripheral smears demonstrate microangiopathic red cell changes (schistocytes).

Conditions Common to Both Children and Neonates

An unusual consumptive thrombocytopenia (Kasabach-Merritt syndrome) is caused by consumption of platelets within the hemangioma. Hemangiomas may be visible on the skin, but imaging studies may be required to detect internal lesions.

Neonates and children are vulnerable to drug-induced thrombocytopenia. When evaluating a neonate with thrombocytopenia, drugs given to mother or neonate can be implicated in this process;

[1]Not FDA approved for this indication.

drug lists of both individuals should be scanned for possible *culprits*.

A variety of genetic syndromes can cause thrombocytopenia in neonates and children. Consultation with an individual familiar with genetic disorders is recommended if such a syndrome is suspected. Many syndromes do comprise prominent nonhematologic clinical features including Wiskott-Aldrich syndrome, Alport syndrome, thrombocytopenia-absent radius syndrome, Fanconi anemia, Turner's syndrome, and a number of chromosomal trisomies. Syndromes in which hematologic findings predominate include May-Hegglin anomaly, congenital amegakaryocytic thrombocytopenia, and Bernard-Soulier syndrome.

Pregnant Patients

Table 7 lists the differential diagnoses. Features that assist in distinguishing gestational thrombocytopenia from ITP are outlined in this table. Patients with preeclampsia, HELLP (hemolysis, elevated liver enzymes, low platelets) syndrome, DIC, and pregnancy-related TTP/HUS can demonstrate thrombocytopenia. Although typical features are listed in Table 7, these conditions can be difficult to distinguish and assistance from a physician skilled in their management should be sought. Issues that must be considered in generating a care plan include safety of the mother, safety of the fetus, optimal delivery method, and the safety of epidural anesthesia.

Transfusion Related

Post-transfusion purpura (PTP) is a rare, but potentially devastating cause of thrombocytopenia found in individuals who lack a common platelet antigen (often HPA-1a). These individuals can develop severe thrombocytopenia following transfusion with blood obtained from an individual with the antigen. Thrombocytopenia typically develops several days after transfusion. Transfusion of platelets lacking the offending antigen may be needed. This entity is similar in pathogenesis to NAIT.

Patients with trauma or other conditions in which massive transfusion support is needed can develop thrombocytopenia partly because of dilution.

von Willebrand Disease

One subtype of the genetic disorder von Willebrand Disease (vWD), namely type IIb vWD, can present with thrombocytopenia. Thrombocytopenia occurs as a result of increased platelet aggregation and clearance. As an important therapeutic agent, 1-deamino-8-D-arginine vasopressin (desmopressin acetate [DDAVP]), has been reported to lead to complications in this subtype of vWD; management should be directed by an individual who is knowledgeable about this syndrome.

TABLE 8 Causes of Disseminated Intravascular Coagulation (DIC)

Sepsis
Acute leukemia, especially promyelocytic
Snake bites
Retained fetus
Malignancy
Transfusion reaction
Placental abruption
Amniotic fluid embolism
Hemangioma
During initial treatment of acute leukemia

KEY DISEASE PROCESSES

Clinical features of DIC, TTP/HUS, and immune thrombocytopenia are delineated in Tables 8, 9, 10, and 11.

The possibility that thrombocytopenia is a manifestation of a disease of the bone marrow should always be considered. Examination of the smear (see Table 6) may reveal abnormalities that suggest a specific bone marrow disorder. If neutropenia and/or anemia are detected, the likelihood of bone marrow process is increased. Patients may also demonstrate constitutional symptoms (fever, weight loss, pain, fatigue).

Medications frequently cause thrombocytopenia. The patient should be questioned carefully regarding prescribed medications, over-the-counter preparations, drug use, and use of alternative/complementary medications. Up-to-date resources regarding medications that can cause thrombocytopenia can be located both in print and on the internet. It is important to note that information regarding the side effects of new medications and alternative/complementary medications may not be readily available or may not exist at all. If a medication has been identified as a likely cause of thrombocytopenia, it should be discontinued if possible. Thrombocytopenia caused by

TABLE 9 Features of Thrombotic Thrombocytopenic Purpura/Hemolytic Uremic Syndrome (HUS)*

1. Symptom pentad: fever, microangiopathic hemolysis (schistocytes), renal dysfunction, neurologic changes, thrombocytopenia. Entire pentad may not be found.
2. PT, APTT are generally normal.
3. Familial forms exist but most cases are sporadic.
4. Individual may have a single episode or a chronic, relapsing form.
5. Condition is potentially life-threatening.
6. Mainstay of therapy is plasma exchange.
7. Platelet transfusions can worsen the syndrome.
8. Syndrome can occur in association with pregnancy, drugs (ticlopidine, quinine, mitomycin C, clopidogrel), infections (*Escherichia coli, Shigella*), immunosuppressive agents used in transplantation.

*HUS is more commonly found in children but can occur in adults as well. In HUS, renal dysfunction is prominent and neurologic manifestations are less common than in TTP.

Abbreviations: APTT = activated partial thromboplastin time; PT = prothrombin time.

TABLE 10 Clinical Features of Immune Thrombocytopenia

1. Disorder is generally self-limited in children.
2. Adults can develop an acute episode or chronic syndrome of immune thrombocytopenia.
3. This disorder is acquired and mediated by antibodies.
4. Immune thrombocytopenia can occur as an idiopathic disorder or in association with pregnancy, medications, lupus, HIV and other infections, and cocaine.
5. Bone marrow, if performed, demonstrates increased megakaryocytes.
6. Platelet size may be increased, and platelet survival may be decreased.
7. Mainstays of therapy include splenectomy, steroids, and immunosuppressive agents.
8. If thrombocytopenia is secondary (see 4 above) discontinuation of offending medication or treatment of underlying condition may be helpful.

heparin is fundamentally different from other drug-induced thrombocytopenias as outlined above.

Hypersplenism can result in thrombocytopenia. Platelet production may be normal, but splenic sequestration reduces the number of platelets in the circulation.

Platelet Function Disorders

Platelet function disorders (thrombocytopathy) should be suspected in any patient who demonstrates *platelet-type* bleeding (see Table 1) but has a normal platelet count. The detection of a prolonged bleeding time or of abnormalities when platelet function is investigated using aggregometry or a platelet function analyzer can assist in confirming the clinical suspicion of a platelet function defect.

Much of the discussion at the beginning of this article outlining an approach to the patient with thrombocytopenia (specifically items 2 through 7 inclusive and item 9) applies equally to the investigation of platelet function disorders. Important disorders that can impair platelet function are described in Table 3. Prominent on this list are genetic disorders, medications, and systemic conditions; the detection of these entities can be greatly facilitated by means of the systematic approach outlined in the approach. Analysis of the smear is of critical importance in the detection of many bone marrow disorders (e.g., leukemia, myeloproliferative disorders, myeloma), congenital thrombocytopathies (e.g., Bernard-Soulier syndrome, May-Hegglin anomaly), and systemic conditions (e.g., liver disease, uremia). As noted earlier, certain disorders can present with both thrombocytopenia and thrombocytopathy (e.g., Bernard-Soulier syndrome, liver disease, type IIb vWD). Concomitant thrombocytosis and thrombocytopathy is a common feature of the myeloproliferative disorders.

TABLE 11 Clinical Features of Liver Disease

1. Myriad causes can be implicated (e.g., hepatitis, ethanol and other toxins, multiorgan failure, malignancy).
2. Complex coagulopathy may be found such as prolonged PT/APTT, thrombocytopenia and abnormal fibrinogen concentration (increased or decreased).
3. Splenomegaly is often present.
4. Platelet function may be abnormal.
5. Abnormal synthetic function of liver may be detected (e.g., decreased albumin).
6. A chronic form of DIC may be present.

Abbreviations: APTT = activated partial thromboplastin time; PT = prothrombin time.

Medications remain an important cause of thrombocytopathy. The discussion of medications and thrombocytopenia is applicable to medication-induced thrombocytopathy.

Thrombocytosis

The patient with thrombocytosis is usually identified by means of a blood count. Key disorders are listed in Table 4. When thrombocytosis is detected, the most important task is to differentiate primary thrombocytosis, caused by a myeloproliferative disorder (MPD) from secondary thrombocytosis. Features that suggest an MPD is present include splenomegaly, immature circulating blood cells, eosinophilia, basophilia, tear drops, nucleated red cells, platelet count of more than 1,000,000 as well as unusual bleeding and/or thrombosis.

Patients with an MPD are vulnerable both to bleeding (generally platelet type; see Table 1) and thrombosis, while, in general, individuals with secondary thrombocytosis are not. The platelets in patients with an MPD are derived from an abnormal clone and may be functionally impaired as a result. In fact, individuals with MPD may develop both bleeding complications and thrombotic complications; both manifestations may even be present simultaneously. Management of this aspect of MPD is often accurately described with the phrase "between a rock and a hard place." Although a wide variety of thrombotic conditions are possible, the clinician needs to be alert for signs of erythromelalgia (ischemia involving fingers or toes) and central nervous system (CNS) dysfunction. Both of these thrombotic manifestations constitute emergencies. Plateletpheresis, antiplatelet agents, anticoagulants, and chemotherapy are the mainstays of therapy for thrombotic complications of MPD. Platelet transfusions (and avoidance of antiplatelet agents) are used to treat surgical and spontaneous bleeding in MPD. The foregoing discussion should make clear that these disorders are best handled by an individual familiar with the treatment dilemmas involved.

This article is dedicated to my husband,
Jerry Elmer.

DISSEMINATED INTRAVASCULAR COAGULATION

METHOD OF

Gail Rock, MD, PhD

Disseminated intravascular coagulation (DIC) is a syndrome characterized by intravascular activation of coagulation occurring secondary to an underlying disorder. As such, DIC can be regarded as a final common pathway of consumptive coagulation that is initiated by a variety of different factors including tissue damage, shock, malignancy, infections, and various obstetrical complications. The systemic activation of the coagulation system results in formation of microthrombi and, ultimately, in consumption and depletion of coagulation proteins and increased degradation of the coagulation factors and protease inhibitors.

Systemic activation of coagulation results in the production of soluble fibrin, which can contribute to multiorgan failure if deposited in organs. Thrombin not only converts fibrinogen to fibrin, but also activates the anticoagulant pathway to limit the size and extent of clot formation. The normally well-tuned balance of these pathways is lost in DIC.

The release of tissue factor (TF) is key to the thrombin generation in DIC with resultant activation of the extrinsic pathway of coagulation. TF interacts with factor VIIa to generate thrombin. The constant generation of thrombin and the final conversion of fibrinogen to fibrin and fibrin-split products are the main determinants of the disease. In obstetrics, DIC is induced through the release of thromboplastin-like substances into the systemic circulation. In trauma there is exposure of TF from damaged surfaces; in sepsis, this is achieved by the upregulation of TF expression and activity in monocytes. Normally, thrombin is bound to antithrombin and is rapidly cleared in the liver or is bound to endothelial thrombomodulin to activate protein C and further limit thrombin production. However, in DIC, the thrombin production overwhelms the ability of the anticoagulant system resulting in enhanced fibrin formation, suppression of fibrinolysis, and direct cell activation. Thrombin generation proceeds via the extrinsic tissue factor-activated, factor-VII route. Simultaneously, thrombin acts to depress the normal inhibitory mechanisms including antithrombin, protein C, and protein S. There is also impaired fibrin degradation caused by high circulating levels of plasminogen activator inhibitor type-1. Platelet function is inhibited by binding of fibrin monomers to the platelet IIb/IIIa receptor. DIC differs from physiologic clotting in that the system ultimately becomes overwhelmed and, if the stimulus continues, the resultant procoagulant activity results in free, circulating, unopposed thrombin and plasmin, the two key substances that are responsible for DIC.

DIC can be unremarkable or, alternatively, can be overwhelming and result in rapid and catastrophic death. A standard definition of DIC has not yet been established; the most common clinical manifestations of DIC are bleeding, thrombosis, and/or both together with subsequent organ dysfunction. It is generally accepted that DIC evolves through three progressive phases.

Phase 1: Activation of Coagulation with Compensation

Few or no clinical signs may be apparent, however, the presence of predisposing diseases associated with DIC should raise suspicion of the syndrome. The prothrombin time (PT), activated partial thromboplastin time (APTT), thrombin time (TT), and platelet count are usually within the normal range. Other more specific laboratory markers such as the thrombin/antithrombin complex (TAT) and prothrombin fragment (F)1.2 may be elevated, but the antithrombin level may be decreased and soluble fibrin may be detectable in the circulation. Most laboratories do not carry out these latter tests, so in the early stages of DIC standard tests are not very useful. Early diagnosis is based on a high degree of clinical suspicion.

Fibrinogen is the final target of the activation process and should be reflective of the consumptive process; however, because fibrinogen is an acute phase reactive protein it may be markedly increased as a result of the underlying disease.

Phase 2: Decompensated Activation of Coagulation

In the next phase, activation exceeds the capability of the normal inhibitory processes to achieve homeostasis. Early on, thrombosis formation is more pronounced, and microthrombi are visible in both the arterial and venous circulation. Fibrinogen may still be normal, and the level of fibrinogen degradation products (FDP) not very high. Subsequently, the patient may bleed from puncture sites and begin to show some degree of organ dysfunction. The PT and the APTT will be prolonged. Sequential analysis, which is the best approach to diagnosis, will show a continuing drop in platelets. Fibrinogen and coagulation factors such as factor V will also continue to drop as the disease progresses. This stage is sometimes marked by accelerated fibrinolysis. With progressive consumption of coagulation factors, bleeding becomes problematic.

Phase 3: Fulminant Disseminated Intravascular Coagulation

In full-blown disease, multiorgan failure caused by fibrin deposition is common. Skin bleeding is often seen, and laboratory assessment will show marked consumption of hemostatic components.

DIC can also be separated into acute and chronic forms. In the chronic form, low-grade activation is effectively balanced by normal inhibitors. This situation is seen, for example, with artificial devices. While not problematic in itself, chronic DIC can become acute in the face of further insult.

Clinical Conditions Associated with Disseminated Intravascular Coagulation

A considerable number of clinical disorders cause DIC. Chief among these are sepsis, obstetrical catastrophes, trauma, and malignancies (Table 1). Bacterial infection, particularly septicemia, which is caused equally by gram-negative and gram-positive bacteria, is the most common cause. Bacterial cell membrane components are involved in these reactions producing an inflammatory response with release of tissue factor and cytokines. Systemic infection by other organisms can also cause DIC. In severe trauma, a combination of factors including release of tissue factor and endothelial cell damage contribute to activation of coagulation within the circulation. DIC is an independent predictor of mortality in patients with both sepsis and severe trauma. The release of tissue factor is a key component in this and explains the fact that the incidence of DIC is high following head injury.

TABLE 1 Clinical Conditions Associated with the Development of Disseminated Intravascular Coagulation

Clinical Condition	Indications
Allergic reactions	Toxic reactions included
Malignancy	Acute leukemia, particularly acute promyelocytic leukemia; solid tumors
Obstetrical catastrophes	Abruptio placentae, amniotic fluid emboli, toxemia of pregnancy, septic abortion, retained dead fetus, uterine rupture
Others	Cardiac bypass surgery, hepatic failure, thermal injury, heat stroke, hypothermia, snake bite
Sepsis	Both gram-negative and gram-positive bacteria, viruses, rickettsia
Transfusion	Acute hemolytic reactions, massive transfusion
Trauma	Especially with brain injury or fat embolism
Vascular abnormalities	Aortic aneurysms

While the mechanism is not yet clearly known, solid tumors and hematological malignancies (particularly promyelocytic leukemia [M3]) can both result in DIC.

Obstetrical problems such as amniotic fluid emboli, abruptio placentae, and septic abortion can cause calamitous DIC. Amniotic fluid alone activates coagulation in vitro; the leakage of thromboplastin-like material from the placenta during placental separation is an important factor. The most common obstetric complication associated with activation of coagulation is preeclampsia, which presents with hemolysis, elevated liver enzymes, and low platelets (the HELLP syndrome).

Vascular disorders, whether congenital or acquired, and various medical procedures such as cardiac bypass surgery can also result in local activation of coagulation that eventually extends into the systemic circulation, causing DIC.

Incidence

The incidence of DIC in various clinical conditions is not easy to establish because of the various presentations of the syndrome. DIC has been reported in 30% to 50% of a series of patients with gram-negative septicemia, and in 50% to 70% of patients with severe trauma where it is closely related to disease severity scores.

Diagnosis

The diagnosis of DIC is primarily based on clinical evidence. The diagnostic laboratory criteria for DIC are not clearly established. A test for soluble fibrin is crucial to the diagnosis, because elevated levels easily confirm DIC. Unfortunately, this test is difficult to perform as appropriate kits are hard to find. No other single test or combination of tests is truly definitive. However, in the context of the underlying disease and using a variety of laboratory tests, the diagnosis is possible. As stated earlier, in the routine setting serial measurements of APTT, PT, TT, platelet count, and antithrombin plus one or two clotting factors along with a test for fibrin degradation products, including FDPs and D-dimer, should permit diagnosis.

In the reference laboratory, tests for fibrin degradation products such as F1.2 give further discrimination from other conditions associated with low platelet counts. Unfortunately, most of these tests are nonspecific and abnormalities can be seen in other disorders including those of extravascular origin. Determination of the level of tissue factor, the thrombin-antithrombin complex, and various factors involved in the fibrinolytic system, such as plasminogen activator inhibitor type 1 (PAI-1), are also useful.

Treatment

The treatment of DIC depends on three considerations:

1. Resolution of the underlying cause or trigger
2. Replacement of depleted blood factors and platelets
3. The use of inhibitors of coagulation and/or fibrinolysis

UNDERLYING CAUSE

The most important issue is to determine and treat the underlying cause. Without this, subsequent treatment of microthrombus formation and depleted coagulation factors is unlikely to be successful. Generalized supportive therapy should also be initiated, including maintenance of blood pressure through adequate volume replacement.

After this is done, the goals of therapy are to inhibit thrombin generation, neutralize the formed thrombin, and block the thrombin receptor-signaling pathway.

PLATELET AND PLASMA TRANSFUSION

Low levels of platelets and coagulation factors increase the risk of bleeding; however, in the early stages of disease they contribute to microthrombus development. This suggests that only when active bleeding occurs or when some invasive procedure is contemplated and the patient is at risk for bleeding should such therapy be administrated. However, it has never been proven in clinical or experimental studies that the infusion of platelets contributes directly to additional microthrombi formation. Therefore, in an actively bleeding patient with a low platelet count, transfusion of missing factors is the rational approach and platelets should be given.

If transfusion of platelets does not result in the anticipated post-transfusion increment, this indicates a continued consumptive process with formation of microthrombi; therefore, additional replacement should not be given unless heparin is also administered.

Large volumes of plasma may be required to overcome the deficiency of coagulation factors. Blood products containing concentrated coagulation factors should not, in general, be used because many of these preparations contain trace amounts of activated factors, which could help to "fuel the fire." Additionally, most blood products are now highly purified and so are not an efficient way of restoring normal hemostatic components. Cryoprecipitate can be used to increase factor VIII (FVIII) and fibrinogen levels, although the fibrinogen concentration in one bag is usually only in the range of 150 mg.

ANTICOAGULANTS

Heparin

Controversy remains regarding the use of heparin in conditions involving bleeding and consumption of coagulation factors. Heparin has been shown to partially inhibit the activation of coagulation in sepsis and in other situations in which DIC occurs. While many uncontrolled case series have claimed that heparin is effective, a beneficial effect of heparin on clinical outcome has never been demonstrated in a controlled trial.

Nonetheless, to prevent thrombotic complications, low-dose heparin should be used. Higher doses of heparin should only be used in patients with overt thromboembolism. Because the deposition of fibrin causes end-organ dysfunction, heparin should be administered at the first overt sign of this happening. Low-dose heparin is generally started at a dose of 500 to 800 units per hour when a consumptive element is present. If purpura fulminans or large vessel thromboembolism occurs without overt bleeding, heparin should be given at full dosage (1000 to 1600 units per hour). Heparin therapy is not warranted in abruptio placentae or other disorders in which bleeding is the major manifestation.

Antithrombin

Many studies have addressed the use of antithrombin III concentrates in patients with DIC. Eventually, patients with DIC generate thrombin in large quantities; therefore, the antithrombin levels decrease and thrombin-antithrombin (TAT) complexes increase. As antithrombin is one of the most important inhibitors of coagulation, replacement of this factor has considerable appeal. Recent trials in patients with sepsis have shown encouraging benefit. Very high doses appear to give more definitive results and improve the DIC score and even organ function. Meta-analysis has shown a statistically significant reduction in mortality (from 47% to 32%). This therapy could be considered when other treatment avenues have not been productive; however, a recent large-scale, randomized, controlled trial indicates no significant reduction in mortality of septic patients treated with antithrombin concentrate. To date it is not clear which patients most benefit from antithrombin III therapy. Another consideration in the use of antithrombin concentrates is the relatively short half-life of the product.

Other Anticoagulants and Fibrinolytics

A number of other anticoagulants are also used in treating DIC. These include protein C, activated protein C, and soluble thrombomodulin. Because an increase in TF is key to the pathogenesis of DIC it would seem logical to use the physiological inhibitor, tissue factor pathway inhibitor (TFPI), for therapy. The use of TFPI has been shown to significantly reduce fibrin deposition in various organs and prevent coagulation factor consumption in animals. Promising results have been found using recombinant TFPI to block endotoxin-induced thrombin generation.

Recombinant nematode anticoagulant protein-2 (rNAPc2), derived from the family of nematoid anticoagulant proteins and directed specifically against the ternary complex between tissue factor, factor VIIa, and factor X, is also being investigated. Hirudin also has considerable appeal as an anticoagulant in DIC because the low levels of antithrombin make interaction with thrombin and heparin less effective. There are presently no large-scale controlled studies using hirudin in humans although one group of patients with malignancy-induced DIC has shown encouraging results.

Antifibrinolytic compounds are effective in treating bleeding patients but are contraindicated in bleeding caused by DIC, because fibrin deposition is an important pathophysiological feature of DIC.

THROMBOTIC THROMBOCYTOPENIC PURPURA

METHOD OF

Kelty R. Baker, MD, and Joel L. Moake, MD

Thrombotic thrombocytopenic purpura (TTP) is a severe microvascular occlusive disorder characterized by systemic platelet aggregation, profound thrombocytopenia, anemia due to red blood cell fragmentation, and organ ischemia. The widespread platelet clumping is often associated with blood platelet counts below 20,000/μL. Schistocytes, or *split* red blood cells, appear on the peripheral blood smear, and indicate the presence of microangiopathic hemolytic anemia. Occlusive ischemia of the brain or the gastrointestinal tract (GI) is common, and renal dysfunction may occur. Serum levels of lactate dehydrogenase (LDH) are extremely elevated, predominantly as a consequence of tissue necrosis. In the past, a pentad of signs and symptoms was often thought necessary to make the diagnosis of TTP, comprised of thrombocytopenia, microangiopathic hemolytic anemia, neurologic abnormalities, renal failure, and fever. In current clinical practice, a triad of thrombocytopenia, schistocytosis, and an extremely elevated serum LDH value is sufficient to suggest the diagnosis of TTP.

Pathophysiology

Normally, circulating von Willebrand factor (vWf) is derived from proteolytic cleavage of unusually large (UL) vWf multimers secreted by the Weibel-Palade bodies of endothelial cells. A vWf-cleaving metalloprotease degrades the ULvWf multimers, which can range in size into the millions of daltons, into smaller vWf multimers. ULvWf multimers bind more avidly than the smaller multimers to the platelet glycoprotein Ibα and glycoprotein IIb/IIIa receptors, and induce the adhesion and aggregation of platelets under conditions of high shear stress. ADAMTS-13, the vWf-cleaving metalloprotease, is *a* *d*isintegrin *a*nd *m*etalloprotease with eight *t*hrombospondin-1-like domains encoded on chromosome 9q34 and produced predominantly in the liver. When this enzyme is absent or inactive, ULvWf multimers remain anchored to the endothelial cells in long strings. Passing platelets adhere via their glycoprotein Ibα receptors to these long ULvWf multimers (platelets do not adhere to the smaller vWf forms that circulate after cleavage of ULvWf multimers). Many additional platelets subsequently aggregate via their activated IIb-IIIa complexes onto the ULvWf multimeric strings. The result is the formation of large, potentially occlusive, platelet thrombi that contain abundant quantities of von Willebrand factor (vWf) antigen, but not fibrinogen.

The activity of ADAMTS-13 is inhibited by ethylenediaminetetraacetic acid (EDTA); consequently, assays of the enzyme must be performed using citrated plasma. Plasma ADAMTS-13 activity in healthy adults ranges from approximately 50% to 178%. Activity is often reduced below normal in liver disease, disseminated malignancies, chronic metabolic and inflammatory conditions, pregnancy, and newborns. Extremely low values (<5% of normal) are found in most patients with familial and acquired thrombotic thrombocytopenic purpura (TTP). This near-absent activity is found at all times in familial TTP, but only during symptomatic episodes of acquired TTP.

Familial TTP is rare. It may appear initially in infancy or childhood and then recur as chronic relapsing TTP episodes at regular intervals of about 3 weeks. Familial TTP patients have homozygous (or double heterozygous) loss-of-function mutations in each of the two 9q34 genes that encode ADAMTS-13. In contrast, acquired TTP is a commonly recognized disorder that occurs in adults and older children. Following successful treatment, 11% to 36% of patients with acquired TTP have recurrent episodes at irregular intervals. In most patients with acquired TTP, immunoglobulin (Ig) G antibodies (presumably autoantibodies) that inhibit plasma ADAMTS-13 activity are produced during initial and recurrent episodes. Acquired TTP is, therefore, often the result of a transient, or intermittently recurrent, defect of immune regulation.

A small fraction of patients treated for arterial thrombosis with the platelet adenosine diphosphate receptor-inhibiting thienopyridine drugs, ticlopidine (Ticlid) or structurally similar clopidogrel (Plavix), develop TTP within a few weeks after the initiation or therapy. Antibodies that inhibit plasma ADAMTS-13 have also been demonstrated in the few patients studied with ticlopidine or clopidogrel-associated TTP. TTP occurs occasionally in pregnancy (especially the last trimester) or in the immediate postpartum period.

Exposure to the following has been associated with a type of thrombotic microangiopathy weeks to months later:

- Mitomycin C
- Inhibitors of the Ca^{2+}-activated phosphatase, calcineurin (cyclosporine or tacrolimus [FK 506])
- Quinine
- Combinations of chemotherapeutic agents
- Total-body irradiation
- Allogeneic bone marrow, kidney, liver, heart, or lung transplantation

The thrombi may be either predominantly renal or systemic. The pathophysiology of this entity is unknown. Bone marrow transplantation-associated thrombotic microangiopathy is not usually associated with an absence or severely reduced level of plasma ADAMTS-13 activity. The classical hemolytic-uremic syndrome associated with Shiga-toxin producing species of enterohemorrhagic *Escherichia coli* and predominantly renal thrombi is also not characterized by absent or severely reduced plasma ADAMTS-13 activity. Effective treatment for these types of thrombotic microangiopathy is not established.

Treatment

Infants or young children (and the rare adult) with familial TTP produce functionally defective ADAMTS-13. They have chronic relapsing TTP episodes that are reversed or prevented by the infusion of normal platelet-poor, fresh-frozen plasma (FFP), cryoprecipitate-poor plasma (cryosupernatant), or solvent/detergent-treated plasma (to inactivate HIV-1, hepatitis B, and hepatitis C viruses), all of which contain functionally active ADAMTS-13. Plasmapheresis is not necessary. The reason why infusion of ADAMTS-13 activity is required only every 3 weeks, approximately, is not known. The plasma $t_{1/2}$ of the infused enzyme is long (approximately 2 days) and perhaps even longer as it attaches to, cleaves, and dissociates from ULvWf multimers secreted from endothelial cells.

ADAMTS-13 has been partially purified from normal human plasma fractions, the sequence determined, and the enzyme produced in active recombinant form. As a consequence, ADAMTS-13 concentrates may soon be available for use in TTP. Because a plasma level of only approximately 5% ADAMTS-13 is sufficient to prevent or truncate TTP episodes in most patients, gene therapy may eventually be a practical means of providing lasting remissions in children with familial TTP.

Adults, along with some older children and adolescents, with acquired TTP require daily plasma exchange. Plasma exchange is the combination of plasmapheresis (which may remove ULvWf multimers and autoantibodies against ADAMTS-13) and infusion of FFP or cryosupernatant (which contain uninhibited ADAMTS-13). Plasma exchange (usually 3 to 4 liters) allows approximately 80% to 90% of patients with acquired TTP to survive an episode, usually without persistent organ damage. Assays of plasma ADAMTS-13 activity are not generally or rapidly available currently, and therefore cannot yet influence emergency clinical decisions. Any patient who develops symptoms and laboratory findings consistent with TTP should have plasma exchange begin as soon as possible.

To achieve a sustained remission, plasma exchange should be continued for more than 3 days after patients attain complete remission (i.e., a normal neurologic status, a platelet count of more than 150,000/μL, a rising hemoglobin value, and a normal serum LDH level). Schistocytes often persist for many days on peripheral blood films, and so cannot be used as a reliable marker for remission. Skipping even 1 day before complete remission may lead to rapid relapse. Neither more than one exchange per day nor more than one plasma volume per exchange has been demonstrated to be beneficial. At least five additional postremission exchanges are currently used empirically in some centers. Following cessation of plasma exchange, platelet counts should be obtained regularly (to detect nascent relapse). If TTP does recur quickly, then the same treatment program should be repeated. If a patient with TTP responds minimally within the first few days of therapy, or actually deteriorates, it may be preferable to substitute cryosupernatant for FFP in the plasma exchange procedures.

Cryosupernatant is at least as effective as FFP in plasma exchange procedures, and is relatively deficient in the largest plasma vWf multimers, as well as fibrinogen and fibronectin, compared to FFP. Solvent/detergent-treated plasma also lacks the large vWf multimers found in untreated plasma; however, it contains a low level of protein S, and has been used in relatively few TTP patients. Transfusions or exchange transfusions with fluids other than plasma, cryosupernatant, or solvent/detergent-treated plasma (e.g., albumin alone or concentrated immunoglobulin) are almost always ineffective. It may be possible to use 5% albumin, followed by FFP or cryosupernatant (each as half of the total volume), as the fluid infused during plasma exchange if plasma products are in short supply; however, experience with this alternative is limited.

If plasma exchange is not immediately available, normal FFP or cryosupernatant should be infused at the rate of about 30 mL/kg per day until plasma exchanges commence or the patient is transferred to a center where plasma exchange is available. The insertion of the appropriate large-bore apheresis catheter, as well as mobilization of blood bank personnel and resources, are not trivial maneuvers, and usually require hours. Plasma infusion alone is less effective than plasma exchange for acquired TTP, and may result in volume overload. Ticlopidine, clopidogrel, quinine, mitomycin, cyclosporine, or any other drug suspected of provoking the episode should be discontinued. Based on a number of clinical reports, we recommend that adult patients with initial or recurrent TTP episodes also receive daily glucocorticoid therapy (e.g., intravenous prednisolone at 1 to 2 mg/kg per day), unless there is a strong contraindication. Glucocorticoids may suppress the production of autoantibodies against ADAMTS-13 in acquired TTP.

Occasionally, patients with acquired TTP and high titers of antibodies to ADAMTS-13 do not respond to glucocorticoids and plasma exchange. It may be possible to suppress the production of autoantibodies against ADAMTS-13 in these patients using agents such as azathioprine (Imuran)[1], cyclophosphamide (Cytoxan)[1], or rituximab (Rituxan)[1]. Especially promising is rituximab, typically given intravenously at 375 mg/m^2 weekly for 4 weeks. Rituximab is a chimeric mouse/human monoclonal antibody directed against the CD20 antigens expressed predominantly on B lymphocytes. Vincristine (Oncovin)[1], which may alter platelet surface vWf receptor exposure as it depolymerizes platelet cytoplasmic microtubules, is occasionally of modest (and transient) use. If the clinical response remains inadequate, then the therapeutic options dwindle to splenectomy, a risky attempt to remove a large mass of immune cells presumed to be responsible for producing ADAMTS-13 autoantibodies.

Depending on the hemoglobin level and intensity of hemolysis, red blood cell transfusions may be required. Circulating erythrocytes increase the lateral movement of platelets toward the vessel wall, and so red cell transfusions should be used generously during the severe thrombocytopenia associated with TTP episodes. In the absence of extensive (or intracranial) hemorrhage, it is prudent to avoid the possible exacerbation of microvascular thrombosis that may follow platelet transfusion. If platelets are required, then slow (instead of bolus) infusion may be safer.

Blockade by acetylsalicylic acid (aspirin) of cyclooxygenase-mediated platelet thromboxane A_2 generation does not inhibit ULvWf-mediated platelet aggregation under flowing conditions. This may explain the lack of consistent therapeutic benefit from aspirin in TTP. Aspirin may exacerbate hemorrhagic complications in severely thrombocytopenic patients, and should be avoided in TTP.

Patients who achieve only a partial response, or worsen during therapy, should be evaluated for concurrent sepsis or superimposed heparin-associated thrombocytopenia (HIT). Sepsis requires appropriate antibiotics and replacement of intravenous catheters (a probable source of infection). HIT is especially likely if LDH values decrease progressively toward normal during treatment, and then do not rise again as platelet counts fall. In such situations, all of the patient's exposure to heparin should be eliminated.

[1]Not FDA approved for this indication.

HEMOCHROMATOSIS

METHOD OF

Chaim Hershko, MD

Early description in the mid-nineteenth century of the combination of cirrhosis, cutaneous hyperpigmentation, pancreatic fibrosis, and diabetes (bronze diabetes) is associated with the names of Trousseau, Troisier, and von Recklinghausen. The term *hemochromatosis* was introduced erroneously by von Recklinghausen who believed that the iron pigment encountered in tissues originated in hemorrhage. Our present understanding of hemochromatosis is largely attributed to the monumental contribution of the English physician Sheldon, who identified hereditary hemochromatosis (HH) in 1935 as an inborn error of metabolism caused by the increased absorption of iron. The introduction of phlebotomy in 1952 has changed the prognosis of HH and remains the mainstay of its management. Simon and associates' discovery in 1975 that the inheritance of HH is closely linked to the human leukocyte antigen (HLA)-A locus on chromosome 6 made definite identification of homozygous relatives of affected probands possible, and paved the way for the identification of the two most common missense mutations, C282Y and H63D, of the major histocompatibility complex (MHC) class I locus on 6p-designated hemochromatosis gene (HFE).

Iron Homeostasis

Despite the abundance of iron in nature, the solubility of its stable ferric form is extremely low. Hence, living organisms were compelled to develop efficient mechanisms for iron transport and storage. There is no mechanism for excreting excess iron, and the inevitable end result of iron absorption exceeding physiologic needs is iron overload.

In recent years a number of key mechanisms have been described that are responsible for adaptation to changing environmental conditions. Production of the iron storage protein, ferritin, and the transferrin receptor (TfR) protein is reciprocally regulated by a translational mechanism in which the iron regulatory protein (IRP) is reversibly bound to the iron response elements (IRE) of their respective mRNAs. A similar iron-dependent translational mechanism may be responsible for the production of divalent metal transporter I (DMT1), which is responsible for the uptake of ferrous iron from the brush border of duodenal enterocytes (Figure 1), and ferroportin (IREGI), which is responsible for the export of ferrous iron through the basolateral membrane of the same cells. The brush border ferric reductase converts ferric to ferrous iron for use by DMT1, and hephaestin, a transmembrane-bound ferroxidase, converts ferrous to ferric iron, creating a concentration gradient of ferrous iron across the cell membrane facilitating iron egress. At low-iron

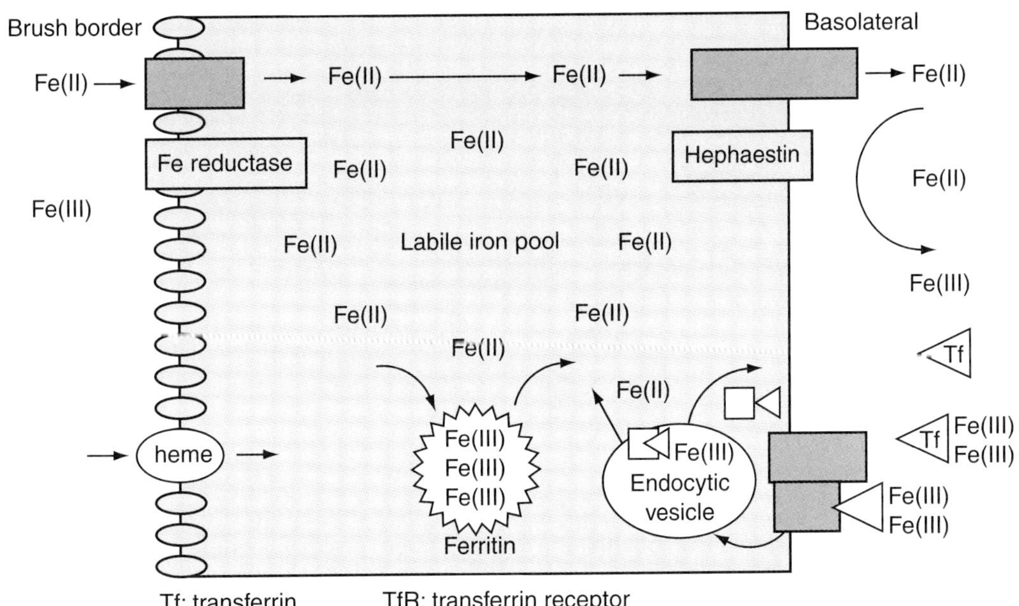

FIGURE 1 Cellular control of iron transport in duodenal enterocyte.

conditions the translation of TfR, DMT1, and ferroportin is enhanced, with the opposite occurring at high-iron conditions. In addition, a new protein, hepcidin, has been described recently and is probably the most important regulator of iron homeostasis. Hepcidin functions as an inhibitor of iron absorption and release from macrophages. Its production is increased by iron overload and inflammation and is suppressed by iron deficiency.

Genetics of Hereditary Hemochromatosis

The HFE protein combines with β_2-microglobulin for presentation on the cell surface. The central role of HFE mutations in the pathogenesis of HH is clearly illustrated by the development of severe hemochromatosis in HFE knockout mice. Although the HFE protein exists in a great variety of tissues, it is most strongly expressed in hepatic parenchymal cells. On the cell surface it is associated with β_2-microglobulin and transferrin receptor and modifies the affinity of the transferrin receptor to diferric transferrin. This can hardly explain its role in the pathogenesis of iron overload. It is quite likely that the HFE protein does not directly regulate iron absorption and release from macrophages, but indirectly through the control of hepcidin production. Both hepcidin and HFE are expressed mainly in hepatic parenchymal cells. Serum hepcidin in HH is inappropriately low, and this may be the cause of increased intestinal iron absorption and the lack of reticuloendothelial iron accumulation characteristic of HH. It is also quite likely that inappropriately low hepcidin production may be the final common pathway of transferrin receptor 2 (a transmembrane protein homologous with transferrin receptor) mutations and other hereditary iron overload syndromes characterized by the HH phenotype.

As expected, mutations of other proteins involved in iron transport and storage may also result in abnormal iron homeostasis. Table 1 describes some of the hereditary iron overload syndromes not associated with the HFE locus. Thus, mutations of hemojuvelin, hepcidin, transferrin receptor 2, ferroportin, L-ferritin IRE, or atransferrinemia may all result in the hereditary hemochromatosis phenotype or inappropriately high serum ferritin. However, in Western populations, HH is attributed in more than 80% of subjects to homozygous C282Y mutation or compound heterozygosity for the C282Y and H63D mutations of HFE. Heterozygosity for either C282Y or H63D is not associated with significant iron accumulation or morbidity.

Diagnosis

Patients with HH may be identified by suggestive clinical features, by family studies of hemochromatotic probands, or by population screening. Despite the increasing sophistication of diagnostic tools, clinical judgment is still an essential part of patient evaluation. Other conditions characterized by abnormal serum ferritin and transferrin saturation such as iron-loading anemias, chronic hepatitis, alcoholic liver disease, nonalcoholic steatohepatitis (NASH), and porphyria cutanea tarda should be considered before embarking on a detailed diagnostic workup for HH. Some of the clinical features of HH are nonspecific,

TABLE 1 Non-HFE Type Hereditary Hemochromatosis

Type 2 Juvenile hemochromatosis	Chromosome 1q	Hemojuvelin.	Clinical symptoms before age 30 caused by cardiac disease and hypogonadism
Hepcidin mutation	Chromosome 19	Hepcidin.	
Type 3 Hemochromatosis: Transferrin receptor 2 mutations	Chromosome 7q22	47% identity with classical transferrin receptor.	Phenotype similar to HFE-associated hemochromatosis
Type 4 Hemochromatosis: Ferroportin mutations	Chromosome 2q	The mechanism of increased iron absorption remains unresolved.	Autosomal dominant; High serum ferritin and near-normal transferrin saturation
Hereditary atransferrinemia	Chromosome 3q21	Increased iron absorption and iron deficiency anemia.	Iron deficiency anemia and severe parenchymal siderosis
Hyperferritinemia Cataract syndrome	Chromosome 19q13	Mutation of L-ferritin IRE and reduced affinity to IRP.	Autosomal dominant; Increased serum ferritin without iron overload

Abbreviation: HFE = hemochromatosis gene.

HFE mutations do not account for all hemochromatotic patients, and homozygosity for the C282Y mutation is not associated with significant clinical disease in the majority of subjects identified by genetic screening.

CLINICAL DIAGNOSIS

A high index of suspicion is required for diagnosis by clinical features. The combination of obscure hepatomegaly with or without abnormal liver enzymes, diabetes, arthropathy with symmetric involvement of proximal interphalangeal, and metacarpophalangeal joints, increased skin pigmentation, cardiomyopathy, or decreased libido are all very suggestive but may be anticipated only at advanced stages of iron accumulation. Consequently in the vast majority of cases, the diagnosis is established by laboratory tests including transferrin saturation, serum ferritin, polymerase chain reaction (PCR) for common HFE mutants, and, optionally, liver biopsy.

Transferrin saturation measured in fasting morning blood samples is a very useful and sensitive test. A transferrin saturation of 60% or more in men and 50% in women, observed on at least two occasions and in the absence of other known causes of increased saturation, is characteristic of HH and permits identification at an early stage. Because of the variability of phenotypic expression of C282Y homozygosity, only 85% of male homozygotes and 44% of female homozygotes will have a transferrin saturation greater than 50%.

Serum ferritin is the next step in the initial diagnostic workup of suspected HH. A value of 300 μg/L or higher is considered evidence of significant iron overload. Quantitative phlebotomy permitting accurate retrospective evaluation of storage iron indicates that 1 μg/L of serum ferritin represents roughly 8 mg of storage iron. However, the limitations of serum ferritin measurements should be kept in mind as inflammation and active liver injury may result in spuriously increased ferritin measurements and coexistent ascorbate deficiency may decrease serum ferritin. It is generally accepted that in patients with serum ferritin above 1000 μg/L, there is an increased likelihood of significant hepatic damage.

Polymerase chain reaction for the common HFE mutants C282Y and H63D is a useful adjunct for evaluating subjects with increased serum ferritin and transferrin saturation. In patients with HH, homozygosity for the C282Y genotype has been found in nearly 100% of subjects in Australia; 90% to 92% in Germany, France, and the UK; 60% to 83% in the United States; and 64% in Italy. Other HFE mutants were compound heterozygotes for C282Y and H63D or the S65C alleles, or homozygotes for H63D. Although useful, identification of common HFE mutations is not obligatory for establishing the clinical diagnosis of HH, and it is even less so in populations wherein the gene frequency of these mutations is low. Conversely, identification of these mutants in probands is of great help in identifying additional subjects with identical genotype within their families.

The importance of *liver biopsy* for the diagnosis and initial evaluation of HH has diminished with the introduction of genetic analysis. In subjects with no abnormality of liver function and with serum ferritin below 1000 μg/L, the risk of significant hepatic fibrosis is minimal and liver biopsy may not be necessary, although this view is not universally accepted. However, in the presence of higher serum ferritins or abnormal liver enzymes, biopsy may yield important additional information. In particular, liver biopsy is the only available method for documenting cirrhosis if this is not indicated by ultrasound, computed tomography (CT), or other imaging techniques. Diagnosing cirrhosis has important prognostic implications, and involves the need of regular screening for hepatocellular carcinoma by repeat ultrasound and α-fetoprotein measurements. Liver biopsy can also be used for measuring liver iron concentrations chemically or by semiquantitative histochemistry, and for examining the cellular distribution of iron, which in HH is predominantly hepatocellular.

Liver iron measurement by noninvasive techniques is another diagnostic tool. The superconducting quantum interface device (SQUID) is the most sensitive, accurate, and reproducible method for liver iron measurement based on the paramagnetic properties of ferritin and hemosiderin. Unfortunately, SQUID is expensive to build and operate and only a few machines are available worldwide, mostly for research purposes. Adaptation of magnetic resonance imaging (MRI) for the measurement of tissue iron is a much less expensive method. Recent improvements in MRI sensitivity and accuracy, based on signal intensity ratio (SIR) or T2*, have greatly improved these techniques and offer both imaging and tissue iron measurements in the liver and other vital tissues, such as the heart. Standardization of these techniques and their simultaneous introduction to multiple regional centers may revolutionize the clinical evaluation of patients with hereditary or transfusional iron overload.

Treatment of Hereditary Hemochromatosis

Although establishing the C282Y genotype is useful, this is not a primary consideration in the selection of patients for therapy. In northern Europe, heterozygosity for the C282Y mutation occurs in 15% and homozygosity in 1 in 200 of the general population. Although most C282Y homozygotes have increased transferrin saturation and some may develop increased iron stores, the prevalence of organ damage in C282Y homozygotes because of iron overload is a topic of current controversy. In addition, in non-European populations, non-HFE–related hereditary hemochromatosis may be predominant. Thus, selection for phlebotomy should be based on clinical assessment and not on genotype. It is generally accepted that men and postmenopausal women with a serum ferritin greater than 300 and women in their reproductive years with ferritin greater than 200 and in whom other causes of increased ferritin (inflammation, hepatitis, etc.) have been excluded, should be treated by phlebotomy.

Therapeutic phlebotomy involves the removal of one unit (450 to 500 mL) of blood weekly, which is the equivalent of 200 to 250 mg of iron. This should be repeated every week until depletion of iron stores indicated by serum ferritin below 30 µg/L and/or mild anemia of 13 g/dL in men and 11 g/dL in women. The rate of blood removal may be higher in men with large body mass and less in small females, elderly subjects, and patients with cardiac or pulmonary problems who tolerate phlebotomy less well. The cumulative volume of blood removed should be monitored. Once iron depletion has been achieved, the cumulative volume measurement may allow retrospective calculation of the initial magnitude of iron stores. Although iron absorption increases with the establishment of iron depletion, the additional daily absorption of 1 or 2 mg of iron is negligible in comparison with the amounts removed. Life expectancy may be substantially decreased in patients in whom iron depletion is not completed within the first year of therapy. Once iron depletion is achieved, phlebotomy should be maintained throughout life at a rate of 2 to 4 units per year, to maintain a serum ferritin of less than 50 µg/L. Chelation therapy has no place in the management of HH with the possible exception of symptomatic cardiomyopathy in which aggressive continuous deferoxamine infusion may rapidly reverse life-threatening cardiac complications.

Drastic dietary restrictions are unnecessary. Red meat should be consumed in moderation, and patients should avoid the ingestion of iron and vitamin C supplements. Alcohol may potentiate hepatic injury. Raw shellfish should be avoided as it may be contaminated by *Vibrio vulnificus*, that may cause fatal infection in iron-loaded hosts.

Effective treatment of HH by phlebotomy before the development of cirrhosis, diabetes, or cardiomyopathy results in normal life expectancy. Table 2 describes the impact of phlebotomy on the various complications of HH and the conditions that may, or may not, be reversed by such treatment. Following iron depletion, serum ferritin normalizes but transferrin saturation usually remains increased.

Treatment of Transfusional Siderosis

In anemic patients requiring long-term blood transfusion, phlebotomy is impractical and only iron chelation therapy is able to remove excess iron. The introduction of deferoxamine (DFO) (Desferal) for regular use in the management of transfusional hemosiderosis has changed the quality of life and life expectancy of many patients with thalassemia. However, effective DFO treatment requires continuous subcutaneous infusion by portable pumps at a dose of 40 mg/kg per day for 8 to 12 hours, 5 days per week, and many patients are unable to cope with the rigorous requirements of such treatment. Patients with thalassemia major and other transfusion-dependent disorders who are able to successfully control iron overload at a safe level with DFO should be encouraged to continue with this approach to chelation therapy.

TABLE 2 Effect of Therapeutic Phlebotomy

Improved	Not Improved
Relief of nonspecific symptoms: malaise, weakness	Hepatic cirrhosis and the associated risk of hepatoma
Abnormal liver function	Joint disease
Control but not resolution of diabetes mellitus	Hypogonadotropic hypogonadism
Reversal of cardiomyopathy	Thyroid disorders
Fading of hyperpigmentation	
Reversal of early pituitary and gonadal dysfunction	

Treatment with the oral chelator deferiprone (DFP)[2] should be considered in patients unable to use deferoxamine or patients with an unsatisfactory response to deferoxamine as judged by liver iron and serum ferritin measurements. At a DFP dose of 75 mg/kg per day, iron stores may decrease in some patients, remain stable in others, and increase in some others. Thus, careful monitoring of iron stores, preferably by measurement of tissue iron and of cardiac function, is important during treatment with DFP as it is with DFO. Enhanced iron excretion can be obtained at higher doses of deferiprone or by combining deferiprone and deferoxamine therapy, and early studies of combined therapy are particularly encouraging, but these approaches have not undergone rigorous long-term testing for complications.

A new and promising orally effective iron chelator, ICL670*, has recently been developed by Novartis, and early clinical studies indicate that at a dose of 20 mg/kg per day it may be as effective as DFO 40 mg/kg per day. It is hoped that a better understanding of the pathophysiology of iron toxicity and the mechanism of iron chelation may promote the development of improved strategies of iron chelation therapy.

[2]Not available in the United States.

*Investigational drug in the United States

HODGKIN'S DISEASE: CHEMOTHERAPY

METHOD OF

George P. Canellos, MD

Hodgkin's disease is a success story of cancer therapeutics with up to 75% to 80% of patients cured of their disease. Chemotherapy, radiation therapy, or the combination of both modalities has contributed to that success. The difficult challenge for the present and future is the modification of the treatment approaches to lessen the toxic side effects of therapy, some of which are in themselves fatal. Thus, there has been an evolution in the last 10 years to using less extensive radiation therapy and minimizing, in the majority of patients, the use of alkylating agents.

Molecular Biology and Histopathology

Progress in defining the cellular origin of the disease has evolved from the study of individual Reed-Sternberg cells obtained by micropipetting techniques. The majority of malignant cells are clonally-derived B cells that have a germinal center or postgerminal center B lymphocyte genotype with rearranged immunoglobulin heavy chains and somatic hypermutations, but without the presence of surface immunoglobulin and other B-cell markers such as CD20. The latter is caused by the absence of key transcription factors that are required for the synthesis of specific proteins.

Thus, the histopathologic terminology which has evolved to include the nodular sclerosis variant, represents up to 90% of cases, and the mixed cellularity variant that is more often seen in older patients is *classic* Hodgkin's disease.

The nodular lymphocyte-predominant disease assumes a different clinical biology in that the median age is 10 to 15 years older, and the disease is usually localized with a very protracted indolent natural history and a low death rate even after relapse. There is also a higher but small likelihood for transformation to large-cell non-Hodgkin's lymphoma. Occasionally nodular lymphocyte-predominant Hodgkin's disease will evolve from a condition known as progressive transformation of germinal centers and occasionally can be confused microscopically with T-cell–rich B-cell lymphoma. Surface markers routinely found in the hematopathology of classic Hodgkin's disease include CD30 (Ki-1 antigen) and CD15, a myeloid marker also known as Leu-M1. These are absent in nodular lymphocyte-predominant disease. It is rare for the classic disease to have CD20 and even rarer to have evidence of T-cell receptor rearrangement (1% to 3%). This leaves the lymphocyte-predominant nodular variant as an almost separate disorder because it has features of an intact germinal center B cell with surface immunoglobulin and the presence of surface markers that characterize such cells—CD20, CD45 (leukocyte common antigen)—which are usually absent or faintly positive in the classic disease.

Clinical Assessment and Staging

The expanded use of systemic therapy has modified the extent of staging techniques required. Beyond the appropriate history and physical examination, a measurement of routine complete blood count and liver function studies have some prognostic value. Interestingly, a bone marrow biopsy, which is so often used in non-Hodgkin's lymphoma staging, is rarely useful in Hodgkin's disease. Clear-cut marrow involvement is extremely rare in localized asymptomatic presentations and, because systemic therapy is used extensively, treatment is not often altered. Although constitutional (B) symptoms (fever, weight loss, night sweats) are noted, they have not assumed a negative prognostic significance in the systemic therapy era.

An elaborate statistical study (1,618 patients) has established the following criteria as independently predictive of a poorer prognosis in patients presenting with advanced disease (stages III, IV):

- Age 45 or above
- Male gender
- Stage IV (extranodal disease)
- Hemoglobin less than 10.5 g
- Leukocytosis 15,000 or greater
- Lymphopenia less than 600 or less than 8% of the white blood cell count
- Albumin less than 4 g (Table 1)

Patients presenting with clinically localized disease but with the above features should also be considered at higher risk. However, even all seven factors combined still yields a 42% progression-free survival. In the localized presentation with bulky nodes, combined modality therapy is required because bulky disease is considered a poor prognostic factor for systemic therapy alone. *Bulk* is variously defined, but is usually greater than 7 to 10 cm, or 33% or greater of the thoracic diameter on an upright chest film. All patients should have a full body computerized axial tomography (CAT) scan. Anatomic abnormalities on the CAT scan can be further assessed with a radionuclide scan with ^{67}gallium or, if available, positron emission tomography (PET) with ^{18}fluorodeoxyglucose. The latter is more sensitive and thus somewhat more liable to false-positives. A more useful role for the radionuclide scans is the assessment of residual masses. As opposed to non-Hodgkin's lymphoma, the clinician should be alerted to the fact that a *positive* PET scan on completion of therapy should be evaluated carefully because a significant percentage (40%) of faintly positive PET scans can revert to normal in time. It is good practice to delay the final PET scan for at least 1 month following completion of therapy to avoid confusion and unnecessary extra therapy.

Treatment

Once the staging assessment is complete, the stage of the disease (based on the Ann Arbor scheme) can be assigned. Because staging laparotomies have not been done for many years, all stages are basically clinical stages. Treatment recommendations are based on evidence, where possible, derived from randomized clinical trials.

TABLE 1 Prognostic Factors in Advanced Hodgkin's Disease and Predicted Progression-Free Survival According to the Number of Factors

Prognostic Factors

Serum albumin <4 g/dL
Hemoglobin <10.5 g/dL
Male gender
Stage IV disease
Age >45 years
White blood count >15,000/mm^3
Lymphocyte count <500/mm^3 or 8% of white count

No. of Factors (From List)	Progression-Free Survival
0-2	88%-70%
3	60%
4	50%-55%
5 or more	~45%

CLASSIC HODGKIN'S DISEASE

Localized Presentations (Stage I/II A or B, Nonbulky)

It is this author's practice to offer systemic therapy alone to younger patients with stages I and II A or B, nonbulky localized disease to avoid the long-term morbidity and potential mortality of radiation therapy, such as radiation-induced cancers that can occur in 20% to 25% of patients followed more than 20 years and cardiovascular damage to coronary arteries and valves. Pilot trials of chemotherapy alone with *A*driamycin (doxorubicin), *b*leomycin, *v*inblastine, and *d*acarbazine (ABVD) have been positive, and a randomized trial from Memorial Sloan-Kettering in 150 patients showed no advantage to adding radiation therapy. Because salvage therapy can be successful in this disease, the omission of radiation in patients without bulk disease who receive a full course of chemotherapy will not, in this author's opinion, compromise survival from Hodgkin's disease and should minimize the long-term risks mentioned above. Because prospective randomized multigroup trials have shown *no* advantage to the addition of alkylating agents contained in *m*echlorethamine, *o*ncovin (vincristine), *p*rocarbazine, and *p*rednisone (MOPP) or MOPP-like regimens given as alternating or hybrid regimens compared with ABVD, the clinician is advised to omit them to diminish the risk of myelodysplasia/leukemia associated with alkylating agents. If systemic therapy alone is to be used, it is uncertain whether a full six cycles of ABVD are required. A Canadian trial testing four cycles is under analysis. Until that issue is clarified, the full six cycles are recommended as that is known to be curative for more advanced stages.

Localized Disease (Stages I/II A or B Bulky)

Localized disease (stages I/II A or B bulky) appears to do well with combined modality therapy. Because radiation therapy is to be added, the ABVD can be abbreviated to four cycles. It is unknown whether fewer cycles can be used, although some phase II series have had two or three cycles of chemotherapy. Following the assessment of response to eliminate the possibility of progressive disease on chemotherapy, the patient would receive involved field radiation therapy. It remains in the future to determine whether radiation can be omitted from patients who achieve a complete response, as assessed by PET scans. This might arise in the circumstance of a young patient in whom radiation therapy poses a risk. At the present time, combined modality is recommended but

TABLE 2 Doxorubicin-Containing Regimens

Drug	Dose (mg/m^2)	Route	Schedule (Days)	RT	Cycle/Length (Days)
ABVD					28
Adriamycin (doxorubicin)	25	IV	1,15		
Bleomycin	10	IV	1,15		
Vinblastine	6	IV	1,15		
Dacarbazine	375	IV	1,15		
EVA				Bulky, residual	28
Etoposide	100	IV	1-3		
Vinblastine	6	IV	1		
Adriamycin (doxorubicin)	50	IV	1		

there may be exceptional circumstances where systemic therapy alone is used.

Advanced Disease (Stages III/IV A or B)

All patients with advanced disease should receive systemic therapy. The current commonly used regimen is ABVD, usually with six or eight cycles (Table 2). Whether eight cycles are needed has not been established in prospective trials, but certainly six cycles should be given. As mentioned above, MOPP or MOPP-like chemotherapy in alternation or hybridized with ABVD does not add a survival advantage and has more toxicity. Furthermore, there is an emerging body of data from the randomized European Organization for Research and Treatment of Cancer (EORTC) trial and from a separate meta-analysis that the addition of radiation therapy to sites of prior bulk disease in patients who achieve a clinically complete remission does not add a survival advantage. The fact that not all patients are cured by ABVD alone justifies new approaches whose ultimate value will require the prospective comparison with a current standard.

There are two systemic therapies currently under investigation. One is the Stanford V regimen, which entails weekly administration of cytotoxic agents such that the regimen is completed in 3 months (Table 3). Patients then receive radiation to primarily involved nodal sites. The initial results from Stanford show a highly favorable progression-free survival at 5 years. It is currently being compared to ABVD with and without radiation in a cooperative Intergroup trial.

The other major treatment is the intensification of the chemotherapy with the addition of the drugs etoposide, cyclophosphamide, procarbazine, and prednisone (BEACOPP) (Table 3). The escalation of BEACOPP doses also produced a remarkable improvement in progression-free survival when compared to a standard COPP (cyclophosphamide, vincristine, procarbazine, prednisone) alternating with ABVD for eight cycles. It is likely that progression-free survival is superior but the escalated doses of BEACOPP do

TABLE 3 Intensive (Investigational) Regimens

Drug	Dose (mg/m^2)	Route	Schedule (Days)	RT	Cycle/Length (Days)
BEACOPP (Escalated BEACOPP)				Bulky, residual	28
Bleomycin	10	IV	8		
Etoposide	100 (200)	IV	1-3		
Adriamycin (doxorubicin)	25 (35)	IV	1		
Cyclophosphamide	650 (1250)	IV	1		
Oncovin (vincristine)	1.4*	IV	8		
Procarbazine	100	PO	1-7		
Prednisone	40	PO	1-14		
G-CSF	-(+)	SQ	8+		
Stanford V				Bulky	12 weeks
Mechlorethamine	6	IV	Wks 1,5,9		
Adriamycin (doxorubicin)	25	IV	Wks 1,3,5,7,9,11		
Vinblastine	6	IV	Wks 1,3,5,7,9,11		
Vincristine	1.4*	IV	Wks 2,4,6,8, 10,12		
Bleomycin	5	IV	Wks 2,4,6,8, 10,12		
Etoposide	60 × 2	IV	Wks 3,7,11		
Prednisone	40	PO	Wks 1-10 qod		
G-CSF			Dose reduction or delay		

*Vincristine dose capped at 2 mg.
Abbreviations: G-CSF = granulocyte colony-stimulating factor; IV = intravenous; PO = oral; RT = radiation therapy; SQ = subcutaneous.

require granulocyte growth factors. Stanford V requires antibiotic and antiviral prophylaxis. There is a small incidence of secondary myelodysplasia when BEACOPP is given in augmented doses. There is also an international randomized trial comparing BEACOPP to ABVD currently underway. The real issue, of course, is the ultimate survival from Hodgkin's disease itself. If the higher progression-free survivorship is 10% to 15% better than ABVD alone, will the longer-term toxicity of added radiation or addition of drugs toxic to marrow stem cells result in treatment-related mortality that will balance the outcomes? The answer is uncertain at the present time.

With effective salvage therapy, especially high-dose chemotherapy and peripheral stem cell support, resulting in approximately 40% to 50% long-term (5 to 7 years), progression-free survival, the overall mortality has decreased even further.

NODULAR LYMPHOCYTE PREDOMINANT DISEASE

Nodular lymphocyte predominant disease is a rare variant (5%) of Hodgkin's disease that often presents as localized nodal disease. Modified or involved fields of radiation therapy have been successful in effecting long-term control. Late relapse in an otherwise unirradiated site can be treated again with radiation therapy. In the circumstance of either presentation with or relapse with advanced disease (stage III or IV), systemic therapy is required. It is the opinion of this author that in contrast to the impact of ABVD in classic Hodgkin's disease (75% to 80% clinically complete remission, with a 65% to 70% long-term, progression-free survival) that regimen is suboptimal and an alkylating agent-containing program is more likely to be effective given the low grade B-cell nature of the disease.

Recently the rituximab anti-CD20 antibody, now widely used in low-grade non-Hodgkin's lymphoma, has been shown to be highly active in most cases of nodular lymphocyte-predominant disease. The remissions are about 12 months or longer in duration but, given the indolent behavior of the disease, the long-term impact of rituximab on survival is uncertain. Whether it will be more effective with chemotherapy remains an unanswered question.

SIDE EFFECTS

The unique feature of ABVD is the rare complication of bleomycin lung toxicity. There is no clear-cut management policy, but pulmonary function studies in alternate cycles in asymptomatic patients is reasonable. Symptoms of cough, dyspnea, and/or radiographic changes suggest bleomycin toxicity. It has been this author's policy to continue the regimen but omit further bleomycin. An alternative could be the etoposide, vinblastine, doxorubicin regimen (EVA), which is also an active regimen (see Table 2).

TABLE 4 Salvage Regimens (Conventional Dose)

EVA (etoposide, vinblastine, doxorubicin)
MINE (mitoguazone, ifosfamide, vinorelbine, etoposide)
Mini-BEAM (BCNU, etoposide, cytosine arabinoside, melphalan)
Dexa-BEAM (dexamethasone, BCNU, etoposide, cytosine arabinoside, melphalan)
VIP (etoposide, ifosfamide, cisplatin)
DNG (liposomal, doxorubicin, vinorelbine, gemcitabine)
ICE (ifosfamide, carboplatin, etoposide)

SALVAGE THERAPY

Patients who relapse from clinically complete remission or who fail to enter an initial complete clinical remission should be considered for high-dose chemotherapy with peripheral or bone marrow stem cell support. As mentioned above, the relatively high long-term, progression-free survival rate justifies the toxicity of the high-dose chemotherapy. An exception to this policy might be the relatively uncommon circumstance of a late-occurring (beyond 12 months) relapse in an isolated nodal site in an asymptomatic patient, which may be managed with conventional dose combination chemotherapy and radiation to the involved site.

Patients who relapse from high-dose chemotherapy can rarely be salvaged with allogeneic bone marrow transplantation. If the disease is refractory to second- or third-line chemotherapy, it is a poor prognostic sign for allotransplantation. Alternative conventional dose regimens, containing known active drugs, have been used as well as single agents, such as vinblastine. More recently gemcitabine has been shown to be an active agent either singly or in combination (Table 4). Most series use these regimens preceding high-dose therapy, thus the real impact of each cannot be compared. All appear to be active. There is no one standard second-line regimen, but early relapse from ABVD would suggest that alkylating agent-containing chemotherapy would be a good preparation before administering high-dose therapy.

HODGKIN'S DISEASE: RADIATION THERAPY

METHOD OF

Chul S. Ha, MD

Considered uniformly fatal even 5 decades ago, Hodgkin's disease is now one of the most curable cancers. Extended field radiation therapy was the first modality shown to cure the disease and has been the standard treatment for early stage disease for nearly 4 decades. However, with the advancement of effective chemotherapeutic agents and recognition of long-term treatment-related complications from radiation therapy, the role of radiation therapy has been evolving during the same time period. This article complements the previous article, *Hodgkin's Disease: Chemotherapy*, with an emphasis on the changing role of radiation therapy in the management of Hodgkin's disease. An overview of the clinical trials assessing the role of radiation therapy is presented.

Establishment of Radiation Therapy as the Standard in the Management of Early Stage Hodgkin's Disease

In the early 1920s, a Swiss radiotherapist, René Gilbert, recognized that with radiotherapy alone it was important to treat contiguous, lymph-node-bearing regions that were not clinically involved. Despite this observation, the administration of low doses of radiation to clinically involved sites remained the standard of care over the next 4 decades. Consequently, Hodgkin's disease was considered incurable. Although M. Vera Peters published in 1950 that early stage Hodgkin's disease could be cured with radiotherapy, physicians remained skeptical. Easson and Russell published the next landmark article in 1963 entitled, "The Cure of Hodgkin's Disease," reemphasizing that radiotherapy could be curative if administered properly. In the 1960s and 1970s, Henry Kaplan at Stanford University helped to refine radiotherapy techniques and, with Saul Rosenberg, helped to popularize the use of radiotherapy for early stage disease. Based on the work described above, the age-adjusted mortality rate for Hodgkin's disease decreased after 1970 for the first time. Since the 1970s, many patients with early stage Hodgkin's disease have been treated with subtotal nodal irradiation (STNI)* alone because radiotherapy remains the single most effective therapeutic agent. STNI is used to treat the mantle, para-aortic, and splenic fields (splenic pedicle if a laparotomy is performed).

Laparotomy (pathologic staging) was an integral part in the staging evaluation of the patients and was used to select early stage patients who could be treated with subtotal nodal radiation therapy with curative intent. However, a European Organization for Research and Treatment of Cancer (EORTC) study randomized patients with clinical stages I and II disease between laparotomy and no laparotomy and demonstrated no difference in the treatment outcomes between the two arms. This study helped establish the use of the STNI in clinically staged patients without a laparotomy.

A more recent source of extensive data on the treatment of patients with clinical stages I and II supra-diaphragmatic Hodgkin's disease comes from the Princess Margaret Hospital. Their actuarial overall survival (OS) was 83%, cause-specific survival 90%, and relapse-free survival (RFS) 72% at 8 years. Local tumor control was 95% with only two true in-field failures. These outcomes are consistent with others' data on similar clinically staged patients treated with extended field radiation therapy.

*This procedure is also known as extended field radiotherapy.

Recognition of the Toxicity of Radiation Therapy

In spite of the high cure rate with radiotherapy alone, a portion of the patients who are cured of Hodgkin's disease unfortunately experience some of the long-term complications of radiotherapy. Though pulmonary and cardiac complications have been reduced greatly because of the improvement of techniques and better understanding of the radiobiologic principles to minimize long-term side effects, the risk of second malignancy still persists and poses an increasingly significant problem for the young patients who are otherwise cured of the disease.

Late complications of mantle irradiation include lung, heart, and thyroid dysfunction; second cancers; and Lhermitte sign. Boivin and colleagues suggested that mediastinal irradiation modestly increases the age-adjusted risk of death secondary to myocardial infarction. Based on an average follow-up of 9.5 years, Hancock and colleagues reported that mediastinal irradiation to total doses of 30 Gy or less, using 1.5 to 2.75 Gy daily, does not increase the patient's risk of cardiac death. However, mediastinal doses greater than 30 Gy increase the relative risk of cardiac death to 3.5. Subcarinal blocking after 30 to 35 Gy reduces the relative risk for cardiac diseases such as congestive heart failure and pancarditis from 5.3 to 1.4, but does not significantly reduce the risk of acute myocardial infarction because the proximal coronary arteries still receive the full dose of radiation. Growth abnormalities are seen in children and adolescents who undergo radiotherapy. The increased risk of second cancers has been well documented. The risk of solid cancers is the main, long-term hazard of radiation therapy. There is an increased incidence of breast cancer in females who are less than 30 years of age at the time of mantle irradiation; the younger the patient and the greater the radiation dose, the higher the relative risk. The cumulative risk of developing a solid cancer (approximately 0.3% to 0.5% per year) such as osteosarcoma or carcinoma of the breast, thyroid, lung, stomach, or colon increases with time, particularly after 10 years. There is also an increased risk of developing non-Hodgkin's lymphoma. After radiotherapy alone, there does not appear to be an increased risk of acute nonlymphocytic leukemia as there is with alkylating-agent chemotherapy.

The Harvard Joint Center for Radiation Therapy reported a retrospective review of 794 patients with pathologic stage IA to IIIB Hodgkin's disease treated between 1969 and 1988. In the study:

- 489 patients were treated with radiotherapy alone.
- 158 patients were treated with radiation therapy and chemotherapy.
- 147 patients were treated with radiotherapy initially, relapsed, and then were treated with chemotherapy.

The 20-year actuarial survival rate was 73%. The absolute excess mortality risk from second malignancy and "not Hodgkin's disease" was higher for the patients treated with combined modality therapy compared to radiotherapy alone. Though the death rate from Hodgkin's disease decreased with time, the risk of death from other causes such as second malignancy and cardiac disease continued to rise. It was projected that the mortality from the second malignancy would surpass that from Hodgkin's disease 15 to 20 years after treatment.

A recent report from the Netherlands Cancer Institute confirmed that the mortality from Hodgkin's disease was negligible after 20 years, but the risk of death from the second malignancy and cardiovascular disease continued to increase.

There have been continuous attempts to reduce the radiation volume and/or dose in order to minimize the risk of radiation without sacrificing the high cure rate. These efforts started in early stage disease whose main treatment was extended-field radiation therapy.

Attempts to Reduce the Volume of Radiation Therapy in the Management of Early Stage Hodgkin's Disease

In an attempt to define a subgroup of patients who could do without the prophylactic para-aortic radiotherapy among the patients with negative laparotomy findings, the EORTC randomized these patients between mantle radiation therapy and mantle plus para-aortic radiation therapy, and found no difference in the RFS or OS. In the next step, the EORTC tried to define a subgroup of patients who could do without the para-aortic and splenic radiation in clinically staged patients, and treated 40 patients with the most favorable prognostic features with mantle radiotherapy alone. The OS was 96% and the RFS 73% at 6 years. However, the majority of the relapses were in the *nodal extension* area, which would have been covered by the para-aortic and splenic fields. This RFS of 73% was felt to be too low, and mantle radiotherapy alone has not been used for any of the EORTC trials subsequently.

The next EORTC trial addressed whether the volume of radiation therapy could be reduced if chemotherapy is used for early stage disease. The patients with favorable prognostic features were randomized between the STNI and six cycles of EBVP (epirubicin [Ellence][1], bleomycin [Blenoxane], vinblastine [Velban], prednisone) followed by involved field (IF) radiotherapy. The RFS at 6 years was 81% for STNI and 92% for EBVP ($p = 0.004$). The OS was 96% for STNI and 98% for EBVP ($p = 0.156$), suggesting a good salvage rate for the patients who relapsed after STNI. This study is one of the first clinical trials to establish combined modality therapy as the standard in the management of early stage Hodgkin's disease.

The EORTC-H9F trial now randomizes patients with very favorable and favorable prognostic features to no radiotherapy, 20 Gy of involved field radiotherapy, or 36 Gy of involved field radiotherapy after six cycles of EBVP.

The ABVD (doxorubicin [Adriamycin], bleomycin, vinblastine, dacarbazine [DIC-Dome]) is the most commonly used chemotherapeutic regimen in the combined modality treatment of Hodgkin's disease. Brusamolino et al has reported a 5-year overall survival of 98% and a relapse-free survival of 97% for 78 patients with stages I and II disease treated with four cycles of ABVD followed by adjuvant limited-field radiation therapy.

The Stanford V (doxorubicin, vinblastine, mechlorethamine [Mustargen], vincristine [Oncovin], bleomycin, etoposide, prednisone with granulocyte colony-stimulating factor) trial is also currently ongoing in combination with involved field radiation therapy for patients with early stage disease.

Attempts to Reduce the Dose of Radiation Therapy

Vijayakumar and Myrianthopoulos have reported, based on a review of the literature, that there is only a 5% likelihood of in-field recurrence after the

[1]Not FDA approved for this indication.

treatment of subclinical disease with radiotherapy alone to 27 Gy. Seydel et al. and Mendenhall et al. have suggested that 20 to 30 Gy is adequate for microscopic disease when patients are treated with radiotherapy alone.

For gross disease, Fletcher and Shukovsky observed a sigmoid dose-response relationship for Hodgkin's disease, which was subsequently corroborated by a number of investigators. Thirty-five Gy resulted in a combined, in-field, and marginal recurrence rate of 5% or less. Vijayakumar and Myrianthopoulos reviewed megavoltage data on 4,117 Hodgkin's disease sites at risk and suggested that, in order to achieve an in-field control rate of 98%, 36.9 Gy and 37.4 Gy are required for disease less than 6 cm and disease greater than 6 cm, respectively. Brincker and Bentzen later reported that the fitting of a dose-response curve to the data compiled by Vijayakumar and Myrianthopoulos results in a plateau in local control at doses greater than 32.5 Gy. In contrast, the Patterns of Care Outcome Study for Hodgkin's disease and the studies by Thar et al., Schewe et al., and Sears et al. failed to demonstrate a benefit to doses greater than 30 Gy. Part of the discrepancy between these studies may be because of the authors' failure to separate marginal from in-field recurrences. In addition, the prescribed dose rather than the minimum dose actually delivered to the tumor was used in the above analyses.

The German Hodgkin's study group (GHSG)-HD4 study randomized pathologic stages I and II A, B patients between 40 Gy of radiotherapy to STNI and 30 Gy to extended field followed by a 10-Gy boost to the involved sites of disease. The 5-year freedom from treatment failure was 82% for the 30 + 10 Gy arm and 70% for 40 Gy arm ($p = 0.026$). The 5-year overall actuarial survival was 97% for 30 + 10 Gy arm and 93% for 40 Gy arm ($p = 0.067$). There was no true in-field failure within the extended field volume in either arm, and it was concluded that 30 Gy is sufficient to control the subclinical disease.

Currently the GHSG uses two or four cycles of ABVD, followed by randomization between 20 and 30 Gy of involved field radiotherapy.

The Role of Radiation Therapy in the Treatment of Intermediate Stage (Unfavorable Stages I and II and Less Advanced Stage III)

The EORTC H8-U study randomized unfavorable groups of patients into three arms:

1. MOPP (mechlorethamine, vincristine, procarbazine [Matulane], and prednisone)/ABV (doxorubicin, bleomycin, vinblastine) six cycles, followed by IF radiotherapy of 36 to 40 Gy
2. MOPP/ABV four cycles, followed by IF radiotherapy of 36-40 Gy
3. MOPP/ABV four cycles, followed by STNI of 36 Gy

The preliminary data showed treatment-failure-free survival rates of 89%, 92%, and 92%, respectively for arms 1, 2, and 3 (no statistical differences). There was no significant difference in overall survival rates either. This suggests that four cycles of MOPP/ABV followed by involved field radiation therapy might be sufficient for this group of patients.

The current EROTC H9-U study also randomizes the unfavorable group of patients into three arms, but with different treatment regimens:

1. ABVD six cycles, followed by IF radiotherapy of 30 Gy
2. ABVD four cycles, followed by IF radiotherapy of 30 Gy
3. BEACOPP (bleomycin, etoposide [VePesid], doxorubicin, cyclophosphamide [Cytoxan], vincristine, procarbazine, and prednisone) four cycles, followed by IF radiotherapy of 30 Gy

Santoro et al. from Milan, Italy, reported on the data of 114 patients who were randomized between ABVD four cycles, followed by IF radiotherapy of 36 Gy and ABVD four cycles, followed by STNI of 30 Gy with a 6-Gy boost to the involved sites. The eligible patients had clinical stage I with a bulky disease, IB, IIA, and IIEA. At 5 years, the complete response rates were 98% for the IF arm compared with 100% with STNI arm. Freedom from progression was 94% for the IF and 95% for STNI, and overall survival was 96% for the IF group and 100% for those treated with STNI. None of these was statistically significant. It was felt that IF radiotherapy was sufficient to treat this group of patients after four cycles of ABVD.

GHSG-HD8 reported on the outcome of the intermediate risk group of patients randomized between two arms:

1. COPP (cyclophosphamide, vincristine, procarbazine, prednisone)/ABVD two cycles, followed by STNI radiotherapy (30 Gy followed by a 10-Gy boost)
2. COPP/ABVD two cycles, followed by IF radiotherapy (30 Gy followed by a 10-Gy boost)

A total of 1,069 patients were randomized. At a median follow-up of 20 months, there was no difference between the arms with RFS of 93% and OS of 98%. The authors concluded that IF radiotherapy is sufficient after the above chemotherapy.

The Role of Radiation Therapy in Advanced Stage (Stages III and IV)

The Southwest Oncology Group (SWOG) did a randomized study between June 1978 and September 1988. Patients with clinical or pathologic stage III or IV disease received six cycles of MOP-BAP (nitrogen mustard, vincristine, prednisone, bleomycin, doxorubicin, procarbazine). The patients who achieved a complete response (CR) were then randomized between two arms:

1. Low-dose involved field radiotherapy (LDIF XRT)
2. No radiotherapy

A total of 530 eligible patients were started with six cycles of MOP-BAP chemotherapy. After treatment:

- 322 of the 530 achieved a CR.
- 135 of 322 were randomized to LDIF.
- 43 of 322 were randomized to no further treatment.
- The remaining 44 were not randomized.

When the analysis was performed with the 278 randomized patients by the intent to treat, the 5-year remission duration estimates were 79% and 68% (p = 0.09) for the LDIF and no treatment arms respectively. However, when the analysis was done with 234 patients who actually received the randomized treatment, the 5-year remission duration rates were 85% and 67% (p = 0.002) for the LDIF and no treatment arms respectively. When the analysis was limited to 169 patients with nodular sclerosis (NS) histology, the 5-year remission duration was 82% versus 60% (p = 0.002) in favor of LDIF. When the analysis was limited to 74 patients with NS histology and bulky disease, the 5-year remission durations were 76% versus 46% (p = 0.006) in favor of LDIF. When the analysis was done for 95 patients with NS histology and nonbulky disease, the 5-year remission duration was 88% versus 68% (p = 0.06) in favor of LDIF. This protocol had difficulty with accrual at the initial phase of the trial, necessitating changes in the design of the trial. However, this trial is of interest because of the significance demonstrated for the benefit of LDIF radiotherapy in subset analysis.

The GHSG-HD3 study asked similar questions with clinical or pathologic stage IIIB or IV disease. Patients were treated with three cycles of COPP/ABVD chemotherapy. Those who achieved a CR were randomized between one of two arms:

1. IF radiotherapy of 20 Gy to initially involved areas
2. COPP/ABVD for one more cycle

Of the 288 patients who were accrued between 1984 and 1988, 171 patients achieved a CR after three cycles of COPP/ABVD. Only 100 out of 171 complete responders were randomized; 51 to the radiotherapy arm and 49 to the additional chemotherapy arm. There was no statistically significant difference in terms of freedom from treatment failure and overall survival between the two arms. Of interest, 21 patients refused any further treatment after achieving a CR to 3 cycles of COPP/ABVD. Their relative risk of failure was 3.67 compared to the patients who received consolidation treatment. Though the number of patients in the study is small, it underscores the importance of consolidation treatment, either radiotherapy or more chemotherapy in this particular group of patients receiving COPP/ABVD chemotherapy. Whether more than six cycles of chemotherapy will eliminate the need for consolidation therapy remains to be seen.

The Groupe d'études des Lymphomes de l'Adulte H89 trial has recently presented its results for stage IIIB-IV Hodgkin's lymphoma. The 418 patients who achieved a complete or partial response to six cycles of ABVPP (doxorubicin, bleomycin, vinblastine, procarbazine, prednisone) or MOPP/ABV were randomized to undergo either two additional cycles of chemotherapy or extended-field radiotherapy of 30 to 40 Gy. The radiation fields were subtotal nodal (mantle, para-aortic, and spleen). However, the inverted Y with spleen fields were used if there was an iliac or inguinal involvement. Though there was a small advantage in disease-free survival (DFS) with the radiotherapy consolidation group (p = 0.07), there was no significant difference in OS. The radiation fields were substantially larger than the involved fields in this study, and this might have led to increased toxicity possibly negating the potential benefit achieved from improved DFS with radiation therapy.

The data from the randomized EORTC trial #20884 were recently reported. Three hundred thirty-three patients with stage III or IV disease who achieved a CR to MOPP/ABV chemotherapy were randomized between no further therapy and involved field radiation therapy. There was no significant difference in event-free survival or OS at 5 years between the two groups of patients.

The Stanford V trial has been recently updated. The eligible patients were between 15 and 60 years of age, with bulky mediastinal disease and/or stage III or IV disease. Patients were given 12 weeks of chemotherapy followed by involved-field radiotherapy of 36 Gy to the pretreatment nodal sites of 5 cm or more and macroscopic splenic disease. A total of 142 patients were accrued. The 5-year survival was 96% and freedom from progression was 89%. An ongoing intergroup trial (E2496) has been initiated based on this outcome to compare Stanford V with ABVD chemotherapy.

Of interest is a preliminary report from four Italian Cooperative Groups that compares ABVD versus Stanford V versus MEC (MOPP/EBV/CAD) (lomustine [CeeNU], doxorubicin [Adriamycin], vindesine) for patients with advanced-stage Hodgkin's disease. IF radiotherapy was delivered to areas with (prechemotherapy) bulky disease or to masses slowly or partially responding to chemotherapy. The overall 3-year survival rates were 94.7%, 95.5%, and 89.9% for ABVD, MEC, and Stanford V, respectively (p = 0.217). The corresponding 3-year failure-free survival rates were 81.4%, 86.6%, and 53.4%. The failure-free survival for the Stanford V regimen was significantly lower (p = 0.0001).

The Role of Radiation Therapy After Partial Response to Chemotherapy in Advanced Hodgkin's Disease

In the EORTC trial #20884 mentioned above, the patients who achieved a partial response (PR) were to receive IF radiotherapy of 30 Gy (with a boost of 4 to 10 Gy as needed) in 1.5 to 2 Gy fraction. Of the 250 partial responders, 227 actually received IF radiotherapy. The 5-year event-free and OS rates for these 250 partial responders were 79% and 87%, respectively. These were not different from the outcomes for the patients who achieved a CR to the induction chemotherapy. This result strongly supports the role of radiotherapy for partial responders to induction chemotherapy, making their prognosis as good as those who achieved an initial CR to induction chemotherapy.

In summary, the mainstay in the management of Hodgkin's disease is chemotherapy. The role of radiation therapy continues to evolve. The extent of the benefit of radiation therapy also depends on the effectiveness of the chemotherapy itself. Radiation therapy is recommended after a PR to chemotherapy in general. The benefit/risk of radiation therapy is probably more pronounced as the number of sites of involvement is smaller and volume of the disease is larger. IF radiation therapy usually implies treating the prechemotherapy tumor volumes with margins. The exact extent of the fields depends on the location of the initial disease, the extent of the residual disease after chemotherapy, if any, and the adjacent organs such as kidneys, heart, and salivary glands. It always needs to be kept in mind to balance the advantages of radiation therapy against added morbidity in doing so.

ACUTE LEUKEMIA IN ADULTS

METHOD OF

Richard A. Larson, MD

After two decades of incremental improvements in therapy, acute myeloid leukemia (AML) and acute lymphoblastic leukemia (ALL) are now curable in approximately 50% of adults with good risk features. An improved understanding of prognostic factors has allowed better risk stratification, and more appropriate management strategies have led to better outcomes for patients with acute leukemia. Recent trials have tested the concepts of dose intensification and the use of multiple non–cross-resistant agents. New drug development has had relatively little clinical impact, except for the introduction of all-trans retinoic acid (ATRA) (tretinoin [Vesanoid]) and arsenic trioxide (Trisenox) for acute promyelocytic leukemia (APL). The appropriate role of hematopoietic stem cell transplantation (SCT) remains to be defined, but progress has been made in elucidating the graft versus leukemia effect of donor lymphocytes. Improved antifungal and antiviral therapies have contributed to better supportive care. The ancillary role of hematopoietic growth factors in antileukemia treatment strategies and in supportive care remains investigational.

Management of acute leukemia remains complex, requiring a multidisciplinary and dedicated team approach for optimal results. Therapy remains hazardous, unpleasant, and costly. Most adult patients with acute leukemia still die from the disease. Progress in understanding the molecular biology of leukemia has not yet translated into improved management and survival. Little progress has been made in improving the survival of poor prognosis groups, especially the elderly, those who develop leukemia after a myelodysplastic syndrome (MDS) or prior cytotoxic exposure (therapy-related leukemia [t-AML]), and those with unfavorable or complex cytogenetic features. Nevertheless, considerable progress has been made. Initial response rates are high. Most patients achieve a remission and recover normal hematopoiesis, at least transiently. The current challenge has shifted to postremission therapy and the ultimate eradication of the disease in order to prevent relapse.

Diagnosis, Classification, and Prognostic Factors

Acute leukemia is a malignant neoplasm of hematopoietic tissue characterized by the clonal accumulation of immature blood cells in the bone marrow. These abnormal cells are generally arrested in the blast stage of the normal maturation pathway. Aberrations in differentiation and function of blood cells are common. Normal hematopoiesis is suppressed.

Acute leukemia usually presents with the clinical features of bone marrow failure. Patients may have infection, anemia, or bleeding. Rare presentations include granulocytic or myeloid sarcoma, and skin or central nervous system (CNS) manifestations. The blood usually shows a leukocytosis with normocytic anemia and thrombocytopenia. Circulating blast cells are often present. Sometimes, however, the leukocyte count may be low. This is a common feature in APL, for example. In rare cases, patients may present with thrombocytosis.

The most precise diagnosis is made by examining the morphology, cytochemistry, immunophenotype, and chromosomal abnormalities of bone marrow and peripheral blood cells. Bone marrow aspiration and biopsy are the standard diagnostic procedures. Aspiration may be difficult or impossible (i.e., a *dry tap*) in patients with very high marrow cellularity (i.e., a *packed marrow*). The World Health Organization (WHO) Classification separates subgroups of AML by recurring cytogenetic features and morphologic characteristics that reflect cell lineage and differentiation

TABLE 1 The World Health Organization Classification of Acute Leukemia

Acute Myeloid Leukemia (AML) with Recurrent Genetic Abnormalities
AML with t(8;21); (AML1/ETO)
AML with abnormal bone marrow eosinophils, inv(16)(p13q22) or t(16;16)(p13q22); (CBFβ/MYH11); FAB M4Eo
Acute promyelocytic leukemia with t(15;17) (q22;q12); (PML/RARα) and variants; FAB M3
AML with 11q23 (MLL) abnormalities
AML with Multilineage Dysplasia
Following a myelodysplastic syndrome (MDS) or myelodysplastic/myeloproliferative disorder
Without antecedent myelodysplastic syndrome
AML and MDS, therapy-related
Alkylating agent-related
Topoisomerase type II, inhibitor-related (some may be lymphoid)
Other types
AML Not Otherwise Categorized
AML minimally differentiated; FAB M0
AML without maturation; FAB M1
AML with maturation; FAB M2
Acute myelomonocytic leukemia (AMMoL); FAB M4
Acute monoblastic and monocytic leukemia (AMoL); FAB M5
Acute erythroid leukemia (AEL); FAB M6
Acute megakaryoblastic leukemia (AMegL); FAB M7
Acute basophilic leukemia
Acute panmyelosis with myelofibrosis
Myeloid sarcoma
Acute Leukemia of Ambiguous Lineage
Undifferentiated acute leukemia
Bilineal acute leukemia
Biphenotypic acute leukemia
Acute Lymphoblastic Leukemia (ALL)/Lymphoblastic Lymphoma
Precursor B-cell ALL
Precursor T-cell ALL

Abbreviation: FAB = French-American-British classification.

(Table 1). Flow cytometric analysis of cell surface markers is widely available and can accurately distinguish myeloid from lymphoid (and B-cell lineage from T-cell lineage) in most cases (Table 2). Clear distinction between AML and ALL is not always possible. Rarely, null, biphenotypic, or bilineal acute leukemias occur.

Cytogenetic analysis of an individual patient's leukemia cells has become an increasingly important component of diagnosis prior to treatment in both AML and ALL. An adequate (more than 2 mL) sample of bone marrow aspirate from a fresh puncture site should be submitted for cytogenetic analysis in all patients suspected of having leukemia. Specific and well-characterized, recurring chromosomal abnormalities facilitate diagnosis, confirm subtype classification, and have major prognostic value for treatment planning (Table 3). This is a work in progress that will expand as additional mutations are discovered, such as the internal tandem duplication of the FLT3 gene or overexpression of the BAALC gene (brain and acute leukemia, cytoplasmic), both of

TABLE 2 Commonly Used Markers for Flow Immunophenotyping in Acute Leukemia

General: CD34, HLA-DR, TdT, CD45
B-cell markers: CD10, CD19, cCD22, CD20, CD79A, CD24
T-cell markers: CD1a, CD2, cCD3, CD4, CD8, CD5, CD7
Myeloid: MPO, CD117, CD13, CD33, CD11c, CD14, CD15
B-lineage ALL phenotypes:
Pro-B: TdT+, CD19/22/79A+, CD10–, cμ–, SIg–
Common precursor-B: TdT+, CD19/22/79A+, CD10+, cμ–, SIg–
Pre-B: TdT+, CD19/22/79A+, CD10+, cμ+, SIg–
Burkitt: TdT–, CD19/22/79A+, CD10+, SIg+
T-lineage ALL phenotypes:
Pro/immature thymocyte: TdT+, cCD3+, CD2/5/7+/–
Common thymocyte: TdT+, cCD3+, CD2/5/7+, CD4+/CD8+, CD1a+
Mature thymocyte: TdT+/–, CD3+, CD2/5/7+, CD4+ or CD8+, CD1a–

Abbreviations: ALL = acute lymphoblastic leukemia; HLA = human leukocyte antigen; HLA-DR = class II gene product; MPO = myeloperoxidase (bone marrow stain); TdT = terminal deoxynucleotidyl transferase.

which are associated with short survival. A current hypothesis for which there is considerable support states that leukemia results from the coincidence of two genetic alterations—one that augments proliferation in progenitor cells or decreases their apoptosis, and a second that blocks cellular differentiation or maturation.

Age is the most important independent patient variable in determining outcome. Treatment results are best in young adults and are considerably poorer in patients older than 60 years. In addition, young or middle-aged adults may benefit from the availability of SCT to rescue patients after suffering a relapse. Older patients have a lower response rate to remission induction chemotherapy and increased treatment toxicity, in part due to their high incidence of co-morbid disorders. The poor survival of older patients, however, is not fully explained by their lower tolerance for intensive treatment. The disease itself appears to have a different natural history in this group. Older patients with AML are more likely to have had a myelodysplastic syndrome (MDS), and are also more likely to have unfavorable cytogenetic features.

Antecedent hematologic disorders such as MDS are a major adverse prognostic factor. Acute leukemia that occurs following treatment with alkylating agents or topoisomerase II inhibitors or radiotherapy for a prior cancer (therapy-related AML [t-AML]) has been well described and has a similarly poor outcome with conventional chemotherapy programs.

General Principles of Therapy

The goal of remission induction chemotherapy is the rapid restoration of normal bone marrow function. The term complete remission (CR) is reserved for patients who have full recovery of normal peripheral blood counts and bone marrow cellularity with less

TABLE 3 Cytogenetic Subsets in Acute Myeloid Leukemia (AML) and Acute Lymphoblastic Leukemia (ALL)

Karyotype	Complete Remission Rate	Remission Duration	Treatment Approach
t(8;21)	High	Long	Standard induction with an anthracycline. Intensive consolidation chemotherapy with high-dose cytarabine (Cytosar-U)[1].
inv(16)(p13q22) or t(16;16)	High	Intermediate to long	Standard induction with an anthracycline. Intensive consolidation chemotherapy with high-dose cytarabine.
t(15;17)	High	Intermediate to long	All-trans retinoic acid (ATRA) (Vesanoid) together with chemotherapy. Arsenic trioxide (Trisenox) at relapse.
t(9;11)	High	Intermediate	Standard induction with an anthracycline. Intensive consolidation chemotherapy with high-dose cytarabine.
del(5q), +13, +8, −7, inv(3), del(12p), t(9;22), or complex abnormalities	Low	Short	New induction regimens, including use of growth factors during chemotherapy or modulators of drug resistance. Allogeneic SCT in first CR.
t(9;22), t(4;11), +8, −7	High	Short	Standard ALL remission induction followed by allogeneic SCT in first CR.
t(8;14) or t(2;8) or t(8;22)	High	Intermediate to long	Short duration, high-intensity chemotherapy with CNS prophylaxis.

[1]Not FDA approved for this indication.
Abbreviations: CNS = central nervous system; CR = complete remission; SCT = stem cell transplantation.

than 5% residual blast cells. Induction therapy aims to reduce the total body leukemia cell population from approximately 10^{12} to below the cytologically detectable level of about 10^{9} cells. This is followed by postinduction or remission consolidation therapy, usually comprising one or more courses of chemotherapy designed at eradication of residual leukemia, allowing the possibility of cure. Multiple chemotherapy drugs in high doses are typically used to prevent the emergence of resistant subclones, and to limit cumulative and overlapping toxicities. The prolonged adjunctive use of lower doses of chemotherapy for remission maintenance lasting 1 to 2 years is commonly used in ALL but has minimal value in AML.

SCT using a human leukocyte antigen (HLA)-identical sibling donor is an established treatment modality in acute leukemia and is indicated for suitable high-risk patients in first remission or for any young or middle-aged patient in first relapse or second remission. Allogeneic SCT (allo-SCT) has two therapeutic components. Intensive myeloablative therapy is used to eradicate all tumor cells, if possible. In addition, T-cells developing from the donor stem cells can produce a graft-versus-leukemia (GVL) immune response that can destroy remaining leukemia cells; this effect has been correlated with improved disease-free survival. Unfortunately, this beneficial immune response is closely associated with acute and chronic graft-versus-host disease (GVHD), a major cause of morbidity and mortality following allo-SCT. GVHD can be reduced by T-cell depletion from the donor marrow, but only at the cost of increased rates of graft failure and leukemia relapse. Because the risk of treatment-related mortality increases with age, many centers restrict allo-SCT to patients less than 60 years old. Recently, however, less intensive, nonmyeloablative preparative regimens have been developed specifically to enable older patients to undergo allo-SCT. The goal here is to engraft the patient with a new immune system and allow the GVL reaction to eradicate residual leukemia. The use of allo-SCT has also been limited in part by donor availability. A patient has only a 25% to 30% chance that a sibling will be HLA identical. Often an HLA-matched but unrelated donor can be found through the National Marrow Donor Registry.

Autologous SCT allows the use of myeloablative therapy in patients who lack an allogeneic marrow donor as well as in older patients. The appropriate role for this treatment modality is controversial. Treatment-related morbidity and mortality are relatively low (<5%), but relapse rates are high, and overall outcomes are not clearly better than in patients who receive intensive but nonablative chemotherapy. The relative contribution to relapse of tumor cell contamination in the reinfused cryopreserved stem cells versus the failure of the high-dose therapy to eradicate all disease in vivo has not been determined. Hematopoietic cells capable of reconstituting bone marrow function can be harvested for autologous transplantation by direct bone marrow aspiration or by apheresis of progenitor cells from peripheral blood. The use of peripheral blood stem cells has not been proven to decrease the risk of relapse compared to bone marrow cells, but it does accelerate the rate of hematopoietic reconstitution.

Remission Induction Therapy for AML

The most common remission induction regimen used for patients with AML is cytarabine (Cytosar-U), given by continuous intravenous (IV) infusion daily for 7 days, plus daunorubicin (Cerubidine)[1], given daily for 3 days (7+3 regimen). Depending on age and patient selection, 60% to 80% of patients achieve a CR. The outcome in general has not been improved by the substitution of other anthracyclines, increasing the dose of cytarabine, or adding a third or fourth drug (Table 4). Current studies are investigating higher doses of anthracyclines and inhibitors of multidrug resistance mechanisms.

Cytarabine in conventional doses of 100 to 200 mg/m^2 per day is generally given by continuous IV infusion for 7 to 10 days. High-dose cytarabine (HiDAC) regimens typically use 1000 to 3000 mg/m^2, given IV over 1 to 3 hours every 12 hours for 8 to 12 doses. HiDAC increases the complete remission (CR) rate to 75% to 90% but at the cost of increased toxicity. Treatment mortality, the rate of early relapse, and overall survival are not clearly improved. In a recent trial, a standard 7+3 regimen was followed immediately by 3 days of high-dose cytarabine. The CR rate was 89% among patients less than 65 years old with no prior myelodysplasia.

Attempts have been made to improve the CR rate of induction therapy by adding potentially non–cross-resistant drugs. Etoposide (VePesid)[1] has activity as a single agent in approximately 25% of patients with previously treated AML. In a randomized trial among newly diagnosed patients, the addition of etoposide at 75 mg/m^2 per day for 7 days to cytarabine and daunorubicin (7+3 regimen) produced increased toxicity but also prolonged remission duration in the etoposide arm. There was no survival benefit. A randomized comparison between cytarabine at standard doses versus high doses, both in combination with daunorubicin and etoposide, showed no improvement in the CR rate or overall survival in the HiDAC arm, although disease-free survival was significantly prolonged.

Gemtuzumab ozogamicin (Mylotarg) is an immunoconjugate that links a monoclonal antibody that binds to CD33, a membrane antigen present on the majority of AML blast cells, with the cytotoxic agent calicheamicin. Approved for use as a single agent in relapsed AML, it is now being studied in combination with 7+3 regimen for newly diagnosed patients. Clinical trials are also testing agents that inhibit antiapoptotic pathways and drug efflux mechanisms that are active in some AML cells.

Acute Promyelocytic Leukemia

Acute promyelocytic leukemia (APL) (French-American-British [FAB] classification M3) is a biologically distinct disease with characteristic

[1]Not FDA approved for this indication.

TABLE 4 Acute Myeloid Leukemia (AML) Remission Induction Chemotherapy Regimens

Drugs	Doses	Comment
Cytarabine (Cytosar-U) Daunorubicin (Cerubidine)	100 mg/m^2 daily as a continuous infusion for 7d 45-60 mg/m^2 IV push on each of the first 3d of treatment	*Standard* induction regimen resulting in approximately 60%-80% remission rate and acceptable toxicity in patients <60 years old.
Cytarabine Daunorubicin	3 g/m^2 twice daily for a total of 12 doses 45 mg/m^2 IV push for 3d following cytarabine	Yields a 90% remission rate, but substantial toxicity precludes postremission therapy in a high proportion of patients.
Cytarabine Idarubicin (Idamycin)	100 mg/m^2 daily as a continuous infusion for 7d 13 mg/m^2 intravenous push on each of first 3d of treatment	Has produced a greater CR rate (88% vs. 70%) compared to cytarabine/daunorubicin in younger patients. Appears superior to daunorubicin in patients with hyperleukocytosis. Overall survival not clearly superior to standard regimen.
Cytarabine Daunorubicin Etoposide (VePesid)[1]	100 mg/m^2 daily as a continuous infusion for 7d 50-60 mg/m^2 intravenous push on each of first 3d of treatment 75 mg/m^2 daily for 7d, or 100 mg/m^2 daily for first 3d	Remission rates similar to standard induction regimen. Remission duration significantly improved but overall survival comparable to standard regimen. May prolong survival in patients <55 years old but at expense of increased toxicity.
Cytarabine Daunorubicin Cytarabine (high-dose)	100 mg/m^2 daily as a continuous infusion for 7d 45 mg/m^2 IV push on each of the first 3d of treatment 2 g/m^2 twice daily on days 8, 9, and 10	High rate of CR after first course in patients <65 years old.

[1]Not FDA approved for this indication.
Abbreviation: CR = complete remission.

clinical, morphological, and cytogenetic features. The cytoplasmic granules in the leukemic blasts contain factors with procoagulant as well as fibrinolytic activity. Disseminated intravascular coagulation at presentation or soon after the initiation of cytotoxic chemotherapy can cause severe hemorrhage in up to 40% of patients and a high mortality rate.

ATRA (tretinoin [Vesanoid]) has proved to be a highly effective remission induction agent, especially when used in combination with anthracyclines such as daunorubicin[1] or idarubicin (Idamycin). ATRA accelerates the terminal differentiation of malignant promyelocytes to mature neutrophils, leading to apoptosis and CR without bone marrow hypoplasia. This effect is a unique consequence of the rearranged PML/RARα gene resulting from the t(15;17), which defines APL. Induction therapy with ATRA and an anthracycline produces CR rates of 80% to 95% in both previously untreated and relapsed patients. Most treatment failure is a result of early mortality. Primary resistance is rare. ATRA is neither immunosuppressive nor myelosuppressive. The coagulopathy of APL typically improves rapidly after initiation of ATRA treatment. The median times to CR range from 38 to 44 days but may take as long as 90 days. As yet, the drug is only available as an oral preparation. The recommended daily dose is 45 mg/m^2.

One serious and specific complication may occur with ATRA treatment of APL. In 25% to 40% of patients, a cytokine release syndrome develops within 2 to 21 days after initiation of treatment. It is characterized by fever, peripheral edema, pulmonary infiltrates and respiratory distress, hypertension, renal and hepatic dysfunction, and serositis resulting in pleural and pericardial effusions. The syndrome is possibly caused by tissue infiltration by maturing malignant promyelocytes, plus the systemic effects of cytokines released from the malignant cells. Many cases are associated with hyperleukocytosis, but the *retinoic acid syndrome* occurs with normal leukocyte counts in 33% of cases. Early recognition and aggressive management with high-dose dexamethasone therapy (10 mg IV every 12 hours for six doses)[3] has been effective. Cessation of ATRA therapy alone does not reverse the syndrome. However, once the complication resolves, ATRA can be restarted in most cases.

Management of the coagulopathy associated with APL may be difficult and should be managed expectantly. Coagulation parameters, including fibrinogen, D-dimer, and platelet levels, should be monitored closely. Platelet transfusions, along with cryoprecipitate or fresh-frozen plasma, are used to maintain the fibrinogen level to more than 100 mg/dL and the platelet count to more than 20,000/μL. The role of heparin has been controversial. Although continuous infusions of 5 to 10 U/kg per hour were widely used in the past and appear effective at stopping the consumption of clotting factors, heparin is rarely indicated today. Inhibitors of fibrinolysis should be considered only for life-threatening hemorrhage because of the risk of thromboses in major vessels.

[1]Not FDA approved for this indication.

[3]Exceeds dosage recommended by the manufacturer.

Postremission Therapy of AML

Additional chemotherapy after a successful remission induction is mandatory to cure AML. The median disease-free survival for patients who receive no additional therapy is only 4 to 8 months. When several courses of consolidation chemotherapy are given, 35% to 50% of young and middle-aged adults remain alive after 2 to 3 years, and the relapse rate is low thereafter.

The same chemotherapy used successfully for remission induction may be repeated for one or more cycles (with or without dose intensification) for consolidation, or non–cross-resistant drugs can be used. There is increasing evidence that high-dose cytarabine (HiDAC) provides the best survival odds for good and intermediate prognosis patients. HiDAC may be effective in eliminating resistant cell populations that survive induction therapy. The Cancer and Leukemia Group B (CALGB) conducted a randomized trial of consolidation therapy using four courses of cytarabine at low (100 mg/m^2/day) or intermediate (400 mg/m^2/day) doses by continuous IV infusions for 5 days, or at high doses (3 g/m^2 IV over 3 hours every 12 hours on days 1, 3, and 5). For patients less than 60 years old with a good or intermediate prognosis, disease-free survival in the HiDAC arm was 46% at 3 years, compared to 35% for the intermediate dose and 31% for the low-dose group ($p = 0.003$). There were relatively few relapses in the HiDAC group more than 2 years after attaining CR. The best consolidation therapy for patients over 60 years old is uncertain; two cycles of daunorubicin (30 to 45 mg/m^2 for 2 days) and cytarabine (100 mg/m^2/day for 5 days) are frequently used. Alternating courses of other two-drug combinations (e.g., etoposide and cyclophosphamide, mitoxantrone [Novantrone] and etoposide, mitoxantrone and cytarabine, or mitoxantrone and diaziquone[1,*]) may provide equivalent disease-free survival.

Most studies reporting on allogeneic or autologous SCT for AML patients in first CR are nonrandomized, and many are retrospective. Considerable selection bias is generated by the delay between remission induction and transplantation, and by the entry requirements in most trials for good performance status. Prospective randomized studies comparing intensive consolidation therapy and SCT for patients in first CR have failed to show a clear survival advantage. In general, allogeneic SCT should be reserved for high-risk AML patients with unfavorable cytogenetic abnormalities or very high initial white blood

[1]Not FDA approved for this indication.

*Investigational drug in the United States.

cell (WBC) counts. However, patients who relapse with AML after intensive chemotherapy treatment should also be candidates for allogeneic SCT.

Treatment for Acute Lymphoblastic Leukemia

Treatment regimens for ALL have evolved empirically into complex schemes that use numerous agents in various doses, combinations, and schedules. Few of the individual components have been tested rigorously in randomized trials. Thus, it is difficult to analyze critically the absolute contribution of each drug or dose schedule to the ultimate outcome. Steady improvements in the cure rate for adults have been achieved through more accurate diagnoses, the use of intensive multiagent chemotherapy, attention to potential sanctuary sites such as the CNS, and the appropriate use of allogeneic SCT. Further progress will require large numbers of uniformly evaluated patients to be entered onto randomized clinical trials, testing various components of the total therapy that have heretofore been added empirically.

In two sequential trials by the CALGB involving 379 adults, a five-drug induction regimen produced a CR rate of 85% and median duration of remission of 28 months. Cyclophosphamide (Cytoxan; 1200 mg/m^2) was given on day 1 with daunorubicin (45 mg/m^2) on days 1, 2, and 3. Vincristine (Oncovin; 2 mg) was given on days 1, 8, 15, and 22 together with 21 days of prednisone (60 mg/m^2). L-asparaginase (Elspar; 6000 units/m^2) was given subcutaneously twice per week starting on day 5. The median duration of remission was 34 months for the 237 patients who rapidly achieved CR within 30 days, compared with 20 months for the 88 patients who required more than 30 days to enter remission. More recent trials have studied higher daunorubicin doses and the substitution of pegylated asparaginase (Oncaspar) and dexamethasone (Decadron). The hyperfractionated cyclophosphamide, doxorubicin, vincristine, Decadron (hyper-CVAD) regimen alternates courses of remission induction chemotherapy with courses combining HiDAC with high-dose methotrexate.

Consolidation and Maintenance

Eradication of subclinical, or *minimal*, residual disease during hematologic remission is the primary aim of the remission consolidation or intensification phases. Once normal hematopoiesis has been restored, patients are good candidates for aggressive attempts for cure. However, it remains controversial as to how intensive this phase of treatment should be, and whether in fact, relative drug resistance can be overcome by myelosuppressive combinations including SCT. Several nonrandomized studies strongly suggest a benefit from intensive multiagent postremission therapy.

Remission maintenance therapy is still a standard component of the management of ALL, although its benefit has not been fully established in adults. Standard outpatient maintenance therapy typically uses oral 6-mercaptopurine (Purinethol; 60 mg/m^2/day) and methotrexate (Mexate; 20 mg/m^2/week) with monthly pulses of vincristine and prednisone for 1 to 3 years. The optimal duration for maintenance treatment is unknown, but typically treatment lasts for 24 to 30 months in total.

CNS Prophylaxis

CNS prophylaxis is an integral step in ALL treatment. The CNS is a common sanctuary for ALL cells as indicated by the frequent involvement of spinal fluid or cranial nerves at the time of relapse. CNS leukemia is more easily prevented than treated. Fewer than 10% of adults with ALL have CNS leukemia at diagnosis. Examination of spinal fluid at diagnosis is not necessary in asymptomatic patients. However, without specific attention to CNS prophylaxis, CNS relapse rates range from 21% to 50%. Cranial neuropathies are common sequelae. Symptoms resulting from increased intracranial pressure include headaches, nausea, vomiting, lethargy, and papilledema, as well as irritability and nuchal rigidity.

Several methods are currently used for prevention of meningeal leukemia. These include, intrathecal (IT) injection of methotrexate or cytarabine, or both, together with hydrocortisone, or intravenous administration of the same chemotherapy agents in high doses with the goal of achieving therapeutic levels in the cerebrospinal fluid (CSF), or cranial irradiation (2400 cGy). Irradiation of the entire spinal cord is quite myelosuppressive and is rarely done.

Use of Hematopoietic Growth Factors

Myelosuppression and the infections that result are common and sometimes fatal complications of intensive chemotherapy. Prolonged myelosuppression can also necessitate long hospital stays and lead to unacceptable delays between scheduled courses of treatment. Such delays diminish dose intensity. With the use of hematopoietic growth factors, neutrophil recovery has been accelerated following chemotherapy for solid tumors as well as after myeloablative therapy and SCT. Several clinical trials now suggest that hematopoietic growth factors may provide important ancillary benefits for adults undergoing treatment for ALL. The major benefit is in older patients.

As yet, growth factors have not had a marked impact on survival or remission duration for patients with AML. Data from several large controlled trials have recently been reported, but the issue remains unsettled. Differences in dose and schedule, and the specific growth factor and chemotherapy agents used, as well as the age group studied prevent firm conclusions. Even though a more rapid recovery of neutrophils has been observed in some trials, the chemotherapy-induced nadir has not been affected, and thus, the incidence of severe infection remains high. At the same time, stimulation of leukemia regrowth by myeloid growth factors appears to be uncommon in vivo. A recent clinical trial suggested that granulocyte colony-stimulating factor (G-CSF) (filgrastim) was beneficial when used following courses of consolidation chemotherapy for AML.

ACUTE LEUKEMIA IN CHILDHOOD

METHOD OF

Raymond J. Hutchinson, MS, MD

The acute leukemias comprise approximately 30% to 35% of all malignant diseases diagnosed in children younger than 15 years of age. Approximately 2400 new cases of acute lymphoblastic leukemia (ALL) are diagnosed annually in the United States among children and adolescents younger than 20 years of age. An additional 800 to 900 cases of acute myelogenous leukemia (AML) are diagnosed annually in U.S. children and adolescents. Of the acute leukemias of childhood, ALL accounts for 75% to 80% of the total and AML for 20% to 25% of the total. Both disease processes continue to be the subject of intense biologic and epidemiologic study and the focus of comprehensive clinical investigation searching for optimal therapy.

The cellular proliferation characteristic of acute leukemias often occurs in association with key molecular events resulting from chromosomal translocations, inversions, and/or additions/deletions with corresponding genetic mutations. Mutations may be germinal arising in utero or acquired occurring in individual somatic cells; individual mutations may be both necessary and sufficient to promote leukemic proliferation or they may be necessary but not sufficient, implying that at least one more genetic event must occur to promote expansion of a preleukemic clone. Certain chromosomal translocations are consistently associated with specific subtypes of acute leukemia and have significant impact upon prognosis and hence upon choice of treatment; for example:

- In ALL, t(9;22), t(4;11), t(12;21), and t(1;19)
- In AML, chromosomal additions, deletions, rearrangements, and translocations such as trisomy 8, monosomies 5 and 7, inversion 16, and translocations t(8;21) and t(15;17)

With further refinements in molecular techniques, the genetic events contributing to or actually responsible for leukemic cell proliferation will be more fully defined. The future holds promise that novel understanding of these events will lead to new treatment approaches that will be much more specific for the leukemia cells than has conventional chemotherapy.

Diagnosis (Table 1)

Patients with acute leukemia are generally well until they or their parents notice the onset of acute symptomatology, including otherwise unexplained fever, bruising, bone pain, and/or lethargy. With persistence of any of these symptoms, medical care is sought. Often the physician notes physical findings, including fever, signs of cutaneous bleeding (petechiae, ecchymoses), splenomegaly, and lymphadenopathy. The astute physician will obtain a complete blood count with a white blood cell (WBC) differential count and a chest radiograph. If two or more blood cell cytopenias are observed (e.g., anemia with leukopenia, leukopenia with thrombocytopenia, etc.), a bone marrow aspirate and biopsy are called for. The bone marrow aspirate typically reveals displacement of normal hematopoietic precursors by leukemic blast cells, which generally have a high nuclear/cytoplasmic ratio, often exhibit nucleoli, and sometimes demonstrate vacuoles in the cytoplasm and occasionally in the nucleus. This test is the definitive test needed to establish the diagnosis of acute leukemia, even in the presence of what appear to be circulating leukemic blasts. When the diagnosis of acute leukemia is apparent, necessary additional studies include examination of the cerebrospinal fluid (CSF) for leukemic blasts; a chest radiograph looking for a mediastinal mass; serum chemistries including blood urea nitrogen (BUN), creatinine, electrolytes, calcium, and phosphorus to assess for tumor lysis syndrome; and coagulation studies (prothrombin time [PT], partial thromboplastin time [PTT]) to rule out a leukemia-associated coagulopathy.

TABLE 1 Diagnostic Approach to Acute Leukemia

History (including a family history of blood disorders) and physical examination
Complete blood count with a manual white blood cell differential count and review of the peripheral smear
Chest radiograph (PA and lateral views)
Serum electrolytes, BUN, creatinine, uric acid, calcium, phosphorus, LDH, ALT, bilirubin
Coagulation studies—prothrombin time, partial thromboplastin time
Varicella titer (immunoglobulin G)
Bone marrow aspirate and biopsy for morphology, cytochemistry, blast cell immunophenotype, blast cell cytogenetics
Lumbar puncture with CSF cell count, morphology on a spun preparation, protein, and glucose

Abbreviations: ALT = alanine aminotransferase; BUN = blood urea nitrogen; CSF = cerebrospinal fluid; LDH = lactate dehydrogenase; PA = posteroanterior.

Classification

The acute leukemias of childhood are initially separated into two broad categories, ALL and AML. Historically, this classification was done by light microscopic histologic review, employing special stains such as periodic acid-Schiff (PAS), myeloperoxidase, and the esterase stains. This classification had significant ramifications as treatment varies widely for these two primary categories of acute leukemia; in addition, treatment outcomes were significantly better for children with ALL than was true for those with AML. In the 1980s, immunophenotyping of leukemic blasts became a mainstay of classification, using monoclonal antibodies, which marked cells expressing their cognate antigen. The antigens were given cluster designation (CD) nomenclature to allow for consistency in analysis and in reporting results (Table 2). Thus, certain CD antigens were characteristic of ALL and others were characteristic of AML:

- ALL—CD2, CD5, and CD7 for ALL of T-cell origin and CD10, CD19, CD20, and CD22 for ALL of pre–B-cell and B-cell origin
- AML—CD11, CD13, and CD33

Establishing the immune phenotype of acute leukemias added greatly to more definitive classification, especially when separating ALL from AML and T-cell ALL from pre–B-cell ALL. Immunophenotypic characterization of acute leukemias enhanced the classification established by the French-American-British (FAB) systems for classifying ALL and AML. The combined approach of using blast cell morphology and blast cell immunophenotype has facilitated the delivery of specific treatment to children with each of the major subtypes of acute leukemia; it has also augmented the application of risk-directed therapies to patients with subclasses of ALL and AML, particularly the former. Further advances in classification have been achieved with refinements in cytogenetic and molecular classification of acute leukemias. Several well-known cytogenetic changes in blast cells are associated with important prognostic differences in outcome; the translocations t(9;22) and t(4;11) impart poor outcomes to those individuals whose leukemia cells contain them, while the t(12;21) translocation imparts a very good prognosis to children with blasts containing that translocation. The same is true in AML, wherein t(8;21), inversion of chromosome 16, and t(15;17) impart favorable outcomes; while monosomy 7, absence of the long arm of chromosome 5, and 11q23 abnormalities signal a poor prognosis. In summary, the classification of childhood acute leukemias, much the same as in adult leukemias, is accomplished using morphology under the light microscope, immunophenotypic features, and blast cell cytogenetic and molecular features; the result of this sophisticated classification impacts both choice of treatment and outcome.

TABLE 2 Immunophenotypes of Major Categories of Acute Leukemia

Phenotype	Antigens Expressed	Frequency
Acute Lymphoblastic Leukemia		
B precursor	CD19, CD20, CD22, CD24, CD10	65%
Pre-B cell	As above plus cytoplasmic immunoglobulin	20%
Mature B cell	CD19, CD20, CD21, surface immunoglobulin	2%
T cell	CD2, CD5, CD7, CD1, CD4, CD8, CD3	13%
Acute Myelogenous Leukemia		
Myeloid	CD11, CD13, CD15, CD33, CD34, CD65	

Supportive Care

Improvements in supportive care continue to enhance outcomes for all patients with acute leukemia. Many of these advances have come in the area of infectious disease. Anti-infective drugs developed for bacteria resistant to conventional antibiotics have made significant inroads in the treatment of both gram-positive and gram-negative infections. New antifungal drugs, in particular, offer promise for some of the most deadly infections that patients with leukemia face. Modified hematopoietic growth factors now allow for fewer painful administrations, while maintaining longer-lasting effects. A new drug designed to reduce uric acid levels has found a place in the management of fulminant tumor lysis syndrome. High-quality transfusional support facilitates oxygen delivery and reduces bleeding in leukemia patients, while minimizing the transmission of infectious agents.

HYPERLEUKOCYTOSIS

At presentation, children with acute leukemia often have WBC counts in excess of 100,000/μL. When they do, consideration is given to leukapheresis or to administration of single-agent corticosteroid therapy to rapidly reduce the blood count and, specifically, the number of circulating leukemic blasts. Hyperleukocytosis may be associated with decreased cerebral and/or pulmonary blood flow, with consequent stroke-like symptoms or respiratory distress and hypoxia. Patients with AML appear to be at higher risk of such adverse physiology than patients with ALL. In general, leukapheresis is recommended when the WBC reaches or exceeds 200,000/μL. The use of single-agent corticosteroids in patients with ALL is discouraged unless part of an established treatment protocol. In fact, indiscriminate use of corticosteroids at the time of diagnosis often precludes patient entry onto one of the current national frontline investigational treatment protocols for ALL.

TRANSFUSION THERAPY

Support of the plasma hemoglobin level and of the platelet count are essential ingredients in the successful management of patients with acute leukemia. Without adequate oxygen delivery, organ dysfunction may occur, impacting negatively upon the patient's ability to tolerate aggressive chemotherapy. Red blood cell (RBC) transfusion, employing irradiated cells, is implemented when the patient's hemoglobin value falls below a value of approximately 8.0 g/dL; in very young children, the threshold for RBC transfusion may be 7.0 g/dL or even somewhat lower. Patient symptoms may also influence the decision of when to transfuse RBCs; dizziness, headache, fatigue, and shortness of breath, when present, should result in a lower threshold for transfusion.

To prevent the bleeding to which thrombocytopenic patients are predisposed, irradiated platelet transfusions are administered to nonbleeding patients for platelet counts below 5,000/µL. For patients who are thrombocytopenic and actively bleeding, there is no specific platelet transfusion threshold; the degree of bleeding drives decisions about the timing of platelet transfusions. For all leukemic patients, transfusions should be done only with irradiated, leukocyte-depleted products, thereby to reduce risks of transfusion-associated graft-versus-host disease (GVHD) and of exposure to transfused cytomegalovirus.

TUMOR LYSIS SYNDROME

When leukemic cell cytoreduction begins with the onset of administration of chemotherapy, byproducts of cell death, including uric acid, potassium, and phosphorus, are released into the blood stream. If the uric acid level exceeds its solubility in the blood, it will precipitate in the form of crystals in the kidneys, resulting in uric acid nephropathy. Thereafter, clearance of potassium and phosphorus in the kidneys can be impaired with threatening consequences for the patient. Allopurinol at 10 mg/kg (maximum dose 600 mg/day) is given orally in two or three divided doses for the first several days of antineoplastic therapy. For most patients, this is sufficient to prevent uric acid nephropathy and tumor lysis syndrome. For patients with:

- Peripheral blood WBC counts in excess of 100,000/mL,
- Significant organomegaly,
- Elevated levels of serum potassium and/or phosphorus, and
- Pre-existent kidney dysfunction,

the uric acid oxidase, rasburicase, may offer the advantage of very rapid reduction of serum uric acid levels, thereby reducing the risk of developing hyperkalemia and subsequently of cardiac arrhythmia. It should be kept in mind, however, that uric acid oxidase is currently very expensive, and for most patients allopurinol is more than sufficient.

INFECTION

Infection remains the primary cause of death in patients with acute leukemia undergoing chemotherapy. When patients are neutropenic with fever, as often occurs during induction, intensification, or reinduction/reintensification therapy, they require rapid evaluation. They should have blood samples and other target fluids/tissues collected for culture, and they should be started promptly on broad-spectrum antibiotic coverage. Most data indicate that chest radiographs are not necessary for febrile patients presenting with no pulmonary symptomatology. Antibiotic coverage typically consists of dual-agent coverage, such as gentamicin and Zosyn, to provide good gram-negative coverage along with reasonable gram-positive coverage. In some centers, single-agent coverage with a drug demonstrating broad-ranging efficacy, such as Cefepime or ciprofloxacin, is initiated, adding additional agents or changing coverage as dictated by culture results and clinical course. Other physicians prefer to add vancomycin initially to achieve excellent gram-positive coverage, important in an era when gram-positive organisms account for a majority of the infections occurring in patients receiving chemotherapy. Usually, the febrile patient is managed as an inpatient for the first 2 days of the illness; however, strategies are being developed and tested, either for total outpatient management of these patients or for rapid discharge from the inpatient unit once initial cultures are negative and fevers disappear. When specific organisms are identified, the therapy should be refined to provide the most active antibiotics for the identified organism. In the face of continuing fevers and neutropenia without positive culture results, antifungal agents, usually amphotericin-B or one of the related lipid formulations, are started. The new agent, voriconazole, offers relatively broad antifungal coverage, while reducing the risk of nephrotoxicity. However, voriconazole interacts with many drugs, altering blood levels of those drugs; it also can cause retinal and liver toxicity. Another new choice among antifungal agents is caspofungin; this agent is well tolerated and has excellent activity against *Candida* and *Aspergillus* infections. Fever occurring during non-neutropenic periods also requires careful management, since many patients have poor cell mediated immunity and often have indwelling plastic central venous catheters. When the latter is the case and also when patients appear ill, it is wise to obtain blood cultures and to initiate antibiotic therapy.

Most patients undergoing therapy for acute leukemia are maintained on prophylactic antibiotics. All patients who are not allergic to trimethoprim-sulfamethoxazole should be placed on this drug at 5 to 6 mg/kg per day (of the trimethoprim component) in two divided doses for 2 to 3 successive days each week in order to prevent *Pneumocystis carinii* pneumonia. For intense induction regimens, the use of oral nystatin (Mycostatin) or of fluconazole reduces the incidence of candidal infections.

GROWTH FACTORS

The hematopoietic growth factor, granulocyte colony-stimulating factor (G-CSF), has been used greatly in patients with solid tumors to facilitate recovery from chemotherapy. However, in patients with acute leukemia, the use of G-CSF and other growth factors has been limited. In part, concerns over expanding leukemic blast cell populations have limited use of G-CSF, particularly for patients with AML. In general, use of G-CSF has largely been limited to treatment of patients when febrile and neutropenic. The development of pegylated growth factors (pegfilgrastim, darbepoetin alfa) offers the prospect of using these agents in children with less discomfort because of the increased interval between injections.

VENOUS ACCESS

The use of indwelling venous access devices has become prevalent in the management of pediatric oncology patients. These catheters offer easy access for blood draws, for administration of chemotherapy and other medications, for transfusions, and for administration of parenteral nutrition, while minimizing pain for the children. Therefore, most leukemia patients have them placed early in the course of their evaluation and before the initiation of therapy. Their use, however, is associated with risks of infection, thrombosis in the used vein, and failure to work properly, most troublesome when patients have low blood counts making line replacement difficult. After the intensive part of therapy has been completed, consideration should be given to removing the catheter, weighing the disadvantages of not having easy venous access against the risk of infection if the catheter remains in place.

Treatment

ACUTE LYMPHOBLASTIC LEUKEMIA

The treatment of ALL has historically been divided into three phases—induction of remission, consolidation or intensification of that remission, and maintenance of the remission. With the advent of reintensifying therapy, additional phases of treatment have come into play (Table 3). One typical scheme of therapy, which is used in the Children's Cancer Group/Children's Oncology Group and is modified from the Berlin-Frankfort-Munster (BFM) Leukemia Study Group, includes induction, intensification, interim maintenance, delayed intensification, and maintenance phases of therapy. Contemporary therapy of ALL produces 70% to 80% 5-year disease-free survival, with outcomes varying according to risk group (Table 4).

Induction

During induction therapy, a combination of vincristine, corticosteroid (prednisone or dexamethasone), and asparaginase (L-asparaginase or PEG-asparaginase) with or without an anthracycline (usually daunorubicin) are employed to achieve several logs of cytoreduction, thereby inducing remission. The induction phase lasts 4 to 6 weeks. Remission is defined by the results of marrow aspiration; individuals with fewer than 5% blasts are considered in complete remission (CR) (M1 status), those with 5% to 24% blasts in partial remission (M2 status), and those with greater than 25% blasts in relapse (M3 status). Typically, remission status also implies that the peripheral blood counts have returned to normal, as has the physical exam.

Approximately 98% of pediatric patients with ALL achieve remission. Early marrow response at day 7 is an important indicator of long-term disease-free survival (DFS). For patients with M_3 marrow status at day 7, intensification of induction therapy with the addition of an anthracycline will often enhance the probability of achieving remission and long-term disease-free survival. If a patient continues to demonstrate M_3 marrow status at day 28 of induction therapy or later, the prognosis with conventional therapy is very poor. These individuals should be considered for alternative induction therapy and for allogeneic hematopoietic stem cell transplantation (HSCT). The use of HSCT for patients with ALL in first CR is limited to individuals with the t(9;22) and t(4;11) translocations, to infants less than 1 year of age, and to patients with high WBC counts (>200,000/mm^3) at diagnosis.

Intensification

Intensification therapy is designed to solidify the remission achieved during induction, with a goal of reducing further the remaining logs of leukemic cells. Various strategies are used in centers around the world. Intravenous cyclophosphamide, pulses of cytosine arabinoside with or without 6-thioguanine, and intravenous methotrexate and/or 6-mercaptopurine have been used. An additional goal of this phase of therapy is the initiation of therapy directed at sanctuary sites of disease, either to prevent central nervous system (CNS) relapse or to treat existent disease in the CNS, in the testes, or in other extramedullary sites. The intensification phase of therapy lasts 4 to 8 weeks.

Interim Maintenance

This phase of therapy is designed to allow a respite from intensive therapy, after induction/intensification but before reintensification, while at the same time providing maintenance therapy that will prevent relapse. This phase of therapy often begins with a dose of vincristine and a pulse of corticosteroid. Oral maintenance agents used include 6-mercaptopurine (or 6-thioguanine) and methotrexate. This phase of therapy lasts for 8 weeks.

Reintensification

During reintensification, induction therapy and intensification therapy are recapitulated, with the goal

TABLE 3 Treatment Approach for Acute Lymphoblastic Leukemia*

Risk Group	Induction	Consolidation	Interim Maintenance
Standard risk	VCR, PRED or DEXA, ASPARA, IT ARA-C/MTX	CYCLO, ARA-C, TG or IDMTX, MP, VCR, PRED/DEXA, IT MTX	VCR, PRED/DEXA, MP, MTX, IT MTX
High risk	VCR, PRED or DEXA, ASPARA, ± DAUNO, IT ARA-C/MTX	CYCLO, ARA-C, TG or IDMTX, MP, VCR, PRED/DEXA IT MTX	VCR, PRED/DEXA, MP, MTX, IT MTX
Very high risk	VCR, PRED or DEXA, ASPARA, ± DAUNO, IT ARA-C/MTX	IFOS, ETOP, IT MTX, ± STI571, HDARA-C, HDMTX	(Proceed to HSCT or to reinduction)
T cell	VCR, PRED, DAUNO, ASPARA, MP, ARA-C, CYCLO, +/– 506U78, IT MTX	MP, HDMTX, IT MTX	(Proceed to reinduction)
Risk Group	**Reinduction/Reintensification**	**Maintenance**	
Standard risk	VCR, DEXA, ASPARA, DOXO, IT MTX, CYCLO, ARA-C, TG	VCR, PRED/DEXA, MP, MTX, IT MTX	
High risk	VCR, DEXA, ASPARA, DOXO, IT MTX, CYCLO, ARA-C, TG	VCR, PRED/DEXA, MP, MTX, IT MTX	
Very high risk	VCR, DEXA, DAUNO, PEG-ASPARA, CYCLO, IT MTX, ± STI571, HDMTX, ETOP, CYCLO, HDARA-C, ASPARA	HDMTX, VCR, DEXA, MP, IT MTX, MTX, ETOP, CYCLO, ± STI571, ± CR XRT	
T cell	VCR, DEXA, DOXO, ASPARA, TG, CYCLO, ARA-C, ± 506U78, IT MTX, CR XRT	VCR, PRED, MP, MTX, ± 506U78	
Risk Group		**Induction/Intensification**	**Reinduction/Reintensification**
Infants		VCR, DEXA, DAUNO, CYCLO, ASPARA, ITT, HDMTX, ETOP	VCR, DEXA, DAUNO, CYCLO, ASPARA, ITT, IT ARA-C, VHDMTX, ETOP
	Consolidation	**Intensification/Maintenance**	**Maintenance**
	ARA-C, ASPARA, VHDMTX, VCR, IT ARA-C,	VCR, DEXA, MTX, MP, IT ARA-C, ETOP, CYCLO	VCR, PRED, MTX, MP

*Recommendations are based upon the following protocols: B-precursor standard risk—Children's Cancer Group (CCG) 1991; B-precursor high risk—CCG 1961; B-precursor very high risk—Children's Oncology Group (COG) AALL0031; infants—CCG 1953; and T cell—COG AALL00P2.

Abbreviations: ARA-C = cytosine arabinoside (Cytosar-U); ASPARA = L-asparaginase (Elspar); CR XRT = cranial radiation therapy; CYCLO = cyclophosphamide (Cytoxan); DAUNO = daunorubicin (Cerubidine); DEXA = dexamethasone; DOXO = doxorubicin (Adriamycin); ETOP = etoposide (VePesid)[1]; HDARA-C = high-dose cytosine arabinoside; HDMTX = high-dose methotrexate; HSCT = hematopoietic stem cell therapy; IDMTX = intermediate dose methotrexate; IFOS = ifosfamide (Ifex)[1]; IT = intrathecal; ITT = triple drug intrathecal (methotrexate, hydrocortisone, cytosine arabinoside); MP = 6-mercaptopurine (Purinethol); MTX = methotrexate, PEG-ASPARA = peg-asparaginase (Oncaspar); PRED = prednisone; STI571 = imatinib (Gleevec)[1]; TG = 6-thioguanine (Tabloid); VCR = vincristine (Oncovin); VHDMTX = very-high-dose methotrexate.

[1]Not FDA approved for this indication.

being eradication of any residual leukemia that has escaped the first three phases of therapy. The initial portion of this therapy includes three weekly doses of intravenous vincristine and doxorubicin, a 3-week course of oral dexamethasone or two 7-day courses of oral dexamethasone (days 1-7 and 15-21), and intramuscular asparaginase. The second segment of therapy consists of a single dose of intravenous cyclophosphamide, eight doses of subcutaneous or intravenous cytosine arabinoside given over 2 weeks, and two 4-day courses of oral 6-thioguanine. This phase of therapy is one in which the risks of low blood counts and infection must be considered; patients often require transfusions and sometimes admission because of fever with neutropenia. The duration of this phase is 7 to 8 weeks.

Maintenance

Maintenance therapy is given over an extended period to bring the total duration of therapy to 2 to 3 years. Monthly pulses of vincristine and prednisone or dexamethasone are complemented with daily oral doses of 6-mercaptopurine and weekly oral doses of

TABLE 4 Risk Classification of B-Cell and T-Cell Acute Lymphoblastic Leukemia

NIH Consensus Risk Definitions		
Standard	WBC <50,000 cells/mm^3 and age 1 to <10 years	
High	WBC ≥50,000 cells/mm^3 or age ≥10 years	
Other Factors Modifying Risk		
Factor	**Better Risk**	**Worse Risk**
Gender	Female	Male
DNA index	>1.16	≤1.16
Cytogenetics	Hyperdiploid	Hypodiploid
	Trisomies 4, 10, 17	t(9;22)
	t(12;21)	MLL gene (11q23) disruption
CSF status	No blasts	Blasts present
Treatment response*	Rapid	Slow

*Determined by bone marrow status at day 7 or 14 or by peripheral blood status at day 7.

Abbreviations: CSF = cerebrospinal fluid; MLL = mixed lineage leukemia; WBC = white blood cell count.

methotrexate. Some maintenance regimens employ pulses of chemotherapy agents rather than continuous oral maintenance agents.

Prophylaxis of Central Nervous System Leukemia

Because of a high propensity for extramedullary recurrence of ALL in the CNS, it is necessary to provide preventative treatment. Historically, this treatment has consisted of a combination of cranial radiation therapy and intrathecal chemotherapy. However, standard-risk patients with ALL do not need to receive cranial radiation therapy, provided the intrathecal therapy is given throughout maintenance therapy. The standard intrathecal medication used is methotrexate; the dose is age-adjusted and ranges from 6 to 15 mg. For patients with high-risk ALL, cranial radiation therapy to a dose of 1260 to 1800 cGy is given along with intrathecal methotrexate.

Treatment of Extramedullary Leukemia

When present at diagnosis, CNS leukemia is managed with cranial radiation of 1800 cGy plus weekly intrathecal methotrexate for at least six doses; intrathecal methotrexate is also continued during maintenance therapy, being given once every 8 to 12 weeks. If the CNS leukemia fails to respond to the single-drug intrathecal methotrexate, triple drug therapy employing cytosine arabinoside, hydrocortisone sodium succinate, and methotrexate should be initiated. With CNS leukemia poorly responsive to intrathecal methotrexate, the radiation field should be expanded to a craniospinal field, using 2400 cGy. Treatment of CNS relapse occurring while on therapy should consist of triple drug intrathecal therapy followed by 2400 cGy craniospinal radiation therapy.

Management of extramedullary leukemia outside of the CNS varies depending upon the location of the relapse, time of occurrence of the relapse, and response to systemic induction therapy. When present at diagnosis, soft tissue leukemia (such as can be seen in the testes, kidneys, ovaries, and skin) often responds well to standard induction therapy; lack of response to induction is managed with radiation therapy of 2400 to 3000 cGy. Extramedullary relapse on therapy should be managed with radiation therapy of 2400 to 3000 cGy plus institution of systemic reinduction therapy. The required total duration of therapy after such an isolated extramedullary relapse is controversial, with most patients receiving therapy for 2 years after relapse.

Treatment of Marrow Relapse

The timing of a marrow relapse of ALL is critical in treatment planning. Early marrow relapses occurring within 18 months of diagnosis carry a poor prognosis, with a high risk of treatment failure following salvage therapy. For patients with early marrow relapse, histocompatibility testing should be done on the patient, the patient's parents, and on any siblings. If a related donor who is compatible at human leukocyte antigens (HLA)-A, -B, -C, and -DR loci can be identified, then plans to undergo HSCT following reinduction therapy should be made. Some oncologists recommend pursuing unrelated donor stem cell transplantation after an early marrow relapse when a matched related donor is unavailable. This entails undertaking an unrelated donor search through the National Marrow Donor Program and other hematopoietic stem cell registries.

For marrow relapses that are either intermediate (18 to 35 months) or late (36 months or more) postdiagnosis, application of reinduction, intensification, and maintenance chemotherapies constitutes the standard approach. Whether hematopoietic stem cell transplantation should be recommended for such patients remains a topic of discussion; clinical trials are needed to define the role of HSCT in the care of intermediate-to-late marrow relapses.

Treatment of Central Nervous System Relapse

Initial, isolated CNS relapses require both regional and systemic therapy. Because most patients experiencing such a relapse currently will not have received cranial radiation therapy as part of their prophylactic regimen, craniospinal radiation therapy to a dose of 2400 cGy is a mainstay of therapy. Typically, patients receive either intrathecal methotrexate or triple intrathecal therapy (methotrexate, hydrocortisone sodium succinate, cytosine arabinoside) for four to six doses to clear the CSF of leukemic blasts.

TABLE 5 Treatment Approach for Acute Myelogenous Leukemia*

Subtypes†	Induction	Consolidation	Intensification
M1, M2, M4-M7	IDAR or DAUNO, ARA-C, ± ETOP, ± TG, ± DEXA, IT ARA-C ± HSS ± MTX	IDAR or DAUNO, ARA-C, ± ETOP, ± TG, ± DEXA, IT ARA-C ± HSS ± MTX, and/or FLUD, ARA-C, IDAR	HDARA-C, ASPARA or MITOX, IT ARA-C ± HSS ± MTX or HSCT
M3	ATRA, DAUNO, ARA-C	DAUNO, ARA-C	ATRA maintenance

*Recommendations are based upon the following protocols: Children's Cancer Group (CCG) 2891, CCG 2961.
†From the French-American-British (FAB) classification system.
Abbreviations: ARA-C = cytosine arabinoside (Cytosar-U); ATRA = all-trans retinoic acid (Vesanoid)[1]; DAUNO = daunorubicin (Cerubidine)[1]; DEXA = dexamethasone; ETOP = etoposide (VePesid)[1]; FLUD = fludarabine (Fludara)[1]; HDARA-C = high-dose cytosine arabinoside; HSCT = hematopoietic stem cell transplantation; HSS = hydrocortisone sodium succinate; IDAR = idarubicin (Idamycin); MITOX = mitoxantrone (Novantrone)[1]; MTX = methotrexate[1]; TG = 6-thioguanine (Tabloid).
[1]Not FDA approved for this indication.

This will then be followed by radiation therapy delivered over 2 to 3 weeks. In addition, systemic chemotherapy is usually given for 2 years as experimental studies following isolated CNS relapse indicate the presence of subliminal disease in the marrow and elsewhere.

Treatment of Testicular Relapse

With testicular relapse, radiation to the testes has been delivered to a dose of 2400 cGy; historically, both testes have been irradiated, even when the relapse appears confined to one testis. However recent data from Holland have challenged the necessity of administering testicular irradiation for late isolated testicular relapses (>8 months after completion of chemotherapy). For some patients with large testicular masses or with slow response to the radiation therapy, the treatment dose has been increased to 3000 cGy. As in isolated CNS relapse, patients with isolated testicular relapse receive systemic chemotherapy for 2 years.

ACUTE MYELOID LEUKEMIA

The management of acute myelogenous leukemia has evolved during the last 20 years to a point where more than 50% of newly diagnosed patients are expected to be alive and disease-free 5 years after diagnosis. The improvement from less than 30% to 50% has occurred because of intensification of therapy, particularly during the consolidation phase of therapy (Table 5). To some degree, the improvement relates to improved algorithms for defining risk groups (Table 6) and predicting outcomes following chemotherapy, with the decision on whether to include hematopoietic stem cell transplantation in therapy being based on the presence or absence of certain high-risk features.

Induction

Once the diagnosis of AML is established, chemotherapy is initiated employing an anthracycline (daunorubicin, doxorubicin, or idarubicin) and cytosine arabinoside with or without other agents, such as etoposide and/or thioguanine. A typical induction course consists of anthracycline daily for 3 days, cytosine arabinoside for 5 to 7 days, and, when used, etoposide or thioguanine for 3 to 4 days. Remissions are successfully induced 80% to 90% of the time.

Consolidation

Once remission is induced, the therapeutic emphasis becomes one of solidifying and maintaining the remission. Most consolidation/intensification strategies center on the use of high-dose cytosine arabinoside with amsacrine, etoposide, mitoxantrone, or L-asparaginase. Often two or three consolidation

TABLE 6 Risk Classification of Acute Myelogenous Leukemia (AML)

Morphologic Classification (FAB)		
M0	Undifferentiated leukemia	
M1	Myeloblastic, no maturation	
M2	Myeloblastic, with maturation	
M3	Promyelocytic, hypergranular type	
M3v	Promyelocytic, microgranular variant	
M4	Myelomonocytic	
M4Eo	Myelomonocytic, with eosinophilia	
M5a	Monocytic	
M5b	Monocytic, with differentiation	
M6	Erythroleukemia	
M7	Megakaryoblastic	
Other Factors Modifying Risk		
Factor	**Better Risk**	**Worse Risk**
White Blood Count	<100,000 cells/mm³	≥100,000 cells/mm³
Chromosomes	t(8;21), t(15;17), Inversion 16	Deletion of 5 or 7
Other	Down syndrome	Secondary AML*, Previous myelodysplasia

*Secondary leukemia occurs following chemotherapy for a prior malignancy.
Abbreviation: FAB = French-American-British.

courses are administered in sequence. Hematopoietic stem cell transplantation is often used as one of these consolidation courses for children who have HLA-matched related donors.

Maintenance

The use of maintenance therapy in AML remains controversial. Randomized studies have failed to demonstrate benefit from maintenance therapy, provided the induction therapy and consolidation therapy are very intense.

Hematopoietic Stem Cell Transplantation

The use of matched related-donor hematopoietic stem cell transplantation in the treatment of newly diagnosed patients with AML, while having found a central role in the United States, is not universally accepted elsewhere for all risk groups. In the United Kingdom, for children with favorable blast cytogenetics (t[8;21], t[15;17], and inv16 with eosinophilia) who also have a rapid early response to chemotherapy, matched related-donor stem cell transplantation is not recommended. The growing trend appears to center on an effort to define high-risk criteria, which, when present, would dictate proceeding with matched related-donor stem cell transplantation in first CR. The use of unrelated donors for HSCT in first CR is limited only to patients with extremely high-risk AML, that is, those with monosomy 7 or 7q–, and those with poor response to induction therapy.

After relapse, stem cell transplantation has a major role in therapy. Both related donors when available and unrelated donors otherwise are used to provide the necessary stem cells. As the prognosis following relapse is so dismal with conventional chemotherapy, little debate surrounds the application of hematopoietic stem cell transplantation to these patients. Typical preparative regimens employed include:

- BuCy4—busulfan for 4 days followed by cyclophosphamide for 4 days
- BuCy2—busulfan for 4 days followed by cyclophosphamide for 2 days
- BAC—busulfan for 4 days followed by cytosine arabinoside for 2 days and then cyclophosphamide for 2 days
- CyTBI—cyclophosphamide for 4 days either before or after total body irradiation (1200 to 1440 cGy in divided doses over 3 to 4 days)

Chloroma

Occasionally patients with AML present with or later develop soft tissue collections of leukemic cells; these collections are called chloromas. At diagnosis, isolated chloromas are managed with systemic chemotherapy, with or without radiation therapy; recent data suggest a similar outcome for those receiving radiation therapy as for those not receiving it. Additional data suggest that the prognosis of patients with isolated chloromas as their presenting feature of AML have better prognoses than do patients presenting with marrow involvement. If a chloroma is present at relapse, local radiation therapy may be appropriate, especially if the relapse occurs while the patient is still receiving chemotherapy.

Relapse

Marrow is the typical site of relapse. Reinduction therapy following marrow relapse typically consists of a combination of high-dose cytosine arabinoside and etoposide, mitoxantrone, and/or L-asparaginase. Amsacrine and idarubicin have been used in place of mitoxantrone. The combination of topotecan and 2-chloro-deoxyadenosine (2-CDA) has activity in relapsed AML. Newer experimental approaches now being evaluated include the use of an anti-CD33 monoclonal antibody conjugated to an antitumor antibiotic (gemtuzumab ozogamicin) and the use of agents that block the activity of mutated FLT3, found in 10% to 15% of childhood AML cases. The use of the latter two biologic therapies requires the expression of CD33 on leukemic blasts for the gemtuzumab and FLT3-ITD (internal tandem duplications) in leukemic cells for the FLT3 mutation blockers. Furthermore, the clinical use of gemtuzumab is limited by an associated risk of veno-occlusive disease of the liver; this is particularly relevant for individuals eligible for HSCT following reinduction therapy, which includes gemtuzumab. Once remission is achieved, stem cell transplantation is an important consideration, using either a matched related donor if available, a mismatched related donor (5/6), or a well-matched unrelated donor (6/6 or 5/6). The availability of cord blood stem cells allows for a greater degree of HLA disparity in the matching process, with less risk of GVHD, but also less benefit from graft-versus-leukemia effect (GVL). The use of cord blood as a stem cell source is limited by the size of the cord blood units available and the weight of the patient, as the cell number per kilogram of weight infused is critical to successful engraftment.

Relapse in Sites Other Than Marrow

CNS relapses require the administration of intrathecal chemotherapy (cytosine arabinoside ± hydrocortisone sodium succinate and methotrexate) and 2400 cGy craniospinal radiation therapy, plus the administration of reinduction and consolidation chemotherapy. Allogeneic stem cell transplantation should be considered for consolidation of remission following a CNS relapse. Similarly, relapse in a soft-tissue site requires radiation at a comparable dose to the affected soft tissues, provided that the field of treatment does not encompass too much normal tissue. Once again, reinduction and reconsolidation chemotherapy are essential, and stem cell transplantation should be considered.

LATE EFFECTS OF THERAPY

The successful management of acute leukemia must take into consideration the side effects of the therapy delivered, as these will significantly impact the quality of life not only during therapy but also after therapy. Oftentimes, the negative impact of therapy is seen years after completion of therapy, and occasionally death results from these late effects of therapy. During treatment, patients experience nausea, vomiting, hair loss, mouth sores, low blood counts with risks of infection and bleeding, liver injury, and renal dysfunction; fortunately, most of these pass quickly and completely once the patient has completed taking the offending drug or receiving radiation therapy. However, deleterious effects on the CNS, such as leukoencephalopathy and radiation injury to the brain, may have lasting ramifications for the patient's well-being. Similarly, growth impairment from radiation therapy; cardiomyopathy from anthracyclines; osteonecrosis from corticosteroids; pituitary, thyroid, and gonadal hormonal insufficiency from radiation therapy; pulmonary injury from chemotherapy or radiation therapy; and the late sequelae of infertility and second malignancy will have lasting impacts on quality of life. As pediatric oncologists achieve improved control of acute leukemia, with higher rates of remission induction and longer disease-free intervals, and, particularly as the long-term cure rate rises, one compelling goal of investigative efforts must be to lessen the long-lasting and late sequelae of treatment. This mission is indeed already being implemented in the management of the lower risk groups of patients with ALL, following trends established in the successful treatment of Wilms tumor and Hodgkin disease. Finally, the establishment of *late effects* clinics in cancer centers around the country allows practitioners to focus on assessing the total impact of the therapy they previously delivered to leukemia patients. With 70% to 80% of children with ALL and 40% to 50% of children with AML surviving for more than 5 years, pediatric oncologists must now deal with treatment-related issues arising in schools and in workplaces, as well as in the homes, of these surviving children. Many of these survivors need guidance and assistance in the educational arena, in job placement, in social adjustment, and in obtaining health insurance coverage. The good news of longer durable remissions and of cures for many patients with acute leukemia must be balanced against the need for achieving greater success in treating high-risk patients with ALL and a majority of patients with AML, as well as against the imperative of evaluating late sequelae of therapy and developing strategies to prevent and assist in managing these problems.

CHRONIC LEUKEMIAS

METHOD OF

Renier Brentjens, MD, PhD, and Mark Weiss, MD

Chronic Lymphocytic Leukemia

Chronic lymphocytic leukemia (CLL), a cancer of B lymphocytes, is the most common adult leukemia. CLL is a disease predominantly of older individuals with a median age at diagnosis of 69.6 years. The disease is quite rare in patients younger than the age of 30, but the incidence increases exponentially between the ages of 30 and 70, leveling off thereafter. The disease is more common in men with a relative risk of 2.8 times that of women. In the United States, the highest incidence of CLL is seen in Caucasians, followed by African-Americans and Hispanics; it is rarely seen in Asians. Approximately 8000 new cases of CLL are diagnosed in the United States annually. To date, the etiology of CLL remains unknown with no environmental or viral exposures having been reliably associated with the disease. While several familial clusters of CLL have been reported, no putative CLL genes have been unequivocally identified.

DIAGNOSIS

CLL is an indolent disease with a relatively long natural history when compared to other malignancies. Overall, the median survival of all patients is 5 years. Patients with CLL have an elevated number of mature B cells in the peripheral blood, usually greater than 10,000/μL, with disease involving the bone marrow and commonly the lymph nodes and spleen.

The diagnosis of CLL is often made incidentally on a routine blood count demonstrating lymphocytosis. Alternatively, patients may present with complications related to lymphadenopathy, splenomegaly, anemia, or thrombocytopenia. At diagnosis, most patients are asymptomatic even when the peripheral blood lymphocyte count exceeds 100,000/mL. Patients with more advanced disease, however, can present with constitutional symptoms including fatigue, weight loss, fevers, and night sweats.

Review of a peripheral blood smear from these patients demonstrates an increase in the number of small, mature-appearing B lymphocytes with a characteristic dense nucleus and a thin rim of clear cytoplasm. Characteristic, although not diagnostic, is the presence of numerous smudge cells on the smear.

The diagnosis of CLL is made by flow cytometric immunophenotyping of the peripheral blood. Flow cytometric analysis reveals a clonal population of

B cells, as determined by restricted expression of either the kappa or lambda light chain on cells that co-express CD5 and the B-cell marker CD19. CLL cells also typically express CD23 and CD20, and they dimly express surface immunoglobulin (sIg). For prognostic analysis, further evaluation at the time of diagnosis includes obtaining baseline serum LDH and β_2 microglobulin levels; as well as quantitative IgG, IgM, and IgA levels. A bone marrow aspirate and biopsy, while not required for diagnosis, may be obtained to provide further prognostic data. Chromosomal analysis using fluorescent in situ hybridization (FISH) should be performed on the tumor cells for diagnostic and prognostic purposes. A baseline computed tomography (CT) scan to assess areas of lymphadenopathy is not required, but may be obtained to determine disease progression over time and to potentially aid in the subsequent diagnosis of transformed disease.

The differential diagnosis of CLL includes several other mature B-cell malignancies such as low-grade lymphomas in leukemic phase, mantle-cell lymphoma (MCL), and B-cell prolymphocytic leukemia (B-PLL). In general, these diagnoses are excluded on the basis of flow cytometric and chromosomal analyses. Most low-grade lymphomas do not express CD5 or CD23, and in contrast to CLL, have bright sIg staining. MCL, a far more aggressive disease, does express CD5 but fails to express CD23. MCL is further distinguished from CLL by immunohistochemistry of the bone marrow biopsy demonstrating an elevated level of expression of cyclin D1, and by cytogenetic analysis demonstrating a characteristic translocation of chromosomes 11 and 14 (t[11;14]). B-PLL is a rare, aggressive variant of CLL. Typically, PLL involves the bone marrow and spleen but not the lymph nodes. Flow cytometric analysis cannot definitively distinguish from CLL, but B-PLL cells typically express higher levels of sIg, and these cells less commonly express CD5 and CD23. The diagnosis of B-PLL is made microscopically as these tumor cells are larger in size than typical CLL cells with the nucleus containing a single, distinct nucleolus.

STAGING AND PROGNOSIS

Currently two well-established staging systems exist for CLL, the Rai and Binet classifications (Table 1). Staging of CLL by these classification schemes allows for a reliable assessment of prognosis. The Rai classification stages patients based on the presence of lymphocytosis, lymphadenopathy, splenomegaly, anemia, and thombocytopenia (see Table 1). The Binet classification is based on the number of lymph node regions involved with disease, and the presence of anemia and/or thrombocytopenia (Table 2).

While disease stage is of prognostic significance, other characteristics of the disease are also of prognostic importance (Table 3). Traditional adverse prognostic features include a lymphocyte doubling time of less than 1 year and an elevated β_2 microglobulin level (>3.5 mg/dL). Modern techniques have illustrated the importance of four new prognostic features. The most important is chromosomal analysis (as determined by FISH). FISH analyses revealing 11q and 17p deletions denote aggressive disease, while trisomy 12 has an intermediate prognosis, and deletion of chromosome region 13q14 (as the sole abnormality) is associated with a relatively good prognosis. Expression of CD38 on more than 30% of tumor cells is a poor prognostic indicator. Somatic mutations in the IgV_H gene are highly predictive of indolent disease, while tumors with an unmutated IgV_H gene have more aggressive disease. Tumor expression of ZAP-70, an intracellular tyrosine-kinase not normally expressed in B cells, is also associated with a poor prognosis relative to tumors that do not express ZAP-70. These last two features (IgV_H somatic mutations and ZAP-70 expression), though powerfully predictive, are currently typically performed in specialized research laboratories and are not widely available at this time.

DISEASE-RELATED COMPLICATIONS

Proper management of CLL requires an appreciation of the complications associated with the disease. Patients with CLL are immune-suppressed and prone to develop life-threatening infections. Infection remains the leading cause of death in patients with CLL. Immune suppression is related both to low levels of immunoglobulins, especially prominent in later stages of disease, and to T-cell and neutrophil dysfunction. For this reason, patients with fever or other evidence of infection should seek immediate medical attention. Such patients should be evaluated with a CBC, blood and urine cultures, and a chest x-ray. Patients typically require broad-spectrum intravenous

TABLE 1 Staging of Chronic Lymphocytic Leukemia: The Rai System

Stage	Clinical Features	Simplified System	3-Year Survival
0	Lymphocytosis only	Low risk	>10y
I	Lymphadenopathy	Intermediate risk	7y
II	Organomegaly		
III	Anemia (HGB <11 g/dL)	High risk	1.5-4y
IV	Thrombocytopenia (platelets <100 K)		

Abbreviation: HGB = hemoglobin.

TABLE 2 Staging of Chronic Lymphocytic Leukemia: The Binet System

Stage	Clinical Features	Median Survival
A	<3 areas of lymphadenopathy*; no anemia of thrombocytopenia	12y
B	≥3 areas of lymphadenopathy*; no anemia of thrombocytopenia	7y
C	Hemoglobin <10 g/dL and/or platelets <100,000/μL	2-4y

*Areas include cervical, axillary, inguinal lymph node regions, the spleen, and the liver.

antibiotics targeting encapsulated organisms (*Pneumococcus*, *Haemophilus influenzae*, and *Klebsiella*) for at least 7 days if a source of infection is identified or if fever persists. Pneumococcal and influenza vaccines are recommended (although many patients cannot produce an adequate antibody response). Patients with frequent infections should be considered for prophylactic monthly intravenous immunoglobulin (IVIG) replacement therapy (400 mg/kg).

Approximately 15% to 20% of patients with CLL will develop disease-related autoimmune complications, most notably autoimmune hemolytic anemia (AIHA) and immune thrombocytopenia (ITP). Although both anemia and thrombocytopenia are indicators of CLL disease progression, autoimmune disease should be excluded before chemotherapy for CLL is initiated. In AIHA, Coombs testing is usually positive, haptoglobin levels are low, and reticulocyte counts are elevated (although not to the degree seen in patients with AIHA but without CLL). In addition, evaluation for other causes of anemia should be performed to exclude other sources of blood loss. The diagnosis of ITP is best established by a bone marrow examination demonstrating an increase in megakaryocytes.

Primary therapy of these autoimmune complications is with corticosteroids. Patients are typically started on 1 mg/kg of prednisone daily until normal red blood cell or platelet levels are restored. Thereafter, corticosteroids are slowly tapered over several months with close monitoring of blood counts.

TABLE 3 Poor Prognostic Features in Chronic Lymphocytic Leukemia

Traditional Features
Advanced disease stage (Rai high risk or Binet C)
Rapid lymphocyte doubling time (<12 months)
Pattern of bone marrow infiltration (diffuse versus other)
β_2 microglobulin levels (>3.5 mg/dL)
Newer Features
Cytogenetics (11q or 17p deletions)
Expression of CD38 (on >30% of tumor cells)
Tumor cells with unmutated IgVH genes
Tumor cell expression of ZAP-70

Abbreviation: ZAP-70 = tyrosine kinase zeta-associated protein of 70 kDa.

Prophylactic antibiotics to prevent PCP and herpes zoster should routinely be administered to patients with CLL receiving corticosteroid therapy.

Treatment failure or relapse of autoimmune disease may respond to therapy with rituximab (Rituxan)[1], 375 mg/m^2 given weekly for four doses. Persistent autoimmune disease despite these interventions may respond to chemotherapy with cyclophosphamide, prednisone, and weekly rituximab. Alternatively, where appropriate, patients may be offered splenectomy in this setting.

In 3% to 5% of patients with CLL, the disease will transform into a more aggressive phenotype (Richter transformation) with histology typically demonstrating diffuse large-cell lymphoma. The diagnosis of transformed disease may be difficult. Often patients will develop B symptoms including weight loss, fevers, and night sweats. Laboratory studies may show an acute elevation of LDH, serum calcium, and/or an M-spike on serum protein electrophoresis. Ultimately, the diagnosis is confirmed on biopsy. However, locating the appropriate site to biopsy is difficult, and the false-negative rate is high with biopsies demonstrating only the underlying CLL. Anatomical sites of transformed disease may be identified by serial CT scans demonstrating areas of rapidly increasing lymphadenopathy over time. Gallium and positron emission tomography may occasionally be helpful in localizing transformed disease. Often, however, transformed CLL is a clinical diagnosis.

THERAPY

Indications for Therapy

In contrast to other malignancies, the most important question to ask in CLL is not *how* to treat, but *when* to treat. Studies comparing early treatment of asymptomatic CLL patients (Binet stage A) with chlorambucil (Leukeran) versus expectant observation until disease became symptomatic demonstrated no survival benefit to early treatment. For this reason, we currently manage patients with expectant observation until the patient develops symptomatic disease or signs of bone marrow failure. Indications to initiate chemotherapy include disease-related anemia (hemoglobin <11 g/dL) or thrombocytopenia (platelets <100,000/μL) in the absence of autoimmune disease, painful (or obstructive) bulky lymphadenopathy, and transformed disease (Table 4). Furthermore, patients with a rapid doubling of their lymphocyte counts (<3 months) when the total lymphocyte counts exceed 100,000/μL may be considered for therapy.

Chemotherapy

Before the introduction of purine analogues, conventional therapy of CLL was restricted to the oral

[1]Not FDA approved for this indication.

TABLE 4 Indications for Treatment of Chronic Lymphocytic Leukemia

Absolute Indications
Bone marrow failure (HGB <10 mg/dL, platelets <100,000/dL)
Transformed disease (Richter transformation)
Bulky, painful, or obstructive lymphadenopathy
Severe B symptoms
Consider Therapy
Treatment-refractory autoimmune disease (AIHA, ITP)
Rapid lymphocyte doubling time (<3 months) with an absolute lymphocyte count >100,000/μL

Abbreviations: AIHA = autoimmune hemolytic anemia; HGB = hemoglobin; ITP = idiopathic thrombocytopenic purpura.

alkylating agents chlorambucil (Leukeran) and cyclophosphamide (Cytoxan) with or without corticosteroids. Unfortunately, while these agents did result in an appreciable degree of partial responses (<50%), complete responses were rarely achieved (<5%). Furthermore, response durations were short and patients soon succumbed to progressive disease. With the discovery that the purine analogue fludarabine (Fludara) had activity in patients previously treated with alkylating agents, this agent was tested as a first-line agent for CLL. In a randomized trial, untreated patients with CLL were randomized to receive fludarabine or chlorambucil as initial therapy. The group randomized to fludarabine had a superior overall response rate (63% versus 37%) and complete response rate (20% versus 3%) when compared to chlorambucil therapy. Response duration was also longer in the fludarabine treatment group (33 months versus 17 months) compared with chlorambucil treatment. Unfortunately, overall survival was not significantly different between the 2 arms of this study. In light of this superior activity, six cycles of fludarabine has become the standard first-line therapy for younger patients with CLL. While superior to alkylating agents in general, fludarabine is associated with a greater degree of myelosuppression. Significantly, fludarabine is also associated with inducing AIHA in up to 10% of treated patients, and may severely exacerbate pre-existing autoimmune disease and should therefore not be used in this setting.

Because of the greater frequency and quality of responses, we prefer fludarabine for initial treatment in most patients with CLL. However, as there has not been a demonstrable survival advantage, we recognize that for selected patients initial therapy with chlorambucil remains an acceptable alternative. Additionally, in patients with fludarabine-refractory disease, or those with a pre-existing autoimmune complication, therapy with cyclophosphamide, vincristine (Oncovin)[1], and prednisone (CVP) is an option. Patients with transformed disease are best treated with rituximab[1], cyclophosphamide, doxorubicin (Adriamycin)[1], vincristine[1], and prednisone (R-CHOP).

[1]Not FDA approved for this indication.

Novel Treatment Strategies

The addition of an alkylating agent to fludarabine has been studied and appears to enhance both the frequency of response as well as the toxicity. Combinations of fludarabine and chlorambucil were abandoned as too toxic to administer. However, with careful attention to dosing, combination therapy with fludarabine and cyclophosphamide can be administered with acceptable safety and significant activity.

Pentostatin (Nipent)[1], a purine analogue with less myelotoxicity than fludarabine, may be a safer alternative for combination therapy. We have recently reported that in a cohort of heavily pretreated patients, 6 cycles of pentostatin with cyclophosphamide therapy resulted in an overall response rate of 74% with a complete response in 19%. Furthermore, severe myelosuppression and infection requiring hospitalization were infrequent when compared to fludarabine-containing combinations.

Antibody Therapy

The anti-CD20 monoclonal antibody rituximab has activity as a single agent in CLL with a response rate of 25%. As rituximab has a favorable toxicity profile, it readily lends itself to combination chemotherapy, and investigators are currently exploring combinations with fludarabine (with or without cyclophosphamide) and pentostatin[1] (with and without cyclophosphamide). In general, the addition of more agents increases both the activity and toxicity of the regimen. Therefore, we favor pentostatin-containing regimens over fludarabine because of what we believe is a more favorable toxicity profile and a more convenient schedule of administration (a 1-day regimen for pentostatin compared with 3 to 5 days for fludarabine regimens). Another monoclonal antibody, alemtuzumab (Campath), has shown promise in CLL, and may have superior activity compared with rituximab. However, alemtuzumab also has greater toxicity and cannot therefore be as readily integrated into combination regimens.

Transplantation

Treatment of CLL with either autologous or allogeneic bone marrow transplantation has been reported. Overall, these therapeutic modalities are associated with a high treatment-related mortality, a high relapse rate, and only a small number of durable remissions. When absolutely necessary, we favor allogeneic over autologous transplantation as this modality is less prone to relapse. Unfortunately, allogeneic transplantation is associated with a high frequency of morbidity and mortality. Reduced-intensity allogeneic transplantation (*mini-transplants*) may ultimately play a bigger role in CLL, but results to date must still be viewed as preliminary. Therefore, at

[1]Not FDA approved for this indication.

this time, stem cell transplantation should be considered experimental and should only be offered in the context of a clinical trial.

CONCLUSIONS

Despite multiple active therapeutic agents to treat CLL, this disease remains incurable. Currently newer investigational treatment combinations, including purine analogues with cyclophosphamide and rituximab, are being investigated in an attempt to optimize response rates and generate durable complete responses. Meanwhile, novel chemotherapeutic and immune-based approaches to treating CLL should be sought in the hope of developing truly curative therapies for this disease.

Chronic Myelogenous Leukemia

Chronic myelogenous leukemia (CML) is a myeloproliferative disease characterized by leukocytosis secondary to a malignant stem cell clone containing the BCR/ABL fusion gene (karyotypic analysis reveals the Philadelphia [Ph] chromosome). The median age of diagnosis is between 50 and 60 with a 1.4:1 male predominance. The cause of CML remains largely unknown; however, the disease incidence is increased after exposure to either high doses of ionizing radiation or benzene.

DIAGNOSIS AND DISEASE PROGRESSION

The diagnosis of CML is made by the presence of leukocytosis with basophilia in the context of the BCR/ABL fusion gene. The BCR/ABL fusion gene is the result of a translocation of the Abelson (ABL) protooncogene on chromosome 9 to the breakpoint cluster region (BCR) gene on chromosome 22, generating the t(9;22)(q34;q11) Ph chromosome (Figure 1). The resulting Bcr-Abl gene product is a constitutively active cytoplasmic tyrosine kinase that drives unregulated cellular proliferation. In CML, this gene most commonly encodes for a 210-kilodalton (p210) fusion protein. The Ph chromosome is also present in approximately 20% of adult patients with ALL, usually encoding a smaller BCR/ABL fusion protein (p190). The Ph chromosome may be identified by routine karyotypic analysis, and with increasing sensitivity, by FISH and polymerase chain reaction (PCR) (Table 5).

CML is a progressive disease with three phases—chronic phase, accelerated phase, and blast phase (or blast crisis). Approximately 90% of patients are diagnosed in the chronic phase of the disease, frequently found incidentally on routine CBC. Patients in chronic phase may present with symptoms including fatigue, weight loss, bone pain, and abdominal discomfort related to splenomegaly. On peripheral blood smears, increased neutrophils in all stages of maturation are evident, with an increase in basophils. Platelets may be normal but often are markedly increased. Although blast cells are commonly seen, they generally account for less than 2% of the total WBC count. A bone marrow evaluation is essential to the staging of CML at diagnosis. In chronic phase, the bone marrow is hypercellular, with increased neutrophils in all stages of maturation. The blast percentage is typically less than 5%. Cytogenetic analysis of the peripheral blood or the bone marrow reveals the presence of the Ph chromosome by karyotype analysis, or the BCR/ABL fusion gene by FISH, but is otherwise normal. With older single-agent palliative therapies, patients typically remained in chronic phase for a median of 4 to 6 years before progression to the more aggressive accelerated and blast phases of CML.

The diagnostic parameters for distinguishing the chronic phase from the accelerated and blastic phases of the disease have traditionally been based

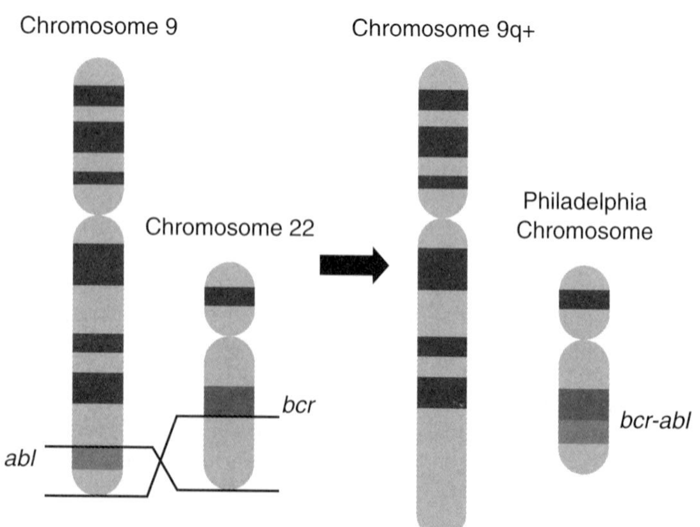

FIGURE 1 The Philadelphia chromosome: t(9;22).

TABLE 5 Detection of the Philadelphia (Ph) Chromosome

Method of Detection	Sensitivity
Cytogenetic analysis	1 Ph^+ cell in 20 normal cells
FISH analysis	1 Ph^+ cell in 500 normal cells
PCR analysis	1 Ph^+ cell in 10^4-10^8 normal cells

on bone marrow blast counts. Various cutoff points have been used in different classification schemes, but typically chronic phase should have less than 5% to 10% blasts on a bone marrow aspirate while blastic disease should be greater than 20% to 30% blasts. Patients with blast counts between these extremes are classified as having accelerated disease. Some authors also recognize other features as indicative of accelerated disease including increasing basophilia, significant thrombocytopenia or thrombocythemia, and the acquisition of additional chromosomal abnormalities by the malignant clone.

Patients with accelerated or blast phase disease have increasing leukocyte counts with worsening fatigue, weight loss, night sweats, bone pain, and abdominal pain related to increasing splenomegaly and splenic infarcts. Marked leukocytosis seen in advanced disease may be associated with thromboses and manifestations of leukostasis including cerebral ischemic events and peripheral neuropathies, gangrene, cardiorespiratory failure, priapism, and bone marrow necrosis. Severe thrombocythemia associated with advanced disease may lead to either thromboses or hemorrhage.

Accelerated phase CML is somewhere between chronic phase disease and blast crisis. In the pre-imatinib era, accelerated disease inevitably led to blast crisis and, therefore, portended a poor prognosis with a median survival of only 0.5 to 1.5 years. Approximately 70% of patients in blast crisis have blast cells of myeloid origin, while 30% are of lymphoid origin. In the pre-imatinib era, patients in blast crisis had a median survival of 3 to 6 months. Those patients with myeloid blast crisis typically had disease that was resistant to chemotherapy and, therefore, an extremely short survival, while patients with lymphoid blast crisis had somewhat more responsive but still ultimately lethal disease in most cases.

Rarely, patients may present in blast crisis, mimicking acute leukemia, without evidence of an antecedent chronic phase of CML. The presence of basophilia in this setting should alert the clinician to the possible diagnosis of CML. Rapid FISH or PCR analysis of the peripheral blood or bone marrow for the BCR/ABL fusion gene prior to treatment will aid in the accurate diagnosis of these patients.

PROGNOSIS

The most important prognostic feature in CML, regardless of therapy, is disease phase. Patients treated in the chronic phase of CML consistently have a longer survival than patients treated in the accelerated phase or blast crisis independent of therapeutic intervention. Historically, several prognostic models have been proposed to further categorize patients into low-, intermediate-, and high-risk groups. As therapy has improved, however, these prognostic models have lost value and have been replaced with newer, more relevant models. The Sokal scale had predictive value for patients treated with conventional single-agent therapies (hydroxyurea [Hydrea] and busulfan [Busulfex]). With the introduction of the disease-modifying agent interferon-alfa (INF-α), the Sokal scale was displaced as a useful tool leading to a new prognostic model, the *EURO formulation*. Both of these models recognized patient age, spleen size, platelet count, and the percentage of myeloblasts in the peripheral blood as having prognostic importance. However, it is not clear whether either of these models will be relevant in the imatinib era.

THERAPY

Response to therapy in CML is classified based on the normalization of peripheral blood counts (hematologic response), as well as the reduction of BCR/ABL-positive cells based on karyotype, FISH, and PCR analyses (Table 6).

Historically, treatment of CML was palliative, using hydroxyurea or busulfan as single-agent therapies. While these agents induced hematologic responses in a majority of patients, cytogenetic responses were rare (1% to 5%) and treatment with these agents failed to delay disease progression or improve overall survival. In the current era of CML therapy, delay in disease progression and improved overall survival are achievable goals. Treatment with allogeneic bone marrow transplantation (allo-BMT), interferon-α (INF-α [2a]), and, most importantly, imatinib mesylate (STI-571, Gleevec) significantly

TABLE 6 Response Criteria to Chronic Myelogenous Leukemia Therapy

Hematologic Response	Normal peripheral blood count WBC count <10 × 10^9/L Platelets <450 ×10^9/L No immature cells
Cytogenic Response	
Major	
Complete	0% Ph^+ chromosome cells by FISH
Partial	1%-35% Ph^+ chromosome cells by FISH
Minor	36%-95% Ph^+ chromosome cells by FISH
Molecular Response	RT-PCR negative for Ph chromosome transcripts on 2 sequential analyses

Abbreviations: Ph = Philadelphia; RT-PCR = reverse transcriptase polymerase chain reaction; WBC = white blood cell.

improves the quality of response and survival of patients with CML.

Allogeneic transplantation was the first therapeutic intervention shown to improve survival for some patients with CML. For carefully selected patients in chronic phase, 5-year survival after a matched related-donor transplant (performed at experienced centers) ranges between 60% to 80%. Results in the accelerated and blast phases are substantially worse. Results with transplants from matched unrelated donors are approximately 5% to 20% worse when compared to transplants from related donors. The success of allogeneic transplantation in CML is related in large part to the graft-versus-leukemia (GVL) effect mediated by donor T cells. For this reason, T-cell depletion of the donor stem cells before transplant results in higher relapse rates. Conversely, treatment of relapsed chronic phase CML after allo-BMT with donor T cells (donor leukocyte infusion [DLI]) results in a 70% to 80% response rate with many patients achieving complete molecular responses. Response rates for patients with relapsed blast crisis treated with DLI are far less remarkable (12% to 28%).

While proponents of allogeneic transplantation argue that this therapy is curative, a recent evaluation by Kiss et al. challenges this assertion, demonstrating continued relapse of disease even beyond 10 years out from transplant. Enthusiasm for allogeneic transplantation must also be tempered by the morbidity and mortality associated with this procedure. Furthermore, because many patients are deemed ineligible for transplantation based on age and associated co-morbidities, less than 50% of patients qualify for transplantation, and of these, only 30% will have a matched related donor.

INF-α (2α), introduced in the mid 1980s, was the first effective disease modifying agent for treatment of CML and prolonged survival compared with hydroxyurea or busulfan. This prolonged survival can be attributed to the ability of IFN-α to induce a major cytogenetic response in a minority of patients. Subsequent studies placed a great deal of attention on improving cytogenetic response rates by combining IFN-α with other agents, most commonly cytarabine (Cytosar-U). All such trials were abruptly halted with the introduction of imatinib (Gleevec).

Imatinib is a small molecule that blocks the activity of the Bcr-Abl tyrosine kinase, thereby inhibiting the proliferation of Bcr-Abl expressing cells. In a phase III comparison of initial therapy with imatinib versus interferon plus cytarabine in chronic phase disease, imatinib was vastly superior to interferon-based therapy with improved disease control (complete cytogenetic responses in 68% vs. 7%) and a far superior toxicity profile (23% of patients treated with interferon discontinued therapy because of intolerance while only 0.7% treated with imatinib discontinued therapy). Patients with accelerated or blast phase disease do not respond as well to imatinib therapy as those in chronic phase and require higher doses (600 mg per day versus 400 mg per day) to achieve optimal responses. At this dose, approximately 80% of patients with accelerated disease achieve a complete hematologic response, while 15% to 21% of patients in blast crisis obtain a complete hematologic response. Furthermore, responses in advanced disease are far less durable than those seen in chronic phase disease. Interestingly, myeloid blast crisis responds better to imatinib therapy than lymphoid blast crisis, the opposite of findings seen with conventional (pre-imatinib) therapy.

Resistance to imatinib, especially prominent in advanced disease, is thought to be mediated, in part, by acquired mutations in the Bcr-Abl protein, inhibiting imatinib binding, or through the amplification of the BCR/ABL gene. Other mechanisms of resistance have been proposed as well. Resistance through the enhanced Bcr-Abl expression may be overcome by escalating the dose of imatinib. In patients with resistant chronic phase disease, escalation of the imatinib dose from 400 mg per day to 800 mg per day may improve the response to treatment. Adding other active agents, including cytarabine and interferon, to imatinib is currently being investigated. Enthusiasm for this approach, however, is tempered by the toxicity these additional agents bring to a treatment that is otherwise essentially nontoxic.

Imatinib is very well tolerated with less than 1% to 3% of patients discontinuing therapy because of adverse events. The most common serious side effect of therapy is myelosuppression, seen more commonly in patients with advanced disease or on doses less than 400 mg per day. Other less common toxicities include hepatotoxicity, fluid retention, skin rashes, muscle cramps, bone pain, nausea, diarrhea, and vomiting.

CONCLUSIONS

Standard therapy for patients with chronic phase CML is with imatinib, 400 mg per day. Allogeneic transplantation is considered an option only if resistance to imatinib therapy is noted despite appropriate dose escalations. Patients with accelerated and blast phase disease are treated with imatinib as well but at higher doses (600 mg per day and 800 mg per day, respectively). Because of the predictably short response duration in this setting, allogeneic transplantation, if available, is offered to these patients after a hematologic response is achieved with imatinib therapy. In those patients with imatinib-refractory disease, more conventional acute leukemia-based chemotherapy regimens are offered followed by allogeneic transplantation, if appropriate.

The introduction of imatinib has revolutionized the treatment of CML, making much of the previous clinical data, prognostic modeling, and therapeutic approaches to this disease obsolete. However, only longer follow-up and further patient experience will

TABLE 7 Median Survival by Chemotherapy in Chronic Myelogenous Leukemia

Treatment	Median Survival
Busulfan (Busulfex)	4y
Hydroxyurea (Hydrea)	5y
Interferon-α (2a [Roferon-A])	6y
Imatinib (Gleevec)	>10y (estimate)

allow us to accurately assess the impact of imatinib therapy on the treatment of CML (Table 7). Nevertheless, it is the very high frequency of complete cytogenetic responses to this treatment that suggests this agent will provide long-term disease control in most patients.

NON-HODGKIN'S LYMPHOMA

METHOD OF

Lawrence Rice, MD, and Uday Popat, MD

Rather than representing a single disease, non-Hodgkin's lymphomas comprise a very diverse spectrum of disorders, varying from the most rapidly growing cancer known to the most indolent of neoplasms having no impact on well-being and requiring no treatment. Together these clonal lymphocyte proliferations comprise 5% of all cancers, ranking fifth in incidence, yet their importance is far greater than their frequency. Reasons for this include that lymphomas have critically accelerated scientific understanding of neoplasia, displaying the roles of oncogenic viruses, specific genetic alterations, and the interplay of tumor with host immune factors. Lymphomas are the most common cancers in adolescents and young adults. Regarding therapy, breakthroughs in lymphomas are being applied to curing cancers more generally. The efficacy of the earliest chemotherapy drugs was established in lymphomas; the principles of combination chemotherapy and of curative radiotherapy were gleaned.

Epidemiology and Genetics

Indolent non-Hodgkin's lymphomas are disorders of older individuals (rare below age 40). While large B-cell lymphomas are also most common after age 65 years, the incidence curve is much flatter because they also represent the most common cancer in adolescents and young adults. Other lymphomas have distinctive epidemiologic patterns, such as T-cell lymphoblastic lymphoma occurring mainly in adolescent and young adult men and primary mediastinal large B-cell lymphoma occurring in young women. Burkitt lymphoma presents as jaw tumors in children in third world countries and is related to Epstein-Barr virus (EBV) infection, but it presents as abdominal masses or leukemia in young adults in developed western countries. Hepatitis C increases the risk for several lymphomas, particularly primary, splenic, marginal-zone B-cell lymphoma. Many lymphomas increase with HIV infection, but Burkitt lymphoma and large B-cell lymphomas with central nervous system (CNS) primaries are particularly common. Mucosa-associated lymphoid tissue (MALT) lymphoma of the stomach is associated with *Helicobacter pylori*.

Lymphomas often display distinctive acquired cytogenetic abnormalities. The abnormal gene products provide clues to pathogenesis and targets for therapy. Examples include Burkitt lymphoma where translocations involve the c-myc oncogene on chromosome 8 and immunoglobulin heavy or light-chain genes. Follicular lymphomas have a characteristic t(14;18), affecting bcl-2 gene regulation of cellular apoptosis. In many lymphomas, cytogenetic patterns provide prognostic information (e.g., small lymphocytic lymphoma) or can help establish the proper diagnosis (e.g., t[11;14] with cyclin D overexpression in mantle-cell lymphoma).

Classification of Lymphomas and Leukemias

Differentiating lymphomas from lymphoid leukemias is arbitrary and semantic, based on whether a clonal neoplasm presents mainly in lymph nodes and tissues or has prominent peripheral blood involvement. Thus, B-cell chronic lymphocytic leukemia and small lymphocytic lymphoma represent different clinical presentations of the same malignant disorder; disease behavior and treatment principles are identical. Similarly, B-cell (L3 type) acute lymphoblastic leukemia and Burkitt lymphoma are the same disorder, as are T-cell acute lymphoblastic leukemia and lymphoblastic lymphoma.

A major advance in understanding and managing non-Hodgkin's lymphomas emerged 35 years ago with the Rappaport classification system. Morphologic parameters, such as whether malignant cells were large or small and whether they showed a nodular (follicular) growth pattern, separated disorders into clinically useful categories predicting disease behavior and responsiveness to therapies. Proliferating alternative classification schemes since then have daunted students and clinicians, becoming an object for satires. Nevertheless, modern classification goes beyond morphology, bringing to bear advances in molecular biology, flow cytometry, and cytogenetics to establish homogeneous disease entities that behave more predictably. Optimizing a patient's treatment requires familiarity with up-to-date classification (Table 1).

Evaluation, Staging, and Prognosis

A thorough history specifically addresses whether the B symptoms of fever, night sweat, and weight loss are present. Physical exam pays extra attention to palpating lymph nodes and abdominal viscera. All patients require a complete blood count (CBC) with differential, blood chemistries including tests of renal function, hepatic function, calcium, lactate dehydrogenase (LDH), and chest radiograph. Essential staging procedures are computed tomography (CT) scans (chest, abdomen, pelvis) and bone marrow. Bone marrow biopsy must be obtained, but bilateral biopsies are not routinely indicated. Nonroutine tests for certain patients and certain disease subtypes include lumbar puncture and gallium scanning. Positron emission tomography (PET) appears promising, and its role is being investigated. The Ann Arbor staging system remains standard: Stage I is involvement of one lymph node region (or IE single extranodal site), Stage II multiple lymph node regions on the same side of the diaphragm, Stage III lymph nodes on both sides of the diaphragm, and Stage IV extralymphatic spread such as to bone marrow, liver or pleura. "A" follows the stage if B symptoms are absent.

TABLE 1 Proposed World Health Organization Classification Scheme for Non-Hodgkin's Lymphoma

B-Cell Neoplasms

Precursor B-cell Neoplasm
- Precursor B-lymphoblastic leukemia/lymphoma

Mature B-cell Neoplasms
- B-cell chronic lymphocytic leukemia/small lymphocytic lymphoma
- B-cell prolymphocytic leukemia
- Lymphoplasmacytic lymphoma
- Splenic marginal zone B-cell lymphoma (± villous lymphocytes)
- Hairy cell leukemia
- Plasma cell myeloma/plasmacytoma
- Extranodal marginal zone B-cell lymphoma of the MALT type
- Nodal marginal zone B-cell lymphoma (± monocytoid B cells)
- Follicular lymphoma
- Mantle cell lymphoma
- Diffuse large-B-cell lymphoma
  - Mediastinal large-B-cell lymphoma
  - Primary effusion lymphoma
- Burkitt lymphoma

T-Cell and NK Cell Neoplasms

Precursor T-cell Neoplasm
- Precursor T-lymphoblastic lymphoma/leukemia

Mature T-cell Neoplasms
- T-cell prolymphocytic leukemia
- T-cell granular lymphocytic leukemia
- Aggressive NK cell leukemia
- Adult T-cell lymphoma/leukemia (HTLV-1–positive)
- Extranodal NK/T-cell lymphoma, nasal type
- Enteropathy-type T-cell lymphoma
- Hepatosplenic $\gamma\delta$ T-cell lymphoma
- Subcutaneous panniculitis-like T-cell lymphoma
- Mycosis fungoides/Sézary syndrome
- Anaplastic large-cell lymphoma, T/null cell, primary cutaneous type
- Anaplastic large-cell lymphoma, T/null cell, primary systemic type
- Peripheral T-cell lymphoma, not otherwise characterized
- Angioimmunoblastic T-cell lymphoma

Abbreviations: HTLV-1 = human T-cell leukemia virus 1; MALT = mucosa-associated lymphoid tissue; NK = natural killer.

The most important factors guiding treatment and prognosis are histology and stage. Age and comorbidities must be considered. An International Prognostic Index (IPI) for large-cell lymphomas has been found applicable to other lymphomas as well. Scores are generated from five parameters consisting of age, stage, number of extranodal sites, performance status, and serum LDH.

Treatment of Some Specific Disease Entities

INDOLENT LYMPHOMAS

The common indolent lymphomas are small lymphocytic lymphomas and grade 1 follicular lymphoma (follicular small cleaved cells), representing more than 33% of non-Hodgkin's lymphomas. The great majority (85% to 90%) present with stage III or IV disease; in fact, 90% to 100% of small lymphocytic lymphomas and 40% to 90% of grade 1 follicular lymphomas have bone marrow involvement, immediately marking them stage IV. Patients with apparent localized presentations are candidates for radiotherapy with curative intent (recognizing that 66% will eventually relapse). Adjuvant chemotherapy is under study for such patients.

Stages III and IV patients cannot be cured with standard therapies, yet median survival for asymptomatic subgroups exceeds 10 years. So, a watch-and-wait approach with no initial therapy is appropriate for most patients, given that the disease is often asymptomatic, is indolent in behavior, is incurable, and is associated with prolonged survival. (One cannot deliver palliative therapy to individuals who are asymptomatic.) Initially untreated patients average four or more years before disease progression mandates treatment, with no decrement in survival attributable to treatment delay. Twenty percent of patients with follicular lymphoma, and a greater number with small lymphocytic lymphoma, may never require treatment even after more than 10 years of follow-up.

Factors that mandate treatment at presentation or during follow-up are mainly related to emerging cytopenias (e.g., significant anemia) or systemic symptoms. Young age and psychoemotional factors can be reasons for early therapy, but most patients readily accept no initial treatment when the rationale is fully explained. A major problem impacting survival is transformation to more histologically aggressive lymphomas (Richter-like syndrome); this may occur in 5% to 10% per year regardless of treatment.

When treatment is warranted, additions to our armamentarium have increased choices, making decisions less clear-cut. Single oral alkylating agents such as cyclophosphamide (Cytoxan) and chlorambucil (Leukeran) were mainstays and remain reasonable choices for many. Response rates are approximately 50%; few patients achieve complete remission, but clinical problems may be dramatically reversed for years. These agents are inexpensive, convenient, and most experience no side effects. Potential toxicities are myelosuppression, leukemogenesis emerging after a few years (in approximately 1%), and bladder toxicity with cyclophosphamide. Cyclophosphamide (often intravenous) is the backbone of the traditional CVP regimen, which is cyclophosphamide combined with vincristine (Oncovin), and prednisone. Adding doxorubicin (Adriamycin; the CHOP regimen) adds toxicity without survival benefit in indolent lymphomas.

Nucleoside analogs, particularly fludarabine (Fludara)[1], are active in these disorders. Response rates may exceed those of alkylating agents at the costs of toxicities and inconvenience (several days monthly of intravenous therapy). Beyond myelosuppression, long-lasting immunosuppression creates significant risks for serious opportunistic infection. Newer combinations such as FC (fludarabine, cyclophosphamide) and FND (fludarabine, mitoxantrone[1] [Novantrone], dexamethasone) reduce the fludarabine dose, reducing toxicities. Spectacular remission rates have been observed with these regimens, making them attractive choices both for initial and salvage therapy.

The promise of monoclonal antibody therapy is being realized in these disorders. Rituximab (Rituxan), an anti-CD20 monoclonal antibody, can be administered singly or in combination with any chemotherapy regimen, either initially or for salvage. It has rapidly become the world's largest selling antineoplastic agent, even though the only cancers for which it is used are B-cell lymphoproliferative disorders. It is remarkably nontoxic, with fever, chill, and manageable hypotension occurring mainly during the first infusion; infectious risks are low. Understandably, regimens such as FC-R and FND-R are becoming popular. Molecular remissions are emerging with these regimens, fueling hopes that curative goals may become realistic. Other monoclonal antibodies for indolent lymphomas are more toxic and are being used for salvage therapy. These include anti-CD52 alemtuzumab (Campath)[1] for small lymphocytic lymphoma, associated with high opportunistic infection risks, and anti-CD20 antibodies conjugated to radioisotopes.

Recurrent or refractory disease is treated with approaches discussed above, but rate and duration of response shorten with each subsequent relapse. To reemphasize, observation without treatment is reasonable for asymptomatic relapse; more harm has resulted from overly aggressive treatment than the reverse. Patients transforming to large-cell lymphoma have a worse prognosis than de novo large cell lymphoma, but some respond to combination chemotherapy with or without stem cell transplants. Transplants, both autologous and allogeneic, have benefited selected patients, but utility is limited by the age of patients, the anticipation of long survival, and the frequency of bone marrow involvement, which could contaminate autografts.

Grade 2 follicular lymphomas are considered indolent, but grade 3 (follicular large cell) should be treated as diffuse large-cell lymphoma because it progresses more rapidly and because long-lasting remissions can be achieved.

DIFFUSE LARGE B-CELL LYMPHOMA

This most common lymphoma subtype comprises another 33% of cases. Unlike indolent lymphomas, these are clinically aggressive with survival of only a few months if untreated. Alkylating agents or monoclonal antibodies used alone are not effective. Contrasting with indolent lymphomas, there is a reasonable possibility of cure with appropriate chemotherapy.

Localized presentations (stage I or II) occur in 30% of large-cell cases. Nonbulky localized disease is treated with three cycles of CHOP (cyclophosphamide, doxorubicin, vincristine, prednisone) or CHOP-R (add rituximab), followed by involved field radiotherapy. A good majority of such patients are cured, as demonstrated in a randomized trial showing this approach superior to 8 cycles of CHOP without radiation.

Patients with stage III or IV disease are given six to eight cycles of CHOP or CHOP-R. Complete response to CHOP will occur in 66%, and 33% will be cured. More intensive regimens like:

- MACOP-B (methotrexate, doxorubicin, cyclophosphamide, vincristine, prednisone, bleomycin)
- ProMACE-CytaBOM (prednisone, methotrexate, doxorubicin [Adriamycin], cyclophosphamide, etoposide-cytarabine, bleomycin, vincristine [Oncovin], mechlorethamine)
- m-BACOD (methotrexate, bleomycin, doxorubicin, cyclophosphamide, vincristine, and dexamethasone)

are more toxic, more difficult to administer, and no more efficacious than CHOP. The addition of rituximab improves survival in patients older than 60, with studies now addressing younger patients.

[1]Not FDA approved for this indication.

A baseline echocardiogram is performed because of the potential cardiotoxicity of doxorubicin. Restaging procedures are usually done after four treatment courses. Two additional courses are delivered after remission is confirmed. Prophylactic intrathecal chemotherapy should be strongly considered with involvement of the testis, ovary, breast, sinuses, bone marrow, more than one extranodal site, or with a high LDH.

Recurrent or refractory disease carries a poor prognosis. Cure is still reasonably possible in candidates for autologous stem cell transplantation (those relatively young without serious co-morbidities). It is very important that they have *chemotherapy-sensitive* relapse; that is, the disease is not progressing during therapy. Common salvage regimens include:

- ICE (ifosfamide [Ifex][1], carboplatin, etoposide)
- ESHAP (etoposide [VePesid][1], methylprednisolone, high-dose cytarabine, cisplatin)
- DHAP (dexamethasone, cisplatin, cytarabine)

Approximately 33% of patients respond, but longer outlook remains bleak unless stem cell transplant ensues (event-free survival improved from 12% to 46% in a randomized study). Patients refractory to salvage therapy may be candidates for investigational agents, allogeneic transplantation, or palliative care. Peripheral T-cell lymphoma and anaplastic large-cell lymphoma are treated similarly to large-cell lymphoma.

LYMPHOBLASTIC AND BURKITT LYMPHOMAS

Lymphoblastic and Burkitt lymphomas represent variant presentations of T-cell and B-cell acute lymphoblastic leukemia (ALL), respectively. They are treated with ALL protocols, which employ vincristine, anthracyclines, cyclophosphamide[1], cytosine arabinoside[1], and methotrexate (e.g., Hyper-CVAD). Prophylactic CNS therapy is mandatory. Care must be taken to avoid the tumor lysis syndrome (especially with Burkitt lymphoma) by vigorous hydration, alkalinization of urine, allopurinol (Zyloprim), and close monitoring. About 33% of patients with these disorders can be cured by chemotherapy (higher in some patient subsets).

LYMPHOMAS RELATED TO INFECTIOUS AGENTS

HIV predisposes to many lymphomas, but particularly to Burkitt lymphoma, and primary CNS large-cell lymphoma. The addition of antiretroviral therapy to chemotherapy improves results. Hepatitis C also predisposes to several lymphomas, particularly primary splenic marginal zone lymphoma. Interferon therapy is highly efficacious for this lymphoma when associated with hepatitis C. (The toxicities of interferon relative to any benefit mitigate against its use in other lymphomas.) With MALT lymphoma of the stomach related to *Helicobacter pylori* infection, eradication of the organism with antibiotics usually results in spontaneous regression of the neoplasm.

[1]Not FDA approved for this indication.

LYMPHOMAS RELATED TO IMMUNE SUPPRESSION OR DEFICIENCY

It has been known for decades that lymphomas complicate primary immunodeficiency disorders. Lymphomas with the AIDS are addressed above. Post-transplant lymphoproliferative disorder is usually (but not always) a monoclonal proliferation of B cells expressing large amounts of EBV DNA. Incidence varies from 1% in renal transplant recipients to 2% to 5% in more heavily immunosuppressed organ transplant recipients. The main therapeutic maneuver is to stop or substantially decrease immunosuppressive therapies. This leads to disease resolution in 50% of patients. Rituximab (Rituxan) may be added, but antivirals have not proven beneficial. The prognosis is poor for patients who progress despite these actions, but some respond well to combination chemotherapy. Immunosuppressive drugs also relate to lymphomas apart from transplantation. Withdrawal of methotrexate from rheumatoid arthritis patients can produce spontaneous lymphoma regression.

Other Treatment Modalities

SURGICAL THERAPY

Surgery has been advocated for isolated extranodal lymphomas, such as stomach or bowel, but its role should be relegated to obtaining biopsy material for diagnosis. Even here, it may be supplanted by needle biopsy with ancillary flow cytometry, histochemistry, and cytogenetics, sometimes allowing definitive diagnosis. (Nonsurgical therapies of gastrointestinal lymphomas do entail a small risk of bowel perforation.)

STEM CELL (BONE MARROW) TRANSPLANT

Autologous stem cell transplants, now usually collected from peripheral blood by cytapheresis, have been favored for lymphomas. This is the preferred therapy (after cytoreduction) for patients with chemotherapy-sensitive relapse where cure remains the goal. *Up-front* use as a form of consolidation/intensification for high risk patients is under investigation. Continuing investigations address the necessity for and means to accomplish purging of tumor cells from autografts. Allogeneic transplants, seeking the advantage of graft-versus-tumor effects, afford a chance of cure for selected patients but with increased risks of toxicity. Toxicities are being reduced by less intensive conditioning regimens.

FUTURE THERAPIES

Tumor vaccines are in clinical trials, and new monoclonal antibodies loom. Molecular advances are bringing to the fore agents such as bcl-2 antisense oligonucleotides, currently in clinical trials.

MULTIPLE MYELOMA

METHOD OF

Robert A. Kyle, MD, and S. Vincent Rajkumar, MD

Multiple myeloma is characterized by the neoplastic proliferation of a single clone of plasma cells producing a monoclonal (M) protein in the serum or urine. In the United States, multiple myeloma constitutes 1% of all malignant diseases and slightly more than 10% of hematologic malignancies. The annual incidence is 4 per 100,000; the incidence in African Americans is twice that in whites. The apparent increase in rate is probably because of increased availability and use of medical facilities and improved diagnostic techniques, particularly in the older population. The median age at diagnosis is 65 to 70 years, and only 2% of patients are younger than 40 years.

Weakness, fatigue, bone pain, recurrent infections, and symptoms of hypercalcemia or renal insufficiency should alert the physician to the possibility of multiple myeloma. Anemia is present in 70% of patients at the time of diagnosis. An M protein is found in the serum or urine in 97% of patients with multiple myeloma. Lytic lesions, osteoporosis, or fractures are present at diagnosis in 80%. Technetium bone scanning is inferior to conventional radiography and should not be used. Magnetic resonance imaging (MRI) or computed tomography (CT) is helpful in patients who have skeletal pain but no abnormality on radiographs or when spinal cord compression is suspected. Hypercalcemia is present in 25% of patients, and the serum creatinine value is 2 mg/dL or greater in almost 20% of patients at diagnosis.

Diagnosis

If multiple myeloma is suspected, the patient should have, in addition to a complete history and physical examination, the following:

- Determination of values for hemoglobin, leukocytes with differential count, platelets, serum creatinine, calcium, and uric acid
- Radiographic survey of bones, including humeri and femurs
- Serum protein electrophoresis with immunofixation
- Quantitation of immunoglobulins
- Bone marrow aspirate and biopsy
- Routine urinalysis
- Electrophoresis and immunofixation of an adequately concentrated aliquot from a 24-hour urine specimen

Measurement of β_2-microglobulin, C-reactive protein, and lactate dehydrogenase values is helpful for prognosis. Cytogenetics and measurement of the plasma cell labeling index are also important from a prognostic standpoint.

Minimal criteria for the diagnosis of multiple myeloma consist of more than 10% plasma cells in the bone marrow or a plasmacytoma and *one* of the following:

- M protein in the serum (usually more than 3 g/dL)
- M protein in the urine
- Lytic bone lesions

In addition, the usual clinical features of multiple myeloma must be present. Metastatic carcinoma, lymphoma, leukemia, and connective tissue disorders may resemble multiple myeloma and must be considered in the differential diagnosis. Patients with multiple myeloma must be differentiated from those with monoclonal gammopathy of undetermined significance (benign monoclonal gammopathy) and smoldering (asymptomatic) multiple myeloma, because they may remain stable for long periods (Table 1). The plasma cell labeling index is helpful in differentiating monoclonal gammopathy of

TABLE 1 Mayo Clinic Criteria for the Diagnosis of MGUS, SMM, and MM

MGUS	Serum monoclonal protein <3 g/dL, bone marrow plasma cells <10%, and absence of anemia, renal failure, hypercalcemia, and lytic bone lesions
SMM	Serum monoclonal protein ≥3 g/dL and/or bone marrow plasma cells ≥10% and absence of anemia, renal failure, hypercalcemia, and lytic bone lesions
MM	Presence of a serum or urine monoclonal protein, bone marrow plasmacytosis and anemia, renal failure, hypercalcemia, or lytic bone lesions; patients with primary systemic amyloidosis and ≥30% bone marrow plasma cells are considered to have both multiple myeloma and amyloidosis

Abbreviations: MGUS = monoclonal gammopathy of undetermined significance; MM = multiple myeloma; SMM = smoldering multiple myeloma.

Modified from Rajkumar SV, Dispenzieri A, Fonseca R, Lacy MQ, Geyer S, Lust JA, et al: Thalidomide for previously untreated indolent or smoldering multiple myeloma. Leukemia 15:1274-6, 2001. Used by permission from Nature Publishing Group.

undetermined significance or smoldering multiple myeloma from multiple myeloma. The patient's symptoms, physical findings, and all laboratory and radiographic data must be considered in the decision to begin therapy. If there are doubts about whether to begin treatment, therapy should be withheld and the patient reevaluated in 2 to 3 months. There is no evidence that early treatment of multiple myeloma is advantageous.

Therapy

If the patient is age 70 years or younger, the physician should consider autologous peripheral blood stem cell transplantation. The hematopoietic stem cells should be collected before the patient is exposed to alkylating agents. Patients older than age 70 years, or younger patients in whom transplantation is not feasible, should be treated with standard alkylating agent therapy.

AUTOLOGOUS PERIPHERAL BLOOD STEM CELL TRANSPLANTATION

In general, if the patient is age 70 years or younger, the physician should seriously consider autologous peripheral blood stem cell transplantation. Some patients older than age 70 years are physiologically younger, whereas some patients younger than age 70 years may have medical problems such as heart disease, pulmonary insufficiency, or renal failure and are not suitable candidates for an autologous stem cell transplant. The patient should first be treated with a chemotherapy regimen that is not toxic to the hematopoietic stem cells. Most physicians initially treat with VAD therapy—vincristine (Oncovin)[1], 0.4 mg/m^2; doxorubicin (Adriamycin)[1], 9 mg/m^2, intravenously each day for 4 days; and dexamethasone (Decadron)[1], 40 mg orally, on days 1 to 4, 9 to 12, and 17 to 20 each month for 3 to 4 months to reduce the number of tumor cells in the bone marrow and peripheral blood. We have found that the oral regimen of thalidomide (Thalomid)[1], 200 mg per day; plus dexamethasone[1], 40 mg per day on days 1 to 4, 9 to 12, and 17 to 20 in odd cycles; and dexamethasone[1], 40 mg per day on days 1 to 4 in the even cycles produces response rates similar to those of VAD, with less toxicity. Venous thrombosis, sedation, constipation, and rash constitute the most frequent side effects of thalidomide. Another option is the use of oral dexamethasone as a single agent. Randomized trials comparing dexamethasone alone to thalidomide plus dexamethasone are ongoing. We proceed with stem cell transplantation even if the patient has not responded to therapy.

Most physicians use granulocyte colony-stimulating factor (G-CSF; filgrastim [Neupogen]) for stem cell collection. After stem cell collection, autologous stem cell transplantation can proceed as soon as the patient has recovered or the transplantation can be delayed and the patient treated with standard alkylating agent therapy, the transplantation being reserved for relapsed disease. There is no difference in overall survival among patients who receive an autologous stem cell transplant immediately after collection and those who receive it at first relapse. We recommend autologous stem cell transplantation as soon as the patient has recovered from the stem cell collection because the patient is saved the inconvenience of prolonged chemotherapy and the potential risk of myelodysplasia from treatment with alkylating agents. Currently, approximately 50% of patients receiving an autologous stem cell transplant are treated as outpatients.

Melphalan (Alkeran), 200 mg/m^2,[3] is the most widely used preparative regimen for autologous stem cell transplantation. Melphalan plus total body irradiation is rarely used because it produces more side effects, particularly mucositis, and is not more effective.

In two studies from France and the United Kingdom, peripheral stem cell transplantation was superior to combination chemotherapy. Progression-free survival was longer and median overall survival was increased by approximately 1 year in the transplant group.

It is not known whether maintenance therapy after transplantation is advantageous. Most physicians do not give therapy after transplantation and simply follow the patient for evidence of relapse. Maintenance options are interferon alfa-2a[1] (Roferon-A) or 2b (Intron A), prednisone[1] every 48 hours, or low-dose thalidomide (Thalomid)[1]; but prospective studies are needed to demonstrate benefit. The role of double or tandem autologous stem cell transplantation is controversial. In a randomized study from France, there was no difference in event-free or overall survival between the single and double autologous stem cell transplant groups when evaluated at 2 years, but at 7 years both event-free and overall survival were superior in the double transplant group. Final results are awaited from this and other randomized trials comparing the two approaches.

Fortunately, the mortality rate with autologous stem cell transplantation is approximately 1%. However, the two major shortcomings are that multiple myeloma is not eradicated even with large doses of chemotherapy and, in addition, the autologous peripheral stem cells are contaminated by myeloma cells or their precursors. In an effort to improve the preparative regimen, the addition of bone-seeking radioisotopes that provide increased radiation to the bone marrow (such as holmium 166 and samarium 153) is being investigated. In an effort to reduce the contamination of hematopoietic stem cells, CD34 selection was studied. Even though contaminating tumor cells were reduced by three logs,

[1]Not FDA approved for this indication.

[3]Exceeds dosage recommended by the manufacturer.
[1]Not FDA approved for this indication.

there was no prolongation of event-free or overall survival with this approach.

SYNGENEIC OR ALLOGENEIC BONE MARROW TRANSPLANTATION

Bone marrow transplantation from an identical twin donor (syngeneic) is the treatment of choice if a donor is available. Results are superior to allogeneic transplantation.

Allogeneic bone marrow transplantation is advantageous in that the graft contains no tumor cells and there is a graft-versus-tumor effect. However, subsequent graft-versus-host disease is troublesome. Furthermore, only 5% to 10% of patients with multiple myeloma are eligible for allogeneic transplantation because a human leukocyte antigen (HLA)-compatible donor is available in only 33% of patients and 90% are age 50 years or older. Currently, allogeneic transplantation is associated with too high a mortality and cannot be recommended. However, promising efforts are under way to reduce allogeneic transplant-related mortality using T-cell depletion or nonmyeloablative regimens.

Nonmyeloablative (*mini-allo*) allogeneic protocols following an autologous stem cell transplantation are being pursued. It is hoped that the benefits of an allograft may be realized while the toxicity associated with the procedure is decreased. The mortality is 10% to 15%, and graft-versus-host disease remains troublesome. Efforts are being made to reduce the toxicity of this approach. Currently, we believe that nonmyeloablative approaches should be limited to protocol studies.

STANDARD ALKYLATING AGENT THERAPY

Alkylating agent-based chemotherapy with oral administration of melphalan and prednisone produces an objective response in 50% to 60% of patients and a median survival of 2 to 3 years. We prefer to give melphalan orally in a dosage of 8 to 10 mg daily for 7 days and prednisone in a dosage of 20 mg three times a day orally for the same 7 days. If the serum creatinine value is more than 2 mg/dL (177 mmol/L), the initial dose of melphalan should be reduced by 25%. Melphalan should be given when the patient is fasting because absorption is reduced after food is eaten. Leukocyte and platelet counts must be determined at 3-week intervals after the start of therapy and the melphalan dosage altered until mid-cycle cytopenia occurs. The melphalan and prednisone regimen should be repeated every 6 weeks. If the neutrophil count is less than 1500/mm^3 or the platelet count is less than 100,000/mm^3 at 6 weeks, chemotherapy should be delayed and the counts determined at weekly intervals until the pretreatment level is reached. If the neutrophil or platelet counts remain low or if the counts are unduly low at 3 weeks, the melphalan dose in the next 7-day course must be reduced. Unless the disease progresses rapidly, at least three courses of melphalan and prednisone should be given before this therapy is abandoned. An objective response may not be achieved for 6 to 12 months, or longer in some patients. The natural course of multiple myeloma is one of progression, and if the patient's pain is alleviated and there is no evidence of progressive disease, the therapeutic regimen is beneficial despite the failure to reach an objective response.

Chemotherapy should be continued for at least 1 year or until the patient is in a plateau state. This is defined as stable serum and urine M-protein levels and no evidence of progression. Continued chemotherapy is not recommended because it may lead to the development of a myelodysplastic syndrome or acute leukemia. Patients should be followed closely during the plateau state, and the same chemotherapy should be reinstituted if relapse occurs more than 6 months later.

Because of the obvious shortcomings of melphalan and prednisone, various combinations of therapeutic agents have been tried. A large meta-analysis, based on data from 6,633 patients in 30 trials comparing melphalan and prednisone with various combinations of chemotherapy, was performed by the Myeloma Trialists Collaborative Group. Although the response rate was higher with combination chemotherapy, there was no survival benefit over melphalan. This meta-analysis also failed to find any category of patients in which combination chemotherapy had a significantly different mortality rate from that with melphalan and prednisone. There was no evidence that poor-risk patients did better with combination chemotherapy than with melphalan and prednisone. Consequently, melphalan and prednisone remain standard treatment outside of clinical trials for patients who are not candidates for autologous stem cell transplantation.

Treatment for Refractory Multiple Myeloma, Including Use of Novel Agents

Almost all patients with multiple myeloma who survive eventually have relapse. If relapse occurs more than 6 months after the plateau state has been reached, the initial chemotherapy regimen should be reinstituted. Most patients will respond again, but the duration and quality of response are usually inferior to the initial response. Patients who are initially refractory or who become refractory to alkylating-agent therapy generally have a low response rate to subsequent chemotherapy and a short survival. The highest response rates in such patients have been with intravenous VAD. VAD given by bolus injection also has been used. Many physicians choose single-agent dexamethasone[1] instead because it accounts for about 80% of the effect of VAD. Methylprednisolone, 2 g intravenously

[1]Not FDA approved for this indication.

three times weekly for a minimum of 4 weeks, is helpful for patients with pancytopenia, and we find fewer side effects than from dexamethasone. Other regimens, including VBMCP (vincristine [Oncovin][1], BiCNU, melphalan, cyclophosphamide [Cytoxan], and prednisone) or VBAP (vincristine[1], BiCNU, doxorubicin [Adriamycin][1] intravenously, and prednisone orally), are useful in relapsed disease. Interferon alfa-2a[1] as a single agent for refractory disease has been disappointing, with objective responses of 10% to 20%.

Novel agents for the treatment of multiple myeloma include thalidomide[1] and its analog CC-5013 (Revlimid)* and the recently approved proteasome inhibitor bortezomib (Velcade, PS-341). Thalidomide is usually given in a dosage of 200 mg daily, with an increase to 400 mg daily as tolerated. Objective responses occur in approximately 33% of patients and last for a median duration of approximately 12 months. The addition of dexamethasone to thalidomide increases the response rate. Side effects from thalidomide include weakness, fatigue, constipation, and somnolence. Rashes, thrombotic events, and sensorimotor peripheral neuropathy are more troublesome side effects.

The immunomodulatory thalidomide derivative CC-5013 (Revlimid)* has shown activity in previously treated patients but is not yet commercially available. Phase II studies produce response in 30% of patients, and constipation, somnolence, and neuropathy have not been observed so far.

Bortezomib produced objective response in 35% of patients with relapsed, refractory myeloma who had received at least two prior therapeutic regimens. It is administered as an intravenous bolus dose of 1.3 mg/m^2 twice weekly for 2 weeks, followed by a 10-day rest period for a maximum of eight 21-day cycles. The median duration of response is approximately 12 months. Adverse events include fatigue, anorexia, nausea and vomiting, fever, diarrhea, constipation, anemia, asthenia, peripheral neuropathy, neutropenia, and thrombocytopenia. The agent has been given accelerated approval by the Food and Drug Administration for the treatment of relapsed, refractory myeloma in patients in whom two or more prior regimens have failed.

Supportive Therapy

RADIOTHERAPY

Palliative radiation in a dose of 20 to 30 Gy should be limited to patients with disabling pain who have a well-defined focal process that has not responded to chemotherapy. Analgesics in combination with chemotherapy usually can control the pain. This approach is preferred to local radiation because pain frequently occurs at another site, and local radiation does not benefit the patient with systemic disease. In addition, the myelosuppressive effects of radiotherapy and chemotherapy are cumulative and may restrict future therapy.

HYPERCALCEMIA

Hypercalcemia must be suspected if the patient has anorexia, nausea, vomiting, polyuria, increased constipation, weakness, confusion, stupor, or coma. If it is untreated, renal insufficiency usually develops. Hydration, preferably with isotonic saline and prednisone (25 mg orally four times daily) is effective in most patients. The dosage of prednisone must be reduced and discontinued as soon as possible. After hydration has been achieved, furosemide (Lasix) may be helpful. If these measures fail, a bisphosphonate such as zoledronic acid (Zometa) or pamidronate (Aredia) should be tried.

RENAL INSUFFICIENCY

Approximately 20% of patients with multiple myeloma have a serum creatinine level of 2.0 mg/dL or more at diagnosis. *Myeloma kidney* and hypercalcemia are the two major causes. Myeloma kidney is characterized by the presence of large, waxy, laminated casts in the distal and collecting tubules. Some light chains are very nephrotoxic, but no specific amino acid sequence of the light chain has been identified.

Dehydration, infection, nonsteroidal anti-inflammatory agents, and radiographic contrast media may contribute to acute renal failure. Hyperuricemia or amyloid deposition may produce renal insufficiency. Nephrotic syndrome rarely occurs in multiple myeloma unless amyloidosis is present.

Maintenance of a high fluid intake producing 3 liters of urine per 24 hours is important for preventing renal failure in patients with Bence Jones proteinuria. Intravenous pyelography or preparation for barium enema can be performed with little risk if dehydration is avoided. If hyperuricemia occurs, allopurinol (Zyloprim), 300 mg daily, provides effective therapy.

Acute renal failure should be treated promptly with appropriate fluid and electrolyte replacement. Patients with acute or subacute renal failure should be treated with VAD or dexamethasone to reduce the tumor mass as quickly as possible. A trial of plasmapheresis is recommended in an attempt to prevent chronic dialysis. Hemodialysis and peritoneal dialysis are equally effective and are necessary for patients with symptomatic azotemia. Renal transplantation for myeloma kidney has been followed by prolonged survival.

ANEMIA

Almost every patient with multiple myeloma eventually becomes anemic. Increase of plasma volume

[1]Not FDA approved for this indication.
*Investigational drug in the United States.

from the osmotic effect of the M protein may produce hypervolemia and spuriously lower the hemoglobin and hematocrit values. Erythropoietin (Epogen, Procrit) reduces the transfusion requirement and increases hemoglobin concentration in more than 50% of patients. Those with low serum erythropoietin values are more likely to respond. Most physicians proceed with a trial of erythropoietin at a dose of 150 U/kg three times weekly or 40,000 units once a week. Darbepoietin, a long-lasting erythropoietin, may be given weekly or biweekly.

SKELETAL LESIONS

Bone lesions manifested by pain and fractures are a major problem. A skeletal radiographic survey should be repeated at 6-month intervals, or sooner if pain develops. Patients should be encouraged to be as active as possible because confinement to bed increases demineralization of the skeleton. Trauma must be avoided because even mild stress may result in a fracture. Fixation of long bone fractures or impending fractures with an intramedullary rod and methyl methacrylate has given excellent results. All patients with multiple myeloma who have lytic lesions, pathologic fractures, or severe osteopenia should receive intravenous bisphosphonates indefinitely. Zoledronic acid (Zometa), 4 mg intravenously over 15 minutes every 4 weeks, or pamidronate (Aredia), 90 mg intravenously over 2 hours every 4 weeks are equally efficacious. Because renal insufficiency or nephrotic-range proteinuria may occur, serum creatinine and 24-hour urine protein monitoring is necessary. Vertebroplasty or kyphoplasty may be helpful for patients with compression fracture of the spine.

INFECTIONS

Bacterial infections are more common in patients with myeloma than in the general population. Pneumococcal and influenza immunization should be given to all patients despite their suboptimal antibody response. Substantial fever is an indication for appropriate cultures, chest radiography, and consideration of antibiotic therapy. The greatest risk for infection is during the first 2 months after initiation of chemotherapy. Prophylactic trimethoprim-sulfamethoxazole[1] (Bactrim, Septra) may be useful during the first 2 months of chemotherapy. Prophylactic daily oral penicillin may benefit patients with recurrent pneumococcal infections. Intravenously administered immunoglobulin[1] may be helpful for patients with recurrent infections, but it is too expensive for long-term therapy.

HYPERVISCOSITY SYNDROME

The symptoms of hyperviscosity may include oronasal bleeding, gastrointestinal bleeding, blurred vision, neurologic symptoms, or congestive heart failure. Most patients have symptoms when the serum viscosity measurement is more than four times that of normal serum, but the relationship between serum viscosity and clinical manifestations is imprecise. The decision to perform plasmapheresis, which promptly relieves the symptoms of hyperviscosity, should be made on clinical grounds rather than on serum viscosity levels. Hyperviscosity is more common in IgA myeloma than in IgG myeloma.

EXTRADURAL MYELOMA (CORD COMPRESSION)

The possibility of cord compression must be excluded if weakness of the legs or difficulty in voiding or defecating occurs. The sudden onset of severe radicular pain or severe back pain is suggestive of compression of the spinal cord. MRI or CT is most helpful for diagnosis. Radiation therapy in a dose of approximately 30 Gy is beneficial. Dexamethasone should be administered during radiation therapy to reduce edema.

EMOTIONAL SUPPORT

All patients with multiple myeloma need substantial and continuing emotional support. The physician's approach must be positive in emphasizing the potential benefits of therapy. It is reassuring for patients to know that some survive for 10 years or more. It is vital that the physician caring for patients with multiple myeloma has the interest and capacity for dealing with incurable disease over the span of years with assurance, sympathy, and resourcefulness.

POLYCYTHEMIA VERA

METHOD OF

Jose F. Leis, MD, PhD

Polycythemia vera (PV) is a clonal chronic myeloproliferative disorder characterized by an elevated red blood cell (RBC) mass that is usually accompanied by leukocytosis, thrombocytosis, and splenomegaly. PV is a rare disorder with an annual incidence of 2.3 per 100,000 in the United States and Western Europe. Median age at diagnosis is in the seventh decade with the disease being rare before the age of 40 years. Patients often present with nonspecific complaints including headaches, fatigue, pruritus, sweat, abdominal distress, and weight loss. However, increasingly more patients whom are asymptomatic are being diagnosed with PV due to the widespread use of laboratory testing during routine examination.

[1]Not FDA approved for this indication.

The most frequent cause of morbidity and mortality in PV is vascular thrombosis. This results as a direct consequence of an increased red cell mass and abnormal platelet metabolism seen in all patients. Patients can present with deep venous thrombosis, pulmonary embolism, or vascular occlusions of the peripheral, cerebral, or coronary vessels. Thromboses in unusual anatomic sites such as the splenic, hepatic (Budd-Chiari syndrome), portal, and mesenteric vessels are not infrequent. Early studies of untreated patients noted a high incidence of thrombotic complications and a median survival of 18 months. Except for a few select cases with allogeneic transplantation, PV remains incurable. However, extended median survivals of greater than 10 years are now routine with optimal management.

Etiology and Pathobiology

X-chromosome inactivation studies using glucose-6-phosphate dehydrogenase (G6PD) polymorphisms and restriction fragment length polymorphisms have clearly demonstrated that PV is due to a clonal proliferation of neoplastic hematopoietic stem cells. The clonal proliferation involves red cells, granulocytes, monocytes, and platelets. Multiple studies have shown that red cell precursors from patients with PV are capable of growing in culture media in an erythropoietin (EPO)-independent manner. In addition these precursors are hypersensitive to other growth factors including stem cell factor, interleukin (IL)-3, granulocyte-macrophage colony-stimulating factor (GM-CSF), and insulin-like growth factor-1. Myeloid and megakaryocytic progenitors also show hypersensitivity to growth factors. This observation has led to the suggestion that a defect in a signaling pathway common to multiple growth factor receptors is at the root of the disease. However, to date no candidate gene or protein has been identified.

The etiology of PV is unknown. Twenty percent of PV patients have cytogenetic abnormalities at diagnosis. The most common cytogenetic abnormality is a deletion in the long arm of chromosome 20. Trisomies of chromosomes 8 and 9 are also relatively common. Recent studies suggest that abnormal karyotype at diagnosis is a poor prognosis indicator and associated with decreased median survival. Chromosomal abnormalities are more common in patients receiving myelosuppressive therapy, and, over the course of the disease, greater than 80% of patients have an abnormal karyotype with more than 10 years follow-up. An intensive search is currently underway to identify the gene(s) involved at the sites of recurrent cytogenetic abnormalities.

Diagnosis

The PV Study Group (PVSG) established the diagnostic criteria for PV in the 1970s. Major criteria included an elevated red cell mass, normal arterial oxygen saturation, and splenomegaly, while minor criteria including thrombocytosis, leukocytosis, elevated leukocyte alkaline phosphatase, and elevated serum vitamin B_{12}. These criteria were limited by the tests available at the time and did not include measurement of serum EPO levels, cytogenetics to establish clonality, ultrasound to evaluate splenomegaly, or EPO-independent colony proliferation. Updated modified criteria have been recently proposed and are shown in Table 1. Molecular assays may soon prove useful in establishing the diagnosis of PV as well. Granulocytes from PV patients overexpress the mRNA for the neutrophil antigen NBI/CD177 (designated PRV-1). Overexpression of PRV-1 is not seen in secondary causes of erythrocytosis and appears to be specific for PV.

TABLE 1 Diagnostic Criteria for Polycythemia Vera (PV)

Category A

1. Elevated red cell mass (>25% above predicted mean or hematocrit >60% in males, >56% in females)
2. Absence of secondary erythrocytosis
3. Palpable splenomegaly
4. Clonal cytogenetic abnormality

Category B

1. Thrombocytosis (platelet count $>400 \times 10^9$/L)
2. Leucocytosis (absolute neutrophil count $>10 \times 10^9$/L; 12.5×10^9/L in smokers)
3. Splenomegaly by radiographic measurement
4. Erythropoietin-independent BFU-E growth or decreased serum erythropoietin level

Diagnosis of PV requires one of the following:
- Category A, numbers 1 + 2 + 3
- Category A, number 4
- Category A, numbers 1 + 2, + two criteria from category B

Abbreviation: BFU-E = burst-forming unit-erythroid.

In establishing the diagnosis of PV it is important to rule out secondary causes of erythrocytosis (Table 2). A detailed history to evaluate for chronic hypoxia (smoking, sleep apnea, or chronic lung disease), renal disease, prior or current thrombosis, and familial erythrocytosis is essential. Nearly 66% of all thrombotic events seen in a large PV study occurred at presentation or in the 2 years preceding diagnosis. Initial evaluation should include a complete blood count (CBC), arterial oxygen saturation, ferritin, vitamin B_{12}, folate, creatinine, liver function tests, uric acid, abdominal ultrasound, serum EPO level, and bone marrow evaluation with cytogenetics. Serum EPO level may be the most useful in differentiating PV from secondary erythrocytosis. Elevated EPO levels are suggestive of secondary erythrocytosis, whereas low-to-normal levels suggest the diagnosis of PV. If the above workup is unrevealing, additional studies may help establish the diagnosis, including:

- EPO-independent burst-forming unit-erythroid (BFU-E) colony growth

TABLE 2 Common Causes of Acquired Secondary Erythrocytosis

Hypoxemia Associated
Chronic lung disease
Sleep apnea
High altitude
Carbon monoxide poisoning
Smoking
Renal Disease
Renal artery stenosis
Renal tumors
Cysts
Diffuse parenchymal disease
Hydronephrosis
Kidney transplantation
Miscellaneous
Liver disease (hepatitis, cirrhosis, hepatoma)
Endocrine (adrenal tumors)
Androgen use
Miscellaneous tumors (uterine fibroids, cerebellar hemangioblastoma, bronchial carcinoma)

- X-chromosome–linked DNA probes, such as the human androgen receptor (HUMARA) gene probe to demonstrate clonal granulocytes (only useful in females)
- EPO receptor mutation analysis

Clinical Course and Complications

Early studies of untreated patients with PV showed a median survival of 18 months with a high incidence of thrombotic events. A large retrospective study by the Gruppo Italiano di Studio sulla PV (GISP) involved 1213 treated PV patients followed over 20 years. It showed a median survival in excess of 15 years with an age- and sex-matched mortality rate that was 1.7 times that of the general population. Death was most frequently caused by thrombotic complications including venous thromboembolic events, myocardial infarction, and ischemic stroke. Prior history of thrombosis and age were most predictive of a vascular event. Major hemorrhage was uncommon and accounted for less than 3% of deaths. The larger prospective European Collaboration on Low-dose Aspirin in PV (ECLAP) Project has recently verified these observations. On the basis of these studies, patients with PV can be stratified into three risk groups for developing thrombotic complications (Table 3).

Nearly 10% to 15% of PV patients progress to the myeloid metaplasia with myelofibrosis (MMM) *spent phase* on average 10 years after diagnosis. The incidence of MMM continues to increase to less than 30% by 20 years. Spent phase is not modified by current therapy and is characterized by increasing splenomegaly, bone marrow fibrosis, leukoerythroblastic peripheral blood features, and pancytopenia. The majority of patients in spent phase die in less than 3 years, frequently from progression to acute monoblastic leukemia (AML).

TABLE 3 Risk of Thrombosis in Polycythemia Vera

	Relative Risk Category		
Risk Factor	**Low**	**Intermediate**	**High**
Age >60 years	–	–	+
History of thrombosis	–	–	+
History of cardiovascular risk factors*	–		+

*Cardiovascular risk factors include smoking, diabetes, hypertension, hypercholesterolemia, and congestive heart failure.

Current Management Strategies

The goal of therapy is threefold:

1. Minimize the risk of thrombotic complications.
2. Decrease the risk of progression to MMM and acute leukemia.
3. Control patient symptoms.

Early randomized studies from the PVSG showed that phlebotomy alone led to improved median survival when compared with alkylating agent therapy or radiation. However, phlebotomy was associated with poor compliance and excess early mortality in the first 3 to 5 years from thrombotic complications. Patients treated with radiation (^{32}P) or alkylating agents had higher rates of leukemic transformation (>10%) and other malignancies. Subsequent PVSG trials focused on hydroxyurea[1] (Hydrea) (HU), an antimetabolite that prevents DNA synthesis by inhibiting the enzyme ribonucleotide reductase, in hope that the agent is nonleukemogenic. Clinical trials using HU[1] have demonstrated rapid responses with a decrease in the incidence of thrombosis. However, lingering questions regarding its leukemogenic potential remain because of studies that show an acute leukemia rate of 5% to 10%. To date no randomized trial comparing HU[1] to phlebotomy alone has been undertaken. Despite the apparent increased incidence of acute leukemia after HU[1] use its lowering of the incidence of thrombosis makes it a useful drug in patients whose disease cannot be controlled with phlebotomy alone. Evidence-based treatment recommendations for patients with PV are shown in Figure 1.

Despite recent advances in our understanding of PV, phlebotomy remains the cornerstone of therapy. The blood volume should be reduced as rapidly as possible to decrease the risk of thrombosis. In patients who are in otherwise good health a suggested approach is to phlebotomize 250 to 500 cc every other day until the hematocrit is less than 45%. Patients with impaired cardiopulmonary status or those over 65 years of age should have phlebotomy every 3 to 4 days with smaller volumes of blood removed. Blood counts should be checked every few weeks, and the hematocrit maintained in the 42% to 45% range. The frequency of phlebotomy will decrease as the patient develops iron

[1]Not FDA approved for this indication.

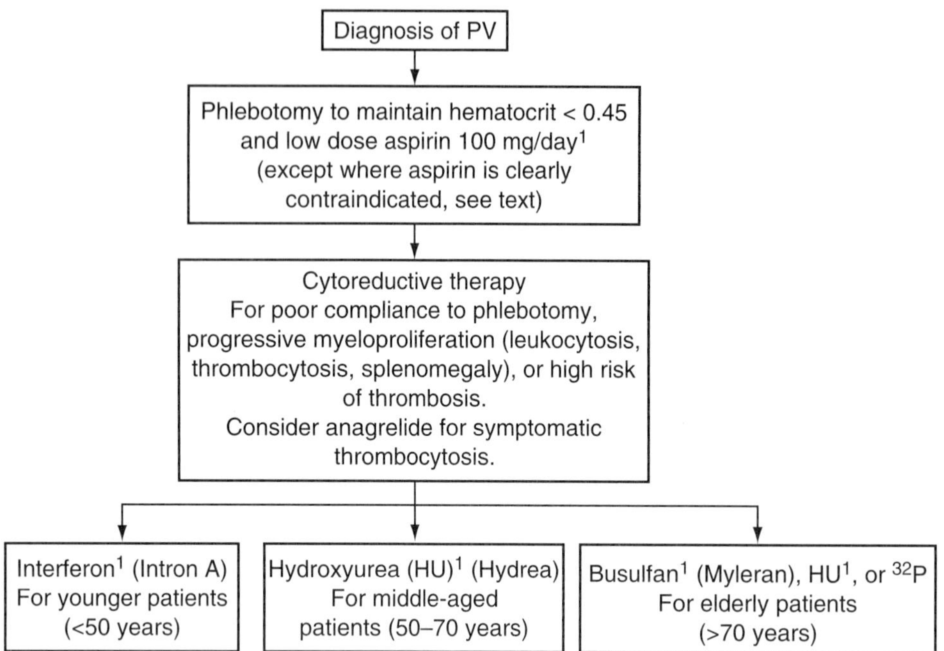

FIGURE 1 Suggested evidence-based treatment algorithm for patients with polycythemia vera (PV).

deficiency. Iron replacement therapy is not recommended as this aggravates erythropoiesis.

Phlebotomy alone has improved survival of patients with PV to 10 to 15 years. However, phlebotomy alone is associated with a higher incidence of early serious thrombotic events and does not control progressive myeloproliferation. Patients with a high risk for thrombotic events, such as those over 65 years of age or those with prior history of thrombosis, should receive myelosuppressive therapy concomitantly with their phlebotomy. HU[1] is the most commonly used cytoreductive agent with a starting dose of 15 to 30 mg/kg per day. Dose is typically decreased to 15 mg/kg per day after 1 week then adjusted weekly to avoid significant leukopenia or thrombocytopenia. The majority of patients exhibit good control of their myeloproliferative disorder with daily doses of 500 to 1000 mg. For patients who do not respond to or do not tolerate HU[1] and elderly patients, oral busulfan (Myleran)[1] at 4 to 6 mg per day for 4 to 8 weeks may be used. Dosing should be stopped when blood counts normalize or platelet count falls below 300,000/mm^3.

Interferon alfa-2b (intron A)[1] (IFN), a biologic response modifier that suppresses hematopoietic progenitor proliferation and antagonizes platelet-derived growth factor (PDGF), has been investigated in several small studies of patients with PV. Clinical trials demonstrated control of erythrocytosis and normalization of the hematocrit in nearly 70% of patients after 6 to 12 months of therapy. In addition, IFN[1]-controlled leukocytosis, thrombocytosis, splenomegaly, and pruritus in the majority of patients enrolled. The incidence of deep venous thrombosis was also significantly decreased. As in chronic myelogenous leukemia (CML), complete cytogenetic responses have been reported. Initial dosing should be 3 million units subcutaneously three times per week with dose adjusted for response and toxicity. IFN[1] therapy appears particularly attractive for young patients with PV as it appears to be nonleukemogenic. Unfortunately, side effects from the drug result in discontinuation of therapy in 20% to 30% of patients.

The role of aspirin[1] in prevention of thrombosis in PV has been clarified by the recently completed ECLAP project. An early randomized study from the PVSG (PVSG-05) suggested an increased risk of bleeding without a reduction of thrombotic complications with the use of aspirin[1] at 900 mg per day. The finding of enhanced thromboxane A_2 biosynthesis in patients with PV suggested that thromboxane-dependent platelet activation might play a role in the increased thrombotic risk. This observation combined with the GISP study, which showed an overall unfavorable impact of myelosuppressive agents, suggested that antithrombotic strategies such as low-dose aspirin should be reexamined. In an intention-to-treat analysis, the ECLAP project enrolled 518 PV patients without a clear indication or contraindication to aspirin therapy in a double-blind, placebo-controlled, randomized clinical trial aimed at assessing the efficacy and safety of low-dose aspirin[1] (100 mg per day) in addition to standard cytoreductive therapy. The use of low-dose aspirin[1] lowered the risk of cardiovascular death, nonfatal myocardial

[1]Not FDA approved for this indication.

[1]Not FDA approved for this indication.

infarction, nonfatal stroke, pulmonary embolism, and major venous thrombosis (relative risk 0.40, 95% CI (confidence interval) 0.18-0.91, p = 0.0277). Total and cardiovascular mortality were also reduced by 46% and 59%, respectively. Major hemorrhage was only slightly increased by aspirin[1] in a nonsignificant manner (relative risk 1.62, 95% CI 0.27-9.71). The investigators concluded that low-dose aspirin[1] should be considered as an evidence-based component of the long-term management of PV except in patients with clear contraindication for its use and that the benefit-to-risk profile of low-dose aspirin[1] in PV is comparable to that seen for the use of low-dose aspirin in prevention of cardiovascular death.

PV patients with thrombosis or hemorrhage in the setting of severe thrombocytosis may benefit from the use of anagrelide (Agrylin)[1], an oral imidazoquinazoline agent that inhibits platelet production through its direct effects on megakaryocyte maturation. Clinical trials of anagrelide in PV have demonstrated that 66% of patients have an excellent response with platelet reduction observed within 1 week and time to complete response generally between days 17 and 25. Starting dose of anagrelide is 0.5 mg four times daily or 1.0 mg twice a day, with the average daily dose to control thrombocytosis in study patients being 2.4 mg per day. Side effects of the anagrelide[1] are primarily cardiovascular, and the drug should be used with caution in patients with known heart disease.

PV is potentially curable if the abnormal clone can be eradicated and replaced by normal stem cells. Allogeneic stem cell transplantation has been used to cure select patients with spent-phase PV. A recent single institution series of 56 patients (median age 39 years) with myelofibrosis receiving related (36) and unrelated (20) donor stem cells after myeloablative therapy demonstrated a 58% 3-year survival. Dupriez score, cytogenetic abnormalities, and degree of marrow fibrosis were the most significant risk factors associated with post-transplant mortality.

Prognostic models have demonstrated that age, anemia, and cytogenetic abnormalities predict poor survival in patients with MMM. This poor prognostic group may benefit the most from allogeneic transplantation. Unfortunately, the majority of patients are not eligible for standard myeloablative transplantations because of their age and increased regimen-related toxicity. Recent reports suggest that nonmyeloablative stem cell transplantation may be effective in these older patients with MMM. Results of ongoing clinical trials will help clarify the role of transplantation in management of PV.

Although PV remains an incurable disease with standard therapies, extended survivals of greater than 10 years can be expected with optimal management. Further progress will depend on a better understanding of the pathobiology of this clonal malignant disorder. An improved understanding of the intracellular signaling pathways involved in the neoplastic process will allow for targeted therapies. In this regard a recent report of two patients with BCR/ABL-negative PV who are having an excellent clinical response to imatinib mesylate (Gleevec)[1] warrants further investigation. The use of low-dose aspirin may have a major impact in the quality of life of patients by decreasing the risk of thrombosis, a major cause of morbidity and mortality. Finally, it is hoped that a better understanding of risk factors for disease progression combined with improved transplant techniques will allow more patients to achieve a cure.

[1]Not FDA approved for this indication.

[1]Not FDA approved for this indication.

THE PORPHYRIAS

METHOD OF

Neville Pimstone, MD, PhD

Key Concepts

1. The human porphyrias are a group of disorders that reflect defective heme biosynthesis. A defective enzyme in one of the eight steps in this process results in a variety of clinical syndromes. As heme is made mainly in the liver and bone marrow, disorders of its biosynthesis present as hepatic or erythropoietic porphyria.
2. The partial deficiency of one of the heme and/or biosynthetic enzymes may be acquired or inherited as an autosomal dominant or an autosomal recessive trait. In autosomal dominant forms, the majority show low clinical penetrance. Individuals who fall into this category are susceptible to develop this clinical disease and are best described as latent or presymptomatic. Although the clinical porphyria syndromes are an interplay of genetic and environmental effects on heme biosynthesis, there are a few purely toxic porphyrias.
3. Porphyrins are oxidized products of the heme precursor porphyrinogens and therefore are not physiological substrates for heme. When these accumulate in the body, they may localize in many areas such as the liver, bone, and the skin; but because of the ability of the porphyrins to absorb sunlight energy, there is damage referred to as the photocutaneous lesions of porphyria in areas where sun strikes the skin.
4. There are five hepatic porphyrias. Three may have photocutaneous problems as part of the clinical presentation. These manifest as blistering of the skin, skin fragility, and the results of healing (i.e., milia and scars). Less frequently,

the skin may become pigmented with increased downy hair production, which is the body's adaptive way to protect itself from sunlight. Because solar energy is needed for the genesis of the skin lesions, these occur usually in the facial area, the scalp, and the "V" areas of the neck and the hands. All cutaneous hepatic porphyrias are clinically indistinguishable.

5. Acute hepatic porphyria is a neurovisceral syndrome with abdominal pain, rapidly progressive neuropathy, mental changes, tachycardia, mild hypertension, and electrolyte disturbances. Two of the four hepatic porphyrias can have cutaneous lesions at the time they develop acute porphyria, or they may present as a purely photocutaneous hepatic porphyria thereby mimicking porphyria cutanea tarda (PCT).
6. PCT, the most common hepatic porphyria, is a defect at the fifth step of heme biosynthesis catalyzed by the enzyme uroporphyrinogen decarboxylase. This is a purely cutaneous porphyria, which is usually sporadic but may be familial. It is most commonly associated with hepatitis C and alcohol use, but may be precipitated by estrogen therapy. It never is complicated with an acute porphyric attack. However, any patient who presents with cutaneous hepatic porphyria may have the predisposition to acute hepatic porphyria (see 5 above).
7. Because induction of hepatic heme metabolism is physiologic after puberty with the normal increased production of sex steroids, acute hepatic porphyria is a postpubertal disease.
8. Acute hepatic porphyria usually is precipitated by a medication that induces drug metabolizing cytochrome P450 hemoproteins in the liver. We do not know whether overproduction of the porphyrinogen precursors delta aminolevulinic acid (ALA) and porphobilinogen (PBG) causes the neurovisceral disorder, or whether this results from heme deficiency.
9. The erythropoietic porphyrias (i.e., congenital erythropoietic porphyria [CEP] and protoporphyria [PP]) result in bone marrow overproduction of porphyrins from birth but present differently. In CEP, the huge outpouring of uroporphyrin I from the bone marrow results in photomutilation. In PP, the photocutaneous sensitivity often presents in childhood in the form of exaggerated sunburn and irritability; only later in life is the repeatedly injured skin pigmented and thickened. Protoporphyrin crystals can also accumulate in the liver presenting as a chronic hepatitis or a cirrhosis, making the liver look chocolate brown in color. Protoporphyrin crystals may seed protoporphyrin gallstones. Indeed, this was how protoporphyria was discovered by a dermatologist in 1961.
10. The diagnosis of human porphyria primarily requires a clinical laboratory that can measure heme precursors. Each porphyria has a unique pattern of heme precursor overproduction. In diagnosing acute attack in hepatic porphyria, it is a common misconception for the physician to request porphyrins to be measured in urine. *This is wrong—the diagnostic heme precursors overproduced during an acute porphyric attack are ALA and PBG, not porphyrins.* In the hepatic porphyrias, a 24-hour urine ALA, PBG, and porphyrin profile, along with a fecal porphyrin profile, distinguishes the acute hepatic porphyrias from PCT. There is increasing evidence that plasma porphyrins may play a more important role in diagnosis. In the erythropoietic porphyrias, CEP is classically associated with large quantities of uroporphyrin I in the urine, whereas no porphyrins occur in the urine of patients with PP. In the latter condition, stool protoporphyrin levels usually are markedly elevated, but the disease can best be diagnosed by measurement of red cell protoporphyrin.
11. The key concepts presented in items 1 to 10 above underscore the plethora of ways that human porphyria may present. Thus, it has become the realm of doctors of various subspecialties, including gastroenterologists, hematologists, dermatologists, neurologists, and psychiatrists. The highlights of the various more common porphyrias is the subject of this article, but I encourage readers to go to the Web site of the American Porphyria Foundation *(www.porphyriafoundation.com)* and/or visit the Web site *www.porphyria-europe.com*, both of which have links to other Web sites, and are reader friendly in that they present data for patients and for physicians. Included in these Web sites are the drugs thought to be suspicious in precipitating an acute porphyric attack.

Types of Porphyria

HEPATIC PORPHYRIAS

Acute Hepatic Porphyrias

There are four acute hepatic porphyrias:

1. ALA dehydratase deficiency porphyria (ADP)
2. Acute intermittent porphyria (AIP)
3. Hereditary coproporphyria (HCP)
4. Variegate porphyria (VP)

The defective enzyme step in heme biosynthesis (Figure 1) determines the pattern of heme precursor overproduction. Usually when an acute attack is precipitated, hepatic heme deficiency (which is presumed to reflect induction of hepatic heme synthesis in the setting of a defect in this pathway) results in an overproduction of only ALA in ADP; whereas both ALA and PBG are high in the other three acute porphyrias. The clinical acute attack and its treatment are the same. Photocutaneous lesions, if present, suggest

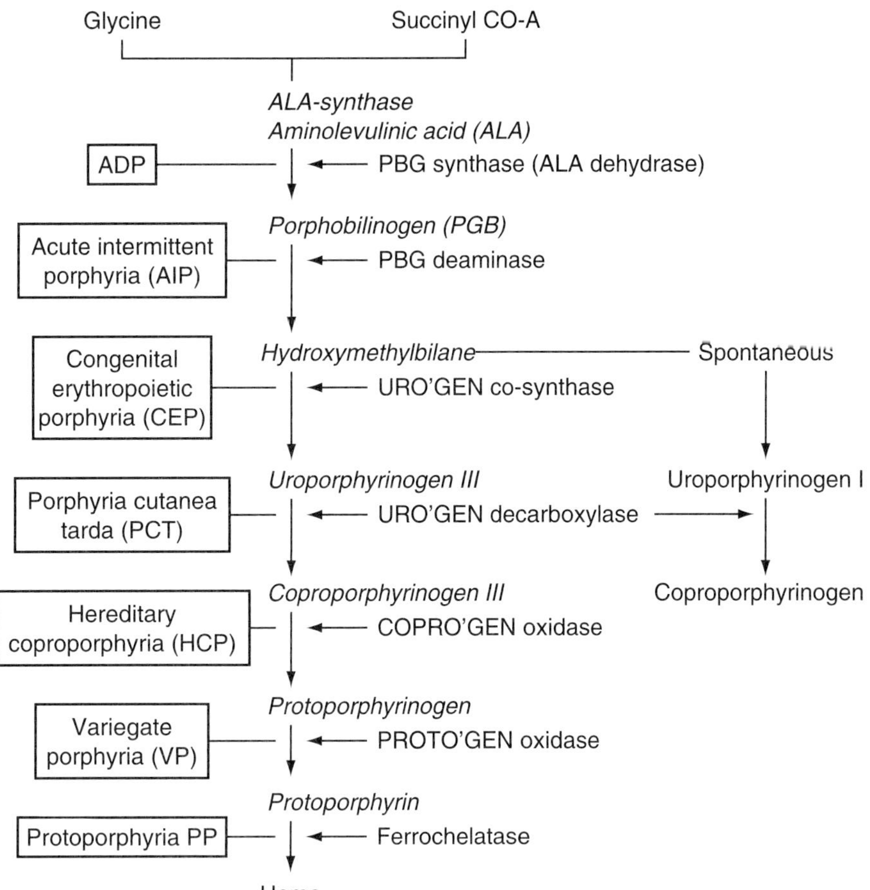

FIGURE 1 The heme biosynthetic pathway. On the right of the pathway are the eight enzymes that catalyze the biosynthesis of heme. In the boxes on the left are the porphyria syndromes relating to the genetic/acquired deficiency of these enzymes.

that the heme biosynthetic enzyme deficiency results in accumulation of porphyrins in the skin.

Acute Attack

Acute neurovisceral attacks of porphyria are usually episodic and may be life-threatening. Attacks are rare before puberty other than in ADP, usually start between the ages of 15 and 35 years, and are more frequent in females. These attacks are often precipitated by drugs, alcohol, calorie restriction, and endocrine factors. Usually after recovery, recurrent acute attacks can be prevented by maintaining a calorie-adequate diet and by avoiding factors that provoke acute attacks. A small percentage of women, less than 10%, may present with recurrent acute attacks that are usually related to the menstrual cycle.

The most common clinical feature is abdominal pain, which occurs in close to 100% of patients. The pain is diffuse and associated with vomiting and constipation; bowel sounds are preserved and there is no evidence of peritoneal irritation. The attacks are usually associated with a mild hypertension, a pulse rate of greater than 80 beats per minute, and hyponatremia; the serum sodium is usually less than 135 mEq/L. Less frequently there are neuropsychological symptoms with memory loss, convulsions, and hallucinations. The most frightening neurological complication is a rapidly progressive polyaxonal peripheral neuropathy that may cause respiratory paralysis requiring mechanical respiration and total body paralysis. This usually recovers 1 to 2 years after the acute attack, during which time urinary ALA and PBG may be normal. The heme precursor profile of the underlying porphyria persists.

Biochemical Diagnosis of Acute Porphyria

Acute hepatic porphyria is accompanied by increased urinary excretion of PBG and, to a lesser extent, ALA; an exception is the rare condition of ADP in which PBG excretion is normal. Thus examination of the urine for excess PBG is essential in diagnosing a suspected acute hepatic porphyria. However, measurement of urinary porphyrins only is unhelpful and may be misleading. In most patients with acute porphyria, 24-hour urine PBG levels are usually 10 times the upper limit of normal. The urine samples may develop a brownish red color on standing, which is produced by condensation of PBG to porphobilin.

In remission ALA and PBG are elevated only in AIP, but may be normal in patients with HCP or VP. All patients should have:

- 24-hour urine testing for ALA, PBG, and porphyrin profile
- A fecal porphyrin profile including request to the clinical lab for coproporphyrin III/I isomer ratio

- Isocoproporphyrin, plasma porphyrin fluorescence, and erythrocyte deaminase activity

If all these tests are normal, patients should be asked to resubmit samples of urine for PBG analysis immediately when symptoms recur. If these tests are still normal, the current or recent symptoms labeled as porphyria are probably incorrect and an alternative cause of the symptoms should be sought.

Treatment of Acute Porphyria

Supportive Treatment. Most patients with acute hepatic porphyria are ill and need to be admitted to a hospital. In milder attacks, the patient may be treated on an outpatient basis. The key to supportive treatment is to maintain nutrition. This is best achieved by a high-protein, high-carbohydrate diet of at least 1000 to 2000 calories per day. If nausea and vomiting precludes oral feeding, calories have to be given IV with dextrose/saline infusions and intermittent boluses of concentrated 50% dextrose, given piggyback to maintain fluid restriction. This nutritional treatment, also known as the glucose effect, is thought to suppress hepatic heme production.

Fluid and electrolyte balance need to be meticulously restored and maintained. If pain is prominent, it can be treated safely with meperidine hydrochloride or morphine. Nausea and vomiting can be controlled with prochlorperazine (Compazine) or chlorpromazine (Thorazine) given orally or by suppository. Hypertension can be treated with β-blockers and encephalopathy with fluid restriction and electrolyte correction. Agitation should be treated with diazepam (Valium) or lorazepam (Ativan), but it should be used with caution. Seizures are difficult to control medically. First correct hyponatremia. Antiseizure drugs have risks. The safer drugs are diazepam, magnesium sulfate, gabapentin (Neurontin), and clonazepam (Klonopin). Diazepam can be given IV.

Cyclic, recurrent acute porphyric attacks are clearly related to female sex steroid changes in their blood, especially progesterone, that induce hepatic heme synthesis. One method of treatment is to administer recurrent intravenous heme, 1 to 2 days mid-cycle with each menstrual cycle. Another is to diminish hormone production by giving analogs of gonadotrophin-releasing hormone[1] (GnRH) to prevent cyclic pituitary release of luteinizing hormone (LH) and follicle-stimulating hormone (FSH). The GnRH analogues may be given orally or by an intranasal route. After 3 to 6 months, osteoporosis is a predictable serious problem. Osteodensitometry should be performed at 6-month intervals to monitor decline in bone mass. The decrease in bone density may be arrested by estrogen orally or as a transdermal patch and/or alendronate sodium (Fosamax).

Specific Treatment. The basis for specific treatment is that there is a presumed hepatic heme deficiency that, by derepressing the heme biosynthetic pathway, results in ALA and PBG overproduction. How this relates to the acute neurovisceral syndrome is unknown, but the standard of care is to replete hepatic heme in the treatment of acute porphyria. This is best achieved by administration of hemin (Panhematin), which comes as a lyophilized powder and is best given in solution at a dose of 3 to 5 mg/kg per day for 4 successive days through a central venous line or a Port-a-Cath. The increased free flow of blood diminishes the most common complication, local phlebitis. This risk is further reduced by mixing equimolar amounts of human serum albumin before infusion; this is stable for 24 hours and is delivered to the liver as metheme-albumin. This should be given early in the acute attacks and is not helpful in reversing long-standing paralysis. Another form of intravenous heme, which is not yet approved by the FDA, is heme arginine (Normosang)[2]. This is reputed to have a lower incidence of phlebitis. Both heme preparations can interfere with coagulation, but this is not usually a problem. Subcutaneous heparin should be avoided during acute attacks.

Most patients improve within 5 days. There has been no study to date comparing intravenous heme treatment to placebo; such a study is unlikely to take place as this treatment predictably lowers the excretion of ALA and PBG in the urine, the markers of acute porphyric activity.

Acute Hepatic Porphyria Syndromes and Their Diagnosis

Acute Intermittent Porphyria (AIP). This is the most common acute hepatic porphyria and results from a defect in the PBG deaminase step in heme biosynthesis (see Figure 1). This may result in acute neurovisceral attacks, which may be sporadic or recurrent. Photocutaneous skin lesions do not occur. It is particularly prevalent in Europe and in the United States, with a gene frequency of one to two per 100,000. It was previously known as Swedish porphyria. The prevalence in northern Sweden is one per 1500 people.

In AIP, increased urine ALA and PBG excretion with normal or near normal fecal porphyrin concentrations are present both in the acute attack and in remission, but ALA and PBG are usually about 10 times greater than baseline in the acute neurovisceral attack.

Variegate Porphyria (VP). VP reflects deficiency of the penultimate step in heme biosynthesis (see Figure 1) catalyzed by the enzyme protoporphyrinogen oxidase (PPOX). This was known as South African genetic porphyria because it is the most common acute hepatic porphyria in that country, where it affects about 10,000 individuals of Dutch descent. (The source of this disease in South Africa traces back to the marriage in 1688 of an orphan girl from Holland who carried the VP gene to one of the free burghers in

[1]Not FDA approved for this indication.

[2]Not available in the United States.

the Dutch Cape Colony.) The gene frequency in South Africans of European descent is 1.5 to 3 per 1000. About 60% of VP patients present with photocutaneous sensitivity alone, 20% with recurrent acute neurovisceral attacks, and 20% with both of the above—hence the name variegate. The photocutaneous changes are identical to those seen in PCT.

In VP, increased urinary excretion of PBG is associated with a unique plasma porphyrin fluorescence emission peak at 624 to 627 nm. This is the best diagnostic marker of VP. Fecal porphyrin analysis may show markedly increased protoporphyrin, usually far greater than twice the coproporphyrin level, and with the coproporphyrin III/I ratio greater than two. The fecal porphyrin profile is not always reliable. In remission, all of the above changes are noted with the exception that urinary PBG excretion is often only slightly increased or normal.

Hereditary Coproporphyria (HCP). HCP is the least common autosomal dominant porphyria and presents similarly to VP. In HCP, there are changes similar to VP, with the following differences:

- The urine contains higher concentrations of coproporphyrin III with lesser amounts of uroporphyrin I from spontaneous nonenzymatic formation from PBG.
- A plasma porphyrin emission peak at 620 nm may be present.
- Fecal coproporphyrin usually exceeds protoporphyrin, and the isomer III/I ratios are greater than two.

Aminolevulinic Acid (ALA) Dehydratase Deficiency Porphyria (ADP). ADP is also known as Doss porphyria and plumboporphyria (lead inhibits the same enzyme). The clinical features in an acute neurovisceral attack in ADP are identical to that seen in AIP. Biochemically, only ALA, not PBG, is overproduced and excreted. There never are any photocutaneous porphyric lesions. It is a very rare autosomal recessive disorder with less than 10 patients been reported since its first description in 1979. It may present in prepuberty.

In the pediatric condition, hereditary tyrosinemia and one of the by-products, succinyl acetone, can also inhibit the dehydratase enzyme causing a similar type of acute hepatic porphyria. It is always important to rule out lead poisoning and to confirm normal blood lead concentrations.

Porphyria Cutanea Tarda (PCT)

PCT is the most common human porphyria and produces a purely cutaneous porphyric syndrome with fragile skin, blistering that can lead to scars and milia, and, more rarely, pigmentation with overproduction of downy hair. Acute attacks never occur. The skin lesions are identical to those seen in two of the four acute hepatic porphyrias. Thus, the physician needs to make a positive diagnosis based on the pattern of heme precursor excretion.

In 80% of patients, a sporadic PCT syndrome is thought to reflect an acquired defect in the fifth heme biosynthetic step, which is catalyzed by the enzyme uroporphyrinogen decarboxylase. In 20%, the disease is familial. In one subtype, caused by ingestion or absorption of toxins such as hexachlorobenzene (the wheat seed fungicide)—ingested by people in Turkey in the 1950s—and the herbicide Agent Orange (tetrachlorodibenzo-*p*-dioxan [TCDD])—from the Viet Nam war period—the deficiency clearly is chemically produced and not genetic. Several thousand Turkish farm dwellers had toxic PCT. Occasionally, estrogen use (contraceptive or in prostate cancer) can be associated with PCT.

Classic PCT is associated with increased total body iron in about 40% of patients, and some are homozygotes for the hemochromatosis (HFE) gene. It is usually a latent disease that becomes clinically overt in response to liver damage, which in the United States most commonly is hepatitis C and alcoholic liver injury. The defective step in heme biosynthesis in PCT is at the level of uroporphyrinogen decarboxylase. This enzyme catalyzes the decarboxylation of 8-carboxyl uroporphyrinogen-7 (hepta)-6 (hexa)-5 (penta)-4 (coproporphyrinogen)-carboxyl porphyrinogens.

Why is PCT most commonly an extrahepatic manifestation of liver injury? The combination of liver cell damage with lipid peroxidation and of increased hepatic iron, a pro-oxidant, causes oxidative stress that may make latent PCT overt. With a defect in uroporphyrinogen decarboxylation, the polycarboxylated porphyrinogen heme precursors may be oxided into porphyrins. These are not physiologic precursors of heme. The porphyrins accumulate in the liver, which is fluorescent in biopsy tissue; they accumulate in the skin, causing photocutaneous sensitivity; and they are excreted in the urine. The urine porphyrin profile of uro-, hepta-, penta-, and copro-porphyrin, with fecal isocoproporphyrin, are diagnostic of PCT. Iron reduction therapy by phlebotomy predictably reverses active PCT. This is the standard of care, although low-dose chloroquine mobilizes hepatic porphyrins, which leads to increased secretion, and can thus also cause remission.

ERYTHROPOIETIC PORPHYRIAS

Congenital Erythropoietic Porphyria (CEP)

Congenital erythropoietic porphyria (CEP) is a condition where ineffective erythropoiesis results in the bone marrow overproduction of isomer I porphyrins (mainly uroporphyrin I), caused by a defect in the fourth heme biosynthetic step catalyzed by the enzyme uroporphyrinogen III synthetase (UROS). This is a rare autosomal recessive condition.

The porphyrins localize in the bones, skin, and teeth; and clinically, most patients present soon after birth. The most striking clinical feature is photomutilating photosensitivity, pigmented teeth that fluoresce under UV light (erythrodontia), and hemolytic anemia.

The bone marrow exhibits normoblast proliferation with some showing bizarre electron microscopic changes. However, porphyrin-laden normoblasts, also known as porphyroblasts, are not necessarily associated with this morphologic change.

This condition is so photomutilating that patients who are exposed to sunlight may lose fingers and facial structures such as the lips, the nose, and the ears. Avoidance from sunlight from youth is the only protection, but most patients cannot remain reclusive to protect themselves, and have serious cutaneous problems. The quality of life may be extremely poor and at this point, bone marrow transplantation is the only effective treatment.

The diagnosis of this disease is confirmed by excessive erythrocyte protoporphyrin with specific excitation and fluorescent peaks, the latter emission peak being 615 to 620, the same as in PCT. The feces have an excess of coproporphyrin isomer I. Examination of the bone marrow by fluorescent microscopy is also diagnostic. An interesting hematologic finding is the reporting of excessive white cells in the peripheral blood following automated analysis. These actually are circulating normoblasts.

Erythropoietic Protoporphyria (EPP)

Erythropoietic protoporphyria (EPP) is a bone marrow porphyria that is autosomal-dominant with low penetrance. In most patients, clinical expression requires co-inheritance of a low-expression allele that is present in about 10% of the general population.

It is the only porphyria that presents with acute photocutaneous sensitivity starting in early childhood that progresses to a thickened hide-like skin from repeated sun trauma. The protoporphyrin is not excreted in the urine but is present in excess in the stool where it is the dominant excreted fecal porphyrin. Erythrocytes have an excess of free protoporphyrin with a fluorescence emission peak of 626 to 634 nm. This is determined by the protein to which protoporphyrin is bound in the plasma; 636 nm reflects protoporphyrin-albumin, and 628 reflects porphyrin-globin, with the latter occurring when there is hemolysis.

A minority, about 2% of patients, have hepatobiliary lesions. Often these run in families suggesting that there may be an inherited defect in the hepatic clearance of protoporphyrin. In the mildest hepatitis phase, the liver has brown pigment granules in hepatocytes that look like hemosiderin. However, the iron stains are negative and the crystals show diagnostic birefringence on polarization microscopy. The protoporphyrin deposition in the liver can lead to fibrosis, cirrhosis, and even liver failure requiring liver transplantation. Plasmapheresis before surgery and special lighting are some of the maneuvers used to circumvent photo necrosis of the abdominal viscera during the surgery.

THERAPEUTIC USE OF BLOOD COMPONENTS

METHOD OF

John M. Fisk, MD, and Edward L. Snyder, MD

Blood component therapy refers to the practice of transfusing only that part of blood indicated to treat a given medical condition. This is the current standard of care and represents best practice in the care of patients who require blood transfusion. Transfusion of whole blood has almost completely been supplanted by component therapy, except in certain specific situations.

With the exception of autologous blood donation, collection of blood from healthy donors in the United States is generally performed by blood collection agencies such as the American Red Cross (ARC), independent blood centers, or hospital-based blood donor services. These operate under a strict set of statutes and regulations provided by the Food and Drug Administration (FDA). Blood collection and processing is considered a manufacturing procedure, which must conform to those FDA regulations under the general title of Good Manufacturing Practices (GMP). Details regarding the technical specifications for blood products and the anticoagulant-preservative solutions used with the various components are given in the *Circular of Information for the Use of Human Blood and Blood Components*. This FDA-approved pamphlet is prepared and updated periodically by the American Association of Blood Banks (AABB), the American Red Cross, and America's Blood Centers; and it functions as the manufacturer's package insert. Copies of this document are available at blood collection agencies or through hospital transfusion services.

Currently, a unit of donated whole blood is processed through a series of centrifugations and other processing steps into a unit of red blood cells, platelets, fresh-frozen plasma, or cryoprecipitated antihemophilic factor (cryoprecipitate). Additionally, plasma may be used to manufacture a variety of derivative products that include coagulation factor concentrates, immune globulins (Ig [Gamimune N]), and plasma volume expanders such as 5% albumin solution. Increasingly, blood component collection is performed on specialized automated apheresis (blood separator) instruments such as those used for preparation of single-donor platelets apheresis (SDP), or single or double units of red blood cells.

A description of each component with indications for transfusion, precautions and contraindications, and dosing and administration guidelines is provided in the following section. Following this is a discussion of additional component processing, performed either at the blood collection center or hospital blood bank, which includes saline washing, leukocyte reduction, and blood irradiation.

Blood Components

WHOLE BLOOD

Description

A unit of whole blood contains approximately 450 to 500 mL of venous blood in 70 mL of a citrate-based anticoagulant solution at an average hematocrit of 40% (range 36% to 44%). It is stored refrigerated at 1°C to 6°C (33.8°F to 42.8°F) with a storage time to expiration that depends on the anticoagulant-preservative solution (21 days for citrate-monobasic sodium phosphate-dextrose [CPD]; 35 days for citrate-monobasic sodium phosphate-dextrose-adenine [CPDA-1]).

Indications

Whole blood provides oxygen-carrying capacity and blood-volume expansion. It has been used to treat massive bleeding in patients who have lost greater than 25% of their total blood volume. Most practitioners, however, use specific component therapy guided by ongoing monitoring of the patient's hematologic status to determine transfusion needs. Fresh whole blood, less than 7 days old, has also been used for neonatal exchange transfusion to help prevent hyperkalemia.

Precautions and Contraindications

Whole blood does not contain viable platelets or granulocytes and is deficient in the labile clotting factors V and VIII. Unless a patient has anemia and concurrent intravascular volume depletion, transfusion of whole blood may result in volume overload, particularly if rapidly infused to patients with poor cardiac function. It is not indicated for the treatment of normovolemic patients with chronic anemia.

Dose and Administration

One unit of whole blood in the adult should raise the hematocrit by approximately 3% and the hemoglobin concentration by 1 g/dL; in pediatric patients, transfusion of 8 mL/kg results in a similar increase. Blood must be transfused through a blood administration set containing a nominal 170 μm (150 to 260 μm) filter. Total infusion time should not exceed 4 hours. An approved volumetric infusion pump and/or blood warmer (40°C [104°F]) may be used for infusion, if desired.

RED BLOOD CELLS

Description

Red blood cells (RBCs) are prepared from whole blood by the removal of 200 to 250 mL of plasma, or they may be obtained by apheresis collection. One unit of RBCs has a volume of 250 to 300 mL and a hematocrit of approximately 75% if stored in CPDA-1 solution, and a volume of 330 mL and hematocrit of approximately 60% if stored in one of the additive solutions (AS-1, AS-3, or AS-5). Additive solutions are anticoagulant-preservative solutions that contain varying concentrations of adenine, which allow increased storage of RBCs to a maximum of 42 days. RBCs are stored refrigerated at 1°C to 6°C (33.8°F to 42.8°F) with a storage time to expiration that depends on the anticoagulation-preservative solution (Table 1). Nearly all hospital transfusion services provide RBCs, rather than whole blood, for the treatment of patients with acute or chronic anemia. RBCs may undergo further processing for specific indications, including leukocyte reduction, irradiation, or saline washing.

TABLE 1 Storage Time to Expiration for Anticoagulant-Preservative Solutions of Red Blood Cells and Platelets

Storage Solution	Used for RBC Storage	Used for PLT Storage	Average Hematocrit in RBC Product Infused	RBC Maximal Storage Time (days)	PLT Maximal Storage Time (days)
AS-1, AS-3, AS-5*	Yes	No	55%	42	N/A
CPDA-1	Yes	Yes	75%	35	5
CPD	Yes	Yes	75%	21	5
CP2D	Yes	Yes	75%	21	5
ACD-A	Yes	Yes	75%	21	5

*Additive solutions; various proprietary formulations are AS-1 (Adsol, Baxter) contains citrate, phosphate, dextrose, sodium chloride, mannitol, and adenine; AS-3 (Nutricel, MedSep) contains citrate, phosphate, dextrose, sodium chloride, and adenine; AS-5 (Optisol, Terumo) contains citrate, phosphate, dextrose, sodium chloride, mannitol, and adenine.

Abbreviations: ACD-A = anticoagulant-citrate-dextrose solution USP Formula A (apheresis products only); AS = additive solution; CP2D = anticoagulant-citrate-phosphate-double-dextrose solution; CPD = anticoagulant citrate-phosphate-dextrose solution; CPDA-1 = anticoagulant citrate-phosphate-dextrose-adenine solution; PLT = platelet; RBC = red blood cell.

Indications

Red blood cell transfusion is indicated in the treatment of patients with symptomatic anemia caused by inadequate oxygen-carrying capacity. There is no single criterion that can be relied upon to determine whether and when a patient requires RBC transfusion. Most practitioners take multiple factors into consideration when making this decision, including the patient's age, acuity of anemia, cardiopulmonary status, metabolic demands, volume status, hemoglobin or hematocrit, presence of co-morbid conditions, whether there is ongoing blood loss, and whether the patient is symptomatic (angina pectoris, tachycardia, tachypnea, lethargy, etc.).

In the hospitalized adult patient, a target hemoglobin of 9 to 10 g/dL has been a generally accepted guideline by most hospital transfusion services. Currently, however, reports of a randomized, prospective study involving intensive care unit patients found that patients who were not transfused until their hemoglobin concentration dropped below 7 g/dL had better outcomes than those transfused at 9 g/dL. Thus, a target hemoglobin of 7 to 8 g/dL or hematocrit of 21% to 24% appears to represent a better transfusion threshold. In the setting of acute hemorrhage—because of trauma, iatrogenic surgical blood loss, or other causes—hematocrit and hemoglobin concentration may not be an accurate measure of RBC loss. Transfusion decisions in this setting require close cardiopulmonary monitoring coupled with frequent clinical assessment.

Transfusion guidelines differ in pediatric patients younger than the age of 4 months. Transfusion of infants in this group with cyanotic heart disease is recommended by some for a hematocrit less than 39% or hemoglobin less than 13 g/dL. For otherwise stable infants, a hematocrit of less than 24% or hemoglobin less than 8 g/dL is used when the patient is symptomatic (tachycardic, tachypneic, recurrent apnea, poor feeding, or decreased vigor). Acute blood loss, greater than 10% of estimated total blood volume, is also an indication for transfusion of RBCs. Most hospital transfusion services have established guidelines for blood component transfusion in both pediatric and adult populations. A sample set of guidelines is provided in Table 2.

TABLE 2 Sample Guidelines for Transfusion of Red Blood Cells

Adults and Children Older Than 4 Months of Age
Symptomatic anemia
Acute blood loss estimated at 30% of total blood volume and not responsive to volume replacement
Hematocrit <24% in patients maintained on chronic transfusion regimen
Hematocrit <24% in preoperative patients with anticipated significant blood loss
Hematocrit <30% in elderly patients with cardiovascular disease
Hematocrit <30% in patients with sickle cell disease and complications (such as cerebrovascular accident, acute chest syndrome, or priapism) or preoperative patients
Infants Younger Than 4 Months of Age
Exchange transfusion
Hematocrit <39% in patients with cyanotic heart disease
Acute blood loss estimated at >10% total blood volume
Hematocrit <24% in stable patients with tachycardia, tachypnea, recurrent apnea, or decreased vigor (failure to thrive)

Precautions and Contraindications

The same precautions and contraindications apply to RBCs as for whole blood. Transfusion of RBCs is not indicated for volume replacement, wound healing, protein nutrition, or when chronic anemia can be corrected with appropriate therapy such as vitamin B_{12}, folic acid, iron, or recombinant erythropoietin (Epogen).

Dose and Administration

One unit of RBCs in the adult should increase the hematocrit by approximately 3% and the hemoglobin concentration by 1 g/dL; in pediatric patients, transfusion of 8 to 10 mL/kg results in an increase in hematocrit of 6% and hemoglobin concentration of 2 g/dL. Blood must be transfused through a blood administration set containing a nominal 170 µm (150 to 260 µm) filter. Total infusion time should not exceed 4 hours. An approved volumetric infusion pump and/or blood warmer (40°C [104°F]) may be used for infusion, if desired.

FROZEN RED BLOOD CELLS

Description

Red blood cells may be frozen to significantly increase storage time. The primary indications for freezing include preservation of units with a rare blood type, autologous units, and stockpiling to provide a frozen reserve. Glycerol, a penetrating cryoprotective agent, is added to the RBC unit prior to freezing to prevent damage during the freezing process. Storage in high-concentration (40 w/v%) glycerol allows units to be stored at –65°C (–85°F) for up to 10 years. Red blood cell units are prepared via thawing and then deglycerolizing to remove the cryoprotectant. This post-thaw processing is often done with the aid of specially designed instruments that partially automate this process. Because deglycerolizing involves use of an *open system* technique, a thawed unit must be transfused within 24 hours of processing, although a new *closed system* process (Haemonetics ACP 215) has recently gained FDA approval for a 2-week post-thaw shelf life. Indications, precautions and contraindications, and dose and administration of frozen RBCs are the same as for nonfrozen RBCs.

PLATELETS

Description

Platelet concentrates (random donor platelets [RDP]) are prepared by centrifugation of whole blood.

One unit of RDP is derived from a single unit of whole blood and must contain 5.5×10^{10} platelets suspended in 40 to 70 mL of plasma at a pH greater than or equal to 6.2. Platelets may also be collected from individual donors via plateletpheresis (single donor platelets [SDP], or apheresis platelets). One SDP unit must contain $\geq 3.0 \times 10^{11}$ platelets suspended in approximately 200 to 300 mL of plasma and is equivalent to 5 to 6 units of RDPs. Platelets are stored at 20°C to 24°C (68°F to 75.2°F) with gentle, continuous agitation, and they have a storage time to expiration of 5 days. The pH must be greater than or equal to 6.2 throughout storage.

Indications

Platelet transfusion is indicated to treat or prevent bleeding caused by abnormally decreased platelet count or abnormally functioning platelets (acquired or congenital). Generally accepted guidelines include prophylactic transfusion for a platelet count less than 10,000/µL in the absence of bleeding (this value ranges from 5000 to 20,000 depending on institutional practice), less than 50,000/µL with active bleeding or anticipated invasive procedure, and less than 100,000/µL with anticipated neurosurgical or ophthalmologic procedures. Platelet transfusion is also indicated for active bleeding or prophylaxis for a planned invasive procedure in patients with congenital or acquired thrombocytopathies. In general, patients with immune thrombocytopenic purpura (ITP) are less likely to bleed at a given platelet count than are patients with chemotherapy-induced thrombocytopenia. Table 3 lists sample platelet transfusion guidelines.

The primary use of SDPs has traditionally been to limit donor exposure in patients requiring long-term platelet support, and who are thereby considered at an increased risk of developing platelet alloimmunization because of the development of anti-HLA (human leukocyte antibody) or platelet-specific antibodies. This practice, while common, is not supported by the findings of the multi-institutional Trial to Reduce Alloimmunization to Platelets (TRAP) Study Group. This study found that leukoreduction, rather than limiting the number of donor exposures, was associated with a decreased risk of platelet alloimmunization.

TABLE 3 Sample Guidelines for Transfusion of Platelets

Adults
Platelet count <10,000/µL without bleeding
Platelet count <50,000/µL with bleeding or planned invasive procedure
Platelet count <100,000/µL and planned neurosurgical or ophthalmologic procedure
Massive blood loss with abnormal bleeding, platelet count pending (as part of concurrent hemostasis workup)
Immediately after cardiopulmonary bypass (CPB) with abnormal nonsurgical bleeding
Premature Infants
In stable condition with platelet count <50,000/µL
In unstable condition with platelet count <100,000/µL

Precautions and Contraindications

Patients with thrombotic thrombocytopenic purpura (TTP) should not be transfused with platelets because of a significantly increased risk of thrombosis. Similarly, platelet transfusion is relatively contraindicated in the setting of heparin-induced thrombocytopenia (HIT), type 2, in the absence of clinically significant bleeding. Platelet transfusion can be considered for these patients, but only if clinically significant bleeding occurs. Response to platelet transfusion may be blunted in a large variety of clinical settings, which are listed in Table 4.

Because platelets must be stored at room temperature (20°C to 24°C [68°F to 75.2°F]) to ensure post-transfusion viability, there is a significantly increased risk of bacterial contamination, as compared with refrigerated blood product storage. For this reason, particular attention must be paid to the development of fever (hyperpyrexia), chills, rigors, or hemodynamic instability (hypotension) during platelet infusion because of the risk of a septic transfusion reaction. Beginning March 1, 2004, bacterial testing of platelets was mandated by voluntary standard-setting organizations to help mitigate this risk.

Dosing and Administration

A conventional platelet dose for an adult is a pool of 4 to 6 RDP units, or 1 SDP unit. The RDP pool size is established by the individual hospital transfusion service. Platelets must be transfused through a blood administration set containing a nominal 170 µm (150 to 260 µm) filter, and RDP must be infused within 4 hours of pooling. Rh-negative patients should receive Rh-negative platelets, if available. Platelets are labeled Rh positive or negative because of red blood cell contamination of the platelet

TABLE 4 Potential Causes of Poor Platelet Transfusion Response

Nonimmune
Fever
Sepsis
Uremia
Disseminated intravascular coagulopathy (DIC)
Drugs (amphotericin, etc.)
Severe viremia
Vasculitis
Following autologous or allogeneic hematopoietic stem cell transplantation
Chemotherapy or radiation therapy
Immune-Mediated
Human leukocyte antibody (HLA) alloantibodies
Platelet-specific antibodies
Circulating immune complexes
Autoantibodies (immune thrombocytopenic purpura [ITP])

concentrates, as platelets do not possess Rh antigens. Rh-negative patients without an anti-D alloantibody may be safely transfused with Rh-positive platelets if Rho (D) immune globulin (RhoGAM) is administered within 72 hours of transfusion. A dose of 300 mg of Rh immune globulin prevents alloimmunization from 15 mL of Rh-incompatible red blood cells or 30 mL of whole blood. Assuming an RDP unit contains approximately 0.1 mL of red blood cells, a dose of Rh immune globulin is generally required very infrequently. Consultation with a blood bank physician is advised in this setting.

The expected post-transfusion platelet count increment is approximately 5000 to 10,000/μL per unit of RDP or 30,000 to 50,000/μL per unit of SDP. When progressive, intermittent, or abrupt deterioration in platelet transfusion effectiveness occurs, a 1-hour post-transfusion platelet count (obtained 10 to 60 minutes following transfusion) should be obtained and a corrected count increment (CCI) calculated.

$$\text{CCI} = \frac{[(\text{Post-tx plt ct}) - (\text{Pre-tx plt ct})] \times \text{BSA}}{\text{Platelets transfused} \times 10^{-11}}$$

where tx = transfusion; plt ct = platelet count

A CCI less than 5000 indicates a potentially platelet-refractory patient who may require additional serologic investigation and may benefit from crossmatch-compatible or HLA-matched SDP transfusion.

GRANULOCYTES

Granulocytes are collected by apheresis techniques from normal volunteer donors—often patient family members. If no granulocyte-stimulating drugs are given to the donor, the yield of granulocytes rarely rises above the minimum acceptable dose of 1×10^{10} neutrophils. To collect a large dose of granulocytes, the donor should receive both granulocyte colony-stimulating factor (G-CSF) (filgrastim [Neupogen]) and dexamethasone. These medications in combination can result in collections of 6 to 8×10^{10} neutrophils or higher. Such doses can provide a measurable increase in granulocytes in an adult recipient. Because some blood collection agencies, however, do not permit the granulocyte donor to receive any medication; many cancer hospitals collect their own granulocytes after obtaining research approval from their institutional review board (IRB). Indications for granulocyte transfusions in patients with a malignancy include:

- Neutropenia (polymorphonuclear neutrophil [PMN] <500/μL)
- Sepsis or infection unresponsive to appropriate antibiotics for more than 24 to 48 hours
- Bone marrow showing myeloid hypoplasia
- Reasonable chance for survival

The granulocyte product, depending on the type of donor premedication, contains from 1 to 8×10^{10} neutrophils in approximately 300 mL of plasma with a 10% to 15% hematocrit. Accordingly, granulocytes must be ABO-compatible and cross-matched with the recipient. The shelf life is 24 hours when stored at room temperature without agitation. Granulocytes should be used as soon as possible after collection, although current transfusion-transmitted disease (TTD) testing makes the logistics for this maneuver somewhat challenging. Granulocytes should be irradiated and infused slowly to avoid a febrile reaction. While granulocytes must be infused through a 170 μm screen filter, leukoreduction filters should *never* be used for infusion, as they will remove the neutrophils. Granulocytes are used primarily for gram-positive sepsis. Gram-negative sepsis and fungal infections have not been shown to respond as well to granulocyte transfusions. If granulocyte transfusions are being considered for a patient, the blood bank director should be consulted.

PLASMA: FRESH-FROZEN PLASMA, THAWED PLASMA, CRYOPRECIPITATE-REDUCED PLASMA

Description

Fresh-frozen plasma (FFP) is prepared from whole blood by centrifugation followed by freezing of the supernatant plasma within 8 hours of collection. It is then stored at −18°C (−4°F), which preserves the activity of the labile coagulation factors V and VIII. One unit of FFP contains from 200 to 250 mL and has a storage time to expiration of 1 year. Fresh-frozen plasma provides all coagulation factors, fibrinogen, antithrombin-III, protein S, protein C, and albumin. In addition to FFP, various other plasma preparations are available.

Thawed plasma is FFP that has been thawed and stored at 4°C (39.2°F) for a maximum of 5 days. The activity levels of factor V and factor VIII decrease over time, although factor V levels do not fall below approximately 65%. Plasma, cryoprecipitate-reduced (cryo-poor plasma or cryosupernatant plasma), is the by-product of the preparation of cryoprecipitated antihemophilic factor (AHF) that has approximately 50% of the fibrinogen and von Willebrand factor (vWf) removed. Its use is generally restricted to the treatment of patients with thrombotic thrombocytopenic purpura (TTP).

Indications

Fresh-frozen plasma is used to treat patients with bleeding because of multiple coagulation factor deficiencies, as occurs in liver disease, vitamin K deficiency, disseminated intravascular coagulopathy (DIC), and dilutional coagulopathy resulting from massive transfusion. FFP is indicated for the emergent reversal of warfarin effect when correction with vitamin K cannot be achieved in sufficient time and for treatment of patients with congenital coagulation factor deficiencies for which no factor concentrate is currently available (such as factors V, X, or XI). Fresh-frozen plasma is used as the replacement solution during plasmapheresis for the treatment of patients with TTP/HUS, while cryosupernatant is generally reserved for use in that subset of TTP patients who fail to respond to repeated exchange with FFP.

Precautions and Contraindications

Plasma is not indicated for uncomplicated intravascular volume expansion when crystalloid or colloid solutions (albumin or plasma protein fraction) will suffice. Thawed plasma should not be the sole plasma-replacement product for patients with consumptive coagulopathies, because of its decreased levels of factors V and VIII, although it may be therapeutic in these cases when used in combination with fresh-frozen plasma. Patients who develop respiratory insufficiency or decreased oxygen saturation during or shortly following plasma transfusion should be evaluated for possible transfusion-related acute lung injury (TRALI)—noncardiogenic pulmonary edema or capillary leak syndrome—because of the well-recognized association of this entity with plasma-containing blood product transfusion.

Dosing and Administration

In patients with coagulation factor deficiencies, a dose of 10 to 20 mL/kg (4 to 6 units in an average-sized adult) will increase the level of all coagulation factors by approximately 20% immediately following transfusion. Patients with vitamin K deficiency can generally be treated with smaller doses. All patients receiving plasma for the correction of coagulopathies should have ongoing laboratory monitoring of their coagulation status (prothrombin time [PT], activated partial thromboplastin time [aPTT], international normalized ratio [INR], or specific factor assay) in order to guide appropriate therapy. Plasma must be transfused through a blood administration set containing a nominal 170 μm (150 to 260 μm) filter.

CRYOPRECIPITATED ANTIHEMOPHILIC FACTOR

Description

Cryoprecipitated antihemophilic factor (AHF) is a plasma derivative that provides a concentrated form of certain coagulation factors. One unit of cryoprecipitated AHF is obtained from one unit of fresh-frozen plasma that has been slowly thawed at 1°C to 6°C (33.8°F to 42.8°F), centrifuged to concentrate the cold precipitated proteins, and had all but 10 to 15 mL of supernatant plasma removed. This product is then refrozen at −18°C (−4°F) and has a storage time to expiration of 1 year. It contains approximately 80 to 120 units of factor VIII (both factor VIII:C and factor VIII:vWf), 20% to 30% of the factor XIII contained in the original unit of FFP, 150 to 250 mg of fibrinogen, and fibronectin.

Indications

The primary indication for cryoprecipitated AHF is the treatment of congenital or acquired fibrinogen or factor XIII deficiency and dysfibrinogenemia (as may be encountered in severe liver disease). It is also indicated in the adjunctive management of bleeding in uremic patients in whom other modalities, such as desmopressin acetate (DDAVP) or hemodialysis, have proven less than fully effective. At present, it is less commonly used as a source of fibrinogen for "fibrin glue" because of the availability of FDA-approved fibrin sealants, such as Tisseel, Crosseal, or Hemaseel.

Precautions and Contraindications

Importantly, cryoprecipitated AHF is no longer indicated for the treatment of patients with factor VIII deficiency (hemophilia A) or von Willebrand disease as specific coagulation factor concentrates, such as Humate-P, Helixate FS, or Advate, are available. Transfusion of ABO-incompatible cryoprecipitated AHF is generally without appreciable clinical sequelae because of the small amount of plasma contained in each unit. However, hemolysis has been reported following infusion of large amounts of cryoprecipitate, and a positive DAT may occur following transfusion of smaller amounts.

Dosing and Administration

In patients with hypofibrinogenemia (fibrinogen <100 mg/dL), each unit of cryoprecipitated AHF should raise the fibrinogen level by 5 to 10 mg/dL. It must be transfused through a blood administration set containing a nominal 170 μm (150 to 260 μm) filter, and infusion must be completed within 4 hours of pooling. Treatment of patients with factor XIII deficiency should be coordinated with the help of a hematologist experienced with this disorder.

Additional Processing

LEUKOCYTE REDUCTION

Description

The goal of leukocyte reduction is to lower the concentration of contaminating white blood cells (Table 5) in RBCs and platelets to less than 5×10^6 leukocytes per component transfused to help prevent a variety of adverse events. The preferred method for achieving leukoreduction is prestorage filtration using third-generation leukoreduction filters processed under current good manufacturing

TABLE 5 FDA and AABB Standards for Blood Banks and Transfusion Services, Leukoreduction

Blood Component	Maximal Allowed Leukocyte Concentration
Red blood cells, leukocyte reduced	<5 × 10^6 per unit
Platelets, leukocyte reduced (RDP)	<8.3 × 10^5 per unit (for a 6 unit pool ≤4.98 × 10^6)
Platelets pheresis, leukocyte reduced	<5 × 10^6 per unit

practice during preprocessing at the blood collection facility. Filtration may also be performed before transfusion at the bedside. Current third-generation leukocyte filters are capable of removing greater than 99.99% (4-log reduction) of leukocytes with less than 10% RBC loss.

Indications

At present, there are no strict indications for the use of leukocyte reduction, although it affords several benefits. These include lower rates of febrile nonhemolytic transfusion reactions by decreasing the number of donor leukocytes that are the target of recipient leukagglutinins, lower rates of transfusion-associated cytomegalovirus (CMV) transmission, and lower rates of HLA-alloimmunization that occurs via stimulation by class I and class II HLA antigens present on donor leukocytes.

CYTOMEGALOVIRUS-REDUCED RISK COMPONENTS

Description

Red blood cells and platelets, but not previously frozen plasma, may transmit CMV from an infective donor to a susceptible recipient because CMV is spread via intact leukocytes. Blood components are generally considered *CMV-reduced risk* (*CMV safe*) if they test CMV-seronegative by an FDA-approved assay method, or if an untested component is leukocyte-reduced by third-generation filtration performed under cGMP.

Indications

Severely immunocompromised, CMV-seronegative patients (Table 6) are at risk for the development of potentially fatal, primary CMV infection and must be transfused with CMV-safe blood components.

TABLE 6 High-Risk Patient Populations Requiring Transfusion of CMV-Safe Blood Components

- CMV-seronegative recipients of allogeneic or autologous hematopoietic progenitor cell (HPC) transplants
- CMV-seronegative recipients of a CMV-seronegative solid-organ transplant
- CMV-seronegative patients receiving immunosuppressive chemotherapy for a hematologic malignancy
- CMV-seronegative patients with a primary immunodeficiency disorder
- CMV-seronegative HIV-infected patients
- CMV-seronegative pregnant women
- CMV-seronegative low-birth-weight (<1200 g) premature infants
- Intrauterine transfusions

GAMMA IRRADIATION

Description

Irradiation involves exposure of blood components to 25 Gy of gamma radiation (15 Gy minimum). This is a dose sufficient to prevent proliferation of viable donor T cells and the development of transfusion-associated graft-versus-host disease (TA-GVHD). Blood components that contain viable T lymphocytes include RBCs, platelets, granulocytes, and nonfrozen plasma. Irradiation may be performed in the hospital blood bank or at blood centers using self-contained blood irradiators with cesium-137 or cobalt-60. Conventional radiation therapy (RT) devices may also be used if proper technical procedures have been established and validated. Irradiated RBCs must be transfused within 28 days or by the originally assigned outdate, whichever comes first, because of radiation-induced damage with potassium leakage and shortened post-transfusion red blood cell survival.

Indications

The sole indication for gamma irradiation is to prevent TA-GVHD in susceptible patients (Table 7). At the doses used, irradiation is ineffective in reducing the viability of transfusion-associated pathogens, such as viruses or bacteria.

SALINE WASHING

Description

Washing of RBCs or platelets with sterile saline is performed to remove donor plasma and is generally

TABLE 7 Patients at Risk for Development of Transfusion-Associated Graft-Versus-Host-Disease (TA-GVHD)

- Intrauterine transfusion
- Neonates receiving exchange transfusion
- Patients with congenital cellular immune deficiencies
- Patients receiving immunosuppressive chemotherapy for hematologic malignancies
- Patients with a history of Hodgkin's disease
- Patients with a history of treatment with purine analogues (such as fludarabine)
- Patients undergoing HPC transplantation
- Patients receiving certain blood products, including:
  - HLA-matched platelets
  - Directed blood donations from family members (blood relatives)
  - Granulocytes

Abbreviations: HLA = human leukocyte antibody; HPC = hematopoietic progenitor cell.

performed in the blood bank using automated blood cell washers. Washing removes approximately 99% of plasma proteins, electrolytes, and antibodies; but it is associated with up to a 20% red blood cell loss and more than a 30% platelet loss. Washing also reduces the number of leukocytes by 90% to 99% in RBCs, but not enough to effectively prevent HLA-alloimmunization. Washed RBCs must be transfused within 24 hours of preparation and washed platelets within 4 hours of preparation.

Indications

Washing is indicated in patients with a history of previous anaphylactic or serious anaphylactoid reaction after transfusion of plasma-containing blood products or in patients with IgA deficiency and anti-IgA antibodies; it may also be beneficial in patients with ahaptoglobinemia and anti-haptoglobin antibodies. Platelets collected from a mother for transfusion to her newborn with neonatal alloimmune thrombocytopenia (NAIT) should be washed to remove maternal antiplatelet antibodies.

Disclaimer

The recommendations and guidelines presented here are intended primarily for educational purposes. All health care providers must acquaint themselves with the local hospital or institutional transfusion policies. Additionally, appropriate consultation with a blood bank or transfusion medicine physician should be sought when questions arise regarding transfusion-related issues in patient care.

ADVERSE REACTIONS TO BLOOD TRANSFUSIONS

METHOD OF

Gerald L. Logue, MD

Transfusion medicine has developed as a clinical discipline with a strong scientific base over the past century. Advances in immunology and blood resource management have allowed transfusion therapy to become standard treatment for many medical conditions. Adverse reactions to blood transfusion therapy range from severe life-threatening emergencies to those posing only minor inconvenience. These reactions may be immediate, occurring during or within hours of transfusion, or delayed, occurring days to months after transfusion.

Immediate Transfusion Reactions

IMMEDIATE HEMOLYTIC TRANSFUSION REACTIONS

Transfusion of ABO-incompatible red blood cells, such as type A or B cells, into a type O recipient, results in the most dangerous and most preventable of immediate reactions. Naturally occurring complement-activating antibodies usually cause rapid intravascular hemolysis producing hemodynamic shock, disseminated intravascular coagulation, and acute renal failure. The prevention of acute hemolytic reactions requires special care to identify the blood drawn from the patient for analysis, as well as the blood products to be transfused. These identification procedures must be taken seriously, because clerical errors account for the majority of acute hemolytic transfusion reactions.

Effective therapy requires rapid diagnosis. All transfusions must be stopped immediately if there is a suspicion of such a reaction. Steps must be taken to identify the cause of this reaction.

Signs and symptoms of an acute hemolytic reaction in a conscious patient include fever, chills, pain at the site of infusion, back or chest pain, flushing, and generalized bleeding. In an unconscious patient, signs may include a falling blood pressure, increased bleeding or oozing, and hemoglobinuria. When an immediate hemolytic transfusion reaction is suspected, a sample of blood should be drawn from the patient and sent immediately to the blood bank with the donor blood. After infusion of ABO-incompatible blood, the plasma is usually red. Fresh urine should be examined for hemoglobin.

If an acute hemolytic reaction is verified, therapy must begin immediately to maintain blood pressure, intravascular volume, blood pH, urine alkalinity, and urine output. Hypotension should be treated with volume replacement, and a screen for disseminated intravascular coagulation should be ordered. If the patient has overt disseminated intravascular coagulation, therapy with cryoprecipitate, 2 to 4 units, should be given if the fibrinogen level is less than 100 mg per dL; platelets, 4 to 6 individual units, should be given if the platelet count is less than 50,000 per mm^3 and fresh-frozen plasma, 1 to 3 units as tolerated by fluid volume status, given if the partial thromboplastin time is elevated. Mannitol or furosemide (Lasix) should be used as necessary to prevent acute tubular necrosis. Urine output and serum electrolyte and creatine levels should be monitored closely. Immediate hemodialysis may be required.

ACUTE FEBRILE REACTIONS

Febrile nonhemolytic reactions are characterized by fever and tachycardia. These reactions occur in previously transfused or multiparous patients and are caused by antileukocyte antibodies. When fever occurs during a blood transfusion, the transfusion should be stopped and the patient studied for a hemolytic reaction. If a hemolytic reaction has not occurred, antipyretics such as acetaminophen may be administered. If a patient has recurrent febrile reactions, it may be necessary to premedicate with antipyretics before the transfusion. White blood cell antibodies can rarely produce a transfusion-associated acute respiratory distress syndrome that is characterized by pulmonary edema with normal cardiac function. Microaggregate filters are useful to prevent febrile transfusion reactions as well as transfusion-associated acute respiratory distress syndrome.

Rarely, blood products become contaminated with bacteria. Some gram-negative organisms such as *Yersinia* spp. and *Pseudomonas* spp. can survive and multiply under refrigerated conditions. If this complication is suspected, the transfusion must be discontinued and the blood product must be cultured and Gram stained immediately. If a contaminated transfusion is suspected, therapy should include support of the patient's blood pressure, kidney function, and tissue oxygenation. Shock, if present, is caused by infusion of endotoxin, but broad-spectrum antibiotics should also be initiated pending the results of culture.

ACUTE URTICARIAL REACTIONS

Hives occur in approximately 3% of patients who receive blood transfusions and usually are caused by a reaction to plasma antigens present in the transfused blood. Such reactions are rarely serious. To treat this reaction, the transfusion is stopped and an antihistamine such as diphenhydramine administered. The patient is then watched carefully for 10 to 30 minutes. If further signs and symptoms of allergic reaction such as dyspnea, wheezing, chills, or fever ensue, epinephrine may be given.

CONGESTIVE HEART FAILURE

Hypervolemia may occur when blood is rapidly given to patients with compromised cardiovascular status. Such patients obviously should receive packed red blood cells rather than whole blood. For patients with severe chronic anemia who have evidence of congestive heart failure, packed red blood cells should be infused slowly with the patient in a semi-upright position. Packed red blood cell transfusions are usually well tolerated, and the increased oxygen-carrying capacity of the blood hastens the patient's overall improvement.

ANAPHYLACTIC REACTIONS

Anaphylactic reactions to blood are extremely rare. Patients who are IgA deficient may experience anaphylactic reactions after receiving blood products. These reactions are caused by antibiotics against IgA, usually in individuals previously exposed to blood products. The incidence of severe IgA deficiency in the general population is approximately 0.1%. If an anaphylactic reaction to blood products is suspected, the patient should have quantitation of serum IgA levels before further transfusion therapy is attempted.

COMPLICATIONS OF MASSIVE BLOOD PRODUCT TRANSFUSION

Other immediate reactions include the potential for citrate toxicity. With massive infusions of large volumes of blood products containing citrate, it is potentially possible to decrease ionized calcium levels. When massive transfusions are being given, it is important to continue careful cardiac monitoring, and if arrhythmias related to calcium occur, it is important that intravenous calcium be administered. Also, hypothermia can be produced with massive blood transfusions of cold blood. Acute vascular hypothermia may affect platelet function and produce cardiac arrhythmias. In all situations of massive transfusion, temperature-controlled warming devices should be used to warm blood before infusion. With large-volume transfusion it is also theoretically possible to produce hyperkalemia by potassium leakage from stored red blood cells. Transfusion-associated hyperkalemia is rare, but in a large-volume transfusion situation, careful monitoring for cardiac arrhythmias related to hyperkalemia is also essential. Dilutional coagulopathy and thrombocytopenia are occasionally seen when massive transfusion requirements are met by transfusion of packed red blood cells alone. It is useful to transfuse fresh-frozen plasma and platelets along with red blood cells if the blood loss exceeds an entire blood volume.

Delayed Transfusion Reactions

A variety of complications may occur days to months after transfusion of blood products. Some of these reactions are immune, but the largest number of reactions occur as the result of the transfusion of infectious agents. The blood supply in the United States is safe because blood is collected from volunteer donors whose history is carefully evaluated and the blood is tested for markers of infectious disease including HIV and hepatitis.

DELAYED HEMOLYTIC TRANSFUSION REACTIONS

Delayed hemolytic reactions occur in patients who have previously been sensitized to minor blood group antigens but whose antibody levels have fallen below detectability by routine screening procedures. After transfusion, an anamnestic antibody response occurs, usually within 2 weeks after transfusion of red blood cells containing the offending antigen. These reactions are characterized by a falling hemoglobin level and a rise in the bilirubin concentration. The direct antiglobulin test may or may not become positive transiently, but plasma antibody against the antigen usually becomes detectable in 1 to 2 weeks. Although the hemolysis remains limited to the transfused cells that possess the antigen, delayed transfusion reactions may rarely produce abrupt intravascular hemolysis with the risk of renal failure. It is important to identify delayed hemolytic transfusion reactions because on subsequent transfusion, the antibody may again have disappeared, and blood bank records are the only method of identifying the antibody and preventing recurrent, delayed hemolytic transfusion reactions.

POST-TRANSFUSION PURPURA

Post-transfusion purpura is a rare, delayed reaction of blood transfusion that occurs most commonly after packed red blood cell transfusions. Patients with post-transfusion purpura usually lack a common "public" platelet antigen such as PL^{A1} (HPA-1A). When these individuals are transfused with the antigen, an immune thrombocytopenic syndrome that destroys the patient's own platelets is triggered. The reaction is characterized by the abrupt onset of severe thrombocytopenia, usually with bleeding, 3 to 14 days after the transfusion of blood products. Treatment is empirical and includes the use of high-dose intravenous immune globulin (2 g/kg) and plasmapheresis.

TRANSFUSION-ASSOCIATED GRAFT-VERSUS-HOST DISEASE

Because blood products contain circulating stem cells, a transfusion recipient, especially if immunocompromised, may be inadvertently engrafted with the donor stem cells and develop graft-versus-host disease. The clinical complex of rash, mucositis, diarrhea, and abnormal liver functions from this disease may not be recognized in transfusion recipients. Although such complications usually occur in patients with recognized immunosuppression, they have been described in patients with no known predisposing conditions. Clinical symptoms usually occur 1 to 2 weeks after transfusion and are almost invariably fatal. Thus, it is extremely important that patients with known or suspected immunodeficiency syndromes receive irradiated blood products. It is also recommended that blood irradiation be used for directed donations from first-degree relatives.

VIRAL AGENTS

Hepatitis Viruses

Hepatitis B and C can be transmitted by transfusion of blood products. Screening of blood for hepatitis B virus is well characterized and effectively eliminates the transfusion of this agent by blood products. Hepatitis C testing eliminates the vast majority of hepatitis C transmissions. Thus, with the advent of rigorous testing for the various hepatitis viruses, the likelihood of transmitting viral hepatitis has been reduced to the range of 1% or less in most areas.

Retroviruses

Human immunodeficiency virus types 1 and 2 (HIV1 and HIV2) and human T-cell lymphotropic virus (HTLV) types I and II may be transmitted by blood products. Prevention of transmission of HIV in blood products is accomplished by several mechanisms. The first includes rigorous questioning to exclude individuals likely to be infected with the virus and immunologic screening, including testing for HIV antibodies and, most recently, HIV antigen testing in transfusion products. These testing procedures make the transmission of HIV by transfusion extraordinarily rare. HTLV screening also occurs. As in other situations described previously, leukodepletion may markedly reduce the transmissibility of agents such as HTLV.

Herpesvirus

The herpesvirus cytomegalovirus and Epstein-Barr virus are known to be transmitted by blood products. Most individuals receiving transfusion therapy are immune to Epstein-Barr virus, so the significance of transmission of this virus is questionable. Cytomegalovirus can also be transmitted by transfusions of blood products, and cytomegalovirus-negative blood is used in certain restricted situations such as for low-birth-weight infants and bone marrow transplant recipients. It is also clear that leukodepletion of blood products markedly reduces the transmissibility of cytomegalovirus infection.

Parvovirus

Parvovirus, an agent that produces erythroid hypoplasia, may be transmitted by transfusion. Parvovirus-induced aplastic anemia is a risk in patients with underlying hematologic diseases with increased red blood cell production such as patients with sickle cell disease. There is no effective method to screen transfusion products for this virus.

TRANSMISSION OF OTHER INFECTIONS

Rare diseases transmitted by transfusion therapy include malaria, trypanosomiasis, babesiosis, and syphilis. Transmission of falciparum, vivax, and ovale malaria has been controlled by deferring the donation of blood by potentially exposed individuals for 6 months. Persons who have been infected with *Plasmodium malariae* are excluded from blood donation because of the high incidence of asymptomatic carriers of this disease. *Trypanosoma cruzi* causes Chagas' disease in Latin America. Transmission in developed countries has occurred through blood donations from immigrants from areas endemic for this agent. Creutzfeldt-Jakob disease could theoretically be transmitted by transfusion, but no cases of such transmission have been clearly proved. Epidemiologic studies continue in this area. Finally, transmission of *Treponema pallidum*, the causative agent of syphilis, is possible through blood transfusion. Current serologic testing includes studies to detect circulating antibodies to these agents. Although some have suggested that syphilis screening is no longer necessary for blood products, it is likely that identifying individuals who have been exposed to syphilis is also a surrogate marker for other sexually transmitted infections and, therefore, a useful means of excluding blood donors who are potentially infectious with retroviruses.

IMMUNE MODULATION

Controversy exists regarding the role of transfusion of blood products in modulation of the recipient's immune system. This immune modulation probably occurs through exposure of the individual to donor leukocytes. Some retrospective clinical studies suggest that recurrence of tumors is increased after resection in individuals who have received blood products. Also, both retrospective and prospective human studies have found an increase in postoperative bacterial infections in individuals receiving transfusion therapy. This increased risk of bacterial infection appears to be reduced with leukodepleted blood products. Clinical studies in this area are continuing. Leukoreduced blood products are also useful for reducing primary HLA alloimmunization in transfusion recipients. Leukoreduction is clearly most beneficial for prevention of recurrent febrile nonhemolytic transfusion reactions as described previously.

IRON OVERLOAD

Chronic transfusion therapy carries the long-term risk of iron overload. Transfusions in the range of 50 to 100 units of red blood cells carry the risk of tissue damage similar to that seen with idiopathic hemochromatosis, including endocrine, hepatic, and cardiac failure. Symptoms of iron overload may be insidious, and the clinical diagnosis may not be established early. The iron chelation agent deferoxamine (Desferal) is available but difficult to use. Clearly, the judicious use of chronic transfusions is indicated, including erythropoietin administration whenever possible.

SECTION 7

The Digestive System

CHOLELITHIASIS AND CHOLECYSTITIS

METHOD OF

Isaac Samuel, MD, and James W. Maher, MD

In the United States, 5% to 15% of adult females and 4% to 10% of adult males harbor gallstones. However, the majority of patients remain asymptomatic throughout their lives.

Etiology and Pathogenesis

The essential etiopathogenic abnormality that results in cholesterol gallstone formation is an imbalance in the relative *biliary composition* of cholesterol, bile salts, and lecithin. Cholesterol precipitates when the amount of bile salts and lecithin are not sufficient to keep it in a soluble phase (micelles or vesicles). This can happen either if the cholesterol composition of bile increases or the amount of bile salts or lecithin in bile decreases. Agglomeration of precipitated cholesterol crystals to form macroscopic stones is the next phase and is called *nucleation*. Mucin formed by the gallbladder epithelium is incriminated as a pronucleating factor, and gallbladder stasis is also implicated as a culprit. The third phase is that of *stone growth* where, in a nucleating environment, the nidus grows by accumulating more cholesterol crystals, bile salts, bile pigments, mucin, and shed epithelial cells. In the United States, mixed cholesterol-pigment stones and pure cholesterol stones constitute the majority (approximately 70%) and the rest are pigment stones. The etiopathogenesis of pigment stones seen in hemolytic anemias is different, as they are composed of bilirubin from the excessive turnover of bile pigments because of the relentless hepatic breakdown of hemoglobin.

Risk Factors

Knowledge of the etiopathogenesis of cholelithiasis improves our understanding of the factors that put individuals at risk of developing gallstones, which are:

- Female sex, multiparity—estrogen reduces the hepatic conversion of cholesterol to bile acids; progesterone promotes gallbladder stasis.
- Age—risk of gallstone formation increases with age.
- Genetic predisposition—patients often give a family history of gallstone disease. The Pima Native Americans have an extremely high incidence of gallstones.
- Obesity—increased cholesterol in bile.
- Rapid weight loss—reduced bile acid secretion and gallbladder stasis.

- Terminal ileal pathology—in Crohn's disease and following terminal ileal resection, the reduced reabsorption of bile salts by the distal ileum interrupts the enterohepatic recirculation of bile salts.
- Central venous nutrition (CVN)—Prolonged dependence on parenteral nutrition is associated with gallbladder stasis and hyperconcentration of bile.
- Increased bile pigments—hemolytic anemias (increased turnover of bilirubin).
- Cirrhosis—incidence of cholesterol gallstones in alcoholic cirrhosis is diminished, but the risk of pigment stones is higher.

Clinical Presentation

Cholelithiasis presents as biliary colic or acute cholecystitis (Table 1), whereas choledocholithiasis manifests as obstructive jaundice, cholangitis, or acute pancreatitis. In **biliary colic,** pain is experienced *in the absence of acute inflammation* of the gallbladder and occurs because of transient cystic duct obstruction by a gallstone (similar to renal colic in nephrolithiasis). The pain typically lasts 1 to 4 hours and subsides because of spontaneous dislodgement of the stone. The pain, which is located in the right upper quadrant or epigastrium, is often brought on by a meal and may be associated with dyspeptic symptoms such as nausea, vomiting, or burping. Mild local tenderness may be elicited but not peritoneal signs such as rebound tenderness. Chronic cholecystitis is a vague term that is used synonymously with recurrent biliary colic. **Acute cholecystitis** is characterized by pain *with acute inflammation* of the gallbladder (similar to acute pyelonephritis in nephrolithiasis). Persistent cystic duct obstruction by a gallstone first promotes a sterile inflammatory reaction to chemicals such as prostaglandins, followed by bacterial overgrowth (e.g., *Escherichia coli, Klebsiella*). The acute inflammation is accompanied by local peritoneal signs, fever, tachycardia, or leukocytosis. The pain lasts hours to days. Signs of peritoneal irritation such as rebound tenderness and a positive Murphy's sign may develop. Murphy's sign is positive when a patient catches the breath against a palpating hand during inspiration. Beware the deceptive presentation of a gangrenous gallbladder in diabetics, which may manifest itself with minimal clinical signs.

TABLE 1 Biliary Colic Versus Acute Cholecystitis: A Comparison of the Contrasting Features of Biliary Colic and Acute Cholecystitis

	Biliary Colic	Acute Cholecystitis
Cystic duct obstruction	Transient	Persistent
Acute inflammation	Absent	Present
Bacterial overgrowth	Absent	Present in the majority
Pain	Brief; 1-4 h	Progressive; hours to days
Rebound tenderness	Absent	Present
Murphy sign	Negative	Usually positive
Tachycardia	Absent	Usually present
Fever	Absent	Usually present
Leukocytosis	Absent	Usually present
Hospital admission	Occasional	Usually the rule
Antibiotics	Not needed	Essential
Cholecystectomy	Less urgent	Ideally within 72 h of onset

Routine Investigations

Leukocytosis is consistent with acute cholecystitis rather than biliary colic. Elevations in serum direct bilirubin, alkaline phosphatase, and gamma-glutamyl transferase (GGT) indicate associated choledocholithiasis. Serum aspartate transaminase and alanine transaminase may be mildly elevated secondary to inflammation of the gallbladder bed and do not correlate with common bile duct obstruction. In obstructive jaundice, urobilinogen is absent in the urine as the exclusion of conjugated bilirubin from the gut prevents formation of urobilinogen. Hyperamylasemia that is greater than three times the basal value suggests acute pancreatitis. Hyperlipasemia is more specific for acute pancreatitis than is hyperamylasemia. Macroamylasemia is a chronic elevation of serum amylase levels because of binding of amylase to macromolecules, such as immunoglobulins or polysaccharides, that prevents renal excretion of amylase; the absence of an elevated urinary amylase differentiates it from hyperamylasemia.

A right upper quadrant ultrasound is the initial investigation of choice to ascertain the presence of gallstones. As most gallstones are radiolucent, radiographic investigations are a waste of time and resources. Ultrasonographic examination is not expensive, does not expose the patient to radiation, is noninvasive, and detects up to 95% of gallstones. The typical appearance of a gallstone on ultrasonographic examination is a hyperechoic area with an acoustic window. Additional findings in acute cholecystitis include edema and thickening of the gallbladder wall, pericholecystic fluid collections, and common bile duct dilatation.

Special Investigations

ERCP (endoscopic retrograde cholangiopancreaticogram) uses a side-viewing endoscope to cannulate the ampulla of Vater, and radiopaque dye is injected retrograde up the biliary tree under fluoroscopic visualization. Dilatation of the common bile duct is evaluated and choledocholithiasis is diagnosed by the presence of filling defects. Endoscopic sphincterotomy and extraction of stones with ERCP are routine procedures in expert hands and are performed before or even after cholecystectomy, making surgical exploration of the common bile duct rarely necessary.

Combined with the appropriate antibiotic therapy, ERCP is also the definitive treatment for acute cholangitis.

HIDA (Hepatoiminodiacetic Acid) Scan

The radionuclide ^{99m}technetium-labeled iminodiacetic acid is injected intravenously and is selectively taken up by the liver and excreted into the biliary tract. In patients in whom the ultrasonogram fails to detect gallstones (e.g., a very small stone) in spite of a strong clinical suspicion of acute cholecystitis, an HIDA scan finding of a nonfilling gallbladder supports the diagnosis. The HIDA scan is also invaluable in detecting bile leaks after cholecystectomy.

Ultrasonography and the HIDA scan have largely replaced the intravenous cholangiogram in most situations. An oral cholecystogram can be useful in biliary colic where ultrasonography was negative (HIDA scan would not show a nonfilling gallbladder if the cystic duct is not actively occluded). ERCP with bile analysis for microlithiasis is indicated if the oral cholecystogram fails to show filling defects suggestive of gallstones. Magnetic resonance cholangiography for detection of common bile duct stones is a developing area. The percutaneous transhepatic cholangiogram is used mainly in biliary tract malignant obstruction with a dilated intrahepatic biliary tree. Computerized tomography (CT) has no place in the routine initial investigation of gallstone problems as most gallstones are radiolucent, but has a useful role in the evaluation of the acute abdomen where it may show inflammatory edema, gas in the gallbladder wall, a dilated common bile duct, or acute pancreatitis.

Differential Diagnosis

Upper abdominal pain of acute onset can be the result of common conditions affecting surrounding organs such as peptic ulcer disease, acute pancreatitis, acute appendicitis, irritable bowel syndrome, renal colic, pyelonephritis, right lower lobe pneumonia, pleurisy, myocardial infarction, and angina pectoris. Obstructive jaundice from choledocholithiasis must be differentiated from biliary tract strictures and obstructions from carcinoma of the head of the pancreas, biliary tract tumors, and periampullary tumors. Applying Courvoisier law, in a patient with obstructive jaundice, if the gallbladder is palpable, it is unlikely to be caused by stones (i.e., think cancer). The underlying principle is that stones cause fibrosis with a nondistensible, or even shrunken, gallbladder.

Treatment

Biliary colic is most often treated in the outpatient setting with analgesia and a diagnostic workup, including right upper quadrant ultrasound and liver function tests, and scheduled for laparoscopic cholecystectomy within 1 to 3 weeks. In the occasional patient the biliary colic is of such severity that the patient needs hospital admission, intravenous fluids and fasting, parenteral analgesia, and urgent laparoscopic cholecystectomy. Antibiotics are not indicated for a clinical diagnosis of biliary colic. In acute cholecystitis the patient is admitted, given intravenous antibiotics in addition to the above measures, followed by laparoscopic cholecystectomy within 3 days (see Table 1). Laparoscopic or even open operations during the second week are more difficult and occasionally dangerous because of the combination of edema and fibrosis of tissues that makes dissection difficult and risks grave injuries to the biliary tract or even large vessels such as the inferior vena cava, portal vein, or hepatic artery. In patients presenting late it is often more advisable to postpone surgery by 6 to 8 weeks, by which time the acute inflammation would have subsided.

Until the late 1980s the traditional management of acute cholecystitis was to treat the initial attack nonoperatively, followed by an elective open cholecystectomy after about 6 to 8 weeks, necessitating a second hospital admission. Over and above the inconvenience and socioeconomic implications of two hospital admissions, this conventional approach was further compounded by the observation that a significant number of patients returned to the hospital with an additional attack of acute cholecystitis during the intervening period. The advent of a laparoscopic approach to cholecystectomy in 1989 dramatically changed this equation. Surgical intervention within the first few days of acute cholecystitis is an advantage for a laparoscopic approach as the edema associated with acute inflammation makes it easier to dissect tissue planes. Furthermore, a second hospital admission for surgery is avoided, and the risk of problems between admissions is altogether eliminated. A laparoscopic approach has several additional advantages such as a shorter hospital stay, expedient return to a normal diet, early ambulation, quicker recovery and return to work, reduced analgesic requirements, better cosmetic results, and the avoidance of incisional hernias.

During cholecystectomy, a selective intraoperative cholangiogram is indicated in patients with a history of jaundice or acute pancreatitis, an obstructive liver function test pattern (elevated plasma direct bilirubin, alkaline phosphatase, or GGT), ultrasonographic or other evidence of a dilated common bile duct, and multiple small stones associated with a wide cystic duct. A cholangiogram can also be a vital aid to delineate the anatomy in difficult cases. Injury to other organs during induction of pneumoperitoneum and unrecognized biliary tract and bowel injuries are rare but serious complications. Postoperative cystic duct leaks manifest within 1 to 2 days with right upper quadrant tenderness, and sometimes fever and jaundice, and are treated with ERCP and stent placement followed by stent removal in three weeks. Severe cirrhotics have a high morbidity and mortality from cholecystectomy and do better with drainage via a cholecystostomy tube placed under ultrasonographic guidance, a modality that also has a useful place in high-risk patients such as in multisystem organ failure, after major surgery, and in patients with significant coexisting conditions.

Complications of Cholelithiasis

Choledocholithiasis may cause obstructive jaundice with dark urine, clay-colored stool, steatorrhea, pruritus, and coagulopathy secondary to reduced vitamin K absorption. ERCP with sphincterotomy or intraoperative common bile duct exploration is required to remove the stones. The former is less invasive but the appropriate expertise must be available. *Acute cholangitis* is an acute inflammation of the biliary tree secondary to choledocholithiasis. The clinical presentation is characterized by Charcot triad (jaundice, pain, fever with chills). *Acute suppurative cholangitis* is a clinical emergency where the biliary tract is filled with pus and presents with Charcot triad plus hypotension and mental confusion (Reynolds pentad). The treatment for suppurative cholangitis consists of fluid resuscitation, broad-spectrum antibiotics, and ERCP with endoscopic sphincterotomy and extraction of stones followed by laparoscopic cholecystectomy, or surgical common bile duct exploration during cholecystectomy. *Acute gangrenous cholecystitis* presents as an acute abdomen and needs broad-spectrum antibiotics and emergent cholecystectomy. *Acute emphysematous cholecystitis* results from anaerobic organisms, affects patients over 60 years of age (especially diabetics), is detected by the presence of gas in the gallbladder wall or lumen, and needs appropriate antibiotics and emergent cholecystectomy. *Gallstone-induced acute pancreatitis* may be mild or severe and needs treatment of acute pancreatitis followed by cholecystectomy with intraoperative cholangiogram on the same hospital admission after the pancreatitis has subsided. If cholecystectomy is postponed for a few weeks, as was the conventional practice, the risk of a second attack of acute pancreatitis is substantial. Gallstone pancreatitis with the stone still impacted at the ampulla is suspected when there are unresolving symptoms or persistent hyperamylasemia or hyperlipasemia. Urgent ERCP with sphincterotomy and extraction of the stone is beneficial in these cases of stone impaction, and also improves the complication rate and mortality in severe cases of gallstone pancreatitis. *Gallstone ileus* is bowel obstruction caused by a gallstone that erodes through the gallbladder wall into the duodenum (sometimes stomach or colon) creating a cholecystoduodenal fistula. A plain radiograph may show the classic triad of bowel obstruction, gas in the biliary tree, and a stone in the right lower quadrant. The stone is removed by enterotomy, but the cholecystoduodenal fistula is dealt with at a later operation if necessary. *Gallbladder cancer* is very rare but infrequently occurs in the absence of gallstones.

Special Considerations

Asymptomatic cholelithiasis patients in the general population do not need surgery. Less than 2% per year of those with gallstones develop symptoms or complications, and the vast majority (more than 66%) remain asymptomatic throughout their lives. In view of these statistics, the general consensus is that prophylactic cholecystectomy for asymptomatic cholelithiasis, even in a diabetic patient, is not indicated as the risk of complications of surgery is greater than the risk of gallstones causing problems. However, there are a few exceptions:

- Patients undergoing bariatric surgery are at high risk of developing symptoms postoperatively during the period of rapid weight loss and therefore should be routinely screened for cholelithiasis prior to bariatric surgery.
- Patients with hemolytic anemias have a more aggressive course of disease progression because of the rapid rate of stone formation.
- Pediatric patients have a potentially longer period to endure and therefore are at greater risk.
- Patients with a porcelain gallbladder have an extremely high risk of developing gallbladder cancer.

Acute acalculous cholecystitis is a recognized clinical entity where an inflamed gallbladder with a clinical picture of acute cholecystitis is seen even in the complete absence of gallstones. It occurs mostly in intensive care patients on parenteral nutrition and can be managed by the placement of a percutaneous cholecystostomy tube and antibiotic administration.

Cholecystodyskinesia is a hypomotility disorder of the gallbladder that presents with a biliary colic-like picture even though gallstones are not present. A diagnosis is made when the gallbladder fails to empty sufficiently under ultrasonography challenged with a fatty meal or HIDA scan with intravenous cholecystokinin stimulation. Carefully selected patients frequently benefit from cholecystectomy.

Bile acid lytic therapy constitutes oral dissolution therapy for gallstones. Ursodeoxycholic acid (Actigall), a bile acid, can dissolve small cholesterol stones in a functioning gallbladder. Prophylaxis with ursodeoxycholic acid[1] has been shown to be effective at reducing the risk of stone formation during rapid weight loss (for example, after bariatric surgery).

Postcholecystectomy syndrome is a term applied in patients with continuing, new, or vague symptoms after cholecystectomy, but following detailed investigation the symptoms are usually found to arise because of a separate disease process and therefore the very existence of such a syndrome is doubted.

[1]Not FDA approved for this indication.

CIRRHOSIS

METHOD OF

David S. Kotlyar, BS, and K. Rajender Reddy, MD

Cirrhosis is the tenth most common cause of death in the United States, and one of the leading causes of death in the world. The condition is characterized by nodular regeneration and fibrosis. Nodular regeneration or fibrosis alone are not synonymous with cirrhosis. The most common causes of cirrhosis include:

- Alcohol abuse
- Infection with hepatitis C virus
- Infection with hepatitis B virus
- Nonalcoholic steatohepatitis
- Cholestatic disorders such as primary biliary cirrhosis and primary sclerosing cholangitis
- Inborn errors of metabolism such as Wilson's disease and hemochromatosis
- Vascular disorders such as hepatic vein thrombosis
- Autoimmune chronic hepatitis

Symptoms and Diagnosis

There are several nonspecific symptoms of cirrhosis including fatigue, malaise, weight loss, skin fragility, easy bruising, and abdominal discomfort. On physical exam there may be jaundice and parotid gland swelling, and the spleen (left upper quadrant) may be enlarged. The right upper quadrant may be tender, and an enlarged liver may be palpable. Also, the patient may have gynecomastia and palmar erythema. There may be spider angiomas on the face, neck, and torso.

If there is dullness upon tapping of the abdomen, or distension of the abdomen, this is an indication that there may be ascites, which suggests the possibility of severe liver disease. Patients may also have slight confusion, which may be a feature of encephalopathy. Generalized pruritus can also be indicative of chronic liver disease, and this is more common in patients with cholestatic liver disease.

Laboratory investigations can further help to narrow down a diagnosis of cirrhosis of the liver. The initial investigations most commonly done are the alanine aminotransferase (ALT) test, the aspartate aminotransferase (AST) test, the serum bilirubin test, and the alkaline phosphatase test. Elevated ALT or AST levels may indicate generalized liver disease, without pinpointing a cause. Cirrhosis may be indicated by the presence of a higher AST over ALT. Additional tests include serum albumin and the measurement of the prothrombin time. In the context of elevated aminotransferase levels, low levels of serum albumin and a prolonged prothrombin time suggest significant liver injury. Blood counts should also be performed; if cytopenia is present it supports portal hypertension secondary to chronic liver disease, which is often cirrhosis. High alkaline phosphatase levels relative to aminotransferase levels strongly suggest a cholestatic process as opposed to hepatocellular injury.

Table 1 lists common causes of cirrhosis and basic diagnostic testing.

Complications

Many patients with cirrhosis have no serious outward complications from the disease. These patients are described as having compensated cirrhosis. For the remaining patients, several classic complications arise, and this is described as decompensated cirrhosis. The major complications include ascites, bleeding from esophageal varices, and hepatic encephalopathy. Other common and serious complications include spontaneous bacterial peritonitis, which may progress to hepatorenal syndrome, and hepatocellular carcinoma.

ASCITES

Manifestations

Ascites is the most common complication to evolve from cirrhosis. In 33% to 50% of patients with compensated cirrhosis, ascites will develop within 10 years. Portal hypertension is a prerequisite for the formation of ascites. In response to portal hypertension, there is vasodilation of the arterioles of the splanchnic circulation, and to compensate, there is activation of the

TABLE 1 Common Causes of Cirrhosis

Condition	Diagnostic Testing*
Hepatitis C	Anti-HCV (EIA), HCV RNA, genotype, quantitative HCV RNA
Hepatitis B	HBsAg, HBeAg, HBeAb, HBV DNA
Autoimmune chronic hepatitis	ANA, ASMA, Anti-LKM, quantitative IgG
Hemochromatosis	Serum iron and total iron binding capacity, serum ferritin, *HFE* gene analysis
Primary biliary cirrhosis	AMA, quantitative IgM
Primary sclerosing cholangitis	p-ANCA, combination of chemical, biochemical, and radiological features
Alcohol abuse	AST/ALT ratio >2:1, ALT and AST usually <500 IU/dL, liver biopsy
Wilson's disease	Serum ceruloplasmin, serum copper, hepatic copper content, Kayser-Fleischer rings

*These are some of the basic tests; further testing may be required based on the clinical situation.

Abbreviations: ALT = alanine aminotransferase; AMA = antimitochondrial antibody; ANA = antinuclear antibody; ASMA = antismooth muscle antibody; AST = aspartate aminotransferase; EIA = enzyme immunoassays; HBeAb = hepatitis B e antibody; HBeAg = hepatitis B e antigen; HBsAg = hepatitis B surface antigen; HCV = hepatitis C virus; IU = international unit; LKM = liver-kidney microsome; p-ANCA = pericytoplasmic antineutrophil nuclear antibodies.

renin-angiotensin system. This causes massive sodium retention, and, when coupled with an increase in hydrostatic pressure in the portal system and a decrease in oncotic pressure due to hypoalbuminemia, leads to ascites. The formation of ascites secondary to cirrhosis is one of the indications for consideration of liver transplant.

Clinical examination is unreliable in the detection of small-to-moderate amounts of ascites, particularly if patients are obese. Therefore ultrasonography is the ideal test to detect small-to-moderate amounts of ascites. Further ultrasonography can be used to rule out thromboses of the hepatic vasculature, and hepatocellular carcinoma. Upon detection of ascites, a paracentesis should be performed and the fluid examined for total protein, polymorphonuclear leukocyte (PMN) count, and albumin. A same-day serum albumin should also be obtained. The serum ascites-albumin gradient (SAAG [serum albumin]-[ascitic albumin]) is an excellent diagnostic tool for confirming portal hypertension as the cause of the ascites (>97% accuracy). A SAAG value of ≥1.1 g/dL is confirmatory for portal hypertension as the cause of ascites. Paracentesis carries a very small risk of bowel perforation or abdominal wall hematoma (<1:1000).

Treatment

Ascites can be graded in severity, and treatment can be tailored based on the grade of ascites. If ascites is solely seen on ultrasound, it is categorized as grade 1. Sodium restriction may be sufficient without the need for diuretics. However, additional diuretics may hasten resolution. If the abdomen becomes distended, then this ascites is categorized as grade 2. Most cases of grade 1 ascites progress to grade 2. Tense ascites is considered grade 3 ascites. Figure 1 is a guide to treatment of ascites.

For ascites of grade 2 or higher, sodium restriction to 2 g (88 mEq) per day is recommended, as well as the initiation of diuretics. The recommended diuretics are oral spironolactone (Aldactone) and furosemide (Lasix)[1] with initial doses of 100 mg and 40 mg, respectively, taken once in the morning. Painful gynecomastia may result from taking spironolactone and if this occurs, amiloride (Midamor)[1] can be substituted (5 to 20 mg/d). However, amiloride[1] is less effective in reducing ascites. If initial doses of spironolactone and furosemide[1] do not resolve the ascites, the dosage can be increased every 3 to 5 days up to a maximum of 400 mg per day for spironolactone and 160 mg per day[3] for furosemide. Grade 3 ascites should be treated first with therapeutic paracentesis, followed by administration of diuretics and salt restriction.

A key indicator of response to diuretics is a random spot urine test to see if the ratio of the sodium-to-potassium concentration has reversed and is greater than 1. If so, then it is approximately 90% certain that the patient is satisfactorily excreting enough sodium (minimum of 78 mmol per day). Ideal target weight loss because of a decrease in ascites should be approximately 0.5 kg per day in patients without edema, and approximately 1 kg per day in patients with leg edema. If it is observed that there is no weight loss, but patients have good sodium clearance, then noncompliance with sodium restriction should be considered and discussed with the patient. Patients who are sensitive to diuretics can be treated with sodium restriction and oral diuretics without the need for therapeutic paracentesis.

Inpatient treatment should be initiated upon the evolution of encephalopathy, bacterial infection, or gastrointestinal hemorrhage. However, if patients do not have these complications, and are steadily losing weight they can be followed in the outpatient setting. Also, fluid restriction is not necessary unless the patient's serum sodium level falls below 120 mmol/L.

If ascites proves resistant to diuretics, two other treatments are available:

1. Serial paracenteses

[1]Not FDA approved for this indication.
[3]Exceeds dosage recommended by the manufacturer.

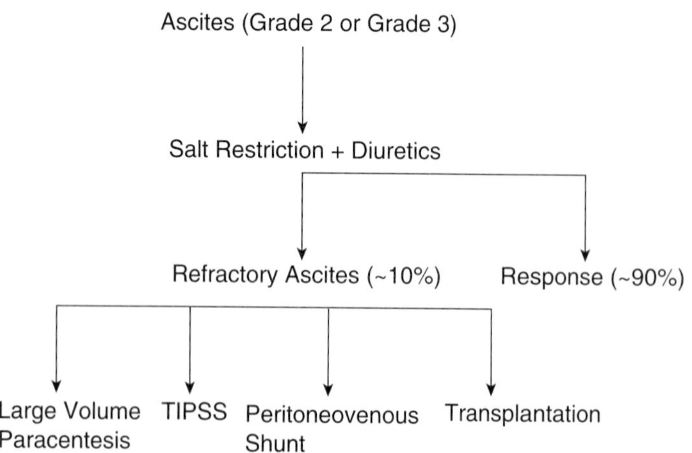

FIGURE 1 A guide to the treatment of ascites.

2. Transjugular intrahepatic portosystemic stent shunt (TIPSS)

Paracentesis is highly effective. Two possible complications are postparacentesis circulatory disturbance (PPCD) and renal impairment. PPCD usually occurs in paracentesis greater than 5 L, and, therefore, in such procedures it is recommended that albumin be given at 8 to 10 g/L of ascites removed.

TIPSS is a radiologically-placed shunt that relieves portal hypertension by shunting blood between the portal vein and the hepatic vein. Ascites resolves in 66% of patients with this procedure. There is no difference in survival between patients who undergo large-volume paracentesis as opposed to TIPSS. Thus, TIPSS is recommended as opposed to large volume paracentesis when it becomes necessary more than two times a month, or if paracentesis is impractical. The major complication to TIPSS is hepatic encephalopathy (20% incidence), particularly in patients with advanced liver disease; it is, therefore, recommended with caution in Child class C patients. Some of the requirements for successful placement of TIPSS include a cardiac ejection fraction of at least 55%, patency of the portal vein, and absence of severe hepatic encephalopathy. Liver transplantation is the only definitive therapy for refractory ascites and should be considered for all appropriate candidates. Another possible treatment for patients ineligible for transplant, TIPSS, or paracentesis is the placement of a peritoneovenous shunt.

ESOPHAGEAL VARICES

Please see the esophageal varices article in this volume for more information.

HEPATORENAL SYNDROME

Approximately 40% of all patients with ascites will develop hepatorenal syndrome (HRS) within 5 years. It occurs when there is continued sodium retention, activation of the renin-angiotensin system, and arterial filling remains too low. The kidneys have an inherent vasodilation system. When this is overcome because of massive systemic vasoconstriction, which commonly occurs with long-term presence of ascites, the renal blood flow and glomerular filtration rates (GFR) plummet, and renal failure evolves. One precipitator of HRS is nonsteroidal anti-inflammatory drugs, such as ibuprofen. These should be scrupulously avoided by a patient with ascites. In the diagnosis of HRS several key criteria are almost always present (Table 2).

There are two types of HRS, type I and type II. In type I HRS, there is a rapid increase in serum creatinine (>2.5 mg/dL within 2 weeks). The prognosis for type I HRS is dismal, with 80% mortality within 2 weeks. Type II HRS is a more slowly progressive form, and can evolve to type I. Type II also has a poor prognosis, with only 50% survival after 6 months.Type II presents with moderate levels of renal deterioration with serum creatinine between 1.5 and 2.5 mg/dL that has evolved in more than 2 weeks time.

The most successful treatment for HRS is liver transplantation, with survival rates greater than 80% over 1 year. The next most effective treatment for type I HRS is albumin infusion (20 to 40 g/d for 20 days) with arterial vasoconstrictors. Albumin, rather than synthetic volume expanders, should be used in this treatment. Octreotide (Sandostatin)[1] at a dose of 200 μg should be given subcutaneously three times per day along with midodrine (ProAmatine)[1] titrated up to 12.5 mg three times per day to achieve an increase in mean blood pressure of 15 mm Hg. TIPSS treatment is experimental for HRS.

HEPATOCELLULAR CARCINOMA

Patients with cirrhosis have a marked increased risk for the development of hepatocellular carcinoma

[1]Not FDA approved for this indication.

TABLE 2 Criteria of the International Ascites Club for Diagnosing the Hepatorenal Syndrome

Major Criteria (All Criteria Must Be Met)	Additional Criteria (Usually Present)
Chronic or acute liver disease with advanced hepatic failure and portal hypertension	Urine volume <500 mL/d
Low glomerular filtration rate, as indicated by a serum creatinine of >1.5 mg/dL or 24 h creatinine clearance <40 mL/min	Urine sodium <10 mEq/L
Absence of shock, ongoing bacterial infection, and current or recent treatment with nephrotoxic drugs; absence of gastrointestinal fluid losses (e.g., vomiting or diarrhea) or renal fluid losses (e.g., overaggressive diuresis)	Urine osmolality greater than plasma osmolality
No sustained improvement of renal function (i.e., a decrease of serum creatinine <1.5 mg/dL or increase in creatinine clearance to >40 mL/min) following removal of diuretic therapy and volume expansion with 1.5 L of normal saline intravenously	Urine red blood cells <50 per high-power field
Proteinuria <500 mg/dL and no ultrasound evidence of either obstructive uropathy or parenchymal renal disease	Serum sodium concentration <130 mEq/L

Source: Arroyo V, Gines P, Gerbes AL, et al: Definition and diagnostic criteria of refractory ascites and hepatorenal syndrome in cirrhosis. International Ascites Club. Hepatology 23(1):164-76, 1996.

(HCC)—10% to 15% of cirrhosis patients develop HCC over a 10-year period. Patients who successfully undergo orthotopic liver transplant (OLT) for HCC that have ideal criteria for transplantation have a 50% to 70% 5-year survival rate.

Screening is best accomplished through both α-fetoprotein (AFP) tests and ultrasound examination of the abdomen every 6 months in the cirrhotic patient. The α-fetoprotein test is less specific, being only definitive for HCC when levels exceed 1000 ng/mL. However, levels of AFP between 300 to 500 ng/mL can be considered suspicious for HCC development. AFP levels are usually elevated in pregnant women and can be elevated in patients with chronic hepatitis. Thus, the specificity of an AFP at low levels is minimal; therefore, there is a dependence on imaging studies and the sequential course of AFP. Other investigational tumor markers are des-γ-carboxyprothrombin (DCP) and lectin-reactive AFP (AFP-L3).

Treatment for HCC includes both surgical and nonsurgical modalities, with surgical treatments being the most successful. Surgery includes resection of the tumor and liver transplantation. Few candidates meet the criteria for successful and safe resection because often they have decompensated cirrhosis, which contraindicates surgical resection. Nonsurgical methods include embolization and ablation of the tumor. Either embolization or ablative therapies might be appropriate in HCC patients with nonresectable tumors. The role of chemotherapy is not clear.

The earlier HCC is detected, the greater the likelihood of successful outcomes with transplantation. To be a candidate for liver transplantation, the patient must have no vascular invasion, no metastatic disease, and no more than three suspected lesions in the liver. If there are multiple lesions, all must be less than 3 cm in diameter; if only one lesion is present, it must be less than 5 cm in diameter.

ENCEPHALOPATHY

Hepatic encephalopathy (HE) is characterized by neurologic and neuromuscular abnormalities, which are primarily caused by accumulation of nitrogenous compounds, endogenous ligands for benzodiazepine receptors, and other unknown neurotoxins released by bacteria from the colon that are not well metabolized by the cirrhotic liver.

HE has five stages, with stage 0 representing no abnormal psychiatric effects of cirrhosis. Patients in stage 0 may have moderate insomnia, with an inversion of the normal night/day sleep cycle. Loss of fine coordination and moodiness indicate a progression to stage 1. Stage 2 patients suffer from ataxia and serious memory problems with possible ankle clonus, while stage 3 patients suffer confusion, incoherence, paranoia, and seizures. Stage 4 patients represent the most severe encephalopathy, with complete coma. Asterixis can be a part of any of these stages.

Precipitating causes of HE include infection, gastrointestinal (GI) bleeding, hypokalemia, progression of cirrhosis, and recent TIPSS placement. Other causes include dehydration or diuretic-induced prerenal azotemia. Use of benzodiazepines, particularly for treatment of stage 0 insomnia, will significantly *worsen* HE and must be avoided. Other tranquilizers and sedatives can have a similar effect and must not be used.

Most cases of HE are avoidable, and a good awareness of the precipitating causes will help prevent it. Reduction and modification of ingested protein (e.g., no red meat) is suggested for patients who manifest features of encephalopathy. An effective treatment for HE is lactulose (Cephulac) with a goal of achieving three to four soft bowel movements a day. Excessive use leading to diarrhea is to be avoided as it can cause prerenal azotemia and other electrolyte imbalances. In patients who have profound encephalopathy and are not able to take medication orally, lactulose can be administered as a retention enema at a dose of 300 mL in 700 mL of tap water, to be administered two to three times per day. Opiate analgesics, calcium, and iron supplements can all exacerbate HE; all should be avoided if possible. Also, antibiotics such as neomycin[1] (1 to 2 g per day) and metronidazole (Flagyl)[1] (250 mg twice daily [bid] or three times a day [tid]) can help alleviate HE and can be used in conjunction with lactulose, particularly in cases where dietary modification and lactulose alone do not adequately treat HE.

SPONTANEOUS BACTERIAL PERITONITIS

Spontaneous bacterial peritonitis (SBP) is a proliferation of bacteria in the ascitic fluid. Hospitalized patients with decompensated cirrhosis have a 10% to 30% chance of SBP. Once it occurs, SBP has approximately 20% mortality per episode. Also, SBP recurs in approximately 70% of patients in 1 year.

Patients with cirrhosis and ascites, and with sudden onset of fever, encephalopathy of unknown origin, abdominal pain, renal failure, acidosis, or peripheral leukocytosis should receive immediate antibiotic therapy *before* the data from paracentesis and ascitic fluid cultures are available. A polymorphonuclear leukocyte (PMN) count of 250 cells/mm^3 suggests SBP. If secondary bacterial infection is suspected, lactate dehydrogenase, total protein, and glucose should be evaluated. Blood and urine cultures should be done and ascites cultures should always be in blood culture bottles.

Treatment involves primarily the antibiotic cefotaxime (Claforan). It is recommended that 2 g of cefotaxime be given intravenously every 8 hours. A paracentesis should be repeated after 48 hours and a PMN count performed again. In SBP the PMN count should be 50% of its previous level, whereas in other sources of peritonitis the PMN count may be higher or unchanged. Treatment with cefotaxime for 5 days is

[1]Not FDA approved for this indication.

sufficient to clear SBP. Alternatively, the patient can take oral ofloxacin (Floxin)[1] if the patient has no vomiting, shock, or hemorrhage; has a serum creatinine of less than 3 mg/dL; and has stage 1 or stage 0 encephalopathy. An optimal dose is 400 mg every 12 hours. Albumin[1] administration has been observed to decrease mortality following an episode of SBP; the suggested dose is 1.5 g albumin/kg of body weight within 6 hours after starting antibiotic therapy, and readministered at 1 g/kg on the third day of treatment.

SBP can be prevented by administration of prophylactic treatment. Norfloxacin (Noroxin)[1] (400 mg/d) is useful and is indicated for patients who have already had an episode of SBP, or who have low ascitic protein levels (<1 g/dL). Norfloxacin[1] prophylaxis has reduced SBP occurrence by 60% and is highly cost-effective. For patients admitted to hospital for cirrhosis and GI hemorrhage, norfloxacin[1] can be given for prevention of SBP twice a day (total of 800 mg per day) for 7 days, or ofloxacin[1] can be given instead (400 mg per day).

SECONDARY BACTERIAL INFECTIONS

Peritonitis can also be caused by other infections from perforations in the gut or from nonperforated infections elsewhere in the peritoneum. If the ascitic fluid protein is more than 1g/dL, the lactate dehydrogenase higher than normal, and glucose less than 50 mg/dL, there is a strong (50%) probability of secondary, rather than spontaneous infection. If the carcinoembryonic antigen (CEA) is more than 5 ng/mL and the ascitic fluid alkaline phosphatase (AP) is more than 240 units/L, there is an 88% chance the infection is caused by a perforation of the gut. For nonperforation, secondary peritonitis, a second PMN count 48 hours later confirms nonperforated secondary peritonitis if:

- The PMN is the same or higher even after antibiotic treatment, and
- The tests for perforated peritonitis (ascites CEA and AP) are negative.

Surgery and antibiotics have a good chance of clearing the infection if it is found in time.

HEPATOPULMONARY SYNDROME AND PORTOPULMONARY HYPERTENSION

Patients with chronic liver disease may have pulmonary manifestations of either hepatopulmonary syndrome (HPS) or pulmonary hypertension (PPH). HPS is characterized by hypoxemia commonly with levels of PO_2 being below 70 mm Hg and can affect as many as 33% of all patients with liver disease. This is as a consequence of inappropriate vasodilation in the lungs. These patients essentially have an intrapulmonary shunt physiology. No effective treatment exists for HPS except for liver transplantation.

[1]Not FDA approved for this indication.

PPH is another lung disorder seen in association with chronic liver disease. Depending on the severity of this manifestation, an overall 30% survival rate over 5 years has been observed. Liver transplantation alone may reverse minor or moderate degrees of pulmonary hypertension. Transplantation is contraindicated in patients with severe pulmonary hypertension because of high postoperative mortality related to cardiac failure. Experimental approaches include vasodilators and combined lung-liver transplant.

Causes and Treatments

HEPATITIS VIRUSES

More information on these viruses and their etiologic outcomes are available in the hepatitis article in this volume.

ALCOHOL

Laboratory features can be specific for alcoholic hepatitis. An AST value more than two times the level of ALT is a good indication of liver damage caused by alcohol. Aminotransferases usually do not exceed 500 IU/L. An AST/ALT ratio of less than 2 indicates that alcohol is unlikely to be the cause of liver injury. One key marker for severity of alcoholic hepatitis is the discriminant function ($4.6 \times [PT_{patient} - PT_{control}]$ + bilirubin). A value greater than 32 predicts 50% mortality in 1 month.

The best treatment for alcoholic liver disease is total abstinence from alcohol. In severe, life-threatening hepatitis caused by alcohol (a discriminant function >32; HE; and the absence of renal failure, infection or pancreatitis) administration of prednisone[1] (40 mg per day for 28 days) is the main treatment. Pentoxifylline (Trental)[1] may also be used (400 mg every 8 hours for 4 weeks), and has significant survival benefit. Liver transplantation is controversial in alcoholic hepatitis.

AUTOIMMUNE HEPATITIS

Autoimmune hepatitis (AIH) is usually progressive, with liver parenchyma destruction and eventual cirrhosis. AIH can be subdivided into three main types. In type I AIH, antibodies to nuclei (ANA or antinuclear antibodies) or to smooth muscle (SMA) are present. In type II AIH, anti-liver/kidney microsome-1 (ALKM-1) antibodies are most common, and in this form, the disease predominantly strikes children or young women. A third type that is associated with anti-SLA (soluble liver antigen) may be a subset of type I.

Other autoimmune diseases such as childhood-onset diabetes and thyroiditis should trigger suspicion

[1]Not FDA approved for this indication.

for AIH. Many patients present asymptomatically. AST, ALT, and bilirubin are commonly elevated in AIH. A particularly indicative diagnostic sign is a high level of globulins, especially IgG. Liver biopsy characteristically shows an increase in plasma cells with other features of chronic hepatitis. In most cases, lifelong therapy with low levels of prednisone[1] or azathioprine (Imuran)[1] are needed to prevent relapses.

For initial induction of remission, adults should be on 20 to 30 mg of prednisone per day, while in children it should be 2 mg/kg per day up to 60 mg per day. Azathioprine (Imuran)[1] can also be given at a dose of 50 mg per day. Once transaminases fall 50%, prednisone[1] can be reduced to 15 mg per day in 5 mg decrements every 2 weeks. Once normalized, both azathioprine[1] and prednisone[1] can be continued at 50 to 75 mg per day and 15 mg per day, respectively, for 2 months. Then prednisone[1] can be held at 12.5 mg per day for 3 months, and then 10 mg per day for the next 3 months. Most patients require a combination of prednisone[1] and azathioprine (Imuran)[1] for a year, at which time attempts can be made to attain remission with azathioprine (Imuran)[1] (2 mg/kg body weight) alone. A full blood count should be performed every 2 weeks to ensure no myelosupression occurs for the first 2 months. There is controversy regarding long-term therapy versus an attempt to discontinue therapy in the hope of sustained remission. Treatment can be stopped, but recurrence rates approach 90% and may need to be aggressively treated.

PRIMARY BILIARY CIRRHOSIS

Primary biliary cirrhosis (PBC) is an autoimmune disease characteristically found in women over 40 years of age. PBC results in progressive granulomatous destruction of bile ducts. Complications of the disease include severe generalized pruritus, osteoporosis, skin xanthomata, sicca disease, vitamin deficiencies, and recurrent urinary tract infection. PBC may progress to cirrhosis, and in some cases liver failure. There are four histologic stages to PBC. First, there is granulomatous destruction of the bile ducts, followed by periportal hepatitis and proliferation of bile ducts. The third stage has fibrous septae and bridging necrosis, while the fourth stage features cirrhosis.

Most patients who are discovered to have PBC have no symptoms. PBC can first be suspected in cases where alkaline phosphatase (AP) is elevated. By cross-checking the γ-glutamyl transpeptidase (γGT), the origin of the rise of AP can be traced to being either of liver or nonliver origin. A positive antimitochondrial antibody (AMA) is seen in 95% of patients with PBC. Markers for autoimmune hepatitis (AIH) such as antismooth muscle antibodies (SMA) are found 25% of the time in PBC patients.

[1]Not FDA approved for this indication.

The first-line treatment for PBC is typically ursodiol (Actigall). It is a safe drug that lowers toxic bile acid levels and has a protective effect on the membranes of liver cells. The typical administration of ursodiol is 13 to 15 mg/kg per day. AP, bilirubin, and γGT all typically fall to normal or near normal levels while a patient takes ursodiol. Immunosuppressive therapy is *not* recommended.

Pruritus is one of the most disabling and difficult-to-manage complications of PBC. For this complication the first-line therapy is cholestyramine (Questran), a bile salt-binding resin. Patients should take cholestyramine 4 hours before taking other medication. The dose is 4 g to be taken before breakfast and dinner with extra doses at bedtime or before lunch. Second-line therapies include naltrexone (ReVia)[1] (50 mg/d) and rifampicin (Rifadin)[1] (150 mg bid). In extreme cases, plasmapheresis can be performed. Liver transplantation is the only definitive therapy for pruritus and can be considered in the rare case of debilitating pruritus.

Bone disease and deficiency of fat-soluble vitamins (A, D, E, and K) may occur in PBC. As a consequence of bone disease fractures of the spine and ribs can occur readily in PBC. Osteopenia can be detected with a bone density scan; between 30% to 50% of patients with PBC have low mineral density in their ribs and vertebrae. To treat this, vitamin D and calcium (1 to 1.5 g/d) are recommended, although only liver transplantation can treat this complication fully. If levels of 25-hydroxy vitamin D are low, supplementation at a dose of 20 μg per day is ideal. Calcitonin (Miacalcin)[1] or alendronate (Fosamax)[1] can also be considered in these patients. Also, malabsorption of the fat-soluble vitamins may occur. It is, therefore, reasonable to place these patients on 400 IU per day of vitamin E. Vitamin A levels can be monitored and if low, up to 15,000 IU per day can be used; otherwise, it is recommended that a maintenance regimen of 5,000 IU per day be used. Vitamin K supplementation is generally not given unless the patient is deeply icteric or has a tendency to bleed from the gums, skin, and so forth.

PRIMARY SCLEROSING CHOLANGITIS

Primary sclerosing cholangitis (PSC) is an uncommon disease (incidence of 10 to 50 cases per million population) affecting both the intra- and extrahepatic bile ducts. In PSC, the bile ducts are intermittently strictured and dilated. In most (70%) cases PSC is accompanied by chronic ulcerative colitis; it is less commonly accompanied by Crohn's colitis. PSC is progressive and eventually leads to portal hypertension, cirrhosis, and liver failure. Patients with PSC have a 15% cumulative risk of eventually developing cholangiocarcinoma.

Patients are predominantly males over 20 years of age. However, women are seen with this condition

[1]Not FDA approved for this indication.

approximately 33% of the time. Many patients present with significant fatigue, intermittent right upper quadrant abdominal pain, generalized pruritus (itching), and jaundice. Approximately 25% of patients have no symptoms. The most common abnormal laboratory finding is often an elevated alkaline phosphatase (AP) in relation to the transaminases. ALT and AST are also usually elevated in this disease to about two to five times normal. The presence of pericytoplasmic antineutrophil nuclear antibodies (p-ANNA, also known as p-ANCA) is associated (70% to 80%) with both PSC and inflammatory bowel disease. Imaging via endoscopic retrograde cholangiopancreatography (ERCP) can confirm PSC by showing multiple strictures in both the extra- and intrahepatic bile ducts.

The progression of PSC is variable, but in general four main stages arise. In the first stage the portal triad becomes inflamed. In the second stage, inflammation spreads to the periportal area, and progresses to septa formation, which is characteristic of the third stage. The fourth stage features regenerative nodules and cirrhosis. These features can be ascertained through biopsy and histology.

Treatment is limited. Currently ursodiol (Actigall)[1] is commonly given for the condition. Doses of 20 to 30 mg/kg per day have shown modest improvement in hepatic biochemical tests. However, unlike in PBC, ursodiol has not been shown to have a benefit on survival when used for patients with PSC. Also, liver transplantation has been successfully accomplished in patients with PSC, but if patients have a cholangiocarcinoma, their outcomes are poor. The overall survival rate after transplant is approximately 70% to 80% after 5 years.

HEMOCHROMATOSIS

Hemochromatosis is defined as excessive iron deposition in major organs such as the kidney and liver. The main cause is hereditary hemochromatosis (HHC), the most common genetic mutation found in people of European descent. Approximately 10% of all northern European men are carriers of the HHC allele. For HHC, there are two main genetic recessive mutations, both on the short arm of chromosome 6. One gene is termed *HFE*.

Iron absorption is usually regulated in normal people where there is little absorption of iron in the gut if serum iron is satisfactory. In HHC, iron absorption is constitutively active, driving serum iron levels too high. In this case, excess iron is stored by the hepatocytes in the liver. Excess iron storage causes eventual activation of hepatic stellate cells initiating the fibrosis-cirrhosis chain of events. Most patients present with liver disease in their forties to fifties. Typical symptoms include severe fatigue, impotence in men, pain in the abdomen, and arthralgia. On exam, patients usually have an enlarged liver and spleen, and skin pigmentation. Cirrhosis is found in more than 60% of patients with HHC. From a biopsy, it is possible to determine the hepatic iron concentration (HIC).

An effective treatment for HHC is serial phlebotomy. By doing phlebotomies, the serum iron decreases, and even severe liver damage can reverse. HHC patients must be rigorously screened for hepatocellular carcinoma. Vitamin C supplements should be avoided, because they increase absorption of iron. Liver transplantation can be considered for patients with end-stage liver disease; however, a careful evaluation is needed for cardiac involvement before determining their candidacy.

[1]Not FDA approved for this indication.

NONALCOHOLIC STEATOHEPATITIS

Nonalcoholic steatohepatitis (NASH) presents almost identically as alcohol-induced hepatitis, with the exception that the patient drinks less than 40 g of ethanol per week. It has been found that NASH is correlated with obesity, hypertriglyceridemia, and with type II diabetes. It can be diagnosed when histology confirms steatosis and inflammation in the absence of the well-recognized causes of liver dysfunction and alcohol abuse. It progresses to cirrhosis between 15% to 40% of the time.

Usually ALT and AST levels are elevated. Interestingly, the ALT level is usually the same or greater than the AST level. This finding is important because it generally rules out alcohol-induced hepatitis. Imaging can also be helpful. First, upon ultrasound examination, the parenchyma of a fatty liver is significantly more echogenic than a normal liver. The first-line treatment for NASH should be weight reduction within 10% of ideal body weight in those who have obesity as an underlying cause for this condition. Weight loss should not exceed 1.6 kg per week. Rapid weight loss, including bariatric surgery in patients with significant fibrosis/cirrhosis, is ill advised as it may precipitate liver failure. On the other hand, bariatric surgery in carefully selected patients in early-stage liver disease is effective. Pilot trials with thiazolidine diones and metformin (Glucophage)[1] (drugs that increase insulin sensitivity), vitamin E (antioxidant), and ursodiol (Actigall)[1], taken 13 to 15 mg/kg per day, have demonstrated limited success in small trials. These, however, should not be considered the standard of care.

OTHER DISEASES

Wilson's Disease (Copper Overload)

Wilson's disease is the inability to properly excrete copper, and thus results in inappropriate copper storage in both liver and central nervous system. Once treatment is initiated the prognosis is excellent.

[1]Not FDA approved for this indication.

TABLE 3 Commonly Used Medications and Procedures for Cirrhosis

Medications and Procedures	Indications	Special Considerations
Diuretics, such as spironolactone (Aldactone) (100-400 mg/d) and furosemide (Lasix)[1] (40-160 mg/d)	Ascites	Avoid prerenal azotemia Emphasize salt restriction (≤2 g/d) Avoid NSAIDs
Lactulose (Cephulac) (30 mL qd-qid)	Hepatic encephalopathy	Avoid red meat Titrate to 2-3 soft bowel movements/d
Norfloxacin (Noroxin)[1] (400 mg/d)	Spontaneous bacterial peritonitis; prevention of recurrence	Consider in patients with low ascites protein to prevent a first episode of SBP
Prednisone[1] and azathioprine (Imuran)[1] (see text for dosing)	Autoimmune hepatitis	Be cautious for bone marrow suppression Steroid side effects
Cholestyramine (Questran) (4-12 g bid, before breakfast and dinner)	Pruritus	GI disturbances possible No other drugs within 4 h
Rifampicin (Rifadin)[1] (150 mg bid)		GI disturbances possible
Ursodiol (Actigall)[1] (see text for dosing)	NASH, cholestatic liver disease	
Phlebotomy	Hemochromatosis	
D-Penicillamine (Cuprimine)	Wilson's disease	Neuropathy Cytopenia Rash
Trientine HCl (Syprine), Zinc[1], BAL	Wilson's disease	Referral needed
Liver transplant	Indicated for decompensated cirrhosis, HCC, fulminant liver failure	Careful selection of candidates by multidisciplinary team at tertiary transplant center
HRS Cocktail: Octreotide (Sandostatin)[1] (200 μg tid subcutaneous), Midodrine (ProAmatine)[1] (12.5 mg tid, orally), Albumin (20-40 g/d for 20 d)	Hepatorenal syndrome	Avoid NSAIDs Consider referral for liver transplant
TIPSS	Refractory ascites, esophageal varices*	Encephalopathy common Use caution in advanced liver disease
β blockers* Esophageal banding	Esophageal varices*	
Pegylated interferon (2a or 2b)† or interferon-α (2a or 2b) Ribavirin (Virazole)	Hepatitis C infection†	
Interferon-α (2a or 2b)† Lamivudine (Epivir) Adefovir (Hepsera)	Hepatitis B infection†	

[1]Not FDA approved for this indication.
*See "Esophageal Varices" article in this volume.
†See "Viral Hepatitis" article in this volume.
Abbreviations: BAL = British anti-Lewisite therapy; GI = gastrointestinal; HCC = hepatocellular carcinoma; HRS = hepatorenal syndrome; NASH = nonalcoholic steatohepatitis; NSAIDs = nonsteroidal anti-inflammatory drugs; qd = once a day; qid = four times a day; SBP = spontaneous bacterial peritonitis; tid = three times a day; TIPSS = transjugular intrahepatic portosystemic stent shunt.

Wilson's disease is quite possible if ceruloplasmin (CP) levels are below 20 mg/dL. Another key diagnostic exam is a slit-lamp examination for Kayser-Fleischer rings. If rings are present with low CP levels, then Wilson's disease is present. If rings are not present, a liver biopsy should be done. Intrahepatic levels of copper greater than 250 μg/g are indicative of Wilson's disease. The drug of choice is D-penicillamine (Cuprimine). Other drugs used are trientine (Syprine) and zinc[1] although the latter is used more as a maintenance therapy. British anti-Lewisite (BAL) therapy is seldom used today.

[1]Not FDA approved for this indication.

α_1-Antitrypsin Deficiency

This deficiency is found in patients with the PiZZ (protease inhibitor phenotype ZZ homozygous) genotype. In this disease, the α_1-antitrypsin deficiency (AT) causes production of a mutant protease inhibitor. This causes liver damage in 10% to 15% of individuals afflicted with this mutation. Most patients with AT-induced liver disease are children. An effective treatment is liver transplantation, and the 5-year survival rate approaches 80%. Hepatocyte transplantation is a theoretical treatment that holds much promise in this disease.

Table 3 summarizes the commonly used treatments for cirrhosis and their indications.

BLEEDING ESOPHAGEAL VARICES

METHOD OF

Greg V. Stiegmann, MD

Esophageal varices are present in 30% to 60% of patients with hepatic cirrhosis. The outlook for these patients can be stratified using the Child-Pugh scoring system (Table 1). Child-Pugh classes A and B patients have relatively well compensated liver disease and approximately 30% have esophageal varices. Their risk of bleeding from esophageal varices is approximately 30% over a 2-year period. Child-Pugh class C patients have poorly compensated liver disease and approximately 60% have esophageal varices. The risk of bleeding for any patient with esophageal varices is directly proportional to the size of the varices. The risk of bleeding is further increased when so-called *red color signs* are observed at endoscopy. These are small, dilated blood vessels on the surface of the varix. Child-Pugh class C patients with large varices and red color signs have approximately 60% risk of bleeding from esophageal varices over a 2-year period.

Pressure within the portal venous system is also related to the risk of bleeding from esophageal varices. Normal portal vein pressures are less than 10 mm Hg. Portal pressure is seldom measured directly. A surrogate for direct portal venous pressure measurement is the hepatic venous pressure gradient (HVPG). This is determined by passing a balloon-tipped catheter (usually via a transjugular route) into one of the hepatic veins and measuring the pressure within the vein. The balloon is then inflated to occlude the vein, and the pressure that results (similar to obtaining a wedged pulmonary artery pressure) is the hepatic venous wedged pressure. This value is subtracted from the free hepatic venous pressure to result in the HVPG. Normal HVPG is 2 to 6 mm Hg. Pressures greater than 12 mm Hg are considered portal hypertension. Patients with HVPG less than 12 mm Hg seldom bleed from esophageal varices. The HVPG is usually an accurate reflection of pressure in the portal venous system in patients with cirrhosis; however, patients who have other causes for esophageal varices (e.g., portal or splenic vein thrombosis) may have normal HVPG pressure determinations.

Bleeding from esophageal varices is currently associated with mortality in 20% to 30% of patients in the year following the index bleed. The risk of dying is directly proportional to the severity of the underlying liver disease (Child-Pugh classification). These results are greatly improved from only a few decades ago (Figure 1) and reflect advances in resuscitation, intensive care, and new pharmacologic, endoscopic, and radiologic treatments. Patients who have one episode of bleeding from esophageal varices have a 70% chance of a second episode of variceal bleeding within 1 year if untreated. There is general agreement that these patients, as well as those with large esophageal varices that have never bled, should be actively treated to prevent an initial or recurrent bleeding episode.

TABLE 1 Child-Pugh Classification*

Parameter	1 Point	2 Points	3 Points
Serum bilirubin (mg/dL)	<2	2-3	<3
Albumin (g/dL)	>3.5	2.8-3.5	<2.8
Prothrombin time (↑,s)	1-3	4-6	>6
Ascites	None	Slight	Moderate
Encephalopathy	None	1-2	3-4

**Grades:* A, 5 to 6 points; B, 7 to 9 points; C, 10 to 15 points.

Acute Bleeding from Esophageal Varices

Hematemesis and melena are the usual clinical presentations of upper gastrointestinal (GI) hemorrhage, including bleeding from esophageal varices. In many cases a history of liver disease or findings of stigmata of cirrhosis/portal hypertension on initial physical examination suggest the possibility of bleeding from esophageal varices. Resuscitation should proceed rapidly with two large-bore intravenous lines; bladder catheterization for monitoring urine output; and transfusion of red blood cells, fresh-frozen plasma, and platelets as needed to achieve hemodynamic stability. Uncooperative patients, such as those with hepatic encephalopathy, may benefit from early endotracheal intubation, both to assure adequate ventilation and to protect against tracheal aspiration. Patients suspected of bleeding from portal hypertensive causes benefit from early administration of drugs that reduce portal venous pressure. Octreotide (Sandostatin)[1] is given intravenously in an initial 50 μg bolus followed by continuous intravenous infusion at 25 to 50 μg per hour. Vasopressin (Pitressin)[1] is an alternative agent that should be given intravenously starting at 0.2 U per minute. The dose may be increased up to 0.4 to 0.6 U per minute. Electrocardiographic monitoring is essential because this drug produces systemic vasoconstriction that can result in myocardial ischemia. Intravenous nitroglycerin is frequently administered in conjunction with vasopressin to lessen these effects. Drugs given to lower portal pressure should be continued for 3 to 5 days after variceal bleeding is controlled. They may be stopped immediately if endoscopic examination finds a nonvariceal (e.g., peptic ulcer, Mallory-Weiss tear) cause of hemorrhage. Patients

[1]Not FDA approved for this indication.

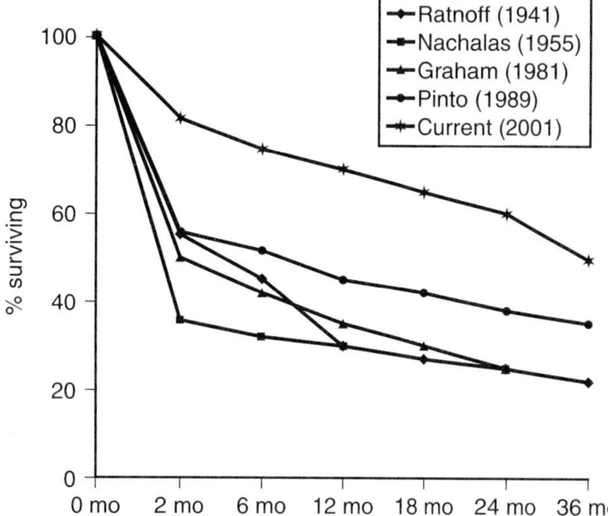

FIGURE 1 Survival after a first bleed from esophageal varices as measured during the past 60 years.
From: Chalasani N, Kahi C, Francois F, et al: Improved patient survival after acute variceal bleeding: A multicenter cohort study. Am J Gastroenterol, 98:656, 2003. Used with permission.

with cirrhosis and acute bleeding from esophageal varices have a high incidence of infection-related complications (e.g., subacute bacterial peritonitis, pneumonia, urinary tract infection) and have better outcomes, including a lower incidence of early recurrent bleeding, when treated with prophylactic antibiotics. Fluoroquinolone drugs, e.g., norfloxacin (Noroxin)[1] or levofloxacin (Levaquin)[1] should be administered intravenously at first and converted to oral administration when feasible. Antibiotic treatment should continue for 5 to 7 days.

Upper GI endoscopy should be performed as soon as possible after the patient with suspected variceal bleeding is hemodynamically stable. Gastric lavage, using a large-bore tube to remove blood and clots from the stomach, may enhance visualization. Uncooperative or combative patients require endotracheal intubation to assure adequate ventilation during endoscopy and to protect their airway. Bleeding from esophageal varices is confirmed if bleeding from a varix is observed directly, if a platelet plug is observed on the surface of a varix, or if large varices are present and no other potential source of bleeding is identified after conducting a complete examination of the stomach and duodenum. A thorough diagnostic endoscopic examination is important because approximately 25% of patients with known esophageal varices and upper GI bleeding have a nonvariceal source of hemorrhage. If bleeding varices are discovered in a patient with no history of liver disease, diagnostic evaluations should be done when bleeding is controlled and the patient has stabilized. These investigations should include an imaging study, such as contrast-enhanced computed tomography (CT), to rule out thrombosis of the portal or splenic vein as the cause of portal hypertension.

[1]Not FDA approved for this indication.

Endoscopic therapy to control variceal bleeding should be started, if possible, at the time of diagnostic endoscopy. Endoscopic band ligation is the preferred treatment (Figure 2) and results in control of bleeding in approximately 90% of cases. Endoscopic sclerotherapy (Figure 3) is also an acceptable treatment for acutely bleeding varices. Sclerotherapy has efficacy similar to band ligation, although it is associated with a higher risk of complications such as esophageal stricture and deep esophageal ulceration.

Patients whose bleeding varices are not controlled by endoscopic/pharmacologic treatment should be considered for transjugular intrahepatic portosystemic shunt (TIPS) (Figure 4). If active bleeding is ongoing, a Sengstaken-Blakemore balloon tamponade tube may be inserted to control bleeding and stabilize the patient (Figure 5). After passage of the tube into the stomach, 50 mL of air is used to inflate the gastric balloon, after which an abdominal radiograph is taken to assure correct position in the stomach. When correct positioning is confirmed, the gastric balloon is inflated to 250 mL and drawn up against the gastroesophageal junction and then secured in place. This maneuver controls bleeding in most situations. If inflation of the esophageal balloon is needed to control bleeding, pressure in the esophageal balloon should not exceed 40 mm Hg as measured by a blood pressure manometer. A nasogastric tube should be passed into the proximal esophagus to aspirate secretions that pool above the inflated balloons of the tamponade tube to prevent tracheal aspiration. Patients treated with balloon tamponade should have definitive portal venous decompression (TIPS) as soon as they are hemodynamically stable.

Prevention of Recurrent Bleeding

The most accurate predictor of future bleeding from esophageal varices is a history of a past episode

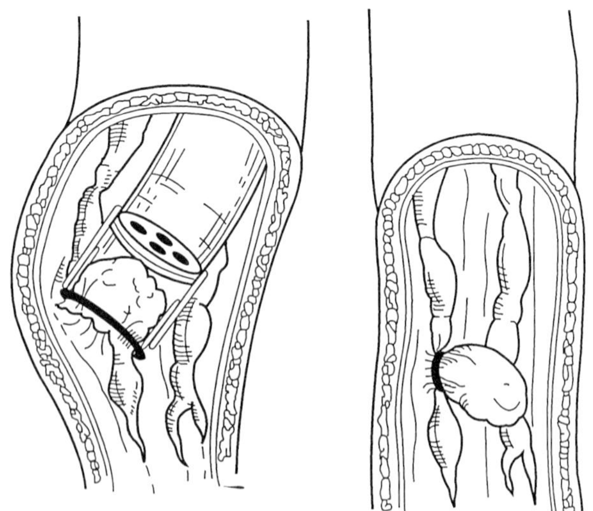

FIGURE 2 Endoscopic band ligation performed with a flexible endoscope. A varix is aspirated into the device using endoscopic suction and ensnared with an elastic band.
From: Schaefer J. In GI/Liver Secrets. Philadelphia, Hanley and Belfus, 1996, p. 355. Used with permission.

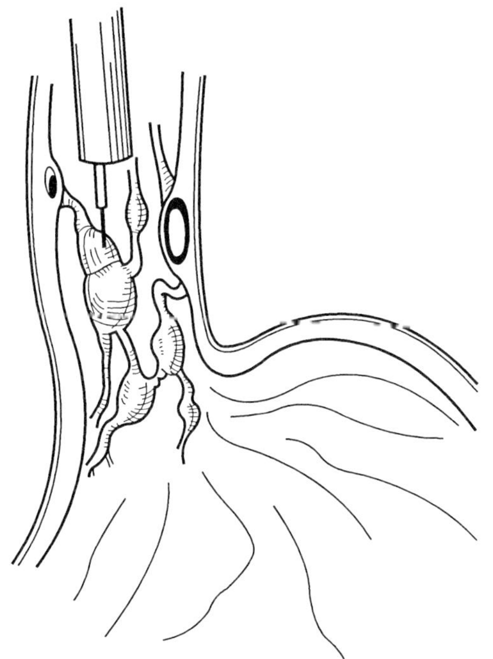

FIGURE 3 Endoscopic sclerotherapy performed with a flexible endoscope. A flexible injection needle is used to inject sclerosant into the varix.
From: Schaefer J. In GI/Liver Secrets. Philadelphia, Hanley and Belfus, 1996, p. 355. Used with permission.

of variceal bleeding. Treatments to prevent recurrent bleeding include pharmacologic, endoscopic, surgical, and radiologic shunt insertion and hepatic transplantation. Drug therapy is based on administration of nonselective β-blocking drugs (e.g., nadolol [Corgard][1]), usually titrated to reduce the resting heart rate by 25%, or to a heart rate of 60 beats per minute. More sophisticated regimens that titrate drug dosage based on measurements of HVPG have been studied and appear to be more effective than relying on reduction in resting pulse rate alone. Agents such as isosorbide mononitrate (Monoket)[1] may be added to the β-blocker regimen to produce further reduction in portal pressure. Problems with pharmacologic therapy include intolerance to side effects of the medication in 10% to 20% of patients and inability for some patients to maintain compliance with the medication schedule. Patients need to continue β-blocker therapy indefinitely because rapid cessation results in a *rebound* effect with increased risk of variceal bleeding. Compliance with β-blocker therapy reduces the risk of recurrent hemorrhage from esophageal varices from 70% to approximately 40% over a 1-year period following an index bleeding episode. Patients treated exclusively with pharmacologic therapy who experience recurrent bleeding from varices should receive endoscopic treatment.

Endoscopic band ligation is the treatment used at most centers to prevent recurrence of bleeding from esophageal varices. Serial endoscopic treatments are done on an outpatient basis at 10 to 14 day intervals until varices in the distal esophagus are obliterated. Obliteration of varices requires an average of 3 to 4 endoscopic treatment sessions. After varices are obliterated, follow-up endoscopy is done every 3 to 6 months to detect and treat any varices that recur. Complications associated with band ligation therapy are few when compared with those resulting from endoscopic sclerotherapy and the number of endoscopic sessions needed to eradicate varices is less. Patients treated with endoscopic band ligation alone have approximately 30% risk of experiencing recurrent bleeding from esophageal varices. Patients treated simultaneously with both β blockade and endoscopic band ligation have approximately 15% risk of recurrent bleeding from esophageal varices. Patients in whom endoscopic therapy fails to control bleeding (e.g., one, or at most two, major episodes of recurrent bleeding from varices after initiation of treatment) should have decompression of their portal hypertension.

Surgical portosystemic shunts are effective at decompressing portal hypertension and preventing recurrent bleeding from esophageal varices. Recurrent variceal bleeding occurs in approximately 10% of patients so treated. Selective shunt operations decompress only the esophageal varices (maintaining high pressure in the portal vein in order to perfuse the liver). Central shunts decompress the entire portal system. The selective shunt is associated with a somewhat lower incidence of hepatic encephalopathy and slightly greater risk of recurrent variceal bleeding than central shunts. Partial (using small diameter vascular grafts) shunt operations aim to lower portal vein pressure enough to prevent

[1]Not FDA approved for this indication.

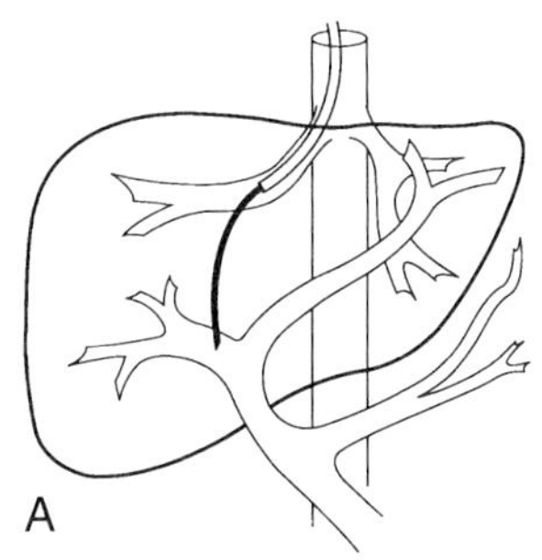

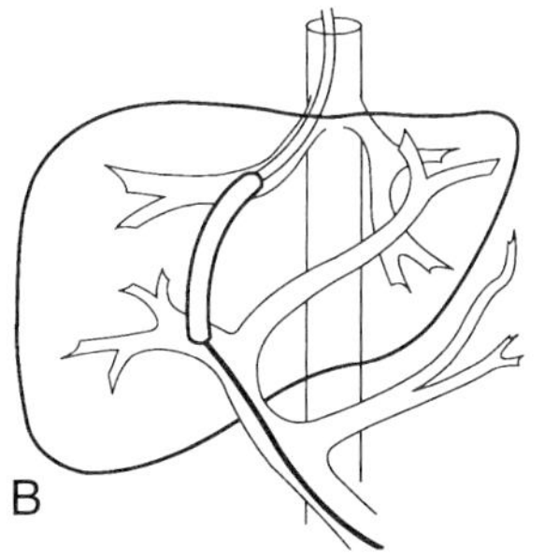

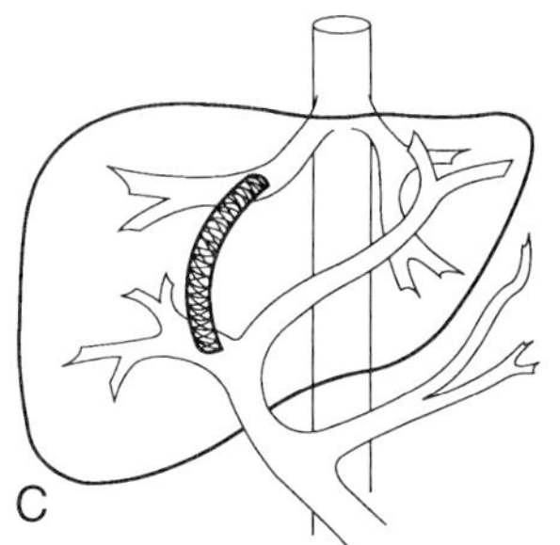

FIGURE 4 Transjugular intrahepatic portal systemic shunt (TIPS). (A) A needle is used to puncture from an hepatic vein into the portal vein. (B) The liver parenchyma is dilated with a balloon catheter. (C) A metal stent is inserted to complete the shunt.
From: McCarter D, and Shonnard K. In GI/Liver Secrets. Philadelphia, Hanley and Belfus, 1996, p. 520. Used with permission.

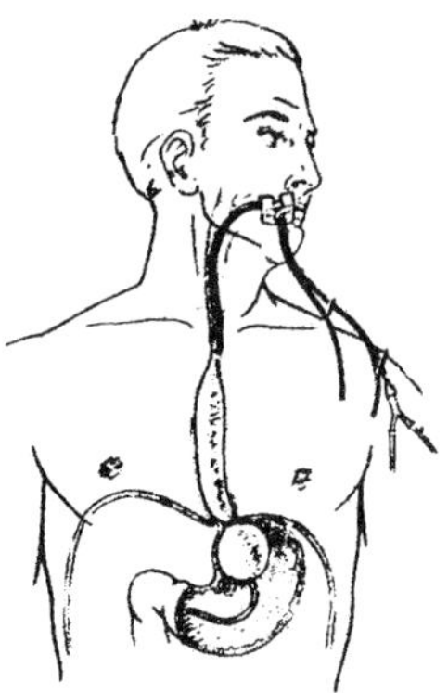

FIGURE 5 Sengstaken-Blakemore balloon tamponade. *From*: Sun JH and Stiegmann GV. In Abernathy's Surgical Secrets. Philadelphia, Hanley and Belfus, 1996, p. 155. Used with permission.

variceal bleeding while still maintaining some portal vein flow to the liver. Failures of endoscopic therapy, good risk patients (Child-Pugh A and B) who live in remote areas, or patients who are not compliant with endoscopic or pharmacologic treatments are the best candidates for elective shunt operations. Central shunt operations should be used sparingly in patients who are candidates for liver transplantation because the subsequent transplant operation is made more difficult as a result of previous dissection in the area of the porta hepatis.

TIPS eliminates the morbidity associated with the laparotomy that is necessary for surgical shunt construction. The trade-off is the need to regularly monitor flow through the intrahepatic stent and revise (usually dilate) the stent in a high percentage of patients. TIPS results in decompression of the entire portal venous system; however, the interventional radiologist can control the magnitude of decompression of the portal system by altering the diameter of the shunt. TIPS is effective in preventing recurrent bleeding from esophageal varices, but the risk of hepatic encephalopathy is similar to that of a surgical shunt. TIPS is best suited for patients who do not want to have pharmacologic/endoscopic therapy or those awaiting liver transplantation and who are willing to return for regular follow-up studies.

Patients who experience bleeding from esophageal varices should all be considered potential candidates for liver transplantation. Most Child-Pugh A and B patients can be managed effectively by the measures outlined above, but progression of liver disease is unpredictable. Patients who remain in Child-Pugh class C after recovery from an episode of bleeding varices are usually candidates for liver replacement provided they meet criteria such as abstinence from alcohol consumption.

Prevention of a First Variceal Bleed

Patients diagnosed with cirrhosis of the liver, who have not experienced upper GI bleeding, should undergo diagnostic upper GI endoscopy to determine presence or absence of esophageal varices. Patients with cirrhosis have approximately a 6% chance per year for developing varices. Treatment to prevent a first episode of variceal bleeding for patients who have small esophageal varices is controversial. These patients may be best served by serial endoscopic examinations with institution of treatment if varices enlarge. Treatment for patients found to have large esophageal varices, and certainly those who have red color signs or who are in Child-Pugh class C (i.e., patients at greater risk for a first variceal bleed) should be recommended. Pharmacologic therapy with β-blocking drugs titrated to reduce the resting pulse rate by 25%, or to a heart rate of 60 beats per minute, reduces the risk for a first variceal bleed from approximately 30% to about 10%. Side effects of the medication and compliance with the medication schedule are the main deterrents to this therapy. Endoscopic band ligation is as effective as β-blocker[1] therapy in lowering the risk of a first variceal bleed. Treatment is done as an outpatient with the goal of obliterating varices in the distal esophagus. When distal esophageal varices are eradicated, surveillance endoscopy should be done at 6- to 12-month intervals to detect and treat recurrent varices. No studies have addressed the efficacy of combining β-blocker therapy with band ligation to prevent a first variceal bleed. Results in patients treated with combined drug and endoscopic therapy to prevent recurrent bleeding from varices suggest that the combined treatment may be advantageous.

[1]Not FDA approved for this indication.

DYSPHAGIA AND ESOPHAGEAL OBSTRUCTION

METHOD OF

Mehnaz A. Shafi, MD, and Gulchin A. Ergun, MD

Swallowing is a fundamental task that is vital for normal health and nutrition. Swallowing disorders adversely affect the quality of life and can result in malnutrition, dehydration, and aspiration pneumonia with associated increased morbidity and mortality.

Dysphagia is the perception of an abnormal swallow. Patients often refer to this as "trouble swallowing" or "food sticking" during swallowing. Pain with swallowing is called odynophagia. Heartburn refers to the sensation of warmth behind the sternum or epigastrium. The combination of heartburn with regurgitation is very accurate in diagnosing gastroesophageal reflux. Dysphagia almost always indicates an organic disease.

Swallowing Physiology

Dysphagia results from propulsive or structural abnormalities of either the oropharynx or the esophagus. Propulsive abnormalities can result from dysfunction of central nervous system (CNS) control mechanisms, intrinsic musculature, or peripheral nerves. Structural abnormalities may result from neoplasm, surgery, trauma, caustic injury, or congenital anomalies. Dysphagia may be broadly classified into two types:

1. Oropharyngeal dysphagia (transfer dysphagia), caused by defects that affect any aspect of the neuromuscular mechanism of the pharynx and upper esophageal sphincter
2. Esophageal (transport dysphagia), caused by disorders affecting peristalsis, or the intrinsic or extrinsic portions of the esophagus. Examples oropharyngeal dysphagia are described in Table 1.

Normal swallowing requires anatomic reconfiguration of the respiratory pathway to a swallowing pathway. This highly organized neural and muscular process involves more than 30 muscles including the tongue, pharynx, and upper esophageal sphincter. It is coordinated by the swallowing center in the brainstem and cranial nerves V, VII, VIII, X, and XII. Once initiated, it takes less than 1 second for a bolus to reach the esophagus and 10 to 15 seconds to complete the swallowing process.

Normal deglutition consists of three phases—oral, pharyngeal, and esophageal. The oral phase is under voluntary control and involves cranial nerves V, VII, and XII. In the mouth, food is chewed to a size and consistency appropriate for passage into the pharynx and esophagus. Once processed, the food bolus is moved to the back of the tongue. The anterior portion of the tongue lifts and retracts, pushing the bolus into the upper pharynx. The soft palate moves upward, sealing off the nasopharynx, and preventing nasal aspiration.

During the pharyngeal phase of swallowing, food is advanced through the pharynx and into the esophagus by sequenced pharyngeal contractions. The larynx and hyoid are pulled upward and forward, opening the cricopharyngeus muscle. The pharyngeal phase requires cranial nerves V, X, XI, and XII and there is simultaneous central inhibition of respiration. Therefore, precise timing and coordination during the oropharyngeal phase are crucial to prevent aspiration.

During the esophageal phase, peristaltic contractions of the esophagus, along with simultaneous relaxation of the lower esophageal sphincter, advance the food distally into the stomach.

TABLE 1 Causes of Oropharyngeal Dysphagia

Neurologic
Stroke
Cerebral palsy
Multiple sclerosis
Polio
Postpolio syndrome
Parkinson's disease
Dementia
Amyotrophic lateral sclerosis
Brainstem tumor
Peripheral neuropathies (botulinum, diabetes mellitus)
Structural
Zenker diverticulum
Cricopharyngeal bar
Oropharyngeal neoplasm
Cervical osteophytes
Cleft palate
Webs
Extrinsic compression
Muscular
Myotonic dystrophy
Muscular dystrophies
Myasthenia gravis
Polymyositis
Sarcoidosis
Paraneoplastic syndromes
Infectious
Diphtheria
Lyme disease
Syphilis
Metabolic
Amyloidosis
Thyrotoxicosis
Cushing syndrome
Iatrogenic
Radiation
Chemotherapy
Postsurgical

Oropharyngeal Dysphagia

Obtaining a careful history is the most critical step in evaluating dysphagia. In oropharyngeal dysphagia, patients accurately recognize that the swallowing dysfunction is in the oropharynx or above the sternal notch. Drooling, a perception of food accumulating uncontrollably in the mouth, or an inability to initiate a pharyngeal swallow may be noticed. Similarly, they may recognize coughing or aspiration before, during, or after a swallow. Typical symptoms of pharyngeal dysfunction also include the need to swallow repeatedly to clear food from the pharynx, a gurgling or wet voice, and, depending upon the cause, nasopharyngeal regurgitation. Globus sensation is a functional complaint and refers to the feeling of a *lump in the throat*. This is usually present continually but disappears during deglutition and should not be confused with dysphagia. Similarly, xerostomia may affect oropharyngeal sensation and create difficulty in manipulating oral contents because of a dry and often sore mouth. This is also often erroneously confused with dysphagia.

Important related symptoms include a history of aspiration pneumonia. Unexplained weight loss may be caused by patients eating less because of the dysphagia. Hoarseness may result from recurrent laryngeal nerve dysfunction. Weakness of the soft palate can cause nasal speech and dysarthria. Medications such as anticholinergics or phenothiazines can contribute to dysphagia by aggravating xerostomia.

Signs of pulmonary or nutritional complications related to dysphagia should be sought on physical exam. The history and physical can indicate blood tests or imaging studies to diagnose systemic diseases such as myasthenia gravis, multiple sclerosis, Parkinson's disease or an oropharyngeal tumor. A careful history and physical examination can suggest the etiology in 80% to 85% of patients.

Barium radiographs, computed tomography (CT) scanning, magnetic resonance imaging (MRI), manometric testing, laryngoscopy, and endoscopy are all used to evaluate dysphagia and are often complementary in the information that they provide. Choosing the testing modality is based upon the likely diagnosis and availability of local expertise. For example, CNS imaging would be selected if a stroke were suspected. Blood and urine studies are indicated for suspected underlying systemic, metabolic, or infectious disorders (e.g., muscle enzymes for inflammatory myopathy, thyroid function tests for thyroid disorders, and acetylcholinesterase antibody for myasthenia gravis).

Videofluoroscopy, also called the modified barium swallow (MBS), is the most sensitive method for detailing the motor events of deglutition. It is designed to identify functional defects in the swallowing process. A set of swallows with varying volume and consistency of oral contrast are imaged, in lateral view, as the contrast moves through the oropharynx, palate, upper esophagus, and proximal airway. Approximately 5 to 30 frames are recorded per second to visualize critical motor events. MBS can identify impaired initiating of pharyngeal swallow, aspiration, and residue within the pharynx. The effect of compensatory maneuvers, such as postural changes during swallowing; rehabilitative and dietary treatments, such as modification of food consistency; and delivery processes may also be observed during this examination.

Nasoendoscopy involves passage of a small endoscope transnasally and directly visualizing the mucosal surfaces of the nasopharynx, oropharynx, and larynx. It is ideal for identifying small intracavity lesions. Swallowing evaluation, detection of aspiration, and laryngeal field sensory assessment can also be done as liquids and solids that are colored with dye are swallowed during direct visualization. An algorithm describing the evaluation and management of oropharyngeal dysphagia is summarized in Figure 1.

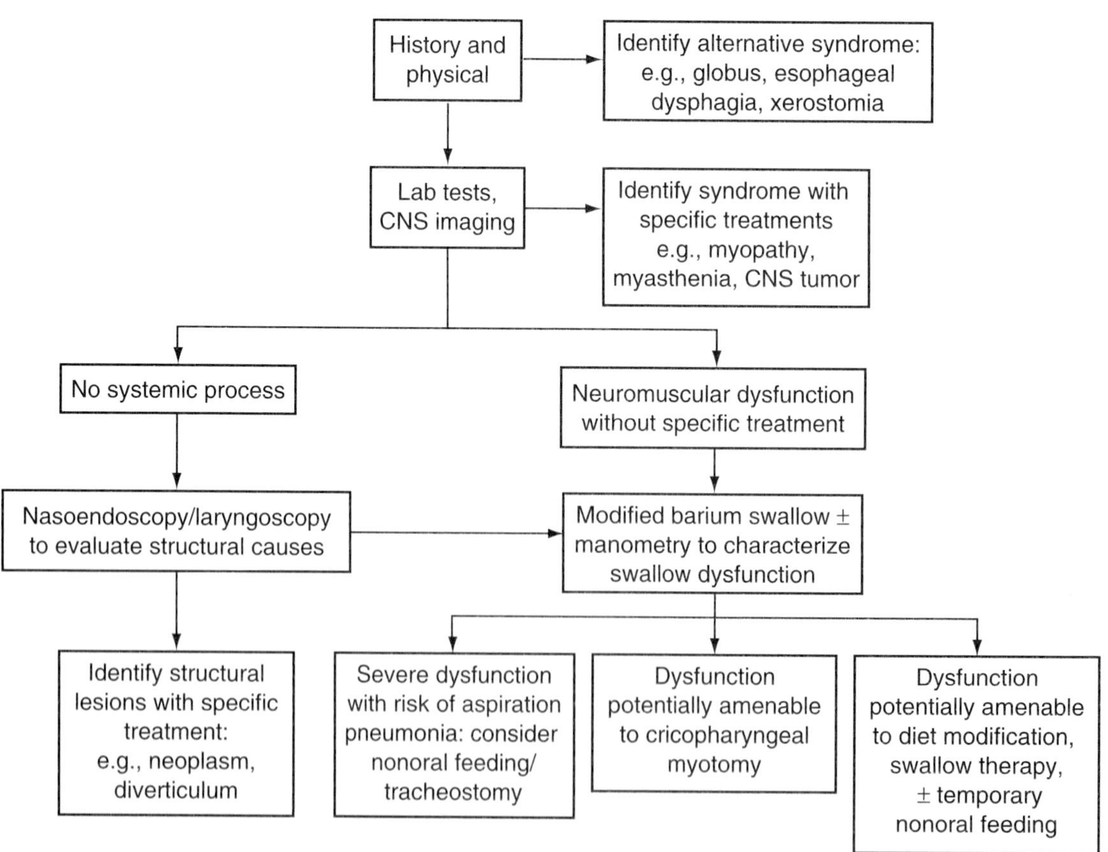

FIGURE 1 Algorithm for evaluation of oropharyngeal dysphagia.
Adapted from: American Gastroenterological Association Technical Review, Cook IJ, Kahrilas PJ. AGA technical review of management of oropharyngeal dysphagia. Gastroenterology 116:455, 1999.

Esophageal Dysphagia

Motility disorders and mechanical obstruction are the most commonly encountered causes of esophageal dysphagia. The etiology is best discerned based upon the history, recognizing that structural lesions are usually painless with progressive dysphagia involving first solids then liquids. Therefore the most important questions to ask during the history are:

- Is the dysphagia for solids or liquids or both?
- Is the dysphagia intermittent or progressive?
- Does the patient have heartburn?
- Does the patient have chest pain?

Dysphagia for both solids and liquids suggests a motility disorder. As the repertoire to esophageal injury is limited, patients with motility disorders may also complain of chest pain. In patients with only solid food dysphagia, a mechanical lesion is likely. Symptoms usually correspond to the caliber of the stricture. Dysphagia is likely when the esophageal lumen is narrowed to 13 mm or less. Intermittent, nonprogressive dysphagia is suggestive of a benign esophageal web or ring. An algorithm for the management of esophageal dysphagia is shown in Figure 2.

If solid food dysphagia is progressive, a peptic stricture or esophageal malignancy should be considered. Weight loss is not common with benign strictures. Ten percent of patients with gastroesophageal reflux disease (GERD) develop benign strictures, hence the importance of ascertaining a prior history of heartburn. Similarly, patients with long-standing GERD are at risk for the development of Barrett esophagus and at an increased risk for the development of adenocarcinoma of the esophagus. Patients with esophageal cancer tend to be older and present with rapidly progressive dysphagia and profound weight loss.

Dysphagia may also be seen with mucosal inflammation. The causes are varied and include erosive reflux esophagitis, although peristaltic dysfunction caused by GERD can also cause dysphagia in the absence of obvious inflammation. Esophagitis caused by pills, infection, or caustic injury can cause dysphagia along with odynophagia. Table 2 lists the causes of esophageal dysphagia.

Diagnostic Tests Used in Evaluation of Esophageal Dysphagia

The goals of imaging studies such as barium radiographs, endoscopy, or CT scanning are to establish site, length, and nature of the obstruction and to form some assessment of the associated esophageal anatomy. A barium esophagram provides different information than an endoscopy. It is a very sensitive method for the detection of structural abnormalities of the esophagus and also provides good qualitative assessment of the motor function of the esophagus and lower esophageal sphincter. It is superior to endoscopy in assessing ring or stricture caliber (particularly if different substances, such as marshmallows or tablets, are used to distend the esophagus), allows visualization of the anatomy distal to the lesion, and evaluates extrinsic compression. Endoscopy, on the other hand, allows for the direct evaluation of the mucosa and allows for tissue biopsy for the exclusion of infection or neoplasm. Mucosal lesions not apparent radiographically may be identified, and therapeutic maneuvers such as esophageal dilation or foreign body removal can be performed.

Small lesions within the wall of the esophagus are often too subtle to be detected by CT or MRI. Because they lack a mucosal element, intramural lesions cannot be evaluated by endoscopy. In such instances, endoscopic ultrasound is a valuable diagnostic tool. Endoscopic ultrasound is a hybrid technology that combines endoscopy with high-frequency ultrasound, which enhances image resolution. Because of its ability to image the gastrointestinal wall and surrounding structures, it has become a well-established method for the evaluation and local staging of various gastrointestinal malignancies including esophageal cancer.

Esophageal manometry allows for quantification of esophageal contractile activity and measures lower esophageal sphincter (LES) pressure, degree of LES relaxation, and the presence or absence of peristalsis. Manometry is used to diagnose an esophageal motility disorder in a patient with esophageal dysphagia once structural abnormalities have been excluded by imaging or endoscopy. The physiologic correlate of esophageal dysphagia, unrelated to intraluminal or extraluminal narrowing, is a peristaltic defect. Failure of the propulsive mechanism may be continuous or intermittent. Peristaltic defects may result from:

- The major motor disorders of the esophagus, achalasia, or diffuse esophageal spasm, in which bolus transport is obviously impaired, or
- Poorly characterized motor disorders such as abnormal LES relaxation, which produces increased intraluminal pressure allowing the formation of pulsion-type esophageal diverticula.

Mechanical Causes of Esophageal Dysphagia

ESOPHAGEAL WEBS AND RINGS

Esophageal webs and rings are thin, circumferential structures that protrude into the lumen. A web is a thin fold that is covered with squamous epithelium. Webs most commonly occur in the cervical esophagus. Patients are often asymptomatic or have mild intermittent dysphagia. Dysphagia is not present if the esophageal diameter is 13 mm or greater. A web is often discovered incidentally on contrast studies.

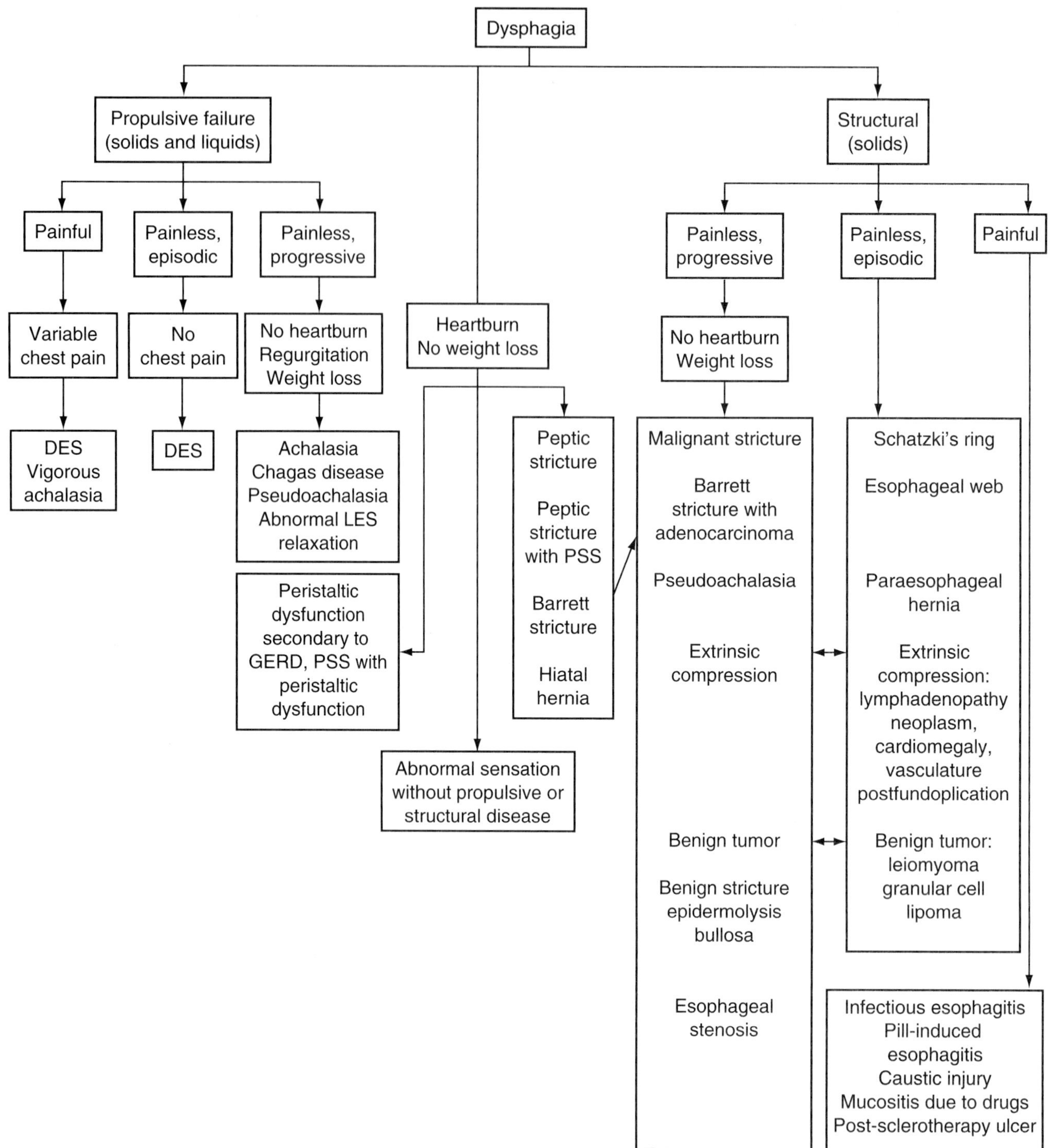

FIGURE 2 Algorithm for evaluation of esophageal dysphagia.
Abbreviations: CMV = cytomegalovirus; GERD = gastroesophageal reflux disease; HSV = herpes simplex virus; LES = lower esophageal sphincter; PPS = progressive systemic sclerosis.
Modified from: Ergun GA: Clinical approach to dysphagia. In: Ertan A (ed): Best Practice of Medicine. Philadelphia, Current Medicine, 2001, XIII:2.1-2.11.

Iron deficiency has been associated with upper esophageal webs (Plummer-Vinson or Paterson-Kelly syndrome).

Schatzki first described esophageal mucosal rings at the gastroesophageal junction that are covered by squamous mucosa above and columnar epithelium below. The pathogenesis of these esophageal rings is unclear, although GERD has been implicated. Muscular rings are much less common than mucosal rings and are characterized by hypertrophic musculature in the distal esophageal body. The caliber of a muscular ring changes during peristalsis,

TABLE 2 Causes of Esophageal Dysphagia

Mechanical

Intrinsic
Peptic stricture
Web or ring
Neoplasm
Foreign bodies
Benign tumor

Extrinsic Compression
Cervical osteophytes
Neoplasm
Goiter
Postfundoplication syndromes

Neuromuscular

Achalasia
Scleroderma
Diffuse esophageal spasm

Mucosal Inflammation

Reflux esophagitis
Infectious esophagitis
Pill induced
Caustic injury
Radiation injury
Bullous dermatologic disease

distinguishing it from a mucosal ring. On barium swallow and endoscopy the appearance is of a thick constriction of variable luminal diameter located above the squamocolumnar junction. The presence of multiple rings should raise suspicion for eosinophilic esophagitis.

Patients with esophageal rings have intermittent dysphagia for solid food. They can present with acute dysphagia after swallowing a large piece of meat (*steakhouse syndrome*) and require prompt endoscopy to remove the food impaction. Patients often learn to chew their food thoroughly or switch to a semisolid diet.

PEPTIC STRICTURES

Peptic strictures are seen in approximately 10% of patients with GERD who seek medical attention. They are also found in other conditions with increased esophageal acid exposure such as scleroderma, Zollinger-Ellison syndrome, and postmyotomy for achalasia. These strictures have been associated with long-standing reflux disease, male sex, and older age. Symptoms of peptic strictures are usually manifestations of slowly progressing from dysphagia for solids to dysphagia for both solids and liquids.

ESOPHAGEAL CANCER

The incidence of esophageal cancer shows marked geographic variation. Ninety percent of new cases arise in the developing countries of Asia, Africa, and South America. The United States, Canada, and most of Western Europe have a lower incidence of about 3 to 4 per 100,000 general population.

Alcohol, tobacco, and lack of vitamins have been implicated in the etiology. Regular alcohol drinkers have six times the incidence of nondrinkers. Alcohol has not been shown to be a direct carcinogen, but increased alcohol intake is associated with decreased consumption of essential nutrients and vitamins, which may play a role as diets deficient in vitamin A, C, and riboflavin have been associated with esophageal cancer.

Most esophageal tumors are squamous in origin. Squamous cell carcinoma, associated with tobacco and alcohol abuse, is common in Asia (China and Singapore), and demonstrates a predilection to African Americans in the United States. Early changes include plaque-like elevations of the mucosa, erosions, and fibrous strictures. Carcinoma in situ is confined to the epithelium and does not penetrate the basement membrane. In intramucosal carcinoma, penetration of the basement membrane, and infiltration of the lamina propria occurs. In submucosal carcinoma, the cancer cells penetrate the muscularis mucosa but do not reach the muscularis propria. Spread occurs by direct invasion to the aorta and bronchial tree. Lymph spread may involve the paraesophageal, mediastinal, and deep cervical lymph nodes with tumors of the lower third of the esophagus spreading to the celiac and splenic nodes. Hematogenous spread can be to the liver, lung, adrenal glands, and kidneys.

Adenocarcinoma involves the lower third of the esophagus and occurs mainly in Caucasian males who have a long history of GERD and underlying Barrett mucosa. The prevalence of adenocarcinoma in patients with Barrett seen at endoscopy is 8% to 15%. Since World War II, the incidence of esophageal cancer has been rising at a rate of 5% per annum.

Other esophageal tumors include verrucous carcinoma which is a variant of squamous cell carcinoma. It grows slowly and locally, rarely metastasizing. Oat cell tumor of the esophagus is histologically identical to the oat cell tumor of the lung. It accounts for approximately 2.5% of all esophageal cancers. These are aggressive and have a poor prognosis. Occasionally primary malignant melanomas may develop in the esophagus. Lymphatic and systemic spread occurs early, and the prognosis is poor. Nonepithelial tumors include leiomyomas, the most common variety, leiomyosarcoma, stromal tumors, lipomas, and lymphoma.

The classic presenting symptom of esophageal cancer is dysphagia. Most esophageal tumors are advanced at the time of presentation. By the time dysphagia is recognized nearly 50% of the esophageal lumen has been compromised. As the tumor grows rapidly, progressive dysphagia, initially for solids and later for liquids, and weight loss are seen. Occasionally solid food becomes impacted above the tumor. These patients frequently have chest pain, odynophagia, and anemia. An achalasia-like syndrome (pseudoachalasia) may be seen in patients with adenocarcinoma of the cardia caused by microscopic infiltration of the myenteric plexus or the vagus nerve. Supraclavicular lymph nodes may occur in particular on the left side of the neck (Virchow node, Troisier sign). Rarely an epigastric mass may be palpable, or transperitoneal spread from a tumor at the gastroesophageal junction may produce ascites or a palpable mass in the pouch of Douglas on rectal exam.

The most appropriate initial investigation is a barium swallow. This gives an assessment of the macroscopic tumor length. Tumors less than 3 cm in length have a 5-year survival rate of 40%, whereas those over 5 cm in length are usually both unresectable and metastatic. Endoscopy is warranted in all patients suspected of esophageal cancer. This enables a positive tissue diagnosis by biopsy or brush cytology. Sampling by both these methods leads to a diagnostic yield in more than 90% of cases. Stenotic areas can be dilated at endoscopy, and local therapy can be given for advanced tumors. CT scans provide information related to the size of the primary tumor and the presence of local and distant metastases. At the time of presentation 30% of esophageal cancers will have metastasized to the liver and 20% to the lung. CT scans are the most accurate modality in detecting distant spread. MRI has not been shown to be superior to CT scanning. Endoscopic ultrasound (EUS) currently provides the most accurate information with regard to local invasion by the primary tumor. The depth of the esophageal wall and extra-esophageal invasion can accurately be imaged by EUS. The overall accuracy of EUS is approximately 90% compared with 60% for CT. In nodal involvement, the accuracy of EUS is 75% and only 50% for CT. Bronchial invasion is seen in 10% of esophageal cancers, usually those in the middle third of the esophagus; bronchoscopy prior to surgery is indicated in such cases.

The only hope for cure is complete surgical resection of the tumor and associated lymph nodes. Carcinoma of the esophagus has the propensity to spread in the submucosal layers of the esophagus, up to 6 cm proximally and 4 cm distally, beyond the macroscopically obvious periphery of the tumor. Surgical resection may be through one of several approaches.

The left thoracotomy and thoracoabdominal approaches are ideal only for small distal tumors. The most widely used surgery for tumors of the middle and lower esophagus is the Ivor Lewis esophagectomy. For extensive and upper esophageal tumors the esophagogastrectomy of McKeown is performed.

Operative mortality for curative resection ranges from 10% to 30%. The stage of disease at the time of treatment is the major determinant of survival. Poor survival rates are because most patients at presentation have advanced disease.

Radiation therapy is used for the management of unresectable esophageal cancer with curative or palliative intent. Factors associated with good response to radiation therapy include female gender, noncircumferential tumors, tumors smaller than 5 cm, and tumors of the upper esophagus. Radiation has been used in combination with surgery and chemotherapy. Combined chemotherapy with radiation has been proven more effective than radiation alone and is currently the standard of care for unresectable esophageal cancer. Preoperative radiation is given to shrink the tumor and sterilize the tumor bed before surgery. Postoperatively radiation is used to control residual disease after surgery. Chemoradiation has also been used preoperatively with clear benefit in select patients although at the cost of increased operative morbidity and mortality. Most regimens use 5-flurouracil (Adrucil)[1] combined with cisplatin (Platinol AQ)[1] or mitomycin C (Mutamycin)[1]. Response rates are 35% to 58% with duration of response under 6 months. Endoluminal brachytherapy can help in palliation of symptoms. Side effects of radiation include esophagitis, stomatitis, neutropenia, and anorexia. Long-term complications include strictures, tracheoesophageal fistulae, and pulmonary fibrosis.

Endoscopic therapy has been used for very early mucosal and submucosal lesions that are less than 2 to 3 cm in size with a 95% 5-year survival following resection. Patient selection must be meticulous. Careful staging with EUS should be done prior to mucosal resection.

Endoscopy has a major role in providing relief of dysphagia for advanced inoperable tumors. Dilation produces short-term relief of dysphagia but requires frequent sessions if used alone. Exophytic tumor masses are most suitable for laser therapy, which may give palliative relief in 70% to 85% of patients with dysphagia. Similar results are seen with thermal therapy such as bipolar circumactive probe (BICAP) heater, which may be used in circumferential stenosing tumors. Photodynamic therapy enables destruction of malignant tissue by using a photosensitizer that destroys tissue when exposed to specific wavelengths at low-intensity light. The principle use is in the treatment of high-grade dysplasia and early adenocarcinoma arising in Barrett metaplasia. Endoscopic placement of flexible, self-expanding metal stents following esophageal dilation can obviate the rapid symptom recurrence caused by malignant strictures. The choice of therapy must, of course, be individualized for each patient.

BARRETT ESOPHAGUS

Barrett esophagus (BE) is the condition in which an abnormal columnar epithelium replaces the stratified squamous epithelium that normally lines the distal esophagus. The abnormal columnar epithelium is a form of incomplete intestinal metaplasia that usually shows evidence of DNA damage, and it appears that most esophageal adenocarcinomas arise

[1]Not FDA approved for this indication.

from the specialized intestinal metaplasia of BE. This is the most severe histologic consequence of GERD because of its association with adenocarcinoma of the distal esophagus.

The prevalence of Barrett esophagus is difficult to determine because most studies suffer from selection bias, but in patients undergoing endoscopy who are symptomatic of GERD, incidence ranges between 6% to 12% for long-segment disease. Short-segment Barrett is more prevalent, although prevalence has ranged from 2% to 12% in patients undergoing routine upper endoscopy. Both short- and long-segment BE affects white men of middle age, although other risk factors include age, obesity, and duration of GERD symptoms.

The annual incidence of esophageal adenocarcinoma in patients with Barrett has been reported to be as high as 1.5%; however, recent publications suggest that this risk has been overestimated because of publication bias and that the actual incidence is closer to 0.5% per year. Recent information suggests that both short- and long-segment cases of Barrett esophagus have similar rates of cancer incidence.

Because BE is thought to be a complication of chronic GERD, gastroenterologists have attempted to use symptoms of GERD as a marker for those at increased risk for the disease. The thinking has revolved around the idea that patients with BE should be enrolled in a surveillance program with the hope of detecting malignancy at an early and curable stage. Unfortunately, endoscopic detection of early adenocarcinoma has been poor. In two large cohorts with esophageal adenocarcinoma, less than 5% had a prior diagnosis of BE. Hence, if the assumption is correct that esophageal adenocarcinoma arises from Barrett esophagus, then why is Barrett esophagus rarely discovered before the cancer diagnosis? Either those with reflux symptoms who are destined to develop adenocarcinoma are not undergoing screening examinations or a large proportion of those who will develop cancer are not having reflux symptoms.

Current practice guidelines recommend that screening for Barrett should be focused on patients with the highest risk—white men aged 50 years or older and/or those with long-standing severe reflux symptoms, typically of greater than 5 years' duration. Moreover, all patients with BE undergo periodic endoscopy for surveillance. For patients without dysplasia, the American College of Gastroenterology suggests that endoscopic surveillance be performed every 3 to 5 years. If dysplasia is found, then the finding should be reviewed and confirmed by another pathologist. Patients with low-grade dysplasia should be treated with high-dose acid suppression with a proton pump inhibitor (PPI) to eliminate the confounding effect of inflammation, and an endoscopy with biopsy should be repeated. If low-grade dysplasia persists, then the patient should undergo endoscopy every 6 months for 1 year, then yearly if no dysplasia is found. If high-grade dysplasia is found, most experts advocate esophagectomy in the healthy patient with minimal surgical risk, although some have questioned this approach because of the variable natural history of high-grade dysplasia and the mortality and morbidity associated with esophagectomy. In patients with unacceptable surgical risk, ablative therapies with thermal, chemical, or mechanical means might be considered.

MUCOSAL INFLAMMATION

Infectious esophagitis is an increasingly common cause of esophageal dysphagia and odynophagia in the immunocompromised host. Although it is rare for a normal host to develop bacterial, fungal, or viral esophagitis, infections with *Mycobacterium tuberculosis*, β-hemolytic streptococci, *Treponema pallidum*, and herpes simplex virus have all been described in patients with normal immunity. The increasing incidence of fungal and viral infections of the esophagus, however, is mainly related to the increased prevalence of organ transplantation with associated immunosuppression and to the increasing incidence of AIDS.

The most common infection in these immunocompromised hosts is candidiasis, although other fungal diseases such as those caused by *Torulopsis glabrata* and actinomycotic infections also occur. Cytomegalovirus esophagitis occurs most often in patients with AIDS and following organ transplantation, causing multiple painful ulcerations. In some instances, HIV itself may be the primary pathogen causing esophagitis, but these patients commonly have multiple concurrent infections with *Candida* species as well as cytomegalovirus or herpes simplex virus.

Patients undergoing radiation for thoracic or head and neck cancers are at risk for developing esophageal strictures. In the acute setting they may develop esophagitis and present with dysphagia and odynophagia. The incidence of radiation strictures depends on the type and dose of radiation, but can be up to 44%. Chronic radiation esophagitis can also develop from prolonged tissue ischemia and radiation fibrosis. The location of the strictures depends upon the site of maximal radiation injury. As a result, proximal strictures are more common in patients receiving radiation for head and neck cancer.

Pill esophagitis is recognized more commonly with almost every pill being described as causing injury. However the most common offenders still include aspirin, tetracycline, doxycycline, quinidine, potassium, alendronate, and nonsteroidal anti-inflammatory drugs (NSAIDs). The mechanism appears to be multifactorial and related to the pill size, shape, coating, and delivery system; but most injury is caused by a local caustic reaction to prolonged contact. Factors such as inadequate fluid consumption with medication intake and recumbency also play a role as both may predispose to lodging in the esophagus and increasing mucosal contact. Recovery usually occurs with withdrawal of the offending agent. Mucosal injury related to doxycycline and iron sulfate usually heals without stricture formation. However, perforation and strictures have been reported with potassium- and quinidine-induced injury. History of known medications causing esophagitis and endoscopy to exclude other lesions are mandatory in making this diagnosis.

Treatment is usually discontinuing the medication or altering the method of delivery into a liquid or suspension. Patients are advised to take their medications with fluids and avoid recumbency for at least 1 hour following ingestion. Symptomatic relief for odynophagia may be provided with viscous lidocaine[1] and acid suppression.

EXTRINSIC COMPRESSION

A number of abnormalities can cause dysphagia by extrinsic compression of the esophagus such as lymphadenopathy from sarcoidosis and mediastinal neoplasms such as thymoma and lymphoma. *Dysphagia lusoria* refers to extrinsic compression caused by the presence of an aberrant right subclavian vein compressing the esophagus. In the elderly, severe atherosclerosis or a large aneurysm of the thoracic aorta can cause impingement on the esophagus and produce dysphagia aortica. Likewise severe enlargement of the left atrium in patients with mitral valve disease may cause dysphagia by external compression.

As an increasing number of antireflux surgeries are performed, dysphagia after fundoplication is increasingly observed, and dysphagia that lasts for more than 3 months has been noted in 12% of patients undergoing laparoscopic fundoplication as compared to those undergoing open fundoplication. The cause of the higher incidence of postoperative dysphagia with the laparoscopic approach is not completely understood. Because the gastric fundus is wrapped around the distal esophagus, possibilities that could contribute to the symptom of dysphagia include creating a wrap that is "too tight" or "too long" despite constructing the wrap over a large esophageal bougie (48 to 60F). Similarly, tight approximation of the diaphragmatic crura, while reducing a hiatal hernia, proximal slippage of the wrap, and the development of a paraesophageal hernia are also causes of dysphagia after fundoplication. Lastly, the development of abnormal esophageal emptying that is simply caused by distorted mechanics at the level of the fundoplication may contribute to the symptom of dysphagia.

Unfortunately, preoperative testing cannot reliably predict postoperative dysphagia; preoperative swallowing difficulty appears to be the single greatest risk factor.

FOREIGN BODIES IN THE ESOPHAGUS

Accidental foreign body ingestion occurs mainly in children. The majority of these foreign bodies are coins. Food impactions are usually seen in edentulous or mentally impaired people. Intentional ingestion is seen in prison inmates and in those with psychiatric disorders.

Meat impaction above an esophageal stricture is the most common cause of acute esophageal obstruction in adults. The classic history is of rapid onset of dysphagia or an inability to swallow saliva, which indicates total esophageal obstruction. Patients may complain of retrosternal pressure and regurgitation of undigested food. Plain neck, chest, and abdominal radiographs should be promptly obtained before any attempt at extraction. They may reveal a radiopaque foreign body or signs of esophageal perforation. A barium swallow should not be done as it can impair endoscopic inspection and retrieval. No treatment is needed in the asymptomatic patient with a history of foreign body ingestion and negative plain radiographs. The majority of foreign bodies pass spontaneously.

Esophageal foreign bodies should be removed within 12 hours to avoid esophageal perforation or pulmonary aspiration. Urgent endoscopy is indicated in the settings of sharp objects, patients with signs of obstruction or pain, and ingestion of disk batteries. Early surgical consult should be obtained if there is any suspicion of perforation.

Endoscopy allows safe retrieval and visual inspection of the esophagus. Use of an overtube to protect the airway is helpful for objects that are small, hard to grasp, or may fragment. Intravenous glucagon[1] may be given to relax the esophagus and allow passage of the foreign body. If adequate endoscopic visualization distal to the impaction is possible, the bolus may be slowly advanced into the stomach with the tip of the endoscope. A food impaction usually consists of meat lodged above a peptic stricture. Dilation of a ring or stricture may be done safely right after the impaction is relieved. Patients in whom the food bolus impaction resolves spontaneously should have elective endoscopy to exclude an underlying stricture or tumor.

Blunt objects that have already entered the stomach can be managed conservatively because most will pass within a week. Weekly radiographs are sufficient in asymptomatic patients. Endoscopic or surgical removal should be considered if the object remains in the same location for more than 1 week; is larger than 2.5 cm, making it less likely to traverse the pylorus; or in patients who develop signs of obstruction or sepsis.

Disk batteries can conduct electricity and pose an additional risk if ingested. Contact of the flat esophageal wall with both poles of the battery conducts electricity that may rapidly result in esophageal necrosis and perforation. These batteries can be removed with a retrieval basket or gently advanced into the stomach. Most disk batteries that have entered the stomach will pass through the remaining gastrointestinal tract without consequence.

[1]Not FDA approved for this indication.

Patients can be followed with a radiograph every 3 to 4 days. Those who develop signs or symptoms of obstruction, necrosis, or have ingested batteries larger than 20 mm in diameter, and those in whom the battery remains in the stomach for longer than 48 hours, require endoscopic removal. Use of emetics and cathartics is of unclear benefit and is not recommended.

Esophageal Motility Disorders

In a clinical setting, esophageal manometry is used to evaluate only limited aspects of esophageal function, namely the integrity of primary peristalsis and LES relaxation, hence the diagnostic yield becomes limited to only a few aberrations such as absent peristalsis, abnormalities of LES tone, or impaired sphincter relaxation. Because of the limited repertoire to injury in the esophagus, each of these motility patterns are nonspecific and potentially caused by more than one disease condition. Despite these limitations, many have sought to classify motility disorders. Using a diagnosis-based method of classification, "classic" motility disorders such as achalasia and diffuse esophageal spasm (DES) account for only a small number of cases. An operationally based classification system is therefore used here to discuss esophageal motility disorders.

IMPAIRED LOWER ESOPHAGEAL SPHINCTER RELAXATION (LES): ACHALASIA, ATYPICAL DISORDERS OF LES RELAXATION

Achalasia is the best-defined major motility disorder of the esophagus. It is an esophageal disorder of unknown cause where there is degeneration of nitric-oxide-producing inhibitory neurons that produce relaxation of the esophageal smooth muscle. It is characterized by the failure of the LES to relax completely—hence the term achalasia, which is derived from the Greek word for *does not relax*. In addition to the failure of the LES to relax completely with swallowing, there is also a lack of peristalsis in the smooth muscle of the esophagus. The symptoms and signs of achalasia are primarily caused by these defects. They often are insidious and gradual in progression. As a result, patients typically experience symptoms for years before seeking medical attention.

The diagnosis is occasionally suggested on a plain radiograph of the chest that shows widening of the mediastinum because of the dilated esophagus, and absence of the normal gastric air bubble caused by the failure of LES relaxation that prevents air from entering the stomach. A barium swallow should be obtained when achalasia is suspected. The barium swallow classically shows a dilated esophagus that terminates in a beak-like narrowing caused by the persistently contracted LES. In some cases, the dilation is so profound that the esophagus assumes a sigmoid shape. Fluoroscopy will show absence of peristalsis in the smooth muscle portion of the esophagus.

Patients with Chagas disease may have clinical features similar to achalasia, but the disease is caused by destruction of the neurons of the myenteric plexus, which is the result of infection by *Trypanosoma cruzi*. Unlike achalasia, Chagas disease is not limited to the esophagus and affects the cardiac conduction system as well as the smooth muscle of the gastrointestinal and genitourinary tracts.

Dysphagia for both solids and liquids is the primary clinical feature. Patients with achalasia may also complain of weight loss, chest pain, regurgitation, heartburn, and globus sensation. Hiccups are common with achalasia and probably result from functional obstruction of the distal esophagus. An abnormality in the belch reflex with impaired LES relaxation can be seen in 85% of patients. Achalasia is an uncommon disorder that has an annual incidence of about 1 case per 100,000 general population. Men and women are affected equally. Although the disease can occur at any age, it is typically diagnosed after the age of 25 years because of its insidious onset of symptoms.

Endoscopic evaluation is required to exclude malignancy at the gastroesophageal junction that could mimic achalasia (pseudoachalasia). Endoscopy typically reveals a dilated esophagus that may contain residual material. The mucosa usually appears normal, although inflammation can result from the retained food. Patients may develop esophageal candidiasis caused by chronic stasis.

Esophageal manometry does not differentiate achalasia from pseudoachalasia. CT scanning may suggest malignancy if there is esophageal wall irregularity or abnormal adenopathy. Endoscopy with biopsy may miss the diagnosis because the tumors are often infiltrative and do not extend through the mucosa to the lumen.

The treatment options for achalasia include medical therapy, pneumatic dilation, surgical myotomy, and botulinum toxin injection of the LES. Nitrates and calcium channel blockers can relax the smooth muscle of the LES but have limited clinical efficacy. Medical therapy is, therefore, used only for patients who are unable to tolerate the more invasive forms of therapy.

Definitive therapy for achalasia requires myotomy of the LES. Endoscopically this can be achieved via pneumatic dilation. This type of dilation cannot be achieved with conventional passive dilations as performed for peptic strictures and is risky because esophageal perforation is the most common serious complication of pneumatic dilation, occurring in about 5% of cases.

In the United States the most popular pneumatic balloon dilator is the Rigiflex (Bard, Boston, MA) balloon dilator, which is passed over a guidewire, positioned fluoroscopically straddling the LES, and inflated until obliteration of the waist or dilation is achieved. Most studies describe good short-term results in 60% to 85% of patients treated with a single session of pneumatic dilation. Approximately 50% of patients with achalasia treated once with pneumatic dilation will require repeated dilation within 5 years, and subsequent pneumatic dilations are less likely to result in a sustained remission. Surgery or other forms of therapy should be considered for patients who have had two or three unsuccessful pneumatic dilations.

Surgery is superior to pneumatic dilation for both the short-term and long-term relief of dysphagia. Laparoscopic surgical myotomy via the modified Heller approach results in excellent relief of symptoms in 70% to 90% of patients with few serious complications. The mortality rate of 0.3% is similar to that for pneumatic dilation. Reflux esophagitis develops in approximately 10% of patients treated by surgery. Surgical myotomy results in excellent remission rates (approximately 85%) at 10 years.

Botulinum toxin (Botox)[1] is a potent inhibitor of the release of acetylcholine from nerve endings. Botulinum toxin injected into the LES of patients inhibits the excitatory acetylcholine-releasing neurons that increase LES smooth muscle tone, producing a reduction in LES pressure. Patients who respond tend to be older and less symptomatic than nonresponders. Compared with pneumatic dilation, botulinum toxin injection is less likely to produce a durable symptom response, however, this approach can be considered for the treatment of patients who have serious co-morbidity and for whom pneumatic dilation or surgical myotomy is not an option.

UNCOORDINATED CONTRACTION: DIFFUSE ESOPHAGEAL SPASM

The patient with suspected esophageal spasm complains of intermittent chest pain and dysphagia to solids and liquids. Unlike achalasia, the esophagus retains the ability to propagate primary peristaltic waves the majority of the time. For this reason, in part, the criteria for diagnosing DES remain variable and confusing. In the unequivocal case, the nonperistaltic, high amplitude, prolonged (uncoordinated) contractions are seen during esophageal manometry and the LES functions normally. Radiographically, DES appears as a *corkscrew* esophagus. However, neither tertiary contractions (nonperistaltic, simultaneous contractions) seen on radiograph nor simultaneous contractions seen on manometry are pathognomonic of esophageal spasm; both are seen with advancing age (presbyesophagus). It is important that such abnormalities be accompanied by symptoms before making a diagnosis of esophageal spasm.

It is important to identify associated underlying disorders that may improve with drug therapy, such as anxiety or depression, although treatment results have been mixed with use of smooth muscle relaxants such as nitrates, CCBs, and antidepressants. Severe cases have been treated with pneumatic dilation or esophageal myotomy, but the literature has been uncontrolled and anecdotal.

[1]Not FDA approved for this indication.

HYPERCONTRACTILE STATES: NUTCRACKER ESOPHAGUS AND ISOLATED HYPERTENSIVE LOWER ESOPHAGEAL SPHINCTER

Hypercontractile disorders such as *nutcracker* esophagus are manometric diagnoses established by the detection of high amplitude (>180 mm Hg), peristaltic contractions in the distal esophagus. However, it is difficult to attribute pain or dysphagia to these findings because their functional significance is uncertain. Bolus transit is usually normal, and there is no established relationship between symptoms and manometric findings over time. Similarly, isolated hypertensive LES with normal relaxation characteristics have unclear significance in that there are no clear clinical or physiological consequences with these manometric abnormalities.

HYPOCONTRACTILE STATES: SCLERODERMA, PERISTALTIC DYSFUNCTION CAUSED BY GASTROESOPHAGEAL REFLUX DISEASE

Scleroderma is the classic example of esophageal hypocontractility with esophageal dysfunction. It is caused by smooth muscle fibrosis and consequent esophageal body atrophy and impaired clearance, often with loss of peristalsis. The proximal esophagus (striated muscle) is spared and exhibits normal motility. The ineffective motility coupled with hypotension of the LES, also caused by smooth muscle fibrosis, results in an increased risk for the development of severe GERD. The GERD is often accompanied by development of erosions (which occurs in up to 50% of patients), peptic stricture, and Barrett esophagus. Most complain of heartburn and regurgitation.

Barium studies show distension of the distal two thirds of the esophagus and poor barium clearance, usually with a patulous and hypotonic LES. The manometric findings are not specific to scleroderma and may be seen in a variety of other disorders including other collagen vascular disorders, rheumatoid arthritis, diabetes mellitus, and amyloidosis, as well as in healthy patients with GERD. In fact, peristaltic defects are commonly encountered in reflux disease. With increasing severity of reflux disease, peristaltic amplitude diminishes; failed peristaltic contractions become increasingly prevalent in association with nonobstructive dysphagia.

Management is directed toward aggressive acid suppression with proton pump inhibitors. Prokinetic agents to improve esophageal dysmotility have not been as successful as improving acid control. Dilation of peptic strictures may be necessary with severe symptoms of dysphagia. Occasionally surgery is considered for intractable esophagitis.

Functional Dysphagia

Functional dysphagia is a diagnosis of exclusion in patients with dysphagia who have undergone a complete diagnostic evaluation without evidence of a structural abnormality, pathologic gastroesophageal reflux, or motility disorder to explain the dysphagia. Diagnostic criteria include at least 12 weeks, in the preceding year, of having a sense of food sticking or passing abnormally through the esophagus.

Symptoms of dysphagia may be intermittent or daily, and may be identical to dysphagia caused by organic disorders. Patients should be reassured, instructed to avoid precipitating factors (if present), and to chew their food well. Treatment with a CCB, anticholinergic agent, anxiolytics, or antidepressants have not proved efficacy. Mechanical interventions such as esophageal dilation with a 50 to 54F Maloney dilator can be tried, although the benefit of this is also unproven.

Dysphagia is considered an alarm symptom and usually implies an organic disorder that should always be evaluated. The clinical history is the most critical component to the evaluation of dysphagia. Once the clinician has attempted to define the likely cause of dysphagia, an evaluation and examination can be thoughtfully tailored to obtaining the definitive diagnosis. In most cases, the cause of dysphagia can be defined and correct therapy can be initiated.

DIVERTICULA OF THE ALIMENTARY TRACT

METHOD OF

Martin Poleski, MD

Diverticula are outpouchings that can be found throughout the gastrointestinal tract, from the pharynx to the rectum. A single outpouching is called a diverticulum. Some diverticula may be present from birth. Diverticula that involve all the layers of the intestinal wall are sometimes called *true diverticula*. An example of this is the congenital Meckel's diverticulum. Most diverticula are acquired through life and represent herniation of the mucosa and submucosa through the muscular wall of the alimentary canal. These have been called *false* or *pseudodiverticula*. The most common example of this is diverticulosis of the colon. These anatomic descriptions of diverticula have little clinical importance. The relevance of diverticula is that they may cause significant symptoms or disease; but, in many cases they are not responsible for a patient's complaints or condition. The astute clinician must decide when the presence of diverticula is the source of discomfort or disease, and when to look elsewhere for the cause of the patient's problem.

Esophageal Diverticula

ZENKER'S DIVERTICULUM

Zenker's, the hypopharyngeal diverticulum, is most common in men older than the age of 70. This represents an outpouching of mucosa and submucosa posterior in the midline between the cricopharyngeus and inferior constrictor muscles. The cause is an incomplete relaxation of the upper esophageal sphincter (UES) muscle, which results in increased pressure during swallowing and herniation of the mucosa. The diverticulum enlarges over a period of time, and symptoms may be mild or severe. Early symptoms are usually those of transient dysphagia. As the diverticular sac enlarges, it retains food contents resulting in gurgling, regurgitation, and aspiration at night leading to some wheezing and coughing. Zenker's diverticulum is usually easily diagnosed with a barium swallow. Endoscopy may be difficult in the presence of a large diverticulum and makes intubation of the esophagus difficult. Blind intubation of the esophagus—as occurs in endoscopic retrograde cholangiopancreatography (ERCP) or transesophageal echocardiography—in the presence of a significant hypopharyngeal diverticulum carries an increased risk of perforation. Symptomatic Zenker's diverticulum is treated with resection and myotomy of the cricopharyngeal muscle; small symptomatic diverticula can be treated by myotomy alone. Asymptomatic Zenker's diverticulum is left alone.

MIDESOPHAGEAL DIVERTICULA

Midesophageal diverticula are usually asymptomatic and are found when investigating for a variety of esophageal complaints. They have been called *traction diverticula* because of their association with underlying necrotic nodal infection, as may occur with tuberculosis. This cause is unusual in western countries today. Most midbody diverticula today may be related to nonspecific motility disorders. Most midesophageal diverticula are not the source of the patient's symptoms. Surgical therapy is rarely indicated.

EPIPHRENIC DIVERTICULA

Epiphrenic diverticula occur just above the esophagogastric junction. They tend to be associated with esophageal spasm or other motor disorders of the lower esophageal sphincter. Successful treatment of the esophageal motor disorder usually resolves all symptoms. Surgery of the diverticulum itself is rarely indicated.

INTRAMURAL ESOPHAGEAL DIVERTICULOSIS

Intramural esophageal diverticulosis is a rare condition that is actually dilated submucosal glands and not diverticula. On barium swallow the glands appear as multiple outpouchings, 1 to 4 mm in size, from the esophageal lumen. They are often noted on an esophagram ordered for a variety of upper gastrointestinal conditions including reflux esophagitis, strictures, caustic ingestion, cancer, and motility disorder. They often do not resolve when the associated condition is treated such as a stricture or reflux esophagitis. Intramural esophageal diverticula may occasionally perforate and present with mediastinitis and free air. These are tiny perforations that can most often be managed medically with antibiotics and by keeping the patient on nothing by mouth (NPO) for a few days.

GASTRIC DIVERTICULUM

Gastric diverticulum (GD) is rare. It is found by chance during upper endoscopy in the retroflexed view at the gastroesophageal junction. Approximately 1 in 500 patients have this finding. GD in the juxtacardiac area may rarely bleed or ulcerate, requiring surgery. The vast majority of these gastric diverticula are asymptomatic.

Diverticula can also develop in the prepyloric area of the stomach. Scarring caused by chronic recurrent peptic ulcer disease is thought to be the cause. *Helicobacter pylori* should be looked for when this deformity is found to prevent recurrent ulceration.

Duodenal Diverticula

Duodenal diverticula in the bulb of the duodenum are also related to recurrent peptic ulcer disease. *H. pylori* should be eradicated if found. Diverticula in the second portion of the duodenum are relatively common, occurring in approximately 6% to 20% of all individuals. They appear most often within a couple of centimeters of the papilla of Vater. They are an incidental finding in many endoscopies or barium meal radiographs. These outpouchings may cause difficulty during ERCP in the small number of people whose papilla empties directly into the diverticulum in the second duodenum and makes cannulation difficult. They have been associated with pancreatitis and cholangitis; but cause and effect are hard to prove. Nonspecific gastrointestinal symptoms have been attributed to duodenal diverticula. In most cases the duodenal diverticulum is an incidental finding unrelated to the patient's complaint. Bleeding, and perforation are rare. Diverticulitis or perforation can be confirmed by a computed tomography (CT) scan. Endoscopy can localize bleeding to this area. Surgery is rarely indicated except for perforation, recurrent bleeding, or diverticulitis.

Meckel's Diverticulum

Meckel's diverticulum usually arises about 100 cm from the ileocecal valve. It arises on the antimesenteric border of the intestine and represents the vestige of the omphalomesenteric duct. Meckel's diverticulum contains all layers of the intestinal wall. The mucosal lining is usually normal ileal mucosa. A significant number contain gastric mucosa capable of secreting acid, and a minority affect other ectopic tissue such as the pancreas, colon, or endometrium.

The ectopic gastric tissue may produce enough acid to cause ulceration and bleeding in the diverticulum or adjacent intestinal mucosa. Bleeding may present as bright red blood and maroon or tarry stool. Hemodynamically significant bleeding usually occurs in childhood; but has been described in all ages. In older individuals, small-bowel obstruction caused by intussusception or bowel wall entrapment is more common than is hemorrhage. Malignancies have rarely been reported. However, approximately 2% of the population may have Meckel's diverticulum and the vast majority are asymptomatic. The ectopic gastric mucosa of Meckel's diverticulum can be diagnosed by a technetium-99 radioisotope scan. The isotope is picked up by gastric mucosa. Selective superior mesenteric angiography can also detect a bleeding diverticulum. The treatment of complications of a Meckel's diverticulum—such as bleeding, intussusception, small bowel entrapment, or malignancy—is surgery.

Small-Bowel Diverticulosis

Small-bowel diverticulosis of the jejunum and ileum occurs particularly in the elderly. Approximately 80% occurs in the jejunum. Their cause is in unknown. They appear to be associated with abnormal gastrointestinal motility, which results in abnormal intraluminal pressure and herniation of mucosa and submucosa through the bowel wall at the mesenteric border. They are also associated with scleroderma. This disease can lead to fibrosis of portions of the intestinal wall and diverticular formation through the weakened wall. Small-bowel diverticula are often asymptomatic. They are seen on small-bowel radiographs. They can predispose to bacterial overgrowth in the small bowel. This situation may cause malabsorption. Patients present with bloating, diarrhea, cramping, and frank fat malabsorption. A therapeutic trial of an antibiotic such as tetracycline[1], 250 mg four times a day, or cephalexin (Keflex)[1] for 1 to 2 weeks will markedly improve the symptoms for several weeks or months. It is often necessary to give repeated courses of antibiotics to control the recurrent overgrowth with resultant symptoms and malabsorption. Rotation of antibiotics may be necessary if resistance occurs. Vitamin B_{12}

[1]Not FDA approved for this indication.

injections are also given monthly because of the decreased absorption of this vitamin. Resection of the diverticula is done in the very rare instances of recurrent diverticulitis or significant hemorrhage.

Colonic Diverticulosis

Colonic diverticulosis may develop in more than 50% of North American people older than the age of 50 years. The vast majority are acquired with aging and are uncommon younger than the age of 40. The etiology is thought to be the low-fiber diet in Western cultures, which results in increase in intracolonic pressure. The increased pressure results in herniation of colonic mucosa and submucosa in the area of weakness caused by the penetration of the circular muscle of the colon by the vasa recta. Abnormalities of collagen and elastin that occur with aging also may contribute to areas of weakness in the colonic wall and diverticulosis. Thickening of the colonic wall is also associated with these outpouchings. Colonic diverticulosis in the past was found to be more than 100 times more common in Western counties than in Asian ones. In Western countries the area most often affected is the sigmoid, whereas in the Orient cecal and ascending colon diverticula are more common. In recent years, epidemiologic studies have shown an increasing incidence of diverticulosis and its complications in Japan. As in the West the incidence is increasing with age; but, the predominant area of involvement remains in the right colon. These findings suggest that Western diet increases the incidence of diverticulosis with aging. Genetic factors may play a role in which part of the colon is involved.

Fortunately, the vast majority of diverticula are asymptomatic. They are frequently seen in normal people undergoing screening for colon cancer. Approximately 10% of people may develop symptoms from the diverticula.

Nonspecific lower abdominal discomfort, bloating, flatulence, and erratic bowel function are common in people with normal colons and irritable bowel. These complaints are also seen in individuals with diverticulosis. It is difficult to say in a patient with uncomplicated diverticulosis whether there is any relationship of the symptoms to the presence of these outpouchings. Both conditions often will respond to a slow increase in fiber, to 20 to 30 g if possible, an increase of fluid intake, and a decrease of fat in the diet. Fiber can be in the form of bran, psyllium, methylcellulose, or other sources. Surgery should not be offered to patients with the above symptoms and uncomplicated diverticulosis.

Uncomplicated diverticulosis is most easily seen with a barium enema. Diverticula can also be seen with a colonoscopy or CT scan.

The most common complications of diverticula are diverticulitis and hemorrhage. Diverticulitis may be accompanied by abscess formation, peritonitis, and free perforation. Massive bleeding from diverticulosis is not an unusual occurrence in the geriatric age group. The hemorrhage is most frequent from right-sided diverticula. Bleeding is thought to be caused by damage to the vasa recta by an adjacent diverticulum. The damaged vessel often ruptures at the neck of the diverticulum. The bleeding is often brisk and sudden in onset. The stool is often maroon or red, depending on the briskness of the hemorrhage and the transit time of the blood. The treatment is stabilization with standard support measures including fluids and transfusion as necessary. Most diverticular bleeding stops spontaneously. Investigation is necessary to exclude other causes. Angiodysplasias of the colon cause hemorrhage from the right side of the colon. Other important causes include malignancy, inflammatory colitis, and ischemic colitis. Once the patient is stabilized, colonoscopy is done after a colonic purge. If the specific bleeding diverticula can be found, injecting epinephrine[1] (1:10,000 or 1:20,000) around the neck of the diverticulum often stops the hemorrhage. If the exact spot of bleeding cannot be found, the most proximal area of residual blood allows localization to the part of the colon that bled. This is helpful if bleeding becomes recurrent and surgery is necessary. If colonoscopy cannot be done or is unhelpful, nuclear scanning techniques using technetium-labeled red blood cells may be able to find the area of bleeding. For massive bleeding at a rate greater than 1 mL per minute, emergency angiography should be considered. Diagnostic angiography not only can identify the cause of hemorrhage, but also offers the option of therapy to stop the bleeding. Infusion of vasoconstrictors such as vasopressin (Pitressin)[1] into the bleeding vessel constricts it and stops bleeding. Often vasoconstrictors work only temporarily, and there is a relatively high recurrence of bleeding. Transarterial selective embolization (TASE) of the affected vessel with Gelfoam, stainless steel, or platinum coils stops bleeding in up to 80% of cases. However, this technique is associated with significant ischemia or necrosis of the bowel and is best reserved for those who are not surgical candidates. Patients who continue to bleed or who have recurrent bleeding should have surgery done to remove the area of bowel where the source of bleeding is suspected.

A large portion of those with colonic bleeding are taking nonsteroidal anti-inflammatory drugs (NSAIDs). These medications should be stopped to decrease the chance of recurrence. If aspirin is necessary for cardiac reasons, the lowest possible therapeutic dose should be used.

Diverticulitis

Diverticulitis is caused by plugging of the diverticulum orifice by a fecalith, resulting in inflammation

[1]Not FDA approved for this indication.

and microperforation. This most often occurs in the sigmoid colon. The bowel wall becomes inflamed and thickened. Patients usually complain of lower abdominal pain; often localized to the left lower quadrant. Fever, nausea, vomiting, and change of bowel movement to constipation or diarrhea may occur. Urinary urgency with dysuria may indicate the inflammatory phlegmon is pressing on the bladder. Colovesical fistulas can occur associated with recurrent urinary tract infection and or pneumaturia. Colovaginal fistulas may complicate the process as well. Physical exam most often reveals left lower quadrant tenderness. If there is severe inflammation, local peritoneal signs may be elicited and a large phlegmon may be felt as fullness or mass in the lower abdomen. On rectal exam, an inflammatory mass can sometimes be felt. Visible rectal bleeding and diverticulitis rarely occur simultaneously. If a right-sided diverticulum becomes inflamed, the condition can be mistaken for appendicitis. Other differentials include perforated colon cancer, inflammatory bowel disease, and urinary tract disease.

Diverticulosis is very common and usually asymptomatic. It is important to confirm the diagnosis of diverticulitis as a cause of lower abdominal pain. Laboratory data will often show a leukocytosis. A CT scan of the abdomen and pelvis with oral and IV contrast is the test of choice during an acute attack if the diagnosis is in doubt. The scan will often demonstrate the inflamed thickened bowel and diverticula.

Complications such as free perforation, abscess formation, and colovesical fistula can be seen on CT scan as well. If the cause of symptoms is not diverticulitis, additional possible diagnoses include inflamed bowel, pancreatitis, and others. Barium enema should not be done during an acute attack of diverticulitis. The test will often be very painful and carries the risk of opening the perforated diverticulum and worsening the process. Regular barium entering the peritoneum can cause a serious peritonitis. Water soluble contrast material studies do not carry the risk of barium in the peritoneum; but still carry the risk of converting a localized, contained infection into general peritonitis because of the pressure of the enema. For the same reason flexible sigmoidoscopy and colonoscopy are not done during the acute episode of diverticulitis.

Treatment of uncomplicated diverticulitis can be done on an outpatient basis. The patient is encouraged to start with a clear fluid diet and advance to a low-residue diet as tolerated. Once the acute episode is resolved, a high-fiber, low-fat diet is encouraged in the hope of preventing further bouts of diverticulitis. Oral broad-spectrum antibiotics are used that cover both anaerobes and gram-negative flora of the gut. The combination of ciprofloxacin (Cipro), 500 mg orally twice daily, or trimethoprim-sulfamethoxazole (160/800) (Bactrim DS)[1] and metronidazole (Flagyl)[1], 250 mg to 500 mg three times daily for 10 to 14 days, often works well. Patients who are more severely ill should be treated with broad-spectrum intravenous antibiotics such as levofloxacin (Levaquin)[1], 500 mg IV daily, with metronidazole[1], 500 mg IV three times a day, or ampicillin sodium/sulbactam (Unasyn)[1] IV. Once a good clinical response is obtained and oral fluids are tolerable, the patient can be switched to the previously mentioned oral regimens. Abscess can be drained percutaneously under CT guidance and a catheter left in place to continue the drainage. Catheter checks can subsequently be done to confirm resolution of the abscess and make sure there is no open connection to the bowel. Indications for surgery during the acute episode include free perforation with generalized peritonitis, failure of the patient to improve, condition of patient worsens, or a bowel obstruction does not resolve. A one-stage procedure with removal of the involved colon and reanastomosis of the bowel can often be done. A staged procedure with a temporary diverting colostomy is performed if significant peritoneal infection is present or primary anastomosis is too difficult for technical reasons. Reanastomosis is usually done in 4 to 6 months. Elective diverticular resection is indicated for patients who have frequent recurrent bouts of diverticulitis or complications such as abscess and colovesical and colovaginal fistulas. If the acute attack does not adequately resolve in a couple of weeks, surgery may be necessary or a repeat CT scan to look for complications not initially noted.

Patients with an uncomplicated episode of diverticulitis should have a colonoscopy or, if that is not possible, a barium enema 5 to 6 weeks after the attack (once the acute symptoms have resolved). This assessment is necessary to make sure the acute inflammation was not caused by a small perforated colon malignancy or other pathology such as inflammatory bowel disease. Inability to adequately asses the colon this way because of stricture or other pathology is an indication to have the involved bowel resected.

[1]Not FDA approved for this indication.

INFLAMMATORY BOWEL DISEASE

METHOD OF

Rahul K. Chhablani, MD, and

Gary R. Lichtenstein, MD

Inflammatory bowel disease (IBD) constitutes multisystem diseases of idiopathic origin. Since Drs. Wilks and Moxon's original description of ulcerative colitis in 1875, and Drs. Crohn, Ginzburg, and Oppenheimer's

[1]Not FDA approved for this indication.

initial description of Crohn's Disease in 1932, much has been learned about these two disorders. Both are found worldwide and spare no socioeconomic group. Recent scientific and technologic advances have not only led to greater understanding of the pathogenesis underlying these disorders, but have also led to the discovery and use of new medications in the treatment of inflammatory bowel disease.

Medical therapies for IBD aim to induce and maintain disease remission; decrease disease-associated complications, including malnutrition, osteoporosis, and colon cancer; and ultimately, improve the patient's quality of life. This article discusses drug therapies, including indications and adverse effects, nutritional therapy, and management strategies for the various site-specific presentations of ulcerative colitis (UC) and Crohn's disease (CD).

Drug Therapy

AMINOSALICYLATES

Sulfasalazine

Sulfasalazine (Azulfidine) is composed of mesalamine (5-aminosalicylate [5-ASA]) joined by an azo-bond to a sulfapyridine moiety. This bond is cleaved by colonic bacterial azo-reductase, separating mesalamine from the sulfapyridine carrier. These molecules inhibit arachidonic acid production; interleukin (IL)-1, IL-2, and nuclear factor-κ B (NF-κB) activity; tumor necrosis factor-α (TNF-α); and reactive oxygen metabolites.

Initially used to treat rheumatoid arthritis by Dr. Nana Svartz of the Karolinska Institute in the 1930s, sulfasalazine[1] was found to reduce diarrhea in patients with coexisting UC. It is now used to treat mildly to moderately active UC and to maintain remission (Table 1). Sulfasalazine is known to benefit patients with mild-to-moderate CD, especially ileocolonic and colonic CD, but not patients with isolated small bowel disease. It is not effective for maintenance therapy of CD, as results from the National Cooperative Crohn's Disease Study (United States) and the European Cooperative Crohn's Disease Studies in the late 1970s and early 1980s failed to show maintenance benefit from reduced doses of sulfasalazine.

The sulfapyridine moiety of sulfasalazine contributes to most of this drug's adverse effects (see Table 1), including headache, nausea, vomiting, pancreatitis, and impaired folate metabolism. Patients on sulfasalazine should receive concurrent folic acid supplementation (1 mg/day).

Sperm abnormalities (dysmorphic sperm and sperm motility abnormalities) are another common, reversible side effect that has been reported with sulfasalazine. Male patients should be informed of the potential adverse effect of reduced fertility prior to using sulfasalazine.

Mesalamine Derivatives

Given the toxicity and the frequent intolerance that many patients experience with sulfasalazine (15% of individuals taking sulfasalazine are unable to tolerate the use of this medication), mesalamine derivatives without the sulfapyridine moiety have been created.

Asacol is made of a special coating that ensures a pH-dependent release in the ileocecal region and allows for approximately 15% to 30% of the mesalamine to be released in the small bowel. Pentasa is composed of sustained-release, ethylcellulose-coated microgranules that allow for equal release of mesalamine in the small bowel (50%) and the colon (50%). Olsalazine (Dipentum) is a mesalamine dimer linked by a diazo bond, formulated as gelatin capsules that is released primarily in the colon. Balsalazide (Colazal), a newer mesalamine derivative, is bound to an inert carrier molecule. Once cleaved from its carrier by colonic bacterial azo-reductase, approximately 99% of the mesalamine is delivered to the colon.

Topical mesalamine can be delivered in the form of enema or suppository. The use of enemas allows mesalamine to be delivered up to the splenic flexure. The suppository is effective in treating disease up to 15 to 20 cm from the anal verge. Topical mesalamine has been proven to be effective in treating distal UC and proctitis. It may be used in patients with colonic CD. However, there have been no randomized, controlled trials to evaluate its efficacy in the setting of colonic CD.

Table 1 lists the indication, dose, route, and adverse effects of these mesalamine derivatives. Neutropenia, agranulocytosis, hypersensitivity reactions (serum sickness, skin rash, pneumonitis, hepatitis, pancreatitis) are rarely seen with mesalamine derivatives. Up to 10% of patients treated with olsalazine experience drug-related diarrhea. This effect is significantly reduced when the drug is taken with meals. Topical mesalamine use has been associated with anal irritation and pruritus, occasionally precluding patients from continuing topical therapy.

CORTICOSTEROIDS

Corticosteroids have multiple effects on the immunomodulatory pathway, including:

- Inhibiting the release of proinflammatory cytokines such as IL-1, IL-2, IL-6, IL-8, γ-interferon, TNF-α
- Down regulating NF-κB activity
- Reducing plasma exudation from postcapillary venules at inflammatory sites
- Interfering with phagocytic activity
- Decreasing chemotaxis of monocytes, eosinophils, and neutrophils

[1]Not FDA approved for this indication.

TABLE 1 Indication, Dose, Route, and Adverse Effects of Drugs Used in Inflammatory Bowel Disease

Agent	Indication	Dose	Route	Adverse Effects
Azo-bonded mesalamine derivatives Sulfasalazine (Azulfidine)	**CD:** *Sulfasalazine:* Induction of remission for mildly to moderately active disease (especially ileocolonic and colonic disease) *Balsalazide and Olsalazine:* No current approved use			
Balsalazide (Colazal) Olsalazine (Dipentum)	**UC:** *Sulfasalazine:* Induction of remission for mildly to moderately active disease Maintenance of remission *Balsalazide:* Induction of remission for active left-sided disease Maintenance of remission *Olsalazine:* Induction of remission for active UC Maintenance of remission for active UC	*Sulfasalazine*: 4 to 6 g/d* 2 to 4 g/d† Balsalazide: 2 to 6.75 g/d Olsalazine: 1.5 to 3 g/d	PO	Sulfasalazine: Nausea, vomiting, anorexia, headache, fever, rash, agranulocytosis pancreatitis, hepatitis, folate malabsorption, sperm abnormalities Balsalazide: Headache, abdominal pain, nausea, vomiting, diarrhea,l arthralgias, respiratory depression Olsalazine: Diarrhea, abdominal pain, cramps
Mesalamine derivatives (Asacol, Pentasa)	**CD:** Induction of remission for mildly to moderately active disease Induction of remission for active disease treated with corticosteroids (reducing steroid dependency) Maintenance of remission (especially surgically induced remission) **UC:** Induction of remission for mildly to moderately active disease Maintenance of remission	4 to 4.8 g/d* 2 to 4.8 g/d†	PO, topical	Nausea, dyspepsia, headache, rare hypersensitivity reactions (fever, rash, agranulocytosis); anal irritation and pruritus possible with topical use
Topical aminosalicylates	**UC:** Induction of remission for acute distal colitis (enema) and proctitis (suppository) Maintenance of remission for acute distal colitis (enema) and proctitis (suppository)	1 to 1.5 g/d	Topical	Anal irritation and pruritus
Corticosteroids	**CD:** *Oral:* Induction of remission for moderately to severely active disease *Topical*[1]*:* Induction of remission of distal Crohn's colitis/proctitis **UC:** *Oral:* Induction of remission for moderately to severely active disease *Topical*[1]*:* Induction of remission of distal ulcerative colitis/proctitis	PO: 40 to 60 mg/d‡ IV: 32 to 60 mg/d Topical: 100 mg§	PO, IV, topical	Fat redistribution, acne, weight gain, mood changes, hyperglycemia, myopathy, osteoporosis; with prolonged use, osteonecrosis, cataracts
Metronidazole (Flagyl)[1]	**CD:** Induction of remission for active colitis Induction of remission for active perianal disease (closure of fistula) Maintenance of remission for surgically induced remission	10 to 20 mg/kg/d	PO	Nausea, abdominal pain, metallic taste; disulfiram-like reaction with concurrent alcohol use; peripheral neuropathy (seen in prolonged use)

Continued

TABLE 1 Indication, Dose, Route, and Adverse Effects of Drugs Used in Inflammatory Bowel Disease—cont'd

Agent	Indication	Dose	Route	Adverse Effects
	UC: No current approved indication			
Ciprofloxacin (Cipro)[1]	**CD:** Induction of remission for active colitis Induction of remission for active perianal disease (closure of fistula) **UC:** No current approved indication	1 g/d	PO	Dyspepsia, diarrhea, headaches, abdominal pain; rarely, hepatotoxicity, seizures, rash, interstitial nephritis, Achilles tendon rupture (unilateral or bilateral)
Azathioprine (Imuran)[1] 6-Mercaptopurine (6-MP Purinethol)[1]	**CD:** Induction of remission for active disease Induction of remission for steroid-dependent disease (allowing for steroid withdrawal) Fistulous disease Maintenance of remission for medically and surgically induced remission **UC:** Induction of remission for active disease Induction of remission for steroid-dependent disease (allowing for steroid withdrawal) Maintenance of remission for medically induced remission	AZA: 2.0 to 2.5 mg/kg/d 6-MP: 1.0 to 1.5 mg/kg/d	PO	Nausea, vomiting, allergic reactions, pancreatitis, abnormal liver function tests, bone marrow toxicity
Cyclosporine[1] Sandimmune, Neoral, Gengraf)	**CD:** Fistulous disease refractory to other medical therapies (antibiotics, AZA/6-MP, infliximab)¶ **UC:** Severe UC refractory to or intolerant of other medical therapies (corticosteroids, AZA/6-MP)	4 mg/kg/d	IV, PO	Hypertension, headache, paresthesias, electrolyte and liver function abnormalities, nephrotoxicity, gingival hyperplasia; rarely, seizures, opportunistic infections
Methotrexate[1] (Rheumatrex, Trexall)	**CD:** Induction of remission for active disease Induction of remission for steroid-dependent disease (allowing for steroid withdrawal) Disease nonresponsive to other medical therapies (infliximab, AZA/6-MP) Maintenance of remission **UC:** No current approved use	25 mg/wk* 15 mg/wk†	PO, IM, SC	Stomatitis, esophagitis, oral ulcerations, nausea, vomiting, diarrhea; bone marrow suppression (anemia, leukopenia, thrombocytopenia); elevated liver function tests, portal fibrosis, and cirrhosis (can be seen in patients who have received cumulative dose of 1.5 g)
Infliximab (Remicade)	**CD:** Induction of remission for moderately to severely active disease Induction of remission for active fistulous disease Maintenance of remission for infliximab-induced remission **UC:** No current approved use	5 mg/kg	IV	Upper respiratory tract infections, headache, nausea, myalgias, vomiting, diarrhea; infusion reaction, possibly delayed hypersentivity response; CHF exacerbation; tuberculosis, histoplasmosis, listeriosis, aspergillosis

[1]Not FDA approved for this indication.
*Dose for induction of remission.
†Dose for maintenance of remission.
‡For ileocecal Crohn's disease; includes budesonide at 9 mg/day.
§Hydrocortisone enema.
¶High relapse rate upon transition to oral cyclosporine.
Abbreviations: 6-MP = 6-mercaptopurine; AZA = azathioprine; CD = Crohn's disease; CHF = congestive heart failure; IM = intramuscular; IV = Intravenous; PO = by mouth; SC = subcutaneous; UC = ulcerative colitis.

Corticosteroids continue to serve as a frequently used therapy for active IBD, regardless of disease distribution. Corticosteroids are not effective for maintenance of remission. Prednisone, in doses equivalent to 40 to 60 mg per day, has been proven effective in treating moderately to severely active UC and CD. Intravenous methylprednisolone, at a dose of 32 to 60 mg daily, is indicated in hospitalized patients with severe UC or CD, or for patients who have failed oral therapy. Hydrocortisone enemas are effective therapy for induction of remission in patients with active UC distal to the splenic flexure, and CD involving the distal colon.

Budesonide (Entocort EC) is a newer corticosteroid that is associated with fewer systemic side effects and less adrenal insufficiency. This is because of its low systemic bioavailability and extensive first-pass metabolism in the liver and erythrocytes. At a dose of 9 mg per day, budesonide is comparable to traditional corticosteroids for the induction of remission for moderately active CD. Studies have not shown oral budesonide[1] to be effective for treating active UC.

There are multiple, potentially serious side effects associated with corticosteroid use (see Table 1), often correlating with dose and duration of therapy. These include the potential of promoting or masking intestinal microperforations. It is critical to evaluate for and exclude the presence of an abscess or other potential sources of infections before using corticosteroids (in the correct clinical setting).

Patients receiving steroids should receive supplemental oral daily calcium (1200 to 1500 mg/day) and vitamin D (400 to 800 IU/day). In addition, patients on chronic steroid therapy should undergo baseline and periodic bone densitometry studies (DEXA scans); in appropriate patients, the use of bisphosphonates may aide in preventing and potentially treating bone loss.

ANTIMICROBIALS

Experimental and clinical evidence indicates that bacterial flora may play a role in the pathogenesis of inflammatory bowel disease. The intestinal mucosal wall, as a result of the inflammatory response, becomes increasingly permeable and vulnerable to bacterial cell wall antigens, like lipopolysaccharides. These antigens are thought to either initiate or sustain an inflammatory response in host tissue. Abnormal intestinal flora has been found in the bowel wall and mesenteric lymph nodes of patients with CD. In addition, diversion of the fecal stream has been shown to delay postoperative recurrence of CD and minimize the severity of inflammation seen in recurrent disease.

Antimicrobials are primarily used in the treatment of active CD and perianal CD, and for maintenance of surgically induced remission. Although clinical trials fail to demonstrate benefit in treating UC, intravenous, broad-spectrum antibiotics are empirically used in patients with severe UC and in those with signs of systemic toxicity or fulminant colitis with or without megacolon.

[1]Not FDA approved for this indication.

The two most commonly used antibiotics for treatment of active CD are metronidazole (Flagyl)[1] and ciprofloxacin (Cipro) (see Table 1). Peripheral neuropathy, commonly seen with prolonged use of metronidazole, is typically reversible if recognized early and the dose is decreased or discontinued. Ciprofloxacin is generally better tolerated; however, Achilles tendon rupture and secondary fungal infections have been reported with ciprofloxacin therapy. A recent study has assessed the efficacy of ornidazole (Avrazor)[2] in the maintenance of postoperative remission. The intention was to use an antibiotic with fewer related adverse events. This antibiotic was effective for the maintenance of postoperative recurrence clinically and endoscopically as long as the medication was taken. There was a significant side-effect profile similar to that of metronidazole. Hence the search for other agents continues.

IMMUNOMODULATORS

Azathioprine and 6-Mercaptopurine

Azathioprine (Imuran)[1] and 6-mercaptopurine (6-MP) (Purinethol)[1] are purine analogues that alter the immune system by inhibiting nucleic acid biosynthesis and the cytotoxicity of natural killer and T cells. Azathioprine is nonenzymatically converted to 6-MP within erythrocytes; 6-MP is then enzymatically cleaved to a group of active end products, called 6-thoiguanine nucleotides. A competing enzyme, thiopurine methyltransferase (TPMT), also converts 6-MP to another metabolite, 6-methylmercaptopurine (6-MMP).

Azathioprine and 6-MP are indicated for induction of remission for active CD and UC, facilitating steroid withdrawal in steroid-dependent UC and CD, and facilitating maintenance of remission in CD and UC. Preliminary data suggest that 6-MP may be effective in preventing postoperative relapse of CD.

In retrospective cohort series, the elevation of this metabolite has been found in association with abnormal alanine aminotransferase (ALT) and aspartate aminotransferase (AST), as well as asymptomatic elevation of serum amylase and lipase. The incidence of lymphoma and leukemia does not seem to be increased in patients with IBD treated with azathioprine and 6-MP.

Bone marrow suppression is a common, dose-dependent toxicity that occurs in 2% to 5% of patients using azathioprine and 6-MP. This potentially significant toxicity should be monitored by

[1]Not FDA approved for this indication.
[2]Not available in the United States.

obtaining complete blood counts biweekly for the first 8 weeks and then every 1 to 3 months for the remainder of therapy.

Methotrexate

Methotrexate[1] (Rheumatrex, Trexall) inhibits the enzymes dihydrofolate reductase and thymidine synthetase, as well as other enzymes critical to DNA synthesis; it interferes with the production of proinflammatory cytokines IL-1, IL-2, TNF-α, and γ-interferon; and it impairs histamine release from basophils and decreases neutrophil chemotaxis.

Methotrexate is primarily indicated for maintenance of remission and induction of remission for active CD or steroid-dependent CD (allowing for steroid withdrawal). It can also be considered in patients with CD that have not adequately responded to azathioprine, 6-MP, or infliximab (Remicade). The route of administration that has been effective for patients with CD is either subcutaneously or intramuscularly. The efficacy of orally ingested methotrexate has not been demonstrated. Randomized clinical trials have yet to demonstrate the efficacy of methotrexate in the treatment or maintenance of UC.

Potential toxicities of methotrexate are listed in Table 1. Many of these can be minimized with folic acid supplementation. Bone marrow suppression can be minimized by the concurrent use of leucovorin (Wellcovorin). Hepatic fibrosis is one of the most serious potential sequela of long-term methotrexate therapy. While the utility of liver biopsy in the management of patients on methotrexate remains controversial, a pretreatment liver biopsy should be considered in patients at increased risk for hepatic toxicity (i.e., obese patients or those who consume alcohol).

During the induction period of treatment, patients should receive frequent evaluations of their complete blood counts and liver function tests, initially perhaps every 2 to 4 weeks. This frequency can be reduced during the maintenance period. While some clinicians recommend follow-up liver biopsy in patients who have received a cumulative dose of 1.5 g, it is currently not recommended universally or widely accepted as the standard of care.

Cyclosporine

Cyclosporine[1] (Sandimmune, Neoral, Gengraf) is a cyclic undecapeptide (polypeptide) that inhibits IL-2 production and T-helper-cell function. It also decreases recruitment of cytotoxic T helper cells and blocks the activity of IL-3, IL-4, γ-interferon, and TNF-α.

Randomized controlled trials do not show cyclosporine to be beneficial in patients with CD; however, data from uncontrolled studies suggest that intravenous cyclosporine may be beneficial in the treatment of fistulous CD unresponsive to corticosteroids, antibiotics, or other immunomodulators such as azathioprine or 6-mercaptopurine. In patients with UC, cyclosporine has been used to treat severe disease that is refractory to corticosteroids; in addition, cyclosporine may be used as a bridge for control of disease until azathioprine or 6-MP reaches therapeutic levels or until elective surgery is performed.

Cyclosporine can be administered orally or parenterally. Its absorption is dependent on several factors, including the small bowel transit time, length of small bowel, and integrity of the intestinal mucosa. The microemulsion formulation of cyclosporine (Neoral, Gengraf, Sandimmune) has similar bioavailability and efficacy to that of intravenous cyclosporine.

Monitoring cyclosporine blood levels is suggested as a means of reducing drug toxicity. Patients receiving oral cyclosporine should have weekly trough cyclosporine levels checked and maintained between 200 and 300 ng/mL, as measured by high-pressure liquid chromatography.

Adverse effects (see Table 1) that may occur with cyclosporine include nephrotoxicity, hypertension, electrolyte abnormalities, seizures, paresthesias, and tremor. Patients receiving cyclosporine may be susceptible to opportunistic infections, therefore *Pneumocystis carinii* pneumonia prophylaxis is recommended with one double-strength dose of trimethoprim-sulfamethoxazole (Bactrim OS) three times a week.

Antitumor Necrosis Factor Therapy

Cytokines, or glycosylated proteins synthesized by various cell types in response to inflammation, can be categorized either as proinflammatory (IL-1, IL-2, IL-6, IL-8, IL-12, TNF-α) or anti-inflammatory (IL-4, IL-10, IL-11, IL-13). An imbalance between the proinflammatory and anti-inflammatory cytokines may play an integral part in the severity of inflammatory bowel disease. Efforts to correct this imbalance have led to the formulation of newer therapy directed at blocking the proinflammatory actions of specific cytokines.

INFLIXIMAB

Infliximab (Remicade) is a chimeric immunoglobulin (Ig) G-1 subclass monoclonal antibody directed against TNF-α. It also inhibits IL-1, IL-6 production, endothelial cell and leukocyte expression of adhesion molecules, fibroblast proliferation, and prostaglandin synthesis. In IBD patients, infliximab reduces TNF-α production and inflammatory cell proliferation in inflamed areas of the intestine. Infliximab is also known to induce apoptosis in lymphocytes and monocytes.

[1]Not FDA approved for this indication.

In 1998, the Food and Drug Administration (FDA) approved infliximab for the treatment of patients with moderately to severely active CD refractory to conventional therapy and with draining enterocutaneous fistulae. Based on recent data, infliximab is indicated for induction of remission for moderately to severely active CD, induction of remission for active fistulous CD, and maintenance of remission in patients with quiescent CD induced by infliximab. Concurrent use of infliximab with azathioprine or 6-MP may be associated with prolonged remission of CD. While infliximab is not FDA approved for the treatment of active UC, preliminary uncontrolled studies show modest benefit in the treatment of severe steroid-refractory UC. Two large randomized, controlled trials are currently being conducted to confirm these preliminary findings.

Infliximab is administered as an infusion and has a rapid onset of action (2 to 4 weeks). The most common adverse effect is headache, seen in approximately 23% of patients. Other effects seen include nausea, vomiting, and abdominal pain (see Table 1). Some patients may develop antibodies against infliximab (formerly known as human antichimeric antibodies [HACA]). Individuals who receive infliximab as an episodic therapy (as opposed to a maintenance therapy given in a specified periodicity) are more prone to develop antibodies against infliximab. The presence of these antibodies at a high level has been correlated with a shorter duration of action and a higher rate of infusion reactions. Individuals who receive infliximab at a specified periodicity after receiving three induction doses (typically at weeks 0, 2, 6) are less likely to develop antibodies than the aforementioned population. Serious infections such as tuberculosis, histoplasmosis, listeriosis, and aspergillosis can occur in patients treated with infliximab. A screening purified protein derivative (PPD) test (and we advocate a chest radiograph as well) is recommended before infliximab therapy is initiated. The long-term risk of developing lymphoma or other malignancies following infliximab therapy is currently being followed. At present, it is believed that the risk of developing lymphoma is not higher in those receiving infliximab than the risk in the general population.

Investigational Therapies

ETANERCEPT AND THALIDOMIDE

Two additional anti-TNF agents that are currently being investigated in the treatment of CD are etanercept (Enbrel) and thalidomide (Thalomid). While etanercept has yet to show benefit in treating CD (when used at a dose of 25 mg twice weekly in a subcutaneous fashion), studies using thalidomide show its benefit in the treatment of intestinal and fistulizing CD that are unresponsive to standard therapies. Neither of these agents can be recommended for the routine care of patients with CD until controlled clinical trials can be completed. Their use should be reserved for clinical trials. The use of thalidomide is complicated by the development of peripheral neuropathy and sedation in a large percentage of treated patients. There currently are second generation thalidomide congeners under investigation that hopefully will not possess the adverse effects seen in the first generation of compounds.

NICOTINE

The observation that smoking appears to have a protective effect in patients with UC has led to therapeutic trials of nicotine in these patients. Based on the results of randomized, placebo-controlled trials, nicotine may be beneficial in patients with active and steroid-dependent UC who recently stopped smoking. Patients who never smoked are frequently unable to tolerate this therapy, given its side effects of nausea and headache. A maintenance trial for patients with ulcerative colitis has failed to demonstrate efficacy over placebo.

HEPARIN

Prothrombic abnormalities within the circulatory system and the presence of inflammatory vasculitis and microthrombi with the bowel mucosa suggest that a hypercoagulable state may contribute to the pathogenesis of IBD. Based on results of several uncontrolled trials, unfractionated heparin (Hepalean) reduces symptoms and improves healing in patients with steroid-resistant UC, but not in treating moderate-to-severe UC. Results from several multicenter, randomized, controlled trials using heparin have failed to demonstrate efficacy for patients with active ulcerative colitis.

PROBIOTICS

Probiotics are living organisms in foods and dietary supplements that help reestablish normal intestinal flora. They create an environment that is unfavorable for the growth of potentially pathogenic bacteria and maintain the integrity of the gut mucosal barrier. In vitro studies suggest that probiotics stimulate the intestinal mucosal immune system by enhancing macrophage and natural killer cell activities, and by augmenting the proliferation of lymphocytes.

Uncontrolled clinical trial results show that probiotics may have a modest benefit in the treatment of CD and in the maintenance of quiescent UC. Placebo-controlled trials are needed before probiotics can be recommended in the management of IBD patients.

Two trials show efficacy of a probiotic called VSL-3 (from VSL Pharmaceuticals, Inc.), which is a conglomerate of three different bacteria. This agent has been shown to lessen the development of pouchitis (inflammation of a surgically created ileoanal pouch after patients have undergone total proctocolectomy) when taken either as postoperative prophylaxis or when taken after an antibiotic-induced remission in patients who have had a chronic course of recurrent pouchitis.

Nutritional Therapy

Total parenteral nutrition (TPN) should be reserved for patients with obstructive CD or CD with a high output fistula. Even though this treatment has not been proven effective in UC, hospitalized patients with severe colitis receiving parenteral therapy who cannot tolerate oral intake or patients who are severely malnourished may benefit from TPN.

Short-chain fatty acids (SCFA) serve as primary energy substrate for colonic mucosal cells, and disrupted delivery of this substrate can result in mucosal inflammation. The primary component of SCFAs is butyrate. Butyrate accounts for approximately 70% of the energy source for the colonocyte. UC patients may have decreased levels of this substrate, and delivery of SCFA in the form of enemas may aid in the treatment of active distal colitis, a finding that has yet to be warranted by large, randomized, controlled clinical trials.

Despite the fact that food may serve as a major source of intraluminal antigens, food elimination diets or highly restrictive diets have not proved effective in the treatment of IBD. Lactose restriction may be helpful in eliminating symptoms that can be confused with those of CD in some patients, but is not mandatory in all patients. Patients with symptomatic fibrostenotic disease may benefit from a low-residue diet and avoidance of particular foods that may cause obstruction, such as nuts, seeds, and corn.

Periodic monitoring of electrolytes and appropriate supplementation of potassium, magnesium, zinc, and vitamin B_{12} may be required in patients with chronic diarrhea or extensive ileal disease, ileal resection, or bacterial overgrowth. Calcium, fat-soluble vitamin, and iron supplementation may be necessary in patients with fat malabsorption and iron deficiency anemia.

Medical Management of Inflammatory Bowel Disease

Appropriate management of ulcerative colitis and Crohn's disease requires defining the extent and severity of disease. While endoscopic evidence is valuable in defining the extent of disease, severity of disease is based on a variety of findings including the patient's symptoms, the impact of disease on daily function, pertinent physical examination findings (e.g., fever, abdominal tenderness), and abnormal laboratory values (e.g., anemia, hypoalbuminemia).

The Truelove and Witts' Activity Index (Table 2) continues to be one of the standard systems used for assessing systemic severity in patients with UC. Patients with toxic megacolon, a life-threatening form of UC, present with signs of toxicity (fever >101°F [38.3°C], tachycardia, abdominal distension, and signs of localized or generalized peritonitis) with leukocytosis (i.e., white blood cell count greater than 11,000 THO/mL) and dilated loops of bowel on plain abdominal radiograph. Standardized instruments (including the Crohn's Disease Activity Index [CDAI]) have been developed to assess disease severity in patients with CD, but most of these are inconvenient for daily practice and are best reserved for clinical trials. From a practical perspective, patients are considered to have mildly to moderately active CD when they are ambulatory; able to tolerate an oral diet; and exhibit no signs of dehydration, toxicity, abdominal tenderness, mass, or obstruction. Patients who have failed treatment for mildly to moderately active disease or patients presenting with fever, weight loss, anemia, nausea, vomiting, abdominal pain, and tenderness (without obstruction) are considered to have moderately to severely active CD. Severe or fulminant CD defines patients with persistent symptoms despite corticosteroid therapy or patients exhibiting high fevers, persistent vomiting, evidence of intestinal obstruction or an abscess, rebound tenderness, cachexia, and profound anemia. Patients are considered to be in remission when they are asymptomatic, either spontaneously or after medical or surgical intervention.

The clinical management of patients with UC and CD classified by extent and severity is discussed below.

TABLE 2 Truelove and Witts' Activity Index for Ulcerative Colitis

Severe
More than six bowel movements a day with blood
Temperature greater than 37°C (98.6°F)
Heart rate greater than 90 beats per minute
Anemia with hemoglobin less than 75%
Erythrocyte sedimentation rate (ESR) greater than 30 mm per hour
Mild
Less than four bowel movements a day without blood
No fever
Heart rate less than 90 beats per minute
Mild anemia
ESR less than 30 mm per hour
Moderate
Features between those of mild and severe

ULCERATIVE COLITIS

Proctitis and Proctosigmoiditis

Patients with proctitis have inflammation limited to the rectum (approximately the distal 15 cm of the colon), while patients with proctosigmoiditis have disease involving the distal 30 to 40 cm of the colon. Symptoms of proctitis include rectal bleeding, tenesmus, and multiple frequent small bowel movements, often associated with mucus. Patients with proctosigmoiditis often have a similar presentation, but may also have minimal systemic symptoms such as fever, weight loss, and anorexia.

Topical aminosalicylates, in the form of twice daily 500 mg mesalamine suppositories (Canasa) or nightly 4 g mesalamine enemas, are among the first-line agents to be considered for treating patients with active proctitis and proctosigmoiditis, respectively (Figure 1). A combination of oral and topical aminosalicylates is usually required for patients who present with severe proctitis or proctosigmoiditis. Treatment is continued for at least 2 to 3 weeks to evaluate for efficacy. For patients who have an inadequate response at this time, another topical aminosalicylate, or hydrocortisone enema (Cortenema[1], 100 mg) can be added to the regimen.

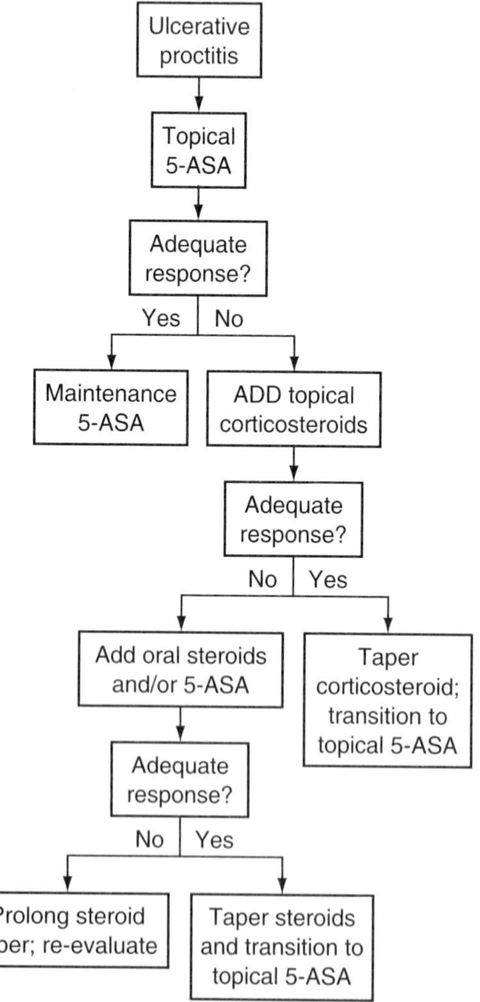

FIGURE 1 Management of ulcerative proctitis and proctosigmoiditis. *Modified from:* Srinivasan R, Su CG, and Lichtenstein GR: Medical Therapy for Ulcerative Colitis. In Lichtenstein GR: The Clinician's Guide to Inflammatory Bowel Disease. Thorofare, NJ, SLACK Incorporated, 2003, pp 255-289. Used with permission.

Corticosteroids (oral prednisone at 40 to 60 mg/day) are often ineffective for treating ulcerative proctitis, but can be used for patients with severe proctosigmoiditis who are symptomatic or have an inadequate response to the aforementioned therapy. A response to corticosteroid treatment is usually seen within 10 to 14 days.

When remission is achieved, corticosteroids should be tapered, as they play no role in the maintenance of disease remission. Patients initially treated with topical corticosteroid preparations should be transitioned to topical mesalamine and gradually tapered off the topical corticosteroid. Maintenance therapy is not required for patients who experienced their first disease exacerbation that responded promptly to treatment. Others patients achieving remission may benefit from maintenance therapy, consisting of continuing the specific combination of mesalamine therapy that was successful in inducing remission. Fewer relapses may occur with twice-daily mesalamine suppositories that compared to once daily doses. Over time, most patients are able to reduce topical mesalamine therapy to once at night and eventually to every third night.

Left-sided Colitis

Ulcerative colitis extending up to but not beyond the splenic flexure (up to 60 cm from the anal verge) is defined as left-sided colitis. These patients often present with bloody diarrhea, tenesmus, and rectal urgency. Initial therapy is determined by the severity of disease symptoms.

Topical therapy with mesalamine enemas, 4 g every hour, can be used as initial therapy for mildly to moderately active disease (Figure 2). Patients with moderately to severely active left-sided colitis may benefit from twice-daily mesalamine enemas with alternating corticosteroid enema, especially in patients who are unable to tolerate aminosalicylate enemas. Combining oral and topical aminosalicylates is usually required for inducing remission in patients with severe left-sided colitis. This combination may be more effective in producing a quicker and more complete relief of symptoms. Therapeutic response should be evident within 4 weeks of therapy and may be seen at maximal doses of aminosalicylates (sulfasalazine [Azulfidine], 6 g/day; oral mesalamine [Asacol] 4 to 4.8 g/day[3]; olsalazine [Dipenum], 3 g/day[3]).

Corticosteroids (e.g., oral prednisone, 40 to 60 mg/day) should be reserved for patients who have an inadequate response to aminosalicylate therapy or patients with severe disease that may benefit from a more rapid response as compared to that of aminosalicylate therapy. When in remission, prednisone

[1]Not FDA approved for this indication.
[3]Exceeds dosage recommended by the manufacturer.

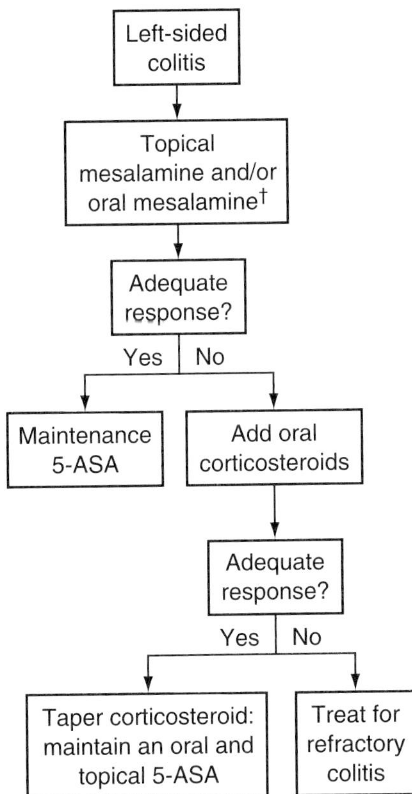

FIGURE 2 Management of left-sided colitis.
Modified from: Srinivasan R, Su CG, and Lichtenstein GR: Medical Therapy for Ulcerative Colitis. In Lichtenstein GR: The Clinician's Guide to Inflammatory Bowel Disease. Thorofare, NJ, SLACK Incorporated, 2003, pp 255-289. Used with permission.

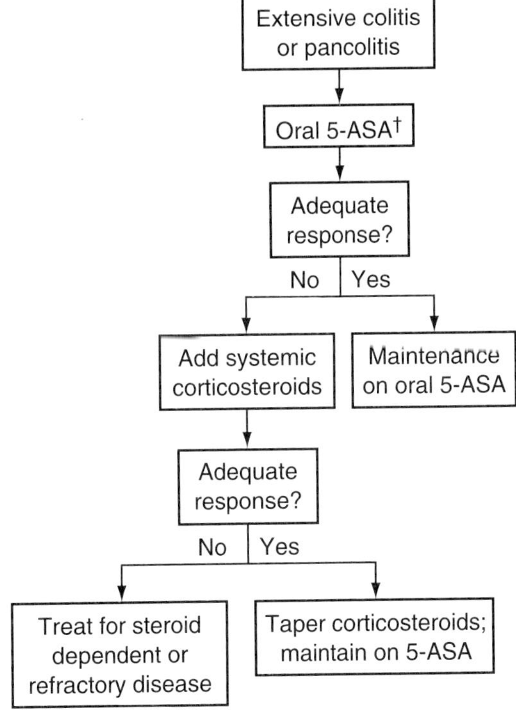

FIGURE 3 Management of extensive colitis or pancolitis.
Modified from: Srinivasan R, Su CG, and Lichtenstein GR: Medical Therapy for Ulcerative Colitis. In Lichtenstein GR: The Clinician's Guide to Inflammatory Bowel Disease. Thorofare, NJ, SLACK Incorporated, 2003, pp 255-289. Used with permission.

should be tapered to reduce steroid-related adverse effects. It is important to ensure that patients have inactive disease before initiating this corticosteroid taper. Even though there are no studies to formally evaluate the rate of corticosteroid taper, a potential regimen may include reducing prednisone by 5 mg per week and then 2.5 mg per week after 20 mg, if deemed appropriate. It is imperative to maintain oral aminosalicylates at their maximal doses while corticosteroids are being tapered.

Once remission is achieved, an oral 5-ASA maintenance therapy with the same drug is recommended. Often, doses similar to what was used to induce remission may be required, as the efficacy of these agents in maintaining remission is dose dependent. A combination of oral and topical mesalamine may be more effective than just oral mesalamine in the maintenance of remission in patients with left-sided colitis.

Extensive Colitis or Pancolitis

Ulcerative colitis that has extended beyond the splenic flexure is termed extensive colitis; when the inflammation reaches the cecum, it is then referred to as pancolitis. For mildly to moderately active disease, oral sulfasalazine (3 to 4 g/day) or mesalamine (2.4 to 4.8 g/day) are the first-line therapy (Figure 3), as the inflammation extends beyond the reach of topical preparations. However, topical aminosalicylates can be added to treat left-sided symptoms such as tenesmus or fecal urgency.

Systemic corticosteroids (oral prednisone, 40 to 60 mg/day) should be used to treat patients who have not achieved remission with maximal doses of oral and topical aminosalicylates. Steroids do not have a role in maintaining remission, but should not be tapered until the symptoms are controlled completely. Long-term maintenance therapy with oral sulfasalazine and the newer mesalamine derivatives at standard maintenance doses should be used once a patient has achieved remission. The addition of maintenance topical 5-ASA may further decrease the risk of disease exacerbation.

Some patients may continue to be symptomatic, despite maximal 5-ASA and oral prednisone therapy. These patients, considered to have refractory disease, may need to be hospitalized and treated with intravenous corticosteroids. The treatment of patients with refractory disease is discussed in the subsequent section on refractory colitis.

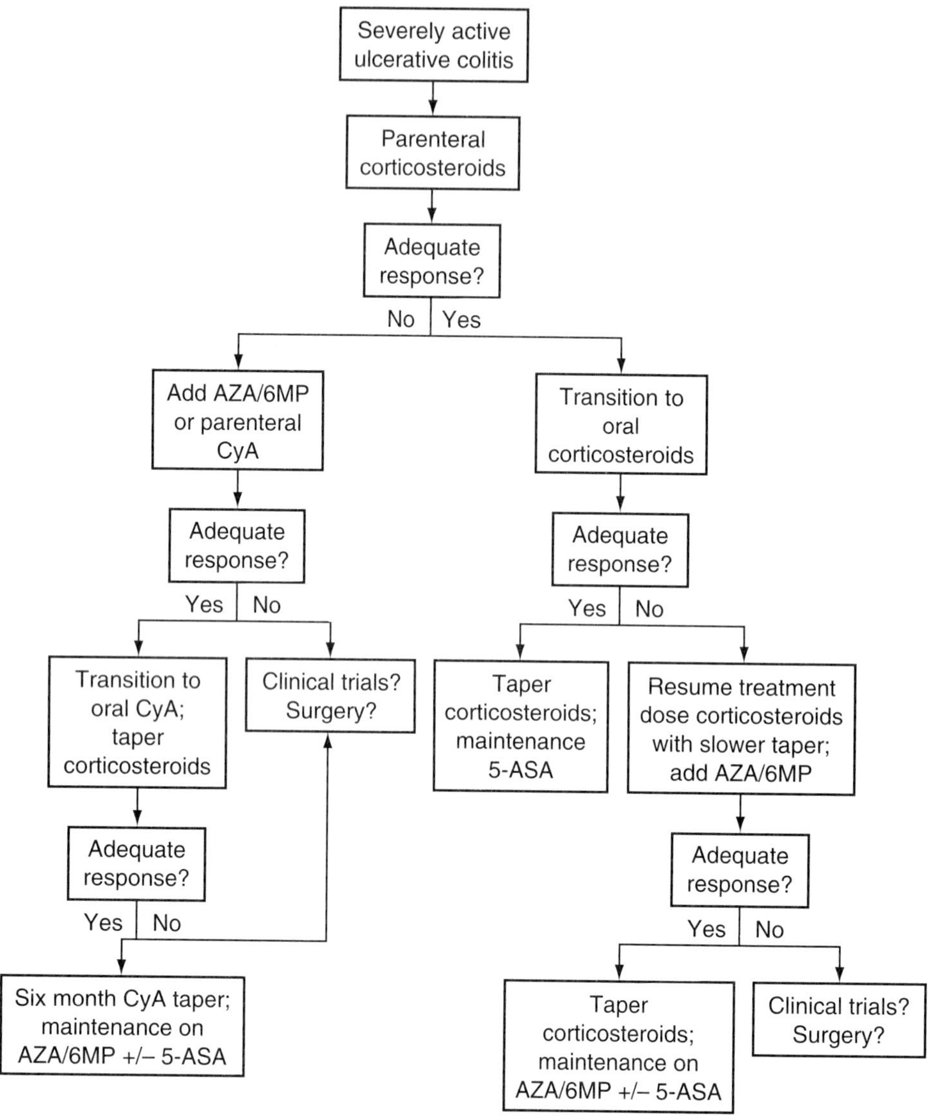

FIGURE 4 Management of severely active ulcerative colitis. *Modified from*: Srinivasan R, Su CG, and Lichtenstein GR: Medical Therapy for Ulcerative Colitis. In Lichtenstein GR: The Clinician's Guide to Inflammatory Bowel Disease. Thorofare, NJ, SLACK Incorporated, 2003, pp 255-289. Used with permission.

Severe Colitis

Patients with severe colitis present with more than six bloody bowel movements per day, fever, hypotension, dehydration, tachycardia, anemia, abdominal pain/tenderness, and an elevated erythrocyte sedimentation rate.

Initial treatment requires hospitalization and initiation of intravenous corticosteroids (prednisolone 40 to 60 mg/day, methylprednisolone 32 to 48 mg/day, or hydrocortisone 300 to 400 mg/day) either as continuous infusion or in divided doses every 8 hours (Figure 4). Topical therapy (hydrocortisone enema [Cortenema], 100 mg every hour) can be offered to patients with significant rectal symptoms such as tenesmus or fecal urgency.

Supportive care with fluid resuscitation, electrolyte repletion, and transfusion to correct anemia should be initiated early in the hospital course. Patients should be placed on bowel rest; anticholinergics, antidiarrheals, and narcotics should be held to decrease the potential for initiation of toxic megacolon. Total parenteral nutrition (TPN) should be used in malnourished patients who do not improve quickly or are unable to tolerate oral intake; as symptoms improve, patients can be transitioned from TPN to a low-residue diet.

Patients should generally improve within 7 days of intravenous corticosteroid therapy. When patients begin to have more formed bowel movements without blood, pain, or urgency and can tolerate oral intake, oral corticosteroids can be substituted (prednisone, 40 mg/day) and aminosalicylate therapy initiated. A slower taper should be initiated if patients remain in remission after the transition to oral steroids. Recurrence of disease at any time during the taper should be treated promptly with increase of steroids to previous dose and a slower taper once symptoms are controlled.

Patients who do not improve during the first week of intravenous corticosteroids generally have a low probability of future improvement; surgical intervention or cyclosporine therapy should be considered to treat these patients. Cyclosporine (Neoral)[1] has several potentially serious adverse effects and its use should be limited to medical centers with access to same-day or next-day cyclosporine levels, and appropriate surgical backup.

Intravenous cyclosporine at a dose of 4 mg/kg per day is given in conjunction with intravenous corticosteroids. Frequent cyclosporine levels should be checked in the treatment phase, and the dose adjusted to maintain a high-pressure liquid chromatography blood level between 250 to 350 ng/mL. Patients receiving cyclosporine should respond within the first 5 days. Surgical intervention should be considered if this response is not seen or if the patient's condition worsens. Patients who respond to and achieve remission on IV cyclosporine should be transitioned to oral cyclosporine twice daily at a total dose twice that of the final IV dose (5 to 7 mg/kg).

Cyclosporine is intended only for short-term use, with long-term maintenance therapy on azathioprine (AZA) (Imuran)[1], 2.0 to 2.5 mg/kg per day, or 6-MP (Purinethol)[1], 1.0 to 1.5 mg/kg per day. The addition of AZA or 6-MP allows for tapering of corticosteroids, improves the potential of long-term maintenance of remission, and reduces the likelihood of future surgery. *Pneumocystis carinii* prophylaxis should be administered to all patients on cyclosporine. Prednisone should first be tapered, followed by cyclosporine over the next 3 to 6 months. AZA or 6-MP should be continued to maintain disease remission.

Fulminant Colitis/Toxic Megacolon

Patients with fulminant colitis present with a toxic appearance and evidence of fever, abdominal tenderness and distention, leukocytosis, and anemia. Rapid extension of inflammation through the bowel wall into the serosa may result in toxic megacolon, manifested by colonic dilatation greater than 6 cm and evidence of systemic toxicity.

Patients should be kept on nothing by mouth (NPO), aggressively fluid resuscitated, and transfused to correct anemia. They should receive perioperative intravenous corticosteroids (methylprednisolone, 40 to 60 mg/day), and broad-spectrum antibiotics. Serial abdominal films should be followed in cases of fulminant colitis to evaluate for colonic dilatation or perforation. Frequently repositioning the patient from supine to decubitus to prone position may aid in passing trapped gas and decompressing the dilated colon. Surgery is indicated in patients with either fulminant colitis or toxic megacolon who do not respond to the aforementioned medical therapy within 72 hours.

[1]Not FDA approved for this indication.

Pouchitis

Approximately 25% of patients with medically uncontrolled UC require surgery. In such cases, a total abdominal colectomy with ileal pouch anal anastomosis (IPAA) is performed. Chronic inflammation of this pouch, or pouchitis, is the most common long-term complication of this procedure. Symptoms of pouchitis include increased stool frequency, hematochezia, fever, abdominal pain, and tenesmus. Up to 50% of patients will develop at least one episode of pouchitis and 15% of these patients will need maintenance therapy and are thought to have chronic pouchitis.

The first-line therapy for the treatment of pouchitis is metronidazole (Flagyl)[1], 10 to 20 mg/kg per day, or ciprofloxacin (Cipro)[1], 1000 mg per day, for a 14-day course (Figure 5). Symptomatic response is usually seen after 1 to 2 days of therapy. Amoxicillin/clavulanic acid (Augmentin)[1] is an alternative antibiotic choice, although there have been no controlled trials using this antimicrobial agent.

[1]Not FDA approved for this indication.

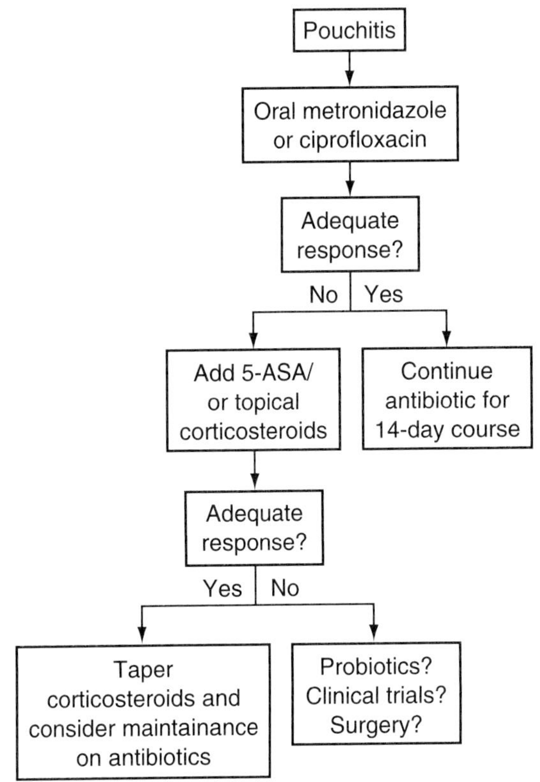

FIGURE 5 Management of pouchitis.
Modified from: Lee T, Buchman AL: Medical Therapy for Ulcerative Colitis. In Lichtenstein GR: The Clinician's Guide to Inflammatory Bowel Disease. Thorofare, NJ, SLACK Incorporated, 2003, pp 125-140. Used with permission.

Patients with pouchitis unresponsive to the 14-day course of metronidazole may benefit from repeating the course of antibiotics. If symptoms still persist, oral or topical mesalamine therapy may be used. Data from uncontrolled studies show that bacterial concentrations in the pouch are sufficient to breakdown the azo bond of sulfasalazine. Other potential investigational agents include topical corticosteroids, probiotics, short-chained fatty acid enemas, and bismuth carbomer enemas. Further research is needed to determine if these agents may be beneficial for select patients.

Some patients may require long-term maintenance therapy on metronidazole. These patients should be closely monitored for adverse effects. Cycling of multiple antibiotics at weekly intervals may help prevent bacterial resistance.

Usually pouchitis is mild and effective to medical therapy, but some patients do not respond to therapy or have frequent recurrences. Occasional complications in these cases include pouch failure requiring removal of the pouch. The risk of dysplasia and malignancy is unclear at this point and warrants further investigation.

CROHN'S DISEASE

Oral Lesions

Aphthous ulcers, deep linear ulcers with associated edema and ulceration are the most common oral manifestations of Crohn's disease. Topical applications of triamcinolone dental paste, hydrocortisone in a pectin or gelatin carrier, or lidocaine lozenges may benefit in reducing the pain and oral discomfort. Refractory disease may require corticosteroids (oral prednisone, 20 mg/day for 1 week), but systemic therapy aimed at treating the underlying Crohn's disease may be required.

Esophagogastroduodenal Crohn's Disease

Fewer than 5% of patients with Crohn's disease present with disease involving the stomach, distal antrum, or duodenum. These patients often present with epigastric pain, postprandial nausea, and vomiting. Because of their distal site of release, aminosalicylates may not be effective, but some patients have been known to occasionally ingest mesalamine in the form of Rowasa enemas. Proton pump inhibitors (omeprazole [Prilosec][1]), 40 mg per day, have been reported to be helpful in inducing and maintaining remission. Moderate-to-severe disease may require treatment with corticosteroids, immunomodulatory agents (azathioprine/6-MP, methotrexate), or infliximab.

Ileocolitis/Colitis

Based on the site of bowel involvement, aminosalicylates are the first-line therapy in mildly to moderately active disease (Figure 6). While Pentasa has historically been used to treat active disease proximal to the terminal ileum, either Pentasa or Asacol can treat distal ileitis and ileocolitis. Once maximal doses are reached, clinical improvement should be seen within 2 to 4 weeks. If not, either ciprofloxacin[1] (1 g/day) or metronidazole[1] (10 to 20 mg/kg/day) should be considered. If patients improve, usually within 3 to 4 weeks, the antibiotic dose can be tapered over the next few weeks to months. Some patients may require long-term antibiotics to maintain disease remission, although no controlled trials have been performed to ascertain the efficacy of antibiotics for maintenance of remission in Crohn's disease.

[1]Not FDA approved for this indication.

Corticosteroids should be reserved for patients whose disease remains unresponsive to aminosalicylate and antibiotic therapy, or who present with moderate-to-severe disease. Oral prednisone (40 to 60 mg/day) or budesonide (9 mg/day) can be administered and tapered slowly once the symptoms are controlled. AZA or 6-MP, when used concomitantly with corticosteroids, may induce remission more rapidly and with lower prednisone doses. Patients who do not respond to the aforementioned therapies should be treated for refractory disease, as described later. Once remission is achieved, corticosteroids should be tapered and patients should be maintained on AZA/6-MP either with or without aminosalicylates.

Severe Crohn's Disease

Patients with severe Crohn's disease often present with fever, abdominal pain and tenderness, bloody diarrhea, hypotension, and leukocytosis. Because of transmural inflammation with serosal involvement, these patients may be prone to microperforation with resulting localized peritonitis.

Patients with severe Crohn's disease should be hospitalized and resuscitated with intravenous fluids. CT of the abdomen should be performed to evaluate for abscess or phlegmon, which requires broad-spectrum antibiotics and, potentially, surgical drainage. Corticosteroids are withheld in this setting.

Once infection is excluded, intravenous corticosteroids (methylprednisolone, 40 to 60 mg/day) should be administered. The addition of AZA or 6-MP to corticosteroid therapy may accelerate remission with lower doses of corticosteroids. Patients who do not respond adequately to this combination therapy should be treated for refractory disease, as discussed later.

Fistulous/Perianal Crohn's Disease

As a result of transmural inflammation, patients with Crohn's disease are prone to developing internal and external fistulas. Internal fistulas often require surgical intervention, as there is little data on the pharmacologic therapy for internal fistulas.

[1]Not FDA approved for this indication.

First-line therapies for perianal fistulas include metronidazole[1] (10 to 20 mg/kg/day) or ciprofloxacin[1] (1 g/day). Combining the two antibiotics may also be effective if monotherapy fails. Antibiotics can be tapered once these fistulas close, although some patients may require chronic antibiotic therapy. AZA[1] or 6-MP[1] can be used to treat fistulous CD that does not respond to antibiotics. Infliximab, infused at a dose of 5 mg/kg at 0, 2, and 6 weeks with subsequent maintenance therapy (usually at 5 mg/kg every 8 weeks thereafter) can be used as an alternative to AZA or 6-MP, or in conjunction with these medications. Because of the significant toxicity of cyclosporine, intravenous cyclosporine[1] (4 mg/kg) should be reserved for patients whose disease remains unresponsive to the aforementioned therapies.

Refractory Disease

Despite the numerous efficacious medical therapies currently available, some IBD patients may

[1]Not FDA approved for this indication.

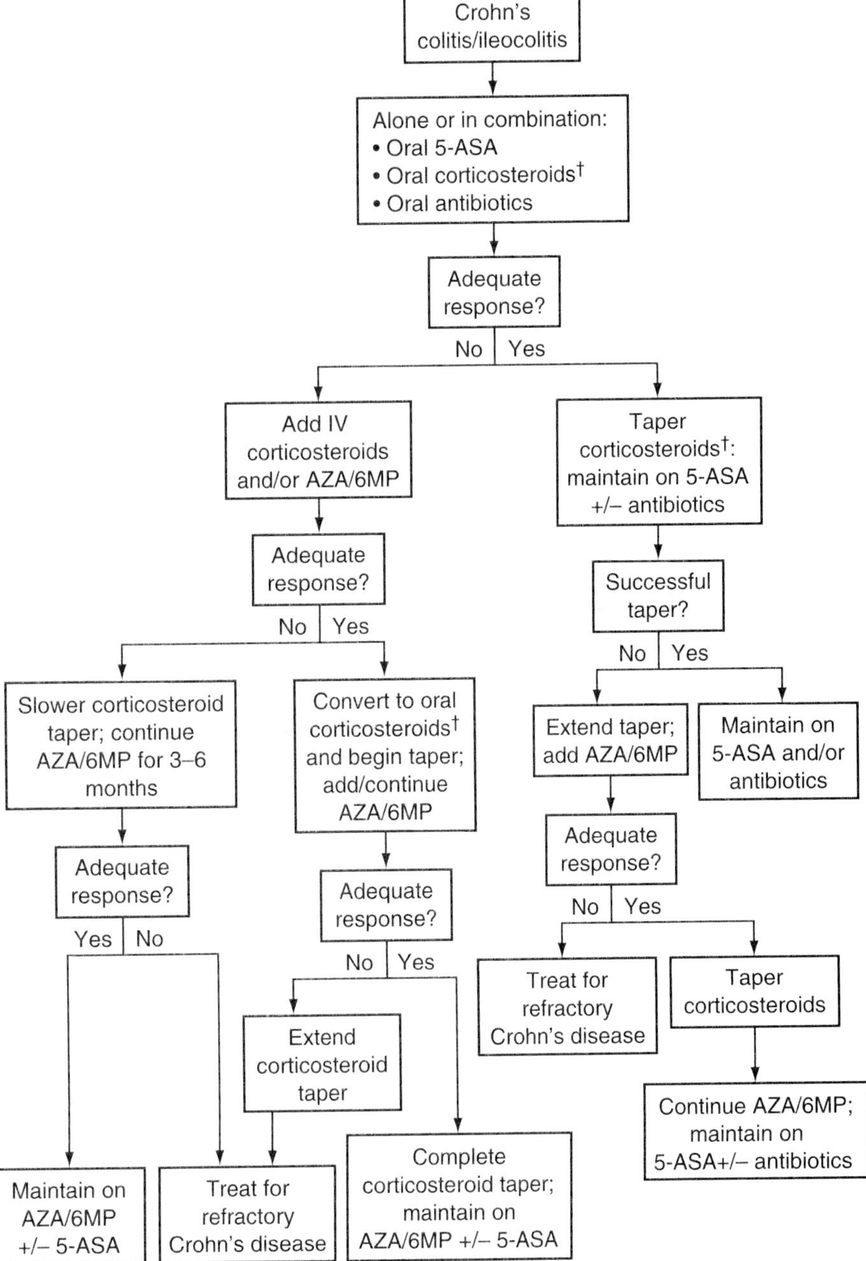

FIGURE 6 Management of Crohn's colitis or ileocolitis.
Modified from: Han P, Cohen RD: Medical Therapy for Ulcerative Colitis. In Lichtenstein GR: The Clinician's Guide to Inflammatory Bowel Disease. Thorofare, NJ, SLACK Incorporated, 2003, pp 343-370. Used with permission.

remain symptomatic while on maximal 5-ASA, antibiotic, and corticosteroid therapy.

Patients who respond to corticosteroids but who are unable to discontinue them are considered to have steroid-dependent disease. Others may have steroid refractory disease, defined as disease that remains active despite high-dose corticosteroids.

The management of refractory UC and CD is outlined in Figures 7 and 8, respectively. While on maximal dose corticosteroids, AZA or 6-MP are initiated at 50 to 100 mg and slowly increased by 25 mg over the next 2 weeks if tolerated to the maximum of 2.5 mg/kg per day for AZA and 1.5 mg/kg per day for 6-MP. Alternatively, AZA or 6-MP can be initiated at maximum doses with careful subsequent monitoring for toxicity. Treatment for at least 3 to 6 months is required to evaluate for an adequate response. Corticosteroids should be tapered if an adequate response is noted on AZA or 6-MP. These agents have several potentially toxic adverse effects, including leukopenia and aminotransferase elevation, which should be closely monitored by following patients' complete blood counts and liver-associated laboratory chemistries. There is conflicting evidence as to the duration of treatment with AZA/6-MP. While some suggest discontinuing AZA/6-MP after 4 years, others recommend continuing AZA/6-MP beyond 5 years—even indefinitely. Lifelong therapy, however, should be reserved for patients with aggressive disease or those who are at high risk for relapse (e.g., patients whose disease began at an earlier age, or who required more than 6 months of immunomodulator therapy to achieve disease remission).

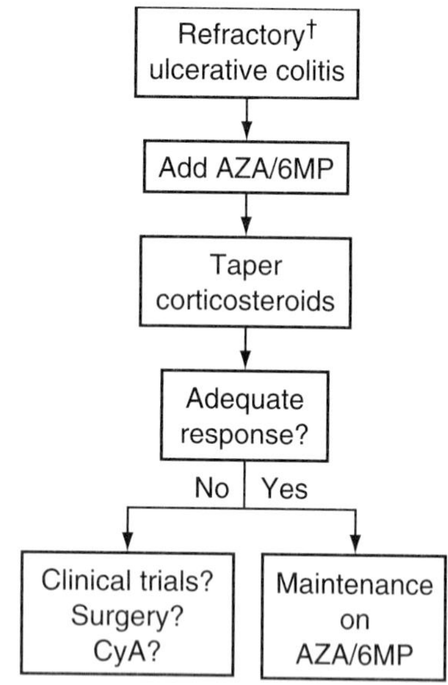

FIGURE 7 Management of refractory ulcerative colitis.
Modified from: Han P, Cohen RD: Medical Therapy for Ulcerative Colitis. In Lichtenstein GR: The Clinician's Guide to Inflammatory Bowel Disease. Thorofare, NJ, SLACK Incorporated, 2003, pp 343-370. Used with permission.

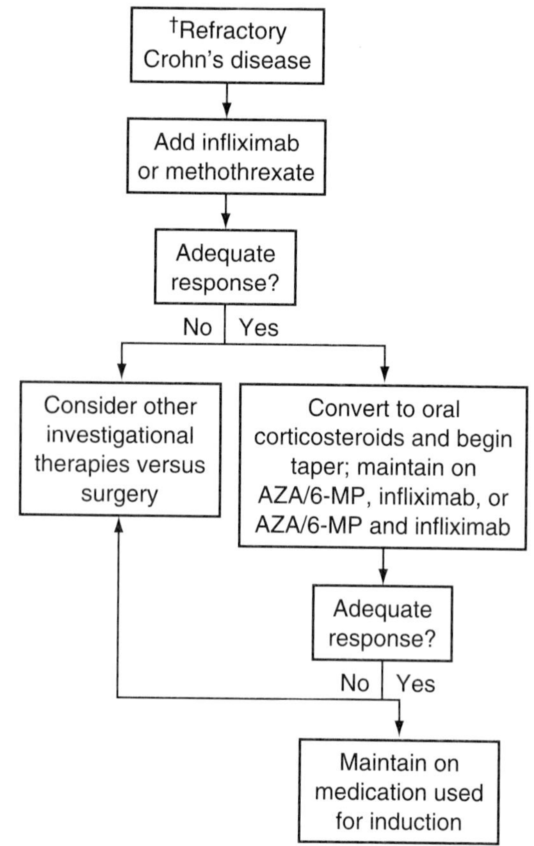

FIGURE 8 Management of refractory Crohn's disease.
Modified from: Han P, Cohen RD: Medical Therapy for Ulcerative Colitis. In Lichtenstein GR: The Clinician's Guide to Inflammatory Bowel Disease. Thorofare, NJ, SLACK Incorporated, 2003, pp 343-370. Used with permission.

Results from a recent study suggest that intravenous cyclosporine may be beneficial in treating steroid-refractory UC. In addition, cyclosporine may serve as a bridge until AZA or 6-MP have reached therapeutic levels or until elective surgery is performed. Cyclosporine has not proven beneficial in the treatment of refractory CD.

Methotrexate, at a dose of 25 mg per week intramuscularly, can be used to treat patients with refractory CD who are intolerant, allergic, or unresponsive to AZA/6-MP. Frequent monitoring of complete blood counts and liver function tests are required to monitor for potential toxicity associated with methotrexate. Methotrexate should be continued for at least 1 to 3 months to assess for an adequate response. If remission and steroid withdrawal are successful, methotrexate can be continued as maintenance therapy at an intramuscular dose of 15 mg per week. Frequent, subcutaneous dosing is administered because of the untested belief that subcutaneous administration is equally as efficacious as intramuscular administration. Randomized clinical trials demonstrated methotrexate to have no benefit in the treatment of UC.

Infliximab can be used to treat patients with refractory CD unresponsive to maximal doses of immunomodulator therapy. Given as 5 mg/kg infusion at 0, 2, and 6 weeks with repeat infusions every 8 weeks thereafter, infliximab has been shown to allow for steroid withdrawal in refractory CD. It also has been shown to prolong disease remission when used concurrently with AZA/6-MP. Patients on infliximab therapy should be monitored for development of infectious complications.

Patients who continue to have active disease despite immunomodulator and infliximab therapy should be evaluated for surgery. However, some patients may choose to participate in ongoing clinical trials of experimental therapies prior to surgery.

As our knowledge expands on the pathophysiology underlying inflammatory bowel disease, better and more efficacious therapies can be expected. The medical therapies and management of site-specific presentations of ulcerative colitis and Crohn's disease aim at inducing and maintaining disease remission, while helping patients maintain an excellent quality of life. Living with inflammatory bowel disease is often challenging, and the Crohn's and Colitis Foundation of America (*www.ccfa.org*) offers social support and educational resources that may help patients cope with these potentially debilitating disorders.

IRRITABLE BOWEL SYNDROME

METHOD OF

James Christensen, MD

Inexplicable gastrointestinal symptoms are generally blamed on the irritable bowel syndrome (IBS)—also called spastic colon, mucous colitis, and functional bowel syndrome. This common diagnosis remains scientifically undefined after more than a century of study. A recent clinical redefinition offers mainly a basis for investigation.

The Clinical Definition

People often blame various unexplained chronic gastrointestinal complaints (abdominal pain, diarrhea, constipation, nausea, vomiting, gas, and bloating) on IBS. Authorities formerly accepted various genitourinary, cardiovascular, and emotional symptoms as those of IBS. The list has shortened over time to the current definition, the Rome II criteria (Table 1), proposed by a panel of authorities convened in Rome to revise previous definitions.

This latest definition requires *abdominal discomfort or pain* that is related to defecation. To support the diagnosis, it also accepts *bloating* and certain *abnormal features of the defecation.*

Centuries of clinical-pathologic correlation taught physicians and surgeons how to interpret abdominal pain by considering certain characteristics—its character, location, chronology, aggravating and relieving factors, and associated symptoms.* The Rome II definition of IBS fails to consider such features.

Clinical–pathologic correlation also taught doctors how to use the characteristics of the stool (consistency, color, presence of overt or occult blood, odor, and daily volume) and the characteristics of disordered defecation (frequency of defecation, changes over time, aggravating and relieving factors, and associated symptoms) to guide the diagnostic process.* The Rome II definition of IBS neglects these matters as well.

The Physiologic Definition

Most physicians and patients accept that IBS reflects dysfunction of the nerves of the gut. However, even the newest information and technologies fail to confirm the theories offered to explain IBS, which are spasm and dysrhythmia in the colon, irritability (hypersensitivity) of the gastrointestinal tract, primary autonomic nerve dysfunction, and food allergy.

The absence of a uniformly accepted clinical definition of the syndrome still limits the selection of patient

*See Web site http://www.vh.org/adult/provider/internalmedicine/BedsideLogic/index.html.

TABLE 1 Rome II Symptom Criteria for a Diagnosis of the Irritable Bowel Syndrome (IBS)

I. At least 12 weeks (not necessarily consecutive) in the preceding 12 months of abdominal pain or discomfort that has two of the following three features:
   1. Relief with defecation
   2. Onset associated with a change in stool frequency
   3. Onset associated with a change in the form (appearance) of the stool

II. Other symptoms not required but supportive:
   1. Abnormal stool frequency (more than three stools per day or less than three stools per week)
   2. Abnormal stool form (lumpy/hard or loose/watery)
   3. Abnormal stool passage (straining, urgency, feeling of incomplete evacuation)
   4. Passage of mucus
   5. Bloating or a feeling of abdominal distension

groups for study. The complexity of gastrointestinal neurophysiology (neurogastroenterology) hampers the search for a pathogenesis. For both reasons, no physiologic definition of IBS has been established.

The Differential Diagnosis

IBS constitutes a set of *symptoms*, which are individual and personal, without *signs*, which are the objective evidence of defined diseases. Thus, the diagnosis is subjective, depending on the communication skills of both patient and physician.

The diagnosis remains a diagnosis of exclusion; that is, the physician must exclude all other reasonable explanations for the symptoms that come to mind. The finding of a rational explanation yields an established and defined pathophysiologic diagnosis based on current knowledge and understanding; the failure to find such a defined disease entity or process leads to the diagnosis of IBS.

The vast array of defined diseases that can produce abdominal pain demands a systematic method for the efficient exploration of the complaint. A thoughtful and thorough analysis of the character, location, chronology, aggravating and relieving factors, and associated symptoms in respect to abdominal pain is the necessary first step in the orderly diagnostic process. A similar analytic method is necessary for all the other gastrointestinal complaints that might be interpreted as a part of IBS, including diarrhea, constipation, nausea, vomiting, gas, and bloating.

Making a diagnosis by exclusion, such as is done with IBS, demands the consideration of such matters as the family history (looking for gastrointestinal cancer or celiac disease, for example), the past medical history (looking for a history of abdominal operations, for example) and the dietary history. The diagnosis also calls for an expert physical examination seeking evidence for all the possibilities suggested by the account of the symptoms. It demands, in sum, the most skillful use of the established clinical methods, the proven methods of history taking and physical examination, to guide the further investigation.

Some authorities suggest certain minor characteristics of the symptom complex that seem to characterize IBS, especially the persistence of the symptoms without change for more than 2 years, the onset of symptoms in young adulthood, and the presence of a family history of the diagnosis of IBS. More usefully, one can take the absence of such *soft* features as warning against the diagnosis.

Beyond the history and physical examination, the modern investigation of gastrointestinal complaints in general commonly employs a battery of blood tests, endoscopic procedures, and radiographic examinations. The routine utilization of the simple lists that some authorities provide as those tests necessary to make a diagnosis of IBS does not substitute for a thoughtful analysis of symptoms and a careful physical examination. Blind routine testing may fail to show the rarer or subtler organic pathology that would explain symptoms otherwise attributed to IBS. With a set of specific organic diagnoses (the differential diagnosis) kept firmly in mind, doctors can direct such investigations more specifically to find disordered function.

Many serious or life-threatening gastrointestinal disorders are signaled by warning signs, such as unexplained weight loss and gastrointestinal bleeding, but such diseases in their early stages can mimic IBS without the warning signs. That is, they can produce only abdominal pain or discomfort coupled with bloating or a disturbed pattern of defecation.

When the most thorough analysis fails to find an explanation for a set of gastrointestinal symptoms, a diagnosis of IBS seems in order. However, even then the physician must not consider IBS to be a single homogeneous entity. It could represent many kinds of neural or neuromuscular dysfunction in the gut, considering how much remains unknown about gastrointestinal physiology. The gut is a mechanical device in which a complex and obscure nervous system drives the musculature. Much remains to be learned about this system before ways can be found to test adequately its manifold operations.

Some Conditions with a High Risk for Misdiagnosis

The risk of an erroneous diagnosis of IBS seems especially likely in some particular conditions (Table 2).

The proliferation of organisms found in the small intestine causes gas, bloating, and abdominal cramps. *Giardiasis* produces such symptoms. The propagation of coliform bacteria in the small intestine, called *small-bowel bacterial overgrowth* (which has several causes, including diabetes), does as well.

Abnormalities in the intestinal epithelium may not be apparent in the usual examinations. Intolerance to dietary lactose from mucosal *lactase deficiency* produces symptoms like those of IBS. Mild *celiac disease* (or *sprue*) may produce mainly abdominal discomfort with little other symptomatology. *Inflammatory bowel disease* can be very subtle, especially lymphocytic colitis and the related disorder, collagenous colitis.

IBS symptoms may arise from unorthodox dietary practices or unrecognized food intolerances that lead to osmotic diarrhea. The most common diet-related cause is *intolerance to fructose*. This natural and poorly absorbed monosaccharide, often called "corn sweetener," now finds such widespread use in the sweetening of commercially prepared beverages and foods that the daily intake can be great. Normal persons may also chronically ingest other sorts of laxative substances, such as the noncaloric sugar alcohol sweeteners (sorbitol, mannitol, and xylitol) and similar artificial sweeteners. Other specific *food intolerances* may be unrecognized by patients. Some common foods such as beans, beer, cabbage, onions,

TABLE 2 Some Conditions Presenting a High Risk of Misdiagnosis as Irritable Bowel Syndrome (IBS)

I. Conditions where diarrhea, constipation, gas, and bloating may be readily misinterpreted as IBS:
   1. Organisms growing in the gut that should not be there:
      a. Giardiasis
      b. Bacterial overgrowth in the small intestine
   2. Abnormalities in the lining of the intestine:
      a. Intolerance to lactose
      b. Celiac disease (sprue)
      c. Inflammatory bowel disease (especially lymphocytic colitis)
   3. Dietary practices:
      a. Intolerance to fructose
      b. Intake of laxative substances (sorbitol, mannitol, xylitol)
      c. Other food intolerances
   4. Unconscious swallowing of air, from:
      a. Poor dentition
      b. Nervous habit
   5. Systemic diseases:
      a. Diffuse systemic sclerosis
      b. Thyroid disease
II. Conditions where abdominal wall pain may be misinterpreted as IBS:
   1. Neuropathies
   2. Trigger points
   3. Incisional neuromas and hernias
III. Conditions where nausea and vomiting may be misinterpreted as IBS:
   1. Disordered emptying of the stomach
      a. The neuropathy of diabetes
      b. Viral neuropathy
   2. Partial small intestinal obstruction

and nuts variably produce gas and bloating in many people. Other foods may produce diarrhea.

Excessive air swallowing sometimes occurs with poor dentition as well as part of a nervous habit. Many *systemic diseases*, such as diffuse systemic sclerosis and thyroid disease, can produce IBS symptoms and remain undiagnosed for many years.

Many people forget that abdominal pain can arise from the abdominal wall as well as from the abdominal cavity. *Sensory somatic neuropathies* (as in complicated diabetes) and *trigger points* in the abdominal wall are common and easily proved with the appropriate techniques of physical examination. Pain from *neuromas* and tiny *hernias* in incisional scars and from rare abdominal wall hernias such as *Richter's hernia* can easily be misconstrued as IBS pain.

Disordered emptying of the stomach is now recognized as common. The abnormality arises from defective operation of the gastric innervation, an *autonomic neuropathy* that is a complication of diabetes or the result of a *viral neuropathy*. Too rapid gastric emptying (dumping) and delayed emptying (gastroparesis) can produce similar symptoms. *Incomplete obstruction of the distal small bowel*, also a mimic of IBS, can be difficult to diagnose.

MAJOR PSYCHOLOGICAL ISSUES

No specific psychopathology correlates with the diagnosis of IBS. The specific psychological determinants that dictate the health-seeking behavior of patients with all sorts of chronic illnesses also determine the health-seeking behavior in IBS.

In the normal mind-body relationship, depression and anxiety can elicit gastrointestinal symptoms that resemble IBS. This normal cause-and-effect relationship makes use of normal physiologic mechanisms. It does not signify gastrointestinal disease and best responds to treatment of the cause.

Many drugs used in modern psychiatry act on neurotransmitter mechanisms in the brain that also operate in the enteric nervous system. Thus, unexplained gastrointestinal symptoms can represent the effects of drugs used to treat emotional and mental disorders.

Management

THE DOCTOR–PATIENT RELATIONSHIP

How does the physician, ethically compelled to explain the pathophysiology of disease to patients, explain IBS? Obviously, when an understood cause of the IBS symptoms is discovered, in the form of a trigger point in the abdominal wall for example, the diagnosis is no longer IBS, and a pathogenesis can be readily explained. In the case of IBS, however, the best that can be done is a general attribution of the symptoms to nerve trouble. Some patients, not accepting uncertainty or confessions of ignorance in their physicians, may seek others who seem to know the truth. This makes for a problematic clinical relationship for which there is no easy solution.

DIETARY ADVICE

Dietary changes should form the mainstay of therapy because they are effective and harmless. This constitutes essentially symptomatic therapy. The commonsense advice to avoid specific foods that worsen symptoms and to take three balanced meals daily may be necessary for those who have unorthodox patterns of eating. When diarrhea is dominant, advice to curtail or eliminate high-fructose beverages and foods (essentially all soft drinks and many "diet" foods) seems reasonable because the intake of large amounts of fructose produces symptoms in normal people. The same can be said of foods prepared as low-calorie sweets for diabetic patients and persons trying to lose weight.

Bulking agents help those with unexplained constipation; they make for normal patterns of defecation in general. Ordinary dietary food fiber may not be enough, and bran supplementation is difficult to make wholly palatable. The many preparations of psyllium seed offer good therapy in the treatment of IBS where defecatory disturbances, both diarrhea and constipation, are troublesome. The dosage can be increased gradually until the desired effect is achieved.

The addition of a small daily dosage of milk of magnesia can soften hard stools when that remains a problem with fiber supplementation.

ANTIDIARRHEAL AGENTS AND ANTICHOLINERGICS

Diarrhea can be controlled temporarily with the synthetic nonabsorbed opioid, loperamide. A particularly thorough search for organic disease should always precede a commitment to the chronic use of loperamide. The addition of bulking agents also may facilitate the treatment of chronic diarrhea.

Preparations of anticholinergic agents have been used in IBS for more than a century for the temporary suppression of abdominal cramps or colicky pain. The side effects of such agents make their chronic administration in IBS unwise.

NEW DRUGS

Some advocates currently promote new agents directed to the neural 5-HT_3 (5-hydroxytryptamine) and 5-HT_4 receptors for serotonin to treat IBS. Their utility remains untested in practice and, because the pathogenesis of IBS remains unknown, there is no logic in their use. Experience to date indicates that alosetron, a 5-HT_3 antagonist, carries some risk of potentially fatal side effects.

HEMORRHOIDS, ANAL FISSURE, ANORECTAL ABSCESS, AND FISTULA

METHOD OF

Mitchell Bernstein, MD

Symptomatic benign anorectal conditions are among the most common reasons that patients seek medical attention. Most commonly these symptoms are attributed to hemorrhoids. While all patients have internal and external hemorrhoids, not all problems are attributable to hemorrhoids and it is important to be aware of other common anorectal conditions that cause symptoms. A simple but directed history often points to the correct diagnosis, and a thorough anorectal examination will confirm it. Treatment is then prescribed accordingly.

History

A simple but directed history is essential to the proper diagnosis of anorectal conditions. The most common anorectal symptoms for which patients seek medical advice, alone or in combination, are bleeding and pain. Careful characterization of these symptoms often yields the correct diagnosis.

Patients that complain of bleeding are often concerned about a colonic malignancy, and a thorough evaluation of the colon is often indicated to exclude this possibility. However, the combination of painless, bright red bleeding with bowel movements (especially in a young individual) is likely to be caused by internal hemorrhoids. Pain and bleeding with bowel movements, however, is likely caused by an anal fissure. Alternatively, perianal pain that is not associated with bowel movements and may have a component of swelling is likely to be a thrombosed external hemorrhoid or abscess.

Physical Examination

With the history strongly suggesting the diagnosis, confirmation of the problem is established with a simple but thorough anorectal examination. Examination of the patient in the prone jack-knife position yields optimal results, however, the lateral decubitus position is adequate. More important than patient position, however, are the proper tools. Good lighting is critical and may be achieved with a headlight or spotlight. A side-viewing anoscope and rigid proctoscope should also be available. Finally, when describing findings related to the anorectum it is useful to describe them using anatomic position (anterior, posterolateral, etc.) rather than using the face of a clock as this reference is dependent on patient position.

Before anoscopy, proctoscopy and digital rectal examination are considered; much information can be gleaned from careful visual inspection of the perineum and perianal region. Excoriation of the perianal skin, erythema of the buttocks or perianal area, external sinuses, and masses or skin tags all can be readily appreciated on visual inspection. Gentle spreading of the buttocks may reveal an anal fissure or a small thrombosed external hemorrhoid not initially appreciated.

Once the perineum has been adequately inspected, the perianal skin and surrounding perineum should be palpated. Discharge (from the anus or external sinuses) and/or tenderness should be noted. A digital rectal examination is performed next. A well-lubricated, gloved finger is slowly inserted. The anal canal and distal rectum is palpated circumferentially. Sphincter tone, motion of the sphincter complex with voluntary squeeze, the presence of masses or sphincter defects all should be noted. The prostate should be felt in men. Upon withdrawal of the gloved finger, the presence of blood, stool or mucus is noted.

Direct visualization of the anal canal is achieved with an anoscope. A side-viewing anoscope is useful in assessing the internal hemorrhoids, the condition of the anal mucosa, as well as the presence of tumors or masses within the anal canal. On occasion, the internal opening of an anal fissure is readily identified. Upon completion of the examination the diagnosis most often has been confirmed and therapy can now be directed.

Hemorrhoids

It is generally agreed upon that hemorrhoids are highly vascular *cushions* of tissue consisting of mucosa and a thick submucosa that contains blood vessels, connective tissue, and smooth muscle. Arterial and venous channels coalesce in specific positions within the anal canal to form three readily identifiable cushions: the left lateral, right anterolateral, and right posterolateral hemorrhoids. Both the portal and systemic systems are involved in drainage of blood from the anal canal with the internal hemorrhoidal plexus draining via the portal system and the external hemorrhoids draining largely through the systemic system.

Hemorrhoidal cushions are present in everyone; however, their exact function remains speculative. Some believe that the hemorrhoidal cushions aid in continence, while others believe that they allow the anal canal to dilate during defection and protect the sphincter muscles and anal canal from trauma during defecation.

External hemorrhoids are located distal to the dentate line. They are covered with anoderm, a modified squamous epithelium devoid of skin appendages. The external hemorrhoids may swell and cause some discomfort, but treatment is generally not necessary unless an acute thrombosis is present. A thrombosed external hemorrhoid manifests itself as a painful, bluish-appearing nodule that is readily visible upon inspection of the perianal region. The nodule is often accompanied by edema of the surrounding tissue. It is the edema causing pressure within the tissues that causes the perianal pain. As the edema subsides the pain slowly abates. However, the nodule is often present for up to 4 weeks as the thrombosis is slowly broken down and absorbed. Accordingly, treatment of a thrombosed external hemorrhoid depends upon the time frame in which medical attention is sought. If seen early in the course of the thrombosis, excisional hemorrhoidectomy can be performed, often with local anesthesia in the office. Alternatively, if the patient is seen several days after the onset of the thrombosis and the pain is improving or no longer present, expectant management is suggested. Following the complete resolution of the thrombosis a small external skin tag often persists.

Internal hemorrhoids are located proximal to the dentate line and are covered by transitional or columnar epithelium. They are often classified according to grade (Table 1), and the grade often dictates treatment. A myriad of complaints are often attributed to hemorrhoids; however, the two most common symptoms that they cause are bleeding and prolapse. Bleeding arises from a break in the lining overlying the hemorrhoids and is characteristically bright red and painless. Blood will often drip into the bowel and appear on the toilet tissue. Prolapse of the hemorrhoidal tissue occurs with straining at defecation. The tissue most often reduces spontaneously, although manual reduction is sometimes necessary. In advanced, chronic states of prolapse the tissue may not reduce and thereby predispose to mucus seepage and subsequent perianal irritation or excoriation. It is important to note that internal hemorrhoids do not cause pain. When pain is a predominant complaint, a search for an associated condition should be undertaken.

The mainstay of treatment of several anorectal conditions is bowel management. A bowel regimen of increased fluid intake and fiber supplementation is recommended. In addition, patients are instructed to minimize time spent in the bathroom (e.g., "take the library out of the bathroom"). With respect to symptomatic internal hemorrhoids, the rationale for adding bulk to the diet is to eliminate straining at defecation. A large, soft stool allows for easier passage and thus reduces straining and engorgement of the hemorrhoidal cushions. A high-fiber diet is effective in the management of grades 1 and 2 internal

TABLE 1 Classification of Internal Hemorrhoids

Degree	Description	Symptoms	Treatment
First	Prolapse of hemorrhoid cushion into the lumen of the rectum and anal canal	Bleeding	Conservative rubber band ligation*
Second	Prolapse out of the anal canal with pressure and spontaneous reduction	Discomfort, swelling, and bleeding	Conservative rubber band ligation;* hemorrhoidectomy excision/stapled
Third	Prolapse out of the anal canal with pressure and requiring manual reduction	Pain when prolapsed and with thrombosis, bleeding	Conservative treatment; hemorrhoidectomy excision/stapled
Fourth	Prolapsed out of the anal canal and unable to be reduced	Severe pain with thrombosis or infarction	Hemorrhoidectomy

*When conservative management fails.

hemorrhoids and may provide adequate relief for patients with grade 3 internal hemorrhoids.

If conservative management fails to provide relief of hemorrhoidal symptoms, several options are available. Treatment often depends on the grade and symptoms of the hemorrhoids as well as patient preference. Rubber band ligation is a simple, effective means of treating bleeding or prolapsing grades 1 and 2 hemorrhoids and selected grade 3 hemorrhoids. Under direct visualization with the aid of an anoscope the hemorrhoidal tissue is grasped, pulled into the ligator, and the rubber band is released at the grasped tissue's base above the dentate line. The incorporated tissue usually sloughs within a week. Although patients experience some discomfort for 24 to 48 hours, the procedure is largely well tolerated. There have been isolated reports of severe pelvic sepsis following rubber band ligation. Potential harbingers of this problem include increasing pain, difficulty voiding, and fever. Patients should be advised to seek immediate medical attention should they experience any of these symptoms.

Excisional therapy, either by stapled hemorrhoidopexy or surgical removal of the hemorrhoidal complexes, is the next line of treatment for symptomatic hemorrhoids. Stapled hemorrhoidopexy is relatively new in the United States, however, it has been performed for many years in Europe. With the aid of an anoscope, a pursestring is applied above the dentate line and a circular stapler is introduced. The pursestring is secured around the stapler, and the device is closed and fired (Figure 1). A 2- to 4-cm napkin ring of mucosa and submucosa is excised, effectively reducing the prolapsing hemorrhoidal tissue as well as interrupting the terminal branches of the hemorrhoidal artery. The internal hemorrhoidal tissue is not excised with this procedure, but the interruption of blood flow and removal of proximal tissue have proven very effective in reducing hemorrhoidal prolapse and, to a lesser extent, bleeding. The procedure does not remove external hemorrhoids or skin tags; however, patients often report a reduction in their size several months following stapled hemorrhoidopexy. Stapled hemorrhoidopexy is associated with significantly less postoperative pain than excisional hemorrhoidectomy.

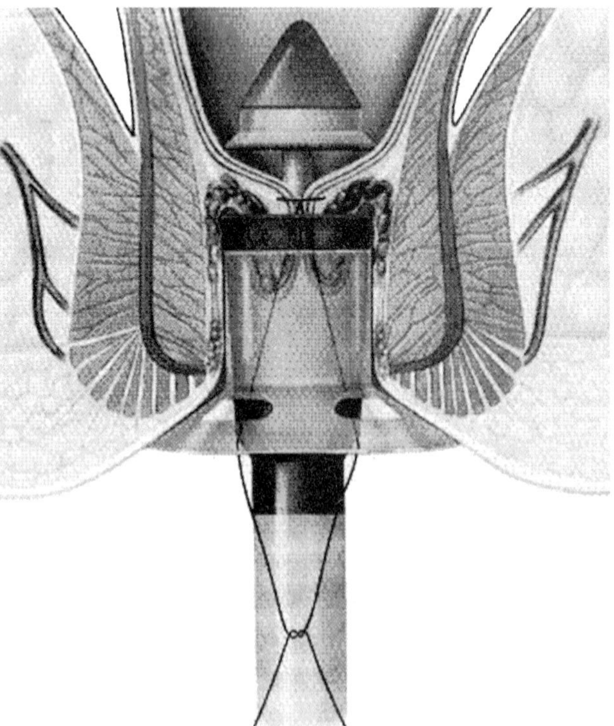

FIGURE 1 Stapled hemorrhoidopexy. The stapler has been inserted and the pursestring secured. (Courtesy of Ethicon Endosurgery.)

Surgical excision of the hemorrhoidal cushions remains a good option for the treatment of symptomatic hemorrhoids unresponsive to conservative measures. Various techniques exist for surgical excision; all involve complete removal of the mucosa and vessel-containing submucosa of all three hemorrhoidal cushions. Although surgical excisions are associated with a significant amount of pain in the postoperative period, for now they remain the gold standard for treatment of symptomatic internal hemorrhoids in the United States.

Anal Fissure

An anal fissure is a cut or tear in the lining of the anal canal. Most commonly located in the posterior midline, it can also be located in the anterior midline of the anus. The fissure causes severe pain with defecation as well as bleeding. The pain is often described as searing or burning in quality and the stool is often streaked with blood. Following the bowel movement, patients may experience a throbbing or aching pain for several hours because of spasm of the underlying internal anal sphincter. The fissure is often caused by hard stool or, alternately, diarrhea.

After eliciting a history suggestive of an anal fissure, the diagnosis can often be confirmed by gentle spreading of the buttocks and eversion of the anal mucosa. An associated sentinel tag may be the first clue to the presence of the fissure. Patients are often too tender for internal examination; if one must be performed, a hypertrophied anal papilla is often noted.

A fissure may be acute or chronic in nature. An acute fissure is initially treated with dietary and hygiene measures. Bowel habits are improved with increased dietary fiber, increased fluid intake, and addition of bulking agents to the diet. Warm baths are helpful in relieving the pain from spasm of the internal anal sphincter. Approximately 66% of patients with an acute fissure will heal their fissure with such treatment. Various chemical agents aimed at relaxing the internal anal sphincter have been introduced into the armamentarium of agents used in treating fissures. The exact role of such agents remains unclear.

Chronic fissures as well as acute fissures that do not heal with conservative management may be treated with surgery. After excluding other etiologies for the fissure (e.g., inflammatory bowel disease, infectious processes), a lateral internal sphincterotomy may be performed. This is a minor operation in which a small portion of the internal anal sphincter is divided. The surgery is effective in relieving pain and bleeding in 90% of patients. Although complications are rare, up to 1% of patients may experience minor disturbances in continence following a sphincterotomy.

Anorectal Abscess and Fistula

The majority of anorectal abscesses result from infection of the anal glands. Anal glands are located within the submucosa and intersphincteric plane at the level of the mid-anal canal. Obstruction of their ducts is thought to lead to subsequent abscess formation. In approximately 33% of patients, drainage of an anorectal abscess will result in a fistula—a small communication from the anal gland from which the abscess arose to the site of drainage.

Pain is the predominant complaint of patients with anorectal abscesses. The pain is persistent and is often exacerbated by bowel movements. In addition, perianal swelling may be reported. Fever may accompany these symptoms. If the abscess has gone on to spontaneously drain, patients will report an improvement in the degree of pain associated with purulent drainage.

On physical examination, a perianal or ischiorectal abscess will often manifest as erythema, swelling, and fluctuance over the abscess. When not present, an intersphincteric or supralevator abscess should be suspected. Digital rectal examination in these cases reveals marked tenderness and a mass bulging into the anorectal lumen.

Anorectal abscesses are classified according to the potential space in which the purulence accumulates (Figure 2). Regardless of where they occur, the treatment of an abscess is drainage. Most perianal and ischiorectal abscesses can be drained in the office setting. Local anesthetic is infiltrated into the site of drainage, and the abscess cavity is unroofed by excising an ellipse of skin. Drainage is performed as close to the anus as possible so that if a fistula forms, a short fistula tract will persist. It is important to remove enough skin to prevent premature closure of the wound and reaccumulation of pus. Antibiotics are rarely needed and are reserved for use in conjunction with drainage in immunocompromised patients.

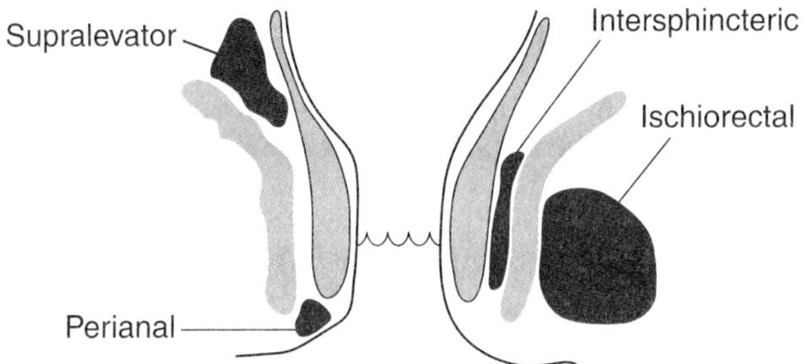

FIGURE 2 Potential spaces in which anorectal abscesses may occur.

Intersphincteric and supralevator abscesses require internal drainage. For an intersphincteric abscess, division of the internal anal sphincter overlying the abscess is performed. An intersphincteric abscess with supralevator extension should be drained into the anal canal to prevent the formation of a high transsphincteric fistula. Alternatively, an ischiorectal abscess that has crossed into the supralevator space should be drained externally to prevent the same high transsphincteric fistula from occurring.

Special mention should be made of a deep-post anal space abscess. Patients will complain of rectal pain that is exacerbated by bowel movements. Often, physical examination is unrevealing with the exception of severe tenderness with digital rectal examination. Alternatively, a deep postanal space may manifest as a horseshoe abscess as pus tracks into the ischiorectal spaces. In both situations drainage is best performed in the operating room. Dividing the lower portion of the internal anal sphincter in the posterior midline opens the deep postanal space. Counterincisions are made over the ischiorectal spaces to facilitate drainage.

Following surgical or spontaneous drainage, most abscesses heal without sequelae. Roughly 33%, however, proceed to fistula formation, which is a tunnel from the internal opening in the anal canal to the external opening at the site of drainage. Fistulas are classified in relation to the sphincter complex. An intersphincteric fistula traverses only the internal anal sphincter and accounts for 70% of anal fistulas. Transsphincteric anal fistulas traverse both the internal and external anal sphincter muscles and are the second most common type of anal fistulas. A suprasphincteric fistula arises in the anal canal, crosses the levator plate and then tracks down to the external opening on the skin. An extrasphincteric fistula is one whose origin is not within the anal canal, but rather starts in the abdomen or pelvis and passes down through the levator muscles and out to the skin. Such fistulae are uncommon and are most often caused by an inflammatory condition such as Crohn's disease or diverticulitis.

Patients with fistulas often complain of intermittent purulent drainage from the external sinus of fistula. They may experience cycles of pain and swelling followed by spontaneous drainage and a decrease in pain. This is caused by healing of the external sinus followed by reformation of a small abscess. When the pressure within the tract is great enough, drainage occurs. Examination will reveal the external opening of the fistula and palpation from the fistula toward the anus may reveal a cord. This represents the chronically inflamed fistula tract. Purulence may be expressed from the external opening with palpation or digital rectal examination. The internal opening of the fistula may be seen on anoscopy as a small punctum or area of inflammation. Gentle probing of the fistula may reveal the complete course of the tract—care should be taken not to force the probe into the anal canal and thereby creat a false passage. Injection of the external opening with hydrogen peroxide often facilitates identification of the internal opening. Complex fistulae may require investigation with endoanal ultrasonography or magnetic resonance imaging to identify the course of the tract or reveal accessory tracts.

Successful treatment of an anal fistula requires identification and elimination of the internal opening of the fistula. Once the internal opening is identified treatment can be planned. The choice of treatment is in part dictated by the amount of sphincter muscle involved. A superficial fistula that involves a small amount of muscle may be treated with a fistulotomy. The tract is unroofed, débrided, and left open to heal by secondary intention. If a significant amount of muscle is involved, a fistulotomy is avoided as division of the muscle may lead to fecal incontinence. Options for treatment of such fistulae include the placement of a seton (suture or vessel loop through the tract), an endorectal advancement flap, or the instillation of fibrin glue.

GASTRITIS AND PEPTIC ULCER DISEASE

METHOD OF

Barry J. Marshall, MD

Gastritis

Gastritis literally means inflammation of the stomach. Gastritis is a nonspecific term because it can be used to describe:

- Symptoms related to the stomach
- An endoscopic appearance of the gastric mucosa
- Histological change characterized by infiltration of the epithelium with inflammatory cells such as polymorphonuclear leukocytes (PMNs)

The last description is the most correct.

CLINICAL GASTRITIS

In lay terms, nausea and vomiting with epigastric pain might be called "an attack of gastritis," even though the exact pathology affecting the stomach is unknown. Use of the term gastritis in this situation is to be discouraged as symptoms correlate rather poorly with actual pathology present in the stomach.

ENDOSCOPIC GASTRITIS

Mucosal Redness (Erythema)

The appearance of the mucosa at endoscopy does not correlate well with the histological diagnosis determined from a biopsy. Confusion can arise because almost every abnormality of the gastric mucosa is called *gastritis* by endoscopists.

The normal color of the gastric mucosa is pink, similar to the palm of your hand. An appearance of redness probably represents increased capillary blood flow in the mucosa, but does not necessarily mean that inflammatory cells are present. When bile is present, the redness often appears to be diffusely present throughout the stomach.

Redness (erythema) in the gastric mucosa may be localized to the antrum or the corpus. It may be homogeneous or mottled, or present in spots from petechia size to a few millimeters. Sometimes redness is present on the top of the gastric folds of the corpus. Often, red streaks radiate upwards from the pylorus. In all cases it is appropriate for the endoscopist to refer to the appearance as *endoscopic gastritis*, accompanied by a description of gastric mucosa. General treatment of endoscopic gastritis is to treat the patient's symptoms, usually with acid reduction therapy and avoidance of foods or medications that might aggravate the problem. Specific treatment of endoscopic gastritis depends on a histologic diagnosis. Therefore, biopsies of the gastric mucosa are necessary.

Surface Irregularity (*Chicken Skin, Gooseflesh, Cobblestones*)

The cause of small lumps on the antral mucosa, which are referred to as *chicken skin, gooseflesh,* and *cobblestones*, is usually *Helicobacter pylori* gastritis.

Erosive Gastritis

Erosions are breaks in the mucosa that do not extend beyond the muscularis mucosa. All lesions less than 1 mm deep are erosions. The distinction between ulcers and erosions might not have much effect on patient management, because both can bleed and both are usually healed with acid blocking therapy.

Umbilicated lumps may be a variant of erosive gastritis. As with all erosive mucosal lesions of the gastrointestinal (GI) tract, viral causes should be considered in immunosuppressed patients.

Atrophic Gastritis and Gastric Atrophy

After many years of chronic gastritis, the gastric mucosa can become atrophic (i.e., thin and translucent), with the submucosal veins easily visible.

In severe cases, the folds normally present in the upper half of the stomach (the corpus) are diminished or absent (gastric atrophy). Acid secretion diminishes and the condition predisposes to adenocarcinoma of the stomach. *H. pylori* and pernicious anemia are the two main causes.

Hypertrophic Gastritis (Ménétrier's Disease)

Rarely, gastric folds are massively increased in size because of hyperplasia and hypertrophy of the specialized acid-secreting mucosa. Excessive mucus secretion leads to a syndrome of hypoalbuminemia with diarrhea, edema, or a hypercoagulable state. *H. pylori* infection is one cause, other cases are idiopathic (so far).

Portal Gastropathy and Angiodysplasia

The red lesions caused by portal gastropathy and angiodysplasia give a pattern of *snake skin* and *watermelon stomach*, respectively when severe. They may cause GI blood loss, but are usually asymptomatic. The former is associated with portal hypertension. The latter is idiopathic and is treated, when necessary, with argon plasma coagulation.

HISTOLOGIC GASTRITIS

Histologic gastritis is present when inflammatory cells infiltrate the mucosa. Diagnostic biopsies for detection of gastritis should be taken from intact mucosa, away from any focal lesion. At least one antrum and one corpus biopsy should be examined by histology because diseases can selectively affect only the mucus-secreting mucosa of the antrum, or only the parietal cell mucosa of the corpus.

If mononuclear cells are increased, *chronic gastritis* is present. If the PMNs are also increased, the gastritis is termed as *active*. In typical *H. pylori* infection, PMNs infiltrate the necks of the mucus-secreting glands of the gastric antrum causing *active chronic gastritis*.

Helicobacter pylori Gastritis

In the first week after infection, many PMNs and a few eosinophils infiltrate the mucosa. These are gradually replaced with the mononuclear cells. The presence of lymphoid follicles is called *mucosa-associated lymphoid tissue* (MALT). Rarely, MALT may become autonomous to form a low-grade, B-cell lymphoma called *MALT lymphoma*. When gastric tissue exists in the duodenal bulb (normally present in approximately 60% of persons), *H. pylori* may also colonize that location leading to active duodenitis.

When *H. pylori* is eradicated with antibiotics, PMNs disappear in a week or so, but reduction in the mononuclear cells is slow, often leaving mild chronic gastritis several years after *H. pylori* has disappeared.

In most countries with a high prevalence of *H. pylori*, gastric cancer is common, although diet probably also modulates the risk so that the association is not universal. Because *H. pylori* causes peptic ulcer and gastric cancer, nearly everyone with *H. pylori* chooses to be treated with antibiotics.

Non-*Helicobacter pylori* Gastritis

Because *H. pylori* is the most common cause of gastritis, and perhaps the most easily treated, non-*H. pylori* gastritis must be diagnosed with caution. Usually the *H. pylori* has been missed because of low numbers of organisms. This occurs when patients have recently taken antibiotics, or are taking proton pump inhibitors (PPIs), or have a patchy infection caused by intestinal metaplasia in the stomach (to which *H. pylori* cannot adhere). Therefore, as well as taking biopsies for urease test, histology, and culture, the physician should check serology before claiming a patient has *H. pylori*-negative histologic gastritis. Laboratory-based serologic tests are quite sensitive so can be used to confirm that *H. pylori* is not present and that the negative biopsy diagnosis is correct.

Rare causes of *H. pylori*-negative histologic gastritis are Crohn's disease, eosinophilic gastritis, gastric MALT lymphoma, as well as (very rarely) other viral and bacterial infections.

NONSTEROIDAL-INDUCED EROSIVE GASTRITIS AND ULCERS

Aspirin and nonsteroidal anti-inflammatory drugs (NSAIDs) are corrosive. Aspirin and NSAIDs inhibit prostaglandin synthesis, which is essential for maintenance of the mucus and bicarbonate barrier in the stomach. The resulting gastric erosions are often asymptomatic but sometimes lead to gastric ulcer or duodenal ulcer.

The harmful effects of NSAIDs and *H. pylori* are not synergistic because *H. pylori* boosts the prostaglandin levels, thus partially negating the deleterious effect of the NSAID.

Eradication of *H. pylori* before or at the beginning of NSAID therapy is worthwhile. Once NSAID patients have developed an ulcer, provided that treatment of the ulcer with a PPI is continued, eradication of *H. pylori* is neither urgent nor essential.

DYSPEPSIA VERSUS GASTRITIS

Dyspepsia is defined here as discomfort in the upper half of the abdomen and lower chest that is somehow related to food. Symptoms and descriptions vary widely so the patient's ethnicity needs to be taken into account when taking a history.

Regurgitation refers to reflux of gastric contents into the mouth without discomfort. Gnawing is a feeling halfway between hunger and nausea, in which case the patient tends to have small snacks to ease the symptom without vomiting. Fullness and bloating are feelings of distension that contribute to early satiety in some patients so that they are unable to finish a normal-sized meal. Burning epigastric and lower thoracic pain that is quickly relieved by antacid is likely to be caused by gastroesophageal reflux disease (GERD), although it is wise to exclude a cardiac cause.

In general, dyspepsia correlates poorly with endoscopic findings. When endoscopy is freely available at no cost to the patient, endoscopy quickly defines a management plan and gives greater patient satisfaction, according to questionnaires given to patients 12 months later. However, endoscopy-first strategies are about 20% more expensive.

The alternative strategy is called *test and treat*, where patients are selected for initial endoscopy only if they have *alarm signs*, are older than 50 years of age, or are in a high-risk category for gastric cancer. Alarm signs are dysphagia, vomiting, weight loss, blood in the stool, a family history of gastric cancer, an abdominal mass, or virtually any abnormal laboratory test.

When dyspepsia is diagnosed but there is no peptic ulcer, the condition is called *nonulcer dyspepsia* (NUD) or *functional dyspepsia*. Many NUD patients actually have GERD. If GERD is suspected, a 7-day trial of double-dose PPI therapy is worthwhile.

For patients not obviously suffering from GERD, the possibility of peptic ulcer should be considered. Because most peptic ulcers are related to *H. pylori* infection, noninvasive tests for *H. pylori* can be used to determine ulcer risk. Patients who are *H. pylori*-negative on serology are unlikely to have peptic ulcer. This means that they can be managed by trial and error until symptoms respond to therapy. On the other hand, patients who are *H. pylori*-positive on serology should be regarded as possible ulcer candidates and should have the bacterium eradicated as the first step in management.

For patients who actually do have an ulcer, antibiotic therapy for *H. pylori* leads to clinical cure in approximately 70% of cases. Of the 30% who do not respond clinically, 50% have persistent *H. pylori* and the remainder have *H. pylori*-negative dyspepsia (GERD, etc.). To differentiate these groups it is necessary to confirm cure of *H. pylori* in all patients who do not completely respond to *H. pylori* eradication. Cure is confirmed with a urea breath test. Follow-up breath test is also necessary in all patients with known peptic ulcer because these patients are at risk of ulcer relapse, with all its possible complications, if *H. pylori* persists. Because a nonendoscopic strategy does not separate ulcer from nonulcer patients at the beginning, there is a case for confirmation of *H. pylori* eradication in all patients, so that ulcer relapse never occurs.

GASTROESOPHAGEAL REFLUX DISEASE

Gastroesophageal reflux disease and symptoms related to the esophagus may be treated initially with acid reduction therapy, as needed. Antacid is used for immediate relief, and histamine-2 receptor antagonists (H_2RAs) or PPIs may be given at the same time to diminish acid secretion over the next few hours. Combinations or these two are available as over-the-counter (OTC) medications in the United States. If dysphagia is present (difficulty swallowing), immediate endoscopy is advised as this could be an early symptom of esophageal cancer or an acid-induced stricture.

If GERD symptoms do not completely respond, or if the patient requires the above treatment on a daily basis, then endoscopy is required. Endoscopy will indicate whether the patient's symptoms correlate with the disease severity. It is important to control both clinical and endoscopic GERD, because continued heartburn raises the lifetime risk of esophageal adenocarcinoma.

GERD patients should be given the following common-sense advice. Eat smaller meals, control obesity, and avoid tight clothing around the abdomen. Avoid liquids with meals, especially tea, coffee, colas, and beer. Do not eat large meals during the working day. Avoid bending or heavy work after meals. Eat the evening meal at least 3 hours before bedtime. Raise the head of the bed and sleep on the left side. Tablets that might damage the esophagus (aspirin, doxycycline, alendronate) should be taken before meals to ensure that they do not linger in the esophagus.

In spite of the above management, many patients continue to have symptoms and endoscopic assessment reveals acid-induced esophageal damage. In this case lifestyle measures are rarely curative and long-term acid reduction with PPI is required. Since PPIs have long half-lives, once-daily therapy is usually sufficient. For severe GERD, start at double the usual dose then decrease after 3 months to a single daily maintenance dose. The aim of medical therapy is complete control of acidic symptoms. Advise patients that long-term medical treatment is usually necessary.

OTHER DYSPEPSIA

Because chronic dyspeptic symptoms unrelated to GERD or ulcer do not have a specific cause or defined therapy, it is worthwhile initially to search for another, more treatable diagnosis. Be certain to exclude cardiac causes of chest pain. Intermittent pain could be esophageal spasm, which can be diagnosed with esophageal manometry. Treat with PPI to abolish any GERD component, smooth muscle relaxants for the acute episode, and calcium channel blockers (CCBs). Note that therapy for angina is quite similar, so cardiac disease needs to be ruled out before treating esophageal spasm. Some of the above medical therapy causes side effects that make treatment hardly worthwhile in patients with intermittent spasm.

EPIGASTRIC DYSPEPSIA AND GASTROPARESIS

Always try to find the definitive causes of epigastric dyspepsia and gastroparesis, as this allows better planning of therapy and more accurate prognosis. Endoscopy often rules out any macroscopic lesion such as an ulcer or a tumor, allowing trials of medical therapy to proceed.

If the patient has symptoms of GERD, but does not respond completely to therapy, he/she may be a rapid metabolizer of PPI. If starting with once-daily omeprazole (Prilosec), double the dose to twice daily, use a more powerful drug (esomeprazole [Nexium]), choose one with a longer half-life (pantoprazole [Protonix]), or a use a drug that is less affected by metabolizer status (rabeprazole [Aciphex]). At endoscopy, avoid PPI on the day of the test and measure gastric-juice pH to see if the patient maintains a pH above 4 for the complete 24 hours after a dose. If pH is above 4.0, then the cause of the continued symptoms might not be acid reflux.

Symptoms of nausea and/or vomiting are unlikely to be caused by esophageal disease. Gastric mucosal problems or gastric outlet obstruction need to be considered. The two should be considered separately because disorders such as acute viral gastroenteritis and food poisoning cause nausea, but motility is normal. Similarly, patients with chronic gastroparesis are worse off if they also have a mucosal disease such as *H. pylori* causing the nausea.

If *H. pylori* is present it should be treated. If patients cannot take antibiotics because of nausea, try to settle them with high-dose PPI as this will suppress *H. pylori* in 50% of cases.

Delayed gastric emptying (gastroparesis) may be diagnosed with an isotope gastric emptying study. When present, gastroparesis is usually a chronic disorder with relapses and remissions. Eradication of *H. pylori* often decreases nausea and settles the condition somewhat, but relapses still occur in most patients. Promotility agents such as metoclopramide (Reglan) and cisapride (Propulsid)* should be used (cisapride is no longer available in the United States because it has caused fatal arrhythmias). Small doses of erythromycin[1] (25 mg per day before meals) may improve gastric peristalsis as this drug is a motilin agonist. As long as obstruction is not present, a soft or liquid diet will usually empty from the stomach, even when motility is poor. Posturing the patient to stay vertical after meals, with an inclination toward the right side, should help gastric contents drain through the pylorus. Avoid uncooked vegetables because skins and salad leaves take many hours to leave the stomach. A low-residue diet is preferred whenever motility is impaired.

Management of Dyspepsia

I usually include a *test and treat* strategy for *H. pylori* as part of any dyspepsia management plan. I also search for and treat GERD with PPI. Lesser symptoms of GERD or vague dyspepsia may respond (if needed) to H_2 blocker such as ranitidine (Zantac), 150 mg once or twice daily. In addition, patients can carry antacid tablets for immediate relief. Antacid-H_2RA combinations are available OTC in the United States, and these are very effective. The complete algorithm for management of dyspepsia is shown as Figure 1.

Peptic Ulcer

Peptic ulcer is usually caused by *H. pylori*, NSAID, or a combination of the two. Rarely, hyperacidity is caused by a gastrinoma (Zollinger-Ellison syndrome) in which case a cause may not be found until serum gastrin is noted to be elevated. In any ulcer situation, resuscitate the patient and control acute bleeding endoscopically. At the first endoscopy, diagnostic biopsies should be taken for *H. pylori* (one urease test, one antrum, and one corpus for histology). If *H. pylori* is present, initiate treatment. *H. pylori* serology should be sent if the bacterium is not detected on biopsy because sometimes the acutely ill patient has taken medication, which suppresses *H. pylori* in the gastric mucosa, but has not eradicated the bacterium.

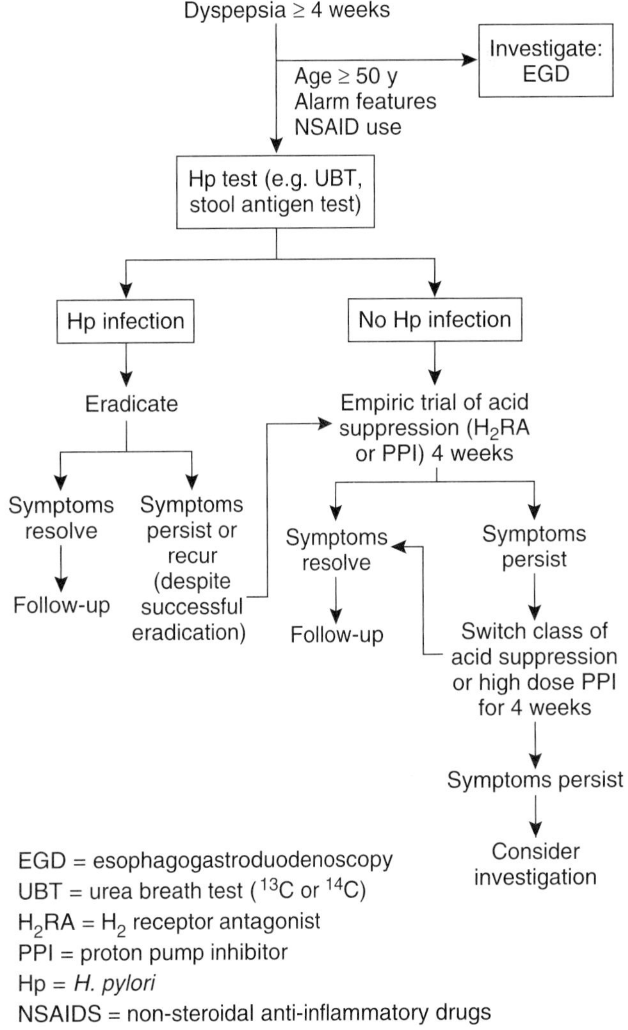

FIGURE 1 Management of uninvestigated dyspepsia.

[1]Not FDA approved for this indication.
*Investigational drug in the United States.

Ulcer patients without *H. pylori* usually have NSAIDs as the cause of the ulcer. In patients who have both *H. pylori* and NSAID, the sensible approach is to treat both. In most cases the NSAID will have been ceased and the patient given intravenous PPI, so antibiotic therapy is not the most important part of the acute therapy. Adding intravenous amoxicillin to an *H. pylori*-positive patient is an option to improve the healing rate of a dangerous ulcer. The normal oral *H. pylori* therapy can be completed a few days later when the patient tolerates a normal diet.

Peptic ulcers almost always heal once the initiating factor has been removed. However, it is usual to give H_2RA or PPI for 8 weeks to ensure a symptom-free healing period. During this time the *H. pylori* can be eradicated. At the end of 8 weeks, PPI can be changed to H_2RA, and a follow-up urea breath test can be done to confirm eradication of the bacterium. A stool antigen test is an alternative.

In patients who are unable to cease their NSAIDs, the drug should be changed to a cyclooxygenase (COX)-2 selective agent. In addition, full-dose PPI should be continued long term. Most ulcers will then heal and not relapse. Low-dose aspirin may remove the benefit of COX-2 selective NSAIDs so the relative benefits of aspirin should be reviewed in all patients. Prostaglandins are not a first choice ulcer therapy because of side effects, such as cramps (in women) and diarrhea; however, they do specifically protect against erosive gastritis and peptic ulcer caused solely by NSAIDs.

TREATMENT FOR *HELICOBACTER PYLORI*

In vitro testing does not correlate with in vivo success, so treatment combinations should be used that have been proven to work in each individual country. Treatment for less than 7 days has a low cure rate, but cure rates from day 7 to day 14 are similar, and more than 14 days of treatment is usually unnecessary. The first drug to use is a PPI in order to render the gastric pH neutral. This enhances the cure rate for the second drug, which is usually amoxicillin (Amoxil). Clarithromycin (Biaxin) is given as the third drug. Treatment and doses vary in each country; doses in Table 1 are typical for the United States and Australia.

TABLE 1 Treatment Options for *Helicobacter pylori*

Group		Duration
A*	BISMUTH	
	Ranitidine bismuth citrate[2] (RBC) 400 mg bid	14 days
	Bismuth subsalicylate (Pepto Bismol)* 525 mg (2 tabs) qid	14 days
	Bismuth subcitrate[1,†] (De-Nol) 120 mg (1 tab) qid	14 days
B	PENICILLIN	
	Amoxicillin 1 g bid	7, 10 or 14 days
C	MACROLIDE	
	Clarithromycin (Biaxin) 500 mg bid	7, 10 or 14 days
	Josamycin[1,2,†] 1000 mg bid	7 days
D	NITROIMIDAZOLE	
	Metronidazole (Flagyl)[1] 500 mg bid or tid	7, 10 or 14 days
	Tinidazole[1,2] 1000 mg od	7, 10 or 14 days
E	TETRACYCLINE	
	Tetracycline[1] 500 mg qid	14 days
F	QUINOLONE	
	Ofloxacin (Floxin)[1] 1000 mg[3] od	7-14 days
	Levofloxacin (Levaquin) 500 mg od	7-14 days
	Ciprofloxacin (Cipro)[1] 500 mg bid	14 days
G	NITROFURANS	
	Furazolidone (Furoxone)[1] 100 mg qid	7, 10 or 14 days
H	ANSAMYCIN	
	Rifabutin (Mycobutin)[1] 150 mg bid	14 days
I	**Proton pump inhibitors** (use double a normal dose)	
	Omeprazole (Prilosec) 20 mg bid	
	Esomeprazole (Nexium) 40 mg bid	
	Lansoprazole (Prevacid) 30 mg bid	
	Pantoprazole (Protonix) 40 mg bid	
	Rabeprazole (Aciphex) 20 mg bid	

[1]Not FDA approved for this indication.
[2]Not available in the United States.
[3]Exceeds dosage recommended by the manufacturer.
*When Pepto Bismol is not available, substitute De-Nol, 1 tablet qid. RBC is not available in all countries.
Side effects are likely as doses of clarithromycin, metronidazole, and furazolidone increase.
Treatment combination priorities are normally: IBC → IBD → IBEG. For penicillin allergy choose ICD or IAED → IFH.
†Investigational drug in the United States.
Abbreviations: bid = twice daily; od = once daily; qid = four times daily; tid = thrice daily.

One month after completing therapy, ensure that the patient is not taking PPI for 7 days, and then perform a urea breath test (UBT). Serology remains positive after treatment so it is not useful to prove eradication. If the UBT shows persistent infection, re-treat with a different regimen. As a second therapy, you may use PPI and amoxicillin again, since *H. pylori* does not develop resistance to amoxicillin. The third drug should change to metronidazole (Flagyl)[1]. Always repeat the UBT after therapy.

If two therapies fail, the *H. pylori* is resistant to both clarithromycin[1] and metronidazole[1]; therefore, alternatives must be chosen. In addition, the motivation of the patient and physician need to be reassessed as compliance may be an issue. A third treatment changes the PPI to a much higher dose and/or a drug less affected by the metabolizer status of the patient. Rabeprazole (Aciphex), 20 mg twice daily, might be a good choice. Amoxicillin is given as before. In addition, add ofloxacin (Floxin)[1] or levofloxacin (Levaquin)[1] plus rifabutin (Mycobutin)[1], with all four drugs being given for 14 days.

An alternative and inexpensive regimen is bismuth (Pepto-Bismol) with tetracycline[1], metronidazole (Flagyl)[1], and a PPI. This is also called *bismuth quad therapy*. It is useful also when patients are allergic to penicillin. Allergic patients might also try PPI with clarithromycin (Biaxin)[1] and metronidazole[1] as the initial therapy. If patients are unable to take oral antibiotics because of nausea, start with a harmless drug such as PPI or bismuth, and then add tetracycline[1] or amoxicillin (Amoxil). After 1 week, by which time symptoms have improved, add the clarithromycin[1] or metronidazole[1]. If all else fails, high-dose PPI will suppress *H. pylori* in 30% to 50% of patients. Alternatively, because biopsy and culture with antibiotic sensitivity testing are necessary, refer patients to a gastroenterologist specializing in *H. pylori*.

After *H. pylori* eradication, symptoms are still present in most patients, but improve gradually over 3 to 6 months. GERD symptoms may temporarily worsen, so I treat these symptoms with H_2 blockers initially because this does not interfere with the follow-up UBT. If symptoms persist then the patient is managed as *H. pylori*-negative dyspepsia as per the algorithm in Figure 1.

[1]Not FDA approved for this indication.

ACUTE AND CHRONIC VIRAL HEPATITIS

METHOD OF

Jacqueline G. O'Leary, MD, and

Lawrence S. Friedman, MD

Viral hepatitis is of particular concern to the primary care physician because of its high prevalence in the general population. There are five classic hepatotropic viruses, designated A, B, C, D, and E. Whereas hepatitis A (HAV) and hepatitis E (HEV) viruses cause only acute hepatitis, hepatitis B (HBV), C (HCV), and D (HDV) viruses may also cause chronic hepatitis. Several other viruses, including hepatitis G virus, transfusion-transmitted virus (TTV), and SEN virus may infect the liver, but there is little evidence that these viruses cause clinical liver disease. Other viruses such as cytomegalovirus (CMV) and Epstein-Barr virus (EBV) lead to systemic illness with varying degrees of hepatic involvement. The focus of this article is on hepatitis A, B, C, D, and E (Table 1).

Acute Viral Hepatitis

HEPATITIS A

Virology

HAV is a positive single-stranded RNA virus classified as a *Hepatovirus* in the picornavirus family. This virus infects humans as well as nonhuman primates and is transmitted by the fecal-oral route. Acquisition of infection is followed by a 2- to 6-week (average 4 weeks) incubation period, with viral shedding starting in the second week and typically declining with the onset of jaundice. HAV causes only acute hepatitis, and after recovery long-lasting immunity develops.

Epidemiology

HAV is common worldwide, with a seroprevalence rate for past exposure of 99% to 100% in countries with poor sanitation and 33% in the United States. Infection in the first few years of life is asymptomatic in 90% of cases, whereas acquisition in adulthood engenders a higher likelihood of symptomatic disease. Risk factors for HAV infection include consumption of contaminated water or shellfish, travel to endemic areas, contact with infected food handlers, household contact, male homosexual activity, and intravenous drug use. The attack rate is 70% to 90% in those exposed, and outbreaks often occur in residential and daycare centers. In 2003, a large food-borne outbreak

TABLE 1 The Hepatitis Viruses

	HAV	HBV	HCV	HDV	HEV
Viral Properties					
Size (nm)	27	42	≈55	≈36	≈32
Nucleic acid	RNA	DNA	RNA	RNA	RNA
Genome length (kb)	7.5	3.2	9.4	1.7	7.5
Classification	Picornavirus	Hepadnavirus	*Flavivirus*	Viroid	*Calicivirus*
Incubation period (days)	15-45	30-180	15-160	21-140	14-63
Transmission					
Fecal-oral	+++	—	—	—	+++
Percutaneous	Rare	+++	+++	+++	—
Sexual (anal intercourse)	+	++	+	++	—
Perinatal	—	+++	+	+	—
Clinical Features					
Severity	Usually mild	Moderate	Mild	May be severe	Usually mild
Chronic infection	No	1%-2%; up to 90% in neonates	85%	Common	No
Carrier state	No	Yes	Yes	Yes	No
Fulminant hepatitis	0.10%	1%	Rare	Up to 20% in superinfection	1%-2% (10%-20%) in pregnant women)
Hepatocellular carcinoma	No	Yes	Yes	Yes	No
Prophylaxis	IG, vaccine	HBIG, vaccine	None	HBV vaccine	None

Abbreviations: HAV, HBV, HCV, HDV, HEV = hepatitis A, B, C, D, E (respectively) virus; HBIG = hepatitis B immune globulin; IG = immune globulin.

in the United States was traced to consumption of green onions imported from Mexico.

Clinical Features

Patients with acute hepatitis A often complain of fatigue, nausea, and vomiting, occasionally accompanied by fever. Extrahepatic manifestations may include rash (14%) and arthralgias (11%). Infrequently occurring immune complex-mediated complications include leukocytoclastic vasculitis, glomerulonephritis, and arthritis. Typical laboratory abnormalities include serum aminotransferase elevations of more than 500 U/L and a rise in the bilirubin level. Liver biochemical elevations generally decline to normal within several weeks, although the bilirubin elevation can last for several months. In rare instances, HAV infection is characterized by profound hyperbilirubinemia (more than 20 mg/dL). Occasionally, biochemical and serologic relapses can occur, but (unless the disease proves fatal) ultimate recovery and seroconversion are inevitable.

The case fatality rate for acute hepatitis A varies with age, from 0.1% in children to 1.1% in adults older than 40 years. In patients with underlying liver disease (e.g., chronic hepatitis C), the mortality rate is higher.

Diagnosis

The diagnosis of acute hepatitis A is based on the detection of immune globulin (Ig) M antibody to HAV (IgM anti-HAV) in serum. IgM anti-HAV typically lasts for 3 to 6 months (rarely longer), after which IgG anti-HAV predominates, persists, and confers long-lasting immunity.

Prevention

Vaccines derived from inactivated virus are effective and provide long-lasting immunity (for at least 20 years). Antibodies develop 2 to 3 weeks after the first dose, and a booster dose is given 6 to 12 months after the initial dose. Persons who should receive the vaccine include travelers to endemic areas, health care providers, military personnel, men who have sex with men, intravenous drug users, inhabitants or staff of residential institutions, and children residing in states with a high incidence of HAV infection.

Immunoprophylaxis with immune globulin, in a dose of 0.02 mL/kg by intramuscular injection, is indicated for unvaccinated intimate (including household and residential) contacts of patients with acute hepatitis A. Because immune globulin provides only temporary passive immunity, recipients also need to be vaccinated.

HEPATITIS B

Virology

HBV is a partially double-stranded DNA virus belonging to the hepadnavirus family. Eight viral genotypes have been identified, A-H. The HBV genome consists of four open reading frames (ORFs): S (surface), C (core), P (polymerase), and X. The S gene encodes three proteins:

- The S protein (hepatitis B surface antigen [HBsAg]) is an envelope protein and also circulates as excess spheres and tubules.
- The L protein plays a role in binding the virus to the hepatocyte.
- The M protein has an unknown function.

The C gene encodes both the nucleocapsid core protein (hepatitis B core antigen [HBcAg]) and its secretory product, e antigen (hepatitis B e antigen [HBeAg]). The P ORF is translated into the HBV DNA polymerase, whereas the X gene encodes a transactivating protein that activates a variety of cellular and viral promoters, including the HBV genome itself.

Several mutations in HBV lead to clinically important viral variants. A mutation in a critical epitope of HBsAg results in decreased affinity of anti-HBs for HBsAg. This mutation accounts for occasional cases of acute hepatitis B following apparently successful vaccine-induced seroconversion. Mutations in the precore or core region lead to lack of production of HBeAg. Patients infected with precore and core variants have high serum levels of HBV DNA despite the absence of HBeAg and the presence of antibody to HBeAg (anti-HBe) in serum. These mutations often arise during the course of chronic infection by wild-type HBV, presumably as a result of immune pressure. The clinical course of infection caused by precore and core mutant viruses is often (but not invariably) characterized by severe chronic hepatitis B, rapid progression to cirrhosis, and only temporary response to antiviral therapy. A mutation of the P gene (the YMDD motif) confers resistance to the antiviral agent lamivudine (see *Chronic Hepatitis B, Treatment*).

Epidemiology

Approximately 300,000 new cases of hepatitis B occur in the United States each year. The majority of cases occur as a result of heterosexual sex (36%), illicit drug use (13%), male homosexual activity (11%), household contact (3%), health care employment (2%), tattoos, acupuncture, and dialysis. Transfusion-associated HBV infection is infrequent with a rate of less than 1 case per 60,000 units of blood transfused. However, household contact transmission may occur through cuts, bites, and sharing of blood-contaminated objects, in addition to sexual relations, because HBV can be found in infectious concentrations in blood, semen, vaginal secretions, and saliva. In endemic areas, such as parts of sub-Saharan Africa, Southeast Asia, and the South Pacific, transmission occurs most commonly during the perinatal period and in infancy. Children born to mothers with high levels of virus in serum have a 70% to 90% acquisition rate; this rate can be decreased to 5% to 10% with active and passive immunization. In endemic areas, HBV carrier rates often exceed 5%, and in some hyperendemic regions rates may exceed 25%.

Clinical Features

After exposure, the incubation period of acute hepatitis B is 2 to 6 months. Acute hepatitis B may be clinically silent in up to 90% of cases, particularly when acquired early in life. In patients who develop acute hepatitis, the risk of fulminant hepatic failure is less than 1%. Infection in immunocompetent adults is associated with clearance of the virus and recovery in more than 98% of cases. By contrast, perinatal transmission or infection in infancy results in chronic infection in up to 90% of cases, and infection in early childhood leads to chronic infection in approximately 30% of cases. Immunocompromised adults also have a high rate of progression to chronic infection. The course of acute hepatitis B may be complicated by immune-complex mediated phenomena, including arthritis, a serum-sickness-like illness, polyarteritis nodosa, and membranous glomerulonephritis with nephrotic syndrome.

Diagnosis

The diagnosis of acute hepatitis B is based on the detection of HBsAg and IgM antibody to HBcAg (IgM anti-HBc) in serum. IgM anti-HBc persists for approximately 6 months. Thereafter, whether the patient has recovered or progressed to chronic hepatitis B, anti-HBc of the IgG class (IgG anti-HBc) predominates and remains detectable indefinitely. With recovery, HBsAg declines in titer and ultimately disappears, with the development of antibody to hepatitis B surface antigen (anti-HBs). Testing for HBeAg is not necessary for the diagnosis of acute hepatitis B, but its persistence for longer than 3 to 4 months signifies an increased likelihood of progression to chronic hepatitis B.

Conventional serologic testing is usually sufficient for the diagnosis of acute hepatitis B; however, in select cases measurement of HBV DNA in serum may be useful, as in patients with undetectable HBeAg (but presence of anti-HBe) despite persistently elevated serum aminotransferase levels. In such instances, the absence of HBV DNA in serum would be consistent with seroconversion from HBeAg to anti-HBe, whereas detection of HBV DNA in serum would suggest evolution to a pre-core or core mutation. Quantitative assays for HBV DNA in serum can also be used to identify patients with chronic hepatitis B who are likely to respond to therapy with interferon α; specifically, persons with high aminotransferase levels and HBV DNA levels less than 200 pg/mL, and especially those with levels less than 100 pg/mL (see *Chronic Hepatitis B, Treatment*).

Prevention

Genetically engineered recombinant HBV vaccines are currently recommended for all infants in the United States as well as all unvaccinated children and high-risk adults, such as health care workers, dialysis patients, intravenous drug users, hemophiliacs, men who have sex with men, sexually promiscuous persons, and contacts of HBV carriers. Standard vaccination consists of three intramuscular injections at 0, 1, and 6 months given in doses (depending on the formulation) of 10 or 20 μg for adults (a double dose is administered to immunosuppressed persons) and 5 or 10 μg for children younger than 10 years. (Thimerosal-free vaccines are recommended for infants younger than 6 months old.) The vaccine failure rate is 5% to 10%. Factors that reduce vaccine responsiveness include age older than 40 years, obesity, smoking, immunosuppression, alcoholism, and chronic renal failure. Adult nonresponsiveness to the HBV vaccine is sometimes genetically determined, whereas perinatal nonresponsiveness is often overcome by revaccination in early childhood. One month after the third vaccine injection, seroconversion can be verified by confirming the presence of anti-HBs in serum.

Although levels of anti-HBs following HBV vaccination decline over time and may fall below the seroprotective threshold, re-exposure to HBV usually leads to an anamnestic response, or, in rare instances, subclinical infection. As a result, routine booster immunization of previously vaccinated persons has not been recommended, except in immunocompromised patients.

For unvaccinated or nonimmune individuals who sustain an exposure to HBV, postexposure prophylaxis with hepatitis B immune globulin (HBIG), in a dose of 0.06 mL/kg for an adult, followed by initiation of the hepatitis B vaccine series is recommended. In an exposed individual who has been vaccinated previously, serum anti-HBs levels should be measured and a vaccine booster dose given to persons with circulating antibody levels less than 10 mIU/mL.

HEPATITIS C

Virology

HCV is a positive single-stranded RNA *Flavivirus* that accounts for the majority of cases previously labeled as non-A, non-B hepatitis. To date, six genotypes of HCV have been defined; these vary in prevalence in different parts of the world and in responsiveness to therapy with interferon α (see *Chronic Hepatitis C, Treatment*). Within each genotype there is considerable genetic variability (quasispecies). During replication, the genome is translated into a single polypeptide that is subsequently cleaved into structural (E1, E2, and nucleocapsid) and nonstructural (helicase, RNA-dependent RNA polymerase, and two proteases) proteins by cellular and viral proteases. Many of these viral products are targets of novel therapeutic agents.

Epidemiology

Like HBV, HCV is a blood-borne infection. Transmission occurs predominantly through exchange of body fluids. In the United States patients with a history of intravenous drug use, blood transfusion, piercings, tattoos, and intranasal cocaine use represent high-risk populations. Outside the United States reuse of medical equipment without proper high-level disinfection is an additional risk factor. Vertical transmission from infected mother to neonate is uncommon, and sexual transmission may occur in heterosexual couples at a rate of approximately 1% per year. The risk of vertical and sexual transmission may correlate with the level of viremia at the time of exposure. Needlestick injuries can lead to infection in health care workers with approximately a 4% risk of transmission. Since 1991, blood has been tested for HCV in the United States, and the risk of HCV infection from a transfusion is now only 1 in 2 million units transfused.

Clinical Features

Acute HCV infection is often asymptomatic, and serum aminotransferase elevations may be mild (100 to 300 U/L). If symptomatic acute hepatitis C develops, it usually occurs 4 to 12 weeks after exposure. Patients with jaundice are more likely to clear the virus spontaneously than are those who remain asymptomatic.

A variety of extrahepatic manifestations of chronic HCV infection have been described. These include cryoglobulinemia, membranoproliferative glomerulonephritis, vasculitis, urticaria, erythema nodosum, lymphocytic sialadenitis, neuropathy, idiopathic pulmonary fibrosis, autoimmune thyroiditis, and lymphoma. Anticardiolipin antibodies have been detected in 20% of patients with chronic HCV infection and may be associated with thrombosis and thrombocytopenia. Other antibodies, such as antinuclear and anti-smooth muscle antibodies, are often detected, although usually in low titers. In addition, the risk of type 2 diabetes mellitus is increased in persons with chronic hepatitis C.

Diagnosis

The diagnosis of both acute and chronic hepatitis C is based on the detection of antibody to HCV (anti-HCV) by enzyme immunoassay (EIA) in serum. However, both false-positive and false-negative results occur. When a false-negative anti-HCV result is suspected, as may occur early in the course of acute hepatitis C, detection of HCV RNA by a qualitative polymerase chain reaction (PCR) assay can confirm the diagnosis. When a false-positive anti-HCV result is suspected, as in patients with hypergammaglobulinemia, HCV RNA will not be found, and a recombinant immunoblot assay (RIBA) for anti-HCV will be negative. Moreover, treatment of the autoimmune disorder or malignancy causing hypergammaglobulinemia will often lead to disappearance of the false-positive anti-HCV EIA result as globulin levels in serum decline.

In any patient with anti-HCV by EIA in serum, HCV RNA by a PCR assay should be ordered to confirm viremia. The qualitative PCR assay for HCV RNA is highly sensitive. A quantitative PCR assay for HCV RNA can be ordered to determine the level of viremia, which correlates inversely with responsiveness to antiviral treatment of chronic hepatitis C.

In approximately 15% of patients with acute hepatitis C, HCV RNA is cleared from serum spontaneously. These patients continue to have anti-HCV in serum (without HCV RNA) and are considered to have resolved infection. (Similarly, patients with chronic hepatitis C who are cured with antiviral treatment will have detectable anti-HCV indefinitely without HCV RNA in serum.) By contrast, approximately 85% of patients with acute hepatitis C progress to chronic hepatitis C with persistence of HCV RNA in serum.

Prevention

Prevention of HCV transmission is accomplished primarily by the avoidance of risk factors. For example, sexually active patients should be advised to use condoms. To date, there is no vaccine or postexposure prophylaxis for HCV infection outside clinical trials. Treatment with interferon α for 4 weeks has been used after needlestick injuries, but the benefit of this approach is uncertain because the risk of HCV transmission by needlestick is low; studies of postexposure treatment with peginterferon[1] are ongoing.

HEPATITIS D

Virology

HDV, or the delta agent, is a positive single-stranded RNA virus (viroid) that requires HBsAg to spread from one hepatocyte to another and is therefore found only in patients infected with HBV.

Epidemiology

HDV is spread through percutaneous routes and sexual contact. Areas of higher prevalence include Eastern Europe, South America, and Western Asia. In the United States HDV is uncommon and found predominantly in intravenous drug users and hemophiliacs.

Clinical Features and Diagnosis

Simultaneous infection with HBV and HDV is called coinfection, whereas acquisition of HDV after HBV is termed superinfection. Although the course of acute HDV/HBV coinfection is similar in severity to that of acute HBV infection alone, HDV superinfection of an HBsAg-positive carrier may be aggressive, leading to the rapid development of cirrhosis.

The diagnosis of HDV infection is based on the detection of antibody to HDV (anti-HDV). In acute HDV/HBV coinfection, anti-HDV may be present in serum only transiently or in low titer. Coinfection classically leads to a biphasic increase in serum aminotransferase levels that is not often seen in acute HBV infection alone. Coinfection may occasionally result in fulminant hepatic failure, although recovery usually leads to resolution of both HBV and HDV infections.

HDV superinfection is typically associated with a uniphasic elevation of serum aminotransferase levels, high and sustained titers of anti-HDV, and subsequent chronicity of both HDV and HBV infections.

Prevention

No specific measures are available to prevent HDV infection in an HBV carrier, but vaccination against HBV protects immunized persons from HDV infection by preventing HBV infection.

HEPATITIS E

Virology and Epidemiology

HEV is a positive single-stranded RNA virus of the *Calicivirus* family. Like HAV, HEV is spread by the fecal-oral route and causes only acute, not chronic, hepatitis. However, unlike HAV infection, person-to-person spread of HEV is uncommon. HEV is an important cause of epidemic (often water borne) acute viral hepatitis as well as sporadic disease in many parts of Central America, Asia, and the Indian subcontinent. The incubation period after infection is 15 to 60 days, and fecal shedding of the virus continues for 4 weeks after patients become symptomatic. Two percent of Wisconsin blood donors were found to be positive for antibodies to HEV, but in most cases the source of the antibody response was unclear.

Clinical Features, Diagnosis, and Prevention

Clinically overt hepatitis E occurs most often in persons 15 to 40 years of age. For unknown reasons, the mortality rate is particularly high (10% to 20%) in pregnant women. Reliable diagnostic tools are not yet widely available. In research settings, patients have been demonstrated to mount a short-lived IgM antibody to HEV (anti-HEV) response and then a sustained IgG anti-HEV response to the virus. Unfortunately, no vaccine or postexposure treatment is currently available.

TREATMENT OF ACUTE VIRAL HEPATITIS

Patients who present with acute viral hepatitis of any cause often have only nonspecific symptoms and signs, which may include fatigue, malaise, nausea, vomiting, fever, and hepatomegaly, with or without jaundice. Patients should be questioned about risk factors for viral hepatitis, and other etiologies of acute hepatitis should be excluded (Table 2). Laboratory evaluation should include viral serologies (see Table 2); complete blood count (CBC); coagulation studies; and

[1]Not FDA approved for this indication.

TABLE 2 Causes of Acute Hepatitis

	Cause	Initial Diagnostic Test
Drugs and toxins	Drug-induced	History
	Toxin-induced (including alcohol)	History
Viral	HAV	IgM anti-HAV
	HBV	HBsAg
	HCV	Anti-HCV
	HDV	Anti-HDV
	HEV	Anti-HEV
	CMV	CMV antigenemia
	EBV	Monospot
	HSV	Culture
Autoimmune	Autoimmune hepatitis	ANA, ASMA
Genetic	Wilson's disease	Ceruloplasmin
Other	Vascular disease	Ultrasound with Doppler or MRI
	Acute biliary obstruction	Ultrasound

Abbreviations: ANA = antinuclear antibody; anti-HCV = antibody to hepatitis C virus; anti-HDV = antibody to hepatitis D virus; anti-HEV = antibody to hepatitis E virus; ASMA = antismooth muscle antibody; CMV = cytomegalovirus; EBV = Epstein-Barr virus; HAV, HBV, HCV, HDV, HEV = hepatitis A, B, C, D, E (respectively) virus; HBsAg = hepatitis B surface antigen; HSV = herpes simplex virus; Ig = immune globulin; IgM anti-HAV = IgM antibody to hepatitis A virus; MRI = magnetic resonance imaging.

serum levels of aminotransferases, bilirubin, albumin, glucose, bicarbonate, and creatinine. Patients without evidence of chronic liver disease, hepatic encephalopathy, hypoglycemia, sepsis, severe coagulopathy (prothrombin time more than 20 seconds), hemorrhage, hypotension, or renal failure can safely be followed as outpatients if they are able to stay hydrated, have social support, and will return for follow-up appointments. Persons who have any of the above complications, are unable to take fluids orally, or lack social support may need to be hospitalized. Virus-specific treatment is generally not indicated or available for acute hepatitis A, B, D, or E, but for acute HCV infection that has not resolved by 3 months, treatment with peginterferon and ribavirin (Rebetol) leads to a 98% cure rate.

Patients with acute viral hepatitis have a small risk of progressing to fulminant hepatic failure (defined as the development of severe coagulopathy and hepatic encephalopathy, in patients without preexisting chronic liver disease, within 8 weeks of the onset of symptoms). Any patient with signs of fulminant hepatic failure should be stabilized and referred to a liver transplant center immediately.

Chronic Viral Hepatitis

Chronic hepatitis is defined as persistent necroinflammation of the liver with elevation of serum aminotransferase levels for more than 6 months (although the diagnosis can often be made on initial evaluation). There are many causes of chronic aminotransferase elevations, including alcohol-induced liver disease and drug-induced hepatitis, which can often be excluded on the basis of the patient's history. If either is found, cessation of the offending agent should be followed by return of aminotransferase levels to normal. Other causes of chronic hepatitis can be categorized as genetic, autoimmune, metabolic, and viral (Table 3). A liver biopsy is often indicated to confirm the diagnosis, determine the grade of inflammatory activity, and assess the stage of fibrosis (Table 4). In occasional cases, more than one cause of liver injury is found.

CHRONIC HEPATITIS B

An estimated 400 million people worldwide and 1.25 million in the United States are chronically infected with HBV. The two major determinants of the evolution of acute hepatitis B to chronic hepatitis B are patient's age at the time of acquisition and the patient's immune status. Whereas more than 98% of cases of acute hepatitis B in immunocompetent adults resolve spontaneously, approximately 90% of cases in neonates progress to chronicity. Chronic infection is also more likely to develop in immunocompromised than in immunocompetent persons.

Traditionally, two stages of chronic hepatitis B are designated as replicative and nonreplicative (Table 5). The replicative phase (or HBeAg-positive chronic hepatitis B) is characterized by the presence in serum of HBsAg, HBeAg, and high levels of HBV DNA ($>10^5$ copies/mL) (see Table 5). (Patients with precore or core mutations will have high HBV DNA levels in serum despite the absence of HBeAg.)

TABLE 3 Causes of Chronic Hepatitis

	Cause	Initial Diagnostic Test
Most common	Alcohol	History
	Drug-induced	History
Viral	HBV	HBsAg
	HCV	Anti-HCV
	HDV	Anti-HDV
Autoimmune	Autoimmune hepatitis	ANA, ASMA
	Primary biliary cirrhosis	AMA
	Primary sclerosing cholangitis	MRCP
Metabolic	Nonalcoholic fatty liver disease	History
Genetic	Hemochromatosis	Iron saturation, ferritin
	Wilson's disease	Ceruloplasmin
	α_1-Antitrypsin deficiency	α_1-Antitrypsin level
Other	Celiac sprue	Transglutaminase antibody

Abbreviations: AMA = antimitochondrial antibodies; ANA = antinuclear antibody; anti-HCV = antibody to hepatitis C virus; anti-HDV = antibody to hepatitis D virus; ASMA = antismooth muscle antibody; HBsAg = hepatitis B surface antigen; HBV, HCV, HDV = hepatitis B, C, D, (respectively) virus; MRCP = magnetic resonance cholangiopancreatography.

TABLE 4 Histologic Grading and Staging of Chronic Hepatitis

Inflammatory Activity			Degree of Fibrosis	
Grade	**Portal**	**Lobular**	**Stage**	**Fibrosis**
0	None or minimal	None		
1	Portal inflammation	Inflammation, no necrosis	1	No fibrosis or limited to expanded portal tracts
2	Mild limiting plate necrosis	Focal necrosis	2	Periportal fibrosis or portal-to-portal septa with intact architecture
3	Moderate limiting plate necrosis	Severe focal cell damage	3	Septal fibrosis with architectural distortion
4	Severe limiting plate necrosis	Bridging necrosis	4	Cirrhosis

The replicative phase of chronic hepatitis B is associated with elevated serum aminotransferase levels and active inflammation on liver biopsy. Such patients are at risk of progressing to cirrhosis and hepatocellular carcinoma (HCC) over time. Hepatic necroinflammation in chronic hepatitis B results from a host immune attack on hepatocytes involving cytotoxic T lymphocytes. Seroconversion from HBeAg to anti-HBe, with a decline in HBV DNA levels, occurs in 9% to 19% of patients per year.

The previously termed *nonreplicative phase* (which may be heralded by a flare in hepatitis activity) is characterized by:

- Presence in serum of HBsAg
- Loss of HBeAg with the appearance of anti-HBe
- Decrease in HBV DNA to low levels ($<10^5$ copies/mL)
- Return of serum aminotransferase levels to normal
- Resolution of inflammation on liver biopsy.

Occasional patients may also have anti-HBs in serum; the anti-HBs is heterotypic to the HBsAg and thus not protective. Patients with HBeAg-negative chronic hepatitis B, normal serum amintotransferase levels, and low HBV DNA levels, are said to be *inactive HBV carriers*. Inactive carriers have a low rate (2%) of progressive liver disease. However, they are still at risk for spontaneous flares of hepatitis associated with an increase in serum aminotransferase levels and active viral replication.

Patients with chronic HBV infection clear HBsAg from serum at a rate of 1% to 2% per year. Patients who clear the virus spontaneously and undergo seroconversion from HBsAg to anti-HBs may still have very low levels of HBV DNA in serum, below the detection threshold of standard assays. Detection of low levels of HBV DNA in serum by PCR signifies ongoing HBV infection with little viral replication. In fact, HBV DNA detectable only by PCR has been shown to persist in serum and peripheral blood mononuclear cells for up to 21 years after otherwise complete clinical and serologic recovery from HBV infection.

An association between HBV and HCC is well established. HBV is thought to lead to HCC as a result of chronic necroinflammatory activity in the liver as well as integration of HBV DNA into the host genome. In endemic areas where HBV infection is acquired at or near birth, the risk of HCC is as high as 25%. Screening for HCC with ultrasound and serum alphafetoprotein testing every 6 months is recommended for all patients with chronic (replicative) hepatitis B as well as inactive carriers older than 40 years of age.

Treatment

The goal of treatment of chronic hepatitis B is suppression of viral replication (with loss of HBeAg and disappearance of HBV DNA in serum), normalization of serum aminotransferase levels, and resolution of hepatic necroinflammatory activity. Approved treatments for HBV infection are interferon α, lamivudine (Epivir), and adefovir dipivoxil (Hepsera) (Table 6). Interferon α was the mainstay of therapy until oral agents, with fewer side effects, became available. Interferon α is still used in a select group of patients. Factors predictive of a response to

TABLE 5 Serologic Patterns Associated with Hepatitis B Infection and Immunization

	HBsAg	anti-HBs	HBeAg	anti-HBe	anti-HBc
Acute hepatitis B	+	–	+	–	IgM anti-HBc +
Inactive carrier	+	–	–	+	IgG anti-HBc +
Chronic hepatitis B (replicative phase or HBeAg-positive chronic hepatitis B)	+	–	+	–	IgG anti-HBc +
Infection with precore/core mutant	+	–	–	+	IgG anti-HBc +
Previous infection	–	+	–	–	IgG anti-HBc +
Immunization	–	+	–	–	–

Abbreviations: anti-HBc = antibody to hepatitis core antigen; anti-HBe = antibody to hepatitis B e antigen; anti-HBs = antibody to hepatitis B surface antigen; HBeAg = hepatitis B e antigen; HBsAg = hepatitis B surface antigen; Ig = immune globulin.

TABLE 6 Drugs Used to Treat Chronic Hepatitis B and C

	Agent	Genotype	Dose	Duration
Hepatitis B	Interferon α-2a (Roferon-A)	All	5 MU subcutaneously daily	4-6mo
	Lamivudine (Epivir)	All	100 mg PO daily	>1y
	Adefovir (Hepsera)	All	10 mg PO daily	>1y
Hepatitis C*	Peginterferon alfa-2a (Pegasys)	1	180 μg subcutaneously weekly	12mo
		2 or 3	180 μg subcutaneously weekly	6mo
	Peginterferon alfa-2b (Peg-Intron)	1	1.5 μg/kg (weight-based) subcutaneously weekly	12mo
		2 or 3	1.5 μg/kg (weight-based) subcutaneously weekly	6mo
	Ribavirin (Rebetrol)	1	weight <75 kg = 1000 mg PO daily	12mo
		1	weight >75 kg = 1200 mg PO daily	12mo
		2 or 3	800 mg PO daily	6mo

*Combine a pegylated interferon α with ribavirin.

interferon α include a baseline serum HBV DNA level less than 200 pg/mL (by a liquid hybridization assay) and serum aminotransferase elevations greater than three times the upper limit of normal. Seroconversion from HBeAg to anti-HBe with normalization of serum aminotransferase levels occurs in up to 37% of interferon α-treated patients. Patients who undergo HBeAg to anti-HBe seroconversion on interferon α usually experience a hepatitis flare, identified by a twofold or more elevation of serum aminotransferase levels, between the second and third month of therapy. The flare is well tolerated in patients with precirrhotic disease, but represents a significant risk in patients with cirrhosis; therefore, patients with HBV infection and cirrhosis should not be treated with interferon α. The standard regimen is 5 million units (MU) of interferon α administered subcutaneously daily for 4 to 6 months. Peginterferon[1] is under study and likely to be as effective as interferon α.

Lamivudine, a nucleoside analogue that inhibits the HBV reverse transcriptase, is an attractive alternative to interferon α because its side effect profile is similar to that of placebo. Therapy with lamivudine, 100 mg orally daily, results in loss of HBeAg in 18% of patients after 1 year and 25% of patients after 2 years. When treatment for 1 year does not result in HBeAg to anti-HBe seroconversion, or in patients infected with HBV containing a precore or core mutation, long-term therapy to suppress HBV DNA may be required. By 2 years of therapy approximately 40% of patients experience a relapse of hepatitis that is usually the result of a YMDD mutation in the HBV polymerase gene that renders the virus resistant to lamivudine.

Adefovir, a nucleotide analogue, may be used as first-line therapy or after lamivudine has failed. The drug can be used in patients infected with the lamivudine-resistant virus. The efficacy of adefovir, 10 mg orally daily, is similar to that of lamivudine, but only 1.7% of patients develop resistance to adefovir over 2 years.

[1]Not FDA approved for this indication.

Nucleoside (or nucleotide) analogues can be discontinued 4 to 6 months after seroconversion from HBeAg to anti-HBe, but reactivation may still occur. New antiviral agents, such as clevudine*, entecavir*, emtricitabine[1], telbivudine*, valtorcitabine*, and tenofovir[1], as well as combination therapy, are under study.

CHRONIC HEPATITIS C

Worldwide, 170 million people are infected with HCV, and in the United States 1.8% of the population is infected. This prevalence reflects the high frequency (85%) of chronic infection following acute hepatitis C. Risk factors for chronicity of HCV infection include male gender, acquisition of infection after age 50 years, certain human leukocyte antigen types, and viral factors.

Persons with chronic hepatitis C are usually asymptomatic. Some patients experience fatigue, malaise, or weakness. The diagnosis of chronic hepatitis C is often made by the incidental finding of elevated serum aminotransferase levels, which are typically 1.3 to 3 times the upper limit of normal. The alanine aminotransferase level is typically higher than the aspartate aminotransferase level until cirrhosis develops, when the ratio tends to reverse. However, patients may have normal serum aminotransferase levels.

Evaluation of the patient with chronic hepatitis C includes a serum HCV RNA level and viral genotype analysis. Determination of the viral genotype is used to plan the duration of antiviral therapy and to assess the likelihood of response. Before treatment, a liver biopsy is generally recommended to assess the grade of inflammation and stage of fibrosis. Characteristic findings on biopsy include a dense portal and periportal inflammatory infiltrate with lymphocytes, accompanied by occasional eosinophils and plasma cells. Typically, lymphocytes extend beyond the limiting plate into the hepatic

*Investigational drug in the United States.
[1]Not FDA approved for this indication.

parenchyma with accompanying hepatocellular necrosis (interface hepatitis). Bile duct abnormalities are common, and macrovesicular steatosis occurs in up to 30% of cases. Fibrosis (initially portal and later bridging) can occur even with relatively mild inflammation.

Approximately 20% of patients with chronic hepatitis C progress to cirrhosis over 20 years. Of those with cirrhosis, 30% develop decompensated disease in 10 years. Host factors that play a role in progression to cirrhosis include male gender, alcohol use, age older than 40 years at acquisition of HCV infection, and human immunodeficiency virus coinfection; other possible risk factors include increased hepatic iron and steatosis. HCV infection is also a risk factor for HCC. In contrast to HBV, which may have oncogenic properties by integrating into the host genome, HCV leads to HCC primarily by causing cirrhosis. After cirrhosis occurs the risk of HCC is 1.4% to 6.9% per year. Therefore, screening of persons with chronic hepatitis C for HCC with ultrasound and α-fetoprotein testing every 6 months is recommended only in those with cirrhosis. Vaccination against HAV and HBV is also recommended for all persons infected with HCV.

Treatment

Successful treatment of chronic hepatitis C with interferon α was first reported in 1986. The treatment half-life of interferon α in serum can be extended by covalent attachment to polyethylene glycol (PEG), and peginterferon significantly improves the sustained virologic response rate (SVR) when compared to treatment with standard interferon α. The SVR can be increased further by adding ribavirin, an oral antiviral agent, to the regimen (see Table 6).

Currently two pegylated formulations of interferon α are available; both are administered subcutaneously once weekly. Peginterferon α-2a (Pegasys, Hoffmann-La Roche, Inc.) consists of interferon α-2a bound to a 40 kD PEG moiety and is prescribed in a fixed dose of 180 μg weekly. Peginterferon α-2b (Peg-Intron, Schering-Plough Corporation) consists of interferon α-2b bound to a 12 kD PEG moiety and is administered in a dose of 1.5 μg/kg (weight-based) weekly. Both formulations of pegylated interferon α are administered with oral ribavirin, 800 to 1200 mg daily in two divided doses (weight-based). The dosing and duration of therapy also depend on the viral genotype. Most patients in the United States are infected with genotype 1 (1a or 1b) and require 1 year of treatment, with a resulting SVR of 46%. Patients infected with genotype 2 or 3 require only 6 months of therapy (as well as a fixed dose of ribavirin of 800 mg daily) and have an 80% SVR. Lower SVRs are often seen in patients with cirrhosis or high viral loads (>850,000 IU/mL) as well as in African Americans. (African Americans infected with genotype 1 HCV who were treated with peginterferon α-2b [PEG-Intron] and ribavirin for 1 year had a SVR of 19% compared with non-Hispanic whites who had an SVR of 52% when treated with the same regimen.) However, the presence of one or more of these factors does not preclude a response to therapy. In patients infected with viral genotype 1, the unlikelihood of an SVR can be predicted at 3 months by lack of a decrease in the HCV RNA level in serum by two logs, in which case treatment can be discontinued. If HCV RNA is undetectable by PCR testing 6 months after completion of therapy, the patient is considered to be a sustained virologic responder.

Side effects of therapy are common. Interferon α can cause cytopenias, and ribavirin invariably causes hemolysis. The hematologic effects of treatment are monitored with a complete blood count every 1 to 2 weeks for the first 2 months and monthly thereafter. Because the correct dose of ribavirin is crucial to achieving an SVR, therapy with erythropoietin may be needed to raise the hematocrit. Neutropenia and thrombocytopenia may result from interferon α and necessitate a dose reduction or occasionally treatment of neutropenia with granulocyte colony stimulating factor. Other side effects of interferon α and ribavirin include flu-like symptoms, fatigue, myalgias, depression, insomnia, irritability, hair loss, nausea, vomiting, headaches, cough, thyroid dysfunction, autoimmune disorders, sexual dysfunction, and retinal damage. Antidepressant therapy may be required for patients who become depressed during interferon α therapy. Contraindications to initiating therapy include a history of myocardial infarction, cardiac arrhythmia, heart failure, poorly controlled seizure disorder, autoimmune hepatitis, hemoglobin less than 11 g/dL, absolute neutrophil count less than 1500/μL, platelet count less than 75,000/μL, severe depression, uncontrolled diabetes, hypersensitivity to the medication, or creatinine clearance less than 50 mL/min. Pregnancy, both during and for 6 months after treatment, should be avoided. In addition, treatment of patients with hepatic decompensation is not recommended outside clinical trials.

Novel therapeutic agents directed against HCV proteins are under study. Several new agents have been designed that inhibit viral translation, the NS3 protease, or the RNA-dependent RNA polymerase.

MALABSORPTION

METHOD OF

Charles E. King, MD

Because we need energy to undergo every metabolic activity of the body, malabsorption of energy-supplying nutrients is a clinically important condition. It can be severe and is more common than is appreciated. It can lead to difficulties as a result of symptoms related to the passage of unabsorbed food through the gastrointestinal tract giving diarrhea. It can also lead to problems of malnutrition and vitamin deficiency. In fact, if malnutrition occurs from malabsorption (or from any other cause such as fasting or during severe illness), protein deficiency can lead to additional malabsorption as a result of enzyme deficiency, cell loss, or both. Thus treatment of malabsorption may require that one treat the secondary malnutrition before the patient can benefit from simplified, specific therapy of the underlying cause of the malabsorption. At times, treatment of the malnutrition may be required before one can even begin testing for the specific causes of malabsorption.

This article is organized in the same way as one would think through the clinical evaluation of malabsorption: (a) Is it present? (b) How can I confirm its presence? (c) How can I diagnose the specific cause? (d) How can I treat the cause(s)? In practical terms, these questions can be answered in a different order; for example, if a therapeutic trial is chosen and successful, this supports the need for continuation of that specific therapy.

General Categories of Malabsorption

Because most ingested nutrients require processing (digestion) prior to absorption, impaired absorption may occur as a result of maldigestion, impaired absorption by the mucosa, impaired exit from the cell following absorption, or a combination thereof. It is helpful to think of maldigestion and postdigestive malabsorption as two broad clinical categories when undertaking the evaluation. Another broad splitting of malabsorption is based on whether only isolated nutrients are malabsorbed (as a consequence of either digestive or absorptive defects) or if generalized malabsorption (e.g., involving carbohydrate, protein, and fat) is occurring (again, as a consequence of either digestive or absorptive defects). Tests performed to evaluate the absorption of various substances enable one to categorize the absorptive problem as either maldigestive or malabsorptive and as either specific or generalized malabsorption. Making these distinctions is discussed in the sections on tests of malabsorption.

Clinical Features

Because ingested nutrients that are not absorbed pass through the small intestine into the colon in larger-than-normal quantities, increased volume and/or watery stool is a frequent presenting feature of malabsorption. This may be manifest as increased frequency of stooling, diarrhea (loose stools), and/or crampy abdominal pain. The failure to absorb energy-rich nutrients can lead to weight loss and fatigue. Poor absorption of protein by-products can lead to malnutrition, with a secondary deficiency of both visceral and serum proteins. Postprandial pain can lead to decreased nutrient intake, further magnifying weight loss and malnutrition. Vitamin malabsorption can be manifest by deficiencies of both water-soluble and fat-soluble vitamins (A, D, E, and K). Diarrhea coupled with malabsorption can lead to high-grade electrolyte disturbances and intravascular volume depletion (with associated renal and vascular dysfunction), as well as deficiencies of micronutrients such as zinc and magnesium. Anemia may be multifactorial, including deficiencies of iron, folate, and/or cobalamin (vitamin B_{12}).

Physiology

FAT ABSORPTION

Triglyceride, the major dietary form of fat, is an important energy source, supplying 9 kcal/g. The assimilation of triglyceride is the most demanding of all nutrients; generalized malabsorption, even when minor, is thus most manifest by the effects of malabsorption of fat. Triglyceride requires digestion by intraluminal lipase, which originates primarily from the pancreas but is also derived from the tongue and stomach. Conjugated bile salts, derived from the liver and stored in the gallbladder, are required for micelle formation to solubilize triglyceride and the products of its digestion (glycerol, free fatty acids, and mono- and diglycerides). Mucosal cells have to not only absorb the fatty acids and glycerol, but also have to repackage the absorbed products back into triglyceride form and form chylomicrons with cholesterol, cholesterol esters, phospholipids, and protein prior to passage into the lymphatics of the chylomicrons (in contrast to the portal venous passage of products of carbohydrate and protein absorption).

Failure to absorb triglyceride leads to loss of 9 kcal/g of energy and to impaired absorption of fat-soluble vitamin A (affecting vision and skin), D (affecting serum calcium and calcification of bone), E (antioxidant deficiency), and K (coagulation factor deficiency). Passage of malabsorbed triglyceride and/or fatty acid to the normal bacterial flora of the colon leads to production of hydroxy-fatty acids (with a castor-oil effect and secretory diarrhea).

CARBOHYDRATE ABSORPTION

Carbohydrates are ingested primarily as complex polysaccharides and disaccharides. Intraluminal carbohydrases break apart the complex carbohydrates sequentially to disaccharides, which are then digested to monosaccharides by mucosal disaccharidases such as lactase, sucrase, isomaltase, and maltase. Once absorbed, the monosaccharides are passed without repackaging directly to the portal venous system.

Failure to absorb carbohydrate most commonly occurs as a result of deficient mucosal disaccharidases, with lactase being the most easily disturbed and clinically apparent disaccharidase deficiency. Malabsorbed carbohydrate that is passed to the bacteria of the colon undergoes breakdown from 6-carbon monosaccharides to twice as many 3-carbon organic acids (which doubles the osmotic effect), ethanol (which leads to electrolyte and water secretion), and gases, such as hydrogen and methane (with secondary abdominal cramping and flatulence).

PROTEIN ABSORPTION

Ingested protein undergoes digestion by proteases and peptidases derived from the stomach and (most importantly) the pancreas. The end products of protein digestion are small peptides containing two to four amino acids (di, tri-, and tetrapeptides) and free amino acids; the ability to absorb incompletely digested products (e.g., dipeptides) makes the absorption of protein less demanding than that of either carbohydrate or fat. Amino acids absorbed from the lumen or produced by the intracellular breakdown of small peptides are passed into the portal venous system, just as occurs with carbohydrates (and in contrast to fat absorption via lymphatic channels).

Failure to absorb protein most commonly occurs as a result of intraluminal protease-peptidase deficiency or marked loss of absorptive cells. Consequences of protein malabsorption lead not only to protein deficiency affecting all parts of the body, but also to worsening mucosal absorption as a result of development of both intraluminal (e.g., pancreatic enzyme) and intracellular (e.g., brush-border) enzyme deficiency.

DIARRHEA BECAUSE OF MALABSORPTION

As noted above, malabsorbed nutrients are passed to the colon, which has a luxuriant bacterial flora (10^{10} to 10^{11} organisms/mL, as contrasted to 10^4 organisms/mL present in the proximal intestinal tract). These bacteria can produce diarrhea by creating an osmotic effect (e.g., breaking down 6-carbon sugars to twice as many 3-carbon by-products); this is exemplified by the osmotic diarrhea one sees when a lactase-deficient subject ingests too much lactose. The second mechanism by which the colonic bacteria can produce diarrhea is through the production of chemicals that cause secretion of water and electrolytes. The production of hydroxy-fatty acids, which mimic castor oil, was noted earlier in the section on fat absorption. Production of ethanol from malabsorbed carbohydrate can also lead to increased secretion of water and electrolytes by the bowel mucosa. Similarly, deconjugation of malabsorbed bile acids can lead to diarrhea from a "Carter's Little Liver Pills" secretory effect on the colon.

Causes of Malabsorption

MALDIGESTIVE MALABSORPTION

The most common cause of maldigestion leading to malabsorption is pancreatic insufficiency. The most common cause of pancreatic insufficiency in the United States is chronic pancreatitis as a result of alcohol-induced injury. Pancreatic duct obstruction as a consequence of malignancy can lead to a similar inadequate flow of pancreatic enzymes to the duodenal lumen. Other less common causes include pancreatic insufficiency caused by surgical resection and/or massive necrosis following acute gallstone, endoscopic retrograde cholangiopancreatography (ERCP)-induced or traumatic pancreatitis. A subtle pancreatic insufficiency can occur in the setting of duodenal–jejunal mucosal atrophy, where inadequate release of cholecystokinin–pancreozymin (CCK-PZ) from enterocytes leads to secondary inadequate release of pancreatic enzymes. As mentioned earlier, protein malnutrition can lead to deficiency of both pancreatic and mucosal enzymes, with consequent maldigestion.

Biliary obstruction, occurring as a result of neoplastic or inflammatory extrahepatic obstruction or intrahepatic cholestatic disease, can lead to decreased triglyceride digestion as a consequence of luminal bile acid deficiency and impaired micelle formation. Abnormal enterohepatic circulation, such as seen in ileal inflammatory disease or following small bowel surgical bypass or resection, can also lead to maldigestion from inadequate levels of conjugated bile salts in the small intestinal lumen. Deconjugation of bile salts by excessive bacteria in the small intestine is one of the mechanisms leading to fat maldigestion and malabsorption in the bacterial overgrowth syndrome. A less common cause of inadequate luminal levels of conjugated bile salts is seen in the setting of massive acid hypersecretion (e.g., Zollinger-Ellison syndrome), where the acid pH precipitates bile salts out of the luminal solution.

MALABSORPTIVE MALABSORPTION

The prototype of malabsorption occurring as a result of mucosal dysfunction is that seen in gluten enteropathy (celiac or nontropical sprue). In this syndrome, injury to cells leads to severe flattening of the mucosa and tremendous loss in villus surface area. In addition to the loss of absorptive columnar epithelial cells, there is a relative increase in secretory crypt cells, with a secondary secretory flux of water and electrolytes to the lumen. The injury is more severe in the proximal small intestine (where highest concentrations of ingested gluten are found after ingestion); thus, nutrients absorbed primarily in the proximal small intestine, such as iron and folic acid, may be severely deranged in this setting. Likewise, because release of the mucosal hormone CCK-PZ occurs primarily in the duodenum and proximal jejunum, secondary depressed luminal bile acid and pancreatic enzyme levels are seen in celiac sprue.

Partial villous atrophy is seen in tropical sprue, where maturation of villi is disrupted probably by a combination of intraluminal toxins (derived in part from ingested bacteria) and vitamin deficiency (particularly folate). A similar picture of partial villous atrophy is occasionally seen in the syndrome of bacterial overgrowth of the small intestine, which may occur as a result of decreased killing of ingested bacteria by acid, slowed small intestinal or gastric motility, and/or altered anatomy (e.g., strictures, small intestinal diverticula, and/or surgical creation of blind intestinal loops). Altered maturation of small intestinal cells, with secondary partial villous atrophy, may occur as a result of any cause of folic acid (dietary, sulfa drugs) or vitamin B_{12} (pernicious anemia, dietary, pancreatic insufficiency, bacterial overgrowth) deficiency. Partial villous atrophy may also be seen during chemotherapy or radiation therapy, during protein malnutrition, or with the use of colchicine. Cell damage can also occur as a result of ethanol intake and from certain drugs, such as neomycin and certain laxatives. Loss of total surface area is also seen with surgical resection of the bowel—the short-bowel syndrome.

The final step of assimilating fat is the passage of triglyceride from the enterocyte into the lymphatics. Marked fat malabsorption may be seen in congenital or acquired dilation of the lymphatics (intestinal lymphangiectasia). Acquired causes include obstruction caused by neoplastic (lymphoma), or infectious (tuberculosis) disease, or in the setting of Crohn's disease. In addition, lymphatic obstruction and decreased surface area are seen in Whipple's disease, where bacilli-laden macrophages swell the enterocyte and obstruct the lymphatics intracellularly.

Clinical Tests to Determine the Presence of Malabsorption

BLOOD TESTS

Screening for malabsorption can be done with commonly used blood tests. Serum iron and folate or red blood cell folate can be used to screen for proximal small-intestinal malabsorption. Serum vitamin B_{12} can screen generally for malabsorption; if it is depressed, this points to long-standing malabsorption leading to depletion of body vitamin B_{12} stores. Vitamin B_{12} malabsorption may be related to gastric hyposecretion of acid and/or intrinsic factor (pernicious anemia or abnormal release of protein-bound B_{12} from foods), pancreatic insufficiency, bacterial overgrowth of the small intestine, ileal disease (e.g., Crohn's disease), or ileal resection. Serum screening for fat malabsorption can be done by determining serum carotene (vitamin A), serum calcium (vitamin D), and prothrombin time and partial thromboplastin time (vitamin K).

FECAL FAT

Because the absorption of fat is more complicated than that of carbohydrate or protein, screening for fat malabsorption is commonly helpful in detecting generalized malabsorption. Staining a microscopic fecal smear with Sudan stain is a useful qualitative screening test for fat malabsorption. It involves the microscopic evaluation of a slide for fat globules when Sudan stain is mixed with stool (staining malabsorbed fatty acids); if negative, a second slide should be examined after the addition of stool, Sudan stain, and ethanol to the slide, and following warming of the slide with a flame to look for malabsorption of undigested triglyceride. When this test is coupled with Wright's stain to look for excessive leukocytes and testing of the stool for reducing substance, one can quickly screen for the most common causes of chronic diarrhea (fat malabsorption with Sudan stain, invasive bacterial or inflammatory bowel disease with Wright's stain, and carbohydrate malabsorption with reducing substance). Although a quantitative 72-hour stool collection for fat analysis is more accurate and reliable than the qualitative Sudan stain, it is not practical for the nonresearch evaluation of malabsorption because of the unpleasantness of handling 3 days of stool collection. When it is performed, however, 24-hour quantitative fat above 6 g (indicating less than 95% fat absorption when 100 g of dietary fat per day is administered for the test) and stool weight greater than 200 g are considered abnormal.

D-XYLOSE ABSORPTION TEST

Measurement of 5-hour urine excretion and 2-hour plasma levels of D-xylose after drinking 25 g of xylose solution is an excellent screen for simple sugar malabsorption. D-xylose is a 5-carbon simple sugar that is absorbed in the proximal small intestine. Because this simple sugar does not require digestion prior to absorption, abnormal values point to mucosal disease, such as gluten enteropathy, or Whipple's disease, and/or bacterial overgrowth of the small intestine. Values can be easily followed to assess response to therapy. The plasma value is particularly helpful as a backup to the 5-hour urine determination when there is unreliable urine collection and/or renal dysfunction.

VITAMIN B_{12} ABSORPTION TEST (SCHILLING TEST STAGE I)

Determination of ^{57}Co excretion in a 24-hour urine sample following the oral administration of ^{57}Co-labeled vitamin B_{12} is a simple and sensitive test of vitamin B_{12} absorption. It involves ingestion of a tracer amount of ^{57}Co-labeled vitamin B_{12}, administration of a parenteral dose of vitamin B_{12} (to "flush" absorbed ^{57}Co-labeled vitamin B_{12} into the urine), 24-hour urine collection (with a backup serum value for possible incomplete urine collection or inadequate renal function), and simple gamma counting of an aliquot of urine for ^{57}Co content. Because test results can be available soon after completion of the 24-hour urine collection, and because vitamin B_{12}

absorption reflects a number of different intestinal functions, this test is excellent to use to screen for malabsorptive disorders. An abnormal Stage I B_{12} absorption test can be followed up with other tests, including administration of gastric intrinsic factor (Stage II) or pancreatic enzymes (Stage III), and/or following antibiotic therapy (Stage IV), to isolate the specific cause of the malabsorptive disorder.

HYDROGEN BREATH TESTS

Ingested carbohydrate that is not absorbed by the small intestine (because of maldigestion and/or altered mucosal absorption) can be metabolized by bacteria in the colon to hydrogen gas. Because approximately 17% of hydrogen produced in the bowel is absorbed and excreted in the breath, a rise in breath hydrogen content can be used to detect malabsorption of carbohydrate. Although originally developed to test for malabsorption of the disaccharide lactose, this technique can be used to test for the malabsorption of simple monosaccharides (e.g., glucose), as well as to test for complex carbohydrate-containing mixtures (e.g., liquid nutritional supplements), to see if they are causing diarrhea or flatulence. A false-negative rise in hydrogen content can occur following recent antibiotic therapy or electrolyte purging of the colon, and altered baseline values of breath hydrogen can occur with cigarette smoking or exercise prior to performance of this test.

Tests to Determine the Cause of Malabsorption

VITAMIN B_{12} ABSORPTION TEST (SCHILLING TEST STAGES II-IV)

As mentioned earlier, an abnormal vitamin B_{12} absorption test can be followed up with other tests, including co-administration of gastric intrinsic factor and/or pancreatic enzymes, or following antibiotic therapy of suspected bacterial overgrowth. Normalization of the ^{57}Co vitamin B_{12} absorption test specifies which gastrointestinal dysfunction or deficiency was causing the vitamin B_{12} malabsorption.

MUCOSAL BIOPSY

Suction biopsy and, more recently, endoscopically obtained mucosal biopsies from the proximal small intestine, allow microscopic evaluation for partial or complete villous atrophy; parasitic or protozoal infestations; presence of macrophages laden with periodic acid-Schiff (PAS)-positive granules (Whipple's disease) or acid-fast staining particles (*Mycobacterium avium-intracellulare*, particularly in the immunodeficient setting); lymphangiectasia; and other infiltrative diseases such as Crohn's disease, lymphoma, eosinophilic gastroenteritis, and amyloidosis. Use of this test should be considered whenever the xylose absorption (or glucose-hydrogen breath) test is abnormal, because mucosal malabsorption is suggested (especially if bacterial overgrowth has been ruled out). Limitations of the test include the expensive nature of biopsy collecting, the spotty character of many of the lesions, and the many different causes of villous atrophy, particularly partial villous atrophy. The recent clinical availability of serum antigliadin antibody and serum tissue transglutaminase testing has decreased the requirement for small intestinal biopsies when gluten enteropathy (celiac sprue) is suspected.

PANCREATIC FUNCTION TESTING

The gold standard of pancreatic function testing—small intestinal intubation to collect secretions for bicarbonate analysis (secretin test) or to analyze enzyme output (CCK-PZ test)—is a very sensitive test but is available only at specialized centers. More practical, but less sensitive, is a determination of urinary excretion of para-aminobenzoic acid (PABA) following administration of PABA conjugated with peptide (bentiromide test). A similar lack of sensitivity is seen with the serum testing of trypsinogen for pancreatic insufficiency. Perhaps the most practical pancreatic function test is assessing clinical improvement (weight gain, improvement in diarrhea) during a therapeutic trial of antecibal pancreatic enzyme supplementation. Although pancreatin tablets are inexpensive, adequate dosing requires six to eight tablets prior to each meal. Newer pancreatic enzyme preparations (e.g., pancrelipase [Creon 20]) protect against acid denaturation in the stomach, are micronized to optimize release in the proximal small intestine, and more predictably improve malabsorption because of pancreatic insufficiency. It should be noted that intensive acid blockade (e.g., proton pump blockers) may actually decrease the effectiveness of enteric-coated pancreatic enzyme preparations; if they are required, moderation to nocturnal H_2 blockade therapy may be desirable.

Tests to Evaluate for Bacterial Overgrowth

Small intestinal intubation with anaerobic collection of jejunal juice for anaerobic and aerobic culturing is the gold standard for detecting bacterial overgrowth of the small intestine. Normal jejunal content of bacteria is 10^4 organisms/mL or less, and includes no coliforms or anaerobic bacteria. When bacterial overgrowth occurs as a result of lessened acid production by the stomach, slowed transit through the stomach and small intestine, or altered anatomy, growth up to 10^7 to 10^8 organisms/mL (including both anaerobic and aerobic bacteria) can be seen. Because specimen collection is time-consuming and good anaerobic–aerobic quantitative culturing is cumbersome, small-bowel culturing is infrequently accomplished in clinical practice.

Because excessive bacteria the small intestine can lead to gas production from the interaction of bacteria and carbohydrate, breath analysis testing has been developed to detect bacterial overgrowth. Breath hydrogen analysis after the ingestion of 50 to 80 g of glucose[1] (which requires no digestion and is avidly absorbed by the small intestine, making colonic bacterial contact with the test sugar less of a problem) is probably the best readily available breath test for bacterial overgrowth. An early rise in hydrogen after the ingestion of lactulose[1] (a disaccharide not digested by mammals) is an alternative breath hydrogen test for bacterial overgrowth of the small intestine. A 15-g xylose hydrogen breath test was recently tested in children with bacterial overgrowth. Tests that detect the production of labeled carbon dioxide (labeled with either radioactive ^{14}C or stable isotopic ^{13}C) as a marker for bacterial overgrowth are more sensitive than the breath hydrogen tests (e.g., 1-g labeled xylose test, labeled bile acid breath test). However, equipment to measure the labeled carbon dioxide is not available in most hospitals, and waiting for test results from a specialized center is less desirable than using the more readily available breath hydrogen results.

Trial of Diet

If lactase insufficiency is suspected (either as an isolated defect or as part of a generalized malabsorption), lactose restriction in the diet, use of lactase-treated milk, and use of lactase tablets with meals containing cheese or other dietary lactose should be encouraged. Ingestion of any nonabsorbed substance in the diet increases the rapidity of passage of the whole meal through the small intestine. This intestinal "hurry" magnifies any defect in digestion or absorption that is already present, increasing overall malabsorption. Obviously, improvement in symptoms (diarrhea, flatulence, cramps) with a trial of lactose restriction and/or lactase supplementation solidifies the diagnosis of lactase insufficiency.

Trial of a gluten-free diet can be made in patients in whom celiac sprue is suspected by either antigliadin antibody testing or mucosal biopsy. A longer period of observation is required with this diet than with the lactose-restricted diet because reversal of the mucosal defect occurs over time. In addition, compliance needs to be as close to 100% as possible, because small amounts of dietary gluten can have deleterious effects on the mucosa for weeks.

Treatment of Malabsorption

Because the primary clinical problems related to malabsorption are caused by side effects from the passage of malabsorbed nutrients to the colon and by deficiencies related to the malabsorption, treatment revolves around three treatment principles: (a) dietary restriction of nutrients that have disturbed absorption, in order to minimize side effect; (b) specific therapy directed at the cause of the malabsorption; and (c) compensation for malabsorbed nutrients by alternative means.

RESTRICTIVE

The first step in treating malabsorption is beginning a diet that does not surpass the quantities of nutrients that can be absorbed by the small intestine. This minimizes colonic bacterial degradation of malabsorbed substances, to minimize diarrhea and electrolyte losses caused by osmotic factors and production of both castor oil-like hydroxy-fatty acids and ethanol. The most extreme example of this restrictive principle is the use of slow-rate, around-the-clock tube feeding of predigested nutrients; this is often required in patients with severe malabsorption, short-bowel syndrome, and/or malabsorption complicated by malnutrition. An intermediate example of the restrictive principle is the use of multiple small oral feedings of liquid nutritionals with limited long-chain triglyceride and limited disaccharides (particularly lactose), possibly supplemented with more easily absorbed medium-chain triglyceride oil. A more easily completed example of this restrictive principle is the use of a lactose-restricted diet for a patient with low-grade, nongeneralized lactose malabsorption. No matter what level of restriction is undertaken, levels of breath hydrogen and symptoms (e.g., diarrhea and cramps) can be used to estimate whether or not the level of restriction is adequate.

COMPENSATORY

Malabsorption of long-chain triglycerides, with secondary calorie deficiency, can be compensated by supplementing the diet with more readily absorbed medium-chain triglyceride. This fat requires no digestion prior to absorption and no re-esterification to triglyceride once absorbed; in addition it is assimilated via the portal venous system rather than via lymphatics. It can thus be helpful in the setting of bile acid deficiency, villous atrophy, and is very important in the setting of lymphatic obstruction.

Digestive abnormalities of protein and carbohydrate can be compensated with liquid nutritional supplements using lactose-free carbohydrate and protein hydrolysate mixtures of amino acids and small peptides.

Compensation for vitamin deficiency accompanying malabsorption may require parenteral administration (e.g., vitamin B_{12} for noncorrectable vitamin B_{12} malabsorption) or the use of water-miscible vitamin formulations of fat-soluble vitamins.

[1]Not FDA approved for this indication.

SPECIFIC

Maldigestion as a consequence of pancreatic insufficiency can usually be adequately treated with antecibal administration of pancreatic enzymes (e.g., pancreatin [Creon], pancrelipase [Pancrease]). Malabsorption as a result of gluten enteropathy responds, albeit slowly, to strict adherence to a diet devoid of gluten. At times, severe involvement with gluten-enteropathy requires administration of corticosteroids during initiation of therapy. Malabsorption because of bacterial overgrowth can usually be managed with combination of periodic oral broad-spectrum antibiotic therapy (e.g., tetracycline[1], amoxicillin[1], chloramphenicol[1]), along with the above-noted restrictive and compensatory therapy. Treatment of Whipple's disease and tropical sprue both involve long-term oral antibiotic therapy. Supplementation of oral folic acid is also given in the setting of tropical sprue.

No matter what therapy is undertaken for malabsorption, success in controlling diarrhea, postprandial pain, and/or fatigue (from loss of nutrients in the toilet bowl) can be extremely gratifying for the health care provider and extremely important in improving the quality of life of the patient.

[1]Not FDA approved for this indication.

ACUTE PANCREATITIS

METHOD OF

Sharon L. Stein, MD, and David W. Rattner, MD

Acute pancreatitis is an inflammatory process with protean manifestations. Acute pancreatitis accounts for over 120,000 hospital admissions annually. The vast majority of cases are mild in nature and self-limiting. Treatment of patients with mild or edematous pancreatitis is largely supportive. However, 10% to 15% of patients with acute pancreatitis progress from mild disease to severe pancreatitis and develop serious complications including shock, respiratory failure, and multiple-organ system failure syndrome. In this subset of patients, mortality rates can be as high as 50%. Death in patients with severe acute pancreatitis is usually as a consequence of sepsis. While the management of mild pancreatitis is straightforward, identification of patients who are at risk to develop more fulminant disease requires knowledge of predictive tests and scoring systems. Identification of high-risk patients mandates monitoring and interventions to manage the potential complications that can ensue. This article reviews the management of mild and severe pancreatitis and highlights the indications for intervention in patients with more severe disease.

Incidence and Etiology

There are many causes of acute pancreatitis. In the United States, cholelithiasis and alcohol abuse are responsible for more than 80% of cases of acute pancreatitis. Since 1901, when Opie first described the autopsy finding of a stone impacted in the ampulla of Vater in a patient with severe pancreatitis, it has been recognized that obstruction of the pancreatic duct by passage of a gallstone can cause pancreatitis. Gallstone pancreatitis occurs in 3% to 5% of patients with cholelithiasis and accounts for 40% to 60% of cases of pancreatitis in the United States. In the past, up to 20% of patients with acute pancreatitis were classified as having idiopathic pancreatitis. However, recent studies that have carefully examined bile from patients with idiopathic pancreatitis demonstrate that most patients thought to have idiopathic pancreatitis have microlithiasis. Passage of these tiny stones in susceptible patients is believed to be sufficient to trigger an episode of acute pancreatitis. This finding has significant clinical ramifications because either cholecystectomy or endoscopic sphincterotomy should be curative. Alcoholic pancreatitis occurs in approximately 10% of patients with chronic alcohol abuse, but can also occur in otherwise healthy individuals following binge drinking. Other causes of pancreatitis include hypertriglyceridemia, viral infections, ampullary stenosis, upper abdominal surgery, and manipulation of the sphincter of Oddi during endoscopic retrograde cholangiopancreatography (ERCP). With the increasing use of endoscopic biliary intervention, post-ERCP pancreatitis is being noted with increasing frequency. Even in the most skilled hands, 1% to 4% of endoscopic procedures involving manipulation of the sphincter of Oddi result in pancreatitis. Table 1 is a more complete list of causes of pancreatitis.

The derangements of cellular processes that lead to acute pancreatitis are incompletely understood. While a variety of agents can cause acute pancreatitis, they all result in certain common alterations of cellular homeostasis. In nearly all experimental models of acute pancreatitis, the secretory pathway of digestive enzymes from the acinar cell is disturbed, resulting in colocalization of trypsinogen with lysosomal enzymes, the rapid accumulation of trypsinogen in the interstitial space, and inappropriate activation of trypsinogen. When trypsinogen is activated either by cathepsin-B in a zymogen granule or by enterokinase in the interstitial space, it cleaves other propeptidases into activated forms. The rapid accumulation of activated enzymes outside the gastrointestinal

TABLE 1 Causes of Pancreatitis

Alcoholic
Gallstones
Choledocholithiasis
Microlithiasis
Obstructive
Pancreatic cancer
Pancreas divisum with stenosis of the minor ampulla
Ampullary stenosis
Traumatic
ERCP/sphincter of Oddi manipulation
Postoperative
Blunt abdominal trauma
Drug induced
Antiretrovirals
Azathioprine/6-MP
Sulfonamides
Thiazides
Furosemide
Estrogen
Tetracycline
Metabolic
Hypertriglyceridemia
Hypercalcemia
Infectious
Viral
Parasitic
Miscellaneous
Cardiopulmonary bypass
Tropical pancreatitis
Autoimmune disorders
Scorpion venom/Gila monster
Idiopathic

Abbreviations: ERCP = endoscopic retrograde cholangiopancreatography; 6-MP = 6-mercaptopurine.

tract leads to inflammation and destruction of tissue in the pancreas and peripancreatic tissue. Tissue injury subsequently results in the release of systemic inflammatory mediators including cytokines, bradykinins, and other vasoactive peptides. These mediators then are responsible for causing the systemic manifestations of acute pancreatitis such as shock and pulmonary injury. The combination of tissue injury and inflammatory mediators also causes profound microcirculatory disturbances in the pancreas adding an ischemic component to the inflammatory process.

A great deal of effort has been made to alter the course of severe acute pancreatitis in both experimental models and clinical studies. Investigators have demonstrated that early interventions resulting in the improvement of the microcirculation can mitigate the progression of early acute pancreatitis to necrotizing pancreatitis. Likewise, inhibition of proinflammatory mediators limits the advancement of mild pancreatitis to necrosis. Unfortunately, clinical trials of therapies effective in the laboratory setting have failed to demonstrate efficacy in humans. The disappointing results of these trials may reflect the difficulty in starting an intervention early enough in the time course of clinical acute pancreatitis as most patients present to the hospital after a minimum of 12 to 24 hours of symptoms.

Diagnosis of Acute Pancreatitis

The typical presentation of acute pancreatitis includes persistent epigastric pain with radiation of pain to the back often accompanied by profuse emesis. Pain may be partially relieved by sitting forward. The differential diagnosis includes perforated duodenal ulcer, intestinal obstruction, acute cholecystitis, mesenteric ischemia, and early appendicitis. Patients may be tender on abdominal exam but in most cases generalized peritoneal signs are absent. Leukocytosis, secondary to inflammatory response, and hemoconcentration, as a result of retroperitoneal third spacing, are often present. In fulminant cases of pancreatitis, the patient may present with signs of shock including tachycardia, hypotension, and fever. Grey-Turner and Cullen's signs (flank and periumbilical ecchymosis, respectively) are classic signs of retroperitoneal hemorrhage associated with pancreatitis, but are seen in fewer than 3% of patients. Up to 20% of patients have atelectasis or pleural effusions, most frequently on the left side. Up to 25% of patients are hypoxic on presentation with PaO_2 less than or equal to 60 mm Hg.

There is no blood test that is both sensitive and specific enough to make a diagnosis of pancreatitis. Rather it is the combination of clinical presentation and laboratory testing that establishes the diagnosis. Serum amylase and lipase are the most commonly used tests to confirm a clinical diagnosis of acute pancreatitis. Hyperamylasemia is usually present, but is not specific for pancreatitis. Elevated serum amylase may be found in other conditions such as disorders of salivary glands, ovaries, bowel infarction, obstruction and perforation. In patients with hypertriglyceridemia, a potential cause of pancreatitis, amylase levels may be falsely normal and urine amylase may be a more sensitive test. The degree of hyperamylasemia also does not correlate with the severity of pancreatitis. In fact, the highest levels of serum amylase are seen with passage of a common duct stone—so-called biochemical pancreatitis—because the degree of pancreatic inflammation is usually negligible. Serum lipase levels are more specific for pancreatitis and generally remain elevated for 7 to 14 days after onset of symptoms. It is important to recognize that at least 10% of patients with pancreatitis have normal pancreatic enzyme levels on presentation. Other markers of pancreatitis, such as C-reactive protein (CRP) and interleukins 6 and 8, are elevated in both humans and laboratory animals with acute pancreatitis. However, despite increased sensitivity and specificity for acute pancreatitis, these markers are not available in most American hospital laboratories at this time, rendering them of limited clinical importance.

Elevated liver function tests are often noted in cases of pancreatitis and should raise suspicion of a gallstone etiology. Serum bilirubin levels greater than 4.0 mg/dL are noted in up to 10% of patients and may be associated with transient jaundice.

Hypocalcemia is noted in up to 25% of patients and is a marker for the severity of disease (Table 2). Hyperglycemia is commonly present, although it is not specific for pancreatitis.

Plain radiographs of the abdomen may show nonspecific intra-abdominal abnormalities such as a dilated loop of bowel in the vicinity of the pancreas, or colonic cut-off sign secondary to inflammation in the colon abutting the inflamed pancreas. Perhaps more importantly, radiographs may be helpful in excluding other causes of abdominal pain, such as duodenal perforation and intestinal obstruction. An abdominal ultrasound to look for gallstones is indicated for all patients. The presence of gallstones, dilated bile ducts, or signs of gallbladder thickening suggest pancreatitis of biliary etiology. A swollen, edematous pancreas may be visualized on ultrasound, but overlying bowel gas frequently prevents good visualization of the pancreas.

A computed tomographic (CT) scan with intravenous (IV) contrast is very sensitive for detecting the presence of pancreatitis, pancreatic edema, and pancreatic necrosis, but CT exams are not routinely required for patients with uncomplicated acute pancreatitis. Pancreatitis is a diagnosis that should be made using clinical and laboratory data. CT scans have not been shown to alter clinical decision making in early pancreatitis of mild to moderate severity. Furthermore, IV contrast has been shown to impair the pancreatic microcirculation in experimental models, raising concern that early CT scans may complicate cases of pancreatitis early on and prolong the hospital course. Given these findings, the International Association of Pancreatology suggests that contrast studies should be reserved for patients whose symptoms have failed to resolve 4 to 5 days after acute presentation or patients with a worsening clinical course. When a patient has pancreatic necrosis documented by CT scan, scans may be repeated as the patient's clinical course progresses and can be used to guide fine-needle aspiration (FNA) after the second week of illness (see later).

TABLE 2 Ranson's Criteria for Predicting Severity of Acute Pancreatitis

Present on Admission
Age >55 years
White blood cells >16,000 μL
Blood glucose >200 mg/dL
Serum lactate dehydrogenase >350 IU/L
SGOT (ALT) >250 IU/dL
Developing During First 48 Hours
Hematocrit fall >10%
Blood urea nitrogen increase >8 mg/dL
Serum Ca^{2+} <8 mg/dL
Arterial Po_2 <60 mm Hg
Base deficit <4 mEq/L
Estimated fluid sequestration >600 mL

Abbreviations: ALT = alanine transaminase; SGOT = serum glutamic-oxaloacetic transaminase.

Evaluation of Severity of Pancreatitis

Two separate criteria are commonly used to correlate clinical findings with patient prognosis. The Ranson/Imrie Criteria (Table 2) allows for evaluation of prognosis 48 hours after presentation. Ranson's criteria correlate well with clinical outcome. Patients with scores <3 have 0.9% mortality rate, whereas patients with scores >6 have a mortality rate approaching 90%. Ranson's criteria are limited by the fact that it takes 48 hours before all criteria can be collected. Therefore, when less than three criteria are present at the time of admission, they may fail to guide clinical decision making. However, when a patient presents with three criteria at admission, there is a high probability the patient has severe pancreatitis. Ranson's criteria are limited in that they are population based and may not be predictive for any single individual. Furthermore, they are a stagnant score that will not be altered by further complicating factors after the initial 48 hours. In practice, Ranson's criteria are most useful in predicting which patients will have an uncomplicated course of pancreatitis.

The Acute Physiology and Chronic Health Evaluation (APACHE) score was developed to correlate clinical findings with prognosis at any time during the clinical course of acute disease. APACHE II, a modification of the original instrument, evaluates 12 prognostic variables. The APACHE II score may be used to evaluate patients with critical care issues with a variety of clinical diagnoses. Scores greater than 13 in patients with acute pancreatitis are linked to poor prognosis. The advantage of this scoring system is that patients may be evaluated and risks stratified at any single moment in time during their hospital course.

Although not routinely recommended, some centers claim that CT scans with intravenous (IV) contrast obtained within 48 hours of the onset of illness are predictive of the severity of pancreatitis. According to criteria first established by Balthazar, if more than 30% of the pancreas is nonperfused, the chances are high that the patient will progress to complicated pancreatitis. These centers then base the need for intensive care unit (ICU) monitoring and use of prophylactic antibiotics on this information. However, not all pancreatologists believe the extent of pancreatic perfusion at this early stage correlates with the ultimate severity of disease and prefer to rely on clinical criteria to identify the cases of pancreatitis needing more intensive monitoring and support.

Management of Pancreatitis

To render timely and effective therapy it is essential to understand the evolution and resolution of pancreatic inflammation. It is most convenient to think of acute pancreatitis in three distinct phases. The first phase lasts from 2 to 7 days and is characterized by the systemic effects of the inflammatory process. In most patients, pancreatitis resolves during this phase. When necrosis develops, patients enter the middle phase in which one must be concerned about pancreatic infection and its management. The middle phase generally begins 7 days into the illness and may extend into the third week. The third phase of acute pancreatitis covers the late complications of necrotizing pancreatitis, such as pancreatic abscess or pseudocyst (Table 3).

EARLY PHASE OF PANCREATITIS

In the first 24 to 48 hours, maintenance of hemodynamic stability is the key task. It is essential to maintain appropriate intravascular volume to prevent sludging and stasis in the pancreatic microcirculation. Ten to 12 L of crystalloid and colloid per day may be required to prevent intravascular depletion secondary to increased vascular permeability and sequestration of fluid in the peripancreatic spaces. Prevention of renal failure is paramount and one should not be concerned about fluid overload at this stage of the illness. Anemia may result from hemodilution or be a harbinger of hemorrhagic pancreatitis. Hemoconcentration implies inadequate fluid resuscitation and is a bad sign. Patients with Ranson's criteria <3 and APACHE II score <13 may be adequately monitored on a routine ward with a Foley catheter and frequent vital signs. More severely ill patients may require invasive monitoring in the intensive care unit.

Volume shifts and emesis may lead to metabolic derangements. Electrolytes should be aggressively repleted. In severe pancreatitis, hypocalcemia may occur. Hypocalcemia is difficult to correct and intervention should be based on the ionized calcium rather than serum calcium levels. Hypomagnesium is particularly common in alcoholic patients and hyperglycemia may occur secondary to hyperglucagonemia. Routine use of nasogastric tubes does not alter the course of pancreatitis; however, in some cases, they are appropriate to empty the stomach and lower the risk of aspiration. Pulse oximetry should be used in all patients with a significant fluid requirement or other signs of hemodynamic instability.

TABLE 3 Interventions in Acute Pancreatitis

Early phase
Aggressive hydration
Prophylactic antibiotics
Endoscopic sphincterotomy for biliary complications
Elective laparoscopic cholecystectomy in those who resolve
Middle phase
Fine-needle aspiration to look for infection
Maintain nutrition
Débridement of infected necrosis
Late phase
Percutaneous drainage of pancreatic abscess
Surgical treatment of mass lesions
Internal drainage of pancreatic pseudocysts—Surgical or endoscopic
Remove gallbladder if stones present
Seek anatomic reason for failure to resolve

Within 48 to 72 hours after onset of pancreatitis, patient stratification will generally occur. Approximately 90% of patients will show clinical improvement with decreased pain, decreased fluid requirements, and hemodynamic stability. In this group, early oral or enteral feedings are appropriate after improvement of pain. Amylase and lipase may remain elevated for 7 to 10 days, but should not dictate timing for resumption of oral intake. Instead, patients should be started on a liquid diet when they are pain free, and the diet subsequently advanced as tolerated.

Although atelectasis and pleural effusions are very common in the first 4 days of illness, patients with severe pancreatitis may progress and develop respiratory failure between 4 and 10 days into the illness. Respiratory failure in these patients is characterized by low pressure pulmonary edema or acute respiratory distress syndrome (ARDS) and is not caused by volume overload during the first few days of illness. It generally fails to resolve with diuresis and ventilatory support may be needed. The course of respiratory failure is usually self-limited unless bacterial superinfection develops.

Patients with evidence of severe pancreatitis on the basis of predictive scoring systems or clinical judgment should be treated with prophylactic antibiotics. There is now good evidence from several randomized prospective trials that appropriate antibiotics decrease both mortality rate and the overall incidence of infection. To be effective, the antibiotics must be concentrated in pancreatic juice and parenchyma. Such antibiotics include the quinolones[1], metronidazole (Flagyl)[1], and the combination imipenem-cilastatin (Primaxin)[1], but do not include the less-expensive and more commonly used drugs such as aminoglycosides[1], cephalosporins[1], and penicillins[1]. The optimal duration of treatment is not known, but most experts give a 2-week course of prophylactic antibiotics. Recently, high-volume centers using these drugs have noted an increased incidence of fungal infections and are adding fluconazole (Diflucan)[1] to the regimen.

GALLSTONE PANCREATITIS

Gallstone pancreatitis is caused by transient obstruction of the pancreatic duct at the ampulla of Vater. Seventy-five percent of offending stones pass within 48 hours and 90% pass within 7 days. Multiple clinical trials have been performed to determine if endoscopic sphincterotomy (ES) in the first 48 hours of illness can alter the severity of pancreatitis. These trials have shown that early ERCP with ES is useful in preventing the biliary complications of pancreatitis, but does not have much, if any,

[1]Not FDA approved for this indication.

impact on the subsequent development of pancreatic necrosis and abscess. Because the majority of patients with gallstone pancreatitis pass their stones promptly, they should first receive supportive treatment for pancreatitis. Patients who show signs of immediate clinical improvement with medical management should undergo a laparoscopic cholecystectomy with intraoperative cholangiogram during their initial hospitalization. If stones are identified at this juncture, a laparoscopic common bile duct exploration can be performed. Patients who fail to improve within 48 hours of presentation, have obstructive jaundice, or have signs of cholangitis represent the subset of patients that require urgent endoscopic intervention. ERCP with ES and stone retrieval can be used to relieve ampullary obstruction, as well as placing a biliary stent to ensure continued decompression. Following endoscopic intervention, cholecystectomy is performed during the initial hospitalization for patients with mild to moderate pancreatitis. In cases of severe pancreatitis, an interval cholecystectomy is universally recommended, after resolution of inflammation and sequelae. Between 25% and 40% of patients who wait 6 weeks for interval cholecystectomy will have symptoms of cholecystitis and 10% will have recurrent pancreatitis.

MIDDLE PHASE OF PANCREATITIS

It is the development of pancreatic and peripancreatic necrosis that serves as the hallmark of severe pancreatitis. In the middle phase of pancreatitis, several possible courses develop: the necrotic tissue remains sterile and is reabsorbed slowly over weeks to months; the necrotic tissue remains sterile but causes symptoms because of mass effect; or the necrotic tissue becomes infected requiring surgical intervention. It is in the middle phase of pancreatitis that CT scans are invaluable. The scans should be obtained with bolus IV contrast so that images are acquired in both the arterial and delayed phase to delineate areas of nonperfusion.

Between 40% and 70% of patients with pancreatic necrosis will develop infection. The incidence of infection is maximal 3 weeks after onset of symptoms. It is likely that the route of infection is translocation from the colon, although hematogenous spread may also occur. Many infections are polymicrobial, often reflective of local colonic flora. *Escherichia coli*, *Klebsiella pneumoniae*, *Enterococci* spp., *Staphylococcus* spp., and *Pseudomonas* spp. are commonly cultured. Anaerobic infections account for less than 10% of infections. In recent studies, an increased incidence of gram-positive organisms and fungal infections have been noted, probably reflecting the more widespread use of prophylactic antibiotics and the use of long-term central venous catheters for administration of parenteral nutrition. Ongoing nutritional status is a concern for these patients. Enteral feedings are helpful in maintaining gut mucosal integrity thereby limiting bacterial translocation. Enteral feedings have clearly been shown not to worsen clinical outcomes. If patients are unable to take oral nutrition, a nasojejunal tube, placed distal to the ligament of Treitz should be used for low-volume continuous feedings. Parenteral nutrition is more expensive, results in further metabolic disturbances, and increases the risk of line sepsis. For these reasons, parenteral nutrition should be reserved for those patients who are unable to tolerate enteral feedings.

Detecting infected necrosis usually requires direct sampling of necrotic tissue by FNA. The only CT finding that will definitively diagnose infected necrosis is extraluminal free air in the pancreatic bed. Clinical findings of leukocytosis, fever, tachycardia, and low systemic vascular resistance can be seen in patients with sterile or infected necrosis. Patients manifesting signs of sepsis after initial response to treatment, experience new-onset organ failure, or any patient whose pancreatitis has not fully responded to supportive care within 2 weeks should undergo a CT scan. If necrosis is identified, FNA should be performed. FNA is the only test that can distinguish sterile from infected necrosis. The sensitivity of FNA is approximately 90% and false negatives are uncommon. There is no increased risk of contamination secondary to this procedure if sterile technique is maintained. Multiple FNAs may be required and should be performed for further clinical deterioration. The presence of infected necrosis mandates surgical débridement.

The indications for surgical débridement of pancreatic necrosis are somewhat controversial. All would agree that infected necrosis needs to be débrided and the infected cavity fully drained. Most would also agree that a clinically stable patient with sterile necrosis who is able to eat does not need débridement. There is only a small risk of late secondary infection of the necrotic tissue in such a patient. There are, however, differing opinions regarding the management of patients who remain in intensive care units with significant amounts of sterile necrosis, and of those who fail to eat after 4 weeks of hospitalization because of mass effect or perigastric inflammation. There is no level one evidence to support the superiority of either conservative management or surgical débridement in such situations. It should be emphasized, however, that sterile necrosis is not a contraindication to surgical débridement. Continuing parenteral nutrition or tube feedings for months is not rational if surgical removal/drainage of an inflammatory mass or fluid collection will relieve obstruction. This can almost always be performed with a low morbidity and mortality rate, particularly after 4 weeks of illness, and can restore the patient to good health.

The third to fourth week after onset of symptoms is generally agreed to be optimal timing for surgical necrosectomy; waiting longer than 4 weeks does not appear to confer any added benefit or reduced morbidity. Waiting until 3 weeks pass allows for optimal tissue demarcation, decreases the risk of intraoperative and postoperative bleeding, and minimizes the loss of viable pancreatic tissue. In some patients with life-threatening infections, débridement must be performed earlier. A recent CT scan with oral and intravenous contrast allows the surgeon to plan approaches to the pancreas and ensure appropriate drainage of all peripancreatic collections. Thoroughness in initial débridement is the most important factor in limiting the need for re-exploration and reducing morbidity and mortality postoperatively. Sparing of viable pancreatic tissue is also critically important. At our institution, the technique of débridement and closed packing is used. After débridement of the peripancreatic tissue through blunt dissection, the remaining cavity is packed with large, stuffed, Penrose drains, as well as closed suction drains. The Penrose drains are left in place for a minimum of 7 days, at which time one drain is removed every other day until none remain. While postoperative pancreatic fistulae are common, they are all controlled through the suction drains and more than 90% close without further surgical intervention. A single surgical intervention is successful in 83% of patients and postoperative mortality is 7% at our institution.

After a severe episode of pancreatitis requiring necrosectomy, nearly 25% of patients require supplemental pancreatic enzymes and 33% of patients develop diabetes. This is surprisingly low when one assesses the extent of necrosis seen on CT scans during the acute phase of their illness. The average length of disability following discharge from the hospital is 4 months.

LATE PHASE OF PANCREATITIS

Patients who were stable throughout the early and middle phase of pancreatitis and who were discharged home, might return with complications after the fourth week of their illness. The most common complications are pancreatic abscess, pancreatic pseudocysts, and failure to progress as a consequence of persistent inflammation. Abscesses generally occur more than 4 weeks after onset of symptoms and present with fever and abdominal pain. As opposed to generalized pancreatic infected necrosis, a pancreatic abscess is a localized, liquefied collection of tissue. CT may be helpful in identifying a well-defined liquid collection that is demarcated from the surrounding viable tissue. The importance of distinguishing pancreatic abscess from pancreatic necrosis is that abscesses can often be drained by percutaneous radiologic intervention, whereas the semisolid nature of pancreatic necrosis generally precludes such an approach. After fluid aspiration, an indwelling catheter is left in place and a minimum course of 2 weeks of appropriate antibiotics is prescribed. Failure to completely resolve with percutaneous drainage necessitates surgical intervention.

Pancreatic pseudocysts are nonepithelized inflammatory pancreatic fluid collections. Patients may complain of abdominal pain or be entirely asymptomatic. Diagnosis is easily made by ultrasound or CT. CT is generally used for initial diagnosis; ultrasound examination is used for follow-up evaluation. Fluid collections seen during the first 3 weeks of pancreatitis should be referred to as acute fluid collections rather than as pseudocysts because most will resolve. Complications of pseudocysts include hemorrhage from erosion into major blood vessels, rupture leading to peritonitis, and secondary infection. Small cysts may be managed expectantly, but cysts larger than 6 cm, those present for more than 6 weeks, and cysts that enlarge in size or are multiple in number have an increased risk of complications. Surgical or endoscopic drainage should be strongly considered. The goal is to allow the cyst wall to mature enough so that it is either adherent to the posterior wall of the stomach or fibrotic enough to allow placement of sutures for an anastomosis. This requires at least 6 weeks from the onset of pancreatitis.

Occasionally patients with acute pancreatitis languish with persistent low-grade inflammation requiring persistent nutritional support and frequent readmission to the hospital. In most cases, this is caused by mass effect from an area of necrosis or a stricture in the main pancreatic duct leading to obstructive pancreatitis. In the former situation, débridement with or without pancreatic resection is needed. Strictures in the pancreatic duct can often be managed by transampullary stents, but one must be cognizant of the possibility that the stricture may caused be a malignancy, particularly if no other cause of the original episode of pancreatitis can be identified.

Conclusion

Acute pancreatitis is generally a self-limiting process, but in its severe form, it can be a life-threatening disease. Patients with necrotizing pancreatitis often require surgical intervention, and those who don't may have a protracted period of recovery. Knowledge of the natural history of disease progression, as well as the timing and indications for intervention, is essential in ensuring proper treatment of patients with acute pancreatitis.

CHRONIC PANCREATITIS

METHOD OF

William H. Nealon, MD

Chronic pancreatitis remains a diagnosis that is likely to create confusion when managed in a clinical setting. Part of this results from an overlapping with a diagnosis of acute pancreatitis. The clinician may not be clear about the distinction between the two diagnoses and management principles are entirely disparate. Chronic pancreatitis for example may present with acute abdominal pain and nausea, as will acute pancreatitis. To make matters worse one may have a diagnosis of chronic pancreatitis and have a separate superimposed episode of acute pancreatitis. In very simple terms, a means of distinguishing these two diagnoses may be applied as follows: almost all episodes of *acute pancreatitis* should, after the acute event have no distinct changes in either the function or the structure of the pancreas. In contrast, *chronic pancreatitis* requires some element of permanent change in the pancreas. These changes may be structural and be no more than simple dilatation of the secondary ductules in the pancreas known as secondary ductular ectasia. Structural abnormalities may extend to massive dilatation of the main pancreatic duct and its side branches, to presence of stones within the ductal system, to significant glandular calcification fibrosis, and possibly to pseudocyst formation. Accompanying the structural changes one may anticipate finding some element of functional derangement. These relate to endocrine and exocrine function. Exocrine dysfunction is manifested by malabsorption, particularly of fat, with a clinical picture of steatorrhea. Endocrine dysfunction is manifested by diabetes. Parenthetically this diabetes is technically considered to be distinct from either type 1 or type 2 diabetes and many have termed it type 3 diabetes or "pancreatogenic" diabetes. From a practical standpoint the importance of this distinction is the fact that most adults who develop glucose intolerance are assumed to have type 2 diabetes and are managed by oral hypoglycemic agents. The diabetes developing in chronic pancreatitis is insulinopenic and therefore must be managed by insulin replacement. It is, unfortunately, common to find that a patient with this diagnosis has been managed by an array of oral agents without success before recognizing that insulin replacement is required. A simple understanding of the roots of the diabetes would help in making a more clear choice of management.

Many believe that chronic pancreatitis means many recurrent episodes of acute pancreatitis. It is estimated that only 10% to 15% of patients with chronic pancreatitis have actually had a history of repeated episodes of acute pancreatitis in the past. One might contrast the diagnosis of chronic bronchitis in which a patient has repeated episodes of acute bronchitis to the diagnosis of chronic pancreatitis which requires the previously mentioned attributes and is completely independent of prior episodes of acute pancreatitis. There is a pattern of disease in which patients have recurrent attacks of acute pancreatitis that is designated *acute relapsing pancreatitis,* not chronic pancreatitis. Considering this fact and the fact that many patients with chronic pancreatitis may present with acute exacerbations it is clear that considerable scrutiny must be applied in evaluating patients with inflammatory diseases of the pancreas. Again, the significance of making this distinction lies in the fact that treatment principles are completely different. Fortunately, imaging techniques have advanced to such a degree that confirmation of this diagnosis is more easily made. It may, however, require a high index of suspicion to establish this diagnosis. The diagnosis of chronic pancreatitis may well have associated abnormalities that are amenable to interventions that might lead to considerable improvement or complete resolution of chronic abdominal problems.

Manifestations of Disease

By far the most common manifestation of chronic pancreatitis is chronic abdominal and mid back pain. In the majority of patients this pain is located in the upper abdomen with radiation to the back. It is often more severe in the left side of the back. It is common for the pain to be worsened by a meal, but not invariably. In spite of ethanol being the mechanism for this disease in the majority of patients, ethanol ingestion does not seem to exacerbate the symptoms of chronic pancreatitis. Because the pain is often registered as severe, nearly all cases that present for care require narcotic analgesics to manage this pain. The entanglement inherent in this fact should be apparent to the reader. If we have a disease that is caused by substance abuse and we have a chronic pain syndrome that requires chronic narcotic use, the risk of narcotic dependence is considerably greater than in other types of chronic pain syndrome where underlying substance abuse personality traits had not preexisted the disease. There are a number of practical issues that arise because of the problem. First, one is asked to interpret the severity of the pain in chronic pancreatitis on the basis of the narcotic need. Because there may be an overlying narcotic dependence and drug-seeking behavior as opposed to pure narcotic use for pain, the careful segregation of these two influences is mandatory. Because the indications for intervention are based upon narcotic needs, among other measures, it is clear that the basis for the narcotic use must be greatly scrutinized. Perhaps even more meaningful to me as a pancreatic surgeon is that success for surgical intervention in chronic pancreatitis requires both relief of the pain and the freedom for the patient from any narcotic need. Because narcotic dependence may cloud the assessment of when a patient can be safely weaned from the patient's narcotics, the definitions for success with operations are profoundly influenced in this matter. It is common, for example, to have what appears to have been an excellent outcome after surgical intervention for chronic pancreatitis only to discover that the process of weaning the narcotics results in an array of complaints as the person is withdrawn from narcotic use. The challenge for all physicians managing patients with this disease is to develop a skill at distinguishing drug-seeking behavior from true pain requiring narcotic support. Unfortunately, no formulas exist to assist one in making this distinction. I will say that with years of experience, certain characteristics may facilitate establishing the distinction. Certainly the patient who is somnolent and repeatedly dozing during the interview is more likely to be, at least in part, suffering from narcotic dependence. Assistance from a psychiatric expert in pain management or an expert in pain management from the anesthesiology department may be of some assistance. A surgeon may need to help the patient with the process of weaning the narcotic dependence after surgery.

Finally, I will mention briefly the concept of pain scales. In the early articles I wrote on this disease, my definition of pain relief was complete absence of pain and the complete absence of any narcotic need. In the following years, many believed that the visual analogue scale was more precise. My concern is that now one may write an article and declare success in treating the pain of chronic pancreatitis because they have taken a person from a pain level of 9 or 10 and converted that to a pain level of 4 or 5. In these patients, it is likely that narcotic analgesia is still required and that the patient is still troubled by pain. I am not suggesting that this is a meaningless improvement, but I believe that the goal of therapy for this disease should be complete abolition of pain. Essentially all invasive interventions applied to chronic pancreatitis have as their primary goal the cessation of all pain.

After pain, other complications of chronic pancreatitis might be seen. Some element of obstruction may occur in various structures associated with the pancreas. First and most obvious is an apparent obstruction or near obstruction of the main pancreatic duct resulting in dilatation in the main pancreatic duct. At times this level of dilatation may result in a diameter in the main pancreatic duct exceeding 20 mm. As is discussed subsequently, there are patients who have normal-sized ducts with chronic pancreatitis. In addition to main pancreatic ductal dilatation, one can anticipate seeing some element of stenosis of the common bile duct as it traverses the intrapancreatic portion of the bile duct. The characteristic picture of this obstruction is an elongated narrowing that is characteristically well beyond the intraduodenal portions of the bile duct. For this reason, it has generally been agreed that these patients should never undergo endoscopic sphincterotomy of the bile duct sphincter in an effort to alleviate the obstruction. An even greater risk arises if one attempts endoscopic retrograde cholangiopancreatography (ERCP) and stent placement in patients with chronic pancreatitis-associated stricture of the bile duct. This intervention is contraindicated at all times. Once a stent has been placed, the patient is essentially condemned to a permanent stent because removal of the stent from the clinically stenotic bile duct invariably results in cholangitis. Unfortunately, leaving these stents in over a long period of time also raises the risk of occlusion of the stent and cholangitis. Thus placement of a stent in the bile duct in a patient with chronic pancreatitis almost certainly commits this patient to operative decompression of the bile duct to free the patient of a need for essentially lifelong dependence on bile duct stents. Interestingly, although the diameter of the narrowed bile duct often appears to be extremely small, jaundice in patients with this bile duct narrowing is exceedingly rare. This may help to distinguish patients with chronic pancreatitis from those who have carcinoma of the pancreas. In chronic pancreatitis, one may anticipate seeing an alkaline phosphatase level of well over 1000 U/L with no hyperbilirubinemia. In contrast, patients with carcinoma of the pancreas may have a bilirubin of greater than 20 U/L with an alkaline phosphatase elevation in the range of 300 or 400 U/L. The chronic narrowing of the bile duct results in a massive elevation of alkaline phosphatase level without jaundice. The only reasonable correction of this narrowing is operative decompression. The use of a self-expanding wall stent would be reserved only for patients who are considered an excessive risk for operative intervention. Stenosis alone is not an indication for decompression. The actual indication for intervention in biliary stenosis with chronic pancreatitis is a chronically elevated alkaline phosphatase level associated with moderate to significant common bile duct dilatation (greater than 12 mm in diameter). Published data confirms that prolonged obstruction of the bile duct results in progressive hepatic fibrosis and operative decompression reverses this process. It is estimated that as many as 50% of patients with chronic pancreatitis have some element of common bile duct narrowing. Only a small percent meet criteria for decompression.

Duodenal narrowing is thought to occur in less than 5% of patients; the percentage of patients who actually require a bypass procedure to manage duodenal narrowing is smaller yet. There are multiple reports of patients who can sustain a colonic narrowing because of chronic pancreatitis. The two mechanisms for this may be an inflammatory mass in the head of the pancreas that compresses the colon or a sufficient inflammation in the blood vessels that supply the colon, particularly the middle colic vessels, which may result in an ischemic narrowing of the colon. Again, these two last complications are uncommon.

Perhaps resulting from a mass compression or from chronic inflammation it is known that venous obstruction and thrombosis is a common feature in chronic pancreatitis. The most common vein to sustain this complication is the splenic vein, and the presence of splenic vein thrombosis in patients with chronic pancreatitis is well recognized. This may result in what has been termed *sinistral portal hypertension,* resulting in varices in the upper abdomen, around the stomach, and in the omentum. This is rarely associated with variceal bleeding; however, there are patients who sustain significant pain from the engorged spleen. This complication is managed by splenectomy. Confirmation of this entity can be made with cross-sectional imaging and does not require arteriography. This thrombosis in no way reflects a hypercoagulable state; consequently, under no circumstance should anticoagulation be considered. In the rare occasion that variceal hemorrhage does occur, splenectomy may be indicated.

Although it is safe to say that pain is the most common manifestation of chronic pancreatitis, I have defined three patterns of pain. There are few studies examining the disparate manifestations of pain in this disease. We published the success rates for operative intervention in patients with the three manifestations of pain patterns that we defined. The first of these manifestations is chronic unrelenting daily abdominal pain that is sufficiently severe to require narcotics for resolution. The second subset of patients suffer from this daily pain but also have intermittent acute exacerbations of their pain, often requiring hospitalization. These episodes are not episodes of acute pancreatitis, but rather are episodes of exacerbation. They are, for example, rarely associated with hyperamylasemia. The third manifestation that we defined is patients who are symptom free except when they have acute exacerbations. Again these acute exacerbations are not episodes of recurrent acute pancreatitis. All of the available literature confirms the success of operative intervention aimed at relieving daily pain. Our study alone confirms the success of operative intervention in reducing the frequency or completely abolishing these acute exacerbations of chronic pancreatitis. It is important to recognize that patients with chronic pancreatitis may present with this particular manifestation. This group of patients may initially be assigned a diagnosis of acute pancreatitis and only with a heightened level of suspicion and further radiographic evaluation can the diagnosis of chronic pancreatitis be established as distinct from recurrent acute pancreatitis.

Functional Derangements

The primary function of the pancreas is in processing nutrients and facilitating absorption with both exocrine and endocrine participation. Thus it should not be surprising that nutritional status and exocrine and endocrine function are significant issues in the management of chronic pancreatitis. Exocrine insufficiency is manifested clinically as steatorrhea and endocrine insufficiency is manifested as diabetes mellitus. A history of weight loss is extremely common in this disease, and very often early management should include addressing possibly unrecognized functional deficits (insulin insufficiency requiring insulin therapy or pancreatic enzyme insufficiency requiring enzyme replacement). At times, dramatic changes can be made in the patient's overall status by simply maximizing the management of these significant medical issues. Interestingly, it is my experience that patients may have maximized their endocrine and exocrine function and still have a persistent nutritional deficit that can be corrected only after decompressive surgery. Again, I stress that the diabetes associated with chronic pancreatitis ("type III" or pancreatogenic diabetes) is insulinopenic. It should therefore be treated only with insulin replacement.

Finally, it must be understood that patients with chronic pancreatitis may also harbor a carcinoma of the pancreas. In my opinion, this may represent two different categories of patients. One is a patient whose clinical or morphologic manifestations of cancer are mistaken for chronic pancreatitis. The other is a patient who has chronic pancreatitis and subsequently develops carcinoma. Data have been gathered to suggest that chronic pancreatitis patients are at higher risk for carcinoma of the pancreas than the general public. Some have theorized that this is related to the fact that most of these patients are also heavy smokers and the connection of cigarette smoking and carcinoma of the pancreas is well established. In either event, attention to the possible coexistence of carcinoma of the pancreas in patients with chronic pancreatitis is mandatory.

Pathophysiology

In general terms, it is understood that the protein-rich juices created by the exocrine pancreas are secreted into the tiny ductules, to the larger ductules, out into the main pancreatic duct, and, finally, on stimulation, to the intestine. The proteins in a normal pancreas remain in the solution very well. There are data to suggest that patients with chronic pancreatitis produce a type of protein that remains poorly in solution and as it precipitates, can serve as a plug in the tiny ductules within the pancreas. Thus it is generally agreed that secondary ductular changes are the first changes seen in chronic pancreatitis, and that these changes support the assumption that the disease begins in these very tiny ductules, where the protein plugging induces a reaction. In experimental animal models, the trigger for fibrosis in the pancreas is obstruction of the main pancreatic duct. Following this logic in the opposite direction, it is possible to speculate that secondary ductular changes can also induce a generalized fibrotic response. Secondary ductular dilatation and plugging can be identified in all patients with chronic pancreatitis. A generalized fibrosis is seen throughout the entire gland, which macroscopically results in a hard, enlarged, white appearance and microscopically manifests dense collagen and an elaborate fibroblastic response. The bicarbonate secretion, which is a product of ductal cells, is admixed with the protein-rich fluid from acinar cells. Precipitation occurs, with calcium carbonate stones developing. Stones form a cast of the secondary ductals, and large intraductal and main pancreatic ductal stones may be seen in this disease. Although the degree of calcification is unpredictable, the presence of calcifications in the glands in patients with chronic pancreatitis is said to occur in approximately 80% of patients. The further detail added by computed tomography (CT) scans has increased the recognized incidence of this association. The amount of fibrosis is also variable. There is a subset of patients who will manifest a large inflammatory mass. In some reports, these masses reached diameters of 20 cm. Although the mass is most commonly seen in the head of the pancreas, one may see significant masses in the body and tail of the pancreas as well. Main pancreatic ductal dilatation is seen in the majority of patients with chronic pancreatitis. Again, the assumption in this manifestation is the presence of a proteinaceous pancreatic juice, which serves to cause an element of obstruction in the distal pancreatic duct. This mechanism triggers the inflammatory response that is seen in the fibrosis of the gland, as well as triggering a proximal dilatation of the pancreatic duct in response to outflow obstruction. Some patients with this disease do not manifest a dilated main pancreatic duct. Although this subset is well recognized, there are insufficient data to define any differences in the disease when it is manifested by a large main pancreatic duct compared to those who have so-called small duct variant of chronic pancreatitis.

There are reports of chronic pancreatitis in patients with completely normal anatomy. There is no worldwide consensus on this entity. Those who have popularized this concept claim that an evaluation of the bicarbonate secretion in patients with chronic pain syndrome may show deficient bicarbonate secretion. These authors, on the basis of this physiologic finding, suggest that a diagnosis of chronic pancreatitis is present with the only abnormality being this reduced production of bicarbonate-rich fluid from the ductal cells of the pancreas. Most believe that structural abnormalities are required in defining chronic pancreatitis.

Pain

The pain of chronic pancreatitis is not easily explained. Recent studies at a microscopic and molecular biologic level show that chronic inflammatory cells do surround the nerves in the pancreas. There are suggestions that monocytes and circulating macrophages may play a role by depositing various cytokines in the microcirculation of the pancreas. Certainly within the body of the pancreas, the question of a localized neuritis seems to be supported by anatomic findings. Mapping the sensory nerves emanating from the pancreas is equally challenging. We do know that the combination of sympathetic and parasympathetic fibers cluster throughout the pancreas and arguments persist as to which of these two paths plays the larger role in carrying sensory signals back to the spinal cord and to the brain. The celiac trunk has been a recognized potential pathway for many years. Operative ganglionectomy and chemical celiac ganglion ablation have been recognized as occasionally effective in abolishing the pain associated with chronic pancreatitis. Transthoracic splanchnicectomy has been reported to have some value in pain reduction in patients with chronic pancreatitis. It is likely that a mixture of innervations through various trunks is the actual pathway for pain impulses to be transported from the pancreas to the brain. For this reason, ablation of individual pathways appears to be insufficient in managing the pain associated with chronic pancreatitis.

In addition, there is evidence that glandular hypertension plays a role in the pathophysiology of pain in chronic pancreatitis. Reber described the syndrome as a "compartment syndrome" of the pancreas. His studies suggest that the high pressures within the pancreas result in a level of localized ischemia in the pancreas. Although the ischemia is insufficient to threaten the viability of the pancreas, it does seem to induce an inflammatory reaction and to perpetuate the signal of pain within the pancreas. The success with decompressive procedures such as the modified Puestow procedure may be attributed to a correction of this glandular hypertension.

Diagnostic Evaluation: Imaging

The number of available modalities for imaging the pancreas in patients with chronic pancreatitis has increased dramatically in the last 15 years. Earlier modalities, such as ultrasound or even simple CT scanning, have been replaced by spiral CT scanning with a focus on the pancreas, as well as by magnetic resonance imaging (MRI), magnetic resonance cholangiopancreatography (MRCP), and endoscopic ultrasound. Each modality provides significant detail regarding the anatomy of the pancreas, as well as of the texture of the parenchyma, and endoscopic ultrasound may even offer options for biopsy. In spite of this, I continue to prefer ERCP in mapping the ductal system as I plan an operative intervention. It is perhaps my bias because MRCP certainly offers very similar information and spiral CT scan also gives an excellent view of the pancreatic duct. Chronic pancreatitis imaging plays two roles. First, to confirm a diagnosis of chronic pancreatitis. As previously stated, structural changes define chronic pancreatitis. The second role is exemplified by an advantage specific to ERCP, for example, when minimal changes, such as secondary ductular ectasia, can only be clearly seen with ERCP.

Management of Chronic Pancreatitis

MEDICAL MANAGEMENT

The mainstay for medical management of chronic pancreatitis is limited to narcotic analgesics to treat the pain. Certainly, maximizing the endocrine and exocrine function for a patient by providing insulin replacement or by providing enzyme replacement is a consideration. Some authors suggest that decreasing the amount of stimulation to the pancreas may reduce the pain. For that reason there have been studies supporting and some failing to see an advantage to either the use of octreotide (Sandostatin)[1], which will suppress pancreatic exocrine stimulation, or to taking oral pancreatic enzymes based upon a theoretical feedback mechanism to reduce stimulation to the pancreas. That in most cases surgery remains the one hope for freeing a patient of a life of daily pain serves as testimony to the fact that medical management of chronic pancreatitis is not yet particularly effective.

SURGICAL MANAGEMENT

One should attempt to preserve as much pancreatic parenchyma as possible because the disease already progresses to insufficiency states. The more pancreas that is removed in a resection, the more one may accelerate the progression to pancreatic insufficiency states. It is my belief that a drainage procedure such as a lateral pancreaticojejunostomy or Puestow procedure is preferable to resectional therapy. Although the criteria for choosing drainage or resection are clear, there does seem to be a predilection toward resection in certain parts of the world and toward drainage procedures in other areas. The primary goal for all operative intervention for chronic pancreatitis is the abolition of chronic unrelenting abdominal pain. The indications for drainage procedure include the presence of this sort of pain combined with anatomic features. It is generally agreed that a dilated main pancreatic duct to a diameter of at least 6 or 7 mm is required for success with an operative drainage of the pancreatic duct. The indication for resection in patients with chronic pancreatitis include so-called small duct chronic pancreatitis or a dominant inflammatory mass in the head of the pancreas, defined as a mass greater than 5 cm in diameter, or a suspicion for malignancy, or a failed prior drainage procedure. Resectional therapy is primarily a pancreaticoduodenectomy. Success rates for pain relief are 60% to 80%.

These procedures are a combination of drainage and resection. Thirty years ago, Hans Beger from Ulm, Germany, developed the procedure that he dubbed the duodenum-preserving pancreatic head resection. This is a drainage procedure for the head of the pancreas after the main body of the pancreatic head has been removed. This procedure also includes decompressing the bile duct by taking the fibrotic rind encasing the bile duct during the pancreatic head resection. Subsequently, Frey developed a procedure in which the body of the pancreas is not divided as it is in a Beger procedure; instead, a large excavation of the head of the pancreas is combined with a drainage procedure such as is seen with the classic Puestow procedure. Both of these procedures have an 80% to 90% success rate for long-term pain relief. More recently, Izbicki from Germany created a V-shaped excavation in the body of the pancreas to create what appears to be a larger duct. He applies this procedure to patients with the small duct variant of chronic pancreatitis. Although his patient series have been small, the data suggest that this can be an effective measure for reducing pain while preserving parenchyma of the pancreas in patients with this variant of disease. Resection of the tail of the pancreas—so-called distal pancreatectomy—is reserved for chronic pancreatitis, which is localized to the body and tail of the pancreas. Unfortunately, the success rates for this modality in achieving long-term pain relief has been the worst of all operative procedures performed for this purpose. Success rates are said to be between 30% and 50%.

Finally, nerve ablation has been applied to this disease for many years. The first operative celiac ganglionectomies were performed with minimal success rates. Subsequently, percutaneous access by CT guidance was used to perform chemical celiac nerve ablation, and more recently endoscopic ultrasound became a useful modality for performing this procedure. The success rates in chronic pancreatitis have always been very low for this procedure. Its success rates are always higher when looking at a group of patients with pancreatic carcinoma who have pain. In all patients these measures are temporary, and recurrence of pain does occur after some months. Transthoracic splenic nerve ablation has also been described and its successes have also been meager.

ENDOSCOPIC MANAGEMENT

In recent years, some attention has been directed toward endoscopic management of chronic pancreatitis. The primary modality for this is the placement of transpapillary stents into the main pancreatic duct. Although the earliest reports on this modality primarily from Kozarek were favorable, there remain considerable questions regarding the applicability of this modality. Perhaps most important is that patients with this disease are typically in their early forties. They require a lifetime of endoscopic stent replacements for management. There are no data to suggest that a temporary stent may result in long-term pain relief for this disease. Some authors suggest that a stent may help to predict the success of drainage procedures and this may well be an example of an opportunity to use pancreatic ductal

[1]Not FDA approved for this indication.

stents as a bridge to operative intervention. Although surgeons for years have known that during an operation one may remove stones from the main pancreatic duct, few surgeons believe that stones alone cause the pain of chronic pancreatitis. It is known that many patients with pancreatic duct stones have chronic unremitting pain that is relieved by a drainage procedure. In spite of the endoscopic literature regarding extraction of pancreatic ductal stones as a definitive measure in the treatment of pancreatic pain, the studies lack long-term follow-up to confirm that long-term pain relief was achieved by stone extraction alone. Although there are reports of pain-free patients after endoscopic removal of stones, the likelihood that stones would recur in patients with these diseases is exceedingly high. Strong support for the use of endoscopic measures, particularly for stone removal, as a definitive measure in the treatment of pain in chronic pancreatitis cannot be given.

GASTRO-ESOPHAGEAL REFLUX DISEASE

METHOD OF

Yuhong Yuan, MD, PhD, and Richard H. Hunt, MD

Gastroesophageal reflux disease (GERD) is a condition where clinically significant symptoms, physical complications, and impairment of health-related well-being are caused by the reflux of gastric contents from the stomach into the esophagus. GERD includes erosive esophagitis (EE) that causes symptoms and/or injury related to the esophageal mucosa, as well as nonerosive esophageal disorders. GERD is an important risk factor for Barrett's esophagus (BE). GERD is also associated with extraesophageal manifestations such as noncardiac chest pain, bronchial wheeze, and laryngitis.

GERD is one of the most common problems seen in medical practice. Heartburn is the most common symptom of GERD, and affects up to 10% of the U.S. population on a daily basis; 14% of adults suffer with GERD symptoms at least once a week, and up to 44% of the population is affected over a 6-month period. In most people, reflux symptoms are short-lived and occur infrequently, so they neither seek medical attention nor are treated in primary care practice with conservative measures. In approximately 20% of cases, however, the condition becomes chronic, and has a significant adverse impact on the quality of life. Although GERD is not a life-threatening condition, severe complications, such as ulceration, stricture, bleeding, or the development of Barrett's esophagus can occur and require specific management.

Pathophysiology

Incompetence of the lower esophageal sphincter (LES) is one of the most important mechanisms in the pathogenesis of GERD. The normal LES opens after the initiation of a swallow to allow food to enter the stomach and then immediately closes to prevent regurgitation of gastric contents, which include gastric acid, digestive enzymes, and often reflux of duodenal contents. The LES maintains a pressure barrier until food is swallowed again. Peristaltic action of the esophagus serves as an additional defense mechanism and propels alkaline salivary secretion and refluxed esophageal contents back into the stomach. Gastroesophageal reflux occurs if the muscular actions of the esophagus or other protective mechanisms fail. However, most patients with GERD have a normal resting LES but an increase in the number of transient lower esophageal relaxations (TLESRs).

Abnormalities such as hiatal hernia and defects in peristaltic function of the esophageal body, poor esophageal clearance, and delayed gastric emptying also play important roles in the pathogenesis of GERD. However, what factors determine the significant clinical impact of GERD remain less clear. Research indicates the importance of the minimal change histologic lesion where nerves lie near the surface of the squamous mucosa because of an increase in cell turnover and thus become exposed to acid that penetrates the mucosal surface, triggering a prolonged and painful symptom response. Mucosal damage and widened intercellular spaces because of acid exposure play a role in the stimulation of sensory nerve endings in the esophagus. Recently, nocturnal GERD symptoms have raised considerable interest. Nocturnal reflux may increase acid contact time with the distal esophageal mucosa, increasing the risk of developing more severe esophagitis, ulceration, or peptic stricture.

Possible mechanisms of heartburn and other esophageal symptoms in patients without erosive esophagitis include nonacid related intraesophageal stimuli; hypersensitivity to minute changes in esophageal pH (>4.0); abnormal acid exposure; and hypersensitivity to reflux events within the "normal" range (pH <4.0). Visceral sensation plays a role in patients with an acid-sensitive esophagus where the dorsal root ganglia (DRGs), spinal cord, and central nervous system are involved in the perception of visceral pain. Psychological factors may also contribute to symptoms in some patients with reflux, particularly in patients without erosive esophagitis. Stress may alter esophageal sensation and psychological factors may alter nociception by influencing cortical processing or descending corticofugal pathways.

Clinical Manifestations and Conditions

The clinical symptoms of GERD are variable and show a wide range of severity. The hallmark symptoms of gastroesophageal reflux are heartburn, a burning sensation in the chest and throat caused by acid and other irritating substances; and regurgitation, a sensation of gastric contents moving in a retrograde manner back up the esophagus. These two symptoms have the highest specificity in the diagnosis of GERD and occur most commonly after food and with recumbency, bending over, or heavy lifting; they often occur after large meals. A cardinal feature of heartburn is relief by antacids or antisecretory treatment. However, the severity of the heartburn does not correlate with the presence or severity of esophagitis. In addition to the discomfort of heartburn, reflux also results in symptoms of esophageal inflammation, such as odynophagia (pain on swallowing) and dysphagia (difficulty in swallowing). Odynophagia results from erosive esophagitis and is most common when the esophagitis is caused by infection or medication damage (pill-induced esophagitis). Dysphagia may be caused by stricture or peristaltic dysfunction, or by esophagitis. When either of these symptoms occurs predominantly, it should raise the possibility of an alternative diagnosis, such as pill-induced esophagitis or achalasia.

Less-common typical symptoms in patients with GERD include dysphagia, especially the difficulty in swallowing solids in those with esophageal strictures. Dysphagia with liquids can occur in patients with achalasia. Some patients may complain of "water brash" (hypersalivation secondary to a vagal reflex) or of globus sensation (a sensation of a lump in the throat).

Although gastric acid is a primary factor in esophageal mucosal damage caused by gastroesophageal reflux, other secretions of the digestive tract, including pepsin, bile, lysolecithin, and pancreatic enzymes, can also be harmful and cause symptoms. GERD can also be associated with a variety of nonspecific upper gastrointestinal symptoms, including nausea, dyspepsia, bloating, belching, and hiccoughs. Less commonly seen in GERD patients is gastrointestinal (GI) bleeding caused by inflammation of the esophagus, although slow blood loss resulting in anemia may occur.

A number of extraesophageal conditions are associated with GERD, including noncardiac chest pain; pulmonary disease particularly nonallergic asthma, chronic bronchitis, aspiration pneumonia, bronchiectasis, and pulmonary fibrosis; ear, nose, and throat (ENT) conditions including hoarseness, chronic cough, laryngitis, pharyngitis, sinusitis, subglottic stenosis, globus sensation, vocal cord granuloma, and laryngeal cancer; sleep apnea; and dental erosions. In contrast to the presentation and manifestations of typical GERD, it is important to emphasize that esophagitis is found in less than 20% of these patients.

There are three major conditions associated with gastroesophageal reflux: erosive esophagitis (EE), endoscopy negative reflux disease (ENRD), and Barrett's esophagus (BE).

EROSIVE ESOPHAGITIS

Erosive esophagitis occurs when gastric acid causes irritation or inflammation in the esophagus. If the damage becomes extensive, erosive esophagitis is observed endoscopically as visible esophageal mucosal injury. Erosive esophagitis can progress to esophageal ulcer, stricture, and bleeding if untreated. Approximately 50% of all patients with GERD in specialist practice, and probably less in community studies, are found to have esophagitis at endoscopy; however, only a small percentage of these patients have severe erosive disease.

ENDOSCOPY NEGATIVE REFLUX DISEASE

ENRD, also called "nonerosive esophageal reflux disorder," is a heterogeneous group of conditions presenting with typical GERD symptoms in the absence of visible esophageal injury at endoscopy. This group can be further divided into nonerosive reflux disease (NERD), with abnormal acid exposure, and functional heartburn, with normal acid exposure. The presence of typical GERD symptoms because of intraesophageal acid exposure without signs of inflammation or erosion in the esophagus at endoscopy is usually referred to as NERD; functional heartburn refers to patients with more than 12 weeks of symptoms in the preceding 12 months, which weeks need not be consecutive, of burning retrosternal discomfort or pain in the absence of pathologic gastroesophageal reflux, achalasia, or other motility disorder with a recognized pathologic basis. In patients with heartburn, approximately 30% to 70% have negative endoscopic findings. Patients with endoscopically negative disease rarely progress to full-blown GERD. Compared to esophagitis patients, those without endoscopic erosive disease tend to be younger, female, nonobese, and without a hiatal hernia. Approximately 50% of patients with ENRD have a normal esophageal acid exposure on pH-metry, but have a similar measurable and substantial impairment of quality of life to those patients with esophagitis. ENRD is also associated with atypical extraesophageal manifestations of gastroesophageal reflux; symptoms can occur without any signs of inflammation or injury to the esophagus, and include chest pain, asthma, chronic cough, and laryngitis.

BARRETT'S ESOPHAGUS

Barrett's esophagus is defined as a change in the esophageal mucosa of any length that can be recognized at endoscopy and is confirmed to have the features of intestinal metaplasia on histological examination of biopsies. This condition is associated with an increased risk of development of adenocarcinoma of the esophagus. Only approximately 10% of patients with gastroesophageal reflux eventually develop Barrett's esophagus, although patients who have had GERD symptoms for many years have a higher risk of developing Barrett's esophagus. It is currently estimated that the risk of developing adenocarcinoma in Barrett's is approximately 0.5% per year. Chronic and severe exposure of the esophageal mucosa to acid reflux is considered to be an important risk factor for the development of Barrett's, which is modified by several genetic factors, including P53, P16, and P17 abnormalities, which determine the individual risk. Patients with Barrett's esophagus have no unique symptoms other than the symptoms of GERD. However, some affected patients are detected by chance with minimal symptoms of GERD. The reduced esophageal acid sensitivity that tends to develop over time in Barrett's esophagus may result in poor recognition and delay in the effective treatment of reflux.

Diagnostic Testing

There is no gold standard test for the diagnosis of GERD because of the wide range of typical, atypical, and extraesophageal symptoms that occur. A careful patient history seeking typical symptoms of heartburn or regurgitation provides for the highest specificity (89% and 95%, respectively) in the diagnosis of GERD. Because of the wide prevalence, empiric therapy with a proton pump inhibitor (PPI) is the most appealing approach in the diagnosis of GERD, because it treats the patient at the same time. The response to a therapeutic trial of a PPI given at least once a day (e.g., omeprazole [Prilosec] 20 mg, lansoprazole [Prevacid] 30 mg, pantoprazole [Protonix] 40 mg, rabeprazole [Aciphex] 20 mg, and esomeprazole [Nexium] 40 mg) for a minimum of 1 to 4 weeks, is as effective as 24-hour intraesophageal pH monitoring for establishing the diagnosis of gastroesophageal reflux. To avoid masking peptic ulcer or malignancy, empiric therapy is recommended in patients younger than age 50 years, who have no alarm signs (e.g., weight loss, iron deficiency, vomiting) as the initial approach. Patients who do not achieve a substantial response to adequate acid suppression therapy and who have a history of symptoms suggestive of GERD complications, have atypical or extraesophageal symptoms that are possibly related to GERD, or have typical symptoms but need objective confirmation of the diagnosis before antireflux surgery, should undergo further investigation, including upper GI endoscopy and 24-hour esophageal pH monitoring. Among all the available tests, only ambulatory 24-hour intraesophageal pH monitoring provides direct evidence of gastroesophageal reflux. Other tests discussed below may reveal esophagitis or impaired lower esophageal sphincter pressure, but these findings are of less value and may give false-negative results especially in patients with ENRD.

AMBULATORY 24-HOUR pH MONITORING

Ambulatory intraesophageal pH monitoring is the most accurate diagnostic test for gastroesophageal reflux and is similar to an empiric trial of PPI treatment, with a high sensitivity (96%) and specificity (96%). This test is performed in an ambulatory setting with a portable data logger to store the pH recordings from an intraesophageal pH probe. The data recorded can be interpreted and analyzed by computer. This technique measures and quantifies the basic pathophysiologic problem of GERD and measurements are quantitatively related to the degree of esophageal mucosal injury. Episodes of gastroesophageal reflux are recorded and with recorded patient response can indicate if symptoms occur during these episodes. The cumulative time the intraesophageal pH is <4 is expressed as a percentage of the total, upright, and supine time; the frequency of the reflux episodes is expressed as the number of episodes per 24 hours; and the duration of the episodes is expressed as the number of episodes longer than 5 minutes per 24 hours and the time in minutes of the longest episode is recorded. However, normal acid exposure values are recorded in approximately 25% of patients with otherwise typical reflux esophagitis and in 30% to 50% of those with ENRD. Compared to healthy controls, ENRD patients have a slightly reduced amplitude of distal esophageal contractions and there is a slight increase in the time the distal esophageal pH is <4.0, but there are no differences in the resting LES pressure. Patients with erosive esophagitis and Barrett's esophagus have significantly higher esophageal acid exposure than do those with ENRD. Unfortunately, 24-hour intraesophageal pH monitoring is considerably less sensitive in patients with extraesophageal manifestations of reflux. Use of dual pH sensors in the proximal and distal esophagus is necessary in some of these patients to detect proximal esophageal or pharyngeal acid exposure. There are some limitations to 24-hour pH intraesophageal monitoring, which is relatively expensive, not always available, and may be poorly tolerated. Moreover, monitoring of the temporal relationship to symptoms must be specifically undertaken.

ENDOSCOPY

Symptom severity does not predict the endoscopic findings in patients with reflux symptoms. Up to 70% of patients with typical symptoms of GERD have a normal esophageal mucosa at endoscopy. Consequently, endoscopy is no longer considered the gold standard for diagnosing GERD because it has a low sensitivity (68%) but high specificity at 96%. However, endoscopy can reveal erosive esophagitis the severity of which can be graded by the Los Angeles classification. This is not necessary for effective therapy, but does predict prognosis. Endoscopy should be undertaken in all patients who have alarm symptoms and most gastroenterologists advocate a once-in-a-lifetime endoscopy to screen for Barrett's esophagus in patients with GERD who cannot be taken off acid-suppressing drugs after 2 to 3 years. There is, as yet, no established guideline for selecting which reflux patients should be screened by endoscopy. However, such patients should be first treated with a PPI to heal erosive or ulcerative changes, which makes evaluation of the columnar epithelium more difficult to recognize and may confound some features of dysplasia.

Some other tests have limited use in GERD diagnosis. Esophageal manometry is useful in the evaluation of motility before antireflux surgery, or to exclude a severe dysmotility syndrome such as achalasia. The Bernstein test (esophageal acid perfusion) helps to determine if symptoms are related to the esophagus and acid reflux and this has a sensitivity of 84% and specificity of 83%. A barium swallow is helpful to show a hiatal hernia, stricture, or reflux into the proximal esophagus, but the sensitivity (40%) and specificity (85%) are low for a diagnosis of GERD.

HELICOBACTER PYLORI AND GERD

The role of *Helicobacter pylori* (*H. pylori*) infection in esophageal disease is controversial. However, the weight of evidence shows that *H. pylori* infection is inversely correlated with GERD, with several studies reporting that *H. pylori* infection is less prevalent in patients with severe GERD, Barrett's esophagus, or adenocarcinoma of the esophagus. Some studies indicate that PPIs have less effect on lowering gastric acid secretion in *H. pylori*-negative patients than in those who are infected. However, this phenomenon is not of any clinical relevance. There is no established agreement to test and eradicate *H. pylori* infection in patients with GERD, although the opinion in Europe is that patients who require treatment with long-term acid suppression should have *H. pylori* infection sought and eradicated if present, to avoid the risk of progression of atrophic gastritis. However, if *H. pylori* infection is found, it should always be eradicated in accordance with existing guidelines.

Treatment

The treatment goals for GERD include effective control of intragastric acidity by raising pH > 4; achievement of rapid onset of symptom relief both during the day and at night; effective healing of erosive esophagitis, both acute and in the long term; and using well-tolerated treatment with flexible dosing options. For the patient, the most important issue is the relief of symptoms. The primary treatment regimens for GERD include lifestyle modification with weight loss, dietary modification, and reduction of any activity that precipitates symptoms, such as stopping smoking and a reduction in alcohol intake. Treatment options include medical therapy, new endoscopic procedures, and surgery.

MEDICAL THERAPY OF GERD

Medical therapies for GERD include antacids, sucralfate (Carafate)[1], promotility agents, histamine H_2 receptor antagonists (H_2RA), and PPIs, but suppression of gastric acid secretion is the mainstay of treatment for GERD. The healing of erosive esophagitis can be predicted by the proportion of time that the intraesophageal pH is raised above 4 throughout the 24-hour period. Today, PPIs are the drugs of choice for gastroesophageal reflux disease. PPIs block the final common pathway of acid secretion by the H^+K^+ adenosine triphosphatase (ATPase) or acid pumps located in the secretory canaliculus of the parietal cells, resulting in a marked decrease in acidity and gastric juice volume both after meals and during the night. With the widespread use of PPIs, the medical treatment of GERD is successful in relieving symptoms, healing esophagitis, esophageal ulcers and preventing complications, such as stricture in the majority of patients. PPIs show significantly higher healing rates and symptom relief than H_2RAs in both erosive esophagitis and endoscopy-negative reflux disorders. In erosive esophagitis patients, PPIs at standard dose, once a day in the morning for 4 to 8 weeks, are the most effective medications, with an 80% to 90% healing rate in patients with erosive esophagitis, in contrast to standard doses of H_2RAs, which are effective in only 40% to 50% of patients. Some patients require an increase in dose of the PPI when the standard dose should be given twice daily to control symptoms, rather than doubling of the single morning dose. This is because the plasma half-life of these prodrugs is short (1 to 1.5 hours) and the acid pumps can be blocked only when they are inserted into the secretory canalicular membrane. The PPIs are all well tolerated in short- and long-term use.

H_2RAs may relieve heartburn and are commonly used for milder reflux symptoms (e.g., cimetidine [Tagamet] 800 mg twice daily [bid], ranitidine [Zantac] 150 mg bid, famotidine [Pepcid] 20 mg bid, nizatidine [Axid] 150 mg bid). However, in long-term therapy H_2RAs are limited by the need for frequent dosing, particularly by tachyphylaxis and by rebound acid hypersecretion. Moreover, they only weakly suppress meal-stimulated acid secretion.

In terms of treatment, NERD should not be considered a milder form of GERD. Patients with NERD are often more difficult to treat than those with erosive esophagitis. Both NERD and complicated

[1]Not FDA approved for this indication.

reflux disease should be treated with high-dose PPIs (standard dose twice daily) for 8 to 12 weeks, and this approach is required in the majority of NERD patients, who will usually respond to such a high-dose regimen.

Prokinetics may help to relieve reflux symptoms particularly by reducing regurgitation and by accelerating gastric emptying. Cisapride (Propulsid)* was the most commonly used drug in this class, before it was taken off the market because of adverse cardiac effects (prolongation of the QT interval and cardiac dysrhythmias). Metoclopramide (Reglan) is a centrally acting dopamine antagonist that has prokinetic effects by increasing contractile motility of the stomach and, to a lesser degree, increasing esophageal motility and LES pressure. However, it is approved only for short-term use (10 mg two to four times daily, 30 minutes before each meal and at bedtime for 4 to 12 weeks). Moreover, metoclopramide can cause drowsiness or restlessness, and is associated with severe extrapyramidal effects, which may be irreversible. Promotility agents seldom work alone, but may be complementary to antisecretory therapy in GERD.

With increasing interest in the role of psychological factors and of visceral hypersensitivity in patients with reflux disease, antidepressants have been used for esophageal symptoms—particularly pain and discomfort. Tricyclic antidepressants[1] in low dose may improve esophageal symptoms without affecting esophageal motility, and selective serotonin reuptake inhibitors (SSRIs)[1] are more likely than nitrates to improve chest pain and dysphagia in patients with diffuse esophageal spasm.

MAINTENANCE THERAPY

Maintenance treatment is needed to achieve long-term remission in most (approximately 80%) patients with erosive esophagitis. Standard-dose PPIs given once daily for 12 months can keep 70% to 90% of patients in remission, while H_2RAs twice daily are able to keep only 15% to 30% of patients in remission. Only approximately 20% of patients have no recurrence 1 year after discontinuing PPI treatment. Full-dose PPIs are associated with the lowest recurrence rates in erosive esophagitis compared to half-dose PPIs, prokinetics, H_2RAs, or placebo. However, some patients may respond to a "step-down" strategy after 8 to 12 weeks of successful initial treatment, to on-demand, alternate-day PPI, or low-dose PPI or H_2RA, although the trial evidence for this approach is not strong. If a patient experiences a recurrence of symptoms after or during step-down therapy, full-dose PPI should be restarted for another 8 to 12 weeks.

Tapering medication before discontinuing treatment is suggested, to avoid rebound acid hypersecretion with H_2RA.

*Investigational drug in the United States.
[1]Not FDA approved for this indication.

The long-term safety of the PPIs is well established over more than 15 years of treatment experience. Assimilation of vitamin B_{12} (cobalamin) from dietary sources requires gastric acid. Reduced serum vitamin B_{12} levels have been documented occasionally during long-term acid suppression therapy with an H_2RA or PPI. This is related to the presence of background atrophic gastritis rather than an effect of treatment. Most patients are unlikely to experience the deficiency because of large body stores of vitamin B_{12}. Vitamin B_{12} status may be monitored in patients taking a PPI for extended periods of time, particularly >3 years.

In Europe, it is recommended that in patients who require long-term PPI treatment, *H. pylori* infection should be sought and treated if present, to avoid the theoretical risk of progression of atrophic gastritis, which is a risk factor for gastric cancer, although no stomach tumors have developed in patients taking long-term antisecretory treatment. No such recommendation has been made in North America.

REFRACTORY PATIENTS

Symptoms can be persistent in a few patients, even on continuing PPI therapy. Possible causes for treatment failure include poor compliance and dosing issues, variation in bioavailability of the PPIs, delayed gastric emptying, inadequate acid control, incorrect diagnosis (e.g., symptoms caused by "nonacid" reflux, pill-induced esophageal injury), acid hypersecretion (Zollinger-Ellison syndrome), the influence of *H. pylori*-associated gastritis, and the like. For poor responders, 24-hour intraesophageal pH-metry should be performed while taking the PPI. Most GERD patients can be treated effectively with currently available PPIs, and twice-daily dosing of a PPI 30 minutes to 1 hour before breakfast and the evening meal effectively controls GERD in the majority of these patients.

Recent research suggests that nocturnal acid breakthrough (NAB) may occur during PPI therapy. NAB is defined as a drop in intragastric pH <4 for 1 hour overnight while on twice-daily PPI therapy. The prevalence of NAB is reported as 70% to 80% in both healthy volunteers and GERD patients, and typically NAB occurs 6 to 7 hours after the evening dose of the PPI and may last 3 to 4 hours. More than 50% of patients with Barrett's esophagus or scleroderma with GERD experience overnight esophageal acid exposure during NAB. However, 96% of GERD patients with NAB have minimal or no esophagitis, but the clinical significance of this observation is not clear. A standard dose of an H_2RA at bedtime (e.g., ranitidine [Zantac] 150 mg, nizatidine [Axid] 150 mg) has been used to control NAB in addition to the once- or twice-daily PPI therapy. However, the benefit of a nocturnal dose of H_2RA is temporary because of tachyphylaxis, and so far there is little or no clinical evidence to support the use this regimen.

ENDOSCOPIC THERAPY FOR GERD

In recent years, endoscopic procedures have been developed for treating reflux disease. Three major endoscopic techniques to reduce acid reflux—the Stretta, EndoCinch, and Enteryx—are approved by the FDA for treating GERD. The Stretta system consists of applying a radiofrequency (RF) current intraluminally to the region of the LES. The radiofrequency ablation results in scarring, causing narrowing or thickening of the LES to reduce reflux and damage of nerves responsible for transient LES relaxations. The Stretta procedure is usually preceded by 24-hour intraesophageal pH monitoring to confirm esophageal acid exposure in patients considered for antireflux surgery but who are unsuitable for general anesthesia or who are at risk of surgery. The Stretta procedure has been followed for up to 12 months, at which time symptom scores and esophageal acid contact time were significantly improved, especially in mild GERD (grades 0 to 1). Patients excluded from clinical trials of the Stretta procedure include those with hiatal hernia, grades 3 to 4 esophagitis, long-segment Barrett's esophagus, or collagen vascular diseases. Approximately 2% of patients have experienced complications, including perforation, bleeding, or mucosal injury. The EndoCinch endoluminal gastric plication technique uses an endoscopic sewing device to create pleats with a series of sutures passed through adjoining folds of the proximal fundus, to tighten the cardiac component of the LES. There are several reports of a benefit in GERD patients. In a multicenter U.S. study of 64 GERD patients, more than 70% of patients reported a significant reduction in GERD symptoms after 6 months. The number of patients requiring medications to control GERD symptoms was reduced by more than 75%. The third procedure, Enteryx, involves injection of a biopolymer, ethylene vinyl alcohol, into the submucosal zone beneath the LES, under fluoroscopic control. After injection, the solvent separates leaving the polymer to solidify into a spongy material that is intended to augment LES pressure and decrease transient LES relaxations. In a 12-month study of 85 patients, 72% had an improvement in their symptom score and 67% of patients were able to discontinue medications. However, persistent acid reflux was noted in 61% of the patients with low-grade inflammation in the distal esophagus, and in 37% of patients at 12 months. Patients with severe erosive esophagitis and hiatal hernia >3 cm were excluded in this trial. The most common side effect was substernal pain, which occurred in more than 90% of patients but usually resolved within 2 weeks.

It is important to emphasize that all these endoscopic procedures for GERD are still new and have been largely performed in patients with mild disease, and that each procedure carries its own risks. Long-term data are not yet available and further evaluation of the safety and efficacy of these endoscopic procedures is needed before introducing them outside the setting of clinical trials.

ANTIREFLUX SURGERY

Fundoplication has been the standard surgical approach for treating GERD. Medical treatment of GERD with PPIs has been demonstrated in good trials to be equal to the success of antireflux surgery in short- and long-term follow-up. Failure to respond to a PPI predicts a poor response to surgery. Predictors for the success of surgery include typical symptoms; a good response to PPI treatment, an abnormal intraesophageal pH study; esophagitis; and for the procedure to be performed by an experienced surgeon. Fundoplication may be done using a laparotomy and thoracotomy, or, more commonly now, a laparoscopic approach. Laparoscopic Nissen fundoplication for GERD is successful in approximately 85% of cases, and can control acid and bile reflux or regurgitation. There is approximately a 9% complication rate and mortality is 0.2%. Dysphagia occurs in approximately 5.5% of patients, and so patient selection and referral to surgical expertise is critical. Esophageal manometry is, in our view, mandatory before fundoplication. Remission rates are similar (at approximately 80%) between open antireflux surgery and treatment with omeprazole after 5 years in esophagitis patients. There is no conclusive evidence that antireflux surgery can induce regression of dysplasia in patients with Barrett's esophagus. The risk of adenocarcinoma in Barrett's esophagus is low and not significantly decreased by a surgical antireflux procedure. In a recent meta-analysis, there was no significant difference in cancer rates between patients who had surgical antireflux procedures and those who were treated medically. Antireflux surgery in the setting of Barrett's esophagus should not be recommended as an antineoplastic measure. Antireflux surgery is presently being challenged by the new endoscopic methods, but it is still too early to say which method is more effective, safe, and longer lasting.

TREATMENT OF EXTRAESOPHAGEAL SYMPTOMS

The extraesophageal manifestations of GERD include pulmonary complaints (e.g., asthma, chronic bronchitis), ENT symptoms (e.g., laryngitis), and symptoms in other systems (e.g., noncardiac chest pain, dental erosions). Although the majority of patients presenting with extraesophageal manifestations of GERD do not have classic heartburn or acid regurgitation, a careful patient history may provide some clues to suggest these extraesophageal symptoms are related to gastroesophageal reflux. For example, GERD-related asthma usually begins in adulthood and there is a lack of family history of asthma and absence of an allergic component; asthma is worsened by eating, exercise, supine posture, theophylline or β_2-agonists; there may be nocturnal respiratory symptoms, as well as other symptoms.

An empiric trial of acid suppression is practical and cost-effective when the clinical history strongly suggests that extraesophageal symptoms are related to gastroesophageal reflux. A full dose of PPI is appropriate given twice daily as described above (e.g., omeprazole [Prilosec] 20 mg twice a day or lansoprazole [Prevacid] 30 mg twice a day) for at least 2 to 3 months. Most patients with reflux-related chest pain respond in 1 to 2 months, but reflux-related asthma or ENT problems usually require at least 3 months of aggressive antireflux therapy. If the extraesophageal symptoms resolve during treatment, the long-term strategy should include a trial of "step-down" in the acid-suppression treatment. If symptoms persist after 3 months of PPI therapy, patients should be referred for diagnostic testing, particularly for ambulatory 24-hour intraesophageal pH monitoring. If tests are positive, patients might require more aggressive acid suppression with higher more frequent dosing of the PPI, and other causes should be investigated in nonresponders with a normal pH profile.

TREATMENT OF GERD IN SPECIAL PATIENT POPULATIONS

Elderly GERD patients usually have less-severe reflux symptoms than younger patients as a consequence of lower pain sensitivity, but treatment of these elderly patients is the same. In elderly patients who cannot swallow capsules or tablets, the choice of a PPI available in granules or fast dissolving formulation (e.g., lansoprazole) is particularly helpful. Granules can be sprinkled on selected soft foods (e.g., lansoprazole, esomeprazole [Nexium], omeprazole) or can be mixed into selected beverages (lansoprazole). Lansoprazole is now available in a fast-dissolving tablet.

Reflux is a common symptom in pregnant women and usually develops as a new symptom, contributed to by the physiologic changes in pregnancy. Lifestyle and dietary modifications, and antacids (e.g., Gaviscon) provide conservative therapy for pregnant women with mild symptoms. H_2RA, sucralfate (Carafate) and most PPIs (except omeprazole, which is under category class C) are still under FDA pregnancy category class B (safe in animal studies but safety not yet proven in humans), although some small case series with omeprazole and lansoprazole have reported safe delivery in humans. Antacids, sucralfate, and H_2RA (with the exception of nizatidine [Axid]) are safe during lactation, but PPIs are not recommended.

TREATMENT OF COMPLICATIONS—BARRETT'S ESOPHAGUS

Medical treatments for the symptoms of Barrett's esophagus are the same as those for GERD. There is little evidence to suggest that PPIs promote regression of Barrett's epithelium, but most patients will be treated with PPIs to control symptoms and to maintain healing. The incidence of esophageal carcinoma in patients with BE is approximately 0.5% per year. Low-grade dysplasia, when detected, is managed by continuing endoscopic surveillance and biopsies every 6 months. Surveillance should be performed every 3 years in patients without dysplasia. Patients with high-grade dysplasia should be managed by esophagectomy, the gold standard. Alternatively, ablation therapy, which removes the target tissue, has been used in Barrett's esophagus with dysplasia and has been reported to be successful in more than half the cases. Ablation combined with photodynamic therapy (PDT) is still experimental and the most commonly used approach for high-grade dysplasia in Barrett's esophagus. However, several trials indicate that patients may have persistent areas of Barrett's and dysplasia as a result of incomplete ablation. Endoscopic mucosal resection (EMR) resects areas of the mucosa identified as dysplastic, and is another experimental method to treat high-grade dysplasia. Chemoprevention therapy with drugs such as the COX-2 inhibitors[1] is also being studied in Barrett's dysplasia. There is no evidence that surgery leads to regression of Barrett's metaplasia.

Conclusion

GERD is a condition caused by the reflux of gastric contents from the stomach into the esophagus. The clinical symptoms of GERD are variable and show a wide range of severity. Suppression of acid secretion is the current mainstay of treatment for GERD. With the widespread use of proton pump inhibitors, the medical treatment of GERD and its complications is successful in relieving symptoms, healing esophagitis, and preventing complications in most of the patients.

[1]Not FDA approved for this indication.

GASTRIC CANCER

METHOD OF

Charu Taneja, MD, and Harold J. Wanebo, MD

The incidence of gastric cancer worldwide is 755,000 cases per year, which is second only to lung cancer. Its incidence is decreasing in the West. There are approximately 21,900 new cases in the United States per year, and it is responsible for 13,500 cancer deaths annually. The current estimated 5-year survival in the United States is less than 20%.

In the United States, gastric cancer is believed to be related to diets rich in nitrosamines. There is a high incidence of gastric cancer in areas where *Helicobacter pylori* is endemic. It is also related to alcohol and tobacco abuse, low socioeconomic status, and African American race. Villous adenomas in the stomach, which account for 2% of gastric polyps, are also associated with gastric cancer, not just in the polyp but elsewhere in the stomach as well. There is also a well-defined co-relation between gastric cancer and prior gastrectomy. Gastric cancer typically appears 1 to 15 years following gastrectomy and is believed to be related to atrophic gastritis and intestinal metaplasia.

Pathologic Types

The most common location (60% to 70%) for gastric cancer has been the antrum, but in recent years, proximal cancers have been increasing. Proximal gastric cancer now accounts for 20% to 40% of all gastric cancers. The incidence of linitis plastica has remained unchanged at 9%. Synchronous gastric cancer is seen in 2% of all cases.

Adenocarcinoma is the most common histologic type of gastric cancer (95%). Others are lymphoma (5%), carcinoid, leiomyosarcoma, and squamous cell carcinoma. Grossly gastric cancer may be either ulcerative (75%), polypoid (10%), scirrhous (10%), or superficial (5%).

Microscopically, the two main types are intestinal and diffuse, the latter of which is more common in the United States. The intestinal type is seen in high-risk, patients older than 65 years of age, is usually well differentiated, and tends to demonstrate hematogenous spread. It usually develops under the risk of dietary and environmental factors and arises in areas of intestinal metaplasia and chronic gastritis. The usual sequence of events is acute or chronic inflammation, then gland loss and mucosal atrophy, followed by dysplasia. It has a better prognosis and has a decreasing prevalence in Western countries.

Diffuse type of gastric cancer is seen in low-risk, younger patients and is more likely to be of a poorly differentiated, signet ring cell type. It usually has lymphatic or contiguous spread. Early gastric cancer is localized to the mucosa and submucosa. It accounts for 40% of cancers in Japan and only 10% in the United States. Despite its name, lymph node metastases are seen in 3% to 5% of all mucosal lesions and up to 20% of all submucosal lesions. The cure rates for early gastric cancer are greater than 90% at 5 years and 80% at 10 years.

Investigations and Preoperative Staging

The diagnosis of gastric cancer is usually made at the time of either upper endoscopy or upper gastrointestinal (GI) series. Barium studies are only 70% to 80% accurate and have a false-negative rate of 10% to 20%. An upper endoscopy is still required for histologic diagnosis. A detailed examination of the mucosa, with 4 to 6 biopsies and/or brushings, is more than 90% accurate in diagnosing cancer. Endoscopic ultrasound is very accurate in preoperative tumor staging but is less useful in evaluation of nodal status. It is not at all useful in the evaluation of distant metastases.

Helical computed tomography (CT) scanning is helpful in diagnosing nodal involvement and liver or lung metastases. The accuracy of CT scanning is 90% in the liver, 60% for nodal involvement, and less than 50% for peritoneal disease. In some studies as many as 60% of patients are understaged by the use of CT scan alone.

LAPAROSCOPY

Laparoscopy is used in patients with T3/T4 lesions to detect peritoneal and liver metastases. The laparoscopic false-negative rate is less than 5%. In a study of 71 patients, 97% were able to undergo laparoscopy and 23% of these had previously unidentified metastases. Only one patient (5%) required surgery at a later date for palliation. The optimal use of helical CT scans with laparoscopy increases the resectability rate to 93%. In a similar study at Memorial Sloan-Kettering of 111 patients with gastric cancer, 94% had accurate staging and unexpected metastatic disease was discovered on laparoscopy in 34% of the patients. Of their patients, 24 patients had laparoscopy alone and were discharged from the hospital within 1 day versus 6.5 days for an exploratory laparotomy. No patient undergoing laparoscopy alone required palliative surgery at a later date. Similarly, data from an Italian study demonstrated that of 100 patients undergoing laparoscopy, 21 patients had widespread metastases and up to 58 were understaged by the preoperative investigations. In this study, the predictive value of laparoscopic staging was 86% in T3/T4 lesions and was more sensitive than other modalities in detecting peritoneal disease.

The addition of peritoneal cytology to diagnostic laparoscopy further increases its value—a positive peritoneal cytology has a similar outcome to that of patients with metastatic disease. Another modality under investigation is positron emission tomography (PET) scanning.

Standard Surgery

The primary mode of treatment remains surgery. Gastric cancer spreads directly into adjacent structures, onto peritoneal surfaces, via lymphatics, and spreads hematogenously to the liver or lung. The nodal metastatic patterns have been well demonstrated by Japanese workers. Although Eastern surgeons and experienced Western gastric surgery centers have long demonstrated superior survival and tumor control rates with extended lymphadenectomy (D2 or D2-4), this has not been confirmed by randomized trial.

ANTRAL OR DISTAL THIRD CANCER

For gastric cancer involving the antrum or distal third (35% of gastric cancers), a radical subtotal (75% to 90%) gastrectomy is recommended, including 3 cm of the duodenum, the omentum, and the hepatogastric ligament. A splenectomy is usually not performed, and reconstruction is either via a roux-en-Y or B2 gastrojejunostomy. A 3- to 6-cm margin should be obtained, and this is confirmed with an intraoperative frozen section. For descriptive purposes, a standard D1 lymphadenectomy includes nodal tissue within 3 cm of the tumor—usually the nodes along the greater and lesser curvatures as well as the supra- and infrapyloric nodes. An extended or D2 lymphadenectomy includes nodes along the celiac artery and the major branches, hepatic, left gastric, and splenic artery. The nodes in the splenic hilum may be locally removed, and a positive biopsy would necessitate a splenectomy.

MIDDLE THIRD CANCER

Middle third or body cancers account for 10% to 30% of gastric cancers, and the standard surgery is a total gastrectomy. A distal subtotal gastrectomy may be considered for intestinal variants. Splenectomy is often required. A D1 lymphadenectomy includes the nodes along the greater and lesser curvatures, supra- and infrapyloric nodes and nodes along the gastric artery. Similarly, a D2 lymphadenectomy includes the nodes along the hepatic, right, and left gastric; celiac arteries; and the splenic hilum and splenic artery. Again, the D2 dissection provides the best staging and may enhance local regional control, although this is not proven.

PROXIMAL GASTRIC CANCER

Surgery for proximal gastric cancers is somewhat controversial. Proximal gastric cancers account for over 35% of all the cancers at this time. With this, there is an increased need for total gastrectomy and splenectomy, which adds considerably to the increased morbidity (10% survival at 5-year follow-up). At least a 10-cm margin is recommended, and these cancers may be approached via either a combined abdominal-left thoracic or abdominal-right thoracic approach. The extent of resection for proximal gastric cancer (total versus proximal gastrectomy) does not affect outcome. A D1 lymphadenectomy includes nodes along both curvatures, right and left cardia nodes, and nodes along the short gastric vessels. A D2 lymphadenectomy additionally includes nodes along the left gastric artery, hepatic artery, splenic artery, celiac artery, and arteries in the splenic hilum, supra- and infrapyloric nodes, and paraesophageal regions. The use of intestinal pouches for reconstruction is a matter of surgical choice, although it has not been confirmed to be of any benefit. Tumors of the gastroesophageal junctions and cardia have a similar prognosis to esophageal cancers, and the surgical approach varies from an Ivor-Lewis esophagogastrectomy to a proximal gastrectomy. This is usually associated with selective conservation of the spleen and has a high incidence of reflux esophagitis. A D2 lymphadenectomy is probably the optimal, though not proven, procedure in most cases.

EXTENT OF GASTRECTOMY

A multicenter Italian study of 618 patients randomized 304 patients to total gastrectomy and 320 patients to a subtotal gastrectomy. There was no difference in overall survival (62% versus 65%). A splenectomy was performed in 18% of patients undergoing a total gastrectomy versus 5% of those undergoing a subtotal gastrectomy. The performance of a splenectomy had no effect on mortality or survival in this study. There was no difference in the extent of lymphadenectomy or incidence of complications. Four patients died following a total gastrectomy (TG), and 7 after a subtotal gastrectomy (STG).

Similar results were reported from a French trial by Gouzi et al. This study examined the role of total versus partial gastrectomy in patients with adenocarcinoma of the gastric antrum. This multicenter trial enrolled 169 patients. The 5-year survival was 48% in both groups. No difference in the morbidity (32% TG versus 34% STG) and mortality (1.3% TG versus 3.2% STG).

ROLE OF LYMPHADENECTOMY STAGING VERSUS THERAPEUTIC

There is extensive data from Japan that suggests a survival benefit for a D2 dissection in patients with intramuscular and serosal lesions. Similarly, Siewert reported that in a nonrandomized prospective trial, there was a survival benefit with extended lymph node dissection (LND). Unfortunately those results have not been duplicated in the West in randomized trials. This could be because of a difference in dissection techniques and pathological analysis.

Cuschieri reported that in a multicenter study involving 32 surgeons and 737 patients; 337 patients were ineligible after laparotomy. Of the 400 patients randomized, there was no survival benefit for an extended LND over a 7-year period. The 5-year survival was 35% for D1 versus 33% D2 lymphadenectomy. Survival from gastric cancer and recurrence-free survival were similar in the two groups. In a multivariate analysis, clinical stages II and III, people over 60 years of age, male sex, and removal of the spleen and pancreas were independently associated with poor prognosis. The complication rate (46% versus 28%) and mortality (13% versus 7%) were increased in patients

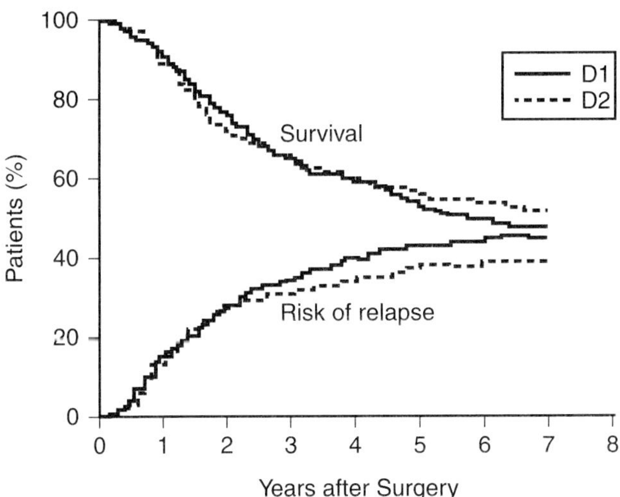

FIGURE 1 Survival and cumulative risk of relapse among patients with R0 (complete) resection, excluding in-hospital deaths. In the sample, 324 patients underwent a D1 and 265 patients had a D2 lymph node dissection.

undergoing a D2 lymphadenectomy. There was no significant difference in the number of nodes removed (17 in D2 versus 13 in D1). In the Japanese literature, an average number of 26 nodes is removed during a D2 lymphoidectomy. There was no difference in the survival of patients undergoing a D2 LND with less or more than 26 nodes removed in the specimen. Of note, 57% of the patients in the D2 group had a distal pancreatectomy and splenectomy versus only 4% of those undergoing a D1 dissection, and this may account for the poorer outcome seen in these patients. Quality control in this study was based on surgeons' operative data forms and pathologic examination of the specimens.

In the Dutch gastric cancer study, the surgeons underwent preprotocol training. There were 8 surgeons at 80 centers in this trial. Of the 711 patients, 285 underwent palliative surgery. A D1 dissection was performed in 380 patients, and 331 had D2 dissections. A D2 dissection increased morbidity (43% versus 25%), length of stay (LOS) in the hospital (16 versus 14 days), and mortality (10% versus 4%). There was no survival benefit (47% for D2 versus 45% for D1 dissection), but the risk of relapse was lower (37% for D2 versus 43% with D1 dissection) (Figure 1). All D2 dissections were performed by "trained surgeons," but in 51% of patients who underwent a D2 dissection, no lymph node (LN) was identified in at least two stations that were supposed to be dissected. In D1 dissections 6% had more nodes taken out than required, and 36% had less nodes taken out than required. All patients in the D2 lymphadenectomy group had distal pancreatectomy with splenectomy, which certainly added to morbidity and improved long-term tumor control.

Although these studies failed to demonstrate a benefit for extended LND, and in fact reported that the in hospital morbidity and mortality were higher, there is a subgroup of patients with positive nodes who might benefit from an extended LND. For this to happen, there should be a margin of negative nodes (i.e., the number of nodes removed should exceed the number of involved nodes). This is expressed in the form of an LN quotient—a ratio of positive-to-negative nodes. An LN ratio less than 0.2 is an independent prognostic factor.

Comparison of United States Data with Japanese and European Data

The overall survival for resected gastric cancer is 19% in the United States and most Western countries (Table 1). Data on the treatment and prognosis of stomach cancer indicate very poor results in the United States. This is in contrast to 45% overall survival in Japanese hospitals. The difference is attributed to the fact that patients in the United States have more advanced disease at presentation (66% versus 52%) and less accurate staging of tumors, as well as worse survival outcome within each stage of disease. In selected centers, however, the outcomes are similar to Japanese data when staging factors are considered. There is a larger percentage of proximal and more diffuse (versus intestinal type) cancers in the United States and other Western countries. There is also the question of whether the disease itself behaves in a biologically different manner in different countries. The United States data on gastric cancer are similar to those from Germany but survival is still approximately 20% less than that seen in Japan (Table 2).

TABLE 1 Comparison of Gastric Cancer Results as Recorded by the American College of Surgeons (ACS) Study and Selected Japanese Hospitals

	Incidence (%)*		Resected Patient Survival (%)†	
	Japan	ACS Study	Japan	ACS Study
Stage I	33.7	17.1	95.6	50.0
Stage II	14.5	16.9	70.1	29.0
Stage III	28.7	35.5	36.3	13.0
Stage IV	23.1	30.5	23.1	3.0
Overall survival	45.4	14	56.3	19

*Number of patients: Japan, 15,589; ACS study, 18,365.
†Number of patients: Japan, 12,535; ACS study, 10,237.
Wanebo HJ, Ann Surg 1993, 218:583.

TABLE 2 Gastric Cancer: Survival in U.S. Versus Japanese Gastrectomy Patients

Stage	Japanese	United States	Japanese/American
II	71%	34%	46%
IIIA	59%	20%	48%
IIIB	35%	8%	18%

Source: Hundahl SA, Phillips JL, Mench HR: The National Cancer Data Base Report on poor survival of U.S. gastric carcinoma patients treated with gastrectomy. Fifth Edition American Joint Committee on Cancer staging, proximal disease, and the "different disease" hypothesis. Cancer 2000; 88:921-932.

Adjuvant Treatment

Adjuvant radiation therapy (RT) adds little to survival (Table 3) but may be used to control pain or bleeding. Some benefit has been shown for neoadjuvant chemoradiation therapy (CRT). A radiation dose of 4000 Gy preoperatively improves 5-year survival from 20% to 30% and is of maximal benefit in T3/T4 cancers.

The recently completed U.S. gastric cancer trial supports the survival benefit of chemoradiation for high-staged gastric cancer. This trial compared adjuvant 4500 cGy plus 5-fluorouracil/leucovorin (5-FU/LV) versus surgery alone in patients with stages Ib to IV M0 gastric cancer who had undergone surgery with curative intent. Of 603 patients, 85% were node positive. The treated patients received 5-FU (Adrucil)[1] (425 mg/m^2) with leucovorin[1] (20 mg/m^2), followed by 4500 Gy RT (1.8 Gy fractions) with concurrent FU (400 mg/m^2 and LV 20 mg/m^2) on days 1 to 4 and the last 3 days of RT. One month after RT, 5-FU (425 mg/M2) and LV (20 mg) were given in two 5-day cycles that were 1 month apart. Three patients (1%) died from the toxic effects of chemotherapy. Grade III chemotoxicity was seen in 41% of patients and grade IV in 32% of patients. Median survival improved from 27 months to 36 months with CRT ($p = 0.005$), and 3-year DFS survival improved from 32% to 49% ($p = 0.001$). The 3-year overall survival improved from 41% to 50% with CRT ($p = 0.03$). Relapse free survival was 44% in the CRT group versus 28% in the surgery alone group. Local relapse decreased from 29% to 19%. Surgical quality control was an issue as lymphadenectomy was minimal in most patients. A D0 lymphadenectomy was done in 54% of patients, D1 in 30%, and D2 in only 10%. In this study, only 18% of patients had more than 15 lymph nodes examined, which is considered a basic requirement for nodal sampling. In spite of poor surgical quality control, the study does support the value of adjuvant chemoradiation.

A similar benefit for adjuvant CRT versus surgery alone was observed in the Italian multicenter trial that used a similar regimen after a D2 dissection—etoposide[1], Adriamycin, and cisplatin[1] (EAP) followed by FU plus folinic acid.

[1]Not FDA approved for this indication.

ADJUVANT CHEMOTHERAPY

Most oncologists believe that gastric cancer is a systemic disease from the outset. One of the popular earlier treatment regimens)—called FAM—combined fluorouracil (Adrucil), doxorubicin (Adriamycin), and mitomycin (Mutamycin). This had an overall 40% response rate with less than 5% complete response. Only 1 in 25 patients with advanced disease benefits from postoperative chemotherapy (CT). The majority of randomized clinical trials do not show any survival benefit for adjuvant chemotherapy. Coombs et al. treated patients with 1 year of FAM versus no postoperative medications and observed no difference in disease free or overall survival. The 5-year survival was 46% with FAM versus 36% for the patients who did not receive FAM treatment. Subset analysis showed no change with node status, but survival was better for T3/T4 cancers (41% versus 23%). An update to the Hermans' paper in 1994, with the addition of two trials to the meta-analysis, did show a survival benefit for adjuvant chemotherapy. Considering that earlier controversy about adjuvant trial benefits are often related to the limitations of underpowered studies, the recent McDonald study is a new beginning even considering its limitations.

Intraperitoneal chemotherapy has been used in patients with T3/T4 tumors with a resultant increase in 4-year survival (58% to 76%), and may be useful in patients at high risk of peritoneal recurrence.

[1]Not FDA approved for this indication.

TABLE 3 Adjuvant Treatment for Gastric Cancer*

Trial	No. of Participants	Chemotherapy Regimen	Survival
Coombs, 1990	281	FAM	Median (mo) or 5-yr (%) 46% versus 35% control (NS)
Italian GITSG, 1988	235	5-FU (Adrucil) + MeCCNU†	NS
Italian GITSG, 1982	142	5-FU+ MeCCNU† ± LEV	46% versus 32% control (NS)
ECOG 3275	180	5-FU + MeCCNU† (Semustine)	37mo versus 33mo control (NS)
Gastric Ca SG, 1999	579	5-FU + Mito + UFT[1,2]	86% versus 83% control (NS)
Estape, 1991	70	Mitomycin C (Mutamycin)	84% versus 48% 10y survival (p <0.01)

*The toxicity for adjuvant therapy is approximately 45% and no difference in recurrence rate or pattern was observed in these studies.
Abbreviations: Ca SG = Cancer Study Group; ECOG = Eastern Cooperative Oncology Group; FAM = fluorouracil (Adrucil), doxorubicin (Adriamycin), and mitomycin (Mutamycin); GITSG = Gastrointestinal Tumor Study Group; LEV = levamisole; MeCCNU = methyl cyclophosphamide, Oncovin, bleomycin, methotrexate, Adriamycin; NS = not significant [difference in results]; UFT = uracil/tegafur.

Among the trials testing intraperitoneal chemotherapy, two trials demonstrated a benefit and another two showed a decrease in intraperitoneal relapse.

ROLE OF NEOADJUVANT THERAPY

Neoadjuvant treatment has been used in unresectable disease in an attempt to downstage tumors and in locally advanced cancers where a complete (R0) resection seems unlikely. In selected cases, up to 50% were clinically and radiologically downstaged, and an R0 resection was possible in 89% of cases. The survival benefit for neoadjuvant CRT appears to be limited to patients who demonstrate a response to it. In a study by Lowy et al., patients were treated with continuous infusion of 5-FU (fluorouracil [Adrucil]) (300 mg/m^2) and 45 Gy RT, followed by restaging, and D2 gastrectomy along with 10 Gy intraoperative radiation therapy (IORT). Progression of disease was present in 17% and 83% could undergo an R0 resection. Of these patients, 11% had a complete remission and 63% had pathologic evidence of a significant treatment effect. The postoperative morbidity was 32% and mortality was 5%. These studies concluded that neoadjuvant therapy may have a role in locally advanced and potentially resectable gastric cancer, but long-term effects on survival are not known.

The incidence of gastric cancer has continued to decline in the United States and in Western countries. The prognosis is largely governed by stage of primary disease and adequacy of primary surgical resection in patients with local regional disease. Adjuvant therapy appears to add survival benefit in completely resected, no residual disease patients. Continued investigation of new agents and therapies is warranted.

NEOPLASMS OF THE COLON AND RECTUM

METHOD OF

Nancy A. Morin, MD, and Philip H. Gordon, MD

Benign Neoplasms

POLYPS OF THE COLON AND RECTUM

The word *polyp* is a descriptive term referring to a projection from the surface of the intestinal mucosa into the bowel lumen regardless of the histologic origin. Polyps can be classified histologically as follows:

- Neoplastic (adenomatous)—sporadic adenomas, adenomas associated with familial adenomatous polyposis syndrome (FAP), adenomas associated with hereditary nonpolyposis colon cancer (HNPCC)
- Hamartomatous—juvenile polyps, Peutz-Jeghers syndrome, Cronkhite-Canada syndrome, Cowden disease
- Inflammatory—inflammatory polyp or pseudopolyp
- Hyperplastic

Submucosal lesions may also present as polyps. These include lipomas, lymphoid nodules, pneumatosis cystoides intestinalis, colitis cystica profunda, fibromas, hemangiomas, endometriosis, carcinoids, and leiomyomas.

Neoplastic Polyps (Adenomas)

Adenomas are neoplastic lesions consisting of dysplastic epithelium with malignant potential. Most adenomas occur sporadically, but 5% to 6% are associated with hereditary syndromes (polyposis syndromes and HNPCC). They are classified according to their physical characteristics (pedunculated or sessile) and the amount of villous component (tubular adenomas, tubulovillous adenomas, and villous adenomas). Tubular adenomas account for 75% of all neoplastic polyps; villous adenomas, 10%; and tubulovillous adenomas, 15%. The villous growth pattern is most prominent in sessile adenomas.

Thirty percent of patients older than the age of 50 years have at least one polyp. It is estimated that 1 in 100 to 200 will ultimately become invasive cancer. Adenomas at high risk of invasive carcinoma include any adenoma with severe dysplasia, adenomas greater than 1 cm, adenomas containing more than 25% villous component, and the presence of more than three synchronous adenomas of any size or type.

DIAGNOSIS OF LARGE-BOWEL ADENOMAS

Adenomas of the large bowel are usually asymptomatic and are frequently discovered during routine barium enema studies or endoscopic examination. They may manifest as a microcytic anemia, bright red bleeding from the rectum, watery diarrhea in a large villous adenoma of the rectum, or, rarely, intermittent abdominal cramps. A polyp up to 8 mm can be removed by biopsy and electrocoagulation and sent for histologic examination. A large polyp should be snared or completely excised and sent for histopathologic examination. Ulcerated lesions should be removed surgically.

MANAGEMENT OF BENIGN ADENOMAS

Most polyps throughout the entire colon and rectum can be excised through the colonoscope with minimal morbidity. Colonic resection, or colotomy, and polypectomy are rarely required and are reserved for cases in which colonoscopic polypectomy cannot be performed, such as lesions that are too large or too flat or when the colonoscope cannot be passed to the site of the polyp. Polyps in the lower third of the rectum can be removed via preanal excision. Patients with a neoplastic polyp have a higher risk of another polyp developing, so follow-up colonoscopy is indicated. After the colon and rectum are cleared of polyps, follow-up colonoscopy every 3 to 5 years is adequate. A large sessile polyp, particularly a villous type, is prone to recur, and follow-up of the polypectomy site should be done every 3 to 6 months the first year, every 6 to 12 months the second year, and every year thereafter to the fifth year. Then colonoscopy every 3 to 5 years is appropriate.

MANAGEMENT OF ADENOMAS WITH INVASIVE CARCINOMA

Invasive carcinoma refers to invasion of malignant cells into or through the muscularis mucosa. Once there is invasion of the submucosa, the risk of nodal metastases increases, and if present, cannot be detected without surgery. Not all adenomatous polyps with invasive carcinoma require bowel resection. Pedunculated polyps with invasive carcinoma have a low risk of lymph node metastasis; complete polypectomy is adequate, unless the cancer is within 2 mm of the cut edge of the stalk, is poorly differentiated, or exhibits lymphovascular invasion. In such cases bowel resection should be considered if the patient is fit for surgery. For a sessile polyp, which by definition has no stalk, the presence of invasive carcinoma has an overall risk of lymph node metastasis of approximately 12%. These patients too should be considered for bowel resection if the patient is in good health. An alternative is local excision followed by adjuvant chemoradiation for lesions in the distal third of the rectum.

FAMILIAL ADENOMATOUS POLYPOSIS

Familial adenomatous polyposis (FAP) is an inherited, non–sex-linked, and mendelian-dominant disease characterized by the progressive development of hundreds or thousands of adenomatous polyps throughout the entire large bowel. The disease has high penetrance, with a 50% chance of development of the disease in a member of an affected family. Colonic polyps begin to develop in early teens. If untreated, colorectal carcinoma develops in most patients by the age of 39 years. FAP accounts for less than 1% of all colorectal carcinomas. There is an attenuated form in which patients reach their 60s with fewer than 100 small adenomas.

Clinical Manifestations and Diagnosis

Symptoms do not usually develop until the full-blown development of polyposis. Bleeding from the rectum and diarrhea are the most common symptoms. The diagnosis is made by endoscopic examination of the colon and rectum or by barium enema studies. It must be confirmed by histologic findings of adenomatous polyps. Nearly two of three patients initially evaluated because of symptoms already have carcinoma.

Molecular Genetics

FAP is caused by a germline mutation that is already present at birth; specifically, a mutation in the tumor suppressor gene adenomatous polyposis coli (APC) located on the long arm of chromosome 5q21. Genetic testing and genetic counseling should be offered to families with FAP. Genetic testing removes the necessity of annually screening at-risk individuals who do not have the gene.

Extracolonic Expressions

Extracolonic expression can occur in any patient with FAP. FAP affects the whole body, and tissues derived from all three germ layers are involved. Endodermal abnormalities include gastric polyps (primarily fundic gland hyperplasia, occasionally antral adenomas), duodenal adenomas and carcinoma, small-bowel polyps, papillary thyroid carcinomas (especially in younger women), and hepatoblastoma. Mesodermal abnormalities include desmoid tumors, osteomas, and dental abnormalities. Ectodermal abnormalities include congenital hypertrophy of the retinal pigmented epithelium (diagnostic of FAP when present), epidermoid cysts, and brain neoplasms.

Differing combinations of the intestinal and extracolonic manifestations have been grouped into syndromes:

- Gardner syndrome—epidermal cysts, desmoids, osteomas, and dental anomalies
- Turcot syndrome—malignant neoplasms of the central nervous system (glioblastomas of the brain)
- Oldfield syndrome—sebaceous cysts

Management

Screening of family members of confirmed polyposis patients is important. Children at risk should be screened annually by sigmoidoscopy starting at age 10 years. If rectal polyps are identified, colonoscopy, esophagoscopy, and biopsy are indicated. Patients with FAP should have prophylactic colectomy. Several options are available:

- *Proctocolectomy with an Ileal Pouch Procedure*—This procedure has become the procedure of choice for most younger patients. The biggest advantage is avoiding a permanent ileostomy but with the benefit of removing all the colon and rectum.
- *Proctocolectomy with Ileostomy*—This procedure is indicated if the patient has carcinoma of the lower part of the rectum, in patients who have a desmoid tumor of the mesentery of the small bowel that

makes the ileal pouch procedure impractical, or in patients who have had fecal incontinence.

- *Colectomy with Ileorectal Anastomosis*—This technique is suitable in patients whose rectum is not carpeted with polyps. The main advantages of this choice are that it is a relatively simple procedure and it has excellent functional results. However, the retained rectum still has a continued risk of carcinoma and requires close follow-up examination.

ADENOMAS ASSOCIATED WITH HEREDITARY NONPOLYPOSIS COLORECTAL CANCER SYNDROMES

Hereditary nonpolyposis colorectal cancer (HNPCC) is inherited as an autosomal dominant pattern with 70% to 80% penetrance. All first-degree relatives of a patient with HNPCC have a 50% risk of carrying one of the deleterious genes. Asymptomatic gene carriers can pass the mutation to their children. It is estimated that approximately 5% of all colorectal carcinomas can be attributed to HNPCC.

The disease, which is heterogeneous, has four major subtypes:

1. *Lynch type I*—site-specific nonpolyposis colorectal carcinoma
2. *Lynch type II*—carcinomas in the colon and extracolonic organs (endometrium, ovary, stomach, urinary tract, among others)
3. *Muir-Torre syndrome*—associated with benign and malignant skin neoplasms
4. *Turcot's syndrome variant*—associated with brain tumors

Despite its name, polyps are a feature of HNPCC with an 8% to 17% incidence in first-degree relatives.

Individuals with HNPCC differ from patients with sporadic carcinomas in several ways. They show an early age of onset (mean 44 years); a predominance of proximal colonic carcinomas; an excess of multiple primary carcinomas; an increase in the proportion of mucinous, poorly differentiated carcinomas; and a higher rate of metachronous lesions that present as early as 1 to 3 years of age. They do, however, have a significantly improved survival rate.

Molecular Genetics

HNPCC is caused by a germline mutation in one of the DNA mismatch repair genes (particularly hMLH1, hMLH2, hMSH6, hPMS1 and hPMS2), leading to replication errors. Adenomas and carcinomas in patients carrying HNPCC gene mutations, therefore, display microsatellite instability.

Clinical Manifestations and Diagnosis

Clinical criteria were established to confirm the diagnosis of HNPCC at a meeting of the International Collaborative Group on HNPCC in Amsterdam in 1990. The criteria, known as the Amsterdam criteria, include:

- At least three relatives with histologically confirmed colorectal carcinoma, one of whom is a first degree relative of the two others.
- At least two successive generations should be affected.
- In one of the relatives, colorectal carcinoma should have been diagnosed when the patient was younger than 50 years of age. FAP must be excluded.

Genetic testing is available for individuals in whom HNPCC is suspected based on the Amsterdam criteria. Once the gene defect for a family is known, testing subsequent family members is virtually 100% accurate. If the test is negative for carrying the gene, the family member's risk drops to that of the general population Young patients with adenomas or colorectal carcinomas that display microsatellite instability are also candidates for genetic testing, especially if another member of the patient's family is affected with colorectal carcinoma.

Management

Screening recommendations for gene carriers include colonoscopy beginning at 20 to 25 years of age, or at least 10 years earlier than the earliest age at which colon carcinoma was diagnosed in a particular kindred, with the procedure repeated every other year until the patient is 30 years of age and then annually. Some authors strongly believe that gene carriers should be offered a prophylactic subtotal colectomy.

For women who are gene carriers, an annual endometrial aspiration and curettage should begin at the age of 30 years. Those patients should be advised of the option of ovarian carcinoma screening with transvaginal ultrasound and the cancer antigen 125 test (CA-125). They should be encouraged to have their children early so they can consider the option of undergoing prophylactic total abdominal hysterectomy and bilateral oophorectomy between the ages of 35 and 40 years. Screening for breast carcinoma should be initiated earlier in life, and urinary and gastric carcinoma screening in both men and women may be recommended.

It is important to determine whether an HNPCC syndrome is present because the operative procedure of choice for the index carcinoma is a subtotal colectomy as opposed to a more limited resection. In the case of a woman who has completed her family, the resection should be extended to a prophylactic hysterectomy and bilateral salpingo-oophorectomy.

Non-Neoplastic Polyps

HYPERPLASTIC POLYPS

Hyperplastic polyps are small, sessile polyps macroscopically indistinguishable from adenomas. Histologic differentiation from neoplastic polyps presents no problem. These lesions are common in adults, particularly in the distal colon and rectum. They do not exhibit any malignant potential.

HAMARTOMATOUS POLYPS

A hamartoma consists of an abnormal mixture of tissues endogenous to the organ, with excess of one or more of these tissues. Hamartomas are found in the various syndromes described below.

Juvenile Polyps

Juvenile polyps are pedunculated, cherry-red polyps that characteristically occur in children. These hamartomas are not premalignant. Bleeding from the rectum is a common finding. A moderate amount of bleeding can occur if the polyp is autoamputated. Intussusception of the colon may occur if the polyp is large. Treatment is by excision or snaring via the colonoscope or proctoscope.

Juvenile Polyposis

Juvenile polyposis syndrome is an uncommon condition, usually presenting in childhood. It occurs sporadically or can be inherited in an autosomal dominant manner, distinct from other polyposis syndromes. Patients usually have 50 to 2200 colorectal polyps and a proportion develop juvenile polyps in the stomach and small bowel. The presence of as few as three juvenile polyps is sufficient for a working diagnosis of juvenile polyposis. The importance of this diagnosis lies in the need for affected individuals to undergo surveillance for colorectal neoplasia because of the presence of synchronous adenomatous polyps. The surgical choices for management are similar to those for FAP.

Peutz-Jeghers Syndrome

Peutz-Jeghers syndrome is a rare, hereditary disorder characterized by gastrointestinal hamartomatous polyposis and mucocutaneous pigmentation. Inheritance is in a mendelian-dominant manner with variable penetrance. The syndrome comprises melanin spots of the buccal mucosa and lips, with involvement of the face and digits to a variable extent. The presence of polyps in the small bowel is a constant finding, but the stomach, colon, and rectum also may be involved. Patients who are the first family member known to have this disease usually present with abdominal pain with or without intestinal obstruction, intestinal bleeding and anemia, or malignancy. The polyp is considered a hamartoma, which generally does not degenerate to malignancy. However, there is a risk of malignant degeneration in the hamartomatous polyps and coexisting adenomas. There is also a risk of extraintestinal neoplasia of the ovary, cervix, testes, breast, pancreas, and fallopian tube. Patients are seen annually with yearly hemoglobin evaluation, breast and gynecologic examination with cervical smears, pelvic ultrasound, and testicular ultrasound. Mammography is performed at 25, 35, and 38 years of age, then every 2 years up to the age of 50, and then every year. Every 2 years, patients undergo esophagogastroduodenoscopy, colonoscopy, and small-bowel contrast studies. Polyps are removed endoscopically. Celiotomy and intraoperative enteroscopy are performed for small-bowel polyps (>1.5 cm) seen on small-bowel radiograph or for unexplained abdominal pain in the presence of polyps.

Cronkhite-Canada Syndrome

Cronkhite-Canada syndrome is an acquired, nonfamilial syndrome characterized by generalized gastrointestinal polyposis associated with alopecia, cutaneous pigmentation, and atrophy of the fingernails and toenails. Colon carcinoma has been reported. Clinical manifestations include vomiting, malabsorption, weight loss, and protein-losing enteropathy caused by chronic diarrhea that may result in cardiac failure and death. The treatment is symptomatic. Bowel resection is reserved for complications such as bowel obstruction.

Cowden Disease

Cowden disease is an uncommon familial syndrome of combined ectodermal, endodermal, and mesodermal hamartomas. Cutaneous and oral verrucous papules are regular and diagnostic findings. The important aspect of this disease is its association with other lesions, particularly carcinomas of the breast, thyroid neoplasms, ovarian cysts, and other gastrointestinal polyps. The polyps are typically small, and the risk of carcinoma is negligible; the removal of these polyps is, therefore, unnecessary. Colonoscopy every 3 to 5 years is encouraged.

INFLAMMATORY POLYPS (PSEUDOPOLYPS)

Inflammatory polyps may look grossly like adenomatous polyps. They are caused by previous attacks of any form of severe colonitis (ulcerative, Crohn's, amebic, ischemic, or schistosomal), resulting in partial loss of mucosa, leaving remnants or islands of relatively normal mucosa. Inflammatory polyps are not premalignant.

Lymphoid Polyps

Benign lymphoid polyps are enlargements of lymphoid follicles within the mucosa or submucosa with the presence of germinal centers. They are commonly seen in the rectum. They may be solitary or diffuse.

Lipomas of the Large Bowel

Lipomas of the large bowel are uncommon fatty neoplasms. In order of frequency, the most common sites are the cecum, ascending colon, and sigmoid colon, with 33% to 50% located in the right, or proximal, portion of the colon. Small and asymptomatic lipomas of the large bowel do not require removal. Symptomatic lipomas should be excised by colotomy or limited colon resection.

Leiomyomas of the Large Bowel

Leiomyomas of the large bowel are rare neoplasms of the smooth muscle of the bowel. They usually occur in the rectum and less commonly in the anal canal. Local excision per anum can be performed for a low-lying lesion that is smaller than 3 cm in diameter. Bowel resection should be performed for larger lesions.

Malignant Neoplasms

Adenocarcinomas of the colon and rectum account for 97% of large bowel malignant neoplasms. The remaining 3% of malignancies include carcinoids, lymphomas, and sarcomas among others.

ADENOCARCINOMA OF THE COLON AND RECTUM

Incidence and Prevalence

Carcinoma of the colon and rectum is the third most common new carcinoma in both sexes—following carcinoma of the prostate and lung in men and the breast and lung in women. Carcinoma of the colon and rectum is also the third most common cause of death in both sexes, also following carcinoma of the lung and prostate in men and the lung and breast in women. The American Cancer Society estimated that in 2003 there would be 147,500 new cases and 57,100 deaths from colorectal carcinoma. However, recent trends reveal a slight decrease in both the incidence and mortality from colorectal carcinoma. This is assumed to be secondary to increased screening rates leading to polypectomy and the diagnosis of cancers at an earlier stage. Still the lifetime risk of developing a colorectal cancer approaches 6%.

Etiology, Pathogenesis, and Genetics

Although neither the etiology nor the pathogenesis of carcinoma of the colon and rectum is known, a number of factors have been considered important in its causation, and certain clinical conditions are thought to be precursors of this malignancy. Most, if not all carcinomas develop from a precursor adenomatous polyp, a situation known as the adenoma–carcinoma sequence. Patients with longstanding ulcerative colitis, Crohn's colitis, and radiation injury to the colon and rectum have an increased risk of carcinoma of the colon and rectum. Dietary factors have been implicated in the etiology of colorectal carcinoma. Prime candidates are diets too high in fat and diets that are fiber-deficient. Other related factors include calcium deficiency, smoking, and a sedentary lifestyle.

The increase in knowledge about the molecular biology of colon and rectal carcinoma has been explosive. It is now known that there are two pathways to colonic neoplasia, depending upon which type of gene has been inactivated. In the first pathway, inactivation of the APC gene (in the 5q21 locus) initiates the multistep neoplastic processes in the pathway from normal mucosa through adenoma to carcinoma and metastases that develop over decades and appear to require at least seven genetic events for completion. Other genes involved in this pathway include K-*ras*, DCC gene, p53, and nm23 genes. This pathway accounts for more than 70% of all colorectal carcinomas, seen in spontaneous colorectal carcinomas (sporadic or familial) and FAP. Mismatch repair gene defects initiate an entirely different sequence of events known as the replication error (RER) pathway. This second pathway to colorectal carcinoma is found in approximately 20% of carcinomas, seen in HNPCC and spontaneous RER carcinoma (sporadic or familial). These carcinomas demonstrate microsatellite instability and altered function of genes that contain or are regulated by microsatellites, such as the transforming growth factor-β (TGF-β) receptor gene.

Clinical Manifestations

The typical symptoms of colon and rectal carcinomas are a change in bowel habits and rectal bleeding, but they do not necessarily indicate an early lesion. The symptoms of abdominal pain, bloating, constipation, and diarrhea are caused by partial bowel obstruction, usually with rather advanced disease. Carcinoma of the rectum may give a feeling of incomplete evacuation or tenesmus. Obstruction is more common in carcinoma of the left, or distal portion of the colon, whereas carcinoma of the right, or proximal part of the colon and the transverse colon is frequently manifested as weakness and anemia. In patients with cardiac disease, the initial symptoms may be angina or heart failure secondary to anemia. Weight loss and poor appetite are signs of advanced carcinoma.

Evaluation

Complete Blood Count

To determine the presence or absence of anemia, a complete blood count is indicated.

Liver Function Tests

Liver function tests often will point to metastatic disease, but a normal liver profile does not rule out hepatic metastases.

Carcinoembryonic Antigen

Carcinoembryonic antigen (CEA) is nonspecific because abnormal levels are also found in other conditions. It has significantly high false-positive and false-negative values. CEA is not useful in screening for large-bowel carcinoma, but it has been shown to have prognostic value. When preoperative CEA results are abnormal, the chance of subsequent recurrence or metastasis is higher than when the results are normal. A routine preoperative CEA determination in patients with colorectal carcinoma should be done as a baseline study. Its main usefulness is for postoperative follow-up.

Colonoscopy

All patients with colorectal carcinoma should have a complete colonic examination to exclude a synchronous carcinoma or adenoma. In the event of an incomplete examination because of colonic obstruction, examination within 6 months of operation is indicated.

Chest Radiography

Chest radiographs should be obtained routinely to rule out pulmonary metastasis.

Ultrasonography

Preoperative assessment of the liver by ultrasound may provide valuable information to consider when recommending the appropriate management of patients with colorectal carcinoma. Intraoperative liver ultrasonography is currently the most accurate method for detecting colorectal metastases.

Computed Tomography of the Abdomen and Pelvis

Computed tomography (CT) is ideally performed routinely for carcinoma of the colon and rectum. CT scanning of the abdomen may help delineate the extent of disease and help plan the extent of the operation should the malignancy invade adjacent structures. In carcinoma of the rectum, it should be performed as part of the preoperative staging because the finding of liver metastases may change the operative treatment.

Endorectal Ultrasound

This technique allows important preoperative staging of carcinoma of the rectum. Endorectal ultrasound can evaluate the depth of invasion and determine the presence of lymph-node metastases, which can also be harvested for biopsy in most cases. If the lesion is T3 or TxN1, preoperative chemoradiation might be considered.

Intravenous Pyelography

Routine use of intravenous pyelography (IVP) is unnecessary unless the patient has evidence of obstructive uropathy, abnormal renal function, a large lesion of the colon near the kidneys, or in case nephrectomy is necessary. For the most part, CT scanning has supplanted the IVP examination.

Cystoscopy

Cystoscopy is indicated when bladder invasion from carcinoma of the rectum is suspected.

Surgical Treatment

Colon

The objective in the treatment of colon carcinoma is to remove the primary lesion along with the surrounding tissue and lymphatic system, draining the carcinoma. If the lesion is adherent to or invading adjacent organs such as the small bowel, ovaries, uterus, or bladder, as much as possible of the adherent organ should be removed en bloc with the colon.

For lesions located in the cecum or ascending colon, a right hemicolectomy to encompass the bowel served by the ileocolic, right colic, and right branch of the middle colic vessels is recommended. For lesions involving the hepatic flexure, a more extended resection of the transverse colon is indicated. For lesions in the transverse colon, a resection to encompass the bowel served by the middle colic vessels or a subtotal colectomy is performed. Splenic flexure lesions require removal of the distal half of the transverse colon and the descending colon. Sigmoid lesions are appropriately treated by excision of the sigmoid colon. Some surgeons prefer more radical excisions, but there is no convincing evidence to suggest that prolonged survival or decreased local recurrence will result. For patients with synchronous polyps in different portions of the colon that cannot be removed colonoscopically, or in patients with HNPCC, a subtotal colectomy should be performed. Other indications for a subtotal colectomy include acute or subacute obstruction, associated sigmoid diverticulosis (symptomatic), prior transverse colostomy for obstruction, young patients (<50 years of age) with a positive family history (controversial indication), and adherence of the sigmoid colon to a cecal carcinoma. For poor-risk patients or patients undergoing palliative resections, segmental resections are more appropriate. The anastomosis can be performed with a hand-sewn technique or a stapling device.

Rectum

Resection of the rectum is technically different from resection of the colon. It is important to sharply mobilize the rectum without breaking its fascial envelope. The distal transection should be at least 2 cm distal to the lower margin of the lesion, and 5 cm for poorly differentiated carcinomas. For carcinoma of the upper portion of the rectum, a rectosigmoid colon resection (anterior resection) is the standard treatment.

The anastomosis can be performed with hand-sewn sutures or a stapling device.

Most carcinomas of the midportion of the rectum can be handled with a low anterior resection. The anastomosis is generally performed with a circular stapling device. If technically impossible, as in patients who have a very narrow pelvis or who are obese, an abdominoperineal resection may be necessary. For carcinoma of the lower part of the rectum in which an adequate distal margin can be achieved, a coloanal anastomosis can be performed; otherwise an abdominoperineal resection is indicated.

In well-selected patients, full-thickness local excision can be performed with a normal margin of about 1 cm. These are patients:

- In whom the carcinoma is within the distal third of the rectum
- In whom the carcinoma is less than one-third of the circumference of the rectal wall
- Who are mobile
- In whom the carcinoma is nonulcerated
- In whom the carcinoma does not deeply penetrate the wall (within the submucosa or into but not through the muscularis propria
- In whom the carcinoma is well or moderately well differentiated, with no suggestion of anal sphincter involvement

Following local excision, if the lesion is deemed incompletely removed or penetrates through the muscularis propria, a radical operative procedure is indicated if the patient is fit for surgery. Because of recent findings that even with adequate local excision the risk of local recurrence is high, postoperative chemoradiation should be considered for lesions penetrating the muscularis propria.

Staging and Prognosis

The TNM (tumor/node/metastasis) system is universally used as the staging system:

- T1 = invasion into the submucosa
- T2 = invasion into the muscularis propria
- T3 = invasion into pericolonic/rectal fat
- N0 = no metastasis
- N1 = metastasis to up to three lymph nodes
- N2 = metastasis to more than three lymph nodes
- M = distant metastasis, for example, to the liver or lung

For practicality in management, stage 1 is a lesion with invasion into the submucosa and muscularis propria without lymph node metastasis; the 5-year survival rate is approximately 70% to 72%. Stage 2 is a lesion with invasion into pericolonic or rectal fat but without lymph node metastasis; the 5-year survival rate is approximately 54% to 80%. Stage 3 is a lesion with lymph node metastasis; the 5-year survival rate is 39% to 44%. Stage 4 is a lesion with distant metastasis; the 5-year survival rate is approximately 7%.

Chemotherapy

Postoperative chemotherapy with 5-fluorouracil (Adrucil) plus leucovorin for a 6-month period is recommended for carcinoma of the colon with lymph node metastasis. This regimen is also applied to carcinoma of the rectum, stages T3/T4N0 and TxN1/2. In the treatment of metastatic disease, several drugs have consistently produced response rates above 15%, but none have produced a clinically significant improvement in overall survival.

Radiotherapy

For colon carcinomas, radiotherapy has limited use, with no truly defined primary or adjuvant role. Patients who undergo resection for large, locally invasive carcinomas with microscopically positive margins have undergone palliative irradiation to the primary site. Radiotherapy for rectal carcinoma lowers local recurrence in stages T3/T4N0 and TxN1/2. Radiotherapy can be delivered preoperatively, postoperatively, or in combination.

Metastatic Disease

In colorectal carcinoma patients, 30% to 70% will develop metastatic disease, predominantly to the liver or the lungs. If left untreated, the 5-year survival is less than 5%. In carefully selected patients, resection of the metastases results in a 5-year survival rate of 22% to 49% for liver disease and 14% to 78% for lung metastases. In addition, concurrent or sequential liver and lung resections are possible with a 5-year survival approaching 30%. Other than systemic chemotherapy, optional therapies for liver metastases include hepatic artery infusion, portal vein embolization, and local destruction using cryosurgical techniques or radiofrequency ablation. There is no long-term data on these options.

Appropriate Follow-Up for Carcinoma of the Colon and Rectum

The goals of follow-up for carcinoma of the colon and rectum are early detection of local recurrences and distant metastases and identification of metachronous carcinomas and adenomas. In general, the investigations include history and physical examination, endoscopy, serum tumor markers, and diagnostic imaging. Because 85% of recurrences occur within 2.5 years, intensive and early follow-up may be beneficial. The American Society of Clinical Oncology recommendations include a history and physical every 3 to 6 months for the first 3 years and a CEA level every 2 to 3 months for at least 2 years. Colonoscopy is recommended every 3 to 5 years. Because chest radiographs are noninvasive and inexpensive, most clinicians order them annually. Other directed evaluations are recommended for symptoms or an elevated CEA.

CARCINOIDS

Carcinoids of the large bowel are uncommon and mostly occur in the rectum, followed by the cecum, and then the rest of the colon. Clinically, the lesion is considered malignant if the invasion is into the muscularis propria or if it is 2 cm or larger. In these circumstances, radical surgery should be considered. Patients with carcinoids of the colon and rectum have a high incidence of other malignancies, particularly adenocarcinoma of the colon. A complete colonoscopic examination is indicated.

LYMPHOMAS

Lymphomas of the colon and rectum are rare and account for approximately 10% of gastrointestinal lymphomas. The cecum is involved more commonly than the left or distal part of the colon or the rectum. Bowel resection is the treatment of choice. Postoperative radiation and chemotherapy are given according to the stage of the disease.

LEIOMYOSARCOMAS

Leiomyosarcoma of the large bowel arises from smooth muscle of the bowel wall and projects either as a submucosal mass into the bowel lumen or on the external surface of the bowel. These malignancies spread by direct extension or via the bloodstream; lymphatic spread rarely occurs. Local excision is reserved for small lesions, but larger lesions require bowel resection or an abdominoperineal resection if they occur in the lower part of the rectum.

INTESTINAL PARASITES

METHOD OF

Linda Yancey, MD, and A. Clinton White, Jr., MD

Although many people in the United States mistakenly think that intestinal parasites are not common, current estimates suggest that half of all people harbor one or more intestinal parasites. Some parasitic diseases have been controlled in the developed world. For example, intestinal helminths such as *Ascaris* and hookworm are rarely acquired in the United States, whereas each infects more than a billion people worldwide. Even in industrialized areas, some infections occur more commonly than appreciated. For example, approximately 33% of the U.S. residents have serologic evidence of prior cryptosporidiosis by the time they reach adulthood. Similarly, colonization with pinworms is common during childhood. Furthermore, global travel and immigration mean that even in nonendemic areas physicians will encounter patients harboring these organisms. The acquisition of most enteric parasites can be minimized by rigorous adherence to personal hygiene and safe eating and drinking habits. In developing countries where safe food and water are not widely available, precautions such as boiling or filtering contaminated water before use, avoiding raw or undercooked food, using proper footwear, and not bathing in fresh water are effective prevention strategies.

In suspected cases the mainstay of diagnosis has been examination of the stool specimens. However, many of the common protozoal parasites are only identified by special stains or immunologic assays. Unfortunately, these tests are often not performed unless specifically requested. The following is a brief overview of a few of the most common intestinal parasites worldwide. Concise and frequently updated guidelines on parasitic diseases are available from the Division of Parasitic Diseases, Centers for Disease Control and Prevention, at their Web site, http://www.dpd.cdc.gov/dpdx/.

Among the more common syndromes caused by intestinal parasites is diarrhea. Diarrheal syndromes can be separated into those associated with watery diarrhea and/or dysentery (Table 1). Bloody mucoid diarrhea is typically associated with colitis. Symptoms often include abdominal pain, tenesmus, hematochezia, and fever. Markers of inflammation such as fecal leukocytes or lactoferrin are often found in stool. Watery diarrhea and malabsorption are typically associated with enteritis. Symptoms include watery stools, cramping, volume depletion, bloating, weight loss, and malodorous stools. Fever, hematochezia, and tenesmus are unusual; and fecal specimens show less pronounced inflammation. Table 1 lists the parasites associated with each of these syndromes.

Protozoan Infections

Common enteric protozoan infections and associated diseases are listed in Table 2, and Table 3 details drug treatments for the various protozoal infections.

TABLE 1 Diarrhea Syndromes Caused by Intestinal Parasites

Bloody Diarrhea/ Dysentery	Watery Diarrhea/ Malabsorption
Entamoeba histolytica	*Cryptosporidium hominis, C. parvum*, other species
Balantidium coli	*Cyclospora cayetanensis*
Trichuris trichiura	*Isospora belli*
Schistosoma spp.	*Giardia lamblia*
Strongyloides	Microsporidia (*Enterocytozoon bieneusi, Encephalitozoon intestinalis*)

TABLE 2 Intestinal Protozoan Infections and Diarrhea

Infection	Parasite	Disease	Comments
Amebiasis	*Entamoeba histolytica*	Amebic dysentery, hepatic amebiasis	Infection may be asymptomatic
Balantidiasis	*Balantidium coli*	Diarrhea, dysentery	Infections are usually asymptomatic
Blastocystosis	*Blastocystis hominis*	Uncertain pathogenicity, diarrhea possible	Most experts do not believe *Blastocystis* is a pathogen
Giardiasis	*Giardia intestinalis*	Acute or chronic enteritis	
Cyclosporiasis	*Cyclospora cayetanensis*	Acute, remittent, or persistent enteritis	
Dientamebiasis	*Dientamoeba fragilis*	Diarrhea, abdominal cramps, flatulence	Not clear if causes enteritis
Cryptosporidiosis	*Cryptosporidium hominis* *Cryptosporidium parvum*	Acute or persistent enteritis, chronic in HIV	Chronic and extraintestinal manifestations in immunodeficiencies
Isosporiasis	*Isospora belli*	Acute, remittent, or protracted enteritis	Chronic enteritis and malabsorption; in AIDS, associated with eosinophilia
Microsporidiosis	*Enterocytozoon bieneusi* and other species	Disease rare in the immunocompetent	Chronic enteritis and extraintestinal manifestations in AIDS

AMEBIASIS

The protozoan *Entamoeba histolytica* causes intestinal amebiasis. Amebiasis is a widespread condition with an estimated 10% of the total world population infected with some type of *Entamoeba* species. In addition to the pathogen *E. histolytica,* the genus also includes *Entamoeba dispar* and *Entamoeba moshkovskii,* which cannot be distinguished from *E. histolytica* on microscopic examination, but which cause only asymptomatic colonization or mild illness. Mexico, South and Central America, the Indian subcontinent, and southern and western Africa have a high prevalence of amebic disease. In developed countries, amebiasis is mainly a disease of immigrants and travelers. Clinical disease is sometimes noted in high-risk groups such as men who have sex with men, locations with poor sanitation, and institutionalized patients.

Infection is acquired by the fecal-oral route including consuming foods or water contaminated with amebic cysts. The cysts are surrounded by a chitinous cell wall, which allows them to remain viable in the environment for up to several weeks. Once in the small bowel, cysts release the trophozoites, which divide, mature, and travel down the gut to the colon, where they live on bacteria and colonic debris. Invasive disease is caused by invasion of the host tissues by the trophozoite forms, which can digest host tissues. They complete their life cycle when they encyst and are passed out of the host with the stool. The trophozoite forms can be excreted during episodes of brisk diarrhea, but they are delicate and do not survive long after leaving the host.

Many infections are asymptomatic. The spectrum of intestinal illness varies from mild diarrhea to severe dysentery. Onset of infection is indolent with symptoms occurring 1 to 4 weeks after acquisition of the parasite. Most patients present with enteric symptoms ranging from mild diarrhea to severe dysentery with abdominal pain and tenesmus. The diarrhea commonly contains blood and mucus but is not usually voluminous. Weight loss is seen in approximately 59% of patients, and fever is present in less than 33%. The more severe presentations (e.g., fulminant colitis, colonic perforation, amebic peritonitis) occur in less than 1% of cases but are associated with a high mortality rate.

Extraintestinal involvement primarily involves the liver. Hepatic amebiasis is caused by digestion of the liver tissue by the invasive trophozoites. The older term, amebic liver abscess, is incorrect in that the infection does not involve abscess formation and the fluid typically contains few white blood cells. Patients often present after an incubation period of weeks to months. The onset can be either indolent or acute. The clinical manifestations are very similar to those of biliary tract infection, with most patients presenting with abdominal pain, weight loss, and fever. Physical examination is characterized by fever and right upper quadrant tenderness. General laboratory tests reveal leukocytosis, often with a left shift and elevations of alkaline phosphatase and transaminases. Ultrasound and computed tomography (CT) scans typically reveal hypodense lesions. Most patients have single lesions with a predominance of involvement of the right lobe.

Distinguishing between *E. histolytica* infections, which require treatment even when not symptomatic, and carriage of its nonpathogenic counterparts (*E. dispar* and *E. moshkovskii*), which require no treatment, has presented a challenge. Amebas containing red blood cells, blood in the stool, or bowel ulcers with amoeba can be presumed to be *E. histolytica*. Serologic tests for antibody to *E. histolytica* can help in invasive infection. However, antibody (especially using older tests) can persist, such that serologic tests are not useful for distinguishing between acute and previous infection. However, the presence of antibody is associated with invasive disease and in the correct context can be diagnostic. Antigen kits have been developed that test for *E. histolytica* specifically.

TABLE 3 Drugs for the Treatment of Protozoan Infections

Infection	Drug	Adult Dosage	Pediatric Dosage
Amebiasis (*Entamoeba histolytica*)			
Asymptomatic:			
Drug of choice	Paromomycin (Humatin)	25-35 mg/kg/d in 3 doses × 7d	25-35 mg/kg/d in 3 doses × 7d
Alternatives	Diloxanide furoate (Furamide)[2]	500 mg tid × 10d	20 mg/kg/d in 3 doses × 10d
	Iodoquinol (Yodoxin)	650 mg tid × 20d	30-40 mg/kg/d (max, 2 g)[3] in 3 doses × 20d
Mild to moderate intestinal disease:			
Drug of choice	Metronidazole (Flagyl) or	500-750 mg tid 10d	35-50 mg/kg/d in 3 doses × 10d
	Tinidazole[2] plus paromomycin or diloxanide[2]	2 g/d × 3d	50 mg/kg (max, 2 g) qd × 3d
Severe intestinal disease, hepatic abscess:			
Drug of choice	Metronidazole or	750 mg tid or 500 mg IV q8h × 7-10d	35-50 mg/kg/d in 3 doses × 7d
	Tinidazole[2] plus paromomycin or diloxanide[2]	2 g/d × 5d	50-60 mg/kg/d (max, 2 g) qd × 5d
Cryptosporidiosis (*Cryptosporidium hominis, C. parvum*, other species)			
Not AIDS:			
Drug of choice	Nitazoxanide	500 mg bid × 3d[3]	100-200 mg bid × 3d
AIDS:			
Drug of choice	Antiretroviral therapy plus Nitazoxanide or Paromomycin[1] plus Azithromycin (Zithromax)[1]	1 g bid × >14d 25-35 mg/kg in 2-3 daily doses 600 mg qd	1 g bid × >14d 25-35 mg/kg in 2-3 daily doses 10 mg/kg/d
Cyclosporiasis (*Cyclospora cayetanensis*)			
Drug of choice for:			
Normal host	TMP-SMZ (Bactrim DS, Septra DS)	160 mg TMP, 800 mg SMZ bid × 7d	5 mg/kg TMP, 25 mg/kg SMZ bid × 7d
AIDS	TMP-SMZ (Bactrim DS, Septra DS)	160 mg TMP, 800 mg SMZ qid × 10d, then bid × 3 wk, then qd	5 mg/kg TMP, 25 mg/kg SMZ × 10d, then bid × 3 wk, then qd
Giardiasis (*Giardia intestinalis*)			
Drugs of choice	Nitazoxanide or	500 mg bid × 3d[3]	100-200 mg bid × 3d
	Metronidazole[1]	250 mg tid × 5d	15 mg/kg/d in 3 doses × 5d
Alternatives	Quinacrine[2] or	100 mg PO tid × 5d (max, 300 mg/d)	2 mg/kg PO tid × 5d (max, 300 mg/d)
	Tinidazole[2] or	2 g once	50 mg/kg once (max, 2 g)
	Furazolidone (Furoxone) or	100 mg qid × 7-10d	6 mg/kg/d in 4 doses × 7-10d
	Paromomycin[1]	25-35 mg/kg/d in 3 doses × 7d	25-35 mg/kg/d in 3 doses × 7d
Isosporiasis (*Isospora belli*)			
Drug of choice for:			
Normal host	TMP-SMZ (Bactrim DS, Septra DS)	160 mg TMP, 800 mg SMZ bid × 7d	5 mg/kg TMP, 25 mg/kg SMZ bid × 7d
AIDS	TMP-SMZ (Bactrim DS, Septra DS)	160 mg TMP, 800 mg SMZ qid × 10d, then bid × 3 wk, then qd	5 mg/kg TMP, 25 mg/kg SMZ × 10d, then bid × 3 wk, then qd
Microsporidiosis			
Encephalitozoon intestinalis:			
Drug of choice	Combination antiretroviral therapy plus albendazole[1]	400 mg bid	15 mg/kg/d dosed bid
Enterocytozoon bieneusi:			
Drug of choice	Combination antiretroviral therapy plus fumagillin[1]	60 mg qd × 21d	

[1]Not FDA approved for this indication.
[2]Not available in the United States.
[3]Exceeds dosage recommended by the manufacturer.
Abbreviations: bid = twice daily; PO = by mouth; qd = daily; qid = 4 times a day; tid = 3 times a day; TMP-SMZ = trimethoprim-sulfamethoxazole.

Antigen can be detected in stool in patients with intestinal infection. In liver disease, blood specimens obtained before treatment also usually contain amebic antigen. The response to empiric therapy with metronidazole is rapid in liver disease and can be helpful in diagnosis.

All persons with *E. histolytica* infection, whether symptomatic or not, require treatment because the asymptomatic carriers can still transmit the disease. However, most patients passing cysts identified as *E. histolytica* may have only *E. dispar* or *E. moshkovskii,* which does not require treatment. Treatment of invasive amebiasis with nitroimidazole (metronidazole [Flagyl], currently available in the United States, and tinidazole [Fasigyn][2], which may soon be available in the United States) results in a 90% cure rate. Side effects of metronidazole consist of a disulfiram-like reaction to alcohol, dizziness, and, rarely, paresthesias and a temporary neutropenia. Even after treatment with metronidazole or tinidazole, more than 50% of patients will have persistent carriage of *E. histolytica* and, like asymptomatic carriers, will require treatment to eradicate the remaining cysts. The drugs of choice for both groups of patients are iodoquinol (Yodoxin), paromomycin (Humatin), and diloxanide furoate[2]. Currently, only paromomycin is readily available in the United States. Nitazoxanide (Alinia)[1], a broad-spectrum antiparasitic agent, may also have activity against amebic cysts. In cases of fulminant amebic colitis, there may be leakage of intracolonic bacteria and broad-spectrum antibiotics can be added to the antiprotozoal regimen.

BALANTIDIUM COLI

Balantidium coli, a ciliated protozoan, is an infectious agent primarily found in domesticated pigs, but, rarely, they cause human colitis especially in those with concurrent disease or immunocompromise. The life cycle is similar to that of *E. histolytica*—it starts with the ingestion of infective cysts that results in a spectrum of disease from asymptomatic carriage to acute bloody diarrhea; rarely, a chronic infection with abdominal pain and diarrhea evolves. Diagnosis, as with most parasitic diseases, is via serial stool analysis for the large, 60 μ, motile-ciliated organisms or their cysts. Tetracycline is the drug of choice, although metronidazole or iodoquinol can also be used.

BLASTOCYSTIS HOMINIS

The protozoan *Blastocystis hominis* is commonly found in stool samples submitted for parasitic examination; its role as a human pathogen remains unclear. For many years it was considered an intestinal commensal and has only recently been studied as a possible cause of infectious diarrhea. Reports of disease related to *B. hominis* have been in the form of case reports and small series, although the literature is mixed with case series that failed to demonstrate pathogenicity in immunocompetent patients. Because the symptoms attributed to blastocystosis (including bloating, abdominal pain, diarrhea, fatigue, and nausea) are found in patients with irritable bowel syndrome (IBS), a link between the disorders has been theorized. However, most experts do not consider *Blastocystis* to be a human pathogen.

Blastocystosis is diagnosed on the basis of serial stool samples, and it is seen in 15% of samples submitted in the United States. Because there remains debate on the pathogenicity of the organism, there are no accepted standards as to what samples, if any, constitute positive specimens. In the vast majority of cases, carriage of the organism is asymptomatic and does not require treatment. Patients with symptoms should be rigorously examined for an alternate diagnosis, as *B. hominis* is often found with other intestinal parasites that are more commonly accepted as pathogenic. Many agents have in vitro activity against *Blastocystis* but none have proven clinical efficacy. Some authorities recommend treatment with metronidazole.

GIARDIA INTESTINALIS

The protozoan *Giardia intestinalis* is found in temperate and tropical regions worldwide. As with other intestinal parasites, giardiasis is more commonly acquired in areas of poor sanitation although outbreaks can be seen in any environment that promotes crowding (such as daycare centers). Travelers to the former Soviet Union and many campgrounds in the western United States are at risk for the infection. *Giardia* infection and malnutrition in children have a close association.

Infection is acquired via the ingestion of infective cysts. Once in the stomach and duodenum, excystation occurs and the motile organisms attach to the bowel wall within the small intestinal crypts. Here they divide and pass down the alimentary tract where encystation occurs. The cysts can survive in cool, moist conditions for long periods of time and are infective to other vertebrates, which serve as reservoirs of infection.

Transmission is via person-to-person spread, waterborne or food-borne routes. Person-to-person spread has been seen in settings such as daycare centers, where fecal contamination of fomites is common, and venereally in male homosexuals. Because the cysts are stable in water and resistant to chlorination, *Giardia* is associated with waterborne outbreaks of diarrhea. The temperatures used to cook food are sufficient to kill *Giardia* cysts, however, raw foods or foods that come into contact with an infective source after cooking can serve as sources of disease.

Giardiasis has a wide range of clinical manifestations ranging from asymptomatic infection, seen in approximately 60% of those infected, to a chronic illness with bloating, wasting, and malabsorption. Patients with defective antibody responses (e.g., common variable immunodeficiency or immunoglobulin [Ig] A deficiency) are predisposed to chronic infection, but chronic infection is also reported in apparently normal hosts. Those who have been previously infected are less likely to develop the characteristic watery, foul-smelling, nonbloody diarrhea with abdominal cramping, flatulence, bloating,

[1]Not FDA approved for this indication.
[2]Not available in the United States.

and nausea. Symptoms develop 1 to 2 weeks after exposure and can last from a week to months. Weight loss and dehydration are commonly seen and, especially in children, can necessitate hospital admission.

Diagnosis is made on the basis of a compatible clinical picture and cysts or trophozoites observed in the stool. Multiple specimens should be examined as the excretion of the parasite can be sporadic in early disease. Stool antigen testing is available and shows promise in improving diagnosis, especially in areas where a trained technician is not available to perform traditional microscopic examinations. However, the immunoassays are not compatible with all stool preservatives and should, ideally, be preformed on fresh or frozen specimens. For a small number of patients, endoscopy may be needed to obtain duodenal samples. Although this technique has a similar yield to stool studies, it can be used to evaluate for alternate diagnosis.

Because asymptomatic infection is common, not all patients with *Giardia* present in the stools require immediate treatment. Certainly any patient with symptoms should be treated. Food handlers and children, especially those in daycare settings and requiring diaper changes, should be treated to prevent the spread of infection. Metronidazole[1] has been the drug of choice for treatment; tinidazole[2] has similar efficacy and may soon be available in the United States. Nitazoxanide (Alinia) has been recently approved for treatment in children. It shows efficacy and tolerability at least as good as metronidazole with a shorter course of treatment (3 days vs. 5 days) and is available in an oral suspension. Metronidazole-resistant cases have been described. They may respond to nitazoxanide or to the addition of quinacrine (Atabrine) to metronidazole. Furazolidone (Furoxone) and the oral, nonabsorbed aminoglycoside paromomycin (Humatin)[1] are somewhat less effective alternative treatments. Furazolidone is available as a suspension. Paromomycin can be used in pregnancy.

Prevention of this, as with other intestinal parasites, hinges on breaking the fecal-oral contamination cycle. While the organism is easily filtered from water, standard chlorination is relatively ineffective in prevention of infection and tap water can be contaminated. Hand washing and hygienic disposal of soiled diapers should be stressed in daycare settings. Travelers should follow standard precautions when in endemic areas. Because of the frequency at which *Giardia* is found in wilderness areas, hikers and campers should filter or boil water before use. Portable, light, and convenient filtration systems with a pore size of less than 2 μm are commercially available at camping supply stores. *Giardia* is sensitive to heat, thus even at high altitudes, bringing water to a boil is an effective treatment.

[1]Not FDA approved for this indication.
[2]Not available in the United States.

THE COCCIDIANS: *CYCLOSPORA CAYETANENSIS* AND *ISOSPORA BELLI*

Cyclospora cayetanensis and *Isospora belli* have been recently recognized as important causes of diarrhea. Identified outbreaks are associated with contaminated water or produce. In contrast to other intestinal parasites, the oocysts are not infectious when shed, but need to sporulate before they become infectious. Approximately 1 week after ingestion of the oocytes some patients experience a flu-like illness with watery diarrhea, fatigue, and malaise. In those with symptoms, illness can range from a brief course to a prolonged picture of chronic diarrhea and abdominal discomfort. Most patients experience a remittent illness lasting several weeks.

Diagnosis is made by stool examination. The oblong oocysts of *Isospora* are larger (typically 10 × 30 to 40 μ) and can often be identified on wet mounts. *Cyclospora* oocysts are smaller (approximately 8 to 10 μ) round, and are more difficult to identify. Either may stain with modified acid-fast stains, although staining of *Cyclospora* is variable. The organisms autofluoresce with ultraviolet (UV) microscopy. Treatment in the form of double-strength trimethoprim-sulfamethoxazole (TMP-SMZ) (Bactrim DS) twice daily for a week is beneficial in immunocompetent patients. Those with symptomatic HIV infection are treated at a higher dose of a double-strength TMP-SMZ four times daily followed by a maintenance dose of TMP-SMZ three times per week. Nitazoxanide is used to treat both *Isospora* and *Cyclospora* and may work in patients who are allergic to sulfonamides. Ciprofloxacin[1] is inferior to TMP-SMZ in AIDS patients with these organisms, but may also have some efficacy.

There have been few outbreaks of *Cyclospora* or *Isospora,* so data on prevention are limited. Because outbreaks of *Cyclospora* are associated with contaminated produce, carefully washing fresh fruits and vegetables could potentially have some benefit. Water purification is also important.

CRYPTOSPORIDIOSIS

Cryptosporidium species are intracellular parasites that inhabit the digestive tract of humans and various other vertebrates. Recent molecular studies demonstrate that humans are infected by several different species, including organisms primarily infecting people (*Cryptosporidium hominis*), ruminants including cattle and sheep (*Cryptosporidium parvum*), dogs, cats, and even turkeys (*Cryptosporidium meleagridis*). Spread is via the fecal-oral route from an infected person or animal, and only a small number are needed to cause disease. Oocysts are very hardy, difficult to kill with common disinfectants, poorly removed by most filtration systems, and persist in the environment for months. Waterborne outbreaks are associated with contaminated drinking

[1]Not FDA approved for this indication.

water and recreational bodies of water such as swimming pools. Person-to-person contact is also a major route of transmission. *Cryptosporidium* is a major agent in persistent diarrhea in children, causing approximately 33% of cases in developing countries and is associated with malnutrition. In the industrialized countries, epidemiologic studies suggest that childhood infection is common, especially in daycare centers. Cryptosporidiosis is mainly diagnosed in immunocompromised hosts and has been the major agent of diarrhea in HIV-positive patients.

Symptoms begin approximately 1 week after ingestion of oocysts and range from asymptomatic infection to severe enteritis. The classic presentation in immunocompetent people is mild to moderate watery diarrhea with associated malaise, crampy abdominal pain, and, less frequently, fever that resolves in 10 to 14 days without therapy. Oocysts are shed after resolution of symptoms and for long periods of time after recovery. In immunocompromised hosts, *Cryptosporidium* can cause a much more protracted syndrome of wasting and prolonged diarrhea. For patients with HIV, a CD4 count below 100 is associated with this chronic infection, whereas those with CD4 counts below 50 are associated with a cholera-like illness with copious stools leading to volume depletion. Extraintestinal manifestations are mainly seen in severely compromised hosts and include biliary involvement.

Diagnosis is usually made by microscopic examination of the stool. *Cryptosporidium* oocysts are difficult to appreciate on routine stool examination. The oocysts can be identified by acid fast staining, immunofluorescence testing, or by antigen-detection methods. Unfortunately, most clinical laboratories do not routinely perform these tests unless requested. Even if tested correctly, multiple stool samples may be needed. In severe disease, however, more oocysts are shed, so the diagnosis may be made based on one sample.

Supportive care remains critically important. Antimotility treatments (e.g., loperamide [Imodium], diphenoxylate/atropine [Lomotil], and tincture of opium), rehydration, nutrition, and immune reconstitution, where possible, are the mainstays of treatment. Antiretroviral therapy is a key component of care in AIDS patients. Nitazoxanide (Alinia) is a broad-spectrum antiparasitic drug. Placebo-controlled trials demonstrate more rapid resolution of cryptosporidiosis in studies of children and adults in Egypt; HIV patients with CD4 counts higher than 50 in Mexico; and hospitalized, malnourished children in Zambia. The latter study shows a significant improvement in mortality rate. However, the drug was not significantly better than placebo in AIDS patients with low CD4 cell counts or in severely malnourished children infected with HIV. Nitazoxanide was approved by the FDA in 2002 for treatment of cryptosporidiosis and giardiasis in children. Paromomycin (Humatin)[1], a nonabsorbable aminoglycoside, has activity against *Cryptosporidium* in vitro and in animal models. However, it has limited efficacy in AIDS patients. The combination of paromomycin and azithromycin (Zithromax)[1] has some activity in AIDS patients.

Cryptosporidium are stable in the environment if kept moist and are completely resistant to potable concentrations of chlorine in water supplies. Those at risk for symptomatic infection should boil or filter all drinking water, especially when traveling to areas with poor public sanitation. They should also avoid contact with farm animals, persons with diarrhea, and recreational water such as public swimming pools. Water filters should be capable of removing particles 1 μ in diameter or less. By contrast, iodine or other common decontaminants do not kill oocysts. In HIV-positive patients on prophylaxis for *Mycobacterium avium,* rifabutin (Mycobutin)[1] decreases the risk of developing cryptosporidiosis.

DIENTAMOEBA FRAGILIS

Dientamoeba fragilis is a small, flagellated protozoan related to *Trichomonas.* It lives in the human large intestine as a trophozoite form. Transmission is via the fecal-oral route. It has been implicated as a cause of diarrhea and other gastrointestinal complaints. Diagnosis depends on demonstration of the trophozoites in stool. Stools need to be examined or placed in preservatives promptly or the organisms may not be visible. The treatment of choice is metronidazole (Flagyl)[1]. Iodoquinol (Yodoxin)[1], paromomycin (Humatin)[1], and tetracycline[1] may also be effective.

MICROSPORIDIOSIS (*ENTEROCYTOZOON BIENEUSI, ENCEPHALITOZOON INTESTINALIS,* OTHERS)

Microsporidia are small obligate intracellular organisms that are transmitted via specialized spores. The thick-walled spores contain a specialized polar tube, that when activated, injects parasite cytoplasm into the host cells, where they enlarge, divide, and form progeny spores. Two microsporidia species cause human enteric infection, *Enterocytozoon bieneusi* and *Encephalitozoon intestinalis* (formerly known as *Septata intestinalis*). Both *E. bieneusi* and *E. intestinalis* cause chronic diarrhea in HIV patients with low CD4 counts. Microsporidia have been reported as a rare cause of diarrhea in otherwise healthy adults. Recent studies have noted asymptomatic carriage is common in developing countries.

Spores can be identified in stool with Weber's modified trichrome or fluorochrome stains that have affinity for chitin (calcofluor, Uvitex 2B), but identification of the specific species requires electron microscopy or polymerase chain reaction (PCR). Infection of immunocompetent individuals is self-limited. AIDS patients with microsporidiosis may improve with

[1]Not FDA approved for this indication.

[1]Not FDA approved for this indication.

effective antiretroviral therapy. Preliminary data suggest that albendazole (Albenza)[1] may be used in the treatment of *E. intestinalis*. *E. bieneusi* responds poorly to albendazole, but, in one study, AIDS and transplant patients with *E. bieneusi* and diarrhea improved with treatment with fumagillin.

Helminth Infections

For most of human history, intestinal helminth infections have been a normal part of life. Even today, most residents of developing countries are intermittently infected. Only during the last part of the twentieth century did intestinal helminths become rare in developed countries. Now most cases in developed countries are seen in immigrants.

Nematodes

ASCARIASIS

Ascaris lumbricoides infection affects an estimated 20% of the world's population. *Ascaris* is found commonly in the tropics where the warm, moist soil conditions are beneficial for year-round transmission. Cases were formerly common in the rural southern United States, but the vast majority of cases in the United States now are in immigrants from developing countries. Children are most commonly affected in endemic areas. Infection is acquired by ingestion of the parasite ova. The eggs are hardy and can survive in moist, shady soil for years. When eggs are ingested, the larvae hatch in the gut, penetrate through the wall of the stomach or small bowel, invade into the bloodstream, and migrate to the pulmonary capillaries. The larvae then exit the vessels and enter the alveoli. After crawling into the respiratory tree, the larvae are coughed up, swallowed, and then mature into adult worms mainly in the jejunum. The mature worms can survive in the intestines for years before being passed in the stool.

Most carriers of disease are asymptomatic or may note mild abdominal symptoms or passing worms in their feces. Most symptomatic infections occur in the minority of patients who develop very heavy infections. During passage of the larvae through the lungs, patients may present with bronchospasms and fleeting pulmonary infiltrates. In patients with a high worm burden, mechanical obstruction of the lumen of the gut with worm balls can occur. The most widespread symptom of infection is the nutritional deficiency. The greater the worm burden the more pronounced the deficiency and, conversely, the more difficult it is for the host to prevent further infestation. Recent studies have documented an adverse effect of worm burden on intellectual development in children in endemic areas.

[1]Not FDA approved for this indication.

Diagnosis is based on stool samples and on the patient reports of adult worms passed in the stool. During the migratory phase, patients may present with eosinophilia and wheezing, but may have negative stool studies. In patients with mature worms, stool examinations are quite sensitive, particularly in patients with heavy worm burdens.

Mebendazole (Vermox)[1] and albendazole (Albenza)[1] are the most widely available treatments (Table 4) and are able to kill adult worms, eggs in the gut, and migratory stages in various tissues. Both are highly effective and reasonably well tolerated. Ivermectin and nitazoxanide are also quite effective. Pregnant patients can be given pyrantel pamoate, which acts as a paralytic agent allowing the worm to be expelled. Because ascaris worms are acquired from the environment, patients living in endemic areas are at a very high risk for reinfection and may require multiple courses of therapy.

Hookworm

More than 1 billion persons are infected with hookworms. The hookworm is found across several continents including the Americas, Africa, and Asia. The two genera that complete their life cycle in humans, *Ancylostoma* and *Necator*, thrive in areas of moist soil that support the development of larvae. The most common species are *Ancylostoma duodenale*, which is found around the Mediterranean Sea and in China and northern India, and *Necator americanus*, which is seen in the western hemisphere. The dog hookworm *Ancylostoma caninum* has also been reported to cause human disease. Hookworms were formerly common in the southern United States, but now most cases are imported.

Eggs hatch in moist soil, undergo several molting steps, and then the mature larvae enter the host through the skin, usually in the area of the foot. They may cause an inflammatory response at the site of entry. The larvae are carried by the circulatory system to the lungs where they become trapped in the pulmonary capillaries, move into the oropharynx, and are swallowed. The larvae mature into adult worms in the proximal small bowel where, with the help of proteases and anticoagulants, they feed on intestinal cells. These actions result in small amounts of blood loss (0.01 to 0.3 mL) for each actively feeding worm leading to iron deficiency anemia in those with high worm burden or low iron stores. Eggs are passed in the stool and contaminate soil. The larvae of *A. duodenale*, but not *N. americanus*, are infectious if consumed orally without the need to pass through the circulatory system and lungs. While all stages of infection can cause symptoms, the major burden of disease is the chronic loss of blood with associated nutritional deficiencies (e.g., iron deficiency anemia).

[1]Not FDA approved for this indication.

TABLE 4 Treatments for Nematode Infections

Infection	Treatment/Drug	Adult Dosage	Pediatric Dosage
Anisakiasis *(Anisakis)*:			
Treatment of choice	Surgical or endoscopic removal		
Ascariasis *(Ascaris lumbricoides,* roundworm):			
Drugs of choice	Albendazole (Albenza)[1] or	400 mg once	200-400 mg once
	Mebendazole (Vermox) or	100 mg bid × 3 d or 500 mg once	100 mg bid × 3d or 500 mg once
	Pyrantel pamoate (Antiminth)	11 mg/kg once (max, 1 g)	11 mg/kg once (max, 1 g)
Enterobiasis *(Enterobius vermicularis,* pinworm):			
Drugs of choice	Albendazole (Albenza)[1] or	400 mg once, repeat in 2 wk	200-400 mg once, repeat in 2 wk
	Mebendazole (Vermox) or	500 mg once, repeat in 2 wk	100 mg bid × 3d or 500 mg once, repeat in 2 wk
	Pyrantel pamoate (Antiminth)	11 mg/kg once, (max, 1 g) repeat in 2 wk	11 mg/kg once, (max, 1 g) repeat in 2 wk
Hookworm (*Ancylostoma duodenale, Necator americanus)*:			
Drugs of choice	Albendazole[1] or	400 mg once	400 mg once
	Mebendazole or	100 mg bid×3 d or 500 mg once	100 mg bid × 3d or 500 mg once
	Ivermectin	150-200 µg/kg once	150-200 µg/kg once
Strongyloidiasis *(Strongyloides stercoralis)*:			
Drug of choice	Ivermectin (Stromectol)	200 µg/kg/d × 1-2d, repeat in 2 wk in hyperinfection	200 µg/kg/d × 1-2d, repeat in 2 wk in hyperinfection
Alternative	Thiabendazole (Mintezol)	50 mg/kg/d in 2 doses × 2 d	50 mg/kg/d in 2 doses × 2d
Trichuriasis *(Trichuris trichiura,* whipworm):			
Drug of choice	Mebendazole	100 mg bid × 3 d or 500 mg once	100 mg bid × 3 d or 500 mg once
Alternatives	Albendazole[1]	400 mg bid × 3 d	400 mg × 3 d
	Nitazoxanide (Alinia)[1]	500 mg bid × 3 d	100-200 mg bid × 3 d

[1]Not FDA approved for this indication.
Abbreviation: bid = twice daily.

In those at risk for anemia and poor nutrition, the impact of infection is related to total worm burden in the patient. Heavy infection also interferes with intellectual development in children. When people are infected with dog or cat hookworms (e.g., *Ancylostoma braziliense*), the larvae are unable to penetrate beyond the skin and form serpiginous areas of inflammation, termed *cutaneous larva migrans*.

Diagnosis relies on the presence of hookworm eggs in serial stool samples. Because of the time required for the larvae to pass through the tissue, blood, and respiratory systems of the host before they arrive and sexually mature in the gut, there is a lag of between 8 to 10 weeks before eggs can be detected in the stool. Eosinophilia is associated with infection and can persist for years in untreated cases, although the response will wane over time.

Treatment is with albendazole (Albenza)[1] or mebendazole (Vermox). Pyrantel pamoate (Antiminth)[1]. Pyrantel pamoate may be used in pregnant patients. Nitazoxanide (Alinia)[1] may also have activity. Cutaneous larva migrans can be treated with ivermectin (Stromectol)[1] or albendazole[1].

[1]Not FDA approved for this indication.

Strongyloidiasis

The helminth *Strongyloides stercoralis* is endemic to the tropical regions of the world. Filariform larvae in the soil pierce intact skin and enter the circulatory system, where they travel to the lung and are caught in the pulmonary capillaries. From there they migrate into the alveoli and up the respiratory tree where they are coughed up and swallowed. In the gut they mature into adult worms that live within the mucosa of the small bowel. Infectious eggs are passed into the bowel where they hatch to release the noninfectious rhabditiform larvae that leave the host in the stool. Once in the soil, the rhabditiform larvae mature into filariform infectious larvae. Some of the larvae mature before passage of the stool. When that occurs, the filariform larvae can penetrate the wall of the gut or perianal

[1]Not FDA approved for this indication.

skin and continue the life cycle leading to chronic infection of the host. In hyperinfection, large numbers of larvae mature and reinvade the host. Hyperinfection is associated with defects in host defenses, and is especially seen with steroid therapy or T-cell lymphotrophic virus type I (HTLV-I) co-infection.

Upon penetration of the skin the larvae may cause a local immune reaction visible as a serpiginous track that follows the migration of the filariform larvae through the dermis. This is termed *larva currens* (literally, larval "running"). The most common site for the reaction is the buttocks and, if identified, is diagnostic for strongyloidiasis. As the larvae pass through the pulmonary tree, they can elicit bronchospasms, fleeting pulmonary infiltrates, and even pulmonary hemorrhage in heavy infection. Once in the gastrointestinal (GI) tract the worms cause nonspecific symptoms of abdominal pain and bloating. Patients with a high worm burden may develop malabsorption and chronic enterocolitis. Hyperinfection syndrome occurs in patients with altered host responses who develop autoinfection with large numbers of filariform larvae. As the larvae migrate, they may drag intestinal bacteria with them, causing sepsis and meningitis, which can be polymicrobial. They can also cause localized symptoms including pulmonary and GI hemorrhage, bowel obstruction, and death.

Diagnosis of strongyloidiasis is difficult. Eosinophilia is usually present except in hyperinfection and can be a clue to infection in suspected cases. However, most patients excrete relatively few larvae, which may not be seen with routine testing. Thus, many patients with strongyloidiasis have negative stool studies. More than three specimens many be required to make the diagnosis. In some patients, duodenal aspirates may improve the diagnostic yield. Serologic tests can be used in suspected cases with negative stool studies. In the hyperinfection syndrome, larvae can be found in stool, sputum and other organs.

Ivermectin (Stromectol) is the drug of choice for treatment of strongyloidiasis and can be given in a single dose for limited infection. Patients with hyperinfection or patients with underlying HTLV-I or chronic steroid therapy should be retreated in 2 weeks. Thiabendazole (Mintezol) was frequently used in the past, but ivermectin is as effective and somewhat better tolerated. Albendazole (Albenza)[1] has been used to treat infection but is less effective. Nitazoxanide[1] may also have some activity.

Trichuriasis

Trichuris trichiura (also called whipworm) is a common intestinal parasite worldwide with more than 1 billion people infected. The organisms are acquired by ingestion of embryonated eggs. The eggs hatch and the larvae mature in the small intestines. The mature worms live in the colon. Most cases are asymptomatic. However, heavy infection may cause bloody diarrhea, growth retardation, poor intellectual development, and rectal prolapse. Diagnosis is by demonstration of the characteristic eggs in stool. Mebendazole and albendazole[1] are treatments of choice. Single-dose therapy, which can be used for *Ascaris* and hookworms, is not effective for *Trichuris*. Nitazoxanide[1] is also effective.

[1]Not FDA approved for this indication.

Enterobiasis (Pinworm)

The pinworm, *Enterobius vermicularis,* is the most common helminthic infection in the United States with more than 20 million cases, mainly in children, reported per year. Infectious eggs are ingested and hatch in the lumen of the gut where they mature into adult worms over a period of weeks. The worms do not penetrate the wall of the gut and live in the large intestine in the area of the cecum. Mature female worms migrate through the anus to deposit their eggs in the perianal area, usually at night when the host is sleeping. The eggs cause perianal itching, which transfers the eggs to the hands of the host where they can be ingested causing a cycle of autoinfection or spread to close contacts. The eggs are delicate and survive only a few days in the environment.

Symptoms of *E. vermicularis* infestation are usually mild with many cases being asymptomatic. Perianal itching is the most common symptom. Occasionally worms can migrate to the female genital tract causing cases of vulvovaginitis and, rarely, salpingitis. Some patients may complain of seeing the adult worms. Case reports describe eosinophilic enterocolitis in patients with high worm burden, but this is a very rare manifestation of infection.

Diagnosis is made by recovering eggs or worms from the perianal area. Because neither worms nor eggs are passed in the feces, stool studies will be negative. The Scotch tape test (consisting of swabbing the perianal skin with cellophane tape and then pressing the tape onto a glass slide) is commonly used for diagnosis. For best yield the samples should be obtained at night or first thing in the morning; three swabs have approximately 90% diagnostic yield.

The treatments of choice are the antihelminthic mebendazole or albendazole[1]. A single dose of these agents has a greater than 95% cure rate, but a second dose in 2 weeks is useful to prevent reinfection. Ivermectin[1] and nitazoxanide[1] have also shown efficacy.

Because *Enterobius* infestations are common in close contacts, the entire household should be treated and all bed clothing and bedding material (including stuffed toys) should be laundered in hot water. Reinfection is common in children, and recurrent infection likely represents a reacquisition of enterobiasis rather than relapse. The teaching of proper hand washing techniques to children is

[1]Not FDA approved for this indication.

beneficial, however, this infection remains very common in children younger than 10 years of age.

Other Nematodes

Humans can occasionally be infected by a number of nematodes for which they are not a normal host. *Angiostrongylus* species are strongylids normally found in rats. In humans, they can cause eosinophilic gastroenteritis and eosinophilic meningitis. Both can be treated with benzimidazoles such as albendazole[1] or mebendazole[1], but there is limited evidence of clinical benefit. Steroids are the treatment of choice for eosinophilic meningitis.

Anisakis is a fish ascarid. Humans are infected by ingestion of infected raw fish. The parasites burrow into the stomach causing a painful syndrome termed eosinophilic gastritis. The infection is self-limited, but resolution is more rapid with endoscopic removal of the worms.

Capillariasis is a rare intestinal infection acquired from ingestion of undercooked fish. The larvae invade the small intestines. The resultant adults can produce eggs and larvae, which can lead to an overwhelming infection associated with diarrhea, abdominal pain, and malabsorption. Treatment with mebendazole[1] or albendazole[1] is associated with improvement.

Cestodes (Table 5)

TAENIA SAGINATA (THE BEEF TAPEWORM)

The beef tapeworm *Taenia saginata* is seen primarily in sub-Saharan Africa and the Middle East, but can occur in any area where raw or undercooked beef is eaten. The disease is acquired by the ingestion of the infective cysticercus in the skeletal muscle of cattle. Once in the human GI, tract the tapeworm attaches to the small bowel, usually in the region of the upper jejunum, and matures over a period of approximately 2 months. The part of the tapeworm that attaches to the intestinal wall is the scolex. A chain of hermaphroditic proglottids, known as the strobila, extend behind the scolex to form the bulk of the tapeworm. Eggs are produced from the proglottids and are passed in the stool. Once in the environment the eggs can last for several years until ingested by cattle. In the bovine intestine, the larvae penetrate the bowel wall and encyst in the muscle.

Mature proglottids break off the end of the tapeworm and can be noticed by the host at time of defecation. The proglottids are motile and cause irritation of the perianal area when they are passed, but most beef tapeworm infections are asymptomatic or produce only vague abdominal discomfort, nausea, or weight loss.

Diagnosis can be made by examination of the stool for eggs or proglottids. Eggs can also be found in the perianal area and may be seen on a cellophane tape test as is used in pinworm infection. Because the eggs of *Taenia saginata* are indistinguishable from the eggs of *Taenia solium,* the pork tapeworm, speciation requires examination of the proglottids or the scolex.

A single dose of praziquantel (Biltricide)[1] is used for treatment after which the entire worm will be passed in the stool. Niclosamide[1,2] is also effective, but is no longer available in the United States. Nitazoxanide[1] is an alternative that has proven effective in

[1]Not FDA approved for this indication.

[1]Not FDA approved for this indication.
[2]Not available in the United States.

TABLE 5 Drugs for the Treatment of Cestode and Trematode Infections

Infection	Drug	Adult Dosage	Pediatric Dosage
Tapeworms (*Taenia* species, *Diphyllobothrium, Dipylidium, Hymenolepis*):			
Drug of choice	Praziquantel (Biltricide)[1]	5-25 mg/kg once	5-25 mg/kg once
Alternative	Niclosamide	2 g once	50 mg/kg once
Alternative for *Hymenolepis* only	Nitazoxanide[1]	500 mg bid × 3d	100-200 mg bid × 3d
Schistosomiasis:			
Drug of choice			
(*S. haematobium. S. mansoni*)	Praziquantel	40 mg/kg/d in 2 doses × 1d	40 mg/kg/d in 2 doses × 1d
(*S. japonicum, S. mekongi*)	Praziquantel	60 mg/kg in 3 doses × 1d	60 mg/kg in 3 doses × 1d
Intestinal and biliary flukes (except for *Fasciola*):			
Drug of choice	Praziquantel	75 mg/kg/d in 3 doses × 1d	75 mg/kg/d in 3 doses × 1d
Lung fluke (*Paragonimus*):			
Drug of choice	Praziquantel	75 mg/kg/d in 3 doses × 2d	75 mg/kg/d in 3 doses × 2d
Fasciola hepatica:			
Drug of choice	Triclabendazole[1,2]	10 mg/kg once	10 mg/kg once

[1]Not FDA approved for this indication.
[2]Not available in the United States.
Abbreviation: bid = twice daily.

limited studies. The cysticerci are temperature sensitive, so cooking meat to 56°C (132.8°F) for 5 minutes or freezing it to –10°C (14°F) for 9 days will prevent infection. The proper disposal of human waste, as in all parasitic infections, can break the cycle of infection.

Taenia solium (The Pork Tapeworm)

The pork tapeworm, *Taenia solium,* is found in areas where pigs are raised with access to human fecal material. It is common in Mexico, Central and South America, sub-Saharan Africa, and southern and Southeast Asia. The life cycle is complicated by the fact that humans can serve as both the definitive and the intermediate host, resulting in two distinct forms of the disease. *Taenia solium* encyst in the skeletal muscles of their intermediate host, the pig. When the cysticerci are ingested by humans, the tapeworm attaches to the jejunum and enlarges to form a segmented worm that can be up to 10 m long. As the worm matures, it will intermittently release the terminal proglottids, which can be passed in the stool. Eggs can be passed in the proglottid or released into the stool. The eggs are infections to both humans and animals. Infection of the intermediate host, pigs, results in the larvae penetrating the wall of the intestine and the completion of the life cycle with encystation in the muscle. If the eggs are consumed by a human, the larvae hatch in the bowel, penetrate the wall, and enter the bloodstream, where they migrate to the tissues. While the larvae can migrate to a large range of tissues, they usually only mature in muscle, the central nervous system, skin, and eyes. These cysticerci can survive for years but eventually die and calcify.

Symptoms of tapeworm infection, taeniasis, are mild and consist mainly of abdominal discomfort, some weight loss, and the passage of proglottids in the stool. Cysticercosis, the invasive infection from ingestion of eggs from a human carrier of the tapeworm, can take a variety of forms depending on the location of the cysticerci and the local immune response. Because the brain is a common site, neurologic manifestations such as new-onset seizures caused by inflammation around the cysticercus, hydrocephalus from mechanical obstruction of the flow of cerebrospinal fluid, and arachnoiditis can all be seen.

Diagnosis of taeniasis is made by identification of the eggs or proglottids in the stool. The adult, intestinal pork tape worm can be effectively treated with a single dose of praziquantel[1]. Niclosamide[2], although not readily available in the United States, is also effective. Prevention of infection centers around proper disposal of waste, both human and animal, careful attention to handwashing technique, and cooking pork sufficiently to kill cysticerci.

[1]Not FDA approved for this indication.
[2]Not available in the United States.

Hymenolepis nana

The dwarf tapeworm is found worldwide in both temperate and tropical countries. Infection with this cestode is the most common of all the tapeworm infestations and is seen at an especially high frequency in institutional settings, because it does not require an intermediate host outside the human. *H. nana* eggs can be acquired from an infected human host or by the ingestion of insects such as larval fleas or mealworms. Once in the intestine, the oncosphere enters the wall of the villi where it develops into a cysticercoid larva; it later migrates back into the lumen of the gut as an adult tapeworm. The eggs are passed in the stool, but they can become infectious prior to exiting the host leading to a cycle of reinfection. Once in the environment, eggs can survive for approximately 10 days and are often passed from person to person.

Infection with *H. nana* is usually asymptomatic. Because the life span of the tapeworm is from 4 to 10 weeks, there is a high spontaneous cure rate. Diagnosis is based upon finding eggs in the stool, and the treatment of choice is one dose of praziquantel (Biltricide)[1]. Prevention is achieve by breaking the chain of person-to-person transmission and a commitment to improved personal hygiene and environmental cleaning.

Other Tapeworms

The *Diphyllobothrium* species of tapeworms is acquired from ingesting undercooked fish infected with larval forms. After ingestion of the larva, the scolex attaches to the small intestines and forms segments or proglottids. The worms can reach a length of several meters. Most patients note no symptoms. They may experience minor intestinal symptoms (bloating, mild abdominal pain, or loose stools). Because *Diphyllobothrium* can compete with the host for vitamin B_{12}, prolonged infection can cause pernicious anemia. Diagnosis is by demonstration of eggs or identification of proglottids in stool. Treatments include praziquantel[1] and niclosamide[2].

Dipylidium caninum is a common intestinal parasite of domestic dogs. Infection is acquired from ingesting fleas, which contain the larval form of the parasite. Humans are accidental hosts, and are also infected by ingestion of fleas. Most human cases are in young children. The main clinical manifestation is passing segments of the parasite, which are similar in size and shape to grains of rice. Diagnosis is made by examination of the proglottids or demonstration of eggs in stool. Treatments are praziquantel[1] and niclosamide[2].

[1]Not FDA approved for this indication.
[2]Not available in the United States.

Trematodes (Flukes) (See Table 5)

SCHISTOSOMIASIS *(SCHISTOSOMA MANSONI, SCHISTOSOMA JAPONICUM, SCHISTOSOMA HAEMATOBIUM)*

Schistosomiasis results from infection with one of the blood flukes of the genus *Schistosoma*. Infection is acquired when people enter water that is contaminated with the freshwater snails, which are intermediate hosts. The cercarial forms penetrate intact skin and then migrate through the bloodstream to the veins draining the intestines (*S. mansoni* and *S. japonicum*) or the urinary tract (*S. haematobium*). There the worms pair up and mate. Eggs shed by the female worm migrate to the intestine or urinary tract, where they induce formation of granulomas, which lead to shedding of the organisms into the stool or urine. Penetration of the skin can cause a localized rash (cercarial dermatitis). Acute schistosomiasis (also termed Katayama fever) develops at the time the parasites begin to lay eggs (2 to 8 weeks postinfection). Patients can present with fever, eosinophilia, diarrhea, and/or an urticarial rash. Other features may include spinal cord involvement or hematospermia. Most of the morbidity, however, results from chronic infections. *S. mansoni* and *S. japonicum* can cause hepatic fibrosis, which can lead to portal hypertension (esophageal varices, hemorrhoids, ascites). They also can cause GI disease with bloody diarrhea and a protein-losing enteropathy. *S. haematobium* can cause chronic urinary tract abnormalities (hematuria, hypotonic bladder, recurrent urinary tract infections, urinary obstruction, and carcinoma of the bladder). Diagnosis of chronic infection depends on demonstration of characteristic eggs in stool or urine. Multiple specimens may be required. Rectal biopsy may be required for diagnosis in some cases. Acute infection may have negative studies for ova, but is often diagnosed by demonstration of specific antibodies. The treatment of choice is praziquantel. Because immature parasites may respond poorly to treatment, patients with acute infection may require a second course of therapy.

Other Flukes

A number of trematodes can infect the human intestines, biliary tract, and even lung. All are associated with freshwater intermediate hosts and are acquired by ingestion. All can be treated with praziquantel with the exception of *Fasciola hepatica,* which responds poorly. Alternative treatments include triclabendazole* (available via compassion use programs). Nitazoxanide[1] may work in chronic infection.

---

*Investigational drug in the United States.
[1]Not FDA approved for this indication.

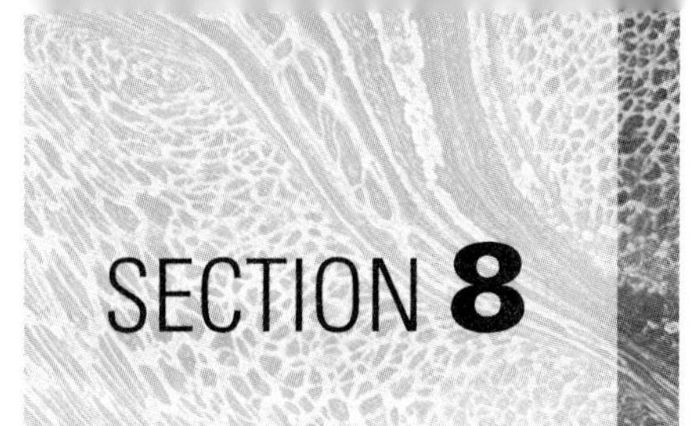

SECTION 8

Metabolic Diseases

DIABETES MELLITUS IN ADULTS

METHOD OF

John B. Buse, MD, PhD

The treatment of diabetes mellitus (DM) has changed more in the last 10 years than between 1922, when insulin was first commercialized, and 1994. This chapter reviews screening and diagnosis, diabetes prevention strategies, treatment of type 1 diabetes, treatment of type 2 diabetes, and screening and treatment of complications and comorbidities of diabetes.

Screening and Diagnosis

Estimates from 2003 suggest that diabetes mellitus afflicts approximately 17 million people in the United States. Approximately 33% are undiagnosed and asymptomatic. In 2002, the term prediabetes was coined to describe those who previously were diagnosed with impaired glucose tolerance and impaired fasting glucose. This group is comprised of an additional 17 million people, almost all of whom are undiagnosed. Table 1 presents glycemic cutpoints for making the diagnosis of these glycemic abnormalities.

How can one go about the process of finding these undiagnosed individuals? There are a number of well-defined risk factors for the development of diabetes. The American Diabetes Association (ADA) suggests screening adults with one or more risk factors. Also, the National Cholesterol Education Program (NCEP) has defined a "metabolic syndrome," as presented in Table 2. There are an estimated 40 million people who meet criteria for the metabolic syndrome; they are at high risk of cardiovascular disease (CVD), defined in this chapter as vascular disorders in the coronary, cerebral, or peripheral beds. The NCEP suggests screening for the parameters of metabolic syndrome to identify high-risk individuals who might benefit from lifestyle intervention as well as control of CVD risk factors.

The most sensitive screening and diagnostic test for diabetes, the oral glucose tolerance test (OGTT) is no longer routinely recommended. When performed, however, it is no longer necessary to draw multiple blood samples during the OGTT; only a single 2-hour sample for plasma glucose after 75 g of oral glucose taken in the fasting state after 3 days on an unrestricted diet (at least 150 g of carbohydrate daily) is required. The ADA recommends that fasting plasma glucose should be the predominant test for the detection of diabetes because of its lower expense and burden. It is approximately 50% less sensitive for the

TABLE 1 Diagnosis of Diabetes and Prediabetes in Nonpregnant Adults (American Diabetes Association Criteria)

	Diabetes Mellitus*	Prediabetes
Fasting plasma glucose	≥126 mg/dL	≥100-125 mg/dL
2-hour plasma glucose in 75-g oral glucose tolerance test	≥200 mg/dL	≥140-199 mg/dL
Random glucose	≥200 mg/dL[†]	

*The diagnosis must be confirmed by a second measurement on a separate day.
[†]To make the diagnosis of diabetes without a fasting value or oral glucose tolerance test, classic symptoms must also be present (polyuria, polydipsia, and weight loss).

diagnosis of diabetes than the OGTT, but those individuals with false-negative tests generally have hemoglobin A_{1c} (HbA_{1C}) of approximately 6% and thus are well controlled in any case. The need for an 8-hour fast still provides a barrier to screening for diabetes in some patients. Recent studies suggest that a random glucose value greater than 120 mg/dL is reasonably sensitive and specific for diabetes and could be used as an initial screening procedure in those unable to fast. Screening should be repeated every one to three years in those whose risk factors persist.

Prediabetes

Prediabetes is a clinical condition associated with a fairly high risk of progressing to diabetes; approximately 5% to 15% of prediabetes patients annually progress to diabetes. There are two issues worth noting in regard to prediabetes. First, people with prediabetes are at increased risk of developing CVD when compared with people with normal glucose tolerance, but are not at increased risk of the eye, kidney, and nerve diseases characteristic of diabetes. There is increasing data to suggest that lipid-lowering therapy and blood pressure control in people with prediabetes is associated with similar benefits with respect to CVD prevention as in diabetic populations. Diet and exercise aimed at producing modest weight loss (5% to 10% of body weight) and including 30 minutes of aerobic and resistance training at least 5 days per week reduces the risk of progression to diabetes by approximately 60%. Various drugs have similar, but generally less robust, benefits, including met-formin (Glucophage),[1] the α-glucosidase inhibitor acarbose (Precose),[1] the thiazolidinedione troglitazone (Rezulin),[1] which is no longer available in the marketplace, and the lipase inhibitor orlistat (Xenical).[1]

Treatment of Diabetes—Targets

The primary goal of diabetes therapy is to prevent diabetes complications and minimize the risk of adverse consequences of therapy. The complications of diabetes include CVD, the leading cause of death in people with diabetes; diabetic retinopathy, the leading cause of adult blindness in the United States; nephropathy, the leading cause of end-stage renal disease requiring dialysis or transplantation in the United States; and neuropathy, a potentially disabling condition that is the leading risk factor for lower extremity amputation in the United States. Table 3 reproduces the ADA's suggested treatment targets for people with diabetes. These are supported by evidence from randomized prospective clinical trials.

[1]Not FDA approved for this indication.

TABLE 2 Risk Factors for Diabetes and Metabolic Syndrome

Diabetes Risk Factors*	Metabolic Syndrome Characteristics[†]
Age ≥45 years	
Body mass index ≥25	Waist >40 inches in men or >35 in women
First-degree relative with diabetes	
Habitual physical inactivity	
High-risk ethnicity (African American, Hispanic American, Native American, Asian American, Pacific Islander)	
History child weighing >9 pounds at birth	
History of gestational diabetes	
Hypertension (≥140/90)	SBP >130 or DBP >85 mm Hg
Triglycerides ≥250 mg/dL	Triglycerides >150 mg/dL
HDL ≤35 mg/dL	HDL <40 mg/dL in men and <50 mg/dL in women
History of polycystic ovarian syndrome	
Prediabetes on previous testing	Fasting plasma glucose >110 mg/dL
History of vascular disease	

*The American Diabetes Association suggests screening everyone older than age 45 years at least every three years. It further suggests screening earlier and perhaps more frequently in younger patients with a body mass index (BMI) >25 and any risk factor.
[†]The National Cholesterol Education Program suggests evaluating these characteristics in people who have uncertain CVD risk who have one or more of the listed features and suggests that the presence of the metabolic syndrome is suggested by having three or more of the five listed features.
Abbreviations: DBP = diastolic blood pressure; HDL = high-density lipoprotein; SBP = systolic blood pressure.

TABLE 3 Treatment Targets for People with Diabetes

Glycemic Control	
Hemoglobin A_{1c}	<7.0% (assuming normal range 4%-6%)
Preprandial plasma glucose	90-130 mg/dL
Peak postprandial plasma glucose	<180 mg/dL
Blood Pressure	
Systolic	<130 mm Hg
Diastolic	<80 mm Hg
Lipids	
LDL	<100 mg/dL
Triglycerides	<150 mg/dL
HDL	>40 mg/dL (>50 mg/dL in women)

Major Types of Diabetes

Gestational diabetes (GDM) refers to the detection of diabetes in women, generally during the second trimester of pregnancy. This chapter will not deal with gestational diabetes other than to point out that pregnant women with marked obesity, a personal history of GDM, glycosuria, or a strong family history of diabetes should undergo glucose testing as soon as possible. Low-risk women must have all the following characteristics: younger than age 25 years, white ethnicity, normal prepregnancy weight, no diabetes among first-degree relatives, no history of abnormal glucose tolerance, and no history of poor obstetric outcome. Otherwise, pregnant women should also be screened between 24 and 28 weeks gestation with a 50-g 1-hour OGTT and/or a 100-g 3-hour OGTT. Meticulous diabetes care in pregnancy is essential for optimal outcomes for mother and child.

Type 1 diabetes (previously known as insulin-dependent diabetes or juvenile-onset diabetes) can occur at any age but is more common among children and young adults. It is characterized by insulin deficiency and affected individuals characteristically have widely fluctuating blood sugars. Diabetic ketoacidosis (DKA) can occur in patients with type 1 diabetes when one or more insulin doses are missed or in the setting of physiologic stress without an adequate compensatory increase in insulin dose. Hypoglycemia is a quite common complication of the treatment of type 1 diabetes. Only 10% of patients with type 1 diabetes have a positive family history in a first-degree relative. Many have another autoimmune endocrine diseases such as hypothyroidism, ovarian failure, adrenal insufficiency, pernicious anemia, vitiligo, and celiac sprue. Although classically believed to be a disease of the young, it is estimated that up to 10% of adults with new-onset diabetes have a slowly evolving form of type 1 DM. Two years after the diagnosis of type 1 diabetes, most patients with type 1 DM will have a stimulated C-peptide of <0.5 μg/L. Islet cell antibodies (ICA), antibodies to glutamic acid decarboxylase (GAD), and other antibodies are often present at diagnosis but are not reliably measured by most commercial laboratories. There are likely environmental triggers to the development of this autoimmune process, although these are poorly understood.

Type 2 diabetes (previously known as non-insulin–dependent diabetes or adult-onset diabetes) generally occurs in adulthood, although it can also develop at any age. Most patients have a first-degree relative with diabetes and most are overweight, generally with a central pattern of obesity. Insulin therapy is often necessary for glycemic control, but DKA does not develop except under extreme physiologic stress or prolonged severe hyperglycemia. Type 2 diabetes is more common in all nonwhite minority groups and tends to occur at an earlier age in these high-risk ethnic groups. It is estimated that 20% to 50% of diabetes cases presenting in teenagers are type 2 diabetes. From recent prospective studies of high-risk groups such as the Pima tribe of Native Americans in Arizona, we understand that diabetes develops as the result of the progressive loss of insulin secretory capacity on the background of insulin resistance, which can be defined as inadequate responses of metabolic proces-ses to physiologic insulin concentrations. Except in the setting of severe uncontrolled diabetes, most patients will have a stimulated C-peptide of >1 mg/L although a more severe insulin deficiency can develop over time.

Associated with insulin resistance are a number of clinical phenotypes that are sometimes discussed together as the metabolic or insulin resistance syndrome. These features include obesity with a central pattern of weight distribution, dyslipidemia, hypertension, hypercoagulability, endothelial dysfunction, and accelerated atherosclerosis. The dyslipidemia is characterized by increased triglycerides, low high-density lipoproteins (HDL), and even though the absolute concentration of low-density lipoproteins (LDL) is the same as the population average, LDL particles are generally small and dense and more prone to oxidation. The pathophysiology of these associations is unknown. Although there is likely a direct contribution of hyperglycemia to cardiovascular risk, a substantial portion of the increased cardiovascular morbidity in diabetes is likely related to this syndrome and its associated features.

There are other conditions in which diabetes is a secondary manifestation and they should be briefly considered at presentation. These include pancreatic disorders (e.g., chronic pancreatitis, cystic fibrosis, hemochromatosis, pancreatic cancer), endocrine disorders (e.g., Cushing's syndrome, acromegaly, hyperthyroidism, pheochromocytoma, glucagonoma), drug-induced disorders (e.g., pentamidine, glucocorticoids, high-dose niacin, α-interferon), as well as in association with certain syndromes (e.g., Down, Turner's, Wolfram, and Prader-Willi syndromes).

At the time of diagnosis of diabetes, a clinical decision needs to be made as to whether the patient has type 1 or type 2 diabetes. Fundamentally, this decision boils down to whether a patient should have insulin therapy initiated at the time of diagnosis. In patients with very high blood glucose (>300 mg/dL), urine ketones or a history of weight loss, it is prudent to assume a diagnosis of type 1 diabetes or at least rather severe insulin deficiency and initiate insulin therapy; once the diabetes is better controlled, further testing and clinical response can help to determine whether patients can be managed without the complex insulin regimens required for the optimal care of type 1 diabetes.

Lifestyle Therapy

All patients with diabetes require lifestyle therapy, including medical nutrition counseling, exercise recommendations, and comprehensive diabetes education. Arguably, over the last 5 years, nothing has changed more fundamentally in diabetes than the emphasis on lifestyle intervention. For decades, health professionals and patients have paid lip service to the notion that lifestyle intervention is important. Clinical trial evidence suggests that each component of lifestyle intervention can contribute to improved outcomes. Furthermore, since passage of the Balanced Budget Act of 1997 and complementary state legislation, lifestyle intervention has been a covered benefit for most people.

Diabetes is a lifelong disease, and health care providers have almost no control over the day-to-day activities of patients. The appropriate role of the health care provider is to serve as a coach to the patient, who has the primary responsibility for the delivery of daily care. This is the fundamental reason why comprehensive patient education in diabetes self-management is a requirement for adequate diabetes care. A certified diabetes educator generally best facilitates this process. Diabetes education programs are being established at a rapid rate; local resources can be identified by contacting the American Association of Diabetes Educators (800-TEAM-UP4) and the ADA (800-DIABETEs). When a treatment plan is not working, identifying barriers to effective management, such as lack of knowledge, lack of time, and lack of resources, and establishing strategies to overcome those barriers, is much more effective than simply labeling patients as noncompliant. Some of the most overlooked contributors to ineffective care are the barriers created by psychiatric, cognitive, and adjustment disorders, which can be responsive to psychosocial therapies.

A comprehensive, individually negotiated nutrition program in which each patient's circumstances, preferences, and cultural background, as well as the overall treatment goals, are considered, is most likely to result in good outcomes. Because of the complexity of both the medical and nutritional issues for most patients, it is recommended that a registered dietitian, with specific skill and experience in implementing nutrition therapy in diabetes management, work collaboratively with the patient and other health care team members in providing medical nutrition therapy. Analogously, physicians and other members of the health care team need to understand the major issues in diabetes and nutrition and support the nutritional plan developed collaboratively. A brief diet history obtained by asking: "What do you eat for breakfast? ...lunch? ...supper? Do you have snacks between breakfast and lunch? ...lunch and supper? ...supper and bedtime? What do you drink during the day?" can be very useful. Ideally, this information should be obtained at each visit, with specific suggestions for changes made that both the patient and provider agree are important and achievable. Easy issues to address include caloric beverages such as juices, which can be replaced quite easily with artificially sweetened alternatives. "Fat-free" and "sugar-free" foods need to be recognized as foods that are not "free." Portion control and recipe modification are excellent dietary techniques. Four- to 6-hour spacing between meals is usually good advice for patients with type 2 diabetes, at a minimum avoiding high-calorie snacks.

Because the bulk of glucose that enters the circulation comes from starches in meals, carbohydrate content of meals should be consistent day to day, or treatment plans developed that allow for variable dosing to compensate for changes in carbohydrate intake. Fat intake is a contributor to obesity and the critical nutrient for cardiovascular risk management. It is generally recommended that people with diabetes consume a diet that is modestly restricted in calories, containing less than 10% of total calories as saturated fat or *trans* fats, and less than 10% as polyunsaturated fat. Some advocate substituting foods high in monounsaturated fatty acids—seeds, nuts, avocado, olives, olive oil, and canola oil—for carbohydrate. Similarly, some would advocate substituting protein for carbohydrate, but the metabolism of protein results in the formation of acids and nitrogenous waste, which may result in bone demineralization and glomerular hyperfiltration. Perhaps the best advice is that the patient with diabetes should consume mixed meals containing carbohydrates, proteins, and fats. The role of vitamins, trace minerals, and nutritional supplements in the treatment of diabetes is poorly understood. There has been one randomized trial to suggest that many patients' diets are deficient in essential vitamins and minerals and that a multivitamin taken daily reduces the risk of infection. Thus, a multivitamin containing at least 400 μg of folic acid is probably reasonable; supplementation with folic acid (1 mg), vitamin B_{12} (400 μg), and pyridoxine (10 mg) reduces the rate of restenosis after coronary angioplasty, presumably by reducing homocysteine levels.

Exercise is perhaps the single most important lifestyle intervention in diabetes because it is associated with improvement in glycemic control, insulin sensitivity, cardiovascular fitness, and remodeling.

Aerobic exercise and resistance (strength) training both have a positive impact on glucose control. Improvements in glycemic control are generally apparent immediately, become maximal after a few weeks of consistent exercise, but only persist for 3 to 6 days after stopping training, hence the rationale for negotiating a minimum of three exercise sessions a week. The key concept is to promote an increase in activity using an approach similar to the one discussed for diet. Goals, methods, intensity, and frequency have to be negotiated with patients. Physicians must screen for complications (neuropathy, nephropathy, retinopathy, vascular disease) and discover ways for patients to be able to exercise safely. Some authorities recommend that all patients older than age 35 years have stress tests before initiating exercise. If the exercise program contemplated does not involve more strenuous (intensity and duration) activity than the patient is accustomed to, screening cardiovascular stress testing is unlikely to be useful. However, when sedentary patients plan to embark on a program of strenuous exercise, stress testing is prudent to evaluate for subclinical coronary disease.

Drug Therapy for Type 2 Diabetes

There are now multiple classes of oral antidiabetic agents available for the treatment of diabetes. Each is effective in lowering glucose. It is useful to consider them based on their mechanisms of action as that helps inform what combinations of agents work well together. Table 4 summarizes the various classes of antidiabetic drugs and their properties. Table 5 lists specific agents with their starting doses, maximal effective doses, maximal doses, and approved combinations.

Although only available in the United States since 1995, metformin (Glucophage) has become the most prescribed antidiabetic agent. Its major activity is to reduce hepatic glucose production. Metformin is generally administered twice daily, although a sustained-release formulation (Glucophage XR), which can be taken once in the evening, is now available. The most common adverse events are gastrointestinal—nausea, diarrhea, crampy abdominal pain, and a metallic taste in the mouth, initially affecting about one third of patients. This gastrointestinal distress can be minimized by starting with a low dose once daily with meals and titrating upward slowly (over weeks) to effective doses. Sustained-release metformin is generally associated with less frequent and severe upper gastrointestinal symptoms, but can increase the frequency of diarrhea. At least 90% tolerate metformin adequately with long-term use. Rare individuals have been reported to develop lactic acidosis, generally in the setting of renal insufficiency, congestive heart failure, and old age. The drug should not be used in males with a serum creatinine ≥ 1.5 μg/dL, in females with a serum creatinine ≥ 1.4 mg/dL, in people with treated congestive heart failure (CHF), or in those older than

TABLE 4 Comparisons of Therapies for Type 2 Diabetes

	Lifestyle	Insulins	Sulfonylureas	Metformin	α-Glucosidase Inhibitors	"Glitazones" Pioglitazone (P) Rosiglitazone (R)	"Glinides" Repaglinide (R) Nateglinide (N)
Target tissue	Muscle/fat	β-Cell supplement	β-Cell	Liver	Gut	Muscle	β-Cell
Δ HbA_{1c} (monotherapy)	Variable	1%->2%	1%-2%	1%-2%	0.5%-1%	0.5%-2%	R: 1%-2% N: 0.5%-1%
Stimulates insulin secretion	No	No	Yes	No	No	No	Yes
Improves insulin sensitivity	Modest	No	No	Modest	No	Yes	No
Severe hypoglycemia	No	Yes	Yes	No	No	No	R: Yes, rare N: No
Weight gain	No	Yes	Yes	No	No	Yes	Yes
Common problem	Recidivism, injury	Hypoglycemia weight gain	Hypoglycemia weight gain	Transient GI	Flatulence	Weight gain, edema, anemia	Hypoglycemia
Rare problem			Sulfa allergy	Lactic acidosis		Congestive heart failure	
Contraindications	None	None	Allergy	Renal failure Liver failure CHF	Intestinal disease	ALT >2.5x normal CHF, class III-IV	
Cost ($ per month)	0–200	15-100+	5-25	20-80	25-50	70-150	50-90
Maximum effective dose		1-2 U/kg/d	1/2 max or double starting	1000 mg bid	50 tid	P: 30-45 mg qd R: 4-8 mg qd	R: 2 mg tid N: 120 mg tid

Abbreviations: ALT = alanine aminotransferase; bid = twice daily; CHF = congestive heart failure; Δ HbA_{1c} = delta hemoglobin A_{1c}; qd = once daily; tid = three times a day.

TABLE 5 Specific Antidiabetic Agents

Class/Agent	Trade Name	Class	Starting Dose	Maximum Effective Dose	Maximum Dose	Approved Combination Therapies
Metformin	Glucophage	Biguanide	500 mg qd or bid	1000 mg bid	850 mg tid	All
Glyburide	DiaBeta, Micronase	Sulfonylurea	1.25-5 mg qd	5 bid	10 bid	M, T, A, I
Glipizide	Glucotrol	Sulfonylurea	2.5-5 mg qd	5-10 mg bid	20 mg bid	M, T, A, I
Sustained-release glipizide	Glucotrol XL	Sulfonylurea	2.5-5 mg qd	5-10 mg qd	20 mg qd	M, T, A, I
Glimepiride	Amaryl	Sulfonylurea	1-2 mg qd	2-4 mg qd	8 mg qd	M, T, A, I
Repaglinide	Prandin	Benzoic acid derivative	0.5-2 mg tid	2-4 mg tid	4 mg qid	M, T
Nateglinide	Starlix	Phenylalanine derivative	60-120 mg tid	120 mg tid	120 mg tid	M
Pioglitazone	Actos	Thiazolidinedione	15 mg qd	Mono: 45 mg qd Combo: 30 mg qd	Mono: 45 mg qd Combo: 30 mg qd	M, S, I
Rosiglitazone	Avandia	Thiazolidinedione	2-4 mg qd	Mono/M: 4 mg bid S/I 4 mg qd	Mono/M: 4 mg bid S/I 4 mg qd	M, S, I
Acarbose	Precose	Alpha-glucosidase inhibitor	25 mg qd-tid	50 mg tid	100 mg tid	M, S, I
Miglitol	Glyset	Alpha-glucosidase inhibitor	25 mg qd-tid	50 mg tid	100 mg tid	S

Abbreviations: A = α-glucosidase inhibitors; bid = twice daily; I = insulin; M = metformin; mono = monotherapy; qd = once daily; qid = four times daily; S = sulfonylureas; T = thiazolidinediones; tid = three times daily.

age 80 years without a documented adequate creatinine clearance. Arguably, metformin has the best record of accomplishment among oral antidiabetic agents in outcome studies. In the United Kingdom Prospective Diabetes Study (UKPDS), among overweight subjects, those randomly assigned to metformin not only had improvements in microvascular complications similar to those of subjects randomly assigned to insulin and sulfonylurea, but also demonstrated a reduction in diabetes-related deaths and myocardial infarction.

The class of drugs with the largest effect to improve insulin sensitivity is the thiazolidinediones, commonly referred to as glitazones. Their activity seems to result from binding and modulation of a family of nuclear transcription factors. They are associated with slow improvement in glycemic control over weeks to months in parallel with an improvement in insulin sensitivity and reduction of free fatty acid (FFA) levels. They are generally well tolerated with weight gain and fluid retention, as well as associated edema formation and hemodilution, as the only significant adverse effects. There is no substantial evidence that pioglitazone (Actos) and rosiglitazone (Avandia) are associated with hepatotoxicity, but they should not be used in patients whose serum alanine aminotransferase (ALT) levels are greater than 2.5 times the upper limit of normal; it is recommended that serum ALT be checked before initiating therapy and intermittently thereafter. Weight gain can be minimized with lifestyle intervention as well as co-administration with metformin. The patients most likely to experience edema are those treated with insulin and those with pre-existing edema. In such individuals it is prudent to initiate therapy at the lowest marketed dose, as well as to instruct them how to assess pitting pretibial edema at home, and to suggest that they make a habit of checking nightly. If they note a pattern of increasing edema, patients can be instructed to restrict sodium intake or to initiate or intensify diuretic therapy. These agents are contraindicated in patients with class III or IV heart failure. There is substantial interest in the possibility that these agents will modulate cardiovascular disease as well as prevent the progressive loss of insulin secreting β cells, arguably the two most challenging aspects of diabetes management. These issues are being explored in a number of clinical trials underway.

There are three classes of insulin secretagogues available: sulfonylureas, repaglinide (Prandin), and nateglinide (Starlix). They all work by modulating the activity of an ion channel on the plasma membrane of β cells, which regulates insulin secretion. Although there are almost a dozen sulfonylureas available, only three are addressed here. Glyburide (DiaBeta, Micronase) is one of the most commonly prescribed insulin secretagogues despite nearly all marketed oral secretagogues having a significantly lower hypoglycemic potential. Furthermore, glyburide seems to interfere with ischemic preconditioning, a protective mechanism in cardiac physiology. Thus several investigators suggest that glyburide should generally be avoided. Glipizide (Glucotrol) is available as a generic tablet as well as a sustained-release formulation (Glucotrol XL). The latter is associated with a low risk of hypoglycemia and weight gain, and is always dosed once daily. Glimepiride (Amaryl) has a similar profile of activity and side effects. These two agents have clear advantages over glyburide and are preferred. Sustained-release glipizide is marginally less expensive than glimepiride. Glimepiride tablets are scored and thus a bit easier to titrate. The sulfonylureas as a class have the distinct advantage over other classes in that they are very inexpensive and arguably may be the most effective oral agents with respect to glucose lowering. In general, dosing at levels twice the starting dose or one half the maximal dose is associated with similar effects as higher doses but with lower hypoglycemic risk.

The "glinide" drugs are also insulin secretagogues. As a consequence of their short half-life, they are generally dosed with each meal. Nateglinide (Starlix) is unique in that it specifically reduces postprandial glucose with very low risk of hypoglycemia. However, nateglinide has minimal effects on fasting glucose, limiting its utility to those patients with essentially normal fasting glucose but inadequate overall control. Repaglinide (Prandin) has a significant fasting effect and thus its overall action is similar to glipizide and glimepiride.

The α-glucosidase inhibitors (AGIs) inhibit the terminal step of carbohydrate digestion at the brush border of the intestinal epithelium. As a result, carbohydrate absorption is delayed and the postprandial rise in glucose is blunted. There are two currently available agents, acarbose (Precose) and miglitol (Glyset). Their use is limited by a number of factors, predominantly gastrointestinal side effects and only modest reductions in blood glucose. These factors should be balanced against the AGIs' ability to lower postprandial glucose, thereby improving glycemia without increasing weight or hypoglycemic risk. To maximize the potential for these agents to be well tolerated, start with a low dose once daily and increase over a period of weeks to months to one-fourth to one-half the maximal dose with each meal.

Insulin has been commercially available since the early 1920s and is still the mainstay of therapy for the majority of people with type 2 diabetes worldwide. Subcutaneous injection of insulin in type 2 diabetes is designed to supplement endogenous production of insulin. There are many formulations of insulin available and Table 6 lists their pharmacologic properties. Adverse events associated with insulin are well known and include weight gain and hypoglycemia. It is interesting that both fast-acting and long-acting insulin analogues provide modest reductions in hypoglycemia. Insulin allergies are rare, as are the chronic skin reactions lipodystrophy and lipohypertrophy. Newer insulin needles cause less discomfort than those previously available because of a finer gauge, shorter length, sharper points, and smoother surfaces. Insulin pens are easy to teach patients to use. Even though most patients find insulin therapy easier and more effective than they believed, there is still substantial resistance to initiating insulin therapy on the part of both patients and providers.

Recent studies document the safety and effectiveness of bedtime NPH (neutral protamine Hagedorn) insulin (Humulin N, Novolin N) and glargine (Lantus) insulin added to oral agents combined with an algorithm for titration based on intermittent telephone contact. In the Treat to Target study, patients added 10 units of NPH or glargine insulin at bedtime and increased the dose by 8 units per week if the average glucose was >180 mg/dL; 6 units per week if the glucose was 140 to 180 mg/dL; 4 units per week if glucose 120 to 140 mg/dL; and 2 units per week if glucose 100 to 120 mg/dL as long as there had been no significant hypoglycemia. An alternative is to have patients monitor their glucose levels at home in the morning on a daily basis, and have patients increase the nightly dose of NPH or glargine insulin 1 unit per day until the morning glucose is generally in the 90 to 130 mg/dL range. In patients with more dramatic hyperglycemia, one can start with a higher dose (e.g., 20 units) and increase more rapidly (3 to 5 units per day) until the fasting glucose is moderately controlled (e.g., <150 mg per day) and then titrate more slowly from there. Many of the patients who achieve control of their fasting glucose will have reasonable control throughout the rest of the day. Most will have elevated glucoses after meals and many will have pre-meal glucoses increasing throughout the day before returning to more normal levels overnight.

TABLE 6 Pharmacology of Insulin

	Onset (min)	Peak (hr)	Duration (hr)	IM/IV Dosing	Forms and Modifiers
Lispro (Humalog)	10-15	1-2	3-5	No	Insulin analogue, monomeric
Aspart (NovoLog)					
Regular (R*)	20-60	1-4	4-10	$t_{1/2}$ IM 20 min, $t_{1/2}$ IV 10 min	None
NPH (N*)	60-180	5-7	13-18	No	Protamine
Lente (L*)	60-240	4-8	13-20	No	Zinc
Ultralente (Humulin U)	60-240	8-12	18-30	No	Zinc
Glargine (Lantus)	~120	None	~24	No	Insulin analogue, precipitates at neutral pH

*Available in Humulin and Novolin brands.
Abbreviations: hr = hours; IM = intramuscular; IV = intravenous; min = minutes.

In this setting, it is possible to try to adjust oral agents, but many will need to take rapid acting insulin with meals to keep the blood sugar down throughout the day. This approach is discussed further in the section on type 1 diabetes.

Perhaps the most common question that arises is how to decide which agent to prescribe when initiating therapy. Each class of drugs has unique advantages and limitations. A growing body of experience indicates that the use of metformin (Glucophage) as initial therapy in combination with diet and exercise can provide impressive lowering of glucose with essentially no risk of hypoglycemia or weight gain. It has been proposed that the use of metformin alone or in combination with a thiazolidinedione may lead to a greater reduction in cardiovascular risk than other approaches, although definitive data are not available. Patients with higher levels of glucose (generally fasting glucose >200 mg/dL) almost always require agents to increase insulin levels; because insulin, sulfonylureas, and glinides provide much faster improvements in overall control than does metformin or glitazones, they may be preferred in such patients as part of initial combined therapy. Metformin combined with sulfonylureas is a well-studied combination that is fairly inexpensive and well tolerated. A thiazolidinedione plus sulfonylurea is another commonly employed combination, which is similarly effective but associated with greater weight gain. In patients who have reasonable control of fasting and preprandial plasma glucose levels (most <130 mg/dL) but with HbA_{1C} >7%, approaches to specifically lower postprandial glucose (nateglinide, α-glucosidase inhibitors or rapid-acting insulin) may be associated with less weight gain and hypoglycemia than using sulfonylureas or long-acting insulins.

Other common questions are whether to add insulin when a patient is failing oral agents, whether to add additional oral agents, and whether to convert to insulin monotherapy. There are adequate data to suggest that combinations of metformin, sulfonylureas, and thiazolidinediones are essentially additive in their effects and can be used together. Furthermore, there are data to suggest that greater glycemic control can be achieved with the combinations of insulin, metformin, and a thiazolidinedione than with insulin alone.

Treatment of Type 1 Diabetes

The treatment of type 1 diabetes requires precise balancing of insulin administered with carbohydrate intake and activity. Fundamentally, when aiming for near-normal glycemia, there are two possible approaches. Classically, providers have prescribed very regular lifestyles in the form of restrictive meal plans, as well as fixed insulin doses to match that lifestyle. Most patients cannot adhere to such consistent lifestyle plans over periods of weeks, months, and years. Currently, most authorities advocate an approach whereby patients can make fairly unrestricted lifestyle choices adjusting insulin doses to match those choices using a "multiple daily injection" (MDI) technique (Figure 1). This technique is an alternative to insulin pump therapy, which does

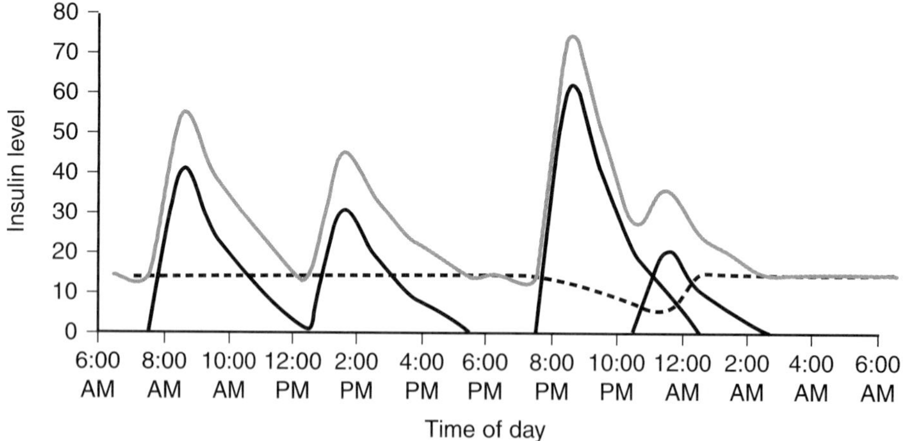

FIGURE 1 Multiple Daily Injection Technique. In this example, basal insulin in the form of glargine insulin is provided as a bedtime injection at 10 PM; its activity is noted here with a *dashed line.* Note the waning of the effect of the glargine in the early evening, which occurs in approximately 10% of patients and can be compensated for by providing extra meal-related insulin at supper or by splitting the insulin dose into a morning and evening injection. Meal-related insulin in the form of lispro or aspart is provided with three meals and a snack (7 AM, noon, 7 PM, and 10 PM in this example) using carbohydrate counting and insulin dose self-adjustment to compensate for dietary intake, as well as glycemic excursion; here, its activity is noted in the *solid line.* Total insulin activity is merely the summation of the activities of these five injections and will vary day to day, largely based on changes in the rapid-acting insulin component as the time, size, and composition of meals, as well as the intensity, frequency, and duration of physical activity changes, here denoted by the *stippled line.*

provide additional flexibility necessary in some patients. In MDI, insulin glargine (Lantus) is often employed to provide the basal insulin needed to prevent hepatic glucose overproduction and a rise in glucose between meals. Basal insulin requirements are about 50% of total daily insulin requirements. In approximately 10% of patients, the duration of glargine is inadequate and glucoses will rise just prior to the injection; in such patients it is sometimes possible to inject glargine about 3 hours after supper and provide a bit of extra insulin with supper to compensate or to just split the glargine into two injections. The dose of glargine is titrated aiming for a normal fasting glucose in the morning and a stable blood glucose throughout the night.

Meal-related insulin requirements are approximately 50% of total daily insulin requirements and allow clearance of meal-related carbohydrate from the circulation; this is usually provided in the form of lispro (Humalog) or aspart (NovoLog) insulin given just before or immediately after meals by using a dietary technique called carbohydrate counting. The carbohydrates in the diet include starchy vegetables (potato, corn, peas), grains, fruit, milk, and sugary snacks and beverages. There are approximately 15 g of carbohydrate in each ADA exchange. Most patients need about 1 unit of insulin for every 15 g of carbohydrate in their diet; a more precise estimate of the "insulin-to-carbohydrate ratio" (the number of grams that 1 unit of insulin would cover) can be obtained by dividing the number 500 by the patient's total daily insulin dose, which is expressed as 1 unit per "x" g carbohydrate. Adding up the grams of carbohydrate in a meal and dividing by the insulin-to-carbohydrate ratio determines the appropriate insulin dose for a given meal. This part of the insulin regimen can be fine-tuned by having patients check blood glucose 2 hours after meals. When meal-related insulin is appropriately dosed, the glucose should not rise by more than 40 mg/dL 2 hours after the meal.

Adjustments can be made for glycemic excursion which occurs as a result of unplanned snacks or miscalculations based on the "rule of 1500." Basically, it is an empirically derived observation that for every unit of additional regular insulin provided, the glucose falls, on average, by a quantity equal to: 1500 ÷ total daily insulin dose. This "insulin sensitivity factor" can be used to derive a simple formula to adjust insulin dose based on pre-meal glucose values such as: correction dose = (current glucose – target glucose) ÷ by the insulin sensitivity factor. The adequacy of this estimate can be assessed by examining whether the glucose returns to target values by the next meal.

So, in the multiple daily injection technique, patients are liberated from a stringent meal plan and administer rapid-acting insulin at each meal based on the food that they consume at that meal and the level of glucose at the time of the meal. As they are taking insulin with each meal, they can also make adjustments for activity, decreasing the insulin dose when prolonged or strenuous activity is planned. Many diabetes educators are quite facile with this technique and can be exceptionally helpful in training, troubleshooting, and dose titrating.

The major complication of therapy for type 1 diabetes is hypoglycemia, which can be severe (requiring the assistance of another), or even fatal, particularly in individuals with risk factors such as prior asymptomatic hypoglycemia, missed meals or snacks, increased activity, lower HbA_{1c} (36% higher for each 1% decrease), long duration of disease, and alcohol use. Raising goals in treatment to >120 mg/dL with an aim of absolutely avoiding any hypoglycemia, especially in mid-sleep, results in a return of symptoms and abatement of asymptomatic hypoglycemia over weeks to months.

MDI regimens and insulin pumps are generally appropriate for all patients with type 1 diabetes and for many patients with type 2 diabetes. Tremendous benefits are seen in patients with erratic glucose control, severe hypoglycemia, recurrent DKA, irregular lifestyles, serious exercise programs, and pregnancy.

Comorbidities and Complications

Complications of diabetes are associated with tremendous cost, disability, and death. A comprehensive program of screening and treatment can prevent poor outcomes. Diabetes, particularly type 2 diabetes, is often accompanied by comorbidities, including hypertension, dyslipidemia, and hypercoagulability, which contribute, to the extreme CVD risk that patients with diabetes face. Diabetes is a cardiovascular risk equivalent (i.e., a person with diabetes and no history of CVD has the same risk of future CVD complications as a person without diabetes who does have a prior history of CVD). As a result, aggressive efforts at CVD risk reduction are indicated. Lifestyle therapy as discussed above is a cornerstone of therapy for these problems. Additional details in this regard are available elsewhere in this text.

The ADA recommends blood pressure treatment with an aim to reduce systolic blood pressure to less than 130 mm Hg and diastolic blood pressure to less than 80 mm Hg. Angiotensin-converting enzyme (ACE) inhibitors, angiotensin-2 receptor blockers (ARBs), thiazide diuretics, and β-blockers reduce the risk of cardiovascular and microvascular complications in diabetes. In general, blood pressure treatment should begin with one of these agents. Most patients with diabetes and hypertension will require multiple agents (an average of three) to achieve blood pressure targets. Particularly effective two-drug combinations include ACE inhibitors or ARBs with thiazide diuretics. There are data demonstrating cardiovascular benefit to calcium channel blockade in the setting of ACE inhibition. The third drug in an antihypertensive regimen might often include a calcium channel blocker or β-blocker. All patients with type 2 diabetes and a history of coronary disease, particularly with a recent history of myocardial infarction should be treated with a cardioselective β-blocker. α-Blockers should not be used as the initial therapy of hypertension. Arguably, achieving blood pressure goals is more important than the details of the antihypertensive regimen selected.

Dyslipidemia affects the majority of people with diabetes. The average LDL in people with diabetes is ~140 mg/dL. Thus, most patients will require treatment with a statin to reach the LDL target of <100 mg/dL. In those patients who are statin intolerant or who do not achieve LDL targets, ezetimibe (Zetia) and/or a bile acid sequestrant such as colesevelam (WelChol) can be added. Niacin preparations, such as extended-release niacin (Niaspan) and fenofibrate (Tricor), also have LDL-lowering properties. These latter two agents are generally employed to reduce triglycerides to goal (<150 mg/dL) and to increase HDL to goal (>40 mg/dL in men and >50 mg/dL in women). Care in combining these classes of drugs is warranted, because there have been rare cases of rhabdomyolysis reported when statins are combined with niacin or fibrates. These severe events seem to be somewhat less common with fenofibrate (Tricor) than with gemfibrozil (Lopid) and are perhaps less common with atorvastatin (Lipitor) and pravastatin (Pravachol) than with simvastatin (Zocor) and lovastatin (Mevacor). Pioglitazone (Actos) and rosiglitazone (Avandia) are quite effective in raising HDL in addition to lowering glucose. Pioglitazone also has a substantial effect in lowering triglycerides independent of improvements in glycemic control. Combined lifestyle intervention and one or more lipid-lowering agents are generally a requirement to managing lipids in people with diabetes.

Aspirin therapy in the form of 81 to 162 mg daily of an enteric-coated preparation is recommended in the secondary prevention of cardiovascular risk in diabetes. Most advocate its use in all adult patients over the age of 21 with diabetes, particularly those patients with cardiovascular risk factors. Arguably, young patients with well-controlled type 1 diabetes and no other cardiovascular risk factors are at low risk and may not benefit from aspirin therapy.

CVD is two to four times more common in people with diabetes than in those without. Approximately 80% of people with diabetes eventually succumb to CVD and its complications. All patients with diabetes should be considered as having CVD, whether it is recognized or not. At each visit, potential symptoms of CVD, such as claudication, transient ischemic attacks, and exertional symptoms, should be elicited. Two recent reports suggest that up to 25% of people with diabetes, a normal electrocardiogram, and no symptoms of cardiovascular disease have abnormal stress-imaging studies. Whether routine screening for flow limiting coronary artery disease will improve outcomes remains unknown. Certainly careful evaluation of any symptoms of CVD is indicated. There is a large and evolving literature regarding optimal techniques of cardiovascular intervention in patients with diabetes. Consultation with a cardiologist is essential in the setting of acute coronary syndromes.

Diabetic retinopathy is the leading cause of blindness in adults. Annual dilated funduscopic examinations are recommended; follow-up evaluation and treatment for abnormalities by ophthalmologists with specific expertise in fluorescein angiography and laser therapy can reduce visual loss. Cataract extraction in the setting of diabetic retinopathy can be associated with visual loss related to macular edema and requires special attention to avoid poor outcomes. Glaucoma seems to be more prevalent in people with diabetes. Expert eye care is essential for optimal outcomes in people with diabetes.

Diabetic nephropathy is the leading cause of end-stage renal disease requiring dialysis or transplantation. Early kidney disease is detectable as an increase in the microalbumin to creatinine ratio on a spot urine sample (>30 μg albumin per mg creatinine). This screening procedure should be performed annually. Patients exhibiting microalbuminuria should be treated with ACE inhibitors or ARBs, and their blood pressure treated to less than 130/80 mm Hg. If the creatinine is increased above normal or if the urinary sediment is active, consultation with a nephrologist or other provider with special expertise in the evaluation of kidney disease may be useful to direct overall treatment and to exclude other causes of kidney disease.

Diabetic neuropathy can be disabling as a consequence of autonomic dysfunction or discomfort. Symptomatic therapy of these various syndromes is beyond the scope of this chapter because there is no single agent that routinely works in even the most affected patients. The insensate foot is the strongest predictor of the risk for foot ulceration and amputation. Annual foot examinations focusing on skin integrity, structural abnormalities, adequacy of perfusion and neurologic function is essential. The Semmes-Weinstein 5.07- or 10-g filament is a particularly essential tool to use to evaluate sensory function, because most patients with insensate feet are unaware of their lack of sensation. People who cannot consistently feel the touch of the 10-g filament are at high risk of ulceration and should enter a comprehensive program of foot care, generally led by a podiatrist or other foot care specialist, including the use of emollients, special shoes, routine nail care, and careful daily self-examinations looking for early lesions.

Summary

Early diagnosis of diabetes and its complications, combined with comprehensive treatment that targets not only glucose but also the associated comorbidities, should lessen the burden of complications on people with diabetes (see Table 3).

DIABETES MELLITUS IN CHILDREN AND ADOLESCENTS

METHOD OF
Laura M. Gandrud, MD, and
Bruce A. Buckingham, MD

Diabetes mellitus is a metabolic disorder resulting from inadequate insulin secretion, insulin action, or both. Lack of insulin action prevents intracellular transport of glucose. Extracellular glucose levels rise, whereas glucose-starved cells depend on fatty acid oxidation to generate energy. There are a number of different forms of diabetes; all result in hyperglycemia. This chapter reviews the pathogenesis, pathophys-iology, and treatment of diabetes in children and adolescents.

Classification and Epidemiology

TYPE 1 DIABETES MELLITUS

Type 1 diabetes mellitus (T1DM) results from destruction of the pancreatic β cells which produce insulin. Individuals with type 1A diabetes have serologic evidence of β-cell autoimmunity, whereas those with type 1B have no serologic markers. T1DM is the second most common chronic disease of childhood; prevalence in the United States is approximately 1 in 350 children. There is a 400-fold variability in the incidence of diabetes in different regions of the world, with the highest rates in Finland, and the lowest in China. The incidence of the disease in children younger than 14 years in the United States is approximately 13.3 per 100,000 per year. The incidence of T1DM has increased sharply throughout the world in the last half of the 20th century, with the highest rates of increase occurring in the populations with the lowest incidence. The annual rate of increase in the incidence of T1DM in children of all ages is approximately 3% to 4%, with an even steeper increase in incidence noted in children younger than 5 years of age.

The autoimmune destruction of β cells is cell mediated and involves CD8 T cells, CD4 T cells, and macrophages. The proinflammatory cytokines interleukin (IL)-1β, interferon (IFN)γ, tumor necrosis factor (TNF)α, and IL-6 are synergistically cytotoxic to β cells. Antibodies are markers of the autoimmune process but are not believed to play a role in the pathogenesis of the disease. Commonly measured antibodies are cytoplasmic islet cell autoantibodies (ICAs), insulin autoantibodies (IAA), glutamine acid decarboxylase (GAD-65), and ICA512/IA-2 (tyrosine phosphatase). Autoantibodies are found in about 90% of Caucasians, 60% of Hispanics, and 40% of African Americans at the onset of diabetes.

There is a genetic predisposition to the autoimmune process. Haplotypes of the major histocompatibility complex (MHC) human leukocyte antigen (HLA) class II genes located on chromosome 6p21 have the most impact on risk. The proteins encoded by the MHC class II genes are located on the surface of immune cells and are involved in presentation of foreign proteins to other cells of the immune system. Haplotypes HLA-DR3 and HLA-DR4 confer the greatest risk, whereas the HLA-DR2 haplotype is protective. Two genes which are not a part of the MHC gene complex have also been linked to an increased risk, IDDM2 on chromosome 11 and IDDM12 on chromosome 2.

Environmental triggers or exposures influence the autoimmune process in genetically vulnerable individuals, although specific triggers have yet to be pinpointed. The increase in incidence of diabetes in genetically stable populations points to the role of external factors in the development of T1DM and the concordance rate among identical twins is only approximately 25% to 50%. A number of retrospective and prospective epidemiologic studies have examined possible triggers, such as infant feeding patterns (cow's milk, cereal), infections (enterovirus), and toxins. The incidence of diabetes is higher in countries with a high consumption of cow's milk containing A1 β casein, and when Finnish children were randomized to a casein hydrolysate they had a lower incidence of diabetes autoimmunity. However the Australian Baby DIAB study followed approximately 500 infants with first-degree relatives who had diabetes, and no association was found between duration of breastfeeding or introduction of cow's milk and the development of autoimmunity to β cells. An association was found, however, between rotavirus infection and the presence of islet cell antibodies. Yet, a prospective study of enteroviral infection in infants (DAISY) did not reveal an association of the infection with autoimmunity measured by serologic studies. Another study of 1183 infants at increased risk of type 1 diabetes was followed to examine the impact of cereal introduction on the development of T1DM. Children exposed to cereal before 3 months and after 7 months of age were at increased risk of developing diabetes or serologic markers of diabetes. Routine childhood vaccination is not associated with an increased risk of developing T1DM.

Based on epidemiologic studies and pilot data, a number of large intervention trials were developed in attempts to prevent T1DM. Interventions have focused on the secondary prevention of further β-cell destruction in individuals with serologic markers of autoimmunity. The Diabetes Prevention Trial (DPT) and the European Nicotinamide Diabetes Intervention Trial (ENDIT) found that neither parenteral insulin, oral insulin, nor nicotinamide lowered the risk of developing diabetes in high to moderate risk individuals. The Trial to Reduce IDDM in Genetically at Risk (TRIGR) is an ongoing randomized controlled trial to evaluate the impact that cow's milk has on the development of diabetes. Infants are randomized to receive casein-based formula (Nutramigen) or cow's milk formula if not receiving breast milk.

Other studies target children and adults who have been newly diagnosed with diabetes. At the time of diagnosis it is estimated that 5% to 10% of the total pancreatic β-cell mass still remains. Interventions involve medications targeted at different levels of the immune response to prevent further β-cell destruction and preserve endogenous insulin production. Conventional immunosuppressant medications such as cyclosporine,[1] prednisone,[1] and azathioprine[1] have been used; however, drug toxicity outweighed the short-term benefit of preserving islet function. New trials are considering drugs such as sirolimus[1] and mycophenolate mofetil[1]. There are also trials of antigen-based therapies such as altered insulin peptides, glutamate decarboxylase (GAD), and heat shock protein, and trials of monoclonal antibodies to deplete specific T-cell populations (anti-CD3, anti-CD20, anti-CD25, and anti-CD52). Results have been promising, but no therapy has resulted in permanent remission of β-cell destruction.

TYPE 2 DIABETES MELLITUS

Type 2 diabetes mellitus (T2DM) results from insulin resistance (IR) and subsequent β-cell secretory failure. The prevalence of T2DM in children is increasing. In Cincinnati, Ohio, in 1994, the incidence of T2DM in children ages 10 to 19 years was 7.2 per 100,000 per year, a tenfold increase in 12 years. Prevalence varies based on ethnic composition of the population studied, with the highest rates in Pima Indians. It is estimated that 8% to 45% of all children diagnosed with diabetes will have T2DM, up from 1% to 2% in the past. The epidemic of T2DM in children is linked to the steep rise in obesity and is a serious public health concern.

Like T1DM, the development of T2DM is related to genetic susceptibility and external factors that affect insulin sensitivity. The disease is multigenic and many loci have been linked to T2DM in adults. There is a first- or second-degree relative with T2DM in 74% to 100% of those diagnosed with T2DM. Obesity increases insulin resistance (IR) and is associated with the development of T2DM. Other factors that increase the risk of developing T2DM include the presence of acanthosis nigricans, polycystic ovarian syndrome (PCOS), being small or large for gestational age (conditions that are associated with IR), and being a member of certain ethnic groups (American Indian, Hispanic American, African American, Asian/South Pacific Islander). T2DM is more frequent in females than in males, and more frequent in adolescents than in children.

IR before the development of T2DM has been documented by an increased early insulin response in hyperglycemic clamp studies. Clinically, this is manifested by impaired glucose tolerance, defined by the American Diabetes Association (ADA) as a 2-hour post-prandial glucose level ≥140 and <200 mg/dL. An impaired fasting glucose is defined as a blood glucose ≥100 and <126 mg/dL. For hyperglycemia to occur, IR must be accompanied by defects of insulin secretion. It is believed that the hyperglycemia is in turn toxic to the β cells, and results in further β-cell dysfunction and worsening hyperglycemia.

MATURITY-ONSET DIABETES OF THE YOUNG

Maturity-onset diabetes of the young (MODY) refers to a heterogeneous group of monogenic forms of diabetes (Table 1). Identified gene mutations affect the enzyme glucokinase or transcription factors in the β cell. Insulin secretion is abnormal; insulin sensitivity is normal. As the gene defects are autosomal dominant, a family history of diabetes is significant. The onset of diabetes in individuals with MODY is typically insidious; diagnosis is often made in puberty. Diagnosis of MODY is important because it has implications on therapy and course of disease. Glycemic control in approximately two thirds of

[1]Not FDA approved for this indication.

TABLE 1 Maturity Onset Diabetes of the Young (MODY)

Type	Gene	Chromosome	Frequency*	Age at Diagnosis	Severity of Diabetes
MODY 1	HNF-4α	20q	Rare	Postpubertal	Severe
MODY 2	Glucokinase	7p	8%-63%	Childhood	Mild
MODY 3	HNF-1α	12q	21%-64%	Postpubertal	Severe
MODY 4	IPF-1	13q	Rare	Early adulthood	Mild
MODY 5	HNF-1β	17	Unknown	Postpubertal	Mild
MODY 6	NeuroD1	2	Rare	Early adulthood	Unknown
MODYX	Unknown	Unknown	15%-45%	Heterogeneous	Mild/heterogeneous

*Percent of MODY families. Distribution is dependent on population studied.
Abbreviations: HNF = hepatic nuclear factor; IPF = insulin promoter factor.
Adapted from Velho G, Robert JJ. Maturity-onset diabetes of the young (MODY): Genetic and clinical characteristics. Horm Res 57(Suppl 1): 29–33, 2002.

individuals with defects of glucokinase (MODY type 2) can be achieved with lifestyle modification, whereas only 2% will require insulin. These individuals have impaired fasting glucose and glucose tolerance may remain intact for years. Other forms of MODY (MODY1 and MODY3) are more severe and often require therapy with oral agents and/or insulin.

OTHER FORMS OF DIABETES

Other disorders result in transient or permanent diabetes, either as a result of insulinopenia, insulin resistance, or both (Table 2).

Pathophysiology and Diagnosis

TYPE 1 DIABETES

Beta-cell destruction begins months to years before the overt signs and symptoms of diabetes develop. When the β-cell mass reaches a critical low, there is no longer enough insulin production to maintain a normal blood glucose level. The intravascular hyperglycemia causes an osmotic diuresis. Polyuria leads to polydipsia, dehydration, weight loss, and electrolyte abnormalities. Without glucose, cells use fat and protein to generate energy. Fatty acid oxidation produces ketones and subsequent acidosis. Approximately one third of children will have diabetic ketoacidosis (DKA) at diagnosis. Additional signs and symptoms of DKA include ileus, abdominal pain, and vomiting. Although polyuria causes potassium and phosphate depletion, significant acidosis results in elevated extracellular potassium levels, as extracellular protons are exchanged for intracellular potassium cations. Mental status changes are caused by dehydration and acidosis. Severe complications of DKA are predominantly caused by cerebral edema and cerebral thromboses; cardiac arrhythmias and cardiac arrest are extremely rare with adequate potassium replacement. Cerebral edema occurs in approximately 1% of children who present with DKA and has been associated with elevated blood urea nitrogen (BUN), low $Paco_2$, and the use of sodium bicarbonate. The etiology of cerebral edema is controversial with possible etiologies including cerebral hypoxia, cerebral ischemia, excessive free water administration, and rapid decreases in the serum glucose with initial therapy.

Diagnosis

Diabetes is defined by the ADA as:

- A casual blood glucose level of ≥200 mg/dL with symptoms of diabetes (polyuria, polydipsia, and weight loss), or
- A fasting glucose ≥126 mg/dL (no caloric intake for more than 8 hours), or
- A 2-hour post-prandial glucose level >200 mg/dL

The initial diagnosis is provisional and must be confirmed by repeat testing. Most children who present with signs and symptoms of diabetes can be screened with a urine dipstick test demonstrating glucosuria and ketonuria. The serum blood glucose confirms the diagnosis. Antibody levels (GAD-65, ICA 512, and IAA) help to differentiate T1DM from T2DM, although approximately 5% to 10% of patients with T1DM may be antibody negative. Children should be screened at diagnosis for other autoimmune disorders such as thyroiditis (free thyroxine [FT_4] and thyroid-stimulating hormone [TSH]) and celiac disease (antitissue transglutaminase and IgA level). Diagnostic studies for pernicious anemia and adrenal insufficiency are performed if suggested by the history or physical examination. If the family history of diabetes is extensive, and the child is not overweight and has negative antibodies, genetic studies can confirm or exclude a diagnosis of MODY.

Extensive education must occur at the time of diagnosis to aid in the self-management of diabetes.

TABLE 2 Etiologic Classification of Diabetes

Etiology	Disorder
Immune-mediated β-cell destruction	Type 1A diabetes
Idiopathic β-cell destruction	Type 1B diabetes
Insulin resistance with relative insulin deficiency	Type 2 diabetes
Genetic defects of β-cell function	MODY, mitochondrial disorders (MELAS,* MERRF†)
Genetic defects of insulin action	Type A insulin resistance, leprechaunism, lipoatrophic diabetes
Disorders of the exocrine pancreas	Cystic fibrosis, pancreatitis, aplasia
Drug induced	Glucocorticoids, nicotinic acid, tacrolimus, cyclosporine, diazoxide
Endocrinopathy	Cushing's disease and syndrome, acromegaly, glucagonoma, hyperthyroidism
Infection	Congenital rubella
Immune mediated	Antibodies to insulin receptor
Genetic syndromes associated with diabetes	Prader-Willi syndrome, Bardet-Biedl syndrome, Turner's syndrome, myotonic dystrophy
Gestational	Gestational diabetes mellitus (GDM)

*Mitochondrial myopathy, encephalopathy, lactic acidosis, stroke-like syndrome.

† Myoclonic epilepsy, ragged red fibers.

Adapted from The Expert Committee on the Diagnosis and Classification of Diabetes Mellitus. Report of the Expert Committee on the diagnosis and classification of diabetes mellitus. Diabetes Care 24(Suppl 1):S5–S19, 2001, with permission. Copyright © American Diabetes Association.

Families must be comfortable with home glucose monitoring and insulin administration. They must be aware of the action profile of each insulin used. They must know the signs, symptoms, and treatment of hypoglycemia and hyperglycemia. Families must learn how and when to administer glucagon and to test for urine ketones. Families are taught carbohydrate counting. A pediatric nutritionist develops a meal plan based on the nutritional needs of the child and in conjunction with the family's usual meal schedule and composition. Families are informed how and when to contact the diabetes care team. Communication and coordination with school administration are necessary to ensure proper management of diabetes while in school.

Management

Insulin Regimen

The inpatient management of DKA is described in another article. After the diagnosis of T1DM, and resolution of ketoacidosis, children begin insulin therapy with multiple daily subcutaneous injections (MDI). The total daily dose (TDD) of insulin used initially depends on the child's age and weight. A child younger than age 7 years requires approximately 0.5 to 1.0 U/kg per day, whereas adolescents may require 1 to 1.5 U/kg per day. Children are often started on a short-acting insulin before breakfast and dinner, and neutral protamine Hagedorn (NPH) insulin in the morning and before dinner or bedtime. Glargine (Lantus) insulin does not have a significant peak and lasts from 20 to 24 hours. It is being increasingly used to avoid nocturnal hypoglycemia. Patients can be started with a dinner or bedtime dose of 0.4 to 0.6 U/kg per day.

Short-acting insulin doses (lispro [Humalog] or aspart [NovoLog] insulin) are ideally adjusted based on carbohydrate intake and the blood glucose before a meal, using a carbohydrate-to-insulin ratio and a correction factor. Dosing of insulin based on carbohydrate intake gives children the flexibility to vary carbohydrate intake from day to day. The carbohydrate-to-insulin ratio is the number of grams of carbohydrates that 1 unit of short-acting insulin will "cover" (roughly 450/TDD). Adjustments of the dose based on the blood glucose allows for correction of high blood glucose. The correction factor is related to insulin sensitivity, and refers to the amount the blood glucose will drop with 1 unit of short-acting insulin (roughly 1700/TDD). Blood glucose testing 2 to 3 hours after an insulin dose for carbohydrate coverage, or for correction of hyperglycemia, can be performed to determine the adequacy of these ratios. Some children require different carbohydrate-to-insulin ratios at different meals, based on circadian changes in insulin sensitivity. Skill in carbohydrate counting is imperative when using a carbohydrate-to-insulin ratio.

The standard insulin regimen using NPH and short-acting insulin often fails to provide ideal control of blood glucose. Unlike beef/pork NPH insulin, recombinant (human) NPH insulin has an earlier peak at 3 to 6 hours and often has minimal activity after 15 hours. This insulin profile results in hypoglycemia in the late morning and overnight, and in hyperglycemia in the late afternoon and before breakfast. Glargine insulin helps to address the short-comings of NPH insulin (Table 3).

Ideally, glargine is used once a day along with a short-acting insulin at the time of carbohydrate intake. To avoid the need for an insulin injection at lunch, many children use glargine instead of NPH at dinner and continue to receive NPH at breakfast along with a short-acting insulin. NPH effectively is only needed to cover lunch as glargine provides coverage in the afternoon and overnight (Figure 1). Glargine cannot be mixed with other insulins, nor given near a simultaneous insulin injection. Intramuscular (IM) injection of glargine has an action profile similar to regular insulin. We recommend giving glargine at dinner as a safety measure, because an accidental IM or intravenous injection at bedtime would result in potentially unrecognized nocturnal hypoglycemia.

In the past 5 years, the use of continuous subcutaneous insulin infusion/pump therapy by children has increased exponentially. Pumps provide continuous short-acting insulin infusion for basal insulin needs, and boluses of insulin are administered for carbohydrate intake or correction of high blood glucose. Bolus doses are calculated using the child's carbohydrate-to-insulin ratio and correction factor described above. Typically, 40% to 50% of the TDD is given as basal insulin. Insulin infusion therapy limits the frequency of hypoglycemia events in adults and children, but may be associated with an increased risk of mild ketoacidosis.

Features of insulin infusion pumps have evolved. A number of pumps allow for basal rates as low as 0.05 units per hour, an attractive feature for young

TABLE 3 Insulin Activity Profiles

Type of Insulin	Onset of Effect	Major Effect	End of Effect
Lispro (Humalog)/Aspart (NovoLog)	10-15 minutes	30-90 minutes	4 hours
Regular (Humulin R, Novolin R)	30-60 minutes	2-4 hours	6-9 hours
NPH (Humulin N, Novolin N)	1-2 hours	3-8 hours	12-15 hours
Glargine (Lantus)	1-2 hours	2-22 hours	24 hours

Adapted from Chase HP. Understanding diabetes. Denver: Children's Diabetes Foundation at Denver, 2002.

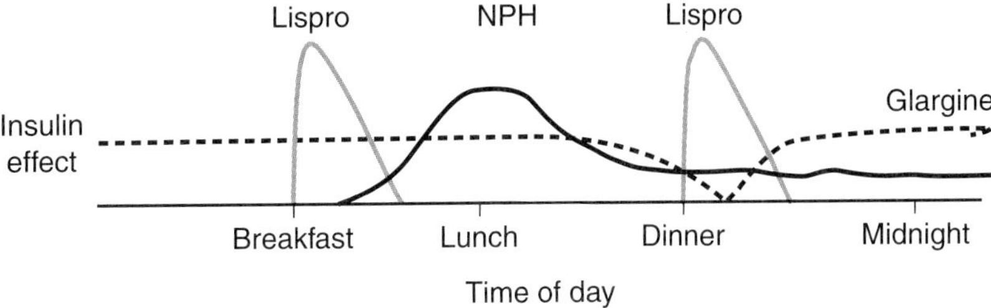

FIGURE 1 Simultaneous use of glargine and NPH insulin.

children who have minimal insulin requirements overnight. Some pumps have a bolus calculator that will calculate the insulin bolus needed after the child or parent enters the number of grams of carbohydrates to be eaten and the current blood glucose level. Pump calculations are based on customizable carbohydrate-to-insulin ratios and correction factors. Alerts remind a child or parent to change an infusion set or bolus at a certain time of day. Pumps are now being integrated with blood glucose meters, so glucose values are automatically entered into the pump. The pump can then suggest a correction bolus based on that blood glucose, subtracting residual insulin activity remaining from a previous correction bolus.

Inhaled insulin has undergone clinical testing and was found to be effective. Inhaled insulin is used in place of short-acting insulin, in conjunction with long-acting insulins such as glargine or NPH. Approval of inhaled insulin by the Food and Drug Administration (FDA) has been delayed because of concern that it may affect pulmonary function. Oral insulin is designed to not be degraded by the digestive enzymes and is absorbed into the portal circulation. Trials to study the effectiveness of oral insulin are under way.

Glucose Monitoring

The Diabetes Control and Complications Trial demonstrated that intensive management, that included at least four blood glucose measurements a day, led to a reduction of long-term microvascular complications in adolescents and adults. The frequency of blood glucose testing correlates directly with glycemic control. At a minimum, fingerstick blood glucose testing must be done before meals, and at bedtime. Blood glucose should be tested before and during strenuous exercise and before driving. Intermittent overnight testing is also recommended, because nocturnal hypoglycemia may be prolonged and damaging, and is often undetected. Reduction of nocturnal hyperglycemia can have a significant impact on overall control. Target blood glucose ranges vary based on age (Table 4). Hypoglycemia can have a long-term effect on the developing brain, thus younger children have higher blood glucose targets. Many blood glucose meters exist. Glucose meters vary in accuracy, size, amount of blood required for testing, speed of obtaining the results, and memory capacity. Most meters can be downloaded to a computer, allowing for evaluation of glucose patterns. The accuracy of the devices can vary tremendously.

TABLE 4 Glycemic and HbA_{1c} Targets Based on Age

	0-2 years old (mg/dL)	3-6 years old (mg/dL)	7-12 years old (mg/dL)	13 years to adult (mg/dL)
Pre-meal glucose	100-180	80-150	70-140	70-140
2-3 hours post-prandial	<200	<190	<180	<180
Before bed	100-200	100-180	90-160	80-150
2-4 AM	>100	>100	>90	>80
HbA_{1c}	<8.5%	<8.0%	<7.5%	<7.0%

Hemoglobin A_{1c} (HbA_{1c}) levels are measured every 2 to 3 months to determine the average blood glucose over this period. Target HbA_{1c} ranges vary by age (see Table 4). HbA_{1c} levels correlate with the long-term risk of developing complications of diabetes, such as early eye changes, retinopathy, and renal failure.

A number of near-continuous glucose monitoring devices have been developed to prevent hypoglycemia while improving overall glycemic control. Ultimately, an accurate glucose sensor will drive insulin infusion pumps, providing an artificial pancreas for the user. In 1999, the Food and Drug Administration (FDA) approved a subcutaneous sensor that measures interstitial glucose levels every 10 seconds and records a glucose value every 5 minutes. The monitor is downloaded to obtain the data collected, much like a Holter cardiac monitor. The FDA approved the first real-time glucose monitor in 2001. This device is noninvasive and withdraws interstitial glucose from the subcutaneous tissue. The glucose concentration is measured and the device reports a glucose value every 10 minutes, which generally reflects the serum glucose level 17 minutes earlier. The device has low and high blood glucose alarms, which are set by the user. Other sensors are in the process of obtaining FDA approval and will likely be available to clinicians and families in the next few years. Studies are underway to assess the accuracy and utility of these devices in children.

Sick Day Management

Illness can cause hyperglycemia as a result of increased insulin resistance, or hypoglycemia as a result of decreased carbohydrate intake. If a child is ill or vomits, determination of the blood or urine ketone level is critical to differentiate DKA from infectious gastroenteritis. After the possibility of DKA is eliminated, the keys to successful management during illness are frequent blood glucose testing and appropriately responding to glucose trends.

In a hypoglycemic child who is vomiting or not eating, the dose of long-acting insulin is reduced by approximately 30%. Families must understand that they should reduce but not omit insulin if the child is not eating. The routine short-acting insulin dose is held, but short-acting insulin is given every 3 hours as needed, based on the blood glucose and the child's correction factor to avoid hyperglycemia and ketone production. Children should sip on sugar-containing liquids to prevent dehydration, starvation ketosis, and hypoglycemia. Families should be prepared with glucose gel and glucagon in the event there is a rapid drop in blood glucose. Small doses of subcutaneous glucagon (20 μg for children ≤2 years of age, 150 μg for children >2 years of age) can be administered en route to the emergency room if the blood glucose falls to dangerous levels in a vomiting child. Evaluation in a clinic or an emergency room and treatment with intravenous dextrose-containing fluids should occur if vomiting or significant hypoglycemia is persistent.

An ill child who is hyperglycemic also requires frequent monitoring of blood glucose and urine or blood ketones to prevent DKA. Long-acting insulin doses should not be reduced, and doses of short-acting insulin should be administered based on the child's correction factor every 2 to 3 hours. The child should drink sugar-free liquids to prevent dehydration. The diabetes care team should be contacted if ketones develop for further management recommendations.

Multidisciplinary Care

Clinic visits with a multidisciplinary diabetes care team should occur quarterly. Blood pressure, growth, and pubertal development are monitored. Poor glycemic control can impair growth and pubertal development and cause weight loss. Examination can reveal early eye changes, lipohypertrophy, hepatosplenomegaly, foot lesions, and evidence of other autoimmune disorders.

HbA_{1c} levels are measured quarterly and thyroid function tests are measured annually. Thyroid antibodies are present in 20% to 30% of children with T1DM, and approximately 5% to 10% of children will require thyroid hormone replacement. After 5 years of diabetes, urine microalbumin is measured annually or more frequently if there is a history of elevation in microalbumin or blood pressure. Angiotensin-converting enzyme inhibitors or angiotensin receptor blockers are used if blood pressure or urine microalbumin levels are elevated. There is about a 6% incidence of celiac disease in children with diabetes, half of which are identified by screening at diagnosis, and the other half can be detected by rescreening 5 years after diagnosis. There is debate whether or not to treat asymptomatic celiac disease. A dilated funduscopic examination by an ophthalmologist is recommended on a yearly basis, beginning 5 years after the diagnosis of diabetes. In children older than age 12 years (or in younger children who are pubertal), the ADA recommends obtaining a lipid panel after diagnosis when glycemic control is achieved. Screening is done at an earlier age if there is a family history of dyslipidemia. Repeat screening occurs every 5 years if the initial values are low and there is no family history of dyslipidemia. Treatment of dyslipidemia involves achievement of glycemic control and lifestyle modification with increased physical activity and dietary changes. If the lipid abnormalities persist after 6 months of good glycemic control and lifestyle modification, medical therapy is recommended for children with low-density lipoprotein (LDL) levels greater than 160 mg/dL and should be considered for children with LDL levels between 130 and 159 mg/dL. Medical therapy includes bile acid sequestrants (resins), statins, or fibric acid medication if triglycerides are elevated (≥1000 mg/dL). Annual influenza vaccination is recommended for all children with diabetes who are older than 6 months of age.

Clinic visits include meeting with a diabetes educator, pediatric nutritionist, and social worker to identify and address the educational, nutritional, and psychosocial issues that may arise. Adolescents need to be counseled about the risks of using alcohol and tobacco. Adolescents who drive must be encouraged to perform blood glucose testing before driving and counseled about the risks of driving while hypoglycemic.

Admissions for DKA in previously diagnosed children are a result of failed insulin delivery, most commonly because of noncompliance or, rarely, an insulin infusion set failure (pump patients). Infrequently, an admission for DKA is associated with an intercurrent illness. Children and adolescents admitted with recurrent DKA should have a psychosocial evaluation by a social worker or child psychologist/psychiatrist.

TYPE 2 DIABETES

Children with type 2 diabetes are typically obese and have acanthosis nigricans (a velvety hyperpigmentation at intertriginous areas), which is associated with insulin resistance. Hyperglycemia results in polyuria, polydipsia, polyphagia, and even weight loss. Twenty percent to 30% of children with T2DM will develop ketoacidosis.

Diagnosis

High-risk children with impaired glucose tolerance or impaired fasting glucose can be identified by an oral glucose tolerance test or a fasting glucose measurement. The most sensitive screening test is a measurement of blood glucose 2 hours after an oral glucose load (75 g or 1.75 mg/kg) or 2 hours postprandial (which can be efficiently and cost-effectively measured at home with the glucose meter of an

TABLE 5 ADA Recommendations for Screening for T2DM

Criteria:
Overweight:
BMI >85th percentile for age and sex or
Weight for height >85th for age and sex or
Weight >120% of ideal body weight
PLUS
Any of the following two risk factors:
Family history of T2DM in a first- or second-degree relative
Member of a high-risk ethnic group (American Indian, Hispanic, Asian/Pacific Islander)
Signs of IR or conditions associated with IR (PCOS, acanthosis nigricans, hypertension, dyslipidemia)
Age of initiation: 10 years or earlier (at onset of puberty if younger than 10 years)
Frequency: Every 2 years
How: Fasting blood glucose

Abbreviations: IR = insulin resistance; PCOS = polycystic ovarian syndrome; T2DM = type 2 diabetes mellitus.
Adapted from the American Diabetes Association: Type 2 diabetes in children and adolescents. Pediatrics 105(3):671–680, 2000, with permission.

affected family member). A study of 167 obese children of multiethnic background identified impaired glucose tolerance in 25% of children (ages 4 to 10 years) and 21% of adolescents (ages 11 to 17 years). Diabetes was diagnosed in four adolescents. Given the ability to identify high-risk individuals, studies in adults have sought to prevent the onset of frank diabetes. Adults with impaired glucose tolerance were randomized to standard care, metformin (Glucophage), and an intense diet and exercise program. The rate of diabetes was significantly reduced in the group who participated in the diet and exercise program, and moderately decreased in the group receiving metformin. The success of interventions and the complications associated with undiagnosed diabetes emphasize the importance of screening to identify high risk children. Table 5 lists the ADA recommendations for screening.

The definitions for diabetes detailed above apply to the diagnosis of T2DM. Insulin, C-peptide, and serologic studies can help differentiate T1DM from T2DM. The HbA_{1c} may demonstrate a history of hyperglycemia, although it may still be normal when post-prandial hyperglycemia is seen with the oral glucose tolerance test (OGTT) and is the least-sensitive screening test. A fasting lipid panel is vital because many children have hypertriglyceridemia and hypercholesterolemia. These studies should be performed after glycemic control is obtained. Liver transaminases should be obtained at diagnosis because many children have nonalcoholic steatohepatitis.

Management

Lifestyle modification is imperative, although less than 10% of children with T2DM will successfully obtain adequate glycemic control with lifestyle modification alone. Medical therapies include insulin and oral medications. Insulin is used initially if the child is significantly hyperglycemic or if ketoacidosis is present. As in adults, oral agents are effective in children with T2DM, often eliminating the need for insulin (Table 6). The most common oral agent used is metformin, a biguanide that inhibits hepatic glucose production and improves insulin sensitivity. In 30% to 70% of patients receiving metformin there is an associated weight loss, and used solely, there is no risk of hypoglycemia. It also improves lipid profiles, as well as improves fertility in women with PCOS. Adolescent females should be aware of this effect and counseled about available birth control. Other oral agents include pioglitazone (Actos) and rosiglitazone (Avandia), which improve insulin sensitivity. Before beginning metformin a serum creatinine level should be obtained. A second oral agent or insulin therapy is required when metformin fails to provide adequate glycemic control. Glitazones (rosiglitazone and pioglitazone) require monitoring of liver function tests.

The glucose monitoring requirements and quarterly clinic visits are similar to those with T1DM. Lifestyle modification should be encouraged at each visit as needed. Surveillance for microvascular complications, such as annual ophthalmologic evaluations and measurement of urine microalbumin, begins at diagnosis. Dyslipidemia screening is performed every 2 years; guidelines for therapy are the same as for children with T1DM.

TABLE 6 Classification of Oral Agents Used to Treat Type 2 Diabetes Mellitus

Class of Drug	Example	Mechanism of Action
Biguanides	Metformin (Glucophage)	Decrease hepatic glucose production; improve insulin sensitivity
Thiazolidinediones	Rosiglitazone (Avandia), pioglitazone (Actos)	Improve insulin sensitivity
Sulfonylureas	Glipizide (Glucotrol), glyburide (Micronase), tolbutamide (Orinase)	Stimulate insulin secretion
Meglitinides	Repaglinide (Prandin)	Stimulate insulin secretion
Glucosidase inhibitors	Acarbose (Precose)	Decrease hydrolysis and adsorption of complex carbohydrates

Adapted from American Diabetes Association. Type 2 diabetes in children and adolescents. Pediatrics 105(3):671–680, 2000, with permission.

Future Therapies

As of October 2002, approximately 15,000 pancreas transplants had occurred in the United States. In 2000-2001, the 1-year graft survival rate in all forms of transplantation (pancreas, pancreas/kidney, pancreas after kidney) was >80%. Improved transplant techniques and immunosuppressive therapy have accounted for a significant improvement in survival of grafts. Children are not candidates for pancreas transplantation at this time given the requirement for immunosuppressive therapy. Additionally, the supply of pancreases is limited, making transplantation an inadequate solution for all individuals with diabetes.

Islet cell transplantation developed in Edmonton, Canada, has resulted in insulin independence in a number of adults with diabetes, but currently children are not candidates for this form of transplantation given the concomitant risks of immunosuppression. The development of glucose responsive, insulin-producing cells from stem cells is promising, and could provide a more widely available transplantation option. Gene therapy is another avenue under study.

Parallel to studies of transplantation, efforts are underway to develop an artificial pancreas. An accurate near-continuous sensor would be linked to an insulin delivery device, and both devices or either device could be implantable. Changes in the rate of insulin delivery would be dictated by glucose trends and a computer driven algorithm. In the United States and Europe, individuals have had intravenous sensor and implantable pumps placed successfully. In an inpatient setting, the sensor data has been used to control insulin infusion rates with promising results.

HYPEROSMOLAR HYPERGLYCEMIC SYNDROME AND DIABETIC KETOACIDOSIS

METHOD OF

Dace L. Trence, MD, and Irl B. Hirsch, MD

Hyperglycemic crises in diabetes mellitus are the end result of progressive metabolic decompensation. The classic forms of hyperglycemic crises, those of diabetic ketoacidosis (DKA) and hyperglycemic hyperosmolar syndrome (HHS), are more clinically overlapping than two distinctly separate entities. In a review of 612 patients with decompensated diabetes, 200 had features of both DKA and HHS. In the same patient, episodes of DKA occurred at times, HHS at other times. For both conditions, treatment goals include correction of the acute metabolic disorder, as well as the volume status of the patient, identification of any precipitating and /or co-morbid condition, facilitating the transition to a long-term treatment plan, and perhaps, most importantly, forming a specific plan to prevent recurrence.

Hyperglycemic Hyperosmolar Syndrome

Hyperglycemic hyperosmolar syndrome is the prototype of hyperglycemic crises in type 2 diabetes. Estimates of death range from as high as 60% to as low as 15%, the latter being related to earlier recognition of illness and, consequently, more prompt initiation of treatment.

A change in sensorium is the typical presentation. HHS can lead to central nervous system irritability, which can present as seizure, hemiparesis, confusion or coma, symptoms likely to result in an evaluation in an acute care setting. However, coma is much less common than previously believed, whereas lethargy and decreased sensorium are more frequently seen.

Physical examination will usually reveal tachypnea and low-grade fever, with normal blood pressure and respiratory rate. If hypotension is present with fever and tachypnea, infection should be suspected, particularly a gram-negative sepsis. Dehydration manifesting as poor skin tissue turgor may be difficult to appreciate in an elderly individual, but can be better appreciated through an examination for dryness of buccal mucous membranes. Abdominal distention with nausea, emesis, and pain can be associated with gastroparesis that is not caused by autonomic neuropathy, but rather by hypertonicity. This typically will resolve spontaneously with fluid treatment. Lethargy and disorientation are common. Focal neurologic signs are common in HHS, believed to reflect cerebrovascular insufficiency in areas of flow insufficiency, and can lead to a diagnosis of suspected acute cerebrovascular accident (CVA), but findings remit with fluid treatment. Seizures can be seen in up to 25% of patients and can be either focal or generalized.

Laboratory findings include plasma glucose >600 mg/dL and serum osmolality >320 mOsm/kg. Mild acidemia is often present, characterized as arterial pH >7.30, and serum bicarbonate (HCO_3) >15 mEq/L. The osmolality is roughly calculated as "effective serum osmolality" from corrected sodium (for glucose), potassium, and glucose (Table 1). Approximately 50% of patients with HHS will have

TABLE 1 Useful Formulas for the Evaluation and Treatment of Hyperglycemic Hyperosmolar Syndrome (HHS)

Calculation of the effective serum osmolality:
Effective Posm = 2 × ([Na^+] + [K^+]) + (glucose in mg/dL/18)
Corrected serum sodium:
Corrected [Na^+] = [Na^+] + 1.6 × ([glucose in mg/dL] − 100)/100

a mild anion gap metabolic acidosis When the acidosis is severe, differential diagnosis should be extended to consider lactic acidosis or other non-HHS entities. Vomiting or use of a thiazide diuretic can cause a metabolic *alkalosis* that can mask the severity of the acidosis. This might be suspected when the combined anion gap and measured bicarbonate combining power (HCO_3) one higher than normal.

Precipitating factors of HHS can be divided into several groupings (Table 2), including infectious, coexisting illness, and medication. Infection is the most frequent with estimates ranging from 32% to as high as 60% in HHS, primarily pneumonia, urinary tract infection, and sepsis. This has led to recommendations to start antibiotic therapy early in HHS treatment protocols, even if an infectious agent or source has not been identified. Others recommend waiting for more definitive evidence, as both fever and leukocytosis can be commonly seen in all episodes of HHS.

Treatment of HHS is targeted to fluid replacement, best done in an inpatient setting. Rapid volume repletion is required both for patient survival as well as to decrease the high risk of thromboembolism. The magnitude of fluid required will vary from individual to individual, but deficits of ~20% to 25% body water, ~12% body weight, or ~9 L are typical in HHS. Initial fluid replacement should consist of 1 to 2 L over the first 2 hours of treatment, followed by 7 to 9 L over the next 2 to 3 days, with specific rate and type of fluid determined individually. Normal saline has the advantage of more rapidly replacing intracellular volume, but increasing the risk of fluid overload in patients with potential cardiac and respiratory compromise, and the consequent complication of adult respiratory distress syndrome. Hypotonic fluids such as 0.45% saline can be more effective at replacing free water loss, but increase the risk of too rapid correction of hypernatremia with the potential for diffuse myelinolysis and death. A compromise is to start fluid replacement with normal saline, of up to 1 L, and then switch to 0.45% saline when urine output is well established. The goal is to replace one half of the free water deficit in the initial 12 hours of therapy, and the remaining one half over the next 12 hours. Once serum glucose drops below 250 mg/dL, it is recommended that glucose be added to the intravenous fluids. The rare reports of cerebral edema in HHS have all occurred when serum glucose fell below 250 mg/dL.

Colloids are not recommended as replacement fluids because they can contribute to an already high plasma viscosity and exacerbate vascular insufficiency, unless shock occurs despite maximal replacement with isotonic fluids. In the established end-stage renal failure patient, fluid replacement has little role and treatment is limited to correction of electrolyte abnormalities and providing insulin.

Once fluid replacement is initiated, attention then should be turned to electrolyte balance. There is a significant expectant diuresis of sodium, potassium, magnesium, calcium, and phosphate in HHS. Replacement of potassium takes precedence, although hyperkalemia is often present initially. Normokalemia or hypokalemia suggest a potassium deficit, minimally between 3 to as much as 10 mEq/kg. Severe hypokalemia is more often associated with a history of use of thiazide diuretic, nasogastric suction, or emesis. Replacement of potassium should not be started until urine output is established. Initial replacement should consist of 20 to 40 mEq/L of infused fluid, targeting a serum potassium level of 3.0 to 5.0 mEq/L. Electrocardiogram (ECG) monitoring is recommended. Potassium can be replaced as potassium chloride. There has been no reported clinical advantage in choosing potassium phosphate or potassium acetate, which have the disadvantage of increased expense. Although phosphate, magnesium, and calcium losses do occur in HHS, there are no data that the replacement of these are routinely necessary.

TABLE 2 Categories of Conditions Associated with Hyperglycemic Hyperosmolar Syndrome (HHS) and Diabetic Ketoacidosis (DKA)

Infection	Co-Existing Illness	Medications	Endocrine	Other
Pneumonia	Renal failure	Diuretics:	Thyrotoxicosis	Heatstroke
Urinary tract	Intestinal obstruction	Thiazide	Glucocorticoid excess	Hypothermia
Sepsis	Acute pancreatitis	Loop		Severe burns
	Myocardial infarct	β-Blockers	Acromegaly	Cardiothoracic surgery
		Cimetidine	Undiagnosed DM	Alcohol
		Calcium channel blockers		Cocaine
		Glucocorticoids		
		Phenytoin		
		Antipsychotics		
		Total parenteral nutrition (TPN)		
		Missed insulin, orals		

Insulin therapy is a secondary adjunct to fluid replacement. Recommended doses are similar to those in DKA. The initial insulin bolus of 0.1 U/kg can be followed by an intravenous infusion of 0.1 to 0.15 U/kg per hour. Starting insulin therapy before fluid therapy can shift 2 to 3 L of fluid from intracellular to extracellular compartments and potentiate hypovolemia, shock, and thromboembolism. Fluids alone can be therapeutic in HHS and can decrease serum glucose by 80 to 200 mg/dL per hour.

Just as there is controversy about the routine initiation of antibiotics, there is also controversy as to the benefit of routine initiation of anticoagulant therapy in this at-risk population for thromboembolic event. Although low-dose heparin has been recommended by some, the disadvantage of starting prophylactic heparin treatment is in potentiating gastrointestinal hemorrhage in the setting of hypertonicity-induced gastroparesis. As a compromise, it has been suggested waiting 1 to 2 days before starting heparin so as to allow gastroparesis to resolve, and then starting heparin only if the patient remains nonambulatory.

Monitoring treatment progress is imperative to successful treatment outcome. Flow sheets, either paper or electronic, are necessary to follow treatment. Coupled with clinical re-evaluation of the patient, this may allow patients with HHS to not need the invasive intervention of Swan-Ganz line placement or intra-arterial catheter, which could potentiate infection. Even bladder catheterization should be avoided if possible.

As important as the treatment of the acute hyperglycemic crisis, is the planning for interventions to prevent the recurrence of HHS. Monitoring hydration status, establishing a routine for home glucose monitoring, and providing education for "sick-day" treatment have been recommended as preventive measures for the recurrence of HHS.

Diabetic Ketoacidosis

The annual incidence of DKA in the United States is approximated at 5 to 8 episodes per 1,000 people with diabetes. DKA can be seen in both type 1 and type 2 diabetes, and can be the presenting condition of either type. Of all hospital admissions for diabetes, 2% to 8% are related to DKA, but with availability of self blood-glucose monitoring, increasingly DKA can be recognized in early stages, and thereby amenable to treatment in an office or urgent clinic setting. However, published mortality rates for DKA have shown little decline from a 2% to 10% range over the past three decades. Mortality rates in patients older than 65 years of age is significant, in excess of 20%.

In contrast to HHS, DKA is associated with typically lower glucose levels, in the 250 to 500 mg/dL range, serum osmolality at 300 mOsm/L, and a pH of <7.30 with ketonemia. In defining predisposing or associated conditions for the development of DKA for patients with type 2 diabetes, suggested associations include higher body mass index (BMI), male sex, history of poorer glycemic control, consistent high carbohydrate intake, and African American, Pacific Asian, and American Indian ethnicities.

Among all patients with DKA, a presenting glucose of <350 mg/dL is seen in 15%. An increased anion gap ($[Na^+]$-$[HCO_3]$-$[Cl^-]$) over 10 mEq/L is common. The use of the anion gap with serum bicarbonate and arterial pH has been proposed as a means of categorizing DKA into mild, moderate, and severe categories, with mild DKA constituting an anion gap of >10 mEq/L, serum bicarbonate 15 to 18 mEq/L, and arterial pH 7.25 to 7.30. Severe DKA is an anion gap of >12, serum bicarbonate <10, and arterial pH <7.00. However, clinical evaluation of sensorium with particular emphasis on degree of mental obtundation must accompany any lab. Plasma osmolality is typically increased but often does not exceed 320 mOsm/kg. Serum ketones are present at >1:2 dilution. New-onset diabetes is the classic etiology to DKA in type 1 diabetes, but in previously diagnosed type 1 diabetes, infection and omission of insulin are the most frequent precipitating factors.

Creatinine levels may be falsely elevated, as automated creatinine measurements are interfered with by ketone bodies, particularly acetoacetate. Serum ketones can be measured qualitatively, except when lactic acidosis or alcohol excess is suspected, as β-hydroxybutyrate is the preferential ketone body formed in these patients. Qualitative assays detect acetoacetate and less so acetone, but not β-hydroxybutyrate, so ketonemia may be underestimated in these patients.

Clinical presentation includes nausea, polydipsia, polyuria, weakness, and fatigue. Abdominal pain may be present with the examination, suggesting ileus. This can lead to confusion over associated metabolic versus precipitating abdominal etiology to pain. Current recommendations are to first treat dehydration and metabolic acidosis, then re-evaluate if abdominal symptoms and findings persist. Up to 25% of patients with DKA will have emesis that may resemble coffee grounds and be guaiac positive. Endoscopy shows this to be caused by hemorrhagic gastritis.

Differential diagnosis to ketoacidosis includes starvation ketosis and alcoholic ketoacidosis, which can be distinguished through clinical history. In these latter conditions glucose levels are typically less than 250 mg/dL. Besides lactic acidosis, an increased anion gap metabolic acidosis can be seen with ingestion of agents such as salicylates, methanol, ethylene glycol, and paraldehyde. Blood levels of lactate, salicylate, and methanol can help to differentiate these conditions. Urine calcium oxalate and hippurate crystals can be sought in ethylene glycol ingestion. Paraldehyde ingestion can be appreciated clinically through its pungent odor on the breath.

Treatment of DKA is focused on hydration, insulin administration, electrolyte balance, and prevention of future episodes. Precipitating causes should be identified and treated concurrently; these are similar to those seen in HHS. Isotonic saline of 1 to 2 L in an adult without cardiac compromise over the first hour should then be followed by re-evaluation of fluid status. Subsequent fluid choice, specifically when to convert to 0.45% normal saline, will be determined by blood pressure stability, presence of normal or elevated corrected sodium, and clinical examination. Typical body fluid deficit in DKA is 6 L, but overaggressive replacement is associated with the risk of cerebral edema, so after the initial fluid load to clinically stabilize, fluid rate should be decreased from 15 to 20 mL/kg per hour to 4 to 14 mL/kg per hour.

Once renal function has been assured, potassium should be added to fluids, as two-thirds potassium chloride and one-third potassium phosphate.

Insulin constant infusion at a rate of 0.1 U/kg per hour should be started in both pediatric as well as adult patients. Adults may receive an intravenous (IV) bolus of 0.15 U/kg after potassium has been documented above 3.3 mEq/L. The targeted decrease of glucose is 50 to 75 mg/dL per hour; if this is not achieved, insulin infusion can be doubled if hydration status is acceptable. With mild DKA, subcutaneous or intramuscular regular insulin given hourly is as effective as intravenous infusion when a priming dose of 0.4 to 0.6 U/kg per hour is first given half subcutaneously and half intramuscularly. Follow-up doses should be decreased to 0.1 U/kg per hour and can all be given in one site.

At a plasma glucose level of 250 mg/dL, the insulin infusion should be decreased to 0.05 to 0.1 U/kg per hour and dextrose added to intravenous fluids, until oral caloric intake is seen and conversion to subcutaneous insulin can be started. Conversion to subcutaneous insulin should be done with some overlap with intravenous infusion. If the patient is NPO (nothing by mouth), insulin infusion should be continued. Once the patient is eating, then an insulin regimen combining basal and prandial insulin should be started, targeting a dose of 0.5 to 1.0 U/kg per day if not previously on insulin, or resuming the patient's previous insulin regimen if taking insulin previously. Because patients with DKA include those with type 2 diabetes, these patients can possibly be discharged on oral antihyperglycemic agents. Previously undiagnosed type 2 diabetics presenting in DKA need particular monitoring post-DKA, because their insulin requirements may drop precipitously posthospitalization. These patients often are unrecognized as having type 2 diabetes until significant hypoglycemia occurs, despite decreasing insulin doses.

DKA treatment complications include cerebral edema, hypoxemia and noncardiogenic pulmonary edema. Cerebral edema occurs in 0.7% to 1.0% of children with DKA. Neurologic deterioration can be rapid, with headache, lethargy, and progressive decrease in arousal leading to seizures, bradycardia and respiratory arrest. Once symptoms progress beyond lethargy, a mortality risk of greater than 70% has been noted and permanent morbidity is seen in 86% to 93% of patients.

As with HHS, prevention of future DKA episodes is a critical part of treatment. Sick-day management should be reviewed and a discussion held regarding blood glucose goals as well as when to use specific supplemental insulin doses of short-acting insulin in illness. This should be coupled with review of the need for increased fluid intake, initiation of carbohydrate and appropriate sodium-containing liquid diet, and when to call the office for help. Education as to the need to continue insulin, even if caloric intake is diminished, the need to check urinary ketones in sustained hyperglycemia, with periodic review of these principles with patients, not only could impact on individual patient morbidity and survival, but also health costs. Repeated admissions for DKA are estimated to cost one of every two health care dollars spent on adults with type 1 diabetes.

GOUT AND HYPERURICEMIA

METHOD OF

Adel G. Fam, MD

Gout is characterized by chronic hyperuricemia, recurrent attacks of acute arthritis provoked by release of monosodium urate crystals into joint cavities, and development in some patients of gross urate deposits (tophi). It chiefly affects men over 40 years of age, and the incidence in women increases after menopause. The overall prevalence of gout is estimated to be 6 per 1,000 men and 1 per 1,000 women. However, recent studies suggest a rising incidence of gout in New Zealand, the United States, and other countries. The reasons for this are unclear, but changing dietary trends, the rising incidence of obesity and insulin resistance syndrome (IRS), increasing longevity, and frequent use of both diuretics and prophylactic low-dose aspirin are implicated.

Gout occurs in three overlapping phases: (a) a long phase of asymptomatic hyperuricemia, (b) a period of recurrent acute gouty attacks separated by symptom-free intervals (interval gout), (c) which is followed in approximately 10% of patients by the development of chronic tophaceous gouty arthritis.

Hyperuricemia, elevated serum urate >7.0 mg/dL (>450 μmol/L) in men and >6.0 mg/dL (>360 μmol/L) in women, is the biochemical hallmark of gout. In the majority of patients, gout is a primary disorder.

Less commonly, hyperuricemia and gout are secondary to purine enzyme defects, myeloproliferative or lymphoproliferative disorders, renal failure, drugs, or other conditions (Table 1). Measurement of 24-hour urinary uric acid (UA) excretion in patients with primary gout, while on a low-purine diet for a week, can often indicate whether the hyperuricemia is the result of overproduction or underexcretion of UA. In the majority of patients (>90%), hyperuricemia results from reduced renal tubular excretion of UA (gouty underexcretors). These patients excrete either normal or reduced amounts of UA (<600 mg per day or <3.6 mmol/L per day on a purine-restricted diet for 1 week). Their urate clearance is reduced <6 mL per minute (normal: 6 to 11 mL per minute). They have a limited capacity to eliminate a urate (purine) load, and excretion of normal amounts of UA is accomplished only at inappropriately high serum urate levels. A genetic basis is suggested by the frequent presence of a similar proximal renal tubular abnormality in first-degree relatives. Whether this underexcretor status is related to structural heterogeneity of a specific proximal renal tubule urate anion exchanger/transporter, URAT1, is unclear.

In a minority of patients (<10%), hyperuricemia results from increased rate of *de novo* purine biosynthesis. These patients excrete excessive quantities of UA: >600 mg per day or >3.6 mmol/L per day on a low-purine diet for 1 week (gouty overproducer/overexcretors). Their UA clearance is either normal or increased with a UA-to-creatinine ratio of >6%. Studies using isotope-labeled UA invariably demonstrate an increased rate of *de novo* purine and UA biosynthesis.

Being a metabolic disorder, gout is significantly influenced by dietary, metabolic, and environmental factors, such as overeating, obesity, dyslipidemia, diabetes mellitus, IRS (metabolic syndrome), and alcohol abuse. Hypertension is also common in patients with gout. Although hyperuricemia and gout are commonly associated with coronary artery disease (CAD), it is unlikely that hyperuricemia per se plays a causal role in the pathogenesis of CAD, and any apparent relation is likely related to the frequent association of hyperuricemia with known risk factors for CAD: IRS, obesity, dyslipidemia, hypertension, and diabetes mellitus. Recent data suggest that hypertriglycidemia, obesity, and hypertension in patients with gout are often part of an underlying IRS or "metabolic syndrome," estimated to occur in 76% to 95% of gout sufferers. Features of the syndrome include overall and abdominal obesity (waist circumference >100 cm, waist-to-hip ratio >0.85), glucose intolerance with resistance to insulin and secondary compensatory hyperinsulinemia, and dyslipidemia characterized by: hypertriglycidemia, increased levels of apolipoprotein B, low-density lipoprotein cholesterol (LDL-C) and atherogenic small dense LDL-C particles, and a decrease in high-density lipoprotein cholesterol (HDL-C) levels. Both hypertension and hyperuricemia are frequently associated with IRS. Hyperinsulinemia has been shown to stimulate renal tubular sodium-hydrogen exchanger, thereby enhancing reabsorption of sodium, chloride, bicarbonate and uric acid.

TABLE 1 Classification of Hyperuricemia and Gout

Primary
Uric acid overproduction: <10%
Uric acid renal underexcretion: >90%
Secondary
Uric Acid Overproduction
Purine enzyme defects:
HGPRT deficiency
PRPP synthetase overactivity
Glucose-6-phosphatase deficiency
Fructose-1-phosphate aldolase deficiency
Increase nucleotide turnover
Myelo- and lymphoproliferative disorders
Hemolytic anemia
Psoriasis
Chemo-/radiotherapy: hematologic malignancies (tumor lysis syndrome)
Excessive dietary purines and ethanol abuse
Uric Acid Renal Underexcretion
Renal failure
Acidosis: lactic, ethanol, diabetic ketoacidosis; dieting
Drugs: low-dose aspirin, diuretics, cyclosporine A, pyrazinamide
Chronic lead nephropathy (saturnine gout)
Uncertain Mechanisms
Hypertension
Hypothyroidism
Preeclampsia and toxemia of pregnancy

Abbreviations: HGPRT = hypoxanthine guanine phosphoribosyltransferase; PRPP = phosphoribosyl pyrophosphate.

Acute Gouty Arthritis

Gouty attacks commonly affect the joints of the lower extremities, particularly the metatarsophalangeal (MTP) joint of the great toe (acute podagra). The intertarsal, ankle, knee, elbow, and wrist joints and olecranon bursae are next in order of frequency. The onset, which typically occurs at night, is rapid; and the acute arthritis often peaks within 24 hours, producing a painful, warm, red, tender, swollen joint, as well as diffuse erythema of the surrounding soft tissues, resembling cellulitis. In the early stages of gout, the attacks are few and far between, with the affected joints returning to normal between attacks. Late in the course of the disease, the acute episodes become more frequent, longer lasting, with a tendency toward incomplete resolution and polyarticular involvement.

Chronic Tophaceous Gouty Arthritis

Before the introduction of effective urate-lowering drugs, approximately 20% to 40% of untreated patients developed chronic tophaceous gouty arthritis. Recent data suggest a much lower incidence (approximately 10% to 20%). However, every so often, one encounters individuals in whom failure to properly diagnose or treat has permitted full expression of the disease. The average time from the initial gouty attack to the development of tophi is 11 years. Tophi are typically located in the peripheral, cooler parts of the body: about the feet, fingers, and knees; in and around bursae (olecranon, prepatellar, and bunion); and in the subcutaneous tissues over the Achilles tendon and ear pinnae. Chronic gouty arthritis is characterized by persistent aching, stiffness, swelling, and often joint deformities. Superimposed episodes of acute gouty inflammation are common. Typical radiographic features include punched out erosions with overhanging margins, and soft-tissue swellings (tophi).

Diagnosis

Although hyperuricemia is a characteristic biochemical marker of gout, it is improper to equate the finding of hyperuricemia with gout. Many individuals who have life-long hyperuricemia do not develop gouty arthritis (asymptomatic hyperuricemia). Serum urate levels may be normal in some patients with gout, particularly during the early phases of gout, following alcoholic excesses or withdrawal of diuretic therapy, and during initial therapy with allopurinol (Zyloprim) or uricosuric drugs.

A firm diagnosis of gout can be established by demonstration of intracellular or extracellular, needle-shaped, negatively birefringent, monosodium urate crystals in joint fluids, bursal effusions, or in aspirates from tophi, using compensated polarized light microscopy. However, this may not be possible in all patients for a number of reasons: absence of a detectable joint effusion or visible tophi, an inaccessible joint, inexperience with either joint aspiration or evaluation of synovial fluid for crystals, or presence of a few urate crystals or crystals too small (<1 μm) to be seen by light microscopy. Under these circumstances, the diagnosis of gout can be made on the basis of a typical clinical history in association with documented hyperuricemia. Between gouty attacks, the diagnosis can sometimes be confirmed by demonstrating urate crystals in fluid aspirates from a previously affected but asymptomatic knee or first MTP joint.

Treatment

Gouty arthritis nearly always occurs in the setting of chronic hyperuricemia. Consequently, management of a patient with gout requires that two objectives be considered independently: (a) immediate control of the acute gouty episode, and (b) long-term treatment of chronic hyperuricemia to prevent both subsequent gout attacks and complications, including chronic tophaceous gouty arthritis, uric acid nephrolithiasis, and urate nephropathy.

ACUTE GOUTY ARTHRITIS

Treatment of acute gouty arthritis consists of rest, splinting of the joint, local ice application, and drug therapy, including nonsalicylate nonsteroidal anti-inflammatory drugs (NSAIDs), colchicine, and corticosteroids (Table 2).

Nonsteroidal Anti-inflammatory Drugs

Cyclooxygenase (COX)-2 nonselective NSAIDs are preferred by most physicians as the drugs of first choice in the treatment of acute gout because they are generally better tolerated and more predictable in their therapeutic effects than is oral colchicine. There is no clear advantage of any one preparation, but a large dose of indomethacin (Indocin), naproxen (Naprosyn), or diclofenac sodium (Voltaren) on the first 1 to 3 days, with a reduction thereafter is generally effective. Whatever drug is used, it should be

TABLE 2 Drugs Used in the Treatment of Acute Gouty Arthritis

Nonsteroidal Anti-inflammatory Drugs	
Nonselective COX-2 inhibitors	
Indomethacin (Indocin)	50 mg qid for 3-6 days
Naproxen (Naprosyn)	500 mg bid or tid for 3-6 days
Diclofenac sodium (Voltaren)	50 mg tid for 3-6 days
Selective COX-2 inhibitors	
Etoricoxib (Arcoxia)[1]	120 mg/d for 3-6 days
Other selective COX-2 inhibitors	Not evaluated
Colchicine	0.6 mg q1-2h until relief occurs, gastrointestinal toxicity or a maximum dose of 4-6 mg/d has been reached
Corticosteroids	
Monoarticular or oligoarticular gouty attacks:	
intra-articular methylprednisolone acetate (Depo-Medrol)	5-40 mg
Polyarticular gouty attacks:	
IM triamcinolone acetonide (Kenalog)	60 mg q1-4d
IM methylprednisolone acetate (Depo-Medrol)	40 mg q1-4d or
IM ACTH (corticotropin)	40-80 IU q6-24h
Ambulatory treatment of gouty attacks:	
oral prednisone	20-40 mg first day, then taper in 4-8 days

[1]Not FDA approved for this indication.

Abbreviations: bid = twice daily; COX-2 = cyclooxygenase-2; IM = intramuscular; qid = four times a day; tid = three times a day.

started as early as possible after the onset of an acute episode. It is important, therefore, to supply the patient with the appropriate NSAID (preferably kept in a convenient pocket, for gout often strikes when the patient is far from home), and instructions on how to self-treat acute flares at the first "twinge" of an attack.

Although adverse reactions (e.g., nausea, dyspepsia, diarrhea, headache, confusion) can occur, the duration of NSAID therapy is usually short, and serious toxicity leading to drug withdrawal (e.g., gastrointestinal [GI] bleeding) is rare (<10% of patients).

A new selective COX-2 inhibitor, etoricoxib (Arcoxia)[1] 120 mg per day, is as efficacious in the treatment of acute gouty arthritis as indomethacin 50 mg thrice daily, with etoricoxib (Arcoxia) demonstrating an improved safety profile. Whether the treatment of acute gout with etoricoxib and other selective COX-2 inhibitors (celecoxib [Celebrex], rofecoxib [Vioxx], valdecoxib [Bextra]), in place of the well-established, conventional NSAIDs, will prove to be more advantageous in terms of efficacy, GI safety, and cost-effectiveness, remains to be established. These promising drugs may, however, be of particular benefit in patients who are intolerant to nonselective NSAIDs and in patients who present with acute gouty attack of several days' duration because a longer course of treatment is likely to be required.

NSAIDs, including selective COX-2 inhibitors, are potentially hazardous and should be used with caution for the treatment of acute gouty events in patients older than 65 years and in patients with co-morbid medical conditions, such as congestive heart failure, renal impairment, peptic ulcer disease, hepatic dysfunction, and anticoagulants.

Colchicine

Although colchicine has traditionally been rooted in the treatment of acute gouty arthritis, in recent years, its use has steadily declined. Drawbacks include (a) slow onset of action, (b) a narrow benefit-to-toxicity ratio, with approximately 80% of patients experiencing GI toxicity (nausea, diarrhea, and abdominal pain) after oral administration, and (c) reduced therapeutic efficacy when administered 24 hours or longer after the onset of acute gouty inflammation—not an infrequent occurrence. It is administered orally in a dose of 0.6 mg every 1 to 2 hours until acute joint pain is relieved, the patient develops GI toxicity, or a maximum of 4 to 6 mg per day has been administered. Colchicine is efficacious in about two thirds of patients. It is primarily useful for patients without renal, hepatic, or bone marrow disease who are intolerant or hypersensitive to NSAIDs.

Recently, the role of intravenous (IV) colchicine in the treatment of acute gout has come under close scrutiny in light of growing concerns about its safety. A major drawback is the drug's potential for serious and sometimes lethal toxicity (bone marrow suppression, oliguric renal failure, hepatic necrosis, diarrhea, seizures, and death), particularly in patients older than 65 years with renal and/or hepatic impairment. This controversy has led to the publication of a set of guidelines for the IV administration of colchicine. However, the guidelines are not widely recognized, inappropriate use of the drug occurs often, and many clinicians advocate restriction of or an outright ban on the use of IV colchicine.

Corticosteroids Including Corticotropin

Intra-articular corticosteroid therapy and both systemic corticosteroids and corticotropin (ACTH)[1], are indicated for the treatment of acute gouty episodes in patients with coexisting medical illnesses, contraindicating the use of both NSAIDs and colchicine (Table 3). Such treatment is also efficacious in the management of acute gout occurring during the postoperative period, for those with NSAID hypersensitivity, and for severe gouty attacks refractory to both NSAIDs and colchicine. Intra-articular corticosteroid injections, such as methylprednisolone acetate (Depo-Medrol) 5 to 40 mg, are particularly useful for the treatment of acute monoarticular and oligoarticular gouty episodes in these patients. However, such therapy is not practical for those with polyarticular gouty attacks. Concern about coexistent joint infection, concomitant anticoagulant therapy, and fear of needle injection may also preclude intra-articular corticosteroid administration. In these clinical situations, intramuscular (IM) triamcinolone acetonide (Kenalog) 60 mg, or IM methylprednisolone acetate 40 mg, repeated every 1 to 4 days as required, can be used to provide rapid control of acute attacks, thereby circumventing delayed absorption after oral administration. IV methylprednisolone sodium succinate (Solu-Medrol) 40 to 160 mg repeated every 1 to 4 days as required, is indicated for those receiving anticoagulant therapy.

TABLE 3 Indications for Corticosteroid Drugs in the Treatment of Acute Gouty Arthritis

Co-morbid medical conditions
Cardiac failure, hypertension
Renal insufficiency
Peptic ulcer, gastrointestinal bleeding
Hepatic insufficiency
Chronic alcoholism
Bleeding diathesis, anticoagulants
Advanced age
Postoperative state
NSAID hypersensitivity
Severe attacks refractory to both NSAIDs and colchicine

Abbreviation: NSAID = nonsteroidal anti-inflammatory drug.

[1]Not FDA approved for this indication.

Oral prednisone, 20 to 40 mg on the first day followed by gradual tapering over 4 to 8 days, is particularly useful for the ambulatory treatment of acute gouty flares in outpatients with co-morbid conditions contraindicating the use of NSAIDs.

Although a number of studies demonstrate the efficacy and safety of IM ACTH (Acthar), 40 to 80 IU repeated every 6 to 24 hours as required, in the treatment of acute gout, there is no convincing evidence that such therapy is superior to corticosteroids. Drawbacks of ACTH therapy include dependence of therapeutic effects on sensitivity of the adrenal cortex (drug may be ineffective in subjects previously treated with corticosteroids); increased release of adrenal androgens and mineralocorticoids, which can lead to fluid overload; and a relatively short duration of action, with a greater potential for rebound attacks and treatment failures compared with IM corticosteroids.

CHRONIC GOUTY ARTHRITIS

Corrective measures constitute sufficient therapy for many patients with infrequent gouty attacks and mild hyperuricemia. These include weight reduction for obesity, elimination of drugs causing hyperuricemia (e.g., low-dose aspirin >325 mg per day, thiazide diuretics), restriction of alcohol intake, and diet modification. The traditional, low-purine diet is rarely recommended because it is not palatable or practical for very long, it is high in both carbohydrates and dairy products rich in saturated fats, and it produces only a 10% to 15% reduction of serum urate. Recent studies suggest a strong association between hyperuricemia/gout and insulin resistance syndrome—abdominal obesity, glucose intolerance with compensatory hyperinsulinemia, hypertension, hyperuricemia, dyslipidemia, and increased risk of coronary heart disease. A pilot study of a weight-reducing diet, restricted in both carbohydrates (40% of energy) and saturated fats, with a proportionate increase intake of protein (30% of energy) and unsaturated fats (30% of energy), resulted in a 37% reduction in serum urate, reduced frequency of gouty attacks, and improvement of IRS with decreased serum triglycerides, low-density lipoprotein C, glucose, and insulin levels. For patients with coexistent hypertension, losartan (Cozaar)[1] may be used given its mild uricosuric effect, and for those with concomitant hyperlipidemia, fenofibrate (Tricor),[1] also a mild uricosuric, may be prescribed.

The frequency of gouty attacks can be reduced by prophylactic administration of colchicine, 0.6 mg once or twice daily. However, such therapy does not correct the hyperuricemia, or prevent the silent progression of tophaceous lesions and cumulative joint damage. It can also lead to a number of toxic reactions, including neuromyopathy, myelotoxicity, alopecia, and malabsorption syndrome.

The ultimate treatment of established gout, requires long-term control of hyperuricemia. Three types of urate-lowering drugs are available: (a) uricostatic drugs (e.g., allopurinol [Zyloprim], a xanthine oxidase inhibitor that decreases uric acid synthesis); (b) uricosuric agents, which act by competitive inhibition of postsecretory renal tubular reabsorption of urate, thus increasing urate excretion and lowering serum urate; and (c) uricolytic drugs, such as uricase (urate oxidase), which catalyze the conversion of UA into the more soluble allantoin.

Not every patient with gout requires treatment with urate-lowering drugs (Table 4). The administration of a drug to normalize serum urate is usually a life-long commitment to regular daily therapy. Frequent measurement of serum urate concentrations is important in monitoring the patient's compliance and the effectiveness of urate-lowering treatment. To prevent further gouty attacks and ongoing joint damage and to ensure resorption of the tophaceous deposits, serum urate should be reduced and sustained to <4 to 6 mg/dL or <250 to 350 μmol/L—well below the concentration at which urate saturates the extracellular fluid: approximately 6.8 mg/dL or 404 μmol/L at 37°C (98.6°F).

Initiation, dose reduction, or interruption of urate-lowering therapy during an acute attack of gout is not recommended; a major change in serum urate levels, induced by starting or stopping allopurinol or a uricosuric drug, can, in theory, worsen an attack already in progress.

The sharp reduction in serum urate level that takes place early in the course of urate-lowering treatment may be associated with flares of gout. These flares may be mistaken for a poor response to treatment. Some physicians advocate prophylactic colchicine, 0.6 mg once or twice daily during the first 1 to 12 months of initiating antihyperuricemic therapy. However, this practice cannot be "routinely" recommended, given the potential toxicity of prolonged colchicine therapy (neuromyopathy, myelotoxicity, alopecia, malabsorption syndrome), and that only about one third of patients develop flares of gouty arthritis after initiation of allopurinol or uricosuric treatment. Instead, many clinicians advocate the temporary use of a supplemental NSAID to control these attacks. Colchicine prophylaxis is of special value, however, in those patients who continue to experience frequent gouty flares precipitated by urate-lowering therapy.

Allopurinol

Allopurinol (Zyloprim) is the urate-lowering drug of choice. As a xanthine oxidase inhibitor, it interferes with the conversion of hypoxanthine to xanthine and of xanthine to UA acid, leading to reductions of serum and urinary urate concentrations, and concomitant increases in serum and urinary hypoxanthine and xanthine concentrations. Allopurinol is rapidly oxidized in the body

[1]Not FDA approved for this indication.

TABLE 4 Urate-Lowering Drugs

Indications for Allopurinol Therapy
Dose: Allopurinol (Zyloprim) 100-600 mg/d (single dose)
Frequent gouty attacks despite corrective measures (>2-4 attacks per year)
Major overproduction of uric acid with hyperuricosuria including HGPRTase deficiency and PRPP synthetase overactivity
Chronic tophaceous gouty arthritis
Gout complicated by urate nephropathy, uric acid, nephrolithiasis, or renal insufficiency
Hyperuricemia secondary to lymphoma, leukemia, and other myeloproliferative disorders treated with cytotoxics or radiotherapy (to prevent tumor lysis syndrome)
Failure of uricosuric drugs
Recurrent calcium oxalate urinary calculi associated with hyperuricosuria
Indications for Uricosuric Drugs
Dose: probenecid (Benemid): 1-2 g/d (divided doses)
Sulfinpyrazone (Anturane): 100-800 mg/d (divided doses)
Patients younger than 60 years of age with primary gout, underexcretion hyperuricemia, normal renal function, and no history of renal calculi or massive tophi
Allergy or intolerance to allopurinol
Combined allopurinol-uricosuric treatment for patients with massive tophaceous deposits
Indications for Uricolytic (Uricase) Therapy
Dose: nonpegylated recombinant uricase (rasburicase [Elitek]): 0.2 mg/kg/d IV infusion for 5-10 days
Short-term prevention and treatment of chemo-/radiotherapy-related malignant hyperuricemia and tumor lysis syndrome in patients with hematologic malignancies (lymphoma, leukemia, myeloma)

Abbreviations: HGPRTase = hypoxanthine guanine phosphoribosyltransferase; IV = intravenous; PRPP = phosphoribosyl pyrophosphate.

to its principal metabolite, oxypurinol, which is also a potent xanthine oxidase inhibitor. The plasma half-life of allopurinol is 1 to 3 hours, whereas that of oxypurinol is 14 to 26 hours. Thus, allopurinol can be administered as a single daily dose. Because oxypurinol is excreted solely through the kidneys, reduction of allopurinol dose is indicated in patients older than 65 years and in those with renal impairment. The starting dose of allopurinol is 50 to 300 mg per day (formulations: 100-mg, 200-mg, and 300-mg tablets), and the total daily dose ranges between 100 mg and 600 mg, with most patients requiring 300 mg per day. Reduction of serum urate concentration is noted within 2 days of starting therapy. The level usually falls to normal within 7 to 21 days, although it may take much longer in patients with extensive tophaceous deposits. Gouty attacks often cease within 3 to 6 months of continuous therapy, whereas dissolution of the tophi may take 6 to 24 months. Discontinuation of allopurinol is followed by a rapid rise of serum urate concentration to pretreatment levels, although recurrence of acute gouty attacks may not occur for long periods. Table 4 outlines specific indications for the use of allopurinol.

Allopurinol is well tolerated by the majority of patients, and adverse reactions are rare (approximately 3.5%). Precipitation of acute gouty arthritis and allergic dermatitis are the most frequent adverse reactions. Cautious reintroduction of allopurinol after cutaneous reactions may be possible using a schedule of gradually increasing doses. An initial oral dose of 50 µg allopurinol daily is progressively increased every 3 to 7 days to 100 µg, 200 µg, 500 µg, 1 mg, 5 mg, 10 mg, 25 mg, and finally to a target dose of 50 to 100 mg daily. Further dose adjustments are based on the patient's serum urate and creatinine levels. This desensitization regimen is particularly useful in patients with renal insufficiency rendering uricosuric drugs ineffective.

Allopurinol hypersensitivity syndrome is a rare (0.1% to 0.4% of patients), life-threatening, toxic reaction characterized by fever, severe dermatitis (toxic epidermal necrolysis, erythema multiforme or exfoliative dermatitis), acute hepatitis, acute interstitial nephritis with renal failure, eosinophilia, and leukocytosis. It occurs most frequently in elderly patients with renal impairment in whom the dose of allopurinol has not been reduced appropriately, resulting in an accumulation of oxypurinol. Allopurinol desensitization is hazardous and is not recommended in these patients.

Uricosuric Drugs

Uricosuric drugs enhance renal excretion of urate, thereby reducing serum urate concentration. The intense initial uricosuria can result in the deposition of UA crystals in renal tubules and formation of urinary calculi, which in turn can cause renal colic or deterioration of renal function. To minimize this risk and to prevent the precipitation of acute gouty attacks associated with rapid decline in serum urate concentrations, uricosuric drugs are started at low doses and gradually increased over 2 to 4 weeks. The risk of UA stones can be further reduced by maintenance of a high urine volume (>2 L per day) and/or alkalization of urine with sodium bicarbonate 1 g 4 times daily, particularly during the first 4 to 6 weeks of therapy when the uricosuria is greatest.

As serum urate normalizes, the intense uricosuria subsides, and renal urate excretion approaches pretreatment levels.

Two uricosuric drugs are used to manage chronic gout. Probenecid (Benemid) is the most frequently used uricosuric. It is administered in a dose of 250 mg twice daily for 1 to 2 weeks, followed by 500 mg twice daily, increasing the dose thereafter to 1000 mg twice daily if required. Sulfinpyrazone (Anturane) 50 to 100 mg is administered twice daily for 1 to 2 weeks, followed by 100 to 200 mg twice daily, increasing to 400 mg twice daily if needed. Side-effects of these drugs include nausea, abdominal pain, allergic rash, and fever.

In the absence of clear-cut indications for treatment with allopurinol (see Table 4), uricosuric drugs can be used in patients younger than 60 years of age with primary gout, underexcretion hyperuricemia, normal renal function, and no gross tophi or a history of urinary calculi. Other indications for uricosurics include patients who are allergic or intolerant to allopurinol, and those with massive tophaceous deposits who may require treatment with both allopurinol to block UA synthesis and a uricosuric to increase UA excretion (see Table 4).

Approximately 75% of patients respond to uricosuric drugs with normalization of serum urate, control of gouty attacks, and resorption of tophaceous deposits. Most failures, in the remaining 25% of patients are caused by declining renal function (uricosurics are ineffective at a creatinine clearance <50 to 60 mL per minute), intolerable side effects (particularly GI events, skin rash), concomitant intake of aspirin >325 mg per day (which antagonizes the uricosuric action), and poor compliance because of multiple daily doses.

Uricolytic Drugs

Uricase, or urate oxidase, is an enzyme that catalyzes the conversion of UA into allantoin, which is 5 to 10 times more soluble than UA and is more readily eliminated by the kidneys. Humans and certain higher primates lack uricase. Both native (nonrecombinant) and recombinant uricases (e.g., rasburicase) have been used as short-term therapy for the prevention and treatment of malignancy-associated hyperuricemia and tumor lysis syndrome, resulting from chemo-/radiotherapy of hematologic malignancies, such as lymphoma, leukemia, and myeloma.

However, long-term uricase therapy for chronic gout is limited by the need for parenteral administration and side effects: pruritus, rash, nausea, headache, myalgia, edema, bronchospasm with respiratory distress, and hemolysis, particularly in patients with glucose-6-phosphate dehydrogenase deficiency. Approximately 10% of patients develop antiuricase antibodies, which can potentially result in declining efficacy.

PATIENTS WITH MASSIVE TOPHACEOUS DEPOSITS

Patients with massive tophaceous deposits who do not respond to either allopurinol or a uricosuric drug alone may benefit from a combination of these drugs. Serum urate concentrations should be kept consistently <5 mg/dL or <300 μmol/L to ensure complete resolution of the tophaceous deposits. Surgical excision of bulky tophi may be required. Other helpful measures include restriction of alcoholic beverages and a weight-reducing diet, restricted in both carbohydrates (40% of energy) and saturated fats, with proportionate increases in intake of proteins (30% of energy) and of unsaturated fats (30% of energy).

PATIENTS WITH GOUT AND RENAL IMPAIRMENT

Uricosuric drugs are generally ineffective in patients with renal insufficiency. Allopurinol therapy in these individuals is associated with an increased incidence of both cutaneous and severe hypersensitivity reactions. To minimize this risk, the drug is introduced in reduced doses, starting at 50 mg every 2 to 3 days, gradually increasing to a maximal daily dose based on the patient's creatinine clearance: 200 mg daily for clearance of 60 mL per minute, 100 mg daily for clearance of 20 mL per minute, and 50 to 100 mg on alternate days for clearance of 10 mL per minute or less.

GOUT IN THE ELDERLY

Co-morbid medical illnesses, including hypertension, cardiac failure, diabetes mellitus, and renal impairment, are common in patients older than 65 years with gout. NSAIDs are potentially hazardous and are not recommended for the treatment of acute gouty episodes in these patients. Oral colchicine is also poorly tolerated by the elderly and is best avoided. Oral, IM, IV, or intra-articular corticosteroids are increasingly being used for treating acute gouty flares in patients older than 65 years with multiple medical conditions, contraindicating NSAID therapy.

Urate-lowering therapy should be approached with caution in the elderly. Because of the frequent presence of concomitant renal impairment, uricosuric drugs are unlikely to be efficacious and are best avoided. Allopurinol therapy is associated with an increased incidence of both cutaneous and severe hypersensitivity reactions. To minimize this risk, the doses of allopurinol must be kept low. A starting dose of 50 to 100 mg on alternate days to a maximum daily dose of 100 to 200 mg is recommended.

GOUT IN THE TRANSPLANT RECIPIENT

Both hyperuricemia and severe tophaceous gouty arthritis occur with increased frequency in cyclosporine-treated kidney, heart, or lung/heart allograft transplant recipients. Cyclosporine induces hyperuricemia by both inhibiting renal tubular urate secretion and enhancing postsecretory tubular urate reabsorption. Concurrent diuretic therapy and coexistent renal insufficiency are important contributing factors.

Both NSAIDs and colchicine are hazardous and are not recommended for the treatment of acute gouty arthritis in these patients. Corticosteroids, administered intra-articularly or systematically, are the preferred drugs. Resistance to ACTH from adrenal suppression by prior or current corticosteroid therapy is common.

Uricosuric drugs are generally ineffective in cyclosporine-treated transplant recipients with renal impairment. Allopurinol is the preferred urate-lowering drug. Its toxicity can be minimized by adjusting the initial dose according to the creatinine clearance.

Because azathioprine (Imuran) is inactivated by xanthine oxidase, inhibition of this enzyme by allopurinol markedly enhances azathioprine toxicity. Thus, in transplant patients receiving both azathioprine and allopurinol, reduction of the initial doses of both drugs by about two-thirds is recommended.

ASYMPTOMATIC HYPERURICEMIA

The exact implications of chronic asymptomatic hyperuricemia remain uncertain. Most individuals do not develop clinical gout, and there is no convincing evidence that hyperuricemia *per se* adversely affects renal function. For these reasons, and because of concerns about cost and potential hazards of unnecessary drug therapy, there seems to be no compelling rationale or clear benefit for treating these individuals with allopurinol. Exceptions include acute urate overproduction due to tumor lysis syndrome, and patients with severe hyperuricemia (>12 mg/dL or >700 μmol/L) and hyperuricosuria who are at increased risk of developing both gout and nephrolithiasis. For most other patients, corrective measures, including weight reduction; correction of an underlying IRS with a weight-reducing, carbohydrate-restricted diet and a proportionate increase in intake of proteins and unsaturated fats; restriction of alcoholic beverages; and elimination of drugs, such as low-dose aspirin (>325 mg per day) and thiazides, are important.

Losartan (Cozaar),[1] an angiotensin II converting enzyme (ACE) receptor antagonist antihypertensive drug, is a mild uricosuric that produces a modest lowering of serum urate. The drug may be particularly useful in treating patients with both hypertension and hyperuricemia, such as those with IRS.

Micronized fenofibrate (Tricor),[1] a lipid-lowering fibric acid derivative, is also a mild uricosuric and a urate-lowering drug. It may be useful in individuals with both dyslipidemia and hyperuricemia, including those with IRS.

[1]Not FDA approved for this indication.

HYPERLIPOPROTEINEMIAS

METHOD OF

John R. Guyton, MD

Treatment of lipid disorders aims mostly at prevention of atherosclerosis, which kills more than one third of all people in industrialized societies. Atherogenesis is promoted by a physiologically high concentration of low-density lipoproteins (LDLs) in the arterial intima. LDL concentration in arterial intima is about equal to plasma concentration, which is approximately 10 times higher than LDL levels in other connective tissues. This is likely a result of the lack of lymphatic vessels in arterial intima, which would otherwise remove excess plasma macromolecules from the tissue space. Thus, it is not surprising that lowering plasma LDL reduces atherosclerotic events in clinical trials by 25% to 40%.

High-density lipoproteins (HDLs) remove cholesterol from the arterial intima and also exert anti-inflammatory effects. Some clinical studies suggest that raising HDL reduces events, but confirmation of an "HDL hypothesis" awaits additional large clinical trials.

Epidemiologic studies suggest additional risk related to plasma triglyceride, lipoprotein(a), and lipoprotein size distributions. However, treatment targeted at these parameters has yet to be validated by adequate clinical outcome trials. Despite the postulated role of lipoprotein oxidation in atherogenesis, large randomized trials have shown no value for antioxidants in cardiovascular risk reduction.

Lipoprotein Metabolism

The plasma lipoproteins (Table 1) transport triglyceride and cholesterol between internal organs—liver and gut—and peripheral tissues such as muscle and adipose tissue. Apolipoproteins on the lipoprotein surface bind to lipid enzymes and cell receptors, and thus target the lipoproteins for uptake or lipid delivery.

Chylomicrons derived from intestinal fat absorption appear in plasma for several hours after fat ingestion. Lipoprotein lipase in peripheral capillaries hydrolyzes triglyceride in the chylomicrons, and the newly released fatty acids are taken up by peripheral tissue

TABLE 1 Four Major Classes of Lipoproteins

	Chylomicrons	Very-Low-Density Lipoproteins (VLDL)	Low-Density Lipoproteins	High-Density Lipoproteins
Major core lipid	Triglyceride	Triglyceride	Cholesteryl ester	Cholesteryl ester
Apolipoproteins	B-48, Cs, E, A-I, A-II	B-100, Cs, E	B-100	A-I, A-II, Cs, E
Density (g/mL)	<0.93	0.93-1.006	1.006-1.063	1.063–1.210
Diameter (nm)	75–1200	30–80	18–25	5–12
Origin	Intestine	Liver	From VLDL, though peripheral/ hepatic processing	Liver, intestine

cells. The chylomicrons shrink in diameter, and the resulting chylomicron remnants circulate to the liver, where they are rapidly taken up by hepatocytes.

Very-low-density lipoproteins (VLDLs) are triglyceride-rich lipoproteins secreted by hepatocytes. Like chylomicrons, VLDLs are metabolized by lipoprotein lipase, delivering fatty acids to peripheral tissues. VLDL remnants (also termed intermediate-density lipoproteins [IDLs]) are partly taken up by hepatocytes and partly processed by hepatic lipase to become LDL. LDLs circulate in plasma for 2 to 3 days until removal by receptor-mediated uptake in hepatocytes and peripheral cells.

Hypertriglyceridemia can be caused by increased production of VLDL or by factors that decrease lipoprotein lipase activity. Obesity drives the production of VLDL by supplying excessive fatty acids to the liver. Lipoprotein lipase activity may be impaired by genetic defects, diabetes mellitus, or ethanol ingestion. Insulin resistance and a high percentage of carbohydrates in the diet also increase plasma triglyceride.

Most cholesterol in body tissues is synthesized de novo; dietary cholesterol makes a small contribution (25% to 30%). The synthetic pathway is dependent on 3-hydroxy-3-methylglutaryl coenzyme A (CoA) reductase. Excess peripheral cholesterol must be transported to the liver, a process termed *reverse cholesterol transport*. The liver eliminates cholesterol through biliary excretion in the form of bile acids and cholesterol.

Heterozygous LDL receptor deficiency occurs in 1 of 500 persons and is characterized by very high LDL cholesterol (usually greater than 220 mg/dL), autosomal dominant inheritance, and sometimes xanthomas of the Achilles and hand extensor tendons. Most adult patients with this condition require two to four medications to achieve adequate LDL control. Another highly atherogenic condition is familial combined hyperlipidemia, which is at least twice as common as LDL receptor deficiency. High cholesterol and triglyceride levels may coexist or present singly in family members.

Lipoprotein(a) is essentially an LDL with an extra glycopeptide, apolipoprotein(a) (apo[a]), attached to apolipoprotein (apo) B through a disulfide bond. Because of apo(a) sequence homology with fibrinolytic enzymes, lipoprotein(a) interferes with physiologic fibrinolysis (but does not inhibit pharmacologic fibrinolysis). Levels of lipoprotein(a) correlate with both atherosclerotic and thrombotic risks. Lipoprotein(a) levels are highly inherited and are largely unaffected by diet and medications; however, niacin and oral estrogens can give 20% to 30% reductions.

The Metabolic Syndrome of Insulin Resistance and Cardiovascular Risk

The metabolic syndrome (Table 2) includes (a) disordered metabolism of body fuels—glucose and fat—featuring insulin resistance and abdominal obesity, (b) atherogenic dyslipidemia as described below, (c) hypertension, and (d) increased procoagulant and proinflammatory factors (not included in the clinical criteria shown in Table 2)—all of which add up to high cardiovascular risk. In overweight subjects, excessive accrual of triglyceride can overwhelm the preferred site of energy storage in small peripheral adipocytes, leading to spillover storage of triglyceride in skeletal myocytes, in hepatocytes, in visceral adipocytes, and in abnormally large peripheral adipocytes. The excessive accumulation of triglyceride in these sites leads to insulin resistance.

The dyslipidemia of the metabolic syndrome consists of high plasma triglyceride, low HDL cholesterol, and small, dense LDL. Most maneuvers that lower plasma triglyceride (e.g., body weight reduction and the administration of fibrates or niacin) increase LDL size and increase HDL cholesterol. However, the oral

TABLE 2 Clinical Identification of the Metabolic Syndrome

Diagnosis of the metabolic syndrome requires any three of the following:

Risk Factor	Defining Level
Abdominal obesity	
Men	Waist circumference >40 inches (>102 cm)
Women	Waist circumference >35 inches (>88 cm)
Triglyceride	≥150 mg/dL
HDL cholesterol	
Men	<40 mg/dL
Women	<50 mg/dL
Blood pressure	≥130/≥85 mm Hg
Fasting glucose	≥110 mg/dL

TABLE 3 National Cholesterol Education Program (NCEP) Risk Categories and Treatment Goals

Risk Category	LDLC Goal	Non-HDLC Goal	LDLC Level at Which to Consider Drug Therapy
Coronary or other clinical atherosclerotic disease, or risk equivalent (10-year risk >20%)*	<100 mg/dL	<130 mg/dL	≥130 mg/dL (100-129 mg/dL: drug optional)
Two or more risk factors (10-year risk ≤20%)	<130 mg/dL	<160 mg/dL	10-year risk 10%-20%: ≥130 mg/dL 10-year risk <10%: ≥160 mg/dL
0-1 Risk factor	<160 mg/dL	<190 mg/dL	≥160 mg/dL (160-189 mg/dL: drug optional)

*Diabetes mellitus is considered risk equivalent with established atherosclerotic disease, because diabetic patients generally have a coronary risk >20% over 10 years.

intake of estrogen or alcohol can raise both triglyceride and HDL cholesterol simultaneously.

Guidelines for Lipid-Lowering Therapy

The guidelines of the U.S. National Cholesterol Education Program (NCEP), revised by the third Adult Treatment Panel in 2001, are the foundation for effective and reasonable lipid-lowering therapy. The guidelines assign patients to three categories of cardiovascular risk (Table 3). Patients with diabetes mellitus are "risk equivalent" to patients with clinical atherosclerotic disease. If two or more risk factors are present in nondiabetic patients (Table 4), the Framingham risk calculation should be performed at the time of initial evaluation of the patient to establish the risk category. A printed point scoring method or a computer (regular personal computer or handheld) program for risk calculation can be downloaded from the NCEP web site at www.nhlbi.nih.gov/guidelines/cholesterol. Nondiabetic patients with one or fewer risk factors are classified in the low-risk category. When significant hyperlipidemia is identified, secondary causes should be investigated (Table 5).

LDL cholesterol (LDL-C) is generally determined through calculation from the relationship (LDL-C = total C − HDL-C − [triglyceride ÷ 5]). A fasting sample is preferred. In a nonfasting sample, the calculated LDL-C can be reduced artifactually by triglyceride-rich postprandial lipoproteins. Therefore, the patient's true LDL-C is at least as high as the estimate obtained by calculation from a nonfasting sample.

Low HDL is at least as strong a predictor of cardiovascular risk as high LDL. However, the clinical evidence for treatment benefit is not as firmly established for HDL as it is for LDL. In primary prevention, isolated low HDL-C generally does not require medication, but should be addressed by lifestyle modification (i.e., smoking cessation, exercise, and perhaps additional dietary monounsaturated fat). When the patient requires medication for lowering LDL-C or non-HDL cholesterol (see below), then it may be appropriate to use medications that also raise HDL-C.

A triglyceride level of 150 mg/dL or higher should lead to screening for the metabolic syndrome (see Table 2) and counseling on therapeutic lifestyle changes, particularly aiming toward weight reduction and exercise. When the triglyceride level is 200 mg/dL or higher, NCEP designates non-HDL cholesterol (total minus HDL cholesterol) as a secondary target of therapy. Non-HDL cholesterol goals are set 30 mg/dL higher than the corresponding LDL cholesterol goals (see Table 3).

Triglyceride levels above 500 mg/dL need consideration of dietary and drug treatment to prevent pancreatitis and other manifestations of the chylomicronemia syndrome—abdominal pain, eruptive xanthomas, aggravation of ischemia, psychological/psychiatric symptoms, and dyspnea. The chylomicronemia

TABLE 4 Atherosclerotic Risk Factors (National Cholesterol Education Program)

Age: male ≥45 years, or female ≥55 years
Hypertension: BP ≥140/90 or on medication
Low HDL cholesterol: <40 mg/dL
Current cigarette smoking
Family history of premature coronary disease in first-degree relative: male <55 years, female <65 years
Negative risk factor: If HDL-C ≥60 mg/dL, then subtract 1 from the number of risk factors counted above.

TABLE 5 Causes of Secondary Dyslipidemia

Condition	LDL effect	VLDL (triglyceride) effect	HDL effect
Hypothyroidism	↑	↑ or 0	
Nephrotic syndrome	↑	↑ or 0	
Cholestasis	↑ LDL or lipoprotein-X*		
Glucocorticoids	↑	↑	
Cyclosporine	↑		
Diuretics	↑ or 0	↑ or 0	
Obesity		↑	↓
Ethanol		↑	↑
Diabetes mellitus		↑	↓ or 0
High glycemic diet		↑	↓ or 0
Renal failure		↑	↓
Oral estrogen		↑	↑
Isotretinoin (Accutane)		↑	
β-Blockers		↑	↓ or 0
Bile acid sequestrants		↑	

*Lipoprotein-X is a disk-shaped particle appearing in advanced cholestasis.

syndrome rarely occurs if the triglyceride level remains below 2000 mg/dL, but triglyceride may increase over a day or two from 500 to 800 mg/dL to 2000 mg/dL or higher. Treatment of severe hypertriglyceridemia requires strong attention to lifestyle and diet (see below), reduction or cessation of alcohol intake, correction of poorly controlled diabetes, and often one or more medications from a list including fibric acid derivatives, fish oil, niacin, and statins.

Dietary Treatment

WEIGHT REDUCTION

A gradual approach targeting a 2- to 4-pound weight reduction per month is best. Weight reduction of 2 pounds requires a negative balance of 230 or more calories per day for an month. After 5% to 10% of body weight is lost, a even greater caloric deficit is needed for further weight reduction, because of a decrease in basal metabolic rate.

The recommended diet for weight reduction is nutritionally balanced with calories proportioned as 50% to 60% carbohydrate, 25% to 35% fat, and 15% protein. However, success with such a diet may be difficult to achieve. I allow and sometimes encourage patients to eat more restrictive diets—either vegetarian or low glycemic (allowing ample meat)—if they are inclined to do so. Short-term use of a very-low-carbohydrate diet (Atkins or South Beach) is *permissible* (while monitoring LDL cholesterol and electrolytes), but data are insufficient to *recommend* these diets. Because of ketosis and diuresis, cessation of diuretics should be considered. Diabetic and hypertensive patients must be monitored very closely if they decide to start a very-low-carbohydrate diet. The safety of this diet in long-term use has not been established.

Short-term weight loss (achieved over 6 weeks) can cause marked reductions in triglyceride, LDL cholesterol, and HDL cholesterol levels. Weight loss accomplished and maintained over 6 or more months gives similar triglyceride reduction, but much more modest reduction of LDL cholesterol, and a rise in HDL cholesterol. The differences between short- and long-term effects might reflect changing distributions of body fat between "preferred" and "spillover" sites as described earlier.

A supportive, but expectant approach is helpful for the patient trying to lose weight. It is not unusual for a person to "get it together" after a year or two, then to drop 10 to 15 pounds, sometimes permanently. Once weight is lost, the characteristics of successful weight maintainers should be discussed with patients. Almost all of these people exercise regularly, most weigh themselves daily, and most eat a low-fat diet.

DIETARY COMPONENTS

The NCEP program of Therapeutic Lifestyle Change (TLC) (Table 6) advises reducing saturated and *trans*-unsaturated fats, because these are the dietary components that contribute most to high LDL-C. Fats that are solid at room temperature, including palm and coconut oils, are saturated, whereas liquid fats (oils) are unsaturated. Hydrogenation of plant oils increases their saturation and also generates *trans* fatty acids. *Trans* fat is particularly bad, because it raises LDL-C but does not raise HDL-C as saturated fat does. Both monounsaturated and polyunsaturated fats are associated with atherosclerotic risk reduction in animal studies and clinical trials.

TABLE 6 Therapeutic Lifestyle Change (TLC) for Atherosclerosis Prevention

TLC diet
Saturated fat <7% of calories, cholesterol <200 mg/d
Consider increased viscous (soluble) fiber (10–25 g/d) and plant stanols/sterols to enhance LDL lowering
Weight management
Increased physical activity

Reducing dietary cholesterol has less impact on plasma cholesterol than reducing saturated and *trans* fats. In vegetarian diets that restrict dietary cholesterol more than the usual recommendation, the impact on plasma cholesterol may be greater.

The TLC program recommends viscous fiber and plant sterol/stanol esters as adjuncts for LDL-C lowering. Viscous fiber, previously known as soluble fiber, includes oat and rice bran, bean fiber, and psyllium (Metamucil and other products). Bloating or flatus can limit this approach. Plant sterol or stanol esters, incorporated into soft margarines (Benecol, Take Control), reduce LDL-C by 8% to 14% through inhibition of intestinal cholesterol absorption.

Many patients with atherosclerosis can make remarkable dietary changes, and they should be encouraged to do so. Studies suggest that intensive dietary changes can relieve anginal symptoms, reverse stenosis, and prevent adverse clinical outcomes in coronary patients. A Mediterranean diet or even a vegetarian/vegan diet may work in motivated patients with advanced atherosclerosis. The best diet for cardiovascular prevention may be low in refined grain products, high in whole grains, vegetables, fruits, and nuts, and adequate in omega-3 fatty acids, while substituting natural poly- and monounsaturated fats for saturated and *trans*-unsaturated (hydrogenated) fats. Furthermore, marked reductions in high glycemic foods and in overall carbohydrate intake may alleviate hypertriglyceridemia, even if body weight remains constant.

Alcohol intake in the range of one to two drinks per day in men and one half to one drink per day in women may reduce coronary risk by as much as 50%. Risk reduction is uncertain in patients with hypertriglyceridemia, however, because ethanol raises triglyceride. Moreover, ethanol can raise blood pressure. One should not recommend drinking for cardiovascular health, because of other risks, but ethanol intake can be approved if it is already part of an established and stable lifestyle.

Nutritional intake of omega-3 fatty acids is associated with 20% to 30% reductions in cardiovascular mortality and 30% to 50% reductions in rates of sudden death. Animal experiments suggest resistance to ventricular fibrillation. A current recommendation is that coronary patients ingest 1 g of omega-3 fatty acids daily from marine sources, either from fatty fish or from capsules. It is reasonable to substitute omega-3 fatty acids from terrestrial sources—flaxseed, walnuts, and canola oil—if fish oil is not tolerated. Fish oil can also be used for triglyceride lowering. Marine, but not terrestrial, omega-3 fatty acids lower plasma triglyceride by as much as 30% to 40%. High daily doses are required (e.g., 5 g omega-3, or 16 typical capsules, or 1 tablespoon of liquid fish oil). Cod liver oil should not be used because of excessive vitamin A.

TABLE 7 Lipid-Modifying Drugs*

Drug Class	LDL Effect	VLDL (Triglyceride) Effect	HDL Effect
Statins	↓ **18%-55%**	↓ 15%-35%	↑ 3%-12%
Niacin	↓ 8%-20%	↓ 10%-30%	↑ **10%-25%**
Fibrates	↑ or ↓ up to 20%†	↓ **40%-50%**	↑ 6%-20%
Bile acid sequestrants	↓ **12%-30%**	0 or ↑	↑ minimally
Ezetimibe (Zetia)	↓ **18%-22%**	↓ minimally	↑ minimally
Fish oil (not flaxseed oil)	0	↓ **up to 35%**	0

*Key therapeutic effects are shown in bold.
†When fibrates are used for hypertriglyceridemia, LDL-C usually increases modestly. In normotriglyceridemic patients, fenofibrate (Tricor) can lower LDL-C by 20%.

Drugs for Lipid Reduction and Atherosclerosis Prevention

The presence of hyperlipidemia warrants consideration of aspirin or other antiplatelet therapy whenever cardiovascular risk is substantial. Aspirin doses between 30 and 325 mg per day are almost equivalent in their ability to inhibit arterial thrombosis.

Common medications for hyperlipidemia include inhibitors of hydroxymethylglutaryl coenzyme A reductase (statins), niacin, fibric acid derivatives, bile acid sequestrants, the cholesterol absorption inhibitor ezetimibe (Zetia), and fish oil (Table 7). Each of these drug classes, except for ezetimibe, has been shown to avert clinical cardiovascular events in randomized trials.

Statins lower LDL-C by 20% to 60% (Table 8 shows the comparative efficacy of various drugs) and lower triglyceride by 15% to 35%. No other drugs have better proven safety or efficacy in reducing cardiovascular events. Hepatic transaminase levels are monitored after initiation of statin therapy or dosage increase, but instances of hepatic failure or fibrosis are almost unknown.

Between 0.5% and 5% of patients may experience myalgia, fatigue, or, rarely, arthralgia related to statin treatment. Myopathy, defined as muscle symptoms plus confirmed serum creatine kinase (CK) elevation of more than 10 times the upper limit of normal, occurs in 0.1% to 0.2% of patients. Rhabdomyolysis, sometimes with death or renal failure, is rarer. Three of the statins—lovastatin (Mevacor), simvastatin (Zocor), and atorvastatin (Lipitor)—are metabolized by the cytochrome P450 3A4 isoenzyme. Rhabdomyolysis has been described with the concomitant use of 3A4 inhibitors such as erythromycin, clarithromycin (Biaxin), cyclosporine (Neoral), nefazodone (Serzone), and azole antifungals. Other statins, including pravastatin (Pravachol), fluvastatin (Lescol), and rosuvastatin (Crestor), are not metabolized by this pathway, but rosuvastatin blood levels are increased by cyclosporine.

A dilemma arises when the patient complains of myalgia, and creatine kinase (CK) levels are normal or less than two to four times the upper limit of normal. CK levels in this low range are usually constitutive or exercise-induced, and rarely correlate with symptoms. In very mild cases, risk-to-benefit considerations may suggest continuing without dose reduction. If symptoms require it, I prefer to reduce the statin dose fourfold (e.g., atorvastatin 5 mg every other day). The dose reduction may be coupled with a switch to a different statin (see Table 8), or nonstatin therapy may be employed, perhaps in combination with a low-dose statin.

TABLE 8 Approximate LDL-C Lowering by Various Statin Doses

Dose (mg) of Statin						
Fluva (Lescol)	Prava (Pravachol)	Lova (Mevacor)	Simva (Zocor)	Atorva (Lipitor)	Rosuva (Crestor)	% LDL-C Reduction
40	20	20	10	—	—	27
80	40	40	20	—	—	34
	80			10	5	
		80	40			41
				20	10	
			80			48
				40	20	
				80	40	55

Niacin, also known as nicotinic acid, is the most effective drug for raising HDL-C. Daily doses of 1000 to 2000 mg raise HDL-C by 10% to 25%. At doses of 1500 to 3000 mg per day niacin reduces triglyceride, LDL-C, and lipoprotein(a) levels. Niacinamide has no lipid-modifying effect. Niacin commonly causes flushing, which should be described when prescribing as a sensation of "prickly heat" usually on the neck and shoulders. Flushing tends to disappear with repetitive use of niacin. Immediate-release niacin is given two to four times per day, with food (best taken two thirds through the meal), at a total daily dose beginning as low as 100 mg and increasing gradually to 1000 to 4000 mg. Sustained-released niacin (also called "flush-free" or "no-flush") is more prone to hepatotoxicity, and the total dose should be limited to 2000 to 2250 mg daily. An extended-release prescription form of niacin (Niaspan), given once daily at bedtime, has well-documented hepatic safety in doses up to 2000 mg. Aspirin 325 mg or another anti-inflammatory drug can be taken 30 minutes before niacin ingestion to reduce flushing. Chewing an 81 mg aspirin tablet might shorten the duration and decrease the severity of flushing once it occurs. Side effects of niacin also include dyspepsia, increased glucose (average 5%), transaminase elevations, atrial fibrillation, peptic ulcer, gout, skin dryness, hypotension (with a severe flush), and visual disturbances (macular edema, rare with doses under 3000 mg per day).

The bile acid sequestrants are nonabsorbed, positively charged polymers that bind negatively charged bile acids in the small intestine, preventing their reabsorption in the terminal ileum. This results in diversion of hepatic cholesterol stores toward bile acid synthesis, ultimately lowering LDL-C by 10% to 30%. Colesevelam (WelChol) has a higher capacity and greater selectivity for bile acids than the older resin polymers—cholestyramine (Questran) and colestipol (Colestid). Triglyceride levels tend to increase, and hypertriglyceridemia is a relative contraindication to the use of bile acid sequestrants. Because of their safety, bile acid sequestrants are recommended for reducing LDL-C in children and in women of childbearing years. Cholestyramine and colestipol are associated with constipation (15% of cases), bloating, and interference with absorption of certain drugs, particularly warfarin (Coumadin), vitamin K (in warfarin-treated patients), digoxin, diuretics, and thyroxine. Take other medications 1 hour before or 4 hours after cholestyramine/colestipol. However, scheduling can sometimes be relaxed, when clinically detectable goals (e.g., blood pressure or lipid goals) are successfully achieved with other medications. Colesevelam has much better gastrointestinal tolerance and almost no drug interactions, but is limited to 15% to 18% LDL-C lowering.

Gemfibrozil (Lopid) and fenofibrate (Tricor) are fibric acid derivatives (or fibrates), which lower plasma triglyceride 40% to 55%—more effectively than any other drug class. HDL-C increases of 6% to 20% can occur. In patients with normal triglyceride levels, fenofibrate reduces LDL-C by 20%. Gemfibrozil improved cardiovascular outcomes in a randomized trial of coronary patients with low HDL-C. Fenofibrate is being tested in two large trials in diabetic patients. Fibrates are largely cleared by the kidney. Doses should be lowered in patients with renal insufficiency. Side effects include dyspepsia, hypersensitivity rash, hepatic transaminase elevations, increased warfarin effect, and increased lithogenicity of bile. Rarely, fenofibrate causes dermal photosensitivity.

Ezetimibe (Zetia) inhibits intestinal cholesterol absorption by binding to a mucosal cell membrane sterol transporter. Ordinarily, the intestine receives 200 to 400 mg dietary cholesterol and 900 mg biliary cholesterol daily. A small amount of ezetimibe is absorbed, but it is rapidly taken up in hepatocytes and excreted in bile, returning to the intestinal lining as an active drug. Ezetimibe at 10 mg daily lowers LDL-C by 18% to 19%. Adding ezetimibe to a statin reduces LDL-C by 20% to 25% from the poststatin baseline. Ezetimibe side effects are minimal and not significantly different from placebo.

Combination drug therapy should be used when LDL-C or non-HDL cholesterol goals are not met by monotherapy, or when cardiovascular risk is high and the presumed additional benefit of raising HDL-C or lowering triglyceride is desired. The best-documented combination regimen for lowering LDL-C is the addition of a bile acid sequestrant to a statin. Ezetimibe-statin combination therapy may equally achieve LDL-C goals. In patients with low HDL-C, the combination of moderate-dose statin with high-dose niacin was associated with a 70% reduction of cardiovascular events in a small study of 160 patients. It is best to

TABLE 9 Some Tips for Lipid Practice

Don't underestimate the impact of diet.
Do expect some (not all!) patients to alter their diet substantially.
Do titrate drug doses upward to meet LDL-C and non-HDL cholesterol goals.
Do remember that non-HDL cholesterol is also a key goal in patients with a triglyceride level of 200 mg/dL or higher.
Do try small statin doses (1/4 usual starting doses) in patients with myalgia and normal or modestly elevated creatine kinase levels.
Don't assume that an alanine transaminase (ALT) elevation is solely caused by a lipid-lowering drug, but stop the drug, aim for 5-10 lb weight reduction to treat fatty liver, and consider restarting the drug if ALT normalizes.
Do use combination therapy when appropriate.
Do develop the ability to prescribe niacin effectively, and always describe flushing before patients experience it.
Do use a fibrate as the initial drug of choice for severe hypertriglyceridemia.
Don't use gemfibrozil with moderate to high statin doses because of substantial myopathy risk.
Don't employ full doses of fibrates in patients with moderate to severe renal insufficiency.
Don't use bile acid sequestrants in patients with severe hypertriglyceridemia.
Do use adequate doses of bile acid sequestrants. In patients with familial hypercholesterolemia, for example, colestipol dosing may reach seven 1-g tablets twice a day.

avoid gemfibrozil-statin combination therapy, unless low statin doses are employed. Fenofibrate-statin regimens have raised no major safety concerns thus far in two large clinical trials. Fish oil, ezetimibe, and/or a bile acid sequestrant can be added safely to any drug regimen, but hepatic monitoring should be performed.

Effective Lipid Practice

An intentional focus on lipid management, often administered by a physician extender, may achieve much better results than usual care. Table 9 incorporates the differentiating features of effective lipid practice into the listed tips.

OBESITY

METHOD OF

Louis J. Aronne, MD

The age-adjusted prevalence of obesity, defined as a body mass index (BMI) ≥30 kg/m^2, has increased from 22.9% in the Third National Health and Nutrition Examination Survey (NHANES III; 1988–1994) to 30.5% in the most recent data from 1999–2000. The prevalence of overweight, defined as a BMI of 25 to 29.9 kg/m^2, also increased slightly during this period from 33% to 34%. As a direct result of this increase, the number of people who suffer from and need treatment for weight-related health conditions continues to increase. It is impossible to find an organ system that is not deleteriously affected by the burden of obesity and related disorders such as diabetes, hypertension, heart disease, hyperlipidemia, osteoarthritis, and a multitude of malignancies. It is for this reason that weight loss is a primary treatment objective for physicians in both the medical and surgical communities.

The most important goal of obesity treatment is to improve the co-morbid conditions associated with obesity, not to reduce weight. The patient and physician should understand that obesity is a chronic disease like diabetes or hypertension that will require long-term management. They should also understand that the efficacy of nonsurgical interventions is limited to a 5% to 15% body weight loss in the majority of successful patients, and that this weight loss is enough to induce better health.

Assessment

The clinical approach to the patient should follow the steps used in the care of any patient with a chronic disease: assessment, classification, and treatment. Assessment includes determining the degree of obesity using BMI and waist circumference, and evaluating the overall health status of the patient. Information collected during the assessment is then used to classify the severity of obesity and related health problems. Decisions about treatment can be made based on the results of the assessment and classification. Table 1 outlines an obesity-specific approach.

HISTORY AND PHYSICAL EXAMINATION

The history is important for evaluating risk and deciding upon treatment. Questions should address age of onset of obesity, minimum weight maintained as an adult, events associated with weight gain, recent weight loss attempts, and previous weight-loss modalities used successfully and unsuccessfully and their complications. For example, loss of weight to below a patient's minimum weight as an adult is unusual, and an earlier age of onset of obesity often, but not always, predicts a less successful outcome.

TABLE 1 Assessment and Management of the Overweight and Obese Patient

Measure height and weight; estimate body mass index.
Measure waist circumference.
Review the patient's medical condition.
Assess co-morbidities:
- How many are present, and how severe are they?
- Do they need to be treated in addition to the effort at weight loss?

Look for causes of obesity, including the use of medications known to cause weight gain.
Assess the risk of this patient's obesity.
Is the patient ready and motivated to lose weight?
If the patient is not ready to lose weight, urge weight maintenance and manage the complications.
If the patient is ready, agree with the patient on reasonable weight and activity goals and write them down.
Use the information you have gathered to develop a treatment plan based on Table 3.
Involve other professionals if necessary.
Don't forget that a supportive, empathetic approach is necessary throughout treatment.

Adapted from the Practical Guide: Identification, evaluation, and treatment of overweight and obesity in adults. NIH Publications No. 00-4084. Bethesda, MD: U.S. Department of Health and Human Services, Public Health Service, National Institutes of Health, National Heart, Lung, and Blood Institute. October, 2000.

A treatment modality that was previously unsuccessful, or during which the patient experienced complications, should generally be avoided. A history of eating disorders, bingeing, and purging by vomiting or laxative abuse may warrant referral to a specialist in these areas. Alcohol and substance abuse require specific treatment. Cigarette smoking can complicate treatment history because weight is often gained on stopping. Although smoking cessation is of paramount importance, implementing a diet and exercise program on or before stopping can minimize weight gain.

Assessing the patient's current level of physical activity is important to determine the starting point for exercise recommendations. Some individuals may be completely sedentary, whereas others are vigorously active. Providing the same recommendation to both patients is inappropriate. Similarly, the patient's level of understanding of nutrition will determine whether a basic or more sophisticated level of nutrition education should be taught. This is crucial toward helping the patient get the most out of each session. Material that is too advanced won't be retained, and material that is too basic will be boring to the patient.

Diseases that may impact on weight, such as polycystic ovarian syndrome and hypothyroidism, require specific treatment, even though that treatment alone may not result in weight loss. In addition, patients may also exhibit substantial weight gain in the months or years before developing overt type 2 diabetes.

The clinician should search for complications of obesity, such as hypertension, type 2 diabetes, hyperlipidemia, coronary heart disease, osteoarthritis of the lower extremities, gallbladder disease, gout, and certain cancers. In men, obesity is associated with colorectal and prostate cancers; in women, it is associated with endometrial, gallbladder, cervical, ovarian, and breast cancers. Signs and symptoms of these disorders, such as vaginal or rectal bleeding, may have been overlooked by the patient and should be carefully reviewed by the physician.

Obstructive sleep apnea is a disorder often overlooked in obese patients. Symptoms and signs include very loud snoring, cessation of breathing during sleep followed by a loud clearing breath, nighttime awakening, daytime fatigue with episodes of sleepiness at inappropriate times, and morning headaches. Associated findings on examination may include enlarged parotid glands, increased neck circumference, hypertension, narrowing of the upper airway, scleral injection and leg edema. Laboratory studies may show polycythemia. If signs of sleep apnea are present, the patient should have a diagnostic sleep study performed. The onset of sleep apnea is sometimes associated with additional weight gain, and the management of sleep apnea may assist with weight loss.

A number of medications may cause weight gain (Table 2). If possible, these medications should be changed to those that do not cause weight gain or that might even induce weight loss. The use of over-the-counter weight-loss remedies and prescribed medications that may interact with planned treatment, such as monoamine oxidase (MAO) inhibitors and other antidepressants, should be reviewed.

TABLE 2 Drugs That Can Promote Weight Gain and Alternatives

Category	Drugs That Can Promote Weight Gain	Alternatives
Psychiatric/neurologic	Phenothiazines Antidepressants Lithium Neuroleptics Antiepileptics	Bupropion, nefazodone topiramate
Steroid hormones	Hormonal contraceptives	Barrier methods of contraception
	Corticosteroids	Nonsteroidal anti-inflammatory agents
	Progestational steroids	Weight loss for menometrorrhagia
Diabetes treatments	Insulin	Metformin
	Sulfonylureas	Acarbose, miglitol
	Thiazolidinediones	Orlistat, sibutramine
Antihistamines	Diphenhydramine, others	Decongestants, inhaled steroids
β-Adrenergic blockers	Propranolol, others	Angiotensin-converting enzyme (ACE) inhibitors, calcium channel blockers

Adapted from Preventing and managing the global epidemic of obesity. Report of the World Health Organization Consultation on Obesity. Geneva: WHO, June 1997.

Height and weight should be measured and the BMI calculated to categorize the severity and risk of obesity. Waist circumference should be assessed using a tape measure (Figure 1). Blood pressure should be checked with an appropriately sized cuff. Other key features include examining the thyroid and looking for manifestations of hypothyroidism; looking for skin tags and acanthosis nigricans around the neck and axilla, which suggest hyperinsulinemia, and identifying leg edema, cellulitis, and intertriginous rashes with signs of skin breakdown. Leg edema may be secondary to right-heart failure or direct compression by an abdominal pannus in the very obese patient.

Type 2 diabetes, gout, hyperlipidemia, and hepatic steatosis are the disorders most often discovered by laboratory evaluation. Other laboratory studies may indicate disorders that may be involved in the induction of obesity and require specific treatment, such as hypothyroidism and hyperinsulinemia. A complete laboratory evaluation might include blood glucose; uric acid; blood urea nitrogen (BUN); creatinine; alanine aminotransferase (ALT); serum aspartate aminotransferase (AST); total and direct bilirubin; alkaline phosphatase; total cholesterol; high-density lipoprotein (HDL); low-density lipoprotein (LDL); triglycerides;

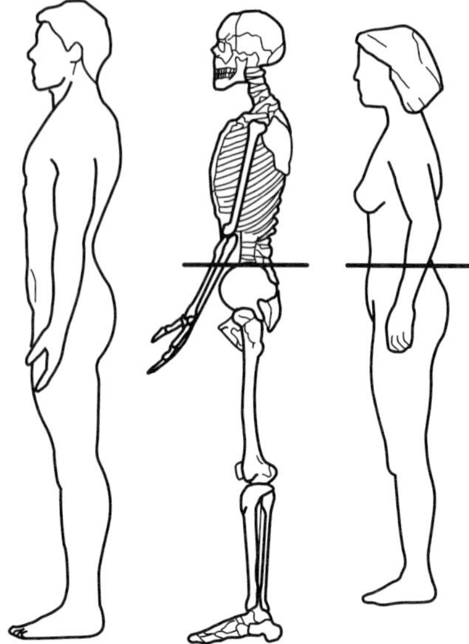

FIGURE 1 Measuring waist circumference. To measure waist circumference, locate the upper hip bone and the top of the right iliac crest. Place a measuring tape in a horizontal plane around the abdomen at the level of the iliac crest. Before reading the tape measure, ensure that the tape is snug, but does not compress the skin, and is parallel to the floor. The measurement is made at the end of a normal expiration.

complete blood count; thyroid-stimulating hormone (TSH); and urinalysis. Measurement of ultrasensitive C-reactive protein may be valuable in that it appears to represent an obesity-related cardiovascular risk factor and responds to weight loss. In some cases, a fasting and 2-hour post-prandial insulin level is of value in diagnosing hyperinsulinism.

Obesity treatment is contraindicated in patients who are pregnant, have anorexia nervosa, or have a terminal illness. Medical or psychiatric illnesses must be stable before weight reduction begins. Furthermore, patients with cholelithiasis and osteoporosis should be warned that these conditions might be aggravated by weight loss.

In almost every case, to succeed the patient must be ready to make the effort to lose weight. If the patient does not wish to lose weight and is not at high risk, weight maintenance should be encouraged. If the patient is at high risk as a result of obesity, the clinician should make an effort to motivate the patient by discussing the medical consequences of obesity. However, negative and pejorative statements should be avoided because they are of no therapeutic value and tend to be demoralizing.

CLASSIFICATION AND TREATMENT

The primary targets for treatment should be those individuals whose health is at risk. This includes overweight patients with a BMI >25, and obese patients with a BMI >30, especially if complications are present. Table 3 outlines a guide to selecting the appropriate treatment based on BMI. Individuals at lesser risk should be counseled about effective lifestyle changes. An initial weight loss of 10% of body weight achieved over 6 months is a recommended target. Even more modest weight loss can reduce visceral fat and improve co-morbid conditions.

TABLE 3 BMI Category

	BMI				
Treatment	**25-26.9**	**27-29.9**	**30-35**	**35-39.9**	**>40**
Diet, exercise, behavior therapy	With co-morbidities	With co-morbidities	+	+	+
Pharmacotherapy		With co-morbidities	+	+	+
Surgery				With co-morbidities	+

+ = Treatment indicated.

Adapted from the Practical guide: Identification, evaluation, and treatment of overweight and obesity in adults. NIH Publication No. 00-4084. Bethesda, MD: U.S. Department of Health and Human Services, Public Health Service, National Institutes of Health, National Heart, Lung, and Blood Institute. October, 2000.

Given the current state of knowledge and the treatments currently available, the goal of obesity treatment should be the lowest weight the patient can comfortably maintain, which in the average patient is approximately 5% to 10% of total body weight or 2 BMI units. Attaining "ideal" body weight, or a loss of 20% to 30% or more of total body weight, is not possible for the vast majority of overweight and obese people. Loss of 5% to 10% of body weight can significantly improve risk factors associated with obesity, even though many patients may be disappointed with not reaching their "dream weight." Focus patients on achievable goals and health benefits such as an improvement in lipids or glucose, improved mobility, reduced waist circumference, or simply compliance with the regimen. Prevention of weight gain is another important treatment goal that should be emphasized, particularly for patients not ready to initiate an active weight-loss program.

At the beginning of treatment, share results of the physical examination and laboratory tests with the patient. Emphasize findings associated with obesity that would be expected to improve with weight loss. The patient should focus on improving these health parameters, rather than achieving a "dream" weight that may not be attainable. Discuss improvements on an ongoing basis. Many patients find this is a helpful motivator.

Monitoring

Patients on a weight-loss regimen should be seen in the office within approximately 2 to 4 weeks of starting treatment to monitor both the treatment's effectiveness and its side effects. Visits every 4 weeks are adequate during the first 3 months if the patient has a favorable weight loss and few side effects. More frequent visits may be required based on clinical judgment, particularly, if the patient has co-morbid conditions. The patient should be weighed each visit, with waist circumference measured less often. Blood pressure and pulse should be monitored if the patient is taking an appetite suppressant. The visit should be used to monitor compliance with the program, provide encouragement, and set new goals. This can be accomplished by reviewing food and exercise records, discussing progress or lack thereof, and solving problems which the patient has encountered. Less frequent follow-up is required after the first 6 months.

Treatment

The foundation of conventional therapy includes behavior and lifestyle changes, exercise, and diet (Table 3). Medications can be used as an adjunct in patients with a BMI of 27.5 to 29.9 who have co-morbidities, and for all patients with a BMI of ≥30. Finally, surgical treatments may be considered for individuals with a BMI of ≥40 kg/m^2 or a BMI of 35 to 40 kg/m^2 if they have co-morbidities.

The use of other health care providers with an interest in obesity treatment, including dietitians, psychologists, nurses, and nurse practitioners, is an efficient way to manage the obese patient. For example, although many physicians feel uncomfortable prescribing a diet, community- or hospital-based dietitians are available to assist with patient education and support.

Other resources available to the patient include commercial and community-based programs such as Weight Watchers, TOPS, and Overeaters Anonymous, and Internet-based programs available at very low cost ($10 to $15 per month). Internet-based support may also be of value as an adjunct for some individuals. Information is available through the NIH *Aim for a Healthy Weight* web site at www.nhlbi.nih.gov/health/public/heart/obesity/lose_wt/ index.htm. More information for the physician is available at naaso.org, the web site of the North American Association for the Study of Obesity.

BEHAVIOR AND LIFESTYLE CHANGE

Behavioral techniques are not used alone, but in conjunction with all other approaches, including diet and exercise, medication, or surgery. The goal of behavior therapy is to overcome barriers to compliance with a regimen of diet and physical activity. Behavior therapy assumes that patterns of eating and physical activity are learned behaviors that can be changed, and that to change these patterns over the long-term, the environment must be modified. In some cases, behavioral therapy is administered on an individual basis; in other cases, as group sessions. Professionals with training in psychology or a related area who can engage a group in a cohesive manner are optimal for leading such groups.

The behavioral techniques that enhance compliance with a program of diet and exercise, include self-monitoring, stimulus control, stress management, reinforcement, cognitive change, relapse prevention, and crisis intervention.

A summary of recent studies combining behavioral treatment with moderate dietary restriction and exercise as part of a comprehensive program showed an 8.5-kg (18.7-lb) average weight loss from an initial average weight of 91.9 kg (202.6 lb) over 21 weeks of treatment with a 22% rate of attrition. A 5.6-kg (12.3-lb) loss was maintained after 1 year of follow-up. Behavior therapy, a structured diet, nutrition education, and increased physical activity is the first-line approach for the vast majority of patients. Longer periods of treatment yield better results, and long-term intermittent treatment is recommended.

DIETARY INTERVENTIONS

No single approach to diet works for everyone. In our opinion, the best approach is to try to customize the diet to "solve" the patient's "problems." For example, a businesswoman eating out almost every meal on the road may benefit from a different approach than a woman who cooks all of the meals for her family. Recent findings suggest that foods with a lower glycemic index (blood glucose rise per ounce of food) may reduce food consumption later in the day, and those with a lower calorie density (number of calories per ounce) such as vegetables, appear to be more filling and may reduce overall food consumption. As a result, the diets used in our program contain a higher percentage of carbohydrate from vegetables and legumes and much less from starch and sugar than those generally published. In general, we recommend an adequate amount of lean protein and large quantities of vegetables as the mainstay of the diet with smaller amounts of whole grains and healthy oil sources.

Formula diets, such as OPTIFAST and HMR can be of value in those individuals who have a medical need to lose weight. A minimum intake of 800 kcal per day is recommended.

Fad diets and other methods that promise a quick, easy way to lose weight with no effort distract the patient from the real task at hand. Although almost any method of unhealthy dieting can reduce weight in the short run, the true test comes long-term. Diets that are too drastic can't be followed long-term; unfortunately, the patient too often bears the blame for the lack of success, adding to a vicious cycle of failure.

EXERCISE

Physical activity should be recommended to all patients. Exercise plays a major role in assisting with weight maintenance, and there is mounting evidence that increased physical activity plays a crucial role in the prevention and management of many chronic diseases even in the absence of weight loss. Aerobic exercise is usually recommended for weight management, but strength training may also be of benefit to build lean body mass. Exercise improves quality of life by enhancing self-esteem, reducing stress, and relieving depression, and is associated with a better weight-loss outcome.

Any physical activity that the patient enjoys and is willing to perform is recommended. For the completely sedentary patient, walking is often the best way to get started. Patients with physical limitations secondary to arthritis or size may start with water exercises, bedside stretching, seated activities, or a program designed by an exercise physiologist or physical therapist. In general, 30 to 45 minutes of exercise 3 to 5 days per week is recommended, although more is better, and greater intensity may be better. Three 10-minute periods of activity yield about the same benefit as a single 30-minute period, and compliance with such a program is better. Increasing activity during daily life, such as climbing stairs instead of taking an elevator, walking or cycling rather than taking a car, and parking further away from the entrance to the mall, can be simple ways to add small periods of physical activity to a busy lifestyle.

MEDICATIONS

Sibutramine (Meridia)

Sibutramine enhances satiety by blocking the reuptake of norepinephrine, dopamine, and serotonin in the central nervous system. A 1-year long placebo-controlled trial demonstrated that of patients receiving 15 mg of sibutramine daily, 65% lost more than 5% of body weight compared with only 29% of patients taking a placebo, and 39% lost more than 10% of their body weight compared with 8% reaching the same mean weight loss in the placebo-treated group. Health benefits demonstrated with the use of sibutramine included reductions in triglycerides, uric acid, total cholesterol, and LDL cholesterol, and an increase in HDL cholesterol. Adverse events observed during randomized trials included dry mouth, constipation, insomnia, increased appetite, dizziness, and nausea. Sibutramine is relatively contraindicated in patients with poorly controlled hypertension and atherosclerotic cardiovascular diseases, including stroke and myocardial infarction. A mean increase in blood pressure of 4 mm Hg has been seen in trials. Approximately 12% of patients have an increase in systolic blood pressure of 15 mm Hg or more; however, less than 1% of patients treated had to be withdrawn from trials as a result of a sustained increase in blood pressure. Of note, a decrease in blood pressure is most often seen in patients who lose more than 5% of body weight and in whom treatment would be most likely to continue. It is recommended that blood pressure and pulse be checked 2 to 4 weeks after the drug is started and then monthly for the first 6 months; thereafter, every 2 to 3 months monitoring is adequate, or more often if indicated.

Orlistat (Xenical)

Orlistat is an inhibitor of pancreatic lipases which prevents the absorption of about one third of dietary fat at a dose of 120 mg three times daily. Analysis of patients completing a 2-year long placebo-controlled trial demonstrated a mean weight loss of 8% after 1 year compared with 4% in the placebo (diet)-treated group. Orlistat slowed down the rate of weight regain in the second year, with a 6% mean weight loss maintained after 2 years of treatment compared with 2% in the placebo-treated group. A 4-year-long placebo-controlled trial of orlistat for the prevention of type 2 diabetes was recently presented. Subjects at risk for type 2 diabetes were treated with a diet and lifestyle program with the addition of orlistat 120 mg orally thrice daily or placebo. Weight loss in the orlistat-treated group was significantly better at both 1 and 4 years. The 4-year incidence of type 2 diabetes was reduced from 9.0% in the placebo group to 6.2% in the orlistat group, a 37% reduction.

Health benefits demonstrated in clinical trials of orlistat include a reduction in LDL and an increase in HDL cholesterol, reductions in blood pressure and fasting insulin levels, improvement in oral glucose tolerance test outcomes, and improved glycemic control in obese diabetics. The gastrointestinal side effects associated with orlistat use are usually mild in intensity, happen early in treatment, and may enhance compliance with a low-fat diet. The administration of psyllium (Metamucil)[1] once in the evening reduces these symptoms by more than 50%. No effects on mineral balance, gallstone, or renal stone formation have been seen. Mild reductions in the levels of vitamin D and beta-carotene were noted in some treated patients during trials and supplementation with a multivitamin taken remotely from a dose of orlistat is recommended.

Phentermine (Ionamin)

Phentermine is a sympathomimetic anorexigenic medication that functions as a norepinephrine-releasing agent. It is the most commonly prescribed weight-loss medication in the United States, representing 31% of prescriptions. A study from 1968 is the only longer-term controlled trial of phentermine. In this study, 64 patients completed 36 weeks of placebo, phentermine, or placebo and phentermine on alternating days. Both phentermine groups lost approximately 13% of their initial weight, whereas the placebo group lost only 5%. Phentermine's main side effects are related to its sympathomimetic proper-ties, such as insomnia, constipation, and dry mouth. Phentermine and other sympathomimetics

[1]Not FDA approved for this indication.

such as diethylpropion (Tenuate) and phendimetrazine (Bontril) have not been studied for long-term safety and efficacy and their use beyond 3 months is "off-label."

Bupropion (Wellbutrin)[1]

Bupropion is an antidepressant that induces weight loss, perhaps because of its mechanism as a norepinephrine and dopamine reuptake inhibitor. Although the mean weight loss seen with bupropion is small, in some patients, bupropion may be preferable to the many other antidepressants that may induce weight gain. Bupropion is contraindicated in patients with epilepsy and may cause anxiety, dry mouth, rash, and, rarely, seizures.

Metformin (Glucophage)[1]

Metformin is a drug used in the treatment of type 2 diabetes that decreases hepatic gluconeogenesis and increases peripheral insulin sensitivity. In general, metformin and α-glucosidase inhibitors should be the first-line drugs in obese diabetic patients. In patients with insulin-resistance syndromes such as polycystic ovarian syndrome and impaired fasting glucose, metformin may help with weight loss.

Topiramate (Topamax)[1]

Topiramate is an antiepileptic agent that reduces body weight in patients with epilepsy, bipolar disorder, binge-eating disorder, and obesity. Topiramate is also being studied for the treatment of migraine headaches, neuropathic pain, and alcoholism. A randomized, double-blind, placebo-controlled, dose-ranging trial of topiramate in overweight and obese subjects showed a mean weight loss from baseline to week 24 of 2.6% in placebo-treated patients and 5% and 6.3% in the groups treated with either 64 and 96, or 192 and 384 mg, respectively. The most common side effects of topiramate were paresthesias (70%), dry mouth (43%), and headache (40%). Other side effects of topiramate include cognitive impairment, renal stones, and, rarely, acute angle glaucoma. If topiramate is used for any indication, small (≤25 mg) doses should be used initially and increased gradually (25 mg every 1 to 2 weeks or less) if clinically necessary and if tolerated by the patient.

Zonisamide (Zonegran)[1]

Zonisamide is a similar antiepileptic drug that induces weight loss. A small placebo-controlled trial was conducted in which the dose of zonisamide was titrated up until a >5% weight loss effect was achieved, requiring an average dose of 427 mg per day. The zonisamide group lost significantly more weight than the placebo-treated group (mean 5.8 kg [22.8 lb] [6.0%] vs. 0.9 kg [2 lb] [1.0%]).

SURGERY

Obesity surgery has increased dramatically in popularity in the past few years. Procedures can be considered in patients with a BMI greater than 40, or between 35 and 40 who fail other methods of treatment, if serious obesity-related complications are present. Careful screening of candidates is required to ensure they are motivated and well-informed about the risks of the procedure as well as the changes in their lives which will occur as a result of the procedure and its long-term effects. These changes may be relatively minor, such as the need for long-term treatment with vitamin and mineral supplements, or could include chronic vomiting, diarrhea after meals, and other problems of malnutrition. Obesity surgery is best performed in specialty centers accustomed to performing procedures on high-risk obese patients. Long-term follow-up is required to ensure the best results and proper nutrition in the postsurgical patient.

The Roux-en-Y gastric bypass is the most common procedure and involves constructing a small proximal gastric pouch as with a gastroplasty whose outlet is a limb of small bowel of varying lengths, creating a Roux-en-Y gastrojejunostomy (Figure 2). Increasing the length of the limb from 75 to 150 cm increases weight loss, as well as long-term side effects and nutrient malabsorption. Laparoscopic and open surgical techniques can be used. The procedure produces malabsorption of food and the dumping syndrome, and is more effective than laparoscopic banding and gastroplasty because it is harder to circumvent, but

[1]Not FDA approved for this indication.

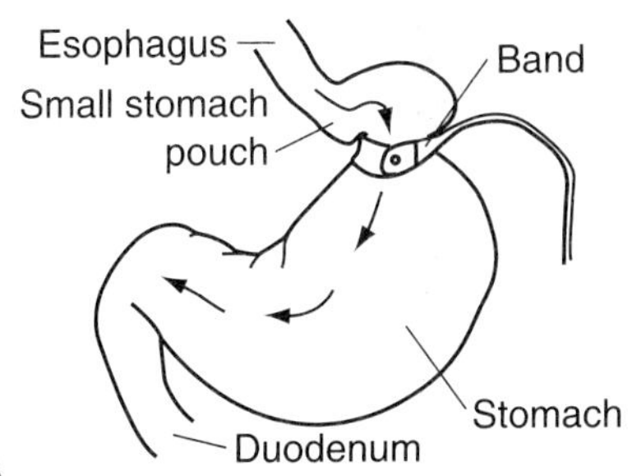

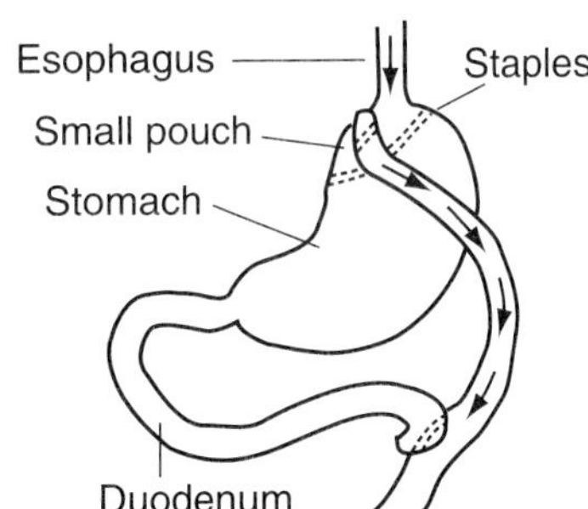

FIGURE 2 Surgical treatments for obesity. A. Laparoscopic adjustable band. B. Roux-en-Y gastric bypass.

the risk of complications is greater. A mean weight loss of 60% to 80% of excess weight can be achieved. Unfortunately, in some surgical series up to 20% of patients ultimately regain all lost weight. Because of the malabsorption of vitamins and minerals, patients need careful nutritional instruction and follow-up, as well as behavioral training. Multivitamin, calcium, iron, and vitamin B_{12} supplementation is recommended long-term.

The vertical-banded gastroplasty (VBG), also known as "stomach stapling" and laparoscopic adjustable silicone gastric banding (LASGB) are solely restrictive procedures. In the VBG, a 30-cc pouch with a restricted outlet is constructed along the lesser curvature of the stomach, reducing the capacity of the stomach 100-fold. LASGB has rapidly replaced VBG as the restrictive procedure of choice. In LASGB, an inflatable device that encircles the stomach is inserted laparoscopically (see Figure 2A). Adjustment of the stoma is readily accomplished by inflating the device with saline through a subcutaneous port. It is less invasive than the VBG because the stomach is not transected or stapled; in most instances, it can also be reversed laparoscopically, if necessary. The amount of weight lost is correlated with the volume of the pouch and diameter of the outlet, with larger volume and diameter yielding less weight loss, but fewer side effects. Patients who have this procedure feel full after eating very small amounts of food, and may vomit if they continue to eat. Within a few months after the procedure, up to 1 cup of food may be eaten at a time. Ingested food is digested in a normal sequence and is fully absorbed, minimizing the risk of malnutrition. In general, 70% of patients maintain a loss of 20% or more of total body weight at the 5-year follow-up. It is not as effective as the gastric bypass in carbohydrate cravers because of the "soft-calorie syndrome," in which highly caloric liquid or meltable foods (e.g., milk shakes or ice cream) are consumed to excess, leading to weight regain. Because of the limited long-term follow-up, many insurance companies consider it to be "experimental."

Conclusion

The obesity epidemic continues to grow at an alarming rate. As the understanding of obesity grows, so, too, will our armamentarium to combat this disease. At that point, obesity will be treated like other chronic diseases. Obesity prevention and treatment may ultimately replace the treatment of its complications.

OSTEOPOROSIS

METHOD OF

Clifford J. Rosen, MD

Osteoporosis is a disease of skeletal fragility that results from a reduction in bone quality and quantity. Some 13% to 18% of women older than age 50 years and close to 5% of men over age 70 years in the United States have osteoporosis, and an additional 37% to 50% of Americans have low bone mass (an independent risk factor for fracture) at the hip. The disease results in more than 350,000 hip fractures alone each year in the United States. Because men and women over the age of 65 are the fastest growing segment worldwide, the annual number of fractures is expected to double by 2025. The estimated annual direct medical cost in 1995 was $13.8 billion for the treatment of osteoporotic fractures in the United States. Although this disorder is multifactorial in origin, and includes changes in bone structure that affect the biomechanics of the skeleton as well as alterations in the cellular components of the bone remodeling unit, the end result is a relentless clinical syndrome of fractures, pain, and disability. Despite the rising prevalence and its impact, major strides have been made in understanding the pathogenesis of this disorder and in developing new treatments that significantly reduce subsequent fracture risk.

Epidemiology

At age 50 years, a white woman in the United States has a 17% chance of sustaining a hip fracture and a 32% chance of vertebral fracture over her lifetime. Hip fractures cause the most morbidity with reported mortality rates of 24% in the first year postinjury. Although some excess mortality may be attributable to deep venous thrombosis and pneumonia rather than the hip fracture itself, up to 50% of patients are unable to walk without assistance and 33% are totally dependent or in a nursing home in the year following a hip fracture. Vertebral fractures are also associated with significant co-morbidities from pain, chronic disability, and reduced quality of life.

Bone density decreases with age and fracture risk rises rapidly. However, age is an independent risk factor for fracture such that for a given bone mineral density measurement (i.e., a T score), the greater the age of the individual the higher the subsequent fracture risk. Given the increased age of the general population (men and women), osteoporosis and fractures are expected to continue to increase. Fracture risk varies by race with hip fracture rates in African American women reported to be one-third those of white women. African American and possibly Hispanic women tend to have higher bone mineral density (BMD) values when compared with white women. However, the BMD differences are less apparent when BMD is corrected for bone size. Despite any apparent BMD artifacts, larger bones may be associated with a lower risk of fracture.

Pathogenesis

The pathogenesis of postmenopausal osteoporosis is complex and multifactorial like many other chronic diseases. It is clear that declining estrogen levels at the time of the menopause are associated with rapid decreases in BMD. Lower estrogen levels in men may also be associated with a greater risk of osteoporotic fracture. However, additional factors that must be considered include genetic background; nutritional status, including vitamin D deficiency; alterations in parathyroid hormone (PTH) levels and the growth hormone–insulin-like growth factor axis; mechanical strain; and factors related to the risk of falling. Secondary causes of osteoporosis must always be considered (Table 1), particularly glucocorticoid excess (endogenous and exogenous), malabsorption states such as nontropical sprue, and malignancies such as myeloma.

TABLE 1 Common Causes of Secondary Osteoporosis

Endocrine
Low testosterone
Low estrogen
Low IGF-I and low estrogen (anorexia nervosa)
Low insulin—type I IDDM
Excess glucocorticoids—Cushing's syndrome or disease
Excess thyroxine
Excess parathyroid hormone
Nutritional
Low IGF-I and estrogen (anorexia nervosa)
Vitamin D deficiency because of malabsorption
Nontropical sprue
Inflammatory bowel disease
Connective tissue disorders involving bowel motility (e.g., scleroderma)
Gastric bypass surgery
Vitamin D deficiency caused by drugs
Glucocorticoids
Anticonvulsants
Vitamin D deficiency caused by liver disease
Primary biliary cirrhosis
Chronic hepatitis
Vitamin D deficiency because of poor sun exposure
Populations in northern latitudes
Nursing home populations
Social states where skin exposure is very limited
Others
Neoplasms
Multiple myeloma
Certain forms of leukemia and lymphoma
Metastatic disease to bone, breast, bowel, thyroid, prostate
Connective tissue disorders
Inflammatory arthritis such as RA, SLE, scleroderma
Postorgan transplantation
Renal calculi as a result of hypercalciuria

Abbreviations: IDDM = insulin-dependent diabetes mellitus; IGF-I = insulin-like growth factor I; RA = rheumatoid arthritis; SLE = systemic lupus erythematosus.

Osteoporosis is a disorder of aberrant bone remodeling. Bone is a metabolically active tissue undergoing constant remodeling during adulthood. The hormonal and cytokine signals for the initiation and maintenance of bone remodeling have recently been identified. They are produced by osteoblasts and influence osteoclast activity and differentiation. These include the interleukins, osteoprotegerin (OPG), receptor activator of nuclear factor-kappa B (RANK), RANK ligand, and macrophage colony-stimulating factor (M-CSF), the latter two being essential for normal bone resorption. Any alteration in the remodeling frequency as a consequence of changes in these cytokines can result in bone loss. On the formation side of the equation, progress has also been made. For example, families have been identified with very high bone mass (more than five standard deviations above age-matched controls) caused by gain of function in a gene found to be related to bone formation (lipoprotein receptor-related protein 5 [LRP5]) through a novel signaling pathway that involves Wnt-related proteins.

Diagnosis

In the absence of clinically available methods to assess bone strength or quality directly, or a history of multiple vertebral or nonspine fractures, the diagnosis of osteoporosis is often made solely on the measurement of BMD. BMD is most frequently measured by dual energy x-ray absorptiometry (DXA). Such measurements are accurate and account for between 70% and 85% of the predicted strength of the bone being measured. Not surprisingly, in postmenopausal women, a strong relationship exists between BMD measurements and fracture risk. A 10% decrease in BMD (1 standard deviation [SD] below the mean) at any site confers a 1.6 to 2.6 relative risk of hip fracture and a 1.7 to 2.3 relative risk of vertebral fracture. Hip or vertebral fractures are best predicted by BMD measured at the hip or vertebrae respectively.

BMD is reported using two scores based on standard deviation measurements: the Z score and the T score. The Z score compares the patient's BMD with the mean value in age-matched subjects. The T score compares the patient's BMD with the mean in a healthy young reference population, assumed to represent a standard for peak bone mass. Both scores may be adjusted for race and gender, although less well-developed nomograms exist other than those for white women. A T score of −2.5 or lower meets World Health Organization (WHO) criteria for osteoporosis and a T score between −2.5 and −1.0 represents osteopenia. However, the categorization of osteopenia may be of limited clinical value because fracture risk may vary widely based on age and other factors for patients in this category. The same T score in an 80-year-old and in a 40-year-old woman has drastically different implications for short-term fracture risk, based on the changes in bone quality that occur with age, yet are distinct from BMD.

BMD measures and their associated T or Z scores at times can be vastly different at anatomic sites in the same individual. This can happen, for example, when spinal BMD measures are falsely elevated by the presence of osteophytes leading to discrepancies with hip BMD measures. However, it is more likely caused by differences in the composition of bone at various sites. Sites rich in trabecular or cancellous bone are highly metabolically active and include the vertebral bodies, proximal femur, calcaneus, and ultradistal radius. Sites that are predominantly cortical bone, such as the distal one-third radius, have lower rates of activation frequencies of bone remodeling units. The femoral neck is a mixture of both trabecular and cortical bone. Conditions associated with estrogen deficiency are more likely to affect sites rich in trabecular bone, such as the spine, whereas conditions associated with PTH excess are more likely to affect cortical bone. These differences should be taken into account when evaluating an individual patient, as well as when analyzing data on the effects of therapeutic agents or medical conditions on bone density.

Single-photon and dual-photon absorptiometry are commercially available but are noted to be less precise and accurate than DXA. Ultrasound is appealing because of low cost and lack of radiation exposure. It correlates with fracture risk but is not standardized and particularly varies across machines. Quantitative CT (QCT) is available clinically and has been used in several clinical trials. It has greater radiation exposure, but is more sensitive for trabecular BMD measurements. Unfortunately, T scores are not equivalent between QCT and DXA; hence, predictions about fracture risk must consider the equipment as well as the site of measurement. Peripheral measurements such as portable DXA of the radius and heel are useful screening tools, but not recommended for follow-up. In addition, there are device-specific thresholds and higher T or Z score thresholds (e.g., T score <-1) which cannot be easily translated to central (hip, spine, and/or radius) measurements.

Secondary causes of osteoporosis should always be considered particularly when the BMD T score (or Z score) is lower than predicted without many risk factors (see below and Tables 1 and 2). A minimal diagnostic work-up for osteoporotic patients is noted in Table 3 and should be considered in everyone undergoing bone density testing. Further follow-up studies are warranted if there are particular abnormalities in the screening tests (see Table 3).

Risk Factors for Low Bone Mass or Fractures

Multiple risk factors have been identified that may contribute to low bone mass and a partial list is included in Table 2. Risk factors consistently found to be associated with osteoporosis include white women, low body weight (<127 pounds) and maternal or personal history of fractures. A history of previous fracture of any type increases the risk of a subsequent fracture at least twofold. A patient with a vertebral fracture will be three to five times more likely to suffer another vertebral fracture within the next year and is also at increased risk of sustaining a hip fracture when compared with women without a vertebral fracture. A hip fracture occurs most typically after sustaining a fall. The risk of fracture from an individual fall is low in women over the age of

TABLE 2 Selected List of Risk Factors for Low Peak Bone Mass or Osteoporosis

Metabolic Conditions
Amenorrhea or history of amenorrhea (>1 year)
Eating disorders
Estrogen deficiency: premature ovarian failure, menopause, surgical oophorectomy
Hyperthyroidism
Hyperparathyroidism
Renal failure
Type I diabetes mellitus
Cystic fibrosis
Malabsorption/Nutritional Conditions
Inflammatory bowel disease (Crohn's disease)
Gluten enteropathy
Gastrectomy
Avoidance of calcium/dairy products
Vitamin D deficiency (lack of sun exposure)
Medications
Glucocorticoid use
Genetic Factors
Personal history of fractures
Family history of osteoporosis
Low body weight
Lifestyle
Smoking
Excess alcohol

TABLE 3 Laboratory Studies for the Evaluation of Osteoporosis

Initial Panel
General chemical profile: calcium, phosphorus, creatinine, uric acid, alkaline phosphatase
Complete blood count
T_4 (thyroxine), TSH (thyroid-stimulating hormone)
Vitamin D status: 25-hydroxyvitamin D
Testosterone (men)
Urinary calcium/creatinine (men)
Serum protein electrophoresis
Erythrocyte sedimentation rate
Follow-up Studies
Leuteinizing hormone (LH)/follicle-stimulating hormone (FSH), prolactin if needed (men especially)
Parathyroid hormone (PTH) (if calcium is increased or urinary calcium is high)
Bone scan (if alkaline phosphatase is high)
Markers of bone turnover (N-telopeptide, osteocalcin)
Liver function studies
Antibodies to determine gluten enteropathy
1,25 Vitamin D (to assess conditions related to increased serum calcium)

70 years (less than 10%), but the likelihood of fracture increases based on specific fall-related factors such as direction (backward and to the side) and potential energy of the fall. Therefore, factors that increase the risk of falling must be considered in the clinical assessment of an individual's risk.

Biochemical markers of bone turnover have been touted as screening tools for risk assessment in postmenopausal women. However in observational trials, only one study has shown that high bone resorption is an independent risk factor for subsequent fractures. Although these serum and urine markers are widely available, the cost-effectiveness of such biochemical tests are still not well defined.

Screening Recommendations

The U.S. Preventative Task Force (USPTF) recommends screening be routinely provided in women older than 65 years of age and in those women 60 to 64 years of age who are at increased risk. Specific risk factors were noted to be difficult to identify but low body weight (<154 lb) was found to be the best single predictor of low bone density. Additionally, the USPTF noted that African American women may be at lower risks than white women as a consequence of higher BMDs and therefore are less likely to benefit from routine screening. The USPTF could make no recommendation for or against routine screening in women younger than 60 years of age or in women 60 to 64 years of age who are not at increased risk.

Therapy for Osteoporosis

When considering treatment options, nonpharmacologic behavior modification, as well as pharmacologic interventions, should be considered. Recent meta-analyses have been published for several therapeutic agents for the treatment of postmenopausal osteoporosis. These treatments are discussed below.

NUTRITIONAL/BEHAVIOR MODIFICATION

Calcium is an accepted adjunct to osteoporosis therapy but controversy continues regarding dosage and duration. A recent meta-analysis of 15 trials (1806 patients) found calcium supplementation to increase BMD slightly at multiple sites whereas only a trend was found in improving vertebral fractures with no clear reduction in nonvertebral fractures. Vitamin D has an important role in enhancing calcium absorption and is derived predominantly from ultraviolet metabolism in the skin rather than nutritional sources. Vitamin D analogs, alfacalcidol and calcitriol (Rocaltrol),[1] are not FDA approved for the treatment of osteoporosis. However, their use is predominantly in conditions where vitamin D metabolism or calcium absorption is altered, such as postorgan transplantation, gastrointestinal malabsorption, or renal insufficiency. Fracture efficacy for vitamin D is limited and conflicting in postmenopausal women. A meta-analysis of various forms of vitamin D therapy suggests overall there may be a reduced incidence of both vertebral and nonvertebral fractures. The National Academy of Science and the National Institutes of Health recommend calcium intakes of 1000 to 1500 mg per day and vitamin D of at least 400 to 800 IU for postmenopausal women, particularly in individuals with little sun exposure. For those individuals with low serum 25-hydoxyvitamin D levels, as well as others at risk, such as nursing home patients, 50,000 units of vitamin D_2 or D_3 administered once weekly will suffice to maintain adequate serum levels and enhance mineralization of newly formed bone. Other nutritional interventions less well studied include adequate vitamin K and protein intakes, predominantly in frail elderly individuals.

HORMONE REPLACEMENT THERAPY

Estrogen therapy has a consistent positive effect across trials in respect to increasing BMD in postmenopausal women. BMD increases nearly 7% at the spine and 4.1% at the femoral neck after 3 years of hormone replacement therapy (HRT). This effect appears to be dose dependent, such that a smaller increase in BMD is seen with lower doses (0.3 mg conjugated equine estrogens [CEE] equivalent) and a greater change seen at higher doses (0.9 mg CEE equivalent). The addition of progesterone and the type of estrogen preparation (e.g., transdermal vs. oral) did not appear to make a difference in these results. It is noted, however, that certain progestogens, such as norethindrone, may have anabolic (bone-forming) properties on bone cells, but the precise roles of these agents have not been definitively established.

The largest and most well known randomized, placebo-controlled trial of HRT is the Women's Health Initiative (WHI). The WHI enrolled 16,608 postmenopausal women (age 50 to 79 years; mean age, 63 years) to evaluate the effects of estrogen-progesterone combination therapy in women with an intact uterus on the primary outcome of coronary heart disease and the primary adverse outcome of breast cancer. The trial was halted early after 5.2 years because of adverse events in cardiovascular mortality and breast cancer end points. But hip and vertebral fractures were reduced by approximately one third even though most of these women were not at high risk. In fact, estrogen-progesterone therapy resulted in five fewer hip fractures per 10,000 person-years of use. However, there were significant risks that outweighed the beneficial effects of HRT on bone, including a greater risk of stroke, heart disease, deep venous thrombosis, breast cancer, and possibly dementia. Given the complexity of decision making regarding estrogen therapy and the consideration of potential

[1]Not FDA approved for this indication.

adverse outcomes, the individual decision rests between the patient and the provider.

SELECTIVE ESTROGEN RECEPTOR MODULATORS

In the wake of the WHI report, there has been an increased interest in alternatives to hormone therapy, particularly in selective estrogen receptor modulators (SERMs) such as raloxifene (Evista) and tamoxifen (Nolvadex). These are novel compounds that interact with the estrogen receptor to selectively induce an agonist or antagonist action in estrogen-responsive target tissues. Raloxifene acts as an agonist on bone and cholesterol metabolism and an antagonist at the breast and appears to have a neutral effect on uterine tissues. The largest randomized placebo-controlled trial of raloxifene, the Multiple Outcome of Raloxifene Evaluation (MORE), studied 7705 postmenopausal women and found a 30% reduction in vertebral fractures with raloxifene when compared with placebo. But there was no decrease in nonvertebral fractures. BMD increases only slightly (by 2%) in the spine and hip with raloxifene use over 3 years. Raloxifene therapy is associated with an increased risk of deep venous thrombosis, leg cramps, and hot flashes. But the number of new breast cancer cases is significantly reduced among users of raloxifene.

BISPHOSPHONATES

Multiple well-designed randomized controlled trials (RCTs) have demonstrated the efficacy of bisphosphonates, specifically alendronate (Fosamax) and risedronate (Actonel), in increasing BMD and reducing vertebral and nonvertebral fractures. Bisphosphonates contain a phosphorus-carbon-phosphorus backbone (pyrophosphate analog) for which additions of various side chains result in different chemical compounds. They have a high affinity for bone hydroxyapatite and are potent inhibitors of bone resorption. They appear to act primarily through reducing the recruitment and action of bone-resorbing osteoclasts. Because their oral bioavailability is low (1% to 3%) and many foods and other nutrient intakes (e.g., calcium) may impair absorption, they should be taken on an empty stomach. Additional recommendations include remaining upright and drinking water to ensure that the tablet does not remain or reflux into the esophagus, which has been reported to cause esophagitis. They have a long half-life in bone, on the order of several years.

Alendronate was the first oral bisphosphonate to be approved for the prevention and treatment of osteoporosis in the United States and elsewhere. A meta-analysis of 11 alendronate randomized trials found that the risk of vertebral fractures in subjects given 5 mg or more of alendronate was reduced by 50%. Nonvertebral fractures were also reduced by 50% in subjects treated with 10 mg or more of alendronate. In addition to those studies, prevention trials demonstrate increased BMD in recently menopausal women (<3 years) without osteoporosis (spine T score >−2) after 3 years of follow-up.

Risedronate is also approved for the prevention and treatment of osteoporosis in the United States and worldwide. Two pivotal trials demonstrated that 5 mg of risedronate daily prevented both vertebral and nonvertebral fractures (41% and 49% relative risk reduction, respectively) in osteoporotic women. Subsequent studies in women over 60 years of age confirm the efficacy of risedronate in reducing spinal and nonspinal fractures, particularly in women with low bone density and previous fractures.

Both alendronate and risedronate are available and approved in once-weekly doses; these doses appear equivalent to daily doses and have better acceptability to patients. Once-weekly alendronate and risedronate are currently the treatments of choice for postmenopausal osteoporosis.

CALCITONIN

Calcitonin, an endogenous peptide that inhibits osteoclast activity, is available in nasal and subcutaneous forms that make it an appealing alternative for women who do not tolerate bisphosphonates or raloxifene. A recent meta-analysis found calcitonin decreased vertebral fractures by approximately 40%. Calcitonin (Miacalcin), however, does not reduce nonvertebral fracture risk. In addition, the largest trial, Prevent Recurrence of Osteoporotic Fractures (PROOF), has come under scrutiny because of the lack of dose-responsiveness and large dropout rates. Calcitonin may have mild analgesic properties although it is not FDA-approved for this indication.

PARATHYROID HORMONE

A new era for management of osteoporosis has begun with the addition of parathyroid hormone (PTH), an anabolic agent directed at stimulating bone formation. PTH is an endogenous 84-amino-acid peptide that has several metabolically active fragments. The human PTH 1-34 fragment was recently developed for clinical use. Although primary hyperparathyroidism or conditions of endogenous sustained excess PTH have been known to contribute to cortical bone loss for decades, it has been intriguing to note that PTH given intermittently can lead to significant increases in BMD, restoration of microarchitecture, and increases in bone size. This paradox is not fully explained but may be a result of intermittent exposure to the medication rather than continuous excess PTH. The changes in BMD at the spine are greater than those achieved with the therapeutic regimens discussed previously, with increased BMD in the order of 7% to 13% after 18 months at the spine, and only modest increases of approximately 3% at the femoral neck. The largest randomized trial to date of PTH (1-34; teriparatide [Forteo]) studied 1637 postmenopausal women with prior vertebral fractures. There was a 65% reduction in vertebral fractures with the 20-μg per day dose, and the effects were more pronounced in women with more than one fracture or more severe fractures. PTH also reduced nonvertebral fragility fractures by 50%. However, PTH in combination with alendronate (Fosamax) offers little additional benefit to alendronate or PTH alone, in both men and postmenopausal women, suggesting that monotherapy is the most rational approach to osteoporosis. Adverse events from PTH may include mild asymptomatic hypercalcemia in a small number of patients. Preclinical studies in rats given long-term PTH at high doses found an increased risk of osteosarcoma, but this has not been observed in any human studies. The FDA approval for teriparatide limits the duration of therapy to 2 years.

SURGICAL PROCEDURES

Timely surgical management of hip fractures is imperative to reduce morbidity and mortality. Surgical procedures such as vertebroplasty and kyphoplasty, developed for the treatment of malignant bone disease, have been recently applied to the management of painful vertebral body fractures in osteoporosis. During vertebroplasty, polymetal methacrylate cement is injected into the vertebral body percutaneously under fluoroscopic guidance and is often done by interventional radiologists. Kyphoplasty involves insertion of a bone tamp (balloon-like catheter) that expands the vertebral body before the injection of cement and is most often performed by orthopedic surgeons. The most notable complication is extravasation of the cement that has the potential to injure or compress adjacent nerve roots. These techniques have been reported to decrease acute pain but no RCTs have been performed and long-term complications have not been adequately assessed.

SUMMARY OF THERAPEUTIC INTERVENTIONS

All patients should be assessed for adequate calcium and vitamin D intake and counseled about exercise and smoking cessation. Any individual with a fracture should receive additional therapy, preferably with a bisphosphonate because of proven efficacy for hip and vertebral fracture reductions. The use of estrogen or estrogen-progesterone therapy continues to be a complex decision that is often based on factors other than osteoporosis benefits. In women who have not yet had a fracture but who have low BMD and risk factors, raloxifene (Evista) or a bisphosphonate may be indicated. Calcitonin (Miacalcin) should be relegated to second-line therapy, but may be used in individuals unable to tolerate other regimens or for treatment of acute pain related to vertebral fractures. Initially, PTH should be reserved for those at greatest risk (continuing fractures) because of its cost. The role of PTH in osteoporosis management, particularly in combination with bisphosphonates or for the first-line management of fracture, is expected to be further clarified. In summary, osteoporosis is a preventable disorder. The greatest challenge remains to identify those at greatest risk of fracture in order to intervene in a timely and cost-effective manner.

PAGET'S DISEASE OF BONE

METHOD OF

Bart L. Clarke, MD

Paget's disease is a progressive focal disorder of bone remodeling caused by increased osteoclast-mediated bone resorption, coupled with increased osteoblast-mediated bone formation. The increased bone turnover results in a disorganized mix of abnormal woven and normal lamellar bone at affected skeletal sites. Bone affected by Paget's disease typically enlarges and becomes structurally weaker, with consequent bone pain, deformity, and fracture.

After osteoporosis, Paget's disease is believed to be the second most common metabolic bone disease. Epidemiologic surveys demonstrate that Paget's disease is relatively common in northern Europe, North America, Australia, and New Zealand, but uncommon elsewhere. The highest prevalence rates are reported from Lancashire, England, where 6.3% to 8.3% of the adult population older than 55 years of age has radiographic evidence of the disease. The prevalence of Paget's disease in the United States population older than 55 years of age is estimated to be 3%, with most affected individuals being of European descent. The most recent estimate of Paget's disease incidence in the United States was 5.4 per 100,000 person-years in the period 1990–1994.

Paget's disease affects slightly more males than females. The average age of diagnosis is in the sixth decade, but it may be diagnosed as early as the second decade. The great majority of patients are asymptomatic and diagnosed incidentally on radiographic studies, but a small percentage has symptomatic disease.

The pathogenesis of Paget's disease remains unknown. Fifteen percent to 30% of patients have a genetic predisposition reflected by positive family history. Transmission within families is typically autosomal dominant. Individuals with affected first-degree relatives have an estimated sevenfold increased risk of developing the disease. Familial Paget's disease is linked to chromosomes 18q, 6, and 5q. Specific genes have not yet been identified in most cases, but the 5q locus maps to a mutation in the sequestasome-1 gene at 5q35-QTER. This gene encodes a ubiquitin-binding protein, which plays a role in the receptor-activated nuclear factor-kappa B (RANK) signaling pathway necessary for osteoclast activation. Although RANK and its ligand (RANKL) are primarily responsible for osteoclast formation and activation, only one mutation has been identified in the RANK gene, in a Japanese family with atypical Paget's disease, and no mutations have been reported in the RANKL gene.

Genetically predisposed individuals apparently develop Paget's disease after chronic paramyxoviral osteoclast infection. Paramyxoviral nucleocapsid RNA transcripts and antigens have been identified within pagetic osteoclasts containing respiratory syncytial virus, measles virus, and canine distemper virus. Osteoclasts experimentally infected with paramyxovirus form multinucleated giant cells quickly, and rapidly resorb bone. Paramyxoviral infections most often occur in childhood, whereas Paget's disease is typically diagnosed in adulthood. Because osteoclasts are not self-renewing cells, it is hypothesized that pluripotent hematopoietic stem cells act as a reservoir of chronic paramyxoviral infection.

Clinical Features and Diagnosis

Paget's disease is typically diagnosed incidentally on radiographic studies. Only a minority of patients has clinical symptoms or signs of disease. Bone involvement may be monostotic or asymmetrically polyostotic. Paget's disease rarely spreads to new bones beyond those involved at diagnosis, although it may progress within affected bones over time. Common sites of involvement include the pelvis, femur, spine, skull, and tibia. Bones of the upper extremities, clavicles, scapulae, ribs, sternum, and facial bones are less commonly involved.

The most common symptom of Paget's disease is bone pain, which may result from Paget's disease activity or from degenerative arthritis in joints adjacent to pagetic bone. Pain caused by microfractures or swelling of cortical bone associated with advancing lytic lesions is usually dull, aching, and localized. Pain may occur at rest, but typically is worse with ambulation or activity. Pagetic bone is often swollen or warm because of increased vascularity. Weight-bearing bones, especially the femur or tibia, may become deformed, causing gait abnormality. Degenerative arthritic changes may occur at joints adjacent to deformity or in the contralateral limb.

Back pain may be caused by pagetic vertebrae, vertebral compression fractures, spinal stenosis, or neural compression. Skull pain may be associated with warmth, tenderness, band-like headache, or increasing head size with frontal bossing or deformity. Hearing impairment may be a result of isolated or combined conductive (caused by otosclerosis) or neurosensory abnormalities. Cranial nerves II, VI, VII, or others may be affected. Platybasia (flattening of the base of the skull) may occur with basilar invagination, resulting in brainstem compression or obstructive hydrocephalus. Facial bone involvement may result in deformity, dental malocclusion, or airway narrowing.

Pagetic bone is susceptible to fracture. Fractures may be traumatic or pathologic, causing considerable blood loss when they occur. Long bones with advancing lytic lesions are most susceptible to fracture. Small asymptomatic cortical fissure fractures along the convex surfaces of bowed lower extremity bones may extend transcortically to cause complete fractures. Vertebral compression fractures may occur. Pagetic fractures typically heal normally, although nonunion may occur rarely.

Malignant transformation occurs in less than 1% of patients with chronic Paget's disease. Affected bone becomes increasingly painful and swollen. Sites most commonly affected are the pelvis, femur, and humerus. Treatment is usually wide local excision of tumor, followed by chemotherapy or radiation therapy. Six-month survival is 50%, with 5-year survival less than 10%. Most Paget's-related malignancies are osteogenic sarcomas, but other types of sarcoma occur. Some patients develop benign giant cell tumors that respond well to glucocorticoids.

Patients with newly diagnosed Paget's disease should have a total-body bone scan, with roentgenograms of affected bones, to document the extent of disease. These studies prevent later confusion concerning new pagetic activity if other bones become symptomatic. Follow-up bone scans or roentgenograms are usually unnecessary unless new or worsening symptoms develop.

Patients with Paget's disease typically have increased serum alkaline phosphatase, reflecting increased osteoblast activity. Because serum alkaline phosphatase derives from several sources, it should be fractionated during the initial evaluation to verify it is bone alkaline phosphatase that is increased. Measurement of markers of bone resorption, such as urinary pyridinoline, deoxypyridinoline, NTx-telopeptide, or CTx-telopeptide, is generally unnecessary. Serum alkaline phosphatase correlates well with activity and extent of disease. Patients with markedly increased serum alkaline phosphatase typically have polyostotic involvement, often including the skull. Patients with mildly to moderately increased serum alkaline phosphatase may have monostotic involvement or mildly active ("burned-out") disease. Patients with long-standing inactive disease or very mild disease may have normal serum alkaline phosphatase. Urinary markers of bone resorption typically decrease by about 50% within days to weeks of starting therapy, whereas serum alkaline phosphatase decreases more slowly.

Serum calcium is normal in Paget's disease except when patients with polyostotic disease are immobilized, or when Paget's disease is associated with primary hyperparathyroidism. Physiologic hyperparathyroidism may develop in 15% to 20% of patients, with normal serum calcium and increased parathyroid hormone and alkaline phosphatase, as a result of increased skeletal demand for calcium. Patients with Paget's disease should maintain a total daily calcium intake of at least 1000 mg, with a vitamin D intake of 400 IU each day.

Treatment

The major indications for the treatment of Paget's disease are relief of bone pain and prevention of fracture or deformity. Asymptomatic individuals generally do not require treatment. Bisphosphonates and subcutaneously injected salmon calcitonin (Miacalcin) are effective in decreasing bone pain and warmth, headache, and low back or hip pain. These agents may improve compressive radiculopathies, slowly progressive brainstem or spinal cord compression, joint pain, or lytic lesions in long bones, thereby preventing pathologic fractures. Bone deformity or hearing loss will generally not improve with treatment, although hearing loss may be slowed.

All agents currently approved by the U.S. Food and Drug Administration for the treatment of Paget's disease suppress osteoclast activity. These include the oral bisphosphonates alendronate (Fosamax), risedronate (Actonel), tiludronate (Skelid), and etidronate (Didronel), and intravenously administered pamidronate (Aredia). Other bisphosphonates are under investigation for use in Paget's disease. Salmon calcitonin (Miacalcin) is approved when given by subcutaneous injection.

BISPHOSPHONATES

The bisphosphonates are very potent, available orally or intravenously, and more effective and less expensive than subcutaneously injected salmon calcitonin. Side effects include upper gastrointestinal (GI) distress, diarrhea, or short-lived bone pain when first starting therapy. Duration of effect of oral bisphosphonates generally depends on duration of treatment. One course, or several courses of cyclical therapy, typically is sufficient to control disease activity. Patients who suddenly develop a marked increase in pain while on therapy should temporarily stop the drug and be evaluated for lytic lesions, impending fracture, or malignancy.

Alendronate (Fosamax) was approved for the treatment of Paget's disease in 1995, and is available in 40-mg tablets, taken as 1 tablet each day for 6 months. A previous clinical trial in patients with moderate to severe Paget's disease showed that serum alkaline phosphatase normalized in 63% of patients, compared with 17% of patients treated with etidronate (Didronel) 400 mg per day, over 6 months. Approximately 85% of patients improved symptomatically with alendronate. No osteomalacia was seen on bone biopsies in 33 patients treated with alendronate for 6 months, and new bone that formed had normal lamellar structure.

Risedronate (Actonel) was approved for treatment of Paget's disease in 1998, and is available in 30-mg tablets, taken as 1 tablet each day for 2 months. Previous clinical trials for 2 or 6 months in patients with moderately active disease showed a nearly 80% reduction in increased alkaline phosphatase, and normalization of bone turnover markers in 50% to 70% of patients.

Tiludronate (Skelid) was approved for use in Paget's disease in 1997, and is available in 200-mg tablets, taken as 2 tablets each day for 3 months. A clinical trial for 3 months in patients with moderately active disease showed normalization of alkaline phosphatase at 6 months in 24% to 35% of patients.

Etidronate (Didronel) was shown to be effective in the treatment of Paget's disease more than 20 years ago, and is available in 200- and 400-mg tablets. Etidronate 5 mg/kg per day for 6 months typically reduces serum alkaline phosphatase by 50%, and improves symptoms in as many as 70% of patients. Etidronate may cause osteomalacia when used in higher doses or for longer than 6 months. Osteomalacia presents with increased bone pain or stress fractures at sites of weakened bone.

Pamidronate (Aredia) was approved in 1995 for use in the intravenous treatment of Paget's disease. The approved regimen is infusion of 30 mg in 500 cc of normal saline or 5% dextrose in water over 4 hours each day on 3 consecutive days. Another commonly used regimen is a single infusion of 60 mg in 500 cc of normal saline over 2 hours. Mild to moderate Paget's disease usually responds to a single infusion of 60 or 90 mg, whereas moderate to severe Paget's disease may require multiple infusions over the course of weeks to months. Side effects of intravenous pamidronate include low-grade fever, myalgias, or bone pain that typically resolves within 48 hours of infusion. Patients may occasionally develop hypocalcemia, hypophosphatemia, hypomagnesemia, or lymphopenia within several days of infusion. Rare patients may develop eye inflammation. Venous irritation may occur if low fluid volumes are infused or the drug is given too rapidly.

SALMON CALCITONIN

Calcitonin is currently available as parenteral synthetic salmon calcitonin and synthetic salmon calcitonin intranasal spray (Miacalcin). Parenteral synthetic salmon calcitonin was shown to be an effective treatment for Paget's disease more than 30 years ago, but is currently used less frequently than bisphosphonates. Salmon calcitonin[1] intranasal spray is approved in the United States for the treatment of osteoporosis, but not for Paget's disease.

Parenteral salmon calcitonin is available in 2-mL vials containing 200 U/mL. The initial dose given for Paget's disease is usually 100 units (0.5 mL) injected subcutaneously each day, with reduction to 50 units (0.25 mL) each day as symptoms improve. Symptoms usually improve within a few weeks of beginning therapy, with biochemical markers improving by 3 to 6 months of treatment. Once improvement has occurred, the maintenance dose may be reduced to 50 to 100 units every other day or three times each week. The initial course of therapy is usually 6 months, although patients with severe involvement may benefit from more prolonged treatment. Despite salmon calcitonin being 20 times more potent than human calcitonin in humans, salmon calcitonin may lose effectiveness over time because of down-regulation of calcitonin receptors or development of neutralizing antibodies. Initial therapy with bisphosphonates does not preclude the use of calcitonin at a later time.

Side effects of parenteral salmon calcitonin include nausea and/or flushing of the face and neck lasting minutes to hours after the injections, and transient hypocalcemia during the first few months of therapy. Patients may minimize nausea or flushing by taking calcitonin at bedtime or with meals, decreasing the dose, or taking aspirin 30 minutes before doses.

OTHER TREATMENTS

Nonspecific treatments used to decrease pain associated with Paget's disease include nonsteroidal anti-inflammatory drugs and narcotics. These may be used alone or in combination with antipagetic agents, especially to decrease arthritic symptoms. Shoe lifts, canes, or walkers may stabilize or improve gait disturbances. Patients should be advised against prolonged immobilization because of the risk of hypercalcemia.

Orthopedic surgery is indicated to stabilize or prevent impending fracture in long bones, or replace joints affected by pagetic arthritis. Deformed bone may be straightened with osteotomy. Neurosurgical decompression may relieve spinal cord compression, neural foraminal syndromes, or basilar skull invagination with neural compromise. All cases of significant neurologic compromise should be referred for immediate neurologic or neurosurgical consultation.

The patient is often best served by a multidisciplinary approach to treatment, which includes the primary physician, endocrinologist, physiatrist, neurologist, orthopedic surgeon, and neurosurgeon as appropriate. The Paget Foundation for Paget's Disease of Bone and Related Disorders (120 Wall Street, Suite 1602, New York, NY 10005–4001; www.paget.org) is an excellent resource for patient information about Paget's disease.

[1]Not FDA approved for this indication.

TOTAL PARENTERAL NUTRITION IN THE ADULT PATIENT

METHOD OF

Eve Callahan, RD, Shannon Daniell, PharmD, and Gordon Jensen, MD, PhD

The concept of total parenteral nutrition (TPN) has its origins with the description of the circulatory system by William Harvey in 1628, leading to the rationale for IV injections and infusions. In 1665, Sir Christopher Wren published studies infusing wine, ale, and opiates in dogs. Peripheral nutrition support using isotonic glucose-protein hydrolysate solutions that could be infused through peripheral veins was developed in the mid 1900s. The disadvantage of these peripheral solutions was difficulty meeting nutrient goals within a reasonable volume, and fluid overload was common.

In the mid 1960s, Dr. Stanley Dudrick and colleagues researched the use of catheters placed in the superior vena cava of beagle puppies for infusion of hypertonic glucose and protein solutions. The beagles were maintained for 36 months receiving hyperalimentation with normal growth and development. The first research establishing that the total nutritional needs of a human patient could be met by an intravenous route was reported by Dudrick and colleagues in 1969. TPN has gained popularity in the past 35 years and has profoundly affected the management of patients with gastrointestinal failure. TPN has greater risk exposure and is more expensive compared with enteral nutritional support. This chapter focuses on indications, implementation, and complications associated with use of TPN. Safe and appropriate administration of TPN requires careful patient selection and follow-up.

Indications for Parenteral Nutrition

Enteral nutrition is the preferred route of nutrition a support, secondary to reduced cost, physiologic presentation of nutrients, maintenance of gut integrity, and reduced serious complications, compared with parenteral nutrition. Research suggests that even a small amount of enteral nutrition will assist in preservation of the enterohepatic circulation and barrier function of the gastrointestinal mucosa. These actions may result in decreased incidence of bacterial translocation and associated sepsis. TPN is indicated when the gastrointestinal tract is not functional or cannot be accessed for placement of an enteric feeding tube safely or when the enteral route cannot adequately meet the nutritional needs of a patient. TPN should be initiated when enteral feeding is not anticipated or established within 7 to 10 days (Table 1).

PERIOPERATIVE SUPPORT IN SEVERE MALNUTRITION

Malnourished surgical patients are at increased risk for postoperative morbidity and mortality. Randomized controlled studies suggest the most benefit may result from providing TPN as nutritional support in the moderately and severely malnourished population preoperatively for 7 to 14 days. The Veterans' Affairs TPN Cooperative Trial found benefit for preoperative TPN among those patients who were severely malnourished (albumin <3.0 g/dL). Mildly and moderately malnourished patients receiving TPN in this study developed an increased rate of infectious complications compared with the control group. Preoperative enteral nutrition support has been found to be equally effective used for 7 to 14 days or longer in malnourished surgical patients if enteral access can be established and such feeds are tolerated preoperatively. Prior studies suggesting adverse outcomes with parenteral compared with enteral support are largely based on antiquated approaches to TPN formulation and administration, including substantial dextrose and lipid doses, rapid infusion rates, and acceptance of hyperglycemia that would be contrary to currently accepted standards of care.

Postoperatively, paralytic ileus is commonly seen after intra-abdominal procedures requiring extensive bowel manipulations. The use of narcotics and other pain medications commonly slows gastrointestinal motility contributing to ileus. TPN should be considered for patients who have ileus with continued NPO (nothing by mouth) status for 7 to 10 days.

INFLAMMATORY BOWEL DISEASE

TPN is used to manage exacerbations of ulcerative colitis, when patients require complete bowel rest and perioperative care. In Crohn's disease, TPN is reserved for complications such as intestinal obstruction, fistula formation, short-bowel syndrome, and severe diarrhea. Otherwise, enteral nutrition support has been successfully used in inflammatory bowel disease for weight stability and maintenance of remission.

TABLE 1 Contraindications to Enteral Nutrition

Contraindications
Diffuse peritonitis
Intestinal obstruction that prohibits use of the bowel
Intractable vomiting
Paralytic ileus
Intractable diarrhea
Gastrointestinal ischemia

Adapted from ASPEN Board of Directors and The Clinical Guidelines Task Force: Guidelines for use of parenteral and enteral nutrition in adult patients. JPEN J Parenter Enteral Nutr 26(1 Suppl):18SA, 2002, with permission from the American Society for Parenteral and Enteral Nutrition (ASPEN). ASPEN does not endorse the use of the material in any other form other than its entirety.

SHORT BOWEL SYNDROME

Short bowel syndrome (SBS) is a malabsorptive condition that results from inadequate intestinal length and/or function. Key determinants of this syndrome include the presence or absence of large-bowel continuity and the fact that the ileum has irreplaceable functions. Nutritional management of these patients is dependent on the physiology and anatomy of the remaining small bowel and the individual patient's condition. Nutritional supplementation by the enteral route is the preferred route when possible. However, patients with extensive bowel resection, those with less than 100 cm of remaining jejunum, may require life-long parenteral nutrition or small-bowel transplantation. Initial management of SBS patients involves the administration of parenteral nutrition and maintenance of normal electrolyte levels. Once the patient is stable, enteral feedings should be slowly initiated. Parenteral supplementation should be gradually tapered as enteral feedings are established. This transition may take as long as 2 years.

ACUTE PANCREATITIS

Severe acute pancreatitis is frequently treated with nutrition support if oral intake is anticipated to be inadequate for 7 to 10 days. Ranson criteria are typically used to classify the severity of pancreatitis and should be used in practice to assess the need for nutrition support. TPN continues to be widely used to manage severe acute pancreatitis. Several studies have described the successful use of nasojejunal or jejunostomy feeding tubes and elemental low fat enteral formulas in patients with mild to moderate pancreatitis. If the patient exhibits signs of feeding intolerance, enteral nutrition should be discontinued and TPN should be initiated.

ENTEROCUTANEOUS FISTULA

Enterocutaneous fistulas may occur as a result of Crohn's disease, abscess, surgery, trauma, ischemia, irradiation, and/or tumor. Many of these patients have pre-existing malnutrition and increased metabolic needs, especially in those with high-output fistulas (>500mL in a 24-hour period). Losses may consist of fluid, electrolytes, protein, vitamins, and minerals resulting in dehydration, acid–base imbalances, calorie and protein malnutrition, and vitamin and mineral depletion. TPN is typically indicated with complete bowel rest in patients with high output enterocutaneous fistulas to improve nutritional status and to promote possible closure of fistulas. Postduodenal enteral feeds can be attempted in malnourished patients with fistulas involving the esophagus, stomach, or duodenum, if expected to have inadequate oral intake for >7 to 14 days.

HEMATOPOIETIC STEM-CELL TRANSPLANTATION

Myeloablative conditioning uses high-dose chemotherapy with or without irradiation during hematopoietic stem-cell transplantation (HSCT). Side effects can include nausea, emesis, diarrhea, mucositis, esophagitis, xerostomia, and odynophagia, resulting in eating difficulties during periods of neutropenia typically lasting 2 to 3 weeks. TPN initiation has been suggested to improve post-transplantation survival, reduction of disease relapse, and shortened hospital stay. Successful enteric tube feeding during HSCT has been described but is limited secondary to gastrointestinal dysfunction and inability to establish enteral feeding access safely.

HYPEREMESIS GRAVIDARUM

Hyperemesis gravidarum (HG) is severe nausea and emesis that can persist throughout gestation in up to 1% of pregnancies. HG typically presents before the 20th week of gestation and is characterized by weight loss >5% of prepregnancy weight, as well as alterations in fluids and electrolytes with acid–base disturbances. Nutrition support is indicated if conventional treatment using antiemetics, IV hydration, and diet modifications are unsuccessful to achieve weight gain. Enteral feedings using a small-bore nasogastric feeding tube and treatment with antiemetics and IV hydration have been successful in some patients. TPN is indicated in HG if enteral feeding is not tolerated.

Technical Aspects of Parenteral Nutrition

Parenteral nutrition may be administered either peripherally or centrally. TPN is hyperosmolar as a consequence of the high dextrose and amino acid contents and must therefore be administered directly into the superior or inferior vena cava to facilitate rapid dilution. Central venous catheters commonly used to administer TPN include triple-lumen catheters, Hickman catheters, peripherally inserted central catheters (PICC), and Port-a-Cath catheters. Catheter type is determined by patient condition, expected duration of therapy, care setting, venous access, and patient or physician preference. Short-term parenteral nutrition can be administered by the peripheral route. This therapy is referred to as peripheral parenteral nutrition (PPN). However, a patient's nutritional needs cannot usually be met using PPN alone unless they are relatively small and can tolerate substantial volume infusion. The limited tolerance of peripheral veins to elevated osmolarity dictates that the PPN solution be limited to contain less than 5% to 10% dextrose and 3.5% to 5% protein (or 600 to 900 mOsm/L). Infusion of a solution that is of greater osmolarity will result in phlebitis and/or infiltration. PPN is contraindicated in patients with volume restriction needs or with limited peripheral intravenous access.

TPN solutions may be standardized or customized for the individual. Standard premixed TPN solutions are available commercially from various manufacturers. These premixed solutions typically contain 5% to 25% dextrose and 2.75% to 5% amino acids. Commercially available solutions may come with electrolytes or may require manual addition of electrolytes. Premixed solutions are generally used in settings where there is a low demand for parenteral nutrition products. Specialized amino acid formulations are available for various disease states and pediatric populations. Individualized solutions are products in which all components are adjusted to meet a specific patient's needs. Standard stock solutions for compounding custom TPN solutions are 10% to 20% amino acids, 70% dextrose, and 20% to 30% lipids.

TPN solutions should always be prepared in a class 100 environment using a laminar flow hood and strict aseptic techniques. Strict adherence to aseptic technique protocols helps to minimize the risk of bacterial contamination of the solution. Additives should always be added in the pharmacy rather than on the floor whenever possible in order to minimize the risk of product contamination. Most medications should not be added to TPN solutions because of incompatibility issues. Medications that have been proven to be compatible in TPN solutions are heparin, regular insulin, H_2-receptor antagonists, and corticosteroids. Lipids may be hung separately as a piggyback to the rest of the TPN formula. Alternatively, lipids may be combined with the formula to create a 3-in-1 admixture. The method of administration of lipids depends on the care setting and institution preference.

Parenteral nutrition therapy is infused on a continuous or cycled basis. A continuous infusion involves the administration of the nutrition solution over a 24-hour period. Long-term TPN patients may benefit from a cycled TPN infusion regimen. A cycled infusion administers the solution over a shorter amount of time, typically 12 hours. A cycled TPN provides more mobility for the patient, allows a more active lifestyle, allows the patient to feel in control of their therapy, and provides a better quality of life. Tolerance should be closely monitored when transitioning to a cycled infusion, especially fluid status and sugars. The rate of the infusion should typically be cut in half or subject to a programmed taper down during the last hour of infusion to prevent hypoglycemia following cessation of the infusion.

Calculating Nutritional Needs

Nutritional requirements should be based on accurate height and weight measurements. In obese

TABLE 2 Energy Needs

• Overnourished/obese	20 kcal/kg (adjusted body weight)
• Maintenance	25 kcal/kg
• Undernourished	30 kcal/kg
• Stressed/critically ill	25 kcal/kg
• BMT/HSCT	27-30 kcal/kg
• Hemodialysis (dry weight used)	
Overnourished/obese	20-25 kcal/kg (adjusted body weight)
Maintenance	30-35 kcal/kg
Undernourished	35-40 kcal/kg
• Peritoneal dialysis (dry weight used)	
Overnourished/obese	20-25 kcal/kg (adjusted body weight)
Maintenance	25-30 kcal/kg
Undernourished	30-35 kcal/kg

Abbreviations: BMT = bone marrow transplant; HSCT = hematopoietic stem-cell transplantation.

TABLE 3 Common Formulas Used in Estimating Energy Expenditure

Harris-Benedict Equation

Males: BEE (kcal) = 66.5 + [13.8 × weight (kg)] + [5 × height (cm)] − 6.8 × age (y)]

Females: BEE (kcal) = 655.1 [9.6 × weight (kg)] + [1.8 × height (cm)] − [4.7 × age (y)]

Long's Activity and Stress Factors

Total estimation of energy requirements = BEE × activity × stress factor

Activity factor:	Confined to bed	1.2	Out of bed	1.3
Stress factor:	Minor operation	1.2	Skeletal trauma	1.35
	Major sepsis	1.6	Major thermal injury	2.1

Abbreviation: BEE = basal energy expenditure

Sources: Harris JA, Benedict FG: Biometric studies of basal metabolism in man. Publication 279. Washington, DC: Carnegie Institute, 1979.

Long CL, Schaffel N, Geiger JW, et al: Metabolic response to injury and illness: Estimation of energy and protein needs from indirect calorimetry and nitrogen balance. JPEN J Parenter Enteral Nutr 3(6):452, 1979.

patients who are >125% of ideal body weight (IBW), the adjusted body weight is used to calculate calorie needs and IBW to calculate protein needs. Ideal body weight can be based on the Metropolitan Life Insurance Table versus optimum weight equations:

(IBW) Men = 106 lb for the first 5 ft + 6 lb for each inch over 5 ft (±10% based on body frame)

(IBW) Women = 100 lb for the first 5 ft + 5 lb for each in over 5 ft (±10% based on body frame)

Adjusted body weight can be calculated using the following formula:

Adjusted Body Weight = IBW + 25% of (Actual Body Weight − IBW)

CALCULATING CALORIE/ENERGY NEEDS

Over- or underfeeding a patient can be detrimental, especially in the critically ill patient. Overfeeding can lead to difficulty weaning from mechanical ventilation secondary to increased carbon dioxide production. Overfeeding is also associated with immunosuppression, hyperglycemia, liver dysfunction, and other metabolic complications. In the severely malnourished person, overfeeding can contribute to refeeding syndrome, which is discussed later in this article. Commonly used methods to estimate calorie requirements include simple weight algorithms (25 to 30 kcal/kg body weight per day (Table 2), the Harris-Benedict equation (Table 3), and indirect calorimetry with portable metabolic cart.

Indirect calorimetry is a technique that measures oxygen consumption ($\dot{V}O_2$) and carbon dioxide production ($\dot{V}CO_2$) to calculate resting energy expenditure (REE) and respiratory quotient (RQ = $\dot{V}CO_2/\dot{V}O_2$). The RQ gives an indication of net substrate oxidation, with RQ >1.0 consistent with carbohydrate oxidation associated with overfeeding, and <0.68 consistent with starvation ketosis. Accurate indirect calorimetry warrants careful steady state measurement and is sensitive to perturbation by gas leaks. It cannot be used with the elevated FIO_2 requirements of many critically ill patients. Nutrition support teams have generally found that estimations of energy needs using simple equations have closely reproduced the results of indirect calorimetry. Consequently, indirect calorimetry is generally reserved for specific clinical situations when estimation of energy requirements may be difficult.

PROTEIN REQUIREMENTS

Promoting maintenance of lean body mass and positive nitrogen balance are desirable goals when estimating a patient's protein needs (Table 4). The degree to which this is feasible depends on the severity of cytokine-mediated stress/inflammatory response. Protein load should be adjusted based on the patient's tolerance and clinical outcome. Most moderate-to-severe stressed patients will generally need on the order of 1.5 g protein/kg body weight per day. Renal or hepatic insufficiency warrants adjustment in protein of the TPN solution. Ideal weight

TABLE 4 Estimation of Protein Needs

Mild stress	1.0 g/kg/day
Moderate stress	1.2-1.5 g/kg/day
Severe stress	1.5-2 g/kg/day
Acute renal failure—no dialysis	0.6 g/kg/day
Hemodialysis	1.1-1.4 g/kg/day
Peritoneal dialysis	1.2-1.5 g/kg/day
Continuous venovenous hemofiltration	1.5 g/kg/day
Liver failure—no encephalopathy	1.2-1.5 g/kg/day
Liver failure—with encephalopathy	0.4-0.6 g/kg/day

should be used to estimate protein needs in the morbidly obese.

The most studied disease specific amino acid formulations are enriched in branch chain amino acids (BCAA). These formulations may be better used in liver failure patients with encephalopathy. Use of BCAA in parenteral and/or enteral formulation has been controversial. The rationale for the use of BCAA is the observed increase in aromatic amino acids in patients with encephalopathy, which might function as false neurotransmitters. BCAA are perhaps most beneficial in chronic encephalopathic patients who are intolerant of standard amino acids and do not respond to standard pharmacotherapies.

CARBOHYDRATE REQUIREMENTS

Dextrose monohydrates are used predominately in TPN solutions as the carbohydrate calorie source. Dextrose monohydrates provide 3.4 cal/g. TPN is typically formulated such that dextrose provides 40% to 55% of total calories. Dextrose infusion should not exceed 5 mg/kg per minute, which is the maximum rate of glucose oxidation. It is prudent to begin with a decreased dextrose load in the TPN formula when the patient has known diabetes mellitus or baseline stress- or medication-related hyperglycemia. Recent studies suggest that tight blood sugar control (80 to 110 mg/dL) is important to prevent poor outcomes in critically ill patients, such that judicious use of parenteral insulin infusion is often indicated in critically ill patients requiring TPN.

FAT REQUIREMENTS

Lipid emulsions are the fat source in TPN. Long-chain fatty acid emulsions derived from soybean oil or a mixture of soybean oil and safflower oil are the only commercially available source of intravenous fat available in the United States at this time. Lipid emulsions provide essential fatty acids and are a concentrated source of calories, providing 9 kcal/g. Lipid emulsions should approximate 20% to 30% of total calories or 0.5 to 1.0 g/kg body weight per day in the TPN solution.

FLUID REQUIREMENTS

A patient's fluid requirements should be individually assessed to meet needs. Physical findings should be noted such as dry mucous membranes and decreased urine output with volume depletion, or edema with volume overload. Typically, a patient's fluid needs can be estimated by providing 30 mL/kg body weight per day for initial fluid needs. Intake and output should be monitored closely, taking into account fluid losses such as vomiting, diarrhea, and fistula drainage.

TPN IMPLEMENTATION

Table 5 outlines the calculation of TPN.

TABLE 5 Calculation of Parenteral Nutrition Formulation

Example: TPN is to provide 2300 kcal with 90 grams of protein daily and 2000 mL of fluid

Amino Acids

Amino acids provide 4.0 kcal/g

90 g protein × 4 kcal/g = 360 kcal protein

A 10% amino acid solution contains 10 g of amino acids per 100 mL

$\frac{\text{90 g protein}}{\text{0.1 g/mL}}$ = 900 mL of 10% amino acid solution

Dextrose

2300 kcal − 360 kcal protein = 1940 kcal total remaining kcal

Dextrose should provide 70% of daily caloric needs

1940 kcal × 0.7 = 1358 kcal provided as dextrose (round to 1360)

Dextrose provides 3.4 kcal/g

$\frac{\text{1360 kcal dextrose}}{\text{3.4 kcal/g}}$ = 400 g dextrose

A 70% dextrose solution contains 70 g dextrose per 100 mL

$\frac{\text{400 g dextrose}}{\text{0.7 g/mL}}$ = 571 mL of 70% dextrose solution

Lipids

The remaining caloric needs are met by providing lipids

2300 kcal total − 360 kcal protein − 1360 kcal dextrose = 580 kcal lipids

Lipids provide 9.0 kcal/g

$\frac{\text{580 kcal}}{\text{9 kcal/g}}$ = 64 g lipids

A 20% lipid emulsion contain 2 kcal/mL

$\frac{\text{580 kcal}}{\text{2 kcal/mL}}$ = 290 mL of 20% lipid emulsion

Final Formulation

290 mL of 20% lipid emulsion + 571 mL of 70% dextrose solution + 900 mL of 10% amino acid solution = 1761 mL total volume of nutrient solutions

2000 mL daily fluid − 1761 mL PN = 239 mL additional fluid required which should be added as sterile water for injection

Monitoring and Management

Monitoring of TPN therapy is important to determine efficacy of therapy, evaluate changes in patient condition, and prevent complications. Patient condition should always dictate monitoring parameters and frequency.

On initiation of therapy, the following parameters should be evaluated: nutritional status, metabolic status, patient weight, vital signs (heart rate, blood pressure, respiratory rate, and temperature), electrolytes (Na, K, CO_2, blood urea nitrogen [BUN], creatinine [Cr], glucose, Ca, Mg, PO_4), and fluid status. These parameters should be monitored daily until the patient is stable. Liver function tests (aspartate aminotransferase [AST], alanine aminotransferase [ALT], alkaline phosphatase [ALP], total bilirubin), prothrombin time (PT), partial thromboplastin time (PTT), and complete blood cell count (CBC) with differential levels should be measured at baseline and weekly thereafter. Long-term monitoring for home TPN can be decreased to weekly or longer depending on patient stability and condition. It is important to remember that critically ill patients will require more frequent monitoring and may necessitate frequent changes to TPN formulation.

Contrary to popular belief, serum albumin is a poor indicator of nutritional status; particularly in the settings of nephropathy, enteropathy, liver disease, and volume overload. Albumin is also an acute-phase protein that is affected by cytokine-mediated inflammatory responses, including injury, stress, or infection. Prealbumin has a shorter half-life, but otherwise suffers many of the same limitations.

Blood glucose levels should be monitored throughout the TPN infusion in order to detect hyperglycemia or hypoglycemia. A blood capillary monitoring device provides a reliable and affordable means of checking levels at the bedside. Blood capillary glucose levels may be obtained every 6 hours for the first 72 hours and then as needed to verify glucose levels obtained by the laboratory.

Triglyceride levels may be obtained before initiation of lipid therapy and periodically during PN therapy. Lipids should be reduced or held in adult patients with triglyceride levels >400 mg/dL. However, weekly lipid infusions may be necessary to prevent essential fatty acid deficiency (EFAD).

Common Complications

Complications of parenteral nutrition therapy may be divided into three classes: mechanical, infectious, and metabolic.

Mechanical complications are usually caused by the insertion of the catheter device. Potential complications associated with the insertion of the central catheter include pneumothorax, arrhythmias, catheter thrombosis, venous thrombosis, and catheter occlusion. A chest x-ray should always be obtained before the use of a central catheter to verify proper placement of the device. Catheter occlusion is the most common mechanical complication.

Catheter-related sepsis is always a concern whenever the venous system is accessed. It is estimated that 90% of nosocomial infections can be attributed to central lines. Potential signs of a catheter-related sepsis are a sudden increase in the patient's usual temperature or new hyperglycemia. Although external signs of catheter infection may be seen, this is often not the case. Sources of the infection may be from endogenous skin flora, contamination of the catheter hub, seeding of the catheter from a distant site, or rarely contamination of the infusate. Strict adherence to aseptic technique helps to minimize the risk of infection. In the event of infection, the venous access device is usually removed, cultures drawn, and antibiotic therapy is initiated. Salvage antimicrobial therapy is sometimes elected for long-term central venous access devices depending on the pathogen.

The reported incidence of metabolic complications in TPN patients is 5% to 10%. Metabolic complications may include intolerances to glucose, protein, or fat; imbalances in potassium, sodium, magnesium, phosphate, calcium or water. Hyperglycemia is the most common complication associated with PN therapy. Van den Berghe and colleagues showed that hyperglycemia is associated with increased infection and mortality in critically ill patients. Therefore, it is important to monitor for hyperglycemia and to adjust the TPN formulation as indicated. Normoglycemic blood glucose levels should be maintained in critical care settings (80 to 110 mg/dL). This may require parenteral insulin drip therapy.

Refeeding syndrome is a potential metabolic complication typically seen in severely malnourished patients. The administration of TPN causes the potassium, magnesium, and phosphorus to shift into the intracellular space, causing a massive depletion within the serum. The electrolyte abnormalities that result can lead to arrhythmias, heart failure, respiratory failure, and death. It is important to realize that refeeding syndrome can occur with oral, enteral, or parenteral feeding. This syndrome can be prevented by the gradual advancement of nutrition support and supplementation of appropriate electrolytes.

Electrolyte adjustments may also be required for a host of other indications. For example, potassium, phosphate, and magnesium are routinely reduced in TPN formulations for patients with renal failure. Patients experiencing renal insufficiency or hepatic failure may require protein restriction. Protein intolerance may be demonstrated by elevated BUN, elevated serum Cr levels, or elevated ammonia levels in combination with encephalopathy. Patients who are adequately dialyzed can generally be administered full goal protein prescriptions. Lipids may be contraindicated in patients with marked hypertriglyceridemia (triglyceride >400 mg/dL). Modest doses of lipids (30 to 40 g once or twice a week) may be adequate to prevent essential fatty acid deficiency.

The lack of enteral nutrients and limited gastrointestinal motility may lead to hepatic steatosis or cholestasis in some TPN patients. Cholestasis ultimately develops in many patients requiring more than 6 weeks of TPN therapy. It is important to transition patients to enteral or oral feeding as soon as possible to prevent the potential development of gallstones associated with cholestasis. A normal bilirubin with mild elevations in alkaline phosphatase and hepatic transaminases may indicate hepatic steatosis (fatty liver). In rare cases, hepatic steatosis may progress to steatohepatitis. To limit hepatobiliary injury, the TPN formulation should be re-evaluated to avoid inclusion of excess lipid and carbohydrate. Cycled TPN infusion and administration of a cholecystokinin-octapeptide may also be considered to limit further injury.

Finally, metabolic bone disease may develop in long-term TPN patients. Metabolic bone disease, including osteoporosis or osteomalacia, may develop as a consequence of the patient's underlying disease, and associated malabsorption of calcium and vitamin D, or the use of predisposing medications (such as corticosteroids), and hypercalciuria. Treatment with bisphosphonate, calcium, and vitamin D[1] may be indicated in long-term TPN patients to prevent the development of metabolic bone disease.

Transitional Feeding

Tapering and discontinuation of TPN are indicated once nutritional needs are met and adequately absorbed through the enteral route. If the patient is establishing oral diet tolerance, 24-hour calorie and protein counts should be monitored closely to assure adequacy of needs. One approach is to reduce macronutrients in the TPN solution by 50% once a patient exhibits initial tolerance to enteral tube feeding and TPN is discontinued when the patient tolerates 75% to 100% of the enteral tube feeding goal.

Home TPN Management

Increasing numbers of patients are receiving TPN in the home setting. Once a patient's medical condition has stabilized and hospitalization is no longer indicated, then TPN can often be managed safely at home. Considerations in effectively managing a patient on home TPN should focus on the patient and/or caregiver's ability to safely operate infusion devices and administer solutions. Education should begin in the inpatient setting and continue in the home setting and focus on aseptic technique, IV line flushing, use of the infusion pump, signs of infection, and monitoring. Electricity, telephone, water, and adequate refrigeration space are required to provide home TPN.

Cycling TPN over 12 hours nocturnally in the home setting is an appropriate goal to enhance mobility and quality of life. This approach may also help to minimize problems with cholestasis. Cycled TPN infusion can begin in the hospital, so tolerance of cycling can be established in a closely monitored setting.

[1]Not FDA approved for this indication.

PARENTERAL FLUID THERAPY FOR INFANTS AND CHILDREN

METHOD OF

Alex R. Constantinescu, MD

Infants and children differ from adults with respect to body composition and energy requirements, and are much more susceptible to fluid and electrolyte imbalances, thus requiring constant modification of therapy and adequate monitoring.

This chapter, in its first part, introduces basic concepts of fluid and electrolyte physiology. The second part describes specific approaches to the diagnosis of major electrolyte abnormalities seen in dehydration states, with emphasis on their therapy.

Physiology

Total body water (TBW) represents approximately 45% to 60% of body weight, in well-demarcated body fluid compartments. The extracellular fluid compartment (ECF) contains one third of TBW (20% of body weight), and the intracellular fluid compartment (ICF) contains two thirds of TBW (40% of body weight). Of the ECF, three fourths is in the interstitium (15% of body weight), and one fourth is in the intravascular compartment as plasma (5% of body weight); 10% of ICF is contained by the red blood cells (RBCs) (4% of body weight). Individuals older than 70 years, females, and obese individuals, as well as patients on dialysis, have less body water and a lower ratio of muscle to adipose tissue.

Infants have 70% of their body weight represented by water. TBW decreases to adult levels by the age of 3 years, with most of this decline being noted in the first year of life. This change in TBW is caused by a shift from a predominantly ECF to a predominantly ICF distribution shortly after birth. Also, there is a rapid turnover of body fluids in these infants, 50% versus <20% of ECF volume per day in adults.

The body fluid compartments are separated by cell membranes, which, in turn, have selective permeabilities. Osmotically active particles are restricted to the ECF or ICF, and account for the tonicity, or "effective" osmolality of these compartments. One can calculate serum osmolality with the following formula:

$$\text{Serum osmolality (mOsm/kg)} = 2[\text{Na}] + \text{glucose}/18 + \text{blood urea nitrogen (BUN)}/2.8$$

Osmotic forces drive the fluid movement between the ICF and ECF, because water diffuses freely and equalizes the osmolalities of the two major water compartments. The normal tonicity is thus maintained by the regulation of water metabolism.

ICF, the larger of the two, has a relatively fixed number of particles (because of the large size of anions and phosphate esters; i.e., adenosine triphosphate [ATP], phospholipids), and any change in ICF osmolality is the result of changes in the ICF water content, with alteration of cell volume (brain cells can defend against cell volume alterations by the synthesis of "idiogenic osmoles").

Sodium, on the other hand, is restricted to ECF, because of active Na transport out of the cells (via Na-K-ATPase); and so are its major coupled anions (Cl^- and HCO_3^-). The ECF volume is determined by body Na content, and is controlled by renal Na excretion.

Another important factor implicated in fluid movement, is the hydrostatic pressure difference, which determines the fluid shift from plasma to the interstitium, and is opposed by the colloid oncotic pressure (exerted by serum albumin), to prevent edema formation.

BRIEF OVERVIEW OF WATER METABOLISM

Once ingested, the water is added to the amount generated from cellular metabolism, and is distributed in the ICF and ECF, with the proportions determined by age, size, and state of hydration. The normal excretion of water can be divided into *fixed* excretion (via stool, sweat, and respiration), also referred to as insensible water losses (IWL), and *variable* excretion (urine).

Infants and children who cannot maximally concentrate their urine (e.g., in nephrogenic diabetes insipidus or renal dysplasia) are at risk of developing severe dehydration; so are those with severe diarrhea or profuse sweating.

The water excretion is determined by glomerular filtration rate (GFR), and if that is normal, by the function of tubular segments. Tubular dysfunctions can be simple or complex, sometimes associated with disturbances in water metabolism. Along the tubular segments, various ion transporters, located at the luminal membrane, determine the final water and electrolyte concentrations required by metabolic homeostasis. The action of antidiuretic hormone (ADH) at the level of the collecting duct is governed by both the intravascular volume and plasma osmolality. This allows maximal urine concentration or dilution, because the clinical condition so mandates by the action of ADH on the aquaporin water channels (AQP-2, AQP-3, and AQP-4). Infants have a reduced concentrating ability contributing to higher losses of fluids, which may be overcome by a reduced GFR (up until 2 years of age).

BRIEF OVERVIEW OF SODIUM METABOLISM

Filtered load of Na contributes, at the level of proximal tubule (PCT), to Na-coupled reabsorption of glucose, amino acids, bicarbonate, and phosphate, and facilitates water reabsorption (ADH-independent mechanism). At the level of the loop of Henle, secondary active Na absorption (via Na-K-2Cl cotransporter) takes place, such that from a normal serum osmolality of 300 mOsm/kg at the beginning of the PCT, it reaches maximal value at the tip of the loop of Henle (~1200 mOsm/kg), only to return to plasma value in the initial portion of the distal convoluted tubule (DCT). Na absorption in this segment mediates calcium and magnesium absorption, the former taking place also in the DCT, via the Na-Ca exchanger, located in the basolateral membrane. At the level of the collecting duct, Na absorption via the epithelial Na channels (ENaC) facilitates K secretion.

The Na absorption is regulated in part by the renin–angiotensin–aldosterone system, and to a smaller extent by sympathetic nervous system (catecholamines) and thyroid hormone. Atrial natriuretic peptide, secreted in cases of intravascular volume expansion, leads to decreased Na reabsorption. Infants have a blunt response to a Na load, being unable to excrete it as quickly as the adults, in part as a result of an immature response to the natriuretic hormones as well as the lower GFR, which, in turn, allows only a small amount of Na to be delivered to the tubular segments.

BRIEF OVERVIEW OF POTASSIUM METABOLISM

Urinary K secretion does not appear until full maturation of tubules, and is mediated by the K channels. Some evidence exists as to K absorption via H-K-adenosine triphosphatase (ATPase). The most important determining factors of K secretion are GFR, urine flow rate, Na absorption, luminal electronegativity, and the aldosterone action. All these factors have to be taken into consideration when assessing a patient with a fluid or electrolyte abnormality.

Maintenance Requirements for Water and Solutes

Organisms lose water and electrolytes constantly through body fluids, which need to be replaced, in proportions dictated by metabolic needs and disease state, to maintain homeostasis. Children have certain important characteristics, which have to be considered when evaluating the state of hydration, as well as when parenteral therapy is prescribed. Some of these are a higher ratio of body surface area (BSA) to body weight (0.043 vs. 0.025 m^2/kg), a higher basal metabolic rate (55 vs. 25 to 30 kcal/kg per day). As to the renal handling of fluids and electrolytes, broad differences result from renal immaturity in infants, a blunt response to Na load, and a reduced buffering capacity (low H and K secretion, lower serum HCO_3^- concentration). These differences will enable us to understand the responses to certain therapeutic maneuvers.

From a practical standpoint, the maintenance requirements are based on body weight, evaporative

TABLE 1 Daily Requirements of Water and Solutes as a Function of Body Weight

Weight	kcal/kg/day (mL/kg/day)	Sodium (mEq/100 mL)	Potassium (mEq/100 mL)
From 0 to 10 kg	100	2-3	2
From 10 to 20 kg	50	2-3	2
Above 20 kg	20	2-3	2

losses, and disease state. It has been established that 100 mL of water are necessary to replace 100 kcal used by metabolic processes. Thus, one can calculate fluid requirements, as well as caloric requirements, based on body weight (Holliday-Segar formula; Table 1) or on body surface area (expressed in m^2, result of square root of [Ht (cm) × Wt (kg) ÷ 3600)]). As an example, a child weighing 15 kg and measuring 100 cm in height has a BSA of 0.64 m^2. The caloric needs based on the Holliday-Segar formula are:

$$\text{Kcal} = 1000 \text{ kcal for first } 10 \text{ kg} + 250 \text{ kcal for next } 5 \text{ kg} = 1250 \text{ kcal}$$

If one uses the "body surface area" method, maintenance requirements would be 2000 kcal/m^2 per day (for patients with isotonic urine), and the result of 1280 kcal is very close to the result obtained with the first method of calculation. Because urine output may vary more compared with the insensible losses, it is prudent to separate the two components, especially in patients who have a pre-existing renal disease with polyuria (such as renal dysplasia or nephrogenic diabetes insipidus) or who are in renal failure with oligoanuria. This way, IWL needing replacement will almost always be 500 to 750 mL/m^2, and the only variable will be the urine output, which can be replaced every 2 to 4 hours. This approach can prevent, in most cases, fluid overload, as well as intravascular volume depletion. Ongoing losses have to be considered and added to the above fluid replacements. Table 2 shows the composition of various sources of fluid loss. We also have to take into consideration the circumstances that could increase the fluid requirements, such as fever (12% higher for each degree above 38°C [100.4°F]), mouth breathing, or decreased urinary concentrating ability.

Table 1 lists the maintenance requirements for electrolytes to help in accurate prescription of solute amounts needed in various clinical conditions. Particular attention has to be given to the prescription of Na, as mEq/100 kcal or mEq/100 mL, *not* mEq/kg, because a total body sodium overload can occur with the latter approach.

Usual parenteral fluids are composed of dextrose (to diminish catabolism), Na and Cl, in various concentrations, as required by age and body weight. Different salts of K (KCl or K phosphate) can be added after documented normal renal function (or after voiding in children without a history of renal disease), and other electrolytes or acid–base imbalances need to be identified and corrected.

TABLE 2 Sources of Fluid and Solute Losses

Source	Na^+ (mEq/L)	K^+ (mEq/L)	Cl^- (mEq/L)	HCO_3^- (mEq/L)
Diarrhea	10-90	10-80	10-110	15-50
Gastric	20-80	5-20	100-150	0
Pancreatic	120-140	5-15	40-80	110-115
Small bowel	100-140	5-15	90-130	30-40
Bile	120-140	5-15	80-120	40
Ileostomy	45-135	3-15	20-115	30
Sweat	30-65	0	30-65	0
Urine	20-100 (~75)	variable	~75	0

TABLE 3 Causes of Dehydration

Decreased Oral Intake
- Nausea/anorexia
- Altered mental capacity
- Immediate postoperative period

Increased Losses

Nonrenal and nongastrointestinal
- Fever
- Burns
- Hyperventilation
- Cystic fibrosis
- Hypermetabolic states
- Bullous or other skin disorders
- Cerebrospinal fluid drainage
- Effusions (pleural, pericardial)
- Peritonitis

Gastrointestinal losses
- Vomiting
- Diarrhea
- Fistulae/ostomies
- Suction/gastrointestinal drainage
- Pancreatitis (mostly third spacing)

Renal losses
- Diuretic use
- Osmotic diuresis
- Diabetes mellitus
- Diabetes insipidus
- Renal dysplasia and other concentrating abnormalities
- Postobstructive diuresis

Evaluation of Hydration Status

An important aspect of clinical pediatric practice is represented by the accurate assessment of hydration state. Because of the extremely sophisticated mechanisms of regulation of water and electrolyte transport and their relative immaturity in infants and children, these young patients are more prone to develop fluid and electrolyte abnormalities than adults. In children, any acute illness can cause a decrease in oral intake that can worsen the dehydration resulting from, most often, a gastrointestinal illness (Table 3 lists the most common causes of dehydration).

Estimation of dehydration can be made from history, physical examination, and laboratory parameters. History can reveal the type and severity of losses such as vomiting and diarrhea, either alone or in combination, blood loss, fever, burns, and the like, as well as the presence of prior renal or cardiac disease.

TABLE 4 Evaluation of Dehydration States

Parameter/ Severity	Mild	Moderate	Severe
Body weight	3%-5% loss	7%-10%	15%
Skin turgor	↓	↓↓	↓↓↓
Membranes	Dry	Very dry	Parched
Skin color	Pale	Gray	Mottled
Urine output	Slight oliguria	Oliguria	Marked oliguria and azotemia
Blood pressure	Normal	Normal, postural hypotension	Hypotension
Pulse	± ↑	↑	↑↑
Capillary refill	<2 seconds	2-3 seconds	>3 seconds
Neurologic status	Normal	Decreased alertness or irritability	Lethargy

A rapid, systematic, clinical evaluation includes assessing the (a) weight, (b) skin turgor and mucous membranes (anterior fontanelle in infants, production of tears or sunken eyes in older children), (c) urine output, and (d) heart rate, blood pressure, and capillary refill, as well as (e) the neurologic status. This "five-point evaluation" allows classification of the dehydration states as mild, moderate, or severe (Table 4). Too often clinicians do not have the previous weight of the patient, and have to estimate the weight loss with the help of these clinical parameters. Other clinical signs can be taken into consideration, such as skin fold (progressive "tenting" with more severe dehydration), skin color (mottled to acrocyanosis as dehydration progresses), respirations (tachypnea as acidosis develops in advanced dehydration), and general appearance (increasingly less active). Urine output in patients with diabetes mellitus or diabetes insipidus should not be used as a criterion of normal hydration state.

Aside from clinical parameters, we often use a combination of laboratory values and ratios that can help us in determining the severity of dehydration (Table 5). It is important to mention at this point that prolonged intravascular volume depletion, or prerenal azotemia, can progress to acute tubular necrosis (ATN), and their distinction sometimes may be difficult. As an example, a serum BUN-to-creatinine ratio may not be as high in ATN as in prerenal azotemia, and if the condition is not accurately assessed by other parameters, may give us a false sense of reassurance and contribute to a delay in vigorous hydration.

TABLE 5 Laboratory Parameters Useful in Assessing the Severity of Dehydration

Laboratory Parameters	Prerenal Azotemia	Acute Tubular Necrosis
Blood urea nitrogen: creatinine ratio	>20	<20
Urine:plasma creatinine ratio	>40:1	<20:1
Urine osmolality	At least 100 m Osm/kg > than plasma osmolality	<350
Urine specific gravity	>1.020	Isostenuria (~1.010)
Urinary Na concentration (mEq/L)	<20	>40
FENa ($U_{Na}/P_{Na} \times P_{cr}/U_{cr} \times 100$)	<1	>1

Based on the serum Na concentration, the dehydration can be isotonic, hypotonic, or hypertonic. The most common is the *isotonic* dehydration, seen in at least two thirds of all cases, characterized by a serum Na concentration of 130 to 150 mEq/L. This is the typical form of dehydration seen in acute gastrointestinal illnesses presenting with vomiting and diarrhea. The next most common is the *hypertonic* dehydration, representing approximately 15% of all cases, seen, for example, in cases of excessive free-water losses (i.e., diabetes insipidus), or excessive electrolyte (Na) intake in children with gastroenteritis. In these cases, the serum Na concentration is above 150 mEq/L. The least-common type is the *hypotonic* dehydration, in which serum Na concentration is less than 130 mEq/L, either because of excessive free-water intake or excessive Na losses.

Na and water abnormalities can occur in cases other than dehydration; Figure 1 is a simple way to conceptualize the changes in water compartment distribution. The normal distribution is seen in panel A. Hypernatremia (depicted in panel B) is characterized by contraction of ICF. In states of hyponatremia caused by gain of electrolyte-free water (panel C), both ECF and ICF expand, as a consequence of free movement of water across the membranes, and in sharp contrast, hyponatremia caused by loss of NaCl (panel D), is characterized by a decrease in both ECF and ICF. If there is isotonic loss of saline (panel E), only ECF contracts, without alteration in ICF, compared with cases of isotonic gain of saline which lead to expansion of ECF only (panel F), without changes in ICF.

Serum osmolality, as well as intravascular volume, are the determinants of water excretion, mediated by thirst and ADH secretion. Both a decrease in plasma osmolality and an increase in circulating volume lead to diminished thirst, lowering the water intake, as well as a low ADH release, leading to decreased water reabsorption. These, in turn, will cause water excretion, in an attempt to bring the plasma osmolality and circulating volume back to normal. The opposite is true as well, inasmuch as when the plasma osmolality is increased or circulating volume is decreased, thirst increases, leading to more water intake, and ADH is released in higher amounts to diminish water excretion. These will lead to water retention, which, in turn, will normalize the plasma osmolality and circulating volume. When the compensatory mechanisms are faulty, one can develop water metabolism abnormalities (hypervolemia or

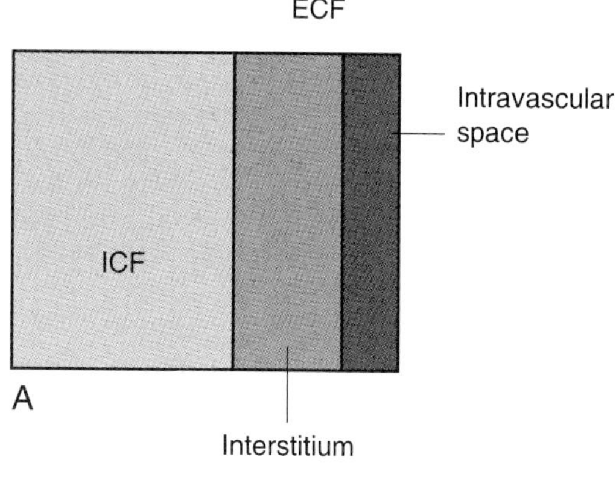

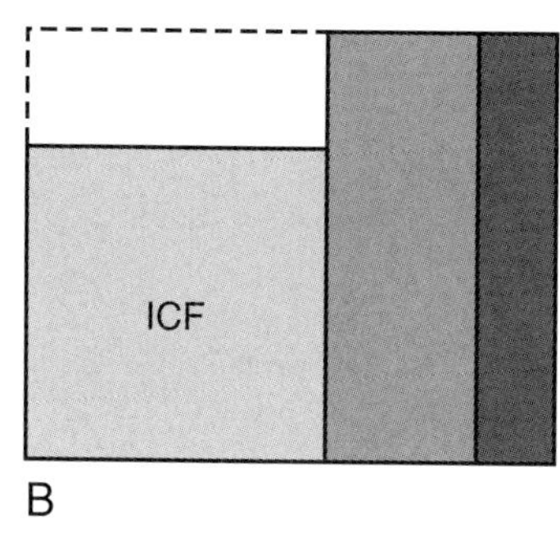

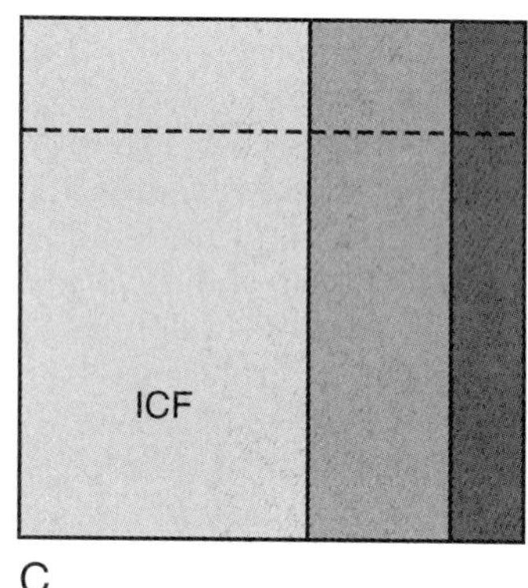

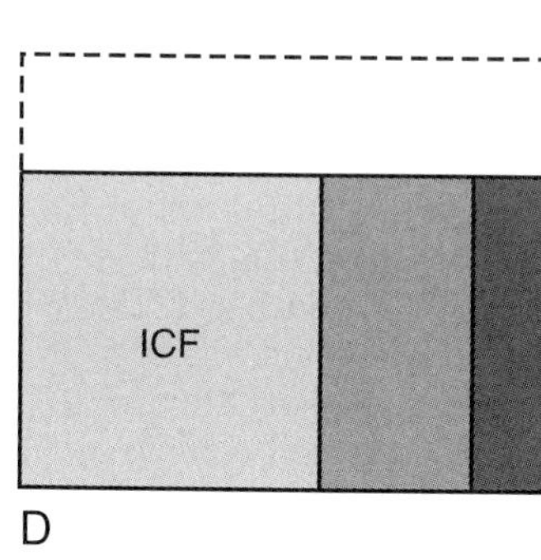
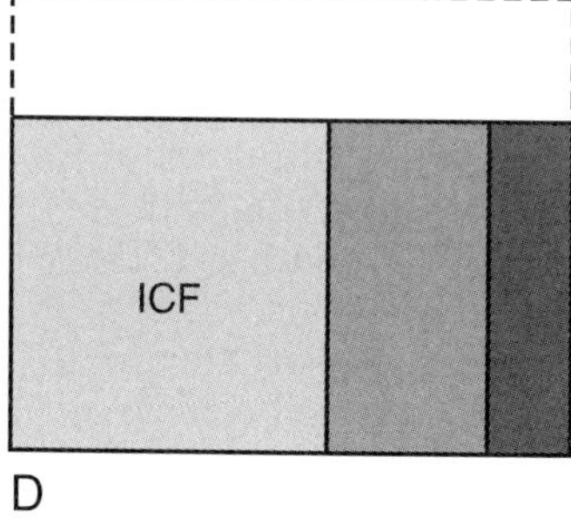

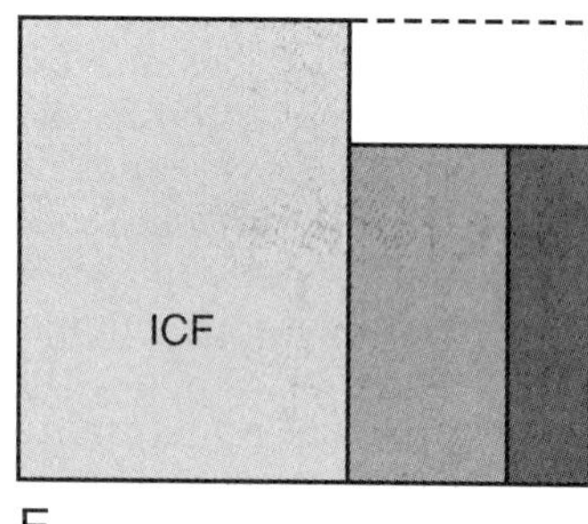

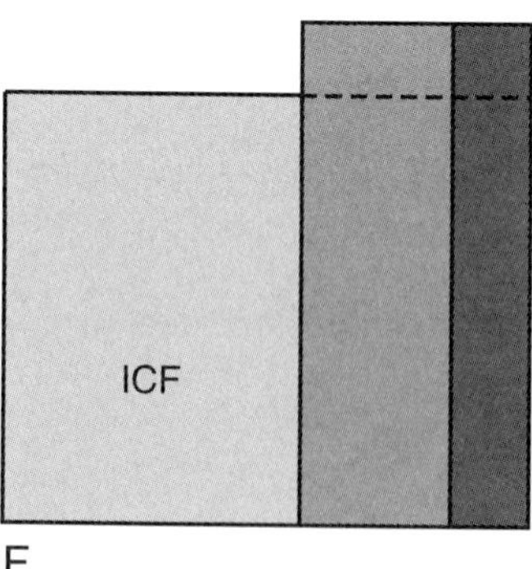

FIGURE 1 Water compartment distribution in states of hypo- and hypernatremia. Panel **A** depicts normal distribution of intracellular fluid compartment (ICF) and extracellular fluid compartment (ECF) made up of intravascular space (represented by plasma) and interstitial fluid compartment. Panel **B** illustrates ICF volume contraction in cases of hypernatremia. The dotted line in panels **B** to **F** represents the normal reference range. Panel **C** is characteristic of a state of free-water gain with subsequent hyponatremia (both ECF and ICF expansion), whereas panel **D** depicts saline loss with subsequent depletion of both ICF and ECF compartments. Isotonic loss of saline (panel **E**) leads to ECF volume contraction, without ICF volume changes, and isotonic gain of saline (panel **F**) determines expansion of ECF, with no alteration of ICF. The *dashed lines* help comparisons with the normal state.

dehydration), as well as abnormal sodium homeostasis: hyponatremia (disorder involving urine dilution, or excess water intake) or hypernatremia (disorder involving urine concentration and/or inadequate sodium or water intake).

Principles of Rehydration in Infants and Children

When faced with a dehydrated patient, based on the severity of the clinical picture, one can decide on the route of rehydration. In a patient with abnormal neurologic status, oral rehydration is not advised, whereas for a child with a mild diarrheal illness without vomiting, intravenous rehydration may not be the first choice. Regardless of the route chosen, the same principles apply: (a) estimate losses, (b) calculate replacement needs by adding maintenance requirements, previous deficits and ongoing losses, and (c) institute a system of monitoring the adequacy of therapy. A simple table can be created, and used as a guide to aide in the prescription of the final solution and help in adjusting the fluid therapy (Table 6).

After identifying a patient in a state of dehydration (based on the clinical and laboratory parameters)

TABLE 6 Guide for Evaluating Water and Solute Needs

	Na	K	H_2O
Deficit	In hyponatremia and isotonic dehydration	In hypokalemia, isotonic or hypertonic dehydration	In hypernatremia and isotonic dehydration
Ongoing losses	Variable	Variable	Stool, vomiting, ileostomy, third spacing
Maintenance	According to Table 1	According to Table 1	According to Table 1
Prior boluses			Usually given in the emergency room, and if substantial, may be subtracted from total needs
Total			
Final solution	D5W with x mL NaCl	+ KCl if needed	
Rate/continuous vs. 2 steps (first 8 h followed by 16 h)			

and classifying the type based on serum Na concentration, the route of rehydration is established.

In isotonic dehydration, it is assumed that ECF volume contraction has occurred and if the patient can tolerate oral fluids, and if the mental status is not altered, 50 or 100 mL of oral rehydration solution per kilogram of body weight can be administered, depending on mild or moderate dehydration state, respectively. It is important to remember that losses in isotonic dehydration involve losses of water *plus* Na (see Table 6). It is advisable that in patients with diarrhea, each stool must be replaced with 10 mL/kg. Various solutions are available, most physiologic ones contain 45 mEq Na/L and contain other electrolytes (such as K, Cl, citrate), as well as glucose. If NaCl losses are larger, the World Health Organization (WHO) solution can be used (it contains 90 mEq Na/L). For severely dehydrated patients, as well as for those with altered mental status, the intravenous route is recommended, because it will provide a faster correction of clinical parameters, improving the outcome. In these latter conditions, plasma expanders (5% albumin) can also be considered, but are less effective than saline infusion. Hypotonic solutions must be avoided because they can cause electrolyte abnormalities, hemolysis, and altered neurologic status.

If the clinical condition requires it, bolus saline (0.9% normal saline contains 154 mEq Na/L) of 20 to 40 mL/kg can be given rapidly, and can be continued at 40 mL/kg per hour until the neurologic status and cardiovascular parameters are stabilized, and urine output has been re-established in patients with oligoanuria. Thereafter, rehydration has to be continued with a solution prescribed based on the maintenance electrolyte needs and the water and electrolyte losses, based on the serum Na concentration (see Table 6). There are two possible methods of rehydration: *continuous* over 24 hours, or a *two-step approach* with the first half of deficit and one third of daily maintenance in the first 8 hours, followed by the other half of deficit and two thirds of maintenance over the next 16 hours. Both approaches have equal effectiveness toward normalization of cardiovascular parameters (blood pressure, heart rate, capillary refill) and urine output, and ongoing losses have to be well documented and replaced with appropriate solutions. Patients with a worse clinical picture may need the two-step approach, as rapid rehydration can be beneficial in these clinical situations.

Potassium is added to a maximum of 40 mEq/L, depending on renal function and needs based on body weight and age. Acid–base abnormalities in dehydration are discussed below. The key to any rehydration is monitoring the electrolyte response to the therapeutic maneuvers, because unknown metabolic disorders may be discovered during these episodes.

Special Situations

Special consideration has to be given to certain electrolyte abnormalities, such as hyponatremia, hypernatremia, and hypokalemia. Acid–base abnormalities can be caused by dehydration, in which case they are transient, or a chronic acid–base abnormality can be brought to medical attention, or aggravated by an episode of dehydration. This section discusses the clinical presentation of these major electrolyte abnormalities, with an emphasis on the appropriate therapy.

HYPONATREMIA

As mentioned at the beginning of the article, hyponatremia can be caused by the gain of free-water, loss of Na alone, or Na loss in excess of water loss. The most common cause of hyponatremia is represented by gastrointestinal losses. Aside from clinical assessment of the severity of dehydration, few key laboratory tests can answer the question as to the pathogenesis and ultimately the etiology. These tests can quickly help in excluding the factitious hyponatremia, seen in patients who have hyperglycemia (correction factor of 1.6 mEq Na/L for each 100 mg glucose/dL, above 100 mg/dL), severe hypercholesterolemia (as in diabetes ketoacidosis) or severe hyperproteinemia (as in multiple myeloma). Other causes of pseudohyponatremia are the use of hyperosmolar substances (e.g., mannitol—it translocates water from ICF to intravascular space, causing dilutional hyponatremia) or hyperviscosity syndrome (laboratory error).

Once determined that the hyponatremia is real, there are multiple approaches to determine the cause, and establish if the hyponatremia is part of an edematous or a nonedematous state. Urine Na (U_{Na}) concentration can help in this regard. The hypervolemic edematous disorders include congestive heart failure, hepatic cirrhosis, and nephrotic syndrome, and are characterized by a U_{Na} of less than 10 mEq/L. The same low U_{Na} can be seen in hypovolemic states (dehydration), such as gastrointestinal losses without bicarbonaturia, or excessive skin losses (cystic fibrosis, ichthyosis, burns). Therefore, U_{Na} concentration can help determine if losses are renal or nonrenal in origin. Renal losses may sometimes represent hormonal imbalances, such as hypothyroidism, hypoaldosteronism (true or pseudohypoaldosteronism), syndrome of inappropriate antidiuretic hormone (SIADH) secretion, and cerebral salt wasting. In addition, hypovolemia during surgery, if not recognized and treated, can lead to excessive Na loss in the postoperative period. Most commonly, however, renal losses are caused by renal disease, such as acute tubular necrosis (ATN), renal dysplasia, obstructive uropathy, tubulopathies (e.g, proximal renal tubular acidosis, Bartter's syndrome), nephrocalcinosis, or diuretic use/abuse. Other nonedematous states have to be considered, such as SIADH and psychogenic polydipsia, based on the higher urine Na concentration in the former, and hyposthenuria with significant pertinent history in the latter. Therapy is different in these two conditions, because fluid restriction is required in SIADH.

The most significant complications of hyponatremia are cerebral edema and generalized seizures, which can be seen at serum Na concentrations below 125 mEq/L. In these cases, the correction has to be made rapidly to bring serum Na just up to 125 mEq/L; this can be done rather quickly with hypertonic saline (0.5 mEq Na/mL), compared with asymptomatic hyponatremic (hypotonic) dehydration, in which case correction can be made over 24 hours. Calculation of deficit is based on volume of distribution, which is TBW (approximately 60% of body weight):

$$\text{Na deficit (in mEq)} = [\text{desired Na} - \text{actual Na}] \times \text{body weight (kg)} \times 0.6$$

For correction of Na in cases of mild hyponatremic dehydration, the desired Na is 140 mEq/L. The deficit has to be added to the daily maintenance and ongoing losses (urine, stool, gastric or intestinal drainage), and rehydration can follow the same principle outlined in isotonic dehydration (continuous, or two-step approach). The rate of rehydration and fluid composition depends on the severity of dehydration (the more severe, the faster the rehydration, to improve the outcome) and the response to initial fluid resuscitation maneuvers. In addition, a too rapid correction can cause cerebral hemorrhage or pontine myelinolysis. Therefore, as a guideline, the rate of correction should be about 12 mEq/L per 24 hours, and 16 to 18 mEq/L per 48 hours. Chronic asymptomatic hyponatremia has to be corrected at an even slower rate.

Particular attention has to be given to patients with renal failure, because they may become fluid overloaded and if the solution is not properly chosen, hyponatremia may in fact worsen. Adequate monitoring requires determination of serum Na concentration at least every 6 hours, to allow for correction of factors that may contribute to inadequate response (previously unknown losses of Na or gain of free-water). This way, iatrogenic hyponatremia can be recognized early and corrected in a timely fashion.

HYPERNATREMIA

As described in Figure 1, hypernatremia (panel B) differs from normal situation (panel A) by the fact that the ICF volume is diminished first, and the cardiovascular parameters are compromised only in late stages, not perceived early on by caretakers. This can explain why these children are brought to the physician's attention in advanced stages of dehydration.

Because of ICF volume depletion, rehydration has to be performed slowly, over 48 to 72 hours, to prevent rapid cell swelling, most importantly, to prevent cerebral edema. The rate of decline in serum Na concentration has to be no more than 0.5 mEq/L per hour (12 mEq/L per 24-hour period). If the initial serum Na is more than 175 to 180 mEq/L, the correction has to take place over a longer time.

Hypernatremic (or hypertonic) dehydration occurs when free-water losses are higher than Na losses. This can be seen in diabetes insipidus (central or nephrogenic; in these cases there is no Na loss), diabetes mellitus (glucose as osmotic diuretic), recovery from renal failure (when urea is the osmotic diuretic), or vomiting and diarrhea (especially if inappropriately prepared formula is given as fluid replacement). Hypernatremia can also occur in cases of administration of hypertonic saline solutions.

After assessing the severity of dehydration, one can calculate the water deficit. There are few ways of determining the result, with two simple ones giving very similar results. A rough estimate can be 4 mL of water per kilogram of body weight, for each mEq Na/L above 145 mEq/L. Another formula is based on water distribution and body weight:

$$\text{Water deficit (in L)} = [(\text{Na}/145) - 1] \times \text{body weight (in kg)} \times 0.6$$

For a 10-kg child, who lost 1 kg and has a serum Na of 160 mEq/L, free-water deficit can be calculated as 15 × 4 mL/kg × 10 kg = 600 mL (0.6 L). The other formula gives a similar result: [(160/145) – 1] × 10 × 0.6 = 0.620 L.

Depending on how large the water deficit is, the length of time needed for correction can be determined. To this, the maintenance fluid *and* electrolytes have to be added (Na and K) for the duration of correction, and a grid similar to that seen in Table 6 can help reach the final composition of intravenous solution needed over those days. The maintenance fluid requirements in these patients, however, have to be decreased by approximately 25%, because of fluid shifts. This will also help prevent a rapid correction of hypernatremia. In the cases of hypertonic dehydration, it is necessary to monitor the electrolytes more often, to adjust the rate of correction, based on the rate of drop in serum Na concentration.

HYPOKALEMIA

Potassium is predominantly an intracellular cation, and if serum concentration is below normal (<3.5 mEq/L), one can speculate significant intracellular losses, making it very difficult to quantify the K losses. In addition to low K intake and increased cell uptake, hypokalemia results from renal and extrarenal losses. States of dehydration associated with hypokalemia can be seen in patients with diarrhea, vomiting, gastric or intestinal fistulae, as well as those taking laxatives or experiencing profuse sweating. These patients will benefit from K supplementation, provided that the renal function is adequate. Table 1 lists the maintenance requirements. In cases of acute dehydration where there is a loss of ICF volume, such as in isotonic and hypertonic dehydrations, one has to calculate the K deficit. It is generally assumed that 20% of the volume lost in these conditions comes from the ICF, and K deficit can easily be calculated for accurate replacement, because K in ICF has a concentration of 150 mEq/L.

ACID–BASE DISTURBANCES IN STATES OF DEHYDRATION

Mild and moderate states of dehydration do not exhibit major acid–base abnormalities. However, severe dehydration, or pre-existing renal disorders may be associated with major disturbances, which can be represented by both acidosis and alkalosis. Significant gastrointestinal (GI) losses (especially in diarrheal disorders) can lead to bicarbonate loss and directly to metabolic acidosis. This acidosis is characterized by a normal anion gap, in contrast to the metabolic acidosis seen in more advanced stages of dehydration, with poor tissue perfusion, where the metabolic acidosis is characterized by a high anion gap (lactic acidosis). The serum anion gap is the difference between Na (as the positive ion) and Cl+HCO_3 (both as the negative ions) (normal: 12 to 15). In cases of high anion gap, fluid resuscitation may suffice, whereas in the cases with normal anion gap, one may consider the addition of sodium bicarbonate or citrate in refractory cases, or those with a prolonged course, not reversed by intravenous fluids, and who continue to have ongoing losses. Attention has to be paid to hyperkalemia, which can be caused by severe metabolic acidosis.

On the other hand, if gastric content (rich in Cl) is lost through vomiting, the patient develops metabolic alkalosis. A similar disorder is seen in patients with cystic fibrosis (loss of NaCl). Both of these conditions can lead to hypokalemia and should respond to appropriate KCl and NaCl supplementation.

SECTION 9

The Endocrine System

ACROMEGALY

METHOD OF

Shereen Ezzat, MD

Regardless of etiology, sustained growth hormone (GH) excess results in physical disfigurement associated with debilitating arthritis, cardiac dysfunction, colonic neoplasia, and reduced survival. This update reflects the current understanding of the pathophysiology of GH hypersecretion as it relates to the diagnosis, complications, monitoring, and treatment of patients with acromegaly.

Diagnostic Studies

The diagnosis of acromegaly rests on the demonstration of excessive, autonomous secretion of GH. Isolated, random sampling of serum GH is usually insufficient to establish the diagnosis, because GH secretion is rhythmic, under dual regulation by the hypothalamus. Growth hormone-releasing hormone (GHRH) stimulates GH synthesis and release, while somatostatin (SS) suppresses its release. SS secretion is also episodic and is increased during fasting, sleep and obesity. In normal individuals sampled during a 12-hour period, at least 75% of serum GH values are below the limits of assay detection (<0.2 ng/mL) and circulating serum GH levels may spontaneously reach several times "the normal range" in healthy individuals. Patients with active acromegaly may have GH levels within the "normal range." Therefore, based on currently available GH assays, the diagnosis of acromegaly requires demonstration of lack of GH suppression to <1 ng/mL following the oral ingestion of 75 g of glucose.

While somatic growth in adults is primarily under the influence of GH, its effects are largely mediated through insulin-like growth factor I (IGF-I), previously known as somatomedin C (Sm-C). This growth factor is produced in most tissues, and acts locally to regulate cell growth and differentiation. Circulating IGF-I is mainly of liver origin and is dependent on GH stimulation. Serum IGF-I levels are usually elevated in most patients with active acromegaly. Poorly controlled diabetes mellitus results in impaired hepatic production of IGF-I. Similarly, IGF-I levels decline with normal aging and during periods of starvation. These conditions can therefore lead to a falsely low IGF-I in patients with active acromegaly. Conversely, IGF-I levels rise during normal pregnancy and puberty, reaching two to three times higher values, resulting in a falsely high IGF-I level in subjects who do not have the disease. With these exceptions, an elevated IGF-I level confirms the diagnosis of acromegaly. Moreover, circulating levels of total IGF-I do not fluctuate as rapidly as GH. Indeed, serial IGF-I levels have proven to be a practical alternative for measuring disease activity in most acromegalic patients.

Monitoring of Disease Activity

Traditional polyclonal radioimmunoassay (RIA) was considered to result in suppression of GH to <2 ng/mL after an oral glucose challenge in normal subjects. This was also accepted as evidence for acromegaly disease remission. Most laboratories now use the more sensitive immunoradiometric assays (IRMA), with a normal cut-off of <1.0 ng/mL following glucose ingestion. With the development of more sensitive IGF-I and IGF-binding protein-3 (IGFBP-3) assays, additional tools are now available to assess the GH/IGF-I axis. Recent studies demonstrate that sensitive GH measurements by IRMA are superior to the RIA method in that overlap between patients with and without active disease is better delineated. Furthermore, while serum IGFBP-3 levels correlate overall with IGF-I levels, total IGFBP-3 levels are not always predictive of disease status. Up to one third of patients with active disease have normal total IGFBP-3 levels. Correlating patients' symptoms with these measurements is necessary especially in the unusual cases where GH and IGF-I measurements provide discordant values.

Treatment Objectives

The aims of treatment in acromegaly include restoration of normal GH secretion and responsiveness to stimulation as well as attainment of a normal age-adjusted IGF-I level. The presence of any mass effect should be relieved. Most important, however, is the prevention, or at least arrest, of long-term complications and excess mortality associated with this condition.

The general consensus is that acromegaly is associated with double the risk of mortality mainly from an increased incidence of cardiovascular disease. Multivariate analysis revealed that survival was significantly influenced by the last known GH, presence of hypertension or cardiac disease at diagnosis, and duration of symptoms prior to diagnosis. Survival among acromegalic patients was reduced by an average of 10 years. A more recent multicenter retrospective cohort study of 1362 patients from the United Kingdom also revealed that the mortality rate for colon cancer was higher than expected. This and another U.S.-based study confirmed that the overall mortality rate in patients with post-treatment GH levels <2.5 ng/mL was comparable with the general population. These data provide the framework for more rational objective measures to validate treatment outcomes. Whether patients with acromegaly have an increased risk of neoplasia in general and colon polyps in particular remains unclear. Furthermore, the influence of treatment on neoplastic disorders in acromegalics remains unproven.

Therapeutic Options

Therapeutic options for the management of acromegaly and/or gigantism include pharmacotherapy, surgery, and/or radiation. Regardless of the approach, it is important to recognize that the criteria that represent biochemical cure may be difficult to achieve. For each type of pituitary adenoma associated with a distinct clinical syndrome, over the years specialists have gravitated in attitude from one end of the spectrum to the other.

SURGERY

Transsphenoidal adenomectomy by an experienced neurosurgeon has traditionally been regarded as the primary form of treatment for acromegaly. A transcranial approach is sometimes necessary for patients with tumors demonstrating extensive suprasellar or parasellar extension. Rapid reduction in GH levels with concomitant improvement in clinical symptomatology can be achieved. GH levels are reduced to a conservative level of <5 ng/mL in up to 80% of patients with microadenomas and in approximately 50% to 60% of those harboring macroadenomas. The frequency of surgical success, however, is closely correlated to the size and degree of invasiveness of the tumor, as well as to the surgical expertise.

PHARMACOLOGIC APPROACHES

The development of somatostatin analogues has resulted in a more aggressive attitude toward the management of patients with persistently active disease. Although somatostatin analogues reduce GH and IGF-I levels and alleviate symptoms in 50% to 70% of patients, tumor-size reduction is limited to at most 30% of patients. These findings have supported the use of these agents as secondary therapy in patients who have had surgery and who continue to have elevated GH and IGF-I levels. In addition, medical therapy has been advocated for acromegalic patients who refuse surgery or who are poor surgical candidates. The controversial issue revolves around whether medical therapy should be considered as *primary* therapy for patients with acromegaly. Limited data from nonrandomized studies demonstrate that somatostatin analogues are effective as long-term agents in normalizing GH and IGF-I levels in approximately two thirds of patients who have not received any other form of treatment including pituitary surgery. The general consensus is that patients with GH-secreting microadenomas should undergo surgery to obtain definitive adenomectomy. For those patients with macroadenomas, medical pretreatment might be considered with the view that the two treatments may synergistically interact. Depending on the response, subsequent surgery should be considered if complete or radical resection is feasible.

Octreotide (Sandostatin) was the first synthetic modified octapeptide analogue of somatostatin that resisted enzymatic degradation and had an extended half-life of nearly 2 hours, lending itself to clinical application for suppression of GH hypersecretion. This agent has now been in use for more than a decade. Its clinical effects, the rapid and significant improvement of most features of the disease, are well described. Mean GH levels decline by more than 25% in 70% of subjects, usually within an hour of administration of 100 μg of octreotide subcutaneously (SC). Maximal suppression is reached within 2 hours and usually lasts for 6 hours. Because the GH response is rapid, this assessment can be done at the outset to identify responsive patients. In subjects whose GH levels return to baseline prior to the end of the dosing interval, the frequency of administration can be increased. To address some of these shortcomings, newer formulations of somatostatin analogues (octreotide, lanreotide[1]) with even longer actions have been developed. Administered as a single intramuscular (IM) injection (10 to 30 mg every 28 days), they result in similar clinical benefits to those achieved with the subcutaneous form. Nevertheless, direct comparison between the SC and long-acting preparations of the somatostatin analogues in controlling acromegaly-related complications has not been demonstrated.

The impact of somatostatin analogues on acromegaly related complications is best studied in terms of impaired cardiovascular function. Glucose-suppressed GH levels to <1 ng/mL together with normalization of plasma IGF-I levels for 1 year are associated with significant improvement, but not complete normalization, of left ventricular ejection fraction. In contrast, persistence of elevated GH was associated with increased systolic blood pressure and impaired cardiac performance.

Somatostatin analogues represent the current agents of choice in the medical treatment of acromegaly. Where they fall within the scheme of management of different patients, however, requires individual assessment. The use of somatostatin analogues is of obvious potential benefit to those patients with persistently nonsuppressible GH and elevated IGF-I levels following pituitary surgery. It may also constitute primary therapy for those who cannot tolerate surgery. Less clear is the potential role of these agents as primary therapy for those with aggressive lesions in whom surgically induced remissions are difficult if not impossible to achieve.

GH-receptor antagonists represent a new class of therapy that has recently been approved. The agent developed competes with natural GH for binding with the GH receptor. Unlike normal GH, this antagonist prevents GH receptor dimerization and signaling, thus blocking GH action and IGF-I generation. Daily SC administration (10 to 20 mg) of the first antagonist (pegvisomant [Somavert]) resulted in normalization of IGF-I levels in more than 80% of acromegalic patients. The long-term effects of this agent on pituitary tumor growth need to be carefully monitored. Furthermore, studies are underway to determine the efficacy of adding this agent to somatostatin analogues compared with treatment with pegvisomant alone.

RADIOTHERAPY

This adjunctive therapeutic option is usually reserved for patients who have failed pituitary surgery and/or medical therapy. It has lost momentum in the last few years as more reports emerge reporting a lack of efficacy in achieving normalization of IGF-I levels. Multiple techniques for irradiation of pituitary tumors have been examined. Conventional external-beam irradiation for a total dose of 4500 rads results in GH reduction in most subjects. GH levels decline by approximately 15% per year, so that values <5 ng/mL are reached by 40% and 70% of subjects after 5 and 10 years, respectively. Tumor growth is arrested, followed by size regression. Adverse effects include transient hair loss and irreversible hypopituitarism. However, IGF-I normalization rates are disappointing. More significant is the finding that a

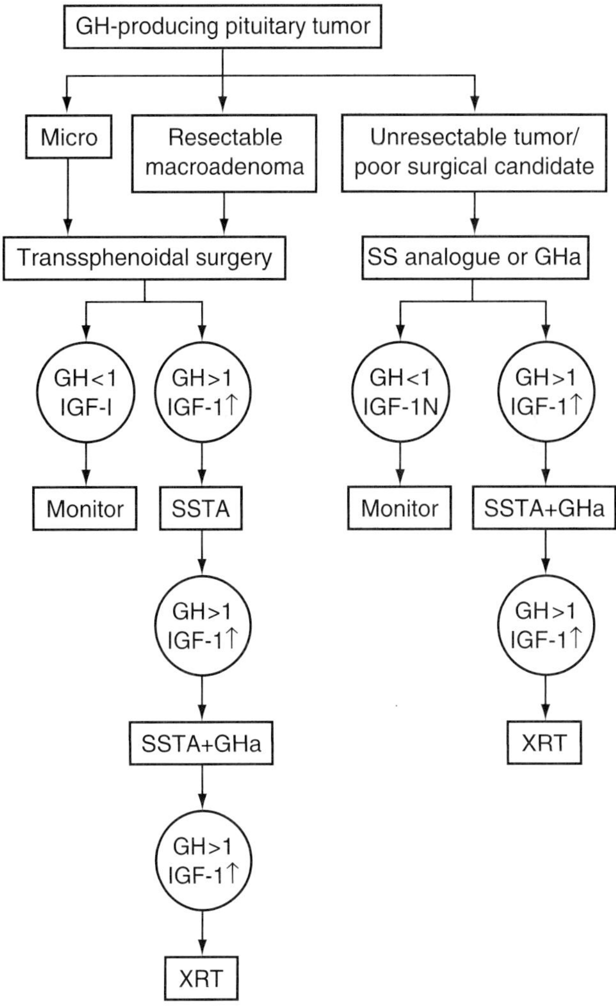

FIGURE 1 A suggested therapeutic algorithm. *Abbreviations:* GH = growth hormone; GHa = growth hormone antagonist; IGF = insulin-like growth factor; SSTA = somatostatin analogue; XRT = external-beam radiation therapy.

[1]Not FDA approved for this indication.

random GH concentration <1.5 ng/mL is associated with a pathologically high IGF-I in nearly one half of patients. Recently, gamma knife stereotactic radiotherapy was investigated. Mean time to normalization of GH and IGF-I levels was 1.5 years in the group treated with the gamma knife compared with approximately 7 years in those treated with fractionated radiotherapy. These early results suggest that the use of stereotactic radiosurgery may become the preferred treatment of choice for patients with surgical and medically refractory disease.

Conclusions

Acromegaly is often a chronic debilitating condition that, if left uncontrolled, is associated with increased morbidity and mortality. The diagnosis is established by documenting autonomous GH hypersecretion and by imaging of the pituitary. Surgical resection of the responsible pituitary adenoma represents the cornerstone of management. This was recently challenged, however, because a strict target of normalization of IGF-I and a glucose-suppressed GH to <1 ng/mL is difficult to achieve by surgery alone. Adjunctive therapy is frequently necessary, as complete resection is often not possible. This has prompted the view that primary medical therapy may be a suitable option to consider for some patients. Persistent disease is now well documented to be associated with increased morbidity and mortality. Figure 1 is a suggested therapeutic algorithm. Somatostatin analogues are of particular benefit to those patients with persistently nonsuppressible GH and/or elevated IGF-I levels following pituitary surgery or during the interim period following radiotherapy. It may also constitute primary therapy for those who decline, are not likely to achieve a remission, or cannot tolerate surgery or irradiation. The use of GH antagonists alone or in combination with somatostatin analogues, while pharmacologically rational, remains to be proven.

ADRENAL INSUFFICIENCY

METHOD OF

David C. Aron, MD, MS

The clinical syndrome of adrenocortical insufficiency results from deficient levels of glucocorticoids and/or mineralocorticoids. Reduced adrenal production of these steroid hormones results from either the destruction/dysfunction of the cortex (primary adrenocortical insufficiency, or Addison's disease) or from deficient pituitary ACTH (adrenocorticotropin) secretion (secondary glucocorticoid insufficiency). Primary adrenocortical insufficiency is uncommon, but readily treatable. Survival now depends primarily upon the underlying cause of the adrenal insufficiency. This section focuses on glucocorticoid deficiency.

Etiology

The etiology of primary adrenocortical insufficiency (Table 1) has changed over time; tuberculosis, once the major cause of adrenocortical insufficiency, has been superseded in frequency by autoimmune adrenalitis. Metastases from an extra-adrenal cancer to the adrenal glands are far more common than clinical adrenal insufficiency, but the latter is more common than previously thought. Primary adrenal insufficiency in AIDS is usually caused by opportunistic infections such as cytomegalovirus and tuberculosis, and adrenocortical insufficiency is usually a late manifestation of HIV infection. As patients with malignant disease and HIV infection live longer, more cases of adrenal insufficiency will be seen. Adrenal hemorrhage typically occurs in the setting of anticoagulant therapy, the postoperative period, or the primary antiphospholipid antibody syndrome. Recent studies point to the possibility of adrenal insufficiency as a consequence of critical illness with severe inflammatory disorders (e.g., septic shock). Glucocorticoid therapy is the most common cause of secondary glucocorticoid insufficiency followed by pituitary tumors (see relevant articles).

Pathophysiology

Clinical manifestations of adrenocortical insufficiency usually occur only after the loss of more than 90% of both adrenal cortices. When adrenocortical destruction is gradual, a phase of decreased adrenal reserve (normal basal steroid secretion,

TABLE 1 Causes of Primary Adrenocortical Insufficiency

Autoimmune
Infectious—tuberculosis, cytomegalovirus, fungi (histoplasmosis, coccidioidomycosis), HIV, sepsis
Cancer—metastases, lymphoma
Adrenal hemorrhage
Infiltrative disorders—amyloidosis, hemochromatosis
Congenital adrenal hyperplasia
Miscellaneous—adrenoleukodystrophy, familial glucocorticoid deficiency and hypoplasia, drugs (ketoconazole, metyrapone, aminoglutethimide, trilostane[2], mitotane, etomidate)

[2]Not available in the United States.

but impaired response to stress) precedes frank adrenal insufficiency. Acute adrenal crisis can be precipitated during this initial phase by the stresses of surgery, trauma, or infection. As destruction of cortical tissue continues, even basal secretion of mineralocorticoids and glucocorticoids becomes deficient, leading to the manifestations of chronic adrenocortical insufficiency. If the destruction is rapid, a patient's first presentation may be crisis or impending crisis.

Clinical Features

The clinical features (Table 2) depend on which steroids are deficient, the magnitude of the deficiency, the rate of development of the deficiency, and the presence or absence of intercurrent illness. Destruction of the adrenals results in deficiencies of both glucocorticoids and mineralocorticoids. In secondary glucocorticoid deficiency, ACTH deficiency is the primary event and leads to decreased cortisol and adrenal androgen secretion; aldosterone secretion is usually normal. Cortisol deficiency causes weakness, fatigue, anorexia, nausea and vomiting, hypotension, hyponatremia, and hypoglycemia. Mineralocorticoid deficiency produces renal sodium wasting and potassium retention and can lead to severe dehydration, hypotension, hyponatremia, hyperkalemia, and acidosis. The chief signs and symptoms of chronic primary adrenocortical insufficiency are weakness and fatigue, weight loss, anorexia, and gastrointestinal disturbances, especially nausea and vomiting, and hyperpigmentation. Hyperpigmentation results from increased ACTH levels and may be generalized or localized to the buccal mucosa and gums, palmar creases, nail beds, or other areas. Hyperpigmentation is increased in sun-exposed areas and accentuated over pressure areas such as the knuckles, toes, elbows, and knees, and may be accompanied by increased numbers of freckles. The gastrointestinal symptoms may mimic a primary intra-abdominal process. Hypotension is seen, most often accompanied by orthostatic symptoms. A minority of patients craves salt. Hypoglycemia is unusual in adults but may be provoked by fasting, fever, infection, or nausea and vomiting. Hypoglycemia occurs more commonly in secondary adrenal insufficiency. Decreased secretion of adrenal androgens can result in loss of axillary and pubic hair in women. Amenorrhea results from weight loss, chronic illness or associated primary ovarian failure. Autoimmune Addison's disease is frequently accompanied by other immune disorders (e.g., hypothyroidism, vitiligo). Hyponatremia and hyperkalemia are classic manifestations of the mineralocorticoid deficiency. Volume depletion results in azotemia. Laboratory findings of glucocorticoid deficiency include eosinophilia, relative lymphocytosis, and hypoglycemia. Acute adrenal (addisonian) crisis occurs in patients with Addison's disease who are exposed to the stresses of infection, trauma, surgery, or dehydration as a consequence of salt deprivation, vomiting, or diarrhea. During this crisis, clinical features of adrenocortical insufficiency are exaggerated (e.g., volume depletion, hypotension); adrenal insufficiency should be considered in any patient with unexplained vascular collapse. Abdominal pain may mimic an acute intra-abdominal emergency. Weakness, apathy, and confusion are usual. Fever occurs as a consequence of infection or glucocorticoid deficiency per se. Shock and coma may rapidly lead to death in untreated patients. The diagnosis of acute adrenal hemorrhage should be considered in the deteriorating patient with unexplained abdominal or flank pain, vascular collapse, hyperpyrexia, or hypoglycemia. Secondary adrenal (glucocorticoid) insufficiency is usually chronic and the manifestations may be nonspecific. However, acute crisis can occur in undiagnosed patients, in corticosteroid-treated patients who do not receive increased steroid dosage during periods of stress, or after surgical removal of a functional adrenal tumor. Features may include weakness, lethargy, easy fatigability, anorexia, nausea, and, occasionally, vomiting, arthralgias, myalgias, and hypoglycemia. Because pituitary secretion of ACTH is deficient, hyperpigmentation is not present. In addition, mineralocorticoid secretion is usually normal so that volume depletion, dehydration, and hyperkalemia are usually absent. Hypotension occurs only in acute presentations. Hyponatremia may occur as a result of water retention and an inability to excrete a water load; there is a lack of glucocorticoid negative feedback on antidiuretic hormone as well as the reduction in glomerular filtration associated with hypocortisolism. Acute decompensation with severe hypotension or shock unresponsive to vasopressors may occur. Patients with secondary adrenal insufficiency commonly have additional features that suggest the diagnosis (e.g. a history of glucocorticoid therapy or manifestations of deficiencies of other pituitary hormones).

TABLE 2 Clinical Features of Adrenocortical Insufficiency

Chronic Primary Adrenocortical Insufficiency	Acute Adrenal Crisis
Weakness, fatigue, anorexia, weight loss	Hypotension and shock
Hyperpigmentation	Fever
Hypotension	Dehydration, volume depletion
Gastrointestinal disturbances	Nausea, vomiting, anorexia
Salt craving	Weakness, apathy, depressed mentation
Postural symptoms	Electrolyte abnormalities—hyperkalemia,
Electrolyte abnormalities—hyperkalemia	Hyponatremia, Hypoglycemia, Hypercalcemia
Hyponatremia, Hypoglycemia, Hypercalcemia	

Diagnosis

Therapy should not be delayed for the purpose of diagnostic testing. In the acutely ill, patient therapy should be instituted at once and the diagnosis established when the patient is stable. The diagnosis of adrenal insufficiency requires the demonstration of inappropriately low cortisol production and involves assessment of the pituitary–adrenal axis Normally, cortisol is secreted episodically from the adrenal cortex with a diurnal rhythm paralleling the secretion of ACTH. Consequently, normal levels of plasma cortisol constitute a broad range; the levels found in adrenal insufficiency may at any given time fall within the "normal" range. The hypothalamic–pituitary adrenal axis responds to "stress" with an increase in CRH (corticotropin-releasing hormone) secretion, followed by an increase in ACTH secretion, followed, in turn, by an increase in cortisol secretion. Such "stress" includes hypotension, hypoglycemia, and a variety of serious illnesses. The diagnostic utility of single plasma cortisol concentrations is limited by the episodic nature of cortisol secretion. However, an unstressed 8 AM plasma cortisol level <3 μg/dL (80 nmol/L) is strongly suggestive of adrenal insufficiency, whereas a level >20 μg/dL (550 nmol/L) at any time, makes clinical adrenal insufficiency highly unlikely. Dynamic testing has been favored over baseline measurements. In fact, severe acute illness constitutes a dynamic test, albeit unplanned. Elevated cortisol levels (>20 μg/dL [550 nmol/L]) would be the normal response. Similarly, ACTH levels should be elevated. Diagnostic tests used when the patient is stable include: ACTH administration which directly stimulates adrenal secretion; metyrapone which inhibits cortisol synthesis, thereby stimulating pituitary ACTH secretion; and insulin-induced hypoglycemia which stimulates ACTH release by increasing CRH secretion.

The rapid ACTH stimulation test measures the acute adrenal response to ACTH and is used to diagnose both primary and secondary adrenal insufficiencies. A synthetic human ACTH (cosyntropin [Cortrosyn]) is administered in a dose of 0.25 mg intramuscularly or intravenously after obtaining a baseline cortisol sample; additional samples are obtained at 30 or 60 minutes following the injection. The peak cortisol response, 30 to 60 minutes later, should exceed 18 to 20 μg/dL (500 to 550 nm/L). Use of a lower dose of ACTH, 1 μg, is thought to be a more sensitive indicator of adrenocortical insufficiency, although this is controversial. A normal response to the rapid ACTH stimulation test excludes both primary adrenal insufficiency (by directly assessing adrenal reserve) and overt secondary adrenal insufficiency with adrenal atrophy. However, a normal response does not rule out partial ACTH deficiency (decreased pituitary reserve). When the diagnosis remains uncertain, metyrapone testing can be used. Metyrapone blocks the pathway of cortisol synthesis, thus stimulating ACTH secretion, which, in turn, increases the secretion and plasma levels of 11-deoxycortisol (a cortisol precursor). A normal response to adequate blockade (cortisol <5 μg/dL [135 nmol/L]) is a plasma 11-deoxycortisol level greater than 7 μg/dL (190 nmol/L) and a plasma ACTH level greater than 100 pg/mL (22 pmol/L). This test is not without risk and it should not be performed in a patient who is already symptomatic from glucocorticoid deficiency. Insulin-induced hypoglycemia tests the entire hypothalamic–pituitary–adrenal system. A normal cortisol response is a peak level greater than 18 to 20 μg/dL (485 to 540 nmol/L) and plasma ACTH >100 pg/mL (22 pmol/L). This test is associated with significant risk and is contraindicated in the presence of ischemic heart disease, cerebrovascular disease, seizure disorder, or in patients with low baseline cortisols (e.g., <3-5 μg/dL). When performed, the patient should be under constant medical supervision. It is rarely necessary in any patient in whom the likelihood of adrenal insufficiency is reasonably high.

If adrenal insufficiency is present, plasma ACTH levels are used to differentiate primary and secondary forms. The normal range for plasma ACTH, using a sensitive immunometric assay (IMA), is 9 to 52 pg/mL (2 to 11 pmol/L). In patients with primary adrenal insufficiency, plasma ACTH levels exceed the upper limit of the normal range (>52 pg/mL [11 pmol/L]) and usually exceed 200 pg/mL (44 pmol/L). Plasma ACTH concentration is usually less than 30 pg/mL (6.8 pmol/L) in patients with secondary adrenal insufficiency. Note that patients with secondary adrenal insufficiency exhibit inappropriately low plasma ACTH levels (i.e., levels are not elevated). A level in the "normal range" is inappropriate for someone with low cortisol levels. Patients with primary adrenal insufficiency should undergo imaging with abdominal computed tomography (CT) scan. CT can detect adrenal calcification and adrenal enlargement. Adrenal calcification is found in approximately 50% of patients with tuberculous Addison's disease and in some patients with other invasive or hemorrhagic causes of adrenal insufficiency. Bilateral adrenal enlargement in association with adrenal insufficiency may be seen with tuberculosis, fungal infections, cytomegalovirus, malignant and nonmalignant infiltrative diseases, and adrenal hemorrhage. Patients with secondary adrenal insufficiency should undergo anatomical evaluation of the hypothalamus and pituitary (e.g., visual field examination, magnetic resonance imaging [MRI]), and functional evaluation to assess for secondary hypothyroidism, gonadal deficiency, and growth hormone deficiency.

Suppression of the hypothalamic–pituitary–adrenal axis may occur with doses of prednisone as low as 5 mg/day, although its development or degree is difficult to predict. In general, patients who develop clinical features of Cushing's syndrome or who have received glucocorticoids equivalent to 10 to 20 mg of prednisone per day for 3 weeks or more should be assumed to have clinically significant axis suppression. Evaluation of response to stress is not performed until glucocorticoids have been tapered to physiologic replacement levels and morning cortisol exceeds 10 μg/mL. Even after the glucocorticoid dose has been reduced to physiologic levels, axis suppression (i.e., secondary adrenal insufficiency) can persist for months to years.

Treatment

The aim of treatment of adrenocortical insufficiency is to produce levels of glucocorticoids and mineralocorticoids equivalent to those achieved in an individual with normal hypothalamic–pituitary–adrenal function under similar circumstances. Treatment for acute Addisonian crisis should be instituted as soon as the diagnosis is suspected. Therapy includes administration of glucocorticoids; correction of dehydration, hypovolemia, hypoglycemia, and electrolyte abnormalities; general supportive measures; and treatment of coexisting or precipitating disorders (Table 3). Cortisol (hydrocortisone hemisuccinate or phosphate) in doses of 100 mg intravenously is given every 6 hours for the first 24 hours. At these high doses hydrocortisone has sufficient sodium-retaining potency so that additional mineralocorticoid therapy is not required in patients with primary adrenocortical insufficiency. The response to therapy is usually rapid, with improvement occurring within 12 hours or less. If improvement occurs and the patient is stable, 50 mg every 6 hours is given on the second day, and in most patients the dosage may then be gradually reduced to approximately 10 mg three times daily by the fourth or fifth day. In severely ill patients, especially in those with additional major complications (e.g., sepsis), higher cortisol doses (100 mg intravenously every 6 to 8 hours) are maintained until the patient is stable. In primary adrenal insufficiency, mineralocorticoid replacement, in the form of fludrocortisone (see below), is added when the total cortisol dosage has been reduced to 50 to 60 mg/day. In secondary adrenocortical (glucocorticoid) insufficiency with acute crisis, only glucocorticoid replacement is needed. Cortisol can be used as above. However, if the salt-retaining properties of high doses of cortisol present a risk (e.g., in a patient with congestive heart failure prone to fluid overload), synthetic steroids with low mineralocorticoid activity, such as prednisolone or dexamethasone, can be used.

Intravenous glucose and saline are administered to correct volume depletion, hypotension, and hypoglycemia. Volume deficits may be severe in Addison's disease, and hypotension and shock may not respond to vasopressors unless glucocorticoids are administered. Hyperkalemia and acidosis are usually corrected with cortisol and volume replacement; however, an occasional patient may require specific therapy for these abnormalities. Therapy for the factors that precipitated the crisis (e.g., infection) is also necessary.

Patients with Addison's disease require life-long glucocorticoid and mineralocorticoid therapy (Table 4). Cortisol (hydrocortisone) is the glucocorticoid preparation of first choice. The basal production rate of cortisol is approximately 8 to 12 mg/m^2 per day. The maintenance dose of hydrocortisone is usually 15 to 25 mg daily in adults. The oral dose is usually divided to more closely mimic normal cortisol secretion. Thrice daily regimens (e.g., 10 mg in the morning, 5 mg in the afternoon, and 5 mg in the evening) are effective in maintaining well-being and normal energy levels. Twice-daily dosing regimens (e.g., 10 to 20 mg in the morning on arising and 5 to 10 mg later in the day) yield satisfactory responses in most patients. Insomnia is a side effect of glucocorticoid administration and can usually be prevented by administering the last dose at 4:00 to 5:00 PM. It is generally expected that the daily dose of hydrocortisone should be doubled during periods of minor stress, and the dose needs to be increased to as much as 200 to 300 mg per day during periods of major stress, such as a surgical procedure.

Fludrocortisone (Florinef) is used for mineralocorticoid therapy; the usual doses are 0.05 to 0.2 mg

TABLE 3 Management of Acute Adrenal Crisis

Glucocorticoid Replacement

1. Administer hydrocortisone sodium phosphate or sodium succinate, 100 mg intravenously every 6 hours for 24 hours.
2. When the patient is stable, reduce the dosage by one half to 50 mg every 6 hours.
3. Taper dosage to maintenance therapy by day 4 or 5 (assuming appropriate clinical response) and add mineralocorticoid therapy as required.
4. Maintain or increase the dose to 200-400 mg/day if complications persist or occur.

General and Supportive Measures

1. Correct volume depletion, dehydration, and hypoglycemia with intravenous saline and glucose.
2. Evaluate and correct infection and other precipitating factors.

TABLE 4 Regimen for Maintenance Therapy of Primary Adrenocortical Insufficiency

1. Hydrocortisone, 10-15 mg in AM, 5 mg in the afternoon, and 5 mg in the evening
2. Fludrocortisone, 0.05-0.1 mg orally in AM
3. Clinical follow-up: maintenance of normal weight, blood pressure, and electrolytes with regression of clinical features
4. Patient education plus identification card, medical alert bracelet or necklace ("dog tag"); useful patient education materials are available from the National Institutes of Health at: http://www.cc.nih.gov/ccc/patient_education/pepubs/mngadrins.pdf
5. Increased hydrocortisone dosage during "stress"; double the oral dose for mild illness; provide patient with injectable form of glucocorticoid for emergency use

per day orally in the morning. Because of its long half-life, a single morning dose is usually sufficient. Approximately 10% of addisonian patients can be managed with cortisol and Adequate dietary sodium intake alone and do not require fludrocortisone. Secondary adrenocortical insufficiency is treated with the cortisol dosages described above for the primary form. Fludrocortisone is rarely required. The recovery of normal function of the hypothalamic–pituitary–adrenal axis following suppression by exogenous glucocorticoids may take weeks to years, and its duration is not readily predictable. Consequently, prolonged replacement therapy may be required. Recent studies have pointed to the potential benefits of dehydroepiandrosterone (DHEA) in doses of 50 mg per day, particularly in women, in terms of improvement in well-being.

Response to Therapy

Traditionally, assessment of the adequacy of glucocorticoid replacement in patients with adrenal insufficiency has involved clinical, but not biochemical measures. These clinical signs include good appetite and sense of well-being. Adequate treatment results in the disappearance of weakness, malaise, and fatigue. Anorexia and other gastrointestinal symptoms resolve, and weight returns to normal. The hyperpigmentation invariably improves but may not entirely disappear. Inadequate cortisol administration leads to persistence of these symptoms of adrenal insufficiency, and excessive pigmentation will remain. Obviously, signs of Cushing's syndrome indicate overtreatment. Patients receiving excessive doses of glucocorticoids are also at risk for increased bone loss and clinically significant osteoporosis. Therefore, the replacement dose of glucocorticoids should be maintained at the lowest amount needed to provide the patient with a proper sense of well-being. Potential risks, especially of overtreatment, have prompted more biochemical testing. Although the use of 24-hour urinary cortisol levels might seem an attractive method for following such patients, there are serious limitations. A very high level of urinary cortisol would suggest over-replacement, but by no means confirm it. Plasma cortisol day curves (i.e., multiple samples for plasma cortisol concentration) have been proposed, but not widely adopted because of their inconvenience, expense, and variation among individuals in terms of the plasma levels of cortisol achieved with orally administered hydrocortisone or cortisol. The use of other glucocorticoids (e.g., prednisone) could not be assessed with these measures. Day curves are reserved for patients who appear to require higher than expected replacement doses. ACTH levels are not useful for monitoring even in treated primary adrenal insufficiency. Plasma ACTH levels fall toward the normal range, but because of the dose and timing of physiologic replacement, plasma ACTH levels usually remain in the high-normal to modestly elevated range. Although undertreatment with mineralocorticoids may lead to fatigue and malaise, adequacy of mineralocorticoid replacement is usually assessed with measurements of blood pressure and electrolytes. Biochemical assessment of the renin–angiotensin system is not routinely performed. With adequate treatment, the blood pressure is normal without orthostatic change, and serum sodium and potassium remain within the normal ranges. Hypertension and hypokalemia result if the fludrocortisone dose is excessive. Some endocrinologists monitor plasma renin activity (PRA) as an objective measure of fludrocortisone replacement.

Prevention of Adrenal Crisis

The development of acute adrenal insufficiency in previously diagnosed and treated patients is almost entirely preventable. Patient education, self-management, and increased glucocorticoid dosages during illness all play roles. The patient should be informed about the necessity for lifelong therapy, the possible consequences of acute illness, and the necessity for increased therapy and medical assistance during acute illness. An identification card or bracelet should be carried or worn at all times. The cortisol dose should be doubled with the development of a minor illness; the usual maintenance dosage may be resumed in 24 to 48 hours if improvement occurs. Increased mineralocorticoid therapy is not required. If symptoms persist or become worse, the patient should continue increased cortisol doses and seek medical attention. Vomiting may result in an inability to ingest or absorb oral cortisol, and diarrhea in addisonian patients may precipitate a crisis because of rapid fluid and electrolyte losses. Patients must understand that if these symptoms occur, they should seek immediate medical assistance so that parenteral glucocorticoid therapy can be given. Patients can be given injectable forms of glucocorticoid (e.g., dexamethasone) as a temporizing measure until medical assistance can be obtained.

TABLE 5 Steroid Coverage for Surgery

1. Correct electrolytes, blood pressure, and volume status if necessary.
2. Administer hydrocortisone sodium phosphate or sodium succinate, 100 mg intramuscularly, preoperatively (on call to operating room).
3. Administer 50 mg intramuscularly or intravenously in the recovery room and then every 6 hours for the first 24 hours.
4. If progress is satisfactory, reduce dosage by one half to 25 mg every 6 hours for 24 hours and then taper to maintenance dosage over 3 to 5 days. Resume previous fludrocortisone dose when the patient is taking oral medications.
5. Maintain or increase hydrocortisone dosage to 200-400 mg/day if fever, hypotension, or other complications occur.

Steroid Coverage for Surgery

The normal physiologic response to surgical stress involves an increase in cortisol secretion. The increased glucocorticoid activity may serve primarily to modulate the immunologic response to stress. Thus, patients with primary or secondary adrenocortical insufficiency scheduled for elective surgery require increased glucocorticoid coverage. This problem is also encountered in patients with pituitary–adrenal suppression caused by exogenous glucocorticoid therapy. Table 5 outlines the principles of management. Recent clinical trials suggest a role for physiologic glucocorticoid replacement therapy in patients with sepsis syndrome.

CUSHING'S SYNDROME

METHOD OF

Susan Samson, MD, PhD, and

Ashok Balasubramanyam, MD

Cushing's syndrome (CS) is an uncommon illness with variable presentation, multiple etiologies, clinical resemblance to common diseases, and complex testing procedures. A reasonable clinical suspicion supported by a systematic diagnostic approach is essential, because random biochemical testing frequently results in equivocal test results that can frustrate both patient and physician. Treatment of a successfully diagnosed patient is usually rewarded by cure or substantial amelioration of a highly morbid condition.

Clinical Suspicion

In keeping with the ubiquitous nature of glucocorticoid signaling, the signs and symptoms of CS are protean (Table 1). No single finding is predominant, nor is one sign or symptom pathognomonic. The most commonly reported features are truncal obesity, facial plethora, and "moon" facies. Hypertension, diabetes mellitus, hirsutism, acne, proximal muscle weakness, skin atrophy, or ecchymoses are frequently present. Muscle atrophy, purple striae, osteoporosis, and nephrolithiasis are present more often in men than in women.

Preclinical and subclinical forms of CS add to the diagnostic challenge. Preclinical CS refers to a mild hypercortisolemic state preceding the development of physical signs. Subclinical CS refers to patients who lack clinical signs of CS but may have metabolic manifestations ascribable to hypercortisolism, including insulin resistance, obesity, and hypertension. Patients with subclinical CS are at increased risk of developing cardiovascular disease and osteoporosis. Subclinical CS frequently is caused by a cortisol-secreting adrenal nodule, and adrenalectomy may ameliorate the metabolic abnormalities, so it should not be overlooked.

Once CS is suspected, the appropriate approach is to employ biochemical tests to (a) confirm hypercortisolism; (b) if necessary, differentiate true CS from pseudo-Cushing's syndrome; (c) determine adrenocorticotropic hormone (ACTH)-dependence or -independence; and (d) if the CS is ACTH-dependent, determine whether ACTH hypersecretion originates from a pituitary tumor or ectopic source. Imaging techniques should be employed only after careful biochemical testing. Even if suspicion of CS has been raised by an incidentally discovered adrenal or pituitary tumor, the same unbiased approach should be followed.

Screening for Hypercortisolism

It is useful to begin the diagnostic process by considering exogenous causes (see Table 1). Glucocorticoid therapy—usually via the oral route, but also with inhaled medications, intra-articular injections, and topical preparations—is the most common cause of CS. A detailed history is usually sufficient to make this diagnosis. Surreptitious use of glucocorticoids by a malingerer is uncommon. If synthetic glucocorticoids are being used, plasma cortisol (and ACTH) levels will be low, because these compounds do not cross-react with the standard assays for cortisol. Gas chromatography or high-performance liquid chromatography (HPLC) may be used to detect them in the urine. If the malingerer is using prednisone or cortisone, diagnosis may be difficult because these compounds can cross-react with standard cortisol assays.

If an exogenous source of CS is unlikely, endogenous hypercortisolism should be confirmed by sensitive tests. Traditional first-line tests exploit three characteristics of the Cushing's state: (a) persistently elevated cortisol secretion, measured as the amount of cortisol in a 24-hour collection of urine; (b) decreased feedback inhibition, detected by a lack of suppression of serum or urine cortisol levels by dexamethasone; and (c) altered diurnal variation, detected by elevated levels of cortisol in the serum or saliva at midnight. No single test is absolutely accurate, and often a combination is needed (Figure 1).

24-HOUR URINE FREE CORTISOL

Cortisol is cleared by renal excretion, largely as free cortisol and as a glucuronidated form after

TABLE 1 Clinical Features of Cushing's Syndrome

System	Signs and Symptoms
General appearance	Central obesity with sparing of extremities Supraclavicular and dorsocervical fat Edema
Skin	"Moon facies" Facial plethora Violaceous striae Ecchymoses Hirsutism Acne Skin atrophy Hyperpigmentation
Cardiovascular	Hypertension Hypercoagulability
Metabolic	Hyperlipidemia Diabetes mellitus Impaired glucose tolerance
Musculoskeletal	Proximal muscle weakness and wasting Osteopenia or osteoporosis
Psychiatric	Depression Cognitive impairment Emotional lability Euphoria Psychosis
Immune	Opportunistic infections Candidal and other fungal infections
Gonadal	Oligomenorrhea Amenorrhea Impotence Decreased libido
Urinary	Nephrolithiasis Polyuria Hypokalemia

conjugation in the liver. The 24-hour urine free cortisol (UFC) test exploits the fact that unbound cortisol, which comprises approximately 5% of total serum cortisol, is freely filtered into the urine. The UFC measurement is not affected by variations in the serum concentration of cortisol binding globulin, such as with elevated estrogen levels. UFC is best measured by HPLC or gas chromatography–mass spectrometry. Immunoassays are less specific and detect cortisol metabolites, thus falsely elevating the reported levels of cortisol. Even with the more precise methods, the "normal" UFC range is broad, from 20 to 140 μg per day, depending on the laboratory and assay used.

A UFC level three- to fourfold higher than the upper limit of normal for the particular laboratory is diagnostic of CS. More moderate elevations are less specific and may be observed in patients with pseudo-Cushing's states (see below), polycystic ovary syndrome, obesity, or eating disorders. Urine volumes above 3 L per day can elevate UFC levels relative to creatinine excretion, as a consequence of increased filtration of free cortisol and a decrease in the proportion metabolized to cortisone by renal 11β-hydroxysteroid dehydrogenase type 2. When the HPLC method is used, falsely elevated UFC measurements also can occur in patients taking fenofibrate, carbamazepine, or digoxin.

Although the sensitivity of UFC for CS is high, a single UFC test may miss the diagnosis in patients who have episodic hypersecretion of cortisol. Hence, three UFC tests should be performed to increase sensitivity to 98% and specificity to 85%. If clinical suspicion remains following a negative result, the UFC test should be repeated weeks or months later.

LOW-DOSE DEXAMETHASONE SUPPRESSION TESTS

These are based on the principle that "physiologic" doses of dexamethasone should greatly diminish endogenous cortisol synthesis by suppressing pituitary ACTH secretion in normal persons, but not in most patients with endogenous CS. In the standard 2-day protocol, dexamethasone 0.5 mg is administered orally every 6 hours for 48 hours, with a 24-hour collection for UFC or 17-hydroxycorticosteroids (17-OHCS) during the second day. Accepted thresholds for probable CS are >10 μg/day for UFC and >2.5 mg/day for 17-OHCS. Because of its low sensitivity and specificity and inconvenience, many clinicians prefer the simpler overnight dexamethasone suppression test. The patient takes 1 mg of dexamethasone between 11 PM and 12 AM midnight, and a fasting plasma cortisol level is measured at 8 AM the next morning. The cut-off value for this screening test depends on the cortisol assay. With the older fluorometric assays of cortisol, normal responses were defined as suppression to <5.0 μg/dL. With the development of more sensitive immunoassays, a cut-off of 1.8 μg/dL is recommended, with a reported sensitivity of 98%. However, the reduced cut-off value sacrifices specificity, and patients with pseudo-Cushing's syndrome, obesity, diabetes, or elevated cortisol-binding globulin as a result of estrogen use may also have morning plasma cortisol levels >1.8 μg/dL following overnight dexamethasone suppression.

MIDNIGHT SERUM OR SALIVARY CORTISOL

In normal persons, the secretion of cortisol is episodic and diurnal; plasma cortisol levels are highest at 7 AM to 8 AM and lowest around midnight (12 AM). Loss of circadian regulation occurs in CS and can be detected by measuring a midnight cortisol level in the plasma. If the blood is collected under controlled circumstances, a midnight cortisol level >7.5 μg/dL is purported to have 100% sensitivity. If the cut-off is raised to 12 μg/dL, sensitivity is lowered but specificity increases. Measurement of midnight salivary cortisol levels is a convenient alternative to midnight cortisol-level measurement. The salivary cortisol concentration reflects plasma levels quite accurately. The sample can be obtained at home (using the commercially available Salivette), stored at room temperature, and measured by enzyme-linked immunoabsorbent assay (ELISA). Cut-off values and diagnostic accuracy vary, hence these should be ascertained from the specific reference laboratory to which

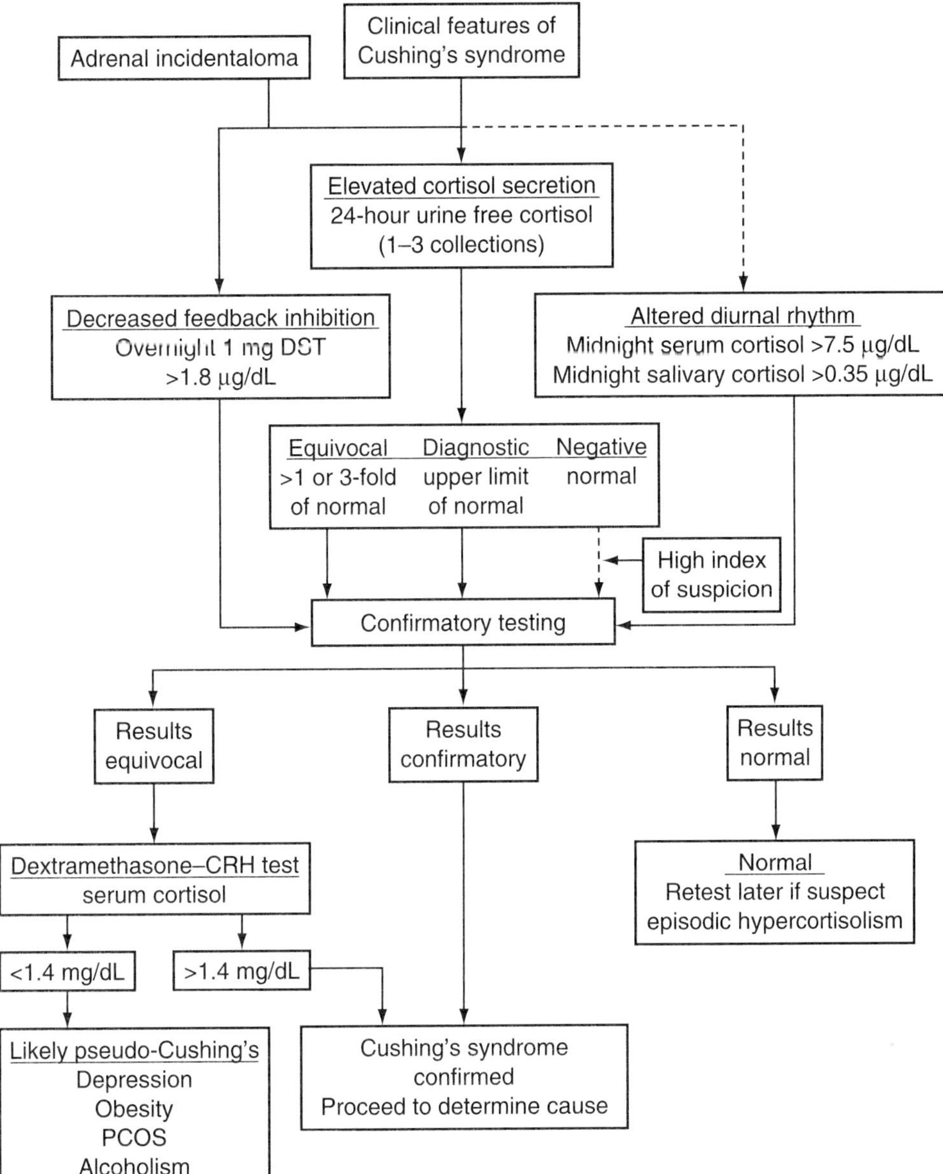

FIGURE 1 Initial evaluation of patients with suspected Cushing's syndrome. See text for steps to follow after confirming the presence of CS. *Abbreviations:* CRH = corticotropin-releasing hormone; DST = dexamethasone suppression test; PCOS = polycystic ovary syndrome.

the sample is sent. A midnight salivary cortisol threshold >0.35 μg/dL has been advocated to diagnose CS, with a diagnostic accuracy similar to that of the 24-hour UFC or midnight cortisol tests in differentiating CS from pseudo-Cushing's syndrome. Hence, the midnight salivary cortisol test may be an appropriate tool to supplement other screening tests.

WHAT TO DO IN THE PATIENT WITH THE INCIDENTAL ADRENAL MASS

The incidence of an unsuspected adrenal mass on abdominal imaging is approximately 1% to 2%, and approximately 15% of these are hormonally active. Subclinical hypercortisolism may occur in 5% to 20% of patients. Therefore, patients with an "incidental" adrenal mass should be screened for CS. The overnight low-dose dexamethasone suppression test has a high sensitivity in this situation, with a cut-off of plasma cortisol <1.8 μg/dL. If the screening test is negative, it is prudent to repeat the test annually for 4 years, especially if the mass is larger than 3 cm and the patient has attendant metabolic risks factors.

Differentiating True Cushing's Syndrome from Pseudo-Cushing's Syndrome

Patients with "pseudo-Cushing's" conditions (Table 2) may respond to the screening tests with values overlapping those for CS. The dexamethasone–corticotropin-releasing hormone (CRH) test is useful to differentiate these persons from those with true CS. A low dose of dexamethasone is administered

TABLE 2 Causes of Hypercortisolism and Cushing's Syndrome

Medications	Exogenous steroids	Iatrogenic: oral, intramuscular, intra-articular, inhaled, topical eye and skin preparations
	Other	Factitious
		Megestrol acetate
Hypercortisolism		Eating disorders
Pseudo-Cushing's syndrome		Acute illness or stress
		Depression
		Alcoholism
		Polycystic ovarian syndrome
		Obesity
Cushing's syndrome		
ACTH dependent	Pituitary	Pituitary adenoma
ACTH independent	ACTH	Corticotroph hyperplasia (ectopic CRH)
	Ectopic	Carcinoid tumors: bronchial, thymic, pancreatic, gastrointestinal
	ACTH	Small cell lung carcinoma
	Ectopic	Medullary thyroid carcinoma
	CRH	Pheochromocytoma
		Pancreatic islet cell tumors
		Uncommon: breast carcinoma, prostate carcinoma, ovarian neoplasms, neuroblastoma
		Bronchial carcinoid
		Pituitary adenoma
		Adrenal adenoma
		Adrenal carcinoma
		Pigmented micronodular adrenal hyperplasia (Carney complex, McCune-Albright syndrome)
		Macronodular adrenal hyperplasia (prolonged ACTH overproduction)
		Adrenal hyperplasia secondary to direct stimulation of aberrant receptors (e.g., by vasopressin, GIP, β-hCG/LH)

Abbreviations: ACTH = adrenocorticotropic hormone; CRH = corticotropin-releasing hormone; GIP = glucose insulinotropic peptide; hCG = human chorionic gonadotropin; LH = luteinizing hormone.

in a sustained fashion to suppress the hypothalamic–pituitary–adrenal axis, and then CRH is administered to stimulate it. The ability of CRH to stimulate ACTH and cortisol production is greater in patients with true CS. Dexamethasone is given orally at a dose of 0.5 mg every 6 hours for 8 doses, starting at 12 noon on day one and ending at 6 AM on day three. Synthetic ovine or human CRH (1 μg/kg up to 100 μg) is administered intravenously at 8 AM on day three, and plasma cortisol levels are measured at baseline and 15 minutes. CS patients will have CRH-stimulated cortisol levels >1.4 μg/dL.

Establishing Adrenocorticotropic Hormone Dependence or Independence

Once endogenous cortisol excess has been confirmed, the next step is to measure the plasma ACTH level, which is elevated in 85% of patients with CS. Of these patients, the majority will have pituitary adenomas, and the rest an ectopic source of ACTH. The blood sample should be drawn at 9 AM, in a tube containing ethylenediaminetetraacetic acid (EDTA) and a protease inhibitor, and then stored on ice or frozen until assayed using a two-site immunoradiometric assay (IRMA).

ACTH INDEPENDENCE

ACTH-independent CS is diagnosed by a fully suppressed undetectable plasma ACTH level (<5 to 10 pg/mL), indicating appropriate negative feedback response by excess cortisol on the pituitary corticotrophs. The usual cause is an autonomously functioning adrenal adenoma or adrenocortical carcinoma. Rarely, bilateral nodular hyperplasia may be the cause, as in inherited diseases such as the Carney complex or McCune-Albright syndrome. CS caused by bilateral hyperplasia rarely occurs as a result of stimulation by vasopressin, β-human chorionic gonadotropin (hCG)/luteinizing hormone (LH), or glucose-dependent insulinotropic polypeptide, because of aberrant expression of the receptors for these hormones on adrenal cortical cells.

If plasma ACTH is fully suppressed, the clinician may proceed to imaging the adrenal glands to identify the lesion. Computed tomography with 4-mm slices at the level of the adrenals is usually adequate to pinpoint a unilateral adrenal tumor or bilateral macronodular hyperplasia. Pigmented micronodular hyperplasia associated with the Carney complex may not be detectable by computed tomography (CT) scan; radiocholesterol scintiscan (^{131}I-6β-iodomethylnorcholesterol), which identifies increased adrenal cortical activity, is a better technique in this instance.

There are two caveats to the assumption that suppressed plasma ACTH is synonymous with a primary adrenal lesion. First, ectopic ACTH-producing tumors occasionally produce bioactive ACTH variants not detected by the IRMA. The diagnosis may be suspected if adrenal imaging fails to demonstrate a nodular lesion, and is confirmed by the use of a radioimmunoassay for ACTH. Second, with prolonged ACTH production by a pituitary adenoma, the adrenal glands may develop macronodular hyperplasia and produce cortisol in a semi-autonomous fashion. In this case, plasma ACTH levels may not be frankly elevated, and even if the pituitary tumor is diagnosed and removed, cortisol hypersecretion may persist. Radiocholesterol imaging may help to demonstrate the autonomous activity.

ACTH DEPENDENCE

Plasma ACTH levels >20 pg/mL are considered unequivocally elevated and signify ACTH-dependent CS. If plasma ACTH is detectable but <20 pg/mL, the CRH-stimulation test should be performed (see below). This is because small or "early" adrenal tumors hypersecreting cortisol may not fully suppress ACTH production, but the patient will show a blunted response to CRH with the peak ACTH level <30 pg/mL.

If Adrenocorticotropic Hormone-Dependent, Is It a Pituitary or an Ectopic Tumor?

If plasma ACTH levels are elevated, the challenge is to differentiate between a pituitary and an ectopic source. Ectopic tumors tend to produce higher plasma ACTH levels, but there is substantial overlap with those observed in pituitary CS.

Imaging of the pituitary gland is indicated in all cases of ACTH-dependent CS. Gadolinium-enhanced T1-weighted magnetic resonance imaging (MRI) has a sensitivity of 35% to 60% in detecting a pituitary adenoma. Because pituitary corticotroph adenoma is the most common cause of CS, the discovery of a pituitary mass in combination with biochemical hypercortisolism would appear to provide an unambiguous diagnosis. However, because of the high prevalence of pituitary "incidentalomas" (up to 15% in the normal population and in those with ectopic ACTH-producing tumors), many specialists advocate further biochemical tests to confirm a pituitary source. The high-dose dexamethasone suppression test and the CRH-stimulation test may be used; if the results remain equivocal, the final arbiter is sampling of blood from the inferior petrosal sinuses.

HIGH-DOSE DEXAMETHASONE SUPPRESSION TEST

This may distinguish pituitary from ectopic ACTH production because pituitary corticotroph adenomas tend to be suppressed by a supraphysiologic dose of exogenous glucocorticoid, while ectopic tumors tend to be nonresponsive. After a baseline 24-hour urine collection for UFC, dexamethasone is administered orally at a dose of 2 mg every 6 hours for 48 hours, with measurement of 24-hour UFC on the second day. Originally, appropriate suppression was considered to be 50% of the baseline UFC level, but 90% suppression may be required for maximum specificity, as some ectopic ACTH-producing tumors (e.g., bronchial carcinoids) may express glucocorticoid receptors and suppress ACTH production significantly. The sensitivity and specificity of this test are 80% for differentiating the possible sources of ACTH.

CRH STIMULATION TEST

This can be used to establish ACTH dependence as well as differentiate pituitary from ectopic ACTH-producing CS. It is based on the principle that pituitary tumors generally express CRH receptors, and, unlike ectopic tumors, respond dynamically to a bolus of CRH by secreting ACTH. CRH (Acthrel)[3] (1 μg/kg up to 100 μg) should be injected intravenously, and blood samples taken at baseline, every 5 minutes for 15 minutes after injection, and then every 30 minutes for a total of 2 hours. The original criterion for a dynamic response (diagnostic of a pituitary source) was a peak rise in plasma ACTH of 35% above the baseline; recently, a threshold of 50% rise, together with a concomitant 20% rise in the plasma cortisol level, was proposed to increase the sensitivity and specificity of this test to 90% and 95%, respectively.

INFERIOR PETROSAL SINUS SAMPLING

Unfortunately, even a combination of the high-dose dexamethasone suppression test and the CRH-stimulation test may not correctly identify the source of excess ACTH in as many as 20% of CS patients. If there is any doubt, inferior petrosal sinus sampling (IPSS) should be performed to confirm a pituitary source of ACTH. IPSS requires the skills of an experienced interventional radiologist; rare complications include pulmonary embolism, vascular damage, and deep vein thrombosis. Blood is sampled for ACTH levels through catheters placed in both inferior petrosal sinuses, which contain venous effluent of the anterior pituitary, and simultaneously from a peripheral vein. An inferior petrosal sinus (IPS)-to-peripheral ACTH ratio >2 at baseline generally is diagnostic of a pituitary source of ACTH. Blood should also be sampled after intravenous CRH administration (1 μg/kg) at 2, 3, 5, 10, and 20 minutes. An IPS-to-peripheral ACTH ratio >3 at any time point after CRH stimulation is also diagnostic. Lateralization of ACTH levels (ratio >1.4 between the two sinuses) may be helpful in localizing the tumor if no adenoma is visualized by MRI.

FINDING AN ECTOPIC ADRENOCORTICOTROPIC HORMONE SOURCE

If biochemical and imaging evidence of pituitary CS are lacking, an ectopic ACTH-producing neoplasm should be sought. The majority of these are lung or

[3]Exceeds dosage recommended by the manufacturer.

bronchial tumors, so the search should begin in the chest and proceed to the neck and abdomen. MRI is a sensitive technique, especially for small bronchial carcinoids. Somatostatin receptor scintography with ^{111}indium-pentetreotide is useful if the lesion is not visible by MRI. ^{18}F-flourodeoxyglucose or $^{11}C_5$-hydroxytryptophan positron emission scanning holds promise to locate "occult" tumors. Endoscopic ultrasound may help to identify a pancreatic lesion.

Treatment

PITUITARY CS

Transsphenoidal resection (TSR) of the pituitary adenoma is the first choice for treatment of Cushing's disease; partial or subtotal hypophysectomy may be required if the adenoma cannot be clearly visualized during surgery. Remission occurs in 75% of patients. Clinically evident regression of CS signs is the foremost indicator of a surgical cure, but this may take months to occur. Biochemical remission is usually assessed using a variety of tests, but none have been shown to be accurate predictors of long-term cure. A useful test is to measure a fasting level of plasma cortisol, just before the morning dose of hydrocortisone replacement. A level <1.8 μg/dL between the 5th and 14th postoperative day is suggestive of remission. A plasma cortisol level <5 μg/dL 3 months following surgery may also predict cure. Consistently normal daytime plasma cortisol and UFC levels have been used to define remission, but recurrence occurs in 25% of patients assessed in this manner. A CRH test performed within 2 weeks of surgery has some predictive value—recurrence is more likely in patients who respond to CRH at this time. Overall, data obtained in the early postoperative period are unreliable in predicting long-term cure, necessitating prolonged follow-up of all patients.

Surgical failure is more likely without definitive preoperative localization of the pituitary adenoma with imaging and IPSS. The rate of false localization by MRI—where location of the pituitary tumor found at surgery differed from that suggested by the scan—has been reported to be as high as 40%. Newer techniques such as intraoperative ultrasound of the pituitary may improve visualization of tumors not detected by MRI, and minimize the amount of normal pituitary tissue removed. Staining the tissue for ACTH helps to confirm removal of the adenoma. Surgical failure is more common with macroadenomas and corticotroph hyperplasia.

For patients not cured by TSR, additional treatment options include external-beam or stereotactic radiation to the sella, bilateral adrenalectomy, and pharmacologic inhibition of adrenal corticosteroid synthesis. Radiation is effective in normalizing cortisol levels in one half of patients, but takes 3 to 12 months for an effect so that adjunctive medical therapies are required. Radiation carries a significant risk of panhypopituitarism within 10 years, as well as the possibility of optic nerve or vascular damage, and secondary brain tumors. High-dose, focused radiation using the gamma knife may limit the adverse effects. Bilateral adrenalectomy carries the risk of Nelson's syndrome, with aggressive and possibly invasive growth of any residual ACTH-producing adenoma because of the lack of negative feedback by cortisol. First-line "adrenolytic" medical therapy (Table 3) includes ketoconazole (Nizoral)[1], metyrapone (Metopirone)[1], and aminoglutethimide (Cytadren). The usual approach is to start with ketoconazole, and if cortisol levels are not normalized, to add metyrapone or aminoglutethimide. Mitotane (Lysodren)[1] should be considered only when the other medications fail, and should be used at lower doses than those for adrenocortical carcinoma. It requires weeks to be effective, and induces adrenal necrosis (see Table 3). The obvious side effect of all these medications is adrenal insufficiency. Less effective agents include mifepristone (Mifeprex)[1], a glucocorticoid receptor antagonist, and cyproheptadine[1], which inhibits pituitary ACTH release.

ADRENAL CUSHING'S SYNDROME

Unilateral adrenalectomy (open or laparoscopic) is indicated for the solitary adrenal adenoma and adrenocortical carcinoma. Because cortisol production by the remaining adrenal gland will be suppressed, patients will need perioperative "stress-dose" corticosteroids. Bilateral adrenalectomy will cure nodular hyperplasia, but necessitate lifelong replacement therapy with corticosteroids and fludrocortisone (Florinef).

The management of subclinical CS with an adrenal mass is controversial. Adrenalectomy can ameliorate metabolic abnormalities in some patients with subclinical CS. Surgery is advocated if follow-up testing reveals hypercortisolism and the plasma ACTH level is suppressed. Patients with adrenal CS who are unable to undergo surgery can be managed medically as discussed above (see Table 3).

TREATMENT OF COMPLICATIONS

In addition to removing the cause of CS, the effects of cortisol excess should be treated. CS patients have a mortality rate four times higher than age- and gender-matched counterparts, mainly as a consequence of increased cardiovascular risk. Even with curative treatment, the vascular and metabolic abnormalities can persist. Because of the high risk of osteoporosis, bone mineral density should be assessed by dual x-ray absorptiometry (DEXA) in all CS patients, and treated according to standard guidelines. Psychiatric complications may also persist. Counseling, psychotherapy, and medical treatment of depression and/or anxiety should be initiated as indicated. Hypogonadotropic hypogonadism is common, and if it lasts for more than

[1]Not FDA approved for this indication.

TABLE 3 Pharmacologic Therapies for Cushing's Syndrome

Drug	Dose	Mechanism of Action	Side Effects
Ketoconazole (Nizoral)[1]	200-400 mg PO bid to tid Maximum 1200 mg/day	Inhibition of cholesterol and cortisol synthesis P450scc CYP11B1 CYP11A1	Adrenal insufficiency Hepatotoxicity Gastrointestinal Pruritus Hepatotoxicity Gynecomastia
Metyrapone (Metopirone)[1]	250 to 750 mg PO tid to qid Maximum 4 g/day[2]	Inhibition of cholesterol and cortisol synthesis (CYP11B1) (CYP11B2)	Adrenal insufficiency Acne Hirsutism Hypertension Hypokalemia Gastrointestinal
Aminoglutethimide (Cytadren)[1]	250 mg PO tid to qid Maximum 1 g/day	Inhibition of cholesterol synthesis (CYP11A1) Inhibition of mineralocorticoid biosynthesis	Adrenal insufficiency Hypoaldosteronism Induces hepatic metabolism enzymes (drug interactions) Ataxia Rash Dizziness Somnolence Leukopenia Hypothyroidism Increased metabolism of dexamethasone
Mitotane (Lysodren)[1]	Start at 500 mg PO qhs and titrate up weekly with addition of 500 mg PO at each meal. Total dose 3-4 g/day	Inhibition of mitochondrial CYP11A1 CYP11B1 Direct inhibition of ACTH secretion by pituitary	Permanent adrenal insufficiency Adrenal atrophy/necrosis Anorexia Gastrointestinal Hypercholesterolemia CNS (dizziness, vertigo, ataxia, somnolence) Rash Arthralgias

[1]Not FDA approved for this indication.
[2]Not available in the United States.
Abbreviations: bid = twice daily; CNS = central nervous system; PO = orally; qhs = at bedtime; qid = four times daily; tid = three times daily.

3 months after treatment, sex hormone replacement may be considered. Replacement of thyroxine for central hypothyroidism is routine; that of growth hormone is more controversial.

DIABETES INSIPIDUS

METHOD OF
Alan G. Robinson, MD

Diabetes insipidus literally means excretion of tasteless urine and is a disorder caused by different diseases that affect the ability of the kidney to produce a concentrated urine because of lack of the hormone vasopressin or lack of response to the hormone. The excretion of a large volume of urine, polyuria, must be distinguished at the outset from frequency, urgency, and urinary symptoms that do not connote a large urine volume. In considering therapy for this disorder, one must have determined the cause among the major differential types of diabetes insipidus: hypothalamic neurohypophyseal diabetes insipidus caused by an inability to secrete (and usually synthesize) vasopressin; nephrogenic diabetes insipidus caused by an inappropriate response to vasopressin at the level of the kidney; transient diabetes insipidus of pregnancy in which there is excessive metabolism of vasopressin; and primary polydipsia in which there is no abnormality of vasopressin but only an inappropriate ingestion of water. It is assumed here that the pathologic cause of the diabetes insipidus has been determined (infiltrated disease, tumor, trauma, idiopathic, renal disease with nephrogenic, etc.) and that the underlying disease has been appropriately treated. It should also be noted that children with diabetes insipidus require special attention and should be seen by a pediatric endocrinologist. The recommendations and dosages described here are for adult patients.

If sufficient water is taken in, lack of vasopressin alone and inability to concentrate the urine does not usually cause any biochemical abnormality in the body. It is, however, inconvenient for the patient to be constantly in need of a large volume of water to drink and to continuously excrete a large volume of urine. A major goal of therapy is to reduce the urine volume and the inconvenience of the patient to a minimum. This assumes that the patient is conscious and able to sense thirst. Patients who are unable to sense thirst constitute a special therapeutic challenge (which is discussed) and patients who are unconscious are at risk for severe dehydration and medical complications from dehydration. It is suggested that patients with diabetes insipidus carry a card or medical alert bracelet indicating the diagnosis and including the name of a physician knowledgeable about the disorder, so in an emergency diabetes insipidus is not confused with diabetes mellitus.

Central Neurohypophyseal Diabetes Insipidus

Table 1 lists the agents available to treat diabetes insipidus.

In the past much was made of distinguishing complete severe hypothalamic diabetes insipidus from partial hypothalamic diabetes insipidus. In fact, whether there is no vasopressin secreted or a small amount of vasopressin secreted that is inadequate to the need has little influence on the recommended therapy. In both cases replacement of vasopressin with desmopressin (DDAVP) is the preferred therapy. Desmopressin (1-[3-mercaptopropanoic acid]-8-D-arginine vasopressin) is a synthetic analogue of arginine vasopressin in which D-arginine is substituted in position 8 and the terminal amine is eliminated. These two changes produce an agent that is nearly 2000 times more specific for antidiuresis than vasopressin. There is considerable variability among patients in response to desmopressin, and it is useful in initiating therapy to determine the duration of a dose by asking the patient to keep a diary recording the volume and time of each voided urine. The patient is allowed ad lib fluid, and when the flow equals that equivalent to what would produce approximately 4 L per day, a dose of desmopressin can be given. Desmopressin reaches a maximum action in 1 to 2 hours and will, in most patients, persist for 6 to 12 hours or longer, depending on the dose and delivery of desmopressin. Once a total duration of action is determined, a dosage schedule can be devised to produce minimum antidiuresis, especially during the important part of the patient's day (e.g., work and/or sleep).

TABLE 1 Therapeutic Agents to Treat Diabetes Insipidus

Water
Water-retaining agents
Arginine vasopressin (Pitressin)
Desmopressin (DDAVP)
Chlorpropamide (Diabinese)[1]
Indomethacin (Indocin)[1]
Natriuretic agents
Thiazide diuretics
Amiloride (Midamor)[1]

[1]Not FDA approved for this indication.

Most patients prefer to begin with the desmopressin tablets available as 0.1- and 0.2-mg tablets. Therapy is begun with a low dose, 0.1 mg or one half of that tablet, and increased as necessary. It is important to note that stepwise doubling of the dose often produces only a modest increase in the duration of the dose of a few hours and no increase in the maximum urinary concentration. Usually a dose is found that can be given two or three times a day and maintain the patient in an asymptomatic state. An occasional early dose or extra dose may be necessary to assure antidiuresis for a specific event.

Desmopressin is also available as an intranasally administered spray (Minerin) or as a liquid that is given with a rhinal catheter. The spray has the disadvantage of less flexibility because it is fixed at 10 μg in a 100-μL spray, and the rhinal catheter has the disadvantage of an inconvenient form of administration. However, the rhinal catheter does allow more variability in the dose that is administered and, for some patients, may be more reliable than the oral medication. Patients should be trained in the appropriate use of the rhinal catheter and it should be noted that the liquid form of desmopressin requires refrigeration for storage.

Parenterally administered desmopressin is available in various sized vials or ampules at a concentration of 4 μg/mL. This is rarely used for routine management of ambulatory patients, but can be administered in a dose of 0.5 to 2 μg total dose given either subcutaneously, intramuscularly, or intravenously in a patient hospitalized for another condition or where there is some other reason that the patient cannot receive desmopressin orally or intranasally. If used for maintenance therapy, a much smaller dose given subcutaneously with an insulin syringe will often suffice.

The complication that must be considered when using desmopressin therapy is hyponatremia, which will occur if a patient drinks excessive amounts of fluid while antidiuretic because of the pharmacologic therapy. This must be considered when allowing the patient to follow a flexible dosage schedule. In addition to checking the patient's symptoms of polyuria and polydipsia, one should regularly check serum sodium to be certain this is maintained within a normal range. When starting therapy, serum sodium should be checked more regularly (i.e., daily). When diabetes insipidus is adequately treated, absence of thirst provides protection against drinking excessively. One can avoid the possibility of hyponatremia by occasionally delaying a dose of desmopressin and allowing the patient to excrete any excess fluid that might have been retained.

Although not approved as an antidiuretic agent, chlorpropamide (Diabinese)[1] increases the action of vasopressin and has been used to treat diabetes insipidus. It must be noted in the record that permission was obtained from the patient to use this agent off-label. Therapy can be initiated with 100 mg per day and increased every 4 days until satisfactory diuresis is maintained. The usual dose is 250 to 500 mg per day. Chlorpropamide is not recommended for children and care must be taken to prevent hypoglycemia especially in patients who are panhypopituitary. Maintenance of regular food intake and routine testing of the blood sugar are required.

There are several clinical situations in which there are special considerations regarding therapy of hypothalamic diabetes insipidus.

HYPOTHALAMIC DIABETES INSIPIDUS AFTER INTRACRANIAL SURGERY

It is important to recognize that after any surgical procedure, if large amounts of fluid are administered, large amounts of urine will be excreted. Consequently, it should always be determined that polyuria persists without administration of large volumes of fluid and in spite of an elevation of serum sodium. If the patient is alert and able to respond to thirst, the usual guidelines for treatment with desmopressin can be instituted and the patient's thirst will be a guide to appropriate therapy. However, if fluids are being administered intravenously, one must check the serum sodium regularly and exercise caution to avoid precipitating hyponatremia. It should also be noted that after pituitary surgery the diabetes insipidus may be transient, and after 5 to 7 days, followed by a phase of uncontrolled release of vasopressin from damaged posterior pituitary neurons. The released vasopressin can produce an antidiuresis and the syndrome of inappropriate secretion of antidiuretic hormone (SIADH) with hyponatremia for several days, which might then be followed by return of diabetes insipidus. The hyponatremia may present quite precipitously with vomiting or seizures and require therapy and fluid restriction to raise the Na^+. Some recent studies report using a continuous intravenous infusion of dilute arginine vasopressin (Pitressin) to control diabetes insipidus postoperatively. Infusions of 0.25 to 2.7 mU/kg/h have been used with the advantage touted that the short half-life of vasopressin (10 to 20 minutes) is an advantage of this form of therapy. The author has no personal experience with this form of therapy, but it is obvious that serum sodium and urine output should be monitored closely.

TRAUMATIC DIABETES INSIPIDUS

Traumatic diabetes insipidus may occur with injury to the head, usually from a motor vehicle accident with injury to the skull and damage or section of the pituitary stalk. The symptoms and course are similar to those of diabetes insipidus after hypothalamic surgery. The risk is that the diabetes insipidus will not be diagnosed in the emergency situation. It is essential also in these situations to consider loss of anterior pituitary function and to treat with appropriate doses of hydrocortisone.

DIABETES INSIPIDUS WITH INADEQUATE THIRST

This produces a difficult management problem. There are reports that chlorpropamide[1] might increase thirst in some of these patients; consequently, a therapeutic trial might be considered to treat both the diabetes insipidus and lack of thirst. There is a special form of partial diabetes insipidus with inadequate thirst in which there is no response of the osmoreceptor to sense thirst or to stimulate secretion of vasopressin, yet the volume/baroreceptors are intact. These patients left to their own devices become hypernatremic but then stabilize at a constant level of hypernatremia because when dehydrated, the stimulation of the baroreceptors stimulate enough vasopressin release to maintain low urine volume. Polyuria may only return when sufficient fluid is given to replace the volume deficit.

In these cases, the most advantageous therapy is to select a dose of antidiuretic agent (usually desmopressin [DDAVP]) that produces chronic antidiuresis and then to vary the amount of liquid given to maintain the patient in a normal sodium balance. A rigid regimen of administered antidiuresis and water intake prescribed every 6 to 8 hours to maintain the required 24-hour intake must be maintained. These patients require frequent measure of serum sodium to insure adequate therapy.

DIABETES INSIPIDUS IN PREGNANCY

Diabetes insipidus in pregnancy may be caused by the action of the normally occurring cysteine aminopeptidase (oxytocinase) that is produced by the placenta and also destroys vasopressin. Normal levels of cysteine aminopeptidase may produce symptomatic diabetes insipidus in patients with otherwise asymptomatic diabetes insipidus (e.g., there is limited ability to concentrate the urine, but a urine volume of 3 to 4 L/day is acceptable to the patient). A rare syndrome of markedly excessive oxytocinase will produce diabetes insipidus in otherwise normal women. Desmopressin is the recommended therapeutic agent, because in the doses used to treat diabetes insipidus desmopressin has minimal oxytocic action on the uterus. It is important that the physician be aware of the expansion of extracellular fluid and the decrease in serum sodium that is normal during pregnancy, and that therapy be sufficient to maintain the normal decrease in serum sodium. As with any patient receiving desmopressin, care should be taken with fluid administration during delivery to avoid producing hyponatremia. With the decrease in oxytocinase after delivery, diabetes insipidus may

[1]Not FDA approved for this indication.

disappear or the patient may become asymptomatic with an acceptable urine volume.

Nephrogenic Diabetes Insipidus

Potential offending agents (e.g., lithium or other drugs) should be discontinued if possible. Potential contributing clinical situations (e.g., hypercalcemia or hypokalemia) should be corrected. Adequate water intake should always be maintained and may be lifesaving in congenital nephrogenic diabetes insipidus. Because these patients will not respond to administered desmopressin, therapy is aimed at reducing urine volume by causing volume contraction. This can be done by reducing total body sodium with diet and a thiazide diuretic. The major action is to decrease the glomerular filtration rate (GFR) and increase proximal sodium and water reabsorption, thus decreasing delivery of fluid to the distal diluting segment. Potassium replacement or co-administration of a potassium-sparing antidiuretic may be useful. Amiloride (Midamor)[1] is a preferred agent and is especially useful in lithium-induced nephrogenic diabetes insipidus because it decreases lithium entry into cells in the distal tubule. Co-administration of indomethacin (Indocin)[1] may be of benefit in these patients, but the possibility of inducing duodenal ulcer and gastrointestinal (GI) hemorrhage requires that this be administered with caution.

Primary Polydipsia

There is no specific treatment for primary polydipsia, but it should be noted that any disorder of the hypothalamus that can cause diabetes insipidus may cause disordered thirst and induce primary polydipsia. In these cases the possible coexistence of diabetes insipidus must be considered and treated if present. The disadvantage of using an antidiuretic agent such as desmopressin in a patient of primary polydipsia is the potential to produce SIADH and hyponatremia. If the disorder is a result of a psychiatric syndrome, treating that syndrome may be helpful. Often there is a habitual lifetime pattern of excessive drinking that is refractory to attempts to restrict fluid.

Managing Diabetes Insipidus in Association with Other Therapy

DIABETES INSIPIDUS WITH PANHYPOPITUITARISM

In diabetes insipidus with panhypopituitarism, remember that patients with hypoadrenalism and hypothyroidism have an inability to excrete water. Therefore, when these deficiencies coexist with diabetes insipidus and are not treated, there may be no polyuria. If a patient with hypothyroidism and hypoadrenalism is replaced with thyroid hormone and hydrocortisone, diabetes insipidus may become manifest. It is important, therefore, for patients with combined anterior and posterior pituitary deficiency to maintain uninterrupted and full replacement for all anterior pituitary deficiencies, as well as treatment of diabetes insipidus.

[1]Not FDA approved for this indication.

SURGICAL PROCEDURES

Routine surgical procedures are often sufficiently limited in time that the patient can have their normal dose of desmopressin and then limit the fluid administered during the procedure to maintain a normal serum sodium. The anesthesiologist and endocrinologist should confer prior to the procedure.

SALINE DIURESIS

Promoting a saline diuresis is necessary for some medical treatments (e.g., chemotherapy) and when a large amount of normal saline is given to a patient taking desmopressin, the fluid may induce natriuresis and hyponatremia (SIADH). Withholding desmopressin to allow return of diabetes insipidus and replacing the urine volume with normal saline will lead to hypernatremia. Continuous ultra low-dose vasopressin (e.g., 0.08 to 0.1 mU/kg/h) is reported to control diuresis while allowing administration of normal saline. Fluid input/output and serum sodium must be monitored carefully.

HYPERTONIC ENCEPHALOPATHY

Hypertonic encephalopathy may occur in the treatment of diabetes insipidus. Usually diabetes insipidus and hypernatremia are known to be acute and treatment with desmopressin and water can be used to bring the sodium back to normal. When the duration of hypernatremia is unknown and is thought to be chronic, the brain may have accommodated to the hypernatremia with production of "idiogenic osmols." Overly rapid normalization of the serum sodium may produce cerebral edema and worsening of the neurologic condition. In such cases, the degree of correction of hypernatremia should not exceed 0.5 mEq/L/h, and the patient should be continuously checked for signs of cerebral edema.

ORGAN DONORS

Organ donors may have diabetes insipidus because diabetes insipidus commonly occurs when a patient becomes brain dead. If the patient is a candidate for organ donation, it is reasonable to consider treatment of the diabetes insipidus with desmopressin to maintain a normal sodium. This is another situation in which continuous administration of low-dose vasopressin intravenously, as described above, may be an appropriate therapy.

HYPERPARATHYROIDISM AND HYPOPARATHYROIDISM

METHOD OF
Jeffrey A. Jackson, MD

Hyperparathyroidism

PRIMARY HYPERPARATHYROIDISM

Primary hyperparathyroidism (PHPT) is a generalized disorder of calcium and phosphate metabolism resulting from an increased production of parathyroid hormone (PTH) caused by an intrinsic abnormality of the parathyroid glands. It is the most common cause of hypercalcemia in nonhospitalized patients. The incidence of PHPT has been declining over recent decades for unclear reasons: from 91 per 100,000 general population in 1979; to about 21 per 100,000 during the period 1983–1992; to 4 per 100,000 in 1992 (in Rochester, Minnesota). Women are more affected than men (3:2 ratio) except in the inherited conditions associated with PHPT; the incidence of PHPT rises with age, especially in postmenopausal women. Over time, the clinical profile of PHPT has shifted from a symptomatic disease with overt bone disease, nephrolithiasis, renal failure and severe hypercalcemia toward an asymptomatic one.

Etiology

Table 1 lists the causes of hyperparathyroidism: 80% to 85% of cases are caused by single adenomas (mostly monoclonal tumors). Multigland hyperplasia may be sporadic but often indicates a hereditary cause (multiple endocrine neoplasia [MEN] syndromes or hereditary PHPT with or without jaw tumors). MEN-1 includes parathyroid hyperplasia and pituitary and pancreatic islet cell tumors, and has been mapped to the MEN-1 tumor-suppressor gene locus (11q13). MEN-2A includes parathyroid hyperplasia, bilateral C-cell hyperplasia and medullary thyroid carcinoma, and bilateral adrenomedullary hyperplasia and pheochromocytomas, and is associated with mutations in the RET proto-oncogene (chromosome 10q). Parathyroid carcinoma is more common in the familial syndromes and accounts for less than 1% of PHPT. It is associated with HRPT2 (hyperparathyroidism 2) gene mutations (chromosome 1q, the same gene associated with hereditary hyperparathyroidism [HPT] and jaw tumors).

TABLE 1 Causes of Hyperparathyroidism

Primary HPT
Single and multiple adenomas
Multigland hyperplasia-sporadic, familial HPT ± jaw tumors, MEN-1, MEN-2A
Parathyroid carcinoma
Familial benign hypocalciuric hypercalcemia
Neonatal primary HPT
Drug-related (chronic lithium)
Secondary HPT
Vitamin D deficiency—nutritional, postgastric surgery, malabsorption syndromes, hepatobiliary disease, drugs (anticonvulsants, sun-blockers, and others)
Chronic renal insufficiency
Vitamin D dependency—defective renal 1α-hydroxylase, defective calcitriol receptor, X-linked hypophosphatemic rickets/bone disease, other causes of prolonged hypophosphatemia or phosphate supplementation
Tertiary HPT
Renal osteodystrophy
? any cause of prolonged secondary HPT

Abbreviations: HPT = hyperparathyroidism; MEN-1 = multiple endocrine neoplasia type 1; MEN-2A = multiple endocrine neoplasia type 2A.

Sporadic PHPT may be associated with prior external head/neck irradiation and chronic lithium therapy. PHPT may often be brought out by the hypocalciuric effects of thiazide diuretics. Familial benign hypocalciuric hypercalcemia (FBHH) should always be distinguished from other causes of PHPT because surgical intervention is unnecessary in these patients.

Clinical Features

Classic symptoms of PHPT (skeletal-osteitis fibrosa cystica or "brown" tumors; renal-nephrocalcinosis and azotemia; gastrointestinal-peptic ulcer disease or pancreatitis [the latter no longer clearly associated with PHPT]) are now rare. These "bones, stones, and abdominal groans" have been replaced by subtle neuromuscular symptoms (muscle weakness or aching) or central nervous system symptoms (depression or reduced sense of well-being)—"psychic moans and fatigue overtones"—although presentation with renal lithiasis is not uncommon. Physical findings are usually sparse; band keratopathy is uncommon. Palpable neck masses are usually of thyroid origin (rarely giant parathyroid adenomas or carcinomas).

Diagnosis

The biochemical hallmarks of PHPT are hypercalcemia and elevated or inappropriate levels of PTH. Measurement of ionized calcium may be useful in the occasional "normocalcemic " patient with mild PHPT. These patients typically have high-normal total serum calcium levels with clinical suspicion of PHPT (history of kidney stones, unexplained osteopenia or hypercalciuria—especially premenopausal women or postmenopausal women on estrogen). Ionized calcium assays may be helpful in hypoalbuminemic or hypoproteinemic patients in whom the formula for "corrected" serum calcium (add 0.8 mg/dL for every 1 g/dL fall in serum albumin) is often inaccurate. Spurious hypercalcemia may occur postprandially or with prolonged tourniquet application during venesection.

Most commercial assays for PTH now measure intact hormone (two-site immunoradiometric assays typically). These assays have no cross-reactivity for PTH-related peptide (PTHrP) and are not affected by renal insufficiency (in which PTH fragments interfere with older assays). The concept of "inappropriate normality" is a crucial one in endocrinology: inappropriately normal PTH levels are seen in 25% to 30% of patients with PHPT, especially in hereditary causes including FBHH. Table 2 lists the nonparathyroid causes of hypercalcemia.

Serum phosphorus tends to be in the lower range of normal, except in azotemic patients. A small increase in serum chloride and decrease in the serum bicarbonate level reflect the renal acid-base effects of PTH. Serum alkaline phosphatase (of osteoblast origin) may be a marker for skeletal involvement. Urinary calcium is typically elevated (>250 mg per 24 hours in women; >300 mg per 24 hours in men) in PHPT. Low levels (<80 to 100 mg per 24 hours) may be the tip-off for FBHH (confirmed by calculating calcium-to-creatinine clearance ratio [<0.01] from spot urine/serum calcium and creatinine). Very high levels (>550 to 600 mg per 24 hours) may indicate coexisting occult nonparathyroid disease or renal hypercalciuria. Circulating 1,25-dihydroxyvitamin D levels are typically normal or elevated in patients with PHPT, in contrast to those with PTHrP excess. Newer bone turnover markers (serum osteocalcin, urinary N-telopeptides, etc.) are typically high in PHPT and seldom clinically necessary.

TABLE 2 Nonparathyroid Causes of Hypercalcemia

Malignant Disease
Parathyroid hormone-related peptide excess (carcinomas of the lung, breast, head and neck, T-cell lymphomas, and others)
Multiple myeloma
Cancers metastatic to bone
1,25-dihydroxyvitamin D excess (rare; lymphomas)
Endocrinopathies/Metabolic Disorders
Hyperthyroidism
Adrenal insufficiency
Milk-alkali syndrome
Hypophosphatemia
Granulomatous Disease (1α-Hydroxylase [Vitamin D] Mediated)
Sarcoidosis
Other: tuberculosis, chronic berylliosis, fungal diseases, etc.
Drug-Induced
Vitamins A and D
Thiazides
Lithium
Aluminum intoxication, etc.
Other
Immobilization with high bone turnover (children, Paget's disease)
Acute and chronic renal failure

In patients with confirmed PHPT, measurement of bone mineral density (BMD) is useful. Patients with PHPT typically have preferential loss of cortical bone (proximal forearm and hip) with sparing of cancellous bone (spine). Dual-energy x-ray absorptiometry (DEXA) of the spine and hip is the most common technique used, although peripheral DEXA or radiogrammetry of the forearm are occasionally obtained. Nephrotomography or ultrasonography may be useful in PHPT patients without stone history to detect silent stones, which may serve as a surgical indication.

Patients with vitamin D deficiency may have masked hypercalcemia and severe PHPT manifestations, particularly bone disease. Patients on thiazide diuretics or lithium may present major diagnostic uncertainty. They usually present with less severe hypercalcemia (usually <13 mg/dL) and low urine calcium, but their PTH levels may be inappropriate or frankly elevated. If there is no clinical urgency, stopping the drugs for several months and retesting will usually clarify the diagnosis.

Treatment

The only cure for PHPT is surgical excision of abnormal parathyroid glands. It is clear that surgery is indicated for all patients with symptomatic PHPT. However, the role of surgical intervention in asymptomatic patients is controversial. The National Institutes of Health (NIH) Workshop on Asymptomatic PHPT in 2002, revised the prior 1990 guidelines for surgical intervention of these patients (Table 3). Surgery is also indicated for any patient in whom surveillance is not desired or possible. With these guidelines, less than 50% of patients will be managed without surgery. For these patients, appropriate long-term surveillance is needed: biannual serum calcium and annual serum creatinine and bone mass measurements. Approximately 15% to 25% of patients followed without surgery will develop evidence of progressive PHPT and require surgery.

Conventional neck surgery for PHPT has involved either bilateral or unilateral explorations usually under general anesthesia by an experienced surgeon (expected cure rate >95%). Recently, minimally invasive parathyroidectomy (MIP) has been developed using preoperative localization techniques—primarily technetium-99m-sestamibi radioisotope scanning plus

TABLE 3 Indications for Surgery in Asymptomatic Primary Hyperparathyroidism

Serum calcium ≥1.0 mg/dL above assay upper limit of normal
24-hour urinary calcium >400 mg
Reductions in age- and gender-matched creatinine clearance by ≥30%
Bone mineral density: T score <−2.5 at any site
Age <50 years

neck ultrasonography—to limit the operative field. The use of an intraoperative gamma probe further minimizes parathyroid surgery in patients in whom preoperative sestamibi scanning detects the parathyroid adenoma. Comprehensive cost analysis and comparative studies of MIP techniques are in process. For patients with multiglandular disease, total parathyroidectomy with a remnant left in situ or autotransplanted in the nondominant forearm is required.

Patients with unsuccessful initial surgery may require extensive localization studies. Radioisotope scanning and ultrasound are followed by computed tomography and magnetic resonance imaging. Invasive localization by arteriography or selective venous sampling for PTH may be required if the noninvasive studies are not definitive.

Postoperatively, PHPT patients may have transient hypocalcemia while the normal previously suppressed parathyroid glands regain calcium sensitivity. "Hungry bone" syndrome with rapid deposition of calcium and phosphate into bone may cause prolonged postoperative hypocalcemia and is still occasionally seen in patients with severe hyperparathyroid bone disease. Postoperative hypoparathyroidism is more commonly seen in patients with prior neck exploration or those undergoing parathyroidectomy with autotransplantation for multiglandular disease. Recurrent laryngeal nerve injuries with vocal cord paralysis are now uncommon complications of parathyroid surgery.

Patients with PHPT who either refuse surgery or cannot have surgery performed because of operative risk (a shrinking population as a result of MIP techniques under local anesthesia) may be considered for medical management. Oral phosphate therapy may reduce serum calcium levels, but PTH levels rise and metastatic calcification may occur if the calcium-phosphorus ion product exceeds 65 to 75. Estrogen[1] may reduce serum and urinary calcium levels and antagonize PTH bone effects, although the findings of the Women's Health Initiative Study (2002) have resulted in patient and physician discomfort with the use of hormone therapy. Progestin-only therapy may attenuate calcium levels. Bisphosphonate therapy—orally with alendronate (Fosamax)[1] 10 mg daily or 70 mg weekly, or risedronate (Actonel)[1] 5 mg daily or 35 mg weekly, or parenterally with pamidronate (Aredia)[1] 60 to 90 mg intravenously every 1 to 3 months, or zoledronic acid (Zometa)[1] 1 to 4 mg intravenously every 3 to 12 months—may improve BMD and stabilize calcium levels. Thiazide diuretics may reduce hypercalciuria and stone risk but potentially may cause worsened hypercalcemia and traditionally are avoided in PHPT patients. New calcimimetic agents with action at the level of the extracellular calcium-sensing receptor may prove to be safe and effective in the future in PHPT (as well as secondary/tertiary HPT).

Hypercalcemic crisis in PHPT is generally a surgical emergency, although aggressive forced saline diuresis along with the use of intravenous bisphosphonates, or less commonly, gallium nitrate or mithramycin (plicamycin [Mithracin])[1], may be temporarily effective in reducing serum calcium levels.

SECONDARY HYPERPARATHYROIDISM

Secondary HPT is characterized by low or normal serum calcium and elevated serum PTH. It is caused most frequently by chronic renal failure with impaired 1α-hydroxylation of 25-hydroxyvitamin D or gastrointestinal malabsorption of vitamin D (as indicated by low 25-hydroxyvitamin D level); other causes are shown in Table 1. Treatment involves control of serum phosphate by nonaluminum phosphate binders, low-phosphorus diets, and aggressive calcium and calcitriol or vitamin D analogue therapy in renal failure patients; vitamin D sterols are used in patients with vitamin D malabsorption. Secondary HPT is an important cause of irreversible bone loss; the subgroup without severe renal impairment may also often require treatment for osteoporosis with oral bisphosphonates—alendronate (Fosamax) or risedronate (Actonel)—or teriparatide (Forteo) once PTH levels have normalized.

TERTIARY HYPERPARATHYROIDISM

Hypercalcemia caused by autonomous secretion of PTH may develop in any patient with prolonged severe secondary HPT over time. It is most commonly seen in chronic renal disease patients (see Table 1) and can be associated with metastatic calcification and calciphylaxis. Total parathyroidectomy with autotransplantation may be necessary in these patients if hypercalcemia and associated symptoms are severe or response to potent vitamin D sterols or analogues (intravenous calcitriol [Calcijex], 1α-hydroxyvitamin D_2 [doxercalciferol-Hectorol], or 19-*nor*-1α-hydroxyvitamin D [paricalcitol-Zemplar]) is inadequate.

Hypoparathyroidism

Hypoparathyroidism is an uncommon and heterogeneous clinical disorder that is caused by inadequate PTH secretion for the maintenance of normal extracellular fluid calcium levels or from impaired PTH action in target tissues.

ETIOLOGY

Table 4 lists the causes of hypoparathyroidism. The most common cause is postsurgical following thyroidectomy, parathyroidectomy, or radical surgery for head and neck cancers.

CLINICAL FEATURES

Increased neuromuscular irritability caused by hypocalcemia is responsible for the symptoms and

[1]Not FDA approved for this indication.

TABLE 4 Causes of Hypoparathyroidism

Parathyroid Gland Destruction
Surgical
Polyglandular autoimmune
Radiation
Infiltration (iron or copper overload, malignancy, granulomatous disease)
Altered PTH Production or Secretion
Primary: calcium sensing receptor mutations, PTH mutations
Secondary: hypomagnesemia, maternal HPT
Impaired PTH Action
Hypomagnesemia
Pseudohypoparathyroidism (with or without Albright's hereditary osteodystrophy)
Drugs: bisphosphonates, calcitonin, mithramycin
Abnormal Parathyroid Gland Development
Isolated hypoparathyroidism
DiGeorge syndrome
Complex genetic syndromes

Abbreviations: HPT = hyperparathyroidism; PTH = parathyroid hormone.

signs of hypoparathyroidism: circumoral and acral paraesthesias; muscle cramps; tetany-carpopedal spasm and laryngeal stridor; impaired consciousness; and convulsions. Symptoms usually occur when the serum calcium is below 7.5 mg/dL. The acute symptoms may be precipitated by pregnancy or lactation, the menstrual cycle, intercurrent illness, exercise, or states of alkalosis. Chronic hypocalcemia may be associated with basal ganglia calcification and occasionally with extrapyramidal manifestations, subcapsular cataracts, eczematous dermatitis, brittle hair and nails, alopecia, and abnormal dentition. Clinical signs can include Chvostek and Trousseau signs and pseudopapilledema. Prolonged QT interval may be present on electrocardiography. Occasionally, hypoparathyroidism may be diagnosed only after the finding of low serum calcium on routine laboratory testing. Polyglandular autoimmune deficiency syndrome (type 1) may also include mucocutaneous candidiasis, Addison's disease, type 1 diabetes, alopecia, steatorrhea, thyroid and gonadal failure, hepatitis, pernicious anemia, and vitiligo. Pseudohypoparathyroidism may present with or without Albright's hereditary osteodystrophy and G-subunit α deficiency (short stature, brachydactyly, subcutaneous ossification, round facies, and dental hypoplasia). Pseudohypoparathyroid patients may also develop primary thyroid and gonadal failure.

DIAGNOSIS

The biochemical hallmarks of hypoparathyroidism are low serum calcium and elevated serum phosphorus in the presence of normal renal function. Measurement of ionized calcium may be useful in hypoproteinemic patients. PTH levels are low or undetectable except in patients with impaired PTH action (hypomagnesemia or pseudohypoparathyroidism) in whom 25-hydroxyvitamin D levels should be normal. Urinary calcium is low reflecting reduced filtered calcium load. Alkaline phosphatase levels are usually normal.

TREATMENT

Correction of hypocalcemia in hypoparathyroidism of any etiology includes oral calcium supplementation (elemental 1 to 3 g daily in divided doses, avoiding calcium phosphate preparations) and vitamin D, except in mild cases, particularly following parathyroid adenomectomy, which may just require temporary calcium supplementation alone. Vitamin D preparations include vitamin D_2 (ergocalciferol [Drisdol]) or D_3 (cholecalciferol [Delta D]) 25,000 to 100,000 units daily; 1α-hydroxyvitamin D_2 (Hectorol) 0.5 to 2.0 µg daily; or calcitriol (1,25-dihydroxyvitamin D_3) 0.25 to 1.0 µg daily. Vitamins D_2 and D_3 are less expensive but have slow onset of action and long duration (because of fat solubility), which can result in prolonged toxicity. This makes the other preparations advantageous and preferable. Requirements for vitamin D are generally lower in pseudohypoparathyroid patients with intact distal renal tubular function than in PTH-deficient patients.

Significant hypercalciuria and risk of nephrolithiasis and nephrocalcinosis may occur with therapy if calcium levels are even brought into the mid-normal (or higher) range as a result of deficient hypocalciuric PTH effect on the kidney. Low-normal serum calcium is generally an appropriate target unless the hypoparathyroid patient is also treated with thiazide diuretics. Thiazides (hydrochlorothiazide 25 to 100 mg daily or potassium-sparing agents) with a low-sodium diet are frequently used to control serum and urinary calcium levels with a cost-effective vitamin D-sparing effect. Phosphate-binding antacids may be required if serum phosphorus levels rise to >6 mg/dL. Once stabilization occurs, serum calcium may be followed at 6- to 12-month intervals with periodic urinary calcium monitoring, if the patient is not treated with thiazide diuretics.

For acute hypocalcemic tetany, bolus intravenous calcium (dosage 2 mg/kg elemental; 90 mg per 10 mL as 10% calcium gluconate) followed by an infusion of 15 mg/kg over 6 to 12 hours is appropriate. Careful observation and monitoring are essential for these patients. Serum magnesium should always be checked in symptomatic hypocalcemic patients. Hypomagnesemia can occur in hypoparathyroid patients, and parenteral magnesium replacement (2 g [16 mEq] $MgSO_4$ infusion every 8 hours) is also appropriate in these patients.

PRIMARY ALDOSTERONISM

METHOD OF
Myron H. Weinberger, MD

Primary aldosteronism is a potentially curable form of hypertension that is being recognized with increased frequency. Estimates of the prevalence of this form of hypertension in an unselected hypertensive population range from 1% to 2% to more than 25% based on different studies. The best explanation for this more than tenfold range of prevalence appears to be the frequency of application and sensitivity of the screening tests used. The increasing recognition of subtle forms of this disorder and the clearer understanding of the many mechanisms by which primary aldosteronism can result, have provided new approaches to its detection and treatment.

Mechanisms

Primary aldosteronism is a collective term for a group of disorders characterized by excessive and unregulated production of mineralocorticoid steroid hormones or inappropriate stimulation of the mineralocorticoid receptor of the kidney. This results in excessive sodium and water reabsorption by the distal portion of the renal tubule and collecting ducts of the kidneys where the mineralocorticoid receptors are located. The mineralocorticoid-induced sodium and water reabsorption occur in exchange for potassium and hydrogen ions that are excreted in the urine. The sodium and water reabsorption expand extracellular fluid volume and raise blood pressure. This is the prototype of "salt-sensitive" hypertension because the blood pressure can be reduced by diuretic administration, restoring the expanded extracellular fluid volume back toward normal, or by drugs that inhibit the production of mineralocorticoids or block stimulation of the mineralocorticoid receptor sites in the kidney. The volume expansion induced by mineralocorticoid excess then suppresses renin release by the kidney that is extremely sensitive to changes in extracellular fluid volume. Thus, the universal hallmark of primary aldosteronism, and one of the most valuable screening tools, is the presence of marked suppression of plasma renin activity that cannot be stimulated into the normal range by typical maneuvers such as a low-sodium diet or diuretic administration. The loss of potassium and hydrogen ions as a result of increased mineralocorticoid receptor activity typically results in hypokalemic alkalosis. However, the ability to identify various forms of primary aldosteronism early in the course of the abnormality makes the dependence on hypokalemic alkalosis less useful as a screening tool.

Most commonly the mineralocorticoid excess results from the inappropriate and usually autonomous excessive production of aldosterone, the primary mineralocorticoid produced by the zona glomerulosa of the adrenal cortex. In rare patients in whom an adrenal biosynthetic defect is present such as the 17α-hydroxylase or 11β-hydroxylase deficiencies, aldosterone cannot be produced, but excessive amounts of a precursor mineralocorticoid, such as desoxycorticosterone, can produce the same biologic results as excessive aldosterone production. Another adrenal enzymatic abnormality has been identified in which a genetic mutation has created a hybrid gene that combines the 11β-hydroxylase and aldosterone synthase genes that produces aldosterone under the control of corticotrophin (ACTH) rather than the normal primary stimulus for aldosterone production, angiotensin II. This results in excessive aldosterone production that can be inhibited by administration of a glucocorticoid (dexamethasone) that acts to decrease ACTH release and thus the subsequent aldosterone production upon which it is dependent. This is a rare, familial disorder usually referred to as dexamethasone-suppressible hyperaldosteronism (DSH) or glucocorticoid-remediable aldosteronism (GRA). Another mechanism for apparent mineralocorticoid excess (AME) is the failure of 11β-hydroxysteroid dehydrogenase to prevent the conversion of cortisol to cortisone. Despite the presence of cortisol in blood concentrations 1000-fold higher than aldosterone, the mineralocorticoid receptor is "protected" from occupancy by cortisol because it is efficiently converted to cortisone by 11β-hydroxysteroid dehydrogenase, and cortisone has virtually no affinity for the mineralocorticoid receptor. In some circumstances, the action of 11β-hydroxysteroid dehydrogenase is inhibited, for example by glycyrrhizic acid, a component of licorice, or by genetic abnormalities, permitting cortisol to occupy and stimulate the mineralocorticoid receptor. Another genetic abnormality producing clinical manifestations that mimic primary aldosteronism was recently elucidated. Liddle's syndrome, a form of salt-sensitive hypertension with marked renin suppression and hypokalemia but with very low levels of aldosterone or other mineralocorticoids, results from a genetic mutation in the β subunit of the epithelial sodium channel. This form of "low-renin" hypertension is responsive to triamterene.

Signs and Symptoms

The symptoms associated with primary aldosteronism are nonspecific. Hypertension is almost always present although in some individuals a marked rise in blood pressure within the normal range has been described. Headaches are a common feature as are fatigue, muscle weakness, and, occasionally, muscle cramps. Rarely, profound muscle weakness, and even tetany, can be observed, but this is usually found in severe cases with marked hypokalemic alkalosis, which can result in decreased ionized calcium levels. Hypokalemia is often but not invariably found and a recent study suggests that 50% of patients with primary aldosteronism may have normal blood potassium levels. Serum sodium levels are typically above 139 mEq/L, but rarely are they above the normal range. Alkalosis, manifest by increased serum bicarbonate values, is often observed and is thought to be the cause of reduced blood magnesium levels, another common finding. Patients often complain of polyuria and particularly of nocturia. The blood pressure elevation can be mild or severe, with many patients presenting with malignant hypertension. Despite severe hypertension and, frequently, a prolonged duration of blood pressure elevation, hypertensive retinopathy is usually not severe, suggesting that vasoactive pressor agents such as angiotensin II and norepinephrine, both of which are suppressed in primary aldosteronism, are required for the vascular changes of severe hypertension to be seen in the eyegrounds. Renal function is typically normal when measured by blood levels of blood urea nitrogen (BUN) or creatinine. However, creatinine clearance is often supranormal, reflecting extracellular volume expansion and glomerular hyperfiltration, in the face of increased renal perfusion pressure and a decrease in angiotensin II-mediated efferent arteriolar tone. Proteinuria may also be present.

Screening and Diagnosis

The traditional use of hypokalemia as a screening test has fallen by the wayside in view of the large numbers of subjects with primary aldosteronism in whom serum potassium levels are not abnormal, as well as a result of the poor specificity of serum potassium in hypertension, because the majority of hypertensives with hypokalemia have secondary aldosteronism from diuretic therapy or renal vascular disease or other forms of hypertension associated with increased renin production. Because of the consistent expansion of extracellular fluid volume in all forms of primary aldosteronism, renin suppression is almost universal, unless the patient has significant renal disease. Consequently, renin suppression is a useful initial screening test. However, as many as 25% or more of the "essential" hypertensive population may also have renin suppression and thus further studies are required. These include the demonstration that aldosterone levels are *not* similarly suppressed. Historically, a 14-day protocol of hospital studies was required to demonstrate both the suppressed and unstimulatable renin levels in combination with the elevated and nonsuppressible aldosterone values, typically measured in a 24-hour urine sample. With the advent of highly sensitive and specific immunologic assay techniques for both renin and aldosterone, it is very simple to screen and diagnose primary aldosteronism with a single blood sample. In 1984, I suggested that the screening and diagnosis of primary aldosteronism could be conducted by measuring plasma renin activity and plasma aldosterone concentration in a single blood sample because renin, but not aldosterone, should be suppressed. Since renin (i.e., angiotensin II) is the primary stimulus of aldosterone production in most individuals, the discrepancy between the two should signal an abnormality. This subsequently proved true and is largely responsible for the marked increase in the frequency of diagnosis of primary aldosteronism. Moreover, some investigators report that this screening test can be conducted even in the presence of antihypertensive medications because those that influence renin and aldosterone should do so in the same direction and thus not create an artificial divergence of values. Additional techniques sometimes used for the demonstration of inappropriate and nonsuppressible aldosterone production include measurement of plasma aldosterone values before and after intravenous administration of 2 L of normal (0.9%) saline over a 4-hour period (8 AM to noon), measurement of aldosterone in a 24-hour urine collection after administration of several days of a high-sodium diet and an exogenous mineralocorticoid such as fludrocortisone (Florinef) orally for 3 days or desoxycorticosterone acetate (DOCA)[1] intramuscularly for 3 days. However, the finding of an aldosterone-to-renin ratio above 30 (disregarding the units of measurement unless they are in molar units) in peripheral vein blood essentially confirms the diagnosis of primary aldosteronism, and, in some cases, ratios above 15 are diagnostic. A few caveats, however, are necessary. Because some laboratories report values of plasma renin activity as being below 0.1 ng/mL, that value cannot be used for the denominator because it will produce a diagnostic ratio when the aldosterone value is only 3 ng/100 mL. Thus, I use a lower value of 0.7 for renin when the laboratory reports a value below their detectability limit. In addition, the value for plasma aldosterone must be 15 ng/100 mL or higher.

Determining the Form of Primary Aldosteronism

In view of the varieties of the abnormalities causing primary aldosteronism and the differences in treatment, it is imperative that further studies to delineate the cause be conducted after the diagnosis is made. In my experience, more than 60% of the patients with primary aldosteronism have a solitary adrenal adenoma. These are generally small, often less than 1 cm in diameter, and difficult to identify with accuracy with anatomic techniques such as computed tomography (CT) scanning. Nonetheless, I do conduct CT scans for comparison with what I consider the "gold standard" for localization: adrenal venous blood sampling. However, for maximal benefit the sampling is conducted during intravenous ACTH

[1]Not available in the United States.

(Cortrosyn) stimulation, administering 25 units of ACTH in 500 mL normal saline beginning 30 minutes before sampling at a rate of 100 mL/h. This minimizes error resulting from episodic secretion of steroids caused by fluctuations in endogenous ACTH release. I measure both aldosterone and cortisol in blood samples to assess purity of nominal adrenal venous samples and to permit correction for dilution of adrenal venous blood by blood from nonadrenal sources. I also obtain a sample from the inferior vena cava remote from the adrenals, representing peripheral venous blood. A ratio of aldosterone to cortisol is determined and the two adrenal samples are compared with each other and with the inferior vena cava sample. Approximately 30% of patients have bilateral adrenal hyperplasia as the cause of primary aldosteronism, whereas others may have unilateral hyperplasia or one of the genetic abnormalities previously mentioned. When the syndrome is the result of unilateral hyperaldosteronism, surgical removal of the involved gland often corrects the metabolic abnormalities and the hypertension. Moreover, the presurgical localization of the abnormality permits the less invasive, laparoscopic approach that I have employed exclusively for the past decade. If the abnormality is caused by bilateral hyperaldosteronism, or if the patient is not a surgical candidate or refuses surgery, medical treatment is available. Spironolactone (Aldactone) is a specific mineralocorticoid receptor antagonist that has been used for almost 40 years. In primary aldosteronism doses of 100 to 800 mg/d[2] are often required, which is frequently associated with undesirable side effects, such as painful gynecomastia and impotence in men, and menstrual irregularities and breast tenderness in women, because of the nonspecific sex hormone receptor effects of the drug. A new, more-selective aldosterone receptor blocker, eplerenone (Inspra) was recently approved by the FDA and appears to be free of these troublesome side effects. Diuretics, usually combined with potassium-sparing agents, particularly amiloride (Midamor), as well as calcium channel entry blockers such as verapamil (Calan) and amlodipine (Norvasc), are also effective in reducing the elevated blood pressure and metabolic abnormalities associated with primary aldosteronism. In the rare cases of DSH/GRA, the above drugs can be used or the glucocorticoid dexamethasone (Decadron) can be given in doses of 0.25 to 0.5 mg every 8 hours. While the latter will reduce the elevated aldosterone production immediately, it takes several weeks for the blood pressure to fall. For long-term treatment the use of potassium-sparing diuretic combinations is preferred to avoid the hyperglucocorticoidism (Cushing's syndrome) associated with chronic steroid administration. Rarely, primary aldosteronism results from adrenal carcinoma. In this situation, excessive production of a variety of steroids is the rule and patients are typically much more ill.

[2]Exceeds dosage recommended by the manufacturer.

DISEASES OF THE PITUITARY GLAND

METHOD OF

Donald Zimmerman, MD

The Hypothalamus

The hypothalamus controls pituitary hormone secretion by two major mechanisms. The first mechanism is by the production of hormones within cell bodies of neurons located in the hypothalamus, and the transport of these hormones down axons that end in the posterior lobe of the pituitary gland. These hormones are then released into the general circulation from nerve endings in the posterior pituitary gland. The second mechanism is by hypothalamic neurons producing signaling molecules (either peptides or biogenic amines) and secreting these molecules into capillary loops that coalesce the portal veins. These veins carry the hypothalamic-stimulating hormones to the pars distalis of the pituitary gland. In this area, the veins give rise to a second bed of capillaries (sinusoids) that facilitate transport of signaling molecules from the hypothalamus into pituitary cells. The hypothalamus produces gonadotropin-releasing hormone (GRH), which regulates pituitary production and secretion of luteinizing hormone (LH) and follicle-stimulating hormone (FSH). It also produces growth hormone-releasing hormone (GHRH), which stimulates pituitary growth hormone production and release, and somatostatin, which inhibits pituitary growth hormone production and release. The hypothalamus produces ghrelin, which also stimulates pituitary growth hormone production release. A large amount of ghrelin is also produced by the stomach. The hypothalamus produces thyrotropin-releasing hormone (TRH), which stimulates pituitary production and release of thyroid-stimulating hormone (TSH), as well as prolactin. Additionally, the hypothalamus secretes dopamine, which inhibits pituitary production and release of prolactin; the dominant effect of the hypothalamus on pituitary prolactin secretion is inhibitory. Finally, the hypothalamus produces corticotropin-releasing hormone (CRH), which stimulates pituitary production and release of adrenocorticotropic hormone. Another stimulant of pituitary production of adrenocorticotropic hormone is vasopressin.

Vasopressin or Antidiuretic Hormone

Vasopressin is secreted by the posterior pituitary gland in response to hyperosmolality of the blood and in response to decreased blood pressure and decreased blood volume.

Vasopressin Excess or Syndrome of Inappropriate Antidiuretic Hormone Secretion

The syndrome of inappropriate antidiuretic hormone secretion (SIADH) is the most common cause of hypoosmolality in individuals with normal blood volume.

Diagnostic Criteria

1. Low plasma osmolality (less than 275 mOsm/kg)
2. Inappropriately elevated urinary concentration (greater than 100 mOsm/kg)
3. Normal plasma volume
4. Increased urine sodium excretion in the face of normal intake of salt and water
5. Absence of other causes of hypoosmolality in the setting of normal blood volume such as hypothyroidism, hypocortisolism, and diuretic use
6. Serum uric acid level less than 4 mg/dL

Causes

1. Medications (carbamazepine and oxcarbazepine, omeprazole, serotonin reuptake inhibitors, vincristine, angiotensin-converting enzyme inhibitors, phenothiazines, and, of course, desmopressin acetate [DDAVP])
2. Pulmonary infections and mechanical ventilation
3. Central nervous system (CNS) abnormalities (path lesions, inflammatory diseases, degenerative or demyelinating diseases, subarachnoid hemorrhage, and head trauma)
4. Non-CNS tumors (lung tumor, nasopharyngeal carcinoma, and leukemia)
5. When central nervous system abnormalities are considered, cerebral salt-wasting must be considered as a possible explanation. In cerebral salt-wasting, patients have evidence of hypovolemia. Thus, elevated vasopressin in this setting is appropriate rather than inappropriate.

Treatment

The treatment of syndrome of inappropriate antidiuretic hormone secretion depends on the severity of the manifestations.

In patients who have mild to moderate hyponatremia and no central nervous system dysfunction, simple fluid restriction may be considered. Fluid restriction may comprise replacing only 90% of a patient's insensible loss plus urine output each hour. To estimate insensible loss, it is reasonable to use 25% to 30% of calculated maintenance requirements.

If patients have severe central nervous system dysfunction thought likely caused by hyponatremia, then one can give 10 to 12 mL/kg of 3% sodium chloride over 60 minutes. Assuming one wants to raise the serum sodium above 125 mEq/L, one can calculate a more precise amount of 3% sodium chloride to give using the equation:

the number of mL of 3% sodium chloride = (the difference between the actual serum sodium and 125 mEq/L) × the patient's body weight in kilograms × 0.6 L/kg.

Finally, in patients with rather severe hyponatremia (less than 125 mEq/L) but no acute neurologic dysfunction, one can use furosemide (Lasix) in a dose of 1 mg/kg every 6 to 12 hours in association with intravenous infusion of normal saline. In patients with normal renal function, 30 to 60 mEq/L of potassium chloride should be added to the normal saline. If one is replacing in these patients the normal saline with potassium chloride, one gives an estimate of insensible loss, which may be 0.3 times the calculated replacement plus 0.5 mL of fluid for every 1 mL of urine calculated each hour.

With all the techniques of raising low serum sodium levels, once the patient's sodium is sufficiently high that the patient is no longer having neurologic symptoms, there is value in continuing the increase in serum sodium at a slow rate of one mEq/L every 2 hours. Slow correction of hyponatremia minimizes the risk of central pontine myelinolysis. A number of vasopressin antagonists are becoming available which will have increasing utility in the treatment of patients with syndrome of inappropriate antidiuretic hormone secretion. These medications may become particularly useful in patients with chronic SIADH. Currently, chronic SIADH is treated mostly with fluid restriction and, in some instances, with demeclocycline (Declomycin)[1] in a dose of 300 mg by mouth twice daily to 4 times daily[3] for adult-sized individuals, and in proportionately lower doses for children. It is important to note that children younger than 8 years of age are susceptible to abnormalities of dental enamel with the use of tetracyclines.

Diabetes Insipidus

Diabetes insipidus results from the inability to secrete vasopressin or antidiuretic hormone or from the inability to respond to vasopressin.

Symptoms

1. Polyuria
2. Polydipsia
3. Nocturia
4. Preference for ice water
5. Failure to thrive and fever in infants

[1]Not FDA approved for this indication.
[3]Exceeds dosage recommended by the manufacturer.

Severe and prolonged hypernatremia may result in central nervous system dysfunction. It is noteworthy that many patients with central diabetes insipidus have associated conditions that also can contribute to their symptomatology.

Associated Conditions

1. Brain tumors (with headaches, vision disturbance, deficiencies in other hypothalamic pituitary axes, hydrocephalus, and seizures)
2. Diabetes insipidus occurring in the setting of Langerhans cell histiocytosis
3. Sarcoidosis
4. Septo-optic dysplasia (associated with optic nerve hypoplasia, occasionally with developmental delay, and with various pituitary hormone deficiencies).
5. Wolfram syndrome (diabetes mellitus, sensorineural deafness, optic atrophy)
6. Nephrogenic diabetes insipidus may occur from genetic causes, which may be x-linked, autosomal dominant, or autosomal recessive. It may also occur in the setting of medullary cystic disease of the kidneys or in the setting of hydronephrosis from a number of causes.

Diagnosis

The diagnosis of diabetes insipidus depends on the demonstration of increased plasma osmolality in association with inability to concentrate the urine. In some patients, the diagnosis may be made by checking the osmolality or specific gravity of a first-voided morning urine in association with serum electrolytes and/or serum osmolality. If plasma osmolality is increased to more than 295 mOsm/kg or if serum sodium is increased to above 145 mEq/L with urine osmolality remaining below 300 mOsm/kg or urine specific gravity remaining below 1.010, then diabetes insipidus is present. In many instances, fasting serum osmolality and/or sodium are not increased. Under these circumstances, a water deprivation study is indicated. During this test, the patient is weighed hourly and the test is terminated if 5% or more of the body weight is lost. When serum osmolality rises above 295 mOsm/kg, blood is drawn for vasopressin levels and urine is obtained to examine concentrating ability. The values may be interpreted as in Table 1.

For patients who have indeterminate results, 5% saline (850 mmol/L) may be given at a rate of 0.05 mL/kg per hour over a period of 2 hours or until plasma osmolality is greater than or equal to 300 mOsm/kg. The plasma vasopressin level is drawn in levels compared with appropriate standards.

Treatment In Children Older Than 1 Year of Age

The standard treatment for diabetes insipidus in individuals older than 1 year of age is desmopressin (DDAVP). The responsiveness that patients manifest to vasopressin is extremely variable. For this reason,

TABLE 1 Urine Osmolality in Diagnosis of Diabetes Insipidus

Urine Osmolality After Fluid Deprivation	Urine Osmolality After Administration of Desmopressin 0.3 μg IM or 5 μg Intranasally	Diagnosis
<300	>750	Central diabetes insipidus
<300	<300	Nephrogenic diabetes insipidus
>750	>750	Primary polydipsia
300–750	<750	Indeterminate

doses are empiric. Typically, treatment is begun with low doses orally of 100 μg twice daily or 2 to 10 μg intranasally once or twice daily. If treatment is initiated subcutaneously, the treatment is usually begun with 0.1 to 0.2 μg subcutaneously each day.

In patients who have diabetes insipidus that does not respond to administration of desmopressin, the diagnosis of nephrogenic diabetes is made. In these individuals, it is important to study the kidneys to learn whether a specific kidney disease is responsible for the problem. Of particular interest is whether such individuals might have hydronephrosis. Individuals who have normal renal function and normal structure on ultrasound study of the kidneys may have genetic causes for nephrogenic diabetes insipidus or may have this condition on the basis of administration of medication. Medications known to produce this include lithium, demeclocycline, and methoxyflurane. Nephrogenic diabetes insipidus may also be caused by hypokalemia and hypercalcemia. In all of these circumstances, one should consider either removing the offending drug or correcting the metabolic disturbance that is producing diabetes insipidus.

Treatment in Infants

Diabetes insipidus in infants may be treated by administering hydrochlorothiazide[1] in a dose of 2 to 4 mg/kg per day. These medications may be used with potassium-sparing diuretics such as amiloride (Midamor)[1], 20 mg/1.73m^2 per day. In patients with nephrogenic diabetes insipidus, prostaglandin synthesis inhibitors such as indomethacin (Indocin) may be used in addition to hydrochlorothiazide in doses of 2 mg/kg per day.

Adrenocorticotropic Hormone (Corticotropin)

Excessive secretion of adrenocorticotropic hormone (corticotropin) (ACTH) produces Cushing's disease. Cushing's syndrome is the clinical condition resulting from glucocorticoid excess. When excessive

[1]Not FDA approved for this indication.

TABLE 2 Clinical Features of Cushing's Disease

Symptom/Sign	Frequency
Weight gain	90%
Growth retardation	83%
Menstrual irregularity	81%
Hirsutism or hypertrichosis	81%
Obesity (BMI > 85th percentile)	73%
Violaceous skin striae	63%
Acne	52%
Hypertension	51%
Fatigue and weakness	45%
Early puberty	41%
Bruising	27%
Mental changes	18%
Delayed bone age	14%
Hyperpigmentation	13%
Muscle weakness	13%
Acanthosis nigricans	10%
Accelerated bone age	10%
Sleep disturbance	7%
Pubertal delay	7%

Abbreviation: BMI = body mass index.

secretion of ACTH by the pituitary causes adrenal hypersecretion of cortisol, the condition is termed *Cushing's disease*. ACTH hypersecretion typically results from a pituitary adenoma but may at times result from hypothalamic hypersecretion of corticotrophin-releasing hormone. Pituitary hypersecretion of ACTH is not autonomous. Rather, it reflects a higher set point of circulating cortisol. Table 2 outlines the clinical features of Cushing's disease.

The diagnosis of Cushing's disease is established by demonstrating hypercortisolism. A 24-hour urine collection is made from measurements of free cortisol and creatinine (the latter to demonstrate a complete urine collection). Age-related normals should be obtained from the laboratory because techniques vary considerably. A second technique of demonstrating hypercortisolism is by determining cortisol levels in plasma or saliva at the time of the diurnal nadir (between 11 PM and midnight). Plasma cortisol levels at this time fall below 5 μg/dL. Of course, the act of drawing blood at midnight is likely to be stressful, particularly in younger children. Stress responses in this age group may produce false-positive test results. Midnight salivary cortisol levels have been studied and appear to have diagnostic accuracy and predictive values similar to those of midnight plasma cortisol levels. A precise diagnostic cut-off level is likely laboratory dependent. A recent report showed excellent diagnostic utility of a salivary cortisol level of 0.35 μg/dL. Another technique for establishing baseline cortisol excess is the low-dose, overnight, dexamethasone suppression test. A dose of 1 mg of dexamethasone per 1.73 m^2 is administered at 11 PM. The following morning, cortisol levels greater than 5 μg/dL indicate hypercortisolemia. Confirmation of hypercortisolemia may require repeat determinations of 11 PM to midnight salivary cortisol or repeat urine free cortisol determinations. This is particularly important, because approximately 10% of individuals with Cushing's syndrome have a periodic, rather than continuous, cortisol hypersecretion.

The standard dexamethasone suppression test is neither more sensitive nor more specific than the overnight test, the midnight plasma, or salivary cortisol test. Typically, this test includes two baseline days during which 24-hour urines are collected and morning and evening plasma cortisols are measured. Low-dose dexamethasone is then administered over a 2-day period (20 μg/kg per day divided into three or four doses). Urines and bloods are again obtained as on the baseline days. Plasma cortisol should fall below 2 μg/dL by the second day and urine 17-hydroxycorticosteroids should decrease by a factor of 50% and urine free cortisol should fall below 20 μg/24 hours in adult-size individuals. To distinguish between hypercortisolism caused by excessive production of ACTH and that caused by autonomous adrenal overproduction of cortisol, ACTH levels are typically suppressed (when two-site immunometric assays are employed) in primary adrenal causes of hypercortisolism, but are within the normal range or higher in ACTH-dependent Cushing's patients. ACTH levels that are greater than 20 pg/mL are strong indicators of an ACTH-dependent mechanism. If the ACTH level does not clearly delineate the involvement or the lack of involvement of ACTH in the mechanism of the patient's disease, then a high-dose dexamethasone suppression test may be employed. Eighty micrograms per kilogram of dexamethasone is administered and urine is collected for 2 days for measurements of 17-hydroxycorticosteroid and urine free cortisol, as well as for creatinine. Blood is drawn for cortisol and ACTH. Typically, both urine free cortisol and serum cortisol are 50% of the baseline or less following 2 days of high-dose dexamethasone administration.

ACTH excess may result from ectopic secretion of ACTH by a number of tumors. Although ACTH production in many of these tumors remains high despite administration of high doses dexamethasone, a number of cases of ectopic ACTH syndrome demonstrate dexamethasone suppressibility. The most reliable method of distinguishing between pituitary and ectopic ACTH production is the inferior petrosal sinus sampling test. An experienced radiologist catheterizes each of the two inferior petrosal sinuses. Blood is drawn in the basal state and 2, 5, and 10 minutes after administration of corticotropin-releasing hormone (Acthrel)* (1 μg/kg). Samples are also drawn at those times from a peripheral venous site. ACTH levels are measured centrally and peripherally. If the ratio of the petrosal sinus sample to the periphery is greater than 3 following CRH administration, then a pituitary source of ACTH is established. If ratios are consistently less than 2, then an ectopic source of ACTH is established.

*Investigational drug in the United States.

Magnetic resonance imaging (MRI) will detect pituitary ACTH-producing tumors in between 35% and 60% of patients with Cushing's disease. It is important to interpret results of MR scanning in light of data indicating the presence of incidental pituitary tumors in at least 10% of normal individuals between 20 and 40 years of age.

Treatment

Treatment of pituitary Cushing's disease consists of transsphenoidal pituitary resection of the corticotrophic tumor. Because these tumors are not visible on MR scans in approximately 50% of patients, some centers employ inferior petrosal sinus sampling to localize the tumors. The criterion often employed is an ACTH ratio of at least 1.4 in comparison with the contralateral petrosal sinus ACTH level. On occasion, the pituitary tumor is not found, and Cushing's disease persists. Under these circumstances, pituitary irradiation may be considered. Alternatively, bilateral adrenalectomy is an option. In the recent past, laparoscopic adrenalectomy has reduced the time of recuperation from surgery. If bilateral adrenalectomy is chosen, then the patient must be monitored carefully for rapid growth of the pituitary tumor (Nelson's syndrome). Serial MR scanning and determinations of ACTH are helpful in such monitoring.

ACTH Deficiency

ACTH deficiency may result from congenital abnormalities of the hypothalamus such as septo-optic dysplasia and holoprosencephaly, congenital abnormalities of the pituitary gland such as mutations in PROP-1, PIT-1 mutations, and mutations in Tbx 19. ACTH deficiency may result from hypothalamic and pituitary tumors, trauma and hemorrhage, as well as granulomatous disease and radiation therapy. Finally, hypothalamic and pituitary corticotrophic axis suppression can be induced by a history of glucocorticoid treatment.

The symptoms of deficient ACTH include hypoglycemia, prostration with intercurrent illness, decreased energy and endurance, orthostatic faintness, anorexia, nausea, vomiting, and skin hypopigmentation.

Low levels of plasma cortisol at 8 AM in association with nonelevated ACTH levels suggest ACTH deficiency. This diagnosis can be confirmed using an insulin tolerance test. Regular insulin, 0.1 U/kg body weight, is given intravenously. Blood glucose is monitored at 15- to 30-minute intervals. Cortisol levels are measured at 30-minute intervals. With sufficient lowering of blood glucose (50% of the basal level), cortisol should rise to at least 18 μg/dL. Two other tests that can be used are the metyrapone test in which metyrapone (Metopirone) is given in a dose of 30 mg/kg at midnight and plasma cortisol and 11-deoxycortisol are measured at 8 AM. A normal morning 11-deoxycortisol is greater than 7 μg/dL. Plasma cortisol should be unstimulated (less than 5 μg/dL). Another test that can be used is the corticotropin-releasing hormone stimulation test. Bovine CRH (Acthrel)* is given in a dose of 1 μg/kg intravenously. Levels of cortisol and ACTH are measured at 15 minutes, 30 minutes, and 60 minutes. Cortisol levels should exceed 20 μg/dL and ACTH levels should exceed 27 pg/mL.

Treatment

Treatment of ACTH deficiency consists of administration of hydrocortisone[1] in a dose of 7 to 10 mg/m^2 per day. In children, this medication is typically divided into doses given three times daily. Typically, the dose given in the morning is the largest dose and that given in the evening is the smallest dose. The adequacy of the dose is typically judged on the basis of the patient's symptoms of energy and presence or absence of symptoms of hypoglycemia.

Thyroid-Stimulating Hormone

Thyroid-stimulating hormone stimulates thyroid hormone synthesis and secretion by the thyroid gland. It is secreted by the anterior pituitary gland in response to stimulation by the hypothalamic hormone, thyrotropin-releasing hormone. Increased thyrotropin releasing hormone occurs in association with central thyroid hormone resistance. Pituitary hypersecretion of thyroid stimulating hormone may also be produced by TSH-secreting tumors. The most sensitive test for the identification of TSH-secreting pituitary adenomas is an elevation of the ratio of serum levels of the α subunit of pituitary glycoprotein hormones to serum TSH levels. This ratio is below 5.7 in patients with normal levels of gonadotropin. These patients also have elevations in the absolute level of the α subunit. Normal values for the α subunit are less than 3 μg/L.

In response to infusion of thyrotropin-releasing hormone 500 μg intravenously, patients with TSH-secreting tumors increase TSH by less than 220%, whereas normal individuals increase TSH by more than 750%.

To confidently diagnose inappropriately elevated TSH, it is important to exclude elevated levels of thyroxine-binding proteins. When levels of thyroxine-binding proteins are elevated, individuals may have hypothyroidism with low levels of free thyroxine but normal or high levels of total thyroxine. Under these circumstances, elevated TSH is an appropriate response to low levels of free thyroxine.

Individuals with TSH excess producing hyperthyroidism have the usual hyperthyroid symptoms such as

[1]Not FDA approved for this indication.
*Investigational drug in the United States.

heat intolerance, tremulousness, insomnia, tachycardia and palpitations, hypersudation, hyperdefecation, attention deficit, and hyperphagia, and menstrual abnormalities in women.

Treatment of TSH-secreting tumors consists of an attempt at removal of the tumor by transsphenoidal surgery. In patients in whom surgical treatment is not curative, external irradiation may be employed. Medical treatment may include octreotide (Sandostatin)[1], which is often effective at doses of 100 to 1500 μg daily.

TSH deficiency may be caused by congenital or genetic abnormalities of the hypothalamus and pituitary such as septo-optic dysplasia and holoprosencephaly. Mutations of Pit-1 or PROP-1 may contribute to multiple pituitary hormone deficiencies, including deficiency of TSH. TSH deficiency may also be caused by mutations in the TSH β subunit gene.

Symptoms

1. Hypothyroid symptoms (decreased energy, cold intolerance, dry hair and skin, decreased appetite, constipation, growth delay in children, and menstrual abnormalities in mature women)
2. In infants, TSH deficiency can give rise to psychomotor delay

TSH/TRH deficiency may result from tumors, trauma, and hemorrhage, as well as from granulomatous diseases and other infiltrative conditions.

Diagnosis

Diagnosis of TSH deficiency is made by finding a low free-thyroxine level in association with a nonelevated level of thyroid-stimulating hormone. It is noteworthy that some patients with TRH deficiency manifest a very slight elevation of immunoassayable thyroid-stimulating hormone. Studies of TSH in these individuals show decreased glycosylation giving rise to decreased bioactivity of the thyroid-stimulating hormone.

Treatment of TSH deficiency comprises administration of L-thyroxine (Synthroid). In infants, L-thyroxine should be given in relatively high doses of 10 to 15 μg/kg per day. The dose should then be rechecked at 1- to 2-week intervals to normalize free thyroxine. In individuals older than 2 years of age, L-thyroxine should be started slowly—particularly in individuals with rather severe hypothyroidism. In children in whom TSH deficiency was treated with L-thyroxine excessively rapidly, hyperthyroid symptoms may occur in association with increased intracranial pressure. In adults, patients may develop hyperthyroid symptoms in association with symptoms of ischemic cardiac disease. Thus, treatment may be initiated in doses of 25 μg daily and slowly increased to achieve normal levels of free thyroxine. It is important to recheck levels of L-thyroxine 5 to 6 weeks after making a change in the dose so that an equilibrium level of circulating hormone can be reached.

[1]Not FDA approved for this indication.

Pituitary Gonadotropins: Luteinizing-Stimulating Hormone and Follicle-Stimulating Hormone

These hormones are secreted in response to hypothalamic secretion of pulses of gonadotropin-releasing hormone (GnRH). Faster pulsations of hypothalamic GnRH induce greater LH than FSH secretion from gonadotropes. Conversely, slower frequencies of hypothalamic GnRH pulsation favor FSH synthesis and secretion. Additionally, the gonadal steroids estradiol and testosterone contribute to determining levels of pituitary LH and FSH secretion. Testosterone decreases gonadotrope production of LH, but does not affect gonadotrope production of FSH. A large percentage of the negative feedback by testosterone occurs at the level of the hypothalamus. Much of the negative feedback of estradiol occurs at the level of the pituitary gonadotrope. Estradiol may also have a positive feedback at both the hypothalamus and pituitary gland. This occurs when estradiol levels are maintained at 500 pg/mL for a period of 36 hours. Pituitary gonadotropins are also regulated by inhibins produced by follicular and luteal cells in the ovary and by the Sertoli cells in the testes. Inhibins specifically suppress pituitary production of FSH without affecting pituitary production of LH.

Overactivity of the hypothalamic–pituitary–gonadal axis may be produced by abnormal migration of the neurons, which produce gonadotropin-releasing hormone. These neurons originate in the olfactory placode and migrate to both the preoptic area and to the medial basal portion of the hypothalamus. The GnRH-secreting neurons are constitutively active. When these neurons are appropriately situated in the hypothalamus, axons from other neurons exert largely inhibitory actions. This inhibition is evident at mid-gestation, as well as in the latter part of infancy. Inhibition is released at the time of puberty. If gonadotropin-releasing hormone neurons are located ectopically (forming hamartomas), then inhibitory influences are absent, and early puberty occurs. Other mechanisms by which inhibitors of gonadotropin-releasing hormone are disturbed include central nervous system tumor, hydrocephalus, a number of conditions such as Rett syndrome, trauma, and hemorrhage. Some individuals with malformations of the brain, such as septo-optic dysplasia or agenesis of the corpus callosum, may experience early puberty on this basis. Finally, on very rare occasions, pituitary adenomas consisting of gonadotropes may produce early puberty.

Recently, loss of the function mutations in a G-protein–coupled receptor, GPR54, have been associated with hypogonadotropic hypogonadism. This receptor is apparently activated by peptides derived from a precursor protein, kisspeptin-1. Patients with X-linked congenital adrenal hypoplasia have hypogonadotropic hypogonadism because of loss of function mutations in the gene for DAX-1. This gene activity is at both the hypothalamic and pituitary levels. Patients with juvenile hemochromatosis develop iron deposition in pituitary gonadotropes in association with hypogonadotropic hypogonadism. Patients with inactivating mutations of KAL-1 have failure of migration of gonadotropin-releasing hormone neurons from their origin in the olfactory placode to the appropriate places within the hypothalamus. Although these neurons make gonadotropin-releasing hormone in the region of the olfactory placode, the concentration of gonadotropin-releasing hormone in blood reaching the anterior pituitary gland is too low to stimulate gonadotrope activity. Patients with septo-optic dysplasia (sometimes associated with mutations in transcription factor HESX1 or LHX3) may have delayed puberty. Mutations may also occur in the gonadotropin-releasing hormone receptor on pituitary gonadotrope. The pituitary transcription factor PROP-1 and the orphan nuclear receptor SF-1 may be mutated and thereby produce hypogonadotropic hypogonadism. Loss of leptin function because of loss of function mutations in the leptin gene, in the leptin receptor gene, or in prohormone convertase 1, may produce hypogonadotropic hypogonadism. Central nervous system tumors, hydrocephalus, cranial irradiation, hemorrhage, and infiltrative diseases may also produce hypogonadotropic hypogonadism. Finally, undernutrition and extremely vigorous activity are associated with hypogonadotropic hypogonadism, perhaps in part because of lower levels of leptin in these individuals.

The clinical presentation varies largely with the severity of the hypogonadism. Some males manifest hypogenitalism at the time of birth. It is noteworthy that patients with hypogonadotropic hypogonadism may have small phalluses but do not have hypospadias. Some hypogonadotropic boys manifest cryptorchidism. If hypogonadotropic hypogonadism has occurred by the time of expected puberty, then secondary sexual characteristics will be either totally absent (particularly in individuals with congenital adrenal hypoplasia in whom even adrenal androgens are absent giving rise to total absence of sex hair), or secondary sexual characteristics are underdeveloped. Frequently, individuals will manifest eunuchoid proportions. At times, hypogonadal males will have a degree of gynecomastia. Sexual function may be decreased in proportion to the completeness of the defect. Infertility is also a major problem.

In infants with micropenis, evaluation depends on the precise timing of the patient's presentation. Male infants tend to have minipuberty beginning at 1 week of life and peaking at 2 months of life. By 6 to 7 months, these individuals manifest little measurable activity of the hypothalamic–pituitary–gonadal axis. If examined within the first 2 to 3 months of life, the basal levels of testosterone and gonadotropins should reflect minipuberty with FSH levels ranging from 0.16 to 4.1 mIU/mL in boys, and from 0.24 to 4 mIU/mL in girls. LH levels range from 0.02 to 7.0 mIU/mL for the first 2 months. Testosterone levels rise from approximately 20 to 50 ng/dL to 60 to 400 mg/dL between the first week and 2 months of life in infant boys. In infant girls, estradiol levels increase to between 0.5 and 5 ng/dL between 1 and 2 months of age and then decline to less than 1.5 ng/dL over the first year of life.

If levels of both sex steroids and gonadotropins are low, this suggests hypogonadotropic hypogonadism. This diagnosis can be bolstered by measuring sex steroid levels following treatment with human chorionic gonadotropin. A frequently used regimen in boys is human chorionic gonadotropin, 33 units per pound, given three times weekly for 3 weeks. Testosterone and dihydrotestosterone may be measured on the day following the final injection. This fairly extensive regimen allows assessment of gonadal responsiveness to human chorionic gonadotropin and, in addition, end-organ responsiveness to testosterone and dihydrotestosterone.

In prepubertal individuals, it is impossible to distinguish between patients with hypogonadotropic hypogonadism and normal children with basal hormone levels (testosterone, LH, FSH, estradiol) or with the use of gonadotropin-releasing hormone testing. At the expected time of puberty, individuals with hypogonadotropic hypogonadism may be difficult to distinguish from those with constitutional delay of growth and development. Both will have prepubertal levels of LH, FSH, and sex steroids. Both will have prepubertal responses to gonadotropin-releasing hormone. In those beyond the expected time of puberty. measurement of body proportions may be useful because teenagers with hypogonadotropic hypogonadism ultimately develop eunuchoid proportions, whereas those with constitutional delay of growth and development do not. Absent a strong family history of pubertal delay, boys who have not begun puberty by 14 years of age and girls who have not begun puberty by 13 years of age need evaluation. Because hypogonadotropic hypogonadism and constitutional delay of growth and development are difficult to distinguish, it is important to perform MR scans of the head to rule out intracranial pathology. This may be less urgent in patients who have a history of marked weight loss or very high activity levels, or in those who have anosmia potentially associated with Kallmann syndrome.

Because of the difficulty in distinguishing constitutional delay of growth and development from hypogonadotropic hypogonadism, it is common to initiate treatment in individuals with marked pubertal delay. Treatment in boys typically consists of testosterone enanthate (Delatestryl), cypionate, or cyclopropionate. Typically, this is begun in a dose of approximately 50 mg intramuscularly every 4 weeks. Transdermal testosterone (Testoderm) may also be given. A dose of 2.5 mg every other night might be useful for the starting dose; it is adjusted once testosterone levels are measured. Very often, this treatment is given for 4 to 6 months and then discontinued to again evaluate the patient's spontaneous puberty. If, within 4 months, the patient is still prepubertal, testosterone treatment can be resumed with a gradual increase in testosterone enanthate doses to 100 and then 200 mg each month. The adult dose of testosterone enanthate is in the range of 200 mg intramuscularly every 2 weeks. This dose can be altered on the basis of circulating levels of testosterone measured 1 week after the injection. Alternatively, transdermal testosterone gel may be used with increasing doses from 2.5 g every day, increasing if needed to 5 g every day and at times 7.5 g every day based on measurements of circulating testosterone levels. Boys who receive testosterone treatment in the setting of constitutional delay of growth and development may be also given an aromatase inhibitor to prevent excessively rapid advancement of skeletal age. This is particularly important for those boys with constitutional delay who also have an element of short stature. Treatment in girls may begin with estradiol (Estrace) in a dose of 0.5 mg daily, ethinyl estradiol in a dose of 5 μg daily, or conjugated estrogens (Premarin) in a dose of 0.3 mg daily. This treatment may be given for a period of 4 to 6 months and then discontinued if it appears that the patient may be entering spontaneous puberty. If, over the ensuing 4 months there is no evidence of spontaneous puberty, and if skeletal age is not advancing excessively, then treatment may be restarted with a gradual increase in dose. It should be noted that as the estradiol increases to 1 mg daily or the conjugated estrogen dose increases to 0.625 mg daily, or the ethinyl estradiol dose to 10 μg daily, then it is necessary to add a progestin such as medroxyprogesterone (Provera) in a dose of 5 mg daily for the first 12 days of each month in order to induce appropriate menstrual flow. The induction of menses is critical for avoiding endometrial hyperplasia. Subsequently, doses of ethinyl estradiol may be increased to 2 mg daily if circulating levels of estradiol are not within the normal range for late puberty. Similarly, conjugated estrogens may be increased to 1.25 mg daily. If menstruation is not induced with medroxyprogesterone 5 mg daily, despite increasing the estrogen dose, then a trial of a higher dose of medroxyprogesterone, such as 10 mg daily, should be considered.

Growth Hormone

Physiology

Pituitary secretion of growth hormone (GH) is directed by three peptides: growth hormone-releasing hormone (GHRH), somatostatin, and Ghrelin. Growth hormone-releasing hormone is produced in the arcuate nucleus of the hypothalamus and is delivered to the anterior pituitary by the hypophyseal portal vessels. Growth hormone-producing pituitary cells respond to GHRH through a G-protein–associated receptor, which is located in the plasma membrane of somatotropes. GHRH triggers somatotrope release of GH. Somatostatin is produced in the periventricular portion of the anterior hypothalamus and is conveyed via the portal system to the anterior pituitary gland. Somatostatin occupies a variety of plasma membrane-associated receptors, which, in turn, activate inhibitory G proteins. Ghrelin is produced both in the hypothalamus and in the stomach. It occupies receptors that are distinct from those that bind GHRH. The magnitude of Ghrelin's contribution to GH regulation is not yet clearly understood.

Growth hormone is a single-chain protein containing 191 amino acids, although 5% to 10% of circulating growth hormone comprises a shorter peptide containing 177 amino acids. Growth hormone is secreted in discrete pulses which are greater in amplitude and frequency in stages 3 and 4 of sleep. Larger pulses also occur postprandially and during exercise and stress. The GH receptor is a member of the cytokine receptor superfamily. All members of this receptor superfamily dimerize in response to the presence of ligand. The dimerized receptor binds to a cytosolic protein, JAK2 (Janus kinase 2); JAK2 contains a tyrosine kinase domain. A number of downstream phosphorylations occur, including phosphorylation of STAT (signal transducer and activator of transcription) proteins 1, 3, and 5.

One of the most important target-tissue responses to growth hormone is transcription of the insulin-like growth factor genes. Insulin-like growth factors are peptides produced in a large number of growth hormone target tissues. A substantial portion of the growth-promoting signal generated by growth hormone is transmitted by production of insulin-like growth factors 1 and 2 (IGF-1 and IGF-2). IGF-1 is generated in tissues such as the liver and transported by the blood to physes (growth centers) of the bones. A portion of insulin-like growth factors appears to be generated within the physes in response to the action of growth hormone at these sites.

Pathophysiology

Growth hormone deficiency may be produced by a number of mechanisms. Genetic abnormalities of hypothalamic function may decrease GHRH production or increase somatostatin production. Midline abnormalities of the hypothalamus such as septo-optic dysplasia may produce growth hormone deficiency among other hormonal abnormalities. "Idiopathic" growth hormone deficiency appears to result most frequently from insufficient GHRH secretion, because GHRH supplementation augments growth hormone secretion and may normalize growth in a large majority of such patients. Irradiation or infiltration of the hypothalamus with histiocytosis or with sarcoidosis can have a similar effect as can tumors of the hypothalamus.

The pituitary gland may fail to respond to GHRH because of inactivating mutations in the GHRH receptor. In other instances, the pituitary has abnormal development that precludes GH secretion. Such abnormal development may occur in response to mutations in their GH gene. A number of genes directing pituitary development, such as PIT-1 and PROP-1, may have inactivating mutations producing growth hormone deficiency among other pituitary defects. Infiltrated diseases such as histiocytosis may interfere with pituitary function as may tumors and vascular malformations. Trauma may interrupt pituitary function. At times this trauma occurs during labor and delivery and disturbs the contiguity of the pituitary stalk.

In some individuals, the secretion of growth hormone is normal, but the responsiveness to growth hormone is attenuated. The most common cause of this is undernutrition, a condition in which GH receptors are down-regulated. In some individuals, the gene for growth hormone receptors has inactivating mutations. GH target tissues are therefore unable to respond to GH and cannot generate insulin-like growth factors and other growth responses.

Diagnosis

The diagnosis of growth hormone deficiency should be suspected in children who have subnormal growth velocity postnatally. Typically, GH deficiency causes little prenatal growth deceleration. Congenitally hyposomatotropic infants grow normally during a substantial portion of infancy and then experience growth deceleration. Acquired GH deficiency may occur at any age and may produce growth deceleration up to the time of closure of the physes.

Subnormal growth may result from abnormalities in the function of virtually any organ system. Among the endocrine abnormalities which can produce poor growth, thyroid hormone insufficiency and cortisol excess are prominent. Thus, poor growth should prompt the physician to obtain a complete history and to perform a thorough physical examination.

Evaluation of the growth pattern is facilitated by obtaining previous height and weight data and by plotting these on appropriate growth charts. In infancy, growth in length and weight may accelerate or decelerate up to 2 to 3 years of age. After 3 years of age, normal growth proceeds at a normal growth velocity such that the patient's height does not cross major percentiles.

Specific patterns can help to determine the cause of poor growth. If weight gain becomes subnormal prior to a decline in growth in height or length, then undernutrition or maldigestion or malabsorption should be suspected. If marked weight gain accompanies a significant decline in growth in length or height, then cortisol excess or thyroid hormone deficiency should be considered.

In screening for GH deficiency, serum levels of IGF-1 and insulin-like growth factor-binding protein-3 (IGFBP-3) should be determined along with baseline GH levels. Measurements of free T_4 (thyroxine) and TSH should be obtained. Additionally, serum electrolytes and tests of liver and kidney function should be performed, in addition to determining levels of calcium and phosphorus. The blood count should be determined and erythrocyte sedimentation rate measured. There is frequently value in performing urine analysis and in studying the stool for occult blood, excess fat, and ova and parasites.

Growth Hormone Deficiency

The diagnosis of growth hormone deficiency is usually established by observing growth deceleration upon plotting the patient's height and weight and by determining IFG-1 deficiency for the patient's age and sex. Other causes of IGF-1 deficiency should be excluded by ascertaining that baseline GH is not high and that GH binding protein is not low (a frequent finding in undernutrition). Additionally, thyroid hormone levels should be normal before diagnosing GH deficiency.

A number of growth hormone provocative tests can be employed, although these are not superior to the diagnostic method noted above. Provocative tests used in children include insulin-induced hypoglycemia, arginine infusion, and clonidine[1] administration. In adults, insulin-induced hypoglycemia or arginine and GHRH may be used.

Treatment

Growth hormone treatment in infants and children is generally started with a dose of 0.3 mg/kg per week administered subcutaneously each day. The dose is adjusted to normalize IGF-1 levels and to stimulate adequate growth. The GH dose in adolescents may be as high as 0.7 mg/kg per week. If the depot preparation is used, then 0.75 mg/kg is given subcutaneously twice monthly. In adults, treatment is begun with 0.006 mg/kg per day and increased to normalize IGF-1 levels. Typically, the maximum dose in adults younger than 35 years of age is 0.025 mg/kg per day; in adults older than 35 years of age, it is 0.0125 mg/kg per day.

Side effects are rare and include pseudotumor cerebri, headache, hyperglycemia, hypothyroidism, exacerbation of scoliosis (in growing children), carpal tunnel syndrome, edema, muscle pain, and increased growth of pre-existing nevi. Concern has been raised about the possibility that the risk of neoplasia might be increased, particularly in individuals in whom high IGF-1 levels are induced.

[1]Not FDA approved for this indication.

Growth Hormone Excess

Growth hormone excess produces gigantism in children and adolescents (whose physes remain open), and acromegaly in adults. Growth hormone excess should be considered in children and adolescents who grow at a velocity that makes them cross major growth percentiles during the interval between 3 years of age and the onset of puberty (typically at 12 years of age in boys and at 10 to 11 years of age in girls). Additionally, children whose height is more than three standard deviations above the mean, or whose predicted adult height is more than two standard deviations above the adjusted mean parental height, should be evaluated for growth hormone excess.

Adults with acromegaly experience enlarging extremities with need for larger shoes, gloves, and rings. They also have coarsening of facial features in conjunction with frontal bossing and progressive prognathia. A large percentage experience arthropathy and hyperhidrosis. Carpal tunnel syndrome is also common. Growth hormone excess may occur in the setting of McCune-Albright syndrome, multiple endocrine neoplasia type 1, or Carney complex.

DIAGNOSIS

Growth hormone excess may be sought with measurement of IGF-1 levels (corrected for age and sex). Oral glucose tolerance testing can demonstrate growth hormone excess in individuals whose GH fails to fall to 1 ng/mL.

Individuals who experience overgrowth as a result of excessive GH secretion in early childhood frequently have excessive hypothalamic GHRH secretion. Those with later onset of GH excess have adenoma formation in approximately 30%. These adenomas form because of an activating somatic mutation in the α subunit of the stimulatory G-protein.

Occasionally GH excess results from excessive GHRH secretion from bronchial carcinoids, small-cell lung cancers, pancreatic endocrine tumors, and medullary thyroid carcinomas.

TREATMENT

The treatment of growth hormone excess depends on the cause. If there is ectopic GHRH secretion, then a search for the source of GHRH should be followed by efforts to surgically remove such tumors.

Individuals with pituitary microadenomas producing GH excess should undergo transsphenoidal tumor removal; 80% of these patients enjoy normalization of IGF-1 following surgery. Macroadenomas produce persistent elevations of GH and IGF-1 in at least 50% of patients taken to surgery. These individuals require radiation therapy and/or administration of octreotide (Sandostatin).

A fraction of patients with GH excess may respond to dopamine agonists such as bromocriptine (Parlodel) (7.5 to 80 mg daily beginning with 2.5 mg daily and gradually increasing) and cabergoline (Dostinex)[1] (beginning with 0.25 mg twice weekly and gradually increasing.)

Octreotide is an analogue of somatostatin. It may be started in doses of 50 μg daily and graduall, increased to a maximum of 1500 μg daily. Frequently, the dose is divided into injections administered subcutaneously every 8 hours. A depot preparation is available, which may be initiated with a monthly dose of 10 mg intramuscularly. Adverse effects of octreotide include cholecystitis, ascending cholangitis, bradycardia, arrhythmias, syncope diarrhea, abdominal pain, flatulence, constipation, nausea and vomiting, hyperglycemia, cholelithiasis, flu-like symptoms, dizziness, headache, arthropathy, and hypothyroidism.

Another medication, pegvisomant (Somavert), is a GH-receptor antagonist that inhibits GH-receptor dimerization. It often is effective in normalizing IGF-1 levels in patients who continue to have elevated IGF-1 levels despite octreotide therapy. Treatment is started with 10 mg subcutaneously each day, which is increased by 5 mg every 4 to 6 weeks, to normalize IGF-1. The maximum dose is 30 mg daily. Side effects include elevated transaminase levels, injection site inflammation, peripheral edema, dizziness, flu-like syndrome, chest pain, paresthesias, nausea, hypertension, and hypoglycemia.

[1]Not FDA approved for this indication.

HYPERPRO-LACTINEMIA

METHOD OF

Shannon Heitritter, MD, and Robert Dluhy, MD

Prolactin is a polypeptide hormone secreted by the lactotroph cells of the anterior pituitary gland. Prolactin secretion is tonically inhibited by dopamine, which reaches the lactotrophs via the hypothalamic–pituitary portal circulation and binds to dopamine subtype 2 (D_2) receptors. The production and secretion of prolactin are stimulated by estrogen and thyrotropin-releasing hormone (TRH).

Etiology

The serum prolactin level may be increased by a prolactin-secreting pituitary adenoma (prolactinoma) or as a result of decreased inhibition by dopamine. The latter may be achieved either by a structural abnormality in the hypothalamus or stalk interrupting the hypothalamic–pituitary system or as a result of the use of medications that deplete or antagonize dopamine action. Table 1 summarizes the physiologic, pathologic, and pharmacologic causes of hyperprolactinemia.

Clinical Presentation

Excess prolactin inhibits gonadotropin-releasing hormone (GnRH) secretion, which leads to a reduction in leuteinizing hormone (LH) and follicle-stimulating hormone (FSH) secretion, resulting in central hypogonadism. In premenopausal women, this manifests as irregular or absent cycles and infertility as a result of anovulation. These women may also experience symptoms of subnormal estrogen concentrations such as vaginal dryness; those with irregular or absent menses may have decreased bone mineral density. Men similarly present with symptoms of hypogonadism, including decreased libido, impotence, infertility, and gynecomastia. Women and, rarely, men may also present with galactorrhea. Postmenopausal women are, by definition, hypogonadal, thus such patients with prolactinomas present with mass effect symptoms such as headaches or visual changes secondary to chiasmatic compression.

TABLE 1 Causes of Hyperprolactinemia

Physiologic	
	Pregnancy, lactation, nipple stimulation, stress, sleep, exercise
Pathologic	
Hypothalamic	Tumors: suprasellar pituitary mass extension (e.g., craniopharyngioma), meningioma, hypothalamic metastases
	Trauma, radiation, infiltrative diseases (e.g., sarcoidosis)
Pituitary	Prolactinoma, growth hormone-secreting pituitary adenoma (acromegaly), macroadenoma (stalk compression), macroprolactinemia
Thyroid	Primary hypothyroidism*
Systemic diseases	Renal failure, cirrhosis, chest wall lesions
Ectopic production	Hypernephroma, bronchogenic carcinoma
Pharmacologic†	
Dopamine store depletors	Reserpine (Serpasil)
Dopamine synthesis inhibitors	Methyldopa (Aldomet)
Dopamine release inhibitors	Opiates: oxycodone (OxyContin)
Dopamine receptor blockers	Benzamines: metoclopramide (Reglan)
	Butyrophenones: haloperidol (Haldol)‡
	Benzisoxazoles: risperidone (Risperdal)‡
	Phenothiazines: prochlorperazine (Compazine)
Estrogens	Oral contraceptive pills
H2 receptor blockers	Ranitidine (Zantac), famotidine (Pepcid)
Others	Antihypertensives: labetalol (Trandate)
	Anticonvulsants: phenytoin (Dilantin)
	Selective serotonin reuptake inhibitors: sertraline (Zoloft), fluoxetine (Prozac)
	Tricyclic antidepressants: Amitriptyline (Elavil), imipramine (Tofranil)

*The incidence of elevated prolactin levels (median: 60 μg/L; range: 10-100 μg/L) in overt hypothyroidism is 20%.
†This list is selective and contains commonly used drugs known to cause hyperprolactinemia.
‡The prevalence of hyperprolactinemia (median: 85 μg/L; range:5-150 μg/L) among patients taking risperidone is 65%, and is 50% among patients taking conventional antipsychotics such as haloperidol.

Diagnosis

The evaluation of hyperprolactinemia begins with a thorough history to determine if physiologic or pharmacologic causes of excess prolactin are present (see Table 1). Initial laboratory investigation should include a repeat prolactin level to confirm the presence of hyperprolactinemia. Prolactin levels of 20 to 150 μg/L are indeterminate and may be found in patients with hyperprolactinemia from any cause; values above 150 to 200 μg /L generally indicate a prolactin-secreting adenoma. A high molecular weight form of prolactin with weak biologic activity, called macroprolactin, can lead to a high prolactin value. The presence of macroprolactinemia, which should be suspected when the prolactin level is elevated out of proportion to a patient's clinical symptoms, can be confirmed with specialized laboratory techniques. Because pregnancy and primary hypothyroidism can cause hyperprolactinemia, it is important to rule out these secondary causes by obtaining β-human chorionic gonadotropin (bHCG) and thyroid-stimulating hormone (TSH) values. Absent such causes, pituitary magnetic resonance imaging (MRI) (with the contrast agent gadolinium) is recommended to identify a prolactin-secreting adenoma or other structural lesion. Prolactin-secreting adenomas are radiologically defined as either microprolactinomas (<1 cm in diameter) or macroprolactinomas (>1 cm in diameter). In patients with macroprolactinomas, it is important to screen for evidence of pituitary hormone deficiencies. In some instances, prolactinomas may not be visualized with current imaging techniques, in which event, the patient is diagnosed with idiopathic hyperprolactinemia.

Objectives of Therapy

The goal of treatment is to normalize the prolactin level and, therefore, to correct the biochemical and clinical consequences of the excess hormone.

TABLE 2 Comparison of the Dopamine Agonists Bromocriptine and Cabergoline

Parameter	Bromocriptine (Parlodel)	Cabergoline (Dostinex)
Biochemical description	Semisynthetic ergot alkaloid	Synthetic ergot derivative
Tablet size	2.5, 5.0 mg	
Frequency of administration	Dose should be divided and given 2 times daily	0.5 mg 1 or 2 times weekly
Initial dose	1.25 mg PO daily, given at bedtime with snack	0.25 mg PO once weekly, given at bedtime with snack
Titration guidelines	Add 1.25 mg in AM after first week; increase daily dose by 1.25 mg each week; repeat prolactin level after 1 month; titrate drug until prolactin normalizes.	Increase biweekly dose by 0.25-0.50 mg each month; repeat prolactin each month and titrate drug until the prolactin level normalizes
Total dose usually required to normalize prolactin	5.0-7.5 mg daily (microprolactinomas) or 7.5-10.0 mg daily (macroprolactinomas)	0.25-0.50 mg twice weekly (for micro- or macroprolactinomas)
Maximum recommended dose	10.0 mg daily	1.0 mg twice weekly
Generic	Yes	No
Monthly cost	7.5 mg daily, $195.50	0.5 mg biweekly, $236.97
Side effects	Nausea, fatigue (if nausea persists, it may be ameliorated with intravaginal administration); postural hypotension may be seen with administration of the first dose	Nausea and fatigue; much less common and milder in severity than with bromocriptine; postural hypotension may be seen with administration of the first dose

This includes restoration of normal gonadal function and fertility (if desired) and the prevention of osteoporosis. If a macroprolactinoma is present, an additional objective is to reduce tumor size and to reverse any mass effects.

Medical Therapy of Hyperprolactinemia

Medical management of both micro- and macroprolactinomas with dopamine agonist therapy is the treatment of choice in most cases. There are two dopamine agonists currently approved by the FDA for the treatment of hyperprolactinemia: bromocriptine (Parlodel) and cabergoline (Dostinex) (Table 2).

Bromocriptine is a semisynthetic ergot alkaloid with a half-life of 6 hours; it binds to anterior pituitary cell-surface D_2 receptors, leading to reductions in the synthesis and secretion of prolactin, and often to a decrease in tumor size. Bromocriptine normalizes prolactin secretion in 82% of patients with microprolactinomas and restores gonadal function in 90%. It normalizes prolactin levels in 80% to 85% of patients with macroprolactinomas. An objective reduction in tumor mass in micro- or macroprolactinomas is reported in 70% to 80% of treated patients. In these responders, maximal tumor diameter is reduced by 56% in patients with microprolactinomas, and in 64% of patients with macroprolactinomas.

Cabergoline, a dopamine agonist with a longer half-life (65 hours), fewer side effects, and greater efficacy than bromocriptine, is currently the first-line therapeutic choice. It normalizes prolactin, restores gonadal function, and leads to significant tumor shrinkage in 82% of patients with macroprolactinomas and in 90% of patients with microprolactinomas. It is also effective in restoring normal prolactin levels in 70% of patients who fail to normalize prolactin levels with bromocriptine therapy. See Table 2 for recommended bromocriptine and cabergoline dosing regimens.

Management of Microprolactinomas

Medical management of microprolactinomas with dopamine agonist therapy is the treatment of choice. Specific management strategies are guided by the clinical presentation and preferences of the patient (Figure 1). Patients with normal menstrual cycles and hyperprolactinemia are not at risk for osteoporosis and thus may be followed with observation alone. Patients with oligomenorrhea or amenorrhea who are not seeking fertility may be treated with a dopamine agonist to normalize prolactin, thus restoring gonadal function for bone protection. An oral contraceptive pill (OCP) is an acceptable alternative to achieve the same endpoint. Patients with microprolactinomas treated with OCPs do not have an increase in tumor size despite the fact that estrogen is known to have a trophic effect on pituitary lactotrophs. Patients who are seeking fertility should be treated with bromocriptine to restore normal cycles and fertility (see below).

Management of Macroprolactinomas

Macroprolactinomas have greater growth potential than microprolactinomas and often have signs of mass effect; therefore, they require treatment at clinical presentation (see Figure 1). Dopamine agonists are the first-line therapy in most cases. In medically treated patients, an MRI should be repeated 6 to 12 months later to assess reduction in tumor size. In the subset of patients with tumors compressing the optic chiasm, however, surgical decompression may be required at the outset.

Surgery

In patients who are refractory to or intolerant of dopamine agonist therapy, transsphenoidal resection

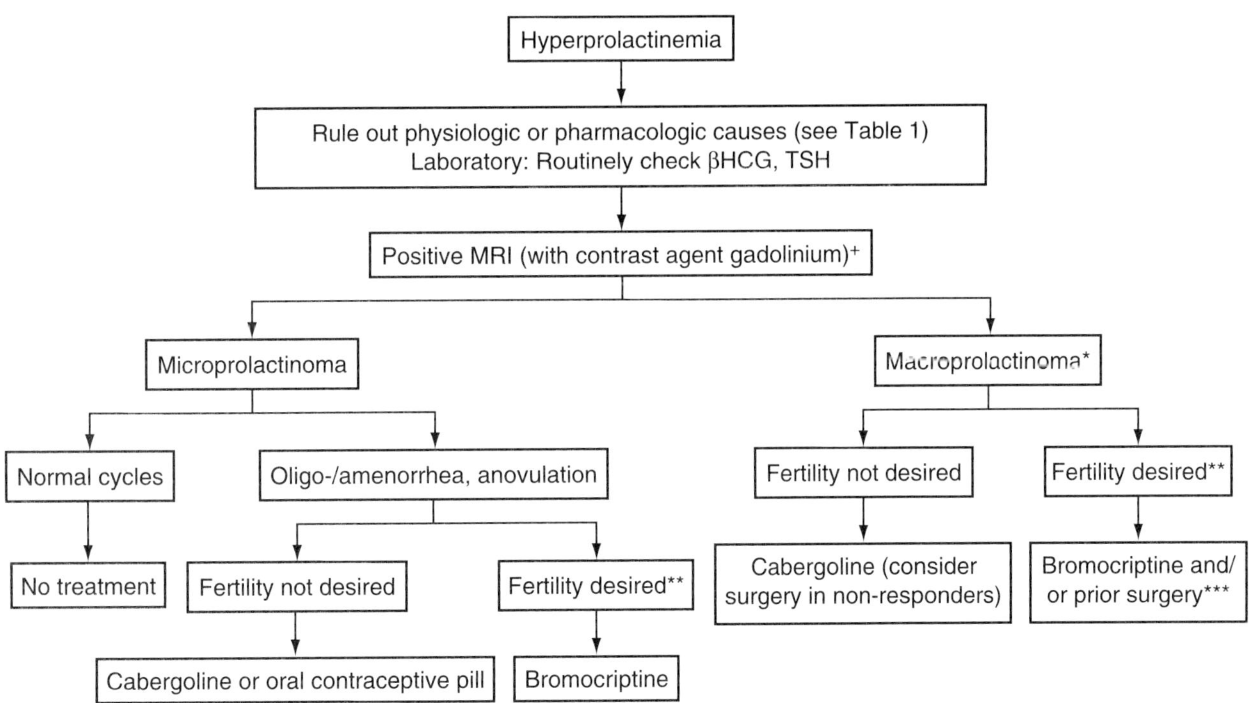

+ Patients who have a normal MRI are diagnosed with idiopathic hyperprolactinemia; they are medically managed in the same way as patients with microprolactinomas.
* In macroprolactinomas, prolactin levels are usually > 200 ug/L.
** When fertility is desired, bromocriptine (Parlodel) is preferred given a greater safety experience with this agent.
*** Patients with macroprolactinomas require medical treatment to reduce tumor volume or surgical treatment to excise the adenoma prior to attempting to conceive.

FIGURE 1 Management of prolactinoma.

(TSPR) should be considered. TSPR normalizes prolactin levels and restores regular cycles in 80% of patients with microprolactinomas, and in 50% of patients with macroprolactinomas. The recurrence rate of hyperprolactinemia, however, is 25% to 50% at 5 years; patients with the highest preoperative prolactin levels have the highest risk of recurrence.

Irradiation

In patients who do not respond to dopamine agonist therapy, or in those patients in whom surgery has debulked tumor volume, radiotherapy should be considered for treating residual mass. While it is effective in stabilizing or decreasing the size of most tumors, there have long-term risk of developing secondary hypopituitarism.

Discontinuation of Medical Therapy

Patients with microprolactinomas who have been treated with cabergoline for 2 years, have normal prolactin levels, and have achieved tumor reductions of 50% or more, should be offered a trial of drug withdrawal. The overall rate of remission in such patients 2 to 5 years after withdrawal of the drug is 69%. Prolactin levels should be followed over time to detect recurrence of hyperprolactinemia.

Patients with macroprolactinomas treated with cabergoline for at least 2 years who have normal prolactin levels and who have demonstrated tumor reductions of 50% or more (with the tumor at a distance of >5 mm from the optic chiasm) have an overall remission rate 2 to 5 years after withdrawal of the drug of 64%. However, because such patients are at risk of tumor re-expansion with associated mass effects, such as visual compromise, we recommend that the drug be gradually tapered to the lowest dose needed to maintain normal prolactin levels. For example, the biweekly dose of 0.25 mg of cabergoline can be decreased every 3 months. A prolactin level is measured after each dose reduction and an MRI is obtained 6 months after the first decrease in medication to evaluate for recurrence of tumor mass.

Management of Prolactinomas in Pregnancy

The treatment and management of micro- and macroprolactinomas when pregnancy is desired differ substantially. In either circumstance, bromocriptine is the preferred dopamine agonist because of a greater safety experience with this agent. While it is known that hyperestrogenemia causes lactotroph hyperplasia, studies have documented that the risk of a microprolactinoma increasing in size significantly during pregnancy is very small (1.6%). Therefore, bromocriptine should be stopped once pregnancy is confirmed. Because of the low risk of tumor growth during pregnancy in these patients, there is no need to perform periodic MRI or visual field testing during pregnancy. However, these studies should be performed in patients with clinical symptoms suggestive of tumor expansion such as visual complaints or headaches.

Patients with macroprolactinomas require medical treatment to reduce tumor volume or surgical treatment to excise the tumor before becoming pregnant. Because these tumors have a risk (13% to 36%) of growth during pregnancy, these patients should undergo a baseline MRI and visual field examination prior to attempting to conceive. If the adenoma does not compress the optic chiasm, bromocriptine may be initiated and continued until the tumor has decreased in size and is contained within the sella turcica. Once this is achieved, the patient may attempt to conceive and should discontinue the bromocriptine with her first missed period. Patients with very large adenomas, or with tumors that compress the chiasm, should undergo primary therapy with TSPR and, possibly, adjunctive radiation before becoming pregnant. During pregnancy, such treated patients should be followed closely for signs or symptoms suggestive of tumor growth such as visual complaints or headaches. In the presence of these symptoms, repeat imaging and visual field examination are indicated. If there is clinical evidence of significant tumor growth or mass effect, the patient should be initially treated with bromocriptine; TSPR may be indicated in nonresponding patients.

HYPOTHYROIDISM

METHOD OF

Peter A. Singer, MD

Hypothyroidism is probably the commonest thyroid disorder encountered in clinical practice. It is estimated that approximately 13 million persons living in the United States have hypothyroidism, or roughly 2% of the population. Hypothyroidism increases in prevalence with increasing age; approximately 10% of 65-year-old women are hypothyroid, and perhaps 15% of 75-year-old women are hypothyroid. Women are affected much more often than men, in a ratio of 8:1 or 9:1. Approximately 95% of hypothyroidism in the United States is from primary thyroid failure, either from chronic autoimmune (Hashimoto's) thyroiditis, or from surgical or radioiodine ablation. There are numerous other causes of hypothyroidism, including transient forms of the disorder associated with either subacute painful thyroiditis, or with postpartum thyroiditis. In addition, certain drugs, including the antiarrhythmic agent amiodarone (Cordarone) and the cytokines interferon-alfa and interleukin-2 (Proleukin), may cause transient hypothyroidism, by causing thyroiditis. Amiodarone, which is heavily iodinated, may cause hypothyroidism by inhibiting thyroid hormone secretion, as may the antidepressant lithium carbonate. Much less common causes of hypothyroidism include congenital hypothyroidism, affecting approximately 1:3500 live births in the United States, and certain rare chronic inflammatory or infiltrative disorders, including hemochromatosis, cystinosis, and Riedel's struma. In geographic areas of iodine deficiency, iodine lack is the principal cause of hypothyroidism; there are no known areas of iodine deficiency in the United States. All of the aforementioned causes of hypothyroidism are termed *primary hypothyroidism*, because of the thyroid gland's deficiency in secreting thyroid hormone. *Secondary hypothyroidism*, on the other hand, occurs when there is a deficiency of thyroid-stimulating hormone (TSH) secretion because of an abnormality of the hypothalamic–pituitary axis, usually from pituitary tumors or craniopharyngiomas, although other disorders may cause deficient TSH secretion. Table 1 lists the different etiologies of hypothyroidism.

Symptom and Signs

The symptoms and signs of hypothyroidism are typically multiple and varied, nonspecific, and often suggestive of other clinical conditions. Symptoms depend on the age of the patient, the severity of the hypothyroidism, and its duration. Young patients typically have fewer symptoms, whereas older individuals are less able to tolerate thyroid hormone deficiency. Typical symptoms of hypothyroidism include fatigue, dry skin and hair, increased need for sleep, cold intolerance, constipation, weight gain, and slowing of intellectual functioning. Increased menstrual flow may also be present. A common misconception among patients (and even many physicians) is that significant weight gain is associated with hypothyroidism; even with overt hypothyroidism, patients gain no more than 10% to 15% over baseline weights, because hypothyroidism is associated with a decreased appetite.

Signs of hypothyroidism may include bradycardia, mild diastolic hypertension, a waxy and pale complexion, puffiness of the eyelids, slowing or even slurring of speech, goiter, muffled heart tones, and delayed

TABLE 1 Causes of Hypothyroidism

Primary Hypothyroidism

Permanent Hypothyroidism

Chronic autoimmune (Hashimoto's) thyroiditis (commonest cause in industrialized countries)
Thyroid ablation (radioactive iodine therapy for hyperthyroidism; thyroidectomy)
External radiotherapy (for head and neck cancer, lymphoma)
Congenital (~1 per 3500 live births in the United States; caused by thyroid agenesis)
Infiltrative disorders (hemochromatosis, amyloidosis, Riedel's thyroiditis, cystinosis, scleroderma, leukemia—all are infrequent to rare)
Iodine deficiency (principally in Asia, Africa, and areas of Latin America)
Iodine excess—from iodine containing medications, such as amiodarone, saturated solution of potassium iodide (occurs in patients with underlying autoimmune thyroid disease)

Transient Hypothyroidism

Subacute painful (viral) thyroiditis
Subacute painless thyroiditis—most frequently postpartum
Drug induced
Interferon-alfa; interleukin-2 (Proleukin); amiodarone (Cordarone) (the drugs induce a thyroiditis-like response)
Exogenous iodides, including amiodarone (euthyroidism returns after drug withdrawal)
Antithyroid drugs—methimazole (Tapazole), propylthiouracil (resolves after medication withdrawal)
Lithium carbonate (Eskalith) (resolves after medication withdrawal; occurs only in patients with underlying autoimmune thyroid disease)

Secondary (Central) Hypothyroidism

Pituitary adenoma, craniopharyngioma
Pituitary apoplexy, Sheehan's syndrome
Lymphocytic hypophysitis
Pituitary irradiation
Cranial radiation
Pituitary stalk section; other major head trauma
Congenital hypopituitarism (rare)
Infiltrative disorders (Langerhans' histiocytosis hemochromatosis)
Granulomatous disorders (sarcoidosis)

deep tendon reflexes. As with symptoms, signs depend on the degree of thyroid hormone deficiency, duration of the disorder, and patient age.

LABORATORY DIAGNOSIS

The serum thyrotropin (TSH) is the cornerstone in the biochemical diagnosis of primary hypothyroidism, and should be the first test employed in screening for hypothyroidism. If the serum TSH is elevated, a serum free thyroxine (FT_4) or its estimate should be obtained, to assess the degree of thyroid deficiency. Mild TSH elevation (i.e., greater than 5 mIU/L and less than 20 mIU/L) associated with a normal FT_4 is termed either *subclinical hypothyroidism, mild hypothyroidism, or mild thyroid failure,* while a low FT_4 associated with an elevation in serum TSH is termed *overt hypothyroidism.* A normal or low serum TSH associated with a low FT_4 suggests secondary hypothyroidism, and in such cases, pituitary imaging with magnetic resonance imaging (MRI) is indicated.

Whether or not to measure thyroid antibodies in patients with elevated TSH levels is a matter of debate. Because most patients with spontaneous hypothyroidism have chronic autoimmune thyroiditis, antimicrosomal (thyroperoxidase [TPO]) antibodies are usually elevated. Thus, if there is clinical and biochemical evidence of hypothyroidism, measurement of antibodies may be superfluous, in terms of treatment, because their presence or absence will not influence the decision to treat. If the TSH is mildly elevated, and the FT_4 is normal, measurement of TPO antibodies may be helpful in determining whether or not there is spurious (transient) TSH elevation; in such cases, TPO antibodies will be negative, and the clinician may wish to defer therapy until persistent TSH elevation has been documented.

It should be noted that there are pitfalls in the interpretation of serum TSH levels. It is most reliable when measured in ambulatory individuals. In hospitalized euthyroid patients, on the other hand, the TSH may be either high or low, depending on the severity of the nonthyroidal illness. Thus, a serum TSH that is mildly abnormal in an ill patient should be repeated following recovery. Serum TSH values may also become mildly elevated with the use of certain drugs, especially by dopamine antagonists such as metoclopramide (Reglan) or domperidone (Motilium)[2]; the degree of TSH elevation with such agents tends to be very mild. Elevated serum TSH levels occur in thyrotoxic patients, such as those with TSH-secreting pituitary adenomas; such patients are clinically and biochemically thyrotoxic, and should not be confused with patients with suspected hypothyroidism. Finally, mild TSH elevations, even in healthy ambulatory individuals, may be transient, and before initiating therapy for hypothyroidism, the serum TSH should be repeated.

Treatment

There is virtual unanimity of opinion among endocrinologists that levothyroxine (L-T4) (Synthroid) is the drug of choice for the treatment of hypothyroidism. Approximately 80% of L-T4 is absorbed from the gastrointestinal tract, and the T_4 half-life of 1 week ensures that a constant level of thyroid hormone in serum can be easily achieved. L-T4 is administered in a daily oral dose, and the goal of therapy is to achieve a normal serum TSH level; while laboratory reference ranges of TSH may be fairly broad, practicing endocrinologists prefer that the TSH be maintained in the range of approximately 0.5 to 2 mIU/L.

The average L-T4 dose for healthy adults is approximately 1.6 μg/kg per day; patients younger than 50 or 55 years of age may be started on full-replacement therapy. Older patients are generally started on doses of between 25 and 50 μg per day. Those with underlying coronary disease, or other significant co-morbidities, such as diabetes mellitus, hypertension

[2]Not available in the United States.

and hyperlipidemia (metabolic syndrome), should be started on doses no greater than 25 μg per day.

After therapy is initiated, patients should be reevaluated in about 6 to 8 weeks, with a clinical examination and serum TSH level. There is little utility in checking the TSH sooner, because serum T_4 and TSH levels take about 6 weeks to equilibrate. If the serum TSH continues to be elevated, the dose of L-T4 should be increased by 25 μg per day, and the patient reevaluated in another 6 to 8 weeks, and every 2 to 3 months thereafter, with 25 μg dose adjustments, until the TSH normalizes. If the TSH level is suppressed, the dose should be decreased, and further adjustments made every few months until normalization of the serum TSH concentration is achieved. Once patients are on a stable dose of L-T4, they may be reevaluated yearly, or more often, as the clinical situation dictates.

Patients should be instructed to take L-T4 on an empty stomach, and to refrain from eating for an hour, as food appears to inhibit L-T4 absorption, albeit slightly. In addition, patients should be instructed to avoid taking iron and/or calcium supplements at the same time as L-T4, because the supplements have a mild inhibitory effect on L-T4 absorption; spacing should be at least 2 hours apart. In addition to interfering with absorption of L-T4, a number of conditions and drugs alter L-T4 dose requirements, and are listed in Table 2.

OTHER CONSIDERATIONS

Pregnancy

Pregnancy increases L-T4 requirements by as much as 40%. The need for the dose increase is multifactorial, in part related to increased T_4 clearance, as well as increased transfer of T_4 to the fetus. The estrogen-mediated increase in thyroxine-binding globulin (TBG) appears to increase T_4 requirements also. It is essential for normal fetal growth and intellectual development that the hypothyroid mother be euthyroid during pregnancy; therefore, once pregnancy is confirmed a maternal serum TSH should be obtained, and then again 4 weeks later. A rise in TSH warrants an immediate increase in L-T4 dose, usually by 25 μg per day. The serum TSH should be checked once each trimester, and the L-T4 dose should be adjusted accordingly. An alternative method is to empirically increase the L-T4 dose by approximately 40% once pregnancy is confirmed, rather than wait for an increase in TSH. In my experience the "40% rule" is inconsistent, and I prefer waiting until an increased dose need is demonstrated. Following delivery, the pre-pregnant dose of L-T4 may be resumed without hesitation.

TABLE 2 Factors Affecting Levothyroxine (L-T4) Dose

Increased L-T4 Dose Requirement
Increase in thyroxine binding globulin (TBG)—pregnancy, estrogen therapy
Weight gain
Impaired gastrointestinal absorption of L-T4
Inflammatory small bowel disease, celiac disease
Vitamins and supplements containing iron, calcium carbonate; aluminum hydroxide gels
Sucralfate (Carafate); bile acid-binding sequestrants (cholestyramine [Questran], colestipol [Colestid])
Diet very high in soy
Drugs increasing L-T4 metabolism—phenytoin (Dilantin), carbamazepine (Tegretol), phenobarbital, rifampin (Rifadin)
Smoking?
Decreased L-T4 Dose Requirement
Decrease in TBG—androgen therapy; nephrotic syndrome
Aging (old age)
Weight loss

Subclinical Hypothyroidism

The issue of whether or not to treat patients with mild TSH elevations and normal FT_4 concentrations is still controversial. Some clinicians use a serum TSH of 10 mIU/L as the lowest cut-off to initiate treatment with L-T4, whereas others suggest treating any patient with an elevated TSH, regardless of the level. I advocate obtaining TPO antibodies in patients with elevated TSHs, and if the antibodies are positive, I encourage L-T4 therapy (usually with a starting dose of 25 to 50 μg/d), because individuals with positive antibodies and TSH levels above the normal range are likely to develop overt hypothyroidism at a rate of about 5% per year. Thus, early initiation of treatment in such patients will avoid the inadvertent development of overt hypothyroidism.

Levothyroxine Product Switching

A common scenario nowadays is product switching by pharmacists, driven by insurance companies' desire to reduce costs. The least expensive preparation is frequently substituted for the product the physician has prescribed. Most endocrinologists strongly urge that patients take a "branded" preparation, and if the product is switched when the prescription is refilled, that the patient be reevaluated with a serum TSH, no sooner than 6 weeks, because the concern is that not all products are bioequivalent.

Other Thyroid Hormone Preparations

In addition to L-T4, there are other thyroid hormone preparations available, including desiccated thyroid, combinations of T_4 and T_3, and T_3 (Cytomel) alone. Some patients have strong preferences for such preparations, and for various reasons, a common one being that they know that T_3 is the biologically active form of thyroid hormone. However, because T_4 is converted to T_3 in peripheral tissues, there clearly is no advantage to the use of T_3-containing preparations. Moreover, there may be disadvantages in their use, including inconsistent bioavailability, and the supranormal increase in serum T_3 levels, which may occur within a few hours after taking them. In patients with underlying heart disease, a significant increase in T_3 concentration may result in angina or arrhythmia. Despite the caveats provided to patients, some are insistent, and believe that they will feel better by taking T_3 alone, or in combinations with T_4. My solution to situations such as these, if my explanation regarding the advantages of L-T4 therapy does not suffice, is to prescribe one of the preparations in a dose tailored to mimic the L-T4 dose. I carefully explain that suppression of TSH must be avoided, and that they may not feel better. It is preferable to ensure some measure of compliance, than to have the patient go untreated.

Treatment of Secondary Hypothyroidism

Patients with secondary hypothyroidism usually have other pituitary hormone deficiencies, and before thyroid hormone therapy is initiated it is imperative that the remainder of pituitary status be evaluated; it is essential that L-T4 not be prescribed unless patients with adrenocorticotropic hormone (ACTH)-cortisol deficiency are also on glucocorticoid therapy. L-T4 therapy alone could precipitate adrenal crisis. Because the serum TSH cannot be used as an endpoint of therapy, the clinician must rely on the serum FT_4 (or estimate) concentration, which should be kept in the upper half of the normal range.

HYPERTHYROIDISM

METHOD OF

Vahab Fatourechi, MD

Epidemiologic studies show that 1.3% of a cross-section of the United States' population older than age 12 years has hyperthyroidism. Of that group, 0.5% have clinical and 0.7% have subclinical hyperthyroidism. Symptoms and signs of hyperthyroidism are quite variable and depend on the degree of excess of circulating thyroid hormones and on the age of the patient. In the subclinical hyperthyroid state, the peripheral thyroid hormone levels (L-thyroxine or T_4 and triiodothyronine or T_3) remain in the normal reference laboratory range. Yet given the nature of sensitive hypothalamic–pituitary–thyroid feedback mechanism and the log–linear relationship between peripheral hormones and thyroid-stimulating hormone (TSH), serum TSH levels may be below lower limit of normal and even be suppressed below the detection level (e.g., <0.01 mIU/L). There is ample evidence for the adverse effects of abnormally low TSH on bone and heart if serum TSH is <0.1 mIU/L. Patients are less likely to have symptoms of hyperthyroidism and other adverse effects when TSH is below normal range but above 0.1 mIU/L (0.1 to 0.3 mIU/L). Overt hyperthyroidism is defined by above-normal laboratory ranges of one or both peripheral thyroid hormones (free T_4 or T_3) and by TSH levels less than 0.1 mIU/L. Clinical signs and symptoms of hyperthyroidism include tachycardia, perspiration, heat intolerance, tremor, and muscle weakness. Patients under the age of 50 years have typical symptoms and older individuals may have atypical symptoms. Weight loss is a common complaint but an occasional young patient may gain weight as a result of an increase in appetite that is disproportionate to the increased metabolic rate. The hyperthyroid person over 60 years of age can be apathetic and may present with atrial fibrillation or unexplained weight loss. Diagnosis of overt hyperthyroidism is based on clinical suspicion, demonstration of suppressed TSH, and high-normal thyroid hormone levels. For diagnosis of subclinical hyperthyroidism other causes of abnormally low TSH such as hypothalamic or pituitary disease, euthyroid-sick syndrome, and recovery from hyperthyroidism should be excluded.

Etiology of Hyperthyroidism

Hyperthyroidism is a syndrome with many causes (listed in Table 1). Etiology should be determined prior to planning treatment. The most common cause of spontaneous hyperthyroidism in a nonendemic goiter area is Graves' disease. Graves' disease has subacute onset and is associated with diffuse goiter and an occasional bruit over the thyroid. Graves' ophthalmopathy occurs in 20% to 40% of the patients. Nodular goiter, either a single hyperfunctioning nodule called *toxic adenoma* or *multinodular toxic goiter* called *Plummer's disease*, is another common cause of hyperthyroidism. In toxic adenoma, an isotopic thyroid scan shows hyperfunction in the nodule and suppression of isotope uptake in the rest of the gland. In multinodular toxic goiter, an isotopic scan shows areas with variable isotope uptake. In nodular goiter, 24-hour radioactive iodine uptake is usually normal. In this condition, as opposed to Graves' disease, TSH-receptor antibodies are negative. Silent autoimmune thyroiditis, postpartum thyroiditis, and subacute thyroiditis are relatively common causes of transient thyrotoxicosis associated with low radioiodine uptake. Rare causes

TABLE 1 Medications Used in the Therapy of Hyperthyroidism

Drug	Starting Daily Dose	Characteristic
Propranolol (Inderal)	60-120 mg	Symptomatic relief
Atenolol (Tenormin)	50-100 mg	Symptomatic relief
Propylthiouracil (PTU)	150-200 mg, twice daily	Blockage of hormone synthesis
Methimazole (Tapazole)	30-40 mg/day	

of hyperthyroidism include TSH-producing pituitary tumor, metastatic follicular cancer of the thyroid, and choriocarcinoma. Exogenous thyroxine therapy either inadvertent or for the management of thyroid cancer is also a common cause of subclinical hyperthyroidism. Surreptitious ingestion of thyroid hormone is an uncommon cause of clinical or subclinical hyperthyroidism.

Management of Graves' Disease

No safe and effective therapy aimed at stopping the autoimmune cascade and arresting generation of thyroid-stimulating immunoglobulins is available. For control of hyperthyroidism of Graves' disease, there are three accepted therapies. Therapy is either aimed at reducing the synthesis and production of thyroid hormones until remission occurs, or at reducing the tissue mass or ablating the thyroid gland (by surgery or radioactive iodine). None of these therapies is ideal. But considering the significant adverse effects and unpredictable course of the disease, one of the three modalities of antithyroid therapy, radioactive iodine therapy, or surgery should be chosen. This decision should be made after considering the clinical circumstances, the severity of disease, the size of the goiter, and the age and preference of the patient. Spontaneous remission can occur occasionally. In long-term follow-up, 20% of patients have developed spontaneous hypothyroidism. However, except in cases of subclinical asymptomatic hyperthyroidism in young individuals, withholding therapy is not an option.

USE OF β BLOCKERS

β-Adrenergic blockers can relieve increased adrenergic activity, which is responsible for tachycardia, tremor, and anxiety. These medications are needed for symptomatic relief until specific therapy lowers the hormone levels. Once biochemical euthyroidism is achieved, β blockers should be tapered off. I administer a sustained-release propranolol (Inderal LA) with a starting dose of 60 to 80 mg. The dose can be doubled to achieve a pulse rate lower than 90 and above 60 beats per minute. Atenolol (Tenormin) 50 to 100 mg per day is an alternative. β Blockers are not recommended as the sole therapy, with the exception of some cases of subclinical hyperthyroidism under observation.

ANTITHYROID THERAPY

Despite possible side effects and low remission rates in Graves' disease (40% to 50%) after an 18-month course of therapy, antithyroid drugs are widely used throughout the world. They are more commonly used as the first choice in Asia and Europe than in the United States. Most endocrinologists in the United States prefer definitive therapy with radioactive iodine (RAI) for adult patients. The reasons for choosing antithyroid drug therapy by some physicians is the higher possibility of avoiding permanent hypothyroidism, concerns about aggravating ophthalmopathy, and patients' fear of radiation exposure.

Childhood, adolescence, and pregnancy are the best indications for antithyroid drug therapy. Two antithyroid drugs are widely used, methimazole (Tapazole) and propylthiouracil (PTU). They both block thyroid hormone formation. Methimazole is the preferred drug because it is faster acting and can be given once daily, as opposed to propylthiouracil, which should be given in divided doses. Methimazole results in euthyroidism earlier and has a more favorable safety profile. Propylthiouracil may partially inhibit T_4 conversion to active T_3; however, the clinical significance of this effect is not known. The usual starting dose of methimazole is 30 to 40 mg per day and for propylthiouracil 300 to 400 mg. For complete blockage of hormone production, doses as high as 60 mg of methimazole and 600 mg of propylthiouracil may be needed. I usually use a daily dose of 20 mg of methimazole for the treatment of small goiters and mild hyperthyroidism and 40 mg for more severe cases and large goiters. There is no benefit in the concomitant use of T_4. I usually obtain a serum free thyroxine (FT_4) level in the first month and serum TSH and free thyroxine monthly thereafter. I advise the patients about the side effects of therapy. I tell them that a skin allergic reaction happens in 2% to 5% of patients. If it happens, I stop therapy and use another modality. If skin eruption occurs with one antithyroid drug, there is a 25% chance of allergy to the other antithyroid drugs. I tell patients that there is a 1 in 1000 chance of agranulocytosis, a serious condition that results in infection. The serious rare side effect of agranulocytosis occurs suddenly and a periodic blood count is not helpful. If sore throat and unexplained fever develop, I advise patients to stop medication and to contact a physician for obtaining a blood count. It is advisable to get a leukocyte count with any new sign of illness. With the understanding that serial blood counts do not predict sudden occurrence of agranulocytosis, I still obtain a monthly complete blood count (CBC) and also serum transaminase (AST) to screen for hepatic toxicity.

Severe hepatic toxicity is rare. I advise patients to stop medication and to seek medical evaluation if abdominal pain, jaundice, or itching occurs. Vasculitis and arthralgia are rare but possible side effects. If encountered, I use another modality of therapy for management of hyperthyroidism. After the first month and after the reduction of free thyroxine to normal range, the dose of methimazole is progressively reduced. Usually serum TSH becomes measurable after 2 to 3 months. I try to keep the TSH level in the mid-to-low normal range. The interval between visits at the stage when the patient is on a low dose of therapy can be increased to 2 to 3 months. I usually stop therapy after 18 months. If recurrence occurs after one course of antithyroid medication, I recommend radioactive iodine therapy for adult patients. Some physicians use a longer course of therapy, especially for children and adolescents. There is evidence to show that the response rate to antithyroid drugs is better and faster in iodine deficient areas. No definitive test or criteria for predicting remission in response to antithyroid medications is available. Small goiter, low requirement of antithyroid medications for maintaining euthyroidism, rapid normalization of serum TSH, and disappearance of TSH receptor antibodies are possible clues for a higher chance of remission.

Antithyroid medications are sometimes used in severe cases of hyperthyroidism for preparation of definitive ablative therapies, such as surgery and radioactive iodine. In our practice, this is rarely necessary except for very severe cases, and β blockers alone are adequate. Patients who have been treated with propylthiouracil may require larger doses of radioactive iodine for therapeutic effect.

RADIOACTIVE IODINE THERAPY

Radioactive iodine (RAI) therapy with ^{131}I has been used since the 1940s and is safe and effective. At the Mayo Clinic we consider RAI therapy the treatment of choice for symptomatic Graves' hyperthyroidism for all adult patients. The reason for preferring RAI over antithyroid therapy is the low remission rate after an 18-month course of antithyroid therapy, relatively high rate of spontaneous hypothyroidism in long-term follow-up of Graves' disease, and unpredictable variation of thyroid function in autoimmune thyroid disease. We also have concerns about the uncommon, but serious, complications of antithyroid therapy.

Radioactive iodine uptake of the thyroid is measured prior to therapy in order to verify diagnosis, to exclude iodine contamination, and to calculate the dose of the RAI based on thyroid weight and 24-hour uptake of radioactive iodine. Attempts to give a small dose of radioiodine to achieve long-term euthyroidism do not usually succeed. Most patients either develop recurrence of hyperthyroidism or eventually become hypothyroid in long-term follow-up. I usually give a relatively large dose calculated on the basis of 200 μCi delivered to 1 g of estimated thyroid tissue. Some clinicians administer a fixed dose of RAI, usually between 5 and 15 μCi. We believe that once the decision is made to treat a patient with Graves' disease, an adequate dose of RAI should be given to make at least an 90% of patients hypothyroid within 3 to 6 months. Hypothyroidism, when it occurs, is treated early and is continued life-long—in short, a serious disease is converted to a stable, more benign, and easily treatable condition. Inability to achieve hypothyroidism in 3 to 6 months may indicate underestimation of the RAI dose or the presence of multinodular goiter.

There is some evidence from randomized studies that there may be a worsening of ophthalmopathy after RAI therapy and that this can be prevented by a concomitant 3-month course of corticosteroid therapy. However, in my opinion, the possibility of this effect is low and, if it happens, it is temporary. I do not administer corticosteroids with RAI therapy unless there is evidence for clinically significant ophthalmopathy and there are risk factors for progression, such as current tobacco use. Ophthalmopathy of Graves' disease may present itself and be progressive at any time after diagnosis, without relationship to the type of therapy. We advise using a relatively large dose of RAI to prevent a need for repeated RAI. We detect and treat hypothyroidism as early as possible.

SURGICAL MANAGEMENT IN GRAVES' HYPERTHYROIDISM

Surgery is usually not indicated for therapy of Graves' hyperthyroidism. The same results can be obtained by RAI therapy without the risks of surgical complications. However, surgery is a safe and effective form of treatment, when performed by an experienced surgeon. Special indications for surgery are a need for rapid control of hyperthyroidism, large goiters, and Graves' disease coexistent with nodular disease. Other indications for surgery include failure of antithyroid drug therapy in children, pregnancy in the second trimester with intolerance to antithyroid mediations, and women of child-bearing age who intend to become pregnant within 6 to 9 months. We prepare patients for surgery with β blockers and iodide such as Lugol or saturated solution of potassium iodide (SSKI), 3 to 5 drops daily for 7 days before the procedure. Iodide reduces blood flow to the gland and lowers levels of thyroid hormones (by acute pharmacologic effects of iodide). Some surgeons leave a part of the thyroid tissue to avoid hypothyroidism. However, this usually results in frequent recurrence of hyperthyroidism and does not eliminate the likelihood of hypothyroidism (50%). In our institution, thyroid surgeons perform a safe, near-total thyroidectomy followed by T_4 therapy for inevitable hypothyroidism. I believe that because of the vascularity of the thyroid gland in Graves' disease, the complications of hypoparathyroidism and recurrent laryngeal nerve damage will be higher than the reported 1% if the surgeon is not experienced in thyroid surgery.

Toxic Nodular Goiter

TOXIC ADENOMA

In this condition, a palpable nodule corresponds to a hot spot in the isotope scan in one lobe, and the other lobe has low or absent uptake of isotope. The likelihood of spontaneous resolution as a result of degeneration and hemorrhage into the nodule is low, and thus antithyroid therapy is not indicated. I prefer surgery in patients younger than 30 years of age or for very large nodules. I advise radioactive iodine therapy (20 to 30 mCi) for older individuals and smaller nodules. Preparation with β blockers is usually adequate. After radioactive iodine therapy or surgery, the function of the contralateral lobe returns to normal. The frequency of hypothyroidism is low after appropriate radioactive iodine therapy. Hypothyroidism does not occur after surgical excision of a single nodule.

MULTINODULAR TOXIC GOITER

The clinical picture and management of multinodular toxic goiter are similar to single toxic nodule. The patients are usually older and the uptake of radioactive iodine may be variable among the nodules. Bilateral excision of nodules is preferable in large nodular goiters if an experienced surgeon is available. Radioactive iodine is also a good option. The required dose of radioactive iodine (^{131}I) is much larger than what is needed for Graves' disease, because of the heterogeneous uptake and larger size of the goiter and also because of lower radioactive iodine uptake. The choice between surgery or radioactive iodine will depend on the patient's preference, age, general medical condition, and access to an experienced surgeon. Preparation with β blockers, with or without antithyroid therapy, is necessary prior to surgery, depending on the severity of the disease.

Postpartum and Silent Thyroiditis

These transient conditions are of autoimmune nature and may be triphasic with hyperthyroid then hypothyroid, followed by a euthyroid state. Destruction of the thyroid results in hormone release, low radioactive iodine uptake of the thyroid, and transient hyperthyroidism. Therapy is symptomatic with β blockers.

Subacute Thyroiditis

Subacute thyroiditis (also called granulomatous or de Quervain thyroiditis) is most likely of viral origin and may be associated with fever. Inflammation of the thyroid results in painful thyroid, release of stored thyroid hormones, low thyroid uptake of radioactive iodine, and a high erythrocyte sedimentation rate. The thyroid is usually very tender on palpation. Therapy is symptomatic, with β blockers, analgesics, and nonsteroidal anti-inflammatory drugs. In cases with significant pain, a short course of corticosteroid therapy may be used.

Hyperthyroidism in Pregnancy

A common cause of hyperthyroidism in pregnancy is Graves' disease. Radioactive iodine is absolutely contraindicated in pregnancy. The usual therapy is propylthiouracil (PTU) because of reports of aplasia cutis in the fetus with methimazole (Tapazole) therapy. Because both PTU and thyroid-stimulating immunoglobulins pass through the placenta, both the mother and the fetus are exposed to the disease process and therapy, and close monitoring of the fetus by an obstetrician is required. Therapy should be with the lowest necessary dose of PTU in order to avoid maternal and fetal hypothyroidism and to avoid the development of goiter in the fetus. There is a high possibility of improvement or remission in the third trimester, resulting in a minimal requirement of antithyroid drugs. If there is intolerance or failure of antithyroid drugs, thyroidectomy in the second trimester can be done safely and should be followed by thyroxine therapy.

Subclinical Hyperthyroidism

Once the diagnosis of subclinical hyperthyroidism is established and a persistent suppression of TSH below 0.1 mIU/L is demonstrated, I treat most patients in the same way as I treat those with clinically overt hyperthyroidism. This recommendation is based on the knowledge of adverse effects of suppressed TSH on the cardiovascular system, the increased risk of atrial fibrillation, and the increased rate of bone loss. In case of nodular goiter, RAI or surgery is chosen. In Graves' disease, RAI is preferable for older patients. In young patients, depending on clinical condition, observation, β blockers, or low-dose antithyroid drug therapy may be tried in the hope of spontaneous remission. Definitive therapy will be needed after a period of conservative therapy if the condition persists. For patients with a serum TSH level of between 0.1 and 0.3 mIU/L close observation is recommended.

TABLE 2 Classification of Thyrotoxicosis According to Radioiodine Uptake of the Thyroid

High Uptake Hyperthyroidism
Graves' disease
Thyroid-stimulating hormone (TSH)-producing pituitary tumor
Chorionic gonadotropin-producing tumor
Normal Uptake Hyperthyroidism
Toxic adenoma
Multinodular toxic goiter (Plummer's disease)
Low Uptake Thyrotoxicosis
Exogenous thyroid hormone
Silent thyroiditis
Postpartum thyroiditis
Subacute thyroiditis
Iodine-induced hyperthyroidism
Uptake Outside of Thyroid Gland
Struma ovary tumor
Metastatic follicular thyroid cancer

Thyroid Storm

This rare condition is an extreme form of thyrotoxicosis, usually precipitated by intercurrent surgical or medical problems. It manifests itself with fever, congestive heart failure, and confusion. Therapy includes supportive care in the intensive care unit; cooling blankets and acetaminophen for fever; high-dose β blockers; 300 to 600 mg of PTU initially, followed by 200 mg every 6 hours. Ten drops of Lugol solution should be given initially, followed by 5 drops given every 6 hours after PTU. I usually give 2 mg of dexamethasone (Decadron) IV every 6 hours. If the patient is unable to take medication orally, it should be given through a nasogastric tube.

THYROID CANCER

METHOD OF

Christopher R. McHenry, MD, FACS, FACE

Thyroid cancer accounts for 1.5% of all cancers in the United States, excluding skin cancer. The incidence of thyroid cancer has been steadily increasing. In 2003, the American Cancer Society estimated that there were 22,000 new cases of thyroid cancer and 1400 deaths per year from thyroid cancer. Thyroid cancer is the most common endocrine malignancy, accounting for more than 95% of all cancers affecting the endocrine organs. The true incidence of thyroid cancer may actually be higher than the actual clinical incidence. Population-based autopsy studies have found occult papillary microcarcinomas in 2% to 13% of thyroid glands examined. Seventy-four percent of the cases of thyroid cancer occur in women.

Histologic Classification

Most thyroid cancers are of follicular cell origin and well differentiated. The median age at the time of diagnosis of differentiated thyroid cancer is 40 to 50 years. Papillary thyroid cancer is the most common, accounting for 75% to 80% of all thyroid malignancies. It includes multiple variants: pure papillary, follicular, tall cell, columnar cell, oxyphilic, diffuse sclerosing, encapsulated, and occult microcarcinomas. The tall-cell variant is notable for a higher incidence of extrathyroidal tumor spread, distant metastases, and mortality, as well as a loss of radioiodine uptake. Papillary carcinoma is characterized by multicentric disease in 25% to 50%, cervical lymph node metastases in 30% to 50%, and systemic metastases in 2% of patients at the time of presentation. It accounts for 90% of radiation-induced thyroid cancer and is familial in 3% of patients. The 20-year survival rate for patients with treated papillary carcinoma is greater than 90%.

Follicular thyroid cancer accounts for 10% to 15% of all thyroid malignancies. It is typically solitary. It often occurs in association with benign thyroid disease and is more common in areas of iodine deficiency. It is known for its propensity to spread hematogenously, most commonly to the lungs and bone. Lymph node metastases are present in only 10% of patients. Invasive follicular carcinoma is defined by the presence of major capsular invasion and angioinvasion. This is in distinction to minimally invasive follicular cancer, which is almost indistinguishable from a benign follicular adenoma except for the presence of minor capsular invasion. Patients with minimally invasive follicular carcinoma have a very indolent course with a near-normal life expectancy. The 10-year survival rate for treated invasive follicular carcinoma is approximately 86%.

Hürthle cell carcinoma is characterized by the presence of encapsulated collections of Hürthle cells. Hürthle cells are identified on the basis of their granular eosinophilic cytoplasm, which corresponds to abundant mitochondria. Hürthle cell carcinomas, which account for approximately 2.5% of all thyroid cancers, have a greater tendency to spread to cervical lymph nodes than follicular carcinomas and a higher incidence of distant metastases. Less than 10% of Hürthle cell cancers concentrate radioiodine, compared with 80% to 90% of patients with papillary or follicular carcinoma. Hürthle cell carcinoma has a higher recurrence rate and a higher 10-year mortality rate (21%) than either papillary or follicular carcinoma.

Anaplastic thyroid cancer accounts for approximately 2% of all thyroid malignancies. It typically occurs in patients older than 60 years of age who have a history of a long-standing goiter that suddenly increases in size. Anaplastic transformation may occur in patients with a pre-existing differentiated carcinoma. It is an extremely aggressive cancer with an overall 5-year survival rate of approximately 3% and a median survival period of only 4 to 6 months. Systemic metastases occur in approximately 75% of patients. However, the cause of death is usually from airway obstruction secondary to extensive local disease.

Medullary thyroid cancer arises from the parafollicular or "C" cells of the thyroid gland. It accounts for 5% of all thyroid cancers and it is usually more aggressive than differentiated thyroid cancer. Medullary thyroid carcinoma does not concentrate radioiodine. Approximately 20% to 30% of medullary carcinomas are familial occurring as a separate entity or as part of the multiple endocrine neoplasia (MEN) type 2 syndromes (Table 1). MEN-type 2 syndromes occur as a result of a germline mutation in the RET (rearranged during transfection) proto-oncogene, which encodes for a tyrosine kinase receptor. All familial medullary carcinomas are autosomal dominant disorders and are typically characterized by multifocal and bilateral disease and associated "C" cell hyperplasia. Twenty-five

TABLE 1 Familial Medullary Thyroid Carcinoma

A. Familial nonmultiple endocrine neoplasia medullary thyroid carcinoma
B. Multiple endocrine neoplasia type 2A
   - Medullary thyroid carcinoma
   - Hyperparathyroidism
   - Pheochromocytoma
   - Lichen planus amyloidosis
   - Hirschsprung's disease
C. Multiple endocrine neoplasia type 2B
   - Medullary thyroid carcinoma
   - Pheochromocytoma
   - Marfanoid body habitus
   - Mucosal neuromas
   - Ganglioneuromatosis of the gastrointestinal tract

percent to 63% of patients with medullary carcinoma have lymph node metastases, which most commonly involve the central compartment of the neck. Lymphatic spread also occurs to the lateral neck and mediastinum. Familial and sporadic medullary thyroid carcinomas are multicentric in 90% and 20% of cases, respectively.

Thyroid lymphoma is rare, accounting for less than 1% of all thyroid malignancies. It is usually a non-Hodgkin's lymphoma, B-cell type. Diffuse large cell lymphoma accounts for more than 50% of all lymphomas. Most lymphomas of the thyroid gland are of intermediate or high grade and arise from mucosa associated lymphoid tissue lymphoma. It is more common in women, and usually occurs during the seventh decade of life. Patients with Hashimoto's thyroiditis are known to have a 70 to 80 times higher risk for developing thyroid lymphoma than the normal population. Patients usually present with a rapidly enlarging goiter that causes compressive symptoms.

Clinical Presentation

Most patients with thyroid carcinoma present with a palpable thyroid nodule. Less often, they may present with an abnormal cervical lymph node; a rapidly enlarging goiter with dysphagia, dyspnea, or hoarseness; an incidentally discovered thyroid nodule on an imaging study of the neck; or as a result of genetic testing in a family with MEN type 2. A family history of thyroid cancer may also be present in patients with familial nonmedullary thyroid cancer, which accounts for 5% of all thyroid cancers. In a patient with a thyroid nodule, associated clinical features that are suggestive of carcinoma include: a prior history of low-dose head or neck irradiation as a child or adolescent, the presence of a firm fixed nodule, a nodule present in association with cervical lymphadenopathy, and vocal cord paralysis as documented by laryngoscopy. A patient with a dominant thyroid nodule and a prior history of head or neck irradiation has an approximate 40% incidence of carcinoma.

Thyroid nodules are common, occurring in 4% to 7% of the population. However, only an approximate 5% of thyroid nodules are malignant. The evaluation of a patient with a thyroid nodule consists of a routine fine-needle aspiration biopsy (FNAB) and a routine serum thyrotropin (TSH) level. FNAB is the mainstay in the diagnosis of thyroid cancer. It has a false-positive rate of 1% to 2% and a false-negative rate of 2% to 5%. Cytologic analyses of FNAB specimens can be classified into one of five categories: malignant (5%), suspicious for papillary cancer (5%), consistent with follicular or Hürthle cell neoplasm (20%), benign (60%), or nondiagnostic (10%). In patients with a FNAB that is malignant, suspicious for papillary cancer, consistent with a Hürthle cell neoplasm, or consistent with a follicular neoplasm or persistently nondiagnostic when the serum TSH level is normal or high, surgical therapy is recommended without any additional testing. In patients with a FNAB that is consistent with a follicular neoplasm or persistently nondiagnostic and a low serum TSH level, an iodine-123 thyroid scan is obtained to distinguish a hyperfunctioning nodule, which is malignant in less than 1% of cases, from a hypofunctioning nodule, which is malignant in 10% to 30% of cases. As a result, patients with a hyperfunctioning nodule and a FNAB that is consistent with a follicular neoplasm or persistently nondiagnostic may be observed or offered nonsurgical or surgical therapeutic options, whereas thyroidectomy is recommended for patients with a hypofunctioning nodule. Finally, patients with a benign FNAB are followed clinically.

Ultrasound may be of value in guiding FNAB for nonpalpable nodules or when repeated palpation-guided FNAB is persistently nondiagnostic. It may also be of value in patients with a FNAB that is malignant or suspicious for papillary cancer to evaluate for associated cervical lymph node disease prior to operation because physical examination is often inadequate for detection of cervical lymph node metastases. When cytologic analysis of a FNAB specimen suggests medullary thyroid cancer, immunohistochemical stains for carcinoembryonic antigen (CEA) and calcitonin should be performed to arrive at a definitive diagnosis. A serum calcitonin and CEA level should also be obtained. In addition, a 24-hour urine for vanilmandelic acid, metanephrine, and normetanephrine, and a serum calcium level should be obtained to screen for pheochromocytoma and hyperparathyroidism, respectively. Pheochromocytoma occurs in 50% of patients with MEN type 2A, and MEN type 2B and hyperparathyroidism occur in 10% to 20% of patients with MEN type 2A.

Familial medullary thyroid cancer may be diagnosed prior to becoming clinically evident by recognition of a marfanoid habitus or mucosal neuromas suggestive of MEN type 2B; genetic testing for the RET protooncogene in a patient with family members known to be affected by MEN type 2; or after diagnosis of other endocrinopathies associated with the MEN type 2 syndromes (Table 1).

Surgical Treatment of Thyroid Cancer

Certain prognostic factors are associated with a higher recurrence and mortality rates. Factors that predict a worse prognosis in patients with differentiated thyroid carcinoma include age older than 40 years in a man; age older than 50 years in a woman; tumor size larger than 4 cm; a high-grade tumor; the presence of extrathyroidal tumor spread; lymph node metastases in an adult patient; systemic metastases; and an incomplete resection. Intraoperatively, patients may be divided into low-risk or high-risk groups based on the presence or absence of various risk factors (Table 2). The recurrence and mortality rates for differentiated thyroid carcinoma in low-risk patients are 5% to 11% and 0.7% to 5%, respectively, compared with 48% and 48%, respectively, in high-risk patients. Risk group definition may be used to determine the extent of thyroidectomy for patients with differentiated thyroid cancer.

Age is the most important prognostic factor for predicting mortality from differentiated thyroid cancer. In patients younger than 45 years of age, the mortality from differentiated thyroid cancer is 1% to 2%. In a review of more than 1500 patients with papillary thyroid carcinoma treated at the Mayo Clinic, the mortality rate was less than 1% in patients younger than 50 years of age, 7% for patients 50 to 59 years of age, 20% for patients 60 to 69 years of age, and 46% for patients older than the age of 70 years. The presence of extrathyroidal tumor spread is the most important prognostic factor for predicting local recurrence. Completeness of resection is also an important prognostic factor for local recurrence and long-term cancer control. Patients with differentiated thyroid cancer and distant metastases have 10-year survival rates of 25% to 40%.

There are no randomized prospective studies evaluating the appropriate extent of thyroidectomy, the necessity of radioiodine, or the management of cervical lymph nodes metastases in patients with differentiated thyroid cancer. Most experts would agree that a thyroid lobectomy and isthmusectomy is appropriate therapy for a papillary microcarcinoma (less than 1 cm in size) and minimally invasive follicular cancer. Most experts would also agree that a total thyroidectomy is the appropriate treatment for patients with high-risk differentiated thyroid cancer (see Table 2). However, considerable controversy exists regarding the treatment of patients with low-risk differentiated thyroid cancer (see Table 2). It is appropriate to treat these patients with a thyroid lobectomy and isthmusectomy. However, in experienced hands, it may be preferable to treat these patients with a total thyroidectomy. Total thyroidectomy is associated with the lowest incidence of local recurrence. It also allows for the most effective use of radioactive iodine postoperatively for the detection and treatment of metastatic disease. Furthermore, serum thyroglobulin is most effectively used as a marker for detection of recurrent cancer following total thyroidectomy. Finally, total thyroidectomy is important in eliminating multicentric disease as well as a 1% risk of anaplastic dedifferentiation.

Enlarged lymph nodes in the central compartment of the neck are removed and submitted for frozen section examination. For documented metastases in the paratracheal lymph nodes, a complete central neck dissection should be performed, removing all lymphatic and fibrofatty tissue between the right and left common carotid arteries from the level of the hyoid bone superiorly to the sternal notch inferiorly. Patients with metastases in the lateral neck nodes that are palpable or identified by ultrasonography are treated with a modified (functional) neck dissection. This involves removal of the upper, mid, and lower anterior cervical and the posterior cervical lymph nodes and associated fibrofatty tissue from the lateral neck. The internal jugular vein, sternocleidomastoid muscle, and the spinoaccessory nerve are all preserved. A modified neck dissection is preferable to a "berry-picking" procedure because of a lower incidence of recurrent nodal metastases.

All patients with medullary thyroid cancer are treated with total thyroidectomy and a routine central neck dissection. Up to 80% of patients have lymph node metastases in the central compartment of the neck. Routine central neck dissection reduces recurrence and improves survival rates, when compared with the removal of lymph nodes, only when they are grossly enlarged. An ipsilateral modified neck dissection is performed in all patients with tumors larger than 2 cm, palpable or microscopic metastases in the central compartment of the neck, or palpable adenopathy in the lateral neck. Some authorities advocate routine bilateral modified neck dissection in all patients with tumors larger than 2 cm in size. Ipsilateral nodal involvement has been reported in up to 80% and contralateral nodal involvement in up to 40% of patients with palpable intrathyroidal primaries. Prior to the surgical treatment of medullary thyroid cancer, all patients should

TABLE 2 Low- and High-Risk Groups for Recurrence and Mortality from Papillary and Follicular Thyroid Cancers

Low Risk
Women <50 years
Men <40 years
Well or moderately well-differentiated tumors
Tumors <4 cm in diameter
Tumor confined to the thyroid gland
No distant metastasis
High Risk
Women ≥50 years
Men ≥40 years
Poorly differentiated tumors, tall cell, columnar cell, or oxyphilic variants of papillary carcinoma
Tumor >4 cm
Local invasion
Distant metastases

undergo appropriate screening to exclude the possibility of a coexisting pheochromocytoma which should be treated prior to thyroidectomy.

For patients with anaplastic carcinoma or lymphoma, the role of surgical intervention is primarily for establishing a diagnosis. Most patients present with locally advanced disease which precludes resection for cure. A tracheostomy may be necessary for patients with impending airway obstruction. Anaplastic thyroid cancer does not produce thyroglobulin nor does it concentrate radioiodine. Most patients with anaplastic thyroid cancer are treated with hyperfractionated radiation in combination with doxorubicin (Adriamycin) with or without cisplatin (Platinol)[1], which are used as radiosensitizers. Rarely, patients may present early with disease limited to the thyroid gland and surgical resection for cure is possible. It is one of the most aggressive of all cancers. Most patients die rapidly from tumor invasion into the aerodigestive tract and less commonly from metastatic disease.

Despite that a diagnosis of lymphoma can be made by FNAB, an open surgical biopsy is often required for specific immunohistochemical studies and definitive classification of a lymphoma. This has important implications in the choice of chemotherapeutic agents used. Once a diagnosis of lymphoma is established, staging is completed to delineate the extent of disease. Most patients are treated with chemotherapy in combination with radiation therapy. The overall 5-year survival rate in patients with lymphoma ranges from 50% to 70%.

Postoperative Management and Follow-Up

The postoperative management of patients with differentiated thyroid cancer consists of administration of thyroid hormone; iodine-131 whole-body scanning for residual normal thyroid tissue and/or metastatic disease; the use of iodine-131 for ablation of residual normal thyroid tissue and/or treatment of metastatic disease; and follow-up physical examination, serum thyroglobulin levels, and iodine-131 whole-body scans for detection of recurrent disease. The use of recombinant human thyrotropin (rhTSH) for diagnostic purposes in patients with thyroid cancer in lieu of thyroid hormone withdrawal is a recent development which avoids hypothyroidism prior to iodine-131 whole-body scans and thyroglobulin monitoring.

TSH promotes the growth of differentiated thyroid cancer cells. As a result, patients with differentiated thyroid cancer are treated with thyroid hormone in dosages that suppress TSH levels. This reduces the recurrence rate and improves survival. L-Thyroxine (Synthroid) is started at a dose of 2 µg/kg and a serum TSH level is measured 6 weeks following the initiation of therapy. In patients without evidence of metastatic disease, the TSH level is maintained just below the lower limit of the normal range, between 0.1 and 0.4 uIU/mL. In patients with metastatic disease, dosages of L-thyroxine (Synthroid) are increased to maintain serum TSH levels <0.1 uIU/mL.

Postoperative iodine-131 whole-body scanning is recommended for all patients with a papillary thyroid cancer larger than 1 cm, a papillary carcinoma of any size with lymph node metastases, invasive follicular carcinoma, and Hürthle cell carcinoma. Patients with residual iodine uptake in the thyroid bed are treated as outpatients with radioiodine ablation using a 30 mCi dose of iodine-131. Total ablation of residual thyroid tissue is achieved in 80% of patients following a 30 mCi dose of iodine-131. If a 30 mCi dose is unsuccessful in ablating all of the residual thyroid tissue, a second 30 mCi dose may be given 6 to 12 months later. It is well recognized that only approximately 10% of Hürthle cell carcinomas concentrate radioiodine but most produce thyroglobulin. As a result, radioiodine ablation of residual normal thyroid tissue is important for effective monitoring of serum thyroglobulin levels for early detection of recurrence.

Differentiated thyroid cancer will recur in 20% to 40% of patients. The incidence of recurrence is greatest within the first 2 years of surgery. However, it is not unusual for recurrence to occur 25 to 30 years after surgery emphasizing the importance of lifelong monitoring. Patients with differentiated thyroid carcinoma are followed at 3 to 6 month intervals with physical examination and a serum thyroglobulin, an antithyroglobulin antibody titer, and TSH levels for the first 2 years, and then yearly thereafter. For iodine-131 whole-body scanning and serum thyroglobulin monitoring to be useful for detection of metastatic disease, all normal thyroid tissue must be gone. This may be accomplished by a total or near total thyroidectomy and iodine-131 ablation.

For optimal sensitivity of radioiodine whole-body scanning and thyroglobulin measurement, the serum TSH level should be >30 uIU/mL to stimulate the residual normal or metastatic thyroid tissue to take up the iodine. Because of the residual circulating thyroid hormone secreted prior to the removal of the thyroid gland, the necessary TSH elevation usually does not occur for at least 4 to 6 weeks after surgery. To minimize the symptoms of hypothyroidism, patients are started on liothyronine (T_3) (Cytomel) 25 µg twice a day, immediately after surgery. T_3 has a half-life of 24 hours, compared with 7 days for L-thyroxine (Synthroid). The shorter half-life of T_3 is advantageous because it reduces the time the patient is hypothyroid prior to iodine-131 whole-body scanning. Two weeks prior to radioiodine scanning, patients are placed on a low-iodine diet and T_3 is discontinued. A serum thyroglobulin level and diagnostic whole-body scan are obtained when the serum TSH level is confirmed to be >30 uIU/mL.

[1]Not FDA approved for this indication.

Metastatic disease, usually involving the lung or bone, occurs in 10% to 15% of patients with differentiated thyroid cancer. Patients diagnosed with metastatic disease are admitted to the hospital, treated with doses of iodine-131 varying from 150 to 200 mCi, and are kept in isolation for 3 days. A follow-up whole-body scan is routinely performed 7 to 10 days after an ablative or therapeutic dose of iodine-131 to evaluate for previously undetected metastases. Approximately 35% to 60% of all metastatic lesions will concentrate iodine-131.

In the absence of normal thyroid tissue, serum thyroglobulin is a sensitive and specific marker for thyroid cancer. A serum thyroglobulin level <3 mg/dL while on thyroid hormone will rule out carcinoma with an approximate 94% sensitivity. However, it has been well documented that a patient with metastatic disease may have an undetectable serum thyroglobulin level while on thyroid hormone, emphasizing the importance of periodic measurement of TSH-stimulated thyroglobulin levels. A serum thyroglobulin level >10 mg/dL after withdrawal of thyroid hormone warrants repeating an iodine-131 whole-body scan. RhTSH may be used as an alternative to thyroid hormone withdrawal to stimulate iodine-131 uptake and thyroglobulin release in euthyroid patients, thus avoiding hypothyroidism. Multiple studies have verified its safety and efficacy in administration prior to radioactive iodine scanning and for measurement of TSH-stimulated thyroglobulin levels. Recently, there were data to suggest that in patients with a TSH-stimulated thyroglobulin level <10 mg/dL (either by withdrawal of thyroid hormone or with the use rhTSH), an iodine-131 whole-body scan is unnecessary.

Patients with medullary thyroid cancer are followed postoperatively with serum calcitonin and CEA levels every 3 to 6 months for the first 2 years and then yearly thereafter. A routine physical examination of the neck is performed, and the patient is evaluated for local recurrence or regional recurrence in the cervical or supraclavicular lymph nodes. Cervical lymph node recurrence is reported to occur in approximately 45% of patients. Systemic metastases, most commonly involving the liver, lungs, and bone, may be very indolent with little change over several years. Patients with MEN type 2 undergo yearly testing for a pheochromocytoma consisting of a 24-hour urine collection for vanilmandelic acid, metanephrine, and normetanephrine. In addition, patients with MEN type 2 also undergo a yearly serum calcium level to screen for the development of primary hyperparathyroidism.

Medullary thyroid cancer, because it arises from the parafollicular cells or C cells of the thyroid gland, does not take up radioiodine. As a result, there is no role for iodine-131 whole-body scanning, ablation, or treatment of metastases. Medullary thyroid cancer also does not produce thyroglobulin nor does TSH affect its growth. As a result, measurement of serum thyroglobulin is not indicated, nor is the use of TSH suppressive doses of thyroid hormone. Patients are started on a normal replacement dose of L-thyroxine (Synthroid), 1.6 μg/kg, postoperatively. Some experts propose that serum testing for the RET proto-oncogene mutations associated with the MEN type 2 syndromes be obtained postoperatively in all patients diagnosed with medullary thyroid cancer. The rationale for this is that up to 30% of patients thought to have sporadic medullary thyroid cancer will turn out to have new germline mutations and are index cases for a new kindred of familial cancer. If a patient has an identified RET mutation, all family members should also be tested for the mutation. The overall 5-year survival rate for all patients with medullary thyroid cancer, including sporadic and familial forms, is 78% to 92% and the 10-year survival rate is between 61% and 75%. Five-year survival rates based on the stage of disease (Table 3) are 100% for Stage I, 90% for Stage II, 86% for Stage III, and 56% for Stage IV.

The most important predictor of outcome in patients with medullary carcinoma is the stage of the disease at presentation (see Table 3). In addition to increasing tumor size, lymph node metastases, and systemic metastases, increasing age is also a negative prognostic factor. Older patients have a higher incidence of lymph node metastases. Male gender, nondiploid DNA tumor ploidy, and decreased calcitonin immunoreactivity have also been cited as factors associated with a worse outcome in patients with medullary thyroid cancer. Among the subtypes of medullary thyroid cancer, familial non-MEN

TABLE 3 Staging of Thyroid Cancer

A. Definitions

Primary Tumor (T)
T_0 = no evidence of primary tumor
T_1 = tumor ≤1 cm
T_2 = tumor >1 cm but ≤4 cm
T_3 = tumor >4 cm
T_4 = tumor extending beyond the thyroid capsule

Nodal Diseases (N)
N_0 = no regional lymph node metastases
N_1 = regional lymph node metastases

Systemic Metastases (M)
M_0 = no distant metastases
M_1 = distant metastases

B. American Joint Committee on Cancer Stage Grouping

Papillary, Follicular, and Hürthle Cell Cancers	**Age <45 Years**	**Age ≥45 Years**
Stage I	Any T, Any N, M_0	$T_1N_0M_0$
Stage II	Any T, Any N, M_1	T_2 or $T_3N_0M_0$
Stage III		T_4 or N_1M_0
Stage IV		Any T, Any N, M_1
Medullary Thyroid Cancer		
Stage I	$T_1N_0M_0$	
Stage II	T_2,T_3,T_4,N_0,M_0	
Stage III	Any T, N_1,M_0	
Stage IV	Any T, any N,M_1	
Anaplastic Thyroid Cancer (all cases are classified as Stage IV)		
Stage IV	Any T, Any N, Any M	

medullary thyroid cancer has the best prognosis, MEN type 2B has the worst prognosis, and sporadic and MEN type 2A medullary thyroid cancers have similar prognoses which are intermediate between the other two subtypes.

PHEOCHROMOCYTOMA

METHOD OF

Jerome M. Feldman, MD

Pheochromocytomas are tumors composed of chromaffin cells that originate from neuroectodermal tissue. The hallmark of pheochromocytomas is the production of catecholamines such as dopamine (DA), norepinephrine (NE), and epinephrine (E). The symptoms of pheochromocytomas are caused by the particular combination of catecholamines they excrete. Sustained secretion of NE can result in sustained hypertension intermittent secretion of NE or E can result in episodic hypertension; sustained secretion of E can result in anxiety and tachycardia; and secretion of DA alone may not produce any vascular symptoms.

Approximately 90% of pheochromocytomas are located in the adrenal glands. The rule of 10% is a handy way to recall some information on pheochromocytomas; 10% are in both adrenal glands (bilateral), 10% are extra-adrenal, and 10% are malignant. This rule of ten can vary from population to population. Patients with multiple endocrine neoplasia (MEN) have a higher percentage of bilateral pheochromocytomas. At Duke Medical Center, which receives many referrals of patients with malignant tumors, more than 10% of pheochromocytomas are malignant.

Medical Management

Once the diagnosis of pheochromocytoma is made, the physician should establish appropriate adrenergic blockade, carry out studies to localize the pheochromocytoma, and then, if possible, have it resected by an experienced surgeon. Occasionally one encounters a patient who is a poor operative risk because of advanced age, other serious illnesses, or the anatomic location of the pheochromocytomas. Although such patients can be managed by chronic medical therapy, there is always the risk that one is following a malignant pheochromocytoma.

The cornerstone of both preoperative and, if necessary, long-term medical management of pheochromocytomas is establishment of adequate α-adrenergic blockade with phenoxybenzamine (Dibenzyline). This drug is given to all patients with NE- and E-secreting pheochromocytomas, even if they do not have sustained hypertension or any hypertension under basal conditions. These nonhypertensive patients may develop dangerous elevations of blood pressure with induction of anesthesia and manipulation of the pheochromocytoma. The initial dose of phenoxybenzamine is 10 mg orally twice a day. The dose is increased by 10 mg per day at 3-day intervals until the patient's blood pressure has been reduced to normal levels. The usual dose for effective α-adrenergic blockades is a daily total of 30 to 60 mg per day given divided into three doses each day. Some patients with pheochromocytoma have required as much as 150 mg per day[3], a dose that is higher than that listed in the manufacturer's official directive. The critical factor is to not increase the dose of phenoxybenzamine until the patient has been on a given dose for 3 days, because it may take this long for it to exert its full effect. If the patient has only intermittent and infrequent bouts of hypertension and one cannot use sustained hypertension as an end point to judge the adequacy of therapy, one will usually give the patient from 30 to 60 mg of phenoxybenzamine per day.

Phenoxybenzamine does not interfere with measurements of vanillylmandelic acid (VMA) and catecholamines when good methodology is employed. The most frequent side effects of phenoxybenzamine are nasal congestion, sedation, dry mouth, and orthostatic hypotension. Orthostatic hypotension is a consequence of relaxation of the patient's chronically constricted blood vessels with a resulting decreased blood volume. If the patient is maintained on a generous salt diet, the contracted blood volume will expand and the orthostatic hypotension will decrease. The patient should be maintained on adequate α-adrenergic blockade for at least 2 weeks prior to surgery.

There are now a number of other medications with α-adrenergic blocking effects, such as phentolamine (Regitine), prazosin (Minipress)[1], terazosin (Hytrin)[1], and doxazosin (Cardura)[1], that have been used in patients with pheochromocytomas. The combination α- and β-blocking agent labetalol (Normodyne, Trandate)[1] has also been used in treating patients with pheochromocytomas. Because we have had good results with phenoxybenzamine, we prefer to use this drug for this important role.

In most patients with pheochromocytoma, β-adrenergic blockade is not as important as the absolutely essential α-adrenergic blockade. However, β-adrenergic blockade is indicated in all patients with pheochromocytomas who have a heart rate greater than 110 beats per minute, a history of arrhythmias, persistent ventricular extrasystoles, or

[3]Exceeds dosage recommended by the manufacturer.
[1]Not FDA approved for this indication.

a pheochromocytoma that is secreting predominantly E. In a substantial number of other patients without these initial findings, the pulse rate will increase to 110 beats per minute after initiation of phenoxybenzamine and these patients should also be treated with α,β-adrenergic blocker. It cannot be emphasized too strongly that one should not initiate therapy with a β-adrenergic blocker until establishing at least a partial α-adrenergic blockade with phenoxybenzamine. If one blocks the vasodilating β-adrenergic effects of catecholamines, one may unmask the vasoconstricting α-adrenergic effects, resulting in a dangerous increase in blood pressure.

Another medication that is now available for clinical use in patients with pheochromocytomas is metyrosine (α-methyl-*p*-L-tyrosine [Demser]). This drug blocks the conversion of tyrosine to L-dopa, the rate-limiting step in the synthesis of catecholamines. The usual initial dose is a 250 mg capsule orally four times a day. The dose is increased by 250 to 500 mg daily until the patient's blood pressure is reduced to the normal range. The usual dose of 1 to 4 g per day is given in four divided doses. Although metyrosine produces an artifactual elevation in urinary catecholamine excretion as measured by fluorometry, most clinical catecholamine measurements are now made by more specific methods that minimize such interference. Metyrosine usually does not interfere with the urinary measurement of VMA or metanephrines. Metyrosine can cause as much as an 80% reduction in the urinary excretion of catecholamines of patients with pheochromocytomas. The side effects reported for metyrosine include sedation in almost all patients and extrapyramidal symptoms in 10% of patients. The latter is probably a result of depletion of DA in the patient's basal ganglia. In addition, occasional patients develop anxiety and psychiatric disturbances, and occasionally crystalluria. Crystalluria can probably be avoided by maintaining a large fluid intake. Metyrosine seems particularly valuable in the patient who is in such poor condition that the patient cannot undergo resection of the patient's pheochromocytoma. In some cases. this is a result of catecholamine-induced myocardiopathy that is improved after chronic metyrosine therapy. The drug is also useful in the patient with an unresectable malignant pheochromocytoma, which is described later. For the time being, it seems prudent in the management of the usual patient with pheochromocytomas to reserve metyrosine for the patients who cannot tolerate phenoxybenzamine (Dibenzyline) because of side effects or when phenoxybenzamine does not adequately control the patient's hypertension in the preoperative period.

Operative Management

In general, we have found either abdominal computed tomography (CT) or magnetic resonance imaging (MRI) to be good techniques for the preoperative localization of pheochromocytomas. Abdominal CT is less expensive and is more acceptable to patients with claustrophobia than MRI. However, MRI is particularly useful in distinguishing right-sided pheochromocytoma that are in contact with the liver from hepatic masses. Because of the possibility of multiple pheochromocytomas or malignant pheochromocytoma, we prefer to also do a more specific imaging procedure with agents more specific for neuroendocrine tumors prior to surgery. We prefer ^{131}I-metaiodobenzylguanidine or iobenguane sulfate ^{131}I injection (^{131}I MIBG) to indium (In)-III pentreotide (OctreoScan) because the former is more specific than the latter. However, there are occasional pheochromocytomas that will concentrate one and not the other of these two agents.

If there is any likelihood that bilateral pheochromocytomas will be found, the patient is given intramuscular injections of cortisone acetate[1] 48 and 24 hours prior to surgery, as well as on the morning of surgery. This is to protect the patient from adrenal insufficiency if they should need bilateral adrenalectomy. This should be done in all cases of pheochromocytoma in patients with multiple endocrine neoplasia type 2, because there is a high frequency of bilateral pheochromocytomas. The patients should receive their phenoxybenzamine and, if warranted, propranolol (Inderal), on the morning of surgery.

The successful removal of a pheochromocytoma remains one of the most demanding surgical procedures. It requires skillful preoperative, intraoperative, and postoperative management with pharmacologic agents, as well as the technical skills of an experienced surgeon and anesthesiologist. When the patient has multiple endocrine neoplasia with medullary carcinoma of the thyroid and pheochromocytomas, it is important to remove the pheochromocytoma and schedule a second operation to remove the thyroid tumor.

In recent years, laparoscopic removal of pheochromocytomas has become the preferred method for removal of pheochromocytomas that are less than 5 cm in diameter. The postoperative hospitalization is usually shorter than after removal by laparotomy. However, laparotomy is preferable for suspected malignant pheochromocytomas, multiple pheochromocytomas, or pheochromocytomas that are more than 5 cm in diameter. Postoperative hypotension can be a problem after removal of the pheochromocytoma. This can be avoided if one allows the patient 2 weeks of therapy with phenoxybenzamine prior to surgery and carefully replaces blood loss with appropriate fluids during surgery. In addition, the anesthesiologist can place the patient in a slightly reverse Trendelenburg position, so that the lower extremities can be used as volume capacitors during surgery. After ligation of the renal veins or removal of the pheochromocytoma, the table can be tilted to the

[1]Not FDA approved for this indication.

horizontal position to increase the circulating blood volume if this proves necessary.

Palpation and resection of the pheochromocytoma result in dramatic increases in the plasma catecholamine concentration with increases in blood pressure and heart rate even in patients with seemingly adequate adrenergic blockade. The hypertensive episodes can be treated by intermittent intravenous injections of the α-adrenergic blocking agent phentolamine. However, phentolamine's hypotensive action can persist for 30 to 60 minutes after the plasma catecholamines have fallen toward the premanipulation level, and, as previously noted, phentolamine (Regitine) has some actions other than α-adrenergic blockade. Thus, one can get into repeated cycles of hyper- and hypotension. The blood pressure surges can be controlled more reliably with sodium nitroprusside (Nipride) drip. The potential side effects of nitroprusside include hypotension and cyanide poisoning. The great advantage of this agent is that its effect rapidly dissipates when its administration is discontinued.

Tachycardia and arrhythmia during surgery can be treated with intravenous injections of small amounts of propranolol. The usual dose of intravenous propranolol in patients with pheochromocytomas is 0.5 to 2.0 mg, with the rate of administration not to exceed 1 mg per minute. This reduces the possibility of lowering the blood pressure and causing cardiac standstill. If a vasopressor should be needed in a patient undergoing surgery for a pheochromocytoma, one should avoid the indirect-acting agents because they can release an unpredictable amount of norepinephrine from the nerve endings of a patient with a pheochromocytoma. Direct-acting vasopressors such as norepinephrine and phenylephrine are the drugs of choice. If the patient has had an adequate preoperative period of α-adrenergic blockade and if fluids and blood are administered appropriately during surgery, it will usually not be necessary to administer vasopressor amines.

Patients who have undergone resections of pheochromocytomas require careful monitoring in the immediate postoperative period. If they have had a bilateral adrenalectomy or unilateral adrenalectomy with significant manipulation of the second adrenal gland, they should be continued on glucocorticoid replacement. In the immediate postoperative period, hypertension may recur; however, this usually reflects fluid shifts and autonomic instability, and does not necessarily indicate a persistent pheochromocytoma. Some patients have developed transitory hypoglycemia. Urinary VMA excretion and sometimes plasma norepinephrine may remain elevated for 3 days after complete removal of all pheochromocytoma tissue. This probably represents elimination of the large stores of extra pheochromocytoma norepinephrine in the tissues of the body. One week or more after surgery the preoperative biochemical tests should be repeated to be certain that they remain hypertensive, either because they have sustained irreversible renal damage or they independently have essential hypertension.

Malignant Pheochromocytoma

About one half of the patients who ultimately prove to have malignant pheochromocytomas appear to have benign tumors at the time of initial diagnosis, while the other half has obviously malignant tumors. Patients with malignant pheochromocytomas have a slow, but usually downhill, course. Eventually metastasis can appear in lung, liver, brain, or bone. Ultimately, the majority of patients with malignant pheochromocytomas die from their tumor.

The bone metastasis can usually be ameliorated by external radiation therapy; the metabolic effects of excessive catecholamine production can be reduced by chronic therapy with phenoxybenzamine, propranolol, or metyrosine. Although not helpful in all patients, the two most useful methods of treating the generalized tumor are therapy with a radiopharmaceutical agent ^{131}I-metaidodobenzylguanidine (iobenguane ^{131}I) therapy and combined chemotherapy. The chemotherapy combination that has been used most successfully is cyclophosphamide (Cytoxan, Neosar)[1], vincristine (Oncovin, Vincasar)[1], and dacarbazine (DTIC-Dome)[1]. Both the ^{131}I-MIBG and the combination chemotherapy should be given in a specialized center.

[1]Not FDA approved for this indication.

THYROIDITIS

METHOD OF

Anthony Toft, MD

Thyroiditis is a nonspecific and somewhat unsatisfactory description of a variety of disparate disorders. Hence, Hashimoto's, postpartum, and silent thyroiditis have an autoimmune basis; de Quervain's and radiation-induced thyroiditis result from an acute inflammatory response; and drug-induced changes in thyroid hormone secretion are poorly understood. Thyroiditis is not an appropriate description of the fibrous replacement of Riedel's thyroiditis, but has been accepted by common usage.

Hashimoto's Thyroiditis

The typical patient with Hashimoto's thyroiditis is a 35- to 45-year-old woman with a small diffuse goiter of rubbery consistency. Thyroid enlargement is often noticed when applying cosmetics, or by friends or relatives. The goiter may be massive, extending into the posterior triangle of the neck and firm, or even hard, in consistency. Pain or discomfort is rare and should raise the possibility of other conditions such as de Quervain's thyroiditis or hemorrhage into a cyst or nodule. The most common biochemical finding is a slightly elevated serum thyrotropin (TSH) of 5 to 10 mU/L (normal: 0.15 to 3.5) with a serum free thyroxine (FT_4) in the lower part of the reference range. However, thyroid function may be normal, or show evidence of overt hypothyroidism. In more than 90% of patients, antibodies are detected in the serum to thyroid peroxidase (microsomes). In 15- to 20-year-olds, these antibodies may be absent, although antinuclear antibodies are often weakly positive. In antibody-negative cases, thyroid ultrasound shows a typical hypoechogenic pattern, which may be useful in differentiating these patients from patients with simple diffuse goiter, if thyroid function tests are normal. Patients with Hashimoto's thyroiditis are at risk of developing other organ-specific autoimmune diseases such as type 1 diabetes mellitus, pernicious anemia, vitiligo, or Addison's disease. Iodine excess, usually in the form of drug treatment with amiodarone (Cordarone), and lithium (Eskalith) may induce hypothyroidism in patients with previously unrecognized or untreated Hashimoto's thyroiditis.

Treatment is with levothyroxine (Synthroid) in a dose sufficient to result in a serum TSH concentration in the lower part of the reference range (e.g., 0.3 mU/L) which not only restores euthyroidism in those presenting with hypothyroidism, but in most cases also results in significant reduction in goiter size, even in those with massive enlargement. Treatment is usually lifelong. Like all patients with hypothyroidism, the dose of levothyroxine may need to be increased during pregnancy by a mean of 50 μg daily, and patients should be aware of the possible need to increase the dose of levothyroxine when taking drugs, such as ferrous sulfate (Feosol), which interfere with its absorption, or antidepressants, such as sertraline (Zoloft), which increase its metabolism. Rarely, hyperthyroidism with high concentrations of TSH-receptor antibody develops after many years of levothyroxine treatment. In such cases, blocking TSH-receptor antibodies are thought to have played a role in the initial development of the thyroid failure. It is in this subgroup of patients in whom ophthalmopathy may be present at the outset.

There is an association between Hashimoto's thyroiditis and both lymphoma and papillary carcinoma of the thyroid. The risk of these conditions is not sufficiently great to justify long-term follow-up in specialist clinics. However, irregularity of the goiter at presentation or increase in size during levothyroxine therapy are indications for further investigation by fine-needle aspiration or surgical resection.

Postpartum Thyroiditis

In patients with underlying autoimmune thyroid disease, often unrecognized, there is likely to be transient disturbance of thyroid function in the first year after delivery. This is caused by a destructive thyroiditis, akin to that which occurs in viral (de Quervain's) thyroiditis. Typically, therefore, there is a period of hyperthyroidism, lasting a few weeks only, that is mild and not requiring treatment other than with a β-blocker, such as long-acting propranolol (Inderal LA) 160 mg daily. This is followed by an equally short-lived and mild hypothyroidism, and then usually by recovery. A small Hashimoto-type goiter may be present and antiperoxidase antibodies are likely to be positive. Pain is not a feature. Postpartum thyroiditis tends to recur after subsequent pregnancies, and the eventual outcome is permanent hypothyroidism some years later in at least 25% of patients.

It is important to decide whether the hyperthyroid patient presenting in the first year after childbirth has postpartum thyroiditis or Graves' disease, because the latter requires therapy. Even patients with a previous history of Graves' disease are as likely to present with postpartum thyroiditis as with a recurrence. The hyperthyroidism of postpartum thyroiditis is usually mild with serum FT_4 concentrations in the range of 30 to 40 pmol/L (normal: 10 to 25), but the best methods of differentiation are measurements of isotope uptake by the thyroid gland and TSH receptor antibodies (Table 1). Characteristically, uptake of iodine-131 or technetium is negligible in postpartum thyroiditis but significant in Graves' disease, but isotope exposure is relatively contraindicated during breastfeeding. The TSH-receptor antibody is not usually present in postpartum thyroiditis, but is detected in some 90% of patients with Graves' disease.

Silent Thyroiditis

This is the term used to describe the disordered thyroid function typical of postpartum thyroiditis, but occurring in patients who have never been pregnant or who are beyond the postpartum period.

TABLE 1 Features That Help to Differentiate Between Postpartum Thyroiditis and Graves' Disease

	Postpartum Thyroiditis	Graves' Disease
Degree of hyperthyroidism	Mild	Variable
Isotope uptake	Negligible	Significant
Thyrotropin-stimulating hormone (TSH) receptor antibody	Usually absent	Present in 90% of cases
Duration of hyperthyroidism	Weeks	Months to years

The presentation is usually to a primary care physician on account of mild hyperthyroidism. By the time specialist investigation has been arranged, thyroid function has often returned to normal or shows evidence of mild thyroid failure. The basis is autoimmune and annual review of thyroid function is advisable. Some patients have repeated episodes over many years, and the expectation is eventual permanent thyroid failure.

de Quervain's Thyroiditis

Subacute or de Quervain's thyroiditis is an inflammatory disorder, probably the result of infection with one of a variety of viruses. The inflamed thyroid is characterized histologically by the presence of multinucleated giant cells and is quite distinct from the lymphocytic thyroiditis of autoimmune thyroid disease.

There is severe pain in the region of the thyroid in the early weeks of the illness, which radiates to the jaws and ears and is made worse by swallowing. There is pyrexia with shivering, myalgia, lassitude, and symptoms of mild hyperthyroidism caused by the release of preformed thyroid hormones. Thyroid tenderness has usually resolved by 8 weeks after the onset of illness, and by 12 to 16 weeks there may be clinical evidence of mild hypothyroidism because the damaged follicles are unable to synthesize new hormone. What is remarkable, given the destructive nature of the inflammatory process, is that recovery occurs in the overwhelming majority of patients.

Uptake of isotope by the thyroid during the phase of hyperthyroidism is negligible for two reasons. First, the damaged follicular cell is unable to trap iodine and, second, there is suppression of endogenous TSH by the elevated serum thyroid hormone concentrations. The erythrocyte sedimentation rate is high and often exceeds 80 mm in the first hour. Serum thyroglobulin concentrations may be increased and antibodies appear transiently in the serum in weak titer to thyroglobulin, thyroid peroxidase, and the TSH receptor in some patients.

In the majority of cases the neck discomfort and associated systemic symptoms such as pyrexia and myalgia respond to salicylates, such as aspirin 600 mg every 4 to 6 hours orally. Occasionally, it is necessary to administer oral prednisolone[1] in a total daily dose of 30 mg for 3 to 4 weeks. Corticosteroids produce relief of symptoms within 24 hours but do not modify the natural history of the disease. Symptoms of mild hyperthyroidism should be controlled with a β-blocker, such as propranolol (Inderal LA) 160 mg daily. Antithyroid drugs are of no benefit because the hyperthyroidism is not caused by excessive synthesis of thyroid hormones. It is not necessary to treat the phase of hypothyroidism, but any evidence of thyroid failure persisting beyond the sixth month should be regarded as permanent.

It should be stressed that subacute thyroiditis is rare, accounting for 3% of all cases of hyperthyroidism presenting to a specialist clinic. Mild forms may not be recognized in primary care or diagnosed as pharyngitis.

[1]Not FDA approved for this indication.

Radiation Thyroiditis

In the first few days after treatment of hyperthyroidism with iodine-131, there may be a transient increase in thyroid hormone concentrations, as a result of radiation damage to the thyroid follicles. This may lead to thyrotoxic crisis in patients with severe hyperthyroidism, but pretreatment with antithyroid drugs will protect against such an outcome, not by preventing the rise in thyroid hormone concentrations, but by ensuring that any increase is from a lower baseline.

Drug-Induced Thyroiditis

Interferon-alfa 2A (Roferon-A), used in the treatment of hepatitis C, and interleukin-2 (Proleukin), used in the treatment of metastatic renal carcinoma, may induce a destructive thyroiditis, particularly in women with underlying autoimmune thyroid disease. The hypothyroidism may prove permanent. Amiodarone (Cordarone), increasingly used in the management of atrial fibrillation, also causes a destructive thyroiditis, the thyrotoxic element of which may be severe and may respond to prednisolone in doses of 40 mg daily for a period of several weeks.

Riedel's Thyroiditis

This is a rare condition of unknown etiology in which there is fibrous replacement of the thyroid extending into adjacent structures. Most endocrinologists will see only one or two cases during their career. The presentation is with a hard goiter, the margins of which are difficult to delineate and which are irregular, raising the clinical suspicion of anaplastic carcinoma. There is usually a degree of mediastinal compression. Hypothyroidism is common, and hypoparathyroidism well recognized. Mediastinal and retroperitoneal fibrosis occurs in up to one third of patients over a 10-year period.

There is no effective treatment, but limited surgical resection is often necessary to alleviate tracheal compression. The antiestrogen tamoxifen (Nolvadex) has been used with some limited success, but its mode of action remains unknown.

SECTION **10**

The Urogenital Tract

BACTERIAL INFECTIONS OF THE URINARY TRACT IN MALES

METHOD OF

John N. Krieger, MD

Urinary tract infections include a spectrum of clinical conditions whose common denominator is invasion of the organs and tissues. Any portion of the urinary tract may be involved, from the renal cortex to the urethral meatus. Infection may occur predominantly at a single site, such as the bladder (cystitis), prostate (prostatitis), kidney (pyelonephritis), or perinephric space (perinephric abscess). The entire urinary tract is at risk for invasion by bacteria when any of its parts has become infected.

Most infections occur by the ascending route, meaning that bacteria from the fecal flora, colonize the perineum, then ascend via the urethra, bladder, and ureter to involve the kidney. On occasion, hematogenous dissemination of bacteria can result in seeding of the urinary tract. Classic examples of hematogenous infection are genitourinary tuberculosis and staphylococcal infection of a renal cyst ("renal carbuncle"). On rare occasions, the urinary tract may be involved by infection from contiguous structures, as may occur in patients with diverticulitis or appendicitis that involves the urinary tract.

Distinguishing Complicated from Uncomplicated Infections

The key issue for therapy is to distinguish uncomplicated (medical) infections from complicated (surgical) infections. An uncomplicated infection occurs in the absence of underlying structural or neurologic disorders of the urinary tract. These infections usually respond well to antimicrobial therapy. Thorough anatomic evaluation and imaging studies are seldom indicated in patients with uncomplicated urinary tract infections. In contrast, complicated infections occur when the urinary tract is repeatedly invaded by bacteria, leaving residual inflammation, or, in cases accompanied by obstruction, stones, foreign bodies, or neurologic conditions that interfere with urinary drainage. Antimicrobial therapy alone is markedly less effective in complicated urinary tract infections. Managing patients with complicated urinary tract infections often requires thorough anatomic evaluation and imaging studies. An important differential point is that patients with complicated infections tend to have persistence of bacteria within the urinary tract in the face of antimicrobial agents to which the bacteria appear to be sensitive in laboratory tests. Often, it is necessary to correct an underlying obstructive lesion or voiding problem to clear the infection. The goal of therapy for any patient with a urinary tract infection should be total elimination of the infecting organism from the urinary tract.

Natural History

In infancy, the incidence of symptomatic urinary tract infections is higher in males than in females. In part, this is related to circumcision status. It appears that bacteria can adhere to the prepuce of uncircumcised male infants and then gain access to the urinary tract. Neonatal circumcision appears to reduce the rate of urinary tract infections in male infants by approximately 90%. After the neonatal period, symptomatic infections in male children and adults are distinctly uncommon until middle age. This is in marked contrast to the situation in females, who experience increasing rates of both symptomatic and asymptomatic infections with a marked increase following initiation of sexual activity, then a continued gradual rise with age. Asymptomatic bacteriuria is also distinctly unusual in males compared with females.

Well-documented urinary tract infections in male children mandate thorough urologic investigation. This is because of the high prevalence of structural genitourinary tract abnormalities in such patients. Often, urinary tract infection represents the key diagnostic presentation for major abnormalities of the urinary tract. For example, vesicoureteral reflux of urine, posterior urethral valves, and other major structural abnormalities often present initially with a bacterial urinary tract infection. Early diagnosis and appropriate therapy offer the best chance for preservation of maximal renal function, although renal scarring may be progressive despite appropriate treatment. Structural urinary tract abnormalities remain a major cause of renal failure in children. Morbidity may be minimized by appropriate evaluation and therapy. Our choice for evaluation of a male child with a urinary tract infection is the combination of renal ultrasound to evaluate the upper urinary tract plus a voiding cystourethrogram to evaluate the lower urinary tract. A voiding cystourethrography should be obtained after resolution of the initial infection because dilation of the upper urinary tract may be exaggerated in the face of recent infection.

Because urinary tract infections are unusual in young men, there are few well-done natural history studies in this population. In patients without obvious neurologic or structural abnormalities, sexual intercourse, particularly among homosexual men and heterosexual men who practice insertive anal intercourse, may be a risk factor. The overall contribution of these practices to bacterial urinary tract infections in adult men is uncertain. Standard urologic teaching is to do a thorough evaluation for structural abnormalities in such patients, including radiographic studies and cystourethroscopy. However, our published experience suggests that previously healthy college-age males with well-documented urinary tract infections have low rates of structural genitourinary tract abnormalities. An excretory urogram with a postvoiding film and a uroflow study are adequate to screen for structural abnormalities in this population. We reserve cystoscopy for those patients who are determined to be at risk for significant abnormalities on the basis of these screening studies and a thorough physical examination. The other major risk factors for urinary tract infections in men are instrumentation of the urinary tract and bacterial prostatitis.

Diagnosis and Localization

Because accurate diagnosis is a prerequisite for appropriate therapy, we recommend culture and sensitivity testing of urine specimens from any male with symptoms or signs suggesting urinary infection. In patients who do not have obstructive lesions, stasis, stones, or foreign bodies, recurrent and persistent urinary tract infections are often related to bacterial prostatitis. Segmented localization cultures can be used to differentiate cystitis and urethritis from bacterial prostatitis. The procedure should be carried out at a time when the patient does not have bacteriuria.

Our procedure for lower urinary tract localization is outlined briefly. After cleaning the glans with sterile water, the first-void urine (initial 5 to 10 mL of voided urine) is collected in a sterile container. Next, a mid-stream specimen is obtained. The patient is asked to stop voiding. Prostatic fluid is expressed by digital prostate massage. The post-void urine (next 5 to 10 mL after the massage) is then collected. Culture and sensitivity testing are then carried out. It is critical to make certain that the laboratory is aware of the purpose of these studies so that the laboratory will evaluate small numbers of uropathogens.

Diagnosis of chronic bacterial prostatitis can be made if the postmassage urine specimen or the expressed prostatic secretion contains a tenfold or greater increase in the concentration of the uropathogen compared with that in the first-void urine specimen. In patients with well-documented bacterial prostatitis, the causative organism is identical to that causing recurrent episodes of bacteriuria.

It is important to recognize that only a small minority of males presenting with symptoms of prostatitis fit into the acute or chronic bacterial prostatitis categories. The great majority of patients with symptoms are classified in the chronic prostatitis/chronic pelvic pain category. In contrast to the recognized benefit of appropriate antimicrobial therapy for patients with acute and chronic bacterial prostatitis, the roles of antimicrobial therapy and other treatments have not been defined for patients with chronic prostatitis/chronic pelvic pain syndrome.

Basic Principles in Therapy

There are three keys to successful therapy for urinary tract infections. First, eliminate or control predisposing factors. For example, we are often asked to manage "resistant urinary infections" in long-term care patients with indwelling catheters. One approach is to change their bladder management from a chronic, indwelling catheter to an intermittent self, or assisted, catheterization program. Other examples include removal of obstructing lesions, stones, or strictures of improved drainage of the lower urinary tract. These measures may be successful in eliminating the focus of infection, even with no antimicrobial therapy. Second, eradicate the infection as soon as possible to prevent colonization of the prostate and other structures. Third, ensure that the infection has been eliminated by obtaining cultures during or immediately after therapy and at follow-up at 1 to 2 months following therapy.

UNCOMPLICATED INFECTIONS

Uncomplicated infections generally present with symptoms of bacterial cystitis, with a combination of urinary frequency, urgency, dysuria, nocturia, suprapubic discomfort, low-back pain, or hematuria. Systemic symptoms of fever, chills, and rigor are absent. Urine culture confirms the diagnosis, with *Escherichia coli* being the most common pathogen. Uncomplicated infections, including those introduced by a single or short course of indwelling urethral catheterization, generally respond promptly to a short course of antimicrobial therapy. The infection may persist and become difficult to eradicate if the prostate becomes colonized or if the patient has a stone or structural abnormality of the urinary tract. Thus, an effort should be made to eliminate predisposing factors while routine therapy is guided by in vitro susceptibility tests.

I prefer oral therapy with one of the agents listed in Table 1. In our geographic area, bacteria causing urinary tract infections have developed substantial resistance to trimethoprim-sulfamethoxazole (Bactrim). Therefore, we usually initiate empiric therapy with a quinolone. Nitrofurantoin (Macrodantin) remains highly effective and is an attractive alternative drug. In general, we recommend that the duration of therapy be at least 2 weeks, although only limited data address this point in males.

COMPLICATED INFECTIONS

Patients with systemic signs or those with a history of structural or neurologic abnormalities merit thorough anatomic investigation of the urinary tract. It is important to do this early in the course of therapy because antimicrobial therapy alone may fail to cure infection and urosepsis may develop unless there is specific management of the underlying problem. Our initial choice for evaluation of these patients is either a computed tomography (CT) scan with contrast or an excretory urogram with post-void film. If an abscess in the retroperitoneal space or the prostate is suspected, CT scanning is superior to the other modalities for diagnosis.

Prolonged courses of therapy are indicated for patients with persistent infections. Often, I have used 3 to 4 months of therapy in this situation. In patients with chronic bacterial prostatitis, elderly patients, or those in nursing homes, continuous therapy may be necessary to suppress bacteriuria, even though eradication may prove impossible. Thus, for patients with recurrent or complicated infections, I recommend an attempt to eradicate the focus of infection, following thorough evaluation of the urinary tract. The therapy is usually with the same drugs listed in Table 1. Our first choice for curative therapy is usually a quinolone. For patients with persistent or frequently relapsing infections, I consider long-term therapy (months or years) using low dosages of antimicrobial drugs for prophylaxis or suppression with periodic monitoring by culture to be sure that the agent continues to be effective. In this situation, our choice

TABLE 1 Oral Antimicrobial Agents Prescribed for Urinary Tract Infections in Adult Males

Antimicrobial Class	Agent	Dosage Frequency
Fluoroquinolone	Ciprofloxacin (Cipro)	250-500 mg twice daily
	Ciprofloxacin (Cipro XR)	500-1000 mg once daily
	Gatifloxacin (Tequin)	200-400 mg once daily
	Levofloxacin (Levaquin)	250-500 mg once daily
	Ofloxacin (Floxin)	200-400 mg twice daily[3]
	Norfloxacin (Noroxin)	400 mg twice daily
Combination agents	Trimethoprim-sulfamethoxazole (Bactrim, Septra, Bactrim DS, Septra DS)	160 mg trimethoprim + 800 mg sulfamethoxazole, twice daily
	Amoxicillin-clavulanic acid (Augmentin)	500-875 mg amoxicillin + 125 mg clavulanate, twice daily
Cephalosporin	Cefaclor (Ceclor)	250-500 mg, 3 times daily[3]
	Loracarbef (Lorabid)	200-400 mg, twice daily[3]
Other antimicrobials	Nitrofurantoin (Macrobid)	50-100 mg per day or twice daily
	Nitrofurantoin (Macrodantin)	50-100 mg, 4 times daily

[3]Exceeds dosage recommended by the manufacturer.

is usually either trimethoprim-sulfamethoxazole (Bactrim) or nitrofurantoin (Macrodantin).

PROSTATITIS

Acute and chronic bacterial prostatitis may present with local urinary tract symptoms characteristic of bacterial cystitis or with systemic signs and symptoms. Acute bacterial prostatitis is usually manifest with the sudden onset of chills, fever, malaise, and low back and perineal pain, as well as difficulty with urination. On rectal examination, the prostate is tense and exquisitely tender. Excessive palpation may induce septicemia. For patients who require hospitalization, my initial choice is the combination of a β-lactam drug and an aminoglycoside until the results of antimicrobial sensitivity testing are available. Following parenteral therapy, the patient is managed with continued antimicrobial therapy for at least 4 weeks, usually employing a quinolone. Patients with acute bacterial prostatitis usually respond well to a variety of antimicrobial agents that penetrate an acutely inflamed prostate. Many of these agents are not effective in chronic bacterial prostatitis.

In contrast to acute bacterial prostatitis, chronic bacterial prostatitis is often insidious in onset. Patients usually have recurrent urinary tract infections and, sometimes, recurrent episodes of acute prostatitis. Between symptomatic episodes, patients may be totally asymptomatic. Diagnosis depends on the localization cultures described earlier. Treatment must be prolonged, because diffusion of antimicrobial agents into the prostates is poor. My initial choice is usually a quinolone, with trimethoprim-sulfamethoxazole (Septra, Bactrim) as a second choice agent. Carbenicillin indanyl sodium (Geocillin) is also approved for this indication, but has not been particularly effective in my experience. It is important not to confuse bacterial prostatitis with chronic prostatitis/chronic pelvic pain syndrome. This is the most common cause of symptomatic prostatitis, but these patients do not have bacteriuria.

LONG-TERM CARE PATIENTS

Long-term care patients, including those with incontinence and indwelling urinary catheters or other devices and chronic asymptomatic bacterial colonization, should not be treated. It is impossible to sterilize the urine permanently in such cases. Furthermore, resistant organisms are likely to emerge, making subsequent therapy difficult. We treat such patients only if they develop acute symptoms referable to the urinary tract, or prior to genitourinary tract procedures. We strongly recommend against obtaining screening cultures in such patients because these cultures often lead to unnecessary therapy that selects resistant bacterial flora. Furthermore, there is evidence that bacterial colonization with relatively "benign" strains can inhibit establishment of symptomatic infections caused by more virulent bacteria.

BACTERIAL INFECTIONS OF THE URINARY TRACT IN WOMEN

METHOD OF
Curtis L. Gingrich, MD

Urinary tract infections (UTIs) are the most common bacterial infections in women and account for more than 8 million office visits and 100,000 hospitalizations a year in the United States. At least one half of all women will experience a UTI during their lifetime. It has been estimated that 30% to 35% of young, sexually active women will have at least one UTI annually and 2% to 4% will have recurrent UTIs. In fact, 30% of all women will have recurrent UTIs during their lifetime. Recurrent infection may represent a failure to completely clear a previously treated UTI, a reinfection by the same organism, or a new infection by a different organism.

Pathogenesis

More than 95% of all UTIs occur through an ascending route. Normal gastrointestinal (GI) flora colonize the vaginal introitus and periurethral region. These bacteria then ascend through the urethra and cause infection of the bladder and occasionally the upper urinary tract. Complete and regular voiding usually removes these organisms and prevents UTI. If this preventive mechanism is altered, whether by anatomic variation, neurologic dysfunction, instrumentation, or voluntary avoidance of urination, the risk for symptomatic infection is increased.

Many factors have been found to increase the risk of developing UTIs. These factors include sexual activity, use of a diaphragm and spermicide or spermicide alone, tampon use, menstruation, pregnancy, history of UTIs, increasing age with estrogen deficiency, and delayed or incomplete voiding. Sexual activity is believed to promote the introduction of GI flora into the periurethral and bladder regions. Young, sexually active females having sexual intercourse three times a week are two to three times more likely to experience a urinary tract infection than are women who are not sexually active. Spermicide use increases the risk of UTI by increasing the vaginal pH and creating an environment more susceptible to *Escherichia coli* colonization. Similarly, estrogen deficiency increases the vaginal pH and allows for a shift in the normal vaginal flora.

An association between Lewis blood group antigen secretion status is also implicated in the causation of UTI. Women who demonstrate lack of secretion of

Lewis blood group antigens from the uroepithelial cells demonstrate increased adherence of uropathogenic *E. coli* as compared with women who secrete such antigens and thus are genetically predisposed to UTI.

Microbiology

The causative agents for UTI have remained consistent and stable. In uncomplicated UTIs, *E. coli* is the causative organism 80% to 90% of the time. *Staphylococcus saprophyticus*, a Gram stain-positive, coagulase-negative organism accounts for 5% to 10% of uncomplicated UTIs. This organism is found more frequently in younger women and displays a late summer and fall preponderance. Other important organisms include *Proteus mirabilis* and *Klebsiella* species. In complicated UTIs, *E. coli* is still the most common organism but *Proteus, Klebsiella,* enterococci, and *Candida* species increase in incidence.

Aside from UTI, other organisms should be considered if the patient fails to respond to conventional therapy. Organisms such as *Chlamydia trachomatis, Neisseria gonorrhoeae*, herpes simplex virus, *Trichomonas vaginalis*, or vaginal candidiasis may cause similar symptoms and should be considered if prompt resolution does not occur with standard antimicrobial treatment. In young, sexually active women with persistent or recurrent dysuria and pyuria but negative urine cultures, chlamydia should be considered. Pregnant women also show an increased risk of UTIs associated with Group B streptococcus.

Diagnosis and Classification of Urinary Tract Infections

The diagnosis of UTI is usually made on the basis of clinical symptoms and the evaluation of a clean-catch midstream urine sample. Reliable methods of evaluation include a urine dipstick measurement for nitrates and leukocyte esterase, as well as microscopic evaluation of the urine sediment for white blood cells and bacteria. The presence of leukocyte esterase in a midstream clean-catch urine specimen has a sensitivity of 75% to 96% and a specificity of 94% to 98% for the presence of UTI. Urine culture may also be obtained, with the acceptable standard of $>10^5$ colony-forming units being positive for infection. This should not be the sole criterion for the diagnosis, however, because up to 50% of women with clinical signs and symptoms of UTI will have a negative urine culture by this standard. Therefore, the diagnosis of UTI is usually made on the basis of clinical history and physical examination, rather than a urine culture. If a urine culture is obtained, any quantitative count of a potential uropathogen, in the presence of clinical signs of a UTI should be considered positive and treated accordingly.

TABLE 1 Factors Associated with Complicated Urinary Tract Infections

Structural	Congenital abnormalities Cystocele Bladder diverticula Bladder outlet obstruction Tumor (renal and bladder) Urolithiasis Stricture of ureter Uterine prolapse Vesicoureteral reflux
Metabolic	Diabetes mellitus Nephrocalcinosis Medullary sponge kidney
Instrumentation	Cystoscopy/ureteroscopy Indwelling bladder catheter Intermittent catheterization Nephrostomy tube Stent placement
Immunocompromise	Congenital/acquired immunodeficiency
Neutropenia	Immunosuppressive therapy Organ transplant
Other causes	Pregnancy Renal abscess Post-void residual >100 mL (neurologic disease, medications) Renal impairment

Once the diagnosis of UTI has been made, the infection should be classified as complicated or uncomplicated. A determination should also be made as to whether the UTI involves only the lower urinary tract or both the lower and upper tracts. The determination of these characteristics will help guide therapy decisions.

UTIs are classified as uncomplicated or complicated based on the presence of associated conditions which make the infection more difficult to treat. Table 1 lists the conditions that, when present, identify the UTI as complicated.

The classification of lower versus upper urinary tract disease is usually based on the clinical presentation. Lower tract infections usually present with the symptoms of dysuria, urgency, frequency, hesitancy and suprapubic tenderness. Hematuria may also be present. Systemic symptoms are usually absent. Upper tract infections usually present with lower tract symptoms, as well as signs of more systemic involvement. These include costovertebral angle tenderness, flank pain, fever, chills, rigors, nausea and vomiting, and, in severe cases, hemodynamic instability.

Management of Urinary Tract Infections

ACUTE UNCOMPLICATED CYSTITIS

Acute uncomplicated cystitis is a common syndrome manifested primarily with symptoms of dysuria, urinary frequency, urgency, and suprapubic tenderness. Symptoms range from mild to severely incapacitating. Table 2 lists the treatment options for this type of infection. Single-dose therapy is not recommended because of its associated high relapse rate. When considering the use of nitrofurantoin (Macrodantin), it should be noted that 3-day therapy produces decreased cure rates; 7 days of nitrofurantoin are required for adequate treatment.

Patients who fail to respond to an empirical 3-day course of therapy should have a urine obtained for culture and susceptibility testing to help guide further therapy. A condition known as *occult pyelonephritis* should be considered in patients who initially respond to therapy, but who have a prompt recurrence of symptoms. These patients should receive a 14-day course of therapy. Also nitrofurantoin (Macrodantin) should not be used when upper tract disease is suspected.

ACUTE UNCOMPLICATED PYELONEPHRITIS

Patients with uncomplicated pyelonephritis usually present with flank pain, nausea and vomiting, fever >38°C (100.4°F), and/or costovertebral tenderness, along with cystitis symptoms. Most young, healthy, nonpregnant women can be treated as outpatients unless they appear ill enough to require hospitalization. Hospitalization should be considered in the following circumstances; inability to take oral medications or maintain oral hydration; uncertainty of diagnosis; concern for patient compliance; and evidence of severe systemic illness with high fevers, severe pain, marked debility, and/or hemodynamic instability. When hospitalization is required, blood cultures should be obtained, because up to 20% of these women will show evidence of bacteremia.

In the outpatient setting, oral fluoroquinolones (see Table 2) are the recommended choice for women with uncomplicated pyelonephritis. Fluoroquinolones achieve high drug concentrations in the renal medulla necessary for the cure of upper tract infections. There has been no proven efficacy of an initial dose of parenteral fluoroquinolone as tissue concentrations are similar for oral and parenteral therapy. The newer fluoroquinolones (sparfloxacin

TABLE 2 Treatment Regimens for Bacterial Urinary Tract Infections in Women

Agent	Dose	Duration (Days)
Acute Cystitis		
First-Line Agents		
TMP-SMX (Septra DS, Bactrim DS)	160/800 mg bid	3-7
Trimethoprim (Proloprim)	100 mg bid	3-7
Nitrofurantoin (Macrodantin, Macrobid)	50-100 mg qid	7
	100 mg bid	7
Fosfomycin tromethamine (Monurol)	3 g	Single dose
Second-Line Agents		
Ciprofloxacin (Cipro)	250 mg bid	3
Norfloxacin (Noroxin)	400 mg bid	3
Levofloxacin (Levaquin)	250 mg qd	3
Ofloxacin (Floxin)	200 mg bid	3
Gatifloxacin (Tequin)	200 mg qd	3
Amoxicillin-clavulanic acid (Augmentin)	500 mg tid	3-7
Cephalexin (Keflex)	500 mg qid	7
Acute Uncomplicated Pyelonephritis		
First-Line Agents		
Ciprofloxacin (Cipro)	250-500 mg bid	10-14
Levofloxacin (Levaquin)	500 mg qd	10-14
Gatifloxacin (Tequin)	400 mg qd	10-14
TMP-SMX (Septra, Bactrim)[1]	160/800 mg bid	14
Trimethoprim (Proloprim)[1]	100 mg bid	14
Second-Line Agents		
Amoxicillin-clavulanic acid (Augmentin)[1]	500 mg tid	14
Cephalexin (Keflex)[1]	500 mg qid	14
Hospitalized Patients*		
Parenteral Therapy		
Ceftriaxone (Rocephin)	1 g qd	
Ampicillin plus gentamicin†		Ampicillin 1-2 g q6h Gentamicin 3-5 mg/kg q24h
Ciprofloxacin (Cipro)	200-400 mg q12h	
Levofloxacin (Levaquin)	250-500 mg q24h	
Piperacillin-tazobactam (Zosyn)†	3.375 g q6-8h	

*Parenteral therapy should continue until the patient shows clinical improvement and can tolerate oral medications.
†Recommended regimen when enterococcus species is suspected.
[1]Not FDA approved for this indication.
Abbreviations: bid = twice daily; qd = daily; qid = 4 times a day; tid = 3 times a day; TMP-SMX = trimethoprim-sulfamethoxazole.

[Zagam][1], trovafloxacin [Trovan][1], and moxifloxacin [Avelox][1]) should be avoided because they do not achieve adequate concentrations in the urine and may not be effective. Trimethoprim (Proloprim)[1], trimethoprim-sulfamethoxazole (Bactrim)[1], and β-lactam medications can be considered, but because there is a higher resistance pattern noted against these agents, they should be used with caution. For most infections a 14-day course of therapy is recommended. A 7- to 10-day course of therapy using the fluoroquinolones can be considered if the upper tract symptoms are mild and there is a rapid response to therapy. However, β-lactam therapy should be continued for 14 days because the 7- to 10-day course is associated with higher-than-acceptable failure rates.

Inpatients should be started on ceftriaxone (Rocephin) if enterococcus is not suspected. If there is concern for enterococcus infection, ampicillin plus an aminoglycoside or piperacillin-tazobactam (Zosyn) should be used. Empirically, aminoglycosides or fluoroquinolones can also be considered (see Table 2). Parenteral therapy should continue until the patient demonstrates clear clinical improvement and is able to tolerate oral therapy. Usually this requires 24 to 48 hours of parenteral treatment. If there has been no improvement within 48 to 72 hours, consideration should be given to imaging of the urinary system to rule out obstruction or abscess formation. Total duration of therapy should be 14 days, possibly longer for more serious infections. The presence of bacteremia does not change the recommended duration of therapy.

In patients who are asymptomatic after treatment, repeat cultures or testing is not indicated. If symptoms recur within 2 weeks and the initial organism is again detected, a renal ultrasound or computed tomographic (CT) scan should be obtained to rule out a complicated infection. Treatment should be undertaken with another antimicrobial agent proven efficacious by susceptibility testing. In patients with upper tract infections that reoccur more than 2 weeks after being free of infection, the infection may be treated as a new and not recurrent infection.

COMPLICATED URINARY TRACT INFECTIONS

Complicated UTIs represent a group of patients with a wide variety of structural or functional abnormalities of the urinary tract (see Table 1). Patients with these conditions should have urine culture and susceptibility testing performed because they are more likely to have infections with organisms such as *Klebsiella, Proteus, Pseudomonas,* or *Serratia* species. *Enterococcus, Staphylococcus aureus,* or *Candida* species are also isolated with greater frequency. Therapy should begin with a broad-spectrum antibiotic, taking into account resistance patterns in a particular community. Therapy should also be directed at correction of the underlying abnormality. Prophylactic antimicrobial therapy is ineffective at preventing recurrence of complicated UTIs.

Special Considerations

ASYMPTOMATIC BACTERIURIA

Isolation of 10^5 colony-forming units (cfu)/mL or more of a uropathogen in two consecutive urine cultures in the absence of symptoms is the criterion used to define asymptomatic bacteriuria. It is commonly found in the elderly, as well as catheterized patients. This condition does not require therapy unless it is detected in pregnant women or in patients with neutropenia, or preceding urogynecologic surgery or renal transplantation. Patients undergoing urologic instrumentation should also be treated if asymptomatic bacteriuria is present.

URINARY TRACT INFECTION IN PREGNANCY

Urinary tract infections during pregnancy warrant special consideration. It has been shown that while the incidence of asymptomatic bacteriuria is similar in the pregnant and nonpregnant patient (4% to 10%), the risk of developing a symptomatic UTI is much higher (20% to 40% vs. 1% to 2%). Symptomatic UTIs in pregnancy are associated with an increased risk of premature birth and other complications in the mother and fetus. Because of this risk, all pregnant women should be screened by urine culture between 12 to 16 weeks gestation. If asymptomatic bacteriuria is found, a 3- to 7-day course of therapy is warranted (Table 3). A repeat urine culture should be obtained approximately 1 week after completion of therapy. If asymptomatic bacteriuria is still present a 7- to 10-day course of therapy should be undertaken and then suppressive therapy should be continued throughout the remainder of the pregnancy (Table 4). Trimethoprim-sulfamethoxazole

TABLE 3 Regimens for Treatment of Urinary Tract Infections and Asymptomatic Bacteriuria in Pregnancy

Agent	Dose	Duration (Days)
First-Line Agents		
Amoxicillin (Amoxil)	500 mg tid	7
Nitrofurantoin (Macrodantin,	50-100 mg qid	7
Macrobid)*	100 mg bid	7
Cephalexin (Keflex)	250 mg qid	7
Second-Line Agents		
TMP-SMX (Septra DS, Bactrim DS)*	160/800 mg bid	7
Amoxicillin-clavulanic acid (Augmentin)	500 mg tid	7

*Avoid use near term in pregnancy.
Abbreviations: bid = twice daily; qid = 4 times a day; tid = 3 times a day; TMP-SMX = trimethoprim-sulfamethoxazole.

[1]Not FDA approved for this indication.

TABLE 4 Prophylactic Antimicrobial Regimens for the Prevention of Reinfection with Urinary Tract Infection

	Dose	
Agent	**Long-Term Low Dose**	**Post-coital***
First-Line Agents		
TMP/SMX (Bactrim, Septra)	80/400 mg qhs or thrice weekly	40/200 mg
Trimethoprim (Proloprim)	100 mg qhs	100 mg
Nitrofurantoin (Macrodantin)	50-100 mg qhs	50-100 mg
Second-Line Agents		
Ciprofloxacin (Cipro)†		125 mg
Norfloxacin (Noroxin)†	200 mg qhs thrice weekly	200 mg
Cephalexin (Keflex)	250 mg qhs	250 mg
Pregnancy Prophylaxis		
Nitrofurantoin (Macrodantin)‡	50-100 mg qhs	
TMP/SMX (Bactrim, Septra)‡	80/400 mg qhs	
Cephalexin (Keflex)		250 mg qhs
Amoxicillin (Amoxil)		500 mg qhs

*Single-dose therapy.
†Not for use during pregnancy.
‡Avoid use near term.
Abbreviations: qhs = at bedtime; TMP-SMX = trimethoprim-sulfamethoxazole.

(TMP-SMX) (Bactrim DS, Septra DS) and nitrofurantoin (Macrodantin) should not be used near term.

RECURRENT UNCOMPLICATED CYSTITIS

Many women experience frequent symptomatic UTIs. Patients with this problem can attempt several nonpharmacologic methods to decrease the need for antibiotics. These include voiding immediately after sexual intercourse and using a non–spermicide-based method of contraception. Ingestion of cranberry juice has been shown in some small studies to be effective in decreasing both bacteriuria and pyuria in an elderly population, but its efficacy in younger women has not been demonstrated. Women who continue to have recurrent symptomatic UTIs may benefit from low-dose suppressive therapy, as shown in Table 4. Antimicrobial prophylaxis is highly effective and is suggested for women with two or more UTIs within 6 months, or who experience more than three infections within 12 months. Although effective, approximately 50% of women who discontinue prophylactic therapy will develop a UTI within 3 months.

URINARY TRACT INFECTION IN THE ELDERLY

Approximately 10% to 15% of community-dwelling women older than age 70 years will have positive urine culture results. In long-term care facilities, 35% to 50% of women will have asymptomatic bacteriuria. The prevalence increases with increasing functional impairment. Asymptomatic UTI in elderly women should not be treated, regardless of whether associated pyuria is present. In the institutionalized population, treatment of asymptomatic bacteriuria does not decrease symptomatic episodes or improve survival. Such treatment is associated with increased occurrence of resistant organisms.

Symptomatic infection in elderly women is treated with similar medications as in younger women. A 7-day course of therapy is recommended, however. Follow-up urine cultures are not recommended for women who remain asymptomatic after therapy.

BACTERIAL INFECTIONS OF THE URINARY TRACT IN GIRLS

METHOD OF

Jack S. Elder, MD

Between 3% and 5% of girls develop a urinary tract infection (UTI). Most commonly, the first UTI occurs by the age of 5 years, with peaks during infancy and toilet training. After the first UTI, 60% to 80% of girls will develop a second UTI within 2 years. UTIs are caused mainly by colonic bacteria, with 75% to 90% caused by *Escherichia coli*, followed by *Enterococcus*, *Klebsiella*, and *Proteus* species. *Staphylococcus saprophyticus* also may be a pathogen.

UTIs have been considered an important risk factor for the development of renal insufficiency or end-stage renal disease. Some have questioned the importance of UTI as a risk factor because only 2% of children with end-stage disease have a history of UTI. This paradox is probably secondary to better recognition of the risks of UTI, prompt diagnosis, and therapy.

Clinical Manifestations and Classifications

There are three forms of UTI: pyelonephritis, cystitis, and asymptomatic bacteriuria.

Pyelonephritis is characterized by any or all of the following: abdominal or flank pain, fever, malaise, nausea, vomiting, and occasionally diarrhea. Some newborns and infants may show nonspecific symptoms such as jaundice, poor feeding, irritability, and weight loss. Involvement of the renal parenchyma is termed *acute pyelonephritis*, whereas if there is no parenchymal involvement, the condition may be termed *pyelitis*. Acute pyelonephritis may result in renal injury, which is termed *pyelonephritic scarring*.

Cystitis indicates that there is bladder involvement and symptoms include dysuria, urgency, frequency, suprapubic pain, incontinence, and malodorous urine. Cystitis does not cause fever and does not result in renal injury.

Asymptomatic bacteriuria refers to a positive urine culture without any manifestations of infection. This condition occurs almost exclusively in girls, is benign, and does not cause renal injury, except in pregnant women, in whom a symptomatic UTI can occur if left untreated.

Pathogenesis and Pathology

Virtually all UTIs are ascending infections, arising from the fecal flora. Pathogens colonize the perineum and enter the bladder via the urethra.

If bacteria ascend from the bladder to the kidney, acute pyelonephritis may occur. Normally, the renal papillae have an antireflux mechanism that prevents urine from flowing in a retrograde direction into the collecting tubules. Some compound papillae, typically located in the upper and lower poles of the kidney, allow intrarenal reflux. Infected urine then stimulates immunologic and inflammatory responses. The result may cause renal injury and scarring. Girls younger than 4 years of age seem most likely to develop renal scarring, although this complication can occur at any age.

The pathogenesis of UTI also is based, in part, on the presence of bacterial pili or fimbriae on the bacterial surface. There are two types of fimbriae: type I and type II. Type I fimbriae are found on most strains of *E. coli* and typically are present in organisms that cause cystitis, whereas type II (or "P") fimbriae are much more likely to cause pyelonephritis.

UTIs are most common in girls younger than age 5 years. Host factors that predispose to UTI include voiding dysfunction, vesicoureteral reflux, constipation, obstructive uropathy, labial adhesion, neuropathic bladder, nonsterile catheterization, sexual activity, and pregnancy.

Diagnosis

A UTI may be suspected based on the symptoms or findings on urinalysis, but a urine culture is necessary for confirmation and appropriate therapy. In toilet-trained girls, a midstream urine sample is usually satisfactory. Most studies fail to show any benefit to formally cleansing the introitus before obtaining the specimen. If the child is not toilet trained, a urine sample obtained by catheterization with a No. 5 or 8 French feeding tube is ideal. This technique can be performed in girls atraumatically. Specimens obtained with a "U-bag" are prone to contamination, although these samples are useful if the culture is negative.

A urinalysis should be obtained from the same specimen as that cultured. Nitrites and leukocyte esterase are usually positive in infected urine. Microscopic hematuria is common in acute cystitis. White blood cell casts in the urinary sediment suggest renal involvement, but these are rarely seen. If the child is asymptomatic and the urinalysis result is normal, it is unlikely that the urine is infected. However, if the child is symptomatic, a UTI is possible, even if the urinalysis result is negative. If the culture shows greater than 100,000 colonies of a single pathogen, or if there are 10,000 colonies and the child is symptomatic, it is considered a UTI.

With acute renal infection, a significantly elevated erythrocyte sedimentation rate and C-reactive protein are common. With a renal abscess, the white blood cell count is markedly elevated to greater than 20,000 to 25,000/mm^3. Because sepsis is common in pyelonephritis, particularly in infants and in any child with obstructive uropathy, blood cultures should be considered.

Treatment

If the child has symptoms of acute cystitis, a urine specimen is obtained for culture and treatment is started immediately. If the symptoms are mild or the diagnosis is doubtful, treatment can be delayed until the culture and sensitivities are known. A 3- to 5-day course of trimethoprim-sulfamethoxazole (Bactrim; Septra) suspension (1 teaspoon twice daily if the child weighs 10 kg; 2 teaspoons daily if the child weighs 20 kg) is effective against most strains of *E. coli*. Nitrofurantoin (Furadantin) (5 to 7 mg/kg per 24 hours in three to four divided doses) is also effective and has the advantage of being active against *Klebsiella* and *Enterobacter* organisms. Nitrofurantoin suspension is tolerated poorly by most children because of its taste and its tendency to cause nausea and vomiting; an alternative is nitrofurantoin macrocrystals (Macrodantin) in capsule form, which can be opened and placed in formula or food. Amoxicillin (Amoxil) (50 mg/kg per 24 hours) is also effective as initial treatment but has no clear advantages over sulfonamides or nitrofurantoin.

In acute febrile infections suggestive of pyelonephritis, a 14-day course of broad-spectrum antibiotics capable of reaching significant tissue levels is preferable. Hospitalization is indicated for children (a) younger than 2 months of age; (b) who are dehydrated and unable to drink liquids; (c) with a complicated UTI (obstructive uropathy, neuropathic bladder); or (d) in whom sepsis is suspected. Parenteral treatment with ceftriaxone (Rocephin) (50 to 75 mg/kg per 24 hours, not to exceed 2 g) or ampicillin (Omnipen; Principen) (100 mg/kg per 24 hours) with an aminoglycoside such as gentamicin (Garamycin) (3 to 5 mg/kg per 24 hours in one to three divided doses) is preferable until cultures and sensitivities are available. Treatment with aminoglycosides is particularly effective against *Pseudomonas,* and alkalinization of urine with sodium bicarbonate increases their effectiveness in the urinary tract. When oral therapy is chosen, third-generation cephalosporins, such as cefixime (Suprax)* (8 mg/kg per 24 hours in one to two doses), is usually effective against a variety of gram-negative organisms other than *Pseudomonas*; an intravenous injection of ceftriaxone (Rocephin) 50 to 75 mg/kg may be given in the office or emergency room, followed by oral therapy. Nitrofurantoin should not be used in children with a febrile UTI because it does not achieve significant renal tissue levels. Children with a renal or perirenal abscess or with infection in obstructed urinary tracts require surgical or percutaneous drainage in addition to antibiotic therapy and other supportive measures.

The oral fluoroquinolone ciprofloxacin (Cipro) is an alternative agent for resistant microorganisms, particularly *Pseudomonas,* in patients older than age 17 years. It also has been used in younger children with cystic fibrosis and pulmonary infection secondary to *Pseudomonas,* and is occasionally used for short-course therapy in children with *Pseudomonas* UTI. The safety and efficacy of oral ciprofloxacin in children are under study.

In a girl with asymptomatic bacteriuria, no treatment is necessary.

A urine culture should be performed 1 week after the termination of treatment of any UTI to ensure that the urine is sterile.

If UTI recurrences are frequent, identifying predisposing factors is beneficial. Establishing more normal patterns of voiding and defecation may be helpful. If there are symptoms of an overactive bladder with frequency and urge incontinence during the day, anticholinergics may be necessary. In addition, prophylaxis against reinfection, using either sulfamethoxazole-trimethoprim (Bactrim) or nitrofurantoin (Macrodantin) is often effective. Cranberry juice has not proved beneficial in preventing UTI. Cystoscopy and measurement of urethral caliber contribute nothing to the therapeutic decisions to be made in girls with a UTI and are contraindicated.

*Discontinued by the manufacturer.

Imaging Studies

The goal of imaging studies in children with a UTI is to identify anatomic abnormalities that predispose to infection. A renal ultrasonogram should be obtained to detect hydronephrosis and other urinary tract abnormalities. Renal ultrasonography is also sensitive for detecting pyonephrosis, a condition that may require prompt drainage of the collecting system by percutaneous nephrostomy.

A fluoroscopic voiding cystourethrogram (VCUG) should be performed in girls with a febrile UTI, girls younger than age 5 years with a UTI (including cystitis), and school-aged girls who have had two or more UTIs. The most common finding is vesicoureteral reflux, which is identified in approximately 40% of patients. The VCUG can be performed while the UTI is being treated. In some institutions, a radionuclide cystogram is performed instead of a contrast VCUG, because there is less radiation exposure to the gonads. However, the contrast VCUG is advantageous because it provides anatomic definition of the bladder, precisely grades reflux, demonstrates paraureteral diverticula, and may reveal upper tract anatomy such as a duplicated collecting system or ectopic ureter.

Some parents question the need for a VCUG if the ultrasonogram is normal. However, ultrasonography is insensitive in detecting reflux; only 40% of children with reflux have any abnormality on the ultrasonogram. In selected cases, oral or nasal[†] midazolam (Versed) (up to 0.5 mg/kg oral route, 0.2 mg/kg nasal route)[3], which causes anterograde amnesia and anxiolysis, may be used. We have found that this medication is efficacious and safe, and that it provides an acceptable experience with VCUG. Vital signs and oxygen saturation are monitored; no anesthesiologist is present.

In selected cases, a dimercaptosuccinic acid (DMSA) or glucoheptonate renal scan may be performed to establish the diagnosis of acute pyelonephritis, which is characterized by photopenia in the area of involvement. In approximately 50% of children with a febrile UTI, the DMSA scan demonstrates parenchymal involvement. In children with grade III, IV, or V reflux and a febrile UTI, 80% to 90% show acute pyelonephritis. If the DMSA scan shows acute pyelonephritis, approximately 50% will acquire a scar at that site over the following 5 months. However, if the DMSA scan is normal during a febrile UTI, no scarring results from that particular infection.

[†]May be compounded by a pharmacist.
[3]Exceeds dosage recommended by the manufacturer.

Computed tomography is another diagnostic tool that can diagnose acute pyelonephritis, but clinical experience with DMSA is much greater.

If vesicoureteral reflux is present, a DMSA scan often is performed to assess whether renal scarring is present. The DMSA is the most sensitive and accurate study for demonstrating scarring. Initial therapy for reflux is generally medical (antibiotic prophylaxis), with surgical therapy, either open or endoscopic, reserved for those who fail medical therapy.

CHILDHOOD ENURESIS

METHOD OF

Julian Wan, MD

Enuresis refers to the socially inappropriate and unplanned for loss of urine control. It becomes a symptom and concern when it occurs beyond the age when normal effective bladder control is expected. Enuresis is classified by the timing and nature of the wetness. *Primary enuresis* refers to children who have never had a prolonged period of dryness. *Secondary enuresis*, in contrast, means that there was a period of control and dryness of at least 6 months duration. Approximately 80% of all cases of enuresis are primary. Secondary enuresis is often attributed to some recent trauma or stress. In practice, the evaluation, treatment, and response are generally no different than those of primary enuresis. The distinction between primary and secondary enuresis is sometimes useful, but is not crucial in selecting a treatment method. When enuresis occurs at night, it is termed *nocturnal enuresis*, and when it occurs in the daytime it is called *diurnal enuresis*, although diurnal enuresis is often used to also describe those patients who are wet both day and night. It was once common to ignore or downplay the situation because there were few effective treatments and just to wait for improvement with time. Today, children have increased social demands to spend time away from home at an earlier age and so it has become a concern for younger children.

Natural History

Most children achieve some degree of toilet training between the ages of 1.5 to 4 years old. Daytime bladder control is usually achieved first along with daytime bowel control. Night-time bowel control comes next, followed by night-time bladder control. Over time, the vast majority of children do achieve full bladder and bowel control. Maturation and growth have strong influences. Nearly 100% of 2-year-olds wet at night. This figure drops to 20% for 5-year-old children. By age 8 years only 5% to 10% are wet, and this percentage continues to decline with an annual spontaneous resolution rate of approximately 15%. This rate accelerates as the child nears puberty, with the percentage of adult enuretics being well under 1%. Because most children will ultimately achieve control without any intervention, many physicians continue to advocate an expectant conservative approach. Parents should be explained the natural history of toilet control and the roles of maturation and growth. It may help them understand that their child may simply not be ready for toilet training. Children with developmental delays may be slower in achieving toilet control. The true functional age as determined by developmental milestones is usually more helpful than the chronological ages.

Evaluation

The evaluation of a child with enuresis requires a careful history and physical examination. The course of the pregnancy and delivery should be noted. The developmental history of the child should be assessed. An inquiry should be made into the child's toilet habits including frequency of urination when awake and bowel habits. Children with urethral strictures or occult posterior urethral valves often report hesitation or straining to void. Constipation is underappreciated as a cause of enuresis. Most normal children have a bowel movement every day or every other day. Children who are constipated are more likely to have dysfunctional voiding and correcting the constipation can in many cases decrease or eliminate the wetting, particularly daytime wetting. The degree of wetting should be noted and it is helpful to record it in terms of the number of days or nights wet per 7-day week. Prior therapy should be noted. The past medical history should specifically inquire about surgeries, medications, and any history of culture-proven urine infection (UTI). Any history of neurologic trauma or disease, such as encephalitis or cerebral palsy, should be pursued. Urinalysis should be done on all patients to rule out possible infection. If the child has an active infection, this has to be treated first before attempting to assess and treat the enuresis. Once treated, all children should undergo a careful investigation for any anatomic or functional conditions that put them at increased risk for UTI.

The physical examination should start with a general assessment of the child. Specific areas to concentrate upon are the neurologic examination, the back, the abdomen, and the genitalia. The finding of a hairy tuft, deep dimple, or deep skin crease, especially over the lower back, is important. It can indicate an underlying spinal abnormality such as a tethered spinal cord. A magnetic resonance imaging scan of the spine is indicated. If a tethered cord or other spinal abnormality is found, neurosurgical referral is necessary. The genitalia should be carefully examined.

In boys, the meatus should be open and without any webbing. Meatal stenosis will present with deflection or splaying of the urine stream. For uncircumcised boys, the foreskin should be pliable and not phimotic. In girls, the introitus should be unobstructed. The labia can be adherent, which can obscure and trap urine behind it into the vagina. If urine is actively welling up into the introitus during the examination, one must suspect the possibility of an ectopic ureter. Girls with a complete ureteral duplication may have an ectopic ureter that drains outside of the bladder and into the introitus, resulting in a persistent leakage. This finding requires surgical treatment. In all children, any findings suggestive of sexually transmitted disease or sexual abuse should be noted and in many jurisdictions even if it is only suspected, must be reported to the appropriate agency.

When to Treat

If the child is otherwise healthy the decision when to treat is one that should be made in conjunction with the patient and family. Nearly all treatment methods require the cooperation of the family and child. In some cases the family is content to wait and see if continence may improve with time, but seek reassurance that there are no underlying physical or psychological problems. Deliberate willfulness or laziness is rarely a cause. A supportive attitude should be recommended to the parents. Draconian punishments rarely work, and can make matters worse, leading, paradoxically, to the creation of psychological problems.

Day-Only Wetting

The child who is wet solely in the daytime but is completely dry at night is an important subset of diurnal enuresis. This finding means that when awake the child is less able to maintain continence than when unconscious and asleep. In nearly all cases, poor toilet habits are the primary cause. Infrequent voiding, use of avoidance maneuvers, and constipation are commonly found. Most parents and children are unable to supply a good toilet history. Adults also have different voiding patterns than children. Typical adults void three to four times during the day while awake. Among normal children who are 6 years old or younger, 10% or fewer void that infrequently. Most void between five and eight times per day. A voiding diary is often necessary to obtain a reliable toilet history. This need not be elaborate and can be a simple chart over 2 to 3 days tracking each and every time the child uses the bathroom. The parents are often surprised at how infrequently the child voids. The term "avoidance maneuver" is used to describe repetitive actions which the child uses to try to inhibit the bladder. The classic example is Vincent's curtsy wherein a girl will roll one leg under herself and sit with the heel pressed up against the perineum. This action and those of other avoidance maneuvers (squirming and twisting with crossed legs, squatting on toys or furniture) help to suppress and dampen the feelings of bladder fullness. Children can become so entranced in play (or video games, television, telephone) that they will begin to squirm and twist about in an effort to continue uninterrupted. With repetition, the avoidance maneuvers become habitual, and the child ultimately fails to perceive the early warning signs of a full bladder. Progressive delay leads finally to wetness. Correcting these habits is achieved by putting the child on a scheduled voiding program. The child is required to try to void at fixed times during the day. The parents are asked to pick six or seven events that punctuate the child's day. For example, breakfast, gym or recess, lunchtime, getting home from school, favorite afternoon activity, dinner time, and bedtime could form one pattern. Association with daily events makes it easier to remember and to maintain compliance. The child must attempt to void at the times selected regardless of how full the child may feel. The parents should not make the mistake of asking if the child feels full and needs to void. If the child's perception of bladder fullness were accurate and the response appropriate, there wouldn't be a problem.

Giggle incontinence is a special form of day only enuresis. Also called *enuresis risoria,* it is a limited condition where the child will wet with laughter, particularly giggling. A typical description is, "I laughed so hard I peed my pants." The usual patient is a pre-teenage girl who will wet when she laughs unexpectedly. Nearly all improve with time, and no specific treatment is necessary. Emptying the bladder regularly, especially before social occasions, seems to be effective in most cases. α-Methylphenidate (Ritalin)[1] has been used for some recalcitrant cases.

Day and Night Wetting

The child who is wet day and night needs to be carefully assessed. A search for the signs or symptoms of a tethered cord should be made. Urinary tract infections should be ruled out. If the child seems otherwise normal, a detailed voiding diary should be obtained. Children who are infrequent voiders and who exhibit avoidance maneuvers need to have these corrected and be started on a scheduled voiding program. Most other children will have urgency or urge incontinence. These patients are placed on a scheduled voiding program and an empirical trial of anticholinergic medication. The primary drug is oxybutynin (Ditropan), which acts on the bladder's smooth muscle. It can have significant side effects, such as dry mouth, constipation, and decreased sweating.

[1]Not FDA approved for this indication.

Other medications which could be used include tolterodine (Detrol)[1], hyoscyamine (Levsin)[1], and dicyclomine (Bentyl)[1], but none of these are specifically approved for this purpose. Although useful, a regular voiding program must be used along with the medication. If the child uses the medication just to delay and defer voiding, the problem will persist. Although both day and night therapy can occur concurrently, usually it is better to emphasize working on day problems first. Children won't become dry at night unless their daytime habits are better. If effective, these children are kept on the treatment plan for 3 to 6 months before being weaned off. For those who are recalcitrant to therapy, further workup with imaging and urodynamics is warranted.

Night-Only Wetting

There are currently three main theories of nocturnal enuresis: (a) failure to concentrate the urine adequately at night, (b) bladder activity and volume mismatch, and (c) impaired nocturnal arousal mechanism. The first notes that some patients lack a normal nocturnal surge in vasopressin. The second postulates that the bladders in these children have not yet achieved a balance of volume and activity. The third observes that some children are heavy sleepers and may not be able to rouse themselves. These are not mutually exclusive and a particular child may fall under two or all three categories. When nocturnal enuresis is secondary, it is worthwhile to inquire about sudden changes in the child's life. A new school, new sibling, moving, divorce, and other social changes are just a few examples. Usually the effect is transient and resolves within a few months. For those that persist, treatment should proceed as if it were primary enuresis.

Behavioral modification, fluid restriction, medications and alarm devices are the main treatment methods. Usually more than one modality is used simultaneously. By the time they seek out medical advice, most parents have already tried several home remedies. Two are worth mentioning because of their common occurrence. The first is night waking: the child is put to bed, and later, when the parents turn in, they wake and toilet the child. Usually this approach fails because many children will wet either before or after they are roused. It is also hard to carry out because it disrupts the family's sleep. The second is daytime holding of urine: this concept is based on the notion that the "bladder is too small and needs to be stretched out." The hope is that by repetitive daytime holding, the bladder enlarges and can hold more urine at night. Intuitively appealing, it rarely works. It may actually deter continence because it promotes daytime avoidance maneuvers. Finally, some parents fear that the use of pads or diapers would deter the development of continence. This belief is groundless, and their use helps to decrease social friction and anxiety by lessening the family's laundry burden.

For very young children (4 years of age or younger) time and patience are usually recommended. If the family feels compelled to act, simple fluid restriction before bed is suggested. All fluids are halted 1.5 to 2 hours before bed. Fruits, vegetables, and other solids that are predominately liquid (ice cream, gelatin, pudding, cereal with milk) are all banned. This should be explained explicitly to the parents and child, who sometime have curious notions of what is or isn't a fluid.

For older children in elementary school, a multiple approach of fluid restriction, regular daytime voiding, and the use of either a wetting alarm or medication is suggested. Regular daytime voiding encourages the child to void five to seven times when awake. It helps to break up any avoidance maneuvers and reminds the child to void before going to sleep. Wetting alarms are behavior-modification devices, and have a sensor that tucks into the child's underwear or pajama bottom. This is linked to an alarm module that attaches to the child's shirt or top. When the sensor becomes wet, the alarm sounds and/or vibrates, and it is hoped that the child wakes sufficiently to finish urinating in the bathroom. There are several models commercially available (Palco Wet Stop, Nytone Enuresis Alarm, Malem Bedwetting Alarm). The chief benefit of the alarms is that when they work, the effect has a low recidivism rate. Approximately 75% of those who respond will still be dry 1 year after the alarm is stopped. Unfortunately, it takes months of use, and some children are heavy sleepers and may not respond at all. They cannot be used discreetly and can wake up other family members. Not all insurance carriers will cover them. The preferred medication is desmopressin acetate (DDAVP) a synthetic version of the posterior pituitary hormone, vasopressin, also known as antidiuretic hormone. Vasopressin concentrates the urine by acting on the kidney to recover free water and by raising the blood pressure. The synthetic version is longer lasting (up to 6 to 8 hours) and has fewer cardiovascular effects. It is available as a pill or nasal spray. Each pill delivers 0.2 mg and the spray delivers 10 μg of the drug. One to three pills or sprays are administered about 30 minutes before bedtime, and must be used with fluid restriction. The drug is well tolerated and has few side effects. Occasionally there are transient headaches, and caution must be taken if the child has any renal problems. If the initial dose of one pill or spray per night is ineffective after 2 to 3 weeks, the dosage is increased to two pills or sprays for another 2 to 3 weeks. This is repeated to three pills or sprays if necessary. It can be used safely for a long time and there are patients who have been using it for years. Once an effective dose has been found, it should be used for at least 3 to 6 months before attempting to wean off. The chief benefits are its discreetness, its ease of use, and its few side effects. Not everyone responds, however, and about one half of the patients who do respond will develop intermittent or complete

[1]Not FDA approved for this indication.

return of nocturnal enuresis 1 year after stopping the medication. Some families opt to use the medication only on sleepovers and other social events.

Patients who do not respond to desmopressin acetate or to alarms are offered imipramine (Tofranil). The drug of choice prior to desmopressin acetate, it is a tricyclic antidepressant and has weak α-adrenergic and anticholinergic effects on the bladder. It affects the brain's sleep cycle. Approximately 50% of children will respond to the medication. The typical dosage is 25 mg taken orally 30 minutes before bedtime and can be raised to 50 mg and 75 mg, depending on the child's size and weight. Caution is necessary because it can have side effects such as blurring of vision and alteration of concentration. Overdose can result in fatal arrhythmias. For this reason, care must be taken to store it securely, and to warn the parents to look for side effects. If effective, the drug is continued for 3 to 6 months before gradually weaning off. For patients who are not responsive to these treatments individually, combination therapy using two drugs and/or devices together can sometimes be effective. Finally, persistently wet patients should undergo further investigations of their bladder by a urologist.

URINARY INCONTINENCE

METHOD OF

Niall T.M. Galloway, MD

Key Points

- Incontinence is a very common condition and patterns of problems run in families.
- There are many contributing causes and most are readily treated.
- Simple treatments are effective, but results are best when the treatment starts early.
- Surgery should be reserved for those with moderate or severe symptoms who have failed conservative therapy.

Definition

The unwanted or involuntary loss of urine that is objectively demonstrable and is a social or hygienic problem.

Significance

- More than 25 million Americans suffer from bladder control problems.
- Incontinence is more common in women than men, but all ages may be affected.
- Incontinence may occur after childbirth or after pelvic surgery (e.g., hysterectomy or prostatectomy).
- Prevalence is greater in the elderly (3% of women age 20 to 29 years, 32% of women >80 years old).

Cost of incontinence can be measured in personal, social, and economic terms.

- Personal issues—loss of confidence, reduced quality of life, negative impact on employment, restriction of activities
- Social—isolation, unable to do sports or exercise, and later not able to go out are often the key factors that push the elderly out of their homes and into residential care
- Economic—$27.8 billion a year estimated to be spent on continence treatments and care for those older than 65 years of age in the United States; more feminine protection products are used to control incontinence problems than for menstrual loss

The Agency for Health Care Policy and Research (AHCPR) developed a *Clinical Practice Guideline for Urinary Incontinence* in 1996, which was published by the U.S. Department of Health and Human Services. This guideline has been accepted widely, for the evaluation and management of urinary incontinence, as a standard for care by medical and nursing practitioners.

Causes

Incontinence can be caused by many factors.

Stress incontinence is used to describe leakage that occurs with coughing, sneezing, or lifting. Stress incontinence implies weakness of the closure mechanism (urethral sphincter muscle). Elements include anatomic displacement of the bladder base, incompetence of the bladder neck, and/or intrinsic urethral sphincter weakness.

Urge incontinence describes leakage that occurs with a strong feeling of needing to go, but the patient is not able to hold on without leaking. Urge leakage is usually more difficult for the patient, because it is unpredictable and often sudden. When urge leakage does occur, it may be a flood (large volume of loss) rather than drops. Urge may be a result of inappropriate contractions of the bladder (overactive bladder) or unwanted relaxation of the pelvic floor and sphincter muscles. Stroke, spinal cord injury, MS (multiple sclerosis), and other nervous system problems can be associated factors.

Overflow incontinence implies that the bladder fails to empty properly. The overfull bladder will spill over as the pressure within exceeds the closure pressure of the urethra. Overflow leakage will occur with any activity by day and at night. Failure to empty the bladder may lead to increased bladder pressures, which will offer resistance to drainage of urine from the kidneys and can lead to kidney damage.

Extraurethral leakage implies that the urine is not leaking from the natural opening of the urethra, but from an abnormal opening. Extraurethral leakage is rare and is usually the result of previous surgery. In adults, there may be a fistula (abnormal opening) from the bladder into the vagina after hysterectomy.

In addition, unwanted urinary leakage can be provoked by other factors that are not related to bladder and urethral function. Epileptic seizures are classically associated with urinary leakage. Coma or excessive sedation can provoke overfilling of the urinary bladder and lead to incontinence. Excessive or inappropriate medications can provoke or exacerbate problems of urinary incontinence. Diuretics can provoke increased urine volume, antihypertensive agents can relax the smooth muscle of the bladder neck and worsen leakage problems. Anti-inflammatory medications and analgesics can provoke incontinence and worsen leakage. Review of medications is always helpful.

There are physical factors in the pelvis that will predispose to incontinence. The bladder shares space in the pelvis with the other pelvic organs, including the colon and rectum, and in women, the uterus and cervix. Enlargement of the uterus during pregnancy will compress the bladder and leave little or no space in the bladder to hold urine. In the final weeks of a pregnancy, urinary symptoms may include increased frequency, nocturia, or urgency, and urinary leakage is a common complaint. The enlarged uterus, crowded with fibroid tumors, can provoke incontinence in the same way. The constipated bowel, loaded with stool, can provoke unwanted urinary leakage at any age, but it is a particularly common cause in the elderly.

Stress and urge incontinence account for at least 80% of urinary incontinence. Extra urethral incontinence is treated by surgical repair of the abnormal opening. Overflow incontinence is treated by intermittent drainage using clean catheterization. If there is an anatomic obstruction that is preventing the flow, such as an enlarged prostate, surgical relief of the obstruction may restore normal voiding and resolve the urinary incontinence.

Signs and Symptoms

A typical patient with stress urinary incontinence is a 57-year-old mother of three with a 7-year history of urinary leakage. At first the episodes of leakage were infrequent and provoked only by vigorous coughing or sneezing, but in the last 2 years, leakage occurs every day and she must wear two or three pads a day for protection. Leakage problems have caused her to stop playing tennis and to avoid vigorous activity. There is a family history of problems—the patient's mother and aunt also experienced bladder control problems.

The symptom is unwanted urinary leakage that occurs with coughing or lifting. Other symptoms may be present, such as skin irritation and dermatitis, or episodes of urinary tract infection. Urinary symptoms of increased urinary frequency and urgency may be prominent. There may be prolapse of the pelvic organs, which may result in an awareness of "something coming down" in the vagina. The patient may see or feel a bulge in the vagina and might complain that the bladder has "dropped down" or "fallen."

Incontinence is not only a complaint and a condition, it is also a clinical sign. When we examine the patient, we should look at the clothing and underwear for signs of wetting or urinary staining. The demonstration of urinary leakage can occur without provocation as the patient moves or turns during clinical examination. If incontinence is less severe, it will be necessary to use some provocation, such as coughing or straining, to provoke urinary leakage. It is important to examine the patient with a full or at least partly full bladder. If incontinence is severe, leakage may be demonstrated with the first cough in the supine position, but if there is no leak in the supine position, you must examine the patient standing. Ideally, the patient should be examined standing on a towel, with one foot raised on a standing stool and one foot on the floor.

Leakage may be provoked by asking the patient to cough gently. For less severe problems, it is necessary to use more vigorous and repeated coughing or straining (Valsalva maneuver) to demonstrate urinary loss. The physician should kneel beside the patient and observe the urethral meatus and vaginal introitus during the efforts to provoke leakage. If leakage occurs, the examining fingers can be used to support the anterior vaginal wall and prevent downward movement of the bladder neck. Repeated provocation will help to determine whether the urinary leakage is or is not controlled by supporting the bladder neck (Marshall test).

Other physical signs and features are commonly associated with incontinence. Recognition of these features will help the physician to develop a management plan to resolve the bladder control problem.

Abdominal distention is very common in incontinence and can be recognized by inspection of the abdomen in the supine position. The patient should be able to push out the anterior abdominal wall and to draw it inward. If there is significant distention, the patient cannot draw the abdominal wall inward from the resting position. This would imply that the abdominal cavity is "full," like a suitcase that is packed too tightly, leaving no space inside. There are five usual causes of distention: fat, fetus, fluid, flatus, and feces. In practice, the most common causes are flatus and feces. Fat is distributed uniformly throughout the body. If the arms, shoulders, and breasts are not heavy with fat, abdominal distention is most unlikely to be a result of fat.

The physician should palpate the abdomen and examine the left and right lower quadrants. The cecum is like the stomach in that it should contain fluid mulch and not solids. The cecum is never palpable in health. If the abdomen is distended and the right colon is palpable, this would imply at least some element of constipation or bowel inertia. Fluid is dull to percussion, and the dullness may be demonstrated to shift when the patient is rolled to one side. Percussion of the abdomen will distinguish the characteristic shifting dullness that suggests the presence of abnormal fluid, such as ascites. Percussion should include the epigastric and suprapubic areas to reveal the presence of a distended bladder.

Hypothyroidism is common in perimenopausal and postmenopausal women. Slowing of the thyroid will contribute to constipation, abdominal distention, and symptoms of urinary incontinence. *Hyperthyroidism* might be found in younger patients. Overactivity of the thyroid is associated with urinary frequency, urgency, and urge incontinence.

The state of hydration is important. Excessive fluid and salt intake can drive urinary symptoms and contribute to problems of polyuria and peripheral edema. Ankle swelling and pitting edema that is evident by day will contribute to excessive fluid mobilization at night when the lower limbs are elevated. This will lead to excessive urine production at night and the need to empty the bladder more often at night (nocturia). In the elderly, this pattern will contribute to problems of nocturnal bedwetting. New onset of bedwetting in adults or the elderly is an important sign and it should prompt the physician to examine the patient to exclude chronic urinary retention, urinary tract infection, renal failure, or fecal impaction.

The patient who is troubled by urinary frequency or incontinence will often try to avoid fluids, which will lead to clinical features of dehydration. The tongue and mucous membranes may be dry, the eyes dark and deeper in the orbits, skin turgor will be increased, and the pulse may be thin and rapid. Examination of the voided urine will reveal small volumes of dark, concentrated, amber-color urine. The specific gravity will be increased (>1.020). Patients complain of fatigue, headache, and abdominal discomfort. When the body is deprived of adequate fluids, extra water is reabsorbed from the colon and the stool becomes more dry and stiff and difficult to evacuate. As the bowel becomes more slow and loaded with stool, so there is more crowding of the bladder, which will worsen symptoms of pelvic pressure, urinary frequency, and incontinence.

Physical characteristics are associated with problems of urinary incontinence. The distended abdomen has been mentioned, but aspects of obesity, gait, posture, and lower extremities are also important. The nerves that are responsible for the activity of the muscles of the pelvic floor are located in the most distal segments of the spinal cord (S2, S3, S4, and S5). These nerves are more caudal in the spinal cord than the nerves for the muscles of the feet and toes (S2 and S3). There may be a history of back or neck problems, including disc disease or spinal stenosis. Examination should include inspection of the back and buttocks. The gluteal form and folds will also reflect the relative strength of the pelvic floor structures.

Inspection of the feet and buttocks is important, because they offer a mirror that will reflect the condition of the muscles of the pelvic floor. The patient who has severe urinary incontinence because of muscle weakness will often have a corresponding pattern of weakness in the intrinsic muscles of the feet. A typical pattern would be flat feet with loss of intrinsic muscles in the lateral toes. This would be marked by an inability to abduct the toes (spread the toes apart in the line of the toes). In health, the toes should lie flat on the floor, like the fingers of a hand palm down on a tabletop. The patient with intrinsic muscle weakness of the sacral segments may have clawing of the toes—hyperextension of the metatarsophalangeal joints and flexion of the interphalangeal joints—so that the toe nails are pointing downward in a vertical direction, instead of horizontal. Lateral deviation of the great toe (hallux valgus) is often present and the lateral toes may be hypoplastic.

Sensory deficits may be recognized by simple clinical examination of the sacral dermatomes. Examine the patient in a lateral position with the knees drawn up. Use two orange sticks held with the tips 4 cm apart to assess two-point discrimination in the perianal and postanal dermatomes. The sensory deficits are typically less marked than the motor deficits.

The physician should complete an examination of the perineum, including inspection with a speculum and bimanual examination. Leakage may be demonstrated by cough in the supine position. Repeated coughing or abdominal straining may be needed to demonstrate leakage if incontinence is not severe. When leakage is not demonstrated in the supine position, examine the patient in a standing position with a full, or at least partly full, bladder. Stand the patient on a towel, with one foot elevated on a low stool. Coughing in this position will usually provoke leakage in the patient with moderate or severe stress urinary incontinence.

Screening and Diagnosis

Prevalence of incontinence is high and many patients will accept symptoms as if incontinence is a normal consequence of childbirth or an expected part of aging, but it is not. Many patients are embarrassed and reluctant to seek help. Many physicians are also embarrassed and reluctant to inquire about these problems, because they may lack interest or awareness about these problems. Some physicians may not have had much training about the assessment and treatments for incontinence. The interest of the physician is often directed to other aspects of health care, and it is easy to miss the opportunity to recognize and resolve urinary leakage problems.

Urinary incontinence is a condition and its symptoms will vary from day to day until the problem becomes severe. Screening may be done as a part of the clinical interview at routine annual visits for cervical smear or other clinical examinations. We must remember that patients are often embarrassed about bladder control problems and may be reluctant to ask their doctor for help. There may be clues in the form of odor, or the presence of pads in the underclothes or urine staining on clothing, bedding, or furniture. The physician must be willing to ask about the problem, but don't ask, "Are you incontinent?" Instead ask, "How much trouble are you having with bladder control?"

When the problem of involuntary leakage has been recognized, it is necessary to distinguish whether the leakage is transient or chronic. Transient leakage will resolve when the provoking factors have been resolved. If incontinence is chronic, the type of incontinence can usually be distinguished by history taking, physical examination, and simple testing to determine whether the bladder is able to empty or not. The physician should consider the reversible factors that might provoke or sustain incontinence. Initial treatment should be directed to resolve the reversible factors.

Prevention and Treatment

It is appropriate to consider how to preserve continence and pelvic health, in the same way that we might modify behaviors, lifestyle, and diet to preserve a healthy heart. Little attention has been paid to strategies that might prevent problems of urinary incontinence in the United States, but other countries do take a more active approach. In France, for example, there is a national program that provides pelvic floor therapy to restore muscle strength after childbirth. The rate of hysterectomy in the women of France is dramatically less than in the United States (1:9).

It has been usual for patients to wait far too long to address the problems of urinary incontinence. Patients may be too embarrassed or mild symptoms may not warrant attention. There may be a fear of surgical treatment and some may not realize that nonsurgical treatments are available and effective. On average, the typical patient will tolerate symptoms of urinary leakage for more than 7 years, before seeking medical attention.

Modification of the diet is appropriate for many patients. Some foods are bladder irritants and will worsen symptoms of urinary frequency urgency and incontinence. These include spicy foods, acidic or citrus fruits, and beverages, including caffeine and alcohol. Patients should be encouraged to drink more water (four to six 8-oz glasses a day) to dilute the urine and improve bowel function. There are no adequate randomized controlled trials to study the impact of these primary management strategies.

The most common cause for incontinence is weakness of the muscles of the pelvic floor. We are not all blessed with the same structures and there are wide differences in pelvic floor muscle strength between one patient and another. There is a tendency for similar structures to be found in members of the same family, and similar symptoms and bladder control problems are shared as a result. It may be easy to dismiss bladder problems as "normal" if several members of the family share the same symptoms.

Pelvic floor muscles can be weakened or damaged by vaginal delivery. As the baby's head passes through the birth canal, the perineum will be stretched and pelvic floor muscles and the pelvic support structures can be torn away from their normal attachments within the pelvis. For some women, the risk of vaginal delivery may be sufficient to warrant cesarean section.

In addition, violent forces on the pelvic floor such as those associated with exceptional stresses of power lifting, gymnastics, or parachute jumping can result in damage to the pelvic floor muscles and the internal attachments of the pelvic support anatomy and pelvic organs. Less dramatic forces are associated with chronic coughing, morbid obesity, and abdominal straining. These activities can also contribute to pelvic floor muscle weakness. We should encourage avoidance of these exceptional and chronic forces in individuals at risk for incontinence problems.

Like other muscles, the pelvic floor muscles can be strengthened by exercise. Kegel exercises are repetitive gripping and tightening contractions of the pelvic floor. These exercises are easy to learn when the pelvic floor is strong, but not so easy when the muscles are weak. These exercises are the time-honored way of treating urinary incontinence by pelvic floor muscle strengthening. Verbal or written instructions alone do not prepare patients adequately. When a trained nurse or therapist provides instruction and coaching with Kegel exercises results are improved.

Postnatal pelvic floor muscle exercises are effective for treating postpartum incontinence. In a randomized controlled trial of 8000 women surveyed 3 months after delivery, 749 reported persistent incontinence and were randomized to instructed pelvic floor muscle exercises and bladder retraining or routine postnatal exercises. At 12 months postpartum, the treatment group showed a significant reduction in stress urinary incontinence.

Biofeedback techniques can be used to help patients to generate more effective contractions and to guide their efforts to target the contractions in the pelvic floor. It is a paradox that the patient with the strongest pelvic muscles (and no symptoms) will master Kegel contractions easily, but those with weaker muscles will find them more difficult to do.

Weighted vaginal cones can be used to help build pelvic floor muscle strength and endurance. This is a classical method of treatment (sometimes referred to as "Chinese eggs"). The patient is taught to insert a graded vaginal weight, starting with a light one and progressing to heavier weights through a range as muscle strength and endurance improves.

Stimulated contractions can be used to strengthen the pelvic floor muscles. If the patient is unable to localize the pelvic floor muscles and cannot generate any useful contraction, electrical stimulation can be used. These treatments use electrodes mounted on a probe that is placed in the vagina or anus or skin patches that are applied to the pelvic floor for stimulation with low-energy direct current. These treatments are widely available in Europe and have an established place in the clinical management of urinary incontinence. The results of electrical stimulation therapy vary from center to center, according to treatment protocols and patient selection. Success with electrical stimulation requires a skilled staff and a motivated patient, but in the best hands, the clinical results are excellent.

Studies have compared electrical stimulation with sham treatment and with pelvic floor exercises alone. Electrical stimulation was associated with improved outcomes for number of leakage episodes, pelvic floor muscle strength, and leakage on pad weight testing. Patients will not always accept electrical stimulation as a treatment option. Some are reluctant to use a probe in the vagina or anus. Some complain of discomfort or irritation with a probe. Even the use of patches on the skin may cause local irritation and skin problems for some patients.

Extracorporeal magnetic innervation is a new technology that uses a pulsed magnetic field flux to induce contractions of the muscles, but without the need for probes or patches and without the need to undress for treatments. The therapy head consists of a magnetic field generator (similar to magnetic resonance imaging) that is built into the seat of a special chair (NeoControl). For treatment the patient sits comfortably, fully clothed, on the chair, and the changing magnetic field will induce effective contractions of the pelvic floor muscles. Treatment is painless and the rate of contractions can be much faster than with conventional Kegels. NeoControl treatments are usually used for 20 minutes twice a week for 8 weeks (see www.neotonus.com for more information).

VAGINAL PESSARY

A formed support can be worn in the vagina to correct prolapse or incontinence. The type and form of the pessary are selected based on the nature of the problem and the shape, internal dimensions, and the size of the vaginal opening. Pessaries for incontinence treatment may include a ring-shaped design with a thickened area that should be positioned beneath the urethra to restore the anterior vaginal wall and bladder neck to a more normal position and to help close the bladder outlet. Some pessaries include the hormone estrogen, which can be absorbed directly with contact to nourish and restore the vaginal mucosa.

Occlusive devices have been developed that offer a physical barrier, which may be a patch over the urethral opening or a plug that can be worn inside the natural opening of the urethra. There is a place for these in selected patients.

Collection and containment systems have a role in managing the problem of leakage until effective treatments are complete or for those who may not be candidates for definitive therapy. External collection systems are to be preferred over internal catheters, which may be associated with problems of urinary infections, stone formation bleeding, and other complications.

MEDICATIONS

There is an important role for medication, particularly in the treatment of urge incontinence. Overactive detrusor contractions can be reduced or eliminated by anticholinergic drugs such as hyoscyamine (Levsin, Levbid)[1], oxybutynin (Ditropan), and imipramine (Tofranil)[1]. The side-effect profile of the traditional anticholinergic medications includes dry mouth and constipation, which may limit the therapeutic benefit. Newer preparations include sustained-release forms (Ditropan XL), which have an improved profile, and newer agents such as tolterodine (Detrol). This is also available as a once-a-day formulation (Detrol LA).

α-Adrenergic agonist medication (phenylpropanolamine)[2] has been used in the treatment of stress urinary incontinence. A randomized controlled trial has compared medication with pelvic floor muscle exercise and revealed no significant benefit of medication over exercise.

SURGICAL TREATMENTS

Bulking agents have an established role in the treatment of stress urinary incontinence. Collagen can be injected at the bladder neck to help close the bladder outlet to prevent unwanted leakage. This is an outpatient treatment that includes cystoscopy to guide the placement of the injections. Collagen treatments can be done without the need for a general anesthetic. Repeat injections may be needed to obtain the best results and further injections may be needed in the future to improve the closure, if the cushions of collagen reduce in size over time. Newer materials have been proposed for use as bulking agents.

NEEDLE-SUSPENSION PROCEDURES AND BURCH PROCEDURE

Early surgical procedures were designed to elevate and fix the bladder neck and urethra in an effort to prevent stress urinary leakage. There is less enthusiasm for these procedures because long-term results are disappointing. New symptoms of voiding difficulty, frequency, urgency, urge leakage, and pain are common after these surgeries. Longer follow-up reveals significant problems with pelvic organ prolapse.

---

[1]Not FDA approved for this indication.
[2]Not available in the United States.

Surgeries can be done using access and exposure that can be from the abdomen, from the vagina, or from both. The development of minimally invasive techniques has led to minimal access procedures that may replace traditional open surgeries. Laparoscopic, vaginal, and endoscopic procedures offer surgical choices for the patient and the surgeon.

Modern techniques reflect a more complete understanding of the mechanisms of pelvic prolapse and incontinence. These techniques recognize that the support structure of the pelvic floor extends to include all of the boundaries of the pelvic floor. If the urethra is not in the correct position, the anterior vaginal wall has lost some of its normal attachments. To correct displacement of the urethra, it is critical to include reattachment of the vaginal wall to its normal attachments within the pelvis. Repair of a lateral detachment of the vagina is called a *paravaginal repair*.

Modern techniques recognize that problems of vaginal prolapse (or bulging from the vagina) rarely include only a single support defect. It is common to find multiple support defects and our surgical repairs should recognize and correct all of the problems in a single procedure. There are patterns of support defect that occur together and can be readily corrected by the appropriate site-specific surgical repairs.

There is fashion in surgery, as in all things, and there is a rush to adopt the newest methods and to be up to date. At the same time, we must remember that the results of our surgical procedures are best judged not early at 2 months or 6 months, but after years. Patients should expect a surgical repair to last and the best repairs should last for years. Any new techniques must be adopted with caution until there is adequate follow-up and long-term outcomes are known. There are significant differences in practice between the urologist and the gynecologist. The urologist tends to favor endoscopic or open surgical procedures, whereas the gynecologist tends to favor vaginal or laparoscopic procedures. There are limited data from randomized comparative studies.

Colposuspension is a surgical procedure that will fix the anterior vaginal wall (adjacent to the bladder neck) to the pelvic bones at Cooper's ligament. This procedure is used by both urologists and gynecologists. Colposuspension has been compared with anterior colporrhaphy (plication of the anterior vaginal wall) and with needle-suspension procedures. After 1 year, results favor colposuspension and the results reveal a stronger difference at 3 years (88% vs. 57%) and 14 years (74% vs. 42%).

Surgical methods that are currently popular include sling procedures that may use the patient's tissue (autologous fascia), or banked tissue (cadaveric fascia), or animal-derived materials (xenograft), or nonbiologic artificial materials (prosthetic sling). Prosthetic slings are associated with unacceptable complications, including erosion and infection. Natural materials are preferred over artificial for sling procedures.

Results of sling procedures may be better when combined with surgical repairs of the associated pelvic support defects, such as paravaginal detachments or vaginal vault prolapse. There is a trend toward minimally invasive surgical procedures, including the use of laparoscopic access for colposuspension and other continence procedures. There are few prospective randomized studies to compare traditional with minimally invasive surgeries. The limited study, that has compared results after 1 and 3 years, suggests that traditional open surgery was significantly more effective.

Clinical Indicators

- Number of leak episodes

The patient should be asked to keep a record of the number of leak episodes and the factors that provoked leak episodes (examples: coughing, sneezing, lifting, a feeling of urgency or leakage without awareness).

- Severity of leakage

The severity of leakage refers to the volume of urine loss (drops, moderate, or a flood of leakage).

- Pad use

The number of pads used per day and the type of pads or protective garment is a useful measure.

- Bladder chart (bladder diary or log)

Patients are given a measuring cup (like an inverted hat that can be placed in the commode) to measure the volume of every void for an interval of 24 hours. Analysis of the chart will reveal the largest voided volume (called the *functional bladder capacity*) and the number of voids by day and at night. Addition of all of the voided volumes will reveal the total urine output in 24 hours. This volume should be in the order of 1.5 to 2 L per day. Patients with urinary frequency and incontinence may have volumes of more than 8 L per day. Dehydrated patients may be oliguric with voided volumes of less than 600 mL per day.

- Incontinence-specific quality of life measures (e.g., I-QOL short survey)

Quality of life measures are useful indicators of the impact of urinary incontinence on our patients. There are validated surveys—both long and short forms—that may be used.

Prognosis

Cure is a reasonable goal for most patients. If incontinence is mild to moderate, leakage can usually be resolved without surgery. Effective nonsurgical treatments include fluid and bowel management, timed or prompted voiding, and pelvic floor muscle strengthening exercises (Kegel). If pelvic floor muscles are weak and the patient is unable to grip effectively with the exercises, biofeedback techniques can be used to improve muscle contraction strength and duration. Electrical stimulation of the pelvic floor muscles can be used if the patient is unable to generate effective contractions. Electrical stimulation involves the use of patches that are placed on the skin of the perineum or probes that are introduced into the vagina or anus. This method involves repeated intervals of stimulation, but when used on a regular treatment regimen, it can be effective. Extracorporeal magnetic innervation is a new technology that uses a pulsed magnetic field flux to induce contractions of the muscles without the need for probes.

Surgery is considered when symptoms have failed to resolve with conservative therapies. Symptoms should be moderate or severe to warrant surgical treatment. There are always risks associated with any type of surgical procedure and the patient and surgeon should weigh the risks and benefits of surgery before electing to proceed. If anatomic defects are responsible, then surgery can be used to correct the defects. Before proceeding with surgery, it is appropriate to consider the role of urodynamic testing. Urodynamic testing is used to define the specific causes of the urinary incontinence and to plan the choice of surgical procedures. There is no single procedure that will be appropriate for all patients, but the principles of effective surgical correction are to define the anatomic defects and to restore normal anatomy by site-specific surgical repairs. Procedures that create compensatory abnormalities (such as sling procedures) should be reserved for those patients with severe defects that cannot be corrected by restoring the normal anatomical relations.

If incontinence is chronic and severe, complete resolution is less likely because of confounding factors such as immobility and irreversible neurological deficits. For the most frail of our elderly patients, cure may not be possible because of the confounding factors and the goal should be to make the problem a manageable one. If incontinence is to be managed, the goal is to reduce the severity of leakage. We need to aim to avoid the complications of incontinence such as urinary infection, dermatitis, and ulceration of the skin. It is important to define the objectives of the management plan with the patient and caregivers. Try to define what is the worst aspect of the problem for the patient. This should be the first target for change in the plan.

Alternative/Complementary Medicine

Bowel management is an important element of pelvic health. The urinary bladder shares space in the pelvis with the bowel (and the uterus) and when the lower bowel is empty, the bladder capacity is optimal and bladder control will be better. There are many complementary and alternative strategies for bowel management. A high-fiber diet is helpful for maintaining stool volume, form, and regularity. The addition of specific foods, such as warm prune juice, prunes, figs, or rhubarb, can act as natural stimulants for the bowel. Natural lubricants, such as olive oil, can improve the bowel pattern. Other oils are more palatable in the form of capsules such as flaxseed oil*[1], fish oil,*[1] or aloe products*[1]. Use of appropriate laxatives, such as herbal remedies, oriental green tea*[1], and similar preparations, is indicated if the simpler measures are insufficient. Suppositories, enemas, or colon cleansing do have a place in bowel management, but the simpler measures are preferred. Physical methods of abdominal palpation and kneading can be helpful to stimulate bowel transit. No randomized controlled trial data is available to compare the outcomes of alternative strategies.

Research Frontiers

SURGICAL TREATMENTS

There is great interest in efforts to make surgical treatments for incontinence less invasive and easier for the patient and the surgeon. The simpler forms of outpatient surgery use some form of fixation staples or screws to attach the soft tissues of the anterior vaginal wall to the bones of the pelvis. These techniques include influence and vesica procedures.

The transvaginal tape (TVT) procedure is a new form of sling procedure that involves the passage of two long needles from a small wound in the anterior vaginal wall beneath the urethra to the abdominal wall. Each needle is attached to the end of a tape of artificial material and as the needles are passed upward, the tape is carried into position. The needles and excess tape are trimmed and the small wounds are closed. This technique is simple to perform and early results are encouraging, but it is too early to predict what the long-term results might be.

Bulking agents have an established role in the treatment of stress urinary incontinence. Collagen was the preferred material to inject at the level of the bladder neck and urethra to help prevent leakage, but newer agents are in development and some are now available. These include artificial substances such as carbon particles and silicone suspension (Macroplastique). Some investigators are using cultured cartilage cells (taken from the back of the patient's own ear) as a bulking material. The cells are grown in tissue culture and then injected in suspension. This technique offers the advantage of using living cells that may be able to remain in place without significant change for years. Long-term results are awaited.

*Available as a dietary supplement.
[1]Not FDA approved for this indication.

BIBLIOGRAPHY

Abrams P, Blaivas JG, Stanton SL, et al: Standardization of terminology of lower urinary tract function. Scand J Urol Nephrol 114(Suppl):5-19, 1988.

Berghmans LCM, Hendricks HJM, Bo K, et al: Conservative treatment of stress urinary incontinence in women: A systematic review of randomized controlled trials. Br J Urol 82:181-191, 1998.

Black NA, Downs SH: The effectiveness of surgery for stress incontinence in women: A systematic review. Br J Urol 78: 497-510, 1996.

Bo K, Hagen RM, Kvarstein B, Jorgensen J, Larsen S: Pelvic floor muscle exercises for the treatment of female stress incontinence. III. Effects of two different degrees of pelvic floor muscle exercises. Neurourol Urodyn 9(5):489-502, 1990.

Bump RC, Hurt WG, Fantl A, Wyman JF: Assessment of Kegel pelvic muscle performance after brief verbal instruction. Am J Obstet Gynecol 165:322-329, 1991.

Burton G: A three year prospective randomized urodynamics study comparing open and laparoscopic colposuspension. Neurourol Urodyn 16:353-354, 1997.

Cammu H, Van Nylen J, Derde MP, et al: Pelvic physiotherapy in genuine stress incontinence. Urology 38(4):332-337, 1991.

Colombo M, Vitobello D, Proietti F, et al: Randomized comparison of Burch colposuspension versus anterior colporrhaphy in women with stress urinary incontinence and anterior vaginal wall prolapse. Br J Obstet Gynaecol 107:544-551, 2000.

Gladzener CMA, Lang G, Wilson PD, et al: Postnatal incontinence: A multicenter controlled trial of conservative treatment. Br J Obstet Gynaecol 105(Suppl 117):47, 1998.

Leach GE, Dmochowski RR, Appell RA, et al: Female stress urinary incontinence clinical guidelines panel: Summary report on surgical management of female stress urinary incontinence. J Urol 158:875-880, 1997.

Simeonova Z, Milsom I, Kullendorf AE, et al: The prevalence of urinary incontinence and its influence on quality of life in women from an urban Swedish population. Acta Obstet Gynecol Scand 78:546-551, 1999.

Wagner TH, Hu TW: Economic costs of incontinence in 1995. Urology 51(3):355-361, 1998.

EPIDIDYMITIS

METHOD OF

J. Curtis Nickel, MD

Epididymitis refers to inflammation of the epididymis, the tubular structure located along the posterior border of the testicle whose function is to facilitate maturation and transport of spermatozoa. *Acute epididymitis* refers to sudden occurrence of pain and swelling of the epididymis associated with acute inflammation of the organ and most commonly adjacent structures (e.g., testes). *Chronic epididymitis* refers to inflammation and pain in the epididymis, with or without swelling and/or induration, persisting for more than 6 weeks.

Classification

Table 1 shows a classification system proposed by the author for epididymitis.

TABLE 1 Classification of Epididymitis

Acute Epididymitis

Secondary to urinary tract infection
Secondary to sexually transmitted disease
Secondary to non-bacterial agents (viral, fungal, parasitic)

Chronic Epididymitis

1. Inflammatory chronic epididymitis
   Infective (e.g., chlamydia)
   Postinfective (e.g., following acute bacterial epididymitis)
   Granulomatous (e.g., tuberculosis)
   Drug induced (e.g., amiodarone [Cordarone])
   Associated with a known syndrome (e.g., Behçet's disease)
   Idiopathic (e.g., no identifiable etiology for inflammation)
2. Obstructive chronic epididymitis (e.g., postinfective or surgical scarring, post vasectomy)
3. Chronic epididymalgia
   Pain but no inflammation
   No identifiable etiology

Pathogenesis

Epididymal inflammation is usually the result of reflux of infection from the bladder, urethra, or prostate via the ejaculatory ducts and vas deferens. The process starts in the tail of the epididymis, then spreads to the body, and, finally, to the head of the epididymis. In infants and boys, acute epididymitis is usually related to a urinary tract infection and/or an underlying congenital anomaly. In prepubertal boys, there is some evidence that a relationship exists between epididymitis and the presence of a foreskin. In men over 50 years, benign prostatic hyperplasia results in urinary obstruction and stasis, and in some cases, urine infection leading to acute bacterial epididymitis. Urethral catheterization is another common cause of acute epididymitis in the older male. In postpubertal males of all ages, epididymal infection is usually associated with bacterial prostatitis. In sexually active men younger than 35 years of age, epididymitis is commonly the result of a sexually transmitted disease.

Chronic epididymitis may result from an inadequately treated acute epididymitis, recurrent epididymitis, obstruction of the genital tract, or immune- or medically related etiologies. In many patients, the etiology of chronic epididymitis and/or chronic epididymalgia is usually unclear.

Microbiology

The most common microorganisms responsible for epididymitis are those microorganisms that are the most common causes of genitourinary infections in the particular age group presenting. For example, the most common causative organisms in the pediatric and elderly age groups are the coliform organisms that cause bacteriuria (e.g., *Escherichia coli*). In men younger than the age of 35 years who are heterosexually active, the most common offending organisms causing epididymitis are usually the same organisms that cause urethritis (e.g., *Neisseria gonorrhea* and *Chlamydia trachomatis*). In homosexual men practicing anal intercourse, *E. coli* and *Haemophilus influenzae* are most commonly responsible. In special cases (especially immune-suppressed patients), viral, fungal, and parasitic microorganisms are implicated in epididymitis.

Diagnosis

The history and physical examination are important for establishing a diagnosis of epididymitis. Pain and swelling of the epididymis are the prominent features of acute epididymitis. Fever and abdominal pain may be present. Physical examination localizes the tenderness to the epididymis. Early on in the acute process, only the tail of the epididymis is tender, but the inflammation quickly spreads to the rest of the epididymis and if it continues to the testicle (which is very common in acute bacterial epididymitis), the swollen epididymis becomes indistinguishable from the swollen, tender testicle (referred to as *epididymo-orchitis*). The spermatic cord is usually tender and swollen in acute epididymitis.

Chronic epididymitis is more difficult to evaluate clinically. Attempts should be made to determine any of the clinical or etiologic factors noted above (and in Table 1), but in many cases, the distinction between chronic epididymitis and epididymalgia (pain without inflammation) may be impossible. The patient usually presents with a long-standing history of pain (waxing and waning or constant) localized to the epididymis. These symptoms may have a significant impact on the patient's quality of life and prevent the patient from doing many of the patient's usual physical activities. The epididymis itself may be enlarged, indurated, or of normal size and configuration.

Laboratory tests should include urethral swabs for culture (and if possible Gram stain) and a midstream urine specimen for culture and sensitivity. If the urethral smear reveals the presence of intracellular gram-negative diplococci, a diagnosis of *N. gonorrhea* is established. If only white cells are seen on the urethral smears, a diagnosis of *C. trachomatis* will be established in 66% of cases. If the diagnosis is uncertain, particularly in boys and young adults, duplex Doppler scrotal ultrasonography should be performed to look for increased blood flow to the infected epididymis. In males younger than 30 years, acute epididymitis can be confused with acute torsion of the testicle or to a lesser extent, testicular tumor.

When an infant or young boy is diagnosed with epididymitis, he should be further evaluated with abdominal/pelvic ultrasound, voiding cystourethrography, and in some cases, cystoscopy.

Treatment

The general principles of therapy include bed rest, scrotal support, hydration, antipyretics, anti-inflammatories, and analgesics. Antibiotic therapy should be employed for acute epididymitis and is ideally based on culture and sensitivity testing, but may be based on microscopic or Gram stain result. For epididymitis associated with cystitis or prostatitis (usually epididymo-orchitis) oral trimethoprim-sulfamethoxazole (TMP-SMX), one double-strength tablet (160 mg TMP and 800 mg SMX [Bactrim DS]) twice daily for 3 to 4 weeks can be administered. Alternatively, an oral fluoroquinolone can be used; for example, ciprofloxacin (Cipro) 500 mg twice daily or levofloxacin (Levaquin) 500 mg once daily. For epididymitis associated with gonococcal urethritis, a single intramuscular dose of ceftriaxone (Rocephin) 250 mg, is indicated. Because *Chlamydia* is associated with gonococcal urethritis 30% to 50% of the time, a 2- to 3-week course of either oral tetracycline, 500 mg four times daily, or oral doxycycline (Vibramycin), 100 mg twice daily, should also be administered. Alternatively, the fluoroquinolones are effective against both *N. gonorrhea* and *C. trachomatis,* and either ciprofloxacin or oral levofloxacin[1] can be given for 2 to 3 weeks. If early testing is negative or results are unavailable, empiric treatment should be initiated and directed at the most likely pathogens based on the available clinical information and the patient's age. Usually a fluoroquinolone is the best agent in this particular scenario (except for young children). Surgical intervention is rarely indicated unless testicular torsion is suspected, abscess formation occurs in the epididymis, or there is a persistent epididymal mass after successful amelioration of symptoms. Such a mass should be evaluated with ultrasound and perhaps surgically removed (most epididymal tumors are benign).

Treatment for chronic epididymitis is supportive. A trial of antibiotic therapy appears to be justified (but no clinical evidence really exists to support this assumption). Anti-inflammatories, analgesics, support, heat therapies, and nerve blocks all have roles in ameliorating symptoms. It is generally believed that the condition is self-limited but could take years (and sometimes decades) to resolve. Epididymectomy is indicated in cases where pain control is refractory to all other measures. It should not be entertained lightly and only in those patients who have had the condition for at least 1 year, because this type of surgery is not always successful in alleviating the chronic pain.

Complications

The two major, early complications from acute epididymitis are abscess formation and testicular infarction. Long-term complications are usually related to the development of chronic epididymitis and include testicular atrophy, infertility, and chronic pain.

[1]Not FDA approved for this indication.

PRIMARY GLOMERULAR DISEASES

METHOD OF

Abhijit V. Kshirsagar, MD, MPH, and

Ronald J. Falk, MD

Glomerulonephritis refers to a disparate group of diseases characterized histologically by glomerular capillary inflammation and by varying degrees of mesangial cellular proliferation. The inflammatory changes lead to a breakdown of the selective permeability capabilities of the kidney. The loss of selective permeability becomes clinically apparent with the onset of proteinuria and hematuria. Loss of renal function may occur depending on the severity and exact location of the inflammatory changes. Glomerular diseases remain an important cause of renal insufficiency, and are the third leading cause of end-stage renal disease (ESRD) in the United States.

Glomerular diseases are often categorized by the presence of *nephritic* or *nephrotic* features (Table 1). Nephritic features include pronounced hematuria, with dysmorphic red blood cells and cellular casts, proteinuria (<3 g per 24 hours), and possibly renal insufficiency. Nephrotic features include pronounced proteinuria (>3 g per 24 hours), lipiduria, oval fat bodies, hypoalbuminemia, hypercholesterolemia, and possibly hematuria and renal insufficiency. Clinical abnormalities, such as hypercholesterolemia, hypoalbuminemia, sodium retention and edema, and hypercoagulability, result directly and indirectly from the glomerular leakage of protein (especially with the nephrotic syndrome). Many glomerular diseases have both nephritic and nephrotic features; this overlap often occurs in the presence of glomerular scarring.

Depending on whether they occur in the absence or presence of a systemic disease, glomerular diseases have also been characterized as either *primary* or *secondary* conditions, respectively. This categorization may be misleading. Most glomerulonephritides are the renal manifestation of a systemic disease. In cases such as lupus or diabetes mellitus, the systemic disease has been well characterized, whereas in other cases, the underlying systemic disease has yet to be determined. Thus, a survey for extrarenal manifestations in the workup of any potential glomerular disease is crucial.

TABLE 1 Tendencies of Glomerular Diseases to Manifest Nephritic or Nephrotic Features

	Nephritic Features	Nephrotic Features
Rapidly progressive glomerulonephritis	++++	+
IgA nephropathy	++++	+
Lupus nephritis	++++	+
Postinfectious glomerulonephritis	++++	+
Membranoproliferative glomerulonephritis	+++	++
Thin basement membrane disease	+++	++
Focal segmental glomerulosclerosis	++	+++
Light chain diseases	+	+++
Membranous nephropathy	+	++++
Diabetic nephropathy	+	++++
Minimal change disease	−	++++

Data from Jennette JC, Falk RJ: Glomerular clinicopathologic syndromes. In Greenburg A, Cheung AK, Falk RJ, Coffman TM, Jennette JC (eds): Primer on Kidney Disease, 3rd ed. London, Academic Press, 2001.

Differential Diagnosis and Diagnostic Strategy

Isolated hematuria or proteinuria, found during a routine clinic visit, may often be the first clue to a potential underlying glomerulopathy. The differential diagnosis of isolated hematuria is broad, and includes glomerular and nonglomerular conditions. Of the latter category, common causes include nephrolithiasis; renal cell cancer; cystitis; prostatitis; urethritis; urologic cancers; renal trauma; exercise hematuria; over-anticoagulation; polycystic kidney disease; renal tuberculosis (in endemic areas); and renal trauma. The differential diagnosis of isolated proteinuria is also broad, and includes postural proteinuria, exercise-induced, overflow (paraproteinemia), tubular, and glomerular sources. Quantification of urine protein excretion greater than 1 g per day (predominantly albumin) is most consistent with a glomerular source. The presence of hematuria and proteinuria together is highly suggestive of a glomerulonephritis. Table 2 lists some conditions that may mimic glomerular diseases.

Once the possibility of a glomerulopathy is considered, timely identification of the lesion is critical. The diagnostic evaluation (Table 3) begins during the first clinical encounter with a thorough history,

TABLE 2 Conditions That May Mimic Glomerular Diseases

Syndrome	Distinguishing Features
Hemolytic uremic syndrome	*Escherichia coli* exposure, diarrhea, thrombocytopenia
Thrombotic thrombocytopenic purpura	Fever, mental status changes, thrombocytopenia
Malignant hypertension	Severely elevated blood pressures, papilledema
Atheroembolic disease	Recent arterial manipulation, livedo reticularis
Interstitial nephritis	Exposure to offending drugs (penicillins, allopurinol, others)

TABLE 3 Suggested Diagnostic Evaluation for Individuals With a Suspected Glomerular Disease

History	Weight loss, fevers, rash, joint involvement, risk factors for exposure to viruses, sinus and upper respiratory infection, hemoptysis, gross hematuria, family history
Physical examination	Blood pressure, retinopathy, rashes/petechiae, tattoo, arthritis, synovitis, edema, lymphadenopathy, hepatomegaly, splenomegaly
Urinalysis	Dipstick hematuria and proteinuria Microscopic: red and white blood cells, casts, oval fat bodies
Laboratory tests	Serum creatinine, urine protein/creatinine C3, C4, ANA, ANCA, hepatitis B and C, cryoglobulins, streptozyme, serum and urine protein electrophoresis
Radiographic studies	Renal ultrasound, chest x-ray
Kidney biopsy	Light, immunofluorescence, electron microphotography

Abbreviations: ANA = antinuclear antibody; ANCA = antineutrophil cytoplasmic autoantibody.

physical examination, and urinalysis. Important information elicited from the history includes the following: the presence of a systemic disease or extrarenal manifestations of disease; family history of renal disease, including proteinuria/hematuria; exposures to environmental toxins or viral illness; and the presence (and duration) of renal insufficiency. The physical examinations helps to confirm suspicions raised by the history; key features of the examination include assessments of blood pressure, joints, skin, oronasopharynx, lymph nodes, abdominal organs, and eyes (retina). Because it is often difficult to perform a dilated funduscopic evaluation, a referral to an ophthalmologist is a suitable alternative. The urine dipstick gives qualitative information on the amounts of proteinuria and hematuria. Microscopic evaluation of a centrifuged urine sample may demonstrate nephrotic/nephritic sediment.

Diagnostic testing obtained after the clinical evaluation includes urine and serum chemistries, serologies, radiographic studies, and possibly a percutaneous kidney biopsy. Timed collection of urine for quantification of proteinuria and glomerular filtration rate may now be obviated by the use of a spot urine protein/creatinine ratio ($U_{P/C}$), and the Cockcroft-Gault or the modified Levey formula, respectively. An important caveat to the use of the $U_{P/C}$ is that it overestimates protein excretion for individuals who weigh much less than 70 kg, and underestimates protein excretion for individuals who weigh much more than 70 kg. Important serologies include complements (C3 or C4, rather than CH_{50}), and tests for systemic disease–antinuclear antibody (ANA), antineutrophil cytoplasmic autoantibody (ANCA), antibodies to hepatitis B and C, rapid plasma reagin (RPR), and serum and urine protein electrophoresis (SPEP and UPEP, respectively). Radiographic studies, such as a chest x-ray, may be necessary if a suspicion of a pulmonary–renal syndrome is raised. Renal ultrasound is not a routine test to workup a suspected glomerulonephritis. It is necessary only when there is a strong likelihood of performing a percutaneous biopsy.

By the end of the diagnostic evaluation, the clinician will have a reasonable estimation of how to classify the suspected glomerulonephritis. Yet classification schemes (see Table 1) are imperfect because of overlapping clinical presentations. The decision to make a referral to nephrology for percutaneous kidney biopsy may become necessary. The gold standard renal biopsy is performed with real-time ultrasound guidance. The tissue is examined under traditional light microscopy, as well as immunofluorescence and transmission electron microphotography. Severe complications of percutaneous biopsies, although quite rare (less than 1 in 2000 cases), include the possibility of nephrectomy and/or death.

Glomerular Diseases with Predominantly Nephritic Features

RAPIDLY PROGRESSIVE GLOMERULONEPHRITIS

The rapidly progressive glomerulonephritides (RPGN) are a group of serious conditions characterized by the rapid loss of renal function within days to weeks. The renal lesions demonstrate aggressive changes: diffuse cellular and mesangial expansion, karyorrhexis, and crescent formation (breakdown of Bowman's capsule). Conditions known to be associated with RPGN are generally divided into three categories: pauci-immune; antiglomerular basement membrane disease; and immune complex disease.

Pauci-Immune Glomerulonephritis

Pauci-immune glomerulonephritis is generally synonymous with small-vessel vasculitis associated with antineutrophil cytoplasmic autoantibodies (ANCA). It is the most common type of RPGN, accounting for approximately 50% of new cases. Disease may manifest primarily in the kidney (microscopic polyangiitis) or concomitantly in the kidney, upper respiratory tract, and lung (Wegener's granulomatosis). Histologically, pauci-immune glomerulonephritis is distinguished from the other types of RPGN by the absence (paucity) of immune complex deposition in the glomerulus.

Pauci-immune glomerulonephritis may affect individuals of all ages, but is most common in middle-age and older adults (i.e., older than age 50 years). It is equally distributed among men and women, and in the United States, the majority of individuals with this condition are white. The prognosis of these conditions is poor without rapid intervention.

The diagnosis of pauci-immune glomerulonephritis is aided by serum ANCA, a test to determine the presence of antibodies to neutrophil antigen. The old classification scheme of C-ANCA and P-ANCA has now been replaced by more specific terminology, PR3-ANCA (serine protease 3) and MPO-ANCA (myeloperoxidase), respectively. Eighty percent of individuals with Wegener's granulomatosis will have high-titer antibodies to PR3-ANCA, whereas 80% of individuals with microscopic polyangiitis will have high titer antibodies to MPO-ANCA. Most individuals also have other symptoms of systemic disease, such as fever, weight loss/malnutrition, and cutaneous rash, as well as localized symptoms (epistaxis, hemoptysis, sinus congestion).

Antiglomerular Basement Membrane Disease

Antiglomerular basement membrane (anti-GBM) disease accounts for approximately 20% of the cases of RPGN. The syndrome is defined by the presence of antibodies to the α_3 chain of type IV collagen. Disease may be limited to the kidney, termed *anti-GBM disease*, or it may involve the kidney and lung, called *Goodpasture's syndrome*. Pulmonary hemorrhage occurs frequently with lung involvement.

Anti-GBM syndrome typically occurs in two distinct age groups. Men younger than age 30 years tend to have both lung and kidney involvement. Women older than age 60 years typically present with renal-limited disease. Histologically, anti-GBM disease is distinguished from the other forms of RPGN by immunohistologic staining that reveals linear IgG along the basement membrane. The vast majority of cases are idiopathic. It has been reported to occur after lung infection and hydrocarbon exposure. It may also occur among individuals who genetically lack type IV collagen (Alport's syndrome) if they receive an unrelated kidney transplant.

High serum antibody titers to glomerular basement membrane help to confirm the diagnosis. Importantly, up to 40% of individuals with anti-GBM disease may also demonstrate ANCA antibodies. The presence of ANCA antibodies suggests a better response to immunosuppressive therapy. Without therapeutic intervention, the prognosis for antiglomerular basement membrane disease is dismal, with nearly all individuals experiencing ESRD or death.

Immune-Complex Glomerulonephritides

The immune-complex glomerulonephritides are a diverse group of conditions accounting for 30% to 40% of the cases of RPGN. They are often seen in the presence of a pre-existing glomerular disease; histopathology is an aggressive variation of the underlying glomerulonephritis. IgA nephropathy, lupus nephritis, membranoproliferative glomerulonephritis, and postinfectious glomerulonephritis all present as an immune-complex RPGN. Diagnostic testing depends on the underlying glomerular disease.

IgA NEPHROPATHY

Worldwide, IgA nephropathy is likely the most common type of nondiabetic glomerular disease. It has a higher predilection for men than women, and its prevalence is highest among Asians and whites. The pathogenesis is unknown. Histologically, IgA nephropathy is defined by the presence of glomerular IgA1 deposits seen on immunofluorescent staining. Light microscopic findings vary from mild mesangial proliferation to extensive crescent formation (much like the variation of its clinical presentation).

The clinical presentation of IgA nephropathy is highly variable. Individuals with IgA nephropathy will typically have persistent microscopic hematuria and proteinuria, with or without renal insufficiency. An important subset of individuals with IgA nephropathy have relapsing and remitting hematuria associated with mucosal stimulation (e.g., upper respiratory infections) termed synpharyngitic hematuria. Diagnosis is made by kidney biopsy. Screening serologies are typically negative. Serum IgA levels are not useful. Many other diseases are associated with IgA1 deposition in the glomeruli, including Henoch-Schönlein purpura; hepatobiliary disease; neoplasia of the lung, larynx, or pancreas; HIV infection; and dermatitis.

The prognosis, like the clinical presentation, is variable. Yet it is now evident that individuals with IgA nephropathy carry a 20% lifetime risk of developing ESRD. The presence of proteinuria, especially greater than 1 g per 24 hours, is a strong risk factor for the progression to ESRD, while a low serum creatinine, and low levels of urine protein excretion are associated with a better prognosis.

POSTINFECTIOUS GLOMERULONEPHRITIS

Postinfectious glomerulonephritis (PIGN) is often considered the prototypical glomerulopathy. It is linked most closely with nephritogenic strains of streptococci (*Streptococcus pyogenes*), although it can be triggered by other species of bacteria, as well as by protozoa and viruses. In the developed world, most potential infections of *S. pyogenes* are treated promptly with appropriate antibiotics. Consequently, occult infections with other bacterial species should be considered (e.g., acute endocarditis [*Staphylococcus aureus* or *Staphylococcus epidermidis*], subacute endocarditis [*Streptococcus viridans*]) in addition to other conditions, such as alcohol abuse and cirrhosis of the liver.

The exact mechanism of injury of postinfectious glomerulonephritis is not known. Histologically, the glomeruli have diffuse proliferative changes in the mesangium and endocapillary space. Immunofluorescent staining reveals extensive IgG and C3 deposition in the subendothelial space and mesangium. The vast majority of PIGN affects children between the ages of 2 and 10 years, yet approximately 10% of new cases develop among individuals older than age 40 years.

Individuals with PIGN typically present with hypertension and nephritic sediment. Renal insufficiency may be present, especially among adults. Important clues to the diagnosis of PIGN include a history of an upper respiratory infection or skin infection 1 to 12 weeks preceding the occurrence of the glomerulopathy. Serologies are notable for decreased complement levels, especially C3, with only slightly depressed or normal levels of C4. Antibodies to streptococcal antigens such as streptolysin O, streptozyme, and hyaluronidase, are elevated. Kidney biopsy confirms the diagnosis.

The prognosis is good for the majority of individuals with PIGN. Most have a spontaneous recovery, and thus, therapy is only recommended for symptoms. Hematuria normalizes by about 6 months. Subnephrotic levels of proteinuria may persist for years. Renal function returns to normal by about 4 weeks. Recent investigation has suggested a 0% to 20% incidence of chronic renal insufficiency; yet it is highly unlikely that this condition progresses to ESRD.

LUPUS NEPHRITIS

Systemic lupus is a common autoimmune disorder known to affect numerous organ systems. Renal involvement typically presents with renal insufficiency and nephritic sediment. Lupus nephritis affects females with a significantly greater frequency than men (9:1), and generally occurs among individuals between the ages of 20 and 40 years. Histologically, lupus nephritis is characterized by five distinct lesions (World Health Organization [WHO] Classes I to V). The grading of these lesions varies according to the extent of mesangial cellular proliferation and immune complex deposition (IgG, IgA, IgM, and complement).

The diagnosis of lupus nephritis is aided by the fact that it is usually associated with other features of systemic lupus, such as rash and/or arthritis. Serum complement levels, both C3 and C4, are typically depressed. Other helpful serologic tests include antibody titers to the nuclear antigen (ANA) and to the double-stranded DNA (dsDNA). The diagnosis is confirmed with a kidney biopsy.

MEMBRANOPROLIFERATIVE GLOMERULONEPHRITIS

Membranoproliferative glomerulonephritis (MPGN) is a relatively rare group of glomerular diseases that has experienced a recent resurgence because of the rise of infection with the hepatitis C (and B) virus. Two distinct subtypes, I and II, exist, as well as a third subtype (III) that shares features of types I and II. Type I disease may be idiopathic or associated with other conditions, including hepatitis B and C virus, cryoglobulins, complement deficiencies, and sickle cell disease. Histologically, light microscopy demonstrates mesangial matrix expansion and hypercellularity, as well as mesangial matrix insertion between the glomerular basement membrane and endothelium. This latter abnormality has been described as "tram-tracking." Immunofluorescence shows granular deposition of C3 in the mesangium and the peripheral capillary loops. Type II disease is considered idiopathic, and differs histologically by the deposition of dense, refractile immune-complex deposits in the glomerular capillary wall. These deposits have a distinctive ribbon-like appearance on light microscopy, while under transmission electron micrography, they have a strong electron-dense property (termed *dense deposit disease*).

Idiopathic type I MPGN typically affects young adults. Secondary forms can occur in any age group. Renal manifestations of viral infections typically occur after 10 to 15 years of infection, and are associated with mild abnormalities of the liver enzymes. Type II disease occurs in children and adolescents.

During the clinical evaluation, it is important to assess for risk factors for viral infections (intravenous drug use, multiple sexual partners, etc.). Serum complement levels are helpful in distinguishing between the two types of MPGN. Type I MPGN is associated with activation of the classical complement pathway, leading to a decrease in C4. Individuals with type II MPGN typically have low levels of C3 because of activation of the alternative complement pathway. Individuals with idiopathic MPGN have a 50% to 60% risk of developing ESRD within 10 to 15 years of diagnosis.

THIN BASEMENT MEMBRANE DISEASE

Thin basement membrane (TBM) disease is often synonymous with benign familial hematuria. As implied by this phrase, the condition is characterized by hematuria with low levels of proteinuria (typically less than 1.5 g per day), normal renal function, and no hypertension. Some authors suggest that thin basement membrane disease is highly prevalent and may affect 5% to 9% of the population. The primary defect in TBM disease is the decreased width of the basement membrane (150 to 225 μm in affected subjects vs. 300 to 400 μm in normal subjects). Clues to the diagnosis of TBM disease may be a family history of hematuria without renal failure. Diagnostic serologies are all negative. The diagnosis is made by kidney biopsy. Loss of renal function is rare, and if it occurs, is generally modest.

Glomerular Diseases with Predominantly Nephrotic Features

FOCAL SEGMENTAL GLOMERULOSCLEROSIS

Focal segmental glomerulosclerosis (FSGS) has been growing in frequency as a cause of nephrotic syndrome over the past decade, and has now surpassed membranous nephropathy as the most

TABLE 4 Summary of the Management of Glomerular Diseases

Condition	Helpful Serologic Tests	Therapy
Pauci-immune RPGN	PR3-ANCA, MPO-ANCA	Pulse and oral steroids, pulse cyclophosphamide (Cytoxan)[1] Plasmapheresis for pulmonary hemorrhage
Anti-GBM RPGN	Glomerular basement membrane antibodies	Pulse and oral steroids, oral cyclophosphamide Plasmapheresis
Immune-complex RPGN	ANA, dsDNA, $\downarrow$C3, $\downarrow$C4	Pulse and oral steroids
IgA nephropathy		Supportive care, possibly prednisone and fish oils[1]
Postinfectious	$\downarrow$C3, Streptolysin O	Supportive care
Lupus nephritis	ANA, dsDNA, $\downarrow$C3, $\downarrow$C4	Classes I and II: supportive care Classes III and IV: pulse and oral steroids, pulse cyclophosphamide[1], MMF (CellCept)[1] Class V: cyclosporine (Neoral)[1]
Membranoproliferative	Type I: hepatitis B/C, $\downarrow$C4 Type II: $\downarrow$C3	Antiviral agents[1] (hepatitis B and C) Possibly prednisone
Thin basement membrane		Supportive care
Focal segmental glomerulosclerosis	HIV	Possibly cyclosporine[1]
Light chain diseases	SPEP, UPEP	Variable—treatment of underlying condition
Minimal change disease	RPR	Oral steroids, cyclophosphamide[1] (rarely)
Membranous nephropathy		Oral cyclophosphamide[1], chlorambucil (Leukeran)[1] alternating with prednisone, possibly cyclosporine[1]
Diabetic nephropathy	HbA_{1C}	Insulin, oral hypoglycemics, biguanides, α-glucosidase inhibitors, thiazolidinediones

[1]Not FDA approved for this indication.

Abbreviations: ANA = antinuclear antibody; dsDNA = double-stranded deoxyribonucleic acid; GBM = glomerular basement membrane; HbA_{1C} = glycosylated hemoglobin; MMF = mycophenolate mofetil; MPO-ANCA = myeloperoxidase-antineutrophil cytoplasmic autoantibody; PR3-ANCA = serine protease 3-antineutrophil cytoplasmic autoantibody; RPGN = rapidly progressive glomerulonephritis; RPR = rapid plasma reagin; SPEP = serum protein electrophoresis; UPEP = urine protein electrophoresis.

common nondiabetic cause. FSGS is defined histologically by the presence of scarring (sclerosis) of parts (segmental) of some (focal) glomeruli. A particularly aggressive variant of FSGS, termed *collapsing*, is characterized by concomitant glomerular capillary collapse.

FSGS may be idiopathic or secondary to another comorbid condition. Important associations include infection with HIV, obstructive sleep apnea, obesity, renal agenesis, loss of nephron mass (i.e., surgical nephrectomy), chronic reflux nephropathy, and possibly intravenous drug use. Individuals with idiopathic FSGS typically present in the second and third decades of life. Most are men, and most are African American. The news media have highlighted several prominent cases among African-American professional athletes. Secondary causes may occur at any time in life, as it depends on the primary disease process.

Diagnosis is made by kidney biopsy. The clinical history, physical examination, and laboratory testing help to distinguish idiopathic from secondary forms of FSGS. The prognosis for idiopathic FSGS is progressive renal insufficiency and possibly ESRD.

LIGHT CHAIN-RELATED GLOMERULAR DISEASES

The light chain-related glomerular diseases include amyloidosis, light chain deposition disease, multiple myeloma, cyroglobinemia, fibrillary glomerulonephritis, and immunotactoid glomerulonephritis. Two other conditions, monoclonal gammopathy of undetermined significance (MGUS) and Waldenström's macroglobulinemia, may cause light chain proteinuria, but are not believed definitively to cause glomerular disease. The majority of all these conditions result from plasma cell dyscrasias, while a minority of conditions are associated with lymphoproliferative disease.

These conditions generally present among middle-age men and women, and do not have a strong racial predilection. Patients present with overflow proteinuria, typically greater than 3.5 g per 24 hours. This overflow proteinuria consists of light chains, rather than albumin, and is therefore not detected by the urine dipstick. Serum and urine protein electrophoresis are both sensitive screening tests for the determination of light chain proteinuria. The prognosis and treatment of these conditions are highly variable, and are beyond the scope of this review.

MEMBRANOUS NEPHROPATHY

Membranous nephropathy is the second most common cause of nondiabetic nephrotic syndrome in adults. The condition is so named because of the appearance of thickened basement membrane on light microscopy. Immunofluorescence reveals granular IgG staining of the basement membrane, and electron microscopy demonstrates electron-dense deposits in the subepithelial space.

Most cases of membranous nephropathy are idiopathic. Important associations are with malignancy (solid tumors), infection with hepatitis B, systemic lupus, nonsteroidal anti-inflammatory drugs, gold salts, and penicillamine. Idiopathic membranous nephropathy has a peak incidence in the middle-age years (older than age 40 years). Secondary causes vary by underlying disease. Diagnosis of membranous nephropathy is made by kidney biopsy. Serologies help to exclude other, secondary causes of the disease.

Left untreated, the natural course of membranous nephropathy is variable. About one third of individuals have spontaneous remission, one third have no change, and one third have progressive loss of renal function. Therapy is therefore directed at those individuals at risk for progressive disease. The presence of the following prognostic factors warrants therapy: male gender, age >50 years, proteinuria >10 g per day, and renal insufficiency.

MINIMAL CHANGE DISEASE

Also called nil disease, minimal change disease (MCD) is characterized by the lack of significant changes on light microscopy and immunohistologic staining. Electron microphotography reveals diffuse effacement of the podocyte foot process.

MCD is primarily a disorder of children, accounting for almost 90% of the cases of nephrotic syndrome in this age group. (In fact, kidney biopsy is often delayed.) It does occur in adults, accounting for up to 20% of cases. A small proportion of adults with MCD develop acute (reversible) renal failure. Most cases of MCD are idiopathic, although it is associated with hematologic malignancy, secondary syphilis, use of nonsteroid anti-inflammatory drugs, and possibly with the use of lithium.

Laboratory testing is not typically helpful in the diagnosis of idiopathic MCD, but may help to exclude other conditions. The diagnosis is made by kidney biopsy. Children typically undergo kidney biopsy only after failing an empiric course of steroids for presumed MCD.

Therapy

Supportive care is recommended for all individuals with glomerular disease. It includes reduction of blood pressure to levels less than 130/85 mm Hg, reduction of urine protein excretion, lipid management, and symptoms relief. Reduction of blood pressure is arguably the single most important therapeutic intervention available. While most antihypertensive agents are equally effective at lowering blood pressure, the angiotensin-converting enzyme inhibitors (ACE inhibitors), and likely the angiotensin II receptor blockers (ARBs) are more effective at lowering urine protein excretion than other classes of agents. Among individuals with sustained hypercholesterolemia, lipid-lowering therapy is strongly recommended to modify cardiovascular risk, and possibly to delay progressive renal insufficiency. Diuretics can be used to reduce edema, but overdiuresis may promote the formation of deep venous thrombosis. Reduction of protein intake has not been convincingly supported by trials in human subjects, and therefore is not routinely recommended as part of supportive care.

Corticosteroids, frequently used as "first-line" drugs in the management of glomerular diseases, act in part by inhibiting several proinflammatory pathways that lead to the activation of T and B cells. High-dose intravenous prednisolone (7 mg/kg per day, maximum daily dose 500 mg, "pulse-dose") followed by 3 to 6 months of oral prednisone (1 mg/kg per day, maximum daily dose 60 mg) is the cornerstone of therapy for RPGN, as well as for class III and class IV lupus nephritis. Oral prednisone is also a mainstay of therapy for MCD among children (1 mg/kg per day, maximum daily dose 60 mg, for 30 days, then tapered) and adults (1 mg/kg per day, maximum dose 60 mg for 8 to 16 weeks, then tapered). Response rates to steroids, as determined by reduction of proteinuria, are higher among children than adults for MCD (90% vs. 60%); furthermore, a significant proportion of adults have recurrence of MCD (30% to 50%), and are either resistant to or dependent on steroids. The efficacy of steroids has not been proven in other glomerular diseases, although some clinicians recommend their use in MPGN, membranous nephropathy, FSGS, and progressive IgA nephropathy.

Cyclophosphamide (Cytoxan)[1] and chlorambucil (Leukeran)[1] are mainstays of cytotoxic therapy. Both agents interfere with the normal function of DNA by alkylation and cross-linking the strands of DNA. Intravenous, monthly cyclophosphamide (0.75 to 1.25 g/m^2) is used to treat pauci-immune glomerulonephritis, as well as class III and class IV lupus nephritis. If patients experience a clinical response, cyclophosphamide may be extended for an additional 18 months, given at an interval of 3 months. Oral cyclophosphamide (2 mg/kg) is given for up to 1 year for individuals with anti-GBM disease; the dose should be adjusted to maintain a white blood cell count >3500 cell/mm^3. Plasmapheresis (one exchange every second day, each exchange consisting of 1 to 1.5 plasma volumes) should be initiated promptly with cytotoxic therapy in the setting of a RPGN with concomitant pulmonary hemorrhage for a total of three to six procedures. Oral cyclophosphamide (1.5 to 2.5 mg/kg per day, along with alternate-day oral prednisone 1 mg/kg per day), or chlorambucil (0.2 mg/kg per day for 28 days alternating with oral prednisone 0.4 mg/kg per day for 28 days) are also recommended for individuals with membranous nephropathy at high risk for progressive disease. Finally, oral cyclophosphamide is suggested for individuals with MCD that are resistant to corticosteroids.

The use of oral cyclosporine (Neoral)[1] in the management of glomerular diseases is growing.

[1]Not FDA approved for this indication.

Cyclosporine inhibits the production of interleukin-2, interleukin-3, and interferon-γ—cytokines necessary for normal T-lymphocyte helper/inducer and cytotoxic cell function. Oral cyclosporine (up to 3.5 mg/kg per day for 1 year) is an alternative therapy for individuals with idiopathic membranous nephropathy who are not tolerating cyclophosphamide or chlorambucil, and a primary therapy for individuals with membranous nephropathy associated with lupus (class V lupus nephritis). Oral cyclosporine (3.5 g/kg per day for 1 year) is also recommended for individuals with FSGS and baseline or progressive renal insufficiency.

Miscellaneous agents are also sometimes used. Mycophenolate mofetil (MMF, CellCept)[1], a potent, noncompetitive, and reversible inhibitor of the eukaryotic inosamine monophosphate dehydrogenase is used as primary therapy (2 g per day orally) for class III and class IV lupus nephritis and as maintenance therapy (1 g per day orally) for individuals with pauci-immune glomerulonephritis after the initial course of intravenous cyclophosphamide. Until recently, N-3 polyunsaturated fatty acids[1], provided in dietary fish oil supplements, were an often recommended therapy for IgA nephropathy because of their nonexistent toxicity. Current trials demonstrate neither a beneficial nor a harmful effect from fish oils.

[1]Not FDA approved for this indication.

PYELONEPHRITIS

METHOD OF

Nayef El-Daher, MD, PhD

Acute pyelonephritis is defined as the acute inflammatory process of the renal parenchyma, caused by microbial agents. Most commonly, it is caused by a bacterial infection from gram-negative organisms. This infection is more difficult to treat compared with a bladder infection, which is usually a superficial infection of the mucosa of the urinary bladder (cystitis).

Etiology

The most common organisms causing community-acquired acute pyelonephritis are gram-negative bacilli. *Escherichia coli* is the most common gram-negative organism causing acute pyelonephritis, accounting for more than 80% of all cases of acute pyelonephritis. Other gram-negative organisms include *Proteus*, *Klebsiella*, and *Pseudomonas* species. Among the gram-positive organisms causing acute pyelonephritis are the *Staphylococcus* species (*Staphylococcus aureus* and *Staphylococcus*-coagulase negative organisms) and enterococci, including vancomycin-resistant enterococci (VRE). The most common organisms causing acute pyelonephritis in hospitalized patients are the gram-negative organisms including *E. coli*, *Proteus*, *Klebsiella*, *Enterobacter*, and *Pseudomonas* species. Among the gram-positive organisms, staphylococci and enterococci are more often isolated. Anaerobic organisms are rarely a pathogen in urinary tract infections, in general. *Staphylococcus saprophyticus* tends to cause acute cystitis in young, sexually active females and rarely causes acute pyelonephritis.

Pathogenesis of Urinary Tract Infection

Urinary tract infections are caused as a result of an interaction between bacterial virulent factors and the host defense mechanisms. There are two possible routes by which bacteria can invade and spread within the urinary tract. The first one is the ascending route and the second is the hematogenous route.

ASCENDING ROUTE

The lower urinary tract (urethra) is usually colonized with bacteria, most commonly gram-negative rods. Any compromise on the host defense (either by instrumentation, obstruction, minor trauma) results in pushing the organism from the distal urethra into the bladder, causing a local inflammation of the superficial mucosa. Subsequently, this infection can be spread upward to involve the ureter and the renal parenchyma. The fact that urinary tract infections are far more common in females than in males supports this theory. The female urethra is shorter and wider compared with that of a male, making contamination more likely. It has been documented that an organism causing urinary tract infections in women colonized the vaginal introitus and the periurethral areas before causing a urinary tract infection. Colonization is usually achieved by adhesive properties of the organisms (adhesins). The adhesins of uropathogenic *E. coli* exist as either pili or as outer membrane proteins.

THE SECOND ROUTE

This is the hematogenous route. Hematogenous spread can cause acute pyelonephritis by seeding the renal parenchyma causing diffuse pyelonephritis with micro- or macro-abscesses. The most common organisms causing this type of acute pyelonephritis are almost always gram-positive (staphylococci and enterococci) as a complication of persistent bacteremia or endocarditis.

Epidemiology

Women are most frequently affected by urinary tract infections and acute pyelonephritis. Acute

TABLE 1 Complicating Factors in Urinary Tract Infection (Pyelonephritis)

Obstruction (foreign body, catheter, stone, etc.)
Urinary tract functional and structural abnormalities
Immunosuppression—"drug-induced," HIV, malignancy, renal transplant
Co-morbidity—diabetes mellitus, pregnancy, sickle cell anemia
Pyelonephritis caused by multi-drug resistance (MDR) organism (e.g., oxacillin-resistant *Staphylococcus aureus* [ORSA])
Others— Surgically created *ileal* loop, male sex

pyelonephritis can be uncomplicated or complicated. Uncomplicated pyelonephritis occurred in a young woman who lacked any evidence of structural, functional, or any co-morbidity *that increased* the risk of having a urinary tract infection (Table 1). Complicated pyelonephritis usually occurs as a result of acute pyelonephritis in an immunocompromised host or in the presence of multiple complicating factors (obstruction, immunosuppression, diabetes mellitus, pregnancy, sickle cell anemia, etc.).

Clinical Presentation

The classical clinical manifestation of a patient with acute pyelonephritis includes fever, chills, flank pain, and frequently lower urinary tract symptoms (e.g., frequency, urgency and painful micturition). A wide spectrum of illness is encountered in patients with acute pyelonephritis ranging from mild illness to severe life-threatening infection with sepsis and septic shock. This spectrum of presentation depends on multiple factors (bacterial and host factors). Only a minority of patients with acute pyelonephritis develop complications, such as intrarenal abscess and/or sepsis or septic shock. In general, a severe manifestation usually is associated with an immunocompromised status in patients with multiple co-morbidities infected by a multiple drug-resistant organism (MDR). Other less frequent symptoms usually include sweats, headache, nausea, vomiting, malaise, abdominal pain, generalized weakness, and dehydration.

Diagnosis

Preferred methods for urine collection include: midstream clean catch, catheterization, and suprapubic aspiration.

Urine analysis, culture, and sensitivity of the causative agents are the cornerstones for the diagnosis of acute pyelonephritis. It should be emphasized that the finding of pyuria is non-specific and a patient with pyuria may or may not have infection. However, the vast majority of symptomatic patients with acute pyelonephritis have pyuria. Microscopic hematuria is usually seen in acute urinary tract infection, mainly hemorrhagic cystitis, but is rarely seen in acute pyelonephritis. The presence of hematuria usually suggests the presence of calculi, tumor, vasculitis, and others. White cell casts in the presence of the acute infectious disease process usually provides strong evidence of acute pyelonephritis. One of the most useful parameters in urine analysis is the presence of bacteria (bacteriuria). The presence of significant bacteria ($>10^5$/mL) on unspun urine indicates the presence of urinary tract infection.

Urine and blood cultures should be considered in every patient presenting with clinical pictures suggestive of acute pyelonephritis. Urine and blood cultures preferably should be done before initiating any antibiotic treatment. Positive blood cultures in the proper clinical setting will confirm the diagnosis of acute pyelonephritis.

Management

Uncomplicated pyelonephritis usually responds to appropriate antibiotic treatment plus hydration in 24 to 48 hours. Usually the patient will experience defervescence and white cell count will normalize. For those patients, switching intravenous antibiotics to oral medication to be continued for 14 to 21 days is appropriate. Follow-up urine culture is not indicated routinely. Follow-up urine culture is required within 1 to 2 weeks of completion of therapy in a pregnant woman, in children, and in patients with recurrent, symptomatic pyelonephritis.

Patients who fail to respond to intravenous antibiotics and hydration (e.g., continue to have fever and repeated positive blood cultures), need further investigation to explore the possibility of complicating pyelonephritis. Those patients should have a computed tomography (CT) scan or perhaps an intravenous pyelography examination to exclude the possibility of urinary obstruction, or intrarenal or perinephric abscess formation. Quick intervention to correct any urinary obstruction is vital. Urology evaluation for possible removal of renal stone and/or tumor or relieving the pressure by an urgent urostomy is vital in the management of acute pyelonephritis. When intravenous antimicrobial therapy fails to treat a patient with acute pyelonephritis due to abscess formation, percutaneous drainage with culture and sensitivity should be tried. Selecting an antimicrobial agent or agents with good activity against the causative organisms with good renal tissue penetration is highly indicated under these circumstances (trimethoprim-sulfamethoxazole [Bactrim] and/or fluoroquinolones). Almost all renal abscesses of less than 5 cm in diameter could be treated medically with no surgical intervention. Renal abscesses of more than 5 cm in diameter need surgical drainage;

percutaneous drainage usually gives an excellent outcome. Nephrectomy is only indicated for treatment of severe life-threatening emphysematous pyelonephritis and in patients with diffuse severely damaged renal parenchyma.

Acute uncomplicated pyelonephritis (mild to moderate) responds well to oral antimicrobial agents. Oral antimicrobial agents currently recommended include trimethoprim-sulfamethoxazole (Bactrim), 800 to 160 mg twice a day, first-generation cephalosporins (Keflex), 500 mg four times a day, amoxicillin/clavulanate (Augmentin), 875 mg twice a day, and fluoroquinolones (e.g., ofloxacin [Floxin], 400 mg twice a day, and ciprofloxacin [Cipro], 500 mg twice a day).

In hospitalized patients with severe complicated pyelonephritis, parenteral therapy should be used. Empirical treatment includes a wide selection of antimicrobial agents: fluoroquinolones (Cipro 400 mg every 12 hours, Floxin 400 mg every 12 hours), third- and fourth-generation cephalosporins (ceftriaxone [Rocephin] 1 g every 24 hours, ceftazidime [Cefizox] 2 g every 8 hours, cefepime [Maxipime] 2 g every 12 hours), ampicillin-sulbactam combination (Unasyn), 3 g every 6 hours, ticarcillin/clavulanate combination, 3.1 g every 4 to 6 hours. All empirical antibiotic treatment should be changed or modified according to culture sensitivity and results. Parenteral antibiotics should be switched to an oral agent once a clinical response has occurred (patient is asymptomatic, white blood cells normalized, and no fever or chills).

TRAUMA TO THE GENITOURINARY TRACT

METHOD OF

Steven B. Brandes, MD

Roughly 10% of all traumas seen in the emergency department involve a urologic organ system. Early diagnosis of injury is essential in order to avoid potentially severe complications.

Kidney Trauma

INCIDENCE AND MECHANISM

The kidney is injured in up to 5% of all trauma cases. Mechanisms of kidney injuries are commonly 80% to 90% blunt and 10% to 20% penetrating. Children are more likely to sustain a blunt renal injury because of the relative large size of the kidney, scant perirenal fat, underdeveloped Gerota's fascia, and incomplete rib ossification. Penetrating kidney injuries are relatively uncommon, with only 7% to 10% of penetrating abdominal wounds involving the kidney. The majority of renal injuries are minor and heal spontaneously. Significant kidney injuries occur in only 4% of blunt, yet 67% of penetrating, renal injuries.

DIAGNOSIS

Signs and Symptoms

Hematuria is the hallmark of renal injury. However, the degree of hematuria often does not correspond or predict the extent of renal injury. Up to 40% of renal pedicle injuries have no hematuria. A history is obtained to quantify the forces involved in the renal injury, such as the vehicle speed and the height of the fall. Falls from height or high-speed motor vehicle accidents imply deceleration injury, and require renal pedicle and ureteropelvic junction (UPJ) evaluation. Patients with trauma to the flank, abdomen or lower chest, flank ecchymosis or tenderness, low posterior rib fractures, and lumbar transverse process fractures should be suspected of having a renal injury. Minor mechanisms of trauma that result in significant renal injury usually occur in a congenitally abnormal kidney.

For a gunshot wound (GSW) to the kidney, it is important to determine if injury is a result of a high- or low-velocity bullet, because a high-velocity bullet usually causes extensive kidney injury and delayed necrosis. The entrance and exit wound sites should be noted. Stab wound (SW) entrance sites posterior to the anterior axillary line (AAL) and below the nipple line are less likely to have associated intraperitoneal organ injury or warrant exploration.

Imaging

Indications for imaging a suspected kidney injury are (a) blunt trauma and gross hematuria; (b) blunt trauma, microscopic hematuria (>5 red blood cells [RBCs]/high-power field [HPF]), and shock (systolic blood pressure <90 mm Hg); (c) major acceleration or deceleration injury; (d) microscopic or gross hematuria after penetrating flank, back, or abdominal trauma, or when the bullet path, as evidenced by entrance and exit sites, is in line with the kidney; (e) pediatric trauma patient with any degree of hematuria; and (f) associated injuries/physical signs suggesting underlying renal injury.

Intravenous urography (IVU) for stable trauma patients, has generally been replaced by abdominal computed tomography (CT) when evaluating for a potential kidney injury. In unstable patients who require celiotomy, however, a one-shot IVU is performed prior to any retroperitoneal hematoma/renal exploration. Intravenous contrast, at 2 mL/kg of body weight, is generally given, followed by a single abdominal radiograph. The one-shot IVU is performed to determine the function of the contralateral kidney, to avoid removing the injured kidney of a solitary kidney patient. Failure to visualize an enhancing kidney or enhancement of only a segment of the kidney suggests significant renal parenchymal or pedicle injury. *Computed tomography* is the imaging study of choice for demonstrating renal parenchymal injury, perirenal/retroperitoneal hematomas, urinary extravasation, injuries to the renal hilum and great vessels, and associated intra-abdominal organ injuries. Renal artery occlusion and renal infarct are noted by lack of parenchymal enhancement or by a "cortical rim sign." *Ultrasonography* (US) is primarily used in Europe for evaluating renal trauma, but is of limited value. US can be useful for demonstrating perirenal fluid collections, but cannot distinguish fresh blood from extravasated urine. *Arteriography* and superselective embolization have important roles in the evaluation and treatment of post-traumatic delayed renal bleeding or arteriovenous fistulas. In recent anecdotal reports, arteriography and endoluminal stent placement have been successful in managing renal artery intimal tears from blunt trauma.

MANAGEMENT

To select nonoperative management, the renal injury needs to be imaged and accurately staged. An incompletely staged renal injury requires surgical exploration. Not all penetrating renal injuries require surgical exploration. Roughly three of four renal gunshot wounds, one of two renal stab wounds, and only 2% of blunt renal injuries demand exploration. Conservative management of renal injuries includes strict bed rest until the urine visibly clears; frequent hematocrit blood draws; transfusions; persistent bleeding demands repeat imaging, arteriography or surgical exploration; and for injuries with urine extravasation, re-image after 3 to 5 days to assess for persistent urinary leak.

SURGERY

Indications for Exploration

Absolute

Persistent and potentially life-threatening renal bleeding is an absolute indication for surgery. Signs of continued renal bleeding are a pulsatile, expanding, or unconfined retroperitoneal hematoma, as well as avulsion of the main renal artery or vein or a massively shattered kidney.

Relative Indications

1. Devitalized renal parenchyma >25%
2. Urinary extravasation in itself does not demand surgical exploration. The majority resolve spontaneously (usually within 72 hours). UPJ avulsion injuries, however, do not heal spontaneously and are best managed by prompt surgical repair.
3. Incomplete staging demands either further imaging or renal exploration.
4. In patients with two normal kidneys, isolated renal artery thrombosis that is not associated with extensive bleeding or urinary extravasation is best managed conservatively, because revascularization rarely preserves significant renal function. Revascularization should be used only for bilateral renal artery occlusion or unilateral occlusion in a solitary kidney.
5. When celiotomy is performed for associated intra-abdominal injuries, it is reasonable to also repair all staged high-grade renal injuries. This should be attempted only by an experienced urologic surgeon; otherwise, poorly controlled bleeding and renal loss may result.
6. High-grade, penetrating renal injuries, particularly from SW, generally should be managed surgically because of the high rate of delayed bleeding.

Technique

The injured kidney is best exposed through a midline transperitoneal incision. Classic teaching dictates that proximal vascular control take place before renal exploration and potential release of the tamponade effect. When consistent proximal vascular control of the renal pedicle is performed, the nephrectomy rate for all renal traumas is low (<15%). Briefly, repair of the damaged kidney requires broad exposure of the kidney and injured area, temporary vascular occlusion for brisk renal bleeding, sharp excision of all nonviable parenchyma, meticulous hemostasis, watertight closure of the collecting system, parenchymal defect closure over collagen or foam bolsters, or coverage with omentum, peritoneum, polyglycolic acid mesh, and or fibrin sealant.

Complications

Complications after renal trauma are most commonly prolonged urinary extravasation, delayed bleeding, arteriovenous fistula, abscess, urinary fistula, and hydronephrosis. Renal vascular hypertension after renal trauma is commonly transient.

Ureter and Renal Pelvis Trauma

MECHANISM

External Trauma

Penetrating ureteral injuries are rare. Mechanism of ureteral injuries are 95% penetrating and 5% blunt. GSW in proximity to the ureter can cause severe ureteral contusion as a consequence of the blast effect. After a deceleration injury, the kidney is often dislocated, and tears typically occur at the UPJ and hilar vasculature. Another mechanism for injury is hyperextension of the back, where the ureter is avulsed, stretched by the lumbar and lower thoracic vertebral bodies. This classically occurs in limber children.

Surgical Trauma

Ureteral injuries usually occur during difficult and/or bloody pelvic operations. Overall, the ureter is injured in only 0.5% to 1.0% of pelvic operations. Iatrogenic ureteral injury most commonly occurs during hysterectomy (especially with the transabdominal approach). Injuries can also occur during urologic, colorectal, and vascular surgeries.

DIAGNOSIS

Successful surgical management of collecting system injuries requires a high index of suspicion, early diagnosis (and thus a low threshold for urinary tract imaging), and an intimate knowledge of ureteral anatomy and blood supply. Hematuria (gross or microscopic) is not a reliable sign and is absent in up to 45% of penetrating and 67% of blunt ureteral injuries. Ureteral injuries are morbid and potentially lethal when unrecognized, and present in a delayed fashion.

Imaging

IVU ability to diagnose a ureteral injury is very variable and thus considered unreliable. Retrograde pyelography (RPG), although accurate in demonstrating presence and location of extravasation, is both time-consuming and cumbersome. RPG has little role in the acute trauma setting. CT has been used with increasing frequency to evaluate ureteral trauma. Medial perirenal extravasation of contrast is the most common finding of renal pelvic/blunt ureteral injury.

The majority of penetrating ureteral injuries, however, are diagnosed intraoperatively. Direct exploration is the most accurate method for diagnosis. Intravenous or retrograde injection of indigotin disulfate sodium (Indigo Carmine) is also helpful in identifying ureteral injury by extravasation of blue dye from the injury site. Ureter injuries are classified by the location of the injury, mechanism, and manner of injury.

Management

General considerations are the patient's overall physical condition, presence of associated injuries, any delay in diagnosis, and the level and full extent of ureteral injury. Promptly diagnosed ureteral injuries, should be explored and surgically reconstructed. Ureteral contusions or bruising because of potential proximity blast injury should be stented and drained. With severe contusions, the ureter should be segmentally resected, débrided, reanastomosed, tension-free over a stent, isolated from associated injuries, and drained.

Distal ureteral injuries (below the iliac vessels) are typically managed by ureteroneocystostomy. With greater distal ureteral loss, a psoas hitch to the ipsilateral psoas minor tendon will usually bridge the gap. A transureteroureterostomy (TUU) is particularly useful when there are associated rectal, pelvic vascular, or extensive bladder injuries. There are multiple relative contraindications to TUU. Ileal interposition, Boari flap, renal displacement, and autotransplantation are best reserved for delayed reconstructive settings. The majority of mid-ureteral injuries can be repaired by primary ureteroureterostomy (UU). In select cases, TUU may also be an option. Injuries to the upper third of the ureter are best repaired by UU. Avulsion of the UPJ is the most common blunt ureteral injury seen, and occurs primarily in children. UPJ lacerations can often be successfully managed expectantly, while avulsion usually demands surgical repair.

When the patient is too unstable to undergo lengthy ureteral reconstruction, a "damage control" approach of temporary cutaneous ureterostomy, or ureteral ligation, followed by percutaneous nephrostomy should be performed. Definitive reconstruction is delayed until the patient has stabilized.

Complications

Delayed recognition of ureteral injuries is common. Delay often results in significant morbidity, including sepsis, abscess, hydronephrosis, loss of renal function, ureteral stricture, fistula, and urinoma.

Bladder Trauma

The majority of bladder injuries are caused by blunt abdominal trauma from motor vehicle accidents and crush injuries. Roughly 90% are associated with pelvic fractures, while 9% to 16% of pelvic fractures have a ruptured bladder. The minority is caused by penetrating trauma. Bladder ruptures are roughly 60% extraperitoneal and 30% intraperitoneal, with the remaining 10% being combined injuries.

MECHANISMS OF INJURY

Intraperitoneal bladder rupture occurs by severe blunt lower abdominal or pelvic trauma to a distended or full bladder. Ruptures are commonly at the dome. Empty bladders are seldom injured. High mortality is a consequence of associated injuries. Extraperitoneal bladder injuries are nearly always associated with pelvic fracture. Injuries are primarily caused by shearing forces, and to a lesser degree by perforation by bony spicules.

SIGNS AND SYMPTOMS

Ninety-five percent of bladder ruptures have gross hematuria, and the remaining 5% have microhematuria. Penetrating bladder injuries have roughly one half microscopic and one half gross hematuria. Symptoms of injury are pelvic or lower abdominal pain and an inability to urinate. Signs of bladder rupture are suprapubic tenderness, low urine output, and gross hematuria. Intraperitoneal bladder rupture that are diagnosed late often present with azotemia, acidosis, hypernatremia, hyperkalemia, and elevated serum urea nitrogen (BUN). Women need a careful pelvic examination for possible vaginal or urethral tears.

IMAGING

Cystography is performed by gravity filling of the bladder with dilute contrast, via a Foley catheter, to at least 300 mL or until extravasation. Postdrainage films are essential, so as not to miss 10% to 15% of injuries. Cystographic injury types include bladder contusion, interstitial rupture, intraperitoneal rupture (contrast outlines loops of bowel or fills cul-de-sac), extraperitoneal rupture (flame-like or star-burst contrast extravasation), or "tear-drop" shaped bladder, because of a pelvic hematoma. *CT cystography* is as accurate as conventional cystography, as long as the bladder is retrograde filled to at least 300 mL or until extravasation.

MANAGEMENT

Figure 1 details the overall evaluation and management of lower urinary tract trauma. For intraperitoneal injuries and all penetrating bladder injuries, each missile tract is explored, debris and devitalized tissue débrided, and injuries closed. After formal bladder repair, the urine is diverted by large-bore Foley catheter and/or suprapubic tube. Blunt extraperitoneal bladder injuries or interstitial ruptures can be successfully managed by catheter drainage. When the abdomen is explored for associated injuries, extraperitoneal bladder ruptures should be repaired. The bladder should be exposed through a midline abdominal incision and the bladder opened at the dome to avoid the pelvic hematoma. Opening the pelvic hematoma may cause bacterial contamination and release the tamponade effect. The bladder neck and ureteral orifices also need inspection for possible injury.

Urethra Trauma

Urethral injuries are relatively uncommon and are usually divided into anterior or posterior injuries. Posterior urethral injuries are caused by pelvic

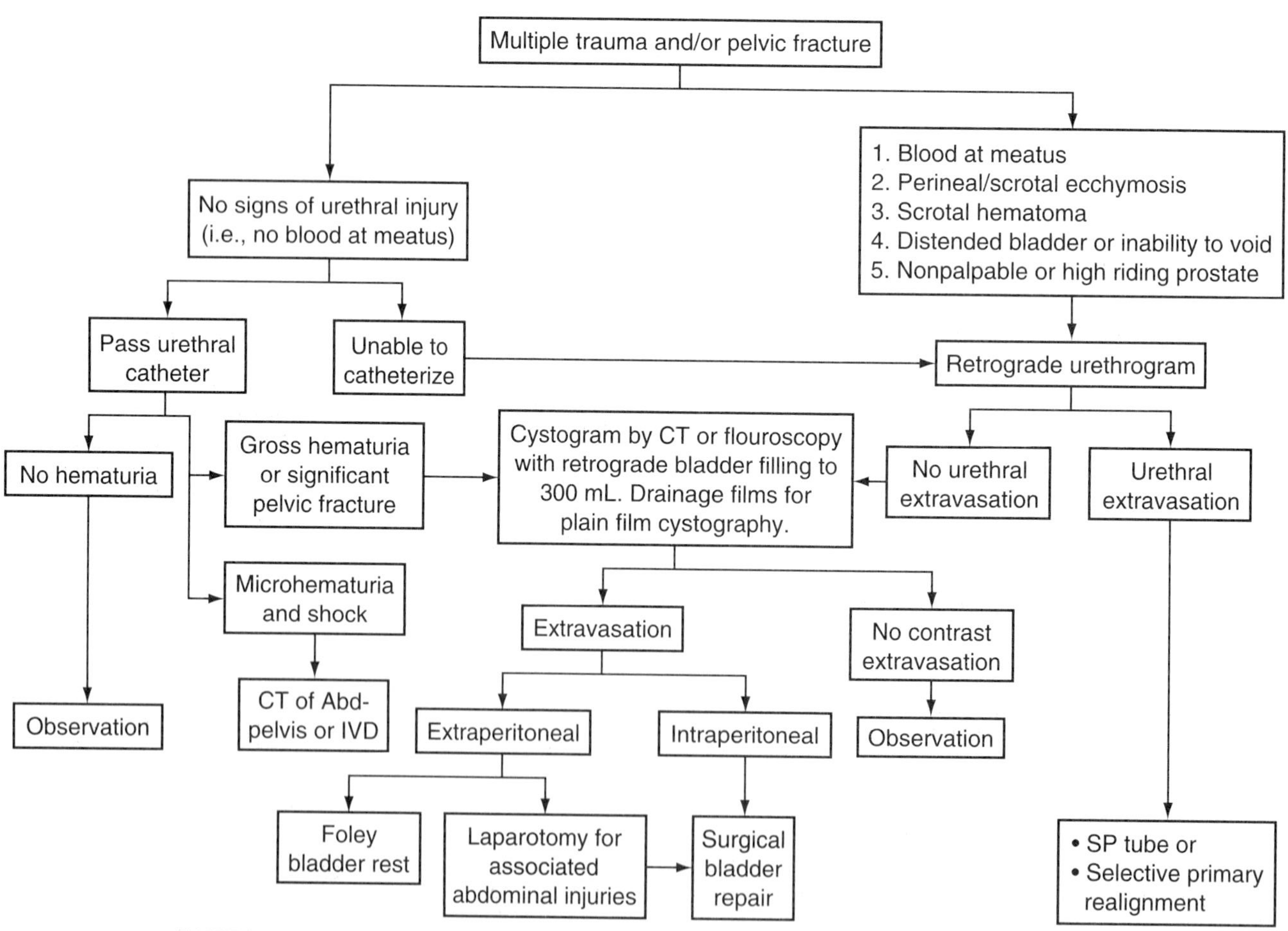

FIGURE 1 Algorithm for multiple trauma and/or pelvic fracture. Abd, abdomen; CT, computed tomography; IVU, intravenous urography; SP, suprapubic.

fracture and anterior urethral injuries to straddle injury. Penetrating injuries are usually caused by a GSW to the anterior urethra. The management goal for urethral injuries is to minimize the chances for the debilitating complications of incontinence, impotence, and urethral stricture.

POSTERIOR URETHRAL INJURIES

The posterior urethra is injured in 3.5% to 15% of pelvic fractures. Of urethral injuries, 73% are complete and 27% are partial transections.

Mechanism

Urethral injuries are mainly the result of shearing forces between a fixed prostate and a mobile bladder, resulting in bladder neck injury, and between a fixed membranous urethra and a mobile bulbar urethra, resulting in membranous urethral injury. In contrast to men, injuries to the female urethra and bladder neck are usually caused by bony fragments.

Signs and Symptoms

When a urethral injury is suspected, avoid catheterization so as not to convert a partial into a complete urethral injury, and to avoid infecting the pelvic hematoma. In the male conscious patient, an inability to pass a catheter is often a result of a contracted external sphincter. With prostatomembranous disruption, the prostate usually feels displaced or nonpalpable. Signs of urethral injury are blood at the meatus (98% sensitive), gross hematuria, perineal ecchymosis/hematoma, scrotal or penile hematoma, difficulty passing a Foley catheter, distended bladder and inability to void, or high-riding prostate. Female urethral injury is suspect when a pelvic fracture presents with vaginal bleeding and laceration, hematuria, labial swelling, or inability to void.

Imaging

On pelvic film, urethral injury is suggested by pelvic ring disruption, and often associated with bilateral pubic rami fractures or vertical shear fractures. Retrograde urethrography (RUG) is the procedure of choice to evaluate for urethral injury. Contrast medium is instilled in small volumes (20 to 30 mL), ideally under fluoroscopy. Grades of injury are determined by retrograde urethrography. The urogenital diaphragm separates the pelvis from the perineum and is the most important landmark.

Management

Management goals for urethral injuries are preserving continence and potency, and avoiding the pelvic hematoma. Despite previous controversy, it is generally felt that the complications of impotence and incontinence result from the initial injury itself and not the management method. The most accepted treatment method is suprapubic tube urinary diversion, followed by delayed urethrotomy or urethroplasty. Primary realignment, however, is a popular management option. If the patient is stable, realignment is performed at the time of injury, and when unstable, delayed a few days. Incomplete lacerations usually heal spontaneously. Male children are typically more susceptible than male adults to bladder neck injuries.

ANTERIOR URETHRAL INJURIES

Blunt anterior urethral injuries are caused by direct injuries to the penis and urethra, have few associated injuries, and have relatively low morbidity rates. Penetrating urethral injuries occur in 18% to 57% of GSWs to the penis and in one half of perineal GSWs.

Signs and Symptoms

Signs of potential anterior urethral injury are history of direct perineal trauma or straddle injury, penetrating wounds to the penis or perineum (i.e., GSW), blood at the meatus (the most important predictor), perineal and/or scrotal swelling/ecchymosis or tenderness (i.e., classic "butterfly sign" hematoma), penile "sleeve-like" hematoma, and inability to void.

Management

Incomplete blunt lacerations are successfully managed with proximal urinary diversion for 2 to 3 weeks. Complete blunt lacerations have a high stricture rate, usually requiring a delayed open surgical repair. For stab wounds and low-velocity GSWs, treatment is primary repair with primary anastomotic urethroplasty. When the urethral injury defect is extensive, the urethra should be marsupialized, the urine diverted, and reconstruction delayed.

Complications

Delay in diagnosis or treatment predisposes the genitalia to abscess formation, sepsis, and fasciitis. Long-term complications are urethral stricture, penile curvature, penile foreshortening, erectile dysfunction, and urinary incontinence.

SUGGESTED READINGS

Bladder

Carroll PR, McAninch JW: Bladder trauma: mechanisms of injury and a unified method of diagnosis and repair. J Urol 132: 254, 1984.

Corriere JN Jr, Sandler CM: Management of the ruptured bladder: 7 years experience with 111 cases. J Trauma 26:830, 1986.

Kidney

Brandes SB, McAninch JW: Reconstructive surgery of the injured upper urinary tract. Urol Clin North Am, 26:183, 1999.

Carroll PR, Klosterman P, McAninch JW: Early vascular control for renal trauma: A critical review. J Urol 141:826, 1989.
Eastman JA, Wilson TG, Ahlering TE: Urological evaluation and management of renal-proximity stab wounds. J Urol 150:1771, 1993.
Haaas CA, Dinchman KH, Nasrallah PF, Spirnak JP: Traumatic renal artery occlusion: A 15-year review. J Trauma 45:557, 1998.

Ureter

Boone TB, Gilling PJ, Husman DA: Ureteropelvic junction disruption following blunt abdominal trauma. J Urol 150:33, 1993.
Brandes SB, Chelsky MJ, Buckman RF, Hanno PM: Ureteral injuries from penetrating trauma. J Trauma 36:766, 1994.
Presti JC, Carroll PR, McAninch JW: Ureteral and renal pelvic injuries from external trauma: Diagnosis and management. J Trauma 29:370, 1989.

Urethra

Colapinto V, McCollum RW: Injury to the male posterior urethra in fractured pelvis: A new classification. J Urol 118:575, 1977.
Webster GD, Mathes GL, Selli C: Prostatomembranous urethral injuries: A review of the literature and a rational approach to their management. J Urol 130:898, 1983.

PROSTATITIS

METHOD OF

Michel A. Pontari, MD

Prostatitis is one of the most commonly seen urologic conditions in both primary care and urology offices. It is estimated that this problem accounts for up to 2 million visits per year to physicians in the United States. The term *prostatitis* refers to a wide array of clinical syndromes, from true bacterial infection, to symptoms of chronic pelvic pain with no identifiable infection, as well as to histologic evidence of prostatic inflammation in the absence of symptoms. This diversity is reflected in the National Institutes of Health (NIH) classification of prostatitis (Table 1).

Category I: Acute Bacterial Prostatitis

Acute prostatitis is characterized by the sudden onset of fever and dysuria. This represents a true acute infection of the prostate, caused by bacteria including *Escherichia coli*, *Klebsiella*, *Enterobacter*, and *Pseudomonas*. Voiding symptoms in addition to the burning with urination can include frequency, urgency, and hesitancy. On physical examination, one should palpate the prostate, but caution should be used to avoid vigorous massage or repeat examinations, which could theoretically produce bacteremia and precipitate urosepsis. The postvoid residual urine should be measured, preferably by ultrasound, to avoid catheterization. Laboratory studies should include both urine and blood cultures, and a white blood cell count.

TABLE 1 NIH Classification of Prostatitis

Category I	Acute bacterial prostatitis
Category II	Chronic bacterial prostatitis
Category III	Chronic pelvic pain syndrome
Category IIIA	Inflammatory
Category IIIB	Non-inflammatory
Category IV	Asymptomatic inflammatory prostatitis

TREATMENT

Patients are generally admitted to the hospital because they are usually acutely ill on presentation. Intravenous (IV) fluids are started as well as IV antibiotics. Traditionally, an aminoglycoside and ampicillin are started. An IV fluoroquinolone is also acceptable. If the patient has a significantly elevated postvoid residual, a suprapubic tube is recommended to avoid a urethral catheter that could exacerbate the infection. If the patient is in retention, I will start an α-blocker[1] to help with urination once the inflammation subsides. I will also use nonsteroidal anti-inflammatory agents to reduce prostate inflammation and help with discomfort. IV antibiotics are continued until the patient is afebrile for 24 hours, or as per indicated by the blood culture results. Oral antibiotic therapy is then started as per the culture and sensitivity and continued for 4 weeks to try to prevent bacterial colonization and chronic bacterial prostatitis. Usually fluoroquinolones are used as the oral agent. If a patient has persistent symptoms and fever, a computed tomography (CT) scan should be performed to rule out a prostatic abscess. If an abscess is present, this should be drained transurethrally.

Category II: Chronic Bacterial Prostatitis

Chronic bacterial prostatitis is characterized by relapsing episodes of urinary tract infections, usually with the same organism seen on urine cultures. These patients are usually asymptomatic between infections. True chronic bacterial prostatitis is relatively uncommon. The presentation is that of a urinary tract infection, with dysuria, frequency, and low back pain. They usually do not have the temperature elevation or toxic appearance of patients with acute bacterial prostatitis. Evaluation includes prostate examination, determination of postvoid residual urine, and a urine culture. If the patient has multiple recurrent infections, I obtain an ultrasound of the kidneys and perform cystoscopy to rule out other causes of recurrent urinary tract infection (UTI) in the male.

[1]Not FDA approved for this indication.

Treatment

Antibiotics are prescribed based on the result of the urine culture. While waiting for the results of the culture, I generally start empiric therapy with either sulfa-based antibiotics or a fluoroquinolone. Treatment should be for 2 to 4 weeks. For cases of more frequent repeat episodes in the absence of an anatomic cause, such as urinary retention, prophylaxis with daily antibiotics can be used for 3 to 6 months.

Category III: Chronic Prostatitis/Chronic Pelvic Pain Syndrome

Patients with category III or chronic prostatitis/chronic pelvic pain syndrome (CP/CPPS) have chronic pelvic pain that can be relapsing and remitting. Sites of discomfort include the penis, suprapubic area, testes, and perineum, as well as dysuria and pain after ejaculation. The name *chronic pelvic pain* indicates that not all discomfort in these men comes from the prostate, and may include the bladder, rectum, penis, or even central nervous system (CNS) as sources of discomfort. Associated systemic symptoms such as fatigue are common, as is erectile dysfunction. Category IIIa is inflammatory CPPS with white blood cells present in either semen, expressed prostatic secretions (EPS), or post-prostate massage urine (VB3). Category IIIb includes individuals without white blood cells in any of these fluids. Clinically, there are no significant differences between categories IIIa and IIIb, therefore it is not necessary to measure white blood cells in these specimens. It is important, however, to obtain a midstream urine culture to rule out a UTI as the source of pelvic pain. Fractionated cultures of VB1 (first 10 mL), VB3, and EPS are not indicated because recent studies show that asymptomatic men have as many localizing bacteria in the prostate as do men with CPPS.

The main tenet of evaluation of men with CPPS is to identify treatable causes of pelvic pain. Unfortunately, in the vast majority of men a clear cause will not be found. In addition to an urine culture, the evaluation should include a thorough history and physical examination. An assessment of symptoms is facilitated by using the NIH-Chronic Prostatitis Symptom Index (NIH-CPSI), a self-administered, validated symptom index. Originally designed as an outcome measure for use in treatment trials, it also is very useful for symptom assessment in the office, and also is now available in Spanish translation. The history should also include history of infections, trauma, or any neurologic disease, including vertebral disc problems. On physical examination, it is important to look for extraprostatic causes of pain, including penile lesions, testicular masses, and perirectal processes. In addition to a urine culture, a urinalysis looking for hematuria is mandatory. Men with irritative voiding symptoms should have a urine cytology sent to rule out carcinoma in situ of the bladder. Another recommended investigation is determination of postvoid residual urine. This is especially important in men over the age of 50, given the greater risk of retention from benign prostatic hypertrophy (BPH) than in younger men with CP/CPPS. Imaging studies should be determined by specific findings, such as looking for midline cysts in men with pain on ejaculation. CT scan should be considered in patients who present with concomitant abdominal pain in addition to the pelvic pain. Urodynamics may be helpful in men with voiding symptoms or elevated residual. Prostate-specific antigen (PSA) is not a part of the standard evaluation of men with CPPS, and an elevated PSA should not a priori be ascribed to prostate inflammation, but should be further evaluated for the possibility of prostate cancer as in any asymptomatic man.

TREATMENT

Men with chronic pelvic pain and symptoms similar to those of a prostate infection are treated with one initial 4-week course of antibiotics, even with a negative urine culture. If they respond, antibiotics are continued for another 2 to 4 weeks. Repeated courses of antibiotics after this initial treatment are not used unless there is a positive urine culture. Second-line therapies in men with persistent symptoms include α-adrenergic blockers[1] and nonsteroidal anti-inflammatory medications. For men with persistent pain, tricyclic antidepressants[1] can be beneficial because of their effect on neuropathic pain. Other pain medications include antiseizure medications[1], and newer non-narcotic analgesics. Urinary frequency and irritative symptoms may be helped by anticholinergic agents and medications used to treat interstitial cystitis such as antihistamines[1] and synthetic heparinoids (Pentosan, Elmiron). Pelvic floor physical therapy may be helpful. For refractory cases, sacral neuromodulation is an option. Surgery on the prostate either transurethrally or to remove the prostate is not recommended.

Category IV: Asymptomatic Inflammatory Prostatitis

Prostatic inflammation is found on many prostate biopsies and specimens from transurethral resections. Patients with asymptomatic histologic prostate inflammation require no further evaluation or specific treatment.

[1]Not FDA approved for this indication.

BENIGN PROSTATIC HYPERPLASIA

METHOD OF

Phuong N. Huynh, MD, MPH, and

Ananias C. Diokno, MD

Epidemiology

Lower urinary tract symptoms (LUTS) suggestive of benign prostatic hyperplasia (BPH) become prevalent in males older than 40 years of age, with 25% experiencing moderate to severe symptoms. The prevalence of these symptoms increases linearly with age, affecting nearly all men who reach average life expectancy. Evidence of BPH is apparent in approximately 50% of men who are 50 years of age and 90% among men 90 years of age. The lifetime incidence of medical or surgical intervention is estimated to be 35% for a 50-year-old male with BPH.

The mechanisms of BPH appear to be multifactorial, and the risk factors for BPH are poorly understood. In addition, strong evidence exists showing a genetic disposition for the development of BPH, while other studies note racial differences in BPH prevalences. Although major complications from BPH are uncommon, LUTS can have a significant impact on the patient's quality of life (QOL).

Pathophysiology

The glandular (stromal and epithelial) portion of the prostate comprises three zones: peripheral (70%), central (20% to 25%), and transitional (5% to 10%), the site of origin of clinical BPH. The nonglandular (fibromuscular) portion comprises the remaining one third of the prostate. Free testosterone is metabolized by the 5α-reductase enzymatic system in prostatic cells to 5α-dihydrotestosterone (DHT), the principal active androgen that binds to androgen receptors (AR). Estrogens are metabolized through peripheral aromatization. Estrogen receptors are found mostly in the stroma, while ARs are found in both epithelial and stromal tissues. Males >50 years of age face a decline in free-testosterone–to–free-estrogen ratio. Estrogens are believed to cause induction of ARs, thereby sensitizing the prostate to free testosterone.

The hyperplastic process is a consequence of an increased number of stromal and epithelial cells. The stroma comprises both collagen and smooth muscles, which are innervated primarily by adrenergic receptors, specifically α_1-adrenoreceptors. Importantly, specific blockade of the isozyme α_{1A}-adrenoreceptors found in the prostatic capsule, adenoma, and bladder neck reduces the dynamic prostatic urethral tone. The static component of outlet obstruction in BPH is caused by hyperplastic tissue overgrowth and subsequent narrowing of the urethral lumen. After conversion by 5α-reductase, specifically the isozyme type 2 in stromal cells, DHT acts in autocrine and paracrine pathways on neighboring epithelial cells, stimulating growth factors and the excretion of expressed proteins. There is strong evidence that the main stromal inhibitory regulation of epithelial proliferation may be defective in BPH. These two enzymatic pathways are the targets of pharmaceutical intervention. Untreated bladder outlet obstruction potentially leads to detrusor hypertrophy, trabeculation, diverticular formation, and eventual detrusor decompensation. Complications of urinary retention include recurrent urinary tract infections, bladder calculi, hematuria, and renal insufficiency.

Diagnostic Evaluation

Although bladder outlet obstruction is most commonly caused by BPH, other pathologies, such as diabetes, cancer, calculi, infections, stricture disease, and neurologic disorders, must be excluded. A detailed medical history with elicitation of specific voiding complaints is performed. The physical examination includes an abdominal examination searching for suprapubic fullness to evaluate for high postvoid residuals or retention. In addition to assessing anal sphincter tone, a digital rectal examination determines the size, consistency, symmetry, and tenderness of the prostate gland. A focus neurologic examination should be performed as well.

The American Urological Association (AUA) Symptom Index or the International Prostate Symptom Score (IPSS) (Figure 1) is an important questionnaire that helps identify patients who need treatment of LUTS and can help monitor their therapeutic response. The assessment quantifies the severity of irritative and obstructive symptoms as mild (0-7), moderate (8-19), and severe (20-35). Complementary to the IPSS is the patient's bothersome factor which is important in determining the timing of treatment initiation.

Urinalysis should be performed to screen for hematuria and infection. Urine cytology is recommended for men with a predominance of irritative voiding symptoms to aid in the diagnosis of bladder carcinoma. Routine measurement of serum creatinine is no longer indicated, but the annual measurement of serum prostate-specific antigen (PSA) should be offered at age 50 years to men with at least a 10-year life expectancy and for whom management would change with the knowledge of prostate cancer. Optional diagnostic tests, including postvoid residual measurements, urinary flow rate, and urodynamic measurements, may be helpful in patients with a complex medical history.

American Urological Association Symptom Index

Question	Not at All	Less Than 1 Time in 5	Less Than Half the Time	About Half the Time	More Than Half the Time	Almost Always
1. During the last month or so, how often have you had a sensation of not emptying your bladder completely after you finished urinating?	0	1	2	3	4	5
2. During the last month or so, how often have you had to urinate again less than 2 hours after you finished urinating?	0	1	2	3	4	5
3. During the last month or so, how often have you found you started again several times when you urinated?	0	1	2	3	4	5
4. During the last month or so, how often have you found it difficult to postpone urination?	0	1	2	3	4	5
5. During the last month or so, how often have you had a weak urinary stream?	0	1	2	3	4	5
6. During the last month or so, how often have you had to push or strain to begin urination?	0	1	2	3	4	5
7. During the last month or so, how many times did you most typically get up to urinate from the time you went to bed at night until the time you got up in the morning?	None	1 Time	2 Times	3 Times	4 Times	5 or More Times
	0	1	2	3	4	5

FIGURE 1 International Prostate Symptom Score.

Treatment

WATCHFUL WAITING

Because BPH is a benign disease, improvement of the patient's QOL is the treatment aim given that the average patient has a remaining life expectancy of 15 to 20 years. AUA treatment guidelines for BPH base the decision to treat upon bothersome factors and IPSS. Watchful waiting is the recommended initial treatment strategy for patients with mild IPSS, and for those patients with moderate to severe symptoms without bother and complications from BPH. Progression of symptomatic BPH is not inevitable; however, the risk of acute urinary retention from untreated BPH is approximately 7% over 4 years. Therefore, the patient is monitored annually by the physician with repeat of the initial evaluation to help assess both prostate volume and risk of BPH progression.

MEDICAL THERAPIES

For patients with IPSS >7 and significant bothersome factors, medical therapy can be offered. α_1-Adrenoreceptor antagonists (Table 1) relax prostatic and bladder neck smooth muscles. Urinary flow rates have been shown to improve 20% to 30% with a significant 20% to 50% improvement in symptom scores. Titration is required of doxazosin (Cardura) and terazosin (Hytrin) because of the adverse effects of orthostatic hypotension and dizziness. These agents are more commonly used for concurrent treatment of hypertension. Uroselective α_1-adrenoreceptor blockers tamsulosin (Flomax) and alfuzosin (Uroxatral) eliminate the need for titration. Treatment of adverse effects from α_1-adrenergic blocker therapy are orthostatic hypotension, dizziness, asthenia, retrograde ejaculation, and nasal congestion.

For patients with LUTS from a demonstrable prostatic enlargement (>40 cm^3), 5α-reductase inhibitors (Table 2) are effective against progression of the disease. They are also partially effective in relieving LUTS, although the effects are usually delayed. 5α-Reductase inhibitors block the conversion of testosterone to DHT in the prostate. Finasteride (Proscar) has been shown to reduce prostate size, increase peak urinary flow rate, and lower serum PSA by 50% at 6 months without masking prostate cancer detection. It also reduces the incidence of acute urinary retention and the probability of surgical intervention. Dutasteride (Avodart) has the same effect as finasteride. Significant but low rates of sexually related adverse effects have been reported for 5α-reductase inhibitors, including erectile dysfunction (8%), decreased libido (6%), and ejaculatory dysfunction (4%). These are reversible and uncommon after 1 year of treatment. Gynecomastia and mastodynia have also been reported.

Combination medical therapy with 5α-reductase inhibitors and α_1-adrenergic blockers has been

TABLE 1 α_1-Adrenergic Blockers for Benign Prostatic Hyperplasia

Alfuzosin (Uroxatral)
Doxazosin (Cardura)
Tamsulosin (Flomax)
Terazosin (Hytrin)

TABLE 2 5α-Reductase Inhibitors

Finasteride (Proscar)
Dutasteride (Avodart)

reported in multiple studies, with the longest follow-up and most definitive results described by the Medical Therapy of Prostatic Symptoms (MTOPS) trial. Combination therapy of doxazosin and finasteride was more effective in relieving symptoms and reducing risk of progression of symptoms than was doxazosin alone with 5 years of follow-up. Furthermore, combination therapy significantly reduced the long-term risk of acute urinary retention by 79% when compared with placebo. Importantly, combination therapy reduced the risk of surgical intervention by 67% when compared with placebo. Therefore, combination therapy benefits those with larger prostate glands and higher PSA values as their risk for progression is significantly higher. These results have been assumed with other α_1-adrenergic blockers and 5α-reductase inhibitors. Adverse effects of combination therapy are similar to the combined profile of monotherapies described above.

PHYTOTHERAPEUTIC AGENTS

Phytotherapy remains popular in Europe, and its popularity is growing in the United States. The mechanism of these herbal treatments is not well elucidated, with the most popular preparations being the saw palmetto berry (*Serenoa repens*)*[1] and the African plum tree bark (*Pygeum africanum*)*[1]. β-Sitosterol is believed to be the active ingredient, and urinary symptoms and flow rates were improved with 20 mg by mouth (PO) three times daily (tid). However, the effectiveness of *S. repens* has not been demonstrated in combination therapy with tamsulosin. Multicenter, randomized, double-blind, placebo-controlled studies remain to be performed for herbal preparations.

Surgical Intervention

MINIMALLY INVASIVE THERAPIES

Invasive therapy should be offered to patients who have moderate to severe LUTS with bother who failed pharmacotherapy and to those patients who are not interested in long-term medical therapy. Transurethral resection of the prostate (TURP) remains the gold standard with which any new therapy for BPH is compared. TURP is efficacious and durable, but is invasive, requiring catheterization and hospitalization with potential serious complications. Minimally invasive procedures (Table 3) are alternatives to circumvent these potential problems and are suitable for poor surgical candidates. Thermal-based therapies including microwaves and radiofrequency (RF) waves produce high temperatures at 45°C to 50°C (113°F to 122°F) to create coagulation necrosis of prostatic tissue (thermotherapy) and passive removal of that tissue. Transurethral microwave therapy (TUMT) is an office-based procedure that uses electromagnetic waves to affect prostatic tissues. In a prospective, randomized trial to TURP, low-energy TUMT produced similar improvements in terms of symptoms, flow rate, and postvoid residual at 12 months, but the TUMT group had a significantly higher rate of prolonged urinary retention. Also, irritative symptoms persisted for weeks in some. High-energy TUMT requires water-conductive cooling of the urethra. It is efficacious for patients with acute urinary retention from BPH, as 94% were able to regain their ability to void at 4 weeks. Improved peak flow rates and symptom scores were observed at 3 months, but there were higher rates of ejaculatory dysfunction (50%). TUMT is more effective than medical therapy, but less effective than TURP. Data on durability (>12 months) remain sparse.

TABLE 3 Minimally Invasive Therapies for Benign Prostatic Hyperplasia

Thermal-based therapies
Transurethral microwave therapy (TUMT)
Transurethral needle ablation (TUNA)
Laser prostatectomy
Visual laser ablation of the prostate (VLAP)
Transurethral evaporization of the prostate (TUEP)
Holmium laser resection/enucleation of the prostate (HoLRP/HoLEP)

Transurethral needle ablation of the prostate (TUNA) is another office-based procedure that uses low-power RF waves to produce thermotherapy of the prostate. A prospective, multicenter study comparing TUNA with TURP showed significant improvements in symptom scores, flow rates, postvoid residuals, and QOL scores at 12 months, although less pronounced than TURP. A catheter was required (41%) on average for 1 to 3 days, but the rate of ejaculatory dysfunction was significantly less than TURP. Incontinence was not reported. Overall, TUNA is a viable minimally invasive alternative to TURP.

Laser energy used for the treatment of BPH can destroy tissue by coagulative necrosis, vaporization, ablation, and resection. Although no tissue is retrieved for pathologic diagnosis, laser therapy is suitable for candidates on anticoagulation therapy. Visual laser ablation of the prostate (VLAP) uses low-power energy to coagulate prostatic tissue, resulting in sloughing. In a meta-analysis comparing VLAP with TURP, the VLAP groups had higher rates of urinary retention (21% vs. 5%) and irritative voiding symptoms (66% vs. 15%). Retrograde ejaculation was 36% to 47% in the VLAP groups. Transurethral evaporization of the prostate (TUEP) uses laser energy to vaporize prostatic tissue. When compared with TURP, TUEP achieved comparable short-term improvements in QOL indices, symptom scores, and flow rates, but had higher rates of urinary retention. Durability of results for TUEP remains in question.

Holmium laser resection/enucleation of the prostate (HoLRP/HoLEP) are popular for very large

*Available as a dietary supplement.
[1]Not FDA approved for this indication.

prostates (>80 g), and these techniques use saline solution, which eliminates the risk for TUR syndrome. As alternatives to TURP and open prostatectomies, both HoLRP and HoLEP retrieve specimens for pathology. In terms of symptoms, continence, urodynamic findings, and potency, HoLRP was equal to TURP at 2-year follow-up. HoLEP removes prostatic glands by enucleating the adenoma, which is then morcellated in the bladder and retrieved for pathologic examination. Similar to TURP and HoLRP, HoLEP requires overnight hospitalization and catheterization. A comparative trial of HoLEP with open prostatectomy found similar urinary flow rates, symptom scores, and QOL indices at 12 months.

STANDARD SURGICAL THERAPY

Standard surgical therapy should be offered to patients who have BPH-related complications or to those who want the most effective treatment initially. Prior medical therapy is not a requirement. TURP is the cornerstone surgical procedure for BPH with lasting results of 10 years on average. Its benefits include satisfaction rates of >75%, with up to 17 years of follow-up. Long-term risks include retrograde ejaculation (75%), bladder neck contractures or urethral strictures (3%), and incontinence (<1%). Short-term complications include urinary retention (10% to 40%), blood transfusions (5%), and TUR syndrome (hypervolemic, hyponatremic state from absorption of the irrigating solution). Retreatment rate is only 5% at 7 years of follow-up.

For smaller prostates (30 g or less), transurethral incision of the prostate (TUIP) is an option. The prostate gland is incised with a Collings knife at the 5- and 7-o'clock positions of the bladder neck. This is an outpatient procedure that provides immediate symptom improvement of 80% to 90%, similar to TURP with shorter duration of catheterization. Compared with TURP, retrograde ejaculation is less common (13% to 20%), but there is a slightly higher rate of secondary procedures.

Open prostatectomy is reserved for glands too large to be removed endoscopically, usually >100 g. Open enucleation is performed through a retropubic or suprapubic infraumbilical incision. This operation entails risks of major surgery but allows treatment of concomitant bladder diverticulum or large bladder calculus. Retrograde ejaculation occurs in almost 100% of patients, but long-term complications, such as incontinence, bladder neck contractures, and erectile dysfunction, are uncommon in 2% to 3% of patients. Its efficacy in terms of symptom score improvement and urinary flow rate is superior to any BPH therapy, including TURP.

ALTERNATIVES TO INVASIVE THERAPY

In patients where medical status excludes surgical intervention, relief of outlet obstruction can be accomplished by other means. Intraprostatic urethral stents are made of titanium and are designed to keep the channel partially patent. Complications include encrustation, obstruction, chronic pain, and infection. Clean intermittent catheterization (CIC) is ideal and is an effective and safe therapy for urinary retention if manual dexterity allows. A chronic indwelling urethral or suprapubic catheter allows relief of outlet obstruction, but bacteriuria from colonization is inevitable, mandating catheter changes at monthly intervals.

Investigational

The Japanese literature describes the use of dehydrated absolute ethanol[1] through transurethral prostatic injections to avoid retrograde ejaculation. Follow-up at 3 months demonstrated symptoms score and flow rate improvement, but durability remains in question. Randomized, long-term studies are pending in the United States. High-intensity focused ultrasound (HIFU) uses high-energy treatment cycles to produce thermotherapy with imaging performed with low-energy cycles. Short-term catheterization is required, and there are symptom and flow rate improvements. Long-term, randomized results are lacking and warranted. Water-induced thermotherapy (WIT) uses an inflatable prostatic urethral balloon to circulate heated water (60°C to 70°C [140°F to 158°F]) to produce conductive heating of prostatic tissue. At 12 months, IPSS improvement was observed, along with improved flow rates and QOL indices. Comparison trials with TURP are lacking. Lastly, interstitial laser coagulation (ILC) delivers Nd:YAG or diode laser energy transurethrally to cause intraprostatic tissue ablation. Symptom improvement may continue up to 6 months after therapy, and the treatment results are comparable to those for TURP at 2 years of follow-up.

LUTS from BPH remain a common problem for men. For those with minimal symptoms, watchful waiting is an acceptable alternative. The refinement of medical therapy and minimally invasive procedures has significant roles in the management of those with significant symptoms and bothersome factors, or complications from BPH. In addition, these options may be optimal for high-risk surgical candidates. TURP remains the gold standard treatment for BPH and should be offered to those who have failed other therapies.

[1]Not FDA approved for this indication.

ERECTILE DYSFUNCTION

METHOD OF

A. Andrew Ray, MSc, MD, and

Gerald Brock, MD

Erectile dysfunction (ED) is the inability to consistently achieve and maintain an erection satisfactory for sexual intercourse. Advances in the understanding of the etiology of ED and the development of effective oral treatments have led to dramatic changes in societal perception of this condition. The Massachusetts Male Aging Study was the first large-scale survey of its kind to prospectively examine the issue of male sexual health. This study conservatively estimated that there are currently more than 18 million men between the ages of 40 and 70 years in the United States suffering with ED, and that approximately 620,000 new cases can be expected each year.

Classically, ED is divided into organic and psychogenic etiologies, with vascular disorders thought to be the primary cause of organic ED. Many of the risk factors are the same as those that cause heart disease. Hypertension, diabetes, smoking, and heart disease are all independent risk factors for erectile dysfunction. Conversely, only maintaining a physically active lifestyle has a protective effect. That men with higher socioeconomic status have a lower incidence of ED likely represents a lower incidence of vascular risk factors in this group. It remains unknown whether lifestyle modification can prevent or even reverse damage to erectile health that has already occurred.

TABLE 1 Risk Factors for Erectile Dysfunction

Vasculogenic	Medication-Induced
Diabetes	Antihypertensives (thiazides, β blockers)
Hypertension	Antidepressants (SSRIs, TCAs, MAOIs)
Heavy smoking	Antiandrogens (spironolactone [Aldactone], ketoconazole [Nizoral])
Heart disease	Antipsychotics
Perineal trauma (straddle injury)	Centrally acting sympatholytics (methyldopa, clonidine [Catapres], reserpine)
Neurogenic	**Other**
Pelvic surgery	*Age*
Prostate disease	Chronic renal failure hypogonadism
Spinal cord injury	Penile deformity (e.g., Peyronie's disease)
Stroke	
Psychogenic	
Depression	
Relationship issues	
Stress	

Abbreviations: MAOIs = monoamine oxidase inhibitors; SSRIs = serotonin reuptake inhibitors; TCAs = tricyclic antidepressants.

Physiology of Erection

Erections are the result of a complex interplay of the neurovascular system. In brief, the penis contains two vascular corpora cavernosal bodies and a ventrally located urinary canal—the spongiosum. Sexual stimulation causes a large increase in penile blood flow, mainly through the paired cavernosal arteries. This process is initiated centrally by dopaminergic action in the medial preoptic area (MPOA) of the hypothalamus. Activation of this area occurs following sexual stimulation in the form of sensory inputs. The MPOA, together with other brainstem nuclei, activates the spinal sympathetic and parasympathetic neurons controlling erection. These nerves emerge from the spinal cord and join to form the pelvic cavernous nerves, which regulate blood flow in the corpora cavernosa by secreting neurotransmitters, the most important of which is nitric oxide (NO). In the corpora, NO causes relaxation of trabecular smooth muscle, facilitating the flow of blood into the penis. Interestingly, the action of increasing blood flow to the penis and relaxing trabecular smooth muscle also causes passive compression of venous outflow. The resulting rise in penile blood pressure causes an erection. Erection rigidity is further intensified through triggering of the bulbocavernosus reflex, usually during the preorgasmic phase. During masturbation or sexual intercourse, this reflex causes the ischiocavernosus muscles at the base of the penis to compress the blood-filled corpora and further impede venous drainage.

A defect in any one of these systems may result in ED. Vascular disease, neurologic dysfunction, and diabetes in particular are thought to be primary contributors. End-organ injury from previous pelvic trauma (straddle injuries), prostate surgery, or pelvic irradiation may also lead to erectile difficulties (Table 1).

Evaluation of Erectile Dysfunction

An algorithmic approach to the diagnosis and treatment of ED has been published (Figure 1).

HISTORY AND PHYSICAL EXAMINATION

In patients undergoing evaluation for ED, a thorough history and physical remains the cornerstone of diagnosis. History provides the greatest amount of information and guides further testing. The clinician should particularly focus on distinguishing ED from other sexual concerns (premature ejaculation and loss of libido). A detailed history should elicit the nature, duration, and severity of the erectile problem.

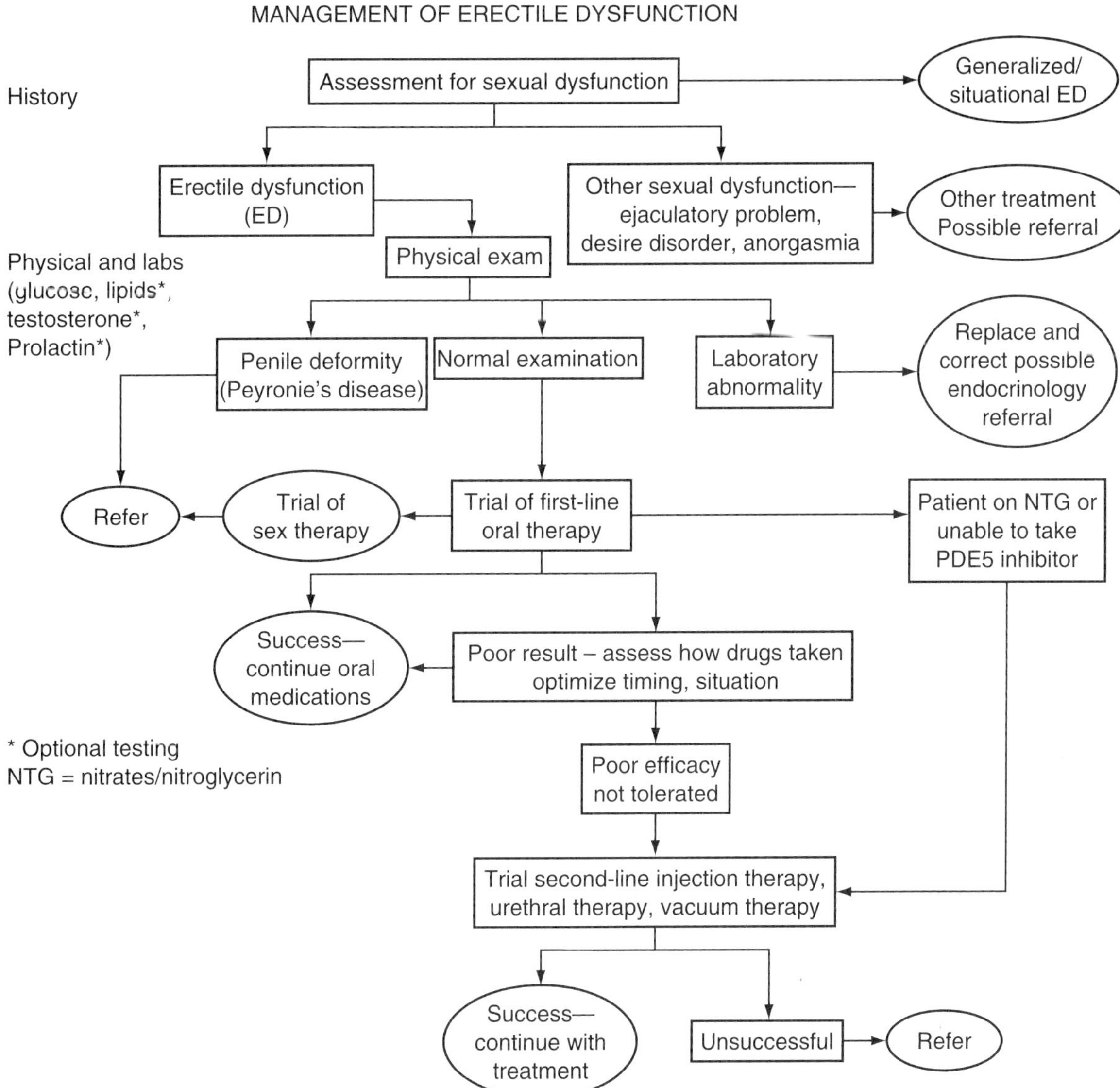

FIGURE 1 Algorithm for the evaluation and management of erectile dysfunction. Adapted with permission from the Canadian Urological Guidelines Committee. Can J Urol 9(4):1583, 2002.

Information about any recent changes in health, medications, or partner, and about any relationship issues, should also be obtained. Use of validated questionnaires, although of great clinical utility in research, are less valuable for the experienced clinician. As previously mentioned, many of the risk factors for ED are the same as those for coronary artery disease. ED may present as the first symptom of systemic illnesses such as diabetes or vascular disease.

The physical examination should include evaluation for gynecomastia, hair distribution, and atrophic testes as evidence of hormonal deficiency. The penis should be examined for deformities such as Peyronie's plaques and chordee. Assessment of femoral and pedal pulses, as well as of perineal sensation, may support a diagnosis of vascular- or neurogenic-induced ED. Finally, because ED may be the reason for presentation to a physician for younger men, a baseline blood pressure should be obtained.

BLOOD WORK

There is no consensus regarding required laboratory testing in the workup of ED; however, guided by the history and physical examination, additional studies may be indicated. Initial laboratory testing should include fasting serum glucose, glycosylated hemoglobin (HGA_{1c}), and fasting lipid profile, as well as morning testosterone in the setting of ED with poor libido. Complete blood count, urinalysis, and hormonal studies, such as thyroid-stimulating hormone (TSH), luteinizing hormone (LH), and prolactin, are optional. If abnormalities are noted, referral to an appropriate specialist should be initiated.

Prostate-specific antigen (PSA) does not form part of the routine workup for ED.

SPECIALIZED TESTING

As surgical interventions become increasingly relegated to third-line treatment, the need for and acceptability of invasive testing are diminished. Thus, initial studies may be reserved for patients who fail first-line treatment or if greater information on etiology is required. Nocturnal penile tumescence (NPT), with a RigiScan device, is a minimally invasive method to assess nighttime erections in the patient's own home. Men without ED usually have between three and five erections per night. Duplex ultrasound can be useful in the assessment of penile circulation and deformity such as Peyronie's disease, but is operator dependent. Other, more invasive testing should be reserved for surgical planning. For example, pudendal arteriography with vasoactive injection is used prior to revascularization surgery. Similarly, in cases of venous leak, DICC (dynamic infusion cavernosometry and cavernosography) can be used to assess the ability of the penis to trap blood and thereby maintain rigidity.

Medical Therapy for Erectile Dysfunction

Originally developed to treat angina, the approval of sildenafil citrate (Viagra) in 1998 revolutionized the treatment of ED. Two other medications (tadalafil [Cialis] and vardenafil [Levitra]) are now approved in many locations worldwide. These agents inhibit phosphodiesterase 5 (PDE5), an enzyme responsible for the breakdown of cyclic guanosine monophosphate (cGMP), an important second messenger in the NO pathway (Figure 2). To date, at least 11 different PDE isoenzymes have been characterized; however, PDE5 is responsible for the majority of cGMP catalytic activity in cavernosal smooth muscle.

SILDENAFIL

Better known as Viagra (Pfizer, Inc.), the safety and efficacy of sildenafil citrate has been replicated in more than 100 clinical trials in a broad spectrum of ED, including both organic and psychogenic types. One large meta-analysis demonstrated that at clinically recommended doses of 50 to 100 mg, 83% of patients on sildenafil were able to achieve at least one erection and 57% of all intercourse attempts were successful as compared with 21% in the placebo group. Sildenafil also benefits specialized populations, including those with spinal injury, hypertension, and diabetes, and following radical prostatectomy. The most common adverse effects are flushing (12%), headache (11%), dyspepsia (5%), and visual disturbances (3%). The visual side effects are related to the binding of retinally expressed PDE6.

Sildenafil is eliminated primarily by hepatic metabolism through the cytochrome P450 system and its elimination half-life ($t_{1/2}$) is approximately 4 hours. To be most effective, sildenafil should be taken on an empty stomach with peak plasma concentrations achieved within 60 minutes for most patients. Patients should initially be given a trial of the medication at 50 mg. This may be increased to 100 mg or decreased to 25 mg, depending on efficacy and side effects. Like all PDE5 inhibitors, its use is contraindicated in men taking organic nitrates.

VARDENAFIL

Vardenafil (Levitra, Bayer Healthcare/GlaxoSmith Kline), another potent and selective PDE5 inhibitor, is effective in treating mild to severe ED of various etiologies including organic, psychogenic, and mixed. Vardenafil is also effective in the treatment of ED secondary to diabetes, traditionally regarded as difficult to treat. Recent studies also suggest a role for vardenafil in the postoperative return of sexual function following nerve-sparing prostatectomy.

Vardenafil is available in 2.5-, 5-, 10-, and 20-mg doses. The suggested starting dose is 10 mg, which can

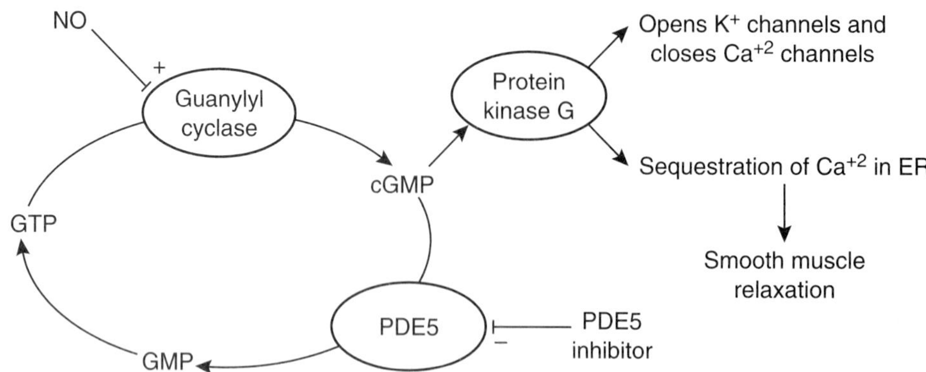

FIGURE 2 The role of cGMP in male erections. Nitric oxide (NO) is synthesized by endothelial-derived nitrous oxide synthase (NOS), activating soluble guanylyl cyclase (sGC). In turn, cGMP activates a biochemical cascade that results in decreased intracellular Ca^{2+} and smooth-muscle relaxation. By inhibiting the breakdown of cGMP, PDE5 inhibitors are able to enhance the erectile response.

be adjusted as necessary. Smaller doses are recommended in those older than 65 years and in patients with hepatic impairment. The onset of action is approximately 20 minutes after ingestion, with peak activity in 45 to 90 minutes. The $t_{\{1/2\}}$ for vardenafil is approximately 4.5 hours and is impaired with liver disease or medications, which affect CYP3A4, CYP3A5, and CYP2C. Vardenafil is well tolerated and its principal side effects are headache (10%), flushing (8%), rhinitis (8%), and dyspepsia (3%). Side effects are dose-related and tend to improve with time. No visual side effects have been reported with this medication.

TADALAFIL

Tadalafil is an oral agent with selective action at the PDE5 isoenzyme. It is being marketed under the brand name Cialis (Lilly ICOS LLC). Randomized, double-blind, placebo-controlled studies show that tadalafil is effective for the treatment of ED across multiple etiologies and independent of age. Tadalafil has an extended half-life (17.5 hours) and is effective in 80% of sexual attempts up to 36 hours following dosage. Tadalafil is effective without regard to food or alcohol intake. Tadalafil is available in 5-, 10-, and 20-mg dosages; however, 10 to 20 mg is most effective. Side effects are proportional to dosage and most commonly involve headache (8%), flushing (6%), dyspepsia (5%), and myalgia (3%). Visual side effects with this medication are rare.

CARDIAC RISK

The safety of PDE5 inhibitors in patients with cardiac conditions has been extensively investigated. In a meta-analysis of 6947 patients taking either sildenafil or placebo, no significant increase in the rate of myocardial infarction or death was observed. Corroborating data have been reported for both tadalafil and vardenafil. Thus, PDE5 inhibitors would appear to be safe for the majority of men with stable coronary artery disease. However, risks should be discussed on an individual basis. Their use is contraindicated in patients taking organic nitrates because of the possibility of profound hypotension.

At the time of writing, no direct head-to-head studies comparing PDE5 inhibitors has been published. As such, it is difficult to directly compare the available agents in terms of efficacy and tolerability. Until this is more completely understood, a common sense approach is best. All agents should be considered first-line, and selection should be based on individual patient factors such as response, side effects, and cost.

Second-Line Therapies

Several options exist for patients who either fail first-line oral therapies, or are unable to tolerate their side effects, or in whom their use is contraindicated. Intracavernosal injection therapy (ICI) with a vasoactive agent such as alprostadil, a synthetic prostaglandin (PG) E_1, acts through the second messenger cyclic adenosine monophosphate (cAMP) to cause smooth-muscle relaxation and venodilation. Marketed as Caverject (Pfizer), alprostadil is the only drug approved by the FDA for this purpose. When used in doses of 10 to 20 µg, it causes erections in 70% to 80% of patients with ED. Patients with vasculogenic ED are the most likely to experience a treatment failure with this therapy. Many urologists use a combination of alprostadil, phentolamine (Regitine),[1] and papaverine[1] for improved results. The most frequently reported side effects include pain at the injection site, hematoma, and priapism. Some patients also develop fibrotic scarring that can result in penile deformity. Alprostadil is also available for direct instillation into the penile urethra (MUSE) where it is transported into the cavernosal tissue through venous channels. MUSE (Vivus, Inc.) has a response rate of approximately 50%, but its use is often limited by penile pain.

Vacuum-constriction devices are another safe and relatively inexpensive option for many patients. Although up to 80% of patients are satisfied with erectile quality; the rate of discontinuation remains high. These devices are often combined with ICI or MUSE for improved performance.

Surgery remains an option for all remaining cases of ED. There is extensive surgical experience with the implantation of both malleable and inflatable devices; however, surgery induces irreversible tissue injury, relegating it to final-option therapy. Despite this morbidity, patient and partner satisfaction is very high, approaching 85%.

Future Directions

The precise cause of ED has yet to be determined at the molecular level and likely varies with different etiologies. As discussed earlier, erections are the result of a complicated interplay between central and peripheral neural transmission and blood flow. While not all the components involved are fully characterized, considerable progress has been made.

Of particular interest, the pathways involving NO and cGMP appear to be important targets for altering the erectile response. Non-NO compounds have already been developed that can activate soluble guanylyl cyclase (sGC), a key step in the NO-mediated cascade. Genetic manipulation through gene transfer techniques also have exciting potential. Adenoviruses have been used to successfully transfer endothelial nitric oxide synthase (eNOS) and improve erectile function in rats. Other experimental models have targeted the expression of NOS, hSlo (a K^+ channel), and vascular endothelial growth factor (VEGF). All show promise for increasing cavernosal pressures.

ED is a common and treatable condition that negatively affects quality of life and for which many patients are reluctant to seek attention. As our population ages,

[1]Not FDA approved for this indication.

the incidence of this condition is likely to increase. Finally, because ED often represents the first symptom of a more serious medical condition, all physicians should be encouraged to address issues of sexual health as part of the routine health review.

ACUTE RENAL FAILURE

METHOD OF

Muhammad G. Alam, MD, MPH,

Mary Jo Shaver-Lewis, MD, and

Sudhir V. Shah, MD

Definition and Epidemiology

Acute renal failure (ARF) can be defined broadly as an abrupt decline in renal function sufficient to result in retention of nitrogenous waste (blood urea nitrogen and creatinine) in the body. Typically, the decline in renal function occurs over hours to days. In general, even a minor decline in renal function is associated with poor patient outcome, thus most experts believe that an increase in serum creatinine of 0.5 mg/dL should be considered as a diagnostic criterion for acute renal failure. A 25% increase in serum creatinine or a 25% decrease in glomerular filtration rate are widely accepted alternative definitions of acute renal failure. The incidence of ARF varies greatly depending on the clinical settings. The incidence of ARF on admission to the hospital is approximately 1% and increases to 2% to 5% during hospitalization. The incidence of ARF is even higher in surgical and medical intensive care units (ICUs) and is reported in up to 30% to 50% of the ICU admissions. Despite major advances in dialysis and intensive care, the mortality rate among patients with severe acute renal failure requiring dialysis has not decreased significantly over the past 50 years. This is partly a result of the age of the patients continuing to rise, and coexisting serious illnesses are increasingly common among these patients. Our efforts should be targeted at the prevention of acute renal failure.

Etiology of Acute Renal Failure

ARF can result from a decrease of renal blood flow (prerenal azotemia), or intrinsic renal parenchymal diseases (renal azotemia), or obstruction of urine flow (postrenal azotemia). Prerenal etiologies are the most common causes of ARF, accounting for 30% to 60% of all cases of ARF. Postrenal causes of ARF are less common in the hospital setting, accounting for 1% to 10% of all causes of ARF, with the remaining cases of ARF caused by intrinsic renal diseases. Table 1 lists the major causes of ARF.

The most common intrinsic renal disease that leads to ARF is an entity referred to as *acute tubular necrosis* (ATN), which designates a clinical syndrome of abrupt and sustained decline in glomerular filtration rate (GFR) occurring within minutes to days in response to an acute ischemic or nephrotoxic event. Its clinical recognition is largely predicated upon exclusion of prerenal and postrenal causes of azotemia, followed by exclusion of other causes of intrinsic ARF (e.g., glomerulonephritis, acute interstitial nephritis [AIN], and vasculitis). Interstitial nephritis is the cause in 10% and acute glomerulonephritis is the etiology in 5% of intrinsic renal azotemia. Although the name *acute tubular necrosis* is not an entirely valid histologic description of this syndrome, the term is ingrained in clinical medicine and is therefore used in this article.

TABLE 1 Causes of Acute Renal Failure

Prerenal Azotemia
Absolute Decrease in Effective Blood Volume
Hemorrhage, skin losses (burns, sweating), gastrointestinal losses (diarrhea, vomiting), renal losses (diuretics, glycosuria), fluid pooling (peritonitis, burns)
Relative Decrease in Blood Volume
Congestive heart failure, sepsis, anaphylaxis, liver failure
Arterial Occlusion
Thromboembolism, aortic dissection
Renal Azotemia
Vascular Causes
Vasculitis, microscopic polyarthritis, malignant hypertension
Acute Glomerulonephritis
Postinfectious glomerulonephritis, antiglomerular basement membrane disease
Acute Interstitial Nephritis
Drugs (antibiotics, nonsteroidal anti-inflammatory drugs, diuretics, allopurinol [Zyloprim])
Infections (streptococcus, pneumococcus, Epstein-Barr virus, CMV, HIV, ehrlichiosis, mycoplasma)
Acute Tubular Necrosis
Ischemic
Severe prerenal azotemia, postsurgical complication
Sepsis syndrome
Nephrotoxic
Exogenous nephrotoxins
Antibiotics (aminoglycosides, cephalosporins, amphotericin B [Fungizone]); iodinated contrast agents; chemotherapeutic agents (cisplatin [Platinol]); solvents (carbon tetrachloride, ethylene glycol)
Endogenous nephrotoxins
Intratubular pigments (hemoglobinuria, myoglobinuria), intratubular proteins (myeloma), intratubular crystals (uric acid, oxalate) tumor lysis syndrome
Postrenal Azotemia
Bladder outlet obstruction, ureteral obstruction (intra- and extraluminal), intratubular obstruction (uric acid, calcium oxalate, acyclovir [Zovirax], methotrexate, indinavir [Crixivan], Bence Jones proteins)

Diagnosis

Despite the exhaustive list of conditions that can cause ARF, a careful history and physical examination and simple laboratory tests often suffice for diagnosis. Correct diagnosis of ARF requires knowledge of the natural history of the different causes of ARF and a systematic approach, which should start by excluding and correcting both prerenal and postrenal causes.

A chart review is important to look for weight loss with negative fluid balance, a drop in blood pressure, evidence of sepsis, or use of contrast media or other nephrotoxins. A careful examination including blood pressure in both supine and standing positions and evaluation of jugular venous distention are important to assess volume status. Funduscopic examination may give clues about cholesterol emboli and endocarditis. Ulceration in the nasal mucosa may point toward illicit drug sniffing or Wegener's granulomatosis. Examination of the heart for pericardial rub or murmur, as well as lung examination, are also important. A careful abdominal examination may uncover a distended, tender bladder, indicating lower urinary tract obstruction. The examination of the prostate and a sterile "in-and-out" diagnostic postvoid bladder catheterization should be performed as a part of the physical examination in all cases of ARF. Table 2 describes the diagnostic evaluations of a patient with ARF.

TABLE 2 Diagnostic Evaluation of a Patient with Acute Renal Failure

Type of Evaluation	Comments
Chart Review	
Previous renal function	Patients with CRI are more susceptible to ARF
Medications	Aminoglycosides are an important cause of ATN (nonoliguric and in the first 2 weeks of therapy); certain antibiotics, NSAIDs, and a host of medications can cause AIN; contrast agents are an important cause of ARF
Start date	
Drug levels	
Nephrotoxins	
NSAIDs	
Aminoglycosides	
Amphotericin B (Fungizone)	
Contrast agent	
Surgery	Cardiac and vascular surgery patients are particularly susceptible to ATN.
Type of surgery	Methoxyflurane (Penthrane) and enflurane (Ethrane), which is related to methoxyflurane but is less toxic, can cause nonoliguric ATN
Hemodynamics	
Blood loss	
Anesthetic used	
Infections	Infection or sepsis can cause ARF even in the absence of hypotension
Fever	
Positive blood cultures	
Hemodynamics	Hypotension can cause prerenal azotemia and ischemic ATN
Blood pressure	
Heart rate	
Weight (in and out)	
Physical Examination	
Volume status	
Edema	Pretibial in ambulatory patients, sacral in bedridden patients
Jugular vein distention	
Crackles	
S_3 gallop	
Skin	
Diffuse rash	Skin rash seen in some drug-induced ARF (e.g., antibiotics and allopurinol [Zyloprim])
Livedo reticularis	
Palpable rash	Atheroembolic disease typically seen after aortic catheterization and vascular surgery Henoch-Schönlein purpura and cryoglobulinemia can lead to palpable rash
Bladder	
Suprapubic fullness	Distended bladder
Bladder catheterization	To assess postvoid residual urinary volume and to relieve obstruction
Urinalysis and Sediment	
Protein and blood	Presence of blood and protein favors glomerulonephritis
Cells	WBCs may be present in AIN and dysmorphic RBCs may be present in glomerulonephritis
Casts	Muddy brown casts are typical for ATN
Urine Indices	See Table 3
Additional Tests	
Ultrasound	Used to rule out obstruction
Radionuclide scans	Useful in the assessment of renal blood flow, obstruction, cortical necrosis, and AIN
Renal biopsy	Indicated only in patients with unexplained ARF or atypical clinical course

Abbreviations: AIN = acute interstitial nephritis; ARF = acute renal failure; ATN = acute tubular necrosis; CRI = chronic renal insufficiency; NSAIDs = nonsteroidal anti-inflammatory drugs; RBCs = red blood cells; WBCs = white blood cells.

Laboratory Tests

Initial laboratory tests include serum chemistries for blood urea nitrogen (BUN), creatinine, sodium, chloride, potassium, and bicarbonate. These tests are important for both the diagnosis of ARF and for assessment of its complications. The BUN and creatinine are used not only for diagnosing ARF, the ratio of BUN to creatinine also helps in the differential diagnosis of ARF. A BUN-to-creatinine ratio of greater than 20:1 is often a result of a prerenal cause of ARF. Other causes of a disproportionate increase in BUN compared with serum creatinine are gastrointestinal bleeding, systemic steroid use, high catabolism as a consequence of the underlying medical condition, or a high-protein diet. An elevated serum creatinine with less of an elevation in BUN suggests enhanced muscle breakdown (i.e., rhabdomyolysis).

A complete blood count may reveal anemia and presence of schistocytes may favor hemolysis, which may be present in hemolytic uremic syndrome, thrombotic microangiopathy, endocarditis, and disseminated intravascular coagulopathy. An elevated creatine phosphokinase (CPK) or myoglobin level favors rhabdomyolysis. Abnormal liver function tests may point toward hepatorenal syndrome, congestive heart failure, or sepsis. Serologic tests (e.g., antinuclear antibody, antiglomerular basement membrane antibody, antineutrophil cytoplasmic antibody test, C3, and C4) are indicated depending upon clinical suspicion.

Urine in Acute Renal Failure

Acute renal failure is traditionally divided into anuric (urine output of <100 mL per day), oliguric (urine output between 100 and 400 mL per day), and nonoliguric ARF (urine output >400 mL per day). Complete anuria (zero urine output) should suggest a diagnosis of obstruction or vascular catastrophe, although it can be seen in ATN and AIN.

In prerenal and postrenal ARF, urine sediment is typically "bland." A moderate number of hyaline and fine granular casts may be seen in prerenal ARF, but coarse granular and cellular casts are infrequent and atypical for prerenal ARF. In ATN, the urine sediment is usually quite characteristic and in 70% to 80% of patients dirty brown granular casts, renal tubular epithelial cells, either free or in casts, can be seen. In AIN, one may see white blood cells (WBC) and WBC casts. The presence of urinary eosinophils strongly suggests AIN, although its absence does not rule out AIN. In ARF associated with intratubular oxalate (e.g., methoxyflurane anesthesia) or uric acid deposition (associated with acute hyperuricemia after chemotherapy of neoplastic disease), the urine sediment contains abundant oxalate or uric acid crystals, respectively.

Urinary indices are often used to distinguish between prerenal azotemia and ATN. In prerenal azotemia, the urinary-to-plasma-creatinine ratio is typically greater than it is in ATN, and urinary sodium concentration is characteristically low. Lately, fractional excretion of urea is also reported to help differentiate pre- versus intrinsic renal azotemia (Table 3). Interpretations of these tests, however, must be made in conjunction with other assessments of the patient because there are clinically important exceptions to these generalizations. For example, certain types of ATN, such as contrast media-induced renal injury, may present with all the clinical characteristics of ATN but with fractional excretions of sodium less than 1%.

Other Diagnostic Tests and Renal Biopsy

If the diagnosis of prerenal azotemia or ATN is reasonably certain and the clinical setting does not require the exclusion of other causes of acute azotemia, generally no further diagnostic evaluation is necessary. Renal ultrasound is commonly used to evaluate for hydronephrosis and obstruction. A high resolution CT scan is considered as a test of choice for suspected urinary tract calculi. Radionuclide scans are available to assess renal blood flow and excretory (secretory) function. The renal scan is also helpful to diagnose acute cortical necrosis. The radionuclide WBC scan has a limited role in diagnosing AIN. Magnetic resonance angiography is recommended to

TABLE 3 Urinary Diagnostic Indices

Indices	Prerenal Azotemia	Acute Tubular Necrosis
Urinary sodium (mEq/L)	<20	>40
Urinary osmolarity (mOsm/kg H_2O)	>500	<450
Fractional excretion of sodium (FE_{Na}) $(U_{Na} \times P_{cr}/P_{Na} \times U_{cr})(100)$	<1%	>1%
Fractional excretion of urea (FE_{UN}) $[(U_{UN}/BUN)(U_{cr}/P_{cr})] \times 100$	<35%	>50%
Urinary creatinine (mg/dL)/plasma creatinine (mg/dL)	>40	<20

Abbreviations: BUN = blood urea nitrogen; U_{Na} = urinary sodium; P_{cr} = plasma creatinine; P_{Na} = plasma sodium; U_{cr} = urinary creatinine; U_{UN} = urinary nitrogen.

evaluate renal arterial or venous thrombosis or obstruction. Renal arterial or venous angiography is recommended when suspicion for vascular obstruction is high. The angiogram gives the advantage of possible intervention at the same time. Because of the invasive nature of the procedure and risk of contrast nephropathy and atheroembolic disease, one must weigh the risks and benefits of the procedure before recommending invasive procedures.

Renal biopsy is rarely required for the workup of ARF. The common indications for renal biopsy in the setting of ARF are (a) unexplained renal failure, (b) suspicion of glomerulonephritis or lupus nephritis as a cause of ARF, and (c) the possibility of interstitial nephritis and continued worsening of renal function despite stopping all possible agents that could lead to AIN.

Prevention of Acute Renal Failure

The steps in the prevention of acute renal failure include identifying the patients at risk, avoiding potentially nephrotoxic agents, and using strategies to prevent renal injury (Table 4). Patients at risk are the elderly, those with pre-existing renal disease, and patients who are volume depleted. Avoidance of nephrotoxic agents is an important aspect of prevention. In instances where it is necessary to use potentially nephrotoxic agents, steps should be taken to reduce the risk of acute renal failure.

Nonsteroidal anti-inflammatory drugs (NSAIDs) can cause interstitial nephritis as direct toxins or ATN via an ischemic mechanism. In prerenal states in which renal perfusion is reduced, intrarenal vasodilator prostaglandin act to buffer the vasoconstrictor effect of angiotensin. Therefore, NSAIDs, by blocking prostaglandin synthesis, can markedly reduce renal blood flow in prerenal patients, leading to ischemic tubular injury. The prevention of NSAID-induced acute ischemic injury depends on eliminating prerenal factors prior to administration, or avoiding their use in patients with fixed reduction in renal perfusion. Similarly, acute renal failure caused by cyclooxygenase-2 inhibitors has been reported with an incidence of ARF similar to that caused by NSAIDs. Diuretics, angiotensin-converting enzyme (ACE) inhibitors, and other vasodilators should be used with caution in patients with suspected true or effective hypovolemia or renovascular disease, because they may convert prerenal azotemia to ischemic ATN and make these patients more susceptible to the adverse effects of nephrotoxins. Careful monitoring of circulating drug levels appears to reduce the risk of cyclosporine (Sandimmune) and tacrolimus (Prograf) nephrotoxicity.

Aminoglycoside antibiotics are a frequent cause of hospital-acquired acute renal failure. A single daily dose is less nephrotoxic and as effective as multiple daily doses. The risk of renal failure with aminoglycosides is increased with prolonged use and nephrotoxicity may occur even when plasma levels are in the therapeutic range. Amphotericin B (Fungizone) is a relatively frequent cause of ARF. Recent studies suggest that amphotericin B in lipid emulsion (Amphotec) is less nephrotoxic than the standard formulation of amphotericin B. Hydration with normal saline prior to amphotericin B infusion decreases the incidence of ARF. In patients at high risk for nephrotoxicity, liposomal amphotericin B is recommended.

Prevention of postsurgical acute renal failure must begin prior to surgery. Recognition of high-risk patients, such as those with pre-existing renal disease, chronic liver disease, cardiac failure, and elderly patients, is the first step. Important preventive measures, such as volume depletion, hypotension during surgery, and nephrotoxic agents, will aid in avoiding additional insults.

TABLE 4 Prevention of Acute Renal Failure

Identify Patient at Risk
Elderly patients
Patients with abnormal renal function and/or diabetics
Patients who are volume depleted
Following vascular surgery
Following trauma
Avoid Nephrotoxic Agents
Nonsteroidal anti-inflammatory drugs
Aminoglycosides
Amphotericin B (Fungizone)
Chemotherapeutic agents (e.g., cisplatin [Platinol-AQ])
Angiotensin-converting enzyme inhibitors in volume-depleted patients
Specific Prevention Strategies
Contrast media
Tumor lysis syndrome
Rhabdomyolysis
Surgical procedures
Avoid multiple insults

PREVENTION OF CONTRAST MEDIUM-ASSOCIATED ACUTE RENAL FAILURE

Risk factors for developing contrast medium-associated nephropathy include chronic renal failure, advanced age, diabetes mellitus, underlying chronic renal insufficiency, congestive heart failure, reduced renal perfusion states, and the total dose of contrast medium used. Several investigators have tried different agents, such as dopamine (Intropin)[1], diuretics, calcium channel antagonists, aminophylline[1], fenoldopam (Corlopam)[1], atrial natriuretic peptide nesiritide[1] (Natecor), and ACE inhibitors, to prevent contrast media-associated nephropathy without significant benefit. To date, only intravenous hydration with saline (1 mL/kg per hour starting 8 hours prior to procedure) shows consistent benefits. Recently, iodixanol (Visipaque), a nonionic, iso-osmolar contrast media, was shown to be beneficial in preventing

[1]Not FDA approved for this indication.

contrast nephropathy in high-risk patients undergoing cardiac catheterization. *N*-acetylcysteine (Mucomyst)[1] is commonly used to prevent contrast nephropathy in high-risk patients. The results of the clinical studies are conflicting and further studies are necessary before recommending the routine use of acetylcysteine to prevent contrast media-induced acute renal failure.

PREVENTION OF ACUTE RENAL FAILURE IN TUMOR LYSIS SYNDROME

Acute renal failure may occur in patients with high turnover malignancies (e.g., acute lymphoblastic leukemia and poorly differentiated lymphomas) who either spontaneously, or more frequently after cytotoxic therapy, release enormous amounts of uric acid precursors leading to uric acid precipitation in the renal tubules. During extensive cell lysis, phosphate and potassium are also released in large amounts, resulting in hyperphosphatemia and hyperkalemia. The peak uric acid level is often greater than 20 mg/dL and a ratio of urinary uric acid-to-creatinine concentrations greater than 1:1 suggests the diagnosis of acute uric acid nephropathy. To prevent uric acid nephropathy in patients likely to develop tumor lysis syndrome, preemptive treatment with allopurinol (Zyloprim), a xanthine oxidase inhibitor, and intravenous hydration are the important measures (Table 5).

PREVENTION OF ACUTE RENAL FAILURE IN RHABDOMYOLYSIS

As soon as diagnosis of rhabdomyolysis is suspected, aggressive optimization of intravascular and extravascular fluid volume by using isotonic normal saline is the most important initial step in preventing acute renal failure (Table 5).

[1]Not FDA approved for this indication.

Conservative Management of Acute Renal Failure

The loss of the excretory function of the kidney makes the patient very vulnerable to derangements in the internal milieu unless special care is taken to monitor the fluid, electrolytes, and nutritional intake of the patient. Daily assessment of patients with particular attention to weight, intake/output, and other laboratory parameters should be performed as described in Table 6.

Management of Volume Homeostasis

An important goal of patient management is to keep the patient euvolemic. Daily measurements of supine and standing blood pressure and pulse, examination of the mucous membranes, skin turgor, examination of the lungs for pulmonary congestion, examination for edema, daily weight, and daily intake and output records are important to assess volume status. In the setting of the intensive care unit, clinical assessment of volume status may be difficult in the presence of surgical wounds, severe pneumonia, or edema caused by capillary leak. Consequently, invasive monitoring, such as central venous pressure or pulmonary capillary wedge pressure monitoring, may be necessary to precisely evaluate volume status.

In addition to urine losses, water losses occur from diffusion and evaporation through the skin and expired water vapor. These losses normally amount to 0.5 to 0.6 mL/kg body weight per hour, or approximately 850 to 1000 mL per day in a 70-kg afebrile resting adult. With fever, insensible water loss increases by approximately 13% for each degree centigrade rise above normal (7% for each degree Fahrenheit). Because insensible loss cannot be determined accurately, daily assessment and modification

TABLE 5 Prevention of Acute Renal Failure in Specific Situations

Tumor Lysis Syndrome

Allopurinol (Zyloprim): 300-600 mg/d starting three days prior to chemotherapy
Forced diuresis: Intravenous normal saline to maintain urine output of more than 5 L/d
Urinary alkalinization: 100 mEq/m^2/d sodium bicarbonate with intravenous fluid to keep urinary pH >7
Intravenous acetazolamide 1 g/m^2 can be used along with sodium bicarbonate; avoid significant metabolic alkalosis

Rhabdomyolysis

Correct intravascular volume depletion: Infuse normal saline as determined by the severity of volume depletion; infuse 200 to 300 mL/h; follow hemodynamics with invasive monitoring when indicated
Alkalinization of urine and use of mannitol: Add 2 ampules of mannitol (25 g in 100 mL) and 2 ampules of sodium bicarbonate (100 mEq in 100 mL), to 800 mL of 5% D_5W (dextrose 5% in water solution) and infuse at a rate of 250 mL/h; if urine output is good, continue infusion until myoglobinuria resolves. If the patient continues to be oliguric, stop fluids and treat as established renal failure

Contrast Media

Hydration: Infuse normal saline 1 mL/kg/h, starting 8 hours prior to procedure
Contrast media: Limit amount of contrast media; iso-osmolar media (iodixanol [Visipaque]) is preferred
Pharmacologic agent: Benefit of *N*-acetylcysteine (Mucomyst)[1] 600 mg twice a day (1 day prior and on the day of procedure) is questionable

[1]Not FDA approved for this indication.

TABLE 6 Daily Assessment of Patients with Acute Renal Failure

Variable	Comments
Weight	Aim for a daily weight loss of 0.5 to 1.0 lb in patients with ATN to prevent fluid retention
JVD, basal crackles	Indicate volume overload or congestive heart failure; restrict volume and consider diuretics or dialysis when indicated
CVP and PCWP	May be indicated in the differential diagnosis of volume overload versus noncardiogenic pulmonary infiltrates; low PCWP (<10) suggests noncardiogenic pulmonary edema (e.g., ARDS)
Intake/output	In euvolemic patients, give the previous day's urine output volume plus 400 mL for insensible loss in stable patients
BUN	When disproportionately high, look for GI bleeding, medications such as steroids, or catabolic states such as sepsis
Serum sodium	Reflects body water status, hyponatremia suggests excess water intake in the face of impaired free water clearance by the kidney
Serum potassium	Hyperkalemia disproportionate to the renal failure suggests tumor lysis or catabolic states such as sepsis; in severe hyperkalemia, electrocardiogram is a better guide for therapy
Total CO_2	Decreases by 1 to 2 mEq/d, stabilizes at 16 to 18 mEq/L, and generally no treatment is required; in case of more severe acidosis, look for other causes such as lactic acidosis, ketoacidosis, or toxin ingestion
Serum calcium	Hypocalcemia is usually asymptomatic and requires no treatment; in hypercalcemia look for hyperparathyroidism or underlying malignancy

Abbreviations: ARDS = acute respiratory distress syndrome; BUN = blood urea nitrogen; CO_2 = carbon dioxide; CVP = central venous pressure; GI = gastrointestinal; JVD = jugular vein distension; PCWP = pulmonary capillary wedge pressure.

of fluid therapy are essential. Water is also continuously generated from endogenous sources by the oxidation of protein (41 mL/100 g), fat (107 mL/100 g), and carbohydrate (55 mL/100 g). Without carbohydrate supplementation, a 70-kg man burns 1 g of protein and 2 g of fat per kilogram of body weight, with the generation of 0.25 to 0.35 mL/kg per hour or approximately 450 mL of water. The addition of 100 g of carbohydrate reduces protein metabolism by 50%, with a small but significant decrease in water generation. Additional carbohydrate will not further reduce protein catabolism. Thus, to balance the difference between insensible water loss and endogenous water production in an afebrile 70-kg man, daily water intake must be limited to 400 mL plus an amount equal to that passed in urine. In hypercatabolic states, such as may occur with severe infections, trauma, or surgery, more water may be generated by enhanced protein and fat catabolism. In the patient maintained with intravenous fluids without protein or fat administration, the physician should target small daily weight losses of 0.2 to 0.3 kg to prevent fluid retention. Patients with evidence of volume depletion should be provided with additional fluid to maintain euvolemia because sustained hypovolemia may delay recovery.

HYPERNATREMIA AND HYPONATREMIA

Abnormal serum sodium concentrations are caused by disorders of water metabolism. Hyponatremia resulting from an excess water intake in the presence of impairment of free water clearance is very common in acute renal failure. Sources for excess water intake that lead to hyponatremia include hypotonic solutions given as 5% dextrose, parenteral medications administered in 5% dextrose, or excess intake of free water with enteral or parenteral feeding. Hypernatremia is uncommon and is usually caused by inappropriate administration of intravenous fluids.

POTASSIUM BALANCE

Hyperkalemia is one of the most serious consequences of acute renal failure, and steps should be taken to prevent hyperkalemia in patients with acute renal failure by potassium intake restriction in the diet to less than 50 mEq per day (Table 7). Cardiac toxicity is the most threatening problem and the electromechanical effects of hyperkalemia on the heart are potentiated by hypocalcemia, acidosis, and hyponatremia. Thus, the ECG, which measures the summation of these effects, is a better guide to therapy than a single K^+ determination. The earliest change is the appearance of a peaked T wave followed by shortening of the QT interval. Later, the P wave may become flat and disappear. The QRS complex becomes wide, followed by ventricular arrhythmia or arrest. The treatment of hyperkalemia depends on the urgency and severity of the problem. In patients with hyperkalemia associated with EKG changes, intravenous calcium infusion in the form of calcium chloride or calcium gluconate immediately antagonizes the

TABLE 7 Prevention of Hyperkalemia in Patients with Acute Renal Failure

Restriction of potassium intake
Omit potassium from parenteral fluids and total parenteral nutrition
Discontinue drugs containing potassium (e.g., penicillin G)
Avoid salt substitutes that contain potassium
Discontinue medications that inhibit potassium excretion
Potassium-sparing diuretics
Nonsteroidal anti-inflammatory drugs
Angiotensin-converting enzyme inhibitors

effect of the potassium on the heart. Potassium can be redistributed from the extracellular to the intracellular space by the administration of insulin and glucose, inhaled or intravenous β-adrenergic receptor agonists, or intravenous sodium bicarbonate. These measures require 30 to 60 minutes before they affect serum potassium and the duration of action is short-lived. Removal of potassium from the body is achieved by the use of cation exchange resin sodium polystyrene sulfonate (Kayexalate), which may be administered orally or rectally. Hyperkalemia that cannot be easily controlled by conservative means is an indication for dialysis.

ACID–BASE HOMEOSTASIS

An individual weighing 70 kg on a normal American diet will produce about 60 to 80 mEq of acid daily that is normally excreted by the kidney to maintain acid–base homeostasis. In patients with acute renal failure, the serum bicarbonate decreases by 1 to 2 mEq per day and stabilizes at about 16 to 8 mEq/L and does not require treatment except as an adjuvant treatment for hyperkalemia. A more rapid or a severe drop is a result of either a very catabolic state related to the underlying disease leading to acute renal failure, infection, or inadequate nutrition. In such patients it is also important to exclude other causes of acidosis, such as lactic acidosis, ketoacidosis, or drug overdose, before it is attributed to acute renal failure. In patients with acute renal failure, dietary protein restriction slows the development of acidosis because acid is generated from protein metabolism. Adequate nonprotein calories must be provided to avoid a catabolic state and should be assessed carefully with the assistance of a dietitian. In the few patients who require the correction of acidosis, sodium bicarbonate can be administered orally or parenterally, depending on the urgency for replacement and the degree of acidosis. Parenteral sodium bicarbonate should be administered in isotonic solution by adding 3 ampules of sodium bicarbonate (50 mEq/50 mL) to 1 L of 5% dextrose in water. Acetate can be added to parenteral nutrition and adjusted to maintain acid–base homeostasis. The disadvantage of sodium bicarbonate or acetate is worsening of volume overload.

CALCIUM AND PHOSPHATE BALANCE

A reduction in the serum calcium concentration is commonly found in patients with acute renal failure and may be particularly severe with rhabdomyolysis and hyperphosphatemia. Hypocalcemia may worsen the cardiac toxicity of hyperkalemia as mentioned above. Hypomagnesemia inhibits synthesis and release of parathyroid hormone and functional hypoparathyroidism may contribute to hypocalcemia. In most patients, hypocalcemia is asymptomatic and does not require specific treatment. Hypercalcemia may occur in the recovery phase of acute renal failure in patients with rhabdomyolysis and generally requires no treatment.

Hyperphosphatemia occurs commonly in acute renal failure but is most severe in tumor lysis syndrome and rhabdomyolysis. Hyperphosphatemia may contribute to secondary hyperparathyroidism and may cause metastatic calcification; consequently, treatment should be given with phosphate binders. Treatment should be given with calcium carbonate (Tums) 0.5 to 1 g with meals or sevelamer (Renagel) 800 to 1600 mg with meals. If calcium phosphate product is high (>70), it is preferable to use sevelamer. Hypophosphatemia is unusual in acute renal failure and is encountered most commonly in patients with burns, patients with a history of alcohol abuse, and some patients on hyperalimentation. Severe hypophosphatemia may affect several organ systems and should be corrected either orally or parenterally.

Hypermagnesemia is common in patients with acute renal failure. High levels occur in patients given magnesium-containing antacids or laxatives. Magnesium can be removed by dialysis. Hyperuricemia is usually modest and has no clinical consequences, and no treatment is usually required. The only exceptions are conditions associated with uric acid nephropathy, such as tumor lysis syndrome, in which case the uric acid levels should be lowered by using hemodialysis.

Nutritional Therapy

Although previous studies suggest that treatment with glucose and essential and nonessential amino acids, as compared with glucose alone or no nutrition, may improve the nutritional status and possible survival, these reports are not conclusive. Nonetheless, a minimum goal of nutritional support is to minimize the catabolic state, and it appears prudent to administer sufficient oral or parenteral nutrition to attain the most optimal nutritional status. The need for nutritional therapy may be particularly important for patients who are wasted or very catabolic. Patients not in hypercatabolic state need protein or amino acids of 0.65 to 1 g/kg per day. Patients on dialysis and in hypercatabolic state need a protein intake of 1.2 to 1.5 g per day. Daily recommended energy intake is 30 to 35 kcal/kg per day. For patients able to receive nutrition by eating, enteral tubes, or gastrostomy, administration of nutrition by these routes is preferred to intravenous administration. Parenteral nutrition is more hazardous, provides greater fluid loads, and is more costly. If oral feeding is not possible, it is reasonable to limit treatment to intravenous fluids for 3 to 5 days. For patients unable to tolerate enteral nutrition for more than 3 to 5 days, total parenteral nutrition should be considered. Adequate supplementation of water-soluble vitamins, trace metals, and folic acid must be provided with all dietary regimens.

Pharmacologic Therapy in Acute Renal Failure

DIURETICS

Whether use of diuretics in acute renal failure affects the outcome favorably is controversial. In fact, recent literature suggests a worse outcome with diuretic use in patients with ARF. Routine use of diuretics in patients with ARF is not recommended. However, patients with evidence of volume overload may warrant a therapeutic trial with diuretics. Furosemide (Lasix) is the most commonly used loop diuretic in patients with acute renal failure. A higher dose in the range of 2 to 10 mg/kg per day intravenously may be required. A maximum single dose of 200 to 250 mg should be given over 20 to 30 minutes to avoid ototoxicity. Continuous infusion of bumetanide (Bumex) produced more sodium excretion and less toxicity than bolus bumetanide. Therefore, continuous infusion should be considered when response to bolus administration is not adequate. Diuretics may convert oliguria to nonoliguric ARF, which makes patient management easier. However, there is no evidence that this is effective in reducing mortality or the need for dialysis.

MANNITOL

Mannitol is an osmotic diuretic and has been used in the prophylaxis and treatment of acute renal failure with the rationale that it prevents cell swelling and decreases intratubular obstruction. Mannitol can be used in conjunction with volume replacement and sodium bicarbonate to prevent acute renal failure related to myoglobinuria and crush syndrome. Mannitol itself can cause acute renal failure and volume overload and routine use is not recommended to prevent or treat acute renal failure.

DOPAMINE (INTROPIN)

Low-dose dopamine (0.5 to 3 μg/kg per minute) dilates renal arterioles and increases renal blood flow and the glomerular filtration rate. Although commonly prescribed, the role of dopamine in the management of acute renal failure is controversial for both the prevention and treatment of acute renal failure. Proponents of dopamine recommend a trial of low-dose dopamine, 1 to 3 μ/kg per minute, in a subset of euvolemic patients with oliguric acute renal failure and believe that dopamine may help to convert oliguric to nonoliguric acute renal failure. The major side effects of dopamine are tachyarrhythmias, pulmonary shunting, and gut and digital necrosis. Fenoldopam (Corlopam)[1], a selective dopamine-1 receptor agonist, also failed to show a beneficial effect in patients undergoing cardiac catheterization in a multicenter trial.

[1]Not FDA approved for this indication.

Conservative Management of Organ System Complications

Extrarenal manifestations of acute renal failure are generally similar to those found in chronic renal failure. Many of the manifestations are the result of volume and electrolyte abnormalities. However, some of these complications are secondary to uremia and may require replacement therapy. Table 8 summarizes the major complications associated with ARF.

INFECTIOUS COMPLICATIONS

Infection is frequently associated with acute renal failure and is a major cause of increased morbidity and mortality. The most common sites for infections include pulmonary, urinary tract, surgical wounds, and peritoneum. Infections related to indwelling venous and arterial catheters can also occur. Because meticulous attention to prevention of infection is crucial, urine catheters should be removed as soon as possible. Similarly, parenteral sites and surgical wounds require extraordinary care in patients with acute ARF. Early recognition and appropriate antibiotic therapy for infections is important in improving the outcome of these patients. The dosage of antibiotics should be adjusted to the degree of renal function.

TABLE 8 Major Complications of Acute Renal Failure

Parameter	Complications
Impairments of Fluid and Electrolyte Excretion	
Water	Hyponatremia
Sodium chloride	Volume expansion Congestive heart failure
Potassium	Hyperkalemia Arrhythmias Muscle weakness
Hydrogen ion	Metabolic acidosis
Phosphate	Hyperphosphatemia Hypocalcemia Metabolic calcification
Magnesium	Hypermagnesemia
Uric acid	Hyperuricemia
Retention of Urea and Other Solutes	Cardiac: uremic pericarditis Neurologic: asterixis, confusion, somnolence, coma, seizures Hematologic: anemia, coagulopathy, bleeding diathesis Infection Gastrointestinal: nausea, vomiting, gastritis, bleeding Skin, pruritus Glucose intolerance
Synthetic Impairment	
1,25-Dihydroxyvitamin D_3	Hypocalcemia
Erythropoietin	Anemia
Impaired Drug Metabolism and Excretion	Drug toxicity, decreased diuretic effectiveness

GASTROINTESTINAL COMPLICATIONS

The major gastrointestinal complications of ARF include symptoms of anorexia and vomiting and upper gastrointestinal bleeding. Gastrointestinal bleeding may be particularly serious in a postoperative or post-traumatic setting. Stress ulcers and gastritis are common and can be prevented by the use of antacids or proton pump inhibitors. Magnesium-containing antacids should be avoided to prevent hypermagnesemia. An increase in serum amylase level may be observed in these patients as amylase is cleared by the kidney. Thus, lipase determination and clinical assessment are often necessary to diagnose acute pancreatitis in the setting of acute renal failure.

CARDIOVASCULAR AND PULMONARY COMPLICATIONS

Cardiovascular problems such as arrhythmia, pulmonary edema, and hypertension are attributable to fluid overload and electrolyte abnormalities. In elderly patients (>70 years of age) there is increased death from myocardial infarction. Uremic pericarditis may rarely complicate the course of acute renal failure. The pericarditis usually resolves with intensive dialysis. If pericardial effusion is present and hemodynamically significant, pericardiocentesis may be required. Pericardial tamponade may not present with the classical clinical findings; therefore, it should be suspected in patients with unexplained hypotension. Pulmonary complications include infection, infiltrates, or hemorrhage associated with rapidly progressive glomerulonephritis. The presence of pulmonary complications adversely affects the prognosis of acute renal failure.

BLEEDING ABNORMALITIES

The most common cause of bleeding abnormalities in acute renal failure is caused by platelet dysfunction associated with prolonged bleeding time. Dialysis usually corrects the disorder. If the bleeding tendency is not corrected or the patient is actively bleeding, the infusion of 10 units of cryoprecipitate, or 1-deamino-8-D-arginine vasopressin (DDAVP)[1] 0.3 μ/kg intravenously can correct the bleeding time abnormality.

ANEMIA

Anemia may occur early in acute renal failure secondary to blood loss, increased hemolysis, or decreased erythropoietin level that occurs rapidly after the onset of acute renal failure. In most patients, asymptomatic anemia does not need treatment. However, patients with coronary heart failure, symptomatic coronary artery disease, or hypoxia may require treatment with blood transfusion. The role of parenteral erythropoietin (Epogen)[1] is not clear but may be useful in prolonged acute renal failure.

[1]Not FDA approved for this indication.

NEUROMUSCULAR COMPLICATIONS

Neuromuscular symptoms such as asterixis, irritability, somnolence, stupor, and coma are found early in the course of acute renal failure and are caused by electrolyte abnormalities such as hypernatremia and hyponatremia, hypocalcemia and hypercalcemia, and hypophosphatemia. Late in the course of the disease, the symptoms are usually a result of uremia. The aim of management is to correct electrolyte abnormalities and uremia by conservative management or dialysis when indicated.

Dialysis Therapy in Acute Renal Failure

Indications for the commencement of renal replacement therapy include diuretic unresponsive volume overload, severe hyperkalemia and metabolic acidosis refractory to conservative measures, uremic pericarditis, and uremic encephalopathy. In addition, most nephrologists initiate dialysis when the BUN reaches approximately 100 mg/dL.

The choice of renal replacement therapy in acute renal failure depends on the patient's circumstances. The main aim of dialysis in patients with ARF is to restore normal electrolytes and acid–base balance, and to remove excess fluid. Intermittent hemodialysis can achieve these goals in hemodynamically stable patients. Most patients typically undergo acute intermittent hemodialysis for 3 to 4 hours daily or on alternate days. Benefits of daily versus intermittent dialysis in the setting of ARF in the ICU are currently under investigation.

There are different methods for continuous renal replacement therapy (CRRT) for hemodynamically unstable patients. Because the process is gradual over a long period, hemodynamic stability can be maintained even if the patient has low blood pressure. Despite the theoretical advantages of CRRT in patients with ARF, there are no controlled studies that show superiority of this technique compared with intermittent hemodialysis or peritoneal dialysis. Recently, hybrid techniques for hemodialysis (slow low-efficiency dialysis [SLED]/daily extended dialysis) in critically ill patients were introduced using standard intermittent hemodialysis equipment but having therapeutic aims in common with CRRT. Typically, dialysis is prescribed for 8 to 12 hours and initial reports suggest that most patients tolerate it well.

There are no studies to indicate the optimal dose of dialysis in patients with acute renal failure and whether early dialysis influences the outcome in ARF. Until such studies are available, the choice of dialysis modality and dose are dependent on individual patient circumstances and local preferences (Table 9).

[1]Not FDA approved for this indication.

TABLE 9 Advantages and Disadvantages of Renal Replacement Therapy

Intermittent Hemodialysis
Advantages
More efficient for solute removal
Short duration
May be performed without heparin
Less complex and rapidly available
No need to train ICU staff
Disadvantages
Large shift in fluid and electrolytes
Risk of cardiac arrhythmias
High incidence of hypotension
Disequilibrium syndrome may occur
Continuous Renal Replacement Therapy (CRRT)
Advantages
Removal of large volumes of fluid
Hemodynamic stability
Permit unlimited nutrition
Removal of larger molecular weight solutes
Disadvantages
Need for anticoagulation
Need training for ICU staff
Prolonged use and may be interrupted by tests
Needs careful follow-up of replacement fluid
Slow, Low-Efficiency Dialysis/Daily Extended Dialysis
Advantages
Short duration compared with CRRT (allows time for out of ICU procedures)
Less complex
Relatively more efficient for solute removal
Hemodynamic stability
Disadvantages
Need for anticoagulation
Need training for ICU staff
Peritoneal Dialysis
Advantages
Hemodynamic stability
No anticoagulation needed
Ability to remove volume easily
Disadvantages
Need surgical insertion of Tenckhoff or acute catheter
Risk of bowel perforation
Technical drainage problems
Risk for peritonitis and exit-site infection

CHRONIC KIDNEY DISEASE

METHOD OF

Todd W.B. Gehr, MD

The term *chronic kidney disease* is the preferred expression to describe patients with all forms of renal disease that progress over an extended period of time, usually months to years. The formerly used terms, chronic renal insufficiency and chronic renal failure, are no longer preferred.

The normal glomerular filtration rate (GFR) averages approximately 130 mL/min/1.7 m^2 in males and 120 mL/min/1.73 m^2 in females. Estimation or direct assessment of GFR remains one of the most important measurements of renal function and is widely used in clinical practice. These normal values of GFR apply to individuals from the teenage years through approximately 35 years of age. Thereafter, GFR declines in most individuals. Whereas the decline was formerly thought to occur at a relatively constant rate of approximately 10 mL per minute per decade, more recent data, obtained in a longitudinal fashion, indicate that this reduction is not so predictable.

The endogenous creatinine clearance (C_{cr}) enjoys widespread use as a reasonable gauge of GFR when great precision is not demanded, which it rarely is in clinical practice. The use of creatinine as a marker of GFR has the advantage that creatinine is endogenously produced and is easily measured by inexpensive methods. Creatinine is freely filtered and not appreciably absorbed. However, creatinine is secreted, and the contribution of secretion to total excretion is greater as the GFR decreases and serum creatinine rises. At GFRs below 40 mL per minute, C_{cr} exceeds inulin clearance, the gold standard, by 50% to 100%. Because cimetidine (Tagamet) competes with creatinine for tubular secretion, administration of cimetidine may increase the accuracy both of C_{cr} in 24-hour collections and of 4-hour, water-loaded clearances. Cimetidine can be administered as a loading dose of 400 mg followed by a dose of 200 mg every 3 hours for the duration of the clearance period.

As a consequence of the practical and technical problems regarding obtaining estimates of GFR by clearance methods, renal function is most commonly estimated by following serum creatinine concentration (SCr). Creatinine is formed nonezymatically from creatine and phosphocreatine in muscle cells and is normally present in the serum at a concentration of 0.8 to 1.4 mg/dL. Because creatinine production is closely related to muscle mass, SCr is generally less in females than in males, and decreases as muscle mass is lost with aging or with debilitating illnesses. The relationship between SCr and C_{cr} can be described by a rectangular hyperbola; however, this relationship applies in the steady state and assumes a constant rate of creatinine production. Thus, a doubling of the SCr reflects a 50% decrease in C_{cr}; a fourfold increase in SCr, reflects a 75% drop in GFR, and so on. It should be appreciated that SCr is an insensitive marker of change early in the course of renal disease. Thus, a 33% fall in GFR may raise the SCr from 0.8 to 1.2 mg/dL, a value that is still within the normal range. If the prior value is not known, this fall in GFR may go unrecognized.

A variety of equations were developed to estimate C_{cr} based on the SCr without collection of urine. These equations generally take into consideration muscle mass (estimated as body weight), sex (males having a higher GFR than females), and age. A commonly used equation is that developed by Crockcroft and Gault:

$$C_{cr} = (140 - \text{age}) \times \text{lean weight in kg}/(72 \times \text{SCr}) \; (\times 0.85 \text{ for females})$$

where age is expressed in years. The reliability of this equation as a measure of GFR has been assessed in a variety of patient groups and these studies show that the accuracy of GFR estimates using this equation is similar to, or greater than, 24-hour C_{cr} and the precision is better. A more accurate estimate of GFR which does not rely on the subject's weight comes from the Modification of Diet in Renal Disease (MDRD) formula and this formula, shown below, is gaining favor for routine use.

$$\text{GFR (mL per minute/} \times 1.73 \text{ m}^2) = 186 \times (\text{SCr})^{-1.154} \times (\text{age})^{-0.203} \times (0.742, \text{ if female}) \times (1.210, \text{ if African-American})$$

No matter what method is employed to either measure or estimate GFR, chronic kidney disease (CKD) is then staged based on this value. The staging system helps to direct the care of these patients. Table 1 depicts this staging system for CKD.

Risk Factors That Predict Progression of CKD

Renal disease often progresses in an inexorable fashion. The hypothesis evoked to explain this is known as the *common pathway theory*. Renal injury resulting in a reduction in nephron mass leads to glomerular hypertension in the remaining nephrons with subsequent increases in glomerular permeability. These factors lead to increased delivery of plasma proteins to the tubular fluid and these proteins evoke an inflammatory response causing tubulointerstitial nephritis, renal scarring, and a vicious cycle of more glomerular capillary hypertension. This process follows a predictable course in individual patients, leading to a reduction in GFR and eventual end-stage renal disease (ESRD). Predicting this decline can be accomplished by measuring changes in the relationship between 1/SCr versus time. Individual patients usually have a fairly constant rate of decline and this rate of decline can be used to predict when a particular patient might reach a particular GFR. Straying away from this constant rate of decline can also be used to predict other more acute factors which might accelerate this decline.

TABLE 1 Stages of Chronic Kidney Disease

Stage	Description	GFR (mL/min/1.73 m²)
1	Chronic kidney damage with normal or increased GFR	>90
2	Mild	60-89
3	Moderate	30-59
4	Severe	15-29
5	Kidney failure	<15 or dialysis

Abbreviation: GFR = glomerular filtration rate.

TABLE 2 Risk Factors for Chronic Kidney Disease Progression

African American, Hispanic race
Diabetes mellitus
Dyslipidemia
High-protein diet
Hypertension
Male sex
Metabolic acidosis
Obesity
Phosphate retention
Proteinuria
Smoking
Type of underlying kidney disease

A number of risk factors have been identified that are important in CKD progression. Table 2 highlights these factors, some of which are modifiable, such as smoking, and some of which are not, such as sex and race. Besides the SCr, the single most useful test employed to predict progressive CKD is the determination of urinary protein excretion. A quantitative protein-to-creatinine ratio in a single voided urine sample closely correlates with 24-hour protein excretion and predicts GFR decline and risk of progression to ESRD. A urinary protein-to-creatinine ratio greater than 1.0 distinguishes progressors from nonprogressors. Another important clinical variable that can predict progression is hypertension. It has been established that the rate of CKD progression can be slowed by strict control of blood pressure.

Treatment of CKD Progression

Treatment of CKD progression has several goals: prevention of additional kidney damage by the underlying disease, slowing the progression of CKD, and preventing complications associated with CKD. Following the institution of specific therapies for the large variety of diseases that cause CKD, therapy is then chosen to slow the progression of CKD in a non–disease-specific manner. These therapies, delineated in Table 3, slow the progression of disease, although none are successful in completely stopping disease progression.

Strict blood pressure control—to less than 135/85 mm Hg in patients without proteinuria, to 130/80 mm Hg in those with proteinuria from 0.25 to 1 g per 24 hours, and to 125/75 mm Hg in those with urinary protein excretion greater than 1 g per day—slows the progression of diabetic and nondiabetic renal disease. It appears that attaining these blood pressure goals results in a reduction in urinary protein excretion regardless of antihypertensive therapy employed.

TABLE 3 Measures Employed to Slow the Progression of Chronic Kidney Disease

Blood pressure control
<135/85 without proteinuria
<125/75 with protein excretion >1 g per day
Angiotensin-converting enzyme inhibitors
Angiotensin receptor blockers
Nonhydropyridine calcium channel blockers
Glycemic control
Treatment of dyslipidemia
Dietary protein restriction
Treatment of anemia

Antihypertensive therapies that decrease proteinuria slow CKD progression although, as mentioned above, it is sometimes difficult to separate the benefit of blood pressure reduction from specific drug effects. It appears, however, that angiotensin-converting enzyme (ACE) inhibitors are more renoprotective than other antihypertensives at similar blood pressure control. It has been more than 10 years since captopril (Capoten) was shown to preserve renal function better than conventional antihypertensives in insulin-dependent diabetics. Ramipril (Altace) has also been shown to preserve renal function in both proteinuric and nonproteinuric CKD. More recently, angiotensin-receptor antagonists employed in type 2 diabetes have been shown to preserve renal function, with results similar to those obtained with ACE inhibitors. With both classes of the drug, GFR falls with the attendant antiproteinuric effects and may be responsible for the beneficial effect. A slight increase in SCr, usually less than 30%, is expected, although a greater increase in SCr may indicate underlying congestive heart failure (CHF), renovascular disease, or dehydration. Even patients with advanced CKD benefit from ACE inhibitors, although care must be exercised to avoid hyperkalemia.

Other therapies directed at preserving renal function have less clear-cut benefits. Strict blood sugar control in diabetes, as shown in the U.K. Prospective Diabetes Trial, decreases the incidence of microvascular complications. Management of hyperlipidemia is probably of benefit although few studies have specifically examined this issue. The treatment of hyperlipidemia with "statins" is not without risk because these drugs can cause rhabdomyolysis and acute renal failure. Finally, dietary protein restriction may be of benefit, although the large prospective trial examining this issue, the MDRD study, was inconclusive. It seems prudent to recommend a protein intake of no more than 1.0 g/kg per day, although malnutrition is important to recognize, prevent, and treat in the setting of CKD.

Diagnosis of CKD

When a patient presents with either a reduction in their GFR and/or an abnormal urinary sediment that suggests renal disease, such as proteinuria, the first objective is to sort out whether the patient has a chronic process (CKD) or has an acute process (acute renal failure [ARF]). A previous SCr or urinalysis is of obvious benefit in making this determination. If unavailable, the presence of small kidneys, the anemia of chronic disease, and the presence of renal osteodystrophy on routine x-ray point to CKD. Unfortunately, the absence of these findings does not eliminate the possibility of CKD. Kidney size is often maintained in diseases such as diabetes and amyloidosis. Anemia is often not present in autosomal dominant polycystic kidney disease, and bone disease is often a late manifestation of CKD.

Although the most common causes of CKD are diabetes and hypertension, multiple diseases can lead to CKD. Similar to the diagnostic strategy employed in the evaluation of ARF, causes of CKD can also be categorized in anatomic terms: glomerular and vascular disease, tubulointerstitial disease, cystic disease, and obstruction of the lower urinary tract. The urinary sediment, particularly the presence of proteinuria, casts, and hematuria, is very helpful in sorting out the many possibilities.

Glomerular diseases, including diabetic nephropathy, represent a diverse group of diseases that may be confined to the kidney, but often are manifestations of systemic disease. The presence of proteinuria is the most important clue for the presence of these diseases. Nephrotic syndrome is defined by a protein excretion of >3.5 g per day, whereas nephritic syndrome is associated with lesser degrees of proteinuria, but by a more active-appearing urinary sediment (red blood cell [RBC], white blood cell [WBC], RBC casts, etc.). Nephritic syndromes usually entail significant inflammation within the kidney and are usually more damaging to the kidney over a shorter period of time.

In the United States, diabetic nephropathy is the most common cause of nephrotic syndrome. It occurs in both type 1 and type 2 diabetes mellitus, and is the leading cause of ESRD. Diabetic nephropathy has a predictable course that starts with the onset of microalbuminuria (30 to 300 mg/g creatinine), progresses to frank proteinuria, and progresses, eventually, to nephrotic syndrome. The onset of proteinuria always precedes the decline in renal function. In the patient with type 1 diabetes, nephropathy usually occurs after 15 to 25 years of the disease. The onset of nephropathy in the type 2 diabetic is unpredictable, but occurs earlier in the course of the disease. Hypertension is a common manifestation of diabetic nephropathy, particularly in the type 2 diabetic. Once nephrotic syndrome occurs, there is a relentless course toward ESRD.

Other causes of nephrotic syndrome are important as they are often manifestations of underlying concomitant disease. Membranous nephropathy is the most common of these and may be idiopathic or a result of infections such as hepatitis B, rheumatologic diseases such as systemic lupus erythematosus, and carcinomas, particularly solid tumors of the gastrointestinal (GI) tract. Focal segmental glomerulosclerosis is also common, particularly in African Americans, and may be idiopathic or secondary to chronic reflux nephropathy, HIV nephropathy, obesity, or intravenous (IV) drug abuse. Minimal change nephropathy, which usually occurs in children, is either idiopathic or secondary to nonsteroidal anti-inflammatory drug (NSAID) use or Hodgkin's disease. Minimal change nephropathy is the most treatable of these causes of nephrotic syndrome. Finally, amyloidosis is increasingly seen and is caused by multiple myeloma or chronic inflammation as a consequence of rheumatoid arthritis, osteomyelitis, or chronic skin infections.

Nephritic causes of CKD are characterized by an active urinary sediment, varying amounts of proteinuria, and usually a more rapid decline in renal function. Vasculitides, such as polyarteritis nodosa, Wegener's granulomatosis, scleroderma, and malignant hypertension, usually have dramatic presentations. The presence of pulmonary, GI, skin, or multiorgan involvement is suggestive of vasculitis. A kidney biopsy is usually necessary to establish the diagnosis although serology may be very helpful. Antineutrophil cytoplasmic antibodies (perinuclear [p-ANCA] and cytoplasmic [c-ANCA]) are particularly helpful in defining the type of vasculitis. Proliferative glomerular diseases also represent a diverse group of diseases such as antiglomerular basement membrane disease (Goodpasture's syndrome when accompanied by pulmonary involvement), postinfectious glomerulonephritis (GN), and lupus nephritis. Hypocomplementemia is present in lupus and postinfectious GN, whereas complements are usually normal in antiglomerular basement membrane GN. Focal proliferative GNs can be idiopathic or be associated with lupus. Membranoproliferative GNs are also hypocomplementemic and most commonly associated with the cryoglobulinemia associated with hepatitis C infection. Hemolytic uremic syndrome in children and thrombotic thrombocytopenic purpura (TTP) in adults cause a necrotizing GN. TTP is associated with bleomycin therapy, calcineurin inhibitor use in transplantation, and AIDS. A common glomerular disease worldwide is IgA nephropathy. In the United States, it is relatively benign, usually presenting in adolescent males. Gross hematuria associated with an upper respiratory infection and normal renal function is the most common manifestation. This same disease can also be a manifestation of Henoch-Schönlein purpura occurring in children. Alport's syndrome and thin basement membrane disease are genetic diseases, often sex-linked, involving abnormal type IV collagen. Although the penetrance can be highly variable, the association of renal failure, hearing loss, and lens ectopia are hallmarks of the syndrome.

Tubulointerstitial diseases of the kidney are less-common causes of CKD, especially with the advent of effective antibiotic therapy used to treat pyelonephritis. Analgesic nephropathy, however, represents a underdiagnosed cause of CKD. It is usually associated with the use of large doses of combination analgesics, particularly combinations containing phenacetin, the precursor of acetaminophen. One recent report in ESRD patients shows a relationship with acetaminophen (Tylenol) use, however. Lithium (Eskalith), lead, and other heavy metals are implicated in this disorder, as is myeloma light-chain disease. Finally, some degree of tubulointerstitial inflammation often accompanies glomerular and/or vascular diseases such as focal and segmental glomerulosclerosis and hypertension. Albuminuria may in and of itself elicit an inflammatory reaction, which may hasten the development of CKD.

Cystic diseases of the kidney are common causes of CKD. Autosomal dominant polycystic disease (ADPKD) is the most prevalent of the inherited polycystic kidney diseases, occurring in between 1 in 400 and 1 in 1000 Americans. Mutations of either of two genes, PKD-1 on chromosome 16 or PKD-2 on chromosome 4, cause the disease. ADPKD is characterized by a progressive replacement of the normal renal parenchyma with large cysts, and the majority of affected individuals will progress to ESRD. Clinical manifestations are often complex with hypertension, hematuria, nephrolithiasis, and back pain commonly occurring. Extrarenal manifestations include liver cysts, aneurysms, particularly of the cerebral circulation, and cardiac valvular abnormalities.

Finally, urinary tract obstruction represents a preventable cause of CKD and should always be considered in the differential diagnosis of any patient with unexplained CKD. Causes can be categorized as intrinsic, arising within the urinary tract or extrinsic, arising outside the urinary tract. Intrinsic causes range from intraluminal precipitation of Bence Jones proteins, medications, or stones to intramural involvement by tumors or infectious processes involving the renal pelvis, ureter, bladder, or urethra. Functional disorders associated with diabetes mellitus, multiple sclerosis, or spinal cord injury can also cause chronic obstruction. Extrinsic causes range from disorders of the female or male reproductive system, such as uterine, ovarian, or prostate cancer, to a variety or gastrointestinal, vascular, or retroperitoneal processes that can lead to compression of the ureters.

Complications of CKD and Treatment of These Complications

Despite severe reductions in GFR occurring in CKD, the kidney is able to adapt surprisingly well to the needs of the body. Only when excessive requirements are imposed on the excretory function of the kidney does decompensation occur. A number of important clinical problems may arise related to water, electrolyte, acid–base, metabolic, and organ-specific disorders.

The ability of the diseased kidney to concentrate and dilute the urine is distinctly abnormal; however, abnormalities in water balance are usually not evident. Patients usually have a normal thirst mechanism, and with appropriate access to fluid will ingest the appropriate amount of water to maintain their serum osmolality. If, however, access to fluid is impaired, then close attention to the fluid prescription is imperative.

Disorders in sodium balance are common in CKD. Sodium retention is the rule with its resulting hypertension, edema, and congestive heart failure. Sodium restricted diets and diuretics are often employed to counter the volume overload encountered in these patients. Rarely, sodium conservation is impaired, leading to volume depletion. Tubulointerstitial diseases may be associated with these salt-wasting states.

Potassium homeostasis is usually maintained until late in the course of CKD. However, hyperkalemia may develop early in the course of CKD in diabetics and in those patients with tubulointerstitial disease. Type 4 renal tubular acidosis (RTA) associated with hyporeninemic hypoaldosteronism, common in diabetics, is associated with hyperkalemia. Increased potassium intake may also overwhelm the normal adaptive mechanisms so patients often require a low-potassium diet. Certain drugs may also be associated with the development of hyperkalemia and include, ACE inhibitors, angiotensin receptor blockers (ARBs), NSAIDs, potassium-sparing diuretics, β blockers, cyclosporine (Sandimmune), and tacrolimus (Prograf). ACE inhibitors and ARBs are sometimes discontinued inappropriately, without employing other methods to treat hyperkalemia. Diuretics, sodium bicarbonate, and sodium polystyrene sulfonate (Kayexalate) can all be used to control potassium homeostasis without discontinuing these other important medications. Although the mineralocorticoid fludrocortisone (Florinef) is sometimes used in patients with hyporenin hypoaldosteronism, care must be exercised in order to avoid fluid overload.

As CKD advances, metabolic acidosis occurs because acid excretion is insufficient to balance the daily endogenous acid production. Typically, the bicarbonate concentration stabilizes between 12 and 20 mEq/L. Bone buffering of the excess acid may exacerbate the bone disease associated with CKD. Chronic metabolic acidosis also leads to muscle breakdown and may contribute to the weight loss and weakness that commonly accompany advanced CKD. The use of alkali therapy is indicated in most patients in order to maintain the bicarbonate concentrate at about 22 mEq/L. Sodium bicarbonate at a daily dose of 0.5 to 1.0 mEq/kg per day is the alkali of choice and is well tolerated. Sodium citrate was commonly used in the past but, when used in conjunction with aluminum-containing phosphate binders, was associated with aluminum toxicity.

Phosphate retention, vitamin D deficiency, and the resulting secondary hyperparathyroidism occur early in progressive CKD. A variety of abnormalities of the bone have been reported, although these abnormalities are most prominent in patients with stage 5 CKD. Osteitis fibrosa cystica (OFS), osteomalacia, and adynamic bone disease may occur at various times in the same patient. OFS is probably the most common disorder, however. High parathyroid hormone concentration can also have a number of untoward effects including cardiac toxicity, extraosseous calcification, pruritus, and is associated with excess mortality. In the early stages of CKD, a phosphate-restricted diet is all that may be necessary to prevent secondary hyperparathyroidism. As CKD progresses, it becomes necessary to decrease phosphate absorption with the use of phosphate binders. Calcium carbonate (Tums) or calcium acetate (PhosLo) are perhaps the most commonly employed binders. Products high in calcium phosphorus may contribute to vascular calcification and the excessive cardiovascular risk of these patients. Therefore, total elemental calcium intake, including binders, should be limited to less than 2000 mg per day. Sevelamer (Renagel), a non–calcium-containing phosphate binder, is often necessary to control serum phosphorus concentrations while limiting calcium intake. As long as phosphate is controlled and calcium is not high, vitamin D is also necessary to treat and prevent secondary hyperparathyroidism. Before starting vitamin D, a serum 25(OH) vitamin D concentration should be measured in order to rule out vitamin D deficiency unrelated to CKD.

Virtually every organ system is adversely affected by advancing CKD (Table 4). Most patients with CKD die of cardiovascular disease. Hypertension and congestive heart failure are almost ubiquitous in this population, with more than 80% of dialysis patients being hypertensive. Left ventricular hypertrophy is present in the majority of these patients, and is exacerbated by anemia. Patients will often go from a state of diastolic dysfunction to one of systolic dysfunction with prolonged burden of hypertension. Coronary artery disease is also common as these patients often exhibit signs of dyslipidemia, chronic inflammation, and thrombotic tendencies. Finally, a late complication of CKD is pericarditis, which presents with a characteristic chest pain and may be accompanied by cardiac tamponade.

Gastrointestinal symptoms are common in CKD with anorexia, nausea, and vomiting, often representing the most prominent symptoms of uremia. With more advanced disease stomatitis, gastritis, and enteritis may be associated with significant blood loss. Peptic ulcer disease occurs in approximately 25% of CKD patients. NSAIDs should be avoided if possible.

Many of the symptoms thought to be related to uremia are actually secondary to the anemia that develops in CKD. The anemia is normocytic and normochromic and is related to the underproduction of red blood cells secondary to reduced erythropoietin production. Complete evaluation of the anemia is

TABLE 4 Major Clinical Abnormalities in Chronic Kidney Disease

Water and Electrolyte Abnormalities
Volume expansion and rarely depletion
Hyperkalemia
Metabolic acidosis
Hyperphosphatemia and hypocalcemia
Cardiovascular Abnormalities
Hypertension
Congestive heart failure
Pericarditis
Arrhythmias
Gastrointestinal Abnormalities
Anorexia, nausea, vomiting
Stomatitis, gastritis, enteritis
Peptic ulcer disease
Bleeding
Hematologic and Immunologic Abnormalities
Normocytic normochromic anemia
Platelet dysfunction
Lymphocytopenia
Increased susceptibility to infection
Neurologic Abnormalities
Headache
Irritability and sleep disorders
Muscle cramps and tremor
Asterixis
Seizures
Peripheral neuropathy
Restless legs
Weakness
Endocrine and Metabolic Abnormalities
Carbohydrate intolerance
Hypertriglyceridemia
Impaired growth
Infertility, sexual dysfunction, amenorrhea
Renal osteodystrophy
Hyperuricemia
Dermatologic Abnormalities
Pruritus
Ecchymoses
Uremic frost

very important since iron deficiency, folate deficiency, and hyperparathyroidism also can aggravate or cause anemia. The management of anemia with the use of recombinant human erythropoietin (Epogen) has dramatically improved the symptomatology associated with CKD. Correction of anemia improves cardiac function, cognitive function, general well-being, and sexual function. A hemoglobin between 11% and 12% is desirable. Higher hemoglobin values are currently not advocated because they may be associated with increased thrombotic events. With the use of recombinant erythropoietin, either oral or intravenous iron is necessary to maintain response. Transferrin saturation of >25% is desirable to assure erythropoietin responsiveness. Ferritin concentrations are often misleading because ferritin is also an acute-phase reactant and is elevated in inflammatory states. Iron can be safely employed as long as the ferritin concentration is <800 mg/dL.

Late in the course of CKD, abnormal bleeding develops as a result of platelet dysfunction. This bleeding tendency often contributes to the increased incidence of gastrointestinal bleeding and contributes to ecchymoses and epistaxis. If bleeding occurs, therapeutic measures may be necessary, including desmopressin (DDAVP)[1], cryoprecipitate, estrogens (Premarin)[1], or dialysis.

Disorders of both the peripheral and the central nervous systems are common with advancing CKD. Apathy, fatigue, impaired memory, and decreased mental capacity are common. With advancing disease mental function deteriorates further progressing from depression, anxiety, and hallucinations to lethargy, stupor, coma, and seizures. Sleep disorders, such as sleep apnea, nightmares, and insomnia, are common. Peripheral neuropathy is usually symmetrical, begins distally, and is dominated by sensory changes such as paresthesias, burning sensations, and pain. Dialysis therapy often controls most of the neurologic complications of CKD.

A variety of metabolic and endocrine disorders accompany CKD. Glucose intolerance develops in most patients and may contribute to the high incidence of diabetes. Insulin clearance is reduced in stage 5 CKD, and reduced insulin doses may be necessary. Lipid abnormalities are also common, with hypertriglyceridemia being the most common. Qualitative alterations in low-density lipoprotein (LDL) levels have also been described. These abnormalities may add to the accelerated atherosclerosis observed in this population.

Protein catabolism with subsequent malnutrition is common in CKD. Indeed, a loss of body weight may be a compelling reason to start renal replacement therapy, even before more significant symptoms occur with CKD. Women may exhibit menstrual disorders as a result of low estrogen and high prolactin levels. Men may have a high incidence of impotence as serum testosterone levels are often low.

Pruritus is practically ubiquitous in CKD. The etiology of pruritus is multifactorial and includes dry skin, secondary hyperparathyroidism, calcium phosphate deposition, anemia, neuropathy, and hypervitaminosis A. Although pruritus is often improved with dialysis, it usually persists. Antihistamines and ultraviolet B (UVB) phototherapy may be effective in controlling this nagging symptom.

Treatment of End-Stage Renal Disease

CKD patients inevitably progress to ESRD and require either dialysis therapy or renal transplantation. Patients who are properly prepared for these options have a reduced mortality and morbidity compared with patients who have had no preparation. Dialysis therapy can be avoided altogether if patients are allowed to explore their transplant options when

[1]Not FDA approved for this indication.

they have stages 3 and 4 CKD. Despite early preparation for renal replacement therapy, a delay in dialysis often occurs as a result of patient and physician reluctance. Most physicians wait for at least mild uremic symptoms to occur, such as nausea, anorexia, and weight loss. Emergent indications for dialysis include hyperkalemia, volume overload, pericarditis, seizures, and severe metabolic acidosis. The early initiations of dialysis may be associated with improved outcomes. Currently, rough guidelines for the initiation of dialysis include a GFR <10 mL per minute for nondiabetics and GFR <15 mL per minute for diabetics.

The exploration by the patient of all options for renal replacement therapy is paramount for them to make their own informed decisions. Transplantation options include cadaveric, living-related, and living-unrelated donor possibilities. The waiting time for cadaveric transplantation often is more than 2 years, so dialysis is usually necessary while the patient waits for the patient's renal transplant. The living-donor option is very attractive and being employed more frequently. Immunosuppressive therapy is not without complications, so patients need to be informed of their risks following transplantation. Despite these risks, transplantation offers a better quality of life and decreased mortality rate compared with patients treated with dialysis.

Once dialysis becomes necessary, patients need to make a choice on the type of dialysis. The types of dialysis include (a) hemodialysis, both in-center hemodialysis and home hemodialysis, and (b) peritoneal dialysis, both continuous ambulatory peritoneal dialysis and continuous cycling or automated peritoneal dialysis. Home hemodialysis usually requires an assistant, although some newer daily hemodialysis techniques may not require an assistant. Peritoneal dialysis is performed at home and does not require an assistant.

The type of dialysis dictates what type of access is necessary to perform the dialysis. An arteriovenous fistula (AVF), placed in the nondominant upper extremity, is the optimal hemodialysis access. Because the AVF takes between 6 and 12 weeks to mature, it should be placed early in stage 4 CKD. This access type has fewer complications, such as infections and thrombosis, and when mature, has a potential to last for the dialysis patient's lifetime. A synthetic arteriovenous graft is necessary if an AVF is not possible, although this type of access often is plagued with complications. Finally, a dual-lumen, tunneled, cuffed catheter may be employed as a bridge to other more permanent access, such as an AVF. These catheters are also used when patients have expended all other access options. Unfortunately, these catheters have a very high incidence of poor function, central thrombosis, and, more importantly, infection. If peritoneal dialysis is contemplated, a peritoneal dialysis catheter can be placed and used almost immediately, although most nephrologists prefer to allow the catheter and exit site to heal for 1 to 3 weeks after placement.

Despite a number of hurdles, many dialysis patients do quite well and adapt to the rigors of the procedure. Unfortunately, dialysis does not optimally control many of the complications of CKD and mortality rates remain high, particularly in diabetics. New dialysis modalities are needed to better care for these patients.

MALIGNANT TUMORS OF THE UROGENITAL TRACT

METHOD OF

Michael S. Cookson, MD, and

Sam S. Chang, MD

Carcinoma of the Prostate

Carcinoma of the prostate (CAP) is the most common cancer in men in the United States, and the second leading cause of cancer death. Each year, there are an estimated 220,900 new cases and 28,900 deaths from prostate cancer. More than 95% of prostatic cancers are adenocarcinomas. The incidence of CAP increases with age. A familial pattern has been identified and the disease is more common in African Americans than in whites. Some studies implicate a high-fat diet as a contributing etiology. Hereditary CAP has been identified in approximately 9% of patients, and may account for as much as 40% of early age of onset cancers. Recently, the Hereditary Prostate Cancer Gene (HPC1) was identified on the long arm of chromosome 1.

Histologically, CAP can be identified at autopsy in more than 75% of men older than age 80 years. Thus, there is a large discrepancy between the microscopic presence of the disease and clinically significant disease. Most men with early stage prostate cancer have no disease-related symptoms. Prostate cancer and benign prostatic hypertrophy (BPH) may occur simultaneously, but there is no apparent causal relationship. Obstructive voiding symptoms or hematuria may be present. Patients with advanced disease may present with pelvic pain, ureteral obstruction, or bone pain from distant metastasis.

Early detection has allowed more patients to be identified with lower-stage clinical disease, with the result that such men have higher recurrence-free survival rates after treatment. Recommendations from groups such as the American Urological Association and the American Cancer Society generally include annual screening with serum prostate-specific antigen (PSA) determination and a digital rectal examination (DRE) for all men older than age 50 years and for all African American men and men with a family history of prostate cancer starting at age 40 years. These recommendations are not uniformly accepted; the U.S. Public Health Service Task Force does not endorse screening for prostate cancer because of a lack of convincing prospective data that screening has an impact on the prostate cancer death rate. The goal of screening is to detect clinically significant prostate cancer in individuals with at least 10 years of life expectancy.

Serum PSA is specific for the prostate but is secreted by both benign and malignant prostatic epithelial cells. PSA may be elevated in men with prostatitis, BPH, or prostate cancer. PSA values differ somewhat depending upon the assay used. In general, a level of <4.0 ng/mL has been considered normal and in younger men a value of >2.5 ng/mL may be considered abnormal. It is important to also point out that approximately 25% of CAP may occur despite what is considered a normal PSA level.

Serum PSA occurs in several forms, with the majority bound to α_1-antichymotrypsin and another that is unconjugated or free. The relative proportion of the two forms can be used to improve the specificity of PSA testing. A greater proportion of free PSA is seen in men with BPH than in those with prostate cancer. In general, a percentage-free fraction of <25% is more commonly associated with prostate cancer than are higher levels. Newer tests, such as complexed PSA, are being used to improve on the specificity of PSA testing.

Most often, transrectal ultrasonography (TRUS) is used for imaging and as a guide for prostate biopsy. TRUS can distinguish the zonal anatomy of the prostate and is an accurate measure of prostate size. Prostatic cancers typically are located in the peripheral zone, and may have a hypoechoic pattern. Because of its lack of sensitivity and specificity, TRUS is not used as a screening test.

The grading of CAP is based upon the degree of differentiation of the tumor. This provides important prognostic information. Most often, the Gleason grading system is used. Tumors with a Gleason score of 2 to 4 are usually considered well differentiated, 5 to 7 moderately differentiated, and 8 to 10 poorly differentiated. Prognosis is strongly linked to grade and Gleason score. Most cancers found through early detection or screening programs are of an intermediate (Gleason score 5 to 7) grade.

Staging of prostate cancer defines the local, regional, and distant extent of disease. The TNM (tumor, node, metastasis) system is used to allow categorization of nonpalpable tumors detected because of PSA or ultrasound abnormalities (stage T1c). The primary staging modality for local disease is DRE. Serum PSA levels correlate only roughly with disease extent. However, bone metastasis is rare in patients with a PSA <20 ng/mL. Radionucleotide bone scanning is the most sensitive method for detection of bone metastases. Bone scan in the absence of symptoms is not required routinely if the PSA value is less than 10 ng/mL and a Gleason score of <7. Computed tomography (CT) scanning is not routinely used because grossly positive nodes are detected rarely with clinically localized tumor.

Lymph node staging is important in selecting patients for therapy. CT scanning may show enlarged lymph nodes in patients with high-volume or high-grade primary tumors. Laparoscopic pelvic lymphadenectomy is feasible and can provide adequate sampling of the pelvic lymph nodes among those not selecting surgery. More commonly, lymph node dissection is performed through an open incision immediately prior to radical prostatectomy.

The optimal therapy for localized prostate cancer is a point of continual controversy and must be individualized. For men with a life expectancy of <10 years, observation alone may be appropriate. Surgery or radiation therapy are the most commonly used treatments. For organ-confined tumors, the 15-year disease-free survival rates are >90% for patients treated with surgery. Moreover, the survival outcomes are similar after radiation therapy or surgery, however randomized comparisons among similar staged patients are lacking. Brachytherapy involves the use of radioactive seeds (iodine 125 or palladium 103) placed into the prostate. This is also a valid option, with similar long-term disease-free survival in low- and intermediate-risk patients. Cryotherapy (i.e., freezing of the prostate) is being investigated, but long-term results are not available.

Radical prostatectomy is accomplished most commonly by a retropubic approach. Currently, laparoscopic and robotic prostatectomies are being performed, with comparable oncologic results as compared with open surgery and the potential for improved functional outcomes. In patients who are sexually active before therapy, potency can be retained in nearly 40% to 60% by preservation of the neurovascular bundles. In patients with organ-confined disease, there is an excellent prognosis, with a life expectancy similar to men without prostate cancer. In patients with positive surgical margins or positive lymph nodes, adjuvant radiation and hormonal therapy may be used, respectively.

Serum PSA should be undetectable after radical prostatectomy because all PSA-producing cells are removed. After radiation therapy, superior results are achieved in patients in whom the PSA level decreases to <1.0 ng/mL. An increasing serum PSA is evidence of tumor recurrence. There is controversy about when to initiate hormonal therapy in men with rising PSA after treatment, although several studies suggest early hormonal therapy may be of benefit for those with more aggressive tumors.

Prostate cancer is a partially androgen-dependent disease. Therefore, the primary treatment for metastatic carcinoma of the prostate is androgen deprivation. Suppression of serum testosterone can be achieved by orchiectomy. Alternatively, medical therapy may be considered. Luteinizing hormone-releasing hormone (LHRH) analogues effectively suppress testosterone to the castrate range within 1 month of administration. LHRH analogues are associated with few serious side effects, but do cause vasomotor hot flashes in approximately two thirds of patients. Loss of libido and impotence are also a consequence of treatment.

The median response to hormonal therapy in patients with metastatic disease is usually around 18 to 24 months. After that time, disease progression often occurs. There are no treatments known to favorably alter the course of the disease after hormonal therapy. However, mitoxantrone (Novantrone) is approved for palliative relief for symptomatic bone pain from prostate cancer. Radiation can also be effective for isolated sites of bone metastasis. Most patients with metastatic carcinoma of the prostate die within 2 to 3 years from the time of diagnosis.

Tumors of the Renal Parenchyma

Malignant tumors of the renal parenchyma are either primary or metastatic. Among the primary renal lesions, the tumors may be either malignant or benign. The most common malignant tumor is renal cell carcinoma (RCC), while other tumor types, such as papillary collecting duct carcinoma, medullary carcinoma, and sarcomas occur infrequently. The most common benign renal tumors are angiomyolipomas and oncocytomas, the latter of which are often indistinguishable from malignant lesions on radiographic imaging. Metastatic lesions such as lung, breast, and ovary may occur, and lymphoma may be present in the kidney.

RENAL CELL CARCINOMA

RCC is the most common primary neoplasm of the kidney and accounts for >85% of all primary renal cancers. In the United States, it is estimated that 31,900 new cases are diagnosed and that about 11,900 patients die of the disease each year. Renal cell carcinoma represents approximately 3% of all adult malignancies. It is a tumor that usually occurs in adults between the ages of 40 and 60 years, although it has been reported in younger age groups. It has a 2:1 male-to-female preponderance, and a well-documented association with von Hippel-Lindau disease.

Renal cell carcinomas arise from the proximal convoluted tubules. The most consistent chromosomal changes in renal cell carcinoma are deletions and translocations of the short arm of chromosome 3. No specific agent is implicated as the cause of RCC. Tobacco smoking poses an approximately twofold relative risk for cigarette smokers. Patients with end-stage renal disease (ESRD) with acquired cystic disease of the kidney (ACDK) have an increased risk of RCC. Of these patients, RCC will develop in 1% to 2%, with younger dialysis patients having the greatest risk. Periodic renal ultrasound every few years is recommended in these patients, with follow-up CT scanning of complex cysts as needed.

Hematuria is the single most common sign, occurring in 29% to 60% of cases. Flank pain and palpable mass occur next most frequently, but the classic triad of hematuria, flank pain, and a palpable abdominal mass are reported in only 10% of cases. Other common signs and symptoms are fever, anemia, and elevated sedimentation rate. While serum lactate dehydrogenase and alkaline phosphatase may be elevated, there are no reliable tumor markers for renal cell carcinoma. RCCs can present only with nonspecific symptoms such as weight loss, fever, or weakness. Most, however, are asymptomatic and detected incidentally on radiographic imaging.

The TNM staging system is currently the most commonly used system to determine the extent of the primary lesion, involvement of contiguous structures, vascular involvement, and whether the tumor has metastasized. It allows for a distinction between venous involvement and nodal invasion and stratifies the extent of each stage. Renal cell carcinomas often will involve the renal vein and vena cava, and may even extend into the right atrium. Five-year survival rates for stages T1N0M0 (<7 cm) and T2N0M0 (>7 cm) are 80% to 90%, for stages T3N0M0, 40% to 60%, and for stages N1-3 and M1 are 10% to 20%.

Radical nephrectomy is the primary treatment of RCC. This classic procedure removes the kidney en bloc within Gerota's fascia, along with the ipsilateral adrenal gland and lymph nodes. Radical nephrectomy traditionally has been performed as an open procedure (flank, transabdominal, or thoracoabdominal incision for very large tumors). Radical nephrectomy has evolved, with adrenalectomy performed for upper pole tumors, very large tumors, or lesions that clearly involve the adrenal gland. If the RCC extends into the renal vein or inferior vena cava, open nephrectomy is usually performed. Rarely, cardiopulmonary bypass is needed to remove the entire tumor thrombus. Hand-assisted laparoscopic nephrectomy and pure laparoscopic nephrectomy are gradually replacing open nephrectomy as less-morbid alternatives to open surgery with equal cancer control.

A partial nephrectomy is performed in patients with solitary kidneys, in those with bilateral RCC, and in patients with compromised renal function. It is also generally agreed that partial nephrectomy or tumor enucleation may be used in patients with lesions of 4 cm or less and a normal contralateral kidney, with local recurrence rates being <5%. Like radical nephrectomy, laparoscopic techniques are emerging as viable alternatives to open surgical removal.

Up to 25% of patients initially seen with symptoms have metastatic disease. Sites of metastasis in decreasing frequency include the lungs, lymph nodes, liver, bone, and adrenal gland. Chemotherapy and radiation have little to no survival benefit, with radiation only palliating painful metastasis. The mainstay of treatment is immunotherapy with 5-year survival rates of 10% to 20%. There is emerging evidence to suggest an improved survival in those undergoing nephrectomy prior to immunotherapy.

BENIGN RENAL TUMORS

Benign solid tumors of the kidney are encountered occasionally. An angiomyolipoma can usually be diagnosed by the characteristic appearance of fat within the lesion on CT scan. Angiomyolipomas may occur as an isolated phenomenon or in association with tuberous sclerosis. Tuberous sclerosis is a disease characterized by mental retardation, epilepsy, and adenoma sebaceum. Approximately 50% of patients with tuberous sclerosis develop angiomyolipomas, and many are bilateral and multifocal. The management of angiomyolipomas is controversial. In asymptomatic lesions of <4 cm in size, observation with annual imaging is reasonable. In patients with an acute bleeding episode, angioinfarction may be used to stabilize the patient. In symptomatic lesions or lesions of >4 cm, surgical excision is considered standard therapy.

Oncocytomas are benign renal tumors that account for between 5% and 10% of solid renal lesions. Renal oncocytomas are more difficult to differentiate from RCC but usually are round, of uniform density and may have a central scar or "spoke-wheel" appearance on CT scan. From a practical standpoint, renal oncocytomas are a pathologic diagnosis and characteristic masses should be considered malignant until proven otherwise. Histologically, they are characterized by eosinophilic granular cells. The cell of origin is thought to be that of distal renal tubules.

METASTATIC RENAL LESIONS

Lung cancer is the most common solid tumor to metastasize to the kidney, although lymphoma, ovarian, bowel, and breast may also be seen. Lymphoma of the kidney is almost always a metastatic manifestation of a systemic disease, and therefore surgical treatment is rarely indicated in the absence of symptoms. However, approximately 15% of renal lymphomas present as solitary masses. It is a challenge to differentiate these tumors from renal cell carcinoma preoperatively.

Tumors of the Renal Pelvis/Ureter

Tumors of the renal pelvis account for approximately 10% of all renal tumors and approximately 5% of all urothelial tumors. Ureteral tumors are even less common, occurring with approximately 25% the incidence of renal pelvic tumors. Ureteral tumors are three times more common in men than in women, and twice as common in whites as in blacks. Cigarette smoking is strongly associated with an increased risk of developing upper tract transitional cell carcinomas. Additionally, analgesic abuse and cyclophosphamide (Cytoxan) are associated with an increased risk.

The risk of upper tract tumors is approximately 4% among those patients with bladder cancer. However, in patients with carcinoma in situ and high-grade urothelial lesions, the risk may approach 20% with long-term follow-up. Conversely, patients with upper tract tumors have a 40% to 70% risk of developing bladder cancer. Therefore, patients with upper tract tumors should undergo periodic surveillance cystoscopy. The incidence of bilateral upper tract tumors is 2% to 5%. In addition to transitional cell carcinomas, squamous cell carcinomas, and adenocarcinomas are included in the differential diagnosis, particularly in a patient with a history of recurrent urinary tract infections or staghorn calculi.

As with renal cell carcinomas, the most common presenting symptom is hematuria. In patients with normal renal function, the diagnostic workup usually includes an intravenous pyelogram (IVP) and urine cytology followed by cystoscopy. However, it must be kept in mind that voided urine cytology may be falsely negative in up to 85% of patients with a low-grade lesion. Approximately 50% to 75% of patients will have a filling defect on IVP. The differential includes tumor, blood clot, fungal ball, sloughed papilla, and a radiolucent stone. A retrograde ureteropyelogram may be helpful in documenting the persistence of the filling defect; however ureteroscopy with biopsy or brushings may be diagnostic. In renal pelvic defects, a noncontrast CT scan with 3 mm cuts through the kidney is usually able to differentiate stone from soft-tissue mass because even radiolucent stones on standard urography are opaque on CT scan. The TNM staging system is recommended for staging.

Patients with low-grade, low-stage lesions do well with conservative or radical treatment. Patients with intermediate- or high-grade tumors are best managed with aggressive surgical resection. Solitary, low-grade, and low-stage upper ureteral tumors may be managed with segmental resection. Similar distal ureteral tumors can be managed with distal ureterectomy and ureteroneocystostomy. Treatment of high-grade and high-stage tumors is nephroureterectomy with removal of a cuff of bladder at the ureteral orifice because of the high incidence of ipsilateral ureteral orifice and bladder involvement. This can be accomplished through a single extended flank of midline incision, but is often performed through two incisions. Currently, hand-assisted laparoscopic nephroureterectomy is the preferred surgical approach allowing for complete tumor removal through a single incision and offers the advantage of quicker convalescence. Successful endoscopic management including percutaneous and retrograde approaches has been reported in selected cases.

Carcinoma of the Bladder

TRANSITIONAL CELL CARCINOMA OF THE BLADDER

Bladder carcinoma is the fifth most common malignancy in the United States with more than 57,000 new cases annually. It is almost three times more common among men than women, and is the fourth most common cancer in men. Because of frequent recurrence, particularly among patients with superficial tumors, bladder cancer is the second most prevalent cancer. Bladder cancer is the fifth most common cause of cancer deaths among men. It is about four times more prevalent among cigarette smokers and is associated with known carcinogens including rubber and oil refinery workers. Patients treated with cyclophosphamide (Cytoxan) have up to a ninefold increased risk of developing bladder cancer, believed to be secondary to acrolein, a urinary metabolite of cyclophosphamide.

Approximately 90% of bladder malignancies are transitional cell carcinoma. Of these, 70% of tumors are papillary, 10% are sessile, and 20% are mixed. Of patients with muscle invasive bladder cancer, approximately 80% to 90% will have invasion on initial presentation. A strong correlation exists between tumor grade and stage, with most well-differentiated tumors being superficial and most poorly differentiated tumors invasive. Carcinoma in situ (CIS) is a poorly differentiated transitional cell carcinoma that is confined to the urothelium. CIS may be found as a solitary or multifocal process and is found in association with invasive carcinoma in approximately 25% of cases. It is associated with a poor prognosis. Between 10% and 20% of patients treated with cystectomy for diffuse CIS are found to have microscopic muscle-invasive disease.

Gross painless hematuria is a common presenting sign. However, approximately 20% of patients may present with only microscopic hematuria. Irritative voiding symptoms such as frequency and urgency may also suggest a malignancy, particularly CIS. Patients suspected of having bladder cancer should undergo evaluations of their upper tracts (IVP or CT scan), cystoscopy, and urine cytology. Transurethral biopsy or resection confirms the diagnosis.

Management of bladder carcinoma depends upon tumor stage. The TNM system is recommended for staging. For most superficial bladder carcinomas, transurethral resection of the tumor is often the only treatment required. However, for CIS or high-grade superficial tumors, tumors that involve the lamina propria (stage T1) and rapidly recurrent tumors, treatment with intravesical agents such as thiotepa (Thioplex), doxorubicin (Adriamycin), and mitomycin-C (Mutamycin)[1] or intravesical bacillus Calmette-Guérin (BCG, Tice) may be indicated.

[1]Not FDA approved for this indication.

Bladder surveillance is mandatory because the recurrence rate in the bladder may be as high as 50% at 5 years. Surveillance protocols include cystoscopy and urinary cytologies every 3 months for the first year, every 4 months for the second year, semiannually in the third year, and annually thereafter. Periodic evaluation of the upper tracts should be performed to rule out an upper tract occurrence.

The risk of progression to muscle-invasive disease is relatively low (less than 10%) for stage Ta tumors, but increases as tumor stage advances (stage T1) or with high-grade lesions. Superficial tumors that progress in stage or fail conservative therapy, and in those that invade the bladder muscle (stages T2 to T3), a radical cystectomy is the treatment of choice.

Each year there are an estimated 12,500 deaths from bladder cancer. Five-year survival rates are approximately 85% to 60% after cystectomy for stages T2a and T2b, respectively. For stages T3a and T3b tumors, the 5-year survival rates decrease to 60% and 40%, respectively, while patients with node-positive disease have a 5-year survival rate of less than 30%. Adjuvant chemotherapy is generally offered to patients at high risk for failure (pathologic stages T3b, T4, and N1/2 disease). The standard regimen over the past decade was and is methotrexate, vinblastine (Velban), doxorubicin (Adriamycin), and cisplatin (Platinol) (MVAC); however, durable complete response rates are less than 15%. There are recent reports of modest survival advantages using MVAC in the neoadjuvant setting.

Urinary diversion may be accomplished with an ileal or colon conduit, which requires wearing of a collection appliance. A continent cutaneous diversion may be created, most often using the right colon with a tapered and catheterizable efferent limb of ileum (Indiana pouch) or with creation of a nipple valve (Koch pouch). Approximately 50% of cystectomy patients undergo continent diversion. An orthotopic neobladder allows creation of a reservoir using detubularized ileum or colon with direct anastomosis to the urethra. With the development of orthotopic urinary diversion, functional status and quality of life among patients following cystectomy have improved significantly.

ADENOCARCINOMA OF THE BLADDER

Adenocarcinomas account for less than 2% of bladder cancers. They are classified into three groups: primary bladder, urachal, and metastatic. Most adenocarcinomas are poorly differentiated and invasive. They are commonly associated with cystitis glandularis, rather than CIS. Adenocarcinomas also are associated with bladder augmentations. Adenocarcinoma is the most common type of cancer in patients with bladder exstrophy. Radical cystectomy with pelvic lymphadenectomy is the treatment of choice.

Squamous Cell Carcinoma of the Bladder

Squamous cell carcinoma accounts for approximately 6% of bladder cancers in the United States, but more than 75% of bladder cancers in Egypt. Chronic bladder inflammation, as occurs with chronic indwelling Foley catheters, recurrent bladder infections, or bladder diverticula are associated with an increased risk of squamous cell carcinoma. Approximately 80% of squamous cell carcinomas in Egypt are associated with *Schistosoma haematobium*. These cancers are known as bilharzial bladder cancers and occur in patients 10 to 20 years younger than those with transitional cell carcinoma. The prognosis for squamous cell carcinoma is generally poor, and radical cystectomy is the standard treatment for patients who are surgical candidates. Chemotherapy, particularly regimens used in transitional cell carcinoma, is ineffective in squamous cell carcinoma. The benefit of neoadjuvant radiation therapy prior to radical cystectomy is unproved in patients with squamous cell carcinoma, with the possible exception of bilharzial cancers.

Urethral Carcinoma

Urethral carcinoma is the only urologic malignancy that is more common in females than in males. It usually occurs after 60 years of age. While the etiology remains undetermined, approximately 50% of cases are associated with urethral stricture. A patient should be evaluated for urethral carcinoma when a urethral mass is palpable, obstruction does not respond to conventional stricture management, a urethral abscess and/or fistula occurs, hematuria is present, or inguinal adenopathy becomes evident. The treatment of the primary tumor is surgical excision. Urethrectomy is performed via a perineal incision. Proximal tumors of the bulbar urethra are managed with cystoprostatectomy and en bloc urethrectomy.

Although the etiology of female urethral carcinoma remains obscure, there is an association with urethral malakoplakia and urethral caruncles. Most patients are white and older than 50 years of age. The usual presenting symptom is a papillary or fungating urethral mass and hematuria. For tumors of the proximal urethral, or in cases of extension into adjacent structures, cystectomy with en bloc urethrectomy and anterior vaginectomy along with pelvic lymphadenectomy are is usually required. Radiation therapy has also been reported to provide local control in select cases. In advanced cases, multimodality treatment with chemotherapy and either surgical excision or radiation therapy provides the best chance for cure, although to date no specific regimen has emerged as standard treatment.

Penile Cancer

Penile cancer is relatively rare in the United States. Poor personal hygiene and retained phimotic foreskin are implicated in the etiology of penile carcinoma. Penile cancer is extremely rare in men who were circumcised at birth. Squamous cell carcinoma of the penis occurs most commonly in the sixth decade of life. The symptoms are related to ulceration, necrosis, suppuration, and hemorrhage of the penile lesion. The clinical evaluation of patients with penile cancer includes physical examination with palpation of the inguinal region, liver function tests, chest radiograph, CT scans of the abdomen and pelvis, and bone scan.

The TNM stage is based primarily on depth of invasion and usually dictates treatment. Small penile cancers limited to the prepuce can be treated by circumcision alone. Partial penectomy with at least a 1-cm margin of normal tissue is used to treat smaller (2 to 5 cm) distal penile tumors. The remaining penis should be long enough to permit voiding in the standing position. The 5-year cure rate for patients treated with partial penectomy is 70% to 80%. Larger distal penile lesions or proximal tumors require total penectomy and perineal urethrostomy. If the scrotum, pubis, or abdominal wall is involved, radical en bloc excision may be necessary.

Many patients will have inguinal lymphadenopathy at presentation. However, inguinal lymph node enlargement before excision of the primary tumor may be the result of infection and not metastatic disease. Thus, clinical assessment of the inguinal region should be delayed 4 to 6 weeks, during which time the patient is treated with antibiotics. If inguinal lymphadenopathy persists or develops, there is a high likelihood of metastatic disease and ilioinguinal lymphadenectomy should be performed. However, if the inguinal lymphadenopathy resolves, prophylactic lymph node dissection may not be necessary. Radiation of the primary tumor and regional lymph nodes is an alternative to surgery in patients with small (≤2 cm), low-stage tumors.

Testicular Cancer

Malignant disease of the testes can be divided into germinal neoplasms, which includes seminomatous and nonseminomatous germ cell tumors (NSGCT) and secondary neoplasms. Ninety-five percent of tumors originating in the testis are germ cell tumors. Fewer than 10% of all germ cell tumors arise from extragonadal primary sites. The mediastinum and retroperitoneum are the most common extragonadal sites. Testicular cancer, although relatively rare, represents the most common malignancy in males in the 15- to 35-year-old age group with 7600 new cases annually.

Testicular cancer has become one of the most curable solid neoplasms and serves as a paradigm for the multimodal treatment of malignancies. The dramatic improvements in survival resulting from the combination of effective diagnostic techniques, improved tumor markers, effective multidrug chemotherapeutic regimens, and modifications of surgical technique have led to a decrease in patient mortality from greater than 50% before 1970 to less than 10% in 1996.

Germ cell tumors are seen principally in whites. Recent data show a white-to-black ratio of approximately 5:1 and a report from the U.S. military showed a relative incidence of 40:1. The cause of germ cell tumors is unknown. Familial clustering has been observed, particularly among siblings. Cryptorchidism and Klinefelter's syndrome are predisposing factors in the development of germ cell tumors arising from the testis and mediastinum, respectively. Orchidopexy performed before puberty may not reduce the risk of germ cell tumors but improves the ability to observe the testis.

A painless testicular mass is pathognomonic of a primary testicular tumor, occurring in a minority of patients. The majority present with diffuse testicular pain, swelling, hardness, or some combination of these findings. Because infectious epididymo-orchitis is more common than tumor, a trial of antibiotics is often undertaken. If testicular discomfort does not abate, or if the findings do not revert to normal within 2 to 4 weeks, testicular sonography is indicated. A radical inguinal orchiectomy with ligation of spermatic cord at the internal ring is required for all patients with suspected testicular tumors.

Regional metastasis first appears in the retroperitoneal lymph nodes below the renal vessels. Right testicular tumors usually metastasize to nodes between the aorta and inferior vena cava (interaortocaval nodes), and left testicular tumors to nodes lateral to the aorta (para-aortic). Left supraclavicular adenopathy and pulmonary nodules may occur with or without retroperitoneal disease. CT scans of the abdomen and pelvis, and chest radiography are required. Lymph nodes in the primary retroperitoneal landing zones that measure between 1 and 2 cm are involved by germ cell tumors in approximately 70% of cases. CT scanning of the chest is required if mediastinal, hilar, or lung parenchymal disease is suspected.

Testicular cancer is one of the few neoplasms associated with accurate serum markers, human β-chorionic gonadotrophin (β-HCG) and α-fetoprotein (AFP). These accurate tumor markers allow careful follow-up and intervention earlier in the course of disease. AFP production is restricted to NSGCT, specifically embryonal carcinoma and yolk sac tumor. Patients with an increased AFP and the finding of pure seminoma on pathology of the orchiectomy specimen should be treated for NSGCT. Increased serum concentrations of β-HCG may be observed in both seminomatous and nonseminomatous tumors. Increased concentrations of β-HCG are seen in 40% to 60% of patients with metastatic NSGCT, and in 15% to 20% of patients with metastatic seminomas. A third serum marker, lactate dehydrogenase is less specific but has independent prognostic value in patients with advanced germ cell tumors. Serum lactate dehydrogenase concentrations are also increased in approximately 60% of patients with NSGCT and in 80% of those with seminomatous germ cell tumors.

Serum tumor marker concentrations are determined before, during, and after treatment. Increased concentrations of AFP, β-HCG, or both, without radiographic or clinical findings, imply active disease and are sufficient reason to initiate treatment if likely causes of false-positive results have been ruled out. The serum half-lives of AFP and β-HCG are 5 to 7 days and 30 hours, respectively. Slow clearance suggests residual active disease.

Seminoma, the most common germ cell histology, has a favorable response to treatment. Therapy for low-stage (stage 1, 2a, or 2b) seminomas following radical inguinal orchiectomy is irradiation to the retroperitoneal and ipsilateral pelvic lymph nodes. Relapse recurs in approximately 4% of patients with stage 1 seminomas, and in 10% of patients with stage 2a or 2b seminomas. Chemotherapy cures more than 90% of patients who have a relapse after radiation therapy. Thus, approximately 99% of patients with low-stage seminomas are cured.

NSGCTs include embryonal cell carcinoma, choriocarcinoma, yolk sac carcinoma, teratoma, and mixed germ cell tumors. The rate of cure for patients with NSGCT in clinical stage 1 exceeds 95%. Twenty percent of patients with stage 1 tumors with no lymphatic or vascular invasion or invasion into the tunica albuginea, spermatic cord, or scrotum are discovered to have regional lymph node or distant metastasis. Surveillance and nerve-sparing retroperitoneal lymph node dissection (RPLND) are standard treatment options for this group of patients. If patients have stage 1 disease confined to the testes, attention must be paid to the surgical pathology. In any patient with embryonal histology or the presence of lymphovascular invasion or extension beyond the tunica albuginea, RPLND is recommended. The rationale for this treatment stems from a 30% relapse rate in stage 1 patients with these findings.

RPLND is a major abdominal operation in which lymph nodes from the retroperitoneum are removed from the renal hilum down to the level of the common iliac artery, with lateral margins confined by the ureters. In the past, this procedure resulted in lack of ejaculation and infertility in 100% of patients. By performing a modified-template RPLND, the contralateral area of aorta below the inferior mesenteric artery is not manipulated. This maneuver serves to preserve the confluence of sympathetic fibers along the aorta that are responsible for ejaculation, with a 60% to 88% rate of preservation of ejaculation and no reports of recurrence for stage 1 disease.

Patients with persistently increased concentrations of AFP, β-HCG, or both, but without other clinical evidence of disease following orchiectomy, usually have systemic disease. These patients should undergo three or four cycles of standard chemotherapy rather than surgery.

Patients with stage 2 NSGCT are treated initially with either RPLND or chemotherapy, depending on the extent of the disease, serum tumor marker concentrations, and the presence or absence of tumor-related symptoms. Asymptomatic patients with solitary retroperitoneal lymph nodes less than 3 cm in diameter as assessed by CT imaging generally undergo retroperitoneal lymph node dissection, whereas those with bulky stage 2 disease (>5 cm) undergo initial chemotherapy. After a properly performed operation, recurrences within the retroperitoneum are rare.

Adjuvant chemotherapy is an important consideration when any lymph node is more than 2 cm in diameter, at least six nodes are involved, or there is extranodal invasion. The majority of patients in this group who relapsed did not receive adjuvant chemotherapy. Although the rate of cure is the same when chemotherapy is withheld until relapse, patients who received adjuvant therapy require fewer cycles of chemotherapy and avoid additional surgery.

Initial chemotherapy is required in approximately one third of patients with germ cell tumors. Because relapse is frequent in patients with clinical stage 2c disease, and in patients with primary retroperitoneal or mediastinal seminomas who receive radiation alone, these patients are treated initially with chemotherapy. Patients also receive initial chemotherapy if they have stage 3 NSGCT or multifocal retroperitoneal lymph node involvement, lymph nodes more than 3 cm in diameter, or tumor-related back pain.

Postchemotherapy RPLND is usually reserved for residual masses (>3 cm) in patients after treatment for seminoma. In NSGCT, the need for postchemotherapy RPLND is controversial. Some groups advocate surgery in all patients with initial bulky retroperitoneal disease, while others advocate observation rather than surgery in patients with >90% shrinkage of retroperitoneal nodes, no residual nodes of >1.5 cm, and with no teratomatous elements in the primary tumor. There is no debate, however, concerning the need for removal of any significant postchemotherapy residual mass.

The first combination chemotherapy regimens containing cisplatin (Platinol), vinblastine (Velban), and bleomycin (Blenoxane) resulted in complete remission in 70% to 80% of patients with metastatic germ cell tumors. Subsequent studies show that prolonged maintenance chemotherapy was unnecessary, and vinblastine was replaced by etoposide (VePesid), which is less toxic and probably more efficacious. Serious adverse effects of combination chemotherapy include neuromuscular toxic affects, death from myelosuppression for bleomycin-induced pulmonary fibrosis, and Raynaud's phenomenon.

Leydig cell tumors comprise between 1% and 3% of all testis tumors. Although the majority of cases have been recognized in men between the ages of 20 and 60 years, approximately 25% have been reported before puberty. The prognosis for Leydig cell tumors following radical inguinal orchiectomy is good because of their generally benign nature.

Gonadoblastomas are rare tumors that occur almost exclusively in patients with some form of gonadal dysgenesis. They constitute approximately 0.5% of all testis neoplasms and occur in all age groups, from infancy to beyond 70 years of age, although the majority occur in individuals younger than 30 years of age. Radical orchiectomy is the first step in therapy. The high incidence of bilaterality (50%) mandates a contralateral gonadectomy when gonadal dysgenesis is present. The prognosis is excellent for patients with gonadoblastoma.

The most common secondary neoplasm of the testis and the most frequent of all testis tumors in patients older than 50 years of age is lymphoma. The median age is approximately 60 years. As with lymphomas elsewhere, patients with poorly differentiated lymphocytic types tend to survive longer than those with histocytic types. Survival is poor with bilateral disease and poor in patients presenting with lymphomas at other sites who later experience a testicular relapse, but among patients with disease apparently confined to the testis, survival appears to be good.

URETHRAL STRICTURE

METHOD OF

Steven M. Schlossberg, MD, and
Gerald H. Jordan, MD

The term urethral stricture relates to an area of narrowing in the anterior urethra. These usually result from tissue injury after local trauma or inflammatory disease. With healing, the scar contracts, decreasing the diameter of the lumen. Areas of the posterior urethra are referred to as *stenoses, distraction defects*, or *contractures*, depending on the location and mechanism of cause (Figure 1). They can involve the prostatic urethra, the membranous urethra, or the bladder neck. Prostatic urethral stenoses or contractures usually occur after surgery for benign or malignant disease of the prostate. Membranous urethral

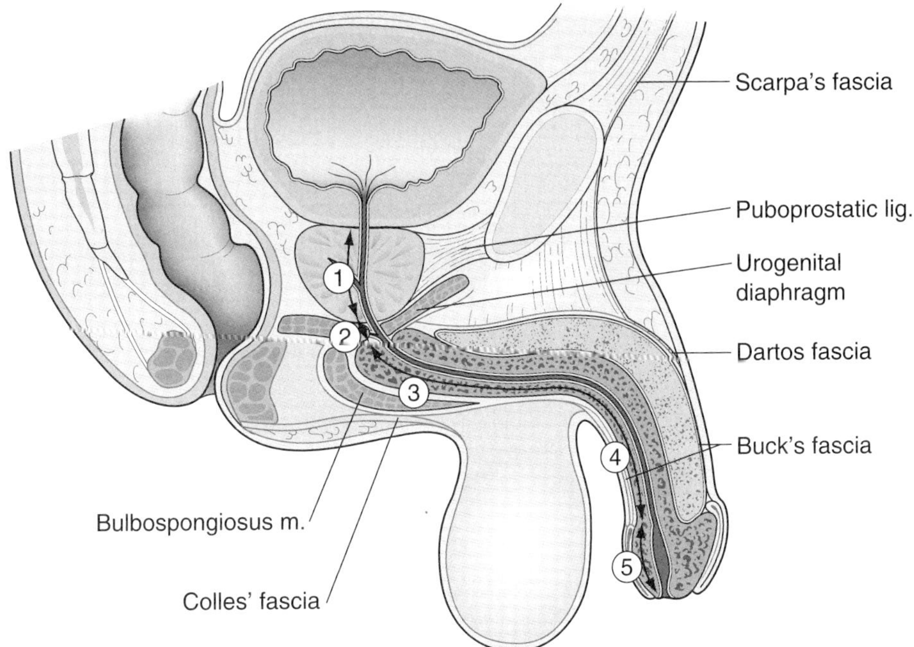

FIGURE 1 Cross-section of the pelvis demonstrating the anatomic divisions of the urethra. 1, Prostatic urethra; 2, Membranous urethra; 3, Bulbous urethra; 4, Pendulous portion of the penile urethra; 5, Fossa navicularis. (From Jordan GH: Urethral surgery and stricture disease. In Droller MJ [ed]: Surgical Management of Urologic Disease. Chicago, Mosby—Year Book, 1992, p. 816.)

distraction defects are inevitably associated with pelvic fracture and attendant urethral injury.

Anterior urethral strictures occur within the area of the urethra that is surrounded by the corpus spongiosum and can be localized to the bulbous urethra, the penile or pendulous urethra, or the fossa navicularis (glandular urethra). Anterior urethral strictures are commonly caused by blunt perineal trauma (occult or recognized), urethral infection (gonorrhea), or instrumentation (urethral catheterization or transurethral surgery). Currently available data do not appear to show any relationship between nonspecific urethritis (*Chlamydia* and *Ureaplasma urealyticum*) and the development of an anterior urethral stricture.

Recently, anterior strictures are much more commonly seen from chronic glanular and meatal inflammation from lichen sclerosus atrophicus (LSA), previously referred to as balanitis xerotica obliterans (BXO). With meatal narrowing, patients can also develop significant stricture disease throughout the anterior urethra. The chronic inflammation and extensive nature of the stricture make these patients extremely difficult to treat.

Although many of the ensuing comments are applicable to all urethral "strictures," the following discussion is mainly concerned with the diagnosis and treatment of anterior urethral strictures in males. Urethral strictures are extremely rare in women.

Diagnosis

Symptoms are related to changes caused by obstruction of the flow of urine. Patients may notice a slow stream, frequency, urgency, nocturia, dysuria, or occasional suprapubic pain. This constellation of symptoms may also suggest prostatic enlargement (bladder outlet obstruction) or prostatic inflammatory processes. Pyuria and recurrent urinary tract infections are common. Recurrent epididymitis in a young patient or the signs and symptoms of recurrent prostatitis should raise the possibility of an undiagnosed stricture. Additionally, in the patient presenting with Fournier's gangrene (rapidly progressive perineal and lower abdominal fasciitis), unsuspected urethral stricture with associated urinary extravasation and undiagnosed perianal abscess must be excluded.

Although the presence of a stricture can be confirmed by the inability to pass a small catheter, the best diagnostic test is a dynamic retrograde urethrogram done with contrast material suitable for intravenous administration. A subsequent voiding cystourethrogram is helpful in determining the length of the stricture. To complete the evaluation, urethroscopy under local anesthesia is helpful. The length, depth, and density of the stricture can be determined from physical examination, the appearance on contrast studies, and the amount of elasticity noted at urethroscopy.

Treatment

Once the diagnosis is made, treatment depends on the "stage" or anatomy of the stricture (Figure 2 and Table 1). Simple procedures can cure a stricture that involves only the urethral epithelium, while more complex strictures usually require open surgical repair. In the past, treatment of urethral strictures was based on the concept of the reconstructive ladder. The simplest treatment was always tried first, and when it failed for the third, fourth, or fifth

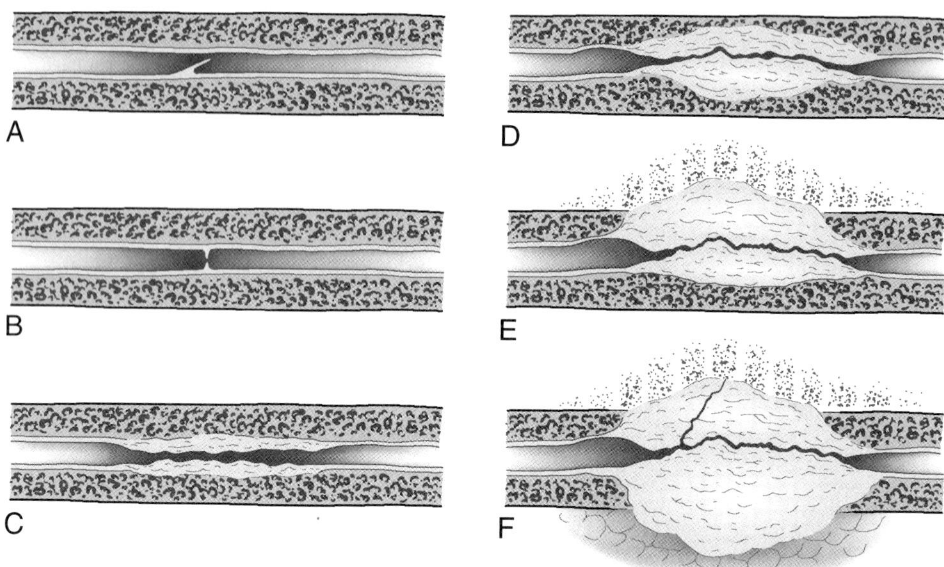

FIGURE 2 Classification of urethral stricture disease according to the anatomy of the stricture as described by Devine. (From Jordan GH: Problems in Urology, Vol. 1. Philadelphia, JB Lippincott, 1987, p. 200.)

time, a more complex procedure was attempted. In addition to complicating treatment in the long run, the "simple" treatment often produced more scarring, thereby increasing the stage of the stricture. Although reasonable in the era of more rudimentary reconstructive techniques, this approach is less acceptable today. With more accurate assessment of the stricture and better surgical techniques, the anatomy of the stricture should determine the appropriate treatment (see Figure 2 and Table 1). However, there is a place for the management, rather than the cure, of a urethral stricture in patients who are poor surgical candidates. As with many other diseases, the patient and physician should discuss the likelihood of success and the treatment-related morbidity that may be obtained with the different therapeutic options.

Urethral Dilation

Dilation is often the first treatment attempted. The goal is to stretch the scar without tearing healthy tissue and producing more trauma. If dilation causes significant bleeding, it has been done too vigorously. A variety of different methods are available for dilating strictures. The initial caliber of the stricture and the experience of the physician often dictates the method chosen. For small-caliber strictures (less than 10 French), and with the advent of guidewire technology, a system is now available that uses a guidewire to traverse the stricture (sometimes passed with the aid of a flexible cystoscope) and a Teflon-coated polyethylene tapered dilator to enlarge the stricture. Our preferred treatment, if possible, is to use a balloon dilator that can be passed with the aid of a guidewire, or a coudé (curved) tip. Because this provides radial dilation without the shearing forces generated by conventional dilators, there possibly are less trauma and pain. Dilation should always be performed with intraurethral lidocaine jelly. Metal sounds or coudé-tip catheters can also be used for larger strictures. Stretching of the scar ideally should be accomplished without tearing. Several sessions may be necessary to obtain a durable and

TABLE 1 Surgical Options for Urethroplasty

Condition	Option
Posterior urethral stricture	1. Open perineal repair 2. Endourethroplasty (stricture <0.5 cm)
Anterior urethral stricture	
Bulbar	
Short (<2.5 cm)	1. Excision and primary anastomosis 2. Patch graft urethroplasty
Long (>2.5 cm)	1. Patch graft urethroplasty 2. Penile hairless scrotal island urethroplasty 3. Graft/flap with partial excision and anastomosis 4. Staged approach with buccal mucosa or split-thickness skin graft
Penile	1. Penile island flap 2. Buccal graft urethroplasty 3. Staged approach with buccal mucosa or split-thickness skin graft

For posterior urethral strictures, short anterior strictures, and penile strictures, the first choice listed is the procedure of choice. For long bulbar strictures, the type of repair is chosen based on stricture anatomy and available tissue.

satisfactory luminal caliber (16 to 18 French). Although dilation may be curative for mucosal strictures, it is often used to manage the stricture; if this is the case, twice a year is an acceptable frequency for the repeat dilation.

Internal Urethrotomy

Transurethral incision of the scar is often attempted as initial therapy or as the next step after dilation for short strictures. Usually performed under general anesthesia or local anesthesia with heavy intravenous sedation, this procedure involves visualizing the stricture cystoscopically and cutting the scar until healthy tissue is seen, allowing the lumen to open to 22 to 24 French in diameter. A urethral catheter is left in place for a variable length of time. Some patients are placed on an intermittent catheterization program to keep the stricture open as the incision heals. The transurethral incision is usually made by the "cold-knife" technique. A specially designed attachment to an operative cystoscope allows the urologist to accomplish a precise and controlled incision. Recently, a variety of different laser techniques have been tried to improve the success over that of conventional internal urethrotomy, but the data suggest that a properly performed laser urethrotomy is no better than a standard approach.

Although internal urethrotomy may be curative, more often it is a form of management that yields a wider caliber stricture. The practice of frequently repeated internal urethrotomy should be condemned except in patients who are not surgical candidates. For a short stricture (less than 1 cm) located in the bulbous urethra, one or two attempts are reasonable. However, if this is not successful, there is a risk that a simple open repair (excision and primary anastomosis) may be converted into a more complex (flap or graft) repair.

Urethral Stent

Stent technology is also available for the treatment of urethral strictures. These stents should be used only in the bulbar urethra for short strictures of less than 3 cm. Because they are designed to be permanent, they should be reserved for elderly patients who are not surgical candidates. Currently, several investigations are underway to evaluate removable stent technology. In this approach, the stricture can be opened and allowed to heal over an indwelling stent that can be removed later. The patient continues voiding normally while the stent is in place.

Open Surgical Repair

The open repair for urethral strictures has evolved significantly over the last 40 years. Currently, almost any urethra can be reconstructed, often in a one-stage operation. The success rate of these procedures is usually in excess of 90%, and in some situations it is in excess of 95%. A small subset of patients may require a staged approach. We have repaired urethras from the meatus to the external sphincter in one stage when there was sufficient healthy tissue. Surgically, it is best to operate on a stable stricture. Therefore, in severe stricture disease requiring dilation every 3 to 4 weeks to prevent urinary retention, a suprapubic cystostomy tube may be needed to allow resolution of the urethral inflammation associated with repeated dilation.

The ideal operation consists of excision of the stricture and repair of the urethra without use of any foreign tissue. Because the corpus spongiosum has inherent elasticity and usually a good blood supply, short strictures (less than 2.5 cm) located from the penoscrotal junction to the membranous urethra can be repaired by excision of the stricture and primary anastomosis. This approach is successful in 96% of cases. If local anatomy is not favorable, addition of tissue as either a graft or a flap is needed.

Grafts are probably the most versatile tissue for urethral repair. The ideal graft source in urethral repair probably is buccal mucosa, although penile skin and bladder mucosa have been used. Hairless extragenital skin should not be used because of less reliable "take" and subsequent poor healing. Currently, buccal grafts are being used much more commonly than flaps (see below). These grafts can be placed either dorsally or ventrally. The dorsal onlay offers the advantage of a stable bed and minimal graft contracture. Some surgeons may prefer ventral placement where the bed of the graft may be the corpus spongiosum. In general, one-stage graft procedures are used to repair bulbar strictures.

Penile island flaps are still the treatment of choice for penile strictures. A better understanding of penile and scrotal blood supply has allowed reconstructive surgeons to generate reliable flaps to repair urethral strictures. In these procedures, the urethra is opened through the stricture into healthy urethra on either side. To compensate for the loss of circumference secondary to the scar, the urethra is patched with an island of skin carried on a vascular pedicle. The ideal donor site is an area of hairless penile skin. Penile island flaps based on a dartos pedicle (axial flaps) can be elevated from the ventral midline with either a longitudinal or a transverse orientation or on the dorsal aspect of the penis in a transverse fashion. Flaps measuring 15 cm in length and 2 cm in width can be mobilized and the penile skin closed primarily.

Although they are not universally accepted, we have found scrotal skin islands to be quite useful in the occasional select patient. Often, a hairless area of scrotal skin can be found and mobilized as an island flap in a similar fashion to a penile skin flap. At times, we have epilated scrotal tissue to enlarge a hairless area, but this is a tedious process that is performed with magnification and usually needs to be repeated at least once. It is imperative that these scrotal islands are properly and aggressively tailored.

A staged repair may be necessary in a small subset of patients. This requires opening the stricture ventrally or, in rare cases, excising the entire corpus spongiosum. Depending upon the location and length, buccal mucosa or a split-thickness skin graft can be placed next to the urethra. The urethra is left open and the patient voids through a perineal urethrostomy. Six months later, when the graft is soft and stable, the urethra is closed. A staged repair is used in patients with a severe and/or long stricture who lack sufficient hairless tissue. A significant number of these patients will have LSA.

URINARY STONE DISEASE

METHOD OF

Andrew B. Joel, MD, and

Marshall L. Stoller, MD

Urinary calculi have plagued humans for centuries. The diagnosis and treatment of urinary stones have advanced significantly since the Egyptians' use of diamond-tipped reeds to fragment bladder stones. New endourologic techniques have replaced open surgery in most cases, and continue to improve patient care. New diagnostic techniques are making it simpler and safer to evaluate patients with urolithiasis.

Clinical Presentation

Patients typically present with colicky flank pain. The pain may radiate to the ipsilateral groin, testis, or labia, and it may be associated with nausea, vomiting, and gross hematuria. Colic can be severe and is characterized by writhing as the patient tries to find a comfortable position, in contrast to intraperitoneal processes, in which the patient tends to lie still. Irritative voiding symptoms are frequent when a stone is lodged in the distal ureter. The stone may cause dysuria and marked urinary frequency and urgency. Clinical presentations can vary, ranging from asymptomatic, incidentally noted calculi to frank urosepsis.

Evaluation

Urinalysis and urine culture may help direct therapy. Microhematuria will be absent in up to 15% of patients presenting with renal colic. Pyuria may be a clue to associated infection. Urine pH may be helpful in predicting stone type: a pH of less than 5.5 is associated with uric acid calculi; a pH of more than 7.2 is associated with struvite (magnesium ammonium phosphate) infection stones. Crystalluria may be a helpful finding if struvite, uric acid, or cystine crystals are present. The ubiquitous nature of calcium oxalate crystals in urine makes their presence nondiagnostic.

A complete blood count is warranted if the patient presents with fever or the diagnosis is in doubt. Measurements of serum electrolytes and creatinine should be obtained. After the acute stone episode has resolved and the diagnosis of urolithiasis is confirmed, an evaluation with determinations of serum calcium, phosphorus, uric acid, and parathormone is performed to rule out obvious medical causes of urolithiasis such as gout, renal tubular acidosis, and hyperparathyroidism.

A plain abdominal radiograph—namely, a kidney ureter bladder film (KUB)—constitutes the simplest initial imaging study. (In female patients, pregnancy status should be ascertained first.) This study helps to pinpoint the location of the calculus, as 85% to 90% of urinary tract calculi are radiopaque. Common sites of stone obstruction include the ureteropelvic junction, as the ureter crosses over the iliac vessels (overlying the sacroiliac joint seen on x-ray film), and the ureterovesical junction.

Intravenous pyelography (IVP) is a standard technique for imaging calculi, evaluating renal anatomy, and obtaining a gross estimate of renal function. It is readily available and is relatively safe and rapid. However, anaphylactic reactions to iodinated contrast material occur in approximately 1 in 10,000 patients. In addition, pregnancy, renal insufficiency, diabetes mellitus, and dehydration are relative contraindications to the use of IVP. Inexperienced technicians, uncooperative patients, and inadequate bowel preparation can result in a suboptimal study.

Renal ultrasonography is useful for patients in whom IVP and computed tomography (CT) are unavailable or contraindicated, and is the examination of choice in pregnant women. It is quick and noninvasive, and avoids ionizing radiation. However, accuracy is operator-dependent and may be limited by body habitus, especially in the obese patient. Doppler techniques improve diagnostic accuracy by measuring the renal artery resistive index and identifying the presence of ureteral jets. Overall, ultrasound and Doppler techniques are best used in conjunction with a scout KUB radiograph and clinical history to help direct the examination.

Noncontrast helical CT scanning is the diagnostic study of choice for imaging calculi in patients with acute renal colic. It is safe and rapid and has a 97% sensitivity and a 96% specificity in detecting ureteral calculi. Advantages include the avoidance of iodinated contrast and improved cost-effectiveness as compared with that for IVP. It also can help diagnose nonrenal causes of abdominal pain.

Contrast CT scans define renal anatomy when planning a surgical approach. A follow-up KUB film obtained after a contrast CT scan can help to further delineate anatomy. Renal scintigraphy may be useful to estimate relative renal function, but caution should be used in the presence of unrelieved obstruction. Because calculi are not visualized with magnetic resonance imaging, this modality is not useful for evaluating patients with suspected urinary calculi.

Treatment

Initial treatment should be directed at hydration to a euvolemic state, pain relief using analgesics, and confirmation of stone passage by straining the urine for calculi (Figure 1). Overhydration inhibits ureteral wall coaptation and weakens the efficiency of ureteral peristalsis. Furthermore, the increased urine production with overhydration results in elevated ureteral and renal pressures, which exacerbate pain. A euvolemic state should be the goal; overhydration does not push calculi down the ureter.

Opiate analgesics are effective in relieving colicky pain. The most commonly used parenteral agents are morphine sulfate and meperidine (Demerol). These agents have no effects on ureteral peristalsis or on intrarenal pressures. Ketorolac (Toradol), a nonsteroidal anti-inflammatory drug, has the advantage of lowering intrarenal pressures by decreasing renal plasma flow. It is effective in relieving renal colic without the sedative side effects associated with opiates. This medication is inappropriate for those patients with underlying renal disease, for patients over 65 years of age, and in pregnancy.

Most patients respond to hydration and analgesics and can be managed expectantly on an outpatient basis while awaiting stone passage. Patients with intractable pain unresponsive to parenteral analgesics, with persistent nausea and vomiting, or with fever should be admitted to the hospital. Adequate urinary drainage from the obstructed renal unit must be obtained in patients with fever and signs of systemic infection using a ureteral catheter or percutaneous nephrostomy tube.

Most calculi less than 6 mm in greatest dimension will pass spontaneously. Symptomatic stones that do not pass spontaneously may necessitate surgical intervention. Surgical treatment depends upon stone location, size, and composition, as well as underlying renal anatomy. Most renal calculi less than 2.5 cm in diameter can be managed with extracorporeal shock wave lithotripsy (SWL). These focused shock waves in diameter used to fragment stones. Small fragments usually pass spontaneously and uneventfully. Lower pole renal calculi greater than 1 cm and other renal calculi greater than 2.5 cm are best managed with percutaneous nephrostolithotomy. Ureteral stones may be managed with in situ SWL or with ureteroscopy and extraction. Endoscopic procedures allow a variety of fragmentation devices, including the ultrasonic, electrohydraulic, pneumatic, and laser lithotrites, to be used. Open surgical treatment is rarely required today and is reserved for patients with unusual anatomy in whom less invasive treatments have failed.

Long-Term Management

After the acute episode has resolved and the patient has passed a calculus or has had it surgically extracted, a thorough medical evaluation should be initiated. The stone should be sent for laboratory analysis. Serum levels of routine electrolytes, creatinine, calcium, phosphate, uric acid, and parathyroid hormone (PTH) should be obtained. A 24-hour urine collection should measure urine volume, pH, specific gravity, calcium, creatinine, citrate, oxalate, phosphate, uric acid, and sodium. The results of the laboratory tests and stone analysis will guide subsequent medical therapy.

MEDICAL THERAPIES

Calcium Urolithiasis

Stone analysis indicating calcium phosphate should raise suspicion of distal renal tubular acidosis (RTA) or primary hyperparathyroidism. Distal RTA can be confirmed by hypokalemia, low serum bicarbonate, and a fasting urinary pH greater than 5.5. Hyperparathyroidism can be confirmed with increased PTH and serum calcium and decreased serum phosphorus levels.

In approximately 75% of cases, stone analysis will reveal calcium oxalate. These stones develop owing to a variety of underlying metabolic defects, which are divided into hypercalciuric and normocalciuric states.

Hypercalciuric States

Absorptive hypercalciuria is subclassified into three types: diet-independent (type I), diet-dependent (type II), and renal phosphate "leak" (type III). All three states are associated with hypercalciuria (defined as the presence of more than 250 mg of calcium in a 24-hour urine specimen). Type I patients have hypercalciuria during both low and high dietary calcium intakes. Serum calcium is normal, and PTH is low or normal. Fasting urinary calcium is normal, but urine calcium levels increase with an oral calcium load. Treatment is usually effective with thiazide diuretics (hydrochlorothiazide[1], 50 mg twice daily). Oral cellulose phosphates (Calcibind) may be used to bind calcium in the gut, rendering it insoluble, thus decreasing urinary calcium levels.

[1]Not FDA approved for this indication.

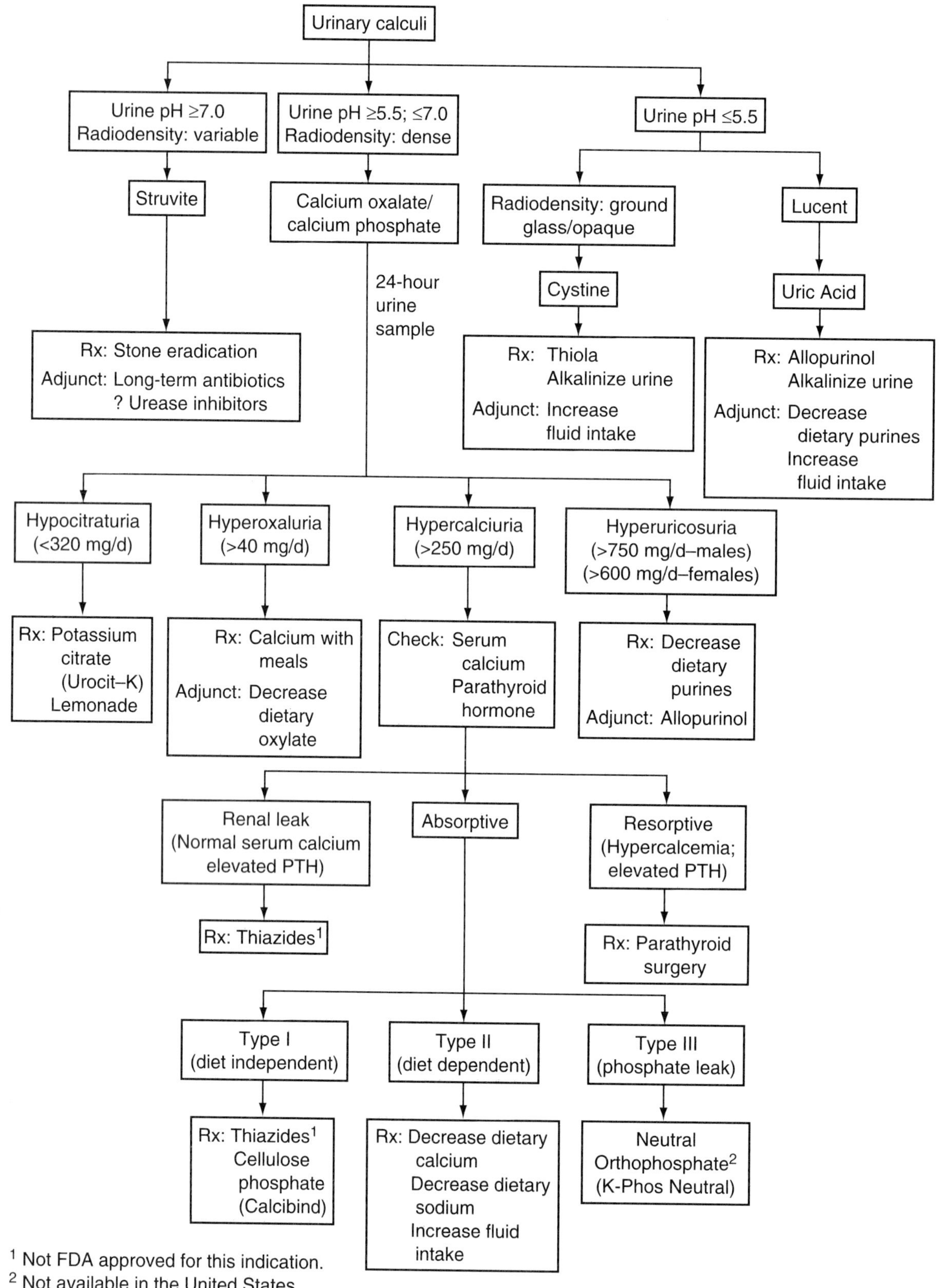

[1] Not FDA approved for this indication.
[2] Not available in the United States.

FIGURE 1 Decision tree for urinary stone disease.

Type II absorptive hypercalciuria patients exhibit hypercalciuria only during periods of increased calcium dietary intake. Therapy is directed at decreasing dietary intake of calcium by 50%, sodium restriction, and hydration adequate to produce 2 L of urine per day.

Type III absorptive hypercalciuria is characterized by high urinary phosphate levels because of a renal phosphate "leak." Serum phosphate concentration is usually less than 2.5 mg/dL. The hypophosphatemia results in increased levels of 1,25-dihydroxyvitamin D. This compound stimulates intestinal phosphate and calcium absorption and renal excretion of calcium. Type III hypercalciuria is treated by adding dietary phosphate in the form of neutral orthophosphate (K-Phos Neutral) 250 mg three times a day, and by titrating the dosage until urinary calcium levels normalize.

Resorptive hypercalciuria is caused by primary hyperparathyroidism. Renal calculi can be the initial manifestation of this disorder. The hypersecretion of PTH results in bone resorption and increased intestinal absorption of calcium, leading to hypercalcemia, hypercalciuria, and hyperphosphaturia. Treatment of this disease is surgical removal of the parathyroid adenoma.

Renal leak hypercalciuria is characterized by impaired renal tubular absorption of filtered calcium. The reduced serum calcium stimulates production of PTH, leading to subsequent stimulation of 1,25-dihydroxyvitamin D. This results in normal serum calcium with normal or increased PTH levels and hypercalciuria. This is effectively treated over the long-term with thiazides.

Hydrochlorothiazide[1] will correct secondary hyperparathyroidism in all of the hypercalciuric metabolic states except resorptive hypercalciuria. This is a clinically useful method of differentiating secondary from primary hyperparathyroidism in patients presenting with urinary stone disease.

Normocalciuric States

When the 24-hour urine collection reveals normal calcium levels (less than 250 mg per day), one or more of three metabolic defects is responsible: hyperuricosuria, hypocitraturia, and/or hyperoxaluria.

Hyperuricosuria is found in up to 20% of patients with calcium oxalate stones. It is characterized by urinary uric acid levels greater than 750 mg per day in men and greater than 600 mg per day in women. It may be seen in patients with primary gout, myeloproliferative states, glycogen storage diseases, and malignancy. Purine overproduction more frequently occurs owing to dietary overindulgence. Monosodium urates may act as a nidus for precipitation of calcium oxalate owing to heterogeneous nucleation. Monosodium urates may also bind urinary inhibitors of calcium stone formation. Treatment involves limiting dietary purines; if this is unsuccessful, administration of allopurinol (Zyloprim) is usually a successful therapy.

Hyperoxaluria is caused by two mechanisms: primary overproduction and increased intestinal absorption. The most common of these is increased absorption, also known as enteric hyperoxaluria. A variety of bowel disorders, such as inflammatory bowel disease, short-gut syndrome, and the decreased absorption in patients who have undergone intestinal bypass, may result in fat malabsorption. Fat saponifies dietary calcium and results in increased levels of free intestinal oxalate, which normally binds with calcium. Free oxalate is readily absorbed. A small increase in absorbed oxalate is more significant in stone formation than is a small increase in absorbed calcium. Restricting dietary intake of oxalate-rich foods is usually unsuccessful. Effective treatment is directed at binding dietary oxalate with calcium supplements at meal time. Mild cases will respond to an intake of calcium-rich foods, such as milk and cheese, at meal times. More severe cases may require use of calcium-containing antacids at meal times.

Citrate is a potent inhibitor of calcium stone formation. Hypocitraturia has been noted in up to 40% of calcium stone formers, often in combination with other disorders. Patients with citrate levels of less than 320 mg per day should be treated with citrate supplements. The simplest and most palatable regimen for many patients is lemonade therapy. Patients are directed to add 4 ounces of lemon juice concentrate to one half gallon of water and sweeten to taste. The lemonade is consumed over the course of the day. This treatment has resulted in significant increases in urinary citrate levels. For patients unable to consume the lemonade, supplementation with potassium citrate (Urocit-K), 60 to 120 mEq per day in divided doses, is recommended.

Presence of Non–Calcium-Containing Stones

Uric acid stones account for approximately 10% of all cases of urolithiasis. Uric acid stones are relatively radiolucent but may contain variable amounts of calcium. Uric acid stones, in contrast to calcium stones, are treatable by dissolution with medical therapy. The dissociation constant of uric acid is 5.75; above this pH, the solubility increases rapidly. If a lucent calculus is noted radiographically, alkalinization therapy using potassium citrate (Urocit-K) is initiated to raise the urinary pH to 6.5 to 7.0. In addition, patients are encouraged to void more than 2 L of urine per day and to decrease dietary purines. Progress with therapy can be monitored using ultrasound or noncontrast CT. Approximately 1 cm of uric acid stone seen on imaging studies can be dissolved in 4 to 6 weeks. Dissolution rapidly increases after performance of SWL, as the stone surface dramatically increases with fragmentation.

Stones containing magnesium ammonium phosphate (struvite) or carbonate apatite are most commonly associated with infection. Struvite calculi

[1]Not FDA approved for this indication.

occur only in the presence of urease-producing microorganisms, which cleave urea to ammonia, resulting in an alkaline urinary milieu. Precipitation of the struvite occurs in urine with a pH of greater than 7.2. *Proteus mirabilis* is the most common organism associated with these stones, but *Pseudomonas*, *Providencia*, staphylococci, *Serratia*, and *Mycoplasma* may also produce the urease responsible for stone formation. The key to therapy is complete stone removal. These stones frequently fill the renal collecting system with a "staghorn" configuration. The large stone size makes SWL a poor choice for stone eradication; percutaneous nephrostolithotomy is often needed for complete stone removal. Antibiotic therapy will be unable to sterilize urine in the presence of residual calculi. Frequently, the extensive nature of the condition dictates that several percutaneous procedures, supplemented with SWL, are needed for complete stone removal. After stone removal patients should be monitored closely for urinary tract infections and stone recurrence.

Cystine stones account for 1% of cases of urolithiasis. Persons with cystinuria have an autosomal recessive disorder affecting the transport of dibasic amino acids. This results in high urinary levels of cystine, which is insoluble at normal urinary pH. The solubility of cystine increases rapidly above a pH of 7.5. Diagnosis of cystinuria is made on the basis of a 24-hour urine analysis; most heterozygotes will excrete more than 200 mg of cystine per day.

The goal of therapy is to keep patients well hydrated with urine production at more than 2 L per day and urine pH at 7.0 to 7.5, using an alkalizing agent such as potassium citrate (Urocit-K). Specific therapy is also aimed at reducing urinary cystine levels to less than 100 mg per day, using agents that increase cystine solubility by creating a mixed disulfide. Penicillamine (Cuprimine) was used in the past, but its association with frequent side effects, including gastrointestinal upset, nephrotic syndrome, dermatitis, and pancytopenia, limited its usefulness. Tiopronin (i.e., α-mercaptopropionylglycine [Thiola]), which also works by binding to the sulfhydryl groups, has fewer side effects and is currently the drug of choice at a dose of 0.5 to 1 g per day in divided doses.

Other Stones

Stones may be composed of a variety of other substances, including matrix, xanthine, triamterene, and indinavir (Crixivan). Indinavir calculi have been cited as a common complication of therapy directed at HIV infection with the protease inhibitor indinavir (Crixivan). Management of these calculi generally consists of temporary cessation of medication with aggressive hydration.

General Dietary Measures

Patients with stones often require dietary manipulation in addition to specific medical therapy. General guidelines include maintaining euvolemia with approximately 1.5 to 2 L of urine output per day; there is little evidence to support the common recommendation of vigorous overhydration. In addition, table salt should be restricted to less than 2 g per day, because sodium exacerbates hypercalciuria. Furthermore, a low-protein diet (protein intake of less than 65 g per day) is recommended to prevent the metabolic acidosis with subsequent mobilization of calcium from bone that occurs after animal protein-rich meals.

Management of urinary stone disease is often frustrating for both the patient and the physician. A recurrence rate of up to 50% in 5 years is noted with no metabolic intervention. Although renal failure is rarely a result of recurrent stone disease, the morbidity and inconvenience for patients are substantial. Many of these episodes can be prevented with a thorough metabolic workup and directed therapy for specific defects.

SECTION 11

The Sexually Transmitted Diseases

CHANCROID

METHOD OF

Ellen S. Rome, MD, MPH

Caused by *Haemophilus ducreyi*, a fastidious gram-negative bacillus, chancroid traditionally has been a disease of Africa and the tropics, with smaller epidemics found in the United States and elsewhere. The estimated incidence worldwide is thought to be about 7 million new cases per year; because of the lack of a good diagnostic test, the true incidence is unknown. Although more cases occur in uncircumcised men, more advanced disease is seen in men who are circumcised, with the male-to-female ratio at 10:1.

Epidemiology

Chancroid has seen a recent resurgence in the United States and worldwide. The most frequent cause of sexually acquired genital ulceration in Africa, chancroid has had its highest prevalences found in southern, central, and eastern Africa. In a recent study of ten cities in the United States, chancroid was confirmed in 12% of genital ulcers in Chicago, and 20% in Memphis. In Jackson, Mississippi, in 1994, an outbreak of genital ulcers included 143 patients tested with a multiplex polymerase chain reaction (PCR) assay. In this study, 56 (39%) were positive for *H. ducreyi*, 44 (31%) for herpes simplex virus, and 27 (19%) for *Treponema pallidum*; 12 (8%) tested positive for more than one organism. Of 136 patients tested for HIV by serology, 14 (10%) were HIV-positive, compared with none of 200 patients without ulcers in their study. Risk factors included sex with a crack cocaine user, exchange of money or drugs for sex, and multiple sex partners.

Epidemiologic evidence from Africa clearly demonstrates that chancroid is a risk factor for the spread of HIV among heterosexuals. Biologic factors may account for this finding. First, the ulcers of chancroid contain CD4+ T cells, and the virus has been isolated from chancroidal ulcers, with these lesions as the probable portal of entry for HIV. Second, HIV-infected partners may have greater numbers of ulcers than non-HIV infected patients. Third, the semen from HIV-positive patients co-infected with chancroid contains a higher viral load of HIV than semen from HIV-infected patients without chancroid. Because chancroid resolves more slowly in HIV-infected patients, antibiotic-treated HIV-positive patients with chancroid may be infectious for a longer period of time. The term *infectious synergy* was coined to describe this risk for coinfection.

Diagnosis

Multiple purulent ulcers with ragged edges and tender inguinal adenopathy are the hallmarks of chancroid, with definitive diagnosis by culture on special media (sensitivity only 80%). Table 1 compares the differentiating features of the genital ulcers seen with herpes simplex, syphilis, and chancroid. In one study, individual signs such as a clean-based ulcer in cases of primary syphilis and undermined lesion borders in cases of chancroid had good sensitivity (82% and 85%, respectively). Similarly, 3+ induration of primary syphilis ulcers had a specificity of 95%, and shallow ulceration in cases of genital herpes had a specificity of 88%. The clinician with a reasonable index of suspicion for chancroid should treat while awaiting culture or diagnostic test results.

Polymerase chain reaction (PCR) is very sensitive for the diagnosis of primary syphilis, chancroid, and genital herpes. Now, with the advances made by DNA amplification strategies, the sensitivity of *H. ducreyi* culture, previously considered the gold standard for diagnosis, has been shown to be only approximately 75% at best.

Elkins and colleagues recently developed a new recombinant protein enzyme immunoassay (rpEIA) for determination of the seroprevalence of chancroid. Three highly conserved outer membrane proteins from *H. ducreyi* strain 35000 were cloned, expressed, and purified from *Escherichia coli* for use as antigens in the rpEIA. This test was designed for use in seroprevalence studies, not for the diagnosis of current infection. The study was limited by the fact that the authors were unable to obtain a reliable history of chancroid from patients studied. Both *H. ducreyi* outer membrane protein (OMP) and lipo-oligosaccharide (LOS) elicit primarily IgG responses that may remain elevated for months. However, it takes several weeks of ulcerative symptoms for patients with a first episode of chancroid to develop an antibody response to *H. ducreyi*. Thus, serology-based approaches currently may have limited sensitivity for the detection of circulating antibodies to *H. ducreyi* in individual symptomatic patients; however, they can be used as a useful tool to perform large scale epidemiologic studies at the community level. Further seroprevalence studies need to be performed to determine the persistence of positive antibodies after treatment along with the effects of reinfection on titers. Commercially available PCR or monoclonal antibody tests may also curb spread of the disease should they become accessible in the future.

TABLE 1 Differential Diagnosis of Genital Ulcers and Nodes

Disease	Ulcer	Lymphadenopathy
Syphilis	Painless chancre	Painless nodes
Chancroid	Painful ulcer	Tender nodes
Herpes simplex virus	Painful vesicle or ulcer	Tender nodes

The incubation period for chancroid is between 4 and 7 days, with the first finding being a small inflammatory papule or pustule containing polymorphonuclear leukocytes. This pustule soon ruptures, exposing the dermis, with formation of an ulcer containing large numbers of *H. ducreyi* and inflammatory cells. *H. ducreyi* prefers to grow at 33°C (91.4°F), perhaps explaining why it does not disseminate and can be cultured only from skin.

Treatment

Table 2 shows the treatment regimens as per the *2002 STD Treatment Guidelines* from the Centers for Disease Control and Prevention. Each regimen appears to be effective against chancroid in the United States, but limited data from Kenya suggest that the ceftriaxone (Rocephin)[1] regimen may not be as effective there as it had been previously. Trimethoprim (Proloprim) resistance has been found in several studies. Penicillin is ineffective as a result of the production of β-lactamase by essentially all strains, and tetracycline resistance is widespread, yet the available antibiotics not yet showing resistance tend to be more expensive and less available. Ciprofloxacin (Cipro)[1] should not be used in pregnant and lactating women, with intermediate resistance to both ciprofloxacin and erythromycin reported worldwide.

Treatment for chancroid is often based on clinical diagnosis because of the lack of rapid diagnostic tests readily available in many clinics and because of the lack of sensitivity of the available tests. Single-dose treatment is usually preferred because of better compliance, reduced costs, and the potential to limit emerging resistance. Patients should be tested for HIV at the time of diagnosis and for HIV and syphilis 3 months after diagnosis, because coinfection rates are high. Persons with HIV do not respond as well to treatment as do those individuals without HIV infection, and uncircumcised males do not respond as well as men who are circumcised. Patients should be reexamined 3 to 7 days after the start of therapy, with

[1]Not FDA approved for this indication.

TABLE 2 Recommended Regimens for Treating Chancroid, as per the Centers for Disease Control and Prevention 2002 STD Treatment Guidelines

Azithromycin (Zithromax)[1], 1 g orally as a single dose
Ceftriaxone (Rocephin)[1], 250 mg intramuscularly as a single dose
Ciprofloxacin (Cipro)[1], 500 mg orally twice a day for 3 days
Erythromycin base (E-Mycin)[1], 500 mg orally four times a day for 7 days

[1]Not FDA approved for this indication.

successful treatment leading to symptomatic improvement by 3 days and objective improvement by 7 days. If no improvement is seen, evaluation for coinfection with either HIV or another STD should occur, along with addressing whether prescribed medicines were actually obtained and ingested. Large ulcers may take 2 weeks to heal. Sexual contacts also need to be treated, with assessment for reinfection or for antimicrobial resistance if the lesion has not resolved.

Chancroid remains a global problem, mainly attacking Africa and Asia, but with outbreaks in the United States and elsewhere. Where chancroid infection occurs, as with syphilis and herpes simplex virus, a portal of entry can increase likelihood of infection with other pathogens, particularly HIV. Moreover, infection with *H. ducreyi* may not occur in isolation, and coinfection can mask accurate diagnosis. Serologic tests for *H. ducreyi* can be useful for epidemiologic survey, but are less helpful to the clinician in the field trying to treat infection. Given the difficulties of accurate culture and lack of accessibility of commercial DNA-amplified tests, the clinician with a high index of suspicion should use an appropriate algorithm for management of infection. Partners should be evaluated and treated accordingly. When chancroid is hard to treat, reassess for co-morbid infection, including HIV. Antibiotic resistance will continue to emerge, making prevention the cornerstone of treatment and prompt treatment with the appropriate drug(s) imperative.

GONORRHEA

METHOD OF

George P. Schmid, MD, MSc

Globally, gonorrhea, a sexually transmitted disease (STD) caused by *Neisseria gonorrhoeae*, is the most important cause of urethritis in men and pelvic inflammatory disease (and its consequences of infertility and ectopic pregnancy) in women. Most cases, however, are asymptomatic or associated with symptoms that are so mild that people do not recognize they have a sexually transmitted infection (STI). Efforts to create a vaccine against *N. gonorrhoeae* have been unsuccessful and control depends upon enhancing safer sexual behaviors to prevent acquisition of infection, screening to detect those who are asymptomatically infected, and appropriate management of detected cases.

Epidemiology

More than 300,000 cases of gonorrhea are reported annually to state health authorities, and *N. gonorrhoeae* is second in frequency only to *Chlamydia trachomatis* among reported communicable infections. Frequency of infection is highest in young persons, 15- to 24-years-old, and approximately equal numbers of reported cases occur in men and women. Prior to the AIDS epidemic, gonorrhea was extremely common in men who have sex with men (MSM). With the adoption of safer sex practices by MSMs, rates plunged. In the past several years, however, the numbers of cases of gonorrhea in MSMs has risen markedly as adherence to safer sex practices has declined. Other groups at risk for gonorrhea include sex workers, those who abuse drugs, and minorities; geographically, gonorrhea is concentrated in large cities and the southeastern United States.

Gonorrhea is efficiently spread. The risk of a woman acquiring *N. gonorrhoeae* from a single act of sex with an infected male is approximately 50%; the risk of a man acquiring *N. gonorrhoeae* from a single act of sex with an infected woman is approximately 20%.

Microbiology and Diagnosis

N. gonorrhoeae is an aerobic, gram-negative bacterium that occurs in pairs (a "diplococcus"), with adjacent, flattened sides. Culture is accomplished using special media (traditionally, Thayer-Martin medium) incubated at 35°C (95°F) to 36°C (96.8°F) in an atmosphere enriched by 3% to 5% CO_2. Recovery rates from infected individuals are highest if specimens, particularly those from women (who have fewer organisms than symptomatic men), are plated directly onto media rather than placed into transport media.

Nonculture diagnostic techniques are replacing culture because of ease of transport and, with some tests, the ability to use noninvasively collected specimens (e.g., urine). Nonculture tests, however, are less sensitive than culture. The initial nonculture test for gonorrhea was an enzyme-linked immunoabsorbent assay (ELISA). This test has been supplanted by more sensitive nucleic acid hybridization and nucleic acid amplification tests, which detect either chromosomal or plasmid DNA, or ribosomal RNA. A considerable advantage of the nucleic acid amplification tests is that they can be used on a broad range of specimens, in particular, urine, making the necessity of an intraurethral swab in men or an endocervical swab in women unnecessary, which is particularly beneficial in screening situations.

In symptomatic men, a Gram stain of urethral secretions remains highly useful and sensitivity of the detection of intracellular diplococci is >95% and 99% specific. For women, a Gram stain of endocervical secretions is only approximately 50% sensitive and other cervical flora can be confused with *N. gonorrhoeae*, decreasing specificity.

In some instances, only culture should be used: in cases of medicolegal importance, to definitively identify *N. gonorrhoeae* and to retain the organism as evidence, and if testing for antimicrobial resistance is desired.

CLINICAL CHARACTERISTICS

Infection may occur at whatever anatomic site sex occurs. The most common site of infection is the urethra in men and the cervix in women. In MSMs, rectal infection occurs in approximately 25% of men with an infection at any site. Approximately 35% to 50% of women with an endocervical infection will also have rectal infection as a result of contamination of the anus by secretions from the vagina. Among persons with infection at any site, pharyngeal infection occurs in approximately 5% of heterosexual men, 15% of heterosexual women, and 15% of MSMs.

The incubation period of gonorrhea is best characterized in men, with a typical incubation period of 3 to 5 days. Women who become symptomatic develop more vague, local symptoms, and the initial symptoms may be caused by pelvic inflammatory disease (PID). In both genders, symptoms may be scant or nonexistent at any site that is infected, and most women, and probably most men, are asymptomatic. Alternately, they may have symptoms that are so mild, that they are overlooked.

Symptoms of urethral infection in men are dysuria and discharge. The discharge is classically purulent (yellow or green), as opposed to the white or clear discharge of nongonococcal urethritis, although testing is required to distinguish the two. Rectal infection (proctitis) in MSMs, when symptomatic, results in anal discharge, discomfort and tenesmus; few women with rectal infection have symptoms. Most pharyngeal infections are asymptomatic, although occasionally pharyngitis of mild to moderate severity occurs.

Complications of infection occur in individuals who are untreated. Disseminated gonococcal infection (DGI), also called *the arthritis–dermatitis syndrome*, occurs in 1% to 2% of infected individuals, and is the commonest cause of septic arthritis in young people. It occurs as a result of bacteremia in individuals typically without genital tract symptoms, and is characterized by moderate fever, tenosynovitis, arthritis and skin lesions (a small number of pustules with a red base on the periphery of the arms and legs); Gram stain of the lesions or joint fluid typically yields the initial diagnosis and culture of these sites (if affected) and blood work should be done. PID occurs in 20% to 40% of untreated women, most commonly during the first few menstrual cycles following infection.

THERAPY

Uncomplicated Genital Tract or Rectal Infection

Uncomplicated infection is effectively treated by a single dose of antimicrobial (Table 1). Quinolone resistance is common in the developing world, particularly Asia, and has appeared in the United States, initially in Hawaii and then in California. In these states, in MSM anywhere in the United States, and for infections acquired in many countries outside the United States, quinolones are not recommended. Resistance to cephalosporins has only rarely been reported.

TABLE 1 Uncomplicated Infection of the Urethra, Cervix, or Rectum*

Ceftriaxone (Rocephin), 125 mg, IM, once; or
Ciprofloxacin (Cipro), 500 mg, PO, once; or
Ofloxacin (Floxin), 400 mg, PO, once; or
Levofloxacin (Levaquin)[1], 250 mg, PO, once;
Each of the above with (unless chlamydial infection excluded):
Azithromycin (Zithromax), 1 g, PO, once; or
Doxycycline (Vibramycin), 100 mg, PO, twice a day for 7 days.

*Cefixime (Suprax), 400 mg, PO, can be used but the distribution of cefixime in the United States has been discontinued by the manufacturer.

[1]Not FDA approved for this indication.

Alternate cephalosporin or quinolone regimens can be used but offer either no advantage over the drugs in Table 1 or have lesser therapeutic experience. Spectinomycin (Trobicin), 2 g, intramuscularly (IM), is highly effective against genital and rectal infections and can be used if cephalosporins or quinolones cannot.

Co-infection by *Chlamydia trachomatis* of individuals with gonorrhea occurs in 10% to 30% of cases. Unless testing for *C. trachomatis* infection is performed, all patients with gonorrhea should be treated for a possible coexisting chlamydial infection with either azithromycin (Zithromax) or doxycycline (Vibramycin).

Cases should be serologically tested for syphilis and offered testing for HIV infection. All cases of gonorrhea confirmed by laboratory testing should be reported promptly to health authorities.

Patients should be counseled about the need to adhere to therapy, possible side effects of medication, the need to return if symptoms do not abate, to refrain from sex until they complete therapy (as do any sex partners), and the need to refer sex partners. Because the onset of symptoms is not always clear and a reliable incubation period difficult to establish, referral of sex partners within the past 60 days is recommended. Partners should be evaluated, tested, and routinely treated. If there has been no sex partner in the last 60 days, the most recent sex partner should be examined.

The effectiveness of recommended regimens is so high (>98%) that patients do not need to return for follow-up but should if symptoms persist. If so, the clinician should consider other causes of symptoms, antibiotic resistance of *N. gonorrhoeae*, and whether the patient adhered to therapy.

Pregnancy

Pregnant women should not be treated with quinolones or tetracyclines. A cephalosporin or spectinomycin should be used, and possible co-infection with *C. trachomatis* treated with erythromycin (E-Mycin) or amoxicillin[1].

[1]Not FDA approved for this indication.

Pharyngeal Infection

Pharyngeal infection is more difficult to cure than anogenital infections. Ceftriaxone (Rocephin) or ciprofloxacin (Cipro) can be used, but cure rates may not exceed 90%. Pharyngeal infection by *C. trachomatis* is uncommon, but co-treatment for *C. trachomatis*—whether an oral or asymptomatic genital infection—is recommended.

Disseminated Gonococcal Infection

Initial hospitalization is advisable, particularly for patients with septic arthritis or other significant illness, a questionable diagnosis, or who may not comply with outpatient therapy. Ceftriaxone (Rocephin) 1 g IM or intravenously (IV) every 24 hours is recommended. Alternately, cefotaxime (Claforan 1 g IV every 8 hours), ceftizoxime (Cefizox 1 g IV every 8 hours), ciprofloxacin (Cipro 400 mg IV every 12 hours), ofloxacin (Floxin 400 mg IV every 12 hours), levofloxacin (Levaquin 250 mg IV daily)[1], or spectinomycin (Trobicin 2 g IM every 12 hours), may be used. Once clinical response has occurred, therapy may be continued for at least one week orally with ciprofloxacin (Cipro) 500 mg twice daily, ofloxacin (Floxin) 400 mg orally (PO) twice daily, or levofloxacin (Levaquin) 500 mg PO once daily.

PID

PID caused by *N. gonorrhoeae* should be treated as described in the pelvic inflammatory disease article.

Complications

Infection rarely causes severe invasive disease (e.g., endocarditis or meningitis) or local disease (e.g., ophthalmitis), and other sources should be consulted.

Infection of Neonates and Children

All neonates should receive ocular prophylaxis against gonococcal ophthalmia with 1% silver nitrate ophthalmic solution or an appropriate topical antimicrobial. Infants born to mothers with cervical infection are at risk of gonococcal ophthalmia or disseminated gonococcal infection and should be evaluated and treated with ceftriaxone (Rocephin), 25 to 50 mg/kg IV or IM, not to exceed 125 mg, once. Infection in older children should prompt an investigation of child abuse. Quinolones are not recommended for children younger than age 18 years, and ceftriaxone (Rocephin) is preferred (125 mg IM unless the child weighs more than 45 kg, in which case, adult doses are used).

[1]Not FDA approved for this indication.

NONGONOCOCCAL URETHRITIS

METHOD OF
John F. Toney, MD

Nongonococcal urethritis (NGU) describes one type of reproductive tract infection seen in men. NGU refers to the large proportion of urethritis not caused by *Neisseria gonorrhoeae*. *Chlamydia trachomatis* has historically been the most common cause of NGU and can be found in 23% to 55% of cases. Undetected genital chlamydia infections are important to recognize and treat because of the potential to cause additional disease in men (epididymitis, Reiter's syndrome) and in their female partners (pelvic inflammatory disease, Reiter's syndrome, and genital tract infection during pregnancy or in the neonate). Additional organisms may also cause NGU; these include other bacteria as well as protozoal or viral etiologies. *Ureaplasma urealyticum*, *Ureaplasma parvum*, *Mycoplasma genitalium*, and *Mycoplasma hominis* have been isolated from the male urethra, most commonly by DNA amplification methodology, such as polymerase chain reaction. Of these organisms, *M. genitalium* causes a significant proportion of nonchlamydial NGU cases, perhaps up to 43% of cases. *Trichomonas vaginalis* and herpes simplex virus (HSV) may also cause NGU; in a minority of patients with genital herpes and urethritis, no external lesions on the penis are found on examination. Of the remaining cases of NGU, the etiologic agents of infection are either poorly characterized or unknown.

The incubation period for NGU is generally 1 to 5 weeks, depending on the organism causing the syndrome. The incubation period for chlamydia is usually 1 to 3 weeks, but for some organisms (such as *M. genitalium*), the incubation time remains unclear.

Diagnosis

NGU is diagnosed if urethritis is present but *N. gonorrhoeae* is not. Although many men have symptoms compatible with urethritis (such as "burning" or "tingling"), these symptoms are not always caused by urethritis. A urethral discharge may be present with NGU; it is commonly scant and more mucoid in appearance when compared with the copious and purulent discharge generally seen with *N. gonorrhoeae*. To evaluate for the presence of urethral disease, urethritis should be documented by any of the following:

- A visible urethral discharge as described above
- A Gram stain or wet preparation microscopic evaluation with four or more white blood cells (WBCs) per oil immersion field

- With the initial few millimeters of voided urine (with no urination in the 2 hours prior), finding 10 or more WBCs per high-power microscopic field
- A positive urine leukocyte esterase test

Always performing a gonococcal and chlamydia test on men with symptoms or signs of urethritis and using other tests as needed help with decisions regarding therapy, partner management, and state or national disease reporting. If urethritis is not documented, tests for *N. gonorrhoeae* and *C. trachomatis* should be performed, and treatment decisions should be based on the clinical and laboratory findings. NGU is a reportable disease in many local public health arenas; clinicians should be familiar with local reporting laws and processes.

Therapy

Treatment should be begun immediately after diagnosis; antibiotic therapy is generally recommended to cover the more common bacteriologic agents associated with NGU (Table 1). When the results of laboratory testing become available, alterations in therapy can be made if necessary.

Patient counseling should also be undertaken at this time. The patient should refer all sex partners within 60 days before the onset of symptoms for evaluation and treatment. Partners of patients with documented chlamydial infection within this time frame should be offered prophylactic antibiotic therapy ("epidemiologically treated") after evaluation. Because the other bacterial causes of NGU are difficult to detect, counseling the patient and the patient's partners can be problematic. For nonchlamydial bacterial NGU, it is unclear if prophylactic antibiotic treatment are useful, and with no specific infectious agent identified, justifying treatment for partners may be confusing for them.

TABLE 1 Initial Therapy for Nongonococcal Urethritis

Preferred Therapy*
Azithromycin (Zithromax), 1 g orally once, *or*
Doxycycline (Vibramycin), 100 mg orally twice a day for 7 d, *or*
Alternative Therapy
Erythromycin base (Ery-Tab), 500 mg orally four times a day for 7 d, *or*
Erythromycin ethylsuccinate (EES), 800 mg orally four times a day for 7 d, *or*
Levofloxacin (Levaquin), 500 mg once a day for 7 d, *or*
Ofloxacin (Floxin), 300 mg twice a day for 7 d

*Therapy selection is based on considerations of efficacy, ease of administration, incidence or severity of side effects, and cost. See MMWR Morbid Mortal Wkly Rep, Vol. 51, 2002.

Routine follow-up for NGU is unnecessary unless symptoms persist or recur. If the latter is noted, these patients should be questioned about adherence to their medical regimen, whether their partner(s) was (were) treated, and whether they have had additional recent sexual contact (especially unprotected intercourse). In these cases, treatment may need to be repeated and the men should be evaluated again for continuing signs of urethritis. The management of patients with continuing symptoms of urethritis but *no* objective signs can be problematic, and it is unclear how best to manage them.

For men with continuing objective signs of urethritis who have successfully completed presumably effective therapy, consideration of antibiotic resistance with genital mycoplasmas should be entertained. A proportion of *U. urealyticum* isolates are resistant to tetracyclines but susceptible to erythromycins. *Mycoplasma genitalium* may not respond to a single dose of azithromycin (Zithromax) or to a 1-week course of tetracyclines or erythromycins, and some experts recommend longer treatment for these bacteria, using a 2- to 4-week course of antibiotics, with erythromycins being the preferred choice.

Another agent causing persistent urethritis is *Trichomonas vaginalis*, which can be difficult to diagnose in men. Testing for this agent should include an intraurethral swab for *Trichomonas* culture, or obtaining a first-voided urine specimen to microscopically examine for *Trichomonas*. A positive test result can be treated with a single 2 g oral dose of metronidazole (Flagyl), which can be given concomitantly with other antibiotics. Additionally, close clinical inspection of the urethral meatal area for erythema or ulceration may suggest herpes simplex virus (HSV) infection. Patients with recurring urethritis without a demonstrable infectious etiology and unresponsive to antibiotic therapy may be considered for the newer type-specific glycoprotein G herpes serology (gG HSV-2) or HSV Western blot testing to evaluate for prior genital herpes exposure.

Other Considerations

Many, if not most, men with urethritis are asymptomatic. These individuals may be detected by the screening studies described above. In these men, however, a Gram stain of urethral secretions may be less sensitive, detecting only approximately 50% of men with gonorrhea. Because *N. gonorrhoeae* is more likely to cause symptomatic infection/urethritis, a greater proportion of men with asymptomatic urethritis will have nongonococcal causes.

DONOVANOSIS

METHOD OF

Nigel O'Farrell, MD

Donovanosis (*Granuloma inguinale*) is an uncommon cause of genital ulceration that is usually sexually transmitted. The causative organism was recently reclassified as *Klebsiella granulomatis*, a gram-negative intracellular pleomorphic bacillus, rather than *Calymmatobacterium granulomatis*. Since the introduction of antibiotics, donovanosis has become uncommon in developed countries, but is still found in diverse developing areas including Papua New Guinea, southern Africa, particularly South Africa, southeast India, and Brazil. In Australia, a recent donovanosis eradication program among aboriginals has reduced cases to a handful. The condition is associated with poor genital hygiene and lower socioeconomic standards, and is more common in uncircumcised men.

The infection usually starts as a papule or subcutaneous nodule that ulcerates after trauma. The incubation period is variable, but is usually around 50 days. The classical lesion is a beefy red ulcer that bleeds readily to the touch. Other types include the hypertrophic, necrotic, and sclerotic variants.

The genital area is usually affected, but nongenital lesions are found in 5% of cases. Inguinal lesions are found in 10% of cases, but inguinal lymphadenopathy is uncommon. In men, common sites of infection are the prepuce, coronal sulcus, frenum, and glans penis; in women, common sites of infection are the labia minora and fourchette. Cervical lesions may mimic carcinoma. Extragenital lesions rarely involve the lips, gums, cheek, palate, pharynx, larynx, and chest. Hematogenous spread to liver and bone is reported. During pregnancy, lesions may develop more rapidly and respond to treatment more slowly. Complications include carcinoma, pseudoelephantiasis and stenosis of the urethra, vagina, and anus.

The diagnosis is usually confirmed by microscopic identification of Donovan bodies in tissue smears prepared carefully as follows. First, a swab should be rolled firmly over an ulcer cleaned previously with a dry swab to remove debris. The swab is then rolled firmly over a slide to spread the material collected from the ulcer. The slide is then stained (rapid Giemsa) and examined by microscopy. Alternatively, a piece of granulation tissue crushed and spread between two slides can be used. Donovan bodies can be seen in large mononuclear cells as gram-negative intracytoplasmic cysts with dark-staining bodies with a safety pin appearance. Histological appearances include chronic inflammation with infiltration of plasma cells and neutrophils. Epithelial changes include ulceration, microabscesses, and elongation of the rete ridges. Cultures have been reported in peripheral blood monocytes and Hep-2 cells in a few centers. Serologic tests have poor specificity, but a polymerase chain reaction test using a colorimetric system was used recently with some success.

Treatment

Azithromycin (Zithromax)[1] has now become accepted as the drug of choice for the treatment of donovanosis. Two effective regimens have been tried in Australia, either 1 g weekly for 4 weeks or 500 mg daily for 1 week. Older, established therapies include trimethoprim-sulfamethoxazole (TMP-SMX, Bactrim DS, Septa DS) 160/800 mg[1] twice daily and doxycycline (Vibramycin) 100 mg twice daily both for 3 weeks or until all lesions are healed completely. Pregnant women should be treated with erythromycin (E-Mycin) 500 mg four times daily until healing is achieved. Rarely, intravenous gentamicin (Garamycin)[1] 1 mg/kg every 8 hours is required. Surgery may be indicated for fistulas and massive tissue destruction. Other effective treatments include ceftriaxone (Rocephin)[1], chloramphenicol (Chloromycetin)[1], ciprofloxacin (Cipro)[1], and norfloxacin (Noroxin)[1].

Patients should be screened for other sexually transmitted infections, counseled about the risks of HIV transmission, and advised to abstain from sexual intercourse until ulcers have been cured. Management should include reassurance that treatments are effective and that ulcers will heal eventually. If sexual partners are identified, they should be examined and offered prophylactic treatment.

[1]Not FDA approved for this indication.

LYMPHOGRANULOMA VENEREUM

METHOD OF

Nigel O'Farrell, MD

Lymphogranuloma venereum (LGV) is a sexually transmitted infection caused by serovars L1-L3 of *Chlamydia trachomatis*, an obligate intracellular bacterium. LGV is uncommon in developed countries and is found mainly in the developing world. Incorrect diagnosis is not uncommon in many areas where diagnostic tests are unavailable. In the past, the condition has been confused with donovanosis (*granuloma inguinale*).

Classical LGV has three stages. After an incubation period of 3 to 12 days, a primary, painless papule, pustule, or small erosion develops that resembles herpes. In men, lesions are found on the glans penis, and in women they are found on the labia or vaginal walls, although primary lesions often go unnoticed.

The primary lesion normally heals in a week and is followed a few weeks later by a secondary stage with painful inguinal and/or femoral lymphadenopathy, systemic symptoms of fever and lassitude, and, occasionally, arthralgia and meningism. Enlargement of femoral and inguinal lymph glands together in men may result in the "groove sign," an indentation along Poupart's ligament. If untreated, buboes in the inguinal region can rupture, leading to protracted healing. Lymph nodes may necrose and form stellate abscesses. Further inflammatory complications include loculated abscesses, fistulas, and sinus tracts. The tertiary (anogenital) stage is defined by the long-term complications of LGV including rectal stricture, fistula formation, and adhesions that follow fibrotic healing of the secondary stage. Most lesions in this category are either in homosexual men or women. Proctocolitis may occur with fever, rectal pain, and abdominal tenderness. Later complications include elephantiasis and chronic edema that can cause gross distortion of the genital anatomy.

LGV is usually diagnosed by using microimmunofluorescence tests that differentiate between chlamydia serovars. High titers with complement fixation tests are also suggestive of LGV. Polymerase chain reaction methods have been used to detect samples from ulcers, but experience of this is limited. Histologic changes include epithelioid and multinucleate giant cells with central necrosis containing neutrophils, plasma cells, stellate abscesses, and macrophages. The differential diagnosis includes other causes of genital ulceration or acute lymphadenitis, including plague, tularemia, tuberculosis, Hodgkin's disease, and cat-scratch disease.

Treatment

Treatment should be given for 21 days with either of the following: doxycycline (Vibramycin) 100 mg twice daily, tetracycline 500 mg four times daily, or for pregnant or lactating women, erythromycin (E-Mycin)[1] 500 mg four times daily. Azithromycin (Zithromax)[1] is probably effective but the optimal dose has not yet been confirmed. Prophylactic treatment should be offered to sexual partners of index cases. Late complications with either fistula, lymphatic obstruction and dilatation, and bowel obstruction may require surgery. Patients with LGV are at risk of other sexually transmitted infections, and should be screened and receive counseling and education about HIV.

[1]Not FDA approved for this indication.

SYPHILIS

METHOD OF

Mrunal Shah, MD

One of the oldest infections known, syphilis dates back more than 500 years. It was known as "The Great Pox" because of its skin manifestations; in contrast to the "small pox" seen around the same time. Studies were done before the use of antibiotics, which is where most of our natural history information comes from. The most recent epidemic occurred in 1990 (20.3 cases per 100,000 population) and has fallen steadily each year since. In the year 2000, the rate was at an all time low of 2.2 cases per 100,000 population. This was a 9.6% drop since 1999. The Centers for Disease Control and Prevention (CDC) hopes to eradicate the disease completely by 2005, but this may be difficult.

Peak ages are 30 to 39 years of age in men and 20 to 24 years of age in women. African-Americans have always had higher incidences than whites. In the 1990s, it was 60:1, but the incidence has since declined to 30:1.

Microbiology

Treponema pallidum is the bacterium responsible for causing syphilis. It is very small, and cannot be detected by ordinary microscopy, a feature that complicates diagnosis. The organism can be seen with darkfield microscopy, a technique that uses a special condenser to cast an oblique light. This allows visualization of a corkscrew-shaped organism with tightly wound spirals. This organism is extremely sensitive to penicillin, as is discussed later in the article. It has a very slow doubling rate, therefore requiring longer courses of treatment.

Pathophysiology

T. pallidum initiates infection when it gains access to subcutaneous tissues through microabrasions that can occur during sexual intercourse. Even though it has a slow doubling time (30 hours), it escapes host immune defenses and leads to the initial ulcerative lesion, the chancre. These can be seen anywhere around the genitalia including the cervix, perianal and rectal areas, and the oral mucosa. Regional lymphadenopathy also can be seen. As the host immune system fights the initial infection, *T. pallidum* is disseminated throughout the host. This is known as latency, as the patient will have no symptoms. There is also vertical spread in utero or during delivery, which is why prenatal panels include screening tests for syphilis.

Clinical Manifestations

The initial clinical manifestation is also called *primary* syphilis. This usually consists of a *painless* chancre at the site of inoculation. Primary syphilis represents a local infection, but quickly becomes systemic with widespread dissemination of the spirochete. Because it is painless, most people do not seek medical attention. Even without treatment, the chancre will resolve in 4 to 6 weeks. It is this painlessness that helps separate it from herpes simplex virus (genital herpes) and *Haemophilus ducreyi* (chancroid).

In approximately weeks to months after the resolution of the chancre, patients will develop *secondary* syphilis, which includes systemic symptoms of rash, fever, headache, malaise, anorexia, and diffuse lymphadenopathy. The rash typically involves the palms and soles but can also include mucosal surfaces. Many patients do not realize that they had these lesions. These symptoms usually resolve spontaneously but can relapse for up to 5 years.

After symptoms resolve, and for up to many years later, the disease goes into *latent* syphilis, which is characterized by a lack of symptoms but seropositive test results. This can be separated into *early* and *late* latent phases based on being potentially infectious in the early phase. This is defined by the United States Public Health Service (USPHS) as infection of 1 year's duration or less. Anything longer is *late* latent.

Finally, for the next 1 to 30 years, untreated patients have a 25% to 40% risk of developing *late* or *tertiary* syphilis. It may involve many tissue types, so the spectrum of disease can be very confusing. Moreover, patients need not have had symptoms of primary or secondary syphilis prior to developing late syphilis. Tissues involved include cutaneous (gumma formation), cardiovascular (aortic disease), and central nervous system (CNS) (tabes dorsalis, meningitis, neurosyphilis) diseases (Table 1).

Diagnosis

The quickest, most direct method of diagnosing primary and secondary syphilis is direct visualization of the spirochete of moist lesions by means of dark-field microscopy. This is difficult and requires using laboratories that perform a high volume of sexually transmitted disease analyses. In general, a moist lesion should be cleaned with saline (not iodine because of bacteriocidal effect). Then, using gauze, the lesion should be unroofed. Any serosanguineous material should be collected on a dry slide for examination.

More common is serologic testing that can be done in most laboratories. The two most common screening tests are rapid plasma reagin (RPR) and the Venereal Disease Research Laboratory test (VDRL). These tests are designed to test for IgM and IgG antibodies against a cardiolipin–cholesterol–lecithin antigen. Positive tests are reported as a dilutional titer. False positives are <1:4, whereas higher titers (1:16 to 1:128) are found in secondary and early latent syphilis. This titer is important as a benchmark to follow treatment. Lack of expected decreases in titer indicate inadequate treatment, false-positive result, re-infection, or late-stage therapy.

Before treatment, a positive screening test needs to be confirmed with specific *T. pallidum* antigen testing, such as the fluorescent treponemal antibody absorption test (FTA-ABS). These tests are expensive and have a high false-positive rate, making them unsuitable as screening tests. They also remain positive for life in most people.

Newer molecular tests include the use of polymerase chain reaction (PCR), which can be used to detect multiple organisms. It has high sensitivity and specificity and can distinguish among *H. ducreyi*, herpes simplex virus, and *T. pallidum*. This test is very expensive and is likely to be available only in specialized laboratories, for now.

TABLE 1 Clinical Manifestations and Treatment of Syphilis

Stage	Clinical Manifestation	Treatment
Primary	Painless ulcer (chancre), adenopathy	Benzathine penicillin G (Bicillin LA), 2.4 million U IM × 1
Secondary (weeks to months)	Rash, mucocutaneous lesions, adenopathy, hepatitis, arthritis, glomerulonephritis, condyloma lata	Benzathine penicillin G, 2.4 million U IM × 1
Latent	Asymptomatic	
Early (<1 year)		Benzathine penicillin G, 2.4 million U IM × 1
Late		Benzathine penicillin G, 2.4 million U IM weekly × 3
Tertiary (late) 1-30 years		
Cutaneous	Gummatous lesions	Benzathine penicillin G, 2.4 million U IM weekly × 3
Cardiovascular	Aortic aneurysm, aortic insufficiency	Benzathine penicillin G, 2.4 million U IM weekly × 3
CNS Neurosyphilis	Tabes dorsalis, Argyll-Robertson pupils, paresis, seizures, subtle psychiatric manifestations, dementia; may be asymptomatic	Aqueous crystalline penicillin G, 18-24 million U/d given as 3-4 million units IV q4h for 10-14 days *or* Procaine penicillin (Wycillin), 2.4 million U qd with probenecid 500 mg PO qid for 10-14 days

Abbreviations: CNS = central nervous system; IM = intramuscularly; IV = intravenously; PO = orally; qd = daily; diq = 4 times a day.
Adapted from the CDC: Guidelines for the treatment of STDs. MMWR Morb Mortal Wkly Rep 51(RR-06):1-80, 2002.

The most significant morbidity of syphilis occurs during the tertiary phase and includes neurosyphilis. *T. pallidum* can be found in the cerebral spinal fluid (CSF) during primary and secondary phases, but usually resolves on its own. Those patients who have an abnormal CSF during the latent phase are at higher risk for symptomatic neurosyphilis, making it helpful to distinguish asymptomatic neurosyphilis. The CDC recommends that CSF testing be done whenever there is clinical evidence of neurosyphilis or vision changes, active tertiary syphilis, treatment failure, or HIV infection. CSF-VDRL is highly specific, but, unfortunately, very insensitive (as low as 30%) and therefore *can rule in* but *cannot exclude* neurosyphilis.

Although the HIV epidemic showed a resurgence of syphilis, it is controversial as to what diagnostic changes occurred in testing. Several studies show contradictory information; one shows that there was an increase in the false-positive rates, whereas a second study showed a decrease in true positive rates, and a third study showed higher false negatives. In any case, testing should still be performed as in non-HIV patients, and followed accordingly.

Pregnancy poses only increased risk, including perinatal death, premature delivery, low birth weight, congenital anomalies, and active congenital syphilis of the neonate. Physical examination and serologic testing should be performed in any female considering pregnancy, or during initial antepartum testing at least. Treatment, discussed below, should be given as if the patient is not pregnant.

Treatment

In all stages, the main reason for treatment is to prevent progression and spread of the disease. Historic treatments included mercury, salvarsan (an arsenic derivative), fever therapy, and malarial injection. Today's treatment has been in use since 1943, since the introduction of penicillin. Because there has been no reported resistance, penicillin remains the treatment of choice, so much so that penicillin-allergic patients have undergone desensitization therapy in order to receive it. Although *penicillin G*, given parenterally, is the preferred drug, the preparation used (benzathine, procaine, crystalline), dosage, and duration of therapy depends on stage and clinical manifestations (see Table 1). *Oral* penicillin is not considered appropriate for treatment. Alternative treatments could include doxycycline (Vibramycin), tetracycline, erythromycin, or ceftriaxone (Rocephin)[1].

Once treatment is started, physicians should be aware of a potential complication called the *Jarisch-Herxheimer* reaction. It is an acute, febrile reaction accompanied by headache and myalgias, which represents treponemal cell death and release of toxins. It peaks within 2 hours and subsides within 24 hours, and is most common in primary and secondary disease.

Follow-up of Treated Patients

Any patient diagnosed with syphilis at any stage should get testing for HIV, and should be retested in 3 to 6 months if a member of a high-risk population. After treatment, repeat serologic testing should be done at 6 and 12 months and titers at 24 months. If there is not at least a fourfold decrease in 6 months, there is likely treatment failure. A lumbar puncture should be done to rule out neurosyphilis, and retreatment with three weekly injections of 2.4 million units of benzathine penicillin (Bicillin LA) is recommended unless there is evidence of neurosyphilis.

Partners of patients diagnosed with syphilis should also be notified and treated. In primary disease, any partner within the previous 3 months should be identified. Empiric treatment is recommended unless there is good follow-up and serologic surveillance.

[1]Not FDA approved for this indication.

SECTION 12

Diseases of Allergy

ANAPHYLAXIS AND SERUM SICKNESS

METHOD OF

Marcia Torres Lima, MD, and Gailen D. Marshall, Jr., MD, PhD

Anaphylaxis

In 1902, Portier and Richet described the experimental induction of hypersensitivity in dogs immunized with the venom from coelenterate invertebrates (sea anemones) while attempting to confer sting prophylaxis. The dogs were sensitized to the venom unexpectedly and had fatal reactions to previously nonlethal doses of the venom. To describe this phenomenon, Portier and Richet proposed the term *anaphylaxis*, which was derived from Greek words ana- (*against*) and phylaxis (*immunity, protection*). Anaphylaxis is an acute, potentially life-threatening clinical condition that is most often caused by a systemic allergic reaction. The term *anaphylaxis* should be reserved only for IgE-mediated systemic reactions as a consequence of release of inflammatory mediators, and *anaphylactoid* should be used to describe systemic reactions from non–IgE-mediated mechanisms that induce mast cell and basophil activation. They are otherwise clinically indistinguishable. The distinction becomes important in therapeutic considerations (see below).

Mast cells are located primarily near mucous membranes and around blood vessels. The skin, conjunctiva, gastrointestinal tract, and upper and lower respiratory systems are the organs that most frequently come in contact with a foreign antigen. Because of their relatively high concentration of mast cells, they are the initial sites of degranulation. IgE is bound to the surface of mast cells by its high-affinity Fc receptor (FcERI). Once antigens cross-link the Fab component, a series of cytoplasmic events take place. Unlike mast cells, basophils commonly circulate in peripheral blood. However, they also have IgE bound to the Fc receptor and can be activated by antigen binding or other physical/chemical factors.

Biochemical mediators and chemotactic substances are released during degranulation of mast cells and basophils. These include preformed granule-associated substances, such as histamine, tryptase, chymase, and heparin; histamine-releasing factor and other cytokines; and newly generated lipid-derived mediators, such as prostaglandin D_2 (PGD_2), platelet-activating factor, leukotriene B_4 (LTB_4), and the cysteinyl leukotrienes (LTC_4, LTD_4, and LTE_4). Eosinophils may play either a direct toxic role (release of cytotoxic granule-associated proteins) or a proinflammatory role (metabolism of vasoactive mediators) to increase vascular permeability, decrease systemic vascular resistance, etc).

Histamine activates H_1 and H_2 receptors. Pruritus, rhinorrhea, tachycardia, and bronchospasm are caused by activation of the H_1 receptors, whereas both H_1 and H_2 receptors mediate headache, flushing, and hypotension. Serum histamine levels correlate with the severity and persistence of cardiopulmonary manifestations but not with formation of urticaria. Gastrointestinal signs and symptoms (abdominal cramping, nausea, vomiting) are associated with histamine more than tryptase levels.

Tryptase is the only protein that is concentrated selectively in the secretory granules of human mast cells. Tryptase levels correlate with clinical severity of anaphylaxis. Postmortem measurements of serum tryptase may be useful in establishing anaphylaxis as the cause of death in subjects experiencing sudden death of uncertain cause.

INCITING ETIOLOGIC AGENTS

In fact, any agent capable of activating mast cells or basophils might potentially cause anaphylaxis or an anaphylactoid reaction. However, as previously reported, multiple mechanisms can be involved in some cases of anaphylaxis. The most common definable causes of anaphylaxis are foods, medications, and insect stings.

The list of foods implicated in anaphylactic reactions is extensive. However, the same few foods, such as peanuts, tree nuts, shellfish, milk, and eggs, are reported to provoke the majority of anaphylactic reactions. In westernized countries, peanuts and tree nuts, fish (cod and whitefish), and shellfish (shrimp, lobster, crab, scallops, oyster) are most often implicated in fatal or near-fatal reactions. These foods also tend to induce a "persistent sensitivity" in the vast majority of patients, in contrast to other foods, such as milk, eggs, and soybeans, which are frequently associated with milder reactions and can usually be "outgrown" by avoidance for 2 to 3 years.

Risk of drug-induced anaphylaxis increases with age, peaking in the elderly, probably as a consequence of the higher proportion of older people who regularly use one or more drugs. In hospital settings, anesthetic agents are commonly used. Muscle relaxants are responsible for the majority of intraoperative anaphylaxis episodes. However, latex also accounts for a significant number of these reactions, and its incidence is actually increasing. There are specific subpopulations who are at increased risk for anaphylaxis to latex: atopic individuals, individuals with increased previous exposure to latex, health care workers who are exposed to latex mainly by inhalation (from glove powder), and possibly patients who have undergone multiple surgical procedures (particularly intra-abdominal) and therefore have been repeatedly exposed to latex intravascularly and/or via genitourinary tract by catheterization. Peptide hormones such as insulin and antidiuretic hormone (desmopressin, DDAVP), enzymes such as streptokinase (Streptase) can induce anaphylaxis. Colloids, opioids, and radiocontrast material can also induce anaphylactoid reactions. Penicillin is a relatively common cause of anaphylaxis; reactions may also be triggered by penicillin derivatives. Up to 10% of those with documented penicillin allergy will also be allergic to cephalosporins (particularly first-generation cephalosporins). The risk of anaphylactoid reactions in those using aspirin and nonsteroidal anti-inflammatory drugs should be considered in general practice. However, the physiopathology of those agents is not completely understood.

Venoms from the stings of bees and wasps are an important cause of anaphylaxis and differentiating between the two is important because immunotherapy is an effective treatment approach in this group. This is accomplished with venom-specific allergen skin test or radioallergosorbent test (RAST).

DIAGNOSIS AND DIFFERENTIAL DIAGNOSIS

It is essential for effective management that a rapid and accurate diagnosis be made and that those who are at greatest risk of reaction be rapidly identified. The most important systems involved are respiratory and cardiovascular. Early signs of anaphylaxis can include flushing and systemic urticaria. However, the clinical manifestations of intraoperative reactions often differ from those of anaphylactic reactions outside of anesthesia. Cutaneous manifestations are less common and cardiovascular collapse may be more common during anesthesia. The diagnosis can be more difficult because patients cannot express symptoms. Anaphylaxis typically begins within 5 to 60 minutes of exposure to the inciting agent. The more rapid the onset of symptoms after exposure, the more severe the clinical reaction is likely to be. Latex-induced anaphylaxis is, however, known to develop more slowly, normally over a period of about 30 to 90 minutes. Table 1 summarizes the main clinical findings. The clinician must be aware of several diseases that may mimic an anaphylaxis reaction (Table 2). Recurrent or biphasic anaphylaxis occurs 8 to 12 hours after the initial attack in up to 20% of subjects who experienced anaphylaxis. Pre-event use of calcium channel blockers, β-adrenergic

TABLE 1 Clinical Findings of Anaphylaxis

Cardiovascular: Feeling of faintness, syncope, and hypotension
Cutaneous: Pruritus, flushing, urticaria, and angioedema
Gastrointestinal: Nausea, vomiting, diarrhea, and abdominal pain
Neurologic: Anxiety, feeling of "impending doom," and loss of consciousness
Oral: Pruritus of lips, tongue, and palate, edema of lips and tongue
Respiratory: Rhinitis, sneezing, "a lump in the throat," dysphagia, dysphonia, hoarseness, stridor, cough, chest tightness, dyspnea, and wheezing

TABLE 2 Differential Diagnosis of Anaphylaxis

Acute or chronic urticaria
Carcinoid syndrome
Globus hystericus
Hereditary angioedema
Mastocytosis
Serum sickness
Vasovagal reaction

antagonists, or angiotensin-converting enzyme inhibitors may increase risk of recurrent anaphylaxis.

If the diagnosis remains uncertain, or if the patient is stabilized before the physical examination, laboratory testing can be done to confirm the diagnosis. Levels of histamine and tryptase change with an anaphylactic event. The concentration of serum histamine rises 5 to 10 minutes after the trigger event, and remains elevated for 30 to 60 minutes. Urinary histamine may remain elevated for several hours after a reaction. Serum tryptase peaks 1 to 1.5 hours after anaphylaxis, and can still be detected as long as 3 to 6 hours later.

TREATMENT

Anaphylaxis is a medical emergency that requires immediate treatment. Rapid assessment and stabilization of the airway, breathing, and circulation are of the greatest importance. The cornerstone of pharmacologic treatment is the administration of epinephrine. The dosage for adults is 0.3 to 0.5 mL of a 1:1000 dilution, and recent research has established the intramuscular route to be superior to the subcutaneous route, and the lateral aspect of the thigh is the site of choice. The dosage for children is 0.01 mL/kg, up to a maximum of 0.3 mL of a 1:1000 dilution. Epinephrine can be reinjected at 10-minute intervals, until improvement occurs. Intravenous epinephrine (1:10,000 dilution) should be administered only in severe hypotensive shock. Continuous hemodynamic monitoring is essential to monitor possible induction of cardiac arrhythmias.

Additional therapy for anaphylaxis includes the use of H_1 antihistamines, diphenhydramine (Benadryl), 1 to 2 mg/kg to a maximal dose of 50 mg, and H_2 antihistamine, ranitidine (Zantac)[1], to 1.5 mg/kg to a maximal dose of 150 mg, each given parenterally. Inhaled β_2-agonists (e.g., albuterol [Proventil]) are useful when bronchospasm is present. Early use of corticosteroids such as intravenous methylprednisolone (Solu-Medrol), 1 to 2 mg/kg, may help to prevent or minimize late-phase reactions. Patients who use β blockers may not respond completely to epinephrine, in which case glucagon should be administered at a dose of 5 to 15 μg/min intravenously.

Anaphylaxis resulting from allergen immunotherapy injections or venom should be also treated by placement of a tourniquet proximal to the injection site or the site of sting.

After appropriate treatment, prevention is of the greatest importance. The first essential step for prevention of anaphylaxis is identification of the inciting agent. Referral of all patients who experienced a generalized reaction to a qualified allergy specialist is the key step to ensuring that patients are appropriately investigated and advised on ways to minimize or prevent future reactions. In case of drug or food allergy, not only must the offending agent be avoided, but the potential for crossreactivity must also be recognized. Allergen immunotherapy should be considered in those with history of venom-induced anaphylaxis.

Patients should be prescribed, and be instructed in the use of, self-injectable epinephrine (EpiPen or EpiPen Jr) and told to keep it with them all the time. They should also wear a Medic Alert bracelet or necklace.

Serum Sickness

Serum sickness was first described in humans by von Pirquet and Schick in 1905, as a syndrome resulting from the repeat administration of heterologous serum (usually equine) as an antitoxin. Hyperimmune antiserum was the major therapeutic option in the preantibiotic era for infectious and toxin-related diseases. It was observed that a significant number of patients developed rash, fever, lymphadenopathy, and arthralgia 7 to 10 days after receiving this treatment for at least the second time. The term *serum sickness* was coined to describe the clinical syndrome. Serum sickness may also occur in response to the administration of foreign proteins such as streptokinase (Streptase), antithymocyte, and antilymphocyte globulins (Atgam), vaccines, and hymenoptera venoms.

The incidence of iatrogenic serum sickness has decreased as a result of the general decline in the need for foreign antisera with the advent of effective immunization procedures, antimicrobial therapy, and the development of specific human immune serum globulins. However, a serum sickness-like reaction that is clinically similar to classic serum sickness may result from the administration of a number of nonprotein drugs.

The immunopathology of serum sickness results from antigen-antibody complex formation in relative antigen excess with foreign protein as the antigen. If the complexes are of an appropriate size and sufficient quantity, they can deposit in endothelial surfaces at a number of tissue sites. Antigen can also combine with specific IgE on mast cells and basophils, leading to the release of platelet-activating factor. Subsequent platelet aggregation triggers its histamine and serotonin release. These substances increase vascular permeability, and thus facilitate the deposition of immune complexes into vascular endothelium. Complement activation by immune complexes results in formation of C3a and C5a, which are

[1]Not FDA approved for this indication.

potent anaphylatoxins. These substances stimulate macrophages, neutrophils, and lymphocytes to release inflammatory toxins. In classical serum sickness reaction, symptoms typically begin 6 to 21 days after drug administration; in previously immunized patients, the reaction may begin as early as 2 to 4 days after initiation of the inciting agent.

The diagnosis is made from the patient's history and by interpreting the appropriate laboratory findings associated with symptoms of rash (urticaria or vasculitis), arthritis, myalgia, and lymphadenopathy. No specific laboratory finding is universally present in serum sickness. However, an elevated sedimentation rate, eosinophilia, and depleted complement levels are often observed. Urinalysis may reveal microscopic hematuria or mild proteinuria. Also, the creatinine and liver transaminases may be transiently elevated.

The removal of the offending agent is the key for the treatment of serum sickness. Mild symptoms can be controlled with an oral antihistamine and nonsteroidal anti-inflammatory agents, whereas severe symptoms often require a course of systemic corticosteroids. Several preparations can be used, such as methylprednisolone (Medrol) 1 to 2 mg/kg per day given orally in twice-daily dosing. Steroids should be given for 3 to 5 days in the majority of cases, although in severe cases, patients may need to be weaned over a 2-week period. Because the cutaneous symptoms of serum sickness may last for several weeks, treatment with antihistamine is recommended for 6 weeks or longer. Hydroxyzine (Atarax), 2 mg/kg per day divided into four doses in children, or 25 mg four times daily in adults, may be used, or diphenhydramine (Benadryl) or the new generation of nonsedating antihistamines, fexofenadine (Allegra) 180 mg per day, loratadine (Claritin) 10 mg per day, or cetirizine (Zyrtec) 10 mg per day, can be used.

ASTHMA IN ADOLESCENTS AND ADULTS

METHOD OF

J. Andrew Grant, MD, and Mark A. Sanchez, MD

Asthma is a disease that affects more than 17 million Americans, costs billions of dollars each year, and causes more than half a million hospital stays. Despite medical breakthroughs and the introduction of new medications, the prevalence has increased dramatically, probably as a result of environmental factors. The mortality in African Americans substantially exceeds that of other ethnic groups and seems to be increasing.

TABLE 1 Systematic Approach to Management of Bronchial Asthma

Establish a diagnosis of asthma and consider the differential diagnosis, triggers, and co-morbid conditions
Educate patients to develop a partnership in asthma management
Assess and monitor asthma severity with symptom reports and periodic measures of lung function
Avoid or control asthma triggers
Establish medication plan for chronic management
Establish plans for managing exacerbations
Provide regular follow-up care
Consider need for consultation and immunotherapy

In 1997, a National Heart, Lung, and Blood Institute Expert Panel Report Update defined asthma as "a chronic inflammatory disorder of the airways in which many cells and cellular elements play a role, in particular, mast cells, eosinophils, T lymphocytes, neutrophils, and epithelial cells. In susceptible individuals, this inflammation causes recurrent episodes of wheezing, breathlessness, chest tightness, and cough, particularly at night and in the early morning. These episodes are usually associated with widespread but variable airflow obstruction that is often reversible either spontaneously or with treatment. The inflammation also causes an associated increase in the existing bronchial hyperresponsiveness to a variety of stimuli." This article addresses diagnosis and treatment for adolescents and adults, and encourages a joint management program for primary care physicians and allergists. Table 1 outlines a systematic approach to management.

Evaluation

MEDICAL HISTORY

Patients typically present with one or more of the classic symptoms of wheezing, shortness of breath, and cough. In 25% to 30% of patients, one of these symptoms is persistent. Other symptoms may include bronchorrhea, chest pain/tightness, hyperventilation, and even hemoptysis. Symptoms may be more severe at night and may appear or worsen with exercise, especially in cold air. Table 2 lists other potential triggers for asthma. Indoor allergens, including house dust mites, cockroaches, fungi (especially *Alternaria*), and cat dander are important triggers of asthma. Many asthma patients have associated rhinosinusitis and eczema. A family history of asthma and/or other atopic disorders is usually present.

PHYSICAL EXAMINATION

"All that wheezes is not asthma and all that is asthma does not always wheeze." Although wheezing is usually the predominant finding on examination, it is not exclusive to asthma. The wheeze is typically high pitched and diffuse. The severity of asthma cannot be

TABLE 2 Potential Triggers for Asthma Attacks

Allergens
House dust mites
Cockroaches
Alternaria
Cats
Other aeroallergens
Respiratory infections
Viral infections are most common, especially rhinoviruses
Sinusitis
Bacterial pneumonia and bronchitis are infrequent
Exercise
Gastroesophageal reflux
Drugs
Aspirin and other nonsteroidal anti-inflammatory drugs
β-Adrenergic antagonists
Angiotensin-converting enzyme inhibitors
Irritants including sulfites and environmental tobacco smoke
Atmospheric pollution and climatic factors
Psychosocial factors
Workplace factors

determined by the degree of wheezing, but the finding suggests narrowing of the airways. The chest may be hyperexpanded and respiratory excursion reduced. Forced expiration is usually prolonged with increased wheezing. Other findings associated with asthma but not exclusive to this disease include eczema, nasal polyps, and features of allergic rhinitis. Severe asthma attacks may present with anxiety, use of accessory muscles, pulsus paradox, and even cyanosis.

LUNG FUNCTION

All patients should have spirometry performed initially and repeated periodically to evaluate the severity of illness and response to interventions. Reduction in the ratio of forced expiratory volume in 1 second to forced vital capacity (FEV_1/FVC) is usually seen. An increase in FEV_1 by 12% or more after a bronchodilator or a course of corticosteroids is the gold standard for diagnosing asthma. The inspiratory/expiratory flow-volume loops may provide confirmation and clues for other potential diagnoses. Spirometry may also indicate if the patient has an underlying restrictive pattern of lung disease. Oxygen saturation should be routinely performed.

Patients who are initially evaluated may have their degree of obstruction monitored at home with peak expiratory flow (PEF). Patients with more-severe asthma have variability in their disease, which can be measured with serial measurements of PEF. The devices are simple and will permit the patient to assess periods of relapse and response to therapy. The downside of PEF monitoring is the dependence on the patient's effort and understanding.

If a diagnosis of asthma cannot be established by reversibility of FEV_1 and in patients with atypical presentations, a challenge procedure to provoke bronchoconstriction is warranted. The most commonly used substance is methacholine (Provocholine); however, inhaled histamine or cold air and exercise are alternatives. In addition, determination of lung volumes and diffusion capacity may be warranted in patients with more complex disease.

OTHER LABORATORY STUDIES

Chest radiographs are usually normal in asthmatic individuals, but should be obtained at baseline to evaluate for other pathology. Other tests that may be useful for evaluation of asthma include a peripheral leukocyte count with a differential. Eosinophilia may be a manifestation of asthma; however, severe eosinophilia may suggest an alternative diagnosis. Elevation of the serum IgE concentration may also be indicative of asthma. Neither eosinophilia nor increased IgE can establish definitely a diagnosis of asthma nor quantify severity. Allergy skin testing by an allergist is useful in patients with moderate to severe asthma in order to determine which aeroallergens are affecting the patient's condition. Where skin testing is not possible, measurement of allergen-specific IgE is indicated. Avoidance measures and behavior modifications should be instituted based on this data. Other tests to consider selectively include cardiac stress evaluation, bronchoscopy, computerized tomography of the lungs, and evaluation for esophageal reflux.

DIFFERENTIAL DIAGNOSIS

A patient presenting with the cardinal symptoms of asthma requires a very careful history, examination, and ancillary tests as outlined above. Table 3 lists some potential etiologies. If asthma is likely, the clinician also must manage co-morbid conditions such as rhinosinusitis, nasal polyposis, and those listed in Table 3.

Management

The first principle in managing patients with asthma is to develop a strong therapeutic relationship.

TABLE 3 Differential Diagnosis of Wheezing, Dyspnea, and/or Cough

Bronchial asthma
Acute viral respiratory tract infection
Chronic obstructive pulmonary disease
Chronic bronchitis
Emphysema
Congestive heart failure
Mechanical obstruction
Foreign body
Malignancy
Vocal cord dysfunction
Tracheomalacia
Sleep apnea
Allergic bronchopulmonary aspergillosis
Pulmonary infiltrates with eosinophilia
Drugs
Nonsteroidal anti-inflammatory drugs
Angiotensin converting enzyme inhibitors
β-Adrenergic blockers
Pulmonary embolism

This should include a specialist such as an allergist for patients with more-severe asthma. The patient should receive instruction about the nature of asthma, how to monitor it at home, methods for avoiding triggers, what to do in case of exacerbations, and information about the proper use of recommended drugs. A written asthma management plan is usually warranted. More severely affected patients should routinely monitor PEF.

CLASSIFICATION OF ASTHMA SEVERITY

Table 4 shows a systematic classification of asthma severity. The severity of the disease dictates the treatment plan recommended (Table 5). Classification is based on several factors, including the nature of symptoms, both daytime and nighttime, frequency of attacks, and lung function including variability. The step chosen is the severest based on the properties in any of the columns. This classification includes characteristics before therapeutic intervention. It is very helpful when planning a therapeutic approach. Patients with mild persistent disease may have severe exacerbations requiring intense treatment.

ASTHMA MANAGEMENT PLAN

Therapy for the treatment of asthma includes, in this order, education, minimizing the provocative factors, pharmacologic therapy, plan for approaching exacerbations, regular follow-up, and immunotherapy (Table 1). Treatment options depend on the severity of the asthma and the success of earlier approaches.

AVOIDANCE AND CONTROL OF ASTHMA TRIGGERS

Table 2 lists potential asthma triggers, and their control is the first principle in therapeutic intervention.

Allergens

A multitude of allergens cause bronchoconstriction and lead to asthma exacerbations in susceptible individuals. These allergens are mostly indoor aeroallergens, including house dust mites, cockroaches, mold (especially *Alternaria*), and animal dander. Pollens and foods are less critical. The most effective way to evaluate for allergens inducing bronchospasm is a thorough history seeking to show relapses with exposure. Allergy skin tests or allergen-specific IgE measurements are confirmatory.

Allergen Avoidance

House dust mites pose a significant problem as their reservoir includes pillows, mattresses, bedding, carpet, and upholstered furniture. These organisms exist in environments with high humidity (>50%). Measures to decrease house dust mites include washing bedding and pillows in hot water (>130°F [54.4°C]) weekly, the use of pillow and mattress covers with an impermeable material, and removal of carpeting and upholstered furniture. If carpet cannot be removed, treatment with tannic acid to denature antigen or acaricides such as benzyl benzoate (Acarosan) to kill dust mites may be helpful. Reducing the humidity to below 50% may prove very effective. Should animal allergens be the culprit, only removal of the animal from the immediate environment is effective, but some animal allergens may still remain for months to years. The use of high-efficiency particulate air (HEPA) filters is ineffective in the treatment of house dust mites, but may offer some benefit for removing animal allergens. Should mold be a factor, water leaks from roofing and plumbing should be repaired. Contaminated areas should be carefully cleaned. Control of cockroaches involves removal of food in open areas and setting of traps. For aeroallergens that are outside, minimal activity should be done outdoors or include the use of a mask during high aeroallergen counts.

Respiratory Infections

Most respiratory infections are viral in nature and will not respond to antibiotics. Antibiotic treatment should be limited to cases of likely bacterial infections, such as cough productive of purulent sputum and active sinusitis.

TABLE 4 Classification of Asthma Severity

Severity of Disease	Daytime Symptom Severity with Activities	Nocturnal Symptoms	Lung Function Parameters
Severe persistent Step 4	Continual Physical activity very limited	Frequent	FEV_1 or PEF ≤60% of predicted PEFR variability >30%
Moderate persistent Step 3	Daily symptoms Activities significantly affected Daily bronchodilator use	More than once weekly	FEV_1 or PEF 60-80% of predicted PEF variability >30%
Mild persistent Step 2	Symptoms more than twice weekly Activities may be affected	More than 2 nights a month	FEV_1 or PEF ≥80% of predicted PEF variability 20%-30%
Mild intermittent Step 1	Symptoms twice a week or less	Twice monthly or less	FEV_1 or PEF ≥80% of predicted PEF variability <20%

Abbreviations: FEV_1 = forced expiratory volume in 1 second; PEF = peak expiratory flow.

TABLE 5 Treatment Recommendations Based on Asthma Severity

Severity of Disease	Daily Controller Treatment
Severe persistent Step 4	High dose ICS, *and* LABA, *and* If indicated, short-acting oral corticosteroid (prednisone 1 to 2 mg/kg/d) for as short a period as possible
Moderate persistent Step 3	Low to medium dose of an ICS, *plus* LABA If LABA is not tolerated, then a low to medium dose of an ICS *plus* a leukotriene modifier or theophylline may be considered
Mild persistent Step 2	First-line therapy is a low-dose ICS A leukotriene modifier is the most frequently used second-line treatment Cromolyn (Intal), nedocromil (Tilade), or sustained-release theophylline (Theo-Dur) are additional alternatives; an LABA should not be used alone
Mild intermittent Step 1	No daily controller medication is usually required; if bronchodilator is required more than twice weekly, consider instituting a controller medication Inhaled short-acting β2-selective agonists are the drugs of choice for quick relief of symptoms and should be used only as needed for maximal efficacy. Ipratropium (Atrovent) may prove useful in some patients and may be added to albuterol. A combination metered-dose inhaler (Combivent) is convenient.

Abbreviations: ICS = inhaled corticosteroid; LABA = long-acting inhaled β_2-agonist.

Exercise

Vigorous exercise in a cold, dry environment is a potent trigger for asthma relapses. The use of masks may be helpful, but is often impractical. Swimming is an alternative form of exercise tolerated by many asthmatic patients. Increasing the regulation of asthma by proper use of asthma controllers is effective, as is the use of bronchodilators prior to exercise.

Gastroesophageal Reflux

Many asthmatics have underlying reflux, which worsens their asthma by irritating the airways through microaspiration and esophageal irritation leading to reflex bronchospasm. Reflux may be asymptomatic, but still a significant factor causing nocturnal or refractory asthma. This condition may interfere with asthma treatment because some drugs, including theophylline (Slo-Phyllin), β agonists, anticholinergics, and oral steroids, may worsen reflux. Therefore, aggressive treatment of reflux with appropriate medications such as proton pump inhibitors initially and H_2 blockers long-term, as well as behavior modification, is encouraged. Rarely is direct measurement of esophageal hyperacidity needed.

Medications

Various medications may trigger bronchoconstriction or inhibit bronchodilation. Nonsteroidal anti-inflammatory drugs (NSAIDs), including both prescribed and over-the-counter agents, are the most common medications that induce bronchoconstriction. Patients with nasal polyps and asthma are especially at risk of having severe bronchospasm to aspirin and other NSAIDs. Medications such as β-adrenergic blockers may cause inhibition of bronchodilators as well as induce bronchospasm with cough. Angiotensin-converting enzyme inhibitors are associated with cough and edema of the airway and may worsen a patient's baseline function.

Irritants and Other Environmental Factors

Chemical substances such as sulfites and cleaning agents cause bronchoconstriction. Air pollution caused by SO_2, NO_2, O_3, diesel exhaust particles, and other particulate matter may cause bronchoconstriction through nonspecific activation of bronchial receptors. Climatic factors may significantly affect the response of asthmatics to environmental pollution. Environmental tobacco smoke may also contribute to bronchoconstriction in this fashion, and really is the only avoidable factor.

Pharmacotherapy

Consideration of triggers is usually insufficient to manage most patients with asthma, and safe and effective drugs are needed. Patients receive various drugs depending on the severity of their disease. Many individuals live with the condition lifelong and are in need of medication daily to maintain optimal control of their condition. Individuals with asthma are also susceptible to attacks, especially if exposed to exacerbating factors (see Table 2), that require medications for instant relief. The National Asthma Education and Prevention Program (NAEPP) established guidelines for treatment of asthma depending on severity (Table 4) with specific recommendations (Table 5). Therapy focuses on controlling the underlying inflammation, in order to reduce bronchial hyperresponsiveness and symptoms, as well as minimizing side effects that may be brought on by asthma drugs. Careful review of the patient's symptoms and objective measures of lung function are important for adjusting medication.

Quick-Relief Asthma Medications

Short-Acting Inhaled β_2-Selective Adrenergic Agonists

This class of medications, which has been a mainstay in asthma therapy, is typically used in its inhaled form through a metered-dosed inhaler (MDI) or via a face mask through a nebulizer machine with a holding chamber or spacer. Albuterol (Proventil) is the most frequently prescribed of these medications. Newer forms of albuterol in an inhaled powder are now available. Once the medication is delivered, onset of action is within 5 minutes and lasts from 4 to 6 hours. The side effects include tremors, restlessness, palpitations, and anxiety. These effects are usually minimal and well tolerated unless the drug is used excessively. In some patients, frequent use may be associated with significant bronchospasm. The nebulized isomer known as levalbuterol (Xopenex) is marketed as causing fewer of these side effects; however, some experts question this advantage. If an individual uses a rescue medication more than twice a week, addition of a controller medication is warranted.

Despite the use of controller medications (discussed below), at times patients are exposed to factors that require the use of quick-relief medications such as albuterol. The anticholinergic drug ipratropium (Atrovent) is also available. Used alone, ipratropium may have minimal effects on asthma, but it does have few side effects. Combined with albuterol in a single unit (Combivent), this formulation offers a distinct advantage for some patients. Oral steroids are also available for quick relief during exacerbations. Their onset of action takes at least 6 to 12 hours and may not be fully appreciated for a few days. A short-course steroid burst is recommended, and prednisone and methylprednisolone (Medrol) at 0.5 to 1 mg/kg per day are the most commonly used drugs. Treatment for 5 days is often effective and tapering is unnecessary.

Asthma Controller Medications

Inhaled Corticosteroids

Inhaled corticosteroids (ICSs) effectively reduce airway inflammation by directly acting on the airways and the responsible cells, including mast cells, epithelial cells, eosinophils, and T cells. One method of producing this beneficial effect is by reducing synthesis of cytokines necessary for asthmatic inflammation. Clinical benefits include improved lung function and measures of quality of life. ICS achieves a dramatic reduction in symptoms and relapses, in the need for quick-relief medications, especially oral steroids, and in the need for emergent care. Finally, use of ICS reduces asthma mortality. The effects of ICS when taken continuously are usually seen in 1 week, with the maximum effect in 4 to 8 weeks. Usually prescribed twice daily, once-daily administration may be adequate when maintenance is achieved. The most frequently used medications are budesonide (Pulmicort), fluticasone (Flovent), flunisolide (AeroBid), beclomethasone (QVAR), and triamcinolone (Azmacort). Fluticasone (Flovent Rotadisk) and budesonide (Pulmicort Turbuhaler) are available in an inhaled powder form, and budesonide is also available in a nebulized form (Pulmicort Respules). When using an MDI, a spacer (AeroChamber, OptiChamber, Ellipse, or InspirEase) is recommended to maximize the amount of medication that reaches the airways and to minimize oropharyngeal exposure. This maneuver usually reduces the major side effects of these medications, which include oral candidiasis (thrush), hoarseness, and sore throat. More serious side effects related to the eye and to skeletal metabolism, as well as suppression of the hypothalamic–pituitary–adrenal axis, are rarely seen with higher doses.

Cromolyn and Nedocromil

Cromolyn (Intal) and nedocromil (Tilade) seem to close cellular chloride channels in inflammatory cells. Their clinical benefits include prevention of cellular activation leading to reduction in airway inflammation, bronchospasm, and hyperreactivity. These drugs may reduce exercise-induced asthma. These drugs both come in MDI form and offer an excellent safety profile. The downside of these medications is that they are probably less effective long-term than ICS. Cromolyn and nedocromil often must be given four times a day, which leads to patient compliance issues.

Leukotriene Modifiers

Leukotrienes are potent mediators that play an important role in asthmatic inflammation and symptoms. Two types of drugs are available to modify their effects, including a 5-lipoxygenase inhibitor zileuton (Zyflo), and the leukotriene receptor antagonists zafirlukast (Accolate) and montelukast (Singulair). These medications improve asthma symptoms and lung function, and reduce exacerbations. They offer an alternative to ICSs, but may not be as effective. Their maximum effect is often seen within the first week of use. The most popular choice in this group currently is montelukast, based on once-daily administration, lack of food effects on absorption, drug interaction, and safety even in small children. The concurrent use of leukotriene modifiers with ICSs leads to improved control of asthma and a decrease in the amount of inhaled steroid in patients taking both medications. Montelukast (10 mg) is administered once daily and zafirlukast (20 mg) twice daily; zafirlukast should not be ingested concurrently with food because it decreases absorption. Zileuton (600 mg tablets) is recommended four times a day and requires hepatic monitoring. Drug interactions with Coumadin and theophylline have been shown in zileuton and zafirlukast.

Long-Acting Inhaled β_2 Agonists

Although available in both inhaled and oral form, the inhaled form is preferred because of lower side effects. These drugs should never be used alone and are best studied in combination with ICSs. This combination is the preferred treatment for moderate and severe persistent asthma. The addition of a long-acting inhaled β_2 agonist LABAs to an ICS is more effective than use of an ICS alone, increasing the dose of an ICS, or adding a leukotriene modifier to an ICS. The two inhaled formulations available are salmeterol (Serevent) and formoterol (Foradil). The effect of a LABA may be seen within 30 minutes, with persistence up to 12 hours, making twice-daily administration satisfactory. These drugs share many properties with the shorter-acting β-agonists. LABAs cause bronchodilation and improved lung function, and also may be beneficial for nocturnal symptoms. Side effects include palpitations, tachycardia, anxiety, and muscle tremor. Caution should also be taken in patients with cardiovascular problems. Clinical trials show a slight increase in mortality in patients using a LABA, so a special warning has been added to labeling.

An inhaled powder form of salmeterol (Serevent) combined with fluticasone (Flovent) is available (Advair Diskus), and is a very popular choice for patients with moderate and severe persistent asthma. Compliance with use of the single unit is superior to use of the two individual components. Advair Diskus is available with several dosages of fluticasone (100, 250, 500 μg) and a fixed dose of (salmeterol 50 μg). It is recommended that Advair be used twice a day. When control of asthma is achieved with higher doses of fluticasone plus salmeterol, the clinician should lower the dose of the steroid to reduce potential side effects. One disadvantage of Advair is that during a relapse, patients should increase their total daily dose of ICSs. This obligates the patient to have a standby ICS unit for this purpose.

Theophylline

Theophylline, a methylxanthine, was the first asthma controller available; the first report of using this potent bronchodilator in asthma was from our institution in 1935. Theophylline and aminophylline were used as the standard of therapy for decades and are still recommended as a second-line therapy. Low cost is an obvious advantage. Theophylline is available in slow-release preparations (Slo-bid) that maintain an effective and reasonably stable blood level. Theophylline offers patients with nocturnal symptoms an alternative, improves mucociliary clearance, and increases contraction of respiratory muscles. The disadvantage of this class of drugs is the narrow window of efficacy versus adverse effects. The metabolism of theophylline is affected by a large number of drugs and food products. The other disadvantage of theophylline is side effects that are similar to other methylxanthines such as caffeine. These effects include nausea, headache, tremor, agitation, tachycardia, nervousness, and insomnia. Seizures and arrhythmias may be seen at higher levels. Levels of theophylline must be checked periodically and the recommended range is from 5 to 15 μg/mL. Patients with a history of cardiac disease should be carefully monitored for tolerance.

Graded Treatment of Asthma

Table 5 outlines the recommended management of patients at different levels of severity.

Mild Intermittent Asthma

Patients with mild intermittent asthma have daily symptoms two times per week or less, or nocturnal symptoms twice a month or less (Table 4). PEF measurement is within the normal range. Patients have inactive asthma, but that may develop symptoms with certain exposures, such as exercise or specific aeroallergens. These individuals require no controller medications, but only need quick-relief medication on an as-needed basis. The preferred treatment is a short-acting, inhaled, β_2-selective, adrenergic agonist. During relapses, a short burst of systemic steroids may be required followed by ICSs until the illness completely clears. The clinician should carefully monitor these relapses and recovery in order to reduce therapy quickly.

Mild Persistent Asthma

Patients with mild persistent asthma have daily symptoms more often than twice a week, but not daily, or nocturnal symptoms more often than twice a month. PEF and FEV_1 measurements are usually in the normal range. Low-dose ICS is the treatment of choice, but many patients respond effectively to a leukotriene modifier, theophylline, cromolyn (Intal), or nedocromil (Tilade). LABA is never indicated alone.

Moderate Persistent Asthma

Moderate persistent asthma is characterized by daily symptoms, or nocturnal symptoms more often than once weekly. The lung function is typically between 60% and 80% of predicted values.

The preferred treatment is low- to medium-dose ICS plus LABA. Some patients will do better with a low- to medium-dose ICS plus a leukotriene modifier or theophylline. A leukotriene modifier may be especially effective in patients with NSAID sensitivity causing asthma.

Severe Persistent Asthma

Patients with severe persistent asthma have daytime symptoms continuously, or frequent nocturnal symptoms. FEV_1 and PEF are usually less than 60% of predicted. The first choice of treatment is high-dose ICSs along with a LABA. If needed, oral corticosteroids also should be given at 1 to 2 mg/kg per day not to exceed 60 mg per day. Ideally, the physician should titrate the dose of oral steroids down as quickly as possible and maintain control of the disease with ICSs. To minimize adrenal suppression, short-acting corticosteroids, such as prednisone or methylprednisolone, should be used.

MANAGEMENT OF RELAPSES

Patients may benefit from a written plan for managing asthmatic relapses. Typically, this is based on changes in PEF. If values fall below 80% of the patient's personal best, it may be appropriate to use quick-relief drugs regularly and to increase the dose of ICS. If PEF falls below 50%, regular albuterol (Proventil) use plus a burst of oral steroids may be warranted. In any case, the patient should be in contact with his or her physician for instructions.

LONG-TERM MANAGEMENT

Patients with asthma should be seen at intervals ranging from monthly to annually depending on disease severity. Spirometry should be repeated at each visit. Symptoms, drug use and effectiveness, PEF monitoring, spacers used with MDIs, relapses, and effective avoidance of triggers should be reviewed. Often these issues can best be approached in consultation with an allergist. Immunotherapy may be warranted in patients not effectively controlled by other measures. Finally, omalizumab (Xolair), a monoclonal antibody against IgE that prevents binding of IgE to its cell receptors, is available for refractory patients. This drug reduces the frequency of asthma relapses and the need for emergent care.

ASTHMA IN CHILDREN

METHOD OF

Jonathan M. Spergel, MD, PhD, and
Matthew I. Fogg, MD

Asthma is the most common childhood chronic disease. However, because there is no specific immunologic, biologic, or physiologic marker for asthma, clinicians must base their diagnosis on a variety of factors, including family history, symptom patterns, risk factors, diagnostic tests, and responses to therapeutic interventions. "Wheezing" in children is not diagnostic of asthma as infants can wheeze from other causes: structural, cardiac, or viral. Approximately 20% of children younger than age 2 years develop wheezing secondary to viral infections and small airways. As their airways enlarge, a majority of children will stop wheezing, with 15% continuing to wheeze into adolescence with the most severe asthma phenotype. Even though many children "outgrow" their wheezing, approximately 30% of children with asthma develop symptoms within their first year of life, 50% by age 2 years, and 80% by the time they start school. Certain risk factors (discussed below) place the early wheezing infant at risk for continued wheezing or asthma.

Epidemiology and Morbidity

Asthma affects 4.8 million (6.9% prevalence) children younger than age 18 years. There is significant morbidity as a result of asthma. The National Health Interview Survey of 17,000 families found that asthmatic children had 10.1 million missed school days, as well as 200,000 hospitalizations, resulting in 1.9 million days of inpatient care. The prevalence of asthma worldwide, like all allergic diseases, has increased over the last 30 to 50 years. The reasons for this increase in prevalence may relate to increased urban living, proximity to coastal regions, changes in native bacteria flora, exposure to endotoxin, and obesity.

Hospitalization and Mortality

Hospitalization rates for children with asthma gradually increased from 1980 to 1996, and leveled off from 1996 to 1999, with greatest increase in rates occurring in children up to 4 years of age and among black children. Male children 5 to 14 years of age were 1.3 times more likely to be hospitalized than were female children of the same age. Similarly, asthma-related deaths increased from 1980 to 1999, peaking in 1996. Higher mortality rates are found in adolescents and black, non-Hispanic children. The individual risk factors for fatal asthma are similar in children and adults (Table 1).

Risk Factors for Developing Asthma

There is no one cause for asthma. Asthma is a classic multifactorial disease with both genetic and environmental factors. Atopy, perinatal, environmental, genetic, and viral factors are all thought to play a role in development of asthma.

ATOPY

Atopy or allergies are a major risk factor for asthma. Eighty percent to 90% of children with asthma have allergies. Fifty percent of children with atopic dermatitis or eczema (allergies of the skin) develop asthma. Additionally, a family history of allergies, including hay fever (allergic rhinitis), is a risk factor for asthma in the child.

TABLE 1 Risk Factors for Fatal Asthma

Prior intensive care unit, hospitalization, or emergency care visit(s) for asthma in the past year	Current use of systemic corticosteroids	Psychiatric disease or psychosocial problems
Noncompliance	Poor access to health care	Passive smoke exposure
Previous near-fatal episodes	Low socioeconomic status	

PERINATAL FACTORS

Prenatal and perinatal risk factors for the development of asthma in inner-city children include lower birth weight and gestational age, oxygen supplementation, and positive-pressure ventilation in the neonatal period. Other risk factors include maternal smoking and no prenatal care.

ALLERGENS

Exposure to high levels of house dust mite antigen in the first year of life increases the risk of developing asthma by the time the child is 5 years of age by threefold. But exposure to animals as a risk factor for asthma is unclear. Studies have found exposure to several cats, dogs or farm animals may decrease the risk for asthma. Nevertheless, once sensitized to animals, exposure to animals is a risk factor for more severe disease and symptoms. These findings indicate that the timing and amount of allergen exposure, as well as the allergen itself, may significantly influence allergic sensitization and possibly asthma as well.

VIRAL INFECTIONS

In infants and children, viruses are the predominant cause of infection-induced wheezing. Lower respiratory tract infections in the first 3 years of life increase the risk of a child developing asthma when evaluated prospectively at both 6 and 11 years of age, with most infections caused by viruses. However, daycare children have an increased number of lower respiratory illnesses and wheezing, but a lower rate of asthma later in childhood. Furthermore, respiratory syncytial virus, the most common cause of bronchiolitis in infancy, was found to be a risk factor for asthma in some studies but not in others. At the current time, it is unclear whether viral infections are a true risk factor for asthma. Again, the exposure and quantity of virus, similar to allergens, have a complex role in the development of asthma.

GENETIC

Family history of asthma or atopy is a marked risk factor for asthma. There is no one individual genetic defect that is responsible for asthma. However, regions have been identified in several genomic screens. The most common identified regions are the cytokine gene cluster of interleukin (IL)-4, IL-13, IL-5, CD14, and granulocyte macrophage-colony-stimulating factor on 5q; major histocompatibility complex (MHC) region on 6p; the high-affinity IgE receptor on 11q13, and chromosomes 12q and 13q. Additionally, genetic polymorphisms in the alpha subunit of the interleukin-4 receptor, the β-adrenergic receptor, ADAM33 gene, and the major cell surface receptor for endotoxin (CD14) may further influence disease expression and responses.

SOCIOECONOMIC

Poverty itself, independent of coexistent factors such as urban living, is not a risk factor for developing asthma. Children living in poverty are more likely to use an emergency department as a primary care source than are children from higher socioeconomic environments. However, sensitization to cockroach allergen, which is more prevalent in inner-city children, is associated with symptomatic asthma.

ENVIRONMENTAL FACTORS

Exposure to cigarette smoke during pregnancy or second-hand smoke during childhood increased the risk of developing asthma by at least twofold. Exposure to pollution (particulate matter, NO_2, and ozone) from living near a busy highway increased individual asthma symptoms, hospital admissions, and incidence of asthma by at least twofold in several studies in the United States, Europe, and Asia.

The Rise of Asthma and Hygiene Theory

The increasing prevalence of asthma in westernized cultures, coupled with evidence that factors such as childhood infections, daycare attendance, and microbe exposure may be protective, led to the initial development and later expansion of the "hygiene hypothesis." The theory is that a decrease in exposure to "good dirt and bacteria" leads to lower expression of cytokines designed to fight these infections (Th1 cytokines) with a concomitant increase in Th2 cytokines that promote allergies. Exposure to these bacteria and their endotoxin induce a switch from the native fetal Th2 milieu to Th1 environment. Other factors that support the "hygiene hypothesis" include (a) decreased asthma rates in individuals with infection from enteric pathogens; (b) decreased asthma rates in children with a greater number of older siblings or who attended daycare during the first 6 months of life with a subsequent increased number of infections; (c) decreased asthma rates with increased environmental endotoxin exposure from farm animals or pets; (d) certain genetic polymorphisms for the major endotoxin receptor CD14 are associated with decreased asthma rates; and (e) frequent oral antibiotic administration with subsequent alterations in gastrointestinal flora is associated with increased asthma rates. However, it is not a straightforward change of Th1 cytokines (interleukin [IL]-2 and interferon [IFN]-γ; proinflammatory) to Th2 cytokines (IL-4, IL-5, and IL-13; proallergic) because proinflammatory diseases, such as diabetes and inflammatory bowel disease, are also on the rise. The latest theory is a loss of function of T regulatory cells, which down-regulate both Th1 and Th2 cellular function leading to an increase of cytokines promoting both types of diseases.

Pathophysiology

The basic finding in asthma is reversible airflow obstruction with airway inflammation. This occurs even in patients with mild asthma and in children. The pathologic changes seen in adult and severe asthma, including connective tissue deposition, intraluminal obstruction, thickened subepithelial collagen, loss of cilia, lymphocyte accumulation, and evidence of mast cell degranulation, have been noted in children as young as 5 years of age.

Additional changes can be seen at the start of persistent symptoms, as bronchoalveolar lavage found increased number of total cells, most significantly lymphocytes, in wheezy infants compared with normal children.

The start of asthma may be *in utero*; all patients at birth have a Th2 phenotype because of placental factors. Furthermore, studies have found a decreased ability to produce IFN-γ production in patients who develop asthma. The decrease in IFN-γ production may shift the lungs toward a Th2 phenotype, resulting in asthma. This process is further propagated in children with atopic dermatitis. In children with atopy and later asthma, the first sign of atopy is often atopic dermatitis. Patients with atopic dermatitis have a Th2 cytokine profile in the skin, as well as systemically. Therefore, patients susceptible to asthma have a Th2 cytokine profile in the lung prior to allergen or viral exposure. The body generates a Th2 response to the allergen or viral stimuli, causing eosinophilia and lymphocyte accumulation. This accumulation along with interaction of the native lung smooth-muscle cells generates the airway obstruction noted in asthma.

Differential Diagnosis

The differential diagnosis of asthma depends on the age of the child. Eighty percent to 90% of asthma patients are atopic and have either allergic rhinitis, atopic dermatitis, food allergy, or a family history of atopy. If a child does not, other diagnosis should be considered. The differential diagnosis for young infants and toddlers includes foreign-body aspiration, gastroesophageal reflux secondary to vagal nerve bronchospasm, viral-induced bronchiolitis, and bronchopulmonary dysplasia. Other rare causes include vascular rings or laryngeal webs, laryngotracheomalacia, tracheal stenosis, bronchostenosis, and enlarged lymph nodes or tumor. Children of any age with frequent lower respiratory infections and wheezing should also be ruled out for cystic fibrosis, dysmotile cilia syndrome, α_1-antitrypsin deficiency, and immunodeficiencies. Vocal cord dysfunction and psychogenic cough should be considered in school-age children or adults with cough who are not responding to therapy.

Diagnosis

HISTORY

A thorough clinical history is extremely important when evaluating a child for the presence of asthma. The patient's baseline level of asthma symptoms is an important factor to consider when making the diagnosis. Specifically, the physician should ascertain the frequency and nature of the symptoms the child is experiencing (Table 2 lists some important questions to ask). Families often may ascribe asthma symptoms to other diseases, such as bronchitis or colds. It is important to ask specifically about cough, wheezing, shortness of breath, chest tightness, and sputum/mucus production. The seasonal pattern of symptoms is important in understanding a patient's disease. A patient whose asthma flares in the early spring may be experiencing allergic reactivity to tree pollens as an asthma trigger, while a patient who gets sicker in the winter may be suffering from recurrent rhinovirus-induced flares or flares induced by an indoor aeroallergen.

When evaluating a child for asthma, it is essential to ascertain what factors cause exacerbations of the child's disease. Precipitating factors that should be asked about include respiratory viruses, indoor and outdoor environmental allergens, changes in

TABLE 2 Key Questions in the Diagnosis of Asthma

Does your child cough, wheeze (a whistling sound when breathing), or have chest tightness or shortness of breath?
Does your child cough or wheeze with exercise, play, and laughter or during temper tantrums?
Does your child cough or wheeze after exposure to pets, dust, or other allergens?
Do colds go right to your child's chest and last longer than 1 week?
Is your child sick all winter with a cold?
Is there a family history of asthma or allergies?
What triggers your child's symptoms—colds, allergens (like the family pet), or exercise?
Is coughing or wheezing keeping you and your child up at night?

environment (i.e., new home or daycare), exercise, irritants (tobacco smoke, perfumes, etc.), changes in weather, foods, medications, and strong emotion. It is also important to ascertain the patient's history of disease. The age of onset of respiratory symptoms, history of emergency visits and hospitalizations, intensive care unit admissions, endotracheal intubations, number of steroid courses, and other respiratory conditions are important factors that help the physician to ascertain the severity of the child's disease. The physician should also attempt to understand the impact of the disease on the life of both the child and the family in terms of missed school for the child or missed work for the caregivers.

The patient's past medical history should be examined, with particular emphasis on symptoms of sinus disease, gastroesophageal reflux, cystic fibrosis, and other allergic diseases, such as rhinitis, conjunctivitis, and atopic dermatitis. As with any medical history, it is important to ascertain a complete family history focusing on atopic diseases in close relatives. A social and environmental history of pets and exposure to cigarette smoke is also important to assess for other asthma risk factors. Finally, the physician should attempt to ascertain the patient's and family's perception of the disease.

PHYSICAL EXAMINATION

A complete and thorough physical examination is essential when evaluating a child for asthma. Attention should be focused on the upper and lower respiratory tracts, as well as on potential allergic disease of other organ systems. Examination of the eyes for conjunctival erythema, cobblestoning, and allergic shiners should be undertaken, as should examination of the nose for mucosal edema, discharge, and an allergic crease, because allergic rhinitis and conjunctivitis are frequent co-morbid conditions with asthma. A purulent nasal discharge and malodorous breath may signify the presence of sinusitis, a condition that may exacerbate asthma. The chest exam should document the patient's respiratory rate, work of breathing, air entry, adventitious breath sounds (wheezes, rales, rhonchi, etc.), symmetry, inspiratory-to-expiratory ratio, and abnormalities of chest configuration (i.e., pectus deformity). An increased anteroposterior diameter of the chest may signify air trapping from asthma. The patient's digits should also be examined for clubbing, which may be seen in a variety of cardiac and pulmonary conditions. The skin should be closely examined for the presence of coexisting atopic dermatitis.

PULMONARY FUNCTION TESTS

While the clinical history and physical exam are extremely important in the diagnosis of asthma, pulmonary function tests, when practical, are extremely important in confirming or excluding the presence of asthma. Pulmonary function tests provide objective data, which can be compared to population normals. The tests take little time, are inexpensive to perform, and can be easily performed in the outpatient setting in children older than 5 years of age. These tests are particularly useful because some families may over- or understate a child's asthma symptoms. Thus, a family who is alarmed that their child is sick and wheezing "all the time" can be comforted by normal spirometry. Conversely, abnormal spirometry documenting the presence of asthma can help a family accept the diagnosis and begin a necessary course of treatment.

Spirometry is an accurate, reproducible way to measure several important pulmonary function parameters. FEV_1 is the forced expiratory volume in 1 second. A postbronchodilator increase of 12% in FEV_1 confirms the diagnosis of asthma. Additionally, spirometry measures the forced expiratory flow from 25% to 75% of forced vital capacity (FVC). This value is known as $FEF_{25\%-75\%}$. A postbronchodilator increase of 25% in $FEF_{25\%-75\%}$ also confirms the diagnosis of asthma. Spirometry also measures the peak expiratory flow rate (PEFR), which some patients can monitor on an outpatient basis. The PEFR is a notoriously effort-dependent and inconsistent value, however. Consequently, patients must be well trained and know a personal-best reference before using peak flows for home monitoring. Spirometry also measures the FVC, which, in conjunction with FEV_1, can be used to distinguish restrictive from obstructive lung disease.

Other measurements of pulmonary function that can be performed include flow-volume loops, plethysmography (which measures lung volumes and airway mechanics), infant pulmonary function tests, and bronchial provocation tests to methacholine (Provocholine), exercise, cold air, or histamine, which tests are available at asthma specialists or children's medical centers. A detailed description of these methods is beyond the scope of this article.

TESTS FOR ALLERGEN-SPECIFIC IgE

Tests for allergen-specific IgE should be performed on all asthmatic children whose disease level is classified as persistent because 80% to 90% of children with asthma have allergies. Tests for allergen-specific IgE can be performed with a skin-prick test by a practicing allergist. *In vitro* tests, such as the radioallergosorbent test (RAST), are also available but are less sensitive and specific than skin-prick tests for aeroallergens.

All patients with persistent asthma should be screened for the presence of allergen-specific IgE because exposure to both perennial indoor aeroallergens (e.g., dust mites, cockroaches, cats, dogs, and molds) and outdoor seasonal aeroallergens (e.g., trees, grasses, and weeds) may cause asthma symptoms. Importantly, removing the offending allergen from the patient's environment may significantly improve asthma symptoms and progression of disease.

Some allergens, such as pollens, are ubiquitous during certain seasons. Complete avoidance of these pollens may not be possible, but immunotherapy to these allergens often significantly reduces asthma symptoms during pollen seasons. Immunotherapy is also possible for some perennial indoor allergens if avoidance measures are unsuccessful.

OTHER LABORATORY TESTS

Routine chest radiography is rarely necessary for the outpatient management of chronic asthma. Additionally, chest radiography should be reserved in acute asthma for situations where complications such as pneumonia, pneumothorax, or pneumomediastinum are suspected. A sweat test for cystic fibrosis should be performed if the patient has atypical symptoms (e.g., failure to thrive, gastrointestinal [GI] malabsorption, pancreatic insufficiency, recurrent pneumonia, or sinusitis) or physical examination findings (e.g., digital clubbing, failure to thrive, nasal polyps) suggestive of cystic fibrosis. Tests for polymorphisms in the β_2-adrenergic receptor are available in some specialized centers. These polymorphisms may be associated with asthma severity and responses to β-agonist medications such as albuterol (Proventil).

Acute and chronic sinusitis may exacerbate or mimic asthma symptoms. Patients who have congestion and a purulent nasal discharge for greater than 10 days should have a sinus computed tomography (CT) scan performed to evaluate for sinusitis. Additionally, some asthmatics may have chronic sinus disease, which makes controlling their asthma difficult. A sinus CT should also be considered for chronic asthmatics that experience a deterioration in symptoms, which does not respond well to aggressive asthma therapy. Another condition that frequently complicates asthma care in children is gastroesophageal reflux disease (GERD). Patients with chronic asthma that fail to respond to therapy, young children and infants with postprandial symptoms, and children with predominantly nocturnal symptoms should be screened for reflux with a barium esophogram and esophageal pH monitoring. Alternatively, some specialists choose to empirically treat for reflux rather than perform diagnostic testing.

Management of Chronic Asthma

The management of chronic asthma requires a proper classification of the patient into a disease severity category. This is best done with the National Asthma Education and Prevention Program (NAEPP) *Guidelines for the Diagnosis and Management of Asthma*. These guidelines classify a patient's asthma by the presence and frequency of day and night symptoms. For children older than age 5 years and adults, spirometry and symptoms are also used to classify the disease. Patients with daytime symptoms more often than twice a week or nocturnal symptoms more frequently than twice a month require low-dose inhaled corticosteroids (ICSs) to control the disease. In addition, a child 5 years or younger with more than three episodes of wheezing in 1 year lasting more than 1 day, and that affects sleep, is classified as mild persistent. In addition, a young child with severe exacerbations less than 6 weeks apart is also considered mild persistent by the NAEPP classifications. Table 3 (and www.nhlbi.nih.gov/guidelines/asthma, appendix A-1) lists the NAEPP guidelines for the management of chronic asthma.

The optimal choice of ICS is a matter of great debate. The choice of ICS is based on a variety of factors including ease of use, bioavailability, potency, and lipophilicity (see www.nhlbi.nih.gov/guidelines/asthma, appendix A-2). The available ICSs (as of January 2004) include beclomethasone (Vanceril), budesonide (Pulmicort), flunisolide (AeroBid), fluticasone (Flovent), and triamcinolone acetate (Azmacort).

TABLE 3 National Heart, Lung, and Blood Institute Asthma Severity Guidelines

Classify Severity Before Treatment or Adequate Control	*Symptoms Day* Symptoms Night	PEF_1 or FEV_1 % of Predicted	Daily Medications
Step 4: Severe Persistent	*Continual* Frequent	<60%	High-dose inhaled corticosteroid (ICS) and long-acting β agonists
Step 3: Moderate Persistent	*Daily* >1 night/week	60-80%	Low- to medium-dose ICS and long-acting β agonists Alternatives: High-dose ICS, low- to medium-dose ICS with theophylline (Theo-Dur) or leukotriene modifiers
Step 2: Mild Persistent	>2×/*week* >2 nights/month	>80%	Low-dose ICS Alternatives: Leukotriene modifiers, theophylline, cromolyn (Intal), or nedocromil (Tilade)
Step 1: Mild Intermittent	<2 *days/week* <2 nights/month	>80%	None

Other preventive medications for the treatment of asthma include leukotriene modifiers (montelukast [Singulair], zafirlukast [Accolate], and zileuton [Zyflo]), theophylline (Theo-Dur, Uniphyl), cromolyn (Intal), salmeterol (Serevent), formoterol (Foradil), and nedocromil (Tilade). Salmeterol, leukotriene modifiers, and theophylline have synergistic or additive effects with ICSs without increasing ICSs adverse events. Because of these factors and ease of use, the combination of fluticasone and salmeterol (Advair) is the preferred therapy in patients with persistent asthma symptoms per the current guidelines. However, salmeterol and formoterol cannot be used as a monotherapy as they have no anti-inflammatory properties as a monotherapy, while the remaining medications can be used as monotherapies. ICSs are more effective than any other preventive medications for the treatment of asthma.

MONITORING PATIENTS ON INHALED CORTICOSTEROIDS

The biggest concern regarding chronic use of ICSs for asthma is the linear growth of children. However, the best studies of this issue show that, while prepubertal children may experience a transient decrease in growth velocity in the first year of therapy on some ICSs, *children on chronic ICS therapy successfully attain predicted adult height*. Furthermore, it should be emphasized that children with chronic asthma may experience impairment in growth based on their chronic disease process. The physician should chart the child's growth at all visits.

Another concern that has been raised regarding ICSs is the effect on bone mineral density (BMD) in growing children. A large study showed that moderate doses of ICSs did not alter BMD in children 5 to 12 years of age with mild to moderate asthma. ICS-induced clinically relevant hypothalamic–pituitary–adrenal (HPA) axis suppression in children on ICSs is exceedingly rare, as ICS therapy does not alter HPA function in a clinically relevant manner in most children. Finally, the available evidence suggests that ICSs *do not* cause cataracts in children.

There is much fear among parents and some physicians regarding the use of ICSs in childhood asthma. Fortunately, the available evidence supports the safety of ICSs for childhood asthma with regard to long-term growth, HPA axis suppression, BMD, and cataract formation. Parental fears regarding these side effects should be alleviated by the data in favor of therapy with the most effective medicine for persistent asthma.

Additionally, support of ICSs is the comparison of daily inhaled versus burst of oral corticosteroids (CSs). The dose of 1 year of low-dose ICSs is one fifteenth of the dose of one course of oral steroids (Table 4). We note that there is a difference between short-burst and chronic medications. However, studies show that as few as four short bursts of oral steroids a year increases fracture rate, so short bursts of corticosteroid are not benign. ICSs show a dramatic decrease in the number of asthma exacerbations, which are typically treated with oral steroids. Therefore, for patients requiring oral steroids more often than once a year, daily preventive ICSs are preferred.

TABLE 4 Daily Inhaled Versus Oral Burst Steroids

Typical 5-day course of oral steroids in a 20-kg child
2 mg/kg a day for 5 days:
2 × 20 × 5 = 200 mg
Total dose: 200 mg
One-year course of low-dose ICS
Assumption: 20% bioavailability of inhaled dose
Fluticasone 44 μg 2 puffs 2× per day for 365 days
44 × 2 × 2 × 365 × 0.2 = 12.8 mg
200 mg/12.8 mg = 15.6 years of daily ICS use

OMALIZUMAB

Omalizumab (Xolair) is the newest therapy for the treatment of asthma. It is a recombinant DNA-derived humanized IgG monoclonal antibody to IgE. The subcutaneously injected monoclonal anti-IgE binds circulating free IgE, thereby blocking IgE binding to the high-affinity receptor $Fc\varepsilon R_1$. Randomized, placebo-controlled trials of omalizumab for chronic asthma in patients 12 to 76 years old showed that omalizumab reduced asthma exacerbations even with the use of lower doses of ICSs. In addition, omalizumab significantly improved peak flow rates and forced expiratory volume at 1 second (FEV_1), although the increase in the latter was small.

Omalizumab is indicated for patients older than age 12 years with moderate to severe persistent asthma (step 3 or 4) who have a positive skin test or *in vitro* reactivity to a perennial aeroallergen and whose symptoms are inadequately controlled on ICSs. The patient's pretreatment IgE level should be between 100 and 700 for omalizumab to be considered. Dosing is based on weight and IgE level.

Omalizumab is generally well tolerated and no drug-related serious adverse effects have been reported. Anaphylaxis has occurred within 2 hours of omalizumab in <0.1% of treated patients. Additionally, malignant neoplasms of different organ systems were observed in 0.5% of patients in the omalizumab group, as compared to 0.2% in the control population. However, the rate of malignancy with omalizumab treatment was no greater than in the general population.

ENVIRONMENTAL CONTROL

Another major treatment for patients with asthma and demonstrable aeroallergen-specific IgE is environmental control. This is particularly important for perennial indoor aeroallergens such as dust mite, cat, dog, cockroach, mouse, and some molds. There is significant evidence that reducing exposure to these allergens in sensitized children will reduce asthma symptoms and improve disease control. Exposure to dust mite allergens can be significantly reduced by using allergy covers for mattresses, box springs, and pillows with frequent washing of all bedding including blankets. If a patient still has significant symptoms after attempts to reduce dust mite exposure, allergen immunotherapy may reduce or eliminate allergic sensitivity to dust mite and alleviate asthma symptoms.

Household pets frequently are a major cause of asthmatic lung inflammation. At a minimum, patients who are sensitized to a pet should never have the pet in their bedroom. Additionally, efforts should be made to limit the animal's exposure to areas where the child plays and areas with carpeting that may act as a reservoir for animal dander. The only proven method to eliminate exposure to pet dander is removal of the pet from the home. Allergen immunotherapy for household pets is controversial. Extermination efforts to reduce exposure to household pests such as cockroaches or mice should be undertaken in all households with children sensitized to these allergens. However, families should be warned not to purchase a cat to eliminate mice, as a child sensitized to mouse will likely become sensitized to cats as well.

Environmental tobacco smoke has been proven to increase the incidence of asthma and otitis media as well as induce airway hyperreactivity, exacerbate lung function, and increase asthma symptoms. Simply stated, children with asthma should never be exposed to tobacco smoke.

IMMUNOTHERAPY

Allergen immunotherapy has been shown to be extremely effective for allergic rhinitis. Its role in asthma care is less clear. A recent meta-analysis performed by the Cochrane group concluded that there is

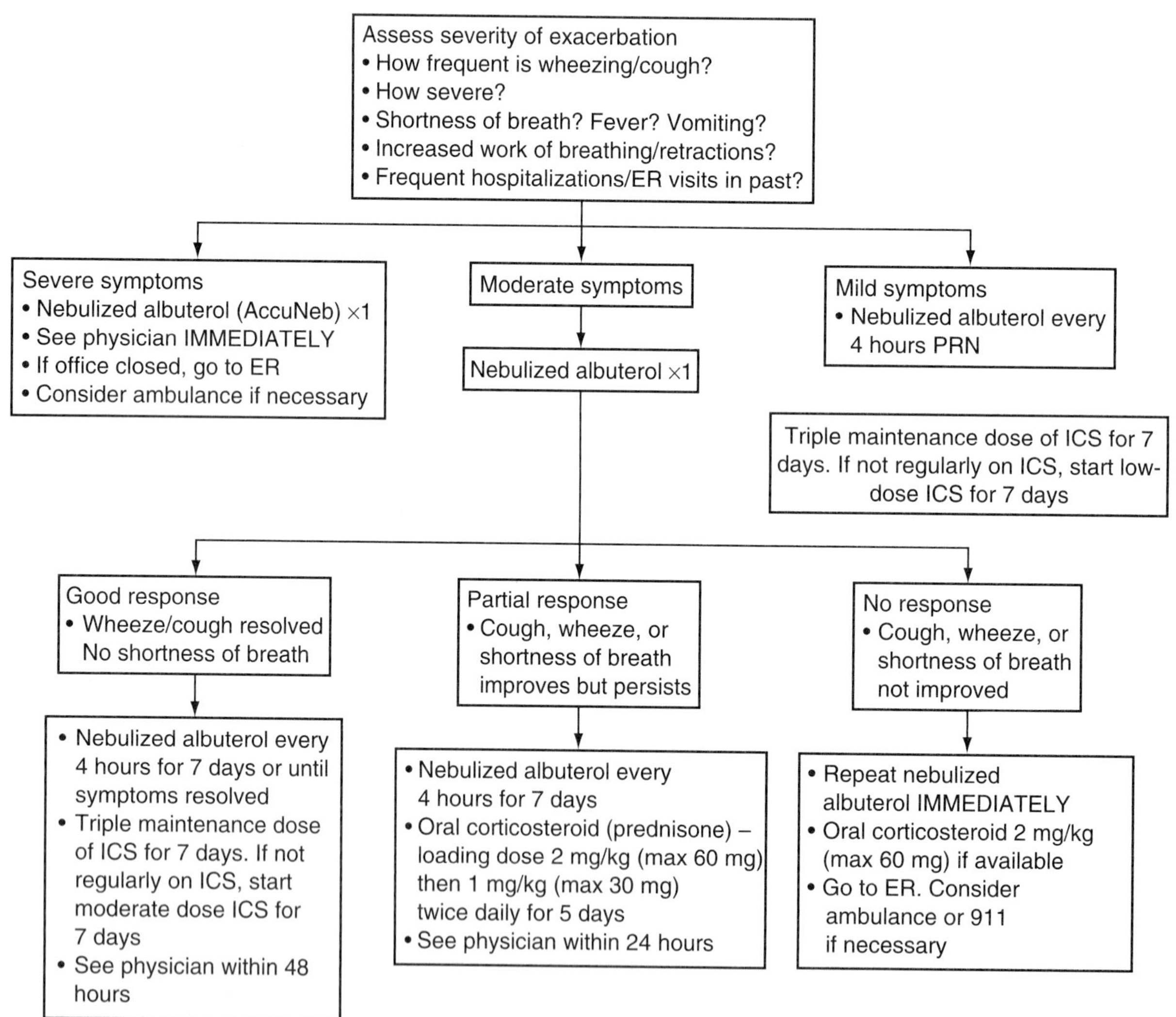

FIGURE 1 Acute asthma exacerbation guidelines for home management based on the current National Asthma Education and Prevention Program of the National Heart, Lung, and Blood Institute.

strong evidence that allergen-specific immunotherapy significantly reduces asthma symptoms, rescue medication use, and airway hyperreactivity. However, the review suggested that these benefits should be weighed against the risks of immunotherapy (anaphylaxis). Given the low risk of anaphylaxis from immunotherapy, it should be considered for patients with documented allergen-specific IgE whose asthma is not well controlled using medications and avoidance measures. It should be strongly considered for asthmatics with significant allergic rhinitis.

EDUCATION

Asthma education for both child and family is an extremely important component of asthma care. Education should address several key issues regarding asthma including: the pathophysiology of disease, symptoms of acute and chronic asthma, the importance of proper medication use and compliance, reduction of allergic and irritant triggers, and when to contact the provider. Patients may not have familiarity with using respiratory devices such as spacers, discus devices, and nebulizers. Effective medicine delivery depends on the technique of medication administration. Teaching families to recognize early symptoms of an acute exacerbation is also important because early recognition of an asthma flare allows a family to intensify asthma treatment before the exacerbation has become severe. Families should also be taught that, under optimal control, asthma should not cause symptoms and should not limit the child's activities or life in any way.

Most patients with asthma should have a written asthma management plan that includes medicines the child should be using every day (if any) as well as how to manage an acute exacerbation. These asthma "action plans" help families treat their children at the onset of an exacerbation. Although there is not a lot of literature in support of the practice, the use of written asthma management plans is very common among asthma specialists and is becoming increasingly common among primary care physicians.

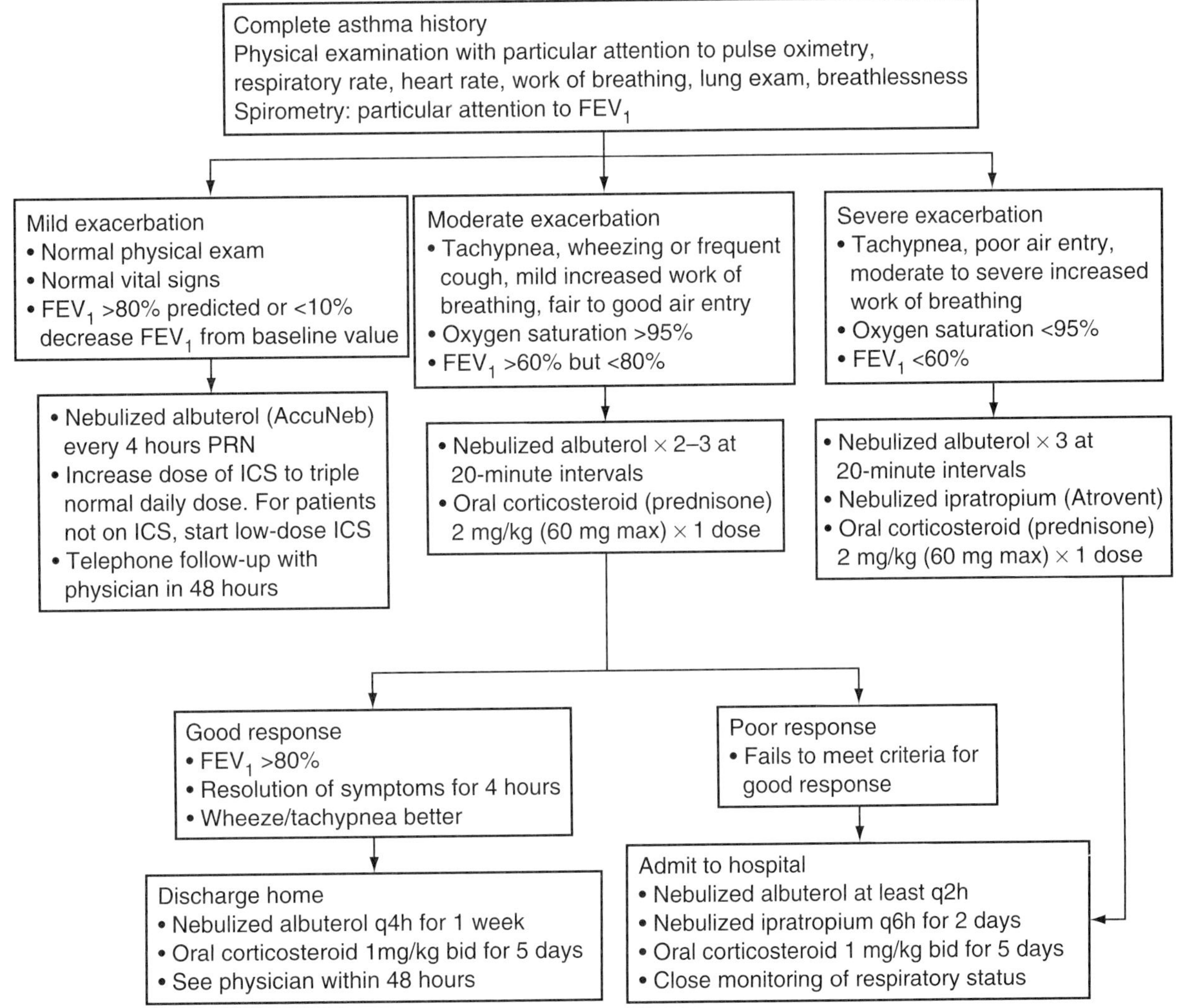

FIGURE 2 Acute asthma exacerbation guidelines for physician office management based on the current National Asthma Education and Prevention Program of the National Heart, Lung, and Blood Institute.

Management of Acute Exacerbations

HOME MANAGEMENT

Home management of asthma exacerbations via telephone is often extremely difficult. Some families are excellent at judging the severity of symptoms with telephone guidance. Others may under- or overestimate the severity of symptoms. For these patients daily peak flow monitoring is helpful. Please see Figure 1 for a childhood asthma home management algorithm. It should be stressed that if the parents are uncomfortable about their child's respiratory status, they should see a physician immediately.

OFFICE MANAGEMENT

Most providers are more comfortable with office management of acute exacerbations because the physician can examine the child and perform spirometry. Figure 2 shows a childhood asthma office/emergency room management algorithm. Antibiotics are not recommended for the acute management of asthma exacerbations in the absence of signs or symptoms of pneumonia.

Asthma is the most common chronic disease of childhood. It is responsible for an enormous amount of health care costs, hospitalizations, emergency department visits, outpatient visits, and mortality. In addition, many children live with poorly controlled or uncontrolled asthma symptoms without access to or treatment with inhaled corticosteroids. Aggressive, early treatment with ICSs of any child with daytime asthma symptoms that occur more often than twice a week, or with nocturnal symptoms that occur more often than twice a month, should be undertaken to improve asthma symptoms and lung function, as well as to reduce the need for acute care and hospitalizations. In addition, allergic triggers and other irritants such as environmental tobacco smoke should be removed from the asthmatic child's home. With good asthma care, the asthmatic child should be able to lead a normal life.

ALLERGIC RHINITIS

METHOD OF

Michael Wein, MD

Rhinitis, an inflammatory disorder of the mucous membranes of the nose and related structures, can be allergic, nonallergic, or both. Rhinitis affects almost 20% of the population in the United States, and the annual economic impact is enormous—billions of dollars spent on prescriptions, office visits, missed work, and lost productivity. Although not associated with hospitalization or surgery, allergic rhinitis significantly impacts quality of life. The increase in allergic diseases has been explained by the *hygiene hypothesis:* a decline in the prevalence of childhood infections and a cleaner home environment results in a shift of T-helper lymphocytes away from expressing the Th1 set of cytokines, which enhance antimicrobial activity, in favor of a second, or Th2, set of cytokines, which up-regulate allergic responses.

Pathogenesis

Sensitization by allergen induces production of allergen-specific IgE by B cells. IgE binds to mast cells in the nasal mucosa. Further allergen exposure triggers the *early-phase* response with release of histamine, chymase, and tryptase, and initiates a *late-phase* response with production of leukotrienes, prostaglandins, cytokines, bradykinin, platelet-activating factor, and other mediators. These mediators produce itching, sneezing, nasal discharge, sinus pressure, and nasal congestion, as well as systemic symptoms of fatigue, irritability, and reduced concentration.

Once the immune system is *primed,* a magnified response may be seen on subsequent exposure with the same amount of allergen. Nonspecific hyperreactivity to a wide range of allergic and nonallergic triggers may also result, which explains the reaction to strong odors, smoke, spicy foods, alcohol, or changes in temperature and relative humidity seen in allergic individuals.

Evaluation of Rhinitis

Most patients present to the physician after antihistamines have failed. At this point a careful and complete history should include the nature of symptoms and their severity, pattern of symptom progression, duration, seasonality, exacerbating and alleviating factors, response to self-treatment, co-morbid conditions, occupational and avocational exposures, medication history, family history, and identification of other notable environmental factors. Published questionnaires can help the physician more rapidly acquire the large amount of data needed to optimally treat rhinitis patients.

The history should include impact on daily activities, and effect of treatment on various symptoms (Table 1). Include questions about anosmia, snoring, sleep problems, fatigue, and cough. The differential diagnosis includes acute infections, structural problems, hormonal factors, and side effects from medications (Table 2).

When history suggests outdoor symptoms, the physician should suspect pollen and mold. Although there is great variability across regions, tree pollen is released during the spring, grass pollen peaks in early summer, and weed pollen peaks in late summer

TABLE 1 Symptoms of Allergic Rhinitis

Primary
Itching of the nose (and eyes, ears, throat)
Sneezing
Rhinorrhea
Nasal congestion
Secondary
Mouth breathing
Headache
Sore throat
Postnasal drip
Cough
Anosmia or hyposmia
Eustachian tube dysfunction
Sleep apnea or sleep disturbance
Fatigue
Halitosis

or early fall. Some species are entomophilous (pollinated by insects and not by wind), so they do not contribute significantly. Pollen levels are tracked by the National Allergy Bureau (http://aaaai.org/nab/index.cfm?p=pollen). Mold or fungi are also found outdoors almost year-round and counts are affected by temperature, humidity, wind, and precipitation. In dry weather *Alternaria* and *Cladosporium* may predominate outdoors; in wet weather *Fusarium*, *Phoma*, and *Cephalosporium* may increase.

When symptoms predominate indoors, mold, pets, or dust mites may be responsible. The growth of indoor mold such as *Penicillium* and *Aspergillus* is influenced by many factors but relative humidity is of primary concern. All warm-blooded animals are capable of producing allergen, including birds and farm animals, but cat allergen is especially ubiquitous, can remain airborne for prolonged periods, and is inadvertently transported to sites without cats, leading to significant levels even in hospital corridors, schools, and shopping malls. The major source of allergen in house dust is the fecal residue of dust mites, which tends to be highest in the bedroom, especially in carpets, bedding, and upholstery. Particles carrying dust mite allergens are relatively heavy and remain airborne for roughly 30 minutes and should be suspected if symptoms worsen shortly after a disturbance such as vacuuming.

Recent ARIA (Allergic Rhinitis and its Impact on Asthma) guidelines discourage the classification of seasonality and distinguish intermittent from persistent rhinitis, with the latter indicating symptoms more than 4 days per week and more than 4 weeks per year (Table 3). This change reflects the concept of a minimal persistent mucosal inflammation in patients who are continuously exposed to relevant allergens. In such patients, even a slight additional swelling of the nasal mucosa might lead to complete obstruction, while the same degree of additional swelling might go unnoticed by patients without baseline edema. Both intermittent and persistent rhinitis can be mild or moderate to severe, with the latter indicating symptoms that interfere with work, school, leisure, or sleep. The temporal nature, severity of rhinitis, and impairment of daily activities are important historical points and should guide therapy. In particular, the physician should consider the impact of disease on quality of life by inquiring about changes in work habits, limitations in recreational activity, social functioning, energy level, mood, ability to concentrate, and sense of well-being.

A history of other allergic diseases, especially asthma, is helpful and relates to the concept of inflammation throughout the airway representing a single allergic disease process. Roughly 50% to 80% of patients with asthma have rhinitis, and 25% of patients with rhinitis have asthma. Exacerbations of rhinitis often trigger asthma while treatment of rhinitis frequently leads to improved control of asthma.

Physical Examination

Physical findings may be nonspecific. Nasal mucosa often appears swollen with a blue tinge and

TABLE 2 Selected Causes of Nasal Symptoms

Allergic sensitivity
Pollen—trees, grasses, weeds
Mold—indoor and outdoor
Dust mites
Animal dander
Cockroaches
Occupational allergens
Infection (viral, bacterial, fungal)
Hormonal (e.g., hypothyroidism, pregnancy, contraceptives)
Anatomic (e.g., septal deviation, concha bullosa, foreign body)
Granulomatous (e.g., Wegener's, midline granuloma, sarcoidosis)
Vasomotor (e.g., temperature, humidity)
Pharmacologic (e.g., antihypertensives, aspirin, rhinitis medicamentosa)
Trauma (e.g., cerebrospinal fluid rhinorrhea)
Neoplastic (e.g., inverted papilloma, squamous carcinoma)
Other (ciliary dysmotility, nonallergic rhinitis with eosinophilia)

TABLE 3 ARIA Symptom Classification*

Frequency	
Intermittent	**Persistent**
<4 days per week *or* <4 weeks per year	>4 days per week *and* >4 weeks per year
Severity	
Mild	**Moderate/Severe**
Normal sleep Normal daily activities No troublesome symptoms	Abnormal sleep Impairs activities, sports, leisure Troublesome symptoms

*Classification is based on untreated patients and adapted from World Health Organization guidelines on Allergic Rhinitis and its Impact on Asthma.

enlarged turbinates. Other findings include conjunctival injection, chemosis, lacrimation, infraorbital creases (Dennie-Morgan lines), infraorbital edema (allergic shiners), middle ear effusion, and a transverse nasal crease from excessive rubbing. Chronic mouth breathing may result in the typical allergic face with a high arched palate, narrow maxillary arch, and greater anterior facial height. Other findings may include nasal polyps and giant papillae or cobblestone appearance of the tarsal conjunctiva.

Diagnostic Testing

Skin testing to detect cell-bound allergen-specific IgE is the best evidence of an allergic basis. Skin testing is accurate, cost-effective, safe, and provides immediate results to guide treatment. Testing can be done with plastic devices rather than needles, rendering the test almost painless. Less accurate and more expensive blood tests to detect circulating IgE are available if the patient has extensive skin disease. Except for very young children, most patients with allergic rhinitis will be found to react to multiple inhalant allergens. Testing blood for total IgE is not very helpful because up to 50% of patients with allergic rhinitis have normal IgE levels and up to 20% of nonallergic patients have elevated total IgE. Blood testing for allergen-specific IgG or IgG_4 antibodies has no value in the diagnosis of allergic rhinitis.

THERAPY

Therapy for rhinitis includes environmental control, pharmacotherapy, and immunotherapy (Table 4). Allergen avoidance should be stressed because it is extremely safe and relatively inexpensive. Reducing exposure to outdoor allergens such as pollen and mold is often impractical, but patients may find improvement if they decrease the time outdoors, especially in the morning or on windy days with low humidity. Physicians should focus on the indoor environment because it is more easily altered. Americans spend a greater portion of time indoors, and the exposure is year-round and at high allergen levels. In addition, reduction of exposure to indoor allergens may reduce reactivity even to outdoor allergens by limiting nonspecific hyperreactivity.

TABLE 4 Management Options for Allergic Rhinitis

Avoidance
Immunotherapy (desensitization with allergy vaccine)
Pharmacotherapy
Intranasal anticholinergics (ipratropium [Atrovent 0.03%])
Intranasal antihistamines
Intranasal cromolyn (NasalCrom)
Intranasal decongestants
Intranasal glucocorticoids
Intranasal saline
Oral antihistamine–decongestant combinations
Oral antihistamines
Oral antileukotrienes
Oral decongestants
Oral glucocorticoids

Avoidance

Emphasis should be placed first on the removal of allergen sources, next on the elimination of reservoirs, and only as a last resort on removal of the free allergen itself. This makes sense because houses usually contain, in total, many milligrams of pure allergens, of which only a few nanograms (i.e., <0.001%) may be airborne at any one time. Allergen is thus replaced even if all the airborne allergen is removed from the air, just as the water is replaced if it is pumped out of a leaking boat.

Indoor mite allergen levels are reduced if relative humidity is kept below 50%. Encasing pillows and mattresses with allergen-impermeable covers, removing carpeting, and laundering with water temperature at least 55°C (130°F) may also decrease mite allergen levels (Table 5). Although mean mite allergen concentrations of 20 to 40 µg/g of dust are often observed, meticulous allergen control to levels below 2 µg/g of dust may result in dust mite skin tests becoming negative over a period of 2 to 3 years.

Many interventions to reduce mite allergens are destined for futility. Washing in 37°C (98.6°F) water with detergent and bleach kills only a portion of dust mites, which can recolonize. Reliance on chemical intervention is not recommended; although benzyl benzoate (Acarosan)[1] kills dust mites, the allergen remains present. Tannic acid denatures mite allergen but the mites are not killed and can produce more allergen. Neither residential air-cleaning devices nor ozone generators have clinical efficacy.

Among pets, cat allergen has been the most intensively studied. Production of allergen varies widely between animals and over time. There are no allergen-free breeds of cats or dogs, although a cat genetically deficient in the major cat allergen has been experimentally designed and bred. Cat shedding of allergen is not reduced by washings, Allerpet-C spray, or acepromazine (Promace)*. Studies demonstrate that

[1]Not FDA approved for this indication.

*Not yet approved for human use in the United States. For animals only.

TABLE 5 Strategies for Avoidance of Indoor Dust Mite Allergens

Decrease ambient humidity below 50%, using a dehumidifier and hygrometer
Encase pillow and mattress in mite-impermeable covers
Remove carpeting
Remove ceiling fans
Remove feather pillows and stuffed animals
Remove upholstered furniture and drapery from bedrooms
Use vacuum and consider high-efficiency particulate air (HEPA) filter attachment
Wash bedding weekly in hot water (at least 130°F [55°C])

using a new high-efficiency particulate air (HEPA) filter vacuum cleaner actually increased inhaled allergen, probably by recruiting allergen from the carpet acting as a reservoir. Even high-quality air filtration is less effective in the presence of carpets. Cat allergen from saliva, urine, and dander is associated with small particles (<5 μm), remains airborne for days, and can be reduced by a combination of a HEPA room air filter, carpet removal, and cat exclusion from the bedroom.

Air conditioners and dehumidifiers may inhibit the growth of indoor mold, such as *Aspergillus* and *Penicillium*. Fungal studies found inconsistencies and inadequacies in exposure and outcome measures, and mold abatement efforts may yield mixed results. Fungicidal agents are commercially available, and as with most allergens, emphasis should be placed on reducing or eliminating the source—eliminate moisture or fungal contamination whenever possible.

Air-treatment devices, especially ionizers and ozone generators, have not shown clinical benefit in well-controlled studies; nevertheless, these products are heavily advertised. Reliance on clean-air delivery rate (CADR) is insufficient. Furthermore, air filters that hang around the neck barely reduce particle concentration in the surrounding air.

Pharmacotherapy

Most patients have already self-medicated with over-the-counter first-generation antihistamines to reduce itching, sneezing, and rhinorrhea with minimal effect on congestion. Although histamine may increase vascular permeability, vasodilation, mucosal blood flow, and goblet cell secretion, histamine is only one of many mediators involved and it is not surprising that symptoms often persist despite antihistamine use. Antihistamines tend to be less effective if taken after exposure to the relevant allergen, and they are also less effective for nonallergic rhinitis. Although may studies show differences in antihistamine-induced wheal suppression, receptor binding affinity, and onset of action, many of these parameters are only weakly associated with clinical efficacy. For example, one pill of astemizole (Hismanal)[2] may eliminate the skin-test wheal response for days with virtually no parallel reduction of symptoms. Studies show that patients are often unaware of cognitive and performance impairment with first-generation antihistamines, leading many to drive cars with reaction times equivalent to someone who is legally drunk. In addition to visual–motor impairment, multiple studies show that first-generation antihistamines impair children's learning and academic performance. It is noteworthy that the time to onset of clinically important relief with nonsedating antihistamines has a median of 60 to 148 minutes, depending on the agent used, quite a bit longer than the first-generation.

[2]Not available in the United States.

It is the safety, side-effect profile, and dosing interval that leads physicians to choose second-generation instead of first-generation antihistamines. Second-generation antihistamines also lack many drug interactions and cause no significant anticholinergic effects. Clinical studies show only minimal improvement when the FDA-recommended dose is exceeded, so there is little reason to ingest more than the recommended dose. Tachyphylaxis generally does not occur, and the peak effect of most occurs at about 5 to 7 hours after a single oral dose. Those with known risk of cardiac arrhythmia have already been withdrawn from the U.S. market. Each has a unique profile; for example, cetirizine (Zyrtec) is technically a second-generation antihistamine despite sedation in 15% of patients, tends to be excreted in the urine rather than metabolized in the liver, and has some interesting anti-inflammatory properties, especially at higher doses (Table 6).

Intranasal antihistamines are at least as effective as oral antihistamines, and may have a somewhat faster onset of action, but 11.5% report somnolence with azelastine (Astelin), the only FDA-approved antihistamine for intranasal use. Third-generation antihistamines such as desloratadine (Clarinex) and tecastemizole (Soltara)[2] may show some mild improvement of congestion, but the latter is not yet FDA approved. Other antihistamines in the pharmaceutical pipeline include levocetirizine (Xyzal)*, oral ketotifen (Zaditor), oxatomide (Tinset)*, levocabastine nasal spray*, and mizolastine (Mizollen)*. Mizolastine is approved for use in Europe, shows significant benefit on congestion, and inhibits the production of leukotrienes.

Oral decongestants reduce congestion, but insomnia and nervousness limit their utility. Phenylpropanolamine was withdrawn from the market because of an association with stroke in women, and pseudoephedrine (Sudafed) and phenylephrine (AH-chew D) must be used with caution in patients with hypertension, glaucoma, thyroid or cardiac disease. The latter medication has extremely poor oral bioavailability.

Nasal decongestants can lead to rapid rebound nasal congestion and tachyphylaxis and should generally be avoided. Nasal cromolyn (NasalCrom) is extremely safe but only minimally effective and must be used four to six times daily. In addition, it is only effective if used before allergen exposure. Nasal ipratropium bromide (Atrovent 0.03%) is very effective for the treatment of rhinorrhea but has no effect on other symptoms.

Leukotriene receptor antagonists are significantly less effective than intranasal corticosteroids for allergic rhinitis, even in combination with antihistamines. Studies show that montelukast (Singulair) is roughly as effective as second-generation antihistamines. Combination of montelukast with antihistamines is

[2]Not available in the United States.
*Investigational drug in the United States.

TABLE 6 Second-Generation Antihistamines

Generic (Trade)*	Minimum Age Indication	Usual Adult Dose	Pregnancy Category	Dose in Renal Impairment	Dose in Hepatic Impairment	Incidence of Somnolence†	Onset of Action	Pediatric Dose
Cetirizine (Zyrtec)	6 months	10 mg qd	B	5 mg qd	5 mg qd	13.7% (6.3%)	<1 hour	2-5, 0.5 tsp (2, 5 mg) qd
Fexofenadine (Allegra)	Age 6 years	60 mg bid or 180 mg qd	C	60 mg qd	NC	1.3% (0.9%)	1 hour	Under 12, 30 bid
Loratadine (Claritin)	Age 2 years	10 qd	B	10 mg qod	10 mg qod	8% (6%)	1-3 hours	Under 6, 1 tsp (5 mg) qd
Azelastine (Astelin)	Age 5 years	2 sprays bid	C	NC	NC	11.5% (5.4%)	2-3 hours	
Desloratadine (Clarinex)	Age 12 years	5 mg qd	C	5 mg qod	5 mg qod	2.1% (1.8%)	<1 hour	

*Levocetirizine (Xyzal) and tecastemizole (Soltara) are not yet FDA approved and are not included in the table.
†Somnolence data in parentheses is for placebo.
Abbreviations: bid = twice daily; NC = no change; qd = daily; qod = every other day.

less effective than nasal corticosteroids alone, and it is not effective in perennial allergic rhinitis. Although it might seem plausible to use antileukotrienes to treat rhinitis when asthma is also present, standard treatment of rhinitis with many other medications has already been shown to improve asthma control and reduce emergency department visits for asthma in a dose-dependent manner.

Intranasal steroids are the cornerstone of pharmacologic management for allergic rhinitis, although they are less effective for ocular symptoms. One study showed that 78% of patients obtain at least moderate relief with nasal corticosteroids, compared with 58% for second-generation antihistamines. In vitro, budesonide (Rhinocort) and fluticasone (Flonase) have the highest pharmacologic potency based on receptor-binding affinity studies and topical vasoconstrictor potency, but this does not correlate directly with clinical efficacy. Mometasone (Nasonex) has the lowest age indication, down to age 2 years, and has extremely low systemic bioavailability. All require prolonged use over weeks to achieve optimal effectiveness, but some studies do show benefit with initial use, suggesting a very limited role for as-needed use. Choosing among the various intranasal steroids also requires a consideration of patient preference as well as characteristics of the preparation itself (Table 7). The dose–response curve for intranasal steroids plateaus, and if a low dose is ineffective, then further increases are likely to increase side effects such as epistaxis without any significant clinical benefit. If one nasal steroid is ineffective, it is unlikely that another will yield significantly better results for the same patient.

The FDA requires all nasal steroids to carry a warning regarding growth suppression. Except for intranasal dexamethasone (Decadron Turbinaire)[2], the risk of significant systemic side effects with nasal corticosteroids are minimal, although testing of corticotrophin releasing hormone can reveal subtle changes in the hypothalamic–pituitary axis. Other demonstrations of systemic side effects with nasal steroids are linear growth suppression in children 6-9 years old with intranasal beclomethasone (Vancenase) taken for 1 year, decreased overnight urinary cortisol levels in healthy volunteers with a 4-day course of fluticasone (Flonase) 200 mg/d, and a slight increase in the prevalence of cataracts with high cumulative lifetime doses (>2000 μg) of inhaled corticosteroids. The physician must watch for rare cases of septal perforation. High doses of inhaled corticosteroid therapy used to treat asthma are another reason to use the lowest effective dose and titrate down whenever possible.

Prolonged use of oral steroids is not a viable option because of the risk of cataracts, osteoporosis, glaucoma, hypertension, glucose intolerance, and aseptic necrosis. Rare individuals may be more susceptible even to intranasal steroids.

[2]Not available in the United States.

Allergen Vaccines (Desensitization)

Allergen immunotherapy is the injection of a vaccine against relevant allergens and is a safe and highly effective treatment to relieve or eliminate allergic rhinitis, is the only treatment able to alter the natural course of the disease, and may even prevent the onset of asthma in some cases. It is usually reserved for patients with persistent symptoms, at least moderate in severity, who have failed other treatment options (Table 8). At the cellular level, allergen vaccination blocks the seasonal rise in IgE, decreases histamine release, prevents recruitment of inflammatory cells, reduces the number of mast cells in tissue, and reduces cytokine production. Clinically, allergen vaccination can improve allergic symptoms, reduce medication usage, and increase pulmonary function. Although effective in 85% to 90% of patients, if a clinical response is not seen within the first 12 months, then immunotherapy is usually stopped. Immunotherapy should not be administered to very young children, to patients using β blockers, or to those experiencing an acute asthma exacerbation because of the risk of anaphylaxis.

TABLE 7 Nasal Corticosteroid Formulations

Generic (Trade)	Minimum Age	Usual Adult Dose per Nostril Spray	Dose Frequency	Intranasal Bioavailability (%)*	Pediatric Dose
Beclomethasone dipropionate (Vancenase AQ 42)	6 years	1 or 2	bid	44	(<12 years, 1 spray bid)
Fluticasone (Flonase)	4 years	1 or 2	qd	0.5-2.0	(4-12 years, 1 spray qd)
Triamcinolone (Nasacort AQ)	6 years	2	qd	46	(6-12 years, 1 spray qd)
Flunisolide (Nasalide, Nasarel)	6 years	2	bid/tid	49	(6-14 years, 1 spray tid)
Mometasone (Nasonex)	2 years	2	qd	0.1	(3-12 years, 1 spray qd)
Budesonide AQ (Rhinocort Aqua)	6 years	1 or 2	qd	34	(Over 6 years no change)

Note that higher doses occur along the plateau of the dose–response curve. As a result, higher than recommended doses tend to cause increasing side effects without much improved therapeutic benefit.

Patients should taper to the lowest effective maintenance dosage to minimize systemic effects. All are Pregnancy Category C, but budesonide nasal spray is Category B. Ciclesonide has not yet been approved by the FDA.

*Bioavailability studies were not based on direct comparison in a single study; data are not to be interpreted otherwise.

Abbreviations: bid = twice daily; qd = daily; tid = three times a day.

TABLE 8 Considerations for Allergen Immunotherapy

Desire for long-lasting relief without medication
Excessive medication usage
Inadequate control with allergen avoidance and pharmacotherapy
Intolerable medication side effects
Unavoidable exposure

Effectiveness requires experienced practitioners exercising careful attention to allergen selection, dosing, and administration. It may be safely continued during pregnancy but should not be initiated in pregnant patients. Data based on Medicare's Resource-Based Relative Value Scale indicate that allergen immunotherapy is cost-effective. After a maintenance level is reached, the frequency of injections can be reduced to one injection every 1 to 3 weeks. A course of 3 to 5 years is usually sufficient to induce a remission that can persist for years, even after injections are discontinued.

Pregnancy

Pregnant patients with rhinitis represent a special challenge, especially because uncontrolled rhinitis may exacerbate asthma and affect pregnancy outcome. Although intranasal cromolyn (NasalCrom) is first-line therapy in this situation, most patients will require additional treatment, either with an antihistamine from Pregnancy Category B (e.g., chlorpheniramine [Chlor-Trimeton], loratadine [Claritin], cetirizine [Zyrtec]) or an intranasal corticosteroid. The most desirable corticosteroids would be either beclomethasone (Vancenase) because of its long record of use, or budesonide (Rhinocort), which was suggested for use in pregnancy by the American College of Obstetrics and Gynecology. Ipratropium (Atrovent nasal spray), lodoxamide (Alomide ophthalmic solution), and montelukast (Singulair) are also Pregnancy Category B, but are not widely used in this situation because of limited clinical experience in pregnancy and less utility than the other options noted above. Avoidance becomes more important in this situation, and as noted patients should not increase or initiate immunotherapy while pregnant.

Future Therapy

The FDA has approved a monoclonal antibody, anti-IgE injection (omalizumab [Xolair])[1], which can reduce asthma exacerbations by more than 40% in patients already treated optimally with inhaled steroids for asthma. Anti-IgE similarly reduces symptoms in patients with rhinitis already treated optimally with allergen immunotherapy. At the time of this writing, it is not expected to be approved for use in allergic rhinitis and I would not recommend off-label use. Perhaps the most exciting rhinitis research involves vaccines using allergen genes, antisense single-stranded DNA, or synthetic CpG deoxynucleotides that mimic microbial DNA and are able to down-regulate Th2 responses through toll-like receptor 9. Future approaches to block the recruitment of inflammatory cells involve monoclonal antibodies directed against chemokines, adhesion molecule antagonists, or interleukins as well as soluble cytokine receptors. One example is the compound R112, an intranasal inhibitor of the tyrosine kinase called Syk. Syk phosphorylates many intracellular signaling proteins and leads to the release of inflammatory mediators. The compound R112 (Rigel Pharmaceuticals, San Francisco, CA) is already in clinical trials and looks promising.

[1]Not FDA approved for this indication.

Summary

Patients with allergic rhinitis experience systemic as well as local symptoms, and the primary complaint is usually either congestion or fatigue. The disease involves multiple mediators and responds best to an approach targeted to reducing inflammation, rather than blocking a single mediator. Even though some nonsedating antihistamines may be available over-the-counter, intranasal steroids are more effective except for ocular symptoms. Leukotriene antagonists are not more effective than antihistamines, and they are less effective than nasal steroids.

If avoidance has failed to provide adequate relief, the patient can (a) use daily nonsedating antihistamine in the morning, (b) add the lowest possible dose of inhaled steroid that is sufficient to provide relief, and (c) avoid known or suspected triggers. Common reasons for lack of a clinical response to treatment are (a) incorrect diagnosis, (b) medication noncompliance, (c) persistent exposure to allergens (e.g., incomplete patient education), and (d) improper selection of medication (e.g., nasal steroids for ocular symptoms). Common reasons for referral to an allergist are (a) pharmacotherapy and avoidance yield poor control or undesirable side effects, (b) co-morbid conditions such as asthma, nasal polyposis, or sinusitis recur, and (c) quality-of-life issues prompt consideration of more intensive treatment, including avoidance or immunotherapy.

ALLERGIC REACTIONS TO DRUGS

METHOD OF

Don McNeil, MD

Drug allergic reactions fall under the broader category of adverse drug reactions (ADRs), which also include toxic drug effects, drug interactions, drug intolerance, and, finally, allergic (or immunologic) drug reactions. Adverse drug reactions are common and often result in only trivial consequences. Some may be severe and life-threatening, and may result from both allergic and nonallergic causes.

The incidence of adverse drug effects is unknown but estimates of 20% of hospital admissions are not unreasonable. A skin rash is the most common manifestation; more importantly, however, severe life-threatening reactions occur, of which only a small portion have an allergic etiology. Most drug reactions are the result of unknown mechanisms. Drug intolerance, drug overdose, and side effects of drugs, as well as drug interactions, all play a significant role. These reactions should be considered both common and predictable.

Although allergic drug reactions are potentially severe, they are also the least common and least predictable. Allergic drug reactions are given particular attention because of the unpredictable, costly, and severe consequences that occasionally arise.

Several mechanisms may play a role in the underlying etiology of immunologic drug reactions. Immediate IgE-mediated reactions represent the classic allergic reaction. This is well characterized and the best understood, but other mechanisms also exist, for example, a cytotoxic reaction in which drug-induced antibodies result in hemolytic anemia. Another example is immune complex formation resulting in organ damage. This is commonly referred to as a "serum sickness" reaction and is characterized by fever, rash, and arthralgia beginning 2 to 4 weeks after initiation of drug. Finally, a delayed-type hypersensitivity reaction occurs when drug-specific T-lymphocytes react. This completes the picture of the four types of immunologic-mediated drug reactions according to the original Gell and Coombs classification. These are referred to as Type I, II, III, or IV reactions, respectively.

Cutaneous reactions comprise the most frequent type of allergic drug reaction. Approximately 94% cause a morbilliform rash and only 5% cause an urticarial reaction. Idiosyncratic reactions are still the most likely cause for a rash and occur much more frequently than a true drug-induced allergic reaction. Ampicillins in conjunction with a viral hepatitis or sulfa drugs taken in the AIDS population are common examples.

Both allergic and nonallergic reactions are known to be associated with severe reactions, including fatalities. Contrast media agents, allergic extracts, anesthetics, and antibiotics are the most commonly implicated drugs. Penicillin remains the most common cause of fatal drug reactions and accounts for up to 75% of these severe drug reactions in the United States.

An allergy to penicillin is the most frequently reported, but as many as 90% of patients labeled "penicillin allergic" are able to tolerate penicillin. This allergy is often mislabeled because of underlying illness or interaction between antibiotic and illness. Unfortunately one-third to one-half of vancomycin (Vancocin) prescriptions in hospitals are given because of a history of "penicillin allergy." This raises the incidence of drug-resistant bacteria because of broad-spectrum antibiotic overuse. The economic impact of treating antibiotic-resistant infections is roughly $4 billion annually.

Pathophysiology

Some drugs are capable of reacting in the body without further alteration in chemical structure, whereas others must first be metabolized to become immunogenic. Many drugs are too small to be immunogenic alone and are incapable of eliciting an immune allergic response. These drugs require binding to a high-molecular-weight protein followed by antigen processing and presentation by the macrophage in the presence of major histocompatibility complex (MHC)-specific antigen to appropriate T-cell receptors.

Penicillin is capable of inducing an allergic reaction in more than one manner. Benzylpenicilloyl, the major penicillin determinant, is able to produce a strong antigenic response. A commercially available product, benzylpenicilloyl-polylysine (PPL) (Pre-Pen), provides the means to reproduce the same allergic response by simple skin testing. Minor determinants are metabolic derivatives of penicillin that may also produce an immune response. The diagnostic capabilities of a penicillin allergy are strengthened by including some measure of the allergic response to the minor determinants when skin testing is conducted for penicillin (Figure 1).

Patients with a history of penicillin allergy but negative skin testing to PPL and the minor determinants rarely experience allergic reactions on re-exposure. If they should occur, these are not fatal, but rather mild and self-limited.

PPL alone will potentially miss a significant percentage of allergic reactions to penicillin. Allergy testing with fresh benzylpenicillin G, aged penicillin (reconstituted more than 24 hours) as well as skin testing with the specific penicillin in question will greatly enhance the likelihood of uncovering of penicillin allergy in a patient with a positive history.

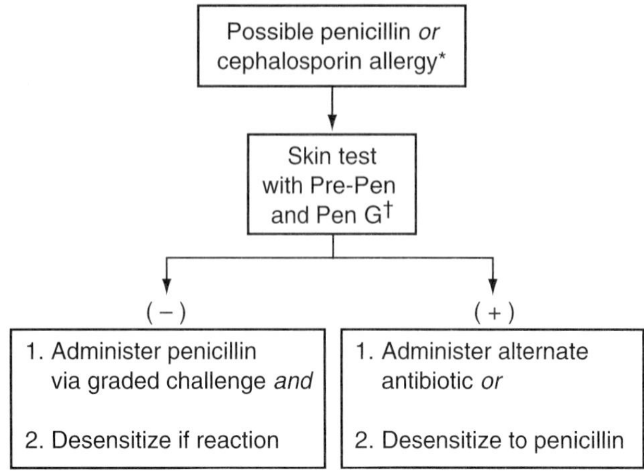

FIGURE 1 Penicillin allergy evaluation.

*Only 10%–20% of patients who report a penicillin allergy are actually allergic.
†Benzylpenicilloyl polylysine (Pre-Pen) and penicillin G (Pen G) will not include all potential penicillin derivatives. The additional benefit of testing with the minor determinant mixture is impractical and usually not available.

Cephalosporins do not provide the same degree of certainty with respect to an allergic evaluation. Cross-reactivity with penicillin allergy patients is known to exist, and although uncommon, it is also unpredictable. To err on the side of safety, a patient with a known penicillin allergy should not be treated with a cephalosporin. A patient with a previous cephalosporin reaction with a negative penicillin skin test cannot safely receive penicillin or another cephalosporin unless further diagnostic measures are taken. This patient may be allergic to a side chain on the cephalosporin that has not been identified by penicillin skin testing. Others recommend a graded oral challenge using a cephalosporin with a different side chain. The latter should be done realizing that standardized procedures have not been developed for this and therefore false negative results may occur.

Successful *desensitization* to penicillin has permitted a similar approach with other drugs. If the drug in question is required, either intravenous or oral drug administration is possible by incremental doses given usually every 15 minutes. A 10,000-fold dilution of the initial dose is usually sufficient to begin, followed by higher doses, 2-fold or greater. The vital signs are monitored throughout the procedure with timely medical intervention if problems arise.

Sulfonamides typically cause cutaneous reactions, infrequently in healthy individuals but extremely common in AIDS patients. Reactions may be relatively benign in nature such as urticaria or fixed-drug eruption, but may also cause more serious reactions (Stevens-Johnson syndrome, toxic epidermal necrolysis). A variety of mechanisms may exist, alone or in combination, using IgE antibody response, T-lymphocytes, and inflammatory cytokines. Because of our inadequate understanding of these mechanisms, there are no universally acceptable means of evaluating sulfonamide hypersensitivity. Unless there has been previously severe reaction, a graded challenge with the drug in question is considered a reasonable alternative (Table 1). Although a theoretical risk exists between sulfonamides and drugs with sulfonamide derivatives (diuretics, COX-2 inhibitors), little data show this is actually true.

Radiographic contrast media (RCM) produce an anaphylactoid reaction by an unknown mechanism. Conventional RCM is hypertonic. The newer nonionic RCM with lower osmolarity are associated with fewer anaphylactoid or allergic-like reactions. Complement system activation, which is capable of causing histamine release, is thought to be the method by which this reaction occurs.

In the continuum of adverse drug effects with suspected hypersensitivity, exposure to *aspirin* and other nonsteroidal anti-inflammatory drugs (NSAIDs) rarely exhibits features that are IgE mediated and allergic in nature, and are more often nonimmunologic mediated. A non–IgE-mediated event must still be approached with caution because the consequences are potentially life-threatening.

More commonly, NSAIDs are associated with the asthma triad syndrome associated with nasal polyps or rhinitis, and severe asthma. This is not an allergic

TABLE 1 Graded Challenge

1. Cautious administration of medications to patient *not* likely allergic to drug.
2. Not to be considered equivalent to desensitization.
3. Used when insufficient evidence available to exclude drug allergy.
4. Medication administered in incremental doses beginning at 1:100 dilution of final dose.
5. Adequate medical resources exist to treat allergic reaction.

drug reaction, but represents a largely unrecognized subpopulation of asthmatics who will benefit by avoiding the use of NSAIDs.

The antibiotic *vancomycin (Vancocin)* causes a reaction referred to as *red man syndrome*. Histamine and other mast cell mediators are released, but not through vancomycin-induced IgE antibody (rare cases have been reported). Most, but not all, cases of the red man syndrome are related to the rate of the infusion, and most will subside once the medication is stopped. A graded challenge with the drug or a full course of desensitization usually permits resumption of treatment.

Angiotensin-converting enzyme (ACE) inhibitors are well known to be associated with cough and angioedema, but like NSAIDs, the mechanism is unknown. Newer ACE inhibitors have been described to cause similar reactions but at a much lower incidence. The symptoms of cough and angioedema may continue to recur for several months and up to a year after the discontinuation of the drug.

As seen from the discussion above, IgE-mediated allergic drug reactions represent only a portion of immune-mediated drug reactions. To assist in the diagnosis, a 7- to 10-day delay in the appearance of the drug reaction after initial treatment or immediate reactivation on re-exposure suggests an immunologic etiology. Oftentimes, only the history will provide this index of suspicion. Confirmation by positive skin testing with the drug in question is highly predictive of IgE-mediated hypersensitivity.

Attempts to label reactions as either IgE- or non–IgE-mediated may prove to be costly, time-consuming, and of no immediate benefit. Non-IgE reactions are capable of eliciting changes in vital signs, pulmonary function, and cutaneous effects similar to anaphylaxis and are referred to as anaphylactoid. These need to be regarded with the same degree of caution as IgE-mediated reactions. Narcotics, radiographic contrast media, and chemotherapeutic agents may directly affect mast cell mediator release with the consequences listed above. Antihistamines and corticosteroids given prior to administration of these drugs are usually sufficient to prevent a re-occurrence, or at least to minimize these reactions.

Drug desensitization is indicated for those patients with positive skin tests who must receive the drug, but should not be assumed to be universally safe or protective. Some chemotherapeutic agents, such as etoposide (VePesid) and teniposide (Vumon), have a much higher incidence of anaphylactoid reactions. Readministration of these drugs in the face of a previous reaction and in spite of prophylactic measures often leads to disappointing results.

Current biologic response modifier agents, as well as others soon to arrive, are associated with adverse reactions. Monoclonal antibodies, T- and B-cell inactivators, and others may prove to have adverse immunologic effects that will only become more apparent with the experience of increased usage.

Evaluation of Drug Allergy in Practice

The importance of a reliable history in a medical evaluation is never more evident than during the initial workup of a suspected drug allergy. The timing of exposure, with the first allergic reaction occurring within days of the priming dose or immediately upon re-exposure, strongly points to an allergic etiology. Multiple exposures to the same drug on previous occasions do not preclude an allergic reaction *de novo*. Similarly, a previous history of an allergic drug reaction does not by itself predict a reoccurrence on re-exposure. The allergic diathesis may wane over time for drugs just as it may occur for other allergens.

Armed with this suggestive drug history and clinical findings such as a rash, fever, bronchospasm, or anaphylaxis, the evaluation becomes more straightforward. In the appropriate clinical setting, eosinophilia will also support a drug-allergic reaction.

Avoiding the implicated drug may be the simplest approach because confirmation of the diagnosis with appropriate skin testing is often unavailable. (Standardized skin testing exists only for penicillin, but even this does not provide 100% reliability.) Skin testing with the drug is questionable, but using both a positive and negative control of histamine and saline may still provide useful information. A positive skin test would certainly discourage use of this drug unless adequate precautions were taken.

If a non–life-threatening history of a reaction exists and the drug cannot be appropriately substituted, the option exists for a graded oral challenge to confirm the diagnosis. This should not be considered to be the same as desensitization because it involves higher doses and exposure over a shorter period of time than would be considered safe in a truly allergic individual. A challenge such as this should be conducted in suitable medical facilities under close medical supervision.

If the drug in question has been shown to cause an allergic reaction but still must be used, then a carefully monitored drug desensitization program should be considered. Under medical supervision, the drug should be administered orally or intravenously beginning with doses that are tenfold more dilute than the final strength. Incrementally higher doses of the drug should be administered every 15 minutes, increasing the dose twofold each time.

Drug-induced skin reactions are common and warrant particular attention. Early recognition is necessary to avoid an incorrect diagnosis and to institute appropriate interventional measures as soon as possible.

The following points will assist the physician in arriving at a correct diagnosis. The *timing of the onset* of the reaction in relation to the time the drug was given provides an important clue. Often signs and symptoms develop 1 to 2 weeks after time of initial drug exposure. Symptoms may develop rapidly on repeat exposure. *Pruritic urticarial lesions* strongly suggest an adverse drug reaction. A *symmetrical or truncal distribution* or a rash that occurs only in sun-exposed areas (polymorphous light eruption) also supports an ADR finding. The *morphology* of the reaction is helpful, although many types occur (lichenoid, morbilliform, eczematous). The *histopathology* of the lesion on skin biopsy may reveal *eosinophils,* which may also be detected in the peripheral blood.

Drugs that commonly cause ADRs tend to be antibiotics. The most common is the morbilliform rash when ampicillin is given in the presence of a viral infection such as infectious mononucleosis or cytomegalovirus. Rarely is this IgE mediated and it should not be regarded as a basis for a history of penicillin allergy. It should also be noted that not all ADRs are caused by prescription medications. A patient may fail to disclose over-the-counter medications that might be responsible (e.g., St. John's wort).

The *response to treatment* may aid in the recognition of an ADR. An incomplete response to topical steroids is typical of an ADR and systemic steroids may turn out to be the therapy of choice. Finally, the *response to withdrawal* of drug may range from a rapid recovery to slow clearing over many weeks, but a favorable response nonetheless.

Table 2 lists several drugs used to treat AIDS/HIV that are worthy of mention. Not all should be considered to be an allergic cause of ADR.

A careful and systematic approach to the patient with a suspected drug allergy will provide valuable information for both the immediate and the long-term management of the patient. A suspected drug allergy that is disproved will facilitate good medical care because unnecessary expense and the risk of further sensitizing the patient to a new medication are spared if the patient is not. On the other hand, a positive screen for a suspected drug allergy will result in a safe alternative. It should be emphasized, however, that neither a family history of a drug allergy nor a patient requesting a "test" for a possible drug allergy without other reason is an indication for further drug allergy evaluation because of the risk of false-negative results.

TABLE 2 Drugs Used to Treat AIDS/HIV

Drug	Reaction
Zidovudine, AZT (Retrovir)	Hyperpigmentation
Zalcitabine, ddC (Hivid)	Oral ulcers
Abacavir (Ziagen)	Severe rash/anaphylaxis
Nevirapine (Viramune)	Toxic epidermal necrolysis
Foscarnet	Urethral ulceration
Trimethoprim-sulfamethoxazole, TMP-SMX (Bactrim)	Morbilliform rash or erythema multiforme

ALLERGIC REACTIONS TO INSECT STINGS

METHOD OF
Debora Ortega-Carr, MD

Responses to insect stings are typically classified as local or systemic reactions. Normally a localized response, such as redness, swelling, and pain and itching, occurs at the sting site. This reaction usually subsides within hours, although some localized erythema may remain for 24 hours. A large local reaction may occur in up to 10% of the population and involve a late-phase inflammatory mechanism that develops over 12 to 24 hours. Pain and induration greater than 5 cm may persist for 5 to 7 days. Systemic reactions are immediate hypersensitivity reactions with manifestations distant from the site of the sting and may include urticaria, angioedema, dyspnea, cough, laryngeal edema, or hypotension. Approximately 50 deaths per year are attributed to insect stings in the United States, but the true incidence of sting-related fatalities is likely higher. Elevated serum tryptase and venom-specific IgE antibodies have been reported in postmortem blood samples in cases of unexpected death in young individuals. Systemic reactions are reported by up to 3% of adults, making stinging insect allergy more common than generally thought.

Allergic or IgE-mediated reactions can result from bites or stings of many kinds of insects, but insects of the order *Hymenoptera* can cause anaphylaxis. These insects include honeybees, yellow jackets, hornets, wasps, and imported fire ants. Recent reports suggest that imported fire ants may pose a greater risk of anaphylaxis for adults living in imported fire ant-endemic regions than the other stinging insects.

Diagnosis

The diagnosis of insect allergy rests on the history as the primary evidence of allergic reactivity, because venom-specific IgE antibodies are also present in a large number of clinically nonreactive individuals. It is important to determine both specific symptoms and the time course of the reaction to determine immediate versus delayed-type hypersensitivity reactions.

The presence of venom-specific IgE antibodies can be demonstrated by skin testing or serologic methods (radioallergosorbent test [RAST]). Commercial venom vaccines are available for honeybee, yellow jacket, hornet, white-faced hornet, and *polistes* wasps. Skin testing with hymenoptera venoms or fire ant whole-body extract is recommended for patients who have had systemic allergic reactions to an insect

TABLE 1 Clinical Recommendations Based on History of Sting Reaction, Age, and Allergy Testing

Reaction to or RAST	Skin Test	Risk of Systemic Reaction	Clinical Previous Sting Recommendation
No reaction	Positive	10-20%	Avoidance
Large local	Positive	5-10%	Avoidance
Cutaneous systemic	Positive	1-10 %	Avoidance
Child			
Adult	Positive	10-20%	Venom immunotherapy
Anaphylaxis	Positive	30-60%	Venom immunotherapy
	Negative	5-10%	Repeat skin test/RAST

Abbreviation: RAST = radioallergosorbent test.

sting, but is not necessary in patients with large local reactions. Because of anergy following systemic reactions, skin testing should be performed at 4 to 6 weeks poststing. Skin testing is performed using a modified intradermal technique, starting with concentrations of .001 µg/mL and increasing concentrations until a positive wheal-and-flare reaction occurs.

Treatment and Prevention of Sting Reactions

Immediate local reactions may be treated with ice, analgesics, and antihistamines. Larger local reactions may benefit from a course of systemic steroids (prednisone) 30 to 60 mg tapering over 4 to 7 days. Topical steroids in limited local reactions have been used anecdotally. Sting sites from imported fire ants should also be observed closely for any sign of secondary infection.

Systemic reactions require epinephrine (1:1000) 0.3 mg in an adult (0.01 mg/kg in children) administered intramuscularly. If necessary the subcutaneous route may be used although the intramuscular route is preferred, the epinephrine may need to be repeated in 10 to 15 minutes. Oxygen, intravenous fluid and airway support should be available if needed. Diphenhydramine hydrochloride (Benadryl) is often administered orally 25 to 50 mg or parenterally 50 mg for more severe reactions. Corticosteroids have no benefit in the acute stage, but are often administered when the patient's condition stabilizes to prevent late-phase reactions. The patient should be monitored for 3 to 6 hours; more than 20% of cases develop recurrent or prolonged reactions. Patients who have accompanying medical conditions such as hypertension or cardiac disease warrant even closer observation, as their response to pressor therapies may be suboptimal.

Future stings may be avoided by reducing exposure. Garbage and outdoor food, especially canned drinks, attract yellow jackets. Perfumes and bright floral clothing should be avoided. Patients should avoid going barefoot outdoors. Patients at risk for anaphylaxis should have a prescription for an epinephrine injection kit with very specific instructions on how and when to use the epinephrine. The EpiPen (0.3 mg of epinephrine) and EpiPen Jr. (0.15 mg of epinephrine) offer a concealed needle and an automatic injection device, which allows them to be injected quickly. The Ana-Kit delivers two doses of 0.3 mL of 1:1000 solution. Having two doses of epinephrine on hand may be preferable in many situations. The EpiPen is also now available in a two-dose pack. Aerosolized epinephrine (Epinephrine Mist) has been helpful in our office in treating laryngeal edema and bronchospasm.

The risk of a systemic reaction to a future sting is assessed by specific details of the patient's history and the presence or absence of IgE antibody to venom (skin testing or RAST) (Table 1). A patient who has experienced a sting-induced systemic reaction should be referred to an allergist. Systemic reactions to insect stings can be prevented with 98% efficacy with venom immunotherapy.

Immunotherapy is given using increasing amounts of venoms (or whole-body extracts in the case of imported fire ants) give weekly for 2 to 6 months until a maintenance dose of 100 µg/mL is reached. Venom injections are given every 4 weeks during the first year of treatment, and then every 6 weeks thereafter. During immunotherapy, systemic reactions occur in 5% to 15% of individuals. Periodic monitoring of venom skin test or RAST sensitivity is recommended to help determine when one may discontinue immunotherapy. The duration of immunotherapy is a matter of clinical judgment. Although the product package insert advises that immunotherapy should continue indefinitely, venom skin tests do become negative in 20% to 25% of patients within 3 to 5 years of therapy. These patients may discontinue immunotherapy with a low risk of anaphylaxis (Table 2). The clinical history of the initial sting reaction and the history of a systemic reaction during immunotherapy are very important factors in determining whether a patient should discontinue immunotherapy after 5 years or continue indefinitely. Recent studies from the Netherlands show that venom immunotherapy provides clinically important improvements in quality of life for 2 of 3 patients treated.

TABLE 2 Patients with a Low Risk for Anaphylaxis

Minimal (<5%)	General adult population
	Patients on venom immunotherapy
	Children with cutaneous systemic reactions
Low (5-10%)	Patients with large local reactions
	Patients who have completed 5 years of venom immunotherapy

SECTION **13**

Diseases of the Skin

ACNE VULGARIS AND ROSACEA

METHOD OF

Julie C. Harper, MD

Acne Vulgaris

Acne vulgaris affects nearly 100% of people at some point during their lifetime. Acne is most commonly observed in adolescence but may also be seen in the neonate and in the adult. In most individuals there is a resolution of acne over time. Even after acne has resolved, many individuals are left with physical and psychosocial scarring. This scarring can be prevented with appropriate diagnosis and management.

PATHOGENESIS

Appropriate treatment of acne rests on a clear understanding of the underlying pathogenesis. Acne vulgaris is a multifactorial disease process. Four key pathogenetic factors are identified in acne vulgaris, including follicular epidermal hyperproliferation, excess sebum production, the presence and activity of the bacteria *Propionibacterium acnes*, and inflammation. The earliest observed histopathologic lesion in acne is the microcomedo. This lesion is characterized only by follicular epidermal hyperproliferation; inflammation and *P. acnes* are not prominent. The factor inciting the follicular epidermal hyperproliferation is not known, but androgen hormones, the inflammatory cytokine interleukin (IL)-1α, and alterations in epidermal lipid components have all been implicated. Although inflammation and *P. acnes* are not prominent early in acne vulgaris their role should not be underestimated. Signs of inflammation including erythema, pain, and swelling are commonly seen in lesions of acne vulgaris. This inflammation occurs secondary to *P. acnes* bacterial cell wall and to its byproducts, which diffuse through the follicular wall into the surrounding dermis. Chemoattractant agents are released that trigger an influx of lymphocytes and neutrophils. In addition, *P. acnes* produces lipases and destructive proteases that further promote inflammation, follicular wall disruption, and potential scarring. Excess sebum is also important in the development of acne and is largely under the control of androgen hormones. In summary, the pathogenesis of acne is multifactorial with the interplay of four key etiologic agents. Understanding the pathogenesis of acne vulgaris is a necessary step in effectively managing the disease.

CLINICAL FEATURES

The primary lesion of acne vulgaris is the microcomedo. This lesion is characterized by noninflammatory plugging of the follicle and is not visible with the naked eye. The microcomedo is the precursor of all other acne lesions. These may include the open and closed comedones, inflammatory papules and pustules, and acne nodules.

Open and closed comedones are noninflamed, small acne lesions averaging only a few millimeters in diameter. The open comedo, or *blackhead*, has a characteristic visible follicular orifice with a dark grey-black keratin plug. The closed comedone is a small, dome-shaped, white papule with a smaller follicular orifice not clinically visible. Both of these lesions are devoid of signs of inflammation.

Inflamed lesions include papules, pustules, and nodules. These lesions are erythematous, raised bumps around the involved follicles and may be pus-filled (pustules). Inflamed acne lesions greater than 5 mm in diameter and encompassing more than one follicle are referred to as acne nodules. Highly inflamed papules and nodules are most susceptible to scarring.

MANAGING ACNE

Acne sufferers should be encouraged to cleanse the skin twice a day. Lukewarm water and a mild, nonabrasive cleanser should be applied to the skin with the fingertips. Rough washcloths and irritating facial scrubs should be avoided. Noncomedogenic moisturizers and cosmetics may be used as needed. A noncomedogenic sunscreen is encouraged for daily use.

Topical Medications

Topical retinoids are the mainstay of acne therapy. Adapalene (Differin), tazarotene (Tazorac), and tretinoin (Retin-A, Retin-A Micro, Avita) are all topical retinoids effective in the treatment of acne vulgaris. Their efficacy is based on their ability to normalize the follicular epidermal hyperproliferation and thus *unplug* the follicles. They rid the skin of the microcomedones, the precursor lesion of all other acne lesions and, therefore, prevent the development of new lesions. Topical retinoids should be applied evenly to the entire affected area once each day after cleansing. To minimize irritation, the skin should be allowed to dry for 10 to 15 minutes before application of the retinoid. A pea-sized amount is sufficient to treat the entire face. A noncomedogenic moisturizer may be applied after the medication. With daily use, 40% improvement can be expected after 2 months of use. Improvement will continue over time, and topical retinoids should be continued as maintenance therapy once clearing has been achieved. Adapalene, tazarotene, and tretinoin are all available in cream and gel formulations.

Benzoyl peroxides are also staples in the treatment of acne vulgaris. They are antimicrobial and very weakly comedolytic and, therefore, target two of the four pathogenetic factors involved in acne. No *P. acnes* resistance to benzoyl peroxide has been identified, while *P. acnes* resistance to other antibiotics used to treat acne is not uncommon. Fortunately, benzoyl peroxides may lessen the development of *P. acnes* resistance to other antibiotics when the two are used in combination, theoretically increasing the efficacy of the topical antibiotic. Benzoyl peroxides are available in many different vehicles including cleansers, creams, gels, and pads. They are also available combined with erythromycin (Benzamycin) and combined with clindamycin (BenzaClin, Duac). These products can be used once or twice a day. A common approach is to prescribe a benzoyl peroxide product for morning application and a topical retinoid at bedtime. This combination therapy alters three of the four etiologic agents at work in acne vulgaris.

Clindamycin (Cleocin T) and erythromycin (Erythra-Derm) are commonly used topically to treat acne. Their pathogenetic target is *P. acnes*, but they are also anti-inflammatory. *P. acnes* resistance to erythromycin and clindamycin has become very common, limiting the utility of these medications as monotherapy. These products can now be used most effectively in combination with a benzoyl peroxide, which assists in the prevention of bacterial resistance. Clindamycin and erythromycin are available as lotions, gels, and solutions. Products combining benzoyl peroxide and topical antibiotics are also available (BenzaClin, Benzamycin, Duac).

Other topical agents used to treat acne vulgaris include azelaic acid (Azelex), salicylic acid, and sodium sulfacetamide preparations. These products are generally considered to be less effective than the topical retinoids, benzoyl peroxides, or topical antibiotics and are reserved for patients who do not tolerate or who do not respond to these more traditional treatments. Salicylic acid is weakly comedolytic, and azelaic acid and sodium sulfacetamide are anti-inflammatory.

Topical medications can be very effective in clearing acne but visible improvement takes time. Noninflammatory, comedonal acne is best treated with a topical retinoid. Mild to moderate inflammatory acne may be treated with a combination of a topical retinoid and a topical antimicrobial. Only 40% improvement is expected after 2 months of treatment. If improvement in inflammatory acne has not been observed after 8 weeks of topical therapy, a systemic antibiotic can be added to the treatment regimen.

Systemic Treatments

Systemic antibiotics are commonly employed in the management of inflammatory acne. They target *P. acnes* and have significant anti-inflammatory properties. Doxycycline (Vibramycin, Adoxa, Doryx) and minocycline (Minocin) are the antibiotics of choice for the treatment of inflammatory acne. Doxycycline is commonly prescribed for acne vulgaris with doses ranging from 75 mg twice a day to 100 mg twice a day. Doxycycline may cause gastroesophageal irritation and should be taken with a full glass of water and with food. Phototoxicity has also been reported with doxycycline, and patients should be instructed to avoid sun exposure while taking the medication. Minocycline is also effective in the treatment of inflammatory acne. Minocycline may be prescribed once or twice a day with daily dosages ranging from 50 to 200 mg. Higher doses may be associated with dizziness and vertigo. There are rare reports of minocycline associated with drug-induced lupus, hepatitis, and acute respiratory distress syndrome (ARDS). *P. acnes* resistance to erythromycin and tetracycline is very common, so these antibiotics have largely been replaced by doxycycline and minocycline as first-line antibiotics in the treatment of acne vulgaris.

As with topical therapy, improvement takes time. Expect only 40% improvement after 8 weeks of therapy. In general, systemic antibiotics should be coupled with a topical retinoid for maximum improvement. Most individuals require treatment with a systemic antibiotic for 4 to 6 months. Once clearing has been achieved, the antibiotic can be tapered and discontinued. The topical retinoid is then continued to maintain clearing.

Isotretinoin (Accutane, Amnesteen) is a systemic retinoid highly effective in the treatment of acne vulgaris. The effectiveness of isotretinoin lies in its singular ability to target all of the four key pathogenetic factors of acne vulgaris. The effectiveness of isotretinoin, however, must be weighed against its potential to cause severe side effects, and its use should be reserved for individuals with severe nodular acne or for moderate to severe acne that is recalcitrant to all other therapy. Potential side effects must be discussed with the patient and a signed consent obtained. Reported side effects include xerosis, cheilitis, hypertriglyceridemia, arthralgias, myalgias, blurred vision, pseudotumor cerebri, depression, and many others. Isotretinoin is also a known teratogen, and pregnancy must be prevented during treatment and for 1 month after discontinuation of the medication. It is imperative that pregnancy be ruled out before initiation of therapy. Two negative pregnancy tests must be obtained before isotretinoin is prescribed. A thorough discussion of the teratogenic effects of the drug is also crucial, and female patients should be instructed to use two forms of birth control during treatment and for 1 month after completing treatment. Once isotretinoin has been prescribed, patients must be seen every 4 weeks; female patients should have a pregnancy test at every visit.

Doses of isotretinoin should begin at 0.5 mg/kg per day or less to prevent early worsening of acne. Doses may be increased to 1 mg/kg after the first month of treatment if tolerated by the patient. A cumulative dose of 120 to 150 mg/kg is necessary to prevent recurrence of the acne; this dose can generally be reached within 5 to 6 months of treatment. Cumulative doses less than the recommended 120 to 150 mg/kg are associated with higher rates of relapse. If these goal dosages are reached, 85% of those treated with isotretinoin will have a durable response. Fifteen percent of individuals will relapse and require additional acne treatment or another course of isotretinoin.

Rosacea

The pathogenesis of acne rosacea is not as well understood as that for acne vulgaris. Vascular instability appears to play a significant role with intermittent blushing evident early in the course of the disease. Over time, the blood vessels become leaky and spill their contents into the surrounding tissue. The result is inflammation and thickening of the skin. Rosacea is characterized by erythema, telangiectases, and inflammatory papules and/or pustules. These changes are most commonly seen on the central third of the forehead, the cheeks, and the chin in individuals with fair, sensitive skin. With time, thickening of the skin and sebaceous tissue of the nose can become disfiguring, resulting in a large, red, bulbous nose referred to as rhinophyma.

Managing rosacea begins with simple, nonirritating skin care. A gentle, nonabrasive cleanser is recommended. α-Hydroxy acids, salicylic acids, and topical retinoids are best avoided in patients with rosacea because of their potential to cause irritation. Sunscreen is recommended for daily use and moisturizers may be used as needed. When possible, individuals with rosacea should avoid exogenous factors that cause them to blush. These may include hot beverages, spicy foods, alcohol, or hot temperatures.

TOPICAL TREATMENT

There are many topical medications available for rosacea. The most commonly prescribed include metronidazole (MetroCream, MetroGel, MetroLotion, Noritate), sodium sulfacetamide (Klaron, Plexion, Rosac), and azelaic acid (Azelex, Finevin, Finacea). Topical metronidazole is available as a lotion, cream, or gel. It is anti-inflammatory and may help reduce redness and inflammatory lesions associated with rosacea. Sodium sulfacetamide is also anti-inflammatory and is available as a cleanser or topical suspension. Several gel formulations of azelaic acid are available that may be helpful in the management of rosacea. In practice, these medications are often used in combination, with one product applied in the morning and a different product applied in the evening.

SYSTEMIC TREATMENT

Systemic antibiotics are often required to control rosacea. Doxycycline[1], minocycline[1], and tetracycline[1] are the most commonly prescribed systemic antibiotics for acne rosacea. Doxycycline and minocycline

[1]Not FDA approved for this indication.

are frequently started at 100 mg twice a day, whereas tetracycline is initiated at 500 mg twice a day. Once improvement has been observed, the dose may be tapered to once a day. Most individuals can discontinue systemic antibiotics after 2 to 4 months and maintain clearing with one of the topical agents described above. The natural course of rosacea is one of relapses and remissions. Topical medications should be used continually for maintenance therapy, but systemic antibiotics should be resumed only when the rosacea flares.

The telangiectases commonly seen in acne rosacea do not respond to treatment with topical or systemic medications. They may be treated with the pulsed-dye laser. Similarly, once the end-stage rhinophyma has developed, topical and systemic medications will not reverse the changes. Surgery, electrosurgery, or laser therapy may help correct the deformity.

DISEASES OF THE HAIR

METHOD OF

Azim J. Khan, MD, Dwight Scarborough, MD, and Emil Bisaccia, MD

Like any other disease entity, diseases of the hair require a thorough history, good physical examination, and sometimes the pertinent laboratory examinations to reach the correct diagnosis. History should always include the duration of onset, the location and the extent of hair loss, family history of similar hair loss, any drug intake, systemic illness, any endocrine abnormality, and history of pulling at the hairs (including compulsive or incidental pulling caused by hair styling and use of hair styling techniques). The examination should include:

- Careful examination of the hair-bearing areas to evaluate the hair density, caliber, and quality
- Examination of the scalp to look for any sign of inflammation and/or scarring
- Examination of the thyroid gland to rule out any thyromegaly
- Examination of the nails

Visual examination of the hair density is usually not very accurate. Approximately 50% of the hairs are generally lost before any hair loss is visually apparent. Parting the hairs at different scalp sites and then comparing the width of the part is more accurate in determining the hair density. Hair density is higher during childhood and decreases with age in both sexes. Crown hair density is usually less than the density at the sides of the scalp.

The history may guide the physician to perform a more detailed examination, including the performing of any pertinent laboratory workup. For example, a case of nonscarring, generalized hair thinning can be a sign of thyroid abnormality, thus necessitating a thyroid-stimulating hormone (TSH) level determination. Similarly a patient with irregular menstruation, acne, and hair loss may require a workup to rule out any androgen excess by performing testosterone and dehydroepiandrosterone sulfate (DHEAS) level tests. A patient with anemia and nonscarring alopecia should be checked for ferritin levels, which is an exceedingly important cause to rule out in most female patients with nonscarring alopecia. In patients with low levels of ferritin (<20 μg/L), generalized thinning of the hair is noted much earlier than the development of anemia. Usually a ferritin level of greater than 40 μg/L is required for the normal growth and development of healthy hairs. Most diseases of the hair can be easily understood and diagnosed by comprehending two vital concepts. The first is the concept of normal hair cycling, and the second involves the clinical classifications of alopecias.

Normal Hair Growth Cycle

On average, a normal scalp contains 100,000 hair follicles. Every hair follicle goes through three phases in its growth cycle:

1. Anagen is the growing phase (lasting an average of 3 years)
2. Telogen is the resting phase (lasting approximately 3 months)
3. Catagen is the destructive phase (lasting approximately 3 weeks)

Approximately 90% of hair follicles on a healthy scalp are in the anagen phase, approximately 10% are in the telogen phase, and less than 1% of hair follicles are in the catagen phase at any given time. It is of note that telogen or catagen hairs are the hairs that fall out spontaneously on a daily basis, and their number usually ranges from 100 to 150 hairs in a normal individual. This is important to know, as many patients may perceive this much hair shedding, which is normal, as pathogenic.

Classifications of Alopecia

Many classifications of alopecia are proposed, but one of the more useful classifications involves dividing the alopecias into scarring and nonscarring categories. On a close visual examination of any area of alopecia, one should be able to discern the presence or absence of hair follicle ostia even if the area is devoid of terminal hairs. If the follicular ostia are present, one of the nonscarring alopecias should be considered in the differential diagnosis. On the other hand, the scarring alopecias are diagnosed by the presence of scar tissue without any follicular ostia visible in it. This distinction is clinically important not only in the diagnosis but also in determining the prognosis of the disease, as most of the scarring alopecias result from severe inflammation of the hair follicle resulting in irreversible damage to the follicle and poor prognosis. Many of the nonscarring alopecias, however, are reversible.

The most common causes of hair loss include androgenetic alopecia (male and female pattern baldness), alopecia areata, trichotillomania secondary to compulsive or incidental hair pulling and traction, telogen effluvium, infections, hair shaft abnormalities, and hereditary and congenital dermatosis, among others. Following are brief descriptions and treatment options for some of the most commonly encountered hair disorders.

NONSCARRING ALOPECIA

Androgenetic Alopecia

Androgenetic alopecia (AGA) is characterized by receding hairline in the frontotemporal fashion in males and generalized thinning of hair in the central scalp in women without any hairline recession. Nonscarring, diffuse, low-density, and thinner caliber hairs, without any distinct patchy hair loss, can easily differentiate AGA from other types of alopecias. Family history on the maternal or paternal side is usually an indicator for AGA. The disease affects at least 50% of men by age 50 and probably a similar percentage of women as well. It can begin at any age after puberty. Testosterone is converted into dihydrotestosterone, which in turn is believed to cause the miniaturization of the susceptible hair follicles in the frontoparietal scalp. The conversion of testosterone into dihydrotestosterone is brought about by enzymatic action of 5α-reductase type II found in hair follicles and prostate glands. Finasteride (Propecia), a 5α-reductase inhibitor, at a dose of 1 mg orally every day, is the most effective FDA-approved treatment for AGA in men that is available today. In placebo-controlled studies, 100% of men noted hair loss in the placebo group whereas 65% in Propecia group had no further hair loss and 35% had retained greater hair density compared to the placebo group. Thus, at the minimum, Propecia can halt or slow the further progression of the hair loss in men. Because finasteride lowers the prostate-specific antigen (PSA) level, a baseline PSA level should be obtained, in case there is a need to follow them in the future. This can be valuable, especially in the middle-aged-to-elderly population who are being monitored for serial PSA levels because of prostatic pathology.

The use of Propecia, however, should not mask the detection of prostate cancer. Some suggest doubling the value of PSA in patients on Propecia for interpretation purposes. Propecia is usually a well-tolerated medication, as it does not affect spermatogenesis or semen production. Sexual side effects encountered in less than 2% of patients are almost always reversible on discontinuation of therapy and resolve in approximately 50% of patients who continue therapy. The benefit of the therapy can be maintained as long as the therapy is continued. Propecia is not recommended for use in females. Pregnant women should not even handle the pills because of possible transcutaneous absorption and possible feminization of the male fetus.

In females, AGA presents as generalized thinning rather than hairline recession and frank baldness. A strong family history of female pattern baldness may predispose patients to this condition at an early age; otherwise this pattern of hair loss is generally seen in perimenopausal patients. If seen in a younger patient, a workup to rule out androgen excess is warranted, especially if other signs of hyperandrogenism (acne, hirsutism) are co-existent. This is done by testing testosterone and DHEAS levels.

Adrenal hyperplasia and polycystic ovary disease are more likely to be encountered in a young patient with AGA as compared to a woman over 65 years of age. Also, female patients thought to have AGA should be ruled out for other systemic causes, such as thyroid abnormality and decreased ferritin level, as generalized hair thinning in female patients is often multifactorial. As opposed to males, multiple therapy options to counteract androgen excess exist for female patients. Most of them, however, are not FDA approved for AGA in particular. Either increasing the estrogen levels or decreasing the androgen levels can be effective. Estrogen-dominant oral contraceptives like Premarin[1] alone or in combination with progesterone (Provera)[1] can be used for estrogen replacement therapy. Antiandrogens like spironolactone (Aldactone)[1], 50 to 200 mg per day, is an effective antiandrogen. Some physicians like to monitor serum K^+ levels, especially if Aldactone is given in higher doses. Dexamethasone[1], 0.125 to 0.25 mg orally at night, can effectively suppress adrenal-based androgen excess. Although effective, none of these treatments is FDA approved for AGA in females.

Telogen Effluvium

Telogen effluvium is a very common nonscarring, generalized alopecia that is caused by a variety of physical or emotional traumas. Usually pregnancy, crash dieting, and intense physical or emotional stress, including major surgeries, are the most frequent causes of telogen effluvium. The diagnosis is usually made clinically on careful history depicting some form of trauma within a few months (6 weeks to 4 months) before the onset of the hair loss. The diagnosis of telogen effluvium can be further strengthened by performing a *hair-pluck* trichogram, a painful procedure that is falling out of favor because of the discomfort it poses to the patient. The test is performed by firmly

[1]Not FDA approved for this indication.

plucking approximately 50 hairs using a hemostat whose jaws are covered with tape to afford a firm grip on the hair. The analysis of the roots of these hairs is easily performed by sandwiching them between two glass slides under a low-power microscope. If the telogen club-shaped hairs are found in more than 10% of the hair sample, it usually indicates telogen effluvium. The plucked anagen hairs are broomstick-shaped and covered with glistening inner and outer hair root sheaths; the plucked telogen hairs are smooth and club shaped at the base. This information is usually helpful in determining the percentage of hairs that are in the anagen versus the telogen phase.

Anagen Effluvium

Most commonly caused by cancer-treating chemotherapeutic agents, anagen effluvium is clinically characterized by marked thinning of the scalp hair, which begins shedding after 1 to 2 weeks of chemotherapy treatment—or other insults like radiation therapy or protein calorie malnutrition—and becomes most evident within 1 to 2 months. Broken hairs show a progressive narrowing of the hair shaft proximally caused by the arrest in keratinization and impaired DNA synthesis, which makes the hair shaft narrow and fragile. A tourniquet band or pressure cuff applied around the scalp during the chemotherapy session is effective in preventing hair loss secondary to chemotherapy. After the cessation of the chemotherapy, hair growth almost always returns to normal.

Alopecia Areata

Alopecia areata (AA) is a cell-mediated, autoimmune disease that presents as patchy round or oval nonscarring hair loss of scalp or any other hair-bearing area. In a small number of patients, a positive family history for alopecia areata can be elicited. Quite often patients give a history of some emotional trauma or stress prior to its onset. The most commonly affected areas include scalp, beard area, eyebrows, eyelashes, and, less commonly, other hair-bearing body areas. If the whole scalp is involved, it is termed as alopecia totalis; if the whole body is involved, the disease is termed as alopecia universalis. The diagnosis is usually clinical except in rare, difficult situations requiring a punch biopsy of the scalp. On close clinical examination, smooth noninflammatory nonscarring patch(es), sometimes containing a few short proximally tapered hairs (exclamation point hairs), are seen. One helpful clue is the presence of nail pitting, which is seen in many patients with alopecia areata. Some related abnormalities include Hashimoto's thyroiditis, vitiligo, and other autoimmune diseases. Many physicians routinely perform a TSH hormone level test to rule out any related thyroid abnormality. Others suggest antithyroid antibody determination to screen patients who may be at risk for hypothyroidism in the future. Mostly, however, alopecia areata occurs without any associated disease. Spontaneous recovery is seen in most patients within a few months even without any treatment. Treatment, however, seems to promote the regrowth of the alopecia patches sooner than spontaneous recovery, and thus is recommended in most cases. If the areas involved are small and few in number, then a potent topical steroid like clobetasol (Temovate Gel)[1], 0.1% gel twice daily, or intralesional triamcinolone acetonide[1], 5 to 10 mg/mL repeated every 6 weeks, can be effective. In resistant cases, or in rapidly spreading larger areas, a short course of oral steroids in tapering doses followed by topical or intralesional steroids can be effective. Small, localized patches in postpubertal patients are usually a good prognostic sign. Poor prognostic signs include prepubertal onset, widespread involvement, alopecia totalis or universalis, involvement of the occipital hairline (ophiasis pattern), and disease process of more than 5-year duration. The challenging nonrespondent cases may require prolonged use of oral steroids, but caution is advised because of the side-effect risks. Other agents shown to be of some benefit in resistant cases include topical sensitizers such as topical 1% anthralin[1] used for 10 to 20 minutes a day and then washed off to produce a local-controlled inflammatory response. Similarly diphencyprone[1], squaric acid dibutylester[1], and dinitrochlorobenzene[1] are some of the local sensitizers that can be considered in resistant cases. Most of these agents, however, are not FDA approved for AA therapy. Also, concern regarding the use of low-level, chronic inflammation-causing sensitizers, reactive lymphoid hyperplasia, and possible mutagenic potential has kept many from using these sensitizing agents. Oral psoralen plus ultraviolet light of A wavelength (PUVA)[1] has also been used in resistant cases with some success.

Whether spontaneous or secondary to treatment, the regrowth is initially fuzzy hairs, usually grey in color, which gradually become thicker and regain the pigment slowly. Many patients with complete recovery may experience recurrences at other areas down the road and should be educated about this possibility. The National Alopecia Areata Foundation is a useful education and support group resource for patients, especially those with severe disease.

Trichotillomania

Trichotillomania is obsessive, compulsive, or habitual picking or plucking of hairs causing traumatic breakage of hair shafts at different lengths. It is usually associated with anxiety, depression, or obsessive–compulsive disorders. If performed repeatedly, it can cause permanent damage to the hair follicle and lead to scarring alopecia. The diagnosis is usually clinical but can be quite difficult in certain cases. Some suggest asking the patient *catch questions* like, "How do you pluck hairs," rather than asking,

[1]Not FDA approved for this indication.

"Do you pluck hairs," as most of the patients deny that they are plucking the hairs at all. Another helpful technique is to shave a small affected area and then watch for the normal hair regrowth as the patient cannot pluck the newly regrowing tiny hairs. A 4-mm punch biopsy can usually confirm the diagnosis in most difficult situations. The characteristic findings include pigmented casts and hemorrhage in the hair follicles, usually without inflammatory changes. Psychotherapy or psychopharmacologic medications are the treatment of choice for this condition. A psychiatric referral can be beneficial in most cases.

CICATRICIAL (SCARRING) ALOPECIA

Cicatricial or scarring alopecia results from the inflammatory destruction of the hair stem cells that reside in the bulge portion of the hair follicle. If this portion is irreversibly destroyed, it can lead to irreversible hair loss and scarring. The end stage in many inflammatory cicatricial alopecias results in a clinical picture termed pseudopelade of Brocq, which refers to the resultant scarring rather than the etiology that caused scarring in the first place. Major causes of cicatricial alopecia are infections (e.g., bacteria-like folliculitis decalvans, viral or fungal), physical injuries (e.g., burns, trauma), congenital defects (e.g., aplasia cutis), neoplasms (e.g., cutaneous T-cell lymphoma), and many inflammatory dermatoses of the scalp (e.g., lupus, lichen planopilaris). To determine the cause of the inflammation that is causing the localized scarring, a culture sensitivity of any suspicious infection for the suspected agent (bacterial, viral, or fungal), as well as a 4-mm punch biopsy, can be extremely helpful. This is especially true if biopsy is obtained early in the course of the disease rather than from an end-stage scar, which is usually nondiagnostic. If diagnosed early, with the appropriate treatment of the underlying cause, the scarring process can usually be halted.

Folliculitis Decalvans

Folliculitis decalvans is characterized by a progressive destruction of the hair follicles secondary to folliculitis. The exact etiology is not known; however, *Staphylococcus aureus* is a common pathogen in many cases. The clinical picture varies according to the extent of the disease but often involves the follicular-based papules and pustules that result in confluent, erythematous plaques sometimes with tufted folliculitis with *doll-like* hairs. In cases with bacterial etiology, long-term antibiotic therapy may halt the process.

Lichen Planopilaris

Also termed as follicular lichen planus, it is a variant of lichen planus. Approximately 50% of the lichen planopilaris patients also have typical cutaneous or oral lichen planus lesions concurrently or prior to the onset of lichen planopilaris. The disease is four times more common in females ages 30 to 70 years old, and usually involves the scalp and eyebrows only. Typical clinical presentations involve the follicular erythema, follicular hyperkeratosis, and, eventually, scarring alopecia if not treated early on. Treatments usually include potent topical steroids or intralesional steroids.

Discoid Lupus Erythematosus

Discoid lupus erythematosus (DLE) is mostly confined to the skin (approximately 95%) without any systemic involvement. In rare instances a larger area, especially below the neck, is also involved; in this case a systemic involvement is more likely. The characteristic erythematous, indurated hypo- or hyperpigmented patches, or plaques with atrophic centers and follicular plugging, are usually seen on the scalp, nose bridge, malar surfaces, and the ears. Scarring alopecia is a common sequela of scalp DLE. Clinical diagnosis can be easily confirmed on biopsy, and treatment with local or intralesional steroids usually suffices. In more resistant cases and in systemic involvement, an antimalarial agent may be helpful.

Hair Shaft Abnormalities

Increased fragility that results from most hair shaft abnormalities is the main cause of alopecia seen in these disorders. A number of inherited hair shaft disorders have been described in many different syndromes involving many systemic complaints. Trichorrhexis nodosa is the most commonly acquired hair shaft abnormality and is caused by chemical or physical damage to the hair shaft. Chronic bending of the weakened hair shaft produces the broomstick appearance that characterizes trichorrhexis nodosa. The diagnosis can be easily performed with light microscopic examination of the hair shaft. Treatment involves avoiding the physical or chemical substances that caused damage to the hair shaft along with gentle handling and aggressive use of gentle hair conditioners. The inherited form of trichorrhexis nodosa is an autosomal dominant condition that is usually found in argininosuccinicaciduria.

CANCER OF THE SKIN

METHOD OF
Leonard H. Goldberg, MD

The three most common skin cancers are basal cell carcinoma (BCC), squamous cell carcinoma (SCC), and melanoma. There is an epidemic of skin cancer with no evidence of slowing in geographic regions with large amounts of sunlight and among populations of light-skinned people.

Diagnosis and Biopsy

The definitive diagnosis of any skin tumor is made by biopsy and histopathologic examination. New skin lesions, especially solitary papules or nodules, ulcers, erosions, and areas susceptible to repeated bleeding, should be carefully examined and adequately biopsied.

Together, 90% of BCCs and SCCs occur on the head and neck in areas that are cosmetically and functionally important. The remainder occur on the sun-exposed areas of the arms, the legs, and, occasionally, the trunk. BCC very rarely metastasizes, whereas SCC metastasizes more frequently, but usually only after the tumor reaches 1 cm in thickness. Metastases are initially to the draining lymph nodes.

Melanoma is usually a pigmented brown or black lesion, and is dealt with elsewhere in this book.

Treatment

Goals of treatment for individual tumors are complete removal of all cancerous tissue, minimization of the amount of normal tissue removed, and achievement of an optimal cosmetic and functional result. Moreover, follow-up visits for treatment of premalignant lesions and for early diagnosis and treatment of new lesions are essential, because patients who have had a skin cancer are more prone to develop other skin cancers of all types—BCC, SCC, and melanoma, as well as leukemia and lymphoma. Follow-up examinations are performed annually, or more frequently in patients in whom active production of new keratoses and tumors is noted. New lesions should be examined, diagnosed, biopsied when necessary, and treated appropriately.

Malignant tumors may be destroyed by any of the following methods.

EXCISIONAL SURGERY

Excisional surgery is the method most often employed for removal of tumors less than 1 cm in diameter. Margins of normal skin of 1 to 4 mm for BCC and of 1 to 5 mm for SCC are excised around the tumor. Tissue is marked with ink or a suture for orientation and sent to the histology laboratory for margin examination and tumor identification, either by frozen section or by paraffin-embedded sections. The resulting defect may be closed primarily or allowed to heal naturally (granulation and epithelialization). Wounds must be cleaned daily with saline, covered with an ointment, and protected by an adequate dressing.

ELECTRODESICCATION AND CURETTAGE

This technique is commonly used by dermatologists to treat nonaggressive BCCs and SCCs. After local anesthesia has been administered, the tumor is scraped away with a sharp curet. The surrounding tissue is then destroyed to a distance of 1 to 2 mm with electrocautery. This process is repeated until a total border of 3 to 4 mm of normal-appearing skin at the edges of the original curetted defect has been destroyed. The resulting defect heals naturally over a 4- to 6-week period, leaving a flat white scar that may be cosmetically prominent. Cure rates of 95% to 98% may be achieved by experienced practitioners. Cure rates drop dramatically for larger BCCs (>1.0 cm), SCCs, recurrent BCCs, infiltrating and morpheaform tumors, and tumors around the eyelids, nose, mouth, and ears. There is no margin control using this technique.

MOHS MICROGRAPHIC SURGERY

Mohs micrographic surgery entails the excision of the tumor and complete microscopic examination of the deep and lateral margins of the excised tissue by frozen section. Areas that are positive for cancer are mapped, selectively re-excised, and examined microscopically until complete excision is ascertained histologically. Loss of normal tissue is minimized, resulting in smaller skin defects, which may be closed cosmetically when possible. Five-year cure rates approximating 100% can be achieved. This method is being used more frequently, especially for removal of larger or recurrent tumors; infiltrative and morpheaform tumors; tumors of the eyelids, nose, mouth, and ears; SCCs; and melanoma.

CRYOSURGERY

Liquid nitrogen at −196°C (−320.8°F) can be used to freeze and kill cells, leaving the inert tissue framework relatively spared. Using spray or direct application of the liquid nitrogen, tumor cells may be frozen to death and the tumors destroyed. Usually, only smaller tumors (<1.0 cm in diameter) are treated with cryosurgery. Debulking the tumor by curettage or shave excision may be done before the application of liquid nitrogen to obtain a specimen for pathology study and for more efficient freezing to the desired depth.

The advantage of this method is the bloodless destruction of the tumor. The disadvantages are subsequent scarring and hypopigmentation, lack of tissue for tumor-free margin verification, and high recurrence rate because of inadequate freezing. Larger SCCs are not treated by this method, because perineural spread may go undetected and untreated.

RADIATION THERAPY

Orthovoltage radiation in fractionated doses applied over 2 to 6 weeks can be used to destroy BCC and SCC. It is well tolerated by frail patients who are poor surgical candidates and may be used to provide palliation for inoperable tumors. Disadvantages include multiple treatment sessions, the lack of tissue for tumor verification or margin control with a corresponding lower cure rate, and, in the long-term, variable cosmetic results due to radiation dermatitis. The advantage of this method is the avoidance of anesthetic or surgery. The effectiveness of other methods of skin cancer treatment has made radiation therapy less popular and less-often used.

PHOTODYNAMIC THERAPY

Photodynamic therapy involves the combination of either the topical application or oral use of a porphyrin derivative to produce photosensitization. The tumor and the surrounding skin, which have absorbed the porphyrin derivative, are then irradiated with an intense light source (red or blue) or laser light (585/595 nm). Light penetration results in photodestruction the tumor cells. Recurrence rates and cosmetic results may vary. This method is used only in specific centers under controlled conditions, with close follow-up of the patients.

Retinoids

Isotretinoin (Accutane)[1] (13-*cis*-retinoic acid) and other retinoids may be used orally in doses of 0.5 to 2 mg/kg per day to suppress the growth of existing tumors and to prevent the development of new tumors. Retinoids are particularly useful for keratoacanthomas, in people with numerous skin cancers, in immunosuppressed patients, and in patients with basal cell nevus syndrome. These agents are quite effective in adequate dosages; however, their usefulness has been limited by problems with dryness of the skin, mucosa of the lips and eyes, increased blood lipids, and, rarely, liver damage and bone spurs.

EXPERIMENTAL THERAPIES

New treatment methods are available for retinoids that avoid the risks of surgery, but, unfortunately, they have lower cure rates than surgical methods of destruction.

Imiquimod (Aldara)[1], 5% cream applied daily for 2 to 16 weeks, may cure superficial BCC. Rest periods between applications may be required to allow resolution of local reactions to the cream, such as itching, erythema, erosions, discharge, and tenderness. Results obtained in selected cases are promising and often surprisingly effective.

Interferon alfa-2b (Intron A)[1] may be injected into smaller tumors and surrounding skin. Nine injections are given over 3 weeks for a total dose of 9 million units. Interferon injections cause fever and chills on the night of the injection. Close follow-up to detect recurrence of the tumor is imperative.

Injections of 5-fluorouracil (Adrucil) or methotrexate (Rheumatrex)[1] into the tumor and surrounding tissue have been used with varying degrees of success. Either single or multiple injections are given. Close follow-up is needed to detect tumor recurrence.

Prevention

The best form of cancer treatment is prevention. Among light-skinned people with ineffective melanin who live in sunny climates, protection should begin in infancy and continue through old age. The cornerstones of prevention are:

- Avoidance of sun exposure, especially at midday
- Adequate clothing (including hats and shirts)
- Use of chemical sunscreen products on sun-exposed areas

Dangerous activities include sunbathing and the use of tanning salons. Reduced dietary fat is associated with a decreased incidence of premalignant lesions and skin cancers. The focus on prevention must be emphasized on an individual level, in the schools, and by local and governmental authorities. Societal lifestyles and habits must be modified to reduce the epidemic of skin cancer.

Regular examination of patients with a personal or family history of skin cancer is important to reveal recurrence of previously treated tumors, the presence of premalignant actinic keratoses, and the formation of new tumors. New tumors must be biopsied and appropriate treatment given. Actinic keratoses and the surrounding cosmetic skin unit can be treated with topical imiquimod (Aldara), 5-fluorouracil (Adrucil) or diclofenac (Solaraze), liquid nitrogen, acid peels, dermabrasion, or laser destruction. Superficial destruction of the premalignant skin surface markedly reduces the formation of new actinic keratoses and malignant tumors.

[1]Not FDA approved for this indication.

CUTANEOUS T-CELL LYMPHOMAS (MYCOSIS FUNGOIDES AND SÉZARY SYNDROME)

METHOD OF

Christiane Querfeld, MD, Timothy M. Kuzel, MD, and Steven T. Rosen, MD

Cutaneous T-cell lymphomas (CTCL) constitute a subset of mostly indolent non-Hodgkin's lymphomas confined to the skin. The malignant T lymphocyte is of the helper/inducer T-cell subset with a $CD4^+$ phenotype with variable expression of CD2, CD3, CD4, CD5, CD7, and CD45RO. Within this disease spectrum, mycosis fungoides (MF) represents the most common form of CTCL with a median age of onset of 55 years, a male predominance of approximately 2:1, and age-adjusted ratio of African Americans to whites of 1.7. It has a yearly incidence of 0.36 cases per 100,000 population that has remained constant over the last decade.

Many factors have been implicated in the etiology of CTCL including microbiologic, environmental, and occupational theories, but none have yet been verified. Neoplastic lesions show characteristic clinical and histologic features in patch, plaque, and tumor stages. However, other variants have been reported, including granulomatous MF, hypopigmented MF, folliculocentric MF, and pagetoid reticulosis.

Sézary syndrome (SS) is the erythrodermic and aggressive variant of CTCL with a leukemic component. Other variants include $CD30^+$ lymphoproliferative disorders, such as lymphomatoid papulosis (LyP) and anaplastic large T-cell lymphoma (ALCL). Their common phenotypic hallmark is the $CD30^+$ T lymphocyte that morphologically resembles Reed-Sternberg cells. LyP is characterized by chronic, recurrent, self-healing, papulonodular, and papulonecrotic skin eruptions with a slight predisposition to develop lymphoid malignancies in up to 20% of cases. Purely cutaneous ALCL presenting with solitary or localized cutaneous nodules appears to have a favorable clinical course and different pathobiology when compared to the systemic form of ALCL involving lymph nodes or viscera. Cutaneous ALCL rarely carries the t(2;5) translocation and is usually anaplastic large cell lymphoma kinase negative. In contrast, cutaneous $CD30^-$ large T-cell lymphomas ($CD30^-$ LTCLs) do not produce T_{H2} cytokines and do not express CD30 antigen. They are aggressive neoplasms usually presenting with solitary, localized, or generalized plaques, nodules, or tumors without spontaneous regression.

Clinical and Pathologic Features

MF is typified by the development of patches, plaques, or tumors. However, the clinical and histologic diagnosis of MF is often difficult to establish, because in the early stages, it may resemble other dermatoses (such as eczematous dermatitis, psoriasis, and parapsoriasis) and histologic features may be nonspecific. SS is characterized by circulating, atypical, malignant T lymphocytes with cerebriform nuclei (Sézary cells) with the presence of erythroderma, disabling pruritus, keratoderma, and lymphadenopathy. Characteristic histologic features of classical MF are:

- A papillary, upper-dermal, bandlike infiltrate with atypical lymphocytes characterized by hyperchromatic, hyperconvoluted nuclei
- Variable findings of inflammatory cells
- Epidermotropism (migration of neoplastic T cells into the epidermis) with infrequently seen Pautrier's microabscesses (clusters of neoplastic T cells) therein

Tumor lesions express more diffuse, superficial, and deep infiltrates with diminished epidermotropism. Biopsies from erythrodermic MF and SS are often nondiagnostic; therefore, diagnosis has to rely on additional methods including immunophenotyping and gene rearrangement studies from skin or peripheral blood samples.

Most MF/SS cases bear the phenotype of the $CD4^+$ T-helper/inducer lymphocyte. Only a minute number of cases are of the cytotoxic/suppressor T-cell subset expressing $CD4^-/CD8^+$ antigen. T-cell clonality is reported in approximately 90% of skin biopsies. In advanced stages, an aberrant phenotype with loss of common T-cell markers, such as CD5 or CD7, is frequent. Patients with advanced-stage MF/SS show a helper T-cell type 1 (Th_1)/(Th_2) imbalance with a predominant type 2 immune response, followed by an impaired cell-mediated immunity. In advanced stages, the number of reactive cytotoxic $CD8^+$ T cells and dendritic cells, which are characteristic in the early patch-stage cutaneous lesions, tends to decrease with the increase of neoplastic $CD4^+$ T cells that is often associated with a decreased response to treatment.

Staging and Prognostic Factors

At present, the classifications developed by the World Health Organization (WHO) and the European Organization for Research and Treatment

TABLE 1 Tumor, Node, Metastasis, Blood (TNMB) Classification for Mycosis Fungoides/Sézary Syndrome (MF/SS)

T (Skin)	
T1	Limited patch/plaque (<10% of BSA)
T2	Generalized patch/plaque (>10% of BSA)
T3	Tumors
T4	Generalized erythroderma
N (Nodes)	
N0	No clinically abnormal peripheral lymph nodes
N1	Clinically abnormal peripheral lymph nodes
NP0	Biopsy performed, not CTCL
NP1	Biopsy performed, CTCL
LN0	Uninvolved
LN1	Reactive lymph node
LN2	Dermatopathic node, small clusters of convoluted cells (<6 cells per cluster)
LN3*	Dermatopathic node, small clusters of convoluted cells (>6 cells per cluster)
LN4*	Lymph node effacement
M (Viscera)	
M0	No visceral metastasis
M1	Visceral metastasis
B (Blood)	
B0	Atypical circulating cells not present (<5%)
B1	Atypical circulating cells present (>5%)

*Pathologically involved lymph nodes.
Abbreviations: BSA = body surface area; CTCL = cutaneous T-cell lymphomas.

of Cancer (EORTC) Cutaneous Lymphoma Project Group provide the most comprehensive definition of CTCL. The recommended staging system is the TNMB (tumor, node, metastasis, blood) that considers the extent of skin involvement, presence of lymph node or visceral disease, and detection of Sézary cells in the peripheral blood (Tables 1 and 2). Routine evaluation should include a complete physical examination, complete blood count with differential and Sézary cell assessment, chemistry panel with lactic dehydrogenase (LDH), skin biopsy for histology, immunophenotyping and gene rearrangement studies, and lymph node biopsies in cases with enlarged nodes at presentation. Imaging studies should be reserved for patients with advanced stages or prominent lymphadenopathy.

TABLE 2 Stage Classification for Mycosis Fungoides/Sézary Syndrome (MF/SS)

Stage	T	N	NP	M
IA	1	0	0	0
IB	2	0	0	0
IIA	1/2	1	0	0
IIB	3	0/1	0	0
III	4	0/1	0	0
IVA	1-4	0/1	1	0
IVB	1-4	0/1	0/1	1

Abbreviations: M = metastases; N = node; NP = performed lymph node biopsy; T = tumor.

The prognosis of early stage MF (T1) is favorable, and survival curves in recently published studies are similar to those of an age-matched general population. However, increasing tumor burden significantly decreases the prognosis. The median survival time of patients who develop extracutaneous disease is approximately 25 months. Several independent prognostic factors have been identified including the presence of visceral and/or lymph node involvement, follicular mucinosis, thickness of tumor infiltrate, and an increase in LDH. A high Sézary cell count, loss of T-cell markers, existence of a peripheral T-cell clone, chromosomal abnormalities in T cells, and transformation to large-cell histology are also independently associated with a poor outcome. Increased density of epidermal Langerhans cells (skin dendritic cells) greater than 90 cells/mm^2 is associated with a better prognosis.

Treatment

The typical clinical course of MF is indolent; however, a subset of patients progress with more aggressive and advanced disease with either cutaneous or extracutaneous tumor manifestations. At present, CTCL are regarded to be incurable. The reason for the slow progression of CTCL is not known; control of tumor growth by tumor-specific immune response is suspected. This is supported by the recognition that cytotoxic CD8$^+$ T lymphocytes, which are present in the dermal infiltrate in early stages of disease, are eliminated with disease progression. In early CTCL, the cell-mediated immune response is usually normal.

Patients with stage IA-IIA disease are ideally treated with topical therapies. Treatment options for early stage MF consist of:

- Topical chemotherapy including steroids, carmustine (BiCNU)[1], nitrogen mustard (Mustargen)[1], or retinoids
- Narrowband-ultraviolet light (UV) B (NB-UVB)
- Photochemotherapy with psoralens and UVA (PUVA)
- Total skin electron-beam irradiation

Systemic therapies are reserved for more advanced stages. Established treatment options include radiation, spot or total skin electron-beam, single-agent or multiagent chemotherapy, extracorporeal photopheresis, interferon-alfa (IFN-α), monoclonal antibodies, recombinant toxins, and, often, combination approaches. Nonrandomized clinical trials have not suggested that any one treatment is preferable. Treatment choice should be made with the patient's preference and practitioner's skill in mind. The toxicity of treatment should not outweigh the cosmetic and functional disability of the disease.

[1]Not FDA approved for this indication.

PHOTOCHEMOTHERAPY

PUVA probably remains the gold standard for the treatment of MF in stages IA to IIA. Several long-term studies confirm the efficacy of this treatment with reported complete remissions in up to 71.4% of patients. Since 1974, PUVA therapy has been widely used in treating psoriasis, vitiligo, and other skin disorders. In 1976, it was introduced for the treatment of MF. After oral ingestion, 8-methoxypsoralen (8-MOP) becomes activated when exposed to UVA light. UVA (320 to 400 nm), with its peak emission wavelength between 330 and 340 nm, penetrates the skin approximately 1 to 2 cm into the mid-dermis. It is thought to act at the nuclear level of cells, inhibiting DNA and RNA synthesis through formation of monofunctional or bifunctional thymine products, induction of gene mutations, or sister chromatid exchanges. However, in vitro studies show that peripheral blood mononuclear cells undergo apoptosis after exposure to PUVA, and immune effects after exposure may be additional mechanisms for crucial benefit.

Initial exposure times of patients are limited to the phototype according to the Fitzpatrick grading system, the ability to tan, and the patient's history of sunburns. The initial UVA dosage is approximately 0.5 J/cm^2 and will be increased per treatment as tolerated or up to the minimal erythema dose. Therapy is typically given three times a week until complete remission is achieved. Additional maintenance therapy can be performed, ranging from 1 week to once every 4 to 6 weeks, to achieve longer remission times.

Other reported side effects of PUVA can be divided into more acute *short-term effects* including nausea from ingestion of psoralen, erythema, pruritus, and photodermatitis; and *long-term effects* such as chronic photodamage and secondary skin malignancies. Despite the increased risk of associated skin cancer after long-term, high-dose exposure to PUVA, practical reasons and the significant efficacy of this treatment as confirmed by several investigative studies make PUVA still attractive. NB-UVB is considered to be less carcinogenic and may be an alternative treatment option in early stage MF. However, the remission time is short. Attempts to reduce UVA exposure and minimize side effects have led to combined regimens with retinoids.

RADIOTHERAPY

CTCL are radiosensitive, and radiation therapy is effective in controlling localized tumors. Total skin electron beam therapy (TSEBT) is a treatment in which ionizing radiation is administered to the entire skin surface, penetrating at least 4 mm into the dermis. The standard total dose is 36 Gy, delivered with electrons of at least 4 MeV energy and fractionated over 8 to 10 weeks. Several techniques, including dynamic rotation, 6-field, or regional patch treatments, are used to administer the electron beam. Proponents of TSEBT point to the durable long-term remissions for early stage disease as a suggestion that this treatment should be used routinely. However, we reserve TSEBT for patients with disseminated plaques or tumors, because of its potential toxicity. Side effects can be significant and consist of erythema, edema, scaling, ulceration, and irreversible loss of skin adnexa. Recently published data of therapeutic efficacy of TSEBT from centers with extensive experience show 60% to 80% complete remission rates among patients from stage IA to IVB, with approximately 26% of them remaining in long-term remission. TSEBT may be repeated for palliative effects, although at reduced doses. Adjuvant therapy including PUVA, photopheresis, and IFN-α may improve the duration of response.

SYSTEMIC CHEMOTHERAPY

Systemic chemotherapy should be restricted to patients with advanced stage disease or with multiple relapsed and refractory plaques and tumors. Established treatment options include single-agent or multiagent chemotherapy including steroids, methotrexate (Rheumatrex), chlorambucil (Leukeran)[1], vincristine (Oncovin)[1], doxorubicin (Adriamycin)[1], cyclophosphamide (Cytoxan)[1], etoposide (VePesid)[1], and alkylators. Combination chemotherapy including cyclophosphamide[1], Adriamycin[1], vincristine[1], and prednisone (CHOP) or CHOP-like therapies has been shown to achieve higher response rates of approximately 70% to 80% of patients. Newer purine analogs such as fludarabine (Fludara)[1] and 2-chloro-deoxyadenosine (cladribine [Leustatin])[1] show initial response rates in 28% to 66% of patients. However, most responses were short-lived and accompanied by harmful side effects related to prolonged immunosuppression. A published study in a limited number of patients demonstrates efficacy of a pegylated liposomal doxorubicin monotherapy with an overall response rate of 88% and a low rate of adverse effects compared with other chemotherapy protocols in patients with CTCL. Temozolomide (Temodar)[1], an oral alkylating agent, has shown activity in patients with relapsed MF and SS, likely due to low levels of the DNA repair enzyme O^6-alkylguanine-DNA alkyltransferase.

BIOLOGIC THERAPIES

Increased understanding of the pathophysiology of the disease has led to attempts to develop agents that may augment the host antitumor response or selectively target the malignant cells.

Retinoids

Retinoids are vitamin A derivatives that have been used therapeutically since the early 1980s.

[1]Not FDA approved for this indication.

Retinoids exert their effects through two basic types of nuclear receptors, the retinoic acid (RAR) and retinoid X (RXR) receptor family. Retinoids inhibit carcinogenesis, suppress benign and premalignant epithelial lesions, and slow tumor growth and invasion in a variety of tissues. The beneficial effects of retinoids in CTCL are established by extensive clinical experience. However, the response rates were modest and duration short. The most common side effects reported are mucous membrane dryness and headache.

The FDA has approved bexarotene (Targretin), a novel synthetic retinoid with increased selectivity, for the treatment of refractory or relapsed CTCL. Two multicenter, phase II-III clinical trials tested bexarotene treatment in early and advanced stages of CTCL patients with reported response rates between 45% and 54% of the patients. At the recommended dose of 300 mg/m^2 daily, it is associated with significant side effects such as hyperlipidemia, hypothyroidism, and cytopenias. Therefore, patients should be monitored closely, and most patients require lipid lowering agents and thyroid hormone replacement. A topical formulation as a 1% gel is also approved. It is indicated for early stage skin disease. A phase II trial demonstrated a 63% overall response rate. Side effects were restricted to the application site and consisted of mild to moderate irritation with erythema in 73% of cases. New insights into the immunomodulatory function of retinoids with potential augmentation or reconstitution of T helper cell type 1 response give implications for combined treatment with interferon-α, denileukin diftitox, or phototherapy. Retrospective comparison data suggest that there is little difference in efficacy between bexarotene (RXR-specific retinoid) and agents such as all-trans retinoic acid (ATRA [RAR-specific retinoid]), but clear differences in toxicity exist.

Interferons

IFN-α is probably the most effective agent in the treatment of CTCL. It was first reported in 1984 for treatment of advanced and heavily pretreated MF/SS. Th_1 cytokines support cytotoxic T-cell–mediated immunity, and, therefore, it has been speculated that IFN-α maintains or enhances a Th_1 cell population balance for an effective and cell-mediated response to malignant T lymphocytes. However, IFN-α also has direct cytotoxic effects against T lymphocytes in vitro. Monotherapy achieved significant response rates in 50% to 80% of patients. The combination therapy of IFN-α and PUVA resulted in high response rates in more than 90% of patients and is superior to other combinations. It is administered subcutaneously, intramuscularly, or intralesionally. IFN-α is initiated at low doses, between 1 and 3 million IU (MIU) three times weekly, with gradual escalation to 9 to 12 MIU daily or as tolerated. Common side effects are flu-like symptoms such as chills, fever, headache, myalgia, and fatigue. With chronic administration, depression, cytopenias, or impaired liver function tests occur. Renal and cardiac dysfunction may rarely occur. Intralesional application may be effective in localized tumors.

Experience with IFN-γ is limited. It has been shown to inhibit Th_2 cytokine production by malignant T cells. In a single trial of 16 CTCL patients with refractory disease, 5 patients showed partial response rates with a median duration of 10 months. The side effects are similar to those of IFN-α.

Extracorporeal Photochemotherapy

Extracorporeal photochemotherapy (ECP), or photopheresis, was originally designed as a modified PUVA treatment. It is a leukapheresis-based method for patients, in which after 8-MOP ingestion, circulating mononuclear cells are exposed to 1- to 2-joule UVA in the machine and returned to the patient. It is performed on two consecutive days every month. Although the mechanism of action is not completely understood, induction of apoptosis with subsequent release of tumor antigens leading to a systemic antitumor response against the malignant T-cell clone is suspected. Studies report response rates between 36% and 64% for patients with advanced disease, especially erythrodermic diseases with circulating neoplastic T cells. Optimal candidates for ECP are patients with SS with modest tumor burden and circulating neoplastic cells and almost normal counts of circulating CD8$^+$ T lymphocytes. Treatment of patients with plaques and tumors has been more disappointing.

Denileukin Diftitox (Ontak)

Denileukin diftitox (Ontak) is a recombinant fusion protein, composed of diphtheria toxin coupled to human interleukin (IL)-2, which is approved for refractory CTCL. It targets the IL-2 receptor (IL-2R), especially the high affinity form on malignant T lymphocytes. Once bound to the IL-2 receptor, it is internalized by endocytosis, and the adenosine 5′-diphosphate (ADP)-ribosyltransferase function of the diphtheria toxin molecule is activated by enzymatic cleavage with subsequent inhibition of protein synthesis and induction of apoptosis. In phase I/II and III trials it showed favorable (30% to 37%) response rates in CTCL patients. These trials were limited to patients with CD25 expression (α chain of IL-2R) in more than 20% of malignant T cells. The quality of life in responding patients was significantly improved. However, adverse effects including acute transfusion-related events such as fever, rash, chills, myalgias, and vascular leak syndrome (VLS) have been reported. VLS occurred in 27% of patients, which may be diminished by premedication with steroids. Bexarotene (Targretin) is known to enhance the expression of the high affinity form of IL-2R in malignant lymphocytes and suggests a rationale for combined treatment of bexarotene with denileukin diftitox.

Alemtuzumab (Campath)

Investigational approaches include monoclonal antibodies such as alemtuzumab[1]. It is a humanized monoclonal immunoglobulin (Ig) G_1 antibody that targets the CD52 antigen that is abundantly expressed on normal and malignant β and T lymphocytes, but not on hematopoietic stem cells. The intensity seems to correlate with the clinical benefits. The mechanism of activity for this antibody is not completely understood, but it is thought to mediate antibody-dependent cellular cytotoxicity, complement-mediated cell lysis, and apoptosis. Alemtuzumab is currently the focus of many clinical trials in hematologic malignancies and has been used in the treatment of lymphomas and lymphoid leukemias. A published phase II trial of alemtuzumab in 22 patients with advanced MF/SS demonstrates a clinical response in 55% of cases, with 32% having complete remissions. The most impressive results are seen in the SS patients. The compound has an acceptable toxicity profile with mostly infusion-related events including fever, rigor, nausea, hypotension, rash, and fatigue. Cytopenias and prolonged immunosuppression require prophylactic antibiotic, antiviral, and antifungal treatment.

At present, there is no cure for CTCL, and stage-dependent therapy is the best approach. Advanced stages are associated with cytokine imbalances resulting in impaired immune responses; however, biologic immune modifiers have the potential to reconstitute the immune function and augment host antitumor response. Combined immunomodulatory regimens in patients with advanced MF/SS may result in sustained remission of disease. The benefits of novel immunomodulatory cytokines, such as recombinant interleukin-12 or vaccines with tumor-associated, antigen-loaded dendritic cells, are currently being evaluated. Cytotoxic chemotherapeutic modalities should be reserved for more advanced disease.

[1]Not FDA approved for this indication.

PAPULOSQUAMOUS ERUPTIONS

METHOD OF

Dana Kazlow Stern, MD, and

Mark G. Lebwohl, MD

Papulosquamous eruptions are a varied group of cutaneous disorders characterized by a common morphologic feature, papules covered with scale. A description of the more common papulosquamous eruptions encountered in clinical practice is provided in this article. Table 1 lists papulosquamous eruptions.

Psoriasis

Psoriasis is a common, chronic, immunologically mediated, relapsing, inflammatory, papulosquamous cutaneous disorder that affects 2% to 3% of the U.S. population and occurs with equal frequency in both sexes. The precise etiology is unknown, although multifactorial inheritance is believed to be of central significance. The average age of onset is 28 years; however, the natural history of psoriasis can vary tremendously. It is characterized clinically by round, well-circumscribed erythematous plaques covered with a grayish silvery white scale. Symptoms, including pruritus, burning, and pain, coupled with the psychological impact of the disease can severely impact patient quality of life. The scalp, extensor surface of the limbs (elbows, knees), and the umbilical and sacral regions are typical areas of involvement. Nail findings can include pitting, onycholysis (detachment of the nail plate from the nail bed), subungual hyperkeratosis, discoloration of the nail bed, and splinter hemorrhage. Between 5% and 42% of psoriasis patients develop psoriatic arthritis. Medications known to exacerbate psoriasis include lithium, antimalarials, angiotensin-converting enzyme (ACE) inhibitors, β-blockers, and withdrawal from systemic steroids. In addition, psoriasis can be exacerbated by emotional stress, and physical trauma can result in the Koebner phenomenon whereby new psoriatic lesions occur at sites of trauma. In addition

TABLE 1 Papulosquamous Eruptions

Psoriasis	Tinea corporis*
Lichen planus	Secondary syphilis
Pityriasis rosea	Lupus erythematosus
Pityriasis rubra pilaris	Lichen striatus
Seborrheic dermatitis	Lichen nitidus
	Parapsoriasis

*Items listed in this column are not discussed in this article.

to classic plaque-type psoriasis, several variants exist including guttate, inverse, pustular, and erythrodermic.

GUTTATE PSORIASIS

The word *guttate* is derived from *gutta,* the Latin word for drop. Guttate psoriasis is characterized by small, droplike, scaling papules that typically erupt abruptly following an upper respiratory infection in patients younger than 30 years. A streptococcal infection should be sought when this occurs. Guttate psoriasis responds particularly well to phototherapy with ultraviolet (UV) B, which may be preferable to topical therapy because of the extensive body surface area involvement associated with this form of psoriasis.

INVERSE PSORIASIS

Inverse psoriasis has a characteristic distribution in skin folds and typically affects the axillae, groin, inframammary folds, intergluteal crease, and umbilicus. The skin appears red and inflamed, and lacks the scaling seen with plaque-type psoriasis. Treatment includes topical corticosteroids, calcipotriene (Dovonex), tars, and anthralin (Psoriatec). Because of the self-occluding anatomic nature of the intertriginous regions, caution should be taken when treating inverse psoriasis with corticosteroids as these areas are particularly sensitive to steroid side effects such as atrophy and formation of striae.

PUSTULAR PSORIASIS

Pustular psoriasis is a rare form of psoriasis that occurs in either an acute, generalized distribution (von Zumbusch type), or as a localized eruption. The von Zumbusch variant, which can be life-threatening, is characterized by tender, painful skin that develops widespread areas of erythema, with pustules that are described as *lakes of pus* that appear in a generalized pattern. Constitutional signs and symptoms such as fever, chills, malaise, anorexia, and nausea accompany these cutaneous manifestations. Patients require supportive care, usually in a hospital setting where they can be treated for infection, fluid loss, and electrolyte imbalance. The localized pattern, in contrast, tends to be more subacute, and does not manifest systemically. The most common cause of pustular psoriasis is withdrawal of systemic corticosteroids. However, many drugs including iodine, lithium, salicylates, tar, anthralin, antimalarials, and minocycline are some of the reported causes.

ERYTHRODERMIC PSORIASIS

Erythrodermic psoriasis is an inflammatory form of psoriasis that appears as fiery erythema and scaling that can affect the entire cutaneous surface and that ultimately becomes exfoliative. Just as in generalized pustular psoriasis, the protective barrier function of the skin becomes compromised, predisposing the patient to infection, electrolyte imbalance, severe dehydration, and an inability to control temperature. It is essentially the same mechanism as a burn injury, and supportive care in a hospital is often required because these complications can be life-threatening. Withdrawal of systemic corticosteroids is the most common precipitator.

TREATMENT

Topical Therapies

Initial treatment of plaque-type psoriasis, for patients with less than 10% body surface involvement, usually involves topical therapies such as corticosteroids, vitamin D analogues, tazarotene (Tazorac), coal tar, anthralin, and salicylic acid. The topical immunomodulators, tacrolimus (Protopic)[1] 0.1% ointment and pimecrolimus (Elidel)[1] 1% cream are also used off-label to treat facial and intertriginous psoriasis.

Topical corticosteroids, available in creams, lotions, ointments, foams, gels, sprays, and occlusive tapes, are the most common therapeutic agents used to treat psoriasis. Steroids are ranked in groups, from I (super potency) to VII (low potency). Choosing the potency compound to use depends on disease location and severity. In general, group I superpotent steroids should be used to treat thick plaques on the trunk and extremities and should be avoided on the face, genitalia, or intertriginous areas. Treatment regimens are usually once or twice daily, limited to 2-week treatment intervals. Ideally, group I corticosteroids should be avoided in children if possible. Ointments, although greasy and messy to apply, tend to be more occlusive and are, therefore, generally more potent than creams and lotions. For very resistant plaques, occlusion with Saran Wrap or other dressings may be used for a maximum of a few days. Lotions, foams, and gels tend to be particularly effective for scalp psoriasis. For psoriasis of the face and intertriginous areas, low-potency topical steroids should be used one to two times daily, though nonsteroidal agents like the topical immunomodulators are preferred. Side effects of topical corticosteroids include atrophy, telangiectasia, striae, folliculitis, perioral dermatitis, and tachyphylaxis. Pulse therapy, sometimes called *weekend therapy* because a superpotent corticosteroid is only applied on weekends, is a popular treatment method used to minimize side effects and prolong psoriasis remissions. Clinically significant hypothalamic–pituitary–adrenal axis suppression is rarely associated with topical application of steroids.

The vitamin D-derived analogue, calcipotriene (Dovonex), is a nonsteroidal topical therapy that induces epidermal differentiation and inhibits keratinocyte proliferation. Calcipotriene is proven

[1]Not FDA approved for this indication.

effective for the treatment of mild to moderate plaque-type and scalp psoriasis without producing any of the side effects associated with corticosteroids. Calcipotriene can be used as monotherapy or in conjunction with topical corticosteroids as sequential therapy, in which potent agents (high-potency topical corticosteroids, for example) are used to initiate disease clearance, and safer, less effective agents are used to maintain disease remission. Calcipotriene can also be used to treat the face and intertriginous areas—sites that are particularly vulnerable to the side effects of topical corticosteroids. Local irritation is the only cutaneous side effect associated with this form of therapy, and can be avoided by diluting the medication with petrolatum.

Tazarotene (Tazorac), a topical retinoid (vitamin A derivative), acts by binding to specific retinoic acid receptors, resulting in normalization of the differentiation and proliferation of the epidermis. Tazarotene is available as a topical gel or cream in 0.05% and 0.1% strengths for the treatment of mild to moderate plaque psoriasis. Applied once daily, usually at bedtime, it can be used to treat most parts of the body, including the face and scalp. The most limiting side effect is local irritation. Treatment in combination with a topical corticosteroid is proven to not only minimize side effects but also to be more effective than tazarotene alone. Retinoids are photosensitizers, so caution should be taken with sun exposure. Because of the teratogenic potential of retinoids, female patients of childbearing potential must use adequate contraception, and pregnancy should be excluded before treatment begins.

Tar and tar-containing products have been used for more than a century for the treatment of psoriasis. Tars are effective, have few side effects, and are considered extremely safe. They are valuable alternatives to corticosteroids for treating intertriginous areas, the face, and scalp disease. It is believed that the more pungent, dark, and cosmetically unacceptable the tar, the more effective the treatment. However, the staining property, odors, and extended treatment times needed to induce a favorable clinical response have made them an unpopular treatment option for patients. Tar products* are available in gels, creams, emollient creams, ointments, and as emulsions that are added to the bath. Coal tars are more commonly used for the treatment of psoriasis than other tar types, and tar shampoos are probably the most commonly used tar products. Shampoos are effective for treating scalp psoriasis, but cause discoloration and have an unpleasant odor.

Anthralin, a hydoxyanthracene derivative, has been used for many years for the treatment of psoriasis but had until recently fallen out of favor because of the unwanted side effects of local irritation and staining associated with it. However, recent novel treatment methods such as short-duration therapy and innovative treatment vehicles have simplified treatment regimens and minimized these side effects. A new formulation of 1% anthralin, which is packaged in a semicrystalline vehicle, releases the anthralin content at skin surface temperatures, resulting in less prohibitive staining. Anthralin can also be used with corticosteroids or calcipotriene as combination therapy.

Combinations of salicylic acid and topical corticosteroids, tar, and anthralin are successfully used to treat thick, scaly plaques associated with psoriasis. It is a particularly useful agent when used in combination with corticosteroids because its keratolytic effect allows greater absorption of other topical therapies. When combined with steroids, the mixture must be compounded by a pharmacist, as premixed combinations are not currently available. Caution should be taken when treating young children and patients with renal/hepatic impairment because of the potential for elevated serum salicylate levels. When considering using salicylic acid as part of a dual treatment regimen, be aware that salicylic acid blocks ultraviolet light and inactivates calcipotriene when applied concurrently.

Phototherapy/Photochemotherapy

UVB therapy, narrowband B therapy, and psoralen plus UVA (PUVA) therapy are the three main types of light therapy used for the treatment of psoriasis. These treatment modalities are ideal for patients with psoriasis who either have widespread disease that is too impractical to treat with topical therapy, or for those whose psoriasis is unresponsive to topical treatments.

Ultraviolet B phototherapy (UVB), or broadband, delivers light in the range 290 to 320 nm. A history of improvement with sun exposure is a useful indication that this form of therapy will be appropriate. Prior application with petrolatum or mineral oil improves treatment efficacy. Treatment is generally three times per week. In addition, combination therapies with a variety of topical and systemic agents have shown additional benefit. For example, topical agents, calcipotriene, and tazarotene are proven to enhance therapeutic efficacy when combined with UVB. Calcipotriene is inactivated by UVA and should, therefore, be applied after phototherapy. Oral retinoids[1] and methotrexate[1] when used with UVB result in increased efficacy and reduce the total dose of systemic agent required. Sunburn is the major potential adverse event associated with UVB therapy.

Narrowband UVB phototherapy (311 nm) is a relatively new phototherapeutic modality that is proven to be superior to broadband and is useful for patients who have not responded sufficiently to broadband. Narrowband light bulbs deliver monochromatic light within the 305 to 315 nm range, exactly the spectrum that is most effective for treating psoriasis.

*May be compounded by pharmacists.

[1]Not FDA approved for this indication.

Although narrowband treatment has demonstrated clinical disease resolution that is superior to broadband, the long-term safety data are not as well known at this time. Narrowband is considered to be safer than PUVA, although it is less clinically effective.

PUVA is a type of photochemotherapy whereby the patient ingests a photosensitizing medication (8-methoxypsoralen)[1], and is subsequently exposed to UVA light (320 to 400 nm). 8-Methoxypsoralen is dosed at 0.4 to 0.6 mg/kg body weight and should be taken 1.5 to 2 hours before UVA phototherapy, depending on the formulation. Treatments are given two or three times per week. Side effects include burning, sun sensitivity, nausea, and vomiting. Nausea can be minimized by late day dosing, dividing doses with food, and, if severe, bath PUVA is available at some centers. It is well known that chronic exposure to PUVA can lead to the development of cutaneous malignancies. Recent evidence also supports an increased incidence of malignant melanoma in patients who had received more than 250 PUVA treatments. As a result of these findings, many dermatologists are advocating PUVA as a combination agent in order to minimize cumulative doses of PUVA. Combining PUVA with oral retinoids[1], often referred to as Re-PUVA, is a method that is viewed as PUVA sparing. In fact, there is some evidence to support that retinoids may be protective against the development of PUVA- and cyclosporine-induced cancers. Contraindications to PUVA therapy include severe hepatic and renal function impairment, and light-aggravated and -induced diseases such as lupus erythematosus, porphyria, and xeroderma pigmentosum. PUVA is contraindicated during pregnancy.

The excimer laser is a relatively new technology that is approved for the treatment of psoriasis. The light that is emitted from this light source is in the UVB range at 308 nm. Because the laser beam can be selectively focused on lesional skin, this treatment modality is able to spare surrounding normal skin from unnecessary light exposure. This advantage, coupled with the need for fewer treatments than with other forms of phototherapy and photochemotherapy, has made the excimer laser a valuable treatment option for treating plaques of limited size.

Systemic Agents

The systemic agents acitretin (Soriatane), methotrexate (Trexall), and cyclosporine (Neoral) are used for moderate to severe plaque-type psoriasis. These agents are particularly effective for the treatment of pustular and erythrodermic psoriasis. Systemic therapies may be associated with varying degrees of long-term toxicity and, therefore, may be inappropriate for long-term monotherapy. To minimize long-term toxicity, these therapies are frequently rotated with UVB and/or PUVA at various clinically appropriate intervals.

[1]Not FDA approved for this indication.

Acitretin, a metabolite of etretinate, is a systemic retinoid that has replaced etretinate for the treatment of psoriasis because of its significantly shorter half-life and similar treatment efficacy. Because acitretin is completely undetectable in serum 3 weeks after treatment is terminated, women are theoretically able to conceive significantly sooner after therapy than they were with the now defunct etretinate. However, women must completely avoid all alcohol, including minute amounts found in cough syrups and food, because in the presence of alcohol acitretin is esterified to etretinate, its active metabolite. It is, therefore, recommended that pregnancy be avoided for 3 years after treatment with acitretin.

The oral retinoids—acitretin (Soriatane), started at 25 mg daily, and isotretinoin (Accutane)[1], started at 1.5 to 2.0 mg/kg per day—are particularly effective as monotherapy for both pustular and erythrodermic psoriasis. Acitretin is modestly effective as monotherapy for the treatment of plaque-type psoriasis in relatively high doses of 50 and 75 mg[3] daily. However, when acitretin is used in combination with UVB or PUVA, clearance of plaque-type psoriasis is expedited and both lower ultraviolet and acitretin doses are needed. Side effects include cheilitis, alopecia, xerosis, hyperostosis, elevation of serum lipids (particularly triglycerides), and elevation of liver function tests. Hypercholesterolemia and hypertriglyceridemia can be treated with atorvastatin (Lipitor). Caution must always be taken when treating women of childbearing potential, as all retinoids are potent teratogens.

Methotrexate is used to treat moderate to severe recalcitrant plaque-type psoriasis; erythrodermic, acute, localized pustular psoriasis; and moderate to severe psoriatic arthritis. Doses are either given as a single weekly oral dose of 7.5 mg to 30 mg per week, or the dose is divided into thirds and given at three 12-hour intervals. Hepatotoxicity and bone marrow suppression are the two most significant side effects. Therefore, before initiation of therapy, a thorough history and physical exam should be done to rule out pre-existing risk factors for liver disease. Additionally, lab work should be performed to exclude severe anemia, leukopenia, thrombocytopenia, renal function abnormalities, and significant liver function abnormalities (including hepatitis A, B, and C). Compete blood count (CBC) with platelet differential and count, renal function tests, and liver chemistries should be monitored throughout the treatment course.

Relative contraindications to methotrexate include active infectious disease, excessive alcohol consumption, hepatitis, and cirrhosis. Pregnancy and nursing are absolute contraindications to treatment with methotrexate. Monitoring hepatotoxicity by performing periodic liver biopsies is advocated for psoriasis patients treated with methotrexate. Rheumatologists do not obtain liver biopsies in rheumatoid arthritis

[1]Not FDA approved for this indication.

[3]Exceeds dosage recommended by the manufacturer.

patients treated with methotrexate, but it is clear that hepatic fibrosis occurs more commonly in psoriasis. Even with normal liver chemistries, liver biopsy is advocated at approximately 1.0 to 1.5 g of cumulative methotrexate and repeated with every additional 1.5 g. There is some evidence supporting the concomitant administration of folic acid (1 to 5 mg per day) to reduce nausea and megaloblastic anemia. The two leading causes of methotrexate overdosage are impaired renal function and concomitant treatment with trimethoprim-sulfamethoxazole (TMP-SMZ; Bactrim). An immediate parenteral or oral dose of leucovorin calcium is the only antidote.

Cyclosporine is an extremely effective immunosuppressive agent approved for the treatment of psoriasis in doses up to 4 mg/kg daily but prescribed up to 5 mg/kg daily[3]. Cyclosporine is an effective agent for plaque-type, erythrodermic, and pustular psoriasis, and is particularly useful for treating acute psoriatic flares because it results in rapid clinical improvement. Because of the concerning side effects of decreased renal function and hypertension, treatment should be initiated only after first trying less toxic therapies, and short-term therapy is ideal when possible.

Before initiation of cyclosporine therapy, baseline monitoring should include a history including a medication history, physical exam, two separate serum creatinine values, chemistry panel including lipid profile, liver function tests, electrolytes, magnesium, and uric acid. Laboratory values should be measured every 2 weeks for at least the month of therapy and monthly thereafter. Patients should be examined for side effects including malaise, nausea, headaches, tremors, sensitivity to extremes of temperature, hypertrichosis, and gingival hyperplasia. The associated hypertension can be effectively treated with a calcium channel blocking agent. Kidney biopsies and drug level monitoring are not routinely performed. Absolute contraindications to cyclosporine include renal disease, poorly controlled hypertension, and severe infections. Long-term treatment with cyclosporine is associated with cyclosporine-induced nephropathy. Therefore treatment periods should be limited and cyclosporine should be used as part of a rotational therapy regimen.

Biologic Agents

Recent advances in the understanding of how T cells play a paramount role in both the development and maintenance of psoriatic plaques has led to an explosive research effort toward the creation and development of biologic agents for the treatment of psoriasis. Psoriasis is now recognized to be a Th_1-mediated T-cell disorder. By selectively targeting specific steps in this T-cell–mediated inflammatory cascade, biologic agents can theoretically control disease with minimal impairment of immune function and few side effects.

Like systemic agents, biologics are generally used to treat psoriasis patients with moderate to severe disease who have not responded to other treatment measures. However, unlike the systemic agents currently in use, biologic agents are neither hepatotoxic nor nephrotoxic. Thus, these new agents represent a significant addition to our current psoriasis therapy armamentarium.

Three types of biologic agents are used for the treatment of psoriasis and psoriatic arthritis:

1. Recombinant human cytokines or growth factors
2. Monoclonal antibodies
3. Fusion proteins

Table 2 shows examples of the latter two kinds of biologics, which are in various stages of approval for psoriasis.

At the time of this publication, alefacept (Amevive), a novel fusion protein, efalizumab (Raptiva), a monoclonal antibody, and etanercept (Enbrel), a dimeric fusion protein are currently the only biologic agents that are FDA approved for the treatment of moderate to severe plaque-type psoriasis in adult patients who are candidates for systemic therapy or phototherapy. Alefacept, efalizumab, and etanercept are safe, tolerable, and effective treatments for psoriasis.

Alefacept is administered as a 15 mg IM weekly dose for 12 weeks. Safety and tolerability profiles were similar to placebo for one or two 12-week courses of alefacept IM. After a 12-week rest period off-drug, a second 12-week course can be administered. Before starting treatment, patients should have a history and physical, as well as laboratory examination of blood including CBC with total lymphocyte and CD4+ T-cell counts. Lymphocyte and CD4+ T-cell counts should be within normal limits before initiating therapy. Current recommendations are to monitor weekly CD4+ counts and to hold therapy if CD4+ counts fall below 250/µL.

Data from four randomized, placebo-controlled, phase III studies show efalizumab to be a safe and effective therapy for the treatment of moderate to severe plaque psoriasis in doses of 1.0 mg/kg per week to 2.0 mg/kg per week. Clinical response was observed as early as 2 weeks after treatment initiation. Additional new and ongoing trials are being conducted to define optimal dosing schedules, determine optimal strategies for withdrawal of therapy, and further support efalizumab as a potential long-term therapy. Adverse events that occurred at least 2% more frequently in efalizumab patients than in the placebo group include infection (mostly upper respiratory), headache, chills, nausea, pain, myalgia, flu syndrome, fever, back pain, and acne. For the third and subsequent doses, the incidence of adverse events was similar to placebo.

Etanercept is indicated for the treatment of moderate to severe plaque-type psoriasis in the dose of 50 mg SC twice weekly for three months followed by a reduction to a maintenance dose of 50 mg per week.

[3]Exceeds dosage recommended by the manufacturer.

TABLE 2 Some of the Well-Known Biologic Agents for the Treatment of Psoriasis and Psoriatic Arthritis

Agent	Type of Agent	Mechanism of Action	Administration	Status
Alefacept (Amevive)	Fusion protein	Blocks T-cell activation; selective reduction of memory effector T cells	IM	Psoriasis—FDA approved for chronic moderate to severe plaque-type psoriasis, January 2003; psoriatic arthritis—phase I
Efalizumab (Raptiva)	Monoclonal antibody	Anti-CD11a, blocks T-cell activation; reduces trafficking of T cells to inflamed skin	SC	Psoriasis—FDA approved for chronic, moderate to severe plaque-type psoriasis, October 2003; psoriatic arthritis—phase II
Etanercept (Enbrel)	Fusion protein	TNF-α inhibitor	SC	Psoriasis—FDA approved for chronic, moderate to severe plaque-type psoriasis, April 2004; psoriatic arthritis—FDA approved, January 2002
Infliximab (Remicade)	Monoclonal antibody	TNF-α inhibitor	IV	Psoriasis—phase III[1]; psoriatic arthritis—phase III[1]
Adalimumab (Humira)	Monoclonal antibody	TNF-α inhibitor	SC	Psoriasis—phase II[1]; psoriatic arthritis—phase III[1]

[1]Not FDA approved for this indication.
Abbreviations: TNF = tumor necrosis factor.

It is also indicated for the treatment of psoriatic arthritis. Over 130,000 patient years of treatment experience (mostly in the rheumatoid arthritis population) have demonstrated etanercept to be safe and effective. Laboratory monitoring is not required during treatment with etanercept. Injection site reactions were the only adverse event that occurred significantly more often in etanercept-treated patients than in placebo-treated patients in controlled clinical trials.

It should be noted that alefacept, efalizumab, and etanercept are fairly new agents without a long history of use, thus limiting our knowledge of the potential long-term side effects of these treatments.

Lichen Planus

Lichen planus is a common papulosquamous disorder of unknown etiology, characterized by small, violaceous, flat-topped, polygonal papules that are extremely pruritic. Lichen planus occurs equally among males and females, and without predisposition to race. Although more than 33% of patients are between 30 and 60 years of age, it does occur, albeit uncommonly, in children. Close examination of individual papules reveals a superficial fine scale that is crossed with gray-white streaks known as Wickham's striae. The eruption tends to occur at the flexor aspects of the upper extremities (especially the wrist), trunk, thighs, shins, buccal mucosa, and glans penis. Scalp involvement can occur as well. Oral involvement occurs on the buccal mucosa or tongue as either an atrophic or ulcerative pattern. Oral disease may occur with or without concomitant cutaneous involvement. Lichen planus can also affect the nails with characteristic nail plate longitudinal grooving and ridging. If nail involvement is severe, the matrix can be destroyed, resulting in pterygium formation. There are several clinical variants of lichen planus including linear, annular, follicular, hypertrophic, atrophic, bullous, and ulcerative forms. (A detailed description of these entities is beyond the scope of this article.)

The pathogenesis of lichen planus is a T-cell–mediated immune response of unknown cause. Although the disease course is highly variable, cutaneous disease tends to resolve in less than 1 year—in contrast to mucous membrane involvement that tends to be chronic and is reported to have a mean duration of 5 years. Because ulcerated lichen planus of the oral mucosa, vulva, and anus is associated with an increased risk of malignant transformation to squamous cell carcinoma, suspicious, erosive, or ulcerated lesions should be biopsied.

There is a well-known association between lichen planus and hepatitis C infection. Because the cutaneous presentation is the same in patients regardless of underlying disease status, hepatitis C should be sought at initial presentation. In addition, many drugs are associated with lichenoid-like eruptions, therefore, a thorough drug history should be taken to rule out drug-induced lichen planus (Table 3).

First-line therapies include class I or II topical corticosteroids, intralesional corticosteroid injections, and antihistamines. Topical corticosteroids should be applied twice daily for 2 to 4 weeks, and concomitant treatment with occlusive dressings is proven to improve efficacy. Intralesional corticosteroid injections are more ideal for limited, recalcitrant, discrete lesions. Oral lesions can be treated with mixtures of high-potency corticosteroids and Orabase, or intralesional

TABLE 3 Medications Associated with Induction of a Lichenoid Eruption

β-Blockers
Methyldopa
Penicillamine (Cuprimine)
Quinidine
Quinine
Nonsteroidal anti-inflammatory drugs (NSAIDs)
Allopurinol (Zyloprim)
Tetracyclines
Furosemide (Lasix)
Hydrochlorothiazide (Esidrix)
Isoniazid (Nydrazid)
Phenytoin (Dilantin)
Hepatitis B vaccination
Angiotensin-converting enzyme inhibitors
Chlorpropamide
Carbamazepine (Tegretol)
Gold
Lithium

injections can be used for unresponsive oral regions. Treatment with high-potency corticosteroids should be limited to prevent unwanted side effects. Pruritus can be quelled with antihistamines such as hydroxyzine (Atarax) in doses of 25 to 100 mg by mouth every 4 to 6 hours.

Second-line therapies—systemic corticosteroids, oral retinoids, and PUVA—are more ideal for widespread disease. Oral prednisone in doses of 30 to 60 mg daily for 2 to 6 weeks is an effective therapy and should be followed by a long taper (2 to 6 weeks) to prevent relapse. Acitretin (Soriatane)[1], in doses of 30 mg daily, also is proven effective for the treatment of cutaneous lichen planus. Isotretinoin (Accutane)[1], in doses of 10 mg orally twice daily for 2 months, shows efficacy for both oral and cutaneous lichen planus with fewer mucocutaneous side effects than with high-dose acitretin. Lastly, there is limited evidence supporting bath PUVA with methoxsalen[1] at 1 mg/L as an effective therapy for lichen planus.

Cyclosporine[1], tacrolimus (FK506)[1], metronidazole[1], TMP-SMX[1], griseofulvin, itraconazole[1], levamisole[1], photodynamic therapy, azathioprine, interferon, and mycophenolate mofetil are some of the many therapies that can be considered third-line therapies for the treatment of lichen planus. These therapies tend to either have limited evidence-based data to support their efficacy, or are more likely to have potentially severe associated toxicities. Cyclosporine, for example, is extremely effective for the treatment of severe lichen planus; however, because of the nephrotoxicity associated with it, this therapy should be reserved for severe, recalcitrant cases.

Pityriasis Rosea

Pityriasis rosea is a self-limited, inflammatory papulosquamous disorder of unknown etiology, characterized by oval, salmon-colored macular and papular lesions that are covered in fine scale. The lesions are distributed with the long axis of the macule parallel to the lines of cleavage, a pattern that is classically described as having a "Christmas tree distribution." Although it can affect any age group, it most commonly occurs in children and young adults; women are more frequently affected. In the United States, it is most prevalent in the spring and fall.

The outbreak usually begins with the appearance of a solitary, pink, herald patch followed in 1 to 2 weeks by a generalized eruption primarily on the trunk, sparing sun-exposed areas. Patients may experience mild constitutional symptoms before the onset, and pruritus tends to occur in most patients. Resolution usually occurs after approximately 6 weeks. Atypical presentations are common in approximately 20% of patients. It is, therefore, important to differentiate pityriasis rosea from a number of other disorders that it resembles such as lichen planus, nummular dermatitis, pityriasis lichenoides, erythema dyschromicum perstans, guttate psoriasis, seborrheic dermatitis, syphilis, tinea versicolor, and tinea corporis. Mycologic examination of skin scrapings and syphilis serology may be warranted to rule out dermatophyte infections and syphilis, respectively.

To date, the etiology of pityriasis rosea remains unknown. It is believed to be caused by a viral infection, although no single causal agent has been identified. In addition, there are reports of medication-induced pityriasis rosea-like eruptions with certain drugs such as captopril (Capoten), metronidazole (Flagyl), ketotifen (Zaditor), arsenicals, gold, bismuth, clonidine (Catapres), and barbiturates. However, there is no evidence to support that pityriasis rosea is drug induced.

Pityriasis rosea is self-limiting. Therefore, treatment is only indicated to relieve pruritus, or as an attempt to expedite disease resolution. First-line therapies include medium potency topical corticosteroids applied twice daily, emollients, and oral antihistamines such as hydroxyzine in doses of 25 mg every 4 to 6 hours. For patients with significant pruritus and extensive disease, UVB phototherapy administered daily for 5 to 10 treatments is proven to ameliorate symptoms and reduce disease severity.

Pityriasis Rubra Pilaris

Pityriasis rubra pilaris (PRP) is a papulosquamous disorder with a clinically distinct presentation characterized by keratotic follicular papules, palmoplantar hyperkeratosis, and generalized red-orange scaling. Follicular papules are topped by a central horny plug, and initially distributed on the dorsum of the proximal phalanges, wrists, neck, and trunk. These characteristic papules are described as looking like goose flesh or as nutmeg grater papules. Eventually the eruption can become diffuse, and any body area may be affected including the nails, mucous membranes, and eyes; however, small areas

[1]Not FDA approved for this indication.

of well-circumscribed uninvolved skin remain spared. As PRP progresses, palmoplantar keratoderma can become severely fissured and painful. In addition, nails can become discolored, thickened, and brittle. Unlike in psoriasis, however, pitting is extremely unusual. In severe cases, a generalized erythroderma may develop, compromising the protective barrier of the skin and predisposing patients to infection, inability to control temperature, and electrolyte imbalances.

The etiology of PRP is unknown. It is classified into several subtypes. The classic adult type is the most common form of PRP. This form presents acutely in adulthood, has the classic aforementioned clinical features, and carries the best prognosis, with 80% of patients going into remission within 3 years. A familial form of the disease with an autosomal-dominant inheritance pattern tends to present in childhood. More recently, there are reports of an HIV-associated form, which is characterized by HIV infection, cutaneous lesions of PRP, nodulocystic and pustular acneiform lesions, hidradenitis suppurativa, and lichen spinulosus.

PRP has a variable clinical response to therapy. Treatment can be challenging and therapeutic response somewhat unpredictable. Medium potency topical corticosteroids applied with bland emollients can help to relieve pruritus. Both retinoids and methotrexate[1] are considered first-line therapies for the treatment of PRP. Isotretinoin (Accutane)[1] in doses of 1.0 to 1.5 mg/kg per day for 3 to 6 months is proven to be a particularly effective treatment. There are also reports of successful treatment with acitretin (Soriatane)[1] combined with UVA phototherapy. As previously mentioned, potential side effects of retinoids include elevation of serum lipids and liver function tests as well as cheilitis, alopecia, xerosis, hyperostosis, and teratogenicity. Methotrexate, in doses of 7.5 to 25 mg weekly for 3 to 4 months, is also a very effective treatment option. Hepatotoxicity and bone marrow suppression are important side effects to be aware of with this type of therapy. Marked clinical improvement can be achieved with azathioprine (Imuran)[1] in doses of 150 to 200 mg daily. Azathioprine can be considered a second-line therapy. Potentially significant side effects associated with azathioprine include myelosuppression, increased malignancy rates, nausea and vomiting, hypersensitivity reactions, and increased susceptibility to opportunistic infections. Clinical responses to cyclosporine (Neoral)[1] are inconsistent. Patients with HIV-associated PRP, although resistant to standard therapies, respond to triple antiretroviral therapy with zidovudine (AZT) (Retrovir)[1], in doses of 250 mg twice daily, lamivudine (3TC [Epivir])[1], in doses of 150 mg twice daily, and saquinavir (Invirase, Fortovase)[1] in doses of 600 mg three times daily. Clinical response is directly related to fall in viral load.

Seborrheic Dermatitis

Seborrheic dermatitis is a common, chronic, papulosquamous disorder characterized by sharply demarcated, greasy, flaky, yellowish, crusted patches overlying red, inflamed skin. It tends to affect sebum-rich areas, with a predilection for the scalp, eyebrows, eyelids, nasolabial folds, beard, postauricular regions, external auditory canal, sternum, axillae, and groin. It can occur in any age group, presenting, for example, on the scalp as cradle cap in infants, and as pityriasis sicca, or dandruff, in adults. It is associated with and may be exacerbated in patients with Parkinson's disease, particularly those with neuroleptic-induced disease, and in patients with HIV.

Although the exact etiology is controversial, seborrheic dermatitis is believed to be associated with the lipophilic yeast *Pityrosporum ovale* (*Malassezia furfur*); however, the mechanism of the disease process remains unresolved. Some argue that *P. ovale* is present in abundance in skin lesions of seborrheic dermatitis patients and, therefore, believe that this yeast is the culprit. Others have challenged this cause and effect relationship by showing that *P. ovale* may be present in profuse levels in patients who have no clinical evidence of seborrheic dermatitis. Some studies demonstrate that it is the higher concentrations of skin lipids in patients with seborrheic dermatitis that result in promotion of growth of the organism and, ultimately, the disease. Yet others believe that seborrheic dermatitis is associated with normal levels of the yeast, and that it is the host's inadequate immune response that is causative.

Seborrheic dermatitis of the scalp responds well to treatment at least two or three times per week with medicated shampoos such as ciclopirox (Loprox), ketoconazole (Nizoral), selenium sulfide (Selsun or Exsel), pyrithione zinc (DHS Zinc or Head & Shoulders), propylene glycol, and coal tar (DHS tar, Neutrogena T/Gel, Polytar). Shampoo should be massaged into a rich lather on the scalp and allowed to remain for 5 minutes before rinsing. A keratolytic agent such as salicylic acid can be of added benefit, by allowing greater penetration of other medications. For treating seborrheic dermatitis of the face, scalp, trunk, and extremities, low potency topical corticosteroids such as hydrocortisone applied once daily for a minimum of three weeks, and antimicrobial preparations such as ketoconazole or ciclopirox gel 0.77% (Loprox) can be helpful. These agents can be used alone or in combination. Ketoconazole, the most commonly prescribed azole, is available as a 2% cream, an oil-in-water emulsion, a foaming gel or, as previously mentioned, as a shampoo. Caution should be taken when treating seborrheic blepharitis with corticosteroids, as steroids in this area may induce glaucoma and cataracts. Instead, the eyelashes should be cleansed with baby shampoo on a cotton-tipped applicator. For severe or refractory seborrheic dermatitis, oral therapies may be more efficacious.

[1]Not FDA approved for this indication.

Oral ketoconazole[1] in doses of 200 mg daily for 1 month is proven to be effective for widespread disease. A number of new potential therapies have recently gained attention including the azoles, fluconazole (Diflucan)[1], metronidazole (Flagyl)[1], ciclopirox (Loprox), tacrolimus (Protopic)[1], and pimecrolimus (Elidel)[1]. Lithium succinate ointment (Efalith)[1] is proven to be effective for facial involvement, and particularly for the treatment of AIDS-related seborrheic dermatitis.

[1]Not FDA approved for this indication.

CONNECTIVE TISSUE DISORDERS

METHOD OF

Edwin A. Smith, MD

Systemic Lupus Erythematosus

Therapies for systemic lupus erythematosus (SLE) vary depending on the clinical manifestations, organ systems involved, and degree of disease activity. Therapy for manifestations in nonvital organs is less toxic than treatments used for visceral (hematologic, renal, cardiopulmonary, or central nervous system [CNS]) involvement (Table 1).

NONVISCERAL MANIFESTATIONS

Constitutional symptoms such as fever, malaise, anorexia, and weight loss are common and may occur independently of, or with, visceral disease. Treatment of the visceral disease results in resolution of the constitutional symptoms. In the absence of visceral involvement, conservative therapy is indicated. Patients should be encouraged to obtain adequate rest and nutrition. Evaluation of fever requires history, physical examination, and laboratory testing to eliminate the possibility of infection, for which SLE patients are at increased risk. Acetaminophen and nonsteroidal anti-inflammatory drugs (NSAIDs) are given for fever. When constitutional symptoms fail to respond and there is weight loss, glucocorticoid therapy with prednisone (10 to 30 mg per day) is justified.

MUCOCUTANEOUS MANIFESTATIONS

Abnormalities of the skin, hair, and mucous membranes are common. Cutaneous eruptions include the classic butterfly malar rash, discoid lupus, subacute lesions, and nonspecific maculopapular rash. Patients must be cautioned to avoid ultraviolet (UV) light exposure. Light-blocking clothing, broad-brimmed hats, and sunscreens with a solar protection factor of 25 or higher provide protection. Topical glucocorticoids are the most effective therapy, and the least potent preparation that is effective should be used. Twice daily 1% hydrocortisone is mild, safe, and often effective for early discoid lesions. Moderately potent preparations such as 0.1% triamcinolone (Kenalog) are necessary for established discoid lesions. Potent fluorinated steroids such as 0.05% fluocinonide (Lidex) or fluocinolone acetonide (Synalar) may be necessary for thick discoid lesions. Intralesional steroid injections into discoid lesions may be effective. Systemic corticosteroids are effective for the malar rash and subacute lesions, but are less effective for discoid lesions. Hydroxychloroquine (Plaquenil), 200 mg orally twice daily, is usually effective but benefit is delayed for 3 to 4 months. Retinal toxicity is rare if the total daily dose remains less than 6.5 mg/kg per day. Patients must have an ophthalmologic examination within a month of starting therapy and annually to monitor for toxicity. Dapsone[1], 25 to 100 mg per day, and low-dose methotrexate (Rheumatrex)[1] may be used in difficult cases. Dapsone has been particularly useful for bullous lupus, lupus panniculitis, and oral ulcers. Patients must be

[1]Not FDA approved for this indication.

TABLE 1 Treatment for Systemic Lupus Erythematosus

Manifestation	Pharmacotherapy
Constitutional	Acetaminophen[1], NSAIDs[1]
Cutaneous	Topical steroids, hydroxychloroquine (Plaquenil), dapsone[1], thalidomide[1] (Thalomid)
Musculoskeletal	NSAIDs, hydroxychloroquine, methotrexate[1] (Rheumatrex), azathioprine[1] (Imuran)
Hematologic	Glucocorticoids, danazol[1] (Danocrine)[1], azathioprine[1], intravenous immunoglobulin[1], cyclophosphamide[1] (Cytoxan)
Antiphospholipid syndrome	Warfarin[1] (Coumadin); heparin[1] and aspirin (in pregnancy)
Cardiopulmonary	Glucocorticoids, azathioprine[1], cyclophosphamide[1], epoprostenol[1] (Flolan), bosentan[1] (Tracleer), treprostinil[1] (Remodulin)
Central nervous system	Antiepileptics[1], neuroleptics[1], glucocorticoids, cyclophosphamide[1], azathioprine[1]
Glomerulonephritis	Glucocorticoids, cyclophosphamide[1], mycophenolate mofetil[1] (CellCept)

[1]Not FDA approved for treatment of SLE.
Abbreviation: NSAIDs = nonsteroidal anti-inflammatory drugs.

monitored closely for hemolytic anemia. For very refractory patients, thalidomide[1] has been used. This known teratogen must be used with utmost caution, with concomitant, diligent contraception; and the patient and physician must follow a strict system for safety called STEPS (System for Thalidomide Education and Prescribing Safety). Doses of 50 to 100 mg per day are used. Drowsiness and peripheral neuropathy are the most common side effects.

MUSCULOSKELETAL MANIFESTATIONS

Arthralgia without synovitis is a frequent complaint and can be controlled with NSAIDs, either nonspecific cyclooxygenase inhibitors or selective cyclooxygenase-2 inhibitors. For true arthritis that is incompletely responsive to NSAIDs, hydroxychloroquine (Plaquenil), 200 mg orally twice daily, can be effective; but its onset of action is often delayed for several months. For refractory arthritis, methotrexate[1], 7.5 to 25 mg once weekly, is used. Patients should receive supplementation with folic acid, 1 mg per day, while taking methotrexate. Monitoring of blood counts and liver functions is required. Azathioprine (Imuran)[1], 50 to 150 mg per day orally, can be quite useful. Patients should have testing for thiopurine methyltransferase activity levels before starting azathioprine, because severe pancytopenia may develop if there is a genetic deficiency of that enzyme. Blood counts should be monitored closely while administering azathioprine. Glucocorticoids (prednisone at 5 to 10 mg per day) are useful while waiting for the delayed response to methotrexate or azathioprine, and to alleviate temporary flares.

HEMATOLOGIC MANIFESTATIONS

Autoimmune cytopenias are common because of autoantibodies to cell membrane components. Lymphopenia alone does not require treatment. Hemolytic anemia in SLE results from antierythrocyte antibodies that activate complement. The opsonized erythrocytes are recognized and removed by the reticuloendothelial cells of the liver and/or spleen. Treatment of hemolysis requires high-dose glucocorticoids. Depending on the clinical severity, this may be 60 mg of prednisone per day in divided doses or pulse therapy (1 g of methylprednisolone IV daily for 3 days followed by the oral prednisone). Once hemolysis is controlled, the prednisone may be tapered by 5 mg per day for 1 week. In patients who are unresponsive to glucocorticoids or for whom the maintenance dose of prednisone cannot be decreased to 15 mg per day or less, other treatment is required. These may include danazol (Danocrine)[1], 300 to 600 mg per day in divided doses, azathioprine (Imuran)[1], 1.5 to 2.0 mg/kg per day, intravenous immunoglobulin (IGIV [Gamimune N])[1], or cyclophosphamide (Cytoxan) at doses similar to those used for renal disease (see below).

Immune thrombocytopenia (ITP) results from antibodies to circulating platelets. The glucocorticoid treatment strategy is the same as for immune hemolysis. If splenectomy is necessary for refractory cases, IGIV[1], 400 mg/kg per day for 5 days, can be used to temporarily raise the platelet count. Platelet counts respond to splenectomy initially, but later recurrence of thrombocytopenia is common. For patients in whom the thrombocytopenia is chronic or in whom glucocorticoid doses cannot be reduced to acceptable levels, treatment with danazol (Danocrine)[1], dapsone, cyclosporine (Neoral), azathioprine (Imuran)[1], or cyclophosphamide (Cytoxan)[1] are all reported to be beneficial.

Thrombotic thrombocytopenic purpura (TTP), a nonimmune thrombocytopenia, also occurs in SLE, but at a lower frequency than ITP. Manifestations include fever, microangiopathic hemolysis, CNS abnormalities, and renal involvement. Treatment of TTP requires plasmapheresis.

Antibodies to phospholipids are associated with thrombocytopenia, thromboembolism, cardiac valvular abnormalities, and spontaneous abortion. These antibodies can be detected by enzyme-linked immunoabsorbent assay (ELISA) tests for antiphospholipid antibodies, or by coagulation tests indicated by the presence of a lupus anticoagulant. Treatment for thromboembolism requires chronic anticoagulation with warfarin (Coumadin) with a target international normalized ratio (INR) of 3.0 to 4.0. For women who have suffered miscarriage, treatment with low-dose aspirin and prophylactic heparin (5000 units subcutaneously twice daily) during pregnancy improves the likelihood of a successful outcome.

CARDIOPULMONARY MANIFESTATIONS

Most SLE patients suffer bouts of pleurisy and/or pericarditis. These are usually transient and can be treated with NSAIDs. Refractory cases may require treatment with moderate doses of glucocorticoids. Although cardiac tamponade is unusual, it does occur, and requires immediate percutaneous drainage. Myocarditis is uncommon, but if present it requires aggressive treatment with glucocorticoids and immunosuppression with azathioprine (Imuran)[1] or cyclophosphamide (Cytoxan)[1]. Pulmonary alveolar hemorrhage is a life-threatening complication that requires treatment with high doses of glucocorticoids as well as immunosuppression with cyclophosphamide (Cytoxan). Plasmapheresis should be initiated early as it appears to improve the outcome. Lupus pneumonitis also requires aggressive therapy with immunosuppressives as well as high-dose glucocorticoids. Pulmonary hypertension occurs in SLE, and treatment should be considered for those with class II, III, or IV symptomatic pulmonary hypertension with calcium channel blockers, anticoagulation, and oral bosentan (Tracleer); or infusions of the prostacyclin

[1]Not FDA approved for this indication.

[1]Not FDA approved for this indication.

analogues epoprostenol (Flolan) or treprostinil (Remodulin), as described below for scleroderma.

NERVOUS SYSTEM MANIFESTATIONS

There are several types of CNS involvement, including seizures, psychosis, chorea, stroke, and myelopathy. In addition, medications used to treat SLE may have CNS side effects, such as aseptic meningitis from NSAIDs, mania from glucocorticoids, and altered cerebral function from seizure medications. Careful history taking, physical examination, laboratory evaluation (including cerebrospinal fluid [CSF] evaluation), and magnetic resonance imaging (MRI) scanning are needed to differentiate the causes of the CNS manifestations. For seizures, antiepileptic therapy is required. A neuroleptic drug such as haloperidol (Haldol), 1 to 4 mg every 12 hours, is used for psychosis. Cerebritis or transverse myelitis must be treated with very-high-dose glucocorticoids, such as methylprednisolone, 1 g intravenously daily for 3 days, followed by prednisone, 60 mg per day orally. When these lesions are unresponsive to glucocorticoid alone, immunosuppressive medications such as cyclophosphamide (Cytoxan)[1] or azathioprine (Imuran)[1] may be useful. Patients with ischemic CNS events and either antiphospholipid antibodies or a lupus anticoagulant should be treated with lifelong anticoagulation to prevent devastating nervous system sequelae.

RENAL MANIFESTATIONS

Involvement of the kidneys is one of the most feared and frequent complications with significant morbidity and mortality. The glomerular lesions result from immune complex deposits with activation of the complement cascade. A membranous glomerulopathy results in the nephrotic syndrome, but it is associated with relative preservation of glomerular filtration rate and only infrequently progresses to end-stage renal disease. In contrast, proliferative glomerulonephritis (focal when fewer than 50% of glomeruli are involved, and diffuse when more than 50% are involved) is manifest as nephritis with hematuria and hypertension, which may progress rapidly to renal failure. This type of severe glomerulonephritis is seen in patients who have circulating antibodies to native DNA and complement consumption. Treatment of proliferative glomerulonephritis is aggressive in an attempt to forestall end-stage renal disease. Initial treatment is with high-dose glucocorticoids (methylprednisolone[1], 1 g intravenously daily for 3 days, followed by prednisone at 60 mg per day). This is supplemented with intravenous cyclophosphamide[1] (0.5 to 1.0 g/m^2 of body surface area in 150 mL of normal saline) monthly for 6 months. During such cyclophosphamide treatment, complete blood counts (CBCs) must be performed 10 to 14 days after each dose and before the subsequent dose. The cyclophosphamide dose is adjusted to lower the nadir white blood cell count (WBC) to between 2,000 and 2,500/mm^3, with a return to normal WBC prior to the next dose. As renal function stabilizes, prednisone may be tapered. The frequency of cyclophosphamide dosing can be decreased to every 3 months when renal function improves and complement and anti-DNA levels have returned to normal. The duration of treatment depends on response, but is often as long as 24 to 36 months. Hemorrhagic cystitis from cyclophosphamide is minimized by hydrating the patient before and during intravenous administration. Treatment with intravenous 2-mercaptoethanesulfonic acid (mesna) at 0, 2, 4, and 6 hours throughout the cyclophosphamide dosing is given to persons who develop cystitis during treatment. Each mesna dose should be 20% of the total cyclophosphamide dose. Nausea resulting from cyclophosphamide can be minimized with granisetron (Kytril), 1 mg IV, or ondansetron (Zofran), 8 mg IV, prior to the cyclophosphamide, and oral doses of either of these antiemetics for 1 day after the chemotherapy.

An alternative to intravenous cyclophosphamide has recently been shown to be as effective. Mycophenolate mofetil (CellCept)[1], 2 to 3 g per day in divided doses, in combination with glucocorticoids, is effective at preventing long-term renal damage and seems to offer the advantage of fewer adverse reactions. However, leukopenia, nausea, diarrhea, and infections are risks.

VASCULAR MANIFESTATIONS

A vasculitis similar to polyarteritis nodosa can occur with fever, malaise, purpura, ulcerative skin lesions, abdominal pain, and wrist and/or foot drop. Sural nerve biopsy can demonstrate vasculitis of the vasa nervorum when nerve conduction velocities are abnormal. Abdominal angiography may show tapering of medium-size vessels with pseudoaneurysm formation in the mesenteric, renal, or hepatic arterial circulation. Treatment is initiated with the same treatment schema as for SLE nephritis, as described above, with high-dose glucocorticoids and monthly doses of intravenous cyclophosphamide (Cytoxan)[1].

REPRODUCTIVE ISSUES

Pregnancies in lupus patients presents specific problems for both maternal and fetal health including fetal loss or preterm birth, intrauterine growth retardation, neonatal SLE, flaring of SLE, hypertension, and/or preeclampsia. Barrier forms of birth control or progesterone-only contraception with medroxyprogesterone (Depo-Provera,) 150 mg IM quarterly, are the preferred methods. Estrogens are avoided because of the risk of SLE flare and thrombotic events. Flares can occur at any time during pregnancy or the postpartum period, and close monitoring for such flares

[1]Not FDA approved for this indication.

[1]Not FDA approved for this indication.

is necessary. Disease flares during pregnancy are best treated with oral glucocorticoids with up to 1 mg/kg per day of prednisone, depending on severity. Cyclophosphamide, methotrexate, and mycophenolate mofetil are absolutely contraindicated during pregnancy. Azathioprine and hydroxychloroquine can be continued through pregnancy if needed to control disease. Any risks associated with these medications are less problematic than untreated SLE flares. SLE patients who have suffered miscarriages as a result of antiphospholipid antibodies or lupus anticoagulant should have prophylaxis during subsequent pregnancies with low-dose heparin (5000 U subcutaneously twice daily) and aspirin (81 mg daily).

Neonatal lupus can occur during fetal development, particularly when there are maternal anti-Ro antibodies. The baby can suffer congenital heart block, rashes, and cytopenias. Screening for heart block with fetal echocardiography is done during the second trimester. If any degree of heart block is demonstrated, the mother should be treated with dexamethasone[1] (which crosses the placenta), 4 mg daily. Unfortunately, third-degree heart block is rarely reversible, and pacing of the neonate is required at time of birth.

Polymyositis/Dermatomyositis

Inflammatory muscle disease can occur with (dermatomyositis) or without (polymyositis) a cutaneous eruption. There is a predominantly proximal muscle weakness caused by inflammatory damage to the myocytes. Three rashes are characteristic of the rash dermatomyositis:

1. Rash over the proximal interphalangeal and metacarpophalangeal joints (Gottron's papules)
2. A purple (*heliotrope*) eruption over the eyelids
3. Erythematous poikiloderma over the upper anterior chest and around over the shoulders (*V and shawl* sign)

Laboratory testing shows elevated muscle enzyme levels (creatine kinase and/or aldolase). Electromyography shows a myopathy, and muscle biopsy shows inflammatory cells and damage to myocytes. These are important tests to eliminate other causes of muscle weakness. Patients who are 50 years of age or older with a diagnosis of dermatomyositis must have a thorough evaluation to exclude an underlying malignancy.

CUTANEOUS MANIFESTATIONS

The rash of dermatomyositis can be treated with topical glucocorticoids of mild to moderate potency, such as hydrocortisone valerate (Westcort), 0.2% applied three times daily. More resistant rash usually responds to hydroxychloroquine (Plaquenil)[1], 200 mg twice daily, or methotrexate (Rheumatrex)[1], 10 to 20 mg once per week.

MUSCULAR MANIFESTATIONS

Initial treatment with high-dose glucocorticoids (prednisone at 1 mg/kg per day orally) gives the best results. Most patients respond to this dose by 1 month with a fall in serum muscle enzyme levels and improvement of weakness. A physical therapy program should be started, with initial emphasis on retaining range of motion and later on muscle strengthening. For patients who do not respond to glucocorticoid treatment and for those who have worsening of the disease as prednisone is tapered, further immunosuppression is required. The two most commonly used drugs are methotrexate[1] and azathioprine[1], with methotrexate having the advantage of faster onset of action. Methotrexate doses for myositis are 15 to 30 mg weekly. Azathioprine (Imuran) is used at 1.5 to 2 mg/kg per day orally. Complete blood counts and liver function testing are required every 6 to 8 weeks. For patients with disease resistance to these immunosuppressive agents, the addition of cyclosporine (Neoral), 2 to 3.5 mg/kg per day in divided doses, has been helpful. Patients taking this latter medicine must be monitored for hypertension and renal insufficiency. For even more refractory disease, intravenous immunoglobulin (Sandoglobulin)[1] at 400 mg/kg per day for 5 days with monthly doses of 1 g/kg has been used with success.

GASTROINTESTINAL MANIFESTATIONS

Involvement of the pharyngeal musculature in patients may cause proximal dysphagia, aspiration, and pneumonia. Attention must be paid to the gag reflex. At times endotracheal intubation is necessary to protect the airway. This problem is rarely severe enough to require feeding tube placement or parenteral nutrition. Some patients have distal esophageal hypomotility, as seen with scleroderma. This may also increase the risk of aspiration. These patients may benefit from a proton pump inhibitor such as omeprazole (Prilosec), 20 mg per day, and/or metoclopramide (Reglan), 10 mg before meals and at bedtime.

PULMONARY MANIFESTATIONS

Dyspnea may be caused by respiratory muscle weakness or pulmonary fibrosis. Respiratory muscle function is monitored with bedside spirometry. Treatment of weakness in these muscles is as above, and attention to carbon dioxide retention and aspiration must be paid. Interstitial lung disease can be fibrotic or inflammatory. Inflammatory disease (demonstrated by *ground glass* opacity on chest computed tomography [CT] scan or by inflammation on

[1]Not FDA approved for this indication.

[1]Not FDA approved for this indication.

bronchoalveolar lavage) may respond to immunosuppression.

Scleroderma (Systemic Sclerosis)

Scleroderma (systemic sclerosis) is a disease with vascular, fibrotic, and immunologic manifestations. Involved organs include the skin, gastrointestinal tract, lungs, heart, and kidneys. No treatment has been shown to specifically alter the course of scleroderma, so treatment is directed at specific organ manifestations.

RAYNAUD'S PHENOMENON

Raynaud's phenomenon is the most common initial manifestation of scleroderma and can lead to ulceration and digital infarctions and gangrene. Avoidance of cold is important—the patient should bundle up well against cold temperatures. Calcium channel blockade with extended-release nifedipine (Procardia-XL)[1], 30 to 90 mg per day, or amlodipine (Norvasc)[1], 5 to 10 mg per day is useful. An antiadrenergic drug such as terazosin (Hytrin)[1], 1 to 5 mg twice daily, may be given in addition to or instead of calcium channel blockers. Low-dose aspirin (81 mg per day) should be used for its antiplatelet effects. Additional antiplatelet treatment with dipyridamole (Persantine) at 50 to 100 mg three times per day can be helpful. When patients develop digital ulcers, the application of nitroglycerin ointment (Nitro-Bid)[1] three times per day at the base of the affected finger is helpful. More resistant ulcers can respond to intravenous prostaglandin such as epoprostenol (Flolan)[1], but this requires central venous administration and is very expensive. There are reports of using sildenafil (Viagra)[1] for finger ulcers at a dose of 50 mg three times per day. Surgical treatment involves the débridement of infected ulcers, which should also be treated with topical antibiotics such as mupirocin (Bactroban). More severe infections require systemic antibiotics, particularly gram-positive coverage with cephalexin (Keflex), 500 mg four times per day, or amoxicillin-clavulanate (Augmentin), 500 mg twice daily. Surgical palmar digital sympathectomy has been used with good results in many patients with recurrent and medically resistant digital ischemia.

CUTANEOUS MANIFESTATIONS

There is no treatment proven to reverse the skin thickening seen in scleroderma. Emollient creams should be used liberally to soften the skin and decrease itching. Antihistamines and doxepin (Sinequan), 50 mg at bedtime, can help alleviate pruritus.

MUSCULOSKELETAL MANIFESTATIONS

An erosive, inflammatory arthritis similar to rheumatoid arthritis can occur, and should be treated with drugs such as methotrexate. In general, glucocorticoids are to be avoided, particularly at higher doses, because they are associated with the development of renal disease.

GASTROINTESTINAL MANIFESTATIONS

The gastrointestinal (GI) tract is involved in all smooth muscle areas. The most frequent clinical manifestation is gastroesophageal reflux caused by poor contractility of the lower esophageal sphincter. This can lead to esophagitis and stricture formation. Dysphagia can be caused by such a stricture or by poor esophageal motility, which leads to slow transit. Patients should be instructed to raise the head of their bed on blocks and to avoid late-evening meals. Nearly all patients require treatment with a proton pump inhibitor such as omeprazole (Prilosec) at 20 mg twice daily. The promotility agent metoclopramide (Reglan), 10 mg orally 30 minutes before meals and at bedtime, can be helpful. Gastric hypomotility can be improved with erythromycin[1], 500 mg four times per day, but dosing can be limited by GI side effects. Intestinal hypomotility can be improved with tegaserod maleate (Zelnorm)[1], 6 mg twice a day before meals. For resistant cases, subcutaneous octreotide (Sandostatin)[1], 50 µg subcutaneously at bedtime, may help increase motility. Jejunoileal hypomotility can result in bacterial overgrowth, resulting in diarrhea. Rotating antibiotic treatment can treat this. Metronidazole (Flagyl) and ciprofloxacin (Cipro) should be included in that rotation. When GI dysmotility is extreme, intravenous hyperalimentation is the only effective supportive measure.

PULMONARY MANIFESTATIONS

Lung fibrosis occurs commonly in scleroderma. Inflammation is sought with CT scan, which may show a ground glass pattern indicative of alveolitis, and with a bronchoalveolar lavage with cell count and differential. For patients in whom inflammation is found, treatment with cyclophosphamide (Cytoxan)[1], 1 to 2 mg/kg per day orally for 2 years, is given. Pulmonary hypertension demonstrated by Doppler echocardiography or right side of the heart catheterization should be treated when symptomatic. Three medications are approved by the FDA for this indication. Two prostacyclin analogues (epoprostenol [Flolan] and treprostinil [Remodulin]) are available. Epoprostenol is given by continuous central intravenous infusion. Frequent upward dosage adjustment is needed, and nearly all patients have neck or jaw pain. Continuous subcutaneous infusion of treprostinil (Remodulin) is started at 1.25 ng/kg per minute with weekly increases by that amount, depending on clinical response. The oral endothelin receptor antagonist bosentan (Tracleer) is an alternative treatment. Bosentan is started at 62.5 mg twice daily

[1]Not FDA approved for this indication.

[1]Not FDA approved for this indication.

for 1 month, at which time the dose can be increased to 125 mg twice daily. Patients must have liver function tests monthly, and elevations of transaminases may require discontinuation or dose reduction. Patients with pulmonary hypertension should be anticoagulated because of the frequent occurrence of pulmonary emboli. Supplemental oxygen should be used for patients with low hemoglobin oxygen saturations, particularly those who desaturate with exercise.

CARDIAC MANIFESTATIONS

Heart involvement is most often conduction abnormalities or dysrhythmias. There may be heart failure. Treatment is with appropriate antiarrhythmics and cardiac pacing, if needed.

RENAL MANIFESTATIONS

The most severe acute manifestation of scleroderma is renal crisis. This is seen early in the disease at a time of rapidly worsening skin disease and has been associated with the use of moderate- to high-dose glucocorticoids. The onset of severe hypertension is abrupt and azotemia develops. There may be associated proteinuria and microangiopathic hemolytic anemia. Before the invention of angiotensin-converting enzyme (ACE) inhibitors, scleroderma renal crisis caused renal failure in all patients and death in many. All patients should be treated with an ACE inhibitor. Because of its short half-life, captopril (Capoten) is used initially so that dose adjustments can be made quickly. An initial dose of 12.5 mg is given orally, and the dose is increased frequently to control blood pressure. Other antihypertensives, particularly calcium channel blockers, should be added to the ACE inhibitor as needed to control blood pressure. The addition of hydralazine (Apresoline), prazosin (Minipress), clonidine (Catapres), and/or minoxidil (Loniten) may be required to control blood pressure. Once control of blood pressure is attained, a switch to a longer-acting ACE inhibitor such as quinapril (Accupril) or benazepril (Lotensin) can be made for the sake of convenience. Diuretics should be avoided as hypovolemia can worsen the renal hypoperfusion seen in this condition. Hemodialysis may be needed to control volume and uremic symptoms. There have been reports of recovery of renal function up to several years after the onset of scleroderma renal crisis, so ACE inhibitor treatment should be continued throughout that period.

Sjögren's Syndrome

Autoimmune destruction of the salivary and lacrimal glands has been termed Sjögren's syndrome. This sicca syndrome may occur as a primary condition or secondary to SLE, rheumatoid arthritis, or scleroderma. The clinical manifestations are dry mouth and dry eyes. Because dental problems are frequent, meticulous oral hygiene and treatment with topical stannous fluoride are required. Patients quickly realize that frequent sips of water offer relief and usually carry water supplementation with them. They often use sugarless lemon drops and chewing gum to stimulate salivary secretion. There are artificial saliva products available (MouthKote, Salivart), but these must be administered frequently to supply relief. Parasympathomimetic drugs including pilocarpine (Salagen), 5 mg orally three times per day, or cevimeline (Evoxac), 30 mg orally three times per day, can stimulate salivary secretion. Patients with glaucoma, iritis, asthma, chronic obstructive lung disease, or congestive heart failure should not use these medications. Side effects can include sweating, flushing, diarrhea, and urinary frequency. Dry eyes are treated with artificial tear supplementation, methylcellulose drops (HypoTears, Refresh Tears), or hydroxypropyl cellulose inserts (Lacrisert) and nighttime ophthalmic petrolatum (Lacri-Lube, Refresh PM). Treatment with topical cyclosporine (Restasis), 1 drop every 12 hours, suppresses lacrimal inflammation and increases tear production. Cigarette smoke and low humidity areas are to be avoided. A trial of obstruction of the nasolacrimal duct with plugs should be made before permanent punctal occlusion is performed.

Some patients with Sjögren's syndrome suffer extraglandular manifestations, including arteritis, interstitial pneumonitis, glomerulonephritis, and peripheral neuropathy. Hydroxychloroquine (Plaquenil)[1], 200 mg twice daily, can help with arthralgia. More severe systemic manifestations may require immunosuppressives such as azathioprine (Imuran)[1] at 1.5 to 2 mg/kg per day or cyclophosphamide (Cytoxan)[1].

Patients with Sjögren's syndrome are at increased risk for B cell lymphomas, usually expressing IgM_k light chains. These lymphomas require radiotherapy and/or chemotherapy as guided by histologic type, location, and extension.

[1]Not FDA approved for this indication.

[1]Not FDA approved for this indication.

CUTANEOUS VASCULITIS

METHOD OF

Thomas M. Bush, MD, and

Matthew H. Kanzler, MD

Cutaneous vasculitis is a form of systemic vasculitis that typically involves the venules, capillaries, and arterioles of the skin. In more severe cases, the kidneys, gastrointestinal (GI) tract, or peripheral nerves may be involved. The hallmark of the disease is palpable purpura—a rash consisting of slightly raised nonblanching papules that usually appear first in the lower extremities (Figure 1). This article covers the clinical presentation, pathology, etiology, differential diagnosis, and treatment of cutaneous vasculitis.

Clinical Presentation

Cutaneous vasculitis usually presents with a crop of lesions in dependent areas, most commonly the lower extremities. The lesions are usually raised, red to light purple in color, and nonblanchable. The papules range from 1 mm to several centimeters in size. They may occasionally be vesicular, ulcerated, or urticarial; and are asymptomatic, mildly pruritic, and occasionally associated with pain or a burning sensation. Although the lesions usually begin on the lower extremities, subsequent crops of eruptions may involve the trunk and arms. Individual lesions usually fade over a period of several weeks, sometimes leaving residual hyperpigmentation.

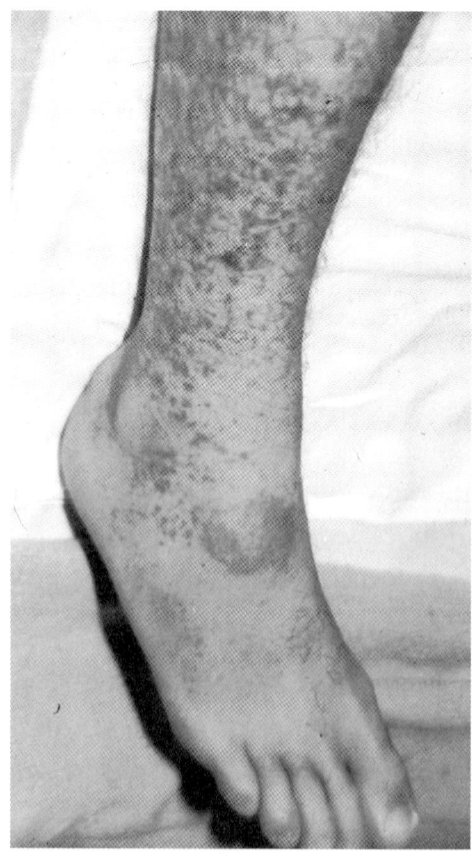

FIGURE 1 Right calf of a patient with palpable purpura.

Typically 50% of patients with cutaneous vasculitis experience an acute or transient course, 30% develop chronic disease, and 20% experience relapsing disease. Approximately 50% of patients with cutaneous vasculitis have systemic involvement of one or more systems. Polyarthritis often presents with tender and swollen joints with painful range of motion. The knees, wrists, and ankles are commonly involved. Nephritis may evolve into chronic renal failure, the most serious long-term sequelae of cutaneous vasculitis. An additional serious complication of cutaneous vasculitis is GI disease. Symptoms may range from mild colicky abdominal pain to rare cases of hemorrhage or intussusception. Unusual complications include peripheral neuropathies or pulmonary hemorrhage.

Pathology

A skin biopsy may demonstrate leukocytoclastic vasculitis—destruction of small postcapillary venules with surrounding nuclear debris from destroyed polymorphonucleocytes, and extravasation of erythrocytes into the surrounding dermis. Direct immunofluorescent studies reveal immunoglobulin (Ig) and/or complement deposition in the vascular walls in approximately 85% of cases. Henoch-Schönlein purpura is notable for the presence of IgA deposited in vessel walls. In typical cases, a skin biopsy is not essential for diagnosis because an experienced clinician can accurately recognize cutaneous vasculitis by its appearance and distribution.

Etiology

Cutaneous vasculitis is considered to be an aberrant immune response that is usually triggered by an infection, exposure to a drug, or an autoimmune disease. The specific etiology of palpable purpura is identified in approximately 50% of cases. Infectious agents are responsible for approximately 20% of cases. There are a wide variety of infections linked to palpable purpura. Bacterial infections associated with cutaneous vasculitis include *Streptococcus*, *Staphylococcus*, and gram-negative organisms. Several viral agents can trigger palpable purpura including HIV, hepatitis B, and hepatitis C. Twenty percent of cases are thought to be triggered by an exposure to a drug. Many drugs are reported to cause palpable purpura, most commonly antibiotics (penicillins, sulfonamides), anticonvulsants, isoniazid (Laniazid), and cardiac medications. Less than 5% of cases are associated with an underlying connective tissue disease such as systemic lupus erythematosus, rheumatoid arthritis, Sjögren's syndrome, and Wegener's granulomatosis. Rarely there have been cases of palpable purpura reported in patients with malignancies, including Hodgkin's disease, mycosis fungoides, and adult T-cell lymphoma.

The most likely cause of transient vasculitis in patients in whom the workup fails to pinpoint an etiology is an undetected viral infection or overlooked medication or chemical ingestion. Chronic vasculitis (months to years) suggests a primary autoimmune disorder if cryoglobulinemia and chronic hepatitis C infection are ruled out.

Differential Diagnosis

The differential diagnosis of purpuric skin lesions includes trauma, pigmented purpuric eruptions (Schamberg's disease), coagulopathies, thrombocytopenia, and embolic or thrombotic disorders. Pigmented purpuric eruptions are benign disorders most commonly presenting on the lower legs as chronic yellow-brown, irregular patches with superimposed pinpoint red macules. These disorders are usually distinctive clinically, and pathology is limited to mild capillaritis of the skin. Purpuras caused by coagulopathies are generally nonpalpable and retiform, branching, or stellate in nature. Associated livedo reticularis and necrosis are common. Thrombocytopenia presents with petechial lesions that are nonpalpable and usually smaller than palpable purpura lesions, in the range of 1 to 5 mm. Coagulopathy panels and platelet counts promptly distinguish these different conditions. It may be more difficult to readily diagnose embolic or thrombotic disorders. Cholesterol emboli may present with a showering of purpuric lesions in the lower extremities. This condition typically follows an invasive vascular procedure and frequently is associated with hypereosinophilia. A skin biopsy may be necessary for establishing a diagnosis based on typical cholesterol clefts. Bacterial sepsis or endocarditis may also present with septic emboli that resemble palpable purpura. Patients with this condition are generally systemically ill and exhibit positive blood cultures.

Henoch-Schönlein Purpura

Henoch-Schönlein purpura (HSP) deserves specific mention because of its history and frequency. Heberden described the first case in a 4-year-old boy in 1801. Schönlein in 1837 and Henoch in 1874 reported additional cases in children. This condition classically presents in children between 5 and 15 years old with palpable purpura, arthritis, nephritis, and colicky abdominal pain. Thirty percent of cases follow an upper respiratory infection, and 10% are associated with the use of β lactam antibiotics. The clinical outcome is excellent in more than 90% of cases without treatment. A few percent will develop persistent renal or gastroenterologic manifestations and may require immunosuppressive therapy. Direct immunofluorescence of skin biopsies demonstrates perivascular IgA deposits.

Cryoglobulinemia

Another important subtype of cutaneous vasculitis is related to hepatitis C and cryoglobulins. Cryoglobulinemia has been identified as a trigger for palpable purpura for many years. It was considered an idiopathic condition until 1990 when Pascual described a link between hepatitis C and essential mixed cryoglobulinemia. It is now well recognized that 40% of patients with chronic hepatitis C infection produce cryoglobulins, which is a type of rheumatoid factor (antibodies that react with the Fc portion of other antibodies) that precipitates in the cold. Ten percent of the patients with cryoglobulinemia develop cutaneous vasculitis with palpable purpura, Raynaud's phenomenon, nephritis, and peripheral neuropathy. It is important to recognize patients who have palpable purpura that is caused by hepatitis C, because the key to their treatment is antiviral therapy.

Treatment

Cutaneous vasculitis is usually a relatively benign condition. The most important intervention is often the recognition and removal of an underlying trigger, such as a medication or infection. Symptomatic improvement may be achieved with leg elevation, nonsteroidal anti-inflammatory drugs, and antihistamines. Persistent palpable purpura without significant internal organ complications may respond to treatment with colchicine[1] (0.6 mg given twice daily), hydroxychloroquine (Plaquenil)[1] (200 mg given at a dose of 6.25 mg/kg per day), or dapsone[1] (100 to 200 mg per day).

Repeated clinical evaluation of patients for indication of renal, GI, or neurologic manifestations is essential. Physical examination and urine analysis for microscopic hematuria and proteinuria should be conducted on a periodic basis until the patient has stabilized. Development of internal organ involvement usually indicates a need for systemic corticosteroid therapy. Prednisone[1] can be started at a moderate dose (0.5 to 1 mg/kg per day), gradually tapering once the patient's symptoms have stabilized. Unfortunately there are no prospective, randomized trials of immunosuppressant medications to guide

[1]Not FDA approved for this indication.

treatment of these patients. If patients develop severe renal disease, more potent immunosuppressive medications such as azathioprine (Imuran)[1] (2 mg/kg per day), methotrexate[1] (7.5 to 15 mg once a week), or cyclophosphamide (Cytoxan)[1] (2 mg/kg per day) may be indicated. Patients with cryoglobulinemia secondary to hepatitis C should be treated with antiviral agents such as interferon-α[1] (3 million units three times a week) and ribavirin[1] (1000 mg per day). In life-threatening cases, prednisone, cyclophosphamide, and plasmapheresis may be indicated.

Cutaneous vasculitis is a relatively common and benign form of vasculitis. It usually presents with palpable purpura but may occasionally progress to involve the joints, kidneys, bowel, or peripheral nerves. The most important step in treating these patients is often the correct identification and treatment of an underlying drug, infection, or connective tissue disease that has triggered the vasculitis. In the majority of patients, the vasculitis will spontaneously resolve and they will not need immunosuppressive therapy. If patients develop internal organ complications, a course of prednisone or other immunosuppressive medication may be indicated.

[1]Not FDA approved for this indication.

DISEASES OF THE NAILS

METHOD OF

Bertrand Richert, MD, PhD

The nail apparatus has a peculiar anatomy responsible for its limited repertoire of clinical expressions. If one is to understand the pathogenesis of diseases affecting the nails then a detailed knowledge of the three-dimensional anatomy and physiology is mandatory. Appropriate treatment of diseases of the nails requires an accurate diagnosis. Any nail sign should prompt examination of the whole integument including hairs and mucous membranes. Questioning should include all medical history and drug intake. Sometimes complementary exams (e.g., radiograph, magnetic resonance imaging [MRI], biopsy) may be needed. And it is of utmost importance to explain to the patient that healing may be expected to take several months, because the full renewal of a fingernail takes 6 months and a great toenail can take up to 18 months to heal.

Infections of the Nails

ACUTE PARONYCHIA

Acute paronychia is an acute infection of the proximal nail fold resulting in swelling and pus collection. The pus may even extend laterally to both lateral nail folds, encircling the nail, giving rise to the so-called "runaround." It mostly results from a staphylococcal infection secondary to a break in the epidermis. In some rare instances it may correspond to a *Fusarium* infection (mold onychomycosis).

Systemic penicillinase-fast antibiotics should be administered in association with soaking in disinfectants (povidone iodine [Betadine] or chlorhexidine [Hibiclens]) and applications of antibiotic ointments (fusidic acid [Fucidin][2], mupirocin [Bactroban]). If there is no obvious improvement within 48 hours, surgery is mandatory in order to avoid any irreversible damage to the matrix. For this procedure, the proximal third of the nail plate is avulsed under proximal digital block, and the pus is harvested for culture. Diabetes and immunosuppression should be searched for.

ONYCHOMYCOSIS

Onychomycosis represents approximately 50% of all nail diseases. Because onychomycosis can present in many guises, it is impossible to determine that a nail dystrophy is an onychomycosis without having performed culture of nail clippings. Moreover, it should be kept in mind that another nail disorder, such as psoriasis or onychogryphosis, may become contaminated with fungi and that treatment of the mycosis may only slightly improve the dystrophy. Approximately 85% of onychomycoses are caused by dermatophytes.

Treatment should be prescribed only after confirmation of the infection. If only the distal third of the distal nail is affected, application of a nail lacquer (amorolfine [Loceryl][2], ciclopirox [Penlac]) should be attempted for 3 to 6 months. If there is improvement with that regimen, it should be carried on for at least 9 months. If there is no improvement or worsening, then combined therapy (débridement, systemic antifungals, and topical antifungals) is advisable. The nail should be largely débrided to remove as much as possible of the fungi. For that purpose, drilling of the infected portion of the nail may be necessary. Chemical avulsion using 40% urea under occlusion during 5 to 8 days is very comfortable. It will soften and detach the entire contaminated nail, allowing a painless removal of the dermatophytoma. In case of matricial involvement (meaning that the infection goes under the proximal nail fold), surgical avulsion is mandatory under local block. Several systemic

[2]Not available in the United States.

antifungals are available and should be prescribed as follows:

- Terbinafine (Lamisil), 250 mg per day for 6 weeks for fingernail infections, and 12 weeks for toenail infections
- Itraconazole (Sporanox), 200 mg twice a day with meals, 7 days a month for 3 months
- Fluconazole (Diflucan), 200 mg once a week until healing is complete

Terbinafine has fewer drug interactions and is more efficient on dermatophytes. Transungual delivery systems (amorolfine[2], ciclopirox) are applied on the remnant nail. Recurrences may be prevented by weekly application of topical antifungal cream in the toe webs and daily antifungal powder in the shoes. The physician should inform the patient that because of the slow growth of the nails, the appearance of their nails may still be abnormal at the end of treatment.

WARTS

Warts are the most common nail tumor affecting the nail apparatus. Although they are mostly localized periungually, they may also be found subungually and, rarely, on the undersurface of the proximal nail fold. Treatment should be adapted to the number of lesions, their location on the nail apparatus, their duration, and the immunologic status of the patient. It should also be cost-effective. Warts often disappear spontaneously in children in a few months or several years, therefore, treatment should not be too aggressive. Spontaneous resolution is far less common in adults and in immunocompromised patients. In adults, any longstanding warty lesions, resistant to proper therapy, should always be biopsied to rule out Bowen's disease.

Treatment includes physical destruction, chemical destruction, and immunomodulation. In children and in adults onychophagia should be discouraged and soles carefully checked for plantar warts. Keratolytics (e.g., DuoFilm) are the first choice treatment especially in children. Their use should be clearly explained to the parents. In most instances, the wart will disappear after several months if the treatment has been done properly. After several weeks, cautious cryotherapy may be performed, especially on the proximal nail fold overlying the matrix. Excessive freezing may result in transitory leukonychia, Beau's line, or permanent nail dystrophy. Application of EMLA (eutectic mixture of local anesthetics) cream (lidocaine, prilocaine) before cryotherapy does not reduce the pain of freezing. In adults the treatment of choice is intralesional injection of bleomycin (Blenoxane)[1] using the bleopuncture technique (multiple punctures to introduce bleomycin within the wart). A Dermo-Jet should never be used in the vicinity of the nail apparatus as it may be responsible for transitory or permanent nail dystrophy. Moreover Raynaud's phenomenon may be a side effect of the technique. Under a digital wing block, a drop of bleomycin solution (1 U/mL) is laid on the wart and pricked into the lesion by multiple rapid punctures with a vaccination needle. The use of a tourniquet may be useful to reduce bleeding during the procedure. Antiseptic dressings are applied for 48 hours. Necrosis of the wart occurs within 1 week and the wart is eliminated in 3 weeks.

Laser treatments (CO_2, erbium-YAG [yttrium-aluminum-garnet], and pulsed-dye lasers) have the same cure rate as the above mentioned treatments; however, their cost limits their use for this condition.

Among the treatments with immunomodulators, imiquimod (Aldara)[1] seems promising but cannot be recommended considering its cost. Efficacy of interferon-alfa[1] and cimetidine (Tagamet)[1] has not yet been proven, and they are not advisable in such a benign condition. Photodynamic therapy is anecdotal considering its very high cost and associated pain.

Virucidal agents, radiotherapy, electrosurgery, and surgery are obsolete treatments for this condition and should not be recommended to the patient.

Nails and Dermatological Diseases

PSORIASIS

Approximately 90% of psoriatic patients experience nail involvement with their disease once in their life. Fingers are more prone to be affected than toenails. In children, 7% to 40% of nail dystrophies are caused by psoriasis. Psoriasis limited to the nails is not rare. The severity of the nail disease is not correlated with that of the skin disease. Nail involvement is more common in cases with concomitant psoriatic arthropathy. Psoriasis may be responsible for several clinical features that may occur simultaneously or separately. Nail psoriasis semiology is proteiform and reflects the location of the disease. It is mandatory to locate it accurately in order to treat it properly. Nail matrix psoriasis presents as pits, which are typically deep, large, and scattered. Rough nails with excessive longitudinal striation and adherent horny scales, called trachyonychia, may also be observed. Beau's line, mottled lunulae, and leukonychia are seldom encountered. Nail bed psoriasis shows with an oily, salmon-colored patch on the medial part of the nail bed. Distal subungual hyperkeratosis and onycholysis are very common. An erythema outlining the onycholysis on its proximal border is very suggestive of psoriasis. Whole matrix involvement results in a crumbling nail.

Treatment is long, tedious, and sometimes unsatisfactory. Because it has an unpredictable course, it is important that doctors and patients have realistic expectations. Lithium and β-blockers may exacerbate psoriasis and should be replaced if possible.

[1]Not FDA approved for this indication.
[2]Not available in the United States.

[1]Not FDA approved for this indication.

Nails should be kept short, and gloves should be worn for any manual work to reduce the potential risk of Koebner phenomenon. Nail matrix psoriasis such as pits, salmon patch, mottled lunulae, or leukonychia should not be treated. In women, nail lacquers should be recommended and artificial nails highly discouraged. Trachyonychia heals spontaneously in several months or years. Intramatrical steroid injections (0.2 to 0.3 mL of triamcinolone acetonide[1] 10 mg/mL) may hasten its resolution in motivated patients. Nail bed psoriasis is the easiest one to treat. Topical drugs may be used, but because they cannot be applied to reach the nail bed through the nail plate or the matrix through the dorsal nail fold, the nail plate must first be clipped away to the most proximal portion of the onycholysis. High potency steroids (clobetasol propionate [Temovate]) may be massaged twice daily or applied under an occlusive material at night. Tazarotene (Tazorac) gel, applied once a day, may be tried. Vitamin D derivatives are useful in reducing the subungual hyperkeratosis and may be used in combination with the two previous ones. Subungual keratosis is most responsive to intralesional steroid therapy. The injection is performed under a local digital block and 0.2 to 0.3 mL of triamcinolone acetonide[1] 10 mg/mL are injected under the nail plate into the nail bed. The procedure may be repeated after 2 to 3 months. Two sessions are usually enough. This technique should be used only if a few nails are involved. If several nails are affected as well as the skin, or if there is a psoriatic arthropathy, systemic treatments should be considered. Acitretin (Soriatane) is effective on the subungual hyperkeratosis. Other forms may worsen from the side effects of the drugs on the nail apparatus. Methotrexate and cyclosporine should be prescribed as first-line therapy when nail psoriasis is associated with psoriatic arthropathy.

LICHEN PLANUS

Nail involvement occurs in approximately 10% of patients who have lichen planus elsewhere. Isolated nail lichen planus is not uncommon. The clinical features of nail lichen planus depend on the location of the disease on the nail apparatus, its severity, and its duration. Nail matrix involvement is frequent and manifests as brittle nails with thinning of the nail plate, excessive longitudinal striation, or deep longitudinal splits (onychorrhexis). Approximately 10% to 15% of all trachyonychias may be caused by lichen planus. The inflammatory process enhances the progressive fusion of the proximal nail fold with the underlying matrix (and even the nail bed), resulting in a projection of the proximal nail fold, called dorsal pterygium, that divides the nail plate in two lateral segments. As the pterygium widens, the lateral nail segments narrow. Involvement of the nail bed is rare, but when it occurs, it leads to a distal subungual hyperkeratosis with or without onycholysis. If diagnosis is made early, the patient may avoid permanent scarring.

The treatment of choice is systemic corticotherapy—oral methylprednisolone[1], 0.5 mg/kg every other day for 6 weeks, then tapering over another 6-week period; or triamcinolone acetonide, 40 mg intramuscularly once a month for 6 to 8 months. Side effects are less frequent with the intramuscular route. If the condition is limited to few nails, intramatrical injection of triamcinolone acetonide[1] (10 mg/mL), 0.2 to 0.3 mL per digit, is recommended. Oral retinoids (acitretin[1], 0.4 mg/kg per day) are an alternative.

ALOPECIA AREATA

Nail dystrophy is commonly reported in association with alopecia areata—its prevalence widely ranges from 7% to 66% according to studies. Its severity is not correlated with the severity of the alopecia areata, and the nail dystrophy does not imply a poor prognosis of the alopecia areata. Nail alterations are two times more frequent in children than in adults. Nail dystrophies mostly reported are pitting and trachyonychia. Patients should be informed that the nail alterations may persist long after total recovery of the alopecia areata.

No treatment is required. Cosmetic care (smoothing nail lacquers) is advisable in women. In very motivated patients, massaging the proximal nail fold twice a day with very potent corticosteroids may hasten healing of the condition. If only a few nails are involved, intramatrical injections of 0.2 to 0.3 mL triamcinolone acetonide[1] 10 mg/mL may be suggested.

Nails and Systemic Diseases

YELLOW NAIL SYNDROME

Yellow nail syndrome affects the nails, the limbs, and the respiratory tract. Patients seek first medical advice for this condition primarily because of the cosmetic appearance of their nails. The nails are thickened, very hard, yellowish, opaque, and show transversal and/or longitudinal over-curvature. *Pseudomonas* contamination may be responsible for a greenish hue. Nail growth is dramatically slowed down or even stopped. Cuticles are absent. Lower limbs are often affected with lymphedema. Cautious exploration reveals an involvement of the upper or lower respiratory tract. Chest radiographs may reveal pleural effusion.

Treatment should address the underlying disease. Oral high doses of vitamin E (800 to 1000 mg per day) may improve the condition and should always be prescribed, considering its innocuousness. Some azole antifungals (itraconazole [Sporanox][1], fluconazole [Diflucan][1]) are proven to stimulate the nail's growth,

[1]Not FDA approved for this indication.

[1]Not FDA approved for this indication.

but their prescription cannot be recommended if there is no concomitant onychomycosis because of their side effects and their cost.

ACROKERATOSIS PARANEOPLASTICA

Acrokeratosis paraneoplastica syndrome (also called Bazex and Dupré syndrome) should be known since it reveals an internal malignancy. The main sign is brittle nails. The nails are invariably involved and are typically the earliest manifestation of the condition. Cautious examination of the integument may reveal symmetric psoriasiform erythematosquamous plaques on the fingers, feet, ears, and nose. An exhaustive search for primary tumor is mandatory.

Treatment is given to the underlying tumor. This paraneoplastic sign may precede the manifestation of the malignancy, disappear with its removal, and reappear with its recurrence. However, the nail involvement may not always clear up with the removal of the tumor, unlike the other skin signs. If the tumor is not removable or if the nails are still affected after the cure of the malignancy, systemic retinoids (acitretin [Soriatane][1]) may be helpful.

Tumors of the Nails

Tumors of the nail apparatus may be difficult to diagnose. Depending on their location, they may be responsible for several clinical features. As a rule, benign lesions induce a deformation of the nail apparatus (exophytic mass lifting up the plate, onycholysis, longitudinal groove resulting from the pressure of the lesion on the matrix, etc.), whereas malignant tumors progressively destroy the nail and its surrounding structures (erosion, bleeding, oozing, etc.).

Any suspicious lesion should undergo medical imaging and/or biopsy. Treatment is surgical and should be performed by surgeons skilled in nail and/or hand surgery.

Trauma to the Nail

SUBUNGUAL HEMATOMA

Subungual hematoma is secondary to an acute trauma. Pain results from the pressure of blood stuck between the nail plate and bone. Evacuation of the hematoma should be performed as soon as possible, ideally within a few hours.

If the hematoma occurs in less than 25% of the visible nail, evacuation of the blood will alleviate pain immediately. Several techniques may be used to trephine the nail plate including a hot paper clip, thermocautery, CO_2 laser vaporization, and others. A compressive dressing should be applied to the nail plate while it readheres to the nail bed.

[1]Not FDA approved for this indication.

If the hematoma involves more than 25% of the nail surface, radiographs are mandatory to rule out a bony fracture. The nail plate should be avulsed to check the integrity of the nail bed and repair any laceration using 6/0 resorbable sutures. The nail plate is cleaned up with hydrogen peroxide, narrowed by several millimeters, perforated with a 3 mm punch in its median portion (to evacuate any oozing), and secured onto the nail bed with stitches in the lateral nail folds. The sutures should be left on for up to 3 weeks. Onychoptosis will follow in most instances.

ONYCHOTILLOMANIA

Onychotillomania refers to the compulsive habit of playing with the nails, leading to several clinical features. Any tool may be used for this purpose, for example, another nail, scissors, and razor blades, among others. In most cases the manipulation is acknowledged by patients or their relatives; but in some instances it is caused by deliberate acts of self-mutilation within the confines of pathomimesis. Various nail dystrophies may be observed (e.g., brachyonychia, partial or even total destruction of the nail plate, subacute paronychia), with the most common being habit tic (washboard nails) and Heller's dystrophy (longitudinal median split with lateral feathery cracks). The existence of a macrolunula should be considered as a clue to onychotillomania.

Treatment is difficult and any *trick* should be attempted. Nail wrapping of the proximal part of the nail plate and the proximal nail fold with adhesive tape 24 hours a day every day for several months may help to stop the habit of pushing back the cuticles. In most instances, the nail will regrow normally but the macrolunula will persist. In case of pathomimesis, fluoxetine (Prozac)[1] or omeprazole (Prilosec)[1] should be prescribed, if possible, with involvement of a psychiatrist.

INGROWN TOENAIL

Ingrown toenail is a very common condition, especially during childhood. It is promoted by improper trimming of the nails (tear off and cutting in the corners) and hyperhidrosis, which is exacerbated by wearing sport shoes. This condition often leads to an inflammatory reaction and development of granulation tissue with concomitant oozing, bleeding, and infection.

Treatment may be conservative at the early stage. Under local block, granulation tissue is curetted and the lateral border of the nail smoothed off (excision of any spicule). Local antiseptics (e.g., povidone iodine [Betadine]) are applied postoperatively twice daily. If this conservative treatment fails or if the condition recurs, a definitive cure should be achieved using partial chemical matricectomy. After local anesthesia and in a bloodless field (tourniquet), the

[1]Not FDA approved for this indication.

lateral fifth of the nail plate is avulsed and the matrix cauterized during 2 to 3 minutes with a Q-Tip dipped into 88% phenol. Postoperative pain is minimal as phenol has anesthetic properties. Oozing will persist into the lateral nail fold for approximately 4 to 6 weeks. Soakings with antiseptics twice daily will prevent infection and enhance healing.

KELOIDS

METHOD OF

Sandra Lee, MD, Cameron K. Rokhsar, MD, and Richard E. Fitzpatrick, MD

Keloids are benign, fibrous proliferations that usually occur at sites of injury or inflammation such as after blunt trauma, surgery, vaccinations, tattoos, burns, body piercings, acne, and varicella infection. They also occur spontaneously without any known antecedent inciting factor. Keloids, by definition, extend beyond the borders of the original wound, do not regress spontaneously, and tend to recur after excision. They can be firm or pliable, erythematous, hyperpigmented or flesh-colored, and can be asymptomatic or elicit burning, pain, or itch. Males and females are equally affected, most frequently between 10 and 30 years of age, with the very young and very old rarely affected. In general, the darker the skin color, the higher the risk for developing keloids. Keloids occur most commonly on the upper anterior and posterior trunk, the proximal upper extremities, and the earlobes. They are commonly compared to hypertrophic scars, which are a distinct clinical, histologic, and pathophysiologic entity (Table 1). Keloids are more resistant to treatment than hypertrophic scars, are often cosmetically disfiguring, and are a source of embarrassment and discomfort for the patient and frustration for the treating physician.

Histologically, keloids are composed of an abundance of fibroblasts creating layers of large eosinophilic acellular collagen bundles interspersed with plasma cells, mast cells, and lymphocytes. There is also an abundance of mucopolysaccharide ground substance.

The etiology for keloids remains elusive. Excessive synthesis of collagens, fibronectin, and proteoglycans by fibroblasts, or deficient matrix degradation and remodeling may lead to keloids, but the mechanisms behind these processes are poorly understood. Keloids have increased prolyl hydroxylase activity, and collagen synthesis rates are reported to be increased by 20-fold. The initiating factors that lead to the formation of keloids are yet to be discovered, and thus we are unable to prevent such lesions from occurring. Although there are many treatment options employed in an attempt to eradicate keloids, unfortunately, there has not been consistent success with any one treatment. Studies provide a variety of information, such as reports of a decrease in apoptosis within keloids, reports suggesting hypoxia may be an inciting factor, and reports that postulate an abnormal immune reaction as the etiology. Most promising are recent studies conducted at the cellular level aimed at characterizing the cytokines and growth factors that are expressed within keloids. Studies have reported increases in hyaluronic acid, transforming growth factor β (TGFβ) types 1 and 2, which stimulate fibroblasts, and tissue plasminogen activator inhibitor type I (PAI-1), which inhibits plasmin, an important regulator of fibrin formation. Recent therapeutic interventions have been directed toward the newer discoveries on the biologic and molecular level.

PRESSURE THERAPY

Pressure therapy is proven successful in lesions that are less than 6 months old. It is believed that pressure augments collagen maturation and induces localized tissue hypoxia, leading to a reduction in keloid height. It is recommended that a pressure

TABLE 1 Differences Between Keloids and Hypertrophic Scars

	Keloids	Hypertrophic Scars
Clinical	Growth of fibrous tissue beyond border of site of injury	Growth confined to site of injury
Timing	Median delay of 30.4 months before keloidal formation	Usually occurs within 4 weeks of injury
Racial predilection	Increased prevalence in higher Fitzpatrick skin types	No racial predilection
Recurrence rate	More likely to recur	Less likely to recur
Regression	Not likely to regress	Possibility for regression
Histology	Large collagen bundles, few macrophages, many eosinophils, mast cells, plasma cells, lymphocytes; associated with mucopolysaccharide ground substance	Collagen only in mid to deep component; contains α-smooth-muscle actin-staining myofibroblasts
Pathophysiology	Fibroblasts produce high levels of collagen, elastin, fibronectin, and proteoglycan, and show abnormal responses to stimulation; collagen I and III production, in particular is increased	Moderate increase in basal level of collagen production, but still responds normally to growth factors

garment (25 to 40 mm Hg) be worn over the areas of concern for 23 to 24 hours per day, continuously for 1 year or more until there is a clinical decrease in inflammation. However, this method is not consistently successful, and the garments can be uncomfortable and decrease mobility.

SURGERY

Primary excision or scar revision has not been very successful, with recurrences being reported in 45% to 100% of patients. Pairing of surgery with cryotherapy, radiation, or intralesional injections of corticosteroid, 5-fluorouracil, or interferon[1] decreases the recurrence rate, although inconsistently.

CORTICOSTEROIDS

Intralesional injection of triamcinolone[1] (10 to 40 mg/mL) is commonly employed for treatment of both hypertrophic scars and keloids. A 50% response rate in keloids studied for a 5-year period is reported as well as a second report of five recurrences in 56 keloids over 4 years. It is more common for intralesional corticosteroid injection to soften or flatten keloids or to provide symptomatic relief rather than to make keloids disappear or decrease in circumference. Multiple injections are necessary, performed at 2- to 4-week intervals, and typically are very painful. Adverse effects include tissue atrophy, telangiectasias, hypopigmentation, necrosis, ulceration, and striae. These side effects have been reported in as many as 40% of patients treated. The mechanism of action of corticosteroids is thought to be through the inhibition of transcription of certain matrix protein genes, such as fibronectin, TGFβ, and other cytokines.

RADIOTHERAPY

Radiation alone has not proven to be successful, but radiation therapy within 10 days of surgical excision has been shown to prevent keloid recurrence. Superficial irradiation has been used at doses of 900 cGy or greater, in fractions. However, the risks may outweigh the benefits with such a treatment because of the carcinogenic potential of radiation therapy.

SILICONE GEL SHEETING

Topical silicone gel sheeting has been a popular treatment modality, primarily because of the low risk for adverse effects. It appears to work through hydration of tissue or elevation of scar temperature. Collagenase activity is known to increase significantly with only 1°F (0.6°C) to 2°F (1.1°C) increases in body temperature. Two months of daily application is recommended, and scars less than 3 years old appear to be more responsive to this therapy.

[1]Not FDA approved for this indication.

CRYOTHERAPY

Cryosurgery is reported to be successful if lesions are less than 1 year old. It is postulated that the ischemic damage triggered by cryosurgery with liquid nitrogen leads to necrosis and decreased bulk of the keloid, resulting in flattening of the lesion. Cryosurgery should be performed with caution on keloids of darkly pigmented individuals because of the risk of irreversible hypopigmentation.

IMMUNOMODULATORS

Imiquimod

Some recent case studies report the shrinking of keloids using imiquimod (Aldara)[1] 5% cream. Imiquimod, which is FDA-approved for the treatment of human papillomavirus infection, has been found to be effective in the treatment of other viral infections of the skin such as common warts and molluscum contagiosum, and in actinic keratosis and superficial nonmelanoma skin cancers. Imiquimod may be useful in treating keloids by stimulating the local increase in interferons, which are believed to increase collagenase activity and reduce collagen formation. When used for treatment of keloids, it is applied twice daily every other day, with application frequency adjusted to avoid a significant inflammatory response.

5-Fluorouracil

Because of the high incidence of side effects coupled with the unpredictable efficacy of intralesional corticosteroids, intralesional 5-fluorouracil (Efudex) (5-FU) has been used for the treatment of both hypertrophic scars and keloids. It is a pyrimidine analogue with antimetabolite activity that inhibits fibroblast proliferation in tissue culture. Its use in keloids has not been particularly successful because of the drug's short duration of action and the need for ongoing painful intralesional injections (50 mg/mL) as often as two to three times per week. Injection frequency is decreased as the response of the keloid progresses. In treatment of symptomatic hypertrophic scars, however, 5-FU is proven to be comparable, if not superior, to intralesional corticosteroids without the associated side effects.

Interferon

Interferon gamma-1b (Actimmune)[1] (IFN-γ), 10 μg one to three times per week, is also used as an intralesional agent for the treatment of keloids, as well as in the prevention of recurrences. IFN-γ inhibits collagen synthesis by transcriptional regulation. All three interferons (IFN-α, IFN-β, IFN-γ) increase collagenase release by fibroblasts, but IFN-γ appears to inhibit collagen synthesis more than the other interferons. However, IFN-γ also increases

[1]Not FDA approved for this indication.

glycosaminoglycan production, while IFN-α and IFN-β decrease glycosaminoglycan synthesis. Studies using interferon alfa-2b (Intron A)[1] (IFN-α2β) with or without antecedent surgical excision report variable success, with recurrence rates ranging from 19% to 50% of patients. In the study, 1 to 3 million units (MU) of IFN-α2β were used at various intervals according to different protocols. Conclusions regarding the success of IFN-γ and IFN-α2β therapy are difficult to analyze, because follow-up has been short-term, many studies were uncontrolled, and treatment regimens differed widely among protocols.

PULSED-DYE LASER

The pulsed-dye laser has been used successfully to treat hypertrophic scars and keloids. The choice of treatment parameters has a significant impact on response, and multiple treatment sessions are necessary, typically 5 to 10. If visible telangiectasias are part of the scar, it appears to be important to eliminate these vessels for successful treatment. There is some suggestion that lower fluences may be more effective than higher fluences in stimulating collagen remodeling, but this remains unclear now. Fluences in the range of 3.0 to 7.0 J/cm^2 have been used. More recently formed lesions appear to respond much better than older lesions.

Keloids have been a treatment dilemma for centuries. Although there are many treatment options, and promising discoveries have been recently made on the cellular level, there still exists no single treatment that is consistently successful. However, general conclusions can be drawn—early treatment appears to be more successful than later treatment, and a multiple modality approach appears to be superior.

[1]Not FDA approved for this indication.

WARTS (VERRUCAE)

METHOD OF

Tamara Salam Housman, MD, and

Phillip M. Williford, MD

Viral warts afflict approximately 10% of the population and are caused by human papillomavirus (HPV). HPV, a nonenveloped, double-stranded DNA virus, is of the papovavirus class and invades both mucous and squamous epithelium. At least 130 known types of HPV have been identified. HPV causes both clinical and subclinical infection and plays a role in certain cutaneous carcinomas, including squamous cell carcinoma (SCCa) of the anogenital area and nail unit. HPV is found in the basal layer of the epidermis but replicates only in the superficial, well-differentiated layer. The subsequent cellular proliferation gives rise to thick, hyperkeratotic lesions generally known as warts.

Cutaneous warts are mainly divided into common warts, plantar warts, flat warts, and genital warts. Common warts account for 70% of all cutaneous warts and are probably associated with HPV types 1, 2, and 4. Two thirds of untreated common warts spontaneously regress within 2 years, but these previously infected individuals have a higher rate of developing new warts than those who were never infected. Treatment of warts with salicylic acid and/or cryotherapy has demonstrated a 60% to 80% cure rate.

Transmission is via skin-to-skin contact, including sexual, and is seen with greater frequency where groups of people are in close contact, including in school-age children, with a frequency of 20% for common warts. Extent of infection is determined by the immune response, and immunocompromised hosts are at increased risk. Symptoms may include pain and bleeding, and warts may interfere with daily functioning, especially if located on the palms, soles, or digits. Warts can be professionally and socially stigmatizing, especially if located on the hands or fingers of patients who must touch others on a daily basis.

Types of Warts

Verrucae vulgares (common warts) are flesh-colored, hyperkeratotic, verrucous, fissured, firm papules that disrupt normal skin lines on fingers and toes. They may be distinguished from calluses and corns by paring down of the stratum corneum (the uppermost horny layer of skin) to reveal thrombosed/ bleeding capillaries seen as brown/black dots. A subtype is a butcher's wart, which is seen on the hands of butchers and fish and meat handlers/packers, and appears as large, cauliflower plaques. Differential diagnoses (DDx) include seborrheic keratosis, molluscum contagiosum, keratoacanthoma, amelanotic melanoma, SCCa in situ, and invasive SCCa. Verrucae vulgares warts are associated with HPV subtypes 1, 2, 4.

Verrucae plantares (plantar warts) are flesh-colored, hyperkeratotic, endophytic papules or plaques located on the soles of the feet that also disrupt normal skin lines and may have thrombosed capillaries manifested as brown/black dots. These can be quite painful and interfere with mobility and daily functioning, especially if located on sites of pressure. A mosaic wart occurs if multiple plantar warts coalesce into a plaque. DDx include callus, corns, exostosis, and acral melanoma. Verrucae plantares warts are associated with HPV subtypes 1, 2, 4, 27, 57.

Verrucae planae (flat warts) are tan- to flesh-colored, flat, sharply demarcated papules located on

TABLE 1 Treatment of Verrucae

Therapy	Available Preparations	Mechanism of Action	Application	Dosage	Disadvantages Adverse Effects
Salicylic acid (keratolytic) (Compound W)	Solution Gel/lotion/cream Plaster Pad 10%-60%	Destruction of infected epidermis; irritation leads to stimulation of immune response.	Patient applied. Adjunct to other treatment modalities. May pare down/shave wart then apply keratolytic to increase penetration.	qhs until clear, usually weeks to months.	Irritation
Cryosurgery	Liquid nitrogen (−196°C [−320.8°F]): cryospray or cotton-tipped applicator	Destruction of infected epidermis; induces inflammation leading to stimulation of immune response.	Physician applied. Paring of thick lesions → liquid nitrogen freeze for 30-60 sec to include a 1-2 mm rim around wart → let thaw → repeat × 2 cycles total. Adjunct to other treatment modalities. Careful with periungual warts, overlying tendons, and on lower extremities.	May repeat q3-4wk.	Pain Erythema Vesicle/bullae Crusting Possible infection Hypopigmentation Scarring (if freeze too deep) Onychodystrophy (if not careful with periungual warts)
Cantharidin[1,2]	Colloidal solution, 0.7%	Destruction of epidermis and leads to blister formation; extract of blister beetle.	Physician applied. Paring of thick lesions. Apply using very fine applicator only to wart then patient is to wash off in 6-8h. Painless—good for children.	May repeat q2-4wk.	Vesicle/bullae Crusting Avoid face or near eyes
Surgical excision Curettage Electrocautery	N/A	Destruction by surgical removal of wart.	Physician applied. Surgical excision of wart or surgical removal by curetting wart then cauterizing the base.	Usually only performed once but may repeat if wart recurs.	Painful (minimal if use local anesthesia but some postoperative pain) Scarring
Trichloroacetic acid (Tri-Chlor) Bichloroacetic acid	Solution, up to 50% concentration	Destruction of infected epidermis.	Physician applied.	Most useful for mucosal warts.	Painful reactions
Lasers: Carbon dioxide Pulsed-dye Erbium:YAG	N/A	Destruction of infected epidermis.	Physician applied.	May repeat q4-6wk.	Expensive Risk of viral spread via laser plume Not superior to conventional therapy
Imiquimod	Cream, 5%	Immunomodulator: indirect in vivo anti-tumor and antiviral effects mediated by induction of cytokines—IFN-α, TNF-α, IL-1, -6, -8, and others.	Patient applied. On nonmucosal skin, including plantar/palmar warts, apply keratolytic, followed by occlusion in P.M., followed by imiquimod in A.M.; may also occlude imiquimod if not getting any erythema. If irritation is severe, stop regimen for few days then resume, if possible. May initiate therapy with cryosurgery followed by keratolytic-imiquimod combination therapy for 6wks then repeat if necessary.	3 times/wk on mucosal skin; 5-7 times/wk on keratinized skin.	Irritation Erythema Pruritus Burning Crusting Infection Scarring

TABLE 1 Treatment of Verrucae—cont'd

Therapy	Available Preparations	Mechanism of Action	Application	Dosage	Disadvantages Adverse Effects
Cimetidine (Tagamet)[1]	Tablets: 200 mg, 300 mg, 400 mg, 800 mg; liquid: 300 mg/5 mL	Immunomodulator: at high doses may enhance immune response.	Patient initiated.	25 to 40 mg/kg daily, divided bid to qid.	True efficacy unclear
DPC[1] SADBE[1] DNCB[1]	Acetone solution, 0.001-2% Acetone solution, 0.01-1%	Immunomodulator: inducing a delayed hypersensitivity reaction thus leading to stimulation of immune response.	Physician applied. Sensitize patient by applying 2%-3% solution of SADBE/DPC to 1 cm area on inner arm → may need to resensitize every 10-14d until get local reaction (erythema/vesicle).	After sensitization, apply to wart using 0.03%-2% solution once per wk until clear.	DNCB—possibly mutagenic May be unable to sensitize some patients Irritation Erythema Vesicle/bullae
Retinoids	Acitretin (Soriatane)[1], 10 mg or 25 mg tabs Isotretinoin (Accutane)[1], 10 mg, 20 mg, 40 mg tabs Topical tretinoin (Retin-A)[1], cream/microgel	Antimitotic: interferes with epidermal differentiation and proliferation.	Patient applied/initiated. Good prevention for immunosuppressed/ immunocompromised patients with multiple warts or EDV. Topical retinoids for flat warts.	Systemic: least effective qd or qod dose. Topical: apply qhs to warts only.	Topical: local irritation, erythema, and dryness Systemic: mucocutaneous dryness, abnormal liver function tests, elevated triglycerides, teratogenicity
Bleomycin (Blenoxane)[1]	Aqueous solution, 0.1% (1 mg/mL)	Antimitotic.	Physician applied. Intralesional.	Single dose of 0.1 mL of 1 unit/mL in 0.1% solution with normal saline (unclear if repeat q2-3wk).	Pain (use with local anesthesia) Tissue necrosis Scarring Loss of nail Raynaud's at local site Possible significant systemic absorption
5-Fluorouracil (Adrucil)	Cream, 5%	Antimitotic: inhibition of DNA and RNA synthesis leading to keratinocyte death.	Patient applied. May be combined with topical tretinoin therapy	Once per wk.	Irritation Erythema Edema

[1]Not FDA approved for this indication.
[2]Not available in the United States.
Abbreviations: DNCB = dinitrochlorobenzene; DPC = diphencyclopropenone; EDV = epidermodysplasia verruciformis; SADBE = squaric acid dibutylester; YAG = yttrium-aluminum-garnet.

the dorsum of hands, distal lower extremities, and face; and are often in a linear arrangement after trauma. DDx include molluscum contagiosum, epidermodysplasia verruciformis, and benign syringomas on the face. Verrucae planae warts are associated with HPV subtypes 3, 10.

Epidermodysplasia verruciformis (EDV) is a rare, autosomal recessive, hereditary disorder presenting with extensive, flesh-colored to pink to tan, round, flat papules on the trunk, hands, upper and lower extremities, and face. These do have malignant potential, especially on the face on sun-exposed areas. Patients with EDV are usually infected with multiple types of HPV. DDx include seborrheic keratosis, actinic keratosis, basal cell carcinoma, SCCa in situ, or invasive SCCa. EDV warts are classified into more than 30 associated HPV subtypes, including types 3, 5, 8, 9, 12, 14, 15, 17, 19-25, 36-38, 47, 49, 50.

Verrucous carcinoma is a slow-growing variant of SCCa arising in three sites:

1. Oral mucosa (oral florid papillomatosis)
2. Anogenital region (giant condyloma of Buschke and Löwenstein)
3. Plantar foot (epithelioma cuniculatum)

Verrucous carcinoma warts are associated with HPV subtypes 6, 11.

Diagnosis

Diagnosis is mainly based on clinical findings. In immunocompromised or immunosuppressed patients, biopsy should be performed in large or suspicious lesions to rule out SCCa.

Therapy

It is well accepted that the treatment of warts must be individualized and that usually more than one therapeutic modality is required to achieve complete resolution (Table 1). Conventional destructive treatments include repeated application of topical chemotherapy (i.e., salicylic acid [Compound W], cantharidin[2], podophyllin [Podofin], 5-fluorouracil [Adrucil], etc.), cryosurgery, surgical excision, curettage and/or electrosurgery, and laser therapy. Other approaches include immunotherapy (i.e., intralesional interferon [IFN] [Alferon N], diphencyprone[2]), tape occlusion, and observation. In 20% of immunocompetent individuals, the warts will spontaneously resolve within 3 months. Cure rates for common and plantar verrucae with salicylic acid vary from 60% to 80%. Also, overall cure rates with cryosurgery range from 60% to 80%; and with carbon dioxide and pulsed-dye laser, they range from 45% to 90%. However, these methods are usually painful and expensive. Nonetheless, with most methods, recurrence is common, and repeat visits to the physician are costly.

[2]Not available in the United States.

Intralesional IFN-α, although promising with a 36% to 62% clearance rate of anogenital warts, requires multiple injections in the physician's office, is expensive, and may cause systemic adverse effects. Imiquimod (Aldara)[1], a self-applied, topical agent that induces interferon production at the site of application, is reported to have a 50% eradication rate in the treatment of genital warts. Other treatments include:

- Hyperthermia with hot water (113°F [45°C]) immersion
- Intralesional injection of *Candida*[1]/mumps[1] antigen
- Photodynamic therapy with aminolevulinic acid (Levulan Kerastick)[1] followed by red light irradiation
- Hypnosis
- Duct tape occlusion

Special attention should be paid to immunosuppressed or immunocompromised patients in whom there is a higher rate of malignant transformation of warts, and in whom warts tend to be more resistant and more numerous, and thus may require systemic retinoids as a maintenance regimen.

[1]Not FDA approved for this indication.

CONDYLOMA ACUMINATA (GENITAL WARTS)

METHOD OF

Kenneth H. Fife, MD, PhD

Genital warts, or condyloma acuminata, are benign tumors of the anogenital epithelium that are highly prevalent in the adolescent and adult populations. They represent what is probably the most common sexually transmitted infection in most developed countries. They are caused by infection with one of several of the human papillomaviruses (HPVs). Approximately five of the more than 80 HPV types have been associated with typical benign genital warts; many other HPV types infect genital epithelium, but they are more often associated with premalignant and malignant conditions (e.g., squamous cell carcinoma of the cervix). Mixed infections with more than one HPV type (sometimes including a cancer-associated type) may be relatively common, although the clinical significance of these mixed infections is not certain. Clinically, genital warts may appear as cauliflower-like growths on the external genitalia, inguinal area, perineum, or perianal area that can range in size from a few millimeters to several centimeters in diameter. They may also appear as keratotic papules in the same anatomic distribution. On mucosal surfaces such as the vaginal wall, cervix, or urethral meatus, they are often soft and sessile. There are usually multiple lesions, although solitary condylomata are occasionally seen. Typical genital warts are relatively easy to diagnose by clinical inspection, but atypical lesions may require biopsy for confirmation. The lesions are usually the color of the surrounding skin or mucous membrane. Pigmented lesions may contain areas of dysplasia and should be biopsied before determining a course of treatment.

Although it is generally accepted that genital warts are acquired by sexual contact with an infected individual, there are few details regarding specific risk factors for acquisition or transmission that are known with certainty. It is clear that HPV can be present in normal-appearing skin, and it is likely that persons with unrecognized or subclinical infection can transmit infection to a sexual partner. There is no evidence that inanimate objects transmit genital HPV infection. The role of condoms in reducing HPV infection is uncertain. It is likely that condoms reduce the risk of HPV transmission to or from epithelium that is exposed to or covered by the condom. However, genital warts (as well as subclinical HPV infections) may occur outside of areas that would normally be protected by a condom, so HPV transmission from or to these sites (such as the inguinal skin) would not be reduced by condom use.

Treatment

Existing therapies for genital warts are suboptimal because of some combination of poor efficacy, slow response, high recurrence rate, high cost, discomfort, and inconvenience. None of the current treatments provides a reliable cure; even surgical treatments that can effectively remove all of the overt growths in most cases cannot eradicate virus in normal-appearing skin. New lesions often develop in these clinically normal areas days or weeks after the overt lesions are removed. Patients should be made aware of these limitations so that they do not have unrealistic expectations. Many patients are struggling to cope with a diagnosis of a sexually transmitted disease and would like a rapid cure. Clinicians need to be sensitive to this concern and approach patients in an open and nonjudgmental fashion. The decision about a treatment plan should be the result of a dialogue between the clinician and the patient so that the patient has some input and understands the plan and the expectations.

Few of the available treatments for genital warts have been subjected to rigorous controlled clinical trials and very few comparative trials of available treatments have been conducted. Among published clinical trials or case series, different definitions of response and recurrence have been used; and the clinical severity, duration, and treatment history of the patients were different or not specified. For that reason, tables (such as the one shown here) that appear to compare therapies cannot be interpreted in that way. Table 1 shows the major treatment modalities and the ranges of efficacy and recurrence rates that have been reported. In this summary, efficacy is defined as complete clearance of all lesions within the anticipated response time of the treatment. Many studies also report partial responders, but those definitions vary so widely that no attempt was made to include them in the table. It is fair to state that no treatment is clearly superior to another.

Available treatment modalities can be divided in a number of ways, but one useful categorization is to think of them as patient-applied treatments and

TABLE 1 Overview of Genital Wart Treatments[a]

Treatment	% Efficacy[b]	% Recurrence[c]	Comments
Podophyllin (Podofin)	19-80	23-70	Slow response, poorly standardized ingredients
Podofilox (Condylox)	37-88	4-38	Patient applied, slow response
Imiquimod (Aldara)	27-54	13-19	Patient applied, slow response, better in women than men
Trichloroacetic acid (TCA)	63-70	6-50	Slow response
Surgical excision	35-72	19-29	Painful, expensive procedure
Cryotherapy (liquid N_2)	27-88	21-79	Painful, multiple treatments
Electrocautery	61-94	22-30	Painful, expensive procedure
CO_2 laser	23-52	60-77	Painful, expensive equipment
Interferon alfa-2b (Intron A)[d]	17-63	9-69	Intralesional injections difficult, expensive
5-Fluorouracil (5-FU) (Adrucil)[1,d]	10-50	45-58	Moderate local toxicity
Cidofovir (Vistide)[1,e]	33	Unknown	Used topically

[1]Not FDA approved for this indication.
[a]Most results are derived from uncontrolled studies on patient populations that were not comparable; direct comparisons of treatments are not valid (see text).
[b]Eradication of warts within a few weeks of therapy (anticipated time of response varies).
[c]Return of visible warts among patients who initially responded.
[d]Not recommended as first-line therapy.
[e]Reformulated from intravenous preparation for topical use.

provider-administered treatments. It is recommended that clinicians who treat patients with genital warts become familiar with at least one patient-applied treatment and one provider-administered treatment so that the patient can have some choices in treatments offered. Some methods require specialized equipment and training and so are not options for all clinicians.

There are currently two patient-applied treatments, podofilox (Condylox), 0.5% solution or gel, and imiquimod (Aldara), 5% cream. Podofilox is a cytotoxic agent that is derived from the same plant source as podophyllin. However, podofilox contains a single chemical compound and so is better standardized. The drug is available as either a solution or a gel. The gel formulation may be easier to apply to lesions, but it has not been shown to be superior to the solution in comparative trials. Either formulation is applied to each lesion twice daily for 3 consecutive days followed by 4 days of *rest*. The application is repeated weekly for up to 8 weeks. Local irritation, burning, and pain are the most common reactions reported. Reported efficacy has been variable in several placebo-controlled clinical trials.

Imiquimod is a cytokine inducer that stimulates production of interferon-α and -γ, interleukin 2, and tumor necrosis factor α, among others. The drug does not directly destroy the wart tissue, but it triggers an inflammatory response that eventually eliminates the wart tissue, when successful. The cream is to be applied to each lesion at bedtime on 3 nonconsecutive nights (e.g., Monday, Wednesday, and Friday) and then washed off in the morning. Treatment should be continued for up to 16 weeks. Most patients require 2 or 3 months to completely respond to imiquimod. More frequent application does not improve the efficacy of imiquimod, but it does increase toxicity. Local itching, burning, pain, and sometimes erosions are reported side effects. Fair-skinned individuals seem to be more likely to have local irritation than do darker-skinned persons. For reasons that are not clear, women respond better to imiquimod than do men. In one study, 72% of women cleared all lesions on imiquimod while only 33% of men did so. Of the patients who do clear completely with imiquimod, the rate of recurrence may be lower than with other treatments. However, this conclusion is based on relatively small numbers of patients and needs to be confirmed in larger studies.

For patient-applied therapy to be successful, the patient must be able to identify all of the lesions to be treated and must be able to reach each lesion to apply medicine. In addition, the patient must be motivated to comply with a treatment course that may last months. This is not always practical; therefore, provider-administered treatments still have a role in the treatment of genital warts. The two treatments that are most widely available to clinicians (and require minimal specialized training to use) are topical application of podophyllin (Podofin) and cryotherapy with liquid nitrogen. Podophyllin resin is a rather crude plant extract that is usually made up as a 20% solution in benzoin. There is significant lot-to-lot variability in the potency of each preparation, and that probably accounts for at least some of the variability in response rate that is reported in the literature. Like podofilox, podophyllin is a cytotoxin that destroys the wart tissue. It is applied by the provider to the lesions once or twice per week and usually requires several weeks for a complete response. It can be moderately irritating, but is usually reasonably well tolerated if the area is washed 8 to 12 hours after drug application.

Cryotherapy is most efficiently employed using a hand-held spray device for liquid nitrogen. Each lesion is sprayed with a stream of liquid nitrogen until all of the tissue is an opaque white color. The lesion is allowed to regain its original color and is frozen a second time. Each lesion is treated in this fashion. The same result can be accomplished using a swab dipped in liquid nitrogen and then applied to the lesion; however, it is sometimes more difficult to achieve complete freezing, especially of larger lesions. This procedure is moderately painful for the patient, especially after the treatment when the lesions fully thaw. Most lesions require weekly treatments for 2 to 4 weeks to achieve complete resolution.

Topical application of trichloroacetic or bichloroacetic acid is also a local cytodestructive treatment. These are caustic chemicals, but the local reactions are usually relatively mild when used carefully. As with the other compounds discussed earlier, repeat treatments at weekly intervals are usually required to achieve maximal response.

A variety of surgical treatments including scissor excision, electrodesiccation, and laser vaporization are also treatment options for clinicians who have the necessary equipment and training. Surgical treatments are the only ones that can clear all lesions (in most cases) with some degree of certainty. However, they are generally expensive and do cause a moderate amount of pain for the patient, depending on the extent of disease.

Two other treatments are sometimes used, but are generally not recommended as first-line therapy: interferon and 5-fluorouracil. Interferon alfa-2b (Intron-A) preparations are licensed treatments for intralesional injection into genital warts. In patients with extensive disease, interferon injections are tedious for the clinician to administer and uncomfortable for the patient. The patient may also suffer systemic interferon toxicities (low-grade fever, myalgias, fatigue) that further reduce its tolerability. Because interferon is also expensive and shows efficacy that is no better than most of the other treatments discussed above, it is usually reserved for refractory cases in which one or more other methods have failed. Topical or intralesional 5-fluorouracil (Adrucil)[1] is used by some practitioners for the treatment of external genital warts. This is another

[1]Not FDA approved for this indication.

cytotoxic agent that can be quite potent. Local reactions can be relatively severe, and patients must be cautioned about these inflammatory and sometimes erosive reactions. The high toxicity potential and modest efficacy of 5-fluorouracil are the major reasons for not recommending it.

The anticytomegalovirus drug cidofovir (Vistide)[1] is reported to have activity against HPV and has been proposed as a treatment for genital warts. The drug is far too toxic when administered systemically to be used for this indication, but topical treatment has been proposed and has been used in a few small series in the literature. However, the drug is only commercially available as an intravenous formulation and must be reformulated to be used topically. Obviously, treatment of external genital warts is not an approved indication for cidofovir.

The treatments discussed in this section are used primarily for the treatment of genital warts on cutaneous epithelium. Most of these methods are even less well studied on mucosal surfaces such as the vagina, cervix, and urethra. Cryotherapy or some type of surgical approach is most commonly used at these sites. Many of the treatments that are irritating on cutaneous epithelium are even more so on mucosal surfaces and must be used with extreme caution, if at all. Similarly, there are few data on the use of any of these treatments in pregnancy. Podophyllin, podofilox, and 5-fluorouracil are potential teratogens and should generally not be used in pregnancy. Cryotherapy and surgery are probably the only treatments that could be considered safe for use in pregnancy.

Although there are a number of treatment options available for the treatment of genital warts, better treatments are still needed. The ideal treatment would be one that was either patient applied or one that required only one clinic visit. Other desirable parameters would be rapid onset of action and high efficacy with a low recurrence rate. A treatment that was low in cost would also be highly desirable. There is still much work to be done in this area.

[1]Not FDA approved for this indication.

MELANOCYTIC NEVI (MOLES)

METHOD OF

Paul Hirsch, MD, JD

Melanocytic nevi (MN), or moles, are benign cutaneous neoplasms of melanocytes that undergo an organized spectrum of clinical and microscopic stages of growth. Nevus cells are nondendritic melanocytes that can synthesize melanin pigment and form clusters or nests. MN are located on any cutaneous surface. Everyone has at least one MN, and the number is dependent on heredity, age, sun exposure, and hormonal influences.

There are various reasons for removing MN. Because MN can be ablated by a variety of methods or techniques, it is essential to have an understanding of the descriptive and microscopic terminologies and a recognition of the factors influencing their growth.

MN may appear at birth or develop over the course of years into adulthood. Those present at birth, or within the first year, are referred to as congenital melanocytic nevi (CMN), and those appearing thereafter are regarded as acquired melanocytic nevi (AMN). Documentation of the origin of a CMN may be difficult if parental history is not available.

It is difficult to clinically differentiate CMN from AMN, except by size. Small CMN can be up to 1.5 cm, while giant CMN can cover large geographic areas of the body. AMN are smaller in size by comparison to CMN. Microscopically, CMN and AMN have some differences; however, they are not specific enough to allow for objective differentiation.

CMN are significant for two reasons. They are potential precursors of malignant melanoma, and they may be cosmetically deforming lesions. It is estimated that the lifetime risk for malignant melanoma in giant MN may be as high as 10%.

Variable amounts of hair are within MN. Greater numbers are found in CMN, especially in the giant CMN.

Although a relatively small proportion of MN are identified in malignant melanoma specimens, it does not appear that most malignant melanomas arise from pre-existing MN.

Classification of Melanocytic Nevi

Classification of MN is based on clinical and histologic features that represent a continum of cutaneous melanocytic maturation. However, the definitive diagnosis can only be made by microscopic examination of the nevus.

CLINICAL

There are four generally recognized clinical types of MN:

1. Flat or macular lesions
2. Elevated or papular lesions
3. Irregular surfaced papular or papillomatous lesions
4. Pedunculated lesions

As a person ages, MN change from the macular to the papular shape. This is a normal growth pattern that correlates with the microscopic distribution of the nevus cells. Therefore, macular lesions are found in a younger person, and as the person ages the MN tend to become more elevated. In all of the clinical types, the characteristics of MN have well-marginated borders, uniformity of pigment, no ulceration, and no inflammation.

MN can be altered by inflammation from a sunburn, local trauma, or folliculitis. These changes may include swelling, redness, pigmentation, and ulceration. Physicians must be aware of these secondary changes in evaluating nevi.

MICROSCOPIC

MN viewed through the microscope are commonly divided into three types:

1. Junction nevus
2. Compound nevus
3. Dermal nevus

Each of these types correlate with the maturation process of cutaneous melanocytes in the formation of an MN.

Correlation of Clinical and Microscopic Findings

The correlation of clinical and microscopic findings for MN is delineated as follows:

- *Junction nevi* are usually macular and uniformly pigmented. The melanocytes are confined to the basal cell level of the epidermis.
- *Compound nevi* may vary from macular to papular, but tend to be more papular than junction nevi. Pigment is variable. Melanocytes are within the basal cell zone of the epidermis and different levels of the dermis.
- *Dermal nevi* are predominantly papular or elevated. They contain variable amounts of pigment. Melanocytes are within varying levels of the dermis and are separated from the epidermis by a zone of uninvolved collagen (grenz zone).

VARIANTS OF MELANOCYTIC NEVI WITH SPECIAL DIAGNOSTIC SIGNIFICANCE

Spitz Nevus

Spitz nevus (juvenile epithelioid nevus or juvenile melanoma) is a particular type of compound nevus commonly occurring in children or young adults and located mostly on the face or extremities. Melanocytes are large and mono- and multinucleated, with bizarre cytologic features that may be incorrectly diagnosed as malignant melanoma. Caution should be used diagnosing this particular nevus in adults older than 30 years of age.

Juvenile Spindle Cell Nevi

Juvenile spindle cell nevi are considered by some authors to be a spindle cell variant of the Spitz nevus. The melanocytes are spindle or fusiform in shape and contain dense deposits of melanin pigment. They may be found on any part of the body.

Dysplastic Nevus

Dysplastic nevus (nevus with architectural disturbance) is a junctional or compound nevus. It has variable clinical features and microscopic cellular atypia. In addition to familial association, dysplastic nevi have occurred as sporadic findings with or without malignant melanoma. Sporadic dysplastic nevi have been identified in approximately 5% of the white population in the United States. Patients with sporadic dysplastic nevi are at a slightly higher risk for malignant melanoma than the general population. Clinical features include a size of 6 to 12 mm in dimension, a shape with poorly defined borders, and a variation of pigmentation. There exists a plethora of opinions regarding the true biologic nature of this nevus. The conundrum is whether this nevus is benign or a precursor for malignant melanoma. In addition to the clinical features, microscopic parameters are still to be determined because of a lack of universal agreement. Because of various uncertainties, it may be prudent to surgically remove these nevi if there is a familial or personal history of malignant melanoma. In the sporadic low-risk group of dysplastic nevi, where there is no history of malignant melanoma, there is no general consensus for the ablation of these nevi.

Blue Nevus

Blue nevus is a blue-black, dome-shaped nevus. The melanocytes are densely pigmented throughout all levels of the dermis and may extend into the subcutaneous fat. They may be mistaken for a malignant melanoma because of their dark color.

Recurrent Nevus

Recurrent nevus (postsurgical melanocytic hyperplasia) is a type of junction or compound nevus appearing in an area of previously and incompletely removed biopsy-proven benign nevus. It may have variable cellular atypia. Some authors have called this type of nevus *pseudomelanoma*. This terminology might be a concern to the physician or patient and should be avoided.

Halo Nevus

Halo nevus (nevus acquisitum centrifugum) is a type of junction or compound nevus surrounded by a halo of depigmentation. This nevus is found mostly on the back and in young adults.

Therapy

Predominant reasons for removing MN are cosmetic, chronic irritation, suspicion of malignant melanoma, or other diagnostic purposes. The specific method used for nevus removal depends on the basic purpose for the ablation. Based on long-term follow-up studies, malignant melanoma has not resulted from partial removal of a biopsy-proven benign MN. All of these studies involved confirmatory biopsy for benignity in the originally treated MN. Because a microscopic confirmatory examination is the only method for accurately determining the actual diagnosis, the procedure selected for removing the MN should consider the submission of a specimen for microscopic examination. One can clinically suspect benignity, but this must be proven by histologic confirmation. Failure to do so may be a detriment to the patient and a potential basis for a lawsuit for medical negligence.

As with all surgical procedures, informed consent with a discussion of scar formation and recurrence should be obtained before the removal of an MN. Attention to these details is extremely important for risk management in preventing a lawsuit. These discussions should be documented at or near the time frame of treatment.

MODALITIES OF THERAPY

MN can be partially or totally excised by various surgical or destructive methods. Before their removal, there should be consideration given to the quality and quantity of the removed specimen for adequate microscopic interpretation.

Surgical techniques include partial or total removal of MN. Partial removal can be accomplished by the shave or curetted technique by ablating the MN at the level of the surrounding skin. Total removal for clearance of margins requires excision of a larger specimen. The control of bleeding and wound repair depends on the amount and depth of the removed specimen. For superficially removed specimens, bleeding can be controlled by application of ferric subsulfate (Monsel's solution) or electrodesiccation. Larger surgical defects require procedures for wound closure.

Destructive methods for removal can be by chemical cauterants, electrodesiccation, cryosurgery, or laser photocoagulation. Use of these destructive techniques could limit the ability to obtain an adequate tissue sample for microscopy.

MN are benign cutaneous pigmented neoplasms having a continuum of maturation with recognizable features. The clinical features of MN are uniformity in shape, size that usually measures 6 mm or less, margination, uniformity of pigmentation, and an absence of inflammation and ulceration. Changes in MN are to be correlated with the patient's personal history. Any definitive diagnosis of MN can only be substantiated by a microscopic examination. The technique selected for removal of MN depends on the reason for their removal. Before removal of the nevus, there should be a discussion with the patient as to possible scar formation and recurrence. This discussion must include written documentation for ample risk management.

MALIGNANT MELANOMA

METHOD OF

Douglas Tyler, MD, and Hilliard Seigler, MD

Malignant melanoma is the ninth most common cancer and is the leading cause of death from cutaneous malignancy. Melanoma ranks second only to adult leukemias in terms of potential life lost. The incidence of melanoma is rising faster than any other malignancy, with the number of new cases doubling over the last 35 years. It is currently projected that 1 in 82 women and 1 in 58 men will develop melanoma in the course of their lifetime. In the United States this accounted for more than 54,000 new cases of melanoma in 2003 and approximately 7600 individuals died from this disease during the same time period.

Diagnosis

Melanoma can have a variety of appearances and be located anywhere on the body. Common clinical features include an asymmetric lesion, a diameter of greater than 6 mm, color variation within the lesion, and border irregularity. Any change in a pre-existing or new nevus is also suggestive of melanoma. Generally, the physician should have a low threshold to diagnostically evaluate skin lesions if melanoma is suspected. The skin lesion in question should be completely removed with an excisional biopsy. The biopsy needs to include the full thickness of the skin into the subcutaneous tissue to allow an accurate measurement of the tumor's thickness. Punch biopsy is a good technique for small lesions, while elliptical excision may be necessary for larger lesions. Shave biopsies should not be done as one risks transecting the melanoma, preventing accurate assessment of its depth.

Pathology

Melanoma has traditionally been broken down into four subtypes based upon pathology and growth pattern:

1. Superficial spreading melanoma (SSM)
2. Acral lentiginous melanoma (ALM)

3. Lentigo maligna melanoma (LMM)
4. Nodular melanoma

SSM accounts for approximately 70% of melanomas, typically arises from a pre-existing nevus, and has a radial growth phase before becoming invasive. ALM accounts for 10% of melanomas and usually arises on the soles, palms, mucous membranes, and subungually. ALM also has a radial growth phase, but it is frequently misdiagnosed early on because the locations at which it develops are not suspected for melanoma. LMM accounts for 5% of melanomas and most frequently arises in the head and neck region. LMM has a slow radial growth pattern and usually develops in older patients from a lentigo maligna precursor lesion. Nodular melanoma is the second most common type of melanoma (15% to 20%), but, unlike the other types mentioned above, it is not associated with a radial growth phase. Nodular melanomas more commonly arise de novo, and a history of rapid onset over several months is not uncommon.

Histologic evaluation of the primary melanoma provides information that is important for determining prognosis and clinical treatment. The Breslow thickness and Clark level are measurements of tumor thickness and histologic depth, respectively. Breslow depth, and to a lesser degree, Clark level are directly associated with prognosis. Other factors that also appear important include ulceration, regression, evidence of lymphatic or vascular invasion, and satellitosis. Each of these is associated with a more aggressive form of melanoma that should be factored into clinical decision making.

Staging

The American Joint Commission on Cancer (AJCC) revised its staging system for melanoma in 2002 (Table 1). The modifications incorporated into the new staging system include subclassification using Breslow categories, which are based upon whole numbers. In addition, the new system takes into account tumor ulceration, which is an independent predictor of survival. It is also becoming clearer that the number of positive lymph nodes, not the size of the largest lymph node, is the most important factor for nodal staging. The presence of satellitosis is also incorporated into the new staging system.

For patients with melanomas less than 4 mm deep, initial staging workup consists of a baseline lactate dehydrogenase (LDH) and chest radiograph. For patients with melanomas greater than 4 millimeters, a more extensive staging workup is performed using chest, abdomen, and pelvic computed tomography (CT) scans or a dual positron emission tomography (PET)/CT scan. Intraoperative lymphatic mapping and sentinel lymph node biopsy for the evaluation of lymph node status in melanoma patients has become a widely accepted staging tool for patients with melanomas greater than 1 mm. It is used in patients with melanomas greater than 4 mm if their imaging

TABLE 1 Pathologic American Joint Commission on Cancer (AJCC) Stage Grouping

Pathologic Stage	TNM	Thickness (mm)	Ulceration	No. Positive Lymph Nodes	Nodal Size	Distant Metastasis
IA	T1a	≤1	No	0	-	-
IB	T1b	≤1	Yes or Clark IV, V	0	-	-
	T2a	1.01-2.0	No	0	-	-
IIA	T2b	1.02-2.0	Yes	0	-	-
	T3a	2.01-4.0	No	0	-	-
IIB	T3b	2.01-4.0	Yes	0	-	-
	T4a	>4.0	No	0	-	-
IIC	T4b	>4.0	Yes	0	-	-
IIIA	N1a	Any	No	1	Micro	-
	N2a	Any	No	2-3	Micro	-
IIIB	N1a	Any	Yes	1	Micro	-
	N2a	Any	Yes	2-3	Micro	-
	N1b	Any	No	1	Macro	-
	N2b	Any	No	2-3	Macro	-
	N2c	Any	Any	0, Satellite or *intransit* present		-
IIIC	N1b	Any	Yes	1	Macro	-
	N2b	Any	Yes	2-3	Macro	-
	N3	Any	Any	4, or Satellite or *intransit* with any number	Micro or Macro	-
IV	M1a	Any	Any	Any	Any	Skin, subcutaneous
	M1b	Any	Any	Any	Any	Lung
	M1c	Any	Any	Any	Any	Other visceral

Abbreviations: TNM = tumor, node, metastasis (classification).
intransit = tumor nodule between primary tumor site and regional nodal basin.

workup is negative, as well as in patients with thin melanomas that are less than 1 mm and that carry poor prognostic features like a discordant Clark level, ulceration, regression, or have a depth between 0.75 to 1 mm. While it has become clear that melanoma does spread in an orderly and predictable fashion through regional lymphatics, most people feel that when tumor cells metastasize from the primary site, they can also shed directly into the bloodstream, either bypassing the lymphatics or floating through them at the same time.

Extensive histologic examination of the sentinel lymph node demonstrates that routine histologic examination of the sentinel lymph node can identify 1 tumor cell in 10,000 lymphocytes. Application of serial sectioning and immunohistochemistry for melanoma-specific markers (monoclonal antibody HMB-45 or S100 protein) can improve tumor detection to 1 tumor cell in 100,000 lymphocytes. Molecular biology techniques using reverse transcriptase polymerase chain reaction (RT-PCR) for detection of messenger RNA (mRNA) for melanoma-associated gene products—such as tyrosinase, glycoprotein (gp)100, melanoma-associated gene (MAGE) 3, or human melanoma peptide antigen MART-1—have the capability of detecting 1 tumor cell in 1,000,000 lymphocytes. Recent studies demonstrate that patients who have a histologically negative, RT-PCR–positive sentinel lymph node have a statistically significant shorter disease-free survival than patients with histologically negative, RT-PCR–negative sentinel lymph nodes. Overall, sentinel lymph node biopsy has emerged as an important staging tool that ensures accurate prognostic and staging information on each patient, as well as identifying a group of patients who may benefit from adjuvant therapy.

Treatment

PRIMARY LESION AND REGIONAL LYMPH NODES

Once the diagnosis of melanoma is made, treatment focuses on appropriately managing the primary lesion to prevent recurrence, and on addressing the status of the lymph nodes in patients thought to be at risk of harboring metastatic disease. The current recommendations for re-excision of primary melanomas are as follows:

- Melanoma in situ should be re-excised with a 5-mm margin.
- Thin melanomas with a Breslow thickness less than 1 mm should be re-excised with a 1-cm margin.
- Intermediate thickness melanomas with a Breslow thickness between 1 and 4 mm should undergo a 2-cm–wide local excision. Although there has been some controversy regarding the size of re-excision margin for thick melanomas carrying a Breslow thickness greater than 4 mm, recent consensus suggests that a 2-cm–wide local excision should be adequate. A recently published study comparing 1- versus 3-cm–wide local excision margins from England failed to provide significant data to change the current 2-cm recommendations.

Evaluation of nodal status is based upon the Breslow thickness, which helps determine the likelihood that the regional lymphatics will be involved.

Melanomas Less Than 1 mm

Although the prognosis for patients with thin melanoma is excellent, approximately 10% of these patients die of their disease. Several studies have tried to determine the characteristics of thin lesions that are more likely to metastasize. Features of regression, ulceration, and/or a discordant Clark level of IV or V are generally associated with a worse prognosis in this subgroup of patients. Intraoperative lymphatic mapping may be another way to further evaluate patients with thin melanomas whose primary tumors have poor prognostic features. Although there are currently no data to suggest this group of patients would receive a survival benefit from a therapeutic lymph node dissection based upon a positive sentinel lymph node, they are candidates for adjuvant therapies in the form of either interferon or immunotherapy trials.

Melanomas Between 1 and 4 mm

Much controversy has surrounded the appropriate management of patients with intermediate thickness melanomas with regard to lymph nodes. It is thought by some that patients in this group have a higher probability of having regional nodal disease (15% to 60%) as compared to distant metastatic disease (8% to 15%), and, therefore, they may in theory benefit from removal of regional lymph nodes. At the time intraoperative lymphatic mapping and sentinel lymph node biopsy was first described, there were only a few retrospective studies that demonstrated a survival advantage to prophylactically or electively removing the regional lymph nodes. In addition to a few large retrospective studies that showed no benefit to elective removal of the regional lymph nodes in this patient population, there were three prospective, randomized clinical trials that failed to show any benefit from early lymph node removal.

To address many of the concerns raised by the initial randomized, prospective, clinical trials, the Intergroup Melanoma Surgical Trial was initiated and accrued 781 patients between 1983 and 1991. This study stratified patients by tumor thickness, ulceration, and site. At the most recent analysis, it has greater than a 5-year follow-up in all patients and a mean follow-up of 10 years. Although there was no overall survival advantage to elective lymph node dissection when the entire group of patients was examined, there did appear to be some groups of patients who benefited from lymph node dissection as identified by subgroup analysis. The analysis of prospectively stratified groups demonstrated significant reductions in mortality for patients with nonulcerated lesions (29%), extremity lesions (27%), and lesions with Breslow thickness between 1 and 2 mm (35%). In addition, although not stratified prospectively, age appeared to be an important factor as patients younger than 60 years of age showed improved survival from elective lymph node dissection.

Although the Intergroup trial demonstrates some survival advantages to certain subgroups of patients with intermediate thickness melanoma, the majority of patients with intermediate thickness melanoma (70% to 80%) do not have micrometastatic disease and thus would not benefit from lymph node dissection. Because lymph node dissection is not without morbidity, many surgeons have been hesitant to perform elective lymph node dissection on all patients to potentially benefit a few. A recent study from the John Wayne Cancer Institute matched more than 500 patients and compared elective lymph node dissection to selective lymph node dissection (i.e., when a lymph node dissection is performed only if the sentinel lymph node is positive). This study suggests that the two procedures were therapeutically equivalent, when no differences in the incidence of tumor-positive dissections, tumor recurrence, or survival were found. Most centers now offer patients with intermediate thickness melanomas a selective lymph node dissection based upon the status of the sentinel lymph node, as this not only provides important prognostic information, but also allows patients to be candidates for adjuvant therapy trials. In addition, it may provide a survival advantage in certain groups in whom a selective lymph node dissection is performed.

Two large clinical trials examining the role of intraoperative lymphatic mapping and sentinel lymph node biopsy in patients with intermediate thickness melanoma have recently closed. The Multicenter Selective Lymphadenectomy trial-I (MSLT-I) randomized patients to wide local excision (WLE) alone versus WLE plus intraoperative lymphatic mapping and sentinel lymph node biopsy. The trial was closed to accrual in March of 2002. If the sentinel lymph node biopsy was positive, patients underwent a completion lymph node dissection.

The Sunbelt Melanoma trial enrolled patients with melanomas greater than 1 mm in depth and incorporated molecular pathologic staging (RT-PCR) in an attempt to determine whether early intervention with lymphadenectomy and/or interferon alfa-2b (Intron-A) will improve survival. This trial was closed at the end of 2003. All patients underwent intraoperative lymphatic mapping and sentinel lymph node biopsy. The sentinel lymph node had a small piece removed for RT-PCR analysis, and the rest of the lymph node was examined with serial sectioning and immunohistochemistry. Patients with a histologically positive sentinel lymph node underwent completion nodal dissection. If the sentinel lymph node was the only positive lymph node, the patient was randomized to observation or adjuvant high-dose interferon for 1 month. If the sentinel lymph node was histologically negative, RT-PCR analysis was performed; and, if positive, patients were randomized to observation, completion lymphadenectomy, or completion lymphadenectomy plus 1 month of high-dose interferon. Preliminary findings from this study suggest that approximately 30% of patients will have a histologically positive sentinel lymph node and that approximately 55% of patients will have a RT-PCR–positive sentinel lymph node. The results of the MSLT-I and Sunbelt trials will not be available for several years, when the data are more mature.

There are currently two large sentinel lymph node trials accruing patients with intermediate thickness melanomas that are focused on examining the need for completion lymph node dissection in patients with a positive sentinel lymph node. The Multicenter Selective Lymphadenectomy Trial-II (MSLT-II) randomizes patients to observation versus completion lymph node dissection, but allows patients to receive any adjuvant therapy; whereas the Florida Melanoma Trial-II randomizes patients to observation versus completion lymph node dissection, but all patients receive 1 year of high-dose interferon. Both of these studies are in their early stages of patient accrual.

Melanoma Lesions Greater Than 4 mm

Most studies suggest that patients with melanoma lesions greater than 4 mm have a very high chance of harboring distant metastatic disease, and as a result no survival benefit has ever been demonstrated for patients undergoing elective regional lymph node dissection. Our approach to this patient population is to perform a staging workup consisting of chest, abdomen, and pelvic CT scan or obtain a dual PET/CT scan. If no metastatic disease is identified, we offer intraoperative lymphatic mapping and sentinel lymph node biopsy to these patients—if they were interested in participating in an adjuvant therapy trial should their sentinel lymph node be positive. The additional benefit of performing a sentinel lymph node biopsy in this patient population is that individuals who have a negative sentinel lymph node have an excellent prognosis, much better than would be expected for the group of patients with thick melanomas as a whole.

ADJUVANT THERAPY

Because patients with metastatic nodal disease have a greater than 50% chance of developing recurrent disease, there has been tremendous effort put into identifying an effective adjuvant therapy to give to patients after lymph node resection. Only one therapy, high-dose interferon alfa-2b (Intron-A), is potentially beneficial for preventing recurrent disease in high-risk melanoma. The Eastern Cooperative Oncology Group (ECOG) 1684 trial, which randomized patients to either high-dose interferon or observation after resection of positive lymph nodes, demonstrates a statistically significant improvement in 5-year, disease-free survival from 26% to 37% and overall survival from 37% to 46%. The follow-up ECOG trial 1690 randomized patients to high-dose interferon, low-dose interferon, or observation after resection. The results on interim analysis (52-month follow-up) demonstrate that high-dose interferon leads to a reproducible improvement in 5-year, disease-free survival. Interestingly, there is no improvement in overall 5-year survival between any of the study arms as the observation group did significantly better in terms of survival in the 1690 trial as compared to the 1684 trial. The reasons for this improvement are still being investigated, but the fact that many patients who recurred in the observation arm were subsequently treated with interferon alfa-2b is a major confounding factor. A more recent trial, ECOG 1694, randomized patients to 1 year of high-dose interferon or 2 years of a ganglioside GM2 vaccine[2]. This trial was stopped early because during an interim analysis the high-dose interferon was found to be associated with significantly improved relapse-free and overall survival. A review of all the interferon data suggests that while it clearly improves relapse-free survival, most studies, if followed long enough, fail to demonstrate a sustained overall survival difference.

Although approved by the FDA for the adjuvant treatment of metastatic melanoma, many physicians suggest adjuvant alternatives other than high-dose interferon to patients. This is because of its controversial survival benefit coupled with the significant side effects indicated by vaccine trials such as ECOG 1684. Vaccine therapies have a lot of appeal to patients because they usually have few side effects and are frequently viewed as a way to potentially help the immune system. While a number of different vaccine strategies have been tried, the observation of an immune response induced by the vaccine has not translated into a survival advantage. Current approaches include:

- Whole-cell vaccines using either allogenic or autologous irradiated cell lines
- Lysate vaccines
- Vaccinia melanoma cell lysate vaccines
- Shed antigen vaccines
- Ganglioside vaccines using purified gangliosides such as GM2 alone or conjugated to the carrier protein keyhole limpet hemocyanin (KLH)
- The adjuvant QS21
- Peptide vaccines
- Dendritic cell vaccines
- DNA vaccines

A number of phase III trials have recently been started or have just completed accrual. To date only one these trials—a small phase III clinical trial of stage III AJCC patients using a shed antigen vaccine—demonstrates a survival advantage in the range of 11 months for patients receiving vaccine therapy.

[2]Not available in the United States.

METASTATIC DISEASE

Treatment options for patients who develop metastatic disease depend upon the pattern of disease. When patients present with metastatic disease, they should undergo an extensive staging workup. This workup traditionally consists of chest, abdomen, and pelvis CT scans along with either magnetic resonance imaging (MRI) or CT scan of the brain. More recently, PET scans have proven to be a more useful tool for staging this patient population. Patients with metastatic disease should initially be considered for surgical resection. Involvement of regional lymph nodes should be treated with surgical resection, because long-term survival occurs in 20% to 25%. A similar observation is seen in patients who undergo pulmonary resection of solitary melanoma metastasis. Patients with solitary lesions in other areas should also be considered surgical candidates, because between 5% to 10% will achieve long-term survival.

Patients with regionally advanced disease in the form of local recurrence or in-transit disease confined to an extremity should be considered for hyperthermic isolated limb perfusion (HILP). HILP with melphalan (Alkeran)[1] is the standard treatment for this group of patients and is associated with response rates of 50% to 80%. Several studies have suggested that the addition of tumor necrosis factor (TNF) to melphalan[1] could improve response rates in patients with large tumors and/or large tumor burdens (greater than 10 nodules). Recently, however, the American College of Surgeons Oncology Group closed its randomized prospective trial comparing HILP with melphalan[1] to HILP with melphalan[1] and TNF[1] in an attempt to better define which subgroups of patients, if any, benefit from the addition of TNF[1] to HILP with melphalan[1]. The interim analysis suggests that there is no difference between the two arms of this study. Another regional treatment called isolated limb infusion (ILI) has also been recently popularized in Australia. In contrast to HILP, ILI consists of a 30-minute infusion in an acidotic, hypoxic extremity using melphalan[1] and dactinomycin (Cosmegen)[1]. While the response rate at the Sydney Melanoma Unit is approximately 85% (41% complete remission [CR] and 44% partial response [PR]), this technique is only currently performed in a few centers in the United States and is currently being validated by a phase II multi-institutional study through the American College of Surgeons Oncology Group.

For patients with widely metastatic disease, the prognosis is poor, with mean survivals measured in the range of 6 to 9 months. A number of treatment options have been used including chemotherapy, biologic response modifiers, and a combination of both. Single-agent therapies, the most effective of which are dacarbazine (DTIC-Dome) and temozolomide (Temodar)[1], have response rates in the 10% to 20% range.

[1]Not FDA approved for this indication.

With multiagent therapy—most notably the Dartmouth regimen (cisplatin[1], DTIC, carmustine [BCNU][1], and tamoxifen[1]) or CVD (cisplatin[1], vinblastine[1] [Velban] and DTIC)—response rates are improved somewhat but no significant changes in overall survival are observed. Combinations of biologic response modifiers with combination chemotherapy have resulted in slightly higher response rates but at the price of higher toxicity. Interleukin-2 alone can produce very durable long-term, complete responses in approximately 5% of treated patients. In general, therapy of advanced disease is mainly palliative with younger patients, usually receiving a cisplatin[1]-based combination therapy protocol, and with older patients, who usually tolerate cisplatin[1] poorly, receiving single-agent therapy.

[1]Not FDA approved for this indication.

PREMALIGNANT LESIONS

METHOD OF

Forrest C. Brown, MD

The most common malignant lesions of the skin are basal cell carcinoma (BCC), squamous cell carcinoma (SCC), and malignant melanoma (MM). Less common tumors are dermatofibrosarcoma protuberans, microcystic adnexal carcinoma, malignant fibrohistiocytoma, and Merkel cell carcinoma. The premalignant expressions of BCC, SCC, and MM skin cancers are discussed in this article; there are no commonly accepted definitions for the premalignant lesions of the less common tumors mentioned above. Additionally, several conditions are not premalignant in themselves, but seem to set the stage for conversion of benign-to-malignant growths.

Nonmelanoma skin cancer is the most commonly occurring group of cancers worldwide. The cost to health care systems has never been accurately quantified, but it is obviously extremely high. Mortality figures for nonmelanoma skin cancer are notoriously flawed, because the recorded lethal event may actually be cardiac arrest or sepsis caused by the debilitated condition and treatment of the skin cancer. With the increasing occurrence rate of nonmelanoma and melanoma skin cancers throughout most of the world—because of increasing carcinogenic exposure of the sun and immune suppression of various causes, both environmental and iatrogenic—these cancers represent an enormous public health problem.

Skin cancers are even more significant because they are so readily curable by early diagnosis and treatment if the mind and eye are schooled to recognize the early and premalignant forms of the tumors. Recognition of an individual likely to have a skin cancer and recognition of premalignant lesions, along with their treatment, are the thrust of this article.

Typically, it is the fair-skinned person with sun exposure who is a likely candidate for both melanoma and nonmelanoma skin cancer. As one moves toward the equator the rate of skin cancer rises significantly in the indigenous population as the intensity of actinic radiation rises. Newer evidence, however, seems to indicate that it is the number of painful sunburns before the age of 20 years that correlates well with nonmelanoma skin cancer; while in melanoma, it may be the total sun exposure, but that is not clear.

Burn scars, long-standing skin ulcers, chronic skin sinuses and infections, as well as areas of chronic edema, are sites where skin cancer frequently develops and may be regarded as occasionally premalignant because of the possibility that these are sites of localized, lowered, or compromised immunity.

Given all these factors, the index of suspicion is highest in a fair-skinned person who has signs of significant sun exposure such as weathered thin skin, increased telangiectasia, rough patches, and pigment irregularities, or in an individual with signs or history of immune depression.

Actinic Keratosis

Actinic keratoses (AK) are separated into two significant but artificial divisions. The first is a very small papular lesion commonly classified as a clinically detectable keratosis, and the second is a larger lesion classified as clinically visible keratosis. This is a significant separation because sun damage in skin may manifest as multiple micro foci of abnormal keratinization that may or may not progress; whereas larger, visible keratoses are more likely to progress on their own to cancer.

The clinically detectable actinic keratosis may be perceived only by touch as a roughness in sun-damaged skin. Often, it is in an area that has received the most sun, such as ears, cheekbones, nose, and upper forehead. Magnified vision reveals surface irregularities and a few small, dilated red vessels. These lesions progress with summer sun exposure, fall dormant in the winter, then grow larger the following summer if sun protection is not provided.

The clinically visible actinic keratosis should be considered as a likely precursor for SCC and BCC. Removal with close follow-up is necessary on all lesions, especially on body areas that receive routine sun exposure such as the face, hands, ears, and back of the neck. Any actinic keratosis that demonstrates increasing thickness or width and/or redness should be removed, as there is evidence that the conversion of a premalignant to a malignant lesion is accompanied by erythema.

Two special forms of actinic keratosis should be recognized, hypertrophic actinic keratosis and proliferative actinic keratosis. Hypertrophic actinic keratosis is a very thick, crusting nodule of approximately 1 cm (or more) that generally occurs on the dorsum of the hands and arms. Nodules of this type are in active transition to malignancy, with approximately 50% showing active foci of either BCC or SCC. Proliferative actinic keratosis is an active, enlarging lesion that is often superficially ulcerated and shows deep proliferation and rapid progression to SCC. Both of these forms require significantly aggressive therapy including wide excision or, alternatively, deep shave excision that encompasses 3 mm of normal skin followed by intense liquid nitrogen spray, which creates an ice front approximately 3 mm beyond the excised margin.

With the exception of hypertrophic actinic keratosis and proliferative actinic keratosis, I have, for many years, treated most actinic keratosis lesions with liquid nitrogen cryospray. It is effective, rapid, and simple. However, this simplicity has led many to undertreat, resulting in treatment failures and recurrences. Liquid nitrogen is not without problems; it may result in significant blistering, scarring, and very noticeable post-treatment hypopigmentation. However, in trained hands it remains very popular for treating a few isolated lesions where hypopigmentation is not a significant consideration.

When treating the face, especially in younger individuals, cosmetic result and treatment morbidity are very important considerations. Even the slightest possibility of a scar or perceived disfigurement is to be avoided, if possible, in the treatment of these epidermal lesions. The nonsteroidal anti-inflammatory agent diclofenac (Solaraze), a recently introduced form of topical therapy, may be used with little or no perceived evidence of treatment except for lesion clearing; however, the treatment regimen requires 3 months.

Topical treatments with either low- or standard-strength 5-fluorouracil (5-FU) (Efudex) usually require a relatively short treatment time (a few weeks), but redness may last significantly longer.

With all self-administered therapies for these premalignant lesions, some very important ground rules must be kept in mind:

- Treat for the full time recommended unless the reaction makes it impossible.
- Never allow these medications to be used ad lib.
- Always biopsy an area that is slow to heal or recurs after treatment.

Physicians should never have a cavalier attitude toward these medications. Numerous reports have been published regarding their improper use; for example, only the tops of unrecognized cancers may be removed by treatment, and large, dangerous subsurface tumors later develop at the lesion sites.

A new treatment that eliminates the dangers of self-directed therapy recently received FDA approval. This treatment, aminolevulinic acid (ALA) (Levulan Kerastick), is a topical, photodynamic therapy. Protoporphyrin IX is created in the cells of the actinic keratosis following exposure to topical ALA after a few hours of incubation. The area is then exposed to coherent light (laser) or noncoherent light (ordinary) for a short time. The photoreaction that occurs destroys very specifically the metabolically active cells of the actinic keratosis. Although there is discomfort during the light exposure, the procedure is popular with many patients because it eliminates the time required to build up to the maximum effect with 5-FU.

The decision to treat actinic keratosis is sometimes questioned. I believe treatment should be given when:

- Lesions are located on areas of the body that continue to receive sun exposure.
- Lesions are showing signs of activity such as thickening or widening.
- Lesions show development of erythema.

DISSEMINATED SUPERFICIAL ACTINIC POROKERATOSIS

Disseminated superficial actinic porokeratosis (DSAP) is an actinic keratosis with a familial history; it probably represents a combination of sun exposure and clones of slightly atypical cells. These lesions appear in individuals after the age of 40 years (primarily in women) on the sun-exposed portions of the extremities. Diagnosis is by pathologic examination, but the lesions are clinically detected by their very definite palpable border and by their erythematous bases. Conversion to squamous cell carcinoma is well documented. Treatment is by liquid nitrogen or by topical treatment; with either, the treatment must be more intense and carried out for a longer period of time than when treating the usual actinic keratosis. Post-treatment erythema may last for many months.

Cutaneous Horn

Cutaneous horn is diagnosed clinically by observing what is at the base of the lesion. Warts, inflamed seborrheic keratoses, Mollusca, hypertrophic actinic keratoses, keratoacanthomas, and squamous cell carcinomas are all possible causes. The treatment is deep shave or excision for diagnosis and appropriate follow-up therapy depending on the microscopic diagnosis.

Nevus Sebaceus

Nevus sebaceus is a congenital lesion occurring primarily on the head and neck that thickens and becomes nodular after puberty. Thereafter, patients should be followed closely, because some percentage develop either BCC or SCC during their lifetime. Excision of the lesion in its entirety is the preferred treatment, but if that is not possible, then any suspicious area should be biopsied.

Premalignant Fibroepithelioma

A premalignant fibroepithelioma is a term coined many years ago by a dermatopathologist for a particular microscopic pattern. It is an unfortunate designation for it is neither premalignant nor a fibroepithelioma; it is a BCC and should be treated accordingly.

Bowen's Disease

Bowen's disease is SCC that has not yet progressed to invasion (SCC in situ). The lesion should be considered malignant and removed. It is tempting to perform only superficial removal because of the intraepithelial nature of the tumor; however, migration down hair follicles is common, and recurrence after such treatments is the usual course. If the lesion is not too large, excision is the best treatment. For larger lesions, destructive therapy followed by excision of any recurrences may be an option. Photodynamic therapy is successful according to some reports. Removal by Mohs micrographic surgery is indicated in areas where tissue conservation is important, such as the face.

Leukokeratosis of the Lip

Leukokeratosis, or leukoplakia, of the lip is the mucosal expression of an actinic keratosis. The entire lip should be considered suspect, because new areas or continuations develop after localized treatment of individual lesions. Carbon dioxide laser ablation of the mucosal surface with healing by second intention is a very effective treatment. Intense liquid nitrogen treatment of the lip usually offers a good result. It is a popular treatment and should be considered before excision and mucosal advancement surgery.

Bowenoid Papulosis

Bowenoid papulosis is multiple papules of histologic Bowen's disease (SCC in situ) that occur in the genital area although a few cases are reported on distant sites. Human papilloma virus has been identified in some cases. Some lesions resolve spontaneously. They should, however, be considered at least premalignant and removed in a simple manner, such as with liquid nitrogen or curettage and desiccation. Recently, excellent response has been reported with the topical immune response modifier imiquimod cream (Aldara).

Special Considerations

The problems of premalignant lesions are very troublesome for the healthy patient, but take on extreme importance in immunosuppressed individuals. In these patients, the biology of a premalignant lesion is so altered that every lesion should be considered as a developing malignant lesion, *not* a premalignant lesion. Therapy as well as the decision to institute therapy should be aggressive to prevent damage by an immunologically unrestrained cancer.

BACTERIAL DISEASES OF THE SKIN

METHOD OF

Michael G. Wilkerson, MD

Bacterial diseases of the skin range (Table 1) from trivial annoyances to life-threatening emergencies that, left unrecognized, result in severe morbidity with loss of limbs and systemic complications. Death may occur in more severe cases, often in otherwise healthy individuals. The skin is the body's first line of defense against an onslaught of microorganisms from the environment including bacteria, fungi, and viruses. Common normal skin flora includes staphylococci, streptococci, diphtheroids, and propionibacteria; and gram-negative bacteria may also be found "below the waist" and in immunocompromised patients. Knowledge of common bacterial flora and their sensitivities to common antibiotics and initial empiric treatment is essential. However, this is changing because of the emergence of bacterial resistance as a result of overuse and incomplete treatment of infections. The most important resistance at this time is methicillin-resistant *Staphylococcus aureus* (MRSA) in the institutional setting, and now community-acquired methicillin-resistant *S. aureus* (CA-MRSA) is becoming more common without obvious nosocomial exposure. Vancomycin-resistant *S. aureus* (VRSA) is also being reported with increasing frequency.

While treatment of skin infections remains empiric, bacterial cultures are becoming increasingly important. Even immunocompetent patients in everyday outpatient settings are at risk because of these evolving resistance patterns.

Bioterrorism with infectious agents, including anthrax, is now a concern. Early recognition and diagnosis may prevent widespread morbidity and mortality.

Impetigo and Ecthyma

Impetigo is a well-known disease even amongst lay people. It is common in school-age children and is

TABLE 1 Bacterial Skin Infections

Infection	Primary Organisms	Recommended Treatments
Impetigo, nonbullous	Group A *Streptococcus* or *Staphylococcus aureus*	Consider bacterial culture. If mild, topical mupirocin (Bactroban) bid × 1 wk. Otherwise, dicloxacillin (Dynapen), cephalexin (Keflex), erythromycin, or clarithromycin (Biaxin).
Impetigo, bullous	*S. aureus* group II	Consider bacterial culture. Treat with dicloxacillin (Dynapen), cephalexin (Keflex), amoxicillin-clavulanate (Augmentin), or clarithromycin (Biaxin).
Folliculitis	*S. aureus* (most common); *Klebsiella, Enterobacter* (long-term acne antibiotics); *Pseudomonas* (hot-tub exposure)	Perform bacterial culture. If superficial: topical mupirocin, erythromycin, clindamycin (Cleocin), and personal hygiene measures. Otherwise, dicloxacillin (Dynapen), cephalexin (Keflex), amoxicillin-clavulanate (Augmentin), clarithromycin (Biaxin). Consider fungal cultures in recalcitrant cases. Hot-tub folliculitis resolves spontaneously.
Cellulitis	β-Hemolytic streptococci; *S. aureus; Haemophilus influenzae* (young children); gram-negatives *below the waist,* especially in immunocompromised patients	Culture by needle aspiration or tissue. Localized, nontoxic presentation: dicloxacillin, amoxicillin-clavulanate (Augmentin), cephalexin (Keflex), and clarithromycin (Biaxin). Progressive, toxic, or immunocompromised: β-lactamase–resistant intravenous antibiotics.
Staphylococcal scalded skin syndrome	*S. aureus* phage group II	β-Lactamase–resistant antibiotics. Mupirocin (Bactroban) for nares.
Necrotizing fasciitis	Polymicrobial infections with aerobic and anaerobic organisms	Surgical consultation; don't delay or wait on imaging studies. Early débridement, broad-spectrum intravenous antibiotics for aerobic and anaerobic bacteria.
Anthrax	*Bacillus anthracis*	Skin biopsy for cultures and immunohistochemical stains. Consult with lab director, pathologist, dermatologist, and public health officials. Ciprofloxacin (Cipro) or doxycycline (Vibramycin), depending on patient age and condition.

easily transmitted. In past years it was thought that much of impetigo was secondary to group A, β-hemolytic *Streptococcus*, however, most cases now involve *S. aureus*. Occasionally, one sees mixed infections of streptococci and *S. aureus*. Impetigo has a predilection for areas of traumatized skin such as contact dermatitis or eczemas. Warm, moist environments, poor living conditions, and close living conditions aggravate impetigo.

Impetigo is classified as bullous or nonbullous. The nonbullous form is much more common (approximately 70% of cases). Bullous impetigo is often linked to the *S. aureus* group II phage. The bullae usually appear on the trunk, buttocks, perineum, or face. A toxin produced by this particular type of *S. aureus* is thought to induce the bullae. Complications of impetigo include glomerulonephritis, septicemia, pneumonia, septic arthritis, osteomyelitis, and necrotizing fasciitis. Nephritogenic strains of *Streptococcus* may produce postinfectious glomerulonephritis after 18 to 21 days, particularly in children 3 to 7 years of age. Unfortunately, antibiotic treatment does not appear to prevent this complication in susceptible individuals.

Ecthyma is a clinical variant of impetigo that affects mainly immunocompromised patients with diabetes, human immunodeficiency virus infection, and neutropenic states from cancer chemotherapy and other immunosuppressants. The same causative organisms as impetigo are found. The lesions are more *punched out* and painful than impetigo and are not responsive to topical therapy.

TREATMENT

Limited superficial impetigo can be treated with topical therapy such as mupirocin (Bactroban) ointment or cream. This product must be applied two to three times a day for 2 to 3 weeks. Bactroban Nasal ointment is helpful for treating the anterior nares, which harbor chronic carriage. In limited disease this treatment is helpful, and avoids use of systemic antibiotics. All known isolates of group A, β-hemolytic *Streptococcus* are sensitive to mupirocin; however, some isolates of *S. aureus* appear to be becoming resistant as use of mupirocin for long time periods occurs. More extensive cases of impetigo and ecthyma should be treated with systemic antibiotics, which are β-lactamase–resistant, such as dicloxacillin (Dynapen), cephalexin (Keflex), amoxicillin-clavulanate potassium (Augmentin), erythromycin (E-Mycin), and clarithromycin (Biaxin). Clindamycin (Cleocin) is an additional consideration, particularly in view of the rapid development of resistance of *S. aureus* to macrolides. Macrolides such as erythromycin and clarithromycin may be used in low-risk individuals, who are penicillin and/or cephalosporin sensitive, for limited disease.

Basic hygiene should be enforced, along with warm compresses to help remove crust, followed by application of mupirocin ointment or cream. In cases of underlying dermatitis, control of the dermatitis is also helpful.

Folliculitis, Furuncles, and Carbuncles

Folliculitis is a common infection involving the hair follicle or pilosebaceous unit. It usually presents as follicular-based yellow pustules. Sometimes these have been excoriated or shaved away, which may make the diagnosis less obvious. Spreading with scratching or shaving is a helpful clue. Patients who shave, work, or exercise in sweaty environments are particularly predisposed.

TREATMENT

Superficial folliculitis frequently responds to changes in local environment, use of topical antibacterial soaps, changes in razors, less frequent shaving, and use of adequate shaving cream or lubricants. Most cases are caused by *S. aureus* and can be treated with topical antibiotics such as mupirocin (Bactroban), erythromycin 2% (A/T/S), or clindamycin 1% (Cleocin T). More severe recalcitrant cases may require systemic β-lactamase–resistant antibiotics. Cultures are now recommended in view of CA-MRSA and nosocomial-acquired MRSA and VRSA. Fungal cultures are also recommended in recalcitrant cases—particularly in patients with tinea pedis, tinea cruris, tinea corporis, and tinea capitis—because of mimicking of bacterial disease by these infections. Less common causes include gram-negative bacteria such as *Klebsiella* or *Enterobacter*, which may be seen as a consequence of antibiotic therapy for acne vulgaris. *Pseudomonas aeruginosa* and *Pseudomonas cepacia* are associated with hot-tub exposure (*hot-tub folliculitis*). Low disinfectant levels in hot tubs need to be addressed before patients reenter the hot tub. Hot-tub folliculitis is usually self-limited and resolves in 7 to 10 days. Proteus is occasionally seen as a deeper, more nodular type of lesion.

Furuncles and Carbuncles

Furuncles are more involved infections of the pilosebaceous unit resulting in indurated, red, painful nodules. Carbuncles are further extensions of this process to include multiple lesions that are interconnected to form multiloculated abscesses. The most common organism is *S. aureus*. Environmental factors including sweating, friction, oils and grease, poor hygiene, pre-existing dermatoses, nutritional factors, and immune status are all-important contributors. The most common areas of involvement include the face, buttocks, thighs, perineum, breast, and axillae. Carbuncles more commonly involve the neck because of the thickness of the skin in this area.

TREATMENT

Good hygiene and warm compresses along with appropriate empiric, systemic, antibiotic therapy will clear most cases. Mupirocin ointment may be applied to the anterior nares, axillae, groin, gluteal cleft, and folds of the neck in patients with recurrent disease to attempt to reduce the carrier state. Use of antiseptic soaps in these patients is discouraged because of lack of efficacy and the potential to develop additional resistance patterns. Large abscesses may require incision and drainage. Bacterial cultures should be obtained, if possible, before institution of therapy and in recalcitrant cases. In immunocompromised patients, including diabetics, fungal and mycobacterial cultures should be considered.

Hidradenitis suppurativa is a condition that at first may resemble chronic furunculosis. Primary involvement is seen in the axillae, nape of the neck, inframammillary, and perineum. These patients form large abscesses, which are usually subcutaneous without evidence of follicular origin. Hidradenitis is treated with incision and drainage, antibiotics, and, in severe cases, extirpation with grafting of the involved skin.

Cellulitis and Erysipelas

Cellulitis is a more invasive infection of the skin and associated soft tissues. Erysipelas is a more superficial form of cellulitis and occurs predominantly on the face and legs. Because of the acute onset and fiery red appearance, it has been called "St. Anthony's fire."

Cellulitis is frequently preceded by some type of superficial injury to the skin. Tinea pedis, dermatitis, varicella, or traumatic injuries are common precipitators. *S. aureus* and β-hemolytic streptococci are the most common causes. *Haemophilus influenzae* (less common since the *H. influenzae* type b [Hib] vaccine) group B streptococci in newborns and pneumonococcal cellulitis in immunocompromised patients also occur. Less common causes include atypical mycobacterium, *Vibrio vulnificus* (from exposure to sea water), and gram-negative bacteria such as *Pseudomonas* and *Klebsiella*.

Localized skin abscesses with necrosis, gangrene, septicemia, ascending lymphangitis, and thrombophlebitis may occur. Anaerobic infections with clostridium originating from soil and bacteroides from fecal material are also seen. Many of these infections are polymicrobial and can be quite aggressive, dissecting along fascial planes.

TREATMENT

Treatment of cellulitis begins with a systemic antibiotic, chosen on an empiric basis, bearing in mind the wound, immune status of the patient, and observed toxicity of the patient. Localized disease may be treated in an otherwise nontoxic healthy individual with oral antibiotics and outpatient follow-up. More aggressive infections in immunocompromised patients require intravenous antibiotic therapy along with incision and drainage and/or débridement if abscesses or necrotic tissue are present. Simpler infections require antibiotics that will cover *S. aureus* and streptococci. In children, *H. influenzae* must be considered, as it is best treated with amoxicillin/clavulanate (Augmentin) or other effective antibiotics. Needle aspiration and tissue cultures are helpful in some cases; however, yield from such procedures is typically less than 10% to 20% recovery of causative organisms. In infections that do not appear to respond or progress despite adequate therapy, the clinician should consider the possibility of resistant organisms, atypical organisms, and necrotizing fasciitis.

Staphylococcal Scalded Skin Syndrome

Staphylococcal scalded skin syndrome (SSSS) is a toxin-mediated manifestation of infection with staphylococci, usually phage group II. It occurs mainly in children and presents with acute fever, skin tenderness, and a scarlatiniform erythema. Flaccid bullae and erosions develop in 1 to 2 days, followed by desquamation.

TREATMENT

Treatment is directed at the *S. aureus* with β-lactamase–resistant antibiotics. Sicker children and adults should be admitted for initial stabilization, then discharged on oral antibiotics once stable. Most cases heal without significant scarring, although darker individuals may have variation of pigmentation that may persist for some time.

Necrotizing Fasciitis

Necrotizing fasciitis is a deep infection of subcutaneous soft tissue involving fascia and fat. It is classified in two categories, type I and type II. Immunocompromised individuals including diabetics, patients with peripheral vascular disease, adolescents, and those over 65 years of age are at increased risk. However, the frequency is increasing in normal individuals including athletes or following minor injuries, varicella, and trauma.

Type I necrotizing fasciitis occurs most commonly after surgical procedures, in diabetic patients, and in patients with peripheral vascular diseases. It is a mixed infection with both aerobic and anaerobic bacteria including *S. aureus*, *Escherichia coli*, group A *Streptococcus*, *Peptostreptococcus* spp, *Prevotella* and *Porphyromonas* spp, *Clostridium* spp, and *Bacteroides fragilis*.

Type II necrotizing fasciitis is caused by group A *Streptococcus* (GAS) and shares clinical features with spontaneous gangrenous myositis. Many of the patients are not as chronically ill as those in type I disease and present from the community following varicella, injection drug use, lacerations, childbirth, surgical procedures, blunt trauma, and exposure to other patients.

Initial presentation of necrotizing fasciitis is not always dramatic and may involve localized swelling of an extremity, followed by dusky, purple, nonblanching skin, and localized tenderness to underlying muscle groups. Patients may be relatively asymptotic, particularly those who are chronically ill, until sepsis and hypotension develop. Laboratory values including leukocytosis and hyperglycemia are usually nonspecific, so a high index of suspicion is necessary to suspect the diagnosis. Most cases progress rapidly to frank septicemia, hypotension, and necrosis. Despite adequate intervention with systemic antibiotics and surgical débridement, mortality may approach 40% to 50%, particularly in patients with multiple underlying medical conditions.

If necrotizing fasciitis is considered in the diagnosis, prompt surgical consult with a surgeon experienced in management of these patients may be lifesaving. Imaging studies may be helpful in some cases, but may delay diagnostic and therapeutic surgical intervention.

Anthrax

Anthrax infections of the skin were considered rare until the occurrence of bioterrorism events during the last few years. Recognizing cutaneous infection requires good diagnostic skills, index of suspicion, and appropriate laboratory evaluation. Early recognition of an outbreak can lead to appropriate lifesaving treatment of the patient involved, and to treatment of asymptomatic, exposed individuals with appropriate antibiotic prophylaxis.

Cutaneous anthrax is caused by *Bacillus anthracis*, a gram-positive, spore-forming bacillus that is named for the Greek word for coal or charcoal, *anthrakos*. The bacillus has two plasmids. One of these codes for a glutamic acid capsule that prevents phagocytosis; the other codes for toxin subunits.

Cutaneous anthrax results from direct inoculation of spores into the skin, usually from minor abrasions to the skin. After a latency period of approximately 5 days (range of 1 to 12 days), a nontender pruritic macule or papule is noted. Within 24 to 48 hours, the lesion progresses to a vesicle or bulla that enlarges up to 2 cm. It ruptures, forms an ulcer, and develops a hemorrhagic crust. Edema and satellite vesicles also ensue. Regional adenopathy, low-grade fever, and malaise may occur. The overlying crust develops into a dark, painless ester. Differential diagnoses include brown recluse spider bite and ulceroglandular tularemia. In anthrax, the edema and painlessness are important differentiating signs. Diagnosis is confirmed by use of cultures and skin biopsy before institution of antibiotic therapy. In suspected cases, consultation with a laboratory director, pathologist, and dermatologist should be obtained to ensure that an adequate sample is obtained and that specimens are handled properly so an accurate positive or negative diagnosis can be made. Public health officials should be alerted in all suspected cases, as they will coordinate public health response and treatment of other potentially exposed patients.

TREATMENT

Once material is obtained by biopsy, treatment of the infection can begin with ciprofloxacin (Cipro) or doxycycline (Vibramycin). Ciprofloxacin is favored in young children, pregnant females, and breast-feeding mothers. Initial therapy in normal adults is ciprofloxacin, 500 mg orally twice daily, or doxycycline, 100 mg orally twice daily. Children should receive ciprofloxacin, 15 mg/kg every 12 hours (not to exceed 1 g per day) or doxycycline, which is given in varying doses depending on age and weight—100 mg every 12 hours in children older than 8 years and weight greater than 45 kg; 2.2 mg/kg every 12 hours if medically indicated rather than ciprofloxacin in smaller children. Pregnant women may be treated with the normal adult dose of ciprofloxacin. Doxycycline is favored in pregnant women only if susceptibilities are known. Immunocompromised patients are treated at the same doses as normal adults. Duration of treatment in all confirmed/suspected cases is 100 days.

HUMAN HERPESVIRUSES

METHOD OF

Sylvia L. Brice, MD

Herpes Simplex Virus Types 1 and 2

Herpes simplex virus types 1 and 2 (HSV-1 and HSV-2) are the most closely related members of the human herpesvirus family (Table 1), and the skin lesions they produce are clinically indistinguishable. Clusters of tense blisters on an erythematous base often quickly evolve into erosions or ulcerations with associated crusting. Lesions may develop at any mucocutaneous site but are typically found in the perioral or anogenital regions. Both HSV-1 and HSV-2 are transmitted by direct mucocutaneous contact with an infected host. Following viral replication in the skin or mucosa, intact viral nucleocapsids travel via sensory neurons to the corresponding dorsal root ganglia to establish latency. Later, a variety of stimuli may trigger reactivation. The virus travels back along the sensory neurons to the mucocutaneous surface to replicate and induce active or subclinical infection. In the case of subclinical infection, no active skin lesions are evident but infectious particles are present, a state known as asymptomatic shedding. While the viral titer is much lower than during clinically active disease, asymptomatic shedding of the virus in oral and genital secretions is thought to be responsible for the majority of cases of HSV transmission.

Primary, initial nonprimary (or first episode), and recurrent are terms used to further define the nature of the HSV infection. A primary infection refers to a patient's first infection with HSV, either type 1 or 2, at any site. These patients are seronegative initially but subsequently develop HSV type-specific antibodies. A patient who is already infected with one HSV type and then develops an infection with the alternate type will experience what is known as an initial/nonprimary or first-episode infection (e.g., the first episode of genital herpes in a patient with a prior history of orofacial herpes). These patients are seropositive for one type-specific HSV antibody (e.g., HSV-1) and later develop antibodies specific for the alternate HSV type (e.g., HSV-2). Finally, a recurrent infection is that which occurs at a site of prior infection. These patients are seropositive for HSV-1 or HSV-2, or both. Because most primary infections, whether oral or genital, are asymptomatic, the first evidence of disease often represents a recurrent or initial/nonprimary infection.

OROFACIAL HERPES SIMPLEX VIRUS

Orofacial HSV, also known as herpes labialis, fever blisters, or cold sores, is commonly acquired during childhood or adolescence. Symptomatic primary disease usually takes the form of gingivostomatitis with or without additional lesions on the cutaneous perioral surfaces. Fever, malaise, and tender lymphadenopathy may also be present. In recurrent episodes, clusters of blisters erupt along the vermillion border of the lips with subsequent erosions and crusting persisting for several days up to 2 weeks. Lesions may develop anywhere in the perioral area, especially on the cheeks. In men, a viral folliculitis of the beard area (herpetic sycosis) may be mistaken for a bacterial process because it is often pustular in nature. The presence of a prodrome and recurrence in the same site are clues to the correct diagnosis. Although recurrent intraoral lesions of HSV may occur, they are uncommon in immunocompetent individuals. Exposure to ultraviolet light is a common trigger factor for herpes labialis as is fever or intercurrent infection.

GENITAL HERPES SIMPLEX VIRUS

When symptomatic, primary genital herpes often involves bilaterally distributed lesions in the anogenital area with associated fever, inguinal adenopathy, and dysuria or urinary retention. Aseptic meningitis

TABLE 1 The Human Herpesviruses

Human Herpesvirus	Alternate Name	Associated Clinical Infection
Human herpesvirus-1 (HHV-1)	Herpes simplex virus type 1	Orofacial herpes, genital herpes, herpetic whitlow, eczema herpeticum
Human herpesvirus-2 (HHV-2)	Herpes simplex virus type 2	Genital herpes, herpetic whitlow, eczema herpeticum, orofacial herpes
Human herpesvirus-3 (HHV-3)	Varicella-zoster virus	Varicella (chickenpox), herpes zoster (shingles)
Human herpesvirus-4 (HHV-4)	Epstein-Barr virus	Infectious mononucleosis, oral hairy leukoplakia
Human herpesvirus-5 (HHV-5)	Cytomegalovirus	Viral exanthem, *blueberry muffin* baby, chronic perianal ulceration in HIV
Human herpesvirus-6 (HHV-6)	None	Roseola infantum (also known as exanthem subitum, sixth disease)
Human herpesvirus-7 (HHV-7)	None	
Human herpesvirus-8 (HHV-8)	Kaposi's sarcoma-associated herpesvirus	Kaposi's sarcoma

may also occur. The lesions often persist for 2 to 3 weeks or longer. Nonprimary infections are usually less severe with fewer constitutional symptoms. Recurrent episodes tend to be milder and shorter in duration. Often, there is a prodrome of tingling or burning followed by the development of localized vesicles that may quickly rupture, leaving nonspecific erosions or ulcerations. The lesions may be anywhere within the anogenital region but tend to recur close to the same area in subsequent episodes. The time between exposure and development of primary disease is estimated to be from 3 to 14 days. However, more often the first clinical indication of disease is a recurrence, which may occur weeks to years after the initial infection. Prior infection with HSV-1 provides some protection against acquisition of HSV-2.

Based on seroepidemiologic evidence, it is estimated that at least 22% of the population in the United States 12 years of age and older is infected with HSV-2. Most of these individuals have not been officially diagnosed with this disease and are not aware that they are infected. Nevertheless, they experience asymptomatic shedding and unknowingly transmit the disease to sexual partners. Interrupting this cycle of transmission has become a major focus among health care givers who work with these patients. A combination of patient education and appropriate use of systemic antiviral agents may gradually have some impact on this epidemic. Recommendations for patients with genital herpes include avoidance of sex with uninfected partners when active lesions or prodromal symptoms are present, and the routine use of latex condoms to minimize transmission during periods of asymptomatic shedding. Chronic suppressive doses of oral antiviral agents (Table 2), including acyclovir (Zovirax), valacyclovir (Valtrex), and famciclovir (Famvir), significantly reduce the frequency of clinical recurrences as well as the rate of asymptomatic shedding and may be recommended together with these other practices to reduce the risk of transmission.

Although HSV-2 is the etiologic agent in a majority of cases of genital herpes infections, an increasing number of genital herpes infections are caused by HSV-1. Symptomatic recurrences and asymptomatic shedding are less frequent with genital HSV-1 infection than with genital HSV-2 infection, and this distinction becomes important for patient counseling and prognosis.

OTHER MUCOCUTANEOUS HERPES SIMPLEX VIRUS INFECTIONS

Eczema herpeticum, also known as Kaposi's varicelliform eruption, represents a cutaneous dissemination of HSV usually seen in patients with atopic dermatitis or other underlying skin disease. Herpetic vesicles develop over an extensive mucocutaneous surface, most often the face, neck, and upper trunk, presumably spreading from a recurrent oral HSV infection or asymptomatic shedding from the oral mucosa. Eczema herpeticum may also develop in the presence of genital HSV. As with other HSV infections, eczema herpeticum may be recurrent. In addition, patients may develop localized, recurrent HSV in previously involved areas. Because of the extensive and inflammatory nature of the process, and the possible secondary bacterial infection, the underlying viral etiology may be obscured. A history of eczema and recurrent HSV in the patient and careful observation for the grouped vesicles or erosions can be key to the correct diagnosis.

Herpetic whitlow refers to HSV infection of the hand, usually one or more distal digits. Previously thought to be limited to health care professionals with exposure to oral secretions of their patients, it is now recognized that autoinoculation from orolabial or genital HSV contributes to a significant number of cases.

Herpes gladiatorum is a problem seen most commonly in athletes who participate in close contact sports such as wrestling. Typically transmitted from active herpes labialis or asymptomatic shedding in oral secretions of an infected opponent, herpes gladiatorum often affects the head, neck, or shoulders and may be recurrent.

TABLE 2 Recommendations for Systemic Antiviral Treatment of Mucocutaneous Herpes Simplex Virus (HSV) Infection

Genital HSV		
Primary/first episode	Acyclovir (Zovirax)	400 mg PO tid or 200 mg PO 5 × per d × 10d (mild to moderate) 5 mg/kg IV q8h × 5d (severe)
	Valacyclovir (Valtrex)	1 g PO bid × 10d
	Famciclovir (Famvir)	250 mg PO tid × 10d
Recurrent episode	Acyclovir	400 mg PO tid or 200 mg PO 5 × d × 5d
	Valacyclovir	500 mg PO bid × 3d
	Famciclovir	125 mg PO bid × 5d
Chronic suppressive therapy	Acyclovir	400 mg PO bid or 200 mg PO tid; adjust up or down according to response (>6 outbreaks per year)
	Valacyclovir	500 mg PO qd (<10 outbreaks per year) 1 g PO qd (10 or more outbreaks per year)
	Famciclovir	250 mg PO bid (6 or more outbreaks per year)
Orofacial HSV		
Recurrent	Acyclovir	400 mg PO 5 × d for 5d; start at prodrome
	Valacyclovir	2 g PO bid ×1d; start at prodrome
	Famciclovir	500 mg PO tid × 5d; minimally more effective than 250 mg PO tid; start at prodrome
Chronic suppressive therapy	Acyclovir	400 mg PO tid (adjust up or down according to response)
	Valacyclovir	500 mg-1 g PO qd
	Famciclovir	250 mg PO bid
Orolabial or Genital HSV in Immunosuppressed Patients		
Recurrent/suppressive	Acyclovir	400 mg PO 5 × d or 5-10 mg/kg IV q8h
	Valacyclovir	500 mg PO bid
	Famciclovir	500 mg PO bid

Abbreviations: bid = twice daily; IV = intravenous; PO = by mouth; qd = daily; tid = three times a day.

Varicella-Zoster Virus (Herpes Zoster)

Varicella-zoster virus (VZV), another member of the human herpesvirus family (see Table 1), produces two specific patterns of disease in the skin. The primary infection results in varicella, also known as chickenpox, a widespread vesicular eruption usually seen in the pediatric population (see Section 2 of this book). Following the primary infection, VZV establishes latency in the dorsal root ganglia until some later point in time when reactivation may occur. The ensuing unilateral dermatomal distribution of blisters, often preceded by neuralgic pain, is known as herpes zoster or shingles. Herpes zoster is especially common in patients over 50 years of age, although it may be seen at any age. It is also seen more frequently in the immunocompromised patient population such as organ-transplant recipients or individuals infected with HIV. Herpes zoster is no longer considered a marker for underlying cancer, and evaluation for occult malignancy in an otherwise asymptomatic individual is not indicated. A single recurrence of herpes zoster, usually in the same dermatome, may occur in up to 4% of zoster patients. Additional recurrences, however, suggest a dermatomal form of HSV, and laboratory assessment for this possibility should be performed.

The most common dermatomes involved with herpes zoster are in the thoracolumbar (T3-L2) and trigeminal (V1) regions. Skin lesions typically evolve from papules to vesicles and pustules, and then crusted erosions, before healing approximately 2 to 4 weeks after onset. The associated neuropathic pain commonly persists after the lesions have healed. If pain continues for more than 1 month after resolution of the skin lesions, it is referred to as postherpetic neuralgia, one of the most common and debilitating complications of this infection.

Several clinical presentations of herpes zoster deserve additional attention. Ophthalmic zoster, with lesions along the tip, side, or base of the nose indicating involvement of the nasociliary branch of the trigeminal nerve (Hutchinson's sign), may be associated with increased risk for ocular complications. Prompt initiation of a systemic antiviral agent (Table 3) and evaluation by an ophthalmologist

TABLE 3 Recommendations for Systemic Antiviral Treatment of Herpes Zoster

Immunocompetent Patients
Acyclovir (Zovirax) 800 mg PO 5 × d for 7-10d
Valacyclovir (Valtrex) 1 g PO tid × 7d
Famciclovir (Famvir) 500 mg PO tid × 7d
Immunosuppressed Patients
Acyclovir 800 mg PO 5 × d for 10d* 10 mg/kg/dose IV q8h × 7-10d*
Valacyclovir 1 g PO tid x 10d*
Famciclovir 500 mg PO tid × 10d*

*Continue until there are no new lesions for 48 hours.
Abbreviations: IV = intravenous; PO = by mouth; tid = three times a day.

are recommended. Disseminated zoster, with more than a few lesions outside the primary and immediately adjacent dermatomes, can be indicative of visceral involvement and its associated complications. The term *zoster sine herpete* is used to describe patients with neuropathic pain resembling zoster but without any skin lesions. The diagnosis can be supported by demonstration of increased immunoglobulin (Ig) G antibody titers between the acute and convalescent phases. Chronic zoster is seen predominantly in HIV-infected individuals. Single or multiple warty growths may persist for weeks or months in areas of skin previously involved by typical lesions of varicella or herpes zoster. Chronic zoster is often acyclovir-resistant. Both tissue biopsy and viral cultures, with further testing for antiviral resistance, may aid in assessment.

Diagnosis

HERPES SIMPLEX VIRUS

Viral culture remains the preferred method for diagnosis of HSV infection. This method is sensitive when specimens are obtained from lesions that have not yet become too dry or crusted, usually during the first 2 to 3 days after onset. An adequate sample, obtained by unroofing the blister and swabbing the base, increases the likelihood of an accurate result. Antigen detection tests may remain positive even after lesions have dried, as long as the specimen includes epithelial cells and not just debris. For this method, a scraping from the lesion is usually smeared on a glass slide to be sent to the laboratory. Not all antigen detection methods are designed to distinguish HSV-1 from HSV-2. The Tzanck smear (cytologic detection) is both insensitive and nonspecific but may be of use in some clinical settings. It does not differentiate HSV types or HSV from VZV. Polymerase chain reaction (PCR) is highly sensitive but not routinely used for diagnosis of mucocutaneous HSV infections.

Serologic testing for HSV was previously of limited use because it could not reliably differentiate HSV-1 from HSV-2. Because they share significant genetic homology, HSV-1 and HSV-2 code for a number of common proteins that are not antigenically distinct. However, they also code for type-specific proteins that can be used to differentiate them. Current tests based on detection of type-specific viral glycoprotein G (gG-based, type-specific assays) are accurate and should be requested for this purpose. A positive HSV-2 serology may be useful in confirming the diagnosis of genital herpes in a patient with a negative viral culture or with unrecognized or asymptomatic disease. Alternatively, a negative serology may exclude the diagnosis of HSV in a patient with chronic, nonspecific oral or genital symptoms.

HERPES ZOSTER

Diagnosis of herpes zoster is often made on clinical grounds alone. A Tzanck smear may provide additional support of the viral etiology. With atypical presentations, however, the diagnosis is best confirmed by either an antigen detection method or viral culture. Both will differentiate VZV from HSV. Samples submitted for viral culture should be obtained from vesicular fluid because dried or crusted lesions are unlikely to yield positive results. Viral cultures are required if there is a need to assess possible antiviral resistance. PCR can be useful for detection of VZV in bodily fluids such as cerebrospinal fluid. VZV serology is rarely useful for diagnosis, because a majority of the population is seropositive.

Treatment

There are three systemic antiviral agents routinely used for the treatment of HSV and VZV infections—acyclovir (Zovirax), valacyclovir (Valtrex), and famciclovir (Famvir). All three are highly effective and generally well tolerated. Because they inhibit only actively replicating viral DNA, they have no impact on latent infection. Recommendations for antiviral treatment of mucocutaneous HSV infections and herpes zoster, localized topical measures, and available formulations are outlined in Tables 2, 3, 4, and 5. Optimal antiviral dosage schedules for less common HSV infections, such as herpetic whitlow, have not been determined. The doses outlined in Table 2 for either episodic or chronic suppressive therapy can be used as a guideline in these cases.

Acyclovir became available more than 20 years ago and continues to be widely used. Inside an infected host cell, acyclovir must be phosphorylated—first by a virally encoded enzyme (thymidine kinase) and then by host-cell enzymes—to the active form of the drug, acyclovir-triphosphate. As a nucleotide analogue, acyclovir-triphosphate is incorporated into replicating viral DNA, abruptly terminating further synthesis of that viral DNA chain. Acyclovir-triphosphate also interferes with viral DNA replication by directly inhibiting viral DNA polymerase. Valacyclovir is an oral prodrug of acyclovir and has a much higher bioavailability. After ingestion, valacyclovir is rapidly metabolized to acyclovir and the subsequent mechanism of action is as just described. Famciclovir is an oral prodrug of penciclovir, designed for greater bioavailability. Similar to acyclovir, penciclovir must first be phosphorylated by viral thymidine kinase and then by cellular enzymes to penciclovir-triphosphate. In this active form, penciclovir-triphosphate interferes with viral DNA synthesis and replication by inhibiting viral DNA polymerase. Famciclovir has both greater bioavailability and a longer intracellular half-life than acyclovir. For all three agents, the required activation by viral thymidine kinase and the preferential inhibition of viral DNA synthesis contribute to the highly specific antiviral activity.

If taken as recommended, acyclovir, valacyclovir, and famciclovir are generally comparable in their safety and effectiveness. Valacyclovir and famciclovir

TABLE 4 Topical Treatment Options for Mucocutaneous Herpes Simplex Virus (HSV) and Varicella-Zoster Virus (VZV) Infections

Topical Treatment	Comment
Cool, moist compresses using tap water or aluminum acetate 1:20 to 1:40 (Burow's solution, Domeboro, Bluboro)	Good for moist, oozing lesions to accelerate drying. Apply wet dressing to involved skin and cover with dry cloth to allow evaporation.
Calamine lotion or similar shake lotion containing alcohol, menthol, and/or phenol; Aveeno colloidal oatmeal	Useful as drying and antipruritic agent. May be applied after wet dressing.
Bacitracin[1], Polysporin, mupirocin[1] (Bactroban)	Use if there is concern for localized secondary bacterial infection.
2% Viscous lidocaine, compounded* suspensions (e.g., Kaopectate or Maalox, diphenhydramine, lidocaine)	Useful for temporary pain relief of oral or genital mucosal involvement.
Acyclovir (Zovirax) ointment	Used together with systemic antiviral agents, may be of benefit to immunocompromised individuals for localized HSV.
Penciclovir (Denavir) cream	May decrease the duration of lesions in herpes labialis by half a day if applied every 2h while awake for 4 days beginning at the first sign of disease.

[1]Not FDA approved for this indication.
*May be compounded by pharmacies.

offer the convenience of less frequent dosing. Dosing for all three should be adjusted in the presence of renal insufficiency (Table 6).

Although antiviral therapy does not decrease the incidence of postherpetic neuralgia, all three agents decrease the time for lesion healing and shorten the overall duration of pain if initiated within 48 to 72 hours after the onset of herpes zoster. Valacyclovir and famciclovir appear to be more effective than acyclovir for this purpose. An otherwise healthy individual younger than 50 years of age with discrete involvement on the trunk and mild to moderate pain may benefit minimally or not at all from this intervention, especially if it is initiated after 72 hours of lesion onset. However, patients who are older than 50 years of age, are immunosuppressed, have involvement in the ophthalmic distribution, or have more extensive lesions or severe pain should receive systemic antiviral therapy, even if the 72-hour deadline has expired. Adequate pain control, often requiring opiates, is also important. The addition of systemic corticosteroids to the antiviral regimen remains controversial. There is evidence to suggest this can lessen the severity of the acute episode but does not decrease the incidence or duration of postherpetic neuralgia. Corticosteroids should not be used without concomitant antiviral therapy.

Despite widespread use of these antiviral agents, antiviral resistance is rarely a problem in the immunocompetent population. However, it does arise in the setting of immunosuppression. The basis for the resistance is most commonly because of a mutation in the gene coding for thymidine kinase. Less commonly, there is a mutation in the viral DNA polymerase. In either case, all three standard drugs become ineffective. Alternative antiviral agents available for treatment of acyclovir-resistant HSV and VZV infections include foscarnet (Foscavir)[1] and cidofovir (Vistide)[1].

Hand Foot and Mouth Disease

Hand foot and mouth disease is typically a disease of childhood. The etiologic agent is an enterovirus, and transmission is via the oral–oral or fecal–oral route. It is highly contagious. Several days after exposure, a prodrome of low-grade fever, malaise, abdominal pain, or respiratory symptoms may develop, followed by the appearance of papulovesicles on the palate, tongue, or buccal mucosa. Similar lesions may subsequently develop on the feet and hands. The eruption persists for 7 to 10 days and then resolves. Treatment is symptomatic.

Parvovirus B19

Cutaneous manifestations of parvovirus B19 infection include the childhood exanthem known as

[1]Not FDA approved for this indication.

TABLE 5 Formulations of Acyclovir, Valacyclovir, and Famciclovir

Drug	Oral	Topical	Intravenous
Acyclovir (Zovirax)	200, 400, 800 mg 200 mg/5 mL suspension	5% Ointment (3 g, 15 g tube)	Yes
Valacyclovir (Valtrex)	500 mg, 1 g	No	No
Famciclovir (Famvir)	125, 250, 500 mg	No	No
Penciclovir (Denavir)	No	1% Cream (1.5 g tube)	No

TABLE 6 Recommended Antiviral Dose Modification in Patients with Impaired Renal Function

Initial Genital HSV		Recurrent Genital HSV	Genital HSV—Chronic Suppression	Herpes Zoster
Acyclovir (Zovirax)				
CrCl >25	200 mg 5 × d	200 mg 5 × d	400 mg q12h	800 mg 5 × d
CrCl 10-24	200 mg 5 × d	200 mg 5 × d	400 mg q12h	800 mg q8h
CrCl <10	200 mg q12h	200 mg q12h	200 mg q12h	800 mg q12h
Valacyclovir (Valtrex)				
CrCl >50	1 g q12h	500 mg q12h	500 mg-1 g q24h	1 g q 8h
CrCl 30-49	1 g q12h	500 mg q12h	500 mg-1 g q24h	1 g q12h
CrCl 10-29	1 g q24h	500 mg q24h	500 mg q24-48h	1 g q24h
CrCl <10	500 mg q24h	500 mg q24h	500 mg q24-48h	500 mg q24h
Famciclovir (Famvir)				
CrCl >60		125 mg q12h	250 mg q12h	500 mg q 8h
CrCl 40-59		125 mg q12h	250 mg q12h	500 mg q12h
CrCl 20-39		125 mg q24h	125 mg q12h	500 mg q24h
CrCl <20		125 mg q24h	125 mg q24h	250 mg q24h

Abbreviation: CrCl = creatinine clearance.

erythema infectiosum (fifth disease) and, less commonly, petechial or purpuric eruptions. The virus is transmitted primarily via respiratory secretions and, to a much lesser extent, through blood or blood products. The host cells for viral replication are erythroid progenitor cells, which subsequently undergo cell lysis.

A child with erythema infectiosum typically develops a low-grade fever and nonspecific upper respiratory symptoms approximately 2 days before the onset of rash. The rash has been described as having a *slapped cheeks* appearance with prominent redness over the malar eminences. This is followed by a pink-to-red lacy or reticular eruption over the trunk and extensor surfaces of the arms and legs. The rash usually lasts a week to 10 days but may transiently recur over months in response to precipitating factors such as sunlight, exercise, and bathing. Diagnosis of erythema infectiosum is usually made on clinical grounds and treatment is symptomatic. By the time the rash appears and the diagnosis has been made, the child is no longer infectious.

Infection with parvovirus B19 in older adolescents and adults often presents with arthralgias or arthritis rather than a rash. In certain patient populations, parvovirus B19 infections may be associated with complications including transient aplastic crisis, chronic anemia, and hydrops fetalis. In these less typical presentations, serology (anti-B19 IgM or documented seroconversion) may be needed for diagnosis. Immunoglobulin intravenous (IGIV [Gamimune N])[1] is used successfully for treatment of chronic/persistent infection in immunosuppressed individuals.

Poxviruses

MOLLUSCUM CONTAGIOSUM

Molluscum contagiosum are benign, umbilicated papules caused by infection with the molluscipoxvirus, a member of the poxvirus family. Lesions are limited to the mucocutaneous surface and typically appear in clusters on the face, trunk, and skin fold areas in children versus thighs, lower abdomen, and suprapubic areas in sexually active adults. Large numbers of lesions in an extensive distribution may be seen in the immunosuppressed population. Transmission routinely occurs by skin-to-skin contact with an infected host, although transmission from contaminated fomites has been reported. Autoinoculation commonly occurs. Diagnosis is usually based on clinical exam, but histopathology of atypical lesions may be used for confirmation. Because molluscum contagiosum tend to be self-limited, treatment is not always required although it may reduce the risk of autoinoculation and transmission to others. Treatment modalities are primarily aimed at lesion destruction, similar to those used for verruca vulgaris. These are outlined in Table 7. In the case of sexual transmission, evaluation for other sexually transmitted diseases may be indicated.

ORF AND MILKER'S NODULES

Orf (also known as ecthyma contagiosum) and milker's nodules are caused by closely related parapoxviruses, members of the poxvirus family. The virus responsible for orf is widespread in sheep and goats, while the virus causing milker's nodules is found in cattle. Transmission to humans is by direct contact with infected animals and is usually seen several days up to 2 weeks after exposure. Orf and milker's nodules most commonly present as one to several nodules on the dorsal aspect of the hands or forearms. Lesions evolve through several clinical stages over a period of 3 to 5 weeks ranging from solid red nodules to vesicular, exudative, or wart-like tumors. As with other poxvirus infections, lesions of orf often demonstrate central umbilication. Regional lymphadenopathy and lymphangitis are commonly seen.

[1]Not FDA approved for this indication.

TABLE 7 Treatment Options for Molluscum Contagiosum

Treatment	Comment
Cryotherapy (liquid nitrogen)	Freeze individual lesions for 5-10 seconds. Repeat PRN in 2-3 weeks.
Curettage	Entire lesion may be removed using a curette. This results in bleeding. Removal of central core with toothpick or other pointed instrument is also effective.
Cantharidin (Cantharone)[1]	Blister-inducing agent. Apply to lesion with toothpick, air dry. Cover with tape or Band Aid. Patient to wash area after 24 hours (or sooner if significant pain).
Podophyllin (25% in tincture of benzoin)[1]	Cytotoxic agent. Apply to lesion with toothpick. Patient to wash off after 4-6 hours. Contraindicated in pregnancy.
Podofilox (Condylox 0.5% gel or solution)[1]	Done by patient. Apply bid for 3 consecutive days per week for 2-4 weeks. Contraindicated in pregnancy.
Salicylic acid/lactic acid (Occlusal, Duofilm)	Done by patient. Apply daily.
Imiquimod (Aldara) 5% cream[1]	Done by patient. Apply daily 5 consecutive days per week. Leave on overnight. Continue for 8-12 weeks.
Cimetidine (Tagamet)[1]	30 mg/kg/d PO for 6-12 weeks. May boost cell-mediated immunity.

[1]Not FDA approved for this indication.
Abbreviations: PO = by mouth; PRN = as needed.

Diagnosis is based on a history of exposure and clinical exam. Tissue biopsy for histopathology or electron microscopy may also be used. The lesions are self-limited and treatment is not routinely required.

PARASITIC DISEASES OF THE SKIN

METHOD OF

H.L. Greenberg, MD, and Harry Sharata, MD, PhD

Parasitic diseases of the skin require the clinician to have a high index of suspicion. Diagnosis is made by obtaining a thorough history, including recent travel (Table 1), and through examination of biopsy specimen and skin scrapings and specialized laboratory studies. A continually updated resource for treatment is available at the Centers for Disease Control and Prevention (CDC) web site, www.cdc.gov/travel/diseases.htm.

Protozoal Infections

Protozoa have a life cycle that includes trophozoite (motile) and cyst (nonmotile) forms. The protozoa which cause cutaneous disease are listed below.

AMEBIASIS

Usually seen in developing countries, *cutaneous amebiasis* is caused by a single-celled organism, *Entamoeba histolytica*. Nonspecific, irregular, and ulcerated, the lesion of amebiasis is often painful. Because of its appearance, cutaneous amebiasis may be confused with syphilis and infectious granulomas. There may also be associated adenopathy, and untreated persons may develop worsening infection or experience spread to internal organs. Transmitted through fecal-oral contact, cutaneous amebiasis may result from anal intercourse in an asymptomatic host, in those with amebic dysentery, or from an abscess located in the anogenital region including the penis, perineum, buttock, or abdomen. Trophozoites may be identified in the ulcer or from stool studies. Treatment includes metronidazole (Flagyl), 750 mg by mouth (PO) twice daily (bid) for 7 to 10 days for extraintestinal disease, followed by iodoquinol (Yodoxin), 650 mg PO three times daily (tid) for 20 days for an intestinal source.

LEISHMANIASIS

Cutaneous leishmaniasis, also known as the *Baghdad boil* or *chiclero ulcer,* is transmitted by an infected sand fly bite. Patients initially present with a papule or nodule that develops into ulcerated sores of different sizes and shapes with raised edges and a central crater, which may be painful. Treatment includes sodium stibogluconate (Pentostam)[1], 20 mg (pentavalent antimony)/kg/d intravenously (IV) or intramuscularly (IM) for 20 to 28 days, available as an Investigational New Drug (IND) from the CDC; itraconazole also has been used at 200 mg PO per day for 28 days.

TRYPANOSOMIASIS

There are three different trypanosomes: *Trypanosoma brucei* variants (*Trypanosoma gambiense* and *Trypanosoma rhodesiense*) and *Trypanosoma cruzi*. Infection with these organisms manifests as two disease variants: Chagas' disease and African sleeping sickness.

[1]Not FDA approved for this indication.

TABLE 1 Cutaneous Parasites and Their Treatment

Class	Disease Name	Geographic Distribution	Causative Organism	Recommended Treatment
Protozoa	Cutaneous Amebiasis	Developing countries	*Entamoeba histolytica*	Metronidazole (Flagy)[1] 750 mg PO tid × 7-10 d
	Leishmaniasis	Africa, Asia Middle East, Central and South America	*Leishmania* species	Sodium stibogluconate (Pentostam)[1] 20 mg/kg/d/ IV or IM × 20-28 d
	Chagas'	Central and South America	*Trypanosoma cruzi*	Nifurtimox (Lampit)[1] 8-10 mg/kg/d PO, qid in divided doses × 120 d
	African sleeping sickness	Africa	*Trypanosoma brucei*	Eflornithine (Ornidyl)[1] 100 mg per kg IV, q6h × 14 d
Helminths	Cutaneous larva migrans	Worldwide	*Ancylostoma braziliense*	Albendazole (Albenza)[1] 400 mg PO × 1 d
			Strongyloides stercoralis	Ivermectin (Stromectol) 200 µg/kg/ PO × 1-2 d
	Dracunculiasis	Rural Africa, Yemen	*Dracunculus medinensis*	Surgical removal, metronidazole (Flagyl)[1] 250 mg tid × 10 d
	Loiasis	Africa	*Loa loa*	Diethylcarbamazine (Hetrazan)[1] 9 mg/kg/d PO in 3 divided doses × 21 d
	Elephantiasis, lymphatic filariasis	Asia, Africa, Caribbean, South America	*Wuchereria bancrofti* and *brugia* species	Diethylcarbamazine[1] 6 mg/kg/d PO in 3 divided doses × 6-12 d
	River blindness	Africa and Latin America	*Onchocerca volvulus*	Ivermectin 150 µg/kg PO q6-12 mo
Arthropoda	Scabies	Worldwide	*Sarcoptes scabiei*	5% permethrin (Elimite) cream +/– ivermectin 200 µg/kg PO × 1 dose
	Body lice	Worldwide	*Pediculus humanus*	Symptomatic, clean clothing
	Pubic and head lice, crabs	Worldwide	*Pediculus pubis* and *P. capitis*	5% permethrin (Elimite), repeat in 1 wk
	Chiggers, tungiasis	Central and South America, Africa	*Tunga penetrans*	Flea removal, symptomatic Rx
	Myiasis	Worldwide	*Dermatobia hominis/botfly*	Surgical removal, topical therapies

[1]Not FDA approved for this indication.
Abbreviations: IV, intravenously; PO, by mouth; q, every; qid, four times daily; tid, three times daily.

Chagas' disease is caused by *T. cruzi*, and is found in Texas, Mexico, Central and South America; transmission is by the reduviid (kissing) bug. Initial infection may be inapparent on the skin or may show a boardlike erythematous induration with a subcutaneous nodule (chagoma). Romaña's sign is seen if the bite is near the eye, yielding eyelid edema and conjunctivitis. Systemic involvement can lead to central nervous system (CNS) disease, dilated cardiomyopathy, mega esophagus, and megacolon. Diagnosis is based on hematologic examination (motile trypomastigotes). Alternatively, the patient may be exposed to laboratory reduviid bugs, which will later be sacrificed and examined for trypomastigotes. Early treatment relieves parasitemia in 2 days with symptomatic improvement in 3 to 10 days and the prevention of systemic sequelae. Treatment efficacy is reduced with visceral involvement. Nifurtimox (Lampit)[1], available through the CDC Parasitic Drug Service, is dosed at 8 to 10 mg/kg/d PO (in divided doses) four times daily for 120 days.

[1]Not FDA approved for this indication.

African sleeping sickness, East and West, is caused by *T. rhodesiense* and *T. gambiense*, respectively, and is found mostly in Africa. Transmission occurs through an infected tsetse fly bite. A painful chancre (red, erythematous nodule) surrounded by a white halo measuring 1 to 3 cm develops at the bite site 50% of the time, usually within 4 to 5 days. As parasitemia develops, the patient may demonstrate generalized pruritic eruptions with erythematous annular plaques, fevers, and posterior cervical adenopathy (Winterbottom's sign) in association with the nodule. Transient edema of eyelids, palms, and soles occurs within weeks to months. Early treatment is essential to prevent CNS involvement including personality changes, slurred speech, seizure, confusion, and sleeping abnormalities. Treatment for *Trypanosoma* infection varies depending on the species; the disease is fatal (within months to years) if not treated. For *T. brucei* or *T. gambiense*, first-line therapy is eflornithine (Ornidyl)[1], available from the World Health Organization (WHO), dosed at

[1]Not FDA approved for this indication.

100 mg/kg IV every 6 hours for 14 days, followed by 75 mg/kg/d PO for 21 to 30 days. *The commercially available topical formulation should not be used to treat trypanosomal disease.* Suramin sodium (Antrypol)[1], available from the CDC Parasitic Drug Service, is used to treat both *T. brucei gambiense* and *T. rhodesiense*. Suramin sodium dosage is 0.2 g IV test dose, followed by 20 mg/kg (maximum dose 1 g) IV on days 1, 3, 7, 14, and 21.

Helminths

ANCYLOSTOMA BRAZILIENSE

Ancylostoma braziliense is the causative agent of cutaneous larva migrans, or creeping eruption. Hookworm larvae (*Ancylostoma*) from contaminated dog or cat feces residing in soil, beach, or other sandy areas penetrate the feet and other skin contact areas. An erythematous papule develops into a wandering, lower epidermal serpiginous tract that can be intensely pruritic in a matter of hours. Associated excoriations from pruritus may become secondarily infected. Once present, larvae progress 1 to 2 cm a day. Another cutaneous larva migrans, *Strongyloides stercoralis*, may progress up to 10 cm a day. Diagnosis is usually clinical; however, a "wet prep" of the tissue may show larvae on microscopy. The larvae die naturally in weeks; however, treatment with albendazole (Albenza)[1], 400 mg PO for 1 day, is effective for *Ancylostoma**. An alternative therapy is mebendazole (Vermox), 500 mg PO for 1 day or 100 mg PO twice daily (bid) for 3 days. Treatment of *Strongyloides* infection includes ivermectin (Stromectol), 200 μg/kg/d PO for 1 to 2 days, or thiabendazole 25 mg/kg/d PO bid for 2 days. Liquid nitrogen application may be used to treat the advancing burrow area.

Infection prevention includes minimizing exposure through protective means including shoes and beach towels. Pet owners should have suspected pets examined and remove fecal matter from areas where human exposure is likely.

DRACUNCULIASIS

Dracunculiasis occurs after consumption of water with microscopic water fleas infected with the larvae of *Dracunculus medinensis*. Larvae are released from the fleas in the intestine, where they mate and develop into worms that travel to and rest in the subcutaneous skin. Within 1 year a blister forms over the now pregnant female worm (now some 70 to 120 cm in length). Once exposed to water, the blister ruptures and the worm releases its larvae. Surgical removal is considered definitive treatment and involves delicately winding the now mature Guinea worm around a small stick as it emerges through the skin. Care is taken to remove the whole worm as residual parasite can lead to inflammation. Metronidazole (Flagyl)[1], 250 mg PO tid for 10 days may be used as adjunctive therapy. Living in an area with good water treatment will prevent infection. Currently, infection is confined to rural African countries and Yemen.

FILARIAL DISEASES

Filarial diseases include infection with *Loa loa* (loiasis), *Onchocerca volvulus* (onchocerciasis), *Wuchereria bancrofti* (filariasis), and *Wuchereria brugia* or (*Wuchereria*) *malayi* (filariasis). Diagnosis is the same in filarial cases and involves a hematologic examination of thick and thin blood sample smears for the presence of microfilariae. Because microfilariae concentrate in the peripheral capillaries, blood draws through finger sticks are recommended. Antigen detection using an immunoassay for filarial antigens may be used for identification, as may an antibody test. However, because of antigenic cross-reactivity and lifelong postexposure positivity, it may not be possible to distinguish between previous and current infection.

LOIASIS

The filarial parasite *L. Loa* causes migratory angioedema, which lasts from hours to days, resulting in localized areas of swelling in the arms, legs, face, and trunk called *Calabar swellings*. In some cases, infection with *L. loa* will have subconjunctival migration of the adult worm visible as a raised serpiginous lesion in the scleral conjunctiva. Transmission occurs via the *Chrysops* fly bite. Treatment is the same as with other filarial diseases and involves diethylcarbamazine (Hetrazan)[1], 50 mg PO on day 1 followed by 9 mg/kg/d PO in three divided doses for 21 days. Encephalopathy has been observed with this medication, and is thought to be a reaction to the release of parasite antigens from microfilarial destruction.

LYMPHATIC FILARIASIS

Lymphatic channel obstruction by microfilarial migration of *W. bancrofti* or *B. malayi* leads to elephantiasis. Mosquitoes pass larvae to the human host; adult worms, measuring 8 to 10 cm, block lymphatics and produce microfilariae. Physical symptoms include massively enlarged extremities with occasional ulcers and sterile abscess formation. Like other filarial diseases, microfilariae are visible in blood samples. Treatment is with diethylcarbamazine (Hetrazan)[1], 6 mg/kg/d PO in three divided doses for 6 to 14 days. Ivermectin[1] 200 μg/kg PO for 1 dose can be used.

[1]Not FDA approved for this indication.

*Investigational drug in the United States.

[1]Not FDA approved for this indication.

ONCHOCERCIASIS

Onchocerca volvulus is a filarial parasite transmitted by the blackfly (genus *Simulium*). Infection is seen in Africa and Latin America, adjacent to rivers where the blackfly larvae develop. The adult worm parasite resides in the subcutaneous tissue where a localized pruritic nodule develops. Adult worms produce millions of microfilariae that spread throughout the subcutaneous tissue and skin, yielding an early maculopapular eruption with an asymmetrical distribution. Later, the eruption becomes hyperpigmented, with loss of skin elasticity, mottling, and atrophy. When infestation is great, there may be microfilariae deposition in the anterior chamber and other areas of the eye leading to chronic inflammation and vision loss, better known as *river blindness*. Treatment is ivermectin (Stromectol), 150 μg/kg PO every 6 to 12 months until free from disease. Unfortunately, ivermectin is only active against the microfilariae because adult worms are resistant to this therapy.

SCHISTOSOMIASIS

The three main *Schistosoma* species infecting humans are *Schistosoma haematobium, Schistosoma japonicum*, and *Schistosoma mansoni*.

Cutaneous schistosomiasis is known as cercarial dermatitis or swimmer's itch. Patients present after skin exposure to water contaminated with larvae (cercariae) from snails or waterfowl. Typically the patient will experience an itching, prickly sensation within minutes of cercariae penetration, sparing covered areas. Within 24 hours, red papules develop and may coalesce into blisters that last 5 to 7 days. This presentation is an allergic reaction, because infection with the nonhuman species of *Schistosoma* is self-limited and does not require specific treatment. Symptomatic treatment with oral antihistamines and topical steroids is all that is needed. Human schistosomiasis is treated with praziquantel (Biltricide), 20 mg/kg two to three times in 1 day.

Seabather's eruption is a closely related cercarial dermatitis occurring in salt water and demonstrating an eruption, confined to the swimsuit area, of pruritic, crusted papules within hours of bathing that resolve in several days. Treatment is the same as for cutaneous schistosomiasis.

Arthropoda

SCABIES

Scabies is a common disease caused by a mite, *Sarcoptes scabiei* (var. *hominis*) (Megnin, 1880). The infestation is usually related to poor hygiene, but is commonly seen in nursing homes, hospital wards, schools, and other close quarters. Transmission may occur through sexual contact and in areas of mite infestation including plush furniture, bedding, carpet, and clothes. Mite survival away from a host may last as long as 3 days. Vacuuming and discarding the used bag is essential. Scabies mites are small, with females measuring 0.4 × 0.3 mm, and males are half that size. Preferential sites of infestation include soft, hairless body parts including intergluteal folds, interdigital webs, genitalia, flexor wrist surface, lower abdomen, and axilla. Infants may have palmoplantar and scalp involvement. Immunosuppressed, debilitated, or institutionalized patients may have a severe and chronic infestation. In Norwegian scabies, numerous mites infest hands, feet, genitalia, and auricles, leading to prominent hyperkeratosis and crusting.

The mite lives in subcorneal burrows a few millimeters long and often attaches to a vesicle at the blind end. Identification of the mite is obtained by pricking the vesicle with a blade, smearing the contents onto a glass slide, adding a drop of 25% KOH, waiting 10 minutes, and then covering with a cover slip. Gentle heating over a flame helps dissolve keratin and release the mite. A chain of dark brown feces (scybala) or egg shells with or without larva are diagnostic (even if the mite is missed). Superficial shave biopsy demonstrates the tissue reaction typical of an insect bite (i.e., patchy lymphocytic infiltrate with eosinophils).

Adults should be treated from the neck down; infants can be treated from the scalp down. Preferred topical therapy is with 5% permethrin (Elimite) topical cream left on for 8 to 10 hours to be repeated in 1 week. An alternative therapy is Crotamiton 10% topical (Eurax) repeated in 24 hours (safety and effectiveness in children not established; treatment in pregnancy is category C). Lindane 1% cream left on 8 to 12 hours is also effective therapy, but has a slight risk of CNS toxicity and seizure; treatment in pregnancy is category B. Patients who are immunocompromised or who fail to resolve may use ivermectin (Stromectol), 200 μg/kg PO for one dose.

Post-scabetic itch may be treated with topical steroids (i.e., triamcinolone or hydrocortisone). Persistent post-scabetic nodules may occur within a year of the original treatment and may be treated with triamcinolone 5 to 10 mg/mL intralesional injection or high-potency topical steroids (e.g., clobetasol [Temovate]) 0.05% ointment or cream bid as needed. Animal scabies are transient bites that manifest as allergic reactions and are not true infestations. Antihistamines and topical steroids may be used to treat both post-scabetic itch and animal scabies.

PEDICULOSIS

Lice are ectoparasites; their only hosts are humans. Lice begin as nits (eggs) cemented to the hair base, becoming nymphs on the hair shaft and growing into adults on the distal hair shaft over a 2- to 3-week period. The louse feeds on blood several times daily. The typical louse bite yields a pruritic red macule with central hemorrhage. There are three types of human lice discussed subsequently: *Phthirus pubis* and *Pediculus humanus* var. *capitis* and *corporis*.

Pediculosis Corporis

Body lice are longer than head and pubic lice. They are seen more commonly in people who wear the same clothing daily, i.e., the homeless, refugees, and soldiers in wartime. Patients may have a wide variety of presentation from papuloerythematous eruptions to urticarial lesions. Involved areas include the buttocks and trunk. Severe cases may have bloody streaks with crusts secondary to deep excoriations. The lice and eggs are not found on the skin itself, but rather in the clothing, often in the seams. After bathing with soap and water, corticosteroid ointments and oral antihistamines may be used to control pruritus. All clothes and bedding will require laundering as detailed later. Incineration of heavily infested clothing may be necessary.

Pediculosis Pubis

Crab lice are broad, crablike, slow-moving organisms infesting the pubic, axillary, eyebrow, and eyelash hair. These organisms are typically transmitted through sexual contact, and workup of other sexually transmitted diseases may be indicated. Patients usually present with intense pruritus, eczematous change, excoriations, and secondary infection of "crabs." Bruise-like blue patches (maculae caeruleae) may be found on the trunk.

Pediculosis Humanus Capitis

Head lice are most commonly seen in children, usually schoolgirls who share combs or brushes. Lice may be confused with dandruff or hair products, such as hairspray. Typically, the occipital scalp shows the most involvement, followed by the posterior and lateral scalp; lesions may extend down the nape of the neck to the upper shoulders in those with longer hair. Pruritus, scalp excoriations, and broken papules are almost always present, and secondary impetigo may occur. Those in close association with the affected patient should also be treated.

PEDICULOSIS THERAPY

Permethrin 5% cream (Elimite) or 1% over-the-counter (Nix) should be applied as a shampoo or lotion and rinsed after 10 minutes with water. Repeat dosing may be needed to kill new progeny in 1 week.

Lindane (Kwell) 1% shampoo is second-line therapy for pediculosis. It is applied to dry hair for 4 minutes, worked into a lather, and rinsed off. A repeat treatment in 1 week may be necessary. There is potential for seizure if toxic amounts of drug are used.

Eyelash involvement is treated with mechanical removal and petrolatum applied to the eyelashes three to five times daily for 1 week. Alternatively, physostigmine (Eserine)[1] 0.25% ophthalmic ointment has been used and is applied three to five times a day for 3 days.

After initial topical therapy, it is important to remove residual nits with a comb/tweezer combination because nits may be viable for up to 1 month. All clothing and bedding that has been in contact with the affected individual is laundered in hot water with detergent, and placed in a hot dryer for at least 20 minutes. Dry cleaning is an acceptable alternative. Items that are plush and not washable should be sealed in plastic for at least 2 weeks prior to usage. Affected contacts need treatment.

[1]Not FDA approved for this indication.

TUNGIASIS

Tungiasis, commonly known as *chiggers* or *jiggers,* is caused by flea infestation with *Tunga penetrans* or the sand flea. In this disease the female flea will penetrate the skin, lay eggs, and produce larvae over a 2- to 3-week period. Development of a painful, necrotic papule or vesicle ensues with a black, necrotic crust. Treatment is flea removal.

MYIASIS

Myiasis is caused by the larvae of the human botfly known as *Dermatobia hominis*. The larvae burrow deep into the skin and the cutaneous reaction is an erythematous papule with central pore. Occasionally the larvae will protrude through the pore. Petroleum jelly or raw bacon/pork fat is placed over the pore, enticing the larvae out. Surgical removal is curative.

FUNGAL INFECTIONS OF THE SKIN

METHOD OF

Phoebe Rich, MD, and Anna Q. Hare, BS

Superficial fungal infections occur when dermatophytes and yeast infect the skin, hair, and nails. Fungal infections are documented by microscopic potassium hydroxide (KOH) stain examination of skin scrapings taken from the scale of the advancing border of the lesion, or by a fungal culture to confirm the presence of the fungal organisms (many nonfungal inflammatory dermatoses mimic fungal infections). This article involves only common superficial fungal infections of the skin caused by dermatophytes, *Pityrosporum*, and *Candida*. Deep fungal infections,

TABLE 1 Location of Common Fungal Infections

Name of Fungal Infection	Location of Fungus on Skin
Tinea pedis	Feet
Tinea corporis	General skin/body/arms/legs
Tinea manuum	Hands
Tinea cruris	Groin
Tinea barbae	Beard
Tinea faciei	Face not beard
Tinea unguium	Nails
Tinea capitis	Scalp

systemic fungal infections, fungal infections of the scalp/hair (tinea capitis), and fungal infections of the nail (onychomycosis) are discussed in other articles.

Dermatophyte Infections of the Skin

Dermatophytes are organisms that invade keratin of the stratum corneum of the skin, the nail bed or plate, and the hair shaft or root. The most common dermatophytes in North America are *Trichophyton rubrum, Trichophyton mentagrophytes, Trichophyton tonsurans*, *Epidermophyton floccosum*, and *Microsporum canis*. It is estimated that approximately 20% of people in the United States have dermatophyte infection, most of which is tinea pedis. Dermatophyte infections are named for the location on the body on which the fungus resides, such as tinea cruris (groin), tinea pedis (feet), tinea corporis (body), tinea manuum (hands), tinea barbae (beard), tinea faciei (glabrous skin of face), and tinea capitis (scalp).

Clinical Manifestations and Differential Diagnosis of Tinea Infections

Tinea pedis can take three forms: moccasin, interdigital, and inflammatory (vesicobullous). Moccasin tinea pedis presents as a fine silvery scale with mild inflammation in a moccasin distribution that includes the plantar surface as well as the heel and sides of the foot. It can be confused with psoriasis or eczema. Interdigital tinea pedis is characterized by a pruritic, scaly infection in the lateral toe web spaces. It may become macerated and malodorous secondary to superimposed bacterial infection in the moist interdigital spaces. Vesicobullous tinea pedis occurs on the sole and lateral foot and toes, and is characterized by small, multilocular vesicles that may coalesce and become pustular. These lesions are very pruritic. The fungal elements are in the roof of the blisters. This form of tinea pedis is often confused with allergic contact dermatitis, dyshydrotic eczema, pustular psoriasis, and even scabies.

Tinea corporis, commonly called ringworm, appears as enlarging annular plaques, often with central clearing. The leading edge of a spreading ring is red and scaly, making it the best place for a KOH specimen to

TABLE 2 Antifungal Drugs Used to Treat Superficial Dermatophyte Infections of the Skin

Drug Class	Drug	Frequency of Dosage	Length of Administration	OTC or Rx
Topical Antifungal Drugs				
Imidazoles				
	Clotrimazole (Lotrimin) 1% cream, solution, lotion	bid	4wk	OTC
	Econazole (Spectazole) 1% cream	qd	1-4wk	Rx
	Ketoconazole (Nizoral) 2% cream, shampoo	bid	1-6wk	Rx
	Miconazole (Lotrimin AF) 1% and 2% aerosols, powder, lotion, solution, aerosol powder	bid	4wk	OTC
	Oxiconazole (Oxistat) 1% cream, lotion	bid	4wk	Rx
	Sulconazole (Exelderm)[2] 1% cream, lotion	bid	4wk	
Benzylamine				
	Butenafine (Mentax) 1% cream	bid	7d	OTC
		qd	14d	
Allylamine				
	Naftifine (Naftin) 1% cream, gel	qd	4wk	Rx
	Terbinafine (Lamisil) 1% cream, solution, spray	bid	1-2wk	OTC
Hydroxypyridine				
	Ciclopirox (Loprox) 0.77% gel, cream, lotion	bid	4wk	Rx
Other				
	Tolnaftate (Tinactin) 1% aerosol, powder, solution	bid	6wk	OTC
Oral Antifungal Medications				
	Griseofulvin oral capsules, 660, 750 mg	daily	4-6wk	Rx
	Fluconazole (Diflucan) oral 50, 100, 150, 200 mg	100 mg wk	4-6wk	Rx
	Itraconazole (Sporanox) oral 100 mg caps	daily	1-2wk	Rx
	Terbinafine (Lamisil) oral 250 mg	daily	2-6wk	Rx

[2]Not available in the United States.
Abbreviations: bid = twice daily; OTC = over-the-counter drug; qd = daily; Rx = prescription drug.

be collected. The differential diagnoses of tinea corporis are eczema, isolated psoriasis, and the herald patch of pityriasis rosea.

Tinea cruris, commonly called jock itch, is predominantly seen in males, although it rarely affects the scrotum or penis. It usually occurs in the inguinal crease and extends onto the thigh with an advancing scaly red border. Occasionally the inguinal lesions are secondarily infected with bacteria. The differential diagnoses of tinea cruris are inverse psoriasis, intertrigo, *Candida*, and erythrasma, which fluoresces coral red with a Wood's lamp. *Candida* infection in the groin appears red and shiny, often has satellite pustules, and may involve the scrotum and penis.

Tinea manuum is not common and is usually overdiagnosed. It occurs in association with moccasin tinea pedis in the form of two-foot, one-hand fungal disease and has the same dry scaly appearance. It is often associated with onychomycosis of the fingernails. The differential diagnoses include psoriasis, atopic eczema, and contact dermatitis. KOH examination will easily confirm the presence of fungus.

Tinea faciei appears as red scaly plaque on the nonbearded areas of the face and is similar in appearance to tinea corporis. The differential diagnoses are contact dermatitis, seborrheic dermatitis, isolated psoriasis, and rosacea.

Tinea barbae occurs in the bearded area of the face in men, and is often contracted from animals. It occurs as inflamed, boggy, pustular lesions that can appear similar to bacterial folliculitis, acne, contact dermatitis, and ingrown hairs in the beard area. The diagnosis is made by KOH and/or culture of the infected hair shaft and root.

Treatment and Prevention of Dermatophyte Infections of the Skin

Unlike dermatophyte infections of hair and nails, which usually require oral antifungal therapy, most superficial dermatophyte infections of the skin can be treated with topical antifungal products. Topical antifungal medications should be used for 7 to 14 days past the resolution of symptoms, usually for a total of 4 to 6 weeks. Topical antifungal medication comes in many vehicles that can be used for different locations of the body. Powder and aerosol forms, for example, are most helpful for moist body areas like skin folds, toe web spaces, and groin; while gel and lotion formulations are more useful in hairy areas like chest and back in men. It is important to continue topical treatment past the point of symptom reduction, and in most cases an additional 4 weeks is required to prevent recurrence. In severe or recalcitrant fungal infections of the skin, such as resistant or recurrent tinea pedis, tinea corporis, or tinea cruris, an oral antifungal medication may be necessary. The drawbacks to the oral medications are their significant cost and potential side effects, including drug–drug interactions, a small (but real) risk of hepatotoxicity, gastric upset, and skin rashes.

The relapse rate for most fungal infections is high, particularly in patients with a genetic predisposition to fungal infections. Once the fungal infection is cleared from the skin, prevention of reinfection and relapse is helpful. Preventative measures are directed at reducing exposure to organisms and changing the local environment to be less favorable for dermatophyte proliferation. Protecting the skin of feet when walking in public showers or around swimming pools minimizes the risk of contracting tinea pedis, and keeping the groin and toe webs dry and cool discourages proliferation of fungi. People who develop frequent recurrences or reinfection bouts of tinea pedis may find it helpful to apply a topical antifungal cream or powder to the feet on a regular basis, even when clinical manifestations are not present.

Tinea Versicolor

Tinea versicolor (pityriasis versicolor) is a common disorder caused by *Pityrosporum* organisms and characterized by small, oval, hyperpigmented and hypopigmented macules with slight, fine scale. The lesions can be tan, brown, or pink and typically located in the sebaceous areas of the trunk, such as the back and chest, although occasionally the lesions are seen on the neck, face, axilla, and extremities. The superficial scaly plaques often coalesce into larger areas that have arcuate outlines. The active acute scaly phase often evolves into hypopigmented macules on the trunk that are accentuated when the skin is exposed to sunlight and tans. The hypopigmentation results from the effect of a dicarboxylic acid byproduct from the *Pityrosporum organism*. The pigmentation is reversible, and the skin color returns to normal after the acute infection is gone.

Pityrosporum can also cause a folliculitis on the chest, neck, and back, usually in women. This condition is characterized by small, superficial pustules surrounding the hair follicles, which are caused by overgrowth of the *Pityrosporum orbiculare* causing inflammation from the byproducts of the yeast growth and fatty acid production.

DIAGNOSIS

The diagnosis of tinea versicolor is made by clinical appearance of the brown, tan, or pink scaly plaques on the trunk and confirmed by the characteristic appearance of the *Pityrosporum* hyphae and spores with a KOH examination. The appearance of the organism on KOH is described as looking like "spaghetti and meatballs" microscopically. If only the hypopigmented phase of the condition is present, the organisms often cannot be found. In *Pityrosporum* folliculitis, only the spore form is seen on KOH examination.

The scaly plaques of tinea versicolor can sometimes be mistaken for pityriasis rosea, guttate psoriasis, dermatophyte infection (ringworm), and seborrheic dermatitis. The hypopigmented macules can look like vitiligo and postinflammatory hypopigmentation. The small pustules of *Pityrosporum* folliculitis are indistinguishable clinically from acne.

TREATMENT

Tinea versicolor is easy to treat but difficult to cure. Many topical medications clear the infection, including topical antifungal medications such as azoles (clotrimazole [Lotrimin], oxiconazole, econazole [Spectazole]), allylamines (terbinafine [Lamisil][1]), and ciclopirox olamine (Loprox) twice daily for 2 weeks. Selenium sulfide (Selsun) lotion or shampoo (2.5% is prescription strength; weaker over-the-counter shampoos include Selsun Blue) is often used by applying it to the skin for 5 to 10 minutes before showering. Ketoconazole (Nizoral)[1] and ciclopirox (Loprox) shampoo[2] are effective when used to lather the skin daily for 1 week. In more extensive or severe cases, an oral antifungal medication such as ketoconazole[1], 200 mg in two tablets taken orally 1 hour before eating, can be prescribed. This very effective single-dose treatment is usually sufficient but can be repeated in 2 weeks if needed. Oral fluconazole (Diflucan)[1], 400 mg single dose, and oral itraconazole (Sporanox)[1], 200 mg daily for 7 days, are very effective. Oral terbinafine (Lamisil)[1] and griseofulvin are ineffective for treatment of tinea versicolor. Salicylic acid[1] in a liquid or bar soap formulation is effective and inexpensive. It is easy to clear tinea versicolor but it is very difficult to prevent recurrences, which often occur every spring in some patients. It may be helpful to use one of the shampoos, soaps, or topical antifungal creams several times a month as a preventative measure.

Candida Infections of the Skin

Candida albicans occurs in the normal healthy gastrointestinal (GI) tract of humans, but is not usually seen on healthy skin as normal flora. *Candida* can infect the skin at the angles of the mouth (perlèche), in the inframammary and inguinal folds, and under the pannus. *Candida* is also seen around the nails (paronychia and onycholysis), and occasionally in other locations such as the finger web spaces and the diaper areas of babies.

Cutaneous *Candida* infections are usually bright red scaly plaques that have satellite pustules. They may or may not be symptomatic. It is important to confirm the diagnosis by KOH and/or culture because the differential diagnoses include many steroid-responsive dermatoses. Monotherapy with cortisone creams usually worsens this infection.

[1]Not FDA approved for this indication.
[2]Not available in the United States.

TREATMENT

Candida albicans can be treated with any of the topical antifungal medications and with oral antifungal fluconazole (Diflucan). Clotrimazole (Mycelex) troches treat perlèche locally. Control of moisture in body folds and an antifungal powder such as Z-Sorb AF may be helpful in prevention in the intertriginous areas. *Candida* as a secondary invader around and under onycholytic nails is best treated by avoidance of excessive water exposure and a topical liquid antifungal applied to the nail bed under the loosened nail plate.

Superficial fungal infections are common and easily treated with topical and oral antifungal medications. It is important to confirm the presence of fungal organisms by KOH or culture, because there are so many steroid-responsive skin disorders that can be indistinguishable from fungal infections of the skin, and cortisone cream used alone usually worsens cutaneous fungal infections.

DISEASES OF THE MOUTH

METHOD OF
Frank C. Powell, MD, and Sharareh Ahmadi, MB

Diseases of the mouth can be a source of misery for both patients and physicians who are unfamiliar with the approach to examination of this area. They may represent a localized anomaly of limited significance or the presentation of potentially life-threatening multisystem disease. Evaluation of a patient with oral lesions requires a systematic approach with resources to appropriate investigations in certain circumstances. Many oral lesions can be diagnosed by obtaining a full history, including family history, drug ingestion, symptoms of concurrent systemic disease, and careful clinical examination carried out in good lighting of the mouth, lips, surrounding skin, and draining lymph nodes. A general physical examination is necessary if an oral presentation of systemic disease is suspected. Occasionally a biopsy is required to provide histologic solution to more difficult problems.

This article should enable physicians to approach the diagnosis and management of the common lesions that affect the lips, oral cavity, and tongue with a degree of confidence. Access to an atlas of oral lesions is essential to those whose experience is limited in this area.

Disorders of the Lips

CHEILITIS

Cheilitis is the term applied to any inflammatory condition involving the lips.

Drug-Induced Cheilitis

Retinoids, such as etretinate[1,2] and isotretinoin[1], cause dryness and cracking of the lips in most patients. The mechanism of this pharmacologic effect is unknown, but is dose related. Patients should be instructed to frequently apply greasy lubricants.

Infective Cheilitis

Recurrent herpes labialis is a common cause of blisters at the mucocutaneous junction. Itchy papules progress to vesicles, pustules, and finally crusts. They occasionally become infected with *Staphylococcus* or *Streptococcus*, resulting in impetiginized lesions. Acyclovir 5%[1] cream should be applied five times daily at the first sign of infection and fusidic acid 2% cream[2] added in the latter stages if impetiginization is suspected.

Herpes zoster and papillomaviruses also affect the lips, which is the most common extragenital site for primary syphilitic lesions. In males these tend to occur on the upper lip and in females on the lower lip. In secondary syphilis, moist, flat, warty lesions (condylomata lata) may appear at the mucocutaneous junctions and commissures.

Actinic Cheilitis

This premalignant condition tends to primarily affect the protuberant lower lip of adults who have had prolonged sun exposure. It is manifested by hyperkeratosis and desquamation. As the condition becomes more established, crusting, erosions, and intermittent bleeding occur. Biopsy may be necessary to evaluate the degree of dysplasia. Treatment with 5% fluorouracil (Efudex)[1], topical tretinoin (Retin-A)[1], CO_2 laser, or 5% imiquimod (Aldara)[1] cream can be effective in clearing lesions of actinic cheilitis, but discomfort and local irritation will be experienced with many of these products. If ulceration or any infiltration suggestive of invasive tumor is detected, surgical excision is the treatment of choice.

Angular Cheilitis

Angular cheilitis (perlèche) is recurrent painful fissures at the commissures of the lips with surrounding erythema and scaling from which *Candida albicans, Staphylococcus aureus*, or streptococci may be cultured. Perlèche may result from mechanical irritation (dentures), nutritional deficiency, or overfolding of the lips, which promotes accumulation of saliva and erosion of intact skin, facilitating the growth of bacteria and yeast in these areas. It is most often seen in the elderly or the immunocompromised patient.

Treatment may require new dentures, miconazole nitrate 2% cream (Monistat)[1], and fusidic acid 2% cream[1,2] applied locally. Plastic surgical correction of overfolding skin may be necessary in some cases.

Exfoliative Cheilitis

Exfoliative cheilitis is characterized by scaling, erythema, and desquamation of the keratinized labial surface and vermilion border caused by repetitive biting, picking, or licking of the lips. In adult patients, underlying psychiatric disturbance or personality disorder may be suspected.

Granulomatous Cheilitis

This is a rare, chronic, soft-to-firm nontender swelling of one or both lips, which shows granulomatous changes on histology. Extraintestinal Crohn's disease and sarcoidosis should be considered in the differential diagnosis. The granulomatous changes may be confined to the lips (Miescher's cheilitis) or be associated with scrotal tongue and recurrent facial palsy (Melkersson-Rosenthal syndrome). The swelling may eventually become permanent. This condition is poorly responsive to therapy. Injection of 1 mL (10 mg) of triamcinolone[1] into the affected lips, repeated every 4 to 6 months, may help. This may be combined with surgical reduction (cheiloplasty).

Contact Cheilitis

This acute weeping dermatitis of the lips is due to irritant or allergic contact factors. Lipstick may be responsible, and following sensitization, its further use is contraindicated. When the dermatitis extends beyond the lips into the oral cavity, toothpaste and mouthwashes should be suspected. Topical triamcinolone acetonide[1] 0.1% in emollient oral paste is useful to treat the dermatitis on the labial and mucosal surfaces.

TUMORS

Benign Tumors

Benign tumors of the lips are relatively common and should be recognized easily by the examining physician.

Mucocele

A labial mucosal cyst presents as a raised, soft, dome-shaped lesion on the lower lip with a slight

[1]Not FDA approved for this indication.
[2]Not available in the United States.

[1]Not FDA approved for this indication.
[2]Not available in the United States.

bluish tinge. It is usually asymptomatic, originates from minor salivary glands or their ducts, and can occur at any age. It appears abruptly, increases in size rapidly, and tends to be persistent. Simple excision is usually curative, and allows confirmation of the benign nature of one of the most common cysts of oral soft tissue.

Fordyce Spots

These represent ectopic sebaceous glands and appear as small, discrete white-to-yellow papules. They commonly occur at the commissures of the lips and on the anterior buccal mucosa. They are asymptomatic and require no treatment.

Malignant Tumors

Squamous Cell Carcinoma

This is the most common malignancy to affect the lip and usually arises in an area of actinic damage. Tobacco smoking is also a major risk factor. Like actinic cheilitis, it is more common in men with outdoor activity and mainly affects the lower lip. Surgical excision following early diagnosis is the preferred mode of therapy because these lesions can metastasize early.

Lentigo Maligna

This is melanoma in situ. It may occur on the labial surface. The lesion requires total surgical excision with long-term follow-up.

Melanoma

This is usually darkish brown to black in color, but amelanotic lesions have been reported. It is rare and has a poor prognosis. Lesions are usually asymptomatic in the early stages, and bleeding may be the first sign. The typical sites of involvement include the lips and gingiva. Asians appear more predisposed to this malignancy than do caucasians.

Vascular Tumors

Venous Lake

This appears as a small, bluish purple, soft swelling, usually on the lower lip of elderly people. The lesion blanches on prolonged pressure. It may bleed after trauma and is treated with electrocautery, argon laser, or surgical excision.

Telangiectasia

These may occur sporadically, or be seen in hereditary hemorrhagic telangiectasia, and in acquired disorders such as the CREST (calcinosis cutis, Raynaud's phenomenon, esophageal motility disorder, sclerodactyly, and telangiectasia) syndrome, chronic liver disease, pregnancy, and post irradiation. If required for cosmetic reasons cauterization or laser therapy is effective.

Pigmentation

Ephelides

Ephelides are sun-induced freckles that occur most frequently in childhood and tend to reduce in number with age. They are usually multiple, uniform light tan color, and less than 1 cm in size with regular outline. They appear and darken with sun exposure and tend to fade in its absence. No treatment is required.

Solar Lentigos

Solar lentigos are more common in older individuals and persist indefinitely. They range in size from 2 mm to 2 cm and are usually tan to dark brown in color. Variation in color or irregularity of outline should raise the suspicion of lentigo maligna and is an indication for histologic evaluation. Nonsun-exposed lentigos may be the component of the LEOPARD (lentigines, electrocardiographic [conduction abnormalities], ocular [hypertelorism], pulmonary [stenosis], abnormal [genitalia], retardation [of growth], and deafness), LAMB (lentigines, atrial myxomas, cutaneous papular myxomas, blue nevi), Carney, or NAME (nevi, atrial myxoma, myxoid neurofibroma, and ephelides) syndromes.

Nevi

Nevi may be found on the keratinized epithelium of the lip, the buccal mucosa, and the hard and soft palates.

Labial Melanotic Macules

Labial melanotic macules are common small, discrete, macular areas of hyperpigmentation ranging from tan to dark brown in color. They may be irregular in outline and can enlarge up to 1 cm in diameter. They mainly affect the lower lip and typically present between the ages of 35 and 42 years. The etiology is unclear, but there may be a genetic predisposition. Malignancy has not been reported to develop in these lesions, but establishing the diagnosis may require a skin biopsy.

Disorders of the Oral Cavity

Stomatitis Medicamentosa

This is a drug eruption affecting the oral mucous membranes, which may represent an idiosyncratic reaction or a toxic or pharmacologic effect. Cytotoxic agents, such as methotrexate (Rheumatrex), may cause ulcerative stomatitis (most marked at sites of trauma). The tendency to develop diphenylhydantoin gingival hyperplasia can be reduced by meticulous oral hygiene, but the fibrotic enlargement may require surgical excision. Gold, penicillamine, and sulfonylureas may cause a lichenoid stomatitis. Pharmacologic reactions to drugs include xerostomia with antihistamines and anticholinergics and hemorrhage with anticoagulants. Elimination of the suspected agent is often sufficient in management.

Stomatitis Nicotina

Stomatitis nicotina causes a grayish-white, wrinkled hard palate with papular swellings, resulting from enlargement of the palatal mucous glands and dilation of their ducts. It is seen in some heavy smokers, and cessation of smoking leads to gradual resolution. No local therapy is required.

Herpes Gingivostomatitis

Herpes simplex virus (HSV) infection is a common infection affecting the oral mucosa. In general, HSV-1 causes primary herpetic stomatitis (and secondary infection of recurrent herpes labialis). Oral infection with HSV-2 may be sexually transmitted in saliva. The incubation period is 3 to 7 days. Many infections with HSV occur in childhood and are subclinical. Symptomatic patients present with malaise, anorexia, fever, cervical lymphadenopathy, and diffuse, purple, boggy gingivitis, with multiple vesicles followed by erosion of the oral mucosa and gingiva. Stomatitis generally resolves in 7 to 10 days, but the virus may remain latent in the trigeminal ganglion. Reactivation can occur following sun exposure, trauma, or immunosuppression. Cytologic smear (Tzanck's preparation) is diagnostic of HSV if large, multinucleated, giant cells are seen. In mild cases, treatment with hydration, analgesics, and antimicrobial mouth washes (e.g., chlorhexidine gluconate 0.2% solution [Peridex]) is sufficient. Topical lidocaine may ease discomfort. In severe cases and in immunocompromised patients, acyclovir (Zovirax), 200 mg five times daily for adults (half dose for children, and double dose for immunocompromised patients) is used for primary infection and prophylactic antiviral drug therapy such as acyclovir, 400 mg twice daily, may suppress frequent recurrent infection.

Herpes Zoster (Shingles)

Mouth ulcers are seen if shingles affects the maxillary or mandibular divisions of the trigeminal nerve. The initial symptoms are paresthesia and severe pain, which may simulate toothache. After 2 to 3 days vesicles with an erythematous base appear in crops along the affected dermatome. Ulcers appear on the site of the mucosa affected, and resolve spontaneously. Postherpetic neuralgia can be distressing. Treatment with acyclovir (800 mg five times daily for 7 to 10 days), valacyclovir (Valtrex) (1 g three times daily [tid] for 7 days), or famciclovir (Famvir) (500 mg three times daily for 7 days) is helpful if initiated early in the process. Tricyclic antidepressants, such as nortriptyline (Pamelor)[1] (10 to 25 mg at night) or gabapentin (Neurontin)[1] (300 mg tid), have been used for postherpetic neuralgia.

[1]Not FDA approved for this indication.

Other Viral Infections

Epstein-Barr virus (EBV) appears in the saliva of patients with infectious mononucleosis and causes palate petechiae and white exudates on edematous tonsils with nonspecific oral ulceration. Oral hairy leukoplakia is seen in severe immunodeficiency, especially HIV infection, as a consequence of opportunistic infection with EBV. Generally, the condition does not require treatment, but zidovudine (Retrovir)[1] or acyclovir[1] (800 mg four times daily) may also be useful, if symptomatic or very florid. Lesions usually recur when treatment is discontinued. Cytomegalovirus may also rarely cause oral ulceration. Herpangina is a self-limiting condition of young children caused by coxsackievirus, manifested by ulcers predominantly on the soft palate. Hand-foot-and-mouth disease is caused by coxsackie A virus. Any area of the mouth (especially the palate) may be involved with vesiculopustules, which superficially ulcerate. The condition is self-limiting. Condyloma acuminatum, verruca vulgaris, and human papillomavirus infection can also affect the oral mucosa and patients present with oral warts.

Candida

Candida albicans is a normal inhabitant of the oral cavity. However, when the patient's mucosal tissue resistance and immune responsiveness are reduced (chronic disease, cancer, diabetes, pregnancy, immunosuppressive or radiation therapy, broad-spectrum antibiotics, and oral contraceptives), it can become a significant pathogen invading the mucosa. The clinical features are creamy, milk-curd exudates on a bright erythematous base, which leaves a raw surface when scraped for culture specimen. In debilitated patients, oral candidiasis may give rise to a generalized erythematous atrophic mucosal inflammation. Chronic candidiasis in denture wearers causes a patchy inflammation of the palatal mucosa with a burning sensation of the roof of the mouth. Hyperplastic lesions may be mistaken for leukoplakia or tumors. Treatment with 1 mL of nystatin (Mycostatin) oral suspension four times daily or ketoconazole (Nizoral) 2% cream four times daily may be helpful. Systemic fluconazole (Diflucan) (100 mg daily for 7 to 10 days) or itraconazole (Sporanox) (200 mg daily for 7 to 10 days) has proved beneficial in many patients with persistent infection despite topical therapy.

Acute Necrotizing Gingivitis (Vincent's Disease)

This is an acute onset of gingival soreness, bleeding, and halitosis caused by a mixed (mainly anaerobic)

[1]Not FDA approved for this indication.

flora consisting of fusiform bacteria and spirochetes. Fatigue, stress, smoking, or immune defects are the main predisposing factors. The mouth ulceration is usually restricted to the interdental papillae. There may be pyrexia and malaise and cervical lymphadenopathy. Management is supportive with improvement of oral hygiene. Regular cleansing with chlorhexidine gluconate 0.2% solution mouthwash and soft toothbrush is very effective. Oral metronidazole (Flagyl)[1], 200 mg three times daily for 7 days, may be required for severe cases.

Syphilis

Primary chancres may involve the palate as small, firm, pink macules or papules, which progress to form painless ulcers. Chancres heal spontaneously in 3 to 8 weeks and are highly infectious. Diagnosis is by dark-ground microscopy and serologic testing and treatment is with appropriate antibiotics.

TUMORS

Benign

Benign tumors are rare in the oral cavity. Multiple neurofibromas may be seen in the oral cavity in von Recklinghausen's disease and in the multiple endocrine adenopathy syndromes (Sipple's syndrome).

Premalignant

Leukoplakia refers to white, keratotic plaquelike lesions seen in the oral cavity. The etiology is unknown. Some may be due to chronic physical (sharp edges of carious teeth) or chemical (tobacco) irritation, or chronic candidiasis. Varying degrees of dysplasia may be seen histologically. Only a small portion of leukoplakias are malignant, but all persistent lesions should be biopsied. Lesions on the tongue and floor of the mouth are more likely to become malignant. Leukokeratoses are small white plaques due to mucosal thickening caused by trauma (cheek biting or sucking of the buccal occlusal linea alba). Single, small lesions can be treated with topical tretinoin (Retin-A)[1]. Surgical excision, electrocautery, or vaporization by CO_2 laser may be indicated if induration or ulceration is apparent.

Erythroplasia is a red, velvety plaque involving the floor of the mouth, tongue, and the soft palate. It occurs with or without leukoplakia and diagnosis should be confirmed histologically. In 90% of cases an in situ or invasive carcinoma is demonstrable. Surgical excision is the treatment of choice. Heavy alcohol consumption and smoking may predispose to erythroplasia.

Malignant Tumor

Squamous cell carcinoma accounts for 90% of the malignant lesions of the mouth. The morphology is varied from asymptomatic red plaque with indistinct borders to white plaque or more florid ulcerations. A high index of suspicion and a willingness to obtain tissue samples promptly are necessary because 60% of oral cancers are advanced at the time of diagnosis and there is only a 30% 5-year survival rate. Extensive and mutilating surgery may be required to remove these lesions once they have developed as an aggressive, invasive state.

[1]Not FDA approved for this indication.

Vascular Lesions

Hemangioma The presence of multiple vascular tufts throughout the oral cavity suggests Rendu-Osler-Weber disease. Port-wine stain of the mucosa may appear as a part of the Sturge-Weber syndrome. Treatment options include surgical excision, corticosteroid injection, and laser ablation.

Kaposi's sarcoma is a multicentric angiogenic tumor associated with HIV infection, presenting usually as red, blue, or purple patches later becoming nodular and ulcerating if traumatized, causing pain. It most commonly affects the junction of the hard and soft palates. Radiotherapy or intralesional injection with recombinant interferon (1 to 3 million units once a week) is the treatment of choice for isolated oral lesions. If disseminated lesions are present, chemotherapy with bleomycin (Blenoxane)[1] (15 mg IV twice a week up to 180 to 200 mg) or interferon-α-2A (3 to 6 million every other day) can be helpful.

Pyogenic granuloma is a pedunculated or sessile, red, painless nodule that grows rapidly and commonly affects the gingiva, lip, or tongue.

Granuloma Gravidarum (Pregnancy Tumor)

Granuloma gravidarum (pregnancy tumor) refers to an interdental pyogenic granuloma-like gingival reaction during pregnancy. Regression may take place spontaneously after delivery. Bleeding may be a problem (caused by trauma associated with eating or brushing of the teeth) and surgical removal may be necessary. Attention to oral hygiene is an important component of the management.

Pigmented Lesions

Pigmentation of the gingiva may be physiologic (in dark-skinned individuals), occur during pregnancy, or while taking oral contraceptive pills. Localized pigmented lesions, such as melanotic macules, and nevi may be found on the buccal and palatal mucosa. Melanoma may occur intraorally, so a high index of suspicion is warranted with early biopsy of unstable or irregularly pigmented lesions.

Generalized Pigmentation

Pigmentation of the oral region may be associated with the disorders listed in Table 1, the drugs listed in Table 2, amalgam tattoo (caused by the presence

[1]Not FDA approved for this indication.

TABLE 1 Generalized Hyperpigmentation of the Oral Cavity

Gastrointestinal polyposis—Peutz-Jeghers syndrome
Cardiomyopathy
Myxoma syndrome
Albright's syndrome
Addison's disease
Acromegaly
Cushing's disease
Nelson's disease
Hyperthyroidism
Hemochromatosis

of foreign material), poor oral hygiene, carotenemia, arsenic poisoning, or scurvy.

Aphthous Ulceration

Recurrent aphthous stomatitis (RAS) is a common and difficult-to-treat ulcer of the oral cavity. Aphthous ulceration may arise in Behçet's disease, Sweet's syndrome, nutritional and mineral deficiencies, and gastrointestinal disorders. Recurrent bouts of rounded, shallow, painful oral ulcers occur at intervals of a few months to a few days. Based primarily on the size of the lesions, aphthous ulcers are classified into three types:

1. **Herpetiform ulcers** are 1 to 2 mm in size and can affect any part of the oral cavity. They often begin as grouped vesicles surrounded by a halo of erythema. These may coalesce into plaques and form ulcers that require weeks to heal. These lesions are not caused by a viral infection.
2. **Minor aphthous ulcers** are the most common form and usually present as recurrent, multiple, small, shallow ulcerations with a yellow pseudomembranous floor on the mucolabial sulci, tongue, and nonkeratinized oral mucosa. Lesions resolve in 7 to 14 days.
3. **Major aphthous ulcers** are recurrent, large, often solitary lesions with a surrounding zone of erythema. They can occur in any area of the mouth, but particularly on the labial mucosa, tongue, or the posterior oral mucosa. Lesions begin as nodules, and subsequently form deep ulcerations, which may extend to involve underlying connective tissue and musculature.

TABLE 2 Drugs Causing Oral Pigmentation

Nicotine	Heroin
Busulfan	Doxorubicin
Bleomycin	Cyclophosphamide
Antimalarial	Phenothiazines
Oral contraceptives	AZT (zidovudine)
Ketoconazole	Minocycline
Tetracycline	Silver
Arsenic	Lead
Gold	Amiodarone
Premarin	Nitrogen mustard
Clofazimine	

Resolution may occur with residual scar with retraction of surrounding tissue. Reduction of trauma, correction of dental defects, and meticulous oral hygiene may help to prevent RAS. Chlorhexidine (Peridex)[1] (0.2% W/W mouth rinse or 1% gel) can reduce the duration of the ulcers. Lidocaine gel applied three times daily can produce transient pain relief. Antihistamine solutions (Bendramine[1] or Chlor-Trimeton[1]) may provide sufficient topical anesthesia to allow eating. Topical tetracycline[1] may reduce healing times and the associated pain. Triamcinolone acetonide (Kenalog)[1], fluocinonide (Lidex)[1], and clobetasol (Temovate)[1], applied at 6-hour intervals, are usually helpful. Sodium cromoglycate lozenges may also provide mild symptomatic relief. Oral prednisolone[1] 30 to 60 mg daily should be reserved for severe cases of major aphthous ulcer. Azathioprine (Imuran)[1], colchicines[1], cyclosporine (Neoral), dapsone[1], and thalidomide[1] have been reported to be effective but toxicity limits their clinical application. β-Blockers (e.g., propranolol)[1], at low dose may have some role in reducing the frequency of recurrence of aphthous ulcers. Women with menstrual-related aphthous ulceration may benefit from an estrogen-dominant[1] oral contraceptive.

Chemical Burns

Salt, gum, escharotics, analgesics, or candy held in prolonged contact with the buccal mucosa and gingiva could cause chemical burn due to necrosis of tissue. These burns can be mistaken for malignant ulceration. Most of these lesions are painless.

Disorders of the Tongue

BLACK HAIRY TONGUE

This condition is the result of hyperplasia of filiform papillae with increased pigment production by bacteria. The cause of the hyperplastic response of the papillae is not known, but it is suspected to relate to the change in microflora population. It often follows a course of antibiotic administration. Gentle cleansing twice daily with a soft-bristled toothbrush and hydrogen peroxide solution is frequently satisfactory. Topical triamcinolone acetonide (Kenalog)[1], applied twice daily after wiping the tongue dry is also effective. A furry tongue may be seen in smokers and patients with febrile illness.

MEDIAN RHOMBOID GLOSSITIS

Median rhomboid glossitis is a dorsal midline plaquelike hypertrophy of the tongue, probably representing a form of chronic hyperplastic candidiasis.

[1]Not FDA approved for this indication.

TABLE 3 Differential Diagnosis of Geographic Tongue

Lichen planus
Leukoplakia
Reiter's syndrome
Pustular psoriasis
Pityriasis rosea
Pityriasis rubra pilaris
Secondary syphilis
Miliary tuberculosis
Drug eruption

GEOGRAPHIC TONGUE

This is a common glossitis, which may be regarded as a variant of normal. There is cyclical atrophy and regrowth of filiform and spongiform papillae, which give the characteristic patchy lesions, surrounded by white keratotic margin. These are often multiple and typically occur on the dorsum of the tongue. Their appearance may vary within days, but the patient is often asymptomatic or experiences mild discomfort with hot, salty, or spicy foods. Geographic tongue is not related to the subsequent development of oral disease, and reassurance is usually the only therapy required, with avoidance of potential irritants. The differential diagnosis of geographic tongue is listed in Table 3.

SCROTAL TONGUE

This is a developmental defect in which the tongue appears enlarged with multiple deep fissures or sulci. It may be seen in association with the Melkersson-Rosenthal syndrome, Sjögren's syndrome, and Down syndrome. Local hygiene is often required to remove food and debris from the fissures.

SMOOTH TONGUE

This condition results from atrophy of the filiform papillae. The smooth tongue may be due to nutritional deficiencies or various systemic conditions (Table 4). There can be considerable discomfort, and a burning sensation may occur spontaneously, or after ingestion of sour, salty, or spicy foods.

TABLE 4 Differential Diagnosis of Smooth Tongue

Iron deficiency anemia
Plummer-Vinson syndrome
Pernicious anemia (Hunter's glossitis)
Riboflavin deficiency
Pellagra (cardinal's tongue)
Celiac disease
Sjögren's syndrome
Malnutrition
Antibiotic therapy
Cardiac failure
Amyloidosis
Syphilis

TABLE 5 Factors Related to Glossodynia

Pernicious anemia
Iron deficiency
Folate deficiency
Antibiotic therapy
Stomatitis medicamentosa
Xerostomia
Trigeminal neuralgia
Vascular thrombosis/spasm
Hiatus hernia
Referred pain from dental disease
Denture sore mouth

GLOSSODYNIA

Glossodynia (paresthesia of the tongue) is a syndrome of burning or stinging sensation of the tongue with no visible lesions. Many patients with this condition suffer from psychiatric disease such as anxiety or depression. These patients should be appropriately investigated, as many will have correctable causative factors (Table 5).

VARICOSITY

Varicose veins on the ventral surface of the tongue are common with aging and are not of any diagnostic significance. Occasionally, a single varix may be noted as a soft purple papule that indents with firm palpation. Varices may also appear on the lateral border of the tongue or labial mucosa. No treatment is necessary once the diagnosis is established.

LYMPHANGIOMA

These lesions are usually solitary, red-yellow nodules that affect the tongue predominantly. They are usually asymptomatic, but as they enlarge in size, pain and discomfort may be felt during speaking, chewing, and swallowing. Surgical excision is the only treatment for symptomatic patients.

Systemic Diseases and the Mouth

HEMATOLOGIC DISEASE

Iron-deficiency anemia causes a smooth tongue. In the Plummer-Vinson syndrome, koilonychia, leukoplakia, and oral and esophageal carcinoma occur in addition to angular stomatitis. A magenta, lobulated tongue with glossodynia may be noted with pernicious anemia. Bleeding from the gingiva may be the initial manifestation of hemorrhagic diseases, whereas patients with polycythemia rubra vera may present with purple engorged gingiva. Patients with leukemia may present with gingival hyperplasia. Neutropenia can cause oral ulceration that may become extensive and necrotic.

Gastrointestinal disease: Both aphthous ulceration and nodular oral lesions, which show noncaseating granuloma, have been recorded in Crohn's disease. In ulcerative colitis, stomatitis and pyostomatitis vegetans may be seen.

Diabetes mellitus: Gingival inflammation, periodontitis, recurrent candidiasis, and glossodynia may be seen.

Lupus erythematosus: The lower lip or the posterior buccal mucosa is most commonly involved, with erythema, superficial ulceration, or hyperkeratosis.

Amyloidosis: Macroglossia and purpuric plaques or nodules may be seen within the tongue and on other mucous membrane in primary amyloidosis.

Scleroderma: In systemic scleroderma, tissues of the mouth and lips become rigid and indurated.

Histiocytosis X: In histiocytosis X, granulomatous nodules may involve the gingiva. Mucous membrane ulceration is also observed.

DERMATOLOGIC DISEASE WITH ORAL MANIFESTATIONS

Pemphigus Vulgaris

A rare autoimmune skin disease, patients with pemphigus vulgaris often present with painful superficial oral erosions, which antedate skin lesions. Blisters in pemphigus are fragile and transient and the patient may be totally unaware of their existence. The most common affected sites are the palate, gingiva, and buccal mucosa (sites of oral trauma). Diagnosis is confirmed by histology and immunofluorescence. Activity of disease is thought to be reflected in the titer of circulating antibody. It is important to exclude malignancy (e.g., lymphoma, leukemia, thymoma, and other solid tumors) because paraneoplastic pemphigus has severe mucocutaneous involvement. Early and aggressive specialist treatment is required.

Bullous Pemphigoid

This entity is more common than pemphigus. Thirty to forty percent of patients may have oral involvement, which usually develops when the disease is established. Intact blisters may be seen in the oral mucosa as tense, fluid-filled blisters. Other oral lesions, such as erosion, ulcer, or desquamative gingivitis, may occur. Diagnosis is confirmed by histology and immunofluorescence. A combination of tetracycline[1] or erythromycin[1] 500 mg four times daily and niacinamide[1] 1500 to 2000 mg per day may control this disease. Specialist referral is advised.

Cicatricial Pemphigoid

Cicatricial pemphigoid is an uncommon variant of bullous pemphigoid, which typically affects the oral and ocular mucosa. Skin lesions are uncommon. In the mouth, there are tense blisters or painful shallow erosions, typically on the gingival, buccal, or labial mucosa.

[1]Not FDA approved for this indication.

Cicatricial pemphigoid is a frequent cause of desquamative gingivitis. Ocular scarring may occur, so early ophthalmologic consultation is advised.

Erythema Multiforme

Erythema multiforme is a reactive process that affects the skin and mucous membranes with an acute, self-limited course. Drugs (e.g., sulfonamides, anticonvulsants, barbiturates, and allopurinol) and infection (e.g., herpes simplex or mycoplasma) are common precipitating factors. In the mouth, the lesions are less distinctive and the labial mucosa is typically involved, but the buccal and palatal mucosa can also be affected. Blisters, erosion, hemorrhagic crusts, or ulcerations may be manifested. Other mucosal surfaces such as conjunctiva and genitalia may be affected. Marked involvement of mucosal surfaces with severe constitutional disturbances is known as the Stevens-Johnson syndrome. Diagnosis is confirmed histologically. Swabs for viral culture may isolate herpes simplex virus, which has also been found with polymerase chain reaction (PCR) in the lesion and blood samples. Treatment is mainly supportive. Continuous oral acyclovir (Zovirax)[1] (400 mg twice daily) or valacyclovir (Valtrex)[1] (500 mg daily) is helpful to prevent recurrent herpes simplex infection. Azathioprine (Imuran)[1] 100 to 200 mg per day can be used in patients with severe mucosal involvement. The use of systemic steroids in this condition is controversial.

Lichen Planus

Oral lichen planus affects 1% to 2% of the general adult population. Typical lesions are striations, papules, plaques, mucosal atrophy, erosions (shallow ulcers), or blisters affecting buccal mucosa, tongue, and gingiva. Lesions are usually bilateral, and erosive lesions are painful and sensitive. There may be skin, genital, and nail involvement. Oral lichenoid lesions may be a complication of systemic medications such as nonsteroidal anti-inflammatory drugs (NSAIDs) and β-blockers. There is ongoing concern that oral lichen planus may be premalignant and biopsy is required to rule out other white or chronic ulcerative lesions, including reactive keratosis, chronic candidiasis, epithelial dysplasia, discoid lupus erythematosus, and malignancy. Treatment should include proper oral hygiene. Localized lesions may be treated with betamethasone propionate ointment[1] (0.05%), applied 3 to 4 times daily. Intralesional triamcinolone acetonide[1] (0.5 mL) can be used for persistent localized lesions. Dexamethasone[1] (0.025 mg) mouth rinse twice daily can be used for generalized lesions. Other topical treatments such as topical tretinoin[1] and cyclosporine[1] have also been used with limited success. Recently, topical tacrolimus (Protopic)[1] 0.1%

[1]Not FDA approved for this indication.

ointment twice daily has been used for treatment of erosive oral lichen planus with limited local or systemic side effects. Short course of systemic steroid is used for lesions that are unresponsive to topical treatment. The combination of systemic and topical steroid therapy is often very effective. Systemic treatment with cyclosporine[1], azathioprine[1], retinoids[1], dapsone[1], and thalidomide has also been reported.

[1]Not FDA approved for this indication.

VENOUS ULCERS

METHOD OF

John Pomann, MD, MS, and David Fivenson, MD

Venous ulcers (also known as venous insufficiency ulcers, stasis ulcers, or varicose ulcers) account for 75% to 85% of ulcers found on the lower leg. They are characterized by irregular margins with exudative, fibrinous bases. The perilesional skin shows features of chronic stasis dermatitis, which are decreased hair on a brawny, erythematous, shiny, indurated base with patches of overlying scale.

In most patients there is a gradual progression that begins with venous insufficiency, followed by venous stasis dermatitis, and ultimately ulceration. A subset of patients develops sunken sclerotic patches on the distal portion of the lower leg (lipodermatosclerosis; hypodermatitis sclerodermiformis) that can result in an inverted *champagne-bottle* deformity of the lower leg if the sclerosis extends circumferentially.

Pathogenesis

The superficial veins of the lower leg connect to the deep veins in the muscular compartments through vessels that perforate the muscular fascia (perforating veins). Normal function of the calf muscle pump allows venous blood to be delivered back toward the heart, while maintaining very low static pressure. Venous valves are a critical component of this pump. They break up a potentially very tall column of fluid (the height from the toe to the head) into much shorter columns arranged in both series and parallel, which greatly decreases the static pressure in each vessel. Because these are one-way valves, any localized increase in tissue pressure (such as from walking) results in directional flow toward the heart. Failure of these valves results in venous reflux and venous hypertension.

Causes of valve failure include congenital weakness, trauma, infection, thrombosis, and hormonal influences. The latter may explain why venous stasis is more common in females. Prolonged standing results in venous filling and dilatation, which tends to open proximal venous valves and permit high pressures to be transmitted to the peripheral leg veins. Thrombophlebitis and deep venous thrombosis (DVT) initially cause obstructive venous insufficiency, which may be followed by permanent valvular destruction and subsequent reflux hypertension.

The mechanism behind the progression from venous hypertension to venous stasis dermatitis to ulceration is less clear. The local tissue physiology apparently changes in a way to prevent efficient healing. This may be secondary to increased vascular permeability, local recirculation of metabolic waste products, decreased oxygenation, deposition of fibrin, and other mechanisms.

Differential Diagnoses

The most frequent causes of lower extremity ulcers include venous stasis, arteriosclerosis, and diabetic neuropathy. If the ulcer is painless, venous, neuropathic, infectious, and neoplastic etiologies are most likely. However, the presence of pain does not rule these out (especially infection). DVT must always be considered, and cannot be excluded based on clinical findings alone. Severe pain points to arterial disease, pyoderma gangrenosum, or atrophie blanche.

Diagnosis

The diagnosis of venous stasis is often made clinically; however, it is important to rule out arterial insufficiency, DVT, or infection, because the presence of these will significantly alter initial therapy.

Plethysmography is used to find the ankle-brachial index (ABI), which is the ratio of the systolic blood pressure measured at the ankle to that measured at the arm. An ABI less than 0.8 indicates moderate arterial insufficiency, in which case compression stockings may further impede arterial inflow, and surgical revascularization should be considered. In patients with calcified vessels (such as diabetics or those with long-standing arteriosclerosis), a false-negative ABI may be reported as incompressible vessels. Transcutaneous oxygen tension may be used to assess arterial sufficiency in this case. After adequate arterial supply is confirmed, compression therapy should be used in all patients with venous stasis ulcers and clinical evidence of edema.

Duplex ultrasound can screen for DVT and also identify specific points of venous reflux. If reflux is most significant in the superficial system, and conservative management is failing, the offending vessels should be surgically removed or ablated (through stripping, sclerotherapy, etc.).

When there is clinical suspicion of infection, tissue should be taken for culture. Cultures taken by swabbing the wound are likely to grow colonizing bacteria, and are therefore not specific for identifying the infectious agent that is impairing healing. A quantitative tissue culture helps identify the offending agent when more than 100,000 organisms are present per gram of tissue. The wound must be thoroughly débrided and irrigated before taking a small sample of healthy-appearing tissue for this quantitative culture. If sinus tracts are present, or when osteomyelitis is otherwise suspected, radiographs should be ordered as part of the initial workup.

Therapy

The mainstay of venous ulcer prevention is compression greater than 30 mm Hg. When an ulcer appears, débridement, appropriate dressing, and surveillance for infection must be included as well.

If the wound is small or improving with therapy, management may be continued in the primary care setting. Initial behavioral interventions include exercising the calf muscles, avoiding prolonged standing, and elevating the legs intermittently throughout the day. Stockings should be worn during the day, and the legs should be elevated at night. Assessment of effective compression therapy should include the fit of the stockings, as well as the patient's ability and willingness to don the stockings. Hardware-donning aids are available, and custom-fitted stockings may be needed. The patient's social support resources (spouse, family, and transportation issues) should be assessed to help predict likelihood of compliance and follow-up.

Traditional, low-profile bandages can be worn under stocking compression if the ulcer is small, or has minimal drainage. To maintain a moist healing environment, petroleum jelly (Vaseline) may be applied to moist wounds, and wound gel may be applied to dry wounds.

Topical antibiotics can be used if there is suspicion of superficial infection. Silver sulfadiazine (Silvadene)[1] may be used in patients without sulfa allergy, providing gram-positive and gram-negative coverage. Mupirocin (Bactroban)[1] covers gram-positive infections, including methicillin-resistant *Staphylococcus aureus* (MRSA), although resistance is emerging. Polymyxin B sulfate provides gram-negative coverage, including *Pseudomonas*. Metronidazole (MetroGel)[1] provides coverage for anaerobic infections. Triple antibiotic ointment should be avoided because it contains neomycin and bacitracin; either of these may cause contact allergy sensitization in this population.

Large chronic ulcers are often more efficiently managed in a specialty clinic, which is stocked with the appropriate supplies and staffed with nurses experienced in the practical aspects of dressings and outpatient wound management.

[1]Not FDA approved for this indication.

DÉBRIDEMENT

Necrotic debris harbors bacteria and creates localized hypoxia and acidosis, which inhibit granulation and epithelialization. All nonviable tissue should be sharply débrided until the healthy base is exposed. Topical anesthesia may or may not be needed. Pinpoint bleeding helps to identify viable tissue during débridement, and superficial red granulation tissue should be left undisturbed. Final rinsing with pressure irrigation may be of benefit. Enzymatic and chemical débridement through daily application of topical papain/urea (Accuzyme)[1] can be used to soften dry wounds, and for patients who cannot tolerate physical débridement. Topical collagenase is a less irritating alternative to papain/urea. Topical antiseptics (alcohol, hydrogen peroxide) are toxic to granulation tissue, and may prolong healing.

CHOICE OF DRESSING AND METHOD OF COMPRESSION

Compression therapy of more than 30 mm Hg is indicated for all venous ulcers that have adequate arterial inflow (ABI >0.8). Ideally, the compression should be graded, with the maximum compression applied distally, starting at the toes. When increased pressure is applied proximally, a tourniquet effect will result, which may further worsen venous stasis. Common clinical examples of this include the swollen foot caused by an elastic leg wrap that began at the ankle instead of the toes, or the constrictive band caused by a patient that has rolled down the proximal portion of a poorly fitted knee-high stocking.

Figure 1 shows the algorithm used by the authors to help select the appropriate dressing, which should function to manage wound drainage, provide a moist (but not wet) environment for healing, and be compatible with compression therapy.

Perilesional skin may be treated with a skin sealant such as zinc oxide to prevent maceration. Topical triamcinolone (Aristocort)[1] 0.1% ointment may be used if there is a component of stasis dermatitis. Tinea pedis should be treated if present.

Frequency of dressing changes is often dictated by the degree of drainage. Wounds with copious drainage on a leg with poorly-controlled edema requires daily absorbent dressing changes until the edema can be better controlled though elastic wraps, elevation, or treatment of the underlying cause. After this, weekly dressing changes may be allowed using a multilayered bandage system over a polyurethane hydrofoam dressing if the drainage is moderate, or a calcium alginate dressing if the drainage remains copious. Patients without family support may require daily home visits

[1]Not FDA approved for this indication.

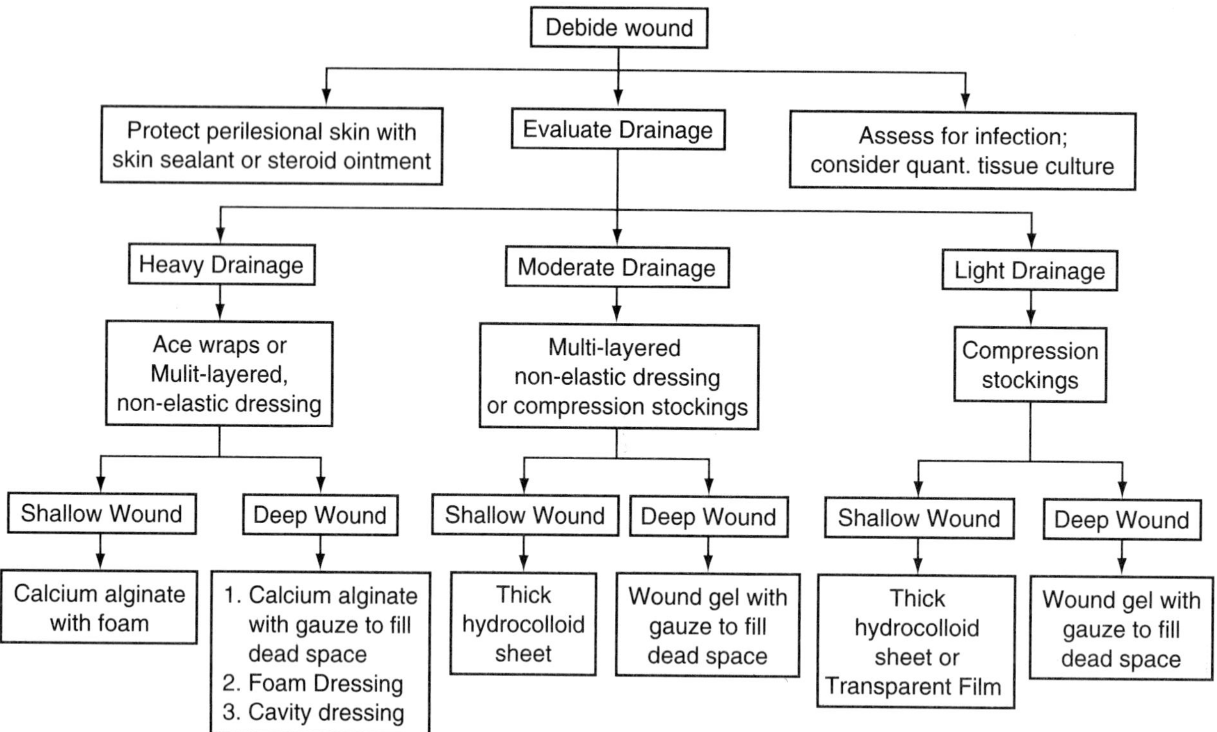

FIGURE 1 Algorithm for managing large venous ulcers.

for dressing changes or weekly clinic visits for reapplication of multilayer bandages until the healing is complete.

Conventional therapeutic support hose should be instituted when drainage is controlled and worn over a hydrocolloid dressing if the drainage is minimal, or an amorphous hydrogel dressing if the wound is dry. Dressings under support hose should be changed daily after bathing, and should not be bulky enough to place undue pressure on the wound.

Wound odor can have a great impact on the patient's quality of life. Dressings that help control odor include metronidazole gel (MetroGel)[1], cadexomer iodine, charcoal compounds, silver-coated dressings, and gauze soaked with 25% strength Dakin's solution[1] (dilute bleach).

Assessment of Therapy

Accurate wound measurement is important in guiding management. The wound is unlikely to resolve if the rate of healing remains less than 0.2 cm per week by week 4 of unaltered treatment. Inadequate healing requires a change in therapy. Vascular surgery may correct any significant reflux in the superficial venous system that has been identified by duplex ultrasound. After the confounding factors have been treated (edema controlled, necrotic tissue débrided, infection resolved, limb revascularized, and so forth), the context of the ulcer's presentation and clinical course may aid in identifying other underlying causes of the wound's persistence.

[1]Not FDA approved for this indication.

Adjuvant Therapies

Pentoxifylline and stanozolol are oral therapies that may modestly improve wound healing in patients whose therapy is already optimized as described above. Hyperbaric O_2, topical platelet-derived growth factor (Regranex)[1], granulocyte-macrophage colony-stimulating factor[1] (GM-CSF), and allogenic (Apligraft) and autologous skin grafting may also favor healing in selected patients.

[1]Not FDA approved for this indication.

PRESSURE ULCERS

METHOD OF

Denis Colin, MD, PhD

Pressure ulcers are chronic wounds caused by a combination of extrinsic and intrinsic factors. Extrinsic causes of pressure damage are pressure, shear, and friction. Pressure is considered the most important factor in the development of pressure ulcers, resulting in localized ischemia of the soft tissue between the bones and the bed or chair surface. Friction and shear occur when the patients slide down the bed or are dragged rather than lifted. Intrinsic factors include patient's age, weight, mobility, nutritional status, continence, and general medical condition. These should all be taken into consideration when assessing risk factors.

Several studies show that at any given time, 3% to 10% of the hospitalized population has a pressure ulcer, and 2.7% develop a new pressure ulcer. Two thirds of pressure ulcers that develop in hospitalized patients occur in elderly patients. Most studies find the prevalence of pressure ulcers in nursing home patients to be 3% to 6%. The elderly are particularly exposed because of tissue changes that occur and coexisting diseases such as ischemic or hemorrhagic cerebral events, consequences of bone fractures, or metabolic diseases, which all reduce their mobility and compel them to permanent chair or bed rest. Pressure ulcers also occur with a higher frequency in neurologically impaired young patients. In spinal-cord-injured patients, the incidence of pressure ulcers is approximately 8% annually, and 25% to 85% develop a pressure ulcer at some time. Although the cause of pressure ulcer occurrence is multifactorial, it is well established that prolonged pressure ischemia will affect the viability of soft tissue and that any occasion of tissue injury (such as transferring) represents a danger. These wounds are likely to occur among underweight patients, the unemployed, smokers, patients having suicide behaviors, people who are incarcerated, or those who have a history of alcohol and drug abuse. Economic studies show that the cost of prevention and treatment of pressure ulcers approaches those of cancer or cardiovascular disease. Patients with pressure ulcers are important users of medical resources. They require 50% more nursing time, remain hospitalized for significantly longer periods, and are associated with higher hospital charges.

It is widely admitted that a large proportion of pressure ulcers are preventable, and identifying patients who are at risk of developing pressure ulcers is a fundamental aspect of prevention. Many scoring systems have been proposed to quantify patients' vulnerability to the development of pressure ulcers. Norton, Braden, and Waterlow scales are the most commonly used pressure ulcer risk calculators. Each of these tools is claimed to have a predictive value and their predictive validity has been investigated within large samples of population. The combination of risk assessment scales and clinical judgment appears to be essential.

Clinical assessment, which should be periodically repeated, must include general medical condition, skin assessment, moistness and incontinence, mobility, pain, and nutrition. A direct causal relationship between nutrition and pressure ulcer development is often related, however, the scientific basis for this assumption is unclear. Studies linking impaired nutrition and a higher incidence of pressure ulcers are very few; still, some authors consider that impaired nutrition may influence tissue vulnerability to extrinsic factors such as pressure. Assessment of nutritional status can be performed using specific tools such as the Mini-nutritional Assessment test or simple measures of height and weight to determine the body mass index (BMI). An undesired weight loss of at least 10% of normal body weight in the past 6 months is generally considered an indicator of malnutrition. Nutritional assessment may also include nutritional intake over the past week; this information may be gathered using 24-hour recall, self- or career-reported food intake records, or through the involvement of a dietician. Biochemical measurements such as serum albumin, hemoglobin, and potassium may be helpful when considering the nutritional status; but it is not certain that biochemical measurements will provide more information than clinical indicators.

When malnutrition exists, nutritional intervention should be considered. The main objective is to correct protein–energy malnutrition through oral feeding. If any limitations on normal food and fluid intake are shown, health providers must consider and change, if necessary, the local environment (e.g., ease of access to food, social and functional issues, and the texture of the diet). If usual feeding and oral supplementation fail to resolve malnutrition, other ways, including tube-feeding, may be undertaken, although the risks associated with these interventions should be considered. It is acknowledged that an individual may require a minimum of 30 kcal per kg body weight per day, with 1.5 g/kg per day of protein required and 1 mL per kcal per day of fluid intake.

Patients at risk should be turned regularly; an important rule is to avoid positioning patients on their trochanters; a semilateral position is highly recommended using positioning devices such as pillows, foams, or specific positioning equipment. Documentation to record repositioning should be completed by the caregivers.

Support surfaces are an important part of clinical management. There are two main approaches in considering support systems. The first is to use a conforming support surface to distribute the body weight over a large area. The second is to use an alternating support, where inflatable cells alternately inflate and deflate. Pressure healing also requires reduction of pressure at the damaged tissue area. Although scientific evidence of support surface efficiency is low, the effectiveness of high specification foam compared to standard hospital foam is demonstrated. As far as treatment is concerned, the evidence of the effectiveness of air-fluidized and low-air-loss equipment is also established. It is difficult, however, to determine the most effective surface for either prevention or treatment. Evaluating support surfaces for clinical use and establishing standards is also difficult. Criteria for evaluation should ideally be evidence based. Randomized, prospective, controlled

TABLE 1 European Pressure Ulcer Advisory Panel (EPUAP) Classification of Pressure Ulcers

Grade	Description
Grade 1	Nonblanchable erythema of intact skin. Skin discoloration, warmth, edema, induration, and/or hardness may also be used as indicators particularly on individuals with darker skin.
Grade 2	Partial thickness loss involving epidermis, dermis, or both. The ulcer is superficial and presents clinically as an abrasion or blister
Grade 3	Full thickness loss involving damage or necrosis of subcutaneous tissue that may extend down to, but not through underlying fascia
Grade 4	Extensive destruction, tissue necrosis or damage to muscle, bone, or supporting structures with or without full thickness skin loss

clinical trials are the gold standard, but they are an unrealistic approach because of cost. Tissue interface pressure measurement is another method. Incorporating shear force into the equation should be done, however, this interesting way of evaluation is still not available. Therefore support surfaces are evaluated in terms of performance. Clinical application of support surfaces begins with a methodological approach to selection of the appropriate support surface. It is important to assess the performance of each type of support surface accurately, identify individual patient's needs, and then select the most appropriate option based on a well-informed, educated approach. Support surfaces used for the prevention and treatment of pressure ulcers may be classified according to their physical form and function. The three physical forms are mattress (or cushion) overlays, mattress (or cushion) replacement, and full-framed specialty beds. The functions may be defined in nonpowered and powered devices.

The priority, when a pressure ulcer has occurred, is to provide adequate pressure relief and further protection of vulnerable areas. Assessment involves the entire person, not only the pressure ulcer. This assessment is essential for an appropriate plan of care and should include physical and psychosocial conditions, hydration, nutrition, level of pain, and the wound itself.

Staging pressure ulcers allows the assessment of the wound and the selection of local treatment (Table 1). Beyond any classification it is important to define location, size, wound bed, exudate, pain, and status of surrounding skin. Pain assessment related to the pressure ulcer is essential. The pain should be managed by eliminating or controlling the source of pain, including covering wounds, adjusting support surfaces, and repositioning the patient. Providing medication or other methods to relieve the pain is also a priority. Caregivers should consider psychological issues that may affect either the patient or his or her family, and treat depression. It is important to establish goals consistent with the values and lifestyle of the individual and his or her family. For example, for terminal patients who are in pain when they move, avoiding pain may be a higher priority than the prevention or management of the pressure ulcers.

A stage 1 pressure ulcer should be protected from further injury from pressure or shearing forces, but usually requires no specific dressing; sometimes a protective dressing of transparent film may be necessary. In a stage 2 pressure ulcer, or a healing-stage 3 or 4 wound, the ulcer base is covered with granulation tissue with an epithelial edge extending from the margins. It is recommended to use a dressing that will keep the ulcer bed continuously moist, while keeping the surrounding intact skin dry. The choice of dressing (Table 2) is determined by clinical judgment, because studies of different types of moist dressings show no difference in pressure ulcer healing outcomes. Wound dead space should be filled with loosely packed dressing material that will absorb excess exudate and can maintain a moist environment. Surface necrosis should be débrided to allow granulation tissue to grow. Appropriate measures may include sharp surgical débridement, hydrogels (dry wound) or alginates (exudative wound), autolysis, or mechanical removal through the use of wet-to-dry dressings, water jets, or whirlpool. Topical antiseptics should not be used. Wounds with extensive subcutaneous tissue damage may require extensive surgical débridement, when appropriate, for the patient's condition and care plan. All devitalized tissue should be removed, and it is recommended that undermined areas be explored and unroofed. Infection of a pressure ulcer can affect treatment. Diagnosis of pressure ulcer infection is suggested by the appearance of a wound that contains necrotic tissue, wound edge erythema, purulent discharge, and foul odor; all of which influence treatment. Systemic antibiotics should be chosen only when there is evidence of a systemic infection, such as cellulitis, osteomyelitis, or sepsis.

Despite the considerable improvement of medical knowledge and its impact on the domain of health in the past 30 years, pressure ulcers remain a major

TABLE 2 Dressings for Different Types of Ulcer

Usual Dressings Categories	Type of Pressure Ulcer
Gauzes	Moderately exudative
Transparent films	Superficial (grade 2)
Hydrocolloids	Exudative (autolytic débridement)
Hydrogels	Dry (autolytic debridement)
Alginates	Exudative (and/or bleeding)
Foams	Exudative (superficial or deep)
Exudates absorbers	Very exudative, foul odor

health care preoccupation. They occur with a worrying frequency, and they are as physically and psychologically painful now as they always were. This severe damage for the patients also includes a heavy economical burden, prolonged hospital stays, and a huge amount of work for the medical staff. Education is probably the most effective way of reducing the incidence of pressure ulcers. There is a requirement for all the caregivers to be aware of the importance of initial and continuous education and to understand their role in improving the patient's quality of life.

Numerous gaps remain in our understanding of effective pressure ulcer prevention and treatment. Moreover the majority of pressure ulcer management is derived from expert opinion rather than empirical evidence. Thus further research is absolutely needed in order to decrease the incidence of this severe disease and improve the quality of life of our patients.

ATOPIC DERMATITIS

METHOD OF

Anthony J. Mancini, MD

Atopic dermatitis (AD) is a genetically-influenced, chronically-relapsing, pruritic skin disorder. It affects 7% to 17% of school-aged children, with 60% of cases beginning within the first year of life. Three criteria are essential to making the diagnosis of AD: (a) a personal or family history of atopy (including AD, asthma, and/or allergic rhinoconjunctivitis); (b) pruritus; and (c) "eczema," which is a nonspecific term for scaly, inflamed, oozing, or crusted skin. Skin findings in patients with AD include scaly, erythematous papules and plaques, often with excoriations, crusting, and fissuring. Subacute AD and chronic AD are marked by lichenification (skin thickening with increased skin markings) and pigmentary alterations (hypo- or hyperpigmentation). Table 1 lists associated skin findings in patients with AD.

TABLE 1 Associated Skin Finding in Patients with Atopic Dermatitis

Finding	Description
Allergic shiners	Blue-gray darkening of infraorbital skin
Ichthyosis vulgaris	Polygonal scaling, mainly lower extremities
Keratosis pilaris	Hyperkeratotic follicular papules, distributed on cheeks (children), lateral arms, and dorsal thighs
Morgan-Dennie folds	Symmetric, prominent folds below margin of lower eyelids
Pityriasis alba	Hypopigmented macules and patches, most often on the face
Skin hyperlinearity	Increased marking on palms and soles
Transverse nasal crease	"Allergic salute"; secondary to nasal rubbing with allergic rhinitis
Xerosis	Dry skin, often diffuse; worse during winter months

The characteristic distribution pattern varies depending on age. In infants, the face and extensor extremities predominate, with sparing of the diaper region. Toddlers and school-aged children tend to have more involvement of the antecubital and popliteal fossae, as well as facial involvement. Older children, adolescents, and adults have a similar distribution, but often with involvement of the neck, hands, and feet. Atopic dermatitis has a profound psychosocial impact on patients and families. It is a source of significant sleep disturbance (both in the patient and the parents), family discord, impaired school performance, social isolation, decreased self-esteem, and negative effects on parental work performance. There are many myths regarding its causes and therapies. Thorough education, anticipatory guidance, and psychosocial support provide the necessary framework for therapeutic success.

Management

The management of AD is multifactorial, and must take into account the various components of the disease. Education is paramount to any therapeutic success, and patient education materials are quite useful to this end. Patients and parents should understand that treatment of AD is supportive and not definitive, and that the natural history is one of a waxing and waning course. Identification of disease "triggers," which is often the primary goal of caretakers, is usually neither practical nor useful. The role of food allergy as an etiologic trigger is exaggerated among laypersons and some practitioners, and is probably associated in only 20% to 25% of patients with moderate-to-severe disease that is recalcitrant to therapy. The risk of blind food eliminations, especially in younger patients, should be underscored, and in patients for whom food allergy is suspected, co-management with an allergist is indicated.

Dry Skin Care

Adequate hydration and lubrication of the skin are important long-term principles of AD therapy. Daily, short (less than 10 minutes) baths or showers are desirable, and have many advantages, including hydration, enhanced medication penetration, bacterial débridement, and bonding between parent and child. Emolliating is vital, and is most effectively achieved with thick creams or greasy ointments. Lotion-based products may be more desirable during the warmer months, especially in humid climates. Emollients should be applied at least twice daily, and as soon as possible after bathing. If anti-inflammatory agents are to be used, they should be applied to affected areas first, followed by the emollient.

Treatment of Inflammation

Controlling inflammation is the primary goal of AD therapy. Topical corticosteroids have long been the mainstay of therapy, and are effective and safe when used appropriately. They are usually applied twice daily, and treatment should be discontinued when the skin feels smooth (regardless of pigmentary changes). Refills should be closely monitored and regular follow-up should be arranged to assess for tachyphylaxis or side effects such as skin atrophy, telangiectases, or striae.

Ointments are usually better tolerated and more effective than creams. If topical steroid agents are used on face or fold regions (groin, axillae), they should be limited to low-strength, nonfluorinated preparations, such as hydrocortisone 1% or 2.5%, desonide 0.05% (DesOwen), or alclometasone 0.05% (Aclovate). Caution should be exercised with use of topical corticosteroids near the eyes. For affected areas on the trunk or extremities, intermediate-strength preparations are appropriate, such as triamcinolone 0.1% (Kenalog) or fluocinolone 0.025% (Synalar)[1]. For more severely involved nonfacial, nonfold areas, more potent preparations such as fluocinonide 0.05% (Lidex), mometasone 0.1% (Elocon), or betamethasone 0.05% (Diprosone) may be indicated. These agents should be used for short, closely monitored periods of time. Scalp dermatitis can be treated with topical corticosteroid solutions, such as fluocinolone 0.01% (Synalar)[1] or hydrocortisone butyrate 0.1% (Locoid). Fluocinolone 0.01% in an oil base (Dermasmooth/FS)[1] and betamethasone 0.12% foam (Luxiq) are other options for the scalp.

[1]Not FDA approved for this indication.

Newer nonsteroidal topical immunomodulators (TIMs) are now available for the treatment of AD. Tacrolimus ointment (Protopic) is available in 0.03% (approved for >2 years) and 0.1% (approved for >15 years) strengths. This product is a topical preparation of the systemic immunosuppressant FK506 (Prograf), and acts via inhibition of T-cell cytokine production. It is applied twice daily to affected areas. Transient stinging with application is common, and sometimes limits its use. Pimecrolimus 1% cream (Elidel) is another nonsteroidal TIM, approved in patients 2 years of age and older. It has a similar mechanism of action, and is also applied twice daily to affected areas. Application site reactions are less common, but it may be less effective in severe disease.

The newer nonsteroidal TIMs offer the advantage of being steroid free, which makes them especially ideal for periorbital therapy. Steroid-related side effects such as striae, atrophy, telangiectasia, and adrenal suppression are not an issue, and there appears to be no systemic immunosuppression when they are used as indicated. Vigilant sun protection is vital while using any topical immunomodulator, and should be stressed with use of these newer agents while long-term safety data are collected.

Treatment of Pruritus

Although topical therapies help to relieve pruritus, additional anti-itch treatment is often necessary. Patients (especially children) with AD often enter a vicious "itch–scratch" cycle, which propagates the disease and contributes to frequent secondary bacterial infection. Abrogation of pruritus is most effectively achieved with the use of oral antihistamine agents. A combination of daytime coverage with a nonsedating agent and nighttime coverage with a traditional (sedating) agent is often useful. Table 2 lists some commonly used antihistamines.

TABLE 2 Antihistamines Used for Atopic Dermatitis

Agent	Dosing	Comment
Cetirizine[1]	5–10 mg qd	
(Zyrtec)[1]	2.5–5 mg qd (2–5 yr)	Liquid: 5 mg/5 mL
Cyproheptadine	4 mg bid-tid	May increase appetite, weight gain
(Periactin)[1]	2 mg bid-tid (2–5 yr)	Liquid: 2 mg/5 mL
Diphenhydramine	25–50 mg tid-qid	Paradoxical hyperactivity in children
(Benadryl)[1]	1 mg/kg qid (children)	Liquid: 6.25 or 12.5 mg/5mL
Doxepin[1]	50–100 mg qhs	
(Sinequan)	5–10 mg qhs (children)	Liquid: 10 mg/1 mL
Hydroxyzine	10–25 mg qid	Author's first choice
(Atarax, Vistaril)	0.5–1 mg/kg qid (children)	Liquid: 10 mg/5 mL
Loratadine[1]	10 mg qd	10 mg "Reditab" available
(Claritin)[1]	5 mg qd (2–5 yr)	Liquid: 5 mg/5mL

[1]Not FDA approved for this indication.
Abbreviations: bid = twice a day; qd = every day; qid = four times daily; tid = three times daily.

Treatment of Infection

Secondary infection with *Staphylococcus aureus* is common in patients with AD, up to 80% of whom may be carriers of this bacteria. Pustules, erosions, and crusting are the hallmarks of secondarily-infected AD. Classic "honey-yellow crusting" of impetigo is unusual. Localized infection may respond well to mupirocin 2% (Bactroban) ointment, but more extensive impetiginization often requires systemic therapy. Consideration for antimicrobial therapy must be balanced by bacterial resistance patterns, and in some instances of mild infection, withholding antibiotic therapy is a viable option. Community-acquired methicillin-resistant *S. aureus* (CA-MRSA) infections are on the increase in the United States, and are being seen in patients who lack traditional risk factors for MRSA infection (hospitalization, frequent antibiotic usage, presence of an indwelling medical device, and so on). These reports highlight the importance of the judicious use of antimicrobials and avoidance of indiscriminate therapy.

When feasible, antibiotic choice should be guided by sensitivity testing of microbial isolates. Cephalexin (Keflex) continues to be a good initial choice for most infections, with an excellent sensitivity profile and a good-tasting suspension for young children. In older individuals, dicloxacillin (Dynapen) tablets are a good initial choice. Macrolide antibiotics have variable effectiveness against *S. aureus*, dependent on regional variation. Clindamycin (Cleocin) may be indicated for resistant organisms, and most CA-MRSA isolates continue to be sensitive.

Eczema herpeticum, representing secondary superinfection of AD lesions with herpes simplex virus, presents with fever and multiple, clustered vesicles or erosions superimposed on lesions of AD. Patients can become quite ill, and therapy with systemic acyclovir (Zovirax) is indicated. Oral therapy is sufficient for mild presentations, but severe or diffuse involvement is best treated by hospitalization with intravenous acyclovir and fluids, as well as pain control.

Table 3 outlines some therapeutic vignettes for differing severities of AD.

Systemic Therapy

Systemic therapies are occasionally necessary for patients with severe AD. Oral prednisone is a very effective therapy, but its use is limited by its long-term toxicities. If a brief course is necessary, it should be tapered gradually over 3 weeks to help prevent the marked rebound seen with more rapid tapers. Oral cyclosporine (2 to 4 mg/kg/day) (Neoral)[1] is an effective therapy for severe AD, but requires close monitoring and has many potential side effects, including hypertension, renal toxicity, gingival hyperplasia, and increased risk of infection. Its use should be limited to patients with severe, recalcitrant disease, and treatment should be discontinued as soon as feasible. Ultraviolet phototherapy (UVB, PUVA, narrow-band UVB) may be useful for some adolescents or adults with chronic refractive disease, but the risks of cumulative ultraviolet exposure make this a less-attractive option for children.

[1]Not FDA approved for this indication.

TABLE 3 Therapeutic Vignettes

The following are examples of appropriate therapies for different severities of disease:

Mild Disease

Daily bathing/emolliating
Alclometasone (Aclovate) 0.05% ointment bid or desonide 0.05% ointment bid

Moderate Disease

Daily bathing/emolliation
Pimecrolimus (Elidel) 1% cream bid (face)
Fluocinolone 0.025% ointment bid (body)
Hydroxyzine (Atarax) bid and qhs as needed for pruritus

Severe Disease with Superinfection

Daily bathing/emolliating
Tacrolimus (Protopic) 0.03% ointment bid (face)
Tacrolimus 0.03% ointment or mometasone 0.1% ointment bid (body)
Cetirizine (Zyrtec)[1] q am
Hydroxyzine after school and qhs as needed for pruritus
Cephalexin (Keflex) tid for 7–10 days
Consider allergy testing

[1]Not FDA approved for this indication.
Abbreviations: bid = twice daily; q am = every morning; qhs = at bedtime; tid = three times a day.

ERYTHEMA MULTIFORME GROUP

METHOD OF

Peter O. Fritsch, MD

The erythema multiforme group comprises acute, self-limited, exanthematic intolerance reactions that result from a cytotoxic immunologic attack on keratinocytes expressing nonself antigens. The morphologic hallmarks are target (or *iris*) lesions (Figure 1) that are stable, circular erythemas or urticarial plaques with central blisters or necrosis and concentric rings of erythema and edema. Two main subsets are recognized:

1. Erythema multiforme proper (EM)—a common, mild, often relapsing eruption strongly linked to herpes simplex virus (HSV) infection

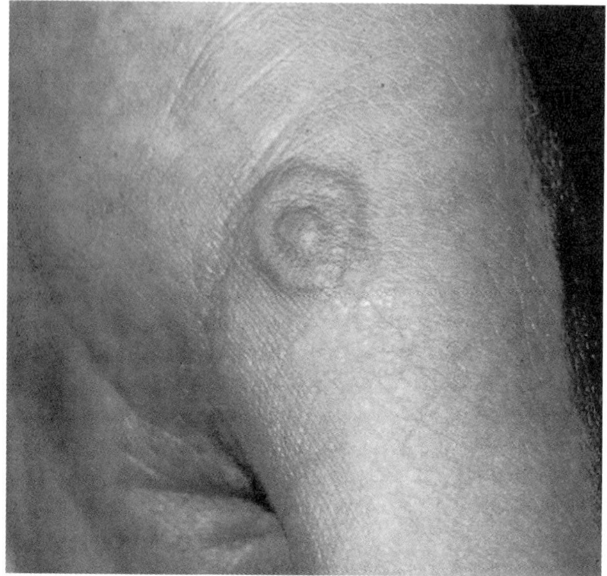

FIGURE 1 A classical target lesion of erythema multiforme, featuring a tense central blister and concentric rings of edema and erythema.

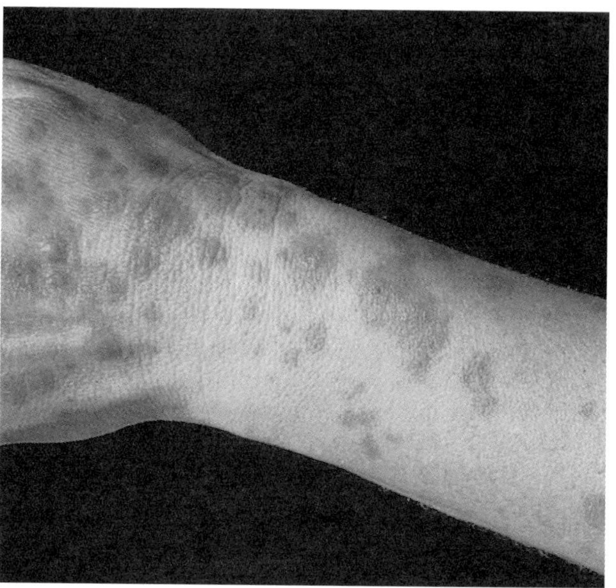

FIGURE 2 Multiple target lesions of wrist and forearms in different stages of development in a patient with erythema multiforme. Note the typical localization (extensor site of extremities).

2. Stevens-Johnson syndrome–toxic epidermal necrolysis complex (SJS–TEN)—an infrequent, severe, mucocutaneous intolerance reaction mostly elicited by drugs

These subsets are considered separate entities (Table 1).

Erythema Multiforme

EM occurs predominantly in young adults. It is relatively common and may account for up to 1% of dermatologic outpatient visits.

CLINICAL FEATURES

Flu-like prodromi are mild or absent. Dozens of target lesions form within a few days, first symmetrically at the distant extensor sites of the limbs (Figure 2) and in the face, then spreading centripctally. Lesions measure from a few millimeters up to 2 cm and show little confluence; the body surface area (BSA) affected is much less than 10%. Histologically, they exhibit intense lymphocytic inflammation with (often individual) keratinocyte necrosis and blister formation. The oral mucosa is involved in up to

TABLE 1 Clinical Features of Erythema Multiforme (EM) and Stevens-Johnson Syndrome–Toxic Epidermal Necrolysis (SJS–TEN)

	EM	SJS-TEN
Etiology	HSV (majority)	Drugs (80%–95%)
Course	Acute, self-limited, recurrent	Acute, self-limited, episodic
Prodromes	Absent or mild	Intensive; skin tenderness
Rash	Disseminated and symmetric on acral extremities, face	Disseminated with confluence; symmetric on face, neck, trunk
Cutaneous lesions	Fixed typical target lesions, blisters; Nikolsky sign negative	Atypical target lesions, central necrosis; Nikolsky sign positive
Mucosal involvement	Frequent, mostly mild; oral mucosa only	Prominent, severe; 2–3 mucosal sites
Body surface affected	<10%	<10% to >80%
Constitutional symptoms	Absent to moderate	Prominent to severe
Pathology	Satellite-cell necrosis of keratinocytes, dermoepidermal blister formation, prominent mononuclear-cell infiltrate, edema	Massive necrosis and sloughing of epidermis, dermal mononuclear infiltrate slight to absent
Internal organ involvement	Absent	Not infrequent
Duration	1–3 weeks	2–6 weeks
Complications	None	Septicemia, pneumonia, heart failure, gastrointestinal hemorrhage
Treatment	Symptomatic	Multidisciplinary
Prophylaxis	Acyclovir	Avoidance of suspected drugs
Mortality rate	0%	1%–50%
Healing	Without scarring	Tendency for mucosal scarring

Abbreviations: HSV = herpes simplex virus.

two-thirds of cases. Constitutional symptoms are mostly absent, and lymphadenopathy is only found with mucosal erosions. Recovery is complete within 2 weeks on average without scar formation.

Recurrences are common and may occur in the majority of cases. The mean number of attacks in recurrent EM per year is 6, and 70% of those recurrences are preceded several days by episodes of recurrent herpes labialis. Frequency and severity tend to improve over time, parallel to the waning of recurrent herpes simplex. Mean total duration of recurrences is close to 10 years.

ETIOLOGY AND PATHOGENESIS

Recurrent EM is strongly linked to HSV infection. It is unclear if this is also true for single-episode EM; other infections may play a role. HSV antigens and DNA fragments (notably viral polymerase) migrate via peripheral blood monocytes from sites of viral replication to the skin, where they can be detected in EM lesions. HSV antigen-expressing epidermal keratinocytes are attacked by cytotoxic effector lymphocytes, and apoptosis of keratinocytes is induced (i.e., satellite-cell or more widespread epidermal necrosis).

LABORATORY

In more severe cases of EM, erythrocyte sedimentation rate (ESR), moderate leukocytosis, and acute phase proteins may be found.

DIFFERENTIAL DIAGNOSES

EM must be distinguished from SJS-TEN, macular–urticarial drug eruptions, some types of urticaria and leukocytoclastic vasculitis, and EM-like disseminated allergic contact dermatitis.

TREATMENT

EM causes little discomfort and often requires topical treatment only, such as shake lotions (e.g., Calamine lotion), ad libitum, and steroid creams (e.g., Locoid cream), twice daily. Analgesics (e.g., acetaminophen [Tylenol], up to 4000 mg/day orally in adults) and antihistamines (e.g., diphenhydramine [Benadryl], up to 200 mg/day orally in adults) have little impact on the course but may reduce symptoms. Painful mouth erosions are soothed by liquid antacids (Maalox)[1], topical glucocorticoids (Kenalog in Orabase), and local anesthetics (Xylocaine mouthwash). Systemic glucocorticoids are considered unnecessary but may be useful in more severe cases (e.g., 40 mg methylprednisolone[1] daily orally with rapid tapering).

In recurrent EM, immediate antiviral treatment with oral acyclovir[1] (Zovirax, 200 mg five times daily for 5 days) or its derivatives valacyclovir[1] (Valtrex, 500 mg twice daily for 5 days) and famciclovir[1] (Famvir, 250 mg twice daily for 5 days) can be tried, but these often fail to prevent EM. With frequent recurrences (>6 per year), continuous administration of low-dose acyclovir (400 to 800 mg per day) or its derivatives for a 6-month period or longer is indicated. This regimen efficiently prevents both HSV and EM, even in some patients in whom HSV is not the proven trigger. No accepted treatment is available for nonresponders, although dapsone, antimalarials, and other medication have been advocated.

[1]Not FDA approved for this indication.

Stevens-Johnson Syndrome–Toxic Epidermal Necrolysis

SJS and TEN are considered the same disease by most authors, differing only in severity (as measured by the maximal BSA involved). According to current parlance, SJS affects less than 10% BSA, and TEN affects more than 30%; cases in between are labeled "SJS–TEN overlap." SJS–TEN is a life-threatening disease of adulthood (with a small peak in childhood), affecting females approximately twice as often as males. The incidence is two to three cases per million population in Europe and the United States; it is up to three orders of magnitude higher in HIV-infected persons.

CLINICAL FEATURES

SJS-TEN usually begins with several days of flu-like prodromi. Patients feel ill and may receive medication that, later, may obfuscate the offending agent. A morbilliform rash appears first on the face, neck, and upper trunk and then rapidly spreads further to partial or total confluence. Individual lesions are flat, pale livid, irregularly shaped, not strikingly concentric, and tender (atypical target lesions). The necrotic epidermis can be sheared off by mild friction (positive Nikolsky sign) (Figure 3); blisters, if present, are flaccid. Maximal expansion is reached within 4 or 5 days; it may cover anywhere between 10% and 90% BSA. In areas of confluence, large sheets of necrotic epidermis slide off (Figure 4), leaving extensive painful oozing erosions. In this stage, SJS-TEN resembles second degree burns. Skin appendages (nails, hair) may be shed (Figure 5). Histopathology shows prominent epidermal necrosis, in contrast to only scanty signs of inflammation.

The rash is paralleled by erosions or shallow ulcers of the oral cavity, less often conjunctiva and anogenital mucosa, coated by hemorrhagic crusts or grayish pseudomembranes. Mucosal lesions are severely painful and may cause eating and breathing difficulties, corneal ulceration, anterior uveitis, urinary retention, and phimosis.

[1]Not FDA approved for this indication.

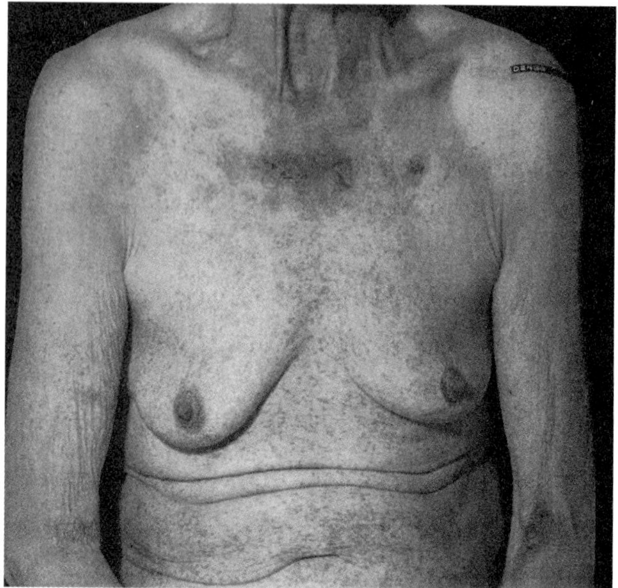

FIGURE 3 Stevens-Johnson syndrome in an elderly woman. Note the exanthem of atypical target lesions of the trunk and the positive Nikolsky sign in the upper chest region.

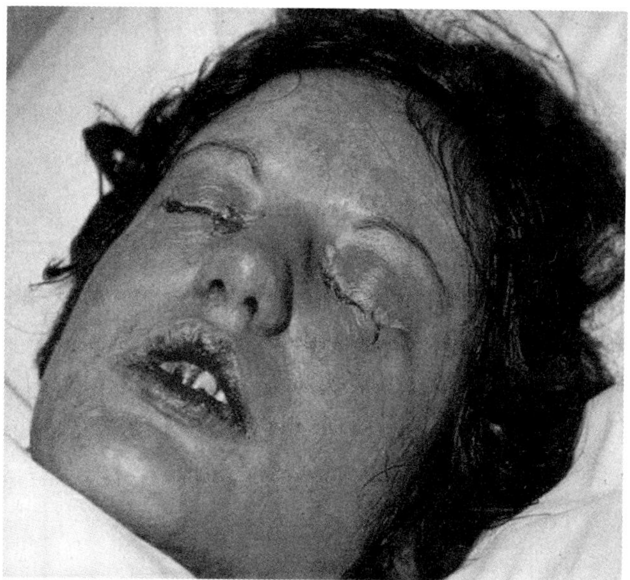

FIGURE 5 Toxic epidermal necrolysis in a young woman. Note the diffuse pale erythema, detachment of necrotic epidermis from the eyelids, shedding of cilia, and hemorrhagic erosions of the lips.

Constitutional signs (fever, prostration, arthralgias) are prominent. Internal organ involvement may be severe, most often affecting the respiratory and gastrointestinal (GI) tracts (e.g., bronchial obstruction, sloughing and expectoration of respiratory tract mucosa, bronchopneumonia, esophageal and GI bleeding, diarrhea, excretion of necrotic intestinal epithelium, colonic perforation). Toxicity, dehydration, and water and electrolyte imbalance may proceed to hemodynamic shock and coma. Except for microalbuminuria, renal complications are rare.

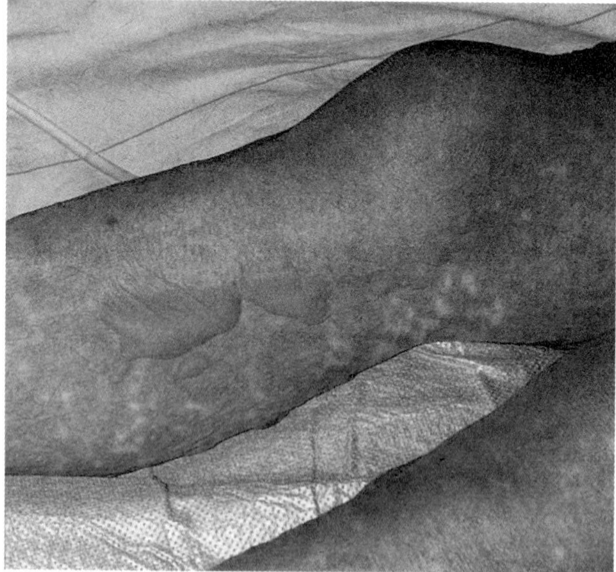

FIGURE 4 Toxic epidermal necrolysis with subtotal confluence. Note the large flaccid blisters.

Following the phase of progression (4 to 5 days), the patient enters the peak phase, which may last up to 2 weeks and bears the highest hazard of systemic complication. Regression is heralded by lightening of erythema and decrease of oozing and skin tenderness. Re-epithelization may take several weeks to be completed. Scarring is a characteristic (up to 30%) late complication of mucosal lesions—symblepharon, ectropion, corneal scarring, and pannus formation may result in blindness; esophageal, bronchial, vaginal, urethral, and anal strictures may also occur.

ETIOLOGY AND PATHOGENESIS

Drug intolerance is the leading causative factor (>80% of cases) (Table 2) of SJS–TEN; a minority of cases are linked to infections (notably *Mycoplasma*).

TABLE 2 Drugs Frequently Associated with Stevens-Johnson Syndrome–Toxic Epidermal Necrolysis (SJS–TEN) (Selection)

Sulfonamides
Nonsteroidal anti-inflammatory drugs
Butazones
Oxicam derivates
Propionic acid derivatives
Anticonvulsants
Hydantoins
Valproic acid
Lamotrigine
Barbiturates
Carbamazepine
Allopurinol
Chlormezanone
Antiretrovirals
Nevirapine
Protease inhibitors

Drugs or their metabolites act as haptens by binding to keratinocyte surfaces; an immunologic assault is carried out by cytotoxic T lymphocytes and activated macrophages. In contrast to EM, there is a drastic overexpression of tumor necrosis factor-α (TNF-α) leading to widespread epidermal necrosis. Genetic or acquired (e.g., in HIV infection) detoxification defects may play additional roles.

DIFFERENTIAL DIAGNOSES

For differential diagnoses, macular drug or infectious exanthemas (Nikolsky negative), generalized fixed drug eruption, and staphylococcal scalded skin syndrome should be sought.

LABORATORY INVESTIGATIONS

Abnormalities include elevated ESR, moderate leukocytosis and fluid-electrolyte imbalances, hypoproteinemia, elevation of liver transaminases, and anemia. Neutropenia is rare and represents an unfavorable prognostic sign. Proteinuria and elevated blood urea nitrogen are seen in approximately 5% of patients. A host of other laboratory signs may occur as systemic complications or secondary infection arise.

TREATMENT

SJS-TEN is an interdisciplinary problem and must be treated in a hospital setting with qualified dermatologic care and access to an intensive care facility. Disease management rests on three cornerstones:

1. Identification and withdrawal of the offending drug
2. Active therapy
3. Supportive measures

The *first step* in treating incipient SJS-TEN involves prompt withdrawal of all non–life-sustaining drugs, which may reduce the death risk by approximately 30%. In absence of appropriate diagnostic tests, the identification of the culprit drug is purely empirical. The most likely candidates are drugs with known high relative risk that the patient began taking in the past 4 weeks. Matters may be obscured by multiple drug intake, drug interactions, and infections.

The *second step* provides treatment. Systemic corticosteroids have long been the therapeutic mainstay, but their use has become controversial. They may well curb disease progression, but they do not shorten the peak and regression phases, and they do increase the risks of infection and of cardiac and metabolic complications. They may be used with caution, if all additional and supportive measures are procured, but they are unacceptable as the sole therapeutic measure. Relatively high initial doses are required (1 to 2 mg/kg methylprednisolone per day orally), and rapid tapering is indicated as progression halts.

Intravenous administration of pooled human immunoglobulins (IVIG [Gamimune N][1]) (0.2 to 0.75 g/kg body weight per day for 4 consecutive days) has emerged as a promising treatment strategy by blocking Fas-Fas ligand (FasL)-mediated apoptosis. Immunoglobulins have a good safety profile and should be regarded as a first-line option even though the optimal regimen has not as yet been determined.

Experimental treatments currently being looked at are immunosuppressants (cyclophosphamide [Cytoxan][1], cyclosporine [Neoral]), antioxidants (acetylcysteine)[1], plasmapheresis, and hemodialysis. All have been used with variable results and are not recommended at present. Experimental use of the TNF-α inhibitor thalidomide (Thalomid)[1] resulted in a significantly increased mortality.

Maintenance of hemodynamic equilibrium and protein and electrolyte homeostasis is important. Blood pressure, hematocrit, blood gases, electrolytes, and serum proteins must be monitored and adjusted appropriately. Fluid replacement regimens, such as those used for burn injuries, are usually not required, however, because the vasculature is not a target tissue in SJS-TEN. Central venous lines and urinary catheters should not routinely be inserted.

Prophylactic antibiotic treatment is used to guard against infections, which pose the most important threat. Bacterial and fungal cultures should be taken at short intervals (2 to 3 times per week) from skin and mucous membranes, blood, and sputum. Prophylactic antibiotic treatment (e.g., sodium penicillin[1], two 10 million units per day) should be initiated from the beginning, and should be adjusted according to the cultured microorganisms.

The *third phase* of treatment provides supportive care, as follows:

- Skin: Patients should be placed on aluminum foil. Loose sheets of detached skin may be removed, but early débridement is not indicated. Erosions should be covered with gauze or hydrocolloid dressings. Allograft skin and biosynthetic dressings have been advocated but are not required as a regular measure.
- Eyes: Steroid and antibiotic collyria should be applied several times a day. Lid–globe adhesions should be cautiously removed with a glass rod to avoid occlusion of the fornices.
- Respiratory tract: Postural drainage and, if necessary, cautious suctioning should be performed.
- Alimentation: A high-calorie, high-protein diet is recommended. Local anesthetic mouth washes before meals are advantageous.

PROGNOSIS

The prognosis for patients with SJS-TEN depends on its severity and the quality of medical care received. Mortality is low (<1%) for SJS and ranges

[1]Not FDA approved for this indication.

from 5% to 50% in TEN. Unfavorable prognostic signs include old age, extensive skin lesions, neutropenia, impaired renal function, and intake of multiple drugs. Fatal outcome is most often caused by septicemia, pneumonia, GI hemorrhage, myocardial infarction, cardiac insufficiency, and, much rarer, by renal insufficiency and hemodynamic shock. Recovery is slow; it may require 3 to 6 weeks or more, depending on the presence of complications.

BULLOUS DISEASES

METHOD OF

Diya F. Mutasim, MD

Autoimmune bullous diseases result from an immune response to molecular components of desmosomes or the basement membrane zone. The various types of pemphigus are caused by antibodies to desmosomal proteins. There is strong direct experimental evidence that antibodies in pemphigus vulgaris (PV), pemphigus foliaceus (PF), and paraneoplastic pemphigus (PNP) cause acantholysis and blister formation by directly interfering with desmosomal function. On the other hand, the subepidermal autoimmune bullous diseases result from antibodies against components of the basement membrane zone. In general, subepidermal vesicles result from activation of complement resulting in a cellular inflammatory infiltrate.

The discussion on drug use in this article is for off-label use. The drugs are not approved nor evaluated by double-blind, placebo-controlled studies for bullous diseases. The quality of evidence-based practice guidelines in bullous diseases is variable but generally low. The reasons for the lack of controlled studies include the rarity of bullous diseases, the potential severe morbidity associated with most cases, and the ethical dilemma of giving placebo to a patient with a serious dermatosis. Most data are derived from case reports and case series. In addition, the experience of the author is expressed in proposed algorithms for the treatment of each disease.

Pemphigus Vulgaris

The aim of therapy in the management of patients with PV is to prevent the appearance of new lesions and produce healing of existing lesions. Successful therapy suppresses the production of pathogenic autoantibodies, therefore, immunosuppressive drugs are used. A positive clinical response is associated with a decrease in or absence of circulating autoantibodies in the serum and then absence of bound autoantibodies in the skin. There has been a dramatic decrease in the mortality of PV because of the increasing availability of immunosuppressive drugs and glucocorticoids, as well as earlier diagnosis and treatment.

The choice of therapy depends to some degree on the severity of the disease at presentation. Other factors that play a role in choosing therapy are patient related (age, general health, and associated medical illnesses such as diabetes, hypertension, or tuberculosis) and drug related (onset of action, efficacy, adverse effects, and cost). Unless there is an absolute contraindication, the initial therapy of PV is systemic glucocorticoid.

Prednisone is the most frequently used agent. The starting dose is 1 mg/kg per day divided into 2 to 3 doses. Most patients obtain remission within 4 to 12 weeks. The dose is maintained for 6 to 10 weeks, then decreased by 10 to 20 mg every 2 to 4 weeks. When the dose is 40 mg daily, the patient is changed to an every-other-day schedule. This is accomplished by keeping the first day's dose at 40 mg and decreasing the second day's dose by 5 to 10 mg every 2 to 4 weeks. When the patient is taking 40 mg every other day, the dose is tapered by 5 mg every 2 to 4 weeks. If there is no recurrence, the patient is maintained on 5 mg daily or every other day for several years. Methylprednisolone (Solu-Medrol), administered intravenously as 1 g per day over a period of 1 to 3 hours for a few (usually 3) consecutive days, is referred to as *pulse steroid therapy*. The goal of this approach is to quickly achieve the immunosuppressive effects of glucocorticoids while avoiding the long-term side effects. Side effects are rare and may include electrolyte imbalance, hypertension, pancreatitis, seizures, and cardiac arrhythmias. Patients with severe PV who did not respond to conventional therapy obtained long-lasting benefits after pulse steroid therapy.

If prednisone fails to induce a remission, or if the patient develops serious adverse effects, adjuvant immunosuppressive drugs may be instituted. Treatment may also be initiated with adjuvant therapy concomitant with steroid therapy to decrease the total dose of glucocorticoid needed. The glucocorticoid is tapered rapidly, and the patient is maintained on the steroid-sparing agent for 18 to 24 months. The most commonly used steroid-sparing immunosuppressive drugs are cyclophosphamide (Cytoxan)[1], azathioprine (Imuran)[1], and mycophenolate mofetil (MMF) (CellCept)[1]. Cyclophosphamide is used at a dose of 2 to 3 mg/kg per day, azathioprine at a dose of 3 to 5 mg/kg per day, and mycophenolate at a dose of 2 to 3 g daily. The addition of cyclophosphamide to prednisone often results in rapid disease control and permits a reduction in the prednisone dose. The use of pulse intravenous cyclophosphamide may decrease adverse effects associated with the oral administration of the drug while maintaining its efficacy. An alternative to cyclophosphamide as a steroid-sparing agent is chlorambucil (Leukeran)[1], particularly in patients who develop

[1]Not FDA approved for this indication.

hemorrhagic cystitis. The dose is 4 mg daily, which may be increased to 10 mg.

Azathioprine is less effective than cyclophosphamide but is more widely used. It is less toxic and therefore requires less monitoring than cyclophosphamide. Because of its relatively lower toxicity, lower risk of sterility, and lower lifetime risk of malignancy, it is indicated in younger individuals. MMF is a generally safe glucocorticoid-sparing agent. It was first used for PV in 1997. Later, its use was reported in a study of 12 patients with PV who had failed combination therapy with prednisone and azathioprine. These patients were given prednisone and MMF (2 g per day). Eleven of the 12 patients improved and did not relapse during the 9- to 12-month follow-up period even with steroid tapering. Although methotrexate (Rheumatrex)[1] is also used as a steroid-sparing agent in PV, it is generally less effective than other agents. The response of PV to cyclosporine (Neoral)[1] is controversial. The literature suggests that cyclosporine is not effective as a single agent but may be beneficial when used as adjuvant to glucocorticoid treatment in long-term maintenance therapy of PV.

High-dose intravenous immunoglobulin (IVIG) (Gamimune N)[1] has a rapid onset of action and appears most effective when used as adjuvant to conventional therapy, especially as a steroid-sparing agent. The mechanism of action of IVIG is not clear. Plasmapheresis has been used in the treatment of severe PV, especially when the disease is refractory to treatment with prednisone and immunosuppressive agents. The effectiveness of plasmapheresis, however,

[1]Not FDA approved for this indication.

is controversial. When used in combination with prednisone, it was not found to be superior to treatment with prednisone alone. In that study, no concomitant immunosuppressive drugs were used. Other studies found it effective at reducing serum levels of autoantibodies and controlling disease activity. To avoid the rebound phenomenon (increased production of autoantibodies), immune suppression (usually with cyclophosphamide) is used concomitantly with plasmapheresis.

For resistant cases of PV consider:

- Experimental therapy with extracorporeal photochemotherapy
- Rituximab (Rituxan)[1] (a mouse and human chimeric monoclonal antibody that is directed against the CD20 antigen on the surface of pre-B cells, B cells, and malignant B cells)
- High-dose intravenous cyclophosphamide (50 mg/kg per day for 4 days) without stem cell rescue
- Immunophoresis

Figure 1 is a proposed algorithm for the treatment of PV.

Pemphigus Foliaceus

The principles and practice of managing PF are similar to those for PV. The aim of therapy is suppression of the production of pathogenic antibodies,

[1]Not FDA approved for this indication.

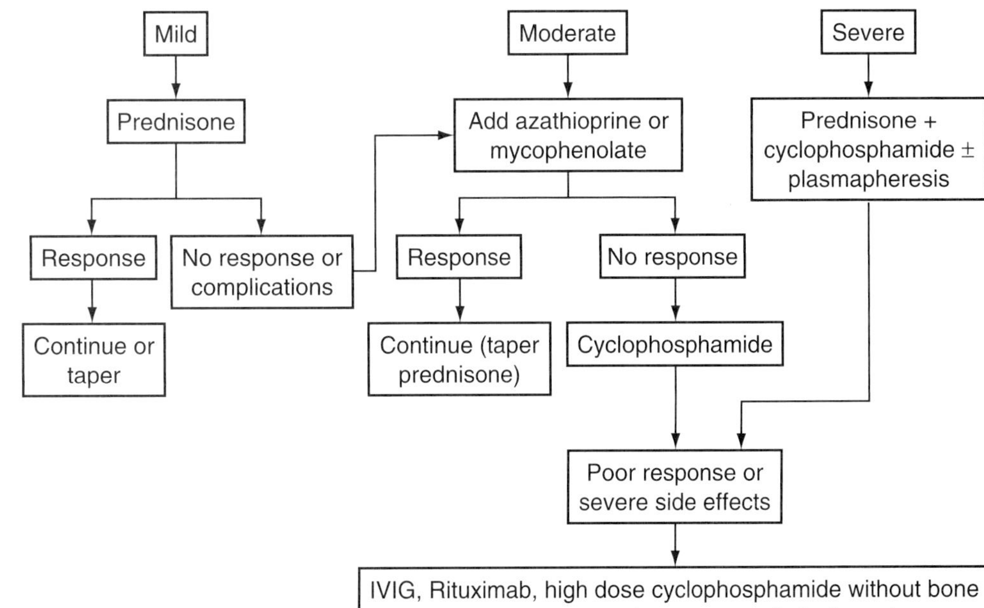

FIGURE 1 Proposed algorithm for the treatment of pemphigus.

cessation of new lesions, and healing of old lesions. This is usually accomplished with the use of systemic glucocorticoids with or without steroid-sparing agents. In addition, dapsone[1], gold[1], and hydroxychloroquine (Plaquenil)[1] have been used with variable success.

Paraneoplastic Pemphigus

The management of PNP consists of the treatment of the underlying neoplasm as well as immune suppression. Surgical excision of benign neoplasms, such as thymoma and Castleman disease, results in clinical and serologic improvement. In patients with malignant neoplasms, treatment of the associated neoplasm may not result in remission. Generally, skin lesions respond more rapidly than mucosal lesions. Systemic glucocorticoids are frequently used as the first-line agent in a dose of 1 to 2 mg/kg per day. Patients usually have a partial response; rarely, there is a complete resolution of lesions. Other immunosuppressive drugs are used with variable success. These include MMF[1], azathioprine[1], and cyclosporine[1].

High-dose cyclophosphamide[1] without stem cell rescue has been reported in a patient with PNP associated with chronic lymphocytic leukemia. The patient received cyclophosphamide, 50 mg/kg per day intravenously on 4 consecutive days. Two months later he had significant improvement of the mucosal disease. Rituximab[1] was effective in a case of PNP associated with CD20-positive follicular lymphoma and in a case of PNP associated with follicular non-Hodgkin's lymphoma. The standard dose is 375 mg/m^2 weekly. Immunophoresis is a procedure that is similar to plasmapheresis in which sheep antihuman IgG bead-formed agarose gel is used to selectively immunoabsorb and remove patients' circulating IgG autoantibodies. Clinical and serologic improvement is reported in a patient after failing systemic glucocorticoid therapy.

Bullous Pemphigoid

Bullous pemphigoid (BP) is a disease that results from an autoimmune response (autoantibodies) and that has prominent inflammatory features (cellular infiltrate). Unlike treating PV, treatment of BP may be accomplished with anti-inflammatory agents. The goal of therapy is to heal the existing lesions and prevent the appearance of new lesions.

Potent topical steroids[1] such as fluocinonide (Lidex) or clobetasol (Temovate) should be considered in the management of patients with localized or limited disease. Most patients with generalized BP require systemic therapy. The most commonly used systemic agents are the glucocorticoids. Prednisone is the most commonly used glucocorticoid, and is sufficient as the only therapy in the majority of cases. The dose is 0.5 to 0.75 mg/kg per day. Unlike PV, higher doses of prednisone are rarely needed. A clinical response is usually obtained within 1 to 3 weeks. The prednisone dose is then gradually decreased by relatively large portions (10 mg) initially and smaller portions (2.5 to 5 mg) later. When the daily dose is 30 to 40 mg, shifting to every other day is attempted to decrease the potential for well-known long-term glucocorticoid side effects. In many patients, prednisone may be completely discontinued after 6 months of therapy. Steroid pulse therapy with methylprednisolone intravenously, 0.5 to 1 g daily for 3 consecutive days, may help control severe disease. Unlike in patients with PV, this therapy is rarely needed in the management of BP.

Immunosuppressive drug therapy is indicated for patients who require a high-maintenance dose of glucocorticoid, for patients who develop glucocorticoid side effects, and for patients whose disease does not respond completely to glucocorticoid therapy. The most commonly used immunosuppressive agents are azathioprine[1], MMF[1], methotrexate[1], and cyclophosphamide[1]. Azathioprine[1] is commonly used in a dose of 2 to 3 mg/kg per day. The dose may be adjusted based on clinical response and side effects. MMF (CellCept)[1] is used in a dose of 30 to 35 mg/kg per day. Mycophenolate and azathioprine are effective both as sole agents or in combination with glucocorticoids. Methotrexate[1] is effective in small doses (up to 12.5 mg/wk) and may be used as sole therapy. Cyclophosphamide[1] is used in a dose of 1 to 2 mg/kg per day.

Tetracyclines or erythromycin, with or without niacinamide, have been used effectively. These agents are known to have anti-inflammatory properties. Initial case reports suggest a moderate beneficial effect of tetracycline with or without niacinamide. A study that compares the effectiveness of the combination of tetracycline and niacinamide versus that of prednisone in the treatment of generalized BP finds that the combination of the two medications is equally effective as prednisone. Tetracycline[1] is given in a dose of 500 mg four times daily and niacinamide in a dose of 500 mg three times daily. Minocycline (Minocin)[1], 100 mg, or doxycycline (Vibramycin)[1], 100 mg twice daily, may be used instead of tetracycline. The use of tetracycline and niacinamide may be indicated in two situations. In mild cases, the combination alone may lead to a clinical remission without use of corticosteroids. In more extensive cases, the addition of this combination of drugs to prednisone may have a steroid-sparing effect.

Dapsone[1] (or sulfapyridine[1,2]) has been used with mild to moderate response. Dapsone is usually started at 50 mg daily and increased by 50 mg increments every week until a beneficial effect is obtained.

[1]Not FDA approved for this indication.

[1]Not FDA approved for this indication.
[2]Not available in the United States.

The mechanism of action of dapsone in BP is not clear. High-dose IVIG[1] is highly effective for selected cases. It is given in a dose of 2 g/kg in a cycle of three to five equally divided daily doses. Patients usually receive two to four cycles (once every 3 to 4 weeks) initially and one to two cycles if their disease recurs. This therapy is extremely expensive and should be reserved for resistant cases. Plasmapheresis is used in severe cases. The procedure should be used in conjunction with immunosuppressive/cytotoxic therapy (e.g., cyclophosphamide) to avoid the rebound phenomenon. Plasmapheresis is costly, time consuming, and produces only temporary benefit.

A recent report reviews the literature and discusses the evidence for treating BP from six randomized, controlled trials comprising 293 patients. No strong recommendations can be made based on the available evidence. In the proposed guidelines, systemic glucocorticoids are the best established treatment. Consideration should be given to potent topical steroids for localized disease. For mild to moderate disease, tetracyclines[1] and niacinamide[1] should be considered. It is recommended that immunosuppressive agents should not be routinely used and should be considered if the glucocorticoid dose cannot be reduced to an acceptable level. Azathioprine (Imuran)[1] is the best established agent, followed by methotrexate (Rheumatrex)[1]. Figure 2 is a proposed algorithm for the treatment of BP.

MUCOSAL PEMPHIGOID

Therapy of mucosal pemphigoid (MP) varies with the sites of involvement, extent, and severity.

[1]Not FDA approved for this indication.

[1]Not FDA approved for this indication.

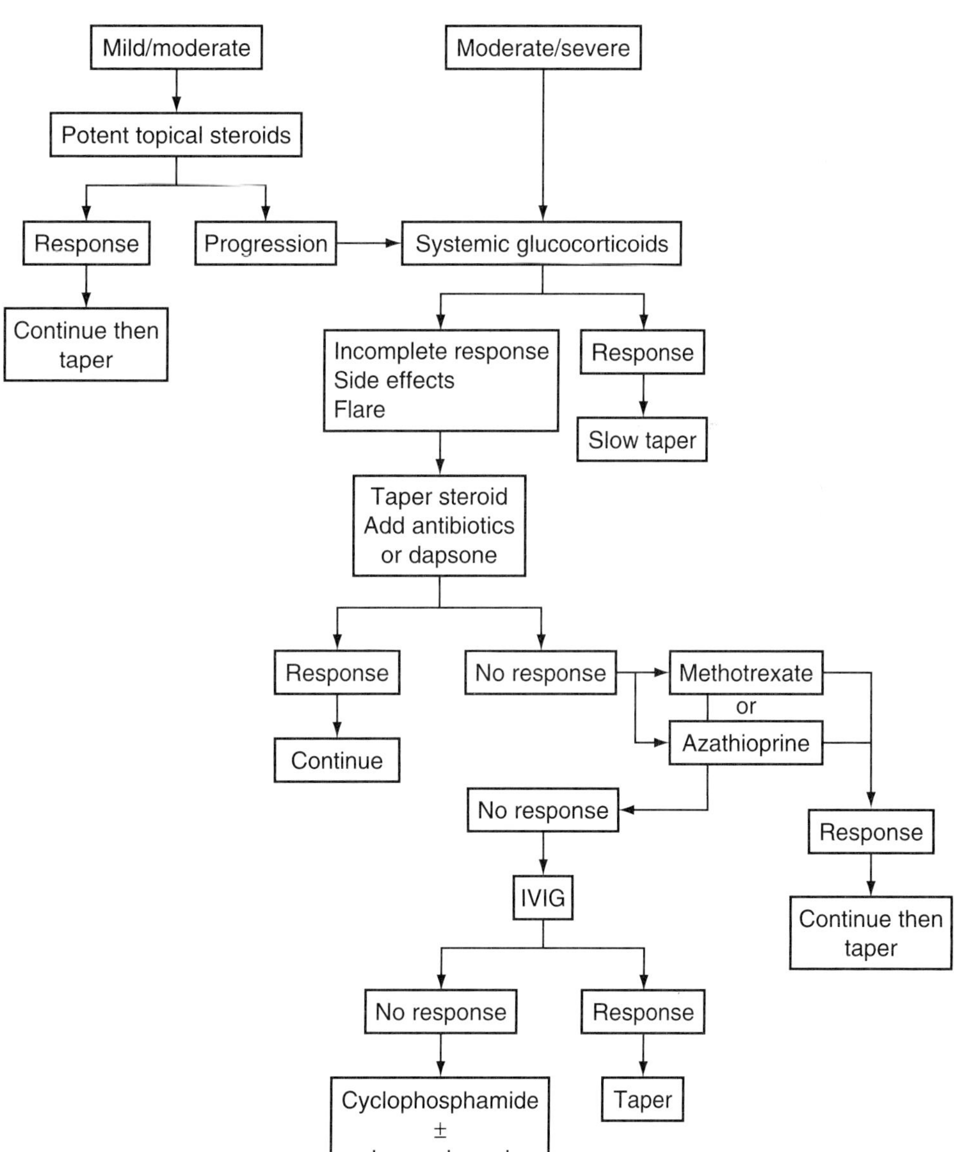

FIGURE 2 Treatment of bullous pemphigoid.

In limited oral disease, local therapy with topical anesthetic agents and topical glucocorticoids in addition to oral hygiene may suffice. The steroid may be applied under occlusion with a prosthetic device or injected intralesionally. Patients with extensive oral involvement may require systemic therapy. Dapsone[1] is effective in some patients. Oral lesions respond faster than ocular lesions. The latter may not respond. The drug is started at 50 mg daily and increased gradually. Tetracyclines[1], with or without niacinamide[1], are effective according to some reports. In severe oral disease as well as patients with ocular, pharyngeal, or laryngeal involvement, systemic glucocorticoids, in combination with cyclophosphamide[1], are indicated. Most of the patients have an excellent response with a prolonged remission after being treated with the combination of prednisone (1 mg/kg per day) and cyclophosphamide (1 to 2 mg/kg per day). Prednisone is used for approximately 6 months while cyclophosphamide is used for 18 to 24 months. Azathioprine[1] and MMF[1] are generally less effective but may be used if there are contraindications to steroid or cyclophosphamide use. High-dose IVIG[1] is sometimes successful in the treatment of patients with MP who are refractory to other therapy. The use of IVIG therapy results in a faster reduction in the level of autoantibody titers. High-dose IVIG results in the induction and maintenance of a sustained clinical and serologic remission. Cases with severe ocular scarring may benefit from cryotherapy ablation of eyelashes. Ocular surgery is contraindicated when the disease is active. Surgical intervention may cause severe flares of the disease. Figure 3 is a proposed algorithm for the treatment of MP.

[1]Not FDA approved for this indication.

[1]Not FDA approved for this indication.

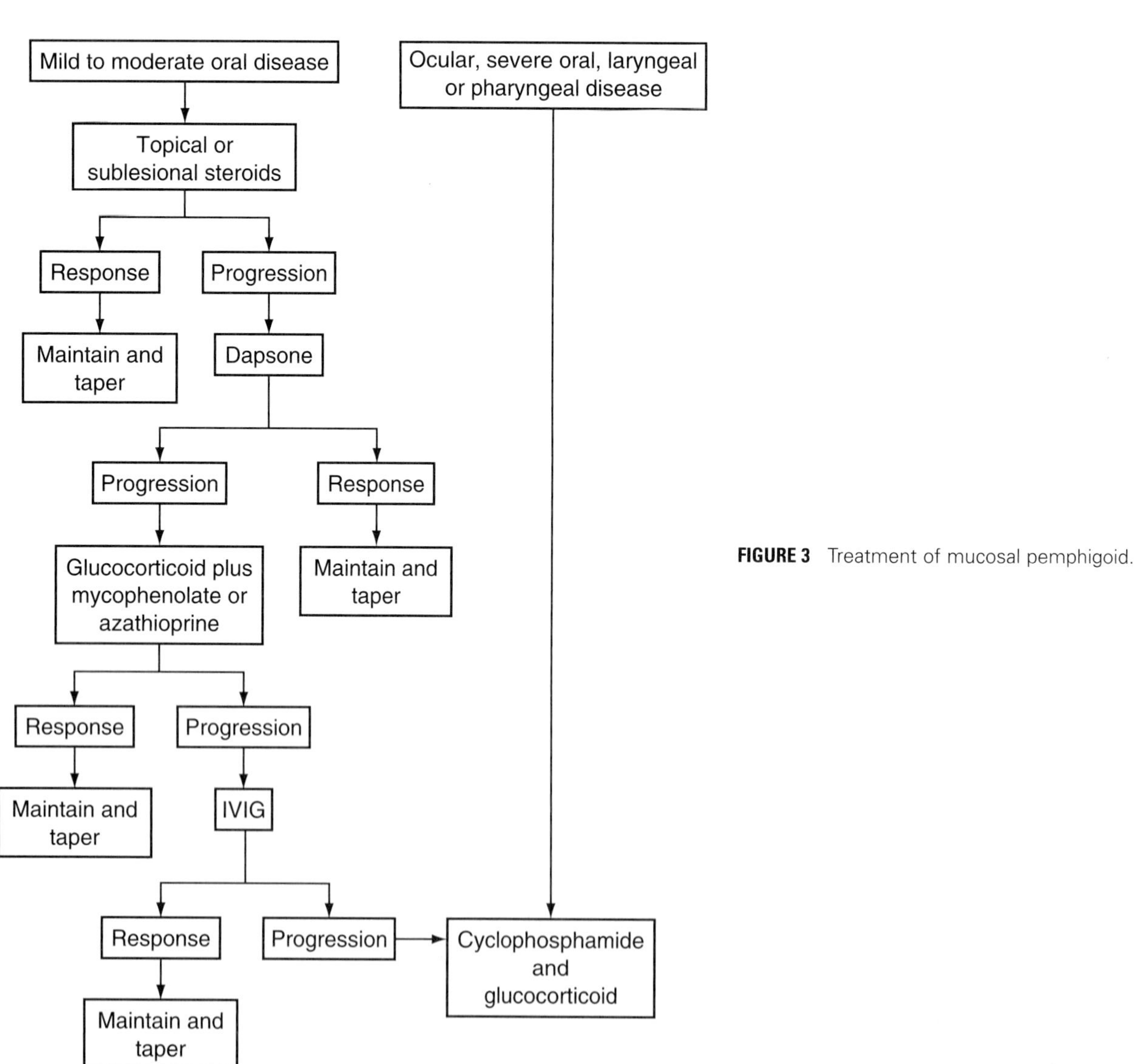

FIGURE 3 Treatment of mucosal pemphigoid.

Epidermolysis Bullosa Acquisita

Unlike other subepidermal autoimmune bullous diseases, epidermolysis bullosa acquisita (EBA) is generally resistant to therapy. The disease waxes and wanes with periods of remission and exacerbation. Trauma is known to contribute to blister formation, especially in the classical form of EBA. The inflammatory form of EBA responds more easily to therapy than the classical form. Because of the neutrophil predominance in the inflammatory form, many patients respond to dapsone[1]. The drug is started at a dose of 50 mg daily and increased by 50 mg every week until clinical remission (usually 100 to 250 mg). The dose is maintained for several months. If the patient remains in remission, the dose may be decreased slowly and ultimately discontinued. Colchicine[1] is reported to be variably effective in a few cases. Patients who do not tolerate or do not respond to colchicine and dapsone may be treated with oral glucocorticoids such as prednisone in a dose of 0.5 to 1 mg/kg per day in divided doses. The response is variable.

If there is no response to glucocorticoids or if the patient develops severe adverse effects, cyclosporine (Neoral)[1] may be initiated and is usually associated with a rapid response with doses ranging from 4 to 9 mg/kg per day. Once disease activity is controlled, the dose is decreased—decrements of 1 mg/kg per day every other week can be instituted until stabilization. Another regimen is to initiate therapy at 2.5 to 3 mg/kg per day and increase the dose by 0.5 to 1.0 mg/kg per day every 2 weeks if needed. Cyclosporine should be discontinued if there is no response in a few weeks.

[1]Not FDA approved for this indication.

The same agents that are used for the inflammatory form of EBA may be used for the classical form. The latter is generally more resistant to treatment. Patients who fail to respond may be treated with immunosuppressive agents such as azathioprine[1] or cyclophosphamide[1] in a manner similar to PV, BP, and MP. Patients who are resistant to these agents may be treated with IVIG alone or in conjunction with plasmapheresis. The advantages of IVIG over plasmapheresis are the rapid onset of action and the lesser degree of invasiveness. Extracorporeal photochemotherapy was effective in four reported cases with refractory EBA. Figure 4 is a proposed algorithm for the treatment of EBA.

Linear Immunoglobulin A Disease

Linear IgA disease (LAD) is mediated by neutrophils. Dapsone[1] is the first-line agent for the treatment of LAD. The drug may be started at 50 mg daily and increased by 50 mg increments every 1 to 2 weeks until an effective dose is reached. Sulfapyridine[1,2] is an alternative agent for patients who cannot tolerate dapsone. The starting dose is 500 mg twice daily and may be increased by 1000 mg every 1 to 2 weeks until adequate disease control. Colchicine, 0.6 mg 2 to three times daily, may be considered. Glucocorticoids may be added if patients do not respond completely to

[1]Not FDA approved for this indication.
[2]Not available in the United States.

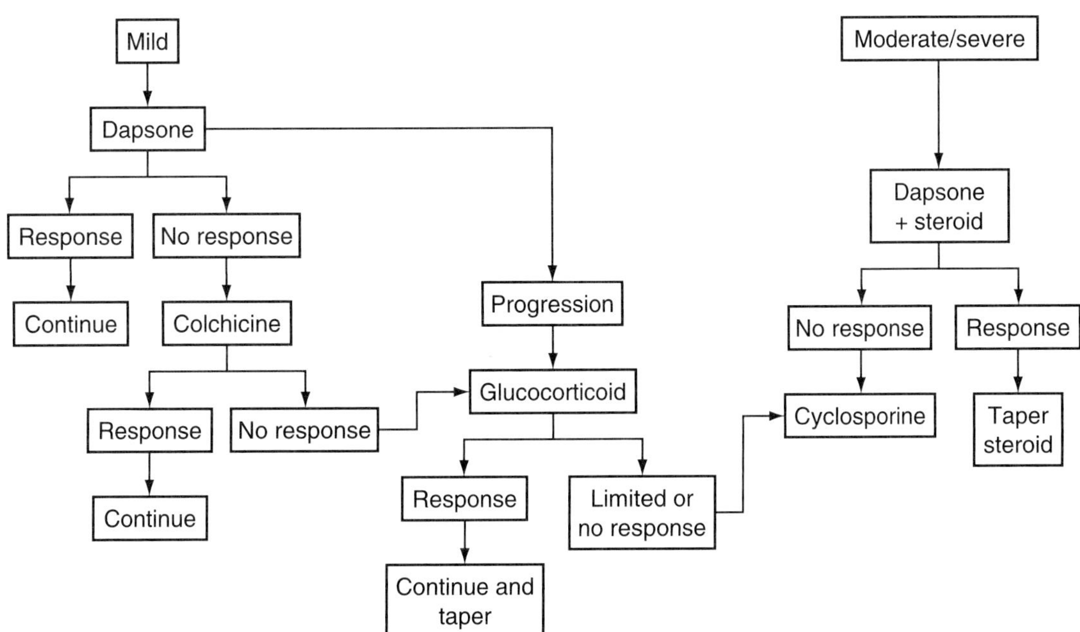

FIGURE 4 Treatment of epidermolysis bullosa acquisita.

dapsone or sulfapyridine. Tetracyclines[1] in combination with niacinamide[1] are reported to be effective. The dose of tetracycline is 500 mg four times daily. Alternatively, doxycycline or minocycline, 100 mg twice daily, may be used. The dose of niacinamide is 500 mg three times daily. Cyclosporine[1] or high-dose IVIG[1] may be used in resistant cases.

Dermatitis Herpetiformis

Dermatitis herpetiformis (DH) results from an immune response to gluten. A gluten-free diet is extremely helpful in the management of patients with DH and is often associated with a marked decrease in the requirement for pharmacologic therapy with drugs such as dapsone[1]. A strict, gluten-free diet may result in complete remission of the disease without requiring dapsone therapy. Reinstitution of a gluten-containing diet results in recurrence of the disease within a few months. The support of a dietician and disease support groups is often helpful. Many patients find a strict gluten-free diet too restrictive and choose pharmacologic therapy. The drug of choice for patients with DH is dapsone. Treatment is initiated with dapsone at 50 mg daily and is increased by 25 mg every week as needed and as tolerated. The average daily maintenance dose is 100 mg. Some patients require slowly increasing doses several years later, which is likely secondary to increased deposition of IgA in the skin that results in increased disease activity.

In patients who are intolerant or allergic to dapsone, therapy with sulfapyridine[1,2] may be considered. The initial dose is 500 mg three times daily and may be increased slowly to 2 g three times daily. The response to sulfapyridine is not as predictable as that to dapsone. Patients who are allergic to dapsone often tolerate sulfapyridine. Patients who are intolerant or allergic to dapsone and sulfapyridine may be treated with colchicine[1], cholestyramine[1], heparin[1], tetracycline[1], and nicotinamide[1]. These agents are much less effective than dapsone and sulfapyridine. Topical steroids are only minimally effective.

The effective management of patients with autoimmune bullous diseases requires knowledge of the pharmacologic effects of the agents used, an accurate diagnosis, knowledge of the pathophysiology of the disease process, and understanding of patient expectations.

[1]Not FDA approved for this indication.

[2]Not available in the United States.

CONTACT DERMATITIS

METHOD OF

James A. Yiannias, MD, and

Stephanie J. Mengden Koon, MD

Dermatitis typically presents as papules and vesicles with weeping and oozing that can become lichenified and scaly when chronic. When this clinical picture is secondary to an exogenous substance coming into contact with the skin, it is termed contact dermatitis. Further delineation leads to irritant-versus-allergic contact dermatitis, although in practice these two categories often overlap.

Irritant contact dermatitis is not an allergic process. It represents damage to the skin often from repeated and cumulative exposure to an agent. Strong irritants may produce findings quickly, whereas weaker irritants require a more prolonged exposure, but neither requires prior sensitization. Decreased barrier function of the skin, for example with frequent hand washing, can either predispose or exacerbate the condition. Examples of irritants include alkalis (present in soaps, detergents, and cleansers), acids (found in germicides, dyes, and pigments), hydrocarbons (petroleum, oils), and solvents.

Allergic contact dermatitis, poison ivy being a classic example, is an immunologic process classified as a type IV, cell-mediated, delayed hypersensitivity reaction. It requires an initial exposure to the contactant in which sensitization occurs but without outward physical effect. Subsequent exposure may elicit a striking response that is not dependent on the amount of the contactant, which may only be minute. The theoretical number of substances that may initiate allergic contact dermatitis is in the thousands, but some are more common than others. A study by the North American Contact Dermatitis Group (NACDG) patch tested patients who were suspected of having allergic contact dermatitis to a screening series of 50 allergens. The top 10 results from 1998 to 2000 were nickel, balsam of Peru, neomycin, fragrance mix, thimerosal, sodium gold thiosulfate 0.5%, formaldehyde, quaternium-15, bacitracin, and cobalt chloride. Every March, *The American Journal of Contact Dermatitis* publishes a "Contact Allergen of the Year," chosen to be a significant clinical allergen by a selection committee of international experts. The allergens recently chosen are disperse blue dye (2000), gold (2001), thimerosal (2002), bacitracin (2003), and cocamidopropyl betaine (2004). Balsam of Peru and fragrance mix are markers for fragrance sensitivity, and thus patients allergic to either one of these should be instructed to use fragrance-free products. Common sources of exposure to nickel include costume jewelry, snaps, zippers, and other metal objects. Clinically relevant sources of gold may be found in jewelry and dental appliances. Cobalt is found with other metals, including zinc, and in items such as jewelry, crayons, hair dye, and antiperspirants. Disperse dyes are used to dye synthetic fabrics, and the allergic patient is thus instructed to wear only natural fibers such as cotton, wool, linen, and silk. Neomycin and bacitracin are topical antibiotics available on their own and in combination with other medications such as polymyxin, antifungals, and corticosteroids. Cocamidopropyl betaine is a non-ionic surfactant found in skin and hair care products such as tearless shampoo. Sources of exposure to formaldehyde include cosmetics, household products, and the resins in plastics and clothing. Quaternium-15 is a formaldehyde-releasing preservative and may be found in cosmetics and industrial products; examples include creams, lotions, shampoos, soaps, paints, paper, inks, and photocopier toner.

The evaluation of a patient with suspected contact dermatitis begins with the history. Once the diagnosis of allergic contact dermatitis is suspected, specific questions directed at the patient's occupation, hobbies, and home routine will be helpful. The person who denies having been outside may have a pet dog that has brushed against poison oak before returning home. Ascertain if there is any relation to sunlight exposure or if the severity abates during a vacation and flares upon returning to work. Examination should note the location and pattern of the eruption. Although eyelid dermatitis may be seen in the atopic individual, it often represents nail polish as the source of the offending allergen. Dyshidrotic eczema presents as vesicles along the lateral aspects of the fingers, whereas eczematous changes along the dorsal hands are more commonly caused by an allergen. Other distributions that serve as clues include postauricular scalp (perfume), perioral (chewing gum, toothpaste), trunk (dyes or finish of clothing), wrist (nickel or chrome), waistline (rubber), feet (shoes), and history or presence of wounds (topical antibiotic ointment).

Patch testing may either confirm or reveal an allergen in a suspected case of allergic contact dermatitis. It involves placement of allergens against the patient's skin for 48 hours, after which an initial reading is done with follow-up readings at 96 hours and sometimes later. If light exposure appears to be a factor, photopatch testing may be done. Preferably the patient should not be taking systemic corticosteroids during patch testing. Because pre-existing dermatitis at the location of the patch test may lead to false-positive results, a large clear area should be chosen, usually the back. Prepared series include the thin layer, rapid-use epicutaneous (TRUE) test, which consists of 24 allergens (see the Web site, www.truetest.com). The customized series such as the North American Contact Dermatitis Group standard screening series, with 65 allergens, and the Mayo Clinic's standard series, with 73 allergens, must be manually assembled.

Many common allergens are not on the TRUE test screening series, including bacitracin. Any series obviously can only contain a limited number of allergens, and the possibility of a false-negative result should be discussed with the patient before initiating the test. In addition to ascertaining degree of positivity, relevance must also be determined. For example, thimerosal (used as a preservative in vaccines, cosmetics, and medications) frequently demonstrates positive reactivity, possibly secondary to childhood vaccination. But when evaluated against the patient's current clinical exposures, a low relevance is often found because thimerosal is rarely used today in topical skin-care products. False-negative results may also be obtained with premature readings; examples of allergens that may not become positive until late include gold, nickel, bacitracin, neomycin, formaldehyde, and textile dyes. Thus, these antigens should be read at 7 to 14 days.

Ideally, the allergen(s) will be identified and then avoided. Realistically, compliance is a challenge. The patient is expected to recognize foreign-sounding chemical names in addition to identifying their synonyms and cross-reactants. In regard to skin-care-product allergy, they must do this by reading long lists of substances on all products they use. To further complicate matters, there are also many nonlabeled items in their environment that they must recognize as being an inducer of contact allergy. Although patients must be proactive concerning environmental allergens, to assist them in skin-care product antigen avoidance, the Contact Allergen Replacement Database (CARD) was created in 1999 and is updated every four months. It includes approximately 2800 ingredients and 2000 individual over-the-counter and prescription products. Once the patient's allergens have been identified with patch testing, he or she can be entered into the database, and a list of products that do not contain the identified substances is generated. The patient should still be aware of their specific allergens, but this list simplifies their task and helps ensure greater compliance with avoidance. In allergic contact dermatitis, the patient should be made aware that even small and infrequent exposures may perpetuate the eczema.

Treatment for severe acute episodes may entail systemic corticosteroids, especially if the eruption is widespread. An appropriate option for an adult includes oral daily prednisone starting at 40 to 60 mg for 5 to 7 days, and then slowly tapering the dose by 5 to 10 mg every 2 to 3 days. Of note, a short course of steroids such as that provided by "dose packs" is too brief in duration, given that contact allergy may persist for several weeks after ceasing allergen exposure. Topical corticosteroids are helpful in hastening resolution after avoidance has been initiated, and may also be used for disease control when the allergen is unknown. Low-potency corticosteroids such as 2.5% hydrocortisone (Hytone) are recommended for the face, neck, axillae, groin, and intertriginous areas. Short-term use of triamcinolone 0.1% (Kenalog) for these areas may be necessary. High-potency steroids such as clobetasol propionate (Temovate) or augmented betamethasone dipropionate (Diprolene) should only be used for a few weeks (avoiding the above-mentioned areas) and then changed to mid-potency steroids (fluocinonide [Lidex]). Symptomatic relief may also be achieved with tap water or Burow's solution compresses. Lubricating moisturizing creams are beneficial but should be free of possible allergens; often the safest is 100% pure petroleum jelly. Steroid-sparing topical immunosuppressants such as tacrolimus (Protopic)[1] and pimecrolimus (Elidel)[1] are also now available for mild to moderate disease. Phototherapy with psoralen plus ultraviolet light (UV) of A wavelength (PUVA), UVB, or narrowband UVB may prove useful. Other systemic therapies include cyclosporine (Neoral)[1] or azathioprine (Imuran)[1], but this would be for the rare and recalcitrant patient. As a last word, it is helpful to instruct the patient in the natural course of healing for the skin. It may take many weeks before the skin reverts to a normal appearance despite successful antigen avoidance, and, in the meantime, extracautious care is required.

An excellent primer for the physician interested in learning more about contact allergy diagnosis and management is Marks JG, Elsner P, DeLeo VA: Contact and Occupational Dermatology, 3rd ed., St Louis, Mosby, 2002.

[1]Not FDA approved for this indication.

SKIN DISEASES OF PREGNANCY

METHOD OF

Wilma F. Bergfeld, MD, and

Melissa Peck Piliang, MD

Many skin findings appear during or are affected by pregnancy. The profound endocrine, metabolic, immunologic, and vascular changes that occur during pregnancy make the woman susceptible to physiologic and pathologic skin changes. Three categories of skin disorders occur during pregnancy:

1. Physiologic changes
2. Skin diseases affected by pregnancy
3. Dermatoses that occur only during pregnancy

These conditions can raise great concern in the patient with regard to the fetus, subsequent pregnancies, and cosmetic appearance. This article reviews the physiologic changes of pregnancy as well as the dermatoses specifically associated with pregnancy.

TABLE 1 Physiologic Changes of Pregnancy

PIGMENTARY
Melasma
Hyperpigmentation
Darkening of freckles, nevi
HAIR
Hirsutism
Prolonged anagen phase
Postpartum telogen effluvium
Postpartum anagen effluvium
VASCULAR
Telangiectasias
Varicosities
Palmar erythema
Gingival hyperplasia
CONNECTIVE TISSUE
Striae gravidarum

Tables 1, 2, and 3 provide lists of skin diseases and conditions affected by pregnancy.

Physiologic Skin Changes of Pregnancy

The physiologic manifestations are normal cutaneous changes that occur in nearly all pregnancies. The hormonal changes associated with pregnancy are significant. Although the influence of individual hormones is not completely understood, it is felt that they are either primarily or secondarily responsible for the cutaneous changes. Pigmentary, hair, connective tissue, and vascular changes are all seen.

PIGMENTARY CHANGES

The two main pigmentary changes seen in pregnancy are hyperpigmentation and melasma. Melasma, also known as the *mask of pregnancy*, is hyperpigmented patches on the face and occurs in

TABLE 2 Skin Diseases Affected by Pregnancy

WORSENED
Urticaria
Systemic lupus erythematosus (SLE)
Scleroderma
Dermatomyositis
Pemphigus vulgaris
Rheumatoid arthritis
Porphyria cutanea tarda
Erythema nodosum
Acanthosis nigricans
Erythema multiforme
Acrodermatitis enteropathica
IMPROVED OR WORSENED
Atopic dermatitis
Psoriasis
Acne vulgaris
Hidradenitis suppurativa
Sarcoidosis

TABLE 3 Dermatoses of Pregnancy

Dermatoses	Time of Onset	Clinical Findings	Fetal Risk	Recurrence (OCP, Subsequent Pregnancies)	Labs	Treatments
PUPPP	3rd trimester (average 35wk)	Polymorphous urticarial papules and plaques; start in striae	None	Unusual	None	Topical steroids Antihistamines Systemic steroids UVB
HG	2nd or 3rd trimester (average 21wk)	Urticarial plaques, tense blisters; start periumbilically	SGA Prematurity Mild, self-limited blisters	Common	Linear IgG on DIF, C3 at BMZ	Topical steroids Antihistamines Systemic steroids Cyclosporine*[1] Azathioprine*[1] Minocycline*[1]
ICP	3rd trimester (average 31wk)	Jaundice, excoriations	Prematurity Fetal distress Fetal death	Common	Increased ALT, AST, Alkaline phosphatase, Bile salt acids	Emollients Topical steroids Antihistamines Systemic steroids Ion exchange resins (cholestyramine, ursodeoxycholic acid)[1]
Prurigo of pregnancy	Any trimester	Pruritic erythematous papules and nodules	None	Unusual	None	Topical steroids Antihistamines

*Postpartum/nonlactating.

Abbreviations: ALT = alanine transaminase; AST = aspartate transaminase; BMZ = basement membrane zone; DIF = direct immunofluorescence (test); HG = herpes gestationis; ICP = intrahepatic cholestasis of pregnancy; IgG = immunoglobulin G; OCP = oral contraceptive pill; PUPPP = pruritic urticarial papules and plaques of pregnancy; SGA = small for gestational age; UVB = ultraviolet B.

[1]Not FDA approved for this indication.

up to 70% of pregnant women. It occurs on the cheeks and around the eyes and mouth. Exposure to ultraviolet (UV) light worsens the condition. It tends to fade postpartum, over many months. Treatment options include hydroquinone, tretinoin (Renova), or a combination of hydroquinone, mid-potency steroid, and tretinoin (Tri-Luma). Sun avoidance and broad-spectrum sunscreens are of utmost importance, as the condition will recur with sun exposure.

There may be a mild accentuation of normally hyperpigmented areas such as the areola, nipples, genital skin, axilla, and inner thighs. Linea nigra is hyperpigmentation of the linea alba. Freckles and nevi frequently darken.

HAIR CHANGES

Hirsutism and a prolonged anagen phase of scalp hair are the primary hair changes seen in pregnancy. Hirsutism, or hair growth in a typical male pattern occurring in a woman, is related to an increase in androgenic hormones. It typically resolves postpartum.

The anagen phase, or growth phase of the hair cycle, is prolonged during pregnancy, which produces thick and luxurious scalp hair. The resultant postpartum telogen effluvium, or shed, is often very distressing to the patient. The shed typically lasts 1 to 5 months, but may last up to 15 months before resolving spontaneously. A search for other triggers of telogen effluvium, including iron deficiency, androgen excess, and thyroid abnormality, should be undertaken. Breast-feeding without nutrient supplementation may be a trigger for a prolonged shed. A significant hair loss is rare.

CONNECTIVE TISSUE CHANGES

Striae gravidarum (striae distensae) are stretch marks that typically occur on the abdomen, buttocks, and upper thighs in up to 90% of women during months 6 and 7 of pregnancy. The development of striae is related to the stretching of the skin that occurs with increased abdominal girth. Pregnancy hormones such as estrogen and relaxin likely contribute. The biggest risk factors are increased fetal and maternal weight gain. Striae are initially pink to violaceous. Over time they fade to become hypopigmented.

VASCULAR CHANGES

The main vascular changes related to pregnancy include palmar erythema, telangiectasias, and varicosities. Palmar erythema is caused by dilation of the peripheral vasculature. Telangiectasias are dilated, tortuous, superficial capillaries that blanch with pressure. The formation of these spider-like macules is caused by estrogen. These vascular abnormalities may or may not persist after pregnancy. If they persist, they can be treated with electrodesiccation or a vascular laser.

Varicosities of the lower extremities are commonly seen after pregnancy. Many factors play a role in the development of varicosities during pregnancy. Increased blood volume, obstruction of venous blood flow by the gravid uterus, and venous valvular incompetence are among the factors postulated to contribute. Wearing support hose during pregnancy can help to decrease the risk of developing varicosities and can decrease associated leg pain and fatigue. Treatment options include sclerotherapy, vein stripping, and vascular lasers.

Dermatoses of Pregnancy

The dermatoses of pregnancy are a heterogenous group of diseases that occur exclusively during pregnancy.

PRURITIC AND URTICARIAL PAPULES AND PLAQUES OF PREGNANCY (PUPPP)

Pruritic and urticarial papules and plaques of pregnancy (PUPPP) is the most common pregnancy dermatosis, affecting between 1 in 130 and 1 in 300 pregnancies. Classically, PUPPP occurs in primigravidas in the third trimester. The mean onset is 35 weeks, but occasionally it appears postpartum. The mean duration is 6 weeks, typically resolving with delivery. It does not usually recur with subsequent pregnancies or oral contraceptives.

The most common clinical presentation is a polymorphous eruption with erythematous, urticarial papules and plaques. Vesicular, purpuric, targetoid, or polycyclic lesions may be seen occasionally. Patients are extremely itchy. The eruption classically begins in abdominal striae and spares the periumbilical area. Over a few days the rash spreads to the thighs, buttocks, breasts, and arms. The face, palms, and soles are spared.

The histopathology of PUPPP is nonspecific, most frequently showing a spongiotic dermatitis with a perivascular or upper dermal lymphocytic infiltrate with eosinophils. Focal parakeratosis or mild acanthosis may be seen. Serologic tests and immunofluorescence are negative.

The etiology of PUPPP has yet to be established, although several theories have been postulated. One theory is that abdominal wall distention leading to striae may cause damage to connective tissue and expose collagen antigens, leading to an inflammatory response. An increased incidence of PUPPP in women with greater maternal and fetal weight gain supports this hypothesis. Aging of the placenta in the third trimester may release a substance into circulation that triggers fibroblast production. The clinical and pathologic findings suggest a hypersensitivity reaction, possibly to estrogen, progesterone, or both.

PUPPP does not harm the mother or the fetus and is self-limited. However, the pruritus may be severe and intractable, causing great distress in the patient. Symptomatic treatment is all that is required. Mentholated topical antipruritic lotions (Sarna or Eucerin Itch-Relief Spray) and topical steroids may provide sufficient relief. A short course of oral steroids is safe and effective for more severe cases. There are reports of cases treated successfully with UVB therapy. The rule is resolution with delivery, and early delivery in cases of intractable pruritus is debated.

HERPES GESTATIONIS

Herpes gestationis (HG), also known as pemphigoid gestationis, is a variant of bullous pemphigoid. HG is rare, occurring in 1 in 50,000 pregnancies. It is most common in the second and third trimester with a mean onset of 21 weeks. There are reports of cases occurring in the first trimester. The eruption can initially present in the postpartum period. HG starts with the sudden onset of extremely pruritic erythematous, edematous, urticarial papules and plaques or papulovesicles. More than 50% of the cases start on the abdomen in the periumbilical area. The lesions rapidly progress to generalized, tense bullae. The face, palms, soles, and mucous membranes are spared.

Histopathologic and immunofluorescence examinations are identical to those performed for bullous pemphigoid. Routine hematoxylin and eosin stain (H&E) reveals bullous lesions with a subepidermal cleft. There is a dermal inflammatory infiltrate with eosinophils. Direct immunofluorescence of perilesional skin shows linear C3 and immunoglobulin (Ig) G along the basement membrane zone. Serologic studies show that the autoantibodies are directed against a 230 kD hemidesmosomal protein, bullous pemphigoid antigen 1 (BPAG1) and a 180 kD transmembrane glycoprotein in the epidermal hemidesmosome (BPAG2).

The clinical course is variable. Often, there is resolution of disease later in gestation only to flare at the time of delivery. There is exacerbation at the time of delivery or immediately postpartum in 75% of cases. Rarely, the disease presents postpartum. Most patients experience spontaneous resolution over weeks to months after delivery. Recurrence with oral contraceptives or menses occurs often. The disease often recurs with subsequent pregnancies, but is much less severe, and disease-free pregnancies have been reported. HG is sometimes associated with prematurity and small-for-gestational-age infants. Neonatal HG is observed in 10% of cases, but the disease is mild and self-limited. There does not appear to be an increased fetal morbidity and mortality.

The mainstay of treatment of HG in pregnant women is systemic steroids at 0.5 to 1.0 mg/kg per day of prednisone[1]. In the postpartum period, steroid-sparing immunosuppressive agents such as azathioprine (Imuran)[1], 150 mg per day, or cyclophosphamide (Cytoxan)[1], 0.5 to 1.0 g/m^2 body surface area can be tried. There are reports of success with minocycline (Minocin)[1], 200 mg per day. To avoid fetal or neonatal

[1]Not FDA approved for this indication.

exposure, the use of cytotoxic agents and minocycline should be limited to the postpartum period. The patient should not breast-feed while taking these medications. Plasmapheresis is reported to be effective.

INTRAHEPATIC CHOLESTASIS

Intrahepatic cholestasis (ICP) occurs in the third trimester in 70% of cases. The mean onset is 31 weeks. The incidence is 0.02% to 2.4% of pregnancies. The cause is a mild intrahepatic bile secretory dysfunction. The main clinical features of ICP are generalized pruritus with or without jaundice, absence of primary skin lesions, serologic evidence of cholestasis, and resolution with delivery.

ICP has no primary cutaneous lesions, but secondary excoriations may occur. The first symptom is moderate to severe pruritus that is worse at night. The pruritus may precede the jaundice by up to 4 weeks. Patients may also have fatigue, anorexia, nausea, and vomiting. Diagnosis is largely clinical, but laboratory studies may reveal elevations in hepatic transaminases, alkaline phosphatase, bile salt acid levels (usually cholic acid), cholesterol, and triglycerides.

The pruritus with ICP resolves within a few days of delivery, but tends to recur with subsequent pregnancies. There are reports of recurrence of cholestatic jaundice with oral contraceptive use. There is increased incidence of prematurity, fetal distress, and fetal death in the infants of women with ICP. Postpartum hemorrhage is increased in these women. Patients with both jaundice and pruritus seem to be at the highest risk of adverse events.

In mild cases, bland emollients and topical antipruritic agents may be sufficient. Low- to mid-potency topical steroids can be tried. Oral antihistamines and oral steroids may be needed in severe cases. UVB phototherapy is reported to be helpful in some cases. Cholestyramine (Questran)[1], a synthetic ion exchange resin that binds bile acids in the gastrointestinal (GI) tract, is effective in some cases. Laboratory values remain abnormal during treatment. Ursodeoxycholic acid (Actigall)[1], 15 mg/kg, both alleviates the pruritus and corrects the laboratory values.

PRURIGO

Prurigo of pregnancy comprises several conditions including Besnier's prurigo gestationis, nurse's early prurigo of pregnancy, and papular dermatitis of Spangler. There is extensive clinical overlap in these conditions and the etiology has not been identified. The unifying clinical presentation is pruritus in a pregnant woman. The incidence of prurigo of pregnancy is 1 in 300 pregnancies. It has been reported in all trimesters of pregnancy.

Clinically, there are pruritic erythematous papules and nodules on the abdomen and extensor extremities. Often, these lesions are excoriated and crusted. They resemble prurigo nodularis of nonpregnant women.

The eruption tends to resolve shortly after delivery, although the condition may persist for weeks to months. There may be postinflammatory hyperpigmentation. Prurigo of pregnancy does not tend to recur with subsequent pregnancies. There is no increase in fetal morbidity or mortality. Mid-potency topical steroids provide symptomatic relief and may be sufficient treatment.

[1]Not FDA approved for this indication.

PRURITUS ANI AND VULVAE

METHOD OF

Lynette J. Margesson, MD, and

F. William Danby, MD

Pruritus is common in perianal and vulvar areas. These two closely associated areas are often considered separately. Here, etiology and investigations are discussed separately, but management issues are combined.

Pruritus Ani

Pruritus ani is itching localized to the anal and perianal area. It affects 1% to 5% of the population, mostly men, with the ratio of men to women of 5:1. The cause is often multifactorial. Fecal soiling or contamination is a major factor.

ETIOLOGY

Etiology is often complex. Occult fecal leakage is very common and complicates other conditions. Leakage affects 2% of the population, 7% of people older than 65 years of age, and even more in parous women. The most common pruritic skin rashes are psoriasis, eczema, contact dermatitis, and lichen sclerosus. Candidiasis is an important contributor. Consider also bacteria, parasites, and HIV and its associations. Anorectal conditions like hemorrhoids and underlying bowel and prostate diseases must be ruled out. Systemic causes of pruritus (e.g., diabetes) can be important. Local factors, particularly hygiene, heat, and sweating, play a role. Psychogenic issues may be important. Always consider the combination of several etiologic factors. Idiopathic pruritus ani is a diagnosis of last resort.

EVALUATION/DIAGNOSIS

Complete history and physical examination, including in-depth information about hygiene, bowel habits, diet, skin disorders, and psychiatric issues, are essential. Accurately identify all topical products used and their ingredients. Rule out tinea infections with potassium hydroxide stain (KOH), look for bacteria and yeast with cultures, and do adhesive tape testing for pinworms. Full-screen patch tests may be indicated. Assess for systemic causes of pruritus. Biopsy any unusual or nonresponsive areas. Do a sigmoidoscopy and/or colonoscopy as indicated.

Pruritus Vulvae

Vulvar pruritus is the most common vulvar complaint, affecting approximately 10% of gynecological patients. It is often a multifactorial problem and can be challenging to manage.

ETIOLOGY

The five most common causes are candidiasis, atopy, contactants, psoriasis, and lichen sclerosus. Other itchy skin rashes are lichen planus, lichen simplex chronicus, and urticaria. Itchy infestations include scabies and pediculosis. Bacterial vaginosis and trichomoniasis cause vulvovaginal itch. Less common causes include human papillomavirus infection, tinea, and neoplasia (vulvar intraepithelial neoplasia and Paget's disease). Consider underlying systemic disease. Psychogenic factors can be a primary or secondary problem. Combinations of these factors are very important (e.g., candidiasis complicating psoriasis).

EVALUATION/DIAGNOSIS

Complete medical history and a full-surface physical examination of the skin, vulva, and vagina are needed. Acquire detailed information about hygiene, sexual habits, and role of menstruation. All topical products and exacerbating factors must be identified. Perform a full-screen patch test, if indicated. Include KOH and culture of the skin plus KOH, culture, and wet preparation of vaginal secretions. Always biopsy questionable or nonresponsive areas. Note that bowel disease can flare the vulva.

Treatment of Pruritus Ani and Vulvae

Almost always there is a combination of factors that need to be managed.

Specifics for pruritus ani:

- Avoid spicy foods and sauces.
- Control stool leakage.
- Control diet to eliminate caustic diarrhea.
- Manage constipation that causes fissuring.
- Adjust laxatives and add bulk-forming agents as needed.

Specifics for pruritus vulvae:

- Clear underlying vaginitis.
- Minimize menstrual flow with birth control pills.
- Use tampons to avoid the potential irritation of wet pads.
- Manage urinary incontinence (essential).

GENERAL MANAGEMENT

Correct epidermal barrier function. Wear only loose cotton clothing. Stop all irritants/allergens. Stop all offending hygiene practices (especially overzealous cleansing).

For open, eroded skin, use cool sitz baths twice a day in plain water. If needed, use a gentle cleanser (unscented synthetic detergent bar) using only bare hands, followed by a good rinse. Gently pat the area to "damp dry," then retard water loss with a *thin* film of plain petrolatum or oily cream. For raw, eroded areas, use zinc oxide ointment.

For episodic itch control, use cool gel packs, kept in the refrigerator, *not* the freezer.

Stress management and good patient education with long-term follow-up are important.

SPECIFIC MANAGEMENT

To help the patient stop scratching:

- Nighttime sedation—hydroxyzine (Atarax) or doxepin (Sinequan) up to 75 mg.
- Morning sedative—citalopram (Celexa)[1] up to 20 mg.
- Topical anesthetic (5% lidocaine ointment)[1] on a cotton ball, as needed, is safe for a limited period of time.

To reduce inflammation:

- Topical corticosteroids may be applied. The potency depends on the degree of inflammation.
- A mild (1% to 2.5%) hydrocortisone ointment may be effective.
- Pramoxine mixed with hydrocortisone (Proctocream-HC) may be of value.
- If the skin is very thick, a superpotent clobetasol (Temovate)[1] or halobetasol (Ultravate)[1] 0.05% ointment can be used for short periods of time, and the potency can later be decreased.
- Topical tacrolimus ointment (Protopic)[1] may be helpful as a steroid sparer.

To treat the infection, use an appropriate oral antibiotic plus oral fluconazole (Diflucan) to prevent secondary candidiasis.

[1]Not FDA approved for this indication.

URTICARIA AND ANGIOEDEMA

METHOD OF
Tariq Mahmood, MD, and
Anuroop Mongia, MD

Urticaria

Urticaria, or hives, is a common disorder affecting 15% to 25% of the general population at some time in their life. The characteristic eruption is marked by a pruritic (at times burning), transient rash that leaves within hours without any scarring. In acute urticaria the episode may last only a few hours to days and is more likely to be associated with an identifiable cause. Urticaria lasting more than 6 weeks is defined as chronic, and the etiologic factors are less likely to be found. Chronic urticaria can last for several years and even decades, thus becoming an annoying condition to the patient.

EPIDEMIOLOGY

The precise prevalence of urticaria is impossible to document, because many cases are never seen by a physician. In a survey of college students, 15.7% had experienced at least one attack of urticaria. Women are affected more commonly and account for 52% to 64% of all cases. Urticaria can occur at all ages; however, approximately 66% of cases occur in young adults between the ages of 20 and 40 years.

PATHOGENESIS

Lewis and Grant, in 1924, were the first to observe the similarity between naturally occurring hives with wheal and flare response caused by the local injection of histamine. Subsequent demonstration of elevated histamine levels in the plasma and involved tissues in several types of urticaria has established the pivotal role of histamine in this disorder. Other mast cell mediators involved in the urticarial response include prostaglandin D_2, leukotrienes C and D, platelet-activating factor, chemotactic factors for eosinophil and neutrophil, as well as additional molecules including histamine-releasing factors (HRF) and bradykinin.

Cutaneous mast cells are located in the loose connective tissue of skin, especially in the perivascular region. They are more abundant around the eyelids, lips, and scalp. Mast cell granules contain preformed mediators, such as histamine and others that are generated on stimulation. A variety of stimuli, both immunologic and nonimmunologic, can lead to the release of mediators from mast cells (Table 1). Foods, drugs, and physical stimuli are relatively common etiologic agents. Owing to the diversity of stimuli capable of inducing the release of mast cell mediators, a thorough history is required to identify the inciting cause in a given patient. Other factors, including heat, fever, exercise, emotional stress, and menstrual changes, tend to exacerbate pre-existing urticaria. Presence of urticaria is dependent on other variables including an increased number of mast cells (e.g., systemic mastocytosis), enhanced release, and impaired clearance of mediators.

TABLE 1 Pathogenesis of Urticaria and Angioedema*

Immunologic Mechanisms
IgE-mediated (require prior exposure and sensitization)
Foods
Drugs
Insect stings
Inhalants
Latex
IgE-receptor autoantibody associated
IgE-autoantibody associated
Anaphylatoxin (C3a, C5a)-mediated
Infections
Hepatitis B, Epstein-Barr virus (EBV), *Streptococcus*
Systemic diseases
Rheumatic diseases
Serum sickness
Neoplastic disorders
Transfusion reactions
Radiographic contrast media (RCM)
Nonimmunologic Mechanisms
Direct mast cell effect
Drugs (opiates, dextran)
Radiographic contrast media
Foods (shellfish, strawberries)
Irradiation
Physical agents (heat, pressure, firm stroking)
Effect on arachidonic acid pathway
Aspirin, other nonsteroidal agents
Undetermined Mechanisms
Idiopathic
Alcohol
Drugs (vancomycin, rifampin, papaverine, others)

*Multiple mechanisms may operate for some agents.

CLINICAL FEATURES

Urticaria usually presents as transient, localized areas of edema within the skin or mucous membranes. The wheals are initially erythematous but soon develop a blanched center. The wheals may vary considerably in size, from 2 to 5 mm to over 30 cm, and may be circular or irregular in shape. Urticarial wheals may occur on any part of the body, though they are more frequent on the trunk. The eruption resolves completely, without scarring, within a few hours. Pruritus is almost always present and is more intense in areas where the skin is tight, such as palms and soles. Pruritus tends to be especially troublesome in the evening and nighttime. Edema of the deeper tissues, referred to as angioedema, can occur concomitantly and may last 2 to 3 days.

The presence of fever and arthralgia should alert the physician to the possibility of an underlying systemic illness. This is seen in cutaneous vasculitis, macroglobulinemia, systemic lupus erythematosus, and delayed pressure urticaria. Acute urticaria typically lasts a few days, is more frequent in individuals with an atopic history, and more likely to be associated with large areas of swelling. Chronic urticaria is defined by its persistence for 6 weeks or more. A vast majority of these patients have an idiopathic disorder that runs a benign course, with waxing and waning, and may last up to 2 decades (average 3 to 5 years). Some of these patients have autoantibodies directed against a subunit of the high-affinity immunoglobulin (Ig) E receptor ($Fc\varepsilon R_{1a}$).

DIAGNOSIS

A detailed history with emphasis on dietary and medicinal consumption, exacerbating factors, and a coexisting or recent medical illness should be obtained in all cases (Table 2 contains a partial listing). Additionally, occupational and hobby exposure, inciting physical stimuli, and a personal or family history of atopy may yield helpful clues. A careful review of systems, including inquiry about the history of infections, connective tissue diseases, and endocrine as well as neoplastic disorders, may uncover potential causative factors. A thorough physical examination, including testing for dermatographism and, where applicable, other physical causes of urticaria, should be performed. A skin biopsy to rule out urticarial vasculitis and the urticarial phase of bullous pemphigoid is needed when atypical features are present. These include absence of, or minimal pruritus, persistence of individual wheals longer than 24 hours, poor response to therapy, and residual pigmentation.

TABLE 2 Systemic Illness Associated with Urticaria

Infections
Viral: hepatitis A or B, infectious mononucleosis
Bacterial: sinusitis, dental abscess, urinary tract infection, *Helicobacter pylori*
Fungal: candidiasis, dermatophytosis
Parasitic: ascariasis, ancylostomiasis, filariasis, strongylosis, trichinosis
Spirochetal: syphilis, Lyme borreliosis
Rheumatic Diseases
Systemic lupus erythematosus
Sjögren's syndrome
Polymyositis
Necrotizing angitis
Cryoglobulinemia
Juvenile chronic arthritis
Rheumatic fever
Endocrine Disorders
Hypothyroidism
Hyperthyroidism
Hyperparathyroidism
Neoplastic Disorders
Lymphoma
Leukemia
Carcinoma (lung, colorectal, ovarian, liver)
Miscellaneous
Pregnancy
Systemic mastocytosis
Urticarial vasculitis
Erythema multiforme

THERAPY

Treatment of urticaria starts with the identification and avoidance of the offending trigger. It is prudent to avoid aggravating factors such as excessive alcohol, overheated surroundings, physical exhaustion, and nonsteroidal anti-inflammatory agents (NSAIDs). Patients with chronic idiopathic urticaria should be educated about their illness and reassured. Medical therapy for amelioration of symptoms is usually required when the inciting cause cannot be identified, as is the case in most patients with chronic urticaria.

Antihistamines are effective in blocking the action of histamine on the target cells in causing vasodilatation and pruritus, but do not alter the course of the disease. Classic or first-generation agents include hydroxyzine (Atarax), diphenhydramine (Benadryl), chlorpheniramine (Chlor-Trimeton) and cyproheptadine (Periactin). These agents are effective but in usual doses may cause sedation, decrease work productivity, and interfere with learning as well as psychomotor performance. A number of oral second-generation H_1 antihistamines such as cetirizine (Zyrtec), 10 mg daily; loratidine (Claritin), 10 mg daily; fexofenadine (Allegra), 180 mg daily; and desloratadine (Clarinex), 5 mg daily are currently available. These agents penetrate poorly into the brain and are less likely to cause sedation or anticholinergic side effects. Fexofenadine is the least sedating even in higher-than-recommended doses.

Therapy should begin with the regular (*not as-needed*) administration of a safe and effective dose of an H_1-antihistaminic agent. Many patients will require a larger-than-recommended dose for amelioration of symptoms. The diurnal periodicity of symptoms in each patient should be kept in mind in prescribing a single daily dose. Combining antihistamines from different chemical groups and using a cocktail of a nonsedating agent in the morning with a sedating antihistamine in the evening (typically 25 to 50 mg of hydroxyzine) can improve efficacy and tolerance. Doxepin (Sinequan)[1], a tricyclic antihistamine, may be warranted in more severe cases. This agent has anxiolytic and antidepressant properties and can be used as a single nocturnal dose of 10 to 25 mg. When adding these agents, patients should be cautioned about the sedative effects and the need to avoid activities requiring a high level of alertness and fine motor skills.

Combination therapy with H_2 antihistamine, cimetidine (Tagamet)[1], 300 mg four times a day, ranitidine (Zantac)[1], 150 mg twice daily, or famotidine

[1]Not FDA approved for this indication.

(Pepcid)[1], 20 mg twice daily, has shown promise in several controlled studies and may be of value in patients whose urticaria is marked by flushing, dermographism, angioedema, or dyspepsia. The addition of an orally administered β-agonist (terbutaline [Brethine])[1], 2.5 to 5 mg four times daily, has been used with some success in patients with persistent urticaria and angioedema.

Systemic corticosteroids, in general, have limited utility in the management of chronic urticaria. A short course with rapid tapering over 1 week to 10 days (prednisone), 0.5 to 1 mg/kg, has been used in occasional patients when rapid control of a resistant episode is desired. Adding a leukotriene antagonist montelukast (Singulair)[1], 10 mg daily, is beneficial both in chronic urticaria as well as in patients in whom urticaria was triggered by the use of NSAIDs. Adding colchicine[1], 0.6 mg twice daily; dapsone[1], 50 to 150 mg daily; sulfasalazine (Azulfidine)[1]; and hydroxychloroquine (Plaquenil)[1] has been effective in selected patient populations.

Cyclosporine (Neoral)[1], intravenous gammaglobulin[1], and plasmapheresis are potential therapeutic options in patients with autoimmune urticaria, who generally tend to have a more refractory course. These therapies are best used in consultation with a specialist who is experienced in treating such cases.

Angioedema

Angioedema is the transient, episodic, bland, nonpruritic swelling of the soft tissues involving the skin and mucosal tissues in the upper airway or intestinal wall. This may coexist with urticaria and/or anaphylaxis where the etiologic agents are similar to the ones described for urticaria. When presenting independently, hereditary angioedema associated with deficiency of the plasma protease inhibitor, C1 inhibitor (C1INH), or a functional defect, or idiopathic cases should be considered. Use of angiotensin-converting enzyme (ACE) inhibitors (e.g., captopril [Capoten], enalapril [Vasotec], fosinopril [Monopril]) or, rarely, ACE-receptor blocking agents (e.g., losartan [Cozaar], valsartan [Diovan]) has been associated with angioedema.

Depending on the site of involvement, angioedema presentation may range from a large, disfiguring swelling of the loose skin to life-threatening swelling of the upper airway. Therapy of nonhereditary angioedema varies based on the severity. In mild cases with frequent recurrence, adequate doses of regularly administered antihistamines, as used in urticaria, may suffice. Elimination of suspected medications and foods is crucial to prevent recurrent episodes.

Moderate angioedema involving the oropharyngeal mucosa should be treated with Medihaler-Epi (4 to 8 puffs) or subcutaneous epinephrine (0.3 mL of 1:1000 solution). All severe cases with or without anaphylaxis should be hospitalized and receive epinephrine, 0.3 mL of 1:1000 solution, repeated every 15 to 20 minutes with a maximum of 1 mL. Intravenous antihistamines such as chlorpheniramine or diphenhydramine and corticosteroids (hydrocortisone 100 to 300 mg) are also given. Patients may require airway support including emergency tracheostomy, oxygen administration, and assisted ventilation. Individuals at risk of recurrent moderate to severe attacks should be educated in epinephrine (EpiPen) self-administration while awaiting emergency care. These patients should carry an identification bracelet and be advised against the use of β-blockers.

[1]Not FDA approved for this indication.

PIGMENTARY DISORDERS

METHOD OF
Robert A. Schwartz, MD, MPH

Cutaneous pigmentation protects man from harmful ultraviolet (UV) light radiation. It results from many factors, including carotenoids and hemoglobin, with the number, size, type, and distribution pattern of melanosomes being an important determinate. Melanin produced in epidermal melanocytes is the main pigment of concern here, although deposition of some medications or their metabolites produce discoloration. A correct diagnosis is mandatory. Pigmentary disorders represent a wide variety of diseases, including tinea versicolor, acanthosis nigricans, Addison's disease, melanoma, onchocerciasis, mycosis fungoides, tuberous sclerosis, and leprosy; the last is a reason for the social stigma of depigmentation in much of the world.

Superficial melanin tends to be seen as tan or brown, whereas deeper deposits often produce a gray or blue-gray hue caused by the Tyndall light scattering effect. Wood's lamp examination may aid in this distinction, separating epidermal melanin, which absorbs it, to appear darker than dermal melanosis, in which light scattering makes the patches less prominent. In general, epidermal melanosis is more amenable to therapy. Both types may be present. In addition, the Wood's lamp long wavelength UV black light examination may be valuable for hypopigmentation in separating total pigment loss from partial forms, detecting the yellowish-green fluorescence of some patches of tinea versicolor, and visualizing depigmented macules (ash leaf spots) in light-complexioned babies with tuberous sclerosis.

Patient education and realistic expectations are critical. All skin products should first be tested by limited application to normal skin that is not cosmetically sensitive and evaluated at 24 and 48 hours.

In addition, effective sunscreens or sunblocks should be employed whenever tretinoin, psoralens, or hydroquinone is used. Therapy for the disorders below is usually directed at improvement rather than cure. Thus, the results may be modest, are usually not permanent, and may require repeat courses of therapy. The risk of side effects needs to be stressed. Tretinoin and hydroquinone may produce irritant or allergic dermatitis, and, rarely, hydroquinone induces exogenous ochronosis, a permanent blue-black hyperpigmentation at the site of application after prolonged and extensive use. Some hydroquinone products contain sodium metabisulfite, a sulfite that can cause allergic reactions, which are sometimes life-threatening and which occur more frequently in asthmatics than nonasthmatics.

Hyperpigmentary Disorders

MELASMA

Clinical Findings

Melasma (chloasma) is a common cutaneous disorder characterized by patchy hyperpigmentation of the face, neck (occasionally), and forearms (rarely). There are three main patterns: centrofacial, malar, and mandibular. It occurs most commonly in women taking oral contraceptives or in those who are pregnant (i.e., *the mask of pregnancy*). It is rare in women with ovarian tumors. It can occur in adolescent girls, boys in puberty, men, and nonpregnant women. Hormonal and genetic factors are important; people of lineage from the Indian subcontinent, China, and Latin America have a propensity for melasma. It tends to darken on solar exposure and fade during winter without it. Hydantoin use may induce a similar eruption.

Treatment

In melasma, epidermal pigmentation, which is often tan in color and appears to darken upon Wood's lamp examination because of epidermal melanin absorption, tends to respond to hydroquinone; whereas bluish-grey dermal pigmentation is much less responsive. Tri-Luma cream (fluocinolone acetonide 0.01%, hydroquinone 4%, tretinoin 0.05%) is a good approach for 8 weeks; it must be used together with an appropriate sunscreen, ideally a sunblock such as Lydia O'Leary's Covermark. Tri-Luma should be used as an initial therapy for approximately 8 weeks. Longer treatment is cautioned due to possible side effects of the steroid component. Treatment can be continued with a hydroquinone (in the morning) and tretinoin (at bedtime) regimen. A combination of hydroquinone 4% cream that contains sunscreen (Solaquin Forte) applied twice daily and 0.1% tretinoin gel (Renova)[1] applied at night for 4 to 6 months may produce substantial lightening, but also can cause irritation, especially when first applied. A similar product is hydroquinone 4% and retinol (EpiQuin Micro), a high-technology effort that is worth trying. Another combination formulation is Alpha Quin HP (hydroquinone 4% cream with glycolic acids and sunscreens). Tretinoin[1] 0.1% cream alone can fade the spots somewhat, but treatment is often protracted. Applying tretinoin cream every other night for the first 2 to 3 weeks and then increasing the frequency of application to nightly can minimize the irritation. Azelaic acid (Azelex)[1] 20% cream applied twice daily with or without 0.1% tretinoin gel for 6 months may also bleach the patches. It can also be combined with hydroquinone 4% cream, with both agents applied twice daily.

It is critical that hormonal therapy, if in use, be discontinued and diligent sun avoidance be followed during therapy. Some hydroquinone products, such as Solaquin Forte, contain sunscreens. All patients with melasma should also use an additional sunscreen agent after treatment. The product should have a sun protection factor (SPF) of at least 15. Water-resistant products are preferred in those who exercise outdoors or sweat heavily (Table 1). If not otherwise contraindicated, oral vitamin C and E supplements may be slightly beneficial.

SOLAR LENTIGO

Clinical Findings

Solar lentigines (also called senile lentigines and liver spots) occur mostly in elderly (60 years of age and older), light-complexioned individuals of European and Oriental lineage, although they often also occur in younger people with marked solar exposure. They begin as tiny macules on the face, shoulders, or dorsal hands, expanding and coalescing into uniformly

[1]Not FDA approved for this indication.

TABLE 1 Sunscreens

Brand Name	Sunscreen Type	Characteristics
Ombrelle 30	Chemical sunscreen	Water-resistant, fragrance-free, wide spectrum of UV protection
Coppertone Sport	Chemical sunscreen	Waterproof, reduced eye stinging
Bull Frog QuikGel	Chemical sunscreen	Greaseless vehicle, waterproof
Olay Complete	Chemical sunscreen, physical blocker	Elegant vehicle, wide spectrum of UV protection
Durascreen 30	Combination chemical and physical sunscreen	Wide spectrum of UV protection, thicker vehicle

Abbreviation: UV = ultraviolet.

brown-colored patches, often with an irregular configuration. Solar lentigo has no malignant potential, but it takes clinical experience to distinguish it from lentigo maligna, an early melanoma.

Treatment

Tretinoin[1] 0.05% emollient cream (Renova) applied sparingly once daily may gradually work. Bleaching creams containing hydroquinone or azelaic acid[1] function slowly and incompletely in most cases. The addition of tretinoin cream may improve the results somewhat. Tri-Luma[1] cream (fluocinolone acetonide 0.01%, hydroquinone 4%, tretinoin 0.05%) is more effective, but must be used together with an appropriate broad-spectrum sunscreen of SPF 30 or higher. A combination of mequinol 2% and tretinoin 0.01% (Solage) has been FDA-approved for solar lentigines. It should not be used in women of childbearing potential, or if other potentially phototoxic oral or topical medications are being used. A comprehensive UV light avoidance plan must be employed. Another combination formulation is Alpha Quin HP (hydroquinone 4% cream with glycolic acids and sunscreens). Liquid nitrogen cryotherapy is effective using a superficial freeze (light pressure with dipped cotton swab for 5 to 7 seconds), but post-therapy hypopigmentation may occur. Mid-depth trichloroacetic acid or glycolic acid chemical peels can lighten or eradicate multiple lesions in a single sitting. The Nd-YAG laser, Q-switched ruby laser, or resurfacing CO_2 laser can also be effective.

DRUG-INDUCED HYPERPIGMENTATION

Clinical Findings

Many medications can produce abnormal skin, nail, and/or oral pigmentation as a result of either deposition of the drug or its metabolites or a drug-induced stimulation of epidermal melanogenesis (Table 2). Some require or are enhanced by UV light exposure. These color alterations range from tan to slate gray to blue-black. Drugs such as 5-fluorouracil (Adrucil), gold, silver, and amiodarone (Cordarone) produce preferential darkening in sun-exposed sites. Other medications such as zidovudine (Retrovir), bleomycin (Blenoxane), doxorubicin (Adriamycin), chloroquine (Aralen), and cyclophosphamide (Cytoxan) also cause pigmented bands in the nails. Minocycline (Minocin; Dynacin) may produce brown-gray discoloration in old acne scars, hyperpigmented patches on the anterior legs, and a generalized brown-gray discoloration.

Treatment and Prevention

In most instances, the dyspigmentation that appears with drugs slowly fades in months to years after use of the drug has been discontinued. However, certain medications such as gold and topical hydroquinone can be responsible for irreversible color changes. The use of sunscreens is encouraged in patients with photo-enhanced, drug-induced hyperpigmentation to minimize additional pigment production.

[1]Not FDA approved for this indication.

TABLE 2 Medication-Induced Pigmentary Abnormalities

Medication	Clinical Characteristics
Busulfan (Myleran)	Generalized increased skin color resembling Addison's disease
Doxorubicin (Adriamycin)	Pigmented nail bands and palmar creases
5-Fluorouracil	Increased pigment in sun-exposed sites
Minocycline (Minocin)	Gray pigment in old scars and/or on the legs or a generalized muddy color
Hydroxychloroquine (Plaquenil)	Brown or gray discoloration of the shins, trunk
Gold (Myochrysine)	Permanent blue-gray color in sun-exposed areas
Estrogen (Premarin)	Melasma
Amiodarone (Cordarone)	Gray discoloration in sun-exposed sites
Zidovudine (AZT) (Retrovir)	Nail pigmentation, diffuse Addison's like pigmentation
Levodopa plus carbidopa (Sinemet)	Diffuse hyperpigmentation

POSTINFLAMMATORY HYPERPIGMENTATION

Clinical Findings

Postinflammatory hyperpigmentation is probably the most common cause of altered skin coloration. This acquired excess of pigment represents the sequela of a variety of skin disorders, traumas, therapeutic interventions, infections, allergic reactions, mechanical injuries, burns, reactions to medications, phototoxic reactions, and inflammatory diseases. Whatever the cause, the underlying process must be effectively treated. The condition results in melanin being released into the dermis, where it is phagocytized by macrophages. The pigment may remain indefinitely and cause macular hyperpigmentation. Superficial melanin tends to be seen as tan or brown, whereas deeper deposits often produce a gray or blue-gray hue.

Treatment

One should attempt to effectively treat underlying skin disorders, avoiding the incited reaction, regardless of etiology. This includes manual manipulation when applicable. Topical tacrolimus[1] 0.03% ointment (Protopic) twice a day for 3 months is now my first choice, because it is also therapy for many of the underlying concerns. Patients should avoid cosmetics. Topical tretinoin[1] 0.1% gel may be effectively employed every other day for 2 weeks and continued

[1]Not FDA approved for this indication.

nightly as tolerated. If the pigment is superficial, the areas can be lightened somewhat with the agents noted earlier for melasma. These agents will not work well in deep dermal melanosis. A combination of hydroquinone 4% cream containing sunscreen (Solaquin Forte), applied twice daily, and 0.1% tretinoin gel (Retin-A)[1], applied at night for 4 to 6 months, can produce substantial lightening. Daily use of sunscreens with an SPF of 15 or greater is essential. Tri-Luma[1] cream (fluocinolone acetonide 0.01%, hydroquinone 4%, tretinoin 0.05%) is another option; it must be used together with an appropriate sunscreen. Another option is a hydroquinone 4% cream combined with hyaluronic acid, 10% glycolic acid, and the sunscreens avobenzone, oxybenzone, and octocrylene (Glyquin-XM). The combination can cause irritation when first used. Applying tretinoin cream every other night for the first 2 to 3 weeks and then increasing the frequency of application to a nightly treatment program can minimize the irritation. Tretinoin alone can fade the spots somewhat, but treatment is often protracted. Laser therapy is ineffective in most cases. Sunscreens are helpful to minimize increased pigmentation in sites that are already too dark.

Hyperpigmentary Disorders

VITILIGO

Clinical Findings

Milk white patches of idiopathic vitiligo affect approximately 1% to 2% of the general population worldwide without racial, sexual, or regional differences. However, they are more pronounced and easily visualized in darker complexioned people, with its visibility enhanced by a tendency of some patches to be surrounded by borders of hyperpigmentation. Because vitiliginous patches do not tan, UV light exposure also emphasizes them when adjacent skin tans normally. Vitiligo reflects total destruction of all melanocytes within the affected epidermis. The hair within vitiligo becomes white if hair bulb melanocytes are destroyed. Vitiligo is most often seen on the face, backs of the hands and wrists, the axillae, the umbilicus, and the genitalia. It tends to be especially prominent around body orifices—eyes, nostrils, mouth, nipples, umbilicus, and genitalia. It begins as small patches and enlarges peripherally with new lesions appearing occasionally. It may coalesce into large patches, or remain localized. Evolving lesions may be hypopigmented initially, especially in dark complexioned persons. Vitiligo may also appear on the arms, elbows, and knees at sites of trauma or sunburn (Koebner phenomenon). Striking, generalized vitiligo after dermatitis medicamentosa may also reflect this circumstance in a predisposed individual.

[1]Not FDA approved for this indication.

Nonsegmental vitiligo is about three times more common than segmental vitiligo; the latter is generally more common in children. Segmental vitiligo tends to have an early onset, spread rapidly into the involved dermatome, stabilize within 2 years, and persist throughout life. The initial involvement is usually solitary. The face is the most common site; trigeminal is the most common dermatome. Nonsegmental vitiligo typically has new patches appearing throughout life, and shows a persistent degree of symmetry in early as well as advanced lesions. Patients should also be evaluated for possible coexistent thyroid disease, as well for a wide range of other occasionally associated autoimmune disorders. Some consider the white halo surrounding the halo nevus and the halo melanoma to represent a type of vitiligo. Halo nevi are not unusual in adolescent girls using birth control pills.

Chemically induced vitiligo may be caused by industrial germicidal phenolic cleansers, rubbers, and plastics; if present, therapy must begin by terminating such exposure.

Treatment

There are multiple options, but no reliable therapy for vitiligo. Many products, such as Dermablend and Covermark, may be recommended for their cosmetic coverup effect, which may provide psychological benefit to the patient, even those who decline therapy after learning that vitiligo will not go away spontaneously and that medical therapy may not be effective. Topical dyes and self-tanning products, such as Vitadye stain, and sun-free tanning products containing dihydroxyacetone, such as Chromelin Complexion Blender, are also good. Regardless of the treatment used, sunscreen use, if it is not already incorporated into one of the above agents, is extremely important—skin with vitiligo is more likely to sunburn than skin with normal pigmentation, and, ultimately, more likely to develop skin cancer. Successful therapy is initially reflected by perifollicular repigmentation after approximately 3 months, which enlarges as melanocytes migrate laterally. Thus, if vitiligo is on the vermillion border of the lip, distal fingers, or penile shaft, or has white hair extruding from it, the patient should be advised that medical therapy will not be successful. In that case surgical repigmentation techniques would be necessary to stabilize vitiligo, although the Koebner phenomenon may limit this approach. Possible surgical techniques are thin-split section grafts or minigrafts of autologous skin or autologous cultured melanocytes into large vitiliginous dermabraded patches.

Topical tacrolimus[1] 0.03% ointment (Protopic) twice a day for 3 months is now my first choice, because cutaneous atrophy and telangiectasia are a risk with topical steroids. With a child having localized

[1]Not FDA approved for this indication.

vitiligo, my next approach is a topical steroid. In children under 10 years of age, hydrocortisone valerate 0.2% cream (Westcort) daily on the face or desonide 0.05% cream daily to the trunk or extremities may be beneficial. For facial and genital vitiligo, use 0.05% fluocinonide cream (Lidex). Elsewhere, clobetasol propionate cream (Temovate) has been employed in patients as young as 5 years of age, with the best results in facial lesions of dark complexioned patients, in whom progressive repigmentation continues after discontinuing therapy. Vitiligo may respond on the face, but rarely does so on hands, elbows, and knees. One can use this steroid for 3 to 4 months, evaluating monthly and stopping if there is evidence of cutaneous atrophy or telangiectasia.

Photochemotherapy for vitiligo is sometimes beneficial in the highly motivated, because responses are often partial and may take years. For localized vitiligo, the topical psoralen methoxsalen (Oxsoralen lotion 0.01) may be applied 30 minutes before UVA exposure and UV light in the A range (PUVA) are used, although blistering can be a problem. Widespread vitiligo requires oral methoxypsoralen, 0.6 mg/kg administered 90 minutes before UVA exposure. This can be done three times a week for 3 to 4 months before perifollicular spots become evident. I do not recommend phototherapy for children under 12 years of age. Vitiligo may respond on the face, but rarely does so on hands, elbows, and knees. Narrowband UVB by itself is another option, and is photochemotherapy using natural sunlight. Patients should be warned that phototherapy has hazards, including carcinogenicity.

If vitiligo involves more than 50% to 75% of the skin, a permanent depigmentation (chemical vitiligo) may be induced, in order to provide uniform coloration. Generalized permanent bleaching can be achieved with monobenzyl ether of hydroquinone 20% cream (Benoquin) twice a day for 6-12 months or longer for adults with generalized vitiligo. Hyperpigmentation from acquired ochronosis is a risk with this therapy, potentially exacerbating the cosmetic problem.

IDIOPATHIC GUTTATE HYPOMELANOSIS

Clinical Findings

Idiopathic guttate hypomelanosis is a common benign condition of unknown etiology in which asymptomatic oval or angular, 2- to 3-mm (or larger) white macules develop. They are persistent, most numerous on the anterior lower extremities, and tend to increase in incidence with age so that senior citizens may have hundreds of them.

Treatment

Therapy for idiopathic guttate hypomelanosis is usually unsatisfactory. Tretinoin[1] 0.1% gel used for 4 to 6 months may partially restore skin color in affected areas. Cryotherapy with liquid nitrogen may be tried, with a gentle, 5-second light freeze sometimes being beneficial. Intralesional triamcinolone[1], 3 mg/mL, may occasionally be beneficial.

[1]Not FDA approved for this indication.

PITYRIASIS ALBA

Clinical Findings

Pityriasis alba (PA) is a relatively common disorder of hypopigmented macules that appears most frequently on the faces of preadolescent children and, occasionally, young adults. It may be the presenting complaint or be an incidental finding. It is a benign, chiefly cosmetic defect that is more prominent in, and problematic for, dark-skinned individuals. The etiology of pityriasis alba is not known precisely, although it has been linked with atopy, and is thought by some to be a postinflammatory reaction in atopic dermatitis. It is usually evident as round-to-oval hypopigmented macules, 0.5 to 5 cm or more in diameter, with borders that are generally well defined but irregular. They are chiefly on the face (forehead and malar ridges), but occasionally are found on the shoulders, upper arms, or legs. They are often two or three in number, but this can vary from 1 to 20 or more. Some become confluent. Initially there is a pink patch with an elevated, slightly erythematous border, which may be slightly pruritic. After a few weeks the erythema fades, leaving a whitish macule, which may be covered with a fine, adherent scale. The late stage is a smooth hypopigmented macule. Repigmentation usually occurs in months to years. All three stages may occur simultaneously; all may be of one stage. The lesions are often most apparent in summer, because of tanning of the surrounding skin. On rare occasions mycosis fungoides may have hypopigmented macules resembling PA. Therefore, long-standing patches unresponsive to therapy may require biopsy.

Treatment

An emollient or bland lubricant, such as petrolatum, may be useful in masking scale; no therapy is overwhelmingly successful. Repigmentation can be sometimes accelerated by the use of a mild to medium strength nonfluorinated topical steroid such as hydrocortisone 1% cream or desonide 0.05% cream. Mild peeling agents may be used with or without these topical steroids. More potent steroids, such as triamcinolone acetonide 0.1% cream and hydrocortisone valerate 0.2% cream, are recommended for nonfacial lesions. Topical tretinoin[1] 0.1% gel applied every other evening may also be useful.

[1]Not FDA approved for this indication.

SUNBURN

METHOD OF

Heidi T. Jacobe, MD

Sunburn is the most conspicuous and common adverse cutaneous reaction to sunlight. Sunburn predominantly affects fair-skinned individuals, although it can occur in any skin type with enough exposure to sunlight. Characteristic clinical findings reflect inflammation in the skin and include erythema, warmth, tenderness, and swelling.

Pathogenesis

Sunburn is caused by ultraviolet radiation (UVR). Most human exposure to UVR is through sunlight. Tanning beds, arc welding apparatus, and unshielded fluorescent and tungsten-halogen lamps also emit UVR and can cause sunburn.

UVR comprises approximately 5% of the solar radiation that reaches the earth's surface. UVR is subdivided into three spectral groups (Figure 1):

1. Ultraviolet C (UVC), 200 to 290 nm
2. Ultraviolet B (UVB), 290 to 320 nm
3. Ultraviolet A (UVA), 320 to 400 nm

These divisions are based on the effect of different ultraviolet light groups on living systems. UVC is divided from UVB because wavelengths from the sun shorter than 290 nm are filtered by the ozone layer of the atmosphere and do not reach the earth's surface. UVC radiation is also called germicidal radiation because it is absorbed by DNA, RNA, and proteins; and it can be lethal to many cells including bacteria. Humans can be exposed to UVC light in the form of germicidal lamps used in industrial and health care settings. UVB radiation is also referred to as the sunburn spectrum because it is the primary cause of sunburn erythema. Approximately half of UVB radiation is absorbed by the stratospheric ozone layer, but depletion of ozone has produced measurable increases in the amount of UVB radiation reaching the earth's surface. UVB is also blocked by window glass. Transmission of UVB rays through the atmosphere fluctuates during the course of the day, with peak transmission occurring between 10 AM and 3 PM. UVA radiation is called black light because it is not visible to the human eye. UVA light is transmitted unfiltered through the atmosphere and window glass. Although UVA radiation is much less efficient at producing sunburn than UVB, large doses can produce a burn, particularly in fair or sun-sensitive individuals. UVA radiation is also linked to the development of melanoma and skin aging. This is of particular concern because tanning beds emit a large amount of UVA light.

Sunburn develops as a result of total dose of UVR and a number of host and environmental factors. The most obvious host factor is the amount of pigment present in the skin. Individuals with blond/red hair, fair skin, and blue eyes are more likely to extensively and severely burn than more darkly pigmented individuals at a given dose of UVR. In addition, sunburn reactions vary with age and anatomic site. The very young and old tend to burn at relatively lower doses of UVR, but have less intense, longer lasting responses. The face, neck, and trunk are more likely to burn than the extremities. Ingestion of photosensitizing medications (Table 1) can also significantly increase the likelihood of developing sunburn even with minimal exposure to UVR. Certain environmental factors also increase the likelihood of sunburn. Water, sand, and snow reflect sunlight, increasing the exposure to UVR. In addition, because water efficiently reflects UVR, clouds do not protect from sunburn. High altitude increases UV irradiation levels. Skin moistened by swimming, sweat, or high humidity is more likely to get burned because of increased transmission of UVR through the skin.

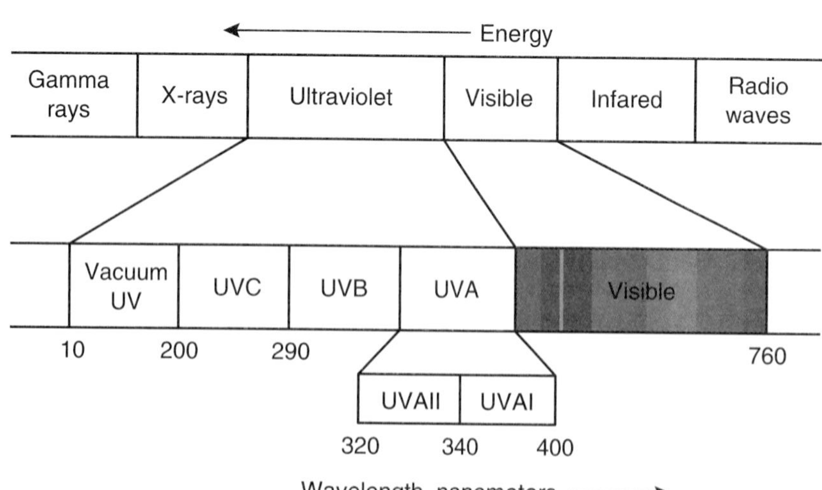

FIGURE 1 Electromagnetic spectrum.

TABLE 1 Systemic Phototoxic Agents

Property	Generic Name (U.S. Trade Name)	Property	Generic Name (U.S. Trade Name)
Antianxiety drugs	Alprazolam (Xanax) Chlordiazepoxide (Librium)	Diuretics	Furosemide (Lasix)* Thiazides Bendroflumethiazide (Naturetin) Chlorothiazide (Diuril*) Hydrochlorothiazide (HydroDIURIL*)
Anticancer drugs	Dacarbazine (DTIC-Dome) Fluorouracil (Efudex, Fluoroplex) Methotrexate (Folex) Vinblastine (Velban)	Dye	Fluorescein (Fluorescite) Methylene blue
Antidepressants	Tricyclics Desipramine (Norpramin) Imipramine (Tofranil)	Food additives	Sulfites
Antifungals	Griseofulvin (Fulvicin-U/F)	Furocoumarins	Psoralens 8-Methoxysalen (Oxsoralen)* Trioxsalen (Trisoralen)*
Antimalarials	Chloroquine (Aralen) Quinine (Quinamm)	Hypoglycemics	Sulfonylureas Acetohexamide (Dymelor) Chlorpropamide (Diabinese) Glyburide (Micronase) Tolazamide (Tolinase) Tolbutamide (Orinase)*
Antimicrobials	Quinolones Ciprofloxacin (Cipro) Enoxacin (Penetrex) Lomefloxacin (Maxaquin)* Nalidixic acid (NegGram)* Norfloxacin (Noroxin) Ofloxacin (Floxin) Sulfonamides Tetracyclines Demeclocycline (Declomycin)* Doxycycline (Vibramycin)* Minocycline (Minocin) Tetracycline (Achromycin)	Hypolipidemics	Fibric acid derivatives Bezafibrate[2] Clofibrate (Atomid-S) Fenofibrate
Antipsychotic drugs	Phenothiazines Chlorpromazine (Thorazine)* Perphenazine (Trilafon) Prochlorperazine (Compazine)* Thioridazine (Mellaril) Trifluoperazine (Stelazine)	NSAIDs	Piroxicam (Feldene) Propionic acid derivatives Ibuprofen (Motrin) Ketoprofen (Orudis) Naproxen (Naprosyn) Tiaprofenic acid†
Cardiac medications	Amiodarone (Cordarone)* Quinidine (Quinidex)	Photodynamic therapy agents	Hematoporphyrin derivative (Photofrin)* Hypericin*
		Retinoids	Isotretinoin (Accutane) Etretinate (Tegison)

[2]Not available in the United States.
*Commonly reported.
†Investigational drug in the United States.

These factors are important considerations not only in the pathogenesis of sunburn, but also when counseling patients regarding sun protection measures.

If UVR dose exceeds the native protective factors of the skin, sunburn occurs. The principal event in sunburn is damage to DNA in skin cells, called keratinocytes, by UVB and short UVA wavelengths. This is followed by inhibition of DNA, RNA, and protein synthesis. Local cutaneous immune responses are also suppressed. Later, DNA repair occurs and cells that cannot be salvaged become apoptotic and are sloughed off (peeling). The salvaged cells increase DNA, RNA, and protein synthesis and new cell formation occurs, peaking at 48 hours. Melanocytes increase pigment formation, eventually producing the hyperpigmentation that follows sunburn. DNA damage also induces the synthesis and release of inflammatory mediators into the skin, such as histamine and prostaglandins, producing the erythema and edema characteristic of sunburn.

Clinical Findings

The sunburn reaction has a characteristic time course. Overexposure to UVB and lower wavelength UVA light produces almost instantaneous erythema. This is replaced by a delayed erythema that starts within a few hours of exposure and peaks 6 to 24 hours later depending on the dose. The severity of the response varies from mild erythema to blister formation accompanied by severe pain. Affected areas are usually limited to sun-exposed sites with a sharp demarcation between sun-exposed and protected sites. The reaction usually begins to subside in 72 hours with the onset of desquamation (peeling) and hyperpigmentation (tanning). Pruritus is not uncommon during this phase.

Prevention and Treatment

The best treatment for sunburn is prevention. Exposure to the sun should be minimized between 10 AM and 3 PM. Use of a wide-brimmed hat protects the head and neck. The weave of the material for the hat should be tight enough that sunlight is not visible through it. Lightweight, cool, sun-protective clothing is also widely available. Umbrellas and canopies composed of sun-protective fabric are ideal for use in areas where other forms of shelter are unavailable.

Sunscreens are also useful for protecting exposed skin. The efficacy of sunscreen is defined by the sun protection factor (SPF). SPF is determined by the ratio of the amount of UVB radiation required to produce erythema in skin treated with 2 mg/cm^2 of sunscreen versus the amount of UVB radiation required to produce erythema in untreated skin. Theoretically, a sunscreen with an SPF of 15 prevents 95% of UVB radiation from reaching the skin, and a sunscreen with an SPF of 30 prevents 97% of UVB rays from reaching the skin. In reality, the SPF is usually much lower. This is because most people apply significantly less sunscreen than is used to determine the SPF. As a result, use of higher SPF sunscreens is beneficial because they are more likely to provide adequate protection. Everyone should wear sunscreen with a minimum SPF of 30 while outdoors. Sunscreen also needs to be reapplied every 2 hours while outdoors and every 1 hour if swimming or heavily perspiring. Sunscreen labels should be checked for both UVB and UVA protective ingredients (Table 2).

TABLE 2 Widely Available Ultraviolet A (UVA) Sunscreen Protective Ingredients

Chemical sunscreen
Benzophenones
Oxybenzone
Sulisobenzone
Dioxybenzone
Other chemicals
Methyl anthranilate
Butylmethoxydibenzoyl methane (avobenzone)
Physical sunblock
Titanium dioxide
Zinc oxide

Once overexposure to sunlight occurs, therapy is guided by the extent and severity of the burn. Very mild sunburns producing only minimal erythema and discomfort rarely require specific treatment. Moderate overexposure manifested by fairly intense erythema, edema, and tenderness can be treated with cool tap water compresses applied for 15 to 20 minutes followed by application of a medium potency topical steroid ointment such as triamcinolone (Aristocort) 0.1% ointment twice a day. Use of aspirin (300 to 600 mg every 4 to 6 hours) or a nonsteroidal anti-inflammatory drug such as ibuprofen (Motrin), 400 to 600 mg every 6 hours, is also helpful in reducing pain and inflammation. In the case of widespread involvement, the patient should soak in a lukewarm bath with oatmeal (Aveeno) for 15 to 20 minutes followed by the application of a medium potency topical steroid ointment immediately after emerging from the bath. Severe, widespread involvement, especially if it is accompanied by systemic symptoms, justifies the addition of oral corticosteroids. Oral prednisone starting at 40 to 60 mg a day and tapered over 7 to 10 days should be adequate. Severely sunburned patients frequently find that wearing clothing and going about their daily activities are exceedingly uncomfortable. If this is the case, a few days of bed rest with the use of soft, loose-fitting bedclothes or sheets is helpful. When desquamation begins, patients should be discouraged from indulging in the temptation to peel the skin off. The pruritus associated with desquamation can be minimized with frequent use of bland emollients like Eucerin, Cetaphil, or Aquaphor. The addition of hydroxyzine (Atarax), 25 to 50 mg orally every 4 to 6 hours, is also helpful.

SECTION 14

The Nervous System

ALZHEIMER'S DISEASE

METHOD OF

Jody Corey-Bloom, MD, PhD

Alzheimer's disease (AD) is the most frequent type of dementia in the United States and Europe, comprising approximately 50% to 80% of elderly subjects presenting with dementing disorders (Table 1). Currently, 4 million individuals in the United States are estimated to have AD, and that number is projected to increase to at least 14 million by the year 2050. AD is a major cause of disability and mortality, and its impact on health care costs, including direct and indirect medical and social service costs, is estimated to be greater than $100 billion per year.

Pathology

The brain of a patient with AD often shows marked atrophy, with widened sulci and shrinkage of the gyri. Microscopically, there is significant loss of neurons, in addition to shrinkage of large cortical neurons. Loss of synapses is believed to be the critical pathologic substrate. The neuropathologic hallmarks of AD are neuritic plaques (NP) and neurofibrillary tangles (NFT), although these lesions are by no means unique to AD and occur in a variety of other neurodegenerative disorders. Classic NP are spherical structures consisting of a central core of fibrous protein known as amyloid that is surrounded by degenerating nerve endings (neurites). NFT are found inside neurons and are composed of paired helical filaments of hyperphosphorylated microtubule-associated tau protein. NP and NFT are not distributed evenly across the brain in AD but are concentrated in vulnerable neural systems. Other pathologic alterations commonly seen in the brains of AD patients include neuropil threads, granulovacuolar degeneration, and amyloid angiopathy.

Pathologic criteria for the diagnosis of AD at autopsy require the demonstration of a sufficient number of NP and NFT on microscopic examination. The most consistent neurochemical change associated with AD has been the well-documented decline in cholinergic activity that has inspired many attempts to treat AD with cholinergic drugs. However, additional deficiencies in glutamate, norepinephrine, serotonin, somatostatin, and corticotropin-releasing factors have also been described.

Epidemiology

Our understanding of the epidemiology of AD has advanced rapidly during the past decade with the recognition of various demographic, genetic, and

TABLE 1 Common Causes of the Dementia Syndrome

Type of Dementia	Incidence
Alzheimer's disease (AD)	50%-80%
Lewy body dementia	20%
AD and vascular dementia (mixed dementia)	10%
Depression	5%-10%
Vascular dementia	5%
Metabolic disorders	<5%
Drug intoxication	<5%
Infections	<5%
Structural lesions	<5%
Dementia 2° to alcohol	<5%
Hydrocephalus	<5%
Parkinson's disease	<5%
Pick's and other frontal dementias	<1%

exposure-related risk factors for its development. Table 2 gives the most important clinical risk factors for the development of AD.

Age is clearly the major risk factor for AD; the overall prevalence of AD after the age of 65 years is approximately 10%. Overall prevalence is, however, much less meaningful than age-specific prevalence. From ages 65 to 85 years, the prevalence of AD doubles approximately every 5 years. Prevalence rises from approximately 2% in people 65 to 69 years of age, to 4% in those ages 70 to 74 years, 8% in those 75 to 79 years, 16% in those ages 80 to 85 years, and approximately 35% to 40% in those older than the age of 85 years.

In addition, genetic influences are important in AD, but their mechanism of action and whether they are operative in all cases of AD remain to be elucidated. In some cases, AD is inherited (familial AD) in an autosomal fashion with the gene linked to markers on three separate chromosomes (1, 14, and 21) (Table 3). Familial AD families are those with multiply affected individuals in which the disease segregates in a manner consistent with fully penetrant autosomal dominant inheritance. Disease onset is usually early in familial AD. Although these cases probably comprise less than 5% of all cases with AD, they have been a source for significant advances in our understanding of its molecular basis.

Recently, the importance of an individual's apolipoprotein E (APOE) gene status has received significant attention as an important genetic susceptibility risk factor for the development of the more

TABLE 2 Risk Factors for Alzheimer's Disease

Age*
Genetic influences*
Apolipoprotein E status*
Female gender
Lack of education
Head trauma
Myocardial infarction

*Highest risk factors.

TABLE 3 Alzheimer's Disease: Genetic Loci

Chromosome	Gene	% of AD	Age at Onset
21	APP	<1	45-60
14	PS-1	1-5	30-60
1	PS-2	<1	50-65
19	APOE	50-60	60+

Abbreviations: AD = Alzheimer's disease; APOE = apolipoprotein E; APP = amyloid precursor protein; PS-1 = presenillin-1; PS-2 = presenillin-2.

typical, or *sporadic*, AD. APOE is a protein involved in cholesterol transport with three possible alleles, ε2 (rare), ε3 (most frequent), and ε4. Individuals who are homozygous and carry two APOE ε4 alleles have an increased probability (>90%) of developing AD by age 85 and do so approximately 10 years earlier than individuals carrying the ε2 or ε3 allelic variants. The exact mechanism by which this occurs remains unsettled; however, because up to 50% of late-onset AD patients do not possess an ε4 allele, APOE genotyping for diagnostic purposes is currently not recommended.

Epidemiologic studies have shown a higher prevalence of family history of AD even in sporadic AD patients. A family history of AD in a first-degree relative increases the risk of developing dementia by approximately fourfold. Other demographic factors, including gender (women may be more susceptible to AD than men) and lack of education, have also emerged as putative risk factors for AD. Head trauma, either a single episode leading to unconsciousness or repeated head injuries as in the case of boxers, appears to be a risk factor for AD. Whether exposure to nonsteroidal anti-inflammatory drugs (NSAIDs) or estrogen *reduces* the risk of developing AD remains unclear.

Clinical Features

The diverse spectrum of symptoms of AD reflects dysfunction of widespread regions of the cerebral cortex. Symptoms begin insidiously and progression is generally gradual and inexorable with occasional pauses. Memory loss is the cardinal and commonly presenting complaint in AD. Initially the patient has difficulty recalling new information, such as names or details of conversations, while remote memories are relatively preserved. With progression, the memory loss worsens to include remote memory (Table 4). Language is frequently normal early in AD, although reduced conversational output may be noted. As dementia progresses, there may be more difficulty with naming and increased loss of fluency. Later, language becomes obviously nonfluent until, terminally, the patient may be reduced to a state of near mutism. Visuospatial impairment in AD results in symptoms such as misplacing objects or getting lost, difficulty with recognizing and drawing complex

TABLE 4 Common Clinical Features of Alzheimer's Disease by Stage

	Early	Intermediate	Late
COGNITIVE			
Memory	Poor recall of new information Remote memories relatively preserved	Remote memories affected	Untestable
Language	Dysnomia Mild loss of fluency	Nonfluent, paraphasias Poor comprehension Impaired repetition	Near mutism
Visuospatial	Misplacing objects Difficulty driving	Getting lost Difficulty copying figures	Untestable
BEHAVIORAL	Delusions Depression Insomnia	Delusions Depression Agitation Insomnia	Agitation Wandering
NEUROLOGIC	Abnormal face-hand test Agraphesthesia Frontal release signs	Abnormal face-hand test Agraphesthesia Frontal release signs	Muteness Incontinence Frontal release signs Rigidity Loss of gait ± myoclonus

figures, and impaired driving. Difficulty with calculation (affecting skills such as handling money), apraxia, and agnosia are further problems that develop in AD. Early in AD, deficits in problem solving, abstraction, reasoning, decision making, and judgment may become apparent, suggesting executive dysfunction as a result of involvement of the frontal lobes. Patients may have difficulty with organizing complex tasks such as a vacation trip, large family meal, or financial and other business deals. Impaired judgment may lead to unusual susceptibility to requests or solicitations and difficulty driving. On the other hand, social comportment and interpersonal skills are often strikingly preserved in AD, and may remain relatively intact long after memory and insight have been lost.

Behavioral or psychiatric symptoms occur frequently in AD. Although major depression is uncommon, depressive symptoms occur in as many as 50% of patients. Delusions are common in AD, although they are rarely as systematized as in schizophrenia. They often have a paranoid flavor, with fears of personal harm, theft of personal property, and marital infidelity. *Phantom boarder* delusions, in which the patient believes that unwelcome individuals are living in the home, and misidentification syndromes also occur. Commonly, television characters are believed real or patients fail to recognize their own reflection in a mirror. Hallucinations, primarily visual, are much less common than delusions, occurring in up to 20% of patients with AD. In addition to depression and psychotic symptoms, patients with AD show a wide range of behavioral abnormalities including agitation, wandering, sleep disturbances, and disinhibition. These often impose a significant burden on caregivers and may precipitate nursing home placement. In contrast to psychotic symptoms, behavioral disturbances are more clearly associated with the degree of dementia.

As neuronal degeneration progresses in AD, all of the above symptoms worsen, and eventually patients become uncommunicative and unable to care for themselves, walk, or maintain continence. They require total care, including feeding, and are often institutionalized. In end-stage AD, death usually results from the complications of being bed bound, such as aspiration pneumonia, urinary tract infections, sepsis, or pulmonary embolism. Although mean survival after symptom onset is highly variable, ranging from 2 to more than 16 years, an excess mortality has consistently been reported. Median duration of survival in most studies has ranged from 5.3 to 5.9 years.

Diagnostic Evaluation

Several criteria have been developed for the diagnosis of AD. The two most widely used are those of the:

1. Diagnostic and Statistical Manual of Mental Disorders, Fourth Edition (DSM-IV)
2. National Institute of Neurological and Communicative Disorders and Stroke and the Alzheimer's Disease and Related Disorders Association (NINCDS–ADRDA) joint task force of 1984

According to DSM-IV, primary degenerative dementia of the Alzheimer type requires an insidious onset, a generally progressive deteriorating course, and exclusion of all other specific causes of dementia. The more detailed NINCDS–ADRDA criteria classify AD into definite, probable, and possible levels of diagnostic certainty. Using NINCDS–ADRDA or other criteria with suitable laboratory and diagnostic studies, at least 85% to 90% accuracy in the clinical diagnosis of AD has been achieved.

No single element of the clinical picture is unique to AD; however, a skillfully taken history may reveal a change from a prior level of performance in several areas of intellectual function (e.g., difficulty recalling details of recent events, diminished attention, language difficulties, visuospatial problems, and impaired judgment). For most patients, an informant should substantiate this information. In taking a history, changes in functional abilities are helpful in confirming the presence of new impairment. Finally, the tempo of cognitive decline is extremely important in the evaluation of the patient with dementia. Acute or subacute onset of disability, a more rapid course, and/or episodic changes along the course suggest possibilities of dementia etiology other than AD.

Cognitive testing should be conducted according to the preference of the individual physician but should include assessment of attention, orientation, recent and remote memory, language, praxis, visuospatial abilities, calculations, and judgment. Brief mental status screening instruments that neurologists have found useful and that may enhance clinical judgment include the Mini-Mental State Examination (MMSE). It should be emphasized, however, that age, education, ethnicity, and language of the respondent can influence responses to mental status test items, and the clinician must make allowances for each of these in assessing patients with cognitive difficulties. Recommended *cut-points* are by no means definitive, and patients who are mildly demented may score in the *normal* range. Test scores do not, of themselves, make a diagnosis of dementia nor do they determine the etiology of the dementing illness. Although not a routine part of the clinical evaluation, neuropsychological testing may be helpful in specific instances, for example, in high-functioning individuals whose history and initial evaluation are borderline or suspicious, or in distinguishing depression from dementia.

The physical neurologic examination is often normal, especially early in AD. However, a thorough examination may reveal significant or lateralizing abnormalities, such as a visual field cut or hemiparesis that may suggest diagnoses other than AD. In intermediate or advanced stages of AD, patients often develop variable features, including extrapyramidal signs (rigidity and bradykinesia), nonspecific gait disturbances leading to an increased risk of falls, and myoclonus.

Currently, there is no laboratory test that can confirm AD during life or permit identification of individuals at risk for the disease. Several promising avenues—genotyping, imaging, other biomarkers—are actively being pursued, and it is hoped that one or several will emerge with the sensitivity and specificity necessary for a diagnostic test. Thus, the primary goal of laboratory testing at present is to exclude other etiologies of mental status impairment. Testing should be designed to systematically evaluate treatable disorders and should include the studies outlined in Table 5. Other tests, while not recommended as routine studies, may be helpful in certain circumstances.

TABLE 5 Laboratory Evaluation of Patients with Dementia

Routinely Obtained	When Clinically Indicated
Complete blood count	Erythrocyte sedimentation rate
Chemistry panel	Urinalysis
Thyroid function tests	Toxicology
Vitamin B_{12} level	Chest radiograph
Computed tomography/magnetic resonance imaging	Heavy metal screen
	Human immunodeficiency virus testing
	Syphilis serology
	Cerebrospinal fluid examination
	Electroencephalogram
	Positron emission tomography/single-photon emission computed tomography

Treatment

ALZHEIMER'S DISEASE–SPECIFIC THERAPIES

Although currently no treatment can either cure or permanently arrest AD, presently available AD-specific therapies are of two types:

1. Symptomatic approaches based on enhancement of neurotransmitter systems
2. Neuroprotective strategies using antioxidant compounds

The most successful cholinergic strategy to date comprises the class of compounds known as cholinesterase inhibitors (Table 6). These agents reduce the metabolism of acetylcholine, thereby prolonging its action at cholinergic synapses in the brain. The three cholinesterase inhibitors currently marketed for the treatment of mild to moderate AD are donepezil (Aricept), galantamine (Reminyl), and rivastigmine (Exelon). As a class, these agents have demonstrated measurable, albeit modest, effects on cognition, behavior, activities of daily living, and global measures of functioning versus placebo in clinical trials. Cholinergic treatment probably does not alter the progression of neurodegeneration in the brain; however, possible long-term benefits of cholinergic therapy may include delayed institutionalization, possible decreased mortality, and economic savings in the cost of patient care. The primary side effects associated with treatment are gastrointestinal (e.g., nausea, vomiting, diarrhea, anorexia, weight loss); not surprisingly, better tolerability is seen if dosing occurs on a full stomach. Insomnia, vivid dreams, and leg cramps are also side effects of treatment.

In the absence of head-to-head comparisons of the cholinesterase inhibitors, the main differences appear to be their side effect profiles, titration schedules, and dosing regimens. Donepezil is administered once daily,

TABLE 6 Features of Cholinesterase Inhibitors Currently Marketed for Alzheimer's Disease

Name (Trade Name)	Class	Selectivity	Time to Maximum Serum Concentration	Metabolism	Daily Dose
Donepezil (Aricept)	Piperidine	Acetylcholinesterase	3-5 h	CYP2D6 CYP3A4	5-10 mg
Galantamine (Reminyl)	Phenanthrene alkaloid	Acetylcholinesterase Allosteric nicotinic modulator	30-60 min	CYP2D6 CYP3A4	8-24 mg
Rivastigmine (Exelon)	Carbamate	Acetylcholinesterase Butyrylcholinesterase	30-120 min	Nonhepatic	3-12 mg

either at bedtime or, alternatively, in the morning if insomnia or nightmares should occur. The initial dose is 5 mg, and patients may be increased to 10 mg after 4 to 6 weeks. Both galantamine and rivastigmine require twice daily dosing, and should be slowly titrated to maximal dosing as tolerated. The recent American Academy of Neurology (AAN) practice parameter on the management of dementia concludes that cholinesterase inhibitors should be considered in patients with mild to moderate AD. This same parameter describes a potential benefit of neuroprotective agents such as alpha tocopherol (vitamin E)[1] and possibly selegiline (Eldepryl), because these compounds reduce functional loss and slow the progression to major milestones in AD. Furthermore, it notes that prospective data do not support the use of anti-inflammatory agents[1], prednisone[1], or estrogen[1] to treat AD.

Recently, the FDA approved an *N*-methyl-D-aspartate (NMDA) receptor antagonist, memantine (Namenda), for the treatment of moderate to severe AD. This compound was very well tolerated in clinical trials. It is recommended that dosing be initiated at 5 mg per day and increased in 5 mg increments to 10 mg twice daily (with a minimum interval of 1 week between dose increases).

ADJUNCTIVE THERAPIES FOR THE BEHAVIORAL SYMPTOMS OF ALZHEIMER'S DISEASE

Because behavioral disturbances impair patients' ability to function, increase their need for supervision, and often influence the decision to institutionalize them, their control is a priority in managing patients with AD. The principal treatable behavioral disturbances in AD are agitation, psychosis, depression, anxiety, and insomnia. Treating behavioral symptoms in AD is probably more of an art than a science. For virtually every group of symptoms, older and newer classes of medications are available, with proven efficacy in patients who are not demented and less clear results in those with AD. Until the appropriate trials are conducted in patients with AD, including comparative studies of different agents, it is recommended that clinicians choose a few medications, know their pharmacokinetic and half-life profiles in depth, and follow the general principles that apply to using any medication in older adult patients. For example, it is important to target therapy clearly by defining the most offending behaviors or symptoms. Precipitating causes of behavioral symptoms (e.g., physical illness or medication side effects) should be treated when present. Environmental modification and nonpharmacologic strategies should be employed whenever possible. For example, mild degrees of pacing or wandering can be channeled into physical activity by simplifying physical surroundings and providing an enclosed yard to walk in. Drugs should be initiated at very low doses and increased slowly, monitoring carefully for common and less-frequent side effects. As much as possible, dose schedules should be simplified with day-by-day pill dispensers, and caregivers should be enlisted to supervise medication compliance. Withdrawal of a drug that has produced symptomatic improvement should always be considered, especially if the targeted symptom is known to be stage-specific.

Treatment of depressive symptoms in AD commonly uses selective serotonin reuptake inhibitors, such as citalopram (Celexa), escitalopram (Lexapro), fluoxetine (Prozac), paroxetine (Paxil), or sertraline (Zoloft) (Table 7). Alternatively, tricyclic antidepressants with low anticholinergic side effects (such as desipramine [Norpramin] or nortriptyline [Aventyl HCL, Pamelor]) or the combined noradrenergic and serotonergic reuptake inhibitor venlafaxine (Effexor) can be tried.

Classes of agents used to treat agitation in AD include antipsychotics, mood-stabilizing anticonvulsants, trazodone (Desyrel)[1], and anxiolytics (Table 8). Although many consider antipsychotics a mainstay in managing agitation, others reserve their use for psychosis, because these agents may produce serious side effects, including parkinsonism, tardive dyskinesia, confusion, and falls. Parkinsonism and tardive dyskinesia may persist for weeks to months after cessation of antipsychotics and, for some, may never remit. Extrapyramidal side effects are more common with typical rather than with atypical antipsychotics, which appear to be better tolerated than traditional agents. Atypical antipsychotics are the treatment of choice for patients with psychotic symptoms. Sedation is the most common side effect reported in patients receiving these agents. The initial antipsychotic dose in AD

[1]Not FDA approved for this indication.

[1]Not FDA approved for this indication.

TABLE 7 Pharmacologic Treatment of Depression

Drug	Recommended Dosage	Potential Side Effects
SSRI		
Citalopram (Celexa)	10 to 40 mg/d	Nausea, insomnia, headache, tremor, restlessness, GI disturbances, sexual dysfunction; paroxetine is more anticholinergic than other SSRIs
Escitalopram (Lexapro)	10 to 20 mg/d	
Fluoxetine (Prozac)	10 to 40 mg/d	
Paroxetine (Paxil)	10 to 40 mg/d	
Sertraline (Zoloft)	25 to 100 mg/d	
Tricyclics		
Nortriptyline (Pamelor)	10 to 100 mg/d	Drowsiness, dizziness, dry mouth, tachycardia
Desipramine (Norpramin)	10 to 100 mg/d	
Other		
Venlafaxine (Effexor)	37.5 to 150 mg/d	Headache, nausea, anorexia

Abbreviations: GI = gastrointestinal; SSRI = selective serotonin reuptake inhibitor.

TABLE 8 Pharmacologic Treatment of Psychosis and Agitation

Drug	Recommended Dosage	Potential Side Effects
Neuroleptics		
Haloperidol (Haldol)[1]	0.5 to 3 mg/d	Parkinsonism
Atypical Neuroleptics		
Risperidone (Risperdal)[1]	0.25 to 3 mg/d	Orthostatic hypotension, nausea
Olanzapine (Zyprexa)[1]	2.5 to 10 mg/d	Weight gain, elevated liver tests
Quetiapine (Seroquel)[1]	12.5 to 200 mg/d	Sedation
Benzodiazepines		
Lorazepam (Ativan)[1]	0.5 to 2.0 mg/d	Lethargy, confusion, dependence, ataxia
Oxazepam (Serax)[1]	10 to 30 mg/d	

[1]Not FDA approved for this indication.

TABLE 9 Pharmacologic Treatment of Anxiety and Insomnia

Drug	Recommended Dosage	Potential Adverse Effects
Tricyclics		
Nortriptyline (Pamelor)[1]	10 to 75 mg qhs; 10 to 20 mg bid	Drowsiness, dizziness, dry mouth, tachycardia
Benzodiazepines		
Lorazepam (Ativan)	0.5 to 1 mg qhs	Lethargy, confusion, dependence, ataxia
Oxazepam (Serax)	10 to 20 mg qhs	
Other		
Trazodone (Desyrel)[1]	12.5 to 75 mg qhs	Orthostatic hypotension
Buspirone (BuSpar)	2.5 to 10 mg bid, tid	Dizziness, headache, insomnia

[1]Not FDA approved for this indication.
Abbreviations: bid = twice daily; qhs = at bedtime; tid = three times daily.

subjects should be low, approximately 25% of that used in young adults, and the total daily dose should be gradually increased as needed, titrating against side effects such as cognitive deterioration, low blood pressure, and parkinsonism.

Most patients with anxiety do not require pharmacologic treatment. For those requiring pharmacologic therapy, however, benzodiazepines should be avoided if at all possible, given their potential deleterious effects on cognition (Table 9). Nonbenzodiazepine anxiolytics such as buspirone (BuSpar) are preferred. For insomnia, it is worthwhile to try nonpharmacologic sleep hygiene measures, including sleep restriction and keeping patients awake during the day as an adjunct to pharmacologic management. If medications are necessary, sedating antidepressants such as trazodone (Desyrel)[1] may be effective choices for promoting sleep in AD, but anticholinergic hypnotics should be avoided.

[1]Not FDA approved for this indication.

INTRACEREBRAL HEMORRHAGE

METHOD OF

Geoffrey Eubank, MD

Stroke is the third leading cause of death in the United States. Ischemic strokes constitute 80% of strokes, and intracranial hemorrhage (ICH) accounts for roughly 15% of strokes (with subarachnoid hemorrhage making up the last 5%). Although ICHs are less common, they carry a larger burden of mortality, with only 38% surviving beyond 1 year. Only 10% to 15% of patients have little or no disability. Approximately 50,000 ICHs occur in the United States each year, and the number is expected to increase gradually because of a number of factors. As age is a significant risk factor, the aging population will contribute to this increase. Changing racial demographics may also play a role, as the condition is 1.4 to 2.0 times more frequent in black and Asian populations.

Nomenclature can be inconsistent in dealing with this subject. In this article, the focus is on spontaneous ICH, to include all hemorrhages not related to trauma or surgery. The term hemorrhagic stroke is avoided as it can refer to a primary intracerebral hemorrhage or to a cerebral infarct with secondary hemorrhage. For the latter, the term cerebral infarct with hemorrhagic conversion is preferred.

Risk Factors

Hypertension is the most important risk factor for stroke, occurring in 50% to 85% depending on the study. Perhaps 50% of patients with ICH have known hypertension, with another 25% thought to have unrecognized hypertension. This risk is further increased in patients who smoke, are 55 years old or younger, and are noncompliant with their medications. Conversely, those who have improved hypertension control have a reduced incidence of ICH, similar to what is seen in ischemic stroke.

Although alcohol in moderate amounts does not increase the risk of stroke in general, the risk for ICH does increase, especially with excessive alcohol use. Alcohol is thought to impair coagulation and perhaps affects cerebral vessel integrity. Another risk factor that is viewed differently for different stroke subtypes is serum cholesterol. Epidemiologic studies have not routinely shown an association between high serum cholesterol and stroke in general. This may be due to the fact that patients with low serum cholesterol tend to have a higher risk of bleeding, which would confound the association of increased serum cholesterol and supposed increased risk of ischemic stroke.

Clinical Features

Stroke is defined as a sudden change in neurologic function caused by an alteration in cerebral blood flow. Certain clinical features can distinguish between the various stroke subtypes as shown in Table 1.

Although Table 1 is not inviolable, it can provide a rapid bedside assessment to direct further history and investigations. Nausea, vomiting, and meningismus are more common in ICH than ischemic infarcts. Seizures are also more common in ICH, occurring in 13% of all cases and 30% to 39% of patients with lobar hemorrhages.

Focal neurologic symptoms depend on the location of the ICH. Hemorrhages usually occur when small penetrating arteries rupture into the brain parenchyma. Table 2 summarizes the relative frequency and common signs on the basis of location.

Secondary deterioration can occur in one quarter of patients. Patients with large hematomas and intraventricular extension of hemorrhage are especially susceptible to deterioration. This can occur within the first few hours (because of rebleeding) or within the first 1 to 2 days (because of edema). Hydrocephalus may occur because of a mass effect, tissue shifts, or obstruction from intraventricular blood.

Causes of Intracranial Hemorrhage

Hypertensive ICH, the most common type of ICH, is thought to be due to degenerative changes leading to rupture of small penetrating arteries or arterioles. The most common locations include the basal ganglia, thalamus, cerebellum, and pons. Lobar ICHs have more heterogeneous causes but are not uncommon with hypertension. Recurrence rate is approximately 2% per year, less with treatment of hypertension.

Cerebral amyloid angiopathy is thought to be due to deposition of β-amyloid in small and medium-sized arteries in the cerebral cortex and leptomeninges, which typically leads to lobar hemorrhages. These tend to be recurrent, up to 10% per year. No specific treatment is available to decrease recurrence. It is a condition primarily of elderly persons, typically 70 years old or older.

Arteriovenous malformations involve the rupture of abnormal small vessels and can occur in various locations. Younger patients without hypertension

TABLE 1 Rapid Stroke Triage Based on Presenting Symptoms

Condition	Headache	Focal Deficit	Decreased Level of Consciousness
Ischemic infarct	−	+	−
Intracerebral hemorrhage	+	+	+
Subarachnoid hemorrhage	+	−	+

TABLE 2 Signs and Symptoms of Intracranial Hemorrhage by Location, Listed in Order of Frequency

Basal Ganglia (40%)
Hemiparesis
Hemisensory loss
Ipsilateral gaze deviation
Dysarthria
Aphasia (left sided)
Neglect/anosognosia (especially right)
Lobar (30%)
Variable, depending on location
Hemisensory loss, hemiparesis, hemianopsia
Neglect, aphasia, dysarthria
Seizures
Cerebellum (15%)
Ataxia, truncal or limb
Nystagmus
Nausea, vomiting
Thalamus (10%)
Hemiparesis
Hemisensory loss
Aphasia
Eye movement abnormalities
Upgaze palsy, skew deviation, and so on
Brainstem (Pons) (5%)
Coma
Quadriparesis
Pinpoint pupils
Gaze palsy, intranuclear ophthalmoplegia
Ataxia

have this as the most common cause of ICH. Risk for recurrence is up to 18%. This can be decreased with surgical excision, embolization, radiosurgery, or a combination thereof. Cavernous malformations bleed because of rupture of capillary-like vessels and have a lower rebleeding rate of 4% to 5%. Depending on location, surgery and/or radiosurgery can be used for treatment. Venous angiomas rarely bleed and when they do the recurrence is less than 0.5%. Treatment is usually not necessary.

Cerebral venous thrombosis can cause ischemic infarcts (venous infarcts), which have a relatively high risk of hemorrhagic transformation. Despite this tendency, the usual treatment is anticoagulation and, in severe cases, transvenous thrombolysis. Anticoagulation is often continued in the presence of associated hemorrhage, although large hemorrhages obviously merit more caution.

Ischemic infarct with hemorrhagic transformation is not uncommon with larger lobar infarctions. Although it is not considered to be a true primary ICH, the appearance of hemorrhage can occasionally cause clinical deterioration or changes in management. This conversion can occur spontaneously with large infarcts. In fact, autopsy studies reveal a high rate of visible hemorrhage, from frank hematoma to petechial hemorrhage. The risk of hemorrhagic conversion is higher with the use of anticoagulants for stroke, especially when boluses are given. Given the lack of proven benefit and increased risk of hemorrhage, most recent reviews on the subject of heparin[1] discourage the routine use of heparin for the treatment of acute cerebral infarct.

Intracranial aneurysms occasionally arise with a prominent ICH but most often with a subarachnoid hemorrhage. This is rare with other causes of ICH. Rebleeding rate is 50% in 6 months, decreasing to about 3% per year. Treatment is accomplished by surgical clipping or endovascular coiling.

Intracranial neoplasms are an uncommon cause of ICH and tend to occur with hypervascular tumors. These can be primary (glioblastoma multiforme) or metastatic (e.g., melanoma, renal cell, bronchogenic).

Coagulopathy as a cause of ICH is usually a result of anticoagulant or thrombolytic therapy but rarely can be a result of hereditary conditions. The risk with anticoagulation increases with age, hypertension, and prior stroke. International Normalized Ratios significantly above normal ranges can also increase the risk. Thrombolytics can cause ICH when used for myocardial infarction (0.5% to 1%) or ischemic infarcts (6% to 7%). When ICH occurs in association with thrombolysis for stroke, it typically occurs in the area of infarct. Otherwise, the ICH tends to be lobar and can be multiple. ICH with thrombolytics (and patients overly anticoagulated) often has a peculiar layered appearance on computed tomography (CT) (hyperdense on the bottom and isodense on top).

Sympathomimetic drugs, such as cocaine, amphetamines, phenylpropanolamine[2], and pseudoephedrine (Sudafed), can precipitate ICH. These agents can cause an abrupt rise in blood pressure, which can overwhelm the cerebral vasculature's autoregulatory capacity. Angiography can show "beading" of vessels, although it is unclear whether this represents a vasculitic pattern versus a vasospastic pattern.

An uncommon cause of ICH is vasculitis. Ischemic infarcts may also occur. Serologic markers may or may not be present. Cerebrospinal fluid is usually abnormal (even without ICH), and angiography can show a beaded appearance. Brain biopsy is often necessary for confirmation. Treatment usually involves long-term immunosuppression.

Age can help determine the likelihood of the cause of ICH. Table 3 illustrates the more common etiologies by age.

Evaluation

A thorough history can help identify conditions associated with ICH (hypertension, malignancy), risk factors for coagulopathy, trauma, and so forth.

Laboratory evaluation should include a complete blood count with platelets, prothrombin time and

[1]Not FDA approved for this indication.
[2]Not available in the United States.

TABLE 3 Etiologies of Intracranial Hemorrhage by Age

Young	Middle Aged	Elderly
Vascular malformation Aneurysm Sympathomimetic agents	Hypertension Vascular malformation Aneurysm	Hypertension Amyloid angiopathy Coagulopathy Vascular malformation Tumor

partial thromboplastin time, erythrocyte sedimentation rate, and renal and hepatic tests. A toxicology screen should be considered, and various coagulation studies can be performed if there is concern regarding a coagulopathy.

Neuroimaging is typically done with CT scanning because of availability, speed, and ease of detection of most hemorrhages. Not only should size and location be considered, but also the presence of intraventricular blood and/or hydrocephalus should be noted. In proper hands, magnetic resonance imaging (MRI) is at least as sensitive as CT, but expertise in identifying blood or blood products at various points in time is mandatory. MRI may be able to identify vascular malformations, tumors, or evidence for old hemorrhage (which could indicate underlying amyloid angiopathy or possible previous hypertensive ICH). Cerebral angiography can help identify underlying arteriovenous malformations. In most cases of unexplained ICH (especially in those who are young and without hypertension), cerebral angiography should be performed. Also, regardless of age or hypertension history, the rare patient who has a primary intraventricular hemorrhage should undergo angiography because of the high rate of abnormalities found (>65%). Those least likely to have significant abnormalities on angiography are those who have all the following characteristics: older than age 45 years, have hypertension, and have an ICH that is not lobar in location (e.g., basal ganglia, thalamus). The timing of angiography depends on the patient's clinical condition and timing of possible surgery.

Management

INITIAL MANAGEMENT IN THE EMERGENCY ROOM OR INTENSIVE CARE UNIT

Initial management in the emergency room centers around initial stabilization of the patient, with attention to airway, breathing, and circulation. Although not every patient needs to be intubated, those who have a significantly decreased level of consciousness and those who have impaired protection of their airway (e.g., because of depressed reflexes) are candidates for intensive airway management. Intubation should be accomplished with short-acting agents (barbiturates, with or without lidocaine). Intubation helps to prevent secondary complications such as hypoxemia, hypercapnia, and aspiration. Ready access for hyperventilation, if needed, would be available.

Reversal of any known coagulopathies should occur as soon as possible. The offending agent (warfarin [Coumadin], heparin, antiplatelet agents, thombolytics) should be discontinued immediately upon diagnosis (or suspicion) of ICH. Depending on the condition, treatments with vitamin K, fresh frozen plasma, platelets, protamine sulfate, and cryoprecipitate may be indicated.

As the risk of deterioration is highest during the first 24 to 48 hours, patients should be monitored in a dedicated intensive care unit. Standard neurologic examination in addition to the Glasgow Coma Scale (GCS) should be performed frequently (e.g., hourly). Patients with a GCS less than 9 or with a clinical condition that is deteriorating because of increased intracranial pressure (ICP) are candidates for invasive ICP monitoring.

MANAGEMENT OF BLOOD PRESSURE

Hemodynamic instability is unusual in the early stages of ICH. The most common hemodynamic parameter deserving of attention is severe hypertension. The development is often due to the underlying etiology (hypertension), compounded by additional contribution of physiologic stress and increased ICP (Cushing's response). Of concern is that increased blood pressure (BP) could lead to expansion of the hemorrhage. On the other hand, patients with increased ICP can have decreased cerebral perfusion pressure, and lowering the mean arterial pressure (MAP) may have a deleterious effect. BP management remains somewhat controversial, although current recommendations suggest a goal of decreasing MAP in patients with values above 130 mm Hg while maintaining cerebral perfusion pressure above 60 mm Hg. Intravenous medications such as labetalol (Normodyne) can be used, although patients who have refractory elevations in BP may require continuous nitroprusside (Nitropress).

OTHER MEDICAL MANAGEMENT ISSUES

Fever should be treated aggressively as it can increase cerebral blood flow as a result of increased metabolic demands. Treatment options include acetaminophen, cooling blankets, and aggressive treatment of infection (empirical therapy for presumed source of infection, e.g., aspiration pneumonia, should be instituted as soon as suspected). Hyperglycemia should also be treated aggressively as evidence has shown that hyperglycemia can have a deleterious effect on patients with stroke. Fluid goals should be to maintain a euvolemic state. Electrolyte or acid-base status should be monitored and corrected to normal values. Agitation may lead to increases in ICP. Treatment with short-acting benzodiazepines or propofol (Diprivan) may be used. Premedicating with analgesics before painful procedures should be considered.

Pneumatic compression devices and subcutaneous heparin can decrease the risk of deep vein thrombosis and subsequent pulmonary embolism. Ulcer prophylaxis should be considered for the critically ill patient. When the patient is clinically stabilized, appropriate therapy (speech, physical, and occupational) should be instituted.

SEIZURE MANAGEMENT

Most seizures with ICH occur within the first 24 hours and are more common with lobar hemorrhages. Controversy exists in terms of prophylaxis, with some advocating prophylaxis with all ICH and others with lobar ICH. Because most seizures occur early, it is reasonable to treat with antiepileptics only if seizures occur. Phenytoin (Dilantin) (with loading doses of 20 mg/kg) is used and maintenance doses can be given to maintain adequate drug levels. Without recurrent seizures, most patients can discontinue phenytoin after 1 month. Late-onset seizures (after the first 2 weeks) often require long-term prophylaxis.

MANAGEMENT OF INCREASED INTRACRANIAL PRESSURE

A mass effect from the hematoma, surrounding edema, and hydrocephalus can all contribute to tissue shifts and increased ICP. ICP monitoring can help direct therapies. Head position is often at 30 degrees, although this can be adjusted to optimize ICP and cerebral perfusion pressure. For patients requiring additional therapy to lower ICP, mild hyperventilation and osmotherapy can be utilized. Ventilation settings can be adjusted with a goal partial pressure of carbon dioxide (PCO_2) of 30 to 35 mm Hg. Osmotherapy is typically accomplished with mannitol. If given urgently, a dose of 1 g/kg can be given, followed by 0.25 to 0.5 g/kg every 4 to 6 hours. Serum osmolality should be monitored and mannitol held if it rises above 315 mOsm/L. Close attention needs to be paid to keeping the patient in a euvolemic state. Limited data are available for high-dose barbiturates or hypothermia at this time to provide firm recommendations.

ROLE OF SURGICAL MANAGEMENT FOR INTRACRANIAL HEMORRHAGE

Surgical evacuation of ICH can decrease mass effect and help remove the neuropathic effects from the hematoma. This benefit can be outweighed by tissue damage caused by the surgical approach, especially for ICH involving the brainstem, thalamus, and basal ganglia. Furthermore, there is a potential for rebleeding when tissue and hematoma are removed (related to loss of local tamponade).

Surgical evacuation of cerebellar ICHs greater than 3 cm (especially those with neurologic compromise, brainstem compression, and obstructive hydrocephalus) should be strongly considered as soon as possible. Consideration for surgical evacuation should be given to younger patients with moderate to large lobar hemorrhages who deteriorate during observation. Stereotactic, endoscopic evacuation can remove hematoma with less tissue damage and holds promise to be more effective than medical therapy alone. Newer techniques, such as instilling local thrombolytics through an indwelling intracranial catheter, have shown benefit in reducing hematoma volume.

ICH remains a condition with high morbidity and mortality. Further studies need to be undertaken to see whether tissue injury can be reduced. The best approach to BP management and many other supportive medical treatments remains uncertain. Newer treatments, such as the neuroprotective drugs being studied now for ischemic stroke, if shown to be beneficial, should be evaluated. Results from trials of newer, less damaging surgical evacuation techniques and local thrombolysis or evacuation will be welcomed to see whether we can improve on the management of this devastating condition.

ISCHEMIC CEREBROVASCULAR DISEASE

METHOD OF

Kenneth Madden, MD, PhD

Ischemic stroke is the third leading cause of death in the United States and is the leading cause of morbidity. Medical care of stroke patients costs many billions of dollars per year, not to mention incalculable costs in patients' quality of life and lost productivity. Traditional care for those affected by stroke has been supportive only, with primary effort directed at rehabilitation of the impaired patient. Basic science research and recent clinical trials, however, have changed the way physicians should approach the stroke patient, with regard to both acute management and prevention of subsequent cerebral infarction.

There are four primary goals for management of the patient with acute stroke. Foremost among these is the need to treat the acute arterial occlusion. Regardless of whether this can be accomplished, identification of the underlying etiology of stroke is the second goal of the patient's physician, both to serve understanding of the condition and to direct specific cerebrovascular prophylaxis. Aggressive identification and modification of the afflicted patient's vascular risk factors are a third goal.

This allows physicians to minimize risk of a subsequent ischemic event involving cerebral, coronary, or systemic vasculature. Finally, physicians should direct early aggressive rehabilitation efforts in order to maximize recovery from stroke. This topic is addressed elsewhere in this text.

Acute Intervention for Stroke

In 1996, recombinant tissue plasminogen activator (rt-PA, Alteplase) was approved for the intravenous treatment of acute ischemic stroke within 3 hours of the onset of ischemic symptoms. Clinical trials have also suggested that thrombolytic medication delivered by the intra-arterial route[1] following symptom onset may also be effective up to 6 hours in improving perfusion to the ischemic cerebral tissue bed and in improving the patient's recovery from acute stroke. Use of these treatments, however, requires a rapid coordinated effort by a team of physicians competent in the neurologic assessment of presenting patients and radiographic interpretation of their cranial imaging. Intra-arterial therapy in particular requires involvement of highly specialized physicians and is probably feasible only in tertiary medical facilities.

An important aspect of each clinical encounter is physician judgment regarding who should and who should not receive consideration for thrombolytic therapy—judgment that should be tempered by careful consideration of clinical trial data. European and Australian clinical trials have demonstrated that alternative thrombolytics such as streptokinase[1] are overly hazardous for use in patients with acute cerebral ischemia. A major North American trial sponsored by the National Institute of Neurological Disorders and Stroke, however, has demonstrated that use of intravenous rt-PA can result in 30% increased likelihood of nearly complete neurologic recovery from stroke, although at the risk of intracranial or major systemic hemorrhage. Physicians must understand that this and subsequent trials have served to identify a subpopulation of patients with acute stroke in which the risk-benefit consideration for this type of therapy is favorable but that treatment of patients who do not mimic characteristics of this population may well be hazardous. In this regard, use of a protocol that identifies patients appropriate for thrombolytics (Table 1) and directs appropriate medication delivery is mandatory.

The most critical aspect of clinical trial data has been time to treatment from symptom onset. Multiple attempts to establish efficacy of intravenous rt-PA beyond the 3-hour time point have been unsuccessful. Secondary analyses of trials have, in fact, suggested a linear relationship between time to treatment and expectation of benefit, with efficacy lost shortly after 3 hours. These data compel treating physicians not only to observe the 3-hour limit but also to initiate therapy as soon as possible within the treatable time frame. For institutions capable of interventional techniques, intra-arterial thrombolytic use or mechanical clot ablation techniques are justified up to 6 hours following onset of ischemic stroke symptoms, although such treatment is still considered investigational.

TABLE 1 Protocol for Use of Recombinant Tissue Plasminogen Activator for Cerebral Ischemia

May consider rt-PA administration:
Ischemic stroke onset <3 h of drug administration
Measurable deficit on NIHSS
Computed tomography without hemorrhage or nonstroke cause of deficit
Age > 18 y
Contraindications for rt-PA:
Symptoms minor or rapidly improving
Seizure at onset of stroke
Suspected aortic dissection associated with stroke
Recent acute myocardial infarction
Suspected subacute bacterial endocarditis or vasculitis
Symptoms suggestive of subarachnoid hemorrhage
Another stroke, serious head trauma, or intracranial surgery within past 3 mo
Major surgery or serious trauma within 14 d
Known history of intracranial hemorrhage, AVM, or aneurysm
Gastrointestinal or urinary tract hemorrhage within 21 d
Arterial puncture at noncompressible site within 7 d
Lumbar puncture within 7 d
Received heparin within 48 h and has elevated PTT
PT >15 s or INR >1.7
Platelet count <100,000/mm^3
Sertum glucose <50 or >400 mg/dL
Sustained systolic blood pressure >185 mm Hg
Sustained diastolic blood pressure >110 mm Hg
Aggressive treatment necessary to lower blood pressure
Probable increased risk of intracranial hemorrhage:
Very large stroke with NIHSS score >22
Computed tomography shows evidence of large MCA territory infarction (sulcal effacement or blurring of gray-white junction in more than one third of MCA territory)

Abbreviations: AVM, arteriovenous malformation; INR, International Normalized Ratio; MCA, middle cerebral artery; NIHSS, National Institutes of Health Stroke Scale; PT, prothrombin time; PTT, partial thrompboplastin time; rt-PA, recombinant tissue plasminogen activator.

Blood pressure management has been a somewhat controversial aspect of thrombolytic protocols. Conventional wisdom in the management of stroke patients dictates that blood pressures be allowed to run well into the hypertensive range during the early phase of their medical care. Greater mean pressures are presumed to drive greater perfusion into ischemic cerebral tissue beds, which have lost autoregulatory capacity. Notably, the limits at which blood pressure elevations achieve maximal benefit before increasing risk for deleterious outcomes such as hemorrhage are unknown. This continues to be an area of clinical research in stroke. The established intravenous rt-PA protocol somewhat arbitrarily

[1]Not FDA approved for this indication.

directs maximum blood pressure limits of 185/110 as exclusion criteria for treatment. Although the appropriateness of these limits remains unproved, they continue as recommended guidelines for both selection of patients and maintenance during the initial time frame following lytic therapy.

Other methods of improving cerebral perfusion to ischemic tissue beds are less proved. For patients who have not received rt-PA, liberalization of blood pressure is recommended, usually by holding antihypertensive medication during the initial phase of hospitalization. Depending on an individual's prior history of hypertension, mean arterial pressures in the range 130 to 150 torr should be allowed. Local tissue edema with associated increased intracranial pressures often accompanies cerebral ischemia and can significantly impair cerebral perfusion. Unfortunately, treatment modalities for this type of cerebral edema are largely ineffective. Hyperventilation reduces intracranial pressures by inducing cerebral vasoconstriction and decreased perfusion, not particularly a desired goal in the setting of stroke. Steroids, although quite effective for the vasogenic edema associated with neoplasm, do not lessen the cytotoxic edema associated with ischemia and may have deleterious effects through induced hyperglycemia. Hyperosmotic agents, such as mannitol, may provide short-lasting benefit but tend to accumulate eventually within the ischemic tissue bed with deleterious consequences. Some authors advocate the use of colloids such as albumin[1] (which may also serve as a free radical scavenger) in combination with furosemide (Lasix) to sustain longer increases in vascular oncotic pressure. Dramatic benefit cannot be expected, however. For overwhelming cerebral edema, hemicraniectomy can be considered at capable institutions.

Supplementation of thrombolytic therapy with medications that may retard neuronal injury associated with ischemia has long been a goal of physicians caring for patients with stroke. Multiple clinical trials investigating potential neuroprotective drugs have been completed. Despite compelling results from tissue culture and animal work, no such agent has demonstrated benefit in the clinical arena. This is still an area of active clinical investigation. Worsening neuronal injury related to hyperthermia or hypoxia can be minimized by close attention to medical conditions such as pneumonia and venous thrombosis as well as through the aggressive use of antipyretics.

Laboratory Investigation of Stroke

The standard investigation into the underlying etiology of cerebral ischemia in individual patients includes cerebral imaging, echocardiography, carotid artery imaging, and interval recording of cardiac rhythm (Table 2). Computed tomography (CT) brain imaging remains the standard initial imaging study for acute cerebral ischemia, as it is a sensitive instrument for the exclusion of hemorrhagic pathology. Magnetic resonance imaging (MRI) is substantially more sensitive for early ischemic injury within brain parenchyma and offers multiple sequences for dating onset of ischemic injury, differentiating ischemia from other pathology, and assessing vessel patency. However, MRI is often less available, less tolerated by patients, and more expensive than CT.

Ultrasonography is the most popular modality for carotid artery assessment. This procedure provides estimates of flow limitations within the common or internal carotid arteries related to atherosclerotic vessel stenosis, as well as B-mode imaging. Elevated flow velocities indicate either increased blood volumes coursing through the insonated vessel or, more commonly, increased resistance to flow as a consequence of vessel narrowing. Rough estimates of the degree of stenosis can be based on peak systolic and end-diastolic flow velocities. Unfortunately, the reliability of carotid ultrasonography varies considerably from institution to institution, secondary to variance in equipment and experience of technician and/or interpreting physician. Decision-making for carotid endarterectomy or other intervention should therefore be based on imaging from vascular laboratories that have demonstrated a high correlation between carotid ultrasonography and the gold standard conventional contrast angiography or on more reliable confirmatory studies.

Magnetic resonance angiography (MRA) provides an alternative noninvasive assessment of the carotid artery and also provides useful information on the entire cranial arterial supply. MRA, however, may also suffer from limited reliability because of tendencies toward overestimation of degree of stenosis in flow-limiting states. Thus, MRA may accurately exclude significant carotid disease but may not have the sensitivity to address particularly relevant

TABLE 2 Laboratory Evaluation of Stroke

Standard Evaluation
Cranial imaging (CT or MRI)
Carotid imaging (ultrasonography, MRA, or contrast angiography)
Transthoracic echocardiography
Cardiac monitoring (in hospital telemetry, Holter monitoring, capture monitor)
Assessment of adequacy of control of vascular risk factors
Stroke in the Young (Additional Considerations)
Prothrombotic laboratory indicators
Transesophageal echocardiography
Toxicology screen (cocaine, amphetamines)
Vascular imaging sensitive for arterial dissection (MRA or contrast angiography)
Cerebral venous imaging (MR venography or contrast angiography)

Abbreviations: CT, computed tomography; MRA, magnetic resonance angiography; MRI, magnetic resonance imaging.

[1]Not FDA approved for this indication.

clinical questions (such as differentiating carotid occlusion from very high grade stenosis or differentiating severity of carotid stenosis best managed by surgical revascularization from that best treated with medical prophylaxis). Such questions may require consideration of contrast angiography despite the approximate 0.5% to 2% morbidity associated with this invasive procedure. Other indications for angiography include concern about vasculitis or other vasculopathies such as arterial dissection. Transcranial Doppler sonography also enables assessment of intracranial arterial blood flow. However, it is more valuable for quantification of vessel stenosis (such as the vasospasm associated with subarachnoid hemorrhage) than documentation of arterial occlusion causing stroke. Absence of flow may be related to limitations of the bony acoustic window instead of true occlusion.

Cardiac dysrhythmias such as atrial fibrillation pose a high risk for systemic and cerebral embolization. Such rhythm disturbances are not uncommonly intermittent. An interval period of cardiac monitoring may be necessary to detect such a condition. Further investigation into possible proximal source of embolism should include transthoracic echocardiography. This noninvasive modality is particularly sensitive for assessment of left ventricular dysfunction, a common cause of local thrombosis and eventual embolization in the aging population. Emboli related to atrial pathology are more common in younger patients with stroke, an occurrence that should prompt the use of a transesophageal method of echocardiography instead.

Stroke in the young often results from mechanisms quite different from those afflicting the aging population and requires investigation into such etiologies as arterial dissection, vasculitis, and prothrombotic state. Laboratory testing for the latter include assays for antiphospholipid antibody, lupus anticoagulant, prothrombotic gene, factor V Leiden, protein C, protein S, homocysteine, and antithrombin III.

Secondary Prevention of Stroke

Active measures to prevent recurrent cerebral thrombotic events should begin with initial contact with the patient. When hemorrhagic pathology has been excluded by imaging, antiplatelet or anticoagulant therapy can be initiated. The value of heparin in the setting of acute stroke has long been debated. Heparin has no thrombolytic activity and cannot affect the primary underlying arterial occlusion. Theoretically, its use may have value in preventing extension of the thrombotic process or preventing recurrent embolization. Clinical trials of acute anticoagulation for stroke do not support the use of heparin as a standard therapy. There may be some benefit, especially for patients with underlying pathologies such as high-grade carotid stenosis, arterial dissection, prothrombotic state, or cardiac embolization. The benefit of sustained anticoagulation, however, is countered by the accumulating incidence of hemorrhage. If heparin[1] is used, therefore, conservative degrees of anticoagulation should be targeted (i.e., activated partial thromboplastin time approximately 1.5 × control), and it should be discontinued immediately after laboratory evaluation excludes the presence of conditions that argue for long-term anticoagulation or immediate carotid endarterectomy. Systemic thrombotic events are also a concern, and pneumatic stockings or other techniques should be utilized to prevent deep venous thrombosis.

The relative merits of carotid endarterectomy have also long been debated as a means of stroke prevention. Clinical trial data have provided justification for endarterectomy by experienced surgeons with demonstrable low surgical morbidity, depending on the severity of stenosis and the symptomatic nature (Table 3). Major reduction in recurrent stroke risk is accomplished by endarterectomy when symptomatic patients have greater than 70% ipsilateral carotid stenosis. Modest surgical benefit can be achieved if symptomatic patients have between 50% and 70% ipsilateral stenosis or if 60% stenosis is identified in an asymptomatic patient. The safety and efficacy of carotid angioplasty with stenting are currently under investigation as an alternative to endarterectomy.

All patients who have suffered a cerebral ischemic event should be considered for a specific vascular prophylactic agent. Aspirin has traditionally been the most widely used drug, and its benefit has now

[1]Not FDA approved for this indication.

TABLE 3 Clinical Trials of Carotid Endarterectomy versus Medical Management

Trial	Stenosis (%)	Stroke Incidence: Surgery (%)	Stroke Incidence: Medical (%)
Symptomatic Trial			
NASCET	70-99	9	26 (2 y)
	50-69	15.7	22.2 (5 y)
	<50	14.9	18.7 (5 y)
ECST	70-99	1.1	8.4 (3 y)
	50-69	10.1	10.5 (3 y)
	30-49	9.8	6.9 (3 y)
	<30	2.7	1.3 (3 y)
VA	>50	7.7	19.4 (1 y)
Asymptomatic Trials			
ACAS	>60	4	6.2 (2 y)
VA	>50	4.7	9.4 (4 y)

Abbreviations: ACAS, Asymptomatic Carotid Atherosclerosis Study; ECST, European Carotid Surgery Trial; NASCET,North American Symptomatic Carotid Endarterectomy Trial; VA, Veterans Affairs Cooperative Study.

been established for both coronary and cerebrovascular disease. Although optimal dosing has not been established, doses of 75 to 325 mg daily are most commonly recommended. Ticlopidine (Ticlid), 250 mg twice daily, is superior to aspirin for stroke prevention, although concerns about hematologic side effects have limited its use. Clopidogrel (Plavix), 75 mg daily, is similar in efficacy to aspirin for cerebrovascular disease but has greater benefit for coronary and peripheral arterial disease. Combined use of drugs with different mechanisms of platelet inhibition provides greater benefit in the prevention of subsequent vascular events. Extended-release dipyridamole-aspirin (Aggrenox), 200/25 mg twice daily, is substantially more effective in preventing recurrent stroke than aspirin alone. Aspirin combined with clopidogrel similarly improves cardiovascular prophylaxis, although its efficacy for cerebrovascular disease remains in clinical trial.

Warfarin (Coumadin) provides no more benefit than aspirin for patients without high risk factors for cardiac embolism but provides dramatically greater benefit if these risk factors are present. Most notably, the high risk of subsequent stroke in patients who have atrial fibrillation is reduced by over 60% using warfarin compared with minimal reduction by aspirin. Similar disparity of benefit may be presumed in patients with other embolism-prone cardiac pathology such as ischemic cardiomyopathy. Warfarin is also recommended for patients in whom a prothrombotic etiology of an ischemic event is suspected. Temporary anticoagulation, with conversion to antiplatelet prophylaxis at 3 to 6 months after the event, is recommended for patients who have had symptomatic arterial dissections.

The most neglected means for lowering the risk of subsequent cerebral infarction is the optimal control of medical conditions such as hypertension, diabetes mellitus, and hyperlipidemia. Aggressive use of angiotensin-converting enzyme inhibitor antihypertensives or statin-type lipid-lowering agents reduces the risk of recurrent vascular events as much as or perhaps more than the use of specific vascular prophylactic drugs. At the minimum, such drugs should be used to target normotension and acceptable lipid profiles and may be considered regardless of blood pressure or lipid status.

REHABILITATION OF THE STROKE PATIENT

METHOD OF

Barbara J. Browne, MD

Every minute in the United States someone experiences a stroke. Four out of five American families' lives will be touched by stroke in some way. Of the 700,000 new stroke survivors per year, 450,000 will be left with a permanent disability. One third of all stroke survivors have another stroke within 5 years. Stroke is the leading cause of adult disability in the United States. Hemiparesis is the most common manifestation. The initial level of stroke severity affects the level and time course of recovery. Most survivors experience some degree of recovery in strength, including those presenting with dense hemiplegia. Of those who survive, 10% experience full or nearly full spontaneous recovery. Another 10% fail to benefit from rehabilitative attempts. The remaining 80% have neurologic impairments that will benefit from rehabilitative intervention. More than 50% of survivors will struggle with chronic impairments in walking and performing basic self-care activities.

The greatest rate of stroke recovery occurs in the first 90 days, but a more protracted recovery may continue for 6 months or longer. The Copenhagen Stroke Study prospectively studied nearly 2000 acute stroke patients. Results demonstrate that 80% of survivors reach their best functional recovery in 6 weeks and 95% in 12 weeks. Patients and families need knowledge of the expected amount and time course of recovery for rational planning of long-term care.

Medical Complications

Survivors of ischemic stroke have a 35% to 65% prevalence of significant coronary artery disease (CAD). Heart disease is the third leading cause of death in the first month following stroke and the leading cause of death among long-term survivors. Uncontrolled hypertension (HTN) is a major modifiable risk factor but should not be quickly lowered immediately following stroke. Initially, blood pressure should be slowly lowered to approximately 180/100 with pre-existing HTN, or 160/95 without pre-existing HTN. Subsequently, blood pressure should be lowered gradually. Precautions for maximal heart rate should be determined individually based on the degree of CAD and age. Patients with congestive heart failure better tolerate exercise in an upright position and should be monitored for a hypotensive response to exercise, which may be a warning of further left ventricular failure.

Given the association between diabetes mellitus (DM), HTN, hyperlipidemia, and CAD; it is not surprising that many stroke survivors also have DM. Frequent adjustment of medications are required because of changes in feeding regimens and activity levels. Lower doses of hypoglycemic agents are commonly needed because of altered diets and intake. Self-administration of insulin is an important goal requiring an interdisciplinary approach. Specialized training to perform one-hand injection techniques can be successful.

Immobility can predispose to decubitus ulcer formation. The most common sites are the sacrum, ischial tuberosities, heels, and posterior scalp. Proper positioning, frequent rotation (every 2 hours in bed), and timely weight shifts in the wheelchair can help prevent breakdown. Minimizing incontinence, maximizing nutrition, controlling spasticity, and using proper transfer techniques are further important adjuncts.

Contractures, or loss of passive joint range of motion, can follow stroke. Important factors include prolonged immobility, paralysis, and muscle imbalance caused by spasticity. The ankles, shoulders, and elbows are most commonly involved; but the hips, knees, wrists, and fingers are certainly at risk too. Preventive measures include proper positioning, daily range of motion, stretching, and the use of orthotic devices. In bed, resting night splints can prevent plantar flexion contractures. Serial casting can reverse a plantar flexion contracture, and the bivalved cast can be used as a splint. Extra caution must be used to avoid skin injury in patients with DM and peripheral vascular disease. Excessive shoulder adduction can be limited by use of pillows to partially abduct the shoulder. Proper wheelchair modifications can prevent kyphosis of the thoracic spine, allow proper lumbar lordosis, and facilitate proper positioning of the shoulder and legs.

Impaired swallowing commonly occurs following stroke, and the resulting aspiration into the lungs can cause pneumonia. Aspiration is most common in brainstem and large-vessel strokes. Aspiration pneumonia is the most common cause of non-neurologic death in the first month following a stroke. All acute stroke patients should initially have nothing by mouth (NPO) until screened for potential risk. Special precautions should also be used for any patient with an impaired level of alertness. Early bedside evaluation can greatly reduce the incidence of aspiration pneumonia. Bedside predictors of aspiration include cough after swallow, wet vocal quality, dysphonia, dysarthria, abnormal gag reflex, lethargy, and inability to follow commands. Up to 60% of stroke patients aspirate silently and require videofluoroscopic study. Videofluoroscopic swallowing studies have identified rates of aspiration as high as 70%. A combination of bedside evaluation and videofluoroscopic study can identify 90% of patients with dysphagia and aspiration. Factors that increase the risk of pneumonia in the context of dysphagia and aspiration include nasogastric feeding, tracheostomy, lethargy, vomiting, and reflux. Stroke patients believed to be at high risk for aspiration should use enteral feedings. Placement of a gastrostomy or jejunostomy tube is done if long-term enteral feeding is anticipated.

Compensatory strategies for dysphagia include chin-tuck with turning the head to the paretic side, upright feeding position, and tactile thermal stimulation to stimulate the swallow reflex. Diet modifications include thickened liquids and pureed solids with progression to soft solids and thinner liquids. Many stroke patients benefit from a quiet, nondistracting dining location that allows quiet observation and assistance. Dehydration and malnutrition can result from use of unpalatable, thickened liquids and lack of feeding assistance. Daily assessment of intake and hydration status should be done to identify patients with poor intake who need supplemental intravenous hydration. Fortunately, most dysphagia patients do eventually recover their ability to safely swallow. The majority of patients who require gastrostomy tubes are relieved of them upon completion of an inpatient dysphagia program.

The risk of thrombophlebitis may be as high as 70% in unprotected stroke patients. At greatest risk are older patients with large strokes, hemorrhagic strokes, severe immobility, infection, prolonged hospitalization, recent surgery, and prior history of deep vein thrombosis. Patients who are walking 100 feet daily are at low risk for developing a venous thrombosis. All other patients should be considered for prophylaxis.

Unfractionated heparin (UH), 5000 units twice a day, produces only a 21% absolute risk reduction for thrombophlebitis. Doses of UH at 5000 units three times a day provide superior protection. Low-molecular-weight heparin (LMWH) may be superior to UH because of superior bioavailability, although it is a more expensive option. An added advantage of LMWH is once daily dosing. Examples include enoxaparin (Lovenox), 40 units once daily, or dalteparin (Fragmin), 5000 units once daily. The addition of antiembolic thromboembolic disease (TED) stockings and pneumatic compression devices may confer additional protection, as well as limit lower limb dependent edema. The safety of UH or LMWH following intracranial hemorrhage has not been well studied. Their use in hypertensive hemorrhage, in which the blood pressure is stable and the cerebral hematoma has been unchanged for 1 week, appears safe. Additionally, low-dose heparin can be used after cerebral aneurysm clipping if the neurologic exam has been stable for 48 hours. Alternatives for patients who cannot be given anticoagulants are intermittent pneumatic compression stockings (IPCSs). IPCSs are most effective when used around the clock, but can be effective when used for 12 hours nightly. They are even more effective when paired with LMWH at prophylactic doses.

Urinary dysfunction (e.g., retention, incontinence, infection) is commonly seen following stroke.

Reports of retention vary from 47% in the first 72 hours to 21% at 3 weeks following a stroke. The neurophysiologic explanation for poststroke detrusor or alexia is unknown, but there is a higher incidence in those with aphasia, cognitive impairment, and lower functional status. Diabetic stroke patients with neuropathy also have higher rates of retention, possibly because of diabetes-related detrusor paresis. Although poststroke urinary retention is generally a transient phenomenon, failure to recognize it can result in damage to the detrusor muscle from over distention. Retention also predisposes the patient to urinary tract infection (UTI). UTI is the most common type of poststroke infection, although it most commonly arises in association with the use of indwelling catheters. Poor mobility, impaired cognition, lethargy, confusion, and impaired bladder function all contribute to incontinence. Indwelling catheters are often needed in the acute poststroke setting to monitor intake and output, and to prevent the negative effects of incontinence. These include poor hygiene, skin injury, poor self-esteem, and added risk of falling from attempts to use the toilet when safe ambulatory skills are not yet established. Removal of the indwelling catheter should be attempted as early as possible to limit the risk of infection; but must be weighed against the risks of incontinence and falls if the patient is unable to perform a safe transfer onto a toilet, use a bedside urinal or call and wait for nursing assistance. Once the catheter is removed, a postvoid residual should be checked to verify adequate emptying. This is easily done using a bedside bladder ultrasound device. When residuals are elevated, bladder scans may have to be monitored every 6 hours with catheterization if indicated. Resolution of retention can be facilitated by avoidance of medications with anticholinergic side effects, voiding in the sitting or standing position, and treatment of UTI, if present. α-Receptor antagonists such as tamsulosin (Flomax), terazosin (Hytrin), or doxazosin (Cardura) may be helpful with underlying outlet obstruction from prostate hypertrophy or in cases of suspected detrusor sphincter dyssynergia[1]. Urodynamic studies with an electromyogram (EMG) recording from the urethral sphincter may provide diagnostic clarification.

Urinary incontinence can be a burden to both the patient and caregiver. Uncontrolled incontinence can be a major factor in institutionalizing a patient for long-term care instead of providing care at home. The pattern of incontinence is that of an *uninhibited neurogenic bladder* in which the desire to void is closely coupled with a detrusor contraction, resulting in incontinence. This can be treated in most cases with a schedule of *time voiding* in which the patient is asked to empty the bladder every 2 to 3 hours during the day and before bedtime. Additionally, judicious use of fluids and avoidance of caffeine and diuretics, when possible, can be very helpful. Anticholinergic medications such as oxybutynin (Ditropan) and tolterodine (Detrol) can increase bladder capacity and reduce the frequency of voiding. Their use can be limited by side effects of dry mouth and sedation. Care must be used if there is a history of glaucoma. An effective combination is oxybutynin, 5 mg at bedtime, with time voiding during the daytime.

[1]Above drugs not FDA approved for this indication.

Management of Spasticity

Spasticity is an expected complication of stroke given the upper motor location of the injury. Spasticity is defined as a velocity dependent resistance to passive range of motion. Typical spasticity patterns in the upper limb involve shoulder adduction with internal rotation and elbow, wrist, and finger flexion. The lower limb develops excessive flexion or extension at the knee, and plantar flexion at the ankle and toes. Involved limbs tend to be flaccid in the initial days following stroke onset. The return of reflexes followed by progressive increased tone can occur over days to weeks. The degree of tone is highly variable as is the point at which it plateaus or resolves. Moderate spasticity can provide greater stability with standing secondary to extensor tone in the lower limb. However, spasticity can impair gait, dressing skills, and hygiene of the hand, axilla, and perineal areas. Additionally, spasticity may cause pain, result in limb contracture, and mask volitional motor recovery.

Several options have emerged as safe and effective treatments for poststroke spasticity. The simplest but least effective agents are oral medications. Tizanidine (Zanaflex) is an α_2 receptor agonist that reduces spasticity by blocking the presynaptic release of excitatory neurotransmitters and facilitating inhibitory neurotransmitters. Its use is limited by its common side effects of sedation, dry mouth, and dizziness. Elevated liver enzymes have been reported and should be monitored periodically. Tolerance is best achieved by starting with low doses of 2 to 4 mg at night and slowly titrating by 2 mg every few days. Doses lower than the recommended 8 mg three times a day and nighttime doses alone are often effective.

Oral baclofen (Lioresal) and diazepam (Valium) are less effective with poststroke spasticity than they are with spinal cord spasticity and often cause unacceptable levels of sedation and confusion.

Dantrolene sodium (Dantrium) is an effective oral treatment that targets the sarcoplasmic reticulum of skeletal muscle. A touted advantage is preservation of cognitive function. Drowsiness and dizziness may occur, although their effect is usually transient. Unacceptable generalized weakness can limit its usefulness. Both fatal and nonfatal hepatitis has been reported at various doses, and the drug should not be given with active hepatic disease. Appropriate titration to the lowest effective dose and monitoring of liver function is needed. Dosing can be started at 25 mg per day and titrated by 25 mg three times a day (tid) up to 100 mg tid if needed.

Stroke patients with focal spasticity can be greatly helped by local muscle injections of botulinum toxin A (BTA) (Botox)[1], which block the release of acetylcholine from the nerve terminal causing a chemical denervation. BTA injections are short-term therapy with reversible effects. BTA requires 14 days to reach a peak effect with duration of 2 to 4 months. Flulike symptoms are the most frequent side effect. Injections should be given no more frequently than every 12 weeks to avoid development of resistance. A more permanent effect can be achieved with the chemoneurolytic agent phenol. Care must be used as phenol-induced neurolysis of mixed nerves, containing both motor and sensory branches, may cause permanent dysesthesia. Phenol is best suited for large muscles such as the hip adductors and extensors, the pectorals, latissimus dorsi, and biceps brachii. Phenol has an immediate onset of action, low cost, and long duration. It should not be used in muscles where further motor recovery is expected to occur.

Before or in conjunction with medication, collaboration with a physical and occupational therapist is essential to achieve and maintain effective functional gains. A skilled therapist can provide stretching, serial casting for contractures, supportive splints, and electrical stimulation to facilitate antagonistic muscle activity. An ankle foot orthosis set in neutral or 5 degrees of dorsiflexion can facilitate knee flexion, control foot drop, and correct minor equinovarus foot position.

Intrathecal baclofen (Lioresal) delivers much lower doses of medication directly into cerebrospinal fluid, thus avoiding lethargy while preserving therapeutic effects. Surgical implantation of the pump delivery system is required. Regular follow-up is needed every 6 to 8 weeks for pump refilling. Dangerous withdrawal symptoms such as seizures can occur if the pump system is not properly refilled or malfunctions. Hence, candidates for pump implantation must have good social support and reliable access to pump refills. Baclofen pump implantation is usually considered after less-invasive options have failed, but the ultimate effectiveness can be superior. Intrathecal baclofen is more effective with lower limb than upper limb spasticity.

Surgery to cut and transfer tendons can also reduce the negative effects of spasticity. Walking ability can be improved with a split anterior tibial tendon transfer (SPLATT). This procedure moves half of the anterior tibial tendon to the outside of the foot limiting excessive inversion and facilitating proper foot position.

Management of Shoulder Pain

Up to 85% of stroke survivors experience some degree of shoulder pain in the paretic limb. Although many different causes have been proposed, the best treatment remains elusive. Poststroke shoulder pain interferes with the rehabilitative process and can prolong the hospital stay. Table 1 provides a summery of the most likely causes of poststroke shoulder pain and potential treatments. Additional use of analgesics is usually necessary. Gabapentin (Neurontin)[1] and tricyclic antidepressants can be especially useful with central or neuropathic pain.

[1]Not FDA approved for this indication.

[1]Not FDA approved for this indication.

TABLE 1 Poststroke Shoulder Pain

Cause	Signs	Diagnosis	Treatment
CRPS I*	Pain with rest and activity Swelling of hand Temperature changes of skin	Painful compression of MCP joints and finger extension Triple phase bone scan	10-14 days of oral steroids Stellate ganglion block
Adhesive capsulitis	Limited external rotation Early scapular motion	Arthrogram	PT/ROM Reduction of internal rotator spasticity Intra-articular steroids†
Impingement syndrome	Pain with abduction of 70 to 90 degrees		Subacromial steroid injection PT/ROM Scapular mobilization reduction of internal rotator spasticity
Rotator cuff tear	Positive abduction and drop arm tests	Radiograph MRI	PT/ROM Steroid injection Surgical repair Reduction of internal rotator spasticity
Inferior subluxation	Acromiohumeral separation	Radiograph	Sling when upright Tray or table support when seated

*CRPS I is also known as reflex sympathetic dystrophy and shoulder hand syndrome

†The efficacy of intra-articular steroid injection in poststroke shoulder pain remains unproven

Abbreviations: CRPS I = complex regional pain syndrome type I; MCP = metacarpophalangeal; MRI = magnetic resonance imaging; PT/ROM = physical therapy/range of motion.

Topical capsaicin (Zostrix)[1] and transcutaneous electrical nerve stimulation (TENS) may be useful adjuncts. Routine use of slings is not beneficial and may encourage disuse and contracture formation. However, limited use of a sling to support a flaccid arm during ambulation may increase comfort. Flaccid shoulder muscles can also lead to painful subluxation. Use of a functional electrical stimulator can reduce the subluxation and alleviate pain. Supportive taping can also reduce subluxation. The use of these measures to prevent the onset of pain in nonpainful shoulder subluxation is not established. Caregivers must be taught proper positioning and transfer techniques to avoid further injury.

Disorders of Mood and Behavior

Depression commonly occurs in stroke survivors. Studies have failed to definitively show a correlation with side or location of the lesion. Distinguishing between a major and minor depression can be difficult, as some symptoms can be a result of the brain lesion itself. Failure to treat poststroke depression can negatively affect rehabilitation outcome. The serotonin-specific release inhibitors (SSRI) are safe and effective agents for treatment and have a side effect profile superior to the tricyclic antidepressants. Fluoxetine (Prozac) alleviates depression and facilitates functional recovery. The psychostimulant methylphenidate (Ritalin)[1] improves mood as well as enhances motor recovery and daily living skill ability. Methylphenidate provides a rapid onset of action, has a good safety profile, is well tolerated, and enables some patients to better participate in therapy during the critical period of inpatient rehabilitation. Use beyond 4 weeks is cautioned because of issues of dependency and unproven long-term benefit. SSRIs are also effective treatment for poststroke emotional lability characterized by socially inappropriate outbursts of crying and sometimes laughter. Excessive lethargy can be treated with more stimulating types of SSRIs. The narcolepsy medication modafinil (Provigil)[1] is used safely with effectiveness. Starting doses are 100 to 200 mg every morning.

Agitation and unsafe behaviors are more commonly seen with strokes involving the frontal lobe or complicating underlying dementia. Training all staff in methods of redirecting agitated patients can be invaluable. However, safe care of an agitated patient often cannot be accomplished without use of antipsychotic medication such as haloperidol (Haldol). Low doses of 0.5 to 2 mg are often effective.

Other Medical Complications

Seizures occurring soon after a stroke (<2 weeks) happen at rates of 2.5% to 15%, with the highest rate occurring in lobar hemorrhages. The risk of recurring early seizures is unclear as is the need for long-term antiepileptic medication. Seizures occurring more than 2 weeks poststroke are related to scar formation, are likely to recur, and can usually be controlled with monotherapy.

[1]Not FDA approved for this indication.

Aphasia occurs in 24% of stroke patients. Broca's aphasia is common in infarctions involving the left middle cerebral artery. Various speech therapy techniques are helpful, although no single approach has proven superior. Case reports have suggested improvements in initiation, content, and fluency using the dopamine agonist bromocriptine (Parlodel)[1] in expressive aphasia. The antiparkinsonian medication amantadine (Symmetrel)[1] may also improve initiation. Blood pressure should be monitored for an orthostatic response with initiating treatment with either medication.

Apraxia, a disorder of learned movement not caused by muscle weakness or sensory loss, is often seen in patients with left middle cerebral artery infarctions. Deficits include difficulty initiating speech, mastication, and use of the paretic and nonparetic upper limbs.

Types of Rehabilitation

Treatment of stroke patients in a dedicated stroke unit during both the acute and rehabilitative stages improves outcome. Conventional methods of rehabilitation include range of motion exercises, mobilization activities, and compensatory techniques. Only 5% of adults recover full use of the paretic upper limb, and 20% fail to recover any functional use. Traditionally, compensatory strategies using the nonparetic limb are emphasized to maximize functional gains quickly. The emphasis on compensatory strategies and belief in the plateau of neural recovery after 3 months has recently been challenged. Several small studies demonstrate functional gains at more than 1 year poststroke. In studies, monkey subjects with chronic stroke demonstrated functional recovery following forced use of the paretic upper limb. A constraint-induced movement technique demonstrates that additional recovery can occur more than 6 months poststroke in certain cases. This technique is based on the theory that there is learned nonuse of the paretic limb that can be reversed with forced use by restraining the unimpaired side. Transcranial dynamic magnetic resonance imaging (MRI) demonstrates activity felt to represent cortical reorganization. Data suggest there is a relationship between the amount of exercise and motor performance of the paretic arm. Initial study protocols cite restraint times of 90% of awake hours with 6 hours per day of training for 10 days. A more recent study finds improved arm function with 2 hours per day combined with intensive therapy. Controlled trials of this

[1]Not FDA approved for this indication.

technique in both subacute and chronic stroke patients are under way. Other promising techniques to enhance recovery include the use of body weight support to enhance recovery of ambulation and functional electrical stimulation to increase muscle strength. Highly repetitive exercises administered by motorized devices may also affect recovery through cortical reorganization. Although still largely experimental, implantable electrodes with neurocontrol systems are being used to enhance function after stroke and spinal cord injury.

Stroke rehabilitation may be provided in several settings. Acute rehabilitation provides 3 hours of therapy per day, 5 to 7 days a week. Care is based on a multidisciplinary team approach usually led by a physiatrist or physician specializing in rehabilitation medicine. Patients receive daily physician visits, and there is a strong emphasis on patient and family training. This level of care is most suitable for patients who require minimal to maximal assistance for mobility and self-care and have the physical and cognitive ability to participate and learn. Patients with language and swallowing impairments also benefit from this intensive level of care.

Subacute and skilled rehabilitation programs provide varying amounts of therapy. Patients may receive single or multiple therapies 1 to 2 hours per day, 3 to 5 days per week. Physician visits are 1 to 3 days per week at the subacute level and monthly at the skilled care level. This level of care is most appropriate for patients with physical or cognitive limitations that preclude participation at a more intensive level.

Outpatient and day programs are appropriate for patients with adequate functional mobility, medical stability, and social supports to manage safely in their homes. Home health programs have the added advantage of teaching patients in their home environment but lack professional equipment and post-rehabilitation care personnel.

Discharge planning should begin during the acute care of the stroke patient. Typically this involves the physician and social worker to assess anticipated need for 24-hour assistance and supervision, available caregiver support, and home accessibility. Further planning occurs throughout the inpatient stay with involvement of the patient and family in setting appropriate goals.

Outpatient follow-up with the rehabilitation physician is generally done at 1 month after discharge. Future visits are done at various intervals as warranted by progress and complications. Patients should retain their primary care physicians for general medical care and medication renewals. Good communication with the primary care physician is essential.

Rehabilitation physician visits should not only address medical and neurologic status but also proper medication usage, daily activity levels, stroke prevention tactics, and compliance with the home exercise program. Direct inquiry about psychosocial issues and depression should be made. All orthotics and equipment should be inspected for fit and stability. The need for further therapy must be assessed. Unfortunately, many patients and families view the reduction or termination of therapy as the end of future progress. The gradual reduction of sessions combined with resumption of leisure activities, and enrollment in community programs for exercise and socialization can ease the transition.

A successful return to work eludes most stroke patients, although it can be an important contributor to life satisfaction. Enrollment in a vocational rehab program can provide training for the patient and employer. A gradual approach with initial part-time hours is most successful.

Driving may be safely resumed in some patients but should be avoided in cases of visual field deficit and neglect. When recovery is incomplete, participation in a driving program for stroke survivors is recommended. Patients with poststroke seizures must be seizure free for 6 to 12 months according to state laws.

Stroke rehabilitation faces both an exciting and challenging future. New information about recovery processes and neural plasticity may change the types and time course of rehabilitative services. The era of managed care will continue to emphasize shorter lengths of stay. The physician caring for a stroke survivor has many responsibilities including prevention of medical complications, assisting patients and families in choosing appropriate therapeutic options, and setting realistic goals. Knowledge of recovery patterns, coordination of care with therapists, consulting physicians, and social workers will greatly assist patients in achieving their maximum functional potential and improve their quality of life.

SEIZURES AND EPILEPSY IN ADOLESCENTS AND ADULTS

METHOD OF

Annemarei Ranta, MD, and

Nathan B. Fountain, MD

Seizures and epilepsy have been long misunderstood by physicians, but a logical framework for the approach to seizures has emerged in recent years. This is especially important today because eight new antiepileptic drugs (AEDs) have been approved for use in the United States since 1993, and their proper use is contingent on a systematic approach.

This chapter follows the systematic analysis that should accompany the approach to treating patients with seizures and epilepsy by dividing the process into five steps. *Step 1* is to confirm that the paroxysmal symptom of concern is a seizure. *Step 2* is to determine the specific type of seizure present, classifying it as focal or generalized in onset. *Step 3* is to determine the neuroanatomic site of seizure onset in order to direct investigations toward identifying pathology at that site. *Step 4* is to identify the etiology, or determine the epilepsy syndrome if the etiology is not identifiable. *Step 5* is to select the appropriate therapy.

Some terms used to describe seizures or epilepsy have definitions that are unique to the study of epilepsy. *Seizures* are behavioral changes that result from abnormal paroxysmal neuronal discharges and are a symptom of an underlying brain problem. A seizure may result from a transient perturbation of neuronal physiology such as during acute head trauma, alcohol withdrawal or hypocalcemia, or a seizure may result from an enduring tendency to seizures, commonly referred to as epilepsy. *Epilepsy*, therefore, is not a single "disease," but instead is any disease characterized by the spontaneous recurrence of seizures. Epilepsy syndromes are diseases that are characterized exclusively or primarily by the occurrence of seizures with few other systemic or neurologic symptoms. When the etiology of seizures is definitely known, for example, when caused by a brain tumor or penetrating brain injury, then classification into an epilepsy syndrome is less important. However, when the etiology is not known because it is not identifiable or the evaluation is incomplete, then classification becomes useful. Patients grouped into a specific epilepsy syndrome are presumed to share a similar pathophysiology and therefore a similar natural history and response to therapy.

Diagnosis

DIFFERENTIAL DIAGNOSIS OF PAROXYSMAL SYMPTOMS

There are several entities that present with symptoms similar to seizures. *Syncope* is commonly accompanied by motor movements, especially clonic or brief tonic arm movements. EEG recording during such "convulsive syncope" or "syncopal seizure" shows profound suppression of brain activity due to cerebral anoxia; it does not show seizure discharges and "convulsive syncope" is not an epileptic seizure. Syncope is distinguished from a true seizure by the presence of presyncopal symptoms (nausea, flushing and lightheadedness), brief loss of consciousness and the return of normal cognition within a few seconds after arousal. *Migraine* headaches may occasionally be accompanied by complex visual phenomena or sensorimotor symptoms that could be confused with seizures. Postictal headaches may be confused with migraine. Complicated migraine with hemiparesis may be mistaken for a postictal paralysis. A history of migraine headaches and preservation of normal consciousness help identify the spells as migraine. Rarely, basilar migraines may be accompanied by loss of consciousness. Transient ischemic attacks (TIAs) should almost never be mistaken for seizures because TIAs cause focal negative phenomena, such as weakness, numbness, aphasia or ataxia, whereas seizures usually cause positive phenomena, such as jerking, tingling, automatisms, or movements. Some movement disorders, sleep disorders, and hypoglycemia may also mimic seizures.

Psychiatric disease can present with symptoms nearly identical to seizures. Anxiety attacks can be characterized by anxiety, palpitation, facial flushing, and incoherence, as can seizure auras. Seizure auras usually progress to complex partial seizures at some point in the evolution of epilepsy and auras are usually more stereotyped than anxiety attacks. *Pseudoseizures*, which have also been termed *psychogenic nonepileptic seizures*, may be identical to seizures in their presentation. However, pseudoseizures are more likely to be long in duration, involve bizarre or unusual symptoms and movements, have pelvic thrusting or thrashing and may be precipitated by psychologically stressful events, and they persist despite AED therapy. Unfortunately, epileptic seizures may also have these characteristics and video/electroencephalograph (EEG) monitoring may be the only way to definitively distinguish seizures from pseudoseizures. Surprisingly, as much as 30% of the patients admitted to inpatient epilepsy units for the diagnosis of spells, end up having pseudoseizures.

SEIZURE CLASSIFICATION

The International League Against Epilepsy (ILAE) has developed a classification of seizures based on the site of seizure origin to facilitate communication (Figure 1). Seizures are divided into *partial* (or *focal*) and *generalized* classes. Consciousness is preserved in partial seizures because only a small region of brain is affected. Consciousness is lost in generalized seizures because the entire cortex is affected. Partial seizures may secondarily generalize. "Primary" generalized seizures involve the whole brain from the onset.

Partial seizures are subdivided into simple partial and complex partial subtypes. *Simple partial seizures* arise in a small region of cortex and give discrete symptoms, depending on the area from which they arise, without altering consciousness. For example, seizures arising in the primary motor cortex in the frontal lobe cause clonic jerking of the contralateral limb, usually the hand. The most common simple partial seizures are indescribable auras arising in the temporal lobe and causing autonomic symptoms.

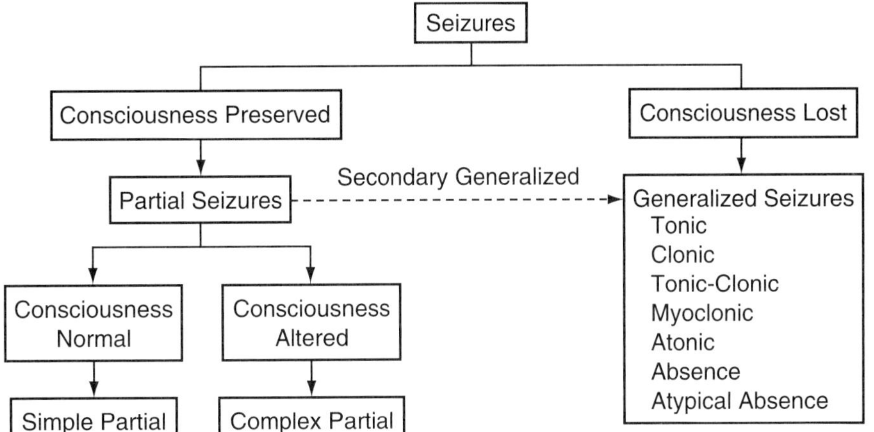

FIGURE 1 Algorithm for seizure classification.

Complex partial seizures (CPS) are characterized by staring with a fixed gaze and lack of distractibility to examiners. Automatisms are common, especially picking or pulling at clothing, lip smacking, and swallowing.

Generalized seizures are classified based on the predominant motor activity. *Generalized tonic–clonic seizures* (GTC) begin with sudden tonic extension of the extremities, often with an expiratory scream, followed by clonic rhythmic jerking of the extremities. Postictally, patients are always unresponsiveness for at least a brief period and usually sleep for minutes to hours. *Tonic seizures* contain only the tonic phase and *clonic seizures* contain only the clonic phase. *Myoclonic seizures* are a brief lightening-like jerk, most commonly of the arms. *Atonic seizures* consist of sudden unprotected falling with loss of muscle tone. *Absence seizures* are associated with nondistractible staring, similar to complex partial seizures, but are very brief, frequent, primarily in children, and associated with a generalized 3 Hz spike and wave pattern on EEG. *Atypical absence seizures* are similar but more prolonged and often accompanied by brief myoclonic jerks or loss of tone and the EEG shows a slow or atypical generalized spike and wave pattern.

ETIOLOGY AND EPILEPSY SYNDROME CLASSIFICATION

The underlying pathology or etiology of seizures ultimately determines the natural history and, to some degree, the response to therapy. The ILAE has established a systematic approach to epilepsy classification to help the clinician with making appropriate decisions regarding the evaluation and treatment of patients with epilepsy (Table 1).

The most important division of epilepsy syndromes is into *focal epilepsies* (or *localization-related)* in which there is pathology localized to one region of the brain, and *generalized epilepsies* in which the pathology is expressed throughout the whole brain. Focal epilepsies generally present with simple partial, complex partial, or secondary GTC seizures. Generalized epilepsies typically present with primary generalized seizures such as absence, primary GTC, atonic, and myoclonic seizures. The epilepsies can be further subdivided into three categories: (a) those that are *symptomatic* of an identified underlying brain lesion; (b) *cryptogenic,* in which an anatomic lesion is suspected, but cannot be identified with current technology; and (c) *idiopathic,* in which an identifiable lesion is neither identified nor suspected.

TABLE 1 Examples of Epilepsy Syndromes in Adolescents and Adults

	Focal (Localization-Related)	Generalized
Idiopathic	Benign childhood epilepsy with centrotemporal spikes Benign occipital epilepsy Autosomal dominant nocturnal frontal lobe epilepsy	Childhood absence epilepsy Juvenile absence epilepsy Juvenile myoclonic epilepsy Epilepsy with GTCs on awakening
Symptomatic	Temporal lobe Frontal lobe Parietal lobe Occipital lobe	Cortical malformations Cortical dysplasias Metabolic abnormalities West's syndrome Lennox-Gastaut syndrome
Cryptogenic	Any occurrence of partial seizures without obvious pathology	West's syndrome (unidentified pathology) Lennox-Gastaut syndrome (unidentified pathology)

Abbreviation: GTCs = generalized tonic–clonic seizures.

The idiopathic syndromes are thought to be caused by inherited abnormalities of neurotransmission without corresponding anatomic lesions. The importance of the latter distinction is that an aggressive search for underlying pathology is not necessary or indicated for idiopathic epilepsies, but is necessary for cryptogenic cases.

One of the most common types of epilepsy encountered in adults is temporal lobe epilepsy (TLE). TLE is characterized by refractory complex partial seizures with occasional secondary generalization, originating in the temporal lobe. If neuroimaging is normal the patient would be said to suffer from a "cryptogenic focal epilepsy," the most common type of epilepsy in adults. Quite frequently, however, magnetic resonance imaging (MRI) demonstrates atrophy and gliosis of the hippocampus in the temporal lobe. Histopathologically, this is represented by neuronal loss and gliosis of the hippocampus and several mesial temporal structures, giving rise to the term "mesial temporal sclerosis." Mass lesions in the temporal lobe may present in a similar manner and include malformations and tumors, such as astrocytomas and dysembryoplastic neuroepithelial tumors (DNET). Patients with such abnormalities on MRI are said to suffer from *symptomatic focal epilepsy.* TLE is an important syndrome to recognize because temporal lobectomy renders >70% of patients essentially seizure-free.

Juvenile myoclonic epilepsy (JME) is an example of a common adulthood idiopathic epilepsy. JME is named for the characteristic onset in adolescence of brief myoclonic arm jerks and GTC seizures. JME is associated with a characteristic EEG pattern of generalized "polyspike and waves" in between seizures. Imaging studies are normal, as is the case for all idiopathic generalized epilepsies. The etiology is undoubtedly an abnormality of neurotransmission and it has been localized to at least two separate chromosomal loci, but the pathophysiology is still unknown. Many other epilepsies are encountered in adults including those that begin in childhood (discussed in the chapter on Epilepsy in Infancy and Childhood), those that are caused by lesions in areas other than the temporal lobe, and other less-commonly encountered, adult-onset, idiopathic, generalized epilepsies.

DIAGNOSTIC EVALUATION

The evaluation of *new-onset seizures* is aimed at finding acute transient causes such as metabolic abnormalities and to exclude acute life threatening etiologies, such as infection, neoplasm, or hemorrhage. Most patients seek emergency care after the first seizure. At that time, it is usually not possible to determine whether this represents epilepsy or an acute medial illness. Consequently, simple screening laboratory tests may be indicated including electrolytes, complete blood count, liver enzymes, and urine drug screen. If central nervous system (CNS) infection is suspected, then lumbar puncture should be performed. An EEG is always indicated because it may reveal interictal epileptiform discharges of the type present in patients with epilepsy but it is not needed acutely. Neuroimaging is always indicated in the evaluation of a partial-onset seizure to exclude acute or serious focal pathology. The imaging technique of choice is an MRI scan, but if unavailable, a noncontrasted head computed tomography (CT) can be substituted in the acute setting. The evaluation of *established epilepsy* is aimed at defining the underlying cause of the epilepsy syndrome, which is usually more subtle. An EEG is always indicated because it may reveal focal epileptiform discharges and assist in classifying the seizure type and epilepsy syndrome. However, a normal EEG does not exclude epilepsy. The first EEG is abnormal in only approximately 40% of patients with clinically definite localization-related epilepsy. The EEG will remain normal in approximately 20% of these patients, even after as many as seven EEGs. The diagnostic evaluation of intractable epilepsy is intertwined with the presurgical evaluation and is discussed below.

Antiepileptic Drug Therapy

PHARMACOKINETIC PRINCIPLES

No logical system has been devised to classify AEDs. One convenient method is to divide them into conventional, new, unconventional, and experimental categories (Table 2). Conventional AEDs are those which were available before the onslaught of new AEDs that were approved starting in 1993. Although there are several conventional AEDs, only phenytoin (Dilantin), carbamazepine (Tegretol), valproate (Depakote), phenobarbital and primidone (Mysoline) are widely used. New AEDs are those that have been approved since 1993. Unconventional AEDs are those that are either outdated, used only in specific circumstances, or primarily used for non–epilepsy-related purposes. This review focuses on the conventional and new AEDs.

The side-effect profile of AEDs is important because conventional AEDs are frequently accompanied by side effects, which often depend on the pharmacokinetics of the drug (Table 3). Half-life is important to AEDs because it determines the dosing interval and is often affected by concomitant AEDs. Infrequent dosing is important to improve compliance, thus long half-life drugs are desirable. Some AEDs have a narrow therapeutic window so that at the peak of the serum level patients may experience side effects. More frequent dosing of smaller amounts may avoid peak dose side effects.

New AEDs have few drug interactions; however, among conventional AEDs, phenobarbital, carbamazepine, and phenytoin are enzyme inducers that can decrease levels of one another and valproate (Table 4). All AEDs necessarily affect the brain so

TABLE 2 Conventional, New, Unconventional and Experimental AEDs

Conventional	New	Unconventional	Experimental
Carbamazepine (CBZ) (Tegretol)	Felbamate (FBM) (Felbatol)	Adrenocorticotropic hormone (ACTH)[1]	Clobazam (Frisium)*,‡
Ethosuximide (ESM) (Zarontin)	Gabapentin (GBP) (Neurontin)	Acetazolamide (Diamox)	Eterobarb‡
Phenobarbital (PB)	Lamotrigine (LMT) (Lamictal)	Amantadine (Symmetrel)[1]	Ganaxolone‡
Phenytoin (PHT) (Dilantin)	Levetiracetam (LEV) (Keppra)	Bromides[1,†]	Losigamone‡
Primidone (PRM) (Mysoline)	Oxcarbazepine (OXC) (Trileptal)	Clomiphene (Clomid)[1]	Nitrazepam (Mogadon)*,‡
Valproic acid (VPA) (Depakene)	Tiagabine (TGB) (Gabitril)	Ethotoin (Peganone)	Piracetam (Nootropil)‡
	Topiramate (TPM) (Topamax)	Mephenytoin (Mesantoin)	Pregabalin‡
	Zonisamide (ZNS) (Zonegran)	Mephobarbital (Mebaral)	Progabide‡
		Methsuximide (Celontin)	Remacemide‡
		Trimethadione (Tridione)	Rotigotine‡
			Retinamide‡
			SPM927 (Harkoseride)‡
			Stiripentol‡
			Vigabatrin (Sabril)*,‡

[1]Not FDA approved for this indication.
*Approved in other countries.
†May be compounded by pharmacists.
‡Investigational drug in the United States.

that pharmacodynamic interactions make CNS side effects of lethargy, ataxia, and blurry vision more common when more than one AED is taken at a time. Even as monotherapy, all AEDs cause CNS side effects at high doses.

There are several principles to guide dosing to avoid problems. When initiating therapy, it is best to "start low and go slow." Most side effects are experienced at the initiation of therapy and can be avoided by starting with a low enough dose and increasing more slowly than recommended by the manufacturer. Table 5 provides general target doses that will usually be therapeutic. However, the "maintenance" doses given cover a wide range because there is no set final dose for any of the AEDs. The only method to determine that a given dose is "therapeutic" is to determine that the seizure frequency has decreased. Serum drug levels are available for conventional and essentially all new AEDs; keeping in mind that oxcarbazepine (Trileptal) and tiagabine (Gabitril) levels are of very limited utility because of their pharmacokinetic properties. In some instances, drug levels can provide a general guide, but many patients will be on a "therapeutic dose" while their blood level is below the usual "normal" range. On the other hand, blood levels can help guide dose increases by warning that toxic side effects may occur with further increases when the blood level is at the upper

TABLE 3 Pharmacokinetics of Conventional and New AEDs

Drug	Metabolized by Inducible Enzymes (Mechanism)	Induces Hepatic Enzymes	Half-Life (Hours)	Protein Bound (%)
Carbamazepine (Tegretol)	Yes (oxidized)	Yes	12-17	76
Ethosuximide (Zarontin)	Yes (oxidized)	No	30-60 (30 in child)	0
Felbamate (Felbatol)	Yes (multiple mechanisms)	No	20-23	25
Gabapentin (Neurontin)	No	No	5-7	<3
Lamotrigine (Lamictal)	Yes (glucuronidated)	No	25 alone or with both 60 with valproate 12 with enzyme inducer	55
Levetiracetam (Keppra)	No	No	6-8	<10
Oxcarbazepine (Trileptal)	Yes (converted to MHD → glucuronidated)	Mixed	9-11 (for MHD)	67
Phenobarbital	Yes (hydroxylated, glucuronidated)	Yes	80-100	45
Phenytoin (Dilantin)	Yes (hydroxylated, glucuronidated)	Yes	22	90
Primidone (Mysoline)	Yes (similar to phenobarbital)	Yes	8-15 (shorter with EI)	20
Tiagabine (Gabitril)	Yes (glucuronidation, oxidation)	No	7-9 (alone) 4-7 (with EI)	96
Topiramate (Topamax)	Yes (hydroxylated, hydrolyzed, glucuronidated)	No	20-24	13-17
Valproic acid (Depakene)	Yes (glucuronidated, oxidized)	No	9-16 (shorter with EI)	70-90 (varies with level)
Zonisamide (Zonegran)	Yes (acetylated, reduced)	No	63	40

Abbreviations: EI = enzyme inducer; MHD = monohydroxy derivative.

TABLE 4 AED Interactions Influencing Serum Concentrations*,†

Drug Added	Serum Level Influenced												
	CBZ	ESM	FBM	GBP	LMT	LEV	OXC	PB	PHT	TGB	TPM	VPA	ZNS
CBZ	↓	↓	↓	–	↓↓	–	↓	–	↑↓	↓↓	↓↓	↓	↓
ESM	?–	–	?–	?–	–	?–	?–	?–	?↑	?–	?–	?–	?–
FBM	↓ epox ↑	?–	–	?–	–	?–	?–	↑	↑↑	?–	?–	↑↑	?–
GBP	–	?–	?–	–	?–	–	?–	–	–	?–	?–	–	?–
LMT	–	–	–	?–	–	–	?–	–	–	?–	?–	↓	?–
LEV	–	?–	?–	–	–	–	?–	–	–	?–	?–	–	?–
OXC	–	?	?–	?–	↓	?–	–	–	–	?	?–	–	?–
PB	↓	↓	↓	–	↓↓	–	↓	–	–	↓↓	↓	↓	↓
PHT	↓	↓	↓	–	↓↓	–	↓	–	–	↓↓	↓↓	↓	↓
TGB	–	?–	?–	?–	?–	?–	?–	?–	–	–	?–	↓	?–
TPM	–	?–	?–	?–	?–	?–	?–	–	↑	?–	–	↓	?–
VPA	↓ epox.↑	↑↓	–	–	↑↑	?↑	–	↑↑	–	–	↓	–	–
ZNS	–	–	?–	?–	?–	?–	?–	–	–	?–	?–	–	–

Abbreviations: CBZ = carbamazepine; ESM = ethosuximide; FBM = felbamate; GBP = gabapentin; LMT = lamotrigine; LEV = levetiracetam; OXC = oxcarbazepine; PB = phenobarbital; PHT = phenytoin; TGB = tiagabine; TPM = topiramate; VPA = valproic acid; ZNS = zonisamide.

*Effect of adding the drug listed in the first column on the blood concentration of the drugs listed in the other columns.

†Clinically significant effects are double arrows; other effects (single arrows) are not usually clinically relevant. Question marks indicate unknown interactions.

limit of the established "therapeutic range." Nonetheless, it is important to increase each drug to the maximum tolerated dose before labeling it ineffective. This usually requires increasing the drug until side effects occur and then reducing the dose by one step. Patients must be informed of this strategy or they may refuse to take the drug, even at a lower dose. If neither seizure control improves nor side effects set in despite high doses of a given AED, checking a serum level can help to uncover noncompliance, a problem especially frequent among adolescents. When substituting one AED for another, it is important to start the second drug and determine that it is effective before gradually withdrawing the first drug. This affords at least some protection from seizures at all times. After a 2-year seizure-free period, a trial of drug withdrawal should be considered in patients who do not have a known continued tendency

TABLE 5 Titration Guidelines for Conventional and New AEDs

			Adult			Child	
Generic Name	Common Brand Name	Dosing Schedule	Initial Dose	Increment (mg)	Maintenance (mg/d)	Initial Dose (mg/kg/d)	Maintenance (mg/kg/d)
Carbamazepine	Tegretol Tegretol XR, Carbatrol	tid-qid bid	200 bid	200 q wk	600-1800	10 qd	10-35 (for age <6 y)
Ethosuximide	Zarontin	qd-bid	250 qd	250 q3-7 d	750	15	15-40
Felbamate	Felbatol	tid	600-1200 qd	600-1200 q1-2 wk	2400-3600	15	15-45
Gabapentin	Neurontin	tid	300 qd	300 q3-7 d	1200-3600	10	25-50
Lamotrigine	Lamictal	bid	25 qd	25 q2 wk	100 with VPA 400 alone 600 with EI	0.15-0.5	0.5-5 with VPA 5 alone 5-15 with EI
Levetiracetam	Keppra	bid	500 bid	500 q wk	2000-4000	20	40-100
Oxcarbazepine	Trileptal	bid	300 qd	300 q wk	900-2400	8-10	30-46
Phenobarbital	(Generic)	qd-bid	30-60 qd	30 q1-2 wk	60-120	3	3-6
Phenytoin	Dilantin Kapseals liquid, Infatab	qd bid-tid	200 qd	100 q5-7 d	200-300	4	4-8
Primidone	Mysoline	tid	125-250 qd	250 q1-2 wk	500-750	10	10-25
Tiagabine	Gabitril	bid-qid	4 qd	4-8 q wk	16-32	0.1	0.4 without EI 0.7 with EI
Topiramate	Topamax	bid	25 qd	25 q1-2 wk	100-400	3	3-9
Valproic acid	Depakene, Depakote Depakote ER	tid-qid bid	250 qd	250 q3-7 d	750-3000	15	15-45
Zonisamide	Zonegran	bid	100 qd	100 q2 wk	200-400	4	4-12

Abbreviations: bid = twice a day; EI = enzyme inducer; qd = every day; qid = four times a day; tid = three times a day; VPA = valproic acid.

for seizures. The risk of seizure recurrence after drug withdrawal is lowest in patients who have a normal MRI and EEG and are not diagnosed with an adult-onset idiopathic epilepsy.

CONVENTIONAL AEDS

Phenytoin (Dilantin) is probably the most widely used and familiar AED despite having the most problematic side effects. The metabolism of phenytoin is saturable which means that it shows zero order kinetics at high blood levels. Very steep elevations in the blood level may occur with even small dose increases when the level is near 20 μg/mL, despite the occurrence of a linear increase in the blood level with dose increases when blood levels are below 20 μg/mL. For example, the blood level may be 10 μg/mL with 200 mg per day, then increase to 15 μg/mL with 300 mg per day, and then increase to 20 μg/mL with 400 mg per day, but with an increase to 500 mg per day, the level may skyrocket to >30 μg/mL if metabolism is saturated. Phenytoin idiosyncratic side effects of hepatitis and blood dyscrasias are rare. One benefit of phenytoin is that Dilantin Kapseals and other slow-release preparations are available so that it can be dosed once per day, unlike other phenytoin preparations, such as the suspension or the Infatab, which must be dosed at least twice a day. Cumulative side effects of phenytoin, which occur over many years, include gum hypertrophy, hirsutism, coarsening of features, ataxia as a consequence of cerebellar atrophy, osteoporosis, and peripheral neuropathy.

Intravenous (IV) phenytoin solution is very basic (pH 11), which frequently causes venous irritation, "purple glove syndrome," and severe acute necrosis leading to amputation. IV phenytoin is mixed in polyethylene glycol causing bradycardia and hypotension, which limits the rate of infusion to less than 50 mg per minute. This can be a significant problem in the treatment of status epilepticus or frequent seizures. Fosphenytoin (Cerebyx) is a phenytoin prodrug in which the phosphate group is rapidly cleaved off upon entering the blood stream yielding phenytoin. It is mixed in an aqueous solution and a more neutral pH, thus it is much better tolerated and can be given as fast as 150 mg per minute.

Carbamazepine (Tegretol), like phenytoin, is metabolized by the liver and induces hepatic metabolism. It also undergoes autoinduction, inducing its own metabolism for up to 3 weeks after initiating it, so that steady-state blood levels are not achieved for several weeks. Carbamazepine has a relatively narrow therapeutic window, with usual therapeutic blood levels of between only 7 μg/mL and 12 μg/mL. It is common to cause acute toxicity (ataxia, diplopia, and lethargy) with only a small increase in the dose. Carbamazepine does not have cumulative side effects, but rarely causes serious idiosyncratic side effects, including blood dyscrasias, hepatitis, and hyponatremia. Mild leukopenia is common and does not require intervention unless the white blood cell count falls below 3000 cells/mm^3. Extended-release preparations (Tegretol XR) that can be dosed twice daily are now available.

Valproic acid (or valproate) is a very useful drug because it is effective for both partial and generalized seizures (see below). It is available as valproic acid (Depakene), sodium divalproex (Depakote), and in an extended-release form (Depakote ER). Valproic acid (Depakene) frequently causes dyspepsia and other gastrointestinal side effects. Sodium divalproex (Depakote) is immediately cleaved to valproate in the stomach, but this preparation is tolerated much better. Valproate is usually dosed three times a day because of its relatively short half-life. Depakote ER was recently approved for once-per-day dosing for migraine headaches, but it is actually released over less than 24 hours, so twice-daily dosing may be more useful for the treatment of epilepsy. Valproate is now available as an IV preparation (Depakon), dosed identical to the oral forms.

Valproate is usually well tolerated but it occasionally causes weight gain, alopecia, tremor, and thrombocytopenia. It can cause potentially fatal hepatitis and pancreatitis. Hepatitis occurs in only 1:40,000 adult patient exposures, but it is much more common in children (as much as 1:500) who are on multiple AEDs and with mental retardation, possibly because they have an undiagnosed metabolic abnormality. It has been suggested that carnitine[1] supplementation may reduce the risk of hepatitis. Although this has not been demonstrated, it is prudent for children with unknown causes of mental retardation on valproate to take carnitine. The overall incidence risk of birth defects associated with valproate is not substantially greater than other AEDs, but it is more often associated with neural tube defects, which are more serious. Folic acid supplementation at 1-5 mg per day can reduce this risk. Women of childbearing potential on valproate should practice an effective method of birth control and take folic acid.

Phenobarbital has fallen out of favor as an AED because it occasionally induces lethargy, depression, and learning difficulties. However, it is usually well tolerated in adults, is effective for partial-onset and primary generalized tonic–clonic seizures, is inexpensive, and can be given IV. It can be dosed once per day and has a very long half-life, which is an advantage in poorly compliant patients. Primidone (Mysoline) is a prodrug of phenobarbital that also has its own antiseizure effects but less often causes lethargy.

Ethosuximide (Zarontin) is unique because it is the only AED that is effective exclusively for absence seizures with no efficacy for other types of seizures. It is usually well tolerated but occasionally causes nausea, anorexia, headache, and blood dyscrasias. It can be dosed once per day because of its very long half-life, but is usually better tolerated twice daily.

[1]Not FDA approved for this indication.

NEW AEDs

Felbamate (Felbatol) was approved in 1993 as the first "new" AED since valproate in 1978. It held great promise because it was highly effective for the most intractable epilepsies, such as the Lennox-Gastaut syndrome, as well as for partial-onset seizures, despite frequent side effects of anorexia, insomnia, and agitation, and the occurrence of frequent AED interactions. However, in 1994, after approximately 100,000 prescriptions had been dispensed, 35 cases of aplastic anemia and 18 cases of fulminant hepatitis were reported. This led to a sudden change in practice and labeling so that it is now only indicated for intractable epilepsy, in cases where the potential benefit outweighs the risk of potentially fatal side effects. Some clinicians obtain written consent from patients prior to its use. Its use should probably be limited to epilepsy centers.

Gabapentin (Neurontin) is very well tolerated and has no pharmacokinetic interactions because it is renally excreted unchanged. It has engendered an unwarranted poor reputation as an AED because some have thought that it is ineffective. Clinical studies examined doses that statistically reduced the frequency of seizures with minimal side effects but were not high enough to determine the maximum tolerated dose; thus it was approved and initially used at relatively low doses of 900 to 1800 mg per day. However, clinical experience suggests that doses of as much as 3600 mg per day may be required to be effective for most patients. On the other hand, high doses may not increase blood levels because drug absorption may be saturated at doses above 4000 mg per day.

Lamotrigine (Lamictal) is particularly useful because it is effective for both partial and generalized seizures. It is severely affected by other AEDs so that its dosing is drastically different depending on concomitant AEDs (see Table 5). When taken alone (or with a combination of an enzyme inducer and inhibitor), the half-life of lamotrigine is approximately 25 hours, but this is reduced to 12 hours when taken with enzyme inducers (such as phenytoin, phenobarbital, carbamazepine), and prolonged to as much as 60 hours when taken with valproate (an enzyme inhibitor). This is important because the anticipated maintenance dose and dose escalation rate will be different depending on the concomitant AED. The only potentially serious side effect of lamotrigine is rash, the occurrence of which is also dependent on concomitant AEDs. Mild rash is common and was present in as many as 1:50 children and 1:1000 adults during initial clinical studies. The rash can be life-threatening in the form of Stevens-Johnson syndrome or toxic epidermal necrolysis but the incidence of the serious rash is probably only approximately 1:40,000. The rash is most likely to occur after the first 3 weeks of therapy but can occur at any time, and is more common with high initial doses and titration rates and when taken with valproate. The titration rates in Table 5 have been used with a very low incidence of rash, probably because the titration rate is so slow; the rate is so slow that patients are unlikely to see an effect for many weeks or months and may require encouragement from the physician. When a rash is reported, the patient must be examined immediately and serious consideration must be given to stopping the drug.

Levetiracetam (Keppra) is approved as add-on therapy for partial seizures in adults and studies in children are ongoing. It is very well tolerated and has not been associated with serious side effects. It can be titrated relatively rapidly so that its effectiveness in a patient can be determined in a few months. It is primarily excreted unchanged with only 24% hydrolyzed before excretion, so it is unlikely to have significant drug interactions.

Oxcarbazepine (Trileptal) was recently approved in the United States, but has been used in Mexico and elsewhere for many years. It is a derivative of carbamazepine. The primary CNS side effects of carbamazepine are caused by epoxide-10,11-carbamazepine, a metabolite produced by oxidation. Oxcarbazepine cannot undergo this conversion and thus does not produce this metabolite. Therefore, it is better tolerated than carbamazepine and is much less likely to cause diplopia and ataxia. The incidence of blood dyscrasias also appears lower than with carbamazepine. It is associated with hyponatremia. It does not induce AED metabolizing liver enzymes (although it does induce other liver enzymes) or undergo autoinduction. The daily dose cannot be directly converted from the carbamazepine dose. It is effective as monotherapy so it is likely that in the future oxcarbazepine will entirely replace carbamazepine.

Tiagabine (Gabitril) is approved as add-on therapy of partial-onset seizures. It is the only AED that was designed for a specific mechanism of action; it inhibits the reuptake of γ-aminobutyric acid (GABA) in the synaptic cleft. It has a very short serum half-life, but it affects the GABA transporter for at least 12 hours so that it can be dosed twice daily. Some patients may require more frequent dosing. It is not associated with any end-organ toxicity, but it can precipitate nonconvulsive status epilepticus in those who are predisposed, usually patients with generalized epilepsy.

Topiramate (Topamax) is effective for partial seizures and some types of generalized seizures, especially the Lennox-Gastaut syndrome. It has acquired an unwarranted reputation for causing cognitive side effects. The source of this is probably the design of clinical studies that appropriately determined the maximum tolerated dose by finding the dose at which an unacceptable frequency of side effects occur. Considering all topiramate clinical studies together, the incidence of subject drop out in those treated with >400 mg per day was twice that of the <400 mg per day group, which was approximately equal to placebo. This indicates that the average maximum tolerated dose is about 400 mg per day.

Topiramate is a weak carbonic anhydrase inhibitor and can cause kidney stones and metabolic acidosis; the use of other carbonic anhydrase inhibitors is relatively contraindicated. Acute narrow-angle glaucoma has been reported in a few cases and requires immediate discontinuation. End-organ toxicities have not been reported with topiramate.

Zonisamide (Zonegran) is the most recently released AED, although it has been available for many years in Japan. It appears to be effective for both focal and some generalized epilepsies. Its pharmacology is not well described, but it is metabolized by multiple mechanisms and has a very long half-life, which may allow it to be dosed once per day. It rarely causes kidney stones. It also may cause oligohidrosis (reduced sweating) and has rarely been associated with blood dyscrasias.

CHOOSING AN AED

Drugs of Choice by Seizure Type and Epilepsy Syndrome

AEDs should be selected based on the epilepsy syndrome or seizure type if the syndrome is not known. All types of *partial-onset seizures* respond to the same medications, so they can be considered together. The available data suggest that all AEDs, except for ethosuximide (Zarontin), are equally effective. Therefore, to select among them, consideration must be given to the relative importance of the side effect profile, dosing interval, pharmacokinetics, and cost for each patient. In general, the new AEDs have less-frequent side effects, daily or twice daily dosing, and simple pharmacokinetics, which suggests that they are more desirable than conventional AEDs. On the other hand, conventional AEDs are familiar, have a proven track record, can often be administered intravenously, and are inexpensive. Most neurologists still prefer to start therapy with a conventional AED, but move quickly to a new AED if necessary. New AEDs are gradually starting to replace conventional AEDs for the initial treatment of partial seizures.

Each type of generalized seizure must be considered individually. *GTC seizures, tonic seizures* and *clonic seizures* seem to respond to the same AEDs as partial-onset seizures, but this may be because historically there was little distinction between primary generalized and secondary generalized seizures during drug development. All conventional AEDs, except ethosuximide, seem to be effective. There have been few published studies of the efficacy of new AEDs, but lamotrigine (Lamictal), felbamate (Felbatol), topiramate (Topamax), and zonisamide (Zonegran) seem to be effective and the others are unknown. *Absence seizures* respond to valproate (Depakote), ethosuximide (Zarontin), and lamotrigine, but not to carbamazepine (Tegretol), gabapentin (Neurontin), or tiagabine (Gabitril). The efficacy of other new AEDs has yet to be demonstrated. *Myoclonic seizures* respond to valproate and lamotrigine, and occasionally to benzodiazepines.

A few epilepsy syndromes in adults and adolescents respond particularly well to specific AEDs. Myoclonic and GTC seizures occurring in *juvenile myoclonic epilepsy* respond very well to valproate or lamotrigine. Atonic, tonic, and atypical absence seizures occurring as part of the *Lennox-Gastaut syndrome* respond very well to valproate, lamotrigine, and topiramate. This is one case where the potential benefit of felbamate usually outweighs the risk. Approximately 30% of patients with *childhood absence epilepsy* have seizures that persist into adulthood, and valproate or lamotrigine is usually a better alternative than ethosuximide when they have GTC seizures in addition to absence seizures.

Special Considerations

Children represent a special population because the seizure types, epilepsy syndromes, etiologies, and pharmacokinetic responses of children are different from adults. This leads to important dosing differences such as dosing based on body weight rather than absolute amounts (see Table 5). Long-term cosmetic cumulative side effects of phenytoin (Dilantin) make it a poor choice for the chronic treatment of children, especially girls. Children are addressed in the chapter on Epilepsy in Infancy and Childhood, but it is important to recognize that many childhood epilepsies persist into adulthood and may evolve.

The elderly deserve special consideration because they are more likely to have side effects, be on multiple medications, and have hepatic and renal impairment. Seizures beginning in late adult life are always partial seizures from acquired etiologies, especially stroke. Phenytoin is particularly poorly tolerated in the elderly, and in addition, may have a prolonged half-life so that levels are unexpectedly high. Some new AEDs are better tolerated and less likely to cause drug interactions. Gabapentin (Neurontin) is particularly desirable because it has no drug interactions. Oxcarbazepine (Trileptal) and levetiracetam (Keppra) are also usually well tolerated.

Women pose several potential difficulties in selecting an AED. Women with epilepsy have increased rates of infertility as a consequence of intrinsic hormone changes, anovulatory cycles, irregular menstrual cycles, and altered sexuality. This can be compounded by the effects of AEDs, especially valproate (Depakote), which is associated with polycystic ovarian disease. Hysterectomy with bilateral oophorectomy may seem like a reasonable treatment for seizures clustering around the menstrual period, but it is usually ineffective and deprives patients of the protective effects of estrogen. Osteopenia is common in postmenopausal women and is augmented by chronic phenytoin use.

Potential teratogenicity is an important consideration for women of childbearing potential but data in humans is only available for the conventional AEDs. The incidence of birth defects in women taking an AED is approximately 5% to 6%, compared to 1% to 2% in the general population. The rate of birth defects appears to be the same for all conventional AEDs. Most birth defects associated with phenytoin (Dilantin), carbamazepine (Tegretol), and phenobarbital are considered mild or cosmetic, but valproate frequently causes neural tube defects. Folic acid reduces the rate of teratogenicity, especially neural tube defects, and is indicated for women on valproate and is good practice for all women of childbearing potential. Some new AEDs are teratogenic in animal models, but the effects in humans are unknown. It is important to monitor blood levels regularly during and immediately after pregnancy due to significant changes in blood volume and metabolism. AEDs are transmitted to infants via breast milk, but the benefits of breast-feeding are probably greater than any potential harm from AED exposure.

Hepatic disease may impair the ability to clear hepatically metabolized drugs (see Table 3). This is particularly a problem for conventional AEDs, which are all hepatically metabolized. Among the new AEDs, gabapentin (Neurontin) is not hepatically metabolized at all and is not affected even by severe liver disease. The new AEDs are not affected until liver disease is severe. The dose reduction of hepatically metabolized AEDs in hepatically impaired patients is determined by the prolongation of clearance, which is different in each patient. Therefore, no standard dosing recommendations can be made.

Renal disease may impair clearance of AEDs eliminated unchanged by the kidneys. All conventional AEDs are primarily deactivated by hepatic metabolism before urinary elimination of inactive metabolites. Therefore, they are not significantly affected by renal disease until end-stage renal disease, in which case the small amount that is normally excreted unchanged may build up. Some new AEDs, such as gabapentin (Neurontin), levetiracetam (Keppra), oxcarbazepine (Trileptal), and topiramate (Topamax), have a significant portion excreted unchanged by the kidneys and therefore require empiric or calculated dose reduction with renal impairment.

A more significant problem in the treatment of renally impaired patients is the removal of free drug during hemodialysis. The amount of drug removed depends on the free fraction, duration and volume of dialysis, and other factors, so that a predictable change in blood levels cannot be determined. After each hemodialysis session, the blood level and effectiveness must be determined in order to decide how much drug must be given until a steady state of post-dialysis dosing is reached. Phenytoin (Dilantin) is not significantly affected by hemodialysis because only 10% exists in the free dialyzable form but free levels should be monitored. A mild to moderate amount of phenobarbital is removed during dialysis, but if the level falls significantly after dialysis, then a bolus can be given. Changes in valproate (Depakote) dosing are usually not necessary because although 20% is removed by dialysis, the half-life increases by 20%, which compensates. Among new AEDs, gabapentin (Neurontin) is the most severely affected; 60% is removed by hemodialysis, but the half-life becomes nearly infinite so that only very small doses are required once the patient becomes anuric, such as only 300 mg after each dialysis.

Refractory Epilepsy

EVALUATION OF INTRACTABLE SEIZURES

The definition of what constitutes refractory epilepsy has evolved in recent years. In statistical terms, patients who continue to have seizures after trying therapeutic doses of two AEDs are very unlikely to respond to additional AEDs, although some do. The definition is becoming increasingly important because refractory patients should be referred to an epilepsy center for diagnosis and consideration of the many therapeutic options now available, including epilepsy surgery to resect the seizure focus, palliative surgery to reduce the severity of some seizure types, unconventional AEDs, and experimental AEDs.

The evaluation of intractable seizures is dependent on a careful history and physical examination directed at elucidating the seizure type, neuroanatomic site of seizure origin, and the epilepsy syndrome or etiology. The most important diagnostic test is prolonged (24 hours per day) simultaneous video and EEG monitoring to capture seizures. Video/EEG is vitally important to determine that the spells in question are indeed seizures, to define the seizure type, and to localize the site of origin. Video/EEG may need to continue for days or weeks to capture enough spells to make a correct diagnosis. Magnetic resonance imaging of the brain using special acquisition protocols to define fine brain anatomy often reveals abnormalities that are not obvious on routine MRI, especially in the temporal lobe where seizures often arise. Positron emission tomography (PET) may reveal focal hypometabolism in the region of seizure onset. Interictal single-photon emission computed tomography (SPECT) occasionally reveals focal hypoperfusion at the focus. To perform an ictal SPECT scan, the radio tracer is injected within 90 seconds of seizure onset and subsequent scanning often reveals focal hyperperfusion in the region of seizure onset. Magnetic resonance spectroscopy is primarily a research tool but can reveal focal changes in the region of the seizure focus. Neuropsychological testing may demonstrate lateralized or localized deficits.

EPILEPSY SURGERY

Surgery to resect the epilepsy focus is the only method of curing epilepsy available today. Successful surgery is, of course, heavily dependent on correctly localizing the seizure focus. Presurgical evaluation is usually carried out in three phases. Phase 1 consists of extracranial monitoring and the noninvasive tests noted above. If the findings yield a general area from which the seizures arise, but do not pinpoint the exact site of onset, then the patient may proceed to Phase 2, which is intracranial EEG monitoring through electrodes placed on or into the brain. Phase 3 is the removal of the seizure focus. Fortunately, most patients do not require intracranial monitoring now because neuroimaging often identifies an anatomic abnormality to corroborate the EEG findings.

Any area of the brain is a candidate for resection, but in reality the vast majority of patients have temporal lobe epilepsy (TLE) and undergo anterior temporal lobectomy (ATL) to remove the anterior 4 to 5 cm of the temporal lobe containing the hippocampus and amygdala. Approximately 70% of patients are essentially seizure free after ATL, and the risk of stroke or other serious complication is less than 1%. Extratemporal resections are more complicated. The seizure focus must be more precisely localized and electrical brain mapping or other methods must be used to ensure that important brain functions will not be removed during surgery. This usually requires intracranial monitoring. Approximately 50% of patients are essentially seizure free. The risk of complications, such as a motor deficit, is only slightly higher than with ATL. More drastic surgeries, such as hemispherectomy or corpus callosotomy are indicated in special circumstances.

Vagus nerve stimulation is a recently developed novel approach to seizure control. A small generator is placed subcutaneously in the left chest wall and wire electrodes are led to the left vagus nerve. The generator supplies a few seconds of current every few minutes at predetermined settings. Its efficacy in blinded controlled trials is about the same as a new AED; it reduces the frequency of seizures by 50% in about half of the subjects.

The treatment of epilepsy is rapidly changing and more complex than in previous years because there are now 14 AEDs to choose from, technologic advances have made diagnostic tests more useful, and epilepsy surgery is safer and more readily available. A systematic approach yields some basic guidelines for therapy (Table 6).

TABLE 6 General Guidelines for Use of New AEDs

Select an AED by seizure type and epilepsy syndrome
Increase dose to maximum tolerated dose (toxicity) before changing
Substitute one drug at a time in attempt to achieve monotherapy
All new drugs are equally efficacious for partial seizures
Select by side effects, dosing, pharmacokinetics, cost
Refer to an epilepsy center for consideration of surgery if seizures are refractory to two AEDs

EPILEPSY IN INFANTS AND CHILDREN

METHOD OF
Edwin Trevathan, MD, MPH

Seizures are the physical manifestation of a sudden surge of abnormal electrical activity in the cerebral cortex. Up to 50% of children who have a single seizure do not have a recurrence. Epilepsy is operationally defined as two or more seizures, excluding febrile seizures, and is the underlying disorder that predisposes the affected individual to have repeated seizures. Epilepsy among adolescents and adults is discussed in the article "Seizures and Epilepsy in Adolescents and Adults"; additionally, neonatal seizures are not reviewed.

Seizure Semiology and Classification

Seizures are classified based upon their electroencephalogram (EEG) and clinical manifestations at the beginning of the seizure. Seizure classification impacts initial treatment decisions. *Partial seizures* are the clinical manifestations of epileptic discharges restricted to a focal region of cortex. *Simple partial seizures* do not impair consciousness, whereas *complex partial seizures* are associated with impaired consciousness. Secondarily generalized seizures start as partial seizures and then spread to encompass both cerebral hemispheres. Once the seizure is secondarily generalized it clinically mimics a primarily generalized seizure. However, the postictal state may be characterized by focal neurologic findings.

Generalized seizures start over both hemispheres simultaneously. *Absence seizures* are genetic disorders associated with a high rate of spontaneous remission by mid-adolescence, and typically begin in children ages 4 to 10 years. Absence seizures last 3 to 10 seconds, may occur more than 100 times daily in untreated children, and are characterized by a sudden onset of staring, unresponsiveness, and subtle eyelid fluttering, with or without stereotypic hand and arm movements. The child instantly returns to normal upon cessation of the absence seizure. Each absence seizure is time-locked with generalized 3-per-second spike and wave discharge on EEG. *Clonic seizures* are manifested by rhythmic bilaterally synchronous flexion of the arms, rhythmic abdominal contractions, and tonic leg extension with loss of consciousness at the onset of the seizure. *Tonic seizures* last a few seconds, with sudden bilateral stiffening/arching of the trunk and back, extension of the extremities, and cyanosis. *Myoclonic seizures* are characterized by very fast, "lightening-like" often asymmetric jerks of the extremities and trunk. *Atonic seizures* produce instantaneous loss of muscle tone with falls, and usually occur in children with other generalized and/or partial seizures.

New-onset seizure(s) may have reversible and treatable causes that must be recognized and treated promptly in order to reduce the risk of permanent brain injury and death (Table 1). This is particularly true when seizures are caused by central nervous system (CNS) infections such as meningitis and encephalitis, and when seizures are caused by hypoxia or hypoglycemia. Clinicians should first stop the seizure and then quickly determine any treatable causes of the seizure (e.g., hypoglycemia, hyponatremia); do not delay seizure treatment while searching for an etiology. Most children with newly diagnosed seizures have no definable cause for their seizure.

Epilepsy Syndromes

The current classification of epilepsy syndromes is based upon a cluster of signs and symptoms, including seizure type, EEG findings, age at onset of seizures, co-morbid conditions, family history of epilepsy, and structural abnormalities on neuroimaging studies (Table 2). *Localization-related epilepsies* are characterized by partial seizures, and syndromes manifested by *generalized seizures* are *generalized epilepsies. Idiopathic epilepsies* are presumed to have a genetic basis, *cryptogenic epilepsies* have an unknown etiology, and symptomatic epilepsies are symptomatic of any underlying brain disorder (e.g., head injury, encephalitis). Some epilepsy syndromes, such as Lennox-Gastaut syndrome, include both generalized and partial seizures. The diagnosis of specific epilepsy syndromes can help the clinician estimate prognosis and choose treatment.

Febrile Seizures

Febrile seizures usually occur in approximately 2% to 5% of otherwise normal children between the ages of 6 months and 6 years, most of whom only have a single febrile seizure. Approximately 90% to 95% of children with febrile seizures never develop epilepsy (two or more afebrile seizures), but prolonged febrile seizures and febrile status epilepticus are associated with an increased risk of temporal lobe epilepsy. Febrile seizures in susceptible children usually occur within the first 24 hours of the illness, when the temperature may rise rapidly. *Simple febrile seizures* are generalized clonic seizures that usually last less than 1 minute and no more than 5 minutes. Febrile seizures that have clearly focal components, are prolonged, are usually referred to as *complex febrile seizures*. Complex febrile seizures may be associated with a higher risk of future epilepsy.

The evaluation of a first febrile seizure should determine (a) that the seizure has stopped (see status epilepticus discussion) and (b) if the child has an underlying treatable infection. A lumbar puncture must be performed immediately and appropriate treatment administered if meningitis is suspected. Children who have experienced multiple febrile seizures, who had a previous normal cerebrospinal fluid (CSF) exam, and who have normal exams need not suffer lumbar punctures after each brief febrile seizure. Daily antiepileptic drugs (AEDs) do not alter the long-term prognosis. Intermittent phenobarbital during febrile illnesses is not effective. Rectal diazepam (Diastat, 0.5 mg/kg per dose) for prolonged seizures (>5 minutes) is probably preferable to daily phenobarbital (5 mg/kg per day). Antipyretic therapy at the onset of febrile illness may reduce the risk of recurrent febrile seizures in susceptible children.

Treatment of Epilepsy in Infants and Children

The decision to begin an AED must balance the risks and benefits of therapy against the risk of subsequent seizures, including the risk of status epilepticus. Among otherwise normal children who have a single seizure, the overall risk of seizure recurrence is about 50%. Most recurrent seizures occur within 6 months of the first seizure. The risk of recurrence is increased among children with remote symptomatic etiology, abnormal EEGs, previous history of febrile seizures, transient postictal focal neurologic abnormalities, and nocturnal seizures. Treatment is usually not started until after the second seizure, unless the initial seizure is prolonged or thought to pose excessive risk.

The first step in choosing the best treatment for childhood epilepsy is classification of the seizure type(s) being treated. AEDs fall into three categories; those effective against partial seizures, those effective against generalized seizures, and those effective

TABLE 1 Potentially Reversible Causes of New-Onset Seizures

Metabolic	Intoxications	Other
Hyponatremia	Antibiotics (e.g., penicillin, isoniazid, ciprofloxacin [Cipro])	Fever
Hypoglycemia	Anticholinergics (antipsychotics, decongestants, tricyclic antidepressants)	Hypertensive encephalopathy
Hypocalcemia	Acute heavy-metal poisoning (arsenic, lead, mercury, thallium)	Hypoxia ± cerebral ischemia
Uremia	Local anesthetics (lidocaine, cocaine)	Sepsis, meningitis
	Salicylates	
	Theophylline	

TABLE 2 Major Pediatric Epilepsy Syndromes

Epilepsy Syndroms	Age Onset	Seizure Types	EEG Findings	Co-morbid Conditions	Treatment	Prognosis
Localization-Related Epilepsies						
Benign rolandic epilepsy	3-11 years	Partial motor, face, mouth tongue	Central-temporal spikes in sleep	Mild learning disorders	Gabapentin, CBZ (Neurontin)	Good
Benign occipital epilepsy	3-11 years	CPS with visual and motor stereotypic signs	Occipital spikes	Migraine	VPA, CBZ	Good
Mesial temporal epilepsy	5-18 years	CPS with aura, mouth/hand automatisms	Normal or anterior temporal spikes	Memory and emotional dysfunction, risk of SUDEP	CBZ, VPA, LTG, LEV, AEDS for partial seizures	Poor if failure of first 2 AEDs
Nocturnal frontal lobe epilepsy	6-17 years	SPS with tonic posturing or 'thrashing' in sleep	Usually normal between seizures	Risk of LD, impulsivity	CBZ, VPA,LTG, LEV, AEDS for partial seizures	Poor if failure of first 2 AEDs
Supplementary motor epilepsy	7-15 years	SPS, bilateral tonic often out of sleep	Often normal between seizures	Risk of LD, impulsivity	CBZ, VPA, LTG, LEV, AEDS for partial seizures	Poor if failure of first 2 AEDs
Generalized Epilepsies						
Childhood absence epilepsy	3-8 years	Absence seizures without aura or postictal state lasting seconds	3 per second spike and wave time-locked with seizures	None	ETH, LTG, VPA	>50% spontaneously remit; some develop JME
Juvenile myoclonic epilepsy (JME)	7-18 years	Absence, myoclonic, GTC	3-4 per second spike and wave	None	VPA, LTG	No spontaneous remission; most with good seizure control
Myoclonic-astatic epilepsy	2-5 years	Myoclonic, atonic	Spike–wave, polyspikes	LD or MR	VPA, ZON	Variable
Syndromes with Both Generalized and Partial Seizures						
Lennox-Gastaut syndrome	1-9 years	Atonic, tonic, atypical absence, GTC, partial	Slow (≤2 hertz) spike–wave	MR, injuries, status epilepticus	VPA, LTG, TPM, ZON, FBM, clobazam	Very poor; up to 30% die by age 25 years
Severe myoclonic epilepsy of infancy	<12 months	Partial and myoclonic seizures with or without fever	Multifocal spikes and generalized polyspikes	High risk for MR	VPA, TPM, ZON, FBM, stiripentol*	Developmental delays and poor seizure control
Acquired epileptic aphasia (Landau-Kleffner syndrome)	12 months to 5 years	Subclinical ± clinical partial	Bilateral focal spikes	Aphasia	Prednisone[1], VPA, ACTH[1]	Poor
Special Syndromes						
Febrile seizures	6 months to 6 years	GTC	Usually normal	None	Usually no treatment; rectal diazepam (Diastat) for prolonged seizures	3%-5% develop epilepsy
Infantile spasms	2-12 mo	Myoclonic	Hypsarrhythmia	MR	ACTH[1], prednisone[1], vigabatrin*, TPM, ZON	High risk for MR

[1]Not FDA approved for this indication.
*Investigational drug in the United States.
Abbreviations: ACTH = adrenocorticotrophic hormone; AED = antiepileptic drug; CBZ = carbamazepine (Tegretol); CPS = complex partial seizures; ETH = ethosuximide (Zarontin); FBM = felbamate (Felbatol); GTCS = generalized tonic–clonic seizure; LD = learning disability; LTG = lamotrigine (Lamictal); LEV = levetiracetam (Keppra); MR = mental retardation; SPS = simple partial seizure; TPM = topiramate (Topamax); VPA = valproic acid (Depakote); ZON = zonisamide (Zonegran)

against both generalized and partial seizures (Table 3). Marketed AEDs effective for partial seizures usually have the same odds of efficacy when administered to newly diagnosed children with partial epilepsy. Therefore, the choice of the first AED should be based upon (a) the anticipated side-effect profile of the AED; (b) interaction of the AED with any concomitant medications; (c) acceptability of the required dose schedule and form (liquid, sprinkles, chewable tablet, etc.) to the patient and family; and (d) cost. Most new AEDs do not have proven advantages over the older and less-expensive AEDs proven in clinical trials among newly diagnosed patients. However, the cognitive effects of phenobarbital and the gingival hypertrophy of phenytoin (Dilantin) should be avoided. Phenobarbital and phenytoin are not usually acceptable as first-line AEDs for epilepsy in developed countries.

Valproate (Depakote), lamotrigine (Lamictal), topiramate (Topamax), zonisamide (Zonegran), and probably felbamate (Felbatol) are effective against both partial and generalized seizures. Among children with both partial and generalized seizures, initial treatment with one of these broad-spectrum AEDs is prudent.

Status Epilepticus

Status epilepticus (SE) is an emergency and is a seizure lasting more than 30 minutes or a series of shorter seizures of a total duration of more than 30 minutes without return to normal between seizures. Prolonged seizures and SE are associated with cardiac and respiratory dysfunction and an increased risk of death. Because almost all seizures that stop spontaneously last less than 5 minutes, any seizure duration of 5 to 10 minutes should be treated as SE (Figure 1). The treatment response to SE should be organized and follow a systematic treatment protocol for optimal results. The most common cause of SE failing to respond to the first intravenous medication is an inadequate dose. Therefore, the current recommendations include administration of an intravenous (IV) (or rectal if IV access is not present) benzodiazepine, followed by a long-acting maintenance AED, typically fosphenytoin (Cerebyx). If the first dose of fosphenytoin at 20 mg phenytoin equivalent (PE)/kg is ineffective, then another 10 mg PE/kg should be given prior to administering the second AED (usually phenobarbital). Phenytoin and fosphenytoin have been reported to exacerbate the generalized seizures associated with juvenile myoclonic epilepsy (JME; see Table 2). Therefore, patients with JME and patients in absence SE should be treated with intravenous valproate (Depacon; see Figure 1).

Up to 25% of patients who are thought to be postictal after cessation of tonic–clonic SE are actually still in nonconvulsive SE (usually complex partial seizures). Prolonged postictal states should trigger an urgent neurology consult with consideration of emergency EEG if the neurologist is uncertain regarding the possibility of ongoing seizures.

General Concepts of Antiepileptic Drug Side Effects

In general, AED side effects can be divided into three broad categories: serious idiosyncratic side effects, dose-related side effects, and teratogenic side effects (Table 4). Teratogenic side effects are reviewed in the article "Seizures and Epilepsy in Adolescents and Adults." *Idiosyncratic side effects* are rare, often serious, and are usually unrelated to the dose. Idiosyncratic side effects may not be reversible upon withdrawal of the drug; therefore, patients take the risk of idiosyncratic side effects when the AED therapy is initiated. The most commonly cited idiosyncratic side effects are bone marrow suppression (aplastic anemia, agranulocytosis) and liver toxicity. *Bone marrow suppression* is most commonly cited in association with carbamazepine (Tegretol) and felbamate (Felbatol), but may occur rarely with most AEDs. Valproate (Depakote) associated idiosyncratic *liver toxicity* among children younger than age 2 years has received much attention. Some experts doubt that this association is causal, and suggest that many (if not most) of these young children who died with valproate-associated liver failure had undiagnosed mitochondrial disorders—children who today are more likely to be diagnosed and either avoid valproate therapy or have their liver failure attributed to their underlying metabolic disorder.

Maintaining good hydration may reduce the risk of kidney stones associated with zonisamide (Zonegran), topiramate (Topamax), and acetazolamide (Diamox). Topiramate is also associated with expressive language difficulties in some children, and may rarely cause closed-angle glaucoma; complaints of eye pain and/or visual loss should prompt immediate ophthalmologic evaluation.

Most routinely used AEDs, with the likely exception of lamotrigine (Lamictal), are associated with osteopenia after several years of use. The frequency of AED-associated osteopenia in childhood is unknown, but future treatment guidelines will likely suggest monitoring for osteopenia and treatment with calcium supplementation for children on long-term AEDs.

Rash is more often associated with AED treatment in children than in adults, probably because children have more rashes than adults. Rashes associated with phenytoin (Dilantin), carbamazepine (Tegretol), and lamotrigine (Lamictal) occur in approximately 1% of children treated. Rarely, serious life-threatening rash, Stevens-Johnson syndrome, or toxic epidermal necrolysis, occurs with AEDs. Rigorous adherence to the lamotrigine slow dose-escalation schedule recommended in the package insert must be followed to reduce excessive risk of serious rash.

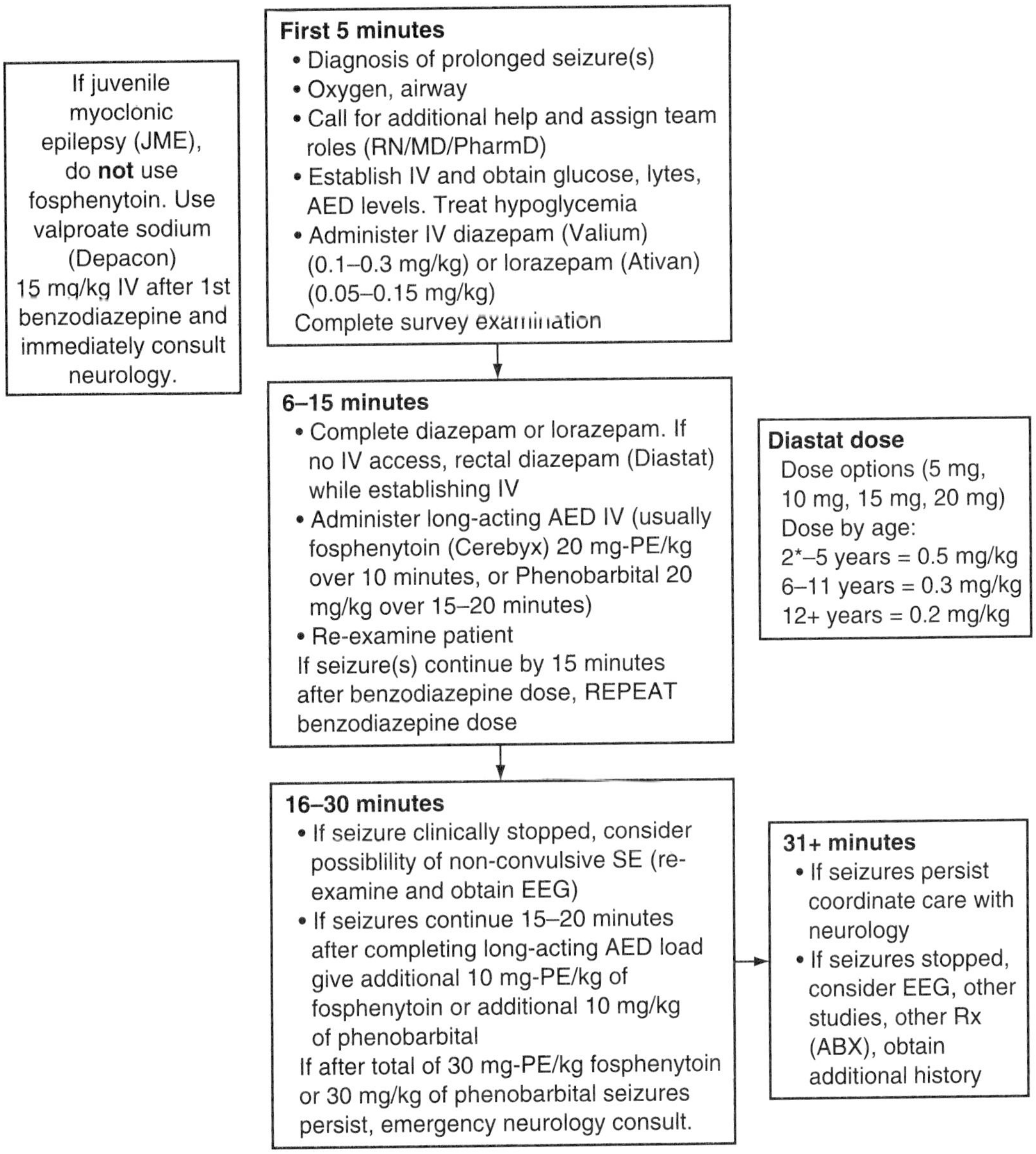

If juvenile myoclonic epilepsy (JME), do **not** use fosphenytoin. Use valproate sodium (Depacon) 15 mg/kg IV after 1st benzodiazepine and immediately consult neurology.

First 5 minutes
- Diagnosis of prolonged seizure(s)
- Oxygen, airway
- Call for additional help and assign team roles (RN/MD/PharmD)
- Establish IV and obtain glucose, lytes, AED levels. Treat hypoglycemia
- Administer IV diazepam (Valium) (0.1–0.3 mg/kg) or lorazepam (Ativan) (0.05–0.15 mg/kg)

Complete survey examination

6–15 minutes
- Complete diazepam or lorazepam. If no IV access, rectal diazepam (Diastat) while establishing IV
- Administer long-acting AED IV (usually fosphenytoin (Cerebyx) 20 mg-PE/kg over 10 minutes, or Phenobarbital 20 mg/kg over 15–20 minutes)
- Re-examine patient

If seizure(s) continue by 15 minutes after benzodiazepine dose, REPEAT benzodiazepine dose

Diastat dose
Dose options (5 mg, 10 mg, 15 mg, 20 mg)
Dose by age:
2*–5 years = 0.5 mg/kg
6–11 years = 0.3 mg/kg
12+ years = 0.2 mg/kg

16–30 minutes
- If seizure clinically stopped, consider possiblility of non-convulsive SE (re-examine and obtain EEG)
- If seizures continue 15–20 minutes after completing long-acting AED load give additional 10 mg-PE/kg of fosphenytoin or additional 10 mg/kg of phenobarbital

If after total of 30 mg-PE/kg fosphenytoin or 30 mg/kg of phenobarbital seizures persist, emergency neurology consult.

31+ minutes
- If seizures persist coordinate care with neurology
- If seizures stopped, consider EEG, other studies, other Rx (ABX), obtain additional history

PE = phenytoin equivalents
* = exceeding manufacturer age recommendation

FIGURE 1 Treatment of status epilepticus.

Dose-related side effects of most AEDs are similar (see Table 4). Levels of most AEDs cross an individual patient-specific threshold that causes sedation or difficulty concentrating, problems with gait instability, and often nausea and dysphoria. Children may also experience rather subtle school difficulties that are manifestations of dose-related AED side effects, although most complaints of learning problems among children with epilepsy and "therapeutic" levels of AEDs are a result of an underlying learning disorder, unrecognized seizures, or both. Phenobarbital, which is almost always sedating among adults and older children, may cause paradoxical "driven" hyperactivity and agitation in young children.

AED serum level monitoring is a useful tool with some AEDs, but clinicians should remember that the normal serum AED values (a) assume that the level obtained is a trough level and (b) are not biologic normal values, but are the statistical normals of serum values from selected patients without overt dose-related side effects. Stopping or holding an AED in a patient without clinical side effects or other significant lab abnormalities because the AED level is elevated is usually a mistake, and places the patient at increased risk of prolonged seizures.

Nonpharmacologic Therapies

Children who do not respond to routine AEDs should be referred to a major pediatric epilepsy center to determine if they are candidates for other

TABLE 3 Antiepileptic Drug Use in Children

Drug (Year of Availability)	Efficacy	Formulation	Doses per Day	Starting Dose (mg/kg/d)	Length of Time to Maintenance	Maintenance Dose (mg/kg/d)	Blood Level (mg/dL)
Phenobarbital (1912)	Partial, GTC	Suspension (20 mg/5 mL) Tabs (15 mg, 30 mg, 60 mg, 100 mg)	qd-bid	3-5	Immediate	3-8	15-40
Phenytoin (1938) (Dilantin)	Partial	Suspension (125 mg/5 mL) Chewable tabs (50 mg) Capsules (30 mg, 100 mg)	qd-tid	4-7	Immediate	4-7	10-20
Primidone (1949) (Mysoline)	Partial	Suspension (250 mg/5 mL) Tabs (50 mg, 250 mg)	bid-tid	5	Average (3-6 weeks)	15	PRM: 4-12 PB: 15-40
Ethosuximide (1958) (Zarontin)	Absence	Suspension (250 mg/5 mL) Caps (250 mg)	qd-bid	10	Average (3-4 weeks)	15-40	40-120
Carbamazepine (1968) (Carbatrol, Tegretol)	Partial	Suspension (100 mg/5 mL) Chewable tabs (100 mg) XR Tabs (100 mg, 200 mg, 400 mg) Sprinkles (100 mg, 200 mg, 300 mg)	bid-tid	5-10	Average (4 weeks)	10-30	6-12
Valproate (1978) (Depakote, Depakene)	Broad spectrum	Suspension (250 mg/5 mL) Tabs (125 mg, 250 mg, 500 mg) ER tabs (250 mg, 500 mg)	bid-tid	10-20	Average (4 weeks)	30-60	50-150
Felbamate (1993) (Felbatol)	Broad spectrum	Suspension (600 mg/5 mL) Tabs (400 mg, 600 mg)	bid-qid	15-20	Average (2-4 weeks)	20-80	18-45*
Gabapentin (1993) (Neurontin)	Partial	Suspension (250 mg/5 mL) Capsules (100 mg, 300 mg, 400 mg) Tabs (600 mg, 800 mg)	tid-qid	15-20	Average (2 weeks)	30-50	5-15*
Lamotrigine (1994) (Lamictal)	Broad spectrum	Chewable tab (2 mg, 5 mg, 25 mg) Tabs (25 mg, 100 mg, 150 mg, 200 mg)	bid	0.2 (with VPA) 0.5 (with CBZ)	Very slow (2-4 months) Slow (2 months)	1-6 5-15	2-20*
Topiramate (1996) (Topamax)	Broad spectrum	Tabs (25 mg, 100 mg, 200 mg) Sprinkle (15 mg, 25 mg)	bid	1-2	Slow (1-3 months)	5-10 (up to 30 if age <3 years)	2-25
Levetiracetam (1999) (Keppra)	Partial	Liquid (500 mg/5 mL) Tabs (250 mg, 500 mg, 750 mg)	bid	10	Average (2-4 weeks)	20-80	20-60*
Oxcarbazepine (2000) (Trileptal)	Partial	Suspension (300 mg/5 mL) Tabs (150 mg, 300 mg, 600 mg)	bid	8-15	Average (3-4 weeks)	20-40	5-50*
Zonisamide (2000) (Zonegran)	Broad spectrum	Capsules (25 mg, 50 mg, 100 mg)	qd-bid	2-4	Average (2-4 weeks)	5-12	10-40

*Relationship between efficacy, dose-related side effects, and blood levels not well-established.

Abbreviations: bid = twice daily; Caps = capsules; CBZ = carbamazepine; ER = extended release; GTC = generalized tonic–clonic seizure; PB = phenobarbital; PRM = primidone; qd = every day; qid = four times a day; tid = three times a day; VPA = valproic acid; XR = extended release.

TABLE 4 Side Effects of Antiepileptic Drugs

Drug	Dose-Dependent	Often Idiosyncratic
Phenobarbital	Lethargy, dizziness, ataxia Cognitive disturbance Hyperactivity, emotional disturbance Sleep disturbance, headache	Rash Megaloblastic anemia Liver toxicity
Phenytoin (Dilantin)	Lethargy, dizziness, ataxia, nystagmus Coarse facies, hirsutism, gingival hyperplasia Osteomalacia	Rash Blood dyscrasias, variable Liver toxicity Lymphadenopathy
Primidone (Mysoline)	Lethargy, dizziness, ataxia Behavioral changes	Rash Megaloblastic anemia, leukopenia
Ethosuximide (Zarontin)	Lethargy, dizziness, ataxia, headache Behavioral changes Nausea, vomiting, stomach pain, hiccups	Rash Blood dyscrasias, variable (rare) Systemic lupus-like syndrome
Carbamazepine (Carbatrol, Tegretol)	Lethargy, dizziness, ataxia, nystagmus, diplopia Nausea, vomiting, abdominal pain Liver toxicity Hyponatremia	Rash Blood dyscrasias, aplastic anemia
Valproate (Depakene, Depakote)	Lethargy, dizziness, ataxia, headache Thrombocytopenia Nausea, vomiting, weight gain Alopecia, tremor	Rash Liver toxicity Pancreatitis
Felbamate (Felbatol)	Ataxia, headache, insomnia Anorexia, abdominal pain	Liver toxicity Aplastic anemia
Gabapentin (Neurontin)	Lethargy, dizziness, ataxia Nausea, vomiting, weight gain	Rash
Lamotrigine (Lamictal)	Lethargy, dizziness, ataxia, diplopia Headache	Rash
Topiramate (Topamax)	Lethargy, dizziness, ataxia, nystagmus Cognitive slowing, language impairment Weight loss Kidney stones	Acute-angle glaucoma
Levetiracetam (Keppra)	Behavioral changes, psychosis Lethargy, dizziness, ataxia	Rash
Oxcarbazepine (Trileptal)	Lethargy, dizziness, ataxia, headache Nausea Hyponatremia	Rash (30% cross-react with carbamazepine)
Zonisamide (Zonegran)	Lethargy, dizziness, ataxia Psychomotor slowing, difficulty concentrating Nausea, anorexia Kidney stones	Rash Oligohidrosis/hyperthermia

therapies, including vagal nerve stimulation (VNS), the ketogenic diet, or resective epilepsy surgery. Among highly selected children who have failed two or more AEDs, epilepsy surgery offers much higher odds of seizure freedom (50% to 80%) than VNS or continued AED trials (odds <10% seizure freedom). VNS may reduce seizure frequency without AED side effects. The ketogenic diet, when administered by an experienced multidisciplinary team that includes dietitians, may significantly reduce seizure freedom among children ages 1 to 10 years who fail routine AEDs.

ATTENTION DEFICIT HYPERACTIVITY DISORDER (ADHD)

METHOD OF

Anouk Scheres, PhD, and
F. Xavier Castellanos, MD

Attention deficit hyperactivity disorder (ADHD), as defined in the fourth edition of the *Diagnostic and Statistical Manual of Mental Disorders* (DSM-IV) of the American Psychiatric Association, is differentiated into three subtypes, predominantly inattentive, predominantly hyperactive/impulsive, and a combination of the two. The diagnosis relies on subjective reports of developmentally inappropriate behavior in the domains of inattention, hyperactivity, and/or impulsiveness that have been present for at least 6 months, and in more than one setting, such as school and home. At least some of the symptoms must be associated with impairment before the age of 7 years, and symptoms must clearly interfere with social, academic, or occupational functioning. The diagnosis does not apply if the symptoms can be better accounted for by a pervasive developmental disorder, schizophrenia, or other psychotic disorders, or by any other specific mental disorder.

The prevalence of ADHD in school-age children is at least 3% to 5%, although some estimates exceed 10%. ADHD is diagnosed more frequently in males than females, with ratios ranging between 2:1 and 9:1 depending on the mode of ascertainment. The diagnosis of ADHD is reached with more difficulty at the extremes of the age distribution. For example, the behavior of preschool-age children is more variable than that of older children, and attention demands on younger children are not as high, which makes it hard to discern attention deficits in very young children. Numerous studies demonstrate that ADHD persists into adulthood, although estimates vary from 4% to 80%. Applying the diagnosis of ADHD to adults is problematic, as the criteria were developed for and field tested with children and adolescents 6 to 14 years of age. Furthermore, retrospective reports of symptoms are unreliable. In practice, many adults are diagnosed after their own children have been determined to have ADHD.

Children are occasionally diagnosed only with ADHD, but 60% to 80% are found to have another disorder as well. The possible co-morbid conditions generally include oppositional defiant disorder, conduct disorder, learning disabilities, and tic disorders. Anxiety or mood disorders may also be present. In some cases, juvenile bipolar (manic–depressive) disorder may initially present as severe ADHD. ADHD also represents a risk for later drug and alcohol abuse, particularly when conduct disorder is also present.

Assessment

There is no objective test for diagnosing ADHD. Rather, the diagnosis is based exclusively on the history of symptoms, derived optimally from more than one informant, such as a parent and a teacher. Children with ADHD are rarely aware of the full impact of their symptoms and their direct assessment is mainly aimed at ruling out alternative diagnoses, such as pervasive developmental disorders or psychotic disorders, and determining whether or not tic disorders or obsessive–compulsive disorder might be present. Standardized parent and teacher rating scales are commonly used to provide a rapid screen for the symptoms associated with ADHD.

The most frequently used questionnaires include:

- The *Child Behavior Checklist*
- The *Teacher Report Form*
- The *Revised Conners Parent and Teacher Rating Scales*
- The *Swanson, Nolan and Pelham (SNAP) Teacher and Parent Rating Scales* (may be downloaded from www.adhd.net)

The *Child Behavior Checklist* and *Teacher Report Form* differ from the others in that they are designed to stratify "externalizing behaviors," such as hyperactivity and aggression, and "internalizing behaviors" that are related to anxiety and mood concerns along a continuum from normal to abnormal, and they are not linked to specific psychiatric diagnoses. They are in wide use around the world and serve as an effective screening tool as well as a tool to assist researchers comparing samples cross-culturally. Conners, SNAP, and similar scales are linked to the *DSM-IV* criteria for ADHD—oppositional defiant disorder and conduct disorder. Raters are asked to indicate how each symptom applies to a child on a 4-point scale, ranging from "not at all" to "very much."

While rating scales are an economical and efficient manner of measuring the severity of behavioral symptoms, at least as rated by observers, they do not suffice for a diagnostic evaluation. The most comprehensive evaluations, such as those performed in research clinics, also use structured or semistructured psychiatric interviews. In structured interviews the interviewer does not interpret the informant's response. In semistructured interviews, interpretation by a clinically astute interviewer is required. Highly structured interviews are more reliable but may be less valid, and semistructured interviews tend to be more valid but less reliable. Structured or semistructured interviews are rarely used in clinical practice, but the goals of reviewing the full range of disruptive behavior disorders, and assessing for the presence of co-morbid learning disorders (mood and anxiety disorders, substance use and abuse, high-risk behaviors), and excluding pervasive developmental disorders and psychotic disorders should be met. Formal psychoeducational evaluation alerts the clinician to the presence of co-morbid learning disorders, which are found in 25% to 40% of children with ADHD, and their extent. Such evaluations should also highlight the individual's cognitive strengths, as those may be easily overlooked. In-person evaluation of the child cannot either confirm or refute a diagnosis of ADHD. However, such examination is generally necessary to assess for the presence of tic disorders, to confirm the social dexterity of the child and thus exclude pervasive developmental disorders, and to probe for the presence of anxiety and mood disorders, including depression, and obsessive–compulsive disorder. It also serves crucially to initiate the therapeutic alliance.

Treatment

Treatment of ADHD can be divided into two categories, pharmacologic (with psychostimulant drugs being the first choice) and psychosocial/behavioral treatments. Neither type of treatment seems to carry over; when treatment stops, the effects on symptoms also stop. The Multimodal Treatment Study of ADHD (MTA) in 579 children with combined-type ADHD compared:

- The effect of medication treatment (mainly psychostimulants, with methylphenidate [Ritalin] being the drug of first choice)
- Intensive behavioral treatments
- The combination of the two
- Community care (which consisted mostly of medication treatment provided by community mental health providers chosen by the parents)

Children in all groups showed reduction of core ADHD symptoms; although medication treatment and combined treatment were equally effective, both were more effective than behavioral treatment alone or community care.

These data suggest that for most children with combined-type ADHD, carefully conducted medication management is likely to be the most cost-effective manner of reducing ADHD symptoms as rated by parents and teachers. The study also demonstrates that medication management in typical community settings produces suboptimal benefits, perhaps because of underdosing, insufficient monitoring, and lack of regular feedback from teachers.

Perhaps not surprisingly, the MTA data continue to provide support for a range of approaches to treatment selection. For many children, psychosocial interventions provided appreciable benefit, and were rated as more acceptable than medication by parents, even when medication produced greater quantitative benefits. Children with a greater burden of risk factors or higher rates of co-morbidity tended to respond best to the combination of optimal medication management and state-of-the-art psychosocial interventions. Unfortunately, such interventions are still mostly unavailable outside the rarefied context of research studies. Thus the challenge to clinicians is how to approximate the effectiveness of optimally delivered treatment within the constraints of usual practice settings. The absence of definitive guidelines regarding optimal treatment means that the parents, along with their child, depending on the child's age, are the ones who select treatment regimens. It is the clinician's task to provide the parents (and preadolescents or adolescents) with relevant information about the known effects of treatments, along with an informed perspective, which can form the basis for collaborative decisions.

PHARMACOLOGIC TREATMENT

The three primary types of medications used to treat ADHD are the psychostimulants, nonstimulant noradrenergic reuptake blockers, and α-agonist antihypertensive agents. Although the specific molecular mechanisms of action differ, all the stimulants increase synaptic levels of dopamine and norepinephrine. Nonstimulants include the tricyclic antidepressants[1], which are now rarely prescribed because of concerns of cardiac toxicity, and the new noradrenergic reuptake inhibitor atomoxetine (Strattera). The antihypertensive agents clonidine (Catapres)[1] and guanfacine (Tenex)[1] also affect noradrenergic neurotransmission via a different mechanism. Methylphenidate (MPH) (Ritalin, Concerta, Metadate CD, Ritalin LA) remains the most common pharmacologic treatment for children with ADHD (Tables 1 and 2). Therapeutic doses of methylphenidate block the dopamine and norepinephrine transporters and result in an increase of synaptic dopamine and norepinephrine. Other psychostimulants used are dextroamphetamine (Dexedrine and Dexedrine Spansules), a mixture of amphetamine salts (Adderall and Adderall XR), and pemoline (Cylert) (see Tables 1 to 3). These psychostimulants are equally efficacious in group comparisons, although not all individuals respond equally to the different types of stimulants. On average, more than 70% of individuals with ADHD are classified as partial or full responders when treated with methylphenidate or one of the amphetamines. When the other type of stimulant is administered, the total response rate increases to more than 90%. Pemoline is now rarely prescribed because of the potential for fatal hepatotoxicity. Placebo response rates vary by study, but are generally between 10% and 20%. A positive response to a stimulant does not confirm the diagnosis of ADHD, as children and adults without ADHD have been shown to also demonstrate improvements in attention and decreases in locomotor activity.

[1]Not FDA approved for this indication.

TABLE 1 Immediate-Release Stimulants for Treatment of Attention Deficit Hyperactivity Disorder

Drug	Doses (mg)	Typical Duration	Schedule
MPH (Ritalin, Metadate, generic)	5, 10, 20	3-4 h	bid-tid
d-MPH (Focalin)	2.5, 5, 10	3-4 h	bid-tid
d-Amphetamine (Dexedrine, generic)	5, 10	4-8 h	qd-bid
d,l-Amphetamine (Adderall, generic)	5, 7.5, 10, 12.5, 15, 20, 30	4-8 h	qd-bid

Abbreviations: bid = two times per day; MPH = methylphenidate; qd = every day; tid = three times per day.

TABLE 2 Extended-Release Methylphenidate for Treatment of Attention Deficit Hyperactivity Disorder

Drug	Method	Immediate Release	Extended Release	Typical Duration
Ritalin SR (20 mg) Metadate SR (10-20 mg)	100% wax matrix	Minimal	More sustained than immediate release	<5 h
Concerta ER (18, 27, 36, 54 mg)	Osmotic system	22% overcoat	78%	10-12 h
Metadate CD (20 mg)	Beads; can sprinkle	30%	70%	8 h
Ritalin LA (20, 30, 40 mg)	Beads; can sprinkle	≈50%	≈50%	8 h

The most notable development over the past several years has been the marketing of long-acting formulations of methylphenidate (Concerta, Metadate CD, and Ritalin LA) and amphetamine (Dexedrine Spansules and Adderall XR). These once-a-day formulations use a variety of different drug delivery systems to extend their effects. Concerta uses an osmotic release system that pumps drug out of the capsule over 10 hours to achieve up to 12 hours of efficacy. The remaining long-acting compounds all use beads that dissolve at different rates once swallowed. Two of the methylphenidate formulations (Metadate CD and Ritalin LA) are designed to provide approximately 8 hours of efficacy. Thus these forms may require a second dose for late afternoon coverage. The long-acting amphetamines are generally only given once per day because their plasma half-lives are up to three times longer than that of methylphenidate. For these reasons, long-acting amphetamines are the most likely compounds to produce substantial suppression of appetite and decreased ability to fall asleep. Finally, the manufacturer of Ritalin has also marketed the *d*-isomer under the brand name Focalin. The chief advantage seems to be that the dosages administered are half those of the racemic parent compound.

Despite the large number of options, many clinicians continue to begin treatment with one of the methylphenidate formulations. The immediate-release methylphenidate formulation is bioequivalent, but many physicians are starting with one of the branded long-acting formulations such as Concerta, Metadate CD, or Ritalin LA. The first of these lasts the longest, providing up to 12 hours of benefit compared to double-blind placebo. However, it comes as a rigid capsule in a limited range of doses (18, 27, 36, or 54 mg). Although higher doses are not yet FDA approved, many adolescents or adults require 72 mg per day. Besides differing in duration of effect, the three formulations differ somewhat in the proportion of methylphenidate that is available for immediate release once swallowed. Concerta has the lowest proportion at 22% of the total dose. By contrast, Metadate CD provides 30% immediate released, and 70% released 4 hours later; and Ritalin LA is designed to release 50% immediately and 50% 4 hours later.

The mixture of *d*- and *l*-amphetamine known as Adderall XR is one of the most commonly prescribed stimulants. It and the long-acting Dexedrine Spansules tend to last much longer than the methylphenidates, and they also tend to have stronger effects on the noradrenergic system.

One of the most interesting developments is the introduction of atomoxetine (Strattera). This selective noradrenergic reuptake inhibitor is significantly more effective than placebo for the treatment of ADHD in children, adolescents, and adults; and it is the first drug approved by the FDA for treating ADHD in adults. Because the drug does not affect striatal dopamine levels, it does not have the same potential to produce substance abuse as the stimulants, and it is not controlled by the Drug Enforcement Administration, as are all the stimulants. Studies by the pharmaceutical company have reported equivalent efficacy to methylphenidate, but this does not seem to match the perception of clinicians in practice. However, Strattera is unquestionably now the first choice for anyone with ADHD and a history of substance abuse. It is also worth considering for individuals with ADHD and a tic disorder such as Tourette's disorder. Because of the potential for gastrointestinal adverse effects, which are generally mild and transient, atomoxetine should be titrated upward more slowly than the stimulants. Interestingly, despite a plasma half-life of less than 6 hours, many individuals seem to be able to take Strattera only once a day. Dosages should be started at no more than 0.5 mg/kg per day for up to 1 week, and increased at weekly intervals until effects are obtained or to a maximum of 1.4 mg/kg per day in children, or to a maximum of 80 mg per day

TABLE 3 Extended-Release Amphetamines for Treatment of Attention Deficit Hyperactivity Disorder

Drug	Method	Immediate Release	Extended Release	Typical Duration	Comments
Dexedrine Spansules (5,10,15 mg)	Beads	≈1/3	≈2/3	8-13	Excretion $t_{1/2}$ >10 h for all amphetamines
Adderall XR (5, 10, 15, 20, 25, 30 mg)	Beads	≈50%	≈50%	12+	Absorption delayed by high-fat breakfast

in those who weigh more than 70 kg. Benefits have been reported for both inattention and hyperactivity/impulsivity symptoms. Additionally, Strattera appears to be effective for improving frustration tolerance and decreasing irritability.

Clonidine (Catapres)[1] and guanfacine (Tenex)[1] are α_2 agonists that are also occasionally used for the treatment of ADHD, although rarely as monotherapy. Clonidine is strongly sedating, and is useful for individuals who have difficulty going to sleep, although care must be taken to monitor potential rebound effects when only bedtime dosing regimens are used. Physicians need to remember that clonidine tablets are 0.1 mg each; usual total daily doses are below 0.25 mg per day. Guanfacine is more selective and consequently much less sedating in low doses (<2 mg per day). Some individuals seem to benefit from even lower doses (as little as 0.5 mg per day) when supplementing a stimulant, although there are no controlled trials to guide such adjunctive treatment.

Some physicians use a range of other options for treating ADHD including bupropion (Wellbutrin)[1] and venlafaxine (Effexor XR)[1]. However, given the wide range of other options, there is much less reason to use these off-label approaches.

Once a drug and a dose are proven to be efficacious in a child, it is important to re-evaluate the effect of the drug regularly (at least once per year)—Is the drug still having a positive effect on the child's behavior, and is medication treatment still needed, or does the dose need to be changed? Especially in adolescents with ADHD, some of the symptoms could decrease naturally without drug use, and therefore a period without medication is recommended in order to reassess the need for medication management. It is also an important means of maintaining the therapeutic alliance with adolescents.

BEHAVIORAL TREATMENT

In addition to medication treatment, behavioral treatment should always be considered. Parents find behavioral treatments intrinsically more satisfying than medications, even though the benefits may not be as large. Although most ADHD can be ascribed to neurobiologic causes, parents and teachers can play an important role in managing the behaviors, or in making them worse. Clinics that specialize in ADHD typically offer parent education classes or groups, which may also be available through parent support groups such as Children and Adults with Attention Deficit Disorder (CHADD).

Child-Focused Behavioral Treatment

Cognitive training and social skills training have been extensively tried in children with ADHD with little meaningful effect on social behaviors or academic achievement. Intensive summer treatment programs are sometimes available and combine intensive behavioral management techniques with the socialization of summer camps. In general, the short-term improvements in summer treatment programs can be large, but evidence is lacking regarding their long-term benefits, as is the case for all interventions for ADHD.

Parent Training

Some degree of parent training is important, regardless of whether the primary treatment is through medications or through behavioral techniques. Typically, parent training programs involve 10 or so group sessions that focus on teaching parents how to manage the behavior of their children. These techniques include setting up school and home daily report cards, rewarding and ignoring the child's behavior, learning how to give effective commands to children, learning how to encourage compliance with instructions, and learning how to use token economies and time-out as a consequence of negative behavior. One of the most important goals of parent training is to help parents to not take their child's ADHD behaviors as personal affronts, and to recalibrate their expectations based on the slower maturation rate of most ADHD children. Such reframing can decrease critical or negative expressed emotion on the part of parents about their children, which seems to mediate many of the poor outcomes of ADHD.

Teacher Consultation

Problem behaviors and situations should be discussed with the child's teacher. Teachers are the most effective observers of the symptoms of ADHD, and of the improvement in symptoms with treatment. They can also notice adverse effects that may be missed by parents and clinicians. Unfortunately, the availability of long-acting medications has made it possible for parents to avoid informing the school and their child's teacher about the diagnosis of ADHD and its treatment. While protection of the child's confidentiality is important, much can be lost when the perspective and insights of an experienced teacher are not available.

When a good working relationship is established amongst parents, teachers, and clinicians, behavioral control can be greatly supported by using a daily report card coupled with home-based rewards, or by the use of a token system in order to reinforce desired behavior within the classroom. During teacher consultation, teachers are advised about several issues such as classroom structure and rules, task demands, clear commands, rewarding and ignoring behavior, individualizing task instructions, token economies, time-out, and others.

ADHD is a common behavioral disorder that needs careful diagnostic assessment, including the use of validated questionnaires and thorough interviews to determine the current and past behavior of the child.

[1]Not FDA approved for this indication.

Information should always be obtained from multiple sources, including parent, child, and teacher reports. ADHD frequently co-occurs with other conduct disorders, (anxiety, learning disorders), and these possible co-morbid conditions also require attention by the clinician. Treatment for ADHD should involve a combination of carefully evaluating the efficacy of pharmacologic treatment (long-acting psychostimulant drugs being the first choice), and behavioral intervention (parent training and teacher consultation), depending on the individual child.

GILLES DE LA TOURETTE SYNDROME

METHOD OF

Ruth Dowling Bruun, MD

Gilles de la Tourette syndrome, more commonly known as Tourette's syndrome (TS) or Tourette's disorder in the United States, is a genetically transmitted, neuropsychiatric disorder. While the diagnostic criteria adhere strictly to characteristics of the movements involved, TS is generally recognized as a heterogeneous disorder, frequently associated with attention-deficit hyperactivity disorder, obsessive–compulsive disorder, and learning disabilities as well as emotional symptoms such as severe mood swings, depression, anxiety, and aggressive outbursts. As such, TS truly bridges the fields of neurology and psychiatry and, in many cases, treatment of the behavioral symptoms may be far more difficult to treat than the tics.

As there is no biologic marker for TS, the diagnosis must be made by observations and a thorough history of symptoms. The *Diagnostic and Statistical Manual of Mental Disorders,* fourth edition, text revision (*DSM-IV-TR*), published by the American Psychiatric Association has set forth criteria for the diagnosis as follows:

- Both multiple motor and one or more vocal tics have been present at some time during the illness, although not necessarily concurrently.
- The tics occur many times a day, usually in bouts, nearly every day or intermittently throughout a period of more than 1 year, and during this period there is never a tic-free period of more than 3 consecutive months.
- The onset is before 18 years of age.
- The disturbance is not caused by the direct physiologic effects of a substance (e.g., stimulants) or a general medical condition (e.g., Huntington's disease or postviral encephalitis).

It should be noted that there is no mention of coprolalia (involuntary utterance of socially unacceptable words and/or phrases) in these criteria. Although coprolalia may be the best known symptom of TS, only a small percentage of people with TS will manifest it. Typical tics are rapid, repetitive, nonrhythmic, meaningless, stereotyped movements or vocalizations. There may also be dystonic, sustained movements, sensations described as "sensory tics," and complex movements that appear to fall somewhere between being tics and obsessive–compulsive symptoms (i.e., the need to do a tic a certain number of times or in a certain way). Tics typically wax and wane in intensity and change in character over time. They are often exacerbated by stress, anxiety or excitement.

When making a diagnosis of TS, it is important to ask about symptoms associated with attention-deficit disorder (ADHD), obsessive–compulsive disorder (OCD), explosive temper outbursts, and other evidences of poor impulse control. If the patient is a child, the possibility of learning problems should also be explored.

Treatment will not provide a cure, only an amelioration of the symptoms. In many cases, if the symptoms are mild, doing a thorough evaluation and educating the patient and his/her family about the disorder may be the only treatment required. Psychotherapy will only be useful for helping the patient to cope with the disability or, by lessening anxiety, may generate some secondary relief of symptomatology.

Pharmacologic intervention should be undertaken only when tics are interfering enough in a person's life to cause significant distress. With all pharmacologic agents used to treat TS there are a few rules that will be helpful when treating the tics:

1. Always start with the smallest dose that can reasonably be given considering the patient and the symptoms.
2. Increase the dose gradually, checking for side effects as well as beneficial effects, with each increment. When (1) and (2) are adhered to, the chance of developing side effects will be considerably diminished.
3. Maintain the patient on the lowest dosage possible. Almost all of the drugs commonly used for tics are primarily used for other conditions, yet effective doses for tic control may be considerably lower than those recommended for other indications.
4. Assure an adequate duration of any drug trial. Some medications (e.g., clonidine [Catapres][1]) may require several weeks to produce their greatest effect.
5. If symptoms are controlled satisfactorily on a certain dose but then become exacerbated, it is best to try to *ride out* the symptom increase for

[1]Not FDA approved for this indication.

a while. Symptoms may spontaneously wane again or there may have been a trigger for the symptom increase that resolves spontaneously (e.g., some viruses may cause temporary exacerbations).

6. When using multiple medications, change only one medication at a time.
7. When discontinuing medications be careful to avoid withdrawal reactions that may worsen the symptomatology.

There is no scientific evidence that any medication is better for vocal tics than motor, or vice versa. Neither is there any way to predict what medication may be more successful for a particular patient. Therefore, the best treatment approach is to first try medications with the lowest potential for harmful side effects. If one can avoid using a neuroleptic, that should be done. If a neuroleptic is necessary, one with less potential for harmful side effects, especially tardive dyskinesia, should be tried first. Thus, although haloperidol (Haldol) is the best known treatment for TS, it is now rarely used by physicians who are experienced in treating the disorder.

Medications (Table 1)

NONNEUROLEPTICS

Clonidine (Catapres)[1] is an α-adrenergic agonist that, in low doses, down-regulates α-adrenergic neurons in the locus ceruleus, decreasing the release of central norepinephrine. Although often less effective for tic suppression then neuroleptics, clonidine also has some beneficial effects on attention deficits, impulsivity, temper outbursts, anxiety, and oppositional behavior. In other words, it may serve as treatment for many of the associated symptoms as well as being a tic moderator. Although not FDA approved for any indication other than hypertension, clonidine has been used as a treatment for TS since 1980 and is in common use in child psychiatry. Side effects are usually few and mild, sedation being the most limiting one. Occasional irritability and insomnia may occur. Serious hypotension is rare if the medication is started at a low dose and raised slowly. Nevertheless, blood pressure should be monitored and electrocardiograms (ECGs) should be done before starting the medication, after increases, and at regular intervals afterwards.

[1]Not FDA approved for this indication.

Clonidine is generally started at a dose of 0.05 mg per day in the evening (0.025 for small children) and increased slowly over a period of several weeks to a maximal daily dosage of 0.1 to 0.5 mg per day (most commonly 0.15 to 3 mg per day). Because the effects on tics and behavior wear off in a few hours, three or four divided doses approximately 4 hours apart are necessary. While sedation may be a problem in the initial period, this usually wears off with time. As full benefits of the drug may not be achieved for several weeks, patience is important for success.

Clonidine is also available in the form of a transdermal patch (Catapres-TTS), which provides a steady flow of medication over the course of a week. The consistency of dosage provided by the patch is often more effective and more convenient than several daily doses of the oral form. The disadvantages of this preparation lie in the difficulty of keeping it on for an entire week and a fairly frequent development of localized skin reactions.

If clonidine is to be discontinued, it is important to do this slowly. A rate of 0.05 mg less per day, every 3 days, is generally safe. Abrupt cessation of the drug, while unlikely to cause rebound hypertension in a normotensive patient, is very likely to cause increased tic movements, irritability, nightmares, and insomnia.

Guanfacine (Tenex)[1], another α-adrenergic agonist, may have better tic suppressing capability and is also somewhat effective for treatment of ADHD. Many clinicians find that guanfacine is preferable to clonidine because it causes less sedation and has a longer half-life. Guanfacine, which is only available in an oral preparation, should be started at 0.5 mg per day and increased slowly, as indicated and/or tolerated, to a maximum of 4 to 5 mg per day in two to three divided doses (most commonly 1.5 to 3 mg per day). The precautions recommended for guanfacine

[1]Not FDA approved for this indication.

TABLE 1 Commonly Used Medications for Tourette's Syndrome

Medication	Typical Daily Dosage	Side Effects
Clonidine (Catapres)[1]	0.15-0.3 mg in 3-4 divided doses	Sedation, BP, ECG changes
Guanfacine (Tenex)[1]	1.5-3 mg in 2-3 divided doses	Sedation, BP, ECG changes
Clonazepam (Klonopin)[1]	1.5-3 mg in 3 divided doses	Sedation
Risperidone (Risperdal)[1]	2-6 mg in 1-2 divided doses	Sedation, weight gain, metabolic changes
Olanzapine (Zyprexa)[1]	2.5-10 mg in 1-2 divided doses	Sedation, weight gain, metabolic changes
Haloperidol (Haldol)	2-6 mg in 1-2 divided doses	Sedation, weight gain, EPS, tardive dyskinesia
Pimozide (Orap)	1-4 mg in 1-2 divided doses	Sedation, weight gain, EPS, tardive dyskinesia, ECG changes

[1]Not FDA approved for this indication.
Abbreviations: BP = blood pressure; ECG = electrocardiogram; EPS = extrapyramidal syndrome.

are similar to those for clonidine. Blood pressure monitoring and ECGs should be done before starting the drug, after increases, and at appropriate intervals thereafter.

Clonazepam (Klonopin)[1], an antiepileptic medication in the benzodiazepine category, may also be effective for tic control. Many patients with relatively mild tics do well on this medication and, although there is a potential for abuse, it has been my experience this is rare in the TS population. Dosage should be started at 0.25 to 0.5 mg and increased to a maximum daily dose of 3 to 4 mg per day (most commonly 1.5 to 3 mg per day), usually in three divided doses. The most common side effect is sedation.

Perhaps the most problematic aspect of clonazepam treatment is the withdrawal associated with cessation of the drug. This medication must be decreased very gradually, sometimes as slowly as 0.25 mg less from the total daily dose every 2 to 3 weeks.

NEUROLEPTICS

Neuroleptics, as a class, act as dopamine antagonists. Because of the danger of tardive dyskinesia as well as extrapyramidal symptoms (EPS), *atypical*, or *new*, neuroleptics are preferable to the older drugs in this class.

Risperidone (Risperdal)[1] is effective for tic control according to a number of studies. This medication can be started at a daily dose as low as 0.25 mg per day and may be raised as high as 12 mg per day. A few patients of adult size may require even higher doses, but this is unusual and most patients achieve tic relief on doses between 2 and 6 mg per day. Risperidone may also be useful for treatment of associated problems such as aggressive behavior and poor impulse control, and as an adjunct to treatment of OCD with selective serotonin reuptake inhibitor (SSRI) medications. It may be administered once or twice a day, as needed. Patients should be monitored for side effects such as akathisia, depression, weight gain, elevated prolactin, hyperglycemia/diabetes, dyslipidemia, and prolongation of the QT_c interval. Unfortunately, teenage boys may develop gynecomastia after long-term treatment on this medication.

Olanzapine (Zyprexa)[1] may also be quite effective for control of tics. Doses may range from 0.5 mg per day to as much as 20 mg per day. Most commonly, doses between 2.5 and 10 mg per day are effective. Although sometimes necessary, higher doses should be avoided if possible because of side effects such as weight gain and metabolic changes.

There are other, more novel neuroleptics including molindone (Moban)[1], ziprasidone (Geodon)[1], quetiapine (Seroquel)[1] and the most recent of this class, aripiprazole (Abilify)[1], which may also be effective for some patients. Ziprasidone may be preferable because of the low associated weight gain. However, in my experience, it is not as effective as risperidone and olanzapine. Aripiprazole is also associated with a low incidence of weight gain. However, its effectiveness for tic control is still largely unproven. In my opinion, clozapine (Clozaril)[1] has no place in the treatment of TS because of the danger of a fatal agranulocytosis.

Of the older neuroleptics, haloperidol (Haldol) has the longest track record for treatment of TS. If it becomes necessary to use this medication, I recommend starting at 0.25 to 0.5 mg per day and increasing the dose very slowly while being alert not only to the more obvious side effects such as extrapyramidal symptoms, but also particularly to depression. Most patients will achieve tic amelioration at doses between 2 and 6 mg per day. The use of antidotes for EPS such as benztropine (Cogentin), may be necessary.

Pimozide (Orap), while still carrying the QT_c interval warning, has been found to be a reasonably safe and effective medication. Treatment with pimozide is usually initiated at 1 mg per day and the dosage gradually increased, with ECG monitoring, to a maximum of 10 mg per day. Most often, doses between 1 and 4 mg per day are effective.

Other, older neuroleptics that may be effective include fluphenazine (Prolixin)[1] and thiothixene (Navane)[1]. Although not generally accepted as a treatment for TS, I have personally had considerable success with thiothixene.

Treatment of PANDAS (pediatric autoimmune neuropsychiatric disorder associated with streptococcal infections) has received considerable attention in the past few years. This is a disorder of young children (prepubertal) that presents with a sudden, dramatic onset of tics and/or OCD symptomatology. It should be considered in the differential diagnosis of prepubertal, relapsing/remitting tics with or without OCD. Throat swabs or, in retrospect, antistreptolysine-O (ASO) and antideoxyribonuclease-B (anti-DNAse-B) titers may also be useful. If there is sufficient evidence for a diagnosis of PANDAS, an antibiotic may be the treatment of choice.

There are a variety of other medications that are effective for tic amelioration. These include, topiramate (Topamax)[1], nicotine preparations[1], donepezil (Aricept)[1], and tetrabenazine[2]. While some of these have been useful when other remedies fail, they should not be considered as first-line drugs.

In addition to treating tics, control of the associated symptoms is usually necessary, and many patients end up with a *cocktail* of three to five different medications. Stimulant medication may cause an exacerbation of tics but do not have any permanent deleterious effect. More often than not, they have no adverse effect on tics, and trials on these medications should not be avoided. The use of SSRI medications for OCD is also frequently indicated and, in fact, I have had a number of patients whose tics were dramatically alleviated by these medications alone.

[1]Not FDA approved for this indication.

[1]Not FDA approved for this indication.
[2]Not available in the United States.

HEADACHE

METHOD OF

Christopher W. Ryan, MD

Headache accounts for more than 10 million office visits annually to primary care physicians. It is the seventh and ninth most frequent presenting symptom among female and male ambulatory patients, respectively. Effective treatment is facilitated by accurate diagnosis, which can usually be accomplished via a thorough interview and a targeted neurologic examination, while keeping diagnostic tests to a minimum. Occasional chronic headaches defy precise classification, but therapeutic measures can still be undertaken.

This discussion focuses on the recognition and management of common chronic headache syndromes. In the case of intracranial mass lesions, significant head trauma, or subarachnoid hemorrhage, attention is appropriately directed to treatment of the underlying serious cause rather than on treatment of the pain per se. Discussion of those treatments is beyond the scope of this article.

Evaluation

THE INTERVIEW

A detailed understanding of the character of the patient's pain is essential. No imaging study or laboratory test can substitute for a vivid mental picture of the patient's experience. This picture can best be painted by inviting the patient to describe his or her experience in an open-ended, narrative fashion. Focused questions can follow, to clarify and verify the details. No one element can be relied upon in isolation to provide a diagnosis; rather, diagnosis depends on the synthesis of all the elements into a coherent, recognizable whole.

Patients and physicians tend to use headache-related terms loosely, without first agreeing upon their definitions. For example, most patients use the term *migraine* to describe an extremely painful headache and call any retrofacial pain *sinus*. However, migraine, properly used, is not a descriptor of intensity of pain, and retrofacial pain often stems from illnesses unrelated to sinusitis. Use of such terms can invite premature and incorrect diagnostic conclusions. Therefore, early in the interview, it is best to avoid them.

Of all the elements in the history, a full description of the time course of chronic headaches is the best aid to diagnosis. A complete temporal description includes the onset of episodes, the frequency of episodes, and the duration of each episode. Patients tend to underestimate the duration of their headache syndrome, identifying the time of onset as the age at which the headaches became particularly bothersome, rather than the age at which they actually began. Meticulous and well-designed questions are needed to define what patients mean by "a while," "all my life," "constantly," and similar catchphrases. The frequency of episodes can be clarified by inquiring about the shortest and the longest intervals that the patient has ever been entirely free of pain. Similarly, the duration can be clarified by inquiring about the shortest and the longest intervals that the patient has ever had continuous pain.

These seemingly minor distinctions are useful clinically. For example, migraines often begin in childhood or adolescence, while temporal arteritis tends to occur in older adults. New-onset migraine is unusual in older adults; significant new headaches in that age group should raise concern for intracranial structural pathology. As Figures 1 through 4 demonstrate, a meticulous dissection of the time course of a patient's chronic headache can suggest a particular diagnosis.

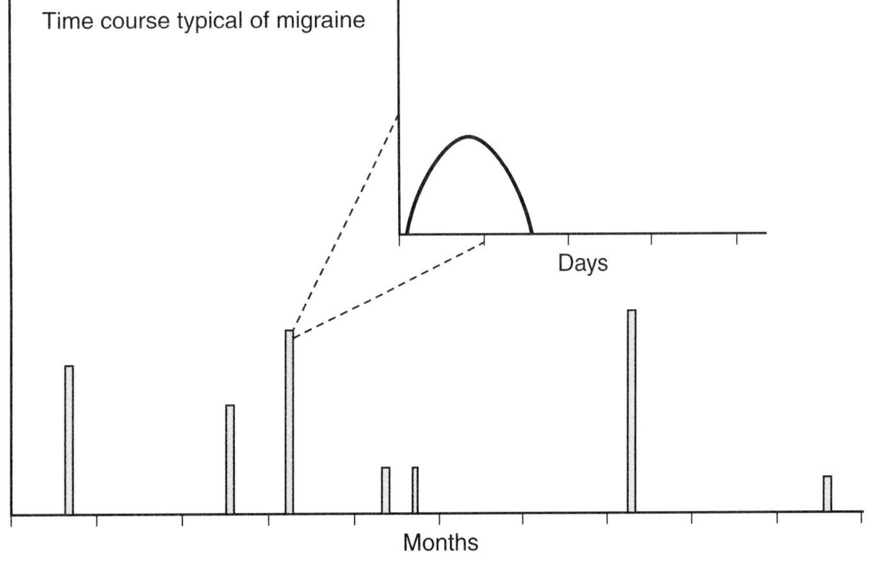

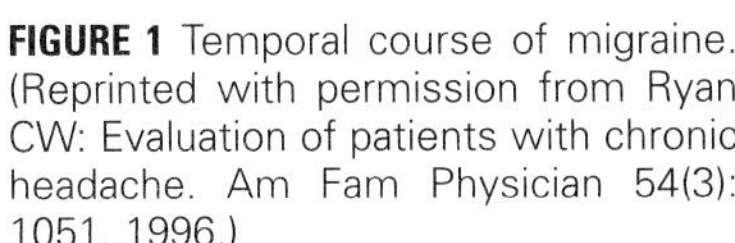

FIGURE 1 Temporal course of migraine. (Reprinted with permission from Ryan CW: Evaluation of patients with chronic headache. Am Fam Physician 54(3): 1051, 1996.)

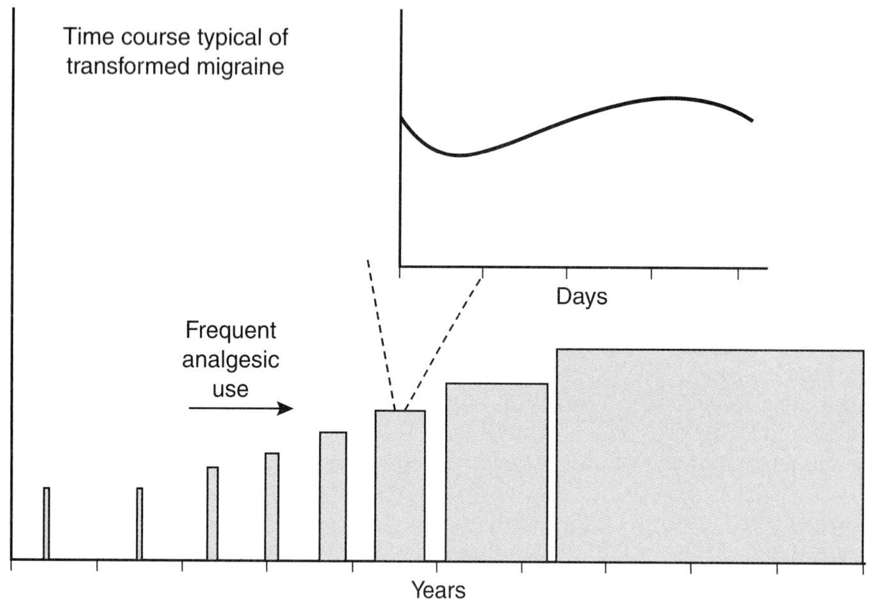

FIGURE 2 Temporal course of transformed migraine. (Reprinted with permission from Ryan CW: Evaluation of patients with chronic headache. Am Fam Physician 54(3):1051, 1996.)

Provoking and relieving factors can also provide clues to etiology. Migraine frequency and intensity can fluctuate with the menstrual cycle and with pregnancy. Certain foods, such as chocolate, can also trigger migraines. Trigeminal neuralgia classically can be triggered by even light tactile stimulation over the involved part of the face.

Symptoms that accompany the headache can provide valuable information. Nausea, vomiting, and visual symptoms occur frequently in migraine. Car sickness, either present or past, is associated with migraines. Unilateral nasal congestion, rhinorrhea, and lacrimation are associated with cluster headache.

Behavioral symptoms can be informative. Migraine sufferers generally prefer lying motionless in dark rooms. Patients with cluster headache often pace around the room, holding or striking the painful area. The wincing movement of the head that accompanies each burst of lancinating pain in trigeminal neuralgia is responsible for its other name, tic douloureux.

A complete list of all the medicines a patient is currently taking should be obtained, because some medicines, such as oral contraceptives, nitrates, and certain antihypertensives, are associated with headache. Quantifying the patient's use of analgesics is challenging but essential, because frequent use of

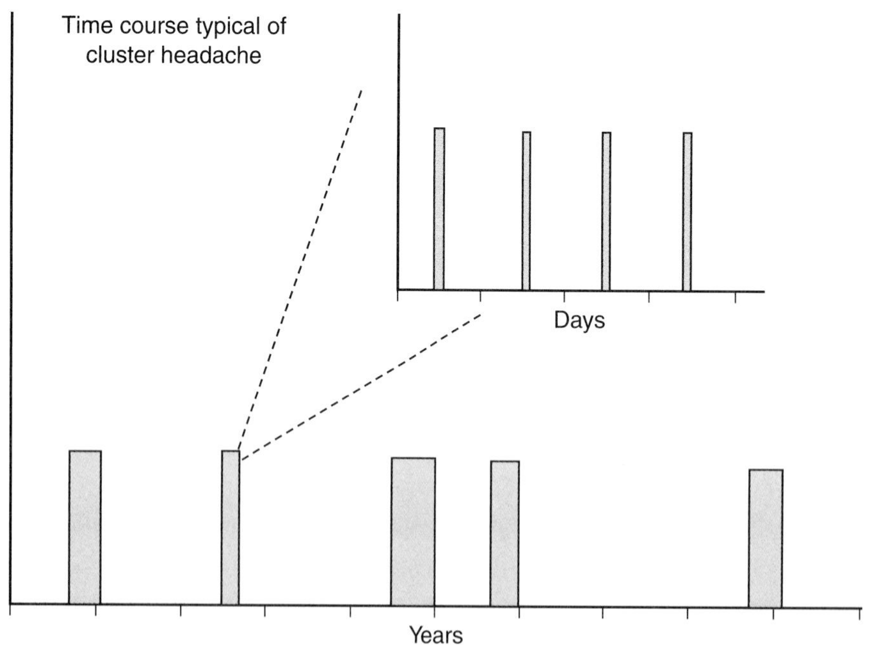

FIGURE 3 Temporal course of cluster headache. (Reprinted with permission from Ryan CW: Evaluation of patients with chronic headache. Am Fam Physician 54(3):1051, 1996.)

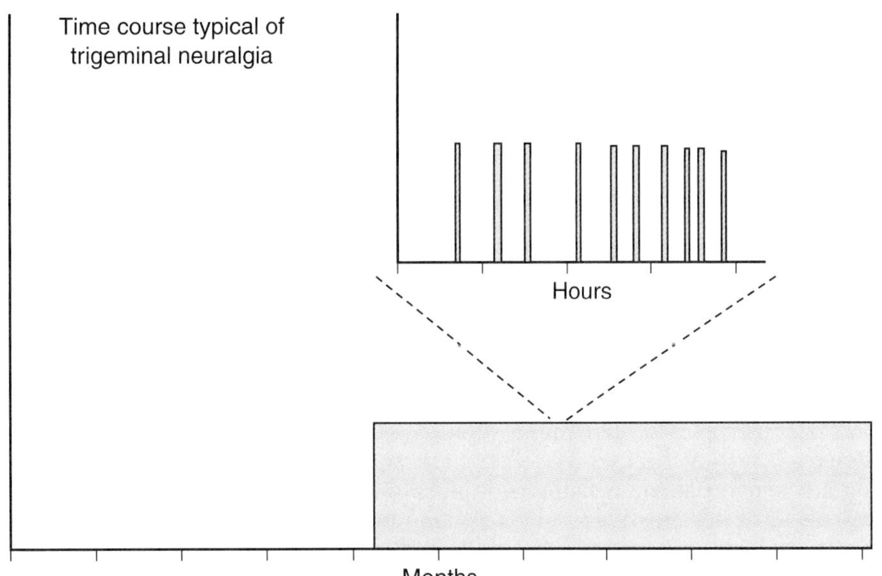

FIGURE 4 Temporal course of trigeminal neuralgia. (Reprinted with permission from Ryan CW: Evaluation of patients with chronic headache. Am Fam Physician 54(3):1051, 1996.)

abortive analgesics, even at customary doses, can convert paroxysmal migraine into chronic daily headache, a phenomenon known as transformed migraine, evolutive migraine, or analgesic rebound headache. Patients should also be asked about their use of caffeine, because caffeine withdrawal can cause headache.

Chronic headache can be associated with depression and is one of the more common ways in which depression presents in the primary care setting. While there may be disagreement as to whether one entity is primary and the other secondary, recognizing their coexistence is important for treatment.

Inquiry about sleep patterns can be useful, because sleep deprivation from any cause can contribute to chronic headache. Sometimes recurrent morning headache in a neurologically normal patient with loud snoring can be a clue to obstructive sleep apnea. Bruxism (clenching or grinding of the teeth during sleep) can be associated with temporomandibular joint dysfunction and tension-type headache. Information about these nocturnal symptoms might best be elicited from the patient's bed partner.

THE PHYSICAL EXAMINATION

A thorough neurologic examination is fundamental in the evaluation of headache, although it is usually normal. Examination of the head and neck occasionally yields other clues. Unilateral mydriasis, conjunctival injection, and nasal congestion can suggest cluster headache. Trigger points on the scalp can suggest a neuralgia, such as of the trigeminal or occipital nerve. Tenderness and induration over the temporal artery is consistent with temporal arteritis. Spontaneous venous pulsations at the optic disc speak reassuringly against the presence of elevated intracranial pressure, although they are not always present even in normal patients.

ANCILLARY TESTING

Any new or evolving focal neurologic abnormality warrants tomographic imaging of the head, to investigate the possibility of an intracranial mass. However, there is little information concerning the utility of computed tomography (CT) and magnetic resonance imaging (MRI) scans in ambulatory family practice patients with headache. In the Ambulatory Sentinel Practice Network, significant abnormalities were found on only 4% to 6% of 293 CT scans in patients with headache. Many of the abnormalities were, in fact, false-positives or incidental findings that did not contribute directly to patient management.

Laboratory tests are rarely helpful. An erythrocyte sedimentation rate (ESR) can be useful in making a diagnosis of temporal arteritis. In the setting of acute headache, lumbar puncture is indicated if there is concern for meningitis or encephalitis. A low serum concentration of ionized magnesium may predict, to some extent, a good response to abortive and preventive treatment with magnesium, but the clinical utility of this requires further study.

General Management Principles

The management of patients with chronic headache can be a vexing problem. It is easy for patients and physicians alike to become demoralized because of the lack of any organic pathology and the low likelihood of definitive cure. However, if suitable goals are negotiated with the patient, management becomes much more satisfying. Emphasis should always be on functional capacity and activities of daily living, rather than on elimination of pain. While eliminating the pain altogether is rarely if ever achievable, reducing the pain almost always is. This involves decreasing the frequency, intensity, and duration of episodes.

A clear distinction should be made between abortive and preventive therapy. For each of the headache syndromes to be addressed, abortive treatments are different from prophylactic ones. Inadvertent overuse of abortive agents, using them essentially as daily preventive agents, can transform intermittent migraines into the much more troublesome transformed migraine. Every abortive analgesic is subject to this phenomenon, including acetaminophen, nonsteroidal anti-inflammatory drugs (NSAIDs), aspirin, opioids, barbiturates, ergotamines, and triptans. The decision to embark on preventive therapy must be individualized, but it should be considered when headaches are occurring roughly twice a month or more.

Analgesic overuse can make otherwise good preventive therapy ineffective. The best solution for analgesic overuse or transformed migraine is abrupt cessation of all abortive analgesics. The patient will likely experience approximately 2 weeks of more severe and frequent headaches, but thereafter will be much improved. Either the headaches will cease altogether, or previously ineffective preventive therapy will regain its effectiveness.

The frequent coexistence of chronic headaches and depression should be addressed. Antidepressant medications can help with both. For this purpose, tricyclic antidepressants have a longer track record of success, but selective serotonin reuptake inhibitors (SSRIs) might be suitable in some circumstances. Sleep interruption because of pain often is an issue, and here again the relatively sedating tricyclic antidepressants can be useful.

Many chronic headache patients have become disheartened by years of medical care and diagnostic workups that were seemingly in vain. Similarly, physicians often are pessimistic about the prognosis for patients with chronic headache, and about their ability to help. Hope can be therapeutic, and it can be restored to both parties in the context of a lasting patient–physician relationship in which the patient plays an active role in his or her recovery. With a sufficient variety of tools in their armamentarium, physicians can be optimistic about achieving improvement in their patients with chronic headaches.

Migraine

DESCRIPTION

Migraine is a systemic phenomenon, with headache as only one of its features. Indeed, in children, migraine can occur without any headache at all, in which case the manifestations consist primarily of cyclical vomiting and abdominal pain. The best and most concise description of migraine is intermittent headache with nausea and vomiting. The headache is often described as throbbing. Common locations for the headache are bifrontal, retrofacial, or hemicranial. More often than not, the headaches are bilateral. Unilateral migraines usually show an incomplete preference for one side, with approximately 5% to 10% of episodes occurring on the contralateral side. Figure 1 shows the typical time course of a migraine. Over time, and often associated with frequent use of abortive analgesics, this temporal pattern can evolve to a continuous daily headache, as demonstrated in Figure 2.

Associated symptoms can include nausea, vomiting, phonophobia, and photophobia. A variety of visual symptoms can occur, such as photopsia (a sensation of flashbulbs going off), scintillating scotomas that wander across the visual field, and fortification phenomenon (roving patterns similar to parapets on the top of a medieval castle.) These can occur before or during the headache.

Migraines are more common among adult women than adult men. Prior to puberty, however, the prevalence is equal in the two sexes. Migraines tend to run in families. There is also an association with childhood motion sickness.

ABORTIVE THERAPY

The availability of an extremely large number of pharmacologic options demonstrates that no single approach is universally effective. Some patients may have concurrent medical conditions that render certain options inadvisable. Other patients may have previously demonstrated a poor response to certain regimens. Thus physicians would do well to have a number of these options at their disposal.

Some of these regimens can be self-administered at home, either orally, nasally, or subcutaneously. Oral regimens are convenient, but they become less effective once the patient has developed the vomiting typical of a migraine episode. Even those that cannot be self-administered can be easily administered in the office setting.

Several of the suggested treatment regimens can result in drowsiness. This adverse effect is, in a way, desired, because migraines often resolve with sleep. Almost any of these abortive treatments can be rendered ineffective if the patient cannot or will not lie down to sleep after returning home.

The wide range of options are reviewed in detail below. But an early and brief discussion of three highly recommended approaches might be useful. These approaches optimize a balance between efficacy (response rates, onset of relief, and duration of effect), safety, convenience, and cost.

1. For a mild episode with little or no vomiting to preclude oral therapy, metoclopramide (Reglan)[1], 10 mg, plus aspirin, 975 mg, provides relief to approximately 55% of patients. The relapse rate is low when the same combination is repeated every 8 hours for three doses per headache episode. Extrapyramidal side effects are a rare complication. The cost to treat one headache is approximately $1.00.

[1]Not FDA approved for this indication.

2. For a moderate episode in which vomiting precludes oral medication, dihydroergotamine (DHE) nasal spray (Migranal) can be self-administered. Intranasal DHE is supplied as a kit containing 4 ampules, with each ampule containing four 0.5-mg sprays. The usual dose to treat one headache is one spray (0.5 mg) in each nostril, repeated 15 minutes later. Local adverse effects include nasal congestion, rhinorrhea, and abnormal tastes. Because it is a potent vasoconstrictor, use of DHE is unwise in patients with coronary artery disease, uncontrolled hypertension, significant risk factors for vascular disease, or pregnancy. The cost to treat one headache is approximately $18.00.
3. For a severe episode with prominent nausea and vomiting, intravenous prochlorperazine (Compazine)[1], in a single dose of 10 mg injected over 2 to 3 minutes, is the most effective, simplest, and least expensive intravenous regimen. Response rates are upwards of 75%. Potential adverse effects include drowsiness and extrapyramidal symptoms. The cost to treat one headache is approximately $3.00.

Other therapeutic options, organized by route of administration, are discussed in the sections below.

Oral Regimens

Simple analgesics such as acetaminophen[1], aspirin, and NSAIDs have proven efficacy in acute migraine. Diclofenac (Cataflam)[1] at a dose of 50 mg is just one example; it provides relief to approximately 75% of patients. The advantage to most of these agents is their ready availability and minimal cost.

Ergotamine tartrate (Ergomar) can be administered orally, in the form of a sublingual tablet of 2 mg, or an oral tablet of 1 mg, combined with 100 mg of caffeine (Cafergot). The main function of the caffeine is to increase intestinal absorption of ergotamine. Response rates exceed 80%. Ergotamines have potential adverse effects typical of potent vasoconstrictors, and they should not be used in patients with coronary artery disease, uncontrolled hypertension, significant risk factors for vascular disease, or pregnancy. The maximum recommended dose of ergotamine is 6 mg a day or 10 mg a week.

Triptans are a group of related serotonin agonists. As a class, they provide relief to approximately 75% of patients within approximately 4 hours. Relapse rates over the ensuing 24 hours range from 20% to 40%, with sumatriptan (Imitrex) at the upper end of that range. Adverse effects include paresthesias, chest pain, nausea, vomiting, and uterine contractions. Use of triptans is unwise in patients with coronary artery disease, uncontrolled hypertension, significant risk factors for vascular disease, or pregnancy. Table 1 contains initial and maximum doses

[1]Not FDA approved for this indication.

TABLE 1 Available Oral Triptan Agents

Drug Name	Brand Name	Initial Dose	Maximum Daily Dose
Sumatriptan	Imitrex	25-100 mg	200 mg
Rizatriptan	Maxalt	5-10 mg	30 mg
Zolmitriptan	Zomig	2.5-5 mg	10 mg
Eletriptan	Relpax	20-40 mg	80 mg
Almotriptan	Axert	6.25-12.5 mg	25 mg
Frovatriptan	Frova	2.5-5 mg	7.5 mg
Naratriptan	Amerge	1-2.5 mg	5 mg

for triptan agents. Irrespective of the particular agent used, the cost of treating one headache, with one dose, is approximately $16.00.

Intranasal Regimens

Sumatriptan (Imitrex) is also available in a nasal spray. The dose is 5 to 20 mg (half in each nostril), with a daily maximum of 40 mg. The cost to treat one headache with one administration is approximately $45.00.

Rectal Regimens

Ergotamine tartrate, 2 mg, combined with caffeine, 100 mg, is available commercially as a suppository (Cafergot Supps). The usual dose is 1 suppository, repeated in 1 hour if necessary, with upper dose limits for the ergotamine similar to those of the oral route.

Subcutaneous Regimens

Sumatriptan (Imitrex) can be administered subcutaneously, either by medical personnel or by the patient, via a commercially-available autoinjector. The usual dose is 6 mg, which may be repeated. Relief is prompt, often beginning within 15 minutes. Approximately 85% of patients are afforded relief within 2 hours. However, relapse rates over the ensuing 24 hours range from 40% to 50%. Potential side effects have been described above. The cost for treating one headache is $25.00 to $50.00, with a two-dose autoinjector costing $100.00.

Dihydroergotamine (D.H.E. 45) can also be administered subcutaneously at a dose of 0.5 to 1 mg. Improvement begins more slowly than with sumatriptan but persists longer, with only an 18% recurrence rate at 24 hours. Also see the *Intravenous Regimens* section below.

Intramuscular Regimens

Ketorolac (Toradol)[1] is a parenteral NSAID. It can be administered intramuscularly for migraine. The usual dose is 15 to 60 mg. The cost for treating a single headache with a 30-mg dose is approximately $10.00.

[1]Not FDA approved for this indication.

Dihydroergotamine (D.H.E. 45) can be given intramuscularly, at doses similar to the subcutaneous and intravenous routes. Also see the *Intravenous Regimens* section below.

Phenothiazines such as prochlorperazine (Compazine)[1], 10 mg, can also be given intramuscularly.

Intravenous Regimens

For severe episodes of migraine, intravenous approaches are often necessary. They also allow replacement of extracellular fluid volume that has usually been lost through vomiting.

Chlorpromazine (Thorazine)[1] has well-documented efficacy in acute migraine. The usual dose is 0.1 mg/kg (7 to 8 mg for an average-sized adult), which can be repeated every 15 to 20 minutes, up to three doses if needed. Potential side effects are similar to prochlorperazine (Compazine)[1], but with orthostatic hypotension being a little more common; thus pretreatment with an intravenous bolus of normal saline is advised. The cost for treating one headache with three doses is approximately $15.00.

Metoclopramide (Reglan)[1] was initially considered a premedication to prevent the nausea typically caused by DHE, however, metoclopramide itself is often effective. The usual dose, either alone or with DHE, is 10 mg. Potential adverse effects are similar to those of phenothiazines.

Dihydroergotamine (D.H.E. 45), preceded by intravenous metoclopramide to prevent nausea and vomiting, is a very effective antimigraine agent. The usual dose is metoclopramide, 10 mg, followed by DHE, 0.5 to 1 mg. In cases of *status migrainous*, or very prolonged and refractory migraine, this combination can be repeated every 8 hours with good result. Potential adverse effects have been described above. The cost to treat one headache is approximately $22.00.

Magnesium[1], in a single dose of 500 to 1000 mg, has yielded some success in preliminary trials. Patients with low serum concentrations of ionized magnesium, or with high ratios of ionized calcium to ionized magnesium, may benefit the most. While still in need of further study before widespread use, intravenous magnesium carries the advantage of minimal adverse effects.

Valproate (Depacon)[1] has been used in a few reported case series. Doses have ranged from 300 to 500 mg. In one randomized, prospective trial, intravenous valproate compared poorly with prochlorperazine. Further study is needed to determine in which clinical scenarios, if any, intravenous valproate is a useful option.

PREVENTIVE THERAPY

If an obvious trigger is discovered on interview, such as a particular food, it should be avoided if possible.

[1]Not FDA approved for this indication.

Maintaining regular sleep patterns, even through the weekend, can be helpful in prevention. Frequent use of any abortive analgesics must be halted.

The most commonly used pharmacologic treatments are tricyclic antidepressants and β-blockers. Either one can yield a 50% reduction in headache frequency, and the choice between them is driven by other considerations such as side effect profiles and concurrent medical problems. Lipid-soluble β-blockers, such as propranolol (Inderal), nadolol (Corgard)[1], and metoprolol (Lopressor)[1], might be more effective than water-soluble versions such as atenolol (Tenormin)[1].

Valproate (Depakote) is a relatively new addition to the preventive armamentarium for migraine. At least three randomized, controlled trials indicate that it too can yield a 50% reduction in frequency and duration of episodes. In some trials, a fixed dose of 400 mg twice daily was used; in others, a starting dose of 250 mg twice daily was titrated to achieve serum levels of 50 to 120 μg/mL. Valproate also seems to be effective in otherwise unclassifiable chronic daily headache.

Methysergide (Sansert)[2] can be used for migraine prevention, in doses ranging from 2 to 8 mg daily. It is usually reserved for patients with particularly severe and intractable migraines, because of the potential for retroperitoneal, pleuropulmonary, and cardiac fibrosis. To reduce the risk of fibrotic complications, uninterrupted treatment with methysergide should not last longer than 6 months; a 1-month drug *holiday* should be scheduled at least every 6 months.

A single trial of riboflavin (vitamin B_2)[1], 400 mg daily, yielded a 50% reduction in headache frequency. Feverfew[1] is a popular herbal preventive agent, but the preparations and the research are both too heterogeneous to draw firm conclusions about its effectiveness.

While there is some early evidence that some patients with migraine are magnesium deficient, trials of oral magnesium[1] for prevention have yielded conflicting results.

Nonpharmacologic strategies for prevention include cognitive–behavioral therapy, hypnosis, and skin-temperature biofeedback. The latter has demonstrated effectiveness equal to that of β-blockers.

Tension Headache

DESCRIPTION

Tension headache usually manifests as a circumferential, band-like squeezing pain. Sometimes it is described in a frontal-to-occipital or a bifrontal distribution. The time course is highly variable—the pain can be intermittent or continuous. Gastrointestinal

[1]Not FDA approved for this indication.
[2]Not available in the United States.

symptoms are characteristically absent, as are focal neurologic symptoms. Many patients describe both tension and migraine headaches, and there is much overlap between the two syndromes, although the pathogenetic relationship remains to be elucidated fully.

ABORTIVE THERAPY

First-line abortive therapy usually involves a simple analgesic such as aspirin, acetaminophen, or a NSAID. However, when tension headaches are frequent, care must be taken to avoid making the situation worse through overuse of these drugs.

Intravenous chlorpromazine (Thorazine)[1], in doses identical to those used for migraine, is also effective in relieving acute tension-type headache.

PREVENTIVE THERAPY

In clinical practice, prevention of chronic tension-type headache, rather than treatment of acute episodes, is more often the issue. Assessing the effectiveness of preventive interventions is complicated by the very high placebo response rate, which is 30% to 40% in most studies and up to 50% in some. As expected from the overlap between the clinical syndromes, there is much overlap in the preventive agents studied for chronic tension-type headache and migraine.

Tricyclic antidepressants[1] have a long history of use in tension-type headache, and some evidence from randomized controlled trials to support their effectiveness. Selective serotonin reuptake inhibitors[1] may also be effective, but the evidence and history behind them are not as strong. Either of these classes of agents may exert their beneficial effect via treatment of an underlying depression, which often accompanies chronic tension headache.

Cognitive behavioral therapy appears to be as effective as antidepressants, and the combination of the two is more effective than either one alone. Instruction in the technique of progressive muscle relaxation is sometimes beneficial.

Most trials of acupuncture that include a sham or blinded placebo arm do not demonstrate any benefit. Controlled trials of injection of botulinum toxin (Botox)[1] into cranial musculature have demonstrated decreases in muscle tension on electromyelogram (EMG) but no corresponding improvement in pain (casting some doubt on the accuracy of the name for this type of headache.)

In some patients, bruxism and temporomandibular joint dysfunction are contributing factors to chronic tension-type headache. In these patients, a nocturnal oral appliance prescribed by their dentist may provide some relief.

[1]Not FDA approved for this indication.

Cluster Headache

DESCRIPTION

Cluster headache derives its name from its temporal course. Patients with cluster headache classically will remain symptom-free for months or years at a time. Symptomatic periods, called *clusters*, last for weeks to months. During clusters, patients will have intermittent headaches. The headaches occur daily or more often, last approximately an hour, and can be extremely intense. In some cases, the headaches occur at precise 24-hour intervals. Figure 3 shows the typical time course of cluster headache. Cluster headache is almost always unilateral, often in a periorbital distribution. Accompanying symptoms can include ipsilateral rhinorrhea, nasal congestion, lacrimation, ptosis, miosis, and anhydrosis (the latter three findings comprising Horner's syndrome). Cluster headache is much more common in men than in women.

MANAGEMENT

Treatment of cluster headache involves three distinct objectives: stopping a particular headache, ending or shortening a cluster period, and preventing cluster periods.

Stopping a Headache

The pain is typically so severe as to render the usual simple analgesics, such as acetaminophen and NSAIDs, ineffective. Inhalation of 100% oxygen relieves the headache promptly. While this is not practical long-term therapy, the response to oxygen can confirm the diagnosis. Ergotamines (IM) and triptan (IM) agents can be effective. Oral or parenteral opioids are sometimes needed.

Ending a Cluster Period

Many different agents have been tried for bringing a particular cluster period to a close, including prednisone, baclofen (Lioresal)[1], valproate (Depakote)[1], carbamazepine (Tegretol)[1], verapamil (Calan)[1], lithium (Eskalith)[1], methysergide (Sansert)[1,2], and others. The evidence supporting any one of these options consists mainly of case series and small, short clinical trials of marginal quality. A tapering course of prednisone is perhaps most commonly used; it is reasonably effective and has the advantage of being familiar to most physicians, both in its actions and its potential adverse effects.

Preventing Further Cluster Periods

Except for corticosteroids, all the agents used to end a cluster period are options for preventing them.

[1]Not FDA approved for this indication.
[2]Not available in the United States.

Similar caveats apply regarding the evidence supporting their use. Lithium[1], the traditional preventive treatment, has a very narrow therapeutic window, with significant toxicity outside that range of serum concentrations. Verapamil[1] and the anticonvulsants[1] are at least as effective, and easier to manage.

Chronic Paroxysmal Hemicrania

DESCRIPTION

Chronic paroxysmal hemicrania bears a resemblance to cluster headache, but it is more prevalent in women. It is convenient (though not necessarily pathogenetically accurate) to think of chronic paroxysmal hemicrania as rapid-cycling cluster headache, with unilateral painful episodes lasting just minutes but reoccurring upwards of 20 times per day.

MANAGEMENT

For the treatment of chronic paroxysmal hemicrania, indomethacin (Indocin)[1] appears to be uniquely effective among the NSAIDs. Conventional doses are used, ranging from 25 to 50 mg three times per day.

Trigeminal Neuralgia

DESCRIPTION

Trigeminal neuralgia is manifested by repetitive, lancinating, unilateral facial pain. It can occur along any of the three major divisions of the trigeminal nerve, although the mandibular division is most commonly involved. The painful episodes, individually, are fleeting but intense. Episodes occur innumerable times throughout the day. Figure 4 shows the typical time course of trigeminal neuralgia. Sometimes episodes can be precipitated by tactile stimulation of the face, such as when washing. They can cause an involuntary wincing movement of the involved side of the face, which leads to the syndrome's other name of tic douloureux (or painful tic).

MANAGEMENT

Anticonvulsants are the mainstay of pharmacologic treatment for trigeminal neuralgia. Carbamazepine (Tegretol) is usually the most effective agent, with one patient expected to achieve at least 50% improvement for every 2 to 3 patients treated. Baclofen (Lioresal)[1], phenytoin (Dilantin)[1], valproate (Depakote)[1], and other anticonvulsants are usually used as second-line drugs. Tricyclic antidepressants can sometimes play a useful secondary role.

[1]Not FDA approved for this indication.

For refractory cases, invasive therapies can be considered. These usually consist of some type of ablation of the trigeminal ganglion, often with a radiofrequency probe.

Temporal Arteritis

DESCRIPTION

The headache from temporal arteritis is just one regional manifestation of a systemic process called giant cell arteritis. As such, temporal arteritis is usually preceded or accompanied by systemic symptoms of fatigue, fever, chills, malaise, myalgias, or weight loss. It is mostly a disease of older adults. There is an incompletely defined relationship with polymyalgia rheumatica. Besides the headache, involvement of other cranial arteries can produce other symptoms, such as jaw claudication or sudden (and irreversible) visual loss. The erythrocyte sedimentation rate is characteristically high.

MANAGEMENT

Corticosteroids are the primary treatment for temporal arteritis. Prompt recognition and treatment of the disease can prevent blindness. Treatment begins with 40 to 60 mg per day of prednisone[1]. After symptoms have abated in approximately 1 month, the dose can be slowly tapered to the minimum necessary to maintain remission. Alternate-day therapy is preferred for maintenance treatment, which can be required for months to years.

Chronic Daily Headache

A formal diagnosis of a headache syndrome can be elusive. A sufficiently skillful interview that covers the entire life course of the patient's headache problems often can disclose evidence of analgesic overuse, and this can provide leverage for therapy. However, some headache syndromes defy classification in spite of optimum diagnostic efforts. Although it is not part of the International Headache Society's classification scheme, the name *chronic daily headache* seems to apply and is appearing more often in the literature. Recently there have been promising reports of the use of valproate (Depakote)[1] for daily maintenance therapy in these patients.

Chronic headache is a vexing and frustrating problem for patients and their physicians alike. Over the years, feelings of despair and futility can settle upon both parties. Yet satisfying improvements can be achieved by following a few simple principles:

- Conduct a detailed and dynamic, patient-centered interview, followed by a targeted physical examination emphasizing the neurologic system.

[1]Not FDA approved for this indication.

- Arrange tomographic imaging of the head if there are new focal neurologic findings.
- Project an attitude of hope.
- Negotiate achievable goals with the patient. While it is rarely possible to put an end to the headaches, it is almost always possible to decrease their frequency, intensity, and duration.
- Make an early and explicit decision regarding the use of preventive medications, to avoid the *slippery slope* of analgesic overuse leading to intractable headache.
- If analgesic overuse and transformed headache have already developed, stop all abortive analgesics and provide appropriate emotional support.

In the context of a long-term relationship, this approach can provide relief for the patient and restore a sense of effectiveness in the physician.

VIRAL MENINGITIS AND ENCEPHALITIS

METHOD OF

Bruce A. Cohen, MD

Viruses are the most common cause of central nervous system (CNS) infections in the United States. Most of the neurotropic viruses responsible for CNS infections may cause either meningitis or encephalitis in a given individual, and in some instances the features of both are combined as a meningoencephalitis. Susceptibility to particular agents and presentations may vary in hosts with immune deficiencies. In approaching a patient suspected to have a viral CNS infection, the physician must consider the clinical presentation, including extraneurologic findings, the season of the year, travel history, any potential environmental exposures, and the status of the patient's immune system.

Clinical Features

Viral meningitis typically presents with fever and headache associated with signs of meningeal irritation. Meningismus may be absent in immune suppressed patients. Fatigue, malaise, photophobia, and myalgias are common. Features of a respiratory or gastrointestinal (GI) infection may precede or accompany the neurologic symptoms including cough, chills, dyspnea, nausea, vomiting, or diarrhea. Irritability is common in infants and small children, and dehydration may lead to lethargy. In older children, adolescents and adults, the sensorium is normal. Clues to specific agents may lie in the associated signs and symptoms of other organ system involvement such as rash and cardiac or hepatic disease.

Viral encephalitis is a febrile illness associated with evidence of brain parenchymal dysfunction, typically including neurologic deficits such as weakness or sensory impairments, changes in sensorium and behavior, seizures, and ataxia in varying combinations. Some viral infections may be associated with a postinfectious encephalitis attributed to an immune response directed against the pathogen that cross-reacts to normal CNS proteins.

Etiologies

Enteroviruses (*Picornaviridae*), which include the echoviruses, coxsackieviruses, numbered enteroviruses, and the polioviruses, are the most common agents causing viral meningitis, accounting for more than 80% of cases. Human-to-human transmission usually occurs through fecal–oral contamination, although some strains may be acquired by inhalation of respiratory droplets. In the United States, the peak incidence for enterovirus infections is in the summer and early fall. Epidemics may occur, and school-age children constitute the majority of cases, although all age groups are affected. Enterovirus 71 is seen in the Asia-Pacific region where it causes hand, foot, and mouth disease and brainstem encephalitis.

Primary infection with enteroviruses occurs in the GI tract. Seeding of the CNS and other organs results from a viremia. A biphasic fever pattern may occur with initial constitutional symptoms followed by a period of improvement and then recurrent fever with the onset of neurologic symptoms. A variety of exanthems may be associated. Coxsackieviruses may cause concurrent myocarditis, pericarditis, pleurodynia, and conjunctivitis. Individuals with hypogammaglobulinemia may develop a chronic, recurrent meningoencephalitis, which may be associated with a dermatomyositis-like rheumatologic syndrome.

The most common cause of viral encephalitis is herpes simplex virus type 1 (HSV-1). A prodromal syndrome of behavior or personality change may evolve over days into fever, seizures, and cognitive and focal neurologic deficits with depressed sensorium. The disease occurs sporadically and has a predilection for the temporal lobes. Herpes simplex virus type 2 (HSV-2) most often causes meningitis, usually in the setting of concurrent genital infection. When associated with primary genital infection, urinary retention may occur. Both HSV-1 and HSV-2 are also associated with recurrent (Mollaret's) meningitis. Encephalitis caused by varicella-zoster virus (VZV) may be seen in association with primary infection (chicken pox) and in older individuals or those with compromised cell-mediated immunity. Reactivation of VZV infection in patients with impaired cell-mediated immunity may be associated with meningitis, meningomyelitis, or meningoencephalitis, which may occur in the absence of the typical dermatomal rash. Human herpes virus 6 (HHV-6) causes exanthem subitum in infants and can cause meningitis and meningoencephalitis with associated febrile seizures. Other herpes viruses are less frequent causes of encephalitis in normal individuals, but they may cause meningitis or encephalitis in patients with AIDS or immune suppression following organ or bone marrow transplantation. *Cytomegalovirus* (CMV) in immunosuppressed patients may produce meningitis, meningomyeloradiculitis, or encephalitis and affect the retina, GI tract, lungs, and adrenal glands. Epstein-Barr virus (EBV) in AIDS patients is associated with primary CNS lymphoma and may be a cause of encephalitis or lymphoproliferative syndrome in immune suppressed individuals. HSV-2, HHV-6, and HHV-7 have also been reported as causes of encephalitis in transplant and AIDS patients.

Arboviruses comprise a variety of pathogens transmitted by arthropod vectors and, therefore, they occur most frequently in summer and fall. The West Nile Virus (WNV), a *Flavivirus* with worldwide distribution carried by birds and spread to humans by mosquitos, has recently become the most prominent arbovirus in the United States. Transmission by blood transfusion and organ transplantation has also been reported. Infants and individuals older than 50 years of age are at increased risk of encephalitis. A poliomyelitis that produces severe flaccid weakness also occurs. Additional CNS syndromes are still being identified. Prodromal fever, headache, anorexia, nausea, vomiting, lymphadenopathy, myalgia, and a maculopapular or roseolar rash on the face and trunk may precede CNS disease.

St. Louis encephalitis (SLE), also a *Flavivirus*, is found particularly in the central and western states but also, occurs throughout North and South America. Encephalitis is more common in older individuals and may be preceded by a prodrome including malaise, fever, headache, myalgias, conjunctivitis, and upper respiratory tract symptoms. Powassan virus is a tick-borne flavivirus that has been reported to cause occasional cases of encephalitis in New York and New England. Eastern equine encephalitis (EEE), a togavirus, is most prevalent in the Atlantic and Gulf of Mexico coastal regions of the United States. Prodromal symptoms include fever, headache, myalgia, lethargy, vomiting, and abdominal pain. Seizures are common and hyponatremia may be seen. Reported mortality is high with neurologic sequelae in many survivors. Western equine encephalitis (WEE) is found in the western United States and Canada and is currently an infrequent cause of encephalitis. The La Crosse virus (LACV) is found in Midwestern and mid-Atlantic states and typically affects children and adolescents. Seizures occur in half the cases, and focal findings may be present with changes on electroencephalogram (EEG) resembling those found in HSV-1 encephalitis. Japanese encephalitis virus (JEV) is one of the most important pathogens causing encephalitis worldwide. Currently it is primarily found in southern and east Asia with occasional cases in the Philippines and Pacific Islands. Clinical features include headaches, nausea, vomiting, behavioral changes, altered sensorium, and seizures. Tremor, choreoathetosis, rigidity, and flaccid paralysis may also be seen. The disease strikes healthy children and young adults, with mortality rates of up to 33% of cases and significant neurologic sequelae in a high proportion of survivors. Nipah virus (NV) occurs in pigs and has recently been found to cause epidemic encephalitis in pig farmers in Malaysia. Cerebellar and brainstem signs and segmental myoclonus are described.

Mumps, a paramyxovirus, is infrequently seen in the United States today; however, meningitis is the most frequent neurologic manifestation. Infection results from inhalation of respiratory droplets and spreads hematogenously. Parotitis is typical but myocarditis, orchitis, oophoritis, and pancreatitis may also be associated.

Lymphocytic choriomeningitis virus (LCMV) is an *Arenavirus* that is transmitted by rodents and may infect field mice, rats, and hamsters. Transmission to humans may occur by exposure to rodent urine through contaminated food or open wounds, and may affect individuals living in less hygienic, impoverished conditions, or who own or work with rodents. The peak incidence occurs in winter. Myocarditis, pericarditis, orchitis, or arthritis may be associated.

The reovirus, which causes Colorado tick fever, is transmitted by a wood tick found in mountainous areas in the western United States. Meningitis is associated with retro-orbital pain and, in some cases, a macular rash. Leukopenia and thrombocytopenia are common, and bleeding complications may result.

Acute infection with HIV may be associated with meningitis as part of a mononucleosis syndrome. JC virus (JCV) infects oligodendrocytes and causes progressive multifocal leukoencephalopathy in immunosuppressed individuals, most commonly in AIDS. Rarely, influenza A and B may cause encephalitis. Influenza A has been associated with a particularly aggressive necrotizing encephalitis. Rabies is rare in the United States where isolated cases of encephalitis have been linked to bat bites.

Postinfectious encephalomyelitis is an acute demyelinating disease that may follow infection with an enterovirus, influenza virus, measles virus, or herpes viruses. It may also be seen following vaccination. Multifocal neurologic symptoms and signs, headache, seizures, or depressed sensorium appear within weeks of the preceding infection or vaccination. The illness is monophasic and may resolve with or without neurologic sequelae.

Diagnosis

A variety of conditions that may mimic viral meningitis or encephalitis need to be excluded in the diagnostic evaluation (Tables 1 and 2).

TABLE 1 Differential Diagnoses of Viral Meningitis

Bacterial meningitis
Parameningeal infections
Sinusitis
Paravertebral abscess
Fungal meningitis
Mycobacterium tuberculosis meningitis
Lymphomatous and carcinomatous meningitis
Syphilis
Lyme disease
Leptospirosis
Parasitic meningoencephalitis
Subarachnoid hemorrhage
Dural sinus thrombosis
Noninfectious inflammatory diseases
Sarcoidosis
Systemic lupus erythematosus
Behçet's disease
Vasculitis
Drug-induced meningitis
Nonsteroidal anti-inflammatory agents
Muromonab-CD3 (OKT-3)
Sulfonamides
Intravenous immunoglobulin
Carbamazepine (Tegretol)
Metronidazole (Flagyl)

Magnetic resonance imaging (MRI) is the imaging study of choice. In viral meningitis, MRI is usually normal although nonspecific enhancement of meninges may be seen following gadolinium contrast infusion. In HSV-1 encephalitis, MRI reveals a lesion with increased signal on T2 sequences and enhancement following gadolinium contrast infusion on T1 sequences, usually in the medial and inferior temporal lobe. In WNV and CMV encephalitis, enhancement of meninges or ventricular ependyma and, in some cases of WNV, lesions in the basal ganglia and thalami may be seen. White matter lesions are found with VZV, JCV, and NV.

Cerebrospinal fluid (CSF) is the most useful examination in evaluating patients with meningitis and encephalitis, and is important both to exclude alternative conditions and to attempt to establish a specific etiologic diagnosis. CSF typically reveals a lymphocytic pleocytosis with less than 1000 cells/mm^3, although higher cell counts may be seen with some arboviruses. An early polymorphonuclear response may be found in the first 24 hours, and CMV is associated with a persistent polymorphonuclear pleocytosis in immunosuppressed individuals. Protein is usually elevated but may be normal in some patients with meningitis. Glucose levels are generally normal but may be depressed with LCMV, mumps, and the herpes viruses. The most sensitive and specific technique for viral diagnosis is detection of genetic material using polymerase chain reaction (PCR) amplification techniques. For RNA viruses, reverse transcriptase PCR (RT-PCR) is used. In HSV-1 encephalitis, PCR has eliminated the need for brain biopsy in most cases.

TABLE 2 Differential Diagnoses of Viral Encephalitis

Bacterial abscesses
Subdural empyema
Brain tumors
Mycobacterium tuberculosis
Fungal infection
Parasitic infections
Rickettsia
Drug intoxication
Delirium tremens
Malignant hyperthermia
Metabolic diseases
Thyroid disease
Electrolyte disorders
Hyperglycemia, hypoglycemia
Hypoxia
Vasculitis
Subdural hematoma
Multiple cerebral infarctions
Syphilis
Sarcoidosis
Paraneoplastic encephalitis
Acute psychosis

Demonstration of virus-specific immunoglobulin (Ig) M responses in blood or CSF, or of fourfold elevations of specific IgG in convalescent compared to acute serum samples, are alternative ways of establishing an etiologic diagnosis. Diagnosis of WNV is established by finding specific IgM in CSF, which appears by the end of the first week. WNV RNA can also be detected by RT-PCR. IgM antibodies to WNV may persist in serum for up to 6 months. IgG antibodies to WNV appear after a week and rise in serum but may cross-react with SLE or JEV and, therefore, must be confirmed with a more specific test such as a plaque neutralization assay. Diagnosis of other arbovirus infections is based on findings of virus-specific IgM antibody in CSF, a fourfold rise in titer of specific viral antibodies in serum, or isolation of the pathogen. Antibodies are less useful for herpes virus infections; in HSV-1 they are not found in the CSF until 10 to 14 days following onset of infection. Enteroviruses may be isolated from stool or throat cultures; however, because viral shedding may persist for weeks after active infection, recovery from these sites is inconclusive unless virus is also recovered from blood or CSF. PCR testing is available for enteroviruses. It has been advocated, despite the benign natural history of enterovirus meningitis in most cases, as cost effective in reducing duration of hospitalization and antibiotic therapy.

In patients with postinfectious encephalitis, CSF reveals a lymphocytic pleocytosis, normal glucose, elevated protein, and myelin basic protein, sometimes with oligoclonal bands.

Electroencephalography may reveal periodic lateralized epileptiform discharges in patients with HSV-1 or LACV, but it is most commonly nonspecific. Brain biopsy is less often pursued since the availability of PCR; however, when a lesion is identified and no specific diagnosis is established, tissue sampling may still be required. (Tables 3 and 4 provide diagnostic studies.)

Treatment

In the immunocompetent individual, most episodes of viral meningitis are self-limited and benign in

TABLE 3 Evaluation of Suspected Viral Meningitis

Cerebrospinal fluid studies
- Opening pressure
- Cell count and differential
- Glucose with matching serum glucose
- VDRL or FTA-ABS
- Gram stain and bacterial culture
- Acid-fast culture and smear, PCR for *Mycobacterium tuberculosis*
- Fungal culture and India ink
- Cryptococcal antigen
- Cytology
- PCR for HSV-1, HSV-2, EBV, VZV, CMV
- RT-PCR for enteroviruses and West Nile virus

Blood studies
- Cultures
- CBC
- Sedimentation rate
- Electrolytes
- Glucose
- Thyroid-stimulating hormone
- Hepatic and renal chemistries
- HIV-1 serology
- Antinuclear antibodies
- VDRL or FTA-ABS
- Protein electrophoresis

Urine drug screen

MRI if indicated to exclude a parameningeal focus, dural venous thrombosis

Abbreviations: CBC = complete blood count, CMV = *Cytomegalovirus*; EBV = Epstein-Barr virus; FTA-ABS = fluorescent treponemal antibody absorption (test); HSV = herpes simplex virus; MRI = magnetic resonance imaging; PCR = polymerase chain reaction; RT-PRC = reverse transcriptase polymerase chain reaction; VDRL = Venereal Disease Research Laboratory (test); VZV = varicella-zoster virus.

TABLE 4 Evaluation of Suspected Viral Encephalitis

Brain MRI
- Cerebrospinal fluid
- Cell count and differential
- Glucose with matching serum glucose
- Protein
- Mycobacterium tuberculosis culture, smear, and PCR
- Fungal culture and antigen studies
- Gram stain and bacterial cultures
- VDRL
- Cytology
- PCR studies for HSV-1, CMV, VZV, EBV, HHV-6, HSV-2, JCV
- RT-PCR for West Nile virus, enteroviruses as indicated
- Antibody studies for arboviruses
- *Borrelia burgdorferi* antibodies (Lyme disease)
- If suspected postinfectious encephalitis: IgG index and oligoclonal bands with matching serum samples

Blood studies
- Serologies for arboviruses, *Toxoplasma gondii*, HIV-1
- Cultures
- CBC
- Sedimentation rate
- Hepatic and renal chemistries
- Electrolytes
- Thyroid-stimulating hormone
- VDRL or FTA-ABS
- Antinuclear antibodies
- Angiotensin-converting enzyme
- Protein electrophoresis
- Paraneoplastic antibody panel

Chest radiograph

Urine toxicology screen

EEG

Imaging of other symptomatic organ systems as indicated

In selected instances, brain biopsy

Abbreviations: CBC = complete blood count, CMV = *Cytomegalovirus*; EBV = Epstein-Barr virus; FTA-ABS = fluorescent treponemal antibody absorption (test); HHV = human herpesvirus; HSV = herpes simplex virus; JCV = JC virus; MRI = magnetic resonance imaging; PCR = polymerase chain reaction; RT-PRC = reverse transcriptase polymerase chain reaction; VDRL = Venereal Disease Research Laboratory (test); VZV = varicella-zoster virus; EEG = electroencephalogram.

their outcome. Coverage with a third-generation cephalosporin such as ceftriaxone (Rocephin), 2 g every 12 hours, or cefotaxime (Claforan), 2 g every 6 hours, and vancomycin, 500 to 750 mg every 6 hours, should be initiated until bacterial meningitis is excluded. Ampicillin may be added if *Listeria monocytogenes* is of concern. Treatment is supportive with administering analgesics and antipyretics, and, particularly in infants and young children, monitoring fluid and electrolyte balance. Pain may be treated with nonsteroidal anti-inflammatory drugs (NSAIDs) and amitriptyline (Elavil) or other tricyclic agents. Although not FDA approved for this use, many physicians combine anticonvulsant agents such as gabapentin (Neurontin), carbamazepine (Tegretol), or lamotrigine (Lamictal) with tricyclics or NSAIDS. In cases of severe pain, short-term use of opiates such as hydrocodone (Norco, Vicodin) may be required. Antiviral therapy is available for the herpes viruses and acyclovir (Zovirax), 200 mg five times daily, or valacyclovir (Valtrex), 1000 mg twice daily, may be given to immunocompetent patients with HSV-2 meningitis complicating genital infection. In immunocompromized patients, HSV-2 meningitis should be treated with high dose intravenous acyclovir as described later for HSV-1 encephalitis.

Acyclovir (Zovirax) is specific therapy for HSV-1 encephalitis in doses of 10 mg/kg intravenously every 8 hours for 14 to 21 days. A similar course of therapy can be used for VZV encephalitis. CMV or HHV-6 meningoencephalitis in immunosuppressed individuals who are not responsive to acyclovir and can be treated initially in individuals with normal renal function using ganciclovir (Cytovene), 5 mg/kg every 12 hours, foscarnet (Foscavir), 90 mg/kg every 12 hours, or for CMV, once weekly cidofovir (Vistide), 5 mg/kg given over 1 hour intravenously in conjunction with 2 g probenecid 3 hours before, and 1 g of probenecid 2 and 8 hours following the infusion. Following successful induction, doses are lowered for maintenance therapy. Careful monitoring of hepatic and renal function is required for all of these agents. Individuals taking cidofovir must have regular monitoring of ocular pressure to prevent blindness related to hypotony. Although no controlled trials are available, some authors recommend initial combined therapy with both ganciclovir and foscarnet in AIDS patients with CMV encephalitis.

Pleconaril is an antiviral agent with efficacy against enteroviruses. While not currently released for use in the United States, it has efficacy for life-threatening enteroviral infections. Ribavirin inhibits WNV and LACV in vitro and is being investigated for therapeutic use. No specific treatment is currently available for other viral encephalitides.

Most neurologists treat patients with postinfectious encephalomyelitis with intravenous methylprednisolone (Solu-Medrol) in typical doses of 1000 mg daily for 5 days, followed by an oral tapering dose, although no controlled trial has been done to support efficacy.

Supportive measures include anticonvulsants to control seizures, control of increased intracranial pressure when required using mannitol, 0.25 to 0.5 g/kg every 3 to 4 hours (adjusting the dose to maintain serum osmolality to between 300 to 320 mOsm/L), management of fluid and electrolyte balance, assisted ventilation as required, prophylaxis for deep vein thrombophlebitis, nutritional support, early initiation of physical therapy to prevent contracture formation, prophylaxis for decubitus, and hygienic measures to limit complicating secondary infections. When the patient is sufficiently stable, more aggressive cognitive and physical rehabilitation measures are initiated.

MULTIPLE SCLEROSIS

METHOD OF

Myla D. Goldman, MD, and

Jeffrey A. Cohen, MD

Multiple sclerosis (MS) is a chronic inflammatory disease of the central nervous system (CNS). The prevalence of MS in the United States is estimated at 250,000 to 350,000 individuals, although there are recent indications that the prevalence may be somewhat higher. The mean age of disease onset is 30 years, with 70% of individuals presenting between 20 and 40 years of age. Women account for approximately 70% of the cases. MS is the most common nontraumatic cause of neurologic disability in young adults. The protean manifestations, clinical heterogeneity, and chronic course after onset in early adulthood make management of MS challenging. Table 1 summarizes the essential features of MS.

TABLE 1 Essential Features of MS

Typical onset age 20 to 40 years (any age possible).
More common in women (approximately 2:1).
Complex genetic susceptibility.
Multifocal inflammatory central nervous system lesions with demyelination and axonal loss.
MRI is useful to detect subclinical pathology, particularly at early stages, both to make the diagnosis and to monitor the disease course.
Protean clinical manifestations.
Marked clinical heterogeneity between patients and in individual patients over time.
RR course at onset In approximately 85% of cases.
Eventual evolution to a SP course in approximately 90% of cases.
Early initiation of disease-modifying treatment is advised for RR-MS.

Abbreviations: MRI = magnetic resonance imaging; MS = multiple sclerosis; RR = relapsing-remitting (multiple sclerosis); SP = secondary progressive (multiple sclerosis).

Etiology and Pathogenesis

The underlying cause of MS remains unknown. The prevailing hypothesis is that MS results from a cell-mediated autoimmune attack directed against myelin antigens. Evidence shows the pathogenesis of the disease to be complex with a number of abnormalities in immune regulation. Recent evidence also supports the involvement of humoral immune mechanisms. Not only is the immunopathogenesis of MS complex, but it appears that there may be four or five pathogenic subtypes, and the predominant immune mechanisms may differ from patient to patient. How this heterogeneity relates to disease course and severity, genetics, imaging characteristics, and response to treatment is the focus of intense study.

MS clearly has a genetic component. The risk of MS in the children of an affected parent is increased approximately 50-fold in comparison to the general population, although it remains relatively low at 3% to 5%. The concordance rate for MS in monozygotic twins is 30% to 50%. While genetic mechanisms are important, their impact on disease expression is not straightforward and involves multiple genes that confer a genetic predisposition and affect the course and severity of disease. A variety of environmental factors also have been implicated as potential causes or triggers of MS in susceptible patients, particularly infectious agents. However, follow-up studies have failed to definitively confirm any of these putative agents. Similar to other autoimmune disorders, MS is more common in women by almost a two to one ratio. This gender effect is mediated at least in part by endocrine factors. The interplay between hormones and the immunopathogenesis of MS is best illustrated during pregnancy when relapse rate is decreased by nearly 50%. In contrast, the year postpartum is a time of increased disease activity.

Historically, demyelination has been emphasized as the main pathophysiologic mechanism producing neurologic manifestations in MS. While inflammatory demyelination and resultant block of nerve conduction in central pathways probably accounts for the reversible manifestations of acute relapses, accumulating evidence suggests that permanent disability results from axonal damage. Axonal damage occurs acutely as a consequence of inflammatory demyelination. Subsequent gradual degeneration occurs in chronically demyelinated fibers and can proceed at least in part in the absence of concomitant inflammation.

Two recent autopsy studies demonstrated that axonal injury is a consistent and prominent feature of active MS lesions. These studies also showed axonal degeneration occurring at a lower rate in axons distant from the site of inflammation. Magnetic resonance spectroscopy studies also demonstrate axonal injury in MS. A number of studies demonstrate reduced levels of the neuronal marker *N*-acetylaspartate in the brains of patients with MS, both in lesions and in white matter that appears normal on routine MR imaging. This reduction in *N*-acetylaspartate begins early in the disease. Cerebral atrophy, from both axonal and myelin loss, can be measured by magnetic resonance imaging (MRI) and is also a frequent finding in patients with long-standing MS. Somewhat surprisingly, considerable atrophy often can be detected in patients with early relapsing-remitting multiple sclerosis (RR-MS) and mild neurologic impairment/disability. These findings have two major implications. First, considerable tissue damage may accumulate subclinically in MS. Second, overt disability probably manifests when ongoing irreversible tissue injury exceeds a critical threshold. These implications support the need to make the diagnosis early in the disease course and consider initiation of treatment before the appearance of significant impairment/disability.

Clinical Features

NEUROLOGIC MANIFESTATIONS

The lesions of MS are multifocal and can occur in any anatomic location within the CNS. Therefore, the possible clinical manifestations are protean. These manifestations vary from patient to patient and in individual patients over time, both in terms of the symptoms present, their anatomic distribution, and their severity.

Visual loss reflects the involvement of the afferent visual system. Unilateral loss of vision caused by optic neuritis is the most common pattern. Involvement of the optic chiasm, optic tract, or optic radiation also can occur. Lesions of the efferent visual system produce abnormalities of eye movement. Diplopia or oscillopsia (jumping vision that may accompany nystagmus) are the most common symptoms.

Motor deficits include weakness, spasticity, and ataxia. Extremity weakness usually is central in character and accompanied by spasticity, hyperreflexia, and abnormal cutaneous reflexes (e.g., Babinski's sign). Involvement of the cerebellum or its afferent or efferent connections leads to appendicular, bulbar, ocular, truncal, or gait ataxia. Weakness or incoordination of bulbar muscle leads to dysarthria or swallowing dysfunction.

Sensory loss can involve any combination of the limbs, trunk, or head in both the small-fiber (light touch, temperature, pain) and large-fiber (vibration, proprioception) modalities. The pattern of sensory involvement can be patchy or simulate a peripheral nerve or dermatomal pattern. Loss of sensation (negative sensory symptoms) often is accompanied by positive sensory phenomena (tingling, prickling, aching). Some patients have neuropathic pain, which can be sharp, lancinating, and paroxysmal, or a more chronic burning hypersensitivity. Other sources of pain include meningeal irritation from adjacent inflammation (e.g., in optic neuritis or transverse myelitis), painful spasms, and musculoskeletal pain from degenerative arthritis and immobility.

Gait impairment and resultant disability is of particular concern because of the impact on quality of life and self-image. Gait dysfunction can result from weakness, spasticity, ataxia, vestibular symptoms, sensory loss, and visual impairment. Identification of the main contributors to gait dysfunction is needed to guide treatment and design compensatory strategies. Evaluation by a physical therapist can help with this determination.

Bladder, bowel, and sexual symptoms are sometimes overlooked by health care providers but can also have an important impact on quality of life. The most common urinary symptoms are increased frequency and urgency, sometimes with urge incontinence, from detrusor hyperactivity (an uninhibited bladder with impaired ability to store urine). Often, in addition to impaired ability of the bladder to store urine, there is hesitancy and a sense of incomplete emptying, reflecting detrusor-sphincter dyssynergia (incoordination between bladder contraction and sphincter relaxation). Occasionally, failure to empty is caused by a flaccid, nonresponsive bladder. Formal urodynamic studies usually are necessary to accurately delineate the pathophysiology of bladder dysfunction. Constipation is the most common bowel symptom, but urgency and incontinence also occur. Erectile dysfunction is common in men, and altered libido is common in both genders. Fatigue, spasticity, altered sensation, bladder symptoms, depression, and medication side effects are important potential contributors to sexual dysfunction.

Cognitive dysfunction occurs in up to 66.6% of patients with MS, most often involving problems with concentration, processing speed, executive function (e.g., complex planning), and visuospatial abilities. Formal cognitive testing usually is necessary to accurately assess the severity of cognitive impairment and delineate the domains involved. Depression also is common in MS. As expected, emotional distress is a common reaction to the diagnosis or subsequent perceived worsening. In addition, patients with

MS appear to be at increased risk for underlying biologic depression.

In several surveys of patients with MS, fatigue was listed as the most troubling symptom. Fatigue in MS has a number of contributing aspects. Medication side effects, sleep disturbance, depression, and other medical conditions all can contribute to fatigue. In addition, there are two aspects of fatigue more directly related to MS. First, patients with MS often experience transient worsening in neurologic function with exertion or increased body temperature, probably reflecting failure of nerve conduction in demyelinated pathways. Second, patients with MS, as in a variety of other immune-mediated and infectious disorders, report chronic lassitude or lack of energy, probably from chronic immune activation and resultant elaboration of immune mediators.

DISEASE COURSE

By convention, MS is classified on the basis of the time course over which clinical manifestations develop (Table 2). This classification system is empiric and, at this point, not based on biologic factors. Therefore, the pathogenic differences between these disease categories remain uncertain. Nevertheless, this classification scheme provides a useful framework for diagnosis, clinical management, and selection of subjects for clinical trials.

Relapsing-Remitting Multiple Sclerosis (RR-MS)

MS initially follows an RR course in approximately 85% of patients. Clinical manifestations of a relapse typically develop over several days to weeks then resolve partially or completely over several weeks to months. Relapses occur on average every 1 to 2 years, although the relapse rate varies markedly both between patients and in individual patients over time.

TABLE 2 Classification of Multiple Sclerosis Based on Clinical Course

Relapsing-remitting (RR)	Symptoms and signs develop in the context of acute relapses followed by partial or complete recovery. Clinical manifestations are stable between relapses.
Secondary progressive (SP)	Gradual worsening following an initially relapsing-remitting course. There may be superimposed relapses or not.
Primary progressive (PP)	Manifestations gradually worsen from disease onset without relapses.
Progressive relapsing (PR)	Manifestations gradually worsen from disease onset with subsequent superimposed relapses.

Adapted from: Lublin FD, Reingold SC: Defining the clinical course of multiple sclerosis: results of an international survey. Neurology 46:907, 1996.

Secondary Progressive Multiple Sclerosis (SP-MS)

Ten to 15 years after disease onset, RR-MS usually evolves into a secondary progressive (SP) phase, in which pre-existing neurologic deficits gradually worsen. The transition from RR-MS to SP-MS is gradual. Early in the transition, there may be relapses superimposed on gradual worsening. However, relapses tend to become less evident over time.

Primary Progressive Multiple Sclerosis (PP-MS)

Approximately 15% of patients have gradually worsening neurologic manifestations (typically those of a myelopathy) from the onset of the disease without acute relapses, the so-called primary progressive (PP)-MS. Compared to patients with relapsing forms of the disease, patients with PP-MS typically are older at onset, more often men, have fewer lesions on an MRI of the brain, and respond less well to disease-modifying therapies.

Progressive-Relapsing Multiple Sclerosis (PR-MS)

Progressive-relapsing (PR)-MS is a rare form of MS in which there is gradual worsening from disease onset with subsequent superimposed relapses. It is suspected that PR-MS in many cases represents SP-MS in which the initial relapses were clinically silent, unrecognized, or forgotten.

PROGNOSIS

MS patients typically have mild manifestations between relapses and minimal residual impairment/disability for the first 5 to 10 years after disease onset. However, in nearly 60%, RR-MS evolves into an SP course with moderate to severe disability within 15 years of onset and, in 90%, 25 years after onset. Thus, the majority of patients become disabled at a relatively young age. A certain proportion of MS patients (10% to 20%) worsen very slowly and exhibit minimal disability even after a prolonged course. Although benign MS does exist, that diagnosis should be made cautiously and most appropriately only in retrospect.

Clinical features that suggest increased risk for disability include:

- Frequent relapses with incomplete recovery
- Evolution from an RR to an SP course
- Progressive course from onset
- Accumulation of disability relatively early after disease onset
- A preponderance of motor or cerebellar manifestations
- Cognitive impairment

The absence of these features plus the presence of a number of other features (e.g., early age of onset, female gender, predominance of visual and sensory relapses, long duration between relapses, and complete recovery from relapses) have been proposed to predict a better prognosis. However, the predictive value of these features for a good prognosis is limited. MRI features that indicate increased risk for future disability include a substantial T_2-hyperintense lesion burden, substantial T_1-hypointense lesion burden, continued radiographic activity such as gadolinium enhancement or development of new lesions, and the presence and progression of atrophy.

Making the Diagnosis of Multiple Sclerosis

Because MS has no absolutely pathognomonic clinical, laboratory, or imaging features, making the diagnosis ultimately remains a clinical decision based on weighing the factors supporting the diagnosis versus those that fail to support the diagnosis or that suggest an alternative one. The potential differential diagnoses of MS are extensive (Table 3). The clinical picture determines how aggressively alternative diagnoses need to be addressed in a particular patient.

Establishing the diagnosis of MS is straightforward when patients exhibit the classic clinical features described above with onset at the appropriate age and developing with an RR or SP course. In this situation, the likelihood of finding another cause is very small, and extensive testing is unnecessary other than cranial MRI and selected blood tests. However, the clinician must remain vigilant for certain *red flags* that suggest an alternative diagnosis needs to be considered (Table 4). In these cases, more extensive testing, guided by the clinical picture, is warranted to provide additional support for the diagnosis of MS and to eliminate other diseases.

TABLE 3 Principal Differential Diagnoses of Multiple Sclerosis

Infection	Lyme disease, syphilis, progressive multifocal leukoencephalopathy, HIV, HTLV-1, herpes zoster, HHV-6
Inflammatory	Systemic lupus, Sjögren's syndrome, vasculitis, sarcoidosis, Behçet's, Susacs syndrome, celiac disease
Genetic and metabolic	Vitamin B_{12} deficiency, lysosomal disorders, adrenoleukodystrophy, mitochondrial disorders, other genetic disorders, CADASIL
Neoplastic	Primary central nervous system lymphoma
Spine disease	Vascular malformations, degenerative spine disease

Abbreviations: CADASIL = cerebral autosomal dominant arteriopathy with subcortical infarcts and leukoencephalopathy; HHV-6 = human herpesvirus-6; HTLV-1 = human T-cell leukemia virus 1.

TABLE 4 Red Flags for the Potential Mistaken Diagnosis of Multiple Sclerosis

- Onset of symptoms before age of 20 years and after age of 40 years
- Very prominent family history
- Atypical course
  - Gradually progressive from onset, particularly in a young patient or with manifestations other than a myelopathy
  - Abrupt onset of symptoms
- Unifocal manifestations (even if relapsing or progressive)
- Presence of neurologic manifestations unusual for MS
- Presence of systemic manifestations
- Missing features, particularly in long-standing or severe disease
  - Absence of visual, sensory, or bladder involvement or abnormal reflexes
  - Normal MRI, cerebrospinal fluid, or evoked potentials
- Atypical response to treatment
  - Lack of any response to corticosteroids
  - Implausibly rapid or dramatic response to corticosteroids or disease-modifying treatments

Abbreviations: MRI = magnetic resonance imaging; MS = multiple sclerosis.

Adapted from: Fox RJ, Cohen JA: Multiple sclerosis: the importance of early recognition and treatment. Cleve Clin J Med 68:157, 2001. Used with permission.

MAGNETIC RESONANCE IMAGING

Cranial MRI is the most useful test in the diagnostic evaluation of MS. It is abnormal in approximately 90% of patients, although it may be normal or the findings nonspecific early in the course. Cranial MRI should include long TR images (T2-weighted or fluid-attenuated inversion recovery [FLAIR]) plus T1-weighted images before and after administration of gadolinium.

Typical findings include multiple ovoid or patchy foci of increased signal on long TR images in the periventricular and subcortical white matter, corpus callosum, brainstem, and cerebellum. Ovoid lesions oriented perpendicular to the lateral ventricles (so-called *Dawson's fingers*) or lesions involving U-fibers underlying cortical sulci are particularly characteristic of MS. Often, one or more (but usually not all) of the T_2-hyperintense lesions exhibit enhancement on T1-weighted images following administration of gadolinium. Gadolinium-enhancement results from increased permeability of the blood–brain barrier and is thought to reflect active inflammation in the lesion. Finally, cortical, corpus callosum, or generalized atrophy is a typical feature, particularly in long-standing MS.

Spinal MRI should be obtained if cranial MRI is negative, the findings are nonspecific, or the patient's principal manifestations localize to the spinal cord. Typical spinal cord lesions in MS are ovoid or patchy and extend for only one or two spinal segments.

CEREBROSPINAL FLUID ANALYSIS

Additional support for the diagnosis of MS can be obtained by examination of the cerebrospinal fluid (CSF). A mild mononuclear cell pleocytosis and modest elevation of total protein are common, though nonspecific, findings. Increased immunoglobulin (Ig) G index, increased calculated IgG synthesis rate, and the presence of oligoclonal bands are more characteristic of MS and reflect intrathecal production of immunoglobulin. CSF examination is not always necessary when the diagnosis can be made with confidence based on clinical features and MRI. However, clinicians should have a low threshold for CSF examination in cases with nondiagnostic or atypical features.

EVOKED POTENTIALS

Evoked potentials are useful to demonstrate lesions in visual, auditory, or somatosensory pathways that cannot be confirmed by clinical examination or imaging studies.

BLOOD STUDIES

Blood studies are obtained to exclude other disorders that can mimic MS (see Table 3). When a patient's clinical and imaging features are typical of MS, only limited blood studies are needed:

- Complete blood count (CBC)
- Erythrocyte sedimentation rate and antinuclear antibody to screen for connective tissue disorders and other inflammatory conditions
- A serologic test for syphilis
- Vitamin B_{12} level
- A thyroid-stimulating hormone level

A low positive antinuclear antibody titer is common in MS and should not prompt concern in the absence of other features suggesting connective tissue disease. When there are clinical, imaging, or CSF findings atypical of MS, more extensive testing is appropriate, guided by the overall picture.

FORMAL DIAGNOSTIC CRITERIA

The diagnosis of MS depends conceptually on demonstrating objective evidence of multifocal lesions of the CNS developing at multiple times, which is well-outlined in the so-called Schumacher criteria. Traditionally, this demonstration depended on clinical history and the neurologic examination. The recently proposed MacDonald criteria include provisions allowing the use of MRI to make this determination, thus facilitating the diagnosis of MS to be made at an early stage.

Symptomatic Management

Patients with MS experience a variety of symptoms and other sequelae that interfere with their daily activities and reduce quality of life. Identification of troublesome symptoms for which effective treatments exist (Table 5) is an important aspect of management. Because medications used to treat some MS symptoms have the potential to exacerbate other symptoms, it is helpful to prioritize which symptoms are most troublesome. The dose and dosing schedule should be tailored to the patient's needs. For example, it sometimes is useful to have patients take a higher dose of medications at bedtime to treat symptoms interfering with sleep and a lower dose during the day to avoid side effects. Because the manifestations of MS evolve over time, symptom management is an ongoing process. Finally, medications are not the only approach to treat the sequelae of MS. Adjunct therapies are a useful addition to medications to treat some symptoms (e.g., use of a stretching program in addition to medications to treat spasticity or counseling in addition to antidepressant medication to treat emotional distress). Also, some sequelae such as employment and family issues, which are common in MS, require approaches other than medication.

Management of Acute Relapses

EVALUATION

The evaluation of a potential relapse focuses on ruling out a *pseudorelapse* and identifying any possible precipitating factor, specifically infection. Patients with MS frequently experience fluctuations in their symptoms. Worsening symptoms lasting only a few minutes or hours do not constitute a relapse. Rather, the new symptom or worsening of pre-existing symptoms should persist for at least 24 hours to constitute a relapse. Also, previous symptoms can reappear or existing symptoms can worsen with increased body temperature from exertion, environment, or fever. In these cases, symptoms revert to their previous baseline with return of body temperature.

The most important precipitating factor to consider when evaluating a potential relapse is infection. First, the fever of an infection can produce a pseudorelapse. Second, treatment of the infection may be required, in addition to treatment of the relapse.

TREATMENT

The initial step in relapse management is treatment of any precipitating conditions (e.g., infection and/or symptoms such as vertigo). Corticosteroid therapy is administered to shorten relapse duration and accelerate recovery. Although, there is the presumption that corticosteroid treatment limits tissue damage and reduces residual impairment, the evidence for this is not convincing. Because most relapses recover spontaneously, mild relapses do not require intervention. However, the occurrence of even mild relapses signals active disease and possibly the need to initiate disease-modifying therapy.

The typical corticosteroid regimen is 500 to 1000 mg of methylprednisolone (Solu-Medrol) administered by

TABLE 5 Pharmacologic Management of Multiple Sclerosis Symptoms

Symptom and Treatment*	Comments
Spasticity	Medication should be combined with a regular stretching program. Consider combination therapy when monotherapy is ineffective. Consider intrathecal baclofen (Lioresal) for severe spasticity inadequately controlled by oral medication.
Baclofen (Lioresol) 5-20 mg bid to qid	Higher doses sometimes are helpful but can exacerbate weakness, ataxia, or fatigue.
Tizanidine (Zanaflex) 4-8 mg tid to qid	Less tendency to produce weakness as compared to baclofen but more sedating.
Gabapentin (Neurontin)[1] 300-900 mg bid to qid	Useful as adjunct therapy for spasticity, particularly when there is concomitant pain or paroxysmal symptoms. Well tolerated but may require high doses. Titrate to avoid sedation.
Diazepam (Valium) 2-10 mg qhs to tid	Useful for nocturnal spasms.
Clonazepam (Klonopin)[1] 0.5-5 mg qhs to tid	Useful for nocturnal spasms.
Dantrolene (Dantrium) 25-100 mg bid to qid	Least cerebral side effects but greatest concomitant weakness. Monitor for hepatotoxicity.
Neuropathic Pain	
Gabapentin (Neurontin)[1] 300-900 mg tid to qid	Useful for neuropathic pain, particularly when there is concomitant spasticity or paroxysmal symptoms. Well-tolerated but may require high doses. Titrate to avoid sedation.
Lamotrigine (Lamictal)[1] 25-200 mg daily to bid	
Topiramate (Topamax)[1] 25-200 mg bid	Cognitive side effects and weight loss may limit utility.
Carbamazepine (Tegretol-XR)[1] 100-600 mg bid	Sedating and may exacerbate ataxia. Extended release form is better tolerated.
Oxcarbazepine (Trileptal)[1] 150-600 mg bid	Sedating and may exacerbate ataxia.
Amitriptyline (Elavil)[1] 25-150 mg qhs	Sedation and anticholinergic side effects may be useful or may be dose-limiting.
Nortriptyline (Pamelor)[1] 25-150 mg qhs	Less sedation and anticholinergic side effects compared to amitriptyline.
Phenytoin (Dilantin)[1] 300-600 mg daily	May exacerbate ataxia.
Paroxysmal Sensory and Motor Disorders	
Gabapentin (Neurontin)[1] 300-900 mg tid to qid	Useful for paroxysmal disorders, particularly when there is concomitant spasticity or neuropathic pain. Well tolerated but may require high doses. Titrate to avoid sedation.
Carbamazepine (Tegretol-XR) 100-600 mg bid	Sedating and may exacerbate ataxia. Extended release form is better tolerated.
Phenytoin (Dilantin)[1] 300-600 mg daily	May exacerbate ataxia.
Fatigue	Medication should be combined with an exercise program. Medication should be administered early in the day.
Amantadine (Symmetrel)[1] 100 mg q AM to bid	Watch for livedo reticularis.
Modafinil (Provigil)[1] 100-200 mg q AM to bid	
Pemoline (Cylert)[1] 18.75-37.5 mg q AM to bid	Hepatotoxicity is rare but must be monitored.
Depression	Combine medications with counseling.
Selective serotonin reuptake inhibitors (SSRIs)	Medications of choice. The energizing effects can be helpful for fatigue.
Tricyclic antidepressants	Useful when there is concomitant pain, detrusor hyperactivity, or sleep disturbance.
Vertigo	
Meclizine (Antivert) 25 mg tid to qid	Sedating

TABLE 5 Pharmacologic Management of Multiple Sclerosis Symptoms—cont'd

Symptom and Treatment*	Comments
Scopolamine patch (Transderm Scop)[1] every 3 days	
Ondansetron (Zofran)[1] 8 mg bid	
Diazepam (Valium)[1] 2-10 mg tid to qid	Sedating.
Ataxic Tremor	Medications are only rarely effective. A selected subset of patients may benefit from surgery, either stereotactic ablation of the ventrolateral thalamic nucleus or implantation of a thalamic stimulator.
Ondansetron (Zofran)[1] 8 mg bid	
Gabapentin (Neurontin)[1] 300-900 mg tid to qid	
Primidone (Mysoline)[1] 100-250 mg tid to qid	
Detrusor Hyperactivity	Fluid restriction in the evening or low-dose desmopressin (DDAVP) acetate may be useful for nocturia, but patients should avoid fluid restriction during the day. Patients on anticholinergic medication need to be monitored for incomplete bladder emptying.
Oxybutynin (Ditropan XL) 5-15 mg daily	Extended-release form is better tolerated.
Tolterodine (Detrol) 2 mg bid	Less systemic anticholinergic side effects as compared to oxybutynin but may not be as potent.
Flaccid Bladder	
Bethanechol (Urecholine) 10-50 mg bid to qid	Intermittent catheterization or urinary diversion often are preferable.
Detrusor-Sphincter Dyssynergia	
Terazosin (Hytrin)[1] 5-10 mg qhs	Often detrusor-sphincter dyssynergia occurs with detrusor hyperactivity. In that setting terazosin or intermittent catheterization can be combined with anticholinergic medication.
Constipation	Medications need to be combined with adequate fluid intake, dietary fiber, and exercise. Avoid anticholinergic medications.
Bulk forming agents	
Lactulose (Kristalose) 10-20 g daily	
Bowel Urgency	
Bulk forming agents	Need to be combined with scheduled voiding. Biofeedback sometimes is useful.
Impotence	
Sildenafil (Viagra) 50-100 mg prn	Largely has replaced other approaches. Need to rule out other medical conditions, emotional factors, effects of other MS symptoms, and medication side effects.

Abbreviations: bid = twice daily; prn = as needed; qhs = at bedtime; qid = four times a day; tid = three times a day.
[1]Not FDA approved for this indication.
*Treatments listed in order of usefulness and general use.
Adapted from: Fox RJ, Cohen JA. Multiple sclerosis: the importance of early recognition and treatment. Cleve Clin J Med 68:157, 2001. Used with permission.

daily intravenous infusion for 3 to 5 days, followed by a tapering dose of oral prednisone over 1 to 2 weeks (e.g., 60 mg per day for 4 days, 40 mg per day for 4 days, 20 mg per day for 4 days). The optimal dose and duration of intravenous methylprednisolone and the need for an oral taper are uncertain. Several studies suggest that comparable doses of oral corticosteroids can be substituted for intravenous methylprednisolone with good tolerability and similar efficacy. This approach, though not standard, certainly reduces cost. Some patients benefit from antacids or gastric acid blocker to lessen gastrointestinal (GI) symptoms and from a sleep medication for insomnia. Corticosteroids typically are administered in an outpatient infusion center or via home health care. Inpatient treatment should be considered for any patient with a concurrent disease that would complicate corticosteroid treatment (e.g., diabetes or severe hypertension), or when the manifestations of the relapse result in loss of independent function.

Rehabilitation can be useful to develop compensatory strategies, restore function, and improve quality of life following an acute relapse. Physical therapy (particularly to address gait impairment), occupational therapy, speech therapy, and swallowing therapy can be helpful in the appropriate clinical setting.

Disease-Modifying Therapy

RELAPSING-REMITTING MULTIPLE SCLEROSIS

It is strongly recommended to initiate disease-modifying therapy once the diagnosis of RR-MS is secure based on the rationale outlined in Table 6. Current therapies target the immune dysfunction in MS and resultant tissue damage in the central nervous system with the goal of reducing or preventing long-term permanent disability. In clinical trials, measures of efficacy have included relapse rate and proportion of relapse-free patients, progression of neurologic impairment and disability, and MRI activity and lesion burden. Based on various combinations of these outcomes, four treatments currently are approved in the United States for standard treatment of RR-MS:

1. Interferon beta-1a by intramuscular injection (IFN-β_{1a} [IM]) (Avonex)
2. IFN-β_{1a} by subcutaneous injection (IFN-β_{1a} [SC]) (Rebif)
3. IFN-β_{1b} SC (Betaseron)
4. Glatiramer acetate (GA) (Copaxone)

The interferons are recombinant products with amino acid sequences identical to or nearly identical to that of human interferon β. The approved doses of the IFN-βs are IFN-β_{1a} (IM) (Avonex), 30 mg IM weekly; IFN-β_{1a} (SC) (Rebif), 22 or 44 μg SC three times per week; and IFN-β_{1b} (Betaseron), 8 million (M)IU (0.25 mg) SC on alternate days. GA is a complex mixture of random polypeptides based on the amino acid sequence of myelin basic protein. The approved dose of GA (Copaxone) is 20 mg SC daily.

TABLE 6 The Rationale for Early Treatment of Multiple Sclerosis (MS)

Most cases ultimately evolve into a progressive course with some degree of permanent disability.
Although benign MS exists, it is uncommon.
The ability to predict prognosis in individual patients, particularly a mild course, is limited.
While clinical relapses are intermittent and impairment/disability is mild early in the disease, inflammatory lesions form almost continuously and irreversible tissue injury accumulates from the earliest stages. Thus, the clinical features present and their severity correlate poorly with the ongoing pathologic process.
Disease-modifying therapies are available that effectively reduce disease activity measured clinically and by MRI in RR-MS, albeit incompletely. It is likely that these agents also reduce the accumulation or irreversible tissue damage and disability. These agents are preventative not restorative.
Extensive experience confirms that, despite troublesome side effects, these agents are safe in general.
These agents exhibit increased effectiveness when started early in the disease.
Accumulating irreversible pathology, decreasing inflammation, increasing complexity of the immunopathogenic process, and evolution of MS into a degenerative process limit the effectiveness of disease-modifying therapies late in the disease.

Although the definitive trials of these drugs examined somewhat different patient populations, had different primary and secondary endpoints, and produced somewhat different results, these agents have, in our view, largely comparable overall effectiveness. All four agents reduced relapse rate by approximately 30% and had beneficial effects on MRI measures of disease activity and lesion accrual. The data for delaying short-term impairment/disability progression was most convincing for IFN-β_{1a} (IM), which produced a 37% reduction in a phase 3 trial. There are data supporting benefit on disability progression for the other three agents also. It is anticipated that the short-term beneficial effects on relapses, impairment/disability progression, and MRI measures demonstrated in clinical trials lasting to 2 to 3 years will translate into meaningful long-term benefit. Data are beginning to emerge that support this expectation.

All of the available agents have limitations. All are expensive, costing approximately $10,000 per year. All are administered by injection one to several times per week, which is inconvenient and unpleasant for patients. Although serious adverse effects are very rare, all of these agents have side effects (Table 7). Patients need to continue these therapies long-term. Patient education before initiation of therapy and aggressive management of side effects are critical to maintaining compliance. In general, we recommend that a neurologist who has familiarity with the use of these therapies be consulted at treatment onset.

The most important limitation of the standard agents used to treat RR-MS is their partial effectiveness. A substantial proportion of patients in the active treatment arms of all of the studies of these agents continued to have relapses or worsening of impairment/disability. The emerging evidence for pathologic heterogeneity in MS suggests that the partial efficacy of these agents may reflect, at least in part, the presence of responders and nonresponders.

Mitoxantrone (Novantrone) was approved in the United States for "reducing neurologic disability and/or the frequency of clinical relapses in patients with secondary-progressive, progressive-relapsing, or worsening relapsing-remitting MS." Mitoxantrone has potent effects on cellular and humoral immunity. Typically in MS it is administered by intravenous infusion at a dose of 12 mg/m^2 body surface area every 3 months. In clinical trials, mitoxantrone led to significant reductions in relapse rate, disability progression, and MRI measures in both RR- and SP-MS. In general mitoxantrone is well tolerated. The most common adverse effects, which are summarized in Table 7, are blue discoloration of the urine and sclera, nausea, transient bone marrow suppression, amenorrhea, and infertility. Because of potential cardiac toxicity, patients with pre-existing cardiac disease should not receive mitoxantrone, and the total cumulative dose should not exceed 140 mg/m^2. Mitoxantrone also has been implicated in increasing risk for secondary leukemia. Mitoxantrone should be administered by clinicians familiar with its use.

TABLE 7 Side Effects of Approved Multiple Sclerosis Disease-Modifying Therapies

Drug and Side Effects	Comments
Interferon-β (Avonex, Betaseron, Rebif)	
Common Side Effects	
Flulike constitutional symptoms	Usually decrease over time. Managed by evening administration and pretreatment with acetaminophen and/or nonsteroidal anti-inflammatory drugs.
Injection site reactions	More frequent with IFN-β_{1b} (Betaseron) (SC) and IFN-β_{1a} (Rebif) (SC) compared to IFN-β_{1a} (Avonex) (IM).
Rare Side Effects	
Thyroid dysfunction	
Depression	
Headache	
Menstrual disorders	
Gastrointestinal symptoms	
Increased spasticity	
Alopecia	
Worsening of psoriasis	
Leukopenia	
Increased hepatic transaminases	
Glatiramer Acetate (Copaxone)	
Injection site reaction	Usually mild.
Postinjection systemic reaction	Noncardiac and nonanaphylactoid. Self-limited flushing, shortness of breath, palpitations, diaphoresis, anxiety.
Hives	Rare.
Mitoxantrone (Novantrone)	
Blue urine and sclera	Lasts 1 to 2 days after infusion.
Leukopenia, thrombocytopenia	Common but usually short-lived and uncomplicated.
Nausea	Usually mild.
Headache	Usually mild.
Alopecia	Usually mild.
Amenorrhea, infertility	Can be irreversible.
Heart failure	Risk related to total cumulative dose. Evaluate cardiac function before and during treatment by radionuclide gated blood pool scan (multigated angiogram [MUGA]). Do not administer mitoxantrone to patients with known heart disease.

Its use should be restricted to patients who are felt to be at substantial risk for future disability because of fulminant disease or disease that remains active despite monotherapy with the standard agents for RR-MS.

The optimal approach for RR-MS patients with modest breakthrough disease on standard therapy and for whom the risk mitoxantrone toxicity is not felt to be justified remains uncertain. Several studies show increased benefit on inflammatory aspects of RR-MS (relapses and MRI measures) with IFN-β administered at higher doses and more frequent dosing. However, the increase in benefit was modest. The potential greater benefit must be weighed against the increased side effects and greater tendency of these IFN-β preparations to elicit neutralizing antibodies. The second general approach would be to change between classes of drug—for example, from IFN-β to GA or vice versa. Although this approach has appeal, its utility is unproven. The third approach is to combine therapy with available agents, such as adding methotrexate (Rheumatrex)[1], azathioprine (Imuran)[1], or corticosteroids to IFN-β or GA. Although combination therapy is effective in other diseases and is frequently employed by clinicians, support for this approach in MS is based on only a small number of preliminary studies. In summary, at the present time, the optimal approach to treat patients with RR-MS and breakthrough disease on monotherapy with standard agents remains uncertain.

CLINICALLY ISOLATED SYNDROMES

The current criteria do not allow the diagnosis of MS to be made at the time of a clinically isolated event (i.e., the first relapse). Evidence of an anatomically and temporally distinct lesion is required. Previous criteria required this additional lesion to manifest as a clinical relapse. The advantage of the new MacDonald criteria is that this lesion can be subclinical and demonstrated by MRI. Even in the absence of additional evidence securing the diagnosis, certain clinical syndromes developing in a young adult should lead a neurologist to strongly suspect the diagnosis of MS, including monocular optic neuritis, partial transverse myelitis, or brainstem syndromes. Individuals with these syndromes should be advised of the possibility of MS, particularly with an abnormal MRI showing lesions in addition to the one accounting for the patient's symptoms. In addition, initiation of disease-modifying therapy should be

[1]Not FDA approved for this indication.

considered, particularly if the initial relapse was severe or recovered incompletely, or if cranial MRI shows a substantial lesion burden. The Controlled High-risk Avonex Multiple Sclerosis Prevention Study trial (CHAMPS) and the Early Treatment Of Multiple Sclerosis (ETOMS) studies show that IFN-β_{1a} effectively decreases clinical and MRI activity when started at the time of a clinically isolated syndrome. IFN-β_{1a} (IM) (Avonex) is approved for this indication.

PROGRESSIVE FORMS OF MULTIPLE SCLEROSIS

IFN-β_{1b} (Betaseron) and mitoxantrone (Novantrone) are approved for the treatment of SP-MS. However, treatment of SP-MS remains problematic. The evidence supporting the benefit of available therapies is less convincing than for RR-MS. The European multicenter study of IFN-β_{1b} shows benefit on impairment/disability progression, relapses, and MRI measures in SP-MS. The North American study of IFN-β_{1b} and studies of IFN-β_{1a} (IM) (Avonex) and IFN-β_{1a} (SC) (Rebif) show benefit on relapse rate and MRI, and the study of IFN-β_{1a} (IM) shows benefit on impairment measured by a new outcome measure, the MS functional composite. However, all three studies fail to show benefit on the traditional measure of impairment/disability, the Expanded Disability Status Scale.

Mitoxantrone is beneficial on relapse rate, impairment/disability progression, and MRI in SP-MS. The risk of serious toxicity, however, limits the use of mitoxantrone to SP-MS patients with relatively rapid progression.

Some studies suggest that every-other-month IV methylprednisolone, low-dose oral methotrexate (Rheumatrex)[1], and glatiramer acetate (Copaxone) may be of benefit in SP-MS. Some studies of intravenous cyclophosphamide (Cytoxan)[1] report benefit in SP-MS, while others have not. Because of its potential toxicity, cyclophosphamide, like mitoxantrone, typically is used to treat rapidly progressive MS.

It appears that later stages of relapsing MS respond less well to immunomodulatory therapies. IFN-β is appropriate as first line therapy. Mitoxantrone is appropriate for patients with rapidly progressive disease that fails to respond to IFN-β. For patients who fail to respond to IFN-β but who are felt not sufficiently severe to warrant mitoxantrone, GA, taken every other month, intravenous methylprednisolone, and low-dose oral methotrexate are reasonable options. Data supporting use of these agents in SP-MS are only preliminary.

Treatment of PP-MS is even more difficult. At present, no agent has been shown to be effective in PP-MS. Several small trials of IFN-β, a small trial of methotrexate, and a large trial of GA failed to show benefit in PP-MS. A trial of mitoxantrone is ongoing.

[1]Not FDA approved for this indication.

Pregnancy

Because MS is more common in women and typically begins in early adulthood, concerns about pregnancy are common. There is no convincing evidence that pregnancy increases the risk of developing MS. Similarly, there is no convincing evidence that single or multiple pregnancies affect the long-term course of the disease or risk for development of permanent disability. However, pregnancy does have effects on the short-term course of the disease and ramifications for its treatment.

Many of the disease-modifying therapies for MS and many of the medications used to treat MS symptoms carry some risk for inducing congenital abnormalities or spontaneous abortion. Therefore, most medications typically are discontinued before attempting a planned pregnancy. Also, it is important to caution female patients with MS to employ effective measures for birth control while on these medications and to notify their physicians immediately if they learn they are pregnant.

A number of studies show that the relapse rate and MRI activity decrease during pregnancy then increase above baseline for 3 to 6 months after delivery. The increased disease activity postpartum suggests that disease-modifying therapy should be restarted soon after delivery in women with previously active disease. In such cases, breast-feeding needs to be avoided or cut short.

MS does not affect fertility or the course of pregnancy. There is no apparent increase in congenital abnormalities or complications of pregnancy, labor, or delivery from MS per se. Normally, no additional precautions or special measures are needed during labor or delivery.

MYASTHENIA GRAVIS AND RELATED DISORDERS

METHOD OF

Robert M. Pascuzzi, MD

Myasthenia gravis (MG) is an autoimmune disorder of neuromuscular transmission involving the production of autoantibodies directed against the nicotinic acetylcholine receptor. Acetylcholine receptor antibodies are detectable in the serum of 80% to 90% of patients with MG. The prevalence of MG is approximately 1 in 10,000 to 20,000. Women are affected approximately twice as often as men. Symptoms may begin at virtually any age with a peak in women in the second and third decades, while the peak in men occurs in the fifth and sixth decades. Associated autoimmune diseases such as rheumatoid arthritis, lupus, and pernicious anemia are present in approximately 5% of patients. Thyroid disease occurs in approximately 10%, often in association with antithyroid antibodies. Approximately 10% to 15% of MG patients have a thymoma, while thymic lymphoid hyperplasia with proliferation of germinal centers occurs in 50% to 70% of cases. In most patients the cause of autoimmune MG is unknown. However, there are three iatrogenic causes for autoimmune MG. D-Penicillamine (Cuprimine) (used in the treatment of Wilson's disease and rheumatoid arthritis) and alfa-interferon therapy are both capable of inducing MG. In addition, bone marrow transplantation is associated with the development of MG as part of the chronic graft-versus-host disease.

Clinical Features

The hallmark of MG is fluctuating or fatigable weakness. The presenting symptoms are ocular in 50% of all patients (25% of patients initially present with diplopia, 25% with ptosis); and by 1 month into the course of illness, 80% of patients have some degree of ocular involvement. Presenting symptoms are bulbar (dysarthria or dysphagia) in 10%, leg weakness (impaired walking) in 10%, and generalized weakness in 10%. Respiratory failure is the presenting symptom in 1% of cases. Patients usually complain of symptoms from focal muscle dysfunction such as diplopia, ptosis, dysarthria, dysphagia, inability to work with arms raised over the head, or disturbance of gait. In contrast, patients with MG tend not to complain of generalized weakness, generalized fatigue, sleepiness, or muscle pain. In the classic case, fluctuating weakness is worse with exercise and improved with rest. Symptoms tend to progress later in the day. Many different factors can precipitate or aggravate weakness, such as physical stress, emotional stress, infection, or exposure to medications that impair neuromuscular transmission (perioperative succinylcholine [Anectine], aminoglycoside antibiotics, quinine, quinidine, botulinum toxin [Botox]).

Diagnosis

The diagnosis is based on a history of fluctuating weakness with corroborating findings on examination. There are several different ways to validate or confirm the clinical diagnosis.

EDROPHONIUM (TENSILON) TEST

The most immediate and readily accessible confirmatory study is the edrophonium (Tensilon) test. To perform the test, choose one or two weak muscles to judge. Ptosis, dysconjugate gaze, and other cranial deficits provide the most reliable endpoints. Use a setting where hypotension, syncope, or respiratory failure can be managed as patients occasionally decompensate during the test. If the patient has severe dyspnea, defer the test until the airway is secure. Start an IV. Have intravenous atropine, 0.4 mg, readily available in case bradycardia or extreme gastrointestinal (GI) side effects occur. Edrophonium, 10 mg (1 mL), is drawn up in a syringe; 1 mg (0.1 mL) should be given as a test dose while checking the patient's heart rate (to ensure the patient is not supersensitive to the drug). If no untoward side effects occur after 1 minute, another 3 mg is given. Many MG patients will show improved power within 30 to 60 seconds of giving the initial 4 mg, at which point the test can be stopped. If after 1 minute there is no improvement, give an additional 3 mg; if there is still no response, 1 minute later give the final 3 mg. If the patient develops muscarinic symptoms or signs at any time during the test (sweating, salivation, GI symptoms), one can assume that enough edrophonium has been given to see improvement in strength and the test can be stopped. When a placebo effect or examiner bias is of concern, the test is performed in a double-blind, placebo-control fashion. The 1 mL control syringe contains either saline, 0.4 mg atropine, or nicotinic acid*, 10 mg. Improved strength from edrophonium lasts for just a few minutes. When improvement is clear-cut, then the test is positive. If the improvement is borderline, it is best to consider the test negative. The test can be repeated several times. Sensitivity of the edrophonium test is approximately 90%. The specificity is difficult to determine, as improvement following IV edrophonium has been reported in other neuromuscular diseases including Lambert-Eaton syndrome, botulism, Guillain-Barré syndrome, motor neuron disease, and lesions of the brainstem and cavernous sinus.

Neostigmine† has a longer duration of effect and, in selected patients, may be an alternative cholinesterase inhibitor (CEI) for diagnostic testing, especially in children. For performance of a neostigmine test, 0.04 mg/kg is given intramuscularly or 0.02 mg/kg intravenously (one time only).

ACETYLCHOLINE RECEPTOR ANTIBODIES

The standard assay for receptor binding antibodies is an immunoprecipitation assay using human limb muscle for acetylcholine receptor antigen. In addition, assays for receptor modulating and blocking antibodies are available. Binding antibodies are present in approximately 80% of all myasthenia patients (50% of patients with pure ocular MG, 80% of those with mild generalized MG, 90% of patients with moderate to severe generalized MG, and 70% of those in clinical remission). By also testing for modulating

*Not available in the United States in parenteral form.
†FDA indicated for treatment but not diagnosis.

and blocking antibodies, the sensitivity improves to 90% overall. Specificity is outstanding with false-positives exceedingly rare in reliable labs. If blood is sent to a reference lab, the test results are usually available within 1 week.

MUSCLE-SPECIFIC KINASE ANTIBODIES

More recently, data show that 25% to 47% of patients who are seronegative for acetylcholine receptor antibodies have muscle-specific kinase (MuSK) antibodies. MuSK antibodies can now be measured by a commercially available immunoprecipitation assay. The clinical features of MuSK-positive patients may differ from non-MuSK MG patients. Such patients, who tend to be younger women (younger than age 40 years), have lower likelihood of abnormal repetitive stimulation and edrophonium test results. Bulbar symptoms are significantly more common at onset of disease in MuSK-antibody-positive patients. MuSK antibodies may also be more commonly associated with patients having weakness of neck extensor, shoulders, or respiratory muscles.

ELECTROPHYSIOLOGIC TESTING

Repetitive stimulation electrophysiologic (EMG) testing is widely available and has variable sensitivity, depending on number and selection of muscles studied and various provocative maneuvers. However, in most labs this technique has a sensitivity of approximately 50% in all patients with MG (lower in patients with mild or pure ocular disease). In general, the yield from repetitive stimulation is higher when testing muscle groups that have clinically significant weakness. Single-fiber EMG (SFEMG) is a highly specialized technique, usually available in major academic centers, with a sensitivity of approximately 90%. Abnormal single-fiber results are common in other neuromuscular diseases, and, therefore, the test must be used in the correct clinical context. The specificity of single-fiber EMG is an important issue because mild abnormalities can clearly be present with a variety of other diseases of the motor unit, including motor neuron disease, peripheral neuropathy, and myopathy. Disorders of neuromuscular transmission other than MG can have substantial abnormalities on SFEMG. In contrast, acetylcholine receptor antibodies (and MuSK antibodies) are not found in non-MG patients. In summary, the two highly sensitive laboratory studies are single-fiber EMG and acetylcholine receptor antibodies; nonetheless, neither test is 100% sensitive.

Prognosis

Appropriate management of the patient with autoimmune MG requires understanding of the natural course of the disease. The long-term natural course of MG is not clearly established other than that it is highly variable. Several generalizations can be made. Approximately 50% of MG patients present with ocular symptoms, and by 1 month 80% have eye findings. The presenting weakness is bulbar in 10%, limb in 10%, generalized in 10%, and respiratory in 1%. By 1 month symptoms remain purely ocular in 40%, generalized in 40%, limited to the limbs in 10%, and limited to bulbar muscles in 10%. Weakness remains restricted to the ocular muscles on a long-term basis in approximately 15% to 20% (pure ocular MG). Most patients with initial ocular involvement tend to develop generalized weakness within the first year of the disease (90% of those who generalize do so within the initial 12 months). Maximal weakness occurs within the initial 3 years in 70% of patients. In the modern era, death from MG is rare. Spontaneous long-lasting remission occurs in approximately 10% to 15%, usually in the first year or two of the disease. Most MG patients develop progression of clinical symptoms during the initial 2 to 3 years. However, progression is not uniform, as illustrated by 15% to 20% of patients whose symptoms remain purely ocular and those who have spontaneous remission.

Treatment

FIRST-LINE THERAPY: PYRIDOSTIGMINE BROMIDE

Cholinesterase inhibitors (CEI) are safe, effective, and first-line therapy in all patients. Inhibition of acetylcholinesterase (AChE) reduces the hydrolysis of acetylcholine (ACh), increasing the accumulation of ACh at the nicotinic postsynaptic membrane. The CEIs used in MG bind reversibly (as opposed to organophosphate CEIs, which bind irreversibly) to AChE. These drugs cross the blood–brain barrier poorly and tend not to cause central nervous system (CNS) side effects. Absorption from the gastrointestinal (GI) tract tends to be inefficient and variable, with oral bioavailability of approximately 10%. Muscarinic autonomic side effects of GI cramping, diarrhea, salivation, lacrimation, diaphoresis, and, when severe, bradycardia may occur with all of the CEI preparations. A feared potential complication of excessive CEI use is skeletal muscle weakness (cholinergic weakness). Patients receiving parenteral CEI are at the greatest risk to have cholinergic weakness. It is uncommon for patients receiving oral CEI to develop significant cholinergic weakness even while experiencing muscarinic cholinergic side effects. Table 1 summarizes the commonly available CEIs.

Pyridostigmine (Mestinon) is the most widely used CEI for long-term oral therapy. Onset of effect is within 15 to 30 minutes of an oral dose, with peak effect within 1 to 2 hours, and wearing off gradually at 3 to 4 hours postdose. The starting dose is 30 to 60 mg three to four times per day, depending on

TABLE 1 Commonly Available Cholinesterase Inhibitors

Cholinesterase Inhibitors	Unit Dose	Average Dose (Adult)	Children's Dose
Pyridostigmine bromide tablet (Mestinon)	60 mg tablet	30-60 mg every 4-6h	Tablet: 1 mg/kg every 4-6h
Pyridostigmine bromide syrup	12 mg/mL	30-60 mg every 4-6h	Syrup: 60 mg/5 mL
Pyridostigmine bromide sustained-release (Mestinon Timespan)	180 mg tablet	1 tablet twice daily	
Pyridostigmine bromide (parenteral)	5 mg/mL ampules	1-2 mg every 3-4h (1/30 of oral dose)	
Neostigmine bromide (Prostigmin)	15 mg tablet	7.5-15 mg every 3-4h	
Neostigmine methylsulfate (parenteral)	0.25-1.0 mg/mL every 2-3h	0.5 mg IM, IV, or SC ampules	For treatment: 0.01-0.04 mg/kg dose, IM, IV, or SC every 2-3h as needed For diagnosis*: 0.1 mg/kg IM or SC once, or 0.05 mg/kg IV once
Edrophonium (Tensilon)	For diagnosis only. See text, page 1067.		For diagnosis: 0.1 mg/kg IV, (or 0.15 mg/kg IM or SC, which prolongs the effect), preceded by a test dose of 0.01 mg/kg

*FDA indicated for treatment, but not for diagnosis.
Abbreviations: IM = intramuscular; IV = intravenous; SC = subcutaneous.

symptoms. Optimal benefit usually occurs with a dose of 60 mg every 4 hours. Muscarinic cholinergic side effects are common with larger doses. Occasional patients require and tolerate more than 1000 mg per day, dosing as frequently as every 2 to 3 hours. Patients with significant bulbar weakness will often time their dose approximately 1 hour before meals in order to maximize chewing and swallowing. Of all the CEI preparations, pyridostigmine has the least muscarinic side effects. Pyridostigmine may be used in a number of alternative forms to the 60 mg tablet. The syrup may be necessary for children or for patients with difficulty swallowing pills. Sustained release pyridostigmine, 180 mg (Mestinon Timespan), is sometimes preferred for nighttime use. Unpredictable release and absorption limit its use. Patients with severe dysphagia or those undergoing surgical procedures may need parenteral CEI. Intravenous pyridostigmine should be given at approximately 1/30 of the oral dose. Neostigmine (Prostigmin) has a slightly shorter duration of action and slightly greater muscarinic side effects.

For patients with intolerable muscarinic side effects at CEI doses required for optimal power, a concomitant anticholinergic drug such as atropine sulfate (0.4 to 0.5 mg orally) or glycopyrrolate (Robinul) (1 to 2 mg orally) on an as needed basis or with each dose of CEI may be helpful. Patients with mild disease can often be managed adequately with CEIs. However, patients with moderate, severe, or progressive disease usually require more effective therapy.

THYMECTOMY: FOR WHOM, WHAT TYPE, AND WHAT TO TELL THE PATIENT TO EXPECT

Association of the thymus gland with MG was first noted around 1900, and thymectomy has become standard therapy for more than 50 years. Prospective, controlled trials have not been performed for thymectomy (although such a trial is currently in the planning stage). Nonetheless, thymectomy is generally recommended for patients with moderate to severe MG, especially those who are inadequately controlled on CEI, and those younger than 55 years of age. All patients with suspected thymoma undergo surgery. Approximately 75% of MG patients appear to benefit from thymectomy. Patients may improve or simply stabilize. For unclear reasons the onset of improvement tends to be delayed by 1 or 2 years in most patients (some patients do not seem to improve until 5 to 10 years after surgery). The majority of centers use the transsternal approach for thymectomy with the goal of complete removal of the gland. The limited transcervical approach has been largely abandoned because of the likelihood of incomplete gland removal. Many centers perform a maximal thymectomy in order to ensure complete removal. The procedure involves a combined transsternal–transcervical exposure with en bloc removal of the thymus. If thymectomy is to be performed, choose an experienced surgeon, anesthesiologist, and center with a good track record and insist that the entire gland is removed.

Which patients do not undergo thymectomy? Patients with very mild or trivial symptoms do not have surgery. Most patients with pure ocular MG do not undergo thymectomy even though there has been some reported benefit in selected patients. Thymectomy is often avoided in children because of the theoretical possibility of impairing the developing immune system. However, reports of thymectomy in children as young as 2 to 3 years of age have shown favorable results without adverse effects on the immune system. Thymectomy has been largely discouraged in patients older than 55 years of age because of expected increased morbidity, latency of clinical benefit, and frequent observation of an atrophic, involuted gland. Nonetheless there are older patients reported to benefit from thymectomy. Major complications from thymectomy are uncommon so long as the surgery is performed at an experienced center with anesthesiologists and neurologists familiar with the disease and perioperative management of MG patents.

Common, although less serious, aspects of thymectomy include postoperative chest pain (which may last several weeks), a 4- to 6-week convalescence period, and cosmetically displeasing incisional scar.

CORTICOSTEROIDS

There are no controlled trials documenting the benefit of corticosteroids in MG. However, nearly all authorities have personal experience attesting to the virtues (and complications) of corticosteroid use in MG patients. In general, corticosteroids are used in patients with moderate to severe, disabling symptoms that are refractory to CEI. Patients are commonly hospitalized to initiate therapy because of the risk of early exacerbation. Opinions differ regarding the best method of administration. For patients with severe MG, it is best to begin with high-dose daily therapy of prednisone[1], 60 to 80 mg per day orally. Early exacerbation occurs in approximately 50% of patients, usually within the first few days of therapy and typically lasting 3 or 4 days. In 10% of cases the exacerbation is severe, requiring mechanical ventilation or a feeding tube (thus the need to initiate therapy in the hospital). Overall, approximately 80% of patients show a favorable response to steroids with 30% attaining remission and 50% marked improvement. Mild to moderate improvement occurs in 15% of patients, and 5% have no response. Improvement begins as early as 12 hours and as late as 60 days after beginning prednisone, but usually the patient begins to improve within 1 or 2 weeks. Improvement is gradual, with marked improvement occurring at a mean of 3 months, and maximal improvement at a mean of 9 months. Of patients having a favorable response, most maintain their improvement with gradual dosage reduction at a rate of 10 mg every 1 to 2 months. More rapid reduction is usually associated with a flare-up of the disease. While many patients can eventually be weaned off of steroids and maintain their response, the majority cannot. They require a minimum dose (5 to 30 mg on alternate days) to maintain their improvement. Complications of long-term high-dose prednisone therapy are substantial, including cushingoid appearance, hypertension, osteoporosis, cataracts, aseptic necrosis, and other well-known complications of chronic steroid therapy. Older patients tend to respond more favorably to prednisone.

An alternative prednisone regimen involves a low-dose, alternate-day, gradually increasing schedule in an attempt to avoid the early exacerbation. Patients receive prednisone, 25 mg on alternate days with increases of 12.5 mg every third dose (approximately every fifth day), to a maximum dose of 100 mg every other day or until sufficient improvement occurs. Clinical improvement usually begins within 1 month of treatment. The frequency and severity of early exacerbation is less than that associated with high-dose daily regimens. High-dose intravenous methylprednisolone (Solu-Medrol)[1] (1000 mg intravenously daily for 3 to 5 days) can provide improvement within 1 to 2 weeks, but the clinical improvement is temporary.

[1]Not FDA approved for this indication.

ALTERNATIVE IMMUNOSUPPRESSIVE DRUG THERAPY

Mycophenolate Mofetil

Mycophenolate mofetil (CellCept)[1] is a purine inhibitor widely used in recent years for the treatment of MG. While prospective, controlled trials are underway, the anecdotal uncontrolled experience suggests that approximately 75% of MG patients benefit from the drug with the typical onset of improvement within 2 to 3 months. The drug is, in general, well tolerated. Typically the drug regimen begins with 250 to 500 mg orally twice daily, and over 2 to 4 weeks the dose is increased to 1000 mg orally twice daily.

Azathioprine

Azathioprine (Imuran)[1] is a cytotoxic purine analog with extensive use in MG (but largely uncontrolled and retrospective). The starting dose is 50 mg orally daily, with complete blood count (CBC) and liver function tests weekly in the beginning. If the drug is tolerated and if the blood work is stable, the dose is increased by 50 mg every 1 to 2 weeks aiming for a total daily dose of approximately 2 to 3 mg/kg per day (approximately 150 mg per day in the average size adult). When azathioprine is first started, approximately 15% of patients will have intolerable GI side effects (nausea, anorexia, abdominal discomfort) that are sometimes associated with fever, leading to discontinuation. Bone marrow suppression with relative leukopenia (white blood cell count [WBC] 2500 to 4000) occurs in 25% of patients but is usually not significant. If the WBC drops below 2500 or the absolute granulocyte count goes below 1000 the drug is stopped (and the abnormalities usually resolve). Macrocytosis is common and of unclear clinical significance. Liver enzymes elevate in 5% to 10% of patients but is usually reversible, and severe hepatic toxicity occurs in only approximately 1%; infection occurs in approximately 5%. There is a theoretical risk of malignancy (based on observations in organ transplant patients), but this increased risk has not been clearly established in the MG patient population.

[1]Not FDA approved for this indication.

Approximately 50% of MG patients improve on azathioprine with onset approximately 4 to 8 months into treatment. Maximal improvement takes approximately 12 months. Relapse after discontinuation of azathioprine occurs in more than 50% of patients, usually within 1 year.

Cyclosporine

Cyclosporine (Sandimmune)[1] is used in patients with severe MG who cannot be adequately managed with corticosteroids or azathioprine. The starting dose is 3 to 5 mg/kg per day given in two divided doses. Cyclosporine blood levels should be measured monthly (aiming for a level of 200 to 300) along with electrolytes, magnesium, and renal function (in general, serum creatinine should not exceed one and one half times the pretreatment level). Blood should be sampled before the morning dose is taken. More than 50% of patients improve on cyclosporine. The onset of clinical improvement occurs approximately 1 to 2 months after beginning therapy and maximal improvement occurs at approximately 3 to 4 months. Side effects include renal toxicity and hypertension. Nonsteroidal anti-inflammatory drugs (NSAIDs) and potassium-sparing diuretics are among the list of drugs that should be avoided while on cyclosporine. In patients on corticosteroids, the addition of cyclosporine can lead to a reduction in steroid dosage (although it is usually not possible to discontinue prednisone).

PLASMA EXCHANGE

Plasma exchange (plasmapheresis) removes acetylcholine receptor antibodies and results in rapid clinical improvement. The standard course involves removal of 2 to 3 liters of plasma every other day or 3 times per week until the patient improves (usually a total of 3 to 5 exchanges). Improvement begins after the first few exchanges and reaches maximum within 2 to 3 weeks. The improvement is moderate to marked in nearly all patients, but usually wears off after 4 to 8 weeks because of the reaccumulation of pathogenic antibodies. Vascular access may require placement of a central line. Complications include hypotension, bradycardia, electrolyte imbalance, hemolysis, infection, and access problems (such as pneumothorax from placement of a central line.) Indications for plasma exchange include any patient in whom a rapid temporary clinical improvement is needed.

HIGH-DOSE INTRAVENOUS IMMUNOGLOBULIN

High-dose intravenous immunoglobulin (IVIG)[1] administration is associated with rapid improvement in MG symptoms in a time frame similar to plasma exchange. The mechanism is unclear but may relate to down regulation of acetylcholine receptor antibody production or, to the effect of anti-idiotype antibodies. The usual protocol is 2 g/kg spread over 5 consecutive days (0.4 g/kg per day). Different IVIG preparations are administered IV at different rates (contact the pharmacy for guidelines). The majority of MG patients improve, usually within 1 week of starting IVIG. The degree of response is variable, and the duration of response is limited, like plasma exchange, to approximately 4 to 8 weeks. Complications include fever, chills, and headache, which respond to slowing down the rate of the infusion and giving diphenhydramine. Occasional cases of aseptic meningitis, renal failure, nephrotic syndrome, and stroke have been reported. Also, patients with selective IgA deficiency can have anaphylaxis, which can be avoided by screening for IgA deficiency ahead of time. The treatment is relatively expensive, comparable to plasma exchange.

GENERAL GUIDELINES FOR MANAGEMENT

1. Be certain of the diagnosis.
2. Conduct patient education. Provide the patient with information about the natural course of the disease (including the variable and somewhat unpredictable course). Briefly review the treatment options pointing out effectiveness, time course of improvement, duration of response, and complications. Provide the patient with educational pamphlets prepared by the Myasthenia Gravis Foundation of America or the Muscular Dystrophy Association.
3. Determine when hospitalization is necessary. Patients with severe MG can deteriorate rapidly over a period of hours. Therefore, those having dyspnea should be hospitalized immediately in a constant observation or intensive care setting. Patients with moderate or severe dysphagia, weight loss, as well as those with rapidly progressive or severe weakness should be admitted urgently. This will allow close monitoring and early intervention in case of respiratory failure, and will also expedite the diagnostic workup and initiation of therapy.
4. Be aware that myasthenic crisis (Table 2) is a medical emergency characterized by respiratory failure from diaphragm weakness or severe oropharyngeal weakness leading to aspiration. Crisis can occur in the setting of surgery (postoperative), acute infection, or following rapid withdrawal of corticosteroids (although some patients have no precipitating factors). Patients should be placed in an intensive care unit (ICU) setting and have forced vital capacity (FVC) checked every 2 hours. Changes in arterial blood gases occur relatively late in neuromuscular respiratory failure. There should be a low threshold for intubation and mechanical ventilation. Criteria for intubation include a drop in the

[1]Not FDA approved for this indication.

TABLE 2 The Acutely Deteriorating Myasthenic Patient

Myasthenic Crisis
Respiratory distress
Respiratory arrest
Cyanosis
Increased pulse and blood pressure
Diaphoresis
Poor cough
Inability to handle oral secretions
Dysphagia
Weakness
Improvement with edrophonium
Cholinergic Crisis
Abdominal cramps
Diarrhea
Nausea and vomiting
Excessive secretions
Miosis
Fasciculations
Diaphoresis
Weakness
Worsening with edrophonium

TABLE 3 Treatment of Myasthenia Gravis

1. Mild weakness: cholinesterase inhibitors
2. Moderate-marked localized or generalized weakness:
   a. Cholinesterase inhibitors, and
   b. Thymectomy for patients under age 55 (complete removal)
3. If symptoms are uncontrolled on cholinesterase inhibitors use immunosuppression
   a. Prednisone if severe or urgent
   b. Mycophenolate mofetil (CellCept)[1] or azathioprine (Imuran)[1]
      Prednisone contraindicated
      Prednisone failure
      Excessive prednisone side effects
4. Plasma exchange or IVIG[1]
   a. Impending crisis, crisis
   b. Preoperative boost (if needed)
   c. Chronic disease refractory to drug therapy
5. If the above fails:
   a. Search for residual thymus tissue
   b. Cyclosporine (Sandimmune)[1]
   c. Long-term high-dose IVIG or PE
   d. Referral to neuromuscular specialty group

[1]Not FDA approved for this indication.
Abbreviations: IVIG = intravenous immunoglobulin; PE = plasma exchange.

FVC below 15 mL/kg (or below 1 L in an average-size adult), severe aspiration from oropharyngeal weakness, or labored breathing regardless of the measurements. If the diagnosis is not clear-cut it is advisable to secure the airway with intubation, stabilize ventilation, and only then address the question of the underlying diagnosis. If the patient has been taking CEI, the drug should be temporarily discontinued in order to rule out the possibility of cholinergic crisis.

5. Screen for and correct any underlying medical problems such as systemic infection, metabolic problems (like diabetes), and thyroid disease (hypo- or hyperthyroidism can exacerbate MG).
6. Be aware of drugs to avoid in MG. Avoid using D-penicillamine (Cuprimine), alfa-interferon, chloroquine (Aralen), quinine, quinidine, procainamide, and botulinum toxin (Botox). Aminoglycoside antibiotics should be avoided unless needed for a life-threatening infection. Neuromuscular blocking drugs such as pancuronium (Pavulon) and D-tubocurarine can produce marked and prolonged paralysis in MG patients. Depolarizing drugs such as succinylcholine (Anectine) can also have a prolonged effect and should be used by a skilled anesthesiologist who is well aware of the patient's MG.

GUIDELINES FOR SPECIFIC THERAPIES (Table 3)

Treatment must be individualized. Mild diplopia and ptosis may not be disabling for some patients, but for a pilot or neurosurgeon, for example, mild, intermittent diplopia may be critical. In similar fashion, some patients may tolerate side effects better than others.

1. Mild or trivial weakness, either localized or generalized should be managed with a CEI (pyridostigmine).
2. Moderate to marked weakness, localized or generalized, should initially be managed with CEI. Even if symptoms are adequately controlled, patients younger than 55 years of age undergo thymectomy early in the course of the disease (within the first year). In older patients, thymectomy is usually not performed unless the patient is thought to have a thymoma. Thymectomy is performed at an experienced center with the clear intent of complete removal of the gland. All patients with suspected thymoma (by chest scan) should have thymectomy, even if their myasthenic symptoms are mild. Unless a thymoma is suspected, patients with pure ocular disease are usually not treated with thymectomy.
3. If symptoms are inadequately controlled on CEI, immunosuppression is used. High-dose corticosteroid therapy is the most predictable and effective long-term option. If patients have severe, rapidly progressive, or life-threatening symptoms the decision to start corticosteroids is clear-cut. Patients with disabling but stable symptoms may instead receive mycophenolate mofetil (CellCept)[1], especially if there are particular concerns about using corticosteroids (i.e., the patient is already overweight, diabetic, or has cosmetic concerns). Patients who respond poorly or have unacceptable complications on steroids are started on mycophenolate.

[1]Not FDA approved for this indication.

4. Plasma exchange or IVIG are indicated in:
   a. Rapidly progressive, life-threatening, impending myasthenic crisis, or actual crisis, particularly if prolonged intubation with mechanical ventilation is judged hazardous.
   b. Preoperative stabilization of MG (such as before thymectomy or other elective surgery) in poorly controlled patients.
   c. Disabling MG refractory to other therapies.
5. If these options fail, azathioprine (Imuran)[1] or cyclosporine (Sandimmune)[1] are used.
6. If the patient remains poorly controlled despite use of the above treatments, then a repeat chest CT scan looking for residual thymus should be performed. Some patients improve after repeat thymectomy. There may be other medical problems (diabetes, thyroid disease, infection, and coexisting autoimmune diseases).
7. Referral to a neurologist or center that specializes in neuromuscular disease is advised for all patients with suspected MG and can be particularly important for complicated or refractory patients.

Other Issues

TRANSIENT NEONATAL MYASTHENIA

Transient neonatal myasthenia occurs in 10% to 15% of babies born to mothers with autoimmune MG. Within the first few days after delivery the baby has a weak cry or suck, appears floppy, and occasionally requires mechanical ventilation. The condition is caused by maternal antibodies that cross the placenta late in pregnancy. As these maternal antibodies are replaced by the baby's own antibodies the symptoms gradually disappear, usually within a few weeks, and the baby is normal thereafter. Infants with severe weakness are treated with oral pyridostigmine, 1 to 2 mg/kg every 4 hours.

CONGENITAL MYASTHENIA

Congenital myasthenia represents a group of rare hereditary disorders of the neuromuscular junction. The patients tend to have lifelong relatively stable symptoms of generalized fatigable weakness. These disorders are nonimmunologic, without acetylcholine receptor antibodies, and, therefore, patients do not respond to immune therapy (steroids, thymectomy, and plasma exchange). Most of these patients improve on CEI. There are many established subtypes of congenital myasthenia, and several are worth noting partly because of specific therapeutic implications.

The fast channel congenital myasthenic syndrome tends to be static or slowly progressive, but it is usually very responsive to combination therapy with 3,4-diaminopyridine[1] (which enhances release of acetylcholine) and pyridostigmine (Mestinon) (which reduces metabolism of acetylcholine).

[1]Not FDA approved for this indication.

Congenital slow-channel myasthenic syndrome typically worsens over years as the endplate myopathy progresses. Although cholinesterase inhibitors typically worsen symptoms, quinidine[1] and fluoxetine (Prozac)[1], which reduce the duration of acetylcholine receptor channel openings, are both effective treatments for slow-channel syndrome.

The congenital myasthenic syndrome associated with acetylcholine receptor deficiency tends to be relatively nonprogressive and may even improve slightly as the patient ages. The disorder typically responds to symptomatic therapy with pyridostigmine and/or 3,4-diaminopyridine. Ephedrine[1] produces benefit in some cases.

Patients with endplate acetylcholinesterase deficiency usually present in infancy or early childhood with generalized weakness, underdevelopment of muscles, slowed pupillary responses to light, and either no response or worsening response with cholinesterase inhibitors. No effective long-term treatment has been described for congenital endplate acetylcholinesterase deficiency.

LAMBERT-EATON SYNDROME

Lambert-Eaton syndrome (LES) (the myasthenic syndrome) is a presynaptic disease characterized by chronic fluctuating weakness of proximal limb muscles. Symptoms (Table 4) include difficulty walking, climbing stairs, or rising from a chair. In LES there may be some improvement in power with sustained or repeated exercise. In contrast to myasthenia gravis, ptosis, diplopia, dysphagia, and respiratory failure are far less common. In addition,

[1]Not FDA approved for this indication.

TABLE 4 Lambert-Eaton Syndrome (LES)

Symptoms
Proximal limb weakness
Legs > arms
Fatigue or fluctuating symptoms
Difficulty rising from a sitting position, climbing stairs
Metallic taste in mouth
Autonomic dysfunction
Dry mouth
Constipation
Blurred vision
Impaired sweating
Signs
Proximal limb weakness
Legs > arms
Weakness on exam is less compared to patient's level of disability
Hypoactive or absent muscle stretch reflexes
Lambert's sign (grip becomes more powerful over several seconds)

LES patients often complain of myalgias, muscle stiffness of the back and legs, distal paresthesias, metallic taste, dry mouth, impotence, and other autonomic symptoms of muscarinic cholinergic insufficiency. LES is rare compared to myasthenia gravis, which is approximately 100 times more common. Approximately 50% of LES patients have an underlying malignancy that is usually small cell carcinoma of the lung. In patients without malignancy, LES is an autoimmune disease and can be associated with other autoimmune phenomena. In general, patients older than 40 years of age are more likely to be men and have an associated malignancy, whereas younger patients are more likely to be women and have no associated neoplasm. LES symptoms can precede detection of the malignancy by 1 to 2 years.

The examination typically shows proximal lower extremity weakness (although the objective bedside assessment may suggest mild weakness relative to the patient's history). The muscle stretch reflexes are absent. On testing sustained maximal grip, there is a gradual increase in power over the initial 2 to 3 seconds (Lambert's sign).

The diagnosis is confirmed with EMG studies, which typically show low amplitude of the compound muscle action potentials and a decrement to slow rates or repetitive stimulation. Following brief exercise, there is marked facilitation of the compound muscle action potential (CMAP) amplitude. At high rates of repetitive stimulation, there may be an incremental response. Single-fiber EMG is markedly abnormal in virtually all patients with LES. The pathogenesis involves autoantibodies directed against voltage gated calcium channels at cholinergic nerve terminals. These IgG antibodies also inhibit cholinergic synapses of the autonomic nervous system. More than 75% of LES patients demonstrate these antibodies to voltage gated calcium channels in serum, providing another useful diagnostic test. In patients with associated malignancy, successful treatment of the tumor can lead to improvement in the LES symptoms. Symptomatic improvement in neuromuscular transmission may occur with the use of cholinesterase inhibitors such as pyridostigmine. 3,4-Diaminopyridine (DAP) increases ACh release by blocking voltage-dependent potassium conductance and thereby prolonging depolarization at the nerve terminal and enhancing the voltage-dependent calcium influx. 3,4-DAP clearly improves most patients with LES with relatively mild toxicity, and is becoming increasingly available, such that it represents first-line symptomatic therapy for LES. The typical beginning dose is 10 mg every 4 to 6 hours, with gradual increases, as needed, up to a maximum of 100 mg per day.

Immunosuppressive therapy is used in patients with disabling symptoms. Long-term high-dose corticosteroids, plasma exchange, and IVIG have all been used with moderate success. In general, the use of these therapies should be tailored to the severity of patient's symptoms.

TRIGEMINAL NEURALGIA

METHOD OF
Ronald I. Apfelbaum, MD

Trigeminal neuralgia, also known as tic douloureux, is a clinical syndrome characterized by repetitive, brief, extremely intense paroxysms of unilateral lancinating facial pain confined entirely to one or more divisions of the trigeminal nerve. The second and third divisions, either alone or in combination, are most commonly affected. The pain is often triggered by cutaneous stimuli such as those provoked by chewing, talking, brushing the teeth, shaving, washing the face, or even a breeze on the face. The patient may experience many attacks daily. Although patients are pain free between attacks, they live in fear of impending pain. The painful spasms infrequently occur at night, and periods of spontaneous remission are common in the natural history. Physical findings are minimal or nonexistent, so an accurate history is paramount for proper diagnosis. Few syndromes in medicine are as consistent from patient to patient and no other condition will have this history. Atypical features or presentations should alert the clinician to question the diagnosis. Although the condition tends to occur more frequently with advancing age, it may begin at any age, afflicting females somewhat more often than males.

Etiology

Trigeminal neuralgia is caused by demyelination at the root entry zone of the trigeminal nerve. This is the region where central myelin derived from oligodendric cells change to peripheral Schwann cell-derived myelin. In the trigeminal nerve this occurs within 5 to 10 mm of the brain stem. Usually demyelination results from extrinsic pressure on the nerve from an ectatic loop of a normal blood vessel, either arterial (approximately 80%) or venous (approximately 20%). Tumors, aneurysms, and vascular malformations can infrequently be the source of compression. Demyelination secondary to multiple sclerosis (MS) can also occur in this region and cause trigeminal neuralgia in approximately 3% of patients with MS, and in approximately 3% of cases of trigeminal neuralgia.

Investigation

Magnetic resonance imaging (MRI) is recommended to detect structural lesions and the changes associated with demyelinating disease. Vascular compression may also be detected at times but often is not, even with thin slices; thus, a *negative* scan does not exclude a vascular compressive etiology.

Medical Therapy

Medical therapy, which will control the pain in more than 90% of the patients, should be tried initially before resorting to any surgical alternatives. Narcotic analgesics rarely are useful because of the extreme intensity and brief duration of pain. Carbamazepine (Tegretol, Carbatrol) and oxcarbazepine (Trileptal)[1] are the most effective therapeutic agents.

Carbamazepine controls the pain in approximately 90% of patients with trigeminal neuralgia. It has some serious side effects, however, and must be used with caution. We recommend starting with 100 mg twice a day, with meals, and then increasing the dose by 100 mg every other day until pain control is achieved or toxicity develops. By gradually increasing the dose, many patients will tolerate fairly large doses of this medication. An average controlling dose is between 400 and 800 mg per day, but some patients will require, and tolerate, twice this dosage. Response to medication and clinical side effects are the most useful dosing indicators. Blood levels do not correlate well with clinical response and hence are not clinically useful. Patients on carbamazepine should have a complete blood count (CBC) and platelet count taken at 2-week intervals initially and then periodically thereafter as long as they are on the medication. In addition to leukopenia and thrombocytopenia, rare aplastic anemias have occurred. Gastrointestinal (GI) upset, lack of coordination, mental obtundation, and liver and renal abnormalities have all been reported. These symptoms often limit the ability to obtain complete control of the pain with the medication. Oxcarbazepine, a newer drug, is a relative of carbamazepine that is reported to have similar clinical effectiveness but fewer side effects.

Phenytoin (Dilantin)[1] is somewhat less effective but may be useful in many patients because it has lower toxicity than carbamazepine. Its best effect seems to be in patients who obtained good relief on carbamazepine but who cannot tolerate it. It also can be helpful when used with carbamazepine. Therapeutic levels of phenytoin (plasma concentration of 10 to 20 μg/mL) can usually be achieved with the administration of 100 mg three to four times per day, after an initial loading dose of double that for the first several days. Plasma level determinations are useful to regulate the dosage. On this regimen, approximately 50% to 67% of the patients achieve satisfactory control. Toxicity may be manifested by nystagmus, ataxia, slurred speech, or mental confusion. Cutaneous eruptions, GI upset, and hematopoietic complications may also occur.

Gabapentin (Neurontin)[1] is widely prescribed for trigeminal neuralgia. This appears to be related to its being another anticonvulsant that is somewhat better tolerated, but also to aggressive pharmaceutical promotion. There is, however, no published data supporting this use except for anecdotal cases. In our experience, it has rarely been effective and never controls the pain of trigeminal neuralgia for any significant period of time.

Several other medications are used as ancillary drugs and may, on rare occasions, provide an additional measure of control, either alone or in conjunction with the aforementioned drugs. Most of these, like the primary drugs, are anticonvulsants, but none are approved for use in trigeminal neuralgia. Some drugs included in this group are clonazepam (Klonopin)[1], lamotrigine (Lamictal)[1], and valproic acid (Depakene)[1]. Baclofen (Lioresal)[1], 20 to 80 mg per day, has been reported to be useful. Our experience with these drugs is limited. In general, they appear to be minor agents that may help an occasional patient but are not as effective as carbamazepine, oxcarbazepine, or phenytoin.

Surgical Therapy

Surgical therapy is usually reserved for patients who have become refractory to medical therapy, whose symptoms are incompletely controlled, or who have developed toxicity necessitating the discontinuance of these drugs. The surgical procedures that have provided long-term relief for this problem in the past involved destruction of portions of the trigeminal pathway. These procedures are now of historical interest only and are rarely indicated. Peripheral nerve injections, avulsions, or section produce only short-term relief and more numbness than percutaneous lesioning. Each has a high incidence of dysesthetic sequelae, which can be very distressing; thus, they are not recommended.

If destructive therapy is required, percutaneous trigeminal neurolysis is the procedure of choice. This can be accomplished using one of the following procedures:

- Radiofrequency energy to produce a thermal lesion
- Glycerol to produce a chemical lesion (chemoneurolysis)
- Balloon compression to produce a mechanical lesion

These procedures, which can be safely performed even on elderly and debilitated patients, involve the selective destruction of portions of the preganglionic trigeminal fibers via a percutaneous technique. Using a brief intravenous anesthetic, a needle electrode is inserted in the cheek, lateral to the mouth, and passed upward through the foramen ovale under radiologic control. For radiofrequency lesioning an electrode is inserted through this needle, and, with

[1]Not FDA approved for this indication.

[1]Not FDA approved for this indication.

stimulation, the electrode position is adjusted to achieve proper localization within the affected trigeminal fibers. A radiofrequency current is then incrementally applied to heat the tip of the electrode, as the patient is repetitively tested, to achieve selective destruction of pain fibers. Usually some touch perception can be preserved.

Serious complications include injury to adjacent neural structures and the carotid artery, but these, fortunately, are rare. More commonly, abnormal dysesthetic sensations (20%), anesthesia dolorosa (1% to 2%), corneal hypesthesia (15% to 20%), and corneal ulceration or keratitis (1%) may occur. Reported recurrences range from 25% to 50%, depending on the duration of the follow-up, but the procedure may be readily repeated without difficulty.

Glycerol chemoneurolysis is performed by quantifying the size of the trigeminal system radiologically with a contrast agent injection, and then filling it with 99.5% anhydrous glycerol[1*]. This procedure, therefore, does not require patient cooperation. Glycerol is a mild neurolytic agent, whose use usually results in minimal facial sensory loss and rare dysesthesia (approximately 1%). Anesthesia dolorosa and corneal ulceration keratitis almost never occur. Pain relief is excellent but recurrences occur more frequently than with radiofrequency lesioning. Three out of four patients will, however, get relief of 3 years or more. Again, the procedure can be easily repeated when needed to treat recurrences.

Although radiofrequency lesioning produces longer relief, we believe that it is preferable to avoid dysesthesia and its complications. *We therefore use glycerol chemoneurolysis as our percutaneous procedure of choice.* It is far easier to treat recurrent pain by repeating the procedure than to try to treat dysesthetic pain and anesthesia dolorosa.

Creating a lesion in the trigeminal root adjacent to the brain stem using focused high-dose radiation (stereotaxic radiosurgery), usually with the gamma knife instrument, has also been recently employed. This seems to help many patients, but it is not as effective as the above procedures, can take up to 5 to 6 months to be effective, and as of yet does not have good long-term follow-up. Sporadic reports of delayed complications and tumor transformation after similar treatment of acoustic nerve tumors are also worrisome. We therefore usually only recommend it in patients who cannot have the other procedures, such as those with bleeding disorders.

For patients younger than 70 years of age who are in good medical condition, *the Jannetta microvascular decompression procedure is the procedure of choice* because it relieves the pain without damaging the nerve, thereby avoiding numbness and dysesthesia. This procedure is based on the observation that the cause of trigeminal neuralgia is compression of the trigeminal nerve at its root entry zone adjacent to the brain stem (except in patients with MS, who have a demyelinating plaque in the same area). The usual cause of this compression is an aberrantly located, elongated, arterial loop, but venous channels and small tumors are also encountered. The procedure involves a limited retromastoid craniectomy and the use of microsurgical techniques. This approach (pioneered by Dr. Peter Jannetta) allows dissection at the root entry zone of the trigeminal nerve and displacement of the offending vascular channel, usually by the insertion of a small synthetic sponge prosthesis interposed between the nerve and artery.

In our personal series of more than 500 patients treated in this manner, the pain of trigeminal neuralgia was fully relieved in 91% and reduced in another 6% of the patients. Recurrences of severe pain refractory to treatment occurred in approximately 1% of our patients per year. At a 14-year follow-up, 81% remained with good pain control. Thus, unlike percutaneous lesioning, a steady increase in the frequency of recurrences with the passage of time has not been observed. Significant complications have included cerebellar hematomas (1.2%), supratentorial strokes (0.6%), transient cranial nerve palsies (up to 3%), and unilateral hearing loss (3%). Five deaths have occurred in our personal series.

The Jannetta microvascular decompression should not be undertaken lightly and requires special microsurgical skill and training. Although it offers major advantages by relieving the pain without sacrifice of trigeminal function (no numbness, dysesthetic sequelae, or corneal anesthesia occurs), it does carry with it a small chance of serious or even lethal complications.

Glossopharyngeal Neuralgia

Glossopharyngeal neuralgia is the exact equivalent of trigeminal neuralgia, involving instead the territory and distribution of the ninth cranial nerve, the glossopharyngeal nerve. Patients experience the same type of brief, severe, lancinating pain as do patients with trigeminal neuralgia, but it is confined to the posterior part of the oral pharynx and posterior aspect of the tongue. Swallowing usually triggers it. Medical therapy as outlined for trigeminal neuralgia is the first line of treatment. If surgery is necessary, the Jannetta microvascular decompression procedure is applicable. If not feasible, section of the ninth nerve and upper fibers of the tenth (vagus) nerve at the jugular foramen in the posterior fossa will usually provide excellent relief.

[1]Not FDA approved for this indication.
*May be compounded by pharmacists.

ACUTE FACIAL PARALYSIS (BELL'S PALSY)

METHOD OF

Bruce J. Gantz, MD, Ted A. Meyer, MD, PhD, and Peter C. Weber, MD

Bell's palsy and *idiopathic facial paralysis* are synonymous terms for acute facial paralysis of unknown etiology. McCormick first postulated that Bell's palsy was caused by the herpes virus in 1972. More recently, Murakami and coworkers (1996) further substantiated this claim when they identified DNA fragments of herpes simplex virus type 1 (HSV-1) in the perineurial fluid of 11 of 14 subjects undergoing facial nerve decompression during the acute phase of the illness. Burgess and colleagues (1994) found HSV-1 DNA in a temporal bone section in the region of the geniculate ganglion in a patient who had died of other causes 6 days after the onset of Bell's palsy. These two independent pieces of evidence strongly support the concept that the facial paralysis known as Bell's palsy is caused by a viral infection that induces inflammatory edema within the facial nerve. The nerve lies within the bony fallopian canal as it traverses the temporal bone. The labyrinthine segment, which has a diameter of approximately 0.6 mm, lies just medial to the geniculate ganglion. As the facial nerve swells, it is constricted to the greatest extent in the labyrinthine segment, and the ensuing neural conduction block causes paralysis of the voluntary facial musculature seen in Bell's palsy. An animal model of Bell's palsy has also been developed by inoculating the auricles and tongues of mice with herpes simplex virus, providing further evidence that a viral infection is an important cause in this disease. Together, this information provides more than circumstantial support for a herpes simplex viral etiology of Bell's palsy. This article highlights the epidemiology, clinical manifestation, evaluation, and treatment of Bell's palsy, taking into account the new information regarding etiology.

Epidemiology

The incidence of Bell's palsy is approximately 30 cases per 100,000 individuals per year, thus making it the most common cause of unilateral facial paralysis. Approximately 40,000 cases occur in the U.S. each year. There appears to be no sex predilection, and the ages range from infant to elderly, with manifestation in the fifth and sixth decades of life most common. Right- and left-side facial palsy occur equally. Recurrence may be unilateral or contralateral in up to 10% of patients, but should alert the physician to perform a rigorous examination to rule out other causes. Pregnancy triples the risk, whereas hypertension and diabetes mellitus are associated with only a small increase in incidence. Roughly 10% have a familial orientation, and 70% relate an upper respiratory tract infection preceding the onset.

Recovery begins within 3 weeks for 85% of the patients, with full recovery occurring in 6 months. Approximately 10% to 15% of patients are troubled with asymmetrical movement, mass movement of all branches, or movement of the mouth when closing the eye (synkinesis). Only 4% to 6% of patients, however, experience severe deformity with minimal return of facial movement. Some of these patients are completely unable to close the eye. Identification of this poor recovery group using electrophysiologic testing must be accomplished within 2 weeks of the onset of complete paralysis. Delay beyond 2 weeks renders approximately 50% of this group with residual facial dysfunction for the rest of their lives.

Evaluation

A detailed history is mandatory for any patient with facial paralysis. Date of onset, duration of associated symptoms, and other precipitating factors are important to document. Many patients report an antecedent viral illness 7 to 10 days before the onset of paralysis. A description of otalgia associated with skin and auricular blebs or blisters is not Bell's palsy but rather herpes zoster oticus (Ramsay Hunt syndrome), which is best treated with antiviral agents (valacyclovir [Valtrex])[1]. The facial paralysis in Bell's palsy may be abrupt or worsen over 2 to 3 days. It is not slowly progressive over weeks to months. Patients with Bell's palsy do not complain of facial twitching, decreased hearing, otorrhea, severe otalgia, or balance dysfunction. It is equally important to rule out recent trauma, tick bites (Lyme disease), or current ear infections.

Physical examination should confirm a facial paralysis of all branches. If the forehead is intact, a central etiology is of concern; whereas involvement of a single branch indicates a parotid tumor or trauma. The middle ear, tympanic membrane, and external canal should be normal. No aural or oral vesicular lesions should be seen. The parotid gland is palpated bimanually to ensure against a deep lobe tumor. All other cranial nerves should function normally, including cranial nerve V, even though patients may complain of vague facial numbness.

Audiometric evaluation is necessary for every patient. Unilateral hearing loss or acoustic reflex decay is suggestive of a cerebellopontine angle tumor and an indication for further retrocochlear evaluation. If vestibular complaints are present, an electronystagmogram (ENG) is performed.

[1]Not FDA approved for this indication.

Although radiographic studies are important in patients with facial paralysis, it is not necessary to image all patients with acute facial paralysis immediately, especially patients with classic symptoms of Bell's palsy. Imaging studies are obtained immediately if the signs and symptoms are not compatible with Bell's palsy or if no return of facial motion is observed at 6 months. Both high-resolution computed tomography (HRCT) and magnetic resonance imaging (MRI) with gadolinium are useful. Computed tomography (CT) allows better visualization of the fallopian canal and associated temporal bone structures. Magnetic resonance imaging can demonstrate inflammatory changes associated with Bell's palsy as well as tumors.

Electrodiagnosis

Electroneurography (ENog) and voluntary electromyography (EMG) are the two electrical diagnostic tests used most often to assess facial paralysis. ENog can estimate the amount of severe nerve fiber degeneration from an injury or conduction block, such as neurapraxia. It takes approximately 3 days for wallerian degeneration to occur after severe injury; therefore, ENog is not performed until more than 3 days after total paralysis. Electrical testing is not employed if a patient exhibits paresis, because the presence of even minimal voluntary motion after 3 days indicates minor injury, with full recovery to be expected.

ENog uses an electrical stimulus to activate the facial nerve as it exits the temporal bone at the stylomastoid foramen. Resulting facial movement generates a compound muscle action potential (CMAP) that is measured with surface electrodes. The amplitude of the CMAP biphasic response correlates with the number of remaining stimulatable fibers. The CMAP from the paralyzed side can be compared with the CMAP of the normal side. The percentage of functioning or degenerated nerve fibers can then be calculated. Degeneration of 90% or more of the fibers indicates poor recovery in more than 50% of patients. Conversely, if 90% of degeneration is not obtained by 2 weeks, a good prognosis is indicated. In addition to the percent of degeneration, the time course of the degeneration is important. Patients reaching 90% degeneration within 5 days have a far worse prognosis than those who exhibit 90% degeneration in 2 to 3 weeks.

If the ENog demonstrates 100% degeneration and no CMAP is discernible, then voluntary EMG testing is performed. EMG measures voluntary motor activity: The patient is asked to make forceful facial muscle contractions, and the single motor unit action potentials are recorded. Because all nerve fibers must synchronously depolarize to generate a CMAP, no response may be seen on ENog, even when polyphasic potentials (a sign of regenerating nerve fibers) are noted on EMG. ENog is also not of benefit in long-standing facial paralysis (>3 weeks) because of polyphasic potentials when degeneration and regeneration are occurring. For similar reasons, ENog is not a useful diagnostic test for facial paralysis caused by tumors.

Treatment Protocols

The management of patients with idiopathic facial paralysis depends on a number of variables. An overview of our treatment protocol is shown in the flowchart in Figure 1. This chart is a general guide. Alterations may be made on an individual basis depending on specific circumstances.

Patients with paresis (partial paralysis) seen within the initial 2 days of onset are treated with oral corticosteroids and antiviral medication. Electrodiagnostic evaluation is not performed until at least 3 days of total paralysis. Prednisone[1] is usually prescribed at 60 to 80 mg per day for 7 days without tapering, and the recommended dosage of valacyclovir (Valtrex)[1] is 500 mg three times per day for 7 days. Patients are re-evaluated within 5 days to assess the progress of the disease. If during the course of treatment complete flaccid paralysis ensues, the patient is managed according to the acute paralysis protocol (see Figure 1). Patients coming to medical attention more than 14 days after onset are followed with only intermittent examinations.

Patients with complete paralysis seen within the first 14 days are started on oral prednisone[1], 60 to 80 mg per day, and valacyclovir (Valtrex)[1], 500 mg three times a day. ENog is obtained no sooner than the third day after the onset of paralysis. If degeneration is less than 90%, medical management is continued for a full 7 days. ENog testing is repeated based on the percentage of degeneration until 2 weeks have elapsed from the date of onset of total paralysis. If more than 90% neural degeneration occurs within the 2-week period after complete paralysis, then surgical decompression of the internal auditory canal, labyrinthine segment, and tympanic portion of the facial nerve through a middle cranial fossa approach is recommended.

Surgical decompression of the facial nerve in Bell's palsy has been controversial since it was reported in 1932. Decompression of the mastoid segment of the nerve provides no benefit to severely degenerated facial nerves compared with the natural history of the disease. Decompression of the nerve medial to the geniculate ganglion, including the meatal foramen, through a middle cranial fossa craniotomy, improves facial nerve return in cases of severe degeneration. We have reported a series of patients with severely degenerated facial nerves that were decompressed through the middle fossa approach (Gantz, et al., 1999). Ninety-one percent of decompressed patients exhibited normal or near-normal return of facial

[1]Not FDA approved for this indication.

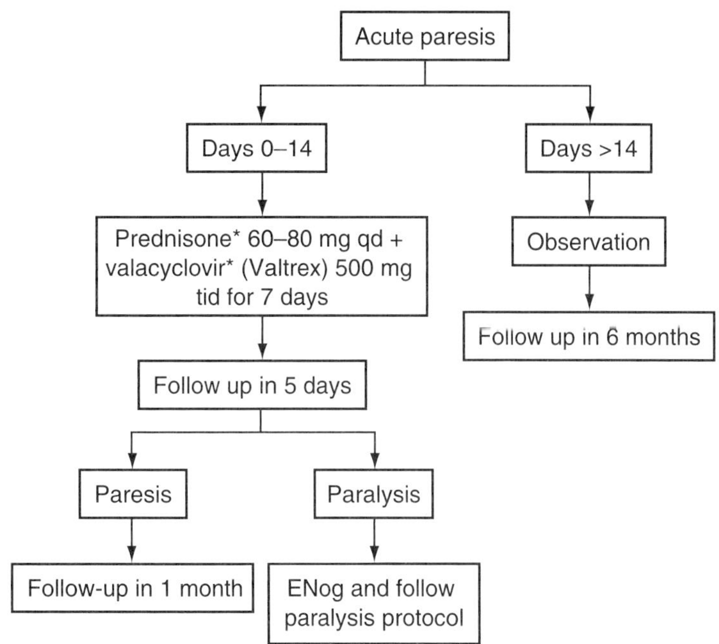

FIGURE 1 Acute facial paralysis flowchart. *Abbreviations*: EMG = electromyography; ENog = electroneurography; MCF = middle cranial fossa.

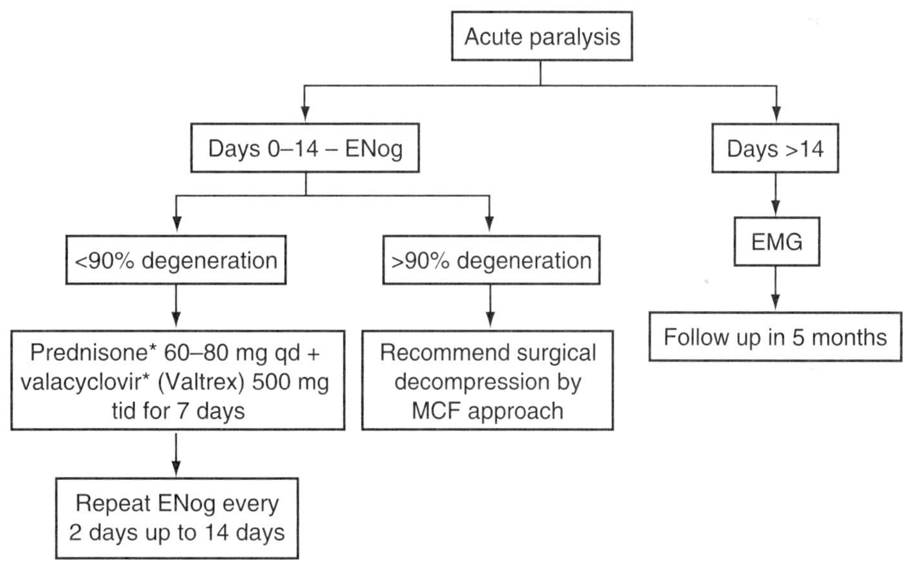

* Not FDA approved for this indication.

function 6 months after the onset of their paralysis. A group of control patients electing not to undergo decompression exhibited normal or near-normal facial function in only 42% of the cases. This study demonstrates that surgical decompression of the meatal foramen and labyrinthine segment of the facial nerve in severely degenerated cases of Bell's palsy provides significantly improved return of facial function compared to those with similar neural degeneration not decompressed ($p = .0002$). Surgical decompression through the middle fossa more than 2 weeks after the onset of paralysis provided results similar to the control group and did not result in improved facial function. If ENog demonstrates 100% degeneration, voluntary EMG is performed to confirm that complete wallerian degeneration has occurred. EMG testing is also performed if patients come to medical attention more than 3 weeks after the onset of paralysis. EMG testing will demonstrate nerve regeneration with polyphasic potentials.

Preventive eye care is mandatory for all patients with Bell's palsy. Failure to keep the eye moist (with drops during the day and ointment/moisture chamber at night) may result in corneal abrasions and ulcers. Any problems that develop with the eye should be managed by an ophthalmologist. Bell's palsy invariably demonstrates some improvement by 6 months. If no movement is identified 6 months after the onset of paralysis, the original diagnosis of Bell's palsy should be questioned and imaging studies, to rule out a neoplastic process, must be performed.

PARKINSONISM

METHOD OF

Dee E. Silver, MD

Idiopathic Parkinson's disease (IPD) is a neurodegenerative disease that is chronic and progressive and may be at least in part a protein deposition disease not unlike Alzheimer's disease and prion diseases. It is best understood and clinically recognized as a syndrome. IPD has a quartet of clinical signs and symptoms, usually with an asymmetrical clinical presentation. Resting tremor is present in 80% of patients. Postural tremor may also be seen in some cases. Bradykinesia/akinesia, rigidity, and, later in the clinical journey, postural instability help make up the four clinical features.

The prevalence of IPD is dependent on age because age is the greatest risk factor for IPD. The term juvenile parkinsonism is used in the rare patients younger than the age of 20 years. Early onset of IPD (ages 20 to 50 years) is less common, and the average age of onset is 60 years. In older age groups (65 years of age and older), it is as common as 1 in 100. There are approximately 1 million IPD patients in North America. There is probably significant underdiagnosis of IPD, because it may have an insidious onset and mild clinical features in the early stages; hence it may be undetectable for many months. Approximately 10% to 20% of IPD patients have a positive family history. Genetics and also environmental factors play a significant role. Hence, etiology is said to have a "double hit" phenomenon. Chromosome 4 has been associated with autosomal-dominant IPD and with mutations for α-synuclein and the ubiquitin-proteasome system. Chromosome 6 is associated with the Parkin gene, which has an autosomal recessive greater than dominant pattern. Clinically, it is a Parkinson's syndrome different from classical IPD. The gene mutations, many probably not yet known, probably lower the threshold for multiple gene interactions and/or for environmental factors to bring about clinical IPD. *N*-methyl-4-phenyl-1,2,3,6-tetrahydropyridine (MPTP), as an exogenous toxin associated with parkinsonism in humans and animals, solidified the environmental association with IPD. Now rotenone in animal models also supports this environmental role in etiology and helps us understand possible mechanisms of cell death. Rural living, well-water consumption, proximity to wood pulp factories, exposure to herbicides and pesticides, and welding are all environmental factors that are possibly associated with the development of IPD. Smoking is associated with reduced incidence of developing IPD, as is coffee drinking, in some Asian populations.

Pathophysiology

The underlying pathophysiology of IPD is not definitely known, but greater understanding is certainly occurring. Initially there is a striatal nigral dopamine-producing cell degeneration, primarily in the substantia nigra. Later there is downstream degeneration in other cells. In areas of cell death there is the presence of α-synuclein–containing Lewy bodies, mainly in the substantia nigra, but also in the cortex and spinal cord. Because the striatal nigral neurons terminate in the caudate and putamen (striatum), there is a deficiency of dopamine in the caudate and putamen. Hence, normal physiologic continuous dopamine stimulation (CDS) at the postsynaptic receptor sites is altered and results in abnormal pulsatile stimulation (PS). The degenerating substantia nigra (SN) with loss of dopamine cells can no longer physiologically manage the levodopa because of loss of presynaptic neuronal capacity. The levodopa can no longer be buffered, and, hence, other cells take up levodopa and release it in a nonphysiologic manner; and then instead of CDS occurring there is PS. This PS seems to be associated with at least two downstream consequences—gene changes, which can be measured by microarray analysis in cells downstream, and glutamate excitotoxicity.

This abnormal excitotoxicity is associated with altered intracellular signaling in cells of the medium spiny neurons in the striatum. Genes dictate protein formation; altered or mutated abnormal genes may give abnormal proteins, which, in turn, cannot be appropriately broken down into amino acids by the ubiquitin proteasome system. Therefore, there may be an abnormal protein deposition. The protein deposition may be part of the process of cell death. The deposition of α-synuclein results in Lewy bodies. The exact mechanism of developing motor fluctuations and dyskinesias is not known, but current thought is that downstream ramifications of PS play a significant role. The downstream changes related to glutamate toxicity are thought to be associated with the development of motor complications, motor fluctuations, and dyskinesias. It is also known that with SN degeneration and dopamine deficiency there develops excessive activity or output from the globus pallidus interna (GPi) and the subthalamic nucleus (STN). This excessive output inhibits thalamic-to-cortical activity resulting in some parkinsonian features. The etiology of cell death is unknown and may well be multifactorial. However, mitochondrial dysfunction (complex I deficiency), excitotoxicity, free radicals and oxidative stress, and ubiquitin proteasome dysfunction with consequent protein deposition may play some role either in an interactive cascade or as a multifactorial mechanism with varying influences.

Differential Diagnosis

The diagnosis of IPD, unless there is a stereotypical asymmetrical presentation, occurs often as a diagnosis by exclusion, and other parkinsonian syndromes must be considered. Essential tremor (ET) is often confused with IPD or vice versa. ET usually starts at a younger age, has a strong positive family history in 70% of the cases, and is usually a postural or kinetic tremor that involves the hands, arms, head, and voice and less likely the chin and lower extremities. The patient usually has a long history of tremor and little or no rigidity or akinesia. Wilson's disease, often with a family history, must be ruled out in those younger than 65 years of age by appropriate laboratory testing. Serum copper and ceruloplasmin levels should be ordered, and liver function tests should be obtained.

Dementia with Lewy bodies (DLB) has a clinical picture of fluctuating levels of somnolence, robust visual hallucinations, dementia, and basal ganglia disease. The clinical course is much shorter than that of IPD, and dementia and behavioral changes become the predominate clinical feature. Frontal temporal dementia, prion disease, normal pressure hydrocephalus, and mass lesions such as subdurals and frontal or deep tumors must be considered in the differential diagnoses in atypical cases of parkinsonism.

Metabolic, infectious, and other neurodegenerative diseases must also be considered. Magnetic resonance imaging (MRI) may need to be done to help rule out other diseases that mimic parkinsonism. Atypical Parkinson's disease (APD) or "parkinsonism plus" syndromes, such as multisystem atrophy (MSA) and progressive supranuclear palsy (PSP), are differential diagnoses with IPD but are usually separated later in the disease's journey by historical and physical findings. APD often has symmetrical rigidity and bradykinesia and, less likely, has resting tremor. It also sometimes has postural tremor and myoclonus. Early presentation of gait disturbance; falling, speech, and swallowing difficulty; and a rapidly progressive course over 5 to 6 years are more likely for APD than IPD. Supranuclear gaze palsy is seen with PSP and involves the vertical then horizontal gaze palsy, usually somewhat early. Dysautonomia—primarily orthostatic hypotension, bladder symptoms, and impotence—are seen in MSA.

Corticobasal degeneration is an APD that is associated with cortical symptoms and dementia, and is noted classically to have an alien limb. Dementia occurs robustly in DLB, but also in PSP, and less commonly, if at all, in MSA. However, 30% of patients with IPD will have dementia later in the disease, usually occurring after 10 years unless dementia of the Alzheimer's type (DAT) or DLB is the etiology of the dementia. APD cases may have a mild, somewhat transient therapeutic response to dopamine agonists (DAs) or levodopa (Dopar), unlike in IPD where there is a robust clinical response. Approximately 10% to 20% of patients with cirrhosis of the liver are said to have a spectrum of symmetrical parkinsonism. These patients will have mild symmetrical rigidity and akinesia with infrequently resting tremor. It is important to detect this parkinsonism in cirrhosis patients, because many will have a significant therapeutic response to levodopa. Drug-induced parkinsonism may be difficult to distinguish from IPD. Drugs such as reserpine, antipsychotics, and antiemetics are most likely to cause this drug-induced syndrome. Atypical neuroleptics such as quetiapine (Seroquel) are less likely to be associated with drug-induced parkinsonism and tardive dyskinesia.

Treatment

Nonpharmacologic therapy for IPD revolves around education for the patient, spouse, and caregiver allowing for better clinical communication, understanding, and compliance. This results in more effective, efficient medical care, better quality of life for the patient, and more cost-effective care. With education there is greater knowledge and understanding of end-dose failure, wearing off, motor fluctuations, and dyskinesias. The patient and caregiver can communicate needed and important information to the physician so the treatment can be individualized and tailored to the patient. Exercise for the patient regardless of the stage of the disease is crucial, not only for rigidity, akinesia, gait, and safety; but also for mental well-being. Clinical experience and studies have documented the significance of the ongoing benefits of regular exercise. Adequate nutrition is also paramount. Support groups are closely related to education and also help caregivers' mental well-being. The caregiver role is difficult and any help is appreciated and needed. Treatment of known or impending co-morbidity in IPD is finally being recognized as important. Aging patients have morbidity and mortality from various diseases related to stroke and central nervous system (CNS) white matter disease, referred to as subacute atherosclerotic encephalopathy (SAE). These two diseases and other vascular diseases are related to diabetes, hypertension, smoking, obesity, hyperlipidemia, and elevated homocysteine levels. Hence, because in the aging IPD patient accumulation of co-morbidity adds to the pathology and disability, it is important to aggressively diagnose and treat the co-morbid diseases.

Pharmacologic therapy can start with any number of drugs, usually depending on the degree of impairment, age, co-morbidity, and state of cognition. Anticholinergic drugs show efficacy in IPD, more so for resting tremor than rigidity and akinesia. Trihexyphenidyl (Artane) is started at 0.5 mg twice daily and then slowly and carefully increased up to 2 mg three times per day or until it is of benefit.

Benztropine (Cogentin) is used at the same dosage. Biperiden (Akineton) is also available. Neuropsychiatric dysfunction (NPD), often heralded by vivid dreams and later associated with agitation, hallucinations, and paranoid ideation, is a contraindication, as is cognitive impairment in the elderly and those that have significant co-morbidity. Adverse events that may occur are confusion, hallucinations, memory impairment, dry mouth, constipation, urinary retention, blurred vision, and tachycardia. Patients with benign prostatic hypertrophy (BPH) and closed-angle glaucoma should be given anticholinergics with caution. Cognitive changes, NPD, or confusion warrant gradual withdrawal of the anticholinergic. Amantadine (Symmetrel), now known as a glutamate antagonist, was first known to reduce presynaptic dopamine uptake and to increase dopamine release. It improves rigidity, akinesia, and, less so, tremor in approximately 60% of patients. It also reduces the severity and presence of dyskinesias probably through its glutamate antagonism. The elderly and patients with cognitive impairment and NPD have more adverse events, which are vivid dreams, hallucinations, confusion, and insomnia. A benign ankle edema and livedo reticularis can occur. Amantadine is often introduced in younger patients to give theoretical neuroprotection and as monotherapy to delay the use of levodopa (Dopar). It is also added to levodopa to reduce dyskinesias in approximately 50% to 70% of patients with IPD. Amantadine also improves activities of daily living (ADL). Amantadine should be slowly withdrawn from patients with adverse events, because often the rigidity, akinesia, and ADL will worsen. It is used at 100 mg once daily, increasing slowly up to 100 mg three times per day; but usually the dose is twice daily, in the morning and at noon.

Dopamine agonists (DAs) directly act on the dopamine receptors and were initially used as adjunctive therapy with levodopa. Studies show their clinical benefits with and without levodopa and the ability to reduce the levodopa dose or delay the need of levodopa. DAs bypass the degenerating SN dopamine neurons and do not require metabolic conversion to an active neurotransmitter. They act directly on the postsynaptic or presynaptic receptor. They also have longer half-lives than levodopa's 90-minute half-life. A shorter drug half-life allows for less CDS and hence more PS. Dopamine agonists are without interference from amino acids at the gastrointestinal (GI) or brain transport sites; so they can be taken with food or protein without affecting transport, unlike with levodopa. Bromocriptine (Parlodel), with a half-life of approximately 5 hours, is a D_2 and D_3 agonist with dosing that ranges from 5 mg to 30 mg, starting at 0.25 mg three times per day. Pergolide (Permax) is a D_1 and D_2 agonist whose half-life is 10 to 18 hours. Usually the starting dose is 0.05 mg three times per day, and it is increased to a total dose of 3 to 5 mg per day. The latter two dopamine agonists are ergots. Ropinirole (Requip) and pramipexole (Mirapex) are nonergot derivatives that are primarily D_2 and D_3 receptor agonists. These drugs in adjunctive studies show improvement in the amount of off time in levodopa-treated patients, and allowed levodopa dose reduction. Also, dopamine agonists show superior antiparkinson effect compared to placebo in levodopa-treated patients. Later studies comparing placebo and DAs in newly diagnosed, untreated IPD patients show DAs give robust clinical benefit. DA monotherapy is now the trend in newly diagnosed IPD patients, sparing and delaying the need for levodopa.

Three placebo-controlled, double-blind trials compare the agonist pramipexole with levodopa against the motor complications of Parkinson's disease (CALM-PD) study (Mirapex) and the O56 (Requip) study. Several key results are noted in both of these studies. Approximately 30% of patients could maintain DA monotherapy for 4 to 5 years. Only a small percent of DA-only treated patients developed dyskinesias at 4 to 5 years (7% to 10%), whereas 50% or more of the patients on levodopa/carbidopa alone developed dyskinesias. Approximately the same percent was true for motor fluctuations, wearing off, and on-off times. However, levodopa gave a slightly more robust clinical benefit with most noticeably better Unified Parkinson's Disease Rating Scale (UPDRS) motor scores. When additional levodopa was added to a DA as compared to levodopa/carbidopa only group, the DA group with added levodopa had less chance of developing dyskinesias compared to the supplemented levodopa group, approximately 25% compared to 50%. Also, the DA group had significantly less disabling dyskinesias compared to the levodopa group. Hence, the studies support using a DA first as monotherapy to allow delaying the need for levodopa, and to delay motor fluctuations and dyskinesias. Imaging tests were also done on patients in these two studies. Positron emission tomography (PET) scans for ropinirole and a 2β-carbomethoxy-3β-(4-iodophenyl) tropane single-photon emission computed tomography (β-CIT SPECT) study for pramipexole both measured different biochemical aspects. The results show 35% (PET scan) and 37% (β-CIT SPECT) relative differences in reduction in loss of uptake for the DA group. This loss of reduction uptake could represent a reduction in the SN neuronal loss when using a DA as compared to levodopa. However, some feel the reason for the reduction in loss of uptake is uncertain or may be a pharmacologic effect. Hence, neuroprotection by a DA cannot be stated with certainty. Further clinical studies are needed.

Ropinirole can be started at 0.25 mg three times per day and increased slowly up to 16 to 20 mg a day. Pramipexole is started at 0.125 mg three times per day and increased to 1.5 to 3 mg per day. Sumanirole*, a new D_2/D_3 agonist, is in clinical trials and looks very promising for efficacy for improving symptoms and disability, and delaying the need for levodopa. It appears to have the same adverse event profile as the other DAs, which are also seen in dopaminergic

---

*Investigational drug in the United States.

medications, most noticeably nausea, vomiting, somnolence, excessive daytime sleepiness (EDS), hallucinations, and postural hypotension. Going low and slow with the dose and titrating carefully helps reduce some of the adverse events. Cognitively impaired and NPD patients have a higher incidence of hallucinations. Rarely, erythromelalgia; ankle edema; and valvular, pulmonary, and retroperitoneal fibrosis can be seen (maybe more so with the ergot DA). Recent case reports show valvular fibrosis occurs with pergolide, however, the frequency is uncertain. This may well be a class effect and will need to be carefully monitored in all patients on DAs.

Apomorphine* is used in Europe and will be in the United States. Apomorphine is a strong D_1/D_2 agonist that is used subcutaneously with an auto-inject pen. Injected subcutaneously, it has clinical benefit in 10 minutes and lasts 20 to 60 minutes. It is a rescue drug used when the patient is having wearing off or just going off. You cannot use it if the patient is allergic to sulfides. Adverse effects seen with apomorphine are somnolence, yawning, rhinorrhea, nausea, dizziness, chest pressure or discomfort, skin nodules, and dyskinesias. Apomorphine may be a drug that will enable some IPD patients to avoid or delay surgery. It may also prove useful in patients where other drugs are not possible because of NPD or cognitive changes. Apomorphine is also being studied as a skin patch and as a nasal spray.

Rotigotine* is a DA skin patch that is being studied and shows clinical benefit. A_2A antagonists have a different mechanism of action but are not yet available for the treatment of IPD. So far studies are promising and demonstrate clinical benefit. It is yet uncertain what effect this class of drugs will have on dyskinesias, probably little or no reduction and in some patients slightly worse.

Levodopa/carbidopa (Sinemet) is the most commonly used form of levodopa. However, it is associated with motor complications, mainly motor fluctuations seen as wearing off, off-on, never on or delayed, on and freezing. Dyskinesia, another motor complication, occurs frequently with levodopa and in the young and advanced patient is the most difficult adverse event to treat and manage. Obviously some development of the motor fluctuations and the dyskinesias is also related to the progressive loss of the dopamine neurons in the SN. The short, 90-minute plasma half-life also is a factor for allowing PS rather than CDS.

Levodopa with carbidopa comes in immediate-release (IR) Sinemet and continuous-release (CR) Sinemet CR forms. Clinical studies show some clinical and probably minor advantages. Sinemet CR was developed to give a more continuous release of the levodopa and hence allow for a smoother levodopa plasma level, hence more CDS and less PS. At 5 years, 25% of the IR and CR patients had dyskinesia, but the clinical study may have had some design flaws. The starting dose should be low, and then increased slowly. In the IR levodopa, one half of a tablet made up of 25 mg carbidopa/100 mg levodopa may be started once a day and gradually increased to three times per day, then to four or five times per day. Doses of more than 600 to 800 mg should be used infrequently and cautiously, and combination therapy would be the ideal therapeutic goal.

Combination therapy is comprised of a DA, levodopa, maybe an anticholinergic, and maybe a monoamine oxidase type B (MAO-B) inhibitor. It is considered ideal to increase the DA to the highest effective yet tolerated dose before maximizing the levodopa dose. Or if levodopa was started first, a DA can be added. As the DA is increased, the levodopa can be gradually reduced. The CR formulation has reduced absorption and hence needs 25% to 30% more levodopa dose to be equivalent to the IR dose. Adverse events with all medications containing levodopa may be nausea, vomiting, hypotension, somnolence, hallucinations, dyskinesia, and motor fluctuations.

Catechol-*O*-methyltransferase (COMT) inhibitors, which should only be used (and only provide benefit) in combination with levodopa, have therapeutic efficacy in IPD. Although tolcapone (Tasmar) improves on time by approximately 2 hours, it can cause drug-induced hepatitis and the FDA has restricted its use significantly. Tolcapone is still available, however, but it must be used cautiously and weekly laboratory tests must be obtained.

Entacapone (Comtan), like tolcapone, inhibits one pathway of levodopa metabolism by COMT inhibition in the plasma and hence reduces the formation of 3-*O*-methyldopa (3-OMD). This gives more available levodopa to the brain and may reduce peripheral dopamine adverse events. Entacapone improves on time by approximately 1.5 hours in fluctuating patients. The plasma levodopa half-life with entacapone COMT inhibition is increased by 75%, area under curve (AUC) is increased by 48%, and there is no change in maximal concentration (C-max); however, the plasma levels gradually increase throughout the day. Hence, entacapone allows for a smoother plasma level, increases the availability of levodopa to the brain, and enhances CDS. This theoretically and ideally reduces the development of motor fluctuations and dyskinesias. Robust evidence of clinical improvement in UPDRS motor scores and ADL, as well as a reduction in levodopa dose requirement is present for fluctuating patients when entacapone is added to levodopa.

Nonfluctuating patients are patients that do not have wearing off, end-dose failure, or dyskinesias. There appear to be more than just the theoretical reasons to use entacapone in nonfluctuating patients, and this is supported by some early studies that show improvement in ADL and other quality-of-life measures. (Even more theoretical would be its use at the time of initiating levodopa therapy in levodopa-naïve patients. This would be done theoretically to try to maximize CDS and reduce PS as soon and as much as possible.) The positive study results with entacapone have led to the development of the triple pill,

*Investigational drug in the United States.

Stalevo. Stalevo contains entacapone, carbidopa, and levodopa. Stalevo allows all the pharmacologic advantages of entacapone with levodopa and carbidopa, along with the ease, convenience, and compliance advantage that one pill obviously offers. Antidotal experience and initial studies with Stalevo show efficacy and patient acceptance and preference with Stalevo. Stalevo may become the first-line drug when initiating levodopa in levodopa-naïve patients.

Entacapone and Stalevo are easy to use and generally well tolerated. However, some adverse events may slightly limit their use in levodopa-naïve patients, mainly diarrhea. Entacapone is associated with a 5% incidence of diarrhea, sometimes transient, yet at times requiring the discontinuance of the drug. Bismuth subsalicylate (Pepto-Bismol) or other antidiarrheal medicines can be used to reduce the initial diarrhea until it dissipates. Also, a benign brownish-yellowish urine discoloration may occur with entacapone and Stalevo. The patient must be warned of this. For the use of entacapone alone when adding to levodopa, dyskinesias are the most common adverse events, because of increased central dopaminergic effect. Occurrence is usually when dyskinesias are already present and/or when the threshold for developing them is low. When switching patients on levodopa to Stalevo, care must be taken to observe for dyskinesia development. Dyskinesias can then be reduced by reducing the levodopa dose by 25%. Entacapone comes in 200 mg tablets and can be cut in half, allowing for either a 100- or 200-mg dose to be given with each levodopa dose. A maximum of 1600 mg can be given a day. Only one tablet should be given with each dose of levodopa. Stalevo is formulated as carbidopa/levodopa/entacapone in the following combinations:

- 50 (12.5/50/200 mg)
- 100 (25/100/200 mg)
- 150 (37.5/150/200 mg)

The Stalevo pill should never be crushed or cut and only one Stalevo pill should be given with each dose. No more than 8 total Stalevo pills per day should be given.

Neuroprotection

Neuroprotection (NP) is a theoretical consideration at the present time. Vitamin E† has been suggested to be neuroprotective, however, this is not confirmed by the Deprenyl and Tocopherol Antioxidative Therapy of Parkinsonism (DATATOP) study. It is probably not easily absorbed into the brain. Coenzyme Q10* is investigated in a small, double-blind, placebo-controlled study at three doses, 300 mg, 600 mg, and 1200 mg. There was a trend to show improvement with coenzyme Q10, however, longer and larger studies are needed, and one multiple drug NP study is ongoing. Selegiline (Eldepryl), a MAO-B inhibitor, certainly was considered to be a potential neuroprotector. The DATATOP study's comparison of vitamin E, selegiline (Eldepryl), and placebo shows symptomatic benefits with selegiline (Eldepryl), but could not in most opinions document neuroprotection. It is started at 5 mg a day in the morning and usually increased to two 5-mg doses taken in the morning and at noon. It is used mostly for symptomatic improvement, but many use it as theoretical NP. There are several new drugs being studied that are MAO-B inhibitors, such as rasagiline.† It is being studied as monotherapy and for NP. Rasagiline is effective in improving symptoms and is also safe and tolerable.

Surgical therapy for IPD (not APD) has been used since 1940 when Meyers at the University of Iowa investigated its use. We now have a better understanding of its limitations, indications, and efficacy. Thalamotomy for essential tremor and pallidotomy for IPD gained acceptance in the 1980s and 1990s. Pallidotomy showed efficacy in IPD, especially for dyskinesias but also somewhat for akinesia, rigidity, and tremor contralaterally. However, when this ablative procedure was done bilaterally, despite robust benefit for dyskinesias, cognitive changes, dysphagia, and dysarthria were more common; this has significantly limited the use of bilateral pallidotomy. Ablation of the STN may have some investigative use and is being used clinically on a limited investigational basis.

Deep brain stimulation (DBS) in the GPi and the STN are the most frequently performed surgical procedures for IPD now. Both sites are shown to be efficacious. However, DBS in the STN may be slightly more beneficial. Tremor, rigidity, akinesia, dyskinesia, and maybe gait can be improved and there is an improvement in UPDRS motor scores and dyskinesia scores. Adverse events are not uncommon, and intracerebral hemorrhage can occur in 0.5% of cases. Infection can be as frequent as 2% to 5%, and electrode and connective wires can be fractured. Eventually batteries will need to be replaced. Also, cognitive changes can occur as well as NPD. Before a patient should be considered a candidate for pallidotomy or DBS he or she should have frequent attempts at optimal pharmacologic management and optimal pharmacologic alteration and individualized tailoring of all medicines. Older patients with significant co-morbidity, cognitive changes, and NPD are generally likely to have significant adverse events and are not candidates for DBS. Patients must be screened for dementia and depression before deciding to do surgery. Most of the clinical series for DBS have been done in patients younger than the age of 70 years. Vivid dreams and hallucinations make it difficult to consider DBS because these often worsen after the surgery. A poor therapeutic response to levodopa indicates a poor surgical response. The patient at best will probably be only as good after the DBS surgery as they were when they were maximally improved on their dopamine agonist and levodopa.

*Available as dietary supplement, and not FDA approved for this indication.

†Investigational drug in the United States.

Dementia in IPD

Cognitive impairment occurs in 30% of patients with IPD, and the first treatment is to slowly and sequentially taper off antiparkinson medicines that may be associated with adverse events such as cognition and NPD. Patients who have IPD and other neurologic diseases must be screened for dementia. The physician must be aware of the patients who are at risk for dementia such as those older than 65 years of age, those with IPD, and those with other neurological diseases. Age is the greatest risk factor for dementia just as it is for IPD. Patients at risk for dementia must be screened for dementia, and the Mini Mental State Examination (MMSE), although not ideal, is easy and quick to use. If antiparkinson drugs must be tapered because of cognitive impairment, they are usually discontinued in the following order:

1. First the anticholinergics amantadine (Symmetrel) and selegiline (Eldepryl)
2. Then the dopamine agonists
3. Lastly the levodopa

In place of these medications, a trial of acetylcholinesterase inhibitors (AChEI) should first be considered. These are donepezil (Aricept)[1], rivastigmine (Exelon)[1], and galantamine (Reminyl)[1]. These would be given not only for cognitive improvement but also for behavior issues. Memantine (Namenda)[1], a glutamate antagonist, may also be considered for improving cognition and behavior in IPD. Memantine can be used in combination with the AChEI; it is uncertain if the combination adds cognitive benefit, but it may allow the AChEI to be better tolerated. Hallucinations and delusions need the same scrutinizing for the tapering off of likely drug offenders as mentioned above.

AChEI can be used for NPD but if it does not help, then atypical neuroleptics such as quetiapine (Seroquel)[1] or clozapine (Clozaril)[1] may be used. Olanzapine (Zyprexa)[1], risperidone (Risperdal)[1], haloperidol (Haldol)[1], perphenazine (Trilafon)[1], and chlorpromazine (Thorazine)[1] will all make the rigidity and akinesia of parkinsonism more pronounced and may well affect the ADL of the patient. Clozapine needs careful weekly laboratory monitoring.

Depression occurs in 30% to 40% of patients with IPD, and it is often closely associated with cognitive impairment. Like with dementia, patients suspected of depression must be screened—the Bender Depression Index is easy to use and is clinically helpful. Evaluation for other causes of depression must be carefully considered. Education and counseling are important in the treatment of depression but usually the tricyclics or selective serotonin reuptake inhibitors (SSRIs) are needed to obtain some relief. Constant awareness of changing and developing symptoms of dementia and depression in a progressive, chronic disease journey brings the realization that repetitive screening is needed.

[1]Not FDA approved for this indication.

Constipation is treated with 8 glasses of water a day and a third to a half a cup of oat bran in the morning. These two are the foundation for resolving constipation. If this does not bring relief, then stool softeners should be added. Lactulose (Cephulac), starting at 1 tablespoon once or twice per day and increasing up to 5 to 6 tablespoons per day, may be needed. Exercise is important also.

Sleep disorders in IPD are common, and excessive daytime sleepiness (EDS) is present in 70% to 80% of IPD patients. A careful workup is needed including screening with the Epworth Sleepiness Scale (ESS). Insomnia or sleep fragmentation is very common. Good sleep hygiene must be established. To help promote sleep, clonazepam (Klonopin)[1] at low doses of 0.25 mg or 0.5 mg at night are of transient benefit. Also, quetiapine (Seroquel)[1] is helpful in refractory insomnia cases. EDS is common in IPD and APD and is associated with reduced activities of daily living and quality of life (QOL). The ESS is of some benefit in detection of EDS, but it is probably of limited benefit for diagnosis of sudden sleep events (SSE). These sudden sleep events can occur at any time but are most concerning when they occur with driving. The patient with IPD, with or without dopaminergic medications, must be warned about sleep disorders and especially SSE. They are more likely to occur in IPD patients on dopaminergic medications, most noticeably the DAs. Not only the patient, but the spouse and other caregivers must be questioned about sleep disorders, especially SSE. For EDS and SSE, modafinil (Provigil)[1] may be considered if caffeine or maybe amantadine (Symmetrel)[1] do not work. Rapid eye movement (REM) behavior disorder (RBD) is an amnestic state when the patient is asleep and where there is acting out of dreams by violent motor activity that may be harmful to the patient or the caregiver. RBD is seen not only in IPD but also DLB. Clearly RBD can precede the onset of IPD. If a diagnosis is made without any clinical features of IPD, the patient must be carefully followed for the development of a neurologic disease. The treatment is clonazepam (Klonopin)[1], 0.5 mg at night, and can be cautiously increased.

Restless legs syndrome (RLS) is sometimes seen in IPD, but it is a separate disorder and is often seen associated with a number of diseases. The symptoms are usually present in the evening or at night, but also sometimes after sitting for a long time. The symptoms are that of an uncomfortable feeling associated with aching, burning, cramping, or dysesthesias. There is an uncontrollable desire to move the legs and with the movement there is some relief of the discomfort. Diagnosis is often delayed and late, but treatment should be as early as possible. The first drugs to use for the treatment of RLS are the DAs. They are given before bedtime or in the early evening. Compared to other medications, the DAs are less likely to cause augmentation, which is an increasingly

[1]Not FDA approved for this indication.

earlier appearance of the symptoms during the day. Levodopa/carbidopa (Sinemet)[1], gabapentin (Neurontin)[1], opiates, or clonazepam (Klonopin) can be tried if DAs fail to treat the symptoms.

Bladder symptoms need to be diagnosed and treated. Nocturia is the most common and earliest urinary symptom. Detrusor hyperactivity is the most common etiology of urinary symptoms in IPD. Awareness of residual bladder volume is important, and if it is more than 200 mL bladder retention may be indicated. Reducing evening and late afternoon fluids is the first step toward improving nocturia and reducing evening urgency and frequency. Regular voiding throughout the day is also very helpful. Oxybutynin (Ditropan), 5 to 10 mg at bedtime or three times per day, can be tried. Tolterodine (Detrol), 4 mg at bedtime, can also be used. Both of these peripherally acting anticholinergics are now in long-acting formulations.

Orthostatic hypotension is not uncommon in IPD and needs to diagnosed and managed. Patients, when examined in the office, must be checked for orthostatic hypotension. It usually occurs asymptomatically first and then becomes symptomatic with dizziness and lightheadedness when standing and falling when getting up. It may also be associated with loss of consciousness when getting up from a reclining position. An overview of the patient's medications is the first step in addressing this problem. Any antihypertensive medication that is not needed should be eliminated. Behavior modification and education is very important for the patient and the caregiver. Next increasing fluid and salt intake is important. Elevation of the bed by 15 to 30 degrees will also be helpful. Fludrocortisone (Florinef)[1] can be initiated at very low doses if orthostatic hypotension is not controlled. The dose is started at 0.1 mg per day and can be carefully and slowly increased up to 0.5 mg per day[3], which is a high dose. Midodrine (ProAmatine), a selective α_1-agonist, can be used starting in the morning with 2.5 mg and increasing up to 5 mg or 10 mg three times per day. It is used mainly in the morning and at noon to avoid evening supine hypertension.

There is a great interest in premorbid personality in IPD, and there is a great deal of uncertainty whether one truly exists. However, it is definitely known that many IPD patients have an impulsive–obsessive personality. Often this does not interfere with their daily lives. The antidotal case reports of sexual misbehavior or excessive sexual appetite and, most recently, excessive gambling may well be an example of inability to control the intrusive abnormal impulsive–obsessive behavior. What the norm is for the same age groups is uncertain for these two behaviors and more studies need to be done.

The treatment of IPD is rapidly advancing and the pathophysiology is now better understood than ever before. Combination therapy using different medications with different mechanisms of action will be the rule.

[1]Not FDA approved for this indication.
[3]Exceeds dosage recommended by the manufacturer.

PERIPHERAL NEUROPATHIES

METHOD OF

Jaya R. Trivedi, MD, and Gil I. Wolfe, MD

The peripheral nervous system is composed of both sensory (afferent) and motor (efferent) components. Most peripheral nerves are mixed and contain both sensory and motor fibers. These fibers can be grouped into three major classes, large myelinated, small myelinated, and small unmyelinated. Motor axons usually are large, myelinated fibers that conduct rapidly (approximately 50 meters per second). Sensory fibers may be any of the three types. Joint position and vibratory stimuli are transmitted to the central nervous system (CNS) by fast-conducting, large-diameter sensory fibers, whereas pain and thermal stimuli are transmitted by smaller, slower-conducting fibers. Autonomic nerves are also small in diameter. Peripheral neuropathies are characterized by impaired function of sensory, motor, or autonomic nerves, either singly or in combination. In reality, most forms of peripheral neuropathy affect more than one type of nerve fiber.

Because there are many causes of peripheral neuropathy, an organized approach is essential if one is to arrive at the correct diagnosis and prescribe the appropriate therapy. A useful approach is to answer four key questions concerning the disorder (Table 1). First, what is the distribution of nerve involvement? Neuropathies may affect distal nerves in a symmetric, glove-and-stocking fashion (polyneuropathies), individual nerves as in carpal tunnel syndrome (mononeuropathies), or multiple nerves in an asymmetrical manner (mononeuropathy multiplex). Second, what classes of nerve fibers are involved? Prominent motor or autonomic involvement provides a useful clue to

TABLE 1 The Diagnostic Approach: Four Key Questions

1. What is the distribution of nerve involvement?
   Symmetrical polyneuropathy
   Mononeuropathy
   Mononeuropathy multiplex
2. What classes of nerve fibers are involved?
   Motor, sensory, autonomic, or combinations
   Small- or large-fiber sensory involvement
3. What is the time course of progression?
   Acute (days to 1mo)
   Chronic (more than 2mo)
4. Is the neuropathy primarily axonal or demyelinating?
   Proximal weakness suggests a demyelinating disorder.

TABLE 2 Causes of Neuropathy with Prominent Motor Involvement

Multifocal motor neuropathy
Guillain-Barré syndrome*
Chronic inflammatory demyelinating polyneuropathy*
Lead intoxication*
Acute porphyria*
Charcot-Marie-Tooth disease (hereditary motor and sensory neuropathy)*

*Sensory signs usually present on examination.

the underlying cause (Tables 2 and 3). When there is severe proprioceptive loss without motor involvement, a short list of large-fiber neuropathies and dorsal root ganglionopathies (sensory neuronopathies) should be considered (Table 4). On the other hand, reduced pinprick or temperature on examination or a history of neuropathic pain should direct attention toward neuropathies with small-fiber involvement. This differential diagnosis includes those neuropathies that cause autonomic dysfunction (see Table 3) in addition to idiopathic polyneuropathies, vasculitis, arsenic and thallium intoxication, and Fabry's disease. Third, is the time course of disease progression acute (<1 month) or chronic (>2 months)? Most neuropathies are chronic disorders; therefore, an acute history helps to limit the differential. Fourth, is the neuropathy primarily axonal or demyelinating? Distal weakness is a common feature of many forms of neuropathy. However, proximal weakness is a strong clinical clue that the neuropathy is demyelinating. The determination that a neuropathy is demyelinating is important, because these disorders are often immune-mediated and can respond favorably to immunotherapies. The clinical suspicion that a neuropathy is demyelinating in nature can be confirmed with nerve conduction studies (NCSs) or nerve biopsy.

Based on the answers to these four questions, the neuropathy can be classified as following one of five major patterns (Table 5). Assigning the neuropathy to one of these patterns will enable the clinician to narrow down the number of potential causes for the neuropathy, thereby minimizing unnecessary and expensive testing. This approach is largely based on elements elicited from the history and physical examination. In all cases, careful documentation of underlying illnesses, toxin or medication exposures, social habits, and family history is essential. Using such a systematized approach, a cause for the peripheral neuropathy can be identified in as many as 75% of patients referred to tertiary clinics. It is important to remember, however, that even the most sophisticated centers fail to uncover an etiology in 10% to 25% of patients with chronic sensory-predominant polyneuropathies.

TABLE 3 Causes of Neuropathy with Prominent Autonomic Involvement

Diabetes mellitus
Amyloidosis (familial and acquired)
Guillain-Barré syndrome
Vincristine (Oncovin) toxicity
Acute porphyria
HIV-related
Idiopathic or paraneoplastic pandysautonomia
Hereditary sensory and autonomic neuropathies

TABLE 4 Causes of Neuropathy with Prominent Proprioceptive Loss

Paraneoplastic (anti-Hu)
Sjögren's syndrome
Idiopathic sensory neuronopathy
Cisplatinum (Platinol) and other analogues
Pyridoxine (vitamin B_6) intoxication
HIV-related sensory neuronopathy
Vitamin E deficiency

Pattern 1: Symmetrical Distal Sensory Loss and Weakness

Peripheral neuropathies that follow this pattern are often referred to as glove-and-stocking neuropathies. They are the most common form of peripheral neuropathy encountered in practice, with a frequency approaching 5% in patients older than 55 years of age. There are many disorders that produce this clinical pattern of distal weakness, sensory loss, and reduced deep tendon reflexes. The majority are axonal disorders, in which the so-called dying back phenomenon first affects the longest, most susceptible fibers. In axonal neuropathies, NCSs demonstrate low or absent sensory or motor amplitudes, or both, whereas conduction velocities are relatively preserved. The axonal degeneration that predominates in this neuropathy pattern is usually the result of a metabolic or toxic insult. Treatment is generally directed at correcting the metabolic abnormality or eliminating exposure to the offending agent.

METABOLIC DISORDERS

Diabetes Mellitus

The most common peripheral neuropathy caused by diabetes mellitus is a mild to moderate distal sensorimotor polyneuropathy that is present in a majority of patients who have had diabetes mellitus for 10 to 25 years. This form of diabetic neuropathy is the most common polyneuropathy in most parts of the

TABLE 5 Five Main Patterns of Peripheral Neuropathy

Symmetrical distal sensory loss and weakness
Symmetrical sensory loss with both distal and proximal weakness
Asymmetrical sensory loss with weakness
Asymmetrical sensory loss without weakness
Asymmetrical weakness without sensory loss

world. In early stages, the neuropathy may be subclinical, and only later do patients notice distal numbness, tingling, or painful paresthesias. Weakness tends to involve only distal musculature and is usually mild. The polyneuropathy can affect small and large-diameter fiber populations to varying degrees. Autonomic involvement characterized by sexual dysfunction, urinary incontinence, distal anhidrosis, orthostatic hypotension, and gastrointestinal (GI) dysmotility may occur. Impotence is the most common autonomic manifestation, affecting 50% of diabetic men. An axonal pattern is usually seen on electrophysiologic studies. The pathogenic basis for diabetic neuropathy remains controversial, although there is evidence that both vascular and metabolic derangements are responsible.

Primary therapy is optimizing blood glucose control with either diet, hypoglycemic agents, or insulin, if needed. Strict control of hyperglycemia by insulin pump or multiple daily injections prevents or even improves neuropathy in insulin-dependent diabetics. To date, clinical trials of various agents, including aldose reductase inhibitors* and neurotrophic factors*, have been disappointing.

Diabetic neuropathic cachexia is an uncommon syndrome seen in diabetics who have had profound weight loss. These patients develop a symmetrical sensory polyneuropathy with severe painful dysesthesias and contact hypersensitivity. Patients tend to be men in their sixth or seventh decade of life. Unlike the more common distal sensorimotor polyneuropathy, diabetic neuropathic cachexia is reversible over a period of weeks to months with strict glucose control. Aggressive pain management, including narcotics, may be required in the acute stage.

Impaired Glucose Tolerance

Impaired glucose tolerance is a milder form of glucose dysmetabolism. Recent studies demonstrate that patients with impaired glucose tolerance are at high risk for developing diabetes mellitus. A sensory-predominant polyneuropathy is associated with impaired glucose tolerance, manifesting as a milder form of diabetic neuropathy. It is largely restricted to small fibers, whereas patients with diabetes have both large- and small-fiber involvement. Two-hour oral glucose tolerance testing is now recommended in all patients with distal axonal sensory or sensorimotor polyneuropathy of unclear etiology.

Uremia

Renal failure, like diabetes, typically causes a distal polyneuropathy with impaired sensory and motor function and reduced tendon reflexes. The frequency of neuropathy is higher in patients with chronic elevations of serum creatinine above 2 mg/dL. Unpleasant paresthesias, described as burning and tingling in the feet and pulling and drawing of the legs, are particularly pronounced in this form of polyneuropathy. Muscle cramping and restless legs are reported by some patients. As the neuropathy progresses, significant distal weakness with foot drop can occur.

Only modest improvements can be expected with hemodialysis, and the neuropathy may continue to progress despite its initiation. Considerable improvement usually follows successful renal transplantation. Therefore, the presence of a clinically significant uremic polyneuropathy may influence treatment decisions in individual patients with chronic renal failure.

Other Metabolic/Systemic Disorders

Axonal polyneuropathy is a complication of a variety of other metabolic disorders. These include the sensory-predominant neuropathies reported in chronic hepatic insufficiency and in hypothyroidism. Glove-and-stocking polyneuropathies are also seen in several inflammatory and vascular disorders including systemic lupus erythematosus, rheumatoid arthritis, Sjögren's syndrome, and sarcoidosis. A distal, symmetric polyneuropathy is present in 10% to 35% of patients with advanced HIV disease. This neuropathy is usually painful, with prominent symptoms of burning, lancinating pain, and pins-and-needles paresthesias.

An axonal sensory-predominant polyneuropathy is also seen with celiac disease, even in the absence of GI symptoms. Patients usually present with distal numbness, burning, tingling, and sensory ataxia. Occasional patients develop distal weakness. NCSs may be normal or reveal an axonopathy. Serologic testing includes antigliadin, endomysial, and transglutaminase antibodies. Diagnosis is confirmed by characteristic histologic findings of villous atrophy, crypt hyperplasia, and inflammatory infiltrates on small bowel biopsy. Treatment focuses on elimination of dietary gluten; this restriction has produced some resolution of symptoms, but without objective neurologic improvement. Immunotherapy has not proven to be beneficial.

Peripheral neuropathies are also a feature of dominantly inherited hepatic porphyrias. These rare disorders should be suspected when altered mentation, abdominal pain, and autonomic dysfunction accompany a motor-predominant neuropathy. A mild, distal, painful sensory neuropathy has been reported in the setting of severe hypertriglyceridemia and may improve with appropriate treatment. Critically ill patients with sepsis, multiorgan failure, and metabolic derangements can develop a severe axonal sensorimotor neuropathy that may delay successful weaning from mechanical ventilatory support. This critical-illness neuropathy can be

*Investigational drug in the United States.

differentiated from other neurologic causes of weakness by electrophysiologic studies.

TOXIC DISORDERS AND MEDICATIONS

Toxins

Alcohol and a variety of toxins are capable of producing peripheral neuropathy. Toxins implicated in the development of peripheral neuropathy are mainly heavy metals (lead, mercury, arsenic, thallium), hexacarbons and solvents (carbon disulfide, *N*-hexane, methyl butyl ketone, acrylamide), and other industrial agents (hexachlorophene, methyl bromide, organophosphates). As with metabolic disorders, toxic neuropathies typically are symmetric and produce distal sensory deficits greater than motor deficits in a length-dependent manner. A less common pattern is selective large-fiber sensory loss from cisplatin (Platinol), methyl mercury, and pyridoxine (vitamin B_6) intoxication. Small-fiber sensory neuropathies may be seen after Kepone, vacor, or ciguatera (reef fish) toxin exposure. As a rule, weakness is not prominent in toxic neuropathies, with *N*-hexane and lead exposures being the exceptions. Prolonged inhalation of *N*-hexane through glue-sniffing can produce marked weakness. Lead neuropathy, now rare because of governmental precautions and regulations, classically appears in adults as a motor neuropathy mainly affecting the upper limbs. Wrist drop is a prominent feature. Interestingly, lead-intoxicated children usually manifest an encephalopathy and not neuropathy. When children do develop the neuropathy, lower extremity weakness predominates.

Treatment of toxic neuropathies involves eliminating exposure to the offending agent. In general, toxic neuropathies continue to progress for several weeks to several months after the chemical exposure has ceased. In most situations, the neuropathy then stabilizes, followed by slow, but steady improvement. In heavy metal intoxication, therapy with the chelating agent D-penicillamine (Cuprimine)[1] at a dose of 250 mg two to four times a day should be considered. Because of potentially life-threatening hematologic and renal complications, patients receiving D-penicillamine should have close monitoring of complete blood counts and urinalysis.

Alcohol

Alcoholic polyneuropathy is a result of chronic overuse, with most patients having consumed more than 100 mL of ethanol daily for at least 3 years. As with other toxic neuropathies, the pattern is a distal sensorimotor polyneuropathy characterized by distal weakness and atrophy with prominent sensory symptoms. Painful paresthesias are common in these patients, mainly involving the feet. Trophic skin changes producing a thin, shiny appearance of the lower legs may be seen. While a direct neurotoxic effect of alcohol remains conjectural, nutritional deficiencies common to alcoholics—especially inadequate intake of the B family of vitamins—are implicated in the generation of the neuropathy. It is known that heavy drinkers who maintain a good diet are less prone to develop the polyneuropathy. Treatment of the neuropathy centers on abstinence from alcohol, resumption of a well-balanced diet, and B vitamin supplementation[1]. The recommended daily doses are 100 mg of thiamine (B_1), 50 mg of pyridoxine (B_6), 100 mg of niacin (B_5), 10 mg of riboflavin (B_2), and 10 mg of pantothenic acid (B_3). Stabilization and even limited recovery can occur with these measures.

[1]Not FDA approved for this indication.

Medications

Many drugs are known to cause peripheral neuropathy (Table 6). As a result, a careful, detailed medication history is an essential component of any peripheral neuropathy evaluation. The majority of drug-induced neuropathies are of the distal, axonal variety with sensory deficits greater than motor deficits. For instance, mild sensory polyneuropathies may be seen from hydralazine (Apresoline), tricyclic antidepressants, and chronic phenytoin (Dilantin) use.

[1]Not FDA approved for this indication.

TABLE 6 Drugs That Cause Peripheral Neuropathy

Antibiotics
Amphotericin B (Fungizone)
Antiretroviral nucleoside analogues
Chloramphenicol (Chloromycetin)
Chloroquine (Aralen)
Dapsone
Ethambutol (Myambutol)
Isoniazid (INH, Nydrazid)
Metronidazole (Flagyl)
Nitrofurantoin (Macrodantin)
Streptomycin
Chemotherapeutic Agents
Cisplatin (Platinol) and other platinum-containing drugs
Misonidazole
Nitrogen mustard
Vinblastine (Velban)
Vincristine (Oncovin)
Sedatives and Hypnotics
Amitriptyline and other tricyclics (Elavil)
Ethchlorvynol (Placidyl)
Monoamine oxidase inhibitors
Miscellaneous
Alcohol
Allopurinol (Zyloprim)
Amiodarone (Cordarone)
Colchicine
Disulfiram (Antabuse)
Ergotamine (Ergomar)
Gold salts (Aurolate)
Hydralazine (Apresoline)
Megadose pyridoxine (Vitamin B_6)
Phenytoin (Dilantin)
Thalidomide (Thalomid)

Chronic metronidazole (Flagyl) therapy produces a painful, sensory neuropathy. However, some medications such as chloroquine (Aralen) and dapsone produce a motor neuropathy. Amiodarone (Cordarone) and perhexiline are known causes of demyelinating neuropathy. Megadose pyridoxine (vitamin B_6), usually greater than 500 mg per day, results in a severe, potentially irreversible sensory neuronopathy with prominent large-fiber deficits and sensory ataxia. This syndrome has been reported at doses as low as 200 mg per day. Interestingly, pyridoxine deficiency can cause a distal, painful, predominantly small-fiber sensory polyneuropathy.

The neuropathies from chemotherapeutic agents are dose-dependent and can lead to disabling symptoms that will limit treatment. Vincristine (Oncovin) and vinblastine (Velban) produce a predominantly sensory polyneuropathy with autonomic dysfunction. With vincristine, paresthesias, often noticed in the fingers before the feet, are a common initial symptom. Weakness can be especially prominent in the fingers and wrists, although it can also affect the distal lower extremities. Cisplatin (Platinol) produces a distal, large-fiber sensory neuropathy with prominent vibratory and proprioceptive loss. Symptoms may begin or progress even after the medication has been stopped.

Several of the antiretroviral agents used to treat HIV infection cause neuropathy. These include the nucleoside analogues didanosine (Videx), stavudine (Zerit), zalcitabine (Hivid), and, less commonly, lamivudine (Epivir). These toxic neuropathies may be clinically indistinguishable from the distal symmetrical polyneuropathy seen in advanced HIV disease. A toxic myopathy is a known complication of zidovudine (Retrovir, AZT).

The treatment of most drug-induced neuropathies centers on discontinuation of the offending medication. In most cases, progression of the neuropathy will slow, followed by stabilization and slow improvement. The improvement in motor strength after stopping chloroquine (Aralen) is at times rapid and dramatic. Pyridoxine deficiency is a complication of isoniazid (INH, Nydrazid) therapy, so patients placed on this drug should be given pyridoxine (vitamin B_6), 50 mg per day, in an effort to prevent neuropathy.

VITAMIN DEFICIENCIES

Vitamin B_{12} Deficiency

Unlike the vitamin deficiency syndromes seen in alcoholics, vitamin B_{12} deficiency is not usually caused by reduced vitamin intake. This condition is usually a result of poor gut absorption from anatomic, autoimmune, or infectious causes. Vitamin B_{12} deficiency produces both central and peripheral nervous system derangements, a condition referred to as subacute combined degeneration. The peripheral neuropathy is characterized by prominent loss of vibration and proprioception in the lower limbs, at times resulting in a sensory ataxia. A superimposed myelopathy may mask the expected hyporeflexia. Babinski signs may be present. This combination of peripheral sensory loss and upper motor neuron signs should raise suspicion of vitamin B_{12} deficiency. Complications of B_{12} deficiency can occur even when B_{12} levels are in the low-normal range. Finding elevated serum homocysteine and methylmalonic acid levels can help establish a diagnosis of B_{12} deficiency in this setting.

Treatment is with intramuscular injections of vitamin B_{12} (cyanocobalamin) and is usually continued indefinitely. The usual dose is 1000 μg daily for 1 week followed by a single 1000-μg injection given on a monthly basis.

Other Vitamin Deficiencies

Other vitamin B deficiency states are rare in developed countries. Niacin deficiency results in pellagra, characterized by diarrhea, dermatitis, and dementia. A peripheral neuropathy may occur along with this classic triad. Niacin, 100 mg three times a day, should be given, but the neuropathy often fails to respond to replacement therapy. Deficiency of thiamine, pantothenic acid, and pyridoxine are also thought to cause peripheral neuropathy. Vitamin B supplementation should follow the guidelines provided in the section on alcoholic neuropathy.

Deficiency of fat-soluble vitamin E is usually secondary to malabsorption. Large-fiber sensory deficits with sensory ataxia may result. The response to vitamin E supplementation is variable, depending on the severity of the associated sensory myelopathy. Oral supplementation of vitamin E can range up to 100 IU/kg per day.

HEREDITARY NEUROPATHIES

Hereditary neuropathies typically follow a symmetrical pattern with distal motor and sensory deficits. Most of these neuropathies fall under the eponym of Charcot-Marie-Tooth (CMT) disease. In a second nomenclature, they are called hereditary motor and sensory neuropathies. There are many forms of hereditary neuropathy, and they are usually classified by the pattern of inheritance, the classes of nerve fibers affected, and whether the nerve injury is predominantly axonal or demyelinating (Table 7). Because as many as 30% of undiagnosed neuropathies may have a hereditary basis, it is important to investigate for clues in the history and examination that suggest the presence of a hereditary disorder before embarking on an expensive evaluation. The presence of high-arched feet (pes cavus), clawed toes, scoliosis, enlarged nerve trunks, Charcot joints, and onset in the first two to three decades of life are strongly suggestive of hereditary neuropathy. A neuropathy that has progressed slowly over several decades should also raise suspicion of

TABLE 7 Classification of Hereditary Motor and Sensory Neuropathies

	Inheritance	Locus	Gene
CMT Type 1 (Demyelinating, Type 1A, Very Common)			
CMT1A*	AD	17p11.2-12	PMP22
CMT1B*	AD	1q22-23	P0
CMT1C	AD	16p13	LITAF
CMT1D*	AD	10q21	EGR2
CMT1E*	AD	1q22	P0
CMT1F	AD	8p21	NF light chain
CMT Type 2 (Axonal, Relatively Common as a Group)			
CMT2A	AD	1p35-36	KIF1B
CMT2B	AD	3q13-22	RAB7
CMT2C	AD	12q23-24	Unknown
CMT2D	AD	7p14	GARS
CMT2E*	AD	8p21	NF light chain
CMT2F	AD	7q11-21	Unknown
CMT2G	AD	3q13.1	Unknown
CMT2I	AD	1q22	P0
CMT2J	AD	1q22	P0
HMSN Type 3† **(Dejerine-Sottas Disease, Severe Demyelinating, Rare)**			
HMSN3A*	AD	17p11.2-12	PMP22
HMSN3B*	AR/AD	1q22-23	P0
HMSN3C	AD	8q23-24	Unknown
CMT Type 4 (Uncommon)			
CMT4A*	AR	8q21.1	GDA P1
CMT4B	AR	11q23	MTMR2
CMT4B2	AR	11p15	SBF2
CMT4C	AR	5q23	KIAA1985
CMT4D	AR	8q24	NDRG1
CMT4E*	AR	10q21	EGR2
CMT4F*	AR	19q13	Periaxin
X-Linked CMT (Type 1 Form, Common)			
CMTX, type 1*	X-semidom	Xq13.1	Connexin 32
CMTX, type 2	XR	Xp22.2	Unknown
CMTX, type 3	XR	Xq26	Unknown
HNPP (Common, Patients Prone to Pressure Palsies)			
HNPPA*	AD	17p11.2-12	PMP22
HNPPB	AD	Unknown	Unknown

*Genetic testing commercially available.
†Classified as HMSN instead of CMT Type 3 to distinguish from allelic CMT Type 1 and 2 forms.
Abbreviations: AD = autosomal dominant; AR = autosomal recessive; CMT = Charcot-Marie-Tooth disease; EGR2 = early growth response 2; GARS = glycyl tRNA synthetase; GDAP1 = ganglioside-induced differentiation-associated protein 1; HMSN = hereditary motor sensory neuropathy; HNPP = hereditary neuropathy with liability to pressure palsies; KIF1B = kinesin family member 1Bβ; LITAF = lipopolysaccharide-induced tumor necrosis factor-α factor; MTMR2 = myotubular-related protein 2; NDRG1 = N-myc downstream-regulated gene 1; NF = neurofilament; PMP22 = peripheral myelin protein 22; P0 = myelin P0 protein; RAB7 = RAS-related GTP binding protein 7; SBF2 = SET binding factor 2; semidom = semidominant; XR = X-linked recessive.

a hereditary process. If the family history is unclear, relatives should be examined and even tested with nerve conduction studies to determine if a familial neuropathy is present. The autosomal dominant forms of CMT represent the most commonly inherited neuromuscular disorders and are divided into demyelinating (CMT type 1) and axonal (CMT type 2) neuropathies on the basis of NCSs. Approximately 1 in every 2500 individuals has autosomal dominant CMT. Symptoms usually begin in the second decade, but there is a large range of phenotypic variability even among members of the same family. At times, relatives may be unaware they have CMT or have had their mild symptoms ascribed to another process. It is estimated that 15% of patients with CMT type 2 present after the age of 50 years. Therefore, a late age of onset does not exclude the possibility of a hereditary neuropathy. Genetic testing is now available through commercial reference laboratories for several forms of CMT (see Table 7).

Other types of hereditary neuropathy are less common (Table 8). The hereditary sensory and autonomic neuropathies (HSAN) mainly affect small myelinated and unmyelinated sensory fibers, resulting in marked loss of pain and thermal sensation. There is variable loss of other sensory modalities. Autonomic dysfunction may also be present. Pressure sores, foot ulcers, and Charcot joints result from repeated trauma to insensitive distal limbs. Familial dysautonomia or Riley-Day syndrome is included in this family of hereditary neuropathies.

There is no specific therapy available for hereditary neuropathies at this time. Ankle-foot orthotic devices have proven very helpful in patients who develop significant foot drop. The vast majority of patients with CMT remain ambulatory to some extent throughout their lives.

CRYPTOGENIC NEUROPATHIES

Up to 33% of polyneuropathies referred to tertiary centers are of undetermined cause. The term cryptogenic sensory polyneuropathy (CSPN) is used to describe this heterogeneous group. These idiopathic neuropathies tend to arise in the sixth to seventh

TABLE 8 Hereditary Disorders That Cause Peripheral Neuropathy

Abetalipoproteinemia (Bassen-Kornzweig syndrome)
Analphalipoproteinemia (Tangier disease)
Fabry's disease
Familial amyloid polyneuropathy
Familial dysautonomia (Riley-Day syndrome; HSAN type 3)
Friedreich's ataxia
Giant axonal neuropathy
Hepatic porphyrias
Hereditary sensory and autonomic neuropathy (HSAN)
Leukodystrophies (with central nervous system involvement)
Mitochondrial disorders
Neuroaxonal dystrophy
Refsum's disease

decade of life and are sensory-predominant, with distal sensory loss primarily affecting vibration and pinprick. The majority of patients have neuropathic pain or complain of tingling. Tendon reflexes may be reduced or intact, and motor involvement, when present, is usually restricted to intrinsic foot and hand muscles. Electrophysiologic and histologic studies are consistent with axonal degeneration. The neuropathy generally is stable to slowly progressive over years. Only rarely do patients have significant motor involvement. Because motor function is relatively preserved, management usually focuses on the neuropathic pain, which is typically the dominant symptom. Pharmacologic approaches to the treatment of neuropathic pain are summarized in Table 9.

Pattern 2: Symmetrical Sensory Loss with Both Distal and Proximal Weakness

The presence of symmetrical proximal weakness in the setting of peripheral neuropathy is strongly suggestive of an acquired, demyelinating process, specifically acute inflammatory demyelinating polyneuropathy (commonly referred to as Guillain-Barré syndrome

TABLE 9 Pharmacologic Therapy for Neuropathic Pain

Therapy	Route	Starting Doses	Maintenance Doses
First Line			
Tricyclic antidepressants[1]	PO	10-25 mg at bedtime	Increase by 10-25-mg increments to 100-150 mg qhs
Gabapentin (Neurontin)[1]	PO	300 mg PO tid	Increase by 300-400-mg increments to 2400-6000 mg daily divided in 3-5 doses
Carbamazepine (Tegretol)[1]	PO	200 mg PO bid	Increase by 200 mg to 200-400 mg 3-4 times/d; follow drug levels on doses greater than 600 mg/d
Tramadol (Ultram)[1]	PO	50 mg PO bid or tid	Increase by 50-mg increments to a maximum of 100 mg qid
Second Line			
Mexiletine (Mexitil)[1]	PO	200 mg once per day	Increase by 50-100 mg increments to a maximum of 300 mg tid
Lamotrigine (Lamictal)[1]	PO	25 mg at bedtime × 2wk	Increase by 25-50 mg increments to 400 mg daily
Venlafaxine XR (Effexor XR)[1]	PO	75 mg/d	Increase by 75-mg increments to 150-225 mg/d
Bupropion SR (Wellbutrin SR)[1]	PO	150 mg/d	Increase to 150 mg bid
Opiate analgesics	PO	Varying doses	After 1-2wk, replace with longer-acting agent on a qd to bid schedule
Topical Agents			
Capsaicin (Zostrix) 0.075%	Topical*	Apply to affected region tid to qid	Continue with starting dose
Lidocaine 5% (Lidoderm patch)[1]	Topical	Apply up to 3 patches, for up to 12h of a 24h period	Continue with starting dose
Salicylate 10%-15%[1]	Topical*	Apply to affected region tid to qid	Continue with starting dose
Menthol 16%/Camphor 3%	Topical*	Apply to affected region tid to qid	Continue with starting dose
Lidocaine 2.5%/Prilocaine 2.5% (EMLA)[1]	Topical	Apply to affected region tid to qid	Continue with starting dose
Ketoprofen 5%/Amitriptyline 2%/Tetracaine 1%	Topical†	Apply to affected region bid	Increase up to a qid schedule
Ketoprofen 10%/Cyclobenzaprine 1%/Lidocaine 5%	Topical†	Apply to affected region bid	Increase up to a qid schedule
Ketamine 5%/Amitriptyline 4%/Gabapentin 4%	Topical†	Apply to affected region bid	Increase up to a tid schedule
Carbamazepine 5%/Lidocaine 5%	Topical†	Apply to affected region bid	Increase up to a qid schedule

[1]Not FDA approved for this indication.
*Available over the counter.
†Must be compounded by pharmacy.
Abbreviations: bid = twice daily; EMLA = eutectic mixture of local anesthetics; PO = orally; qhs = at bedtime; qid = four times daily; tid = three times daily.

[GBS]), or chronic inflammatory demyelinating polyneuropathy (CIDP). These disorders actually represent polyradiculoneuropathies, and the propensity for nerve root involvement results in the marked proximal weakness that can involve the truncal and cranial musculature. In demyelinating neuropathies, the NCS demonstrates markedly slowed conduction velocities. In addition, prolongation of distal latencies and F waves, conduction block, and temporal dispersion of evoked responses may be observed.

GUILLAIN-BARRÉ SYNDROME

GBS is the most common cause of acute flaccid generalized weakness in industrialized countries. It is a monophasic illness that usually begins with acral paresthesias and back pain. Over several days GBS progresses to cause ascending weakness that varies from mild to a severe quadriplegia, with patients requiring ventilatory support. The motor features usually predominate over any sensory loss. The majority of patients have had a mild viral upper respiratory infection, *Campylobacter jejuni*-related GI illness, or surgery in the 4 weeks before onset of neurologic symptoms. GBS has also been associated with lymphoma and leukemia as well as a variety of viral infections including HIV, hepatitis, Epstein-Barr virus, and cytomegalovirus. The time-course from onset to a clinical plateau is usually several days and, by definition, does not exceed 4 weeks. Cranial weakness with bulbar symptoms is common. Reflexes are depressed or absent. Approximately 20% of GBS patients have autonomic instability that usually consists of labile hypertension, tachycardia, or urinary dysfunction. Life-threatening cardiac arrhythmias and ileus can occur.

The diagnosis of GBS can be confirmed with cerebrospinal fluid (CSF) studies, demonstrating an elevated protein without pleocytosis, the classic albuminocytologic dissociation. The CSF protein may remain normal in the first week. In addition, HIV-associated GBS patients may have a moderate pleocytosis. In most cases, NCSs demonstrate multifocal demyelination. Patients with severe axonal degeneration have a more prolonged illness and are less likely to have a complete recovery. Treatment with plasmapheresis (250 mL/kg over several exchanges) or intravenous immunoglobulin (IVIG) (Gamimune N)[1], according to several studies, accelerates the recovery phase and shortens hospital stays. These treatments are summarized in Table 10. Plasmapheresis and IVIG may be withheld in patients who have minor deficits or are improving spontaneously. Corticosteroids used alone have demonstrated no benefit. Diligent supportive care, including good pulmonary toilet, physical therapy to prevent contractures, and measures to prevent decubitus ulcers, is important.

CHRONIC INFLAMMATORY DEMYELINATING POLYNEUROPATHY

CIDP, like GBS, usually presents as a motor predominant neuropathy with prominent proximal weakness. Unlike GBS, CIDP is a progressive neuropathy and is rarely associated with antecedent illnesses or respiratory failure. Occasionally CIDP can present in

[1]Not FDA approved for this indication.

TABLE 10 Standard Immunotherapy for Immune-Mediated Neuropathies

Therapy	Neuropathy Types	Route	Starting Doses	Maintenance Doses
Prednisone[1]	CIDP, VN	PO	60-100 mg/d for 4wk	60-100 mg qod, reducing dose by 10 mg q2-4wk; in diabetics, consider daily dosing to simplify glucose control
Methylprednisolone[1]	CIDP, VN	IV	1 g daily or qod for a total of 3-5 doses	1 g q2-4wk
Azathioprine (Imuran)[1]	CIDP	PO	50 mg/d	Increase by 50 mg increments q2-4wk to 2-3 mg/kg/d
Cyclophosphamide (Cytoxan)[1]	CIDP, VN, MMN	PO	50 mg/d	Increase to 1.5-2 mg/kg/d
Cyclophosphamide	CIDP, VN, MMN	IV	0.5-3 g/m²	Repeat dose monthly for 6 mo
Cyclosporine (Neoral, Sandimmune)[1]	CIDP	PO	100 mg bid	Increase by 100 mg increments to 3-6 mg/kg/d on a bid schedule
IVIG[1]	GBS, CIDP, MMN	IV	0.4 g/kg/d for 5d	0.4-1 g/kg as a single dose q4-8wk as needed
Plasmapheresis	GBS, CIDP, MMN	IV	Exchange total of 250 mL/kg plasma over 7-14d	Total exchanges of 50-250 mL/kg may be repeated prn
Rituximab (Rituxan)[1]	MMN, IgM-associated neuropathy	IV	375 mg/m² q wk × 4wk	Repeat 375 mg/m² as needed 9-15 mo later

[1]Not FDA approved for this indication.
Abbreviations: CIDP = chronic inflammatory demyelinating polyneuropathy; GBS = Guillain-Barré syndrome; IVIG = intravenous immunoglobulin; MMN = multifocal motor neuropathy; prn = as needed; q = every; qod = every other day; VN = vasculitic neuropathy.

the pattern of a mononeuropathy multiplex, large-fiber neuropathy with sensory ataxia, pure motor neuropathy, or small-fiber neuropathy. The diagnosis is based on an electrophysiologic pattern of multifocal demyelination, elevated CSF protein, and, when necessary, nerve biopsy. The treatment of CIDP is based on immunomodulating therapies, which are summarized in Table 10. CIDP does respond to corticosteroids. Plasmapheresis is generally reserved for refractory patients.

PARAPROTEIN-ASSOCIATED NEUROPATHY

A chronic polyradiculoneuropathy that in some cases is indistinguishable from CIDP is associated with a monoclonal protein. The M-protein may be immunoglobulin (Ig) G, A, or M, and should prompt investigation for an underlying lymphoma, myeloma, amyloidosis, or other lymphoproliferative disorder. However, the majority of patients have a monoclonal gammopathy of undetermined significance (MGUS). Approximately 10% of MGUS patients develop neuropathy, and it is thought that the paraprotein represents antibodies directed against peripheral nerve components. Some studies have shown that demyelinating features are more frequent in patients with an IgM paraprotein, 50% of whom have reactivity to myelin-associated glycoprotein.

Treatment of MGUS-associated neuropathy can be challenging, but patients may respond to similar approaches to those used in CIDP including prednisone, IVIG (Gamimune N)[1], and plasmapheresis. Patients with IgG or IgA paraproteins may respond better to plasmapheresis than those with an IgM. In unresponsive patients, a combination of prednisone with melphalan (Alkeran)[1] or chlorambucil (Leukeran)[1] may be considered. Rituximab (Rituxan)[1] has recently been used with success in a small series of patients with IgM paraproteins. In the less common situation where an isolated plasmacytoma is present (as in osteosclerotic myeloma), the neuropathy may respond to excision of the bony lesion, irradiation, or chemotherapy.

Pattern 3: Asymmetrical Sensory Loss with Weakness

MONONEUROPATHIES

A mononeuropathy implies injury to a single nerve and is typically the result of direct trauma causing focal compression. Sensory and motor fibers are usually involved together, although there are situations where sensory or motor function is affected in isolation. Individual nerves are susceptible to compression at specific sites—the median nerve at the carpal tunnel in the wrist, the ulnar nerve at the cubital tunnel in the elbow, the radial nerve at the spiral groove of the humerus, and the peroneal nerve at the fibular head. These mononeuropathies are a common clinical problem in otherwise healthy individuals. When chronically compressed, these mononeuropathies can be managed by avoiding activities that make the nerves vulnerable to injury and with orthotic devices. In more severe cases, surgery may be necessary to decompress the nerve. The greatest success is with carpal tunnel release for median mononeuropathies at the wrist. Diabetics are prone to develop mononeuropathies from nerve infarction. The third and sixth cranial nerves and thoracic roots are especially prone to this type of injury. In most cases, diabetic mononeuropathies resolve spontaneously over several months.

[1]Not FDA approved for this indication.

MONONEUROPATHY MULTIPLEX

When the asymmetrical pattern involves multiple nerves, a mononeuropathy multiplex is present. This distinctive pattern is the result of damage to individual peripheral nerves and is unlike the length-dependent, symmetric neuropathies covered earlier. Initially, conditions that typically affect sensory and motor fibers together are discussed here. The differential diagnosis is restricted when sensory or motor fibers are involved in isolation, and these scenarios are discussed in later sections.

Vasculitic Neuropathies

When the individual neuropathies develop abruptly, a vasculitic disorder needs to be considered. The diagnosis can be confirmed by sensory nerve biopsy. A variety of diseases are known to produce vasculitic neuropathy. These include polyarteritis nodosa (PAN), Churg-Strauss syndrome, rheumatoid arthritis, systemic lupus erythematosus, Sjögren's syndrome, Wegener's granulomatosis, and giant cell arteritis. PAN is the most common cause of nerve vasculitis. Vasculitic neuropathies are treated with a combination of corticosteroids and cyclophosphamide (Cytoxan)[1]. Doses for these medications are provided in Table 10.

Diabetes may also produce a mononeuropathy multiplex pattern. Most commonly, these take the pattern of a proximal diabetic neuropathy, also called diabetic amyotrophy or Bruns-Garland syndrome. These motor-predominant neuropathies tend to occur in older, noninsulin-dependent diabetics and classically involve the femoral nerve, affecting the lower extremities more than upper extremities. Severe pain usually precedes by several days the onset of weakness and muscle atrophy. In most cases, there is a prominent asymmetry, although patients who develop bilateral involvement are well documented. There is growing evidence that both inflammatory and ischemic

[1]Not FDA approved for this indication.

vascular injury is involved in the pathogenesis, prompting some investigators to use corticosteroids and immunomodulating agents in the management of these patients. To date, no randomized, controlled trials have been completed. In most cases, spontaneous improvement can be expected over several months.

Cryoglobulinemia causes vessel occlusion by precipitation of proteins on exposure to cold, resulting in nerve infarction. Essential (idiopathic) cryoglobulinemia can be managed by avoidance of cold exposure. Other forms of cryoglobulinemia, such as those associated with plasma cell dyscrasia and paraproteins, require aggressive treatment aimed at the underlying disease.

Infectious Causes

A mononeuropathy multiplex pattern may also arise from infectious processes. Leprosy, although uncommon in industrialized countries, is a frequent cause of neuropathy worldwide. In the lepromatous form, *Mycobacterium leprae* infects peripheral nerves diffusely and causes extensive axonal loss, primarily in cooler parts of the face and limbs where the mycobacterium thrives. On a superficial level, nerve involvement may resemble a glove and stocking pattern, however, close examination often reveals an irregular pattern of sensory loss. In the tuberculoid form, the nerve damage follows the classic mononeuropathy multiplex pattern. Superficial nerves are thickened and may be palpable. Lyme disease may cause a polyradiculoneuropathy or mononeuritis multiplex. Systemic treatment for these infections is covered elsewhere in this book.

Multiple Pressure Palsies

When the mononeuropathy multiplex develops in a more slowly progressive fashion, nerve entrapment or pressure palsies should be considered. Conditions that predispose individuals to multiple nerve entrapments include rheumatoid arthritis, hypothyroidism, acromegaly, amyloidosis, and sarcoidosis. A remarkable feature of sarcoidosis is multiple fluctuating and remitting cranial neuropathies. Multiple pressure palsies may also represent an inherited trait. Hereditary neuropathy with liability to pressure palsies (HNPP) is referred to as tomaculous neuropathy in the older literature, after the sausage-like myelin expansions seen histologically. The focal neuropathies of HNPP can be managed with bracing and by educating patients to avoid situations and positions that predispose them to develop pressure palsies, such as leaning on their elbows or crossing their legs. Genetic testing is available for the most common form of HNPP (see Table 7).

In addition to the activity avoidance, splinting, and surgery used for compressive mononeuropathies, the management of multiple pressure palsies should include treatment of any underlying predisposing condition. In the case of sarcoidosis, corticosteroids are believed to abbreviate the course of neuropathy and prevent the development of new nerve injuries.

Pattern 4: Asymmetrical Sensory Loss without Weakness

Compressive mononeuropathies may occasionally spare motor fibers and manifest only sensory deficits. For instance, carpal tunnel syndrome may involve sensory fibers in isolation both clinically and on electrodiagnostic studies. However, pure, asymmetric sensory deficits should alert the clinician to the possibility of a sensory neuronopathy, where the site of injury is in the dorsal root ganglia. Sensory neuronopathies often present initially as an acute to subacute asymmetrical process. Large-fiber sensory function is primarily affected, and over time the deficits may become confluent, producing a symmetrical pattern. Symptoms include limb numbness and tingling associated with gait clumsiness, sensory ataxia, and falling. The sensory ataxia is exacerbated by restriction of visual cues, as occurs in a dark environment or when patients close their eyes. The differential diagnosis for sensory neuronopathies is relatively limited (see Table 4). In the paraneoplastic form, the large-fiber sensory deficits may predate diagnosis of the cancer by several years. The underlying malignancy is usually small cell carcinoma of the lung, but other solid tumors have been described. Anti-Hu antibodies are a marker of paraneoplastic sensory neuronopathy, and when not present, this form of neuropathy is essentially excluded and other causes should be considered. On the other hand, when anti-Hu antibody testing is positive, an aggressive search for an underlying neoplasm is indicated, with repeat screening every 6 to 12 months if the initial search is unrevealing. Testing for anti-Hu antibodies is available through several reference laboratories.

Pattern 5: Asymmetrical Weakness without Sensory Loss

In most cases, this rare pattern is produced by motor neuron disease, specifically amyotrophic lateral sclerosis (ALS). Patients with ALS may initially have only lower motor neuron signs, but the majority of cases will present with or develop upper motor neuron findings over time. Motor neuron disorders are a topic to themselves and will not be discussed further in this article.

Multifocal Motor Neuropathy

A motor neuropathy that produces an asymmetrical pattern of motor deficits has been described in the last 2 decades and is of particular importance, as it can mimic ALS but has a more favorable prognosis and can respond to immunotherapy. Multifocal motor neuropathy (MMN) presents with asymmetric distal weakness greater than proximal weakness that tends to begin in the upper extremities. Muscle atrophy and fasciculations are typical features, leading to the confusion with ALS. MMN can be distinguished from other forms of motor neuropathy by the presence of demyelinating features on NCSs. Conduction block has been heralded as the electrophysiologic marker for the neuropathy, but this feature cannot be demonstrated in all patients. The majority of patients also have high titers for the anti-ganglioside antibody, anti-GM1. However, anti-GM1 seropositivity is not essential for the diagnosis, and patients who are seronegative appear to respond equally well to immunotherapy. First-line treatment is IVIG (Gamimune N)[1], with cyclophosphamide (Cytoxan)[1] and plasmapheresis reserved for nonresponders. As discussed earlier, lead intoxication produces a motor neuropathy that often presents with asymmetrical wrist drop.

Treatment

In many forms of neuropathy, there is no specific therapy available. However, general supportive measures can help patients maximize function and alleviate symptoms. Range-of-motion exercises can prevent joint contractures in weakened limbs, ankle-foot orthotic devices can prevent tripping in patients with foot-drop, and canes and walkers can enhance stability and preserve ambulation. Good foot hygiene and well-fitted shoes are of extreme importance in insensitive feet, especially in diabetic neuropathy. Severe generalized weakness as seen in GBS requires intensive care, with frequent repositioning and foam supports to prevent decubitus ulcers and compressive neuropathies; splinting to prevent contractures; and prophylactic measures for deep venous thrombosis.

IMMUNOTHERAPY

A variety of immunotherapies are available to treat immune-mediated neuropathies. These medications and procedures are mainly used in acute and chronic inflammatory demyelinating polyneuropathies, vasculitic neuropathy, and neuropathies associated with inflammatory disorders such as connective tissue disease. The immunotherapies are summarized in Table 10.

PAIN MANAGEMENT

Neuropathic pain is a prominent feature of several peripheral neuropathies including diabetic neuropathy, uremic neuropathy, HIV- and alcohol-associated neuropathies, and idiopathic polyneuropathies. The pain may be described as burning, stinging, needle-like, stabbing, throbbing, or aching. Pain management should begin with a concerted effort to identify the underlying cause of the neuropathy, as directed therapy may improve the symptoms. If the pain persists or no etiology is identified, a number of agents are available to treat neuropathic pain. In addition, simple measures such as soaking feet in cold water followed by application of petroleum jelly or lotions may provide some relief. The pharmacotherapy for neuropathic pain is summarized in Table 9. Placebo-controlled trials have been conducted for the oral agents and for topical capsaicin (Zostrix) and lidocaine patches (Lidoderm)[1], in some cases with varying conclusions regarding efficacy. No specific guidelines exist for choosing one agent over another, but treatment must be individualized, with medications chosen that are most likely to be tolerated by the patient, as adverse events are common, especially in elderly patients.

Treatment of neuropathic pain is challenging, with considerable variability in an individual's response to the various agents and even to different drugs in the same class. General recommendations for a successful trial require that the patient and physician agree that the goal is to find an effective medication with tolerable side effects, understand that responses vary considerably between patients and that pain relief is rarely complete, and initiate medications at low doses and titrate them slowly until an adequate clinical response is observed or intolerable side effects appear. An oral drug trial of at least 4 to 6 weeks is recommended before moving to another medication. Capsaicin cream (Zostrix) should be continued for at least 3 to 4 weeks, and patients should be warned that burning may worsen initially. Polypharmacy with oral agents should be reserved for those instances where one drug provides partial relief but higher doses produce intolerable side effects. Topical agents are often used as adjunctive therapy.

AUTONOMIC COMPLICATIONS

Postural hypotension, impotence, gastroparesis, diarrhea, and sphincter disturbances are potential complications of autonomic neuropathy. Postural hypotension can be managed with fludrocortisone (Florinef)[1], 0.1 mg twice a day, or midodrine (ProAmatine), 10 mg three times a day. Sildenafil (Viagra) can improve the impotency caused by autonomic neuropathy. The usual dose is 50 mg approximately 1 hour before sexual activity. The reader should refer to other sources for treatment of gastroparesis and diarrhea.

[1]Not FDA approved for this indication.

[1]Not FDA approved for this indication.

ACUTE HEAD INJURIES IN ADULTS

METHOD OF
Scott A. Rutherford, AFRCS, and
Paul A. Leach, MRCS

The management of an adult with a head injury is something that the majority of medical practitioners will encounter by virtue of its high incidence. While the management of more severe injuries is undoubtedly better undertaken in specialized centers, it is imperative that all doctors recognize head-injured patients, as well as understand aspects of their long-term care. The term head injury has been largely superseded by the more descriptive term traumatic brain injury (TBI), to which we will make reference in this article.

Epidemiology

Approximately 1 million patients will present to hospitals in the United Kingdom (UK) each year with TBI, with the figure in the United States proportionately higher. Approximately 70% are adults 16 years of age or older, and 15% to 20% require admission. The outcome of even a mild TBI can be very disruptive. Some 63% of adults with a moderate TBI and 85% with a severe TBI remain disabled 1 year after their injury, and even patients with minor TBI may experience long-term problems such as headache, memory loss, and poor concentration (13% to 15%), often delaying a return to work.

The mortality rate overall is low (6 to 10 per 100,000 patients), but in total amounts to many thousands of deaths per year. The death rate from TBI following motor vehicle accidents has fallen in the past 30 years with the introduction of occupant-protective devices, seat belts, and alcohol limits, but this remains the most common cause of TBI, particularly in younger people. Falls are the leading cause of TBI in the elderly. Population characteristics of a certain region can alter the epidemiologic profile of TBI. For example, in the area we serve, which has a higher proportion of deprived communities than the national average, there is an increased prevalence of vulnerable road users (i.e., pedestrians and cyclists), interpersonal violence, and chronic diseases. This increases both the incidence and the morbidity and mortality of TBI. Other factors cited as more prevalent in adults sustaining a TBI (especially severe TBI) are poor social background, alcoholism, drug abuse, and poor educational attainment.

The costs of TBI are vast, both because of the mortality and the long-term disability that can result. Significant behavioral, cognitive, emotional, and physical impairment leads to loss of employment, breakdown of relationships, and dependence on social services.

Classification

The main classification of TBI rests on grading of the severity. Although historically this has been done by duration of coma or duration of post-traumatic amnesia, there is now global acceptance of severity grading based on the post-resuscitation Glasgow Coma Score (GCS) (Table 1):

- A mild TBI has a GCS between 13 and 15. There is usually unconsciousness for less than 15 minutes, and most will make a full neurologic recovery.
- Moderate TBI refers to patients with a GCS between 9 and 12, and there is often unconsciousness for more than 15 minutes.
- Severe TBI results in a postresuscitation GCS between 3 and 8.

With these definitions, 90% of emergency room patients with TBI have mild TBI, 5% have moderate TBI, and 5% severe TBI. In the UK approximately 10% of an emergency room's total workload will be patients with TBI.

Pathophysiology

Traumatic brain injury is broadly divided into primary and secondary injury. The primary injury occurs at the time of impact, and apart from preventative measures, there is no treatment that can influence the extent of this injury. Secondary brain injury develops in the time after the primary injury, sometimes within a matter of minutes if other systemic injuries are severe, or more commonly in the days and weeks after TBI. If there is a severe primary injury and/or early secondary injury, death typically results before hospital care can be initiated. It has in fact been estimated that more than two thirds of people who die from TBI do so before reaching the hospital.

Once the brain is injured, even to a relatively minor degree, it becomes far more susceptible than a normal brain to further damage caused by fluctuations in blood pressure or oxygenation. Secondary insults to an injured brain include hypotension, hypoxia, and raised intracranial pressure. It is imperative that all patients with a TBI have resuscitation aimed to counter these insults from the outset of their management. As such, the early management of a patient with a likely TBI is more appropriately focused on general resuscitation

TABLE 1 Glasgow Coma Score for Adults

	Score	Response	Description
Eye Opening			
	4	Spontaneously	Eyes open when the patient is at rest
	3	To speech	Eyes open when the patient is spoken to
	2	To pain	Eyes open to stimulus not inflicted to the face
	1	None	Both eyes remain closed to painful stimulus
If the eyes are unable to open because of swelling, this must be documented and the eye score is invalid.			
Verbal Response			
	5	Oriented	Patient knows who he or she is, the time/date.
	4	Confused	Talking/answers questions, but confused and disoriented.
	3	Inappropriate words	Recognizable, but inappropriate words.
	2	Incomprehensible sounds	Grunts/groans, but no actual words.
	1	None	No sounds at all.
If speech is impossible because of injury or intubation, this must be documented.			
Motor Response			
	6	Obeys commands	Appropriately responds to simple commands.
	5	Localizes to pain	Localizes to painful stimulus above eye.
	4	Normal flexion	Flexes arm normally to above clavicle, but does not reach stimulus.
	3	Abnormal flexion	Decorticate flexion of all arm joints, not reaching above clavicle.
	2	Extension	Extends arms to side of body.
	1	None	No response.
The best response in the upper limbs is recorded. For patients not responding to verbal command, a central painful stimulus is applied to the supraorbital nerve, with the arms positioned across the body so that the elbows are flexed to 90°.			

and maintenance of ventilation and circulation, rather than specific measures to deal with the primary cranial damage (Advanced Trauma Life Support [ATLS] system).

Management Principles

PREHOSPITAL ASSESSMENT AND CARE

The aims of the early management of any patient with TBI are:

- General ATLS resuscitation if required (securing airway, breathing, circulation, and cervical spine)
- Assessing the severity of the TBI, which determines further hospital management
- Continued measures to prevent, detect, and correct secondary brain insults
- Identifying associated injuries

Prompt resuscitation in the field, rapid evacuation from the scene of injury, and sophisticated critical care management in the hospital have been shown to reduce mortality significantly, largely because these measures address the principles above.

In less severe injuries, we suggest that the guidelines in Table 2 be followed for referring a patient to the hospital after an injury. This entails taking a brief history of the mechanism of injury and conducting a

TABLE 2 Indications for Referral to the Hospital of Patients with Traumatic Brain Injury

Indication	Examples
Impaired consciousness (GCS <15) at any time since injury	
Amnesia for the incident or subsequent events	
Neurologic symptoms	Severe and persistent headache Nausea and vomiting Irritability or altered behavior Seizure
Clinical evidence of a skull fracture	CSF leak Periorbital hematoma
Significant extracranial injuries	
A concerning mechanism of injury	High energy injury (fall from height) Possible penetrating brain injury Possible nonaccidental injury (in a child)
Continuing uncertainty about the diagnosis after first assessment	
Medical co-morbidity	Anticoagulant use Alcohol abuse
Adverse social factors	No one able to supervise the patient at home

limited neurologic examination. Other than the GCS, it is important to note pupillary size and reactivity, any limb weakness, and any external evidence of head trauma.

Patients with a TBI who present with any of the following risk factors should have full cervical spine immobilization attempted if possible:

- GCS less than 15 at any time since the injury
- Neck pain or tenderness
- Focal neurologic deficit
- Paresthesia in the extremities
- Any other clinical suspicion of cervical spine injury

MANAGEMENT OF MILD TRAUMATIC BRAIN INJURY

Mild traumatic brain injury comprises the vast majority of patients seen in the hospital with a brain injury. They should be promptly assessed by triage personnel, who should establish their risk for a clinically important brain injury and/or cervical spine injury. There has recently been a shift of emphasis away from simple observation for neurologic deterioration to early predictive imaging. This reduces the time to detection of life-threatening complications and is associated with better outcomes.

Within the group of mild TBI, some authorities advocate differentiating patients with a GCS of 13 to 14 (mild) from those with a GCS of 15 (minor), because of the difference it makes in the need for and the urgency of imaging. The rate of computerized tomography (CT) scan abnormalities in GCS 13 patients is 28%, GCS 14 is 16%, and GCS 15 (with loss of consciousness) is 3%. The clinically important subgroup of GCS 15 patients are those with a skull fracture. If a fracture is present, the risk of an intracranial hematoma rises from a 1 in 31,300 chance (adults with TBI with GCS 15 and no skull fracture) to 1 in 81 chance.

The topic that has recently received a lot of attention within the UK is the selection of patients for CT scanning of the head following TBI. The National Institute for Clinical Excellence (NICE) in the UK recently issued guidelines to this effect, and these are summarized in Table 3. These consign the use of skull radiographs to the detection of nonaccidental injury in children and to those few institutions where CT scanning resources are limited or unavailable. In this setting, skull radiographs together with inpatient observation can still be employed in the management of minor TBI. The indications for skull radiograph in this situation are:

- Violent mechanism of injury (e.g., blow to the head with a hard object, struck by a vehicle)
- Loss of consciousness or amnesia at any time
- Boggy scalp hematoma
- Clinically compound, depressed skull fracture

It should, however, be mandatory that CT scanning be readily available on a 24-hour basis to emergency rooms responsible for assessing patients with TBI.

The management algorithm for a patient with a minor TBI is shown in Figure 1. In summary, the only patients fit for immediate discharge from the emergency room are those with a GCS of 15 and no or minimal symptoms, or those with a GCS of 15 with some other risk factor in whom a CT scan has been shown to be normal. It is important that the appropriate advice is given to these patients and/or their caregivers, both in verbal and written forms, and that a responsible individual will remain with the patient for the first 48 hours. The key information that should be conveyed is shown in Table 4.

Patients identified as requiring a period of observation locally (persistent GCS 13 to 14 with normal CT scan) should be admitted and have half-hourly observations performed (GCS, pulse, blood pressure, respiratory rate, pupillary size, and response) for the first 6 hours or until their condition is stable. The minimum stay should be 24 hours, and they should only be discharged at this stage if recovered to GCS 15 and minimally symptomatic.

In combative patients with a GCS of 13 or 14, other possible causes for agitation should be sought

TABLE 3 National Institute for Clinical Excellence (NICE) Guidelines for Cranial CT Scanning of Patients with Traumatic Brain Injury

Time Scale of CT Scan	Indication
Within 1 hour of request	GCS <13 at any point since injury GCS = 13 or 14 at 2 hours after injury Suspected open or depressed skull fracture Any sign of basal skull fracture More than one episode of vomiting Age ≥65 years (providing there was some loss of consciousness or amnesia) Post-traumatic seizure Coagulopathy (providing there was some loss of consciousness or amnesia) Focal neurologic deficit
Within 8 hours of injury	Amnesia >30 minutes of events before impact Dangerous mechanism of injury (providing there was some loss of consciousness or amnesia)

Abbreviation: CT = computed tomography.

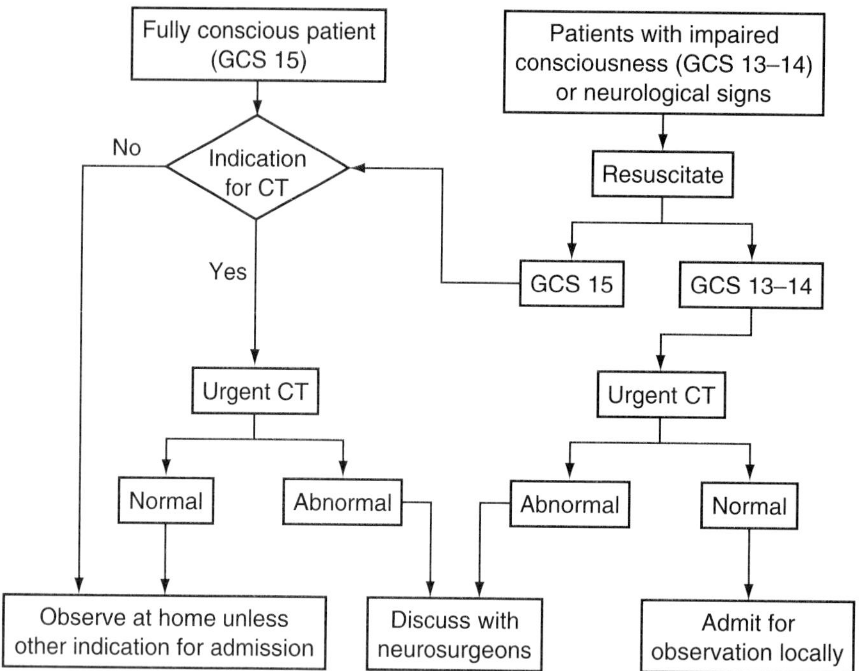

FIGURE 1 Guidelines for the initial triage of traumatic brain injuries in adults. *Abbreviations*: CT = computed tomography; GCS = Glasgow Coma Score.

such as hypoglycemia, hypoxia, drug intoxication, and post-ictal states. These patients might require intubation before their CT scan. The drunk patient with a mild TBI remains a difficult problem. Usually drunk patients do not become agitated, and, therefore, aggres-sive behavior may be caused by other factors such as listed above. If these are excluded and their GCS does not return to 15 within 2 hours of the injury, they should then undergo CT scanning. Measuring serum alcohol levels may be useful if alcohol consumption is uncertain.

If the CT scan reveals any sort of abnormality, it is recommended that the case be discussed with a neurosurgeon. Patients with contusions or extra-axial (epidural or subdural) hematomas should be admitted to the neurosurgical unit, where a further decision will be made as to whether the patient is observed or taken for surgery. In those with a hematoma, we will have a low threshold for rescanning them if there is any deterioration, and often will evacuate the hematoma for symptom control even if the GCS does not fall.

MANAGEMENT OF MODERATE TRAUMATIC BRAIN INJURY

Patients with a GCS of 9 to 12 are much less common than mild TBI, and they will all require a CT scan of their head. The general principles of early management once again apply as laid out in the ATLS system. Not all patients with moderate TBI require intubation. Those with an isolated head injury (particularly if CT scan is normal) who are maintaining their own airway and breathing normally can simply be carefully observed. The following patients should, however, be intubated:

- Penetrating TBI
- Associated major injury to the chest and/or abdomen
- A deteriorating GCS
- When neurosurgery is anticipated
- Combative patients who are endangering themselves and others

Approximately 40% of patients with a moderate TBI have abnormal CT findings, and 8% require surgery.

Cervical spine imaging is an important element in the management of patients in this category. With a significantly impaired conscious level, all these patients must be assumed to have a cervical spine injury by the same impact that resulted in their head injury until proven otherwise. In regards to clearing the cervical spine radiologically, it should be borne in mind that a plain lateral cervical radiograph identifies only 75% of fractures, and even a three-view cervical spine series (lateral, anteroposterior, and odontoid peg views) will still miss 7% of fractures. We, therefore, recommend that all these patients have lateral and anteroposterior radiographs, CT of occipital condyles to C2, CT of C7-T1 if not clearly seen on plain radiographs, and CT of any other suspicious areas.

The further neurosurgical treatment of patients with moderate TBI, whether it is surgery or conservative management in an intensive care unit, overlaps considerably with that of patients with a severe TBI. This is dealt with in the following section.

TABLE 4 Advice to Patients with Mild Traumatic Brain Injury Prior to Discharge

Advice	
Symptoms requiring urgent medical help	Unconsciousness, or lack of full consciousness Any confusion Any drowsiness Any problems understanding or speaking Any loss of balance or problems walking Any weakness in one or more arms or legs Any problems with eyesight Very painful headache that will not go away Any vomiting Any fits Clear fluid coming out of ear or nose Bleeding from one or both ears New deafness in one or both ears
Symptoms that you should not worry about	Mild headache Feeling sick (without vomiting) Dizziness Irritability or bad temper Problems concentrating or problems with your memory Tiredness Lack of appetite Problems sleeping
Things that will help you get better	Do not stay at home alone for the first 48 hours. Do make sure you stay within reach of a telephone and medical help. Do have plenty of rest and avoid stressful situations. Do not take any alcohol or drugs. Do not take sleeping pills, sedatives, or tranquilizers unless given by a doctor. Do not play any contact sport for at least 3 weeks. Do not return to your normal school or work activity until you feel you have completely recovered. Do not drive a car, motorbike, or bicycle or operate machinery unless you have completely recovered.

MANAGEMENT OF SEVERE TRAUMATIC BRAIN INJURY

Patients with severe TBI should, whenever possible, be treated in an intensive care unit that has on-site neurosurgical facilities. If such a facility is unable to take the patient because all the beds are full, head injured patients who do not have a mass lesion can be managed in a non-neurosurgical intensive care unit (ICU). However, a recent study in the UK that included more than 3500 patients indicates that the patients managed in the non-neurosurgical ICU have a significantly higher mortality than their counterparts managed in specialist neurosurgical intensive care units.

After discussion with both the intensive care physicians and the neurosurgeons, the patient should be transferred as soon as their general condition allows. This again requires application of ATLS guidelines, which are especially important in the setting of severe, often multisystem injury:

- Airway management—usually the patient is intubated and ventilated.
- Breathing—exclusion of life-threatening chest injuries, securing of endotracheal tube, use of high-flow oxygen.
- Circulation—insertion of two large-bore peripheral cannulas, administration of intravenous resuscitation fluids, continuous invasive arterial blood pressure monitoring
- Cervical spine control and neurologic assessment.
- Secondary survey.

The need for a safe but swift transfer is to enable access to neurosurgical facilities if surgical intervention is needed and also to prevent secondary brain injury. Up to one half of patients have an episode of hypoxia, and up to one third have an episode of hypotension at some point from the time of the accident to the completion of definitive treatment. Both of these factors have a significant effect on overall morbidity and mortality, and it is, therefore, paramount to maintain adequate blood pressure and oxygenation at all times.

Cerebral Perfusion Pressure

During the first few hours and days following a severe TBI, cerebral blood flow (CBF) is reduced and cerebral metabolism increased. Together these can lead to cerebral ischemia, and, therefore, it is essential to maintain a good cerebral perfusion pressure to prevent secondary brain injury. Cerebral perfusion pressure is calculated as follows:

Cerebral perfusion pressure (CPP) =
Mean arterial blood pressure (MAP) −
Intracranial pressure (ICP)

We aim to maintain mean arterial blood pressure above 90 mm Hg and the intracranial pressure below 20 mm Hg, therefore, maintaining a cerebral perfusion pressure of at least 70 mm Hg. It may be necessary to use vasopressive agents such as norepinephrine (Levophed) to maintain an appropriate MAP, but not before the patient has had restoration of their intravascular volume. If this is to be measured accurately, the patient must have a central venous line allowing the central venous pressure (CVP) to be continuously measured. A urinary catheter must also be placed.

Ventilation

Most patients with a severe TBI are sedated, intubated, and ventilated for transfer and are usually kept in that manner at least in the initial stages of their care. It is important to maintain good oxygenation, with a PO_2 above 11 kPa. The patient will need regular monitoring of arterial gas tensions, regular chest toilet, daily chest physiotherapy, and early detection and treatment of ventilator-associated pneumonia.

In our unit we aim for early tracheostomy as this can aid with chest toilet and often helps the patient wean from the ventilator, therefore enabling an earlier discharge from the intensive care unit.

Hyperventilation causes cerebral vasoconstriction and, therefore, decreased CBF, which if prolonged, will lead to cerebral ischemia. Recent studies show that prolonged periods of hyperventilation (up to 5 days) are associated with poorer outcomes. Our policy is to keep the PCO_2 between 4.0 and 4.5 kPa. However, severe hyperventilation will reduce ICP in the short term and can be effective in an emergency situation while awaiting more definitive treatment (e.g., an acute neurologic deterioration resulting in a unilateral dilated pupil).

Intracranial Pressure Monitoring

Although this is the cornerstone of management of patients with severe TBI, no randomized, prospective, controlled study of ICP monitoring has been undertaken to provide grade 1 evidence of improved outcomes. Despite this fact, the general consensus supported by the American Association of Neurological Surgeons is that ICP monitoring is appropriate in such patients.

In our unit we aim to keep the ICP below 20 to 25 mm Hg. This can be achieved with various methods of medical treatment, with or without surgical treatment, depending on CT scan findings. The basic management strategy is outlined in Figure 2, with our management subdivided into three levels of intensity of ICP treatment.

Level 1 treatment:

- Sedatives—patients can be kept at various levels of anesthesia depending on ICP and the stage of their recovery. Sedatives not only slow cerebral metabolism but also have analgesic properties which both help to lower ICP. Our regime consists of propofol (Diprivan) and a short acting opiate such as alfentanil (Alfenta). Care should be taken as propofol can cause hypotension. With a climb in ICP it is always prudent to check the level of sedation.
- Position—ensure that the head is in a neutral position with no pressure on the neck veins, and that the patient is head up at an angle of 30°.
- Temperature—core temperature should be continuously measured and any pyrexia should be treated with antipyretics (acetaminophen [Tylenol]) in the first instance, and, if resistant, with active cooling measures. Overcooling is not beneficial, so we aim for normothermia. Causes for the pyrexia should be sought. The correlation between core and brain temperature is unclear, although work in our unit is ongoing in this field.
- Oxygenation—maintain good gas exchange with a PCO_2 between 4.0 and 4.5 kPa and a PO_2 above 11 kPa.
- Mean arterial blood pressure—aim for a CPP of 70 mm Hg.

If the ICP is refractory to all these maneuvers, then the on-call neurosurgeon should be contacted and a repeat CT scan considered. If this again shows no mass lesion, then we step up to the next level of ICP management.

Level 2 treatment:

- Mannitol—This is an osmotic diuretic that works in two ways. First it expands the intravascular space and, therefore, increases CBF. Second it also has a direct osmotic effect on cerebral tissue drawing fluid into the intravascular space. Both these effects cause a drop in ICP. We give a bolus of 0.5 to 1.0 g/kg over 15 to 20 minutes. The patient must have a urinary catheter in place and have fluid replacement to maintain euvolemia. We do not use a continuous infusion as there is a theoretical risk of reverse osmotic shift. This is because of mannitol opening the blood–brain barrier and accumulating in the brain, thus exacerbating cerebral edema and increasing ICP. It is also important to monitor electrolytes and serum osmolality, and we do not give mannitol if the serum osmolality is above 320 mOsm.
- Cerebrospinal fluid (CSF) diversion—If the most recent CT scan shows any dilatation of the ventricular system, we advocate insertion of an external ventricular drain. This can be left open, draining at a preset level, or intermittently opened when ICP rises above a given limit.
- Muscle relaxants—These are useful for transfers either between hospitals or for a trip to the CT scanner. We also use them for resistant intracranial hypertension. Disadvantages include masking any seizure activity, muscle breakdown, and an increased incidence of pneumonia.

Level 3 treatment:

- Barbiturate coma—Barbiturates lower cerebral metabolic rate of oxygen and CBF by up to 50%, thus decreasing cerebral blood volume and, therefore, ICP. There is some evidence that part of their effect is as an inhibitor of lipid peroxidation, which lowers the amount of free radicals produced. We use a single bolus dose of thiopental (Pentothal), 250 mg over 5 minutes, and then a continuous infusion if ICP responds. Serum blood levels do not correlate with effect or

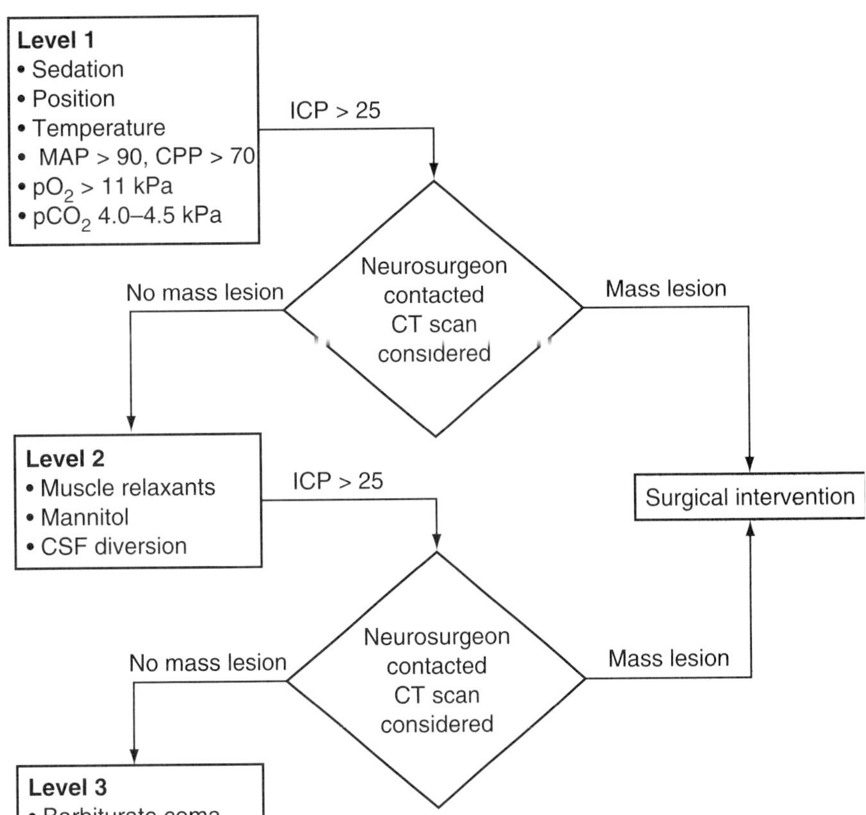

FIGURE 2 Management of raised intracranial pressure (ICP) in severe traumatic brain injury. *Abbreviations*: CPP = cerebral perfusion pressure; CT = computed tomography; CSF = cerebrospinal fluid; MAP = mean arterial pressure.

outcome, and if electroencephalographic recordings are made when burst suppression is reached, then an increase in dose imparts no further benefit. Caution should be taken as these agents can cause systemic hemodynamic instability and suppression of leukocyte activity.

If maximal medical management for raised ICP has been reached, then some units will embark on decompressive craniectomies. There is no convincing evidence that these aggressive surgical maneuvers improve outcome, and, hence, they have not gained universal acceptance.

The use of corticosteroids in severe TBI has failed to show any effect on ICP or any improvement in outcome, and, therefore, have no role in the management of these patients. We also do not routinely use prophylactic antibiotics for base of skull fractures.

Other considerations that must not be overlooked when managing someone with severe TBI are:

- Control of blood sugar—Hyperglycemia is associated with a worse prognosis. We maintain the blood sugar tightly between 6 and 8 mmol/L.
- Nutrition—Proper nutrition should be instigated as soon as possible via a nasogastric tube (or an orogastric tube if there is clinical or radiologic evidence of a base of skull fracture). A regime should be devised in conjunction with the dietician and should be started with a gastric-protective agent. We consider early gastrostomy or jejunostomy if there is an anticipated delay in resumption of normal oral intake.
- Thromboembolic prophylaxis—Severe TBI has a systemic procoagulant effect, which together with long periods of immobility predisposes to thromboembolic events. All of our patients are fitted with graded thromboembolic deterrent stockings from the time of admission, and we begin prophylactic low-molecular-weight heparin (LMWH) as soon as we feel it is safe to do so.
- Cervical spine control—If a cervical spine injury is known or suspected, the patient must be log rolled. While sedated, we remove their hard collar to avoid compression of the great neck veins that might cause a rise in ICP, but we keep in place sandbags on either side of the head.
- Treatment of seizures—Seizures are either early (within 7 days of injury) or late (after 7 days). Seizure activity can cause secondary brain injury because of increased metabolic activity, hypoxia, and raised ICP and should be treated promptly. Evidence suggests prophylactic anticonvulsants do not improve outcome or reduce the risk of late seizures, and so are not routinely used. If seizures occur, we treat them with either carbamazepine (Tegretol) or sodium valproate (Depakote), and always consider a repeat CT scan. Late seizures should be treated in the same way as any other nontraumatic seizure.

SURGICAL TREATMENT OF TRAUMATIC BRAIN INJURY

Epidural Hematoma (Figure 3)

Epidural hematoma classically presents with a brief loss of consciousness followed by a lucid interval followed in turn by a delayed neurologic deterioration, although this is only true in up to one third of patients. Epidural hematomas typically do not occur in conjunction with significant primary brain injury, but can threaten major secondary brain injury as they rapidly enlarge. They must, therefore, be diagnosed and treated with all possible haste. These hematomas are nearly always associated with a fracture of the skull vault, usually disrupting the middle meningeal artery, but can also be caused by venous bleeding. Small hematomas in a patient with a GCS of 15 are often described as fracture hematomas and can be treated conservatively within a neurosurgical unit.

Evidence shows that outcome is significantly improved if definitive surgical intervention is commenced within 2 hours of a neurologic deterioration.

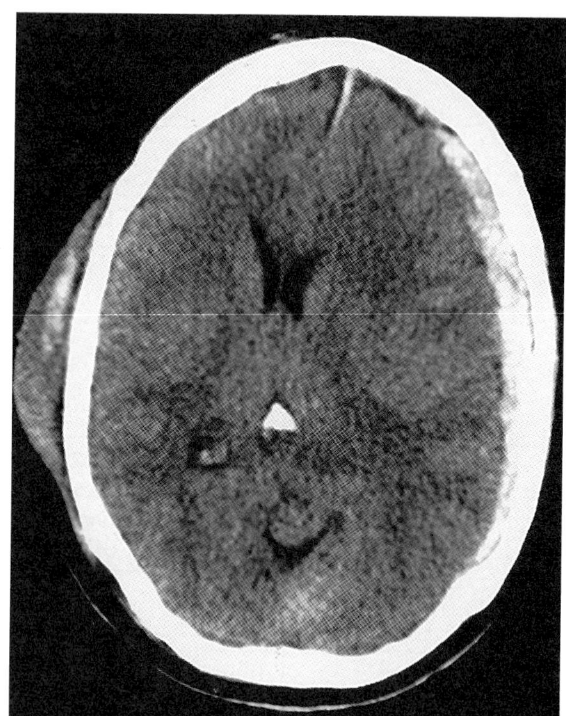

FIGURE 4 Computed tomography (CT) scan showing an acute subdural hematoma, the shape of which is in stark contrast to Figure 3. The midline shift is disproportionate to the thickness of the subdural, indicating generalized swelling of that hemisphere. Note that this is a contrecoup injury with the scalp swelling contralateral to the intracranial damage.

Acute Subdural Hematoma (Figure 4)

Up to one third of patients with severe TBI have an acute subdural hematoma. These are associated with a worse outcome than epidural hematomas as they are a consequence of a severe primary brain injury. They are usually caused by a tear on the cortical surface and associated with marked cerebral swelling and mass effect. The majority of patients with acute subdural hematomas present in coma (GCS ≤ 8). Outcome, although poor, improves if surgery occurs within 4 hours of injury.

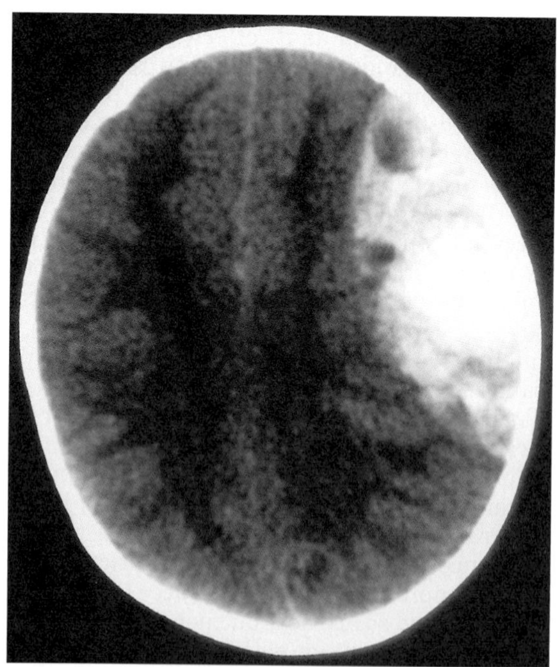

FIGURE 3 Computed tomography (CT) scan of a young adult with an epidural hematoma. The hematoma has the classical biconvex shape, and there is marked mass effect and midline shift.

Parenchymal Brain Injury (Figure 5)

Contusion injury is seen in up to one third of people with severe TBI and can be either single or multiple, as a result of a coup or contrecoup injury. They usually expand and swell over the first 72 hours after injury and may cause refractory rises in ICP, necessitating resective brain surgery.

Posterior Fossa Injury

This is relatively rare and, if present, is usually in the form of an epidural hematoma. As the posterior fossa is small, it does not tolerate mass lesions well, and the time frame for surgery is, therefore, significantly reduced.

Cerebral Spinal Fluid Diversion

As mentioned above, we have a low threshold for diversion of CSF if a scan shows any amount of ventricular dilatation in a patient with an ICP that is difficult to manage.

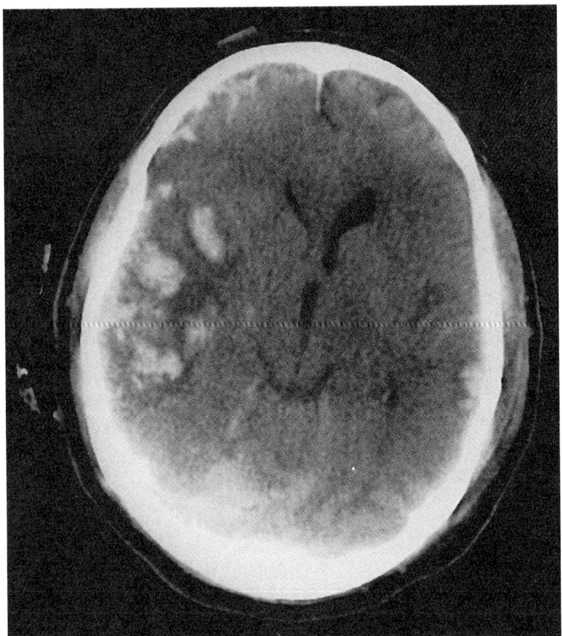

FIGURE 5 Computed tomography (CT) scan demonstrating contusion brain injury in the right temporal lobe. This is evidenced by the mixed density changes (part hemorrhagic and part low density) in this region. There are smaller contusions elsewhere, along with blood on the tentorium giving the veiled appearance posteriorly.

Depressed Skull Fractures

Any skull fracture is associated with a higher incidence of intracranial pathology, and patients should always be admitted for observation. Not all depressed skull fractures require surgery, with the principle indications being a heavily contaminated overlying wound, a significantly depressed fragment of bone, or poor cosmesis. We cover all open depressed skull fractures with prophylactic antibiotics.

Outcome

Head injury accounts for 1% of all deaths, but 20% of deaths between the ages of 5 and 45. Patients suffering mild brain injury can have organic problems such as poor attention, memory, and concentration as well as emotional distress. As many as 75% will have persistent headaches 3 months after their injury. All of these neuropsychologic symptoms can have a detrimental effect on the individual's relationships, social interactions, and ability to work.

Most studies looking at outcome after moderate and severe TBI use the Glasgow Outcome Scale, which was first described in 1975 and is shown in Table 5. Approximately 30% to 40% of patients can be described as having a good recovery or moderate disability at one year after injury. This scale has been criticized because of its subjectivity, and its assessment of final outcome at 1 year is potentially premature.

Factors that are associated with poor outcome are:

- GCS of 8 or less
- Pupillary changes, especially bilaterally unreactive pupils
- Age older than 65 years
- An episode of hypotension and/or hypoxia
- Traumatic subarachnoid blood

Although 90% of neurosurgically managed patients are independently mobile at 1 year, only 1 in 6 patients with severe TBI are back in their job at 5 years, often because of significant cognitive and behavioral deficits.

Mortality rates associated with severe TBI have been reduced over the last 30 years. This is a result of improved prehospital resuscitation, rapid transfers to local hospitals and neurosurgical units, increased availability of CT scanning and improved critical care management. The widespread use of ICP monitoring may have also played a role.

All of these major advances have largely come about from the simple principles of reducing the threat of secondary insults to an injured brain. Future advances will have to focus on how to modify the brain's response to injury, and further clarify what aspects of management do truly limit secondary brain injury. From such evidence-based data, more rigorous guidelines of TBI care can be developed nationally and internationally. Wide dissemination and implementation of these guidelines should then allow standardization of care, which in turn will facilitate conduction of further trials to continue refining practice.

TABLE 5 Glasgow Outcome Score

Score	Rating	Definition
5	Good recovery	Resumption of normal life despite minor deficits
4	Moderate disability	Disabled but independent, work in sheltered setting
3	Severe disability	Conscious but severely disabled, dependent for daily support
2	Persistent vegetative state	No conscious behavior
1	Death	

ACUTE HEAD INJURIES IN CHILDREN

METHOD OF
Chang-Yong Tsao, MD, and Warren Lo, MD

Moderate and Severe Acute Head Injury in Children

Head injuries of all types affect 100,000 to 200,000 children per year, with an incidence of 193 to 367 per 100,000 of children 0-19 years of age. Traumatic brain injury (TBI) is considered severe when the Glasgow Coma Score (GCS) (Table 1) is 8 or less, and moderate when the GCS is 9 to 12. Severe to moderate TBI accounts for 40% to 50% of all deaths in children. One peak incidence occurs in early childhood due to nonaccidenal TBI. Another peak incidence occurs in mid-to-late adolescence because of motor vehicle accidents, sports injuries, and assaults.

While acute TBI may be a penetrating injury, in 95% of children it is closed. Focal injuries including epidural, subdural, subarachnoid, and intracerebral hematomas occur less often in children (15% to 20%) than in adults (30% to 42%). Skull fracture can occur in 5% to 25% of children who suffer from focal TBI. Diffuse injury occurs in 44% of children with severe TBI, and may be complicated by cerebral edema and increased intracranial pressure. The primary pathologic feature of TBI is axonal injury, which is caused by rotational acceleration and deceleration. TBI may disrupt blood vessels, resulting in epidural, subdural, or subarachnoid hematomas. After acute TBI, hypotension, hypoxemia, and cerebral edema can cause secondary injuries that extend the initial damage. Loss of cerebral autoregulation and blood–brain barrier breakdown may contribute to cerebral edema and increased intracranial pressure, which produce further injury.

Evaluation and Treatment

Cervical spine immobilization should be maintained throughout the evaluation and stabilization of any child with head trauma. Minimizing secondary brain injury is essential. After acute TBI, many patients hypoventilate or become apneic; therefore, endotracheal intubation and ventilatory support may be necessary to prevent hypoxia and hypercarbia. Oxygenation should be optimized without reducing P_{CO_2} below 30 mm Hg, which decreases cerebral perfusion. Administration of isotonic fluids then blood products may be necessary to maintain normal blood pressure and cerebral perfusion. TBI usually does not cause hypotension so signs of shock should lead to an urgent search for another injury, usually in the abdomen. Inotropic or vasoactive drugs may be necessary to maintain cerebral perfusion when there is persistent hypotension despite appropriate fluid and blood product therapy.

Brain computed tomography (CT) imaging is necessary to detect significant subdural or epidural bleeding because emergency evacuation is life saving. Intracranial pressure monitoring is necessary when severe brain edema is suspected, and should be considered if the GCS is less than 8. If herniation is impending, hyperventilation to reduce the P_{CO_2} to 30% to 35% mm Hg is indicated. Once other injuries have been stabilized and the patient is adequately monitored, intermittent mannitol boluses (0.25 to 0.50 g/kg) may be needed to keep intracranial pressure under 15 to 20 mm Hg, to treat severe brain edema and prevent herniation. Barbiturate coma may be used to treat intractable intracranial hypertension. Some centers use systemic hypothermia to treat increased intracranial pressure, but the data are still preliminary.

When shaken baby syndrome is suspected (the classic CT finding is multiple subdurals of differing ages), ophthalmologic consultation to detect multiple retinal hemorrhages and skeletal radiograph survey for the detection and staging of fractures

TABLE 1 Glasgow Coma Scale for Children

Score	Eyes Open	Best Verbal Response in Adults	Best Verbal Response in Children <36 mo	Best Verbal Response in Infants and Preschoolers	Best Motor Response
6	—	—	—	—	Obeys commands
5	—	Oriented and converses	Smiles, interacts	Babbles/gestures	Localizes painful stimuli
4	Spontaneously	Disoriented and converses	Cries, interacts	Cries for needs	Flexion withdrawal
3	To verbal command	Inappropriate words	Consolable, moans	Cries, nonspecific	Flexion abnormal
2	To painful stimuli	Incomprehensible sounds	Irritable, restless	Sounds	Extension
1	No response	No response	No response	No response	No response

are indicated. A child abuse team, if available, should also be consulted.

Spinal cord injury should be ruled out in severe TBI patients. This is done with prompt cervical spine radiograph or CT imaging, and patients must be maintained in spinal immobilization in the acute setting. If visceral organ injuries are suspected, general surgeons or a surgical trauma service should be consulted. Although long-term treatment is beyond the scope of this review, rehabilitation with multiple disciplines—including physical, occupational, and speech/language therapy—and psychology should be started as soon as possible to optimize the extent of recovery.

Post-traumatic seizures may occur in three forms. Acute generalized tonic–clonic seizures can occur at the time of impact. Treatment with anticonvulsants requires judgment, for these acute seizures may not recur, and anticonvulsants are not always indicated acutely. Early post-traumatic seizures occur in the first week after TBI, and have an incidence of 4% to 25%. These are often generalized tonic–clonic seizures, but may be partial seizures. A load with intravenous 15 to 20 mg/kg phenytoin (Dilantin) followed by maintenance at 4 to 6 mg/kg/day can treat early post-traumatic seizures. Phenobarbital, diazepam (Valium), or lorazepam (Ativan)[1] may be needed if phenytoin fails to control these early post-traumatic seizures. Late post-traumatic seizures occur more than 1 week after TBI, with an incidence of 9% to 42%, and 68% of late post-traumatic seizures occur in the first 2 years after TBI. Approximately 1% to 2% of patients with closed TBI and 50% of patients with penetrating TBI will develop post-traumatic seizures. Approximately 25% of patients who experience early post-traumatic seizures develop epilepsy later, especially those with depressed skull fracture, intracranial hemorrhage, cerebral contusion, or gunshot wounds. Prophylactic treatment with anticonvulsants does not prevent the development of late post-traumatic seizures.

Outcome

Mortality and morbidity of TBI are affected by the mechanism and severity of TBI, secondary brain injury, other organ injury, and age. Only 20% of children with severe TBI achieve good neurologic outcome, and the majority have chronic problems including emotional, behavioral, speech, gait, hearing, visual difficulties, or seizures. Even children with *good* outcomes may have substantial functional morbidity. Children suffering from shaken baby syndrome frequently have diffuse and multiple injuries resulting in a 20% mortality. Of shaken baby survivors, 50% have sequelae, including impaired motor, cognitive, language, visual, and behavior problems. The mortality of adolescents with severe TBI caused by motor vehicle collisions ranges from 59% to 90% because of the effects of multiple traumas. School-aged children with focal and less severe head injury experience a lower mortality rate. Coma of less than 24 hours is rarely associated with permanent neurologic sequelae, but few of those who remain in coma more than 3 weeks have good neurologic function. Variable outcome is seen with coma lasting from 1 to 3 weeks.

Mild Traumatic Brain Injury

Mild TBI is more common than severe TBI. While there is no standard definition of mild TBI, most investigators define mild TBI as a GCS ranging from 13 to 15, together with a normal neurologic exam. In some studies subjects have been included who have a loss of consciousness lasting 60 minutes or less, or post-traumatic amnesia lasting 24 hours or less. Given these parameters, the incidence of TBI affecting all ages, and managed with outpatient care, ranges from 390 to 540 per 100,000 cases.

EVALUATION

CT brain scan is the preferred method to detect intracranial lesions, because CT is sufficiently sensitive and is more available than magnetic resonance imaging (MRI). Of note, MRI can detect structural lesions even when the CT scan is normal, although these lesions do not require intervention. While skull radiographs are excellent for detecting fractures, they cannot detect intracranial lesions, and are of less use when a CT scan is available. There are no large prospective studies of children with mild TBI that answer which child should undergo a CT scan. In one study of 5000 children and adults, no patient with a GCS of 15 and no loss of consciousness had an intracranial lesion that required surgical intervention. In two large studies of children with mild TBI and a GCS of 15, one study found 5% of the patients had intracranial lesions. The other study found 16% of the patients had an intracranial lesion even though there was no loss of consciousness, and 2% of the patients required neurosurgical or medical intervention. If the patient had a brief loss of consciousness or amnesia (<60 minutes), the risk of an intracranial lesion ranged between 0% to 7%, but the risk of an intracranial lesion requiring neurosurgical intervention remained less than 1%. A GCS of 13 or 14 increases the risk of a significant intracranial lesion. In one study of 209 children with GCS scores of 13 to 14, 27% had intracranial lesions, and 2.5% required neurosurgical intervention. Based upon these data, one may recommend the following evaluation of mild TBI. A child who has a GCS of 15, a normal neurologic exam, and no history of amnesia or loss of consciousness is unlikely to have an intracranial lesion that requires intervention, and likely can be observed conservatively with careful follow-up. In the special case of a child who is 2 years

[1]Not FDA approved for this indication.

of age or less who has suffered a skull fracture, a CT brain scan should be performed to look for intracranial lesions even if the exam is normal. When there is a definite history of loss of consciousness or amnesia, a CT scan should be considered. If an intracranial lesion is detected, the child will need closer observation, more likely in an inpatient setting, even though the need for intervention may be low. If the GCS is 13 to 14, or if the neurologic exam is abnormal, then a CT scan should be performed and the patient should be closely observed, most likely as an inpatient, for clinical deterioration.

MANAGEMENT

If an intracranial lesion is identified, monitoring for a deteriorating level of consciousness and other signs of increased intracranial pressure is warranted. If this occurs, then the child should be managed as described above. Neurosurgical consultation is important when an intracranial lesion is identified; however, not all lesions require surgical treatment, and some may be managed medically.

Acute seizures occurring after TBI often imply a severe or moderate injury, but seizures can occur immediately after mild TBI. If a child has a brief, single seizure after TBI, a CT scan is indicated. If the scan is normal, if the child has a normal neurologic exam, and if the child has returned to normal, it may not be necessary to treat with an antiepileptic medication because the risk of seizure recurrence is low. If there is a reliable caregiver, the child may be observed at home instead of being admitted to an inpatient unit.

OUTCOME

After mild TBI, children may complain of headaches, dizziness, and fatigue, but these symptoms typically subside by 3 months, although exceptions occur. The risk of chronic sequelae following mild TBI appears to be low. The incidence of chronic headache following mild TBI is unknown, and reports of chronic post-traumatic headaches after mild TBI tend to be small, retrospective, and uncontrolled. There is considerable controversy regarding the cognitive and behavioral outcomes of mild TBI. Behavior problems and cognitive impairment in children with mild TBI tend to be small, retrospective, and uncontrolled. There is considerable controversy regarding the congnitive and behavioral outcomes of mild TBI. Behavior problems and cognitive impairment in children with mild TBI tend to be associated with pre-existing learning problems, pre-existing neurologic or psychiatric disorders, family stressors, or socioeconomic disadvantages, but may also reflect the result of a brain injury. Management by establishing the premorbid baseline and educating the caregivers about the outcome and course of mild TBI can reduce long term concerns.

BRAIN TUMORS

METHOD OF

Ashwatha Narayana, MD

Primary brain tumors accounted for an estimated incidence of 18,000 diagnosed new cases and 13,500 deaths in the year 2002 in the United States. Several histopathologically different tumors arise in the brain, reflecting the diversity of phenotypically distinct cells within the central nervous system (CNS) that have a capacity for neoplastic transformation. Gliomas, the most common tumors, are considered first in this article. Many of the principles of brain tumor management are discussed here. Less common tumors are also briefly presented. The article closes with a discussion on the management of metastatic brain tumors.

Gliomas

INCIDENCE

Malignant gliomas make up 35% to 45% of primary brain tumors, and of these, nearly 85% are glioblastoma multiforme. The incidence of anaplastic astrocytoma peaks in children younger than 10 years of age and then remains constant in each subsequent decade of life. In contrast, the incidence of glioblastoma multiforme increases dramatically after the age of 40 years. Low-grade astrocytomas make up 5% to 15% of primary brain tumors and 67% of low-grade gliomas, the remainder of low-grade gliomas being mixed oligoastrocytomas (19%) and oligodendrogliomas (13%). Unlike their malignant counterparts, low-grade gliomas are most common between the ages of 20 and 40 years and rarely occur after the age of 50 years.

GENETICS AND ETIOLOGY

Genetic abnormalities have been demonstrated for 50% to 75% of adult astrocytomas. It is hypothesized that a *p53* gene mutation is associated with the transition to grade II tumors. Malignant progression to anaplastic astrocytoma is associated with loss of heterozygosity (LOH) for chromosomes 9p, 13q, or 19q, and *CDK4* gene amplification. Subsequent LOH on chromosome 10 and amplification of the epidermal growth factor receptor genes characterize further progression to glioblastoma multiforme. A second, *p53*-independent pathway that leads more directly to glioblastoma multiforme development has also been documented.

Losses of genetic information from chromosomes 1p and 19q are commonly seen in oligodendroglioma specimens, whereas losses on 17p and *p53* gene mutations are notably less frequent, suggesting that early events in their oncogenesis are distinct from those associated with astrocytic tumors.

Although some environmental factors have been linked with brain tumor development, they do not appear to be responsible for most brain tumors. Radiation-induced gliomas have been reported, mainly in children with acute leukemia who received prophylactic cranial irradiation and chemotherapy. The hereditary syndromes that are associated with an increased risk of brain tumors are neurofibromatosis-1, neurofibromatosis-2, tuberous sclerosis, Li-Fraumeni syndrome, familial polyposis, Turcot's syndrome, Gardner's syndrome, and von Hippel-Lindau disease.

Pathology

Central nervous system tumors are generally classified as follows (Table 1):

- Gliomas
- Neuronal/glioneuronal neoplasms
- Embryonal neoplasms
- Meningeal neoplasms
- Miscellaneous nonglial neoplasms

Reliance on a pathologic classification of brain tumors is a requisite for treatment. Indeed, histopathology is

TABLE 1 Histopathology of Brain Tumors

Major Classification	Variants	WHO Grades
Glioma:		
Astrocytic, circumscribed	Pilocytic astrocytoma	I
	Subependymal giant cell astrocytoma (SEGA)	I
	Pleomorphic xanthoastrocytoma (PXA)	II
Astrocytic, diffuse	Astrocytoma	II
	Anaplastic astrocytoma	III
	Glioblastoma multiforme	IV
Oligodendroglial	Oligodendroglioma	II
	Anaplastic oligodendroglioma	III
Mixed gliomas	Oligoastrocytoma	II
	Anaplastic oligoastrocytoma	III
Ependymal	Subependymoma	I
	Myxopapillary ependymoma	I
	Ependymoma	II
	Anaplastic ependymoma*	III
Choroid plexus	Choroid plexus papilloma	I
	Choroid plexus carcinoma*	III
Cranial and peripheral nerve tumors	Schwannoma	I
Neuronal and glioneuronal tumors	Gangliocytoma/ganglioglioma	I–III
	Desmoplastic infantile ganglioglioma (DIG)	I
	Dysplastic cerebellar gangliocytoma	I
	Central neurocytoma	I
	Dysembryoplastic neuroepithelial tumor	I
	Paraganglioma	I
Pineal parenchymal tumors (PPT)	Pineocytoma	II
	PPT with intermediate differentiation	III
	Pineoblastoma	IV
Embryonal tumors	Medulloepithelioma*	IV
	Primitive neuroectodermal tumor (PNET)*, including medulloblastoma and variants*	IV
	Atypical teratoid/rhabdoid tumor (AT/RT)	IV
	Cerebral neuroblastoma/ganglioneuroblastoma	IV
	Ependymoblastoma*	IV
	Olfactory neuroblastoma (esthesioneuroblastoma)	IV
Meningeal tumors	Meningioma	I
	Atypical meningioma	II
	Anaplastic (malignant) meningioma	III
Germ cell tumors	Hemangiopericytoma†	II–III
	Germinoma	NA
	Mature teratoma	NA
	Nongerminomatous germ cell tumors	NA
Tumors of the sellar region	Craniopharyngioma, adamantinomatous	I
	Craniopharyngioma, papillary	I
Hemopoietic neoplasms	Primary CNS lymphoma (PCNSL)	NA
	Secondary lymphoma/leukemia	NA
	Histiocytic tumors and histiocytoses	NA
Secondary tumors/metastases	Carcinomas and sarcomas	NA

*Indicates tumors with a tendency to disseminate throughout the central nervous system.
†Origin of hemangiopericytoma is uncertain.
Abbreviations: NA = not applicable; WHO = World Health Organization.

more important than anatomic staging in determining the clinical behavior and prognosis of these tumors. Neuropathologists do not uniformly agree on a uniform classification system for astrocytic gliomas. The World Health Organization system is the one used most often, and it divides astrocytic tumors into four grades, from grade I, corresponding to pilocytic astrocytomas, to grade IV, corresponding to the glioblastoma multiforme.

Low-grade astrocytomas are well-differentiated tumors that display increased cellularity compared with normal brain tissue and have mild to moderate nuclear pleomorphism (Figure 1). The cytoplasmic processes that extend from the astrocytes contain a characteristic filamentous protein, glial fibrillary acidic protein (GFAP), which provides an immunohistochemical marker for these tumors. Over time, at least 50% of these tumors transform into more anaplastic lesions. The characteristic histopathologic features of anaplastic astrocytomas include moderate hypercellularity, moderate cellular and nuclear pleomorphism, variable mitotic activity, and microvascular proliferation. The presence of tumor necrosis is the hallmark that distinguishes anaplastic astrocytoma from glioblastoma multiforme (Figure 2).

Oligodendrogliomas, on the other hand, are composed of small, uniform cells with round central nuclei and distinct cytoplasmic borders. Formalin fixation causes a perinuclear halo that produces a *fried egg* or *honeycomb* appearance. The cells lack fibrillary cytoplasmic processes. Calcification is a frequent feature.

Clinical Presentation

The presenting symptoms and signs of brain tumors include those associated with a mass effect and increased intracranial pressure, and those that are focal. The most common presenting symptom with gliomas is headache. Approximately 33% of adult patients with low-grade astrocytomas and 20% of patients with malignant tumors present with seizures, but are otherwise neurologically intact. Others exhibit a slowly progressive neurologic syndrome consisting of headache, vomiting, motor deficit, visual or sensory loss, language disturbance, or personality change. Symptoms may be present for months or years before a diagnosis is made.

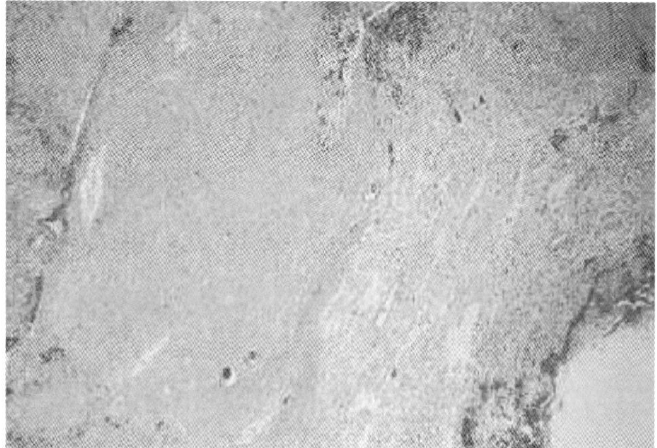

FIGURE 1 Low-grade astrocytoma showing mildly increased cellularity with uniform cells and nuclei.

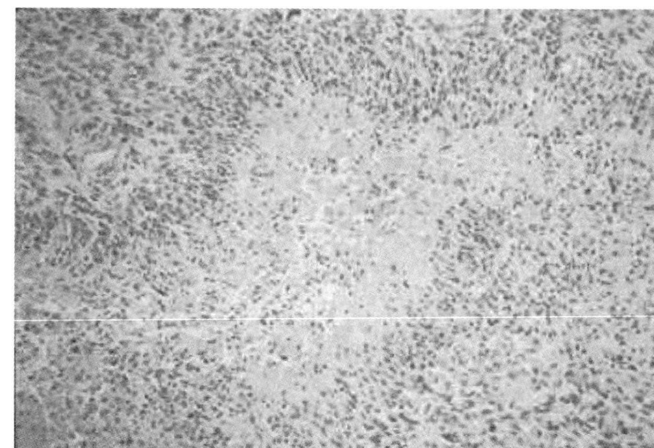

FIGURE 2 Glioblastoma multiforme with the hallmark features of necrosis with peripheral pseudopalisading of neoplastic nuclei.

Routes of Spread

The most common route of spread for gliomas is through local extension. As they enlarge, malignant gliomas extend directly into adjacent lobes and disseminate along anatomically defined nerve fiber pathways. Multicentric gliomas are found in less than 5% of patients. Dissemination by seeding through the cerebrospinal fluid (CSF) pathways occurs in approximately 10% of cases but is usually a late event. Metastases rarely arise outside the CNS.

Diagnostic Studies

Computed tomography (CT) and magnetic resonance imaging (MRI) play an indispensable role in the management of brain tumors. CT is a reliable screening and diagnostic method for suspected supratentorial brain tumor lesions. MRI is now more frequently used in patients with malignant brain tumors, and has become the screening procedure of choice for diagnosing and localizing tumors in the brain stem, posterior fossa, and spinal cord. Ordinary astrocytomas appear as diffuse, poorly defined, low-density, nonenhancing lesions (Figure 3). Approximately 40% of ordinary astrocytomas enhance, and calcification is found in 10% of cases. While the majority of malignant gliomas enhance with contrast media, as many as 30% of anaplastic astrocytomas present as nonenhancing lesions (Figure 4). In both low-grade and malignant gliomas, parenchymal infiltration by isolated tumor cells may be present in regions of T_2-weighted abnormality that appear normal on CT.

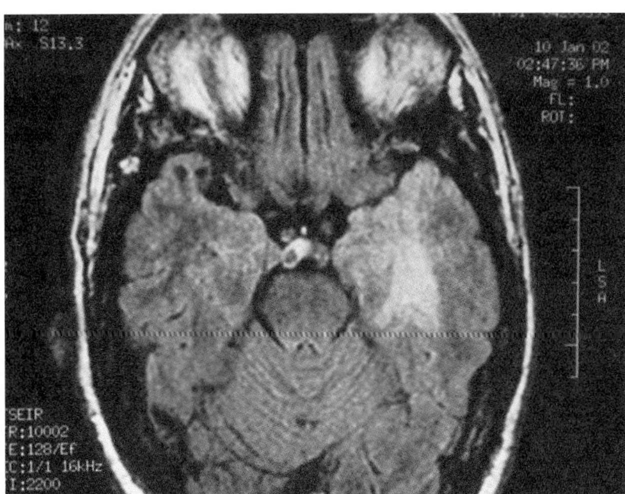

FIGURE 3 Axial MRI of low-grade astrocytoma of left temporal lobe.

Positron emission tomography (PET), single photon emission computed tomography (SPECT) with thallium-201 (^{201}Tl), and magnetic resonance spectroscopy (MRS) are other imaging approaches used in brain tumor management.

Staging

There is no accepted staging system for primary brain tumors. The American Joint Committee on Cancer had proposed a staging scheme for primary brain tumors based on tumor size, metastases, and tumor grade; however, the system was not generally adapted to clinical use, and was subsequently discontinued.

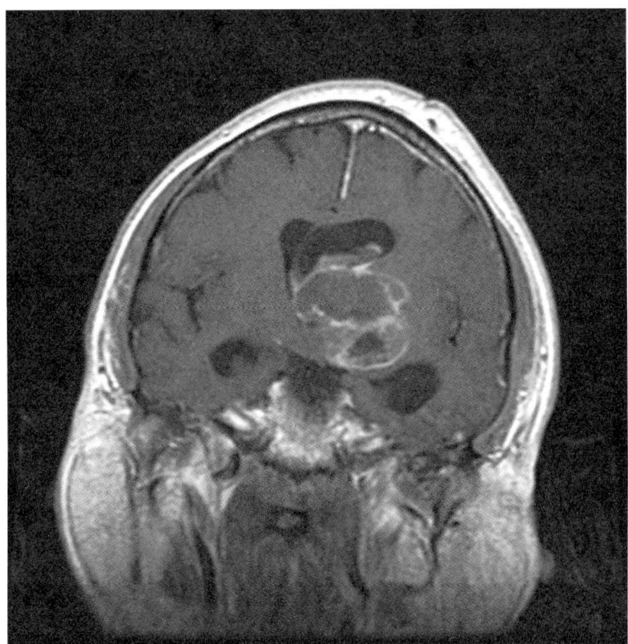

FIGURE 4 Coronal MRI of high-grade astrocytoma of left internal capsule and brainstem region.

Prognostic Factors

Age, histologic appearance, Karnofsky performance status (KPS), mental status, duration of symptoms, neurologic functional class, extent of surgery, and radiation dose are significant partitioning covariates in clinical trials. This information is important for interpreting correctly the results of studies comparing different treatment regimens and for assessing the potential of new therapeutic methodologies.

STANDARD THERAPEUTIC APPROACHES FOR GLIOMAS

Surgery

The combination of surgery, radiation therapy, and chemotherapy represents the standard approach to the treatment of gliomas. The goals of surgery are to provide a histologic diagnosis, to alleviate intracranial hypertension and focal neurologic deficits caused by a mass effect, and to permit rapid corticosteroid dose tapering. Pilocytic astrocytomas are relatively well circumscribed, and 60% to 80% are amenable to total removal. Resection of the more common diffuse astrocytomas is limited by the lack of clear demarcation between the infiltrating tumor and normal brain tissue. There is evidence that suggests that patients with more complete resections live longer and have an improved functional status compared with those who undergo a biopsy or partial resection only. Advances in neurosurgery, including diagnostic ultrasound, lasers, ultrasonic tissue aspirators, cortical mapping, functional imaging, and computer-assisted stereotactic laser techniques, have improved the ability of neurosurgeons to remove intracranial tumors radically.

Radiation Therapy

Limited radiation fields are used for the treatment of gliomas. Three-dimensionally designed complex treatment plans with multiple fields are used whenever appropriate to limit the high-dose volume and to minimize the risk of long-term radiation sequelae. Doses of 50.4 to 54 Gy are usually recommended for low-grade gliomas and 59.4 to 60 Gy for high-grade gliomas. Rapid fractionation schemes (such as 30 to 36 Gy) may be appropriate for some elderly or poor-performance-status patients with glioblastoma multiforme who have relatively short survival expectancies.

In low-grade gliomas, the role of radiation therapy is being debated. Although it has been shown to improve disease-free survival, overall survival is not altered indicating that deferring postoperative therapy is an option for a select group of patients. There is also evidence suggesting that lower doses of radiation therapy are probably as effective as higher doses of radiation for low-grade gliomas.

Randomized trials provide seminal evidence that external beam irradiation favorably affects the outcome of malignant gliomas. These trials demonstrate both a significant survival advantage and the ability to maintain a full or partial working capacity for irradiated patients.

Chemotherapy

Chemotherapy has little established role in adult low-grade astrocytomas. However, adjuvant chemotherapy is part of the standard therapeutic regimen for malignant gliomas. The addition of chemotherapy to radiation therapy improves 1-year survival by 10% and 2-year survival by 8.6%. The nitrosoureas, especially carmustine (BCNU) are the most active single agents. No benefit of chemotherapeutical agents such as tirapazamine (Triazone)*, topotecan (Hycamtin)[1], paclitaxel (Taxol)[1], β-interferon (β-IFN)[1], and thalidomide (Thalomid)[1] was noted when used with standard radiation in clinical trials. Temozolomide (Temodar)[1] is an alkylating agent that has shown some promise in gliomas. Anaplastic oligodendrogliomas are chemosensitive tumors. PCV chemotherapy regimen has produced response rates of 50% to 75% in both recurrent and newly diagnosed anaplastic oligodendrogliomas.

Some of the newer biologic agents being presently explored in gliomas include tyrosine kinase inhibitors, matrix metalloproteinase inhibitors and antitenascin antibodies.

Outcome

The 5-year recurrence-free survival rates of patients with low-grade astrocytomas or mixed oligoastrocytomas who undergo total or radical subtotal tumor resection range from 52% to 95%. The median survival times for high-grade gliomas using conventional radiation therapy alone or with chemotherapy consistently range from 9 to 14 months. The median survival for patients with glioblastoma multiforme is 10 to 12 months, and the 3-year survival rate is only 6% to 8%. The median survival for patients with anaplastic astrocytoma is 36 months, and the 3-year survival rate is approximately 50%.

Uncommon Primary Brain Tumors

PRIMARY CENTRAL NERVOUS SYSTEM LYMPHOMA

Primary CNS lymphomas (PCNSLs) represent approximately 2% to 5% of all intracranial neoplasms. During the last 2 decades, the incidence is increasing in both the AIDS and immunocompetent general populations. PCNSLs most frequently arise in the supratentorial paraventricular region of the brain. Multifocal tumors are present at diagnosis in 25% to 50% of immunocompetent patients and in 60% to 80% of AIDS patients. Cytologic examination of cerebrospinal fluid reveals malignant cells in up to 66.6% of immunocompetent patients and in nearly all AIDS patients. The neoplastic cells are similar to those of non-Hodgkin's lymphoma, arising in extranodal sites. Single or multiple uniformly contrast-enhancing lesions in the paraventricular regions, basal ganglia, thalamus, or corpus callosum on MRI are characteristic findings.

The role of surgery is to establish a tissue diagnosis only. Primary CNS lymphomas respond dramatically to corticosteroid therapy. At least 90% of patients improve clinically, whereas 40% of lesions shrink considerably. Whole-brain irradiation with corticosteroids has been the standard treatment for PCNSL. Recommended doses range from 36 to 45 Gy. Several reports document improved survival when chemotherapy is added to radiation therapy. The outcome is better with high-dose methotrexate-based regimens, often combined with intrathecal chemotherapy.

Survival times for primary CNS lymphoma with no treatment or steroids alone are approximately 1 to 4 months. The median survival for radiotherapy alone varies from 12 to 20 months. Median survival times for treatment programs that include high-dose methotrexate-based chemotherapy range from 33 to 42 months.

EPENDYMOMA

Ependymomas represent approximately 5% of all intracranial gliomas. The incidence peaks at 5 years and again at 34 years of age. Of these, 60% to 70% of ependymomas arise in the infratentorial brain. Ependymomas are separated into low-grade and high-grade lesions. The 5-year survival for low-grade tumors ranges from 60% to 80%, whereas it varies from 10% to 47% for high-grade tumors. Supratentorial ependymomas generally have a poorer prognosis than their infratentorial counterparts.

Most ependymomas cannot be completely excised because of their location and growth characteristics. Postoperative irradiation improves local tumor control and survival and is an accepted part of the standard treatment for these tumors. Although most ependymomas are slow-growing, others are more aggressive and may disseminate throughout the cerebrospinal fluid pathways. Current therapy for high-grade ependymomas after surgical debulking is with local fields to a dose of 59.4 Gy. The value of chemotherapy in adults with ependymomas and anaplastic ependymomas is not well defined.

BRAIN STEM GLIOMA

Brain stem gliomas account for less than 2% of brain tumors. Children constitute approximately

*Investigational drug in the United States.
[1]Not FDA approved for this indication.

66.6% of the cases that are reported. Diagnostic imaging is sufficient for the majority of the cases. The role of surgery is minimal and is limited to biopsy only if there are questions about the diagnosis. Radiation therapy alone by conventional fractionation to 54 Gy in symptomatic or large brain stem lesions is recommended. Chemotherapy has not shown any benefit in the management of brain stem gliomas. The median survival time for brain stem glioma is 9 to 12 months.

MEDULLOBLASTOMA

Medulloblastoma accounts for 33.3% of pediatric brain tumors and is the most common tumor arising in the posterior fossa in children. It arises from the roof of the fourth ventricle or from the vermis. The presenting symptoms include headache, vomiting, and imbalance. On microscopic examination, small blue undifferentiated cells are noted, which are consistent with primitive neuroectodermal tumors. CSF involvement is noted in 25% to 40% of the patients. Five-year survival rates range from 50% to 80%, and 10-year rates vary from 40% to 55%.

Surgery involves maximal resection of the tumor. Radiation therapy to the entire craniospinal axis is essential. The dose to the craniospinal axis is 23.4 to 36 Gy. A boost of 18 to 31.4 Gy is given to the posterior fossa to bring the total to 54 Gy. The role of chemotherapy is to decrease the craniospinal radiation dose and to improve the survival in poor-risk patients. Combinations of vincristine (Oncovin), lomustine (CCNU) and cisplatin (Platinol)[1] have been used.

Brain Metastases

EPIDEMIOLOGY

Metastases to the brain occur in as many as 30% of patients with systemic cancer and represent the most common type of intracranial tumor. Brain metastases exert a profound effect on the quality and length of survival, and, despite the best current management, they represent the direct cause of death in 25% to 30% of affected patients. Melanoma and carcinomas of the lung, breast, and colorectum have a higher propensity to metastasize to the brain. Approximately 50% of patients present with a solitary lesion. Most brain metastases, particularly those that arise from primary sites other than the lung, occur at a late stage when metastatic dissemination is present elsewhere in the body.

STANDARD TREATMENT APPROACHES

Because the majority of patients with metastatic brain lesions have or will soon develop widely disseminated disease, treatment is dictated by the need to achieve immediate short-term palliation and the desire for durable symptom-free remission. The median survival of patients with symptomatic brain metastases is approximately 1 month without treatment and 2 months with corticosteroid administration. Survival is longer and the quality of life better if brain metastases are treated.

Corticosteroids

Corticosteroids rapidly ameliorate many symptoms of brain metastasis and should be used at the onset for all symptomatic patients. Symptomatic but stable patients can begin with approximately 16 mg of dexamethasone (Decadron) daily in two to four divided doses. Patients who are receiving whole-brain irradiation should receive steroids for at least 48 hours before treatment. Steroid tapering may begin during week 2 of radiotherapy. For patients receiving 16 mg of dexamethasone, the drug should be tapered by 2 to 4 mg every fifth day.

Surgery

Surgery is used to establish the diagnosis of metastatic brain disease when it is uncertain and as a treatment for single metastases. Surgery can provide better local control and immediate relief of neurologic signs and symptoms caused by a mass effect. Surgically treated patients also live longer, have fewer recurrences of cancer in the brain, and enjoy a better quality of life compared with those treated by radiotherapy alone. However, only 10% of patients are ideal candidates for surgical extirpation.

Whole-Brain Radiation Therapy

Radiotherapy is the appropriate treatment for most patients with brain metastases, including those with multiple lesions and those with single metastases who are not candidates for surgery. The standard approach is to treat the whole brain to 30 Gy in 10 daily fractions over 2 weeks. Depending on the symptom, the response rate varies from 70% to 90%. Overall, neurologic function is improved in 50% of patients. The median survival with radiation therapy is 4 to 6 months. Overall, 75% to 80% of remaining life is spent in an improved or stable neurologic state.

Stereotactic Radiosurgery

Stereotactic radiosurgery (SRS) is an excellent alternative to surgical extirpation of solitary and multiple brain metastases. The procedure involves the delivery of a single large dose of radiation to a small volume of region in the brain under stereotactic frame guidance. The available data from the largest SRS series show a local control of approximately 90%

[1]Not FDA approved for this indication.

and a median survival of 9 months. These survival results are comparable to those observed for surgical resection.

Chemotherapy

Chemotherapy can be considered in selected patients who progress locally after whole-brain irradiation. Systemic chemotherapy has a response rate of 25% to 50%. Recently, temozolomide (Temodar)[1] is promising both as an adjuvant to whole-brain radiation therapy and in patients who have failed radiation therapy.

[1]Not FDA approved for this indication.

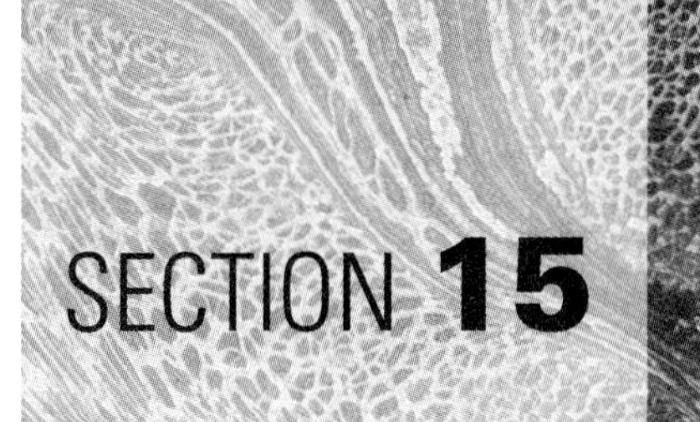

The Locomotor System

RHEUMATOID ARTHRITIS

METHOD OF

G. Andres Quiceno, MD, and John J. Cush, MD

Rheumatoid arthritis (RA) is a chronic, progressive, systemic inflammatory disease in which the synovial joints are the primary targets. The prevalence of RA is very consistent around the world, affecting about 1% of the population. Women are affected three times more often than men. The age of distribution is unimodal, with a peak incidence during the fourth and fifth decades of life. The classic presentation of RA is a symmetric polyarthritis, most commonly involving the small joints of the hands and feet. Often the arthritis is accompanied by systemic symptoms characterized by fatigue, low-grade fever, anemia, serositis, and systemic vasculitis.

The etiology of this malady is unknown, but it is presumed that RA is secondary to a persistent immunologic response to an unknown antigen. There is a genetic predisposition for the development of RA. First-degree relatives develop RA at a frequency that is four times the rate in the general population. RA is associated with certain alleles of the class II major histocompatibility complex (MHC). HLA-DR4 and HLA-DR1 are associated with more severe disease in people with RA. Patients with these shared epitopes have a higher risk of persistent, erosive disease.

RA increases mortality. Life expectancy is shortened by 7 years in males and 3 years in females. The cause of death often results as a consequence of infection, heart disease, respiratory failure, renal failure, or gastrointestinal disease. Because RA is a chronic disease, it has an important socioeconomic impact. Disability rates in the United States and Europe range from 22% to 85% and 31% to 80%, respectively.

Because of the long-term effects of RA and the negative impact on quality of life, early diagnosis and prompt treatment are important. The primary goals of treatment are the alleviation of pain, reduction of inflammation, preservation of muscle strength and joint function, prevention of joint damage, and preservation of normal activities.

Treatment of RA

Historically, RA has been managed with symptomatic therapies, such as analgesics, nonsteroidal anti-inflammatory drugs (NSAIDs), and, when necessary, the use of disease modifying antirheumatic drugs (DMARDs). This approach is based on studies from the 1950s and 1960s that underestimated the long-term complications of RA. However, cohort studies done in the 1980s emphasized the severity of the complications from RA and proved that these approaches to treatment had no effect on the long-term outcome and complications of the disease. The data obtained from Early Arthritis Clinic studies showed that early, aggressive treatment improves the long-term prognosis of patients with RA.

The advent of new therapies, their early use, and the focus on early diagnosis and treatment have led to a remodeling of the traditional treatment pyramid. In the last decade, the recommended treatment has changed significantly after the realization that early diagnosis and treatment were critical in the short and long-term. New DMARDs, such as leflunomide, tumor necrosis factor (TNF) inhibitors, and an interleukin-1 receptor antagonist, were recently introduced.

NONSTEROIDAL ANTI-INFLAMMATORY DRUGS

NSAIDs reduce the signs and symptoms of inflammation. They effectively and rapidly control the symptoms of RA, but they do not prevent future complications of RA. These medications selectively inhibit cyclooxygenase and suppress the synthesis of prostaglandins from arachidonic acid. Prostaglandins are proinflammatory lipids that, in some tissues, have homeostatic and cytoprotective functions. In the kidney, prostaglandins regulate blood flow at the glomerular level. They are key players in platelet aggregation and have a cytoprotective function in the gastric mucosa.

The cyclooxygenase 1 (COX-1) isoenzyme is present in platelets, vascular endothelial cells, and stomach and kidney collecting tubule cells, and produces the prostaglandins that protect the gastric mucosa from gastric acids. The proinflammatory effects are regulated by the induction of cyclooxygenase 2 (COX-2), while the gastrointestinal adverse effects are associated with the inhibition of COX-1.

NSAIDs are still very important in the treatment of arthritic and inflammatory conditions and are among the most prescribed medications around the world. However, they are associated with significant gastrointestinal (GI) toxicities. Approximately 40% of the patients who chronically use NSAIDs will develop asymptomatic ulcers. Serious complications, such as hemorrhage, perforation, and death, are less common, but the incidence is approximately 1.5% per year.

Several strategies can be employed to reduce the risk of these GI complications from NSAIDs. Misoprostol (Cytotec), at doses of 400 μg to 800 μg, reduces the risk of ulcers. At higher doses (800 μg), there is a statistically significant decrease in the incidence of gastric ulcers, as compared to lower doses. More side effects, such as diarrhea, nausea, and abdominal pain, are seen with the higher doses. H_2-receptor antagonists have also been studied. At standard doses, they do not offer GI protection, but at double the standard dose, they decrease the relative risk of gastric ulcers by 56%.

Proton pump inhibitors (PPIs) significantly reduce the risk of duodenal ulcers (relative risk [RR] = 0.19; 95% confidence interval [CI]: 0.09 to 0.37) and gastric ulcers (RR = 0.40; 95% CI: 0.32 to 0.51), as compared to placebo. Misoprostol (Cytotec), high doses of H_2-receptor antagonists, and PPIs should be employed to protect patients at high risk for GI toxicity from NSAIDs. Patients older than age 65 years and those with concomitant medical problems or with a previous history of GI bleeding are at highest risk.

With the discovery of the COX-2 enzyme and further use of COX-2 inhibitors, such as celecoxib (Celebrex), rofecoxib (Vioxx), and valdecoxib (Bextra), this class of medications is one of the most commonly prescribed for RA. Randomized, controlled trials show that celecoxib reduces the symptoms of RA to a similar degree as that of traditional NSAIDs, such as naproxen (Naprosyn), diclofenac (Voltaren), and ibuprofen (Motrin). When compared with placebo, 51% of the patients who received celecoxib, at a dose of 200 mg by mouth twice daily, obtained an improvement by ACR (American College of Rheumatology) 20 criteria. The ACR 20 criteria response represents a 20% improvement in the number of swollen and tender joints, plus a 20% improvement in 3 of 5 of the following core measures: patient and physician global assessments, pain, functional status, and an acute-phase reactant measurement. ACR 50 and 70 represent, respectively, a 50% and 70% improvement in the same parameters.

There were fewer GI adverse events, defined as gastric and duodenal perforation, gastric outlet obstruction, or upper GI bleeding, in the celecoxib (Celebrex) group (32 of 3987 patients), as compared with the combined group of ibuprofen (Motrin) and diclofenac (Voltaren) (51 of 3981 patients) at 26 weeks. When the data at 12 months were reviewed, the event rates for GI adverse effects were not significantly different between the diclofenac (Voltaren), ibuprofen (Motrin), and celecoxib (Celebrex) groups. A partial explanation for these findings is that the patients with a cardiovascular indication for aspirin use were allowed to continue on it.

In general, celecoxib (Celebrex) is equivalent, but not superior, to naproxen (Naprosyn), diclofenac (Voltaren), and ibuprofen (Motrin) in the treatment of RA. At 6 months, the CLASS (Celecoxib Long-Term Arthritis Safety Study) studies suggested that there is less GI toxicity with celecoxib (Celebrex), but these benefits were not evident at 12 months. All these factors should be considered when making decisions about therapy because of the significant difference in cost between the traditional NSAIDs and COX-2 inhibitors.

The VIGOR (Vioxx Gastrointestinal Outcomes Research) study showed that rofecoxib (Vioxx) dosed at 50 mg a day improved patients' global assessments of disease activity and the patients reported similar functioning (Health Assessment Questionnaire [HAQ] score), as compared with naproxen (Naprosyn), but these differences were not statistically significant. Rofecoxib (Vioxx) showed a relative risk reduction of 54% for gastric perforations, GI obstructions, and GI bleeding, as compared with naproxen (Naprosyn) 1 g per day. For patients at low risk for GI bleeding, the difference between both treatments for GI adverse events was not statistically significant. However, patients taking rofecoxib (Vioxx) had a higher incidence of serious thrombotic cardiovascular events, and post-hoc analysis of the data revealed that these patients had indications for aspirin prophylaxis but aspirin use was excluded in the trial. The results of the CLASS study suggest that the benefit of reduced GI toxicity seen with coxibs may be diminished when aspirin is co-prescribed.

The newest medication in the group of the COX-2 inhibitors is valdecoxib (Bextra). In a randomized, double-blind, placebo-controlled trial, single daily doses of valdecoxib at 10, 20, and 40 mg a day demonstrated an efficacy superior to placebo and similar to naproxen (Naprosyn).

DISEASE-MODIFYING ANTIRHEUMATIC DRUGS AND COMBINATION THERAPY

The modern approach to RA differs from the previous concept of gradualism. The current goal is to suppress inflammation as soon as the diagnosis of RA is confirmed and to continue to quell disease activity in the long term. This approach is supported by the American College of Rheumatology. The current DMARDs have a low risk of complications when the recommended monitoring is followed. Early control of the disease seems to improve the long-term prognosis, decreases mortality, and, as was shown with methotrexate, will decrease the rate of disability. Medications that show evidence of decreased radiographic joint disease progression include methotrexate (Rheumatrex), leflunomide (Arava), sulfasalazine (Azulfidine), etanercept (Enbrel), infliximab (Remicade), adalimumab (Humira), and anakinra (Kineret).

Hydroxychloroquine (Plaquenil), an antimalarial medication, has been used in early, mild disease because it is relatively safe. Many patients, however, have only a modest clinical response. The mechanism of action is probably interference with antigen processing, leading to reduced stimulation of CD4+ T cells and down-regulation of the autoimmune response. The recommended dose is 200 mg twice a day or 400 mg once a day orally.

Sulfasalazine (Azulfidine) was first used in the early 1940s. Uncontrolled trials demonstrated clinical efficacy that was later confirmed with controlled trials. Sulfasalazine (Azulfidine) delays radiographic progression of disease when compared with placebo. Its efficacy is similar to gold and methotrexate (Rheumatrex), but it commonly has more adverse effects than methotrexate (Rheumatrex). The most common side effects are GI intolerance, elevation in transaminases, rash, neutropenia, aplastic anemia, agranulocytosis, hemolysis, and infertility in males. The recommended dose varies from 0.5 g to 3 g a day. This medication is very popular in Europe and is less commonly used in the United States.

Methotrexate (Rheumatrex) is an antimetabolite analogue of folic acid. Several double-blind, placebo-controlled trials have demonstrated its efficacy and a meta-analysis showed that methotrexate significantly decreased the number of swollen and tender joints, joint pain, morning stiffness, and delayed radiographic disease progression. Because of these studies, methotrexate (Rheumatrex) is considered the gold standard for treatment of RA. In general, methotrexate (Rheumatrex) is better tolerated than other DMARDs, except leflunomide (Arava), in which the tolerance is equivalent. Adverse effects that can be prevented with folic acid supplementation include stomatitis, GI intolerance, and bone marrow suppression. Hepatitis can be prevented with frequent monitoring of liver function. Methotrexate (Rheumatrex) is teratogenic and considered category X in pregnancy; male and female patients should be advised to use appropriate contraception. The effective doses range from 7.5 mg to 30 mg a week and can be administered orally or by intramuscular or subcutaneous injection.

Leflunomide (Arava) is an antiproliferative isoxazole compound. In a placebo-controlled trial, leflunomide (Arava) was compared to methotrexate (Rheumatrex) and placebo for 52 weeks. The results showed an ACR 20 response in 52% of patients on leflunomide, in 48% of patients on methotrexate, and in 26% of patients on placebo. An ACR 50 response was obtained in 34%, 23%, and 8% of the patients for leflunomide, methotrexate, and placebo, respectively. Leflunomide (Arava) is efficacious for up to 2 years in patients with active RA. Leflunomide (Arava) has also been studied in combination with methotrexate (Rheumatrex); the combination showed significant clinical improvement. Common adverse effects of leflunomide (Arava) are diarrhea, dyspepsia, abdominal pain, hypertension, rash, alopecia, and elevation of liver enzymes. Because the medication has an enterohepatic cycle, it has a prolonged half-life and, in the case of significant toxicity, it can be washed out with cholestyramine or charcoal. Leflunomide can be dosed at 10 to 20 mg a day orally. This medication is teratogenic and patients should be advised to use contraception.

Combination therapy is the most aggressive approach used to treat RA. A randomized, controlled trial of methotrexate (Rheumatrex) 7.5 to 17.5 mg per week, sulfasalazine (Azulfidine) 500 mg twice daily, and hydroxychloroquine (Plaquenil) 200 mg twice daily was compared with methotrexate (Rheumatrex) alone and with the combination of sulfasalazine (Azulfidine) and hydroxychloroquine (Plaquenil). After 24 months, 77% of patients receiving triple therapy, 40% of the patients receiving sulfasalazine (Azulfidine) plus hydroxychloroquine

(Plaquenil), and 33% of the patients receiving methotrexate (Rheumatrex) achieved a clinically significant response. The group that received the combination therapy did not show increased toxicity.

Cyclosporine (Neoral) plus methotrexate (Rheumatrex) was studied in a 6-month, randomized, double-blind trial on patients with partial response to methotrexate (Rheumatrex). The cyclosporine (Neoral) dose was 2.5 to 5 mg/kg plus methotrexate (Rheumatrex) at a dose of 15 mg per week or less. More patients treated with methotrexate (Rheumatrex) plus cyclosporine (Neoral) (48%) achieved an ACR 20 than did the patients treated with methotrexate (Rheumatrex) alone (16%). But patients in the combination group had significantly increased levels of serum creatinine.

BIOLOGICS IN THE TREATMENT OF RA

Unfortunately, many patients are unable to tolerate DMARDs or they fail to maintain response in the long-term. Fortunately, newer classes of treatments are available that target cytokines such as tumor necrosis factor-α (TNF-α) and interleukin 1 (IL-1) that have been implicated in the pathogenesis of RA. Three TNF-α blockers and an IL-1 receptor antagonist (IL-1ra) are approved for the treatment of RA in the United States.

Infliximab (Remicade) is a human–mouse chimeric anti–TNF-α monoclonal antibody that is used in the treatment of RA and Crohn's disease. At a dose of 3 mg/kg every 8 weeks, 53% of patients achieved an ACR 20 response, compared to 20% of the controls at the 6-month analysis. ACR 50 responses were significantly improved compared with controls; at 3 mg/kg every 8 weeks, 26% of patients obtained an ACR 50, compared to 5% of controls. ACR 70 was obtained in 8% of the patients versus none in the control group.

Adverse events at 6 months included infections that required antibiotics in 31% of the patients on infliximab (Remicade) versus 21% of the controls. Serious infections occurred in 3.7% of patients treated with infliximab (Remicade) versus 5% of the control patients with a relative risk (RR) of 0.7 (95% confidence interval [CI] 0.3 to 1.8), which is not statistically significant. From these data we can conclude that infliximab (Remicade) is efficacious and well tolerated in the treatment of RA. It is important to consider the potential adverse effects, such as opportunistic infections, including *Mycobacterium tuberculosis* (TB) and fungal infections. Patients should be screened for latent TB infection with a tuberculin skin test.

Etanercept (Enbrel) consists of the extracellular portion of the human p75 TNF-α receptor linked to the Fc portion of human IgG1. Thus, etanercept (Enbrel) blocks the interaction of TNF with the TNF receptor in the cell, thereby modulating the inflammatory and immune response mediated by TNF-α. In clinical trials, 59% of patients taking etanercept (Enbrel) achieved an ACR 20 response, as compared with 11% of patients on placebo. When etanercept (Enbrel) was combined with methotrexate (Rheumatrex), 71% of the patients obtained an ACR 20 response, as compared with 27% of patients on methotrexate (Rheumatrex) plus placebo.

The recommended dose is 25 mg injected subcutaneously twice a week. The most common side effect is injection-site reaction, but like all medications of this group, there is a concern of infection.

Adalimumab (Humira) is a fully human anti–TNF-α monoclonal antibody that was evaluated on patients whose disease activity was not controlled with standard antirheumatic therapy. In this 24-week, double-blind, placebo-controlled study, 67.2% of the patients in adalimumab (Humira) achieved an ACR 20 response, versus 14.5% in the placebo group. Of the patients in the treatment group, 55.2% obtained an ACR 50 versus 8.1% in the control group, and ACR 70 was obtained in 26.9% of the adalimumab-treated patients versus 4.8% in the placebo group. At 24 weeks, there were no statistically significant differences in adverse events between adalimumab (Humira) and placebo (86.5% vs. 82.7%), serious adverse events (5.3% vs. 6.9%), or severe life-threatening events (11.9% vs. 15.4%). The recommended dose is 40 mg injected subcutaneously every other week.

Anakinra (Kineret) is a recombinant IL-1ra, which is approved for the treatment of RA as monotherapy or in combination with methotrexate. Four different trials showed that anakinra is efficacious as monotherapy or when combined with methotrexate (Rheumatrex).

The most common adverse event is injection-site reactions, which, in general, are mild and transient. In combination with methotrexate (Rheumatrex), the rate of adverse events is similar to monotherapy. Fifty-one percent of the anakinra-treated patients obtained an ACR 20 response at week 24 and 46% of these patients maintained this response at week 48. The recommended dose is 100 mg injected subcutaneously once a day.

JUVENILE ARTHRITIS

METHOD OF

Andreas Otto Reiff, MD

Juvenile arthritis (JA) is the most common rheumatic condition in childhood, with an estimated annual incidence of 0.8 to 22 per 100,000 children, and a prevalence of approximately 7 to 400 per 100,000 children. The wide range can to some extent be explained by significant geographic and ethnic variability and the use of different classification systems. The American

TABLE 1 Differential Diagnostic Considerations in Juvenile Rheumatoid Arthritis

Inflammatory	Musculoskeletal
Acute rheumatic fever	Chondromalacia patellae
Dermatomyositis	Fibromyalgia syndrome
Inflammatory bowel disease	Growing pains
Kawasaki disease	Hypermobility syndrome
Mixed connective tissue disease	Legg-Calvé-Perthes disease
Psoriatic arthritis	Osgood-Schlatter disease
Reiter's disease	Reflex sympathetic dystrophy
Scleroderma	Trauma and overuse syndrome
Sjögren's syndrome	**Other**
Systemic lupus erythematosus	Bleeding diathesis (hemophilia with hemarthrosis)
Transient synovitis of the hip	Histiocytosis
Infectious	Immune deficiency (congenital and acquired)
Lyme disease	Neoplasm (neuroblastoma, acute leukemia, hematologic malignancy)
Postinfectious arthritis secondary to *Yersinia* or *Shigella*	Pigmented villonodular synovitis
Septic arthritis	Sarcoidosis
Viral-associated arthritis	Sickle cell disease

Data from Siegel DM, Baum J. Juvenile arthritis. Prim Care 20:883-893, 1993.

College of Rheumatology (ACR) diagnostic criteria for JA require age at onset before 16 years, inflammation of one or more joints for at least 6 weeks, and exclusion of other causes of arthritis.

The pathogenesis of JA remains unknown. Associations between JA subtypes and specific human leukocyte antigen (HLA) loci suggest a genetic predisposition.

The differential diagnosis of JA is extensive and encompasses other rheumatic and musculoskeletal conditions, diseases, infectious processes, and malignancies, which are reviewed in Table 1.

Because of a different nomenclature for JA in Europe (juvenile chronic arthritis [JCA] or juvenile idiopathic arthritis [JIA]) and the United States (juvenile rheumatoid arthritis [JRA]), the International League of Associations of Rheumatologists (ILAR) has proposed reclassification of childhood arthritis based on the identification of more clinically homogeneous arthritis groups. In addition to the three traditional subtypes (oligoarticular-, polyarticular-, and systemic-onset JIA), the ILAR criteria also recognize psoriatic arthritis, enthesitis-related arthritis, and nonclassifiable forms of childhood arthritis. However, these new criteria continue to evolve and have not yet been implemented by the American College of Rheumatology. Although the term JRA is still commonly used, many pediatric rheumatologists have now adopted the ILAR criteria as the current classification (Table 2).

JA Subtypes

As a consequence of space constraints, this article focuses on the three major genetically distinct JA subtypes (*pauciarticular-* or *oligoarticular-onset*, *polyarticular-onset*, and *systemic-onset*), which are based on the initial clinical presentation, including number of inflamed joints, presence of fever, rash, and other systemic manifestations during the first 6 months of the disease course (Table 3). Table 2 summarizes the key characteristics of JA subtypes.

Approximately 50% of all children with JA present with *pauciarticular-* or *oligoarticular-onset*, involving one to four joints during the first 6 months after disease onset. This subtype particularly affects large joints in an asymmetric pattern and is usually not accompanied by significant extra-articular symptoms.

There are two recognized subgroups of pauciarticular disease: the early childhood-onset subgroup, with persistent arthritis in four or fewer joints, and the extended oligoarticular form, affecting a cumulative of five or more joints after the first 6 months of disease and frequently representing a challenging patient group.

Children with early childhood-onset pauciarticular JA who are antinuclear antibody (ANA)-positive (75% to 85%) have an approximately 30% risk for developing chronic uveitis, which can result in significant loss of vision or blindness.

Approximately 40% of children with JA present with *polyarticular-onset* disease, involving five or more joints. This subtype of JA is more commonly observed in females and is generally characterized by symmetric arthritis of either small or large joints. Systemic manifestations are variable and the risk of uveitis in this subgroup is approximately 5%.

Polyarticular-onset JA is further divided into two major subgroups on the basis of the rheumatoid factor (RF) status. The more common RF-negative polyarticular-onset JA affects younger patients and is less likely to involve the small joints. Usually 25% of these children are ANA positive. Conversely, RF-positive polyarthritis, associated with HLA-DR4, is seldom seen in children younger than 8 years of age and bears a striking resemblance to adult-onset RA. Most of the children in this subgroup are also ANA positive, and rheumatoid nodules may be present. Early erosions are more common in RF-positive patients than in those with the RF-negative subtype.

TABLE 2 Classification of Juvenile Arthritis

ACR (JRA)*	EULAR (JCA)†	ILAR (JIA)‡	ILAR Definition	%	RF	ANA	Peak Onset (y)	M:F	Articular Characteristics	Extra-articular Features
Systemic arthritis	Systemic arthritis	Systemic arthritis	Arthritis with or preceded by fever of 2 wks plus 1 of the following: rash, lymphadenopathy, serositis hepato-/splenomegaly	10-20	–	– (0-10%)	No peak	1:1	Multiple joint involvement; myalgia, arthralgia, or transient arthritis In late phase, symmetric involvement of large and small joints	Fever, rash, serositis, lymphadenopathy, hepatosplenomegaly, other systemic features
Polyarticular arthritis	Polyarticular arthritis *RF negative*	Polyarticular arthritis *RF negative*	Arthritis of ≥5 joints during first 6 mo; RF negative on 2 occasions (at least 3 months apart)	20-30	–	+ (25%)	2	1:3		Mild or absent systemic symptoms
	RF positive	*RF positive*	Arthritis of ≥5 joints during first 6 mo; RF positive on 2 occasions (at least 3 months apart)	5-10	+	+ (75%)	>8	1:6	Symmetric involvement of large and small joints plus cervical spine	Systemic symptoms generally mild, rheumatoid nodules in some
Pauciarticular arthritis	Oligoarthritis	Oligoarthritis *Persistent* *Extended*	Arthritis of 1-4 joints during first 6 months Affecting only 4 joints during disease course Affecting 5 or more joints after 6 mo	30-40	–	+ (50%)	1-2 (early onset)	1:5	Asymmetric large joint involvement	Systemic symptoms usually absent, high risk of chronic uveitis (ANA positive)
Spondyloarthritis		Enthesitis-related arthritis	Arthritis and/or enthesitis with at least 2 of: sacroiliac tenderness and/or inflammatory spinal pain, HLA B27+; first- or second-degree relative with history of HLA B27-associated disease	10-15	–	–	>8 (late onset)	10:1	Asymmetric large joint involvement, especially hips and sacroiliac joints	Acute uveitis, occasional fever, anemia (HLA-B27+)
		Psoriatic arthritis	Arthritis and psoriasis, or arthritis and at least 2 of: dactylitis, nail abnormalities, first-degree relative with history of psoriasis	~3	–	–	7-11	0.95:1	Scattered asymmetric oligoarthritis of large and small joints	~3
		Nonclassifiable arthritis	All forms of arthritis that do not meet criteria for other categories	~10	–	?	?	?		~10

*Cassidy JT, Levinson JE, Bass JC et al: A study of classification criteria for a diagnosis of juvenile rheumatoid arthritis. Arthritis Rheum 29:274-281, 1986.
†European League against Rheumatism: EULAR bulletin No. 4: Nomenclature and Classification of Arthritis in Children. Basel, National Zeitung A, 1977.
‡Petty RE et al: Revision of the proposed classification criteria for juvenile idiopathic arthritis: Durban 1997. J Rheumatol 22:1566-1569, 1995.
Abbreviations: ANA = antinuclear antibody; ILAR = International League of Associations of Rheumatologists; JRA = juvenile rheumatoid arthritis; JCA = juvenile chronic arthritis; JIA = juvenile idiopathic arthritis; RF = rheumatoid factor.

TABLE 3 Laboratory Studies in Juvenile Rheumatoid Arthritis

	Systemic Onset	Polyarticular	Pauciarticular
ANA	N	N, ↑	↑↑
CRP	↑↑	↑↑, ↑	N, ↑
ESR	↑↑	↑↑	N, ↑
Hemoglobin/ hematocrit	↓↓	N	N
Platelets	↑↑	N	N
RF	N	↑	N
WBC count	↑↑	↑	N

Abbreviations: ↑ = mild to moderately elevated; ↑↑ = extremely elevated; ↓ = mild to moderately decreased; and ↓↓ = extremely decreased; ANA = antinuclear antibody; CRP = C-reactive protein; ESR = erythrocyte sedimentation rate; N = normal or absent; RF = rheumatoid factor; WBC = white blood cell.

Data from Siegel DM, Baum J. Juvenile arthritis. Prim Care 20:883-893, 1993, with permission.

The remaining 10% to 20% of children present with *systemic-onset* JA (SOJA). Although SOJA can occur at any age, it usually affects children less than 10 years of age. Systemic symptoms may precede the development of arthritis by weeks or even years. The diagnosis of SOJA requires a history of arthritis in any number of joints and at least 2 weeks of daily monophasic or biphasic fever accompanied by at least one of the following:

- Salmon-pink rash on the trunk or overlying the joints
- Hepatosplenomegaly
- Lymphadenopathy
- Serositis

Other rare manifestations include pericarditis and central nervous system (CNS) involvement. Approximately 80% of these children develop severe, treatment-resistant polyarticular-course arthritis. Children with systemic JA have an increased risk of mortality and account for the majority of children with JA who suffer from long-term disability when compared to other forms of JA.

JA Prognosis

If not treated early and aggressively enough, JA can have potentially devastating, lifelong consequences. Abnormalities include arrested or asymmetric skeletal development, retarded linear growth, and persistence of infantile proportions. Localized growth disturbances can lead to considerable deformities. Delays in gross and fine motor skills are common. Other possible sequelae include osteopenia, pericarditis, and chronic eye disease.

The once prevalent view that children typically "grow out of" JA is challenged by several recent epidemiologic studies. In summary, these studies describe 984 children with JA (approximately 60% with pauciarticular-onset, 30% with polyarticular-onset, and 10% with systemic-onset JA) with a mean age at onset of 7.5 years, followed over a mean of 20.5 years. Forty-seven percent of these patients still had active arthritis at a mean age of 30 years, 46% reported significant difficulty in daily life, and 22% had undergone JA-related surgery. Additionally there were statistically significant differences for disability, pain, fatigue, physical functioning, and level of employment in patients with JA when compared to a healthy control population. Increased rates of depression and academic, as well as psychosocial, difficulties were also observed in children with JA, depending on their degree of disability. Systemic-onset, polyarticular-course and polyarticular-onset JA, particularly in females, appear to have the worst prognosis of the three subtypes.

JA Management

Notably, long-term damage in children with JA rarely arises from overly aggressive therapy; rather, it arises from an overly conservative and cautious approach in the early stages of the disease. In addition to pharmacotherapy, early aggressive physical and occupational therapy remain one of the cornerstones of JA treatment. High-risk patients, such as children with systemic-onset polyarticular-course or early erosive RF-positive disease, should be identified near the beginning of the disease course and should receive disease-modifying antirheumatic drug (DMARD) therapy within the first 3 months after disease onset.

JA PHARMACOTHERAPY

Nonsteroidal Anti-Inflammatory Drugs

Nonsteroidal anti-inflammatory drugs (NSAIDs) are commonly used as first-line agents. Ibuprofen, naproxen, and tolmetin are currently the only FDA-approved NSAIDs for JA. NSAIDs with a longer half-life and less-frequent dosing, such as naproxen, are often preferred by children and are available in suspension form. *Cyclooxygenase-2 inhibitors* are available as a treatment alternative. A recent 12-week multinational trial in 310 children with pauci- and polyarticular-onset JA demonstrated that particularly the higher dose of rofecoxib (0.6 mg/kg/d) was safe and as effective as naproxen in achieving JRA30 response rates (30% improvement in a composite score of Parent/Patient's Assessment of Overall Well-Being, Investigator's Global Assessment of Disease Activity; functional ability [Childhood Health Assessment Questionnaire (CHAQ)]); number of joints with active arthritis and with limited range of motion; and erythrocyte sedimentation rate). Interestingly, there was no difference in the gastrointestinal tolerability profile when compared to naproxen.

Corticosteroids

For some JA subtypes, especially in children with monoarticular disease, treatment may be initiated with intra-articular injections of triamcinolone hexacetonide, which can result in dramatic symptomatic improvement and even remission.

Systemic steroids may still be required for treating difficult JA, especially in children with systemic-onset disease. However, long-term use should be avoided because of numerous, well-recognized adverse effects (e.g., growth arrest secondary to premature epiphyseal closure, avascular necrosis, osteoporosis, Cushing's disease).

Methotrexate (Rheumatrex)

Methotrexate (MTX) is still considered the gold standard for most cases of JA and is frequently used in combination with other DMARDs. A survey of studies of methotrexate in JA demonstrated that only 60% of children respond to a standard dose of 0.5 mg/kg once weekly and clinical remission is achieved in merely 50% of children after a year of therapy. Relapse rates after discontinuation of MTX are high. The systemic-onset subtype appears to be even less responsive to MTX than the other subtypes. Methotrexate is equally safe and effective whether administered orally or by intramuscular (IM) or subcutaneous (SC) injection, and is usually given in conjunction with weekly folinic[1] or daily folic acid[1] supplementation. Hepatic and pulmonary toxicity, although rare in children, require regular patient monitoring.

Cyclosporine A (Neoral)[1]

Cyclosporine A is effective in the treatment of refractory JA, and can be useful in children with systemic-onset disease, but renal toxicity and secondary infections remain a concern. In an open prospective study of 34 patients with JA, 66% withdrew from therapy because of inefficacy or side effects. In general, the benefit of cyclosporine was mainly limited to a steroid-sparing effect and controlling fever. Effects on joints, laboratory parameters, and uveitis were less clear. Combination therapy of MTX with cyclosporine A may be superior to monotherapy with either agent alone.

Cyclophosphamide (Cytoxan)[1]

Although cyclophosphamide is frequently used in pediatric systemic lupus erythematosus (SLE), only one study of four children with systemic JA has been published. After 12 to 20 pulses of intravenous cyclophosphamide (500 to 1000 mg/m^2), three children achieved remission and all four children were able to discontinue concomitant corticosteroids with subsequent increase in their linear growth.

[1]Not FDA approved for this indication.

Leflunomide (Arava)[1]

This selective pyrimidine synthesis inhibitor is comparable in efficacy to sulfasalazine and MTX in RA. In a recent 16-week, double-blind, controlled pediatric trial, the safety and efficacy of leflunomide was compared to MTX. Ninety-four children (47 per arm) with active polyarticular-course JA between the ages of 3 and 17 years were enrolled. Both leflunomide and MTX were highly effective and well tolerated. Efficacy favored MTX, which was statistically superior to leflunomide in achieving JRA30 response rates (see above). The most frequently observed side effects for both drugs included nausea, diarrhea, abdominal pain, headache, nasopharyngitis, and alopecia. Elevations of liver enzymes were reported in 7 children treated with leflunomide and in 15 children treated with MTX. Leflunomide may be an effective and well-tolerated alternative to MTX in children who have failed or cannot tolerate MTX. Because of the long half-life and potential teratogenic effects, leflunomide should be cautiously used in females of childbearing age and treatment with cholestyramine is recommended prior to pregnancy.

BIOLOGIC RESPONSE MODIFIERS

Etanercept (Enbrel)

Etanercept is composed of two human soluble tumor necrosis factor (TNF)-α receptors (p75) and a naturally occurring TNF-neutralizing protein fused to the Fc portion of human immunoglobulin G1. Etanercept binds and inhibits both TNF and lymphotoxin (LT)-α, formerly known as TNF-β, both of which have been implicated in the pathogenesis of JA.

In a two-part, open-label study of 69 children with polyarticular-course JA, who were refractory or intolerant to MTX, 0.4 mg/kg of etanercept injected SC twice weekly (maximum 25 mg per dose) resulted in significant improvement in the JRA30 response rates (see above). At the end of 90 days of etanercept therapy (part 1 of the study), 51 children (74%) had a 30% improvement, 44 children (64%) had a 50% improvement, and 25 children (36%) had a 70% improvement relative to baseline. Efficacy was sustained for up to 2 years during the extension of the trial with no increase in rates of adverse events. Etanercept is well tolerated with injection-site reactions being the most frequently reported adverse event. The FDA has approved etanercept for patients with moderate to severe JA. In addition, etanercept has also been successfully used in the treatment of refractory uveitis in children.

Infliximab (Remicade)[1]

Infliximab, a chimeric (mouse/human) monoclonal TNF antibody, is usually administered intravenously every other month and requires concomitant MTX to

[1]Not FDA approved for this indication.

suppress antibody formation. Encouraging results in several small, uncontrolled trials in JA have been reported. Serious infections, especially early clusters of tuberculosis, remain a concern and limit the use of this drug. In addition, occurrence of neutralizing anti-infliximab antibodies, SLE-type autoimmune features, and severe infusion reactions in response to the drug have been observed.

A multinational trial with infliximab in JA is currently underway.

Anakinra (Kineret)[1]

In addition to TNF, interleukin 1 (IL-1) plays a central role in the pathogenesis of arthritis. In a recent international multicenter, open-label study, 82 children with polyarticular-course JA were treated with anakinra at 1 mg/kg per day SC for 12 weeks. Of the 82 children enrolled, 72 (88%) completed the 12-week open-label phase and 46 (58%) showed signs of clinical improvement in JRA30 response rates when compared to baseline. Interestingly, children with systemic-onset JA showed a more favorable response than children with polyarticular- or oligoarticular-onset JA (79% vs. 67% vs. 52%). There was no difference in outcome in children with or without concomitant MTX. The most common adverse events were injection-site reactions (70%). In two children isolated neutrophil counts <1.5 with no clinical sequelae were observed. No deaths, malignancies, opportunistic infections, or treatment-associated laboratory abnormalities were seen.

Anti-IL-6 Receptor Antibody

Recent studies suggest that IL-6 and IL-18 are pivotal cytokines in the pathogenesis of systemic arthritis, unlike in oligo- or polyarticular JA where TNF appears to be the predominant proinflammatory cytokine. This is supported by the observation that less than 50% of children with acute systemic JA respond to TNF antagonists. In a recent phase II dose escalation trial with an anti-IL6 receptor antibody monoclonal receptor antagonist (MRA), 11 children with treatment-resistant systemic JA were treated with up to 8 mg/kg of MRA given intravenously every other week. A dramatic treatment response with a 70% improvement in the JRA core set criteria was observed in 7 of 11 children after 2 weeks. It appeared that 8 mg/kg was the most efficacious dose. None of the children experienced a disease flare during the study and none withdrew because of adverse events. Future trials with this promising agent are planned.

AUTOLOGOUS BONE MARROW TRANSPLANTATION

Recent data from several small studies support autologous bone marrow transplantation as a

[1]Not FDA approved for this indication.

treatment option for children with severe treatment-refractory JA. The concept is to achieve immunologic tolerance through the aggressive elimination of autoreactive B- and T-cell clones, with subsequent infusion of the patient's own purged bone marrow containing immunologically naïve stem cells. Applying slightly differing treatment regimens, approximately 45 children with refractory, predominantly systemic JA have been transplanted to date.

The largest series reported 31 children with treatment refractory JA (25 with systemic onset and 6 with polyarticular onset), who had progressive disease despite treatment with NSAIDs, MTX[1], prednisone, cyclosporine[1], or intravenous (IV) cyclophosphamide[1]. Treatment included antithymocyte globulin (ATG)[1], high-dose cyclophosphamide and total-body irradiation (4 Gy single fraction). After a mean follow-up of 33 months (range: 8 to 60 months), 17 children (55%) were considered to be in drug-free remission, while 7 children (22.5%) relapsed. Four children (13%) never responded to therapy. Three children died as a result of overwhelming infections or macrophage-activation syndrome (MAS). These findings suggest that autologous bone marrow transplantation may be a viable option for patients with refractory JA. However, with a mortality risk of approximately 10% and an expected response rate of approximately 50%, this method should be reserved for children with most severe disease.

Conclusion

With the availability of new JA outcome data, childhood arthritis can no longer be considered a benign disease. Early, aggressive pharmacologic intervention is a critical component of optimal disease management to prevent further disease progression, restore range of motion in the joints, and promote normal growth and development. Physicians treating children with JA need to recognize that children are not small adults and often respond less favorably to conventional RA therapy. Notably, agents used for adult RA, such as D-penicillamine[1], gold[1], and hydroxychloroquine[1] as monotherapy, have failed to demonstrate any greater benefit than placebo in children with JA.

Although the diverse nature of JA precludes a one-treatment-fits-all approach, children at risk for poor disease outcome should be identified early and receive DMARDs within the first 3 months of disease onset. High-risk patients include those with severe, erosive polyarticular disease, systemic-onset, polyarticular-course disease, and extended pauciarticular disease.

New agents that may have potential in the treatment of JA are rapidly becoming available, but, for most of them, data are sparse in pediatric populations. Although MTX is still considered the gold standard for most cases of JA, biologic agents such as etanercept

[1]Not FDA approved for this indication.

have considerably raised the treatment standard and may therefore offer a significant improvement in prognosis. In contrast to adults, the effect of biologic response modifiers on radiographic progression in children is yet undetermined. To date, etanercept is the only new agent to receive FDA approval for the treatment of JA.

In addition to the agents previously discussed, other new therapeutic strategies are currently in early phases of clinical trials. These include combination therapies of biologic agents (anti-TNF/anti-IL6)*, selective inhibitors of intracellular inflammatory pathways (p38 MAP Kinase inhibitors)*, and anti–B-cell therapy (anti-CD20, rituximab)*.

*Investigational drug in the United States.

ANKYLOSING SPONDYLITIS

METHOD OF

Sterling G. West, MD

Ankylosing spondylitis (AS) is the prototypic member of the seronegative spondyloarthropathies, which as a group constitute the second most common form of inflammatory arthritis. This family of disorders shares clinical, radiologic, pathologic, and genetic features (Table 1). AS typically presents as an inflammatory arthritis of the sacroiliac joints and spine that most likely results from an interaction between an environmental trigger and susceptibility genes. The severity of disease presentation and subsequent course is influenced by the patient's gender, ethnicity, and genetic background. Treatment is most successful when aggressively started early in the disease course.

Epidemiology

Ankylosing spondylitis is strongly associated with the HLA-B27 class I major histocompatibility antigen in all populations. Therefore, ethnic groups with a high frequency of HLA-B27 have a higher prevalence of AS. Among whites in the United States, up to 1.0% have AS, while American blacks have a much lower frequency. The male-to-female ratio is 3:1, with males having more severe back disease and females presenting more commonly with peripheral arthritis. The majority of patients have onset of symptoms in late adolescence and early adulthood. Onset after age 45 years is rare. Various criteria have been proposed for the classification of AS but are not useful to diagnose individuals with early or atypical disease presentations.

TABLE 1 Characteristics of the Spondyloarthropathies

DEMOGRAPHIC
Onset younger than age 40 years
Males affected more than females
Whites more than other races
CLINICAL
Sacroiliitis with constant or alternating buttock pain and stiffness
Spondylitis with low back pain, night pain, and morning stiffness (>1 hour)
Oligoarticular peripheral arthritis and dactylitis (sausage digits) with asymmetric lower extremity predominance
Enthesitis causing heel pain, plantar fasciitis, and pain at other insertion sites
Overlapping extraarticular manifestations, including mucous membrane lesions, clinical/subclinical bowel disease, acute anterior uveitis, psoriasiform skin lesions, and aortitis
LABORATORY
Absence of rheumatoid factor and antinuclear antibodies
RADIOGRAPHIC
Radiographic sacroiliitis ± spondylitis
Enthesopathic calcifications
PATHOLOGIC
Inflammation of entheses
Inflammatory synovitis
GENETIC
Association with HLA-B27 antigen
Familial aggregation

Clinical Features

Most patients with AS present with the insidious onset of low back pain and stiffness. Many patients complain of bilateral buttock pain, back symptoms that interrupt sleep, and prolonged morning stiffness for more than an hour. Unlike patients with mechanical back pain, AS patients may have improvement in their pain and stiffness during the day with use. Physical examination shows tenderness to direct pressure over the sacroiliac joints and/or with stressing maneuvers (Gaenslen's and Patrick's tests). Examination of the axial skeleton shows loss of spinal mobility in all planes (Schober test, lateral bending, and lateral rotation). The cervical spine can also be involved. With longer disease duration, loss of lumbar lordosis, thoracic spinal kyphosis, and restriction of chest expansion (<2.5 cm) may be seen. Neurologic examination is normal.

Many patients have additional musculoskeletal complaints. Enthesitis, which is caused by inflammation at the insertion site of a ligament or tendon into bone, can cause juxtaarticular pain at the costochondral junctions, spinal processes, iliac crests, or Achilles tendon and plantar fascia insertions of the heel, as well as other attachment sites. Enthesitis can be the presenting presentation of patients, particularly in children (juvenile-onset AS).

Peripheral arthritis may be a prominent and early manifestation. Up to one-third of patients will develop hip and less commonly shoulder involvement within the first 10 years of disease onset. Hip involvement is typically bilateral and more common to occur in patients developing AS in adolescence or late teenage years. Glenohumeral joint involvement is unusual, although erosive enthesopathy of the supraspinatus tendon insertion is characteristic. Other peripheral joint involvement, particularly of the lower extremity, is common and may be the initial presentation in juvenile-onset AS, women, and patients with subclinical inflammatory bowel disease.

The most common extraarticular manifestation is acute anterior uveitis, occurring in 25% to 40% of patients. This is usually unilateral and can precede or follow the onset of musculoskeletal symptoms by months to years. Subclinical gastrointestinal mucosal lesions resembling Crohn's disease can be found on ileocolonoscopy in up to 50% of AS patients, especially in those with peripheral arthritis. Osteoporosis caused by inflammation and spinal immobility is common and may predispose the patient to spinal fractures. Diagnosis may be hampered by a falsely elevated bone mineral density of the lumbar spine as a consequence of overlying ligamentous calcifications. Aortitis causing aortic insufficiency (1% of patients), upper lobe pulmonary fibrosis, cauda equina syndrome caused by adhesive arachnoiditis, and renal amyloidosis are rare manifestations, occurring primarily in patients with long-standing AS. Each of these extraarticular manifestations will require assessment and therapy by specialists skilled in the care of these complications.

Investigations

RADIOLOGY

The diagnosis of AS is confirmed by the development of sclerosis and erosions in both sacroiliac joints. Radiographic changes in the spine manifest as anterior squaring of the vertebral body and calcification of the annulus fibrosis causing marginal syndesmophytes. Whereas all patients will develop radiographic sacroiliitis by age 40 years, only 66% will have radiographic changes in the spine and less than 10% will develop a "bamboo" spine. Unfortunately, radiographic changes can take years to develop, which may delay an early diagnosis. Magnetic resonance imaging (MRI) will show sacroiliac joint inflammation and osteitis associated with spinal enthesitis early in the disease course before radiographs become abnormal. However, MRI scans are expensive and are rarely necessary to confirm a clinical diagnosis of AS.

LABORATORY TESTS

An elevated erythrocyte sedimentation rate or serum C-reactive protein is present in up to 70% of AS patients, but do not always follow the disease activity. Rheumatoid factor and antinuclear antibody tests are negative. Testing for the presence of the HLA-B27 antigen is unnecessary in patients with typical symptoms and radiographs for AS. When clinical suspicion for AS is high but radiographs are normal, the presence of HLA-B27 enhances the likelihood of a correct diagnosis. Conversely, in patients with ill-defined back pain, testing for HLA-B27 antigen may be misleading and should be avoided.

Etiology

The etiopathogenesis of AS is postulated to be caused by an environmental trigger in a genetically predisposed host. The environmental trigger is unknown but postulated to be an ubiquitous antigen such as enteric bacteria in the gastrointestinal tract. The major genetic association is with HLA-B27. The concordance rate for HLA-B27–positive monozygotic twins is 60% to 75%, whereas for HLA-B27–positive dizygotic twins it is only 15% to 25%, clearly supporting a role for additional genetic loci.

The risk for AS varies among ethnic and racial groups but approximates the frequency of HLA-B27. HLA-B27 is present in 6% to 14% of all normal whites, but present in more than 90% of white AS patients. Thus, an HLA-B27–positive individual has a 50 to 100 times increased relative risk for developing AS. However, the overall absolute risk for developing AS in an HLA-B27–positive individual without a family history of AS is only 2% to 5%, whereas for an individual with a family history, the risk is 20% to 33%. Therefore, the majority of HLA-B27–positive individuals never develop AS, further supporting other genetic influences. In addition, the variability in disease severity among patients with AS suggests that while some genes (i.e., HLA-B27) contribute to a person's susceptibility to develop this disease, other genes determine the risk of having a severe disease course.

Differential Diagnosis

In some case series, approximately 5% of patients presenting to a primary care clinic with low back pain were found to have ankylosing spondylitis. Separating inflammatory from noninflammatory (mechanical) back pain is crucial to starting therapy in an early stage of disease. The following features are useful to identify patients with ankylosing spondylitis:

- Insidious onset of discomfort
- Age at onset before age 40 years
- Persistence of symptoms for more than 3 months
- Association with nighttime and morning pain and stiffness (>1 hour)
- Improvement in symptoms with exercise

- Limited motion of low back in all three planes
- No neurologic abnormalities

In the patient with early disease who has suggestive signs and symptoms but negative sacroiliac joint radiographs, HLA-B27 testing and/or an MRI scan may be helpful in selected cases. Other features suggesting a spondyloarthropathy (see Table 1) can also help make a confident diagnosis of AS.

Prognosis

Ankylosing spondylitis can have a variable disease course, ranging from mild to severe. In most patients, a predictable pattern of disease is established within the first ten years. Overall, more than 70% of patients continue to be able to work, and life expectancy is not shortened. Patients with mild disease restricted to the sacroiliac joints and controlled symptomatically with nonsteroidal anti-inflammatory medications (NSAIDs) are able to maintain full functional and employment capacity. However, in an individual patient, disease activity may fluctuate. AS does not spontaneously go into remission.

Up to 30% to 40% of patients will have a more aggressive disease course. These patients can be identified by the following clinical findings:

- Hip disease or
- Three of the following:
  Onset younger than age 16 years
  Limitation of spine motion
  Oligoarthritis
  "Sausage" digit
  High erythrocyte sedimentation rate or C-reactive protein
  Poor efficacy of NSAIDs

Patients with hip disease or patients with three or more of the other clinical variables, even without hip disease, will have a severe outcome (specificity 97.5%, sensitivity 50%). These patients need to be recognized early, followed closely, and treated aggressively.

The presence of HLA-B27 does not adversely affect the musculoskeletal prognosis. However, HLA-B27–positive patients are at increased risk to develop uveitis and aortitis. Patients who have severe radiographic changes of "bamboo" spine (10% of all patients) are more likely to have neurologic sequelae, including cauda equina syndrome or spinal cord injury from spinal fractures as a consequence of falls. Patients with a family history of AS usually have a more benign disease than do patients without a family history (sporadic disease).

Treatment

The primary objectives of any treatment program are to:

- Educate the patient and family
- Relieve pain
- Decrease inflammation
- Maintain good posture and function

The earlier in the disease course treatment is instituted, the better the outcome.

GENERAL APPROACHES

All patients and their families should be educated about the disease process and objectives of therapy. This will improve patient compliance with medications and physical therapy. All patients should be encouraged to stop smoking, because obstructive lung disease will add to the respiratory compromise caused by restriction of lung function caused by limited costovertebral joint motion. When appropriate, genetic counseling should inform the family that the risk of transmitting the HLA-B27 antigen is 50%, and those children who are HLA-B27–positive have a 20% to 30% chance of developing AS. Thus, the overall risk is, at most, 1 in 6, with offspring of diseased women being at highest risk. Additional educational materials can be obtained by writing the Spondylitis Association of America, 14827 Ventura Boulevard, Suite 222, Sherman Oaks, California 91403 (phone: 1-800-777-8189).

SPECIFIC APPROACHES

Treatment of AS patients should be individualized based on disease activity, presence of poor prognostic factors, concurrent illnesses, and the patient's risk tolerance for medication side effects. Most patients benefit from an exercise program and NSAIDs.

Physiotherapy

Physical therapy and exercise delay ankylosis, improve posture, and maintain joint range of motion. Particular attention should be given to neck and back extension exercises, such as wall pushups and prone lying, deep breathing exercises, and shoulder and hip range of motion exercises. Swimming is the best overall exercise to achieve these goals. Additionally, the AS patient should be encouraged to sleep with a small pillow under his or her head to lessen the forward flexion of their neck at night.

Medications

Medications used in AS include NSAIDs, sulfasalazine (Azulfidine)[1], methotrexate (Rheumatrex)[1], and antitumor necrosis factor-α (TNF-α) therapy (Table 2). Narcotic analgesics and prolonged oral corticosteroids should be avoided. Most patients with active AS benefit from an NSAID, which lessens pain and stiffness and enables them to participate in physical therapy. Indomethacin (Indocin) has anecdotally

[1]Not FDA approved for this indication.

TABLE 2 Medications Used in Therapy of Spondyloarthropathies

Drugs (Trade Name)	Dose and Dosage	Toxicities	Monitoring
Sulfasalazine (Azulfidine, Azulfidine EN-tabs)[1]	500 mg/tab; 1000-1500 mg twice a day	Skin rash, nausea Myelosuppression Hepatitis Oligospermia (reversible)	CBC, AST twice a month until stable dose, then every 3 months
Methotrexate (Rheumatrex, Trexall)[1]	2.5 mg/tab; 7.5-20 mg weekly Can be given by injection	Myelosuppression Pulmonary infiltrate Hepatic fibrosis Birth defects Infection Lymphoma (rare) Avoid in alcoholic patients or renal insufficiency	CBC, AST, albumin, creatinine every 4-8 weeks Use with folate 1 mg/d
Etanercept (Enbrel)	25 mg subcutaneously twice a week	Infection-site reaction Same as infliximab	Baseline PPD CBC monthly for 3 months, then every 3 months
Infliximab (Remicade)	Loading dose, then 3-10 mg/kg intravenously every 1-2 months	Infusion reaction TB reactivation Opportunistic infection Rarely lupus-like syndrome, aplastic anemia, demyelination, heart failure, lymphoma	Same as etanercept

[1]Not FDA approved for this indication.
Abbreviations: AST = aspartate aminotransferase; CBC = cell blood count with platelets; PPD = purified protein derivative; TB = tuberculosis.

been most effective at doses of 50 mg three times a day or 75 mg slow-release (SR) capsules twice a day. Many other NSAIDs, including the new cyclooxygenase-2 inhibitors, have been used with variable success. When maximum doses of NSAIDs are ineffective, additional medication may be helpful. For patients with persistent isolated sacroiliitis or peripheral oligoarthritis, intraarticular steroids may be used. We use fluoroscopy to guide injections into the sacroiliac joints to assure proper needle placement. Injections of enthesitis of Achilles or patellar tendon insertion should only be done by experienced physicians (if at all) because of the risk of tendon rupture.

Patients with persistently active disease and poor prognostic indicators should be treated more aggressively. Oral corticosteroids should generally be avoided, although a few patients with severely active disease may benefit from a 6-week course of tapering prednisone or a single intravenous pulse of 500 mg of methylprednisolone (Solu-Medrol), while a second-line agent is being started. Sulfasalazine (Azulfidine)[1] and methotrexate (Rheumatrex)[1] have both been used successfully to control peripheral arthritis. Sulfasalazine is started at 500 mg a day and incrementally increased weekly by 500 mg, to as high as 1500 mg twice a day. Patients with gastrointestinal side effects may be able to tolerate Azulfidine EN-Tabs (delayed release). Methotrexate is also useful for peripheral arthritis. Patients start at 7.5 mg weekly and can be titrated monthly to as high as 20 mg weekly. All patients should be on folate 1 mg per day to lessen side effects. Table 2 outlines common side effects and a monitoring schedule.

There is no evidence that either sulfasalazine or methotrexate improves or prevents progression of the spine disease, which is a hallmark of AS. Recently, the anti–TNF-α agents etanercept (Enbrel) and infliximab (Remicade)[1] were shown, in controlled trials, to have significant efficacy in treating both the spinal disease and peripheral arthritis of patients with AS. Studies using adalimumab (Humira)[1] are ongoing and are expected to yield similar results. Etanercept is a soluble TNF-α receptor, given 25 mg subcutaneously twice a week. Infliximab is a chimeric mouse–human monoclonal anti–TNF-α antibody, given 5 mg/kg intravenously at baseline, 2, and 6 weeks, and then every 4 to 8 weeks thereafter. Patients on infliximab must also be on methotrexate to avoid the formation of neutralizing antichimeric antibodies. MRI of the sacroiliac joints and spine of AS patients treated with anti–TNF-α therapy show objective improvement of inflammation in the sacroiliac joints and spinal entheses, with more than 80% responding to therapy and at least half experiencing >50% relief of their symptoms and improvement in function. Response to anti–TNF-α agents occurs quickly, frequently within the first 1 to 2 months of therapy, but the effect is quickly lost upon discontinuation. Extra-articular manifestations, such as refractory uveitis, can also respond to these agents. Although these biologic agents are effective, their indiscriminate use is discouraged because of

[1]Not FDA approved for this indication.

[1]Not FDA approved for this indication.

cost concerns and a lack of long-term safety data. Table 2 lists potential side effects and a monitoring schedule. However, the 30% of AS patients who demonstrate poor prognostic signs, who have failed NSAIDs, with or without sulfasalazine/methotrexate for 3 to 4 months, should be placed on one of these agents. The use of thalidomide (Thalomid)[1], which is a weak TNF-α inhibitor and thus effective in some AS patients, should be avoided because it causes a painful neuropathy in many patients with long-term use.

Specific Clinical Situations

Osteoporosis occurs frequently in patients with AS and, when demonstrated, should be treated with calcium, vitamin D, and a bisphosphonate such as alendronate (Fosamax, 70 mg per week) or risedronate (Actonel, 35 mg per week). For patients unable to tolerate an oral bisphosphonate, pamidronate (Aredia)[1], 30 mg intravenously over 2 hours every 3 months, can be used. Notably, pamidronate at doses of 60 mg a month decreases AS symptoms by 35% within 6 months of therapy. Sleep disturbance is common in AS patients as a consequence of nighttime pain and may be helped with low-dose tricyclic antidepressants such as amitriptyline (Elavil)[1] or trazodone (Desyrel)[1] 50 mg at night. Pregnancy is a difficult situation because medications must be stopped, and AS does not remit during pregnancy. For many, use of NSAIDs, sulfasalazine, and the addition of corticosteroids may be necessary after the first trimester to control severe symptoms. Cesarean section may be necessary in patients with severe hip disease.

Surgery

Patients with long-standing disease that remains active can still benefit from physical therapy and medications. However, severe spinal deformities, C1-C2 cervical spine instability, and hip disease may need surgical correction to improve function. Wedge osteotomy of the spine is indicated for patients with flexion deformities preventing the ability to look forward. Cervical fusion is necessary for the few patients with atlantoaxial subluxation and spinal cord compromise. Total hip replacement is indicated in AS patients with severe pain and/or poor hip mobility. Total hip replacement is usually successful, with <10% of patients requiring revision at 10 years. However, patients with AS are at higher risk (30%) of developing heterotopic ossification following joint replacement. Use of indomethacin, bisphosphonates, or perioperative radiation (single 7 Gy fraction within 4 hours of surgery) may lessen this complication. AS patients requiring surgery should have preoperative evaluation of their temporomandibular joints and cervical spine, which can interfere with intubation, as well as their thoracic chest expansion, which can be decreased, putting them at risk for postoperative pneumonia.

[1]Not FDA approved for this indication.

MUSCULOSKELETAL DISORDERS IN THE JAW–FACE AND NECK

METHOD OF

Per-Olof Eriksson, DDS, PhD, and

Hamayun Zafar, PT, PhD

Anatomic structures are more diverse in the orofacial region than in any other region. No other location expresses so many systemic and local diseases as does the oral cavity. It serves as a focal point of interest to more medical and dental specialties than any other single part of the body. Intraoral and dental diseases are the most common cause of jaw–face pain. However, a number of possible etiological factors have to be considered in patients seeking care for pain and functional impairment in the jaw–face–head region. It is generally known that jaw–face pain and dysfunction may originate from dental, neurologic, otolaryngologic, vascular, cervical spine, metaplastic, infectious or systematic diseases. Outside the dental profession, it is less known that longstanding pain and disturbed function in the jaw–face are often due to musculoskeletal disorders, which in fact are as prevalent as the two other major dental diseases, caries and periodontitis, and therefore constitute a significant health problem. Thus, the dental profession is responsible for three major "dental" diseases which can explain jaw–face pain and dysfunction.

This article focuses on assessment and management of musculoskeletal disorders in the jaw–face region. It highlights the functional interaction between the jaw and the neck sensorimotor systems in health and disease. The article begins with a brief review of the development and maturation of structure and function of the orofacial region. Finally, the human jaw–face muscles show unique fiber types and contractile proteins, both for the extrafusal and the intrafusal (muscle spindles) fibers, and changes with aging in fiber type and myosin compositions are opposite those of limb muscles.

Development and Maturation of Structure and Function of the Jaw–Face Region

It is generally agreed that there is an orderly development and maturation of motor control, including postural control, in a cephalocaudal direction. First comes the ability to stabilize the head, followed by stabilization of the shoulder, trunk, and hips, to allow control of the lower limbs. Similarly, development is directed proximal–distal, which means that the child first learns to control proximal body segments such as the trunk, shoulders and hips, and after that hand movements.

The orofacial muscles are the first to develop in the body, in keeping with the cephalocaudal sequence of fetal development, and facial premuscle masses are formed between the gestational ages of 8 and 9 weeks. Muscular response to a stimulus first develops in the perioral region, and has been elicited at 7.5 weeks' gestational age, as a result of tactile cutaneous stimuli applied to the lips, indicating that the trigeminal nerve is the first cranial nerve to become active. Stroking the face of the 7.5-week-old embryo produces a reflex bending of the head and upper trunk away from the stimulus, an avoiding reaction, as a total neuromuscular response. Stimulation of the lips at 8.5 weeks' gestational age results in incomplete but active reflex opening of the mouth. Swallowing begins at 12 weeks' gestational age in association with extension reflexes, and occurs when the fetus drinks the amniotic fluid in which it is bathed. Tongue movements may begin at 12.5 weeks' gestational age and lip movements at 14.5 weeks' gestational age. The earliest "functional movements" include oral actions, such as suckling and swallowing, and full swallowing and suckling permitting survival occurs at only 32 to 36 weeks of fetal age. Head movements remain strongly associated with mouth movements even into the postnatal period, whereby perioral stimulation leads to ipsilateral head rotation, which in the infant is associated with suckling. Respiratory movements may be elicited by stimulation as early as 13 weeks, but spontaneous rhythmical respiration necessary for survival does not occur until much later. Increasingly complex muscle movements, producing mastication and speech, depend upon development of the appropriate reflex proprioceptive mechanisms. All of the complex interrelated orofacial movements of suckling, swallowing, and breathing are reflex in origin rather than learned, and constitute unconditioned congenital reflexes necessary for survival. Conditioned acquired reflexes develop with maturation of the neuromuscular system and are generally learned, habits. The conversion of the (a) infantile swallowing, using predominantly facial nerve muscles, into mature swallow when molar teeth have erupted and the trigeminal nerve muscles come into action, (b) infantile suckling into mastication, and (c) infantile crying into speech, are all examples of the substitution of conditioned reflexes acquired with maturation for the unconditioned congenital reflexes of the neonate. Superimposed upon these reflex movements are voluntary activities under conscious control that are acquired by learning and experience.

Pain and Dysfunction in the Jaw–Face Region

A number of diseases may give rise to similar symptoms and signs of pain and dysfunction in the jaw–face region. Assessment and management and treatment outcome are therefore related to the profession of the care provider. Thus, pain experienced in the ear may be of muscular origin, referred to the ear region from adjacent painful jaw muscles. If such pain is interpreted as being caused by infection instead of dysfunction, treatment will fail instead of being beneficial and cost-effective for patient and society.

Symptoms and signs of musculoskeletal disorders in the jaw–face region originate preferentially in the temporomandibular joint (TMJ) and the jaw–face–head muscles. Typically, they include feelings of fatigue and stiffness in the jaw and face; pain in the jaw, face, ear, head, and neck regions; sounds in the TMJ; limitation of mandibular movements; tenderness to palpation above the TMJ and jaw muscles. Pain is aggravated during jaw movements. These joint and muscle problems hamper unrestrained motor control with regard to amplitude, speed, force, coordination, direction and endurance of movement, and may result in difficulties in gaping, biting, chewing, swallowing, i.e., eating behavior, yawning, and speech.

Terminology, Epidemiology, Sex Differences

Musculoskeletal disorders in the jaw–face region are generally termed *craniomandibular disorders* (CMD) or *temporomandibular disorders* (TMD). Epidemiologic studies report a high prevalence of signs and symptoms of CMD, although prevalence rates vary. Recent data, including mild symptoms and signs, reveal average values for perceived and clinically assessed CMD to be 30% and 44%, respectively. Severe pain and dysfunction, which need treatment, are estimated to occur in the range of 5% to 10% of the adult population. There is a strong female preponderance among patients seeking care for CMD, and symptoms and signs of CMD are more frequent and severe, and more long-lasting in women than in men. No conclusive explanation for gender differences in CMD has as yet been reported. This is in accordance with what is known for musculoskeletal disorders in other body regions.

Etiology and Treatment of Craniomandibular Disorders

Knowledge about mechanisms behind musculoskeletal disorders is in general limited. Consequently, treatment and preventive care are hampered. This is the case also for musculoskeletal disorders in the jaw–face region. Generally, it is a matter of load and capacity and both central and peripheral factors seem to be of importance. Central factors include lifestyle related psychogenic muscular tension and stress induced clenching of the jaws. Peripheral factors include the stability of the bite, i.e., the relation between the lower jaw, mandibular teeth and the upper jaw, skull or "head–neck" teeth at rest and during jaw movements. Psychogenic tension and jaw clenching in a bite that lacks stability may to various degrees give rise to overload of dental and musculoskeletal components, and accordingly result in pain and dysfunction.

Studies on treatment outcome present both dental and nondental therapies, and between 65% and 95% of CMD patients who seek care for the first time are reported to improve. Treatment usually includes (a) counseling, (b) jaw exercises for tension relief and to regain movement skills, (c) a decrease of load on dental, muscle, and joint tissues by improving bite stability, which can be fulfilled by using reversible methods (e.g., intraoral appliances, bite splints) and irreversible methods (e.g., dental fillings and selective grinding of teeth), (d) drugs for relief of pain and tension, and (e) TMJ surgery when pain and dysfunction are caused by internal derangement.

Functional Coupling Between the Jaw and the Neck Regions

A line of evidence from neuroanatomic and neurophysiologic studies in animals demonstrates close connections between the trigeminal and the neck neuromuscular systems. In people, a functional coupling between the craniomandibular and the cervical spine regions is suggested by intimate anatomic and biomechanical relationships, by findings of reflex activities in the neck muscles following electrical stimulation of trigeminal nerve branches, and from observations of simultaneous activation of jaw and neck–shoulder muscles during mandibular movements. The earliest reflex found in the human embryo is the trigeminal-neck reflex, which consists of contraction of neck muscles elicited by light touch of the perioral region. Thus, previous studies in animals and people indicate a close functional linkage between the jaw and the neck regions. However, systematic studies of integrated mandibular and head–neck behavior during natural jaw function are lacking.

In a series of studies in people, using optoelectronic wireless technique for three-dimensional movement recording and electromyography, we showed concomitant and well-coordinated mandibular and head–neck movements during both single and rhythmic jaw opening–closing tasks (Figure 1). We also demonstrated that such movements are invariant in nature. The findings led us to propose a new concept for natural jaw function. In this concept, "functional jaw movements are the result of jointly activated jaw as well as neck muscles, leading to simultaneous movements in the temporomandibular, atlanto-occipital and cervical spine joints." We also suggested, based on our results, that these jaw and head–neck movements have neural commands in common and are preprogrammed. Furthermore, our findings, when combined with observations in ultrasonographic studies on human fetal yawning, that mouth opening–closing is accompanied by head extension–flexion movements, respectively, indicate that a functional connection between the jaw and the neck in natural jaw function is innate. Thus, based on results from studies in animals and people, "natural jaw function," by definition, includes integrative jaw–neck behavior.

Significance of Functional Coupling Between the Jaw and the Neck

Connections between the trigeminal system and neck motoneurons are of importance for head withdrawal reactions in all species. Any sudden or unexpected stimulus in the orofacial region leads to fast head aversion, hence paralleling the flexor reflex of the limbs. Such connections are also likely to be critical for coordinating jaw and head–neck motions, in timing of jaw opening and closing with head–neck movements during daily activities such as eating and communication.

Free neck movements are a prerequisite for natural maximal gaping. A reduced head extension ability may limit the three-dimensional space for the mandibular movement, due to impingement of the mandible with suprahyoid and airway structures. A connection between the jaw and the neck motor systems is probably of importance to allow simultaneous mandibular and head–neck movements, aimed at optimizing both the magnitude of the gape and the positioning of the gape in space. From an evolutionary perspective, such a mechanism, to optimally direct the jaw motor system, i.e., the mouth or the gape, in basic actions such as feeding, attack, and defense behavior, is probably of great survival value, e.g., during catching of prey.

Craniomandibular Disorders and Pain and Dysfunction in the Neck

Clinical trials demonstrate an association between CMD and neck symptoms, that pain and dysfunction in the neck are often present in patients with CMD. It is also known that patients with neck problems may have signs and symptoms of CMD. In fact, randomized controlled trials show that treatment of CMD in patients who were on sick leave for neck–shoulder pain and dysfunction, but who also had CMD, gave relief of both CMD and neck–shoulder symptoms. Notably, treatment outcome was measured in terms of reduced number of days on sick leave and use of medical services. The treatment consisted of improvement

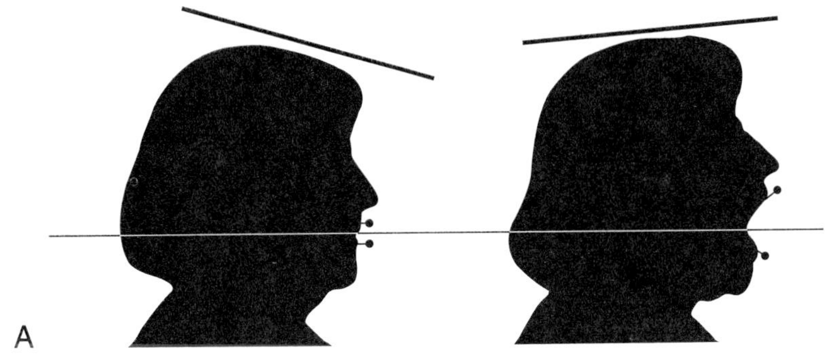

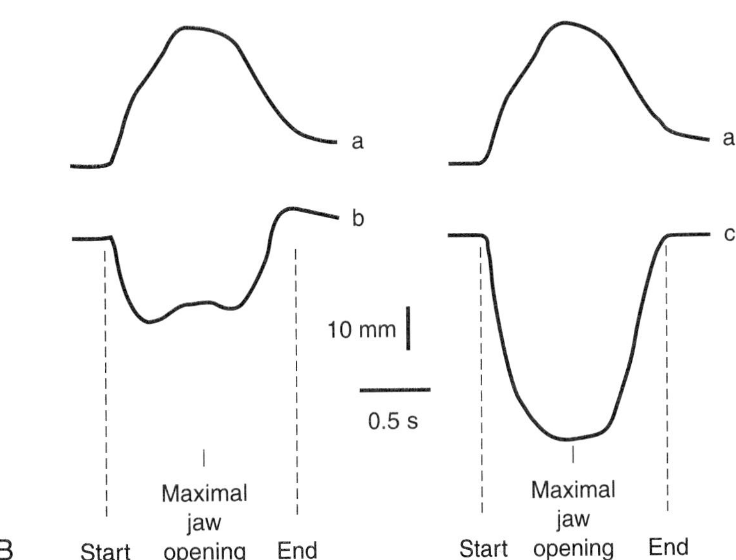

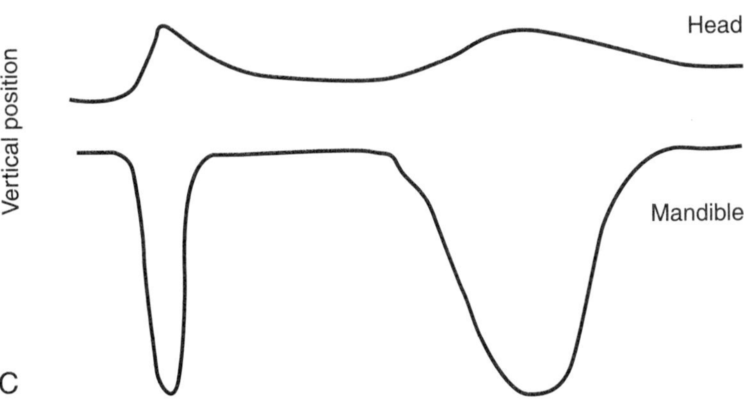

FIGURE 1 **A**, Head position at rest (*left*) and at maximal jaw opening (*right*). Note change in head position indicated by reference line above the head and recording markers attached to the upper and lower frontal teeth. Note also the relatively unchanged midposition of the gape at maximal jaw opening, indicated by the horizontal reference line. **B**, Movement trajectories in vertical dimension over time of the mandible (*b, c*) and the head (*a*) for a maximal jaw opening–closing movement. Start and end of movement are labeled. The *left panel* (*b*) illustrates the mandibular movement "in space," i.e., the trajectory is the result of the combined mandibular and head–neck movements. The *right panel* (*c*) shows the magnitude of the mandibular movement after mathematical compensation for head movement, i.e., in relation to the head. **C**, Movement trajectories in vertical dimension over time of head–neck and mandibular movements at fast (*left*) and slow (*right*) jaw opening–closing tasks, and after mathematical compensation for head movements. Note simultaneous start of mandibular and head movements.

of bite stability by selective grinding of the lower and upper teeth. Such adjustment of peripheral input probably influences the relation between the mandible and the head–neck biomechanically, by changing the functional load on jaw and neck components, and with regard to integrative sensorimotor control of the jaw and neck.

Craniomandibular Disorders in Whiplash-Associated Disorders

Trauma to the neck from a motor vehicle accident or some other type of head–neck trauma, generally called whiplash trauma or injury, may lead to a condition comprising a number of symptoms and signs in the neck and head termed *whiplash-associated disorders* (WAD). Studies indicate that such head–neck trauma can result in pain and dysfunction in the jaw–face region (i.e., CMD), although the matter is under debate.

Our studies on integrated jaw–neck motor control in healthy subjects and in WAD patients have led to an explanatory model for the development of CMD in subjects who have met with whiplash injury. Given that natural jaw actions require a healthy state with unrestricted motion of both the temporomandibular joint and the atlanto-occipital and cervical spine joints, it can be assumed that an injury to or disease of any of these three joint systems might derange natural jaw motor control. Furthermore, such a functional impairment would be reflected by disturbed jaw–neck behavior, which could be detected by recording and analyzing concomitant mandibular and head–neck movements during natural jaw actions. We recently tested this hypothesis by studying integrative jaw–neck function in patients suffering from WAD and pain and dysfunction in the jaw–face. The results show an association between neck trauma and disturbed jaw–neck function, indicating that coordinated jaw–neck motor control during both single and rhythmic jaw opening–closing movements indeed can be disturbed following neck injury. Thus it can be proposed that *cervicocraniomandibular disorders* (CCMD) is an appropriate term for the clinical condition comprising both jaw–face and head–neck pain and dysfunction.

Treatment Model for Improvement of Mandibular and Head–Neck Mobility

Our studies on integrative jaw–neck function include measurement of magnitude, temporal coordination, speed, and spatiotemporal consistency of concomitant mandibular and head–neck movements. By applying the methods we developed for analysis of healthy jaw–neck behavior in investigations of patients, we have found signs of disturbed jaw–neck function in individuals suffering from WAD. Based on the findings in healthy subjects and in patients, we developed a new model for treatment of pain and dysfunction in the jaw–face and WAD. This treatment approach is aimed at improving both mandibular and head–neck mobility, thereby regaining natural jaw function. The model is based on the fact that motor control starts to develop and mature in the jaw–orofacial region (as described above), and that data from numerous studies in animals and people suggest a close linkage between the jaw and the neck sensorimotor systems in natural jaw function. Consequently, treatment for improving jaw function should include the neck. Our studies to test this treatment model in patients with jaw–face pain and dysfunction and WAD show improvement of both jaw and neck function, results that merit further studies in randomized clinical trials.

Figure 2 shows a typical example, data from a female patient, 30 years of age, who had met with a car accident and developed WAD 4 years before she was referred to the department of Clinical Oral Physiology, Umeå University Hospital, Umeå, Sweden for assessment and management of pain and dysfunction in the jaw and face. The patient had received all care and treatment for WAD available according to routines used by the health care system. Our examination revealed severely impaired jaw and neck function and widespread pain in all body regions. The initial, pretreatment, investigation of concomitant mandibular and head–neck movements during jaw opening–closing tasks, using our routine protocol and optoelectronic wireless three-dimensional movement recording technique, verified the functional impairment of jaw–neck behavior. As seen in Figure 2 the follow-up recordings after 4 and 7 months show an increase in magnitude of movement amplitudes of both the mandibular and the head–neck movement. In addition, the speed of movement increased. The figure also illustrates that functional impairment, as well as change in behavior in response to treatment, can be measured and documented qualitatively and quantitatively by objective recording methods.

Treatment Regimen for Craniomandibular Disorders and Whiplash-Associated Disorders

The general aim of the treatment regimen was to regain natural jaw function by "reprogramming" faulty jaw–neck sensorimotor behavior. In short, this was performed by (a) education, advice, and instructions with regard to anatomy, physiology, pathophysiology, and treatment; (b) specific jaw–neck exercises, including mandibular and head–neck movements to gain successive increase in movement amplitude and speed in very minor steps, i.e., to slowly "reteach" the neuromuscular system to execute coordinated mandibular and head–neck movements in

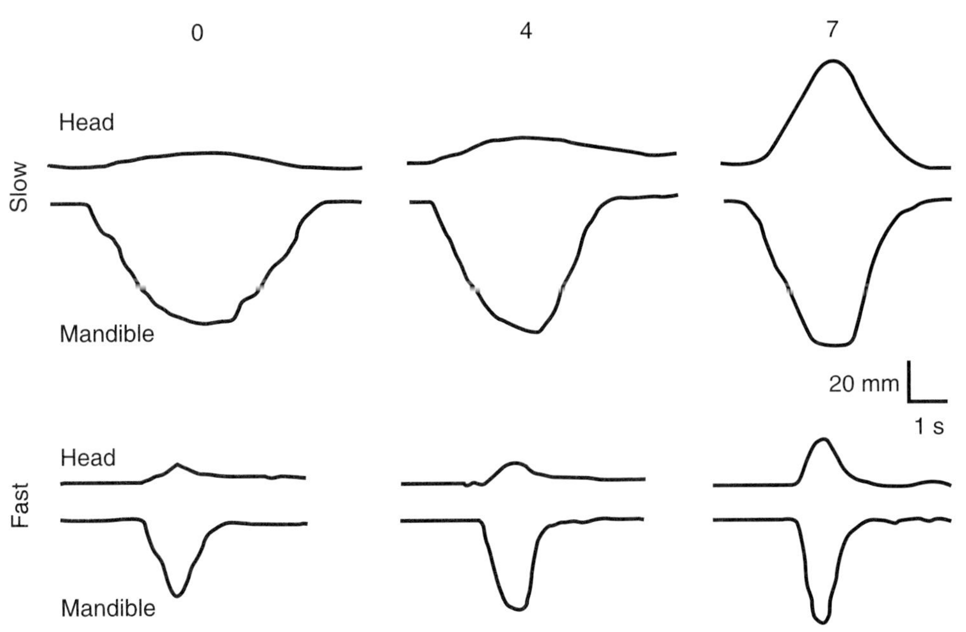

FIGURE 2 Repeated movement recordings in a female patient, 30 years old, suffering from whiplash-associated disorders and pain and dysfunction in the jaw–face. Trajectories for the vertical dimension over time of mandibular and head–neck movements at slow (*upper panel*) and fast (*lower panel*) maximal jaw opening–closing tasks. Initial, pretreatment, recording (0), and recordings after 4 and 7 months of treatment. Note post-treatment increase in amplitude and speed for both mandibular and head–neck movements, and for both slow and fast jaw opening–closing tasks.

a cost-effective way; and (c) a custom-made intraoral appliance (bite splint) attached to the upper teeth for day and night use, to change biomechanical relations, reducing detrimental load on sensitized components of the jaw–neck motor system and give pain relief, and to modulate sensorimotor settings for control of jaw–neck behavior and disturb jaw-clenching habits.

Summary

- Because different diseases in the jaw–orofacial region may give rise to similar symptoms, proper examination and diagnosis must precede treatment.
- Musculoskeletal disorders in the jaw–face region, generally termed craniomandibular disorders (CMD), are as prevalent as the two major dental diseases, caries and periodontitis, and constitute a significant health problem.
- There is a strong female preponderance among patients seeking care for CMD, and symptoms and signs are more frequent, severe, and longer-lasting in women than in men.
- Between 65% and 95% of CMD patients who seek care for the first time are reported to improve.
- A new concept for natural jaw function suggests that "functional jaw movements" are the result of jointly activated jaw and neck muscles, leading to simultaneous movements in the temporomandibular, atlanto-occipital, and cervical spine joints, and that these jaw and head–neck movements have neural commands in common, are preprogrammed, and are innate. Accordingly, natural jaw function, by definition, includes integrative jaw–neck behavior.
- A new explanatory model for the development of pain and dysfunction in the jaw–face in subjects with whiplash-associated disorders (WAD) proposes because natural jaw actions require a healthy state of the temporomandibular, atlanto-occipital, and cervical spine joints, it can be assumed that an injury to or disease of any of these three joint systems might derange natural jaw motor control.
- Based on findings of disturbed jaw–neck function in WAD, a new treatment model is suggested for patients with jaw–face pain and dysfunction and WAD, The rationale behind this approach is that intervention of jaw function by definition includes neck function. Results from implementation of this treatment model, showing improvement of magnitude and speed for both mandibular and head–neck movements, are reported.
- Finally, an appropriate term for the clinical condition comprising both jaw–face and head–neck pain and dysfunction is cervicocraniomandibular disorders (CCMD).

BURSITIS, TENDINITIS, MYOFASCIAL PAIN, AND FIBROMYALGIA

METHOD OF

Daniel J. Clauw, MD

Approximately 10% of the population suffers from chronic widespread pain, and approximately 20% suffers from chronic regional pain. In population-based studies, chronic pain is about 1.5 times more common in women than in men. In clinical samples, an even higher proportion of individuals seen for chronic pain are women, because women are more likely to seek health care than men.

In general terms, there are three reasons for chronic pain: (a) regional (e.g., tendinitis or bursitis) or widespread (e.g., rheumatoid arthritis or systemic lupus erythematosus) inflammation; (b) damage to peripheral tissues (e.g., osteoarthritis, neuropathy), and (c) "central pain" (i.e., myofascial pain, fibromyalgia). This article focuses on the diagnosis and management of regional inflammatory conditions and central pain syndromes.

Diagnostic Considerations

A careful musculoskeletal history and examination remains the most important diagnostic test for musculoskeletal pain. In contrast to other fields of medicine, where proliferation in technology has largely rendered a physical examination obsolete, in musculoskeletal medicine, technology confuses as much as it helps. For example, a high proportion of the healthy, asymptomatic population has a positive antinuclear antibody (as high as 20% have a 1:40 titer), positive rheumatoid factor, or abnormal results of imaging studies (50% of individuals older than age 60 years has one or more bulging disks on magnetic resonance imaging [MRI]). Worse yet, there is typically a poor correlation between what is seen on imaging studies and the degree of pain an individual is experiencing. Therefore, the musculoskeletal history and examination must enable the clinician to arrive at the diagnosis or, at worst, a very narrow differential diagnosis, and then, if necessary, further diagnostic testing can be used to confirm these findings.

In diagnosing the above conditions, the physical examination looking for specific areas of tenderness is vitally important. In a regional inflammatory condition such as bursitis, the individual typically is only tender over the affected bursae. In tendinitis, the tendon may be tender, but more typically the pain can be exacerbated by maneuvers that stretch or use the tendon. In myofascial pain, the individual is tender over an entire region of the body that is typically muscular, whereas in fibromyalgia, the tenderness extends throughout the entire body.

Bursitis and Tendinitis

Although the body has more than 150 bursae, and even more tendons, only a few commonly become painful. Although the terms *tendinitis* and *bursitis* are used in this article because these remain the preferred semantic terms, the reader should be aware that in many cases there is no actual evidence of inflammation (i.e., *-itis*) when these regions are carefully studied. In some cases the pain may be from accumulation of fluid, or from more regional neurologic processes that remain poorly understood at present. Also, when there is inflammation, it is typically of the tendon sheath (i.e., tenosynovitis) rather than the tendon *per se.*

HAND/WRIST

Perhaps the most common tendinitis or tenosynovitis in the hand is a "trigger finger," or flexor tenosynovitis. Individuals usually present with a painless complaint of their fingers "locking" in a flexed position, although they can typically extend the finger forcefully by pulling on it. In many cases, if the finger is forcefully flexed and extended while palpating the flexor tendon, the "triggering" can be palpated, and/or a lump can be detected. When the extensor tendons of the hand are affected by tenosynovitis, the typical presentation is of a mass on the dorsum of the hand or wrist. Such a mass is typically filled with very viscous fluid (it feels this way on examination) that moves when the individual flexes and extends the digits. Less-common problems are De Quervain's tenosynovitis, which affects the tendon that extends the thumb, and acute calcific periarthritis, which presents as an acutely inflamed tendon in the hand, typically in females.

ELBOW

Arthritis of the elbow is exceedingly rare. Three alternative and common causes of elbow pain are olecranon bursitis and medial and lateral epicondylitis. In olecranon bursitis, individuals present with swelling over the olecranon process; in some cases this can be quite large. If this swelling is painless and there is no evidence of inflammation (e.g., warmth, redness, overlying open wound) on examination, this may just represent post-traumatic olecranon bursitis, and no specific treatment is necessary. On the other hand, infection and crystals (e.g., uric acid or calcium pyrophosphate) can both cause an inflammatory olecranon bursitis; if inflammation is present on examination, the bursae must be aspirated and treated appropriately. Lateral epicondylitis ("tennis elbow") and medical epicondylitis ("golf elbow") are common conditions that present with elbow pain, but in fact typically occur because of overuse at the wrist. Overuse of the wrist extensors can lead to lateral epicondylitis, where individuals will have pain at the insertion of these muscles at the lateral epicondyle. This pain will be exacerbated by having the individual hyperextend the wrist and forcefully opposing this motion. The "opposite" condition is medial epicondylitis, in which individuals have pain at the medial epicondyle, worsened by opposition against wrist flexion.

SHOULDER

Again, arthritis of the shoulder is exceedingly uncommon. Most pain in this region occurs because of pathology in the rotator cuff structures, or, less commonly, in the acromioclavicular joint. Because the rotator cuff muscles are responsible for abducting and externally rotating the arm, individuals will give a history of difficulty lifting their arm over their head, brushing their hair, reaching into the back seat of a car, and the like. One useful test is to ask the individual to stand with both arms at the sides and slowly abduct the "painful" arm, informing the examiner when pain occurs. In isolated rotator cuff problems (without concurrent adhesive capsulitis), individuals will typically have a "painful arc" from approximately 20 to 110 degrees of motion. Another useful test for rotator cuff pathology is to examine for evidence of impingement, by holding firmly over the acromial process as the arm is abducted. Finally, careful palpation in the shoulder region can identify discrete evidence of bursitis, such as subacromial (palpated in midline, in the "notch" between the acromial process and the head of the humerus) or subdeltoid bursitis.

HIP

The most common soft-tissue problem to affect this region is trochanteric bursitis. Individuals typically complain of pain in the hip, and note that the pain is worst when they lie on that side in bed or change position. In contrast, pathology of the hip joint is more likely painful in the groin, and typically is worse with weight-bearing or rotating the hip. Individuals with trochanteric bursitis have significant pain directly over the greater trochanter, which is the most lateral portion in this region if an individual is standing upright. A less-common area of bursitis is the buttock region, especially ischiogluteal bursitis.

KNEE

There are several soft-tissue rheumatism problems that can occur in the knee region and "simulate" (or occur concurrently with) osteoarthritis. The anserine bursa is located on the medial portion of the knee, approximately 3 cm below the true knee joint. This will be extremely painful to touch if inflamed. Two other commonly inflamed bursae are in the anterior midline, just above and below the patellae. Prepatellar bursitis is similar to olecranon bursitis, in that infection needs to be excluded, especially if there is a history of trauma or an abrasion. Infrapatellar bursitis is sometimes called "housemaid's knee" because it commonly occurs because of prolonged kneeling.

FOOT/ANKLE

Pain in the Achilles region can either occur because of Achilles tendinitis or retrocalcaneal bursitis. In the former, there is pain throughout the entire tendon that is worsened by dorsiflexing the ankle, whereas in the latter, the pain is more localized to a discrete region (i.e., the bursae) over the tendon. Retrocalcaneal bursitis is often caused or exacerbated by wearing shoes that apply pressure to this region.

TREATMENT

For both bursitis and tendinitis, in addition to treating the problem, it is also important to attempt to address the underlying cause. Most of these conditions occur because of "overuse," although it is sometimes very difficult to determine the precise nature of the problem. Sometimes the inciting action can be elucidated by asking patients to record what they are doing when pain occurs. In other cases, the overuse is much more subtle, e.g., a leg-length discrepancy or pain in the contralateral foot leading to trochanteric bursitis.

If the inciting event can be identified, cessation or correction of this activity (sometimes combined with the use of a nonsteroidal anti-inflammatory drug [NSAID]) is frequently all that is necessary to treat tendinitis or bursitis. In more refractory cases of tendinitis, splinting (e.g., of the wrist for medial or lateral epicondylitis), physical therapy (especially in regions such as the shoulder where immobility may lead to a "frozen shoulder"), or injection with corticosteroids can all be effective and necessary. Corticosteroid injections are quite safe and efficacious, but should be avoided in large, weight-bearing tendons (e.g., Achilles), and probably should not be given frequently (e.g., more than twice over a few weeks/months).

Myofascial Pain

There are two broad schools of thought within the myofascial pain field. The older view is that myofascial pain represents a "peripheral" problem of muscle, and can be detected by the presence of "trigger points" and "taut bands" in muscle. Trigger points are not the same as tender points; when such regions are palpated, individuals will typically experience pain not just at the area of palpation, but also referred to a different (typically adjacent) region. The other "school" feels that myofascial pain is just a regional variant of fibromyalgia. This theory suggests that although pain may be located in one region of the body, in many cases there is more widespread evidence of pain amplification (i.e., tenderness not just where the individual is experiencing pain) and accompanying somatic symptoms (e.g., fatigue, sleep disturbance, headaches). These views are not mutually exclusive. In fact, it is likely that there are some individuals with myofascial pain who have a more peripheral problem (regional pain, regional tenderness, no other symptoms) and some who have a regional form of fibromyalgia.

For those with more peripheral syndromes, there are a variety of therapies that can be helpful. A number of "manual therapies," such as myofascial release therapy or deep massage, "spray and stretch" techniques (a freezing spray is applied and then the region is stretched), chiropractic manipulation, and acupuncture, may be of benefit. Injections may also be helpful, although "dry" needling is likely as beneficial as injection of anesthetics and/or corticosteroids. The injection of botulinum toxin type A (Botox)[1] may be effective in some instances.

With respect to pharmacologic therapy, NSAIDs may be tried. Muscle relaxants, such as cyclobenzaprine (Flexeril)[1], best tolerated if given as a single dose of 5 to 20[3] mg a few hours before bedtime, or others can also be of benefit. It is particularly important that individuals with acute or subacute myofascial pain retain their normal activities and exercise. This is best understood in low back pain, where we know that rest and cessation of routine exercise leads to a much higher rate of chronicity of symptoms. This suggests that our generic advice that people should "rest" or take off work when they have such problems may be ill-advised.

Fibromyalgia

Diffuse pain is a defining symptom of fibromyalgia, and also occurs in a number of other settings. The diagnostic evaluation of an individual with diffuse pain varies depending on the duration of symptoms, and the findings in the history and physical examination. Diffuse pain that has been present for years is likely to be caused by fibromyalgia, especially if there are accompanying symptoms such as fatigue, memory difficulties, and sleep disturbance, and the individual is tender on examination. In this setting, a minimal workup is necessary.

In contrast, an individual who has diffuse pain for weeks or months needs a more extensive evaluation. In performing the evaluation, particular attention should be focused on the onset and character of the pain, accompanying symptoms, and "exposures" that could be causing the symptoms (especially to both prescription and over-the-counter drugs and supplements). The examination should focus on identifying signs of inflammation (e.g., synovitis), or other findings (e.g., objective weakness) that are not seen in fibromyalgia.

At a minimum, individuals who present with chronic, widespread pain should have a complete blood count, liver and kidney function tests, thyroid-stimulating hormone (TSH), and sedimentation rate (or C-reactive protein) performed during the course of their illness. Because fibromyalgia occurs less frequently in males, some physicians suggest more aggressive diagnostic testing when a male presents with symptoms consistent with fibromyalgia (especially for conditions that are more common in males, such as sleep apnea and hepatitis C infection).

The overlap between fibromyalgia and autoimmune disorders deserves special mention. Many individuals early in the course of autoimmune disorders may present with symptoms reminiscent of fibromyalgia, but a larger problem is that many patients with nonspecific symptoms of fibromyalgia have laboratory testing performed that suggests they may have an autoimmune disorder (e.g., positive antinuclear antibody [ANA] or rheumatoid factor). Symptoms that can be seen in both fibromyalgia and autoimmune disorders include arthralgias, myalgias, and fatigue, as well as morning stiffness and a history of subjective swelling of the hands and feet. In addition, a Raynaud-like syndrome (characterized by the *entire hand* turning pale or red instead of just the digits), malar flushing (in contrast to a fixed malar rash), and livedo reticularis are all common in fibromyalgia, and can mislead the practitioner to suspect an autoimmune disorder.

FIBROMYALGIA SYNDROME

Clinical Features

To fulfill the American College of Rheumatology criteria for fibromyalgia, an individual must have both a *history* of chronic widespread pain involving all four quadrants of the body (and the axial skeleton), and the presence of 11 of 18 "tender points" on *physical examination.* These criteria were never intended to be strictly applied to individual patients as diagnostic criteria. In clinical practice, most individuals who have chronic widespread pain, and no inflammatory or mechanical damage that can account for the pain, probably have fibromyalgia. Finding tenderness in multiple locations and/or multiple somatic symptoms (fatigue, insomnia, headache, irritable bowel or bladder) makes it more likely this is the correct diagnosis.

Although both pain and tenderness are defining features of fibromyalgia, the latter is rarely a presenting complaint. The pain of fibromyalgia frequently waxes and wanes, may be quite migratory, and may be accompanied by dysesthesias or paresthesias following

[1]Not FDA approved for this indication.

[3]Exceeds dosage recommended by the manufacturer.

a nondermatomal distribution. In some instances, patients present with "aching all over," whereas in other instances, patients experience several areas of chronic regional pain. In this setting, regional musculoskeletal pain typically involves the axial skeleton, or areas of "tender points," and may originally be diagnosed as a local problem (e.g., low back pain, lateral epicondylitis). Regional pain involving nonmusculoskeletal regions is also common, including a higher-than-expected prevalence of both tension and migraine headaches, temporomandibular dysfunction (or temporomandibular joint) syndrome, noncardiac chest pain, irritable bowel syndrome, a number of entities characterized by chronic pelvic pain, and plantar or heel pain.

In addition to pain and tenderness, many individuals with these illnesses experience fatigue (thus many also meet criteria for chronic fatigue syndrome), memory difficulties, fluctuations in weight, heat and cold intolerance, and the subjective sensation of weakness. Patients with fibromyalgia and related illnesses also display a wide array of hypersensitivity symptoms, ranging from adverse reactions to drugs and environmental stimuli, to vasomotor rhinitis, and hyperacusis. Individuals also suffer from a number of symptoms of "functional" disorders of visceral organs, including a high incidence of recurrent noncardiac chest pain, heartburn, palpitations, mitral valve prolapse, esophageal dysmotility, and irritable bowel symptoms. Neurally mediated hypotension and syncope also occur more frequently in these individuals. Similar syndromes characterized by visceral pain and/or smooth-muscle dysmotility are also seen in the pelvis, including dysmenorrhea, urinary frequency, and urinary urgency, interstitial cystitis, endometriosis, and vulvar vestibulitis or vulvodynia.

The physical examination is generally unremarkable in fibromyalgia, other than finding tenderness. The tenderness may be virtually anywhere, and is not just confined to tender points. The former concept of "control points," previously described as areas of the body that should not be tender, has been abandoned.

Laboratory testing should be used judiciously. Even if the individual has acute or subacute onset of symptoms, ordering serologic assays such as ANA and rheumatoid factor should generally be avoided unless there is strong evidence for an autoimmune disorder.

Treatment

General Approach

At present, the treatment of fibromyalgia is as much art as science. Once an individual with this diagnosis is identified, the practitioner first has to consider whether to "label" the individual. For the majority, this label will help them understand their symptoms and the most appropriate treatment, but there may be some individuals for whom this is harmful.

The practitioner should schedule a prolonged visit, or series of visits, when this diagnosis is considered. This "up-front" time is extremely useful for both patients and providers, as it helps the physician understand precisely what is bothering the patient, and assists the patient in understanding the goals and rationale of treatment. The physician should explore the symptoms that are most bothersome, the impact of these symptoms are having on various aspects of the patient's life, their perception about what is causing these symptoms, and the stressors that may be exacerbating the problem.

Education

Some patients who present with symptoms of fibromyalgia want only to be told that this is a benign, nonprogressive condition. These patients generally have milder symptoms that have been present for some time, and they possess adequate strategies for improving symptoms and maintaining function. The physician should describe this condition in terms the patient feels most comfortable with, and then refer the patient to reputable sources of information such as the Arthritis Foundation, several national patient support organizations, or up-to-date web sites (e.g., www.med.umich.edu/painresearch).

Pharmacologic Therapies

Tricyclic compounds, notably amitriptyline (Elavil)[1] and cyclobenzaprine (Flexeril)[1], are the most extensively studied agents for the treatment of fibromyalgia and other central pain syndromes. To increase the tolerance of cyclobenzaprine and amitriptyline, these compounds should be administered several hours before bedtime, begun at low doses (10 mg or less), and increased very slowly (10 mg every 1 to 2 weeks) until the patient reaches the maximally beneficial dose (up to 40 mg of cyclobenzaprine or 70 to 80 mg of amitriptyline).

Because of the side effects of tricyclics, recent studies have examined the efficacy of better tolerated compounds in these conditions. Selective serotonin reuptake inhibitors (SSRIs) are not as effective analgesics as tricyclic antidepressants (TCAs), but can be a useful adjunct in fibromyalgia, especially if the individual has depression. Using either a SSRI or a mixed reuptake inhibitor such as venlafaxine (Effexor)[1] (37.5 or 75 mg extended-release capsule given in the morning, or as a split dose in the morning and early afternoon) with a low dose of a TCA at night is quite useful for many patients. If individuals have excessive side effects from TCA, alternative compounds to use for insomnia include zolpidem (Ambien), zaleplon (Sonata), and trazodone (Desyrel) (50 to 200 mg at bedtime). If patients need additional analgesia despite TCA and a mixed reuptake inhibitor, compounds such as gabapentin (Neurontin)[1] (up to 2400 mg per day with a higher percentage of dosage in the evening), tramadol (Ultram)[1], or tizanidine

[1]Not FDA approved for this indication.

(Zanaflex)[1] can be useful. For patients in whom fatigue and/or cognitive difficulties are problematic, activating compounds such as venlafaxine (Effexor)[1], bupropion (Wellbutrin)[1], and modafinil (Provigil)[1] may be useful, as may long-acting amphetamines. In persons with symptoms suggestive of autonomic dysfunction, such as orthostatic intolerance, vasomotor instability, or palpitations, increased fluid and sodium/potassium intake, and/or low doses of β blockers, might be of benefit.

Nonpharmacologic Therapies

As individuals experience chronic pain and fatigue, they typically become less active, reduce or eliminate exercise, become withdrawn or isolated, and find difficulty functioning in roles at home and work. Any of these behavioral responses to symptoms can, in and of themselves, worsen pain and other symptoms. So the physician must dually address (a) *symptom* improvement primarily with pharmacologic therapy, and (b) *functional* improvement with nonpharmacologic therapies such as cognitive behavioral therapy (CBT) and aerobic exercise.

Cognitive behavioral therapy refers to a structured education program that focuses on teaching individuals skills that they can use to improve their illness. CBT is effective in improving patient outcomes in nearly every chronic medical illness, including fibromyalgia, and needs to be tailored to the specific condition being treated. The skills most commonly associated with CBT for pain include relaxation training, activity pacing, pleasant activity scheduling, visual imagery techniques, distraction strategies, focal point and visual distraction, cognitive restructuring, problem solving, and goal setting. A goal of CBT is to allow patients to gain more control of their illness, and to give them the tools to accomplish this.

Aerobic exercise has likewise been demonstrated to be effective at improving outcomes for a wide range of conditions, including fibromyalgia. The reason for the benefit is likely multifactorial, because aerobic exercise has an analgesic as well as antidepressant effect, and can enhance the sense of well-being and control. Patients may experience a worsening of symptoms immediately after exercise, and thus fear that any form of exercise will exacerbate their condition. To reduce the pain associated with exercise, low-impact exercises such as aquatic exercise, walking, swimming, or stationary cycling are recommended. Just as with medication, a "start low, go slow" approach appears to be most effective, with a gradual progression in exercise intensity and a focus on adherence to a lifelong program being of paramount importance.

Several different types of complementary therapies are used by physicians and patients to treat fibromyalgia. Some of these are physical modalities such as trigger-point injections, myofascial release therapy (or other "hands-on" techniques), acupuncture, and chiropractic manipulation, each of which has some data supporting efficacy.

Because there are very few controlled trials that can guide the practitioner in how to grapple with these treatment modalities, a general approach is suggested. The practitioner should first evaluate the safety of the proposed treatment, and point out to the patient any potential harmful effects. The physician should then consider whether this treatment is reinforcing a maladaptive belief, that in the long run will be harmful to the patient (e.g., a treatment program of prolonged bed rest, or of isolation). If the treatment is neither harmful nor maladaptive, then the practitioner may suggest that the patient conduct the equivalent of a clinical trial on themselves (as is done in "n of 1" trials). In this setting, the patient begins a single treatment (keeping all other variables constant) and determines if the treatment is beneficial. If the patient judges the treatment to be helpful, then the treatment should be discontinued to determine if the symptoms worsen. If the treatment withstands this test of efficacy, a placebo effect cannot be excluded, but in clinical practice, especially in an enigmatic condition such as fibromyalgia, it is difficult to argue with success.

[1]Not FDA approved for this indication.

OSTEOARTHRITIS

METHOD OF

George E. Ehrlich, MD

In some respects, the term *osteoarthritis* is a misnomer because it refers only to a subset of joint changes—those accompanied by inflammation. An older, and still popular name in some parts of the world, is osteoarthrosis, which implies a condition of the joints without inflammation, and perhaps this should be revived for a majority of cases, in which pain is minimal at worst. A former synonym, degenerative joint disease, has been largely discarded, as it implies a specificity that cannot be supported. The confusion arises from the fact that no adequate definition of the term exists, and osteoarthritis occurs in almost all individuals past middle life, as well as in many individuals who are younger, but symptomatic osteoarthritis afflicts only a minority of these. Part of the reason why no adequate definition exists derives from the roentgenographic criteria: a narrowing of "joint space" implies loss of cartilage (there is no real space in a joint, only the distance between the bones, composed of cartilage, which is radiolucent unless it contains crystals or metabolic derivatives), but other attributes, such as marginal osteophytes, are part of the repair process, and geodes (cysts in the subchondral bone) may even be part of the pathogenesis. The pathologist's definition includes diminished cartilage, fibrillation of cartilage, cartilaginous debris, the osteophytes and geodes, eburnation (smoothing of exposed bone denuded of its cartilage), and, in many instances, angiogenesis and increased vascularity. The clinician is confronted chiefly by symptomatic osteoarthritis, although roentgenograms taken for any purpose that include diarthrodial joints may disclose joint changes that can delude one into attributing symptoms to these; this is particularly true of spinal changes at the discs and intervertebral neural foramina.

From the standpoint of therapy, only symptomatic osteoarthritis requires treatment, and even much of that remains under dispute. Prevention would obviously be best, if it could be achieved, but in such a slowly developing process as osteoarthritis, it would require a lifetime of effort and may still not be attainable. Osteoarthritis, then, is not a disease but a final common pathway for all insults, overuse and abuse of a joint, begun by trauma, diseases of metabolism, heritable and genetic predisposition, hormonal influences, and inflammatory diseases of the joints. The initial insult may well have occurred in childhood, but the expression as osteoarthritis takes years to develop (faster when the insult is severe, as in athletic injury, slower if because of repetitive minor trauma, and slower yet if the inception was minimal). But when it becomes symptomatic, osteoarthritis fits the definition of disease and challenges treatment paradigms.

Osteoarthritis must be viewed as a reparative process, as confirmed by its antiquity: it is found in skeletons of prehistoric animals and early hominids; it afflicted all vertebrates that lived long enough. At that, it is not a manifestation of aging, only a slowly developing process that requires time and is, therefore, more common in elderly individuals. Weather changes influence symptoms but not the process itself. There is no particular geographic predilection. Although some patterns are more common in some populations (e.g., interphalangeal osteoarthritis, which, except as a consequence of trauma, is rarely found in Africans and east Asians), that applies chiefly to interphalangeal osteoarthritis in which rows of joints are involved, and not to single large joints. Obesity has been cited as a precursor, a reasonable contention for affliction of weight-bearing joints, but equally true for interphalangeal osteoarthritis, where it should theoretically play no role. Increased bone density seems to parallel osteoarthritis, but whether causal or consequential needs to be determined (similarly, osteoporosis and osteoarthritis tend to be mutually exclusive, but again cause and effect are problematic). Some investigators have looked for causes in the bone: subchondral microfractures and bone marrow edema have been cited, but again the relationship to expression remains controversial. Table 1 lists some of the known precursors and Table 2 lists some of the presumed risk factors. Ultimately, osteoarthritis is thought to be a disease of chondrocyte fatigue, accelerated when the effete chondrocytes can no longer replace proteoglycans, leading to structural alterations. Chondrocalcinosis, with deposition of hydroxy apatite or calcium pyrophosphate dihydrate, commonly accompanies symptomatic osteoarthritis, but may play more of a role in causing symptoms than contributing to pathogenesis. Although some would classify osteoarthritis as primary or secondary, it probably is always secondary, even if the inception is remote in the past and long forgotten. Remember that osteoarthritis is not an acute disease, even if punctuated by acute painful episodes in approximately 15% to 20% of those in whom roentgenographic evidence of osteoarthritis exists.

TABLE 1 Precursors of Osteoarthritis

Congenital, hereditary, inborn	Slipped femoral epiphysis, Legg-Calvé-Perthes disease Bone dysplasias ? Kashin-Beck disease, ? Mseleni joint disease, ? familial Mediterranean fever
Metabolic	Ochronosis, hemochromatosis, calcium pyrophosphate deposition disease, gout
Traumatic	Acute (e.g., athletic injury) or chronic (repetitive trauma)
Endocrine	Diabetes mellitus, acromegaly, ? obesity (cofactor?)
Idiopathic joint disease	Rheumatoid arthritis, septic arthritis
Vascular	Avascular necrosis
Neurologic	Charcot joint, Charcot-Marie-Tooth disease
Bone disease	Paget's disease (osteitis deformans)

TABLE 2 Risk Factors

Aging	Time duration; weak muscle control (lower extremities)
Sex predilection	Women: interphalangeal osteoarthritis, knees in valgus
Obesity	May be cofactor (interphalangeal, knees in women)
Genetics	Symmetrical Heberden's nodes, Ehlers-Danlos syndrome, genetic collagen abnormalities
Endocrine	Elevated growth hormone concentrations (postmenopause?)
Diet?	
Bone density	Increased bone density; osteopetrosis
Race	Site predilections that may be racially related
Occupation	Jackhammers and similar tools, habitual usage (e.g., specific finger joints in knitting shop workers; elbows in foundry workers, knees in professional football running backs, shoulders in baseball pitchers, etc.)
Avocation	Knees and hips in joggers and runners on hard surfaces (not those who continue but those who drop out)
Inflammation	Calcium pyrophosphate dihydrate, hydroxy apatite, other crystal depositions
Trauma	Acute and severe, repetitive but mild to moderate

Regional Issues

Patterns differ and give clues to pathogenesis. The knees are more frequently afflicted in women, perhaps because the broader pelvis leads to genu valgum and predisposes to knee afflictions. However, although cartilage loss on the gliding surface of the patella generally results in symptoms, even major cartilage loss in the opposing surfaces of the femur and tibia may not, and the anatomic features fail to correlate with symptomatic expression. Although proprioceptive changes were thought to play a role in the pathogenesis of knee osteoarthritis, recent studies refute this contention.

The hips tend to be more often afflicted in men. The classic FABERE maneuver (flexion, abduction, external rotation, and extension) reveals limitations of motion and elicits pain. However, in time, knee and hip osteoarthritis is nearly equal in the sexes.

Osteoarthritis of the distal interphalangeal (DIP) joints (Heberden's nodes) and proximal interphalangeal joints (PIP), usually symmetrical, occurs in white women at about the time of menopause (earlier after total hysterectomies) and implies genetic predisposition; nonsymmetrical involvement of these joints is often a consequence of specific traumas or work exposure. The symmetrical variety often bares erosive changes at the joint margins, and is accompanied by the traditional signs of inflammation at presentation: redness, heat, swelling, pain, and functional deficits. The joints at the bases of the thumbs (first carpometacarpal, or trapeziometacarpal joints) tend also to be involved, and even the metacarpophalangeal joints, which rarely develop osteoarthritis in other circumstances. In these women, accompanying osteoarthritis at other joints is unrelated to the heredofamilial variety, bearing a casual, not causal, relationship.

The encroachment of osteophytes on the intervertebral foramina in the movable sections of the spine (cervical and lumbar) leads to referred pain in the areas served by the appropriate nerves. The shoulders are rarely a site of osteoarthritis, but sometimes severe destructive changes (the Milwaukee shoulder) do occur. Elbows are generally spared, but "cystic" protrusions through the joint capsules of distended fluid-filled joints lead to antecubital "cysts," the corollaries of the popliteal cysts at the knees; the latter can rupture, simulating thrombophlebitis in the calves. Wrists and ankles are almost always spared, because the mosaic distribution of the small bones diffuses forces. The first metatarsophalangeal joint is subject to osteoarthritis (the bunion) but rarely other joints of the toes (thought to be spared because shoes act as splints).

Although several studies claim that jogging and running do not predispose to osteoarthritis, these studies dealt with individuals who habitually exercised and not with those who dropped out along the way, so they may well not conclusively prove the advantages of exercise for the majority of patients.

I have left out the molecular biology, the catalytic enzymes and debris, and even the synovial fluid changes, as these are of greater interest to the investigator than to the clinician responsible for counseling and treating patients. They are giving us some clues to better treatments in the future, however, and a later version of this article might well give them more prominence. Of greatest importance is not necessarily to ascribe symptoms to osteoarthritis detected on imaging; false attributions can delay correct diagnoses and appropriate treatment.

Management

PREVENTION

As osteoarthritis is the culmination of all life events at the joints, it cannot really be prevented. Attempts to use bovine cartilage extracts and other substances failed to retard progression and have been largely abandoned. However, as osteoarthritis is consequent to trauma or inflammation, aggressive treatment of this initial insult might delay its onset years later, but this remains unproven. Attention must be paid to the risk factors (see Table 2), minimizing them as much as possible; weight reduction obviously decreases the load on knee and hip joints in overweight individuals. Keeping joints supple through exercising and not exposing them to shear factors (particularly in sports), jogging on soft surfaces rather than on unyielding pavement, wearing supportive footwear (spike heels may not lead to osteoarthritis *per se* but can lead to accidents that do, and flat heels put excessive strain on the calf muscles and later the knees), and in general maintaining physical fitness are all helpful. Despite recently published studies that isometric exercises, especially of the quadriceps, probably cannot prevent osteoarthritis of the knees, these apply chiefly to x-ray changes and not to symptoms; it is still wise to recommend exercises that strengthen the muscles that move a joint, because function will be retained even if the anatomic changes continue. Osteoarthritis found on x-rays taken for another purpose, if asymptomatic, requires no treatment; the old dictum, "treat the patient, not the x-ray," applies. Architectural barriers should be avoided; ramps are particularly troublesome for knee and hip osteoarthritis, especially descending (that applies to stairs as well, as descent requires knee extension, which increases joint discomfort).

Symptomatic osteoarthritis occasions discomfort at times of weather changes, but the symptoms are often mild and tolerated. Many people treat themselves for these, before seeing a physician. It is important to know what they may be taking, as they often do not consider these as medicines, and potential drug interactions can occur.

COMPLEMENTARY AND ALTERNATIVE TREATMENTS

Analgesics, such as acetaminophen (Tylenol and many unbranded generics) and aspirin, and several nonsteroidal anti-inflammatory drugs are readily available on supermarket shelves and pharmacies. In these days of global travel and ethnic migrations, other approaches also are common. Ayurvedic medicine is another system, popular in Southeast Asia and spreading from there; its medicines are based on plant extracts. Ayurvedic schools are found in India and the medicines themselves are carefully prepared and tested. The most popular treatment for osteoarthritis is composed of winter cherry, Indian frankincense, turmeric, and ginger (Artrex).

Herbal medicines available chiefly in health food stores have become popular throughout the United States. These are exempted by law from testing and approval by the FDA, and their safety and efficacy remain problematic. Potential interactions with prescribed drugs have not been studied. Ginger is especially popular, but among the other preparations are boron[1], borage oil[1], evening primrose oil[1], and avocado soybean saponifiables[1], all of which are claimed to be anti-inflammatory.

Yoga is currently being studied as a potential treatment for knee osteoarthritis, and acupuncture is said to provide considerable pain relief. Chiropractic adjustment is popular, especially for back pain attributed to osteoarthritis. However, the placebo effect is very striking in most osteoarthritis; even follow-up telephone calls from the doctor's office inquiring about the health of the patient lead to improvement. But do not slight the placebo effect; it is, after all, an effect.

GENERAL PRINCIPLES

A recent symposium on osteoarthritis concluded that osteoarthritis is all about biomechanics, and normalization thereof yields better results than drug therapy (that means splints, braces, canes, shoe corrections, abolition of unsound architectural and style features). Joint damage is not the main determinant of pain, but psychosocial factors, compensation systems, and inaccurate labeling play a major role. And people who have osteoarthritis, because of the long duration of its inception, tend to be elderly and therefore more likely to tolerate drug therapy and surgery poorly, and because many have concurrent problems under treatment, are prone to untoward drug interactions.

As stated, only approximately 15% to 20% of individuals have sufficient pain to seek medical attention. This pain waxes and wanes, and considerable controversy addresses the best approaches to treatment. A much-cited study compared acetaminophen 4 g per day with ibuprofen 1200 and 2400 μg a day during a span of 4 weeks, and concluded that there was no difference in results. However, the span is short, and proves only that analgesics are analgesic. Most patients prefer a nonsteroidal anti-inflammatory drug (NSAID), especially in anti-inflammatory dosage, as confirmed in epidemiologic and observational studies. Physical and occupational therapy can help joint-sparing mobility; ergonomic principles help at the work site; and sexual counseling, for those afflicted with hip involvement in particular, should be part of the treatment program.

For inflammatory erosive osteoarthritis of the fingers, the overnight wearing of nylon and spandex stretch gloves can inhibit nodose deformities if started early enough, before these excrescences become bony and function is compromised.

DRUG THERAPY

The severe pain of osteoarthritic joints—knees, hips, and fingers, chiefly—may be the result of secondary inflammation, caused by cartilaginous debris inciting cytokine response. A whole array of nonsteroidal anti-inflammatory drugs is available by prescription (from indomethacin [Indocin] and ibuprofen [Motrin, Advil, unbranded generics] through naproxen [Naprosyn] and diclofenac [Voltaren], with doses usually lower than those for rheumatoid arthritis), and others, not available in the United States, may be taken by patients who purchased them abroad (e.g., tiaprofenic acid*). These inhibit cyclooxygenase, an enzyme necessary for prostaglandin synthesis that has been found to have at least two components, COX-1, the constitutive that helps protect against gastric erosion and other consequences, and COX-2, which is evoked by inflammatory mediators and may lead to adverse gastric mucosal effects (a COX-3 has been proposed as well). To avoid the latter complication, misoprostol (Cytotec) may be prescribed or incorporated into a combination formulation with diclofenac (Arthrotec), but that is not without its own complications, namely, diarrhea and cramps. To avoid the adverse effects, a series of selective (at least in recommended dosage) COX-2 inhibitors were developed: celecoxib (Celebrex, 200 μg per day) and valdecoxib (Bextra, 10 μg per day). Lumiracoxib (Prexige)*, 100 to 200 μg per day, was recently approved for short-term relief in osteoarthritis abroad. As of this writing, recommended doses may vary, so the package insert should always be consulted to determine the current appropriate dose. Etoricoxib (Arcoxia)[2] is on the horizon and appears to be stronger. Gastric mucosal protection appears to be better, but there are renal consequences associated with its use and other problems are imputed. It must be stated that compounds considered safer are usually

[1]Not FDA approved for this indication.

*Investigational drug in the United States.
[2]Not available in the United States.

given to the patients most at risk, so the profiles do not address comparable populations. Moreover, the coxib NSAIDs are currently more expensive and not approved by all medical payment plans. Other NSAIDs, such as sulindac (Clinoril) and nabumetone (Relafen), are prodrugs, converted after absorption and hepatic biotransformation. Etodolac (Lodine) seems to work by a different mechanism; nimesulide is popular in Europe under a variety of trade names, but not available in the United States, is more COX-2 selective but less expensive, and may be brought back by travelers. Licofelone[2] is awaiting approval in Europe. The choice of NSAIDs is relatively arbitrary; patients may respond well to one and not to another. In most instances, the most severe symptoms can be brought to a level patients will tolerate within a few days to weeks, and long-term therapy may not be necessary.

Aspirin, once the mainstay of treatment, has largely been superseded. Gastrointestinal intolerance, irreversible inhibition of platelet aggregation, and animal studies that show it to be deleterious to cartilage may be the reasons, but nonacetylated salicylates, such as salsalate (Disalcid) and choline magnesium trisalicylate (Trilisate), and simple analgesics, such as propoxyphene (Darvon)[1] and tramadol (Ultram), alone or in combination, are given alone or with NSAIDs. Narcotics are best avoided because of the potential for addiction.

Gastric mucosal erosions are found by endoscopy but usually do not translate into clinical problems. Similarly, elevation of hepatic enzymes is noncongruent with hepatotoxicity. Adverse effects on gastric mucosa are the most common; however, liver, kidneys, and bone marrow complications, although uncommon, need also to be guarded against.

In most parts of the world, NSAIDs are available in creams and ointments for topical administration. The FDA is not convinced that this is more than a placebo effect so these formulations are not currently available in the United States. However, topical capsaicin, the spice in pepper plants, has been approved for use in osteoarthritis and is available under a number of trade names over the counter (a prescription no longer is necessary). During the initial period of administration, localized burning is usual. Capsaicin is also available on a patch, which is especially popular in Asia.

INTRA-ARTICULAR THERAPY

For nearly 50 years, cortisol derivatives have been injected into joints, usually after removal of the excess synovial fluid through arthrocentesis. When even symptomatic osteoarthritis was deemed not to be inflammatory, many clinicians cautioned that the resultant lack of pain indicated an insensitivity that could lead to further joint destruction, similar to the neuropathic Charcot joint. This fear has not been borne out and now arthrocentesis and corticosteroid instillation, preferably of a depot compound, in appropriately calibrated dosage, depending on the size of the joint, can effect long-lasting relief. However, patients should be admonished not to overuse the joint, at least for the first 3 days, as the lesions have not healed, even if the symptoms have abated. A general rule for counseling: do no more than when it hurt.

On the assumption that lubrication of the joint is impaired and corticosteroids are strictly palliative, preparations of hyaluronate have been approved for intra-articular instillation. While this procedure is called viscosupplementation, there is as yet little evidence that the instilled material is long retained in the joint or that it improves lubrication. Nevertheless, the results usually are as good as those with corticosteroids, and the duration of effect often long lasting. The two preparations currently available are sodium hyaluronate (Hyalgan) and hylan G-F 20 (Synvisc), administered as a short series of three to five weekly injections; why they should work is problematic, and some controlled trials concluded that they were no more effective than placebo. But this has been claimed for many preparations, as the placebo effect on pain is quite potent. Functional impairment remains, in most instances, especially at the hip, but often also at the knee. Hyaluronic acid is not indicated for interphalangeal injection, although small doses of corticosteroid into these tiny joints can sometimes lead to dramatic relief.

GLUCOSAMINE AND CHONDROITIN SULFATE

Oral glucosamine[1] is said to be as analgesic as NSAIDs and acetaminophen. Multicenter controlled trials seem to agree, but there is still much skepticism about this treatment. There is no rationale to explain why it should be analgesic, but all studies show glucosamine to be superior to placebo or reference compounds, even if not statistically in all cases. It appears to be harmless, with no untoward interactions, and the hypothesis that it might aggravate diabetes mellitus has not been borne out. Most preparations are available over the counter, but some glucosamine sulfate formulations are by prescription only (e.g., Dona[2]). The likelihood exists that any patient with symptomatic osteoarthritis is taking glucosamine, and so are many rheumatologists, empirically trusting that it has a salutary effect. Chondroitin sulfate[1] has not been shown to add anything, except in some poorly designed studies. However, the combination of glucosamine and chondroitin sulfate is marketed more frequently than either compound alone. And whole shelves in markets and pharmacies are devoted to these.

[1]Not FDA approved for this indication.
[2]Not available in the United States.

[1]Not FDA approved for this indication.
[2]Not available in the United States.

DISEASE MODIFICATION

By the time osteoarthritis becomes symptomatic and fulfills roentgenographic criteria, it is already well established. Thus, it is too late to think of "disease modification," as is now possible in rheumatoid arthritis. Nevertheless, the search for disease-modifying osteoarthritis drugs (DMOADs) goes on. All the compounds cited as possible DMOADs have been tested in animals only; no satisfactory assessment exists for studies in humans. Tetracycline derivatives, such as doxycycline[1], seem to have merit. Drugs that work on the inner mechanisms of cells, such as chloroquine (Aralen)[1], are also under study on theoretical grounds, but have not yet proved themselves. Antioxidant vitamins, tamoxifen (Nolvadex)[1], nitric oxide inhibitors, metalloproteases, and the aforementioned nutraceuticals have all been mentioned, but no reliable protocol exists that can measure their effect on cartilage and the joint. Specialized radiography that requires positioning is too crude for the purpose; magnetic resonance imaging and ultrasound have yet to be validated and standardized for this condition.

Studies are currently underway in Europe of diacerein (Diadar)[2] and growth factors, including insulin-like growth factor β, somatomedins, fibroblast growth factor, chondrocyte growth factor, and cartilage-derived and transforming growth factors. The problem of what to study and what outcome measures to use, and the duration of the trial, also bedevil these studies. While it is true that these are experimental treatments, not currently in use, and may never come to pass, they are mentioned here to counter the argument that the neurologist diagnoses untreatable disease, the rheumatologist treats untreatable disease. If not these, other treatments deriving from our better understanding of arthritis and its pathogenesis surely are in the offing. Included among these are mesenchymal stem cells that can produce site-specific tissue, thus restoring lost cartilage and bone; but how can that be done while mechanical impediments remain? The same is true for gene manipulation, and if new cartilage and bone are created, even with no counterpressures, how will the new attach to the older remnants and what will determine that? Cartilage transplants and chondrocyte transfer and stimulation are also being investigated. A polymer of glucosamine is available (Polynag).

[1]Not FDA approved for this indication.
[2]Not available in the United States.

SURGERY

Surgery is the consequence of failure of medicine. Our inability to effect healing and repair leads to treatments that would be forestalled if we could anticipate who, and under what circumstances, develops symptomatic disease and offer appropriate medical treatments. Barring that, the surgical treatment of osteoarthritis has made remarkable progress during the past 40 years. By and large, the osteotomies that were formerly performed have faded into well-deserved oblivion. Arthroscopy was hailed as a less invasive way to deal with motion-impeding osteophytes and derangements and meniscal tears, especially if combined with lavage, but the results do not materially differ from those achieved with placebos. Indeed, removal of the meniscus seems to hasten the development of the ultimate osteoarthritic lesion. The major advance was the total joint replacement, first for hips, then knees and even fingers and other small joints of the hands. These have given back life content and quality of life, to myriad recipients, more than 100,000 people annually in the United States alone! While surgery is clearly not a last resort, it has successfully addressed the functional deficits and pains and permitted recipients to resume their life styles. Shut-ins are liberated. Despite the trepidation of orthopedists, travel, skiing, tennis, golf, become achievable, even with bilateral surgery. Newer materials and methods of bonding have improved the longevity of these interventions.

Osteoarthritis remains an enigma, despite the major scientific advances of the past few years. Paradoxically, we have become more effective in treating advanced osteoarthritis and symptomatic disease (because of our better understanding of inflammation and the recognition that it plays a major role in evoking symptoms) than in addressing the variety of presentations. Symptomatic relief is achievable; restoration of function also; roentgenographic and pathologic changes may fulfill the definition but do not necessarily demand treatment. The removal of infectious and other killer diseases that curtailed life expectancy in the past has paradoxically resulted in the emergence of more chronic disorders. As stated in the World Health Organization's catalogue of disabilities, the killer diseases remove the consumer shortly after the consumer ceases to be a producer; the crippling diseases leave the consumer long after the consumer ceases to be a producer. The expense and increased suffering require a humane and scientifically sound understanding.

POLYMYALGIA RHEUMATICA AND GIANT CELL ARTERITIS

METHOD OF

Peter J. Embi, MD, MS, and

Gary S. Hoffman, MD, MS

Polymyalgia rheumatica (PMR) and giant cell arteritis (GCA) are closely related, immune-mediated, inflammatory conditions of the elderly. They likely represent extremes of the same disease spectrum and may coexist, with approximately 40% of GCA patients developing PMR and approximately 10% of PMR patients developing GCA.

The incidence of both conditions increases with age. Average age of onset is about 70 years, and occurrence before age 50 years is rare. Caucasians, and specifically those of Scandinavian ancestry, are afflicted more commonly; people of African and Asian descent develop the diseases only rarely. Women are affected approximately twice as often as men.

Although the cause or causes of PMR and GCA remain unknown, their etiology is likely multifactorial, with an interplay of age, environmental, and genetic factors contributing to disease onset and severity.

Polymyalgia Rheumatica

The term *polymyalgia rheumatica* was proposed in 1957, but it was first described as "senile rheumatic gout" in 1888, illustrating its long-recognized propensity to affect the elderly. Although diagnosis can be challenging, treatment is very gratifying given its dramatic response to corticosteroids.

The typical patient is an elderly caucasian who describes the subacute onset and persistence of aching and stiffness in the shoulders (70% to 95%), neck and pelvic girdle (50% to 70%). Discomfort tends to be symmetric, and radiation of pain distally into the proximal arms and thighs may be noted. Symptoms worsen with movement and are typically most severe in the morning for the first hour or more after awakening. Patients may have difficulty performing daily activities such as dressing, brushing hair, or rising from a seated position. Systemic symptoms such as fever, malaise, anorexia, and weight loss are noted in approximately 33% of patients.

Examination often reveals limited active range of motion as a consequence of pain. However, barring the co-morbidities of true shoulder and hip arthritis, passive range of motion is usually normal. In contrast to polymyositis, PMR does not cause true muscle weakness, only subjective symptoms of weakness. Distal extremity findings occur in up to 50% of patients and may include modest swelling of knees, wrists and metacarpophalangeal joints, carpal tunnel syndrome, diffuse soft-tissue swelling, and pitting edema of the dorsal hands, ankles, and feet. However, one must be wary, because frank synovitis is far more likely to be associated with rheumatoid arthritis or other inflammatory arthropathies than with PMR.

Laboratory studies reveal an erythrocyte sedimentation rate (ESR) greater than 40 mm/h in more than 90% of patients. Other findings of systemic inflammation often include elevated C-reactive protein (CRP), normocytic normochromic anemia, elevated platelet count, and elevated alkaline phosphatase. Of note, muscle enzymes such as creatine kinase are normal.

Differential diagnostic considerations include malignancies, chronic infections, and other rheumatic conditions such as rheumatoid arthritis, the latter of which can sometimes be difficult to differentiate from PMR at presentation.

THERAPY

The cornerstone of PMR treatment is corticosteroids, typically with prednisone starting at 10 to 20 mg daily. Although it can happen, failure of such therapy to cause near-total symptom relief within a few days is unusual and should prompt reconsideration of the diagnosis. Gradual decline in acute-phase reactants is also expected, although lab tests should not be the primary gauge of treatment adequacy.

If response is achieved, the initial dose is typically maintained for 1 month before being tapered gradually by approximately 2.5 mg decrements every 2 to 4 weeks. Most patients require 6 months to 2 years of low-dose corticosteroid therapy. Disease flares with corticosteroid tapering are common.

Because PMR may precede the development of GCA, physicians and patients should remain vigilant for the development of GCA symptoms. The development of such symptoms, especially visual disturbances, should prompt immediate medical evaluation and escalation of corticosteroid dose.

Giant Cell Arteritis

GCA is the most common form of vasculitis affecting adults in Western countries. It is an inflammatory vasculopathy of medium- and large-size arteries. Although widespread arterial involvement may occur, aortic arch vessels and cranial arteries are preferentially targeted, as suggested by the condition's other name, temporal arteritis. Involvement of the thoracic aorta occurs in at least 15% of patients.

As with PMR, the typical GCA patient is an elderly caucasian. Symptom onset is usually gradual, but may be sudden and severe. Manifestations resulting from systemic inflammation occur in approximately 50% of patients and include fever, malaise, fatigue, and weight loss. Vascular symptoms relate to the consequences of arterial inflammation, namely occlusion or aneurysm of involved vessels.

Classic symptoms of cranial involvement include headache, scalp tenderness (temporal or occipital), visual symptoms (transient or persistent blindness, diplopia), "jaw" (masseter muscle) claudication, or stroke. If aortic branch vessels are involved, symptoms of upper extremity claudication may occur. As many as 40% of patients may not present with classic symptoms and may instead manifest such features as cough, throat pain, fever of unknown origin, or pain elsewhere in the head and neck (tongue, cheeks, etc.). Any such symptoms in an elderly person with an elevated ESR should raise the possibility of GCA.

Examination may reveal a normal or thickened, nodular, tender or pulseless temporal artery. Asymmetry of pulses or blood pressures in the extremities, bruits over subclavian or carotid arteries, or the murmur of aortic insufficiency suggest involvement of the aorta and/or its branches. PMR features may be present in approximately 50% of patients.

Laboratory findings are similar to those found in PMR. ESR is elevated in the vast majority of patients, and elevated CRP, platelet count, alkaline phosphatase, and anemia may be noted. Elevated interleukin-6 levels appear to be a sensitive indicator of active disease, but most labs do not yet offer measurement of this marker.

Temporal artery biopsy prior to initiating therapy is ideal, but this is often not possible or prudent. Positive findings may be noted on biopsies obtained 2 weeks or longer into treatment, but the goal should be to biopsy as soon as possible after starting therapy. A specimen 2 cm in length optimizes chances for a positive result. Unilateral biopsies performed in such a manner are positive in 50% to 80% of affected individuals. While some researchers claim that bilateral biopsies increase the yield by approximately another 10%, other researchers do not endorse this approach.

THERAPY

Once a diagnosis of GCA is made, treatment with corticosteroids should begin immediately. Although lower doses may be effective in some patients, most authorities employ 40 to 60 mg of prednisone daily. The higher dose is preferred when ocular, neurologic, or other serious manifestations are present. In the setting of recent (<48 hours) blindness, many authorities advocate use of intravenous (IV) methylprednisolone (Solu-Medrol), 1000 mg per day for 1 to 3 days. However, the utility of this approach has not been evaluated in randomized, controlled trials. The initial effective oral dose is usually maintained for 1 month before gradual tapering is started. As with PMR, treatment with low-dose corticosteroids is often necessary for 1 to 2 years or longer.

Current evidence does not support the use of cytotoxic agents to help reduce total corticosteroid dose or to improve patient outcomes. Newer biologic agents are undergoing investigation and may prove effective. However, for now, corticosteroids are the mainstay of treatment.

Patients should be monitored long-term for late vascular complications. Aortic aneurysms (thoracic >> abdominal) are much more likely to occur in GCA patients than in the general population, and up to half of these aneurysms may go on to rupture, even years after apparent disease "resolution."

Finally, the use of prolonged corticosteroids in this population is associated with significant morbidity, including osteoporosis, and should prompt appropriate screening for and treatment of such conditions.

OSTEOMYELITIS

METHOD OF

Edward J. Septimus, MD

Despite recent advances in antimicrobial therapy and surgical techniques, osteomyelitis continues to pose a challenge to clinicians. The condition may at times be difficult to diagnose, yet if undiagnosed, it may progress to a chronic stage, with serious short- and long-term consequences to the patient. Osteomyelitis is usually caused by microorganisms that reach the bone by one of three routes: hematogenous, contiguous focus of infection, or direct inoculation secondary to trauma or surgery.

Osteomyelitis can be classified as acute or chronic depending on the presentation and clinical findings. If the initial acute episode of osteomyelitis is diagnosed early and appropriate antimicrobial therapy administered, the infection usually can be eradicated with minimal residual sequelae. However, if treatment is delayed, bone necrosis can occur, making eradication of the infection much more difficult and leading to the chronic phase of osteomyelitis, which is characterized by draining sinuses and recurrent episodes. Many investigators resist the word cure in osteomyelitis, because infection can recur years after apparently successful treatment.

An alternative classification system has been proposed by Cierny and Mader (Table 1). This classification system takes into account the anatomic extent of disease and the status of the host. There are four anatomic types combined with three physiologic host stages.

Stage 1 is termed medullary osteomyelitis associated with early hematogenous osteomyelitis. Most of these cases can be treated with antibiotics alone. In stage 2, or superficial osteomyelitis, the infection usually results from a contiguous soft-tissue infection.

TABLE 1 Cierny-Mader Classification System

Anatomic Type
Stage 1, medullary osteomyelitis
Stage 2, superficial osteomyelitis
Stage 3, localized osteomyelitis
Stage 4, diffuse osteomyelitis
Physiologic Class
A host: normal host
B host
Systemic compromise (Bs)
Local compromise (Bl)
C host: treatment worse than the disease
Systemic (Bs)
Malnutrition
Renal, liver failure
Diabetes mellitus
Chronic hypoxemia
Immune deficiency
Malignancy
Extremes of age
Immunosuppression
Tobacco use
Intravenous drug use
Local Compromise (Bl)
Chronic lymphedema
Venous stasis
Major vessel compromise
Arteritis
Extensive scarring
Radiation fibrosis
Small-vessel disease
Complete loss of local sensation

TABLE 2 Microbiology

Group or Condition	Organism(s)
Neonates*	*Escherichia coli, Staphylococcus aureus, Streptoccus agalactiae*
Children*	*S. aureus,* streptococci
Adults*	*S. aureus,* Enterobacteriaceae
Sickle cell*	*Salmonella* spp., *S. aureus*
Intravenous drug abuse*	*S. aureus, Pseudomonas aeruginosa* Enterobacteriaceae, fungi
Open fracture	*S. aureus,* Enterobacteriaceae
Puncture of foot	*P. aeruginosa*
Animal or human bite	*Pasteurella multocida* *Eikenella corrodens*
Rheumatoid arthritis	*S. aureus*
Foreign body	Coagulase-negative staph, propionibacterium
Vascular insufficiency	Mixed aerobic/anaerobic bacteria
Diabetic foot lesion	Mixed aerobic/anaerobic bacteria
Decubitus ulcers	Mixed aerobic/anaerobic bacteria
Immunocompromised	Fungi, Group G strep, Enterobacteriaceae

*Hematogenous.

Necrosis is limited to exposed surfaces at the base of the wound. Stage 2 osteomyelitis generally requires superficial débridement, appropriate antimicrobial therapy, and coverage with a local or microvascular flap. Stage 3, or localized osteomyelitis, is defined by full-thickness cortical necrosis. This usually results from trauma, but can also result from evolving stage 1 and 2 disease. Stage 3 osteomyelitis requires débridement and appropriate antimicrobial therapy. Surgery does not usually result in instability of the infected bone. Stage 4, or diffuse osteomyelitis, represents necrosis through and through with loss of bone stability. Stage 4 requires débridement, dead space obliteration with bone stabilization, and appropriate antimicrobial therapy.

In the alternative classification system, patients are classified as A, B, or C hosts. A hosts are those patients with no underlying metabolic or immunologic disorders. B hosts are patients with localized or systemic diseases. It is important to improve factors and diseases to make a B host more like an A host. The last category, C hosts, represents patients for whom the treatment of the bone infection is worse than the disease itself.

Acute Hematogenous Osteomyelitis

More than 80% of cases of acute hematogenous osteomyelitis occur in the long bones of people younger than age 20, with a second smaller peak in persons older than 50 years of age in whom the primary focus is the axial skeleton. In children, the site of involvement is characteristically the metaphysis of rapidly growing long bones. Several factors appear to contribute to this predilection: high blood flow in the metaphyseal region, sluggish blood flow in the postcapillary venous sinusoids, and reduced active phagocytic cells lining the capillary loops. Trauma also may cause local hemorrhage and further impair bacterial clearance. Most children present with fever, pain on motion, and local tenderness. A history of prior trauma to the affected limb is present in approximately one third of patients. *Staphylococcus aureus, Streptococcus pyogenes,* and *Haemophilus influenzae* are the most common organisms isolated (Table 2). However, the incidence of *H. influenzae* is decreasing because of the new *H. influenzae* vaccine now given to children.

Neonatal osteomyelitis presents with few systemic symptoms. Fever is often absent. Local findings may include some swelling and failure to move the affected extremity. Joint involvement is present in 60% to 70% of cases because of the absence of epiphyseal plates in this age group. Group B streptococcus, *S. aureus,* and *Escherichia coli* are the most frequently reported organisms.

Acute hematogenous osteomyelitis in adults is different from that in children in that it usually affects the vertebral spine and infrequently the long bones. The prevalence of vertebral osteomyelitis in adults is attributed to the fact that organisms can reach the vertebral spine directly from segmental arteries supplying the vertebrae, which bifurcate to supply two adjacent vertebral bodies. Therefore, the disease frequently involves the intravertebral disc and the two adjacent vertebral bodies. The lumbar vertebrae are most commonly involved, followed by the thoracic and cervical vertebrae. The disease usually begins insidiously with progressive, dull, continuous back pain.

Less commonly, the back pain may be of rapid onset, occasionally accompanied by neurologic symptoms. On physical exam, localized pain and tenderness of the involved site are present in more than 90% of patients. Some patients may also have severe muscle spasm over the affected area. Fever and elevated white blood cell count are documented in a minority of patients. If the infection extends posteriorly, compression of the cord may develop, necessitating emergency surgical decompression. In the normal host, *S. aureus* is the most commonly documented organism (see Table 2). In intravenous drug abusers, *Pseudomonas aeruginosa* and *S. aureus* are the most common, and in patients with urinary tract infections, Enterobacteriaceae spp. are the most common organisms.

Contiguous Osteomyelitis

Contiguous osteomyelitis is caused by secondary extension of a soft-tissue infection into adjacent bone. The majority of patients in this category have diabetes mellitus or peripheral vascular disease. Most patients are generally older than 40 years of age. Patients usually present with local erythema and swelling in the affected area of variable duration. Unlike hematogenous osteomyelitis, in which a single organism is usually identified, osteomyelitis secondary to a contiguous focus often is associated with multiple pathogens. *S. aureus* is still the most common organism, but aerobic gram-negative bacilli and anaerobes also may be cultured (see Table 2). Other examples of contiguous osteomyelitis include decubitus ulcers with osteomyelitis of the sacrum and heels and mandibular osteomyelitis secondary to odontogenic infections.

Direct Inoculation

Osteomyelitis secondary to direct inoculation can result from open fractures, puncture wounds, and orthopedic surgery. Open fractures pose a particular challenge. By definition, the wound is contaminated, which increases the risk for infection. The bacteriology in this setting can be very diverse and polymicrobial. Puncture injuries of the foot, especially by stepping on a nail, have been associated with osteomyelitis because of *Pseudomonas aeruginosa*. Animal bites, especially from cats, can result in osteomyelitis because of *Pasteurella multocida*, and osteomyelitis secondary to human bites, especially from closed-fist injuries, is associated with osteomyelitis because of *Eikenella corrodens* (see Table 2).

Diagnosis

To manage patients with any form of osteomyelitis, the need for accurate microbiology cannot be overemphasized. In acute hematogenous osteomyelitis, blood cultures may be positive in up to 50% of patients. If a joint effusion is present, an arthrocentesis should be performed to obtain fluid for analysis, including culture. If blood cultures are negative, a needle aspirate of the affected area may yield the pathogen; however, if this is negative, a percutaneous or open biopsy may be necessary to determine the pathogen. This is especially important in vertebral osteomyelitis, where a broad range of organisms may be involved. Other laboratory data may be of limited value. Leukocytosis may be present and the sedimentation rate and C-reactive protein are usually elevated, but these tests are not specific for the diagnosis of osteomyelitis.

In patients with contiguous osteomyelitis, surface cultures of decubitus ulcers and diabetic/vascular ulcers may be misleading, making biopsies or aspirates imperative. Sinus tract cultures are reliable for *S. aureus* but not for predicting gram-negative organisms causing osteomyelitis. For patients with osteomyelitis resulting from direct inoculation, deep cultures by aspiration, biopsy, or intraoperative samples are preferred (Table 3).

Imaging Studies

One of the problems in making an early diagnosis of osteomyelitis by plain radiographs is that radiographic findings are normal in the early stages of disease. At least 50% of the bone must be destroyed before radiographs show typical lytic changes. Radiographic improvement can lag behind clinical response as well. In contiguous osteomyelitis and chronic osteomyelitis, the radiographic changes may be very subtle. Comparison with prior radiographs can be very useful.

The use of ^{99m}technetium scans (bone scans) has provided clinicians with a sensitive study for demonstrating early inflammatory disease. Bone scans may be positive as early as 24 hours after the onset of symptoms. A positive bone scan is not pathognomonic for osteomyelitis because a positive bone scan can be seen with fractures, tumors, infarcts, and trauma. It is less specific in settings of complicated disease (i.e., overlying cellulitis, trauma, diabetic feet). Gallium scans show increased uptake in areas of neutrophils, macrophages, and tumors. Gallium does not distinguish bone inflammation from cellulitis well.

TABLE 3 Methods for Confirming Diagnosis of Osteomyelitis

Procedure	Sensitivity (%)	Specificity (%)
Blood culture	50	>95
Arthrocentesis	75	>95
Needle aspiration	60	>95
Surgical bone biopsy	90	>95
Wound or sinus tract	100	25-90

TABLE 4 Imaging Studies for Osteomyelitis

	Sensitivity (%)	Specificity (%)
Bone scan		
Uncomplicated	94	95
Complicated	95	33
Gallium scan	81	50-70
Indium scan	88	80
MRI	95	88

Indium-labeled white cell scans also have decreased sensitivity and specificity compared with bone scans in uncomplicated cases. Patients with chronic osteomyelitis often have negative indium scans. Computed tomography (CT) can play a role in the diagnosis of osteomyelitis. CT can show medullary destruction and necrotic bone, but image distortion can occur because of artifacts caused by bony fragments or metal. Magnetic resonance imaging (MRI) has become the imaging study of choice in difficult cases. MRI can differentiate bone and soft-tissue infection, often a problem with other radionuclide studies. The typical appearance of osteomyelitis is an area of abnormal marrow with decreased T_1-weighted images and increased T_2-weighted images (Table 4).

Treatment

In acute hematogenous osteomyelitis in children and vertebral osteomyelitis, treatment is primarily medical. In acute hematogenous osteomyelitis in children, surgical intervention is indicated if the patient does not respond within 2 to 3 days to appropriate antimicrobial therapy. In vertebral osteomyelitis, open surgical intervention is usually not necessary unless there is an extension of the infection, such as a paravertebral or epidural abscess, especially with any neurologic symptoms. After the organism has been identified, appropriate susceptibility studies should be performed to determine the most suitable antibiotic (see the following section). The patient should be treated for 4 to 6 weeks with intravenous therapy or 4 to 6 weeks after the last major surgical intervention. Oral antibiotics have been used successfully in treating hematogenous osteomyelitis in children; however, this should be conducted under carefully controlled situations. It is still recommended that the patient receive 1 to 2 weeks of intravenous therapy before changing to an oral drug.

In contiguous and chronic osteomyelitis, the major problem is infected necrotic bone with poor blood supply. Control of infection is difficult until adequate débridement and drainage has been accomplished and infected hardware removed if present. Management of dead space to replace dead tissue and fibrosis with well-vascularized tissue is critical to long-term success. Muscle flaps may be used to fill in dead space and provide adequate wound closure. The patient should be treated with 4 to 6 weeks of antibiotic therapy after the last major débridement.

Antibiotic-impregnated beads have been used to deliver a high concentration of antibiotics to the affected site and temporarily fill in dead space. The beads are usually removed within 2 to 4 weeks. Hyperbaric oxygen therapy may have a role where marginal or low oxygen tensions are present.

As discussed previously, establishment of the microbiologic diagnosis cannot be overemphasized (Table 5). The most common organism is *S. aureus*. For oxacillin (methicillin)-sensitive strains, treatment with nafcillin (Unipen)[1], cefazolin (Ancef), or clindamycin (Cleocin) is preferred. For osteomyelitis resulting from oxacillin-resistant *S. aureus*, treatment is more problematic. Vancomycin (Vancocin) remains the drug of choice with or without rifampin (Rifadin). Trimethoprim-sulfamethoxazole TMP-SMX (Bactrim)[1] plus rifampin[1], clindamycin (if susceptible), or linezolid (Zyvox)[1] offer alternatives. Ciprofloxacin (Cipro) plus rifampin for staphylococcal infections related to orthopedic implants given for 3 to 6 months has been very effective. Penicillin or clindamycin remain the drugs of choice for the beta-hemolytic *Streptococcus*.

[1]Not FDA approved for this indication.

TABLE 5 Initial Antimicrobial Choice for Osteomyelitis (Adult Dose)

Organism	Antibiotic of Choice	Alternative(s)
Staphylococcus aureus, oxacillin sensitive	Nafcillin[1] (Unipen) 2 g q4-6h	Cefazolin (Ancef)
S. aureus, oxacillin resistant	Vancomycin (Vancocin) 1 g q12h	TMP-SMX (Bactrim) + rifampin (Rifadin) or linezolid (Zyvox)
Enterococcus spp.	Ampicillin[1] 2 g q6h	Vancomycin or linezolid[1]
Beta-hemolytic *Streptococcus*	Penicillin[1] 2 MU q4-6h or clindamycin (Cleocin) 600-900 mg q8 h	Cefazolin
Enterobacteriaceae	Ceftriaxone (Rocephin) 1-2 g daily	Quinolone
Pseudomonas spp.	Ceftazidime (Fortaz) 2 g q8h or piperacillin/tazobactam[1] (Zosyn) 4.5 g q6h	Ciprofloxacin (Cipro) or imipenem (Primaxin) and cilastatin
Anaerobes	Metronidazole (Flagyl) 500-750 mg q8h	Clindamycin or imipenem and cilastatin or ampicillin/sulbactam (Unasyn)

[1]Not FDA approved for this indication.

For osteomyelitis resulting from gram-negative organisms, therapy should be based on the sensitivities of the infecting organism. For polymicrobial infections with anaerobic and aerobic pathogens, an effective anaerobic drug should be part of the antimicrobial regimen, such as metronidazole (Flagyl), clindamycin, imipenem (Primaxin), or a beta-lactam beta-lactamase inhibitor (e.g., ampicillin/sulbactam [Unasyn], piperacillin/tazobactam [Zosyn]).

Quinolones have been used with increasing frequency in the treatment of osteomyelitis. The published success for osteomyelitis resulting from quinolone-susceptible Enterobacteriaceae is more than 90%; however, the success for *Pseudomonas aeruginosa* and *S. aureus* is less than 80%. Furthermore, the development of resistance to quinolones on therapy has been observed with both *P. aeruginosa* and *S. aureus*.

Prevention

Antimicrobial prophylaxis with an antistaphylococcal agent given preoperatively (within 1 hour before the surgical incision) for patients undergoing either joint replacement or open reduction and internal fixation for closed fractures has been shown to reduce the incidence of postoperative surgical site infections. Antimicrobial prophylaxis has also decreased infection rates in patients with compound or open fractures.

Patients with diabetes mellitus can reduce the risk for osteomyelitis with tight glycemic control and meticulous foot care.

COMMON SPORTS INJURIES

METHOD OF

Scott W. Pyne, MD

Participation in sport has a broad range of definitions in most patient populations. Any activity in a group or individual setting that requires physical exertion can be loosely defined as sport, whether or not it is associated with a team, competition, or occupation. Exercise is sport and exercise is an important part of maintaining personal and population health. An ounce of prevention is worth a pound of cure and physicians should advise their patients about exercise- and sports-specific safety, as well as provide care after injuries occur. Injuries can generally be classified as acute, where the time and circumstance of the injury are clearly identifiable, or chronic, which gradually progress without a recalled episode of trauma.

The evaluation, diagnosis, and treatment of common sports injuries require a basic understanding of applied functional anatomy of the area injured. Most consternation in the treatment of active adults and children arises when the physician is confronted with an acute or chronic problem that the physician cannot clearly define. The understanding of the sport or activity, its rules of play, and the level of performance required for participation, often allow for a better appreciation of how or why an injury occurred. Most common sports injuries have classic mechanisms and historical findings that the athlete will freely reveal if guided along the appropriate line of questioning. Assisted by this information, the diagnosis is often apparent before the physical exam is performed. The physical exam of musculoskeletal injury follows a common theme regardless of the body part injured. All injured areas should be inspected for deformity, swelling, ecchymosis, assessed for range of motion, strength, neurologic function, and joint stability, and palpated for tenderness or crepitus. The exam is completed with a few body-part-specific tests. The evaluation can guide the decision for specific imaging tests to best define the injury and provide appropriate treatment. Plain radiographs are most valuable in the initial evaluation and can be augmented with bone scan, ultrasound, computed tomography (CT), and magnetic resonance imaging (MRI), as appropriate.

The treatment of most musculoskeletal injuries is easily remembered by PRICEMM, *p*rotection, relative *r*est, *i*ce, *c*ompression, *e*levation, *m*edications, and *m*odalities. Protection from further injury may involve splinting, taping, bracing, or casting, and does not necessarily require removal from sports participation. Athletes, as a rule, do not like to rest. It is important not to lose focus on what activities the athlete can do despite the athlete's injury. Athletes who are permitted to safely exercise while injured feel better about their recovery process, maintain a higher level of physical fitness, and follow medical recommendations to a greater degree. Ice is a valuable tool for decreasing swelling, inflammation, and pain. It should be applied for no more than 15 to 20 minutes every 1 to 2 hours to prevent cold injury to the skin or superficial nerves. Compression and elevation of the injured area above the heart effectively decreases swelling. Medications, primarily nonsteroidal anti-inflammatory drugs (NSAIDs), to decrease pain and inflammation are also commonly used. Physical therapists and certified athletic trainers are invaluable partners in the recovery of musculoskeletal injuries and can assist through the use of reconditioning exercise and modalities of ultrasound, electrical stimulation, iontophoresis, and phonophoresis.

Head Injuries

The degree and extent of head injuries can be prevented by the proper use of helmets. Biking, skateboarding, rollerblading, skiing, and snowboarding, as well as collision sports, can result in lacerations, abrasions, and concussions, as well as more serious cerebral and intracranial hemorrhage or contusion. The evaluation, treatment, and rehabilitation of concussion have received close scrutiny over the past several years. An individual who sustains a closed head injury with or without loss of consciousness that results in an alteration of their mental processing capabilities can generally be considered to have suffered a concussion. The classification systems for concussion are numerous and often vary as to the severity, degree, and treatment of this injury. The International Concussion in Sport Group was established to provide recommendations addressing the improvement of safety and health of athletes who suffer concussive injuries.

An athlete who has sustained a concussion should have a full history and physical exam, including a neurologic exam, recognizing that the same impact that created the concussion may also have injured the cervical spine. Any findings suggestive of additional injury should be further explored using appropriate imaging studies. Symptoms of concussion include headache, dizziness, difficulty concentrating, antegrade or retrograde amnesia, and emotional lability. Brain functioning can be further evaluated by Mini Mental State Examination, sideline assessment of concussion (SAC), or more formal neuropsychological testing. Individuals demonstrating a progressive decline in their mental function should be aggressively evaluated for more severe cerebral injury. Athletes should not be permitted to return to collision activity until their symptoms have completely resolved and they are able to exert themselves without recurrence of these symptoms. Currently several guidelines regarding return to play are available to help physician decision making; additionally, the role of neuropsychological testing is an exciting area of research. The primary goal of concussion management is to protect athletes from the potential adverse cumulative effects of repeated injury and a conservative approach ensuring full resolution of symptoms prior to return is best.

Shoulder

The shoulder is a joint that sacrifices stability for mobility. Anatomically, the scapular glenoid and humeral head articulation can be envisioned as a golf tee and a golf ball. The golf ball is held to the golf tee by dynamic stabilizers, rotator cuff and periscapular muscles, and passive stabilizers, glenohumeral ligaments through the glenoid labrum. The rotator cuff muscles (supraspinatus, infraspinatus, teres minor, and subscapularis [SITS]) actively stabilize just as you would actively tense your muscles for an impending automobile accident. The glenohumeral ligaments through the glenoid labrum passively stabilize the shoulder just as a seatbelt would in the automobile analogy.

The origin and attachment of these muscles help to recall their names and functions. The supraspinatus, originating posteriorly *above* the scapular *spine,* elevates and abducts the humerus. The infraspinatus and teres minor muscles, originating posteriorly *below* the scapular *spine,* externally rotate the humerus. The subscapularis muscle, originating along the anterior aspect or *underneath* the *scapula,* between it and the thoracic wall, internally rotate the humerus. Injuries to the rotator cuff muscles can be demonstrated by weakness and/or pain upon manual muscle testing. Of the four, the supraspinatus is the most often injured, which can occur acutely or chronically. Supraspinatus tendinopathy, partial or complete tear, may initially respond to rest, NSAIDs, and muscle-strengthening exercises focused on increasing the strength and tone of the shoulder internal and external rotators and scapular stabilizers. Corticosteroid injection, additional imaging studies, and surgical consultation can be considered in injuries not responding to 6 to 8 weeks of conservative treatment.

Subacromial impingement is commonly seen following repetitive overhead or throwing activity and may represent supraspinatus tendinopathy, subacromial bursitis, long head of the biceps brachii tendinopathy, or any combination of these. The most marked physical finding is increasing pain with overhead motion and special tests, Hawkins and Neer signs, that decrease the subacromial space and compress these structures. Treatment involves avoidance of offending activities, NSAIDs, internal rotator, external rotator, and scapular stabilizer strengthening, and ice. A corticosteroid and anesthetic injection into the subacromial space is often both therapeutic and diagnostic. In unresponsive cases, especially those in association with subacromial spurring or a down-sloping acromion, surgical referral may be necessary.

The glenohumeral labrum–ligament complex may be injured acutely, as with a dislocation, or chronically, with repeated episodes of stressing these structures, such as throwing or volleyball spiking. There is wide individual variation in shoulder laxity, which only becomes clinically concerning when it is associated with pain and decrease of function. Patient symptoms often occur in the position of abduction and external rotation and may reveal reproducible painful clicking or clunking with certain motions. Clinical evaluation requires placing the rotator cuff muscles at rest or at a mechanical disadvantage. Apprehension, O'Brien's sign, and manual translation of the humeral head on the glenoid are a few of the tests performed. The initial treatment for ligamentous instability is identical to that for other shoulder complaints, with the primary goal of optimizing rotator cuff and scapular stabilizer function. Those unresponsive to 6 to 8 weeks of conservative therapy should be considered for further imaging studies and/or surgical consultation.

A dislocated shoulder should be reduced as quickly as possible. The initial clinical evaluation should include inspection and palpation for evidence of a fracture or neurovascular compromise to the extremity. Most dislocations can be reduced without delay for radiographs or sedation. Postreduction radiographs and repeat examination to include neurovascular testing should be performed. Initial treatment involves rest in a sling for up to 3 weeks, followed by rehabilitative exercises to strengthen the dynamic stabilizers of the shoulder. Surgical referral may be indicated, depending on the patient's age, circumstances of the injury, anticipated future physical demands and repeated dislocations.

Knee Injuries

Knee injuries are all too common in many sports. By remembering the functional anatomy of the knee and reviewing the mechanism of injury, many diagnoses are clearly established. The knee is supported medially by the medial collateral ligament (MCL) and laterally by the lateral collateral ligament (LCL). Acute injury to the MCL via a valgus stress on the knee is far more common than injury to the LCL with a varus stress. Injuries of the MCL are graded according to their laxity, with valgus stress testing at 0 and 30 degrees of flexion from grade 1 with no laxity, to grade 3 with complete instability and extensive joint effusion. Grades 1 and 2 MCL injuries can be treated conservatively and most patients can resume normal activities in 3 to 4 weeks. The treatment for isolated grade 3 injuries is less clear, with some clinicians recommending conservative protection and gradual rehabilitation as with grade 1 and 2 injuries, limited flexion bracing at 30 degrees, or surgical evaluation. The extra-articular LCL is easily palpable as it traverses from the proximal fibula to the lateral femur. Tenderness in this area and associated varus instability support the diagnosis. Treatment consists of PRICEMM and gradual activity advancement with the assistance of a physical therapist or a certified athletic trainer to surgical referral for complete tears. LCL injuries are often confused with irritation of the iliotibial band as it crosses the lateral femoral epicondyle to insert on the proximal lateral tibia. Iliotibial band syndrome (ITBS) is an overuse injury, rarely associated with a traumatic event, common with running, hiking, and marching, and usually presents after prolonged activity with sharp pain over the lateral knee when the knee is repeatedly flexed between 20 and 30 degrees. These diagnoses can be differentiated through history and area of tenderness. Treatment for ITBS also begins with PRICEMM, correction of training errors, and a gradual resumption of activities.

The anterior cruciate ligament (ACL), which runs from the anterior medial tibia to the posterolateral femur, is the primary anterior stabilizer of the tibia. It is often injured in noncontact situations during abrupt knee twisting or hyperextension. Athletes and others close to the injured commonly report an audible pop and associated instability. The knee also develops an effusion over an interval of a few hours. Instability commonly persists with pivoting activities. The classic physical exam finding described by Lachman is an increase anterior tibial translation without palpable end-point while the knee is flexed at 10 to 20 degrees. Initial treatment is PRICEMM followed by physical therapy or certified athletic trainer-assisted range of motion and hamstring strengthening exercises. Most athletes sustaining an ACL injury should be afforded the opportunity to discuss their injury and desires with an orthopedic surgeon. Nonoperative management includes strengthening, avoidance of reinjury, and specialized bracing.

The patella is a common site of overuse injury in the knee. Retropatellar pain often develops insidiously and increases with activities increasing forces between the patella and corresponding femoral groove such as running and climbing or descending stairs. Patients also may complain of pain with prolonged sitting. The knee exam is generally benign except for pain under the patella that can be increased with tests that increase patellofemoral compressive forces. The evaluation is completed with examination of gait and foot dynamics. Patients with increased foot motion or overpronation may note improvement of their knee symptoms with appropriate footwear or orthotics. Additional treatment consists of a flexibility program, concentrating on the hamstrings, quadriceps strengthening, and gradual resumption of activities. Occasionally a knee sleeve may decrease symptoms; less commonly, surgical evaluation for realignment of the patella is indicated.

Leg Pain

Leg pain in runners, joggers, and walkers is common. This pain is frequently labeled as medial tibial stress syndrome (MTSS), a catchall diagnosis that simply describes varying degrees of pain and pathology over the posterior medial tibia and that is associated with increased activity or physical stress. This discomfort follows a continuum that may only be bothersome after exercise to that which interferes with activities of daily living. Shin splints is a term used to describe the mildest form of MTSS, and its etiology most likely involves a pull from the myofascial attachment of the leg muscles to the posterior tibia. Shin splints respond to PRICEMM and gradual return to training.

Stress fractures of the lower extremity occur most commonly in the tibia, but can be seen in the fibula, metatarsal, femur, and pelvis. They present with an insidious onset of pain associated with increased training frequency, duration, and intensity. The pain is usually well localized, increases with continued activity, and may persist at rest. A high level of clinical suspicion according to the clinical history and physical exam is most useful. Radiographs of the area may be normal, demonstrate periosteal thickening or elevation, or reveal a completed fracture.

Treatment focuses on activity restriction to ensure the pain is not increased and may involve crutches, casting, or bracing. With the resolution of pain, a gradual reconditioning program can be started. Additional imaging study options include repeat radiographs in 10 to 14 days after activity limitations, bone scan, and magnetic resonance imaging.

Patients with an essentially normal exam who complain of tightness, pain, numbness, and weakness only with exercise, may have chronic exertional compartment syndrome, resulting from increased pressure in the fascial bound compartments of the lower leg. In addition, their history reveals the onset of symptoms generally at a set time or distance into a run that resolve over 15 to 30 minutes following exercise. The diagnosis can be confirmed by the comparison of pressure testing of the fascial compartments before and after exercise. Treatment involves activity limitation to a degree that does not cause symptoms or surgical compartment releases.

Distance Event Injuries

With the ever-growing participation in marathons, triathlons, and road races, a discussion of sports injuries would not be complete without the mention of exercise-associated collapse. The care of a collapsed athlete in a field setting with very few medical resources available can be daunting to even the most experienced clinician. A common evaluation and initial treatment sequence can be used for collapsed athletes in this setting. All cases of collapse should initially be evaluated according to basic life support principles. Of athletes who collapse without cardiopulmonary arrest, the most common etiology is positional hypotension associated with the abrupt cessation of exercise and loss of the secondary pump action of contracting leg muscles. These athletes generally have a normal mental status and respond rapidly while in the supine position with their legs and pelvis elevated.

Athletes presenting with collapse and mental status alteration ranging from confusion, emotional lability, combativeness, and obtundation to unconsciousness are of greater concern. Additional evaluation of a core body temperature via rectal temperature is important in determining the etiology and guiding treatment. Exertional heat stroke generally presents with temperatures greater than 103°F (39.4°C) and often in excess of 108°F (42.2°C). The most important treatment step is to cool the body as rapidly as possible with ice-water immersion. Hyponatremia is exertional collapse with similar presentation and normal core temperature that is caused by the sum of overhydration, increased sodium losses in sweat, and decreased renal excretion of free water. It may represent a less-common diagnosis, but it is an area of growing concern and research. Untreated hyponatremia can lead to seizure, pulmonary and cerebral edema, coma, and death. Early identification and rapid transfer to an appropriate site of care are the most important steps.

Common sports injuries can best be diagnosed, treated, and reconditioned by understanding the athlete, the functional anatomy of the injured part, and the mechanism by which the injury occurred, and performing a consistent, focused physical exam. PRICEMM remains the initial treatment for most injuries, followed by an active reconditioning plan focused on the restoration of full range of motion, strength, and stability. The value of partnering with a physical therapist or a certified athletic trainer in the care of musculoskeletal injury cannot be overemphasized.

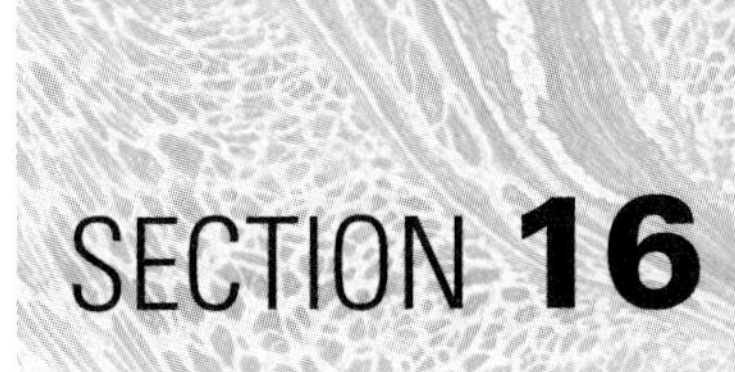

SECTION **16**

Obstetrics and Gynecology

ANTENATAL CARE

METHOD OF

Alex C. Vidaeff, MD, MPH, and Susan M. Ramin, MD

The introduction of antenatal care is attributed to the efforts of Ballantyne, circa 1913, at the University of Edinburgh. Since then to the present, antenatal care is considered a self-evident part of health services that is traditionally focused on health education and promotion at an individual level. Frequently discussed aspects of this approach are the number and timing of routine visits, as well as the content of the visits.

Number and Timing of Antenatal Visits

There is no unanimity of opinion as to the timing of the first prenatal visit or the total number of antenatal visits. However, it seems reasonable to initiate care at sometime during the first trimester to help establish gestational dating and to identify major problems or habits (i.e., smoking, alcohol, drugs, and medications) that might impact pregnancy. This is also the ideal time for certain antepartum tests and to discuss the option of pregnancy termination if so indicated. As pointed out by the American College of Obstetricians and Gynecologists (ACOG) and the American Academy of Pediatrics (AAP), "early and ongoing risk assessment should be an integral component of perinatal care."

The average number of visits in developed countries is between 11 and 14. A commonly followed schedule is monthly visits until 32 weeks, then every 2 weeks until 36 weeks, and weekly thereafter. Importantly, as summarized by ACOG and AAP, a woman's individual needs and risk status should dictate the extent and timing of antenatal visits. In a systematic review sponsored by the World Health Organization (WHO), a reduced number of visits were not associated with worse outcomes, unless the number of visits was less than four. With a reduced number of visits, it is important to schedule them adequately, so that important testing milestones (triple serum screening, glucose tolerance test) can be observed.

Content of Antenatal Visits

Routine antenatal care includes a series of screening tests, early diagnostic strategies, health behavior interventions, and patient education specific to pregnancy. Such education should include information regarding pregnancy changes and discomfort, nutrition and weight gain, fetal movements, plans for labor and birth, use of safety belts, infant feeding, promotion of breastfeeding, and worrisome signs and symptoms. It may be conducted by nonphysician care providers, or in childbirth education classes.

Health behavior interventions (or health promotion) address nutritional requirements and tend to identify barriers to adequate nutrition. Social behavior is also assessed, such as smoking, alcohol use, problem drinking, and domestic violence. Generally speaking, pregnancy may be the best time for behavioral modifications. It has been reported, as an example, that pregnant women are more receptive to smoking-cessation information and advice.

Early diagnosis strategies may be a significant benefit of prenatal care. For example, early diagnosis, evaluation, and treatment of hypertension, renal disease, diabetes, thrombophilias, and multiple gestation may lead to improved outcome.

The majority of screening tests (Table 1) are performed at the first or second antenatal visit. Some screening tests may impact disease modification at the population level. For example, testing for rubella immune status with postpartum vaccination of susceptible mothers can eliminate congenital rubella syndrome. Moreover, screening for the presence of hepatitis B surface antigen (HBsAg) is of neonatal benefit, because perinatal hepatitis B can be prevented by administering hepatitis B immune globulin (BayHep B) and hepatitis B vaccine (Recombivax HB) after birth. Vaccination of susceptible household members and sexual contacts can also be implemented for positive HBsAg cases. Ascertaining the blood group and Rh factor along with screening for atypical blood group antibodies detects the rare instances of isoimmunization. More importantly, it allows for low-cost treatment with Rh_0(D) immune globulin (RhoGAM) in nonisoimmunized, possibly incompatible pregnancies. This strategy has almost eliminated erythroblastosis fetalis from modern obstetrics.

Screening all pregnant women for sexually transmitted diseases (syphilis, gonorrhea, chlamydial cervicitis, and HIV) is also recommended as part of routine prenatal care and forms the basis of well-established perinatal disease prevention programs. In areas of excess prevalence, repeat testing in the third trimester may be indicated. At the same time with the cervical cultures, a Papanicolaou (Pap) smear should be obtained. For many women, pregnancy occasions their first Pap smear ever.

Screening for anemia is also conducted at the first antenatal visit. Anemia is defined as a hemoglobin level lower than 11 g/dL (hematocrit <33%) in the first and third trimester, and hemoglobin level lower than 10.5 g/dL (hematocrit <32%) in the second trimester. It should be treated with iron supplementation as indicated, or with folic acid in the rare cases of different etiology, without iron deficiency. Although common practice, the routine prescription of vitamin supplements in pregnancy has little, if any, scientific justification.

It is also recommended that all pregnant women be screened for gestational diabetes (GD) at 24 to 28 weeks gestation with a 1-hour glucose screen. Improved outcomes attributable to screening for and managing GD with normal fasting glycemia have not been clearly demonstrated, although such women are at increased risk of preeclampsia and having a macrosomic infant. Moreover, it is important to identify women with fasting hyperglycemia, because they may require insulin. Screening may be performed earlier in women with the following risk factors:

- First-degree relative with diabetes mellitus
- Previous pregnancy complicated by gestational diabetes, fetal macrosomia, or unexplained stillbirth

If the results of screening are all normal, the patient should be rescreened between 24 and 28 weeks. The 50 g glucose screening load can be administered irrespective of time of day, without any prerequisites. According to the American Diabetes Association and

TABLE 1 Routine Antenatal Laboratory Screening Panel

First Visit	16-20 Weeks	24-28 Weeks	35-37 Weeks
CBC VDRL or RPR Rubella serology Hepatitis B surface antigen HIV antibody testing Blood group and Rh type Blood group antibody screen Pap smear Cervical culture for gonococci and *Chlamydia* Urine culture, urinalysis	Genetic serum screen	1h (50 g) glucose screen	GBS culture

Abbreviations: CBC = complete blood count; GBS = group B streptococcus; RPR = rapid plasma reagent (test); VDRL = Venereal Disease Research Laboratory (test).

the Fourth International Workshop-Conference on Gestational Diabetes, the cutoff used to define an abnormal screen is 130 to 140 mg/dL. After an abnormal screening test, the definitive diagnostic test is the 100 g, 3-hour glucose tolerance test (GTT). The National Diabetes Data Group–recommended cutoff values for the 3-hour, 100 g GTT are 105, 190, 165, and 145. The cutoff values recommended by Carpenter and Coustan are even lower (95, 180, 155, and 140). At least two abnormal values out of four on a 3-hour GTT are necessary for the diagnosis of gestational diabetes. Significant fasting hyperglycemia (>130 mg/dL), even as a single abnormality, may also justify the diagnosis of gestational diabetes. Most capillary glucose meters lack the precision needed for screening and diagnosis of GD, and should not be used for this purpose.

Group B streptococcus (GBS) is the most common infectious cause of neonatal morbidity. Recently, the Centers for Disease Control and Prevention (CDC) recommended routine culture screenings at 35 to 37 weeks as the best screening protocol to prevent neonatal GBS sepsis. The ACOG (2002) supports this recommendation. Proper collection for culture (swab of both the vaginal introitus and anal area) and proper laboratory processing (broth enhancement) are essential. Administration of intrapartum prophylactic antibiotics as per protocol, using penicillin or ampicillin, markedly decreases the risk of transmission of GBS from a colonized mother to her infant. Two practical aspects require attention. First, antenatal cultures obtained more than 5 weeks in advance do not reliably predict which patients remain colonized during the intrapartum period. The second practical aspect concerns patients allergic to penicillin. Cefazolin (Ancef) is recommended for women with penicillin allergy if they are not at high risk for anaphylaxis. Clindamycin (Cleocin) or erythromycin are suitable only if the GBS isolate is susceptible to these antibiotics. It is advisable to obtain antibiotic sensitivities at the time of the GBS culture for patients allergic to penicillin and at high risk for anaphylaxis, so that in labor not all of them will be treated with vancomycin (Vancocin).

Although it has been suggested that screening for maternal hypothyroidism at the first prenatal visit may lead to a reduction in the incidence of neurodevelopmental deficits in children, universal screening has not yet been adopted, and the ACOG considers that it is premature to adopt such a policy. Equally controversial is the need for bacterial vaginosis (BV) screening. BV is associated with an increased risk of preterm delivery, but a 2003 Cochrane review found that the rate of preterm delivery was not influenced by the treatment of BV. If used, screening should be only in women at high risk for preterm delivery.

Other Content of Prenatal Visits

An early first prenatal visit is very important for adequate dating. A bimanual examination at this time can reveal size-date discrepancies, and help correlate size with the ability to detect fetal heart tones. A size-date discrepancy is an indication for an ultrasound examination. Changes in estimated date of delivery need to be clearly documented and explained to the pregnant woman. A targeted ultrasound may be performed at 18 to 20 weeks gestation for fetal anatomy. The art of monitoring fetal growth or estimating fetal weight by clinical means should not be abandoned in favor of repeat ultrasound examinations. Only 65% of fetal weights estimated by ultrasound are within 10% of the actual weight. Especially with larger fetuses, the ultrasound measurements tend to underestimate. There is very good evidence that ultrasound is no better than clinical palpation (Leopold's maneuvers) and uterine fundus measurements. Only in specific situations, such as obesity, uterine myomas, and hydramnios, is exclusive clinical examination suboptimal, and ultrasound monitoring of fetal growth required. Uterine height after 20 weeks is expected to equal gestational age in weeks. Differences of more than 2 cm should prompt an ultrasound evaluation to rule out erroneous dating, multiple pregnancies, hydramnios, oligohydramnios, fetal macrosomia, or fetal growth restriction. If the ultrasound findings are normal, and the difference in measurement is attributed to maternal body habitus or uterine myomas, it is helpful to remember the extent of the difference (as a baseline). Further ultrasound examinations are indicated only for fundal height measurements in excess of that initial baseline difference. Insufficient maternal weight gain would be another indication for ultrasound to evaluate for intrauterine growth restriction.

At antenatal visits, the routine practice is to assess fetal heart tones, fundal height, maternal weight, maternal blood pressure, and to check for urine protein and glucose. Multinational randomized trials show that routine digital examinations during pregnancy are of no benefit. Digital examination of the cervix may be of benefit at term to help guide the practitioner regarding induction of labor.

Hypertensive disorders in pregnancy are among the leading causes of maternal and perinatal mortality, accounting for 15% of maternal deaths and 4% of perinatal deaths. Routine blood pressure measurement and dipstick urinalysis to detect proteinuria are helpful in the timely detection of preeclampsia. Edema and excessive weight gain are no longer considered as diagnostic criteria for preeclampsia by the National High Blood Pressure Education Program Working Group on High Blood Pressure in Pregnancy. Maternal weighing at each visit remains important for monitoring the maternal nutritional status and fetal growth. A weight gain of less than 2 pounds or more than 6.5 pounds per month should be scrutinized, and nutritional consult should be considered. The recommended weight gain in pregnancy is approximately 35 pounds for nonobese women and 10 to 20 pounds for obese women.

Proteinuria present on dipstick urinalysis should be confirmed by a 24-hour urine collection. However, a recent prospective observational study concludes that in the absence of hypertension, routine urinalysis at each prenatal visit is a poor predictor of preeclampsia. Urinalysis may also be useful in the diagnosis of overt diabetes in pregnancy. However, glycosuria may be observed in approximately 2% of singleton pregnancies and correlates poorly with blood glucose levels. It has also been suggested that urinalysis for nitrates and leukocyte esterase in pregnancy may assist in the detection of asymptomatic bacteriuria. It is important to detect and treat asymptomatic bacteriuria in pregnancy because 30% of them may progress to pyelonephritis. How effective this strategy is in asymptomatic women beyond the first visit, when a routine urine culture is sent to screen for the same thing (i.e., asymptomatic bacteriuria), is questionable. Women with abnormal dipstick results, including the presence of leukocytes, nitrites, or blood, should have the sample sent for culture and sensitivity. Women with proteinuria and/or hematuria at their first visit may have underlying renal disease, and should be further investigated.

Genetic Screening (Including Screening for Neural Tube Defects)

Antenatal genetic screening is also part of routine antenatal care. The aim is to identify a patient at increased risk of having a fetus with a congenital disorder so that diagnostic tests can be offered. Once the diagnosis is established, the patient can be counseled regarding the various options available to her. The psychological value of knowing and being prepared for a disabled child should also be considered along with other options.

The first prenatal screening test to be introduced into clinical practice was maternal serum α-fetoprotein (MSAFP). An elevated level is associated with neural tube defects (NTDs), as well as other anomalies, such as ventral defects, congenital nephrosis, and fetal demise. A low level indicates an increased risk for Down syndrome. The sensitivity of the test for fetal aneuploidy has been increased by combining it with other biochemical markers in maternal serum, specifically, human chorionic gonadotropin (hCG) and estriol (E3). The resulting triple screen regimen (MSAFP, hCG, E3) was widely adopted in the United States as screening for chromosomal abnormalities and NTDs in the second trimester. More recently, first trimester genetic screening by ultrasound and multiple serum markers has been introduced. A first-trimester nuchal translucency sonogram in combination with early maternal serum markers (pregnancy-associated plasma protein A and free β-hCG) and computer-assisted risk calculations achieve a 90% discovery rate. An abnormally high nuchal translucency measurement is also associated with an increased risk of a major heart defect.

In addition to the aforementioned routine screening, women over the age of 35 years, or couples with a history of chromosomal anomalies or other hereditary conditions, should be offered genetic counseling before undergoing such testing. Women need to be counseled regarding both false-positive and false-negative result possibilities. Results should not be reported unless and until access to an immediate follow-up discussion is available.

Prepregnancy Counseling

Ideally, antenatal care should start with a visit before pregnancy. A maternal medical history, family history, and a genetic evaluation at this point will aid in the identification of hereditary risks for abnormalities, and may alleviate the ethical burden associated with genetic testing later in pregnancy. Some ethnic or geographic extraction groups are at increased risk for specific genetic conditions such as cystic fibrosis, Tay-Sachs disease, hemoglobinopathies, or inborn errors of metabolism.

For example, African American women should be tested for sickle cell trait, the most common hemoglobinopathy in the United States. African American women and Asian women are also at increased risk of thalassemias. β-Thalassemia may be a risk for women of Mediterranean descent. Jewish patients (especially Ashkenazi Jews) should be counseled about Tay-Sachs, Canavan disease, Gaucher's disease, and Niemann-Pick disease, whereas northern Europeans have the highest risk for cystic fibrosis. It is recommended that cystic fibrosis screening be offered to whites, because 90% of cystic fibrosis mutations are in whites, and that other groups be informed of this test's availability. The risk of Tay-Sachs disease is also higher in French Canadian and Cajun populations, and Jewish patients have a moderately increased risk of cystic fibrosis.

Folic acid intake is recommended for all reproductive-age women capable of becoming pregnant. It is effective in reducing the risk of NTDs and congenital heart disease in offspring if used before conception and through the first trimester (approximately 1 month before and 3 months after conception). The recommended daily dose in the general population is 0.4 mg folic acid. For women at high risk for NTD, such as those with a previously affected child, or those taking anticonvulsant medications, the preventive dose should be 10 times higher (4 mg daily).

The prepregnancy visit is also an opportunity to assess environmental and work hazards, as well as possible teratogen exposures. Rubella serologic status may be determined and immunization offered to seronegative individuals. In women with occupational risk for contracting *Cytomegalovirus* (CMV) (child care facilities, dialysis units), it is important to determine their serologic status prior to pregnancy. Susceptible women can take precautionary measures and seroconversion during pregnancy can be ascertained, allowing an adequate counseling regarding fetal risks. Health care workers or women from areas that have a high risk for tuberculosis may have a Mantoux skin test with purified protein derivative. This is also an ideal time to screen for diabetes and to achieve normoglycemic control, if necessary, to decrease the risk of congenital anomalies.

Antenatal care is an essential component in the management of the pregnant woman and her fetus. Although there have been few or limited scientific studies addressing the benefits of antenatal care, there can be little doubt that antenatal care at the very least offers the clinician the opportunity to detect, prevent, and treat various disease conditions. The currently recommended routine tests may need to be modified on a regional or population basis, taking into account the prevalence of various targeted conditions, to allow a rational delivery of care and reduce wastage. The ultimate purpose is to balance immediate and long-term health consequences for children and mothers with the costs incurred by individuals and society.

ECTOPIC PREGNANCY

METHOD OF

Ertug Kovanci, MD, and John E. Buster, MD

Management of ectopic pregnancy has changed dramatically. For decades, emergency laparotomy was the only option until modern diagnosis techniques enabled treatment before tubal rupture and even before symptoms. Although surgery remains the only option for hemorrhage, neglected cases, and medical therapy failures, medical management is the first choice treatment for minimum morbidity and mortality, preservation of fertility, and control of costs.

Epidemiology

The number of ectopic pregnancies in the United States in recent years is unknown. It remains the leading cause of first trimester mortality, accounting for approximately 6% of all pregnancy-related deaths between 1991 and 1999. Hospitalizations for ectopic pregnancies steadily increased through 1989, then declined between 1990 and 1999. The increased hospitalizations reported in the 1980s is attributed to increased prevalence of risk factors including chlamydia infections and tubal sterilization. Early detection and intervention with the advent of sensitive β human chorionic gonadotropin (β-hCG) assays and transvaginal ultrasound has enabled outpatient management, which, in turn, has led to the recent drop in hospitalizations.

Any condition that causes tubal epithelial damage should be considered a risk factor for ectopic pregnancy. Table 1 summarizes major risk factors.

Diagnosis

With identification of risk factors, serial β-hCG measurements, and transvaginal ultrasound, clinicians frequently diagnose ectopic pregnancy before symptoms. When symptoms occur, complaints of lower abdominal pain and vaginal bleeding are the classical presentations. Physical findings may include abdominal tenderness, rebound, cervical motion, and adnexal tenderness with or without a mass. Diagnosis is established through algorithms that use serial β-hCG measurements, transvaginal ultrasound, and uterine curettage (Figure 1). An intrauterine pregnancy should be seen on ultrasound above a threshold β–hCG titer, the discriminatory zone. This zone is usually between 1500 and 2000 IU/mL (International Reference Preparation [IRP]) for transvaginal ultrasound. If no intrauterine gestational sac is detected above the discriminatory zone, pregnancy is clearly nonviable and uterine curettage should be performed to rule out incomplete abortion. Dilatation and curettage (D&C) under local anesthesia is the preferred method.

TABLE 1 Risk Factors for Ectopic Pregnancy

Strong Association	Odds Ratios	Weak Association	Odds Ratios
Tubal ligation	9.3	Cigarette smoking	1.6-3.9
Previous ectopic pregnancy	8.3-76.6	Multiple sexual partners	1.6-2.1
Tubal surgery	4.0-21.0	First intercourse <18 years of age	1.6
In utero DES exposure	5.6	Appendectomy/abdominal surgery	1.4
Use of intrauterine device	4.2-45.0		
Assisted reproductive technology	4.0		
Maternal age ≥40 years	2.9		
Infertility	2.5-3.6		
Previous pelvic infections	2.5-3.8		

Abbreviation: DES = diethylstilbestrol.

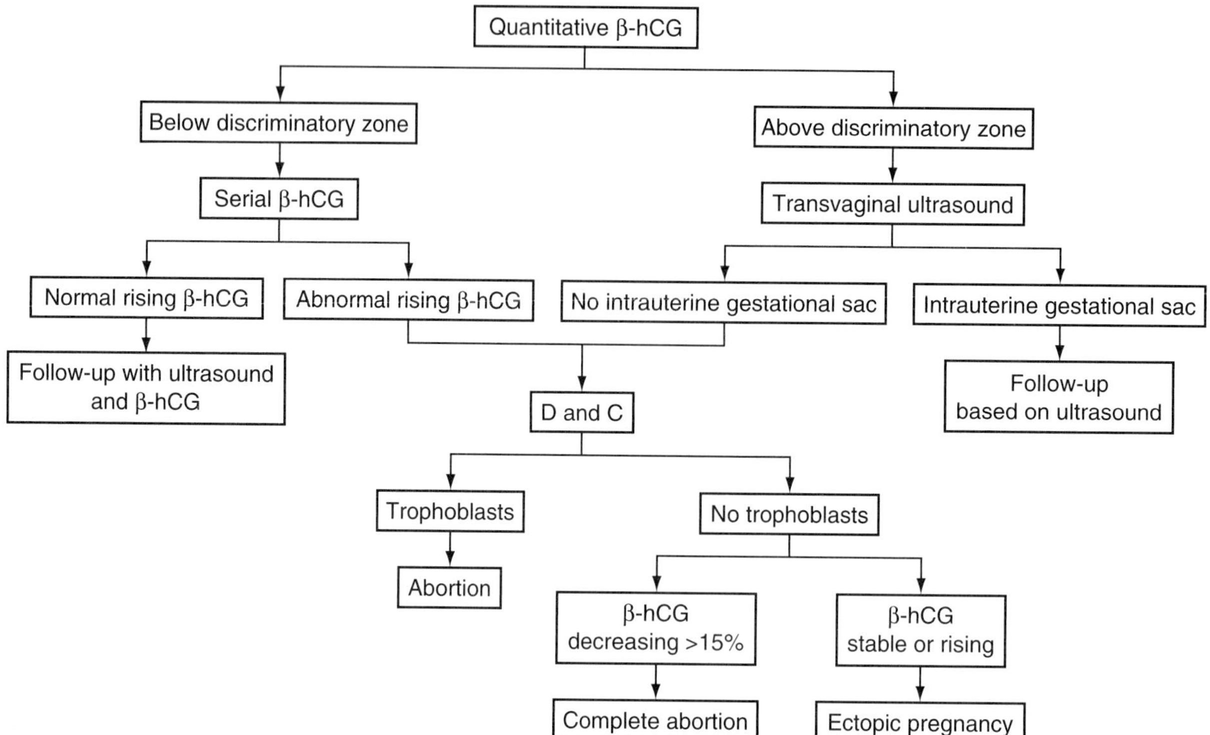

FIGURE 1 Diagnostic algorithm for ectopic pregnancy.

The β-hCG level rises at least 50% every 2 days in normal pregnancy. If a slow rise or a plateau is detected during serial β-hCG measurements, a nonviable pregnancy such as missed abortion or ectopic pregnancy is declared. In this case, D&C is performed even though the β-hCG level is below the discriminatory zone. However, when there is uncertainty, a repeat ultrasound or additional β-hCG measurements should be obtained to avoid D&C in a normal intrauterine pregnancy.

Transvaginal ultrasound has limitations. Identification of a gestational sac with a fetal pole and heart beat outside the uterus is diagnostic but not common. A hypoechoic area in the endometrial cavity may be seen because of blood or fluid accumulation; it may falsely diagnose an intrauterine pregnancy. Similarly, a complex-appearing adnexal mass, such as hemorrhagic corpus luteum, may lead to false diagnosis of ectopic pregnancy.

When the combination of abnormally rising β-hCG and no intrauterine gestational sac by ultrasound is encountered, approximately 40% of patients will have a nonviable intrauterine pregnancy. Thus, D&C is essential to avoid misdiagnosis.

Laparoscopy is rarely needed for diagnosis.

Treatment

MEDICAL THERAPY

Medical therapy is the first choice in hemodynamically stable patients with no contraindications to methotrexate (MTX) (Rheumatrex)[1]. MTX inhibits dihydrofolate reductase, which results in the depletion of methylene tetrahydrofolate and formyl tetrahydrofolate, cofactors in the biosynthesis of thymidylate and purines, causing cell death. Rapidly proliferating trophoblasts are highly susceptible to MTX. Overall success rates for MTX and conservative surgery (i.e., laparoscopic salpingostomy) are comparable at 89% and 93%, respectively. Tubal patency and subsequent intrauterine pregnancy rates are also similar. Medical therapy is less expensive than surgery. MTX also avoids the morbidity of surgery and anesthesia.

MTX can cause bone marrow suppression, hepatotoxicity, alopecia, photosensitivity, stomatitis, nausea, vomiting, febrile morbidity, and pulmonary fibrosis. Life-threatening neutropenia and febrile morbidity have been reported rarely. Side effects can be minimized by administering folinic acid, active form of folic acid (leucovorin, citrovorum factor, Wellcovorin). Once the diagnosis of ectopic pregnancy is made, pelvic examinations and ultrasound scans should be deferred. Transient separation pain (<12 hours) is commonly encountered during therapy. A baseline laboratory workup including complete blood count (CBC), liver function tests, blood urea nitrogen (BUN), creatinine, and blood type should be obtained before MTX is commenced.

Contraindications to MTX include ectopic size greater than 4 cm, blood dyscrasias, hepatic

[1]Not FDA approved for this indication.

dysfunction, and renal disease. A positive fetal heart beat, β-hCG level greater than 10,000 mIU/mL, and rapidly increasing serial β-hCG measurements should prompt cautious monitoring of the patient, as they are associated with increased risk of rupture.

Two MTX regimens are in common use (Table 2):

1. *Single-Dose MTX Regimen*: MTX is administered intramuscularly. Dosage is determined by body surface area at 50 mg/m^2. Folinic acid rescue is not needed. A baseline β-hCG level should be obtained on the day of treatment and should be repeated on days 4 and 7 thereafter. If 15% decline is not detected between days 4 and 7, MTX injection should be repeated. β-hCG titers should be followed weekly after therapy until it is negative. Single injection is more convenient for the patient and the physician than the multiple dose regimen. A meta-analysis shows that odds ratio of treatment failure for a single-dose regimen is 1.71 (95% CI 1.04 to 2.82) compared to the multiple dose regimen. The overall success rate for the single-dose regimen was approximately 88.1% in this meta-analysis.

2. *Multiple-Dose MTX Regimen*: MTX is administered intramuscularly every other day for a maximum of 4 doses. Dosage is 1.0 mg/kg of the patient's weight. Overall success rate is approximately 92.7%. Folinic acid rescue is given intramuscularly every other day starting the day after the first MTX injection for a total of 4 doses. MTX therapy can be stopped once a 15% decline in β-hCG levels is reached. Weekly β-hCG levels should be monitored after completion of therapy. If β-hCG titers do not decline by 15%, another course of MTX therapy can be started.

SURGERY

Surgery is the first choice for ruptured ectopic pregnancies. A laparotomy is justified in hemodynamically unstable patients. Laparoscopy is the preferred method for stable patients. Laparoscopic salpingostomy has approximately a 92% success rate. Weekly β-hCG measurements are recommended after conservative surgery. Subsequent intrauterine and ectopic pregnancy rates are 61% and 15.5%, respectively, comparable to systemic MTX treatment. In case of a persistent ectopic pregnancy after salpingostomy, systemic MTX is highly successful (97%). Laparoscopic conservative surgery is indicated for patients who refuse or cannot use MTX. However, when the opposite tube is damaged, subsequent ectopic pregnancy rate can be as high as 52%. Laparoscopic salpingectomy may be considered if the ipsilateral tube is severely damaged.

EXPECTANT MANAGEMENT

Numerous studies report patients who were managed expectantly with success rates—from 46.7% to 100%. If β-hCG titers are declining and are less than 1000 mIU/mL, success rate is higher. Expectant management may be considered in patients with low β-hCG levels that are declining.

TABLE 2 Methotrexate[1] Protocols

	Single Dose			Multiple Dose	
	Studies	**Treatment**		**Studies**	**Treatment**
Day 1	β-hCG CBC Platelet count LFT RFT	MTX 50 mg/m^2 IM	Day 1	β-hCG CBC Platelet count LFT RFT	MTX 1 mg/kg IM
Day 4	β-hCG		Day 2		Folinic acid (leucovorin) 0.1 mg/kg IM
Day 7	β-hCG CBC Platelet count LFT RFT		Day 3	β-hCG	MTX 1 mg/kg IM
Weekly	β-hCG until negative		Day 4		Folinic acid 0.1 mg/kg IM
			Day 5	β-hCG	MTX 1 mg/kg IM
			Day 6		Folinic acid 0.1 mg/kg IM
			Day 7	β-hCG	MTX 1 mg/kg IM
			Day 8	CBC Platelet count LFT RFT	Folinic acid 0.1 mg/kg IM
			Weekly	β-hCG until negative	

[1]Not FDA approved for this indication.

Abbreviations: CBC = complete blood count; hCG = human chorionic gonadotropin; IM = intramuscular; LFT = liver function test; MTX = methotrexate; RFT = renal function test.

Management Highlights

- Serial β-hCG measurements, transvaginal ultrasound, and uterine curettage facilitate early diagnosis of ectopic pregnancy and enable timely treatment with few complications.
- MTX and laparoscopic salpingostomy have similar success and subsequent intrauterine pregnancy rates. MTX is the first choice for treatment, as it avoids morbidity of surgery and anesthesia and is less expensive. Surgery is performed for ruptured ectopic pregnancies, or when MTX is contraindicated.
- A multiple-dose MTX regimen is superior to a single-dose regimen, because it has a lower failure rate. However, a single-dose regimen is used more frequently than a multiple dose regimen because of convenience. Side effect profiles are very similar for both regimens.

VAGINAL BLEEDING IN LATE PREGNANCY

METHOD OF

Jami Star Zeltzer, MD

Vaginal bleeding in late pregnancy complicates approximately 6% of pregnancies and is associated with increased maternal and fetal morbidity and mortality. Excluding labor, the most likely causes are placenta previa and placental abruption, followed by uterine rupture and vasa previa; less common etiologies include trauma, cervical lesions, and coagulopathy. The primary focus in obstetric hemorrhage, regardless of cause, is maternal hemodynamic assessment and stabilization. Given the extraordinary blood flow to the uterus at term (600 to 800 mL/min), exsanguination can occur rapidly. Additionally, redistribution of maternal blood flow may lead to fetal hypoxia.

Early maternal signs of hemodynamic compromise include tachycardia and tachypnea; later, hypotension, weakened pulses, and oliguria ensue, along with evidence of fetal compromise. Further decompensation can ultimately result in the death of both mother and fetus. Guidelines for restoration of maternal circulating volume are approximately 3 mL of intravenous crystalloid, (i.e., normal saline or Ringer's solution) per 1 mL of blood lost (often underestimated). Laboratory evaluation includes a complete blood count, blood type, and cross-match; in the setting of thrombocytopenia (less than 100,000 platelets), coagulation studies (prothrombin time [PT], partial thromboplastin time [PTT], fibrinogen, fibrin degradation products [FDPs]) are recommended. Packed red blood cells, fresh-frozen plasma, platelets, and/or cryoprecipitate are given to maintain maternal hemoglobin near 10 g/dL and correct coagulopathy (unlikely if whole blood is observed to clot in less than 8 minutes). Additional measures include administration of oxygen, lateral displacement of the uterus and, rarely, vasopressors. Fetal evaluation and treatment, including consideration of delivery, follow stabilization of the mother.

Placenta Previa

Placenta previa, or the implantation of the placenta adjacent to or covering the internal os, complicates approximately 0.5% of all deliveries. The degree of placenta previa may be:

- Complete (internal os covered entirely)
- Partial (portion of internal os covered)
- Marginal (placental edge at cervix or less than 2 cm away)
- Low lying (not a true previa, where the placental edge implants in the lower uterine segment but doesn't reach the cervix)

Table 1 lists the risk factors. The pathophysiology appears to involve endometrial damage, with resulting limitation of healthy uterine tissue for implantation.

The hallmark symptom is painless vaginal bleeding, presumably initiated by development of the lower uterine segment. Usually, this occurs by 29 to 30 weeks of gestation, although in approximately 33% of cases, there is no bleeding until labor. The first bleed may be self-limited, but rebleeding complicates approximately 60% of cases. The diagnosis is often made in the absence of symptoms on routine ultrasound. The incidence of placenta previa is 5% to 10% in mid-gestation; this resolves in most cases with development of the lower uterine segment (*placental migration*). When asymptomatic, expectant management is appropriate, although vaginal precautions after 28 weeks gestation may be advised.

When a patient presents with third-trimester bleeding, speculum exams are contraindicated until placenta previa is ruled out. The most accurate method of diagnosis is transvaginal ultrasound, which is safe in experienced hands; transperineal or transabdominal

TABLE 1 Risk Factors for Placenta Previa

Advancing maternal age
Ethnic background (increased in Asians)
Multiparity
Multiple gestation
Previous curettage
Prior cesarean section (increases with number of sections)
Prior placenta previa
Smoking

ultrasound carry greater risks of false-positive and false-negative results.

Observation in the hospital is recommended following a bleed, during which time approximately 50% of patients will deliver. Steroids are indicated for enhancement of fetal lung maturation. Tocolysis can be administered if the mother and fetus are stable, preferably with magnesium sulfate to minimize cardiovascular effects. Outpatient management is acceptable if bleeding ceases, as long as the patient is compliant and has ready access to a hospital. Serial ultrasound assessment is recommended because there is an increased risk of intrauterine growth restriction. Transfusion should be offered to maintain hemoglobin greater than 10 mg/dL.

Urgent delivery by cesarean section is indicated when there is ongoing maternal hemorrhage or evidence of fetal compromise. In the stable patient, a planned cesarean section can be performed at 35 to 36 weeks, generally after an amniocentesis is performed to confirm fetal lung maturity. Vaginal delivery is preferable in the setting of fetal demise; it may be attempted if delivery is imminent, or with marginal previa, although a *double setup* for emergent cesarean section is advised.

Placenta previa predisposes to postpartum hemorrhage, either from atony of the lower uterine segment or inability to remove the placenta because of absence of the decidua basalis. The most common form of this latter condition is placenta accreta, where the trophoblast adheres to the myometrium. Less common forms include placenta increta (the trophoblast invades the myometrium) and placenta percreta (trophoblast invades uterine serosa and/or adjacent organs). The primary risk factor for placenta accreta is the number of previous cesarean sections, with an incidence approaching 40% in patients with two prior cesarean sections and a placenta previa. Other risk factors include age, parity, and history of curettage. Color Doppler ultrasound and magnetic resonance imaging (MRI) are helpful but not always definitive for diagnosis. If placenta accreta is suspected, preparations can be made for scheduled delivery with trained personnel and blood products available. At delivery, the placenta should be left in place if a cleavage plane cannot be developed easily. Cesarean–hysterectomy is often required for hemostasis, although conservative management, including preoperative and intraoperative selective embolization and/or use of methotrexate, has been reported. With placenta percreta, bladder invasion may require cystoscopy and urologic repair.

Vasa Previa

Vasa previa is a rare condition (estimated 1 in 2500 deliveries) in which fetal blood vessels cross over the membranes in advance of the presenting part. This is most often associated with velamentous insertion of the umbilical cord (vessels reach the placenta after coursing through the membranes rather than by direct insertion); Table 2 lists the risk factors. Vasa previa carries a profound risk of fetal mortality from exsanguination, particularly at the time of membrane rupture (fetal blood volume at term is approximately 250 mL). Even in the absence of bleeding, vessel compression may result in compromise of the fetal circulation.

TABLE 2 Risk Factors for Vasa Previa

Bilobed placenta
In vitro fertilization
Low-lying placenta
Multiple pregnancy
Succenturiate lobe
Velamentous insertion of umbilical cord

Signs include hemorrhage, as well as fetal heart rate abnormalities. A high index of suspicion is required, and advances in imaging techniques (color Doppler, transvaginal ultrasound) make prenatal diagnosis possible. If there is unexplained bleeding, an Apt test or Kleihauer-Betke test can identify fetal red blood cells. If the diagnosis of vasa previa is strongly suspected at term, or if hemorrhage is significant, prompt cesarean delivery is recommended, followed by neonatal resuscitation.

Uterine Rupture

Most often reported following prior cesarean section, uterine rupture can also occur in an unscarred uterus (1 in 8000 to 1 in 15,000 deliveries). This phenomenon implies complete separation of the uterine wall (as compared to uterine dehiscence), with or without expulsion of the fetus. Table 3 lists risk factors and differential diagnoses.

Common signs and symptoms include abdominal pain/tenderness and vaginal bleeding; additional complaints include epigastric or shoulder pain, abdominal distention, and constipation. The fetal tracing may show sudden variable decelerations or abrupt and prolonged bradycardia, often accompanied by recession of the presenting part. Maternal and

TABLE 3 Uterine Rupture

Risk Factors	Differential Diagnoses
Previous cesarean section (especially classical)	Appendicitis
Use of oxytocin, prostaglandins, or misoprostol	Biliary colic
Multiparity	Pancreatitis
Midforceps application	Peptic ulcer disease
Breech version/extraction	Intestinal obstruction
Placental abruption	Ovarian torsion
Shoulder dystocia	Placental abruption
Placenta percreta	Urinary tract disorders
Müllerian duct anomalies	
History of pelvic radiation	

fetal morbidity and mortality are high, particularly with delayed diagnosis. Treatment is urgent cesarean delivery, with repair of the uterus and/or hysterectomy as needed. Repeat cesarean section is advised in future because of the risk for recurrence.

Placental Abruption

Abruption of the placenta, or separation of the normally implanted placenta before birth, complicates 1% to 2% of pregnancies. Bleeding into the decidua basalis, with subsequent separation of varying amounts of placental tissue from the endometrium, may result in fetal compromise and/or demise. The exact pathophysiology is unclear. Table 4 lists the risk factors.

Vaginal bleeding in the second half of pregnancy is assumed to be caused by placental abruption, once placenta previa and other rare causes are ruled out. Concealed hemorrhage, present in 10% to 20% of cases, can complicate the diagnosis. Abdominal pain, back pain, uterine contractions (often described as low amplitude, high frequency), hypertonus, uterine tenderness, and/or idiopathic premature labor may be present. While ultrasound can identify placenta previa, it cannot be relied upon to definitively diagnose abruption, as clot is sonographically visible in less than 50% of cases. The differential diagnoses include uterine rupture, appendicitis, and chorioamnionitis, as well as other causes of abdominal pain.

Most commonly, bleeding is not profuse and, if the episode is self-limited, expectant management of a preterm gestation includes observation, serial fetal growth assessment, fetal well-being testing, and steroid therapy to accelerate fetal lung maturation. With ongoing significant blood loss, stabilization of the mother, fetal assessment, and laboratory evaluation are indicated. Coagulopathy is rare in the absence of fetal demise. If tocolysis is required, magnesium sulfate is preferred, as β-sympathomimetics may mask maternal cardiovascular decompensation.

Vaginal delivery is appropriate if mother and fetus are stable. Amniotomy may decrease extravasation of blood into the myometrium by head compression. Not uncommonly, effacement will precede dilatation; oxytocin (Pitocin) is acceptable for labor dysfunction. In the event of an intrauterine demise, vaginal delivery is preferred. Acute hemorrhage requires immediate cesarean delivery, with blood and coagulation factor replacement as needed.

Potential complications of abruption include hemorrhagic shock, disseminated intravascular coagulation (unlikely unless there is greater than 2000 mL blood loss and/or fetal demise), ischemic necrosis of maternal organs (especially kidney), and Couvelaire uterus (extravasation of blood into uterine muscle). Recurrence is approximately 5% to 15%, increasing with each subsequent event. There are no known preventive measures other than correcting modifiable risk factors.

TABLE 4 Risk Factors for Placental Abruption

Chorioamnionitis
Cocaine use
Ethnic background (highest in blacks)
Hypertension
Male fetal gender
Multiple gestation
Parity
Polyhydramnios (rapid decompression at membrane rupture and/or therapeutic amniocentesis)
Preterm premature rupture of membranes
Previous cesarean section
Smoking
Trauma, including domestic violence
Unexplained elevated second trimester alpha-fetoprotein
Uterine anomalies/short umbilical cord

HYPERTENSIVE DISORDERS OF PREGNANCY

METHOD OF

Joanie Hare-Morris, MD

Toxemia of pregnancy is an old term that presumed that circulating toxins were responsible for the hypertensive disorders of pregnancy. This archaic term was discontinued because it neither described nor revealed the etiology of this complex disorder of pregnancy. Hypertensive disorders occur in 6% to 8% of all pregnancies, more commonly in 2% to 7% of nulliparous women, 14% of twin gestations, and up to 18% of those with previous history of preeclampsia. Around the world, a woman dies every hour because of a hypertensive disorder of pregnancy and its complications. This multisystem dysfunction may produce significant morbidity including seizures, cerebral hemorrhage, blindness, acute renal failure, disseminated intravascular coagulation, liver hemorrhage, and pulmonary edema. The fetal/placental unit may also be jeopardized with intrauterine growth restriction and abruptio placentae, leading to premature delivery, stillbirth, or even neonatal death.

The proper diagnosis, management, and treatment must occur because of the rapid, aggressive, and progressive effects of hypertensive disorders of pregnancy. It is imperative that any practitioner of obstetrics is knowledgeable and familiar with these diseases. More importantly, that practitioner should recognize that the ultimate cure is delivery of the fetus and placenta; however, delivery may not be the best thing for the fetus due to prematurity. This article reviews the hypertensive disorders of pregnancy and discusses the diagnosis, management, and various treatment modalities.

Definitions and Classifications

Hypertension is defined in the nonpregnant population as systolic blood pressure of 140 and/or a diastolic blood pressure of 90 mm Hg or greater. Accurate diagnosis of hypertension requires proper measurement of blood pressure. The patient should be seated or, if applicable, lying in the left lateral position, and the arm should be at the level of the heart. A sphygmomanometer (manual or electronic) device should be used, and the appropriate cuff size is imperative for accurate blood pressure measurements. Korotkoff phase V (disappearance of the sound) should be used for the diastolic blood pressure.

The hypertensive disorders of pregnancy include gestational hypertension, preeclampsia/eclampsia, chronic hypertension, and superimposed preeclampsia with hypertension (Table 1). Gestational hypertension and preeclampsia/eclampsia account for 70% of the hypertension of pregnancy; whereas 30% is a result of chronic hypertension and superimposed preeclampsia with hypertension.

GESTATIONAL HYPERTENSION

Gestational hypertension is defined as a newly diagnosed hypertension of pregnancy that occurs after 20 weeks of gestation or postpartum in a woman known to be normotensive, without proteinuria. Hypertension is noted on two occasions 6 hours apart. More importantly, gestational hypertension resolves by 12 weeks postpartum, and it may also be predictive of future chronic hypertension.

PREECLAMPSIA

Traditionally, preeclampsia was defined by the triad of hypertension, proteinuria, and edema. Recently, edema was discarded as a diagnostic criterion because it is a nonspecific finding that occurs in most normal pregnant women. Preeclampsia is presently defined by the dyad of hypertension (blood pressure >140/90 mm Hg) and proteinuria (300 mg over 24-hour or more urine collection and/or 1+ or greater on semiqualitative dipsticks) that occurs after 20 weeks of gestation. Preeclampsia rarely occurs before 20 weeks of gestation. If present prior to 20 weeks of gestation, it is associated with a molar pregnancy and/or fetal hydrops. Recent studies find that urinary dipstick determinations correlate poorly with the 24-hour urine collections. Therefore, the definitive test to diagnose proteinuria should be quantitative protein excretion in a 24-hour period. A 24-hour urine specimen also evaluates the creatinine clearance, which may be decreased in severe preeclampsia.

Preeclampsia may be further classified into mild and severe categories (Table 2). Severe preeclampsia is diagnosed if there is severe hypertension and severe proteinuria. Severe preeclampsia may also involve multiorgan dysfunction such as pulmonary edema, oliguria, epigastric pain, or persistent severe central nervous system symptoms such as headache or scotoma. Laboratory tests, including the platelet count, liver function studies, serum creatinine, lactic acid dehydrogenase, and coagulation studies, may help in the diagnosis and management of these patients with severe preeclampsia.

ECLAMPSIA

Eclampsia is defined as severe preeclampsia accompanied by seizures unrelated to other cerebral

TABLE 1 Definitions of Hypertensive Disorders in Pregnancy

Gestational Hypertension
New-onset hypertension (blood pressure >140/90 mm Hg) after 20 weeks of gestation
Absence of proteinuria or other signs of preeclampsia
Blood pressure normal by 12 weeks postpartum
Preeclampsia/Eclampsia*
Hypertension after 20 weeks of gestation
Proteinuria >300 mg in 24h urine specimen collection
Chronic Hypertension
Hypertension (bp >140/90 mm Hg) present before pregnancy or before 20 weeks of gestation
Hypertension diagnosed after 20 weeks of gestation and persisting more than 12 weeks postpartum
Superimposed Preeclampsia
In presence of hypertension, new-onset proteinuria >300 mg/24h after 20 weeks of gestation
An exacerbation of hypertension and/or new-onset proteinuria or increase of existent proteinuria

*New-onset tonic–clonic seizures not attributable to any other cause.

TABLE 2 Diagnostic Criteria for Preeclampsia

Mild Preeclampsia
Blood pressure ≥140 mm Hg after 20 weeks of gestation
Proteinuria ≥300 mg over 24h urine specimen collection
Severe Preeclampsia
Blood pressure ≥160 mm Hg systolic or ≥110 mm Hg diastolic recorded on two occasions 6h apart with bed rest
Proteinuria ≥5 g/24h
Oliguria (500 mL/24h)
Serum creatinine >1.2 mg/dL
Cerebral visual disturbances/scotoma
Severe headache
Pulmonary edema
Epigastric/right upper quadrant pain/nausea and vomiting
Eclampsia new onset seizures
HELLP syndrome
Hemolysis
Microangiopathic anemia
Schistocytes peripheral smear
Increased lactic dehydrogenase >600 IU/L
Elevated liver function
Increased aspartate transaminases ≥72 IU/L
Increased lactic dehydrogenase >600 IU/L
Low platelets (thrombocytopenia) <100,000/mm^3

conditions with signs and symptoms of preeclampsia. Early writings of the Egyptians warned of the dangers of convulsions during pregnancy. Eclampsia occurs in 0.2% to 0.5% of all deliveries. Approximately 75% of eclamptic seizures occur before delivery. Approximately 50% of postpartum eclamptic seizures occur in the first 48 hours after delivery, but seizures may occur as late as 6 weeks postpartum. The pathophysiologic events leading to seizures remain unknown.

CHRONIC HYPERTENSION

Chronic hypertension is classified as preexisting hypertension present before 20 weeks of gestation and hypertension that persists 42 days postpartum. The severity of chronic hypertension is associated with the duration of hypertension and the presence of end organ damage. It may be diagnosed in women who present before 20 weeks of gestation with blood pressures greater that 140/90 mm Hg on two separate occasions. However, when presenting for late prenatal care after 20 weeks of gestation, hypertension may be masked because of the normal physiologic changes of pregnancy, in which a decrease in the systolic and diastolic blood pressures occurs in the second trimester. This normal physiologic process results in blood pressures returning to baseline by the third trimester, which may cause confusion when diagnosing gestational hypertension versus chronic hypertension. Thus, early prenatal care is crucial for all pregnant women.

After 20 weeks of gestation, chronic hypertension may worsen because of poor compliance, or development of hypertensive crisis. Chronic hypertension is associated with increased maternal and perinatal morbidity and mortality. Perinatal mortality is three to four times higher in pregnancies complicated by chronic hypertension than in the general population.

SUPERIMPOSED PREECLAMPSIA WITH HYPERTENSION

Superimposed preeclampsia is defined as the development of preeclampsia in a patient with chronic hypertension but without proteinuria. Approximately 15% to 30% of patients with chronic hypertension may develop preeclampsia, which increases the morbidity for the fetus and mother. In superimposed preeclampsia, the patient may develop severe exacerbation of hypertension, proteinuria (500 mg in 24-hour urine collection test) or multisystem organ involvement.

Pathophysiology of Hypertensive Disorders of Pregnancy

There are numerous published clinical reports that attempt to decrease the incidence and/or severity of preeclampsia. Table 2 lists the risk factors associated with the development of preeclampsia, which include low-dose aspirin[1], heparin[1], calcium[1], fish oil[1], zinc[1], and low-salt and high-protein diets. However, none of the studies are conclusive in ameliorating or preventing preeclampsia.

The etiology of preeclampsia is even more confusing. It is a multisystem disorder involving vasoconstriction of the maternal vasculature, hypercoagulability, and placental trophoblastic invasion. Many theories on the possible etiology have been published including an imbalance between thromboxane-prostacyclin, endothelial cell injury, genetic factors, dietary factors, and altered vascular reactivity. Recent studies suggest that preeclampsia results from abnormal placental development, involving the maternal spiral arteries and decidua coupled with suboptimal maternal compensatory response.

In normal pregnancy, the proliferating trophoblasts of the placenta invade the decidua and the adjacent myometrium. Subsequently, the spiral arteries evolve from a muscular into thin-walled, low-resistance vessel, allowing increased perfusion to the placenta that is independent of maternal vasoactive control. In contrast to the normal pattern, in preeclampsia there appears to be inadequate invasion of the trophoblast, and the spiral arteries retain their muscular walls. The result is vascular resistance that prohibits the passive flow of blood. This leads to endothelial dysfunction producing thrombus formation, vasospasms, and increased vascular permeability. These vascular changes result in the myriad of maternal complications seen in preeclampsia in pregnancy.

Because there is no single screening test available and reliable for predicting preeclampsia, various predisposing factors for preeclampsia have been established (Table 3).

[1]Not FDA approved for this indication.

TABLE 3 Predisposing Factors to Preeclampsia

African American race
Antiphospholipid syndrome
Chronic hypertension
Diabetes
Fetal triploidy or trisomy 13
Hydatidiform mole
Low socioeconomic status
Maternal age <20 or >35 years of age
Multiple gestation
Nonimmune fetal hydrops
Nulliparity/primigravida
Obesity
Polyhydramnios
Preeclampsia in first-degree relative
Preeclampsia in prior pregnancy
Prolonged interval between pregnancies
Renal disease
Systemic lupus erythematosus
Thrombophilia

Management and Treatment of Hypertensive Disorders of Pregnancy

Once the diagnosis of a hypertensive disorder in pregnancy is established, the decision to deliver immediately or to continue the pregnancy is dependent on the severity of the disease, the status of the mother and fetus, and the fetal gestational age. The definitive cure in most scenarios is delivery, especially for the mother. The ultimate goal is to prevent eclampsia or the morbidity/mortality associated with severe preeclampsia, chronic hypertension, and superimposed preeclampsia. However, for the fetus the goal is to deliver a live, mature newborn that does not require intensive and/or prolonged neonatal care.

Fetal evaluation is performed with nonstress testing, serial ultrasounds for growth, amniotic fluid assessment, and biophysical profile. If mild preeclampsia does not progress, delivery of the fetus should occur after 37 weeks of gestation. If the fetus has had less than 34 weeks of gestation, a tertiary hospital is recommended, and antenatal steroid therapy should be given to accelerate the lung maturation. Betamethasone (Celestone Soluspan)[1], 12 mg intramuscularly every 24 hours for two doses, or dexamethasone (Decadron)[1], 6 mg every 12 hours for four doses, is recommended. Steroid therapy decreases the incidence of neonatal respiratory distress syndrome and intraventricular hemorrhage. However, immediate delivery is necessary if the fetus has a nonreassuring nonstress test, oligohydramnios, intrauterine growth restriction, biophysical profile of 4 or less, and/or reversal of diastolic flow of the umbilical artery seen in Doppler ultrasonography.

Treatment and Management of Mild and Severe Preeclampsia

The treatment of preeclampsia may range from bed rest at home, hospitalization, antihypertensive therapy, magnesium sulfate therapy, and, ultimately, delivery. Bed rest is the initial intervention prescribed when preeclampsia is diagnosed. In mild preeclampsia before 37 weeks of gestation, outpatient management of the patient on bed rest may be an optional treatment. Weekly to biweekly office visits are recommended to assess blood pressure, urine protein, laboratory data, and maternal symptoms. In women with mild preeclampsia, the goal is early detection of severe preeclampsia.

The goal in the management of severe preeclampsia is to observe the development of organ dysfunction; however, this may be controversial because of the increased morbidity and mortality of the mother and fetus. Consultation with a maternal–fetal medicine specialist may also be advantageous. Daily blood pressure monitoring, laboratory data, and fetal assessment should be performed. Delivery should be imminent if progression occurs that would disrupt the maternal or fetal environment (Table 4). Maternal indications for immediate delivery include severe preeclampsia; multisystem organ dysfunction; eclampsia; or the hemolysis, elevated liver enzymes, low platelets (HELLP) syndrome.

Preeclampsia management is controversial for patients who are early in the gestation period (24 to 32 weeks). It has been reported that prolongation of pregnancy in such patients could occur with serial laboratory data, bed rest, magnesium sulfate, antihypertensive therapy, and fetal monitoring.

Magnesium sulfate has been used in antepartum, intrapartum, and postpartum management to prevent convulsions in patients with severe preeclampsia. Magnesium has been used in the United States for more than 50 years for seizure prophylaxis. The mechanism of decreasing or blocking seizure potential is still not quite understood; however, recent studies show that magnesium sulfate decreases the initial and/or repeated seizure rate in women with preeclampsia. It is a better anticonvulsant compared to phenytoin (Dilantin) in the Magpie study.

Treatment and Management of Chronic Hypertension

Hypertension in pregnancy is different because the duration of therapy is shorter, the benefits to the mother may not be obvious during the short time of treatment, and the drug exposure includes both mother and fetus. In this respect, one must balance the potential short-term maternal benefits against possible short- and long-term benefits and risks to the fetus and infant. Most women with chronic hypertension during pregnancy have mild, essential,

TABLE 4 Indications for Delivery in Patients With Preeclampsia

Maternal
Eclampsia
Epigastric pain
HELLP syndrome
Oligoria (<500 mL/24h)
Persistent or severe headache
Persistent SBP >160, DBP >110 mm Hg in 24h period
Pulmonary edema
Rising serum creatinine
Fetal
Abnormal fetal heart rate testing
Reversal of diastolic flow in the umbilical artery on Doppler ultrasound
Small-for-gestational-age fetus with failure to grow on serial ultrasound

Abbreviations: DBP = diastolic blood pressure; SBP = systolic blood pressure.

[1]Not FDA approved for this indication.

uncomplicated hypertension and are at minimal risk for maternal and perinatal complications within the short frame of pregnancy. However, the following characteristics indicate possible high risk for increased maternal and perinatal complications related to hypertension:

- Maternal age older than 35 years
- African American race
- Obesity
- Insulin-dependent diabetes
- Renal dysfunction
- Cardiomyopathy
- Hypertension for more than 15 years
- Connective tissue disorders
- Thrombophilias
- Lower socioeconomic class

The major benefit of antihypertensive therapy to the mother and the fetus would be the reduction of the incidence of superimposed preeclampsia. Antihypertensive therapy is used to prevent cerebrovascular and cardiovascular complications such as encephalopathy, hemorrhage, hypertensive crisis, and congestive heart failure in the mother. Ideally, antihypertensive therapy should begin before pregnancy, as well as an extensive evaluation of workup of the etiology, severity, and presence of target organ damage of chronic hypertension.

Antihypertensive Therapies

Methyldopa (Aldomet) has been the gold standard in the treatment of chronic hypertension in pregnancy because of long follow-up time of fetuses exposed in utero. Recently, nifedipine (Procardia), a calcium channel blocker, and labetalol (Normodyne), a β-blocker, have had data reporting the lack of adverse effects on the fetus and the mother in pregnancy. Angiotensin-converting enzyme (ACE) inhibitors have adverse effects on the fetus, such as oligohydramnios and renal failure and are contraindicated in pregnancy. Table 5 lists the antihypertensive agents used for chronic hypertension during pregnancy.

Once the decision for delivery has been established, vaginal delivery should be the route of choice and cesarean performed only in the presence of the appropriate indicators. Induction of labor should be expeditious and aggressive within a predetermined time frame. If this timetable is not achieved, then one should move toward cesarean delivery to decrease the risk to mother and fetus. Fetal monitoring in labor is imperative, preferably internal monitoring, to closely observe the beat-to-beat variability of the fetal heart. Magnesium sulfate may decrease the beat-to-beat variability when used intrapartum. Cesarean should be reserved for the usual indicators, but cesarean should be expedited if there is evidence of hepatic capsular hematoma because of the risk of liver rupture or if adequate fetal monitoring is not available.

Emergencies of Hypertensive Disorders of Pregnancy

Hypertensive disorders in pregnancy still remain one of the most common causes of maternal morbidity and mortality in the world. Severe hypertension should be aggressively treated if the systolic blood pressure is 160 mm Hg and/or diastolic blood pressure is greater than 105 mm Hg. The objective of treating acute severe hypertension is to prevent the progression to complications such as hypertensive emergency, hypertensive encephalopathy, stroke, acute left ventricular failure, and abruptio placentae leading to disseminated intravascular coagulopathy (DIC). Initial treatment may begin with intravenous hydralazine (Apresoline), a direct arteriolar vasodilator that causes a secondary baroreceptor-mediated sympathetic discharge resulting in tachycardia and increased cardiac output. Labetalol (Normodyne) can also be administered intravenously to control blood

TABLE 5 Antihypertensive Drugs Used During Pregnancy

Drug	Category	Dosing
Chronic Hypertensive Management		
Methyldopa (Aldomet)	Central α-adrenergic agonist	Initial: 250 mg bid; Max: 3000 mg/d
Labetalol (Normodyne, Trandate)	β-Blocker	Initial: 10 mg bid; Max: 300 mg bid
Nifedipine (Procardia, Adalat)	Calcium channel blocker	Initial: 30 mg XL qd; Max: 90 mg XL bid
Acute Hypertensive Management		
Hydralazine (Apresoline)	Arteriolar vasodilator	Initial: 5-10 mg IV q15min
Labetalol (Normodyne)	β-Blocker	Initial: 20 mg IV then double the dose q10min max as needed
Sodium nitroprusside (Nipride, Nitropress)	Vasodilator	Initial: 0.25-5 μg/kg/min, increase 0.25 μg/kg/min q5min as needed
Nitroglycerin (Tridil, Nitrostat)	Venodilator	Initial: 0.5 μg/min, then double the dose q5min as needed

Abbreviations: bid = twice daily; IV = intravenous; q = every; qd = every day; XL = extended release.

pressure in the acute setting. Labetalol is a nonselective β-blocker and postsynaptic α_1-adrenergic blocking agent. Nifedipine (Procardia) can be administered orally. The bite-and-swallow technique* to lower blood pressure acutely is not recommended by the manufacturer.

Eclampsia

Eclampsia may be mistaken for hypertensive encephalopathy. There is a poor correlation between occurrence of seizures and severity of hypertension. Eclamptic seizures are tonic–clonic, lasting 1 to 2 minutes, and are without focal deficits and localizing symptoms. During the convulsion, the most important measure is to ensure the patient's safety, prevent injury, minimize trauma, prevent aspiration, and maintain airway. Seizure-induced complications include tongue biting, aspiration, broken bones, and head trauma.

Fetal bradycardia frequently accompanies maternal seizures and usually responds to maternal stabilization. It may result from respiratory and lactic acidosis that develops during the apneic phase. However, persistent fetal bradycardia may be indicative of a placental abruption. Vaginal delivery is associated with less morbidity and should be attempted when feasible. Cesarean delivery should be entertained if the cervix is unfavorable, induction efforts are failing, recurrent seizures are occurring (10% of eclamptic women will have recurrent seizures), or the mother is experiencing uncontrolled hypertension.

Magnesium sulfate is effective and safe for seizure prophylaxis and treatment in pregnancy. Magnesium sulfate is usually administered intravenously as a loading dose of 6 g over 20 minutes followed by a constant infusion of 2 g per hour; however, it may also be administered intramuscularly (Table 6).

TABLE 6 Magnesium Sulfate Administration in Hypertensive Disorders of Pregnancy*†

Intravenous Infusion	
NORMAL RENAL FUNCTION	
Loading dose: 4-6 g over 10-15 min	
Maintenance infusion: 1-2 g/h	
OLIGURIA	
Loading dose: 4 g over 15 minutes	
Maintenance infusion: 1 g/h	
Intramuscular Injection	
Loading dose: 5 g in each buttock (10 g total)	
Maintenance infusion: 5 g in one buttock every 4h	
Frequent Evaluation of Patient	
Measure magnesium level every 4-6h	
Maintain magnesium level between 4 and 7 mEq/L	
Patellar reflex present	
Respiratory rate	
Pulmonary auscultation	
Pulse oximetry	
Urine output	
Magnesium Levels	
5-7 mg/dL	Therapeutic range
8-12 mg/dL	Loss of deep tendon reflexes
10-12 mg/dL	Mental status changes
15-17 mg/dL	Respiratory impairment
30-3 mg/dL	Cardiac arrest

*Magnesium is usually discontinued 24h after delivery.
†When magnesium toxicity occurs, calcium gluconate or calcium chloride, 1 gm (one ampule) can be used IV to reverse the toxicity.

Hemolysis, Elevated Liver Enzymes, and Low Platelets Syndrome

HELLP syndrome is an extremely dangerous subtype of severe preeclampsia. This atypical form of preeclampsia is diagnosed by clinical and laboratory evidence including thrombocytopenia, increased concentrations of serum aspartate transaminases (AST), and lactic dehydrogenase (LDH), which are evidence of hepatic dysfunction and red-cell destruction. The most feared consequences of HELLP syndrome are subcapsular bleeding and hepatic rupture. HELLP syndrome can be a challenge to diagnose because the signs and symptoms of preeclampsia may appear late in its disease course and because the patient's presentation may resemble other disorders. Imitators of the *great masquerader*, HELLP syndrome, include acute fatty liver of pregnancy (AFLP), thrombotic thrombocytopenic purpura (TTP), and hemolytic uremic syndrome (HUS). These disorders share common signs and symptoms and all may be easily misdiagnosed (Table 7). AFLP usually responds to timely delivery and intensive medical support; whereas TTP and HUS have a maternal mortality that exceeds 50% if not treated by plasmapheresis, which has nearly a 90% success rate.

Patients diagnosed with HELLP syndrome are associated with a high maternal morbidity and mortality rate. Once the diagnosis of HELLP syndrome is made, an accepted plan of management is to stabilize the patient and proceed to an expeditious delivery. High-dose intravenous dexamethasone (Decadron), 10 mg every 12 hours, has been proposed as a therapy for potential arrest and reversal of the progression of HELLP syndrome.

The route of delivery is dependent upon the degree of laboratory abnormalities, status of the cervix, and on the presentation and condition of the fetus. The rationale for this strategy is that, regardless of gestational age, the maternal risks of prolonging the pregnancy in the face of this potentially lethal and unpredictable disease are unacceptable. The disease may progress with astonishing and frightening rapidity, and culminate in maternal death.

HELLP syndrome, a relatively frequent and potentially lethal presentation of severe preeclampsia, requires a high index of suspicion. Management is stabilization followed by expeditious delivery.

The etiology and pathogenesis of the hypertensive disorders of pregnancy continue to remain unknown.

*Not recommended by the manufacturer.

TABLE 7 Comparison of HELLP, TTPHUS, and AFLP

	HELLP Syndrome	Thrombotic Thrombocytopenia & Hemolytic Uremic Syndrome (TTP/HUS)	Acute Fatty Liver of Pregnancy (AFLP)
Hypertension	Present	Normal	Normal
Proteinuria	Present	Normal	Normal
Thrombocytopenia	Present	Present	Normal
Lactate dehydrogenase	Increased	Increased	Increased
Anemia	Present	Present	Present
Bilirubin	Increased	Increased	Increased
Aspartate transaminase	Increased	Normal	Increased
Fibrinogen	Normal	Normal	Decreased
Antithrombin III	Decreased	Normal	Decreased
Ammonia	Normal	Normal	Increased
Glucose	Normal	Normal	Decreased
Creatinine	Increased	Increased	Increased

Abbreviation: HELLP = hemolysis, elevated liver enzymes, low platelets.

There are neither proven therapies nor preventive methods to avert preeclampsia and all of its serious side effects. These potential catastrophic outcomes result in significant maternal and fetal morbidity and mortality unless the proper antenatal and/or postnatal diagnosis is made. Antihypertensive therapy remains controversial in mothers with mild hypertension, with questions concerning the benefit/risk to the fetus. Magnesium sulfate is definitely the anticonvulsant for prophylaxis and treatment of eclampsia. The practitioner must be consciously aware that diagnosis and appropriate management is the mainstay of a successful outcome.

POSTPARTUM CARE

METHOD OF

Ana M. Vidal, MD, and George R. Saade, MD

The postpartum period, or puerperium, is traditionally defined as the first 6 weeks after delivery. It is the time period in which the woman begins her physiologic return to her prepregnancy state.

Postpartum Physiology

The postpartum period is the time for the maternal adaptations to pregnancy to return gradually to the prepregnancy state. The first most notable change is the contraction of the uterus immediately after delivery of the placenta, when the fundus can be palpated at the level of the umbilicus. The uterus regains its nonpregnancy size at about 4 weeks postpartum. The gestationally regulated cardiovascular changes continue during the first 48 hours after delivery. Cardiac output increases further as a result of an increase in stroke volume in response to the increase in venous return, which is precipitated by the contraction of the uterus and the relief of inferior vena cava compression. The immediate postpartum period is, therefore, a critical time for women at risk for cardiac decompensation, such as those with valvular heart disease. The cardiovascular system is back to a normal state by 2 to 6 weeks postpartum. Mobilization of extracellular fluid and diuresis is also prominent during the first 2 to 5 days postpartum. Women who are at risk for voiding difficulty, such as those who had epidural analgesia or prolonged labor, should be monitored for urinary retention and promptly catheterized if needed. Abdominal wall stretching requires several weeks for recovery, a process that can be accelerated by exercise.

General Care Measures

During the first few hours after delivery the woman should be watched with vital signs taken every 15 minutes, the amount of vaginal bleeding noted, and uterine tone checked. If so desired, she may begin breast feeding, which may help increase uterine tone. The woman should be instructed on proper perineal care. Ice bags may be applied initially to ease perineal swelling; and after 24 hours warm compresses, baths, or topical anesthetics may be used. The diet may be unrestricted if there are no complications likely to necessitate intervention and anesthesia. Analgesia should be provided as needed, usually starting with nonsteroidal anti-inflammatory drugs (NSAIDs). Occasionally, narcotics may be required, especially if delivery was complicated. Before discharge from the hospital or birthing center, immunizations should be checked to see if they are current, and women who are rubella nonimmune should also receive vaccination. Typically, infants are now routinely immunized for hepatitis B, but mothers are vaccinated only if at high risk for exposure. Women who are Rh negative with an Rh positive infant should receive Rh_0 immune globulin (RhoGAM), 300 μg intramuscularly (IM). Hospitalization for an uncomplicated vaginal delivery is usually 48 hours. Before discharge mothers should be given warning signs to return to the hospital should they have excessive vaginal bleeding or fever, or develop leg pain or swelling, chest pain, or shortness of breath.

Lactation

Nursing should be encouraged starting in the antepartum period. Colostrum can typically be expressed for 2 to 3 days postpartum. The first breast milk (colostrum) is protein rich and provides antibodies that the infant cannot yet produce and are not found in cow's milk or formula. Infants who are breast fed have a lower incidence of inner ear infections and diarrheal illnesses as compared to bottle-fed infants. Breast-feeding also improves bonding between mother and infant in those first few days.

Breast engorgement may occur around day 2 or 3, and can be painful. This can be relieved with frequent feedings and analgesics. Some women may experience nipple cracking and pain, which may be relieved with regular cleansing of the nipple and areola with soap and water, allowing the nipple to air dry. The woman should continue to take prenatal vitamins and iron supplementation (Prenatal Plus) as well as increase caloric intake by 640 kcal per day while breast-feeding. Although a woman may not menstruate during the period of breast-feeding, this does not guarantee anovulation, and contraception should be used if needed. Progesterone-only methods are preferred for women who are nursing.

Mastitis may occur in a nursing mother. Symptoms include fever, erythema of the breast, mastalgia, and malaise. It is commonly caused by inoculation with staphylococcal organisms from the infant's oral cavity. Treatment is usually on an outpatient basis and includes penicillin or cephalosporin, such as dicloxacillin, 500 mg orally four times a day; analgesia; and continued breast-feeding. If a breast abscess is suspected, the patient should be admitted to the hospital, breast-feeding discontinued, intravenous antibiotics administered, breast ultrasound performed, and surgical drainage considered.

Contraindications to breast-feeding include HIV infection, breast abscess, severe maternal illness, active herpes infection of the breast, and maternal ingestion of certain medications (Table 1). For these women, breast engorgement can occur and be painful. Binding of the breasts with an elastic bandage or tight fitting brassiere helps to suppress milk production. Medical treatment to suppress lactation is generally avoided and unnecessary.

TABLE 1 Common Medications Contraindicated During Breast-Feeding

Medication	Reason
Alprazolam (Xanax)	Fetal weight loss, lethargy, and probable withdrawal
Atorvastatin (Lipitor)	Excreted into breast milk of rats
Bromocriptine (Parlodel)	Suppress lactation
Cocaine	Cocaine intoxication
Lithium (Eskalith)	Increased blood levels in infants
Metronidazole (Flagyl)	Mutagenic and carcinogenic in test species; avoid breast-feeding for 24h after taking 2 g oral dose
Methotrexate (Rheumatrex)	Possible immune suppression, neutropenia, unknown effect on growth
Radioactive iodine	Concentrated in breast milk and uptake by infant's thyroid gland observed

Counseling Issues

There is no definite time after delivery when coitus may be resumed, and this issue should be guided by amount and type of vaginal bleeding or lochia, as well as the patient's comfort. If breast-feeding, the woman should be counseled that she may experience vaginal dryness and atrophy due to suppression of estrogen.

A common patient question is when normal menstruation will resume. A woman should expect to have a small amount of bleeding intermittently starting after delivery. Lochia is a vaginal discharge composed of blood and decidua. The lochia is bloody in the first 3 to 4 days after delivery, becoming more watery and eventually white. On average, lochia persists for up to 1 month, but may persist up to 6 weeks in some women. If a woman does not breast feed, the first normal menses typically occurs 6 to 8 weeks postpartum. In nursing women, normal menses may not occur as long as they are nursing. Ovulation, however, may not be suppressed completely by lactation alone.

Ideally contraception should be initially presented antenatally, but definitely reviewed post partum. In lactating women, progestin-only contraceptives, whether in pill form (Micronor) or injection (Depo-Provera), will not interfere with nursing. Estrogen-containing oral contraceptives can be used in nursing mothers but should be started after lactation has been established. Intrauterine devices are typically placed at the 6-week postpartum visit to avoid increased risk of expulsion or perforation if inserted earlier when the uterus is larger and the cervix dilated. Barrier methods such as diaphragms should also be fitted at the 6-week postpartum visit when the vagina should have achieved its definitive shape and form.

A weight loss of 8 to 9 kg (17.6 to 19.8 lb) can be expected from delivery of the baby, expulsion of the placenta, and diuresis during the first postpartum week. Most women can expect to return to near prepregnancy weight by approximately 6 months, but most can expect a surplus of 1.4 kg (3 lb) to remain.

Complications

POSTPARTUM HEMORRHAGE

Postpartum hemorrhage is defined as a 10% drop in hematocrit or a need for erythrocyte transfusion. Postpartum hemorrhage can be early (within the first 24 hours) or late (after 24 hours but less than 6 weeks). The most common cause of early hemorrhage is uterine atony; and late hemorrhage is usually caused by subinvolution of the placental site, infection, and retained products of conception. A woman with hemorrhage should be stabilized with volume and blood product replacement as needed, followed by search for and correction of the cause. Medical treatment initially involves using intravenous oxytocin (Pitocin), methylergonovine maleate (Methergine), and prostaglandins. Surgery (typically curettage, or, rarely, hysterectomy) is reserved for cases refractory to medical management.

INFECTION

The most common source of postpartum infections is endomyometritis. Cesarean delivery is the most common predisposing factor. The diagnosis is based on physical findings of fever, uterine tenderness, parametrial tenderness, and purulent lochia. Endometritis is polymicrobial, and therapy should cover both aerobic and anaerobic bacteria. Other causes of postpartum infection include urinary tract infections, mastitis, and, rarely, episiotomy breakdown.

POSTPARTUM MOOD CHANGES

Postpartum blues is the most common of the mood changes occurring in an estimated 50% to 80% of women postpartum. These women experience emotional lability, anxiety, and fatigue. The condition is transient and can be managed by close observation and reassurance. If the symptoms persist for more than 2 weeks, then postpartum depression is likely and medical therapy may be needed. Postpartum depression in a prior pregnancy is the most common predisposing factor, with a 30% risk of recurrence in a future pregnancy. Postpartum psychosis is a rarer event, occurring in 1 of 1000 deliveries with a recurrence also of approximately 30%.

RESUSCITATION OF THE NEWBORN

METHOD OF
Jeffrey D. Merrill, MD, and
Roberta A. Ballard, MD

The transition from intrauterine to extrauterine life involves remarkable physiologic changes as the fetus moves from the warm, protected, supportive environment within the mother, and becomes an independent newborn infant. Also remarkable is the fact that at least 90% of infants make this transition without any major assistance in the form of resuscita-tion. However, 5% to 10% of newborn infants require some assistance at birth, and approximately 1% of infants require a more extensive skilled resuscitation.

Neonatal Resuscitation Program

Guidelines for resuscitation of the adult were recommended in 1966 by the National Academy of Sciences, and subsequently, in 1978, a working group of the American Heart Association Emergency Cardiac Care Committee was formed to address issues of pediatric resuscitation. It became clear that resuscitation of the newborn required a different emphasis than that for the adult, namely a focus on ventilation rather than on cardiac dysfunction such as cardiac arrest or fibrillation. In 1985, the American Academy of Pediatrics (AAP) joined the American Heart Association (AHA) in a joint commitment to develop a Neonatal Resuscitation Program (NRP), to teach the principles of resuscitation of the newborn. By the end of 1998, at least 1 million providers were trained in the techniques of neonatal resuscitation. Statewide implementation of NRP instruction and certification is associated with an improvement in Apgar scores of high-risk neonates. The evaluation of both the science and technique of neonatal resuscitation has involved periodic international cardiopulmonary resuscitation and emergency cardiac care conferences. Based on these conferences, a textbook has been developed with guidelines, most recently for the year 2000.

Transition From Fetal to Neonatal Circulation

In utero, the placenta serves as the gas exchange organ for the fetus, and as a result of constricted pulmonary arterioles with high pulmonary vascular resistance, only a very small portion of the cardiac output flows through the lungs. Two right-to-left shunts exist in utero. The first shunt from the right atrium to the left atrium through the foramen ovale serves to direct the more highly oxygenated umbilical venous return toward the systemic circulation of critical organs such as the heart and brain. The second right-to-left shunt directs less oxygenated blood from the pulmonary artery to the aorta across the patent ductus arteriosus, and back to the placenta for gas exchange.

The fetus accommodates well in utero to a normal PaO_2 between 20 and 25 mm Hg. Fetal adaptation to relative in utero hypoxia includes the presence of fetal hemoglobin, with higher affinity to oxygen than adult hemoglobin and greater uptake at the placenta. In addition, oxygen demand is reduced given the neutral thermal environment and lack of respiratory work. The fetus has greater resistance to tissue acidosis as compared to the adult, and, through bradycardia and an exaggerated *diving reflex*, diverts blood flow to critical organs in times of crisis.

Immediately following delivery, with clamping of the umbilical cord, the low resistance placental circulation is removed and respiration is initiated by the fetus. Expansion of the lung promotes an immediate drop in pulmonary vascular resistance, and pulmonary blood flow is propagated by further ventilation and oxygenation. Increased pulmonary venous return elevates left atrial filling pressure, exceeding right atrial pressure and functionally closing the foramen ovale. As pulmonary vascular resistance decreases and systemic vascular resistance increases, right-to-left shunting across the patent ductus arteriosus also ceases.

Asphyxia is defined as a combination of hypoxemia, hypercapnia, and metabolic acidemia. If there is failure to establish spontaneous ventilation after birth, the aggressive cycle of worsening hypoxemia, hypercapnia, and metabolic acidemia evolves, causing pulmonary vascular resistance to remain high, the ductus to remain widely patent, and the resulting right-to-left shunts to continue. A number of factors that are of maternal or placental origin, as well as fetal origin, may contribute to the occurrence of asphyxia in the perinatal period by interrupting in the establishment of the normal neonatal circulation.

NRP Resuscitation Guidelines

INITIAL ASSESSMENT

Earlier guidelines from NRP suggested a very *hierarchical* approach, first evaluating pulmonary status, then cardiac status, and then perfusion. The more recent guidelines stress a more *integrated* approach in which the resuscitation team takes into account neonatal risk factors, activity after birth, and cardiopulmonary status simultaneously. Upon initial assessment, if the infant is:

- Born at term
- Active
- Breathing with good tone and color
- Clear of meconium

then routine care is indicated. If all of these conditions are not met, one should proceed to the first steps of resuscitation, including positioning the infant under a radiant warmer, clearing the upper airway of secretions, drying, stimulating, and providing blow-by oxygen as necessary.

THERMOREGULATION

The current guidelines continue to emphasize close attention to neonatal body temperature during resuscitation. Newborns have significant heat losses, particularly evaporative heat losses, after delivery. These heat losses are compounded in smaller preterm infants by the large body-surface-area-to-body-weight ratio, and may cause a large increase in oxygen consumption from unnecessary thermoregulatory work. While routinely avoiding significant hypothermia remains important, there is preliminary evidence suggesting that hypothermia may be neuroprotective in asphyxiated infants. While randomized trials continue to address this possible clinical intervention in asphyxiated term infants, the NRP algorithm currently recommends avoidance of hyperthermia during resuscitation.

INFANT WITH MECONIUM-STAINED AMNIOTIC FLUID

The philosophy of approach to infants born through meconium-stained fluid has changed. Previously, the recommendation was to intubate and suction the trachea of all infants born through meconium-stained fluid. Recent evidence suggests that automatic intubation and suctioning of the trachea does not lead to an improvement in the incidence of meconium aspiration syndrome in healthy, vigorous infants. The latest recommendations are to perform direct tracheal suction only if the infant has depressed respiratory drive, bradycardia, or poor muscle tone.

ASSISTED VENTILATION

If, after initial assessment the infant remains apneic or with a heart rate less than 100 beats per minute, positive pressure ventilation is indicated. *Effective* ventilation is the single most important step in resuscitation of the depressed newborn. Evidence exists that the reversal of hypoxia, acidosis, and bradycardia is dependent on adequate expansion of the lung.

Adequate lung inflation not only improves gas exchange, but stimulates further pulmonary vasodilation and surfactant release. The initial ventilation of a gasless, fluid-filled lung may require relatively higher inflation pressures with longer inspiratory times.

The optimal concentration of supplemental oxygen to be used in neonatal resuscitation remains controversial. Saugstad and co-investigators report evidence that room air is as efficient as 100% oxygen for resuscitation of newborn infants, with a shorter time to initiation of spontaneous respiratory effort. In addition, markers of oxidative stress are higher, and persist longer after resuscitation with 100% oxygen than room air. Follow-up between the ages of 18 and 24 months was performed, and there was no significant difference in growth or neurologic handicap in infants resuscitated in room air versus 100% oxygen. Additional studies are being undertaken to determine both efficacy and safety of resuscitation with room air rather than 100% oxygen. In the meantime, the NRP algorithm continues to recommend use of 100% oxygen. However, if oxygen is not available, positive pressure ventilation may be initiated with room air for depressed neonates.

Assisted ventilation should continue until the heart rate is higher than 100 beats per minute, and the infant demonstrates spontaneous respirations. If bag and mask ventilation persists for several minutes, one should place an orogastric tube to suction air. Endotracheal intubation should be considered if the need for assisted ventilation persists for several minutes without signs of improvement. If poor respiratory effort continues and there is a history of maternal narcotic administration within four hours of delivery, one should consider naloxone (Narcan) administration to the neonate. This is contraindicated in neonates born to opiate-addicted mothers.

CHEST COMPRESSIONS

The majority of neonates in need of resuscitation will respond to ventilatory maneuvers alone. However, if the heart rate remains below 60 beats per minute despite 30 seconds of *effective* ventilation, chest compressions should be administered in a ratio of three compressions to one breath. Based on animal studies of systemic perfusion with mechanical compressions, the two-thumb and circling hands method of chest compression is preferred over the two-finger method. The depth of compression is one third to one half the anterior–posterior diameter of the chest.

EPINEPHRINE

The dose of epinephrine suggested is 0.01 to 0.03 mg/kg and should be administered if the heart rate remains less than 60 beats per minute after at least 30 seconds of *effective* ventilation and chest compressions. Epinephrine may be given either IV or via endotracheal tube. Although higher IV doses of epinephrine have been shown to increase coronary perfusion and cardiac output in adults and older children, the benefit of this effect is not clear in neonates, and higher doses are associated with a significant increase in postresuscitative hypertension and possible increased risk of intracranial hemorrhage. Similarly, although higher doses of endotracheally administered epinephrine may provide higher systemic levels, they are associated with a significant prolongation of the aforementioned postresuscitative hypertension, as compared to standard dose endotracheal epinephrine. Therefore, standard dose epinephrine is recommended regardless of route of administration.

CARDIOVASCULAR SUPPORT

Most infants are not hypovolemic in the delivery room. In cases where volume is indicated, volume expansion may be accomplished with isotonic saline or Ringer's lactate solution. If one suspects severe hemorrhage with anemia, transfusion of type O-negative packed red cells should be considered. It is no longer appropriate to use albumin-containing solutions as the fluid of choice for initial volume resuscitation and expansion. Volume replacement should be administered slowly, as neonatal cerebral vasculature may be maximally dilated in cases of shock, and rapid replacement may be associated with an increased risk of intracranial hemorrhage. In cases of sepsis or severe asphyxia with myocardial failure, one should consider pressor administration to maintain renal perfusion and/or systemic vascular support.

SODIUM BICARBONATE ADMINISTRATION

Administration of sodium bicarbonate in delivery room resuscitations continues to be controversial. One may consider bicarbonate administration in cases of *severe* metabolic acidosis, but only after establishment of *effective* ventilation. Diluted (4.2%) preparations should be used and given slowly, as rapid administration of sodium bicarbonate is associated with intracranial hemorrhage, particularly in premature infants.

PRETERM INFANTS

Preterm infants present a special challenge in the resuscitation room. One must consider the cause of preterm delivery and its impact on the degree of resuscitation required, given the high incidence of perinatal asphyxia from conditions such as placental insufficiency, placental abruption, chorioamnionitis, and infection. In addition, one must consider the range of sizes of resuscitative equipment required for various sized infants as well as age-specific changes to resuscitation guidelines for those infants who are extremely immature.

Extremely premature infants are prone to anatomic airway obstruction from floppy pharyngeal structures, which may impede efforts of assisted bag and mask ventilation. The younger and more immature premature infants have a higher likelihood of respiratory failure and surfactant deficiency. It is known that infants who are at risk for respiratory distress syndrome benefit from prophylactic surfactant (Survanta) given soon after delivery, rather than rescue surfactant treatment at a later point based on severity of pulmonary disease. It is also known, however, that bronchopulmonary dysplasia is associated with intubation and prolonged mechanical ventilation, and, therefore, many nurseries are proceeding to earlier use of nasal continuous positive airway pressure (CPAP) in the delivery room. Studies demonstrate that earlier delivery of surfactant via endotracheal tube, followed by rapid extubation to nasal CPAP, may benefit a premature infant who is likely to progress to respiratory failure, yet reduce the risk of later bronchopulmonary dysplasia.

If preterm infants are intubated, one must avoid overdistention and hyperventilation with hypocarbia. Excessive ventilator pressures increase the risk of lung injury and may compromise cardiac output. An increased incidence of white matter lesions (periventricular leukomalacia) has been reported in premature infants with prolonged periods of hypocarbia. One must also avoid hyperoxygenation given the increased risk of later lung disease and retinopathy of prematurity in preterm infants exposed to excessive oxygen concentrations.

DURATION AND LIMITS TO RESUSCITATION

For infants that continue with absent heart rate despite effective ventilation, compressions, and medication administration, resuscitative efforts should rarely be continued beyond 15 minutes. The incidence of death or irreversible neurologic damage in survivors of this group of neonates is unacceptably high.

While studies demonstrate survival of infants whose birth weight is less than 750 g (26.4 oz) requiring chest compressions and/or epinephrine during initial resuscitation, the incidence of severe intracranial hemorrhage and/or periventricular leukomalacia increases significantly after such an event. In addition, the gestational age limit of viability is controversial and probably represents a range of extremely immature gestational ages and associated circumstances rather than a single line at a single gestational age. It is clear that the survival for less than 23 weeks gestation and birth weight of less than 400 g (14.1 oz) is exceedingly low, and one should consider counseling parents before the delivery about comfort-care-only measures.

PITFALLS TO AVOID IN RESUSCITATION

In resuscitating a newborn infant, the team should be aware of a number of potential pitfalls that may occur either with lack of skilled staff or over-vigorous resuscitation of the newborn:

- Avoid panic around intubation. Concentrate on the technique of bag and mask ventilation if an endotracheal tube cannot be placed.
- Don't focus excessively on the use of medications or cardiac resuscitation. Remember that the most likely cause of neonatal depression is pulmonary and one must establish effective ventilation before moving to cardiac resuscitative maneuvers.
- Remember that the fetal lung is fluid-filled before delivery and that normal absorption of clear lung fluid is into the lung and the circulation. Thus avoid excessive suctioning of clear fluid.
- Avoid the use of excessive inspired oxygen concentrations, particularly in the preterm infant at risk for retinopathy of prematurity, and in asphyxiated infants. Such infants may often be resuscitated with 40% oxygen or less.
- Avoid the use of excess ventilatory pressure when expanding the lungs, particularly in the preterm infant. Overexpansion of the lung may set up processes contributing to bronchopulmonary dysplasia or lead to pneumothorax.
- Avoid over-ventilation and hypocapnia as well. There is evidence that a low PCO_2 may have a significant detrimental effect on the neonatal brain.
- Be sure to monitor oxygenation in term or post-term infants, particularly in those stained with meconium, who may have some early evidence of elevated pulmonary vascular resistance.

The most important aspects of safe resuscitation of the newborn infant remain an in-depth understanding of maternal and neonatal physiology, a team approach to management of the mother, delivery of her newborn infant at an optimal location with appropriate equipment and skilled personnel available to intervene as necessary to make sure the infant has a successful transition to extrauterine life.

CARE OF THE HIGH-RISK NEONATE

METHOD OF

Caraciolo J. Fernandes, MD

High-risk neonates may broadly be defined as newborn infants requiring a level of care that is greater than that which is routinely provided for the uncomplicated term birth. The care of these infants should ideally be in a hospital adequately equipped and staffed to care for such infants. While the birth of such high-risk infants cannot be predicted with certainty, careful attention to the maternal and fetal history (where available) can identify maternal and fetal conditions that suggest a need for infants to be delivered at a hospital capable of providing a higher level of care (Table 1). Transport of a high-risk

TABLE 1 Identifying the High-Risk Neonate

Prior to Birth

MATERNAL CONDITIONS
Age (>40 years, <16 years)
Detrimental habits (smoking, drug and/or alcohol abuse)
Medical conditions
  Diabetes mellitus, hypertension, chronic heart and/or lung disease, kidney diseases/urinary tract infections, blood disorders (thrombocytopenia, anemia, blood group incompatibilities)
Obstetric conditions
  Prior stillbirth/fetal loss/early neonatal death, prior birth of a high-risk infant, antepartum hemorrhage, premature rupture of membranes, serious infection during pregnancy, placental anomalies (previa, polyhydramnios or oligohydramnios, pregnancy-induced hypertension, group B *Streptococcus* carrier)
Poor socioeconomic status (poverty, malnutrition)

FETAL CONDITIONS
Congenital anomalies
Hydrops
Intrauterine growth retardation
Macrosomia
Multiple gestation

During Birth

Abnormal fetal heart rate patterns
Abnormalities of presentation (transverse lie, breech, etc.)
Chorioamnionitis or systemic maternal infection
Complications of maternal medical disease
Foul-smelling or meconium-stained amniotic fluid
Instrumented delivery (forceps, vacuum, or cesarean)
Narcotic administered to mother within 4 hours of birth
Premature labor
Prolapsed cord
Uteroplacental bleeding

After Birth

Birth depression
Macrosomia
Postmature infant
Premature and/or low-birth-weight infant
Respiratory depression and/or distress
Seizures

neonate in utero before birth is preferable to having a high-risk neonate be born in a setting that is ill-equipped to care for it, necessitating its subsequent transport after birth to a tertiary care setting. Unfortunately, not all high-risk infants are identified before birth, and infants are often delivered in situations that are not optimal for their successful management, which increases the potential for adverse outcomes. As such, health care workers who care for pregnant women and newly born infants are best advised to ensure that persons skilled in basic neonatal resuscitation are present at every delivery. Infants that need a higher level of care can then be rapidly stabilized and transported to the tertiary care facility.

Delivery Room Management

NEONATAL RESUSCITATION

To be able to deliver the highest standard of care, caregivers must understand perinatal physiology, the principles of resuscitation, and have mastered specific technical skills needed to care for high-risk neonates. The Neonatal Resuscitation Program (NRP) sponsored by the American Academy of Pediatrics/American Heart Association presents a logical, coordinated approach to neonatal resuscitation, and it is highly recommended that anyone involved in the delivery room care of the newborn be familiar with and able to execute the resuscitation protocol. Because, despite one's best efforts, high-risk deliveries cannot be predicted with certainty, the labor and delivery areas must maintain a state of constant readiness; appropriate personnel must be readily available, and supplies and equipment must ideally be checked at least every shift, and replaced after use or if found faulty. Further information regarding the neonatal resuscitation can be found in the article on resuscitation of the newborn elsewhere in this book.

PERINATAL PHYSIOLOGY

In utero, the placenta is the organ of respiration and the lungs are filled with fluid. Because the lung does not function to oxygenate the blood in utero, oxygenated blood from the placenta enters the right atrium via the inferior vena cava, is shunted through the foramen ovale into the left heart, and distributed to the brain and peripheral circulation. The right heart primarily receives blood with a lower oxygen content, which is ejected into the pulmonary artery, and then diverted via the ductus arteriosus to the aorta rather than the high-resistance lungs. This blood is then distributed to the placenta via the aorta and umbilical arteries to receive oxygen and nutrients, and to release carbon dioxide and waste products.

At birth, the newborn infant transitions from an intrauterine to extrauterine environment, in which the lung is the organ of respiration. With the newborn's first few breaths, certain cardiopulmonary adaptations rapidly occur that make this transition successful. First, the lungs expand as they are filled with gas; fetal lung fluid gradually leaves the alveoli by moving into the extra-alveolar interstitium, and is eventually cleared by lung lymphatic vessels. At the same time, the pulmonary vascular resistance decreases rapidly and pulmonary blood flow correspondingly increases. These changes are associated with an increase in the partial pressure of oxygen in the alveoli and arterial circulation from the fetal level (approximately 25 mm Hg) to approximately 50 to 70 mm Hg. With clamping of the umbilical cord, the systemic vascular resistance increases. Even though the foramen ovale and ductus arteriosus remain anatomically open, the decrease in pulmonary vascular resistance and the increase in systemic vascular resistance effectively reverse the direction of blood flow through these two shunt pathways. However, if pulmonary vascular resistance remains elevated, blood shunts right-to-left through the foramen ovale and ductus arteriosus, mimicking the fetal circulatory pathways and impairing oxygen delivery. Hypoxia, acidosis, and hypothermia are common causes of elevated pulmonary vascular resistance; hence, it is apparent that attention to prevention of hypoxia, acidosis, and hypothermia at birth will help assure a smooth transition to normal postnatal circulation.

Fortunately, the first few breaths of most newborn infants are effective and allow the cardiopulmonary adaptations previously discussed to take place. However, in certain situations, the transition from in *utero* to *ex utero* does not occur smoothly, and the infant may need to be helped if it is to survive without sequelae. For example, some infants are asphyxiated *in utero* and are born with ineffective respiratory efforts, others are delivered by cesarean section and may have tachypnea associated with delayed clearing of fetal lung fluid, while yet others may have aspirated meconium-stained amniotic fluid that compromises their ventilation. Premature infants may lack surfactant, which may lead to hyaline membrane disease.

ASSESSMENT AND STABILIZATION

While the reader is referred to the article on neonatal resuscitation, a brief overview is presented here with reference to personal practices of the author regarding specific situations. Review of the perinatal history often prepares the caregivers for certain planned interventions. The birth of a premature infant presents risks of complications of prematurity that are inversely correlated with the infant's gestation age; such problems include, e.g., hyaline membrane disease, intraventricular hemorrhage, and hypotension. Similarly, the infant of a diabetic mother has an increased risk of macrosomia, birth trauma, dystocia, asphyxia, hypoglycemia, cyanotic congenital heart disease, and caudal regression. As such, prior knowledge of certain specific details pertaining to the infant may launch a series of interventions that are best drafted as a protocol for use of the health care team, so as to allow the team to function optimally because all members will know what is expected of them in the given situation. Copies of the mother's medical record with details of the pregnancy, labor, and pertinent medical history are usually presented to the pediatrician or neonatologist, either before or at the time of the infant's birth. Ideally, in the case of a high-risk birth, the obstetrician will communicate his or her concerns regarding the infant to the personnel assuming care of the newborn. However, in an emergency situation, it might be prudent for the pediatrician/neonatologist to seek out such information if it is not presented to him or her.

The neonatal resuscitation flow diagram (Figure 1) outlines the steps detailed for resuscitation of the infant at birth. The first box of questions helps decide which infants are in need of assistance and which may safely be expected to complete normal transition with the mother. The main emphasis of the new NRP is that of timely interventions involving attention to the ABCs of resuscitation in a given sequence of interventions. If one remembers that one of the prime goals of resuscitation is to get oxygen to the infant's brain, the steps involved in resuscitation become logical, sequential interventions. Adequacy of airway patency is a vital prerequisite to ventilation, and adequacy of ventilation is a vital prerequisite of cardiac compressions. As, for the most part, cardiac compromise of the neonatal heart is usually caused by hypoxia and rarely a result of ischemic heart damage, attention to obliterating hypoxemia usually results in the recovery of the depressed neonate. For the same reasons, gasping respiratory efforts of compromised neonates may signify need for positive pressure ventilation. Drugs are rarely needed in neonatal resuscitation. Ongoing assessment of the neonate is vital, and additional interventions are instituted according to the response to the prior interventions.

While large preterm infants and term infants are intubated if increased work of breathing or apnea is observed, the extremely premature infant (<28 weeks) is often intubated electively to ensure adequacy of supportive care, as the risks of the complications of prematurity are high. In some instances, the medium-sized premature infant (28 to 32 weeks) may do well with only the provision of continuous distending airway pressure via nasal prongs, which allows the maintenance of the infant's functional residual capacity of the lung and possibly to prevent the development of respiratory distress syndrome.

The Apgar score, a universally used method of assessing the infant's adaptation to extrauterine life, was developed by Dr. Virginia Apgar. The score reflects the infant's status at 1 and 5 minutes of life, and is composed of five components (Table 2):

1. Heart rate
2. Respiratory effort
3. Muscle tone
4. Reflex irritability
5. Skin color

While the 1- and 5-minute Apgar scores may be used as reflections of how well an infant tolerated the birth process and responded to resuscitative efforts respectively, they are not used to determine one's interventions for resuscitation. In addition, they may be *abnormal* in premature infants who typically have lower tone and less robust reflexes than the term infant, and in infants whose mothers may have been given certain anesthetic medications immediately before birth. The delivery room assessment of the newborn typically involves a quick review of the history, a brief physical examination to discover any life-threatening malformations and/or disease, and determination of a plan of care for the infant. Vital initial assessments are the determination of the infant's gestational age and whether or not intrauterine growth has been appropriate. While a formal gestational age assessment using a scoring

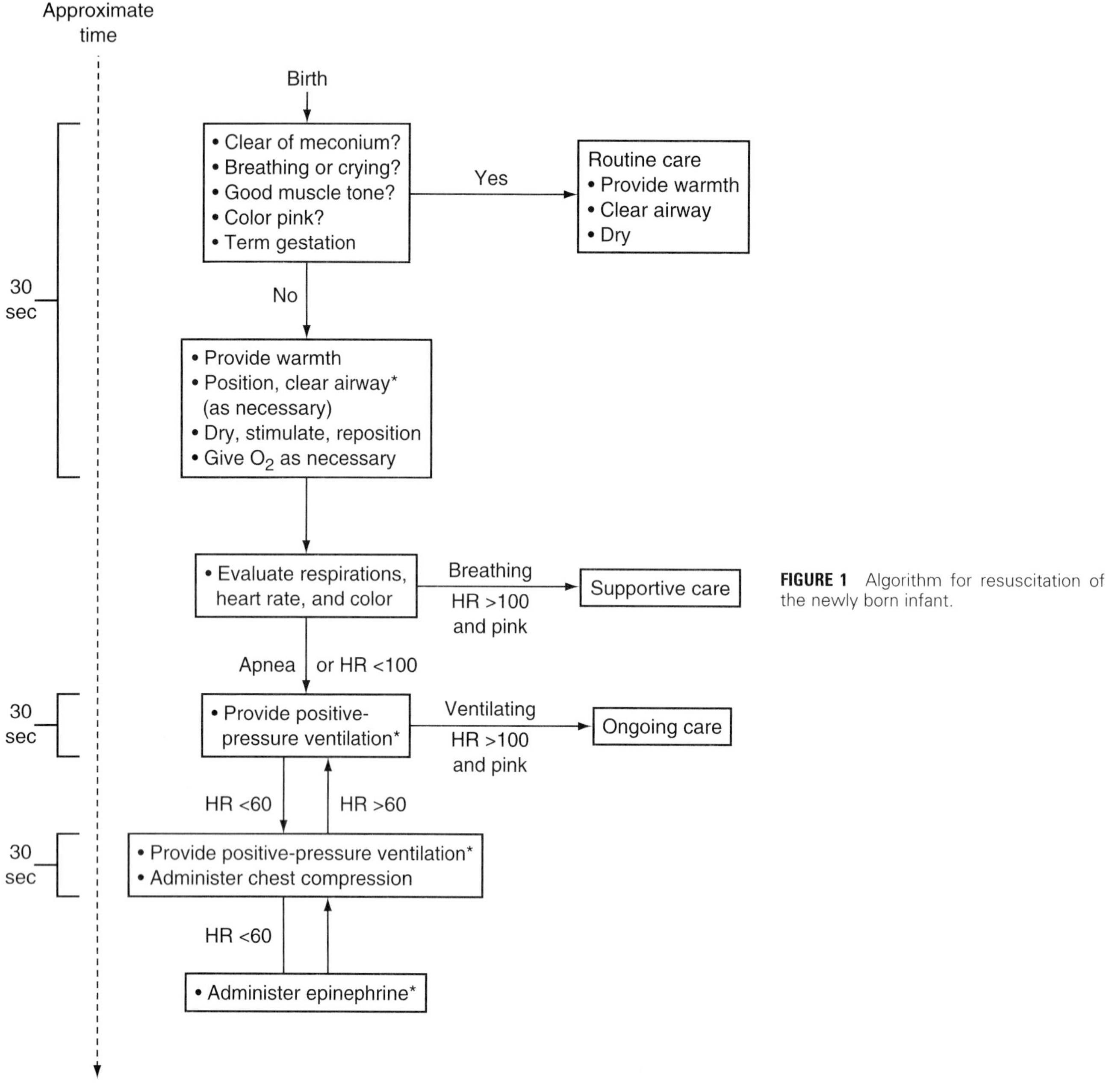

FIGURE 1 Algorithm for resuscitation of the newly born infant.

system such as the Ballard score (Figure 2) is commonly done as part of the nursing admission protocol in many nurseries, most experienced perinatal physicians are able to rapidly and adequately estimate the infant's gestational age and appropriateness of growth during a routine physical examination. This is useful to categorize the newborn as appropriate for gestational age (AGA), small for gestational age (SGA), or large for gestational age (LGA), as each category has its own associated potential problems that can be anticipated. Newborn infants may also be classified according to birth weight—normal birth weight (>2500 g), low birth weight (LBW) (<2500 g), very low birth weight (VLBW) (<1500 g), and extremely low birth weight (ELBW) (<1000 g).

The rapid assessment should include a complete set of vital signs (temperature, heart rate, respiratory rate, blood pressure), pulse oximetry (if available), determination of the presence of cyanosis and/or respiratory distress, level of activity, tone, and responses to the environmental stimuli (light, sound and touch). These assessments assist the caregivers in determining whether the infant is adapting appropriately to the extrauterine environment and what

TABLE 2 The APGAR Scoring System

Component	0	1	2
Heart rate	Absent	<100 beats per minute	>100 beats per minute
Respiratory effort	Apneic	Shallow, irregular, gasping	Vigorous cry
Reflex irritability	Absent	Grimace	Active avoidance
Muscle tone	Flaccid	Weak, passive	Active movement
Skin color	Pale, cyanotic	Pale, acrocyanotic	Pink

Adapted from: Gowen CW Jr. Care of the high-risk neonate. *In* Rakel RE: Conn's Current Therapy 1995. Philadelphia, WB Saunders Co., 1995, p. 964.

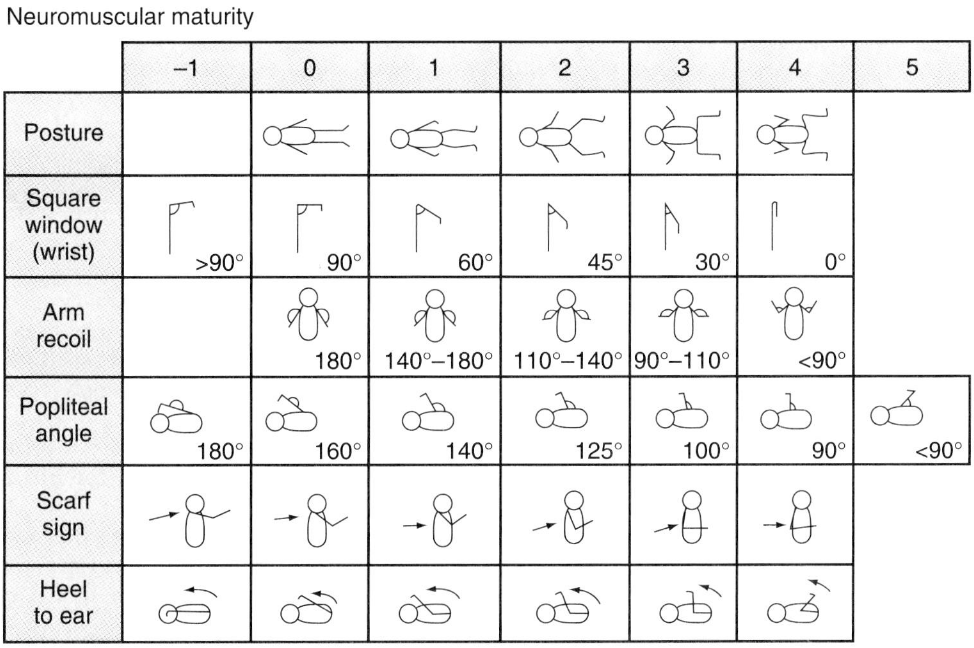

Neuromuscular maturity

	–1	0	1	2	3	4	5
Posture							
Square window (wrist)	>90°	90°	60°	45°	30°	0°	
Arm recoil		180°	140°–180°	110°–140°	90°–110°	<90°	
Popliteal angle	180°	160°	140°	125°	100°	90°	<90°
Scarf sign							
Heel to ear							

Physical maturity

Skin	Sticky friable transparent	Gelatinous red translucent	Smooth pink, visible veins	Superficial peeling and/or rash, few veins	Cracking pale areas rare veins	Parchment deep cracking no vessels	Leathery cracked wrinkled
Lanugo	None	Sparse	Abundant	Thinning	Bald areas	Mostly bald	
Plantar surface	Heel-toe 40-50 mm:–1 <40 mm:–2	>50 mm no crease	Faint red marks	Anterior transverse crease only	Creases ant. 2/3	Creases over entire sole	
Breast	Imperceptible	Barely perceptible	Flat areola no bud	Stippled areola 1–2 mm bud	Raised areola 3–4 mm bud	Full areola 5–10 mm bud	
Eye/ear	Lids fused Loosely:–1 Tightly:–2	Lids open pinna flat stays folded	Sl. curved pinna; soft; slow recoil	Well-curved pinna; soft but ready recoil	Formed and firm instant recoil	Thick cartilage ear stiff	
Genitals male	Scrotum flat, smooth	Scrotum empty faint rugae	Testes in upper canal rare rugae	Testes descending few rugae	Testes down good rugae	Testes pendulous deep rugae	
Genitals female	Clitoris prominent labia flat	Prominent clitoris small labia minora	Prominent clitoris enlarging minora	Majora and minora equally prominent	Majora large minora small	Majora cover clitoris and minora	

Maturity rating

Score	Weeks
–10	20
–5	22
0	24
5	26
10	28
15	30
20	32
25	34
30	36
35	38
40	40
45	42
50	44

FIGURE 2 The Ballard scoring system.

support it might need. The presence of cyanosis, low oxygen saturations (<90%), respiratory distress (flaring of the ala nasi, grunting, suprasternal/substernal/intercostal retractions, or tachypnea), or hypotension suggests the need for immediate supportive intervention. Normal heart rate is generally between 120 to 160 beats per minute (with a range from 80 to 180 beats per minute). A slow heart rate in a sleeping term infant that rapidly increases following stimuli is likely to be normal. Normal respiratory rate in a newborn is generally between 40 to 60 breaths a minute. When examining neonates, it is best to proceed in a systematic and orderly fashion, generally from top-down (head to toe), and least invasive to most invasive (observation, auscultation, and, last, palpation).

While many clinical findings are similar to those in the older infant and child, some details of the examination are specifically relevant to the neonatal period only, and are commented on herein (from top-down). The head should be examined for the presence of molding (that may alter its shape), bruising or the presence of a cephalhematoma (which should be differentiated from a caput as the former does not cross suture lines). The size and shape of the anterior and posterior fontanelles and any overriding of the sutures should be noted. Abnormalities of the shape, size and position of the ears, eyes, nose, and mouth are often noted in many syndromes. However, characteristics of the face (forehead, eyes, nose, and ears) should be compared to the parents before one determines that an infant has *dysmorphic* facies. Presence of other dysmorphic features of the neck (webbed, short), trunk (widely spaced nipples), limbs (poly or syndactyl), spine (myelomeningoceles), heart (abnormal heart sounds or murmurs associated with defects), and others are clues to the existence of a dysmorphic syndrome. Ears are generally said to be "low set" if they are below an imaginary line joining the outer canthus of the eye and the occiput. The eyes are examined for the presence of a *red reflex*, which is normal; inability to elicit a red reflex may be noted with the presence of a cataract (suggestive of a metabolic or infectious disease) or intraocular tumor (like a retinoblastoma). Subconjunctival hemorrhages, while alarming to parents, are fairly common and generally resolve without any problems in a few days.

Mild flaring of the ala nasi is often seen as part of normal transition, but the infant should be closely monitored for other signs indicative of respiratory distress. A feeding tube is commonly passed through both nares into the hypopharynx to check for patency of the choanae. The oral cavity should be inspected and palpated for the presence of palatal clefts. Symmetry of movement of the mouth and eyes provide clues to facial palsies resulting from traumatic and/or instrumented deliveries. The infant's neck should be examined for any masses, and the clavicles for the presence of fractures (that may be seen with term LGA infants). Observation of the chest of the noncrying infant for symmetry of movement, presence of retractions, and position of the cardiac impulse may provide clues to the presence of lung or heart disease. Heart sounds are best auscultated for over the left sternal border. Transient systolic murmurs associated with a closing ductus arteriosus may be heard in the immediate newborn period. However, the presence of abnormal heart sounds or a murmur should prompt the measurement of upper and lower limb blood pressure to evaluate for possible coarctation of the aorta or similar obstructive lesion. Similarly, coarse breath sounds or rales on auscultation of the lungs in an otherwise well appearing infant are occasionally heard as part of the transitional state, and usually do not herald more sinister processes. Nevertheless, caregivers should ensure that breath sounds are bilaterally equal, and other signs of respiratory disease do not exist or appear subsequently.

Examination of the abdomen is typically noncontributory; the liver can usually be palpated just below the right costal margin, but the spleen is usually not palpable. A scaphoid abdomen is associated with congenital diaphragmatic hernia, as the abdominal contents are displaced into the chest cavity. If abdominal masses are detected on palpation, further investigations are indicated. The umbilical cord should be examined for meconium staining and inflammation, and the number of blood vessels. A single umbilical artery is seen in some syndromes. The anal orifice should be examined for location and patency. Genitalia of both male and female infants provide clues to help estimate the infant's gestational age. The presence of hypospadias or cryptorchidism in the term male is reason for referral to a urologist. The female infant often has a creamy white vaginal discharge, which is normal.

The back and spine should be carefully examined and palpated for spina bifida (or meningomyeloceles), sacral dimpling, and sinus tracts. Mongolian spots are hyperpigmented patches commonly seen on the lower back in darker pigmented populations. Examination of the hips for clicks and clunks suggestive of developmental dysplasia of the hip should be a part of the routine examination, although it is not typically done in the delivery room. Extremities should be evaluated for the presence of anomalies or abnormalities (such as talipes) secondary to intrauterine positioning. Mottling of the skin is commonly seen in infants that are cold or have problems with perfusion, while erythema toxicum is a rash common and peculiar to newborns.

Neurologic examination of the newborn infant differs from that of the older child in that most of it is done by observation of the infant's tone, activity, responses to various stimuli, and one's ability to elicit various neonatal reflexes. Neonatal reflexes that are usually elicited are the startle reflex, Moro reflex, rooting and sucking reflexes, and plantar and palmar grasp. In general, a complete and thorough examination of the newborn is done on admission to the neonatal unit. However, the delivery room assessment helps one decide what interventions need to be effected immediately, and what can wait until the infant is transported to the nursery. Parents should ideally be spoken to in the delivery room to update them as to the status of their infant, and what (if any) issues need immediate intervention. Many first-time parents worry needlessly over items that have no long-term significance, such as prominent cranial molding or transient skin rashes. If, as part of the initial assessment and stabilization, it is determined that an infant is a healthy term infant (see Figure 1), the infant only needs routine newborn care, i.e., keeping the infant's airway clear of mucus and ensuring it is dry and warm. The infant may be transported with the mother to the level I nursery.

If the infant displays abnormal pathophysiology, the infant should be rapidly stabilized and a decision made as to whether it needs to be transported to a tertiary care facility (Figure 3). Interventions that may be needed include provision of supplemental oxygen, support of respiration for respiratory distress and/or apnea (ventilator therapy), provision of intravenous fluids for an energy source or blood pressure support (intravenous [IV] dextrose, normal saline bolus), and antimicrobial therapy to counteract an infection (evaluation of sepsis and antibiotic therapy). Laboratory evaluations that may be performed in the delivery room include determination of arterial and/or venous blood gases (following insertion of umbilical catheters), blood glucose, and hematocrit. An evaluation for sepsis typically includes a complete blood count with a differential leukocyte count, platelet count, and blood culture; a lumbar puncture is usually performed in symptomatic infants. Radiologic studies are occasionally performed for determination of intrathoracic pathophysiology and for evaluation for positioning of catheters and endotracheal tubes. Details of various conditions are described later in this article.

TRANSPORT

If an infant needs to be transported to a tertiary care facility, the earlier the facility is contacted and made aware of the infant the better it is. Timely involvement of the subspecialty physicians allows them to participate in the care of the infant before transport. Most regional centers have complete neonatal transport teams and neonatologists available 24 hours a day to provide telephonic consultation and assistance both before and during the transport. The transport team usually includes a nurse, a respiratory

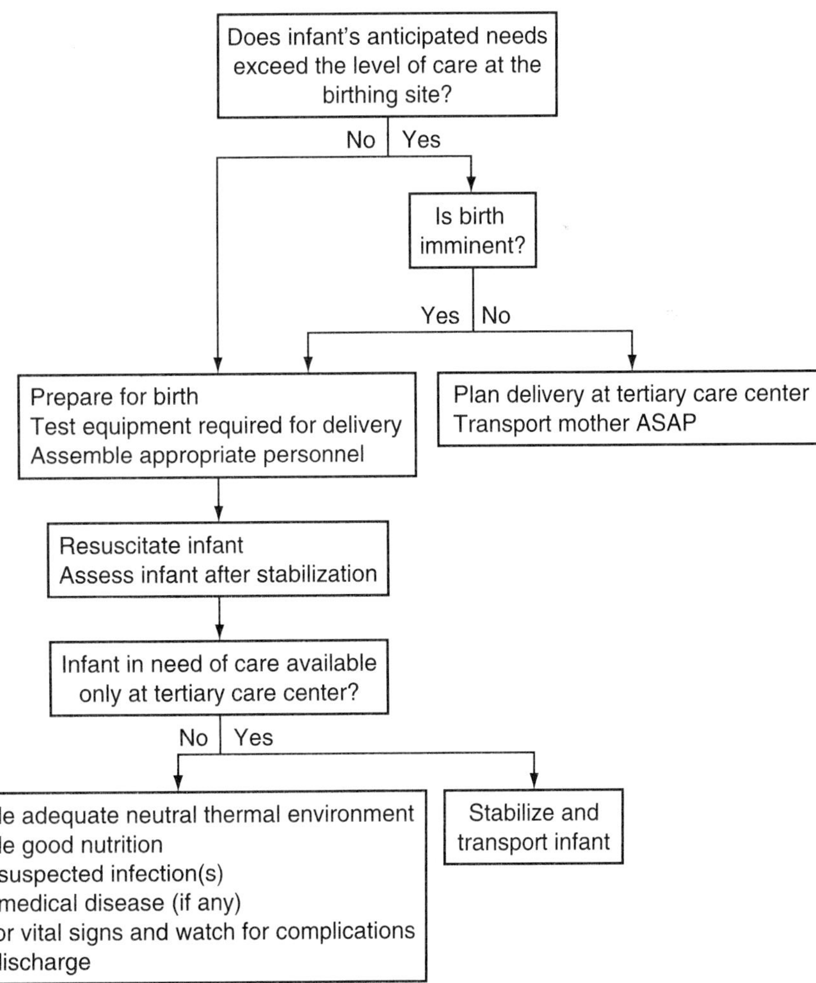

FIGURE 3 Algorithm for deciding care for the high-risk neonate.

therapist, a neonatal nurse practitioner, and/or a physician.

General Management

THERMOREGULATION

One of the foremost concerns with the birth of a high-risk infant is the provision of a *neutral thermal environment*, which is the thermal environment required to permit the neonate to maintain a normal body temperature with a minimum expenditure of energy. This varies with gestational age, size, and chronologic age of the infant. The large surface area relative to body weight and poor insulation (fat stores) of premature infants make them particularly susceptible to cold stress. Estimated heat loss in newborn infants at birth can be as high as 200 kcal/kg per minute, which is far above their maximal heat production. Failure to dry an infant to minimize heat loss and to provide an external heat source can result in hypothermia with the development of acidosis. Initially, we attempt to maintain a newborn infant's temperature usually with an overhead warmer with a servocontrolled radiant heater, which is regulated by a thermostat set to maintain the skin temperature in the range of 36.2°C to 36.5°C (97.2°F to 97.7°F). The radiant heater allows maximal access to the infant with adequate provision of heat. For ELBW infants, who are at greatest risk of evaporative heat loss, the use of a *plastic wrap* blanket provides additional benefit. Following stabilization and transport of the infant to the nursery, a double-walled incubator may also be used for the same purposes.

RESPIRATORY SUPPORT

Following establishment of a neutral thermal environment, ensuring adequate oxygenation and ventilation is of paramount importance. The general goal is to support the infant's respiration (and oxygen and carbon dioxide levels in the blood) with the least amount of support that one has to administer, so as to minimize the risks of hyperoxia, barotrauma, and volutrauma. Many infants with mild respiratory distress and transient tachypnea of the newborn can be managed with humidified oxygen provided by an oxygen hood. Clinical examination and blood gas estimation help decide which infants may need ventilator support. Ventilator strategies are best decided by considering the pathophysiology of the disease process, its natural history, and responses to interventions. Time-cycled, pressure-limited ventilators are the most commonly used standard ventilator in most nurseries, although some centers prefer to use high-frequency oscillators as an initial therapy for premature infants. High-frequency oscillatory ventilators are also commonly used following failure of conventional ventilation, with air leak syndromes, persistent pulmonary hypertension, pulmonary hypoplasia, and congenital diaphragmatic hernia. Volume-cycled ventilators are more commonly used in chronically ventilated older infants with bronchopulmonary dysplasia. All infants needing oxygen therapy or ventilatory support of any kind should be monitored closely by means of a cardiorespiratory monitor, a transcutaneous pulse oximeter, and periodic arterial blood gas estimations. Typical goals (on arterial blood gases) are:

- pH—7.30 to 7.45
- P_{CO_2}—35 to 50 torr
- pO_2—50 to 80 torr

However, these goals may need to be altered in light of the postulated pathophysiology of the disease and what is feasible with the least amount of risk. Infants with respiratory disease typically have some response in oxygenation (pO_2) following institution of the following maneuvers:

- Institution of oxygen
- Institution of continuous positive airway pressure (CPAP)
- Institution of ventilator therapy

Infants who remain hypoxemic despite attainment of adequate ventilation (i.e., low P_{O_2} with normal P_{CO_2}) may have either cyanotic heart disease or persistent pulmonary hypertension (PPHN), both of which are best managed at tertiary care centers that routinely care for such infants. Some infants with PPHN may respond to inhaled nitric oxide (INO_{MAX}) administered via the ventilator circuit, while others may not, necessitating the use of extracorporeal membrane oxygenation (ECMO).

FLUID AND ELECTROLYTES

Following establishment of a neutral thermal environment and adequate oxygenation and ventilation, provision of adequate fluid and nutrition is vital to

TABLE 3 Fluid Requirements in the Newborn Period*

	Birthweight (g)				
	≤1000	1000-1250	1250-1500	1500-2000	≥2000
Day 1	120-100	100-80	80	80-65	65
Day 2	130-120	120-100	100	100-80	80
Day 3	140-130	130-120	120	120-100	100
Day 5	150	150	150	150	150

*Values given are total daily intake (mL/kg/d).

the well-being of the infant. Many factors need to be considered when determining fluid therapy for a sick neonate. The most immediate concerns are the need for fluid boluses for blood pressure support and those for correction of hypoglycemia. For routine maintenance fluids, the following guidelines are offered (Table 3 gives fluid administration practices at our institution), keeping in mind that therapy must be individualized depending on the infant's particular circumstances. When possible, the enteral route is preferred for the administration of both fluid and nutrition; however, problems common to the high-risk neonate often dictate that intravenous therapy be started initially. The choice of fluid on the first day of life is intravenous dextrose (without any added electrolytes) to provide a glucose infusion rate of 4.5 to 6 mg/kg per minute. When possible (if not contraindicated), total parenteral nutrition (TPN) may be preferable even on the first day of life for premature infants, although electrolyte supplements are usually omitted from this *early* TPN. Maintenance electrolytes are typically added to the fluids after urine output (losses) and kidney function are established, usually by 24 hours of life—sodium (2 to 3 mEq/kg per day) and potassium (1 to 2 mEq/kg per day). Serum electrolytes are usually monitored at least once daily and more frequently in the extremely premature or critically ill infant. Generally accepted normal values are:

- Serum sodium—130 to 150 mEq/dL
- Serum potassium—3.5 to 5.5 mEq/dL

Calcium, another commonly monitored serum electrolyte, exists in the serum in ionized and non-ionized states; hypocalcemia is generally defined as a total serum calcium level less than 7.0 mg/dL (in preterm infants) and less than 8.0 mg/dL (in term infants). Although total serum calcium is commonly monitored, it is the ionized fraction that is vital for homeostasis and prevention of the symptoms of hypocalcemia. Hence, we typically monitor the ionized form, and treat LBW infants if they are symptomatic or have an ionized calcium less than 0.8 mmol/L, and larger infants if they are symptomatic or have an ionized calcium less than 1.0 mmol/L. Symptomatic infants are treated with a 100 mg/kg bolus of calcium gluconate given as a slow infusion with cardiac monitoring to observe for bradycardia. Asymptomatic infants are treated by addition of calcium gluconate (300 to 500 mg/kg per day) to the daily intravenous fluids. Close monitoring of weight, daily fluid intake and output, and serum electrolytes help guide subsequent fluid therapy. Frequency of laboratory monitoring is dependent on expected changes, which depend on the infant's gestation, size, and ongoing losses associated with any disease.

BLOOD PRESSURE SUPPORT

Hypotension is a common problem in preterm infants and sick, term newborns. Normal values for blood pressure are dependent on the infant's gestational and chronologic age. As a general rule, we expect very preterm infants (24 to 30 weeks) to have a mean blood pressure in the high 20s to low 30s mm Hg range, and term infants to have a mean blood pressure approximately 45 mm Hg. Irrespective of the exact number, adequacy of tissue/organ perfusion is confirmed by clinical examination and documentation of urine output. If blood pressure support is needed, a normal saline volume bolus (10 mL/kg) may be attempted if the history suggests loss of blood volume as is seen with placenta previa or abruptio placentae. If the volume bolus fails to increase the blood pressure, an intravenous dopamine (Intropin) infusion is initiated at 5 μg/kg per minute, and titrated up to 20 μg/kg per minute until the blood pressure is in the expected normal range. In patients whose blood pressure remains a concern despite use of volume boluses and inotropic (dopamine) support, intravenous steroids (hydrocortisone [Solu-Cortef][1] or dexamethasone [Decadron][1]) may be considered.

NUTRITION

Attention to adequate nutrition for the high-risk infant is vital if the neonate is to do well and be discharged in a timely fashion. In infants able to tolerate enteral feeds, enteral nutrition is always preferable to intravenous nutrition. If oral feedings are not contraindicated and a near-term or term infant may be expected to feed well *PO* (per oral), we attempt a test feed, usually administered by an experienced nurse, to determine what volume of feed the infant may consume per feed. If not contraindicated, *PO ad lib* feeds of the formula of choice may be written for the infant. In infants who consume only part of their expected feed (for total daily requirement), the balance of the fluid and nutritional intake is made up by the administration of intravenous nutrition. In infants who do not feed well orally or are not expected to feed well orally (such as very preterm infants), we usually begin with gavage feedings of 20 mL/kg per day of expressed breast milk (EBM) or the formula of choice, and advance daily in steps of 20 mL/kg per day as long as feedings are tolerated, until full enteral feedings are achieved. In infants weighing less than 2000 g (approximately 4.5 pounds), a 24-calorie preterm formula is the formula of choice; when expressed mother's milk is used, it is fortified with a human milk fortifier once 100 mL/kg per day of feeds are tolerated. Tolerance of feedings is determined by monitoring the amount of gastric residuals, presence of emesis, stooling frequency, and abdominal examination. Adequate nutritional intake typically implies approximately 160 mL/kg per day of 24-calorie preterm formula, or at least 180 mL/kg per day of fortified human milk or term formula. Occasionally,

[1]Not FDA approved for this indication.

infants with bronchopulmonary dysplasia may be fluid restricted to 130 to 150 mL/kg per day, and may need additional supplements to ensure adequate nutrition.

In infants too sick to tolerate enteral feeds, parenteral nutrition is generally begun between the first and third day of life. The volume of parenteral nutrition delivered is decided by taking into account the total fluid requirements for the day, and adjusting for other fluid intake derived from administration of medications, blood products, enteral feeds, and so on. Amino acids are provided to deliver 3 to 3.5 g/kg per day; while glucose infusions typically provide at least 4.5 to 6 mg/kg per minute initially, and are increased daily as tolerated to approximately 11 mg/kg per minute (16 g/kg per day). The parenteral solutions also contain a mixture of electrolytes, calcium, phosphorus, other minerals, and multivitamins to ensure daily requirements are met. Lipid infusions are generally started, at the same time as the TPN, at 5 mL/kg per day of a 20% solution, and increased in steps to 20 mL/kg per day. Serum triglyceride levels are monitored as an indicator of tolerance of the lipid infusion.

LABORATORY INVESTIGATIONS

Laboratory tests ordered depend on the clinical status of the infant and the differential diagnoses being considered in the case of the high-risk neonate. As mentioned earlier, typical tests ordered in the delivery room include a hematocrit, blood glucose, and blood gases. An investigation for sepsis usually includes a complete blood cell count (CBC) with differential and platelet count, and tracheal and blood cultures. Other typical admission tests include determination of the infant's blood type and Coombs' test. In sick neonates in the nursery, routine daily tests typically include serum electrolytes, blood urea nitrogen (BUN), creatinine, glucose, bilirubin, and hematocrit. In the very sick or very preterm infant that may have high ongoing losses (*third spacing*, or insensible fluid losses), some tests such as electrolytes may be done more than once per day. Generally, urine specimens are evaluated by a dipstick for glucosuria every shift, as hyperglycemia is common in the very sick or very preterm infant, and such infants may need treatment with insulin. Conversely, frequent monitoring for hypoglycemia may be needed in infants born to diabetic mothers as they have too high insulin levels, and may need infusions of glucose to prevent hypoglycemia. As the serum chemistry profile of the infant typically reflects the mother's for the first 24 hours after birth, such tests are best deferred to the second day of life, except in the very preterm (e.g., 23- to 26-week-gestation neonate) or very sick infant (e.g., suspected inborn error of metabolism, possible kernicterus) whose metabolic parameters are expected to change very rapidly.

Specific Problems of the High-Risk Neonate

NEUROLOGIC

Seizures

As in older children and adults, seizures in the neonate constitute an emergency. However, unlike older children and adults, seizures in neonates do not typically present with the classic tonic–clonic activity seen in older patients. Seizures in neonates may be classified as myoclonic, clonic, tonic, or subtle; the last is the most common type seen in the very preterm neonate. Subtle seizures may manifest as tonic eye deviations, sucking and smacking movements of the mouth and lips, and *bicycling* and *swimming* movements of the extremities. Seizures can also present as apnea or autonomic dysfunction with blood pressure changes. As in older patients, the causes of seizures are many, and treatable causes should always be sought first. In the neonate, specific causes that bear mentioning include:

- Metabolic problems (such as hypoglycemia and hypocalcemia)
- Infectious causes (meningitis and encephalitis, especially with a maternal history suggestive of infection)
- Congenital anomalies with intracranial malformations
- Central nervous system (CNS) pathology (such as intraventricular hemorrhage or hypoxic-ischemic encephalopathy)

As it is often difficult to differentiate jitters from seizures by clinical examination alone, an electroencephalogram should be obtained if seizures are suspected. Management typically includes simultaneous investigation to determine the cause of the seizures and initiation of measures to control the seizures. Specific therapy (when possible) such as correction of hypoglycemia or hypocalcemia is always preferable to nonspecific anticonvulsant therapy; when anticonvulsants are used, typically phenobarbital is the first drug of choice, followed by phenytoin (Dilantin), and/or lorazepam (Ativan).

Intracranial Hemorrhage

Intraventricular hemorrhage (IVH) is a serious concern in preterm infants, and varies inversely with gestational age. Most such hemorrhages occur in the first 3 to 5 days of life, and are more likely in critically ill infants that are hypotensive or need substantial ventilatory support. While most intraventricular hemorrhages are diagnosed during routine head ultrasound screening, severe intraventricular and intraparenchymal hemorrhages may be associated with seizures, hypotension, a fall in hematocrit, or abnormalities of tone or activity. A commonly used classification of intracranial hemorrhages is that of Papile, which grades the hemorrhages from 1 (least severe) to 4 (most severe). In an attempt to minimize the risk of an intraventricular hemorrhage, most centers practice some form of "minimal stimulation" care for very preterm infants in the first few days of life; such care seeks to minimize interventions (such as excessive tracheal suctioning, rapid fluid boluses, etc.) that might lead to swings in blood pressure that might lead to rupture of fragile intracranial blood vessels, and bleeding. Once an intracranial hemorrhage is discovered, the infant is monitored closely by serial measurement of the head circumference and ultrasonography to identify early complications such as posthemorrhagic hydrocephalus. Prognosis varies with severity of the hemorrhage, although less severe hemorrhages (grades 1 and 2) usually resolve without sequelae.

Periventricular Leukomalacia

Periventricular leukomalacia is a lesion of white matter commonly seen in sick preterm infants. The pathogenesis of the lesion consists of an ischemic necrosis of the periventricular white matter followed by possible progression to cavitation, cyst formation, and subsequent enlargement of ventricles. Risk factors are similar to those associated with IVH, and include prematurity, hypotension, and hypoxemia. Sequelae, which depend on the degree of neurologic involvement, may not be discovered until many months later, and include diplegic cerebral palsy and varying degrees of intellectual dysfunction.

Hypoxic–Ischemic Encephalopathy

Hypoxic–ischemic encephalopathy is a result of prepartum, intrapartum, or perinatal asphyxia, and is most commonly seen in full-term or post-term infants. The pathogenesis involves a sequence of cerebral insults that occur initially with hypoxemia and ischemia, and next by oxygenation and reperfusion of the ischemic tissue. Cerebral edema and hemorrhagic infarctions may be seen on cranial imaging. Management is essentially supportive. Long-term outcomes depend on the degree of cerebral insult, but many infants have some degree of intellectual and/or motor impairment. Although electronic fetal heart rate monitoring during labor is now routinely done in an attempt to identify infants at risk of perinatal asphyxia, it has not been uniformly successful in predicting the birth of a depressed infant in a timely fashion; hence, it is vital that every birth be attended by personnel trained in neonatal resuscitation.

RESPIRATORY

Respiratory Distress Syndrome

Respiratory distress syndrome (RDS), or hyaline membrane disease, is the result of decreased amounts of pulmonary surfactant, and occurs commonly in very preterm infants (less than 28 to 30 weeks gestation). Like intraventricular hemorrhage, its incidence varies inversely with gestational age. It may also be seen in infants of diabetic mothers, and following perinatal asphyxia. In recent years, its incidence has diminished following the increasing use of antenatal steroids and postnatal prophylactic surfactant administration in very preterm infants. For infants who exhibit signs and symptoms suggestive of hyaline membrane disease, early administration of artificial surfactant (Survanta) intratracheally may abort or ameliorate the progression of the disease. Additional treatment is essentially supportive with the provision of supplemental oxygen, CPAP support, and positive pressure ventilation. As hyaline membrane disease cannot be definitely differentiated from group B streptococcal pneumonia radiologically, infants with RDS are generally also treated with antibiotics for a possible sepsis–pneumonia.

Bronchopulmonary Dysplasia

Bronchopulmonary dysplasia (BPD), or chronic lung disease (CLD), is mostly seen in preterm infants treated with ventilatory support. Like IVH and RDS, it varies inversely with gestational age, and may be seen in up to 30% to 40% of extremely preterm infants (23 to 24 weeks gestation). BPD has classically been defined as the need for oxygen therapy more than 28 days after birth; however, most recent literature defines it as need for supplemental oxygen at 36 weeks corrected gestational age. The latter definition is preferable as it takes into account that lung maturity is different in preterm infants of differing gestational ages. While an infant may not be officially labeled as having BPD until much later in life, current thinking holds that the pathogenesis of the disease is initiated in the first few days of life. Radiologic changes that may be noted include atelectasis alternating with areas of overdistention or pulmonary interstitial emphysema. Infants are typically ventilated for long periods of time, and therapy is essentially supportive with attention to good nutrition to promote (lung) growth. Other therapies include modest fluid restriction, diuretics, and a variety of inhalers.

Apnea of Prematurity

Apnea is classically defined as a cessation of breathing for longer than 20 seconds, and needs to be differentiated from the brief pauses commonly seen with normal periodic breathing that may be seen in both preterm and term infants. Apnea is a common problem of premature infants, and is inversely correlated with gestational age. Apnea may be caused by an immature central control of breathing, obstruction because of poor pharyngeal tone, or both. It may be accompanied by bradycardia (heart rate <80 beats per minute), and/or a drop in oxygen saturations.

Apnea of prematurity is essentially a diagnosis of exclusion; other more serious causes of apnea (infection, metabolic disease, intraventricular hemorrhage, hyperthermia, and seizures) should always be considered in an infant with a new-onset apnea. If a specific etiology is discovered, it should be addressed simultaneously with addressing the apnea itself to ensure the best possible outcome. The goal in management of apnea of prematurity is to support the infant's (inadequacy of control of) breathing until it has matured developmentally, and apnea is no longer a concern. If apneic episodes are brief and/or infrequent, and either resolve spontaneously or respond promptly to tactile stimulation, all the infant may need is close monitoring for worsening of symptoms. If the episodes are frequent, especially if the infant is less than 30 weeks gestation, we usually attempt pharmacologic therapy with caffeine citrate (Cafcit) (20 mg/kg loading dose IV or orally, followed by 5 mg/kg once daily). Side effects with caffeine are rarely seen, but may include tachycardia and jitteriness. In premature infants less than 32 weeks gestation, obstructive apnea may be minimized by the use of nasal CPAP (NCPAP). If multiple episodes occur acutely or despite pharmacologic therapy and NCPAP, an infant may need intermittent mandatory ventilation. As the infant matures, need for positive pressure and/or pharmacologic support for control of breathing diminishes. We usually discontinue caffeine once infants have achieved a corrected gestational age of 34 weeks. Infants are generally monitored for apnea until serum caffeine levels have been deemed to be subtherapeutic and apnea is no longer noted. While cardiorespiratory monitoring for apnea at home may be considered in patients with a history of severe apnea (if desired by the parents), it has not been shown to lower the incidence of the sudden infant death syndrome. If undertaken, such patients should be enrolled in a program especially designed for home monitoring, and managed by a physician (typically a pulmonologist).

Pulmonary Hypertension

Pulmonary vascular pressures are normally elevated in utero, as the placenta (not the lung) is the organ of respiration. The elevated pulmonary pressures ensure that blood that returns to the heart from the body is diverted via the foramen ovale and ductus arteriosus to the systemic circulation. While the suprasystemic pulmonary resistance is desirable before birth, it necessarily needs to fall after birth if the newborn lung is to become the organ of respiration. In the normal newborn, as effective first few breaths cause the lungs to expand, pulmonary vascular resistance decreases rapidly and pulmonary blood flow correspondingly increases. Associated increases in the partial pressure of oxygen in the alveoli and arterial circulation from the fetal level (approximately 25 mm Hg to approximately 50 to 70 mm Hg) stimulate pulmonary vasodilation, as oxygen is a potent pulmonary vasodilator. Failure of the pulmonary vascular resistance to fall normally should result in a condition termed *persistent pulmonary hypertension of newborn* (PPHN), in which blood bypasses the lungs and fails to get oxygenated, causing hypoxemia to develop. As hypoxia, acidosis, and hypothermia are common causes of persistently elevated pulmonary vascular resistance, it is apparent that attention to prevention of these entities at birth will help assure a smooth transition to extrauterine life. While PPHN is typically a disease of full-term and post-term infants, it may occasionally be seen in premature infants. While the cause of PPHN is not known in some cases, a condition termed as primary PPHN, in some instances PPHN may be secondary to other pathophysiologic processes, such as perinatal hypoxemia associated with fetal distress, meconium aspiration syndrome, sepsis–pneumonia, and so on. In infants with symptoms suggestive of lung disease, the maneuvers listed in the Respiratory Support section earlier should be attempted to improve oxygenation. Infants that fail to respond to such maneuvers either have PPHN or congenital cyanotic heart disease, which can only be differentiated reliably by cardiac echocardiography. Treatment is generally supportive, while appropriate investigations to determine a primary cause are initiated. Management includes treatment for and correction of abnormal pathophysiology (if present) that may contribute to the development of PPHN, such as sepsis, hypotension, hypoglycemia, hypocalcemia, acidosis, and polycythemia. Infants are usually given IV fluids/TPN, placed on nothing-by-mouth (NPO) status, and ventilated in an attempt to improve oxygenation. The mean airway pressure and oxygen index (a calculated measure of what ventilator pressures it takes to oxygenate the infant) are generally monitored to determine whether the infant is improving or deteriorating. Occasionally infants may respond to respiratory alkalosis, although such responses are usually transient. Following the discovery that INO_{MAX} is a specific pulmonary vasodilator, centers that are equipped with nitric oxide therapy will initiate it when the oxygen index is greater than or equal to 25. Other therapies attempted in patients with refractory PPHN include ECMO and high-frequency oscillatory ventilator (HFOV). Ideally infants that need such support have already been transported to a tertiary care center.

CARDIAC

Patent Ductus Arteriosus

If, after birth, the ductus arteriosus fails to close as it normally should, blood may flow from the systemic circulation into the pulmonary vascular bed, causing an increase in the pulmonary blood flow. This patent ductus arteriosus (PDA) is typically seen in the more premature infant. Its incidence is inversely correlated with gestational age. Hemodynamically significant patent ductus arteriosus with left-to-right shunts usually presents within the first week of life when the pulmonary vascular resistance is falling. Clinical signs suggestive of a PDA include a wide pulse pressure (usually greater than 20 mm Hg, and caused by a fall in diastolic BP), an *active* or hyperdynamic precordium, *bounding* or especially vigorous pulses, and a murmur. As the murmur heard depends on size of the PDA, the pressure gradient across the PDA, and the turbulence caused, it may vary from absent, to only mid-systolic, to holosystolic, to continuous. Other findings that may be present include metabolic acidosis, need for increasing ventilatory support, and hemorrhagic pulmonary edema. A PDA can only be diagnosed definitively by cardiac echocardiography. Pharmacologic treatment with indomethacin (Indocin I.V.) is generally successful in closing a majority of the PDAs of the mid-size premature infant that are diagnosed in the first few days of life. Surgical ligation of PDAs may be necessary in the sick very preterm neonate, or if pharmacologic therapy fails or is contraindicated.

Congenital Heart Disease

Congenital heart disease is said to occur in approximately 8 in every 1000 live births. With the advent of antenatal ultrasonography, many lesions are diagnosed antenatally allowing antenatal transport of the mother and fetus to a tertiary care center equipped for the care of the high-risk neonate. Age at presentation and diagnosis of cardiac anomalies not diagnosed antenatally depends on the type of lesion and index of suspicion of the caregiver examining the infant postnatally. Some lesions (pulmonary stenosis, pulmonary atresia, tricuspid atresia, transposition of the great vessels, total anomalous pulmonary venous return) can be obvious at birth or shortly thereafter, as they may present with one or more identifying symptoms: cyanosis, a loud murmur, or cardiac failure leading to respiratory distress. Other lesions (severe coarctation of the aorta, interrupted aortic arch, hypoplastic left heart syndrome) may not be suspected until later when the ductus arteriosus begins to close, which may not be until after the infant is discharged. Management of these patients is particularly complicated by the fact that they may present with severe shock and respiratory distress that mimics a gram-negative septic shock. Morbidity and mortality in the latter group directly depends on how fast the infant can be returned to a facility able to correctly diagnose and treat the lesion. Lesions such as ventricular septal defects may present with a murmur and/or cardiac failure (detected on routine follow-up examination), which depend on the size of the lesion(s) and the rapidity and degree of fall of pulmonary vascular resistance. Management at the outlying facility is generally aimed at stabilization of the infant, initiation of prostaglandins (Prostin VR Pediatric), if appropriate (to reopen the ductus), and prompt transfer/referral of the infant to a tertiary care center.

GASTROINTESTINAL

Necrotizing Enterocolitis

Necrotizing enterocolitis (NEC) is an inflammatory disease of the bowel of unknown, but likely, multifactorial etiology resulting from a combination of gut immaturity, altered gut perfusion, and infectious agents. It is most commonly seen in premature infants weighing less than 1500 g (3.3 lb), but can also occur in older premature infants, and rarely in term infants. The incidence of NEC is approximately 8% to 10% of infants less than 1500 g.

Symptoms and signs suggestive of NEC include those of feeding intolerance, such as increased gastric residuals, emesis, abdominal distention, and bloody stools. As the disease progresses, signs of systemic instability are seen including apnea, bradycardia, respiratory distress, hypotension, and lethargy; specific abdominal symptoms of advanced NEC include abdominal tenderness, guarding, and decreased bowel sounds. Abdominal radiographs will show pneumatosis intestinalis, intrahepatic portal air, and pneumoperitoneum. Therapy is aimed at providing bowel rest, treating a possible infection, and general supportive care. Hence, if NEC is suspected, the infant is made NPO, an orogastric tube is placed to decompress the stomach, intravenous fluids (and later parenteral nutrition) are initiated, and broad-spectrum antimicrobial therapy is begun. Severe NEC is often associated with respiratory compromise (necessitating the use of a ventilator), hypotension (necessitating the use of fluid boluses and inotropic infusions), and thrombocytopenia (which is treated with transfusions of platelets). Typical laboratory investigations include those for suspected infection, and serial abdominal radiographs for signs confirmatory of NEC and its complications. Surgical consultation is always desirable in cases of confirmed NEC, in view of the high risk of gut necrosis and/or perforation, necessitating the need for surgery. In the absence of the need for surgery, medical treatment is generally continued for 10 to 14 days, after which feeds are reinitiated and advanced cautiously as tolerated.

HEMATOLOGIC

Anemia

Anemia is common amongst the neonatal intensive care unit (NICU) population, especially in the very sick or very preterm infant. Anemia that presents at birth may be caused by blood loss (placental abruption, twin-to-twin transfusion, or fetoplacental/fetomaternal blood loss), or hemolysis (commonly because of blood group incompatibility); decreased red cell production is extremely rare, and usually associated with a variety of dysmorphic syndromes. Detailed analysis of the maternal obstetric, medical, and family history usually provides clues to the diagnosis. Initial laboratory tests generally include a CBC with a peripheral smear, blood group, Coombs' test, and a reticulocyte count. Other specific tests depend on the diagnoses suggested by the clinical history, infant's examination, and initial laboratory tests such as an osmotic fragility test if there is a family history of gallstones suggestive of hereditary spherocytosis, a Kleihauer-Betke test on the mother with suspected fetomaternal transfusion, and others. Treatment is essentially directed at correcting the infant's hemodynamic instability (if any) while treating the anemia as needed. Acute blood loss in the infant may present with hypotensive shock, and may necessitate rapid reconstitution of the circulating blood volume; chronic blood loss may present with severe anemia without any hemodynamic instability, and may be treated either with multiple small red cell transfusions or a partial exchange transfusion.

Polycythemia

Polycythemia, defined as a central hematocrit greater than 65% to 70%, may be seen following maternal pregnancy-induced hypertension, maternal diabetes, delayed clamping of the umbilical cord, or twin-to-twin transfusion. Polycythemia increases the viscosity of the blood, which predisposes the infant to develop a stroke, NEC, pulmonary infarction, and respiratory distress. On clinical examination, polycythemic infants may appear plethoric or cyanosed. Because of the vagaries of peripheral heel-stick sampling, polycythemia should only be diagnosed on a free-flowing venous sample. Treatment, directed at lowering the central hematocrit to approximately 50% by a partial exchange transfusion, is generally reserved for the symptomatic infant with central hematocrit greater than 65% or an asymptomatic neonate with a central hematocrit greater than 70%.

Hyperbilirubinemia

Hyperbilirubinemia or jaundice is a very common problem in newborns. Some degree of jaundice may be seen in approximately 66% of term newborn infants and the majority of premature infants in the first few days of life. Physiologic jaundice in the newborn period is a result of an increased bilirubin load (caused by breakdown of the large red cell mass), coupled with an inability of the liver to metabolize the bilirubin, and an increased enterohepatic circulation. Physiologic jaundice generally peaks on or before the fourth day of life in full-term infants and the seventh day of life in preterm infants; the peak levels are approximately 10 to 12 and 12 to 15 mg/dL in the term and preterm, respectively. Concerns related to hyperbilirubinemia are linked to the possible development of kernicterus with concomitant brain damage. Use of early and intensive phototherapy when serum bilirubin levels exceed normal physiologic peak levels has decreased the need for exchange transfusion in recent times. While the American Academy of Pediatrics has a policy statement (available on their Web site) regarding the management of jaundice in healthy term and near term infants, no evidence-based guidelines exist for management of jaundice in the sick and/or very preterm infant, and the care of such infants is best overseen by a neonatologist. Given that kernicterus is a preventable complication of hyperbilirubinemia, provided jaundice is recognized and treated in a timely fashion, it is of paramount importance that health care personnel are aware of the risk factors associated with severe hyperbilirubinemia and kernicterus. As visual examination often underestimates the level of hyperbilirubinemia, serum bilirubin levels should be checked when severe jaundice is suspected. Common clinical risk factors for severe hyperbilirubinemia include:

- Jaundice in the first 24 hours
- Visible jaundice before early (<48 hours) discharge
- Previous sibling with neonatal jaundice
- Gestation less than 38 weeks
- Exclusive breast-feeding
- Asian race
- Male sex
- Maternal age greater than 25 years
- Failure to respond to parental concerns regarding jaundice, poor feeding, and lethargy

Phototherapy is generally initiated when serum bilirubin levels exceed the physiologic range, and cause a concern for kernicterus. Infants who are at a higher risk for the need of an exchange transfusion are best transferred to a tertiary care center, as preparation for an exchange transfusion is an involved process best handled by neonatologist.

SEPSIS

Although the incidence of confirmed neonatal infections is reported variably as 0.1% to 1% of all live births, depending on the population studied, the incidence of suspected sepsis is substantially higher. Because of its relatively immunocompromised state, the premature infant is considered to be at a higher risk for acquiring infections, which is thought to be inversely related to gestational age. Approximately 33% of infants with sepsis have concurrent meningitis, although meningitis without culture-positive bacteremia has been reported. Common organisms that infect both term and preterm infants include group B *Streptococcus* (GBS), *Escherichia coli* (and other gram-negative bacteria), *Listeria monocytogenes*, *Staphylococcus aureus*, and enterococci; whereas coagulase-negative *Staphylococcus* (including *Staphylococcus epidermidis*) usually presents as a nosocomial infection in small premature infants, especially ones that have indwelling catheters. Maternal factors that increase the risk of infection include fever (maternal temperature greater than

38°C [100.4°F] is considered suggestive of infection), prolonged rupture of membranes (greater than 24 hours), chorioamnionitis, maternal colonization with GBS, and preterm labor. Because of the great risk of neonatal morbidity and mortality associated with GBS and the high prevalence of vaginal GBS colonization (20%), current obstetric practice often includes routine screening of pregnant women for GBS colonization at approximately 36 weeks, and treating them with antibiotics during labor. This strategy has been endorsed by the American College of Obstetrics and Gynecology, the American Academy of Pediatrics, and the Center for Disease Control and Prevention, and has resulted in a substantial decrease in the incidence of early onset GBS infection over the past decade. Neonatal infections are often classified as early onset (within the first week of life) and late onset (beyond the first week of life) to differentiate between the common modes of presentation. While early onset infections are usually generalized, late-onset infections may present primarily with meningitis. Symptoms and signs of infection in a neonate are nonspecific, and may include respiratory distress, apnea, poor feeding, feeding intolerance, temperature instability, hypotension, metabolic acidosis, hyperglycemia, lethargy, and seizures. Unfortunately, there are no good clinical or biochemical tests to definitely exclude infection in a symptomatic neonate, and culture of the blood to identify possible bacteremia remains the gold standard to diagnose neonatal infection. Laboratory tests usually obtained as part of an evaluation for sepsis include:

- CBC with differential count and platelet count
- Blood culture
- Cerebrospinal fluid examination (Gram stain, culture, cell count, and biochemical analyses)
- Urine examination (in infants greater than 72 hours old)

Other investigations, such as blood glucose, ionized calcium, chest radiograph, and others, may be obtained (depending on the clinical presentation), as the clinical presentation of sepsis is similar to that of other etiologies. Initial empiric treatment depends on the bacterial flora known to cause early onset infections in the given population, and generally includes ampicillin and an aminoglycoside (often gentamicin [Garamycin]) or cephalosporin. The initial antibiotic choice in the case of suspected nosocomial infection is a combination of vancomycin (Vancocin) and gentamicin (Table 4 gives doses used at our institution). If the blood culture proves to be negative, antibiotic therapy is generally discontinued after 48 to 72 hours. If the blood culture is positive, antimicrobial choices or changes from the initial regimen are dictated by results of the culture sensitivities of the particular organism to various antibiotics tested. Additional management includes general supportive measures such as respiratory support, correction of hypotension, and correction of any abnormalities in fluids and electrolytes. The length of antibiotic therapy depends on the type of infection and the organism isolated, and can vary between 10 days for a *simple* bacteremia to 21 days for gram-negative meningitis. As inborn errors of metabolism can present with symptoms indistinguishable from those of sepsis, it is prudent to check serum ammonia and lactate levels as part of the evaluation for sepsis in infants after the third day of life. Timely identification and appropriate management of infants with such metabolic disorders can make a significant difference in their ultimate neurodevelopmental outcome.

CONGENITAL ANOMALIES

Major congenital anomalies occur in 2% to 4% of live births. With appropriate prenatal care, significant medical and surgical abnormalities are increasingly being diagnosed antenatally, and both parents and physicians can prepare for the birth of the child. When life-threatening anomalies are known to exist, the infant is best delivered in a tertiary care center. When an infant with a previously undiagnosed congenital malformation is born, depending on the

TABLE 4 Common Antibiotic Dosages for the Newborn

Ampicillin			
Initial dose	100 mg/kg	q 8h	
If LP negative	50 mg/kg	q 8h	
Cefotaxime (Claforan)			
≤7 days	50 mg/kg	q 12h	
>7 days	50 mg/kg	q 8h	
Gentamicin (Garamycin)	<30 weeks PCA	30-37 weeks PCA	>37 weeks PCA
≤7 days	3 mg/kg q 24h	3 mg/kg q 18h	2.5 mg/kg q 12h
>7 days	3 mg/kg q 18h	2.5 mg/kg q 12h	2.5 mg/kg q 8h
Therapeutic levels—peak: 5-12 μg/mL, trough: <2 μg/mL			
Vancomycin (Vancocin)	<30 weeks PCA	30-37 weeks PCA	>37 weeks PCA
≤7 days	20 mg/kg q 24h	15 mg/kg q 18h	15 mg/kg q 12h
>7 days	20 mg/kg q 18h	15 mg/kg q 12h	15 mg/kg q 8h
Therapeutic levels—peak: 20-40 μg/mL, trough: 5-15 μg/mL			

Abbreviations: LP = lumbar puncture; PCA = postconceptional age; q = every.

nature of the anomaly, the child may or may not need to be transferred to a tertiary care center immediately. If the infant is clinically stable, telephonic consultation with the appropriate specialist can sometimes aid in planning the subsequent care. In some cases, the infant may need to be transferred for comprehensive evaluation and treatment, while occasionally all that is needed is ensuring appropriate follow-up appointments with relevant specialists. Appropriate genetic and emotional counseling of the parents is vital for optimal management of both the current and future pregnancies.

SURGICAL EMERGENCIES

Most surgical emergencies in the early newborn period are secondary to a life-threatening congenital anomaly. Commonly encountered problems include congenital diaphragmatic hernia, gastrointestinal obstruction, abdominal wall defects, tracheoesophageal fistula, and neural tube defects. As described above, such problems are best managed at a tertiary care center, and infants should be quickly stabilized and transported to the regional center. Telephonic consultation with pediatric surgeons before transfer helps optimize care of the infant as the appropriate support staff can be mobilized to care for the patient, as well as specific interventions to support the infant may be initiated as desired by the specialist. Again, irrespective of what the emergency is, the parents need emotional support and adequate information regarding their infant's condition.

Discharge Planning

Discharge planning ideally begins at admission. Health care personnel that practice *family-centered* care realize that an infant ultimately will go home with his/her parents, and involving parents in their newborn's care and decision-making increases the likelihood that care initiated in the hospital will be continued at home. Parents should be informed of their child's clinical status and the plans of care on a regular (preferably daily) basis. Questions should be expected and even encouraged. Closer to the discharge date, the parents should be actively involved in learning the specific tasks necessary to care for the infant, as well as familiarize themselves with any specialized equipment the child may need at home. Treatment plans for complex conditions are best made at multidisciplinary meetings, where the different subspecialists can jointly discuss the infant's needs and family's abilities to care for the infant. Follow-up visits for subsequent care are best made by the health care team before the child's discharge to home. On discharge, care of the infant is essentially transferred from the hospital physician to a designated primary care pediatrician; telephonic and written communication between the two is essential to ensure continuity of care. Appropriate intrahospital care of the high-risk neonate is just the first step of the continuing ongoing management of an infant that will likely need greater medical attention than the average child. Good outcomes can only result from careful attention to the little details.

NORMAL INFANT FEEDING

METHOD OF

Shirley H. Huang, MD, and

Virginia A. Stallings, MD

Infancy is the period from birth to 1 year of age, which is characterized by remarkable growth and development. During this time period, the goals of infant feeding are to meet nutrient requirements, to provide appropriate foods in accordance with the infant's developmental stage and nutrient needs, and to establish a pattern of optimal growth and nutritional status to support lifelong normal development and health. This article focuses on the nutritional and feeding issues of the term infant.

Important Developmental Milestones

Knowledge of the neuromuscular and digestive development of infants is vital to the understanding of the basis for food and feeding recommendations. Neuromuscular development begins in utero as the fetus swallows amniotic fluid and exhibits the sucking reflex. The mature nutritive suck-swallow pattern is established at 33 to 34 weeks gestational age. The infant progresses from the extrusion reflex of early infancy to the ability to swallow nonliquid foods at 4 to 5 months of age. The baby lifts her head and neck in prone position at 2 months, reaches at 4 months, sits unsupported with good head control at 6 months, and exhibits the pincer grasp at 9 months. At 5 to 6 months of age, infants indicate a desire for food by opening their mouths and leaning forward, and indicate disinterest or satiety by leaning back and turning away. These motor and communications skills aid in solid and textured food introduction with minimal risk of aspiration, help promote cup usage and finger feeding, and provide a means for the infant to indicate hunger and satiety.

Gastrointestinal (GI) processes for digestion of complex foods mature during the first year of life. Nevertheless, newborn infants are fully capable of digesting and absorbing all the constituents of human milk and infant formula in amounts needed to support growth and development. When solids are introduced at 4 to 6 months of age, the ability to digest and absorb carbohydrates, proteins, and fats is mature, and the renal concentrating ability in most infants permits the excretion of hyperosmolar loads without excessive water loss. Intestinal enzymes and bacteria efficiently metabolize lactose, the principal carbohydrate in human milk and many formulas. Glucoamylase helps to digest milk at 1 month of age, and increasing levels of salivary and pancreatic amylase aid the digestion of cereals when introduced at 4 to 6 months of age. Protein digestion is relatively well developed in infancy, although trypsin and chymotrypsin activities increase during the first 4 months of life. In contrast to the digestion of protein, the digestion and absorption of fats are less well developed in early infancy. Nonetheless, babies absorb the fat from human milk better than from cow milk. The current recommendations of the American Academy of Pediatrics (AAP) for the introduction of complementary solid foods at 4 to 6 months are based on individual aspects of the infant's developmental progress in eating-related skills.

Nutritional Requirements

The energy and nutrient needs for rapid growth differentiate nutritional requirements in infancy from all other ages. Water requirements for infants, provided by human milk or infant formula, are much greater than for adults because of high insensible losses from the larger proportional surface area and higher percentage of body water. The healthy infant's absolute requirement for water is approximately 100 mL/kg per day after the neonatal period. A higher amount is needed during periods with water losses, increased metabolic rate, and increased susceptibility to dehydration, such as with fever, vomiting, and/or diarrhea. Energy requirements per unit of body weight are three to four times that of an adult because of the infant's relatively higher resting metabolic energy needs and rapid growth and development—108 kcal/kg per day for 0 to 6 months of age and 98 kcal/kg per day for 6 to 12 months of age, versus 30 to 40 kcal/kg per day for an adult.

The protein requirement, including essential amino acids per unit of body weight, is also greater than that of the older child and adult. The recommended daily allowance (RDA) for protein is approximately 2.2 g/kg per day during the first 6 months of life and 1.6 g/kg per day from 6 to 12 months of age. Fat is the major source of energy for infants, providing 50% per day of energy in human milk and 40% to 50% per day in formulas. According to the recently revised Dietary Reference Intakes (DRI), the adequate intake of n-6 polyunsaturated fatty acids is 4.4 to 4.6 g per day, or 6% to 8% per day of total calories; and n-3 polyunsaturated fatty acids is 0.5 g per day, or 1% per day of total calories. Although the minimum requirement of the essential fatty acid linoleic acid (the parent n-6 fatty acid) in infant formulas is 2.7% per day of total calories (U.S. Food and Drug Administration [FDA], 2000), there is no minimum requirement for the essential fatty acid α-linolenic acid (the parent n-3 fatty acid). However, vegetable oils that contain α-linolenic acid are used in these formulas. In contrast to the requirements for essential amino acids and fatty acids, there appears to be no absolute requirement for carbohydrates as long as there are adequate sources of fat and protein that supply energy through ketones or minimal amounts of essential glucose via gluconeogenesis. The lower limit of dietary carbohydrate compatible with life or for optimal health in infants is unknown. Nonetheless, the recommended adequate intake for infants based on the average intake of carbohydrate consumed from human milk and complementary foods is 60 g per day for 0 to 6 months of age and 95 g per day for 7 to 12 months of age. Furthermore, vitamins and minerals also have recommended intake levels established in the DRI.

Infant Feeding

BREAST-FEEDING

The AAP recommends human milk as the preferred feeding for all infants, including premature and sick newborns, with few exceptions. National surveys in 2001 showed that the initiation of in-hospital breast-feeding in the United States reached the highest levels recorded to date at approximately 65% to 70% per day, and is projected to meet the *Healthy People 2010* goal of 75% per day. Continued breast-feeding at 6 months also reached highest levels at 27% to 33% per day, although significant gains are required before reaching the *Healthy People 2010* goal of 50% per day. This is especially true for women who are black, teenagers, primiparous, less than high school educated, or enrolled in the Supplemental Nutrition Program for Women, Infants and Children (WIC).

The AAP recognizes human milk as the primary food source in achieving optimal infant and child health, growth, and development. Thus, breast-feeding should begin as early as possible after birth and be offered to newborns every 2 to 3 hours until satiety, usually 10 to 15 minutes on each breast. Exclusive breast-feeding is recommended for the first 6 months. Breast-feeding should continue until 12 months of age, and thereafter for as long as mutually desired.

Human milk is uniquely superior for infant feeding and exhibits many nutritional benefits. It contains hormones, immune factors, growth factors, enzymes, and viable cells, most of which cannot practically be added to infant formulas. The composition of human milk varies among individuals and with the stages of lactation. Colostrum is the breast secretion during the last part of pregnancy and for the first 4 days after delivery. It contains more protein, calcium, minerals and immunologic factors than mature human milk. Mature milk is established by the third or fourth week postpartum and contains constituents different from cow milk. Human milk contains less protein (1.0% to 1.5% of volume) than cow milk (3.3%). Human milk protein consists of approximately 75% whey proteins, largely α-lactalbumin, and 25% casein, whereas cow milk composition is approximately reversed. Other human milk proteins, such as lactoferrin, lysozyme, and secretory immunoglobulin A, appear to protect infants against GI and upper respiratory infections. Lactose is the principal carbohydrate of both human and cow milk with slightly higher concentrations in human milk. Human milk also contains carbohydrate polymers and glycoproteins that contribute to intestinal microbial defense. Furthermore, the fat content in human milk is higher during the latter portion of a single nursing session, which may influence the satiety of the infant. Although both human and cow milk contain mainly triglycerides, they are more readily digested in human milk. Human milk also contains long-chain metabolites of linoleic and linolenic acid, which are important fatty acid constituents in the developing retina and the nervous system. Human milk provides all of the vitamins that an infant needs, with the exception of vitamin K and, potentially, vitamin D. In human milk, the calcium-to-phosphorus ratio of 2:1 (versus 1.2:1.0 in cow milk) is favorable for calcium absorption, and iron is readily absorbed and adequate for the first 6 months.

Other compelling health benefits of breast-feeding are well documented. There is strong evidence that human milk decreases the incidence and/or severity of diarrhea, lower respiratory infection, otitis media, bacteremia, meningitis, urinary tract infection, and necrotizing enterocolitis. There are also possible protective effects against sudden infant death syndrome, insulin-dependent diabetes mellitus, inflammatory bowel disease, and asthma and allergic diseases (including food allergies, atopic dermatitis, and allergic rhinitis). The enhancement of cognitive development is also proposed. Moreover, the extent and duration of breast-feeding are reported to be inversely associated with the risk of obesity in later childhood. Mothers benefit as well, including less postpartum bleeding, increased weight loss, prolonged contraceptive effect, and reduced risk of ovarian and premenopausal breast cancer. Furthermore, there are also reduced health care costs and employee absenteeism for care attributable to child illness, as well as savings of at least $400 during the first year that would be spent for infant formula.

INFANT FORMULAS

Iron-fortified infant formulas are appropriate substitutes for human milk when one chooses not to breast feed. The composition of formulas continues to evolve in an effort to provide health, growth, and developmental outcomes similar to those seen in a breast-fed infant. Although no infant formula has the exact composition of human milk, parents should be assured that formula-fed infants grow and develop into healthy children.

Formulas that are available in the United States for term infants generally can be classified into four categories based on the protein source:

1. Cow milk-based formulas
2. Soy protein-based formulas
3. Hydrolysate-based formulas
4. Free amino acid-based formulas

The Infant Formula Act of 1980, amended in 1986, established minimum levels for 29 nutrients and maximum levels for 9 nutrients. Average daily requirements for vitamins and minerals are met when infants are given a minimum daily intake of 25 oz of standard formula with a concentration of 20 kcal per ounce. Aside from the protein source, the carbohydrate, fat and electrolyte components differ in various formulas. Specialized formulas have been developed for infants with certain medical conditions, such as metabolic disorders.

As it is common for families to consider changing formulas with symptoms of intolerance, the AAP recommendations clarified some of the issues of allergy and formulas. Lactose intolerance is very rare in healthy term infants. Most infants with a documented immunoglobulin (Ig) E-mediated allergy to cow milk protein will do well on soy protein or hypoallergenic (extensively hydrolyzed or free amino acid-based) formulas. Infants with documented cow milk protein-induced enteropathy or enterocolitis frequently are sensitive (cross-reactive) to soy protein and should be given a hypoallergenic formula. High-risk infants for the development of allergy, identified by a strong family history, may benefit from hypoallergenic formulas as a supplement to breast-feeding during the first year of life.

Recently, there have been several nutritional modifications of infant formulas to more closely approach human milk composition as new components and functions of human milk are determined. *First*, interest has recently focused on the importance of long-chain fatty acids. Docosahexaenoic acid (DHA) and arachidonic acid (AA) are available in formulas in the United States. Infant formulas have historically only contained the precursor essential fatty acids, α-linolenic acid and linoleic acid, from which formula-fed infants synthesize DHA and AA, respectively. DHA and AA are found in cell membranes, especially those of the central nervous system and retina. Studies have indicated that infants who were fed formulas without DHA and AA had significantly less erythrocyte DHA and AA compared to those who are breast-fed. These data suggest that formulas containing only the precursor essential fatty acids are not as effective in meeting the essential fatty acid requirements as those with the DHA and AA added.

However, current randomized clinical trials show limited evidence for benefit of visual or general development of term infants despite increases in DHA and AA in red blood cells. The long-term effects remain to be determined through longer and larger trials.

Second, since 1989, an increasing number of U.S. infant formulas have provided nucleotides. Nucleotides are nonprotein nitrogen compounds present in higher amounts in human milk than in cow milk-based formulas. Although studies have reported beneficial effects of nucleotide supplementation on immune function, iron absorption, lipid metabolism, and intestinal flora and function, the clinical and health benefits of nucleotides remain controversial.

Third, formulas try to mimic the GI flora of breast-fed infants by the addition of probiotics, such as lactobacilli, or prebiotics, such as oligosaccharides. Lactobacilli are bacteria not present in human milk. Special preparation of the formula is necessary to keep the bacteria live for administration. The addition of probiotics to infant formula decreases the incidence and severity of diarrhea. Oligosaccharides are normally found in human milk. In the prebiotic concept, the addition of oligosaccharides to formulas result in a gut flora similar to that of breast-fed infants. There is limited evidence for health-promoting effects such as protection against invasive microorganism translocation and colonization and possible roles in immunity and allergy.

COMPLEMENTARY FOODS

Complementary foods are introduced when the infant is developmentally ready and the nutrients in human milk become growth limiting. At approximately 4 to 6 months of age, foods are introduced one at a time at weekly intervals to identify possible food intolerance. Iron-fortified foods are important initial complementary food choices, and the gradual addition of pureed individual vegetables, fruits, and meats sets the pattern for a diverse diet. At 9 months of age, the infant accepts finely chopped foods and teething biscuits. Foods such as hot dogs, nuts, grapes, raw carrots, popcorn, and round candies should never be fed to infants because of the risk of aspiration and choking. Honey should not be used to sweeten foods because of the risk of botulism. Cow milk also should not be introduced before 12 months of age because of the low concentration and bioavailability of iron, possible gastrointestinal bleeding, and the high renal solute load of cow milk protein. Fruit juice is introduced with cup feeding after 6 months of age and should be limited to 4 to 6 oz per day. Healthy infants usually require no supplemental water, except in hot weather or other conditions that promote dehydration.

SUPPLEMENTATION

Under usual circumstances, the healthy, full-term infant requires little vitamin or mineral supplementation. The AAP recommends that all infants receive a single, intramuscular dose of vitamin K at birth to prevent vitamin K deficiency bleeding; oral administration has recently been questioned because of concerns of inadequate prevention of the late-onset type of vitamin K deficiency bleeding. Vitamin D should be given to breast-fed infants by 2 months of life, as well as to infants who take less than 500 mL per day of vitamin D-fortified formula. This is especially important for infants who are dark-skinned or exposed to minimal sunlight. Although iron absorption from human milk is excellent, the infant's body iron stores diminish during the first 4 months of life and the iron requirements for growth are high. Thus, the breast-fed infant requires additional iron sources after 4 to 6 months of age. Moreover, vitamin B_{12} must be provided to the breast-fed baby when the mother is a vegan who consumes no animal products. Fluoride supplements are also recommended for all infants after 6 months of age when the local water supply is insufficient in fluoride.

Infant Growth

NORMAL GROWTH

Assessing the nutritional status of an infant includes the evaluation of normal growth and body composition as well as the early detection and treatment of nutritional deficiencies and excesses. Growth assessment is an essential part of pediatric care because both medical and social problems adversely affect growth. Weight, length, and head circumference should be plotted on the revised growth charts (Centers for Disease Control and Prevention, 2000). These charts are based on populations with a better representation of both breast- and formula-fed infants and more diverse ethnic and economic backgrounds. A newborn's weight may decrease 10% per day below birth weight in the first week of life and should regain or exceed birth weight by 2 weeks of age, gaining approximately 15 to 30 g per day during the first 9 months of life. In addition, there is much discussion regarding the pattern of growth in breast-fed versus bottle-fed infants during the first year of life. In general, exclusive breast-feeding may accelerate weight and length gain in the first few months and then decline slowly thereafter. Some studies show that there is no difference in weight or length by 12 months in breast-fed versus bottle-fed infants; others show that breast-fed infants tend to weigh less. Currently, it is unclear whether there are long-term consequences caused by these differences in patterns of growth over the first year of life. Nonetheless, human milk is considered the ideal food for infants.

UNDERNUTRITION

The analysis of growth patterns provides critical information for the recognition of failure to thrive (FTT), or the failure to maintain the expected rate of growth over time. Although there are no universal criteria for the definition of FTT, most clinicians carefully evaluate a child when the weight is below the third or fifth percentile or drops more than two percentile channels. Length and head circumference are usually affected later than weight in more severe and chronic cases. Despite disagreement over the definition of FTT, all agree that it describes a sign of something to further evaluate, not a diagnosis. Labeling a child with FTT has little value when the etiology is not determined and proper therapeutic efforts initiated. Categorizing the infant's condition as organic (medical) or nonorganic (nonmedical) FTT may be helpful, although the practical therapeutic distinctions often are blurred. Regardless of the cause of FTT, prompt attention to nutritional rehabilitation is essential for the infant. A multidisciplinary team approach involving the physician, nutritionist, psychologist, social worker, and other community services is often required and optimal.

OVERNUTRITION

In an era in which the prevalence of obesity is increasing in the United States, several critical periods, including early infancy, are postulated in the development of childhood- or adolescent-onset obesity. For example, high infant weight-for-age or rapid rate of weight gain during the first few months of life may be associated with obesity in childhood as well as young adulthood. At present, there are no known safe and effective interventions in early infancy to prevent adulthood obesity. The health supervision visit (well baby visit) is a time to identify patients at risk by virtue of family history, weight status, and socioeconomic, ethnic, cultural, and environmental factors. As evidenced by the new AAP recommendations for pediatric overweight and obesity prevention, we continue to strive for optimal nutrition and growth during this important period by promoting healthy eating patterns to prepare the infant for a healthy lifestyle later in life.

DISEASES OF THE BREAST

METHOD OF

D. Scott Lind, MD

The majority of women will see a health professional for a breast-related complaint during their lifetime. Therefore, all clinicians must have a working knowledge of the evaluation and management of breast disorders. Unfortunately, it is becoming increasingly difficult for the practitioner to stay current with the complex, contemporary management of breast disease. Furthermore, many of the standard textbooks devoted to breast problems are disease-focused rather than patient management-focused, which limits their clinical utility. This article outlines, in a manner relevant to the practicing clinician, the evaluation and management of the most common clinical presentations for patients with breast disease such as a palpable mass, an abnormality detected by breast imaging, nipple discharge, and breast pain or mastalgia. In addition, specific breast disease problems are also discussed.

Palpable Mass

The presence of palpable breast mass compels the clinician to exclude or establish a diagnosis of cancer. A dominant breast mass is defined as a discrete lump that is distinctly different from the surrounding breast tissue. Overall, approximately 10% of dominant breast masses are malignant. The incidence of cancer in a dominant breast mass increases with age so that more than 30% of masses in women 55 years of age and older are malignant.

The first step in the evaluation of any breast complaint is a complete history and focused physical examination. Important elements of the history include questions related to the mass itself (how long the abnormality has been present, whether any change has been observed, fluctuation of the mass with the menstrual cycle), and the presence of associated symptoms, if any. The risk factors for breast cancer should also be noted including the reproductive history—the age at menarche and menopause, parity, and the age at first full-term pregnancy. A personal or family history of breast, ovarian, and endometrial cancer and the use of oral contraceptives or postmenopausal estrogen should also be determined. Because the majority of women with breast cancer have no obvious risk factors, all breast masses should be thoroughly evaluated regardless of the presence of risk factors.

Physical examination includes inspection of the breast for any asymmetry, skin or nipple retraction, erythema, or peau d'orange. The mass should be characterized with respect to its size, location, consistency, margins, and mobility. Although certain physical findings, such as skin changes, irregular borders, firmness, irregular margins, and immobility increase the likelihood of cancer; the absence of these findings does not exclude the diagnosis of cancer.

Diagnostic mammography is the first imaging study employed to evaluate palpable breast abnormalities. Diagnostic mammography, as opposed to screening mammography, is performed when a breast abnormality is already present. It is a more comprehensive examination and consists of multiple specialized images such as magnification views or spot compression views. The classic mammographic

TABLE 1 American College of Radiology Breast Imaging Reporting and Data System (BI-RADS)

Category	Assessment	Description/Recommendation
0	Need additional imaging evaluation	Recommend additional imaging.
1	Negative	There is nothing to comment on. Routine screening.
2	Benign finding	A negative mammogram, but the interpreter may wish to describe a finding. Routine screening.
3	Probably benign finding	A very high probability of benignity. Short interval follow-up suggested to establish stability.
4	Suspicious abnormality	Probability of being malignant. Biopsy should be considered.
5	Highly suggestive of malignancy	High probability of being cancer. Appropriate action should be taken.

characteristics of a malignant mass include a speculated appearance with pleomorphic microcalcifications. It is important to note, however, that a normal mammogram does not exclude the diagnosis of malignancy.

Cysts are a common cause of dominant breast lumps, particularly in premenopausal women. Ultrasonography is useful in differentiating a cystic from a solid lesion. Sonographically, simple cysts tend to be oval or lobulated and anechoic with well-defined borders. Asymptomatic simple cysts require no further intervention. Symptomatic cysts can be treated by fine-needle aspiration (FNA). If the aspirate is nonbloody, then the fluid should not be sent for cytologic analysis because diagnostic yield for cancer is low. If the aspirate is bloody, it should be sent for cytologic examination. Women should be followed 4 to 6 weeks after cyst aspiration to determine whether the cyst has recurred. If a simple cyst recurs after aspiration, it should be excised. Complex cysts with indistinct walls or intracystic solid components have a higher incidence of carcinoma and, therefore, they should be biopsied either by image-guided methods or surgical excision.

FNA is also appropriate for sufficiently large, solid, dominant masses; but it requires an experienced cytopathologist. A nondiagnostic cytologic evaluation necessitates re-aspiration, core-needle biopsy, or surgical excisional biopsy. The presence of malignant cells requires surgical referral for definitive therapy. Atypical or suspicious cytology results should be followed by core-needle biopsy or excisional biopsy. Unless the clinical exam, FNA, and mammogram are convincingly negative for malignancy (i.e., negative triple test), a negative FNA should be followed by tissue acquisition by core or excisional biopsy.

Abnormality Detected by Breast Imaging

The increasing use of screening mammography has led to a dramatic rise in the number of nonpalpable breast lesions requiring tissue acquisition. Because primary care practitioners order most screening mammograms, they must be capable of evaluating women who have an abnormal result.

Generally, 5% to 10% of all screening mammograms are abnormal, and 10% of women with abnormal mammograms have breast cancer. The American College of Radiology recommends one of six assessments for interpretation of a screening mammogram (Table 1). Women with either a negative or benign assessment (Breast Imaging Reporting and Data System [BI-RADS] 1-2) should undergo routine screening mammography in 1 to 2 years. Women with BI-RADS 3 results should have a repeat study in 6 months, at which time the mammographic abnormality is assessed for stability.

In the past, the preferred biopsy method for non-palpable, mammographically detected lesions was needle-localized surgical biopsy. This procedure is initially performed in the breast-imaging suite where a wire is placed in the breast adjacent to the imaged abnormality. The patient is then transferred to the operating room where the surgeon uses the wire as a guide to remove the abnormality. A mammogram of the excised lesion is performed to confirm its removal (i.e., specimen mammogram). More recently, stereotactic and ultrasound-guided percutaneous core biopsy devices have virtually replaced wire-guided diagnostic surgical procedures because they are minimally invasive, less expensive, and more expedient. It is important, however, to verify concordance between the breast imaging abnormality and the pathologic analysis of the specimen retrieved. Patient follow-up should be based on the pathologic findings and the breast imaging appearance.

The possibility of occult invasive cancer must be considered when ductal carcinoma in situ (DCIS) is diagnosed by core biopsy. In addition, atypical ductal, lobular, and papillary lesions and radial scar diagnosed by core biopsy require subsequent wire-localized excisional biopsy to exclude sampling error. In summary, close communication between the clinician, breast imager, and pathologist is necessary to ensure the optimal patient outcome.

Nipple Discharge

Nipple discharge or galactorrhea is a common breast complaint occurring in approximately 20% to 25% of women. While the incidence of cancer in women with nipple discharge is low, it produces significant anxiety because of the fear of possible breast cancer. Galactorrhea can be a complex diagnostic challenge for the clinician, and it requires a thorough history, focused physical examination, and the appropriate use of diagnostic studies.

Similar to any breast complaint, the first step in the evaluation of nipple discharge is a complete history and focused physical examination. The history should evaluate associated risk factors for breast cancer such as a family history of breast or ovarian cancer, reproductive and menstrual history, and any previous breast biopsies and associated medications. The symptom of nipple discharge should be evaluated with respect to its duration, character (i.e., bloody, nonbloody, milky), location (i.e., unilateral, bilateral), and precipitating factors (i.e., spontaneous versus expressed). Because endocrine imbalances such as hypothyroidism or hyperprolactinemia produce galactorrhea, symptoms indicative of these conditions, such as lethargy, constipation, cold intolerance, and dry skin, should be elicited. The patient should also be questioned regarding symptoms of an intracranial mass (i.e., prolactinoma) such as headache, visual field disturbances, and amenorrhea.

Numerous medications are associated with galactorrhea, including several antidepressants such as fluoxetine (Prozac), buspirone (BuSpar), alprazolam (Xanax), and chlorpromazine (Thorazine). Other classes of drugs associated with nipple discharge include antihypertensives, H_2 receptor antagonists, and any antidopaminergic medications such as metoclopramide (Reglan) and chlorpromazine (Thorazine).

A focused physical examination is the next step in the evaluation of nipple discharge and obviously a detailed breast exam is essential. If nipple discharge is not immediately apparent, the clinician should attempt to elicit the discharge by gentle squeezing of the nipple. The clinician should attempt to determine if the discharge is isolated to a single duct or involves multiple ducts. Attention should also be paid to detecting physical findings suggesting endocrine imbalance such as thyromegaly (hypothyroidism) or visual field deficits (prolactinoma).

The diagnostic evaluation of nipple discharge is predicated on the findings from the history and physical examination. Galactorrhea is physiologic during pregnancy, and it can occur as early as the second trimester and continue as late as 2 years postpartum. Therefore, the evaluation of nipple discharge in women of childbearing years should include a pregnancy test. Elevated thyroid-stimulating hormone (TSH) levels associated with hypothyroidism can increase prolactin secretion and produce galactorrhea. Therefore, women with nipple discharge should have thyroid function tests performed. When the clinician's suspicion for a prolactinoma is sufficiently high, serum prolactin level should be checked. If the serum prolactin level is elevated the patient should have magnetic resonance imaging (MRI) of the head (i.e., sella turcica) to determine if a prolactin secreting pituitary tumor is present.

Mammography is the first imaging study performed to evaluate nipple discharge. Mammography may reveal nonpalpable masses or microcalcifications that require biopsy. Because most pathologic causes of nipple discharge are located close to the nipple, magnification views of the retroareolar region may assist in identifying pathology. The absence of any mammographic abnormalities, however, should not lead to a false sense of security; further evaluation is required.

The role of exfoliative cytology in the management of nonlactational galactorrhea is unclear. Although cytology can be diagnostic of cancer, it is limited by its low sensitivity. The high false-negative rate mandates further evaluation when cytology is negative or nondiagnostic. The diagnostic yield of cancer may be increased when the discharge is bloody, unilateral, and spontaneous.

Galactography or ductography consists of mammography performed after cannulating the offending lactiferous duct and filling it with contrast medium. Ductography can only be performed in the presence of active discharge, and it requires identification and cannulation of the secreting duct. Not infrequently, ductography is technically impossible or the images are not interpretable secondary to incomplete ductal filling or contrast extravasation. Solitary papillomas, the most common cause of abnormal nipple discharge, typically present as a ductal cutoff or filling defect by ductography. Unfortunately, a normal galactogram does not exclude pathology, and it requires further evaluation.

Recent advances in endoscopic technology have made visualization and biopsy of the mammary ducts possible. Flexible fiberoptic ductoscopy is a new technique that may permit direct identification and treatment of ductal pathology. At present, this technology is only available at a few centers and, like all new technological procedures, there is a learning curve associated with its use. Further experience with this investigational technique is required to determine its precise role in the evaluation and management of nipple discharge.

After a thorough history, focused physical examination, and appropriate diagnostic studies, persistent pathologic nipple discharge requires surgical therapy. Surgery can resolve the discharge and provide a diagnosis. Ductal excisions can usually be performed under local anesthesia supplemented with intravenous sedation (monitored anesthesia care [MAC]). The traditional surgical management of pathologic nipple discharge is a central duct excision. Central duct excision effectively removes all of the central lactiferous ducts and sinuses, thereby preventing further discharge. Single duct excision or microdiscectomy can be performed when the offending duct is clearly identified. The advantage of this procedure is that it conserves breast tissue with minimal deformity. The nipple–areola complex remains intact, thereby maintaining the patient's ability to breast-feed. On the other hand, single duct excision may result in a greater likelihood of recurrence of the discharge than with central duct excision.

In summary, nipple discharge (or galactorrhea) is a common breast complaint among women. While the incidence of cancer in women with nipple discharge is low, this clinical presentation requires a thorough history, focused physical examination, and the appropriate use of diagnostic studies. Surgical therapy includes duct excision that can provide both effective treatment and diagnosis. Recent technological advances in diagnostic imaging and endoscopy may permit a more rational, less radical surgical approach to this clinical entity.

Mastalgia

Breast pain, or mastalgia, is one of the most common medical complaints for which women seek medical attention. Although pain is not usually a presenting symptom for breast cancer, it still requires a comprehensive evaluation.

The elements of the history that are important in the evaluation of breast pain are the location, character, severity, and timing of the pain. It is important to determine if the pain is arising from the breast or chest wall. The etiologies of chest wall pain that can mimic breast pain include costochondritis, pleurisy, or myalgias. Breast pain occurring in a predictable pattern just before the menstrual cycle is called cyclical mastalgia, and it is probably hormonally mediated.

Women with mastalgia also require a thorough breast exam followed by a mammogram. If the physical examination and mammogram are normal, then the management of mastalgia consists of reassurance and symptomatic treatment of the pain. The majority of women are satisfactorily treated with nonsteroidal pain medications, and they experience a high spontaneous resolution rate. A relatively small percentage of women have persistent breast pain that significantly interferes with their lifestyle. Several lifestyle interventions have been proposed as effective breast pain treatments. Dietary measures, such as the avoidance of methylxanthines (coffee, tea, sodas), are not evidence-based. Some data suggest that an over-the-counter preparation, evening primrose oil (γ-linolenic acid)[1], may be an effective treatment with relatively few side effects.

More aggressive management of refractory breast pain includes endocrine therapy with bromocriptine (Parlodel)[1], danazol (Danocrine)[1], or tamoxifen (Nolvadex)[1]. Unfortunately, the use of these medications is limited by their side effects. Bromocriptine is an ergot alkaloid that acts as a dopaminergic agonist that suppresses prolactin secretion. Danazol, a synthetic derivative of testosterone, is the only medication approved by the FDA for the treatment of refractory breast pain. Side effects of Danazol treatment include menstrual irregularity, acne, weight gain, and hirsutism. The synthetic estrogen response modifier (SERM), tamoxifen, has been used in the treatment of breast pain; but its use is also limited by hot flashes, deep venous thrombosis, pulmonary emboli, and an increased incidence of uterine cancer.

[1]Not FDA approved for this indication.

HIGH-RISK PATIENT

Despite significant progress, at least 33% of women with breast cancer will ultimately die from their disease. This harsh reality has led to efforts toward primary prevention in high-risk women. In the past, precise predictors of breast cancer risk were lacking. Recently, however, genetic testing and the use of mathematical models have significantly improved our ability to define breast cancer risk. The two most commonly used models for predicting breast cancer risk are the Gail and Claus models. Both models have limitations, and the risk estimates derived from the two models may differ for an individual patient. The Gail model is based on family history in a first-degree relative, late age at childbirth, early menarche, and multiple previous benign breast biopsies. Unfortunately, the Gail model brings into play only a limited amount of family history information, and it does not use data regarding ovarian cancer or lobular carcinoma in situ. The Claus model addresses some of these deficiencies and it includes the number, type, and age of onset of affected relatives.

Researchers have identified the *BRCA1* and *BRCA2* genes associated with an inherited predisposition to breast and ovarian cancers. While family history is an important breast cancer risk factor, only approximately 5% of all breast cancers are caused by germline mutations in the *BRCA1* and *BRCA2* genes. Testing is commercially available to detect mutations in these breast cancer susceptibility genes.

While the lifetime risk of breast and ovarian cancers is substantially elevated for carriers of *BRCA1*- and *BRCA2*-altered genes, recent studies suggest that risk is not as high as earlier estimates. Specific gene mutations have been identified in different ethnic and geographic groups such as Ashkenazi (Eastern European) Jews and Icelandic populations, and each mutation probably confers differing degrees of risk.

Women at high-risk for breast cancer currently have three possible management options:

1. Increased surveillance
2. Risk-reduction or prophylactic surgery
3. Chemoprevention

Currently, no evidence-based data exists for comparing these management strategies.

Presently, intensive surveillance consists of frequent breast imaging and clinical breast exam. This management strategy is dependent upon patient compliance and the efficacy of early detection of breast cancer in high-risk women.

Recent data confirming the efficacy of prophylactic mastectomy and the use of minimally invasive

[1]Not FDA approved for this indication.

oophorectomy techniques have led to a renewed interest in these risk-reduction strategies. There remains, however, no clear consensus on the indications for these procedures. The benefits of prophylactic mastectomy must be weighed against the irreversibility and psychosocial consequences of the procedure. The side effects of oophorectomy include the premature onset of menopause with the associated morbidity of increased osteoporosis and cardiovascular disease.

The Breast Cancer Prevention Trial (BCPT) has shown that tamoxifen (Nolvadex) reduces the risk of developing breast cancer in women at increased risk for the disease. In this study, there was a slightly increased risk of developing endometrial carcinoma with tamoxifen. Studies examining the chemopreventative effects of newer selective estrogen response modifiers (SERMs) with fewer side effects than tamoxifen are ongoing (Study of Tamoxifen and Raloxifene [STAR] trial).

Patient counseling is critical in the decision-making process for high-risk women. Each woman will make a personal, well-informed decision based on the amount of risk she is willing to accept. Further research is required to answer many remaining questions regarding the optimal management strategy in women at high risk for breast cancer.

Breast Cancer

With the exception of skin cancer, breast cancer is the most common malignancy in American women. In the typical primary care practice of 1000 patients, it is estimated that one case of breast cancer will be diagnosed every 1 to 2 years. The decision-making process related to the management of breast cancer has become extremely complex. In general, the surgical management of breast cancer is becoming less radical and less invasive, while more women are being treated with combined modality therapy.

DUCTAL CARCINOMA IN SITU

Ductal carcinoma in situ (DCIS) is a noninvasive neoplasm of ductal origin in which malignant cells are confined to the basement membrane. DCIS represents a heterogeneous group of lesions with diverse malignant potential. Before the widespread use of screening mammography, DCIS made up a small percentage of all breast cancer and it was usually detected as a palpable mass. With the extensive use of screening mammography, the detection of DCIS has increased dramatically to over 50,000 cases annually. There is no clear consensus on the optimal classification of DCIS. Traditional pathologic classification of DCIS based on microscopic morphology includes five subtypes—comedo, papillary, micropapillary, solid, and cribriform. Comedo-type DCIS appears to be more aggressive, with a higher probability of associated invasive ductal carcinoma. Local therapy for DCIS consists of breast-conserving therapy (segmental mastectomy with radiation) or mastectomy.

INVASIVE CANCER

The options for surgical management of invasive breast cancer are the same as for noninvasive breast cancer. Criteria for breast-conserving therapy depend on the relationship between the size of the lesion and the size of the breast, the mammogram, and the patient preference. The presence of multifocal disease, collagen vascular disease, prior therapeutic chest wall radiation, and the first and second trimester of pregnancy are contraindications to breast-conserving therapy. Radiation therapy (as part of breast-conserving therapy) consists of postoperative external-beam radiation to the entire breast with a boost to the tumor bed delivered daily, usually over a 5-week period. Time and travel issues related to several weeks of conventional radiotherapy have led to studies investigating partial breast or limited-field radiation therapy after breast-conserving surgery. Data from randomized prospective trials is required before this technique can be recommended in women with early stage breast cancer.

SENTINEL LYMPH NODE BIOPSY

The histologic status of the axillary nodes is the single most important predictor of outcome in breast cancer. Traditionally, axillary dissection has been a routine part of the management of breast cancer. Axillary dissection-guided subsequent adjuvant therapy provided local control, and it may have contributed a small overall survival benefit. Unfortunately, axillary dissection can be associated with sensory morbidities and lymphedema.

Sentinel lymph node (SLN) biopsy is a minimally invasive, less morbid, and accurate method of determining occult lymph node metastasis. Sentinel lymph node biopsy is based on the principle that the sentinel node is the first node of tumor spread, and, if the sentinel node is tumor free, then the patient can be spared the morbidity of an axillary dissection. The technique has been validated, and surgeons competent in SLN biopsy should be able to identify the SLN with an accuracy of more than 85% and a false-negative rate of less than 5%. While the technique of SLN biopsy is evolving, the most common method of identifying the SLN employs a vital dye and a radionuclide. At the time of breast surgery, the sentinel node can be examined by frozen section or imprint cytology. If metastases are present in the sentinel node, axillary node clearance can subsequently be performed, thus avoiding the need for a second surgical procedure. There is a learning curve for the procedure and, therefore, the success rate varies with the surgeon's experience.

There remain several controversial issues surrounding sentinel node biopsy, such as the value of axillary dissection in the presence of a positive sentinel node and the clinical significance of micrometastases. These issues will be clarified when data from ongoing clinical trials become available.

BREAST RECONSTRUCTION

Despite the fact that the majority of women are candidates for breast conserving surgery, some women require or prefer mastectomy. Advances in reconstructive techniques have made breast reconstruction increasingly popular. Reconstruction may be done at the time of the mastectomy (immediate reconstruction) or later (delayed reconstruction). Prosthetic reconstruction involves the use of an implant to restore the breast contour. Although it is technically the simplest type of reconstruction, implants can lead to complications such as contracture, infection, and rupture that may necessitate further surgery. Autologous reconstruction involves the transfer of the patient's own tissue to reconstruct the breast. Tissue from a number of sites has been used for breast reconstruction including the transverse rectus abdominis, latissimus dorsi, and others.

Skin-sparing mastectomy with immediate reconstruction consists of resection of the nipple areolar complex, any existing biopsy scar, and the breast parenchyma, followed by immediate reconstruction. The generous skin envelope that remains optimizes the cosmetic result after breast reconstruction. The procedure is oncologically safe with no increased incidence of local recurrence. In general, immediate reconstruction should be reserved for patients at low risk for postoperative adjuvant therapies because of the effect of radiation on patients undergoing prosthetic reconstruction capsular contracture.

ADJUVANT SYSTEMIC THERAPY

Hormone Therapy

Breast cancer has long been known to be sensitive to hormonal therapy. Many adjuvant trials, including a meta-analysis, have confirmed the overall survival benefit of tamoxifen (Nolvadex) in estrogen receptor (ER)-positive patients. The optimal duration of adjuvant tamoxifen appears to be 5 years. As mentioned earlier, the use of tamoxifen is associated with several side effects including endometrial cancer. The value of screening techniques such as endometrial biopsy or transvaginal ultrasound in the early detection of uterine cancer remains unclear. Tamoxifen may be associated with additional beneficial effects. Recent data suggest that aromatase inhibitors are an additional group of endocrine agents with beneficial effects in the treatment of breast cancer. These agents act by inhibiting aromatase, which is the rate-limiting enzyme in the synthesis of estrogen. The Anastrozole or Tamoxifen Alone or in Combination (ATAC) trial demonstrates with relatively short follow-up that anastrozole (Arimidex) provides superior disease-free survival benefit with less toxicity than tamoxifen in the adjuvant treatment of ER-positive postmenopausal women. Although additional follow-up is required, anastrozole can be considered an alternative to tamoxifen in this group of patients. Anastrozole (Arimidex) should not be used in premenopausal women because it inadequately suppresses ovarian estrogen secretion.

Chemotherapy

As a result of many clinical trials demonstrating a survival benefit, more and more women are receiving adjuvant cytotoxic chemotherapy. Polychemotherapy regimens are proven superior to single-agent therapy. Anthracycline-based combination chemotherapy may be more effective that nonanthracycline regimens (i.e., cyclophosphamide, methotrexate, 5-fluorouracil [CMF]). Some evidence suggests that HER-2/neu expression may predict anthracycline responsiveness. Data are also emerging that newer agents, such as the taxanes (paclitaxel [Taxol] and docetaxel [Taxotere]), have potent antitumor activity. Adjuvant chemotherapy is effective in postmenopausal women but consideration must be given to co-morbid conditions. While preoperative (neoadjuvant) chemotherapy has no proven survival benefit, tumor response may permit breast conservation in patients who would not otherwise be candidates for the procedure.

BREAST CANCER FOLLOW-UP

Little evidence-based data exist to direct the clinician regarding the optimal post-treatment surveillance strategy for breast cancer patients. As a result, there is extensive variation in practice patterns related to the use of follow-up tests for these patients. Exhaustive post-treatment testing does not seem warranted in early stage breast cancer patients. There is no evidence to support the use of routine bone scans, computed axial tomography (CAT) scans, positron emission tomography (PET) scans, brain imaging, and serum tumor markers in asymptomatic patients after treatment for early stage breast cancer. The use of such intensive surveillance was based on the presumption that detecting disease recurrence at its earliest stage would offer the chance of cure, improved survival, or at least improved quality of life. Because patients detect the majority of recurrences themselves, clinicians need to further educate patients regarding the symptoms of recurrent disease. A thorough history and physical examination by a clinician and mammography will detect the majority of breast cancer recurrences. In addition, breast cancer patients are at increased risk for developing a second primary cancer, so mammographic screening is important in this high-risk population. While some practice guidelines exist for the appropriate use of tests in the management of breast cancer patients, the effect of these guidelines on practice patterns remains limited.

ENDOMETRIOSIS

METHOD OF

G. David Adamson, MD

Endometriosis is an enigmatic disease affecting approximately 7% of reproductive-age women—that is, approximately 5 million women in the United States. Most of these women do not know they have endometriosis, although many may suffer significant symptoms ranging from pelvic pain to infertility. Because our understanding of the clinical presentation, diagnosis, and management of endometriosis has improved dramatically in the past few years, physicians can now provide better care for patients who may suffer from this potentially debilitating and chronic disease.

Definition

Endometriosis is the presence of endometrial tissue, consisting of endometrial glands and stroma, in ectopic locations. This tissue reacts to estrogen and progesterone. The usual location is in the pelvis, but endometriosis has also been found in omentum, small intestine, appendix, anterior abdominal wall, surgical scars, diaphragm, lung, urinary tract, musculoskeletal, and neural systems. The tissue can be very diverse histologically and can appear to be proliferative, secretory, or menstrual.

Prevalence and Incidence

The prevalence and incidence of endometriosis depends on the population of women being studied. The range is 1% to 50% depending on the surgical series. It is reported to occur in 10% to 15% of women undergoing diagnostic laparoscopy, 2% to 5% of women undergoing tubal sterilization, 30% to 40% of infertile women having laparoscopy, and 14% to 53% of women with pelvic pain.

Pathogenesis and Pathophysiology

There are several theories that attempt to describe the pathogenesis of endometriosis. The most popular are retrograde menstruation through the fallopian tubes, metaplasia, activation of embryonic rests of müllerian tissue, hematogenous and lymphatic spread, or by direct placement in wounds. Each of these and other possible etiologies may contribute variably to endometriosis in different patients. Altered immunity may also play a role. There are numerous factors that appear to affect whether a woman will have this disease, how severe the disease will be, what symptoms she will have, and how well she will respond to treatment. These factors include:

- Genetics (An affected sister or mother doubles the risk.)
- Hormonal status (Higher estrogen levels and prolonged heavy menses increases risk.)
- Lifestyle (Low weight and smoking reduce risk by decreasing estrogen levels.)
- Contraceptive use (Oral contraceptives possibly reduce progression of disease.)
- Obstetric history (Pregnancy and lactation reduce risk.)
- Anatomic factors (Cervical stenosis increases risk.)
- Treatment history (Prior medical or surgical treatment reduces risk.)
- Race
- Possibly, exposure to environmental toxins, especially those which are estrogenic

Endometriosis is thought to cause reproductive dysfunction by resulting in cyclic bleeding at the time of menses, which leads to an inflammatory reaction, fibrosis, and adhesions. This may cause distorted anatomy, endocrinopathies (such as increased prostaglandin production), altered pelvic physicochemical milieu, abnormally functioning immune system, interference with sperm function, and, possibly, an altered process of embryo implantation. It is certain there is an association between endometriosis and pain and endometriosis and infertility. Studies collectively demonstrate higher pregnancy rates following ablation and generally lower fecundity than the nonendometriosis population. While a cause–effect relationship has not been definitively proven for endometriosis and infertility, many clinicians believe one likely exists.

Clinical Presentation

Endometriosis presents primarily as pelvic pain in approximately 50% of patients, infertility in approximately 25%, pain and infertility in approximately 25%, and ovarian endometrioma in less than 5% of cases. There is also a large incidence of asymptomatic disease, from 1% to 40%. Endometriosis may occur anytime after puberty, including adolescence.

Pain symptoms of endometriosis often do not correlate well with severity of disease. Pain may occur as a result of secretion of irritating factors (e.g., histamine), adhesions that cause scarring or retraction, leaking endometriomas, compression of other visceral structures (e.g., bowel), compression of uterosacral nodules, and/or invasion of the urinary or gastrointestinal (GI) tract. Endometriosis is associated with infertility in patients with all stages of disease. Patients who have endometriomas, extensive endometriosis lesions and/or adhesions, or extensive invasive disease have a poorer prognosis than patients without these lesions. Endometriosis may also be associated with intraluminal fallopian tube pathology. Studies overall do not support an association between endometriosis and increased spontaneous abortion rates.

Endometriosis lesions occur throughout the pelvis. They tend to be more frequently in the posterior cul-de-sac and the ovary, and less frequently on the fallopian tubes. Endometriosis is almost certainly a progressive disease, but the rate of progression and nature of lesions varies from patient to patient.

Adhesions develop as a result of the inflammatory process caused by long-standing endometriosis, with more extensive and dense adhesions developing over time. Complete cul-de-sac obliteration can result from long-standing invasive and adhesive disease or may result from abnormal müllerian development.

Diagnosis

The diagnosis of endometriosis is suggested by several symptoms, including dysmenorrhea, dyspareunia (especially with aching following coitus), dyschezia, dysuria, mittelschmerz, or focal or generalized pelvic pain. Hematuria and hematochezia may also be symptoms of endometriosis. Approximately 30% of patients with endometriosis do not have any pain. Signs of endometriosis include tenderness or nodularity in the posterior cul-de-sac, especially on the uterosacral ligaments, anterior cul-de-sac nodularity, adnexal masses from endometriomas, and reduced mobility or fixation of the pelvis because of pelvic adhesions. The location of tenderness often corresponds to the location of the pain. Pelvic examination should be performed at the time of menses because disease is more easily identified.

Tests that may assist in the diagnosis of endometriosis include ultrasonography to evaluate the adnexa for endometriomas and the uterus for myomas or adenomyosis. A cancer antigen (CA)-125 test may occasionally be helpful in following the course of endometriosis after diagnosis and treatment, but the high false-positive and false-negative rate give it little utility in the initial diagnostic workup.

Currently the only definite test for pelvic endometriosis is diagnostic laparoscopy. Biopsy of lesions is almost always desirable to confirm the diagnosis of endometriosis and should always be performed if the surgeon is uncertain of the diagnosis. Preoperative consultations with gastroenterologists, urologists, general surgeons, or other specialists as indicated should be scheduled to help ensure that laparoscopy produces maximum benefits for the patient.

The differential diagnoses include pelvic inflammatory disease, ectopic pregnancy, adenomyosis, myomas, benign ovarian tumors, malignant ovarian tumors (rare), hernias, abdominal wall trigger points, interstitial cystitis, irritable bowel syndrome, pelvic pain of undetermined etiology, and normal pelvis. It should be emphasized to patients that diagnosis requires laparoscopy but that endometriosis is not always found at laparoscopy even when it has been suggested by the history, physical examination, and preoperative testing. The degree of pain frequently does not correlate with the extent of disease, but pain does seem to be present more often when the patient has invasive, nodular lesions, or endometriomas.

It is estimated that the diagnosis of endometriosis is missed in more than 7% of patients at laparoscopy, and the extent of disease is underestimated in as many as 50% of patients. Subtle lesions can be missed even by experienced laparoscopists. Other lesions such as old suture, ovarian cancer, carbon deposits from prior laser surgery, and hemangiomas may look like endometriosis. The surgeon must recognize the classical powder burn or blueberry lesion; white scar tissue that may be older, less endocrinologically active disease; clear or slightly brown-colored papillary lesions; or strawberry or flame-like lesions, which are more recently developed and have more endocrinologic, immunologic, and inflammatory activity. Peritoneal pockets may also be associated with endometriosis. There is frequently a delay of many years in the diagnosis of endometriosis, leading to much patient discomfort and poor quality of life. It is imperative for clinicians to consider and rule out endometriosis in women presenting with pelvic pain. It is also important to remember that endometriosis can present even in young adolescent girls.

INDICATIONS FOR LAPAROSCOPY

One indication for laparoscopy to diagnose endometriosis is infertility of more than 1 year duration without other symptoms, or possibly after 6 months if the patient has symptoms or is older than age 35 years. Evaluation for other female factors and sperm quality should be performed before laparoscopy. Patients with pelvic pain who have not responded after 3 months of nonsteroidal anti-inflammatory drugs (NSAIDs) and/or 3 months of oral contraceptives are candidates for laparoscopy. Patients with an adnexal mass suspected of being an endometrioma should have laparoscopy if the lesion does not resolve by 3 months, or sooner if there are concomitant symptoms such as pain or other factors that make surgery appropriate.

CONTRAINDICATIONS TO SURGERY

Contraindications to surgery include multiple repeat operations at short intervals to treat lesions. If appropriate surgery is performed, it is uncommon for endometriotic lesions to recur within a few months. Repeat surgery for adhesiolysis is sometimes indicated in selected patients, usually those who are younger than 30 with infertility of less than 3 years' duration. Repeat surgery may occasionally be indicated after 1 to 2 years if symptoms recur and are not treatable with medical therapy. Laparoscopy may be repeated to perform gamete intrafallopian transfer (GIFT) in highly selected patients. Surgery should not be performed in patients with unacceptably high medical or surgical risks. Laparoscopy should not be performed in patients at high risk for bowel injury unless an open technique or a technique designed to avoid bowel injury is used. Laparotomy is an appropriate approach for many surgeons when laparoscopy may be too hazardous or the surgeon may not have the requisite skills or facilities to perform operative laparoscopy.

Management Options

Managing the patient with endometriosis requires evaluation of her reproductive goals. She may be a teenager desiring future pregnancy, a woman planning immediate pregnancy, or a woman who has completed her childbearing and/or does not desire future pregnancy. Patients may present with undiagnosed pelvic pain or pain associated with recurrence of endometriosis after prior treatment. The objectives of therapy are to remove or destroy implants, relieve symptoms, maintain or restore fertility, and avoid or delay recurrence of the disease. Several management options are available.

NO TREATMENT

In some cases, no treatment may be necessary; however, the patient should be observed every several months and have limited use of analgesics and NSAIDs. These may be especially helpful for women with dysmenorrhea associated with endometriosis.

OVARIAN SUPPRESSION TREATMENT

Medical therapy to suppress ovarian function can consist of oral contraceptives (OCs), progestins, danazol (Danocrine), or gonadotropin-releasing hormone (GnRH) agonists. Oral contraceptives can be given cyclically, but many patients do better with continuous active ingredient tablets for 3 months, followed by withdrawal, and then repetition. Monophasic OCs are superior to triphasic OCs. The best dosage to begin with is usually 35 μg of ethinyl estradiol, but this can be decreased if the patient is symptomatic with headaches or increased breakthrough bleeding. Norethindrone (Ortho Micronor), 0.35 to 0.7 mg daily, may be added if the patient is still symptomatic with bleeding. Transdermal estradiol (Estraderm)[1], 0.05 mg or 0.1 mg twice weekly, may also be used if this is better tolerated. Treatment lasts 3 to 6 months. Progestins such as medroxyprogesterone acetate (Provera)[1], 30 mg every day, alone suppress gonadotropin secretion and ovarian function, but can be associated with breakthrough bleeding, mastalgia, bloating, weight gain, and depression. They may be useful in a few women who cannot tolerate oral contraceptives. Treatment is relatively inexpensive.

Danazol (Danocrine), 200 to 400 mg twice a day, is an ethisterone derivative that functions primarily by suppressing follicle-stimulating hormone (FSH) and luteinizing hormone (LH) from the pituitary gland, thereby creating a hypoestrogenic state. However, danazol is also associated with androgenic side effects, including weight gain, vasomotor instability (hot flashes), muscle cramps, acne, edema, hirsutism, reduced breast size, vaginitis, and sweating. It is contraindicated during pregnancy and lactation, and in women with undiagnosed abnormal genital bleeding or markedly impaired hepatic, renal, or cardiac function. These pharmacologic effects are reversed within 2 months of discontinuing treatment.

GnRH agonists are synthetic decapeptides. Nafarelin acetate (Synarel), 200 μg nasal spray used twice a day, is a superactive, hydrophobic stimulatory analog of GnRH that is 200 times more potent than naturally occurring GnRH, and is delivered in a metered nasal spray pump. Leuprolide acetate (Lupron Depot) is much more commonly used, given as a single monthly 3.75 mg intramuscular injection. The GnRH agonists result in an initial stimulation of the pituitary gland with release of FSH and LH, and a consequent increase in serum estradiol levels to approximately 100 pg/mL. However, continued use of GnRH agonists leads to down-regulation and desensitization of the pituitary gland after 7 to 14 days, and the inability to release FSH and LH. This produces hypoestrogenemia (estradiol less than 40 pg/mL) and resultant amenorrhea, which permits regression of endometriosis and relief of symptoms. The GnRH agonists do not have any known direct effects on the ovary. Treatment costs approximately $3000 for 6 months.

Side effects include hot flashes in approximately 90% of patients, decreased libido, vaginal dryness, headaches, emotional lability, and insomnia. Cardiovascular and liver enzyme parameters show favorable changes relative to danazol. The major concern with GnRH agonists is the loss of bone density, approximately 3% to 8%, which occurs over 6 months of drug therapy, with a 2% to 3% loss persisting approximately 1 year following treatment. The FDA and others' consensus is that this is not clinically significant in women who have no evidence of bone disease, and it is not generally necessary to perform an evaluation of bone density before initiating treatment. While only one 6-month course of GnRH agonist is FDA approved, studies have shown that 3 months of treatment, both initially and for subsequent retreatment if symptoms recur, is as effective as 6 months of treatment, and is associated with less bone loss. Patients should generally undergo dual-photon absorptiometry (DPX) and have normal bone density before GnRH agonist retreatment, and should be fully informed of the potential risks. Subsequent symptoms may also be treated with oral contraceptives, danazol, and/or surgery.

Hot flashes can be effectively managed with norethindrone (Ortho Micronor)[1], 0.35 mg per day.

[1]Not FDA approved for this indication.

[1]Not FDA approved for this indication.

Higher doses of norethindrone may provide some protection against bone loss, but have an unfavorable side effect profile for liver and cardiovascular systems, and patients are often very symptomatic. Low doses of conjugated estrogen (Premarin)[1], 0.6 mg per day, or estradiol (Estrace)[1], 1.0 mg per day, which are also used as *add-back* therapy to reduce bone loss, show some promise. Add-back therapy for 6 to 12 months with norethindrone[1], 2.5 mg per day, alendronate (Fosamax), 10 mg per day, and calcium, 1000 mg per day, appears to have reasonable long-term efficacy in limiting bone loss; but long-term safety concerns await further data. Some advocate using GnRH agonists for initial treatment of pelvic pain not responding to NSAIDs or oral contraceptives and without a diagnostic laparoscopy to confirm the disease. This treatment approach has developed because of the cost and risk of laparoscopy, and because GnRH agonist treatment is effective in the treatment of carefully selected pain patients who have not undergone laparoscopy. However, many clinicians feel the cost of GnRH treatment, the bone loss attendant with treatment, and the potential need for multiple courses of treatment over a long period of time, make this approach inappropriate for many pain patients. This is especially so for younger patients in whom diagnosis is important for long-term management decisions.

SURGICAL TREATMENT

Diagnostic laparoscopy provides a relatively safe and simple method of diagnosing endometriosis. When appropriate, operative laparoscopy enables treatment to be initiated and possibly completed at the same time. Surgical therapy is usually conservative, consisting of excision, laser vaporization, or electrosurgical fulguration of endometriosis. Adjunctive procedures such as salpingo-ovariolysis may also be performed. Additional, occasionally indicated, but still controversial, procedures for pain include uterosacral nerve ablation, or, for severe midline dysmenorrhea, presacral neurectomy. In cases of advanced disease, radical surgery comprising hysterectomy and/or bilateral salpingo-oophorectomy may be required. Laparoscopic treatment of endometriosis requires a surgeon who is familiar with the pathophysiology of endometriosis, and who can integrate this knowledge with surgical judgment and technique. Medical and surgical treatment modalities sometimes have the same results, but surgical treatment completed at the time of diagnosis has a distinct advantage over medical therapy because of decreased time, cost, and side effects. The patient can also be spared a second operation (laparotomy) if operative laparoscopy can be performed at the time of diagnosis. Operative laparoscopy offers several advantages to laparotomy, primarily because of better visualization, less tissue trauma, and much shorter recovery time. However, tactile sense is less than that which can be obtained digitally at laparotomy. It is more important to give the patient the best operation possible in the particular surgeon's hands rather than to compromise by performing a poor operation at laparoscopy. The guiding surgical principle is complete removal of all endometriosis lesions, fibrosis, and adhesions, including those requiring deep dissection. The prevention of postoperative adhesions is based primarily on meticulous surgical technique.

COMBINED TREATMENTS

Laparoscopic treatment of endometriosis may sometimes be combined with medical therapy involving danazol (Danocrine) or GnRH agonists. The purpose of combined treatment is to improve treatment success or facilitate surgical procedures. Preoperative medical treatment suppresses ovulation so that functional cysts are not present or confused with endometriosis. Metastatic or extensive superficial disease is suppressed and becomes atrophic. The reduced vascularity in the pelvis may result in reduced inflammation and postoperative adhesions, although this has not been proven. There may be a slight reduction in endometrioma size. Other uses of GnRH agonists prior to surgery include reduction of symptoms, increased time for adequate preoperative evaluation, easier scheduling of surgery, and even delay or avoidance of surgery for a woman nearing menopause. Potential disadvantages of preoperative medical treatment include the changed appearance of endometriosis, which might make it more difficult to diagnose; drug cost and side effects; delay of diagnosis; and delay in attempting pregnancy. Postoperative medical treatment with GnRH agonists may be indicated if complete resection of disease has not been accomplished, for treatment of microscopic or metastatic disease, or for treatment of pain. Preoperative or postoperative treatment is usually given for 2 to 6 months, but 3 months is adequate for most patients. A very successful treatment approach is to use oral contraceptives continuously for 12 weeks (four packages of oral contraceptives), withdraw for 1 week, and then repeat the 3 months of treatment. This cycle can be continued even to menopause or to the time of attempting pregnancy. It is the most cost-effective approach for many patients.

The approach to each patient must be individualized depending on her symptoms, signs, age, type and extent of disease, and the desire for fertility. Many patients prefer no treatment or medical treatment before electing surgery. However, surgery is often the most appropriate approach. Most patients prefer to retain as many of their reproductive organs as possible, but for some oophorectomy and/or hysterectomy is a better option. Laparoscopy is generally the preferred surgical approach, but laparotomy may be appropriate for some cases, especially those requiring

[1]Not FDA approved for this indication.

extirpation of large endometriomas, extensive enterolysis, enterostomy, or bowel resection. Alternatives to treatment, or treatment in combination with surgery, such as the use of GnRH agonists preoperatively to treat severe endometriosis, should be considered.

It is critical that physicians recognize the degree to which endometriosis can physically and emotionally disrupt patients' lives, and provide comprehensive understanding and an empathetic management approach. Attention to healthy lifestyle with respect to diet, exercise, sleep, and stress reduction through mind–body techniques can be very helpful. Psychological support through information can be obtained from organizations such as the Endometriosis Association (414-355-2200), RESOLVE (the National Fertility Association) (617-623-1156), and the American Society of Reproductive Medicine (205-978-5000). Personal or group counseling may also be helpful, especially for the patient with chronic pain. Some patients may seek nontraditional and unproven approaches to treatment such as acupuncture, herbal medicine, or special diets. Management in these chronic, complex situations should focus on alleviation of symptoms and improved quality of life. A comprehensive evaluation of gastrointestinal, genitourinary, musculoskeletal, neurologic, and psychologic systems may be indicated. Referral to a pain clinic may be helpful for further treatment including biofeedback strategies, nerve blocks, psychotherapy, or other pain management techniques. Treatment of reactive depression is often necessary and often requires a multidisciplinary approach. A comprehensive long-range treatment approach needs to be individualized for each patient. A complete cure can sometimes only be achieved by total hysterectomy and bilateral salpingo-oophorectomy.

Comparison of Treatment Outcomes

PAIN

No treatment and/or mild analgesics or NSAIDs may be entirely appropriate for women younger than 30 with minimal symptoms or for women who have just completed a course of medical treatment. Women who remain symptomatic with minimal or mild pain may frequently be successfully treated with cyclic oral contraceptives, and this treatment should be attempted in most women. For women who have persistent pain, treatment with progestins, danazol (Danocrine), or GnRH agonists have similar efficacy with approximately 80% to 90% of patients having significant relief.

In one study, which is representative of those in the literature, nafarelin acetate (Synarel) at both high (400 μg twice daily) and low (200 μg twice daily) doses, as well as danazol (Danocrine, 400 mg twice daily), provided significant relief of several types of pain associated with endometriosis during 6 months of daily treatment (Table 1). This beneficial effect persisted after the end of drug treatment, but 6 months after treatment was completed, approximately 66.6% of patients experienced a return of dysmenorrhea; however, pelvic pain was reported by only approximately 50% and dyspareunia by approximately 33.3% of subjects. Dysmenorrhea returns with menses and presumably the cyclic release of endometrial prostaglandins. Generalized pelvic pain and dyspareunia may depend upon the reestablishment of endometrial implants. Patients with severe disease or large endometriomas tend to have an earlier recurrence. Danazol and GnRH agonists should generally not be used in the treatment of

TABLE 1 Reports of Specific Types of Pain in Patients with Laparoscopically Diagnosed Endometriosis Treated with Nafarelin Acetate or Danazol*

	Pain Reports (%)									
	Dysmenorrhea			Dyspareunia				Pelvic		
Treatment	N	Absent	Present	N	Absent	Present	Not Reported	N	Absent	Present
Nafarelin (Synarel) 800 μg	45			26				40		
Admission		0	100		0	100	0		0	100
Treatment†		100	0		62	31	8		65	35
Post-treatment‡		36	64		62	35	4		45	55
Nafarelin 400 μg	45			31				37		
Admission		0	100		0	100	0		0	100
Treatment†		98	2		65	32	3		57	43
Post-treatment‡		33	67		71	29	0		49	51
Danazol (Danocrine)	34			23				28		
Admission		0	100		0	100	0		0	100
Treatment†		94	6		70	17	13		64	36
Post-treatment‡		50	50		65	30	4		50	50

*All subjects reported pain on admission.
†Treatment was continued for 6 months.
‡Post-treatment period was 6-month follow-up.
Data from: Adamson GD, Kwei L, Edgren RA: Pain of endometriosis: Effects of nafarelin and danazol therapy. Int J Fertil 39(4):215, 1994.

endometriosis unless the diagnosis has been confirmed at laparoscopy.

Laparoscopic and laparotomy treatments are also effective for treating pelvic pain, with approximately 90% of patients showing significant clinical improvement following complete resection of disease. Approximately 90% should have reasonable symptom relief at 5 years and 50% at 10 years if the disease is completely resected. Patients with more severe disease are at higher risk of recurrence than those with mild disease. In vitro fertilization (IVF) can be used effectively to treat infertile patients with endometriosis following failed prior infertility treatment. IVF is also frequently appropriate in women older than age 35 years with extensive endometriosis and/or adhesions who do not have pelvic pain or endometriomas and for whom the prognosis following surgery would be limited, and for those with multiple infertility factors.

Hysterectomy is the definitive treatment for patients with recurrent or intractable pain associated with endometriosis. In young women of reproductive age removal of one or both ovaries is controversial, although the ovaries are the most common site of endometrial implants and the growth of endometrial implants is driven by cyclic ovarian activity. An ovarian cystectomy for endometrioma is usually the most appropriate approach. If a hysterectomy is warranted, all remaining ovarian tissue should be removed at the same time.

Hysterectomy combined with oophorectomy for endometriosis results in a very high probability of *cure*. There is a small recurrence rate in the range of 5% to 8%. When recurrence does occur, it may be because of residual endometriosis, recurrent endometriosis, ovarian remnant syndrome, adhesions, or other nongynecologic problems. This recurrence rate may be reduced by meticulous resection of all endometriosis at the time of hysterectomy and by oophorectomy at the time of hysterectomy. The use of hormone replacement therapy (HRT) and its duration should be dependent on patient symptomatology, as there is almost certainly no cardiovascular benefit and slightly increased risk of cardiovascular and other adverse events. If HRT is used, it can be started immediately postoperatively.

INFERTILITY

For minimal and mild disease, a prospective randomized study demonstrates that laparoscopic treatment of endometriosis results in higher pregnancy rates at 9 months than no treatment. The pregnancy rate by 3 years is not different from the pregnancy rate with no treatment, laparoscopy, and laparotomy when 3-year estimated cumulative life-table pregnancy rates are calculated (Table 2). Likewise, no treatment or surgery is superior to ovarian suppression for minimal and mild endometriosis

TABLE 2 Estimated Cumulative Life Table Pregnancy Rates by Treatment Group for Different Stages of Endometriosis

	Entire Patient Population					Endometriosis-Only Subset				
	No.	No. Pregnant in 3y	Pregnant*			No.	No. Pregnant in 3y	Pregnant*		
Minimal/Mild			1y (%)	2y (%)	3y (%)			1y (%)	2y (%)	3y (%)
No treatment	15	10	53.3 ± 12.9	66.7 ± 12.2	66.7 ± 12.2	13	9	61.5 ± 13.5	69.2 ± 12.8	69.2 ± 12.8
Medical treatment	44	20	26.5 ± 7.2	53.0 ± 8.9	62.3 ± 9.3	32	13	25.6 ± 8.4	47.7 ± 10.2	55.2 ± 11.2
Laparoscopy	241	122	43.6 ± 3.5	59.6 ± 3.8	67.8 ± 4.1	134	70	45.5 ± 4.7	60.4 ± 5.1	70.3 ± 5.4
Laparotomy	46	28	55.7 ± 7.9	65.6 ± 7.9	74.3 ± 8.1	13	6	38.0 ± 15.1	50.4 ± 6.4	64.5 ± 16.8
Moderate/Severe†										
Laparoscopy	120	52	29.1 ± 4.5	50.8 ± 5.6	62.2 ± 6.2	48	25	32.2 ± 7.5	70.0 ± 9.0	82.0 ± 8.5
Laparotomy	102	37	23.8 ± 4.5	36.7 ± 5.3	44.4 ± 5.6	15	5	20.0 ± 10.3	26.7 ± 11.4	33.3 ± 12.2

*Values are estimates ± standard error.

†Eleven patients treated nonsurgically have been excluded from the entire patient population. Three patients treated nonsurgically have been excluded from the Endometriosis-only subset.

Data from: Adamson GD, Hurd SJ, Pasta DJ, Rodriguez BD: Laparoscopic endometriosis treatment: Is it better? Fertil Steril 59(1):35, 1993.

associated with infertility. Meta-analysis shows that there is no statistically significant difference in crude pregnancy rates between no treatment and medical treatment (Figure 1). Therefore, no treatment is appropriate for selected patients younger than 30 with minimal or mild disease and short duration of infertility, although superior pregnancy rates can be achieved with laparoscopic surgery. Controlled ovarian hyperstimulation with clomiphene citrate (Clomid, Serophene), 100 mg every day from cycle days 3 through 7 for 3 to 6 months, and intrauterine insemination (IUI) improves pregnancy rates in this group. This treatment may also be a reasonable initial treatment approach before laparoscopy in younger women with no known significant infertility factors even when endometriosis is suspected. It has been clearly demonstrated that gonadotropin and IUI treatment for 3 to 6 months is an effective way to treat many endometriosis patients who have already had surgical ablation of their disease, with pregnancy rates per month being approximately 15% versus 4% in untreated patients. However, gonadotropin treatment should only be performed by physicians experienced in its use because of the serious and unwanted complications of multiple pregnancy and ovarian hyperstimulation.

Ovarian suppression for minimal and mild endometriosis results in, at best, negligible improvement in ultimate pregnancy rates and is associated with additional cost and undesirable side effects. Ovarian suppression merely delays the possibility of pregnancy by the duration of the therapy. Ovarian suppression alone should not be used to treat minimal and mild endometriosis when the only symptom is infertility.

Preoperative ovarian suppression should probably be reserved for patients with severe symptomatology, to facilitate surgery scheduling when necessary, or for patients with known severe disease where ovarian suppression may allow for a better pelvic milieu for reconstructive surgery. It is unknown what, if any, effect preoperative ovarian suppression has on subsequent pregnancy rates. Ovarian suppression for 6 to 12 weeks before ovarian stimulation for IVF may improve success rates in patients with severe endometriosis. Postoperative ovarian suppression may be indicated for patients with severe refractory pelvic pain or in whom disease has not been completely extirpated, but it should be avoided whenever possible in infertility patients because of the inability to conceive while taking the medication. Postoperative ovarian suppression does not improve pregnancy rates (see Figure 1). Overall, the available data do not support the routine perioperative use of GnRH agonists or other hormonal therapies, but these may be of value in selected patients.

A recent review of laparoscopic treatment of endometriosis reports pregnancy rates for minimal and mild disease after laparoscopic electrocoagulation of 64% and 52%, respectively. Treatment with CO_2 laser vaporization results in a 59% pregnancy rate for minimal and 58% for mild disease. (Table 2 reflects the author's experience.) It is not known whether patients with extensive and/or invasive peritoneal disease alone will have pregnancy rates (PRs) higher or lower than those reported in these studies. Surgical treatment is required for more advanced endometriosis with invasive nodular disease, endometriomas, and adhesions.

Infertile women with endometriosis can be treated at laparoscopy if the equipment and skill of the surgeon permit. In every analysis, laparoscopy group PRs are equal to or higher than other treatment options whether in the entire population (n = 579), the endometriosis-only subset with at least one normal tube and fimbria and normal male (n = 258), patients with minimal or mild endometriosis, or in patients with moderate or severe endometriosis. Furthermore, even when significant variables were controlled for, laparoscopy group PRs were equal to or higher than other treatments.

Patients with minimal or mild endometriosis undergoing assisted reproductive technology (ART) have similar rates to patients with other diagnostic categories. Those with moderate or severe disease probably have slightly reduced PRs, possibly because of reduced ovarian response to gonadotropins secondary to endometriomas or prior ovarian surgery. Live birth rate per retrieval depends on patient age,

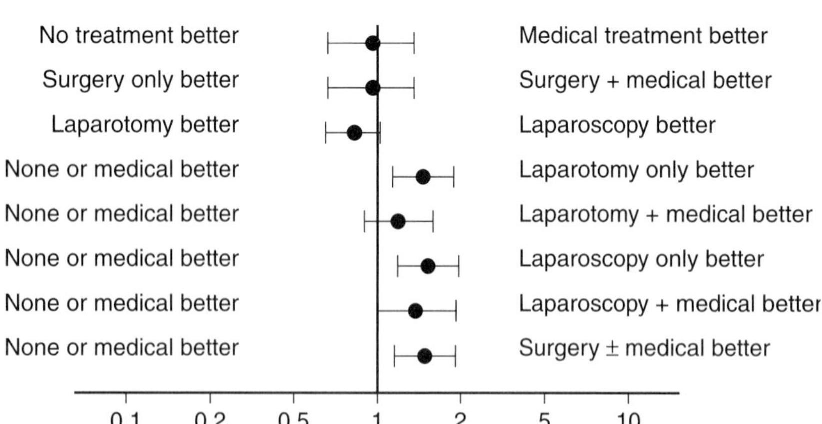

FIGURE 1 Summary of meta-analysis estimates of relative risk of pregnancy (point estimate and 95% confidence interval). (From: Adamson GD, Pasta DJ: Surgical treatment of endometriosis-associated infertility: meta-analysis compared with survival analysis. Am J Obstet Gynecol 171:1488, 1994.)

ranging from approximately 40% per cycle at 30 years of age to 20% per cycle at 40 years of age.

ENDOMETRIOMAS

Endometriomas cannot be successfully treated medically, and if left untreated are thought generally to enlarge and potentially destroy more ovarian tissue, and/or cause pelvic pain and reduced fertility. Surgical removal can be accomplished at least as well by laparoscopy as it can by laparotomy by an experienced surgeon. Postoperative pregnancy rates are approximately 40% to 50% by 2 years. Many surgeons favor complete ovarian cystectomy as opposed to less extirpative procedures, such as cyst drainage or coagulation of the endometrioma cyst wall; both are associated with higher recurrence rates, but may also be associated with less ovarian damage. Recurrence rates are approximately 10% to 15% following cystectomy. Oophorectomy is rarely indicated except for a nonfunctional ovary or for older women who have completed their childbearing.

Algorithm for Management of Endometriosis

Laparoscopy is required to diagnose endometriosis. Whether the patient's symptoms are pain or infertility, surgical treatment involving complete laparoscopic resection of the disease should be performed at the time of diagnosis if the surgeon is capable of so doing. The only exception to this approach is the young woman whose only symptoms are infertility and

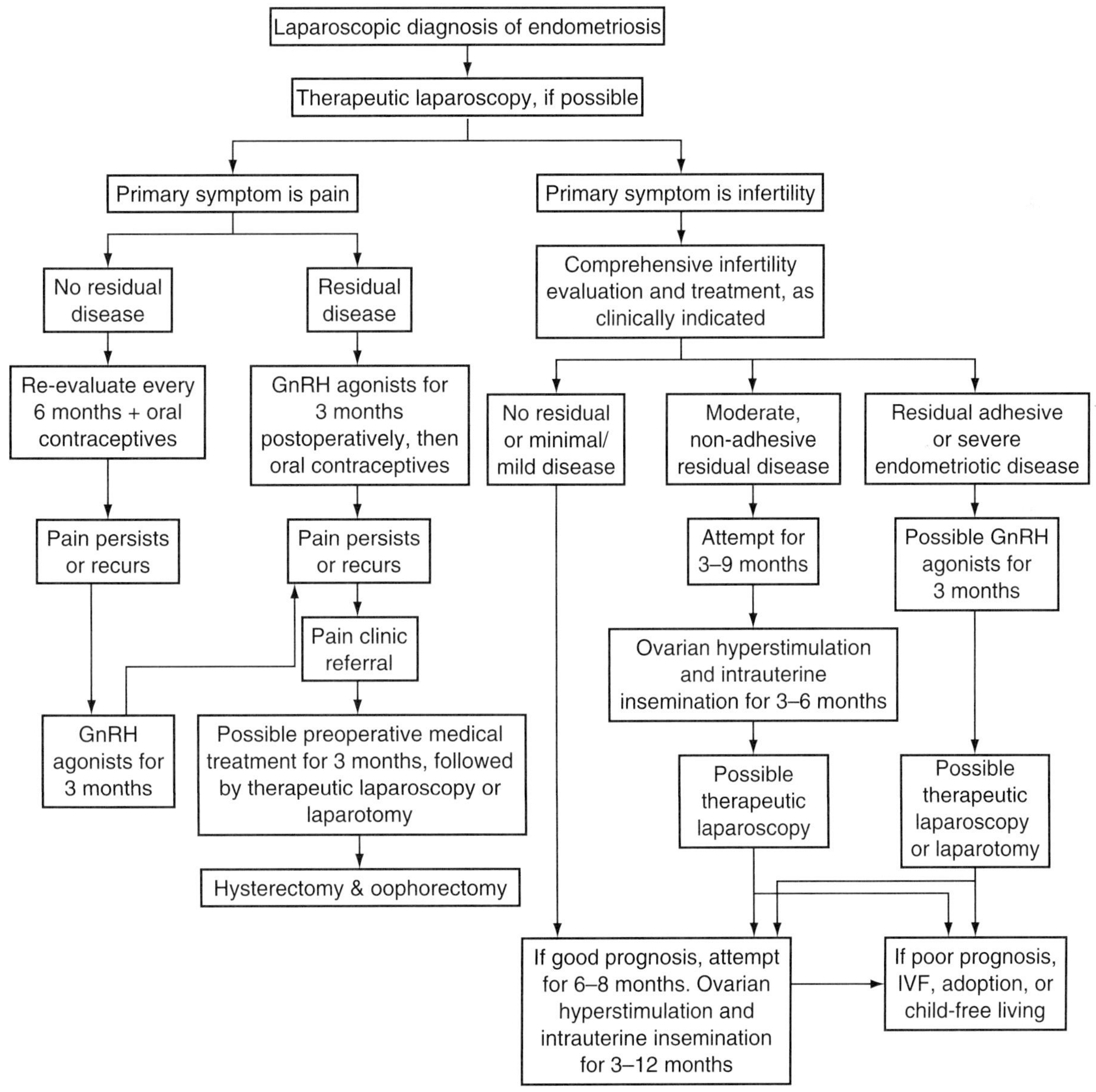

FIGURE 2 Postlaparoscopy management of endometriosis. (From Adamson GD: Laparoscopic treatment of endometriosis. In Adamson GD (ed): Endoscopic Management of Gynecologic Disease. Philadelphia, Lippincott-Raven, 1995, pp 147-187.)

extensive superficial peritoneal and/or ovarian disease. Treatment of such lesions may increase pregnancy rates but also may result in pelvic adhesions. Pain patients should generally receive oral contraceptives continuously postoperatively. For infertility patients, controlled ovarian hyperstimulation and intrauterine insemination postoperatively for 3 to 6 months with clomiphene (Clomid) and/or 3 to 6 months with gonadotropins will increase pregnancy rates.

If the patient has adequate surgical extirpation of the disease, no further postoperative medical treatment is indicated (except for continuous oral contraceptives), either for pain patients or infertility patients. If pain recurs, GnRH agonists should usually be the first line of treatment. For infertile patients who fail to conceive, a second-look laparoscopy at 6 to 18 months may be indicated in selected patients younger than 30 with no other infertility factors. If extensive endometriosis, adhesions, or tubal abnormalities are found, in vitro fertilization (IVF) should be considered within 0 to 12 months following surgery.

If the patient does not have operative laparoscopy at the time of diagnosis, or has incomplete resection of endometriosis, patients with pain have the option of a repeat laparoscopy or laparotomy, most likely by a more experienced surgeon specializing in endometriosis. Another option is use of GnRH agonists or danazol (Danocrine) for 3 to 6 months. GnRH agonists are generally preferred because of their more favorable side effect profile. Failure to manage pain with surgical and/or medical treatment should result in referral to pain specialists for a comprehensive approach to the pain. Such an option should be discussed with the patient at her first consultation and integrated into the treatment plan.

For infertility patients who have not had operative resection or inadequate resection, minimal and mild disease (no adhesions, no invasive lesions, no endometriomas) need no further treatment. Patients with moderate or advanced disease should be referred for laparoscopy or, occasionally, laparotomy. Medical treatment should not be used.

Infertile patients who do not conceive within approximately 6 to 15 months should have a repeat laparoscopy for treatment and/or assisted reproductive technologies such as IVF and/or GIFT (Figure 2), depending on the patient's age and other infertility factors.

The Future

We have much to learn about endometriosis. More detailed evidence-based meta-analysis and prospective randomized studies are being performed to help improve our clinical guidelines. Basic research currently underway should give us a better understanding of β3 integrins and immunology and, hopefully, lead to new therapeutic approaches. New drugs such as GnRH antagonists and aromatase inhibitors might bring new therapeutic approaches. Add-back therapy might be further improved. IVF results will hopefully continue their upward trend. An international study to determine the genetic basis of endometriosis is currently underway, and hopefully will lead to much more successful treatment, and possibly prevention, in the years ahead.

DYSFUNCTIONAL UTERINE BLEEDING

METHOD OF

Ronald D. Miller, MD, and

Deborah M. Miller MB, ChB

Dysfunctional uterine bleeding (DUB) is abnormal vaginal bleeding that occurs in the absence of other medical or pathologic illness. DUB results from hormonal abnormalities, often as a result of anovulatory menstrual cycles, and it is always a diagnosis of exclusion. Excessive vaginal bleeding is considered to be bleeding for more than 7 days, with blood loss exceeding 80 mL per menstrual cycle, or a menstrual cycle less than 21 days. For many patients it can be debilitating, distressing, and a significant distraction from normal life, yet it is often overlooked by health care professionals.

The hormonal causes of DUB are related to abnormalities within the hypothalamic-pituitary-ovarian axis. Abnormal bleeding is a result of estrogen withdrawal or excessive estrogen, without modulation from progesterone, and is most frequently caused by anovulatory cycles. Anovulation, a failure of the ovary to expel the developing ovum, results in the lack of secretion of progesterone, which would take place in a normal menstrual cycle. Continuous, unopposed estrogen results in excessive endometrial growth and vascular proliferation. This leads to variable and often excessive vaginal bleeding, manifested either by regular periods with significant menorrhagia or irregular periods with either moderate or severe bleeding. The etiology, and therefore management of DUB, differs for different stages of life—childhood, adolescence, adult reproductive years, and menopause.

Etiology

Table 1 summarizes the multiple causes and differential diagnoses to be considered in genital tract bleeding. As DUB is a diagnosis of exclusion, it is important to consider the many possible etiologies of suspected uterine bleeding. In all women with reproductive capacity, pregnancy should be considered, especially in the less obvious adolescent and perimenopausal years.

TABLE 1 Differential Diagnoses

Diagnosis	Childhood*	Adolescence*	Reproductive Years*	Menopause*
Dysfunctional uterine bleeding	0	3	3	3
Anovulatory cycle	0	2	3	1
Polycystic ovarian syndrome	0	1	2	N/A
Premature ovarian failure	0	0	0	3
Menopause				
Pregnancy	0	2	3	1
Intrauterine	0	2	2	1
Ectopic	0	3	3	1
Incomplete abortion				
Nongenital tract bleeding	2	2	2	2
Urinary tract	2	2	2	2
Anus	1	1	1	2
External dermatologic lesions				
Inflammation				
Infectious	1	1	1	1
Sexually transmitted disease				
Other organisms	1	1	1	1
Streptococcus, Staphylococcus, Shigella, enteric organisms (e.g., *Escherichia coli*)				
Dermatologic conditions	1	1	1	1
Trauma	2	1	1	1
Foreign bodies	2	2	1	1
Straddle injuries	1	1	1	1
Sexual abuse/assault				
Benign tumors				
Vagina	1	1	2	2
Polypoid lesions	1	1	2	2
Papillomatous lesions				
Cervix	1	1	3	3
Polypoid lesions				
Uterus	1	1	3	3
Polypoid lesions	0	1	3	3
Submucous fibroids				
Malignant tumors				
Vagina	0-1	1	1	1
Carcinoma	0-1	1	1	1
Sarcoma				
Cervix	0-1	1	2	2
Carcinoma				
Uterus	0-1	1	2	3
Carcinoma	0-1	1	1	1
Sarcoma				
Metabolic/hormonal	1	2	2	3
Estrogen-containing medication	0	1	2	2
Hypothyroidism	0	1	2	2
Renal disease	0-1	0-1	0-1	0-1
Adrenal disease				
Hematologic				
Coagulopathies	1	1	1	1
Liver disease	0	2	1	1
Von Willebrand disease	0	1	1	1
Factor XI deficiency	0	1	1	1
Platelet abnormalities				
Thrombocytopenia				
Platelet function defects	0	1	1	1
Bernard-Soulier syndrome	0	1	1	1
Glanzmann thrombasthenia				
Medications	0	1	1	1
Chemotherapy	0	1	1	1
Anticoagulants	0	1	1	1
Hematologic malignancies				

*0 = Not possible; 1 = possible; 2 = likely; 3 = common; N/A = not applicable.

CHILDHOOD

Prepubescent females with genital bleeding without evidence of development of secondary sexual characteristics (Tanner stage 1) are unlikely to manifest endogenous estrogen as a cause for bleeding, and alternative causes should be considered. Likely causesin this age group are trauma (straddle injuries), child abuse, foreign body, and accidental ingestion of exogenous estrogen (e.g. taking mother's birth control pills). Vaginitis, dermatologic conditions, and a nongenital source of bleeding should also be considered.

ADOLESCENCE

Menstrual abnormalities can have a significant psychosocial and educational impact in adolescents. As many of the likely causes of uterine bleeding in this age group may be difficult to diagnose, DUB should be used only as a diagnosis of exclusion, and it should not be assumed that bleeding is functional or physiologic unless other pathology is first ruled out. Diagnosis may be difficult, as an accurate history may be hard to elicit in adolescents and family history may not be available. It is important to rule out pregnancy (regardless of stated sexual history) and also to consider that symptoms could be the initial presentation of hematologic conditions such as von Willebrand disease or rarer coagulopathies. Studies show that 13% to 20% of women with menorrhagia meet the criteria for diagnosis of von Willebrand disease and many of these will present at the time of onset of menses. Anorexia nervosa and strenuous exercise most often cause amenorrhea, but they can also cause anovulation with resulting DUB.

ADULT REPRODUCTIVE YEARS

Approximately 6% to 10% of all adult women have chronic anovulation, usually associated with polycystic ovarian syndrome (PCOS) and hyperandrogenic symptoms. A thorough evaluation is warranted, including testing for thyroid abnormalities or premature ovarian failure, if indicated. While tumors are relatively uncommon in this age group, they remain an important consideration and should not be overlooked.

PERIMENOPAUSAL/POSTMENOPAUSAL

The probability for malignancies of the genital tract increases in the perimenopausal and postmenopausal years, and underlying nonhormonal causes need to be fully evaluated. Declining ovulatory function is the most common cause of DUB in this age group. This is because of a decrease in ovarian function represented by an increase in anovulatory cycles, which results in unopposed estrogen stimulation of the endometrium. As in all patients with the potential for pregnancy, this should be ruled out early in the investigation.

Diagnosis

The importance of history and clinical examination is paramount in the management of patients who present with abnormal uterine bleeding in order to tailor investigations appropriately.

HISTORY

A thorough medical history is crucial and should include the age of the patient, age of menarche, and age of development of secondary sexual characteristics. A family history of menstrual abnormalities, bleeding disorders, and endocrine disorders should also be included. A history focused on the complaint of abnormal vaginal bleeding should include onset and frequency of bleeding as well as the nature of bleeding (regular/irregular, heavy/light, presence or absence of clots, number of days of bleeding, amount and type of tampons or pads used). A sexual history and history of perineal trauma should also be obtained.

EXAMINATION

In the clinical exam it is important to note vital signs, general skin condition, height and weight, and presence of any abnormal physical findings such as hirsutism. In adults the clinical exam should include a comprehensive pelvic examination with close observation of external genitalia, vagina, and cervix. If the patient is bleeding at the time of examination, it is important to determine the origin of bleeding: is it through the cervix (uterine in origin), from the cervix, or from vaginal sites? The pelvic exam should include the routine assessment of pelvic organs with any abnormality of uterus or adnexa. A rectal exam is helpful with respect to ascertaining extragenital sites of bleeding, such as hemorrhoids or rectal mass. At the time of the exam a Papanicolaou smear as well as any other cultures indicated should be performed.

In children and adolescents, the exam should include Tanner staging. An external exam is usually well tolerated, but an internal exam should be deferred or limited, taking into account the child's maturity level, parental preference, and tolerance of procedures. If additional information is needed, a pelvic ultrasound or examination under anesthesia should be considered to minimize the impact of investigations on the child.

Investigations

The investigation of the diagnosis for DUB should include:

- *Pregnancy exclusion*: A pregnancy test is essential as this is the most important diagnosis to rule out.
- *Blood tests*: A complete blood count can give an indication of the severity of the bleeding as well as the urgency of any interventions. If indicated, hormonal studies, thyroid studies, follicle-stimulating hormone (FSH), luteinizing hormone (LH), and

progesterone should be included. If evidence of hirsutism is present, dehydroepiandrosterone (DHEA) and testosterone should be obtained. Consider liver function and coagulation studies, especially in adolescents or those with significant menorrhagia of unknown etiology.

- *Ultrasound*: An ultrasound can assist in defining uterine abnormalities and assess the adnexa (including ruling out ectopic pregnancy).
- *Dilatation and curettage (D&C)*: A D&C can be both diagnostic and curative and should include tissue sampling.
- *Tissue sampling*: Tissue collected via D&C, hysteroscopy, or endometrial biopsy should be considered, especially in women older than 40 years of age.
- *Menstrual diary*: For ongoing assessment, a menstrual diary is a useful tool and should include days of bleeding, amount of flow (spotting, light, medium, heavy), as well as the number and type of pads/tampons used.

Treatment

The treatment regimen will depend on the severity of bleeding, age of the patient, and suspected underlying etiology of dysfunctional uterine bleeding (Table 2). Any life-threatening bleeding should be treated promptly. Long-term goals of treatment should also take into account any risk factors, contra-indications, and other goals of treatment such as desire for fertility or contraception. If other pathologies are suspected, the patient should be appropriately treated or referred for necessary diagnosis and treatment.

A conservative hormonal therapy plan is optimal. Various hormonal combinations and lengths of treatment may be indicated to control bleeding (see Table 2). In most women with significant bleeding, monophasic oral contraceptive pills (OCPs)[1] are preferable, with a usual starting dose of 35 μg ethinyl estradiol, although this should be increased to 50 μg ethinyl estradiol if bleeding is severe or not controlled at the lower dose. In milder cases, or after bleeding is controlled in more severe cases, options include progesterone-only compounds or continuing with a combined OCP. The extended cycle OCP, which contains levonorgestrel and ethinyl estradiol (Seasonale)[1] in a newly formulated 3-month preparation, has potential compliance benefits and may be preferable to some patients; however, it has not yet been used extensively for DUB. As with all prescriptions for OCPs, the relative contraindications that should be considered are smoking, hypertension, hyperlipidemia, diabetes, migraine headaches, venous thromboembolism, sickle cell disease, and concomitant medications such as anticonvulsants and antibiotics. Certain medications, especially antibiotics, can decrease the efficacy of the OCP; this should be considered if these medications are being used for contraception in addition to

TABLE 2 Treatment of Dysfunctional Uterine Bleeding (DUB)

Treatment
Immediate Management Options
Medical
TREATMENT OF ACUTE/SEVERE HEMORRHAGE
Admit to hospital
Fluids
Blood transfusion if indicated
HORMONAL THERAPY
Combined oral contraceptive
Ethinyl estradiol 35 μg/norethindrone 1 mg (e.g., Norinyl 1 + 35, Ortho-Novum 1/35)
q6h × 2d followed by
q8h × 1d followed by
q12h × 1d followed by
q24h × 3-6d
High-dose combined oral contraceptive
Ethinyl estradiol 50 μg/norethindrone 1 mg (e.g., Norinyl 1 + 50, Ortho-Novum 1/50)
q6h × 2d followed by
q8h × 1d followed by
q12h × 1d followed by
q24h × 3-6d
Intravenous estrogen
Conjugated estrogen (Premarin) 25 mg IV q4-6h
ANTIEMETIC IF HORMONAL THERAPY INDUCES NAUSEA
Surgical
Dilatation and curettage (D&C)
Intermediate/Long-Term Management Options
Medical
MODIFY/ARREST EXCESSIVE BLEEDING
Combined monophasic estrogen/progestin OCP (many brands available including Ortho-Cyclen, Norinyl 1 + 35)
Extended-cycle combined estrogen/progestin OCP
Levonorgestrel/ethinyl estradiol (Seasonale)
Cyclic progestin
Medroxyprogesterone acetate (Provera) 5-10 mg PO qd, second half of menstrual cycle
Norethindrone (Aygestin) 2.5-10 mg PO qd, 5-10d, second half of menstrual cycle
Continuous systemic progestin
Depot medroxyprogesterone acetate (Depo-Provera) 150 mg IM q3mo
Continuous local progestin
Levonorgestrel-releasing intrauterine system (Mirena)
Combined estrogen/progesterone HRT (postmenopausal women); many brands available including Prempro, Activelle, CombiPatch
Estrogen-only HRT (postmenopausal/posthysterectomy); many brands available including Estrace, Premarin, Ortho-Est
Nonsteroidal anti-inflammatory drugs (NSAIDs)
Mefenamic acid (Ponstel) or Naproxen (Naprosyn) 250-500 mg PO tid
Ibuprofen (Motrin) 400-800 mg PO q8h
TREAT ANEMIA/IRON DEFICIENCY
Iron Therapy 60-180 mg elemental iron PO daily
Surgical
D&C
Endometrial ablation (postreproductive patients only)
Hysterectomy (postreproductive patients only)

Abbreviations: HRT = hormone replacement therapy; IM = intramuscularly; IV = intravenously; OCP = oral contraceptive pill; PO = orally; q = every; qd = every day; tid = three times a day.

[1]Not FDA approved for this indication.

treating DUB. If hormonal therapy does not correct DUB, re-evaluation of the diagnosis is indicated.

Adolescents can be expected to need treatment for 6 months to 2 years, until regular ovulation is established. Treatment for perimenopausal/postmenopausal women should be individualized; and results can be achieved with low-dose cyclical combined estrogen and progesterone (OCPs), cyclic progestogens, or cyclic hormone replacement therapy. Current evidence suggests increased risks associated with long-term use of hormonal therapy in postmenopausal women, and it is, therefore, prudent to consider minimizing the duration of treatment with hormonal therapy.

Nonsteroidal anti-inflammatory drugs (NSAIDs)[1] can be used as a sole or adjuvant to hormonal therapy, especially for ovulatory DUB. The exact mechanism of action in DUB is not entirely understood, but most likely acts to decrease bleeding by decreasing levels of vasodilating prostaglandins.

Where pregnancy is desired, especially in the presence of anovulation and PCOS, clomiphene citrate (Clomid)[1], 50 mg orally for 5 days beginning on day 3, 4, or 5 of the menstrual cycle should be considered. See the article devoted to PCOS for a more in-depth discussion.

Surgery is considered when there is inadequate response to hormonal therapy. Surgical options include dilatation and curettage, which is frequently a valuable tool for both diagnostic and therapeutic purposes. It is very effective in both the acute and long-term management of DUB. For long-term management where future pregnancy is not desired, endometrial ablation or hysterectomy are additional treatment options. Endometrial ablation, while not definitive therapy, has a high rate of satisfaction among patients with DUB.

There is increasing interest in the use of herbal supplements for the treatment of gynecologic disorders. While there are several that may be helpful in the treatment of specific symptoms of menopausal women, only the Mexican wild yam (*Dioscorea villosa*)[1] or yam extracts are purported to be of help specifically for menstrual disorders. However, studies show that these products contain no therapeutic bioavailable compounds, although some preparations have been *laced* with progesterone. There are very little data supporting the value of herbal supplements in the treatment of menstrual disorders, the safety of these preparations has not been established, and they are, therefore, not currently recommended by the American College of Obstetrics and Gynecology.

In all women, treatment should be guided by severity of symptoms, etiology, desire for fertility, response to previous treatments, and patient preference for type of treatment. It is also important to bear in mind that these conditions are not merely bleeding from the genital tract, but can also have a significant psychosocial impact. Appropriate reassurance and explanation should be provided and frequent follow-up care is essential.

[1]Not FDA approved for this indication.

AMENORRHEA

METHOD OF

Dan Gehlbach, MD

Menstruation is the cyclic shedding of the uterine endometrium, recognized as vaginal bleeding. Menarche, the onset of menstruation, is the culmination of puberty, marking the beginning of the reproductive years, while the cessation of menses represents the onset of menopause. Menstruation requires a dynamic interaction between the ovary, pituitary and hypothalamus, a functional endometrium, and a patent outflow tract. Amenorrhea, or the absence of menstruation, can be either physiologic (such as during pregnancy or lactation), or pathologic.

Amenorrhea can also be classified as primary (menses has never started) or secondary (menses began and then stopped). Primary amenorrhea is defined as the absence of menarche by age 16, while secondary amenorrhea is the interruption of menses for 3 months in women with regular menstrual cycles or for 6 months in those without. Evaluation for primary amenorrhea should also be considered at age 14 years if there are no signs of secondary sexual development.

Because there are so many organ systems involved in menstruation, the evaluation for amenorrhea can be quite complicated. This article reviews the more common causes of amenorrhea and lays out a rational approach to its evaluation.

The Outflow Tract

The uterine endometrium proliferates in response to estradiol, which is produced during follicular growth; is converted to a secretory stage under the influence of progesterone, which is produced by the corpus luteum following the release of a mature oocyte; and is shed when progesterone levels fall if pregnancy does not occur.

Primary amenorrhea may result from a reproductive malformation causing obstruction of the outflow tract. Congenital absence of the uterus and vagina, also known as müllerian agenesis or Mayer-Rokitansky-Küster-Hauser syndrome, is one of the more common causes of primary amenorrhea. Patients have normal external genitalia and secondary sexual development, but the vagina is markedly shortened and the uterus absent. This condition must be differentiated from androgen insensitivity, in which a defect in the androgen receptor leads to a failure of masculinization. Although these patients have a 46,XY karyotype, they are unable to differentiate into a male phenotype and present as females who lack a uterus and vagina and who have scant or absent sexual hair.

Obstruction of menstrual flow can be caused by a transverse vaginal septum or an imperforate hymen.

Patients may give a history of cyclic pelvic pain, and blood trapped behind the obstructing membrane is often palpable as a vaginal mass.

Intrauterine adhesions (Asherman's syndrome) may lead to amenorrhea by replacing the endometrium or obstructing the lower uterine segment. It typically results from instrumentation of the uterine cavity, most commonly when performed in the immediate postpartum period or when the procedure is complicated by infection.

Last, but certainly not least, pregnancy is one of the most common reasons for secondary amenorrhea and should be tested for regardless of the sexual history or method of contraception.

The Ovaries

Follicles in the ovary respond to follicle-stimulating hormone (FSH) by undergoing differentiation and maturation; release of the oocyte is triggered by a surge of luteinizing hormone (LH). The number of oocytes reach their peak during fetal life, and the supply steadily dwindles thereafter. The average age of menopause is approximately 50 years; menopause before age 40 is called premature ovarian failure. There are a number of reasons for ovaries to fail prematurely. Physical agents such as radiation, chemotherapy, or surgical procedures involving the ovaries and/or their blood supply can all lead to premature ovarian failure. Hot flashes, vaginal dryness, and other symptoms of hypoestrogenism are often present at the time the ovaries stop estrogen production. If the ovarian failure occurs prior to puberty, secondary sexual development (breast growth, female fat distribution) does not take place.

The most common cause of primary amenorrhea is gonadal dysgenesis, also known as Turner's syndrome. These patients are typically short (<150 cm in height [4 ft 9 in]), and may have other stigmata such as a webbed neck, shield chest, cubitus valgus, and coarctation of the aorta. Nearly half will have a 45,X karyotype, while the others will be mosaic or have a normal karyotype but are missing just a part of the X chromosome; these patients are more likely to be of normal stature and to have normal pubertal development and even menarche before developing amenorrhea. A small number may carry a Y chromosome and thus be at risk for gonadal tumor formation.

Central Nervous System

Follicular growth and maturation are controlled by FSH and LH, which are produced in the anterior pituitary. Their secretion is stimulated by gonadotropin-releasing hormone (GnRH), which is produced by cells in the arcuate nucleus of the hypothalamus. This center is also called the GnRH pulse generator because secretion is pulsatile in nature, and the pulse amplitude and frequency determine the differential production and release of the gonadotropins. Circulating levels of steroid hormones as well as input from higher centers in the brain influence the GnRH pulse generator.

Polycystic ovary syndrome (PCOS) is one of the leading causes of secondary amenorrhea, and in some extreme cases may even cause primary amenorrhea. Ovarian dysfunction is caused by an interruption of the normal hormonal feedback signals that are required for ovulation. Chronic anovulation and hyperandrogenism are the hallmarks of this common syndrome, which affects 5% to 10% of women. PCOS should be suspected in any woman with irregular or absent periods who also has acne, hirsutism, or obesity. Because their ovaries are continuously producing estrogen, these patients are at risk for development of endometrial hyperplasia or even neoplasia. Many also have insulin resistance, which predisposes them to the development of diabetes, hypertension, hypercholesterolemia, and heart disease.

PCOS cannot be diagnosed without excluding other causes of anovulation and androgen excess. Thyroid dysfunction, either hypo- or hyperthyroidism, is a relatively common cause of ovulatory dysfunction, as is hyperprolactinemia, which may or may not be accompanied by galactorrhea. Late-onset congenital adrenal hyperplasia, caused by a partial deficiency of the enzymes responsible for cortisol production, leads to overproduction of androgens at puberty that closely mimics PCOS. Androgen-secreting tumors of the ovary or adrenal are rare, and tend to have a more abrupt onset and rapid progression of symptoms as well as show signs of virilization, such as clitoromegaly, deepening of the voice, or male-pattern balding. Cushing's syndrome (hypercortisolism) is sometimes found in older women who have hypertension, striae, and signs of both cortisol and androgen excess.

Pituitary adenomas can interfere with the production of FSH and LH. Prolactinomas are the most common, and hyperprolactinemia is usually accompanied by amenorrhea and galactorrhea. Pituitary dysfunction may arise from the empty sella syndrome, in which a herniation of the subarachnoid fluid through a defect in the sellar diaphragm compresses the pituitary tissue. Sheehan's syndrome refers to infarction of the pituitary in the postpartum period caused by excessive blood loss; in addition to amenorrhea, these patients are unable to lactate. Tumors of the hypothalamus, such as craniopharyngiomas, or transsection of the pituitary stalk caused by a whiplash injury, can interfere with the transport of gonadotropin-releasing hormone (GnRH) to the pituitary. A variety of central nervous system (CNS) disorders can affect the GnRH pulse generator. Eating disorders, such as anorexia nervosa or bulimia, should be considered in young slender girls who have an altered perception of their body image (i.e., consider themselves to be overweight despite a normal or asthenic figure). Exercise-induced amenorrhea can be seen in those involved in intense exercise, such as running or weight training. Psychogenic amenorrhea, resulting from either physical or emotional stress, can sometimes result in prolonged amenorrhea. Pseudocyesis is an unusual psychiatric disorder in which the person believes they are pregnant, leading to amenorrhea and even abdominal distention.

Primary amenorrhea in association with pubertal failure may be caused by a failure of migration of the GnRH-producing neurons to the arcuate nucleus during fetal development. Known as isolated gonadotropin deficiency, it is also called Kallmann's syndrome when accompanied by anosmia.

Evaluation

A thorough history and confirmatory physical examination will suggest the diagnosis in most cases. Inquire about the prior menstrual history in those with secondary amenorrhea, or pubertal progression (or lack thereof) in those with primary amenorrhea. Ask specifically about her level of exercise, changes in weight or eating habits, perception of body image, history of head trauma, symptoms of hirsutism, acne, galactorrhea, method of contraception, and associated medical conditions.

Physical examination should include assessment of height, weight, and body mass index. Look for signs of hyperandrogenism, such as acne, hirsutism, acanthosis nigricans (velvety pigmentation in skin folds), temporal balding, and clitoromegaly. If the complaint is primary amenorrhea, use Tanner staging to determine the degree of pubertal development. Pelvic examination should look for abnormalities of the external genitalia. A blind vagina could be because of an obstructing membrane or absence of the uterus; if a vaginal mass is present, bulging of the membrane with Valsalva maneuver suggests an imperforate hymen rather than a transverse vaginal septum. An enlarged uterus should be considered pregnant until determined otherwise.

Obstruction of the outflow tract or absence of the uterus should be confirmed with either a pelvic ultrasound or magnetic resonance imaging (MRI). All patients with an absent uterus should have a karyotype to identify those with androgen insensitivity syndrome, as these patients will require removal of the gonads because of their increased risk of neoplasia.

If the outflow tract is normal, evaluation is focused on determining the estrogen status. The traditional approach has been a progestin challenge. Administration of medroxyprogesterone acetate (Provera), 10 mg for 5 days, will normally result in a withdrawal bleed within 7 days if the uterus has been adequately primed with estrogen. A simpler method is to measure serum estradiol, which is performed simultaneously with measurement of other hormones that are commonly involved in amenorrhea, including human chorionic gonadotropin (hCG), thyroid-stimulating hormone (TSH), prolactin, FSH, LH, testosterone, and dehydroepiandrosterone sulfate (DHEAS) (Table 1). Such an approach dramatically shortens the time required for evaluation.

TABLE 1 Tests for the Evaluation of Amenorrhea

For those with outflow tract obstruction:	
Pelvic ultrasound or MRI	
Karyotype if uterus is absent	
For those with a normal outflow tract:	
β hCG, TSH, prolactin, FSH, LH, estradiol, total or free testosterone, DHEAS	
Additional testing as indicated:	
Androgen excess	17-OH-P
History of uterine trauma	Hysterosalpingogram
Low estradiol level, normal FSH	MRI or CT of pituitary and hypothalamus
Pubertal failure	Karyotype

Abbreviations: 17-OH-P = 17 α-hydroxyprogesterone; CT = computed tomography; DHEAS = dehydroepiandrosterone sulfate; FSH = follicle stimulating hormone; hCG = human chorionic gonadotropin; LH = luteinizing hormone; MRI = magnetic resonance imaging; TSH = thyroid-stimulating hormone.

If the estradiol level is low and FSH and LH are high, the diagnosis is ovarian failure. Gonadal dysgenesis is the most likely diagnosis when primary amenorrhea is associated with pubertal failure, which is confirmed by a karyotype; those with a normal karyotype and no stigmata of Turner syndrome should have an MRI of the hypothalamus to look for isolated gonadotropin deficiency. Occasional patients with secondary amenorrhea may be a Turner mosaic, and a small number will have a Y chromosome present as well, which will require removal of the gonads.

If the estradiol level is low and the FSH and LH are low or even in the low-normal range, a CNS cause is likely and either a computed tomography (CT) or an MRI of the pituitary and hypothalamus should be ordered to look for a possible organic lesion, such as a craniopharyngioma or pituitary adenoma. If the imaging study is normal, the diagnosis is hypothalamic amenorrhea, and therapy is directed at the specific cause, such as a reduction in exercise or correction of an eating disorder. Psychogenic amenorrhea is a diagnosis of exclusion, and the stress that caused the amenorrhea may not be recognizable. Hormone replacement is required for all of these conditions to prevent osteoporosis, which may be given in the form of steroid contraception.

If the estradiol level is normal and hyperandrogenism is present, whether clinically or biochemically, the most common diagnosis is PCOS. A 17α-hydroxyprogesterone (17-OH-P) is an appropriate screening test for late-onset congenital adrenal hyperplasia, and a value above 200 ng/dL should be followed by an adrenocorticotropic hormone (ACTH) stimulation test for confirmation. Patients with PCOS may be treated with steroid contraception unless they are trying to conceive, in which case ovulation induction is the treatment of choice. Consideration should also be given to testing for insulin resistance and checking for hypercholesterolemia, which are frequently part of the syndrome.

DYSMENORRHEA

METHOD OF

Joyce Olutade, MD, MBBS

Dysmenorrhea, defined as painful menstruation, affects approximately 50% of women of reproductive age and 60% to 80% of female adolescents in the United States. The result is a loss of approximately 600 million work hours annually in the United States, severely limiting school attendance and work or physical activities in approximately 10% to 45% of those affected. Dysmenorrhea is subdivided into two types, primary and secondary dysmenorrhea.

Primary Dysmenorrhea

Primary dysmenorrhea starts within 6 to 12 months of menarche when ovulatory cycles have been established. The pain begins a few hours before or on the first day of menses and is most intense during the first 2 days of the menstrual period. It is a crampy, midline lower abdominal pain caused by uterine ischemia, which results from hypercontractility of the myometrium and increased uterine pressure. Prostaglandin $F_{2\alpha}$ and prostaglandin E_2 from secretory endometrium induce these uterine contractions. Vasopressin and leukotrienes also cause uterine contractions. Other symptoms of primary dysmenorrhea including headaches, low back pain, diarrhea, nausea, and vomiting are also attributable to the increased prostaglandin production. Menorrhagia is not a common feature of primary dysmenorrhea.

DIAGNOSIS

A thorough medical and gynecologic history and a pelvic examination help to establish the diagnosis of primary dysmenorrhea. Age at menarche; onset of menstrual pain in relation to menarche; the duration of the menstrual cycle and menstrual period; the intensity, location, and duration of the pain; the presence of intermenstrual bleeding; the intensity of the flow; and other associated symptoms are important elements of the menstrual history. The speculum and bimanual pelvic examination are usually normal in primary dysmenorrhea.

TREATMENT

Primary dysmenorrhea is treated with nonsteroidal anti-inflammatory drugs (NSAIDs), combined oral contraceptives (OCPs), or a combination of both. NSAIDs are prostaglandin synthetase inhibitors (Table 1). More recently, cyclooxygenase-2 (COX-2) selective inhibitors have been approved for the treatment of primary dysmenorrhea (Table 2). NSAIDs (including COX-2 selective inhibitors) reduce endometrial hypercontractility through their antiprostaglandin effect. There are several classes of NSAIDs. The NSAIDs, which are considered first-line medications for treating primary dysmenorrhea, belong to two main classes, propionic acid derivatives and fenamates. The former include ibuprofen (Motrin), ketoprofen (Orudis), and naproxen (Naprosyn). Fenamates include mefenamic acid (Ponstel), flufenamic acid[1], and meclofenamate. Fenamates work by inhibiting prostaglandin production and by directly blocking the effect of already formed prostaglandins. One review found that naproxen, ibuprofen, mefanamic acid, and aspirin were all effective in treating primary dysmenorrhea; but ibuprofen has the best risk–benefit ratio. COX-2 selective inhibitors have a similar pain control profile as naproxen sodium. Other studies report fenamates to be more effective than propionic acid derivatives. NSAIDs should be started at the onset of menses. If a patient fails to respond to one class of NSAIDs, an agent from another class should be selected.

[1]Not available in the United States.

TABLE 1 Nonsteroidal Anti-inflammatory Drugs (NSAIDs) for Treatment of Dysmenorrhea

	Formulation (mg)	Dosage
Propionic Acids		
Ibuprofen (Motrin, Advil)	200, 400, 600, 800	400 mg every 4-6h; max 2400 mg/d
Ketoprofen (Orudis, Oruvail)	12.5, 25, 50, 75,100	25-50 mg PO every 6-8h; max 300 mg/d
Naproxen (Naprosyn)	250, 375, 500	500 mg first dose, then 250 mg every 6-8h prn; max 1250 mg/d
Naproxen sodium (Anaprox)	275, 550	550 mg PO first dose, then 275 mg PO every 6-8h; max 1375 mg/d
Fenamates		
Mefenamic acid (Ponstel)	250	500 mg first dose, then 250 mg PO q6h prn; max 3d
Meclofenamate	50, 100	100 mg PO tid; max 300 mg/d × 6 days

Abbreviations: max = maximum; PO = orally; prn = as needed; qd = once daily; tid = three times a day.

TABLE 2 Cyclooxygenase-2 (COX-2) Selective Inhibitors

Drug	Formulation (mg)	Dosage
Celecoxib (Celebrex)	100, 200, 400	400 mg PO first dose, then 200 mg PO twice a day; may take additional 200 mg on day 1
Rofecoxib (Vioxx)	12.5, 25, 50 or 25/5 mL (suspension)	50 mg PO once a day; max 50 mg/d × 5 days
Valdecoxib (Bextra)	10, 20	20 mg PO bid

Abbreviations: bid = twice daily; max = maximum; PO = orally.

Oral contraceptives may be used as first-line medications in sexually active females who also desire contraception. NSAIDs may not be effective in approximately 30% of women. Oral contraceptives alone or in combination with NSAIDs may be beneficial in such women. If dysmenorrhea persists after a 3- to 6-month trial of second-line agents, then evaluation for possible secondary dysmenorrhea should be initiated. COX-2 selective inhibitors are beneficial in women who are unable to take NSAIDs because of peptic ulcer disease. NSAIDs should always be taken with food. Adverse effects of NSAIDs include dyspepsia, gastrointestinal (GI) bleeding, hepatotoxicity, acute renal failure, and bronchospasm. COX-2 selective inhibitors have a similar adverse profile as other NSAIDs except for a lower incidence of gastrointestinal bleeding and gastritis. Precautions for NSAIDs include history of GI bleeding, peptic ulcer, hypertension, congestive heart failure, renal and hepatic insufficiency, and aspirin- or NSAID-induced asthma.

By inhibiting ovulation and causing endometrial thinning, oral contraceptives reduce the production of prostaglandins and, consequently, decrease dysmenorrhea. A 2003 Cochrane review of medium-dose estrogen (35 to 50 μg) and first- or second-generation progestogens found them to be more effective than placebo for treating dysmenorrhea. The failure rate of the first- and second-line medications is approximately 20% to 25%.

Secondary Dysmenorrhea

Secondary dysmenorrhea is painful menstruation associated with underlying pathologic conditions. It tends to occur several years after the onset of menarche. The pain usually starts 2 to 3 days before the onset of menstruation and lasts throughout the menstrual period. It may also persist several days afterward. Excessive prostaglandin production also occurs in secondary dysmenorrhea. Menorrhagia is usually associated with secondary dysmenorrhea. Table 3 lists the major gynecologic disorders associated with secondary dysmenorrhea. Nongynecologic disorders such as inflammatory bowel disease, psychogenic disorders, irritable bowel syndrome, and uteropelvic junction obstruction may cause secondary dysmenorrhea.

Adenomyosis has the classic features of dysmenorrhea, menorrhagia and a uniformly enlarged uterus. The pain is limited to the menstrual period and occurs in women older than 35 years of age. The diagnosis may be confirmed by magnetic resonance imaging (MRI). A total hysterectomy is the only definitive treatment. Endometrial polyps cause irregular vaginal bleeding and dysmenorrhea and are best diagnosed by sonohysterography.

ENDOMETRIOSIS

Endometriosis is a disorder in which endometrial glands or stroma are found outside the uterine cavity and musculature. Dysmenorrhea from endometriosis may result in lower abdominal, lower back, or deep pelvic pain. The pain usually starts several years after menarche. Primary or secondary infertility, dyspareunia, menorrhagia, and shorter menstrual cycles are important clinical features. Endometriosis may occur in adolescents, approximately 3 years after menarche. A bimanual examination may reveal palpably enlarged ovaries and a fixed, retroverted uterus with tender nodularity in the uterosacral ligament. Magnetic resonance imaging and pelvic ultrasonography may be helpful, but the gold standard for confirmation of endometriosis is laparoscopy.

A complete review of the treatment of endometriosis is beyond the scope of this article and is discussed in a separate article of this book. Dysmenorrhea secondary to endometriosis may be treated medically or by surgery. Medical therapy includes the use of NSAIDs[1], oral contraceptives[1], danazol (Danocrine), gonadotropin-releasing hormone agonists, and injectable medroxyprogesterone[1]. A Cochrane review found that a combination of laparoscopic laser ablation, adhesiolysis, and uterine nerve ablation relieved pelvic pain in women with minimal, mild, and moderate endometriosis. Lysis of adhesions and excision, vaporization, or coagulation of macroscopic

[1]Not FDA approved for this indication.

TABLE 3 Major Gynecologic Causes of Dysmenorrhea

Endometriosis	Endometrial polyps
Pelvic inflammatory disease	Adenomyosis
Cervical stenosis	Pelvic adhesions
Ovarian cysts	Congenital obstructive müllerian malformations

endometriosis during laparoscopy may help relieve dysmenorrhea in 70% to 80% of treated women.

PELVIC INFLAMMATORY DISEASE

Pelvic inflammatory disease (PID) should be suspected as a cause of secondary dysmenorrhea in any sexually active female who exhibits high-risk sexual behavior. An intrauterine contraceptive device may predispose a female to acquire PID. Chronic endometritis resulting from PID may cause intermenstrual bleeding, menorrhagia, postcoital bleeding, and dysmenorrhea. The Centers for Disease Control and Prevention's (CDC) minimum criteria for the diagnosis of PID are uterine/adnexal tenderness and/or cervical motion tenderness. A speculum examination may reveal a mucopurulent cervical or vaginal discharge or may be normal. The treatment of PID is covered in a separate article of this book. Broad-spectrum antimicrobial agents, which include *Neisseria gonorrhoeae, Chlamydia trachomatis,* anaerobes, gram-negative bacteria, and streptococci, are used in the treatment of PID. NSAIDs are useful for relieving the associated dysmenorrhea.

CERVICAL STENOSIS

Cervical stenosis, which may be congenital or secondary to cervical instrumentation, conization, radium application, laser or electrical cauterization, or infection, causes severe menstrual pain in some women. The stenosis is usually at the level of the internal cervical os. Menstrual flow is impeded, causing a buildup of menstrual blood within the uterine cavity with a resulting increase in intrauterine pressure. The occurrence of hypomenorrhea and menstrual pain lasting throughout the menstrual period in a female with a history of cervical instrumentation is highly suggestive of cervical stenosis. Some women may be amenorrheic but experience severe cyclical lower abdominal or pelvic pain. A speculum examination may reveal a scarred external cervical os. The inability to pass a cervical probe of a few millimeters' diameter through the internal cervical os is diagnostic. The diagnosis may be established using hysterosalpingography.

Cervical os dilatation relieves the resulting dysmenorrhea, but the effect is often temporary, necessitating repeated attempts to dilate the cervical os.

Complete curettage of endometrial polyps, preferably during hysteroscopy, cures the majority of cases.

PSYCHOGENIC DISORDERS

Some women experience severe menstrual pain for secondary gain, a conditioned behavior for control and reward. A personality profile test will help confirm the diagnosis of conditioned behavior. Women with conditioned behavior need the help of psychologists for definitive diagnosis and behavior modification.

Stress and tension both worsen menstrual pain. Relaxation techniques, counseling, and antidepressants are useful in such cases.

Alternative Therapies for Primary and Secondary Dysmenorrhea

A Cochrane review of herbal therapies for primary and secondary dysmenorrhea shows that vitamin B_1[1], 100 mg daily, is effective for treating dysmenorrhea. Magnesium[1] is more effective than placebo, but the effective dose is unknown. Uterine nerve ablation and presacral neurotomy are more effective in relieving primary dysmenorrhea than no treatment, but nerve interruption surgery is not recommended. Transcutaneous electrical nerve stimulation is effective for treating primary dysmenorrhea. Acupuncture may be beneficial, but spinal manipulation is not useful.

[1]Not FDA approved for this indication.

PREMENSTRUAL SYNDROME*

METHOD OF

Susan Thys-Jacobs, MD

Premenstrual syndrome (PMS) is a very common problem that affects approximately 40 million young women in the United States, disrupting their emotional and physical well-being. PMS is widely recognized as a recurrent, cyclical disorder related to and restricted to the latter half of the menstrual cycle, disappearing soon after the onset of menstruation. It is characterized by a complex group of signs and symptoms that may include depression, mood swings, irritability, fatigue, abdominal discomfort, and changes in appetite (Table 1). More than 150 symptoms have been described in PMS, partially explaining the difficulty of defining and studying this syndrome. The four main categories of symptoms include: negative affect, water retention, pain, and appetite changes. Although many women experience only mild symptoms, as many as 30% to 50% suffer from troublesome symptoms. Surveys indicate that approximately 5% of North American women consider their symptoms to be severe enough to have a substantially negative impact on their health and social well-being. This latter group has been referred

*This article is a modified version of a previously published manuscript that appeared in J Am Coll Nutr 19:220-227, 2000.

TABLE 1 Common Symptoms of Premenstrual Syndrome

Emotional/Negative Affect	Bloating/Water Retention
Anger/irritability	Abdominal bloating
Depression/sadness	Breast swelling and tenderness
Mood swings/crying spells	
Tension/nervousness	**Appetite Changes**
Pain	Cravings for salt and sweets
Abdominal cramps	Increased or decreased appetite
Generalized aches and pains	
Headache	

TABLE 2 Clinical Features of Hypocalcemia

Anxiety
Depression
Fatigue
Impaired memory and intellectual capacity
Muscle cramps
Neuromuscular irritability
Paresthesias
Personality disturbances
Tetany

Modified from: Kenneth Becker (Ed.). *Hypocalcemia in Principles and Practices of Endocrinology and Metabolism* (3rd ed.). Lippincott Williams & Wilkins, 2001.

to as severe PMS or premenstrual dysphoric disorder (PMDD).

Etiology

The pathogenesis of the cyclical mood and somatic changes in PMS is poorly understood. Numerous theories concerning the etiology of this syndrome have been proposed including hormonal imbalances such as an abnormal estrogen–progesterone ratio, progesterone deficiency, vitamin B_6 deficiency, and altered endogenous opiates. Most theories have been disproved, the remainder are unproven. What is known is that PMS is related to the hormonal rhythmicities of the menstrual cycle and occurs in ovulatory women, despite the unsuccessful attempts to identify differences in basal levels and pulsatility of the ovarian steroid hormones and pituitary gonadotropins between women with and women without PMS. Ovarian steroid hormones appear important in the pathogenesis of PMS and influence menstrual symptoms as well as calcium and vitamin D metabolism. Suppression or cessation of ovarian function resulting in estrogen deficiency—permanently because of menopause, temporarily because of amenorrhea, as with the administration of gonadotropin-releasing hormone agonists (Lupron)[1], or following oophorectomy—significantly diminishes and may even abolish PMS symptoms. Serotoninergic dysregulation appears to be important in the pathophysiology of the syndrome, and this is well supported by the many clinical trials demonstrating the efficacy of the serotonin reuptake inhibitors in the management of both PMS and PMDD.

Evidence now strongly suggests that PMS is associated with a calcium and vitamin D deficiency state, which is clinically unmasked during the latter half of the menstrual cycle when estradiol and progesterone predominate. The symptoms of PMS are strikingly similar to those of hypocalcemia (Table 2) and respond to calcium and vitamin D therapy. Supplemental calcium[1] alleviates symptoms such as irritability, depression, anxiety, social withdrawal, headache, and cramps. Calcium results in a beneficial clinical response in the treatment of premenstrual symptomatology in a number of studies and significantly benefits all four major categories of PMS (i.e., emotional or negative affect symptoms, bloating or water retention symptoms, food cravings, and pain symptoms), reducing overall symptoms by 50%. These clinical trials in conjunction with recent epidemiologic evidence linking lower dietary calcium and vitamin D intakes with PMS symptoms support the role of calcium in PMS and menstrual health. Calcium may ultimately affect monoamine metabolism and reverse the serotoninergic dysregulation, thus providing a biochemical basis for the therapeutic benefit in PMS trials. In addition, variations in calcium and the calcium-regulating hormones (parathyroid hormone [PTH], 25-hydroxyvitamin D, 1,25-dihydroxyvitamin D, and ionized calcium) accompany normal ovarian steroid hormone fluctuations during the menstrual cycle. Exaggerated cyclical fluctuations of the calcium-regulating hormones across the menstrual cycle may explain many of the features of PMS. PMS may truly represent one of the most classic manifestations of a mineral deficiency syndrome.

Premenstrual Assessment and the Diagnosis of Premenstrual Syndrome

The key to diagnosis of PMS is the relationship of luteal to postmenstrual symptoms, although this relationship has been evaluated and measured differently by various authors. There is as yet no objective biochemical marker in the diagnosis of PMS, and the diagnosis depends on the menstrual pattern of symptoms cited by the woman. A prospective assessment of symptoms is recommended but not required for PMS and is strongly advised in PMDD. There is currently no uniform standard assessment of menstrual cycle symptomatology. However, the assessment can be accomplished with a menstrual calendar, daily rating scale, visual analogue scale, or symptom diary (Table 3) for at least 2 months. For PMS, current National Institute of Mental Health recommendations

[1]Not FDA approved for this indication.

TABLE 3 PMS Diary*

Date				Are you presently menstruating? Yes No
Rate the Average Intensity of Discomfort You Experienced During the Previous 24 Hours				
PMS/Menstrual Symptoms	**Absent (0)**	**Mild (1)**	**Moderate (2)**	**Severe (3)**
1. Mood swings/crying spells				
2. Depression/sadness/feelings of hopelessness				
3. Anxiety/tension/nervousness				
4. Decreased interest in usual activities				
5. Difficulty concentrating				
6. Fatigue				
7. Increased/decreased appetite				
8. Insomnia/hypersomnia				
9. Sense of being out of control				
10. Abdominal bloating				
11. Abdominal cramps and discomfort				
12. Headache				
13. Breast tenderness/fullness				
14. Generalized aches and pains				

*Modified version of the PMS Diary. From Thys-Jacobs S, Alvir JM, Fratarcangelo P: Comparative analysis of three PMS assessment instruments—the identification of premenstrual syndrome with core symptoms. Psychopharmacol Bull. 1995;31:389-396.

suggest a 30% change from luteal phase to postmenstrual phase to meet criteria of PMS. This can be measured by comparing the average symptoms' scores 6 days premenstrually to scores 5 to 10 days postmenstrually. Of course, other diagnoses such as major depression, generalized anxiety, thyroid disease, and other endocrine disorders should be excluded. Of note is that the International Classification of Diseases (ICD)-10 does not require prospective confirmation or a requirement for functional impairment for the diagnosis of PMS, although it would be prudent to document the pattern of symptoms. Whether severe PMS or PMDD is a distinct and separate entity from PMS or is even a disease remains a controversial issue. However, a diagnosis of PMDD does require prospective symptom confirmation with specific inclusion criteria of an affective/emotional component with evidence of functional impairment (Table 4).

Current Treatments in Premenstrual Syndrome

There is no one, established therapy for PMS. A variety of treatments have been proposed over the years including lifestyle and dietary modifications, hormonal therapies, and pharmacologic interventions. The majority have proven ineffective or only temporizing, while other treatments have proven scientific efficacy. Some popular methods of treatment that have failed scientifically rigorous evaluation include progesterone therapy[1], monamine oxidase inhibitors[1],

[1]Not FDA approved for this indication.

bromocriptine (Parlodel)[1], and evening primrose oil[1]. In general, the current approaches in the treatment of PMS include calcium supplementation[1], the selective serotonin receptor reuptake inhibitors (SSRIs), and the gonadotropin-releasing hormone agonists[1]. Table 5 lists possible and proven treatments.

For some women, recommending lifestyle changes or pharmacologic interventions are not satisfactory

[1]Not FDA approved for this indication.

TABLE 4 Criteria for Premenstrual Dysphoric Disorder

A. The presence of 5 or more of the following symptoms during the week before menses, with remission within the first few days after menses. One symptom must include an emotional component from items 1-4:
  1. Depression or hopelessness
  2. Anxiety or tension
  3. Mood lability or mood swings
  4. Anger or irritability
  5. Decreased interest in usual activities
  6. Difficulty in concentrating
  7. Fatigue or lack of energy
  8. Change in appetite
  9. Increased or decreased in sleep
  10. Sense of being out of control
  11. Other physical symptoms (headache, breast tenderness)

B. Evidence of functional impairment; symptoms must interfere with work or usual activities.

C. Not an exacerbation of another disorder.

D. Prospective confirmation over 2 consecutive months.

Source: The criteria are modified from the American Psychiatric Association: Diagnostic and Statistical Manual of Mental Disorders, 4th ed. Washington, DC: Author, 1994.

TABLE 5 Current Treatments of PMS

Treatment	Dose
Chasteberry[1]	4-20 mg daily
Calcium (elemental)[1]	500 mg twice daily
Calcium carbonate (Tums)	
Calcium citrate (Citracal)	
Calcium citrate/malate	
Vitamin D[1]	
Cholecalciferol–D_3	1000-2000 IU daily
Ergocalciferol (Drisdol)–D_2	50,000 IU weekly
Calcium (elemental) and vitamin D combined	
Premcal Light	500 mg calcium/500 IU vitamin D_3 twice daily
Regular	500 mg calcium/750 IU vitamin D_3 twice daily
Extra strength	500 mg calcium/1000 IU vitamin D_3 twice daily
Osacal	500 mg calcium/200 IU vitamin D_3 twice daily
Magnesium (elemental)[1]	200-400 mg daily
Magnesium aspartate	
Magnesium oxide (Mag-Ox)	
Antidepressants	
Selective serotonin reuptake inhibitors	
Fluoxetine (Sarafem)	20 mg daily
Escitalopram (Lexapro)[1]	10-20 mg daily
Sertraline (Zoloft)	25-100 mg daily
Paroxetine (Paxil)[1]	10-30 mg daily
Selective serotonin and norepinephrine reuptake inhibitors	
Venlafaxine (Effexor)[1]	75-150 mg daily
Gonadotropin-releasing agonists	
Leuprolide (Lupron depot)[1]	3.75-7.5 mg monthly; 11.25 to 22.5 mg every 3mo 30 mg every 4mo
Goserelin (Zoladex) implant[1]	3.6 mg every 28d 10.8 mg every 3mo

[1]Not FDA approved for this indication.

for a natural biologic process. Herbal products are sought by many women for PMS symptom relief as these remedies are considered more natural. However, some of the botanical therapies can be quite toxic such as blue cohosh[1] or dong quai[1], which is considered unsafe during pregnancy. Of the herbal therapies, chasteberry[1], also known as *Vitex agnus-castus*, appears to demonstrate some efficacy, while other data show conflicting results. It appears to diminish follicle-stimulating hormone (FSH) with decreases in estrogen synthesis and at higher doses may inhibit prolactin levels. One large clinical trial demonstrates total relief of PMS symptoms in more than 33% of the women treated. The use of chasteberry should be avoided during pregnancy and during breast-feeding.

Initially advising dietary and lifestyle modifications by increasing daily dietary calcium intake and an adequate aerobic exercise program will often alleviate PMS symptomatology. Calcium (elemental calcium)*[,1] at 1000 mg (500 mg in the form of calcium carbonate twice daily is the most convenient) and vitamin D_3–cholecalciferol*[,1] at 1000 to 2000 international units (IU) daily should be recommended to all women initially, and may be all that is required in those women with mild or even moderate symptoms. The potential for dietary supplements other than calcium to reduce PMS symptoms is less convincing. Magnesium*[,1] at a dose of 200 to 400 mg daily may alleviate PMS symptoms. Facchinetti in 1991 observed that 360 mg of magnesium reduced affective symptoms, while Walker in 1998 noted a reduction in bloated symptoms but not in mood symptoms. Scientific evidence on vitamins E*[,1] and B_6*[,1] is very limited. Evening primrose oil[1], which is a rich source of γ-linolenic acid, had been suggested as a possible treatment, but two well-designed studies did not demonstrate efficacy. In a rigorous, double-blind study, progesterone therapy was not found to be better than placebo and is currently not advocated for PMS.

The antidepressants classified as SSRIs are effective, specifically in severe PMS or premenstrual dysphoric disorder. Fluoxetine (Sarafem), sertraline (Zoloft), paroxetine (Paxil), and fluvoxamine (Luvox) all appear to have similar beneficial effects. These antidepressants are usually administered daily, but intermittent therapy during the luteal phase of the cycle is efficacious. Side effects of the SSRIs may include anxiety, nervousness, insomnia, nausea, tremor, and somnolence.

Gonadotropin-releasing agonists (GnRH agonists) (Lupron, Zoladex) produce hypogonadotropic hypogonadism or a form of medical oophorectomy. These agents are effective, because they obliterate the normal menstrual cycle. Although they reduce PMS symptoms, the hypoestrogenic side effects and potential bone loss are of major concern. Other side effects include hot flashes, emotional lability, and insomnia. These latter drugs should be administered with great caution, and careful monitoring is highly recommended. Of all the potential remedies, GnRH agonists as well as surgical ovariectomy should be considered last. If long-term therapy is required, add-back therapy with hormone replacement is strongly recommended.

Management of Premenstrual Syndrome

It is important to document PMS symptomatology prospectively with a menstrual calendar or symptom diary for at least 2 months. The initial evaluation of the PMS should include instruction on the use of daily diaries, and an exclusion of conditions that may compound or emulate PMS symptomatology, such as

[1]Not FDA approved for this indication.

*Available as a dietary supplement.
[1]Not FDA approved for this indication.

thyroid disease and depression. Laboratory evaluation consists of a baseline complete blood count (CBC), chemistries with total serum calcium, and a thyroid function panel. A calcium profile including a serum 25-hydroxyvitamin D, intact parathyroid hormone, and 24-hour urine calcium excretion should be obtained for women with moderate to severe symptoms. The acquisition of a calcium profile and urine calcium can be extremely helpful in the management of these women and often guides therapy. Hypocalciuria, when present, may indicate a malabsorption syndrome such as celiac sprue or lymphoma, and hypercalciuria may indicate that the woman has primary hyperparathyroidism or, more commonly, idiopathic hypercalciuria. Not every woman with PMS requires such an expensive laboratory evaluation. However, one can often readily treat with just the serum 25-hydroxyvitamin vitamin D concentration alone. A realistic approach is to empirically treat the woman following a 25-hydroxyvitamin D level by supplementing the diet with calcium (elemental calcium) at 1000 mg and vitamin D_3–cholecalciferol at 1000 to 2000 IU daily. Vitamin D deficiency has become more commonly recognized as a consequence of dietary deficiency and inadequate production of vitamin D by the skin. Vitamin D at 2000 IU daily in a premenopausal woman is safe. The majority of women with PMS experience a sense of well-being and relief within 1 to 2 months of treatment. For those who do not experience relief, the calcium profile along with serum 25-hydroxyvitamin D (25[OH]D), intact parathyroid hormone and 24-hour urine calcium excretion should be obtained. While a normal 25-hydroxyvitamin D concentration has been of some controversy recently, levels of 25(OH)D at 35 to 40 ng/mL appear adequate and optimal. To correct for inadequate levels of vitamin D, the following replacement regimen may be administered:

- If the 25(OH)D concentration is less than 20 ng/mL, prescribe vitamin D_3–cholecalciferol, 4000 IU daily, or ergocalciferol (Calciferol), 50,000 IU thrice weekly for 1 month. The level of 25(OH)D should be repeated in 1 and 6 months or as necessary with adjustments in dosage to achieve a 25(OH)D level of 35 to 40 ng/mL.
- If the 25(OH)D concentration is more than 21 ng/mL and less than 40 ng/mL, prescribe vitamin D_3–cholecalciferol, 2000 IU daily, or ergocalciferol, 50,000 IU weekly. The level of 25(OH)D should be repeated at 1 and 6 months or as necessary with adjustments in dosage to achieve a 25(OH)D level of 35 to 40 ng/mL.
- If the 25(OH)D concentration is more than 40 ng/mL and normal, prescribe vitamin D at 1000 IU.
- Note that a daily maintenance dose of vitamin D may vary from 1000 IU to 4000 IU daily to achieve a 25(OH)D level of 35 to 40 ng.

Dietary modifications may be helpful as well, and adding dairy products such as yogurt or milk can reduce the total supplemental calcium while maintaining the total dietary calcium. As an example, one cup of skim milk contains 302 mg of elemental calcium, 1 ounce of Swiss cheese contains 272 mg of elemental calcium, 3 ounces of sardines contains 372 mg of elemental calcium, and ½ cup of cooked collards contains 168 mg of calcium. Substituting one daily yogurt and one glass of skim milk for a 500 mg calcium tablet can reduce the number of calcium supplements required while preserving total calcium intake. Increases in both dietary and supplemental calcium may cause an initial exacerbation of PMS physical symptoms, such as menstrual cramps. Women should be alerted to this initial symptom eruption, but comforted that continual treatment usually results in an overwhelming sense of balance and resolution of the majority of their symptoms within 2 to 3 months. Constipation and nausea are very common complaints that women cite with calcium supplementation. The addition of magnesium to the diet often alleviates this complaint, and ingesting the calcium supplements with meals, and not on an empty stomach, usually resolves the nausea.

In conclusion, PMS is a very common disorder among women of reproductive age, with many women experiencing emotional and physical symptoms of varying degrees. When recognized, women should be reassured that there is a probable biochemical reason for their symptoms, that this is not a psychological disorder, and that treatment for PMS is available. Evidence strongly suggests that PMS is a calcium and vitamin D deficiency syndrome. Dietary modifications with increases in total daily calcium intake may be all that is necessary. Adequate calcium and vitamin D supplementation with daily calcium intake at 1000 mg and vitamin D_3 at 1000 to 2000 IU will relieve the majority of symptoms in women with PMS. The remainder should have additional hormonal and biochemical investigations to elucidate the etiology of persistent symptoms. For women who do not adequately respond to adequate calcium and vitamin D replacement therapy, pharmacologic intervention may be required.

MENOPAUSE

METHOD OF

Jan L. Shifren, MD, and

Isaac Schiff, MD

Menopause, the permanent cessation of menstruation, occurs at a mean age of 51 years. The age at menopause appears to be genetically determined and is unaffected by race, socioeconomic status, age at menarche, or number of prior ovulations.

Factors that are toxic to the ovary often result in an earlier age of menopause; women who smoke experience an earlier menopause, as do many women exposed to chemotherapy or pelvic radiation. Despite a great increase in female life expectancy, the age at menopause has remained remarkably constant. A woman in the United States today will live approximately 30 years, or greater than a third of her life, beyond the onset of menopause.

Options for caring for menopausal women have increased greatly since estrogen therapy (ET) was first introduced in the 1960s. With respect to hormone use, there are many choices of hormone type, dose, and method of administration. Not only have new forms of estrogens and progestins been introduced, but novel ways of combining the two hormones are available. In addition to hormones, selective estrogen receptor modulators (SERMs) and bisphosphonates are available. Women are requesting more information on complementary and alternative therapies, which are being studied more carefully.

Health Concerns After Menopause and Treatment Options

VASOMOTOR SYMPTOMS

Vasomotor symptoms affect up to 75% of perimenopausal women. They last for 1 to 2 years after menopause in the majority of women, but may continue for up to 10 years. Hot flashes are the primary reason women seek care at menopause and request hormone therapy (HT). Hot flashes not only disturb women at work and interrupt daily activities, but also disrupt sleep. Many women complain of difficulty concentrating and emotional lability during the menopausal transition. Treatment of vasomotor symptoms should improve these cognitive and mood symptoms if they are secondary to sleep disruption and resulting daytime fatigue. The incidence of thyroid disease increases as women age; therefore, thyroid function tests should be checked if vasomotor symptoms are atypical or resistant to therapy.

Treatment

Systemic estrogen therapy is the most effective treatment available for vasomotor symptoms and associated sleep disturbance. Vasomotor symptoms appear to be the result of estrogen withdrawal, rather than simply low estrogen levels. Abruptly stopping hormone treatment may result in a return of disruptive vasomotor symptoms; therefore, if cessation of HT is desired, it is important to reduce the dose slowly over several months. This recommendation is based on clinical experience, as few controlled trials have examined the optimal way to cease HT use. When a woman chooses not to take estrogen or when it is contraindicated, progestin therapy alone is an option. Medroxyprogesterone acetate (MPA; Provera)[1] and megestrol acetate (Megace)[1] effectively treat vasomotor symptoms. Several drugs that alter central neurotransmitter pathways also are effective (Table 1). Clonidine (Catapres)[1] may be used orally or as a weekly transdermal patch. Potential side effects include orthostatic hypotension and drowsiness.

Interestingly, selective serotonin reuptake inhibitors (SSRIs) and other antidepressants also are effective. Menopausal women experienced significant reductions in both hot flash frequency and severity in double-blind, randomized, placebo-controlled trials of paroxetine (Paxil CR)[1] (12.5 and 25 mg per day), fluoxetine (Prozac)[1] (20 mg per day), and venlafaxine (Effexor)[1] (75 mg per day). The improvement in vasomotor symptoms was independent of any significant change in mood symptoms. Possible side effects include fatigue, dry mouth, nausea, and decreased libido.

Many menopausal women are interested in trying nutritional and vitamin supplements for relief of hot flashes. Many of these therapies claim to relieve hot flashes, but rarely are studied in controlled trials. Options include dietary soy[1] and related compounds, vitamin E[1] (800 IU per day), black cohosh[1], evening primrose oil[1], and others. Uncontrolled studies of acupuncture, exercise, and paced respiration demonstrate an improvement in vasomotor symptoms. Lifestyle interventions including wearing light, layered clothing, avoiding hot beverages, and the liberal use of desk fans and air conditioners should be encouraged.

UROGENITAL ATROPHY

Urogenital atrophy results in vaginal dryness and pruritus, dyspareunia, dysuria, and urinary urgency. These are common complaints of menopausal women that respond well to therapy.

Treatment

Systemic estrogen therapy is very effective for the relief of vaginal dryness, dyspareunia, and urinary symptoms. Another option for women who should not (or choose not) to use standard estrogen therapy is topical application. Low doses of estrogen cream

[1]Not FDA approved for this indication.

TABLE 1 Alternative Treatments for Hot Flashes

Drug*	Suggested Dose
Venlafaxine (Effexor)	37.5-75 mg XR/day
Fluoxetine (Prozac)	20 mg/day
Paroxetine (Paxil)	10-20 mg/day or 12.5-25 mg CR/day
Clonidine (Catapres)	0.1 mg/week patch
Gabapentin (Neurontin)	300-900 mg/day

*None of these medications is FDA approved for the treatment of hot flashes.
Abbreviations: CR = controlled release; XR = extended release.

(Estrace, Premarin) are effective when used only one to three times weekly. An estradiol vaginal tablet (Vagifem) inserted twice weekly is available, as is an estrogen-containing vaginal ring (Estring) that is placed in the vagina every 3 months. Lubricants are a nonhormonal alternative for reducing discomfort with intercourse when urogenital atrophy is present.

OSTEOPOROSIS

Osteoporosis affects approximately 8 million women in the United States, with an additional 15 million women at risk for the disease. As therapy is most likely to benefit those at highest risk, it is important to review a woman's risk factors for osteoporosis when making treatment decisions, and to consider bone mineral density screening for high-risk women. Nonmodifiable risk factors include age, Asian or white race, family history, small body frame, early menopause, and prior oophorectomy. Modifiable risk factors include decreased intake of calcium and vitamin D, smoking, and a sedentary lifestyle. Medical conditions associated with an increased risk of osteoporosis include hyperthyroidism, hyperparathyroidism, chronic renal disease, and diseases requiring systemic corticosteroid use.

Treatment

Counseling women to alter modifiable risk factors is important for both the prevention and treatment of osteoporosis. Many women have diets deficient in calcium and vitamin D and will benefit from dietary changes and supplementation. Reducing the risk of osteoporosis is another of the many health benefits of smoking cessation and regular exercise. Hormone therapy is very effective at both preventing and treating osteoporosis. The Women's Health Initiative (WHI) randomized, controlled trial confirms a significant 34% reduction in hip fractures in healthy women receiving HT after a mean follow-up of 5 years.

Bisphosphonates, including alendronate (Fosamax) and risedronate (Actonel), specifically inhibit bone resorption and are very effective for both osteoporosis prevention and treatment. SERMs are compounds that act as both estrogen agonists and antagonists, depending on the tissue. Raloxifene (Evista) is a SERM that has been approved for both the prevention and treatment of osteoporosis. Raloxifene has estrogen-like actions on bone and lipids, without stimulating the breast or endometrium. Calcitonin nasal spray (Miacalcin) and parathyroid hormone injections (teriparatide [Forteo]) are other therapies for osteoporosis.

CARDIOVASCULAR DISEASE

Cardiovascular disease is the leading cause of death for women, accounting for approximately 45% of mortality. Nonmodifiable risk factors include age and family history. Modifiable risk factors include smoking, obesity, and a sedentary lifestyle. Medical conditions associated with an increased risk of heart disease include diabetes, hypertension, and hypercholesterolemia.

Treatment

Advising women to alter modifiable risk factors and adequately treating diabetes, hypertension, and hypercholesterolemia are important measures in reducing the risk of heart disease. In the past, prevention of heart disease was thought to be a potential benefit of hormone therapy use. Epidemiologic studies report an approximately 50% decrease in heart disease in women who use HT. Observational studies are prone to bias, however, and women who choose to use hormones are generally at lower risk for heart disease than those who do not.

However, the WHI randomized, controlled trial of combination hormone therapy versus placebo showed that not only does HT *not* prevent heart disease in healthy women, it actually increases it slightly (Table 2). The WHI trial enrolled approximately 16,000 women nationwide, between the ages of 50 to 79 years. The average age of women in the study was 63 years. The major goal of the WHI clinical trial was to determine whether combined estrogen and progestin HT (Prempro) prevented heart disease and fractures, and whether there were associated risks. After an average of 5 years of follow-up, heart disease and stroke were significantly increased in HT users by 29% and 41%, respectively. Venous thromboembolic events (VTEs) were increased twofold. Approximately 11,000 women without a uterus participated in a

TABLE 2 WHI & WHIMS Results: Risks per 10,000 Person-Years Attributable to Estrogen Plus Progestin

Excess Risk	
Coronary heart disease	+7
Stroke	+8
Pulmonary embolism	+8
Invasive breast cancer	+8
Dementia*	+23
Reduced Risk	
Colorectal cancer	−6
Hip fracture	−5

*Dementia was assessed in a subset of women from the WHI trial, ages 65 years or older. Increased risk of dementia was statistically significant when data from both estrogen plus progestin and estrogen alone trials pooled.

Abbreviations: WHI = Women's Health Initiative; WHIMS = Women's Health Initiative Memory Study.

Adapted from: Writing Group for the Women's Health Initiative Investigators: Risks and benefits of estrogen plus progestin in healthy postmenopausal women: Principal results from the Women's Health Initiative randomized, controlled trial. JAMA 288:321-33, 2002.

Shumaker S, Legault C, Rapp S, et al: Estrogen plus progestin and the incidence of dementia and mild cognitive impairment in postmenopausal women. JAMA 289:2651-62, 2003.

separate WHI study and were randomized either to estrogen alone (Premarin) or placebo (Table 3). After an average follow-up of 7 years, there was no increased risk of heart disease in estrogen users. Estrogen use did have adverse vascular effects, increasing the risk of stroke by 39% and VTEs by 33%.

There is no role for estrogen therapy in the prevention of coronary heart disease (CHD), not only in healthy women, but also in women with established heart disease. The Heart and Estrogen/progestin Replacement Study (HERS), a randomized, placebo-controlled trial of HT (Prempro) for secondary prevention of heart disease, also did not demonstrate any reduction in CHD events overall. The risk of cardiovascular events actually was greater in HT users during the first year of treatment.

Of note, the WHI trials and the HERS study examined only treatment with conjugated equine estrogens and medroxyprogesterone acetate. The effects of other oral estrogens, transdermal estradiol, cyclic HT, or therapy with other progestins may be different. Without data from randomized controlled trials, the conservative approach is to assume that the risks of various HT regimens in menopausal women are similar.

Raloxifene (Evista)[1] has several beneficial effects on lipids, but whether these effects will translate into a reduced incidence of heart disease currently is being studied. Interestingly, in a secondary analysis of results from a randomized, controlled trial of raloxifene (Evista) versus placebo in more than 7000 women with osteoporosis, there were no significant differences between groups in coronary and cerebrovascular events. Among a subset of approximately 1000 women with increased cardiovascular risk at baseline, the women who received raloxifene experienced a significant 40% reduction in cardiovascular events.

[1]Not FDA approved for this indication.

TABLE 3 WHI & WHIMS Results: Risks per 10,000 Person-Years Attributable to Estrogen Alone in Women with Hysterectomy

Excess Risk	
Stroke	+12
DVT	+6
Dementia*	+12
Reduced Risk	
Hip fracture	−6
No Difference	
Coronary heart disease	
Invasive breast cancer	
Colorectal cancer	

*Dementia was assessed in a subset of women from the WHI trial, ages 65 years or older. Increased risk of dementia was statistically significant when data from both estrogen plus progestin and estrogen alone trials pooled.

Abbreviations: WHI = Women's Health Initiative; WHIMS = Women's Health Initiative Memory Study.

Adapted from: The Women's Health Initiative Steering Committee. Effects of conjugated equine estrogen in postmenopausal women with hysterectomy: The Women's Health Initiative randomized controlled trial. JAMA 291:1701-1712, 2004.

Shumaker SA, Legault C, Kuller L, et al. Conjugated equine estrogens and incidence of probable dementia and mild cognitive impairment in postmenopausal women. JAMA 291:2947-2958, 2004.

BREAST CANCER

Breast cancer is the most common cancer in women and is the second leading cause of cancer death. The lifetime risk of developing invasive breast cancer is 12%; therefore, any therapies that reduce or increase this risk will have a major impact on women's health. Risk factors for breast cancer include age, early menarche, late menopause, family history, and prior breast disease, including epithelial atypia and cancer. Oophorectomy and a term pregnancy before the age of 30 are associated with reduced risk. Many of these risk factors are consistent with the hypothesis that prolonged estrogen exposure increases the risk of breast cancer.

Long-term use of hormone therapy is associated with an increased risk of breast cancer. Observational studies demonstrate a relative risk of approximately 1.3 with long-term HT use, generally defined as greater than 5 years. The WHI HT trial found a significant 26% increase in the risk of invasive breast cancer in women assigned to HT after approximately 5 years of use. Interestingly, the WHI trial of estrogen alone in women with prior hysterectomy demonstrated no increased risk of breast cancer after an average of 7 years of estrogen use.

The SERM, tamoxifen (Nolvadex), is an estrogen antagonist in the breast used in the treatment of estrogen-receptor-positive breast cancer. Tamoxifen also is approved for the prevention of breast cancer in high-risk women, resulting in an approximately 50% reduction in the risk of disease. Raloxifene (Evista) also may reduce the risk of breast cancer, although it is not approved for this indication. Postmenopausal women receiving raloxifene as part of a large osteoporosis treatment trial experienced a 76% reduction in the risk of invasive breast cancer compared to placebo-treated women.

There are risks associated with SERM use. Tamoxifen and raloxifene increase the risk of VTEs approximately threefold, similar to the increased risk seen in HT users. Hot flashes are increased with raloxifene and tamoxifen use, and raloxifene is associated with leg cramps. Tamoxifen acts as an estrogen agonist in the endometrium, increasing the risk of endometrial polyps, hyperplasia, and cancer, while no endometrial stimulation is seen with raloxifene.

Treatment

Screening mammography annually for women older than the age of 50 years reduces breast cancer mortality, according to several large studies. Women at increased risk for breast cancer are advised not to use HT, or to use it only short term. Women at high risk also may elect tamoxifen therapy.

ENDOMETRIAL CANCER

The use of unopposed estrogen is associated with an increased risk of endometrial hyperplasia and cancer. Combination estrogen–progestin therapy, therefore, is recommended for all women with a uterus. Treatment may be provided in a sequential manner, with estrogen daily and progestin for 12 to 14 days of each month, or in a continuous-combined fashion with estrogen and a lower dose of progestin daily. Sequential regimens result in regular, predictable vaginal bleeding. The benefit of continuous-combined regimens is that approximately 60% to 70% of women will experience amenorrhea by the end of one year of therapy; the problem is that the bleeding that does occur is irregular and unpredictable. Several combination therapies may have a lower incidence of bleeding, including norethindrone acetate (NETA) with either ethinyl estradiol (FemHRT) or estradiol (Activella), or low-dose conjugated equine estrogens and MPA (Prempro 0.45/1.5 or 0.3/1.5).

ALZHEIMER'S DISEASE

Alzheimer's disease is the most common form of dementia. Women are at greater risk for developing the disease than men, and the number of affected Americans is expected to double to more than 8 million by the year 2010. Several small trials and observational studies, often of women who initiated HT early with the onset of menopausal symptoms, suggest that hormone therapy use may decrease the risk of Alzheimer's disease. A randomized, controlled study in women with mild to moderate Alzheimer's disease, however, demonstrated that 1 year of estrogen treatment did not slow disease progression nor improve cognition. The effect of HT on cognitive function in women without dementia was studied in the WHI Memory Study (WHIMS), a randomized, double-blind, placebo-controlled trial of women ages 65 years and older enrolled in the WHI trial. In contrast to the findings of observational studies, women randomized to estrogen therapy in WHIMS experienced a significant twofold increased risk of dementia.

Contraindications to HT use include known or suspected breast or endometrial cancer, undiagnosed abnormal genital bleeding, active thromboembolic disorders, and active liver or gallbladder disease. Relative contraindications include heart disease, migraine headaches, a history of liver or gallbladder disease, previous breast or endometrial cancer, or prior thromboembolic events.

Summary

There are many options available to address the quality of life and health concerns of menopausal women. Currently, the primary indication for hormone therapy is the alleviation of hot flashes and associated symptoms. Women need to be informed of the potential benefits and risks of all therapeutic options and care should be individualized based on a woman's needs and preferences.

VULVOVAGINITIS

METHOD OF

David A. Baker, MD

Vulvovaginitis brings large numbers of women to see their health care provider. Over the last several decades with the availability of numerous over-the-counter preparations, most patients medicate themselves to treat their symptoms. However, it is clear that the majority of patients make the wrong diagnosis. They use the wrong medications and delay bringing their symptoms and complaints to the attention of the clinician; as a result, many women will experience complications from their vaginal infection. Therefore, the clinician needs to take this condition (vulvovaginitis) seriously and view the patient as one with a significant medical, physiologic, and social problem that may lead not only to significant medical conditions and complications but also to significant interpersonal problems.

An accurate diagnosis is required to provide proper and correct treatment of this condition. Symptoms presented to the health care provider by phone can be very nonspecific and may lead to an improper diagnosis and treatment. The three major categories of vaginitis in the United States (Figure 1) are those caused predominately by candidiasis, trichomoniasis, and bacterial vaginosis (BV). Of these three abnormal symptomatic manifestations, BV is the most common in the United States. Many patients mistake BV for *Candida* infections and take over-the-counter antifungal preparations, which are costly and ineffective. Patients do not appreciate the significance of this most common condition: BV may lead to important medical complications not only during pregnancy but also when the patient is not pregnant. Of the three conditions, the only one that is considered a sexually transmitted disease (STD) is trichomoniasis. BV is associated with other STDs.

The goal of therapy is to not only treat or control the organism that is abnormally colonizing or growing in the vagina but also return the vagina to normal vaginal colonization. This objective may be difficult, and one of the major problems of recurrent vaginal infection is our inability to colonize the lower genital tract with healthy bacteria. The normal vagina has an acidic pH that is produced by a combination of normal host flora and the species

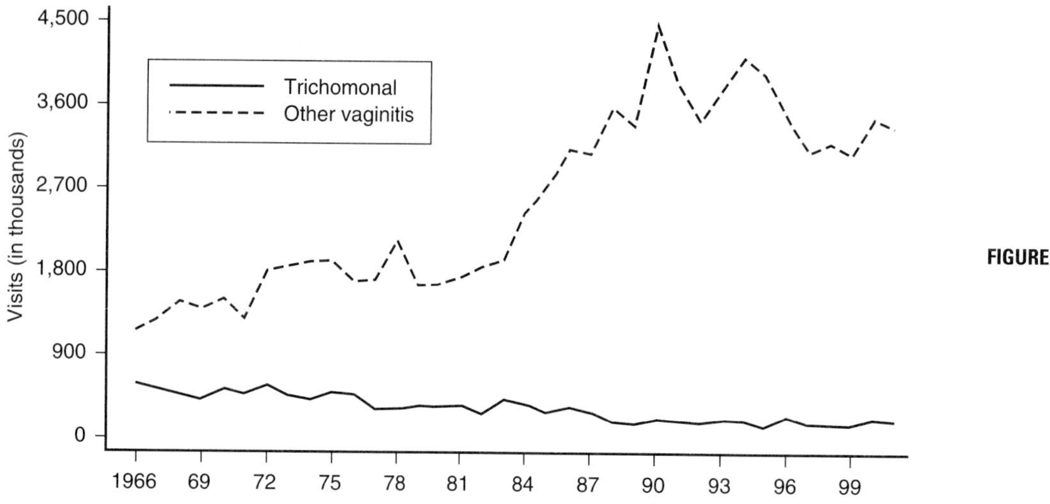

FIGURE 1.

Lactobacillus, which produces lactic acid. The importance of *Lactobacillus* strains that produce not only lactic acid but also hydrogen peroxide cannot be overemphasized; they maintain the lower genital tract flora and act as a protective barrier to the acquisition of certain STDs, including HIV. It is therefore the goal of the treating clinician to eradicate the patient's symptoms, control the abnormal vaginal colonization, and try to propagate normal lower genital tract flora. Women with normal lower genital tract flora containing lactobacilli producing lactic acid and hydrogen peroxide were less likely to contract chlamydiosis, trichomoniasis, and symptomatic candidiasis. In addition, the prevalence of gonorrhea, chlamydiosis, and trichomoniasis was significantly lower in women who had normal vaginal *Lactobacillus* flora during pregnancy.

Bacterial Vaginosis

The term given to abnormal colonization of the lower genital tract with anaerobic bacteria is bacterial vaginosis. However, a more meaningful definition of BV may be one that includes an inflammatory component of this anaerobic bacterial overgrowth. Currently, approximately 50% of women in the United States who visit a clinician for treatment of vaginitis have BV. It is a polymicrobial infection involving an increase in anaerobic bacteria, loss of the normal *Lactobacillus* flora, and consequently, an imbalance in the vaginal ecosystem. The absence or a decreased number of lactobacilli facilitates the overgrowth of pathogenic organism, which are predominately anaerobic bacteria.

The exact factors that trigger the overgrowth of anaerobic bacteria are still not fully understood. Douching can lead to a disturbance in the delicate balance of lower genital tract organisms. Other risk factors for BV include trichomoniasis, other STDs, early sexual experience, multiple sexual partners, and the use of an intrauterine contraceptive device.

DIAGNOSIS

Proper diagnosis is important for the treatment and eradication of BV. The diagnosis can be made during vaginal examination and does not require expensive and elaborate techniques. The current 2002 Centers for Disease Control and Prevention (CDC) STD treatment guidelines require three of the following symptoms or signs for diagnosis: a homogeneous, white, noninflammatory discharge that coats the vaginal walls smoothly; the presence of clue cells on microscopic examination; a pH of vaginal secretions of less than 4.5; and a fishy odor of the vaginal discharge before or after the addition of 10% KOH (the whiff test). Gram stain is an acceptable laboratory method for diagnosing BV. However, culture is not recommended as a diagnostic tool. In addition, cervical Papanicolaou (Pap) tests have limited clinical utility for the diagnosis of BV because of low sensitivity. Other commercially available tests add to the cost and rarely aid the clinician in diagnosing this vaginal infection.

TREATMENT

The goal of therapy is to not only control this anaerobic infection but also relieve vaginal symptoms, lessen the risk of infectious complications after procedures, and reduce the risk of development of other infectious complications, HIV, and other STDs. All women who have symptomatic disease require treatment. Because of the increased risk of postoperative infectious complications associated with BV, it is suggested that before surgical procedures are performed on women, they be screened and treated for BV, in addition to undergoing other routine prophylactic measures.

BV during pregnancy has been associated with adverse pregnancy outcomes, including preterm labor, premature rupture of membranes, and postpartum infections. Therapy during pregnancy has the potential of reducing these potential risks, as well as reducing the risk of acquiring STDs and HIV during pregnancy. The CDC has given recommendations for the treatment of nonpregnant and pregnant women with BV (Table 1). Patients need to be informed that clindamycin (Cleocin) cream and ovules are oil-based preparations that may interfere with the efficiency of latex condoms and diaphragms. In addition, oral and topical metronidazole (Flagyl) regimens are equally efficacious. Studies of vaginal clindamycin cream appear to demonstrate that it is less efficacious than metronidazole regimens. Short-course therapy for BV in the form of metronidazole, 2 g orally in a single dose, has been proposed. The clinician must recognize that metronidazole, 2 g in a single dose, is an alternative regimen because of its lower efficacy in the treatment of BV. Unfortunately, at the current time, no preparation, either intravaginal or oral, is able to induce reversion to the normal lower genital tract vaginal flora.

BV is not considered an STD, and therefore routine treatment of sex partners is not currently recommended. When using clindamycin and metronidazole, one must differentiate between side effects and allergic reactions. Metronidazole gel (MetroGel) may be appropriate for patients who have side effects with oral metronidazole, but it should not be used in a patient allergic to metronidazole.

Oral regimens are recommended (see Table 1) for pregnant women. Topical clindamycin (Cleocin vaginal cream) is contraindicated in pregnancy because of the potential overgrowth of gram-negative aerobic bacteria (*Escherichia coli*) in the vagina. Patients who have BV should be offered testing for HIV and other STDs. Patients with HIV should be screened and treated for BV with the same regimens as those who are HIV negative.

TABLE 1 Bacterial Vaginosis: Treatment Regimens

Recommended Regimens, Nonpregnant
Metronidazole (Flagyl), 500 mg orally twice a day for 7 d
or
Metronidazole (Metro-Gel), 0.75% gel, 1 full applicator (5 g) intravaginally once a day for 5 d
or
Clindamycin (Cleocin), 2% cream, 1 full applicator (5 g) intravaginally at bedtime for 7 d
Alternative Regimens, Nonpregnant
Metronidazole, 2 g orally in a single dose
or
Clindamycin, 300 mg orally twice a day for 7 d
or
Clindamycin ovules, 100 g intravaginally once at bedtime for 3 d
Recommended Regimens, Pregnant
Metronidazole, 250 mg orally three times a day for 7 d
or
Clindamycin, 300 mg orally twice a day for 7 d

Note: Patients should be advised to avoid consuming alcohol during treatment with metronidazole and for 24 hours thereafter. Clindamycin cream and ovules are oil based and might weaken latex condoms and diaphragms: Refer to condom product labeling for additional information.

From Centers for Disease Control and Prevention: Sexually transmitted diseases treatment guidelines 2002. MMWR Morb Mortal Wkly Rep 51:42–48, 2002.

Trichomoniasis

The incidence of trichomoniasis has slowly declined in the United States since the mid 1960s and has remained at a low level over the past decade. Trichomoniasis is caused by the protozoan *Trichomonas vaginalis*. Women who are infected usually have a vaginal discharge and specific symptoms, in contrast to men, who are generally asymptomatic. *T. vaginalis* is a pear-shaped flagellated protozoon that is usually identified in wet mounts by a rapid swaying motion and the presence of polymorphonuclear leukocytes. Growth is typically enhanced by anaerobic conditions and an elevated pH. The incubation period ranges from 4 to 28 days. The clinician needs to recognize that infection with this organism occurs not only in the vagina but also in the urethra, Skene's glands, and the bladder. In men, the urethra is the most common site. However, the prostate and epididymis may also be infected, and the organism may be detected in semen and urine. Trichomoniasis is an STD transmitted through sexual contact, with infection documented in 85% of female partners of infected men. Risk factors for trichomoniasis are the presence of other STDS, an increased number of sexual partners, the presence of BV, smoking, and a vaginal pH over 4.5.

DIAGNOSIS

The patient usually has a discharge, odor, and vulvar itching with or without dysuria. The discharge is yellow-green with a frothy appearance. Further evaluation of the patient reveals that the pH of the vagina is over 4.5, the amine test may be positive, and on wet preparations, the organism and an increase in the white blood cell count (greater than 10 per high-power field) are usually found. Wet preparations and Pap smears have an approximately 50% to 60% sensitivity and greater than 90% specificity. Other techniques are in development that should better enable the clinician to diagnose this infection. Trichomoniasis in pregnant women has been associated with adverse pregnancy outcomes, specifically, preterm rupture of membranes, preterm labor, and preterm delivery. In addition, studies have shown that the presence of trichomoniasis is associated with an increased risk of acquiring HIV, so patients in whom trichomoniasis has been diagnosed should be screened for other STDs, and HIV testing should be encouraged.

TREATMENT

Current CDC treatment guidelines are presented in Table 2. The metronidazole regimen recommended has resulted in cure rates of approximately 90% to 95%. Because trichomoniasis is an STD,

TABLE 2 Trichomoniasis: Treatment Regimens

Recommended Regimen
Metronidazole (Flagyl), 2 g orally in a single dose
Alternative Regimen
Metronidazole, 500 mg twice a day for 7 d

From Centers for Disease Control and Prevention: Sexually transmitted diseases treatment guidelines 2002. MMWR Morb Mortal Wkly Rep 51:42-48, 2002.

treatment of sexual partners is mandatory. Metronidazole gel has an efficacy of approximately 50% for the treatment of trichomoniasis. Because the organism may be found in locations other than the vagina, such treatment is less efficacious and not recommended. Women who fail oral therapy may repeat a 7-day course of therapy with topical metronidazole. Because metronidazole is currently the only approved therapy in the United States, patients with allergic reactions to metronidazole may be managed by desensitization. Newer medications and therapies for this condition are in development and may be of assistance in patients with allergic reactions or the emerging problem of metronidazole-resistant trichomoniasis.

Candidiasis

Most patients think that their symptoms are associated with a yeast infection, but in reality, studies show that 75% of patients with chronic candidiasis have another etiologic agent for their problems. However, candidiasis is still one of the most common vaginal infections and is usually treated initially with over-the-counter or alternative regimens. Patients who cannot control the infection or experience recurrent symptoms generally seek medical assistance. The CDC has classified vulvovaginal candidiasis (VVC) as uncomplicated VVC or complicated VVC (Table 3). This classification is based on clinical findings, microbiology, host factors, and response to therapy. Approximately 10% to 20% of women will have complicated VVC.

TABLE 3 Classification of Vulvovaginal Candidiasis (VVC)

Uncomplicated	Complicated
Sporadic or infrequent VVC	Recurrent VVC
or	*or*
Mild-to-moderate VVC	Severe VVC
or	*or*
Likely to be *Candida albicans*	Non-*albicans* candidiasis
or	*or*
Nonimmunocompromised women	Women with uncontrolled diabetes, debilitation, or immunosuppression or those who are pregnant

From Centers for Disease Control and Prevention: Sexually transmitted diseases treatment guidelines 2002. MMWR Morb Mortal Wkly Rep 51:42–48, 2002.

DIAGNOSIS AND TREATMENT

Pruritus and an inflammatory reaction suggest the diagnosis of candidal vaginitis. A white, cheesy discharge is usually what drives the patient to buy an over-the-counter antifungal preparation. The clinician needs to use additional modalities for diagnosis, including a wet preparation with 10% KOH, Gram stain or culture, and determination of vaginal pH (less than 4.5). Because a significant number of

TABLE 4 Vulvovaginal Candidiasis: Recommended Treatment Regimens

Intravaginal Agents
Butoconazole (Mycelex), 2% cream, 5 g intravaginally for 3 d*
or
Butoconazole 2% cream, 5 g (butoconazole—sustained release), single intravaginal application,
or
Clotrimazole (Gyne-Lotrimin), 1% cream, 5 g intravaginally for 7-14 d*
or
Clotrimazole, 100-mg vaginal tablet for 7 d
or
Clotrimazole, 100-mg vaginal tablet, 2 tablets for 3 d
or
Clotrimazole, 500-mg vaginal tablet, 1 tablet in a single application
or
Miconazole (Monistat), 2% cream, 5 g intravaginally for 7 d*
or
Miconazole, 100-mg vaginal suppository, 1 suppository for 7 d*
or
Miconazole, 200-mg vaginal suppository, 1 suppository for 3 d*
or
Nystatin, 100,000-U vaginal tablet , 1 tablet for 14 d
or
Tioconazole (Vagistat), 6.5% ointment, 5 g intravaginally in a single application*
or
Terconazole (Terazol), 0.4% cream, 5 g intravaginally for 7 d
or
Terconazole, 0.8% cream, 5 g intravaginally for 3 d
or
Terconazole, 80-mg vaginal suppository, 1 suppository for 3 d
Oral Agent
Fluconazole (Diflucan), 150-mg oral tablet, 1 tablet in single dose

Note: The creams and suppositories in these regimens are oil based and may weaken latex condoms and diaphragms. Refer to condom product labeling for further information.

*Preparations for intravaginal administration of butoconazole, clotrimazole , miconazole, and tioconazole are available over the counter (OTC). Self-medication with OTC preparations should be advised only for women in whom VVC has previously been diagnosed and who have a recurrence of the same symptoms. Any woman whose symptoms persist after using an OTC preparation or who has a recurrence of symptoms within 2 months should seek medical care. Unnecessary or inappropriate use of OTC preparations is common and can lead to a delay in treatment of other etiologies of vulvovaginitis that could result in adverse clinical outcomes.

From Centers for Disease Control and Prevention. Sexually transmitted disease treatment guidelines 2002. MMWR Morb Mortal Wkly Rep 51:42–48, 2002.

women are colonized with *Candida*, culture in the absence of symptoms is not clinically relevant. Most patients with uncomplicated VVC have no precipitating factor; however, VVC commonly develops after antibiotic use. The CDC has recommended numerous regimens (Table 4) for the treatment of uncomplicated VVC, including 14 topical regimens and 1 single-dose oral regimen. VVC is not acquired through sexual activity, and therefore treatment of the partner is not usually recommended.

Complicated VVC is usually defined as four or more episodes of symptomatic VVC each year and should occur in only a small percentage of women. Most patients with recurrent VVC have no apparent predisposing or underlying conditions. Culture may be important in determining the appropriate treatment and management of these patients. Non-*albicans* species of *Candida* are found in only 10% to 20% of patients with recurrent VVC. Different therapeutic regimens for a longer duration may be of benefit in treating recurrent VVC. The use of antifungals for maintenance therapy or in specific daily or weekly recommended regimens can be considered for up to 6 months. However, side effects and the toxicity of oral medications need to be taken into account. Once maintenance therapy is discontinued, VVC will recur in upward of 40% of women.

Nonfluconazole azole drugs are recommended as first-line therapy for non-*albicans* VVC. In this specific clinical situation, 600 mg of boric acid[2] by capsule intravaginally once daily for 2 weeks may be beneficial.

Specific investigation to evaluate for pregnancy, HIV infection, and systemic immunocompromising conditions such as diabetes is important in managing vulvovaginitis.

[2]Not available in the United States. May be compounded by pharmacists.

CHLAMYDIA TRACHOMATIS

METHOD OF

Catherine Stevens-Simon, MD

The Scope of the Problem

Responsible for more than 3 million infections each year in the United States, *Chlamydia trachomatis* poses a public health problem of epidemic proportions. Because of the large reservoir of undiagnosed, asymptomatic infections, the number of reported cases significantly underestimates the true prevalence of this infection. Nonetheless, *C. trachomatis* is not only the most commonly reported bacterial sexually transmitted disease (STD) in the United States, but also the nation's most commonly reported bacterial infection. It is difficult to give meaningful prevalence figures, as the proportion of infected individuals depends on the characteristics of the population studied and how they are studied. In addition, while passive surveillance systems indicate that the prevalence of this infection has risen precipitously over the last decade, studies conducted at sentinel surveillance sites demonstrate a decline; which suggests that expanded screening, increased reporting, and improved test sensitivity mask a true decrease in prevalence in some sectors of American society. The epidemiologic characteristics and clinical manifestations of chlamydial infections in the United States reflect the fact that most infections are sexually transmitted and prevalent stereotypes have an affinity for columnar epithelium. Teenage girls are most susceptible to these infections because:

- At their age, the columnar epithelium is prominent on the ectocervix.
- Some experience a high level of unprotected, serially monogamous sexual activity with older males whose sexual risk profiles they rarely investigate.

With these two factors combined, teenage girls are at maximal biological and social risk. While the national prevalence of chlamydial infections in this population is unknown, school and clinic-based studies suggest a range of 8% to 26% (compared to 3% to 5% in sociodemographically similar young adult women), with the highest age-specific prevalence reported among 14- to 15-year-olds. Although readily eradicable, the economic and human costs of these infections are staggering. Annual expenditures are estimated to exceed $1.5 billion, with 75% of the cost devoted to treating sequelae of cervical infections that were initially uncomplicated. Because the majority of severe consequences of untreated infections occur in women, and as much as 66.6% of tubal factor infertility and 33.3% of ectopic pregnancies in the United States are attributed to chlamydial infections; it is estimated that every dollar spent on screening and treating asymptomatic young females and their sex partners saves approximately $12. While this uniquely positions primary health care providers to prevent the costly sequelae of chlamydial infections, given their prevalence among teenagers, expansion of screening and treatment programs to nontraditional settings such as schools, juvenile detention centers, and drug treatment facilities is likely to be a critical component of any national strategy to control this infection.

Clinical Presentation

Chlamydial infections are an excellent example of the dependence of the clinical manifestations of disease on the intrinsic properties of the pathogen and host. In western industrialized countries, virtually all chlamydial infections are either sexually transmitted or vertically transmitted at birth. They are caused by nonlymphogranuloma venereum stereotypes that have an affinity for columnar epithelium and can only survive by a cytotoxic, replicative cycle that evokes a variable immune response in the host. Hence, in the United States the endocervix, urethra, rectum, and conjunctiva are preferentially affected; and clinical manifestations range from asymptomatic to florid inflammatory conditions with severe reproductive consequences. Chlamydia should be suspected in:

- Women and men with dysuria and pyuria
- Women with dyspareunia; abnormal vaginal discharge; postcoital, irregular menstrual, or *breakthrough* contraceptive bleeding; and lower abdominal or pelvic pain
- Infants with conjunctivitis or a staccato cough

However, these signs and symptoms are neither a sensitive nor a specific indication of infection. Indeed, because nearly 90% of chlamydial infections are asymptomatic and *C. trachomatis* is isolated from less than 33.3% of women with mucopurulent cervicitis and less than 50% of men with nongonococcal urethritis, such complaints are unreliable predictors of infection.

In women the most common sign is mucopurulent cervicitis, a nonspecific clinical syndrome characterized by erythema, edema, and friability of the ectocervix and purulent endocervical exudate. Mucopurulent cervicitis, however, is also caused by other STDs and noninfectious factors (i.e., cyclical fluctuations in gonadal hormones), which increase the size of the cervical ectropion or the resident population of cervical leukocytes. Other clinical manifestations of lower genital tract chlamydial infections in women include urethritis and bartholinitis. Although pelvic inflammatory disease (PID) is a polymicrobial infection, *C. trachomatis* is also often involved and, conversely, PID is the most common complication of chlamydial cervicitis. The estimated incidence ranges from 10% to 40% in untreated women. Young age and prolonged or recurrent infection significantly increase, whereas treatment of asymptomatic infections significantly decrease both disease severity and sequela, such as salpingo-oophoritis, perihepatitis (Fitz-Hugh-Curtis syndrome), infertility, ectopic pregnancy, and chronic pelvic pain. Adverse outcomes associated with chlamydial infections during pregnancy include preterm labor, premature rupture of the placental membranes, low-birth-weight delivery, neonatal death, postpartum or postabortal endometritis, and vertical transmission to infants. In the infected infants, 30% to 50% develop conjunctivitis, 15% to 20% develop nasopharyngitis, and 5% to 10% develop pneumonia.

In males the most common clinical manifestation is urethritis, the symptoms of which typically commence 1 to 3 weeks after exposure and range from mild dysuria to frank penile discharge. Other clinical syndromes in men include epididymitis, prostatitis, acute proctocolitis, and Reiter's syndrome (urethritis, conjunctivitis, arthritis, and mucocutaneous lesions). These suppurative complications rarely require inpatient therapy and are far less common than those encountered in females. Nonetheless, sequelae ranging from urethral strictures to infertility do occur. Nongenital clinical manifestations such as conjunctivitis, tenosynovitis, and arthritis are uncommon among adults in the United States.

Diagnosis and Screening

In the United States, testing for both symptomatic and asymptomatic chlamydial infections is done with ligase chain reaction (LCR), polymerase chain reaction (PCR), and other nucleic acid amplification techniques (NAATs), because they do not require the presence of intact organisms. Urine, cervical, vaginal, or urethral fluids can be used as the analyte for these tests; specimens are stable and easy to transport; and results can be obtained within a day. This is a major advantage over the stringent collection, transport, and 3-day growth period culturing requirements associated with this fastidious organism. Although nonculture, non-NAATs, and rapid diagnostic tests capable of making a diagnosis within 30 minutes are available, these assays are too insensitive to be recommended for routine testing.

The signs and symptoms of chlamydial infection are nonspecific and often persist for weeks after documented eradication of the pathogen. Because of this, leukocyte, esterase-positive urine dip sticks, leukocyte-laden vaginal wet mounts, and endocervical Gram stains should be regarded as no more than a trigger for testing. Although concerns about the consequences of underdiagnosis and undertreatment typically overshadow concerns about the consequences of overdiagnosis and overtreatment, therapeutic decisions should not be based on these poorly standardized tests. Indeed, given their low positive predictive value for chlamydial infections, the adverse psychological effects of being diagnosed with an STD, and the serious public health problems the indiscriminate use of antibiotics creates—even in settings where the prevalence of chlamydial infections is high and patient follow-up is uncertain, and in resource-poor clinics where NAATs are unavailable—enthusiasm for the practice of diagnosing chlamydial infections empirically must be tempered by the knowledge that to prevent one individual from suffering the sequelae of an untreated infection, hundreds will needlessly suffer the adverse psychosocial consequences of an STD diagnosis. This is true even when the diagnosis is made based on characteristic symptom complexes, suggestive leukocyte esterase urine dip sticks, and/or vaginal wet mounts. Thus, with sensitivities and specificities fluctuating approximately 98% on male urethral and urine specimens as well as on female cervical specimens, NAATs are currently the best chlamydial tests available. However, because the sensitivity of these assays for detecting infections in women is significantly lower when urine (80% to 95%) or patient- or provider-collected vaginal fluid (70% to 85%) is the analyte, endocervical specimens should be used, except in screening situations where it is impractical to perform pelvic examinations. Every case diagnosed on a urine or vaginal specimen is a bonus.

Despite consensus about how to screen, there continues to be uncertainty about whom to screen and how frequently to screen them. Pregnant women and sexually active women younger than 25 years of age are the only groups for whom there is good evidence that the benefits of screening outweigh the harms. Specifically, when prevalence rates exceed 2%, testing and treating these individuals for asymptomatic chlamydial infections is a cost-effective preventative measure that:

- Averts PID and associated medical complications.
- Reduces transmission to sex partners.
- Reduces the risk of acquiring HIV.
- Lowers the prevalence of chlamydia in the community.

It is unlikely that these benefits reflect factors other than screening (i.e., increased condom use), as knowledge of sexual risk behavior adds nothing to the predictive algorithm that includes age and prior STD history. However, because of the highly infectious nature of this bacterium, the lack of a vaccine, and the failure of the human immune system to build up resistance to the bacteria, reinfection of effectively treated individuals tends to diminish short-term efficacy, making long-term, periodic screening a prerequisite of cost efficacy.

The only other caveat is that most cost-effectiveness analyses are based upon culture-proven disease, and may, therefore, reflect a larger inoculum than infections diagnosed by NAAT assays, which can detect extremely low levels of viable and nonviable organisms. Thus, further research is needed to determine if and how inoculum size affects disease presentation and to define the clinical and public health significance of NAAT-detectable infections. Specifically, studies comparing transmission rates and the clinical consequences of infections that are detected only by NAAT assay versus those that are detected by traditional assays are still needed to prove that routine, periodic, urine-based screening of asymptomatic individuals is a cost-effective way to control chlamydial infections at the population level. Moreover, because identifying infected individuals is only the first step in effective disease control, it is also important to demonstrate that once identified, the majority of these asymptomatically infected individuals and their sex partners can be contacted and treated. The randomized trial data that determine how frequently community members should be screened to lower chlamydial infections at the population level are lacking; however, observational studies consistently indicate that among sexually active teens the median time between first and repeat infections is approximately 6 months. Based on these data, biannual screening seems reasonable for females at this age (<25 years). Because the risk of reinfection is inversely related to age, however, it is unclear if this recommendation should be extended to young adults. Nevertheless, a history of prior infection predicts reinfection regardless of sexual risk behavior, and repeat infections are implicated in the pathogenesis of upper genital tract damage. It may be wise, therefore, to rescreen all women who have been treated for chlamydial infections at 6-month intervals.

Finally, with the exception of age, no single demographic or behavioral risk factor or combination of risk factors consistently identifies a group of young, sexually active females who should *not* be screened. The utility of more selective screening is limited by the high proportion of missed infections.

Parallel evidence to support screening asymptomatic males may be lacking, because before the introduction of urine screening men were not routinely tested for chlamydial infection. However, because:

- the cost of treating males is lower than the cost of treating females,
- a greater proportion of infected males are symptomatic than females, and
- the harm associated with misdiagnoses is not inconsequent,

it will undoubtedly be more difficult to justify routine, periodic male screening. Specifically, false-negative test results create a reservoir of untreated disease that is likely to contribute disproportionately to the spread of *C. trachomatis*. Also, the psychosocial consequences of false-positive test results can range from dysphoric feelings and decreased self-esteem to the disruption of romantic relationships and domestic violence. Moreover, if treatment is initiated inappropriately, the adverse effects of drug reactions and bacterial resistance caused by antibiotic overuse must be taken into account. Thus, until more data become available, the United States Preventive Services Task Force recommends symptom-based screening for all males and for females older than 25 years of age who do not exhibit other characteristics associated with a high prevalence of chlamydial infections (i.e., unmarried status, African American race, a history of STDs, a history of new or multiple sex partners, cervical ectopy, and inconsistent condom use).

Treatment

Recommendations for antibiotic treatment of chlamydial infections depend on the clinical syndrome. The options for outpatient therapy of uncomplicated

TABLE 1 Recommended Treatment Regimens by Clinical Syndrome

Asymptomatic, Cervicitis, Urethritis*

First-Choice Regimen
Azithromycin (Zithromax), 1 g orally in a single dose
or
Doxycycline (Vibramycin), 100 mg orally twice a day for 7d

ALTERNATIVE REGIMENS (ONE OF THE FOLLOWING)
Erythromycin base (E-Mycin), 500 mg orally four times a day for 7d
Erythromycin ethylsuccinate (E.E.S.), 800 mg orally four times a day for 7d
Ofloxacin (Floxin), 300 mg orally twice a day for 7d
Levofloxacin (Levaquin)[1], 500 mg orally for 7d

Epididymitis

Ceftriaxone (Rocephin)[1], 250 mg intramuscularly (single dose)
or
Doxycycline[1], 100 mg orally twice a day for 7d

Outpatient Pelvic Inflammatory Disease

Ofloxacin, 400 mg orally twice a day for 14d
or
Levofloxacin[1], 500 mg orally for 14d
with or without
Metronidazole (Flagyl), 500 mg orally twice a day for 14d

ALTERNATIVE REGIMENS
Ceftriaxone, 250 mg intramuscularly (single dose)
or
Cefoxitin (Mefoxin), 2 g intramuscularly (single dose)
plus
Probenecid, 1 g orally
plus
Doxycycline, 100 mg orally twice a day for 14d
with or without
Metronidazole, 500 mg orally twice a day for 14d

Inpatient Pelvic Inflammatory Disease[†]

Cefotetan (Cefotan), 2 g intravenously every 12h
or
Cefoxitin, 2 g intravenously every 6h
plus
Doxycycline[1], 100 mg orally or intravenously every 12h

ALTERNATIVE REGIMENS
Clindamycin, 900 mg intravenously every 8h
plus
Gentamicin[1], 2 g/kg of body weight loading dose, then 1.5 mg/kg of body weight every 8h. Treatment should be continued for 24 to 48h after significant clinical improvement occurs and then should consist of oral therapy with Doxycycline, 100 mg orally twice a day for 14d or Clindamycin, 450 mg orally 4 times a day, for a total of 14d.

[1]Not FDA approved for this indication.
**Pregnancy*: Doxycycline, erythromycin estolate (Ilosone), and ofloxacin are contraindicated and repeat testing 3 weeks after completion of therapy is recommended, as antibiotics may be less efficacious.
HIV Infection: Patients who have chlamydial infection and who also are infected with HIV should receive the same treatment regimen as those who are HIV-negative.
[†]Studies indicate that the efficacy of inpatient and outpatient treatment is comparable in terms of fertility and other long-term health outcomes (e.g., ectopic pregnancy and chronic pelvic pain). Therefore, inpatient therapy is no longer recommended except for individuals who do not respond to outpatient regimes or develop tuboovarian abscesses or other manifestation of severe upper genital tract disease.

genital tract infections in males and females are summarized in Table 1. However, because humans do not develop a natural immunity to chlamydia, treated patients remain at risk for reinfection. For this reason therapy should not be considered complete until all recent sexual contacts have been treated and the patient has been counseled about future disease prevention. It is estimated that 70% of the male partners of females with chlamydial cervicitis are infected, and, conversely, that approximately 30% of the female partners of chlamydia-infected males are infected. Treatment is recommended for the most recent sex partner and all other individuals who had sexual contact with the infected person during the 60 days preceding the onset of symptoms or diagnosis. Also, partners should abstain from sexual intercourse for a week after they complete treatment.

While patient-delivered partner treatment is as effective as partner notification, partners are more likely to be treated if informed by physicians rather than by the patients. This is because only 65% (approximately) of females with known chlamydial infections refer their sex partners for therapy, and even fewer (approximately 45%) infected males do so. Because the cure rate for single-dose azithromycin (Zithromax) therapy is close to 100% and the medication can easily be administered under medical supervision, a test of cure 3 weeks after treatment—NAATs remain positive for this long despite successful eradication of infection—is only recommended for pregnant women (among whom antibiotic efficacy may be reduced) and when compliance is in doubt.

Approximately 50% of all chlamydial infections occur in previously treated persons. Demographic characteristics, such as age and a past history of chlamydial infection, are better predictors of infection than behavioral risk factors, such as multiple sexual partners and the failure to use condoms consistently. Being involved with a sexual network in which chlamydia is hyperendemic appears to put individuals at greater risk for infection than unsafe sexual behavior in the general population. Hence, to control the spread of *C. trachomatis* it may be necessary to:

- Extend screening and treatment beyond recent partners to include the group of core-transmitters in the infected individual's sexual network.
- Help STD patients learn to choose less risky sex partners by promoting sexual health communication within partnerships.

Although the debate about the content and duration of counseling necessary to achieve this goal is ongoing, there is a growing consensus that brief (5 minutes), personalized (provider-delivered–client-centered) counseling sessions—aimed at personal risk reduction and increasing awareness of partner risk behavior—are more effective than the conventional didactic approach to STD prevention education. They are certainly as effective as more prolonged sessions, which are difficult to conduct in busy public health clinics.

PELVIC INFLAMMATORY DISEASE

METHOD OF

Lydia A. Shrier, MD, MPH

Pelvic inflammatory disease (PID), which is an infection of the female upper genital tract, may include parametritis, endometritis, acute salpingitis, oophoritis, tuboovarian abscess (TOA), and pelvic peritonitis.

Risk factors for PID include young age, at risk sexual behaviors (unprotected intercourse, multiple sexual partners, and intercourse during menses), smoking, and douching. Bacterial vaginosis may facilitate ascension of pathogenic organisms from the lower genital tract. Cervical ectopy, commonly seen in young women, may increase their risk of PID because pathogens readily adhere to the columnar cells exposed on the exocervix. Cervicitis with *Neisseria gonorrhoeae* or *Chlamydia trachomatis* is clearly associated with PID. Invasive procedures, such as a therapeutic abortion or insertion of an intrauterine device within the past 30 days, increase the risk of PID. Recent studies have not found an association between the use of any hormonal contraception and PID. Scarring and impaired local barriers to infection from one episode of PID places a woman at risk for future episodes. PID is associated with black race, low socioeconomic status, and substance abuse.

PID is a polymicrobial infection that may involve *C. trachomatis, N. gonorrhoeae, Mycoplasma hominis, Ureaplasma urealyticum,* nontypable *Haemophilus influenzae*, aerobes, and anaerobes (especially with TOA and with more severe PID). Lower genital tract test results do not correlate well with the presence of upper tract infection.

Infection occurs by direct canalicular spread from the endocervix along the endometrial surface to the tubal mucosa. The end of the tube may become blocked with pus, leading to pyosalpinx or TOA if the ovary is also involved. Mechanisms of ascension include direct migration or transport via attachment to sperm or with refluxed menstrual blood. Chlamydial and gonococcal PID commonly occur within 7 days of the onset of menses. This is likely because of loss of the protective cervical mucus plug; sloughing of the endometrium, which produces a *stickier* surface for bacteria; and the presence of menstrual blood, a good culture medium.

Although symptoms have poor sensitivity and specificity for PID, it is useful to elicit history of:

- Lower abdominal and/or pelvic pain
- New or malodorous vaginal discharge
- Dysuria or urinary frequency
- Dyspareunia
- Onset of symptoms within 1 week of menses
- Increased or irregular menstrual flow
- Increased menstrual cramps
- A sexual partner with recent urethritis

Women with PID may also complain of fever, chills, nausea, vomiting, diarrhea, or constipation. The severity of the patient's presentation does not correlate with the severity of the pelvic infection. In fact, subclinical infection accounts for the majority of cases of PID.

The diagnosis of PID is generally made on the basis of nonspecific clinical criteria. Physical examination should include vital signs, abdominal examination, and pelvic examination with visualization and a bimanual examination. Adnexal tenderness, if present, may be unilateral or bilateral. Wet preparations and pH of vaginal secretions and specimens to test for *N. gonorrhoeae* and *C. trachomatis* should be obtained. In most cases of PID, mucopurulent cervical discharge or white blood cells (WBCs) on a saline preparation of vaginal fluid is present. A pregnancy test is essential. Urinalysis, a complete blood count with WBC differential, and erythrocyte sedimentation rate or C-reactive protein level are useful in specifying the diagnosis. However, it is important to note that all tests can be normal in a woman with PID.

Recognizing that many episodes of PID go undiagnosed, the Centers for Disease Control and Prevention (CDC) has recommended new, less stringent criteria for the diagnosis of PID (Table 1). While these new guidelines increase the sensitivity of clinical diagnosis,

TABLE 1 2002 CDC Criteria for the Diagnosis of Pelvic Inflammatory Disease (PID)

Minimum Criteria

Empiric treatment of PID should be initiated in sexually active at-risk women if at least one of the following criteria are met and no other cause(s) for the illness can be identified:

- Uterine/adnexal tenderness *or*
- Cervical motion tenderness

Additional Criteria

These criteria may be used to enhance the specificity of the minimum criteria, but are not required to diagnose PID:

- Oral temperature >101°F (>38.3°C)
- Abnormal cervical or vaginal mucopurulent discharge
- White blood cells on saline microscopy of vaginal secretions
- Elevated erythrocyte sedimentation rate
- Elevated C-reactive protein
- Laboratory documentation of cervical infection with *Neisseria gonorrhoeae* or *Chlamydia trachomatis*

Definitive Criteria

- Endometrial biopsy with histopathologic evidence of endometritis
- Transvaginal sonography or magnetic resonance imaging techniques showing thickened, fluid-filled tubes with or without free pelvic fluid or tuboovarian complex
- Laparoscopic abnormalities consistent with PID

specificity is reduced and clinicians must be sure to consider exhaustive differential diagnoses, including other gynecologic, gastrointestinal, urinary tract, orthopedic, rheumatologic/autoimmune, and psychiatric disorders. Clinicians must balance the consequences of misdiagnosing PID (e.g., cost, risk of missing other diagnoses, unnecessary exposure to antibiotics, stigma, bias toward diagnosing PID again) with the consequences of missing the diagnosis of PID and exposing the patient to undue risk of the serious complications and sequelae associated with PID.

Ultrasonography may be useful if:

- The clinician cannot adequately assess adnexae on examination
- An adnexal mass or fullness is palpated
- There is otherwise suspicion for an ovarian cyst, ectopic pregnancy, or TOA

However, a normal ultrasonographic examination does not eliminate the diagnosis of PID. Laparoscopy may be indicated if the diagnosis is very uncertain or if the patient does not respond to appropriate treatment for PID.

Hospitalization and parenteral therapy is not superior to outpatient management with oral and intramuscular therapy. A woman with suspected PID should be hospitalized if:

- A surgical emergency cannot be excluded.
- She is pregnant.
- She has severe illness, nausea/vomiting, high fever.
- She cannot follow or tolerate an outpatient treatment regimen.
- Oral therapy has been attempted and failed to produce clinical improvement.
- TOA is present.

In addition, hospitalization may be considered for women who are less than 15 to 17 years of age, have had a gynecologic surgical procedure within the previous 14 days, have had a previous episode of PID, or have other extenuating medical or social circumstances. If a woman is to be treated as an outpatient, the clinician should assess her ability to fill prescriptions, abstain from sexual intercourse, notify her partner(s) of the need for treatment, abstain from use of illicit substances and other risk behaviors, and maintain personal safety. The patient's living situation, financial situation, and medical insurance status should also be assessed.

The recommended parenteral and oral treatment regimens are presented in Table 2. With the oral regimens, some experts recommend the inclusion of metronidazole for better coverage of anaerobic organisms, although compliance may be reduced and there is the potential for more side effects. Metronidazole should be included in the treatment regimen if bacterial vaginosis is also diagnosed.

If the patient is treated as an outpatient, she should be reassessed in 48 to 72 hours; hospitalization should be considered if there is no clinical improvement or if she is not able to tolerate/follow the outpatient regimen. Regardless of the regimen used, if there is not substantial clinical improvement within 72 hours, the clinician should reconsider the diagnosis and evaluate for complications. Patients need to complete the full course of treatment regardless of their STD test results. HIV testing and counseling should be recommended and hepatitis B vaccination status determined. All sexual partners from at least the previous 60 days need to be treated for both *N. gonorrhoeae* and *C. trachomatis*, regardless of their symptoms or test results. The patient should be rescreened for reinfection in 3 to 4 months.

The complications of PID include Fitz-Hugh-Curtis perihepatitis and TOA. The patient with perihepatitis may have left upper quadrant abdominal pain or back pain, leukocytosis, an elevated erythrocyte sedimentation rate that is out of proportion with the severity of their presentation, and increased liver transaminases. The management of patients with PID and perihepatitis is no different from that

TABLE 2 Parenteral and Oral Treatment Regimens for Pelvic Inflammatory Disease (PID)

Parenteral Regimens
REGIMEN A
Cefoxitin (Mefoxin), 2 g IV q6h
or
Cefotetan (Cefotan), 2 g IV q12h
plus
Doxycycline (Vibramycin), 100 mg IV or PO q12h
REGIMEN B
Clindamycin (Cleocin) 900 mg IV q8h
plus
Gentamicin loading dose 2 mg/kg then 1.5 mg/kg IV or IM q8h (single daily dosing may be substituted)
Patients should be treated parenterally for at least 24h after demonstrating clinical improvement, then discharged to home on doxycycline, 100 mg PO bid, to complete 14 days of antibiotic treatment. If the patient is pregnant, erythromycin, 500 mg PO qid for 14 days should be given instead of doxycycline.
Oral Regimens
REGIMEN A
Ofloxacin (Floxin), 400 mg PO bid × 14 days
or
Levofloxacin (Levaquin), 500 mg PO qd × 14 days
with or without
Metronidazole (Flagyl), 500 mg PO bid × 14 days
REGIMEN B
Ceftriaxone (Rocephin), 250 mg IM in a single dose
or
Cefoxitin (Mefoxin), 2 g IM in a single dose, and probenecid, 1 g PO administered concurrently in a single dose
or
Another third-generation cephalosporin
plus
Doxycycline 100 mg PO bid × 14 days
with or without
Metronidazole, 500 mg PO bid × 14 days

Abbreviations: bid = twice daily; IM = intramuscular; IV = intravenous; PO = orally; q = every; qd = every day; qid = four times per day.

of PID alone. TOA requires prolonged parenteral therapy and if it ruptures, it is a surgical emergency. Women who have had PID have an increased risk of ectopic pregnancy, infertility, chronic pelvic pain, dyspareunia, pelvic adhesions, and recurrent PID.

Primary and secondary prevention efforts are essential to reducing the burden of PID. Routine STD screening lowers the incidence of PID, and prompt recognition and treatment of PID decreases the risk of sequelae.

UTERINE LEIOMYOMA

METHOD OF

Dylan R. Wells, MD, and

Frank W. Ling, MD

Leiomyoma are benign tumors that arise from smooth muscle cells. Commonly referred to as *myomas* or *fibroids*, they constitute the most common class of female pelvic neoplasms. They are present in approximately 30% to 35% of females of reproductive age, with a propensity for African American women versus white women in a 2:1 ratio.

These tumors are generally firm and well circumscribed, being composed of interdigitating smooth muscle cells separated by fibrous connective tissue. Primarily arising from the uterine corpus, myomas may also originate from the uterine cervix, ovaries, and oviducts, or from the various ligamentous attachments to the uterus. At the uterine corpus, they occur in one of three primary locations:

1. Submucosal—projecting into the uterine cavity
2. Intramural—arising or contained within the myometrium
3. Subserosal—projecting into the pelvis or abdominal cavity

Furthermore, subserosal fibroids may outgrow their blood supply and detach from the uterine serosa, implanting on adjacent tissues in a parasitic fashion. Such unfortunate secondary locations may include portions of the upper or lower gastrointestinal (GI) or urinary tracts, or the peritoneum overlying major vascular structures.

Although the majority of women with myomas are asymptomatic, up to 40% will ultimately present with common symptoms of abnormal uterine bleeding, reproductive disturbance, or pelvic pain and pressure-related complaints.

Etiology and Pathophysiology

Individual myomas arise from a single progenitor myocyte. The proposed theory of myoma formation is that of excessive cell growth and replication following genetic mutation. Deletions and translocations involving chromosomes 7, 12, and 14 within the smooth muscle cell result in clonal expansion. Under the influence of estrogen, progesterone, and localized growth factors, the myoma enlarges into a clinical entity.

Approximately 75% of patients with fibroids present with multiple tumors. They range in size from a few millimeters to large, multinodular lesions occupying the balance of the abdominal cavity. They may hemorrhage, ulcerate, or undergo various forms of histologic breakdown, including hyaline, calcific, fatty, myxomatous, edematous, or carneous (infarcted or red) degeneration. Rarely, malignant transformation into or de novo formation of a leiomyosarcoma may occur. Overall incidence ranges from 0.2% to 0.7%, with the classic presentation being that of a rapidly expanding myoma or growth of a myoma during the postmenopausal period.

The question as to why some women form fibroids while others do not remains to be completely answered. Similarly, why some women with small fibroid tumors become symptomatic while others with much larger tumors deny complaints is also a matter of some debate.

Symptomatology

Symptomatic uterine leiomyoma are the primary indication for 33.3% to 50% of hysterectomies performed each year in the United States. Potential symptoms include heavy, prolonged vaginal bleeding (menorrhagia and hypermenorrhea, respectively) and intermenstrual spotting (metrorrhagia). The resultant expansion of intracavitary surface area due to myoma growth can alter contraction of the endometrial vessels during menses. Often a complication of submucosal fibroids, larger intramural myomas may also induce unpredictable or excessive bleeding. In addition, passive congestion, necrosis, and ulceration of the endometrium overlying the myoma can cause intermenstrual bleeding and dysmenorrhea (excessively painful menstruation).

Pelvic pain and pressure-related symptoms involving surrounding organs are also common. Urinary frequency or discomfort, constipation, dyspareunia (painful intercourse), and ureteral compression have all been discovered concurrently with pelvic myomas. Patients with degeneration or torsion of a myoma can present with fever, leukocytosis, and acute abdominal pain, particularly in the pregnant patient.

Other pregnancy complications may occur such as preterm labor, abnormal formation or placement of the placenta, abnormal fetal lie, and postpartum hemorrhage. Patients may also suffer from recurrent pregnancy loss as a result of large or strategically located submucosal or intramural fibroids. Conversely, the infertile woman may present with occlusion or altered motility of the fallopian tubes.

Myomas generally regress in size and symptomatology following menopause with the decline of circulating steroid hormone levels.

Diagnosis

The patient presenting with a pelvic mass poses a significant diagnostic challenge to the primary care physician and gynecologist alike. Other particularly worrisome etiologies include cervical, tubal, and ovarian malignancy, in addition to a number of GI and lower urinary tract lesions. Nonetheless, a timely and accurate diagnosis and plan of care is essential in both the outpatient and acute care settings.

The diagnosis of uterine leiomyoma is best made by performing a thorough history and physical examination. An enlarged, irregular uterus on rectovaginal or bimanual examination is the standard presentation. Generally firm and nontender, the fibroid uterus will vary in its mobility within the pelvis depending on its overall volume as well as on the size and location of individual myomas. A smooth, mobile, and somewhat tender uterus calls the additional diagnoses of intrauterine gestation and adenomyosis into question. Screening for pregnancy is simple enough in most settings. Adenomyosis describes the growth of endometrial glands into the uterine myometrium, potentially causing significant dysmenorrhea and heavy, but regular uterine bleeding.

Pelvic imaging using various methodologies confirms the diagnosis of leiomyoma. Transvaginal ultrasonography is relatively inexpensive; is reliable in diagnosing the size, location, and number of uterine fibroids; and thus should be considered the initial imaging technique of choice. The addition of saline-infusion sonography has improved the detection of submucosal fibroids and endometrial polyps.

Computed tomography (CT) often identifies myomas incidentally on a pelvic study, and magnetic resonance imaging (MRI) is particularly useful in aiding the diagnosis of adenomyosis with or without the presence of fibroids. Hysterosalpingography employs serial radiograph technology with dye instillation, providing information not only on uterine filling defects, but also on tubal patency. Although somewhat uncomfortable, this method holds particular weight in both the workup and treatment of the infertility patient. Office hysteroscopy allows for precise medical and surgical planning based on outpatient visualization of submucosal fibroids.

Laboratory testing that may aid management includes a hemoglobin level, with platelet count and coagulation studies obtainable from the patient with a prolonged history of abnormal bleeding. Office endometrial biopsy will assist in excluding concurrent endometrial hyperplasia or malignancy. Ancillary studies such as intravenous pyelography and a barium enema may be obtained when a patient with a pelvic mass presents with the findings of constipation or hydronephrosis, or when the mass is of uncertain origin.

Treatment

The treatment of uterine leiomyoma depends on the severity of symptoms, if any, the response to previous medical or surgical treatments, and the patient's age and desire for future fertility. Treatment options include medical, surgical, radiologic, and genetic modalities.

Expectant management is the treatment of choice in patients with minimal to no symptoms and small myomas (less than an 8- to 10-cm aggregate uterine size). Repeat examinations are recommended at least annually or with initial symptomatic complaint.

Medical therapy is based on the finding that fibroids tend to grow in the presence of estrogen and progestins, and shrink in the presence of androgens. However, low-dose oral contraceptives can be given without significant change in uterine volume. In the patient without contraindications, both the volume of the monthly menses and the incidence of intermenstrual bleeding may be reduced by:

- A monophasic, combined oral contraceptive pill containing 20 to 35 μg of ethinyl estradiol (such as Alesse[1] or Levlen[1]), administered once daily, or
- Cyclic luteal phase progestins, such as medroxyprogesterone acetate (Provera)[1], 5 to 10 mg on cycle days 15 to 25

Combined with a nonsteroidal anti-inflammatory medication on either a scheduled or symptomatic basis for pelvic pain and dysmenorrhea, many patients may avoid further medical or surgical management.

If the above fails, a trial of gonadotropin-releasing hormone (GnRH) agonist therapy may be given in selected cases. In the preoperative state, a 40% to 50% reduction in uterine volume and improvement in pretreatment anemia can be expected after 3 months administration of leuprolide acetate (Lupron Depot), 3.75 mg administered monthly via IM injection, which potentially will facilitate myomectomy or vaginal hysterectomy shortly thereafter. The perimenopausal patient may be bridged into the menopausal state with this treatment, potentially avoiding surgical intervention. *Add-back* medical therapy for the menopausal state induced by GnRH agonists may be necessary with prolonged use. The antiprogestin mifepristone (RU-486)[1] could potentially work to reduce uterine volume, but further clinical studies are required before recommending this.

As alluded to previously, hysterectomy remains the definitive surgical option for symptomatic

[1]Not FDA approved for this indication.

leiomyomas. However, the range of operative management also encompasses several uterine-conserving techniques, either proven or promising.

Laparotomy with myomectomy, as with the other uterine-conserving techniques, is the procedure of choice in the woman who desires to maintain her fertility. Operative goals include minimizing the number and size of uterine incisions, avoiding posterior or cornual incisions (site of tubal implantation), and maintaining the incisions superficial to the endometrial cavity. Risks include excessive blood loss, adhesion formation, and a 2% possibility of conversion to hysterectomy.

Laparoscopic myomectomy is useful for the small- to medium-sized fibroids, which are subserosal or intramural in position. Removal by sharp dissection, endocoagulation, or laser is recommended. Larger fibroids may prove difficult to remove without extensive morcellation; experience with this technique as well as that of laparoscopic suturing for layered closure of the myoma bed or the incidental extension into the endometrial cavity is imperative. Risks include a 15% possibility of conversion to laparotomy and extensive postoperative adhesion formation.

Laparoscopic myolysis and cryolysis employ bipolar endocoagulation or liquid nitrogen probes, respectively, to penetrate the fibroid and cause shrinkage. Risks are similar to laparoscopic myomectomy in addition to the postoperative pain of a degenerating mass that remains in the abdomen.

Hysteroscopic myomectomy is used for submucous myomas with less than 50% intramural extension. Using an electrocautery resectoscope, laser, or myolytic technique, up to 85% of patients experience relief from abnormal bleeding. Risks include uterine perforation and systemic fluid overload.

Vaginal myomectomy is specifically reserved for the prolapsing cervical or lower uterine submucosal myoma. Transection and ligation of the myoma stump, followed by hysteroscopy to evaluate for concurrent lesions, is the suggested course. Importantly enough, 20% to 25% of patients who undergo conservative surgery for uterine fibroids subsequently require further operative management. As an alternative to surgery, much attention has been focused on uterine artery embolization (UAE). Occlusive particles of compounds such as polyvinyl alcohol foam, metal coils, and silicone spheres are injected under fluoroscopic guidance into the uterine arteries in attempts to reduce or eliminate the blood supply to larger fibroids. Symptomatic improvement in 80% to 90% of patients has been seen, although the postoperative pain and potential need for subsequent surgical intervention remain. Other risks include adverse effects on the endometrium and ovarian function. UAE thus remains relatively contraindicated in the patient desirous of future fertility.

Finally, new research in gene therapy holds hope for transferring therapeutic DNA into myoma cells to affect their regression via corrective, immunotherapeutic, or cytotoxic means.

ENDOMETRIAL CANCER

METHOD OF

James J. Burke II, MD, and

Donald G. Gallup, MD

Endometrial cancer is the most common gynecologic cancer in the United States, with an estimated 40,100 new cases reported each year. Although approximately 80% of these cases are diagnosed as stage I disease, 6800 women will succumb to their disease annually.

Endometrial cancer is subdivided into two histologically and clinically separate groups. Type I endometrial cancer is directly related to an increased estrogenous state. This type of endometrial cancer is the most common and is usually found at an earlier stage, and treatment results in a more favorable outcome. Type II endometrial carcinoma is a more virulent type of carcinoma characterized by early metastasis, and it typically has a worse prognosis.

Epidemiology, Clinical Features, and Diagnosis

TYPE I ENDOMETRIAL CARCINOMA

Endometrial carcinoma is a heterogeneous mix of several histologic types with various clinical outcomes. This more common type of endometrial carcinoma represents approximately 90% of all endometrial cancers and is associated with a hyperestrogenic state. Table 1 lists risk factors associated with type I endometrial carcinoma. In the 1970s, it was found that giving estrogen preparations without progestin for hormone replacement therapy led to at least a six times greater chance of endometrial carcinoma developing. Similarly, women who are obese have an increased risk of endometrial carcinoma as a result of peripheral conversion of androstenedione to estrone in peripheral adipose tissue by 5α-reductase enzyme

TABLE 1 Risk Factors for the Development of Endometrial Carcinoma

Risk Factors	RR
Overweight (age 50–59)	
By 20–50 lb	3
By >50 lb	10
Nulliparity vs. multiparity	5
Menopause after age 52	2
Diabetes	3
Unopposed estrogen replacement	6
Combination OCP	0.5

Abbreviations: OCP, oral contraceptive preparation; RR, relative risk.

activity. Finally, women who have untreated atypical endometrial hyperplasia, a well-known precursor to type I endometrial carcinoma, have a 29 times greater chance of endometrial carcinoma developing. Hence, intervention when this precursor is found can prevent endometrial cancer.

Although 90% of women with this type of carcinoma initially have painless, postmenopausal vaginal bleeding or some form of vaginal discharge, most postmenopausal vaginal bleeding is related to conditions other than malignancy. Nonetheless, all postmenopausal bleeding needs further evaluation. The gold standard is endometrial biopsy, usually carried out in the office with minimal patient discomfort. However, should the results of this type of in-office biopsy still be equivocal or performance of the biopsy not be possible because of cervical stenosis, formal fractional dilation and curettage should be performed. Another modality used for assessment of postmenopausal bleeding is transvaginal ultrasound to measure the thickness of the endometrium. Endometrial stripes found to be thicker than 5 mm require endometrial sampling because of the higher likelihood of malignancy.

TYPE II ENDOMETRIAL CARCINOMA

Unlike type I endometrial carcinoma, type II is not related to an increased estrogenic state and encompasses several histologic variants that are quite aggressive. These carcinomas tend to have either serous, papillary serous, or clear cell histology and typically occur in women older than age 70 years. Fortunately, carcinomas of these types account for less than 10% of all endometrial cancers; but unfortunately, they contribute the majority of deaths from endometrial cancer. Because of the aggressive nature of these cancers, most have metastasized before initial evaluation and diagnosis and spread in a fashion similar to ovarian carcinoma.

As with type I endometrial carcinoma, type II carcinomas are commonly manifested as painless, postmenopausal vaginal bleeding or vaginal discharge. However, patients may have no bleeding at all but instead have nonspecific gastrointestinal symptoms such as nausea and vomiting, constipation, early satiety, abdominal bloating, and abdominal pain. All these symptoms point to intra-abdominal metastasis, common with this type of endometrial carcinoma. In these patients, early computed tomography (CT) can aid in the diagnosis. Even when these carcinomas have not spread and are limited to the endometrium or endometrial polyps, the risk of recurrence is high.

Staging and Treatment

STAGING

Recognizing that clinical staging did not take into account pathologic or surgical prognostic information, the Gynecologic Oncology Group (GOG) conducted two large prospective surgical staging trials in the 1980s. In 1988, the Fédération Internationale de Gynécologie et d'Obstétrique (FIGO) adopted the surgical staging of endometrial cancer (Table 2). Surgical staging involves obtaining pelvic washings, extrafascial hysterectomy, bilateral salpingo-oophorectomy, and lymph node sampling from the pelvic and paraaortic regions. In addition, if high-risk histology or gross spread of disease is present at the time of surgery (common with type II endometrial cancers), removal of the omentum is recommended. Table 3 shows the typical stage distribution for endometrial carcinoma.

TABLE 2 FIGO Surgical Staging Classification for Endometrial Carcinoma

Stage IA	Tumor limited to the endometrium
Stage IB	Invasion to less than half the myometrium
Stage IC	Invasion equal to or more than half the myometrium
Stage IIA	Endocervical glandular involvement only
Stage IIB	Cervical stromal invasion
Stage IIIA	Tumor invading the serosa of the corpus uteri and/or adnexa and/or positive cytologic findings
Stage IIIB	Vaginal metastases
Stage IIIC	Metastases to the pelvic and/or paraortic lymph nodes
Stage IVA	Tumor invasion of the bladder and/or bowel mucosa
Stage IVB	Distant metastases, including intra-abdominal metastasis and/or metastasis to the inguinal lymph nodes

Abbreviation: FIGO, Fédération Internationale de Gynécologie et d'Obstétrique.

ADJUVANT THERAPY

Radiotherapy is currently the mainstay of adjuvant therapy for early stage endometrial carcinoma at risk for recurrence. Several trials have examined hormonal therapy or chemotherapy in an adjuvant setting for early stage disease, but none has shown any benefit in reducing recurrences.

Although 75% of endometrial carcinomas are found to be confined to the uterus after surgical staging, some of these patients will be at risk for recurrence and failure with surgical treatment only (Figure 1). Patients found to be at high risk for recurrence are treated with whole-pelvic radiotherapy after surgery, whereas patients who are at "intermediate" risk usually do not need radiotherapy, provided that they have

TABLE 3 Distribution of Endometrial Cancer by Stage

Stage I	72.8%
Stage II	10.9%
Stage III	13.1%
Stage IV	3.2%

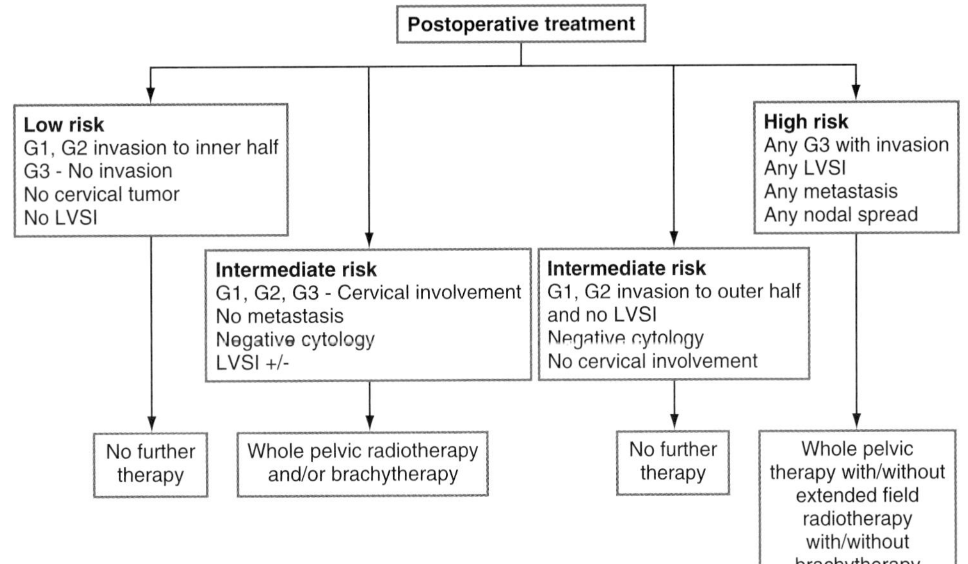

FIGURE 1 Postoperative treatment scheme at Memorial Health University Medical Center for surgical stage I endometrial carcinoma. G, grade; LVSI, lymphovascular space involvement.

been surgically staged. However, any adjuvant therapy for this group of patients remains controversial.

ADVANCED-STAGE OR RECURRENT DISEASE

A study conducted by the GOG showed that 36% of patients who were found to have metastasis to the para-aortic lymph nodes (stage IIIC) and were treated with radiotherapy were tumor free at 5 years. Similarly, if only pelvic lymph node metastasis (stage IIIC) was found and treated with radiotherapy, 72% would be alive at 5 years.

For serous or clear cell carcinomas found to have extrauterine spread at the time of surgery, "debulking" the metastasis and treating with chemotherapeutic regimens used for ovarian cancer have been shown to increase progression-free survival in several case series. Patients with gross intra-abdominal spread of endometrioid carcinoma generally have a grim prognosis and have not been shown to have prolonged survival with radiotherapy or chemotherapy. Therefore, these patients should be offered participation in clinical trials.

In most patients in whom cancer recurs, it will do so within 3 years of initial treatment. Unfortunately, if the recurrence is any place other than the pelvis (vaginal apex), the likelihood of long-term cure is poor. Depending on the location of the recurrence, radiotherapy, surgery, hormonal therapy, or chemotherapy can be used. Progestins have been studied for the treatment of recurrent disease but have demonstrated modest responses of limited duration.

FOLLOW-UP

Of the endometrial carcinomas that recur, most will do so within the first 3 years after treatment. Typically, the site of recurrence is in the pelvis, with the vaginal apex being the most common location. Unfortunately, a number of patients will have recurrence at distant sites, and the chest and upper part of the abdomen are the most common areas. Thus, patients treated for endometrial carcinoma are usually monitored closely for 5 years. At Memorial Health University Medical Center, we use an assessment program in which patients are seen every 3 months for the first year, every 4 months for the second year, and every 6 months until 5 years has elapsed since completion of treatment. In addition, a Papanicolaou (Pap) smear is performed at every visit, and chest radiographs are obtained annually for the first 2 years. Furthermore, annual mammography as well as counseling for screening colonoscopy is carried out. CT scanning is not generally used for surveillance in follow-up because of its high cost and low yield of detection. However, patients with abdominal symptoms may be assessed with CT because the likelihood of finding pathology is greater. For patients with advanced disease or high-risk histologic features, serum measurement of cancer antigen (CA) 125 may be considered. Table 4 shows 5-year survival rates of patients with endometrial carcinoma by stage.

TAMOXIFEN (NOLVADEX)

The National Surgical Adjuvant Breast and Bowel Project (NSABP) conducted a prevention trial with

TABLE 4 Endometrial Cancer: Five-Year Survival Rate by Stage

Stage	5-Year Survival Rate
Stage IA	91%
Stage IB	88%
Stage IC	81%
Stage II	72%
Stage III	51%
Stage IV	9%

tamoxifen, known as the P-1 trial. In this randomized, double-blind, prospective trial, women with high-risk family histories were treated with tamoxifen or placebo for 5 years. The trial demonstrated a 49% reduced risk for breast cancer, but a 2.5 times greater risk for endometrial carcinoma. Most of the endometrial carcinomas detected were stage I carcinomas, were of endometrioid histology (type I endometrial carcinoma), and were successfully treated with surgery. Additionally, other nonmalignant endometrial abnormalities were detected.

In addition to the use of tamoxifen for prevention of breast cancer, many women who have receptor-positive breast carcinomas are using tamoxifen for adjuvant treatment.

The question arises of how one monitors patients taking tamoxifen? The consensus has been to not perform transvaginal ultrasonography or endometrial sampling in women who are asymptomatic. However, women who are taking tamoxifen and experience vaginal bleeding need to have an immediate evaluation by endometrial sampling to rule out endometrial carcinoma.

Although endometrial carcinoma remains the most common gynecologic malignancy in the United States, it is also the most curable because of its low stage at diagnosis. Surgery remains the primary treatment modality for this type of carcinoma, with adjuvant radiotherapy reserved for patients at high risk for recurrent disease after surgery. Chemotherapeutic and hormonal agents have been used to palliate advanced-stage or recurrent disease, but durable, long-term survival has not been demonstrated. Finally, women who are taking tamoxifen for prophylaxis or adjuvant treatment of breast carcinoma need no special surveillance for the development of endometrial carcinoma. However, should any postmenopausal or abnormal vaginal bleeding occur in this group of women, immediate evaluation by endometrial sampling is required.

CANCER OF THE CERVIX

METHOD OF

Larry J. Copeland, MD, and

Alberto Selman, MD

Cervical cancer is a serious health problem, with a worldwide incidence of approximately one-half million new cases annually, second only to breast cancer. Most cases occur in countries where no effective screening is available. Squamous cell carcinoma is the most common malignant cervical tumor, but the incidence of adenocarcinomas has been rising during the past few decades. Cervical cytology (Papanicolaou [Pap] smear) screening has led to an increase in the diagnosis of preinvasive lesions and a resultant decrease in the diagnosis of invasive cancer in developed countries. Risk factors include exposure to human papillomavirus, smoking, and immune-system dysfunction.

Cervical cancer remains a clinically staged malignancy according to the Fédération Internationale de Gynécologie et d'Obstétrique (International Federation of Gynecology and Obstetrics) (FIGO) staging system. Only if the rules for clinical staging are strictly observed is it possible to compare results using different modalities of treatment. Treatment failure is best predicted by early lymph node or distant organ involvement that may be undetectable by standard radiographic methods. Given the importance of lymph node metastasis, many believe that cervical cancer should be surgically staged (surgical and pathologic data are important for precise analysis of survival and prognostic risk factors).

Treatment of invasive cervical cancer is dependent on the extent of disease (stage). Most women with early stage tumors are cured with either radiotherapy or surgery (Table 1). Results of randomized clinical trials show that for women with locally advanced cancers, chemoradiotherapy should be regarded as standard care (Table 2). Treatment of recurrent cervical cancer remains largely ineffective, with single digit extended survival.

Microinvasive Cervical Cancer

Because rates of parametrial and pelvic lymph node involvement are negligible, in general, patients with stage IA-1 can be treated with simple hysterectomy without nodal dissection or, in selected cases, with conization of the cervix. Patients with stage IA-2 disease (risk of up to 5% of developing lymph node metastasis) should undergo radical hysterectomy and pelvic lymphadenectomy.

Early Stage Disease (Stage IB-IIA)

Carcinoma of the cervix may be treated surgically or by radiation therapy. Radiation is suitable for the majority of patients, while surgery is reserved for patients medically fit with small tumors (<4 cm). In this setting, both modalities have equivalent therapeutic efficacy. Treatment choice is, therefore, driven by side effects. In young or older patients, surgery allows true surgical pathologic definition of the extent of disease, shorter treatment time, preservation of healthy ovaries, and maintenance of a pliable, healthy vagina. The advantages of radiation therapy are that it is mostly an outpatient procedure and it is better suited for patients who are poor operative candidates. In patients undergoing radical hysterectomy, 15% to

TABLE 1 Radical Hysterectomy Versus Radiation in Early Stage Cervical Cancer (Stages I-IIA)

	Radical Hysterectomy	Radiation Therapy
Advantages	Possible to preserve ovarian function Improved coital function	Can treat virtually any lesion Avoid surgery in patients who have poor operative risk
Disadvantages	As single modality, applicable only to tumors confined to cervix Some degree of bladder dysfunction occurs in most patients	Vaginal scarring interferes with coital function Greater incidence of delayed complications, often years after treatment
5-Year disease-free survival	90%	85%
Major complications	12%-14%	3%-5%

20% of them require adjuvant whole pelvic radiotherapy and chemotherapy for poor prognostic features such as lymph node involvement, positive surgical margins, deep cervical invasion, and lymph vascular space involvement. Patients treated with both modalities have a higher incidence of short- and long-term morbidity.

Locally Advanced Cervical Carcinoma

Radiation was, until recently, the key and only modality for routine treatment of locally advanced cervical carcinoma (tumor whose size exceeds that which can be treated successfully with surgery alone). A National Cancer Institute Clinical announcement (1999), identified five randomized trials in locally advanced cervical cancer, all demonstrating that concurrent cisplatin-based chemotherapy along with radiation therapy yields better outcomes than radiation therapy alone (see Table 2).

Surgical Staging

Surgical staging for more advanced carcinoma of the cervix prior to definitive radiotherapy remains controversial. Surgical removal of lymph nodes is the most sensitive and specific way to detect lymph node metastasis. The information gained from lymph node dissection can be applied to designing better radiation fields as well as to removing microscopically positive lymph nodes and possibly debulking macroscopically positive lymph nodes. The use of lymphadenectomy for patients with bulky or locally advanced cervical cancer leads to improved survival rates. Originally performed transperitoneally, it carried an unacceptable high morbidity when combined with radiation therapy. However, when approached extraperitoneally the morbidity associated with combined modality is significantly reduced. Whether or not this holds true for the laparoscopic approach remains to be seen.

Fertility-Sparing Surgery

COLD-KNIFE CONIZATION

Fertility-preserving treatment is considered for selected patients with FIGO stage IA1 squamous cell cervical cancer, for whom the rates of parametrial and pelvic lymph node involvement are negligible. The fertility rate is not affected by conization, but the risk of spontaneous second-trimester loss and prematurity are greater. This increased risk appears to be related to the amount of cervical tissue removed by conization.

RADICAL VAGINAL TRACHELECTOMY PRECEDED BY LAPAROSCOPIC PELVIC LYMPHADENECTOMY

This surgical procedure has the advantage of preserving the uterine body, which in turn allows the preservation of childbearing potential.

TABLE 2 Randomized Studies of Concurrent Cisplatin-Based Chemoradiation in Cervical Carcinoma

Author	Drugs	Number	Survival C/RT	Survival RT	P
CRT versus RT					
RTOG 9001	CF	386	73%	58%	0.004
GOG 123	C	369	84%	68%	0.008
SWOG 8797	CF	241	81%	63%	0.01
CRT					
GOG 85	CF versus H	388	50.8% CF	39.8% H	0.018
GOG 120	C versus. H	526	64% C	39% H	0.002
GOG 120	CHF versus H		66% CHF	39% H	0.002

Abbreviations: C = cisplatin (Platinol-AQ); CRT = chemoradiation; F = 5-fluorouracil (5-FU); H = hydroxyurea (Hydrea); GOG = Gynecologic Oncology Group; RT = radiation therapy; RTOG = Radiation Therapy Oncology Group; SWOG = Southwest Oncology Group.

Laparoscopic pelvic lymphadenectomy (LPL) is indicated when the patient desires preservation of fertility, in stage IA1 (with vascular space involvement), IA2 or IB1 (squamous cell carcinoma or adenocarcinoma), when any lesions present are 2 cm or less in diameter, and when there is limited endocervical involvement (determined by magnetic resonance imaging and colposcopy). Radical vaginal trachelectomy (RVT) is feasible when there is no evidence of lymph node metastasis, as determined by frozen section at laparoscopy, and when the upper endocervical margins are free of tumor, as determined by frozen section of the trachelectomy specimen.

Among the group of more than 200 women who have undergone this operation, more than 50 healthy babies have been born so far, the majority by elective cesarean section at term. The preliminary data collected on LPL-RVT make it clear that the subsequent recurrence rate is not higher than the rate observed after radical hysterectomy.

Recurrent Cervical Cancer

Despite advances in early detection, surgical treatment, and radiation therapy, cervical cancer still recurs. Recurrence rates of up to 10% for early tumors and 20% to 40% for more advanced lesions have been reported. Early detection, leading to better prognosis, is not achieved by routine follow-up in the vast majority of patients. Symptoms (87%), and signs (9%) are the most important diagnostic tools to detect recurrent disease (Table 3). Vaginal cytology plays little role in the detection of recurrent disease. Although vaginal cytology has a high specificity, sensitivity is poor.

The prognosis of patients with recurrent cervical cancer after primary therapy is invariably poor regardless the type of initial treatment. Pelvic recurrences are treated with radiation therapy and chemotherapy, if not already given, but patients already irradiated have only chemotherapy or exenteration as options.

CHEMOTHERAPY FOR ADVANCED OR RECURRENT CERVICAL CANCER

Multiple clinical trials have evaluated chemotherapy for cervical cancer, but all have met with poor response rates. The response of recurrent cervical cancer to chemotherapy is poor, and its use should be considered palliative. Cisplatin (Platinol-AQ) has response rates of 20% to 38% in recurrent carcinomas of the cervix; however, median survival is short at 6 months. Combination chemotherapy regimens have been evaluated in recurrent cervical cancer, and response rates of up to 50% have been noted. Nevertheless, no significant difference in overall survival has been shown, and toxicity is greater with combination regimens.

TABLE 3 Signs and Symptoms of Recurrent Cervical Cancer

Chest pain
Cough
Hemoptysis
Leg edema (excessive and often unilateral)
Pelvic and/or thigh-buttock pain
Progressive ureteral obstruction
Supraclavicular lymph node enlargement (usually left side)
Weight loss (unexplained)

INDICATIONS FOR PELVIC EXENTERATION

Pelvic exenteration has been used for central pelvic recurrences. Rarely, young patients with fistulas or purulent tumors but who do not meet the typical criteria undergo exenteration for short-term palliation.

PRIMARY FACTORS AFFECTING MANAGEMENT OPTIONS FOR RECURRENT CARCINOMA OF THE CERVIX

Prior Treatment

Treatment of recurrent cervical cancer is influenced by the nature of the primary therapy. Patients who initially undergo surgery are candidates for radiotherapy and chemotherapy; patients who initially receive radiotherapy should be considered for surgery or chemotherapy, depending on the location of recurrence. Most recurrences occur in patients with advanced-stage disease. Because these patients have been treated with primary pelvic irradiation, they are no longer candidates for this modality if the recurrence is in the pelvis.

After radical hysterectomy, approximately 25% of recurrences occur locally in the upper part of the vagina or the area previously occupied by the cervix. The location of recurrence after radiation therapy showed a 27% occurrence in the cervix, uterus, or upper vagina; 6% in the lower two thirds of the vagina; 43% in the parametrial area, including the pelvic wall, 16% distant; and 8% unknown. Less than 15% of patients with recurrent cervical cancer develop pulmonary metastasis.

Anatomic Involvement

Recurrent cervical cancer may occur in one of three sites. Most commonly, it occurs in the pelvis on the sidewall, presumably in lymph-node-bearing areas. Recurrence may also be seen in distant sites, such as para-aortic or other distal lymph node metastasis, or bony metastasis, most commonly in vertebral bodies. A few patients have a central pelvic recurrence.

Patients with locally recurrent disease after simple or radical hysterectomy should be treated with pelvic radiation, resulting in anticipated survival at 5 years of 22% to 44%. The role of concomitant chemotherapy in these cases has not been defined, but chemotherapy is usually recommended.

Because of constraints involving the radiation tolerance of other pelvic structures, such as the small intestine, bladder, and rectum, re-irradiation is generally not possible in patients with persistent or recurrent cervical cancer after maximal radiation. In these patients, therapy is dependent upon the site and extent of the disease. Patients with distant metastases are essentially incurable and are candidates for palliative chemotherapy only. With the advent of sophisticated methods of radiation therapy, including improved methods of brachytherapy and supervoltage external irradiation therapy, patients with pure central recurrence have become a rarity. For this small subset of patients, exenterative surgery remains the treatment modality that offers the best opportunity for curative potential. In selected cases, the successful completion of a pelvic exenteration is associated with a 5-year survival rate of 20% to 60%. Occasionally, however, there are patients with small central recurrences (≤2 cm in diameter) whose disease could conceivably be cleared by a less extensive procedure such as radical hysterectomy.

An operative technique for the resection of different types of pelvic sidewall recurrences has now been developed, known as laterally extended endopelvic resection (LEER). Exenteration en bloc with the parietal endopelvic fascia and the adjacent pelvic wall muscles leads to clear margins in the majority of cases. In cases of resections with microscopic residual disease, guide tubes for postoperative brachytherapy are implanted on the tumor bed at the pelvic wall. By transposition of nonirradiated autologous tissue from the abdominal wall or from the thigh, a compartmentalization of the tumor bed is achieved. This pelvic wall plasty also provides therapeutic angiogenesis and creates a protective distance of several centimeters to the remaining hollow organs in the pelvis. The complete therapy is known as combined operative radiotherapeutic treatment (CORT). The rate of severe complications is 25%. Local control rates between 80% and 90% and 5-year survival rates between 30% to 40% can be achieved. However, this therapeutic approach remains investigational.

Isolated lung metastases from pelvic malignancies have responded in very selected cases to lobectomy. A surgical attack for isolated pulmonary recurrence should be considered, especially if the latent period has been longer than 3 years.

CONFIRM DIAGNOSIS

In most cases, the diagnosis of recurrent cervical cancer should be confirmed histologically. Despite extensive investigation including computed tomography (CT) scans, CT-guided biopsies, lymphangiogram, examination under anesthesia, and tru-cut biopsies; preoperative confirmation of tumor recurrence and resectability may remain unsettled. Exploratory laparotomy is thus the logical next step, but unfortunately, inoperable disease is frequently discovered then. Indeed, in most series, the reported rate of aborted exenteration varies between 40% and 63%, depending upon extent of the preoperative investigation.

SURGICAL OPTIONS FOR RECURRENT CERVICAL CANCER

The criteria for various surgical options in recurrent cervical cancer are:

- Radical hysterectomy (type 2 or 3)—If limited to cervix, less than 2 cm, original stage IB or IIA
- Pelvic exenteration—If central recurrence not amenable to radical hysterectomy
- Radical surgical resection combined with intraoperative radiation therapy (IORT) (excluding normal tissues from the treatment area)—Patients with locally recurrent cervical cancer after definitive radiotherapy, disease involving the pelvic sidewalls and/or nodal draining areas.
- Laterally extended endopelvic resection (LEER), sacral resections, hemipelvectomy, and CORT (for positive or close margins)—If extending to pelvic sidewall

Future Directions

Primary prevention of cervical cancer through modifying sexual behavior that transmits human papillomavirus (HPV) infection should remain a priority as research in behavioral interventions. Vaccines against portions of the HPV are also under investigation and may offer some opportunity for greater intervention in the area of prevention, an approach that could result in significant decline in mortality in the underdeveloped countries.

Advances in imaging methods and in contrast agents, along with advances in the combined use of the two, are expected to make imaging technologies more valuable in cervical cancer assessment.

The most significant research priorities on invasive cervical cancer are large, group-randomized trials of management strategies for microinvasive disease, development of fertility-sparing procedures, identification of candidates for chemotherapy, and development of innovative approaches to exenteration.

NEOPLASMS OF THE VULVA

METHOD OF

Gary C. Reid, MD

Vulvar neoplasms can be either benign or malignant in nature. The advantage the physician has in evaluating a patient's complaints is that vulvar neoplasms are readily visible on the skin surface and can be easily biopsied to help in the diagnosis. There has been an increase in the frequency of high-grade preinvasive vulvar intraepithelial neoplasia (VIN). Yet, the incidence of invasive vulvar carcinoma remains constant, presumably because of treatment of the preinvasive lesions.

Classification

The current classification of vulvar neoplasms (Table 1) was established in 1989 by the International Society for the Study of Vulvar Disease (ISSVD). It was designed to eliminate confusing previous terminology such as *vulvar dystrophies, vulvar dysplasia, leukoplakia,* or *carcinoma in situ*. The new classification separates the neoplasms with atypia from the nonneoplastic epithelial disorders.

Diagnosis of Vulvar Neoplasms

Symptoms and treatment of each vulvar neoplasm is discussed later, but the general examination and biopsy can be applied to any of the vulvar lesions. When a patient presents with vulvar complaints, the entire vulva including the labia minora, clitoris, vestibule, and anus should be visualized because lesions may be multifocal. Examination of the vagina and anus are important because vulvar neoplasms—in particular lichen sclerosis, VIN, or cancer—can extend to these areas. It is important to determine the full extent of the lesion and clearly inform the patient of the location so that the patient can properly apply any treatment such as creams/ointments. Failure of treatment can easily occur by a patient placing a cream in the incorrect location on the vulva. Depending on the clinical presentation, colposcopy of the vulva should be performed. Five percent acetic acid (vinegar) is applied to the vulva and anus before colposcopic examination. Dysplastic lesions may appear as white lesions with distinct borders and vascular abnormalities such as punctations.

Once the areas are selected for biopsy, the skin is injected with 1% lidocaine (Xylocaine). A Keyes punch biopsy is used to obtain a circumscribed area of the lesion with a depth of approximately 3 mm, and the base is cut with the aid of forceps and iris scissors (Figure 1).

TABLE 1 Classification of Vulvar Disease

Nonneoplastic Epithelial Disorders of Skin and Mucosa
Lichen sclerosis (formerly lichen sclerosis et atrophicus)
Squamous hyperplasia (formerly hyperplastic dystrophy)
Other dermatoses
Mixed Nonneoplastic and Neoplastic Epithelial Disorders
Intraepithelial Neoplasia
SQUAMOUS INTRAEPITHELIAL NEOPLASIA
VIN I (mild dysplasia)
VIN II (moderate dysplasia)
VIN III (severe dysplasia/carcinoma in situ)
NONSQUAMOUS INTRAEPITHELIAL NEOPLASIA
Paget's disease
Tumors of melanocytes, noninvasive
Invasive Tumors

From Committee on Terminology. International Society for Study of Vulvar Disease. Int J Gynecol Pathol 8:83, 1989. Used by permission.

Nonneoplastic Epithelial Disorders

LICHEN SCLEROSIS

Lichen sclerosis of the vulva is usually seen in postmenopausal women, but can occur in younger women. Lichen sclerosis currently is not thought to be a precancerous lesion, but it is common to find lichen sclerosis present in conjunction with vulvar cancer. It is a chronic disease with no known etiology that, in severe cases, can be frustrating or debilitating for the patient. Pruritus is the most common symptom. The affected skin of the vulva appears white and thin like parchment or can have a crinkled appearance. The skin affected can extensively involve the entire vulva and perianal areas. The labia minora frequently appears absent or shortened from agglutination or synechia. In advanced cases, phimosis of the clitoris, narrowing of the vaginal introitus, and skin fissures occur. All of these changes can result in dyspareunia and decreased frequency of intercourse. The microscopic appearance is epithelial thinning with the hallmark of flattened rete pegs. Approximately 30% of women with lichen sclerosis also have concomitant squamous cell hyperplasia mixed elsewhere on the vulva. Currently, high-potency steroids such as clobetasol propionate (Temovate)[1], 0.05%, is the treatment of choice with a 75% response rate, versus a 20% response rate for testosterone cream[1,*]. Clobetasol can be applied to the vulva twice daily for

[1]Not FDA approved for this indication.
*May be compounded by pharmacists.

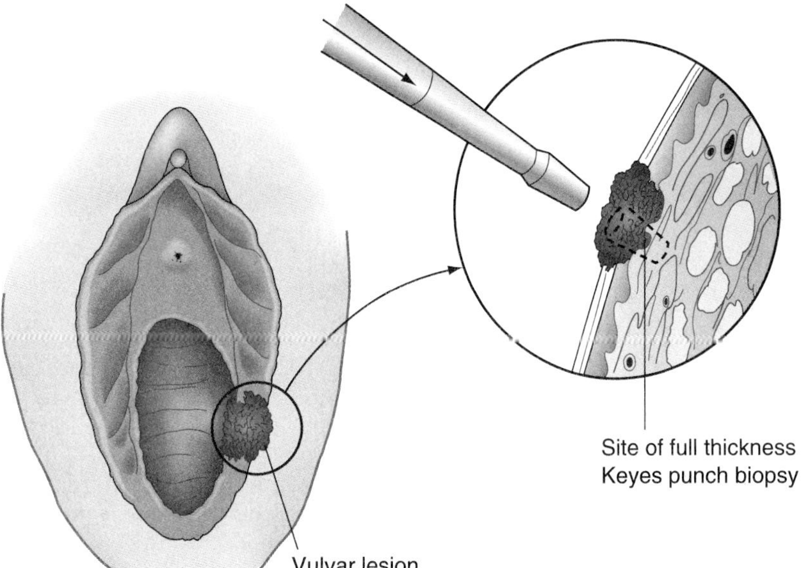

FIGURE 1 The Keyes punch biopsy is performed to ensure full thickness through the vulvar lesion to allow measurement of tumor thickness or invasion.
(Adapted from Reid GC: Surgical aspects of vulvar melanoma, in Gershenson DM (Ed.): Operative Techniques in Gynecologic Surgery, vol 4, no. 3. Phildelphia, WB Saunders, 1998, p 23. Used with permission.)

8 to 10 weeks, after which a maintenance dose is applied 1 to 4 times per month. If symptoms stop, treatment can then be discontinued. However, lichen sclerosis is a chronic disease that frequently needs maintenance steroids to control symptoms. The appearance of the vulva rarely returns to normal and the goal of therapy is to prevent symptoms and progression of the disease.

SQUAMOUS CELL HYPERPLASIA

Squamous cell hyperplasia (SCH) can occur in premenopausal and postmenopausal women, and the etiology is unknown. Like lichen sclerosis, pruritus is common. SCH can affect all areas of the vulva, but is frequently more localized and better defined than lichen sclerosis. The vulva can have a white or dusky red appearance. Biopsy is important to differentiate from lichen sclerosis or even carcinoma.

Treatment is topical steroids. Fluorinated steroids such as desoximetasone (Topicort)[1], 0.25% twice daily for 1 month, help control symptoms of pruritus. Treatment can be stopped if symptoms resolve and the vulva appears normal. Intermittent maintenance use is frequently needed to keep the symptoms under control. Because of the potential risk of atrophy from prolonged steroid use, the fluorinated steroids can be replaced with hydrocortisone cream (Hytone) that is used two times per week as maintenance.

Intraepithelial Neoplasia of the Vulva

VULVAR INTRAEPITHELIAL NEOPLASIA

The incidence of VIN has doubled in the last 2 decades, but the incidence of invasive vulvar cancer has remained stable. Human papillomavirus (HPV) is associated with VIN, particularly types 16 and 18. Yet it has not been conclusively established that VIN lesions progress to invasive lesions.

[1]Not FDA approved for this indication.

More than 30% of women with VIN present with symptoms of pruritus, burning, or pain. A past history of condyloma is common. The lesions are frequently multifocal but can be a single, isolated lesion. VIN most often is white, but dark- or pigmented-appearing lesions also occur. Colposcopic examination with biopsy is the key to accurate diagnosis and to determine disease extent.

Treatment

Surgical treatment with CO_2 laser or local excision are mainstays of treatment. If the VIN lesion is a single, small lesion, a wide local excision may be preferred, because further histologic assessment can be done and primary suture closure gives a shorter healing time than CO_2 laser.

Currently, CO_2 laser for diffuse or multifocal lesions has replaced skinning vulvectomy, because the normal vulvar anatomy can be preserved. CO_2 laser has the advantage over surgical excision with less scarring and good cosmetic results, but has the disadvantage of prolonged healing and postoperative discomfort. Postoperatively, 1% silver sulfadiazine (Silvadene)[1] cream is applied frequently along with analgesics for patient comfort. In a prospective, randomized study on the use of interferon-alfa 2 (Intron A)[1], 1 million units injected subcutaneously (in the thigh) three times per week for 8 to 12 weeks postoperatively significantly reduced the recurrence of VIN.

CONDYLOMA

Condyloma acuminata is sometimes considered to be a variant of VIN I. Its treatment options are more

[1]Not FDA approved for this indication.

TABLE 2 Condyloma Treatment Options

Type	Method	Dose
Cytotoxic agent	Podophyllin (Podocon-25)	1 time weekly
Acid	Trichloroacetic acid (Tri-Chlor 80%)	1 time weekly
Immune response modifier	Imiquimod cream (Aldara)	3 times per week until clear, maximum 16 weeks
Antimitotic drug	Podofilox (Condylox)	Twice daily for 3 consecutive days each week, maximum 4 treatments
Surgical	CO_2 laser	

numerous than treatments available for VIN II and VIN III (Table 2). CO_2 laser may be avoided with the use of imiquimod (Aldara), or podofilox (Condylox). Both imiquimod (Aldara) and podofilox (Condylox) have the potential side effects of skin irritation, burning, and tenderness, which may limit treatment in some women. In the advanced or resistant condyloma, CO_2 laser may be the best treatment method. The treatment decided upon depends on the location and extent of the condyloma, along with the patient's wishes.

PAGET'S DISEASE

Paget's disease is characterized by the presence of Paget's cell, usually located within the epithelium. The lesions appear red and eczematoid and are frequently misdiagnosed as eczema. Approximately 15% of women with vulvar Paget's disease have an underlying adenocarcinoma. Because of this, wide local excision is the treatment of choice because it allows further histologic evaluation for the entire lesion. Paget's disease frequently extends beyond the visible lesion margins. Thus, in surgery it is recommended to obtain a frozen section for analysis of the peripheral margins to ensure complete resection.

Invasive Carcinoma of the Vulva

Cancers of the vulva may include squamous cell, adenocarcinoma, melanoma, sarcoma, and Bartholin gland carcinomas. Ninety percent of vulvar cancers are squamous in origin and most commonly occur in the elderly (60 to 80 years of age).

The etiology of squamous cell vulvar cancer is uncertain, but there is a strong association with HPV (Table 3). HPV has been isolated in invasive cancer (50%) and carcinoma in situ (80%), with the most common HPV being type 16. An association between vulvar condyloma and the later occurrence of vulvar cancer has been demonstrated, along with an increased relative risk with smoking (Table 4). However, currently there is no definite cause-and-effect relationship between HPV and vulvar cancer, as compared to HPV causing cervical cancer.

The majority of patients present with vulvar pruritus, mass, or pain. Although vulvar cancer is easily visible, unfortunately it is often not diagnosed until it has reached advanced stages, either because of patient delay in seeking medical help or because of physician delay by using inappropriate ointments for months before a biopsy is performed.

TABLE 3 Vulvar Cancer Etiology

Not Related	Associated With
Hypertension	Human papillomavirus (HPV)
Diabetes	Smoking
Obesity	
Lichen sclerosis	
Granulomatous infections	
Herpes simplex	
Syphilis	

DIAGNOSIS AND SPREAD PATTERN

Biopsy must be done of any suspicious vulvar lesion whether it is exophytic, ulcerative, white, red, or pigmented. Vulvar cancer occurs most frequently on the labia majora, but it can involve or originate anywhere on the vulva. Usually the borders of the cancer are distinct and its size and involvement of urethra, vagina, and anus need to be assessed for staging (Table 5) and treatment planning.

The lymphatic drainage of the vulva goes to the inguinal lymph nodes (Figure 2). The superficial inguinal lymph nodes located above the cribriform fascia are probably the initial nodal group involved. The deep nodes located below the fascia, including Cloquet's node, are the last of the inguinal nodes to

TABLE 4 Vulvar Cancer Relative Risk

	Vulvar Cancer	
	In Situ	Invasive
History of Condyloma		
No	1.0	1.0
Yes	18.50	14.55
Smoking Status		
Nonsmoker	1.0	1.0
Current smoker	4.65	1.19
Former smoker	1.78	.40

Data from Briton LA, Nasca PC, Mullin K, et al: Case-control study of cancer of the vulva. J Obstet Gynecol 75:859, 1990. Used by permission.

TABLE 5 Vulvar Staging

FIGO Stage	TNM	Clinical/Pathologic
Stage 0	Tis	Carcinoma in situ
Stage I	T1N0M0	≤2 cm, no nodal metastasis
IA	T1aN0M0	≤2 cm, ≤1.0 mm invasion, no nodal metastasis
IB	T1bN0M0	≤2 cm, >1.0 mm invasion, no nodal metastasis
Stage II	T2N0M0	>2 cm, no nodal metastasis
Stage III	T3N0M0	Tumor any size with either:
	T3N1M0	1. Unilateral groin node metastasis
	T1N1M0	2. Tumor spread to lower urethra, vagina, or anus
	T2N1M0	
Stage IV	T1N0M0	Tumor invades any of the following:
	T2N2M0	1. Upper urethra, bladder mucosa, rectal mucosa, pelvic bone
	T3N2M0	2. Bilateral groin node metastasis
	T4, any N, M	
Stage IVb	Any T, N, M	Any distant metastasis including pelvic nodes

Abbreviations: FIGO = International Federation of Gynecology and Obstetrics; is = in situ; TNM = tumor, node, metastasis.

be involved before spread to the pelvic nodes. If the lesion is on one side of the vulva, spread is to the ipsilateral inguinal nodes, and involvement of the contralateral nodes is unusual.

LYMPH NODE RISK FACTOR AND LYMPHEDEMA

The incidence of lymph node metastasis is related to tumor size, tumor thickness, depth of invasion, grade, and lymph vascular space involvement (Tables 6 and 7). Generally, the risk of lymph node metastasis increases in conjunction with increasing size and depth of the tumor. As expected, survival decreases with nodal involvement (Table 8). The accurate assessment of inguinal lymph node involvement is critical in vulvar cancer survival, because if patients develop recurrence in the groin nodes it is nearly always fatal.

Although inguinal lymph node dissection is important in treatment, it can result in lymphedema of the lower extremity (up to 30% to 40% of cases). This is a frustrating problem for patients. Support hose, low-dose prophylactic antibiotics to prevent lymphangitis, and use of pneumatic hose can improve symptoms. To prevent lymphedema, inguinal sentinel node biopsy is being evaluated by the Gynecologic Oncology Group (GOG) to determine if inguinal lymphadenectomy can be avoided. As in breast cancer, the concept of the sentinel node is that it represents the first lymph node where metastatic spread to regional inguinal lymph nodes would occur. If the sentinel node is negative, it is thought the remaining nodes would be negative and can be left in place. Preliminary data with both isosulfan blue dye intraoperatively and radioisotope injection (technetium-99) indicates that inguinal sentinel nodes can be identified. If the current GOG studies confirm the feasibility of inguinal sentinel node biopsy for vulvar cancer, the morbidity of inguinal lymphadenectomy hopefully can be markedly reduced.

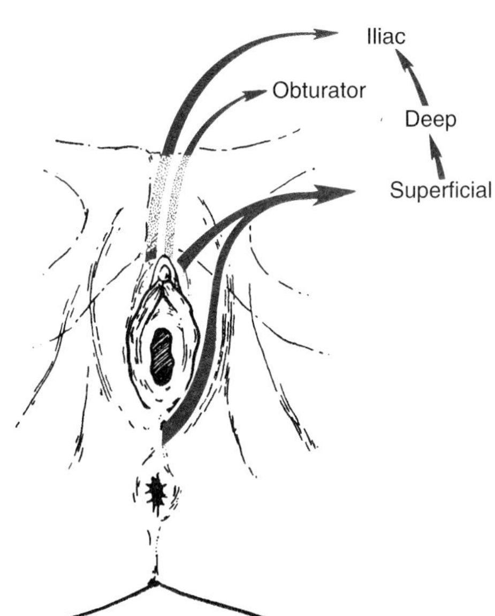

FIGURE 2 Lymphatic spread of vulvar malignancy.
(Adapted from DiSaia PJ, Creasman WT (Eds.): Clinical Gynecologic Oncology, 6th ed. St. Louis, Mosby, 2002, p 16. Used with permission.)

TABLE 6 Groin Node Metastasis Related to Tumor Diameter

Tumor Diameter (cm)	Positive Groin Nodes (%)
<1.0	18.0
1.1-2.0	19.4
2.1-3.0	31.4
3.1-4.0	54.3
4.1-5.0	39.6
>5.0	51.8
Total	34.2

Data from Homesly HD, Bundy BN, Sedlis A, et al: Prognostic factors for groin node metastasis in squamous cell carcinoma of the vulva (a Gynecologic Oncology Group Study). Gynecol Oncol 49:279, 1993. Used with permission.

TABLE 7 Groin Node Metastasis Related to Tumor Thickness (Invasion)

Tumor Thickness (mm)	Positive Groin Nodes (%)
≤1 mm	2.6
2	8.9
3	18.6
4	30.9
5	33.3
>5	47.9
Total	34.4

Data from: Homesly HD, Bundy BN, Sedlis A, et al: Prognostic factors for groin node metastasis in squamous cell carcinoma of the vulva (a Gynecologic Oncology Group Study). Gynecol Oncol 49:279, 1993. Used with permission.

Treatment

MICROINVASIVE VULVAR CANCER

Microinvasive vulvar cancer is defined as invasion of 1 mm or less, with lesions less than 2 cm in size, and no lymphvascular space involvement. The risk of lymph node metastasis is minimal. Treatment is wide local excision with a 2-cm margin, and lymph node dissection is not needed. The patient is spared the risk of lymphedema.

Stage I and Stage II Vulvar Cancers

Treatment of early vulvar cancers is radical vulvectomy and inguinal lymphadenectomy. If the lesion is on one side of the vulva, a hemivulvectomy and ipsilateral lymphadenectomy are performed. The goal of surgical therapy is to remove the cancer entirely, assess for lymph node spread, and spare as much vulvar anatomy as possible without undermining survival. This approach reduces morbidity and helps with psychosexual recovery. However, if the cancer involves the midline structures such as the clitoris, then radial bilateral vulvectomy and bilateral inguinal lymphadenectomy are indicated.

TABLE 8 Vulvar Cancer Survival Related to Nodal Status

No. Positive Nodes	Relative 5-Year Survival
0	90.9%
1-2	75.2%
3-4	36.1%
5-6	24.0%
<7	0%
Laterally	
Unilateral positive	70.7%
Bilateral positive	25.4%

Data from Homesley HD, Bundy BN, Sedlis A, et al: Assessment of current International Federation of Gynecology and Obstetrics staging of vulvar carcinoma relative to prognostic factors for survival (a Gynecologic Oncology Group Study). Am J Obstet Gynecol 164:997, 1991. Used with permission.

Stage III and Stage IV Vulvar Cancers

Advanced-stage vulvar cancers present special problems for the patient and gynecologic oncologist. When tumor involves the lower urethra or vagina, these areas can frequently be included in the radical vulvectomy resection. But involvement of the anus, upper urethra, sphincter, bladder, or rectal mucosa require exenteration with vulvectomy and associated ileostomy or colostomy. Recently these advanced vulvar cancers have been treated with chemoradiation. Initially a bilateral inguinal lymphadenectomy is performed to assess node status. Then treatment of the advanced vulvar cancer with concomitant radiation and cisplatin (Platinol-AQ)[1], 40 mg/m^2 weekly, is administered. After radiation if any residual cancer is present, it frequently has regressed in size away from the anus or bladder and these structures can be spared in postradiation resection.

Lymph Node Involvement

If lymph nodes are positive, postoperative radiation to the groin and hemipelvis will improve survival rates, especially if more than one node is involved. Of patients with positive groin nodes, the GOG demonstrated in a randomized study that postoperative groin radiation has a better 2-year survival rate (68%) versus pelvic node dissection (54%). Currently radiotherapy is given after lymphadenectomy with positive nodes if there is more than one micrometastasis (<5 mm), one macrometastasis, or extra capsular lymph node spread. The drawback of combining inguinal lymphadenectomy with postoperative radiotherapy is increased incidence of lymphedema.

Survival

Table 9 gives the 5-year survival rates for vulvar cancer based on stage. Lymph node involvement is a very important prognostic indicator of survival in vulvar cancer. If lymph nodes are negative, the 5-year survival rate is 90% regardless of stage, but if lymph nodes are positive, survival decreases to 57%. The number and locations of lymph nodes

[1]Not FDA approved for this indication.

TABLE 9 Vulvar Cancer 5-Year Survival Rates

Stage	Percentage
Stage I	98%
Stage II	85%
Stage III	74%
Stage IV	31%

Data from Homesley HD, Bundy BN, Sedlis A, et al: Assessment of current International Federation of Gynecology and Obstetrics staging of vulvar carcinoma relative to prognostic factors for survival (a Gynecologic Oncology Group Study). Am J Obstet Gynecol 164:997, 1991. Used with permission.

TABLE 10 Staging Systems for Vulvar Melanomas

Level	Clark	Breslow	Chung
I	Intraepithelial	<0.76 mm	Intraepithelial
II	Into the papillary dermis	0.76-1.50 mm	<1 mm superficial penetration
III	Filling the dermal papillae	1.51-2.25 mm	1-2 mm into subepithelial tissue
IV	Into the reticular dermis	2.26-3.0 mm	Penetration >2 mm
V	Into the subcutaneous fat	>3 mm	Into subcutaneous fat

are also important, because patients with one microscopically positive lymph node have a good prognosis; but if 3 or more lymph nodes are involved, prognosis is poor (see Table 8). Also, prognosis is poor if tumor breaks through the capsule of the lymph node. If pelvic nodes are involved, survival is very poor at 11%.

Verrucous Carcinoma

Verrucous carcinoma is an indolent, warty, cauliflower-like cancer. It may mimic condyloma acuminatum. It has a pushing border that is locally destructive but rarely metastasizes. This latter characteristic is important in the treatment, because a radical local excision without lymph node dissection is the usual treatment. Radiation therapy is contraindicated for verrucous carcinoma because it can result in more rapid and aggressive growth.

Basal Cell Carcinoma

Basal cell carcinoma behaves much like basal cell carcinoma elsewhere on the body. It is usually well circumscribed, less than 2 cm, and appears on the labia majora. It rarely metastasizes, and wide local excision is the treatment of choice.

Melanoma

Vulvar melanoma is rare, but is the second most common type of vulvar malignancy. Melanoma may arise from a preexisting pigmented nevus. Thus, it is suggested that any pigmented lesion on the vulva be biopsied or excised. The types are superficial spreading, lentigo maligna, and nodular, with the latter being the most aggressive, frequently metastasizing. Many patients have no symptoms, but a few may have pruritus or bleeding. The lesions may be raised, ulcerated, and some are nonpigmented.

Staging for vulva melanoma is related to the depth of invasion as with melanomas elsewhere (Table 10). Treatment is surgical in nature, but the scope of the surgery is somewhat controversial. Most authors agree that if invasion is superficial (level I or II) that wide local excision without lymphadenectomy is adequate treatment. If invasion is deeper, then lymphadenectomy is frequently performed because of increasing risk of metastasis. Survival is related to depth of invasion. The Mayo Clinic reports 10-year survival rates for Clark levels as follows:

- I = 100%
- II = 100%
- III = 83%
- IV = 65%
- V = 23%

Nodular melanoma has a decreased 5-year survival compared to superficial spreading of 35% versus 71%, respectively. Using the Breslow method, other authors report approximately:

- 100% survival for lesions less than 1.5 mm
- 65% to 70% survival for lesions of 1.5 to 4 mm
- 25% to 35% survival for deep lesions more than 4 mm

Other Vulvar Malignancies

Other, more rare cancers of the vulva include Bartholin's gland cancer, adenocarcinomas, adenosquamous carcinomas, and sarcomas. Treatment for most is radical surgical resection with inguinal lymph node dissection.

CONTRACEPTION

METHOD OF

Heather Paladine, MD, and

M. Patrice Eiff, MD

Knowledge of contraception is essential for any health care provider who sees women and men of reproductive age. There are more than 3 million unintended pregnancies in the United States per year and approximately 50% of these are caused by contraceptive failures. Recent developments in contraception have made many new options available, which allows the contraceptive method to be tailored to individual patient's needs and preferences, which should improve efficacy (Table 1).

TABLE 1 Contraceptive Failure Rates (Percentage of Users Who Become Pregnant in 1 Year of Use)

Contraceptive	Actual Use	Ideal Use
No method	85%	85%
Natural family planning/ fertility awareness	25%	1-3%
Male condom	15%	2%
Female condom	21%	5%
Diaphragm	16%	6%
Cervical cap		
Parous women	32%	6%
Nulliparous women	26%	6%
Spermicide only	29%	15%
Combination hormone oral contraceptives	8%	0.3%
Ethinyl estradiol/ norelgestromin patch (Ortho Evra)	N/A	0.3%-0.8%
Ethinyl estradiol/etonogestrel ring (NuvaRing)	N/A	0.6%
Progestin-only oral contraceptives (Micronor)	8%	0.3%
DMPA injection (Depo-Provera)	3%	0.3%
Copper IUD (ParaGard)	0.8%	0.6%
Levonorgestrel IUD (Mirena)	0.1%	0.1%
Vasectomy	0.15%	0.1%
Tubal ligation	0.5%	0.5%
Essure device	N/A	0.2%
Lactational amenorrhea (for 6 months following delivery only)	2%	0.5%

Abbreviations: DMPA = depot medroxyprogesterone acetate; IUD = intrauterine device.

Abstinence, Natural Family Planning, and Fertility Awareness

Abstinence, natural family planning, and fertility awareness rely on the avoidance of intercourse during the fertile period of a woman's menstrual cycle. This *rhythm*, or calendar, method relies on regular menstrual cycles to determine fertile and infertile days, and has an estimated failure rate of 25% per year with typical use, compared with an 85% conception rate for couples using no method of contraception. Other methods use basal body temperature charting and/or the consistency of cervical mucus to determine fertile days. Yearly pregnancy rates with perfect use of these methods range from 1% to 3%. Natural family planning allows couples to avoid the need to use hormonal and barrier contraceptives and, for many couples, its use agrees with their religious beliefs. Another advantage is the ability to use the same systems to plan a pregnancy when conception is desired. However, these systems are limited by lower effectiveness than most other methods of contraception, and are very user-dependent. These methods work best when a couple undergoes specific training and is committed to natural family planning.

Barrier Methods and Spermicides

A variety of barrier methods are available for both men and women. All have the advantage of avoiding systemic hormone use, and only need to be used when intercourse is desired rather than continuously. Male and female condoms are the only forms of contraception that protect against sexually transmitted diseases (STDs) as well as pregnancy. Condoms also are available without a prescription, which increases their ease of use.

The typical use failure rate is 15%, with a failure rate of 2% for perfect use. Both latex and polyurethane male condoms are available. Polyurethane condoms are appropriate when one member of the couple has an allergy to latex; however, they are more prone to slippage. Female condoms allow women to have more control over barrier contraception and STD prevention, but the effectiveness is lower (failure rates 21% per year for typical use and 5% for perfect use). Because of the higher cost and failure rate of the female condom, the male condom is generally preferred for women whose partners are willing to use it.

Diaphragms and cervical caps are latex or silicone barriers that are placed in the vagina before intercourse and also serve as reservoirs for spermicide. The cervical cap is a soft plastic cup that covers the cervix and blocks semen from contact with the os. Two versions are available in the United States, the standard Prentif cap and the newer FemCap. The FemCap is nonlatex and has a rim designed to cover the vaginal fornices. Efficacy is decreased in parous women (see Table 1).

Both the cervical cap and diaphragm can be placed before intercourse and must be left in place for at least 6 hours. Both have the advantages of being nonhormonal, easily reversible, and not dependent on the woman's partner. The main disadvantage of both methods is the failure rate, which is higher than the rate with hormonal contraception or IUDs. Although the data are unclear, the cervical cap may increase the risk of cervical dysplasia in the first few months after initiation, and a Papanicolaou (Pap) test is recommended after 3 months of use. The risk of cervical dysplasia is not increased after 1 year of use. The cervical cap and diaphragm may increase the frequency of urinary tract infections. Both methods are available by prescription only, and, except for the FemCap, both the cervical cap and diaphragm must be fitted by a medical provider. The FemCap comes in three standard sizes depending on whether a woman has never been pregnant, has had a previous pregnancy, or has had a vaginal delivery.

Spermicides with nonoxynol 9, in the form of vaginal suppositories, jelly, foam, gel, and film, are available over the counter in the United States. A spermicide-containing sponge was also previously available and may be an option again in the future. Although nonoxynol 9 is more effective when used in addition to barrier methods of contraception, some women may choose to use spermicide alone as a contraceptive. The typical use failure rate is 29%; perfect use failure rate is 15%. Spermicides can increase the risk of HIV transmission by causing vaginal irritation, and the effect on transmission rates of other STDs is unclear.

Combination (Estrogen and Progesterone) Hormonal Contraceptives

Oral contraceptive pills (OCPs) were FDA approved in the United States in 1960 and have a long history of use and safety. Recently, combination hormone (estrogen and progesterone) contraceptives have become available in several other delivery systems including injection, skin patch, and vaginal ring. These new methods share many of the advantages and disadvantages of OCPs but also have unique factors related to their delivery methods. All of these methods function by inhibition of ovulation, thickening of cervical mucus and endometrial atrophy.

The benefits of OCPs are well described in the medical literature. OCP use decreases menstrual bleeding and cramping, makes menstrual bleeding more regular, reduces the risk of ovarian and endometrial cancer, decreases the incidence of ovarian cysts, and can be used to treat acne* and hirsutism[1].

The disadvantages of OCPs are also well known. Because they contain estrogen, OCPs create a hypercoagulable state, increasing the risk of deep venous thrombosis. The risk is increased approximately twofold in the average user, but the risk may be significantly higher in users who have inherited tendencies toward hypercoagulation, such as factor V Leiden deficiency. Because the hypercoagulable state may also increase the risk of myocardial infarction and stroke, OCP use is contraindicated in women older than 35 who smoke cigarettes. One percent of OCP users develop hypertension. The association between OCP use and breast cancer has been controversial, but the most recent data conclude that OCPs do not cause breast cancer, even in women with a positive family history. The typical use failure rate is 8%, with a perfect use failure rate of 0.3%.

More than 50 brands of OCPs are marketed in the United States, allowing health care providers to tailor the specific estrogen and progesterone, and the dose of each, to individual users. All OCPs share the disadvantage of requiring daily pill taking for effectiveness. Although the new delivery systems for combination estrogen/progesterone contraceptives (such as the patch and vaginal ring) have not been proven to increase compliance; this is a theoretical benefit of these new contraceptives.

[1]Not FDA approved for this indication.

*Not FDA approved for this indication except for Ortho Tri-Cyclen and Estrostep.

The ethinyl estradiol/norelgestromin (Ortho Evra) patch has become popular with women since its release in 2001. The incidence of irregular bleeding with this method is similar to OCPs, but the rate of nausea is less. A unique disadvantage is the possibility of patch allergy or problems with adhesion. This method is too new to cite typical use failure rates, but rates in studies range from 0.3% to 0.8% per year.

An ethinyl estradiol/etonogestrel vaginal ring (NuvaRing) provides another route for combination hormonal contraception. This 5.4 cm flexible ring is inserted in the vagina for 3 weeks, and then removed for 1 week, during which the woman should have menstrual-like bleeding. Unlike the diaphragm and cervical cap, exact placement in the vagina is not important. The ring may cause increased vaginal discharge, although not an increased rate of infections, and some women may be uncomfortable with vaginal placement of the ring. Failure rates of this new method are unconfirmed but reported to be approximately 0.3%.

Recently, extended or continuous contraception has become more popular and widely known. In surveys, many women (especially younger women) would prefer less frequent or no menses. Extended contraception has been shown to be safe and well accepted by women and decreases overall vaginal bleeding with long-term use. Extended contraception has also been used to decrease pain from endometriosis and menstrual migraines. Monophasic OCPs, the ethinyl estradiol/norelgestromin patch, and the ethinyl estradiol/etonogestrel vaginal ring can all be used. A dedicated OCP product (Seasonale) is available, providing continuous hormonal contraception for 84 days followed by a 6-day, pill-free interval. Disadvantages of extended contraception include a greater cost and higher chance of irregular bleeding, although this generally improves with time. Studies demonstrate no increased risk of endometrial hyperplasia with extended contraception.

An estradiol cypionate/medroxyprogesterone acetate (Lunelle) contraceptive injection was FDA approved in October 2000, but is currently not available because of problems with the formulation. Its function is similar to other combination hormone contraceptives; the delivery system requires a monthly injection in a health care provider's office.

Progestin-Only Methods

Progestin-only contraceptives are available in several forms, including pills, injections, and implants. Progestin-only OCPs (Micronor) work primarily by thickening cervical mucus. Ovulation is inhibited in approximately 50% of cycles. Although progestin-only OCPs have a higher failure rate than combination hormone OCPs in studies, this is very dependent on regular pill-taking at the same time (within 3 hours) each day. The typical use failure rate is 8%, with a perfect use failure rate of 0.3%. Progestin-only

OCPs are a good option for women who would like to take pills but cannot take estrogen (such as lactating women or those with hypercoagulable states). Although they do decrease menstrual bleeding and cramping, cycle control is not as good as with combination OCPs. Progestin-only OCPs are taken daily, with no pill-free interval.

Depot medroxyprogesterone acetate (DMPA or Depo Provera) injections provide a more effective form of progestin-only contraception. The DMPA injection works through several mechanisms, including inhibiting ovulation, thickening cervical mucus, and causing atrophy of the endometrium. A visit to a medical office is required every 11 to 13 weeks for the injection. A major advantage of this method is that it is less user-dependent than OCPs or barrier contraceptives. The first-year typical use failure rate is 3%, with a perfect use failure rate of 0.3%. Amenorrhea is a common side effect with long-term use of the DMPA injection and may be preferred by patients. DMPA injection has additional benefits in women with certain medical conditions; it reduces pain in endometriosis, raises the seizure threshold in women with epilepsy, and reduces the risk of sickle cell crisis by 70%.

The major disadvantage of DMPA injection is irregular bleeding, causing many women to discontinue this method in the first year. This method is also associated with weight gain, with an average of 5.4 pounds in the first year and 16.5 pounds after 5 years of use. Progesterone side effects are possible and headaches, depression, and acne may occur. DMPA injection is not a good choice for women who are planning a pregnancy in the near future because it is not immediately reversible and the average time for return to fertility is 10 months. It may take as long as 18 months after discontinuation for regular cycles to return.

The six-rod levonorgestrel implant (Norplant) is no longer available in the United States. A two-rod implant (Jadelle)[1] was FDA approved in 1996, but is not yet being marketed. The Norplant implant had a user-independent failure rate of 0.05%, but irregular bleeding and difficulty with removal limited use. The new two-rod implant (Norplant II)[1] and a one-rod etonogestrel implant (Implanon)[1] currently used in Europe have fewer difficulties with removal. The progestin-only implants thicken cervical mucus (within 24 hours), inhibit ovulation, and produce an atrophic endometrium. The two-rod levonorgestrel implant is effective for 5 years; the one rod etonogestrel implant works for 3 years.

Intrauterine Devices

Intrauterine devices (IUDs) offer extremely effective, reversible contraception options. New data and new developments in IUDs mean that many women are now candidates for this method who were previously thought to be ineligible. The two IUD models available in the United States are the copper IUD (ParaGard) and the levonorgestrel IUD (Mirena).

The primary mechanism of action of the copper IUD is spermicidal; it causes a sterile inflammatory reaction in the uterus and interferes with sperm motility. The typical use failure rate in the first year is 0.8%, and the perfect use failure rate is 0.6%. The copper IUD is very cost-effective when used long term and provides effective contraception for 10 years. The high efficacy and lack of hormones make it a valuable option for women who cannot or do not wish to use hormonal methods of contraception. This is also an easily reversible form of contraception with fertility returning rapidly after removal.

The disadvantages of the copper IUD are increased risk of bleeding and infection. Menstrual bleeding and cramping are increased, although this may be mitigated by the use of NSAIDs during menses. Pelvic inflammatory disease risk is increased in women at risk for STDs, especially in the first 20 days after insertion. When pregnancies do occur, approximately 5% will be ectopic pregnancies, but overall the risk for ectopic pregnancy is decreased compared with women not using contraception. Nulliparity is not a contraindication in patients at low risk for STDs. Wilson's disease is a rare contraindication for copper-containing IUDs.

The levonorgestrel IUD (Mirena) primarily functions by thickening cervical mucus and reducing sperm motility. The typical use failure rate and perfect use failure rate are not significantly different from the copper IUD. In contrast to the copper IUD, the levonorgestrel IUD markedly reduces menstrual bleeding and approximately 20% of women will become amenorrheic with long-term use. Patients should be counseled about the increased incidence of irregular bleeding in the first 6 months after insertion. Progesterone side effects such as acne or headaches are possible but rare in the first few months of use.

Postcoital Contraception

Postcoital contraception refers to methods that can be used after intercourse has occurred. They are not recommended as primary methods of contraception, but serve as backup (*emergency*) methods for the less effective barrier methods of contraception and protection for episodes of unplanned intercourse or rape. Postcoital contraception works by delaying ovulation or by interfering with transport of sperm and ova. The most common method involves 0.75 mg levonorgestrel tablets, marketed in the United States as Plan B. Although the labeling instructs patients to take the first dose within 72 hours and the second dose 12 hours later, both doses can be taken together without reduction in efficacy. Although the pregnancy rate is not significantly higher if the medication is

[1]Not FDA approved for this indication.

taken 5 days after intercourse rather than three, it is important to counsel patients that the efficacy is generally higher the sooner the pills are taken. The World Health Organization estimates that 89% of pregnancies that would be expected after a single act of intercourse can be prevented with use of levonorgestrel postcoital contraception.

The only contraindications to levonorgestrel postcoital contraception are established pregnancy, allergy to the ingredients, and undiagnosed vaginal bleeding. Because relatively few patients will have these contraindications, many health care providers give advance prescriptions of levonorgestrel for patients to have on hand if needed. Some states allow pharmacists to counsel and dispense postcoital contraception without a prescription. Nausea is fairly common with the levonorgestrel regimen (23%), and the subsequent menstrual period may occur earlier than expected. Progesterone-only OCPs can also be used for postcoital contraception, but a total of 40 pills (yellow Ovrette pills)[1] are needed. Use of combination estrogen/progesterone emergency contraception, either as the dedicated product Preven or using combination hormone OCPs[1], is associated with a lower efficacy and higher rates of nausea and vomiting. Prescription of a prophylactic dose of an antiemetic is recommended when combination hormone postcoital contraception is used.

The copper IUD (ParaGard)[1] can also be used as postcoital contraception when inserted within 5 days of intercourse. Because of the greatly increased cost when compared with levonorgestrel pills, insertion of the IUD is generally only recommended for women who want to use this as an ongoing method. The failure rate of the copper IUD is less than 1% when used in this manner. The levonorgestrel IUD (Mirena)[1] has not been found to be effective for postcoital contraception.

Male and Female Sterilization

Vasectomy and tubal ligation are popular methods of contraception in the United States. They have the advantage of high efficacy rates and no user dependence, but they do require surgical procedures and should be considered permanent.

Although vasectomy has a higher efficacy and is safer than surgical tubal ligation, it is less commonly performed in the United States. Vasectomy is an outpatient office procedure usually performed under local anesthesia. It involves ligation or cauterization of the vas deferens, preventing sperm transport. The procedure does not interfere with hormones or sexual function. The first year perfect use failure rate for vasectomy is 0.1% but the typical use failure rate is somewhat higher at 0.15%, because some men may not delay intercourse until their sperm count is verified to be zero. Other disadvantages are mainly short-term complications around the time of the procedure, such as pain, infection, or bruising; but long-term pain and patient regret are possible.

Tubal ligation is performed either as laparoscopic surgery or as a postpartum mini-laparotomy. First-year typical and perfect use failure rates are the same at 0.5%, but pregnancy is possible many years after the surgery. These lower failure rates are for postpartum partial salpingectomy and Filshie clip ligation; other variations of the procedure have higher failure rates. Although rare, when pregnancy does occur, an ectopic pregnancy is more likely. Because of the need for an operating room and general or regional anesthesia, tubal ligation is quite expensive when compared with vasectomy and carries more surgical risks. The risk of major complications (bleeding, anesthesia complications, damage to other organs) is 1.5% for minilaparotomy and 0.9% for laparoscopy. Patient regret is also a possible complication for this form of permanent contraception. Long-term studies have not shown an increase in menstrual irregularities or pain following tubal ligation.

Recently, a procedure for transcervical tubal occlusion with coiled spring implants (Essure) has been FDA approved in the United States. The implant is hysteroscopically inserted into the fallopian tube, and local tissue growth then causes tubal occlusion over a period of 3 months. The failure rate in initial studies was 0.2%. The procedure can be done in an ambulatory setting and requires only local anesthesia. Most women were able to return to work or their usual activities the same or the following day. Because of the cost of the implants, the tubal occlusion procedure is more expensive than vasectomy. The primary disadvantage is the need for the woman to use alternate contraception for 3 months following the procedure, and then return for a hysterosalpingogram to verify tubal closure. Approximately 15% of women will have to return for a second procedure because one or both of the implants cannot be placed correctly or is expelled. Because this is a newer procedure, the degree of reversibility is unknown, but it will probably be more difficult to reverse than standard tubal ligation. This method may not be effective in immunosuppressed women.

Postpartum Contraception

Following delivery, most women will experience a delay in return of regular ovulation. Breast-feeding delays ovulation; the average time to ovulation is 189 days for breast-feeding women and 45 days for non–breast-feeding women. Women who wish to rely on lactational amenorrhea as a form of contraception must be exclusively breast-feeding on demand, amenorrheic (considered as having no vaginal bleeding after 8 weeks postpartum), and have an infant less than 6 months old. If these three criteria are met, the perfect use failure rate is 0.5% for the first 6 months and the typical use failure rate is 2%.

[1]Not FDA approved for this indication.

Barrier methods of contraception have the advantage of not interfering with breast milk production, and may be used together with lactational amenorrhea to provide additional protection against pregnancy. Male and female condoms can be used once lochia stops. Diaphragms and cervical caps must be refit after delivery, usually after 4 to 6 weeks.

Progestin-only methods, including pills, implant, and injection, may be used immediately following delivery with minimal effect on lactation. However, the WHO recommends delaying use for 6 weeks in lactating women because of unknown effects on the newborn.

Combination hormone contraceptives, including pills, patch, vaginal ring, and injection, may decrease the volume of breast milk when lactation is not firmly established. Most authorities recommend waiting until 6 weeks postpartum to prescribe these methods.

Both copper and levonorgestrel IUDs can be inserted either immediately after delivery of the placenta, or 6 weeks post partum. Neither interferes with breast-feeding.

Tubal ligation can be done in the first 48 hours after delivery or as an interval procedure at 6 weeks postpartum. The newer hysteroscopic tubal occlusion can only be performed as an interval procedure.

Contraceptive counseling must take into account the preferences of the patient, safety, side effects, efficacy, and noncontraceptive benefits. Multiple new contraceptive methods allow health care providers to tailor their recommendations to fit patient circumstances. The goal is to assist patients in choosing the contraceptive method that they are most likely to use correctly and consistently.

SECTION 17

Psychiatric Disorders

ALCOHOL USE DISORDERS

METHOD OF

Raymond F. Anton, MD

An Institute of Medicine analysis suggests that although alcohol dependence is a serious disease, considerably more people who do not meet dependence criteria abuse alcohol regularly or drink at levels harmful to their health. Lifetime and current prevalence of alcohol abuse is approximately 9% and 3%, respectively, while for alcohol dependence it is 14% and 4.4%, respectively. Men account for up to 75% of identified individuals. Currently there are approximately 15 to 20 million Americans with diagnosable alcohol disorders. It is estimated that alcohol-induced problems account for at least 15% of health care expenditures and cost the U.S. economy close to 175 billion dollars in medical costs, loss of life and property, and reduced productivity. At least 20% of new ambulatory care patients, 43% of emergency department cases, and 20% to 50% of inpatient admissions have past or current alcohol problems, many of which are not documented in the clinical record.

Despite the documented reduction in coronary artery disease attributed to low/moderate (two or fewer drinks daily) alcohol consumption, heavier alcohol consumption (four to six drinks per day) is known to increase blood pressure and the risk of cerebral vascular accidents, liver disease, and some carcinomas.

Taken together, these data make a strong case for improved recognition of heavy drinking. Recent increases in treatment options make recognition and diagnosis of alcohol use disorders even more compelling, especially in relationship to health care cost containment.

Detection and Diagnosis

Both verbal and written screens and blood tests show acceptably high accuracy in the detection of early stage problem drinking, long before diagnostic criteria may be met. In particular, a positive answer on at least two of the four CAGE questions (Table 1) indicates the need for further evaluation. (CAGE is derived from words taken from each question—cut down, annoyed, guilty, and eye-opener.) The Alcohol Use Disorders Identification Test (AUDIT), a 10-item questionnaire developed by the World Health Organization (WHO), aids in the identification of harmful alcohol consumption in health care settings. Blood tests have also been widely used as indicators of heavy alcohol consumption. In particular, serum g-glutamyltransferase (GGT) is used extensively. If nonalcoholic hepatobiliary disease and certain medications (such as anticonvulsants) are not present, GGT levels above approximately 50 IU may indicate heavy alcohol consumption. A new test that measures a carbohydrate-deficient variant of serum transferrin (CDT) is a relatively sensitive marker of persistent heavy

TABLE 1 CAGE Questions

Have you ever felt that you should cut down on your drinking?
Have people annoyed you by criticizing your drinking?
Have you ever felt guilty about your drinking?
Have you ever had a drink the first thing in the morning to steady your nerves or get rid of a hangover (eye-opener)?

TABLE 2 Definition of a Standard Drink; Safe and Heavy Drinking Levels

Standard Drink
1.5 ounces of hard liquor (spirits)—80 proof (alcohol concentration 40%).
5 ounces of wine (normal alcohol concentration 10%-12%).
12 ounces of beer (normal alcohol concentration 4%-5%).
Safe Drinking Levels
Less than, or equal to, 2 drinks per day (no more than 14 drinks per week) for men; less than, or equal to, 1 drink per day (no more than 7 drinks) a week for women. In the elderly and in those taking certain medications safe levels may be lower. Any alcohol consumption during pregnancy can be considered unsafe.
Heavy Drinking Levels
Five or more drinks per day for men and four or more drinks per day for women.

(four to six drinks daily) alcohol consumption, particularly in men. CDT, which is becoming more widely available in the United States, is more specific than GGT in that elevated levels of CDT occur primarily in relationship to drinking even within individuals with nonalcoholic liver disease. Elevations in CDT appear to occur largely independent of GGT and, as such, they can be used in a complementary fashion. Both GGT and CDT can be used to monitor increases or decreases in drinking over time, similar to how hemoglobin A_{Ic} is used to monitor glucose control.

The most important way to detect heavy alcohol use is to actually ask about it. While a substantial minority of patients may not provide an accurate answer, many will. Many heavy drinkers present with symptoms associated with their alcohol use, such as GI complaints, hypertension, gout, traumatic falls, and accidents; or they may have elevated uric acid, macrocytic red blood cell indices, elevated liver function tests, or psychiatric complaints of insomnia, depression, anxiety, and irritability. All of these should trigger an automatic questioning of alcohol consumption. While there are specific criteria for diagnosable alcohol abuse and dependence available, if alcohol is leading to health or social harm, a person is simply drinking too much and needs to cut down or stop. The core features of alcohol abuse are frequent heavy drinking occasions, which lead to consequences (falls, fights, domestic arguments, arrests or driving under the influence citations [DUIs]). Alcohol dependence is characterized by almost daily drinking with loss of control (inability to cut down or stop), drinking more than intended (can't have just one or two drinks), or a build-up of tolerance (needs more alcohol to get high or feel relaxed). Some people report morning shakes or other symptoms of physical dependence if the problem is more serious.

The starting point with almost any heavy drinker (with or without alcohol abuse or dependence) is simple *advice* to cut down or quit, with appointments provided for monitoring progress. If a health care professional advises them to do so, a substantial number of individuals will cut down or quit, especially if they have not lost complete control over their drinking. It is useful to ask a person to monitor his or her own alcohol use by writing down how many standard drinks of alcohol they consume every day (a daily diary). Table 2 provides the definition of a standard drink. Counsel patients that many people are unaware of how much liquor or wine they might actually pour in a glass. So ask them to measure a standard amount that they might ordinarily drink with a measuring cup. Also be aware that beer comes in different size cans and alcohol concentrations—so inquire as specifically as possible.

In addition to advice, educating a patient about how alcohol may be causing or augmenting their health problems as well as a review of the long-term risks of heavy consumption could be quite helpful. Objective evidence such as blood tests (GGT, mean corpuscular volume [MCV], uric acid, CDT) or other physical signs or symptoms of harmful alcohol use allow for a focused dialogue regarding the harmful effects of alcohol. Discussions about alcohol use should be no different than discussing the role of diet and exercise in cholesterol control. An empathetic, educational, and motivational approach will serve many patients quite well. The setting of defined goals (abstinence versus reduction), monitoring with feedback, and modification of the treatment plan, if initial goals are not met, as part of a brief intervention approach to alcohol management should be standard practice.

Assessment and Treatment of Alcohol Withdrawal

Alcohol withdrawal (AW) may be one of the most serious acute medical consequences of chronic heavy consumption. It is characterized by autonomic hyperactivity, tremulousness, anxiety and agitation, and cognitive disturbances (illusions and hallucinations). In its more serious form, delirium tremens (DTs) and seizures can occur. Although the probability of AW symptoms increases with the amount of alcohol consumption before cessation, and also with increasing age, there is considerable variation in both the emergence and level of alcohol withdrawal symptoms. It is estimated that only approximately 10% to 20% of chronic heavy alcohol consumers will need medical intervention for alcohol withdrawal. The probability of alcohol withdrawal seizures, which normally occur in approximately 5% to 15% of alcoholics in withdrawal, is increased in individuals experiencing repeated medical detoxifications and by the presence of current medical illnesses. The Clinical Institute Withdrawal Assessment—Alcohol revised (CIWA-Ar), a 10-item rating scale, has become a standard instrument for the evaluation of the severity of alcohol withdrawal.

Many alcohol-dependent individuals can be managed with social support during the cessation of drinking, but many others benefit from pharmacologic intervention that is increasingly being provided to outpatients. According to the American Society of Addiction Medicine criteria, inpatient detoxification should be reserved for those with a history of complicated alcohol withdrawal (DTs and seizures), significant medical problems (e.g., pancreatitis, hypertension), those who have little social support or live distant to the clinical facility, and individuals who have failed outpatient detoxification. Individuals who have other co-morbid substance abuse and psychiatric disorders might also fit into this category.

Hydration, electrolyte replacement, and thiamin supplementation are standard practice for severe inpatient or emergent care alcohol withdrawal management. Medical management of alcohol withdrawal in health care facilities requires frequent nursing observation to avoid underdosing or overdosing with the recommended medications. Outpatients should be seen daily for 2 to 3 days to evaluate safety and tolerability of the prescribed treatment, and on-call medical services should be available. Although most of the acute symptoms of alcohol withdrawal will ameliorate in the first 48 hours after the cessation of drinking, some symptoms (insomnia, anxiety, tremor) may linger for up to 5 to 7 days and beyond. Patients and their families should be alerted that seizures may occur later than 48 hours after the cessation of drinking, and cardiac arrhythmias may occur at extended times after the end of medical detoxification.

Benzodiazepines are the most widely studied and clinically used treatment for uncomplicated alcohol withdrawal. Table 3 contains several standard alcohol withdrawal protocols. Care must be used on an outpatient basis because benzodiazepines can cause sedation, act synergistically with alcohol, and be abused by alcoholics. Lower doses, frequent prescriptions of fewer pills, daily clinic attendance, and use of significant others for dosage administration and transportation can all minimize outpatient iatrogenic complications.

Other agents that lack some of the disadvantages of benzodiazepines, such as abuse liability and cognitive suppression, may be used. The noradrenergic α_2 agonist clonidine (Catapres)[1] and the β-adrenergic antagonist atenolol (Tenormin)[1] may be used. In general, these drugs are superior to placebo and may be better than benzodiazepines in suppressing some autonomic symptoms (like high blood pressure and heart rate) evident during alcohol withdrawal. However, AW seizures may occur when these agents are used as monotherapy.

[1]Not FDA approved for this indication.

TABLE 3 Treatment of Alcohol Withdrawal

Fixed-Schedule Regimens for Common Withdrawal

Chlordiazepoxide (Librium), 50 mg PO q6h for 4 doses, then 25 mg q6h for 8 doses.
Diazepam (Valium), 10 mg PO q6h for 4 doses, then 5 mg q6h for 8 doses.
Lorazepam (Ativan)[1], 2 mg PO q6h for 4 doses, then 1 mg q6h for 8 doses.
Carbamazepine (Tegretol)[1] 200 mg PO q6h, taper over 4-5 days.
Provide additional medication as needed when symptoms are not controlled (i.e., CIWA-Ar >8-10) with above.

Symptom-Triggered Regimens for Common Withdrawal

Monitor patient every 4-8h by means of CIWA-Ar until score has been ≤8-10 for 24h; use additional assessments as needed.
Administer one of the following medications every hour when CIWA-Ar ≥8-10:
Chlordiazepoxide, 50-100 mg PO
Diazepam, 10-20 mg PO
Lorazepam[1], 2-4 mg PO
Repeat CIWA-Ar 1h after every dose to assess need for further medication.

For Patients with Agitation or Delirium

Lorazepam[1], 1-4 mg IV q5-15min, or lorazepam, 1-4 mg IM q30-60min, until calm, then q1h prn to maintain light somnolence.
Diazepam, 5 mg IV (2.5 mg/min). If the initial dose is not effective, repeat the dose in 5-10 min. If a second dose of 5 mg is not satisfactory, use 10 mg for the third and fourth doses q5-10 min. If not effective, use 20 mg for the fifth and subsequent doses until sedation is achieved. Use 5-20 mg q1h prn to maintain light somnolence.
Haloperidol (Haldol)[1], 0.5-5 mg IV/IM q30-60 min prn for severe agitation (only to be used as adjunctive therapy with sedative/hypnotics).
Haloperidol, 0.5-5mg PO q4h prn for agitation not controlled by sedative/hypnotics alone.

[1]Not FDA approved for this indication.
Abbreviations: CIWA-Ar = Clinical Institute Withdrawal Assessment–Alcohol, revised; IM = intramuscular; IV = intravenous; PO = orally; prn = as needed; q = every.
Modified from: Rakel RE, Bope ET (Eds.): Conn's Current Therapy 2003. Philadelphia, Elsevier, 2003, p 1179. Used with permission.

The anticonvulsant and mood stabilizing agent carbamazepine (Tegretol)[1] is as least as efficacious as the benzodiazepines oxazepam (Serax) and lorazepam (Ativan)[1] in suppressing alcohol withdrawal symptoms. Consider the use of carbamazepine in the treatment of AW in individuals who have had multiple previous detoxifications, who had a seizure during a past AW, who have concomitant psychiatric pathology such as affective disturbances, and in situations where neurocognitive suppression and abuse of benzodiazepines may be of concern. While there was no reported worsening of liver function or clinically significant neutropenia in the AW studies, these may occur when carbamazepine[1] is used. Also, benzodiazepines can be used to supplement the effects of carbamazepine[1] as required.

[1]Not FDA approved for this indication.

It is important to reiterate with patients that alcohol detoxification is not a treatment for alcoholism per se. It allows a patient to achieve sobriety in the short term, but for the vast majority of patients an extended course of relapse prevention treatment is indicated.

TREATMENT OF ALCOHOL DEPENDENCE

Alcohol dependence is characterized by persistent high levels of alcohol use that is uncontrolled, is automatic, has compulsive features, and develops over a long period of time. Many of these behaviors have a neurobehavioral basis. Alcoholism, therefore, can be described as an acquired brain dysfunction with specific neurochemical and neuroanatomical pathways playing crucial roles. While brief interventions in medical care settings (described previously), various self-help groups (Alcoholics Anonymous), and counseling techniques (relapse prevention therapies) are successful in a number of individuals, it is becoming increasingly clear that pharmacologic intervention combined with efforts at behavioral change offer the highest rates of success. When there is a co-morbid psychiatric disorder (depression, anxiety, psychosis) present, referral to a psychiatrist or addiction specialist is indicated.

PHARMACOTHERAPY OF PRIMARY ALCOHOLISM

Aversive agents, such as disulfiram (Antabuse), make people feel ill if they consume alcohol, whereas newer medications work on brain mechanisms to reduce *craving*, promote abstinence, and/or reduce heavy drinking episodes.

Disulfiram

Disulfiram (Antabuse) has limited effectiveness because only very compliant individuals may benefit from its use. While information is scarce, disulfiram is unlikely to reduce craving and, therefore, people often discontinue its use. Techniques to enhance compliance, such as monitored ingestion, could increase its effectiveness.

Naltrexone

The opiate antagonist drug naltrexone (ReVia) is approved by the FDA for the treatment of alcohol dependence. Studies indicate that it is most efficacious when used along with specific relapse prevention counseling techniques; however, some smaller studies indicate that it can be used along with support for abstinence, or with brief counseling, in heavy drinkers. After a few days of abstinence, naltrexone can be started at 25 mg per day, and after several days maintained at 50 to 100 mg once per day. A reduction in both craving and relapse drinking is reported with this agent when used over a 3- to 6-month period. Longer periods of maintenance may be useful for some individuals. Nausea, abdominal pain, headache, and fatigue may occur but generally dissipate during continued treatment. Because naltrexone blocks central nervous system (CNS) opiate receptors, individuals dependent on opiates could experience a severe withdrawal syndrome. Naltrexone is also contraindicated in those requiring opiates for pain relief.

Promising Drugs

Acamprosate[2] (calcium-acetyl-homotaurinate) appears to modulate the excitatory glutamate amino acid system (*N*-methyl-D-aspartate [NMDA] receptor) in the brain. Acamprosate could hypothetically *reset* this neurochemical system after alcohol withdrawal to reduce craving and relapse drinking. A number of studies in Europe indicate the potential efficacy of acamprosate. Because of its pharmacokinetic profile, acamprosate must be taken at least twice daily. It is currently being evaluated in the United States.

Recently, in a single-site trial, *topiramate* (Topamax)[1] reduced drinking and craving and promoted abstinence. This medication must be titrated over 6 weeks to a target dose of 300 mg. However, caution should be taken until the results of a larger multisite study, currently under way, are available.

The combination of *naltrexone* (ReVia) and *acamprosate*[2] may be more potent than either drug alone. A large National Institutes of Health (NIH)-sponsored trial is currently under way to evaluate this possibility.

The treatment of co-morbid alcoholism and major depression is a common problem. It is clear that selective serotonin reuptake inhibitors (SSRIs) are well tolerated by depressed alcoholics and are useful for treating depressive symptoms. However, studies to date have been equivocal about the effect of these medications in reducing alcohol intake and promoting abstinence. Often depressive symptoms will diminish without specific treatment if abstinence is achieved. Therefore, whenever possible, the primary goal should be the maintenance of 7 to 14 days of abstinence before consideration of specific antidepressant therapy.

---

[1]Not FDA approved for this indication.
[2]Not available in the United States.

DRUG ABUSE

METHOD OF

Joyce A. Tinsley, MD

The U.S. Department of Health and Human Services reported that in 2001 nearly 7% of the population, or 16 million Americans age 12 and older, were actively using illegal drugs. The combination of drug and alcohol use costs taxpayers a staggering sum; an estimated $143 billion per year is spent on associated health care costs, extra law enforcement, motor vehicle accidents, crime, and lost productivity. The president's fiscal year 2003 budget included $4.4 billion for all substance abuse–related activities, with $127 million earmarked for treatment services. The abuse of legal drugs, such as prescription medications and nicotine, is also a serious problem. Nicotine dependence is responsible for more morbidity and mortality than any other abused substance and is so highly addictive that quitting eludes many who try to stop.

Many addicts in need of treatment do not get it. Reasons for this include a lack of treatment and recovery resources, the stigma surrounding drug use, and pessimism about recovery from addictions. Unfortunately, much of the clinical pessimism about addiction treatment is based on an inadequate or outdated knowledge base. At a minimum, clinicians should be familiar with the common drugs of abuse; signs of intoxication, withdrawal, and overdose; management of simple detoxification; and contemporary treatment options.

Diagnosis

In the *Diagnostic and Statistical Manual of Mental Disorders, 4th ed., Text Revision* (DSM-IV-TR), published by the American Psychiatric Association, disorders are classified as either *abuse* or *dependence* (Table 1).

TABLE 1 DSM IV-TR Diagnostic Criteria

Substance Abuse

A maladaptive pattern of use leading to clinically significant impairment and distress in at least *one* of the following areas within a 12-month period:

1. Failure to fulfill major role obligations at work, school, or home
2. Use in physically hazardous situations
3. Substance-related legal problems
4. Use despite social or interpersonal problems exacerbated by use of the substance

Substance Dependence

A maladaptive pattern of use leading to impairment and distress in at least *three* of the following areas within a 12-month period:

1. Tolerance—need for increasing amounts to achieve intoxication or desired effect *or* diminished effect with continued use of the same amount.
2. Withdrawal—development of characteristic withdrawal symptoms *or* use of the same or related substance to relieve or avoid withdrawal symptoms.
3. The substance is used in larger amounts or over longer time periods than intended.
4. Inability to cut down or control use.
5. Significant time is spent in activities related to obtaining the substance or recovering from its effects.
6. Social, occupational, or recreational activities are given up or reduced.
7. Use continues despite knowledge of harmful physical or psychological effects.

Adapted from: American Psychiatric Association: Diagnostic and statistical manual of mental disorders 4th ed., text revision (DSM-IV-TR). Washington, DC: Author, 2000. Used with permission.

These criteria may be applied to any drug within the major classes of addictive substances. Inherent to the definition of dependence is the concept of impaired control. In other words, the addict cannot predictably control when or how much of a substance he or she will use. In both abuse and dependence, the individual continues to use the substance even though it causes problems in one or more important life areas. The diagnosis is based on behaviors surrounding the drug abuse rather than the amount consumed. Substance dependence, synonymous with addiction, is the more advanced disorder.

It is often challenging to diagnose drug abuse. Patients may be hesitant to reveal illegal drug abuse or the misuse of prescription drugs. Clinicians should ask questions that are perceived to be nonjudgmental. For instance, asking, "Has anyone ever been concerned about your drug use?" is less likely to be met with resistance than initial questions that ask about quantity or frequency of use. Supplemental history from significant others and objective data from urine drug screens can help clarify the diagnosis. Some addicts readily admit their addictions. For instance, heroin users have been known to overestimate their use in order to receive a more generous opiate dose for detoxification or maintenance. Heroin and cocaine addicts with advanced dependence often acknowledge their addictions because of devastating social, legal, or physical consequences. In addition, a majority of cigarette smokers express a desire to stop smoking and attempt to get help.

Nicotine

Nicotine dependence is similar to other drug addictions in that it is best viewed as a chronic disease that requires ongoing attention. It is the addiction on which primary care clinicians may have the greatest impact. An estimated 25% of adults in the United States smoke cigarettes, and 70% of current smokers would like to quit. In view of the lethal nature of smoking, the high percentage of smokers who want to quit, and the number of individuals affected, the clinician should be prepared to encourage smoking cessation.

The nicotine withdrawal syndrome is a serious obstacle for patients who want to stop smoking. Withdrawal symptoms often begin within hours after the last cigarette, peak within 2 to 3 days, and may continue for several weeks. Nicotine cravings last much longer. Early abstinence is characterized by irritability, anxiety, restlessness, depressed mood, inattention, and insomnia. A nicotine replacement product is effective in ameliorating many of the withdrawal symptoms.

Brief counseling improves smoking cessation rates, especially when directed toward the patient's unique situation. The U.S. Public Health Service recommends easy-to-follow strategies that clinicians can use in counseling patients to quit smoking (Table 2). The "5 As" represent a strategy particularly helpful to the clinician who wants to initiate discussion about a patient's tobacco use. The "5 Rs" may be used if the patient lacks motivation to stop smoking. Finally, an action plan known by the mnemonic STAR is a guide for those ready to make a quit attempt.

There is solid evidence that several medications are effective in improving smokers' quit rates (Table 3). Unless there are contraindications to the use of these medications, a first-line agent, either a nicotine replacement product or bupropion (Zyban), should be recommended to patients who want to stop smoking. If initial agents are ineffective or contraindicated, the clinician should consider recommending a second-line agent, specifically clonidine (Catapres)[1] or nortriptyline (Pamelor)[1]. The Public Health Service provides additional information to clinicians who want to learn more about how to help patients stop smoking on their Web site *http://www.surgeon-general.gov/tobacco*.

Marijuana

Marijuana, or cannabis, is the most commonly used illegal drug in the United States. Despite purported medical uses, it is not a benign substance. Individuals who become addicted often experience impairment in multiple life areas. The active ingredient in marijuana is tetrahydrocannabinol (THC). THC is classified as a hallucinogen, which it can be in large quantities or in highly sensitive individuals. More often intoxication brings relaxation, euphoria, a dreamy state, time-space distortion, and impaired attention. Perceptual disturbances may impair driving. Anxiety and paranoia are also common effects. Like other addictive substances, marijuana abuse can interfere with the assessment and treatment of psychiatric symptoms. No specific medical management is warranted for either cannabis intoxication or withdrawal.

Teenagers are among the most vulnerable users. Common signs of problematic use during adolescence include changes in sleeping and eating habits, declining school performance, changes in the adolescent's peer group, and moodiness. Physical signs include increased appetite, dry mouth, and injected conjunctiva. The University of Michigan's Monitoring the Future survey of U.S. high school students has been tracking teenage substance use for the past 25 years. In 2000, they found that by the age of 18 years, 80% of U.S. youth had used alcohol and 54% had used illicit drugs. Their drug of choice was marijuana. One in five high school seniors and nearly as many tenth graders reported marijuana use during the previous month. Treatment for marijuana abuse and dependence in adolescents or adults consists of psychotherapeutic approaches.

Cocaine and Other Stimulants

Cocaine is a highly addictive drug that is extracted from the coca leaf. Amphetamine, which is structurally similar to cocaine, is a synthesized product used to suppress hunger, improve energy or alertness, and improve mood. The euphoria that cocaine elicits is probably caused by increased dopamine activity. Physical effects include elevated heart rate and blood pressure, mediated by stimulation of the sympathetic nervous system. All stimulants possess these qualities, though in varying degrees and with variable risks. In overdose, these effects are intensified so that myocardial infarction, arrhythmia, stroke, and psychosis may occur. In those situations, therapeutic measures are supportive and aimed at reversing specific ill effects.

Physiologic withdrawal is not a major problem, and no medical management is indicated. However withdrawal from cocaine produces symptoms known

[1]Not FDA approved for this indication.

TABLE 2 Office-Based Interventions for Smoking Cessation

Initial Intervention: 5 As	Motivational Intervention: 5 Rs	Action Plan: STAR
Ask about tobacco use. **Advise** the patient to quit. **Assess** readiness to quit. **Assist** in the quit attempt. **Arrange** follow-up.	**Relevance:** Why stop? **Risks:** Personalize them. **Rewards:** Potential benefits. **Roadblocks:** Identify and address barriers. **Repetition:** Repeat message at the next visit.	**Set** a quit date. **Tell** others of plan. **Anticipate** difficulties. **Remove** tobacco products.

Adapted from: U.S. Public Health Service: Treating tobacco use and dependence—clinician's packet. A how-to guide for implementing the public health service clinical practice guideline. March 2003. http://www.surgeongeneral.gov/tobacco/clinpack.html

TABLE 3 Pharmacotherapy of Smoking Cessation

	Instructions	Dose	Advantages	Disadvantages
Nicotine gum/over-the-counter (Nicorette)	Chew until peppery taste, then *park* between cheek and gum.	2 or 4 mg per piece. Maximum 24 pieces per day. Use for up to 6 mo.	Flexibility with scheduled and/or prn doses to relieve cravings. Delivery is more rapid than the patch.	Incomplete absorption when chewed incorrectly. Cannot eat or drink while using. Caution with dental or jaw problems.
Transdermal nicotine patch/over-the-counter (Nicoderm)	Apply to skin daily. Available as 16-h or 24-h patch. Do not smoke while using.	Start 21 mg × 6 wk (14 mg if weight <100 lb or smoking <½ ppd). Taper to 14 mg, then 7 mg × 2-4 wk. Use for 2-3 mo total.	Easy to use. Few side effects. Releases steady dose of nicotine to reduce cravings. Can use in combination with gum.	Releases nicotine more slowly. No response for sudden cravings. Can cause skin irritation. Consider lower dosing in known cardiac disease.
Nasal spray/prescription (Nicotrol NS)	Use every 1-2 h. Take deep breath, spray into each nostril, and exhale through mouth.	From 8 to 40 times per day. Use for 3 mo with gradual taper.	Fastest delivery of nicotine. Good at reducing sudden cravings.	Nose and sinus irritation common at first. Caution with allergies or asthma.
Nasal inhaler/prescription (Nicotrol Inhaler)	Inhale nicotine by bringing inhaler to mouth when desired.	From 6 to 16 cartridges per day for first 3-6 wk. Use for 3 mo with gradual taper.	Delivers nicotine as quickly as gum. Satisfies hand-to-mouth habit. Few side effects.	May cause mouth or throat irritation. Caution with asthma or chronic lung disease.
Bupropion HCl/prescription (Zyban)	Take 1 pill in the morning,1 in late afternoon. Start 2 wk before quit date.	150 mg SR bid. Continue for 7 to 12 weeks after quitting.	Easy to use, few side effects. May be more helpful when used with the patch.	Contraindicated in seizure, eating disorders, patients taking Wellbutrin or MAOIs, pregnancy, or breast-feeding.

Abbreviations: bid = twice daily; MAOIs = monoamine oxidase inhibitors; ppd = packs per day; prn = as needed; SR = slow release.
Adapted from: American Cancer Society: Set yourself free; deciding how to quit, a smoker's guide. 1999.

as a *crash*. A crash may begin within hours of the last use and intensify over the next several days. During this time the addict feels extreme fatigue. Depression can be severe and carries a risk of suicidal ideation and behavior. Relapse is common during withdrawal because return to use provides quick and reliable relief.

The person who abuses cocaine may use it by snorting, injecting, or smoking. The rate at which the drug reaches the brain correlates with its addictive potential. Therefore, users with more advanced addictions commonly report a progression from snorting to intravenous use or the most rapid form of administration, smoking crack cocaine. Intravenous users are at risk for contracting hepatitis and HIV, as well as developing phlebitis and endocarditis. Treatment relies on psychotherapeutic approaches such as self-help, contingency management, and cognitive-behavioral therapy. Despite multiple medication trials, no drug effectively treats cocaine dependence.

Opiates

Among the opiates, heroin may be the most widely recognized drug of abuse. In 2000, there were an estimated 1,000,000 heroin addicts. There is concern that this number will increase because heroin has become less expensive in some parts of the country. All opiates have some abuse potential depending upon a specific drug's potency and its route of administration. Not only are illicit opiates abused, but the abuse of opiate analgesics such as methadone, hydromorphone (Dilaudid), oxycodone (OxyContin), and fentanyl (Duragesic) is also common.

Signs of intoxication include sedation, mild euphoria, pinpoint pupils, bradycardia, and low blood pressure. Overdose on drugs within the opiate class produces a reduced level of consciousness that may progress to coma and respiratory depression. When overdose is suspected, naloxone (Narcan), a synthetic opioid antagonist, can be administered to reverse the opiate's effects; the initial dose of 0.4 mg intravenously (IV) (0.01 mg/kg) can be repeated every 2 to 3 minutes as clinically indicated. Naloxone may be administered intramuscularly or subcutaneously if necessary. If the patient does not respond to a dose of 5 to 10 mg, opiate overdose is doubtful.

There is a well-defined withdrawal syndrome that occurs when an opiate is discontinued in one who is physiologically dependent (Table 4). Symptoms of withdrawal from a short-acting drug such as heroin begin within a few hours; withdrawal symptoms from a long-acting opiate such as methadone begin within 3 to 4 days. Opiate withdrawal is not a medical emergency in otherwise healthy adults. However, it is uncomfortable and may be a strong trigger for continued drug use.

TABLE 4 Symptoms of Opiate Withdrawal

	Objective	Subjective
Early	Lacrimation Rhinorrhea Diaphoresis Yawning	
Middle	Dilated pupils Piloerection	Restlessness Irritability Insomnia
Late	Tachycardia Increased blood pressure Vomiting Diarrhea Mood lability	Bone pain Nausea Abdominal cramps Depression

There are several ways to address opiate withdrawal. In the context of a prescription medication being stopped too abruptly, the simplest approach is to restart the medication and reduce it more slowly. Planned detoxification is often accomplished by substituting methadone (Dolophine), a long-acting opioid agonist, for the shorter-acting opiate. With this method, the patient is stabilized on a methadone dose that blocks significant withdrawal. A dose of 40 mg given in divided doses during the day is adequate to block significant withdrawal symptoms in most patients. The stabilizing dose is tapered over several days. Clonidine (Catapres)[1] is a nonopiate that can be used to treat opiate withdrawal. It is a centrally acting a_2-agonist that reduces autonomic symptoms such as vomiting, diarrhea, and sweating (Table 5).

Methadone maintenance is the mainstay treatment for dependence on illicit opiates. The Food and Drug Administration (FDA) approved methadone for opioid maintenance therapy in 1972. Federal regulations placed tight restrictions on methadone programs that include special state and federal licensing. These restrictions have had an unintended effect of limiting treatment access for some opiate-addicted patients. Methadone maintenance treatment is criticized for a number of reasons:

- There is a risk that dispensed methadone will be sold on the street.
- Daily administration is inconvenient for patients.
- Some facilities offer inadequate adjunctive psychosocial or therapy services.

Despite concerns, methadone maintenance is effective in reducing criminal activity among heroin addicts, in decreasing the risk of HIV and hepatitis acquired through needle-sharing, and in returning some addicts to functional lifestyles.

Another synthetic opiate agonist, levomethadyl (Orlaam), is approved for maintenance therapy. This agent is also federally regulated. It has an advantage of a long half-life, allowing for less frequent dosing than methadone. However, it can prolong the QT interval, and this may account for the reluctance of some approved facilities to prescribe it.

Alternatively, an opiate antagonist may be useful for treatment of opiate addiction. Naltrexone (ReVia) blocks the euphoric effects of opiates. This medication should only be prescribed once a patient is opiate-free for 7 to 10 days, in order to avoid a precipitated withdrawal syndrome. The typical dose of naltrexone is 50 mg daily, often initiated at 25 mg daily to reduce the risk of sedation and nausea. One group that has benefited from naltrexone maintenance is health care professionals who participate in a comprehensive recovery plan and are carefully monitored by state licensing boards.

Buprenorphine (Subutex) is a mixed opioid agonist–antagonist that was recently approved for the treatment of opiate addiction. A product (Suboxone) that combines buprenorphine with the opioid-antagonist naloxone reduces the risk of medication diversion for intravenous use. Office-based clinicians, including primary care physicians, may prescribe buprenorphine for treatment of opiate addiction after taking an approved training course and receiving a special waiver from the Drug Enforcement Agency. It is unclear to what extent approval of this newest agent will improve the care of opiate addicts. The potential advantages include greater convenience for patients, decreased risk of drug diversion, additional options for less severely addicted individuals, and fewer federal regulations for practitioners.

Patients at greatest risk for prescription opiate dependence include those who abuse other substances and those with a history of illicit opiate abuse. Patients with chronic pain are at risk for opiate dependence when increasing doses of medication are needed to control pain. It is advisable for clinicians who are unsure about prescribing opiates to seek the opinions of other professionals, especially when treating patients with chronic, nonmalignant pain.

Benzodiazepines

Benzodiazepines are used most often in the outpatient setting for the treatment of anxiety and insomnia. They have replaced barbiturates as the sedative–hypnotic of choice because of a greater safety profile in overdose. Benzodiazepines act on the brain's γ-aminobutyric acid (GABA) receptors, which results in relaxation and mild sedation. Signs of intoxication with benzodiazepines are similar to those experienced with alcohol, with higher doses producing greater sedation, slurred speech, and ataxia. However, benzodiazepines may be used as anesthetics, whereas alcohol is lethal in very high doses. In serious overdoses where benzodiazepines are suspected to play a role, the benzodiazepine antagonist flumazenil (Romazicon) may be administered at a dose of 0.2 mg IV over 30 seconds and repeated up to a 3 mg total dose. There is a risk of seizures in sedative-dependent individuals and in

[1]Not FDA approved for this indication.

TABLE 5 Opioid Treatment Summary*

Treatment of Opioid Overdose

Drug	Administration
Naloxone (Narcan)	Initial dose 0.4 mg IV (0.01 mg/kg) Repeat every 2-3 minutes as indicated by symptoms Reevaluate diagnosis if no response to 5-10 mg total

Sample Methadone Detoxification†

Day	Drug	Administration
Day 1	Methadone 40 mg (Dolophine)	Give initial dose of methadone 20 mg Additional doses of 10 or 20 mg may be given if withdrawal symptoms persist after 4 hours Maximum 40 mg total dose
Day 2-3	Methadone 25-30 mg	Reduce dose by 25% daily
Day 4	Methadone 20 mg	
Day 5	Methadone 10 mg	
Day 6	Methadone 5 mg	
Day 7	Discontinue	

Sample Clonidine Detoxification‡

Day	From Short-Acting Opioid	With or Without Naltrexone (ReVia)Induction	From Methadone
Day 1-2	0.3-0.6 mg	12.5 mg	0.3-0.6 mg
Day 3	0.3-0.8 mg	25 mg	0.4-0.6 mg
Day 4-5	0.6-1.2 mg Then reduce total daily dose by 50% each day, not to exceed 0.4 mg/d	50 mg Continue maintenance therapy	0.5-0.8 mg
Day 6-10			0.6-1.2 mg Then reduce total daily dose by 50% each day, not to exceed 0.4 mg/d

*All treatment must be individualized to meet specific patient needs and adjusted based on response to treatment.
†May be used in combination with clonidine (Catapres) or other as-needed medications. Catapres is not FDA approved for this indication.
‡Give a test dose of clonidine 0.1 mg. Continue only if blood pressure >85/55. Clonidine 0.1-0.2 mg every 2-4 hours, hold for systolic blood pressure <85 or diastolic blood pressure <55.

patients taking benzodiazepines as part of an antiepileptic regimen.

Benzodiazepines are effective in treating alcohol withdrawal. The symptoms of sedative withdrawal and alcohol withdrawal are similar—insomnia, anxiety, tachycardia, elevated blood pressure, and fever. In addition, seizures and delirium can be serious sequelae of an untreated alcohol- or sedative-withdrawal syndrome. Whereas opiate withdrawal is not a life-threatening condition unless it occurs in the context of medical frailty, untreated benzodiazepine withdrawal may result in death.

When a patient is addicted to a benzodiazepine and needs detoxification, it is common practice to substitute a long-acting benzodiazepine for a short-acting one. Table 6 gives an approximation of equivalent doses to ease the conversion from one medication to another. Once the patient is comfortable on the long-acting benzodiazepines, the dosage is gradually reduced and discontinued. However withdrawal does not always go smoothly and medication adjustments may be needed. The reduction schedule varies depending upon the severity of the addiction, the duration of benzodiazepine use, and the dosage used.

Hospitalized patients who are addicted to high doses of benzodiazepines often do well when converted to an equivalent dose of a long-acting agent such as clonazepam (Klonopin) or chlordiazepoxide (Librium). Then the dose may be reduced on a 10% per day schedule. In these patients it is necessary to monitor vital signs every 4 hours and have additional doses of benzodiazepine ordered for signs of withdrawal. Such signs include tremulousness, diaphoresis, blood pressure higher than 150/100, and heart rate more than 100. Outpatients may require several weeks to months for detoxification. Some treatment centers use anticonvulsants, specifically valproic acid (Depakote)[1] and carbamazepine (Tegretol)[1], to prevent or minimize withdrawal symptoms.

Other Drugs of Abuse

Clinicians may deal with any number of abused substances. The popularity of particular drugs changes over time. However, there are several types

[1]Not FDA approved for this indication.

TABLE 6 Approximate Benzodiazepine Dose Equivalency

Generic Name (Trade Name)	Dose Equivalents (mg)*	Short- or Long-Acting
Alprazolam (Xanax)	1	Short
Chlordiazepoxide (Librium)	25	Long
Clonazepam (Klonopin)	0.5	Long
Diazepam (Valium)	10	Long
Flurazepam (Dalmane)	30	Long
Lorazepam (Ativan)	2	Short
Oxazepam (Serax)	30	Short
Prazepam (Centrax)	10	Long
Temazepam (Restoril)	20	Short
Triazolam (Halcion)	0.25	Short

*Doses are approximately equivalent to phenobarbital 30 mg.

of substances that come up frequently enough to warrant inclusion here. One example is the inhalants. The agents that make up this group are inexpensive and accessible in common household products such as glue, shoe polish, paint thinners, aerosols, and correction and cleaning fluids. Intoxication on these agents most resembles alcohol intoxication. Acute overdose is rare but can result in death from asphyxiation or cardiac arrhythmia. The brain, kidneys, and liver are susceptible to damage from repeated inhalant exposure. The result over the long term may be chronic delirium, psychosis, or renal failure. An estimated 15% of young adults have tried an inhalant. However, it is estimated that less than 1% are addicted to inhalant use.

Hallucinogens are another group of abusable drugs. Management of intoxication on these drugs is supportive in most cases. Lysergic acid diethylamide (LSD) is a well-known drug in this class. Like most hallucinogens it produces visual hallucinations and increases sensory awareness. Intoxication can also cause dilated pupils, facial flushing, tachycardia, and increased blood pressure. 3,4-Methylenedioxymethamphetamine (MDMA), or ecstasy, may be classified as either a hallucinogen or a stimulant because it has properties of both. It is generally considered a dangerous drug because of its potential for long-term brain damage. It may also be toxic to the heart and liver.

Phencyclidine (PCP) intoxication can have a frightening presentation. The patient may become agitated and unpredictable, requiring physical and chemical restraints to ensure the safety of the patient and those around him or her. Medication may not be necessary if the patient is placed in a quiet, supportive setting. If medications are used, benzodiazepines are typically chosen first. If antipsychotics are required, agents with low anticholinergic activity are preferred. Toxic doses of PCP can produce a life-threatening condition with severe autonomic instability in which hypertension, hyperthermia, convulsions, and coma may become serious medical management problems.

Treatment

While medication management is increasingly important in the treatment of alcohol and drug dependence, nonpharmacologic approaches are the mainstay of substance abuse treatment. Alcoholics Anonymous (AA) helped many alcoholics recover before physicians had treatment techniques to offer. AA remains a proven resource, and other self-help groups are modeled after it. Narcotics Anonymous (NA) and Cocaine Anonymous (CA), similar to AA, are pivotal in the recovery of some drug abusers. The caveat is that one group may be very different from another.

There are significant problems in some self-help groups. Patients may have concerns about heavy cigarette-smoking in meetings, about attendees who actively use or sell drugs, and about criticism of prescribed psychotropic medications. Therefore, when a patient finds one group unsatisfactory for some reason, the clinician can suggest he or she try another group. Some patients object to the religious tone of traditional 12-step groups. For these individuals alternative groups such as Women for Sobriety and Rational Recovery may be more acceptable. In addition, self-help groups are free of charge, which is a factor for some patients.

Most professional addiction treatment occurs in an outpatient setting. However, higher levels of care are available in hospital, residential, or partial hospital programs if there are chaotic living situations, or pressing psychiatric or other medical needs. Social interventions are crucial for patients faced with unemployment, legal consequences, and housing dilemmas. Psychiatric

TABLE 7 Benzodiazepine Treatment Summary*

Treatment of Overdose

Drug	Administration
Flumazenil (Romazicon)	Initial dose 0.2 mg IV over 30 seconds Repeat every minute up to a 3 mg total dose. Re-evaluate diagnosis if no response after 3-5 minutes.

Detoxification Guidelines

Day	Action
Day 1	Long-acting benzodiazepine until symptom control is achieved. Common upper limits are clonazepam (Klonopin) 6-8 mg per 24 hours or chlordiazepoxide (Librium) 400 mg per 24 hours.
Day 2–Completion	Taper by 25% every 1-2 days Monitor vital signs every 4 hours Have PRN doses available, i.e., clonazepam, 1 mg, chlordiazepoxide, 25 mg, for signs or symptoms of withdrawal (tremulousness, diaphoresis, systolic blood pressure >150, diastolic blood pressure >100, or heart rate >100). Consider adding anticonvulsants.

*All treatment must be individualized to meet specific patient needs and adjusted based on response to treatment.

disorders occur with a high frequency in drug abusing populations, and both disorders should be treated to optimize the patient's chances for recovery. Therefore, a multidisciplinary approach to treatment often works best.

Psychiatric symptoms in patients who abuse drugs are easy to recognize. Mood lability, depression, and anxiety are common. The challenge lies in sorting out whether these symptoms are caused by the use of a mood altering substance or represent a separate mood or anxiety disorder. Psychiatric expertise may be needed to assist in sorting out this diagnostic dilemma. Patients with schizophrenic and bipolar disorders are also at high risk for drug abuse, which can exacerbate psychoses.

The cognitive aspects of professional treatment often include educational, motivational, cognitive–behavioral, relapse prevention, and 12-step strategies. Most treatment programs try to get the patient to more fully recognize the problems associated with his or her drug use, identify reasons to change, acknowledge obstacles to sobriety, become aware of triggers to relapse, and consider ways to build a sober support network. Patients with addictive disorders do get better, and treatment of patients with drug abuse can be highly rewarding. It is important to recognize this problem as one of many chronic, relapsing conditions seen in medicine today.

ANXIETY DISORDERS

METHOD OF

Lawrence R. Wu, MD

Feeling anxious or requests for a "nerve pill" are among the most common chief complaints encountered in a primary care practice. The National Co-morbidity study estimates that 25% of the general population experiences pathologic anxiety at some time during their lifetime. Anxiety disorders are associated with increased medical use and expenditures. More often than not, anxiety disorders are likely to manifest with somatic symptoms in the primary care setting.

The spectrum of anxiety disorders includes panic disorder and agoraphobia, generalized anxiety disorder (GAD), obsessive-compulsive disorder (OCD), phobic disorder (including social phobia), and post-traumatic stress disorder (PTSD). Making a specific diagnosis within this spectrum is essential because each of these disorders responds to specific pharmacotherapy and psychotherapy.

In many situations, anxiety can be adaptive. Some stress is necessary to improve performance in our daily lives, resulting often in personal growth and development. When anxiety interferes with the functions of daily living, causes distress, or is difficult to control, anxiety is pathologic and requires treatment.

The approach to anxiety should recognize that anxiety and depression are often co-morbid conditions. Selective serotonin reuptake inhibitors (SSRIs), which were designed to treat depression, are also effective for many anxiety disorders. In spite of the availability of these medications (Table 1), psychotherapy is the preferred initial treatment for post-traumatic stress disorder and phobia disorders.

Assessment and Diagnosis

Symptoms of anxiety should prompt a mental status exam and brief physical exam to assess for organic causes. Expressing interest and a willingness to listen to the patient are essential for diagnosis and are often therapeutic for the patient. The duration and frequency of symptoms, the quality of the distress, the precipitating events or cues (if any), associated symptoms, and relieving factors should be elicited from the patient. Associated symptoms can be somatic as well as psychiatric.

Asking the patient about any situations that they tend to avoid, the effect of the worry on behaviors, and the quality of sleep can clarify the specific type of anxiety present. Intensive feelings of fear or doom suggest a panic disorder, whereas reminders and intrusive thoughts about a terrible event in the past point to PTSD. Avoidance of people or anxiety performing in front of people is the hallmark of social phobia disorder, whereas recurrent thoughts or behaviors that are strange to the patient or others suggest OCD.

As with all psychiatric complaints, patients should be assessed for thoughts of harming themselves or others and the ability to perform the activities of daily living in their current situation. Questioning the patient about signs and symptoms of depression is recommended, because depression is often a coexisting or the primary psychiatric disorder.

Assessing for anxiety is also recommended when patients complain of multiple, unexplained somatic symptoms. Concurrent attention to the mental health evaluation is recommended in situations where the provider is investigating for physical causes of anxiety.

Review of the patient's medicines, use of illicit drugs (and/or alcohol), and past medical history will often reveal physical causes of anxiety. Hyperthyroidism and pulmonary disorders, particularly hypercapnia, can cause symptoms of anxiety. Medications that can cause anxiety include albuterol, theophylline, and sympathetic nervous system agonists. Weight loss, tachycardia, or heat intolerance on history/physical exam should be a clue to hyperthyroidism.

TABLE 1 Common Medications Used in the Treatment of Anxiety

Medication	Starting Dose (mg)	Therapeutic Range (mg/d)	Common Side Effects	Indications (Underline Indicates FDA Approved)
Selective Serotonin Reuptake Inhibitors				
Citalopram (Celexa)	10	10-60	Nausea, somnolence, dry mouth	PD/AG, OCD, PTSD, SP, GAD
Escitalopram (Lexapro)	10	10-20	Nausea, ejaculation failure, insomnia	<u>GAD</u>
Fluoxetine (Prozac)	5-10	10-80	Nausea, anorexia, insomnia, somnolence	<u>OCD</u>, <u>PD/AG</u>, PTSD, SP, GAD
Fluvoxamine (Luvox)	50	50-300	Nausea, insomnia, somnolence, headache	OCD, PD/AG, PTSD, SP, GAD
Paroxetine (Paxil)	10	10-50	Nausea, somnolence, ejaculation failure	<u>OCD</u>, <u>PD/AG</u>, <u>SP</u>, <u>PTSD</u>, <u>GAD</u>
Sertraline (Zoloft)	25	25-200	Nausea, insomnia, ejaculation failure	<u>OCD</u>, <u>PD/AG</u>, <u>PTSD</u>, <u>SP</u>, GAD
Novel Antidepressants				
Venlafaxine (Effexor XR)	37.5	37.5-225	Nausea, dry mouth, insomnia, dizziness	<u>GAD</u>, <u>SP</u>, PD/AG
Tricyclic Antidepressants				
Clomipramine (Anafranil)	25	25-250	Weight gain, sedation, dry mouth	<u>OCD</u>, PD/AG, PTSD, GAD
Imipramine (Tofranil)	10-25	150-300	Sedation, dry mouth	PD/AG, GAD, PTSD
Other Medications				
Buspirone (BuSpar)	7.5 bid	15-60	Dizziness, nausea	<u>GAD</u>
Propranolol (Inderal)	20	20-160	Depression, sedation	Performance anxiety
Hydroxyzine	25	50-100	Dry mouth, somnolence	<u>Anxiety</u>
Benzodiazepines				
Alprazolam (Xanax)	0.25 tid	4	Drowsiness, withdrawal	<u>GAD</u>, <u>PD/AG</u>, PTSD
Clonazepam (Klonopin)	0.25 bid	1	Somnolence, fatigue, depression	<u>PD/AG</u>, GAD, PTSD
Lorazepam (Ativan)	0.5 tid	6	Sedation, dizziness	GAD, PDAG, SP

Abbreviations: AG = agoraphobia; bid = twice daily; GAD = generalized anxiety disorder; OCD = obsessive-compulsive disorder; PD = panic disorder; PTSD = post-traumatic stress disorder; SP = specific phobia; tid = three times a day.

The diagnoses of specific anxiety disorders are based on clinical criteria adapted from the *Diagnostic and Statistical Manual of Mental Disorders*, 4th edition (DSM-IV)—Primary Care Version (Tables 2 through 6). These criteria assume that the provider has made a clinical judgment that the patient's symptoms are not caused by a physical disease and not solely caused by another mental health disorder. The clinician must be vigilant and consider that the patient will often have two or more psychiatric disorders.

Approach to Treatment

Successful treatment of anxiety in the primary care setting requires an interested health provider who is comfortable with the multiple modalities required to treat the anxious patient. Reassurance to the patient is necessary. The patient is told that anxiety is common and treatable and is reassured that asking for help is a positive first step. Cognitive restructuring and simple coping techniques can be taught by the interested primary care clinician and are covered in more detail, later. Certain aspects of lifestyle improve anxiety. For example, light aerobic exercise improves self-efficacy and can decrease anxiety.

The selective serotonin reuptake inhibitors are the mainstay of the treatment of anxiety. SSRIs are effective for OCD, panic disorders, phobias, PTSD, and GAD (see Table 1). Doses of SSRIs for anxiety disorders must be started at lower doses than are used for depression, to minimize the short-term agitation sometimes experienced with these medications. The patient should be counseled that side effects often

TABLE 2 Features of Generalized Anxiety Disorder

A. Excessive anxiety and worry, occurring >50% days over ≥6 months, causing distress or impairment in social, occupational, or other important areas of functioning.
B. Person finds it difficult to control the worry.
C. Anxiety and worry are associated with ≥3 out of the following 6 symptoms:
   1. Restlessness
   2. Fatigue
   3. Difficulty concentrating or mind going blank
   4. Irritability
   5. Muscle tension
   6. Difficulty sleeping or restless unsatisfying sleep

TABLE 3 Features of Panic Disorder with Agoraphobia

A. Recurrent unexpected panic attacks. Panic attacks are periods of intense fear or discomfort, in which ≥4 of the following symptoms abruptly appear and peak within 10 minutes:
   Palpitations, sweating, trembling, shortness of breath or smothering, feeling of choking, chest pain/discomfort, nausea/abdominal distress, feeling dizzy or faint, feelings of unreality, fear of losing control, fear of dying.
B. At least one of the attacks is followed by ≥1 month of ≥1 of the following:
   Worry about having additional attacks, worry about the consequences of the attack, change in behavior related to the attacks.
C. Agoraphobia is anxiety about being in places or situations from which escape or help may be difficult to obtain, such as being out of the home alone, or in crowds.

diminish with time, and that empirical switching to another SSRI may be necessary. Venlafaxine (Effexor XR), a novel antidepressant, has been approved for the treatment of GAD, and there is now evidence that chronic use of SSRIs is just as effective for GAD as benzodiazepines. Once stabilized, the duration of treatment is usually 6 to 12 months, at which time patients should be tapered from their medications. Patients with recurrent symptoms will likely need long-term pharmacologic treatment.

Although tricyclics have been used with success in anxiety disorders, drowsiness, anticholinergic side effects, and toxicity have made these medications less popular. Imipramine (Tofranil)[1] is effective for panic disorder and preferred if a sedating medication is required.

Benzodiazepines are the oldest class of medications used to treat anxiety (see Table 1). Although they have the advantage of rapid onset of action, they carry the risks of dependence, sedation, falls in the elderly, and road traffic accidents. Withdrawal syndromes resulting in rebound anxiety, even reactions as severe as delirium tremens, are possible. The prescribing

[1]Not FDA approved for this indication.

TABLE 4 Features of Specific Phobia

A. Marked and persistent fear that is excessive or unreasonable, is recognized as such by the patient, and is cued by a specific precipitant (flying, heights, closed spaces, for example).
B. Exposure to the precipitant invariably provokes an immediate anxiety response, such as a panic attack.
C. The phobic situation is avoided and such avoidance interferes significantly with social, occupational, or other important areas of functioning.
D. Types of phobias may be classified into specific animal type, natural environment type, blood-injection-injury type, situational type, or other type. Social phobia is the fear of one or more social or performance situations in which the person is exposed to unfamiliar people or to scrutiny by others.

TABLE 5 Features of Post-traumatic Stress Disorder

A. Person has experienced a **traumatic event** that involved actual or threatened death/serious injury to self or others with a response of fear, helplessness, or horror.
B. The traumatic event is **persistently re-experienced** in recurrent and intrusive recollections of the event, recurrent distressing dreams, perceptions of reliving such as dissociative flashback episodes, intensive psychological distress or physiological reactions when exposed to cues that may represent the event.
C. Persistent **avoidance** of the stimuli associated with the trauma and **numbing** of general responsiveness, as in efforts to avoid thoughts/conversations associated with the trauma, efforts to avoid activities/places/people that arouse recollections, inability to recall an important aspect of the event, markedly diminished interest in significant activities, feeling of detachment or estrangement from others, restricted range of expressed emotions, and/or sense of foreshortened future such as not expecting to have a career or marriage.
D. Persistent symptoms of increased arousal such as difficulty falling asleep, irritability or outbursts of anger, difficulty concentrating, hypervigilance, exaggerated startle.
E. Duration of disturbances in B, C, D is >1 month and interferes with social, occupational, or other important areas of functioning.

provider must inform the patient and family about these risks. Benzodiazepines should be avoided in patients with a past history of substance abuse, personality disorder, and/or dosage escalation. These medications are ideal for patients who experience infrequent bouts of anxiety or episodes of anxiety-related insomnia. Shorter acting benzodiazepines such as clonazepam (Klonopin)[1] have been studied for use in specific anxiety disorders, while little research has been done using older benzodiazepines (with longer half-lives) in specific anxiety disorders.

Buspirone (BuSpar) is a nonbenzodiazepine indicated for generalized anxiety disorder. In head-to-head trials, it works as well as benzodiazepines for GAD, but it has a slower onset of action and is not sedating. It is, therefore, less useful for the anxious patient who needs a sedative. It does not impair alertness and lacks abuse potential.

β-Blockers are effective and the preferred treatment for performance anxiety such as public speaking. These medications are taken before the anxiety-provoking

[1]Not FDA approved for this indication.

TABLE 6 Features of Obsessive-Compulsive Disorder

A. Patients may have either obsessions or compulsions. Obsessions are recurrent thoughts, impulses, or images that cause marked anxiety or distress that are experienced as intrusive. Compulsions are ritualistic behaviors or mental acts that are performed in response to an obsession or according to rules that must be applied rigidly.
B. The obsessions or compulsions are excessive, occupy more than 1 hour per day, are distressing, and interfere with a person's social, occupational, or other important areas of functioning.

event. β-Blockers are rarely effective for other forms of anxiety.

Although monoamine oxidase inhibitors have been effective for anxiety, their interaction with common foods (and medicines such as meperidine [Demerol]), causing malignant hypertension, have limited their use to psychiatrists familiar with their use and only after other medications have failed.

Kava kava (*Piper methysticum*)[1], an alternative medicine and an extract of the oceanic kava plant, is superior to placebo in treating GAD. Case reports of liver toxicity and skin reactions have limited its use.

Recent studies have shown that gabapentin (Neurontin)[1], 600 to 1800 mg per day, can be effective as monotherapy or as an adjunct for the treatment of GAD. Use of this medication should be limited to practitioners familiar with the medication, and it should be a second-line therapy.

Treatment of Specific Anxiety Disorders

Table 2 lists the criteria for GAD. While some complain of worry, patients with GAD are most likely to present with somatic symptoms in the primary care setting. Many of these patients will readily admit to worry and stresses, when asked. Most primary care clinicians can provide simple supportive therapy consisting of listening empathetically to the patient's perception of stresses. Disabling episodes of anxiety may require a short course of benzodiazepines for stabilization. Persistent anxiety will require chronic treatment with buspirone (BuSpar) or an SSRI, starting at a low dose. Venlafaxine (Effexor XR), a novel antidepressant, is effective and has been FDA approved for GAD. Dosing of venlafaxine starts at 75 mg per day and is titrated upward to 225 mg per day. Cognitive behavior therapy (as described later) is helpful and may require referral.

Panic disorder is distinguished from GAD in that the panic disorder requires at least four somatic symptoms (see Table 3). Although these symptoms often warrant a search for a physical condition, the patient should be concurrently educated about the possibility of panic disorder and its treatability. Patients younger than 35 years of age who have unexplained, recurrent physical symptoms are more likely to have panic. Coexisting depression is common with panic disorders, as is agoraphobia. Patients with panic disorder benefit from medication with adjunctive psychotherapy. Infrequent panic attacks can be treated with benzodiazepines such as alprazolam (Xanax) or clonazepam (Klonopin)[1]. Chronic or frequent attacks can be treated with SSRIs or tricyclic antidepressants. Because side effects of these classes of medications can be particularly troubling to these patients, especially stimulation from SSRIs, initial dosing should begin at significantly lower doses than doses used for depression.

[1]Not FDA approved for this indication.

Imipramine (Tofranil)[1] and clomipramine (Anafranil)[1] are the best studied among TCAs and should be started at 10 mg per day, with increases of 10 mg dosing every 3 to 4 days. Among SSRIs, paroxetine (Paxil) should be started at 10 mg per day, fluoxetine (Prozac)[1] at 10 mg per day, or sertraline (Zoloft)[1] at 25 mg per day. Although monoamine oxidase inhibitors (MAOIs) are effective for panic, severe interactions with foods and other medications limit their use, and they should be used only by psychiatrists. Supportive therapy by the provider can be effective in establishing trust between the provider and patient. Cognitive behavioral approaches, exposure therapy (if there is a feared stimulus), and relaxation therapy can be helpful in relieving milder panic attacks.

Table 4 lists the criteria for a simple phobia. An example of a common phobia is fear of flying. Initial therapy should consist of psychotherapeutic approaches because they provide longer lasting benefits than medications. Cognitive behavioral therapy consists of reviewing maladaptive automatic thoughts, analyzing assumptions, role playing, and having successful encounters with phobic situations. Social skills training may be required for patients with social phobia. Patients with phobias should be referred for such therapy with experienced providers. SSRIs, which improve social anxiety among patients with social phobia, include paroxetine (Paxil), sertraline (Zoloft), and Venlafaxine (Effexor XR)[1].

Lifetime risk of PTSD is estimated to be 1% to 14%. High-risk populations include victims of sexual assault and war veterans. Table 5 lists the criteria for PTSD. Psychotherapy should be the initial approach to PTSD. Supportive therapy consisting of empathic listening in the setting of a safe environment can be provided by the primary care physician, even in the context of a short visit. Persistent symptoms require referral to a more experienced therapist. SSRIs can decrease intrusive recollections and numbing. Medications should also be directed at co-morbid depression, panic, or phobias, if needed.

OCD begins most often in adolescence or early adulthood. Table 6 gives the DSM-IV criteria of OCD. A combination of behavioral therapy and medication is necessary for this disorder, yielding greater benefit than either modality alone. Behavioral therapy from an experienced therapist is useful for compulsive conditions. Although clomipramine (Anafranil) was the first medication useful for OCD, paroxetine (Paxil), sertraline (Zoloft), and other SSRIs are just as useful to decrease compulsions and intrusive obsessions. In OCD, medications may need to be prescribed at higher doses than for other forms of anxiety. Therapeutic benefits of medications make require 8 to 12 weeks.

Patients should be referred to more experienced mental health providers when the treatment modality exceeds the experience or interest of the primary care provider. Examples of such situations include

[1]Not FDA approved for this indication.

the need for psychotherapy, patients who threaten harm to themselves or others, patients unable to care for themselves, or those who fail to respond to pharmacotherapy as expected.

BULIMIA NERVOSA

METHOD OF

James E. Mitchell, MD, and

Tricia Cook Myers, PhD

Bulimia nervosa is an eating disorder that was first described as a discrete, common diagnostic entity by Gerald Russell in 1979. The disorder is characterized by binge-eating episodes, during which the individual consumes large amounts of food in a short period of time, frequently followed by self-induced vomiting or other compensatory behaviors, such as laxative abuse. Table 1 gives the *Diagnostic and Statistical Manual of Mental Disorders*, 4th ed. (DSM-IV) criteria for bulimia nervosa.

Most patients with bulimia nervosa who have been described in the literature, and in particular those who have been the focus of treatment research, have been of the purging subtype; very little is known about nonpurging patients who engage in other types of compensatory behaviors, such as excessive exercise or fasting, although these patients are occasionally seen in clinical practice.

In addition to the abnormal eating and compensatory behaviors, most of these patients can also be characterized by evidencing certain distinct psychological symptoms. In particular, most of them are very preoccupied with body weight and shape, and most fear that they are or will become overweight, despite the fact that most are of normal or low weight. These symptoms are similar to those seen in anorexia nervosa, although usually not as severe.

The disorder has been described in all socioeconomic groups. It does appear, however, to be seen most commonly among women in industrialized societies in which a high value is placed on slimness as a model of attractiveness for young women, and where food is freely available to the general population. Prevalence studies suggest that 1% to 2% of women in such societies develop the full disorder, while approximately 4% to 5% develop partial syndromes. Prevalence studies in preindustrial countries suggest that bulimia nervosa occurs rarely, but may be increasing in prevalence, with patients in these settings more likely to present with atypical characteristics. Also, recent data suggest that bulimia nervosa is more common in urban than rural areas.

The median age of onset of bulimia nervosa is approximately 18 years of age, but it can occur anytime during adolescence or young adulthood; it is rare for patients to report an age of onset beyond age 40 years. It is interesting that the age of onset clusters around the age of 18 years, this being the time when many young women are leaving home and going into the work force or to college. This crucial period of role transition seems to be a high-risk time for the development of this disorder.

TABLE 1 Diagnostic Criteria for Bulimia Nervosa

A. Recurrent episodes of binge-eating. An episode of binge-eating is characterized by both of the following:
   1. Eating, in a discrete period of time (e.g., within any 2-hour period), an amount of food that is definitely larger than most people would eat during a similar period of time and under similar circumstances.
   2. A sense of lack of control over eating during the episode (e.g., a feeling that one cannot stop eating or control what or how much one is eating).

B. Recurrent inappropriate compensatory behavior in order to prevent weight gain, such as self-induced vomiting; misuse of laxatives, diuretics, enemas, or other medications; fasting; or excessive exercise.

C. The binge-eating and inappropriate compensatory behaviors both occur, on average, at least twice a week for 3 months.

D. Self-evaluation is unduly influenced by body shape and weight.

E. The disturbance does not occur exclusively during episodes of anorexia nervosa.

Specify Type of Bulimia Nervosa

Purging type: During the current episode of bulimia nervosa, the person regularly engages in self-induced vomiting or the misuse of laxatives, diuretics, or enemas.

Nonpurging type: During the current episode of bulimia nervosa, the person uses other inappropriate compensatory behaviors, such as fasting or excessive exercise, but does not regularly engage in self-induced vomiting or the misuse of laxatives, diuretics, or enemas.

Diagnostic Criteria

As summarized in Table 1, the hallmark of the disorder is the binge-eating episode. Although at times these appear to be precipitated by discrete cues such as stressful events or unpleasant emotions, often the binge-eating episodes become an institutionalized activity, occurring usually late in the day when the individual returns home from work or school.

The caloric content of binge-eating episodes can vary dramatically, but commonly as many as 3000 to 5000 calories or more are consumed. The most frequently ingested binge-eating foods include those that are easily prepared and that tend to be high in fat and carbohydrates, ice cream being the most common binge food. These same foods tend to be avoided at times when the individual is not binge-eating.

Many individuals describe feeling "out of control" while binge-eating. After binge-eating they then engage in some compensatory behaviors, most often self-induced vomiting. At other times they may ingest drugs as a way of attempting to precipitate weight loss, for example, take large numbers of laxatives or diuretics, both of which result in a decrease in body weight through the loss of fluid rather than ingested calories. Rarely, patients with bulimia nervosa use ipecac to induce vomiting, which is particularly dangerous given the dose-dependent cardiomyopathy that this agent can cause.

Co-morbidity

Although some individuals with bulimia nervosa are relatively free of other problems, it is more common to encounter co-morbid psychopathologic conditions in these patients. Most often seen are affective disorders, particularly recurrent depression. The prevalence of anxiety disorders appears high as well. Co-morbid substance abuse problems also have received considerable attention, because they markedly complicate the treatment of patients. These patients appear to be at increased risk for the abuse of both typical substances of abuse (such as alcohol) and atypical substances of abuse (such as laxatives, diuretics, diet pills, and ipecac). Screening for both types of problems should be part of a routine evaluation.

Bulimia nervosa has also been associated with certain personality disorders, particularly Cluster B, Axis II disorders such as borderline personality disorder. Such individuals generally are characterized by poor insight, problems with affect regulation, impulsivity, and difficulties with interpersonal relationships.

Medical Complications and Medical Management

Most patients with bulimia nervosa are at a relatively normal body weight, and one does not usually see the marked physical changes associated with starvation that one encounters with anorexia nervosa patients. However, despite a grossly normal body weight, many patients with bulimia nervosa evidence subtle changes suggestive of malnutrition, including, on screening laboratory examination, elevations in β-hydroxybutyric acid and free fatty acid levels, and fasting hypoglycemia. Interestingly, brain imaging studies using computed tomography (CT) or magnetic resonance imaging (MRI) have demonstrated pseudoatrophy in some patients with bulimia nervosa, again suggesting problems with malnutrition, although the degree of atrophy is usually less severe than in anorexia nervosa.

On physical examination there are a few clues that are useful in making this diagnosis. The best area of focus is the teeth. Recurrent episodes of vomiting are associated with decalcification of the dental surfaces that are exposed to the vomitus, and the majority of patients who have been actively vomiting for more than 4 years have obvious evidence of enamel erosion. Interestingly, the amalgams or fillings are relatively resistant to the acid and therefore often project above the surface of the teeth.

Some patients with bulimia nervosa evidence salivary gland hypertrophy, often involving the parotid glands, which at times can be dramatic and which may persist intermittently for several months during recovery. Some patients with bulimia nervosa also show callus or scar formation on the dorsum of the hand or knuckles, resulting from trauma to these areas when using the hand to stimulate the gag reflex to induce vomiting.

On laboratory testing, patients with bulimia nervosa not uncommonly evidence fluid and electrolyte abnormalities. Metabolic alkalosis and hypochloremia are most commonly seen, and hypokalemia is occasionally seen. Edema generally is suggestive of laxative or diuretic abuse, both of which result in reflex fluid retention.

Many patients with bulimia nervosa have a variety of gastrointestinal complaints including constipation, diarrhea, bloating after eating, abdominal pain, and dyspepsia. Gastric dilation and rupture have also been reported and, although rare, may be the leading cause of death in these patients. Various subtle endocrine abnormalities have been described in bulimic patients.

Etiology

There are three variables that correlate highly with the development of the disorder:

1. Female sex: bulimia nervosa is rare in males, who account for only 2% to 8% of the cases.
2. Age of onset in teen to early adult years: bulimia nervosa seems to develop in the context of dieting during adolescence or early adulthood, and rarely outside of this context.
3. Cultural variables: bulimia nervosa and other similar eating disorders appear to exist almost exclusively in societies in which a high positive value is placed on slimness as a model of attractiveness, and where obesity is disparaged.

However, all three of these variables identify a very large group of girls and women, most of whom do not develop full-blown eating disorders or bulimia nervosa. The reason why some move from experimentation to ongoing problems is unclear, although genetic studies suggest there may be genetic diathesis for the development of this disorder.

Other risk factors appear important, including a history of sexual abuse in childhood, a history of excessive weight prior to illness onset, and overweight parents. It is possible that certain physiologic changes that develop in the course of the eating disorder perpetuate the behavior. For example, recent studies suggest that metabolism of serotonin, a neurotransmitter involved in appetite and impulse regulation, may be abnormal in patients with bulimia nervosa. Also, elevated levels of the peptide ghrelin, known to increase appetite, have been found in bulimic patients. Bulimic patients may also have impaired satiety responses, including impaired peripheral release of satiety hormones such as cholecystokinin. Additionally, gastric capacity is increased in bulimic patients, which may further alleviate fullness after normal intake.

Diagnosis and Treatment

The most important ingredient in the diagnosis of eating disorders is a high index of suspicion. Disorders of mood and eating are common enough in adolescent girls and young adult women that questions about such problems should be included in the routine evaluation of such patients. The physician should routinely inquire about the presence of binge-eating, protracted fasting, and compensatory behaviors such as self-induced vomiting. Also, it is useful to inquire about body image. A straightforward, nonjudgmental approach will increase the likelihood of a valid response.

Most patients with bulimia nervosa can be successfully treated out of the hospital. However, they tend to be somewhat difficult to work with for many health professionals, and the available treatment studies suggest that they do best in structured programs that use techniques designed specially to treat this group. Hospitalization may be considered in patients who fail to respond to outpatient treatment, who are co-morbidly depressed to the point where suicide is of concern, or for whom mental instability is a problem.

The treatment literature on bulimia nervosa has centered on the parallel development of two strategies—pharmacologic strategies, primarily using antidepressant drugs, and psychotherapy or counseling approaches. We discuss each in turn.

PHARMACOTHERAPIES

Many placebo-controlled, double-blind antidepressant trials of bulimia nervosa have been published, and the results are fairly consistent in showing that antidepressant drugs do have a potent and significant suppressant effect on binge-eating and purging behavior. The available studies suggest that individuals who are not depressed at baseline may respond equally well to antidepressant treatments, suggesting that the mechanism of action may be other than the antidepressant effect. Many tricyclic antidepressant compounds and monoamine oxidase (MAO) inhibitors have been used experimentally. However, in recent years, the serotonin reuptake inhibitors have become the agents of choice, mainly because they appear to be equally as efficacious as the older agents, but better tolerated. The agent that has been studied in the most subjects, including in two large multicenter trials, is fluoxetine hydrochloride (Prozac); this drug appears to work optimally in these patients at dosages higher than those usually employed in the treatment of depression (e.g., 60 mg per day).

Although there are dramatic and significant reductions in the frequency of target eating behaviors with antidepressant treatment, and impressive improvement in symptoms of mood, many patients with bulimia nervosa remain symptomatic despite antidepressant treatment. This raises questions as to whether or not antidepressants are in themselves a sufficient treatment for these patients.

Several studies have examined the combined use of antidepressants and psychotherapy, and these studies suggest that for eating disorder symptoms, certain psychotherapy approaches are probably superior; however, there is some evidence that on certain variables, such as depression, anxiety, and in some eating disorder symptoms, the combination is best. Therefore, consideration should be given to treatment with combined drug therapy and psychotherapy when both are available.

PSYCHOTHERAPY

Paralleling the interest in antidepressant treatment, a fairly large treatment literature on psychotherapy approaches has developed. Initial studies compared active treatments with waiting-list control groups or minimal interventions; more recently psychotherapy studies have progressed to the point at which active treatments are being compared and dismantling studies are being undertaken. The results of these studies are quite consistent in showing that cognitive behavioral therapy (CBT) techniques, delivered in either group or individual formats, appear to be as effective as or more effective than the comparison treatments that have been used. There are a number of common elements among these CBT treatments:

1. There is strong emphasis on nutritional counseling. In many of the programs patients are given a structured meal-planning system at the beginning of treatment and strongly encouraged to eat regular, balanced meals, while treatment focuses on the problem of dietary restraint as a precipitant to binge-eating.
2. Other behavioral techniques are employed, such as examining cues associated with binge-eating and the consequences of the behavior (both positive and negative). Many of these programs also focus on cognitive restructuring techniques around weight and shape concerns and irrational beliefs about food and dieting.
3. Self-monitoring is also very useful. Research shows that simply having patients record when

and how much they are binge-eating can be very helpful in teaching them to gain control of the behavior.
4. Family involvement may be useful, particularly for younger patients who are living at home.

One other form of structured psychotherapy, interpersonal therapy (IPT) has also been shown to be effective in two additional studies.

COURSE AND OUTCOME

Unfortunately, many patients with bulimia nervosa go untreated and have the illness chronically or in a chronic relapsing fashion over many years. Carefully designed research studies show that using structured techniques, 40% to 70% of patients with bulimia nervosa can learn to control their eating behavior during the course of a relatively short-term therapy (e.g., 3 to 4 months). However, 15% to 20% of these patients will later relapse, usually within 6 months after treatment. Long-term follow-up, at 10 to 15 years following evaluation, suggests that upwards of 80% of individuals eventually improve significantly or completely recover.

DELIRIUM

METHOD OF

Ondria C. Gleason, MD

Delirium is an alteration in mental state caused by an underlying medical problem or effect of medication or substance. The presence of delirium often indicates a more severe form of medical illness and is associated with increased morbidity and mortality. Delirium can mimic a number of primary psychiatric conditions. Table 1 lists its characteristic signs and symptoms.

TABLE 1 Signs and Symptoms of Delirium

Disturbance of consciousness with impaired attention
Cognitive dysfunction
Memory impairment and disorientation may incorrectly be attributed to dementia unless reliable history is obtained regarding the timing of the onset of symptoms
Acute onset
Symptom onset must be obtained from a reliable source
Fluctuating course throughout the day
Agitation
Apathy and withdrawal
Most evident in the hypoactive form of delirium; easily confused with depression due to the associated blunted affect, decreased appetite, decreased motivation and disrupted sleep pattern
Sleep disturbance
Intermittent daytime sleepiness; nighttime agitation
Emotional lability
Wide range of emotions may be observed during the course of delirium, including anxiety, sadness, and euphoria
Perceptual disturbances
Visual and auditory hallucinations; delusions, often a product of disorientation and memory impairment

Differentiation from Primary Psychiatric Disorders

Visual hallucinations suggest an underlying metabolic disturbance or adverse effect of medication or substances and may be formed (people, animals) or unformed (lines, lights).

In delirium, the electroencephalogram (EEG) will show a diffuse background slowing, which may be described as "medication effect" or "encephalopathy" by the neurologist. Delirium tremens is an exception, where fast activity is observed. The EEG may detect seizure activity, both ictal and postictal states, as well as nonconvulsive status epilepticus, all of which could be underlying causes of delirium. Normal EEG results would be expected in patients with psychotic disorders or depression; however, slowing can be seen in dementia.

Finally, the acute onset and fluctuating nature of delirium are key features in distinguishing delirium from primary psychiatric disorders. It is important to interview family members or caregivers to determine the time of onset of symptoms and how the patient is different from the baseline cognitive state. Any psychiatric symptom arising in a person older than age 50 years without a prior psychiatric history, or the development of new or different symptoms in a patient with a preexisting psychiatric illness, should prompt a thorough medical workup.

There are three subtypes of delirium: hypoactive, hyperactive, and mixed. The hyperactive subtype is characterized by agitation and may be accompanied by disorientation, delusions, and hallucinations. This presentation may be confused with schizophrenia, agitated dementia, or a psychotic disorder. The patient with hypoactive delirium is subdued, confused, disoriented, and apathetic, and the delirium may be misdiagnosed as depression. The mixed subtype is characterized by fluctuations between both hyperactive and hypoactive symptoms.

High-Risk Patients and Potential Settings

Some patient populations have especially high rates of delirium. For example, more than 50% of postoperative patients develop delirium and up to 60% of all nursing home residents older than age 75 years have delirium. Table 2 lists patient subgroups and medical conditions where the risk for delirium is increased. It is important to recognize dementia as a

TABLE 2 Risk Factors for Delirium

Abrupt discontinuation of alcohol or drugs
Burns
Cardiac disease
Children
Elderly
Hip fracture
HIV
Kidney disease
Liver disease
Malnourishment
Multiple medical problems
Multiple medications
Parkinson's disease
Poststroke
Postsurgical states
Pre-existing dementia
Terminally ill
Transplant

risk factor for delirium and to understand that many geriatric patients will have both dementia and delirium. Such understanding helps one avoid attributing the confusion and agitation associated with a delirium to a pre-existing dementia and forgoing a search for, and potential correction of, an underlying medical condition or discontinuation of a problematic medication.

Screening Tools

Formal testing of memory and orientation is important because these deficits may not be obvious with casual observation. The Folstein Mini Mental Status Examination (MMSE) is useful in screening for deficits in orientation, attention, memory, language, and visuoconstructional abilities. Serial administrations of the MMSE are useful in assessing cognitive improvement.

Indication of Underlying Medical Problem

The underlying cause of a delirium should be sought as aggressively as one would in any other organ system failure. Nearly half of all elderly patients will have two or more conditions responsible for the delirium. Table 3 outlines a plan of assessment for patients with delirium.

Course

The course of delirium may last several hours to several months. With appropriate identification and correction of the underlying etiology, most patients will experience complete remission, although full recovery may lag behind corrected laboratory abnormalities or medical problems by several days.

TABLE 3 Assessment of Patients with Delirium

History*
Time of onset of symptoms
Description of symptoms
Past medical history
Past psychiatric history
Medication history, including the use of over-the-counter medications and herbals
Alcohol and illicit substance use
Physical Examination
Mental Status Examination
Include brief cognitive tests such as the Folstein Mini Mental Status Examination
Basic Laboratory Tests
Urinalysis
Blood chemistries (electrolytes, blood urea nitrogen, creatinine, glucose, calcium, aspartate aminotransferase, albumin, bilirubin, alkaline phosphatase, magnesium, Venereal Disease Research Laboratory [VDRL])
Complete blood count
Drug screen
Serum drug levels (e.g. lithium, digoxin, theophylline, anticonvulsants)
Oxygen saturation level or arterial blood gases
Additional Tests, as Indicated
Lumbar puncture
Electroencephalogram
Magnetic resonance imaging or computed tomography of the brain
B_{12} and folate levels
Urine porphyrins
Ammonia level
HIV
Erythrocyte sedimentation rate
Lupus erythematosus panel
Antinuclear antibody
C-reactive protein

*In most cases information from a collateral source is necessary.

Less likely to recover are elderly patients and those with HIV. Without proper recognition and management, progression to stupor, coma, or death may occur.

Management

During the search for the underlying medical condition, an antipsychotic may be used to control agitation and hallucinations and to clear the patient's sensorium (i.e., improve attention abilities and level of orientation). Haloperidol (Haldol)[1] has been the drug most studied for symptomatic management of delirium. There is emerging data regarding the use of the newer atypical antipsychotics, risperidone (Risperdal)[1], olanzapine (Zyprexa)[1], and quetiapine (Seroquel)[1], consisting of a few case reports and small studies. The results have generally been favorable, although a poorer response to olanzapine (Zyprexa), compared to haloperidol (Haldol), has been observed in hospitalized cancer patients who were older than 70 years

[1]Not FDA approved for this indication.

of age and had a history of dementia, central nervous system metastases or hypoxia as etiologies of the delirium, hypoactive subtype and more severe delirium. Theoretically, risperidone (Risperdal) may be the most advantageous of the atypical antipsychotics due to less anticholinergic activity and lower incidence of sedation.

Haloperidol (Haldol) can be started at 1 to 2 mg twice a day and every 4 hours as needed. The medication can be given orally, intramuscularly, or intravenously (not FDA approved). The intravenous route produces a lower incidence of extrapyramidal side effects; however, it does carry a risk for the development of torsades de pointes, making it preferable that patients be on a cardiac monitor. Elderly patients should be started on lower doses, such as 0.5 to 1.0 mg twice a day and every 4 hours as needed.

Risperidone (Risperdal) can be initiated at 0.5 mg twice a day and 0.5 mg every 4 hours as needed up to 4 mg a day. Olanzapine (Zyprexa) can be started at 2.5 to 5 mg at bedtime and 5 mg every 4 hours as needed up to 20 mg. Quetiapine (Seroquel) can be started at 25 to 50 mg twice a day and every 4 hours as needed for agitation or psychosis. An effort should be made to increase dosage in increments of 25 to 50 mg per day, up to a maximum dose of 600 mg.

For all antipsychotics, the response to the drug as well as the total daily dosage, including as needed medication, used should be monitored at least every 24 hours. The scheduled antipsychotic dose should be increased if as needed medication is necessary on a regular basis. Once the patient's cognitive state stabilizes, the antipsychotic should be continued over the next few days and then tapered and discontinued. The physician should not be too quick to discontinue the antipsychotic as soon as the patient's mental state clears because this apparent improvement may simply be a normal fluctuation of the patient's delirium.

Environmental Interventions

Proximity of the nursing station to the patient's room allows for closer monitoring of the delirious patient. The presence of a family member or close friend can be helpful; however, in more severe cases, a 24-hour sitter may be necessary. Nursing staff and family should be instructed to reorient the patient several times a day to the date, day of the week, time, location, city, state, and reason for hospitalization. A calendar and clock should be visible to the patient. The overall environment should not be overstimulating, with too many lights and beepers, nor should it be too understimulating, with no cues as to the time of day or situation. Routine vital signs throughout the night should be obtained only if necessary, to avoid sleep deprivation that may worsen delirium.

Physical restraints should be avoided, if possible. In the cognitively impaired patient, the use of restraints may increase agitation and injury risk. However, if the patient's behavior suggests likelihood of injury to self or others, and more conservative measures are ineffective, restraints can be used with caution. While restrained, the patient should be closely monitored and restraints should be discontinued as soon as possible. Practitioners need to regard hospital policy and other regulations regarding use of restraints.

Education

Education about the nature of delirium and its association with an underlying medical etiology is important, for both the patient and the family. The patient and the family should be advised that the symptoms of delirium are expected to resolve, unless there is reason to believe otherwise. Obtaining a neurology consult can be helpful in identifying the underlying etiology of the delirium, and psychiatric consultation can aid in managing the behavioral disturbances associated with delirium, as well as distinguishing delirium from a primary psychiatric disorder.

MOOD DISORDERS

METHOD OF

Michael J. Burke, MD, PhD

This article reviews the diagnosis and treatment of mood disorders focusing on major depressive disorder. As a group, mood disorders represent a collection of prevalent, serious, yet highly treatable medical conditions. Untreated, mood disorders can be debilitating and cause considerable functional impairment for the individual. A potential outcome for untreated mood disorders is death by suicide, which continues to rank in the top ten causes of death for most age groups. As an indication of the prevalence of mood disorders, in most medical settings antidepressant medications fall in the list of the top ten most frequently prescribed drugs.

Making the Diagnosis

There are several types of mood disorders, which are described in the *Diagnostic and Statistical Manual of Mental Disorders* (DSM-IV). Essentially when a patient presents with the complaint of "depression," or when depressive symptomatology is a focus of clinical attention, there are a number of possible diagnoses (Table 1). In addition to major depressive disorder (MDD), other considerations include bipolar affective disorder and whether the

TABLE 1 Differential Diagnosis for Major Mood Disorders

Bipolar disorder (type I) (Depressed, Hypomanic, Manic, or Mixed Episode)
Bipolar disorder (type II) (Depressed, Hypomanic)
Cyclothymic disorder
Dysthymic disorder
Major depressive disorder (Single Episode, Recurrent)
Mood disorder due to a general medical condition
Substance-induced mood disorder

depressive symptoms are a manifestation of some underlying general medical condition or are substance induced. Substance-induced mood disorders may be related to drugs of abuse (e.g., cocaine) or prescription medications (e.g., prednisone).

Mood disorders are syndromal diagnoses. In this sense, a mood disorder diagnosis represents a collection of specific signs and symptoms occurring together (Table 2). Not all patients with mood disorders will display or endorse all possible signs and symptoms (e.g., diagnostic criteria) for a particular mood disorder. This is where the clinician's experience and judgment come into play in formulating a diagnosis.

The patient's age may affect how they present with a mood disorder. Over the years a belief evolved that mood disorders would more likely present in children and adolescents as behavioral disturbances. The thought has been that youth may lack the ability to express how they feel, hence irritability and oppositional behavior may be the most prominent presenting symptoms of their mood disorder. Although it is still recognized that behavioral disturbance may bring a child with a mood disorder to clinical attention, the clinician needs to elicit additional diagnostic criteria to support a mood disorder diagnosis (see Table 2).

The elderly patient (i.e., older than 65 years of age) with a mood disorder presents another set of diagnostic challenges. On presentation, the elderly patient with a mood disorder may focus on somatic complaints, directing the clinical evaluation toward insomnia because of back pain or weight loss, and may not be forthcoming with complaints of low mood, feelings of hopelessness, and suicidal thoughts. Hence, when the clinician has a suspicion of a mood disorder in an elderly patient, the clinician must be fairly rigorous in exploring for depressive symptomatology. Regardless of the age of the patient, the approach to diagnosing a mood disorder should always include a thorough history and physical exam, with close attention to family history and medication use. The issue of substance abuse should be explored. It may be necessary to seek collateral history particularly in the case of adolescents and children, the elderly, or when the patient is hesitant about entertaining the possibility of a mood disorder diagnosis.

Treatment of Depressive Disorders

Once the clinician has made a depressive disorder diagnosis, the next consideration is treatment. When the diagnosis is substance-induced depressive disorder or depression secondary to a general medical condition, the focus of treatment is to address the underlying cause. In the case of a substance-induced depression, suspected drugs should be discontinued, and if substance abuse is identified chemical-dependency treatment is indicated. For depression secondary to a general medical condition, the focus of treatment would be correcting the general medical condition (e.g., optimizing blood sugar regulation in a diabetic). Because of the relatively low toxicity of newer antidepressant medications, the present practice would support consideration of their use while correction of the underlying causes of the mood disorder is ongoing. However, this decision should be made on a case-by-case basis.

PHARMACOTHERAPY FOR DEPRESSIVE DISORDERS

In the last 20 years there has been a dramatic evolution of the antidepressant armamentarium.

TABLE 2 Diagnostic Criteria for Depressive and Manic Episodes

Major Depressive Episode	Manic Episode
FIVE OR MORE OF THE FOLLOWING SYMPTOMS PRESENT DURING A 2-WEEK PERIOD	FOUR OR FIVE OF THE FOLLOWING SYMPTOMS PRESENT DURING A 1-WEEK PERIOD OR ANY DURATION IF HOSPITALIZATION IS REQUIRED
Depressed or irritable mood*	Elevated, expansive, or irritable mood*
Diminished interest or pleasure (anhedonia)*	Inflated self-esteem or grandiosity
Disturbance in appetite	Decreased need for sleep
Insomnia or hypersomnia	Hyperverbal
Psychomotor agitation or retardation	Racing thoughts, flight of ideas
Fatigue or loss of energy	Distractibility
Feelings of worthlessness or guilt	Increased activity or psychomotor agitation
Diminished ability to concentrate	Excessive involvement in pleasurable activities with risk for painful consequences
Recurrent thoughts of death, suicidal ideation, suicide attempt	

*For a major depressive episode diagnosis, the symptom of either depressed mood or anhedonia must be present. For a manic episode diagnosis, the altered mood symptom must be present.

The number of antidepressant medications has increased significantly and, more importantly, the newer agents have superior safety and tolerability profiles than their predecessors. Approximately 20 years ago, antidepressant medications fell into two general categories: the tricyclic antidepressants (TCAs) and the monoamine oxidase inhibitors (MAOIs). These two classes of antidepressant drugs had significant safety risks and were often difficult for patients to tolerate. Today, TCAs and MAOIs are relegated to third- and fourth-line antidepressant treatment options and their use is increasingly rare. The presumed antidepressant mechanism of TCAs and MAOIs was their effects on three neurotransmitters: norepinephrine, serotonin, and dopamine. Of note, despite the improved clinical profile of newer antidepressants, their therapeutic effects are still attributed to activity on these same three neurotransmitters.

Table 3 lists currently available antidepressant medications, the recommended daily dose range for treating depressive disorders, and presumed mechanism of antidepressant activity. The approach to conceptualizing antidepressants based on their pharmacodynamic profiles is reminiscent of how antihypertensive agents are organized and provides a basis for treatment selection. As an illustration, when a patient cannot tolerate a particular antidepressant or response is inadequate, the clinician selects an alternative agent that targets a different neurotransmitter or affects the same neurotransmitter through another mechanism.

Antidepressant Treatment Selection

Over the years, a number of antidepressant treatment algorithms have been published to assist with the selection of antidepressant medications in treatment-naïve patients. The tolerability and safety features of the individual antidepressants principally support these algorithms as no particular antidepressant medication or class of antidepressants has been found to have consistently superior efficacy. Hence efficacy in and of itself is not a feature that assists in treatment selection.

First-Line Antidepressants

Most published algorithms would list the selective serotonin reuptake inhibitors (SSRIs) as the first-line antidepressant of choice for the treatment-naïve patient. This first-line position for the SSRIs is based in part on broad clinical experience with this group of agents over the last decade. SSRIs are well tolerated. There may be some transient gastrointestinal adverse effects during the initiation of treatment, but for most patients these tend to resolve quickly, and there is limited risk of serious adverse effects. There are data to support that lack of response to one SSRI does not predict lack of response to another drug in the class. Hence, it has become common practice for patients to have sequential trials of more than one SSRI when the initial drug choice does not produce the desired response. For the SSRIs, sexual adverse effects (e.g., delayed time to orgasm, anorgasmia), when they occur, may lead to drug discontinuation. This adverse effect appears to be concentration dependent and may resolve if the drug dose can be lowered. Patients who experience sexual adverse effects with one SSRI are likely to experience them with other drugs in the class. For these patients, switching to an antidepressant medication without prominent serotonin reuptake inhibition would be indicated.

Second-Line Antidepressants

In patients who do not have an optimal response or can't tolerate SSRIs, second-line antidepressant agents would include venlafaxine (Effexor), mirtazapine (Remeron), and bupropion (Wellbutrin). In general, all of these agents are well tolerated and relatively safe, and for a given patient they might be considered first-line treatments. However, each of these drugs has some at least potential disadvantages relative to SSRIs. Venlafaxine (Effexor) is a potent serotonin and norepinephrine reuptake inhibitor. There is some belief that by virtue of targeting two neurotransmitters this agent may carry some advantages over SSRIs. Theoretically the potentiation of norepinephrine by venlafaxine may enhance the benefit of this medication for some patients. Some data suggest that in severely ill patients venlafaxine may have greater efficacy than SSRIs. However, norepinephrine potentiation is also associated with potential adverse effects related to autonomic arousal including increased blood pressure, palpitations, and diaphoresis. In the case of children and adolescents and physically healthy adult patients, the effects of norepinephrine potentiation may be tolerated without incident. But for patients who already have medical problems such as high blood pressure or palpitations, venlafaxine may aggravate these conditions. Patients who experience prominent sexual adverse effects associated with SSRIs may experience them with venlafaxine, which is also a potent serotonin reuptake inhibitor.

Bupropion (Wellbutrin) is a medication that is relatively safe and can be very well tolerated. Bupropion is a norepinephrine and dopamine reuptake inhibitor with little or no effect on central serotonin activity. Hence it is particularly useful for those patients who cannot tolerate the adverse effects related to serotonin potentiation (e.g., sexual dysfunction). Because of the potentiating effects on norepinephrine and dopamine, bupropion may be experienced by the patient as activating and has the potential to cause adverse effects related to autonomic arousal. Data suggest that preexisting cardiac arrhythmias may be aggravated by bupropion. Unique to bupropion with a mechanism that is not well understood is the risk of seizures. Although the seizure risk may be reduced with the sustained release formulations, bupropion is contraindicated in patients with seizure disorders

TABLE 3 Antidepressant Pharmacotherapy: Presumed Mechanism of Action, Dose Range, and Clinical Comments

Drug Name	Presumed Mechanism of Action	Daily Dose Range (mg/d)	Remarks
First-Line Agents			
Fluoxetine (Prozac)	SSRI	10-80	Potent inhibitor of CYP 2D6; now available in generic form
Paroxetine (Paxil)	SSRI	10-60	Potent inhibitor of CYP 2D6; most likely SSRI associated with withdrawal syndrome on abrupt discontinuation
Paroxetine (Paxil CR)	SSRI	25-62.5	Controlled-release formulation; potent inhibitor of CYP 2D6; reduced risk of SSRI withdrawal syndrome relative to immediate-release formulation is unclear
Sertraline (Zoloft)	SSRI	25-200	
Fluvoxamine (Luvox)	SSRI	50-300	Potent inhibitor of CYP 1A2 and 2C19; only SSRI with recommended BID dosing
Citalopram (Celexa)	SSRI	20-60	
Escitalopram (Lexapro)	SSRI	10-20	S-enantiomer of citalopram
Second-Line Agents			
Venlafaxine (Effexor)	SSNRI	37.5-375	Divide daily dose as bid or tid; associated with autonomic arousal, may cause or aggravate hypertension
Venlafaxine (Effexor XR)	SSNRI	75-225	Extended-release formulation; once-a-day dosing; associated with autonomic arousal, may cause or aggravate hypertension
Bupropion (Wellbutrin)	NE and DA reuptake inhibitor	300-450	See PDR for strict dosing guidelines; can induce seizures; may aggravate pre-existing arrhythmias; not to be used with Zyban (bupropion HCl)
Bupropion (Wellbutrin SR)	NE and DA reuptake inhibitor	150-400	Sustained-release formulation; bid for doses exceeding 150 mg; can induce seizures; may aggravate pre-existing arrhythmias; not to be used with Zyban (bupropion HCl)
Bupropion (Wellbutrin XL)	NE and DA reuptake inhibitor	150-450	Alternative extended-release formulation; given as single daily dose; not to be used with Zyban (bupropion HCl)
Mirtazapine (Remeron)	SE receptor (2A, 2C, 3) antagonist; NE potentiation as α_2-antagonist	15-45	Dosed at bedtime; prominent antihistaminic effects of sedation and weight gain
Third-Line Agents			
Tricyclic Agents (TCA)	Within TCA class each agent varies in relative potency as reuptake inhibitors of NE and SE		Cardiotoxic; lethal in overingestion; rarely used today; titrate dose in small increments based on TDM
Amitriptyline (Elavil)		150-300	
Nortriptyline (Pamelor)		50-150	
Desipramine (Norpramin)		75-300	
Clomipramine (Anafranil)[1]		100-250	
Monoamine Oxidase Inhibitors (MAOI)	Irreversibly inhibits enzyme that metabolizes SE, NE and DA		Rarely used today; requires restriction of diet and of other medications to avoid hypertensive crisis and hyperserotonergic syndrome
Phenelzine (Nardil)		30-90	
Tranylcypromine (Parnate)		20-60	
Nefazodone (Serzone)	SE receptor (2A) antagonist	300-600	Bid dosing; potent inhibitor of CYP 3A4; α_1 blockade may cause orthostasis; the manufacturer of Serzone has withdrawn the drug from Canadian, European, and U.S. markets after reports of serious hepatic effects including liver failure; see June 4, 2004, FDA guidelines for use

[1]Not FDA approved for this indication.

Abbreviations: CYP = cytochrome P450 isoenzymes, inhibiting these isoenzymes is the basis for potentially serious drug interactions; DA = dopamine; MOA = mechanism of action; NE = norepinephrine; PDR = *Physician's Desk Reference;* SE = serotonin; SSNRI = selective serotonin and norepinephrine reuptake inhibitor; SSRI = selective serotonin reuptake inhibitor; TDM = therapeutic drug monitoring; BID = twice a day dosing.

and its use should be scrutinized in patients with a history of head injury.

Mirtazapine (Remeron) is a unique antidepressant that is not a reuptake inhibitor but has effects on both serotonin and norepinephrine. It acts as a serotonin receptor antagonist, and it potentiates norepinephrine by blocking presynaptic α_2-adrenergic receptors. Mirtazapine has predictable sedation and weight gain associated with its use, which is thought to be associated with the drug's potent antihistamine activity (i.e., H_1 blockade). For this reason, it is dosed at bedtime. These effects of the antidepressant may be beneficial in some patients (e.g., depressive syndrome with prominent anorexia and insomnia), but may be perceived by other patients as problematic.

Third-Line Antidepressants

At one time the cornerstones of antidepressant pharmacotherapy, TCAs and MAOIs have now been relegated to a "last resort" position in the antidepressant armamentarium. Their use is rare and usually confined to complicated cases where all other treatment trials have been ineffective and the patient is under the direct care of a psychiatrist. At one time considered to be more effective than "newer" antidepressants, there are at present no data to suggest that under routine circumstances TCAs or MAOIs have superior efficacy compared to other agents; hence it is difficult to justify exposing patients to the risks associated with their use.

Nefazodone (Serzone) is one of the newer antidepressants from the 1990s that until recently was considered a relatively safe, well-tolerated drug with a presumed mechanism of blocking serotonin receptors. Because of its half-life, nefazodone required twice daily dosing, which was considered a disadvantage, but it appeared to be free of the adverse sexual effects seen with SSRIs. It is a relatively potent inhibitor of the cytochrome P450 isoenzyme 3A4 and hence presented risk of interaction with other drugs requiring this enzyme for their metabolism.

Reports of adverse hepatic effects, including liver failure, led to nefazodone's being removed from the Canadian and European markets in November 2003. In May 2004, Bristol-Myers Squibb pulled Serzone from the U.S. market. It is possible that generic nefazodone may remain available in the United States. However, because the serious risk of hepatic failure associated with nefazodone is now recognized, it is anticipated that the use of this drug will be limited and only in rare, exceptional cases would nefazodone be initiated as antidepressant therapy. It is possible that in some cases where patients have only been responsive to nefazodone and have been stable on the drug for a period of time, the decision may be made to continue the therapy. However, any use of nefazodone should require informed consent by the patient and close monitoring according to FDA guidelines. Patients with liver disease or elevated liver enzymes should not receive nefazodone.

Other Considerations in Treatment Selection

This discussion of antidepressant treatment selection has focused on the treatment-naïve patient. In the case of patients with recurrent mood disorders, a thorough history will identify antidepressant medications that were well tolerated and helpful to the patient in the past. In such cases, the recommendation would be to resume whatever medicine had been effective for the patient in treating prior mood disorder episodes. Another useful piece of history relevant to treatment selection is whether or not the patient has other family members who have been treated for mood disorders and what their response to particular antidepressant agents has been. A general belief is that if one family member has responded well to a particular antidepressant agent, the patient seeking treatment may also respond to that agent.

What has become clear in the last decade is that in addition to targeting neurotransmitters, a number of antidepressants also have effects on hepatic enzyme activity, specifically the cytochrome P450 (CYP) isoenzymes. In principle, drugs that affect a particular CYP isoenzyme activity will alter the metabolism of other medications the patient may be taking that are substrates for that isoenzyme. A detailed discussion of pharmacokinetic drug interactions involving CYP isoenzymes is outside the scope of this article. There are numerous references available and most, if not all, pharmacy departments at this time have computer software that will identify potential pharmacokinetic drug interactions and can provide a resource as to whether or not a particular drug has an effect on CYP isoenzymes. Among currently popular antidepressant medications, fluoxetine (Prozac) and paroxetine (Paxil) are considered to be relatively potent inhibitors of CYP 2D6 and therefore have a likelihood of altering the plasma concentration of other drugs the patient may be taking that require CYP 2D6 for their metabolism. As mentioned earlier, nefazodone (Serzone) is a relatively potent inhibitor of CYP 3A4. A number of other antidepressant agents are recognized to have mild to moderate effects on CYP isoenzymes but the clinical significance of this is not clear.

An Antidepressant Treatment Trial

One can conceptualize an antidepressant treatment trial as having four principal considerations. These can be referred to as the four "Ds": diagnosis, drug, dose, and duration. For this discussion, we assume that the diagnosis of a depressive disorder for which antidepressant medication is indicated has been made. The next step is to select an antidepressant medication. As discussed, antidepressants that are currently available can be generally organized into first-line, second-line, and third-line agents. For a treatment-naïve patient, it is most likely that the clinician would select a first-line antidepressant agent. Knowledge that the patient had a preferential response to a particular antidepressant in the past, or has a family member who had a preferential response to a particular antidepressant, may influence the treatment selection.

Once an antidepressant is selected, the next issue is dosing. Prior to the 1990s, antidepressant therapy often involved a lengthy process of dose titration, typically starting at very low doses to minimize toxicity and then advancing in small increments over time. In the 1990s, with the advent of better-tolerated, less-toxic antidepressant agents, oftentimes the starting dose was the effective dose. Perhaps the best illustration of this phenomenon is the SSRIs, where the starting doses were the effective doses for many patients. After a decade of experience with the newer antidepressant agents, there is now a recognition that dose titration in and of itself is not necessarily a practice to be avoided and may offer certain advantages to patients. Recently, several antidepressants have become available in lower-dose formulations so that these agents can be initiated at a low dose, even if it is only for a few days or a week, to improve tolerability and positively influence treatment compliance. Some patients will respond optimally to lower doses than were previously believed to be the effective, but other patients will require higher than the usually effective dose. Where a particular patient falls in this dose–response spectrum only becomes apparent during a dose titration process.

Once an antidepressant medication has been initiated, the question becomes how long a treatment trial should continue before the clinician makes the decision to change the dose or switch to another antidepressant medication. The guidelines for duration of a treatment trial have shifted over the last decade. At one time, the recommendation was that all patients should be maintained for 6 to 8 weeks at the usually effective dose of a medication (e.g., fluoxetine 20 mg per day) before considering dose titration. The principle underlying this approach was that the antidepressant-induced biologic changes in the central nervous system might take several weeks to occur. This principle has not been challenged, but data now suggest that those patients who go on to have an optimal response to an antidepressant medication are most likely to show at least a partial response by 2 to 4 weeks at the usually effective dose. Hence, in current practice the response of the patient should be factored into the decision to titrate dose or change medication. By the 2- to 4-week mark in a treatment trial, if the patient has been in the range of the usually effective dose and is showing marginal beneficial response and no adverse effects, it would be reasonable to consider advancing the medication dose. Keep in mind that there is broad variability among patients in the plasma drug concentrations achieved at a given antidepressant dose. Hence, it is quite possible that a patient on a usually effective antidepressant dose may for a variety of reasons develop a plasma drug concentration that is much less than expected and outside the range of concentration that is associated with optimal response.

By the 4-week mark in a treatment trial, if the selected antidepressant agent has been titrated without appreciable benefit but also without appreciable adverse effects, it would be reasonable to advance the dose further. If the selected antidepressant dose is already at the recommended maximum dose, or adverse effects prohibit further dose escalation, considerations include using an augmentation strategy or changing drugs. Common augmentation strategies for antidepressant medications include low-dose thyroid hormone on the order of 25 to 50 μg per day or low-dose lithium (Eskalith)[1] therapy on the order of 300 or 600 mg a day. Low-dose stimulants such as methylphenidate (Ritalin)[1] have also been used as an augmentation strategy. In general, the thought is that augmentation strategies should show added benefit within a relatively short period of time, on the order of 1 to 2 weeks.

Another option for the patient who has had only marginal benefit to antidepressant therapy by the 4 to 6 week mark in the treatment trial is change to a different antidepressant medication. Before switching to an alternative antidepressant the clinician should assess whether the patient has had an adequate dose titration and has been compliant with the treatment trial. In some cases, the clinician may decide to assay the plasma level of the antidepressant drug to assess whether the particular patient has a drug concentration much lower than would be predicted based on the antidepressant drug dose. A plasma drug level can provide the necessary data to direct either further dose titration or a drug change.

In general, 40% to 60% of patients will have an optimal response to an antidepressant treatment trial. These numbers suggest that a high percentage of patients will not have an optimal response and ultimately will receive sequential antidepressant treatment trials. When selecting an alternative antidepressant for a patient who has not had an optimal response during a current treatment trial, there are a number of options. There are data to suggest that patients who do not respond optimally to one SSRI will go on to have a desired response to a second SSRI. For better or worse, it has become common practice for patients to have multiple, sequential treatment trials with SSRIs. For a patient who has not responded optimally to trials of two SSRIs, although one could generate a rationale for proceeding with another SSRI treatment trial, it would be reasonable to consider selecting an antidepressant with a different mechanism of action. Popular non-SSRI antidepressant choices include venlafaxine (Effexor), bupropion (Wellbutrin), and mirtazapine (Remeron).

In the primary care setting it is not unreasonable to expect that ambulatory patients may undergo multiple sequential antidepressant treatment trials until an optimal response is achieved. Over the last several

[1]Not FDA approved for this indication.

years, primary care clinicians have become increasingly effective in their use of the newer antidepressant agents. That said, there may come a time when it would be most appropriate to refer a patient for psychiatric specialty care. Marginal response to antidepressant treatment trials with ongoing significant functional impairment, the onset of psychotic symptoms, or when the clinician is considering the use of a third-line antidepressant medication (e.g., TCA, MAOI) are all reasons to obtain psychiatric consultation. For those patients expressing suicidal ideation or with a significant suicide risk profile (Table 4), a psychiatric referral is the appropriate strategy.

A FINAL WORD ON ANTIDEPRESSANT PHARMACOTHERAPY

In the spring of 2004, the FDA issued a Public Health Advisory cautioning clinicians, patients, and families about the need to closely monitor all patients being treated with antidepressant drugs. Although a causal role for antidepressants has not been established, this advisory arose from ongoing concern about the potential for emerging suicidality or worsening of depressive symptoms in patients taking antidepressants. It is likely that within the year, the FDA will propose labeling changes for most antidepressant drugs that reflect this advisory.

NONPHARMACOLOGIC THERAPY FOR DEPRESSIVE DISORDERS

Psychotherapy

Although pharmacotherapy is the principal treatment intervention for patients with depressive disorders, psychotherapy should always be a consideration. Psychotherapy can be considered an adjunct to pharmacotherapy. It can be considered for those patients who prefer not to take medications, and it may be particularly suitable for patients with mild depressive symptomatology. Specifically, data support cognitive behavioral therapy (CBT) and interpersonal therapy (IT) as effective interventions for patients with milder depressive symptomatology. There is a belief that CBT and IT may have additive benefits for patients taking antidepressant medication. Both CBT and IT require a practitioner who has received special training. When referring a patient for one of these particular types of psychotherapy, the clinician should inquire about the background and training of the therapist. In contrast to less well defined psychotherapy approaches that may have been used in the past, both CBT and IT as practiced today are characterized by setting specific treatment goals and timelines for achieving those therapeutic goals.

Even in those cases where the clinician has not selected specific psychotherapies for the patient, ideally some form of generic supportive psychotherapy should be available to accompany pharmacotherapy. Elements of this generic supportive psychotherapy would include psychoeducation about mood disorders and antidepressant medications, helping the patient recognize personal strengths, helping the patient prioritize what can sometimes be complex biopsychosocial problems, and in some cases offering guidance to assist with problem solving. This form of supportive psychotherapy can certainly be delegated to a "therapist," but it can also be accomplished by a practiced clinician with relative efficiency.

TABLE 4 "SAD PERSONS" Scale for Assessment of Suicide Risk

S	Sex: Males are more likely than females to kill themselves by 3:1.
A	Age: Older more than younger, especially white males.
D	Depression: A depressive episode precedes suicide in up to 70% of cases.
P	Previous attempt(s): Most people who die of suicide do so on their first or second attempt. Patients who make multiple (4+) attempts have an increased risk of future attempts.
E	Ethanol use: Recent onset of ethanol use or other sedative–hypnotic drug use increases risk.
R	Rational thinking loss: Profound cognitive slowing, psychotic depression, and pre-existing brain damage.
S	Social support deficit: Social withdrawal, disconnected from family and friends, unemployed.
O	Organized plan: Person has gone beyond thinking of death and considered a plan for suicide.
N	No spouse: The absence of a spouse or significant other is a risk factor.
S	Sickness: Intercurrent medical illnesses.

Electroconvulsive Therapy

Perhaps the most effective treatment for depressive disorders is electroconvulsive therapy (ECT). ECT has been used for decades to treat mood disorders and its efficacy and safety are supported by a wealth of data. Despite its effectiveness, ECT is not considered a first-line therapy for most patients with depressive disorders and this is principally because of the risks associated with the general anesthesia required for the treatments. ECT is indicated for patients with severe depressive symptoms, significant functional impairment, psychotic symptoms, and catatonia. There are no absolute contraindications to ECT and it has been used effectively in the frail elderly as well as in pregnant patients. In the primary care setting, the severity of depressive symptomatology or lack of response to multiple treatment trials are usually the basis for consideration of ECT. Whenever considering ECT, it is reasonable to first obtain a psychiatric consultation, which will either offer further support for pursuing ECT or suggest alternative treatment strategies that should be implemented prior to further consideration of ECT.

There are other nonpharmacologic interventions either available or in development for the treatment of mood disorders. These include transcranial magnetic stimulation (TMS), vagal nerve stimulation (VNS), light therapy, and herbal/homeopathic remedies.

In different parts of the country there are clinics that specialize in light therapy, and light sources are commercially available for patients to use in treating mood disorders. Light therapy is indicated as an adjunct to pharmacotherapy or for those patients with mild to moderate depressive symptoms who decline drug therapy. It has often been used for patients who have a seasonal variation to their depressive symptoms. Further information about light therapy is available through multiple sources, including the Internet.

TMS and VNS are still considered investigational treatments for depression and as such their use is confined to clinical trials at research centers. A multicenter trial of VNS to treat depression has been recently completed and the data are currently under review by the FDA. Homeopathic, herbal, and "traditional medicine" therapies for depression are available; however, they tend to lack rigorous scientific data to support their efficacy and safety and hence are not considered as part of the standard of care of treating mood disorders.

Treatment of Bipolar Mood Disorders

Although unipolar depressive disorders are more common, no discussion of mood disorders would be complete without some review of bipolar disorders. Bipolar affective disorder (BAD), formerly referred to as manic-depressive illness, can carry considerable morbidity for the patient and represents a particular challenge for the treating clinician. Ideally, clinicians in any medical setting should be familiar with the various presentations of BAD. Increasingly, efforts to manage BAD in the primary care setting are being made.

BIPOLAR DEPRESSION

When a patient presents with a depressive episode, there may be no prior history of a bipolar diagnosis. In such cases, the clinician would proceed with antidepressant treatment as discussed above. The important point to keep in mind is that any antidepressant agent has the potential to induce a manic or "mixed" episode in a vulnerable patient (i.e., a patient with a bipolar diathesis), where "mixed" refers to a state in which the patient meets DSM-IV criteria for both a depressive and manic episode. Hence, part of routine management in the treatment of depression is to monitor for the possible cycling of a patient from a depressive episode into a manic or mixed episode. During the antidepressant treatment trial, if the clinician has a suspicion that the patient may be cycling into mania, it would be reasonable to obtain a psychiatric consultation.

Alternatively, a patient may present with a depressed episode and a prior history of BAD. This history would suggest that the patient is at risk for cycling if an antidepressant medication is initiated and hence a principal concern in treatment planning is to prevent cycling from occurring (i.e., mood stabilization). The standard approach to treating depression in the bipolar patient would be to implement a mood-stabilizing medication (e.g., lithium, valproic acid[1], carbamazepine[1]) in conjunction with an antidepressant medicine. It does not appear that any particular antidepressant medication carries less risk of inducing cycling to a manic or mixed episode in a vulnerable bipolar patient. Hence, the guidelines discussed previously with regard to antidepressant treatment selection still apply. There has been some suggestion that bupropion (Wellbutrin) may have advantages in treating depression in bipolar patients by virtue of a decreased risk of inducing cycling. However, the data to support the advantages of bupropion are limited and there is no consensus that this medication should have a particular first-line position in treating bipolar depression.

Recent industry-sponsored controlled trials suggest that the atypical antipsychotic agents olanzapine (Zyprexa) and ziprasidone (Geodon)[1] may have mood-stabilizing properties and could be used in either the treatment of bipolar depression along with an antidepressant or as monotherapy in the treatment of mania. Also in the last few years, a number of new anticonvulsant agents have been studied for mood stabilizing properties. However, the two most frequently prescribed mood stabilizers remain lithium and valproic acid (Depakote)[1], which would be considered the first-line agents for treating either bipolar depression or bipolar mania. In addition to pharmacotherapy, bipolar depression can also be treated by ECT. Because of the recognized challenge of treating bipolar depression, when this diagnosis is being considered, it is reasonable to refer the patient to a psychiatrist. Once a bipolar patient is stable and euthymic, it is possible that ongoing care could be managed in a primary care setting.

BIPOLAR MANIA

In addition to depressive episodes, bipolar patients may present with hypomania, mania without psychosis, or mania with psychosis or in what is referred to as a mixed state, where the patient exhibits symptoms of both mania and depression simultaneously. The cornerstone therapy for any one of these presentations is a mood-stabilizing agent. As discussed, first-line mood-stabilizing agents include lithium, valproic acid (Depakote)[1], and carbama-zepine (Tegretol)[1]. It is important to recognize that these drugs may take days to weeks to bring about the desired clinical outcome and often adjunctive therapy with other classes of drugs will be necessary initially to help control the patient's symptoms. It is not uncommon that patients in a manic episode may require a mood stabilizing agent, an antipsychotic

[1]Not FDA approved for this indication.

drug, and a benzodiazepine. Depending on the severity of symptoms, a second mood stabilizer may be indicated.

Patients who are identified to be in a manic or mixed state should be referred for psychiatry specialty care as soon as possible. Temporizing acute interventions until the patient can be seen by a psychiatrist might include benzodiazepines for insomnia and atypical antipsychotic agents for agitation. Lorazepam (Ativan)[1] 1 to 2 mg or clonazepam (Klonopin)[1] 1 to 2 mg are reasonable sleep aids. Olanzapine (Zyprexa) 5 mg twice daily or risperidone (Risperdal)[1] 1 mg twice daily are possible acute interventions for agitation. However, because of the number of variables that must be considered when instituting therapy for patients in a manic episode or mixed state, if the patient cannot be referred immediately, it would be reasonable to obtain a phone consultation with a psychiatrist and review the patient's particulars to formulate a treatment strategy and discuss whether hospitalization is indicated. If lithium is selected, it is important to assess the patient's renal function before initiating the medication. If either valproic acid[1] or carbamazepine[1] is selected, it is appropriate to assess the patient's liver function and hematologic status by obtaining liver function tests and a complete blood count (CBC) before initiating therapy. One advantage of the first-line mood-stabilizing agents is that they have established plasma level ranges associated with optimal response and toxicity. A typical strategy is to initiate the mood stabilizers at low to moderate doses, allow the patient to achieve steady-state blood levels, assess the plasma concentration, and then adjust the medication accordingly.

Mood disorders, both unipolar and bipolar, are relatively prevalent medical conditions that may occur in any clinical setting. Mood disorders are serious medical conditions that can cause significant morbidity for patients and carry a significant risk of mortality either through suicide or accident. Currently, pharmacotherapy is the principal intervention for major mood disorders. Psychotherapy is used for milder symptomatology and as an adjunct to pharmacotherapy. Increasingly, mood disorders are being managed in the primary care setting. When patients are not responding optimally to antidepressant treatment, when the symptomatology is particularly severe, when the patient is at risk for suicide, or when the patient presents with a manic episode or mixed state, it is advisable to obtain psychiatric consultation and refer the patient for specialty care.

SCHIZOPHRENIA

METHOD OF

Robert R. Conley, MD, and

Deanna L. Kelly, PharmD

Schizophrenia is one of the most challenging and complex psychiatric disorders that afflicts humans. The core symptoms of this illness are highly variable among people with schizophrenia. They include hallucinations, delusions, disorganized speech and behavior, inappropriate affect, cognitive deficits, and impaired psychosocial functioning. The onset of symptoms in most cases is insidious, usually preceded by a prodromal phase characterized by gradual social withdrawal, diminished interests, changes in appearance and hygiene, changes in cognition, and bizarre or odd behaviors. One percent of the population will suffer from this disorder, with symptoms usually first in late adolescence/early adulthood. Symptoms generally appear in males earlier in life than they appear in females. Most people with the disorder require treatment with antipsychotics and comprehensive care over the course of their lives. This article focuses on the pharmacologic aspects of the treatment of schizophrenia. Neurobiologic and clinical aspects of these treatments are also reviewed.

Pathophysiology

The most common neuropathologic theory associated with the etiology of schizophrenia involves the dopaminergic system. This hypothesis was formed in the late 1950s when it was discovered that antipsychotic drugs are postsynaptic dopamine antagonists. It has been observed that drugs that increase dopamine (e.g., cocaine, amphetamines) enhance or produce positive psychotic symptoms (delusions, hallucinations, suspiciousness, disorganized thinking) and drugs such as antipsychotics, which decrease dopamine, decrease or stop positive symptoms. There is much evidence supporting the dopamine hypothesis, particularly in areas of the brain with dopamine$_2$ receptors. Increased glucose metabolism in the basal ganglia and decreased metabolism in the frontal cortex may be indicative of dopaminergic hyperactivity and hypoactivity in these regions, respectively. Positron emission tomography (PET) studies that measure receptor densities using dopamine$_2$-specific ligands, such as raclopride, show increased densities of dopamine$_2$ receptors in the basal ganglia and decreased densities in the prefrontal cortex. Other direct evidence supporting the validity of the dopamine hypothesis comes from postmortem evaluation of tissues and plasma. Investigators have measured the amount of dopamine and its metabolites, such as homovanillic acid (HVA). Brain tissue from people with schizophrenia has increased presynaptic dopamine and/or HVA levels in areas of the mesocortical and mesolimbic systems when compared to normal controls.

The hypothesis that the dopamine system explains schizophrenia symptoms is far from complete, however. Recently, it has been suggested that combined dysfunction of the dopamine and glutamate transmitter systems may better explain this disorder. There has also been a great deal of speculation regarding the role of serotonin receptor antagonism in regard to antipsychotic effects. Many traditional antipsychotics are highly active at serotonin receptors, but this property does not distinguish the clinical effects of these drugs in a meaningful way. The serotonin hypothesis of psychosis actually predates the dopamine hypothesis, largely because of lysergic acid diethylamide (LSD), a drug with psychotomimetic properties that releases serotonin. Interest in this theory was reinvigorated by the finding that clozapine, which has a 100-fold selectivity for serotonin compared to dopamine receptors, is highly efficacious. The other second-generation antipsychotics also have high serotonin-to-dopamine binding ratios. Serotonin receptor binding may be important to these drugs' actions, possibly by stimulating dopamine activity in mesocortical pathways. However, a compelling theory relating dopamine and serotonin receptor affinities does not yet exist.

Genetic Predisposition

The genetic component of this hypothesis is that there is a lesion present at birth with the potential for *N*-methyl-D-aspartate (NMDA) receptor hypofunction, and this may not trigger psychopathologic or neuropathologic processes until late adolescence, at which time it would begin to trigger schizophrenic symptoms. There is fairly strong evidence that schizophrenia is at least partially genetic in nature. For example, the risk of developing schizophrenia if a first-degree relative or both parents are diagnosed is 10% and 40%, respectively. Many genes have weakly been associated with the development of schizophrenia. However, there is probably no one schizophrenia gene. The possible genetic effects are either a susceptibility to schizophrenia with a certain gene or a combination of several genes necessary to develop the disorder. The chromosomes with the most significant evidence include 5, 6, 8, 10, 13, 15, and 22. Environmental stimuli or triggers may contribute to the expression of symptoms.

Clinical Presentation

Schizophrenia is a chronic disorder of thought and affect and a significant disturbance in the individual's ability to function in society and develop interpersonal relationships. The clinical presentation of this disorder can be extremely varied and, despite the attempts to portray a stereotype in the media, the stereotypic schizophrenic individual does not exist. In the 1970s, Strauss and others suggested that schizophrenic symptoms fell into three specific symptoms complexes—positive symptoms, negative symptoms, and disorders of relating. Carpenter and others further characterized these three symptom domains into psychotic disturbances, cognitive dysfunction, and negative symptoms.

PSYCHOTIC SYMPTOMS

The acute psychotic symptoms include hallucinations (distortions or exaggeration of perception) and delusions (fixed false beliefs). Hallucinations may occur as auditory, visual, olfactory, gustatory, or tactile, but auditory hallucinations are the most common type in people with schizophrenia. Voices frequently occur and are distinct from the person's own thoughts. The content of hallucinations is variable, but is often threatening or commanding. Delusions are erroneous beliefs that usually involve a misinterpretation of perceptions or experiences and often are bizarre in nature and involve suspiciousness on the part of the patient.

COGNITIVE SYMPTOMS

Subtle disturbance in associative thinking may develop years before disorganized thinking (formal thought disorder). Inferences about thought are based primarily on the individual's speech. Thinking and speech are frequently incomprehensible to others and often are illogical. Characteristics of formal thought disorder include loosening of associations, tangentiality, thought blocking, concreteness, circumstantiality, and perseveration. Additionally, the average intelligence quotient (IQ) in people with a schizophrenia diagnosis is 80 to 84, with the presence of prominent memory and learning difficulties.

NEGATIVE SYMPTOMS

Primary negative symptoms or deficit symptoms are quite ubiquitous in schizophrenia, however, they are difficult to evaluate because they occur in a continuum with normality, are nonspecific, and are often caused by medication side effects (secondary negative symptoms), mood disorder, environmental understimulation, or demoralization. The best test for establishing true negative symptoms is to examine their persistence for a considerable period of time despite efforts directed at resolving the other causes. Approximately 10% to 15% of people with schizophrenia may exhibit the majority of psychopathology as negative symptoms; these people may be referred to as having a deficit syndrome. Negative symptoms include impoverished speech and thinking, lack of social drive, flatness of emotional expression, and apathy.

PRESENTATION OF SYMPTOMS

People with a diagnosis of schizophrenia may be uncooperative, hostile, and verbally or physically aggressive because of their misinterpretation of reality and, often, because of command hallucinations. Difficulty with anxiety may be exhibited because of positive symptoms and suspiciousness. Because of negative and depressive symptoms, people with schizophrenia may have impaired self-care skills and may be dirty and unkempt. Sleep and appetite are often disturbed. People with schizophrenia often have difficulty living independently in the community and have difficulty forming close relationships with others. Additionally they have problems with initiating or maintaining employment and are often noncompliant with medications, increasing their risk for relapse.

Diagnosis

The commonly accepted diagnostic criteria for schizophrenia comes from the *Diagnostic and Statistical Manual of Mental Disorders, 4th ed., Text Revision* (DSM-IV-TR). The essential features are a mixture of characteristic signs and symptoms that have been present for a significant portion of time during a 1-month period (or a shorter time if successfully treated), with some signs of the disorder persisting for at least 6 months. These signs and symptoms are associated with marked social or occupational dysfunction, are not accounted for by a mood disorder, and are not caused by the direct physiologic effects of a substance or a general medical condition. Differential diagnoses of psychotic signs and symptoms may include the following:

- Schizoaffective disorder
- Mood disorders
- Dementia
- Delirium
- Drug intoxication
- Pervasive developmental disorders
- Neurologic conditions (neoplasm, migraines, epilepsy)
- Medical conditions (fluid or electrolyte imbalances, metabolic conditions, autoimmune disorders)

Course and Prognosis

Although the course of schizophrenia is variable, the long-term prognosis for independent function is often poor. This illness is marked by intermittent acute psychotic episodes and a downward decline in psychosocial functioning. A patient may become more withdrawn, bizarre, and nonfunctional over many years. Complete return to full premorbid functioning is not common in this disorder. Many of the more dramatic and acute symptoms will disappear with time, but severe residual symptoms may persist. Family and friends may find this illness difficult to interpret and understand. Involvement with the law is fairly common for misdemeanors such as vagrancy, loitering, and disturbing the peace. The overall life expectancy is shortened primarily because of suicide, accidents, and the inability for self-care. The lifetime risk of suicide for schizophrenia is 10% to 13%. People with schizophrenia who have fewer acute psychotic episodes and those who are treated very early in their course of illness may have a better prognosis. Persistent compliance with a tolerable drug regimen also improves prognosis.

Pharmacologic Treatment

Antipsychotic drugs are used to treat nearly all forms of psychosis, including schizophrenia, schizoaffective disorder, affective disorders with psychosis, and dementias. Antipsychotic medications are the primary pharmacologic treatment of schizophrenia. Approximately 20 antipsychotics are available in the United States, of which 6 are termed atypical or second-generation antipsychotics (SGAs). Adjunctive medications may be appropriate in some people and include anticholinergic medications, mood stabilizers, benzodiazepines, β-blockers, and antidepressants. The basis for adjunctive use includes the treatment of side effects, refractory symptoms, agitation, anxiety, depression, or mood elevation.

FIRST-GENERATION ANTIPSYCHOTICS

Antipsychotic drugs have been in clinical use since the 1950s, when chlorpromazine was synthesized in France. It was first used as a preanesthetic agent. Within 2 years of use, it was found to be effective in the treatment of people with psychosis. Many other similar medications followed in the next decade. These medications were commonly referred to as neuroleptics, which meant *causing a neurologic disorder*. This name came about because of the profound extrapyramidal motor side effects (EPS) they produced. Many believed the induction of motor side effects was necessary, however, for efficacy of the medications. All of the first-generation antipsychotic (FGA) agents available are high affinity D_2 receptor antagonists (e.g., haloperidol [Haldol], chlorpromazine [Thorazine]). These agents block 65% to 80% of D_2 receptors in the striatum during chronic treatment and block dopamine in the other dopamine tracts as well. While differing in potency and side effect profiles, all FGA agents are generally equivalent in efficacy when used in equipotent doses (300 to 600 chlorpromazine [CPZ] units). All, however, may cause significant extrapyramidal symptoms (EPS) (pseudoparkinsonism, dystonia, and akathisia) and tardive dyskinesia (TD). EPS has a pervasive negative impact on treatment and adherence. Furthermore, worsening of negative symptoms and cognition as well as an increased risk for TD has led to a new class of antipsychotic medications.

SECOND-GENERATION ANTIPSYCHOTICS

Over the past decade, six atypical or novel antipsychotics have been introduced in the United States—clozapine (Clozaril), risperidone (Risperdal), olanzapine (Zyprexa), quetiapine (Seroquel), ziprasidone (Geodon), and aripiprazole (Abilify). What principally distinguishes these newer antipsychotic agents from the FGAs is their ability to induce an antipsychotic effect with a much lower risk of causing EPS. These agents produce a similar if not better response than the FGAs for positive symptoms, and they may provide better efficacy in other domains such as negative symptoms, cognition, and mood. Table 1 lists the recommended dosing for adult schizophrenia patients. Similar efficacy is observed among different antipsychotics in people with treatment-responsive schizophrenia. Clozapine, however, has superior efficacy in people who are treatment-resistant and has a response rate of approximately 30% to 60% in this population.

While SGAs are moving into first-line therapy in schizophrenia, it is noteworthy that treatment with this class of medications is not without side effects. Appropriate monitoring and attention should be paid to the development of side effects and these should be minimized and addressed. Some important differences include:

- Clozapine and olanzapine are associated with the greatest gains in weight and metabolic disturbances (elevations in glucose and lipids).
- Risperidone is associated with the highest risk for dose-dependent EPS and sexual dysfunction.
- Quetiapine is associated with a moderate degree of early and transient sedation.
- Ziprasidone has a tendency to prolong the QTc.
- Aripiprazole is associated with gastrointestinal disturbances.

Side effect profiles for SGAs are listed in Table 2.

Although multiple treatment modalities are important in schizophrenia, antipsychotics remain the

TABLE 1 Dosing Recommendations for Second-Generation Antipsychotics*

Agent	Initial Target Dose	Maximal Dose Likely to be Beneficial	Comments
Clozapine (Clozaril)	400 mg/d	500-600 mg/d	Plasma level ≥350 ng/mL is most effective.
Risperidone (Risperdal)	2-4 mg/d	6 mg/d	Long-acting injectable available for every 2wk dosing; liquid and fast dissolving formulations available.
	15-20 mg/d	30-40 mg/d[3]	>20 mg/d is outside product labeling; fast dissolving formulation available.
Quetiapine (Seroquel)	400-600 mg/d	800-1200 mg/d[3]	>800 mg/d is outside product labeling.
Ziprasidone (Geodon)	100-120 mg/d	160-200 mg/d[3]	>160 mg/d is outside product labeling; IM preparation available.
Aripiprazole (Abilify)	15-30 mg/d	30 mg/d	

[3]Exceeds dosage recommended by the manufacturer.
*Lower doses should be used in children, in those over 55 years of age, in other diagnoses, in vulnerable populations, and as adjunct treatment.

TABLE 2 Side Effect Profiles of Second-Generation Antipsychotics*

	Clozapine	Risperidone	Olanzapine	Quetiapine	Ziprasidone	Aripiprazole	Haloperidol
Anticholinergic side effects (dry mouth, constipation, blurry vision, urinary hesitancy)	+++	±	++ (higher doses)	±	±	±	±
EPS at clinical doses	±	+	±	±	±	±	++
Dose-dependent EPS	0	++	+	0	+	±	+++
Orthostatic hypotension	+++	++	+	++	+	+	+
Prolactin elevation (hormonal and sexual side effects)	0	+++	+	±	+	0	++
QTc prolongation	+	±	±	±	+	±	±
Sedation	+++	+	+	++	+	+	+
Seizures	++	±	±	±	±	±	±
Weight gain	+++	++	+++	++	+	+	±
Glucose dysregulation	++	±	++	±	±	±	±
Lipid abnormalities	+++	±	+++	+	±	±	±
GI disturbances	+	±	±	±	±	+	±

*0 = absent; ± = minimal; + = mild or low risk; ++ = moderate; +++ = severe.
Abbreviations: EPS = extrapyramidal motor side effects; GI = gastrointestinal.

cornerstone of treatment. Second-generation antipsychotics do provide advantages over FGAs but are much more costly than FGAs. Some evidence, however, does suggest that SGAs are cost-effective as compared to FGAs. To maximize the benefits of SGAs, the dose of these medications should be carefully adjusted to maximize efficacy and minimize side effect occurrences. Proper monitoring of side effects should be implemented. Because each pharmacologic treatment has its own unique profiles, clinicians should now attempt to optimize antipsychotic therapy for each patient in a highly individualized way.

PANIC DISORDER

METHOD OF

Alexander Bystritsky, MD, PhD, and

Kira Williams, MD

Diagnosis

Panic disorder (PD) and related agoraphobia (AG) are very prevalent and disabling conditions affecting 3% to 8% of the world population. Panic disorder is characterized by sudden episodes of acute apprehension or intense fear that occur *out of the blue* without any apparent cause–panic attacks. Intense panic usually lasts no more than a few minutes, but, in rare instances, can return in *waves* for a period of up to 2 hours. During the panic itself, any of the symptoms listed in Table 1 may occur.

The attack is spontaneous, unexpected, and occurs for no apparent reason. The word *agoraphobia* means fear of open spaces; however, under many instances agoraphobia is a fear of panic attacks. Patients suffering from agoraphobia are afraid of being in situations from which escape might be difficult, or in which help might be unavailable if they suddenly had a panic attack. Many agoraphobics not only fear having panic attacks but also fear embarrassment should they be seen having a panic attack. It is common for the agoraphobic to avoid a variety of situations (Table 2). The fear usually results in travel restrictions, or a need to be accompanied by others when leaving home. They may avoid certain situations such as waiting in a line, being in crowded places (malls, theaters) and even using transportation, including driving a car. In the end, agoraphobic patients often end up completely housebound.

TABLE 1 Symptoms of Panic Attack

Dizziness, unsteadiness, or faintness
Fear of dying
Fear of going crazy or losing control
Feeling of choking
Feeling of unreality—as if you're *not all there*
Heart palpitations—pounding heart or accelerated heart rate
Hot and cold flashes
Nausea or abdominal distress
Numbness, pain, or tingling in hands, feet, arms, legs, fingers, toes, lips, face
Pain or discomfort in chest, upper back, shoulder blades
Shortness of breath or a feeling of being smothered
Sweating
Trembling or shaking

Impact and Cost

Panic attacks are very common events. Some studies show that lifetime prevalence of panic or panic-like episodes is somewhere from 15% to 45%. Panic disorder, characterized by frequent, disturbing panic attacks accompanied by at least 1 month of persistent fear of having another attack is less frequent. Epidemiologic studies throughout the world indicate the lifetime prevalence of PD (with or without AG) ranges between 1.5% and 3.5%. Twice as many women as men suffer from panic disorder. Studies have suggested high co-morbidity, showing that 63% to 73% of PD patients have had at least one other mental health condition, including major depressive disorder, obsessive–compulsive disorder, or another anxiety disorder during their lifetime. Panic patients also tend to seek relief from their anxiety by self-medicating with alcohol and drugs (prescription and/or illicit). The professional life of a PD patient is also likely to suffer. The majority of these patients admit that the quality of their work diminished as a result of their anxiety. Those who are financially dependent and those who receive either welfare or disability benefits constitute a considerable 27% of all PD patients. Furthermore, there seems to be a lower life expectancy among PD patients because of an increased risk of developing some cardiovascular disease or because of suicidal behavior, although the evidence for this is not consistent. The actual costs of panic disorder are difficult to evaluate because they are indirect and hidden, but it is estimated that they are quite extensive. Because of the physical nature of panic attack symptoms, most PD patients repeatedly consult their family physicians, internists or other health professionals. Current estimates of cost of these conditions in U.S. society are more than $44 billion per year, a figure comparable to the cost of cardiovascular disorders.

TABLE 2 Some of the More Common Situations Feared by Agoraphobics

Being at home alone
Crowded public places such as grocery stores, department stores, restaurants
Enclosed or confined places such as tunnels, bridges, or the hairdresser's chair
Public transportation such as trains, buses, subways, planes

TABLE 3 Differential Diagnosis and Co-morbidity of Panic Disorder

1. Cardiac conditions
   a. Arrhythmias[a,c,d]
   b. Supraventricular tachycardia[a,c,d]
   c. Mitral valve prolapse[b,c,d]
2. Endocrine disorders
   a. Thyroid abnormality[a,b,c,d]
   b. Hyperparathyroidism[b,c,d]
   c. Pheochromocytoma[d]
   d. Hypoglycemia[a,c,d]
3. Vestibular dysfunctions[a,b,c,d]
4. Seizure disorders (temporal lobe epilepsy)[a,b,c,d]
5. Other psychiatric conditions
   a. Affective disorders
      (1) Major depression[d,e,f]
      (2) Bipolar disorder[b,d,e,f]
   b. Other anxiety disorders
      (1) Acute stress disorder[a,b,c,d,e,f]
      (2) Obsessive–compulsive disorder[a,b,c,d,e,f]
      (3) Post-traumatic stress disorder[a,b,c,d,e,f]
      (4) Social phobia[a,c,d,e,f]
      (5) Specific phobia[a,c,d,e,f]
   c. Psychotic disorders[a,d,e,f]
   d. Substance abuse and dependence
      (1) Withdrawal from central nervous system depressants[a,b,c,d,e,f]
         (a) Alcohol abuse (present in 40% of panic disorder patients)
         (b) Barbiturates
      (2) Stimulants[a,b,c,d,e,f]
         (a) Cocaine
         (b) Amphetamines
         (c) Caffeine
      (3) Cannabis[a,b,c,d,e,f]
      (4) Hallucinogens[a,b,c,d,e,f]

[a]The disorder can mimic panic disorder (PD).
[b]The disorder can cause or worsen panic disorder through a variety of physiologic mechanisms.
[c]The disorder's symptoms could serve as triggers of panic attacks.
[d]The disorder could coexist with PD as an independent disorder.
[e]The disorder could be a co-morbid disorder with symptoms that intermingle with PD.
[f]The disorder could lead to PD or be a sequela of PD.

Differential Diagnoses

Table 3 summarizes the differential diagnoses for PD. The relationship between panic disorder and the other disorders listed in the table can be very complex, for example:

- Another disorder can mimic PD.
- Another disorder can cause or worsen PD through a variety of physiologic mechanisms.
- Another disorder's symptoms could serve as triggers of panic attacks.
- Another disorder could coexist with PD as an independent disorder.
- Another disorder could be a co-morbid disorder with symptoms that intermingle with PD.
- Another disorder could lead to PD or be a sequela of PD.

One such example of this interaction is cardiac arrhythmias. Although it is uncommon, an arrhythmia can coexist with panic disorder as an independent condition, and a sudden increase of heart rate could potentially provoke panic in a patient with PD. However, arrhythmia accompanied by fear could mimic a panic attack, and patients with potentially dangerous arrhythmias may receive inappropriate treatment as the result of misdiagnosis. Another possible association is mitral valve prolapse (MVP) in patients with panic, which is a frequent finding thought to be of doubtful clinical significance. However, recent research suggested that it is possible that these two disorders in some patients are linked genetically (via chromo-some 13) in a syndrome characterized by β-adrenergic hyperactivity, MVP, panic, and kidney problems. Careful initial medical and psychiatric evaluation is recommended in panic patients. However, prolonged and repetitive testing should be discouraged.

Theoretical Framework

Different theories, including cognitive–behavioral and biomedical, have been used in an attempt to describe the biologic mechanisms of panic. A brief synthesis of these theories reveals that panic disorder is likely a combination of:

- An increase in alarm reaction
- An error in information processing (catastrophic thinking)
- Abnormal coping strategies to relieve anxiety and provide a sense of security (safety rituals and avoidance)

The disorder represents a sequential process where the symptoms start with the physical symptoms of panic and progress through the stages of abnormal thinking, rituals, and, finally, avoidance (Table 4). These symptom clusters may be wired

TABLE 4 Theory of Panic

Stages of Panic Disorder	Neuronal Circuits	Possible Treatments
Panic attacks (alarm reactions)	Periaqueductal gray amygdala, hippocampus	SSRI, SNRIs, benzodiazepines Interoceptive exposure
Catastrophic thoughts (abnormal information processing)	Orbital frontal cortex, cingulum, hippocampus	SSRI, SNRI, cognitive restructuring, neuroleptics
Precaution rituals and avoidances	Prefrontal and temporal cortex	SSRI, SNRI, neuroleptics Exposure and response prevention

Abbreviations: SNRI = serotonin-norepinephrine reuptake inhibitor; SSRI = selective serotonin reuptake inhibitor.

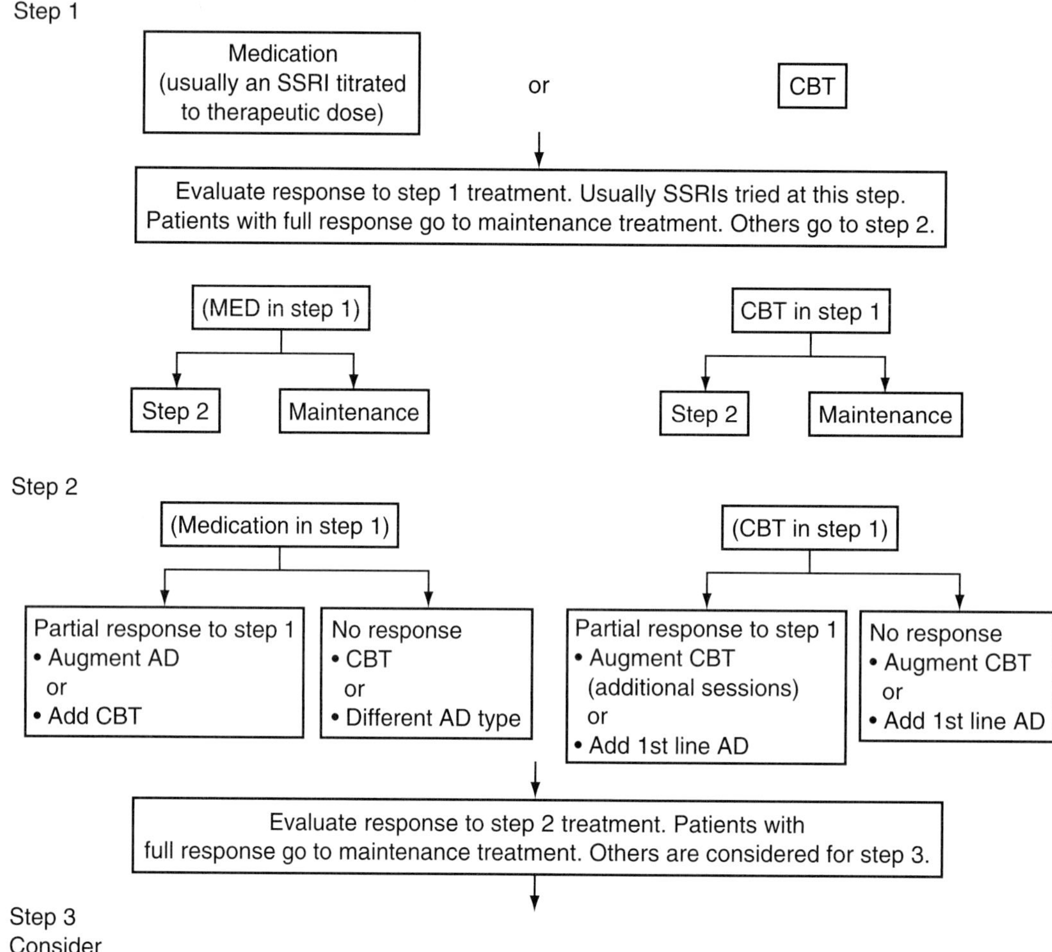

FIGURE 1 Treatment of panic disorder. AD = antidepressant; CBT = cognitive behavior therapy; MED = medication; PTSD = post-traumatic stress disorder; SSRI = selective serotonin reuptake inhibitor.

through different neuronal circuits and respond preferentially to different treatments. However, this theoretical framework is incomplete, as the intricacy of the neuronal circuits and neurotransmitters is not fully understood.

Treatment Algorithm

The treatment of PD is a stepwise process that starts with treatments of proven efficacy that are capable of ameliorating symptoms and decreasing avoidance behaviors. Figure 1 provides an algorithm of the treatment steps.

Step 1 starts with a first-line medication of a selective serotonin reuptake inhibitor (SSRI) or a therapeutic approach with cognitive behavior therapy (CBT). Both treatments have demonstrated efficacy between 70% and 90% in multiple studies. The treatment choice is based on the initial patient session with the physician, in which patients usually express their preference for either medication or psychotherapy. When availability and cost of the therapy is an issue, medication is the simplest way of treating PD. If, after two trials, the SSRI is deemed unsuccessful, step 2 begins.

Step 2 should start with a discussion with the patient about his/her preference for adding another medication or switching to another treatment modality (e.g., psychotherapy).

Step 3 involves treatment with more intensive CBT or with medications or combinations of treatments that have not yet been tried. Unusual and alternative treatments may be considered at that point (an expert consultation is usually recommended).

BEHAVIORAL THERAPY

Behavior therapy can be effective in as few as four sessions and can significantly reduce a patient's distress. Table 5 gives the stages of CBT. The treatment is based on desensitizing patients to their internal sensations and external phobic situations via exposure, reduction of catastrophic thinking, and improvement in coping strategies. However, patients who have very severe anxiety accompanied by depression are frequently unable to follow the therapist's instructions and may need to be started on antidepressants early.

TABLE 5 Cognitive Behavioral Therapy

Assessment
Cognitive restructuring (de-catastrophizing thinking)
Coping enhancement
Education
Exposure and response prevention (to phobic situations)
Interceptive exposure (exposure to internal sensation)
Relapse prevention
Self-monitoring

MEDICATION

Selection of medication depends on whether patients have received prior pharmacotherapy for the treatment of a mood or anxiety disorder, on their previous reaction to medication, and on the severity and acuity of their panic state. An SSRI is the treatment of choice for patients who have never received pharmacotherapy and have at least moderate severity of illness. In addition to treating anxiety, SSRIs will treat a co-morbid major depressive episode (MDE) and lower the risk of future MDEs. All of the SSRIs are thought to be effective in the treatment of the four major anxiety disorders (including PD, obsessive–compulsive disorder, generalized anxiety disorder, and social anxiety disorder) and have little differences except for subtle differences in side-effect profiles and differences in their effects on the cytochrome P450 liver enzyme system (Table 6). In general, selection among antidepressants should be based on the patient's anxiety symptom profile (one should avoid medications with side effects that mimic panic symptoms) and a history the side effects of medications previously taken. Table 7 can be used as a guide. For example, in the patient with severe insomnia, one might select a sedating tricyclic, such as nortriptyline (Pamelor)[1], or perhaps mirtazapine (Remeron)[1]. Paroxetine (Paxil), fluvoxamine (Luvox)[1], or citalopram (Celexa)[1] would be the SSRI of choice

[1]Not FDA approved for this indication.

TABLE 6 Antidepressants Used in Treatment of Panic

Antidepressant	Anxiolytic Efficacy*	Advantages	Disadvantages
Fluoxetine (Prozac)	Panic† and PTSD	Generic form Long half-life (no withdrawal)	Most stimulating Longer half-life
Fluvoxamine (Luvox)[1]	Panic, GAD, and SAD	No P450 2D6 effects	Effects on P4501A$_2$, 2C9, and 3A4 Short half-life—worse withdrawal
Paroxetine (Paxil)	Panic†, GAD†, SAD†, PTSD†	Least stimulating No P4503A4 effects	Most anticholinergic Most sedating
Sertraline (Zoloft)	Panic†, GAD, SAD†, PTSD†	Least P450-2D6 effects Minimal P450-3A4 effects Intermediate half-life (less withdrawal)	Most diarrhea
Citalopram (Celexa)[1] Escitalopram (Lexapro)[1]	Panic	No P450 effects	Least studied
Venlafaxine ER (Effexor XR)[1]	Panic, GAD†, SAD†, PTSD	No P450 effects	Short half-life Withdrawal with missed dose or sudden discontinuation—increased BP at >225 mg
Nefazodone (Serzone)[1]	No controlled studies Open reports in panic, PTSD, SAD	Sedation, can take at bedtime	Prominent P450 3A4 effects Rare reports fatal hepatotoxicity
Mirtazapine (Remeron)[1]	No controlled studies Rare open reports	Sedation	Oversedation Increased appetite and weight gain Rare agranulocytosis
Nortriptyline (Pamelor)[1]	No controlled trials, but for other TCAs (imipramine), controlled evidence in panic, GAD, PTSD	Sedation, can take at bedtime	Too many SEs

[1]Not FDA approved for this indication.
*Data obtained from randomized clinical trials.
†FDA approved for this indication.
Abbreviations: BP = blood pressure; GAD = generalized anxiety disorder; PTSD = post-traumatic stress disorder; SAD = social anxiety disorder; SEs = side effects; TCAs = tricyclic antidepressants.

TABLE 7 Adverse Effects of the Antidepressants*

Adverse Effect	Fluoxetine (Prozac)	Sertraline (Zoloft)	Paroxetine (Paxil)	Fluvoxamine (Luvox)	Citalopram (Celexa) or Escitalopram (Lexapro)	Nortriptyline (Pamelor)	Venlafaxine†
Headache	↑	-	-	-		↓	-
Agitation/anxiety	↑↑	↑	-	-	↑	-	↑
Tremor	↑	↑	↑	-		↑↑	↑↑
Insomnia	↑↑	↑↑	-	-		↓	↑↑
Drowsiness	↑	↑	↑↑	↑↑		↑↑	↑↑
Fatigue	↑	-	↑↑	-		↑↑	↑
Confusion	-	-	-	-		-	-
Dizziness	-	-	↑	-		↑	↑
Anticholinergic‡	-	-	↑	-		↑↑↑	-
Sweating	-	-	-	-		↑↑	↑↑
Weight gain	↑	↑	↑	↑		↑↑	↑
Gastrointestinal	↑	↑↑	-	↑↑		-	↑↑
Sexual	↑↑	↑↑	↑↑	↑	↑	↑	↑↑

*↑ indicates the drug increases the occurrence of the adverse effect; ↓ indicates that it decreases the occurrence.
†Can increase blood pressure; must be monitored.
‡Anticholinergic side effects include dry mouth, constipation, urinary hesitancy or retention, blurred vision.

for patients with prominent activation. For the patient with prominent gastrointestinal (GI) side effects, one would avoid sertraline (Zoloft), and paroxetine would be the SSRI of choice. For patients with prominent palpitations and problems with weight gain, one would avoid tricyclics, paroxetine, and mirtazapine.

Benzodiazepines are not the first choice because of tolerance, dependency potential, and possible interference with CBT (especially with as-needed use). They should be reserved for emergency situations (initial panic attacks), for the reduction in extreme anxiety, or infrequent phobic situations (airplanes, elevators, etc.) before the beginning of the CBT. Finally, they can be used for maintenance of chronic patients with unremitting anxiety. If the benzodiazepines are used chronically, they should be prescribed using a pharmacokinetically appropriate schedule to minimize daily withdrawal or interdose anxiety. As-needed use of benzodiazepines should be avoided and history of alcohol and drug abuse should be assessed before beginning treatment.

TREATMENT RESISTANCE

If the patient is nonresponsive or has side effects to two prior SSRI trials, the choice is then between:

- A serotonin–norepinephrine reuptake inhibitor (SNRI)
- A newer antidepressant (e.g., venlafaxine [Effexor][1], nefazodone [Serzone][1], mirtazapine [Remeron][1])
- A tricyclic
- A g-aminobutyric acid (GABA) agent (e.g., gabapentin [Neurontin][1]) (step 2)

[1]Not FDA approved for this indication.

A final consideration (step 3) involves the management of anxiety and other symptoms with a concomitant medication that would not ordinarily be a first-line treatment choice for anxiety disorders. This involves the use of sedating atypical neuroleptics such as olanzapine (Zyprexa)[1] and quetiapine (Seroquel)[1]. At this point one could consider the use of monoamine oxidase inhibitors (MAOIs), which boast very impressive data supporting their efficacy. These medications require dietary restrictions and stopping concomitant antidepressants. Combining intensive CBT (several times a week) with medication augmentation strategies may also bring a desired effect. Other strategies are under development for the treatment of this resistant population, but none of them have moved past an early experimental stage.

Long-Term Management

While in some patients panic attacks stop in the course of a few months, PD is usually a chronic, waxing and waning condition. Some patients may completely recover, while others may be left with symptoms of other disorders initially masked by the panic attacks. If CBT is initiated, it is important to coordinate the medication treatment with the therapy. Completely blocking anxiety may impair patients' learning in therapy and discourage them from developing new coping techniques. Gradual reduction and stopping medication can be attempted after 2 or 3 months of complete resolution of symptoms. Approximately 20% of patients will not respond to any treatment and need to be maintained in the most comfortable state with medication or therapy or a combination thereof.

[1]Not FDA approved for this indication.

SECTION 18

Physical and Chemical Injuries

BURNS

METHOD OF

Lee D. Faucher, MD

Every year, approximately 1.4 million people suffer burn injuries in the United States; 45,000 of them require hospital admission and 5000 die. Approximately 50% of those hospitalized go to specialized burn centers and 50% go to the other 5000 hospitals throughout the United States. The most current burn care resource directory of the American Burn Association (ABA) lists 131 burn care facilities in the United States, 42 of which are verified burn centers by the ABA and American College of Surgeons Committee on Trauma.

The quality of care during the first several hours after a burn injury has a significant impact on long-term outcome. This article focuses on the first 24 hours of burn care.

The ABA offers an Advanced Burn Life Support Provider Course that is designed to provide physicians, nurses, nurse practitioners, physician assistants, and paramedics with the ability to assess and stabilize patients with serious burns during the first critical hours following injury and also to identify patients who require transfer to a burn center (Table 1). Additional information about the course can be found on the ABA Web site, *www.ameriburn.org*.

Today, more patients are surviving than ever before after sustaining much larger burns. This is most likely because of our better understanding of burn physiology, early excision and grafting of the burn, and initiation of early and adequate nutrition. As a result, we face new challenges in getting those who sustain extensive burns back into society and returning them to the level of function they had before their injury.

There have been many advances in burn prevention over the past 60 years. Household smoke detectors have saved countless lives since being introduced and are attributed with the reduction in the number of massive burns and overall burn-related mortality. Still, 90% of burns are thought to be preventable, and most are caused by carelessness.

Initial Evaluation

PRIMARY SURVEY

The initial evaluation of a burn patient is the same as for any patient involved in trauma. The immediate priority is the airway, followed by breathing, circulation, disability, and exposure.

TABLE 1 Burn Center Referral Criteria

Partial thickness burns greater than 10% total body surface area.
Burns that involve the face, hands, feet, genitalia, perineum, or major joints.
Third-degree burns in any age group.
Electrical burns, including lightning injury.
Chemical burns.
Inhalation injury.
Burn injury in patients with preexisting medical disorders that could complicate management, prolong recovery, or affect mortality.
Any patients with burns and concomitant trauma (such as fractures) in which the burn injury poses the greatest risk of morbidity or mortality. In such cases, if the trauma poses the greater immediate risk, the patient may be initially stabilized in a trauma center before being transferred to a burn unit. Physician judgment is necessary in such situations and should be in concert with the regional medical control plan and triage protocols.
Burned children in hospitals without qualified personnel or equipment for the care of children.
Burn injury in patients who will require special social, emotional, or long-term rehabilitative intervention.

Airway

The airway must be assessed immediately and, if compromised, treated immediately. Simple procedures such as the chin lift with jaw thrust may be all that is needed. If the airway is still not functional, endotracheal intubation should be performed. The cervical spine must be protected at all times during this and following treatments.

Breathing

Bilateral chest wall motion does not guarantee adequate ventilation and oxygenation. Auscultation of bilateral breath sounds, cutaneous signs of oxygen delivery, and objective measurements of oxygen delivery and carbon dioxide removal are necessary. Any patient involved in an enclosed-space fire needs to remain on 100% inspired oxygen until the serum carbon monoxide level returns to normal. Patients with circumferential full-thickness burns to the entire torso need to be monitored closely for adequacy of ventilation, because these may impair ventilation.

Circulation

Adequacy of circulation is measured with palpation of the pulse, blood pressure, and capillary refill. Intravenous access is gained with placement of two large-bore catheters placed under unburned skin, if possible. The catheters can be placed through the burn if necessary, but they should be sutured securely in place. When pulses distal to a burned area are not palpable, a Doppler ultrasound should be used to evaluate blood flow to this area.

Disability, Neurologic Deficit

Burn patients are most often alert and oriented. If not, reasons include unknown head trauma, hypoxia, hypercarbia, poisoning, and substance abuse. Treatment of depressed mental status should follow trauma protocols.

Exposure and Environment Control

It is important to remove all involved clothing and remove any source of further thermal damage. All constrictive jewelry should also be removed. The patient should be kept warm and dry. The room should be warmed to minimize conductive heat loss, and intravenous fluids should be warmed.

SECONDARY SURVEY

After completion of the primary survey, and when resuscitation measures are established, a formal head-to-toe examination follows. Because the burn injury is highly visible, a thorough examination is necessary to ensure that an injury is not overlooked.

History

It is important to gain as much information as possible regarding the injury and the patient's medical history. Many times conditions worsen in patients with large burns, and obtaining this information later is not possible. After obtaining the complete medical, surgical, family, and social history, questions should be focused on the injury itself. The patient needs to be asked, "What was the cause of the burn? What time did it occur? Was it in an enclosed space? Did clothing catch fire? Was there any fuel source involved? Was there an explosion? Was anyone else involved? What has been done to the burned area?"

Physical Examination

The head-to-toe survey is of utmost importance to evaluate the patient for any other signs of trauma. Inspection of the skeleton and joints can reveal fractures. The skin should be examined for signs of penetrating injuries, especially in situations of known trauma or explosion. It is also important to obtain the patient's weight as soon as possible after admission.

Inhalation Injury

Inhalation injury is acute respiratory tract damage caused by toxic inhalants, superheated gases, or steam. The injury manifests itself over the first 5 days after the burn injury and creates difficulty with oxygenation and ventilation. Direct burns to the posterior pharynx can create edema, such that the upper airway is occluded because of the soft tissue edema. Inhalation injury can be thermal airway tissue damage, carbon monoxide (CO) poisoning, or both. Whenever there is a question of airway security or potential loss of the airway because of edema or injury, the patient should be intubated.

Most of the fatalities at the scene of structural fires are caused by CO poisoning. Carbon monoxide has a 200 times greater affinity to hemoglobin than oxygen. The oxygen–hemoglobin dissociation curve loses its sigmoidal shape and shifts to the left. This further impairs oxygen availability to the tissue. Levels of CO greater than 60% are usually fatal. It takes approximately 80 minutes for a person breathing room air to reduce the CO level of 60% to a safer level of 20%. The addition of 100% oxygen can reduce that time to 20 minutes. Patients with high levels of CO usually have normal partial pressure of oxygen in the alveoli (PAO_2) and hemoglobin saturation. The reported cherry-red discoloration of the skin is not always present. The only abnormal objective finding is the elevated level of CO.

Direct injury to the airway can occur in patients involved in an enclosed-space fire. The injury rarely occurs below the level of the glottis because of the respiratory tract's efficient heat exchange mechanism. It is rare for an inhalation injury to occur in other circumstances. Other signs of an inhalation injury include burns to the face, singed facial and nasal hairs, and carbonaceous sputum. Additional signs include a hoarse voice, signs of hypoxemia, dysphagia, and the use of accessory muscles of respiration.

The noxious chemicals in smoke create the injury below the level of the glottis. The injury causes severe inflammation, with hypersecretion of fluid and significant edema formation. The transudative effusion that occurs releases potent smooth muscle constrictors. The exudative materials form casts that cannot be expelled because of the narrow airways. This leads to a progressive inability to adequately oxygenate and ventilate the patient.

The treatment of inhalation injury is mainly supportive. The airway needs to be secured, pulmonary toilet maintained, pneumonia treated when it arises, and the ventilator managed by a physician with experience in burn injuries.

Burn Extent and Depth

The severity of a burn provides information on need for surgical intervention, need for specialized care, and mortality. Extent and depth are two factors that provide most of the information. The extent of the burn is an estimate of the area burned as a percentage of the total body surface area. The burned area is examined, excluding first-degree burns, and mapped onto a chart. The most commonly used device to estimate the total body surface area burned is the rule of nines (Figure 1). The Lund and Browder chart (Table 2) can give a more accurate calculation of the total body surface area burned. An estimate of the area burned for each part of the body, totaled using the age-appropriate column, will give the sum of the partial and full thickness burns. A computerized version is available for use online at *www.sagediagram.com*.

Depth of burn is what determines wound management, need for skin grafting, and possibility of rehabilitation difficulties. The depth of burn usually does not have an impact on the body's physiologic response to injury. Burns to the deep fascia, muscle, and fat—fourth-degree burns—can require greater resuscitative efforts.

A burn can only become deeper as time progresses, and no burn is homogenous in its level of injury. Three zones of injury surround a burn. There is an inner area called the zone of coagulation. In this area there may be no blood flow, and the cells have undergone coagulation necrosis. The area that surrounds the zone of coagulation is the zone of stasis. In this area there is a marked decrease in blood flow, and these cells are at risk of death from ischemia. Surrounding the zone of stasis is the zone of hyperemia. This area most often heals in 7 days and is at much less risk of cell loss. Preventing the zone of stasis from becoming a zone of coagulation, which will extend the injury, is the primary goal of resuscitation and wound care.

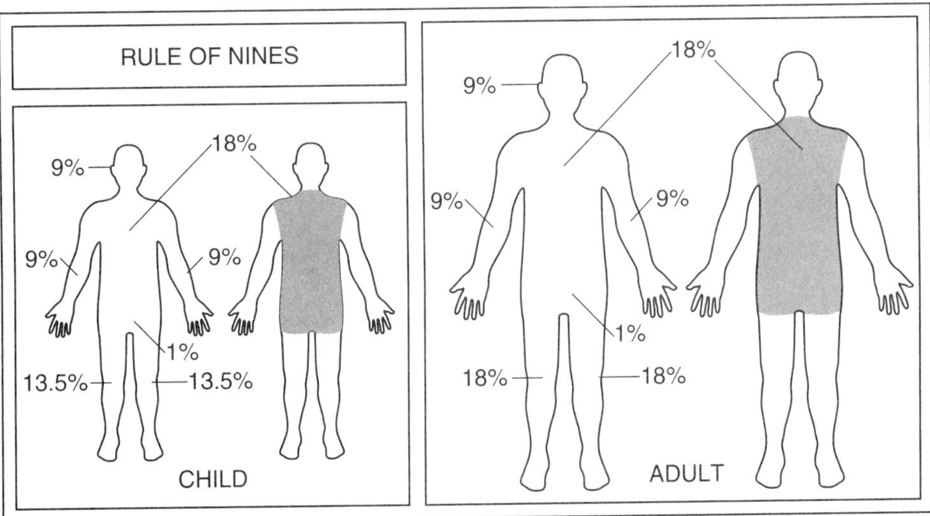

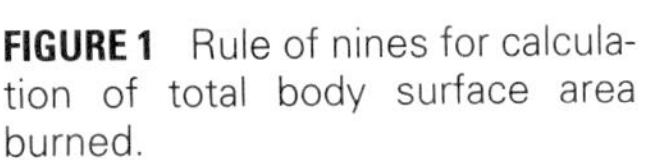
FIGURE 1 Rule of nines for calculation of total body surface area burned.

TABLE 2 Lund and Browder Chart

Area	0-1y	1-4y	5-9y	10-14y	15y	Adult
Head	19	17	13	11	9	7
Neck	2	2	2	2	2	2
Anterior thorax	13	13	13	13	13	13
Posterior thorax	13	13	13	13	13	13
Right buttock	2.5	2.5	2.5	2.5	2.5	2.5
Left buttock	2.5	2.5	2.5	2.5	2.5	2.5
Genitalia	1	1	1	1	1	1
Right upper arm	4	4	4	4	4	4
Left upper arm	4	4	4	4	4	4
Right lower arm	3	3	3	3	3	3
Left lower arm	3	3	3	3	3	3
Right hand	2.5	2.5	2.5	2.5	2.5	2.5
Left hand	2.5	2.5	2.5	2.5	2.5	2.5
Right thigh	5.5	6.5	8	8.5	9	9.5
Left thigh	5.5	6.5	8	8.5	9	9.5
Right leg	5	5	5.5	6	6.5	7
Left leg	5	5	5.5	6	6.5	7
Right foot	3.5	3.5	3.5	3.5	3.5	3.5
Left foot	3.5	3.5	3.5	3.5	3.5	3.5
Total						

A first-degree burn does not stimulate the body's physiologic response to injury and, therefore, is not included in the calculation of total body-surface-area burn. First-degree burns can be quite painful, and patients may need to be admitted for pain control. These burns heal in 3 to 4 days without scarring. Many times, nonsteroidal anti-inflammatory medications (NSAIDs) can be quite helpful for pain control.

A second-degree burn involves only part of the dermis. There is usually blistering of the skin and visible fluid loss from the injured areas. The injured area can be red or pink and may blanch with pressure. It may be painful to the touch. If these burns heal within 14 days, there is minimal to no scarring. Burns that take longer than 5 weeks to heal most often will result in significant visible scars and can lead to function-limiting contractures. Most burn surgeons will excise and graft burns that will take longer than 2 weeks to heal.

A third-degree burn destroys the entire dermis and thus the ability for the skin to heal. These burns can range in color from bright red to charred and blackened. They do not blanch with pressure and are most often insensate. A full-thickness burn will develop an eschar that is dead, structurally intact tissue that will eventually separate from the underlying viable tissue.

A fourth-degree burn extends through the subcutaneous layer to the underlying bone, muscle, or fibrous structures. If the skin of this area remains intact, it is most often depressed, charred, and blackened. This degree of burn is the most difficult to manage because it will create a more vigorous physiologic response and require greater resuscitative efforts. It also becomes more difficult to obtain adequate skin graft coverage and may require a flap or tissue transfer, and there is an increased likelihood of amputation for extremity burns.

Resuscitation

The goal of resuscitation of a thermally injured patient is the same as in any other injured patient, to maintain tissue perfusion and oxygen delivery to the tissues. Thermally injured patients, especially those with an inhalation injury, can require a staggering amount of intravenous fluid to maintain perfusion. Our first understanding of the extensive fluid needs came from studying those injured in the Rialto Theater fire in 1921 and the Cocoanut Grove nightclub fire in 1942. There have been many weight-based formulas developed for the resuscitation of the thermally injured patient since the original Evans' formula of 1952. Therefore, no matter the formula chosen, effective resuscitation needs to maintain adequate urine output and avoid systemic acidosis.

The hemodynamic effects of a thermal injury create both a hypovolemic shock and a cellular shock. The result is decreased cardiac output, extracellular fluid, plasma volume, and oliguria. The cellular shock leads to increased vascular permeability, and as a result a large volume of fluid shifts into the extravascular space. The exact mechanism of the postburn vascular change is unknown.

The Parkland formula is the most commonly used formula for the resuscitation of burn patients. Once the patient's weight and total body surface area burned are known, the resuscitation volume can be calculated. The patient is given a volume of intravenous lactated Ringer's of 4 mL/kg body weight per percent body surface area burned. One half of this volume is given in the first 8 hours and the other half over the next 16 hours. For example, an 80-kg person with a 50% burn would get a total volume of 16,000 mL given at a rate of 1000 mL per hour for 8 hours, followed by 500 mL per hour for the next 16 hours.

Urine output needs to be maintained at a rate of at least 30 mL per hour, and the fluids can be adjusted to meet these needs. Oliguria is always the result of inadequate fluid resuscitation; diuretics are contraindicated.

Wound Care

The optimal outcome of treating burn patients is returning a thermally injured patient to the functional status he or she had before the injury. This begins with proper wound care upon admission. Circumferential, full-thickness burns of the extremities can lead to a compartment syndrome. The risk for compartment syndrome increases as resuscitation continues. The circumferential eschar does not permit normal tissue expansion as the burn edema progresses. Indications for escharotomy include signs of decreased distal circulation, symptoms of compartment syndrome, or elevated compartment pressures. An escharotomy is a bedside procedure using a knife, or most commonly an electrocautery device. The preferred incision sites for escharotomies are the medial and lateral aspect of the extremities. Chest escharotomies start from the midclavicular line, proceed down to the anterior axillary line, then continue to approximately the tip of the twelfth rib. A transverse incision is also made at the level of the xiphoid (Figure 2). The eschar is incised through the damaged skin, but not into the subcutaneous layer. Great care must be taken to avoid neurovascular bundles, tendons, and boney prominences. Hemostasis is a must.

If the patient is to be transferred to a burn center within 24 hours of injury, it is not necessary to undergo débridement and antimicrobial coverage of the wounds. The priority is to keep the patient warm and dry. Wound care begins with simple washing of the wound with soap and water. Removal of the blistered and burned skin can be quite painful, and patients usually require higher doses of narcotics than are recommended for their weight. To débride the wounds effectively, the patient's pain control needs must be met.

It is important to remove all tissue that can be easily removed to facilitate application of the topical agent. There are many agents from which to choose; silver sulfadiazine cream (SSD) is the most commonly used agent to treat burn wounds. Apply SSD as a thin paste to all affected areas and cover with a light gauze dressing. The purpose of the dressing is to hold the SSD in place. Any exposed areas can be covered with more SSD. Daily wound care consists of removal of the bandage and washing the wound with soap and water to remove the bacteria-laden SSD. More tissue loss can occur as the eschar separates, and this should be débrided. This process of daily wound care limits bacterial overload and decreases the risk of wound infection. All burn wounds become colonized with skin flora within the first few days, followed by gastrointestinal flora.

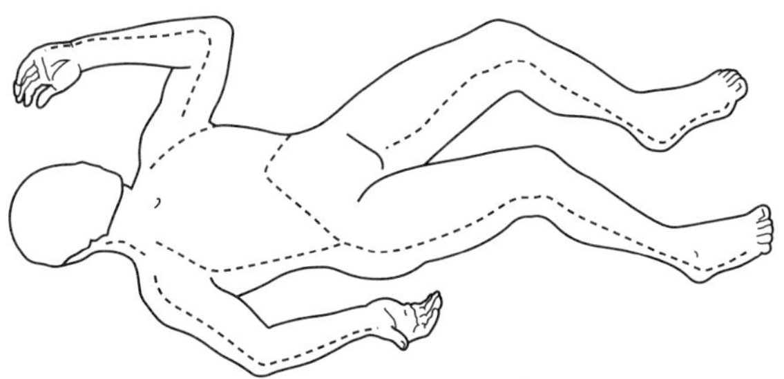

FIGURE 2 Anatomic positions for escharotomies.

As the burn heals and the eschar has sloughed, the SSD can be discontinued and petroleum jelly-based products can be used. The same daily wound care is needed until the wound is fully healed.

Other Burns

Scald and flame burns account for 75% of admissions to burn centers. Scald burns account for 70% of admissions in patients younger than 2 years of age. The incidence decreases with age. Flame is the etiology for 50% to 60% of burns in patients who are 5 through 70 years of age.

CHEMICAL

Chemical burns affect approximately 5% of all patients admitted to burn centers and are most common in middle-aged adults. The severity of a chemical burn is directly related to length of exposure to the agent. Prompt treatment can drastically minimize the depth of the burn.

Treatment of chemical burns begins with the ABCs as outlined above. This is followed by the removal of all clothing that may contain the offending compound. The caregiver must be properly protected to avoid injury during treatment. Once the clothing is removed, the injured areas need to be flushed with copious amounts of water. There should be no attempt at neutralizing the compound because the most common byproduct of a chemical reaction is heat. This would compound the chemical burn with a thermal burn and could increase the depth of injury. Water irrigation should continue until the patient feels relief or until the patient has been evaluated in a burn center.

ELECTRICAL

Electrical burns are the cause of approximately 5% of the admissions to burn centers and are most common in middle-aged adults. The true extent of an electrical injury is hard to diagnose, as the amount of visible cutaneous damage is only a small fraction of the overall tissue destruction. Similar to other burns, tissue destruction is proportional to the amount of current and duration of contact. A high-voltage burn is caused by voltage greater than 1000 volts and is the most concerning. The damage caused by passage of current is related to the Joule effect. Electrical energy is converted to heat by tissue resistance. The amount of electrical energy of a given voltage is indirectly proportional to the cross-sectional area of the body part. This explains why extremities can be destroyed and the trunk is spared.

The management begins with the ABCs and a close inspection for contact points to identify the burns. All circumferential clothing and jewelry should be removed. The burn size is estimated and resuscitation begun. The urine needs to be closely monitored to look for signs of myoglobinuria. If myoglobinuria is present, the intravenous fluid rate should be increased to achieve a urine output of at least 100 mL per hour. This will prevent myoglobin deposition in the renal collecting tubules that could lead to renal failure.

Signs of shock, progressive acidosis despite aggressive fluid resuscitation, and increased pain are signs of severe muscle destruction and require immediate operative exploration. Fasciotomies are often required to relieve extremity compartment syndrome. Patient symptoms or elevated compartment pressure indicate the need for compartment release. Fasciotomies are best done by a surgeon in the operating room. Upper extremity fasciotomies often require a carpal tunnel release, and, in the lower extremity, all four compartments require release.

The need for cardiac monitoring after electrical injury is highly controversial. A patient without electrocardiogram conduction abnormalities on admission will not develop delayed cardiac problems. An abnormal admission electrocardiogram is often seen, but large studies do not demonstrate a benefit in prolonged cardiac monitoring.

Outpatient Burn Care

Approximately 33.3% of all burns are managed without admission to a hospital. Several conditions need to be met before outpatient management is considered (Table 3). In the outpatient setting, the same principles apply for initial wound care as described above. The first step is to cleanse the wound thoroughly with soap and water, then cover the wound with appropriate antimicrobial cream. Next, a light dressing is applied to hold the cream in place. The patient then needs instructions on proper range of motion therapy and a clear understanding of the risks of failing to comply. There is no role for prophylactic antibiotics, as they have not been shown to improve outcome and can lead to the development of resistant organisms. A follow-up appointment is made and enough supplies and pain medications are given to the patient to last until the next appointment.

After the burn is healed, there is still remodeling of the skin structure occurring for a period of up to 18 months. Healed burned skin must be protected from the sun with liberal use of sun block at all times. A sunburn in a healed burn undergoing cellular change can trigger changes in pigment deposition and leave the area lighter or darker than normal.

TABLE 3 Outpatient Management Criteria

Intravenous fluid resuscitation is not necessary.
The patient is able to consume adequate oral intake.
The patient is able to return for follow-up.
The patient understands the need for aggressive physical therapy.
Oral medications control pain.
The patient has adequate family/friend support.

Consultation with a burn care specialist is recommended if any complications arise during outpatient management.

Rehabilitation

Rehabilitation of burn patients begins the day of injury and never really ends. Burn centers have physical and occupational therapists with expertise in the needs of burn patients. Therapy begins with range-of-motion exercises with every joint, burned or unburned. This helps to minimize edema, promote blood flow, and minimize nosocomial complications, such as pneumonia and deep venous thrombosis. Patient ambulation is begun as soon as possible and bed rest is minimized around the grafting procedures.

Approximately 5 days after skin grafting, patients begin aggressive range-of-motion exercises that concentrate on the grafted sites. All scars shrink, and the shrinking can lead to deformities that can cause loss of function. Only aggressive therapy can overcome these natural effects to maintain full function and return patients back to their preinjury level of function.

HIGH-ALTITUDE SICKNESS

METHOD OF

James S. Milledge, MD

High-altitude sickness is caused by hypoxia because of the low barometric pressure of altitude. The same sickness can be induced by lowering the partial pressure in a chamber by lowering either the pressure or the percentage of oxygen in the gas breathed. What is crucial is the partial pressure of oxygen in the inspired air as was first shown by Paul Bert more than 120 years ago.

Many other clinical conditions may be encountered on mountains because of cold, infections, and others; and the hypoxia of altitude causes other changes such as weight loss, psychomotor dysfunction, and reduced physical performance, but these are not considered in this article. The high-altitude illnesses discussed in this article are:

1. Acute mountain sickness (AMS)—simple or benign; high-altitude cerebral edema (HACE); and high-altitude pulmonary edema (HAPE)
2. Subacute mountain sickness (S-AMS)
3. Chronic mountain sickness

Acute Mountain Sickness

AMS affects otherwise fit people if they go up to altitude too fast. When a person goes rapidly to altitude, there is usually a delay of from 6 to 24 hours before symptoms are felt. Headache is usually the first symptom followed by general malaise, loss of appetite, nausea, and vomiting. Sleep is disturbed. The symptoms get worse, typically peaking on the second or third day at altitude and remitting by day five. Recurrence at that altitude is not seen but may well recur on going to a higher altitude. Treatment is not really necessary but analgesics can be given for the headache and voluntary hyperventilation helps temporarily.

The incidence of AMS depends upon the rate of ascent and the height reached. An incidence of 25% was found in Colorado ski resorts at 1900 to 2940 m (6233.6 to 9645.7 ft) where people typically drive in a day from low altitude. In Europe, climbers walking to mountain huts have an incidence of 9% at 2850 m (9350.4 ft), 13% at 3050 m (10,006 ft), and 34% at 3650 m (11,975 ft). An incidence of 95% has been reported in tourists flying directly to Shayangboche (3800 m [12,467 ft]) in the Everest region of Nepal. A history of previous AMS is predictive of likely future trouble and vice versa, but there are many exceptions and any infection, especially of the respiratory tract, is a risk factor. All ages, all races, and both sexes can be affected. Possibly older people are at lower risk. Previous altitude experience may be protective to a degree. People born and raised at altitude seem less at risk.

Various drugs (Table 1) can mitigate the severity of AMS, of which acetazolamide (Diamox) is the best studied and most used. Acetazolamide probably works by promoting bicarbonate excretion, thus stimulating ventilation and improving blood gases, giving a sort of artificial acclimatization. The dose used in trials was 250 mg 2 or 3 times a day, but usually a dose of 125 mg twice a day is now recommended so as to lessen side effects. These consist of tingling in the fingers and toes and occasionally around the mouth. Most find these side effects to be unimportant, but a substantial minority find them very unpleasant. Subjects should also be warned that the drug is a mild diuretic. They should try the drug at home before using it at altitude to see if the side effects are acceptable. Dexamethasone, 2 to 4 mg orally every 6 hours which is recommended for cerebral edema, is also protective for simple AMS. Unlike acetazolamide, however, it does not improve blood gasses. Theophylline is beneficial in a dose of 350 mg slow release (250 mg in patients <70 kg [154.3 lb]) twice daily. It is best if drugs are started 24 hours before ascent, but some benefit can be gained even if drugs are started after symptoms begin. The best way to prevent AMS is to plan to ascend sufficiently slowly to avoid it (see Table 1). A rule of thumb that has been suggested is:

- If above 3000 m (9842.5 ft), each night should be no higher than 300 m (984.3 ft) above the last.
- Have a rest day every 2 to 3 days (2 nights at the same altitude).

However, there is such variability in susceptibility that this rule will be unnecessarily slow for many and too fast for some. An additional rule is needed—do not ascend further with symptoms of AMS.

TABLE 1 Recommendations for the Prevention and Treatment of Acute Mountain Sickness (AMS)

	AMS Simple	HACE	HAPE
Prevention	Gain height slowly* Go no higher if symptomatic Take acetazolamide (Diamox) or dexamethasone (Decadron)[1]	Same as for AMS	Same as for AMS
Treatment	Self-limiting If needed, acetaminophen (Tylenol)[1], acetazolamide, or dexamethasone[1]	DESCENT Dexamethasone[1], 4-8 mg every 6 hours Pressure bag	DESCENT Nifedipine (Procardia)[1], 20 mg every 6 hours Pressure bag

[1]Not FDA approved for this indication.
*Suggested maximum rate of ascent is:
Above 3000 m (9842.5 ft), gain no more than 300 m (984.3 ft) a day.
Take a rest day (no height gain) every 2-3 days.
Abbreviations: AMS = acute mountain sickness; HACE = high-altitude cerebral edema; HAPE = high-altitude pulmonary edema.

High-Altitude Cerebral Edema

HACE is a potentially lethal condition that develops from simple or benign AMS. The setting and the initial symptoms are the same but instead of resolving, the symptoms progress with the addition of more serious neurologic signs. Often the first of these is the development of unsteadiness (ataxia) on walking and later even on sitting. There may be mood changes. In the context of AMS these early signs are all too easily missed because patients may complain only of a headache and want to be left alone in their bedroom or tent. They may insist that they are "fine," because loss of insight is part of the symptomatology. The patient may then start hallucinating and on examination may be found to have up-going plantar reflexes and papilledema. Occasionally there are ocular palsies. In untreated cases coma follows and death in a few hours or days. The picture is often complicated by the presence of HAPE.

Prevention of HACE is the same as for AMS (see Table 1):

- Gain altitude slowly.
- Do not go higher with symptoms.
- Go down if symptoms get worse.

As with AMS, all ages and races and both sexes are at risk. The incidence is on the order of 1% to 2% of lowlanders going to altitudes above 3000 to 4000 m (9842.5 to 13,123 ft).

Treatment of HACE is to get the patient down to a lower altitude as soon as possible. If evacuation is impossible or delayed, dexamethasone is beneficial. The dose suggested is 4 to 8 mg initially followed by 2 to 4 mg every 6 hours until there is relief of symptoms. Recompression in a portable pressure chamber (Gamow or CERTEC bag) for an hour is likely to help and may make it possible for the patient to walk down instead of being carried, a great help in difficult terrain. However, relapse is likely if the patient is not evacuated to lower altitude, and it is stressed that these measures should not take the place of evacuation to lower altitudes.

High-Altitude Pulmonary Edema

HAPE is the other lethal form of AMS. It is now thought that some degree of subclinical pulmonary edema may be quite common on arrival at altitude during the period of risk of AMS. But in the majority of people this resolves over the next few days. However, in perhaps 1% to 3% of people the condition becomes progressive. The symptoms of simple AMS usually precede those of HAPE, although these may be quite mild. To these are added increased breathlessness and a cough, which is dry at first and later productive of white frothy sputum becoming blood-tinged as the condition progresses. The patient, if climbing, falls behind his or her companions and is easily exhausted. There may be chest discomfort, a rapid pulse, fast breathing rate, and a mild pyrexia. The oxygen saturation (on pulse oximetry) is lower than normal for the altitude from an early stage in the condition. On listening at the lung bases, crackles are heard, and as the condition progresses these are audible without a stethoscope as the patient literally drowns in his or her own secretions. Death can come in a matter of hours from first symptom.

Patients with HAPE have a very high pulmonary artery pressure, and a loud pulmonary second heart sound may be detected. They have a greater than normal pulmonary artery pressor response to hypoxia especially during exercise. Individual susceptibility is marked, that is, once a patient has had one attack the risk is high for subsequent attacks on going to altitude. All ages and races and both sexes are at risk, but possibly youth is a greater risk factor.

Treatment, as for HACE, is first and foremost to get the patient down. If this is not possible or while awaiting evacuation, nifedipine, 20 mg by mouth, is beneficial. This can be repeated every 6 hours if necessary. It is thought to act by reducing the pulmonary artery pressure. Cold, by causing peripheral vasoconstriction and so increasing central blood volume, is a risk factor, so keeping the patient warm is important. Oxygen, if available, certainly helps, as does treatment in a Gamow or CERTEC recompression bag and, as in HACE, may improve the patient's condition sufficiently to make evacuation easier. However, it is not a substitute for evacuation to lower altitude. Infection may be a factor in causing the condition in some cases, so antibiotics are often given, but the mechanism is not essentially infective.

Although individual susceptibility is clear and trouble on future altitude trips is likely, it must be said that having had an attack on an expedition and gone down, many climbers have then acclimatized more slowly and succeeded in climbing their peak, for example at Mt. McKinley in Denali National Park, Alaska (6194 m [20,321.5 ft]).

Subacute Mountain Sickness

Two forms of S-AMS have been reported, adult and infantile. The infantile form was found in Han Chinese babies born in Lhasa (3700 m [12,139 ft]). They present within the first few months of life with dyspnea, cough, irritability, sleeplessness, and signs of cyanosis, edema of the face, oliguria, tachycardia, liver enlargement, crackles in the lungs, and fever. The condition was usually fatal in a few weeks if the babies were kept at altitude. The adult form was reported in Indian soldiers encamped at approximately 6000 m (19,685 ft) or higher in Kashmir for more than 6 months. They presented with cough, dyspnea, and effort angina. The signs were of dependent edema. They had cardiomegaly, right ventricular enlargement, and, in most cases, pericardial effusion. The pulmonary artery pressure was elevated. Recovery was rapid on descent to low altitude.

Both forms seem to represent the human form of brisket disease, a condition affecting cattle taken to high altitude. The mechanism seems to be right-heart failure caused by chronic pulmonary hypertension resulting from hypoxia.

Chronic Mountain Sickness (CMS)

Chronic mountain sickness (CMS) is a condition affecting long-term or lifelong residents at high altitude. It was first described in people native to high altitude in the Andes, but has since been reported in Tibet and from high altitude towns in the United States (e.g., Leadville, Colorado). In Tibet it is much more common in immigrant Han Chinese than Tibetan people.

The symptoms are rather vague and include complaints of headache, dizziness, somnolence, fatigue, difficulty in concentration, and even hallucinations. Poor exercise tolerance is common but dyspnea is not a prominent complaint. On going down to low altitude the symptoms disappear. The underlying problem is excessive production of red cells with very high hemoglobin concentrations; 23 g/dL is not uncommon. The normal hemoglobin is higher at altitude but patients with CMS have values much higher than normal for that altitude. Patients are also more hypoxic and so appear markedly cyanotic.

Treatment of choice is relocation to low altitude. This is often not possible, however, for economic reasons. Repeated venesection of a unit of blood is beneficial but must be repeated every 2 to 4 months.

DISTURBANCES CAUSED BY COLD

METHOD OF

Major (res) Andrew W. Kirkpatrick, CD, MD, and

Colonel Ian B. Anderson, CD, MDCM

Hypothermia is a physical state that can manifest as a patient's sole and life-threatening problem or can secondarily complicate the treatment and management of other serious medical and surgical illnesses. Localized manifestations of cold disorders involve tissue injuries ranging from completely reversible exposures, such as frostnip, to full thickness necrosis in severe frostbite. Systemic hypothermia has fascinated clinicians for millennia. It is a proverbial double-edged sword. It decreases the metabolic requirements and efficiency of enzyme systems, but it decreases oxygen demands and may protect the brain. In specific, controlled situations there may be benefits in both tolerating and inducing hypothermia in the critically ill. Conversely, hypothermia can, in and of itself, be fatal and is accepted as a harbinger of death in trauma. After exhaustive review and participating in research regarding the physiologic effects of hypothermia, the authors remain uncertain how to best answer the question, "is hypothermia harmful to the sick patient?" We believe the most practical answer depends on the circumstances, hemodynamic stability, and, particularly, whether the patient is actively bleeding.

Localized Cold Injuries

FROSTNIP AND CHILBLAINS

Frostnip is a reversible condition that results from exposure to subfreezing and freezing environments; and manifests as cold, whitened areas, typically on the face, ears, or extremities. Chilblains (or pernio) appears as red, itchy lesions, usually on the dorsum of the foot. Rewarming and protection from further injury are definitive.

IMMERSION (TRENCH) FOOT

We have not personally seen immersion (trench) foot, which is mostly reported in the military literature and is the result of prolonged exposure to cold but nonfreezing water temperatures. The feet were typically immersed in cold water with a resultant direct cold injury that may involve demyelination and muscle necrosis. The military literature has emphasized that prevention is paramount, and currently such injuries would raise concerns over the leadership of the involved personnel if not explained by unavoidable circumstances.

FROSTBITE

This serious tissue injury reflects the local effects of temperatures cold enough to freeze tissue water. There are marked pathophysiologic similarities between these injuries and those seen in burns and ischemia/reperfusion injuries. In civilian practice, alcohol and drug use, poor planning, vehicular accident or failure, and psychiatric illness figure prominently as causal in recreational and urban cold injuries. Extracellular ice initially causes an intracellular osmotic dehydration, damages cell membranes, and initiates cell death. Intracellular ice may further mechanically disrupt cells. Repeated cycles of thawing and freezing are markedly deleterious and hasten progressive thrombosis. A progressive ischemia occurs with arrest of dermal blood flow, endothelial injury, release of inflammatory mediators, and edema formation. Both the temperature gradient and duration of exposure relate to the severity, but the duration of exposure more directly correlates with the degree of injury than the ambient temperature. The initial signs of frostbite involve a feeling of numbness, with hard, insensitive, whitened blanched areas of skin. Favorable early signs include preservation of sensation to pinprick and deformability.

Field care of frostbite involves rewarming the involved part—once only! This may entail avoiding rewarming altogether and simply ensuring protection from mechanical trauma until transport or shelter is available. When definitive rewarming can be carried out, it is done with warm water heated to 40°C to 42°C (104°F to 107.6°F). Rewarming should be continued until the part is red/purple and pliable. Analgesics should be liberally administered, and we use narcotics as well as ibuprofen (Motrin), both for analgesia and to inhibit the inflammatory cycle. Aloe vera (Dermaide Aloe)[1,*] may be used as a topical inhibitor of thromboxane. Tetanus toxoid (Td) is given according to tetanus status as these are tetanus-prone wounds, but we do not prophylactically prescribe antibiotics. Although the procedure is controversial, superficial clear blisters may be débrided, but large hemorrhagic blisters are left intact. True classification can only be applied after rewarming, and is done in degrees, as follows:

- First-degree injury involves a white plaque with surrounding erythema.
- Second-degree injury shows clear or milky blisters surrounded by erythema and edema.
- Third-degree injury presents hemorrhagic blisters with subsequent black eschar.
- Fourth-degree injury produces complete necrosis and tissue loss.

Daily hydrotherapy will assist the débridement and demarcation. Demarcation of the extent of tissue loss often takes weeks. Physiotherapy is important for future functional recovery. We undertake no elective surgical interventions during this time period, although compartment syndromes may necessitate escharotomy or fasciotomy, and sepsis may warrant earlier amputation. Others have suggested that technetium scintigraphy and magnetic resonance scanning may allow an earlier demarcation of ischemic soft tissue, but this remains inconclusive.

Systemic Hypothermia

DEFINITIONS

Hypothermia is considered to be:

- Mild at temperatures of 35°C to 32°C (95°F to 89.6°F)
- Moderate at temperatures of 32°C to 28°C (89.6°F to 82.4°F)
- Severe at temperatures of less than 28°C (82.4°F)

This classification applies well to accidental systemic hypothermia and suggests treatment strategies. In the mild cases the normal homeostatic thermoregulatory mechanisms remain functional and the patient may still generate a spontaneous heat flux. In moderate hypothermia, this capacity is lost. In severe hypothermia, unconsciousness is generally present, shivering is absent, and spontaneous cardiac arrhythmias are commonly present.

After multisystem trauma, hypothermia is considered any temperature below 36°C (96.8°F). Intraoperative decision making considers any temperature below 34°C (93.2°F) to be severe and a trigger for abbreviated *damage control* surgical techniques aimed at staging definitive surgery to a later period when thermoregulation has been restored. The classic categories thus appear inconsistent with current concepts of hypothermia in trauma. We classify posttraumatic hypothermia as types I to IV:

- Type I is 36°C to 34°C (96.8°F to 93.2°F)
- Type II is 34°C to 32°C (93.2°F to 89.6°F)
- Type III is 32°C to 28°C (89.6°F to 82.4°F)
- Type IV demonstrates a temperature of less than 28°C (82.4°F).

Hypothermia can also be considered exogenous, being solely the result of environmental cooling; or endogenous, as a result of metabolic failure from medical conditions such as neurologic injuries and illnesses, hypothyroidism, adrenal insufficiency, hypopituitarism, or sepsis (in which it is a poor prognostic sign). In reality, it is often hard to separate the two. For example, a drug overdose may induce coma (endogenous) but may leave one immobilized in a cold room (exogenous).

PATHOPHYSIOLOGY

Systemic hypothermia affects every organ system and decreases the metabolic activities of every cell, although heat will not be lost or conserved equally throughout the body because of variations in organ composition, insulation, metabolic activities, and, particularly, the structure of the thermal core (heat is preferentially conserved) versus the thermal shell (heat is not preferentially conserved). Physiologic responses will also differ depending on the degree of hypothermic stress. The initial responses seen are reflexive, counter-regulatory responses that attempt to restore body heat, as well as the typical responses to any serious stress. Sudden cooling will stimulate arousal with induced shivering, with an increased heart rate, blood pressure, and respiratory rate and depth. As the degree of hypothermia increases, however, consciousness is progressively lost, and blood pressure and cardiac output diminish. Tissue perfusion progressively diminishes as blood viscosity increases secondary to a cold-induced diuresis, peripheral vasospasm intensifies, and there is a shift away from oxygen release in the oxyhemoglobin dissociation curve. A serum hyperkalemia is expected.

[1]Not FDA approved for this indication.
*Available as alternative medicine.

Electrical conduction in all pathways is slowed, which in the heart manifests as both atrial and ventricular irritability, with ventricular fibrillation common below 30°C (86°F). As the coagulation system constitutes a series of enzymatic reactions, it should be expected that profound changes occur in blood clotting, with coagulopathies occurring, that are further exacerbated by a cold-induced platelet dysfunction.

The end result—that a patient may be in an unresponsive, apneic, pulseless, seemingly brain dead state, yet remain fully viable with appropriate care—is a sobering thought that should guide clinical decision making.

TRAUMATIC VERSUS NONTRAUMATIC HYPOTHERMIA

The basic role of hypothermia in critical illness remains somewhat uncertain. Shock is a progressive lethal condition, in which a cumulative irreversible oxygen debt may accumulate. If a subject is not actively hemorrhaging, hypothermia may actually benefit survival and has been induced experimentally for this purpose. Alternatively, in victims of hemorrhagic shock, control of hemorrhage is unlikely unless co-incident, hypothermia-induced coagulopathies are reversed by rewarming. We thus feel the distinction between hypothermia with and without hemorrhage is crucial.

PREHOSPITAL CARE

The basic dictum is that "no patient is dead, until warm and dead." In order to reasonably manage resources and avoid unnecessary risk to caregivers, exceptions to this are obvious unsurviveable injuries, known hyperkalemia (>10.0 mmol/L), and a known period of anoxia prior to cooling. When in doubt, the victim should be transported to definitive medical care to allow an attempt at resuscitation, or at least accurate measurement of the core temperature. Remarkable survivals are reported in seemingly *dead* individuals with accidental hypothermic exposures, particularly, but not limited to, children. One of our own younger brothers is a living example. Because of their high surface-to-mass ratio, children cool rapidly after complete immersion, which coupled with a pronounced conservation of brain blood flow with cool water immersion (so called "diving reflex"), has led to remarkable survivals with completely normal neurologic recovery. Although the exact mechanism is controversial, even modest cooling of the brain imparts cerebral protection in excess of that predicted by reduced oxygen consumption alone.

When first approaching the severely hypothermic patient, basic tenets of advanced life support should be applied. Traumatic injury should be suspected whenever the circumstances are uncertain. As always, the airway takes precedence. If the patient is unconscious and not protecting the airway, one should be established through whatever means the rescuer is most familiar. Endotracheal intubation is the most definitive, despite the theoretical risks of inducing fibrillation if this has not already occurred. Oxygen should be administered and hyperventilation should be avoided. Intravenous access should be obtained, and warmed intravenous fluids (such as normal saline containing 5% dextrose) should be administered, because the patient will be inherently volume contracted. If vigorous shivering is present, passive (endogenous) rewarming can be maximized by drying and insulating the patient. Theoretically, active external rewarming methods may attenuate the shivering response in such patients. In more severely hypothermic patients without shivering this is not a concern, although core temperature afterdrop, and cardiovascular rewarming stresses are.

Potentially the most difficult determination is whether there is a spontaneous circulation present or not. If spontaneous cardiac rhythm is not seen electrocardiographically, or if this is not available, one should feel for a carotid pulse for at least 1 minute before determining that the pulse is not present. If it is not, and adequate ventilation has been secured, then standard cardiopulmonary resuscitation (CPR) should be instituted and not be interrupted until the patient has been rewarmed. Although our opinion is controversial, we believe that patients with severe hypothermia and cardiovascular collapse requiring CPR should not be rewarmed until they can be definitively rewarmed in a hospital setting, preferably using an extracorporeal circulation. The prime reason is to conserve the hypothermic neuroprotection in a transport setting where rewarming attempts are likely to be limited. Trauma systems and regional coordination are important in assuring the most expedient transport to this level of care. Defibrillation may be attempted, but the arrested, cold myocardium is likely to respond only to rewarming.

HOSPITAL CARE

While obtaining pertinent history and physiologic data from the prehospital care personnel, the clinician should simultaneously reassess the patient's cardiorespiratory status. Treatment of co-incident injuries or illnesses may dominate the resuscitation in complicated hypothermia. In such cases, it is crucial that the temperature be measured early and with a low reading thermometer at a central site, which will reflect the thermal core rather than peripheral tissue. Rectal temperature is easier to obtain but will lag behind the esophageal temperature during non–steady state conditions. The greatest inaccuracy may occur during transition from cooling to warming, when cardiac temperatures are rising, but the rectal temperature is still falling.

In any critically ill patient, nasogastric tubes are required to prevent aspiration. Indwelling bladder catheters greatly assist in assessing hemodynamic responses to resuscitation. Standard blood assays should be obtained including blood count, glucose, creatinine, and electrolytes including the magnesium, calcium, and phosphate. Arterial blood gasses and coagulation studies are routinely determined at 37°C (98.6°F). The coagulation studies may thus be falsely reassuring, while interpreting the uncorrected blood gases is clinically appropriate. Cultures for infection and toxicology studies should be liberally obtained.

THE PATIENT WHO IS NOT BLEEDING

If hypothermia appears to be the primary medical concern, treatment may focus solely on rewarming. A careful reassessment and detailed history should be obtained when possible, with a high suspicion for other systemic illnesses if the etiology of the hypothermic presentation is not fully explained. Rewarming strategies can be considered passive or active, whereas active rewarming can be further considered either internal or external (Table 1). While also therapeutic, the provision of warmed IV fluids (and blood if necessary), coverage with warm blankets and/or convective air, and ventilation using warmed gases if intubated, should be routine.

The conscious patient with mild hypothermia can be passively rewarmed. To use passive rewarming, all wet clothing should be removed, and the patient fully covered with warm blankets. They should be frequently reassessed, but may be permitted access to warm oral fluids. These patients are typically expected to make an otherwise uneventful recovery with the clinical outcome determined by the nature of the inciting event. With moderate hypothermia, treatment decisions are based on whether the patient is hemodynamically stable. Rewarming the thermal shell before the core may lead to continued core cooling (afterdrop) as the cool periphery is washed out, as well as hemodynamic instability (rewarming shock) as the periphery is reperfused. Methods of preferential core rewarming include peritoneal or pleural lavage, which may be thermally effective; or bladder, colonic, or gastric lavages, which are limited by the smaller volumes employed. If the patient is either severely hypothermic or unstable, then cardiac bypass is the best method of rewarming as it can provide hemodynamic support. If cardiac bypass is not available, other extracorporeal circuits such as continuous venovenous renal replacement technology or continuous arteriovenous rewarming, which involves perfusing a standard blood rewarmer with systemic blood pressure, may provide faster rewarming of the thermal core.

TABLE 1 Classification and Methods of Rewarming

Passive Rewarming
- Blankets
- External insulation to prevent further heat loss and encourage a positive heat flux
- Warm environment

Active Rewarming

Active External
- Convective air rewarming
- Heating pads
- Radiant heat
- Warm water immersion
- Warming blankets

Active Internal

Intracorporeal
- Airway rewarming with heated ventilatory gasses (40°C-45°C [104°F to 113°F])
- Warm bladder irrigation
- Warm colonic or gastric lavage
- Warm peritoneal dialysis
- Warm pleural dialysis
- Warmed intravenous fluids and blood infusions (40°C-42°C [104°F to 107.6°F])

Extracorporeal
- Cardiopulmonary bypass with heparin
- Centrifugal vortex blood pumps without systemic heparin
- Continuous arteriovenous rewarming technology
- Hemodialysis equipment
  - Continuous renal replacement technology (e.g., venovenous)
  - Intermittent hemodialysis technology

CARE OF THE HYPOTHERMIC BLEEDING PATIENT

The appreciation of the danger of the *hypothermia, coagulopathy, acidosis syndrome* in multisyndrome trauma patients is considered a major advance in trauma care. This aptly named syndrome is the overt manifestation of the patient's physiologic exhaustion, and if ignored constitutes a preterminal state. The trigger temperature for recognition of this lethal syndrome is 34°C (93.2°F), a temperature that would only be considered *mild* hypothermia in the nontrauma setting. As per all medical settings, prevention is preferable to treatment, and all injured patients should be considered to be at risk for hypothermia from both endogenous and iatrogenic causes. A crucial aspect of prevention is hemorrhage control at the earliest time to prevent ongoing requirements for resuscitation.

If the patient manifests type II or greater posttraumatic hypothermia (<34°C [93.2°F]) during surgery, the interventions should use damage control procedures to control hemorrhage and enteric spill and thus facilitate transportation to the critical care unit for ongoing resuscitation and rewarming. Uncontrolled bleeding unresponsive to damage control precludes leaving the operating room, however, and may reflect the most devastating effects of posttraumatic hypothermia. In such settings, we aggressively treat grade II hypothermia with all measures described in Table 1 commensurate with the anatomic injuries and surgical exposure.

Once grade III hypothermia (<32°C [89.6°F]) is manifest, we also employ a centrifugal vortex blood pump and heparin-bonded circuitry to rewarm before reoperating or transferring to the critical care unit. While previous familiarization with this equipment is required, noncardiac surgeons can effectively use this circulatory technology with either open or percutaneous access techniques.

DISTURBANCES CAUSED BY HEAT

METHOD OF

John F. Coyle II, MD

Heat stroke is an illness caused by failure of thermoregulation, with elevation of core temperature to 40.6°C (105°F) or more, associated with central nervous system dysfunction. Heat stroke has traditionally been subdivided into *exertional* and *classic* (or nonexertional) forms.

Exertional Heat Stroke

Exertional heat stroke is a sporadic illness triggered by exercise in warm environmental conditions that add to the thermal load produced by muscular contraction. It mainly strikes manual laborers, soldiers in training, and athletic competitors; indeed, it is the third leading cause of death among high school and college athletes in the United States. Exertional heat stroke may occur at mod-erate temperatures, especially if humidity is high. However, both exertional and classic heat strokes are most likely to develop in conditions of high heat. The incidence of heat stroke increases exponentially when heat stress exceeds a boundary value. Appearance of the first case should sound an alarm that conditions have become dangerous, and more cases should be anticipated. The typical heat stroke victim is highly motivated, poorly conditioned, obese, and not acclimatized. Fatigue and sleep deprivation are commonly encountered, and recent or ongoing febrile or dehydrating illness increases risk. Dehydration may play a role, especially if severe. The use of certain medicines also increases risk, most notably those that decrease cardiac output (β-blockers), promote dehydration (diuretics), affect hypothalamic control (major tranquilizers, neuroleptics, alcohol), inhibit sweating (anticholinergics, tricyclic antidepressants, antihistamines), or increase thermogenicity (amphetamines, cocaine).

Prevention is the ideal treatment. Since behavior is the most powerful thermoregulatory mechanism, education and empowerment have the greatest preventive potential. To avoid exertional heat stroke, organizers should schedule vigorous exercise in the coolest hours of the day (shortly after dawn or after nightfall, in difficult seasons). Exercise level should be governed by athlete fitness, acclimatization, hydration status, and freedom from intercurrent illness. Clothing should be appropriate for exercise conditions. Medication use that might interfere with effective thermoregulation should be recognized, and medical personnel must be charged with the responsibility for stopping any participant who appears to be decompensating.

Triage of those with exertional heat stroke is highly variable. Runners who are plunged unconscious into an ice water bath at the end of a race often respond promptly to treatment, reawaken, and are sometimes sent home without hospitalization. A less-favorable response necessitates hospital admission.

Classic (Nonexertional) Heat Stroke

Classic (nonexertional) heat stroke usually occurs during heat waves that cause passive warming by exposure to unrelenting hot and humid conditions, afflicting urban dwellers who are elderly, infirm, solitary, and poor. Heat waves tend to be "silent and invisible killers of silent and invisible people." Their housing lacks air-conditioning or they do not use it because of expense or confusion. Alcoholism and chronic illness, especially mental illness, predispose people to heat stroke. Young children are susceptible, reflecting their high surface-to-volume ratio, relatively inefficient sweat glands, and dependent status. Classic heat stroke requires preventive measures at the community level. Those with chronic illness and substance abuse history are at highest risk, and may be most difficult to contact. Although ventilation fans are of little help in hot and humid conditions, a few hours spent in air-conditioned rooms each day can significantly reduce the likelihood of heat stroke. Whether this is primarily a physiologic or a sociologic effect is unclear. Patients with classic heat stroke usually respond slowly to treatment and require hospital admission.

Pathophysiology

The pathophysiology of heat stroke is incompletely understood. Although a vast number of runners in a marathon may develop dehydration and a high core temperature, very few proceed to heat stroke. Excessive heat is a noxious agent that causes direct cell injury. The severity of heat stroke is related to the degree and duration of temperature elevation above 41.6°C (106.9°F). Exercise lowers the thermal threshold for heat stroke because of hormonal effects and competing demands of organ systems, as blood flow is directed away from the viscera to the active muscles and the skin. Gut ischemia may result in release of bacterial polysaccharides into the blood. What happens next is a complex interplay of factors including cytokines, bacterial polysaccharides, and heat shock proteins. As endothelial abnormalities accumulate, there is precipitation of a cascade of events including activation of the coagulation system and vascular dilatation, resulting in hypotension and coagulation disorders. These events in many respects mimic sepsis.

Because the brain is extremely sensitive to heat stress, the first signs of heat stroke are neurologic. Judgment is impaired, and the chance for self-diagnosis is greatly reduced. After loss of consciousness, muscular activity is markedly diminished, but temperature may remain elevated for hours.

Multisystem injury may follow, with the possibility of neurologic, pulmonary, cardiac, hepatic, renal, vascular, hematologic, and immunologic damage. A high percentage of classic heat stroke patients will suffer infection within 36 hours of hospital admission.

Treatment

Treatment of heat stroke can be summarized easily:

- Immediately lower rectal temperature to 39°C (102.2°F)
- Support organ systems injured by heat, hypotension, inflammation, and coagulopathy

There is a *golden hour* after the onset of heat stroke in which therapy can be extremely effective. When treating a patient outside of the hospital, the patient should be moved to a shaded area, his or her clothes should be removed, and he or she should be covered with water and fanned. When resources become available, the simplest treatment appears to be cold-water immersion in a shallow tub, with patient head, arms and lower legs outside the tub. The high efficiency of this method comes from two properties of water—it has 25 times the thermal conductivity of air, and it makes perfect contact with all skin surfaces. In addition, the hydrostatic properties of water tend to reduce the risk of hypotension. Other methods of cooling include skin wetting with fanning, application of total-body ice packs (24 ice packs, with special emphasis on the neck, armpits and groin) or use of a body-cooling unit (evaporation and convection).

Assessment of the patient with presumed heat stroke should be delayed pending initiation of cooling. Determination of rectal temperature, heart rate, and blood pressure can be carried out after the patient is being cooled. Oral and tympanic membrane temperatures cannot be used, as they may be misleadingly low. Rectal temperature should be measured every 5 to 10 minutes, and the patient should be removed from cooling when 39°C (102.2°F) is reached, to avoid overshoot hypothermia. Hydration with normal saline or lactated Ringer's solution should be started after initiation of cooling, and most patients will require 1 liter in the first hour of treatment. Further rehydration will need to be guided by estimated water losses, and in difficult cases placement of a central venous monitoring catheter may be needed. Overhydration may promote cerebral edema, pulmonary edema, and hyponatremia.

Seizures occur commonly, and these should be managed with diazepam (Valium), 5 mg intravenously (IV). Shivering may also be treated with diazepam. The patient must be monitored closely with use of this medication, which occasionally promotes hypotension. Hypotension should be treated with cooling and volume expansion. If blood pressure remains depressed, pressors may be needed. For patients with prolonged exertional heat stroke, mannitol, 0.25 g/kg, or furosemide (Lasix), 0.5-1 mg/kg, should be given after volume expansion has been carried out to minimize the adverse effects of rhabdomyolysis on renal function.

In patients with severe multiorgan damage, disseminated intravascular coagulation (DIC) is a common finding. Bleeding in DIC should be treated with transfusion of fresh-frozen plasma, cryoprecipitate, and platelet concentrates as needed. There is no role for heparin or thrombolytics in DIC in this setting. Adult respiratory distress syndrome tends to occur in conjunction with DIC, and prolonged ventilator support may be required. Hepatic failure in heat stroke is usually transient. Renal failure may necessitate emergency hemodialysis. There is no evidence-based support for use of anti-inflammatory agents or antipyretic agents in heat stroke. Use of strategies that have been helpful in sepsis may ultimately find a role in treatment of heat stroke, but such treatments should be considered experimental at this time.

Prognosis can be estimated by time to recovery of consciousness (shorter is better) and elevation of liver enzymes (lactate dehydrogenase [LDH] at 24 hours <3 times normal is a good prognostic sign).

Heat stroke should usually be regarded as an accident, like drowning. The population at highest risk is readily defined, but because of the rarity of this ailment it is difficult to maintain a high level of preparedness for its prevention and treatment. Once encountered, heat stroke must be treated with much the same urgency as cardiac arrest, since prompt cooling can sometimes make the crisis little more than an inconvenience. After the process of systemic injury becomes established, heat stroke's cascade of microvascular dysfunction can take on a life of its own, eventuating in a desperate struggle against multisystem failure and a high mortality rate.

SPIDER BITES AND SCORPION STINGS

METHOD OF

Lucinda S. Buescher, MD

Spider Bites

More than 30,000 species of spiders exist; most are venomous, but few are considered a hazard to human beings. When someone encounters a spider with chelicerae (jaws) long enough to penetrate the skin, the envenomation may be painful but is rarely dangerous. The site of the bite is usually erythematous, edematous, and tender. Minor spider bites are sufficiently treated with gentle wound cleansing, resting and elevating the affected body part, applying cold compresses, using nonsteroidal anti-inflammatory agents for pain and swelling, administering tetanus prophylaxis (if indicated), and prescribing antibiotics if secondary infection is suspected. It is crucial for the patient to bring in the spider for identification whenever possible because significant morbidity can result from bites by species of *Loxosceles* (fiddleback or violin spiders) and *Latrodectus* (widow spiders).

LOXOSCELES ENVENOMATION

Although the brown recluse spider, *Loxosceles reclusa*, is the most notable and widespread of this genus, at least four other species in the United States are known to cause cutaneous necrosis (necrotic arachnidism). These spiders are most prevalent in the south-central United States but have been reported in most states. They prefer a warm, dry habitat outdoors in a protected niche, but as they migrate north, they move indoors. These spiders spin inconspicuous matted webs. As its name implies, the spider is reclusive and is a nocturnal feeder. Encounters with human beings are rare, and bites usually result when the spider is trapped against the skin (often after occupying clothing left on the floor overnight).

Loxosceles spiders are tan or gray and have a distinctive dark brown, violin-shaped marking on the dorsal cephalothorax (*L. unicolor* has a very subtle marking). Another distinguishing feature is the presence of six eyes, rather than the usual eight found in most arachnids. The body measures 10 to 15 mm in length, and its leg span may be greater than 25 mm.

The actual *Loxosceles* bite usually goes unnoticed and often occurs on the lower abdomen, thigh, or axilla. Six to 12 hours after the bite, local signs and symptoms appear, including pruritus, pain, edema, erythema, and induration. A pustule or vesicle may appear at the bite site. When necrotic arachnidism is imminent, the center of the lesion becomes mottled dark blue or purple, surrounded by a white halo and finally a large area of reactive erythema, which is somewhat irregular in configuration because of gravitational effects. Over the ensuing 2 or 3 days, the darkened skin progresses to frank cutaneous necrosis, with stellate ulceration and eschar formation, often requiring months to heal.

Systemic signs and symptoms such as headache, malaise, arthralgias, myalgias, fever, and a generalized, faintly papular eruption may accompany many bites, but viscerocutaneous loxoscelism is rare. This syndrome affects primarily children, who may present with massive hemolysis. This can eventuate in renal failure, which may not appear until 2 to 3 days after the bite. Other findings include leukocytosis, leukopenia, thrombocytopenia, disseminated intravascular coagulation, convulsions, and coma.

Venom isolated from *L. reclusa* contains numerous enzymes, but that responsible for cutaneous necrosis and hemolysis is sphingomyelinase D. This enzyme binds to target cell membranes and causes structural alterations that presumably initiate an inflammatory reaction. Neutrophil activation is essential for the development of cutaneous inflammation and necrosis after envenomation; complement, arachidonic acid metabolites, and lymphokines are also likely participants.

Treatment

Because most *Loxosceles* bites are trivial, the same initial care noted earlier will suffice (i.e., cleansing, rest, elevation, cool compresses), and this approach should be employed until the lesion resolves. These measures should greatly diminish pain, but analgesics are often required. Administration of tetanus toxoid may be indicated, and antibiotics are necessary if wound infection is suspected.

Perhaps the most important management aspect in cases of cutaneous necrosis is careful consideration of the differential diagnosis. The definitive diagnosis of an arachnid bite is made only when there is identification of a captured spider. Other causes include trauma, infection (e.g., with herpesviruses or bacteria), and pyoderma gangrenosum.

Surgical excision and grafting are rarely necessary and are contraindicated in the early stages of necrosis, when graft failure is likely. Surgical intervention should be reserved for late eschars that fail to heal by secondary intention.

Patients with suspected systemic loxoscelism may have hemolysis and renal compromise. Treatment is supportive. Serial laboratory evaluations should include complete blood cell counts and urinalysis. Hydration is essential to maintain adequate renal perfusion. Systemic steroids may minimize hemolysis (especially in children) and may protect renal function. Treatments for viscerocutaneous loxoscelism such as dapsone,[1] hyperbaric oxygen, and antivenin are occasionally reported to be useful, but none of these have proved beneficial in controlled clinical trials.

LATRODECTUS ENVENOMATION

Five widow spiders inhabit the United States. *Latrodectus mactans* is the most common species and can be found throughout the country, especially in the southern states. *Latrodectus variolus* is the northern black widow, and *Latrodectus hesperus* is the western black widow. These three species are all similar in appearance. The brown widow (*Latrodectus geometricus*) may be found in Florida and California, whereas the red widow (*Latrodectus bishopi*) is limited to Florida. These spiders establish webs in dark, protected spaces indoors and out.

Female black widow spiders are shiny, with the characteristic, but variable, red or orange hourglass

[1]Not FDA approved for this indication.

marking on the abdomen. Mature arachnids have a 3- to 4-cm leg span. Males are approximately half this size; thus, their bites rarely result in significant symptoms.

The actual bite by a mature female widow is mild. A blue or red macule surrounded by a white halo and a faint urticarial eruption may ensue. Other local signs include piloerection, focal perspiration, and lymphangitis.

Neurotoxic signs and symptoms may begin within an hour, peak by 6 hours, and usually remit after 24 hours. Severe cramps and muscle contractions gradually spread from the inoculation site; that is, patients with an upper extremity bite will suffer from pleuritic pain and respiratory difficulty, whereas those with lower extremity bites may have abdominal rigidity mimicking an acute abdomen, but distention and severe tenderness will be lacking. Some authorities suggest that burning of the volar feet is a characteristic symptom of latrodectism. Additional findings are headache, anxiety, dizziness, diaphoresis, nausea, vomiting, salivation, lacrimation, respiratory distress, fever, priapism, hyperactive deep tendon reflexes, urinary retention, tachycardia, tremors, hypertension, paresthesias, and coma. Death is rare, occurring in less than 1% of patients bitten.

α-Latrotoxin, a neurotoxin, is the venom released by black widow spiders. It induces a massive, calcium-dependent release of acetylcholine and catecholamines from synaptic terminals and blocks transmitter reuptake as well.

Treatment

Early application of ice packs to the bite site may slow the absorption of venom. Tetanus immunization status should be assessed, and the patient should be monitored for signs of shock. Pain relief is the focus of management, and patients require oral or, occasionally, intravenous analgesics (e.g., morphine or fentanyl). Sedatives (e.g., benzodiazepines) may also be beneficial. Some pain may persist for several weeks and may necessitate appropriate outpatient management. Suspected cellulitis at the bite site requires systemic antibiotics.

Antivenin (produced in horses) is available and is not species-specific. Because antivenin can cause anaphylaxis and serum sickness, it is reserved for those patients with potential for severe complications (e.g., infants, young children, pregnant women, the elderly, and patients with hypertensive heart disease or respiratory distress). Those patients at risk of complications should be hospitalized and monitored for renal failure, convulsions, cardiac and respiratory failure, cerebral hemorrhage, and local cellulitis.

Scorpion Stings

Scorpions have a crablike appearance, with pincers on the front appendages, a segmented body and tail with a bulbous terminal segment, and a distal curved stinger. They vary in size from 2 to 10 cm. *Centruroides exilicauda* (*Centruroides sculpturatus*) is the only deadly species in the United States. It is yellowish-brown and less than 6 cm in length. This arthropod resides in southern Arizona, western New Mexico, and Mexico. The common striped scorpion *Centruroides vittatus* is the most commonly encountered scorpion in southwestern states and has an extremely painful, nonfatal sting.

Scorpions are known to burrow into small crevices only to emerge at night to feed on insects and spiders. They may enter homes, especially attics that provide cool, dark niches. They may appear around sinks, bathtubs, and toilets in their quest for water.

Most scorpion stings cause immediate sharp pain and local edema and erythema, but unless the patient has an allergy to the venom, stings are rarely of medical importance. Regional lymph node enlargement, local itching, paresthesias, fever, nausea, and vomiting may follow. The more deadly species inject venom with greater neurotoxic and hemolytic activity. Systemic effects may not appear until 2 to 20 hours after envenomation. The patient may experience drowsiness, partial paralysis, muscle twitching, sialorrhea, perspiration, hypertension, tachycardia, and convulsions. Death may result from respiratory paralysis, peripheral vascular failure, or myocarditis.

TREATMENT

To minimize the absorption of venom, patients should remain calm and should apply ice and pressure to the sting site. Antivenin (produced at Arizona State University by inoculation of goats with *C. sculpturatus* venom) is species-specific and can be administered in cases of severe envenomation and in young children, but it is not FDA approved. There is a high incidence of allergic hypersensitivity and serum sickness to the antivenin. Midazolam (Versed) bolus followed by continuous infusion (to induce a light sleep state) can suppress involuntary movements. This approach requires prior assurance of adequate airway, breathing, and circulation and then continuous cardiopulmonary monitoring.

Supportive measures and careful monitoring for relapse and deterioration are mandatory. Oxygen and positive-pressure breathing may be necessary for patients with impending respiratory failure. Tachycardia and severe hypertension may require temporary treatment with β-blockers and α-blockers, respectively. Antiepileptic drugs are indicated to control seizures. Opiates and other narcotics are contraindicated because they have a synergistic effect with the venom.

SNAKEBITE

METHOD OF

Richard W. Carlson, MD, PhD, and

John Khazin, DO

Because of the historical mystique and symbolism, many people have a natural curiosity about serpents. Snakebites have been associated with many misconceptions, which have led to errors in diagnosis and management. Bites by venomous snakes may cause trivial injuries or multisystem organ failure and death. The role of the clinician is to identify and quantify envenomation and to use appropriate measures to manage the direct and secondary effects of the poisoning.

Approximately 500,000 snakebites are reported worldwide each year, and venomous snakes are found on every continent. There are approximately 3000 species of snakes of which approximately 10% are venomous. In North America, several thousand individuals are treated for snake venom poisoning each year. Fewer than 10 deaths result from these injuries annually.

The predominant native venomous snakes in North America are the dozen or so species of rattlesnakes (genus *Crotalus*), pygmy rattlesnakes (massasauga, genus *Sistrurus*), and the other pit vipers, the cottonmouths and copperheads (genus *Agkistrodon*). The only native elapids are the eastern and western coral snakes (genera *Micrurus* and *Micruroides*, respectively). The eastern and western diamondback rattlesnakes (*Crotalus adamanteus* and *Crotalus atrox*) are among the largest venomous snakes in North America and account for most fatal snakebites.

Bites by exotic, non-native snakes in North America occur sporadically, as a result of contact with animals in zoos or private collections. To optimize management of bites by non-native species, as well as for general information and guidance for other species, it is useful to contact a local or regional poison control center.

This review focuses on the management of crotalid envenomation in North America. Individuals at risk for snake bite can be identified by proximity and behavior. Outdoor enthusiasts or those working in a snake's habitat are at risk for an unprovoked attack. As rural habitats are altered for new homes and commercial developments, construction workers and homeowners may also encounter venomous snakes. In such instances bites usually involve the lower extremity. Bites involving the face or other structures occur in small children or individuals who are playing with or trying to capture the animal. In fact, one of the more common snakebite scenarios involves attempted capture or intentional handling. Furthermore, many bites are complicated by alcohol intoxication or other recreational drug use.

Venom Delivery and the Composition of Venom

The pit vipers possess large, erectile fangs and are generally heavy-bodied snakes. They have a well-developed venom apparatus and can inject a large amount of venom via canaliculated upper maxillary teeth or fangs. The orifice of the venom canal is located proximal to the tip of the fang. When a snake strikes, variable amounts of venom may be introduced into the target, usually into the superficial skin structures.

Venom is produced by modified salivary glands and contains multiple toxic substances including a variety of peptides, proteins, and enzymes, many of which are classified as metalloproteins. The metalloproteins participate in the proteolytic destruction of the extracellular matrix and basement membranes of small blood vessels, and produce myonecrosis. Thrombin-like enzymes are present, which can stimulate fibrinogenolysis. Together with other venom fractions, these components affect the intrinsic and extrinsic coagulation cascade and produce a disseminated intravascular coagulation–like (DIC-like) condition. In addition, thrombocytopenia may be prominent following envenomation by certain species of crotalids. Venom components are also involved in the processing of various cytokines, including tumor necrosis factor.

Accordingly, local tissue injury as well as systemic findings may develop. For pit viper bites involving humans, approximately 20% are *dry bites* in which no venom is introduced into the victim. It is therefore crucial to evaluate and observe each bite for signs and symptoms of envenomation.

Clinical Evaluation: Estimation of Snakebite Severity

Envenomations are graded by evaluating local as well as systemic effects of toxicity. Additional factors affecting severity include the age of the victim and medical co-morbidities. Numerous grading systems of envenomation exist. For the purposes of this article, four categories are presented.

DRY BITE OR NONENVENOMATION

A dry bite is a documented bite by a venomous snake with fang marks, but no evidence of envenomation. No local edema, necrosis, or systemic findings develop aside from trauma induced by the fangs.

MINIMAL ENVENOMATIONS

These are characterized by edema, pain, bruising, and the potential development of bullae. No systemic toxicity or laboratory abnormalities are present.

MODERATE ENVENOMATIONS

These bites exhibit evidence of local changes that may include the findings listed above, as well as local neuromuscular alterations. Laboratory abnormalities including thrombocytopenia may be present, but systemic findings are generally mild or absent. Despite a minimal envenomation, patients such as children, the elderly, or the chronically ill may be graded as a moderate envenomation because of the overall increased risk.

SEVERE ENVENOMATION

This category of severity includes signs and symptoms of systemic toxicity with or without local changes. These injuries may be life-threatening. Features of severe envenomation may include hypotension, tachycardia, arrhythmias, hypovolemia with marked hemostatic defects, and respiratory failure. Central nervous system dysfunction can also occur.

One subset of a severe envenomation follows direct intravenous introduction of the poison. These cases may be associated with rapid development of systemic toxicity, with potential for a fatal outcome. Expedient, aggressive therapy is indicated.

Laboratory Abnormalities

Hallmarks of crotalid toxicity are disturbances of hemostasis. A DIC-like syndrome may develop because of activation of fibrinogen by thrombin-like components of venom, as well as fibrinogenolysis. If there is a decline of fibrinogen, together with elevated fibrin products and other specific factor deficiencies, more extensive monitoring of coagulation parameters is indicated.

Platelet counts may also be affected. In some instances the development of thrombocytopenia may be an indicator of the quantity of venom received. Accordingly, thrombocytopenia is a marker of systemic toxicity, and serial platelet counts may be useful to assess progression of the poisoning.

Creatine phosphokinase (CPK) levels are helpful to assess muscle damage. An escalating trend of CPK may indicate the development of a compartment syndrome and warrants ongoing evaluation that may include measurement of intracompartmental pressures.

Treatment

FIELD TREATMENT

Incision of the wound and extraction of venom are no longer indicated. Current care includes supportive measures and transport to a medical facility. Supportive measures should include rest, removal of binding garments or jewelry, and maintenance of the extremity in a slightly dependent position. Physical activity should be minimized. Tourniquets or local ice packs are not indicated and may be harmful.

It is helpful for field personnel to delineate the area of swelling or other local changes with a pen or marker. Circumferential measurements of an affected limb and descriptions of the wound site are also useful.

Rescue personnel should identify the snake if possible. However, capture of venomous snakes should be attempted only by trained personnel.

HOSPITAL THERAPY

Snakebite treatment has been a subject of controversy for decades. Exotic and unproven modalities of treatment such as cryotherapy and electric shock have been used with disastrous results. Wide local excision and extensive débridement may be unnecessary and result in disfigurement. Because death from crotalid envenomation is rare, practitioners should avoid unproven or experimental therapies.

Minimal envenomations may be observed for at least 12 hours and patients possibly discharged if no signs of progressive toxicity are observed. Patients with a moderate envenomation or greater, or with significant co-morbidities, should be admitted to a monitored setting. Antivenin treatment carries a risk of a systemic hypersensitivity and may lead to anaphylaxis. Accordingly, administration of antivenin should only occur in a monitored setting.

ANTIVENIN THERAPY

Patients with moderate or severe envenomation are candidates for antivenin therapy. Traditionally, antivenin therapy used an equine-based polyvalent antivenin, which is no longer in production. Recently the polyvalent immune Fab, ovine-based CroFab preparation has been approved by the FDA. There are no direct comparisons between the two preparations. However, the ovine product is likely to provoke fewer allergic reactions and may have increased efficacy. Currently, CroFab is the only preparation manufactured in the United States.

In the CroFab preparation, antibodies to venom undergo molecular processing, resulting in the cleavage of the Fc fragment from the antibody molecule, leaving the high-affinity Fab portion as the active agent. The Fc portion triggers much of the adverse effects seen with the equine preparation. Some risk of hypersensitivity still remains with CroFab, but the incidence appears to be much less (5% to 7% systemic reaction).

The initial dose of CroFab should be administered as soon as possible, usually within 6 hours. Skin testing for CroFab antivenin is not required. Table 1 provides dosing recommendations.

With the use of CroFab, recurrence or initial onset of defibrination and thrombocytopenia may be seen 2 to 5 days after the last dose of antivenin. Therefore, all patients including those who did not initially manifest thrombocytopenia or coagulopathy should be evaluated for the development of subsequent hemostatic changes. Management of late hemostatic changes should be tempered by severity, and delayed antivenin therapy may be indicated.

TABLE 1 Children and Adults: CroFab Crotalidae Polyvalent Immune Fab–Ovine Treatment

Initial: 4-6 vials; observe patient for 1 hour following completion of the first dose; if initial control* is not achieved after the first dose, an additional 4-6 vials may be repeated until initial control of the envenomation syndrome is achieved
After initial control is established: 2 vials every 6 hours for up to 18 hours (3 doses); an additional 2-vial dose may be administered if deemed necessary based on clinical response

*Initial control is defined as complete arrest of local manifestations of venom effects, and returning of hematologic values toward normal.
Adapted from: CroFab package insert.

Transfusion of blood products such as platelets and fresh-frozen plasma (FFP) is controversial. Some authorities believe that replacement of factors has no effect in correcting the coagulopathy because venom components may destroy them as they are given. However, in the presence of severe bleeding with thrombocytopenia, hypofibrinogenemia, or hyperfibrinogenolysis, the replacement therapy is warranted. Further administration of CroFab may also be indicated.

A complication of limb envenomation is the development of a compartment syndrome. Serial measurements of limb circumference and intracompartmental tissue pressure measurements may help guide the practitioner to assess this threat, and serial measurements of CPK are likely to correlate with ongoing muscle injury. The need for fasciotomy is uncommon.

Routine antimicrobial therapy has not been shown to be helpful. Wound infections should be treated with broad-spectrum antimicrobials. The presence of anaerobic organisms should be considered when selecting an antimicrobial regimen.

Patients should be discharged on rest and refrain from work, sports, and physical activity for several days. Most patients with crotalid envenomation recover with few residual effects. Further investigation into the biochemistry and pharmacology of venom components may lead to safer and more convenient treatment formulations in the future.

MARINE TRAUMA, ENVENOMATIONS, AND INTOXICATIONS

METHOD OF

Charles K. Brown, MD

Our planet is 71% water. Four-fifths of all organisms reside there and many have unique methods of attack and defense. Although references date to ancient times, and some of the most potent toxins known are marine in origin, it has only been in the last several decades that physicians have scientifically approached the management of injuries and illnesses produced by marine creatures. As humans increase their encounters with the marine environment, the risk of hazardous encounters with ocean-dwelling organisms increases as well. Air travel rapidly moves both people and seafood internationally, virtually eliminating regional illnesses and intoxications. Physicians will encounter patients presenting after marine injuries or intoxication and must be prepared to rapidly diagnose and treat life-threatening envenomations and intoxications.

The number of potentially hazardous organisms is enormous, yet the various syndromes may be categorized and often treated similarly (Table 1). Patients present with generally one of three encounter types:

1. Traumatic incidents
2. Toxic ingestions
3. Venomous bites, stings, or skin exposures (by far the most common)

Traumatic incidents require basic and advanced trauma care and the general principles of advanced trauma life support apply. Toxic ingestions are mostly self-limited gastrointestinal (GI) illnesses requiring supportive care, unless the patient has co-morbid conditions that are affected and require specific measures. Some ingestions and envenomations have life-threatening cardiovascular, respiratory, and/or neurologic symptoms. Care for these patients requires analgesia and intensive support of airway and respiratory functions unless an antidote is available. Skin exposures are usually an irritant causing acute dermatitis, and local care is required.

Shark

Shark attacks are overly dramatized but uncommon; less than 100 proven shark attacks and 12 deaths have been recorded in the United States since 1926, with 100 to 150 reported but unproven

TABLE 1 Symptoms of Envenomation or Intoxication

Symptom	Scorpion Fish	Sting-ray	Cat-fish	Weever-fish	Sea Snakes	Jelly Fish	Urchins	Star-fish	Sponges	Cone Shells	Octopus	Ciguatoxin	Scom-broid	Putter Fish	Mollusk	Shell-fish
Pain	X	X	X	X	X	X	X	X	X	X	X					
Radiation	X	X	X	X			X				X					
Ischemia/cyanosis	X	X	X	X						X						
Erythema	X		X	X		X	X	X	X		X		X			
Edema	X	X	X	X		X	X	X	X	X	X					
Vesicles	X					X			X		X		X oral	X oral		
Necrosis	X		X	X					X							
Cellulitis	X															
Nodes	X		X					X								
FB granuloma							X	X								
Bleeding							X				X					
Dye							X									
Urticaria					X	X	X				X		X			X
Fever	X			X		X										
Rash	X															
Headache	X	X		X		X							X	X		
Nausea/vomiting	X	X		X	X	X	X	X		X	X	Also cramps/ diarrhea	X	X		Also cramps/ diarrhea
Restlessness	X															
Delirium	X			X		X										
Anxiety	X				X											
Euphoria					X						X					
Weakness		X	X		X	X	X					X		X		
Fasciculations/tremors	X	X	X								X			X	X	
Myalgia/muscle cramps		X	X		X	X	X				X	X				
Hemoglobinuria					X											
Myoglobinuria					X											
Vertigo/ataxia		X				X	X				X	X		X	X	

Paresthesias/ dysesthesias	X		X			X	X	X	X	X	X		X	X	X
Paralysis	X	X			X	X	X	X	X	X			X	X	X
Seizures	X	X		X		X					X		X	X	
Aphasia				X		X	X		X	X					
Dysphasia					X								X		
Diplopia									X	X	X				
Trismus					X										
Dysphagia					X				X				X	X	
Ptosis					X										
Coma						X			X				X		
Respiratory distress	X	X	X	X		X	X		X	X	X	X	X	X	X
Bradycardia	X	X													
Tachycardia	X	X													
Arrhythmias	X	X		X		X							X	X	
Hypotension	X	X	X	X											
Diaphoresis	X	X		X	X						X		X		
Congestive heart failure	X														
Syncope	X	X	X	X			X								
Death	X	X	X			X	X		X				X		X
Chest pain	X														
Tetanus risk	X														
Conjunctivitis						X									X
Corneal ulcers						X									

From: Olshaker JS, Deniz T: Emergency Medicine Clinics of North America: Environmental Emergencies, vol 10, no. 2. Philadelphia, WB Saunders, May 1992. Used with permission.

attacks annually worldwide. Inhabiting coastal waters of North America, South Africa, and southern Australia, the sharks most often implicated in human attacks are the great white, blue, mako, bull, and grey reef sharks.

Safe water conduct is paramount in the prevention of shark attacks. Recommendations include avoiding shark-infested waters, especially at night or dusk, and turbid waters near waste outlets and deep channels; and never swimming with open wounds or in isolated areas. It is controversial whether menstruating females are at higher risk of attack. Bright, reflective swim wear and equipment are attractants. Captured fish should be tethered or stored away from divers. Chemical shark repellants have not been successful, and an electrical device is being developed

Patient management centers on basic trauma care—airway, breathing, bleeding control, and management of hypovolemic shock. Medications include tetanus immune globulin (BayTet), 250 units IM, tetanus toxoid (Td), 0.5 mL IM for patients older than 7 years of age, and prophylactic trimethoprim-sulfamethoxazole DS (TMP-SMX) (Bactrim DS), 1 tablet orally twice daily for 7 to 10 days, or ciprofloxacin (Cipro), 500 mg orally twice daily for 7 to 10 days. Imipenem cilastatin (Primaxin), 250 to 1000 mg IV every 6 to 8 hours, or a third-generation cephalosporin such as ceftriaxone (Rocephin), 1 to 2 g IM/IV every 24 hours, or ceftazidime (Fortaz) 1 to 2 g IM/IV every 8 to 12 hours are additionally indicated for established infections. Wounds are prone to contamination with aerobes and anaerobes, including *Aeromonas*, *Vibrio*, and *Clostridia*. Wound care must include vigorous irrigation, débridement, and exploration. Wounds are usually packed open, and delayed primary closure is used.

Barracuda

The great barracuda, *Sphyraena barracuda*, is the only species that has been implicated in human attacks. Solitary fish are the rule, but occasionally schools are involved in attacks. Their wide mouth is filled with large, knifelike teeth. The Atlantic range is from Brazil to Florida, and the Indo-Pacific range is from the Red Sea to Hawaii. All attacks occur in tropical seas. An attack is swift and fierce, often occurring out of confusion and in murky waters. The large, knifelike teeth produce straight or V-shaped lacerations often in rows (versus an arcuate shark bite). They are attracted to the same stimuli as sharks, and avoidance is the best means of prevention. Patients should be managed as victims of penetrating trauma, analogous to shark bites.

Moray Eel

These powerful bottom dwellers of tropical, subtropical, and temperate waters may reach 10 feet in length. Living under rocks or coral and in holes or crevices, they evade confrontation unless cornered. Their narrow, viselike jaws and sharp, fanglike teeth inflict severe lacerations through biting and holding. The moray eel may need to be beheaded or have its jaw broken to release the victim. Treatment is analogous to shark bites.

Giant Grouper

Species of the family *Serranidae* (sea bass, grouper) inhabit tropical and temperate seas; the giant grouper grows to 12 ft in length and can weigh 1000 lb. These curious, pugnacious, voracious feeders are feared because of their large size, boldness, and cavernous jaws. They inhabit old wrecks and caverns and lurk behind rocks. Treatment is the same as for shark bites.

Others

Sea lions can be aggressive, particularly mating males and females with pups. Bites can result in significant wounds. As this is a mammalian bite, rabies prophylaxis may be necessary. Rabies immune globulin, human (Imogam, Rabies-HT, or BayRab), 20 IU/kg with as much as possible infiltrated around the wound, and then rabies vaccine (Imovax rabies vaccine), 1 mL IM deltoid on days 0, 3, 7, 14, and 28. The killer whale, *Orcinus orca*, inhabits all oceans and grows to 30 ft in length. Although no documented attacks have occurred, a human could easily be mistaken for a sea lion. Needlefish (family *Belonidae*) are slender, lightening-quick surface swimmers that resemble freshwater gar. They inhabit tropical waters and attain lengths of 6 to 7 feet, often leaping out of the water and unintentionally spearing people. Treatment is according to the nature and location of the wound.

Envenomations and Intoxications

Marine zootoxins are of three types:

1. *Oral*—bacterial products, and products of decomposition
2. *Parenteral*—venoms produced in specialized glands and injected with specialized devices
3. *Crinotoxin*—venoms produced in specialized glands and administered without injection (i.e., slime)

All venoms are poisons, but not all poisons are venoms. Venoms are of large molecular weight with vasoactive compounds and proteolytic enzymes, whereas poisons are smaller protein or polypeptide metabolic byproducts of animals or plants. Both can cause widespread immunologic, cardiovascular, and neurologic dysfunction. Venoms and poisons can frustrate researchers, as both lack sufficient immunogenicity to foster development of antitoxins and antivenoms.

BONEY FISH

Boney fish, which cause envenomation, include lionfish, scorpion fish, stone fish, weever fish, and catfish. There are at least 200 species of fish that envenomate victims by their spines. The boney fish generally have heat-labile, short-chain polypeptide toxins that are present in the fish up to 24 hours after its death. The family *Scorpaenidae* is the most dangerous, composed of 30 genera and 350 species, at least 80 of which are known to cause venomous injuries. Other vertebrate envenomations occur from stingrays and sea snakes.

SCORPION FISH

Scorpion fish inhabit warm, shallow reef waters in a worldwide distribution and public and private aquariums. Less venomous varieties are seen on the west and southeast U.S. coasts. These bottom dwellers have very effective camouflage. The scorpion fish are divided into three genera, *Scorpaena* (sculpin, bullrout, and scorpion fish); *Synanceja* (stonefish); and *Pterosis* (zebrafish, lionfish, and butterfly cod). The stonefish, inhabiting Indo-Pacific waters, are the most lethal. Stonefish venom, similar to cobra venom, can precipitate cholinergic and adrenergic discharges, acting primarily on muscle. An estimated 300 scorpion fish envenomations occur annually in the United States.

The degree of envenomation depends upon the species, the number and location of stings, the amount of venom injected, and the general health of the patient. Pain is severe and immediate, radiating up the extremity. Stonefish envenomation may cause pain severe enough to produce delusions and may, although rarely, persist for days. Pain peaks at 60 to 90 minutes and may last 6 to 12 hours. The site is initially ischemic and pale and then cyanotic with erythema, edema, and possible vesicle formation leading to ulceration. Many systemic autonomic and neurologic manifestations can occur. The paresthesias and numbness often persist for weeks, and the wound is often present for months. With stonefish envenomation, dyspnea, hypotension, and cardiovascular collapse have been reported within 1 hour and death usually occurs within 6 hours without treatment.

Immerse the affected limb in hot water (113F° [45°C]) for 30 to 90 minutes or until pain is relieved. The extremity may be reimmersed if pain persists. Local anesthetic infiltration or regional nerve block with 1% to 2% plain lidocaine or 0.25% plain bupivacaine (Marcaine) may be needed. Cryotherapy is contraindicated. Wounds should be copiously irrigated with warm saline and explored and all slime and debris removed. The wound should be left open and treated with antibiotics if deep wounds are present on the hand or foot. Stonefish equine antivenom is obtained from Sea World in San Diego and Cleveland, Sharp Cabrillo Hospital in San Diego, and the Steinhart Aquarium in San Francisco. Antivenom, 1 mL, should neutralize 10 mg of venom. Anaphylaxis and serum sickness are possible, and sensitivity testing using 0.02 mL of 1:10 antivenom dilution intradermally should be done. Give 2 mL IM or IV if envenomation is severe, repeating as needed; one vial should handle two stings.

STINGRAYS

Stingrays are the most commonly encountered venomous fish, with approximately 2000 stings reported annually. Rays burrow in sand beneath shallow water, and, when startled, they defensively hurl their tails upward, their barbs causing venom-laden lacerations and punctures. Secondary infection is common. The venom is highly unstable and very heat labile. It includes a number of toxic compounds, including phosphodiesterases and 5′-nucleotidases, which produce varying degrees of cardiovascular and neurologic disturbance in addition to severe pain. Its effects do not appear to be caused by paralysis of neuromuscular transmission. The mechanism is unclear.

Injuries occur most commonly on the lower extremities followed by the upper extremities, abdomen, and thorax. Abdominal and thoracic wounds may cause major organ trauma. Symptoms are immediate and may persist for several days. Initial treatment, after addressing any life threats, should include rapid irrigation of the wound with cold, sterile saline or water solution to provide mild anesthesia, local vasoconstriction, and removal of sheath contents left in the wound and explorations. Other suggested treatments include superficial venous and lymphatic occlusion with a wide constriction band released for 90 seconds every 10 minutes and/or mechanical suction if immediately applied. The wound should be soaked in hot water (113°F [45°C]) for 30 to 90 minutes. Pain control may be augmented with infiltration locally of 1% to 2% plain lidocaine or 0.25% plain bupivacaine (Maracaine). Cryotherapy is contraindicated. Narcotics are a useful adjunct for pain control (morphine IM/IV 0.1 mg/kg per dose titrated to analgesic effect). The wound should be débrided and packed open. Antibiotic prophylaxis is recommended. Steroids and antihistamines are without evidence of efficacy.

CATFISH

More than 1000 species of freshwater and saltwater catfish exist. *Plotosus lineatus* (oriental catfish) envenomation may cause significant systemic as well as local symptoms. The venom contains dermatonecrotic, vasoconstrictive, and other bioactive agents. Both freshwater and saltwater venoms are heat labile, unaffected by freezing and poorly antigenic; they behave similar to mild stingray venom and are treated similarly, but they cause much less severe symptoms.

An instantaneous stinging, throbbing, or burning sensation occurs and usually resolves in 30 to 60 minutes. Occasionally, pain lasts 48 hours. The wound appears ischemic, and swelling can be significant. Gangrene has been reported. When infection occurs there is a high incidence of *Aeromonas* species, which is resistant to TMP-SMX (trimethoprim-sulfamethoxazole, Bactrim) and tetracycline, so antibiotics should be adjusted accordingly. There are no antidotes. The spines are radiopaque and must be sought after as foreign bodies.

WEEVERFISH

Also known as adder-pike, sea dragon, sea cat, and stang; weeverfish are small (<46 cm), stout-bodied fish inhabiting flat sandy or muddy-bottomed bays. The victims are usually professional fisherman or wading vacationers who have caught it in a net or disturbed the fish. They are the most venomous fish found in the temperate zone, inhabiting the Mediterranean Sea, East Atlantic Ocean, and European coastal waters. Generally sedentary, they will strike very accurately if provoked. The spines can penetrate a leather boot and result in substantial punctures. Venom contains 5-hydroxytryptamine, two peptides, and a mucopolysaccharide among other biogenic compounds.

The puncture results in an intense burning pain that is difficult to control. Pain is instantaneous and described as burning or crushing, quickly spreading throughout the entire limb. Pain peaks at 30 minutes and usually lasts 24 hours, but it can persist for several days and produce delirium and syncope. An initially pale and edematous puncture site develops erythema, warmth, ecchymosis, and significant edema. Total healing time may take months. A broad array of systemic symptoms may accompany envenomation, and secondary infection is common. As with stingrays, no commercial antidote is available and treatment is essentially the same. Narcotics are poorly effective. Occasionally, spines may be found in the wound. Prevention is primarily avoidance, wearing sufficiently protective footwear, and never handling live weeverfish. The fish can survive for hours out of water and should still be handled with extreme caution.

SEA SNAKES

The most dangerous sea snake is *Enhydrina schistosa*. They are close relatives of the cobra and krait, and all 52 species are venomous. At least seven have been implicated in fatalities. They are native to Indo-Pacific waters but have been found in the Gulf of California. There are no sea snakes in the Atlantic Ocean or Caribbean.

Sea snakes have a patchy, finlike tail, are generally nonaggressive, and are encountered during summer months or when entangled in fishing nets. Sea snakes have two to four maxillary fangs, each associated with paired venom glands. The fangs are short and easily dislodged; hence, most bites are without envenomation. The venom, containing neurotoxins and acting at both presynaptic and postsynaptic terminals, is more potent than that in any terrestrial snake. The presynaptic toxins initially release acetylcholine, then block resynthesis of acetylcholine both in the peripheral and autonomic nervous systems. The postsynaptic toxins attach irreversibly to the acetylcholine receptor at the motor endplate, blocking neuromuscular transmission. Myotoxins, including phospholipase A, cause striated muscle necrosis and myoglobin release, which may occur as early as 30 minutes and as late as 8 hours after the bite. Many tissue-toxic enzymes, hemotoxins, direct cardiotoxins, and vasoactive compounds are also present.

When bitten, the patient is initially asymptomatic and without pain. Symptoms can develop within 5 to 10 minutes and are usually present within 2 hours after the bite and certainly by 6 to 8 hours later. Usually one to four (but up to 20) hypodermic-like punctures are found. Painful, stiff muscle movements and myoglobinuria are the hallmarks of envenomation. Initial systemic complaints are a thick tongue, euphoria, malaise, and anxiety progressing to dysarthria, ophthalmoplegia, ptosis, trismus, and ascending flaccid or spastic paralysis. The causes of death are usually respiratory failure or aspiration (bulbar paralysis), hyperkalemia, or acute renal failure from hemoglobinuria or myoglobinuria. Early congestive heart failure and late acute renal failure have been noted, and intensive supportive respiratory and circulatory care is often needed. Diagnosis is based upon several factors:

- Whether the bite occurred when the patient was in the water
- Initial absence of pain
- Multiple tiny fang marks
- Identification of the snake
- Characteristic symptoms of painful muscle movement, lower extremity paralysis, trismus, and ptosis.

If no symptoms occur by 6 to 8 hours, then no envenomation has occurred.

Treatment is similar to that for elapid bites, with dependent pressure immobilization to localize the venom and minimize systemic distribution. The patient should remain quiet and warm. Incision and drainage is generally not recommended and cryotherapy is contraindicated. An equine polyvalent antivenom[1] obtained from *Enhydrina schistosa* and *Notechis scutatus* is available and is indicated in the presence of envenomation. Administration is effective up to 24 to 36 hours after envenomation and should begin promptly. After anaphylaxis skin testing, at least one and up to 10 ampules may be required. Polyvalent tiger snake antivenom[1] is an accepted alternative, beginning with one ampule and titrating the dose to the clinical situation. Respiratory and renal function must be closely monitored, as mechanical ventilation may be required and hyperkalemia secondary to rhabdomyolysis is not uncommon.

[1]Not FDA approved for this indication.

Hemodialysis has been reported effective in two cases but is not an established mode of therapy for venom removal.

Infectious Agents

Infection is a hazard with any marine wound and should be treated appropriately. *Vibrio* species are part of coastal flora and are an established source of extraintestinal infections. These are potential pathogens for severe wound infection, bacteremia, and sepsis. *Vibrio vulnificus* can cause wound infection in any patient or primary septicemia in patients with underlying chronic disease such as diabetes, leukemia, chronic renal failure, steroid-dependent asthma, and, especially, chronic liver disease. Infections with this organism are most common during the warmer months and can be caused by ingesting seafood. A variety of local manifestations occur, but the more severe infections have necrotic features; a pustular bullous eruption occasionally progresses to necrotizing fasciitis. These patients appear toxic, and examination reveals extensive necrotic tissue. Wounds have intense pain, swelling, and cellulitis that can rapidly progress to bullae and massive swelling. Gangrene has been reported. Treatment combines aggressive wound care, including débridement of necrotic tissue and antibiotic therapy. A combination of cefotaxime (Claforan), 1 to 2 g IM/IV every 6 to 8 hours, and minocycline (Minocin), 200 mg IV or orally initially, then 100 mg every 12 hours, are effective in vitro.

Primary septicemia is associated with ingestion of contaminated shellfish, especially oysters. *Vibrio* enter through the GI mucosa, and asymptomatic carriage is possible. Clinically, findings vary from abrupt onset of fever and chills with abdominal pain, nausea, vomiting, and diarrhea; to bullae, hypotension, and hypoperfusion states. Mortality approaching 50% has been reported. The onset of fever and chills is abrupt. Secondary skin lesions appear within 24 hours and are associated with extreme pain. Treatment of sepsis includes antibiotics, vasopressors, and intense supportive care. More than 90% mortality has been reported when hypotension occurred within the first 12 hours. Treatment combines aggressive wound care including débridement of necrotic tissue and antibiotic therapy as noted above.

Aeromonas hydrophilia can cause wound infections, GI symptoms, or septicemia. Initially cellulitic soft tissue infection can progress to fasciitis, gas forming infection, or sepsis. Fever, chills, hypotension, or jaundice are common with septicemia. Immunosuppressed patients or those with chronic liver disease are most susceptible. A host of antibiotics are effective.

There have been several large outbreaks of hepatitis A from raw clam and oyster ingestion since the 1960s. Norwalk virus causes a self-limited although potentially severe gastroenteritis after consumption of contaminated shellfish. Nine marine species of *Vibrio* are associated with human infection, including *Vibrio cholera*. Cholera can surface virtually anywhere because of both rapid worldwide transport of raw seafood and increased world travel. Cholera produces a life-threatening enteritis that may progress to hypovolemia, acidosis, or acute renal failure. *Vibrio parahaemolyticus* causes 50% of food poisonings worldwide and is associated with improperly cooked crustaceans (especially shrimp). Tetracycline (Sumycin), 250 to 500 mg orally four times per day may abbreviate this illness if given within the first 48 hours. *Erysipelothrix rhusiopathiae* causes fish handler's disease, which is manifested by a characteristic ring lesion around the contaminated puncture and is best treated with oral penicillin (Pen VK), 250 to 500 mg four times per day, or ciprofloxacin (Cipro). Botulism may result from ingestion of improperly processed fish and roe. *Campylobacter*, *Salmonella*, *Shigella*, and *Escherichia coli* are only occasionally traced to seafood. Several helminthic infections are possible, primarily from the consumption of raw fish.

Venomous Invertebrates

Humans are frequently exposed to venomous invertebrates. Coelenterates of the phylum Cnidaria are commonly encountered when swimming in salt or brackish water. Stings are the most common injury. Classes are *Scyphozoa* (true jelly fish), *Hydrozoa* (Portuguese man-of-war, blue bottle), and *Anthozoa* (sea anemones, soft coral). These organisms envenomate prey through nematocysts bathed in venom. Composition varies among species and has direct and indirect effects on the autonomic nervous system and end organs, particularly the heart, central nervous system, skin, and vascular system. The venom has been shown experimentally in animals to produce a general destabilizing action upon the cell membrane.

COELENTERATES

Both living and dead jelly fish as well as separated tentacles can cause envenomation. The sting produced is a linear painful erythematous eruption, which may blister and persist for 7 days. Jellyfish produce three grades of envenomation, mild, consisting solely of skin irritation; intermediate, producing stinging, pruritus, paresthesias, throbbing, and central radiation; and severe, with systemic symptoms involving multiple organ systems. Neurologic, cardiovascular, respiratory, musculoskeletal, gastrointestinal, and ocular reactions may occur. Chronic manifestations may include keloids, hyperpigmentation, flat atrophy, contractures, gangrene, urticaria, muscle spasm, autonomic nerve paralysis, bladder paralysis, and mononeuritis. Cutaneous lesions should be sought in cases of unexplained water-related collapse or near drowning. In these circumstances, scraping fresh skin wheals with a scalpel or the edge of a glass slide or using tape to lift off nematocysts may help make the diagnosis.

Probably the most dangerous jellyfish is the box jellyfish or sea wasp, *Chironex fleckeri*, of the South Pacific, found mainly in Australian waters off northern Queensland. A much less lethal variety is found in the Chesapeake Bay. Larger specimens can inject more than 10 mL of venom, causing cardiorespiratory death in less than 1 minute and an overall mortality of 15% to 20%. More than 70 documented fatalities have been reported from Australia. *C. fleckeri* toxin's dominant active components are proteinaceous. An active musculotoxic agent and a vasopermeability toxin, possibly serotonin, have been isolated. Sea wasp antivenom made from sheep serum is available and should be used for all *Chironex* envenomations. It is best given IV (20,000 units [1 vial] over 5 minutes), but three vials can be administered IM. The same anaphylactic precautions as with other animal-based antivenoms should be observed. Clinically, if patients have more than one half of one limb involved or loss of consciousness, then immediate transport to a hospital for antivenom is indicated.

The Irukandji syndrome has been reported from stings of the *Cubozoa* class of jellyfish (*Carukia barnesi*). Stings are characterized by rapidly developing pulmonary edema leading to acute respiratory failure in young healthy people. Although the pathophysiology is unclear, the symptoms are similar to unchecked catecholamine release.

All patients with suspected *Chironex* envenomation should be observed for 6 to 8 hours after treatment because rebound phenomena have been reported. Pain control becomes a major hurdle once the nematocysts are removed. Narcotics are generally required and should be used as needed. Methocarbamol (Robaxin) (1 g slowly), diazepam (Valium), or other muscle relaxants can be used to alleviate cramps. A 10% calcium gluconate solution (5 to 10 mL IV) is effective in relieving muscle spasms if given acutely.

Portuguese man-of-war (*Physalia physalis*) are found in the Gulf of Mexico and off Florida from July to September. Consisting of a floating sail (up to 30 cm across) and a number of tentacles up to 30 m in length, these creatures contain up to several million nematocysts. The Pacific blue bottle (*Physalia utriculus*) is smaller, having only one tentacle up to 15 m in length. *Physalia* toxin is proteinaceous and induces histamine release and prostaglandin-induced vasodilatation and is believed to act at the level of the sarcolemma. This action may be blocked by nonsteroidal anti-inflammatory drugs (NSAIDs). Hemolysis, caused by toxin interaction with the red blood cell membrane, can occur. Clinically, *Physalia* envenomations are similar to those from lesser jellyfish but carry much more likelihood of a severe reaction. Acute renal failure was reported in a patient after experiencing a severe *Physalia* sting. A severe hemolytic reaction occurred and was suspected of causing pigment-induced nephropathy. Erythema nodosum has also been reported and may recur up to 4 weeks later.

Treatment of a jellyfish sting is controversial on many points and must be somewhat species specific, but all authorities seem to agree on one point: Do not immerse the area in fresh water. Initial seawater rinsing is recommended to maintain isosmolar conditions. Current recommendations to inactivate nematocysts still present on the skin include application of 5% acetic acid solution (vinegar) for 30 seconds or until pain subsides. Stingose (aluminum sulfate surfactant) or, as a last resort, isopropyl alcohol (40% to 70%) may also be used. Do not rub the wound as this may discharge more nematocysts or induce skin trauma. Some argue that Stingose is ineffective. For moderate to severe or large surface area stings, a pressure immobilization technique is used after vinegar application. A cloth or gauze, approximately 6 to 8 cm by 6 to 8 cm by 3 cm (thick), is applied over the sting tightly but not so tight as to occlude arterial inflow. The area of the sting is believed to become locally ischemic and venous and lymphatic obstruction may preclude systemic absorption of the venom. The extremity and patient are immobilized and transported to medical care. For minor stings, after deactivation, with care for yourself, a baking soda or sand/mud paste or shaving cream may be applied, followed by gentle shaving to remove attached nematocysts. Tetanus prophylaxis should be current. Mild topical steroids and antihistamines may be indicated for symptomatic relief. Local or topical anesthetics may be soothing when used after removal of nematocysts, but a paradoxic reaction has been reported to topical benzocaine (Americaine). There is no basis for prophylactic antibiotic administration. A popular but unproven method is application of Adolph's Meat Tenderizer (papain) or Pepsi-Cola. Study of optimum methods is ongoing.

Other invertebrates causing human envenomation include the Anthozoa class (sea anemones, corals) and Echinodermata (sea urchins, starfish, sea cucumbers). These are usually encountered by skin divers or tide pool scavengers. Sea anemones are flower-like sessile creatures, ranging from a few millimeters to 0.5 m in diameter. After encountering the hell's fire anemone (*Actinodendron plumosum*), the origin of the name becomes readily apparent.

Fire coral (*Millepora* species) are found on rocks, pilings, and other coral and are not true corals. They resemble a tiny brush, usually 7 to 10 cm in length, but can grow to 2 m. An initial stinging or burning pain on contact is often followed by severe pruritus and urticaria. Rubbing the area worsens envenomation. Untreated, pain will resolve in 90 minutes and wheals will flatten within 24 hours and resolve within 1 week. Residual hyperpigmentation may persist up to 8 weeks. Treatment for both *Anthozoa* and *Millepora* stings is analogous to jelly fish stings. Persistent rash may respond to a 2-week tapered course of prednisone.

Contact with hard corals causes lacerations contaminated by debris and abundant marine microorganisms. Wounds may heal poorly, leaving a scar or forming a granuloma. Treatment includes aggressive cleansing with saline and hydrogen peroxide, appropriate débridement, and application of topical antibiotic to cover marine organisms mentioned previously. The term *coral reef granuloma* is a misnomer; actually it is a tropical streptococcal or staphylococcal pyoderma with wound hyperplasia.

SPINY INVERTEBRATES

There are 6000 species of sea urchins; 80 are known to be poisonous or venomous. They are covered with spines or triple-jawed pedicellaria, and both can envenomate. Most spines are solid, producing only punctures and retained foreign bodies. Some are hollow and attached to a poison sac. Pedicellaria have flexible heads containing pincers or jaws that open on contact. Penetration of the spines into the skin produces the major injury and can lead to infection by marine organisms or impalement of deeper structures (i.e., nerves and joints). The hand is particularly vulnerable. Pain from the puncture is similar to an insect sting with surrounding edema and erythema. A large number of urchin toxins have been identified; many mediators are histamine- or kinin-like. Some species secrete an acid mucopolysaccharide. There is no known antivenom. The wound may be stained black or purple by dye within the spines and give a false impression of a retained foreign body. Spines are radiopaque. Infrequently, systemic symptoms occur with multiple embedded or undetected spines. Local pain may persist for days. One Pacific urchin, *Tripneustes*, secretes a neurotoxin with a predilection for facial and cranial nerves. Pedicellaria envenomations are more severe; symptoms are primarily neurologic.

Pain may resolve in 1 hour, whereas muscular weakness or paralysis may last for up to 6 hours. A delayed reaction may manifest 2 or more months after injury. It may consist of either localized granuloma formation or a diffuse inflammatory process, most often fusiform, with swelling and discoloration. Bone destruction may occur. Local nodules are usually 2 to 5 mm in diameter, pink to cyanotic in color, centrally umbilicated, and may have a keratotic surface. Pain and suppuration are not present unless the nodules occur on a weight-bearing surface. It remains undefined whether these are local allergic reactions or granulomatous inflammation.

Therapy is supportive and generally symptomatic. Treatment of sea urchin injuries consists of immediate hot water (113°F [45°C]) immersion, careful removal of attached pedicellariae and embedded spines, and prevention of cellulitis or synovitis by débridement. Pedicellariae must be removed or envenomation will continue. Infection is common and antibiotic prophylaxis is indicated. Analgesics may be needed for several days. If delayed nodules or cysts appear, excision is indicated, as they rarely heal spontaneously. Intralesional steroids have not been studied formally but are recommended with variable success. Prevention of echinoderm-mediated injuries includes careful stepping and use of protective footwear in shallow water.

Starfish, like sea urchins, are bottom dwellers. Only a few noxious species exist. The most studied starfish, the Crown-of-Thorns sea star (*Acanthaster planci*), inhabits warm waters from Polynesia to the Red Sea and is particularly venomous. Foreign body granulomata may form. Treatment of starfish envenomation includes hot water immersion to relieve pain, topical treatment of the contact dermatitis (a useful agent is calamine lotion with 0.5% menthol)*, and supportive symptomatic treatment for the self-limited systemic reaction. The spines are a radiopaque foreign body. Local or regional anesthetic injections may be required for pain control or substituted for narcotics.

OTHER INVERTEBRATES

Sea cucumbers are free-living, bottom dwelling, sausage shaped echinoderms encountered at all depths. Holothurin is extruded defensively, causing an intense dermatitis or conjunctivitis on contact. Blindness can occur if the cornea is contacted and injured. Underwater swimming near sea cucumbers may cause symptoms as a result of the high concentrations of holothurin in the water. Some cucumber species eat nematocysts and may secrete this venom as well. Ingestion of the sea cucumber can cause death, as holothurin is a potent cardiac glycoside. Local care includes acetic acid or isopropyl alcohol detoxification of the venom and removal of the slime by hot soapy water. Topical steroid therapy for dermatitis is indicated. If the eye is involved, topical anesthesia, copious irrigation, fluorescein staining, and immediate ophthalmologic consultation are recommended. Severe reactions may respond to systemic corticosteroids.

At least 13 species of sponges cause irritant dermatitis on contact. A slimy surface liquid contains the crinotoxin. Identified toxins include halitoxin, okadaic acid, and subcritine. Species common to American waters include *Tedaria ignis* (fire sponge), *Fibula nolitangere* (poison bun sponge), and *Microciona prolifera* (red sponge). The Mediterranean red sponge and the tropical Pacific Hawaiian fire sponge are particularly noteworthy. Dermatitis also may be produced from silica or calcium spicule penetration of the skin. Skin lesions can progress to bullae and desquamation over several days. Stinging may increase over the first 2 or 3 days and persist for weeks. Plaques and papules may persist for several months. Eye contact may produce iritis and corneal lesions. Erythema multiforme and anaphylaxis are most common after contact with *Fibula* species.

Removal of the foreign body spicules may be accomplished with adhesive tape, rubber cement, or a facial peel. Acetic acid or isopropyl alcohol soaks for 10 to 30 minutes should be applied 3 times daily. Topical steroids may help the secondary inflammation but should be applied after the initial acetic acid soak.

*May be compounded by pharmacists.

Antihistamines and topical anesthetics are other soothing measures. Severe secondary reactions may require systemic corticosteroid administration. Tetanus immunization should be current. Infected wounds should be cultured and appropriate antibiotics administered.

Marine annelids are segmented marine worms known a bristle worms. Easily detachable projections attached to the worm's parapodia penetrate the skin. These are difficult to remove and produce an intense inflammation with erythema, pruritus, swelling, and paresthesia. Some worms can also bite. Treatment consists of spine removal analogous to that for sponges. Hot water (113°F [45°C]) immersion for 30 minutes may provide pain relief. Secondary infection and cellulitis are not uncommon.

Ichthyosarcotoxism

This term refers to a variety of conditions arising from fish flesh. Ninety-nine percent of toxins involve the viscera, skin, or mucus membranes of the organisms ingested. Rarely are the gonads or blood of the organism involved. Three classes of illness can occur, allergic, toxic, and infectious. The risk of eating seafood and becoming ill is low, with most episodes consisting of self-limited GI illness. Although we discuss a sample of these syndromes, the reader is referred to other more detailed sources for definitive information on this vast topic. The differential diagnoses for nontraumatic marine-borne illness are extensive. This discussion centers primarily on toxins ingested from seafood and includes toxins associated with shellfish, scombroid fish, and marine animals of the *Gymnothorax* and *Tetraodon* genus as well as several other serious but less common entities.

CIGUATERA

Ciguatoxin is endemic in warm water bottom dwelling shore and reef fish. These fish are found in the temperate zone but worldwide accounts of toxicity exist for the majority of fish-borne illness. More than 500 species have been associated with ciguatera including barracuda, sea bass, parrot fish, red snapper, grouper, amber jack, moray eel, porgy, trigger fish, surgeon fish and wrasse. Ciguatera is the most common type of nonbacterial food poisoning in the United States and accounts for 10% to 15% of the food poisoning cases reported to the Centers for Disease Control and Prevention. Hawaii and Florida account for more than 90% of the U.S. cases, but the Caribbean and South Pacific regions are also significant sources. Patients most commonly present during the spring and summer months.

Ciguatoxin is found in blue-green algae, protozoa, and free living dinoflagellates, which serve as the main food source for small herbivorous fish. These fish in turn are the major food source for larger carnivorous fish, and the toxin becomes more and more concentrated in tissue as it moves up the food chain. The toxin is believed to be elaborated by the dinoflagellate, *Gambierdiscus toxicus*. It is now believed that this toxin causes inhibition of voltage-dependent sodium cell-membrane channels. Toxicity patterns may be confusing, with local variation in the same geographic area. Ciguatoxin has a low molecular weight and can cross the placenta. Children born of mothers affected late in pregnancy may manifest bizarre movements in utero and facial palsies may be present after delivery.

Patients become ill after eating either fresh or improperly frozen fish prepared by any method. Most patients experience symptoms 2 to 6 hours after ingestion, with 75% by 12 hours and 100% by 36 hours. Symptoms are acute in onset, consisting of a constellation of GI and neurologic complaints. The neurologic symptoms are predominantly dysesthesias and paresthesias but also include a strange metallic taste and perioral and oral tingling and numbness. Also described is an odd temperature reversal sensation. Patients state that their skin is burning but feels cold underneath; or cold food is perceived as hot and vice versa. Severe headache and a feeling of loose painful teeth are often present. Deaths are very unusual and are caused by respiratory paralysis and seizures, possibly hypoxic. Delayed or protracted symptoms, consisting of itching, hiccoughs, and dysesthesias may last for days or weeks, proportional to the amount of toxin ingested.

Laboratory testing is of no diagnostic help but can eliminate other possibilities. An immunoassay is available to commercially test fish for presence of the toxin. Treatment is primarily supportive and symptomatic. Gut emptying and decontamination with charcoal are recommended, but this seems illogical in the face of nausea, vomiting (40% of patients), and diarrhea (70% of patients). Atropine is indicated for bradycardia. Intravenous mannitol[1] provided rapid relief of both GI and neurologic symptoms within minutes in one study of 24 patients. The mechanism of mannitol efficacy is unknown, but hypotheses include competitive inhibition of the toxin's effect on the sodium channel and neutralization of the toxin. Hospital admission is indicated if the diagnosis is uncertain or if significant volume depletion is present. Gastrointestinal symptoms resolve more slowly than do the neuromuscular symptoms. Dopamine (Intropin)[1] at an appropriate dose or calcium gluconate are recommended for treatment of shock. Paresthesias may respond to a course of amitriptyline (Elavil)[1], starting at 25 to 100 mg orally at bedtime, increasing to 50 to 300 mg per day. Chronic symptoms may respond to acetaminophen (Tylenol)[1] or indomethacin (Indocin)[1], 25 to 50 mg orally or rectally three times per day. There is no immunity.

Recurrences are common and increasingly severe; they may be prevented by intake of a high-protein, high-carbohydrate diet that avoids fish, nuts, and ethanol for 3 to 6 months after symptom resolution.

---

[1]Not FDA approved for this indication.

SCOMBROID POISONING

Scombroid poisoning, called saurine poisoning in Japan, occurs when spoiled fish are eaten. These fish include the large dark meat yellow fin, blue fin, and albacore tuna; wahoo; bonito; mackerel; and skip jack—all of which live in temperate or tropical waters. Also frequently implicated are the nonscombroid mahi-mahi, sardine, anchovy, herring, bluefish, and amber jack. The syndrome is entirely preventable and results when bacteria proliferate on warm or improperly refrigerated freshly killed fish. These organisms elaborate histidine decarboxylase, which converts histidine to histamine, saurine, and other heat-stable compounds. The extent of spoilage correlates with histamine levels. The appearance, taste, and smell of the fish generally is unremarkable, but a pungent peppery taste has been noted.

A scombroid outbreak in San Francisco in 1977 revealed an uneven distribution of histamine in the flesh of an individual fish, which may explain why a variable occurrence of disease among people eating the same fish can occur. The differential diagnoses encountered in a patient with flushing as a prominent symptom are lengthy, and coincident ethanol consumption must be taken into consideration.

Symptoms of scombroid poisoning often occur within minutes but may take several hours to develop. Very similar to allergic reactions, symptoms are histamine-mediated. Treatment consists of gut decontamination and supportive symptomatic care as indicated for hypotension, bronchospasm, nausea, or vomiting. The following have been used successfully, but significant improvement will occur spontaneously within a matter of hours:

- Antihistamines, including both H_1 (diphenhydramine [Benadryl]), 5 mg/kg per day orally or IV, and H_2 (famotidine [Pepcid]), 20 mg IV every 12 hours or 20 mg orally twice daily
- Epinephrine, 0.01 mg/kg with a maximum dose of 0.5 mg
- Parenteral steroids (dexamethasone [Decadron]), 0.5 mg/kg every12 hours with a maximum dose of 10 mg

Diagnosis is ordinarily clinical but can be confirmed by elevated serum and urine histamine levels.

Mollusks

Some 45,000 species of mollusks exist worldwide, comprising the single largest group of potentially toxic marine invertebrates. Most intoxications result from ingestion of toxic *Pelecypods* (oysters, clams, scallops, etc.), whereas relatively few true envenomations occur. Toxins implicated in envenomation and intoxication by both mollusks and neurotoxic fish species are very similar and produce toxicity by inactivating the voltage-dependent sodium membrane channels. The effect is very much like curare's. Neuromuscular paralysis is the result; the most urgent is respiratory muscle paralysis. If not treated promptly, respiratory failure and anoxia will occur followed by brain damage and ultimately death. Patients are alert, mentating normally unless anoxia has occurred.

Cone shells include 300 species, 18 of which are implicated in human envenomations. Comparable in size to hymenoptera toxins, these toxins are neurotoxic. Two major types have been isolated, a presynaptic ω-conotoxin, which affects calcium-mediated acetylcholine release, and μ-conotoxin, which directly modifies sodium influx channels in muscle cells, thereby abolishing action-potential propagation.

The puncture may resemble a minor bee or wasp sting but *Conus geographus* can cause death within a few hours. The initial local symptoms of burning, local cyanosis, and numbness rapidly advance to severe neurologic symptoms including respiratory paralysis. No antivenom is available, and treatment is entirely empiric and symptomatic. Some relief may be offered by hot water immersion at 113°F (45°C). For severe envenomations the treatment is supportive and primarily respiratory with symptoms resolving completely in 6 to 8 hours. Prevention is by patient education.

Octopi are actually shy, reclusive creatures that usually pose no threat to humans. The venomous octopi are small, less than 20 cm in diameter. The blue-ringed octopus (*Hapalochlaena maculosa*) of Australia is the most well known. Yellow-brown and inconspicuous when docile, it develops brilliant iridescent blue rings when threatened. Another dangerous species is *Octopus joubini*, which is native to the Caribbean. All octopi less than 20 cm in diameter should be handled only with protective gloves.

The bite frequently manifests as two small puncture wounds. The patient may be totally unaware of being bitten or have a mild bee sting–like burning. The maculotoxin injected appears to block peripheral nerve transmission. The blue-ringed octopus also secretes tetrodotoxin and is the only creature known to envenomate with tetrodotoxin. Initially, the wound is numb and often blanched, but this is followed quickly by pain that may persist for up to 6 hours. More serious envenomations involve neurotoxic symptoms, with oral and facial numbness occurring within 10 to 45 minutes. Muscle weakness is next, with death being caused by respiratory failure. Treatment is supportive and based on individual symptoms, as there is no antivenom available. First aid is pressure immobilization dressing. Hot water is without benefit. Symptoms begin to resolve 4 to 10 hours after the bite and recovery may take 2 to 4 days unless anoxia has occurred. Intensive respiratory support is crucial to survival. A monoclonal rabbit serum immunoglobulin (Ig) G antibody is being developed.

Tetraodon Poisoning

Tetraodon poisoning occurs after ingestion of fish of the order *Tetraodontiformes*, which inhabit both fresh and saltwater. They have no geographic restriction but are encountered most frequently off Japan, California, Africa, Australia, and South America. More than 100 species known regionally by different names and *fugu* (a specific preparation of pufferfish considered a delicacy in Japan) are capable of producing intoxication. Other sources include ocean sunfish, blue-ringed octopus, and certain species of newts and salamanders. Tetrodotoxin is a heat-stable (except at alkaline pH), basic, water-soluble, nonprotein compound. Geographic variations in toxicity occur. Tetrodotoxin effects are similar to saxitoxin's (toxic shellfish), with sodium-fast channel blockade-induced paralysis, direct chemoreceptor trigger-zone stimulation (resulting in emesis), and respiratory depression secondary to a direct medullary effect. Tetrodotoxin relaxes vascular smooth muscle and blocks the preganglionic cholinergic motor and sensory nerves and sympathetic nervous system. Symptoms occur within minutes and may progress to ascending paralysis and respiratory death. Toxicity is significant, with an estimated 50% to 60% mortality even when appropriate therapy is given. Complete paralysis with fixed, dilated pupils and normal mentation occurs until anoxia ensues.

Respiratory support is essential. There have been two reports of successful reversal of respiratory and motor paralysis with edrophonium (Tensilon)[1], 10 mg IV after a 1 mg test dose.

Toxic Shellfish

Shellfish poisoning occurs from eating healthy mollusks from the temperate zone (clams, oysters, mussels, and scallops) that have ingested and filtered large amounts of dinoflagellates. Shellfish are a major source of seafood during the *non-R months*. The *red tide* intermittently found worldwide is because of the presence of dinoflagellate blooms. Not all red tides are toxic and toxic dinoflagellates are not necessarily associated with red tides. These toxins are similar to tetrodotoxin and other neurotoxins. A single mussel may contain 10 mg of toxin, and ingestion of less than six clams can be lethal. Saxitoxin, one of the best characterized, is a potent paralytic neurotoxin concentrated in the gills and digestive glands of shellfish. Saxitoxin is a heat-stable, water-soluble acetylcholinesterase inhibitor rapidly absorbed from the GI tract, which acts on the peripheral and autonomic nervous systems. A murine bioassay is used to detect the toxin, as no laboratory test to do so exists.

PARALYTIC SHELLFISH POISONING

Symptoms occur dramatically and rapidly (30 minutes) after eating a saxitoxin-containing mollusk. They are related to the amount ingested and the method of food preparation; increased toxicity exists with raw food. Oral and perioral dysesthesias and burning progress rapidly caudally. A number of neurologic symptoms occur, and patients may describe a sensation of their body "floating." Flaccid paralysis and respiratory failure may ensue. Similar to tetraodon intoxication, the patient may remain awake. Treatment consists of gut decontamination and supportive ventilatory care. Untreated, up to 75% will die within 12 hours.

NEUROTOXIC SHELLFISH POISONING

Ptychodiscus brevis toxin ingestion causes a milder form of paralytic shellfish poisoning. Onset may be delayed up to 3 hours. Neurologic symptoms resemble early paralytic shellfish poisoning and ciguatera. Paralysis is rare. Only a few patients have symptoms after the first 24 hours. Treatment consists of the standard methods of gut decontamination and supportive care, particularly respiratory support. The fatality rate is reported to be 8% to 9%, with death occurring in 1 to 12 hours from respiratory failure. Patients surviving beyond 12 to 18 hours have a good prognosis for complete recovery.

Gymnothorax Intoxication

Intoxication from *Gymnothorax* genus (moray, conger, and anguillid eels) results from a neurotoxin present in the viscera, muscles, and gonads that does not affect the fish itself. The heat-stable toxin produces a ciguatoxin-like syndrome. A toxidrome of cholinergic symptoms and hemolysis may be separate from, or coincide with, the neurotoxicity. Treatment is purely supportive, with deaths occurring from respiratory paralysis and seizures.

When humans encounter marine creatures, a variety of maladies may occur, ranging from dermatitis to life-threatening trauma, allergy, envenomations, or intoxications. The physician should be prepared to recognize quickly and address appropriately the potential life threats. These are primarily neurologic, respiratory, and cardiovascular. A high degree of suspicion for these illnesses is needed. Intoxications may be especially confounding, but the treatment is essentially identical, that is, supportive.

Although most of the syndromes are self-limited and treatment supportive, time is of the essence if neuromuscular paralysis, hypotension, or respiratory compromise is present.

Much folklore exists regarding detection and prevention of these entities and should be regarded as such. The last several decades have seen a marked increase in our knowledge base regarding these fascinating envenomations and intoxications. Research in the next several decades probably will produce a variety of diagnostic and therapeutic tools that will further our understanding of and ability to specifically manage these syndromes.

[1]Not FDA approved for this indication.

MEDICAL TOXICOLOGY: INGESTIONS, INHALATIONS, AND DERMAL AND OCULAR ABSORPTIONS

METHOD OF

Howard C. Mofenson, MD, Thomas R. Caraccio, PharmD, Michael McGuigan, MD, and Joseph Greensher, MD

Introduction and Epidemiology

According to the national Toxic Exposure Surveillance System (TESS), almost 2.4 million potentially toxic exposures were reported last year to Poison Control Centers throughout the United States. Poisonings were responsible for almost 1100 deaths and more than 500,000 hospitalizations. Poisoning accounts for 2% to 5% of pediatric hospital admissions, 10% of adult admissions, 5% of hospital admissions in the elderly (>65 years of age), and 5% of ambulance calls. In one urban hospital, drug-related emergencies accounted for 38% of the emergency department visits. An evaluation of a medical intensive care unit and step-down unit over a 3-month period indicated that poisonings accounted for 19.7% of admissions.

The largest number of fatalities resulting from poisoning reported to the TESS are caused by analgesics. The other principal toxicologic causes of fatalities are antidepressants, sedative hypnotics/antipsychotics, stimulants/street drugs, cardiovascular agents, and alcohols. Less than 1% of overdose cases reaching the hospitals result in fatality. However, patients presenting in deep coma to medical care facilities have a fatality rate of 13% to 35%. The largest single cause of coma of inapparent etiology is drug poisoning.

Pharmaceutical preparations are involved in 40% of poisonings. The number one pharmaceutical agent involved in exposures is acetaminophen. The severity of the manifestations of acute poisoning exposures varies greatly depending on whether the poisoning was intentional or unintentional. Unintentional exposures make up 85% to 90% of all poisoning exposures. The majority of cases are acute, occurring in children younger than 5 years of age, in the home, and resulting in no or minor toxicity. Many are actually ingestions of relatively nontoxic substances that require minimal medical care. Intentional poisonings, such as suicides, constitute 10% to 15% of exposures and may require the highest standards of medical and nursing care and the use of sophisticated equipment for recovery. Intentional ingestions are often of multiple substances and frequently include ethanol, acetaminophen, and aspirin. Suicides make up 52% of the reported fatalities. About 25% of suicides are attempted with drugs. Sixty percent of patients who take a drug overdose use their own medication and 15% use drugs prescribed for close relatives. The majority of the drug-related suicide attempts involve a central nervous system (CNS) depressant, and coma management is vital to the treatment.

Assessment and Maintenance of the Vital Functions

The initial assessment of all patients in medical emergencies follows the principles of basic and advanced cardiac life support. The adequacy of the patient's airway, degree of ventilation, and circulatory status should be determined. The vital functions should be established and maintained. Vital signs should be measured frequently and should include body core temperature. The assessment of vital functions should include the rate numbers (e.g., respiratory rate) and indications of effectiveness (e.g., depth of respirations and degree of gas exchange). Table 1 gives important measurements and vital signs.

Level of consciousness should be assessed by immediate AVPU (Alert, responds to Verbal stimuli, responds to Painful stimuli, and Unconscious). If the patient is unconscious, one must assess the severity of the unconsciousness by the Glasgow Coma Scale (Table 2).

If the patient is comatose, management requires administering 100% oxygen, establishing vascular access, and obtaining blood for pertinent laboratory studies. The administration of glucose, thiamine, and naloxone, as well as intubation to protect the airway, should be considered. Pertinent laboratory studies include arterial blood gases (ABG), electrocardiography (ECG), determination of blood glucose level, electrolytes, renal and liver tests, and acetaminophen plasma concentration in all cases of intentional ingestions. Radiography of the chest and abdomen may be useful. The severity of a stimulant's effects can also be assessed and should be documented to follow the trend.

The examiner should completely expose the patient by removing clothes and other items that interfere with a full evaluation. One should look for clues to etiology in the clothes and include the hat and shoes.

TABLE 1 Important Measurements and Vital Signs

Age	Body Surface Area (m^2)	Weight (kg)	Height (cm)	Pulse (bpm) Resting	Blood Pressure			Respiratory Rate (rpm)
						Hypertension		
					Hypotension	Significant	Severe	
Newborn	0.19	3.5	50	70-190	<60/40	>96	>106	30-60
1 mo–6 mo	0.30	4–7	50–65	80–160	<70/45	>104	>110	30–50
6 mo–1 y	0.38	7–10	65–75	80–160	<70/45	>104	>110	20–40
1–2 y	0.50–0.55	10–12	75–85	80–140	<74/47	>112/74	>118/82	20–40
3–5 y	0.54–0.68	15–20	90–108	80–120	<80/52	>116/76	>124/84	20–40
6–9 y	0.68–0.85	20–28	122–133	75–115	<90/60	>122/82	>130/86	16–25
10–12 y	1.00–1.07	30–40	138–147	70–110	<90/60	>126/82	>134/90	16–25
13–15 y	1.07–1.22	42–50	152–160	60–100	<90/60	>136/86	>144/92	16–20
16–18 y	1.30–1.60	53–60	160–170	60–100	<90/60	>142/92	>150/98	12–16
Adult	1.40–1.70	60–70	160–170	60–100	<90/60	>140/90	>210/120	10–16

Data from Nadas A: Pediatric Cardiology, 3rd ed. Philadephia, WB Saunders, 1976; Blumer JL (ed): A Practice Guide to Pediatric Intensive Care. St Louis, Mosby, 1990; AAP and ACEP: Respiratory Distress in APLS Pediatric Emergency Medicine Course, 1993; Second Task Force: Blood pressure control in children–1987, Pediatr 79:1, 1987; Linakis JG: Hypertension. In Fliesher GR, Ludwig S (eds); Textbook of Pediatric Emergency Medicine, 3rd ed. Baltimore, Williams & Wilkins 1993.

TABLE 2 Glasgow Coma Scale

Scale	Adult Response	Score	Pediatric, 0–1 Years
Eye Opening	Spontaneous	4	Spontaneous
	To verbal command	3	To shout
	To pain	2	To pain
	None	1	No response
Motor response			
To verbal command	Obeys	6	
To painful stimuli	Localized pain	5	Localized pain
	Flexion withdrawal	4	Flexion withdrawal
	Decorticate flexion	3	Decorticate flexion
	Decerebrate extension	2	Decerebrate flexion
	None	1	None
Verbal response: adult	Oriented and converses	5	Cries, smiles, coos
	Disoriented but converses	4	Cries or screams
	Inappropriate words	3	Inappropriate sounds
	Incomprehensible sounds	2	Grunts
	None	1	Gives no response
Verbal response: child	Oriented	5	
	Words or babbles	4	
	Vocal sounds	3	
	Cries or moans to stimuli	2	
	None	1	

Data from Teasdale G, Jennett B: Assessment of coma impaired consciousness. Lancet 2:83, 1974; Simpson D, Reilly P: Pediatric coma scale. Lancet 2:450, 1982; Seidel J: Preparing for pediatric emergencies. Pediatr Rev 16:470 ,1995.

Prevention of Absorption and Reduction of Local Damage

EXPOSURE

Poisoning exposure routes include ingestion (70%), dermal (8%), ophthalmologic (5%), inhalation (6%), insect bites and stings (4%), and parenteral injections (0.4%). The effect of the toxin may be local, systemic, or both.

Local effects (skin, eyes, mucosa of respiratory or gastrointestinal tract) occur where contact is made with the poisonous substance. Local effects are nonspecific chemical reactions that depend on the chemical properties (e.g., pH), concentration, contact time, and type of exposed surface.

Systemic effects occur when the poison is absorbed into the body and depends on the dose, the distribution, and the functional reserve of the organ systems. Shock and hypoxia are part of systemic toxicity.

DELAYED TOXIC ACTION

Therapeutic doses of most pharmaceuticals are absorbed within 90 minutes. However, the patient with exposure to a potential toxin may be asymptomatic at this time because a sufficient amount has not yet been absorbed or metabolized to produce toxicity at the time the patient presents for care.

Absorption can be significantly delayed under the following circumstances:

1. Drugs with anticholinergic properties (e.g., antihistamines, belladonna alkaloids, diphenoxylate with atropine [Lomotil], phenothiazines, and tricyclic antidepressants).
2. Modified release preparations such as sustained-release, enteric-coated, and controlled-release formulations have delayed and prolonged absorption.
3. Concretions may form (e.g., salicylates, iron, glutethimide, and meprobamate [Equanil]) that can delay absorption and prolong the toxic effects. Large quantities of drugs tend to be absorbed more slowly than small quantities.

Some substances must be metabolized into a toxic metabolite (acetaminophen, acetonitrile, ethylene glycol, methanol, methylene chloride, parathion, and paraquat). In some cases, time is required to produce a toxic effect on organ systems (Amanita phalloides mushrooms, carbon tetrachloride, colchicine, digoxin [Lanoxin], heavy metals, monoamine oxidase inhibitors, and oral hypoglycemic agents).

Initial Management

1. Stabilization of airway, breathing, and circulation and protection of same.
2. Identification of specific toxin or toxic syndrome.
3. Initial treatment: D50W; consider thiamine, naloxone (Narcan), oxygen, and antidotes if needed.
4. Physical assessment.
5. Decontamination: Gastrointestinal tract, skin, eyes.

DECONTAMINATION

In the asymptomatic patient who has been exposed to a toxic substance, decontamination procedures should be considered if the patient has been exposed to potentially toxic substances in toxic amounts.

Ocular exposure should be immediately treated with water irrigation for 15 to 20 minutes with the eyelids fully retracted. One should not use neutralizing chemicals. All caustic and corrosive injuries should be evaluated with fluorescein dye and by an ophthalmologist.

Dermal exposure is treated immediately with copious water irrigation for 30 minutes, not a forceful flushing. Shampooing the hair, cleansing the fingernails, navel, and perineum, and irrigating the eyes are necessary in the case of an extensive exposure. The clothes should be specially bagged and may have to be discarded. Leather goods can become irreversibly contaminated and must be abandoned. Caustic (alkali) exposures can require hours of irrigation. Dermal absorption can occur with pesticides, hydrocarbons, and cyanide.

Injection exposures (e.g., snake envenomation) can be treated with venom extracts. Venom extractors can be used within minutes of envenomation, and proximal lymphatic constricting bands or elastic wraps can be used to delay lymphatic flow and immobilize the extremity. Cold packs and tourniquets should not be used and incision is generally not recommended. Substances of abuse may be injected intravenously or subcutaneously. In these cases, little decontamination can be done.

Inhalation exposure to toxic substances is managed by immediate removal of the victim from the contaminated environment by protected rescuers.

Gastrointestinal exposure is the most common route of poisoning. Gastrointestinal decontamination historically has been be done by gastric emptying: induction of emesis, gastric lavage, administration of activated charcoal, and the use of cathartics or whole bowel irrigation. No procedure is routine; it should be individualized for each case. If no attempt is made to decontaminate the patient, the reason should be clearly documented on the medical record (e.g., time elapsed, past peak of action, ineffectiveness, or risk of procedure).

Gastric Emptying Procedures

The gastric emptying procedure used is influenced by the age of the patient, the effectiveness of the procedure, the time of ingestion (gastric emptying is usually ineffective after 1 hour postingestion), the patient's clinical status (time of peak effect has passed or the patient's condition is too unstable), formulation of the substance ingested (regular release versus modified release), the amount ingested, and the rapidity of onset of CNS depression or stimulation (convulsions). Most studies show that only 30% (range, 19% to 62%) of the ingested toxin is removed by gastric emptying under optimal conditions. It has not been demonstrated that the choice of procedure improved the outcome.

A mnemonic for gathering information is STATS:

S—substance
T—type of formulation
A—amount and age
T—time of ingestion
S—signs and symptoms

The examiner should attempt to obtain AMPLE information about the patient:

A—age and allergies
M—available medications
P—past medical history including pregnancy, psychiatric illnesses, substance abuse, or intentional ingestions
L—time of last meal, which may influence absorption and the onset and peak action
E—events leading to present condition

The intent of the patient should also be determined.

The Regional Poison Center should be consulted for the exact ingredients of the ingested substance and the latest management. The treatment information on the labels of products and in the Physician's Desk Reference are notoriously inaccurate.

Ipecac Syrup

Syrup of ipecac–induced emesis has virtually no use in the emergency department. Although at one time it was considered most useful in young children with a recent witnessed ingestion, it is advised only within 1 hour of ingestion of known agents only when a toxic amount is involved. Current guidelines from the American Association of Poison Control Centers has significantly limited the indications for inducing emesis because the risk most often exceeds the benefit derived from this procedure. The Poison Control Center should be called before one induces emesis.

Contraindications or situations in which induction of emesis are inappropriate include the following:

- Ingestion of caustic substance
- Loss of airway protective reflexes because of ingestion of substances that can produce rapid onset of CNS depression (e.g., short-acting benzodiazepines, barbiturates, nonbarbiturate sedative-hypnotics, opioids, tricyclic antidepressants) or convulsions (e.g., camphor [Ponstel], chloroquine [Aralen], codeine, isoniazid [Nydrazid], mefenamic acid, nicotine, propoxyphene [Darvon], organophosphate insecticides, strychnine, and tricyclic antidepressants)
- Ingestion of low-viscosity petroleum distillates (e.g., gasoline, lighter fluid, kerosene)
- Significant vomiting prior to presentation or hematemesis
- Age under 6 months (no established dose, safety, or efficacy data)
- Ingestion of foreign bodies (emesis is ineffective and may lead to aspiration)
- Clinical conditions including neurologic impairment, hemodynamic instability, increased intracranial pressure, and hypertension
- Delay in presentation (more than 1 hour postingestion)

The dose of syrup of ipecac in the 6- to 9-month-old infant is 5 mL; in the 9- to 12-month-old, 10 mL; and in the 1- to 12-year-old, 15 mL. In children older than 12 years and in adults, the dose is 30 mL. The dose can be repeated once if the child does not vomit in 15 to 20 minutes. The vomitus should be inspected for remnants of pills or toxic substances, and the appearance and odor should be documented. When ipecac is not available, 30 mL of mild dishwashing soap (not dishwasher detergent) can be used, although it is less effective.

Complications are very rare but include aspiration, protracted vomiting, rarely cardiac toxicity with long-term abuse, pneumothorax, gastric rupture, diaphragmatic hernia, intracranial hemorrhage, and Mallory-Weiss tears.

Gastric Lavage

Gastric lavage should be considered only when life-threatening amounts of substances were involved, when the benefits outweigh the risks, when it can be performed within 1 hour of the ingestion, and when no contraindications exist.

The contraindications are similar to those for ipecac-induced emesis. However, gastric lavage can be accomplished after the insertion of an endotracheal tube in cases of CNS depression or controlled convulsions. The patient should be placed with the head lower than the hips in a left-lateral decubitus position. The location of the tube should be confirmed by radiography, if necessary, and suctioning equipment should be available.

Contraindications to gastric lavage include the following:

- Ingestion of caustic substances (risk of esophageal perforation)
- Uncontrolled convulsions, because of the danger of aspiration and injury during the procedure
- Ingestion of low-viscosity petroleum distillate products
- CNS depression or absent protective airway reflexes, without endotracheal protection
- Significant cardiac dysrhythmias
- Significant emesis or hematemesis prior to presentation
- Delay in presentation (more than 1 hour post-ingestion)

Size of Tube

The best results with gastric lavage are obtained with the largest possible orogastric tube that can be reasonably passed (nasogastric tubes are not large enough to remove solid material). In adults, a large-bore orogastric Lavacuator hose or a No. 42 French Ewald tube should be used; in young children, orogastric tubes are generally too small to remove solid material and gastric lavage is not recommended.

The amount of fluid used varies with the patient's age and size. In general, aliquots of 50 to 100 mL per lavage are used in adults. Larger amounts of fluid may force the toxin past the pylorus. Lavage fluid is 0.9% saline.

Complications are rare and may include respiratory depression, aspiration pneumonitis, cardiac dysrhythmias as a result of increased vagal tone, esophageal-gastric tears and perforation, laryngospasm, and mediastinitis.

Activated Charcoal

Oral activated charcoal adsorbs the toxin onto its surface before absorption. According to recent guidelines set forth by the American Academy of Clinical Toxicology, activated charcoal should not be used routinely. Its use is indicated only if a toxic amount of substance has been ingested and is optimally effective within 1 hour of the ingestion. Because of the slow absorption of large quantities of toxin, activated charcoal may be beneficial after 1 hour postingestion.

Activated charcoal does not effectively adsorb small molecules or molecules lacking carbon (Table 3). Activated charcoal adsorption may be diminished by milk, cocoa powder, and ice cream.

There are a few relative contraindications to the use of activated charcoal:

1. Ingestion of caustics and corrosives, which may produce vomiting or cling to the mucosa and falsely appear as a burn on endoscopy.
2. Comatose patient, in whom the airway must be secured prior to activated charcoal administration.
3. Patient without presence of bowel sounds.

Note: Activated charcoal was shown not to interfere with effectiveness of *N*-acetylcysteine in cases of acetaminophen overdose, so it is no longer contraindicated as was thought in the past.

The usual initial adult dose is 60 to 100 g and the dose for children is 15 to 30 g. It is administered orally as a slurry mixed with water or by nasogastric or orogastric tube. *Caution:* Be sure the tube is in the stomach. Cathartics are not necessary.

Although repeated dosing with activated charcoal may decrease the half-life and increases the clearance of phenobarbital, dapsone, quinidine, theophylline, and carbamazepine (Tegretol), recent guidelines

TABLE 3 Substances Poorly Adsorbed by Activated Charcoal

C	Caustics and corrosives
H	Heavy metals (arsenic, iron, lead, mercury)
A	Alcohols (ethanol, methanol, isopropanol) and glycols (ethylene glycols)
R	Rapid onset of absorption (cyanide and strychnine)
C	Chlorine and iodine
O	Others insoluble in water (substances in tablet form)
A	Aliphatic hydrocarbons (petroleum distillates)
L	Laxatives (sodium, magnesium, potassium, and lithium)

indicate there is insufficient evidence to support the use of multiple-dose activated charcoal unless a life-threatening amount of one of the substances mentioned is involved. At present there are no controlled studies that demonstrate that multiple-dose activated charcoal or cathartics alter the clinical course of an intoxication. The dose varies from 0.25 to 0.50 g/kg every 1 to 4 hours, and continuous nasogastric tube infusion of 0.25 to 0.5 g/kg/h has been used to decrease vomiting.

Gastrointestinal dialysis is the diffusion of the toxin from the higher concentration in the serum of the mesenteric vessels to the lower levels in the gastrointestinal tract mucosal cell and subsequently into the gastrointestinal lumen, where the concentration has been lowered by intraluminal adsorption of activated charcoal.

Complications of treatment with activated charcoal include vomiting in 50% of cases, desorption (especially with weak acids in intestine), and aspiration (at least a dozen cases of aspiration have been reported). There are many cases of unreported pulmonary aspirations and "charcoal lungs," intestinal obstruction or pseudoobstruction (three cases reports with multiple dosing, none with a single dose), empyema following esophageal perforation, and hypermagnesemia and hypernatremia, which have been associated with repeated concurrent doses of activated charcoal and saline cathartics. Catharsis was used to hasten the elimination of any remaining toxin in the gastrointestinal tract. There are no studies to demonstrate the effectiveness of cathartics, and they are no longer recommended as a form of gastrointestinal decontamination.

Whole-Bowel Irrigation

With whole bowel irrigation, solutions of polyethylene glycol (PEG) with balanced electrolytes are used to cleanse the bowel without causing shifts in fluids and electrolytes. The procedure is not approved by the U.S. Food and Drug Administration for this purpose.

Indications

The procedure has been studied and used successfully in cases of iron overdose when abdominal radiographs reveal incomplete emptying of excess iron. There are additional indications for other types of ingestions, such as with body-packing of illicit drugs (e.g., cocaine, heroin).

The procedure is to administer the solution (GoLYTELY or Colyte), orally or by nasogastric tube, in a dose of 0.5 L per hour in children younger than 5 years of age and 2 L per hour in adolescents and adults for 5 hours. The end point is reached when the rectal effluent is clear or radiopaque materials can no longer be seen in the gastrointestinal tract on abdominal radiographs.

Contraindications

These measures should not be used if there is extensive hematemesis, ileus, or signs of bowel obstruction, perforation, or peritonitis. Animal experiments in which PEG was added to activated charcoal indicated that activated charcoal-salicylates and activated charcoal-theophylline combinations resulted in decreased adsorption and desorption of salicylate and theophylline and no therapeutic benefit over activated charcoal alone. Polyethylene solutions are bound by activated charcoal in vitro, decreasing the efficacy of activated charcoal.

Dilutional treatment is indicated for the immediate management of caustic and corrosive poisonings but is otherwise not useful. The administration of diluting fluid above 30 mL in children and 250 mL in adults may produce vomiting, reexposing the vital tissues to the effects of local damage and possible aspiration.

Neutralization is not proven to be either safe or effective.

Endoscopy and surgery have been required in the case of body-packer obstruction, intestinal ischemia produced by cocaine ingestion, and iron local caustic action.

Differential Diagnosis of Poisons on the Basis of Central Nervous System Manifestations

Neurologic parameters help to classify and assess the need for supportive treatment as well as provide diagnostic clues to the etiology. Table 4 lists the effects of CNS depressants, CNS stimulants, hallucinogens, and autonomic nervous system anticholinergics and cholinergics.

Central nervous system depressants are cholinergics, opioids, sedative-hypnotics, and sympatholytic agents. The hallmarks are lethargy, sedation, stupor, and coma. In exception to the manifestations listed in Table 4, (a) barbiturates may produce an initial tachycardia; (b) convulsions are produced by codeine, propoxyphene (Darvon), meperidine (Demerol), glutethimide, phenothiazines, methaqualone, and tricyclic and cyclic antidepressants; (c) benzodiazepines rarely produce coma that will interfere with cardiorespiratory functions; and (d) pulmonary edema is common with opioids and sedative-hypnotics.

The CNS stimulants are anticholinergic, hallucinogenic, sympathomimetic, and withdrawal agents. The hallmarks of CNS stimulants are convulsions and hyperactivity.

There is considerable overlapping of effects among the various hallucinogens, but the major hallmark manifestation is hallucinations.

Guidelines for In-hospital Disposition

Classification of patients as high risk depends on clinical judgment. Any patient who needs cardiorespiratory support or has a persistently altered mental

TABLE 4 Agents with Central Nervous System (CNS) Effects

Agents	General Manifestations	Agents	General Manifestations
CNS Depressants		**Hallucinogens**	
Alcohols and glycols (S-H) Anticonvulsants (S-H) Antidysrhythmics (S-H) Antihypertensives (S-H) Barbiturates (S-H) Benzodiazepines (S-H) Butyrophenones (Syly) β-Adrenergic blockers (Syly) Calcium channel blockers (Syly) Digitalis (Syly) Opioids Lithium (mixed) Muscle relaxants Phenothiazines (Syly) Nonbarbiturate/benzodiazepine glutethimide, methaqualone, methyprylon, sedative-hypnotics (chloral hydrate, ethchlorvynol, bromide) Tricyclic antidepressants (late Syly)	Bradycardia Bradypnea Shallow respirations Hypotension Hypothermia Flaccid coma Miosis Hypoactive bowel sounds	Amphetamines[‡] Anticholinergics Cardiac glycosides Cocaine Ethanol withdrawal Hydrocarbon inhalation (abuse) Mescaline (peyote) Mushrooms (psilocybin) Phencyclidine	Tachycardia and dysrhythmias Tachypnea Hypertension Hallucinations, usually visual Disorientation Panic reaction Toxic psychosis Moist skin Mydriasis (reactive) Hyperthermia Flashbacks
		Anticholinergics	
		Antihistamines Antispasmodic gastrointestinal preparations Antiparkinsonian preparations Atropine Cyclobenzaprine (Flexeril)	Tachycardia, dysrhythmias (rare) Tachypnea Hypertension (mild) Hyperthermia Hallucinations ("mad as a hatter")
CNS Stimulants			
Amphetamines (Sy) Anticholinergics* Cocaine (Sy) Camphor (mixed) Ergot alkaloids (Sy) Isoniazid (mixed) Lithium (mixed) Lysergic acid diethylamide (H) Hallucinogens (H) Mescaline and synthetic analogs Metals (arsenic, lead, mercury) Methylphenidate (Ritalin) (Sy) Monoamine oxidase inhibitors (Sy) Pemoline (Cylert) (Sy) Phencyclidine (H)[†] Salicylates (mixed) Strychnine (mixed) Sympathomimetics (Sy) (phenylpropanolamine, theophylline, caffeine, thyroid) Withdrawal from ethanol, β-adrenergic blockers, clonidine, opioids, sedative–hypnotics (W)	Tachycardia Tachypnea and dysrhythmias Hypertension Convulsions Toxic psychosis Mydriasis (reactive) Agitation and restlessness Moist skin Tremors	Mydriatic ophthalmologic agents Over-the-counter sleep agents Plants (*Datura* spp)/mushrooms Phenothiazines (early) Scopolamine Tricyclic/cyclic antidepressants (early)	Mydriasis (unreactive) ("blind as a bat") Flushed skin ("red as a beet") Dry skin and mouth ("dry as a bone") Hypoactive bowel sounds Urinary retention Lilliputian hallucinations ("little people")
		Cholinergics	
		Bethanechol (Urecholine) Carbamate insecticides (Carbaryl) Edrophonium Organophosphate insecticides (Malathion, parathion) Parasympathetic agents (physostigmine, pyridostigmine) Toxic mushrooms (*Clitocybe* spp.)	Bradycardia (muscarinic) Tachycardia (nicotinic effect) Miosis (muscarinic) Diarrhea (muscarinic) Hypertension (variable) Hyperactive bowel sounds Excess urination (muscarinic) Excess salivation (muscarinic) Lacrimation (muscarinic) Bronchospasm (muscarinic) Muscle fasciculations (nicotinic) Paralysis (nicotinic)

Abbreviations: H = hallucinogen; S-H = sedative–hypnotic; Sy = sympathomimetic; Syly = Sympatholytic; W = withdrawal.
*Anticholinergics produce dry skin and mucosa and decreased bowel sounds.
[†]Phencyclidine may produce miosis.
[‡]The amphetamine hybrids are methylene dioxymethamphetamine (MDMA, ecstasy,"ADAM") and methylene dioxyamphetamine (MDA, "Eve"), which are associated with deaths.

status for 3 hours or more should be considered for intensive care.

Guidelines for admitting patients older than 14 years of age to an intensive care unit, after 2 to 3 hours in the emergency department, include the following:

1. Need for intubation
2. Seizures
3. Unresponsiveness to verbal stimuli
4. Arterial carbon dioxide pressure greater than 45 mm Hg
5. Cardiac conduction or rhythm disturbances (any rhythm except sinus arrhythmia)
6. Close monitoring of vital signs during antidotal therapy or elimination procedures
7. The need for continuous monitoring
8. QRS interval greater than 0.10 second, in cases of tricyclic antidepressant poisoning
9. Systolic blood pressure less than 80 mm Hg
10. Hypoxia, hypercarbia, acid–base imbalance, or metabolic abnormalities
11. Extremes of temperature
12. Progressive deterioration or significant underlying medical disorders

Use of Antidotes

Antidotes are available for only a relatively small number of poisons. An antidote is not a substitute for good supportive care. Table 5 summarizes the commonly used antidotes, their indications, and their methods of administration. The Regional Poison Control Center can give further information on these antidotes.

Enhancement of Elimination

The acceptable methods for elimination of absorbed toxic substances are dialysis, hemoperfusion, exchange transfusion, plasmapheresis, enzyme induction, and inhibition. Methods of increasing urinary excretion of toxic chemicals and drugs have been studied extensively, but the other modalities have not been well evaluated.

In general, these methods are needed in only a minority of cases and should be reserved for life-threatening circumstances when a definite benefit is anticipated.

DIALYSIS

Dialysis is the extrarenal means of removing certain substances from the body, and it can substitute for the kidney when renal failure occurs. Dialysis is not the first measure instituted; however, it may be lifesaving later in the course of a severe intoxication. It is needed in only a minority of intoxicated patients.

Peritoneal dialysis uses the peritoneum as the membrane for dialysis. It is only 1/20 as effective as hemodialysis. It is easier to use and less hazardous to the patient but also less effective in removing the toxin; thus it is rarely used except in small infants.

Hemodialysis is the most effective dialysis method but requires experience with sophisticated equipment. Blood is circulated past a semipermeable extracorporeal membrane. Substances are removed by diffusion down a concentration gradient. Anticoagulation with heparin is necessary. Flow rates of 300 to 500 mL/min can be achieved, and clearance rates may reach 200 or 300 mL/min.

Dialyzable substances easily diffuse across the dialysis membrane and have the following characteristics: (a) a molecular weight less than 500 daltons and preferably less than 350; (b) a volume of distribution less than 1 L/kg; (c) protein binding less than 50%; (d) high water solubility (low lipid solubility); and (e) high plasma concentration and a toxicity that correlates reasonably with the plasma concentration. Considerations for hemodialysis and hemoperfusion are cases of serious ingestions (the nephrologist should be notified immediately), and cases involving a compound that is ingested in a potentially lethal dose and the rapid removal of which may improve the prognosis. Examples of the latter are ethylene glycol 1.4 mL/kg 100% solution or equivalent and methanol 6 mL/kg 100% solution or equivalent. Common dialyzable substances include alcohol, bromides, lithium, and salicylates.

The patient-related criteria for dialysis are (a) anticipated prolonged coma and the likelihood of complications; (b) renal compromise (toxin excreted or metabolized by kidneys and dialyzable chelating agents in heavy metal poisoning); (c) laboratory confirmation of lethal blood concentration; (d) lethal dose poisoning with an agent with delayed toxicity or known to be metabolized into a more toxic metabolite (e.g., ethylene glycol, methanol); and (e) hepatic impairment when the agent is metabolized by the liver, and clinical deterioration despite optimal supportive medical management. Table 6 gives plasma concentrations above which removal by extracorporeal measures should be considered.

The contraindications to hemodialysis include the following: (a) substances are not dialyzable; (b) effective antidotes are available; (c) patient is hemodynamically unstable (e.g., shock); and (d) presence of coagulopathy because heparinization is required.

Hemodialysis also has a role in correcting disturbances that are not amenable to appropriate medical management. These are easily remembered by the "vowel" mnemonic:

A—refractory acid–base disturbances
E—refractory electrolyte disturbances
I—intoxication with dialyzable substances (e.g., ethanol, ethylene glycol, isopropyl alcohol, methanol, lithium, and salicylates)
O—overhydration
U—uremia

TABLE 5 Initial Doses of Antidotes for Common Poisonings

Antidote	Use	Dose	Route	Adverse Reactions/Comments
***N*-Acetyl cysteine (NAC, Mucomyst):** Stock level to treat 70 kg adult for 24 h: 25 vials, 20%, 30 mL	Acetaminophen, carbon tetrachloride (experimental)	140/mg/kg loading, followed by 70 mg/kg every 4 h for 17 doses.	PO	Nausea, vomiting. Dilute to 5% with sweet juice or flat cola.
Atropine: Stock level to treat 70 kg adult for 24 h: 1 g (1 mg/mL in 1, 10 mL)	Organophosphate and carbamate pesticides: bradydysrthythmics, β-adrenergics, calcium channel blockers	*Child:* 0.02–0.05 mg/kg repeated q5–10 min to max of 2 mg as necessary until cessation of secretions *Adult:* 1–2 mg q5-10min as necessary. Dilute in 1–2 mL of 0.9% saline for ET instillation. *IV infusion dose:* Place 8 mg of atropine in 100 mL D_5W or saline. Conc. =0.08 mg/mL; dose range = 0.02–0.08 mg/kg/h or 0.25–1 mL/kg/h. Severe poisoning may require supplemental doses of IV atropine intermittently in doses of 1–5 mg until drying of secretions occurs.	IV/ET	Tachycardia, dry mouth, blurred vision, and urinary retention. Ensure adequate ventilation before administration.
Calcium chloride (10%): Stock level to treat 70 kg adult for 24 h:10 vials 1 g (1.35 mEq/mL)	Hypocalcemia, fluoride, calcium channel blockers, β-blockers, oxalates, ethylene glycol, hypermagnesemia	0.1–0.2 mL/kg (10–20 mg/kg) slow push every 10 min up to max 10 mL (1 g). Since calcium response lasts 15 minutes, some may require continuous infusion 0.2 mL/kg/h up to maximum of 10 mL/h while monitoring for dysrhythmias and hypotension.	IV	Administer slowly with BP and ECG monitoring and have magnesium available to reverse calcium effects. Tissue irritation, hypotension, dysrhythmias from rapid injection. Contraindications: digitalis glycoside intoxication.
Calcium gluconate (10%): Stock level to treat 70 kg adult for 24 h: 20 vials 1 g (0.45 mEq/mL)	Hypocalcemia, fluoride, calcium channel blockers, hydrofluoric acid; black widow envenomation	0.3–0.4 mL/kg (30–40 mg/kg) slow push; repeat as needed up to max dose 10–20 mL (1–2 g).	IV	Same comments as calcium chloride.
Infiltration of calcium gluconate	Hydrofluoric acid skin exposure	Dose: Infiltrate each square cm of affected dermis/ subcutaneous tissue with about 0.5 mL of 10% calcium gluconate using a 30-gauge needle. Repeat as needed to control pain.	Infiltrate	
Intra-arterial calcium gluconate	Hydrofluoric acid skin exposure	Infuse 20 mL of 10% calcium gluconate (not chloride) diluted in 250 mL D_5W via the radial or brachial artery proximal to the injury over 3–4 hours.		Alternatively, dilute 10 mL of 10% calcium gluconate with 40–50 mL of D_5W.

Continued

TABLE 5 Initial Doses of Antidotes for Common Poisonings—cont'd

Antidote	Use	Dose	Route	Adverse Reactions/Comments
Calcium gluconate gel Stock level: 3.5 g	Hydrofluoric acid skin exposure	2.5 g USP powder added to 100 mL water-soluble lubricating jelly, e.g., K-Y Jelly or Lubifax (or 3.5 mg into 150 mL). Some use 6 g of calcium carbonate in 100 g of lubricant. Place injured hand in surgical glove filled with gel. Apply q4h. If pain persists, calcium gluconate injection may be needed (above).	Dermal	Powder is available from Spectrum Pharmaceutical Co. in California: 800-772-8786. Commercial preparation of Ca gluconate gel is available from Pharmascience in Montreal, Quebec: 514-340-1114.
Cyanide antidote kit: Stock level to treat 70 kg adult for 24 h:2 Lilly Cyanide Antidote kits	Cyanide Hydrogen sulfide (nitrites are given only) Do not use sodium thiosulfate for hydrogen sulfide Individual portions of the kit can be used in certain circumstances (consult PCC)	Amyl nitrite: 1 crushable ampule for 30 secs of every min. Use new amp q3min. May omit step if venous access is established.	Inhalation	If methemoglobinemia occurs, do not use methylene blue to correct this because it releases cyanide.
	Cyanide Hydrogen sulfide (nitrites are given only) Do not use sodium thiosulfate for hydrogen sulfide Individual portions of the kit can be used in certain circumstances (consult PCC)	Sodium nitrite: *Child:* 0.33 mL/kg of 3% solution if hemoglobin level is not known, otherwise based on tables with product. *Adult:* up to 300 mg (10 mL). Dilute nitrite in 100 mL 0.9% saline, administer slowly at 5 mL/min. Slow infusion if fall in BP.	IV	If methemoglobinemia occurs, do not use methylene blue to correct this because it releases cyanide.
	Do not use sodium thiosulfate for hydrogen sulfide Individual portions of the Kit can be used in certain circumstances (consult PCC)	Sodium thiosulfate: *Child:* 1.6 mL/kg of 25% solution, may be repeated every 30–60 min to a maximum of 12.5 g or 50 mL in adult. Administer over 20 min.	IV	Nausea, dizziness, headache. Tachycardia, muscle rigidity, and bronchospasm (rapid administration).
Dantrolene sodium (Dantrium): Stock level to treat 70 kg adult for 24 h: 700 mg, 35 vials (20 mg/vial)	Malignant hyperthermia	2–3 mg/kg IV rapidly. Repeat loading dose every 10 minutes, if necessary up to a maximum total dose of 10 mg/kg. When temperature and heart rate decrease, slow the infusion 1–2 mg/kg every 6 hours for 24–28 h until all evidence of malignant hyperthermia syndrome has subsided. Follow with oral doses 1–2 mg/kg four times a day for 24 h as necessary.	IV/PO	Hepatotoxicity occurs with cumulative dose of 10 mg/kg. Thrombophlebitis (best given in central line). Available as 20 mg lyophilized dantrolene powder for reconstruction, which contains 3 g mannitol and sodium hydroxide in 70-mL vial. Mix with 60 mL sterile distilled water without a bacteriostatic agent and protect from light. Use within 6 hours after reconstituting.

Deferoxamine (Desferal): Stock level to treat 70 kg adult for 24 h: 17 vials (500 mg/amp).	Iron	IV infusion of 15 mg/kg/h (3 mL/kg/h: 500 mg in 100 mL D_5W) max 6 g/d Rates of >45 µg/kg/h if cone >1000 µg/dL.	Preferred IV: avoid therapy >24 h	Hypotension (minimized by avoiding rapid infusion rates) DFO challenge test 50 mg/kg is unreliable if negative.
Diazepam (Valium) Stock level to treat 70 kg adult for 24 h: 200 mg, 5 mg/mL; 2,10 mL	Any intoxication that provokes seizures when specific therapy is not available, e.g., amphetamines, PCP, barbiturate and alcohol withdrawal. Chloroquine poisoning.	Adult, 5–10 mg IV (max 20 mg) at a rate of 5 mg/min until seizure is controlled. May be repeated 2 or 3 times. Child, 0.1–0.3 mg/kg up to 10 mg IV slowly over 2 min.	IV	Confusion, somnolence, coma, hypotension. Intramuscular absorption is erratic Establish airway and administer 100% oxygen and glucose.
Digoxin-specific Fab antibodies (Digibind): Stock level to treat 70 kg adult for 24 h: 20 vials.	Digoxin, digitoxin, oleander tea with the following: (1) Imminent cardiac arrest or shock, (2) hyperkalemia >5.0 mEq/L. (3) serum digoxin >5 ng/mL (child) at 8–12 h post ingestion in adults, (4) digitalis delirium, (5) ingestion over 10 mg in adults or 4 mg in child, (6) bradycardia or second- or third-degree heart block unresponsive to atropine, (7) life threatening digitoxin or oleander posioning.	(1) If amount ingested is known total dose × bioavailability (0.8) = body burden. The body burden + 0.6 (0.5 mg of digoxin is bound by 1 vial of 38 mg of FAB) = # vials needed. (2) If amount is unknown but the steady state serum concentration is known in ng/mL: Digoxin: ng/mL: (5.6 L/kg Vd) × (wt kg) = µg body burden. Body burden + 100 = mg body burden/0.5 = # vials needed. Digitoxin body burden = ng/mL × (0.56 L/kg Vd) × (wt kg) Body burden + 1000 = mg body burden/0.5 = # vials needed. (3) If the amount is not known, it is administered in life-threatening situations as 10 vials (400 mg) IV in saline over 30 min in adults. If cardiac arrest is imminent, administer 20 vials (adult) as a bolus.	IV	Allergic reactions (rare), return of condition being treated with digitalis glycoside. Administer by infusion over 30 min through a 0.22-µ filter. If cardiac arrest imminent, may administer by bolus. Consult PCC for more details.
Dimercaprol (BAL in peanut oil): Stock level to treat 70 kg adult for 24 h: 1200 mg (4 amps—100 mg/mL 10% in oil in 3 mL amp)	Chelating agent for arsenic, mercury, and lead.	3–5 mg/kg q4th usually for 5–10 d	Deep IM	Local infection site pain and sterile abscess, nausea, vomiting, fever, salivation, hypertension, and nephrotoxicity (alkalinize urine).

Continued

TABLE 5 Initial Doses of Antidotes for Common Poisonings—cont'd

Antidote	Use	Dose	Route	Adverse Reactions/Comments
2,3 Dimercaptosuccinic acid (DMSA succimer): 100 mg/capsule: 20 capsules	Used as a chelating agent for lead, especially blood lead levels >45 μg/dL. May also be used for symptomatic mercury exposure	10 mg/kg 3 × daily for 5 days followed by 10 mg/kg 2 × daily for 14 days.	PO	Precautions: monitor AST/ALT; use with caution in G6PD-deficient patients. Avoid concurrent iron therapy. Relatively safe antidote, rarely severe, uncommon minor skin rashes may occur.
Diphenhydramine (Benadryl) Antiparkinsonian action. Stock level to treat a 70 kg adult for 24 h: 5 vials (10 mg/mL, 10 mL each)	Used to treat extrapyramidal symptoms and dystonia induced by phenothiazines, phencyclidine, and related drugs.	Children: 1–2 mg/kg IV slowly over 5 minutes up to maximum 50 mg followed by 5 mg/kg/24 h orally divided every 6 hours up to 300 mg/24h *Adults:* 50 mg IV followed by 50 mg orally four times daily for 5–7 days Note: Symptoms abate within 2–5 min after IV.	IV	Fatal dose: 20–40 mg/kg. Dry mouth, drowsiness.
Ethanol (ethyl alcohol): Stock level to treat 70 kg adult for 24 h:3 bottles 10% (1 L each)	Methanol, ethylene glycol	10 mL/kg loading dose concurrently with 1.4 mL/kg (average) infusion of 10% ethanol (consult PCC for more details)	IV	Nausea, vomiting, sedation. Use 0.22 μm filter if preparing from bulk 100% ethanol.
Flumazenil (Romazicon): Stock level to treat 70 kg adult for 24 h: 4 vials (0.1 mg/mL, 10 mL)	Benzodiazepines (may also be beneficial in the treatment of hepatic encephalopathy)	Administer 0.2 mg (2 mL) IV over 30 sec (pediatric dose not established. 0.01 mg/kg), then wait 3 min for a response, then if desired consciousness is not achieved, administer 0.3 mg (3 mL) over 30 sec, then wait 3 min for response, then if desired consciousness is not achieved, administer 0.5 mg (5 mL) over 30 sec at 60-sec intervals up to a maximum cumulative dose of 3 mg (30 mL) (1 mg in children). Because effects last only 1–5 hours, if patient responds monitor carefully over next 6 hours for resedation. If multiple repeated doses, consider a continuous infusion of 0.2–1 mg/h.	IV	Nausea, vomiting, facial flushing, agitation, headache, dizziness, seizures, and death. It is not recommended to improve ventilation. Its role in CNS depression needs to be clarified. It should not be used routinely in comatose patients. It is **contraindicated** in cyclic antidepressant intoxications, stimulant overdose, long-term benzodiazepine use (may precipitate life-threatening withdrawal), if benzodiazepines are used to control seizures, in head trauma.
Folic acid (Folvite): Stock level to treat 70 kg adult for 24 h:4 100-mg vials	Methanol/ethylene glycol (investigational)	1 mg/kg up to 50 mg q4h for 6 doses.	IV	Uncommon
Fomepizole (4-MP, Antizol): Stock level to treat 70 kg adult: 4 1.5-mL vials (1 g/mL)	Ethylene glycol Methanol	Loading dose: 15 mg/kg (0.015 mL/kg) IV followed by maintanence dose of 10 mg/kg	IV	Suggested: co-administer folate 50 mg IV (child1 mg/kg), thiamine 100 mg/d (child 50 mg), and pyridoxine 50 mg IV/IM q6h until intoxication is resolved.

		(0.01 mL/kg every 12h for 4 doses, then 15 mg/kg every 12h until ethylene glycol levels are <20 mg/dL. Fomipazole can be given to patients undergoing hemodialysis (dose q4h).		Monitor for urinary oxalate crystals. Adverse reactions include headache, nausea, and dizziness. Antizole should be diluted in 100 mL 0.9% saline or D_5W and mixed well. Antizole should not be given undiluted.
Glucagon: Stock level to treat 70 kg adult for 24 h: (10 vials, 10 units)	β-Blocker, calcium channel blocker	3–10 mg in adult, then infuse 2–5 mg/h (0.05–0.1 mg/kg in child, then infuse 0.07 mg/kg/h) Large doses up to 100 mg/24h used	IV	Use D_5W, not 0.9% saline, to reconstitute the glucagon (rather than diluent of Eli Lilly, which contains phenol). Vomiting precaustions.
Magnesium sulfate: Stock level to treat 70 kg adult for 24 h: approx 25 g (50 mL of 50% or 200 mL of 12.5%)	Torsades de pointes	*Adult*: 2 g (20 mL or 20%) over 20 min. If no response in 10 min, repeat and follow by continuous infusion 1 g/h. *Children*: 25–50 mg/kg initially and maintenance is (30–60 mg/kg/24h) (0.25–0.5 mEq/kg/24h) up to 1000 mg/24h. (Dose not studied in controlled fashion.)	IV	Use with caution if renal impairment is present.
Methylene blue: Stock level to treat 70 kg adult for 24 h: 5 amps (10 mg/10 mL)	Methemoglobinemia	0.1–0.2 mL/kg of 1% solution, slow infusion, may be repeated every 30–60 min	IV	Nausea, vomiting, headache, dizziness.
Naloxone (Narcan): Stock level to treat 70 kg adult for 24 h: 3 vials (1 mg/mL, 10 mL)	Comatose patient; decreased respirations <12; opioids	In postoperative opioid depression reversal, IV 0.1–0.5 μg/kg every 2 min as needed and may repeat up to a total dose of 1 μg/kg In **suspected overdose**, administer IV 0.1 mg/kg in a child younger than 5 years of age up to 2 mg, in older children and adults administer 2 mg every 2 min up to a total of 10–20 mg. Can also be administered into the endotracheal tube. If no response by 10 mg, a pure opioid intoxication is unlikely. **If opioid abuse** is suspected, **restraints** should be in place before administration; **initial dose** 0.1 mg to avoid with-drawal and violent behavior. The initial dose is then doubled every minute progressively to a total of 10 mg. **A continuous infusion** has been advocated because many opioids outlast the short half-life of naloxone (30–60 min). The **naloxone infusion hourly rate** to produce a response is	IV, ET	**Larger doses** of naloxone may be required for more poorly antagonized synthetic opioid drugs: buprenorphine (Buprenex), codeine, dextromethorphan, fentanyl, pentazocine (Talwin), propoxyphene (Darvon), diphenoxylate, nalbuphine (Nubain), new potent "designer" drugs or long-acting opiolds such as methadone (Dolophine). **Complications**. Although naloxone is safe and effective, there are rare reports of complications (<1%) of pulmonary edema, seizures, hypertension, cardiac arrest, and sudden death. The infusions are titrated to avoid respiratory depression and opioid withdrawal manifestations. Tapering of infusions can be attempted after 12h and when the patient's condition is stable.

Continued

TABLE 5 Initial Doses of Antidotes for Common Poisonings—cont'd

Antidote	Use	Dose	Route	Adverse Reactions/Comments
		equal to the effective dose required (improvement in ventilation and arousal). An additional dose may be required in 15–30 min as a bolus.		
Physostigmine (Antilirium): Stock level to treat 70 kg adult for 24 h: 2–4 mg (2 mL each)	Anticholinergic agents (not routinely used, only indicated if life-threatening complications).	*Child*: 0.02 mg/kg slow push to max 2 mg q30–60 min; *Adult*: 1–2 mg q5 min to max 6 mg.	IV	Bradycardia, asystole, seizures, bronchospasm, vomiting, headaches. Do not use for cyclic antidepressants.
Pralidoxime (2PAM, Protopan): Stock level to treat 70 kg adult for 24 h: 12 vials (1 g per 20 mL)	Organophosphates	Child ≤12 y, 25–50 mg/kg max (4 mg/min); >12 y, 1–2 g/dose in 250 mL of 0.9% saline over 5–10 min. Max 200 mg/min. Repeat q6–12h for 24–48h. Max adult 6 g/d. Alternative: Maintenance infusion 1 g in 100 mL, of 0.9% saline at 5–20 mg/kg/h (0.5–12 mL/kg/h) up to max 500 mg/h or 50 mL/h. Titrate to desired response. End point is absence of fasciculations and return of muscle strength.	IV	Nausea, dizziness, headache; tachycardia. muscle rigidity, bronchospasm (rapid administration).
Pyridoxine (vitamin B_6): Stock level to treat 70 kg adult for 24 h: 100 mg/mL 10% solution. For a 70 kg patient, 10 g = 10 vials	Seizures from isoniazid or *Gyromitra* mushrooms; ethylene glycol	*Isoniazid: Unknown amt ingested*: 5 g (70 mg/kg) in 50 mL D_5W over 5 min + diazepam 0.3 mg/kg IV at rate of 1 mg/min in child or 10 mg dose at rate up to 5 mg/min in adults. Use different site (synergism). May repeat q5–20 min until seizure controlled. Up to 375 mg/kg have been given (52 g). *Known amount*: 1 g for each gram isoniazid ingested over 5 min with diazepam (dose above) *Gyromitra mushroom*: Child 25 mg/kg or 2–5 g, adults IV over 15–30 min to max 20 g. *Ethylene glycol*: 100 mg IV daily.	IV	After seizure is controlled, administer remainder of pyridoxine 1 g/1 g isoniazid total 5 g as infusion over 60 min. Adverse reactions uncommon; do not administer in same bottle as sodium bicarbonate. For *Gyromitra* mushrooms, some use PO 25 mg/kg/d early when mushroom ingestion is suspected.
Sodium bicarbonate ($NaHCO_3$): Stock level to treat 70 kg adult for 24 h: 10 ampules or syringes (500 mEq)	Tricyclic antidepressant cardiotoxicity (QRS >0.12 sec; ventricular tachycardia, severe conduction disturbances); metabolic acidosis; phenothiazine toxicity	1–2 mEq/kg undiluted as a bolus. If no effect on cardiotoxicity, repeat twice a few minutes apart	IV	Monitor sodium, potassium, and blood pH because fatal alkalemia and hyponatremia have been reported.
	Salicylate: to keep blood pH 7.5–7.55 (not >7.55) and urine pH 7.5–8.0. Alkalinization recommended if salicylate conc. >40 mg/dL in acute poisoning and at lower levels if symptomatic in chronic	*Adult* with clear physical signs and laboratory findings of acute moderate or severe salicylism: Bolus 1–2 mEq/kg followed by infusion of 100–150 mEq $NaHCO_3$ added to 1 L of 5%		Monitor both urine and blood pH. Do not use the urine pH alone to assess the need for alkalinization because of the paradoxical aciduria that may occur. Adjust the urine pH to 7.5–8 by $NaHCO_3$ infusion.

	intoxication. 2 mEq/kg will raise blood pH 0.1 unit	dextrose at rate of 200–300 mL/h *Child*: Bolus same as adult followed by 1–2 mEq/kg in infusion of 20 mL/kg/h 5% dextrose in 0.45% saline. Add potassium when patient voids. Rate and amount of the initial infusion, if patient is volume depleted: 1 h to acheive urine output of 2 mL/kg/h and urine pH 7–8. In mild cases without acidosis and urine pH >6 administer 5% dextrose in 0.9% saline with 50 mEq/L or 1 mEq/kg $NaHCO_3$ as maintanence to replace on going renal losses. If acidemia is present and pH <7.2, add 2 mEq/kg as loading dose followed by 2 mEq/kg q3 to 4h to keep pH at 7.5–7.55. If acidemia is present, recommend isotonic $NaHCO_3$, 3 ampules to 1 L of D_5W @ 10–15 mL/kg/h or sufficient to produce normal urine flow and a urine pH of 7.5 or higher.		After urine output established, add potassium 40 mEq/L.
	Long-acting barbiturates: Phenobarbital and primidone (Mysoline) Note: Alkalinization is ineffective for the short- or intermediate-acting barbiturates	$NaHCO_3$: 2 mEq/kg during the first hour or 100 mEq in 1 L of D_5W with 40 mEq/L potassium at rate of 100 mL/h in adults. Adequate potassium is necessary to accomplish alkalinization	IV	Additional sodium bicarbonate and potassium chloride may be needed. Adjust the urine pH to 7.5–8 by $NaHCO_3$ infusion.
Thiamine 100 mg/mL, 2 vials	Thiamine deficiency, ethylene glycol poisoning, alcoholism	100 mg IV followed with 100 mg V/IM for 5–7 days in an alcoholic and followed by 100 mg/d orally.	IV/IM	
Vitamin K_1 (Aqua Mephyton) 10 mg/1–5 mL; 5 mg tablets	Warfarin anticoagulant or rodenticide toxicity	Oral 0.4 mg/kg/dose child, 10–25 mg adults. If evidence of bleeding administer vitamin K_1 SC, IV 0.6 mg/kg/dose child and up to 25–50 mg adults for 6 hours depending on severity.	PO/SC, IV	Give vitamin K daily until PT/INR are normal. Examine stools and urine for evidence of bleeding.

Abbreviations: ALT = alanine aminotransferase; amp = ampule; AST = aspartate aminotransferase; BAL = British anti-Lewisite; BP = blood pressure; Ccnc. = concentration; ECG = electrocardiogram; ET = endotracheal; G6PD = glucose-6-phosphate dehydrogenase; IM = intramuscular; IV = intravenous; PCC = poison control center; PO = oral; PT = Prothrombin time; SC = subcutaneous.

TABLE 6 Plasma Concentrations Above Which Removal by Extracorporeal Measures Should Be Considered

Drug	Plasma Concentration	Protein Binding (%)	Volume Distribution (L/kg)	Method of Choice
Amanitin	NA	25	1.0	HP
Ethanol	500–700 mg/dL	0	0.3	HD
Ethchlorvynol	150 μg/mL	35–50	3–4	HP
Ethylene glycol	25–50 μg/mL	0	0.6	HD
Glutethimide	100 μg/mL	50	2.7	HP
Isopropyl alcohol	400 mg/dL	0	0.7	HD
Lithium	4 mEq/L	0	0.7	HD
Meprobamate (Equanil)	100 μg/mL	0	NA	HP
Methanol	50 mg/dL	0	0.7	HD
Methaqualone	40 μg/dL	20–60	6.0	HP
Other barbiturates	50 μg/dL	50	0-1	HP
Paraquat	0.1 mg/dL	poor	2.8	HP > HD
Phenobarbital	100 μg/dL	50	0.9	HP > HD
Salicylates	80–100 mg/dL	90	0.2	HD > HP
Theophylline		0	0.5	
Chronic	40–60 μg/mL			HP
Acute	80–100 μg /mL			HP
Trichlorethanol	250 μg /mL	70	0.6	HP

Abbreviations: HD = hemodialysis; HP = hemoperfusion; HP > HD hemoperfusion preferred over hemodialysis.

Note: Cartridges for charcoal hemoperfusion are not readily available anymore in most locations, so hemodialysis may be substituted in these situations. In mixed or chronic drug overdoses, extracorporeal measures may be considered at lower drug concentrations.

Data from Winchester JF: Active methods for detoxification. In Haddad LM; Winchester JF (eds). Clinical Management of Poisoning and Drug Overdose, 2nd ed. Philadelphia, WB Saunders, 1990; Balsam L, Cortitsidis GN, Fienfeld DA: Role of hemodialysis and hemoperfusion in the treatment of intoxications. Contemp Manage Crit Care 1:61, 1991.

Complications of dialysis include hemorrhage, thrombosis, air embolism, hypotension, infections, electrolyte imbalance, thrombocytopenia, and removal of therapeutic medications.

HEMOPERFUSION

Hemoperfusion is the parenteral form of oral activated charcoal. Heparinization is necessary. The patient's blood is routed extracorporeally through an outflow arterial catheter through a filter-adsorbing cartridge (charcoal or resin) and returned through a venous catheter. Cartridges must be changed every 4 hours. The blood glucose, electrolytes, calcium, and albumin levels; complete blood cell count; platelets; and serum and urine osmolarity must be carefully monitored. This procedure has extended extracorporeal removal to a large range of substances that were formerly either poorly dialyzable or nondialyzable. It is not limited by molecular weight, water solubility, or protein binding, but it is limited by a volume distribution greater than 400 L, plasma concentration, and rate of flow through the filter. Activated charcoal cartridges are the primary type of hemoperfusion that is currently available in the United States.

The patient-related criteria for hemoperfusion are (a) anticipated prolonged coma and the likelihood of complications; (b) laboratory confirmation of lethal blood concentrations; (c) hepatic impairment when an agent is metabolized by the liver; and (d) clinical deterioration despite optimally supportive medical management.

The contraindications are similar to those for hemodialysis.

Limited data are available as to which toxins are best treated with hemoperfusion. Hemoperfusion has proved useful in treating glutethimide intoxication, phenobarbital overdose, and carbamazepine, phenytoin, and theophylline intoxication.

Complications include hemorrhage, thrombocytopenia, hypotension, infection, leukopenia, depressed phagocytic activity of granulocytes, decreased immunoglobulin levels, hypoglycemia, hypothermia, hypocalcemia, pulmonary edema, and air and charcoal embolism.

HEMOFILTRATION

Continuous arteriovenous or venovenous hemodia filtration (CAVHD or CVVHD, respectively) has been suggested as an alternative to conventional hemodialysis when the need for rapid removal of the drug is less urgent. These procedures, like peritoneal dialysis, are minimally invasive, have no significant impact on hemodynamics, and can be carried out continuously for many hours. Their role in the management of acute poisoning remains uncertain, however.

PLASMAPHERESIS

Plasmapheresis consists of removal of a volume of blood. All the extracted components are returned to the blood except the plasma, which is replaced with a colloid protein solution. There are limited clinical data on guidelines and efficacy in toxicology. Centrifugal and membrane separators of cellular elements are used. It can be as effective as hemodialysis or hemoperfusion for removing toxins that have high protein binding, and it may be useful for toxins not filtered by hemodialysis and hemoperfusion.

Plasmapheresis has been anecdotally used in treating intoxications with the following agents: paraquat (removed 10%), propranolol (removed 30%), quinine (removed 10%), L-thyroxine (removed 30%), and salicylate (removed 10%). It has been shown to remove less than 10% of digoxin, phenobarbital, prednisolone, and tobramycin. Complications include infection; allergic reactions including anaphylaxis; hemorrhagic disorders; thrombocytopenia; embolus and thrombus; hypervolemia and hypovolemia; dysrhythmias; syncope; tetany; paresthesia; pneumothorax; acute respiratory distress syndrome; and seizures.

Supportive Care, Observation, and Therapy for Complications

ALTERED MENTAL STATUS

If airway protective reflexes are absent, endotracheal intubation is indicated for a comatose patient or a patient with altered mental status. If respirations are ineffective, ventilation should be instituted, and if hypoxemia persists, supplemental oxygen is indicated. If a cyanotic patient fails to respond to oxygen, the practitioner should consider methemoglobinemia.

HYPOGLYCEMIA

Hypoglycemia accompanies many poisonings, including with ethanol (especially in children), clonidine (Catapres), insulin, organophosphates, salicylates, sulfonylureas, and the unripe fruit or seed of a Jamaican plant called ackee. If hypoglycemia is present or suspected, glucose should be administered immediately as a intravenous bolus. Doses are as follows: in a neonate, 10% glucose (5 mL/kg); in a child, 25% glucose 0.25 g/kg (2 mL/kg); and in an adults, 50% glucose 0.5 g/kg (1 mL/kg).

A bedside capillary test for blood glucose is performed to detect hypoglycemia, and the sample is sent to the laboratory for confirmation. If the glucose reagent strip visually reads less than 150 mg/dL, one administers glucose. Venous blood should be used rather than capillary blood for the bedside test if the patient is in shock or is hypotensive. Large amounts of glucose given rapidly to nondiabetic patients may cause a transient reactive hypoglycemia and hyperkalemia and may accentuate damage in ischemic cerebrovascular and cardiac tissue. If focal neurologic signs are present, it may be prudent to withhold glucose, because hypoglycemia causes focal signs in less than 10% of cases.

THIAMINE DEFICIENCY ENCEPHALOPATHY

Thiamine is administered to avoid precipitating thiamine deficiency encephalopathy (Wernicke-Korsakoff syndrome) in alcohol abusers and in malnourished patients. The overall incidence of thiamine deficiency in ethanol abusers is 12%. Thiamine 100 mg intravenously should be administered around the time of the glucose administration but not necessarily before the glucose. The clinician should be prepared to manage the anaphylaxis that sometimes is caused by thiamine, although it is extremely rare.

OPIOID REACTIONS

Naloxone (Narcan) reverses CNS and respiratory depression, miosis, bradycardia, and decreased gastrointestinal peristalsis caused by opioids acting through μ, κ, and δ receptors. It also affects endogenous opioid peptides (endorphins and enkephalins), which accounts for the variable responses reported in patients with intoxications from ethanol, benzodiazepines, clonidine (Catapres), captopril (Capoten), and valproic acid (Depakote) and in patients with spinal cord injuries. There is a high sensitivity for predicting a response if pinpoint pupils and circumstantial evidence of opioid abuse (e.g., track marks) are present.

In cases of suspected overdose, naloxone 0.1 mg/kg is administered intravenously initially in a child younger than 5 years of age. The dose can be repeated in 2 minutes, if necessary up to a total dose of 2 mg. In older children and adults, the dose is 2 mg every 2 minutes for five doses up to a total of 10 mg. Naloxone can also be administered into an endotracheal tube if intravenous access is unavailable. If there is no response after 10 mg, a pure opioid intoxication is unlikely. If opioid abuse is suspected, restraints should be in place before the administration of naloxone, and it is recommended that the initial dose be 0.1 to 0.2 mg to avoid withdrawal and violent behavior. The initial dose is then doubled every minute progressively to a total of 10 mg. Naloxone may unmask concomitant sympathomimetic intoxication as well as withdrawal.

Larger doses of naloxone may be required for more poorly antagonized synthetic opioid drugs: buprenorphine (Buprenex), codeine, dextromethorphan, fentanyl and its derivatives, pentazocine (Talwin), propoxyphene (Darvon), diphenoxylate, nalbuphine (Nubain), and long-acting opioids such as methadone (Dolophine).

Indications for a continuous infusion include a second dose for recurrent respiratory depression, exposure to poorly antagonized opioids, a large overdose, and decreased opioid metabolism, as with impaired liver function. A continuous infusion has been advocated because many opioids outlast the short half-life of naloxone (30 to 60 minutes). The hourly rate of naloxone infusion is equal to the effective dose required to produce a response (improvement in ventilation and arousal). An additional dose may be required in 15 to 30 minutes as a bolus. The infusions are titrated to avoid respiratory depression and opioid withdrawal manifestations. Tapering of infusions can be attempted after 12 hours and when the patient's condition has been stabilized.

Although naloxone is safe and effective, there are rare reports of complications (less than 1%) of pulmonary edema, seizures, hypertension, cardiac arrest, and sudden death.

AGENTS WHOSE ROLES ARE NOT CLARIFIED

Nalmefene (Revex), a long-acting parenteral opioid antagonist that the Food and Drug Administration has approved, is undergoing investigation, but its role in the treatment of comatose patients and patients with opioid overdose is not clear. It is 16 times more potent than naloxone, and its duration of action is up to 8 hours (half-life 10.8 hours, versus naloxone 1 hour).

Flumazenil (Romazicon) is a pure competitive benzodiazepine antagonist. It has been demonstrated to be safe and effective for reversing benzodiazepine-induced sedation. It is not recommended to improve ventilation. Its role in cases of CNS depression needs to be clarified. It should not be used routinely in comatose patients and is not an essential ingredient of the coma therapeutic regimen. It is contraindicated in cases of co-ingestion of cyclic antidepressant intoxication, stimulant overdose, and long-term benzodiazepine use (may precipitate life-threatening withdrawal) if benzodiazepines are used to control seizures. There is a concern about the potential for seizures and cardiac dysrhythmias that may occur in these settings.

Laboratory and Radiographic Studies

An electrocardiogram (ECG) should be obtained to identify dysrhythmias or conduction delays from cardiotoxic medications. If aspiration pneumonia (history of loss of consciousness, unarousable state, vomiting) or noncardiac pulmonary edema is suspected, a chest radiograph is needed. Electrolyte and glucose concentrations in the blood, the anion gap, acid–base balance, the arterial blood gas (ABG) profile (if patient has respiratory distress or altered mental status), and serum osmolality should be measured if a toxic alcohol ingestion is suspected. Table 7 lists appropriate testing on the basis of clinical toxicologic presentation. All laboratory specimens should be carefully labeled, including time and date. For potential legal cases, a "chain of custody" must be established. Assessment of the laboratory studies may provide a clue to the etiologic agent.

ELECTROLYTE, ACID-BASE, AND OSMOLALITY DISTURBANCES

Electrolyte and acid–base disturbances should be evaluated and corrected. Metabolic acidosis (usually low or normal pH with a low or normal/high $Pa{CO_2}$ and low HCO_3) with an increased anion gap is seen with many agents in cases of overdose.

TABLE 7 Patient Condition/Systemic Toxin and Appropriate Tests

Condition	Tests
Comatose	Toxicologic tests (acetaminophen, sedative-hypnotic, ethanol, opioids, benzodiazepine), glucose.
Respiratory toxicity	Spirometry, FEV_1, arterial blood gases, chest radiograph, monitor O_2 saturation
Cardiac toxicity	ECG 12-lead and monitoring, echocardiogram, serial cardiac enzymes (if evidence or suspicion of a myocardial infarction), hemodynamic monitoring
Hepatic toxicity	Enzymes (AST, ALT, GGT), ammonia, albumin, bilirubin, glucose, PT, PTT, amylase
Nephrotoxicity	BUN, creatinine, electrolytes (Na, F, Mg, Ca, PO_4), serum and urine osmolarity, 24-hour urine for heavy metals if suspected, creatine kinase, serum and urine myoglobin, urinalysis and urinary sodium
Bleeding	Platelets, PT, PTT, bleeding time, fibrin split products, fibrinogen, type and match

Abbreviations: ALT = alanine aminotransaminase; AST = aspartate aminotransaminase; BUN = blood urea nitrogen; ECG = electrocardiogram; FEV_1 = forced expiratory volume at 1 second; GGT = γ-glutamyltransferase; PT = prothrombin time; PTT = partial thromboplastin time.

The anion gap is an estimate of those anions other than chloride and HCO_3 necessary to counterbalance the positive charge of sodium. It serves as a clue to causes, compensations, and complications. The anion gap (AG) is calculated from the standard serum electrolytes by subtracting the total CO_2 (which reflects the actual measured bicarbonate) and chloride from the sodium: $(Na - [Cl + HXO_3]) = AG$. The potassium is usually not used in the calculation because it may be hemolyzed and is an intracellular cation. The lack of anion gap does not exclude a toxic etiology.

The normal gap is usually 7 to 11 mEq/L by flame photometer. However, there has been a "lowering" of the normal anion gap to 7 ± 4 mEq/L by the newer techniques (e.g., ion selective electrodes or colorimetric titration). Some studies have found anion gaps to be relatively insensitive for determining the presence of toxins.

It is important to recognize anion gap toxins, such as salicylates, methanol, and ethylene glycol, because they have specific antidotes, and hemodialysis is effective in management of cases of overdose with these agents.

Table 8 lists the reasons for increased anion gap, decreased anion gap, or no gap. The most common cause of a decreased anion gap is laboratory error. Lactic acidosis produces the largest anion gap and can result from any poisoning that results in hypoxia, hypoglycemia, or convulsions.

Table 9 lists other blood chemistry derangements that suggest certain intoxications.

TABLE 8 Etiologies of Metabolic Acidosis

Normal Anion Gap Hyperchloremic	Increased Anion Gap Normochloremic	Decreased Anion Gap
Acidifying agents	Methanol	Laboratory error†
Adrenal insufficiency	Uremia*	Intoxication—bromine, lithium
Anhydrase inhibitors	Diabetic ketoacidosis*	Protein abnormal
Fistula	Paraldehyde,* phenformin	Sodium low
Osteotomies	Isoniazid	
Obstructive uropathies	Iron	
Renal tubular acidosis	Lactic acidosis†	
Diarrhea, uncomplicated*	Ethanol,* ethylene glycol*	
Dilutional	Salicylates, starvation solvents	
Sulfamylon		

*Indicates hyperosmolar situation. Studies have found that the anion gap may be relatively insensitive for determining the presence of toxins.
†Lactic acidosis can be produced by intoxications of the following: carbon monoxide, cyanide, hydrogen sulfide, hypoxia, ibuprofen, iron, isoniazid, phenformin, salicylates, seizures, theophylline.

Serum osmolality is a measure of the number of molecules of solute per kilogram of solvent, or mOsm/kg water. The osmolarity is molecules of solute per liter of solution, or mOsm/L water at a specified temperature. Osmolarity is usually the calculated value and osmolality is usually a measured value. They are considered interchangeable where 1 L equals 1 kg. The normal serum osmolality is 280 to 290 mOsm/kg. The freezing point serum osmolarity measurement specimen and the serum electrolytes specimens for calculation should be drawn simultaneously.

The serum osmolal gap is defined as the difference between the measured osmolality determined by the freezing point method and the calculated osmolarity. It is determined by the following formula:

$$(\text{Sodium} \times 2) + (\text{BUN}/3) + (\text{Glucose}/20)$$

(where BUN is blood urea nitrogen).

TABLE 9 Blood Chemistry Derangements in Toxicology

Derangement	Toxin
Acetonemia without acidosis	Acetone or isopropyl alcohol
Hypomagnesemia	Ethanol, digitalis
Hypocalcemia	Ethylene glycol, oxalate, fluoride
Hyperkalemia	β-Blockers, acute digitalis, renal failure
Hypokalemia	Diuretics, salicylism, sympathomimetics, theophylline, corticosteroids, chronic digitalis
Hyperglycemia	Diazoxide, glucagon, iron, isoniazid, organophosphate insecticides, phenylurea insecticides, phenytoin (Dilantin), salicylates, sympathomimetic agents, thyroid, vasopressors
Hypoglycemia	β-Blockers, ethanol, insulin, isoniazid, oral hypoglycemic agents, salicylates
Rhabdomyolysis	Amphetamines, ethanol, cocaine, or phencyclidine, elevated creatine phosphokinase

This gap estimate is normally within 10 mOsm of the simultaneously measured serum osmolality. Ethanol, if present, may be included in the equation to eliminate its influence on the osmolal gap (the ethanol concentration divided by 4.6; Table 10).

The osmolal gap is not valid in cases of shock and postmortem state. Metabolic disorders such as hyperglycemia, uremia, and dehydration increase the osmolarity but usually do not cause gaps greater than 10 mOsm/kg. A gap greater than 10 mOsm/mL suggests that unidentified osmolal-acting substances are present: acetone, ethanol, ethylene glycol, glycerin, isopropyl alcohol, isoniazid, ethanol, mannitol, methanol, and trichloroethane. Alcohols and glycols should be sought when the degree of obtundation exceeds that expected from the blood ethanol concentration or when other clinical conditions exist: visual loss (methanol), metabolic acidosis (methanol and ethylene glycol), or renal failure (ethylene glycol).

A falsely elevated osmolal gap can be produced by other low molecular weight un-ionized substances (dextran, diuretics, sorbitol, ketones), hyperlipidemia, and unmeasured electrolytes (e.g., magnesium).

Note: A normal osmolal gap may be reported in the presence of toxic alcohol or glycol poisoning, if the parent compound is already metabolized. This situation can occur when the osmolal gap is measured after a significant time has elapsed since the ingestion. In cases of alcohol and glycol intoxication, an early osmolar gap is a result of the relatively nontoxic parent drug and delayed metabolic acidosis, and an anion gap is a result of the more toxic metabolites.

The serum concentration is calculated as mg/dL = mOsm gap × MW of substance divided by 10.

RADIOGRAPHIC STUDIES

Chest and neck radiographs are useful for suspected pathologic conditions such as aspiration pneumonia, pulmonary edema, and foreign bodies and to determine the location of the endotracheal

TABLE 10 Conversion Factors for Alcohols and Glycols

Alcohols/Glycols	1 mg/dL in Blood Raises Osmolality mOsm/L	Molecular Weight	Conversion Factor
Ethanol	0.228	40	4.6
Methanol	0.327	32	3.2
Ethylene glycol	0.190	62	6.2
Isopropanol	0.176	60	6.0
Acetone	0.182	58	5.8
Propylene glycol	not available	72	7.2

Example: Methanol osmolality. Subtract the calculated osmolality from the measured serum osmolarity (freezing point method) = osmolar gap × 3.2 (one-tenth molecular weight) = estimated serum methanol concentration.
Note: This equation is often not considered very reliable in predicting the actual measured blood concentration of these alcohols or glycols.

tube. Abdominal radiographs can be used to detect radiopaque substances.

The mnemonic for radiopaque substances seen on abdominal radiographs is CHIPES:

C—chlorides and chloral hydrate
H—heavy metals (arsenic, barium, iron, lead, mercury, zinc)
I—iodides
P—PlayDoh, Pepto-Bismol, phenothiazine (inconsistent)
E—enteric-coated tablets
S—sodium, potassium, and other elements in tablet form (bismuth, calcium, potassium) and solvents containing chlorides (e.g., carbon tetrachloride)

TOXICOLOGIC STUDIES

Routine blood and urine screening is of little practical value in the initial care of the poisoned patient. Specific toxicologic analyses and quantitative levels of certain drugs may be extremely helpful. One should always ask oneself the following questions: (a) How will the result of the test alter the management? and (b) Can the result of the test be returned in time to have a positive effect on therapy?

Owing to long turnaround time, lack of availability, factors contributing to unreliability, and the risk of serious morbidity without supportive clinical management, toxicology screening is estimated to affect management in less than 15% of cases of drug overdoses or poisonings. Toxicology screening may look specifically for only 40 to 50 drugs out of more than 10,000 possible drugs or toxins and more than several million chemicals. To detect many different drugs, toxic screens usually include methods with broad specificity, and sensitivity may be poor for some drugs, resulting in false-negative or false-positive findings. On the other hand, some drugs present in therapeutic amounts may be detected on the screen, even though they are causing no clinical symptoms. Because many agents are not sought or detected during a toxicologic screening, a negative result does not always rule out poisonings. The specificity of toxicologic tests is dependent on the method and the laboratory. The presence of other drugs, drug metabolites, disease states, or incorrect sampling may cause erroneous results.

For the average toxicologic laboratory, false-negative results occur at a rate of 10% to 30% and false-positives at a rate of 0% to 10%. The positive screen predictive value is approximately 90%. A negative toxicology screen does not exclude a poisoning. The negative predictive value of toxicologic screening is approximately 70%. For example, the following benzodiazepines may not be detected by some routine immunoassay benzodiazepine screening tests: alprazolam (Xanax), clonazepam (Klonopin), temazepam (Restoril), and triazolam (Halcion).

The "toxic urine screen" is generally a qualitative urine test for several common drugs, usually substances of abuse (cocaine and metabolites, opioids, amphetamines, benzodiazepines, barbiturates, and phencyclidine). Results of these tests are usually available within 2 to 6 hours. Because these tests may vary with each hospital and community, the physician should determine exactly which substances are included in the toxic urine screen of his or her laboratory. Tests for ethylene glycol, red blood cell cholinesterase, and serum cyanide are not readily available.

For cases of ingestion of certain substances, quantitative blood levels should be obtained at specific times after the ingestion to avoid spurious low values in the distribution phase, which result from incomplete absorption. The detection time for drugs is influenced by many variables, such as type of substance, formulation, amount, time since ingestion, duration of exposure, and half-life. For many drugs, the detection time is measured in days after the exposure.

Common Poisons

ACETAMINOPHEN (PARACETAMOL, *N*-ACETYL-PARAAMINOPHENOL)

Toxic Mechanism

At therapeutic doses of acetaminophen, less than 5% is metabolized by P450-2E1 to a toxic reactive oxidizing metabolite, *N*-acetyl-p-benzoquinoneimine

(NAPQI). In a case of overdose, there is insufficient glutathione available to reduce the excess NAPQI into nontoxic conjugate, so it forms covalent bonds with hepatic intracellular proteins to produce centrilobular necrosis. Renal damage is caused by a similar mechanism.

Toxic Dose

The therapeutic dose of acetaminophen is 10 to 15 mg/kg, with a maximum of five doses in 24 hours for a maximum total daily dose of 4 g. An acute single toxic dose is greater than 140 mg/kg, possibly greater than 200 mg/kg in a child younger than age 5 years. Factors affecting the P450 enzymes include enzyme inducers such as barbiturates and phenytoin (Dilantin), ingestion of isoniazid, and alcoholism. Factors that decrease glutathione stores (alcoholism, malnutrition, and HIV infection) contribute to the toxicity of acetaminophen. Alcoholics ingesting 3 to 4 g/d of acetaminophen for a few days can have depleted glutathione stores and require *N*-acetylcysteine therapy at 50% below hepatotoxic blood acetaminophen levels on the nomogram.

Kinetics

Peak plasma concentration is usually reached 2 to 4 hours after an overdose. Volume distribution is 0.9 L/kg, and protein binding is less than 50% (albumin).

Route of elimination is by hepatic metabolism to an inactive nontoxic glucuronide conjugate and inactive nontoxic sulfate metabolite by two saturable pathways; less than 5% is metabolized into reactive metabolite NAPQI. In patients younger than 6 years of age, metabolic elimination occurs to a greater degree by conjugation via the sulfate pathway.

The half-life of acetaminophen is 1 to 3 hours.

Manifestations

The four phases of the intoxication's clinical course may overlap, and the absence of a phase does not exclude toxicity.

- Phase I occurs within 0.5 to 24 hours after ingestion and may consist of a few hours of malaise, diaphoresis, nausea, and vomiting or produce no symptoms. CNS depression or coma is not a feature.
- Phase II occurs 24 to 48 hours after ingestion and is a period of diminished symptoms. The liver enzymes, serum aspartate aminotransferase (AST) (earliest), and serum alanine aminotransferase (ALT) may increase as early as 4 hours or as late as 36 hours after ingestion.
- Phase III occurs at 48 to 96 hours, with peak liver function abnormalities at 72 to 96 hours. The degree of elevation of the hepatic enzymes generally correlates with outcome, but not always. Recovery starts at about 4 days unless hepatic failure develops. Less than 1% of patients with a history of overdose develop fulminant hepatotoxicity.
- Phase IV occurs at 4 to 14 days, with hepatic enzyme abnormalities resolving. If extensive liver damage has occurred, sepsis and disseminated intravascular coagulation may ensue.

Transient renal failure may develop at 5 to 7 days with or without evidence of hepatic damage. Rare cases of myocarditis and pancreatitis have been reported. Death can occur at 7 to 14 days.

Laboratory Investigations

The therapeutic reference range is 10 to 20 μg/mL. For toxic levels, see the nomogram presented in Figure 1.

Appropriate and reliable methods for analysis are radioimmunoassay, high-pressure liquid chromatography, and gas chromatography. Spectroscopic assays often give falsely elevated values: bilirubin, salicylate, salicylamide, diflunisal (Dolobid), phenols, and methyldopa (Aldomet) increase the acetaminophen level. Each 1 mg/dL increase in creatinine increases the acetaminophen plasma level 30 μg/mL.

If a toxic acetaminophen level is reached, liver profile (including AST, ALT, bilirubin, and prothrombin time), serum amylase, and blood glucose must be monitored. A complete blood cell count (CBC); platelet count; phosphate, electrolytes, and bicarbonate level measurements; ECG; and urinalysis are indicated.

Management

Gastrointestinal Decontamination

Although ipecac-induced emesis may be useful within 30 minutes of ingestion of the toxic substance, we do not advise it because it could result in vomiting of the activated charcoal. Gastric lavage is not necessary. Studies have indicated that activated charcoal is useful within 1 hour after ingestion. Activated charcoal does adsorb N-acetylcysteine (NAC) if given together, but this is not clinically important. However, if activated charcoal needs to be given along with NAC, separate the administration of activated charcoal from the administration of NAC by 1 to 2 hours to avoid vomiting.

N-Acetylcysteine (Mucomyst)

NAC (Table 11), a derivative of the amino acid cysteine, acts as a sulfhydryl donor for glutathione synthesis, as surrogate glutathione, and may increase the nontoxic sulfation pathway resulting in conjugation of NAPQI. Oral NAC should be administered within the first 8 hours after a toxic amount of acetaminophen has been ingested. NAC can be started while one awaits the results of the blood test for acetaminophen plasma concentration, but there is no advantage to giving it before 8 hours. If the acetaminophen concentration result after 4 hours following

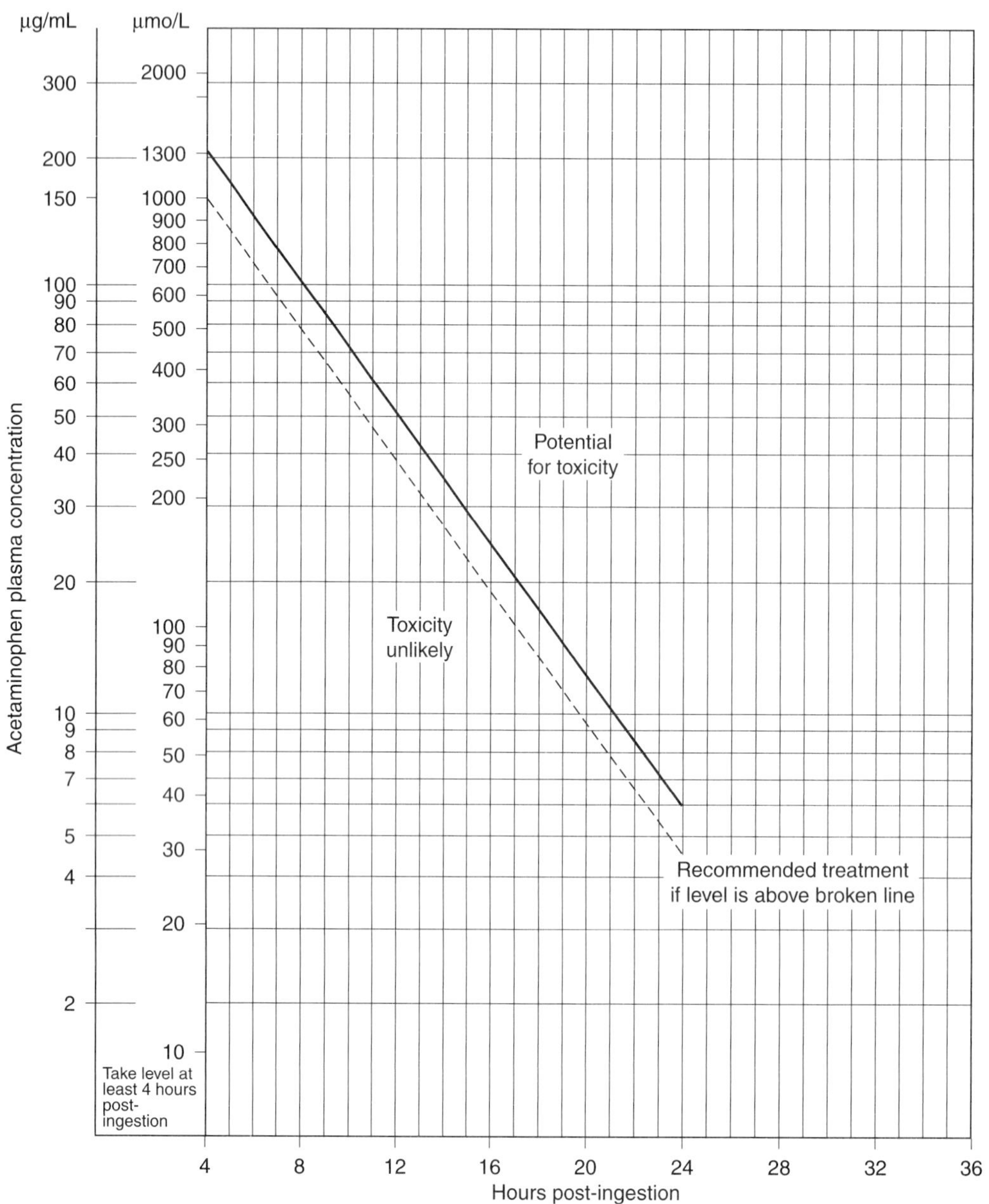

FIGURE 1 Nomogram for acetaminophen intoxication. *N*-acetylcysteine therapy is started if levels and time coordinates are above the lower line on the nomogram. Continue and complete therapy even if subsequent values fall below the toxic zone. The nomogram is useful only in cases of acute single ingestion. Levels in serum drawn before 4 hours may not represent peak levels. (From Rumack BH, Matthew H: Acetaminophen poisoning and toxicity. Pediatrics 55:871, 1975.)

TABLE 11 Protocol for *N*-Acetylcysteine Administration

Route	Loading Dose	Maintenance Dose	Course	FDA Approval
Oral	140 mg/kg	70 mg/kg every 4 h	72 h	Yes
Intravenous	150 mg/kg over 15 min	50 mg/kg over 4 h followed by 100 mg/kg over 16h	20 h	Yes

ingestion is above the upper line on the modified Rumack-Matthew nomogram (see Figure 1), one should continue with a maintenance course. Repeat blood specimens should be obtained 4 hours after the initial level is measured if it is greater than 20 mg/mL, which is below the therapy line, because of unexpected delays in the peak by food and co-ingestants. Intravenous NAC (see Table 11) is approved in the United States.

There have been a few cases of anaphylactoid reaction and death by the intravenous route.

Variations in Therapy

In patients with chronic alcoholism, it is recommended that NAC treatment be administered at 50% below the upper toxic line on the nomogram.

If emesis occurs within 1 hour after NAC administration, the dose should be repeated. To avoid emesis, the proper dilution from 20% to 5% NAC must be used, and it should be served in a palatable vehicle, in a covered container through a straw. If this administration is unsuccessful, a slow drip over 30 to 60 minutes through a nasogastric tube or a fluoroscopically placed nasoduodenal tube can be used. Antiemetics can be used if necessary: metoclopramide (Reglan) 10 mg per dose intravenously 30 minutes before administration of NAC (in children, 0.1 mg/kg; maximum, 0.5 mg/kg/d) or ondansetron (Zofran) 32 mg (0.15 mg/kg) by infusion over 15 minutes and repeated for three doses if necessary. The side effects of these antiemetics include anaphylaxis and increases in liver enzymes.

Some investigators recommend variable durations of NAC therapy, stopping the therapy if serial acetaminophen blood concentrations become nondetectable and the liver enzyme levels (ALT and AST) remain normal after 24 to 36 hours.

There is a loss of efficacy if NAC is initiated 8 or 10 hours postingestion, but the loss is not complete, and NAC may be initiated 36 hours or more after ingestion. Late treatment (after 24 hours) decreases the rates of morbidity and mortality in patients with fulminant liver failure caused by acetaminophen and other agents.

Extended relief formulations (*ER* embossed on caplet) contain 325 mg of acetaminophen for immediate release and 325 mg for delayed release. A single 4-hour postingestion serum acetaminophen concentration can underestimate the level because ER formulations can have secondary delayed peaks. In cases of overdose of the ER formulation, it is recommended that additional acetaminophen levels be obtained at 4-hour intervals after the initial level is measured. If any level is in the toxic zone, therapy should be initiated.

It is recommended that pregnant patients with toxic plasma concentrations of acetaminophen be treated with NAC to prevent hepatotoxicity in both fetus and mother. The available data suggest no teratogenicity to NAC or acetaminophen.

Indications for NAC therapy in cases of chronic intoxication are a history of ingestion of 3 to 4 g for several days with elevated liver enzyme levels (AST and ALT). The acetaminophen blood concentration is often low in these cases because of the extended time lapse since ingestion and should not be plotted on the Rumack-Matthew nomogram. Patients with a history of chronic alcoholism or those on chronic enzyme inducers may also present with elevated liver enzyme levels and should be considered for NAC therapy if they have a history of taking acetaminophen on a chronic basis, because they are considered to be at a greater risk for hepatotoxicity despite a low acetaminophen blood concentration.

Specific support care may be needed to treat liver failure, pancreatitis, transient renal failure, and myocarditis.

Liver transplantation has a definite but limited role in patients with acute acetaminophen overdose. A retrospective analysis determined that a continuing rise in the prothrombin time (4-day peak, 180 seconds), a pH of less than 7.3 2 days after the overdose, a serum creatinine level of greater than 3.3 mg/dL, severe hepatic encephalopathy, and disturbed coagulation factor VII/V ratio greater than 30 suggest a poor prognosis and may be indicators for hepatology consultation for consideration of liver transplantation.

Extracorporeal measures are not expected to be of benefit.

Disposition

Adults who have ingested more than 140 mg/kg and children younger than 6 years of age who have ingested more than 200 mg/kg should receive therapy within 8 hours postingestion or until the results of the 4-hour postingestion acetaminophen plasma concentration is known.

AMPHETAMINES

The amphetamines include illicit methamphetamine ("Ice"), diet pills, and formulations under various trade names. Analogues include MDMA (3,4 methylenedioxymethamphetamine, known as "ecstasy," "XTC," "Adam") and MDA (3,4-methylenedioxyamphetamine, known as "Eve"). MDA is a common hallucinogen and euphoriant "club drug" used at "raves," which are all-night dances. Use of methamphetamine and designer analogues is on the rise, especially among young people between the ages of 12 and 25 years. Other similar stimulants are phenylpropanolamine and cocaine.

Toxic Mechanism

Amphetamines have a direct CNS stimulant effect and a sympathetic nervous system effect by releasing catecholamines from α- and β-adrenergic nerve terminals but inhibiting their reuptake.

Hallucinogenic MDMA has an additional hazard of serotonin effect (refer to serotonin syndrome in the SSRI section). MDMA also affects the dopamine system in the brain. Because of its effects on 5-hydroxytryptamine, dopamine, and norepinephrine, MDMA can lead to serotonin syndrome associated with malignant hyperthermia and rhabdomyolysis, which contributes to the potentially life-threatening hyperthermia observed in several patients who have used MDMA.

Phenylpropanolamine stimulates only the β-drenergic receptors.

Toxic Dose

In children, the toxic dose of dextroamphetamine is 1 mg/kg; In adults, the toxic dose is 5 mg/kg. The potentially fatal dose of dextroamphetamine is 12 mg/kg.

Kinetics

Amphetamine is a weak base with pKa of 8 to 10. Onset of action is 30 to 60 minutes, and peak effects are 2 to 4 hours. The volume distribution is 2 to 3 L/kg.

Through hepatic metabolism, 60% of the substance is metabolized into a hydroxylated metabolite that may be responsible for psychotic effects.

The half-life of amphetamines is pH dependent—8 to 10 hours in acid urine (pH <6.0) and 16 to 31 hours in alkaline urine (pH >7.5). Excretion is by the kidney—30% to 40% at alkaline urine pH and 50% to 70% at acid urine pH.

Manifestations

Effects are seen within 30 to 60 minutes following ingestion.

Neurologic manifestations include restlessness, irritation and agitation, tremors and hyperreflexia, and auditory and visual hallucinations. Hyperpyrexia may precede seizures, convulsions, paranoia, violence, intracranial hemorrhage, psychosis, and self-destructive behavior. Paranoid psychosis and cerebral vasculitis occur with chronic abuse.

MDMA is often adulterated with cocaine, heroin, or ketamine, or a combination of these, to create a variety of mood alterations. This possibility must be taken into consideration when one manages patients with MDMA ingestions, as the symptom complex may reflect both CNS stimulation and CNS depression.

Other manifestations include dilated but reactive pupils, cardiac dysrhythmias (supraventricular and ventricular), tachycardia, hypertension, rhabdomyolysis, and myoglobinuria.

Laboratory Investigations

The clinician should monitor ECG and cardiac readings, ABG and oxygen saturation, electrolytes, blood glucose, BUN, creatinine, creatine kinase, cardiac fraction if there is chest pain, and liver profile. Also, one should evaluate for rhabdomyolysis and check urine for myoglobin, cocaine and metabolites, and other substances of abuse. The peak plasma concentration of amphetamines is 10 to 50 ng/mL 1 to 2 hours after ingestion of 10 to 25 mg. The toxic plasma concentration is 200 ng/mL. When the rapid immunoassays are used, cross-reactions can occur with amphetamine derivatives (e.g., MDA, "ecstasy"), brompheniramine (Dimetane), chlorpromazine (Thorazine), ephedrine, phenylpropanolamine, phentermine (Adipex-P), phenmetrazine, ranitidine (Zantac), and Vicks Inhaler (L-desoxyephedrine). False-positive results may occur.

Management

Management is similar to management for cocaine intoxication. Supportive care includes blood pressure and temperature control, cardiac monitoring, and seizure precautions. Diazepam (Valium) can be administered. Gastrointestinal decontamination can be undertaken with activated charcoal administered up to 1 hour after ingestion.

Anxiety, agitation, and convulsions are treated with diazepam. If diazepam fails to control seizures, neuromuscular blockers can be used and the electroencephalogram (EEG) monitored for nonmotor seizures. One should avoid neuroleptic phenothiazines and butyrophenone, which can lower the seizure threshold.

Hypertension and tachycardia are usually transient and can be managed by titration of diazepam. Nitroprusside can be used for hypertensive crisis at a maximum infusion rate of 10 μg/kg/minute for 10 minutes followed with a lower infusion rate of 0.3 to 2 mg/kg/minute. Myocardial ischemia is managed by oxygen, vascular access, benzodiazepines, and nitroglycerin. Aspirin and thrombolytics are not routinely recommended because of the danger of intracranial hemorrhage. It is important to distinguish between angina and true ischemia. Delayed hypotension can be treated with fluids and vasopressors if needed. Life-threatening tachydysrhythmias may respond to an α-blocker such as phentolamine (Regitine) 5 mg IV for adults or 0.1 mg/kg IV for children and a short-acting β-blocker such as esmolol (Brevibloc) 500 μg/kg IV over 1 minute for adults, or 300 to 500 μg/kg over 1 minute for children. Ventricular dysrhythmias may respond to lidocaine or, in a severely hemodynamically compromised patient, immediate synchronized electrical cardioversion.

Rhabdomyolysis and myoglobinuria are treated with fluids, alkaline diuresis, and diuretics. Hyperthermia is treated with external cooling and cool 100% humidified oxygen. More extensive therapy may be needed in severe cases. If focal neurologic symptoms are present, the possibility of a cerebrovascular accident should be considered and a CT scan of the head should be obtained.

Paranoid ideation and threatening behavior should be treated with rapid tranquilization using a benzodiazepine. One should observe for suicidal depression that may follow intoxication and may require suicide precautions.

Extracorporeal measures are of no benefit.

Disposition

Symptomatic patients should be observed on a monitored unit until the symptoms resolve and then observed for a short time after resolution for relapse.

ANTICHOLINERGIC AGENTS

Drugs with anticholinergic properties include antihistamines (H_1 blockers), neuroleptics (phenothiazines), tricyclic antidepressants, antiparkinsonism drugs (trihexyphenidyl [Artane], benztropine [Cogentin]), ophthalmic products (atropine), and a number of common plants.

The antihistamines are divided into the sedating anticholinergic types, and the nonsedating single daily dose types. The sedating types include ethanolamines (e.g., diphenhydramine [Benadryl], dimenhydrinate [Dramamine], and clemastine [Tavist]), ethylenediamines (e.g., tripelennamine [Pyribenzamine]), alkyl amines (e.g., chlorpheniramine [Chlor-Trimeton], brompheniramine [Dimetane]), piperazines (e.g., cyclizine [Marezine], hydroxyzine [Atarax], and meclizine [Antivert]), and phenothiazine (e.g., Phenergan). The nonsedating types include astemizole (Hismanal), terfenadine (Seldane), loratadine (Claritin), fexofenadine (Allegra), and cetirizine (Zyrtec).

The anticholinergic plants include jimsonweed (*Datura stramonium*), deadly nightshade (*Atropa belladonna*), henbane (*Hyoscyamus niger*), and antispasmodic agents for the bowel (atropine derivatives).

Toxic Mechanism

By competitive inhibition, anticholinergics block the action of acetylcholine on postsynaptic cholinergic receptor sites. The toxic mechanism primarily involves the peripheral and CNS muscarinic receptors. H_1 sedating-type agents also depress or stimulate the CNS, and in large overdoses some have cardiac membrane–depressant effects (e.g., diphenhydramine [Benadryl]) and α-adrenergic receptor blockade effects (e.g., promethazine [Phenergan]). Nonsedating agents produce peripheral H_1 blockade but do not possess anticholinergic or sedating actions. The original agents terfenadine (Seldane) and astemizole (Hismanal) were recently removed from the market because of the severe cardiac dysrhythmias associated with their use, especially when used in combination with macrolide antibiotics and certain antifungal agents such as ketoconazole (Nizoral), which inhibit hepatic metabolism or excretion. The newer nonsedating agents, including loratadine (Claritin), fexofenadine (Allegra), and cetirizine (Zyrtec), have not been reported to cause the severe drug interactions associated with terfenadine and astemizole.

Toxic Dose

The estimated toxic oral dose of atropine is 0.05 mg/kg in children and more than 2 mg in adults. The minimal estimated lethal dose of atropine is more than 10 mg in adults and more than 2 mg in children. Other synthetic anticholinergic agents are less toxic, and the fatal dose varies from 10 to 100 mg.

The estimated toxic oral dose of diphenhydramine (Benadryl) in a child is 15 mg/kg, and the potential lethal amount is 25 mg/kg. In an adult, the potential lethal amount is 2.8 g. Ingestion of five times the single dose of an antihistamine is toxic.

For the nonsedating agents, an overdose of 3360 mg of terfenadine was reported in an adult who developed ventricular tachycardia and fibrillation that responded to lidocaine and defibrillation. A 1500-mg overdose produced hypotension. Cases of delayed serious dysrhythmias (torsades de pointes) have been reported with doses of more than 200 mg of astemizole. The toxic doses of fexofenadine (Allegra), cetirizine, and loratadine (Claritin) need to be established.

Kinetics

The onset of absorption of intravenous atropine is in 2 to 4 minutes. Peak effects on salivation after intravenous or intramuscular administration is at 30 to 60 minutes.

Onset of absorption after oral ingestion is 30 to 60 minutes, peak action is 1 to 3 hours, and duration of action is 4 to 6 hours, but symptoms are prolonged in cases of overdose or with sustained-release preparations.

The onset of absorption of diphenhydramine is in 15 minutes to 1 hour, with a peak of action in 1 to 4 hours. Volume distribution is 3.3 to 6.8 L/kg, and protein binding is 75% to 80%. Ninety-eight percent of diphenhydramine is metabolized via the liver by *N*-demethylation. Interactions with erythromycin, ketoconazole (Nizoral), and derivatives produce excessive blood levels of the antihistamine and ventricular dysrhythmias.

The half-life of diphenhydramine is 3 to 10 hours.

The chemical structure of nonsedating agents prevents their entry into the CNS. Absorption begins in 1 hour, with peak effects in 4 in 6 hours. The duration of action is greater than 24 hours.

These agents are metabolized in the gastrointestinal tract and liver. Protein binding is greater than 90%. The plasma half-life 3.5 hours. Only 1% is excreted unchanged; 60% of that is excreted in the feces and 40% in the urine.

Manifestations

Anticholinergic signs are hyperpyrexia ("hot as a hare"), mydriasis ("blind as a bat"), flushing of skin ("red as a beet"), dry mucosa and skin ("dry as a bone"), "Lilliputian type" hallucinations and delirium ("mad as a hatter"), coma, dysphagia, tachycardia, moderate hypertension, and rarely convulsions and urinary retention. Other effects include jaundice (cyproheptadine [Periactin]), dystonia (diphenhydramine [Benadryl]), rhabdomyolysis (doxylamine), and, in large doses, cardiotoxic effects (diphenhydramine).

Overdose with nonsedating agents produces headache and confusion, nausea, and dysrhythmias (e.g., torsades de pointes).

Laboratory Investigations

Monitoring of ABG (in cases of respiratory depression), electrolytes, glucose, and the ECG should be undertaken. Anticholinergic drugs and plants are not routinely included on screens for substances of abuse.

Management

For patients in respiratory failure, intubation and assisted ventilation should be instituted. Gastrointestinal decontamination can be instituted. Caution must be taken with emesis in cases of diphenhydramine (Benadryl) overdose because of the drug's rapid onset of action and risk of seizures. If bowel sounds are present for up to 1 hour after ingestion, activated charcoal can be given. Seizures can be controlled with benzodiazepines (diazepam [Valium] or lorazepam [Ativan]).

The administration of physostigmine (Antilirium) is not routine and is reserved for life-threatening anticholinergic effects that are refractory to conventional treatments. It should be administered with adequate monitoring and resuscitative equipment available. The use of physostigmine should be avoided if a tricyclic antidepressant is present because of increased toxicity. Urinary retention should be relieved by catheterization to avoid reabsorption of the drug and additional toxicity.

Supraventricular tachycardia should be treated only if the patient is hemodynamically unstable. Ventricular dysrhythmias can be controlled with lidocaine or cardioversion. Sodium bicarbonate 1 to 2 mEq/kg IV may be useful for myocardial depression and QRS prolongation. Torsades de pointes, especially when associated with terfenadine and astemizole ingestion, has been treated with magnesium sulfate 4 g or 40 mL 10% solution intravenously over 10 to 20 minutes and countershock if the patient fails to respond.

Hyperpyrexia is controlled by external cooling. Hemodialysis and hemoperfusion are not effective.

Disposition

Antihistamine H_1 Antagonists

Symptomatic patients should be observed on a monitored unit until the symptoms resolve, then observed for a short time (3 to 4 hours) after resolution for relapse.

Nonsedating Agents

All asymptomatic children who acutely ingest more than the maximum adult dose and all symptomatic children should be referred to a health care facility for a minimum of 6 hours' observation as well as cardiac monitoring. Asymptomatic adults who acutely ingest more than twice the maximum adult daily dose should be monitored for a minimum of 6 hours. All symptomatic patients should be monitored for as long as there are symptoms present.

BARBITURATES

Barbiturates have been used as sedatives, anesthetic agents, and anticonvulsants, but their use is declining as safer, more effective drugs become available.

Toxic Mechanism

Barbiturates are γ-amino butyric acid (GABA) agonists (increasing the chloride flow and inhibiting depolarization). They enhance the CNS depressant effect of GABA and depress the cardiovascular system.

Toxic Dose

The shorter-acting barbiturates (including the intermediate-acting agents) and their hypnotic doses are as follows: amobarbital (Amytal), 100 to 200 mg; aprobarbital (Alurate), 50 to 100 mg; butabarbital (Butisol), 50 to 100 mg; butalbital, 100 to 200 mg; pentobarbital (Nembutal), 100 to 200 mg; secobarbital (Seconal), 100 to 200 mg. They cause toxicity at lower doses than long-acting barbiturates and have a minimum toxic dose of 6 mg/kg; the fatal adult dose is 3 to 6 g.

The long-acting barbiturates and their doses include mephobarbital (Mebaral), 50 to 100 mg, and phenobarbital, 100 to 200 mg. Their minimum toxic dose is greater than 10 mg/kg, and the fatal adult dose is 6 to 10 g. A general rule is that an amount five times the hypnotic dose is toxic and an amount 10 times the hypnotic dose is potentially fatal. Methohexital and thiopental are ultrashort-acting parenteral preparations and are not discussed.

Kinetics

The barbiturates are enzyme inducers. Short-acting barbiturates are highly lipid-soluble, penetrate the brain readily, and have shorter elimination times. Onset of action is in 10 to 30 minutes, with a peak at 1 to 2 hours. Duration of action is 3 to 8 hours. The volume distribution of short-acting barbiturate is 0.8 to 1.5 L/kg; pKa is about 8. Mean half-life varies from 8 to 48 hours.

Long-acting agents have longer elimination times and can be used as anticonvulsants. Onset of action is in 20 to 60 minutes, with a peak at 1 to 6 hours. In cases of overdose, the peak can be at 10 hours. Usual duration of action is 8 to 12 hours. Volume distribution is 0.8 L/kg, and half-life is 11 to 120 hours. The pKa of phenobarbital is 7.2. Alkalinization of urine promotes its excretion.

Manifestations

Mild intoxication resembles alcohol intoxication and includes ataxia, slurred speech, and depressed cognition. Severe intoxication causes slow respirations, coma, and loss of reflexes (except pupillary light reflex).

Other manifestations include hypotension (vasodilation), hypothermia, hypoglycemia, and death by respiratory arrest.

Laboratory Investigations

Most barbiturates are detected on routine drug screens and can be measured in most hospital laboratories. Investigation should include barbiturate level; ABG; toxicology screen, including acetaminophen; glucose, electrolyte, BUN, creatinine, and creatine kinase levels; and urine pH. The minimum toxic plasma levels are greater than 10 μg/mL for short-acting barbiturates and greater than 40 μg/dL for long-acting agents. Fatal levels are 30 μg/mL for short-acting barbiturates and 80 to 150 μg/mL for long-acting agents. Both short-acting and long-acting agents can be detected in urine 24 to 72 hours after ingestion, and long-acting agents can be detected up to 7 days.

Management

Vital functions must be established and maintained. Intensive supportive care including intubation and assisted ventilation should dominate the management. All stuporous and comatose patients should have glucose (for hypoglycemia), thiamine (if chronically alcoholic), and naloxone (Narcan) (in case of an opioid ingestion) intravenously and should be admitted to the intensive care unit. Emesis should be avoided especially in cases of ingestion of the shorter-acting barbiturates. Activated charcoal followed by MDAC (0.5 g/kg) every 2 to 4 hours has been shown to reduce the serum half-life of phenobarbital by 50%, but its effect on clinical course is undetermined.

Fluids should be administered to correct dehydration and hypotension. Vasopressors may be necessary to correct severe hypotension, and hemodynamic monitoring may be needed. The patient must be observed carefully for fluid overload. Alkalinization (ion trapping) is used only for phenobarbital (pKa 7.2) but not for short-acting barbiturates. Sodium bicarbonate, 1 to 2 mEq/kg IV in 500 mL of 5% dextrose in adults or 10 to 15 mL/kg in children during the first hour, followed by sufficient bicarbonate to keep the urinary pH at 7.5 to 8.0, enhances excretion of phenobarbital and shortens the half-life by 50%. Diuresis is not advocated because of the danger of cerebral or pulmonary edema.

Hemodialysis shortens the half-life to 8 to 14 hours, and charcoal hemoperfusion shortens the half-life to 6 to 8 hours for long-acting barbiturates such as phenobarbital. Both procedures may be effective in patients with both long-acting and short-acting barbiturate ingestion. If the patient does not respond to supportive measures or if the phenobarbital plasma concentration is greater than 150 μg/mL, both procedures may be tried to shorten the half-life.

Bullae are treated as a local second-degree skin burn. Hypothermia should be treated.

Disposition

All comatose patients should be admitted to the intensive care unit. Awake and oriented patients with an overdose of short-acting agents should be observed for at least 6 asymptomatic hours; overdose of long-acting agents warrants observation for at least 12 asymptomatic hours because of the potential for delayed absorption. In the case of an intentional overdose, psychiatric clearance is needed before the patient can be discharged. Chronic use can lead to tolerance, physical dependency, and withdrawal and necessitates follow-up.

BENZODIAZEPINES

Benzodiazepines are used as anxiolytics, sedatives, and relaxants.

Toxic Mechanism

The GABA agonists produce CNS depression and increase chloride flow, inhibiting depolarization.

Flunitrazepam (Rohypnol; street name “roofies”) is a long-acting benzodiazepine agonist sold by prescription in more than 60 countries worldwide, but it is not legally available in the United States.

Toxic Dose

The long-acting benzodiazepines (half-life >24 hours) and their maximum therapeutic doses are as follows: chlordiazepoxide (Librium), 50 mg; clorazepate (Tranxene), 30 mg; clonazepam (Klonopin), 20 mg; diazepam (Valium), 10 mg in adults or 0.2 mg/kg in children; flurazepam (Dalmane), 30 mg; and prazepam, 20 mg.

The short-acting benzodiazepines (half-life 10 to 24 hours) and their doses include the following: alprazolam (Xanax), 0.5 mg, and lorazepam (Ativan), 4 mg in adults or 0.05 mg/kg in children, which act similar to the long-acting benzodiazepines.

The ultrashort-acting benzodiazepines (half-life <10 hours) are more toxic and include temazepam (Restoril), 30 mg; triazolam (Halcion), 0.5 mg; midazolam (Versed), 0.2 mg/kg; and oxazepam (Serax), 30 mg.

In cases of overdose of short- and long-acting agents, 10 to 20 times the therapeutic dose (>1500 mg diazepam or 2000 mg chlordiazepoxide) have been ingested with resulting mild coma but without respiratory depression. Fatalities are rare, and most patients recover within 24 to 36 hours after overdose. Asymptomatic unintentional overdoses of less than five times the therapeutic dose can be seen. Ultrashort-acting agents have produced respiratory arrest and coma within 1 hour after ingestion of 5 mg of triazolam (Halcion) and death with ingestion of as little as 10 mg. Midazolam (Versed) and diazepam (Valium) by rapid intravenous injection have produced respiratory arrest.

Kinetics

Onset of CNS depression is usually in 30 to 120 minutes; peak action usually occurs within 1 to 3 hours when ingestion is by the oral route. The volume distribution varies from 0.26 to 6 L/kg (LA, 1.1 L/kg); protein binding is 70% to 99%. For flunitrazepam, the onset of action is in 0.5 to 2 hours, oral peak is in 2 hours, and duration 8 hours or more. The half-life of flunitrazepam is 20 to 30 hours, volume distribution is 3.3 to 5.5 L/kg, and 80% is protein bound. Flunitrazepam can be identified in urine 4 to 30 days after ingestion.

Manifestations

Neurologic manifestations include ataxia, slurred speech, and CNS depression. Deep coma leading to respiratory depression suggests the presence of short-acting benzodiazepines or other CNS depressants. In elderly persons, the therapeutic doses can produce toxicity and can have an additive effect with other CNS depressants. Chronic use can lead to tolerance, physical dependency, and withdrawal.

Laboratory Investigations

Most benzodiazepines can be detected in urine drug screens. Quantitative blood levels are not useful. Some of the immunoassay urinary screens cannot detect all of the new benzodiazepines currently available. A consultation with the laboratory analyst is warranted if a specific case occurs in which the test result is negative but benzodiazepine use is suspected by the patient's history. Situations in which benzodiazepines may not be detected include ingestion of a low dose (e.g., <10 mg), rapid elimination, and a different or no metabolite. Some immunoassay methods can produce a false-positive finding for the benzodiazepines when nonsteroidal anti-inflammatory drugs (tolmetin [Tolectin], naproxen [Aleve], etodolac [Lodine], and fenoprofen [Nalfon]) are used. If this is a concern, the laboratory analyst should be consulted.

In cases in which "date rape" drugs such as flunitrazepam are suspected, a police crime or reference laboratory should be consulted for testing.

Management

Emesis and gastric lavage should be avoided. Activated charcoal can be useful only if given early before the peak time of absorption occurs. Supportive treatment should be instituted but rarely requires intubation or assisted ventilation.

Flumazenil (Romazicon) is a specific benzodiazepine receptor antagonist that blocks the chloride flow and inhibitor of GABA neurotransmitters. It reverses the sedative effects of benzodiazepines, zolpidem (Ambien), and endogenous benzodiazepines associated with hepatic encephalopathy. It is not recommended to reverse benzodiazepine-induced hypoventilation. The manufacturer advises that flumazenil be used with caution in cases of overdose with possible benzodiazepine dependency (because it can precipitate life-threatening withdrawal), if cyclic antidepressant use is suspected, or if a patient has a known seizure disorder.

Disposition

If the patient is comatose, he or she must be admitted to the intensive care unit. If the overdose was intentional, psychiatric clearance is needed before the patient can be discharged.

β-ADRENERGIC BLOCKERS (β-BLOCKER)

β-Blockers are used in the treatment of hypertension and of a number of systemic and ophthalmologic disorders. Properties of β-blockers include the factors listed in Table 12.

Lipid-soluble drugs have CNS effects, active metabolites, longer duration of action, and interactions (e.g., propranolol). Cardioselectivity is lost in overdose. Intrinsic partial agonist agents (e.g., pindolol) may initially produce tachycardia and hypertension. Cardiac membrane depressive effect (quinidine-like) occurs in cases of overdose but not at therapeutic doses (e.g., with metoprolol or sotalol).

TABLE 12 Pharmacologic and Toxic Properties of β-Blockers

Blocker	Maximum Solubility	Therapeutic Plasma Level	Lipid Solubility	Intrinsic Sympathomimetic Activity (Partial Agonist)	Membrane Stabilizing Effect		Cardiac Selectivity
					β-Selective		α-Selective
					β_1	β_2	
Acebutolol (Sectral)	800 mg	200–2000 ng/mL	Moderate	+	+	+	+
Alprenolol[2]	800 mg	50–200 ng/mL	Moderate	2+	+	–	–
Atenolol (Tenormin)	100 mg	200–500 ng/mL	Low	–	–	2+	–
Betaxolol (Kerlone)	20 mg	NA	Low	+	–	+	–
Carteolol (Cartrol)	10 mg	NA	No	+	–	–	–
Esmolol (Brevibloc) (Class II antidysrhythmic, IV only)			Low	–	–	+	–
Labetalol (Trandate)	800 mg	50–500 ng/mL	Low	+	+/–	–	+
Levobunolol (AKBeta eyedrop) (Eye drops 0.25% and 0.5%)	20 mg	NA	No	–	–	–	–
Metoprolol (Lopressor)			Moderate	–	–	2+	–
Nadolol (Corgard)	320 mg	20–40 ng/mL	Low	–	–	–	–
Oxyprenolol[2]	480 mg	80–100 ng/mL	Moderate	2+	+	–	–
Pindolol (Visken)	60 mg	50–150 ng/mL	Moderate	3+	+/-	–	–
Propranolol (Inderal) (Class II antidysrhythmic)	360 mg	50–100 ng/mL	High	–	2+	–	–
Sotalol (Betapace) (Class II antidysrhythmic)	480 mg	500–4000 ng/mL	Low	–	–	–	–
Timolol (Blocadren)	60 mg	5–10 ng/mL	Low	–	+/–	–	–

[2]Not available in the United States.

α-Blocking effect is weak (e.g., with labetalol or acebutolol).

Toxic Mechanism

β-Blockers compete with the catecholamines for receptor sites and block receptor action in the bronchi, the vascular smooth muscle, and the myocardium.

Toxic Dose

Ingestions of greater than twice the maximum recommended daily therapeutic dose are considered toxic (see Table 12). Ingestion of 1 mg/kg propranolol in a child may produce hypoglycemia. Fatalities have been reported in adults with 7.5 g of metoprolol. The most toxic agent is sotalol, and the least toxic is atenolol.

Kinetics

Regular-release formulations usually cause symptoms within 2 hours. Propranolol's onset of action is 20 to 30 minutes and peak is at 1 to 4 hours, but it may be delayed by co-ingestants. The onset of action with sustained-release preparations may be delayed to 6 hours and the peak to 12 to 16 hours. Volume distribution is 1 to 5.6 L/kg. Protein binding is variable, from 5% to 93%.

Metabolism

Atenolol (Tenormin), nadolol (Corgard), and santalol (Betapace) have enterohepatic recirculation. The duration of action for regular-acting agents is 4 to 6 hours, but in cases of overdose it may be 24 to 48 hours. The duration of action for sustained-release agents is 24 to 48 hours.

The regular preparation with the longest half-life is nadolol, at 12 to 24 hours, and the one with the shortest half-life is esmolol, at 5 to 10 minutes.

Manifestations

See "Toxic Properties" and Table 12.

Highly lipid soluble agents produce coma and seizures. Bradycardia and hypotension are the major cardiac symptoms and may lead to cardiogenic shock. Intrinsic partial agonists initially may cause tachycardia and hypertension. ECG changes include atrioventricular conduction delay or asystole. Membrane-depressant effects produce prolonged QRS and QT interval, which may result in torsades de pointes. Sotalol produces a very prolonged QT interval. Bronchospasm may occur in patients with reactive airway disease with any β-blocker because the selectivity is lost in overdose. Other manifestations include hypoglycemia (because β-blockers block catecholamine counter-regulatory mechanisms) and hyperkalemia.

Laboratory Investigations

Measurements of blood levels are not readily available or useful. ECG and cardiac monitoring should be maintained, and blood glucose and electrolytes, BUN, and creatinine levels should be monitored, as well as ABG if there are respiratory symptoms.

Management

Vital functions must be established and maintained. Vascular access, baseline ECG, and continuous cardiac and blood pressure monitoring should be established. A pacemaker must be available. Gastrointestinal decontamination can be undertaken initially with activated charcoal up to 1 hour after ingestion. MDAC is no longer recommended, based on the latest guidelines. Whole-bowel irrigation can be considered in cases of large overdoses with sustained-release preparations, but there are no studies evaluating the efficacy of intervention.

If there are cardiovascular disturbances, a cardiac consultation should be obtained. Class IA antidysrhythmic agents (procainamide, quinidine) and III (bretylium) are not recommended. Hypotension is treated with fluids initially, although it usually does not respond. Frequently, glucagon and cardiac pacing are needed. Bradycardia in asymptomatic, hemodynamically stable patients requires no therapy. It is not predictive of the future course of the disease. If the patient is unstable (has hypotension or a high-degree atrioventricular block), atropine 0.02 mg/kg (up to 2 mg) in adults, glucagon, and a pacemaker can be used. In case of ventricular tachycardia, overdrive pacing can be used. A wide QRS interval may respond to sodium bicarbonate. Torsades de pointes (associated with sotalol) may respond to magnesium sulfate and overdrive pacing. Prophylactic magnesium for prolonged QT interval has been suggested, but there are no data. Epinephrine must not be used because an unopposed α effect may occur.

Hypotension and myocardial depression are managed by correction of dysrhythmias, Trendelenburg position, fluids, glucagon, or amrinone (Inocor), or a combination of these. Hemodynamic monitoring with a Swan-Ganz catheter or arterial line may be necessary to manage fluid therapy.

Glucagon is the initial drug of choice. It works through adenyl cyclase and bypasses catecholamine receptors; therefore, it is not affected by β-blockers. Glucagon increases cardiac contractility and heart rate. It is given as an intravenous bolus of 5 to 10 mg[3] over 1 minute and followed by a continuous infusion of 1 to 5 mg/h (in children, 0.15 mg/kg followed by 0.05 to 0.1 mg/kg/h). In large doses and in infusion therapy D_5W, sterile water, or saline should be used as a dilutant to reconstitute glucagon in place of the 0.2% phenol diluent provided with some drugs. Effects are seen within minutes. It can be used with other agents such as amrinone.

Amrinone (Inocor) inhibits phosphodiesterase enzyme, which metabolizes cyclic AMP. It is administered as a bolus of 0.15 to 2 mg/kg (0.15 to 0.4 mL/kg) intravenously, followed by infusion of 5 to 10 μg/kg/min.

[3]Exceeds dosage recommended by the manufacturer.

Hypoglycemia should be treated with intravenous glucose. Life-threatening hyperkalemia is treated with calcium (avoid if digoxin is present), bicarbonate, and glucose or insulin. Convulsions can be controlled with diazepam or phenobarbital. If bronchospasm is present, β_2 nebulized bronchodilators are given.

Extraordinary measures such as intra-aortic balloon pump support can be instituted. Extracorporeal measures can be undertaken. Hemodialysis for cases of atenolol, acebutolol, nadolol, and sotalol (low volume distribution, low protein binding) ingestion may be helpful, particularly when there is evidence of renal failure. Hemodialysis is not effective for propranolol, metoprolol, and timolol.

Prenalterol[2] has successfully reversed both bradycardia and hypotension but is not currently available in the United States.

Disposition

Asymptomatic patients with history of overdose require baseline ECG and continuous cardiac monitoring for at least 6 hours with regular-release preparations and for 24 hours with sustained-release preparations. Symptomatic patients should be observed with cardiac monitoring for 24 hours. If seizures or abnormal rhythm or vital signs are present, the patient should be admitted to the intensive care unit.

CALCIUM CHANNEL BLOCKERS

Calcium channel blockers are used in the treatment of effort angina, supraventricular tachycardia, and hypertension.

Toxic Mechanism

Calcium channel blockers reduce influx of calcium through the slow channels in membranes of the myocardium, the atrioventricular nodes, and the vascular smooth muscles and result in peripheral, systemic, and coronary vasodilation, impaired cardiac conduction, and depression of cardiac contractility. All calcium channel blockers have vasodilatory action, but only bepridil, diltiazem, and verapamil depress myocardial contractility and cause atrioventricular block.

Toxic Dose

Any ingested amount greater than the maximum daily dose has the potential of severe toxicity. The maximum oral daily doses in adults and toxic doses in children of each are as follows: amlodipine (Norvasc), 10 mg for adults and more than 0.25 mg/kg for children; bepridil (Vascor), 400 mg for adults and

[2]Not available in the United States.

more than 5.7 mg/kg for children; diltiazem (Cardizem), 360 mg for adults (toxic dose > 2 g) and more than 6 mg/kg for children; felodipine (Plendil), 40 mg for adults and more than 0.56 mg/kg for children; isradipine (DynaCirc), 40 mg for adults and more than 0.4 mg/kg for children; nicardipine (Cardene), 120 mg for adults and more than 0.85 mg/kg for children; nifedipine (Procardia), 120 mg for adults and more than 2 mg/kg for children; nimodipine (Nimotop), 360 mg for adults and more than 0.85 mg/kg for children; nitrendipine (Baypress)[2], 80 mg for adults and more than 1.14 mg/kg for children; and verapamil (Calan), 480 mg for adults and 15 mg/kg for children.

Kinetics

Onset of action of regular-release preparations varies: for verapamil it is 60 to 120 minutes, for nifedipine 20 minutes, and for diltiazem 15 minutes after ingestion. Peak effect for verapamil is 2 to 4 hours, for nifedipine 60 to 90 minutes, and for diltiazem 30 to 60 minutes, but the peak action may be delayed for 6 to 8 hours. Duration of action is up to 36 hours. The onset of action for sustained-release preparations is usually 4 hours but may be delayed, and peak effect is at 12 to 24 hours. In cases of massive overdose, concretions and prolonged toxicity can develop.

Volume distribution varies from 3 to 7 L/kg. Hepatic elimination half-life varies from 3 to 7 hours. Patients receiving digitalis and calcium channel blockers run the risk of digitalis toxicity, because calcium channel blockers increase digitalis levels.

Manifestations

Cardiac manifestations include hypotension, bradycardia, and conduction disturbances occurring 30 minutes to 5 hours after ingestion. A prolonged PR interval is an early finding and may occur at therapeutic doses. Torsades de pointes has been reported. All degrees of blocks may occur and may be delayed up to 16 hours. Lactic acidosis may be present. Calcium channel blockers do not affect intraventricular conduction, so the QRS interval is usually not affected.

Hypocalcemia is rarely present. Hyperglycemia may be present because of interference in calcium-dependent insulin release. Mental status changes, headaches, seizures, hemiparesis, and CNS depression may occur.

Laboratory Investigations

Specific drug levels are not readily available and are not useful. Monitor blood sugar, electrolytes, calcium, ABG, pulse oximetry, creatinine, and BUN, and also use hemodynamic monitoring, ECG, and cardiac monitoring.

Management

Vital functions must be established and maintained. Baseline ECG readings should be obtained and continuous cardiac and blood pressure monitoring maintained. A pacemaker should be available. Cardiology consultation should be sought.

Gastrointestinal decontamination with activated charcoal is recommended. If a large dose of a sustained-release preparation was ingested, whole-bowel irrigation can be considered, but its effectiveness has not been investigated.

If the patient is symptomatic, immediate cardiology consult must be obtained, because a pacemaker and hemodynamic monitoring may be needed. In the case of heart block, atropine is rarely effective and isoproterenol (Isuprel) may produce vasodilation. The use of a pacemaker should be considered early.

Hypotension and bradycardia can be treated with positioning, fluids, and calcium gluconate or chloride, glucagon, amrinone (Inocor), and ventricular pacing. Calcium salts must be avoided if digoxin is present. Calcium usually reverses depressed myocardial contractility but may not reverse nodal depression or peripheral vasodilation. Calcium chloride can be given in a 10% solution, 0.1 to 0.2 mL/kg up to 10 mL in an adult, or calcium gluconate in a 10% solution 0.3 to 0.4 mL/kg up to 20 mL in an adult. Administration is intravenous, over 5 to 10 minutes. One should monitor for dysrhythmias, hypotension, and the serum ionized calcium. The aim is to increase calcium 4 mg/dL to a maximum of 13 mg/dL. The calcium response lasts 15 minutes and may require repeated doses or a continuous calcium gluconate infusion 0.2 mL/kg/h up to maximum of 10 mL/h.

If calcium fails, glucagon can be tried for its positive inotropic and chronotropic effect, or both. Amrinone (Inocor), an inotropic agent, may reverse the effects of calcium channel blockers. An effective dose is 0.15 mg to 2 mg/kg (0.15 to 0.4 mL/kg) by intravenous bolus followed by infusion of 5 to 10 μg/kg/min.

In case of hypotension, fluids, norepinephrine (Levophed), and epinephrine may be required. Amrinone and glucagon have been tried alone and in combination. Dobutamine and dopamine are often ineffective.

Extracorporeal measures (e.g., hemodialysis and charcoal hemoperfusion) are not useful, but extraordinary measures such as intra-aortic balloon pump and cardiopulmonary bypass have been used successfully.

For cases of calcium channel blocker toxicity that fail to respond to aggressive management, recent studies demonstrate that insulin and glucose have therapeutic value. The suggested dose range for insulin is to infuse regular insulin at 0.5 IU/kg/h with a simultaneous infusion of glucose 1 g/kg/h, with glucose monitoring every 30 minutes for at least the first 4 hours of administration and subsequent glucose

---

[2]Not available in the United States.

adjustment to maintain euglycemia (70 to 100 mg/dL). Potassium levels should be monitored regularly, as they may shift in response to the insulin.

Disposition

Patients who have ingested regular-release preparations should be monitored for at least 6 hours and those who have ingested sustained-release preparations should be monitored for 24 hours after the ingestion. Intentional overdose necessitates psychiatric clearance. Symptomatic patients should be admitted to the intensive care unit.

CARBON MONOXIDE

Carbon monoxide is an odorless, colorless gas produced from incomplete combustion; it is also an in vivo metabolic breakdown product of methylene chloride used in paint removers.

Toxic Mechanism

Carbon monoxide's affinity for hemoglobin is 240 times greater than that of oxygen. It shifts the oxygen dissociation curve to the left, which impairs hemoglobin release of oxygen to tissues and inhibits the cytochrome oxidase enzymes.

Toxic Dose and Manifestations

Table 13 describes the manifestations of carbon monoxide toxicity. Exposure to 0.5% for a few minutes is lethal. Sequelae correlate with the patient's level of consciousness at presentation. ECG abnormalities may be noted. Creatine kinase is often elevated, and rhabdomyolysis and myoglobinuria may occur.

The carboxyhemoglobin (CoHB) expresses in percentage the extent to which carbon monoxide has bound with the total hemoglobin. This may be misleadingly low in the anemic patient with less hemoglobin than normal. The patient's presentation is a more reliable indicator of severity than the CoHB level. The manifestations listed in Table 13 for each level are in addition to those listed at the level above. The CoHB may not correlate reliably with the severity of the intoxication, and linking symptoms to specific levels of CoHB frequently leads to inaccurate conclusions. A level of carbon monoxide greater than 40% is usually associated with obvious intoxication.

TABLE 13 Carbon Monoxide Exposure and Possible Manifestations

CoHB Saturation (%)	Manifestations
3.5	None
5	Slight headache, decreased exercise tolerance
10	Slight headache. dyspnea on vigorous exertion, may impair driving skills
10–20	Moderate dyspnea on exertion, throbbing, temporal headache
20–30	Severe headache, syncope, dizziness, visual changes, weakness, nausea, vomiting, altered judgment
30–40	Vertigo, ataxia, blurred vision, confusion, loss of consciousness
40–50	Confusion, tachycardia, tachypnea, coma, convulsions
50–60	Cheyne-Stokes, coma, convulsions, shock, apnea
60–70	Coma, convulsions, respiratory and heart failure, death

Kinetics

The natural metabolism of the body produces small amounts of CoHB, less than 2% for nonsmokers and 5% to 9% for smokers.

Carbon monoxide is rapidly absorbed through the lungs. The rate of absorption is directly related to alveolar ventilation. Elimination also occurs through the lungs. The half-life of CoHB in room air (21% oxygen) is 5 to 6 hours; in 100% oxygen, it is 90 minutes; in hyperbaric pressure at 3 atmospheres oxygen, it is 20 to 30 minutes.

Laboratory Investigations

An ABG reading may show metabolic acidosis and normal oxygen tension. In cases of significant poisoning, the ABG, electrolytes, blood glucose, serum creatine kinase and cardiac enzymes, renal function tests, and liver function tests should be monitored. A urinalysis and test for myoglobinuria should be obtained. Chest radiograph can be useful in cases of smoke inhalation or if the patient is being considered for hyperbaric chamber. ECG monitoring should be maintained, especially if the patient is older than 40 years, has a history of cardiac disease, or has moderate to severe symptoms. Which toxicology studies are used is based on symptoms and circumstances. CoHB should be monitored during and at the end of therapy. The pulse oximeter has two wavelengths and overestimates oxyhemoglobin saturation in carbon monoxide poisoning. The true oxygen saturation is determined by blood gas analysis, which measures the oxygen bound to hemoglobin. The co-oximeter measures four wavelengths and separates out CoHB and the other hemoglobin binding agents from oxyhemoglobin. Fetal hemoglobin has a greater affinity for carbon monoxide than adult hemoglobin and may falsely elevate the CoHB as much as 4% in young infants.

Management

The first step is to adequately protect the rescuer. The patient must be removed from the contaminated area, and his or her vital functions must be established.

The mainstay of treatment is 100% oxygen via a non-rebreathing mask with an oxygen reservoir or endotracheal tube. All patients receive 100% oxygen until the CoHB level is 5% or less. Assisted ventilation may be necessary. ABG and CoHB should be monitored and the present CoHB level determined. *Note:* A near-normal CoHB level does not exclude significant carbon monoxide poisoning, especially if the measurement is taken several hours after termination of exposure or if oxygen has been administered prior to obtaining the sample.

The exposed pregnant woman should be kept on 100% oxygen for several hours after the CoHB level is almost 0, because carbon monoxide concentrates in the fetus and oxygen is needed longer to ensure elimination of the carbon monoxide from fetal circulation. The fetus must be monitored, because carbon monoxide and hypoxia are potentially teratogenic.

Metabolic acidosis should be treated with sodium bicarbonate only if the pH is below 7.2 after correction of hypoxia and adequate ventilation. Acidosis shifts the oxygen dissociation curve to the right and facilitates oxygen delivery to the tissues.

The decision to use the hyperbaric oxygen chamber must be made on the basis of the ability to handle other acute emergencies that may coexist in the patient and of the severity of the poisoning. The standard of care for persons exposed to carbon monoxide has yet to be determined, but most authorities recommend using the hyperbaric oxygen chamber under any of the following conditions:

- If the patient is in a coma or has a history of loss of consciousness or seizures
- If there is cardiovascular dysfunction (clinical ischemic chest pain or ECG evidence of ischemia)
- If the patient has metabolic acidosis
- If symptoms persist despite 100% oxygen therapy
- In a child, if the initial CoHB is greater than 15%
- In symptomatic patients with preexisting ischemia
- If there are signs of maternal or fetal distress regardless of CoHB level (infants and fetus are a special problem because fetal hemoglobin has greater affinity for carbon monoxide)

Although controversial, a neurologic-cognitive examination has been used to help determine which patients with low carbon monoxide levels should receive more aggressive therapy. Testing should include the following: general orientation memory testing involving address, phone number, date of birth, and present date; and cognitive testing, involving counting by 7s, digit span, and forward and backward spelling of three-letter and four-letter words. Patients with delayed neurologic sequelae or recurrent symptoms up to 3 weeks may benefit from hyperbaric oxygen chamber treatment.

Seizures and cerebral edema must be treated.

Disposition

Patients with no or mild symptoms who become asymptomatic after a few hours of oxygen therapy and have a carbon monoxide level less than 10%, and normal physical and neurologic-cognitive examination findings can be discharged, but they should be instructed to return if any signs of neurologic dysfunction appear. Patients with carbon monoxide poisoning requiring treatment need follow-up neuropsychiatric examinations.

CAUSTICS AND CORROSIVES

The terms *caustic* and *corrosive* are used interchangeably and can be divided into acids and alkalis. The U.S. Consumer Product Safety Commission Labeling Recommendations on containers for acids and alkalis indicate the potential for producing serious damage, as follows:

- Caution—weak irritant
- Warning—strong irritant
- Danger—corrosive

Some common acids with corrosive potential include acetic acid, formic acid, glycolic acid, hydrochloric acid, mercuric chloride, nitric acid, oxalic acid, phosphoric acid, sulfuric acid (battery acid), zinc chloride, and zinc sulfate. Some common alkalis with corrosive potential include ammonia, calcium carbide, calcium hydroxide (dry), calcium oxide, potassium hydroxide (lye), and sodium hydroxide (lye).

Toxic Mechanism

Acids produce mucosal coagulation necrosis and may be absorbed systemically; they do not penetrate deeply. Injury to the gastric mucosa is more likely, although specific sites of injury for acids and alkalis are not clearly defined.

Alkalis produce liquefaction necrosis and saponification and penetrate deeply. The esophageal mucosa is likely to be damaged. Oropharyngeal and esophageal damage is more frequently caused by solids than by liquids. Liquids produce superficial circumferential burns and gastric damage.

Toxic Dose

The toxicity is determined by concentration, contact time, and pH. Significant injury is more likely with a substance that has a pH of less than 2 or greater than 12, with a prolonged contact time, and with large volumes.

Manifestations

The absence of oral burns does not exclude the possibility of esophageal or gastric damage. General clinical findings are stridor; dysphagia; drooling; oropharyngeal, retrosternal, and epigastric pain; and ocular and oral burns. Alkali burns are yellow, soapy, frothy lesions. Acid burns are gray-white and later form an eschar. Abdominal tenderness and guarding may be present if perforation has happened.

Laboratory Investigations

If acid ingestion has taken place, the patient's acid–base balance and electrolyte status should be determined. If pulmonary symptoms are present, a chest radiograph, ABG measurement, and pulse oximetry are called for.

Management

It is recommended that the container be brought to the examination, as the substance must be identified and the pH of the substance, vomitus, tears, or saliva tested.

If the acid or alkali has been ingested, all gastrointestinal decontamination procedures are contraindicated except for immediate rinse, removal of substance from the mouth, and dilution with small amounts (sips) of milk or water. The examiner should check for ocular and dermal involvement. Contraindications to oral dilution are dysphagias, respiratory distress, obtundation, or shock. If there is ocular involvement one should immediately irrigate the eye with tepid water for at least 30 minutes, perform fluorescein stain of eye, and consult an ophthalmologist. If there is dermal involvement, one should immediately remove contaminated clothes and irrigate the skin with tepid water for at least 15 minutes. Consultation with a burn specialist is called for.

In cases of acid ingestion, some authorities advocate a small flexible nasogastric tube and aspiration within 30 minutes after ingestion.

Patients should receive only intravenous fluids following dilution until endoscopic consultation is obtained. Endoscopy is valuable to predict damage and risk of stricture. The indications are controversial, with some authorities recommending it in all cases of caustic ingestions regardless of symptoms, and others selectively using clinical features such as vomiting, stridor, drooling, and oral or facial lesions as criteria. We recommend endoscopy for all symptomatic patients or patients with intentional ingestions. Endoscopy may be performed immediately if the patient is symptomatic, but it is usually done 12 to 48 hours postingestion.

The use of corticosteroids is considered controversial. Some feel they may be useful for patients with second-degree circumferential burns. They recommend starting with hydrocortisone sodium succinate (Solu-Cortef) intravenously 10 to 20 mg/kg/d within 48 hours and changing to oral prednisolone 2 mg/kg/d for 3 weeks before tapering the dose. We do not usually recommend using corticosteroids because they have not been shown to be effective.

Tetanus prophylaxis should be provided if the patient requires it for wound care. Antibiotics are not useful prophylactically. Contrast studies are not useful in the first few days and may interfere with endoscopic evaluation; later, they can be used to assess the severity of damage.

Emergency medical therapy includes agents to inhibit collagen formation and intraluminal stents. Esophageal and gastric outlet dilation may be needed if there is evidence of stricture. Bougienage of the esophagus, however, has been associated with brain abscess. Interposition of the colon may be necessary if dilation fails to provide an adequate-sized passage.

Management of inhalation cases requires immediate removal from the environment, administration of humid supplemental oxygen, and observation for airway obstruction and noncardiac pulmonary edema. Radiographic and ABG evaluation should be obtained when appropriate. Intubation and respiratory support may be required.

Certain caustics produce systemic disturbances. Formaldehyde causes metabolic acidosis, hydrofluoric acid causes hypocalcemia and renal damage, oxalic acid causes hypocalcemia, phenol causes hepatic and renal damage, and picric acid causes renal injury.

Disposition

Infants and small children should be medically evaluated and observed. All symptomatic patients should be admitted. If they have severe symptoms or danger of airway compromise, they should be admitted to the intensive care unit. After endoscopy, if no damage is detected, the patient may be discharged when he or she can tolerate oral feedings. Intentional exposures require psychiatric evaluation before the patient can be discharged.

COCAINE (BENZOYLMETHYLECGONINE)

Cocaine is derived from the leaves of *Erythroxylum coca* and *Truxillo coca*. "Body packing" refers to the placement of many small packages of contraband cocaine for concealment in the gastrointestinal tract or other areas for illicit transport. "Body stuffing" refers to spontaneous ingestion of substances for the purpose of hiding evidence.

Toxic Mechanism

Cocaine directly stimulates the CNS presynaptic sympathetic neurons to release catecholamines and acetylcholine, while it blocks the presynaptic reuptake of the catecholamines; it blocks the sodium channels along neuronal membranes; and it increases platelet aggregation. Long-term use depletes the CNS of dopamine.

Toxic Dose

The maximum mucosal local anesthetic therapeutic dose of cocaine is 200 mg or 2 mL of a 10% solution. Although CNS effects can occur at relatively low local anesthetic doses (50 to 95 mg), they are more common with doses greater than 1 mg/kg; cardiac effects can occur with doses greater than 1 mg/kg.

The potential fatal dose is 1200 mg intranasally, but death has occurred with 20 mg parenterally.

Kinetics

Cocaine is well absorbed by all routes, including nasal insufflation, and oral, dermal, and inhalation routes (Table 14). Protein binding is 8.7%, and volume distribution is 1.5 L/kg.

Cocaine is metabolized by plasma and liver cholinesterase to the inactive metabolites ecgonine methyl ester and benzoylecgonine. Plasma pseudocholinesterase is congenitally deficient in 3% of the population and decreased in fetuses, young infants, the elderly, pregnant people, and people with liver disease. These enzyme-deficient individuals are at increased risk for life-threatening cocaine toxicity.

Ten percent of cocaine is excreted unchanged. Cocaine and ethanol undergo liver synthesis to form cocaethylene, a metabolite with a half-life three times longer than that of cocaine. It may account for some of cocaine's cardiotoxicity and appears to be more lethal than cocaine or ethanol alone.

Manifestations

The CNS manifestation of cocaine ingestion are euphoria, hyperactivity, agitation, convulsions, and intracranial hemorrhage. Mydriasis and septal perforation can occur, as well as cardiac dysrhythmias, hypertension, and hypotension (with severe overdose). Chest pain is frequent, but only 5.8% of patients have true myocardial ischemia and infarction. Other manifestations include vasoconstriction, hyperthermia (because of increased metabolic rate), ischemic bowel perforation if the substance is ingested, rhabdomyolysis, myoglobinuria, and renal failure. In pregnant users, premature labor and abruptio placentae can occur.

Body cavity packing should be suspected in cases of prolonged toxicity.

Mortality can result from cerebrovascular accidents, coronary artery spasm, myocardial injury, or lethal dysrhythmias.

Laboratory Investigations

Monitoring of the ECG and cardiac rhythms, ABG, oxygen saturation, electrolytes, blood glucose, BUN, creatinine, and creatine kinase levels should be maintained. One should monitor cardiac fraction if the patient has chest pain, as well as the liver profile, and the urine for myoglobin. Intravenous drug users should have HIV and hepatitis virus testing.

Urine should be tested for cocaine and metabolites and other substances of abuse, and abdominal radiographs or ultrasonogram should be ordered for body packers. If the urine sample was collected more than 12 hours after cocaine intake, it will contain little or no cocaine. If cocaine is present, cocaine has been used within the past 12 hours. Cocaine's metabolite benzoylecgonine may be detected within 4 hours after a single nasal insufflation and for up to 114 hours. Cross-reactions with some herbal teas, lidocaine, and droperidol (Inapsine) may give false-positive results by some immunoassay methods.

Management

Supportive care includes blood pressure, cardiac, and thermal monitoring and seizure precautions. Diazepam (Valium) is the drug of choice for treatment of cocaine toxicity agitation, seizures, and dysrhythmias; doses are 10 to 30 mg intravenously at 2.5 mg per minute for adults and 0.2 to 0.5 mg/kg at 1 mg per minute up to 10 mg for a child.

Gastrointestinal decontamination should be instituted, if the cocaine was ingested, by administration of activated charcoal. MDAC may adsorb cocaine leakage in body stuffers or body packers. Whole-bowel irrigation with polyethylene glycol solution (PEG) has been used in body packers and stuffers if the contraband is in a firm container. If the packages are not visible on plain radiographs of the abdomen, a contrast study or CT scan can help to confirm successful passage. Cocaine in the nasal passage can be removed with an applicator dipped in a non–water-soluble product (lubricating jelly) if this is done within a few minutes after application.

In body packers and stuffers, venous access must be secured, and drugs must be readily available for treating life-threatening manifestations until the contraband is passed in the stool. Surgical removal may be indicated if the packet does not pass the pylorus, in an asymptomatic body packer, or in the case of intestinal obstruction.

Hypertension and tachycardia are usually transient and can be managed by careful titration of diazepam. Nitroprusside may be used for severe hypertension. Myocardial ischemia is managed by oxygen, vascular

TABLE 14 The Different Routes and Kinetics of Cocaine

Type	Route	Onset	Peak (min)	Half-life (min)	Duration (min)
Cocaine leaf	Oral, chewing	20–30 min	45–90	NA	240–360
Hydrochloride	Insufflation	1–3 min	5–10	78	60–90
	Ingestion	20–30 min	50–90	54	Sustained
	Intravenous	30–120 sec	5–11	36	60–90
Free base/crack	Smoking	5–10 sec	5–11	—	Up to 20
Coca paste	Smoking	Unknown	—	—	—

access, benzodiazepines, and nitroglycerin. Aspirin and thrombolysis are not routinely recommended because of the danger of intracranial hemorrhage.

Dysrhythmias are usually supraventricular (SVT) and do not require specific management. Adenosine is ineffective. Life-threatening tachydysrhythmias may respond to phentolamine (Regitine) 5 mg IV bolus in adults or 0.1 mg/kg in children at 5- to 10-minute intervals. Phentolamine also relieves coronary artery spasm and myocardial ischemia. Electrical synchronized cardioversion should be considered for patients with hemodynamically unstable dysrhythmias. Lidocaine is not recommended initially but may be used after 3 hours for ventricular tachycardia. Wide complex QRS ventricular tachycardia may be treated with sodium bicarbonate 2 mEq/kg as a bolus. β-Adrenergic blockers are not recommended.

Anxiety, agitation, and convulsions can be treated with diazepam. If diazepam fails to control seizures, neuromuscular blockers can be used. The EEG should be monitored for nonmotor seizure activity. For hyperthermia, external cooling and cool humidified 100% oxygen should be administered. Neuromuscular paralysis to control seizures will reduce temperature. Dantrolene and antipyretics are not recommended. Rhabdomyolysis and myoglobinuria are treated with fluids, alkaline diuresis, and diuretics.

If the patient is pregnant, the fetus must be monitored and the patient observed for spontaneous abortion.

Paranoid ideation and threatening behavior should be treated with rapid tranquilization. The patient should be observed for suicidal depression that may follow intoxication and may require suicide precautions. If focal neurologic manifestations are present, one should consider the possibility of a cerebrovascular accident and obtain a CT scan.

Extracorporeal clearance techniques are of no benefit.

Disposition

Patients with mild intoxication or a brief seizure that does not require treatment who become asymptomatic may be discharged after 6 hours with appropriate psychosocial follow-up. If cardiac or cerebral ischemic manifestations are present, the patient should be monitored in the intensive care unit. Body packers and stuffers require care in the intensive care unit until passage of the contraband.

CYANIDE

Hydrogen cyanide is a byproduct of burning plastic and wools in residential fires. Hydrocyanic acid is the liquefied form of hydrogen cyanide. Cyanide salts can be found in ore extraction. Nitriles, such as acetonitrile (artificial nail removers) are metabolized in the body to produce cyanide. Cyanogenic glycosides are present in some fruit seeds (such as amygdalin in apricots, peaches, and apples). Sodium nitroprusside, the antihypertensive vasodilator, contains five cyanide groups.

Toxic Mechanism

Cyanide blocks the cellular electron transport mechanism and cellular respiration by inhibiting the mitochondrial ferricytochrome oxidase system and other enzymes. This results in cellular hypoxia and lactic acidosis. *Note:* Citrus fruit seeds form cyanide in the presence of intestinal β-glucosidase (the seeds are harmful only if the capsule is broken).

Toxic Dose

The ingestion of 1 mg/kg or 50 mg of hydrogen cyanide can produce death within 15 minutes. The lethal dose of potassium cyanide is 200 mg. Five to 10 mL of 84% acetonitrile is lethal. Infusions of sodium nitroprusside in rates above 2 μg/kg per minute may cause cyanide to accumulate to toxic concentrations in critically ill patients.

Kinetics

Cyanide is rapidly absorbed by all routes. In the stomach, it forms hydrocyanic acid. Volume distribution is 1.5 L/kg. Protein binding is 60%. Cyanide is detoxified by metabolism in the liver via the mitochondrial thiosulfate-rhodanase pathway, which catalyzes the transfer of sulfur donor to cyanide, forming the less toxic irreversible thiocyanate that is excreted in the urine. Cyanide is also detoxified by reacting with hydroxocobalamin (vitamin B_{12a}) to form cyanocobalamin (vitamin B_{12}).

The cyanide elimination half-life from the blood is 1.2 hours. The elimination route is through the lungs.

Manifestations

Hydrogen cyanide has the distinctive odor of bitter almonds or silver polish. Manifestations of cyanide intoxication include hypertension, cardiac dysrhythmias, various ECG abnormalities, headache, hyperpnea, seizures, stupor, pulmonary edema, and flushing. Cyanosis is absent or appears late.

Laboratory Investigations

The examiner should obtain and monitor ABGs, oxygen saturation, blood lactate, hemoglobin, blood glucose, and electrolytes. Lactic acidemia, a decrease in the arterial-venous oxygen difference, and bright red venous blood occurs. If smoke inhalation is the possible source of cyanide exposure, CoHB and methemoglobin (MetHb) concentrations should be measured.

Cyanide levels in whole blood, red blood cells, or serum are not useful in the acute management because the determinations are not readily available.

Specific cyanide blood levels are as follows: smokers have less than 0.5 μg/mL; a patient with flushing and tachycardia has 0.5 to 1.0 μg/mL, one with obtundation has 1.0 to 2.5 μg/mL, and one in coma or who has died has more than 2.5 μg/mL.

Management

If the cyanide was inhaled, the patient must be removed from the contaminated atmosphere. Attendants should not administer mouth-to-mouth resuscitation. Rescuers and attendants must be protected. Immediate administration of 100% oxygen is called for and oxygen should be continued during and after the administration of the antidote. The clinician must decide whether to use any or all components of the cyanide antidote kit.

The mechanism of action of the antidote kit is twofold: to produce methemoglobinemia and to provide a sulfur substrate for the detoxification of cyanide. The nitrites make methemoglobin, which has a greater affinity for cyanide than does the cytochrome oxidase enzymes. The combination of methemoglobin and cyanide forms cyanomethemoglobin. Sodium thiosulfate provides a sulfur substrate for the rhodanese enzyme, which converts cyanide into the relatively nontoxic sodium thiocyanate, which is excreted by the kidney.

The procedure for using the antidote kit is as follows:

Step 1: Amyl nitrite inhalant perles is only a temporizing measure (forms only 2% to 5% methemoglobin) and it can be omitted if venous access is established. Alternate 100% oxygen and the inhalant for 30 seconds each minute. Use a new perle every 3 minutes.

Step 2: Sodium nitrite ampule is indicated for cyanide exposures, except for cases of residential fires, smoke inhalation, and nitroprusside or acetonitrile poisonings. It is administered intravenously to produce methemoglobin of 20% to 30% at 35 to 70 minutes after administration. A dose of 10 mL of 3% solution of sodium nitrite for adults and 0.33 mL/kg of 3% solution for children is diluted to 100 mL 0.9% saline and administered slowly intravenously at 5 mL/min. If hypotension develops, the infusion should be slowed.

Step 3: Sodium thiosulfate is useful alone in cases of smoke inhalation, nitroprusside toxicity, and acetonitrile toxicity and should not be used at all in cases of hydrogen sulfide poisoning. The administration dose is 12.5 g of sodium thiosulfate or 50 mL of 25% solution for adults and 1.65 mL/kg of 25% solution for children intravenously over 10 to 20 minutes.

If cyanide symptoms recur, further treatment with nitrites or the perles is controversial. Some authorities suggest repeating the antidotes in 30 minutes at half of the initial dose, but others do not advise this for lack of efficacy. The child dosage regimen on the package insert must be carefully followed.

One hour after antidotes are administered, the methemoglobin level should be obtained and should not exceed 20%. Methylene blue should not be used to reverse excessive methemoglobin.

Gastrointestinal decontamination of oral ingestion by activated charcoal is recommended but is not very effective because of the rapidity of absorption. Seizures are treated with intravenous diazepam. Acidosis should be treated with sodium bicarbonate if it does not rapidly resolve with therapy. There is no role for hyperbaric oxygen or hemodialysis or hemoperfusion.

Other antidotes include hydroxocobalamin (vitamin B_{12a}) (Cyanokit), which has proven effective when given immediately after exposure in large doses of 4 g (50 mg/kg) or 50 times the amount of cyanide exposure with 8 g of sodium thiosulfate. Hydroxocobalamin has FDA orphan drug approval.

Disposition

Asymptomatic patients should be observed for a minimum of 3 hours. Patients who ingest nitrile compounds must be observed for 24 hours. Patients requiring antidote administration should be admitted to the intensive care unit.

DIGITALIS

Cardiac glycosides are found in cardiac medications, common plants, and the skin of the Bufo toad.

Toxic Mechanism

Cardiac glycosides inhibit the enzyme sodium/potassium-adenosine triphosphatase (NA^+, K^+, ATPase), leading to intracellular potassium loss and increased intracellular sodium, and producing phase 4 depolarization, increased automaticity, and ectopy. There is increased intracellular calcium and potentiation of contractility. Pacemaker cells are inhibited, and the refractory period is prolonged, leading to atrioventricular blocks. There is increased vagal tone.

Toxic Dose

Digoxin total digitalizing dose, the dose required to achieve therapeutic blood levels of 0.6 to 2.0 ng/mL, is 0.75 to 1.25 mg or 10 to 15 μg/kg for patients older than 10 years of age; 40 to 50 μg/kg for patients younger than 2 years of age; and 30 to 40 μg/kg for patients 2 to 10 years of age.

The acute single toxic dose is greater than 0.07 mg/kg or greater than 2 or 3 mg in an adult, but 2 mg in a child or 4 mg in an adult usually produces only mild toxicity. One to 3 mg or more may be found in a few leaves of oleander or foxglove. Serious and fatal overdoses are more than 4 mg in a child and more than 10 mg in an adult.

Acute digitoxin ingestion of 10 to 35 mg has produced severe toxicity and death. Digitoxin therapeutic steady state is 15 to 25 ng/mL. In cases of chronic or acute-on-chronic ingestions in patients with cardiac disease, more than 2 mg may produce toxicity; however, toxicity can develop within therapeutic range on chronic therapy.

Patients at greatest risk of overdose include those with cardiac disease, those with electrolyte abnormalities (low potassium, low magnesium, low T_4, high calcium), those with renal impairment, and those on amiodarone (Cordarone), quinidine, erythromycin, tetracycline, calcium channel blockers, and β-blockers.

Kinetics

Digoxin is a metabolite of digitoxin. In cases of oral overdose, the typical onset is 30 minutes, with peak effects in 3 to 12 hours. Duration is 3 to 4 days. Intravenous onset is in 5 to 30 minutes; peak level is immediate, and peak effect is at 1.5 to 3 hours.

Volume distribution is 5 to 6 L/kg. The cardiac-to-plasma ratio is 30:1. After an acute ingestion overdose, the serum concentration is not reflective of tissue concentration for at least 6 hours or more, and steady state is 12 to 16 hours after last dose.

Sixty percent to 80% of the parent compound is excreted unchanged in the urine. The elimination half-life is 30 to 50 hours.

Manifestations

Onset of manifestations is usually within 2 hours but may be delayed up to 12 hours.

Gastrointestinal effects of nausea and vomiting are frequently present in cases of acute ingestion but may also occur in cases of chronic ingestion. The "digitalis effect" on ECG is scooped ST segments and PR prolongation; in cases of overdose, any dysrhythmia or block is possible but none are characteristic. Bradycardia occurs in patients with acute overdose with healthy hearts; supraventricular tachycardia occurs in patients with existing heart disease or chronic overdose. Ventricular tachycardia is seen only in cases of severe poisoning.

The CNS effects include headaches, visual disturbances, and colored halo vision. Hyperkalemia occurs following acute overdose and correlates with digoxin level and outcome. Among patients with serum potassium levels of less than 5.0 mEq/L, all survive. If the level is 5 to 5.5, 50% survive, and if the level is greater than 5.5, all die. Hypokalemia is commonly seen with chronic intoxication. Patients with normal digitalis levels may have toxicity in the presence of hypokalemia.

Chronic intoxications are more likely to produce scotoma, color perception disturbances, yellow vision, halos, delirium, hallucinations or psychosis, tachycardia, and hypokalemia.

Laboratory Investigations

Continuous monitoring of ECG, pulse, and blood pressure is called for. Blood glucose, electrolytes, calcium, magnesium, BUN, and creatinine levels should also be monitored. An initial digoxin level should be measured on patient presentation and repeated thereafter. Levels should be measured more than 6 hours postingestion because earlier values do not reflect tissue distribution. Digoxin clinical toxicity is usually associated with serum digoxin levels of greater than 3.5 ng/mL in adults.

An endogenous digoxin-like substance cross-reacts in most common immunoassays (not with high-pressure liquid chromatography) and values as high as 4.1 ng/mL have been reported in newborns, patients with chronic renal failure, patients with abnormal immunoglobulins, and women in the third trimester of pregnancy.

Management

A cardiology consult should be obtained and a pacemaker should be readily available.

In undertaking gastrointestinal decontamination, excessive vagal stimulation should be avoided (e.g., emesis and gastric lavage). Activated charcoal should be administered, and if a nasogastric tube is required for the activated charcoal, pretreatment with atropine (0.02 mg/kg in children and 0.5 mg in adults) should be considered.

Digoxin-specific antibody fragments (Fab, Digibind) 38 mg binds 0.5 mg digoxin and then is excreted through the kidneys. The onset of action is within 30 minutes. Problems associated with Fab therapy are mainly from withdrawal of digoxin and worsening heart failure, hypokalemia, decrease in glucose (if the patient has low glycogen stores), and allergic reactions (very rare). Digitalis administered after Fab therapy is bound and may be inactivated for 5 to 7 days.

Absolute indications for Fab therapy include the following:

- Life-threatening malignant (hemodynamically unstable) dysrhythmias
- Ventricular dysrhythmias, unstable severe bradycardia, or second- or third-degree blocks unresponsive to atropine or rapid deterioration in clinical status
- Life-threatening digitoxin and oleander poisonings
- Relative indications for Fab therapy include the following:
- Ingestions greater than 4 mg in a child and 10 mg in an adult
- Serum potassium level greater than 5.0 mEq/L
- Serum digoxin level greater than 10 ng/mL in adults or greater than 5 ng/mL in children 6 hours after an acute ingestion
- Digitalis delirium and thrombocytopenia response

Digoxin-specific Fab fragments therapy can be administered as a bolus through a 22-μm filter if the case is a critical emergency. If the case is less urgent, then it can be administered over 30 minutes. An empiric dose is 10 vials in adults and 5 vials in a child for an unknown amount ingested in a symptomatic patient with history of a digoxin overdose.

To calculate the dose in the case of a known ingestion, the following equation is used:

$$\text{Amount (total mg)} \times (0.8) = \text{body burden}$$

If liquid capsules were taken or the substance was given intravenously the 80% bioavailability figure is not used. Instead, the body burden divided by 0.5 (0.5 mg digoxin is bound by 1 vial of 38 mg of Fab) equals the number of vials needed.

If the amount is unknown but the steady state serum concentration is known, the following equations are used:

For digoxin

$$\text{Digoxin ng/mL} \times (5.6 \text{ L/kg Vd}) \times (\text{wt kg}) = \text{mg body burden}$$

$$\text{Body burden} \div 1000 = \text{mg body burden}$$

$$\text{Body burden}/0.5 = \text{number of vials needed}$$

For digitoxin

$$\text{Digitoxin ng/mL} \times (0.56 \text{ L/kg Vd}) \times (\text{wt kg}) = \text{mg body burden}$$

$$\text{Body burden} \div 1000 = \text{mg body burden}$$

$$\text{Body burden}/0.5 = \text{number of vials needed}$$

Antidysrhythmic agents or a pacemaker should be used only if Fab therapy fails. For ventricular tachydysrhythmias, electrolyte disturbances should be corrected by the administration of lidocaine or phenytoin. For torsades de pointes, magnesium sulfate 20 mL 20% IV can be given slowly over 20 minutes (or 25 to 50 mg/kg in a child), titrated to control the dysrhythmia. Magnesium should be discontinued if hypotension, heart block, or decreased deep tendon reflexes are present. Magnesium is used with caution if the patient has renal impairment.

Unstable bradycardia and second-degree and third-degree atrioventricular block should be treated by Fab first. A pacemaker should be available if necessary. Isoproterenol should be avoided because it causes dysrhythmias. Cardioversion is used with caution, starting at a setting of 5 to 10 joules. The patient should be pretreated with lidocaine, if possible, because cardioversion may precipitate ventricular fibrillation or asystole.

Potassium disturbances are caused by a shift, not a change, in total body potassium. Hyperkalemia (>5.0 mEq/L) is treated with Fab only. Calcium must never be used, and insulin/glucose and sodium bicarbonate should not be used concomitantly with Fab because they may produce severe life-threatening hypokalemia. Sodium polystyrene sulfonate (Kayexalate) should not be used. Hypokalemia must be treated with caution because it may be cardioprotective. Treatment can be administered if the patient has ventricular dysrhythmias or a serum potassium level less than 3.0 mEq/L and atrioventricular block.

Extracorporeal procedures are ineffective. Hemodialysis is used for severe or refractory hyperkalemia.

One must never use antidysrhythmic types Ia (procainamide, quinidine, disopyramide [Norpace], amiodarone [Cordarone]), Ic (propafenone [Rythmol], flecainide [Tambocor]), II (β-blockers), or IV (calcium channel blockers). Class Ib drugs (lidocaine, phenytoin [Dilantin], mexiletine [Mexitil], and tocainide [Tonocard]) can be used.

Disposition

Consultation with a poison control center and a cardiologist experienced with digoxin-specific Fab fragments is warranted. All patients with significant dysrhythmias, symptoms, elevated serum digoxin concentration, or elevated serum potassium level should be admitted to the intensive care unit.

ETHANOL

Table 15 lists the features of alcohols and glycols.

Toxic Mechanism

Ethanol has CNS depressant and anesthetic effects. Ethanol stimulates the γ-aminobutyric acid (GABA) system. It promotes cutaneous vasodilation

TABLE 15 Summary of Alcohol and Glycol Features

	Methanol	Isopropanol	Ethanol	Ethylene Glycol
Principal uses	Gas line antifreeze, Sterno, windshield de-icer	Solvent jewelry cleaner, rubbing alcohol	Beverage, solvent	Radiator antifreeze, windshield de-icer
Specific gravity	0.719	0.785	0.789	1.12
Fatal dose	1 mL/Kg 100%	3 mL/kg 100%	5 mL/kg 100%	1.4 mL/kg
Inebriation	±	2+	2+	1+
Metabolic change		Hyperglycemia	Hypoglycemia	Hypocalcemia
Metabolic acidosis	4+	0	1+	2+
Anion gap	4+	±	2+	4+
Ketosis	Ketobutyric	Acetone	Hydroxybutyric	None
Gastrointestinal tract	Pancreatitis	Hemorrhagic gastritis	Gastritis	
Osmolality*	0.337	0.176	0.228	0.190

*1 mL/dL of substances raises freezing point osmolarity of serum. The validity of the correlation of osmolality with blood concentrations has been questioned.

(contributes to hypothermia), stimulates secretion of gastric juice (gastritis), inhibits the secretion of the antidiuretic hormone, inhibits gluconeogenesis (hypoglycemia), and influences fat metabolism (lipidemia).

Toxic Dose

A dose of 1 mL/kg of absolute ethanol (100% ethanol, or 200 proof) gives a blood ethanol concentration of 100 mg/dL. A potentially fatal dose is 3 g/kg for children or 6 g/kg for adults. Children are more prone to developing hypoglycemia than adults.

Kinetics

Onset of action is 30 to 60 minutes after ingestion; peak action is 90 minutes on empty stomach. Volume distribution is 0.6 L/kg. The major route of elimination (>90%) is by hepatic oxidative metabolism. The first step is by the enzyme alcohol dehydrogenase, which converts ethanol to acetaldehyde. Alcohol dehydrogenase metabolizes ethanol at a constant rate of 12 to 20 mg/dL/h (12 to 15 mg/dL/h in nondrinkers, 15 to 30 mg/dL/h in social drinkers, 30 to 50 mg/dL/h in heavy drinkers, and 25 to 30 mg/dL/h in children). At very low blood ethanol concentration (<30 mg/dL), the metabolism is by first-order kinetics. In the second step, acetaldehyde is metabolized by acetaldehyde dehydrogenase to acetic acid, which is metabolized by the Krebs cycle to carbon dioxide and water. The enzyme steps are nicotinamide adenine dinucleotide-dependent, which interferes with gluconeogenesis. Less than 10% of ethanol is excreted unchanged by the kidneys. The relationship between blood ethanol concentration (BEC) and dose (amount ingested) can be calculated as follows:

BEC (mg/dL) = amount ingested (mL) × % ethanol product × SG (0.79) / Vd (0.6 L/kg) × body wt (kg)

Dose (amount ingested) = BEC (mg/dL) × Vd (0.6) × body wt (kg) / % ethanol × specific gravity (0.79)

Manifestations

Table 16 lists the clinical signs of acute ethanol intoxication.

Chronic alcoholic patients tolerate higher blood ethanol concentration, and correlation with manifestations is not valid. Rapid interview for alcoholism is the CAGE questions:

- C—Have you felt the need to Cut down?
- A—Have others Annoyed you by criticism of your drinking?
- G—Have you felt Guilty about your drinking?
- E—Have you ever had morning Eye-opening drink to steady your nerves or get rid of a hangover?

Two affirmative answers indicate probable alcoholism.

TABLE 16 Clinical Signs in the Nontolerant Ethanol Drinker

Ethanol Blood Concentration (mg/dL)*	Manifestations
>25	Euphoria
>47	***Mild incoordination,*** sensory and motor impairment
>50	Increased risk of motor vehicle accidents
>100	Ataxia (legal toxic level in many localities)
>150	***Moderate incoordination,*** slow reaction time
>200	Drowsiness and confusion
>300	Severe incoordination, stupor, blurred vision
>500	***Flaccid coma,*** respiratory failure, hypotension; may be fatal

*Ethanol concentrations sometimes reported in %.

Note: mg% is not equivalent to mg/dL because ethanol weighs less than water (specific gravity 0.79). A 1% ethanol concentration is 790 mg/dL and 0.1% is 79 mg/dL. There is great variation in individual behavior at different blood ethanol levels. Behavior is dependent on tolerance and other factors.

Laboratory Investigations

The blood ethanol concentration should be specifically requested and followed. Gas chromatography or a breathanalyzer test gives rapid reliable results if no belching or vomiting is present. Enzymatic methods do not differentiate between the alcohols. ABG, electrolytes, and glucose should be measured, the anion and osmolar gaps determined (measure by freezing point depression, not vapor pressure), and a check for ketosis made.

Management

The examiner should inquire about trauma and disulfiram use. The patient must be protected from aspiration and hypoxia. Vital functions must be established and maintained. The patient may require intubation and assisted ventilation.

Gastrointestinal decontamination plays no role in the management of ethanol intoxication.

If the patient is comatose, glucose should be administered intravenously, 1 mL/kg 50% glucose in adults and 2 mL/kg 25% glucose in children. Thiamine, 100 mg intravenously, is administered if the patient has a history of chronic alcoholism, malnutrition, or suspected eating disorders to prevent Wernicke-Korsakoff syndrome. Naloxone (Narcan) has produced a partial inconsistent response but is not recommended for known alcoholics.

General supportive care includes administration of fluids to correct hydration and hypotension and correction of electrolyte abnormalities and acid–base imbalance. Vasopressors and plasma expanders may be necessary to correct severe hypotension. Hypomagnesemia is frequent in chronic alcoholics. In case of hypomagnesemia, a loading dose of 2 g magnesium sulfate 10% is administered by intravenous solution over 5 minutes in the intensive care unit with blood pressure and cardiac monitoring and calcium chloride 10% on hand in case of overdose. This is followed with constant infusion of 6 g of 10% solution over 3 to 4 hours. Caution must be taken with the use of magnesium if renal failure is present.

Hypothermic patients should be warmed. See the section on disturbances caused by cold.

Hemodialysis can be used in severe cases when conventional therapy is ineffective (rarely needed).

Repeated or prolonged seizures should be treated with diazepam (Valium). The brief "rum fits" do not need long-term anticonvulsant therapy. Repeated seizures or focal neurologic findings may warrant skull radiographs, lumbar puncture, and CT scan of the head, depending on the clinical findings. Withdrawal is treated with hydration and large doses of chlordiazepoxide (Librium) 50 to 100 mg or diazepam (Valium) 2 to 10 mg intravenously; these doses may be repeated in 2 to 4 hours. Very large doses of benzodiazepines may be required for delirium tremens. Withdrawal can occur in presence of elevated blood ethanol concentration and can be fatal if left untreated.

Chest radiograph is warranted to determine whether aspiration pneumonia is present. Renal and liver function tests and bilirubin level measurement should be made.

Disposition

Clinical severity (e.g., intubation, assisted ventilation, aspiration pneumonia) should determine the level of hospital care needed. Young children with significant unintentional exposure to ethanol (calculated to reach a blood ethanol concentration of 50 mg/dL) should have blood ethanol concentration obtained and blood glucose levels monitored for hypoglycemia frequently for 4 hours after ingestion. Patients with acute ethanol intoxication seldom require admission unless a complication is present. However, intoxicated patients should not be discharged until they are fully functional (can walk, talk, and think independently), have suicide potential evaluated, have proper disposition environment, and have a sober escort.

ETHYLENE GLYCOL

Ethylene glycol is found in solvents, de-icers, radiator antifreeze (95%), and air-conditioning units. Ethylene glycol is a sweet-tasting, colorless, water-soluble liquid with a sweet aromatic fragrance.

Toxic Mechanism

Ethylene glycol is oxidized by alcohol dehydrogenase to glycolaldehyde, which is metabolized to glycolic acid and glyoxylic acid. Glyoxylic acid is metabolized to oxalic acid via a pyridoxine-dependent pathway to glycine and by thiamine and magnesium-dependent pathways to α-hydroxy-ketoadipic acid. The metabolites of ethylene glycol produce a profound metabolic acidosis, increased anion gap, hypocalcemia, and oxalate crystals, which deposit in tissues (particularly the kidney).

Toxic Dose

The ingestion of 0.1 mL/kg 100% ethylene glycol can result in a toxic serum ethylene glycol concentration of 20 mg/dL. Ingestion of 3.0 mL (less than 1 teaspoonful or swallow) of a 100% solution in a 10-kg child or 30 mL of 100% ethylene glycol in an adult produces a serum ethylene glycol concentration of 50 mg/dL, a concentration that requires hemodialysis. The fatal amount is 1.4 mL/kg of 100% solution.

Kinetics

Absorption is via dermal, inhalation, and ingestion routes. Ethylene glycol is rapidly absorbed from the gastrointestinal tract. Onset is usually in 30 minutes but may be delayed by co-ingestion of food and ethanol. The usual peak level is at 2 hours. Volume distribution is 0.65 to 0.8 L/kg.

For metabolism, see *Toxic Mechanism.*

The half-life of ethylene glycol without ethanol is 3 to 8 hours; with ethanol, it is 17 hours, and with hemodialysis it is 2.5 hours. Renal clearance is 3.2 mL/kg/minute. About 20% to 50% is excreted unchanged in the urine. The relationship between serum ethylene glycol concentration (SEGC) and dose (amount ingested) can be calculated as follows:

0.12 mL/kg of 100% = SEGC 10 mg/dL

Manifestations

Phase I

The onset of manifestations is 30 minutes to several hours longer after ingestion with concomitant ethanol ingestion. The patient may be inebriated. Hypocalcemia, tetany, and calcium oxalate and hippuric acid crystals in urine can be seen within 4 to 8 hours but are not always present. Early, before metabolism of ethylene glycol, an osmolal gap may be present (see *Laboratory Investigations*). Later, the metabolites of ethylene glycol produce changes starting 4 to 12 hours following ingestion, including an anion gap, metabolic acidosis, coma, convulsions, cardiac disturbances, and pulmonary and cerebral edema. Because fluorescein is added to some antifreeze, the presence of fluorescence may be a clue to ethylene glycol exposure. However, it has been shown that fluorescent urine is not a reliable indicator of ethylene glycol ingestion and should not be used as a screen.

Phase II

After 12 to 36 hours, cardiopulmonary deterioration occurs, with pulmonary edema and congestive heart failure.

Phase III

Phase III occurs 36 to 72 hours after ingestion, with pulmonary edema and oliguric renal failure from oxalate crystal deposition and tubular necrosis predominating.

Phase IV

Neurologic sequelae may occur rarely, especially in patients who fail to receive early antidotal therapy. The onset ranges from 6 to 10 days after ingestion. Findings include facial diplegia, hearing loss, bilateral visual disturbances, elevated cerebrospinal fluid pressure with or without elevated protein levels and pleocytosis, vomiting, hyperreflexia, dysphagia, and ataxia.

Laboratory Investigations

Blood glucose and electrolytes should be monitored. Urinalysis should look for oxalate ("envelope") and monohydrate ("hemp seed") crystals. Urine fluorescence is not reliable as a screen. ABG, ethylene glycol, and ethanol levels, plasma osmolarity (using freezing point depression method), calcium, BUN, and creatinine should be measured. A serum ethylene glycol concentration of 20 mg/dL is toxic (ethylene glycol levels are very difficult to obtain). If possible, a glycolate level should be obtained. Cross-reactions with propylene glycol, a vehicle in many liquids and intravenous medications (phenytoin [Dilantin], diazepam [Valium]), other glycols, and triglycerides may produce spurious ethylene glycol levels. False-positive ethylene glycol values may occur with colorimetric or gas chromatography using an OV-17 column in the presence of propylene glycol.

The following equations can be used to calculate the osmolality, osmolal gap, and ethylene glycol level:

$$2(\text{Na+ mEq/L}) + (\text{Blood glucose mg/dL})/20 + (\text{BUN mg/dL})/3 = \text{Total calculated osmolality (mOsmL/L)}$$

$$\text{Osmolar Gap} = \text{measured osmolality (by freezing point depression method)} - \text{calculated osmolality}$$

A gap greater than 10 is abnormal. *Note:* if ethanol is involved, add ethanol level/4.6 to the calculated equation.

An increased osmolal gap is produced by the following common substances: acetone, dextran, dimethyl sulfoxide, diuretics, ethanol, ethyl ether, ethylene glycol, isopropanol, paraldehyde, mannitol, methanol, sorbitol, and trichloroethane. Table 10 gives the conversion factors for these substances.

Although a specific blood level of ethylene glycol in milligrams per deciliter can be estimated using the equation below, this is not considered to be a reliable method and should not take the place of obtaining a measured ethylene glycol blood concentration.

$$\text{osmolar gap} \times \text{conversion factor} = \text{serum concentration}$$

Caution: The accuracy of the ethylene glycol estimated decreases as the ethylene glycol levels decrease. The toxic metabolites are not osmotically active, and patients presenting late may show signs of severe toxicity without an elevated osmolar gap.

The anion gap can be calculated using the following equation:

$$\text{Na} - (\text{Cl} + \text{HCO}_3) = \text{anion gap}$$

The normal gap is 8 to 12. Potassium is not used because it is a small amount and may be hemolyzed. Table 8 lists factors that may account for an increased or a decreased anion gap.

Management

Vital functions should be established and maintained. The airway must be protected, and assisted ventilation can be used, if necessary. Gastrointestinal decontamination has a limited role. Only gastric aspiration can be used within 60 minutes after ingestion. Activated charcoal is not effective.

Baseline measurements of serum electrolytes and calcium, glucose, ABGs, ethanol, serum ethylene glycol concentration (may be difficult to obtain readily in some institutions), and methanol concentrations should be obtained. In the first few hours, the measured serum osmolality should be determined and compared to calculated osmolality (see osmolality equation, earlier). If seizures occur, one should measure serum calcium (preferably ionized calcium) and treat with intravenous diazepam. If the patient has hypocalcemic seizures, he or she should also be treated with 10 to 20 mL 10% calcium gluconate (0.2 to 0.3 mL/kg in children) slowly intravenously, with the dose repeated as needed. Metabolic acidosis should be corrected with intravenous sodium bicarbonate.

Ethanol therapy should be initiated immediately if fomepizole (Antizol) is unavailable (see next paragraph). Alcohol dehydrogenase has a greater affinity for ethanol than ethylene glycol. Therefore, ethanol blocks the metabolism of ethylene glycol. Ethanol therapy is called for if there is a history of ingestion of 0.1 mL/kg of 100% ethylene glycol, serum ethylene glycol concentration is greater than 20 mg/dL, there is an osmolar gap not accounted for by other alcohols or factors (e.g., hyperlipidemia), metabolic acidosis is present with an increased anion gap, or there are oxalate crystals in the urine. Ethanol should be administered intravenously (the oral route is less reliable) to produce a blood ethanol concentration of 100 to 150 mg/dL. The loading dose is 10 mL/kg of 10% ethanol intravenously, administered concomitantly with a maintenance dose of 10% ethanol of 1.0 mL/kg/h. This dose may need to be increased to 2 mL/kg/h in patients who are heavy drinkers. The blood ethanol concentration should be measured hourly and the infusion rate should be adjusted to maintain a blood ethanol concentration of 100 to 150 mg/dL.

Fomepizole (Antizol, 4-methylpyrazole) inhibits alcohol dehydrogenase more reliability than ethanol and it does not require constant monitoring of ethanol levels and adjustment of infusion rates. Fomepizole is available in 1 g/mL vials of 1.5 mL. The loading dose is 15 mg/kg (0.015 mL/kg) IV; maintenance dose is 10 mg/kg (0.01 mL/kg) every 12 hours for four doses, then 15 mg/kg every 12 hours until the ethylene glycol levels are less than 20 mg/dL. The solution is prepared by being mixed with 100 mL of 0.9% saline or D_5W (5% dextrose in water). Fomepizole can be given to patients requiring hemodialysis but should be dosed as follows:

Dose at the beginning of hemodialysis:

- If <6 hours since last Antizol dose, do not administer dose
- If >6 hours since last dose, administer next scheduled dose

Dosing during hemodialysis:

- Dose every 4 hours

Dosing at the time hemodialysis is completed:

- If <1 hour between last dose and end of dialysis, do not administer dose at end of dialysis
- If 1 to 3 hours between last dose and end of dialysis, administer one half of next scheduled dose
- If >3 hours between last dose and end of dialysis, administer next scheduled dose

Maintenance dosing off hemodialysis:

- Give the next scheduled dose 12 hours from the last dose administered

Hemodialysis is indicated if the ingestion was potentially fatal; if the serum ethylene glycol concentration is greater than 50 mg/dL (some recommend at levels of >25 mg/dL); if severe acidosis or electrolyte abnormalities occur despite conventional therapy; or if congestive heart failure or renal failure is present. Hemodialysis reduces the ethylene glycol half-life from 17 hours on ethanol therapy to 3 hours. Therapy (fomepizole and hemodialysis) should be continued until the serum ethylene glycol concentration is less than 10 mg/dL, the glycolate level is nondetectable (not readily available), the acidosis has cleared, there are no mental disturbances, the creatinine level is normal, and the urinary output is adequate. This may require 2 to 5 days.

Adjunct therapy involving thiamine, 100 mg/d (in children, 50 mg), slowly over 5 minutes intravenously or intramuscularly and repeated every 6 hours and pyridoxine, 50 mg IV or IM every 6 hours, has been recommended until intoxication is resolved, but these agents have not been extensively studied. Folate, 50 mg IV (child 1 mg/kg), can be given every 4 hours for 6 doses.

Disposition

All patients who have ingested significant amounts of ethylene glycol (calculated level above 20 mg/dL), have a history of a toxic dose, or are symptomatic should be referred to the emergency department and admitted. If the serum ethylene glycol concentration cannot be obtained, the patient should be followed for 12 hours, with monitoring of the osmolal gap, acid–base parameters, and electrolytes to exclude development of metabolic acidosis with an anion gap. Transfer should be considered for fomepizole therapy or hemodialysis.

HYDROCARBONS

The lower the viscosity and surface tension of hydrocarbons or the greater the volatility, the greater the risk of aspiration. Volatile substance abuse has produced the "Sudden Sniffing's Death Syndrome," most likely caused by dysrhythmias.

Toxicologic Classification and Toxic Mechanism

All systemically absorbed hydrocarbons can lower the threshold of the myocardium to dysrhythmias produced by endogenous and exogenous catecholamines.

Aliphatic hydrocarbons are branched straight chain hydrocarbons. A few aspirated drops are poorly absorbed from the gastrointestinal tract and produce no systemic toxicity by this route. However, aspiration of very small amounts can produce chemical pneumonitis. Examples of aliphatic hydrocarbons are gasoline, kerosene, charcoal lighter fluid, mineral spirits (Stoddard's solvent), and petroleum naphtha. Mineral seal oil (signal oil), found in furniture polishes, is a low-viscosity and low-volatility oil with minimum absorption that never warrants gastric decontamination. It can produce severe pneumonia if aspirated.

Aromatic hydrocarbons are six carbon ring structures that are absorbed through the gastrointestinal tract. Systemic toxicity includes CNS depression and, in cases of chronic abuse, multiple organ effects such as leukemia (benzene) and renal toxicity (toluene). Examples are benzene, toluene, styrene, and xylene. The seriously toxic ingested dose is 20 to 50 mL in adults.

Halogenated hydrocarbons are aliphatic or aromatic hydrocarbons with one or more halogen substitutions (Cl, Br, Fl, or I). They are highly volatile and are abused as inhalants. They are well absorbed from the gastrointestinal tract, produce CNS depression, and have metabolites that can damage the liver and kidneys. Examples include methylene chloride (may be converted into carbon monoxide in the body), dichloroethylene (also causes a disulfiram [Antabuse] reaction known as "degreaser's flush" when associated with consumption of ethanol), and 1,1,1-trichloroethane (Glamorene Spot Remover, Scotchgard, typewriter correction fluid). An acute lethal oral dose is 0.5 to 5 mL/kg.

Dangerous additives to the hydrocarbons can be summed up with the mnemonic CHAMP: C, camphor (demothing agent); H, halogenated hydrocarbons;

A, aromatic hydrocarbons; M, metals (heavy); and P, pesticides. Ingestion of these substances may warrant gastric emptying with a small-bore nasogastric tube.

Heavy hydrocarbons have high viscosity, low volatility, and minimal gastrointestinal absorption, so gastric decontamination is not necessary. Examples are asphalt (tar), machine oil, motor oil (lubricating oil, engine oil), home heating oil, and petroleum jelly (mineral oil).

Laboratory Investigations

The ECG, ABG, pulmonary function, serum electrolytes, and serial chest radiographs should be continuously monitored. Liver and renal function should be monitored in cases of inhalation of aromatic hydrocarbons.

Management

Asymptomatic patients who ingested small amounts of aliphatic petroleum distillates can be followed at home by telephone for development of signs of aspiration (cough, wheezing, tachypnea, and dyspnea) for 4 to 6 hours. Inhalation of any hydrocarbon vapors in a closed space can produce intoxication. The victim must be removed from the environment, have oxygen administered, and receive respiratory support.

Gastrointestinal decontamination is not advised in cases of hydrocarbon ingestion that usually do not cause systemic toxicity (aliphatic petroleum distillates, heavy hydrocarbons). In cases of ingestion of hydrocarbons that cause systemic toxicity in small amounts (aromatic hydrocarbons, halogenated hydrocarbons), the clinician should pass a small-bore nasogastric tube and aspirate if the ingestion was within 2 hours and if spontaneous vomiting has not occurred. Some toxicologists advocate ipecac-induced emesis under medical supervision instead of small-bore nasogastric gastric lavage; we do not.

Patients with altered mental status should have their airway protected because of concern about aspiration. The use of activated charcoal has been suggested, but there are no scientific data as to effectiveness and it may produce vomiting. Activated charcoal may, however, be useful in adsorbing toxic additives such as pesticides or co-ingestants.

The symptomatic patient who is coughing, gagging, choking, or wheezing on arrival has probably aspirated. The clinician should provide supportive respiratory care and supplemental oxygen, while monitoring pulse oximetry, ABG, chest radiograph, and ECG. The patient should be admitted to the intensive care unit. A chest radiograph for aspiration may be positive as early as 30 minutes after ingestion, and almost all are positive within 6 hours. Negative chest radiographs within 4 hours do not rule out aspiration.

Bronchospasm is treated with a nebulized β-adrenergic agonist and intravenous aminophylline if necessary. Epinephrine should be avoided because of susceptibility to dysrhythmias. Cyanosis in the presence of a normal arterial Pa_{O_2} may be a result of methemoglobinemia that requires therapy with methylene blue. Corticosteroids and prophylactic antimicrobial agents have not been shown to be beneficial. (Fever or leukocytosis may be produced by the chemical pneumonitis itself.)

Most infiltrations resolve spontaneously in 1 week; lipoid pneumonia may last up to 6 weeks. It is not necessary to surgically treat pneumatoceles that develop because they usually resolve. Dysrhythmias may require α- and β-adrenergic antagonists or cardioversion.

There is no role for enhanced elimination procedures.

Methylene chloride is metabolized over several hours to carbon monoxide. See treatment of carbon monoxide poisoning. Halogenated hydrocarbons are hepatorenal toxins; therefore, hepatorenal function should be monitored. *N*-acetylcysteine therapy may be useful if there is evidence of hepatic damage.

Extracorporal membrane oxygenation (ECMO) has been used successfully for a few patients with life threatening respiratory failure. Surfactant used for hydrocarbon aspiration was found to be detrimental.

Disposition

Asymptomatic patients with small ingestions of petroleum distillates can be managed at home. Symptomatic patients with abnormal chest radiographic, oxygen saturation, or ABG findings should be admitted. Patients who become asymptomatic and have normal oxygenation and a normal repeat radiograph can be discharged.

IRON

There are more than 100 iron over-the-counter preparations for supplementation and treatment of iron deficiency anemia.

Toxic Mechanism

Toxicity depends on the amount of elemental iron available in various salts (gluconate 12%, sulfate 20%, fumarate 33%, lactate 19%, chloride 21% of elemental iron), not the amount of the salt. Locally, iron is corrosive and may cause fluid loss, hypovolemic shock, and perforation. Excessive free unbound iron in the blood is directly toxic to the vasculature and leads to the release of vasoactive substances, which produces vasodilation. In cases of overdose, iron deposits injure mitochondria in the liver, the kidneys, and the myocardium. The exact mechanism of cellular damage is not clear but is thought to be related to free radical formation.

Toxic Dose

The therapeutic dose is 6 mg/kg/d of elemental iron. An elemental iron dose of 20 to 40 mg/kg may produce mild self-limited gastrointestinal symptoms, 40 to 60 mg/kg produces moderate toxicity, more than 60 mg/kg produces severe toxicity and is potentially lethal, and more than 180 mg/kg is usually fatal without treatment. Children's chewable vitamins with iron have between 12 and 18 mg of elemental iron per tablet or 0.6 mL of liquid drops. These preparations rarely produce toxicity unless very large quantities are ingested and have never caused death.

Kinetics

Absorption occurs chiefly in the upper small intestine. Ferrous (+2) iron is absorbed into the mucosal cells, where it is oxidized to the ferric (+3) state and bound to ferritin. Iron is slowly released from ferritin into the plasma, where it binds to transferrin and is transported to specific tissues for production of hemoglobin (70%), myoglobin (5%), and cytochrome. About 25% of iron is stored in the liver and spleen. In cases of overdose, larger amounts of iron are absorbed because of direct mucosal corrosion. There is no mechanism for the elimination of iron (elimination is 1 to 2 mg/d) except through bile, sweat, and blood loss.

Manifestations

Serious toxicity is unlikely if the patient remains asymptomatic for 6 hours and has a negative abdominal radiograph. Iron intoxication can produce five phases of toxicity. The phases may not be distinct from one another.

Phase I

Gastrointestinal mucosal injury occurs 30 minutes to 12 hours postingestion. Vomiting starts within 30 minutes to 1 hour of ingestion and is persistent; hematemesis and bloody diarrhea may occur; abdominal cramps, fever, hyperglycemia, and leukocytosis may occur. Enteric-coated tablets may pass through the stomach without causing symptoms. Acidosis and shock can occur within 6 to 12 hours.

Phase II

A latent period of apparent improvement occurs over 8 to 12 hours postingestion.

Phase III

Systemic toxicity phase occurs 12 to 48 hours postingestion with cardiovascular collapse and severe metabolic acidosis.

Phase IV

Two to 4 days postingestion, hepatic injury associated with jaundice, elevated liver enzymes, and prolonged prothrombin time occur. Kidney injury with proteinuria and hematuria occur. Pulmonary edema, disseminated intravascular coagulation, and *Yersinia enterocolitica* sepsis can occur.

Phase V

Four to 8 weeks postingestion, pyloric outlet or intestinal stricture may cause obstruction or anemia secondary to blood loss.

Laboratory Investigations

Iron poisoning produces anion gap metabolic acidosis. Monitoring should include complete blood cell counts, blood glucose level, serum iron, stools and vomitus for occult blood, electrolytes, acid–base balance, urinalysis and urinary output, liver function tests, and BUN and creatinine levels. Blood type and match should be obtained.

Serum iron measurements taken at the proper time correlate with the clinical findings. The lavender top Vacutainer tube contains EDTA, which falsely lowers serum iron. One must obtain the serum iron measurement before administering deferoxamine. Serum iron levels of less than 350 μg/dL at 2 to 6 hours predict an asymptomatic course; levels of 350 to 500 μg/dL are usually associated with mild gastrointestinal symptoms; those greater than 500 μg/dL have a 20% risk of shock and serious iron toxicity. A follow-up serum iron measurement after 6 hours may not be elevated even in cases of severe poisoning, but a serum iron measurement taken at 8 to 12 hours is useful to exclude delayed absorption from a bezoar or sustained-release preparation. The total iron-binding capacity is not necessary.

Adult iron tablet preparations are radiopaque before they dissolve by 4 hours postingestion. A "negative" abdominal radiograph more than 4 hours postingestion does not exclude iron poisoning.

Patients who develop high fevers and signs of sepsis following iron overdose should have blood and stool cultures checked for *Yersinia enterocolitica*.

Management

Gastrointestinal decontamination should involve immediate induction of emesis in cases of ingestions of elemental iron of greater than 40 mg/kg if vomiting has not already occurred. Activated charcoal is ineffective. An abdominal radiograph should be obtained after emesis to determine the success of gastric emptying. Children's chewable vitamins and liquid iron preparations are not radiopaque. If radiopaque iron is still present, whole-bowel irrigation with polyethylene glycol solution should be considered. In extreme cases, removal by endoscopy or surgery may be necessary because coalesced iron tablets produce hemorrhagic infarction in the bowel and perforation peritonitis.

Deferoxamine (Desferal) in a dose of about 100 mg binds 8.5 to 9.35 mg of free iron in the serum. The deferoxamine infusion should not exceed 15 mg/kg/h or 6 g daily, but faster rates (up to 45 mg/kg) and larger daily amounts have been administered and tolerated in extreme cases of iron poisoning

(>1000 mg/dL). The deferoxamine-iron complex is hemodialyzable if renal failure develops.

Indications for chelation therapy are any of the following:

- Very large, symptomatic ingestions
- Serious clinical intoxication (severe vomiting and diarrhea [often bloody], severe abdominal pain, metabolic acidosis, hypotension, or shock)
- Symptoms that persist or progress to more serious toxicity
- Serum iron level greater than 500 mg/dL

Chelation should be performed as early as possible within 12 to 18 hours to be effective. One should start the infusion slowly and gradually increase to avoid hypotension.

Adult respiratory distress syndrome has developed in patients with high doses of deferoxamine for several days; infusions longer than 24 hours should be avoided.

The endpoint of treatment is when the patient is asymptomatic and the urine clears if it was originally a positive "vin rosé" color.

For supportive therapy, intravenous bicarbonate may be needed to correct the metabolic acidosis. Hypotension and shock treatment may require volume expansion, vasopressors, and blood transfusions. The physician should attempt to keep the urinary output at greater than 2 mL/kg/h. Coagulation abnormalities and overt bleeding require blood products or vitamin K. Pregnant patients are treated in a fashion similar to any other patient with iron poisoning.

Hemodialysis and hemoperfusion are ineffective. Exchange transfusion has been used in single cases of massive poisonings in children.

Disposition

The asymptomatic or minimally symptomatic patient should be observed for persistence and progression of symptoms or development of toxicity signs (gastrointestinal bleeding, acidosis, shock, altered mental state). Patients with mild self-limited gastrointestinal symptoms who become asymptomatic or have no signs of toxicity for 6 hours are unlikely to have a serious intoxication and can be discharged after psychiatric clearance, if needed. Patients with moderate or severe toxicity should be admitted to the intensive care unit.

ISONIAZID

Isoniazid is a hydrazide derivative of vitamin B_3 (nicotinamide) and is used as an antituberculosis drug.

Toxic Mechanism

Isoniazid produces pyridoxine deficiency by increasing the excretion of pyridoxine (vitamin B_6) and by inhibiting pyridoxal 5-phosphate (the active form of pyridoxine) from acting with L-glutamic acid decarboxylase to form γ-aminobutyric acid (GABA), the major CNS neurotransmitter inhibitor, resulting in seizures. Isoniazid also blocks the conversion of lactate to pyruvate, resulting in profound and prolonged lactic acidosis.

Toxic Dose

The therapeutic dose is 5 to 10 mg/kg (maximum 300 mg) daily. A single acute dose of 15 mg/kg lowers the seizure threshold; 35 to 40 mg/kg produces spontaneous convulsions; more than 80 mg/kg produces severe toxicity. A fatal dose in adults is 4.5 to 15 g. The malnourished patients, those with a previous seizure disorder, alcoholic patients, and slow acetylators are more susceptible to isoniazid toxicity. In cases of chronic intoxication, 10 mg/kg/d produces hepatitis in 10% to 20% of patients but less than 2% at doses of 3 to 5 mg/kg/d.

Kinetics

Absorption from intestine occurs in 30 to 60 minutes, and onset is in 30 to 120 minutes, with peak levels of 5 to 8 μg/mL within 1 to 2 hours. Volume distribution is 0.6 L/kg, with minimal protein binding.

Elimination is by liver acetylation to a hepatotoxic metabolite, acetyl-isoniazid, which is then hydrolyzed to isonicotinic acid. In slow acetylators, isoniazid has a half-life of 140 to 460 minutes (mean 5 hours), and 10% to 15% is eliminated unchanged in the urine. Most (45% to 75%) whites and 50% of African blacks are slow acetylators, and, with chronic use (without pyridoxine supplements), they may develop peripheral neuropathy. In fast acetylators, isoniazid has a half-life of 35 to 110 minutes (mean 80 minutes), and 25% to 30% is excreted unchanged in the urine. About 90% of Asians and patients with diabetes mellitus are fast acetylators and may develop hepatitis on chronic use.

In patients with overdose and hepatic disease, the serum half-life may increase. Isoniazid inhibits the metabolism of phenytoin (Dilantin), diazepam, phenobarbital, carbamazepine (Tegretol), and prednisone. These drugs also interfere with the metabolism of isoniazid. Ethanol may decrease the half-life of isoniazid but increase its toxicity.

Manifestations

Within 30 to 60 minutes, nausea, vomiting, slurred speech, dizziness, visual disturbances, and ataxia are present. Within 30 to 120 minutes, the major clinical triad of severe overdose includes refractory convulsions (90% of overdose patients have one or more seizures), coma, and resistant severe lactic acidosis (secondary to convulsions), often with a plasma pH of 6.8.

Laboratory Investigations

Isoniazid produces anion gap metabolic acidosis. Therapeutic levels are 5 to 8 μg/mL and acute toxic levels are greater than 20 μg/mL. These levels are not readily available to assist in making decisions in acute overdose situations. One should monitor the blood glucose (often hyperglycemia), electrolytes (often hyperkalemia), bicarbonate, ABGs, liver function tests (elevations occur with chronic exposure), BUN, and creatinine.

Management

Seizures must be controlled. Pyridoxine and diazepam should be administered concomitantly through different IV sites. Pyridoxine (vitamin B_6) is given in a dose of 1 g for each gram of isoniazid ingested. If the dose ingested is unknown, at least 5 g of pyridoxine should be given intravenously. Pyridoxine is administered in 50 mL D_5W or 0.9% saline over 5 minutes intravenously. It must not be administered in the same bottle as sodium bicarbonate. Intravenous pyridoxine is repeated every 5 to 20 minutes until the seizures are controlled. Total doses of pyridoxine up to 52 g have been safely administered; however, patients given 132 and 183 g of pyridoxine have developed a persistent crippling sensory neuropathy.

Diazepam is administered concomitantly with pyridoxine but at a different site. They work synergistically. Diazepam should be administered intravenously slowly, 0.3 mg/kg at a rate of 1 mg/min in children or 10 mg at a rate of 5 mg/min in adults. After the seizures are controlled, the remainder of the pyridoxine is administered (1 g/1 g isoniazid) or a total dose of 5 g.

Phenobarbital or phenytoin are ineffective and should not be used.

In asymptomatic patients or patients without seizures, pyridoxine has been advised by some toxicologists prophylactically in gram-for-gram doses in cases of large overdoses (<80 mg/kg per dose) of isoniazid, although there are no studies to support this recommendation. In comatose patients, pyridoxine administration may result in the patient's rapid regaining of consciousness. Correction of acidosis may occur spontaneously with pyridoxine administration and correction of the seizures. Sodium bicarbonate should be administered if acidosis persists.

Hemodialysis is rarely needed because of antidotal therapy and the short half-life of isoniazid, but it may be used as an adjunct for cases of uncontrollable acidosis and seizures. Hemoperfusion has not been adequately evaluated. Diuresis is ineffective.

Disposition

Asymptomatic or mildly symptomatic patients who become asymptomatic can be observed in the emergency department for 4 to 6 hours. Larger amounts of isoniazid may warrant pyridoxine administration and longer periods of observation. Intentional ingestions necessitate psychiatric evaluation before the patient is discharged. Patients with convulsions or coma should be admitted to the intensive care unit.

ISOPROPANOL (ISOPROPYL ALCOHOL)

Isopropanol can be found in rubbing alcohol, solvents, and lacquer thinner. Coma has occurred in children sponged for fever with isopropanol. See Table 10 for ethanol features of alcohols and glycols.

Toxic Mechanism

Isopropanol is a gastric irritant. It is metabolized to acetone, a CNS and myocardial depressant. It inhibits gluconeogenesis. Normal propyl alcohol is related to isopropyl alcohol but is more toxic.

Toxic Dose

A toxic dose of 0.5 to 1 mg/kg of 70% isopropanol (1 mL/kg of 70%) produces a blood isopropanol plasma concentration of 70 mg/dL. The CNS depressant potency is twice that of ethanol.

Kinetics

Onset of action is within 30 to 60 minutes, and peak is 1 hour postingestion. Volume distribution is 0.6 kg/L. Isopropyl alcohol metabolizes to acetone. Its excretion is renal.

Note: The serum isopropyl concentration and amount ingested can be estimated using the same equation as is used in ethanol kinetics and substituting the specific gravity of 0.785 for isopropyl alcohol.

Manifestations

Ethanol-like inebriation occurs, with an acetone odor to the breath, gastritis, occasionally with hematemesis, acetonuria, and acetonemia without systemic acidosis.

Depression of the CNS occurs: lethargy at blood isopropyl alcohol levels of 50 to 100 mg/dL, coma at levels of 150 to 200 mg/dL, potentially death in adults at levels greater than 240 mg/dL.

Hypoglycemia and seizures may occur.

Laboratory Investigation

Monitoring of blood isopropyl alcohol levels (not readily available in all institutions), acetone, glucose, and ABG should be maintained. The osmolal gap increases 1 mOsm per 5.9 mg/dL of isopropyl alcohol and 1 mOsm per 5.5 mg/dL of acetone. The absence of excess acetone in the blood (normal is 0.3 to 2 mg/dL) within 30 to 60 minutes or excess acetone in the urine within 3 hours excludes the possibility of significant isopropanol exposure.

Management

The airway must be protected with intubation, and assisted ventilation administered if necessary. If the patient is hypoglycemic, glucose should be administered. Supportive treatment is similar to that for ethanol ingestions.

Gastrointestinal decontamination has no role in the treatment of isopropanol ingestion. Hemodialysis is warranted in cases of life-threatening overdose but is rarely needed. A nephrologist should be consulted if the blood isopropanol plasma concentration is greater than 250 mg/dL.

Disposition

Symptomatic patients with concentrations greater than 100 mg/dL require at least 24 hours of close observation for resolution and should be admitted. If the patient is hypoglycemic, hypotensive, or comatose, he or she should be admitted to the intensive care unit.

LEAD

Acute lead intoxication is rare and usually occurs by inhalation of lead, resulting in severe intoxication and often death. Lead fumes can be produced by burning of lead batteries or use of a heat gun to remove lead paint. Acute lead intoxication also occurs from exposure to high concentrations of organic lead (e.g., tetraethyl lead).

Chronic lead poisoning occurs most often in children 6 months to 6 years of age who are exposed in their environment and in adults in certain occupations (Table 17). In the United States, the prevalence in children aged 1 to 5 years with a venous blood lead greater than 10 μg/dL decreased from 88.2% in a 1976-1980 survey to 8.9% in a 1988-1991 survey as a consequence of measures to reduce lead in the environment, particularly leaded gasoline. However, an estimated 1.7 million children between 1 and 5 years of age and more than 1 million workers in over 100 different occupations still have blood lead levels greater than 10 μg/dL.

Toxic Dose

In cases of chronic lead poisoning, a daily intake of more than 5 μg/kg/d in children or more than 150 μg/d in adults can give a positive lead balance. In 1991, the Centers for Disease Control and Prevention (CDC) recommended routine screening for all children younger than 6 years of age. In children a venous blood level greater than 10 μg/dL was determined to be a threshold of concern. The average venous blood level in the United States is 4 μg/dL. In cases of occupational exposure (see Table 17), a venous blood level greater than 40 μg/dL is indicative of increased lead absorption in adults.

Toxic Mechanism

Lead affects the sulfhydryl enzyme systems, the immature CNS, the enzymes of heme synthesis, vitamin D conversion, the kidneys, the bones, and growth. Lead alters the tertiary structure of cell proteins by denaturing them and causing cell death. Risk factors are mouthing behavior of infants and children and excessive oral behavior (pica), living in the inner city, a poorly maintained home, and poor nutrition (e.g., low calcium and iron). The CDC questionnaire given in Table 18 is recommended at every pediatric visit. If any answers to the CDC questionnaire are "positive," a blood screening test for lead should be administered. To be more accurate, however, identifying lead exposure studies have suggested that the questionnaire will have to be modified for each individual community because it has had poor sensitivity (40%) and specificity (60%) as it stands.

Table 19 lists sources of lead. The number one source is deteriorating lead-based paint, which forms leaded dust. Lead concentrations in indoor paint were not reduced to safer (0.06%) levels until 1978. Lead can also be produced by improper interior or exterior home renovation (scraping or demolition). It is found in pre-1960 built homes. The use of leaded gasoline (limited in 1973) resulted in residue from leaded motor vehicle emissions. Lead persists in the soil near major highways and in deteriorating homes and buildings. Vegetables grown in contaminated soil may contain lead.

Oil refineries and lead-processing smelters produce lead residue. Food cans produced in Mexico

TABLE 17 Occupations Associated with Lead Exposure

Lead production or smelting	Demolition of ships and bridges
Production of illicit whiskey	Battery manufacturing
Brass, copper, and lead foundries	Machining/grinding lead alloys
Radiator repair	Welding of old painted metals
Scrap handling	Thermal paint stripping of old buildings
Sanding of old paint	Ceramic glaze/pottery mixing
Lead soldering	
Cable stripping	
Worker or janitor at a firing range	

Modified from Rempel D: The lead-exposed worker. JAMA 262:533, 1989.

TABLE 18 CDC Questionnaire: Priority Groups for Lead Screening

1. Children age 6–72 months (was 12–36 months) who live in or are frequent visitors to older, deteriorated housing built before 1960.
2. Children age 6–72 months who live in housing built prior to 1960 with recent, ongoing, or planned renovation or remodeling.
3. Children age 6–72 months who are siblings, housemates, or playmates of children with known lead poisoning.
4. Children age 6–72 months whose parents or other house hold members participate in a lead-related industry or hobby.
5. Children age 6–72 months who live near active lead smelters, battery recycling plants, or other industries likely to result in atmospheric lead release.

TABLE 19 Sources of Lead

Product	Lead Content (%) by Dry Weight
Paint	0.06
Solder	0.6
Plastic additives	2.0
Priming inks	2.0
Plumbing fixtures	2.0
Pesticides	0.1
Stained glass came	0.1
Wine bottle foils	0.1
Construction material	0.1
Fertilizers	0.1
Glazes, enamels	0.06
Toys/recreational games	0.1
Curtain weights	0.1
Fishing weights	0.1

contain lead solder (95% do not in United States). Lead water pipes (until 1950) and lead solder (until 1986) deliver lead-containing drinking water (calcium deposits, however, may offer some protection). Water at a consumer's tap should be contain less than 15 parts per billion (ppb) of lead (Table 20).

For occupational exposure, see Table 17. The Occupational Safety and Health Administration (OSHA) standards require employers to provide showering and clothes changing facilities for personnel working with lead; however, businesses with fewer than 25 employees are exempt from the regulation. The OSHA lead standard of 1978 set a limit of 60 μg/dL for occupational exposure to lead. At a blood lead level of 60 μg/dL, a worker should be removed from lead exposure and not allowed back until his or her lead level is below 40 μg/dL. Many authorities believe that this level should be lower. The lead residue on the clothes of the workers may represent a hazard to the family. Other occupations that are potential sources of lead exposure include plumbers, pipe fitters, lead miners, auto repairers, shipbuilders, printers, steel welders and cutters, construction workers, and rubber product manufacturers.

Leaded pots to make molds for "kusmusha" tea represent lead exposure. Imported pottery lined with ceramic glaze can leach large amounts of lead into acids (e.g., citrus fruit juices).

Hobbies associated with lead exposure are listed in Table 21. Some "traditional" folk remedies or cosmetics that contain lead include the following:

- "Azarcon por empacho" ("Maria Louisa" 90 to 95% lead trioxide): a bright orange powder used in Hispanic culture, especially Mexican, for digestive problems and diarrhea.
- "Greta" (4% to 90% lead): a yellow powder "por empacho" ("empacho" refers to a variety of gastrointestinal symptoms), used in Hispanic cultures, especially Mexican.
- "Pay-loo-ah": an orange-red powder used for rash and fever in Southeast Asian cultures, especially among Northern Laos Hmong immigrants.
- "Alkohl" (Al-kohl, kohl, suma 5% to 92% lead): a black powder used in Middle Eastern, African, and Asian cultures as a cosmetic and an umbilical stump astringent.
- "Farouk": an orange granular powder with lead used in Saudi Arabian culture.
- "Bint Al Zahab": used to treat colic in Saudi Arabian culture.
- "Surma" (23% to 26% lead): a black powder used in India as a cosmetic and to improve eyesight.
- "Bali goli": a round black bean that is dissolved in "grippe water," used by Asian and Indian cultures to aid digestion.

Cases of substance abuse involving lead poisoning have been reported, in which the patient sniffs

TABLE 20 Agency Regulations and Recommendations Concerning Lead Content

Agency	Specimen	Level	Comments
CDC	Blood (child)	10 μg/dL	Investigate community
OSHA	Blood (adult)	60 μg/dL	Medical removal from work
OSHA	Air	50 μg/m³	PEL*
	Air	0.75 μg/m³	Tetraethyl or tetramethyl
ACGIH	Air	150 μg/m³	TWA†
EPA	Air	1.5 μg/m³	Three-month average
EPA	Water	15 μg/L (ppb)	5 ppb circulating
EPA	Food	100 μg/d	Advisory
FDA	Wine	300 ppm	Plan to reduce to 200 ppm
EPA	Soil/dust	50 ppm	
CPSC	Paint	600 ppm (0.06%) by dry weight	

Abbreviatons: ACGIH = American Conference of Governmental Industrial Hygienists; CDC = Centers for Disease Control and Prevention; CPSC = Consumer Product Safety Commission; EPA = Environmental Protection Agency; FDA = Food and Drug Administration; OSHA = Occupational Safety and Health Administration.

*PEL = permissible exposure limit (highest level over an 8-hour workday).

†TWA = time-weighted average (air concentration for 8-hour workday and 40 hour workweek).

TABLE 21 Hobbies Associated with Lead Exposure

Casting of ammunition	Print making and other fine arts (when lead white, flake white, chrome yellow pigments are involved)
Collecting antique pewter	Liquor distillation
Collecting/painting lead toys (e.g., soldiers and figures)	Hunting and target shooting
Ceramics or glazed pottery	Painting
Refinishing furniture	Car and boat repair
Making fishing weights	Burning/engraving lead-painted wood
Home renovation	Making stained leaded glass
Jewelry making, lead solder	Copper enameling
Glass blowing, lead glass	
Bronze casting	

leaded gasoline or uses improperly synthesized amphetamines.

Kinetics

Absorption of lead is 10% to 15% of the ingested dose in adults; in children, up to 40% is absorbed, especially in cases of iron deficiency anemia. With inhalation of fumes, absorption is rapid and complete. Volume distribution in blood (0.9% of total body burden) is 95% in red blood cells. Lead passes through the placenta to the fetus and is present in breast milk.

Organic lead is metabolized in the liver to inorganic lead. Its half-life is 35 to 40 days in blood; in soft tissue, the half-life is 45 days and in bone (99% of the lead), the half-life is 28 years. The major elimination route is the stool, 80% to 90%, and then renal 10% (80 g/d) and hair, nails, sweat, and saliva. Nine percent of organic lead is excreted in the urine per day.

TABLE 22 Summary of Lead-Induced Health Effects in Adults and Children

Blood Lead Level (μg/dL)	Age Group	Health Effect
>100	Adult	Encephalopathic signs and symptoms
>80	Adult	Anemia
	Child	Encephalopathy Chronic nephropathy (e.g., aminoaciduria)
>70	Adult	Clinically evident peripheral neuropathy
	Child	Colic and other gastrointestinal symptoms
>60	Adult	Female reproductive effects CNS disturbance symptoms (i.e., sleep disturbances, mood changes, memory and concentration problems, headaches)
>50	Adult	Decreased hemoglobin production Decreased performance on neurobehavioral tests
	Adult	Altered testicular function Gastrointestinal symptoms (i.e., abdominal pain, constipation, diarrhea, nausea, anorexia)
	Child	Peripheral neuropathy*
>40	Adult	Decreased peripheral nerve conduction Hypertension, age 40–59 years Chronic neuropathy*
>25	Adult	Elevated erythrocyte protoporphyrin in males
15–25	Adult	Elevated erythrocyte protoporphyrin in females
>10	Child	Decreased intelligence and growth Impaired learning Reduced birth weight* Impaired mental ability
	Fetus	Preterm delivery

*Controversial.

From Anonymous: Implementation of the Lead Contamination Control Act of 1988. MMWR Morb Mortal Wkly Rep 41:288, 1992.

Manifestations

Adverse health effects are given in Table 22 and include the following.

Hematologic

Lead inhibits γ-aminolevulinic acid dehydratase (early in the synthesis of heme) and ferrochelatase (transfers iron to ferritin for incorporation of iron into protoporphyrin to produce heme). Anemia is a late finding. Decreased heme synthesis starts at >40 μg/dL. Basophilic stippling occurs in 20% of severe lead poisoning.

Neurologic

Segmental demyelination and peripheral neuropathy, usually of the motor type (wrist and ankle drop) occurs in workers. A venous blood level of lead greater than 70 μg/dL (usually >100 μg/dL), produces encephalopathy in children (symptom mnemonic "PAINT": P, persistent forceful vomiting and papilledema; A, ataxia; I, intermittent stupor and lucidity; N, neurologic coma and refractory convulsions; T, tired and lethargic). Decreased cognitive abilities have been reported with a venous blood level of lead greater than 10 μg/dL, including behavioral problems, decreased attention span, and learning disabilities. IQ scores may begin to decrease at 15 μg/dL. Encephalopathy is rare in adults.

Renal

Nephropathy as a result of damaged capillaries and glomerulus can occur at a venous blood level of lead greater than 80 μg/dL, but recent studies show renal damage and hypertension with low venous blood levels. A direct correlation between hypertension and venous blood level over 30 μg/dL has been reported. Lead reduces excretion of uric acid, and high-level exposure may be associated with hyperuricemia and "saturnine gout," Fanconi's syndrome (aminoaciduria and renal tubular acidosis), and tubular fibrosis.

Reproductive

Spontaneous abortion, transient delay in the child's development (catch up at age 5 to 6 years), decreased sperm count, and abnormal sperm morphology can occur with lead exposure. Lead crosses the placenta and fetal blood levels reach 75% to 100% of maternal blood levels. Lead is teratogenic.

Metabolic

Decreased cytochrome P450 activity alters the metabolism of medication and endogenously produced substances. Decreased activation of cortisol and decreased growth is caused by interference in vitamin conversion (25-hydroxyvitamin D to 1,25 hydroxyvitamin D) at venous blood levels of 20 to 30 μg/dL.

Other Manifestations

Abnormalities of thyroid, cardiac, and hepatic function occur in adults. Abdominal colic is seen in children at doses greater than 50 μg/dL. "Lead gum lines" at the dental border of the gingiva can occur in cases of chronic lead poisoning.

Laboratory Investigations

Serial venous blood lead measurements are taken on days 3 and 5 during treatment and 7 days after chelation therapy, then every 1 to 2 weeks for 8 weeks, and then every month for 6 months. Intravenous infusion should be stopped at least 1 hour before blood lead levels are measured. Table 23 gives a classification of blood lead concentrations in children.

One should evaluate CBC, serum ferritin, erythrocyte protoporphyrin (>35 μg/dL indicates lead poisoning as well as iron deficiency and other causes), electrolytes, serum calcium and phosphorus, urinalysis, BUN, and creatinine. Abdominal and long bone radiographs may be useful in certain circumstances to identify radiopaque material in bowel and "lead lines" in proximal tibia (which occur after prolonged exposure in association with venous blood lead levels greater than 50 μg/dL).

Neuropsychological tests are difficult to perform in young children but should be considered at the end of treatment, especially to determine auditory dysfunction.

TABLE 23 Classification of Blood Lead Concentrations in Children

Blood Lead (μg/dL)	Recommended Interventions
<9	None
10–14	Community intervention Repeat blood lead in 3 months
15–19	Individual case management Environmental counseling Nutritional counseling Repeat blood lead in 3 months
20–44	Medical referral Environmental inspection/abatement Nutritional counseling Repeat blood lead in 3 months
45–69	Environmental inspection/abatement Nutritional counseling Pharmacologic therapy DMSA succimer oral or $CaNa_2EDTA$ parenteral Repeat every 2 weeks for 6–8 weeks, then monthly for 4–6 months
>70	Hospitalization in intensive care unit Environmental inspection/abatement Pharmacologic therapy Dimercaprol (BAL in oil) IM initial alone Dimercaprol IM and $CaNa_2EDTA$ together Repeat every week

Abbreviations: BAL = British anti-Lewisite; $CaNa_2EDTA$ = Edetate calcium disodium; DMS = dimercaptosuccinic acid; IM = intramuscular.

Management

The basis of treatment is removal of the source of lead. Cases of poisoning in children should be reported to local health department and cases of occupational poisoning should be reported to OSHA. The source must be identified and abated, and dust controlled by wet mopping. Cold water should be let to run for 2 minutes before being used for drinking. Planting shrubbery (not vegetables) in contaminated soil will keep children away.

Supportive care should be instituted, including measures to deal with refractory seizures (continued antidotal therapy, diazepam, and possibly neuromuscular blockers), with the hepatic and renal failure, and intravascular hemolysis in severe cases. Seizures are treated with diazepam followed by neuromuscular blockers if needed.

Lead does not bind to activated charcoal. One must not delay chelation therapy for complete gastrointestinal decontamination in severe cases. Whole-bowel irrigation has been used prior to treatment. Some authorities recommend abdominal radiographs followed by gastrointestinal decontamination if necessary before switching to oral therapy. Chelation therapy can be used for patients in whom venous blood level of lead is greater than 45 μg/dL in children and greater than 80 μg/dL in adults or in adults with lower levels who are symptomatic or who have a "positive" lead mobilization test result (not routinely performed at most centers) (Table 24).

Succimer (dimercaptosuccinic acid, DMSA, Chemet), a derivative of British anti-Lewisite (BAL), is an oral agent for chelation in children with a venous blood level of greater than 45 μg/dL. The recommended dose is 10 mg/kg every 8 hours for 5 days, then every 12 hours for 14 days. DMSA is under investigation to determine its role in children with a venous blood level less than 45 μg/dL. Although not approved for adults, it has been used in the same dosage. Monitoring should be maintained by CBC, liver transaminases, and urinalysis for adverse effects.

TABLE 24 Pharmacologic Chelation Therapy of Lead Poisoning

Drug	Route	Dose	Duration	Precautions	Monitor
Dimercaprol (BAL in oil)	IM	3–5 mg/kg q4–6h	3–5 days	G6PD deficiency Concurrent iron therapy	AST/ALT enzymes
$CaNa_2EDTA$ (calcium disodium. versenate)	IM/IV	50 mg/kg per day	5 days	Inadequate fluid intake Renal impairment	Urinalysis, BUN Creatinine
D-Penicillamine (Cuprimine)	PO	10 mg/kg per day increase 30 mg/kg over 2 weeks	6–20 weeks	Penicillin allergy Concurrent iron therapy; lead exposure Renal impairment	Urinalysis, BUN Creatinine, CBC
2,3-Dimercap-tosuccinic acid (DMSA; succimer)	PO	10 mg/kg per dose tid, 10mg/kg per dose bid 14 days	19 days	AST/ALT Concurrent iron therapy G6PD deficiency lead exposure	AST/ALT

Abbreviations: ALT = alanine aminotransferase; AST = aspartate transaminase; BAL = British anti-Lewisite; bid = twice daily; BUN = blood urea nitrogen; CBC = complete blood count; G6PD = glucose-6-phosphate dehydrogenase; IM = intramuscular; IV = intravenous; PO = oral; tid = three times daily.

D-Penicillamine (Cuprimine) is another oral chelator that is given in doses of 20 to 40 mg/kg/d not to exceed 1 g/d. However, it is not FDA approved and has a 10% adverse reaction rate. Nevertheless, D-penicillamine has been used infrequently in adults and children with elevated venous blood lead levels.

Edetate calcium disodium (ethylene diaminetetra-acetic acid or $CaNa_2EDTA$ Versenate) is a water-soluble chelator given intramuscularly (with 0.5% procaine) or intravenously. The calcium in the compound is displaced by divalent and trivalent heavy metals, forming a soluble complex, which is stable at physiologic pH (but not at acid pH) and enhances lead clearance in the urine. EDTA usually is administered intravenously, especially in severe cases. It must not be administered until adequate urine flow is established. It may redistribute lead to the brain; therefore, BAL may be given first at a venous blood lead level of greater than 55 μg/dL in children and greater than 100 μg/dL in adults. Phlebitis occurs at a concentration greater than 0.5 mg/mL. Alkalinization of the urine may be helpful. $CaNa_2EDTA$ should not be confused with sodium EDTA (disodium edetate), which is used to treat hypercalcemia; inadvertent use may produce severe hypocalcemia.

Dimercaprol (BAL) is a peanut oil–based dithiol (two sulfhydryl molecules) that combines with one atom of lead to form a heterocyclic stable ring complex. It is usually reserved for patients in whom venous blood lead is greater than 70 μg/dL, and it chelates red blood cell lead, enhancing its elimination through the urine and bile. It crosses the blood–brain barrier. Approximately 50% of patients have adverse reactions, including bad metallic taste in the mouth, pain at the injection site, sterile abscesses, and fever.

A venous blood lead level greater than 70 μg/dL or the presence of clinical symptoms suggesting encephalopathy in children is a potentially life-threatening emergency. Management should be accomplished in a medical center with a pediatric intensive care unit by a multidisciplinary team including a critical care specialist, a toxicologist, a neurologist, and a neurosurgeon. Careful monitoring of neurologic status, fluid status, and intracranial pressure should be undertaken if necessary. These patients need close monitoring for hemodynamic instability. Hydration should be maintained to ensure renal excretion of lead. Fluids, renal and hepatic function, and electrolyte levels should be monitored.

While waiting for adequate urine flow, therapy should be initiated with intramuscular dimercaprol (BAL) only (25 mg/kg/d divided into 6 doses). Four hours later, the second dose of BAL should be given intramuscularly, concurrently with $CaNa_2EDTA$ 50 mg/kg/d as a single dose infused over several hours or as a continuous infusion. The double therapy is continued until the venous blood level is less than 40 μg/dL.

As long as the venous blood level is greater than 40 μg/dL, therapy is continued for 72 hours and followed by two alternatives: either parenteral therapy with two drugs ($CaNa_2EDTA$ and BAL) for 5 days or continuation of therapy with $CaNa_2EDTA$ alone if a good response is achieved and the venous blood level of lead is less than 40 μg/dL. If one cannot get the venous blood lead report back, one should continue therapy with both BAL and EDTA for 5 days. In patients with lead encephalopathy, parenteral chelation should be continued with both drugs until the patient is clinically stable before changing therapy. Mannitol and dexamethasone can reduce the cerebral edema, but their role in lead encephalopathy is not clear. Surgical decompression is not recommended to reduce cerebral edema in these cases.

If BAL and $CaNa_2EDTA$ are used together, a minimum of 2 days with no treatment should elapse before another 5-day course of therapy is considered. The 5-day course is repeated with $CaNa_2EDTA$ alone if the blood lead level rebounds to greater than 40 μg/dL or in combination with BAL if the venous blood level is greater than 70 μg/dL. If a third course is required, unless there are compelling reasons, one should wait at least 5 to 7 days before administering the course.

Following chelation therapy, a period of equilibration of 10 to 14 days should be allowed and a repeat venous blood lead concentration should be obtained. If the patient is stable enough for oral intake, oral succimer 30 mg/kg/d in three divided doses for 5 days followed by 20 mg/kg/d in two divided doses for 14 days has been suggested, but there are limited data to support this recommendation. Therapy should be continued until venous blood lead level is less than 20 μg/dL in children or less than 40 μg/dL in adults.

Chelators combined with lead are hemodialyzable in the event of renal failure.

Disposition

All patients with a venous blood lead level of greater than 70 μg/dL or who are symptomatic should be admitted. If a child is hospitalized, all lead hazards must be removed from the home environment before allowing the child to return. The source must be eliminated by environmental and occupational investigations. The local health department should be involved in dealing with children who are lead poisoned, and OSHA should be involved with cases of occupational lead poisoning. Consultation with a poison control center or experienced toxicologist is necessary when chelating patients. Follow-up venous blood lead concentrations should be obtained within 1 to 2 weeks and followed every 2 weeks for 6 to 8 weeks, then monthly for 4 to 6 months if the patient required chelation therapy. All patients with venous blood level greater than 10 μg/dL should be followed at least every 3 months until two venous blood lead concentrations are 10 μg/dL or three are less than 15 μg/dL.

LITHIUM (ESKALITH, LITHANE)

Lithium is an alkali metal used primarily in the treatment of bipolar psychiatric disorders. Most intoxications are cases of chronic overdose. One gram of lithium carbonate contains 189 mg (5.1 mEq) of lithium; a regular tablet contains 300 mg (8.12 mEq) and a sustained-release preparation contains 450 mg or 12.18 mEq.

Toxic Mechanism

The brain is the primary target organ of toxicity, but the mechanism is unclear. Lithium may interfere with physiologic functions by acting as a substitute for cellular cations (sodium and potassium), depressing neural excitation and synaptic transmission.

Toxic Dose

A dose of 1 mEq/kg (40 mg/kg) of lithium will give a peak serum lithium concentration about 1.2 mEq/L. The therapeutic serum lithium concentration in cases of acute mania is 0.6 to 1.2 mEq/L, and for maintenance it is 0.5 to 0.8 mEq/L. Serum lithium concentration levels are usually obtained 12 hours after the last dose. The toxic dose is determined by clinical manifestations and serum levels after the distribution phase.

Acute ingestion of twenty 300-mg tablets (300 mg increases the serum lithium concentration by 0.2 to 0.4 mEq/L) in adults may produce serious intoxication. Chronic intoxication can be produced by conditions listed below that can decrease the elimination of lithium or increase lithium reabsorption in the kidney.

The risk factors that predispose to chronic lithium toxicity are febrile illness, impaired renal function, hyponatremia, advanced age, lithium-induced diabetes insipidus, dehydration, vomiting and diarrhea, and concomitant use of other drugs, such as thiazide and spironolactone diuretics, nonsteroidal anti-inflammatory drugs, salicylates, angiotensin-converting enzyme inhibitors (e.g., captopril), serotonin reuptake inhibitors (e.g., fluoxetine [Prozac]), and phenothiazines.

Kinetics

Gastrointestinal absorption of regular-release preparations is rapid; serum lithium concentration peaks in 2 to 4 hours and is complete by 6 to 8 hours. The onset of toxicity may occur at 1 to 4 hours after acute overdose but usually is delayed because lithium enters the brain slowly. Absorption of sustained-release preparations and the development of toxicity may be delayed 6 to 12 hours.

Volume distribution is 0.5 to 0.9 L/kg. Lithium is not protein bound. The half-life after a single dose is 9 to 13 hours; at steady state, it may be 30 to 58 hours. The renal handling of lithium is similar to that of sodium: glomerular filtration and reabsorption (80%) by the proximal renal tubule. Adequate sodium must be present to prevent lithium reabsorption. More than 90% of lithium is excreted by the kidney, 30% to 60% within 6 to 12 hours.

Manifestations

The examiner must distinguish between side effects, acute intoxication, acute or chronic toxicity, and chronic intoxications. Chronic is the most common and dangerous type of intoxication.

Side effects include fine tremor, gastrointestinal upset, hypothyroidism, polyuria and frank diabetes insipidus, dermatologic manifestations, and cardiac conduction deficits. Lithium is teratogenic.

Patients with acute poisoning may be asymptomatic, with an early high serum lithium concentration of 9 mEq/L, and deteriorate as the serum lithium concentration falls by 50% and the lithium distributes to the brain and the other tissues. Nausea and vomiting may occur within 1 to 4 hours, but the systemic manifestations are usually delayed several more hours. It may take as long as 3 to 5 days for serious symptoms to develop. Acute toxicity and acute on chronic toxicity are manifested by neurologic findings, including weakness, fasciculations, altered mental state, myoclonus, hyperreflexia, rigidity, coma, and convulsions with limbs in hypertension. Cardiovascular effects are nonspecific and occur at therapeutic doses, flat T or inverted T waves, atrioventricular block, and prolonged QT interval. Lithium is not a primary cardiotoxin. Cardiogenic shock occurs secondary to CNS toxicity. Chronic intoxication is associated with manifestations at lower serum lithium concentrations. There is some correlation with manifestations, especially at higher serum lithium concentrations. Although the levels do not always correlate with the manifestations, they are more predictive in cases of severe intoxication. A serum lithium concentration greater than 3.0 mEq/L with chronic intoxication and altered mental state indicates severe toxicity. Permanent neurologic sequelae can result from lithium intoxication.

Laboratory Investigations

Monitoring should include CBC (lithium causes significant leukocytosis), renal function, thyroid function (chronic intoxication), ECG, and electrolytes. Serum lithium concentrations should be determined every 2 to 4 hours until levels are close to therapeutic range. Cross-reactions with green-top Vacutainer specimen tubes containing heparin will spuriously elevate serum lithium concentration 6 to 8 mEq/L.

Management

Vital function must be established and maintained. Seizure precautions should be instituted and seizures, hypotension, and dysrhythmias treated. Evaluation should include examination for rigidity and hyperreflexia signs, hydration, renal function (BUN, creatinine), and electrolytes, especially sodium. The examiner should inquire about diuretic and other drug use that increase serum lithium concentration, and the patient must discontinue the drugs. If the patient is on chronic therapy, the lithium should be discontinued. Serial serum lithium concentrations should be obtained every 4 hours until serum lithium concentration peaks and there is a downward trend toward almost therapeutic range, especially in sustained-release preparations. Vital signs should be monitored, including temperature, and ECG and serial neurologic examinations should be undertaken, including mental status and urinary output. Nephrology consultation is warranted in case of a chronic and elevated serum lithium concentration (>2.5 mEq/L), a large ingestion, or altered mental state.

An intravenous line should be established and hydration and electrolyte balance restored. Serum sodium level should be determined before 0.9% saline fluid is administered in patients with chronic overdose because hypernatremia may be present from diabetes insipidus. Although current evidence supports an initial 0.9% saline infusion (200 mL/h) to enhance excretion of lithium, once hydration, urine output, and normonatremia are established, one should administer 0.45% saline and slow the infusion (100 mL/h) for all patients.

Gastric lavage is often not recommended in cases of acute ingestion because of the large size of the tablets, and it is not necessary after chronic intoxication. Activated charcoal is ineffective. For sustained-release preparations, whole-bowel irrigation may be useful but is not proven. Sodium polystyrene sulfonate (Kayexalate), an ion exchange resin, is difficult to administer and has been used only in uncontrolled studies. Its use is not recommended.

Hemodialysis is the most efficient method for removing lithium from the vascular compartment. It is the treatment of choice for patients with severe intoxication with an altered mental state, those with seizures, and anuric patients. Long runs are used until the serum lithium concentration is less than 1 mEq/L because of extensive re-equilibration. Serum lithium concentration should be monitored every 4 hours after dialysis for rebound. Repeated and prolonged hemodialysis may be necessary. A lag in neurologic recovery can be expected.

Disposition

An acute asymptomatic lithium overdose cannot be medically cleared on the basis of single lithium level. Patients should be admitted if they have any neurologic manifestations (altered mental status, hyperreflexia, stiffness, or tremor). Patients should be admitted to the intensive care unit if they are dehydrated, have renal impairment, or have a high or rising lithium level.

METHANOL (WOOD ALCOHOL, METHYL ALCOHOL)

The concentration of methanol in Sterno fuel is 4% and it contains ethanol, in windshield washer fluid it is 30% to 60%, and in gas-line antifreeze it is 100%.

Toxic Mechanism

Methanol is metabolized by alcohol dehydrogenase to formaldehyde, which is metabolized to formate. Formate inhibits cytochrome oxidase, producing tissue hypoxia, lactic acidosis, and optic nerve edema. Formate is converted by folate-dependent enzymes to carbon dioxide.

Toxic Dose

The minimal toxic amount is approximately 100 mg/kg. Serious toxicity in a young child can be produced by the ingestion of 2.5 to 5.0 mL of 100%

methanol. Ingestion of 5-mL 100% methanol by a 10-kg child produces estimated peak blood methanol of 80 mg/dL. Ingestion of 15 mL 40% methanol was lethal for a 2-year-old child in one report. A fatal adult oral dose is 30 to 240 mL 100% (20 to 150 g). Ingestion of 6 to 10 mL 100% causes blindness in adults. The toxic blood concentration is greater than 20 mg/dL; very serious toxicity and potential fatality occur at levels greater than 50 mg/dL.

Kinetics

Onset of action can start within 1 hour but may be delayed up to 12 to 18 hours by metabolism to toxic metabolites. It may be delayed longer if ethanol is ingested concomitantly or in infants. Peak blood methanol concentration is 1 hour. Volume distribution is 0.6 L/kg (total body water).

For metabolism, see *Toxic Mechanism*.

Elimination is through metabolism. The half-life of methanol is 8 hours, with ethanol blocking it is 30 to 35 hours, and with hemodialysis 2.5 hours.

Manifestations

Metabolism creates a delay in onset for 12 to 18 hours or longer if ethanol is ingested concomitantly. Initial findings are as follows:

- 0 to 6 hours: Confusion, ataxia, inebriation, formaldehyde odor on breath, and abdominal pain can be present, but the patient may be asymptomatic. Note: Methanol produces an osmolal gap (early), and its metabolite formate produces the anion gap metabolic acidosis (see later). Absence of osmolar or anion gap does not always exclude methanol intoxication.
- 6 to 12 hours: Malaise, headache, abdominal pain, vomiting, visual symptoms, including hyperemia of optic disc, "snow vision," and blindness can be seen.
- More than 12 hours: Worsening acidosis, hyperglycemia, shock, and multiorgan failure develop, with death from complications of intractable acidosis and cerebral edema.

Laboratory Investigation

Methanol can be detected on some chromatography drug screens if specified. Methanol and ethanol levels, electrolytes, glucose, BUN, creatinine, amylase, and ABG should be monitored every 4 hours. Formate levels correlate more closely than blood methanol concentration with severity of intoxication and should be obtained if possible.

Management

One should protect the airway by intubation to prevent aspiration and administer assisted ventilation as needed. If needed, 100% oxygen can be administered. A nephrologist should be consulted early regarding the need for hemodialysis.

Gastrointestinal decontamination procedures have no role.

Metabolic acidosis should be treated vigorously with sodium bicarbonate 2 to 3 mEq/kg intravenously. Large amounts may be needed.

Antidote therapy is initiated to inhibit metabolism if the patient has a history of ingesting more than 0.4 mL/kg of 100% with the following conditions:

- Blood methanol level is greater than 20 mg/dL
- The patient has osmolar gap not accounted for by other factors
- The patient is symptomatic or acidotic with increased anion gap and/or hyperemia of the optic disc.

The ethanol or fomepizole therapy outlined below can be used.

Ethanol Therapy

Ethanol should be initiated immediately if fomepizole is unavailable (see *Fomepizole Therapy*). Alcohol dehydrogenase has a greater affinity for ethanol than ethylene glycol. Therefore, ethanol blocks the metabolism of ethylene glycol.

Ethanol should be administered intravenously (oral administration is less reliable) to produce a blood ethanol concentration of 100 to 150 mg/dL. The loading dose is 10 mL/kg of 10% ethanol administered intravenously concomitantly with a maintenance dose of 10% ethanol at 1.0 mL/kg/h. This dose may need to be increased to 2 mL/kg/h in patients who are heavy drinkers. The blood ethanol concentration should be measured hourly and the infusion rate should be adjusted to maintain a concentration of 100 to 150 mg/dL.

Fomepizole Therapy

Fomepizole (Antizol, 4-methylpyrazole) inhibits alcohol dehydrogenase more reliably than ethanol and it does not require constant monitoring of ethanol levels and adjustment of infusion rates. Fomepizole is available in 1 g/mL vials of 1.5 mL. The loading dose is 15 mg/kg (0.015 mL/kg) IV, maintenance dose is 10 mg/kg (0.01 mL/kg) every 12 hours for 4 doses, then 15 mg/kg every 12 hours until the ethylene glycol levels are less than 20 mg/dL. The solution is prepared by being mixed with 100 mL of 0.9% saline or D_5W. Fomepizole can be given to patients requiring hemodialysis but should be dosed as follows:

Dose at the beginning of hemodialysis:

- If less than 6 hours since last Antizol dose, do not administer dose
- If more than 6 hours since last dose, administer next scheduled dose

Dosing during hemodialysis:

- Dose every 4 hours

Dosing at the time hemodialysis is completed:

- If less than 1 hour between last dose and end dialysis, do not administer dose at end of dialysis
- If 1 to 3 hours between last dose and end dialysis, administer one half of next scheduled dose
- If more than 3 hours between last dose and end dialysis, administer next scheduled dose

Maintenance dosing off hemodialysis:

- Give the next scheduled dose 12 hours from the last dose administered

Hemodialysis increases the clearance of both methanol and formate 10-fold over renal clearance. A blood methanol concentration greater than 50 mg/dL has been used as an indication for hemodialysis, but recently some toxicologists from the New York City Poison Center recommended early hemodialysis in patients with blood methanol concentration greater than 25 mg/dL because it may be able to shorten the course of intoxication if started early. One should continue to monitor methanol levels and/or formate levels every 4 hours after the procedure for rebound. Other indications for early hemodialysis are significant metabolic acidosis and electrolyte abnormalities despite conventional therapy and if visual or neurologic signs or symptoms are present.

A serum formate level greater than 20 mg/dL has also been used as a criterion for hemodialysis, although this is often not readily available through many laboratories. If hemodialysis is used, the infusion rate of 10% ethanol should be increased 2.0 to 3.5 mL/kg/h. The blood ethanol concentration and glucose level should be obtained every 2 hours.

Therapy is continued with both ethanol and hemodialysis until the blood methanol level is undetectable, there is no acidosis, and the patient has no neurologic or visual disturbances. This may require several days.

Hypoglycemia is treated with intravenous glucose. Doses of folinic acid (Leucovorin) and folic acid have been used successfully in animal investigations to enhance formate metabolism to carbon dioxide and water. Leucovorin 1 mg/kg up to 50 mg IV is administered every 4 hours for several days.

An initial ophthalmologic consultation and follow-up are warranted.

Disposition

All patients who have ingested significant amounts of methanol should be referred to the emergency department for evaluation and blood methanol concentration measurement. Ophthalmologic follow-up of all patients with methanol intoxications should be arranged.

MONOAMINE OXIDASE INHIBITORS

Nonselective monoamine oxidase inhibitors (MAOIs) include the hydrazines phenelzine (Nardil) and isocarboxazid (Marplan), and the nonhydrazine tranylcypromine (Parnate). Furazolidone (Furoxone) and pargyline (Eutonyl)[2] are also considered nonselective MAOIs. Moclobemide[2], which is available in many countries but not the United States, is a selective MAO-A inhibitor. MAO-B inhibitors include selegiline (Eldepryl), an antiparksonism agent, which does not have similar toxicity to MAO-A and is not discussed. Selectivity is lost in an overdose. MAOIs are used to treat severe depression.

Toxic Mechanism

Monoamine oxidase enzymes are responsible for the oxidative deamination of both endogenous and exogenous catecholamines such as norepinephrine. MAO-A in the intestinal wall also metabolizes tyramine in food. MAOIs permanently inhibit MAO enzymes until a new enzyme is synthesized after 14 days or longer. The toxicity results from the accumulation, potentiation, and prolongation of the catecholamine action followed by profound hypotension and cardiovascular collapse.

Toxic Dose

Toxicity begins at 2 to 3 mg/kg and fatalities occur at 4 to 6 mg/kg. Death has occurred after a single dose of 170 mg of tranylcypromine in an adult.

Kinetics

Structurally, MAOIs are related to amphetamines and catecholamines. The hydrazine peak levels are at 1 to 2 hours; metabolism is hepatic acetylation; and inactive metabolites are excreted in the urine. For the nonhydrazines, peak levels occur at 1 to 4 hours, and metabolism is via the liver to active amphetamine-like metabolites.

The onset of symptoms in a case of overdose is delayed 6 to 24 hours after ingestion, peak activity is 8 to 12 hours, and duration is 72 hours or longer. The peak of MAO inhibition is in 5 to 10 days and lasts as long as 5 weeks.

Manifestations

Manifestations of an acute ingestion overdose of MAO-A inhibitors are as follows:

Phase I

An adrenergic crisis occurs, with delayed onset for 6 to 24 hours, and may not reach peak until 24 hours. The crisis starts as hyperthermia, tachycardia, tachypnea, dysarthria, transient hypertension, hyperreflexia, and CNS stimulation.

---

[2]Not available in the United States.

Phase II

Neuromuscular excitation and sympathetic hyperactivity occur with increased temperature greater than 40°C (104°F), agitation, hyperactivity, confusion, fasciculations, twitching, tremor, masseter spasm, muscle rigidity, acidosis, and electrolyte abnormalities. Seizures and dystonic reactions may occur. The pupils are mydriatic, sometimes nonreactive with "ping-pong gaze."

Phase III

CNS depression and cardiovascular collapse occur in cases of severe overdose as the catecholamines are depleted. Symptoms usually resolve within 5 days but may last 2 weeks.

Phase IV

Secondary complications occur, including rhabdomyolysis, cardiac dysrhythmias, multiorgan failure, and coagulopathies.

Biogenic interactions usually occur while the patient is on therapeutic doses of MAOI or shortly after they are discontinued (30 to 60 minutes), before the new MAO enzyme is synthesized. The following substances have been implicated: indirect acting sympathomimetics such as amphetamines, serotonergic drugs, opioids (e.g., meperidine, dextromethorphan), tricyclic antidepressants, specific serotonin reuptake inhibitors (SSRI; e.g., fluoxetine [Prozac], sertraline [Zoloft], paroxetine [Paxil]), tyramine-containing foods (e.g., wine, beer, avocados, cheese, caviar, chocolate, chicken liver), and L-tryptophan. SSRIs should not be started for at least 5 weeks after MAOIs have been discontinued.

In mild cases, usually caused by foods, headache and hypertension develop and last for several hours. In severe cases, malignant hypertension and severe hyperthermia syndromes consisting of hypertension or hyperthermia, altered mental state, skeletal muscle rigidity, shivering (often beginning in the masseter muscle), and seizures may occur.

The serotonin syndrome, which may be a result of inhibition of serotonin metabolism, has similar clinical findings to those of malignant hyperthermia and may occur with or without hyperthermia or hypertension.

Chronic toxicity clinical findings include tremors, hyperhidrosis, agitation, hallucinations, confusion, and seizures and may be confused with withdrawal syndromes.

Laboratory Investigations

Monitoring of the ECG, cardiac monitoring, CPK, ABG, pulse oximeter, electrolytes, blood glucose, and acid–base balance should be maintained.

Management

In the case of MAOI overdose, ipecac-induced emesis should not be used. Only activated charcoal alone should be used.

If the patient is admitted to the hospital and is well enough to eat, a nontyramine diet should be ordered.

Extreme agitation and seizures can be controlled with benzodiazepines and barbiturates. Phenytoin is ineffective. Nondepolarizing neuromuscular blockers (not depolarizing succinylcholine) may be needed in severe cases of hyperthermia and rigidity. If the patient has severe hypertension (catecholamine mediated), phentolamine (Regitine), a parenteral β-blocking agent, 3 to 5 mg intravenously, or labetalol (Normodyne), a combination of an α-blocking agent and a β-blocker, 20-mg intravenous bolus, should be given. If malignant hypertension with rigidity is present, a short-acting nitroprusside and benzodiazepine can be used. Hypertension is often followed by severe hypotension, which should be managed by fluid and vasopressors. *Caution:* Vasopressor therapy should be administered at lower doses than usual because of exaggerated pharmacologic response. Norepinephrine is preferred to dopamine, which requires release of intracellular amines.

Cardiac dysrhythmias are treated with standard therapy but are often refractory, and cardioversion and pacemakers may be needed.

For malignant hyperthermia, dantrolene (Dantrium), a nonspecific peripheral skeletal relaxing agent, is administered, which inhibits the release of calcium from the sarcoplasm. Dantrolene is reconstituted with 60 mL sterile water without bacteriostatic agents. Glass equipment must not be used, and the drug must be protected from light and used within 6 hours. Loading dose is 2 to 3 mg/kg intravenously as a bolus, and the loading dose is repeated until the signs of malignant hyperthermia (tachycardia, rigidity, increased end-tidal CO_2, and temperature) are controlled. Maximum total dose is 10 mg/kg to avoid hepatotoxicity.

When malignant hyperthermia has subsided, 1 mg/kg IV is given every 6 hours for 24 to 48 hours, then orally 1 mg/kg every 6 hours for 24 hours to prevent recurrence. There is a danger of thrombophlebitis following peripheral dantrolene, and it should be administered through a central line if possible. In addition one should administer external cooling and correct metabolic acidosis and electrolyte disturbances. Benzodiazepine can be used for sedation. Dantrolene does not reverse central dopamine blockade; therefore, bromocriptine mesylate (Parlodel) 2.5 to 10 mg should be given orally or through a nasogastric tube three times a day.

Rhabdomyolysis and myoglobinuria are treated with fluids. Urine alkalinization should also be treated.

Hemodialysis and hemoperfusion are of no proven value.

Biogenic amine interactions are managed symptomatically, similar to cases of overdose. For the serotonin syndrome cyproheptadine (Periactin), a serotonin blocker, 4 mg orally every hour for three doses, or methysergide (Sansert), 2 mg orally every 6 hours for three doses, should be considered. The effectiveness of these drugs has not been proven.

Disposition

All patients who have ingested more than 2 mg/kg of an MAOI should be admitted to the hospital for 24 hours of observation and monitoring in the intensive care unit because the life-threatening manifestations may be delayed. Patients with drug or dietary interactions that are mild may not require admission if symptoms subside within 4 to 6 hours and the patients remain asymptomatic. Patients with symptoms that persist or require active intervention should be admitted to the intensive care unit.

OPIOIDS (NARCOTIC OPIATES)

Opioids are used for analgesia, as antitussives, and as antidiarrheal agents and are illicit agents (heroin, opium) used in substance abuse. Tolerance, physical dependency, and withdrawal may develop.

Toxic Mechanism

At least four main opioid receptors have been identified. The μ receptor is considered the most important for central analgesia and CNS depression. The κ and δ receptors predominate in spinal analgesia. The σ receptors may mediate dysphoria. Death is a consequence of dose-dependent CNS respiratory depression or secondary to pulmonary aspiration or noncardiac pulmonary edema. The mechanism of noncardiac pulmonary edema is unknown.

Dextromethorphan can interact with MAOIs, causing severe hyperthermia, and may cause the serotonin syndrome (see *Selective Serotonin Reuptake Inhibitors*). Dextromethorphan inhibits the metabolism of norepinephrine and serotonin and blocks the reuptake of serotonin. It is found as a component of a large number of nonprescription cough and cold remedies.

Toxic Dose

The toxic dose depends on the specific drug, route of administration, and degree of tolerance. For therapeutic and toxic doses, see Table 25. In children, respiratory depression has been produced by 10 mg of morphine or methadone, 75 mg of meperidine, and 12.5 mg of diphenoxylate. Infants younger than 3 months of age are more susceptible to respiratory depression. The dose should be reduced by 50%.

Kinetics

Oral onset of analgesic effect of morphine is 10 to 15 minutes; the action peaks in 1 hour and lasts 4 to 6 hours. With sustained-release preparations, the duration is 8 to 12 hours. Opioids are 90% metabolized in the liver by hepatic conjugation and 90% excreted in the urine as inactive compounds. Volume distribution is 1 to 4 L/kg. Protein binding is 35% to 75%. The typical plasma half-life of opiates is 2 to 5 hours, but that of methadone is 24 to 36 hours. Morphine metabolites include morphine-3-glucuronide (inactive) and morphine-6-glucuronide (active) and normorphine (active). Meperidine (Demerol) is rapidly hydrolyzed by tissue esterases into the active metabolite normeperidine, which has twice the convulsant activity of meperidine. Heroin (diacetylmorphine) is deacetylated within minutes to 6-monacetylmorphine and morphine. Propoxyphene (Darvon) has a rapid onset of action, and death has occurred within 15 to 30 minutes after a massive overdose. Propoxyphene is metabolized to norpropoxyphene, an active metabolite with convulsive, cardiac dysrhythmic, and heart block properties. Symptoms of diphenoxylate overdose appear within 1 to 4 hours. It is metabolized into the active metabolite difenoxin, which is five times more active as a regular respiratory depressant agent. Death has been reported in children after ingestion of a single tablet.

Manifestations

Initially, mild intoxication produces miosis, dull face, drowsiness, partial ptosis, and "nodding" (head drops to chest then bobs up). Larger amounts produce the classic triad of miotic pupils (exceptions below), respiratory depression, and depressed level of consciousness (flaccid coma). The blood pressure, pulse, and bowel activity are decreased.

Dilated pupils do not exclude opioid intoxication. Some exceptions to the miosis effect include dextromethorphan (paralyzes iris), fentanyl, meperidine, and diphenoxylate (rarely). Physiologic disturbances including acidosis, hypoglycemia, hypoxia, and postictal state, or a co-ingestant may also produce mydriasis.

Usually, the muscles are flaccid, but increased muscle tone can be produced by meperidine and fentanyl (chest rigidity). Seizures are rare but can occur with ingestion of codeine, meperidine, propoxyphene, and dextromethorphan. Hallucinations and agitation have been reported.

Pruritus and urticaria are caused by histamine release by some opioids or by sulfite additives.

Noncardiac pulmonary edema may occur after an overdose, especially with intravenous heroin abuse. Cardiac effects include vasodilation and hypotension. A heart murmur in an intravenous addict suggests endocarditis. Propoxyphene can produce delayed cardiac dysrhythmias.

TABLE 25 Doses and Onset and Duration of Action of Common Opioids

Drug	Adult Oral Dose	Child Oral Dose	Onset of Action	Duration of Action	Adult Fatal Dose
Camphored tincture of opium	25 mL	0.25–0.50 mL/kg (0.4 mg/mL)	15–30 min	4–5 h	NA
Codeine	30-180 mg	0.5-1 mg/kg	15–30 min	4–6 h	800 mg
	>1 mg/kg is toxic in a child, above 200 mg in adult >5 mg/kg fatal in a child				
Dextromethorphan	15 mg 10 mg/kg is toxic	0.25 mg/kg	15–30 min	3–6 h	NA
Diacetylmorphine; street heroin is less than 10% pure	60 mg	NA	15–30 min	3–4 h	100 mg
Diphenoxylate natiopine (Lomotil)	5–10 mg	NA	120–240 min	14 h	300 mg
	7.5 mg is toxic in a child, 300 mg is toxic in adult				
Fentanyl (Duragesic)	0.1–0.2 mg	0.001-0.002 mg/kg	7–8 min	Intramuscular: 1/2-2 h	1.0 mg
Hydrocodone with APAP (Lortab)	5-30 mg	0.15 mg/kg	30 min	3-4 h	100 mg
Hydromorphone (Dilaudid)	4 mg	0.1 mg/kg	15–30 min	3-4 h	100 mg
Meperidine (Demerol)	100 mg	1-1.5 mg/kg	10–45 min	3-4 h	350 mg
Methadone (Dolophine)	10 mg	0.1 mg/kg	30–60 min	4-12 h	120 mg
Morphine	10–60 mg	0.1-0.2 mg/kg	<20 min	4-6 h	200 mg
	Oral dose is 6 times parenteral dose, MS Contin sustained release prep				
Oxycodone APAP (Percocet)	5 mg	NA	15–30 min	4-5 h	NA
Pentazocine (Talwin)	50–100 mg	NA	15–30 min	3-4 h	NA
Propoxyphene (Darvon)	65–100mg	NA	30–60 min	2-4 h	700 mg

Fentanyl is 100 times more potent than morphine and can cause chest wall muscle rigidity. Some of its derivatives are 2000 times more potent than morphine.

Laboratory Investigations

For patients with overdose, one should obtain and monitor ABG, blood glucose, and electrolyte levels; chest radiographs; and ECG. For drug abusers, one should consider testing for hepatitis B, syphilis, and HIV antibody (HIV testing usually requires consent). Blood opioid concentrations are not useful. They confirm diagnosis (morphine therapeutic dose, 65 to 80 ng/mL; toxic, <200 ng/mL), but are not useful for making a therapeutic decision. Cross-reactions can occur with Vick's Formula 44, poppy seeds, and other opioids (codeine and heroin are metabolized to morphine). Naloxone 4 mg IV was not associated with a positive enzyme multiplied immunoassay technique urine screen at 60 minutes, 6 hours, or 48 hours.

Management

Supportive care should be instituted, particularly an endotracheal tube and assisted ventilation. Temporary ventilation can be provided by a bag-valve mask with 100% oxygen. The patient should be placed on a cardiac monitor, have intravenous access established, and have specimens for ABG, glucose, electrolytes, BUN, and creatinine levels, CBC, coagulation profile, liver function, toxicology screen, and urinalysis taken.

For gastrointestinal decontamination, emesis should not be induced, but activated charcoal can be administered if bowel sounds are present.

If it is suspected that the patient is an addict, he or she should be restrained first and then 0.1 mg of naloxone (Narcan) should be administered. The dose should be doubled every 2 minutes until the patient responds or 10 to 20 mg has been given. If the patient is not suspected to be an addict, then 2 mg every 2 to 3 minutes to total of 10 to 20 mg is administered.

It is essential to determine whether there is a complete response to naloxone (mydriasis, improvement in ventilation), because it is a diagnostic therapeutic test. A continuous naloxone infusion may be appropriate, using the "response dose" every hour. Repeat doses of naloxone may be necessary because the effects of many opioids can last much longer than naloxone does (30 to 60 minutes). Methadone ingestions may require a naloxone infusion for 24 to 48 hours. Half of the response dose may need to be repeated in 15 to 20 minutes, after the infusion has been started.

Acute iatrogenic withdrawal precipitated by the administration of naloxone to a dependent patient should not be treated with morphine or other opioids. Naloxone's effects are limited to 30 to 60 minutes (shorter than most opioids) and withdrawal will subside in a short time.

Nalmefene (Revex), an FDA-approved long-acting (4 to 8 hours) pure opioid antagonist, is being investigated, but its role in cases of acute intoxication is unclear and it could produce prolonged withdrawal. It may have a role in place of naloxone infusion.

Noncardiac pulmonary edema does not respond to naloxone, and the patient needs intubation, assisted ventilation, positive end-expiratory pressure, and hemodynamic monitoring. Fluids should be given cautiously in patients with opioid overdose because opioids stimulate the antidiuretic hormone.

If the patient is comatose, 50% glucose (3% to 4% of comatose opioid overdose patients have hypoglycemia) and thiamine should be given prior to naloxone. If the patient has seizures that are unresponsive to naloxone, one administers diazepam and examines for metabolic (hypoglycemia, electrolyte disturbances) causes and structural disturbances.

Hypotension is rare and should direct a search for another etiology. If the patient is agitated, hypoxia and hypoglycemia must be excluded before opioid withdrawal is considered as a cause. Complications to consider include urinary retention, constipation, rhabdomyolysis, myoglobinuria, hypoglycemia, and withdrawal.

Disposition

If a patient responds to intravenous naloxone, careful observation for relapse and the development of pulmonary edema is required, with cardiac and respiratory monitoring for 6 to 12 hours. Patients requiring repeated doses of naloxone or an infusion, or those who develop pulmonary edema, require intensive care unit admission and cannot be discharged from the intensive care unit until they are symptom free for 12 hours. Intravenous overdose complications are expected to be present within 20 minutes after injection, and discharge after 4 symptom-free hours has been recommended. Adults with oral overdose have delayed onset of toxicity and require 6 hours of observation. Children with oral opioid overdose should be admitted to the hospital for observation because of delayed toxicity. Some toxicologists advise restraining a patient who attempts to sign out against medical advice after treatment with naloxone, at least until the patient receives psychiatric evaluation.

ORGANOPHOSPHATES AND CARBAMATES

Cholinergic intoxication sources are insecticides (organophosphates or carbamates), some medications, and some mushrooms. Examples of organophosphate insecticides are malathion (low toxicity, median lethal dose [LD_{50}] 2800 mg/kg), chlorpyrifos, which has been removed from market (moderate toxicity), and parathion (high toxicity, LD_{50} 2 mg/kg). Carbamate insecticides include carbaryl (low toxicity, LD_{50} 500 mg/kg), propoxur (moderate toxicity, LD_{50} 95 mg/kg), and aldicarb (high toxicity, LD_{50} 0.9 mg/kg). Pharmaceuticals with carbamate properties include neostigmine (Prostigmin) and physostigmine (Antilirium). Cholinergic compounds also include the "G" nerve war weapons tabun (GA), sarin (GB), soman (GB), and venom X (VX).

Toxic Mechanism

Organophosphates phosphorylate the active site on red cell acetylcholinesterase and pseudocholinesterase in the serum, neuromuscular and parasympathetic neuroeffector junctions, and in the major synapses of the autonomic ganglia, causing irreversible inhibition. There are two types of organophosphate intoxication: (a) direct action by the parent compound (e.g., tetraethylpyrophosphate, or (b) indirect action by the toxic metabolite (e.g., parathoxon or malathoxon).

Carbamates (esters of carbonic acid) cause reversible carbamylation of the active site of the enzymes. When a critical amount, greater than 50%, of cholinesterase is inhibited, acetylcholine accumulates and causes transient stimulation at cholinergic synapses and sympathetic terminals (muscarinic effect), the somatic nerves, the autonomic ganglia (nicotinic effect), and CNS synapses. Stimulation of conduction is followed by inhibition of conduction.

The major differences between the carbamates and the organophosphates are as follows: (a) carbamate toxicity is less and the duration is shorter; (b) carbamates rarely produce overt CNS effects (poor CNS penetration); (c) carbamate inhibition of the acetylcholinesterase enzyme is reversible and activity returns to normal rapidly; (d) pralidoxime, the enzyme regenerator, may not be necessary in the management of mild carbamate intoxication (e.g., carbaryl).

Toxic Dose

Parathion's minimum lethal dose is 2 mg in children and 10 to 20 mg in adults. The lethal dose of malathion is greater than 1375 mg/kg and that of chlorpyrifos is 25 g; the latter compound is unlikely to cause death.

Kinetics

Absorption is by all routes. The onset of acute ingestion toxicity occurs as early as 3 hours, usually before 12 hours and always before 24 hours. Lipid-soluble agents absorbed by the dermal route (e.g., fenthion), may have a delayed onset of more than 24 hours. Inhalation toxicity occurs immediately after exposure. Massive ingestion can produce intoxication within minutes.

Metabolism is via the liver. With some pesticides (e.g., parathion, malathion), the effects are delayed because they undergo hepatic microsomal oxidative metabolism to their toxic metabolites, the -oxons (e.g., paroxon, malaoxon).

The half-life of malathion is 2.89 hours and that of parathion is 2.1 days. The metabolites are eliminated in the urine and the presence of p-nitrophenol in the urine is a clue up to 48 hours after exposure.

Manifestations

Many organophosphates produce a garlic odor on the breath, in the gastric contents, or in the container. Diaphoresis, excessive salivation, miosis, and muscle twitching are helpful clues to diagnosis.

Early, a cholinergic (muscarinic) crisis develops that consists of parasympathetic nervous system activity.

DUMBELS is the mnemonic for defecation, cramps, and increased bowel motility; urinary incontinence; miosis (mydriasis may occur in 20%); bronchospasm and bronchorrhea; excess secretion; lacrimation; and seizures. Bradycardia, pulmonary edema, and hypotension may be present.

Later, sympathetic and nicotinic effects occur, consisting of MATCH: muscle weakness and fasciculation (eyelid twitching is often present), adrenal stimulation and hyperglycemia, tachycardia, cramps in muscles, and hypertension. Finally, paralysis of the skeletal muscles ensues.

The CNS effects are headache, blurred vision, anxiety, ataxia, delirium and toxic psychosis, convulsions, coma, and respiratory depression. Cranial nerve palsies have been noted. Delayed hallucinations may occur.

Delayed respiratory paralysis and neurologic and neurobehavioral disorders have been described following certain organophosphate ingestions or dermal exposure. The "intermediate syndrome" is paralysis of proximal and respiratory muscles developing 24 to 96 hours after the successful treatment of organophosphate poisoning. A delayed distal polyneuropathy has been described with ingestion of certain organophosphates, such as triorthocresyl phosphate, bromoleptophos, and methomidophos.

Complications include aspiration, pulmonary edema, and acute respiratory distress syndrome.

Laboratory Investigations

Monitoring should include chest radiograph, blood glucose (nonketotic hyperglycemia is frequent), ABG, pulse oximetry, ECG, blood coagulation status, liver function, hyperamylasemia (pancreatitis reported), and urinalysis for the metabolite alkyl phosphate paranitrophenol. Blood should be drawn for red blood cell cholinesterase determination before pralidoxime is given. The red blood cell cholinesterase activity roughly correlates with clinical severity. Mild poisoning is 20% to 50% of normal, moderate poisoning is 10% to 20% of normal, and severe poisoning is 10% of normal (>90% depressed). A postexposure rise of 10% to 15% in the cholinesterase level determined at least 10 to 14 days after the exposure confirms the diagnosis.

Management

Protection of health care personnel with clothing (masks, gloves, gowns, goggles) and respiratory equipment or hazardous material suits, as necessary, is called for. General decontamination consists of isolation, bagging, and disposal of contaminated clothing and other articles. Vital functions should be established and maintained. Cardiac and oxygen saturation monitoring are needed. Intubation and assisted ventilation may be needed. Secretions should be suctioned until atropinization drying is achieved.

Dermal decontamination involves prompt removal of clothing and cleansing of all affected areas of skin, hair, and eyes. Ocular decontamination involves irrigation with copious amounts of tepid water or 0.9% saline for at least 15 minutes. Gastrointestinal decontamination, if the ingestion was recent, involves the administration of activated charcoal.

Atropine sulfate can be given as an antidote. It is both a diagnostic and a therapeutic agent. Atropine counteracts the muscarinic effects but is only partially effective for the CNS effects (seizures and coma). Preservative-free atropine (no benzyl alcohol) should be used. If the patient is symptomatic (bradycardia or bronchorrhea), a test dose should be administered, 0.02 mg/kg in children or 1 mg in adults, intravenously. If no signs of atropinization are present (tachycardia, drying of secretions, and mydriasis), atropine should be administered immediately, 0.05 mg/kg in children or 2 mg in adults, every 5 to 10 minutes as needed to dry the secretions and clear the lungs. Beneficial effects are seen within 1 to 4 minutes and maximum effect in 8 minutes. The average dose in the first 24 hours is 40 mg, but 1000 mg or more has been required in severe cases. Glycopyrrolate (Robinul) can be used if atropine is not available. The maximum dose should be maintained for 12 to 24 hours, then tapered and the patient observed for relapse. Poisoning, especially with lipophilic agents (e.g., fenthion, chlorfenthion), may require weeks of atropine therapy. An alternative is a continuous infusion of atropine 8 mg in 100 mL 0.9% saline at rate of 0.02 to 0.08 mg/kg/h (0.25 to 1.0 mL/kg/h) with additional 1 to 5 mg boluses as needed to dry the secretions.

Pralidoxime chloride (Protopam) has both antinicotinic and antimuscarinic effects and possibly also CNS effects. Successful treatment with pralidoxime chloride may allow a reduction in the dose of atropine. Pralidoxime acts to reactivate the phosphorylated cholinesterases by binding the phosphate moiety on the esteritic site and displacing it. It should be given early before "aging" of phosphate bond produces tighter binding. However, recent reports indicate that pralidoxime chloride is beneficial even several days after the poisoning. Improvement is seen within 10 to 40 minutes. The initial dose of pralidoxime chloride is 1 to 2 g in 250 mL 0.89% saline over 5 to 10 minutes, maximum 200 mg/minute, in adults or 25 to 50 mg/kg, maximum 4 mg/kg/minute, in children younger than 12 years of age. The dose can be repeated every 6 to 12 hours for several days. An alternative is a continuous infusion of 1 g in 100 mL 0.89% saline at 5 to 20 mg/kg/h (0.5 to 12 mL/g/h) up to 500 mg/h and titrated to desired response. Maximum adult daily dose is 12 g. Cardiac and blood pressure monitoring are advised during and for several hours after the infusion. The end point is absence of fasciculations and return of muscle strength.

Contraindicated drugs include morphine, aminophylline, barbiturates, opioids, phenothiazine, reserpine-like drugs, parasympathomimetics, and succinylcholine.

Noncardiac pulmonary edema may require respiratory support. Seizures may respond to atropine and pralidoxime chloride but often require anticonvulsants. Cardiac dysrhythmias may require electrical cardioversion or antidysrhythmic therapy if the patient is hemodynamically unstable. Extracorporeal procedures are of no proven value.

Disposition

Asymptomatic patients with normal examination findings after 6 to 8 hours of observation may be discharged. In cases of intentional poisoning, the patients require psychiatric clearance for discharge. Symptomatic patients should be admitted to the intensive care unit. Observation of milder cases of carbamate poisoning, even those requiring atropine, for 6 to 8 hours symptom-free may be sufficient to exclude significant toxicity. In cases of workplace exposure, OSHA should be notified.

PHENCYCLIDINE (ANGEL DUST)

Phencyclidine is an arylcyclohexylamine related to ketamine and chemically related to the phenothiazines. Originally a "dissociative" anesthetic banned in United States since 1979, it is now an illicit substance, with at least 38 analogs. It is inexpensively manufactured by "kitchen chemists" and is mislabeled as other hallucinogens. Improper phencyclidine synthesis may release cyanide when heated or smoked and can cause explosions.

Toxic Mechanism

The mechanism of phencyclidine is complex and not completely understood. It inhibits some neurotransmitters and causes a loss of pain sensation without depressing the CNS respiratory status. It stimulates α-adrenergic receptors and may act as a "false neurotransmitter." The effects are sympathomimetic, cholinergic, and cerebellar.

Toxic Dose

The usual dose of phencyclidine mixed with marijuana joints is 100 to 400 mg of phencyclidine. Joints or leaf mixtures contain 0.24% to 7.9% of PCP, 1 mg of PCP/150 leaves. Tablets contain 5 mg (the usual street dose). CNS effects at doses of 1 to 6 mg include hallucinations and euphoria, 6 to 10 mg produces toxic psychosis and sympathetic stimulation, 10 to 25 mg produces severe toxicity, and more than 100 mg has resulted in fatalities.

Kinetics

Phencyclidine is a lipophilic weak base, with a pKa of 8.5 to 9.5. It is rapidly absorbed when smoked and snorted, poorly absorbed from the acid stomach, and rapidly absorbed from the alkaline middle small intestine. It has an enterogastric secretion and is reabsorbed in the small intestine. The onset of action when smoked is 2 to 5 minutes, with a peak in 15 to 30 minutes. With oral ingestion, the onset is in 30 to 60 minutes and when taken intravenously it is immediate. Most adverse reactions in cases of overdose begin within 1 to 2 hours. Its duration of action at low doses is 4 to 6 hours and normality returns in 24 hours; in large overdoses, fluctuating coma may last 6 to 10 days.

Volume distribution is 6.2 L/kg. Phencyclidine concentrates in brain and adipose tissue. Protein binding is 70%. The route of elimination is by gastric secretion, liver metabolism, and 10% urinary excretion of conjugates and free phencyclidine. Renal excretion may be increased 50% with urinary acidification. The half-life is 1 hour (in cases of overdose, it is 11 to 89 hours).

Manifestations

The classic picture is bursts of horizontal, vertical, and rotary nystagmus, which is a clue to diagnosis (occurs in 50% of cases), miosis, hypertension, and fluctuating altered mental state. There is a wide spectrum of clinical presentations.

Mild intoxication with 1 to 6 mg produces drunken and bizarre behavior, agitation, rotary nystagmus, and blank stare. Violent behavior and sensory anesthesia make these patients insensitive to pain, self-destructive, and dangerous. Most are communicative within 1 to 2 hours, are alert and oriented in 6 to 8 hours, and recover completely in 24 to 48 hours.

Moderate intoxication with 6 to 10 mg produces excess salivation, hypertension, hyperthermia, muscle rigidity, myoclonus, and catatonia. Recovery of consciousness occurs in 24 to 48 hours and complete recovery in 1 week.

Severe intoxication with 10 to 25 mg results in opisthotonus, decerebrate rigidity, convulsions, prolonged fluctuating coma, and respiratory failure. Patients in this category have a high rate of medical complications. Recovery of consciousness occurs in 24 to 48 hours, with complete normality in a month. Medical complications include apnea, aspiration pneumonia, cardiac arrest, hypertensive encephalopathy, hyperthermia, intracerebral hemorrhage, psychosis, rhabdomyolysis and myoglobinuria, and seizures. Loss of memory and "flashbacks" last for months. Phencyclidine-induced depression and suicide have been reported.

Fatalities occur with ingestions of greater than 100 mg and with serum levels greater than 100 to 250 ng/mL.

Laboratory Investigations

Marked elevation of creatine kinase level may occur. Values greater than 20,000 units have been reported. Urinalysis should be monitored and urine tested for myoglobin. One should monitor the blood for creatine kinase, uric acid (an early clue to rhabdomyolysis), BUN, creatinine, electrolytes (hyperkalemia), blood glucose (20% of patients have hypoglycemia), urinary output, liver function tests, ECG, and ABG if the patient has any respiratory manifestations. Measurement of phencyclidine in the gastric juice is called for because concentrations are 10 to 50 times higher than in blood or urine. Phencyclidine blood concentrations are not helpful. Phencyclidine may be detected in the urine of the average user for 10 days to 3 weeks after the last dose. In chronic users, it can be detected for over 1 month. The analogs of phencyclidine may not produce positive test results for phencyclidine in the urine. Cross-reactions with bleach and dextromethorphan may cause false-positive urine test results on immunoassay, and cross-reaction with doxylamine may produce a false-positive finding on gas chromatography.

Management

The patient should be observed for violent, self-destructive, bizarre behavior and paranoid schizophrenia. Patients should be placed in a low sensory environment and dangerous objects should be removed from the area.

Gastrointestinal decontamination is not effective because phencyclidine is rapidly absorbed from intestines. Overtreating the mild intoxication should be avoided. There is insufficient evidence to support the use of MDAC. In cases of severe toxicity (stupor or coma), continuous gastric suction can be tried (with protection of the airway) because the drug is secreted into the gastric juice. The value of this procedure is controversial because of limited data.

The patient must be protected from harming himself or herself or others. Physical restraints may be necessary, but they should be used sparingly and for the shortest time possible because they increase risk of rhabdomyolysis. Metal restraints such as handcuffs should be avoided. For behavioral disorders and toxic psychosis, diazepam is the agent of choice. Pharmacologic intervention includes diazepam (Valium) 10 to 30 mg orally or 2 to 5 mg intravenously initially and titrated upward to 10 mg; however, up to 30 mg may be required. "Talk down" technique is usually ineffective and dangerous. Phenothiazines and butyrophenones should be avoided in the acute phase because they lower the convulsive threshold; however, they may be needed later for psychosis. Haloperidol (Haldol) administration has been reported to produce catatonia.

Seizures and muscle spasm are managed with diazepam, from 2.5 mg up to 10 mg. Hyperthermia (>38.5°C [101.3°F]) is treated with external cooling measures. Hypertension is usually transient and does not require treatment. In the case of emergent hypertensive crisis (blood pressure >200/115 mm Hg) nitroprusside can be used in a dose of 0.3 to 2 μg/kg/min. Maximum infusion rate is 10 μg/kg/min for only 10 minutes.

Acid ion trapping diuresis is not recommended because of the danger of myoglobin precipitation in the renal tubules. Rhabdomyolysis and myoglobinuria are treated by correcting volume depletion and insuring a urinary output of greater than 2 mL/kg/h. Alkalinization is controversial because of reabsorption of phencyclidine.

Hemodialysis is beneficial if renal failure occurs; otherwise, the extracorporeal procedures are not beneficial.

Disposition

All patients with coma, delirium, catatonia, violent behavior, aspiration pneumonia, sustained hypertension greater than 200/115, and significant rhabdomyolysis should be admitted to the intensive care unit until asymptomatic for at least 24 hours. If patients with mild intoxication are mentally and neurologically stable and become asymptomatic (except for nystagmus) for 4 hours, they may be discharged in the company of a responsible adult. All patients must be assessed for suicide risk before discharge. Drug counseling and psychiatric follow-up should be arranged. Patients should be warned that episodes of disorientation and depression may continue intermittently for 4 weeks or more.

PHENOTHIAZINES AND NONPHENOTHIAZINES (NEUROLEPTICS)

Toxic Mechanism

Neuroleptics have complex mechanisms of toxicity, including (a) block of the postsynaptic dopamine receptors; (b) block of peripheral and central α-adrenergic receptors; (c) block of cholinergic muscarinic receptors; (d) quinidine-like antidysrhythmic and myocardial depressant effect in cases of large overdose; (e) lowering of the convulsive threshold; (f) effect on hypothalamic temperature regulation (Table 26).

Toxic Dose

Extrapyramidal reactions, anticholinergic effects, and orthostatic hypotension may occur at therapeutic doses. The toxic amount is not established, but the maximum daily therapeutic dose may result in significant side effects, and twice this amount may be potentially fatal. Chlorpromazine (Thorazine), the prototype, may produce serious hypotension and CNS depression at doses greater than 200 mg (17 mg/kg) in children and 3 to 5 g in an adult. Fatalities have been reported after 2.5 g of loxapine (Loxitane) and mesoridazine (Serentil) and 1.5 g of thioridazine (Mellaril).

Kinetics

These agents are lipophilic and have unpredictable gastrointestinal absorption. Peak levels occur

TABLE 26 Neuroleptics and Properties

Compound	Antipsychotic	Anticholinergic	Extrapyramidal	Hypotensive and Cardiotoxic	Sedative
Phenothiazine					
Aliphatic Chlorpromazine (Thorazine) Promethazine (Phenergan)	1+	3+	2+	2+	3+
Piperazine Fluphenazine (Prolixin) Perphenazine (Trilafon) Prochlorperazine (Compazine) Trifluoperazine (Stelazine)	3+	1+	3+	1+	1+
Piperidine Mesoridazine (Serentil) Thioridazine (Mellaril)	1+	2+	1+	3+	3+
Nonphenothiazine					
Butyrophenone Haloperidol (Haldol)	3+	1+	3+	1+	1+
Dibenzoxazepine Loxapine (Loxitane)	3+	1+	3+	1+	2+
Dihydroindolone Molindone (Moban)	3+	1+	3+	1+	1+
Thioxanthenes Thiothixene (Navane) Chlorprothixene (Taractan)	3+	1+	3+	3+	1+

1+ = very low activity; 2+ = moderate activity; 3+ = very high activity.

2 to 6 hours postingestion and have enterohepatic recirculation.

The mean serum half-life in phase 1 is 1 to 2 hours and the biphasic half-life is 20 to 40 hours. Volume distribution is 10 to 40 L/kg; protein binding is 92% to 98%. Chlorpromazine taken orally has an onset of action in 30 to 60 minutes, peak in 2 to 4 hours, and duration of 4 to 6 hours. With sustained-release preparations, the onset is in 30 to 60 minutes and duration is 6 to 12 hours.

Elimination is by hepatic metabolism, which results in multiple metabolites (some are active). Metabolites can be detected in urine months after chronic therapy. Only 1% to 3% is excreted unchanged in the urine.

Manifestations

In cases of phenothiazine overdose, anticholinergic symptoms may be present early but are not life-threatening. Miosis is usually present (80%) if the phenothiazine has strong α-adrenergic blocking effect (e.g., chlorpromazine), but anticholinergic activity mydriasis may occur. Agitation and delirium rapidly progress into coma. Major problems are cardiac toxicity and hypotension. The cardiotoxic effects are seen more commonly with thioridazine and its metabolite mesoridazine. These agents have produced the largest number of fatalities in patients with phenothiazine overdose. Cardiac conduction disturbances include prolonged PR, QRS, and QTc intervals, U- and T-wave abnormalities, and ventricular dysrhythmias, including torsades de pointes. Seizures occur mainly in patients with convulsive disorders or with administration of loxapine. Sudden death in children and adults has been reported.

Idiosyncratic dystonic reactions are most common with the piperidine group. Reactions are not dose-dependent and consist of opisthotonos, torticollis, orolingual dyskinesia, or oculogyric crisis (painful upward gaze). These reactions are more frequent in children and women. Neuroleptic malignant syndrome occurs in patients on chronic therapy and is characterized by hyperthermia, muscle rigidity, autonomic dysfunction, and altered mental state. There is one case reported with acute overdose. The loxapine syndrome consists of seizures, rhabdomyolysis, and renal failure.

Laboratory Investigations

Monitoring should include arterial blood gases, renal and hepatic function, electrolytes, blood glucose, and creatine kinase and myoglobinemia in neuroleptic malignant syndrome. Most of these agents are detected on routine screening. Quantitative serum levels are not useful in management. Cross-reactions with enzyme multiplied immunoassay technique tests occur with cyclic antidepressants. Phenothiazines give false-negative results on pregnancy urine tests using human chorionic gonadotropin as an indicator, and give false-positive results for urine porphyrins, indirect Coombs test, urobilinogen, and amylase.

Management

Vital functions must be established and maintained. All overdose patients require venous access,

12-lead ECG (to measure intervals), cardiac and respiratory monitoring, and seizure precautions. One should monitor core temperature to detect poikilothermic effect. If the patient is comatose, intubation and assisted ventilation may be required, as well as 100% oxygen, intravenous glucose, naloxone (Narcan), and thiamine.

Emesis is not recommended. Activated charcoal can be administered if ingestion was within 1 hour. MDAC has not been proven beneficial. A radiograph of the abdomen may be useful, if the phenothiazine is radiopaque. Haloperidol (Haldol) and trifluoperazine (Stelazine) are most likely to be radiopaque. Whole-bowel irrigation may be useful when a large number of pills are visualized on radiograph or if sustained-release preparations were taken, but whole-bowel irrigation has not been evaluated in patients with phenothiazine overdose.

Convulsions are treated with diazepam or lorazepam (Ativan). Loxapine (Loxitane) overdose may result in status epilepticus. If nondepolarizing neuromuscular blockade is required, pancuronium (Pavulon) or vecuronium (Norcuron) should be used (not succinylcholine [Anectine], which may cause malignant hyperthermia), and EEG should be monitored during paralysis.

Patients with dysrhythmias should be monitored with serial ECGs. Unstable rhythms can be treated with electrical cardioversion. Class 1a antidysrhythmics (procainamide, quinidine, and disopyramide [Norpace]) must be avoided.

Hypokalemia predisposes to dysrhythmias and should be corrected aggressively. Supraventricular tachycardia with hemodynamic instability is treated with electrical cardioversion. The role of adenosine has not been defined. Calcium channel and β-blockers should be avoided.

Prolongation of the QRS interval is treated with sodium bicarbonate 1 to 2 mEq/kg by intravenous bolus over a few minutes. Torsades de pointes is treated with magnesium sulfate IV 20% solution 2 g over 2 to 3 minutes. If there is no response in 10 minutes, the dose is repeated and followed by a continuous infusion of 5 to 10 mg/min or given as an infusion of 50 mg/minute for 2 hours followed by 30 mg/minute for 90 minutes twice a day for several days, as needed. The dose in children is 25 to 50 mg/kg initially and maintenance dose is 30 to 60 mg/kg per 24 hours (0.25 to 0.50 mEq/Kg per 24 hours) up to 1000 mg per 24 hours. Serum magnesium levels should be monitored.

To treat ventricular tachydysrhythmias in a stable patient, lidocaine is used. If the patient is unstable, electrical cardioversion is used. Patients with heart block with hemodynamic instability should be managed with temporary cardiac pacing.

Hypotension is treated with the Trendelenburg position and 0.9% saline. If the condition is refractory to treatment or there is a danger of fluid overload, vasopressors are administered. The vasopressor of choice is α-adrenergic agonist norepinephrine (Levophed), titrated to response. Epinephrine and dopamine should not be used because β-receptor stimulation in the presence of α-receptor blockade may provoke dysrhythmias and phenothiazines are antidopaminergic.

Hypothermia and hyperthermia are treated with external warming and cooling measures, respectively. Antipyretic drugs must not be used.

Management of the neuroleptic malignant syndrome includes the following actions:

- Immediately discontinuing the offending agent
- Hyperventilating the patient, using 100% humidified, cooled oxygen at high gas flows (at least 10 L/min) because of rapid breathing
- Administering a benzodiazepine to control convulsions and facilitate cooling measures
- Initiating appropriate mechanical cooling measures, which may include intravenous cold saline (not lactated Ringer's), ice baths, cold lavage of the stomach, bladder, and rectum, and a hypothermic blanket
- Correcting acid–base and electrolyte disturbances and treating significant hyperkalemia with hyperventilation, calcium, sodium bicarbonate, intravenous glucose, and insulin; hemodialysis may be necessary

In addition, dysrhythmias usually respond to correction of the underlying acid–base disturbances and hyperkalemia. If antidysrhythmic agents are required, calcium channel blockers must be avoided because they may precipitate hyperkalemia and cardiovascular collapse. Dantrolene sodium (Dantrium), which is a phenytoin derivative, inhibits calcium release from the sarcoplasmic reticulum and results in decreased muscle contraction. Dantrolene acts peripherally and does not reverse the rigidity or psychomotor disturbances resulting from the central dopamine blockade; it therefore is often used in combination with bromocriptine. Bromocriptine mesylate (Parlodel) acts centrally as a dopamine agonist, as does amantadine hydrochloride (Symmetrel). Bromocriptine and dantrolene have been reported to be successful in combination with cooling and good supportive measures in malignant hyperthermia.

Dosing for these agents is as follows: dantrolene sodium at 2 to 3 mg/kg IV as a bolus, then 1 mg/kg/minute to a maximum of 10 mg/kg or until the tachycardia, rigidity, increased end-tidal CO_2, and temperature elevation are controlled. *Note:* Hepatotoxicity occurs with doses greater than 10 mg/kg. To prevent symptom recurrence, 1 mg/kg should be administered every 6 hours for 24 to 48 hours after the episode. After that time, oral dantrolene can be used at a dose of 1 mg/kg every 6 hours for 24 hours as necessary. The patient should be observed for thrombophlebitis following intravenous dantrolene. It is best administered via a central line. Bromocriptine mesylate at 2.5 to 10 mg orally or via a nasogastric tube, three times a day, should be used in combination with dantrolene.

Idiosyncratic dystonic reaction can be treated with diphenhydramine (Benadryl) 1 to 2 mg/kg/dose intravenously over 5 minutes up to maximum of 50 mg intravenously; a response is noted within 2 to 5 minutes. This can be followed with oral doses for 4 to 6 days to prevent recurrence.

Extracorporeal measures (hemodialysis, hemoperfusion) are not effective in removing these agents.

Disposition

Asymptomatic patients should be observed for at least 6 hours after gastric decontamination. Symptomatic patients with cardiotoxicity, hypotension, and convulsions should be admitted to the intensive care unit and monitored for 48 hours.

SALICYLATES (ACETYLSALICYLIC ACID, SALICYLIC ACID)

Toxic Mechanism

The primary toxic mechanisms include (a) direct stimulation of the medullary chemoreceptor trigger zone and respiratory center; (b) uncoupling oxidative phosphorylation; (c) inhibition of the Krebs' cycle enzymes; (d) inhibition of vitamin K dependent and independent clotting factors; (e) alteration of platelet function; and (f) inhibition of prostaglandin synthesis.

Toxic Dose

Acute mild intoxication occurs at a dose of 150 to 200 mg/kg, moderate intoxication at 200 to 300 mg/kg, and severe intoxication at 300 to 500 mg/kg. Acute salicylate plasma concentration greater than 30 mg/dL (usually >40 mg/dL) may be associated with clinical toxicity. Chronic intoxication occurs at ingestions greater than 100 mg/kg/d for more than 2 days because of accumulation kinetics. Methyl salicylate (oil of wintergreen) is the most toxic form of salicylate. A dose of 1 mL of 98% contains 1.4 g of salicylate. Fatalities have occurred with ingestion of 1 teaspoonful in children and 1 ounce in adults. It is found in topical ointments and liniments (18% to 30%).

Kinetics

Acetylsalicylic acid and salicylic acid are weak acids with a pKa of 3.5 and 3.0, respectively. Acetylsalicylic acid is absorbed from the stomach, from the small bowel, and dermally. Onset of action is within 30 minutes. Methyl salicylate and effervescent tablets are absorbed more rapidly. Salicylate plasma concentration is detectable within 15 minutes after ingestion and peaks in 30 to 120 minutes. The peak may be delayed 6 to 12 hours in cases of large overdose, overdose with enteric-coated or sustained-release preparations, and development of concretions. The therapeutic duration of action is 3 to 4 hours but is markedly prolonged in cases of overdose.

Volume distribution is 0.13 L/kg for salicylic acid but increases as the salicylate plasma concentration increases. Protein binding is greater than 90% for salicylic acid at pH 7.4 and a salicylate plasma concentration of 20 to 30 mg/dL, 75% at a salicylate plasma concentration greater than 40 mg/dL, 50% at a salicylate plasma concentration of 70 mg/dL, and 30% at a salicylate plasma concentration of 120 mg/dL.

The half-life for salicylic acid is 3 hours after a 300 mg dose, 6 hours after a 1 g overdose, and greater than 10 hours after a 10-g overdose. Elimination includes Michaelis-Menten hepatic metabolism by three saturable pathways: (a) glycine conjugation to salicyluric acid (75%); (b) glucuronyl transferase to salicyl phenol glucuronide (10%); and (c) salicyl aryl glucuronide (4%). Nonsaturable pathways are hydrolysis to gentisic acid (<1%). Ten percent is excreted unchanged.

Acidosis increases the severity of the intoxication by increasing the non-ionized salicylate that can cross membranes and enter the brain cells. In kidneys, the un-ionized salicylic acid undergoes glomerular filtration, and the ionized portion undergoes tubular secretion in proximal tubules and passive reabsorption in the distal tubules. Renal excretion of salicylate is enhanced by alkaline urine.

Manifestations

The ingestion of concentrated topical salicylic acid preparations (e.g., wart remover) can cause mucosal caustic injury to the gastrointestinal tract. Occult salicylate overdose should be considered in any patient with unexplained acid–base disturbance.

The manifestations of acute overdose of salicylates are as follows:

Minimal Symptoms

Tinnitus, dizziness, and deafness may occur at high therapeutic salicylate plasma concentrations of 20 to 30 mg/dL. Nausea and vomiting may occur immediately because of local gastric irritation.

Phase I. Mild manifestations occur at 1 to 12 hours after ingestion with a 6-hour salicylate plasma concentration of 45 to 70 mg/dL. Nausea and vomiting followed by hyperventilation are usually present within 3 to 8 hours after acute overdose. Hyperventilation, an increase in both rate (tachypnea) and depth (hyperpnea), is present but it may be subtle. It results in a mild respiratory alkalosis with a serum pH greater than 7.4 and urine pH greater than 6.0. Some patients may have lethargy, vertigo, headache, and confusion. Diaphoresis may be noted.

Phase II. Moderate manifestations occur at 12 to 24 hours after ingestion with a 6-hour salicylate plasma concentration of 70 to 90 mg/dL. Serious metabolic disturbances, including a marked respiratory alkalosis with anion gap metabolic acidosis, dehydration, and urine pH less than 6.0, may occur. Other metabolic disturbances include hypoglycemia or hyperglycemia, hypokalemia, decreased ionized calcium, and increased BUN, creatinine, and lactate. Mental disturbances (confusion, disorientation, hallucinations) may occur. Hypotension and convulsions have been reported.

Phase III. Severe intoxication occurs more than 24 hours after ingestion with a 6-hour salicylate plasma concentration of 90 to 130 mg/dL. In addition to the above clinical findings, coma and seizures develop and indicate severe intoxication. Pulmonary edema may occur. Metabolic disturbances include metabolic acidemia (pH <7.4) and aciduria (pH <6.0). In adults, alkalosis may persist until terminal respiratory failure.

In children younger than 4 years of age, a mixed metabolic acidosis and respiratory alkalosis develop earlier (within 4 to 6 hours) than in adults because children have less respiratory reserve and accumulate lactate and other organic acids. Hypoglycemia is more common in children.

Fatalities occur at 6-hour salicylate plasma concentrations greater than 130 to 150 mg/dL and result from CNS depression, cardiovascular collapse, electrolyte imbalance, and cerebral edema.

Chronic salicylism is more serious than acute intoxication and the 6-hour salicylate plasma concentration does not correlate well with the manifestations in both acute and chronic cases of intoxication. Chronic intoxication usually occurs with therapeutic errors in young children or the elderly with underlying illness, and the diagnosis is delayed because it is not recognized. Noncardiac pulmonary edema is a frequent complication in the elderly. The mortality rate is about 25%. Chronic salicylate poisoning in children may mimic Reye syndrome. It is associated with exaggerated CNS findings (hallucinations, delirium, dementia, memory loss, papilledema, bizarre behavior, agitation, encephalopathy, seizures, and coma). Hemorrhagic manifestations, renal failure, and pulmonary and cerebral edema may occur. The metabolic picture is hypoglycemia and mixed acid–base derangements. A chronic salicylate plasma concentration greater than 60 mg/dL with metabolic acidosis and an altered mental state is very serious.

Laboratory Investigations

All patients with intentional salicylate overdoses should have acetaminophen plasma level measured after 4 hours.

One should continuously monitor ECG, urine output, urine pH, and specific gravity. Every 2 to 4 hours in cases of severe intoxication, salicylate plasma concentration, glucose (in a case of salicylism, CNS hypoglycemia may be present despite normal serum glucose), electrolytes, ionized calcium, magnesium and phosphorous, anion gap, ABGs, and pulse oximeter should be monitored. Daily monitoring of BUN, creatinine, liver function tests, and prothrombin time should take place.

The therapeutic salicylate plasma concentration is less than 10 mg/dL for analgesia and 15 to 30 mg/dL for anti-inflammatory effect. Cross-reaction with diflunisal (Dolobid) will give a falsely high salicylate plasma concentration. The Done nomogram is not considered accurate in evaluating acute or chronic salicylate intoxications.

Management

Treatment is based on clinical and metabolic findings, not on salicylate levels. Continuous monitoring of the urine pH is essential for successful alkalinization treatment. One should always obtain an acetaminophen plasma level.

Vital functions must be established and maintained. If the patient is in an altered mental state, glucose, naloxone, and thiamine are administered in standard doses. Depending on the severity, the initial studies include an immediate and a 6-hour postingestion salicylate plasma concentration, ECG and cardiac monitoring, pulse oximeter, urine (analysis, pH, and specific gravity), chest radiograph, ABGs, blood glucose, electrolytes and anion gap calculation, calcium (ionized), magnesium, renal and liver profiles, and prothrombin time. Gastric contents and stool should be tested for occult blood. Bismuth and magnesium salicylate preparations may be radiopaque on radiographs. Consultation with a nephrologist is warranted in cases of moderate, severe, or chronic intoxication.

For gastrointestinal decontamination, activated charcoal is useful (each gram of activated charcoal binds 550 mg of salicylic acid) if a toxic dose was ingested up to 4 hours postingestion. MDAC is not recommended for salicylate intoxication.

Concretions may occur with massive (usually >300 mg/kg) ingestions. If blood levels fail to decline, prompt contrast radiography of the stomach may reveal concretions that have to be removed by repeated lavage, whole-bowel irrigation, endoscopy, or gastrostomy.

Fluids and electrolyte treatment of salicylate poisonings is given in Table 27. For shock, perfusion and vascular volume should be established with 5% dextrose in 0.9% saline, then the treatment can proceed with correction of dehydration and alkalinization.

For cases of acute moderate or severe salicylism (see Table 27), adults should receive a bolus of 1 to 2 mEq/kg of sodium bicarbonate ($NaHCO_3$) followed by an infusion of 100 to 150 mEq $NaHCO_3$ added to 500 to 1000 mL of 5% dextrose and administered over 60 minutes. Children should receive a bolus of 1 to 2 mEq/kg of $NaHCO_3$ followed by an infusion of 1 to 2 mEq/kg added to 20 mL/kg of 5% dextrose administered over 60 minutes. Potassium is added after the patient voids. The goal is to achieve a urine output of greater than 2 mL/kg/hr and a urine pH of

TABLE 27 Fluid and Electrolyte Treatment of Salicylate Poisoning

Type of Salicylism	Metabolic Disturbance	Blood pH	Urine pH	Hydrating Solution	Amount of $NaHCO_3$ (mEq/L)	Amount of Potassium (mEq/L)
Mild	Respiratory alkalosis	>7.4	>6.0	5% Dextrose, 0.45% saline	50 (adult) 1 mEq/kg (child)	20
Moderate Chronic Child <4 Years	Respiratory alkalosis Metabolic acidosis	>7.4 or <7.4	<6.0	5% Dextrose in water	100 (adult) 1–2 mEq/kg (child)	40
Severe Chronic Child <4 years	Metabolic acidosis Respiratory alkalosis	<7.4	<6.0	5% Dextrose in water	150 (adult) 2m Eq/kg (child)	60
CNS depressant co-ingestant	Respiratory acidosis	<7.4	<6.0	5% Dextrose in water	100-150*	60

*Correct hypoventilation.

Modified from Linden CH, Rumack BH: The legitimate analgesics, aspirin and acetaminophen. In Hansen W Jr (ed): Toxic Emergencies. New York, Churchill Livingstone, 1984.

greater than 8. The initial infusion is followed by subsequent infusions (two to three times normal maintenance) of 200 to 300 mL/h in adults or 10 mL/kg/h in children. If the patient is acidotic and has a serum pH of less than 7.15, an additional 1 to 2 mEq/kg of $NaHCO_3$ is given over 1 to 2 hours; persistent acidosis may require 1 to 2 mEq/kg of bicarbonate every 2 hours. The infusion rate, the amount of bicarbonate, and the electrolytes should be adjusted to correct serum abnormalities and to maintain the targeted urine output and urinary pH. Diuresis is not as important as the alkalinization. Careful monitoring for fluid overload should take place for patients at risk of pulmonary and cerebral edema (e.g., the elderly) and because of inappropriate secretion of the antidiuretic hormone.

In patients with mild intoxication who are not acidotic and have a urine pH greater than 6, 5% dextrose in 0.45% saline should be administered as maintenance to replace ongoing fluid loss. Some toxicologists may consider adding sodium bicarbonate 50 mEq/L or 1 mEq/kg in some cases.

To achieve alkalinization, sodium bicarbonate is administered to produce a serum pH 7.4 to 7.5 and a urine pH greater than 8. Carbonic anhydrase inhibitors (acetazolamide [Diamox]) should not be used. If the patient is acidotic, additional bicarbonate may be required. About 2 mEq/kg raises the blood pH 0.1. In children, alkalinization may be a difficult problem because of the organic acid production and hypokalemia. Hypokalemic and fluid-depleted patients cannot be adequately alkalinized. Alkalinization is usually discontinued in asymptomatic patients with a salicylate plasma concentration less than 30 to 40 mg/dL but is continued in symptomatic patients regardless of the salicylate plasma concentration. A decreased serum bicarbonate but normal or high blood pH indicates respiratory alkalosis predominating over metabolic acidosis, and the bicarbonate should be administered cautiously. An alkalemic pH of 7.40 to 7.50 is not a contraindication to bicarbonate therapy because these patients have a significant base deficit in spite of elevated blood pH.

Potassium is added, 20 to 40 mEq/L, to the infusion after the patient voids. In cases of severe, late, and chronic salicylism, 60 mEq/L of potassium may be needed. When the serum potassium is below 4.0 mEq/L, 10 mEq/L should be added over the first hour. If the patient has hypokalemia less than 3 mEq/L and flat T waves and U waves, 0.25 to 0.5 mEq/kg up to 10 mEq/h is administered. Potassium should be administered under ECG monitoring. Serum potassium is rechecked after each rapidly administered dose. A paradoxical urine acidosis (alkaline serum pH and acid urine pH) indicates that potassium is probably needed.

Convulsions are treated with diazepam or lorazepam, but hypoglycemia, low ionized calcium, cerebral edema, and hemorrhage should first be excluded with a CT scan. If tetany develops, the $NaHCO_3$ therapy is discontinued and calcium gluconate 0.1 to 0.2 mL/kg 10% administered.

Pulmonary edema management consists of fluid restriction, high FIO_2, mechanical ventilation, and positive end-expiratory pressure.

Cerebral edema management consists of fluid restriction, elevation of the head, hyperventilation, osmotic diuresis, and administration of dexamethasone. Vitamin K_1 is administered parenterally to correct an increased prothrombin time (>20 seconds) and coagulation abnormalities. If the patient has active bleeding, fresh plasma and platelets are administered as needed. Hyperpyrexia is managed by external cooling measures, not antipyretics.

Hemodialysis is the choice for removal of salicylates because it corrects the acid–base, electrolyte, and fluid disturbances as well. The indications for hemodialysis include the following:

- Acute poisoning with salicylate plasma concentration greater than 100 mg/dL without improvement after 6 hours of appropriate therapy

- Chronic poisoning with cardiopulmonary disease and a salicylate plasma concentration as low as 40 mg/dL with refractory acidosis, severe CNS manifestations (coma and seizures), and progressive deterioration, especially in elderly patients
- Impairment of vital organs of elimination
- Clinical deterioration in spite of good supportive care and alkalinization
- Severe refractory acid–base or electrolyte disturbances despite appropriate corrective measures

Disposition

There are limitations of salicylate plasma levels and patients are treated on the basis of clinical and laboratory findings. Patients who are asymptomatic should be monitored for a minimum of 6 hours, and longer if enteric-coated tablets or massive overdose was taken or if there is suspicion of concretions. Those who remain asymptomatic with a salicylate plasma concentration less than 35 mg/dL may be discharged following psychiatric evaluation, if indicated. Chronic salicylate-intoxicated patients with acidosis and an altered mental state should be admitted to the intensive care unit. Patients with acute ingestion and a salicylate plasma concentration less than 60 mg/dL and mild symptoms may be able to be treated in the emergency department. Patients with moderate and severe intoxications should be admitted to the intensive care unit.

SELECTIVE SEROTONIN REUPTAKE INHIBITORS

Selective serotonin reuptake inhibitors (SSRIs) are primarily prescribed as antidepressants. SSRIs include fluoxetine (Prozac), paroxetine (Paxil), and sertraline (Zoloft).

Toxic Mechanism

The SSRIs interfere with the neuron reuptake of serotonin (5-hydroxytryptamine) at the presynaptic ganglia sites in the brain, increasing the activity of serotonin. SSRIs should not be used within 5 weeks of when a MAOI is given, nor should MAOI therapy be initiated or discontinued within 5 weeks of SSRI therapy.

Toxic Dose

The therapeutic oral dose of fluoxetine is 20 to 80 mg/d. No toxicity is seen in children with up to 3.5 mg/kg/dose orally. A fatal dose for adults is 6 g. The therapeutic dose for paroxetine is 20 to 50 mg/d. In 35 adult patients, none developed serious side effects after the ingestion of 10 to 1000 mg, and a study involving 35 children failed to demonstrate serious adverse effects at doses less than 180 mg. The therapeutic dose for sertraline is 50 mg to 200 mg/d. Patients have ingested up to 2.6 g without serious side effects. Overdose involving children who ingested less than 100 mg failed to cause adverse events.

Kinetics

Fluoxetine is well absorbed from the gastrointestinal tract, and has a peak plasma concentration at 6 to 8 hours. Volume distribution is 20 to 42 L/kg; 95% is protein bound. The half-life is 4 days (for the demethylated active metabolite norfluoxetine, the half-life is 7 to 15 days). Elimination is 80% renal. Fluoxetine and other serotonin inhibitors are inhibitors of the cytochrome P450, CYP 2D6 enzyme. Therefore interactions may occur with many other medications, such as antidysrhythmic class IC drugs (quinidine), phenytoin (Dilantin), haloperidol, lithium, tricyclic antidepressants (TCAs), β-blockers, codeine, and carbamazepine (Tegretol).

Paroxetine is almost completely absorbed from the gastrointestinal tract, with a peak in 2 to 8 hours. Protein binding is greater than 90%; volume distribution is 13 L/kg. Paroxetine undergoes extensive first-pass liver metabolism by oxidation and methylation to inactive metabolites. It inhibits the P450 system (see fluoxetine metabolism). The average half-life is 21 hours.

Sertraline peaks in 8 to 12 hours. Its volume distribution is 20 L/kg and protein binding is 98%. The average half-life of sertraline is 26 hours. It is metabolized to form a less-active metabolite, *N*-desmethylsertraline (half-life of 62 to 104 hours).

Manifestations

All SSRIs may cause serotonin syndrome, a potentially life-threatening reaction, if they are administered concurrently with an MAOI. Serotonin syndrome is caused by cerebral serotonergic stimulation and can cause severe hyperthermia, myoclonus, rhabdomyolysis, confusion, tremors, and a variety of psychological disturbances. In addition, cardiovascular complications and extrapyramidal side effects, including akathisia, dyskinesia, and Parkinson-like syndromes may occur. Also, increased suicidal ideation, seizures, sexual disorders, and hematologic disorders (platelet serotonin activity blockade leading to prolonged bleeding times) may develop. Inappropriate secretion of antidiuretic hormone resulting in hyponatremia may occur when SSRIs are administered to the elderly. This effect is usually seen within the first week of therapy.

Overdose effects are similar to the serotonin syndrome.

Laboratory Investigations

One should obtain a complete blood count (CBC), electrolytes, glucose levels, a coagulation profile, liver function tests, creatine kinase level, and an ECG.

Management

There is no specific antidote to SSRI intoxication.

Initial management consists of stabilizing vital functions, including thermoregulation. Supportive therapy and anticipation of potential life-threatening manifestations (hypotension, hyperthermia, seizures, coma, disseminated intravascular coagulation, ventricular tachycardia, and metabolic acidosis), are essential. Vital signs, EEG, creatine kinase, and blood chemistry should be monitored.

Benzodiazepines are administered to prevent and control muscle hyperactivity (diazepam [Valium] for seizures, clonazepam [Klonopin] for myoclonus). If benzodiazepine therapy fails to control muscle activity or seizures, anesthesia or nondepolarizing neuromuscular blockade may be necessary.

Electrolyte abnormalities and acid–base balance should be corrected. Fluids are used to maintain a urine output of greater than 2 mL/kg/h if there is a risk of myoglobinuria.

There are no data to support the use of gastrointestinal decontamination, although activated charcoal may be used if an ingestion has occurred within 1 hour. Hemodialysis and charcoal hemoperfusion are unlikely to be beneficial. Haloperidol (Haldol), phenothiazines, and other highly protein-bound drugs are to be avoided.

Benzodiazepine and cooling therapy can be used for hyperthermia. Serotonin antagonists, such as cyproheptadine (Periactin), may be useful in treating serotonin syndrome, although there are no controlled data. Dantrolene (Dantrium) and bromocriptine (Parlodel) are not recommended and may actually precipitate serotonin syndrome.

Disposition

Cases of ingestions in children up to 5 years of age of less than 180 mg of paroxetine (Paxil), less than 3.5 mg/kg of fluoxetine (Prozac), or less than 100 mg of sertraline (Zoloft) can be observed at home. Symptomatic patients should be admitted to the intensive care unit until asymptomatic for 24 hours. Asymptomatic patients should be observed for 6 hours. All patients should be assessed for risk of suicide before discharge. When taken chronically, SSRIs may increase cholesterol and triglycerides and decrease uric acid, so these test results should be followed.

THEOPHYLLINE

Theophylline (Slo-Phyllin) is a methylxanthine alkaloid similar to caffeine and theobromine. Aminophylline is 80% theophylline. Theophylline is used in the acute treatment of asthma, pulmonary edema, chronic obstructive pulmonary disease, and neonatal apnea.

Toxic Mechanism

The proposed mechanisms of action include phosphodiesterase inhibition, adenosine receptor antagonism, inhibition of prostaglandins, and increase in serum catecholamines. Theophylline stimulates the central nervous, respiratory, and emetic centers and reduces the seizure threshold. It has positive cardiac inotropic and chronotropic effects, acts as a diuretic, relaxes smooth muscle, and causes peripheral vasodilation but cerebral vasoconstriction. Gastric secretions, gastrointestinal motility, lipolysis, glycogenolysis, and gluconeogenesis are all increased.

Toxic Dose

A single dose of 1 mg/kg produces a theophylline plasma concentration of approximately 2 μg/mL. The therapeutic range usually is 10 to 20 μg/mL. An acute, single dose greater than 10 mg/kg causes mild toxicity, a dose greater than 20 mg/kg causes moderate toxicity, and a dose greater than 50 mg/kg causes serious, possibly fatal toxicity. Fatalities occur at lower doses in patients with chronic toxicity, especially those with risk factors (see *Kinetics*).

Kinetics

The pKa is 9.5. Absorption from the stomach and upper small intestine is complete and rapid, with onset in 30 to 60 minutes. Peak theophylline plasma concentration occurs within 1 to 2 hours after ingestion of liquid preparations, 2 to 4 hours after ingestion of regular tablets, and 7 to 24 hours after ingestion of slow-release formulations. Volume distribution is 0.3 to 0.7 L/kg. Protein binding is 40% to 60% in adults, mainly to albumin (low albumin increases free active theophylline).

Elimination is 90% by hepatic metabolism to an active metabolite, 2-methyl xanthine. The half-life is 3.5 hours in a child and 4 to 6 hours in an adult. The half-life is shorter in smokers and patients taking enzyme-inducing drugs. Only 8% to 10% of the drug is excreted unchanged in the urine.

Risk factors that produce a longer half-life include age younger than 6 months or older than 60 years, use of enzyme-inhibitor drugs (calcium channel blockers, oral contraceptives, cimetidine [Tagamet], ciprofloxacin [Cipro], erythromycin, macrolide antibiotics, isoniazid), illness (persistent fever >38.9°C [>102°F]), viral illness, liver impairment, heart failure, chronic obstructive pulmonary disease, and influenza vaccination.

Manifestations

Acute toxicity generally correlates with blood levels; chronic toxicity does not (Table 28).

In the case of an acute, single, regular-release overdose, vomiting and occasionally hematemesis occur at low theophylline plasma concentrations. CNS stimulation includes restlessness, muscle tremors, and protracted tonic–clonic seizures, but coma is rare. Convulsions are a sign of severe toxicity and usually are preceded by gastrointestinal symptoms (except with sustained-release and chronic

TABLE 28 Theophylline Blood Concentrations and Acute Toxicity

Plasma Concentration (μg/mL)	Toxicity Degree	Manifestations
8–10	None	Bronchodilation
10–20	Mild	Therapeutic range: nausea, vomiting, nervousness, respiratory alkalosis, tachycardia
15–25		35% have mild manifestations of toxicity
20–40	Moderate	Gastrointestinal complaints and central nervous system stimulation Transient hypertension, tachypnea, tachycardia; 80% will have some manifestations of toxicity
60	Severe	Convulsions, dysrhythmias
100		Hypokalemia, hyperglycemia Ventricular dysrhythmias protracted convulsions, hypotension, acid–base abnormalities

intoxications). Cardiovascular disturbances include cardiac dysrhythmias (supraventricular tachycardia) and transient hypertension with mild overdoses, but hypotension and ventricular dysrhythmias with severe intoxications. Rhabdomyolysis and renal failure are occasionally seen. Children tolerate higher serum levels, and cardiac dysrhythmias and seizures occur at theophylline plasma concentrations greater than 100 μg/mL. Possible metabolic disturbances include hyperglycemia, pronounced hypokalemia, hypocalcemia, hypomagnesemia, hypophosphatemia, increased serum amylase, and elevation of uric acid.

Chronic intoxication, defined as multiple doses of theophylline over 24 hours, or cases in which interacting drugs or illness interfere with theophylline metabolism are more serious and difficult to treat. Cardiac dysrhythmias and convulsions may occur at theophylline plasma concentrations of 40 to 60 μg/mL and there is no correlation with TPC. The seizures occur without warning and are protracted and repetitive and may produce status epilepticus. Vomiting and typical metabolic disturbances do not occur.

Differences with slow-release preparations are that few or no gastrointestinal symptoms occur, peak concentrations and convulsions may be delayed 12 to 24 hours postingestion, and convulsions occur without warning.

Laboratory Investigations

Monitoring includes vital signs, pulse oximeter, ABG, hemoglobin, hematocrit (for gastrointestinal hemorrhage), ECG and cardiac monitor, renal and hepatic function, electrolytes, blood glucose, acid–base balance, and serum albumin. Gastric contents and stools should be tested for occult blood. Samples for theophylline plasma concentration measurement should be drawn within 1 to 2 hours after ingestion of liquid preparations, 2 to 4 hours after ingestion of regular-release formulations, and 4 hours after ingestion of slow-release formulations. One should check the serum albumin level because a decrease in albumin levels may cause manifestations of toxicity despite normal theophylline plasma concentration. A single theophylline plasma concentration reading may be misleading; therefore, theophylline plasma concentration measurement should be repeated every 2 to 4 hours to determine the trend until a declining trend is reached and then monitored every 4 to 6 hours until it is below 20 μg/mL.

Management

Vital functions must be established and maintained. If the patient is in a coma or has convulsions or vomiting, he or she should be intubated immediately. The theophylline plasma concentration is obtained and repeated every 2 to 4 hours to determine peak absorption, and a theophylline bezoar should be considered if the theophylline plasma concentration fails to decline. Consultation with a nephrologist about charcoal hemoperfusion is recommended.

Gastrointestinal decontamination is warranted in the case of an acute overdose, but emesis must not be induced. Activated charcoal is the choice decontamination procedure in a dose of 1 g/kg to all patients, followed with MDAC 0.5 g/kg every 2 to 4 hours until the theophylline plasma concentration is less than 20 μg/mL. MDAC is effective in treating acute, chronic, and intravenous overdoses. Activated charcoal shortens the half-life of theophylline by about 50% and may be indicated up to 24 hours following ingestion.

Whole-bowel irrigation with polyethylene-electrolyte solution has been recommended for cases of massive overdose, possible concretions, and ingestion of sustained-release preparations. If intractable vomiting occurs, the antiemetic metoclopramide (Reglan) (0.1 mg/kg adult dose), droperidol (Inapsine) (2.5 to 10 mg IV), or ondansetron (Zofran) (8 to 32 mg IV) is administered. Ondansetron, however, inhibits metabolism of theophylline after a few doses.

Convulsions are controlled with lorazepam (Ativan) or diazepam (Valium) and phenobarbital. Phenytoin (Dilantin) is ineffective. The convulsions in patients with chronic intoxication are often refractory and may require, in addition to anticonvulsants, neuromuscular paralyzing agents, sedation, assisted ventilation, and EEG monitoring.

Hypotension is treated with fluids and vasopressors, if necessary. Norepinephrine (Levophed) 0.05 μg/kg/min is preferred as the vasopressor over dopamine.

Supraventricular tachycardia with hemodynamic instability requires cardioversion. Low-dose β-blockers may be used but should not be used in patients with reactive airway disease or hypotension. Adenosine (Adenocard) is ineffective. For ventricular dysrhythmias, electrolyte disturbances should be corrected. Lidocaine is the treatment of choice but has the potential to cause seizures at toxic concentrations. Cardioversion may be needed.

Hematemesis is managed with sucralfate (Carafate) 1 g four times daily and/or Maalox TC 30 mL every 2 hours and blood replacement, if necessary. H_2 antihistamine blockers that are enzyme inhibitors are not used.

Fluid and metabolic disturbances should be corrected. Hyperglycemia does not require insulin therapy. Hypokalemia should be corrected cautiously, as it may be largely an intracellular shift and not total body loss. Usually adding 40 mEq potassium to a liter of fluid will suffice. The serum potassium level must be monitored closely.

Charcoal hemoperfusion is the management of choice for patients with serious intoxications. Hemoperfusion can increase the clearance twofold to threefold over hemodialysis, but hemodialysis can be used if hemoperfusion is not available. Criteria for charcoal hemoperfusion are as follows:

- Life-threatening events such as convulsions or dysrhythmias
- Intractable vomiting refractory to antiemetics
- Acute intoxications with a theophylline plasma concentration greater than 80 µg/mL or greater than 70 µg/mL 4 hours after overdose with a sustained-release formulation and greater than 40 µg/mL in the case of chronic intoxication
- Acute or chronic overdoses with a theophylline plasma concentration greater than 40 µg/mL, especially if the patient has risk factors that lengthen the half-life of the drug (see Kinetics).

Disposition

Patients with mild symptoms and a theophylline plasma concentration less than 20 µg/mL can be treated in emergency department and discharged when asymptomatic for a few hours. Any patient with acute ingestion and a theophylline plasma concentration greater than 35 µg/mL should be admitted to a monitored bed with seizure precautions and suicide precautions, if needed. If neurologic or cardiotoxic effects or a theophylline plasma concentration greater than 50 µg/mL is present, the patient should be admitted to the intensive care unit. A patient with an overdose of a sustained-release preparation, regardless of symptoms or initial theophylline plasma concentration, requires admission, monitoring, activated charcoal, and MDAC. In patients on chronic therapy, toxicity may occur at a lower theophylline plasma concentration, and these patients should not be discharged until they are asymptomatic for several hours.

TRICYCLIC AND CYCLIC ANTIDEPRESSANTS

Historically, tricyclic antidepressants are an important cause of pharmaceutical overdose fatalities. The mortality rate was reduced from 15% in the 1970s to less than 1% in the 1990s because of a better understanding of the pathophysiology of these agents and improvements in management (Table 29).

Toxic Mechanism

The major mechanisms of toxicity of the tricyclic antidepressants are (a) central and peripheral anticholinergic effects; (b) peripheral α-adrenergic blockade; (c) quinidine-like cardiac membrane stabilizing action blockade of the fast inward sodium channels; and (d) inhibition of synaptic neurotransmitter reuptake in the CNS presynaptic neurons. The tetracyclics, monocyclic aminoketones, and dibenzoxazepines possess convulsive activity and less cardiac toxicity in overdose than the older tricyclic antidepressants. Triazolopyridine has less serious cardiac and CNS toxicity.

Toxic Dose

The therapeutic dose of imipramine (Tofranil) is 1.5 to 5 mg/kg; a dose greater than 5 mg/kg may be mildly toxic; 10 to 20 mg/kg may be life threatening, although less than 20 mg/kg has produced few fatalities; greater than 30 mg/kg carries a 30% mortality rate; and at a dose greater than 70 mg/kg, patients rarely survive. In children 375 mg and in adults as little as 500 mg have been fatal. In adults, five times the maximum daily dose is toxic and 10 times is potentially fatal. Although major overdose symptoms are associated with plasma concentrations greater than 1 µg/mL (>1000 ng/mL), plasma tricyclic levels do not correlate well with toxicity; clinical signs and symptoms should guide therapy.

The relative dosage or potency equivalents are as follows: amitriptyline (Elavil) 100 mg = amoxapine (Asendin) 125 mg = desipramine (Norpramin) 75 mg = doxepin (Sinequan) 100 mg = imipramine (Tofranil) 75 mg = maprotiline (Ludiomil) 75 mg = nortriptyline (Pamelor) 50 mg = trazodone (Desyrel) 200 mg. This allows one to determine an equivalent dosage of an agent compared with another (see Table 29).

Kinetics

The tricyclic and cyclic antidepressants are lipophilic. They are rapidly absorbed from the alkaline small intestine, but absorption may be prolonged and delayed in cases of massive overdose owing to anticholinergic action. Onset varies from less than 1 hour (30 to 40 minutes) to, rarely, 12 hours. The peak serum levels are reached in 2 to 8 hours and the peak effect is in 6 hours but may be delayed 12 hours because of erratic absorption. The clinical effects correlate poorly with plasma levels.

Cyclic antidepressants are highly protein-bound to plasma glycoproteins, 98% at a pH 7.5 and 90% at 7.0. Volume distribution is 10 to 50 L/kg. The elimination route is by hepatic metabolism. The tertiary amines

TABLE 29 Cyclic Antidepressants, Daily Dose and Their Major Properties

Generic Name	Adult Daily Dose (mg)	Therapeutic Range (ng/mL)	Half-life (hours)	Toxicity*		
				ANTICHOL	CNS	CARDIAC
Tertiary Amines						
Amitriptyline (Elavil)	75–300	120–250	31–46	3+	3+	3+
Imipramine (Tofranil)	75–300	125–250	9–24	3+	3+	2+
Doxepin (Sinequan)	75–300	30–150	8–24	3+	3+	2+
Trimipramine (Surmantil)	75–200	10–240	16–18	3+	3+	2+
Secondary Amines						
Nortriptyline (Pamelor)	75–150	50–150	18–93	2+	3+	3+
Desipramine (Norpramin)	75 200	75–160	14–62	1+	3+	3+
Protriptyline (Vivactil)	20–60	70–250	54–198	2+	3+	3+
Newer Cyclic Antidepressants						
Teracyclic			30–60	1+	2+	3+
Maprotiline (Ludiomil)	75–300	—	30–60	1+	2+	3+
Trizolopyridine, a noncyclic, produces less serious cardiac and CNS toxicity						
Trazodone (Desyrel)	50–600	700	4–7	1+	1+	1+
Monocyclic Aminoketone						
Bupropion (Wellbutrin)	200–400	—	8–24	1+	3+	1+
Dibenzazepine						
Clomipramine (Anafranil)	100–250	200–500	21–32	2+	2+	2+
Dibenoxazepine						
Amoxapine (Ascendin)	150–300	200–500	6–10	1+	3+	2+

*Antichol = anticholinergic effect; CNS = central nervous system effect primarily seizures; Cardiac = cardiac effect.
Other drugs with similar structures are cyclobenzaprine, a muscle relaxant (similar to amitriptyline), and carbamazepine, an anticonvulsant (similar to imipramine); however, they cause less cardiac toxicity.

are metabolized into active demethylated secondary amine metabolites. The active secondary amine metabolites undergo a 15% enterohepatic recirculation and are metabolized over a period of days into nonactive metabolites. The intestinal bacterial flora may reconstitute the metabolites, which are active.

The half-life varies from 10 hours for imipramine to 81 hours for amitriptyline and 100 hours for nortriptyline. The active metabolites have longer half-lives.

Only 3% of the ingested dose is excreted in the urine unchanged.

Manifestations

There are reports of asymptomatic patients who, upon arrival to an emergency department, suddenly have a seizure, develop hemodynamically unstable dysrhythmias, and die shortly thereafter from ingestion of a tricyclic antidepressant. Most patients with severe toxicity develop symptoms within 1 to 2 hours, but symptoms may be delayed 6 hours after overdose.

Small overdoses produce early anticholinergic effects, agitation, and transient hypertension, which are not life-threatening. Large overdoses produce depression of the CNS and myocardium, convulsions, and hypotension. Death can occur within the first 2 to 6 hours following ingestion.

Some ECG screening tools for predicting cardiac or neurologic toxicity from ingestion of a tricyclic antidepressant have been developed: (a) A QRS greater than 0.10 second may produce seizures, and if greater than 0.16 second, 50% of patients may develop ventricular dysrhythmias (20% of these may be life-threatening) and seizures; (b) a terminal 40 msec of the QRS axis greater than 120 degrees in the right frontal plane may be associated with toxicity; or (c) a large R wave greater than 3 mm in ECG lead aVR may predispose the patient to toxicity. The quinidine cardiac membrane stabilizing effect produces depression of myocardium, conduction, and ECG changes. The peripheral α-adrenergic blockade produces hypotension.

The secondary amines are metabolized to inactive metabolites. The tetracyclics produce a high incidence of cardiovascular disturbances and seizures. Monocyclic aminoketones produce seizures in doses greater than 600 mg. Dibenzoxazepines produce a syndrome of convulsions, rhabdomyolysis, and renal failure.

Laboratory Investigations

If the patient has altered mental status or ECG abnormalities, ABG, ECG, chest radiograph, blood glucose, serum electrolytes, calcium, magnesium, blood urea nitrogen, and creatinine levels, liver profile, creatine kinase level, urine output, and, in severe cases, hemodynamic monitoring are indicated. Levels of the tricyclic and cyclic antidepressants less than 300 ng/mL are therapeutic; levels greater than 500 ng/mL indicate toxicity, and levels greater than 1000 ng/mL indicate serious poisoning and are associated with QRS widening.

Management

Vital functions must be established and maintained. Even if the patient is asymptomatic, intravenous access should be established, vital signs and neurologic status monitored, and baseline 12-lead ECG and continuous cardiac monitoring obtained for at least 6 hours from admission or 8 to 12 hours postingestion. QRS interval should be measured on a limb lead ECG every 15 minutes for 6 hours postingestion.

For gastrointestinal decontamination, emesis should not be induced and gastric lavage should not be used. Activated charcoal is preferable. If the patient is in an altered mental state, the airway must be protected. Activated charcoal 1 g/kg is recommended up to 1 hour postingestion. Benefit from MDAC has not been demonstrated.

Alkalinization does not control seizures; diazepam or lorazepam should be used. Status epilepticus may require high-dose barbiturates or neuromuscular blockers with intravenous diazepam. If not successful, the patient can be paralyzed with short-term nondepolarizing neuromuscular blockers such as vecuronium (Norcuron), intubation, and assisted ventilation. A bolus of sodium bicarbonate is recommended as an adjunct to correct the acidosis produced by the seizures.

Sodium bicarbonate is administered in a dose of 1 to 2 mEq/kg undiluted as a bolus and repeated twice a few minutes apart, if needed, for "sodium loading" and alkalinization, which may increase protein binding from 90% to 98%. The sodium loading overcomes the sodium channel blockage and is more important than the alkalinization. Indications include (a) a QRS complex greater than 0.12 second, (b) ventricular tachycardia, (c) severe conduction disturbances, (d) metabolic acidosis, (e) coma, and (f) seizures. A continuous infusion of sodium bicarbonate is of limited usefulness for controlling dysrhythmias. Bolus therapy should be used as needed.

Hyperventilation alone has been recommended, but the pH elevation is not as instantaneous and there is compensatory renal excretion of bicarbonate; therefore, we do not recommend it. The combination of hyperventilation and sodium bicarbonate has produced fatal alkalemia and is not recommended. One should monitor serum potassium level (the sudden increase in blood pH can aggravate or precipitate hypokalemia), serum sodium, and ionized calcium levels (hypocalcemia may occur with alkalinization) and blood pH.

Specific cardiovascular complications should be treated as follows: Hypotension is treated with norepinephrine, a predominantly α-adrenergic drug, which is preferred over dopamine. Hypertension that occurs early rarely requires treatment. Sinus tachy cardia usually does not require treatment. Supraventricular tachycardia in a patient who is hemodynamically unstable requires synchronized electrical cardioversion, starting at 0.25 to 1.0 watt-second per kg, after sedation. Ventricular tachycardia that persists after alkalinization requires intravenous lidocaine or countershock if the patient is hemodynamically unstable. Ventricular fibrillation should be treated with defibrillation. Torsades de pointes is treated with magnesium sulfate IV 20% solution, 2 g over 2 to 3 minutes, followed by a continuous infusion of 1.5 mL 10% solution or 5 to 10 mg per minute. For the treatment of bradydysrhythmias, atropine is contraindicated because of the anticholinergic activity. Isoproterenol 0.1 μg/kg/ minute, used with caution, may produce hypotension. If the patient is hemodynamically unstable, a pacemaker is used.

Extraordinary measures, such as aortic balloon pump and cardiopulmonary bypass, have been successful.

Investigational treatments include FAB fragments specific for tricyclic antidepressant, which have been successful in animals. Prophylactic $NaHCO_3$ to prevent dysrhythmias is also being investigated.

Physostigmine has produced asystole, and flumazenil has produced seizures. Both are contraindicated.

Disposition

A patient with an antidepressant overdose who meets any of the following criteria should be admitted to the intensive care unit for 12 to 24 hours: (a) ECG abnormalities except sinus tachycardia, (b) altered mental state, (c) seizures, (d) respiratory depression, and (e) hypotension. Low-risk patients include those in whom the above symptoms are absent at 6 hours postingestion, those who present with minor transient manifestations such as sinus tachycardia who subsequently become and remain asymptomatic for a 6-hour period, and asymptomatic patients who remain asymptomatic for 6 hours. These patients may be discharged if the ECG remains normal, they have normal bowel sounds, and they undergo psychiatric disposition.

Even if the patient is asymptomatic upon presentation to the health care facility, intravenous access should be established, vital signs and neurologic status monitored, a baseline 12-lead ECG obtained, and cardiac monitoring continued for at least 6 hours. *Caution:* in 25% of fatal cases, the patients were initially alert and awake at presentation. However, in most cases of fatality initially deemed as sudden cardiac death, the patient, upon reexamination, actually had symptoms that were missed.

Children younger than 6 years of age with nonintentional (accidental) exposures to amitriptyline (Elavil), desipramine (Norpramin), doxepin (Sinequan), imipramine (Tofranil), or nortriptyline (Aventyl) in a dose less than 5 mg/kg, who are asymptomatic and have what are deemed reliable caregivers, can be observed at home, with close poison control follow-up for 6 hours. Parents or caregivers should be given instructions regarding signs and symptoms to be alert for. Children who are symptomatic, or who ingested greater than 5 mg/kg, should be referred to the emergency department for monitoring, observation, and activated charcoal treatment.

SECTION 19

Appendices and Index

REFERENCE INTERVALS FOR THE INTERPRETATION OF LABORATORY TESTS

METHOD OF

William Z. Borer, MD

Most of the tests performed in a clinical laboratory are quantitative; that is, the amount of a substance present in blood or serum is measured and reported in terms of concentration, activity (e.g., enzyme activity), or counts (e.g., blood cell counts). The laboratory must provide reference intervals to assist the clinician in the interpretation of laboratory results. These reference intervals represent the physiologic quantities of a substance (concentrations, activities, or counts) to be expected in healthy persons. Deviation above or below the reference range may be associated with a disease process, and the severity of the disease process may be associated with the magnitude of the deviation. Unfortunately, a sharp demarcation rarely exists to distinguish between physiologic and pathologic values, and the time of transition between the two is often gradual as the disease process progresses.

The terms *normal* and *abnormal* have been used to describe laboratory values that fall inside and outside the reference range, respectively. Use of these terms is inappropriate because no good definition of normality exists in the clinical sense and the term *normal* may be confused with the statistical term *gaussian*. Reference ranges are established from statistical studies in groups of healthy volunteers. These study subjects must be free of disease, but they may have lifestyles or habits that result in variations in certain laboratory values. Examples of these variables include diet, body mass, exercise, and geographic location. Age and gender may also affect reference values.

When the data from a large cohort of healthy subjects fit a gaussian distribution, the usual statistical approach is to define the reference limits as 2 standard deviations (SD) above and below the mean. By definition, the reference range excludes the 2.5% of the population with the lowest values and the 2.5% with the highest values. Nongaussian distributions are handled by different statistical methods, but the result is similar in that the reference range is defined by the central 95% of the population. In other words, the probability that a healthy person will have a laboratory result that falls outside the reference range is 1 in 20. If 12 laboratory tests are performed, the probability that at least one of the results will be outside the reference range increases to about 50%, which means that all healthy persons are likely to have a few laboratory results that are unexpected. The clinician must then integrate these data with other clinical information, such as the history and physical examination, to arrive at an appropriate clinical decision.

The reference intervals for many tests (especially enzyme and immunochemical measurements) vary with the method used. Accordingly, each laboratory must establish reference intervals that are appropriate for the methods used.

SI Units

During the 1980s, a concerted effort was made to introduce SI units (le Système International d'Unités). The rationale for conversion to SI units is sound. Laboratory data are scientifically more informative when the units are based on molar concentration rather than on mass concentration. For example, the conversion of glucose to lactate and pyruvate or the binding of a drug to albumin is more easily understood in units of molar concentration. Another example is illustrated as follows:

CONVENTIONAL UNITS

1.0g of hemoglobin:

- Combines with 1.37 mL of oxygen
- Contains 3.4 mg of iron
- Forms 34.9 mg of bilirubin

SI UNITS

4.0 mmol of hemoglobin:

- Combines with 4.0 mmol of oxygen
- Contains 4.0 mmol of iron
- Forms 4.0 mmol of bilirubin

The use of SI units would also enhance the standardization of nomenclature to facilitate global communication of medical and scientific information. The units, symbols, and prefixes used in the international system are shown in Tables 1, 2, and 3.

Unfortunately, problems have arisen with the implementation of SI units in the United States. The introduction of this system in 1987 prompted many medical journals to report laboratory values in both SI and conventional units in anticipation of complete conversion to SI units in the early 1990s.

TABLE 1 Base SI Units

Property	Unit	Symbol
Length	Meter	m
Mass	Kilogram	kg
Amount of substance	Mole	mol
Time	Second	s
Thermodynamic temperature	Kelvin	K
Electrical current	Ampere	A
Luminous intensity	Candela	cd
Catalytic amount	Katal	kat

TABLE 2 Derived SI Units and Non-SI Units Retained for Use with SI Units

Property	Unit	Symbol
Area	Square meter	m^2
Volume	Cubic meter	m^3
	Liter	L
Mass concentration	Kilogram/cubic meter	kg/m^3
	Gram/liter	g/L
Substance concentration	Mole/cubic meter	mol/m^3
	Mole/liter	mol/L
Temperature	Degree Celsius	C = K − 273.15

The lack of a coordinated effort toward this goal forced a retrenchment on the issue. Physicians continue to think and practice with laboratory results expressed in conventional units, and few, if any, hospitals or clinical laboratories in the United States use SI units exclusively. Complete conversion to SI units is not likely to occur in the foreseeable future, but most medical journals will probably continue to publish both sets of units. For this reason, the values in the tables of reference ranges in this appendix are given in both conventional units and SI units.

Tables of Reference Intervals

Some of the values included in the tables that follow have been established by the Clinical Laboratories at Thomas Jefferson University Hospital in Philadelphia and have not been published elsewhere. Other values have been compiled from the sources cited in the suggested readings. These tables are provided for information and educational purposes only. Laboratory values must always be interpreted in the context of clinical data derived from other sources, including the medical history and physical examination. One must exercise individual judgment when using the information provided in this appendix.

TABLE 3 Standard Prefixes

Prefix	Multiplication Factor	Symbol
yocto	10^{-24}	y
zepto	10^{-21}	z
atto	10^{-18}	a
femto	10^{-15}	f
pico	10^{-12}	p
nano	10^{-9}	n
micro	10^{-6}	µ
milli	10^{-3}	m
centi	10^{-2}	c
deci	10^{-1}	d
deca	10^{1}	da
hecto	10^{2}	h
kilo	10^{3}	k
mega	10^{6}	M
giga	10^{9}	G
tera	10^{12}	T

SUGGESTED READINGS

Bick RL (ed): Hematology: Clinical and Laboratory Practice. St Louis, Mosby–Year Book, 1993.

Borer WZ: Selection and use of laboratory tests. In Tietz NW, Conn RB, Pruden EL (eds): Applied Laboratory Medicine. Philadelphia, WB Saunders, 1992, pp 1-5.

Campion EW: A retreat from SI units. N Engl J Med 327:49, 1992.

Drug Evaluations Annual. Chicago, American Medical Association, 1994.

Friedman RB, Young DS: Effects of Disease on Clinical Laboratory Tests, 3rd ed. Washington, DC, AACC Press, 1997.

Henry JB: Clinical Diagnosis and Management by Laboratory Methods, 19th ed. Philadelphia, WB Saunders, 1996.

Hicks JM, Young DS: DORA 97-99: Directory of Rare Analyses. Washington, DC, AACC Press, 1997.

Jacob DS, Demott WR, Grady HJ, et al (eds): Laboratory Test Handbook, 4th ed. Baltimore, Williams & Wilkins, 1996.

Kaplan LA, Pesce AJ: Clinical Chemistry: Theory, Analysis, and Correlation, 3rd ed. St Louis, Mosby-Year Book, 1996.

Kjeldsberg CR, Knight JA: Body Fluids: Laboratory Examination of Amniotic, Cerebrospinal, Seminal, Serous and Synovial Fluids, 3rd ed. Chicago, ASCP Press, 1993.

Laposata M: SI Unit Conversion Guide. Boston, NEJM Books, 1992.

Scully RE, McNeely WF, Mark EJ, McNeely BU: Normal reference laboratory values. N Engl J Med 327:718-724, 1992.

Speicher CE: The Right Test: A Physician's Guide to Laboratory Medicine, 3rd ed. Philadelphia, WB Saunders, 1998.

Tietz NW (ed): Clinical Guide to Laboratory Tests, 3rd ed. Philadelphia, WB Saunders, 1995.

Wallach J: Interpretation of Diagnostic Tests: A Synopsis of Laboratory Medicine, 6th ed. Boston, Little, Brown, 1996.

Young DS: Effects of Preanalytical Variables on Clinical Laboratory Tests, 2nd ed. Washington, DC, AACC Press, 1997.

Young DS: Effects of Drugs on Clinical Laboratory Tests, 4th ed. Washington, DC, AACC Press, 1995.

Young DS: Determination and validation of reference intervals. Arch Pathol Lab Med 116:704-709, 1992.

Young DS: Implementation of SI units for clinical laboratory data. Ann Intern Med 106:114-129, 1987.

Reference Intervals for Hematology

Test	Conventional Units	SI Units
Acid hemolysis (Ham test)	No hemolysis	No hemolysis
Alkaline phosphatase, leukocyte	Total score, 14-100	Total score, 14-100
Cell counts		
Erythrocytes		
Males	4.6-6.2 million/mm³	4.6-6.2 × 10^{12}/L
Females	4.2-5.4 million/mm³	4.2-5.4 × 10^{12}/L
Children (varies with age)	4.5-5.1 million/mm³	4.5-5.1 × 10^{12}/L
Leukocytes, total	4500-11,000/mm³	4.5-11.0 × 10^{9}/L
Leukocytes, differential counts*		
Myelocytes	0%	0/L
Band neutrophils	3-5%	150-400 × 10^{6}/L
Segmented neutrophils	54-62%	3000-5800 × 10^{6}/L
Lymphocytes	25-33%	1500-3000 × 10^{6}/L
Monocytes	3-7%	300-500 × 10^{6}/L
Eosinophils	1-3%	50-250 × 10^{6}/L
Basophils	0-1%	15-50 × 10^{6}/L
Platelets	150,000-400,000/mm³	150-400 × 10^{9}/L
Reticulocytes	25,000-75,000/mm³ (0.5-1.5% of erythrocytes)	25-75 × 10^{9}/L
Coagulation tests		
Bleeding time (template)	2.75-8.0 min	2.75-8.0 min
Coagulation time (glass tube)	5-15 min	5-15 min
D Dimer	<0.5 μg/mL	<0.5 mg/L
Factor VIII and other coagulation factors	50-150% of normal	0.5-1.5 of normal
Fibrin split products (Thrombo-Welco test)	<10 μg/mL	<10 mg/L
Fibrinogen	200-400 mg/dL	2.0-4.0 g/L
Partial thromboplastin time, activated (aPTT)	20-25 s	20-35 s
Prothrombin time (PT)	12.0-14.0 s	12.0-14.0 s
Coombs' test		
Direct	Negative	Negative
Indirect	Negative	Negative
Corpuscular values of erythrocytes		
Mean corpuscular hemoglobin (MCH)	26-34 pg/cell	26-34 pg/cell
Mean corpuscular volume (MCV)	80-96 μm³	80-96 fL
Mean corpuscular hemoglobin concentration (MCHC)	32-36 g/dL	320-360 g/L
Haptoglobin	20-165 mg/dL	0.20-1.65 g/L
Hematocrit		
Males	40-54 mL/dL	0.40-0.54
Females	37-47 mL/dL	0.37-0.47
Newborns	49-54 mL/dL	0.49-0.54
Children (varies with age)	35-49 mL/dL	0.35-0.49
Hemoglobin		
Males	13.0-18.0 g/dL	8.1-11.2 mmol/L

Continued

Reference Intervals for Hematology—cont'd

Test	Conventional Units	SI Units
Females	12.0-16.0 g/dL	7.4-9.9 mmol/L
Newborns	16.5-19.5 g/dL	10.2-12.1 mmol/L
Children (varies with age)	11.2-16.5 g/dL	7.0-10.2 mmol/L
Hemoglobin, fetal	<1.0% of total	<0.01 of total
Hemoglobin A_{1C}	3-5% of total	0.03-0.05 of total
Hemoglobin A_2	1.5-3.0% of total	0.015-0.03 of total
Hemoglobin, plasma	0.0-5.0 mg/dL	0.0-3.2 µmol/L
Methemoglobin	30-130 mg/dL	19-80 µmol/L
Erythrocyte sedimentation rate (ESR)		
Wintrobe:		
Males	0-5 mm/h	0-5 mm/h
Females	0-15 mm/h	0-15 mm/h
Westergren:		
Males	0-15 mm/h	0-15 mm/h
Females	0-20 mm/h	0-20 mm/h

*Conventional units are percentages; SI units are absolute cell counts.

Reference Intervals* for Clinical Chemistry (Blood, Serum, and Plasma)

Analyte	Conventional Units	SI Units
Acetoacetate plus acetone		
Qualitative	Negative	Negative
Quantitative	0.3–2.0 mg/dL	30-200 µmol/L
Acid phosphatase, serum (thymolphthalein monophosphate substrate)	0.1-0.6 U/L	0.1-0.6 U/L
ACTH (see Corticotropin)		
Alanine aminotransferase (ALT), serum (SGPT)	1-45 U/L	1-45 U/L
Albumin, serum	3.3-5.2 g/dL	33-52 g/L
Aldolase, serum	0.0-7.0 U/L	0.0-7.0 U/L
Aldosterone, plasma		
Standing	5-30 ng/dL	140-830 pmol/L
Recumbent	3-10 ng/dL	80-275 pmol/L
Alkaline, phosphatase (ALP), serum		
Adult	35-150 U/L	35-150 U/L
Adolescent	100-500 U/L	100-500 U/L
Child	100-350 U/L	100-350 U/L
Ammonia nitrogen, plasma	10-50 µmol/L	10-50 µmol/L
Amylase, serum	25-125 U/L	25-125 U/L
Anion gap, serum calculated	8-16 mEq/L	8-16 mmol/L
Ascorbic acid, blood	0.4-1.5 mg/dL	23-85 µmol/L
Aspartate aminotransferase (AST), serum (SGOT)	1-36 U/L	1-36 U/L
Base excess, arterial blood, calculated	0±2 mEq/L	0±2 mmol/L
Bicarbonate		
Venous plasma	23-29 mEq/L	23-29 mmol/L
Arterial blood	21-27 mEq/L	21-27 mmol/L
Bile acids, serum	0.3-3.0 mg/dL	0.8-7.6 µmol/L
Bilirubin, serum		
Conjugated	0.1-0.4 mg/dL	1.7-6.8 µmol/L
Total	0.3-1.1 mg/dL	5.1-19.0 µmol/L
Calcium, serum	8.4-10.6 mg/dL	2.10-2.65 mmol/L
Calcium, ionized, serum	4.25-5.25 mg/dL	1.05-1.30 mmol/L
Carbon dioxide, total, serum or plasma	24-31 mEq/L	24-31 mmol/L
Carbon dioxide tension (P_{CO_2}), blood	35-45 mm Hg	35-45 mm Hg
β-Carotene, serum	60-260 µg/dL	1.1-8.6 µmol/L
Ceruloplasmin, serum	23-44 mg/dL	230-440 mg/L
Chloride, serum or plasma	96-106 mEq/L	96-106 mmol/L
Cholesterol, serum or EDTA plasma		
Desirable range	<200 mg/dL	<5.20 mmol/L
Low-density lipoprotein (LDL) cholesterol	60-180 mg/dL	1.55-4.65 mmol/L
High-density lipoprotein (HDL) cholesterol	30-80 mg/dL	0.80-2.05 mmol/L
Copper	70-140 µg/dL	11-22 µmol/L
Corticotropin (ACTH), plasma, 8 AM	10-80 pg/mL	2-18 pmol/L

Reference Intervals* for Clinical Chemistry (Blood, Serum, and Plasma)—cont'd

Analyte	Conventional Units	SI Units
Cortisol, plasma		
8:00 AM	6-23 μg/dL	170-630 nmol/L
4:00 PM	3-15 μg/dL	80-410 nmol/L
10:00 PM	<50% of 8:00 AM value	<50% of 8:00 AM value
Creatine, serum		
Males	0.2-0.5 mg/dL	15-40 μmol/L
Females	0.3-0.9 mg/dL	25-70 μmol/L
Creatine kinase (CK), serum		
Males	55-170 U/L	55-170 U/L
Females	30-135 U/L	30-135 U/L
Creatinine kinase MB isoenzyme, serum	<5% of total CK activity <5% of ng/mL by immunoassay	<5% of total CK activity <5% of ng/mL by immunoassay
Creatinine, serum	0.6-1.2 mg/dL	50-110 μmol/L
Estradiol-17β, adult		
Males	10-65 pg/mL	35-240 pmol/L
Females		
Follicular	30-100 pg/mL	110-370 pmol/L
Ovulatory	200-400 pg/mL	730-1470 pmol/L
Luteal	50-140 pg/mL	180-510 pmol/L
Ferritin, serum	20-200 ng/mL	20-200 μg/L
Fibrinogen, plasma	200-400 mg/dL	2.0-4.0 g/L
Folate, serum	3-18 ng/mL	6.8-4.1 nmol/L
Erythrocytes	145-540 ng/mL	330-120 nmol/L
Follicle-stimulating hormone (FSH), plasma		
Males	4-25 mU/mL	4-25 U/L
Females, premenopausal	4-30 mU/mL	4-30 U/L
Females, postmenopausal	40-250 mU/mL	40-250 U/L
Gastrin, fasting, serum	0-100 pg/mL	0-100 mg/L
Glucose, fasting, plasma or serum	70-115 mg/dL	3.9-6.4 nmol/L
γ-Glutamyltransferase (GGT), serum	5-40 U/L	5-40 U/L
Growth hormone (hGH), plasma, adult, fasting	0-6 ng/mL	0-6 μg/L
Haptoglobin, serum	20-165 mg/dL	0.20-1.65 g/L
Immunoglobulins, serum (see table of Reference Intervals for Tests of Immunologic Function)		
Iron, serum	75-175 μg/dL	13-31 μmol/L
Iron-binding capacity, serum		
Total	250-410 μg/dL	45-73 μmol/L
Saturation	20-55%	0.20-0.55
Lactate		
Venous whole blood	5.0-20.0 mg/dL	0.6-2.2 mmol/L
Arterial whole blood	5.0-15.0 mg/dL	0.6-1.7 mmol/L
Lactate dehydrogenase (LD), serum	110-220 U/L	110-220 U/L
Lipase, serum	10-140 U/L	10-140 U/L
Lutropin (LH), serum		
Males	1-9 U/L	1-9 U/L
Females		
Follicular phase	2-10 U/L	2-10 U/L
Midcycle peak	15-65 U/L	15-65 U/L
Luteal phase	1-12 U/L	1-12 U/L
Postmenopausal	12-65 U/L	12-65 U/L
Magnesium, serum	1.3-2.1 mg/dL	0.65-1.05 mmol/L
Osmolality	275-295 mOsm/kg water	275-295 mOsm/kg water
Oxygen, blood, arterial, room air		
Partial pressure (Pa_{O_2})	80-100 mm Hg	80-100 mm Hg
Saturation (Sa_{O_2})	95-98%	95-98%
pH, arterial blood	7.35-7.45	7.35-7.45
Phosphate, inorganic, serum		
Adult	3.0-4.5 mg/dL	1.0-1.5 mmol/L
Child	4.0-7.0 mg/dL	1.3-2.3 mmol/L
Potassium		
Serum	3.5-5.0 mEq/L	3.5-5.0 mmol/L
Plasma	3.5-4.5 mEq/L	3.5-4.5 mmol/L
Progesterone, serum, adult		
Males	0.0-0.4 ng/mL	0.0-1.3 mmol/L
Females		
Follicular phase	0.1-1.5 ng/mL	0.3-4.8 mmol/L
Luteal phase	2.5-28.0 ng/mL	8.0-89.0 mmol/L

Continued

Reference Intervals* for Clinical Chemistry (Blood, Serum, and Plasma)—cont'd

Analyte	Conventional Units	SI Units
Prolactin, serum		
Males	1.0-15.0 ng/mL	1.0-15.0 μg/L
Females	1.0-20.0 ng/mL	1.0-20.0 μg/L
Protein, serum, electrophoresis		
Total	6.0-8.0 g/dL	60-80 g/L
Albumin	3.5-5.5 g/dL	35-55 g/L
Globulins		
α_1	0.2-0.4 g/dL	2.0-4.0 g/L
α_2	0.5-0.9 g/dL	5.0-9.0 g/L
β	0.6-1.1 g/dL	6.0-11.0 g/L
γ	0.7-1.7 g/dL	7.0-17.0 g/L
Pyruvate, blood	0.3-0.9 mg/dL	0.03-0.10 mmol/L
Rheumatoid factor	0.0-30.0 IU/mL	0.0-30.0 kIU/L
Sodium, serum or plasma	135-145 mEq/L	135-145 mmol/L
Testosterone, plasma		
Males, adult	300-1200 ng/dL	10.4-41.6 nmol/L
Females, adult	20-75 ng/dL	0.7-2.6 nmol/L
Pregnant females	40-200 ng/dL	1.4-6.9 nmol/L
Thyroglobulin	3-42 ng/mL	3-42 μg/L
Thyrotropin (hTSH), serum	0.4-4.8 μIU/mL	0.4-4.8 mIU/L
Thyrotropin-releasing hormone (TRH)	5-60 pg/mL	5-60 ng/L
Thyroxine (FT_4), free, serum	0.9-2.1 ng/dL	12-27 pmol/L
Thyroxine (T_4), serum	4.5-12.0 μg/mL	58-154 nmol/L
Thyroxine-binding globulin (TBG)	15.0-34.0 μg/mL	15.0-34.0 mg/L
Transferrin	250-430 mg/dL	2.5-4.3 g/L
Triglycerides, serum, after 12-h fast	40-150 mg/dL	0.4-1.5 g/L
Triiodothyronine (T_3), serum	70-190 ng/dL	1.1-2.9 nmol/L
Triiodothyronine uptake, resin (T_3RU)	25-38%	0.25-0.38
Urate		
Males	2.5-8.0 mg/dL	150-480 μmol/L
Females	2.2-7.0 mg/dL	130-420 μmol/L
Urea, serum or plasma	24-49 mg/dL	4.0-8.2 nmol/L
Urea, nitrogen, serum or plasma	11-23 mg/dL	8.0-16.4 nmol/L
Viscosity, serum	1.4-1.8 × water	1.4-1.8 × water
Vitamin A, serum	20-80 μg/dL	0.70-2.80 μmol/L
Vitamin B_{12}, serum	180-900 pg/mL	133-664 pmol/L

*Reference values may vary, depending on the method and sample source used.

Reference Intervals for Therapeutic Drug Monitoring (Serum or Plasma)*

Analyte	Therapeutic Range	Toxic Concentrations	Proprietary Name(s)
Analgesics			
Acetaminophen	10-40 μg/mL	>150 μg/mL	Tylenol Datril
Salicylate	100-250 μg/mL	>300 μg/mL	Aspirin Bufferin
Antibiotics			
Amikacin	20-30 μg/mL	Peak >35 μg/mL Trough >10 μg/mL	Amkin
Gentamicin	5-10 μg/mL	Peak >10 μg/mL Trough >2 μg/mL	Garamycin
Tobramycin	5-10 μg/mL	Peak >10 μg/mL Trough >2 μg/mL	Nebcin
Vancomycin	5-35 μg/mL	Peak >40 μg/mL Trough >10 μg/mL	Vancocin
Anticonvulsants			
Carbamazepine	5-12 μg/mL	>15 μg/mL	Tegretol
Ethosuximide	40-100 μg/mL	>250 μg/mL	Zarontin
Phenobarbital	15-40 μg/mL	40-100 ng/mL (varies widely)	Luminal

Reference Intervals for Therapeutic Drug Monitoring (Serum or Plasma)*—cont'd

Analyte	Therapeutic Range	Toxic Concentrations	Proprietary Name(s)
Phenytoin	10-20 μg/mL	>20 μg/mL	Dilantin
Primidone	5-12 μg/mL	>15 μg/mL	Mysoline
Valproic acid	50-100 μg/mL	>100 μg/mL	Depakene
Antineoplastics and Immunosuppressives			
Cyclosporine	100-300 ng/mL	>400 ng/mL	Sandimmune
Methotrexate, high-dose, 48h	Variable	>1 μmol/L, 48h after dose	
Tacrolimus (FK-506), whole blood	3-20 μg/L	>15 μg/L	Prograf
Bronchodilators and Respiratory Stimulants			
Caffeine	3-15 ng/mL	>30 ng/mL	Elixophyllin
Theophylline (aminophylline)	10-20 μg/mL	>30 μg/mL	Quibron
Cardiovascular Drugs			
Amiodarone (obtain specimen more than 8h after last dose)	1.0-2.0 μg/mL	>2.0 μg/mL	Cordarone
Digoxin (obtain specimen more than 6h after last dose)	0.8-2.0 ng/mL	>2.4 ng/mL	Lanoxin
Disopyramide	2-5 μg/mL	>7 μg/mL	Norpace
Flecainide	0.2-1.0 μg/mL	>1 μg/mL	Tambocor
Lidocaine	1.5-5.0 μg/mL	>6 μg/mL	Xylocaine
Mexiletine	0.7-2.0 μg/mL	>2 μg/mL	Mexitil
Procainamide	4-10 μg/mL	>12 μg/mL	Pronestyl
Procainamide plus NAPA (N-acetyl procainamide)	8-30 μg/mL	>30 μg/mL	
Propranolol	50-100 ng/mL	Variable	Inderal
Quinidine	2-5 μg/mL	>6 μg/mL	Cardioquin Quinaglute
Tocainide	4-10 ng/mL	>10 ng/mL	Tonocard
Psychopharmacologic Drugs			
Amitriptyline	120-150 ng/mL	>500 ng/mL	Elavil Triavil
Bupropion	25-100 ng/mL	Not applicable	Wellbutrin
Desipramine	150-300 ngmL	>500 ng/mL	Norpramin
Imipramine	125-250 ng/mL	>400 ng/mL	Tofranil
Lithium (obtain specimen 12h after last dose)	0.6-1.5 mEq/L	>1.5 mEq/L	Lithobid
Nortriptyline	50-150 ng/mL	>500 ng/mL	Aventyl Pamelor

*Values may vary depending on the method and sample collection device used. Always consult the reference values provided by the laboratory performing the analysis.

Reference Intervals* for Clinical Chemistry (Urine)

Analyte	Conventional Units	SI Units
Acetone and acetoacetate, qualitative	Negative	Negative
Albumin		
Qualitative	Negative	Negative
Quantitative	10-100 mg/24h	0.15-1.5 μmol/d
Aldosterone	3-20 μg/24h	8.3-55 nmol/d
δ-Aminolevulinic acid (δ-ALA)	1.3-7.0 mg/24h	10-53 μmol/d
Amylase	<17 U/h	<17 U/h
Amylase/creatinine clearance ratio	0.01-0.04	0.01-0.04
Bilirubin, qualitative	Negative	Negative
Calcium (regular diet)	<250 mg/24h	<6.3 nmol/d
Catecholamines		
Epinephine	<10 μg/24h	<55 nmol/d
Norepinephine	<100 μg/24h	<590 nmol/d
Total free catecholamines	4-126 μg/24h	24-745 nmol/d
Total metanephrines	0.1-1.6 mg/24h	0.5-8.1 μmol/d
Chloride (varies with intake)	110-250 mEq/24h	110-250 mmol/d
Copper	0-50 μg/24h	0.0-0.80 μmol/d
Cortisol, free	10-100 μg/24h	27.6-276 nmol/d

Continued

Reference Intervals* for Clinical Chemistry (Urine)—cont'd

Analyte	Conventional Units	SI Units
Creatine		
Males	0-40 mg/24h	0.0-0.30 mmol/d
Females	0-80 mg/24h	0.0-0.60 mmol/d
Creatinine	15-25 mg/kg/24h	0.13-0.22 mmol/kg/d
Creatinine clearance (endogenous)		
Males	110-150 mL/min/1.73 m^2	110-150 mL/min/1.73 m^2
Females	105-132 mL/min/1.73 m^2	105-132 mL/min/1.73 m^2
Cystine or cysteine	Negative	Negative
Dehydroepiandrosterone		
Males	0.2-2.0 mg/24h	0.7-6.9 μmol/d
Females	0.2-1.8 mg/24h	0.7-6.2 μmol/d
Estrogens, total		
Males	4-25 μg/24h	14-90 nmol/d
Females	5-100 μg/24h	18-360 nmol/d
Glucose (as reducing substance)	<250 mg/24h	<250 mg/d
Hemoglobin and myoglobin, qualitative	Negative	Negative
Hemogentisic acid, qualitative	Negative	Negative
17-Hydroxycorticosteroids		
Males	3-9 mg/24h	8.3-25 μmol/d
Females	2-8 mg/24h	5.5-22 μmol/d
5-Hydroxyindoleacetic acid		
Qualitative	Negative	Negative
Quantitative	2-6 mg/24 h	10-31 μmol/d
17-Ketogenic steroids		
Males	5-23 mg/24h	17-80 μmol/d
Females	3-15 mg/24h	10-52 μmol/d
17-Ketosteroids		
Males	8-22 mg/24h	28-76 μmol/d
Females	6-15 mg/24h	21-52 μmol/d
Magnesium	6-10 mEq/24h	3-5 mmol/d
Metanephrines	0.05-1.2 ng/mg creatinine	0.03-0.70 mmol/mmol creatinine
Osmolality	38-1400 mOsm/kg water	38-1400 mOsm/kg water
pH	4.6-8.0	4.6-8.0
Phenylpyruvic acid, qualitative	Negative	Negative
Phosphate	0.4-1.3 g/24h	13-42 mmol/d
Porphobilinogen		
Qualitative	Negative	Negative
Quantitative	<2 mg/24h	<9 μmol/d
Porphyrins		
Coproporphyrin	50-250 μg/24h	77-380 nmol/d
Uroporphyrin	10-30 μg/24h	12-36 nmol/d
Potassium	25-125 mEq/24h	25-125 mmol/d
Pregnanediol		
Males	0.0-1.9 mg/24h	0.0-6.0 μmol/d
Females		
Proliferative phase	0.0-2.6 mg/24h	0.0-8.0 μmol/d
Luteal phase	2.6-10.6 mg/24h	8-33 μmol/d
Postmenopausal	0.2-1.0 mg/24h	0.6-3.1 μmol/d
Pregnanetriol	0.0-2.5 mg/24h	0.0-7.4 μmol/d
Protein, total		
Qualitative	Negative	Negative
Quantitative	10-150 mg/24h	10-150 mg/d
Protein/creatinine ratio	<0.2	<0.2
Sodium (regular diet)	60-260 mEq/24h	60-260 mmol/d
Specific gravity		
Random specimen	1.003-1.030	1.003-1.030
24-h collection	1.015-1.025	1.015-1.025
Urate (regular diet)	250-750 mg/24h	1.5-4.4 mmol/d
Urobilinogen	0.5-4.0 mg/24h	0.6-6.8 μmol/d
Vanillylmandelic acid (VMA)	1.0-8.0 mg/24h	5-40 μmol/d

*Values may vary, depending on the method used.

Reference Intervals for Toxic Substances

Analyte	Conventional Units	SI Units
Arsenic, urine	<130 μg/24h	<1.7 μmol/d
Bromides, serum, inorganic	<100 mg/dL	<10 mmol/L
Toxic symptoms	140-1000 mg/dL	14-100 mmol/L
Carboxyhemoglobin, blood	Saturation, percent	
Urban environment	<5%	<0.05
Smokers	<12%	<0.12
Symptoms		
Headache	>15%	>0.15
Nausea and vomiting	>25%	>0.25
Potentially lethal	>50%	>0.50
Ethanol, blood	<0.05 mg/dL <0.005%	<1.0 mmol/L
Intoxication	>100 mg/dL >0.1%	>22 mmol/L
Marked intoxication	300-400 mg/dL 0.3%-0.4%	65-87 mmol/L
Alcoholic stupor	400-500 mg/dL 0.4%-0.5%	87-109 mmol/L
Coma	>500 mg/dL >0.5%	>109 mmol/L
Lead, blood		
Adults	<20 μg/dL	<1.0 μmol/L
Children	<10 μg/dL	<0.5 μmol/L
Lead, urine	<80 μg/24h	<0.4 μmol/d
Mercury, urine	<10 μg/24h	<150 nmol/d

Reference Intervals for Tests Performed on Cerebrospinal Fluid

Test	Conventional Units	SI Units
Cells	<5 mm³; all mononuclear	$<5 \times 10^6$/L, all mononuclear
Protein electrophoresis	Albumin predominant	Albumin predominant
Glucose	50-75 mg/dL (20 mg/dL less than in serum)	2.8-4.2 mmol/L (1.1 mmol/L less than in serum)
IgG		
Children <14 y	<8% of total protein	<0.08 of total protein
Adults	<14% of total protein	<0.14 of total protein
IgG index		
$\left(\frac{\text{CSF / serum IgG ratio}}{\text{CSF / serum albumin ratio}}\right)$	0.3-0.6	0.3-0.6
Oligoclonal banding on electrophoresis	Absent	Absent
Pressure, opening	70-180 mm H_2O	70-180 mm H_2O
Protein, total	15-45 mg/dL	150-450 mg/L

Reference Intervals for Tests of Gastrointestinal Function

Test	Conventional Units
Bentiromide	6-h urinary arylamine excretion >57% excludes pancreatic insufficiency
β-Carotene, serum	60-250 ng/dL
Fecal fat estimation	
Qualitative	No fat globules seen by high-power microscope
Quantitative	<6 g/24h (>95% coefficient of fat absorption)
Gastric acid output	
Basal	
Males	0.0-10.5 mmol/h
Females	0.0-5.6 mmol/h
Maximum (after histamine or pentagastrin)	
Males	9.0-48.0 mmol/h
Females	6.0-31.0 mmol/h
Ratio: basal/maximum	
Males	0.0-0.31
Females	0.0-0.29
Secretin test, pancreatic flud	
Volume	>1.8 mL/kg/h
Bicarbonate	>80 mEq/L
D-Xylose absorption test, urine	>20% of ingested dose excreted in 5h

Reference Intervals for Tests of Immunologic Function

Test	Conventional Units	SI Units
Complement, serum		
C3	85-175 mg/dL	0.85-1.75 g/L
C4	15-45 mg/dL	150-450 mg/L
Total hemolytic (CH_{50})	150-250 U/mL	150-250 U/mL
Immunoglobulins, serum, adult		
IgG	640-1350 mg/dL	6.4-13.5 g/L
IgA	70-310 mg/dL	0.70-3.1 g/L
IgM	90-350 mg/dL	0.90-3.5 g/L
IgD	0.0-6.0 mg/dL	0.0-60 mg/L
IgE	0.0-430 ng/dL	0.0-430 μg/L

Lymphocytes Subsets, Whole Blood, Heparinized

Antigen(s) Expressed	Cell Type	Percentage (%)	Absolute Cell Count
CD3	Total T cells	56-77	860-1880
CD19	Total B cells	7-17	140-370
CD3 and CD4	Helper-inducer cells	32-54	550-1190
CD3 and CD8	Suppressor-cytotoxic cells	24-37	430-1060
CD3 and DR	Activated T cells	5-14	70-310
CD2	E rosette T cells	73-87	1040-2160
CD16 and CD56	Natural killer (NK) cells	8-22	130-500
Helper/suppressor ratio: 0.8-1.8			

Reference Values for Semen Analysis

Test	Conventional Units	SI Units
Volume	2-5 mL	2-5 mL
Liquefaction	Complete in 15 min	Complete in 15 min
pH	7.2-8.0	7.2-8.0
Leukocytes	Occasional or absent	Occasional or absent
Spermatozoa		
Count	60-150 × 10^6 mL	60-150 × 10^6 mL
Motility	>80% motile	>0.80 motile
Morphology	80-90% normal forms	>0.80-0.90 normal forms
Fructose	>150 mg/dL	>8.33 mmol/L

TOXIC CHEMICAL AGENTS REFERENCE CHART: SYMPTOMS AND TREATMENT

METHOD OF

James J. James, MD, DrPH, MHA, and
James M. Lyznicki, MS, MPH

Toxic chemical agents are poisonous vapors, aerosols, gases, liquids, or solids that have toxic effects on people, animals, or plants. Most of these agents are liquid at room temperature and are disseminated as vapors and aerosols. They may be released as bombs, sprayed from aircraft and boats, or disseminated by other means to intentionally create a hazard to people and the environment. Some of these agents are highly toxic and persistent, features that can render a site uninhabitable and require costly and potentially hazardous decontamination and remediation. Health effects range from irritation and burning of skin and mucous membranes to rapid cardiopulmonary collapse and death.

Efficient deployment of hazardous materials (HazMat) teams is critical to control a chemical agent attack. Although all major cities and emergency medical systems have plans and equipment in place to address this situation, physicians and other health professionals must be aware of principles involved in managing a patient or multiple patients exposed to these agents. Chemical weapon agents have a high potential for secondary contamination from victims to responders. This requires that medical treatment facilities have clearly defined procedures for handling contaminated casualties, many of whom will transport themselves to the facility. Precautions must be used until thorough decontamination has been performed or the specific chemical agent is identified. Health care professionals must first protect themselves (e.g., by using protective suits, respiratory protection, and chemical-resistant gloves), because secondary contamination with even small amounts of these substances (particularly nerve agents such as VX) may be lethal.

Primary detection of exposure to chemical agents will be based on the signs and symptoms of the victim (Table 1). Confirmation of a chemical agent, using detection equipment or laboratory analyses, will take considerable time and will not likely contribute to the early management of mass casualty victims. Several patients presenting with the same symptoms should alert physicians and hospital staff to the possibility of a chemical attack. If a chemical attack occurs, most victims will likely arrive within a short time. This situation differentiates a chemical attack from a biological attack involving infectious microorganisms. Additional diagnostic clues include:

- Unusual temporal or geographic clustering of illness
- Any sudden increase in illness in previously healthy persons
- Sudden increase in nonspecific syndromes (e.g., sudden unexplained weakness in previously healthy persons; dimmed or blurred vision; hypersecretion, inhalation, or burn-like syndromes)

A coordinated communication network is critical for transmitting reliable information from the incident scene to treatment facilities. Any suspicious or confirmed exposure to a chemical weapons agent should be reported to the local health department, local Federal Bureau of Investigation office, and the Centers for Disease Control and Prevention (1-770-488-7100).

TABLE 1 Quick Reference Chart on Chemical Weapons Agents

Chemical Agent	Diagnostic Considerations	Treatment Considerations*
Cyanides Cyanogen chloride (CK) Hydrogen cyanide (AC)	Symptom onset: rapid, seconds to minutes. Odor: bitter almonds, musty, or chlorine-like. Nonspecific hypoxic and hypoxemic symptoms. Binds cellular cytochrome oxidase-causing chemical asphyxia. Respiratory: shortness of breath, chest tightness, hyperventilation, respiratory arrest. GI: nausea, vomiting.	Immediate treatment of symptomatic patients is critical. Antidote: sodium nitrite and sodium thiosulfate; repeat one-half of initial doses of both agents in 30 minutes if there is inadequate clinical response. Amyl nitrate capsules are available for first aid until intravenous access is achieved. Cyanide antidote kits are commercially available. Investigational in the United States, available in Europe: hydroxycobalamin (vitamin B_{12a}) administered with thiosulfate.

Continued

TABLE 1 Quick Reference Chart on Chemical Weapons Agents—cont'd

Chemical Agent	Diagnostic Considerations	Treatment Considerations*
	Cardiovascular: ventricular arrhythmias, hypotension, cardiac arrest, shock. CNS: anxiety, headache, drowsiness, weakness, apnea, convulsions, seizure, coma. CNS effects may be confused with carbon monoxide and hydrogen sulfide poisoning. Metabolic acidosis and increased concentration of venous oxygen (patient also may present with cyanosis). Laboratory testing: cyanide, thiocyanate, serum lactate levels; venous and arterial partial oxygen pressure.	Activated charcoal for oral exposure. Mechanical ventilation as needed. Circulatory support with crystalloids and vasopressors. Metabolic acidosis corrected with IV sodium bicarbonate. Seizures controlled with benzodiazepines.
Incapacitating Agents Agent 15 3-Quinuclidinyl benzilate (BZ)	Symptom onset: hours 0-4h: parasympathetic blockade and mild CNS effects. 4-20h: stupor with ataxia and hyperthermia. 20-96h: full-blown delirium. Resolution phase: paranoia, deep sleep, reawakening, crawling, climbing automatisms, eventual reorientation. Odorless. Competitive inhibitor of acetylcholine muscarinic receptor. Mydriasis, blurred vision, dry mouth, dry skin, possible atropine-like flush, initial rise in heart rate, decreased level of consciousness, confusion, disorientation, visual hallucinations, impaired memory.	Antidote: physostigmine salicylate (Antilirium). Supportive care, intravenous fluids.
Nerve Agents Cyclohexyl sarin (GF) Sarin (GB) Soman (GD) Tabun (GA) VX	Symptom onset: vapor (seconds), liquid (minutes to hours). Odor: none (GB, VX); fruity (GA); camphor-like (GD). Most toxic of known chemical agents. Irreversible acetylcholinesterase inhibitors. Eyes: lacrimation, miosis. Respiratory: rhinorrhea, bronchospasm, respiratory failure. Gastrointestinal: hypersalivation, nausea, vomiting, diarrhea. Skin: localized sweating. Cardiac: sinus bradycardia. Skeletal muscles: fasciculations followed by weakness, flaccid paralysis. CNS: loss of consciousness, convulsions, apnea, seizures.	Antidote: Atropine and pralidoxime chloride (Protopam chloride, 2-PAM); additional doses until bronchial secretions are cleared and ventilation improved. Early administration of 2-PAM is critical to minimize permanent agent inactivation of acetylcholinesterase (i.e., *aging*). Benzodiazepines to control nerve agent-induced seizures. Airway and ventilatory support as needed. Atropine, pralidoxime, and diazepam are available in autoinjector kits through the U.S. military.

TABLE 1 Quick Reference Chart on Chemical Weapons Agents—cont'd

Chemical Agent	Diagnostic Considerations	Treatment Considerations*
	May be confused with organophosphate and carbamate pesticide poisoning. Laboratory testing: erythrocyte or serum cholinesterase activity to confirm exposure.	
Pulmonary or Choking Agents Acrolein Ammonia (NH_3) Chlorine (CL) Chloropicrin (PS) Diphosgene (DP) Nitrogen oxides (NO_x) Perfluoroisobutylene (PFIB) Phosgene (CG) Sulfur dioxide (SO_2)	Symptom onset: rapid or delayed; 1-24h (rarely up to 72h). Odor (CG): freshly mown hay or grass. Easily absorbed via mucous membranes of eyes, nose, oropharynx. Degree of water solubility of the agent influences onset and severity of respiratory injury. Eye and airway irritation, dyspnea, chest tightness, rhinorrhea, hypersalivation, cough, wheezing. High-dose inhalation may produce laryngospasm, pneumonitis, and acute lung injury with delayed onset (≤48h) of acute respiratory distress syndrome. Chest radiograph: hyperinflation, noncardiogenic pulmonary edema. May be confused with inhalation exposure to industrial chemicals (e.g., HCl, Cl_2, NH_3).	No specific antidote. Supportive measures; specific treatment depends on the agent. IV fluids for hypotension; no diuretics. Ventilation with or without positive airway pressure. Bronchodilators for bronchospasm. Methylprednisolone may be effective in preventing noncardiogenic pulmonary edema.
Riot Control Agents Mace (CN) Tear gas (CS)	Symptom onset: immediate. Odor: apple blossom (CN); pepper (CS). Metallic taste. SN_2 alkylating agents. Burning and pain on mucosal membranes and skin. Eyes: irritation, pain, tearing, blepharospasm. Airways: burning in nose and mouth, respiratory discomfort, bronchospasm (may be delayed 36h). Skin: tingling, erythema. Nausea and vomiting common. CN can cause corneal opacification. No specific laboratory tests.	Supportive care. Irrigation as necessary. Persons with asthma, emphysema may need oxygen, inhaled bronchodilators, steroids, assisted ventilation. Lotions, such as calamine, for persistent erythema.
Vesicant or Blister Agents	Symptoms onset: immediate (L, CX); delayed 2-48h (H, HD). Primary liquid hazard. May be confused with skin exposure to caustic irritants (e.g., sodium hydroxide, ammonia). Intracellular enzyme and DNA alkylating agents.	Immediate decontamination. Thermal burn-type treatment; supportive care. Symptomatic management of lesions.

Continued

TABLE 1 Quick Reference Chart on Chemical Weapons Agents—cont'd

Chemical Agent	Diagnostic Considerations	Treatment Considerations*
Sulfur mustard (H) Distilled mustard (HD)	Odor: garlic, horseradish, or mustard.	No specific antidote.
	Skin: erythema and blisters (may be delayed ≤8h), pruritus.	Skin: silver sulfadiazine.
	Eye: irritation, conjunctivitis, corneal damage, lacrimation, pain, blepharospasm.	Eye: homatropine ophthalmic ointment.
	Respiratory: mild to marked acute airway damage, pneumonitis within 1-3d, respiratory failure.	Pulmonary: antibiotics, bronchodilators, steroids.
		Colony stimulating factor may be helpful for leukopenia.
	Gastrointestinal effects (nausea, vomiting, diarrhea) may be present.	Systemic analgesic and antipruritics.
	Bone marrow stem cell suppression leading to pancytopenia and increased susceptibility to infection.	Early use of positive-end expiratory pressure or continuous positive airway pressure.
	Fever, sputum production.	Maintain fluid and electrolyte balance (do not excessively fluid resuscitate as in thermal burns).
	Combination with Lewisite (called mustard-Lewisite or HL) results in rapid effects of Lewisite and delayed effects of mustard agents.	
Lewisite (L)	Odor: fruity or geranium.	Antidote: British antilewisite (BAL or dimercaprol).
	More volatile than mustard.	
	Damages eyes, skin, and airways by direct contact.	
	Skin: gray area of dead skin within 5min, erythema within 30min, blistering 2-3h, immediate irritation or burning pain on contact, severe tissue necrosis.	
	Eyes: pain, blepharospasm, conjunctival, and lid edema.	
	Airway: pseudomembrane formation, nasal irritation.	
	Intravascular fluid loss, hypovolemia, shock, organ congestion, leukocytosis, miosis, immediate pain on contact.	
Phosgene Oxime (CX)	Odor: freshly mown hay.	No antidote.
	Urticant, nonvesicant agent.	Parenteral methylprednisolone may be effective in preventing noncardiogenic pulmonary edema.
	Vapor extremely irritating; vapor and liquid cause tissue damage upon contact.	Experimental: aerosolized dexamethasone and theophylline for pulmonary involvement.
	Immediate burning, irritation, wheal-like skin lesions, eye and airway damage, conjunctivitis, lacrimation, lid edema, blepharospasm.	
	No distinctive laboratory findings.	

TABLE 1 Quick Reference Chart on Chemical Weapons Agents—cont'd

Chemical Agent	Diagnostic Considerations	Treatment Considerations*
Vomiting (Arsine-Based) Agents Adamsite (DM) Diphenylchlorarsine (DA) Diphenylarsine cyanide (DC)	Symptom onset: All rapidly acting within minutes. Odor: none (DA); garlic (DC); burning fireworks (DM). Primary route of absorption is through respiratory system. Arsine gas depletes erythrocyte glutathione and causes hemolysis. Eyes: conjunctival irritation, tearing, and blepharospasm. Airways: sneezing, mucosal lung irritation, edema, progressive cough, wheezing. Cardiac: tachypnea, tachycardia. Gastrointestinal: intestinal cramps, emesis, diarrhea. Skin: erythema, edema at the site of dermal contact. CNS depression, syncope. Chest radiograph to rule out chemical pneumonitis.	Supportive care. Monitor for hemolysis. Wheezing or dyspnea; may need albuterol inhalation. Eye irrigation (water, normal saline, lactated Ringer's solution) in patients sustaining ocular exposure. Treat repetitive emesis with IV hydration and antiemetics. Blood transfusion may be required. Exchange transfusion may be required. Hemodialysis may be useful in decreasing arsenic level and treating renal failure.

*Different situations may require different treatment and dosage regimens. Please consult other references as well as a regional poison control center (1-800-222-1222), medical toxicologist, clinical pharmacologist, or other drug information specialist for definitive dosage information, especially dosages for pregnant women and children.
Abbreviations: CNS = central nervous system; GI = gastrointestinal.

BIOLOGIC AGENTS REFERENCE CHART: SYMPTOMS, TESTS, TREATMENT

METHOD OF

James J. James, MD, DrPH, MHA, and

James M. Lyznicki, MS, MPH

Biologic weapons are devices used intentionally to cause disease or death through dissemination of microorganisms or toxins in food and water, by insect vectors, or by aerosols. Potential targets include human beings, food crops, livestock, and other resources essential for national security, economy, and defense. Unlike nuclear, chemical, and conventional weapons, the onset of a biological attack will probably be insidious. For some infectious agents, secondary and tertiary transmission may continue for weeks or months after the initial attack.

Initial detection of an unannounced biologic attack will likely occur when an astute health professional notices an unusual case or disease cluster and reports his or her concerns to local public health authorities. Physicians and other health professionals should be alert to the following:

- Unusual temporal or geographic clustering of illnesses
- Sudden increase of illness in previously healthy persons
- Sudden increase in nonspecific illnesses (e.g., pneumonia, flu-like illness; bleeding disorders; unexplained rashes, particularly in adults; neuromuscular illness; diarrhea)

To enhance detection and treatment capabilities, physicians and other health professionals in acute care settings should be familiar with the clinical manifestations, diagnostic techniques, isolation precautions, treatment, and prophylaxis for likely causative agents (e.g., smallpox, pneumonic plague, anthrax, viral hemorrhagic fevers). Table 1 provides a quick summary of diagnostic and treatment considerations for various infectious and toxic biological agents. For some of these agents, delay in medical response could result in a potentially devastating number of casualties. To mitigate such consequences, early identification and intervention are imperative. Front-line physicians must have an increased level of suspicion regarding the possible intentional use of biologic agents as well as an increased sensitivity to reporting those suspicions to public health authorities, who, in turn, must be willing to evaluate a predictable increase in false-positive reports.

Medical response efforts require coordination and planning with emergency management agencies, law enforcement, health care facilities, and social services agencies. Health care agencies should ensure that physicians know whom to call with reports of suspicious cases and clusters of infectious diseases, and should work to build a good relationship with the local medical community. Resource integration is absolutely necessary to:

- Establish adequate capacity to initiate rapid investigation of an outbreak
- Educate the public
- Begin mass distribution of antibiotics and vaccines
- Ensure mass medical care
- Control public anger and fear

In an epidemic, overwhelming numbers of critically ill patients will require acute and follow-up medical care. Both infected persons and the *worried well* will seek medical attention, with a corresponding need for medical supplies, diagnostic tests, and hospital beds. The impact—or even the threat—of an attack can elicit widespread panic and civil disorder, overwhelm hospital resources, and disrupt social services.

Any suspicious or confirmed exposure to a biologic weapons agent should be reported immediately to the local health department, local Federal Bureau of Investigation office, and the Centers for Disease Control and Prevention (1-770-488-7100).

TABLE 1 Quick Reference Chart on Biological Weapon Agents

Disease/Agent	Diagnostic Considerations	Treatment Considerations*	Prophylaxis
Bacteria			
Anthrax *Bacillus anthracis*	Incubation period: 1-5d (perhaps ≤60d)†. <u>Cutaneous</u> Evolving skin lesion (face, neck, arms), progresses to vesicle, depressed ulcer, and black necrotic lesion. Lethality: 20% if untreated, otherwise rarely fatal. <u>Gastrointestinal</u> Nausea, vomiting, abdominal pain, bloody diarrhea, sepsis. Lethality: approaches 100% if untreated but data are limited; rapid, aggressive treatment may reduce mortality. <u>Inhalational</u> Abrupt onset of flu-like symptoms, fever with or without chills, sweats, fatigue or malaise, non- or minimally productive cough, nausea, vomiting, dyspnea, headache, chest pain, followed in 2-5d by severe respiratory distress, mediastinitis, hemorrhagic meningitis, sepsis, shock§.	Combination therapy of ciprofloxacin (Cipro) or doxycycline (Vibramycin) plus one or two other antimicrobials should be considered with inhalational anthrax‡. Penicillin should be considered if strain is susceptible and does not possess inducible β-lactamases. If meningitis is suspected, doxycycline (Vibramycin) may be less optimal because of poor CNS penetration. Steroids may be considered for severe edema and for meningitis.	Ciprofloxacin (Cipro) or doxycycline (Vibramycin) with or without vaccination; if strain is susceptible, penicillin or amoxicillin (Amoxil) should be considered. Inactivated vaccine (licensed but not readily available); six injections and annual booster.

TABLE 1 Quick Reference Chart on Biological Weapon Agents—cont'd

Disease/Agent	Diagnostic Considerations	Treatment Considerations*	Prophylaxis
	Widened mediastinum on chest radiograph is characteristic for inhalational and occasionally GI anthrax[‖]. Lethality: Once respiratory distress develops, mortality rates may approach 90%; begin treatment when inhalational anthrax is suspected, do not wait for confirmatory testing[¶]. Gram stain and culture of blood, pleural fluid, CSF, ascitic fluid, vesicular fluid or lesion exudate; sputum rarely positive; confirmatory serologic PCR tests and available through public health laboratory network Incubation period: 5-60d (usually 1-2mo).		
Brucellosis *Brucella abortus* *Brucella canis* *Brucella melitensis* *Brucella suis*	Nonspecific flu-like symptoms, fever, headache, profound weakness and fatigue, GI symptoms such as anorexia, nausea, vomiting, diarrhea, or constipation. Osteoarticular complications common. Lethality: less than 5% even if untreated; tends to incapacitate rather that kill. Blood and bone marrow culture (may require 6wk to grow *Brucella*); confirmatory culture and serological testing available through public health laboratory network.	Doxycycline (Vibramycin) plus streptomycin or rifampin (Rifadin). Alternative therapies: Ofloxacin (Floxin) plus rifampin (Rifadin). Doxycycline (Vibramycin) plus gentamicin (Garamycin). TMP-SMX (Bactrim, Septra) plus gentamicin (Garamycin).	Doxycycline (Vibramycin) plus streptomycin or rifampin (Rifadin). No approved human vaccine.
Inhalational (pneumonic) tularemia *Francisella tularensis*	Incubation period: 3-5d (range of 1-21d). Sudden onset of acute febrile illness, weakness, chills, headache, generalized body aches, elevated WBCs. Pulmonary symptoms such as dry cough, chest pain or tightness with or without objective signs of pneumonia. Progressive weakness, malaise, anorexia, and weight loss occurs, potentially leading to sepsis and organ failure. Largely clinical diagnosis. Lethality: ≈30%-60% fatal if untreated. Culture of blood, sputum, biopsies, pleural fluid, bronchial washings (culture is difficult and potentially dangerous); confirmatory testing available through public health laboratory network	Streptomycin or gentamicin (Garamycin). Alternative therapies: Ciprofloxacin (Cipro). Doxycycline (Vibramycin). Chloramphenicol (Chloromycetin).	Tetracycline. Doxycycline (Vibramycin). Ciprofloxacin (Cipro). Live attenuated vaccine (USAMRIID, IND) given by scarification; currently under FDA review; limited availability.

Continued

TABLE 1 Quick Reference Chart on Biological Weapon Agents—cont'd

Disease/Agent	Diagnostic Considerations	Treatment Considerations*	Prophylaxis
Pneumonic plague *Yersinia pestis*	Incubation period: 1-10d (typically 2-3d). Acute onset of flu-like prodrome: fever, myalgia, weakness, headache; within 24h of prodrome, chest discomfort, cough, and dyspnea. By day 2 to 4 of illness, symptoms progressing to cyanosis, respiratory distress, and hemodynamic instability. Lethality: Almost 100% if untreated; 20%-60% if appropriately treated within 18-24h of symptoms. Begin treatment when diagnosis of plague is suspected; do not wait for confirmatory testing. Gram stain and culture of blood, CSF, sputum, lymph node aspirates, bronchial washings; confirmatory serological and bacteriologic tests available through public health laboratory network.	Streptomycin; gentamicin (Garamycin). Alternative therapies: Doxycycline (Vibramycin). Tetracycline. Ciprofloxacin (Cipro). Chloramphenicol (Chloromycetin) is first choice for meningitis except for pregnant women.	Tetracycline. Doxycycline (Vibramycin). Ciprofloxacin (Cipro). Inactivated whole-cell vaccine licensed but not readily available; injection with boosters vaccine not effective against aerosol exposure.
Rickettsia			
Q-Fever *Coxiella burnetii*	Incubation period: 2-14d (maybe ≤ 40d). Nonspecific febrile disease, chills, cough, weakness and fatigue, pleuritic chest pain, pneumonia possible. Lethality: 1-3%. Fatalities are uncommon even if untreated but relapsing symptoms may occur. Isolation of organism may be difficult; confirmatory testing via serology or PCR available through public health laboratory network.	Tetracycline. Doxycycline (Vibramycin).	Tetracycline. Doxycycline (Vibramycin). Inactivated whole-cell vaccine (IND). Skin test to determine prior exposure to *C. burnetii* recommended before vaccination.
Viruses			
Smallpox Variola major virus	Incubation period: 7-17d. Prodrome of high fever, malaise, prostration, headache, vomiting, delirium; followed in 2-3d by maculopapular rash uniformly progressing to pustules and scabs, mostly on extremities and face. Requires astute clinical evaluation; may be confused with chickenpox, erythema multiforme with bullae, or allergic contact dermatitis. Lethality: 30% in unvaccinated persons.	Supportive care. Cidofovir (Vistide) shown to be effective in vitro and in experimental animals infected with surrogate orthodox virus.	Live attenuated vaccinia vaccine derived from calf lymph; given by scarification (licensed, restricted supply). New vaccine being developed from tissue culture. Vaccination given within 3-4d following exposure can prevent, or decrease the severity of disease.

TABLE 1 Quick Reference Chart on Biological Weapon Agents—cont'd

Disease/Agent	Diagnostic Considerations	Treatment Considerations*	Prophylaxis
	Pharyngeal swab, vesicular fluid, biopsies, scab material for electron microscopy and PCR testing through public health laboratory network. Notify CDC Poxvirus Section at 1-404-639-2184.		
Viral Encephalitis Eastern (EEE) Western (WEE) Venezuelan (VEE)	Incubation period: 2-6d (VEE); 7-14d (EEE, WEE). Systemic febrile illness, with encephalitis developing in some populations. Generalized malaise, spiking fevers, headache, myalgia. Incidence of seizures and/or focal neurologic deficits may be higher after biological attack. WBC count may show striking leukopenia and lymphopenia. Clinical and epidemiologic diagnosis. Lethality: <10% (VEE); 0% (WEE); 50%-75% (EEE). Confirmatory test and viral isolation available through public health laboratory network.	Supportive care. Analgesics; anticonvulsants, as needed.	Several IND vaccines, poorly immunogenic, highly reactogenic.
Viral Hemorrhagic Fevers (VHFs) Arenaviruses (Lassa, Junin, and related viruses) Bunyaviruses (Hanta, Congo-Crimean, Rift Valley) Filovirus (Ebola, Marburg) Flaviviruses (yellow fever, dengue, various tick-borne disease viruses)	Incubation period: 4-21d. Fever with mucous membrane bleeding, petechiae, thrombocytopenia, and hypotension in patients without underlying malignancies. Malaise, myalgias, headache, vomiting, diarrhea possible. Lethality: Variable depending on viral strain; 15%-25% with Lassa fever to ≤90% with Ebola. Confirmatory testing and viral isolation available through public health laboratory network. Call CDC Special Pathogens Office at 1-404-639-1115.	Supportive therapy. Ribavirin (Virazole) may be effective for Lassa fever, Rift Valley fever, Argentine hemorrhagic fever, and Congo-Crimean hemorrhagic fever.	Ribavirin (Virazole) is suggested for Congo–Crimean hemorrhagic fever and Lassa fever. Yellow fever vaccine is the only licensed vaccine available. Vaccines for some of the other VHFs exist but are for investigational use only.
Biological Toxins			
Botulism *Clostridium botulinum* toxin	Symptom onset: 1-5d (typically 12-36h). Blurred vision, diplopia, dry mouth, ptosis, fatigue. As disease progresses, acute bilateral descending flaccid paralysis, respiratory paralysis resulting in death. Clinical diagnosis. Lethality: 60% without ventilatory support. Serum and stool should be assayed for toxin by mouse neutralization bioassay, which may require several days.	Intensive and prolonged supportive care; ventilation may be necessary. Trivalent equine antitoxin (serotypes A,B,E—licensed, available from the CDC) should be administered immediately after clinical diagnosis. Anaphylaxis and serum sickness are potential complications of antitoxin. Aminoglycosides and clindamycin (Cleocin) must not be used.	Pentavalent toxoid (A-E), yearly booster (IND, CDC). Not available to the public. Antitoxin may be sufficient to prevent illness following exposure, but is not recommended until patient is showing symptoms.

Continued

TABLE 1 Quick Reference Chart on Biological Weapon Agents—cont'd

Disease/Agent	Diagnostic Considerations	Treatment Considerations*	Prophylaxis
Enterotoxin B *Staphylococcus aureus*	Symptom onset: 3-12 h. Acute onset of fever, chills, headache, nonproductive cough. Normal chest radiograph. Clinical diagnosis. Lethality: probably low (few data available for respiratory exposure). Serology on acute and convalescent serum can confirm diagnosis.	Supportive care.	No vaccine available.
Ricin toxin *Ricinus communis*	Symptom onset: ≤ 6-24 h. Weakness, nausea, chest tightness, fever, cough, pulmonary edema, respiratory failure, circulatory collapse, hypoxemia resulting in death (usually within 36-72 h). Clinical and epidemiological diagnosis. Lethality: mortality data not available but is likely to be high with extensive exposure. Confirmatory serologic testing available through public health laboratory network.	Supportive care. Treatment for pulmonary edema. Gastric decontamination if toxin ingested.	No vaccine available.
T-2 Mycotoxins *Fusarium* *Myrothecium* *Trichoderma* *Stachybotrys* Other filamentous fungi	Symptom onset: minutes to hours. Abrupt onset of mucocutaneous and airway irritation and pain. May include skin, eyes, and GI tract; systemic toxicity may follow. Lethality: severe exposure can cause death in hours to days. Consult with local health department regarding specimen collection and diagnostic testing procedures; confirmation requires testing blood, tissue, and environmental samples.	Clinical support. Soap and water washing within 4-6 h reduces dermal toxicity; washing within 1h may eliminate toxicity entirely. No effective medications or antidotes.	No vaccine available.

*Different situations may require different dosage and treatment regimens. Please consult other references and an infectious disease specialist for definitive dosage information, especially dosages for pregnant women and children.

†Data from 22 patients infected with anthrax in October and November 2001 indicate a median incubation period of 4d (range: 4-7d) for inhalational anthrax and a mean incubation of 5d (range: 1-10d) for cutaneous anthrax.

‡Other agents with in vitro activity suggested for use in conjunction with ciprofloxacin (Cipro) or doxycycline (Vibramycin) for treatment of inhalational anthrax include rifampin (Rifadin), vancomycin (Vancocin), imipenem (Primaxin), chloramphenicol (Chloromycetin), penicillin, ampicillin, clindamycin (Cleocin), and clarithromycin (Biaxin).

§Limited data from the October and November 2001 anthrax infections indicate hemorrhagic pleural effusions to be strongly associated with inhalational anthrax; rhinorrhea was present in only 1 in 10 patients.

‖Chest radiograph abnormalities include paratracheal and hilar fullness and may be subtle. Consider chest computed tomography if diagnosis is uncertain.

¶Limited data from the 2001 terrorist-related anthrax infections indicate that early treatment significantly decreased the mortality rate.

Abbreviations: CDC = Centers for Disease Control and Prevention; CNS = central nervous system; CSF = cerebrospinal fluid; GI = gastrointestinal; IND = investigational new drug; PCR = polymerase chain reaction; TMP-SMX = trimethoprim-sulfamethoxazole; USAMRIID = U.S. Army Medical Research Institute of Infectious Diseases; WBC = white blood cell.

Adopted from: American Medical Association: Biological Weapons: Quick Reference Guide. Chicago: Author, 2002. Available at http://www.ama-assn.org/ama1/pub/upload/mm/415/quickreference0902.pdf.

SOME POPULAR HERBS AND NUTRITIONAL SUPPLEMENTS

METHOD OF

Miriam M. Chan, RPH, PharmD

Herb/Nutritional Supplement	Common Uses	Reasonable Adult Oral Dosage*	Precautions and Drug Interactions
Black cohosh root	Commonly used to relieve menopausal symptoms, such as hot flashes. Also used to treat premenstrual discomfort and dysmenorrhea	20 mg bid of the rhizome extract standardized to triterpene glycosides The German guidelines do not recommend its use for >6mo	Black cohosh has an estrogen-like effect and has been shown to decrease luteinizing hormone Large doses may induce miscarriage and it is contraindicated during pregnancy It may cause GI disturbances, headache, and hypotension
Bilberry fruit	Often used orally to improve visual acuity and to treat degenerative retinal conditions Also used orally to treat chronic venous insufficiency, varicose veins, and hemorrhoids Approved in Germany to use orally for acute diarrhea, and topically for mild inflammation of the mucous membranes of mouth and throat	For eye conditions and circulation, 80–160 mg tid of the extract standardized to at least 25% anthocyanosides For diarrhea, 20–60 g/d of the dried, ripe berries or as a tea preparation (5–10 g of crushed dried berries in 150ml water, brought to a boil for 10 min, then strained) For external use, 10% decoction	No known side effects reported with bilberry fruit and extract However, bilberry leaf taken in large quantities or with long-term use has been shown to cause wasting, anemia, jaundice, acute excitation, disturbances of tonus, and death in animals The anthocyanidin extracts from bilberry may increase the risk of bleeding in those taking warfarin or other blood thinners.
Chamomile flower	Used orally to calm nerves and treat GI spasms and inflammatory diseases of the GI tract Used topically to treat wounds, skin infections, and skin or mucous membrane inflammation	1 Cup of freshly made tea three or four times daily (1 tbsp or 3 g of dried flower in 150 mL boiling water for 5–10 min)	Chamomile may cause an allergic reaction, especially in people with severe allergies to ragweed or other members of the daisy family (e.g., echinacea, feverfew, and milk thistle). It should not be taken concurrently with other sedatives, such as alcohol or benzodiazapines.
Chaste tree berry (Chasteberry, Vitex)	For normalizing irregular menstrual periods and relieving premenstrual complaints For relieving menopausal symptoms For restoring fertility in women For treating acne associated with menstrual cycles Also for increasing breast milk production in lactating women	For menstrual irregularities and premenstrual complaints, 30–40 mg/d of the dried berries or an equivalent amount of aqueous-alcoholic extracts (50–70% v/v) Dried fruit extract, standardized to 0.6% agnusides, is used in doses of 175–225 mg/d For other conditions, no established dosage documented	Chaste tree berry can have uterine stimulant properties and should be avoided in pregnancy. Women with hormone-dependent conditions (e.g., breast, uterine, and ovarian cancer, and endometriosis and uterine fibroids) and men with prostate cancer should avoid chaste tree berry, because it contains progestins.

Continued

Herb/Nutritional Supplement	Common Uses	Reasonable Adult Oral Dosage*	Precautions and Drug Interactions
			Side effects include intramenstrual bleeding, dry mouth, headache, nausea, rash, alopecia, and tachycardia. High doses (≥480 mg/d extract) can paradoxically decrease lactation. Chaste tree berry is thought to have dopaminergic effects and may interact with dopamine antagonists, such as antipsychotics and metoclopramide. Chaste tree berry may also decrease the effects of oral contraceptives and hormone replacement therapy.
Chondroitin	For osteoarthritis, commonly used in combination with glucosamine	400 mg tid; chondroitin derived from bovine cartilage may carry a potential risk of contamination with diseased animals	Occasional mild side effects include nausea, indigestion, and allergic reactions
Chromium	For diabetes For hypercholesterolemia Commonly found in weight-loss products Also promoted for body building	For diabetes, 100 µg bid for ≤4mo or 500 µg bid for 2 mo For hypercholesterolemia, 200 µg tid for 500 µg bid for 2-4 mo For body building, 200-400 µg/d Chromium picolinate has been used in most studies, even though the chloride form is also available.	Adverse effects are rare, but they may include headaches, insomnia, sleep disturbances, irritability, and mood changes. Some patients may also experience cognitive, perceptual, and motor dysfunction. Long-term use of high doses (600-2400 µg/day) can cause anemia, thrombocytopenia, hemolysis, hepatic dysfunction, and renal failure. There have been two case reports of interstitial nephritis. A few studies suggest that chromium may cause DNA damage. Chromium competes with iron for binding to transferrin and can cause iron deficiency. Antacids, H_2 blockers, and proton pump inhibitors can decrease the absorption of chromium.
Coenzyme Q10	As adjunctive treatment for congestive heart failure, angina, and hypertension Also used for reducing cardiotoxicity associated with doxorubicin	For heart failure, 100 mg/d in two or three divided doses For angina, 50 mg tid For hypertension, 60 mg bid	Mild adverse events include gastric distress, nausea, vomiting, and hypotension Doses >300 mg/d may cause elevated liver enzymes Coenzyme Q10 may reduce the anticoagulation effects of warfarin. Oral hypoglycemic agents and HMG-CoA reductase inhibitors may reduce the serum coenzyme Q10 levels.
Creatine	To enhance muscle performance, especially during short-duration, high-intensity exercise	A loading dose of 20 g/d for 5-7 d followed by a maintenance dose of ≥2 g/d An alternative dosing of 3 g/d for 28 d has been suggested.	Creatine can cause gastroenteritis, diarrhea, heat intolerance, muscle cramps, and elevated serum creatinine levels.

Herb/Nutritional Supplement	Common Uses	Reasonable Adult Oral Dosage*	Precautions and Drug Interactions
			Creatine is contraindicated in patients taking diuretics. Concurrent use with cimetidine, probenecid, or nonsteroidal anti-inflammatory drugs increase the risk of adverse renal effects. Caffeine may decrease creatine's ergogenic effects.
Dong quai root	Commonly used for the relief of premenstrual and menopausal symptoms Also used as a "blood tonic" and a strengthening treatment for the heart, spleen, liver, and kidneys	For premenstrual and menopausal symptoms, 3-4 g/d in three divided doses For other conditions, no established dosage documented	Dong quai should not be used in pregnant women due to its uterine stimulant and relaxant effects Women with hormone sensitive conditions (e.g., breast, uterine, and ovarian cancer, endometriosis, and uterine fibroids) should avoid dong quai because of its estrogenic effects. Drinking the essential oil of dong quai is not recommended because it contains a small amount of carcinogenic constituents. Dong quai contains psoralens that can cause photosensitivity and photodermatitis. Dong quai also contains natural coumarin derivatives that can increase the risk of bleeding in those who are taking anticoagulant or antiplatelet drugs.
Echinacea	As an immune stimulant, particularly for the prevention and treatment of the common cold and influenza Supportive therapy for lower urinary tract infections Used topically to treat skin disorders and promote wound healing	300 mg tid of *E. pallida* root or 2-3 mL tid of expressed juice of *E. purpurea* herb Do not use for >8wk because echinacea may suppress immunity if used long term.	Echinacea should not be used in transplant patients and those with autoimmune disease or liver dysfunction. Allergic reactions have been reported. Adverse events are rare and may include mild GI effects. It should be discontinued as far in advance of surgery as possible. Echinacea may decrease effectiveness of immunosuppressants.
Ephedra (ma huang)	For diseases of the respiratory tract with mild bronchospasm Commonly found in weight-loss products Also marketed as a stimulant for performance enhancement	1 tsp or 2 g of dried herb (15-30 mg of ephedrine) in 240 mL boiling water for 10 min	Ephedra contains ephedrine, which has sympathomimetic activities; consequently, it should not be used in patients who have cardiovascular disease, diabetes, glaucoma, hypertension, hyperthyroidism, prostate enlargement, psychiatric disorders, or seizures. Serious adverse effects, including seizures, arrhythmias, heart attack, stroke, and death, have been associated with the use of ephedra; as a result, the FDA has recently

Continued

Herb/Nutritional Supplement	Common Uses	Reasonable Adult Oral Dosage*	Precautions and Drug Interactions
			announced plans to ban the sale of ephedra products in the United States by the year 2004. Because of the cardiovascular effects of ephedrine, patients taking ephedra should discontinue use at least 24 h before surgery. Concurrent use of ephedra and digitalis, guanethidine, monoamine oxidase inhibitors, or other stimulants, including caffeine, is not recommended.
Evening primrose oil	For premenstrual syndrome (PMS), especially if mastalgia is present Licensed in the United Kingdom for the treatment of atopic eczema Also used for other medical conditions, including rheumatoid arthritis, menopausal symptoms, Raynaud's phenomenon, Sjögren's syndrome, and diabetic neuropathy	For PMS, 2-4 g/d For atopic eczema, 6-8 g/d For rheumatoid arthritis, 2.8 g/d These doses are based on products standardized to 9% γ-linolenic acid. The daily dose can be given in divided doses.	Evening primrose oil may increase the risk of pregnancy complications. Side effects may include indigestion, nausea, soft stools, and headache. Seizures have been reported in patients with schizophrenia who were taking phenothiazines and evening primrose oil concomitantly. Evening primrose oil may interact with anesthesia and cause seizures. Concomitant use of evening primrose oil with anticoagulant and antiplatelet drugs can increase the risk of bleeding.
Fenugreek seed	For diabetes and hypercholesterolemia Also for constipation, dyspepsia, gastritis, and kidney ailments Approved in Germany to use orally for loss of appetite and topically as a poultice for local inflammation	For a loss of appetite, 1-2 g of the seed tid or 1 cup of tea (500 mg seed in 150 mL cold water for 3 h) several times a day Maximum 6 g/d For other conditions, no established dosage documented For topical use, 50 g powdered seed in 1/4 L of hot water to form a paste	Fenugreek may cause uterine contraction and should be avoided in pregnancy. Individuals who have allergies to peanuts or soybeans may also be allergic to fenugreek. Fenugreek can cause diarrhea and flatulence; it may also make the urine smell like maple syrup. Hypoglycemia may occur if fenugreek is taken in large amounts. Repeated external applications can result in undesirable skin reactions. Fenugreek contains small amounts of coumarins and may interact with anticoagulants and antiplatelet drugs. The high mucilage content of fenugreek can affect the absorption of oral drugs; therefore, fenugreek should not be taken within 2 h of other drugs.
Feverfew	For migraine headache prophylaxis For treatment of fever, menstrual problems, and arthritis	50-125 mg qd of the encapsulated dried leaf extract standardized to at least 0.2% parthenolide	Feverfew may induce menstrual bleeding and is contraindicated in pregnancy.

Herb/Nutritional Supplement	Common Uses	Reasonable Adult Oral Dosage*	Precautions and Drug Interactions
			Fresh leaves may cause oral ulcers and GI irritation. Sudden discontinuation of feverfew can precipitate rebound headache. Feverfew may interact with anticoagulants and potentiate the antiplatelet effect of aspirin.
Garlic	To lower blood pressure and serum cholesterol To prevent artherosclerosis	Fresh clove: 1 (4 g)/d Tablet: 300 mg bid to tid standardized to 0.6%-1.3% allicin	Intake of large quantities can lead to stomach complaints. Garlic has antiplatelet effects, so patients should discontinue use of garlic at least 7 d before surgery. Concomitant use of garlic and anticoagulants may increase the risk of bleeding.
Ginger root	As an antiemetic For prevention of motion sickness	Fresh rhizome: 2-4 g/d Powdered ginger: 250 mg three to four times daily Tea: 1 cup tea tid (0.5-1 g dried root in 150 mL boiling water for 5-10 min)	Ginger should not be used in patients with gallstones because of its cholagogic effect. It may inhibit platelet aggregation; cases of postoperative bleeding have been reported. Large doses of ginger may increase bleeding time in patients taking anti-platelet agents.
Ginkgo biloba leaf	To slow cognitive deterioration in dementia To increase peripheral blood flow in claudication To treat sexual dysfunction associated with the use of SSRIs	60-120 mg bid of extract Egb 761 standardized to 24% flavonoids and 6% terpenoids	Adverse effects are rare and may include mild stomach or intestinal upset, headache, or allergic skin reaction Ginkgo can inhibit platelet aggregation; reports of spontaneous bleeding have been published. Patients should discontinue ginkgo at least 36 h before surgery. Concurrent use of ginkgo and anticoagulants, antiplatelet agents, vitamin E, or garlic may increase the risk of bleeding.
Ginseng root	As a tonic during times of stress, fatigue, disability, and convalescence To improve physical performance and stamina	Root: 1-2 g/d Tablet: 100 mg bid of extract standardized to 4%-7% ginsenosides A 2- to 3-week period of using ginseng followed by a 1- to 2-week "rest" period is generally recommended. Ginseng is commonly adulterated, especially Siberian ginseng products	Ginseng has a mild stimulant effect and should be avoided in patients with cardiovascular disease. Tachycardia and hypertension can occur. Overdosages can lead to "ginseng abuse syndrome," characterized by insomnia, hypotonia, and edema. Ginseng has estrogenic effects and may cause vaginal bleeding and breast tenderness. Ginseng has been shown to inhibit platelets, so patients should discontinue ginseng use at least 7 d before surgery. Ginseng should not be used with other stimulants.

Continued

Herb/Nutritional Supplement	Common Uses	Reasonable Adult Oral Dosage*	Precautions and Drug Interactions
			Patients taking antidiabetic agents and ginseng should be monitored to avoid the hypoglycemic effects of ginseng. Ginseng may interact with warfarin and cause a decreased international normalized ratio. Siberian ginseng may increase digoxin levels. There have been reports of a drug interaction between ginseng and phenelzine (a monoamine oxidase inhibitor) resulting in insomnia, headache, tremulousness, and manic-like symptoms.
Glucosamine	For osteoarthritis	500 mg tid with meals Glucosamine is available in the form of sulfate, hydrochloride, or n-acetyl salt. Glucosamine sulfate is the form that has been used in most clinical studies.	Side effects are generally limited to mild GI symptoms, including stomach upset, heartburn, diarrhea, nausea, and indigestion. Glucosamine derived from marine exoskeletons may cause reactions in people allergic to shellfish. Glucosamine may raise blood glucose level in patients with diabetes.
Hawthorn leaf with flower	Commonly used in Germany to increase cardiac output in patients with New York Heart Association stage I and II heart failure	160-900 mg water-ethanol extract (30-169 mg procyanidins or 3.5-19.8 mg flavonoids) divided into 2-3 doses	Side effects include GI upset, palpitations, hypotension, headache, dizziness, and insomnia. Concomitant use with CNS depressants may have additive CNS effects. Hawthorn may potentiate effects of digoxin and vasodilators.
Horse chestnut seed	To relieve symptoms of chronic venous insufficiency	250 mg bid of extract standardized to 50 mg aescin in delayed-release form It is unsafe to ingest the raw seed, which contains significant amounts of the most toxic constituent, esculin	Mild GI symptoms, headache, dizziness, and pruritis have been reported. Ingestion of high doses may cause renal, hepatic, and hematologic toxicity. Concomitant use with anticoagulants may increase the risk of bleeding. Horse chestnut may potentiate the effects of hypoglycemic drugs.
Kava kava	As an anxiolytic for nervous anxiety, stress, and restlessness As a sedative to induce sleep	Herb and preparations equivalent to 60-120 mg kava pyrones/d Most clinical trials have used 100 mg tid of extract standardized to 70% kava pyrones for anxiety disorders	Kava should not be used by patients with depression and pregnant or nursing women. Kava may affect motor reflexes and judgment, so it should not be taken while driving and/or operating heavy machinery. Accommodative disturbances have been reported. Kava may exacerbate Parkinson's disease. Extended use can cause a temporary yellow discoloration of skin, hair, and nails.

Herb/Nutritional Supplement	Common Uses	Reasonable Adult Oral Dosage*	Precautions and Drug Interactions
			Reports have linked kava use to at least 25 cases of severe liver toxicity. Kava has been shown to have additive CNS depressant effects with benzodiazapines, alcohol, and herbal tranquilizers. Kava may also potentiate the sedative effects of anesthetics, and so, patients taking kava should be discontinued at least 24 h before surgery.
Melatonin	For jet lag, insomnia, shift-work disorder, and circadian rhythm disorders Also for other medical conditions, including depression, multiple sclerosis, tinnitus, headache, and cancer	For jet lag, 5 mg at bedtime for 2-5 d beginning the day of return For sleep disorders, 0.3-5 mg taken 2 hrs before bedtime Avoid melatonin from animal pineal gland due to possibility of contamination	Avoid use in pregnancy because melatonin decreases serum luteinizing hormone concentrations and increases serum prolactin levels. The common adverse reactions include headache, transient depressive symptoms, daytime fatigue and drowsiness, dizziness, abdominal cramps, irritability, and reduced alertness. Concomitant use of melatonin with alcohol, benzodiazepines, or other CNS depressants may cause additive sedation. Melatonin can affect immune function and may interfere with immunosuppressive therapy. Concomitant use with other herbs that have sedative properties (e.g., chamomile, goldenseal, hop, kava, valerian) may produce additive CNS-impairing effects.
Milk thistle fruit	As a hepatoprotectant and antioxidant, particularly for the treatment of hepatitis, cirrhosis, and toxic liver damage Used in Europe for the treatment of hepatotoxic mushroom poisoning from *Amanita phalloides*	Average daily dose is 12-15 g of crude drug or formulations equivalent to 200-400 mg of silymarin	Adverse effects are rare but may include diarrhea and allergic reactions Milk thistle may potentiate the hypoglycemic effect of antidiabetic agents.
Red clover flower	Commonly used for conditions associated with menopause, such as hot flashes, cardiovascular health, and osteoporosis Also used for premenstrual syndrome, benign prostate hyperplasia, and cancer prevention Used topically to treat psoriasis, eczema, and other rashes	For hot flashes, 40 mg/d of the isoflavones extract (Promensil™) For other conditions, no established dosage documented	Red clover has estrogenic activity and should be avoided during pregnancy and lactation. Women with hormone-dependent conditions (e.g., breast, uterine, and ovarian cancer, endometriosis, and uterine fibroids) and men with prostate cancer should also avoid taking red clover. Side effects include headache, myalgia, nausea, and rash. Red clover contains coumarin derivatives and may increase the risk of bleeding in those who are taking anticoagulants or antiplatelet drugs.

Continued

Herb/Nutritional Supplement	Common Uses	Reasonable Adult Oral Dosage*	Precautions and Drug Interactions
			Preliminary report suggests that red clover may antagonize the effects of tamoxifen. Some evidence suggests that red clover can increase levels of drugs that are metabolized by the cytochrome P450 3A4 isoenzyme (e.g., lovastatin, ketoconazole, itraconzaole, fexofenadine, and triazolam).
SAMe (S-adenosyl-L-methionine)	For treatment of osteoarthritis, depression, fibromyalgia, and liver disease	For osteoarthritis, 200 mg tid For depression and fibromyalgia, 800 mg bid For liver disease, 600-800 mg bid	Common side effects include flatulence, nausea, vomiting, and diarrhea. SAMe can cause anxiety in people with depression and hypomania in people with bipolar disorder. Concurrent use of SAMe and other antidepressant may cause serotonin syndrome.
Saw palmetto berry	To treat symptomatic benign prostatic hyperplasia and irritable bladder	160 mg bid of extract standardized to 85%-95% fatty acids and sterols	Adverse effects are rare but may include headache, nausea, and upset stomach. High doses can cause diarrhea.
St. John's wort	Effective for the treatment of mild to moderate depression May have anti-inflammatory and anti-infective activities	300 mg tid of hypericum extract standardized to 0.3% hypericin	St. John's wort should not be used in pregnancy. Side effects include dry mouth, GI upset, dizziness, fatigue, and constipation. St. John's wort may induce photosensitivity, especially in fair-skinned individuals. It may cause serotonin syndrome if use with other antidepressants, including SSRIs, or other serotonergic drugs. It has been shown to induce the cytochrome P450 3A4 isoenzyme and decrease blood levels of many drugs such as indinavir, nevirapine, cyclosporine, digoxin, theophylline, simvastatin, oral contraceptive pills, and warfarin. St. John's wort should be discontinued at least 5 d before surgery to avoid any potential drug interactions.
Soy	Commonly used for cholesterol reduction in combination with a low fat diet Also used for menopausal symptoms and for preventing osteoporosis and cardiovascular disease in postmenopausal women	For lowering cholesterol, 25-50 g/d of soy protein For hot flashes, 20-60 g/d of soy protein For osteoporosis, 40 g/d of soy protein containing 90 mg isoflavones	Soy may cause GI side effects such as constipation, bloating, and nausea. Allergic reactions such as rash and itching have been reported. Soy may inhibit the effects of estrogen replacement therapy. Soy may reduce the absorption of zinc, iron, or calcium supplements.
Valerian root	Used as a mild sedative for insomnia and anxiety	2-3 g of dried root or 1-3 mL of tincture, qd to several times/d	Valerian has a bad odor and can cause morning drowsiness.

Herb/Nutritional Supplement	Common Uses	Reasonable Adult Oral Dosage*	Precautions and Drug Interactions
		Two clinical trials have found 400-450 mg of the root extract effective for insomnia	Long-term administration may lead to paradoxical stimulation including restlessness and palpitations. Because of the risk of benzodiazepine-like withdrawal, valerian should be tapered over a period of several weeks before surgery. It may potentiate the sedative effect of CNS depressants (e.g., benzodiazapines, alcohol) and other herbal tranquilizers.

*Doses presented in the table are adapted from the German Commission E Monographs and/or data from clinical trials. Products from different manufacturers vary considerably. A reliable product should have a label clearly stating the botanical name of the herb and milligram amount contained in the product. Standardized extracts should be used whenever possible and are often disclosed on the label of quality products.

CNS, central nervous system; GI, gastrointestinal; HMG-CoA, 3-hydroxy-3-methylglutaryl coenzyme A; SSRIs, selective serotonin reuptake inhibitors.

NEW DRUGS IN 2003 AND AGENTS PENDING FDA APPROVAL

METHOD OF

Miriam M. Chan, RPH, PharmD, and

Kristin Casper, PharmD

TABLE 1 New Drugs Approved in 2003

Generic Name	Trade Name (Manufacturer)	Strength	Dosage Form	Normal Dosage Range	Pregnancy Rating*	FDA Approval Date	Indication	Classification
Abarelix	Plenaxis (Praecis)	113 mg/vial (yields 100 mg/2 mL when reconstituted)	Injection	100 mg IM on day 1, 15, 29 (week 4) and every 4 weeks thereafter	X	11/03 (only physicians who have enrolled in the Plenaxis Safety Program may prescribe Plenaxis)	Palliative treatment for men with advanced symptomatic prostate cancer in whom LHRH agonist therapy is not appropriate, who refuse surgical castration, and who have one or more of the following: 1, Risk of neurological compromise due to metastases; 2, ureteral or bladder outlet obstruction caused by local encroachment or metastatic disease; or 3, severe bone pain from skeletal metastases persisting on narcotic analgesia	Gonadotropin-releasing hormone antagonist
Agalsidase beta	Fabrazyme (Genzyme)	35 mg/vial	Injection	1 mg/kg per IV infusion q 2 wk	B	4/03	Use in patients with Fabry disease to reduce globotriasylceramide deposition in capillary endothelium of the kidney and certain other cell types	Recombinant human α-galactosidase A enzyme
Alefacept	Amevive (Biogen)	7.5, 15 mg/vial	Injection	7.5 mg IV bolus or 15 mg IM once weekly × 12 wk	B	1/03	Treatment of adult patients with moderate to severe plaque psoriasis who are candidates for systemic therapy or phototherapy	Immunosuppressive dimeric fusion protein
Alfuzosin	Uroxatral (Sanofi-Synthelabo)	10 mg	Extended-release tablet	10 mg qd	B	6/03	Treatment of the signs and symptoms of benign prostatic hyperplasia	Selective alpha$_1$-adrenoreceptors antagonist
Alpha$_1$-proteinase inhibitor (Human) (A$_1$-PI)	Zemaira (Aventis Behring)	Single use vial containing the labeled amount of A$_1$-PI	Injection	60 mg/kg once weekly, given as IV infusion over approximately 15 min	C	7/03	Chronic augmentation and maintenance therapy in adults with A$_1$-PI deficiency and clinical evidence of emphysema	Alpha$_1$-proteinase inhibitor
Antihemophilic factor (recombinant) plasma/albumin-free method (rAHF-PFM)	Advate (Baxter)	250, 500, 1000, 1500 units/vial	Injection	Dose based on desired or expected factor VIII increase	C	7/03	Hemophilia A for prevention and control of bleeding episodes; in perioperative management of hemophilia A; can be of therapeutic value in patients with acquired Factor VIII inhibitors not exceeding 10 Bethesda units/mL	Antihemophilic agent
Aprepitant	Emend (Merck)	80, 125 mg	Capsule	125 mg taken 1 h prior to chemotherapy (Day 1) and 80 mg once daily in the morning on Day 2 and 3	B	3/03	Use in combination with other antiemetic agents to prevent acute and delayed nausea and vomiting associated with highly emetogenic chemotherapy	Human substance P/Neurokinin 1 receptor antagonist

Atazanavir	Reyataz (Bristol-Myers Squibb)	100, 150, 200 mg	Capsule	400 mg once daily taken with food	B	6/03	In combination with other antiretroviral agents for the treatment of HIV-1 infection	Antiretroviral agent, protease inhibitor
Bortezomib	Velcade (Millenium)	3.5 mg/vial	Injection	1.3 mg/m²/dose given as an IV bolus twice weekly × 2 wk (Day 1, 4, 8, and 11) followed by a 10-day rest period (Day 12 to 21)	D	5/03	Treatment of multiple myeloma in patients who have received at least two prior therapies and have demonstrated disease progression on the last therapy	Proteasome inhibitor
Ciprofloxacin/dexa-methasone	Ciprodex (Alcon)	0.3%/0.1% in 5, 7.5 mL Drop-Tainer System	Otic sus-pension	4 drops into affected ear(s) bid × 7 d	C	7/03	Treatment of acute otitis media in pedriatic patients (≥6 mo of age) with tympanostomy tubes or acute otitis externa in children (≥6 mo of age) and adults	Antibiotic and corticosteroid combination
Daptomycin	Cubicin (Cubist)	250, 500 mg/vial	Injection	4 mg/kg IV infusion over 30 min once daily for 7–14 d	B	9/03	Treatment of complicated skin and skin structure infections caused by susceptible aerobic gram-positive organisms	Antibiotic, cyclic lipopeptide
Desirudin	Iprivask (Aventis)	15 mg/vial	Injection	15 mg SC q 12 h with initial dose given up to 5 to 15 min before surgery, but after induction of regional block anesthesia, if used	C	4/03	Prophylaxis of deep vein thrombosis (DVT), which may lead to pulmonary embolism, in patients undergoing elective hip replacement survey	Anticoagulant, antithrombin agent
Efalizumab	Raptiva (Genentech)	125 mg/vial	Injection	A single 0.7 mg/kg SC conditioning dose followed by weekly SC doses of 1 mg/kg (max 200 mg/dose)	C	10/03	Treatment of adults (≥18 y) with chronic moderate to severe plaque psoriasis who are candidates for systemic therapy or phototherapy	Immunosuppressive, recombinant humanized IgG 1 kappa isotype monoclonal antibody
Emtricitabine	Emtriva (Gilead Sciences)	200 mg	Capsule	200 mg qd	B	7/03	In combination with other antiretroviral agents for the treatment of HIV-1 infection in adults	Antiretroviral agent, nucleoside reverse transcriptase inhibitor
Enfuvirtide	Fuzeon (Roche)	108 mg/vial (yields 90 mg/ml when reconstituted)	Injection	90 mg SC bid	B	3/03	In combination with other antiretroviral; agents for the treatment of HIV-1 infection in treatment-experienced patients with evidence of HIV-1 replication despite ongoing antiretroviral therapy	Antiretroviral agent, fusion protein inhibitor

Continued

TABLE 1 New Drugs Approved in 2003—cont'd

Generic Name	Trade Name (Manufacturer)	Strength	Dosage Form	Normal Dosage Range	Pregnancy Rating*	FDA Approval Date	Indication	Classification
Epinastine HCl	Elestat (Allergan)	0.05% in 8, 15 mL bottle	Ophthalmic solution	1 drop in each eye bid	C	10/03	Prevention of itching associated with allergic conjunctivitis	Ophthalmic antihistamine
Estradiol topical emulsion	Estrasorb (Novavax)	4.35 mg estradiol/ 1.74 g pouch	Topical emulsion	Apply 2 pouches once daily to thighs and calves, with excess amount to buttocks	Not rated	10/03	Treatment of moderate to severe vasomotor symptoms associated with menopause	Estrogen therapy
Ethinyl estradiol/ levonor-gestrel	Seasonale (Barr)	0.03 mg/ 0.15 mg/tab (13-week supply/pack)	Tablet	1 active tablet qd × 84 d followed by 1 inert tablet qd × 7 d	X	9/03	Prevention of pregnancy in women who elect to use oral contraceptives as a method of birth control	Oral contraceptive
Fosamprevavir calcium	Lexiva (Glaxo SmithKline)	700 mg	Tablet	Therapy-naïve patients: 1400mg bid (without ritonavir); 1400mg qd (with ritonavir 200 mg qd); 700 mg bid (with ritonavir 100 mg bid)	C	10/03	In combination with other antiretroviral agents for the treatment of HIV infection in adults	Antiretroviral agent, protease inhibitor
Gatifloxacin	Zymar (Allergan)	0.3% in 2.5, 5 mL dropper bottle	Ophthalmic solution	Day 1 and 2: 1 drop in affected eye(s) q 2 hours while awake up to 8 times/d; Days 3 through 7: 1 drop up to 4 times/d while awake	C	3/03	Treatment of bacterial conjunctivitis for susceptible strains of bacteria	Antibiotic, fluoroquinolone
Gefitinib	Iressa (AstraZeneca)	250 mg	Tablet	250 mg qd	D	5/03	As monotherapy for the treatment of patients with locally advanced or metastatic non-small cell lung cancer after failure of platinum-based and docetaxel chemotherapies	Antineoplastic, tyrosine kinase inhibitor
Gemifloxacin	Factive (Genesoft)	320 mg	Tablet	320 mg qd	C	4/03	Treatment of acute bacterial exacerbation of chronic bronchitis and community-acquired pneumonia (of mild to moderate severity)	Antibiotic, fluoroquinolone
Ibandronate	Boniva (Roche)	2.5 mg	Tablet	2.5 mg qd	C	5/03	Treatment and prevention of osteoporosis in postmenopausal women	Bisphosphonate
Influenza virus vaccine	FluMist (MedImmune/ Wyeth)	0.5 mL	Nasal spray	0.5 mL/dose; children 5-8 y not previously vaccinated: 2 doses per season; previously	C (Not recom-mended for pregnant women)	6/03	Immunization for the prevention of disease caused by Influenza A and B viruses in healthy children and adolescents 5-17 y and healthy adults 18-49 y	Attenuated live vaccine

				vaccinated children 5-8 y and patients 9-49 y: 1 dose per season				
Laronidase	Aldurazyme (BioMarin)	2.9 mg/5 mL vial	Injection	0.58 mg/kg IV infusion once q wk	B	4/03	Treatment of Hurler and Hurler-Scheie forms of mucopolysaccharidosis I (MPSI); treatment of Scheie form of MPSI in patients with moderate to severe symptoms	α-L-iduronidase enzyme
Memantine	Namenda (Forest Labs)	5, 10 mg	Tablet	5 mg qd up to 10 mg bid	B	10/03	Treatment of moderate to severe dementia of the Alzheimer type	NMDA-receptor antagonist
Miglustat	Zavesca (Actelion)	100 mg	Capsule	100 mg tid	X	7/03	Treatment of adult patients with mild to moderate type 1 Gaucher disease when enzyme replacement therapy is not a therapeutic option (e.g., because of constraints such as allergy, hypersensitivity, or poor venous access)	Enzyme inhibitor of glucosylceramide synthase
Moxifloxacin	Vigamox (Alcon)	0.5% in 3 mL Drop-Tainer	Ophthalmic solution	1 drop to the affected eye(s) tid for 7 d	C	4/03	Treatment of bacterial conjunctivitis for susceptible strains of bacteria	Antibiotic, fluoroquinolone
Omalizumab	Xolair (Genentech/ Novartis)	202.5 mg/ vial (yields 150 mg/1.2 mL when reconstituted)	Injection	150-375 mg SC q 2 or 4 wk (Individualized based on pretreatment IgE serum levels and body weight; adjust dose during treatment for significant change in body weight only)	B	6/03	Treatment of moderate to severe, persistent allergic asthma not adequately controlled with inhaled corticosteroids in adults and adolescents ≥12 y	Monoclonal antibody, anti-asthmatic
Oxybutynin transdermal system	Oxytrol (Watson)	3.9 mg/d	Trans-dermal patch	Apply twice weekly to abdomen, hip or buttocks	B	2/03	For the relief of symptoms of bladder instability/treatment of overactive bladder associated with voiding in patients with uninhibited and reflex neurogenic bladder (e.g., urgency, frequency, urinary leakage, urge incontinence, dysuria)	Antispasmodic, anticholinergic
Palonosetron	Aloxi (MGI Pharma)	0.25 mg/5mL	Injection	0.25 mg IV 30 min prior to chemotherapy administration (day 1 of each cycle)	B	7/03	Prevention of acute (within 24 h) and delayed (2-5 d) nausea and vomiting associated with initial and repeat courses of moderately and highly emetogenic cancer chemotherapy	Antiemetic, selective 5-HT_3 receptor antagonist

Continued

TABLE 1 New Drugs Approved in 2003—cont'd

Generic Name	Trade Name (Manufacturer)	Strength	Dosage Form	Normal Dosage Range	Pregnancy Rating*	FDA Approval Date	Indication	Classification
Pegvisomant	Somavert (Pharmacia)	10, 15, 20 mg/vial	Injection	Loading dose: 40 mg SC; Maintenance dose: 10 mg SC qd	B	3/03	Treatment of acromegaly in patients who have had an inadequate response to surgery and/or radiation therapy and/or other medical therapies, or for whom these therapies are not appropriate.	Growth hormone receptor antagonist
Prussian blue (insoluble)	Radiogardase (HEYL Chemis-chpharma)	500 mg	Capsule	Children 2-12 y: 1 gm tid, Children >12 y and adults: 3 gm tid	C	10/03	Treatment of known or suspected internal contamination with radioactive cesium and/or radioactive or nonradioactive thallium to increase rate of elimination	Antidote for contamination
Rosuvastatin	Crestor (AstraZeneca)	5, 10, 20, 40 mg	Tablets	5-40 mg qd	X	8/03	Used with dietary therapy to reduce elevated total cholesterol, LDL-C, Apo B, non-HDL-C, and TG levels and to increase HDL-C in patients with primary hypercholesterolemia and mixed dsylipidemia; used with diet therapy to reduce TG levels (Fredrickson Type IV); used to reduce LDL-C, total cholesterol, and ApoB in patients with homozygous familial hypercholesterolemia	Antihyperlipidemic agent, HMG-CoA reductase inhibitor
Sertaconazole nitrate	Ertaczo (Mylan Pharmac-euticals)	2% in 15, 30 g tube	Cream	Apply bid for 4 wk	C	12/03	Topical treatment of interdigital tinea pedis caused by *Trichophyton rubrum, Trichophyton mentagrophytes,* and *Epidermophyton floccosm* in immunocompetent patients ≥12 y	Antifungal, imidazole
Tadalafil	Cialis (Lilly)	5, 10, 20 mg	Tablet	5–20 mg taken prior to anticipated sexual activity, not more than once daily	B	11/03	Treatment of erectile dysfunction	Phosphodiesterase Type 5 enzyme inhibitor
Testosterone buccal system	Striant (Columbia Labs)	30 mg/buccal system	Transbuccal tablet	1 buccal system applied to gum region bid (12 h apart)	X	6/03	Replacement therapy in males with congenital or acquired primary hypogonadism or hypogonadotropic hypogonadism	Sex hormone, androgen

Tositumomab and Iodine^{131} I-Tositumomab	Bexxar (Corixa/GSK)	Dosimetric kit (step 1), Therapeutic kit (step 2)	Injection	Dosimetric kit on day 1 followed by Therapeutic kit 7-14 d later	X	6/03	Treatment of patients with CD20 positive, follicular, non-Hodgkin's lymphoma, with or without transformation, whose disease is refractory to rituximab and has relapsed following chemotherapy	Antineoplastic radioimmunotherapeutic monoclonal antibody
Vardenafil	Levitra (Bayer)	2.5, 5, 10, 20 mg	Tablet	5-20 mg taken 60 min prior to anticipated sexual activity, not more than once daily	B	8/03	Treatment of erectile dysfunction	Phosphodiesterase Type 5 enzyme

*FDA Pregnancy Categories

A- Adequate studies in pregnant women have not demonstrated a risk to the fetus in the first trimester of pregnancy, and there is no evidence of risk in later trimesters.

B- Animal studies have shown an adverse effect, but adequate studies in pregnant women have not demonstrated a risk to the fetus during the first trimester of pregnancy, and there is no evidence of risk in later trimesters.

C- Animal studies have shown an adverse effect on the fetus, but there are no adequate studies in humans; the benefits from the use of the drug in pregnant women may be acceptable despite its potential risks.

D- There is evidence of human fetal risk, but the potential benefits from the use of the drug in pregnant women may be acceptable despite its potential risks.

X- Adverse reaction reports indicate evidence of fetal risk; the risk of use in a pregnant woman clearly outweighs any possible benefit.

No drug should be administered during pregnancy unless it is clearly needed and potential benefit outweighs potential hazard to the fetus, regardless of the pregnancy category.

TABLE 2 Agents Pending FDA Approval

Generic Name	Trade Name (Manufacturer)	Indication
AFO150 (perfluorohexane emulsion)	Imavist (Alliance Pharmaceuticals)	Ultrasound contrast agent
Artesunate	No current trade name (World Health Organization)	Treatment of malaria
Cilomilast	Ariflo (GlaxoSmithKline)	Treatment of patients with COPD
Clofarabine	No current trade name (ILEX)	Treatment of refractory or relapsed pediatric acute lymphoblastic leukemia
Darifenacin	Enablex (Novartis)	Treatment of overactive bladder
Duloxetine	Cymbalta (Eli Lilly)	Treatment of depression
Etoricoxib	Arcoxia (Merck)	Treatment of arthritis pain
Everolimus	Certican (Novartis)	Prevention of rejection after heart and kidney transplantation
Insulin detemir	No current trade name (Novo Nordisk)	Long-acting insulin analog for the treatment of diabetes mellitus
Lanthanum carbonate	Fosrenol (Shire)	Treatment of hyperphosphatemia in patients with end-stage renal disease
Lecanidipine	Zanidip (Forest Laboratories)	Treatment of hypertension
Lumiracoxib	Prexige (Novartis)	Treatment of osteoarthritis, rhematoid arthritis, acute pain, and dysmenorrhea
Norastemizole	Soltara (Sepracor)	Treatment of allergic rhinitis
Parecoxib sodium	No current trade name (Pharmacia)	Management of acute pain
Pleconaril	Picovir (VioPharma)	Treatment of viral respiratory infection in adults
Pramlinitide acetate	Symlin (Amylin Pharmaceuticals)	Treatment of patients with diabetes mellitus using insulin
Prasterone	Prestara (Genelabs Technologies)	Treatment of mild-to-moderate systemic lupus erythematosus on low-dose glucocorticoids
Prostatic acid phosphatase	Provenge (Dendreon)	Treatment of androgen-independent prostate cancer
Ranolazine	Ranexa (CV Therapeutics)	Treatment of androgen-independent prostate cancer
Rifaximin	Lumenax (Salix Pharmaceuticals)	Treatment of traveler's diarrhea
Solifenacin	Vesicare (Yamanouchi Pharma America)	Treatment of overactive bladder (urinary frequency, urgency, and incontinence)
Telithromycin	Ketek (Aventis)	Treatment of community acquired pneumonia in patients 18 years and older
Tibolone	Xyvion (Akzo Nobel)	Treatment of osteoporosis
Tiotropium	Spiriva (Boehringer Ingelheim)	Treatment of patients with chronic obstructive pulmonary disease
Ziconotide	Prialt (Elan)	Treatment of chronic pain

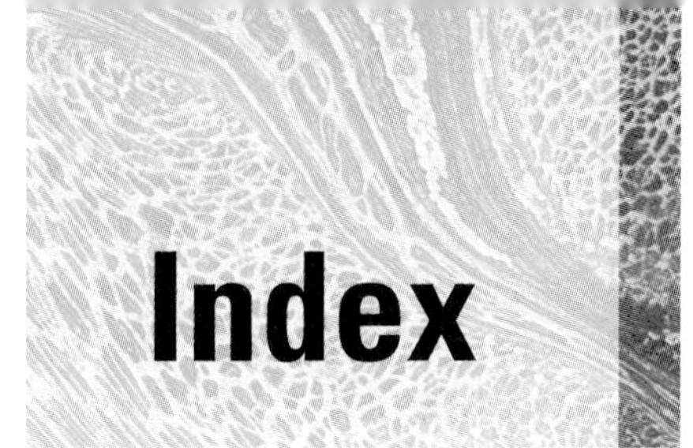

Index

Note: Page numbers followed by the letter f refer to figures; those followed by t refer to tables. Drugs are listed under the generic name.

B

C

D

G

M

Q

U

W